MOSBY'S
MEDICAL & NURSING
DICTIONARY

MOSBY'S MEDICAL & NURSING DICTIONARY

SECOND EDITION

ILLUSTRATED

Forty-four page full-color atlas of human anatomy

Managing Editor, Second edition

Walter D. Glanze

Revision Editor

Kenneth N. Anderson

Consulting Editor and Writer

Lois E. Anderson

Editor in Chief, First edition

Laurence Urdang

Managing Editor, First edition

Helen Harding Swallow

THE C. V. MOSBY COMPANY

ST. LOUIS • TORONTO • PRINCETON 1986

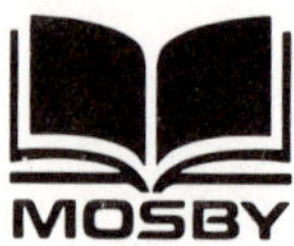

A TRADITION OF PUBLISHING EXCELLENCE

Editor: Nancy L. Mullins
Assistant editor: Maureen Slaten
Editing supervisor: Lin A. Dempsey
Production: Jeanne Genz, Mary Granger Stueck, Suzanne C. Glazer

Publisher: Thomas A. Manning
Editor-in-chief: Alison Miller

Printed in the United States of America

The C.V. Mosby Company
11830 Westline Industrial Drive, St. Louis, Missouri 63146

Library of Congress Cataloging-in-Publication Data
Main entry under title:

Mosby's medical and nursing dictionary.

1. Medicine—Dictionaries. 2. Nursing—Dictionaries.
I. Glanze, Walter D. II. Anderson, Kenneth N.
III. Anderson, Lois E. IV. C.V. Mosby Company.
V. Title: Medical & nursing dictionary. VI. Title:
Mosby's medical and nursing dictionary. [DNLM:
1. Dictionaries, Medical. 2. Nursing—dictionaries.
WY 13 M894]
R121.M89 1986 610'.3'21 85-21617
ISBN 0-8016-5195-6

TS/R/R 9 8 7 6 5 4 3 2 02/B/277

STAFF

SECOND EDITION

Managing editor:
Walter D. Glanze

Revision editor:
Kenneth N. Anderson

Consulting editor and writer:
Lois E. Anderson

Associate editor:
Frank R. Abate, A.B., M.A., Ph.D.

Chief writer:
Barbara Guidos, B.A., M.A.

Programing and composition by:
Typographic Sales, Inc.

Pronunciation editor:
Walter D. Glanze

Artists:
Ernest W. Beck, B.S., M.A., Medical Illustrator
Glenna Deutsch
John Hagen
David Mascaro
Jeanne Robertson
Karen Waldo
Marcia Williams, Marcia Williams Medical Illustrations

FIRST EDITION

Editor in Chief:
Laurence Urdang

Managing Editor:
Helen Harding Swallow, B.A., R.N., M.S.N., CNM

Chief Writers:
Barbara Guidos, B.A., M.A.
John Bernard Landry, B.A.
Elsie Rosner, B.S., M.A.

Writers:
Janice M. Bohall, R.N. • Lawrence S. Carlton, M.D., F.A.C.P., Senior Attending Physician in Medicine, Physician Coordinator, Nurse Practitioner Program, Hartford Hospital, Hartford, Connecticut • Mary Lee Evans, R.N., M.S.N., Assistant Professor, College of Nursing, University of Rhode Island, Kingston, Rhode Island • Janet I. Hirsch, R.N., M.S., Ed.D., Associate Professor of Nursing, University of Rhode Island, Kingston, Rhode Island • John Hoover, B.S., Pharmacist • Aaron Klein, B.A., M.S. • Leslie L. Lewis, L.L.B., AMWA, Life Fellow, associated with Rush-Presbyterian-St. Luke's Medical Center, Chicago, Illinois • Willard J. Morse, Jr., M.D., F.A.C.O.G., Attending Obstetrician-Gynecologist, Women's and Infant's Hospital, Providence, Rhode Island; Medical Director, New Beginnings Birth Center, Warwick, Rhode Island • Penelope Steiner, B.A., B.S., M.Ph., Instructor, State University of New York, Downstate Medical Center, Brooklyn, New York • Roberta E. Weisbrod, Ph.D.

Pronunciation Editor:
Antoinette Baicich d'Oronzio, B.A., M.A.

Editorial Assistants:
Elsie P. Chapman, A.S.
John J. Czepiel, B.A.
Joyce P. Donovan, B.A.
Jesse White-Fresé, A.S.C.

Typographic and systems design by:
Laurence Urdang

Programing and composition by:
Alexander Typesetting, Inc.

CONTENTS

EDITOR'S FOREWORD

It would take many centuries just to read the medical literature published in a single year. The importance of having access at least to the *language* of this vast and vital field is obvious, and this access, in our fast-paced world, seems to be best provided in a single source that sorts what is immediately relevant from what is incidental to the needs of its users.

Mosby's Medical and Nursing Dictionary offers this kind of relevant knowledge and does it reliably and in clear language. But reliability and clarity must be matched by recency: This thoroughly revised edition—besides including over 3000 new entries and many novel features—has been computerized for ongoing revision. The changes and additions are constantly maintained, which means that this dictionary is up to date not only from edition to edition but continuously from printing to printing.

Many of the 3000 new entries and many of the changes in former entries are meant to appeal to both nursing and the allied health professions. The consultant board has been expanded to 54, representing not only diverse specialties but Canadian and international interests as well. Two large new categories of entries were added: dental terms and computer terms. These entries were identified as significant additions to expand the usefulness of the dictionary in allied health, and responding to the prevalence of computer technology throughout all of health care. There is also greater emphasis on geriatrics and on radiology. More metric equivalents are given. The defining syntax and terminology, clear as they were in the first edition, were made even more accessible to more readers, and the choice of language takes increasingly into account that we live not in a "man's world" but in a human world.

The revised edition has an entirely different pronunciation system, basically a system that most readers know from their use of popular English dictionaries, especially the major college or desk dictionaries.

Illustrations and tables were added and updated throughout. The 44-page color atlas of human anatomy is now totally in four colors and presented in the front of the dictionary for easy access. The 342-page appendices comprise 16 major categories, including a geriatrics section, a section on understanding and using medical terminology and, particularly relevant in today's changing health care economic environment, a list of DRG's. Also featured in the appendices are complete anatomy tables, normal laboratory values, drug names and drug interactions, nutrition, health history, the Washington development guide, a unique table of communicable and infectious diseases, the DSM-III classification, a complete patient education section, a list of burn centers, directories of nursing associations in the United States and Canada, and other valuable reference matter.

All the virtues of the first edition have been retained. To name a few: Among the entries on diseases, drugs, and procedures, there are at least 1000 that have separate paragraphs with pragmatic and nursing-significant headings such as "methods," "adverse effects," "nursing considerations," and "outcome criteria." The patient's right to be informed of all procedures and their rationale is given due attention. "Every effort has been made," Laurence Urdang wrote in the Foreword to the first edition, "to present the most up-to-date information in understandable English, using full sentences, without recourse to a skimpy, telegraphic style that may create ambiguity and interfere with clarity." Meanings within the same entry are clearly discriminated. The large amount and the nature of combining-form entries give the reader additional access to the meanings of defined terms and defining terms, as well as access to thousands of further terms that are not included in this dictionary and that, to a large extent, are not found in any other reference work. The many (10,000) cross-references from definition to definition are well chosen and contribute to the dictionary's encyclopedic dimensions. As with the first edition, *Mosby's Medical and Nursing Dictionary* continues to serve nursing and the allied health professions as the most comprehensive, authoritative, and up-to-date dictionary available.

It is impossible to acknowledge specifically all the contributions that many people have made to this project. But the editors are especially grateful for the guidance of Nancy L. Mullins, Editor, The C.V. Mosby Company, who supervised both editions; her common sense and wisdom have been a major ingredient in the development and completion of this dictionary.

Walter D. Glanze

EDITOR'S FOREWORD

TO FIRST EDITION

The second half of the twentieth century has seen an information explosion many times greater than that which characterized the sixteenth and seventeenth centuries in Europe. The enormous number of professionals and spcialists in virtually every field of activity has contributed to new ideas, and new ideas breed new language. Communication among professionals of all persuasions and between professionals and the lay public cannot take place without language, and it is specifically in the lexicon—the word stock—of language that the communication of new ideas is documented.

Some people think that dictionaries represent the judgment of editors as to what the words of a language ought to mean. But that notion is erroneous: the meanings of words are established by the convention of their users. It is the lexicographer's profession to interpret those conventions, to examine the ways the language is used, and to describe the meanings of the words and expressions in keeping with those ways. It is an ancillary, though customary function of the compiler and editor of dictionaries to define the terms, occasionally—depending on the kind of dictionary being prepared—to show how they are pronounced, where they originated, how and under what circumstances they are used, and to give other information about them. The technique of defining, or of describing what a term means by interpreting its various senses in language that is simpler than the term being defined, is one of the chief functions of the lexicographer. The writing of definitions is, essentially, an art, not a science. To be sure, there are certain conventions that may be followed and certain structures (and strictures) to be observed, but in the final analysis, it must be the user of the dictionary who decides the success of the work.

Mosby's Medical and Nursing Dictionary is an entirely new work, not based on a long line of dictionaries published over the last decades. Such a project presents certain difficulties to its compilers and editors; on the other hand, it provides the opportunity to take a fresh look at the style of defining, unhampered by a style established dozens of years earlier that is probably inappropriate to the needs of users today. The concept of an encyclopedic format suggests thorough coverage—that is, tending toward explanatory presentation of information rather than toward dry, brief, terse definitions such as those found in ordinary dictionaries. In this sense, definitions in this dictionary usually include more information than do general dictionaries, whose users are most often satisfied with relatively succinct definitions of technical terms, understanding that if they want fuller information, they must go to specialized works.

We believe that in *Mosby's Medical and Nursing Dictionary* we have compiled, written, and edited a reference book of consummate usefulness to nurses as well as to other health professionals. Its definitions are full; the breadth of coverage is as complete as is practical while retaining a convenient size and affordable price. Every effort has been made to present the most up-to-date information in understandable English, using full sentences, without recourse to a skimpy, telegraphic style that may create ambiguity and interfere with clarity. The illustrations, tables, and appendices supplement the text.

Many, many people have been involved in the various states of preparing the dictionary, but none more important to its successful culmination than Thomas A. Manning, Publisher. We are grateful to him and to Nancy L. Mullins, Editor, not only for all their help but for their forbearance during some of the more difficult periods of compilation.

Laurence Urdang

CONSULTANTS

Donna C. Aguilera, Ph.D., F.A.A.N.
Consultant in Clinical Psychology,
Beverly Hills, California

Kathleen G. Andreoli, D.S.N., F.A.A.N.
Vice President for Educational Services,
Interprofessional and International Programs;
Professor of Nursing,
The University of Texas
Health Science Center at Houston,
Houston, Texas

Miriam G. Austrin, R.N., B.A.
Allied Health Care Consultant;
Past Coordinator-Director,
Medical Assistant Program,
St. Louis Community College,
St. Louis, Missouri

Diane M. Billings, R.N., M.S.Ed.
Associate Professor of Nursing,
Indiana University School of Nursing,
Indianapolis, Indiana

Violet A. Breckbill, R.N., Ph.D.
Dean and Professor, School of Nursing,
State University of New York at Binghamton,
Binghamton, New York

Carolyn H. Brose, Ed.D., R.N.
President, Nu-Vision, Inc.,
Liberty, Missouri

Charlene D. Coco, R.N., M.N.
Assistant Professor of Nursing,
Louisiana State University Medical Center
School of Nursing, Associate Degree Program,
New Orleans, Louisiana

Mary H. Conover, R.N., B.S.
Instructor of ECG and Arrhythmia Workshops,
West Hills Hospital,
Canoga Park, California,
and throughout the western United States

Helen Cox
Principal Nurse Educator, School of Nursing,
St. Vincent's Hospital,
Ascot Vale, Victoria,
Australia

Joyce E. Dains, R.N., M.S.N.
Assistant Professor of Nursing,
The University of Texas
Health Science Center at Houston,
Houston, Texas

Rene A. Day, R.N., M.Sc.
Associate Professor, Faculty of Nursing,
University of Alberta,
Edmonton, Alberta,
Canada

Claire M. Fagin, Ph.D., F.A.A.N.
Dean and Professor,
University of Pennsylvania
School of Nursing,
Philadelphia, Pennsylvania

A. Jolayne Farrell, R.N., M.P.H.
Gerontological Consultant,
Toronto, Ontario,
Canada

William F. Finney, M.A., R.T.
School of Allied Medical Professions,
The Ohio State University,
Columbus, Ohio

Marilyn E. Flood, R.N., Ph.D.
Associate Director of Nursing,
University of California Hospitals,
San Francisco, California

Catherine Ingram Fogel, R.N.C., M.S.
Associate Professor,
School of Nursing,
Department of Primary Care,
University of North Carolina,
Chapel Hill, North Carolina

Anne Gray, M.Ed., B.A., Dip.N.Ed.
Head, Department of Nursing,
Kuring-gai College of Advanced Education,
Lindfield, New South Wales,
Australia

Janet Gray, B.S.N., M.A.
Nursing Assistant Program, Wascana Institute,
Regina, Saskatchewan,
Canada

Consultants

Susan J. Grobe, R.N., Ph.D.
Associate Professor,
The University of Texas at Austin,
Austin, Texas

Maureen W. Groër, R.N., Ph.D.
Professor of Nursing,
University of Tennessee, Knoxville,
College of Nursing,
Knoxville, Tennessee

Jane Hirsch, R.N., M.S.
Assistant Director of Nursing,
Assistant Clinical Professor,
Department of Biodysfunction,
School of Nursing,
University of California,
San Francisco, California

Eugene M. Johnson, Jr., Ph.D.
Professor,
Department of Pharmacology,
Washington University Medical School,
St. Louis, Missouri

Virginia Burke Karb, R.N., M.S.N.
Assistant Professor,
University of North Carolina at Greensboro,
School of Nursing,
Greensboro, North Carolina

Judith Belliveau Krauss, R.N., M.S.N.
Associate Dean and Associate Professor,
Psychiatric Mental Health Nursing,
Yale University School of Nursing,
New Haven, Connecticut

Mavis E. Kyle, R.N., M.H.S.A.
Assistant Dean, Associate Professor,
College of Nursing,
University of Saskatchewan,
Saskatoon, Saskatchewan,
Canada

Linda Armstrong Lazure, R.N., M.S.N.
Creighton University
School of Nursing,
Omaha, Nebraska

Maxine E. Loomis, R.N., Ph.D., F.A.A.N.
Professor and Assistant Dean for
Professional Development,
University of South Carolina
College of Nursing,
Columbia, South Carolina

Jannetta MacPhail, R.N., Ph.D., F.A.A.N.
Dean and Professor,
Faculty of Nursing,
The University of Alberta,
Edmonton, Alberta
Canada

Ann Marriner, R.N., Ph.D.
Professor,
Graduate Department of Nursing Administration
and Teacher Education,
Indiana University
School of Nursing,
Indianapolis, Indiana

Edwina A. McConnell, R.N., M.S.
Independent Nurse Consultant,
Madison, Wisconsin

Janice M. Messick, R.N., M.S., F.A.A.N.
Consulant,
Laguna Hills, California

Patricia A. Mickelsen, Ph.D.
Associate Director,
Clinical Microbiology Laboratory,
Stanford University Hospital,
Stanford, California

Susan I. Molde, R.N., M.S.N.
Associate Professor,
Yale University School of Nursing,
New Haven, Connecticut

Mary N. Moore, Ph.D., R.N.
School of Nursing,
University of Pennsylvania,
Philadelphia, Pennsylvania

Helen K. Mussallem, O.C., B.N., M.A., Ed.D., O.St.J., LL.D., D.Sc., F.R.C.N., M.R.S.H.
Special Advisor to National and International
Health-Related Agencies;
Former Executive Director,
Canadian Nurses Association,
Ottawa, Ontario,
Canada

Susan Jenkinson Neuman, R.N., B.A.
Nursing Practice Officer,
College of Nurses of Ontario,
Toronto, Ontario,
Canada

Marie L. O'Koren, R.N., Ed.D., F.A.A.N.
Dean, School of Nursing,
The University of Alabama in Birmingham,
Birmingham, Alabama

Kathleen Deska Pagana, R.N., M.S.N.
Instructor of Nursing,
Lycoming College,
Williamsport, Pennsylvania

Ann M. Pagliaro, R.N., M.S.N.
Associate Professor, Faculty of Nursing,
The University of Alberta,
Edmonton, Alberta
Canada

Anne Griffin Perry, R.N., M.S.N.
ANA-Certified Adult Nurse Practitioner;
Associate Professor,
Graduate Nursing Program—Cardiopulmonary Option,
School of Nursing,
St. Louis University,
St. Louis, Missouri

Susan Foley Pierce, R.N., M.S.N.
University of North Carolina,
Chapel Hill, North Carolina

Patricia A. Potter, R.N., M.S.N.
Clinical Director of Surgical Nursing,
Barnes Hospital,
St. Louis, Missouri

Jack D. Preston, D.D.S.
Harrington Professor of Esthetic Dentistry;
Director, Advanced Education in Prosthodontics,
University of Southern California
School of Dentistry,
Los Angeles, California

Ginette Rodger, R.N., B.ScN., M.N.Adm.
Executive Director,
Canadian Nurses Association,
Ottawa, Ontario,
Canada

Charlotte Searle, D.Phil., R.N.
Professor and Head,
Department of Nursing Science,
University of South Africa,
Pretoria, South Africa

Kay See-Lasley, M.S., R.Ph.
Medical Editorial Consultant,
Writer/Consultant in Medicine and Christian Literature,
Board Member, Chairman of Missions,
Christian Pharmacy Fellowship International,
Lawrence, Kansas

Susan Budassi Sheehy, R.N., M.S.N., C.E.N.
Clinical Nurse Specialist,
Emergency and Ambulatory Services,
St. Joseph Hospital and Health Care Center,
Tacoma, Washington;
Associate Professor of Clinical Nursing,
Department of Physiological Nursing,
University of Washington School of Nursing,
Seattle, Washington

Sandra L. Siehl, R.N., M.S.N.,
Oncology Clinical Nurse Specialist,
The Jewish Hospital of St. Louis,
Washington University Medical Center,
St. Louis, Missouri

Margretta M. Styles, R.N., Ed.D., F.A.A.N.
University of California,
San Francisco, California

June D. Thompson, R.N., M.S.
Assistant Professor of Nursing,
The University of Texas
Health Science Center at Houston,
Houston, Texas

Diana M. Uhler, R.N.
Department of Dermatology,
Gundersen Clinic, Ltd.,
La Crosse, Wisconsin

Lerma Ung
Senior Lecturer,
Department of Clinical Nursing,
Phillip Institute of Technology,
School of Nursing,
Bundoora Campus,
Bundoora, Victoria,
Australia

Lucille Whaley, R.N., M.S.
Pediatric Nurse Specialist;
Formerly Professor of Nursing,
San Jose State University,
San Jose, California

Bethany L. Wise, M.S., M.T.(ASCP)CLS
Instructor,
Medical Technology Division,
School of Allied Medical Professions,
The Ohio State University,
Columbus, Ohio

CREDITS

Appreciation is expressed to the following Mosby authors whose titles provided a valuable resource toward the compilation of this dictionary:

Anthony, C.P., and Thibodeau, G.A.: Textbook of anatomy and physiology, ed. 11, 1983.

Austrin, M.G.: Young's learning medical terminology, ed. 5, 1983.

Barnard, K.E., and Erickson, M.L.: Teaching children with developmental problems: a family care approach, ed. 2, 1976.

Bauer, J.D., Ackermann, P.G., and Toro, G.: Clinical laboratory methods, ed. 8, 1974.

Beck, E.W.: Mosby's atlas of functional human anatomy, 1982.

Bergerson, B.S.: Pharmacology in nursing, ed. 14, 1979.

Billings, D.M., and Stokes, L.G.: Medical-surgical nursing: common health problems of adults and children across the life span, 1982.

Bower, F.L., and Bevis, E.O.: Fundamentals of nursing practice: concepts, roles, and functions, 1979.

Brooks, S.M., and Paynton-Brooks, N.: The human body: structure and function in health and disease, ed. 2, 1980.

Budassi, S.A., and Barber, J.M.: Emergency nursing: principles and practice, 1981.

Budassi, S.A., and Barber, J.M.: Mosby's manual of emergency care: practices and procedures, ed. 2, 1983.

Butler, R.N., and Lewis, M.I.: Aging and mental health, ed. 3, 1982.

Campbell, J.M., and Campbell, J.B.: Laboratory mathematics: medical and biological applications, ed. 3, 1984.

Conover, M.B.: Understanding electrocardiography: physiological and interpretive concepts, ed. 4, 1984.

Fogel, C.I., and Woods, N.F.: Health care of women: a nursing perspective, 1981.

Goth, A.: Medical pharmacology: principles and concepts, ed. 11, 1984.

Groer, M.W., and Shekleton, M.E.: Basic pathophysiology: a conceptual approach, ed. 2, 1983

Hahn, A.B., Barkin, R.L., and Oestreich, S.J.K.: Pharmacology in nursing ed. 15, 1982.

Hilt, N.E., and Cogburn, S.B.: Manual of orthopedics, 1980.

Iorio, J.: Childbirth: family centered nursing, ed. 3, 1975.

Jensen, M.D., and Bobak, I.M.: Maternity and gynecologic care: the nurse and the family, ed. 2, 1985.

Kaye, D., and Rose, L.F., editors: Fundamentals of internal medicine, 1983.

Lawrence, R.A.: Breastfeeding: a guide for the medical profession, 1980.

Malasanos, L., et al.: Health assessment, ed. 2, 1981.

McClintic, J.R.: Human anatomy, 1982.

Parcel, G.S.: Basic emergency care of the sick and injured, ed. 2, 1982.

Pasquali, E.A., et al.: Mental health nursing: a holistic approach, ed. 2, 1985.

Phibbs, B.: The human heart: a consumer's guide to cardiac care, 1982.

Phipps, W.D., Long, B.C., and Woods, N.F.: Medical-surgical nursing: concepts and clinical practice, ed. 2, 1983.

Pierog, S.H., and Ferrara, A.: Medical care of the sick newborn, ed. 2, 1976.

Rosen, P., et al.: Emergency medicine: concepts and clinical practice, Vol. 1, 1983.

Saxton, D., Pelikan, P., Nugent, P., and Needleman, S.: Mosby's Assesstest, 1985.

Schottelius, B.A., and Schottelius, D.D.: Textbook of physiology, ed. 18, 1978.

Smith, A.L.: Microbiology and pathology, ed. 12, 1980.

Tucker, S.M., et al.: Patient care standards, ed. 3, 1983.

U.C.S.F.: Mosby's manual of clinical nursing procedures, 1981.

Warner, C.G.: Emergency care: assessment and intervention, ed. 3, 1983.

Whaley, L.F., and Wong, D.L.: Nursing care of infants and children, ed. 1 and 2, 1979, 1983.

Whaley, L.F., and Wong, D.L.: Essentials of pediatric nursing, ed. 2, 1985.

Williams, S.R.: Nutrition and diet therapy, ed. 4, 1981.

GUIDE TO THE DICTIONARY

A. ALPHABETIC ORDER

The entries are alphabetized in dictionary style, that is, letter by letter, disregarding spaces or hyphens between words:

analgesic	**artificial lung**
anal membrane	**artificially acquired immunity**
analog	**artificial pacemaker**

(Alphabetized in telephone-book style, that is, word by word, the order would be different: **anal membrane / analgesic / analog; artificial lung / artificial pacemaker / artificially acquired immunity.**)

The alphabetization is alphanumeric; that is, words and numbers form a single list, numbers being positioned as though they were spelled-out numerals: **Nilstat / 90-90 traction / ninth nerve** (An example of the few exceptions to this rule is the sequence **17-hydroxycorticosteroid / 11-hydroxyetiocholanolone / 5-hydroxyindoleacetic acid,** which can be found between the entries **hydroxochloroquine sulfate** and **hydroxyl,** not, as may be expected, **17-. . .** in letter "S," **11-. . .** in letter "E," and **5-. . .** in letter "F.")

Small subscript and superscript numbers are disregarded in alphabetizing: **No / N_2O / nobelium**

For the alphabetization of combining forms, see F below.

B. COMPOUND HEADWORDS

Compound headwords are given in their natural word order: **abdominal surgery,** not **surgery, abdominal; achondroplastic dwarf,** not **dwarf, achondroplastic.**

When appropriate, a reference is made elsewhere to the nonalphabetized element; the entry **dwarf,** for example, shows this indirect cross-reference: ". . . Kinds of dwarf include **achondroplastic dwarf,** . . ." (followed by 16 more terms ending in "dwarf").

There are few exceptions to this natural word order; nearly all of these concern formal classifications, for example: "**comfort, alteration in: pain,** a nursing diagnosis accepted by the Fourth National Conference on the Classification of Nursing Diagnoses . . ."

(NOTE: In this guide, the term "headword" is used to refer to any alphabetized and nonindented definiendum, be it a single-word term or a compound term.)

C. MULTIPLE DEFINITIONS

If a headword has more than one meaning, the meanings are numbered and are often accompanied by an indication of the field in which a sense applies: "**fractionation, 1.** (in neurology) . . . **2.** (in chemistry) . . . **3.** (in bacteriology) . . . **4.** (in histology) . . . **5.** (in radiology) . . ."

Smaller differences in meaning are occasionally separated by semicolons: "**enervation, 1.** the reduction or lack of nervous energy; weakness; lassitude, languor. **2.** removal of a complete nerve or of a section of nerve."

Words that are spelled alike but have entirely different meanings and origins are usually given as separate entries, with superscript numbers: "**aural**[1], of or pertaining to the ear or hearing . . ." followed by "**aural**[2], of or pertaining to an aura."

For reference entries that appear in the form of numbered senses, see the example of **hyperalimentation** at E below.

D. THE BOLDFACE ELEMENTS OF AN ENTRY

After the entry headword, which has large boldface type, the following elements may occur in boldface, in this order.

In large boldface:

- HEADWORD ABBREVIATIONS: **central nervous system (CNS)**

A corresponding abbreviation entry is listed: "**CNS,** abbreviation for **central nervous system.**" (For abbreviation entries, see F below.)

Occasionally the order is reversed: "**DDT (dichlordiphenyltrichloroethane),**" with a corresponding reference entry: "**dichlordiphenyltrichloroethane.** See **DDT.**" (For reference entries, see E below.)

In smaller boldface (all others):

- PLURAL OR SINGULAR FORMS that are not obvious.

The first form shown is the more common except when plurals are of more or less equal frequency: "**carcinoma,** *pl.* **carcinomas, carcinomata**"; **cortex,** *pl.* **cortices**"; "**data,** *sing.* **datum**"

A reference entry is listed only when the terms are alphabetically separated; for example, there are several entries between **data** and "**datum.** See **data.**"

■ HIDDEN ENTRIES, that is, terms that can best be defined in the context of a more general entry. For example, the definition of the entry **equine encephalitis** continues as follows: " . . . **Eastern equine encephalitis (EEE)** is a severe form of the infection . . . **western equine encephalitis (WEE),** which occurs . . . **Venezuelan equine encephalitis (VEE),** which is common in . . ."

The corresponding reference entries are "**eastern equine encephalitis.** See **equine encephalitis.**"; "**western equine encephalitis.** See **equine . . .**"; and so forth. For further reference, from the abbreviations **EEE, WEE,** and **VEE,** see F below.

■ INDIRECT CROSS-REFERENCES to other defined entries, shown as part of the definition and usually introduced by "Kinds of": "**dwarf,** . . . Kinds of dwarfs include **achondroplastic dwarf, Amsterdam dwarf,** . . . , and **thanatophoric dwarf.**"

The entry referred to may or may not show a reciprocal reference, depending on the information value.

■ SYNONYMOUS TERMS, preceded by "Also called," "Also spelled," or, for verbs and adjectives, "Also": "**abducens nerve,** . . . Also called **sixth nerve.**"

A corresponding reference entry is usually given: "**sixth nerve.** See **abducens nerve.**"

Occasionally the synonymous term is accompanied by a usage label: "**abdomen,** . . . Also called *(informal)* **belly.**"

If a synonymous term applies to only one numbered sense, it precedes rather than follows the definition, to avoid ambiguity: "**algology, 1.** the branch of medicine that is concerned with the study of pain. **2.** also called **phycology.** the branch of science that is concerned with algae." (Whenever a synonymous term *follows* the last numbered sense, it applies to all senses of the entry.)

■ (DIRECT) CROSS-REFERENCES, preceded by "See also" or "Compare," referring to another defined entry for additional information: "**abdominal aorta,** . . . See also **descending aorta.**"

The cross-reference may or may not be reciprocal.

Cross-references are also made to illustrations, to tables, to the color atlas, and to the appendixes.

For cross-references from an abbreviation entry (with "See"), see F below.

■ PARTS OF SPEECH related to the entry headword, shown as run-on entries that do not require a separate definition: "**abalienation,** . . . —**abalienate,** *v.*, **abalienated,** *adj.*"

E. REFERENCE ENTRIES

Reference entries are undefined entries referring to a defined entry. There, they usually correspond to the boldface terms for which reference entries are mentioned at D above.

However, many of the less frequently used synonymous terms are listed as a reference only; at the entry referred to, the reader's attention is not drawn to them with "Also called."

A reference entry may also refer to a defined entry for other reasons: A particular lightface term in the definition is occasionally referred to: "**motion sickness,** . . . air sickness . . . "—with the reference entry "**air sickness:** See **motion sickness.**" Or a reference is made to give additional access to a definition or to part of a definition: "**congenital condition.** See **congenital anomaly.**"—although the latter entry does not literally mention "congenital condition," and is not a synonymous term.

Some reference entries appear in the form of a numbered sense of a defined entry: "**hyperalimentation, 1.** overfeeding or the . . . in excess of the demands of the appetite. **2.** See **total parenteral nutrition.**" The latter entry says "Also called **hyperalimentation.**"

If two or more alphabetically adjacent terms refer to the same entry or entries, they are styled as one reference entry: "**coxa adducta, coxa flexa.** See **coxa vara.**"

A reference entry that would be derived from a boldface term in an immediately adjacent entry is not listed again as a headword; it becomes a "hidden reference entry": "**acardius amorphus,** . . . Also called **acardius anceps.**" But **acardius anceps** is not listed again as a reference entry because it would immediately *follow* the entry, the next entry being **acariasis.** Likewise: "**acoustic neuroma,** . . . Also called **acoustic neurilemmona, acoustic neurinoma, acoustic neurofibroma.**" But the three synonymous terms are not listed again as reference entries because they would immediately *precede* the entry, the entry ahead being **acoustic nerve.** Therefore:

If a term is not listed at the expected place, the reader might find it among the boldface terms of the immediately preceding or the immediately following entry.

F. OTHER KINDS OF ENTRIES

■ ABBREVIATION ENTRIES: Most abbreviation entries, including symbol entries, show the full form of the term in boldface: "**ABC,** abbreviation for **aspiration biopsy cytology.**" "**H,** symbol for **hydrogen.**" Implied reference is made to the entries **aspiration biopsy cytology** and **hydrogen** respectively.

Abbreviation entries for which there is no corresponding entry show the full form in italics: "**CBF,** abbreviation for *cerebral blood flow*." "**f,** symbol for *respiratory frequency*."

A combination of abbreviation entry and reference entry occurs when the abbreviation is that of a boldface or lightface term appearing under another headword. For example, the hidden entries at D above (in addition to the reference entries shown there), are also referred to in the following manner: "**EEE,** abbreviation for **eastern equine encephalitis.** See **equine encephalitis.**" An example with a lightface term: "**HLA-A,** abbreviation for *human leukocyte antigen A*. See **human leukocyte antigen.**" The latter entry says ". . . They are HLA-A, HLA-B, HLA-C . . . "

■ COMBINING FORMS: For a definition, see the entry **combining form.** The large amount and the nature of combining-form entries are an important feature of this dictionary. Through the combining forms the reader has additional access to the meanings of headwords and the words used in defining them. But the combining forms give also access to thousands of terms that are not included in this dictionary (and, to a large extent, are not found in any other reference work). For example, the combining-form entries **xylo-** and **-phage** (plus **-phagia, phago-,** and **-phagy**) may lead to the meaning of "xylophagous," namely, "wood-eating."

Combining-form headwords consisting of variants are alphabetized by the first variant only. For example, "**epi-, ep-,** a combining form meaning 'on, upon' . . ." is followed by **epiblast** (notwithstanding "**ep-**"). The other variant or variants are listed in their own alphabetical place as reference entries referring to the first variant: "**ep-.** See **epi-.**"

■ ENTRIES WITH SPECIAL PARAGRAPHS: Among the entries on diseases, drugs, and procedures, at least 1000 feature special paragraphs. These paragraphs are headed as follows.

For disease entries: "observations," "intervention," and "nursing considerations."

For drug entries: "indications," "contraindications," and "adverse effects."

For procedure entries: "method," "nursing orders," and "outcome criteria."

G. FURTHER COMMENTS

■ ETYMOLOGY is shown only in entries where it contributes immediately to a better understanding of the meaning: "**lysergide,** . . . Also called **LSD** (an abbreviation of the original German name, *Lyserg-Säure-Diäthylamid),* **lysergic acid diethylamide,** *(slang)* **acid.**" "**hangnail,** . . . painful . . . ("Hang" is not related to the verb but is an old English word for pain.) . . ."

■ EPONYMOUS TERMS THAT END IN "SYNDROME" OR "DISEASE" are given with an apostrophe (and "s" where appropriate) if they are based on the name of one person: **Adie's syndrome; Symmers' disease; Treacher Collins' syndrome** (the ophthalmologist Edward Treacher Collins). If they are based on the names of several people, they are given without apostrophe: **Bernard-Soulier syndrome; Brill-Symmers disease.**

■ ABBREVIATIONS AND LABELS IN ITALIC TYPE: The abbreviations are *pl.* (plural), *npl.* (noun plural), *sing.* (singular); *n.* (noun), *adj.* (adjective), *v.* (verb). The recurring labels are *slang, informal, nontechnical, obsolete, archaic; chiefly British, Canada, U.S.*

■ DICTIONARY OF FIRST REFERENCE for general spelling preferences is *Webster's New Collegiate Dictionary;* thereafter: *Webster's Third New International Dictionary.* End-of-line hyphenation of technical terms follows *The Medical & Health Sciences Word Book* (Houghton Mifflin).

H. PRONUNCIATION

■ SYSTEM: See the pronunciation key. The pronunciation system of this dictionary is basically a system that most readers know from their use of popular English dictionaries, especially the major college or desk dictionaries. All symbols for English sounds are ordinary letters of the alphabet with few adaptations, and with the exception of the schwa, /ə/ (the neutral vowel).

■ ACCENTS: Pronunciation, given between slants, is shown with primary and secondary accents, and a raised dot shows that two vowels or, occasionally, two consonants, between the slants are pronounced separately:

anoopsia /an′ō•op′sē•ə/
cecoileostomy /sē′kō•il′ē•os′təmē/
methemoglobin /met′hēməglō′bin, met•hē′məglōbin/

Without the raised dot, the second /th/ in the last example would be pronounced as in "thin." (The pronunciation key lists the following paired consonant symbols as representing a single sound: /ch/, /ng/, /sh/, /th/, /*th*/, /zh/, and the foreign sounds /kh/ and /*kh*/—if no raised dot intervenes.)

■ TRUNCATION: Pronunciation may be given in truncated form, especially for alternative or derived words:

defibrillate /difī′brilāt, difib′-/
bacteriophage /baktir′ē•əfāj′, . . . —**bacteriophagy** /-of′əjē/, *n.*

In the last example, the reader is asked to make the commonsense assumption that the primary accent of the headword becomes a secondary accent in the run-on term:

/baktir′ē•of′əjē/.

■ LOCATION: Pronunciation may be given for any boldface term and may occur anywhere in an entry:

aura /ôr′ə/, **1.** *pl.* **aurae** /ôr′ē/, a sensation . . . **2.** *pl.* **auras,** an emanation of light . . .
micrometer, 1. /mīkrom′ətər/, an instrument used for . . . **2.** /mī′krōmē′tər/, a unit of measurement . . .

Occasionally it is given for a lightface term:

b.i.d., (in prescriptions) abbreviation for *bis in die* /dē′ā/, a Latin phrase meaning . . .
boutonneuse fever . . . , an infectious disease . . . a tache noire /täshnô•är′/ or black spot . . .

■ LETTERWORD VERSUS ACRONYM: For definitions of these terms, see the entries **letterword** and **acronym** in this dictionary. If the pronunciation of an abbreviation is not given, the abbreviation is usually a letterword:

ABO blood groups [read /ā′bē′ō′/, not /ā′bō/]

If the pronunciation is an acronym, this is indicated by pronunciation:

AWOL /ā′wôl/

Some abbreviations are used as both:

JAMA /jä′mä, jam′ə, jā′ā′em′ā′/

■ FOREIGN SOUNDS: Non-English sounds do not occur often in this dictionary. They are represented by the following symbols:

/œ/ as in (French) **feu** /fœ/, **Europe** /œrôp′/; (German) **schön** /shœn/, **Goethe** /gœ′tə/
/Y/ as in (French) **tu** /tY/, **déjà vu** /dāzhävY′/; (German) **grün** /grYn/, **Walküre** /vulkY′rə/
/kh/ as in (Scottish) **loch** /lokh/; (German) **Rorschach** /rôr′shokh/, **Bach** /bokh, bäkh/
/*kh*/ as in (German) **ich** /i*kh*/, **Reich** /rī*kh*/ (or, approximated, as in English **fish:** /ish/, rīsh/)
/N/ This symbol does not represent a sound but indicates that the preceding vowel is a nasal, as in French **bon** /bôN/, **en face** /äNfäs′/, or **international** /aNternäsyōnäl′/.
/nyə/ Occurring at the end of French words, this symbol is not truly a separate syllable but an /n/ with a slight /y/ (similar to the sound in "onion") plus a near-silent /ə/, as in **Bois de Boulogne** /bo͞olō′nyə/, **Malgaigne** /mälgā′nyə/.

Because this work is a subject dictionary rather than a language dictionary, certain foreign words and proper names are rendered by English approximations. Examples are **Müller** /mil′ər/ (which is closer to German than /mY′lər/), **Niemann** /nē′mon/ (which is closer than /nē′män/), **Friedreich** /frēd′rīsh/ (which is close enough for anyone not used to pronouncing /*kh*/), or **jamais vu,** for which three acceptable pronunciations are given: /zhämävY′/ (near-French) and the approximations /zhämävē′/ and /zhämävo͞o′/ (/-vē′/ being much closer to French than /-vo͞o′/). Depending on usage, a foreign word or name may be given with near-native pronunciation, with entirely assimilated English pronunciation (as **de Quervain's fracture** /də kərvānz′/), or with both (as **Dupuytren's contracture** /dYpY•itraNs′, dēpē•itranz′/ or **Klippel-Feil syndrome** /klipel′fel′, klip′əlfīl′/).

At any rate, the English speaker should not hesitate to follow whatever is usage in his or her working or social environment.

Many of the numerous *Latin* terms in this dictionary are not given with pronunciation, mainly because there are different ways (all of them understood) in which Latin is pronounced by the English speaker and may be pronounced by speakers elsewhere. However, guidance is given in many cases, often to reflect common usage.

■ LATIN AND GREEK PLURALS: The spelling of Latin and Greek plurals is shown in most instances. However, when the plural formation is regular according to Latin and Greek rules, the pronunciation is usually not included. Therefore, the following list shows the suggested pronunciation of selected plural endings that are frequently encountered in the field of medicine.

PLURAL ENDINGS	EXAMPLES
-a /-ə/	**inoculum,** *pl.* **inocula** /inok′yo͞olə/
-ae /-ē/	**vertebra,** *pl.* **vertebrae** /vur′təbrē/
-ces /-sēz/	**thorax,** *pl.* **thoraces** /thôr′əsēz/
	apex, *pl.* **apices** /ā′pisēz/
-era /-ərə/	**genus,** *pl.* **genera** /jen′ərə/
-ges /-jēz/	**meninx,** *pl.* **meninges** /minin′jēz/
-i /-ī/	**calculus,** *pl.* **calculi** /kal′kyəlī/
	coccus, *pl.* **cocci** /kok′sī/
-ia /-ē•ə/	**criterion,** *pl.* **criteria** /krītir′ē•ə/
-ides /-idēz/	**epulis,** *pl.* **epulides** /ipyo͞o′lidēz/
-ina /-ənə/	**foramen,** *pl.* **foramina** /fəram′ənə/
-ines /-ənēz/	**lentigo,** *pl.* **lentigines** /lentij′ənēz/
-omata /-ō′mətə/	**hemotoma,** *pl.* **hematomata** /hē′mətō′mətə/
-ones /-ō′nēz/	**comedo,** *pl.* **comedones** /kom′ədō′nēz/
-ora /-ərə/	**corpus,** *pl.* **corpora** /kôr′pərə/
	femur, *pl.* **femora** /fem′ərə/
-ses /-sēz/	**analysis,** *pl.* **analyses** /ənal′əsēz/
-udes /-o͞o′dēz/	**incus,** *pl.* **incudes** /inko͞o′dēz/
-us /-o͞os/	**ductus** (/duk′təs/), *pl.* **ductus** /duk′to͞os/

NOTE: Notwithstanding the listing of Latin and Greek plurals in this dictionary, and notwithstanding the foregoing examples, in most instances it is acceptable or even preferable to pluralize Latin and Greek words according to the rules of English words. (For certain kinds of entries, both the English and the foreign plurals are given in this dictionary, usually showing the English form first, as, for example, in nearly all **-oma** nouns: **hematoma,** *pl.* **hematomas, hematomata.**)

W.D.G.

PRONUNCIATION KEY

Vowels

SYMBOLS	KEY WORDS
/a/	h**a**t
/ä/	f**a**ther
/ā/	f**a**te
/e/	fl**e**sh
/ē/	sh**e**
/er/	**air**, f**err**y
/i/	s**i**t
/ī/	**eye**
/ir/	**ear**
/o/	pr**o**per
/ō/	n**o**se
/ô/	s**aw**
/oi/	b**oy**
/o͞o/	m**o**ve
/o͝o/	b**oo**k
/ou/	**ou**t
/u/	c**u**p, l**o**ve
/ur/	f**ur**, f**ir**st
/ə/	(the neutral vowel, always unstressed, as in) **a**go, foc**u**s
/ər/	teach**er**, doct**or**

Consonants

SYMBOLS	KEY WORDS
/b/	**b**ook
/ch/	**ch**ew
/d/	**d**ay
/f/	**f**ast
/g/	**g**ood
/h/	**h**appy
/j/	**g**em
/k/	**k**eep
/l/	**l**ate
/m/	**m**ake
/n/	**n**o
/ng/	si**ng** dri**n**k
/ng·g/	fi**ng**er
/p/	**p**air
/r/	**r**ing
/s/	**s**et
/sh/	**sh**oe, lo**ti**on
/t/	**t**one
/th/	**th**in
/*th*/	**th**an
/v/	**v**ery
/w/	**w**ork
/y/	**y**es
/z/	**z**eal
/zh/	a**z**ure, vi**si**on

For /œ/, /Y/, /kh/, /*kh*/, /N/, and /nyə/, see FOREIGN SOUNDS, p. xviii.

COLOR ATLAS OF HUMAN ANATOMY

SKELETAL SYSTEM

ANTERIOR VIEW OF SKELETON

Axial skeleton is shown in blue. Appendicular system is bone colored.

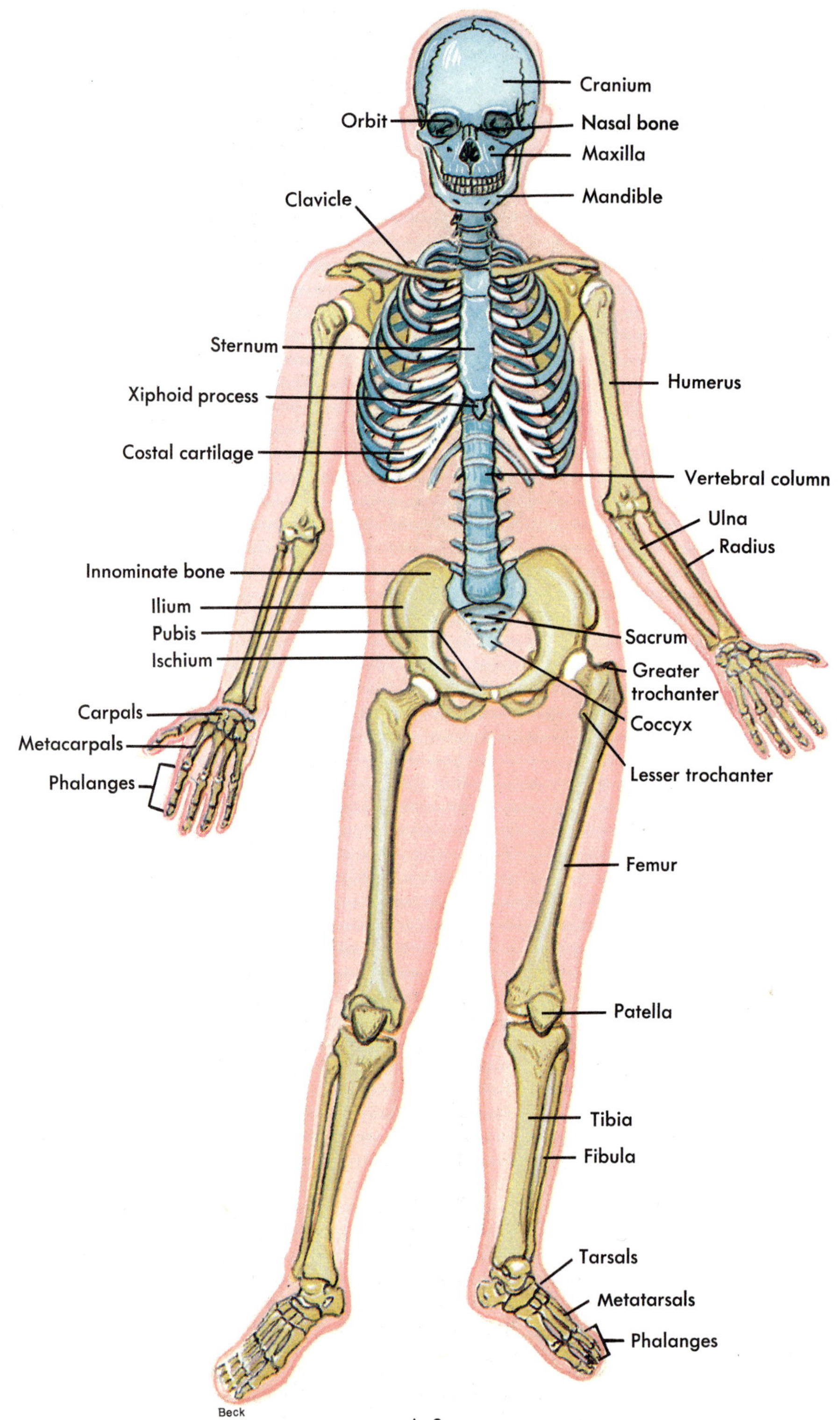

POSTERIOR VIEW OF SKELETON

Axial skeleton is shown in blue. Appendicular system is bone colored.

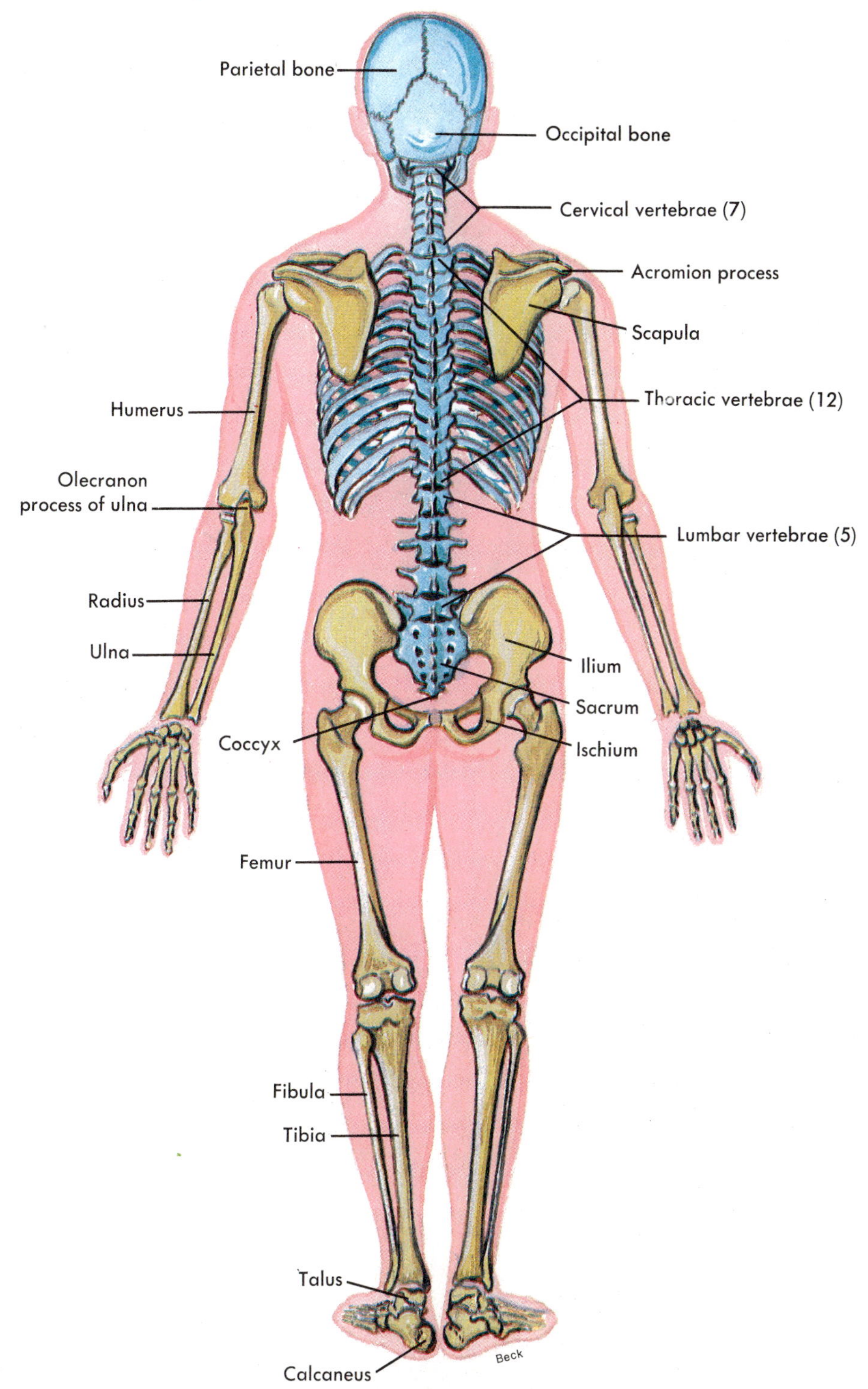

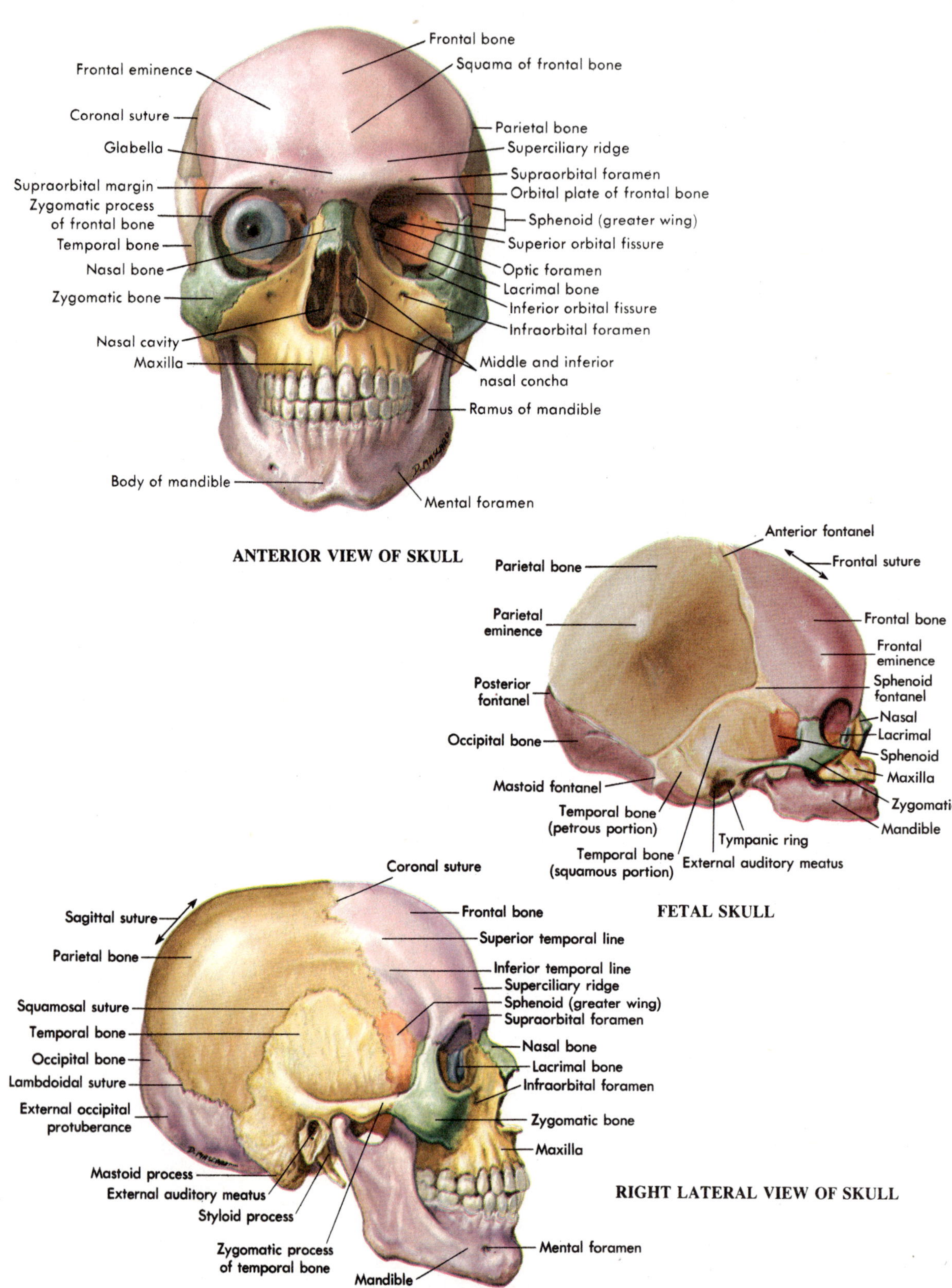
Frontal bone
Squama of frontal bone
Frontal eminence
Coronal suture
Parietal bone
Glabella
Superciliary ridge
Supraorbital foramen
Supraorbital margin
Orbital plate of frontal bone
Zygomatic process of frontal bone
Sphenoid (greater wing)
Temporal bone
Superior orbital fissure
Nasal bone
Optic foramen
Lacrimal bone
Zygomatic bone
Inferior orbital fissure
Infraorbital foramen
Nasal cavity
Maxilla
Middle and inferior nasal concha
Ramus of mandible
Body of mandible
Mental foramen
Anterior fontanel
Parietal bone
Frontal suture
Parietal eminence
Frontal bone
Frontal eminence
Posterior fontanel
Sphenoid fontanel
Nasal
Lacrimal
Occipital bone
Sphenoid
Maxilla
Mastoid fontanel
Zygomatic
Temporal bone (petrous portion)
Mandible
Tympanic ring
Temporal bone (squamous portion)
External auditory meatus
Coronal suture
Sagittal suture
Frontal bone
Superior temporal line
Parietal bone
Inferior temporal line
Superciliary ridge
Squamosal suture
Sphenoid (greater wing)
Supraorbital foramen
Temporal bone
Nasal bone
Occipital bone
Lacrimal bone
Lambdoidal suture
Infraorbital foramen
External occipital protuberance
Zygomatic bone
Maxilla
Mastoid process
External auditory meatus
Styloid process
Zygomatic process of temporal bone
Mental foramen
Mandible

ANTERIOR VIEW OF SKULL

FETAL SKULL

RIGHT LATERAL VIEW OF SKULL

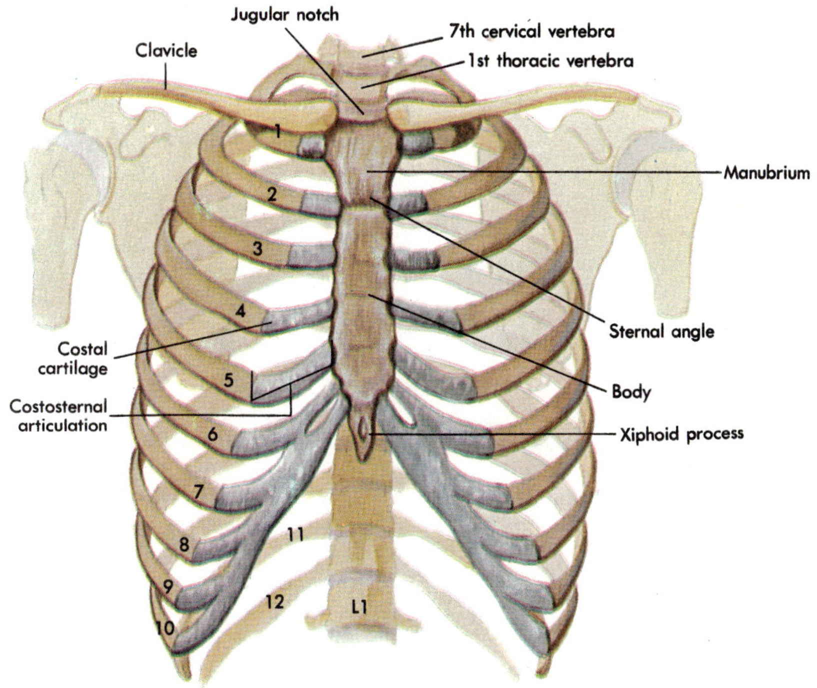

THORAX AND RIBS

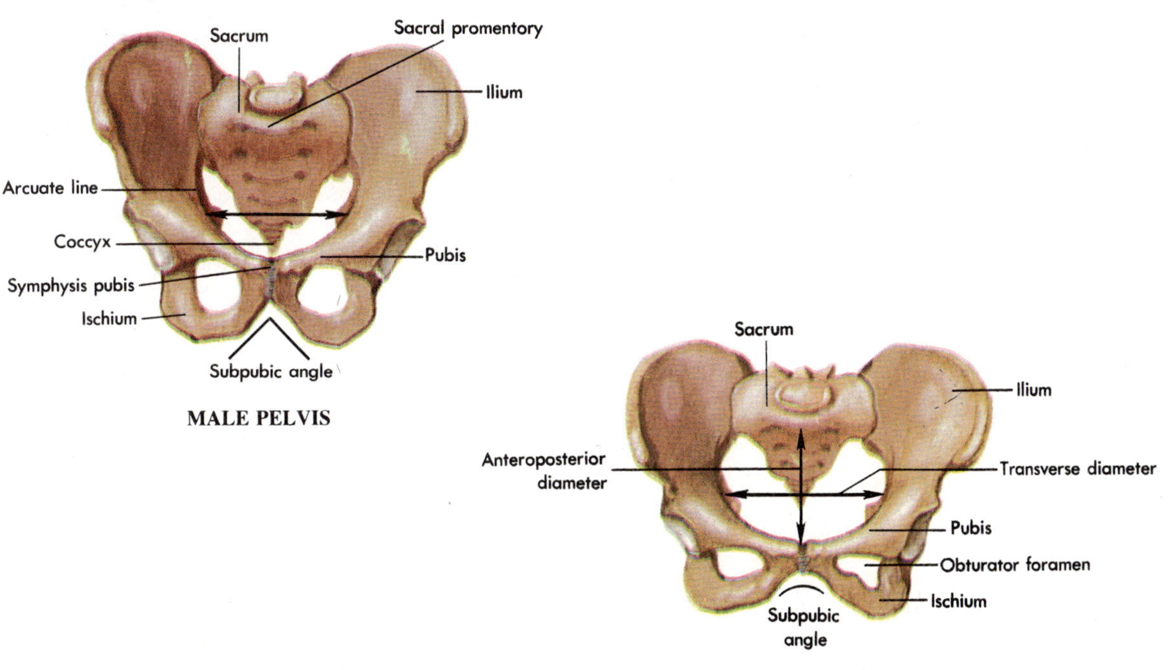

MALE PELVIS

FEMALE PELVIS

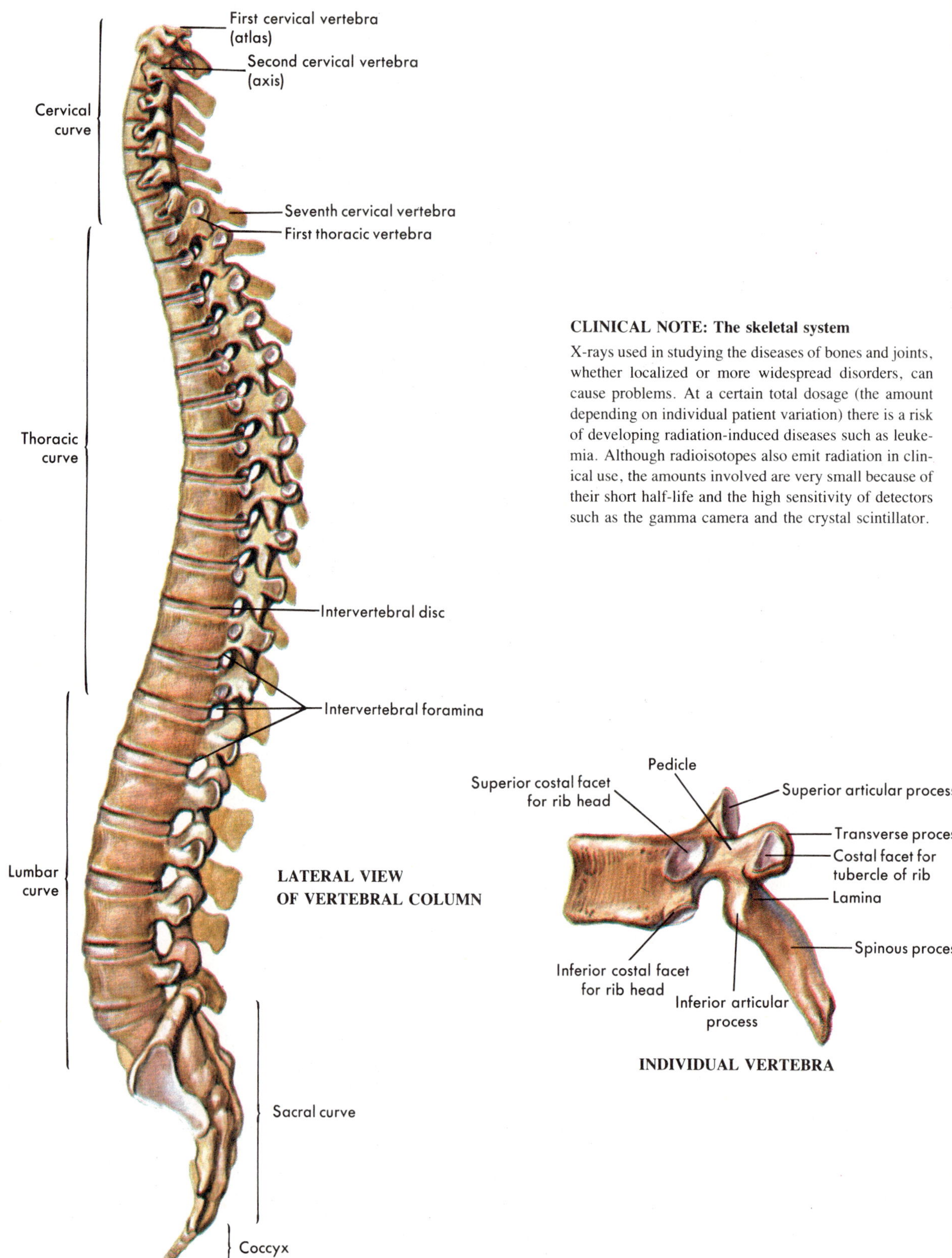

LATERAL VIEW OF VERTEBRAL COLUMN

INDIVIDUAL VERTEBRA

CLINICAL NOTE: The skeletal system

X-rays used in studying the diseases of bones and joints, whether localized or more widespread disorders, can cause problems. At a certain total dosage (the amount depending on individual patient variation) there is a risk of developing radiation-induced diseases such as leukemia. Although radioisotopes also emit radiation in clinical use, the amounts involved are very small because of their short half-life and the high sensitivity of detectors such as the gamma camera and the crystal scintillator.

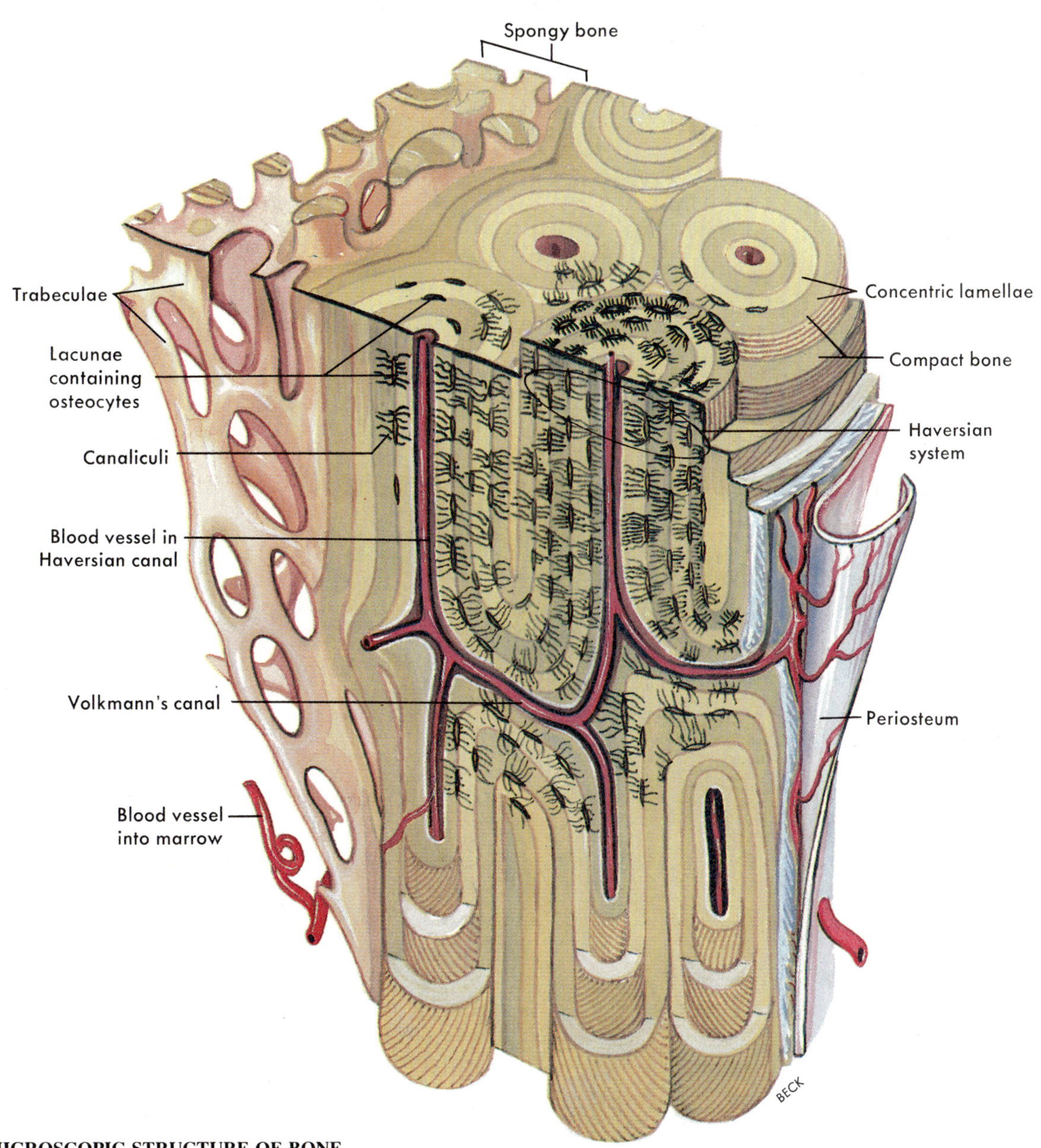

MICROSCOPIC STRUCTURE OF BONE

Haversian systems, several of which are shown here, compose compact bone. Note the structures that make up one haversian system: concentric lamellae, lacunae, canaliculi, and a haversian canal. Shown bordering the compact bone on the left is spongy bone, a name descriptive of the many open spaces that characterize it.

MUSCULAR SYSTEM

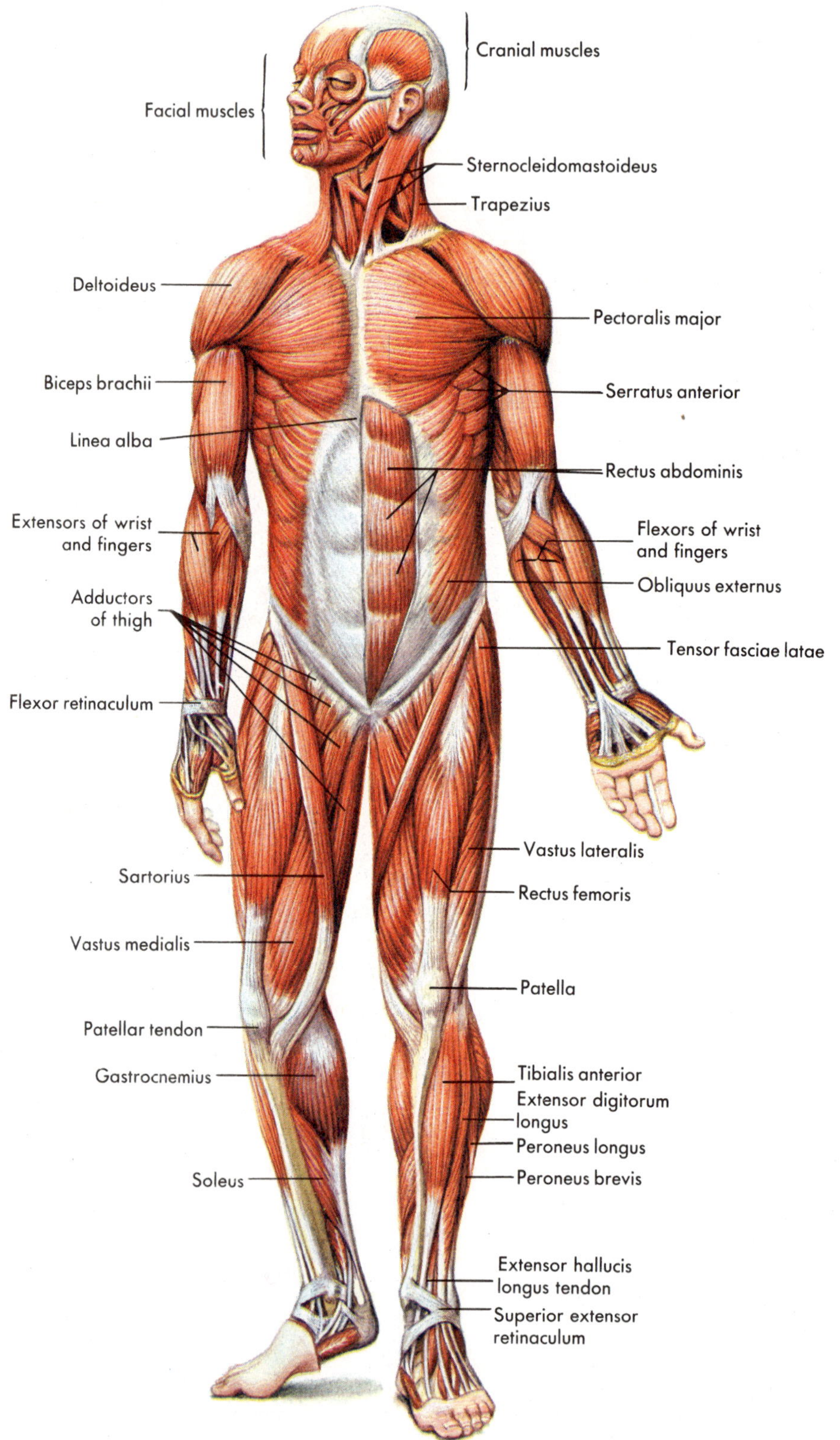

Cranial muscles
Facial muscles
Sternocleidomastoideus
Trapezius
Deltoideus
Pectoralis major
Biceps brachii
Serratus anterior
Linea alba
Rectus abdominis
Extensors of wrist and fingers
Flexors of wrist and fingers
Obliquus externus
Adductors of thigh
Tensor fasciae latae
Flexor retinaculum
Vastus lateralis
Sartorius
Rectus femoris
Vastus medialis
Patella
Patellar tendon
Gastrocnemius
Tibialis anterior
Extensor digitorum longus
Peroneus longus
Soleus
Peroneus brevis
Extensor hallucis longus tendon
Superior extensor retinaculum

ANTERIOR VIEW

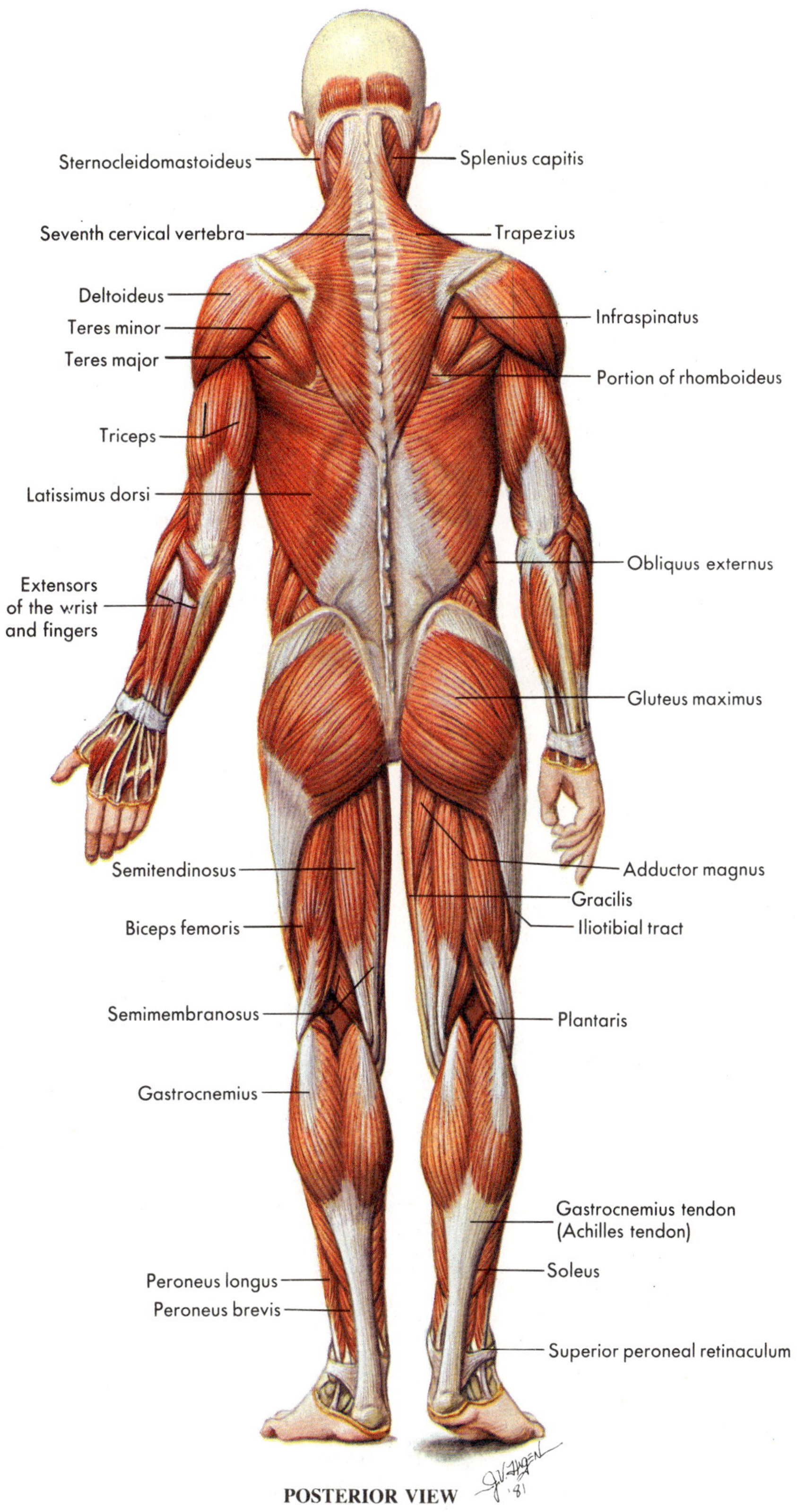
Sternocleidomastoideus
Splenius capitis
Seventh cervical vertebra
Trapezius
Deltoideus
Teres minor
Infraspinatus
Teres major
Portion of rhomboideus
Triceps
Latissimus dorsi
Obliquus externus
Extensors
of the wrist
and fingers
Gluteus maximus
Semitendinosus
Adductor magnus
Gracilis
Biceps femoris
Iliotibial tract
Semimembranosus
Plantaris
Gastrocnemius
Gastrocnemius tendon
(Achilles tendon)
Soleus
Peroneus longus
Peroneus brevis
Superior peroneal retinaculum

POSTERIOR VIEW

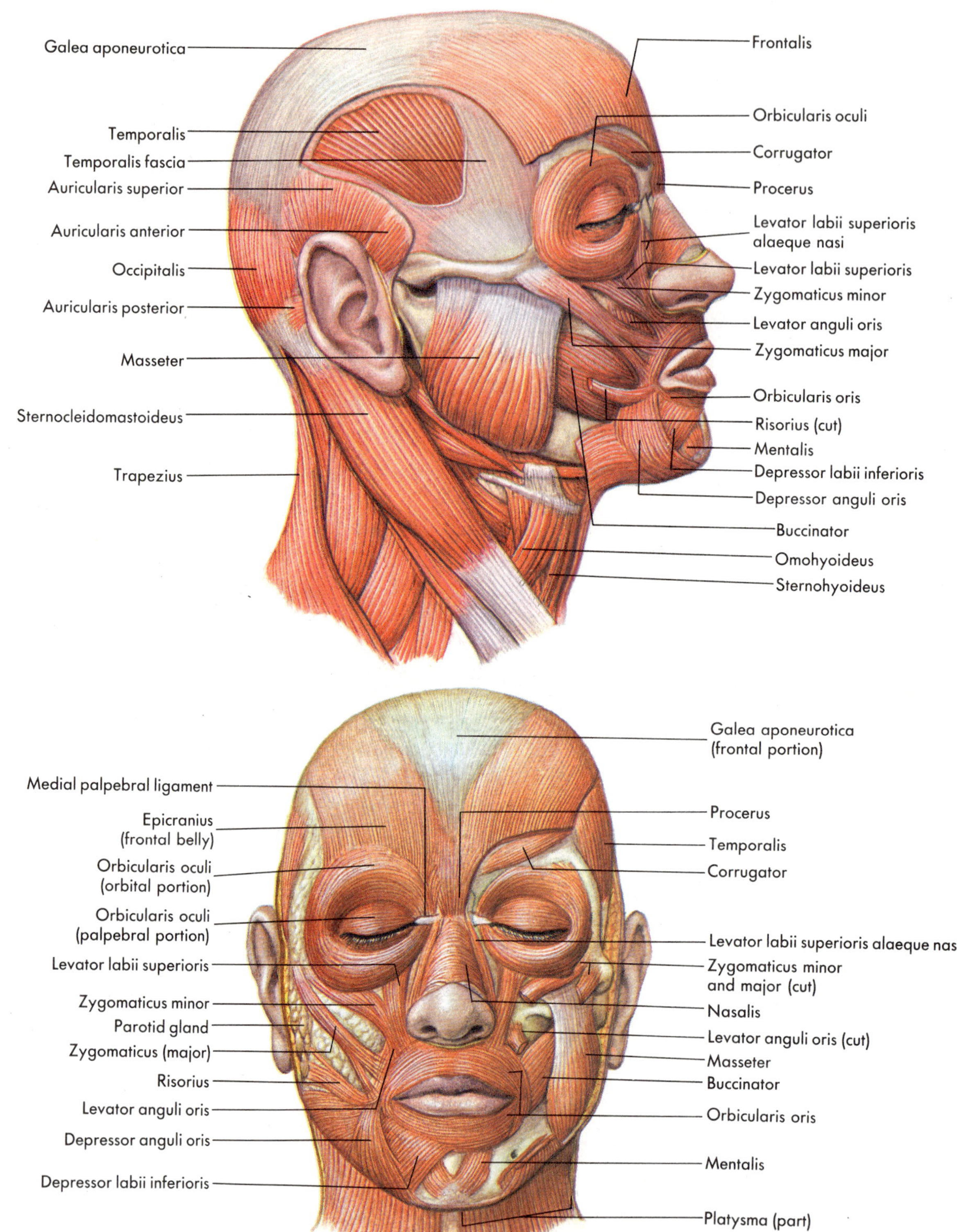
Galea aponeurotica
Temporalis
Temporalis fascia
Auricularis superior
Auricularis anterior
Occipitalis
Auricularis posterior
Masseter
Sternocleidomastoideus
Trapezius
Frontalis
Orbicularis oculi
Corrugator
Procerus
Levator labii superioris alaeque nasi
Levator labii superioris
Zygomaticus minor
Levator anguli oris
Zygomaticus major
Orbicularis oris
Risorius (cut)
Mentalis
Depressor labii inferioris
Depressor anguli oris
Buccinator
Omohyoideus
Sternohyoideus
Medial palpebral ligament
Epicranius (frontal belly)
Orbicularis oculi (orbital portion)
Orbicularis oculi (palpebral portion)
Levator labii superioris
Zygomaticus minor
Parotid gland
Zygomaticus (major)
Risorius
Levator anguli oris
Depressor anguli oris
Depressor labii inferioris
Galea aponeurotica (frontal portion)
Procerus
Temporalis
Corrugator
Levator labii superioris alaeque nasi
Zygomaticus minor and major (cut)
Nasalis
Levator anguli oris (cut)
Masseter
Buccinator
Orbicularis oris
Mentalis
Platysma (part)

LATERAL AND ANTERIOR VIEWS OF MUSCLES OF FACE AND ANTERIOR CRANIUM AND SEVERAL MUSCLES OF MASTICATION

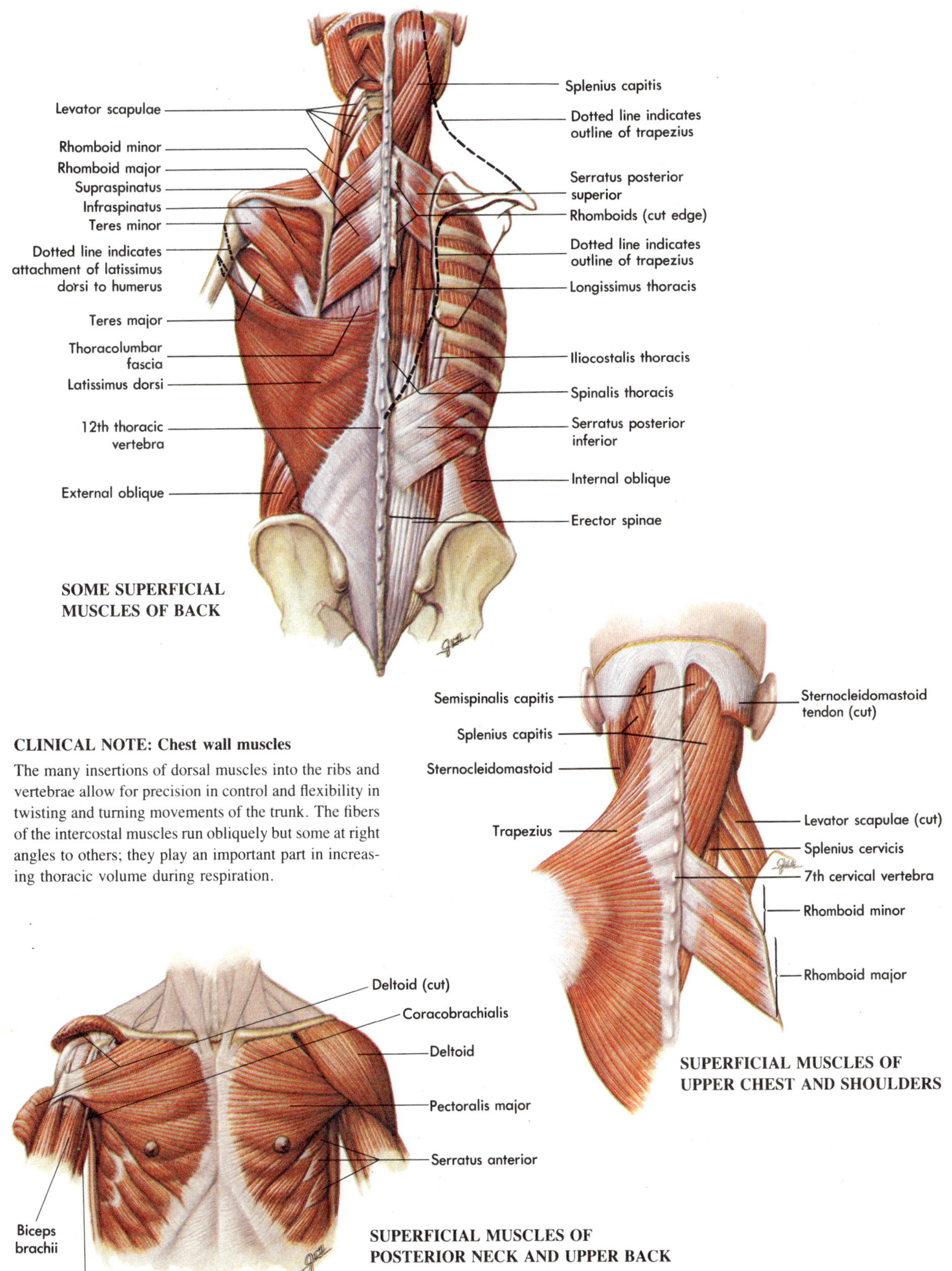

SOME SUPERFICIAL MUSCLES OF BACK

SUPERFICIAL MUSCLES OF UPPER CHEST AND SHOULDERS

SUPERFICIAL MUSCLES OF POSTERIOR NECK AND UPPER BACK

CLINICAL NOTE: Chest wall muscles

The many insertions of dorsal muscles into the ribs and vertebrae allow for precision in control and flexibility in twisting and turning movements of the trunk. The fibers of the intercostal muscles run obliquely but some at right angles to others; they play an important part in increasing thoracic volume during respiration.

CIRCULATORY SYSTEM

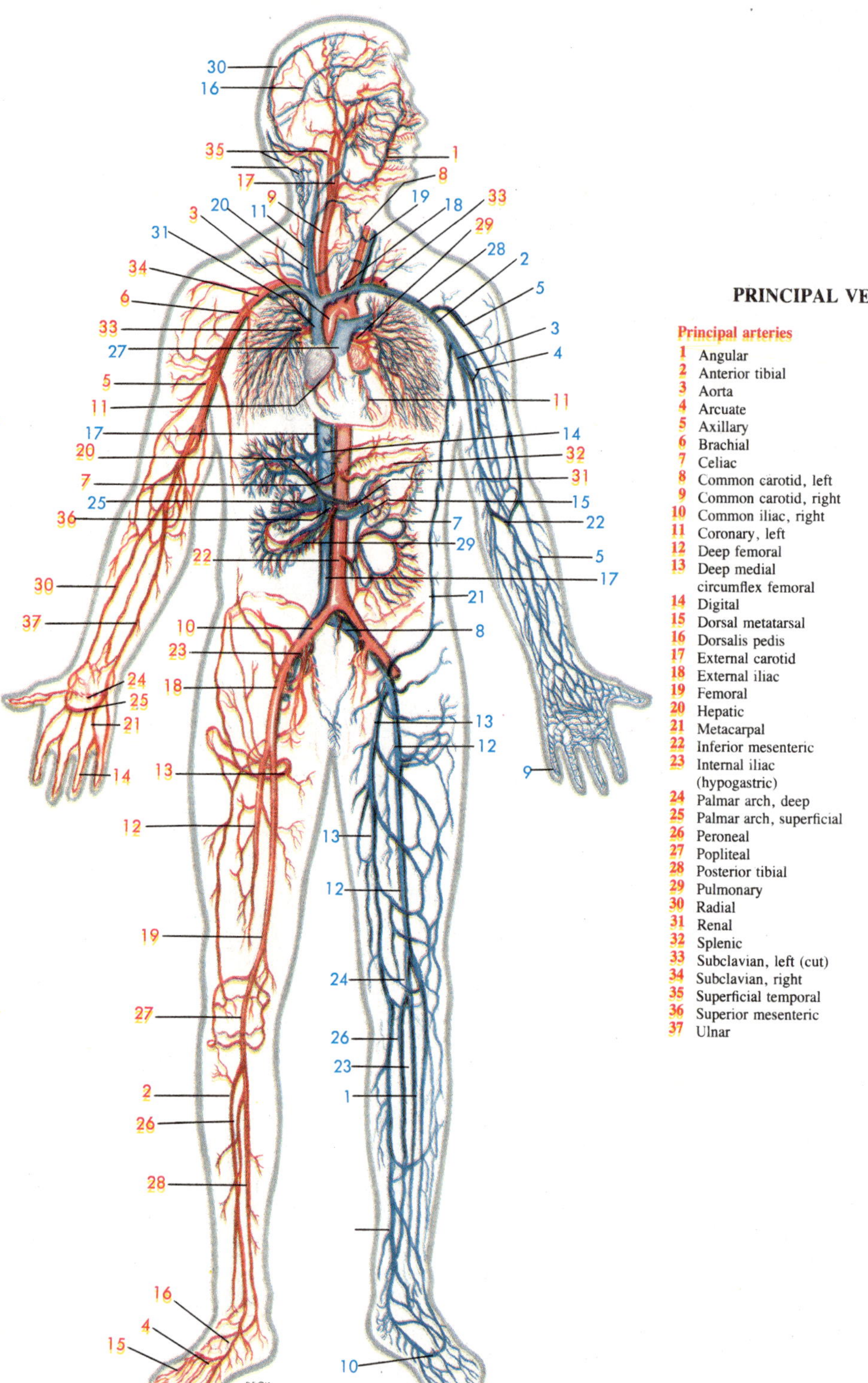

PRINCIPAL VEINS AND ARTERIES

Principal arteries

1 Angular
2 Anterior tibial
3 Aorta
4 Arcuate
5 Axillary
6 Brachial
7 Celiac
8 Common carotid, left
9 Common carotid, right
10 Common iliac, right
11 Coronary, left
12 Deep femoral
13 Deep medial circumflex femoral
14 Digital
15 Dorsal metatarsal
16 Dorsalis pedis
17 External carotid
18 External iliac
19 Femoral
20 Hepatic
21 Metacarpal
22 Inferior mesenteric
23 Internal iliac (hypogastric)
24 Palmar arch, deep
25 Palmar arch, superficial
26 Peroneal
27 Popliteal
28 Posterior tibial
29 Pulmonary
30 Radial
31 Renal
32 Splenic
33 Subclavian, left (cut)
34 Subclavian, right
35 Superficial temporal
36 Superior mesenteric
37 Ulnar

Principal veins

1 Anterior tibial
2 Axillary
3 Basilic
4 Brachial
5 Cephalic
6 Cervical plexus
7 Colic
8 Common iliac, left
9 Digital
10 Dorsal venous arch
11 External jugular
12 Femoral
13 Great saphenous
14 Hepatic
15 Inferior mesenteric
16 Inferior sagittal sinus
17 Inferior vena cava
18 Brachiocephalic, left
19 Internal jugular, left
20 Internal jugular, right
21 Lateral thoracic
22 Median cubital
23 Peroneal
24 Popliteal
25 Portal
26 Posterior tibial
27 Pulmonary
28 Subclavian, left
29 Superior mesenteric
30 Superior sagittal sinus
31 Superior vena cava

Aorta
Left pulmonary artery
Left pulmonary veins
Left atrium
ircumflex branch of
eft coronary artery
reat cardiac vein
Oblique vein
osterior vein of
left ventricle
Left ventricle
Apex
Azygos vein
Superior vena cava
Right pulmonary artery
Right pulmonary veins
Right atrium
Right auricle
Inferior vena cava
Small cardiac vein
Right coronary artery
Coronary sinus
Right ventricle
Posterior interventricular sulcus
Middle cardiac vein
Right interventricular artery

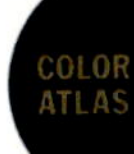

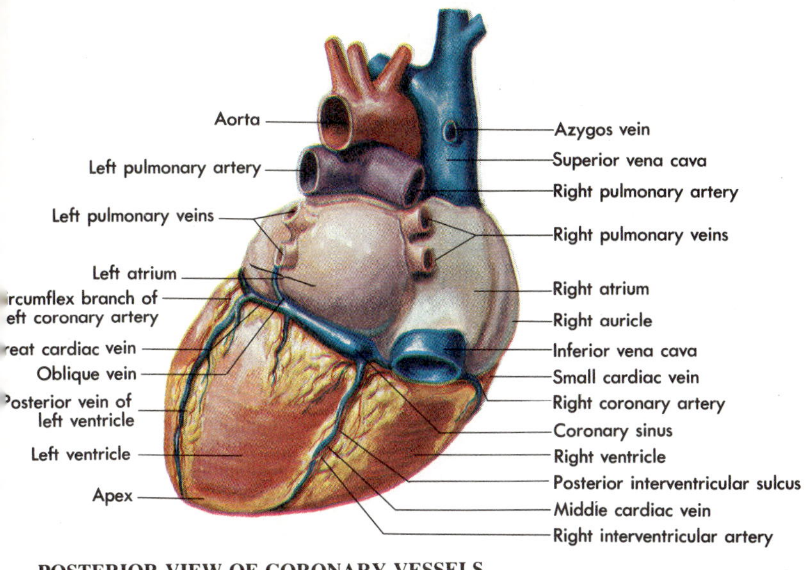

POSTERIOR VIEW OF CORONARY VESSELS

Brachiocephalic artery
Left common carotid artery
Right common
carotid artery
Right internal
jugular vein
Right subclavian
vein
Left subclavian artery
Aortic arch
Ligamentum arteriosus
Pulmonary trunk
Superior vena cava
Left pulmonary arteries
Right pulmonary
arteries
Left pulmonary veins
Right pulmonary veins
Pulmonary valve leaflet
Right atrium
Aortic valve (dotted lines)
Left atrium and mitral valve
Section of right
ventricle intact
Chordae tendineae
Papillary muscle
Tricuspid valve
Left ventricle
Right ventricle
Interventricular septum
Inferior vena cava
Myocardium
Papillary muscle

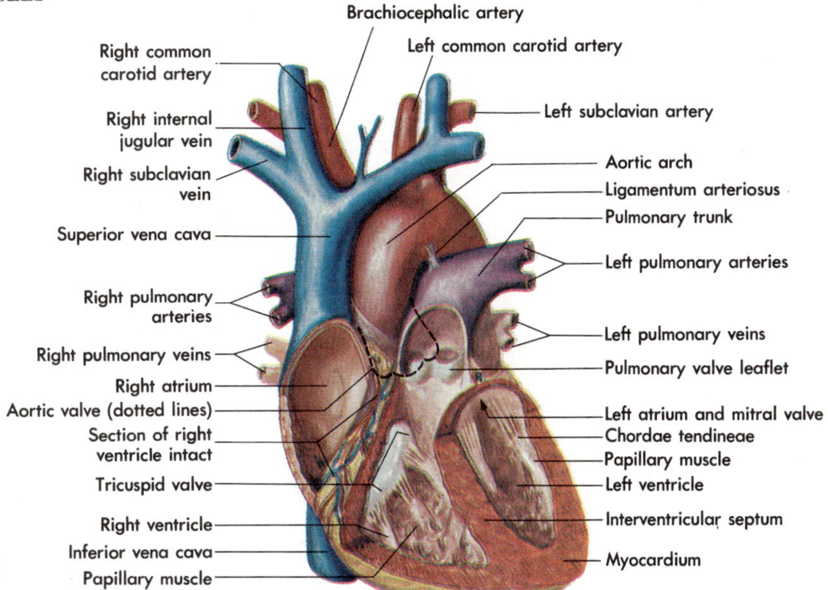

HUMAN HEART IN FRONTAL SECTION

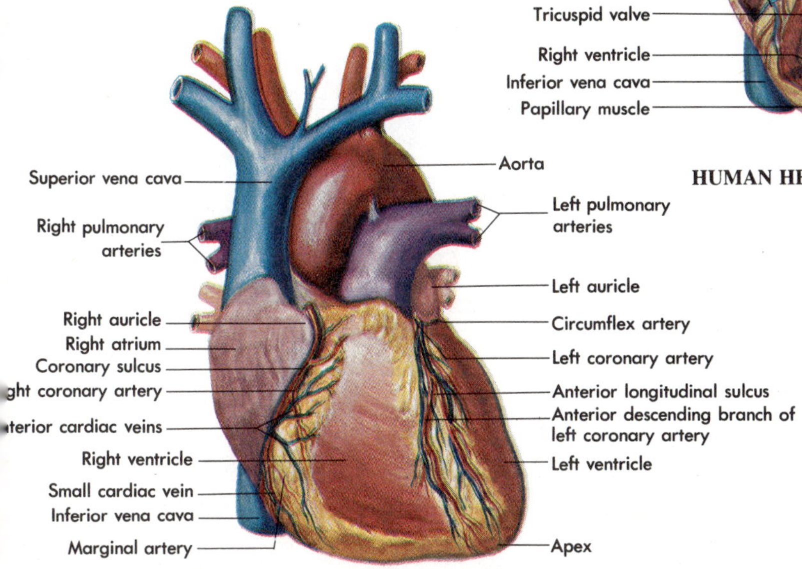

Aorta
Superior vena cava
Right pulmonary
arteries
Left pulmonary
arteries
Left auricle
Right auricle
Circumflex artery
Right atrium
Left coronary artery
Coronary sulcus
ght coronary artery
Anterior longitudinal sulcus
terior cardiac veins
Anterior descending branch of
left coronary artery
Right ventricle
Left ventricle
Small cardiac vein
Inferior vena cava
Marginal artery
Apex

ANTERIOR VIEW OF CORONARY VESSELS

Transverse cervical artery
Suprascapular artery
Descending scapular artery
Acromial branch
Axillary artery (rib 1 to teres tendon)
Posterior humeral circumflex artery
Anterior humeral circumflex artery
Subscapular artery
Brachial artery
Inferior thyroidal artery
Common carotid artery
Thyrocervical trunk
Subclavian artery
Brachiocephalic artery
Highest thoracic artery
Internal thoracic artery
Thoracoacromial artery
Thoracic branch
Lateral thoracic artery

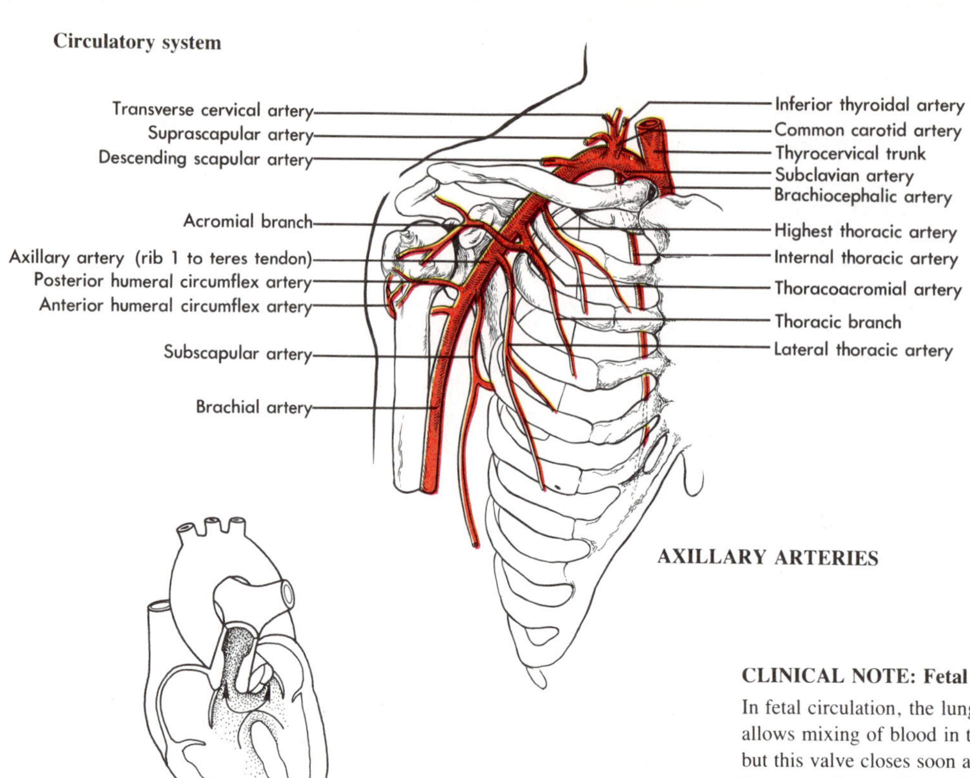

AXILLARY ARTERIES

TETRALOGY OF FALLOT

CLINICAL NOTE: Fetal circulation

In fetal circulation, the lungs are inactive. A flap valve allows mixing of blood in the left ventricular chamber, but this valve closes soon after the first breath is taken. Some cardiac malformations cause cyanosis due to improper oxygenation of arterial blood. Tetralogy of Fallot is an example. The stenosed pulmonary artery, ventricular septal defect, poorly positioned aorta, and right ventricular hypertrophy are all characteristic but are usually correctable by surgery.

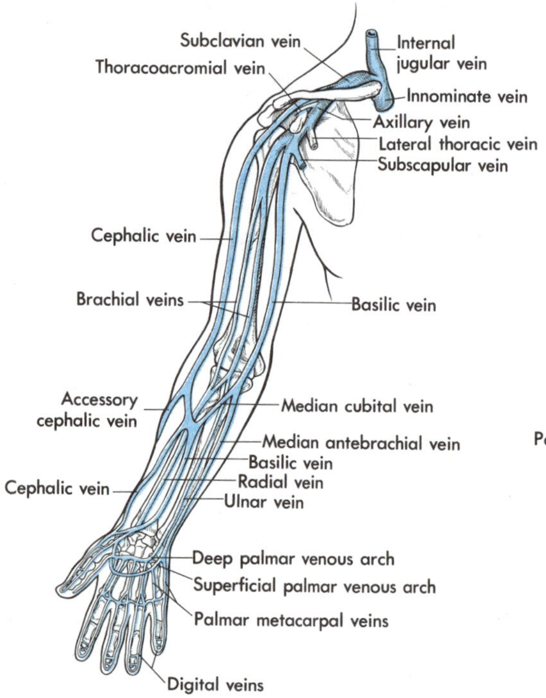

Subclavian vein
Thoracoacromial vein
Internal jugular vein
Innominate vein
Axillary vein
Lateral thoracic vein
Subscapular vein
Cephalic vein
Brachial veins
Basilic vein
Accessory cephalic vein
Median cubital vein
Median antebrachial vein
Basilic vein
Radial vein
Cephalic vein
Ulnar vein
Deep palmar venous arch
Superficial palmar venous arch
Palmar metacarpal veins
Digital veins

MAJOR VEINS OF UPPER APPENDAGES

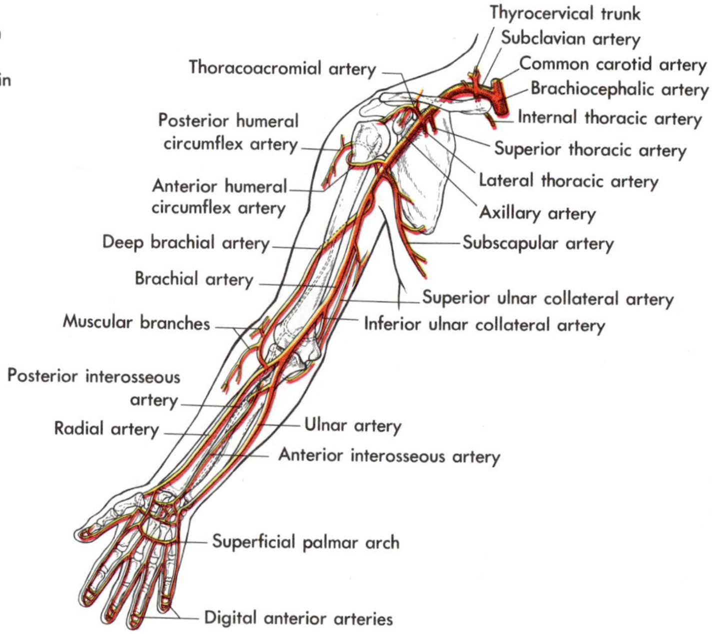

Thyrocervical trunk
Subclavian artery
Common carotid artery
Brachiocephalic artery
Thoracoacromial artery
Internal thoracic artery
Posterior humeral circumflex artery
Superior thoracic artery
Lateral thoracic artery
Anterior humeral circumflex artery
Axillary artery
Deep brachial artery
Subscapular artery
Brachial artery
Superior ulnar collateral artery
Muscular branches
Inferior ulnar collateral artery
Posterior interosseous artery
Radial artery
Ulnar artery
Anterior interosseous artery
Superficial palmar arch
Digital anterior arteries

MAJOR ARTERIES OF UPPER APPENDAGES

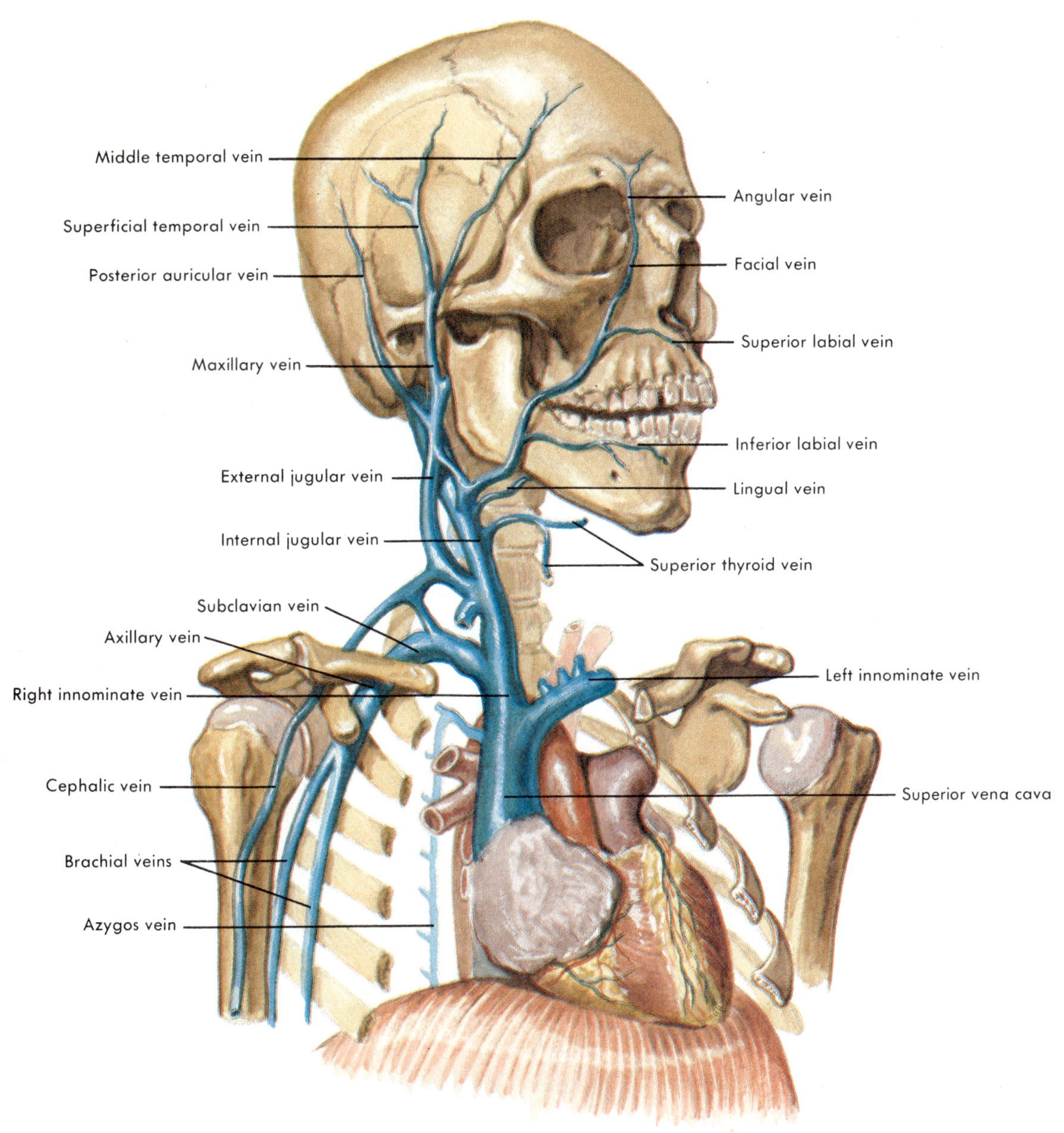
Middle temporal vein
Superficial temporal vein
Posterior auricular vein
Maxillary vein
External jugular vein
Internal jugular vein
Subclavian vein
Axillary vein
Right innominate vein
Cephalic vein
Brachial veins
Azygos vein
Angular vein
Facial vein
Superior labial vein
Inferior labial vein
Lingual vein
Superior thyroid vein
Left innominate vein
Superior vena cava

VEINS FORMING SUPERIOR VENA CAVA

ENDOCRINE SYSTEM

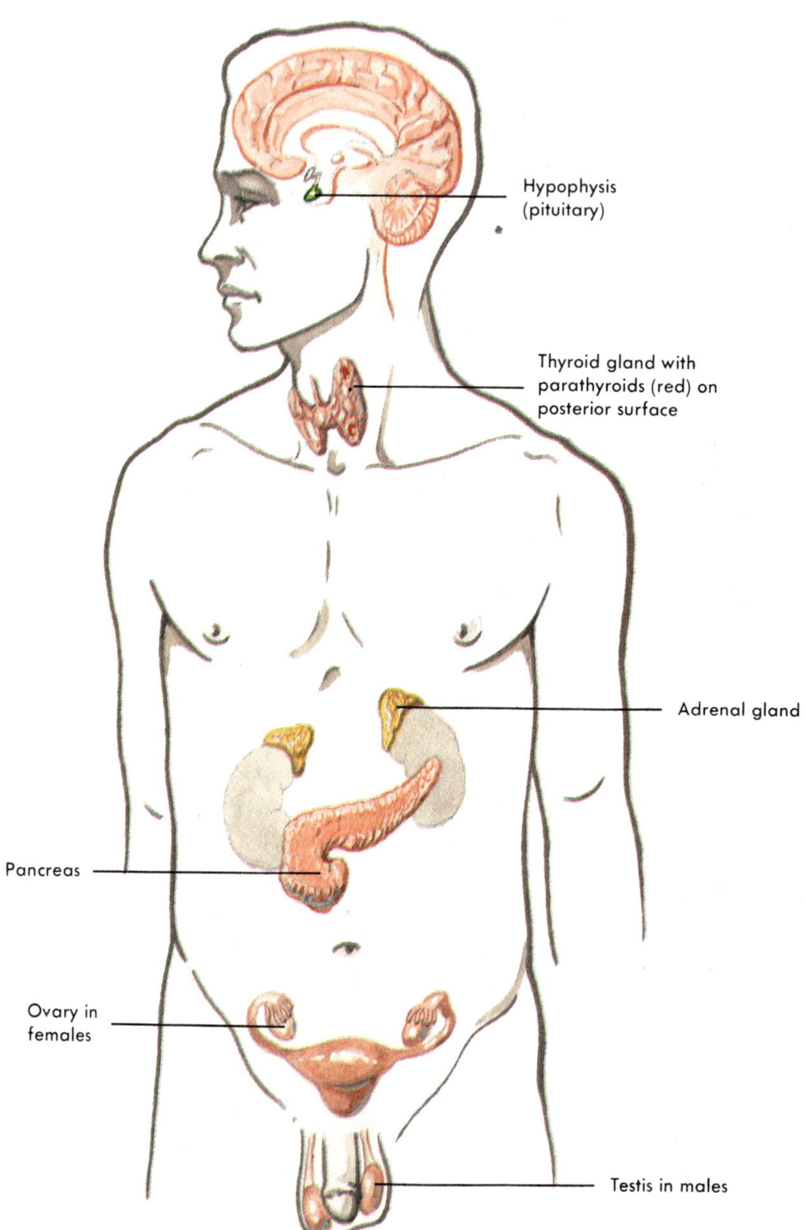

ENDOCRINE SYSTEM

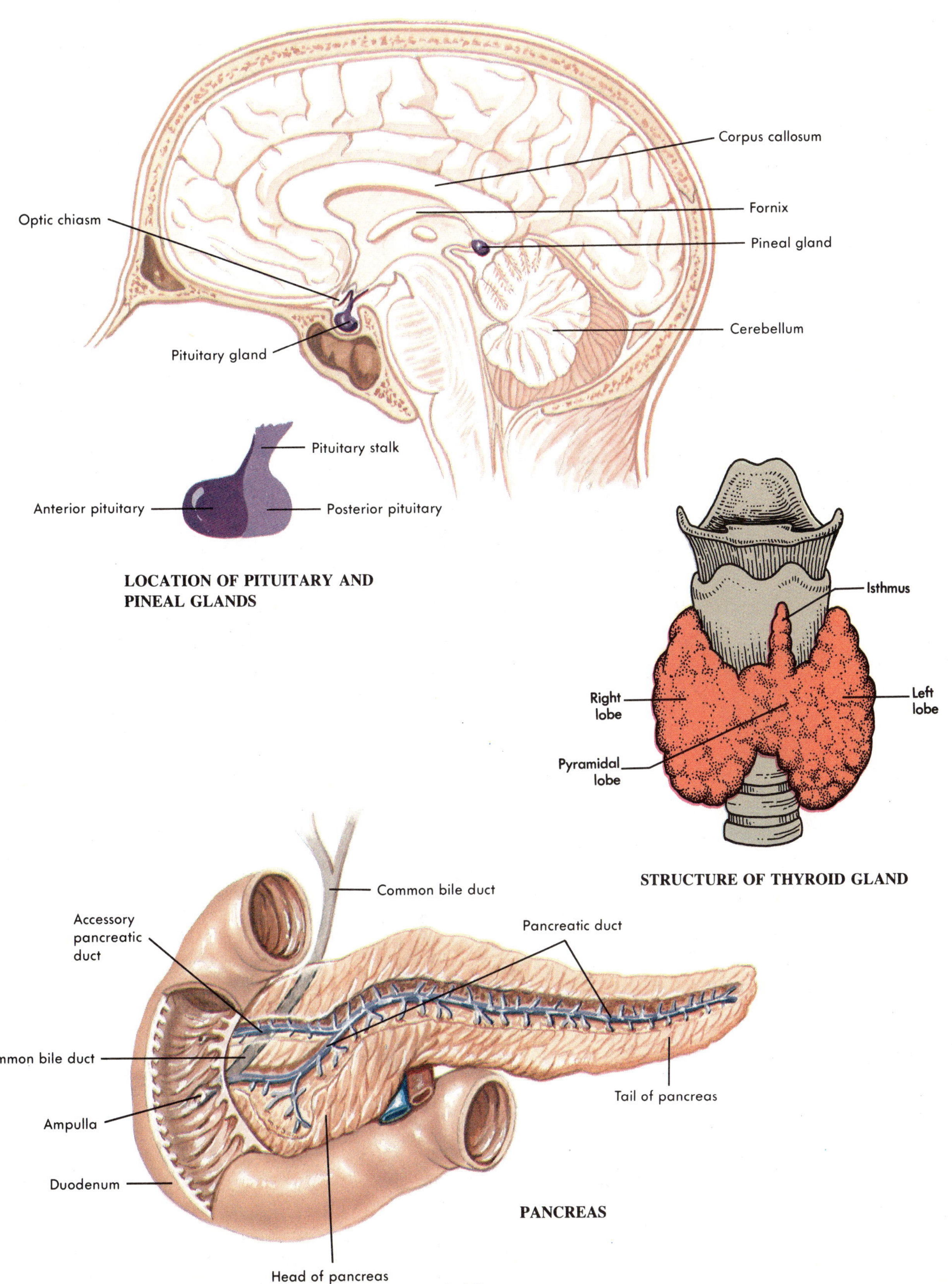

LOCATION OF PITUITARY AND PINEAL GLANDS

STRUCTURE OF THYROID GLAND

PANCREAS

LYMPHATIC SYSTEM

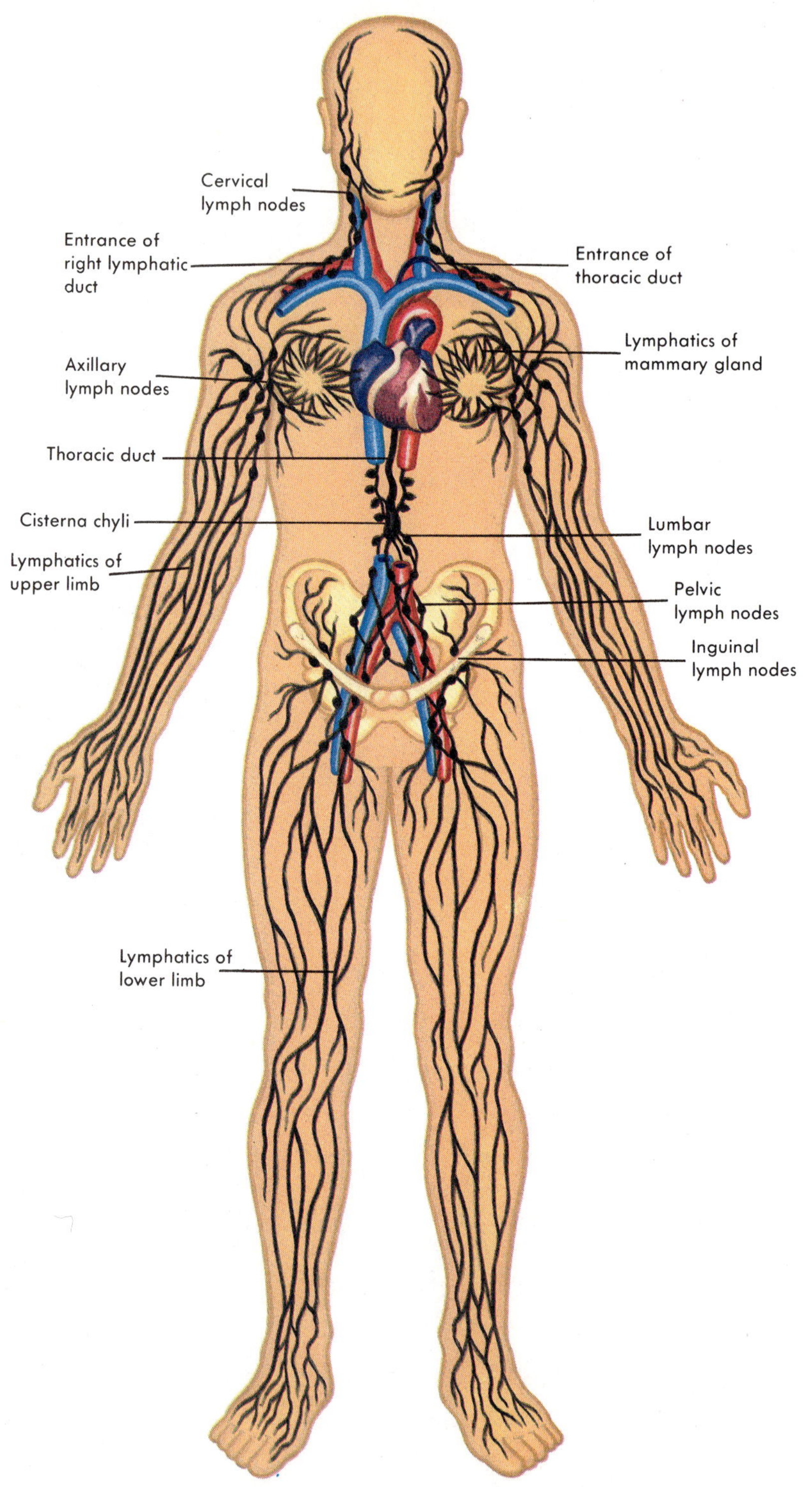

LYMPHATIC SYSTEM

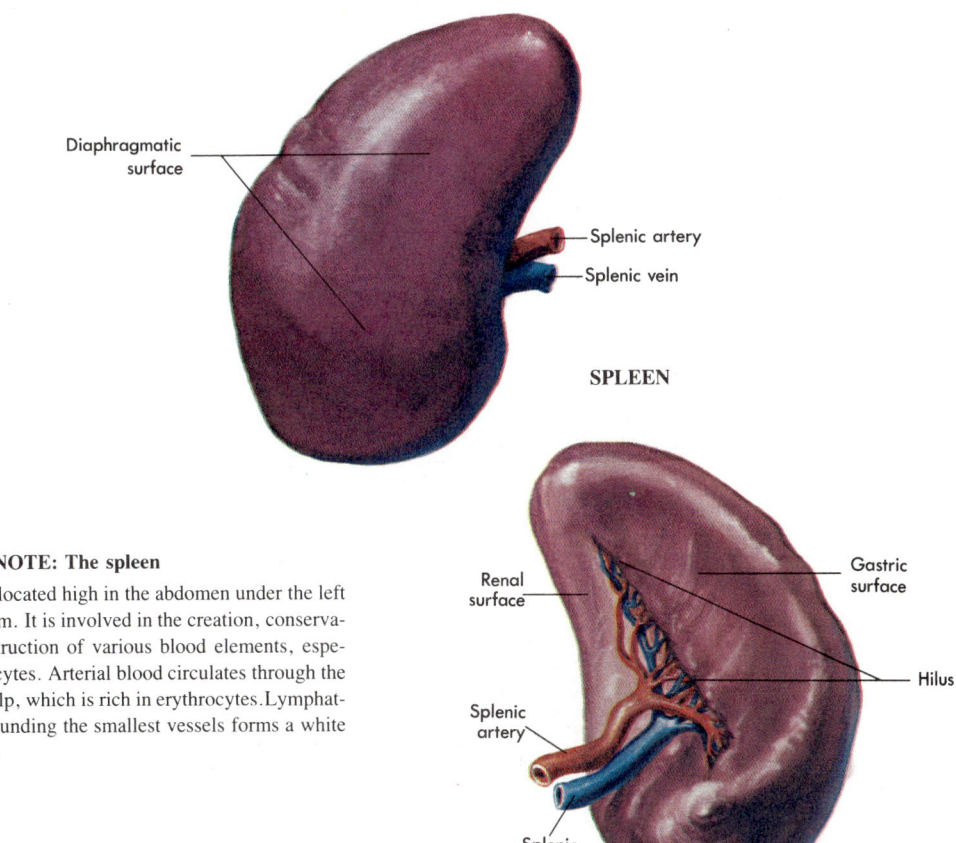

Diaphragmatic surface
Splenic artery
Splenic vein

SPLEEN

Renal surface
Gastric surface
Hilus
Splenic artery
Splenic vein

CLINICAL NOTE: The spleen

The spleen is located high in the abdomen under the left hemidiaphragm. It is involved in the creation, conservation, and destruction of various blood elements, especially erythrocytes. Arterial blood circulates through the red splenic pulp, which is rich in erythrocytes. Lymphatic tissue surrounding the smallest vessels forms a white pulp material.

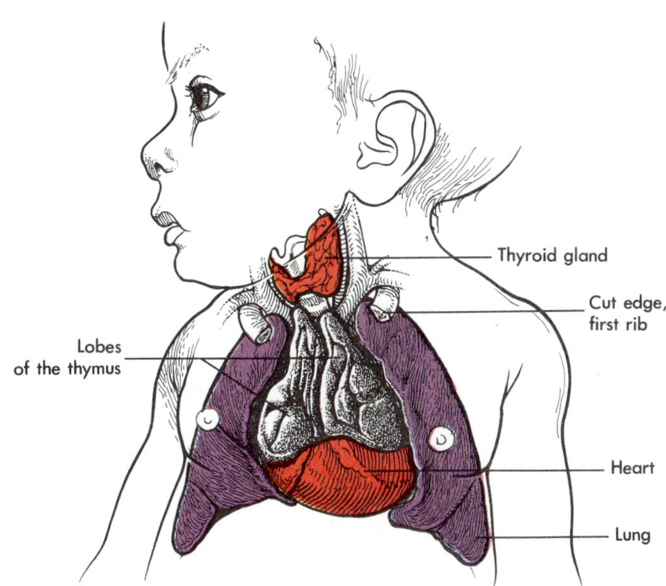

LOCATION AND GROSS ANATOMY OF THYMUS

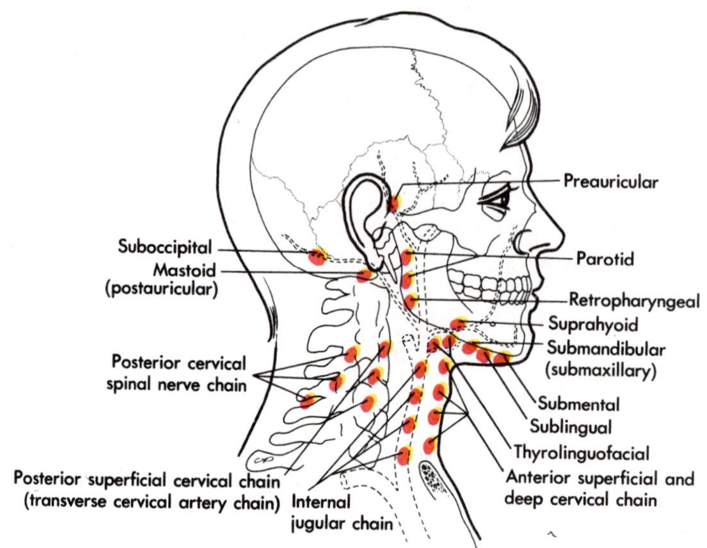

LYMPHATIC DRAINAGE SYSTEM OF HEAD AND NECK

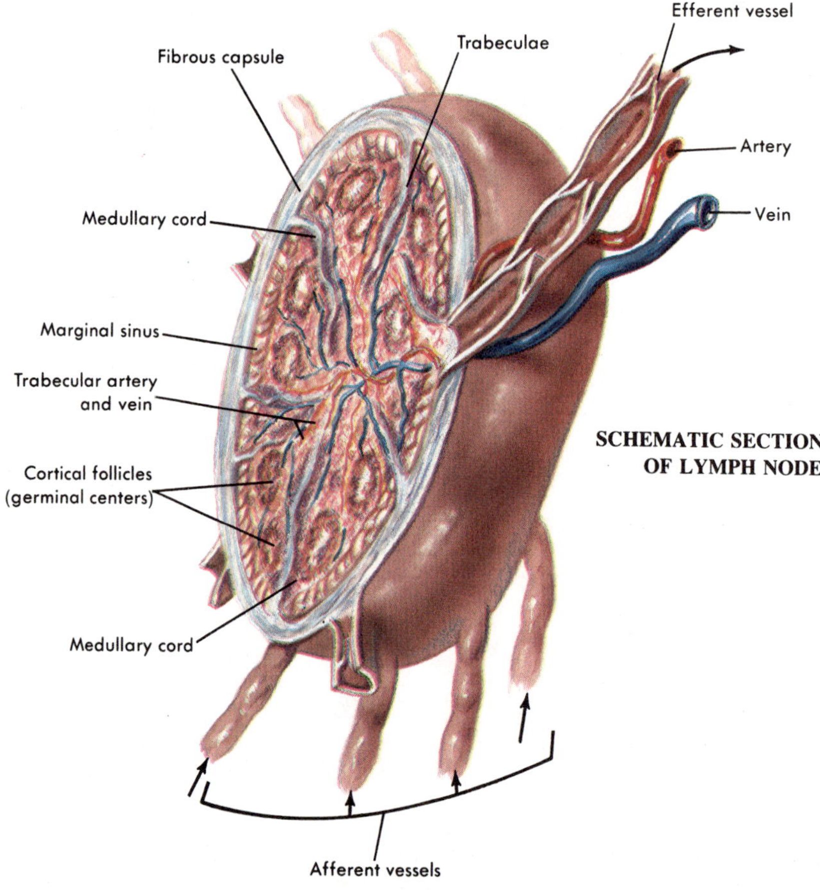

SCHEMATIC SECTION OF LYMPH NODE

NERVOUS SYSTEM

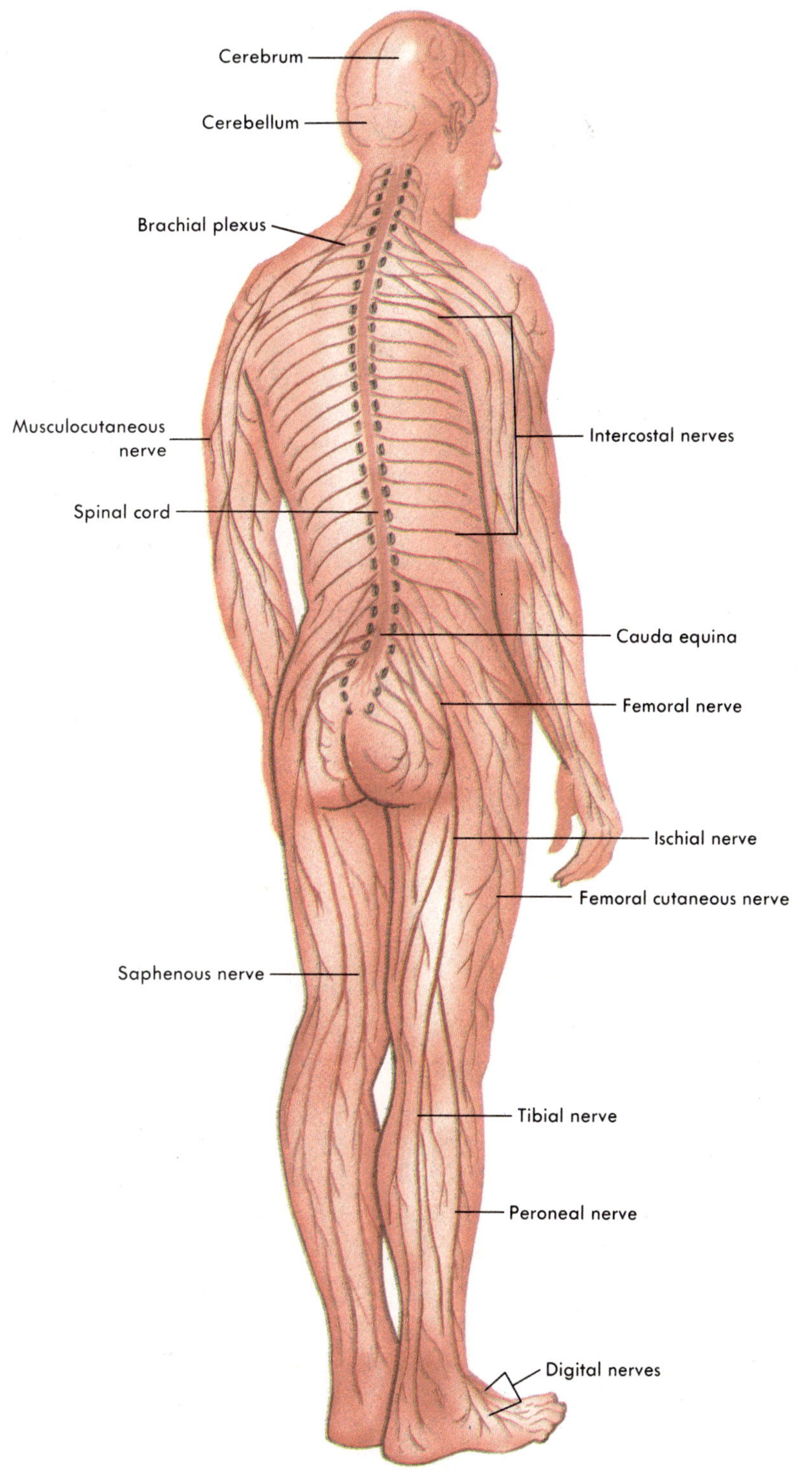

SIMPLIFIED VIEW OF NERVOUS SYSTEM

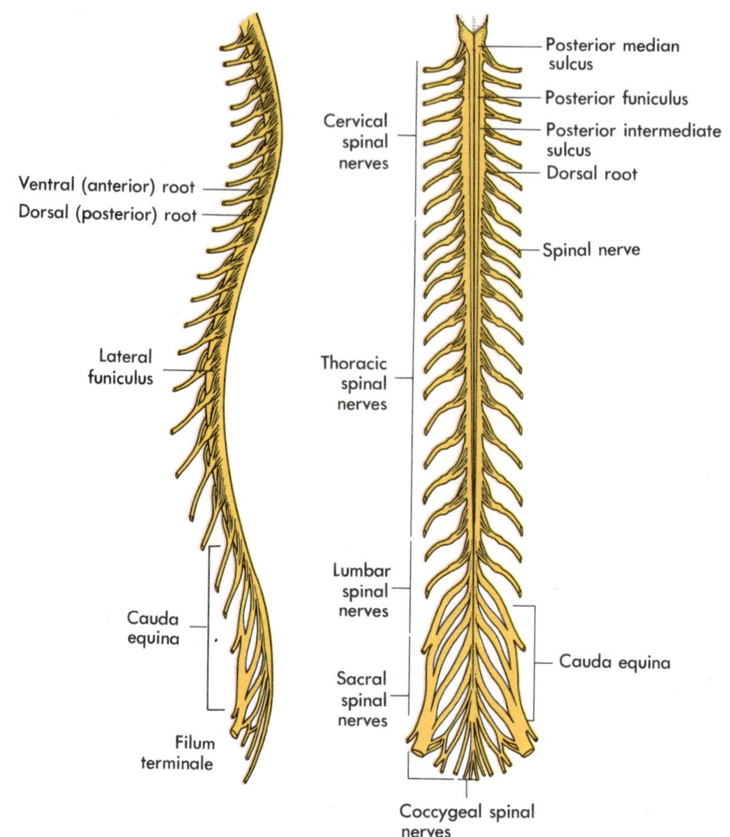
Ventral (anterior) root
Dorsal (posterior) root
Lateral funiculus
Cauda equina
Filum terminale
Posterior median sulcus
Posterior funiculus
Posterior intermediate sulcus
Dorsal root
Spinal nerve
Cervical spinal nerves
Thoracic spinal nerves
Lumbar spinal nerves
Sacral spinal nerves
Cauda equina
Coccygeal spinal nerves

TWO VIEWS OF GROSS ANATOMY OF SPINAL CORD

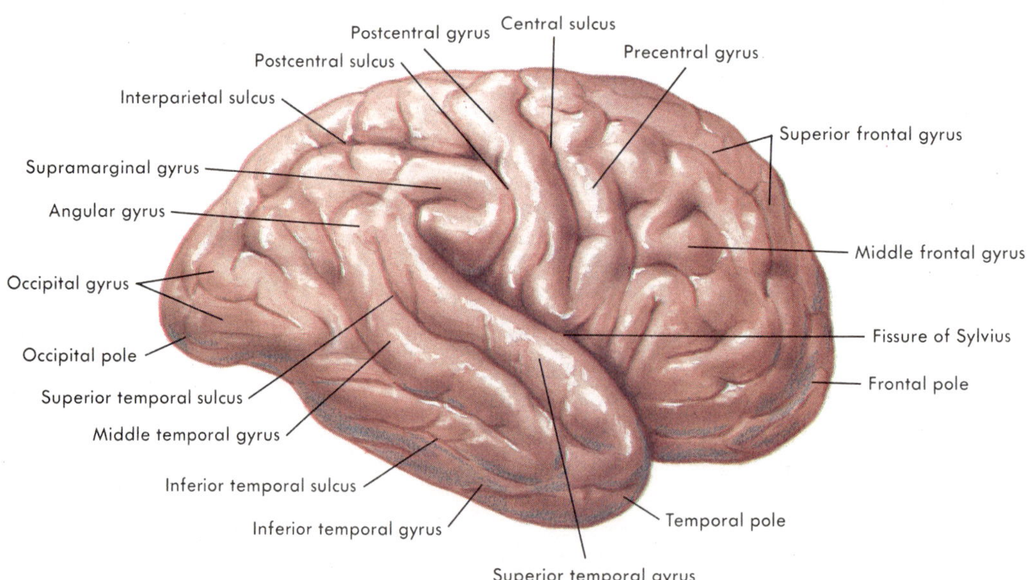
Postcentral gyrus
Central sulcus
Postcentral sulcus
Precentral gyrus
Interparietal sulcus
Superior frontal gyrus
Supramarginal gyrus
Angular gyrus
Middle frontal gyrus
Occipital gyrus
Occipital pole
Fissure of Sylvius
Frontal pole
Superior temporal sulcus
Middle temporal gyrus
Inferior temporal sulcus
Inferior temporal gyrus
Temporal pole
Superior temporal gyrus

SURFACE ANATOMY OF CEREBRAL CORTEX

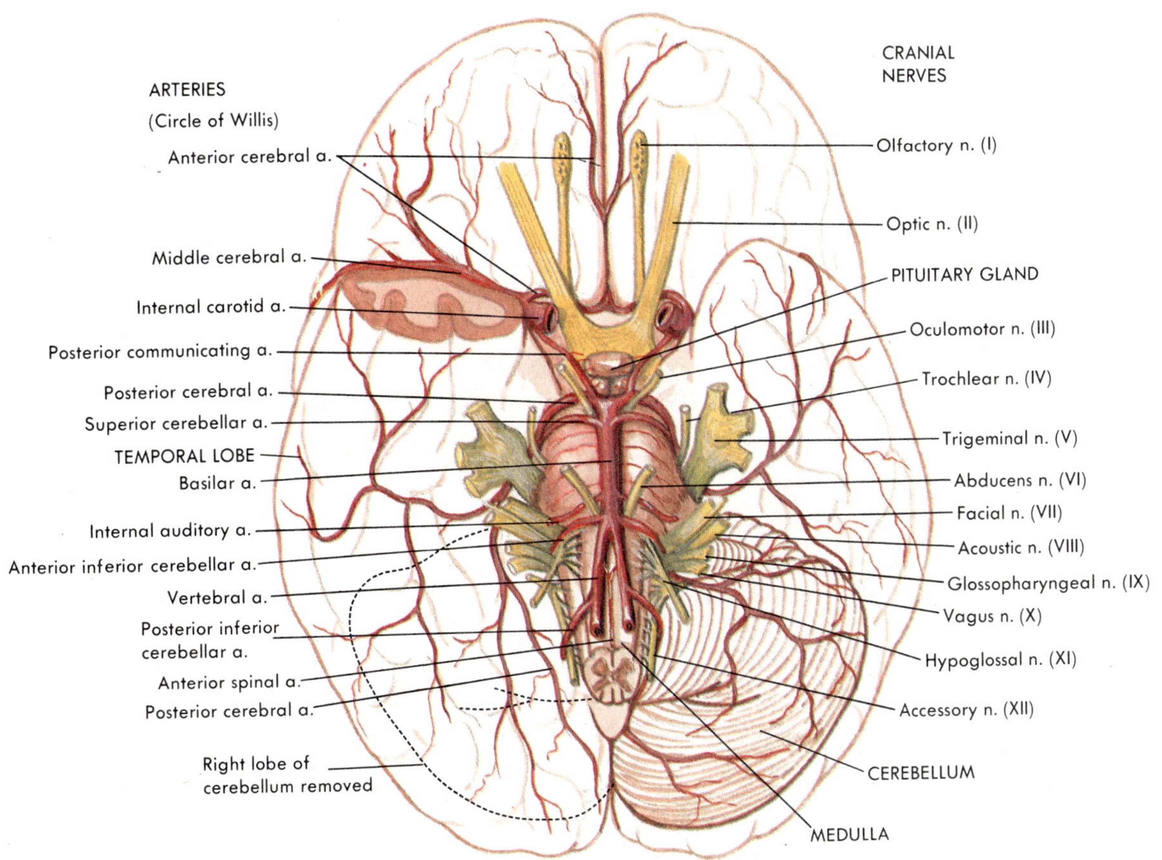
ARTERIES
(Circle of Willis)
Anterior cerebral a.
Middle cerebral a.
Internal carotid a.
Posterior communicating a.
Posterior cerebral a.
Superior cerebellar a.
TEMPORAL LOBE
Basilar a.
Internal auditory a.
Anterior inferior cerebellar a.
Vertebral a.
Posterior inferior cerebellar a.
Anterior spinal a.
Posterior cerebral a.
Right lobe of cerebellum removed
CRANIAL NERVES
Olfactory n. (I)
Optic n. (II)
PITUITARY GLAND
Oculomotor n. (III)
Trochlear n. (IV)
Trigeminal n. (V)
Abducens n. (VI)
Facial n. (VII)
Acoustic n. (VIII)
Glossopharyngeal n. (IX)
Vagus n. (X)
Hypoglossal n. (XI)
Accessory n. (XII)
CEREBELLUM
MEDULLA

BASE OF BRAIN

ANATOMY OF CEREBELLUM

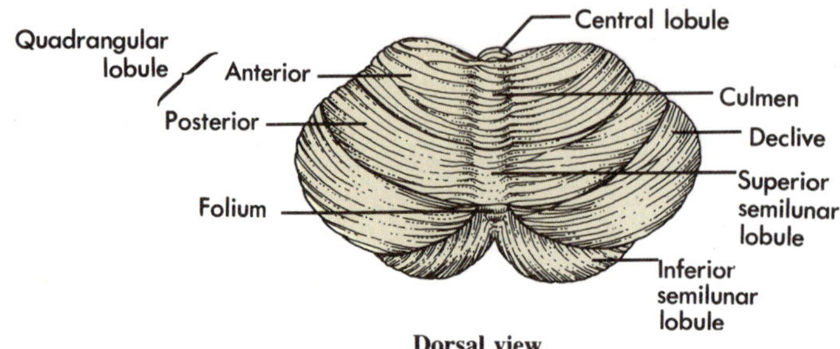

Dorsal view

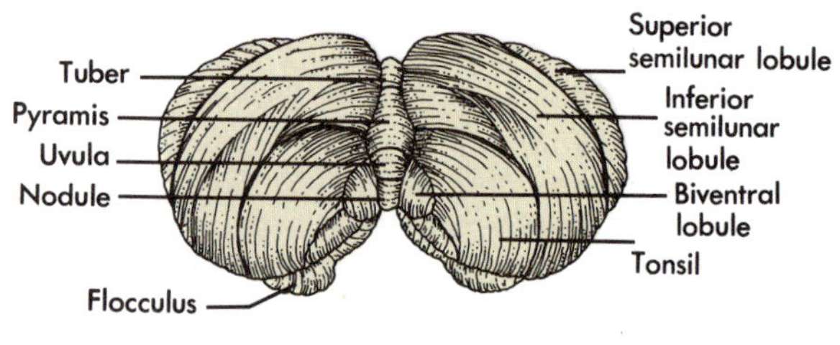

Ventral view

Input	Sensor	Integrator	Effector	Output
External environment: Light, Sound, Temperature, Barometric pressure, Trauma	Sight, Hearing, Taste, Smell, Touch		Skeletal muscle, Smooth muscle	Contraction or relaxation
Internal environment: Muscular work, Visceral activity, Body chemistry, Trauma (pain)	Internal sensors		Exocrine glands, Endocrine glands	Secretion

COMPONENTS OF NERVOUS SYSTEM

CLINICAL NOTE: The neuron

The neuron is the basic excitable cell unit of the nervous system. Neurons display a variety of shapes and sizes. Usually they have a large number of dendritic processes but a single axonal extension. Axons appear elongated; bundles of axons, called tracts, make up the white matter that surrounds the gray matter of spinal nerve cells.

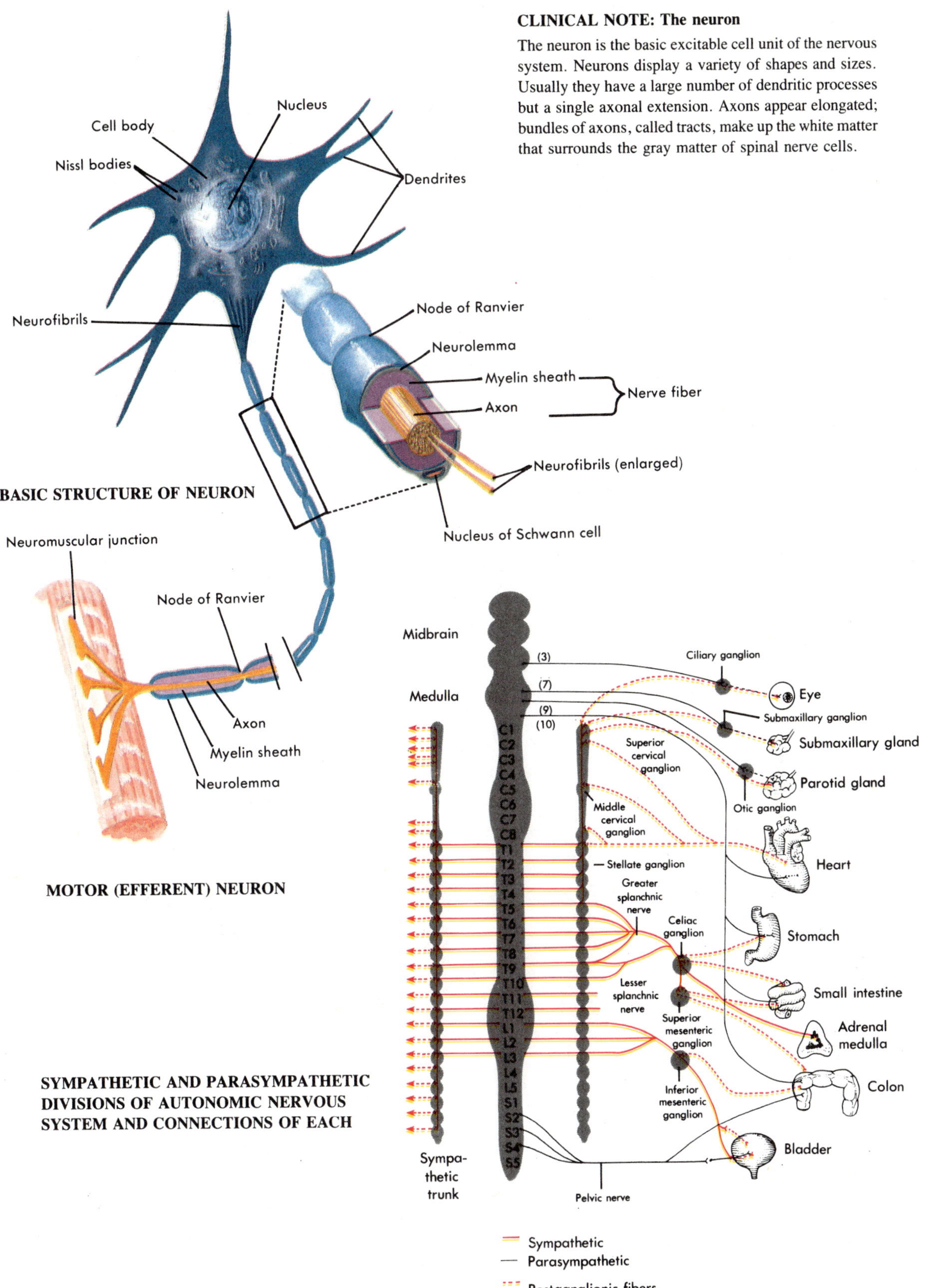

BASIC STRUCTURE OF NEURON

MOTOR (EFFERENT) NEURON

SYMPATHETIC AND PARASYMPATHETIC DIVISIONS OF AUTONOMIC NERVOUS SYSTEM AND CONNECTIONS OF EACH

RESPIRATORY SYSTEM

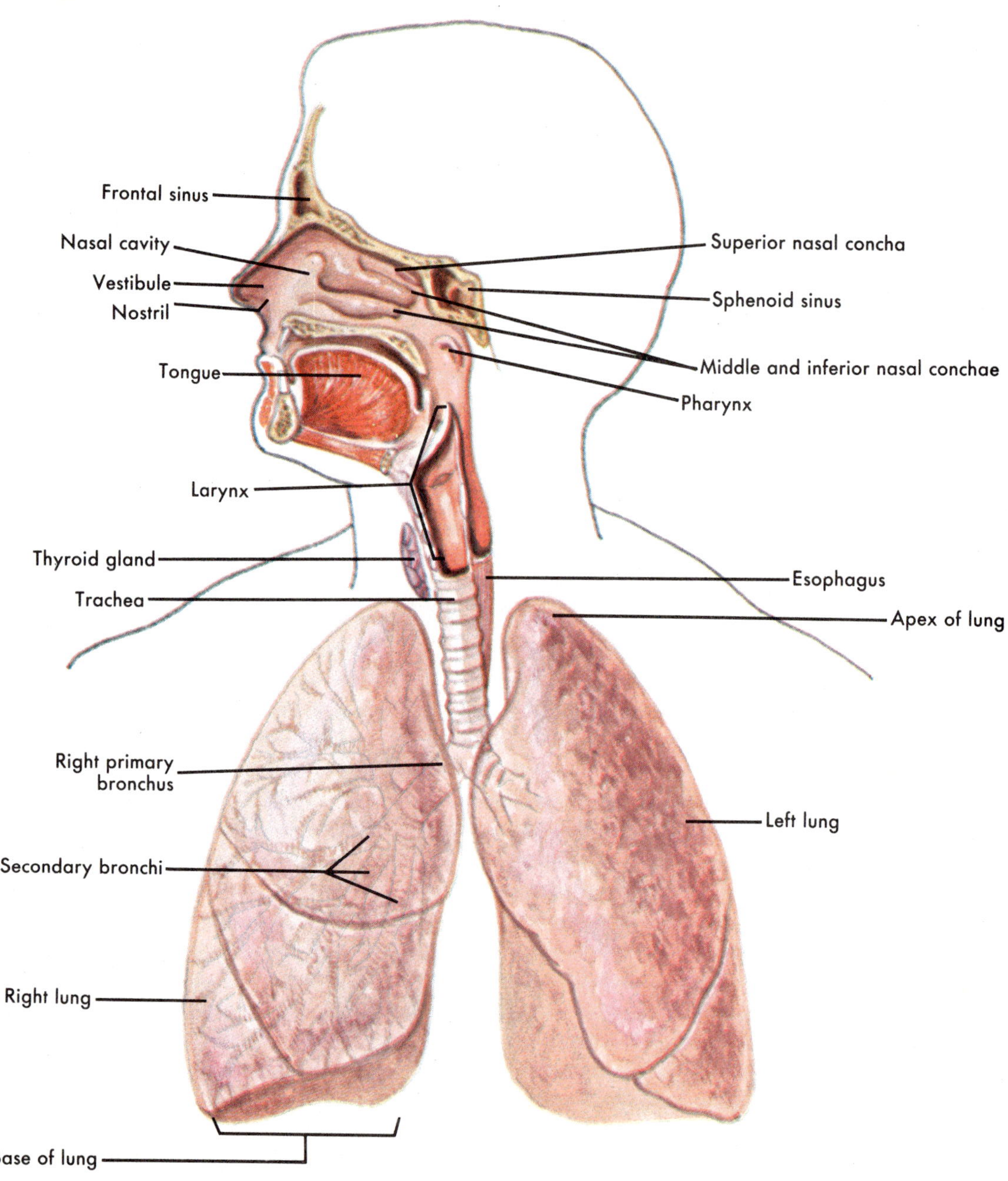

ORGANS OF RESPIRATORY SYSTEM
AND ASSOCIATED STRUCTURES

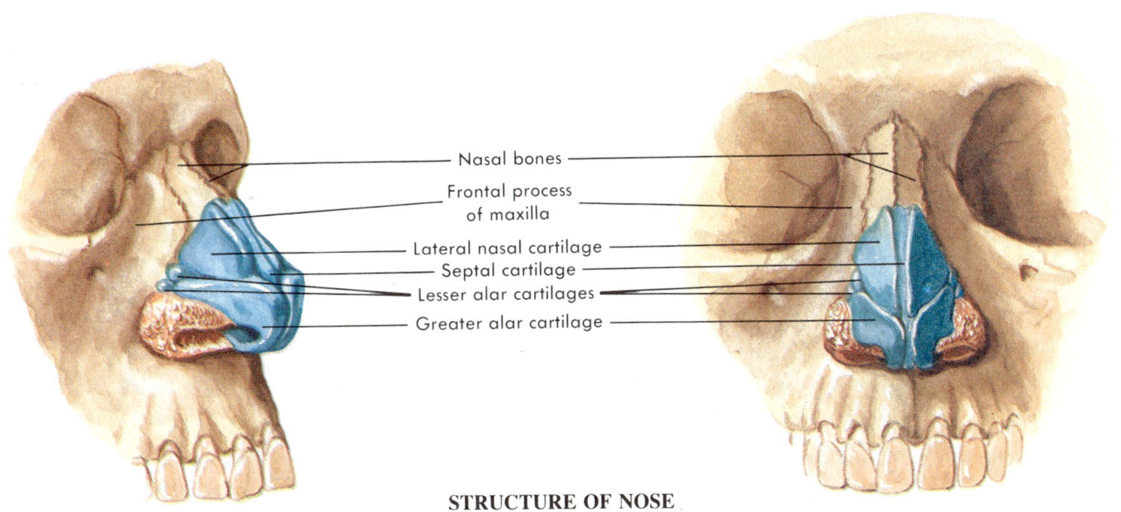

STRUCTURE OF NOSE

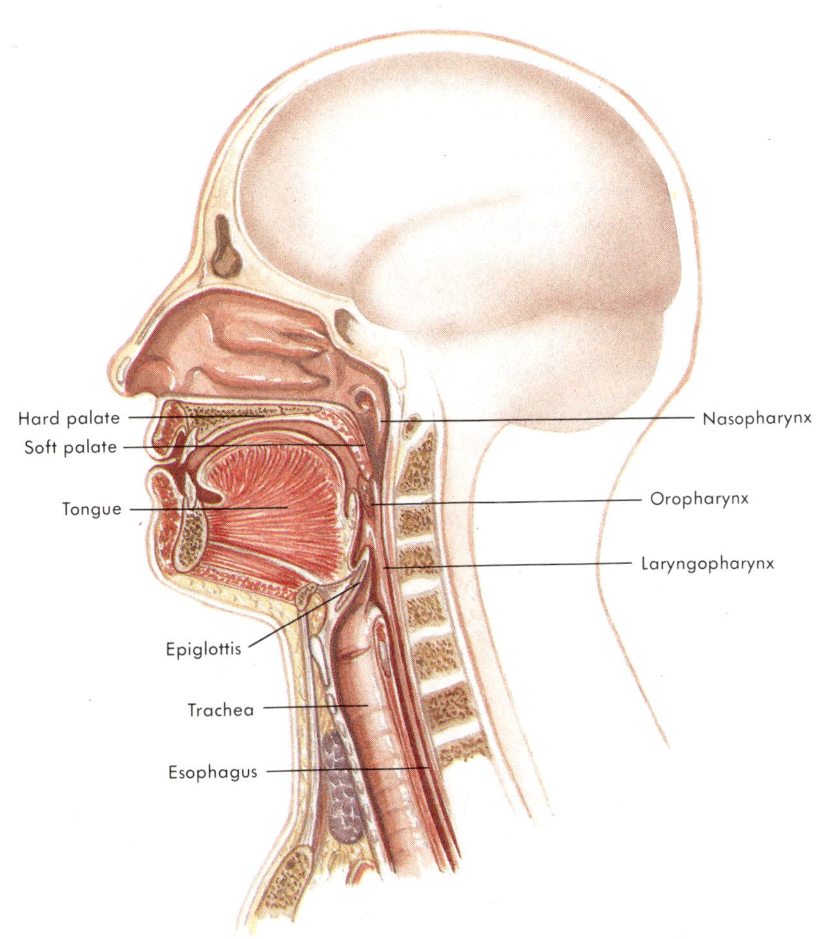

STRUCTURES OF NASAL PASSAGES AND THROAT

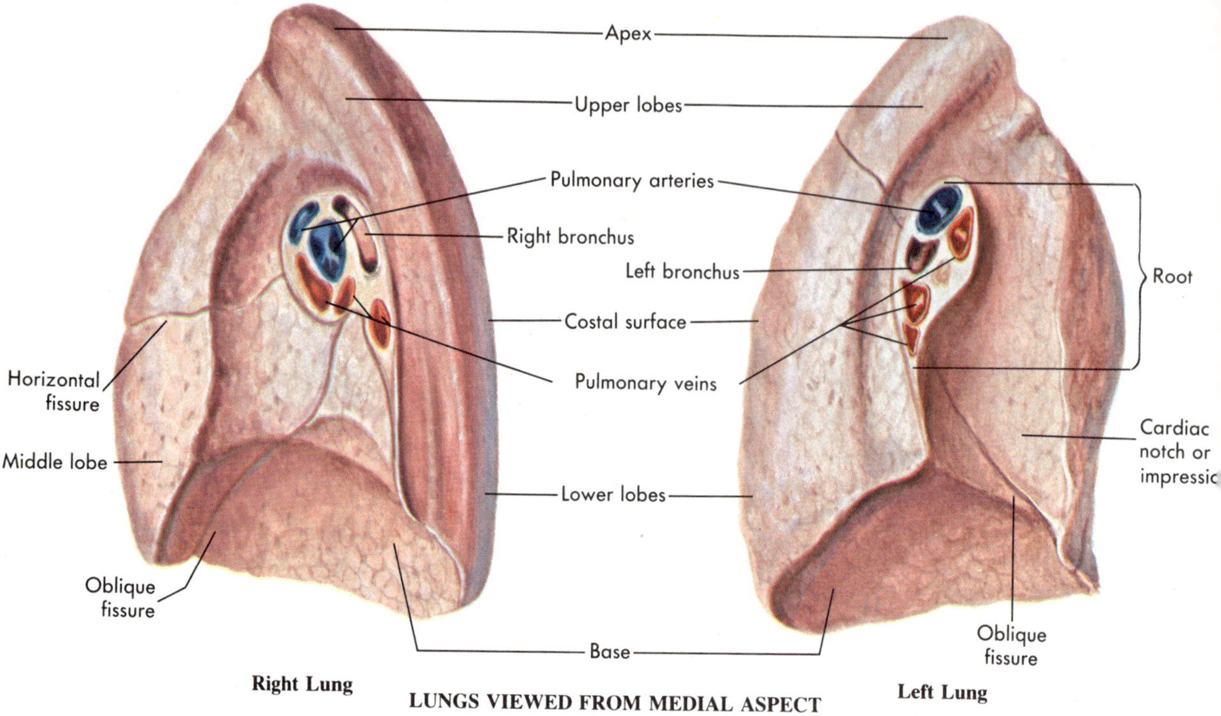

Apex
Upper lobes
Pulmonary arteries
Right bronchus
Left bronchus
Root
Costal surface
Pulmonary veins
Horizontal fissure
Middle lobe
Cardiac notch or impressio
Lower lobes
Oblique fissure
Base
Oblique fissure
Right Lung
Left Lung

LUNGS VIEWED FROM MEDIAL ASPECT

Capillaries
O_2
CO_2
Terminal bronchiole
CO_2
Alveoli
Arteriole
O_2
Venules
Vein
Artery

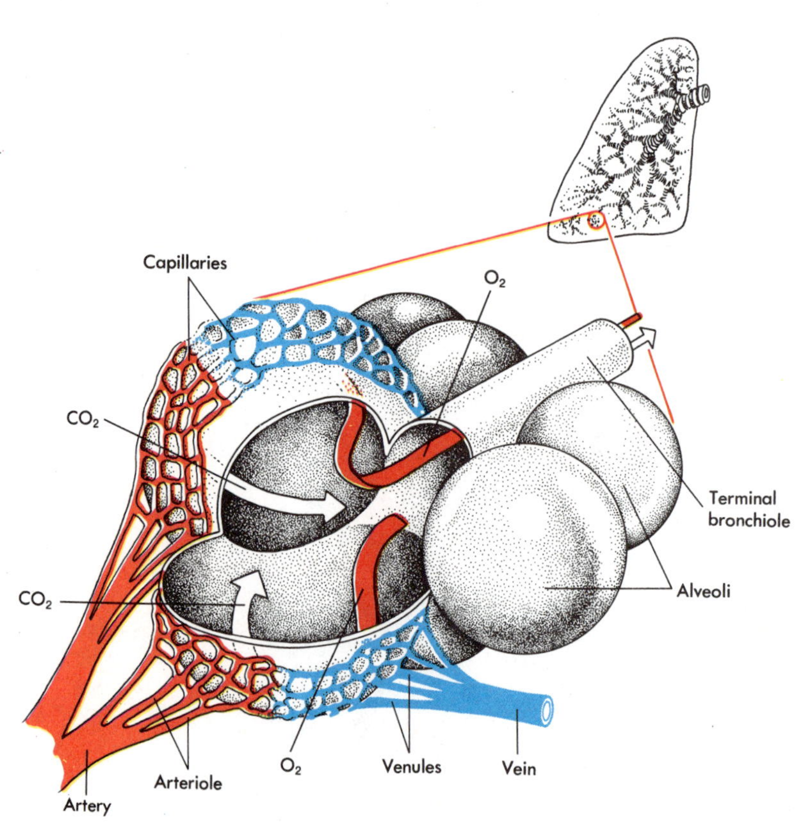

ANATOMY OF AIR-EXCHANGING SURFACE OF LUNGS

CLINICAL NOTE: Respiratory muscles

Unlike cardiac muscle, respiratory muscles are skeletal and striated and possess no inherent rhythm. The periodic nature of respiratory movements results instead from the activity of certain pontine and medullary cells belonging to the reticular formation. Some stimulate breathing movements, others the opposite (inspiratory and expiratory centers).

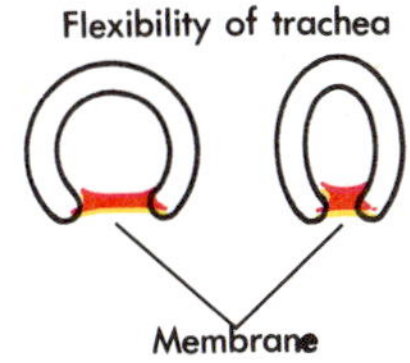

FLEXIBILITY OF TRACHEA

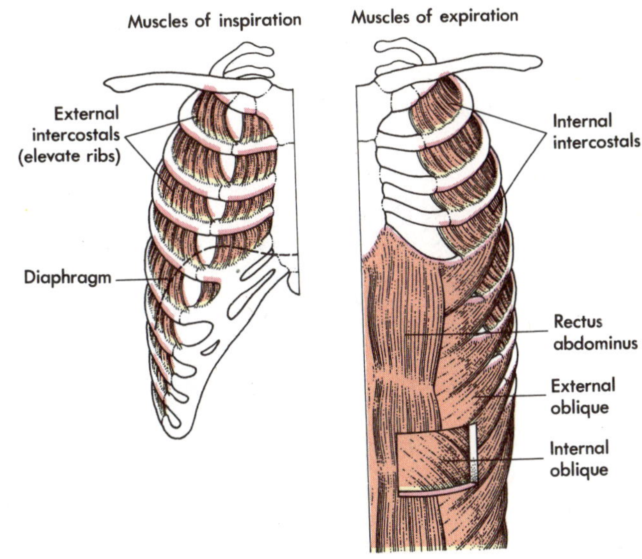

MECHANICS OF RESPIRATION: Muscles required for inspiration and expiration

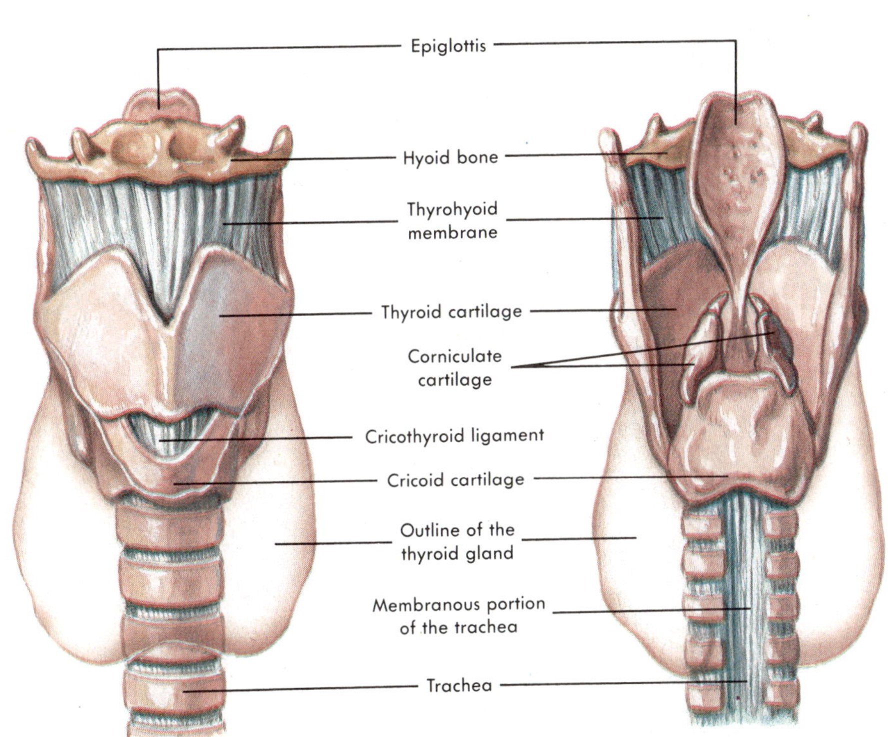

CARTILAGINOUS STRUCTURE OF LARYNX AND UPPER TRACHEA

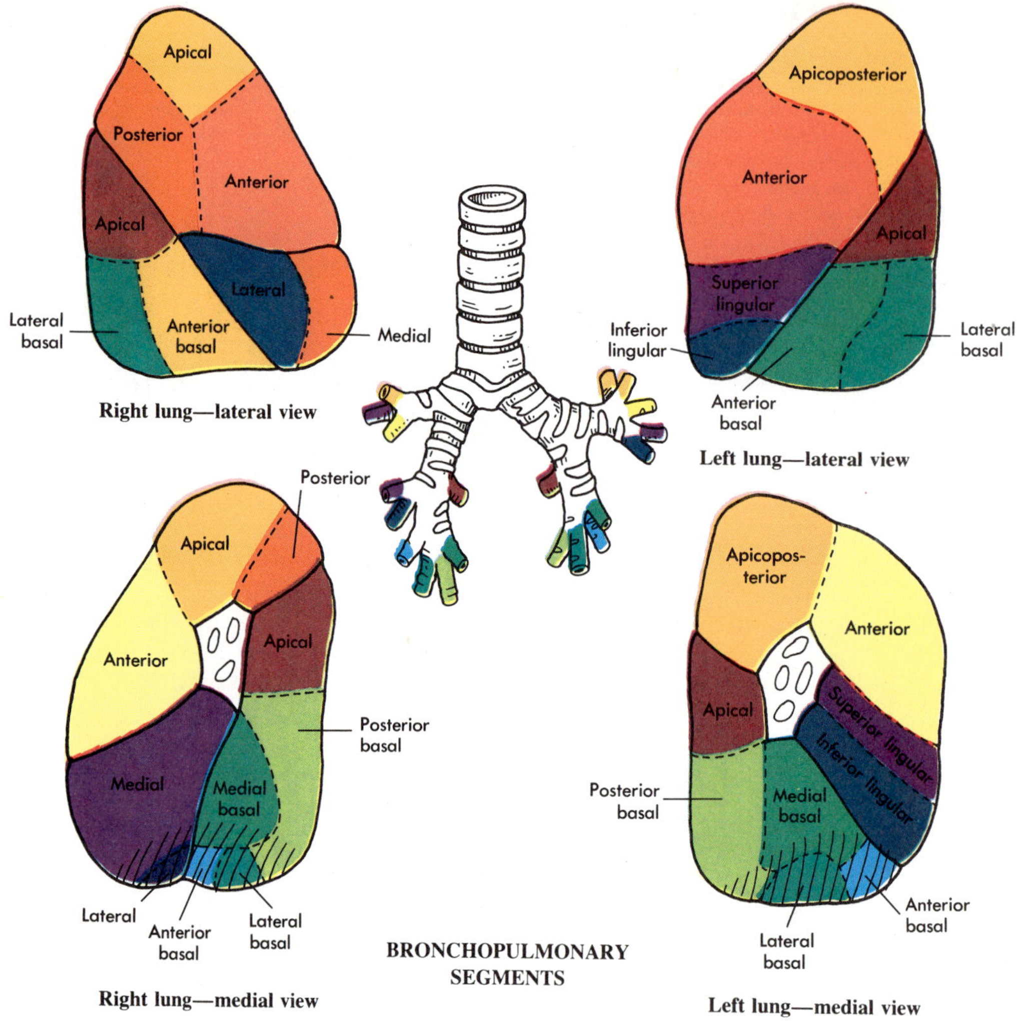

Apical
Posterior
Anterior
Apical
Lateral
Lateral basal
Anterior basal
Medial
Right lung—lateral view
Apicoposterior
Anterior
Apical
Superior lingular
Inferior lingular
Lateral basal
Anterior basal
Left lung—lateral view
Posterior
Apical
Anterior
Apical
Posterior basal
Medial
Medial basal
Lateral
Anterior basal
Lateral basal
Right lung—medial view
Apicopos-terior
Anterior
Apical
Superior lingular
Inferior lingular
Posterior basal
Medial basal
Anterior basal
Lateral basal
Left lung—medial view

BRONCHOPULMONARY SEGMENTS

Trachea
Right bronchus
Left bronchus
Pulmonary arteries
Superior pulmonary veins
Inferior pulmonary veins

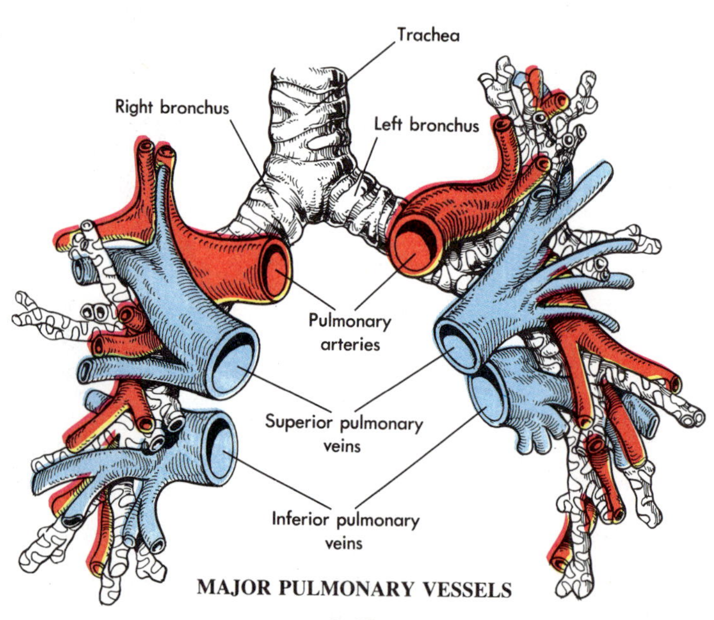

MAJOR PULMONARY VESSELS

DIGESTIVE SYSTEM

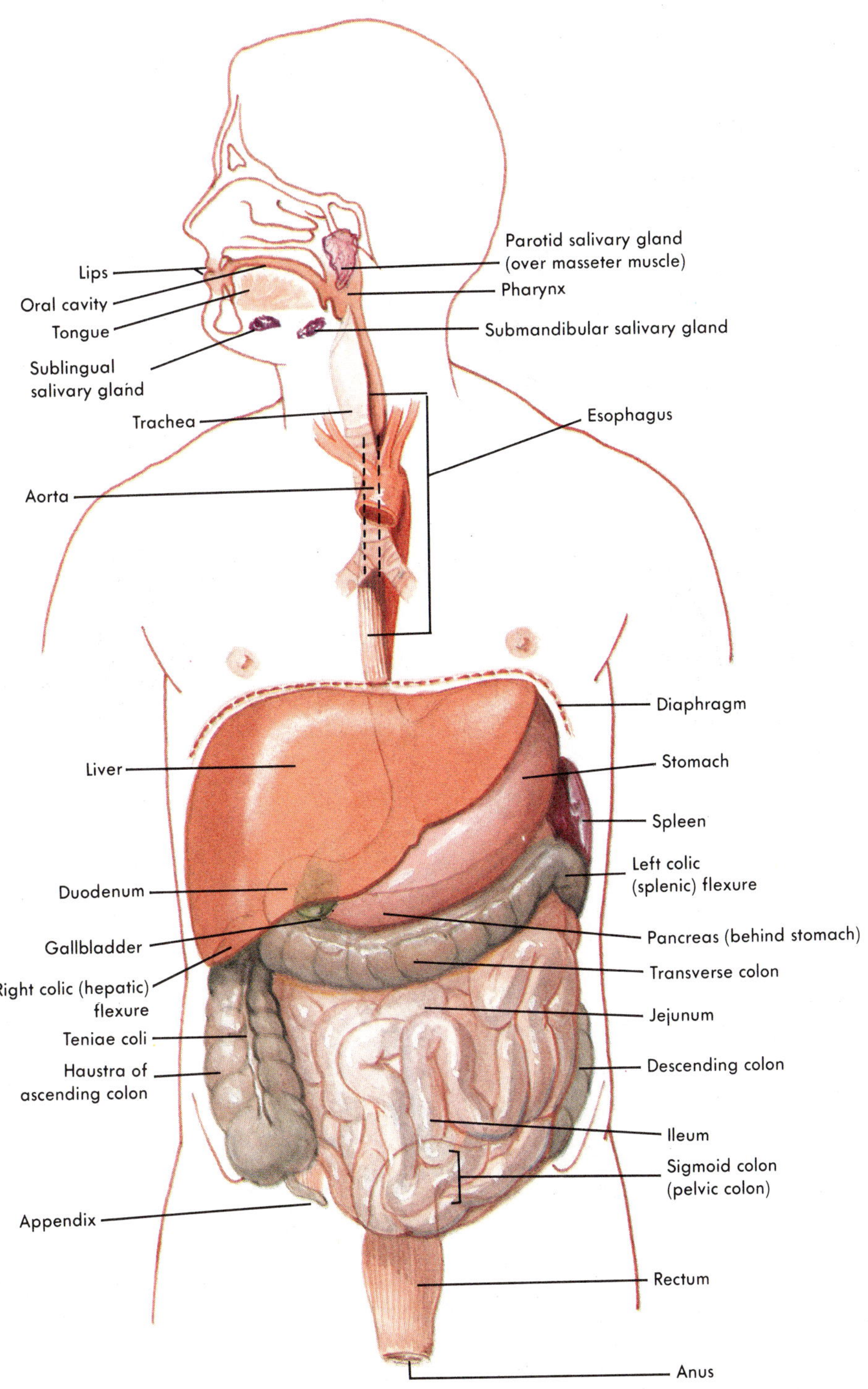

ORGANS OF DIGESTIVE SYSTEM AND
SOME ASSOCIATED STRUCTURES

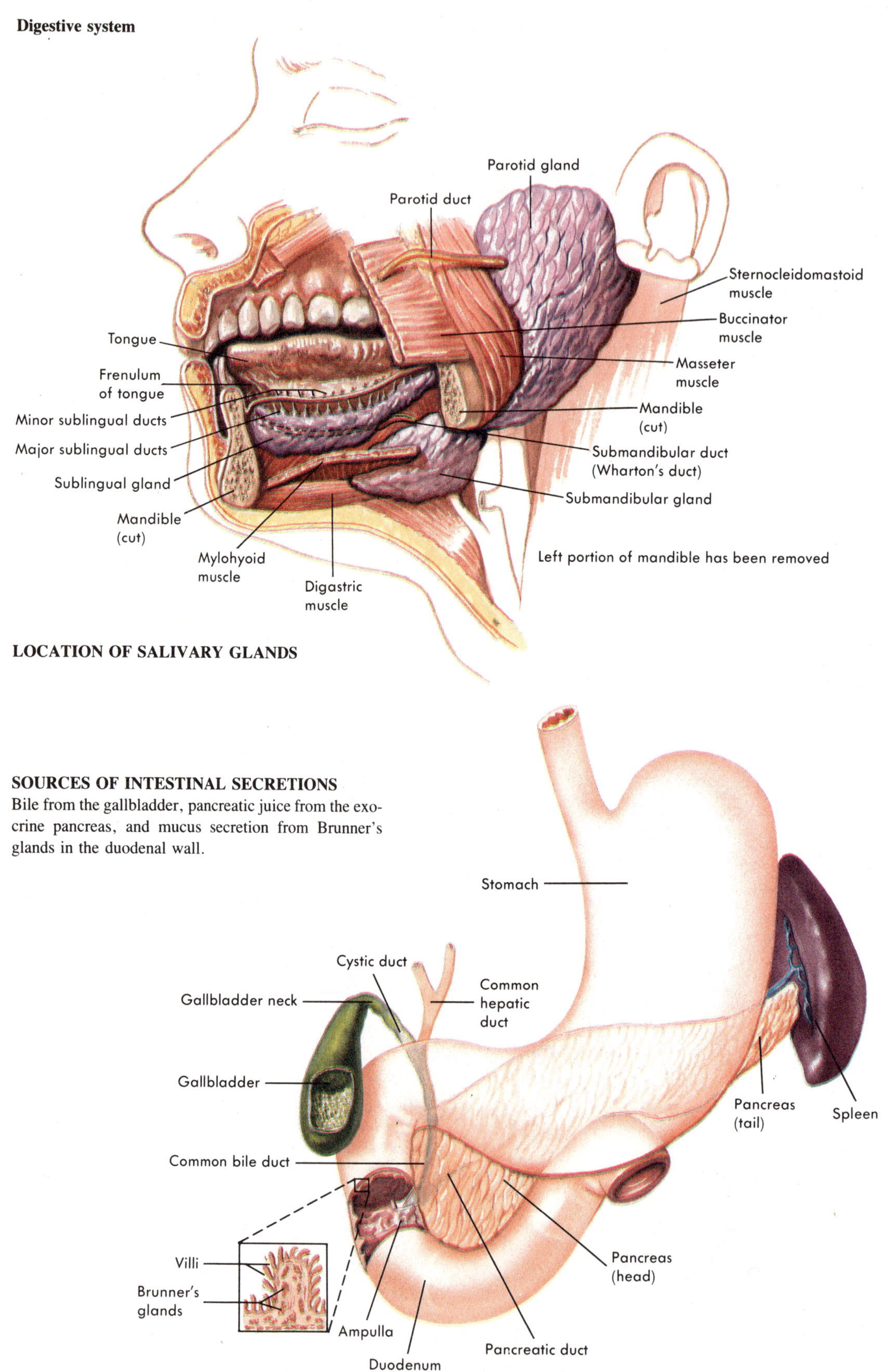

LOCATION OF SALIVARY GLANDS

SOURCES OF INTESTINAL SECRETIONS

Bile from the gallbladder, pancreatic juice from the exocrine pancreas, and mucus secretion from Brunner's glands in the duodenal wall.

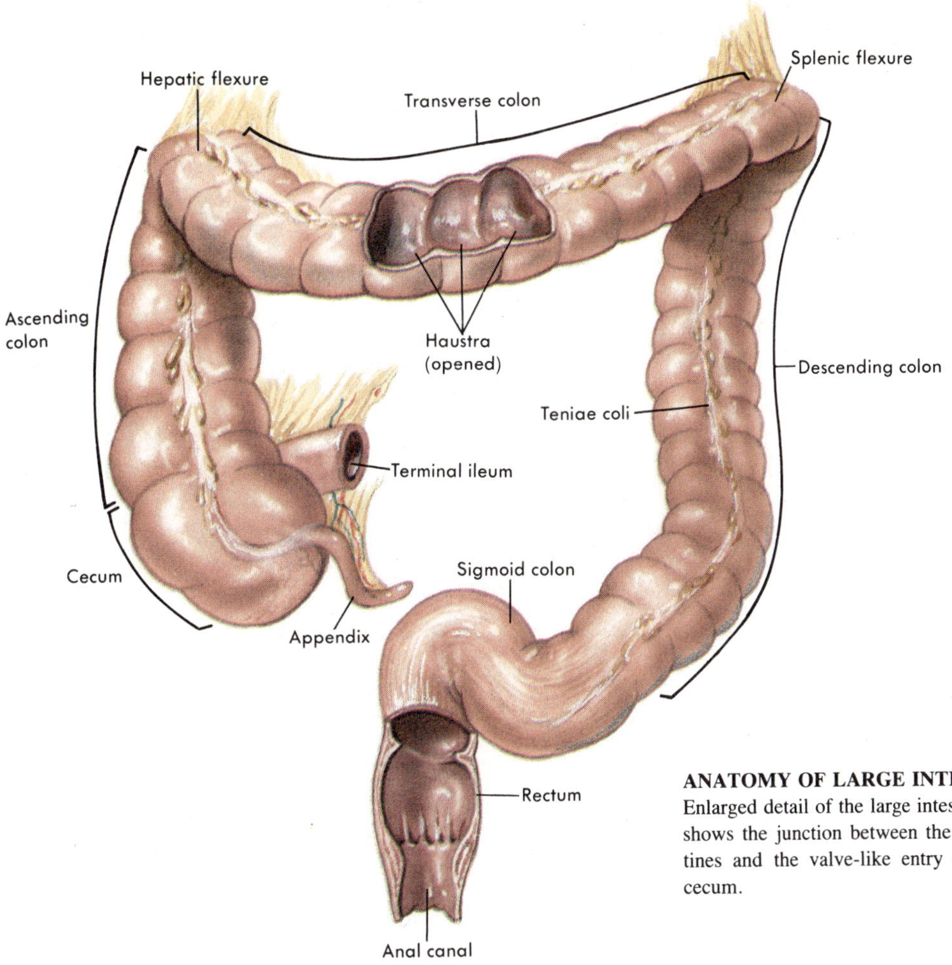

Hepatic flexure
Transverse colon
Splenic flexure
Ascending colon
Haustra (opened)
Descending colon
Teniae coli
Terminal ileum
Cecum
Sigmoid colon
Appendix
Rectum
Anal canal

ANATOMY OF LARGE INTESTINE

Enlarged detail of the large intestine, rectum, and anus shows the junction between the large and small intestines and the valve-like entry of the ileum into the cecum.

Teniae coli
Haustra
Ascending colon
Ileocecal valve
Terminal portion of ileum
Cecum
Appendix
Orifice to appendix

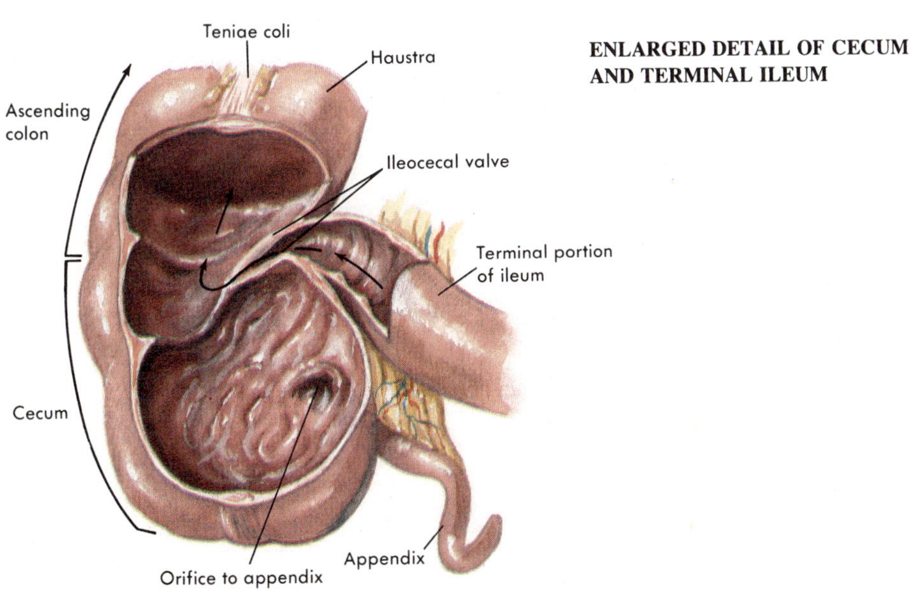

ENLARGED DETAIL OF CECUM AND TERMINAL ILEUM

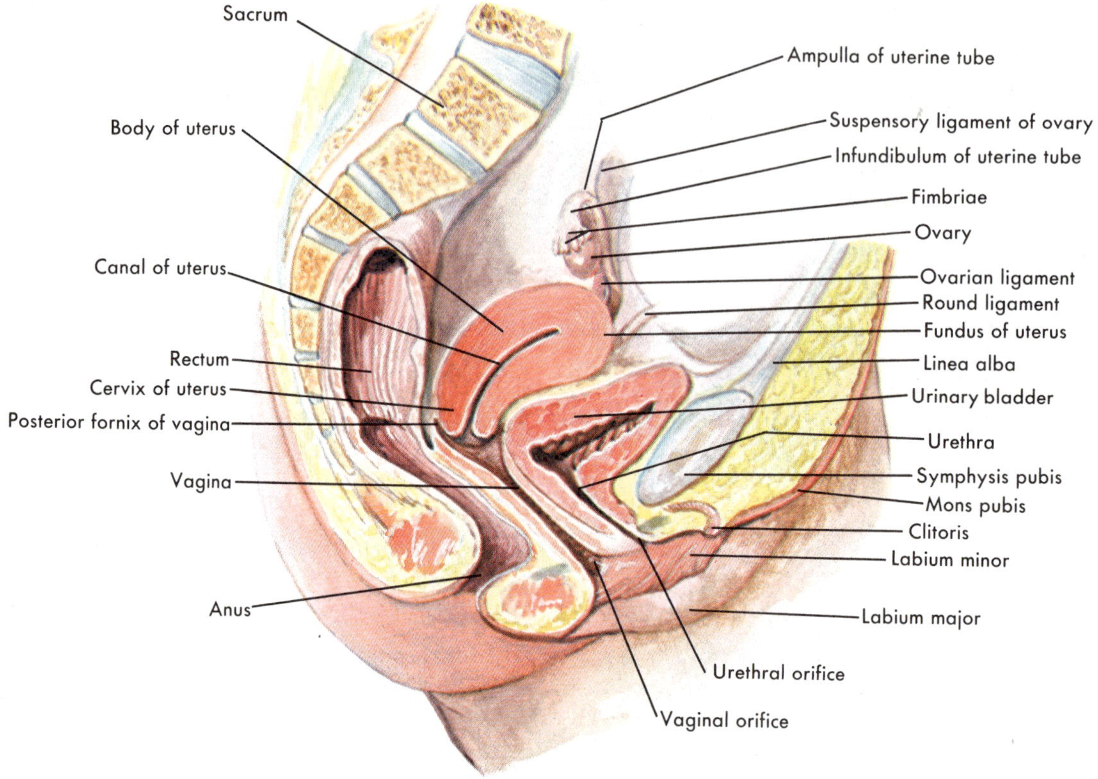

Sacrum
Body of uterus
Canal of uterus
Rectum
Cervix of uterus
Posterior fornix of vagina
Vagina
Anus
Ampulla of uterine tube
Suspensory ligament of ovary
Infundibulum of uterine tube
Fimbriae
Ovary
Ovarian ligament
Round ligament
Fundus of uterus
Linea alba
Urinary bladder
Urethra
Symphysis pubis
Mons pubis
Clitoris
Labium minor
Labium major
Urethral orifice
Vaginal orifice

FEMALE REPRODUCTIVE ORGANS AND ASSOCIATED STRUCTURES

Mons pubis
Labia minora
Vestibular bulb
Greater vestibular (Bartholin's) gland
Anus
Sacrotuberous ligament
Clitoris
Urethral orifice
Vaginal orifice
Ischiocavernosus muscle
Transversus profundus muscle
Bulbocavernosus muscle
Levator ani muscle
Sphincter ani muscle
Gluteus maximus muscle
Coccyx

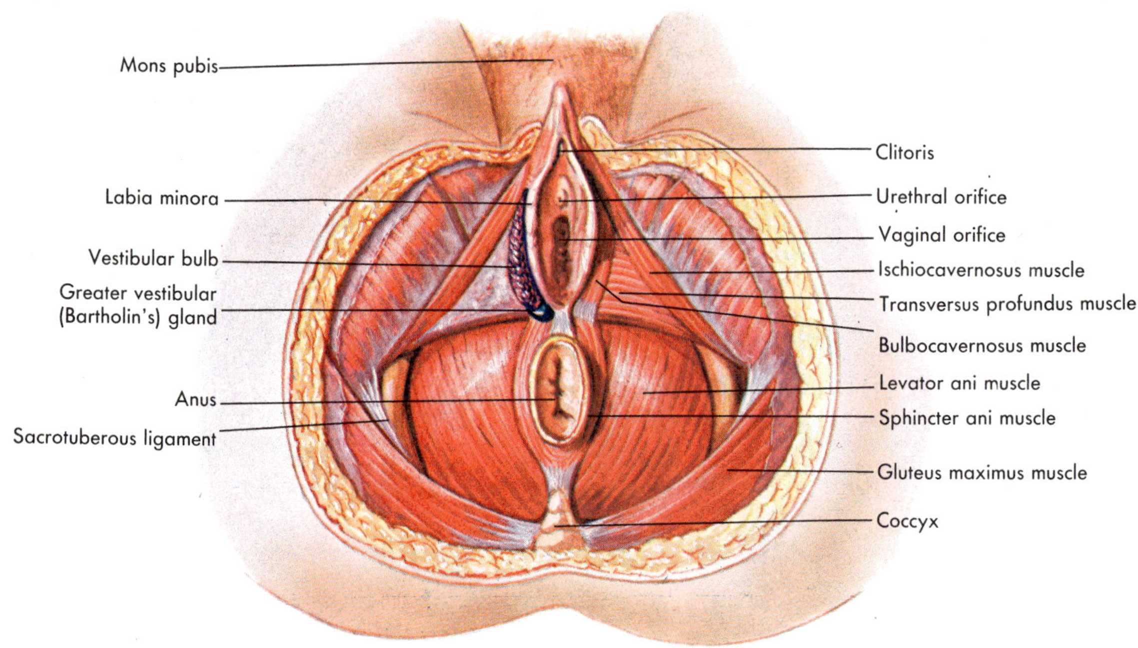

FEMALE PERINEUM

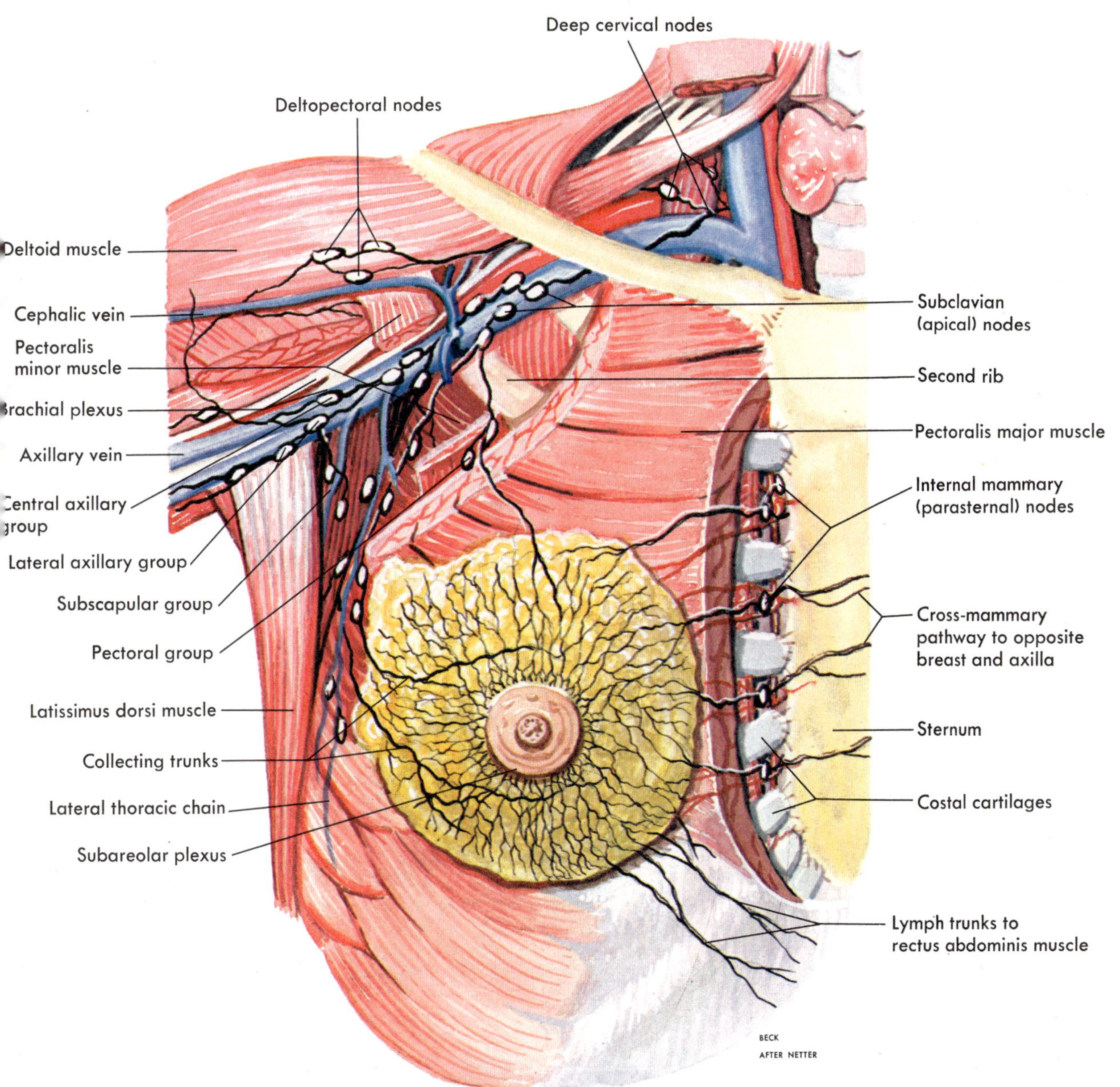

Deep cervical nodes
Deltopectoral nodes
Deltoid muscle
Cephalic vein
Pectoralis minor muscle
Brachial plexus
Axillary vein
Central axillary group
Lateral axillary group
Subscapular group
Pectoral group
Latissimus dorsi muscle
Collecting trunks
Lateral thoracic chain
Subareolar plexus
Subclavian (apical) nodes
Second rib
Pectoralis major muscle
Internal mammary (parasternal) nodes
Cross-mammary pathway to opposite breast and axilla
Sternum
Costal cartilages
Lymph trunks to rectus abdominis muscle
BECK
AFTER NETTER

LYMPHATIC AND RETICULOENDOTHELIAL SYSTEM

CLINICAL NOTE: Female reproductive system

Immense structural changes occur within the uterus during pregnancy. However, if fertilization does not take place, then the endometrial lining is shed cyclically under hormonal control in the phenomenon of menstruation.

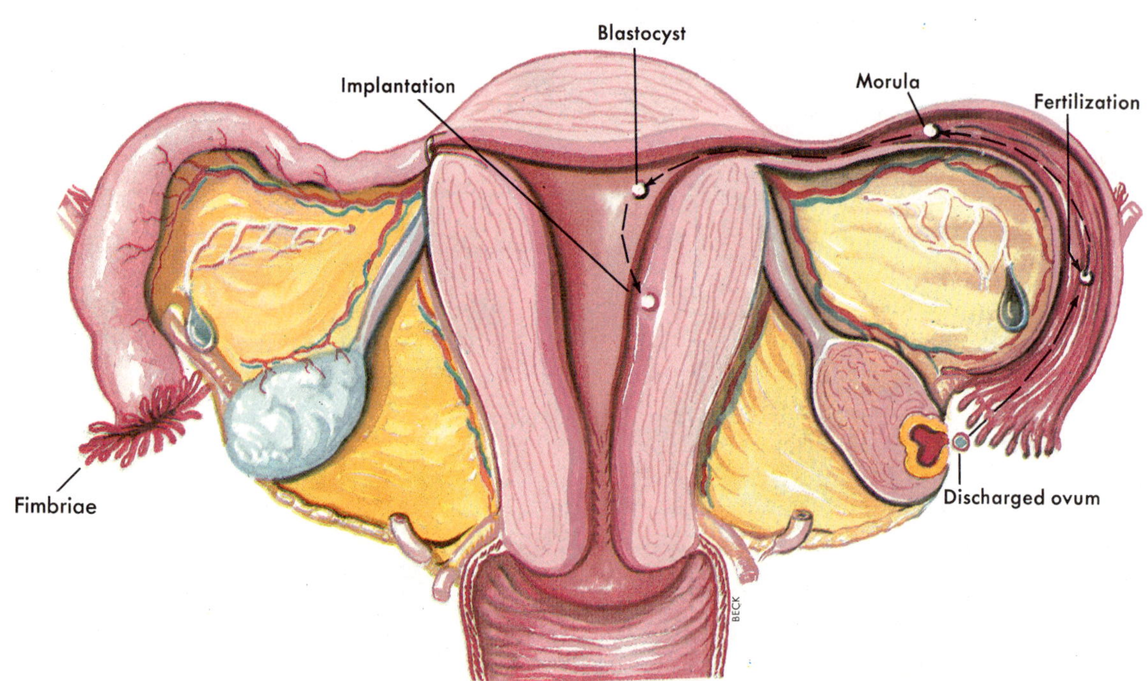

APPEARANCE OF UTERUS AND UTERINE TUBES FROM FERTILIZATION TO IMPLANTATION

Fertilization occurs in the outer third of the uterine tube. Development reaches the blastocyst stage after the embryo has entered the uterus.

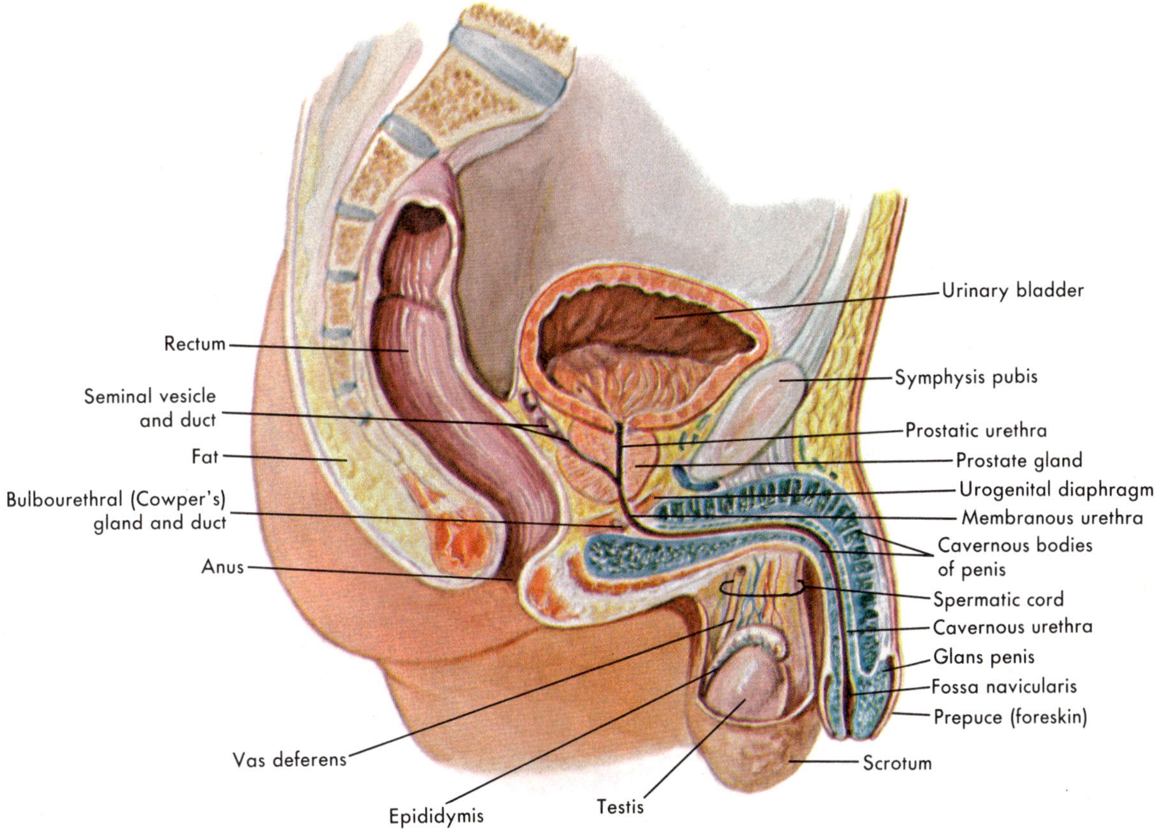

Urinary bladder
Rectum
Symphysis pubis
Seminal vesicle
and duct
Prostatic urethra
Fat
Prostate gland
Urogenital diaphragm
Bulbourethral (Cowper's)
gland and duct
Membranous urethra
Cavernous bodies
of penis
Anus
Spermatic cord
Cavernous urethra
Glans penis
Fossa navicularis
Prepuce (foreskin)
Vas deferens
Scrotum
Epididymis
Testis

MALE REPRODUCTIVE ORGANS AND ASSOCIATED STRUCTURES

Acrosome
Principal
piece
Head
Nucleus
Middle piece
End
piece
Front
Side

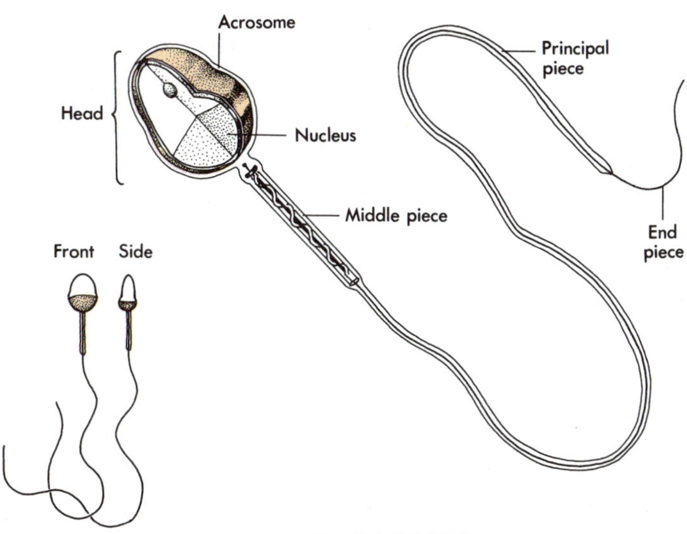

ANATOMY OF A SPERM

URINARY SYSTEM

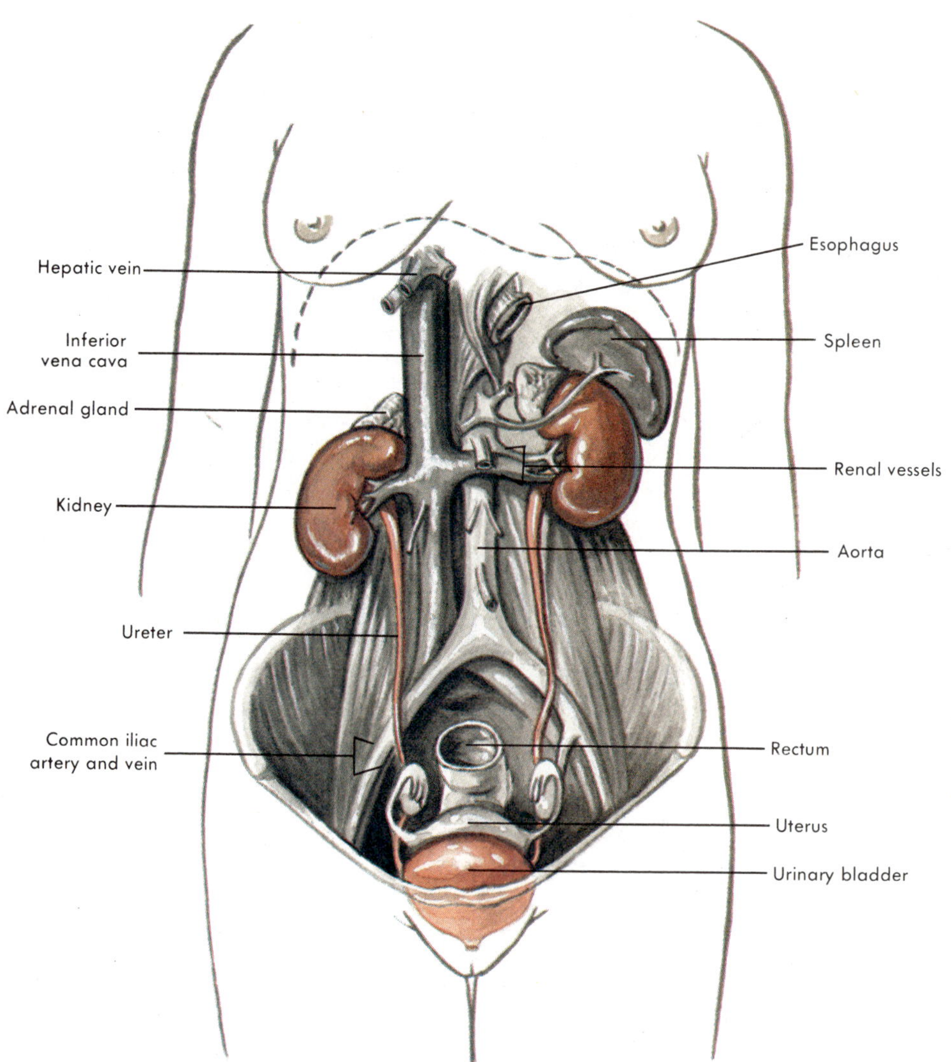

URINARY SYSTEM AND SOME ASSOCIATED STRUCTURES

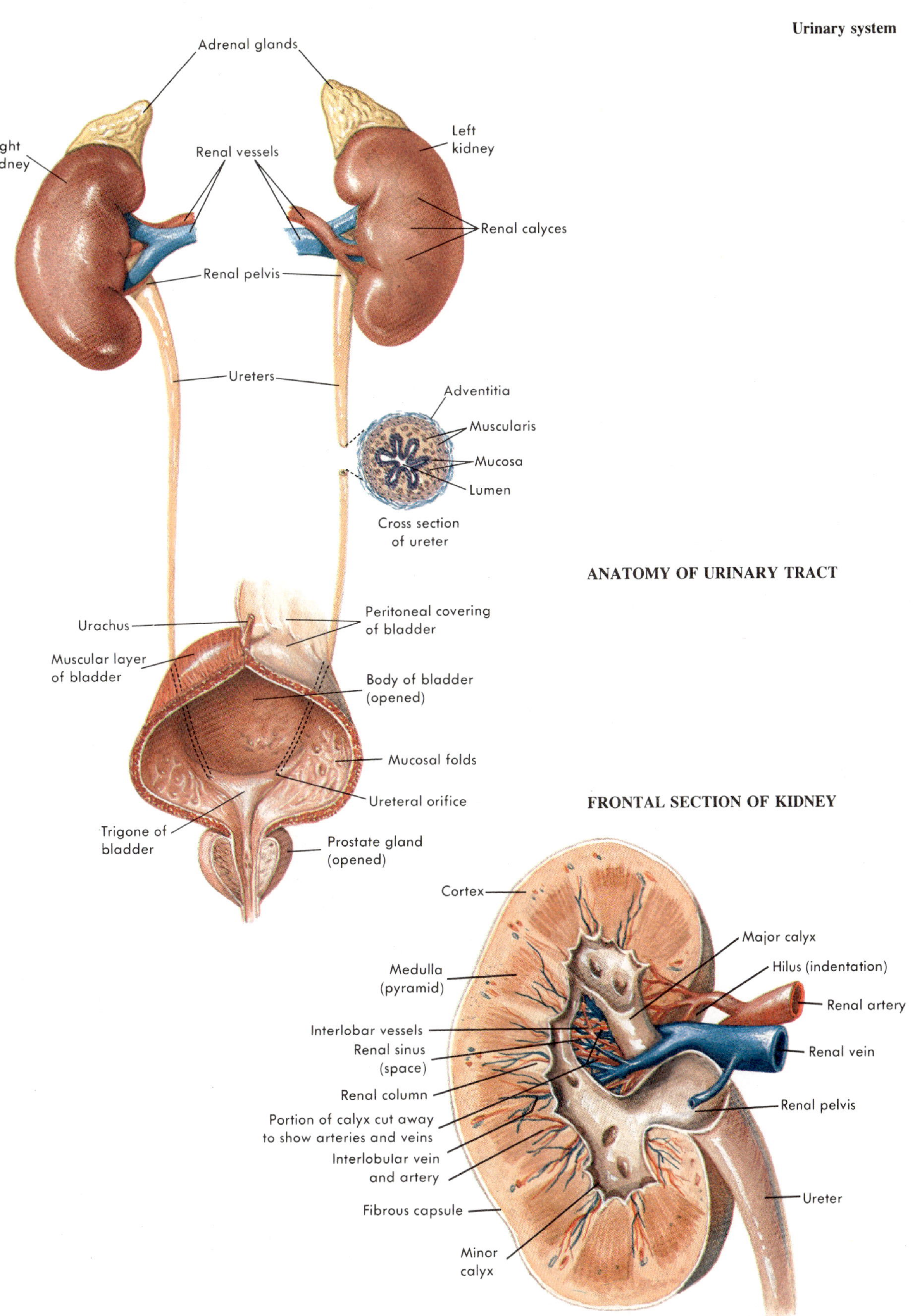
Adrenal glands
Right kidney
Renal vessels
Left kidney
Renal calyces
Renal pelvis
Ureters
Adventitia
Muscularis
Mucosa
Lumen
Cross section of ureter
Urachus
Peritoneal covering of bladder
Muscular layer of bladder
Body of bladder (opened)
Mucosal folds
Ureteral orifice
Trigone of bladder
Prostate gland (opened)
Cortex
Major calyx
Hilus (indentation)
Medulla (pyramid)
Renal artery
Interlobar vessels
Renal sinus (space)
Renal vein
Renal column
Renal pelvis
Portion of calyx cut away to show arteries and veins
Interlobular vein and artery
Ureter
Fibrous capsule
Minor calyx

ANATOMY OF URINARY TRACT

FRONTAL SECTION OF KIDNEY

SPECIAL SENSES

Hearing

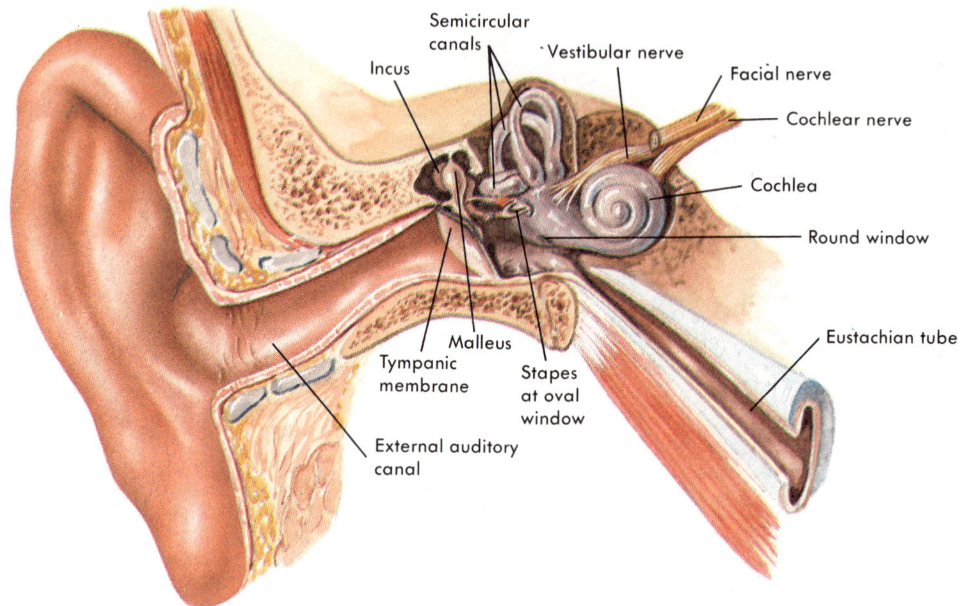

GROSS ANATOMY OF THE EAR IN FRONTAL SECTION

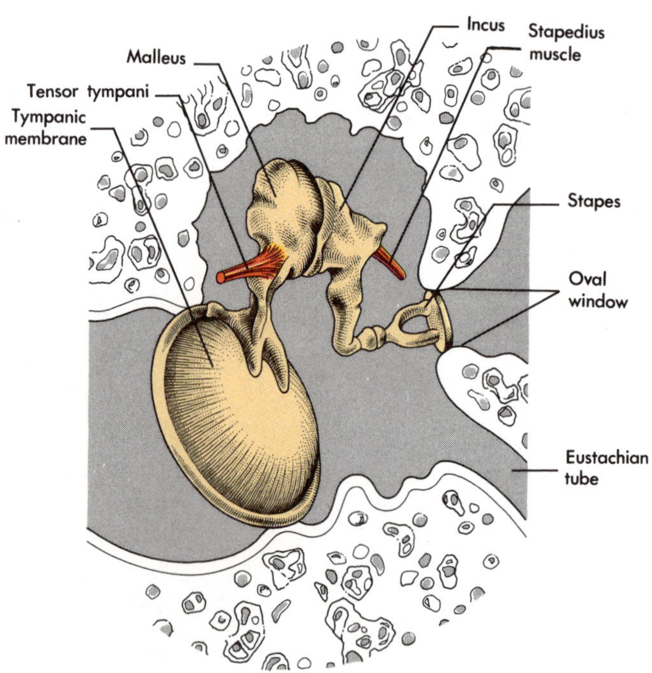

IMPEDENCE-MATCHING COMPONENTS OF INNER EAR

Sight

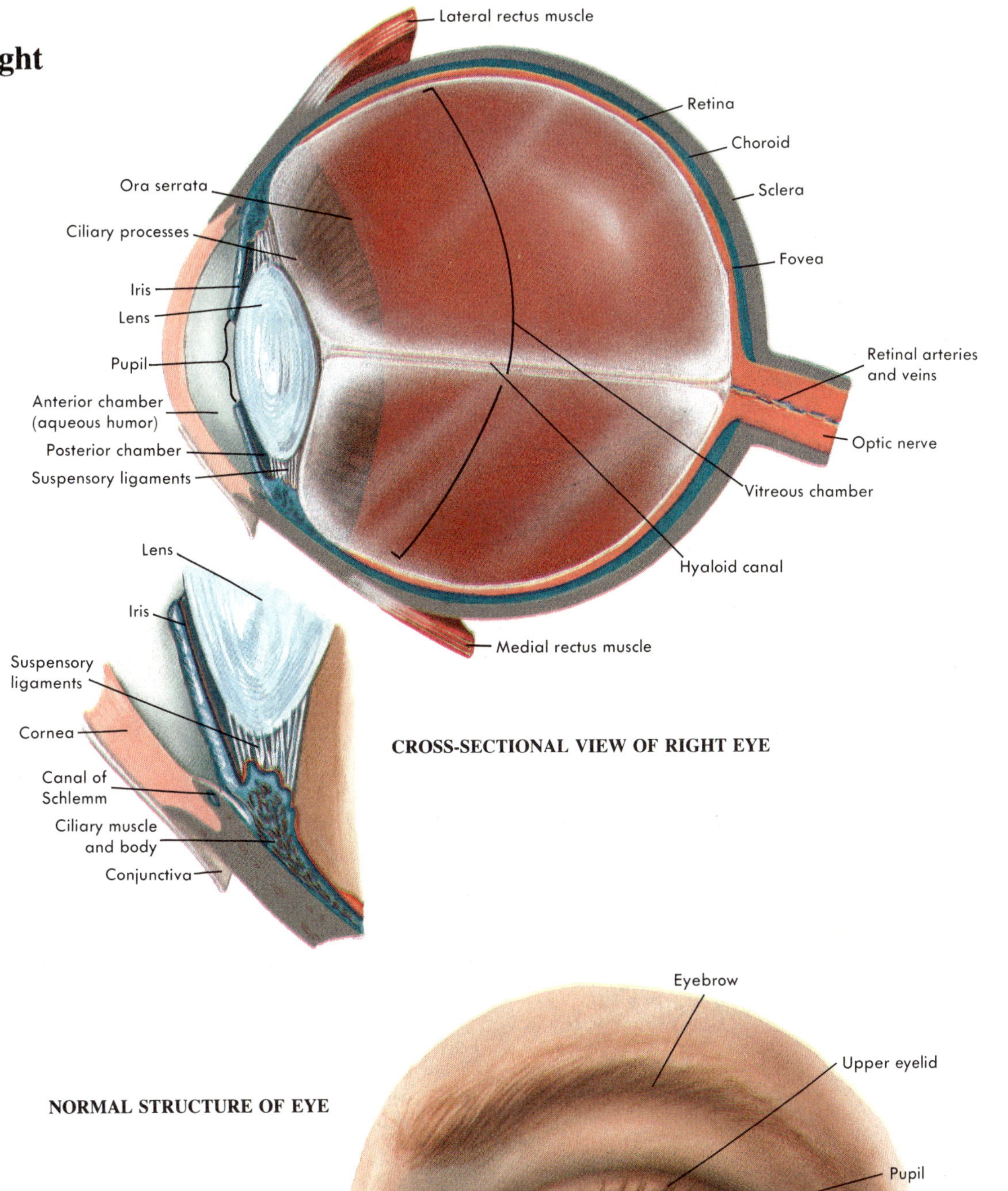

CROSS-SECTIONAL VIEW OF RIGHT EYE

NORMAL STRUCTURE OF EYE

Taste and Smell

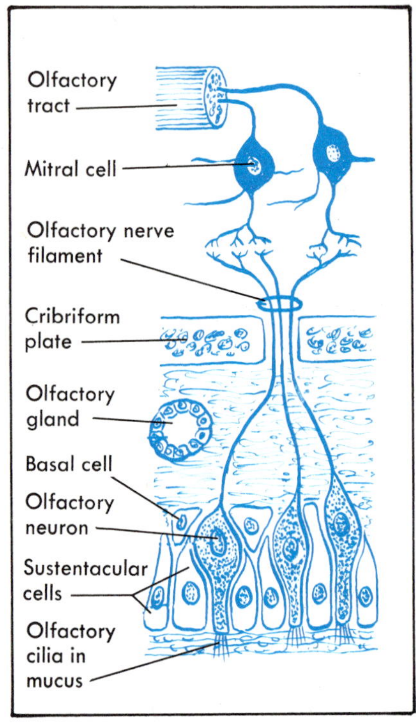

SCHEME OF CELL AND FIBER ARRANGEMENT IN OLFACTORY EPITHELIUM

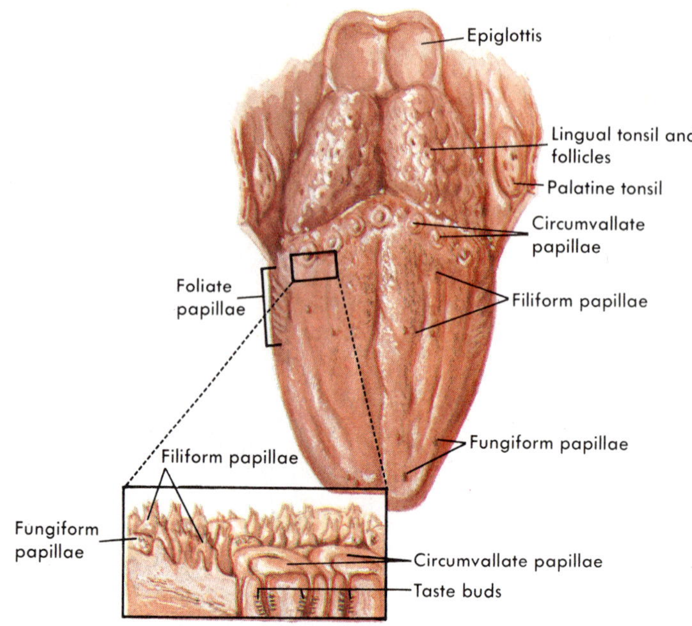

PAPILLAE ON TONGUE AND LOCATION OF TASTE BUDS

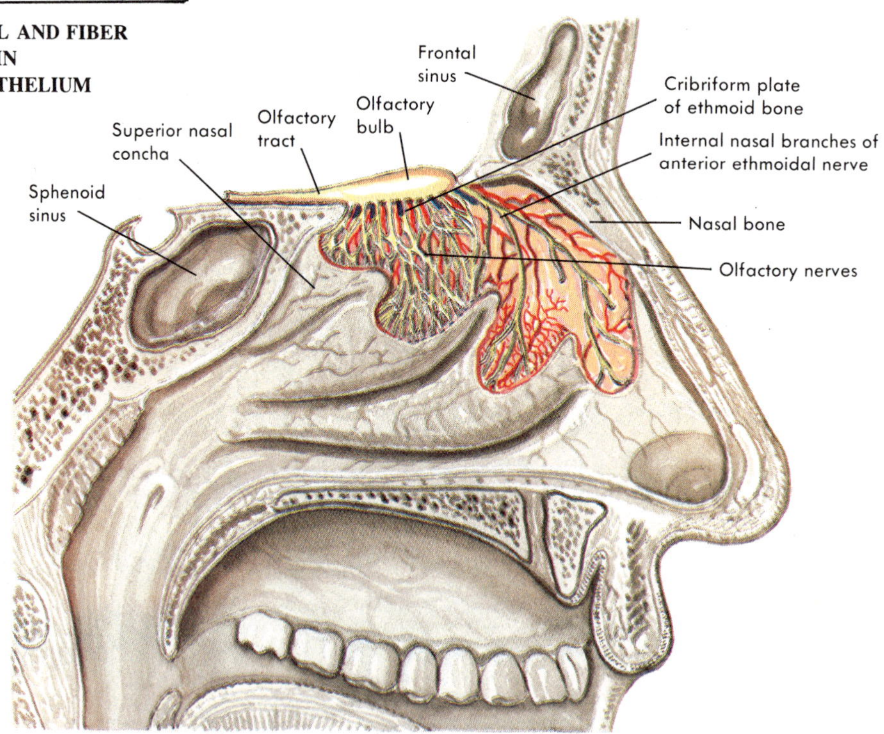

OLFACTORY NERVE DISTRIBUTION TO MUCOSA OF NASAL CAVITY

SKIN

Protection and Touch

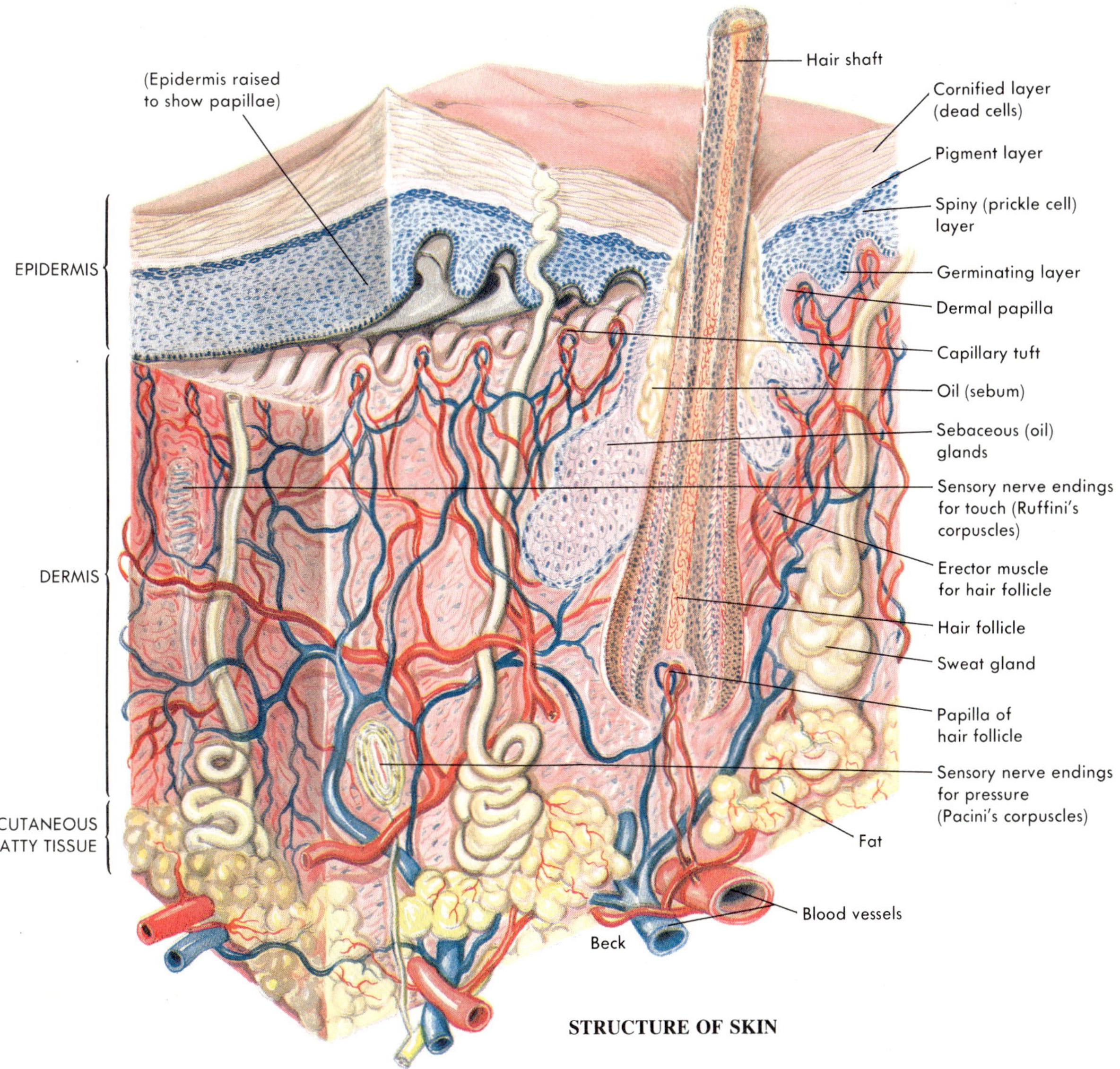

(Epidermis raised to show papillae)
EPIDERMIS
DERMIS
SUBCUTANEOUS FATTY TISSUE
Hair shaft
Cornified layer (dead cells)
Pigment layer
Spiny (prickle cell) layer
Germinating layer
Dermal papilla
Capillary tuft
Oil (sebum)
Sebaceous (oil) glands
Sensory nerve endings for touch (Ruffini's corpuscles)
Erector muscle for hair follicle
Hair follicle
Sweat gland
Papilla of hair follicle
Sensory nerve endings for pressure (Pacini's corpuscles)
Fat
Blood vessels
Beck

STRUCTURE OF SKIN

Common Skin Disorders

CLINICAL NOTE: Skin disorders

Skin problems may result from various causes, such as parasitic infestations, fungal, bacterial, or viral infections, reactions to substances encountered externally or taken internally, or new growths. Many of the skin manifestations have no known cause; others are hereditary.

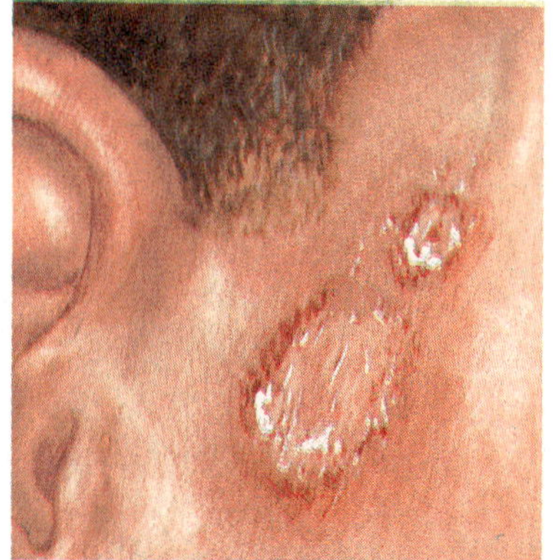

TINEA CORPORIS (RINGWORM)

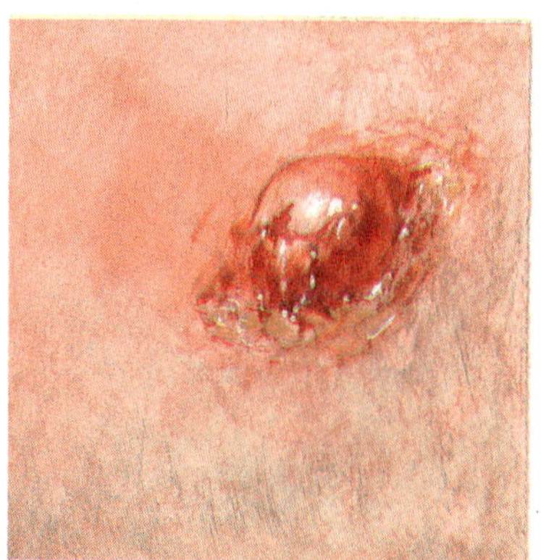

SQUAMOUS CELL CARCINOMA

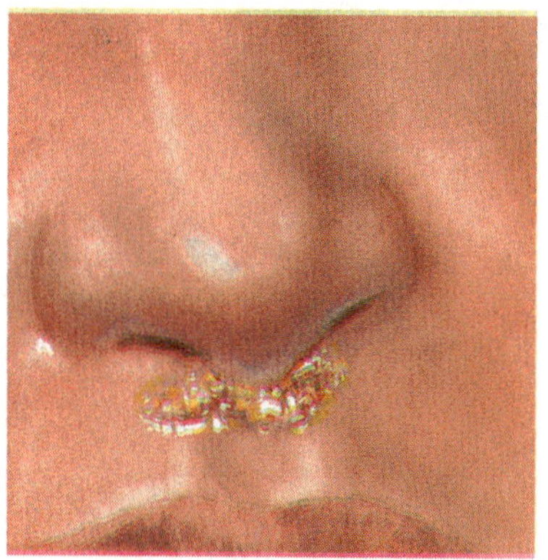

IMPETIGO CONTAGIOSA

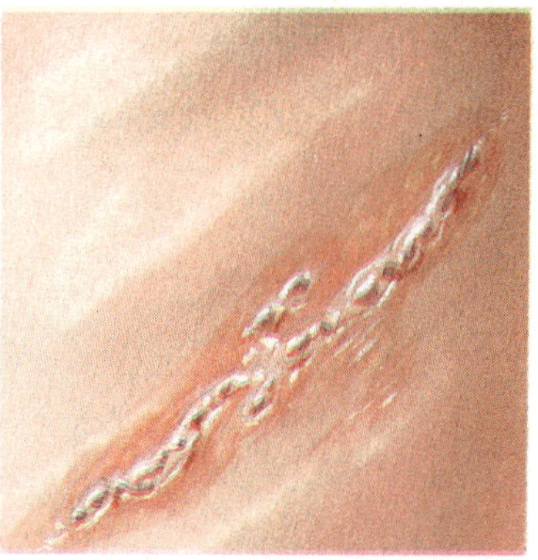

HERPES ZOSTER (SHINGLES)

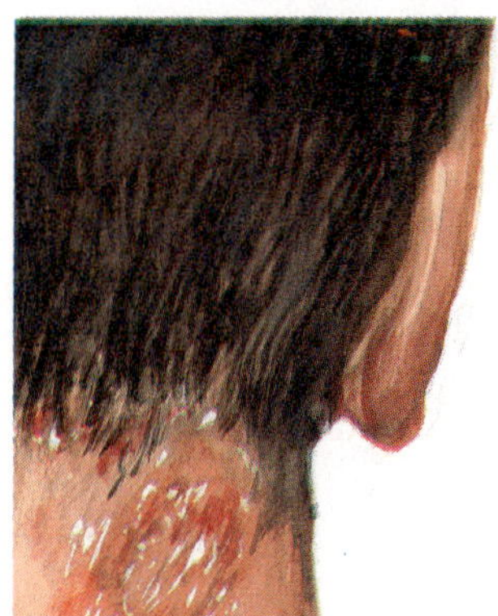

DERMATITIS

a, symbol for **arterial blood.**

A, **1.** abbreviation for **accommodation. 2.** symbol for **alveolar gas. 3.** abbreviation for **ampere. 4.** abbreviation for **anterior. 5.** abbreviation for **atomic weight. 6.** abbreviation for **axial. 7.** symbol for **mass number.**

Å, symbol for **angstrom.**

a-, a combining form meaning 'without, not': *abacterial, abaptiston, abasia.*

AA, **1.** abbreviation for **achievement age. 2.** abbreviation for **Alcoholics Anonymous. 3.** abbreviation for **amplitude of accommodation.**

āa, āā, ĀĀ, (in prescriptions) abbreviation for *ana,* indicating an equal amount of each ingredient to be compounded.

AAAI, abbreviation for **American Academy of Allergy and Immunology.**

AACN, **1.** abbreviation for **American Association of Colleges of Nursing. 2.** abbreviation for **American Association of Critical Care Nurses.**

AAIN, abbreviation for **American Association of Industrial Nurses.**

AAMC, abbreviation for **American Association of Medical Colleges.**

AAN, abbreviation for **American Academy of Nursing.**

AANA, abbreviation for **American Association of Nurse Anesthetists.**

AANN, **1.** abbreviation for **American Association of Neuroscience Nurses. 2.** abbreviation for **American Association of Neurosurgical Nurses.**

AANNT, abbreviation for **American Association of Nephrology Nurses and Technicians.**

AAOMS, abbreviation for **American Association of Oral and Maxillofacial Surgeons.**

AAPA, abbreviation for **American Academy of Physicians' Assistants.**

AAPB, abbreviation for **American Association of Pathologists and Bacteriologists.**

AAPMR, abbreviation for **American Academy of Physical Medicine and Rehabilitation.**

AART, abbreviation for **American Association for Respiratory Therapy.**

AAUP, abbreviation for **American Association of University Professors.**

AAV, abbreviation for **adenoassociated virus.**

Ab, abbreviation for **antibody.**

ab-, abs-, a combining form meaning 'from, off, away from': *abarthrosis, abarticulation, abaxial.*

abacterial /ab′aktir′ē•əl/, any atmosphere or condition free of bacteria; literally, without bacteria.

abaissement /ä′bāsmäN′/, a falling, lowering, or depressing; in ophthalmology, the displacement of a lens.

abalienation /abāl′yənā′shən/, **1.** a state of physical deterioration or mental decay. **2.** a state of insanity. –**abalienate,** *v.,* **abalienated,** *adj.*

abandonment of care, (in law) wrongful cessation of the provision of care to a patient, usually by a physician.

abarthrosis. See **synovial joint.**

abarticular /ab′ärtik′yŏŏlər/, **1.** of or pertaining to a condition that does not affect a joint. **2.** of or pertaining to a site or structure remote from a joint.

abarticulation, **1.** dislocation of a joint. **2.** a synovial joint.

abasia /əbā′zhə/, the inability to walk, as in paralytic abasia that paralyzes the leg muscles. **–abasic, abatic,** *adj.*

abaxial /abak′sē•əl/, **1.** of or pertaining to a position outside the axis of a body or structure. **2.** of or pertaining to a position at the opposite extremity of a structure.

Abbe-Estlander operation /ab′ē-est′-/, a surgical procedure that transforms a full-thickness section of one oral lip to the other lip, using an arterial pedicle for ensuring survival of a graft.

Abbokinase, a trademark for a plasminogen activator (urokinase).

Abbot pump /ab′ət/, a small portable pump that can be adjusted and finely calibrated to deliver precise amounts of medication in solution through an intravenous infusion set. It is similar to a Harvard pump, but the flow rate may be increased or decreased by smaller increments.

ABC, abbreviation for **aspiration biopsy cytology.**

abdomen /ab′dəmən, abdō′mən/, the portion of the body between the thorax and the pelvis. The abdominal cavity contains the lower portion of the esophagus, the stomach, the intestines, the liver, the spleen, the pancreas, and other visceral organs. The walls of the abdominal cavity are lined with the parietal layer of the peritoneum, a serous membrane. The covering, or outermost layer of each organ, is formed by the visceral layer of the peritoneum. A small amount of serous fluid in the space between the membranous layers allows the organs to slide freely, as in the normal process of digestion, evacuation, and breathing. Also called *(informal)* **belly.** See also **abdominal regions.** –**abdominal** /abdom′-/, *adj.*

abdominal actinomycosis. See **actinomycosis.**

abdominal aorta, the portion of the descending aorta that passes from the aortic hiatus of the diaphragm into the abdomen, descending ventral to the vertebral column, and ending at the fourth lumbar vertebra where it divides into the two common iliac arteries. It supplies many different parts of the body, as the testes, ovaries, kidneys, and stomach. Its branches are the celiac, superior mesenteric, inferior mesenteric, middle suprarenal, renal, testicular, ovarian, inferior phrenic, lumbar, middle sacral, and common iliac arteries. See also **descending aorta.** Compare **thoracic aorta.**

abdominal aponeurosis, the conjoined tendons of the oblique and transverse muscles of the abdomen.

abdominal bandage, a broad supportive bandage commonly used after abdominal surgery.

abdominal binder, a bandage or elasticized wrap that is applied around the lower part of the torso to support the abdomen. An abdominal binder is sometimes applied after abdominal surgery to decrease discomfort, thereby increasing a patient's ability to begin ambulatory activities and accelerate convalescence. A kind of abdominal binder is the **Scultetus binder.**

abdominal delivery, the delivery of a child through a surgical incision in the abdomen. The procedure performed may be any of the several kinds of cesarean section.

abdominal fistula, an abnormal passage from an abdominal organ to the surface of the body. In a colostomy, a passage from the bowel to an opening on the surface of the abdomen is created surgically.

abdominal hernia, a hernia in which a loop of bowel protrudes through the abdominal musculature, often through the site of an old surgical scar. Also called **ventral hernia.** See also **hernia.**

abdominal hysterectomy, the excision of the uterus through the abdominal wall.

abdominal pain, acute or chronic localized or diffuse pain in the abdominal cavity. Abdominal pain is a significant symptom because its cause may require immediate surgical or medical intervention. The most common causes of severe abdominal pain are inflammation, perforation of an intraabdominal structure, circulatory obstruction, intestinal or ureteral obstruction, or rupture of an organ located within the abdomen. Specific conditions include appendicitis, perforated gastric ulcer, strangulated hernia, superior mesenteric arterial thrombosis, and small and large bowel obstruction. The differential diagnosis of the cause of acute abdominal pain requires localization and characterization of the pain by means of light and deep percussion, auscultation, and palpation and by abdominal, rectal, or pelvic examination. Direct physical examination may be supplemented by various laboratory and radiologic examinations. Aspiration of peritoneal fluid for bacteriologic and chemical evaluation is sometimes indicated. Conditions producing acute abdominal pain that may require surgery include appendicitis, acute or severe and chronic diverticulitis, acute and chronic cholecystitis, cholelithiasis, acute pancreatitis, perforation of a peptic ulcer, various intestinal obstructions, abdominal aortic aneurysms, and trauma affecting any of the abdominal organs. Gynecologic causes of acute abdominal pain that may require surgery include acute pelvic inflammatory disease, ruptured ovarian cyst, and ectopic pregnancy. Abdominal pain associated with pregnancy may be caused by the weight of the enlarged uterus; rotation, stretching, or compression of the round ligament; or squeezing or displacement of the bowel. In addition, uterine contractions associated with premature labor may produce severe abdominal pain. Chronic abdominal pain may be functional or the result of overeating or aerophagia. When the symptoms are recurrent, an organic cause is considered. Organic sources of abdominal pain include peptic ulcer, hiatus hernia, gastritis, chronic cholecystitis and cholelithiasis, chronic pancreatitis, pancreatic carcinoma, chronic diverticulitis, intermittent low-grade intestinal obstruction, and functional indigestion. Some systemic conditions may be responsible for abdominal pain. Examples of these include systemic lupus erythematosus, lead poisoning, hypercalcemia, sickle cell anemia, diabetic acidosis, porphyria, tabes dorsalis, and black widow spider poisoning.

abdominal pregnancy, an extrauterine pregnancy in which the conceptus develops in the abdominal cavity after being extruded from the fimbriated end of the fallopian tube or through a defect in the tube or uterus. The placenta may implant on the abdominal or visceral peritoneum. Abdominal pregnancy may be suspected when the abdomen has enlarged but the uterus has remained small for the length of gestation. Abdominal pregnancies constitute approximately 2% of ectopic pregnancies and approximately 0.01% of all pregnancies. The condition results in perinatal death of the fetus in approximately 90% of cases, maternal death in approximately 6%. Because of its rarity, the condition may be unsuspected, and diagnosis is often delayed. Ultrasound or x-ray visualization showing gas in the maternal bowel below the fetus is diagnostic of the condition. Surgical removal of the placenta, sac, and embryo or fetus is necessary, but the procedure is often complicated by massive bleeding, and, as the placenta tends to adhere firmly to the peritoneum and to the bowel, complete removal is seldom possible. Postoperative sequelae may include necrotization of retained placental tissue, infection, continued bleeding, and sterility.

abdominal pulse, the pulse of the abdominal aorta.

abdominal reflex, a superficial neurologic reflex obtained by firmly stroking the skin of the abdomen, normally resulting in a brisk contraction of abdominal muscles in which the umbilicus moves toward the site of the stimulus. This reflex is lost in diseases of the pyramidal tract. See also **superficial reflex.**

abdominal regions, the nine topographic subdivisions of the abdomen, determined by four imaginary lines, in a tic-tac-toe pattern, imposed over the anterior surface. The upper horizontal line passes along the level of the cartilages of the nine ribs; the lower along the iliac crests. The two vertical lines extend on each side of the body from the cartilage of the eighth rib to the center of the inguinal ligament. The lines, which are drawn straight or curved in an alternate formation, divide the abdomen into three upper, three middle, and three lower zones: right hypochondriac, epigastric, and left hypochondriac regions (upper zones); right lateral, umbilical, and left lateral regions (middle zones); right inguinal, pubic, and left inguinal regions (lower zones).

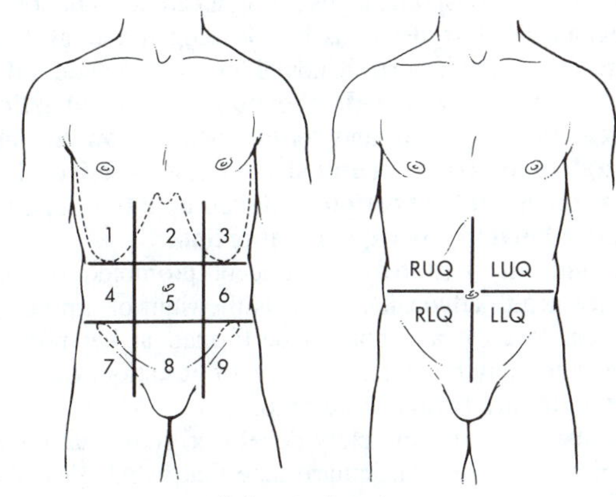

Abdominal regions

abdominal surgery, any operation that involves an incision into the abdomen, usually performed under general anesthesia. Before surgery a complete blood count, a type and crossmatch of the blood, and a urinalysis are done. Often an enema is given. The skin is shaved and cleansed from the nipple line to the pubis. A barbiturate is often given at bedtime; food and fluids by mouth are forbidden after the midnight before surgery. Shortly before surgery a barbiturate or tranquilizer and a narcotic are usually given, along with an anticholinergic agent, such as atropine. Postoperatively, the nurse ensures that the airway is open, checks tubes and catheters, connects drainage tubes to collection containers, and checks the dressing for excessive bleeding or drainage. Close observation of vital signs is essential. A careful record is kept of fluid intake and output. The patient is turned and is helped to cough and breathe deeply every hour. Medication is given as needed for relief from pain. Some kinds of abdominal surgery are **appendectomy, cholecystectomy, colostomy, gastrectomy, herniorrhaphy,** and **laparotomy.** See also **acute abdomen.**

abdominal tenaculum. See **tenaculum.**

abdomino-, a combining form meaning 'pertaining to the abdomen': *abdominocentesis, abdominoscopy, abdominothoracic.*

abdominocentesis. See **paracentesis.**

abdominocyesis /abdom'inōsī•ē'sis/, an abdominal pregnancy.

abdominoscopy /abdom'inos'kəpē/, a procedure for examining the contents of the peritoneum in which an electrically illuminated tubular device is passed through a trocar into the abdominal cavity. See also **endoscopy, laparoscopy, peritinoscopy.**

abducens nerve /abdo͞o'sənz/, the sixth cranial nerve. It arises in the pons, near the fourth ventricle, leaves the brainstem between the medulla oblongata and pons, and passes through the cavernous sinus and the superior orbital fissure. It controls the external rectus muscle, turning the eye outward. Also called **abducent nerve, nervus abducens.**

abduction, movement of a limb away from the body. Compare **adduction.**

abduction boots, a pair of orthopedic casts for the lower extremities, available in both short-leg and long-leg configurations, with a bar incorporated at ankle level to provide hip abduction. Abduction boots are used for postoperative positioning and immobilization after hip adductor releases and to promote proper positioning during healing after surgery to repair structures in the lower extremities.

abductor, a muscle that draws a body part away from the midline, or one part from another. Compare **adductor.**

Abernethy's sarcoma /ab'ərnē'thēz/, a malignant neoplasm of fat cells, usually occurring on the trunk.

aberrancy. See **aberrant ventricular conduction.**

aberrant /aber'ənt/, **1.** of or pertaining to a wandering from the usual or expected course, as various ducts, nerves, and vessels in the body. **2.** (in botany and zoology) of or pertaining to an abnormal individual, as certain atypical members of a species.

aberrant goiter, an enlargement of a supernumerary or ectopic thyroid gland.

aberrant ventricular conduction (AVC), the temporary abnormal intraventricular conduction of a supraventricular impulse, usually associated with a change in cycle length. This conduction is fairly common after a very early premature atrial beat and is most often conducted with a right bundle branch block. Also called **aberrancy, ventricular aberration.**

aberration, **1.** any departure from the usual course or normal condition. **2.** abnormal growth or development. **3.** (in psychology) an illogical and unreasonable thought or belief, often leading to an unsound mental state. **4.** (in genetics) any change in the number or structure of the chromosomes. See also **chromosomal aberration. 5.** (in optics) any imperfect image formation caused by unequal refraction or focalization of light rays through a lens.

abetalipoproteinemia /əbā'təlīp'ōprō'tinē'mē•ə/, a rare inherited disorder of fat metabolism, characterized by acanthocytosis, low or absent serum betalipoproteins, and hypocholesterolemia. In severe cases steatorrhea, ataxia, nystagmus, motor incoordination, and retinitis pigmentosa occur. Also called **Bassen-Kornzweig syndrome** /-kôrn′zwīg/.

abient /ab′ē•ənt/, characterized by a tendency to move away from stimuli. Compare **adient.** **–abience,** *n.*

ability, the capacity to act in a specified way because of the possession of appropriate skills and mental or physical fitness.

abiogenesis /ab′ē•ōjen′əsis/, spontaneous generation; the theory that organic life can originate from inanimate matter. Compare **biogenesis.** **–abiogenetic,** *adj.*

abiosis /ab′ē•ō′sis/, a nonviable condition or a situation that is incompatible with life. **–abiotic,** *adj.*

abiotrophy /ab′ē•ot′rəfē/, a premature depletion of vitality or the deterioration of certain cells and tissues, especially those involved in genetic degenerative diseases. **–abiotrophic** /ab′ē•ətrō′fik/, *adj.*

ablation /ablā′shən/, an amputation, an excision of any part of the body, or a removal of a growth or harmful substance.

ablatio placentae. See **abruptio placentae.**

ablepsia /əblep′sē•ə/, the condition of being blind. Also called **ablepsy.**

ABMS, abbreviation for **American Board of Medical Specialties.**

abnerval current, an electric current that passes from a nerve to and through muscle.

abnormal behavior, maladaptive acts or activities detrimental to the individual and to society. The acts range from the transitory inability to cope with a stressful situation to persistent bizarre or destructive behavior or total disorientation and withdrawal from the realities of everyday life. See also **behavior disorder.**

abnormal psychology, the study of mental disorders and maladaptive behavior, including neuroses and psychoses, and of normal phenomena that are not completely understood, such as dreams and altered states of consciousness.

ABO blood groups, the most important of several systems for classifying human blood based on the antigenic components of the red blood cell. The ABO blood group is identified by the presence or absence of two different antigens, A or B, on the surface of the erythrocyte. The four blood types in this grouping, A, B, AB, and O, are determined by and named for these antigens. Type AB indicates the presence of both antigens; type O the absence of both. Corresponding antibodies, anti-A and anti-B agglutinins, can be found in the plasma of type O blood. The plasma components of type A and type B blood are, respectively, devoid of anti-A and anti-B agglutinins; both agglutinins are absent from type AB blood plasma. In addition to its significant role in blood banks and transfusion therapy, the ABO blood grouping contributes to forensic medicine, genetics, and, together with the less important blood groups, to anthropology and legal medicine. See also **blood group, Rh factor, transfusion.**

aboiement /ä′bô•ämäN′/, an involuntary making of abnormal, animal-like sounds, such as barking. Aboiement may be a clinical sign of Gilles de la Tourette's syndrome.

abort, **1.** to deliver a nonviable fetus; to miscarry. See also **spontaneous abortion.** **2.** to terminate a pregnancy before the fetus has developed enough to live ex utero. See also **induced abortion.** **3.** to terminate in the early stages or to discontinue before completion, as to arrest the usual course of a disease, to stop growth and development, or to halt a project.

aborted systole, a contraction of the heart that is usually weak and is not associated with a radial pulse.

abortifacient /əbôr′tifā′shənt/, **1.** producing abortion. **2.** an agent that causes abortion.

abortion, the spontaneous or induced termination of pregnancy before the fetus has developed enough to be expected to live if born. Kinds of abortion include **habitual abortion, infected abortion, septic abortion, threatened abortion,** and **voluntary abortion.** See also **complete abortion, criminal abortion, elective abortion, incomplete abortion, induced abortion, spontaneous abortion, therapeutic abortion.**

abortion on demand, a concept promoted by prochoice health advocates that it is the right of a pregnant woman to have an abortion performed at her request. That right may be limited by time of gestation, or it may pertain to any period of gestation.

abortus, any incompletely developed fetus that results from an abortion, particularly one that weighs less than 500 g.

abortus fever, a form of brucellosis, the only one endemic to North America. It is caused by *Brucella abortus,* an organism so named because it causes abortion in cows. Infection in humans results from the ingestion of contaminated milk from cows infected with *B. abortus,* from handling infected meat, or from skin contact with the excreta of living infected animals. Streptomycin and tetracycline are usually prescribed together as treatment. Also called **Rio Grande fever.** See also **brucellosis.**

abouchement /ä′bōōshmäN′/, the junction of a small blood vessel with a large blood vessel.

aboulia. See abulia.

abrachia /əbrā′kē•ə/, the absence of arms. **–abrachial,** *adj.*

abrasion, a scraping, or rubbing away of a surface by friction. Abrasion may be the result of trauma, as a skinned knee; of therapy, as in dermabrasion of the skin for removal of scar tissue; or of normal function, as the wearing down of a tooth by mastication. Compare **laceration.** See also **bruxism, friction burn.** **–abrade,** *v.,* **abrasive,** *adj.*

abreaction an emotional release resulting from mentally reliving or from bringing into consciousness, through the process of catharsis, a long-repressed, painful experience. See also **catharsis.**

abrosia /əbrō′zhə/, a condition caused by fasting or abstaining from food. See **anoxia.**

abruptio placentae, separation of the placenta implanted in normal position in a pregnancy of 20 weeks or more or during labor before delivery of the fetus. It occurs approximately once in 200 births, and, because it often results in severe hemorrhage, it is a significant cause of maternal and fetal mortality. Hypertension and preeclampsia are associated with increased rates of occurrence, but in many cases there is no explanation. Complete separation brings about immediate death of the fetus. Bleeding from the site of separation causes abdominal pain, uterine tenderness, and tetanic uterine contraction. Bleeding may be concealed within the uterus or may be evident externally, sometimes as sudden massive hemorrhage. In severe cases, shock and death can come in minutes. Cesarean section must be performed immediately and rapidly. Extensive extravasation of blood within the wall of the uterus may deplete fibrinogen, prolong clotting time, bring about intractable bleeding, and, by damaging the musculature of the uterus, prevent the uterus from contracting well after delivery. Hysterectomy may be necessary to prevent exsanguination. Partial separation may cause little bleeding and may not interfere with fetal oxygenation. If the pregnancy is near term, labor may be permitted or induced by means of amniotomy. A premature pregnancy may be allowed to continue under close observation of the mother at bed rest. The nurse must be alert to the possibility that bleeding is present but concealed internally and that if all the blood can escape, there may be little pain. Also called **ablatio placentae, accidental hemorrhage.** Compare **placenta previa.** See also **Couvelaire uterus.**

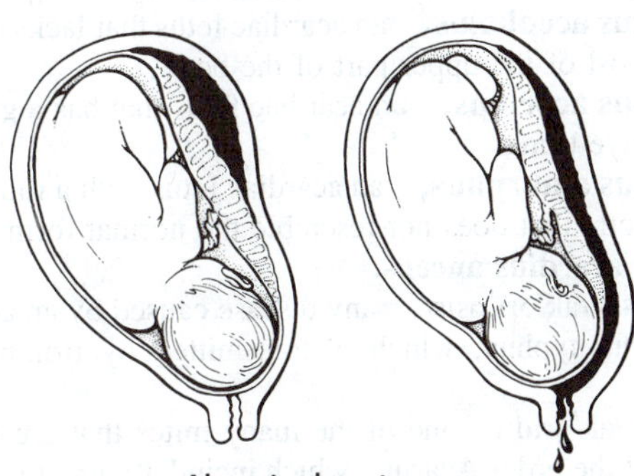
Abruptio placentae

abscess, a cavity containing pus and surrounded by inflamed tissue, formed as a result of suppuration in a localized infection (characteristically, a staphylococcal infection). Healing usually occurs when an abscess drains or is incised. If an abscess is deep in tissue, drainage is made by means of a sinus tract that connects it to the surface. In a sterile abscess, the contents are not the result of pyrogenic bacteria.

absent without leave (AWOL) /ā′wôl/, describing a patient who leaves a psychiatric facility without authorization.

absolute alcohol. See **dehydrated alcohol.**

absolute cephalopelvic disproportion. See **cephalopelvic disproportion.**

absolute growth, the total increase in size of an organism or a particular organ or part, as the limbs, head, or trunk.

absolute refractory period. See **refractory period.**

absorb, **1.** the act of taking up various substances; for example, the tissues of the intestines absorb fluids. **2.** the energy transferred to tissues by radiation, as an absorbed dose of radioactivity.

absorbable gauze, a gauzelike material, produced from oxidized cellulose, that can be absorbed. It is applied directly to bleeding tissue for hemostasis.

absorbance, the degree of absorption of light or other radiant energy by a medium through which the radiant energy passes. It is expressed as the logarithm of the ratio of light transmitted through a pure solvent to the intensity of light transmitted through the medium. Absorbance varies with such factors as wavelength, the solution, concentration, and path length.

absorbed dose, (in radiotherapy) the energy imparted by ionizing radiation per unit mass of irradiated material at the place of interest. The SI unit of absorbed dose is the gray, which is 1 joule/kg and equals 100 rad.

absorbent dressing, a dressing of any material applied to a wound or incision to absorb secretions.

absorbent gauze, a gauze for absorbing fluids. The form, weight, and use vary. Gauze may be a fine fabric in rolled single layers for spiral bandages, or it may be a thick, many-layered pad for a sterile pressure dressing.

absorbifacient /absôr′bifā′shənt/, **1.** any agent that promotes or enhances absorption. **2.** causing or enhancing absorption.

absorption, **1.** the incorporation of matter by other matter through chemical, molecular, or physical action, as the dissolving of a gas in a liquid or the taking up of a liquid by a porous solid. **2.** (in physiology) the passage of substances across and into tissues, as the passage of digested food molecules into intestinal cells or the passage of liquids into kidney tubules. Kinds of absorption are **agglutinin absorption, cutaneous absorption, external absorption, interstitial absorption, intestinal absorption, parenteral absorption,** and **pathologic absorption. 3.** (in radiology) the process of absorbing radiant energy by living or nonliving matter with which the radiation reacts.

absorption rate constant, a value describing how much drug is absorbed per unit of time.

absorption spectrum, the range of electromagnetic energy that is used for spectroanalysis, including both visible light and ultraviolet radiation; also, a graph of spectrum for a specific compound.

absorptivity, absorbance divided by the product of the concentration of a substance and the sample path length.

abstinence, voluntary avoidance of any substance or the performance of any act for which the person has an appetite.

abstract /ab′strakt, abstrakt′/, a condensed summary of a scientific article, literary piece, or address.

abtraction, a condition in which the teeth or other maxillary and mandibular structures are below their normal position or away from the occlusal plane.

abstract thinking, the final stage in the development of the cognitive thought processes in the child. During this phase, thought is characterized by adaptability, flexibility, and the use of concepts and generalizations. Problem solving is accomplished by drawing logical conclusions from a set of observations, as making hypotheses and testing them. This type of thinking appears from about 12 to 15 years of age, usually after some degree of education. Compare **concrete thinking, syncretic thinking.**

abulia /əbo͞o′lyə/, a loss of the ability or a reduced capacity to function voluntarily or to make decisions. Also spelled **aboulia.**

abuse, **1.** improper use of equipment, a substance, or a service, as a drug or program, either intentionally or unintentionally. **2.** to attack or injure. A kind of abuse is **child abuse.** See also **drug abuse.**

abuse of process, a civil action for damages in which it is alleged that the legal process has been used in a manner not contemplated by law. This action might be brought by a health practitioner attempting to countersue a patient or by a psychiatric patient attempting to demonstrate wrongful confinement.

abutment, a tooth, root, or implant for the support and retention of a fixed or movable prosthesis. Compare **multiple abutment.** See also **intermediate abutment.**

abutment tooth, a tooth selected to support a prosthesis.

Ac, symbol for **actinium.**

AC, abbreviation for **alternating current.**

ac-. See **ad-.**

a.c., (in prescriptions) abbreviation for *ante cibum,* a Latin phrase meaning "before meals." The times of administration are commonly 7 AM, 11 AM, and 5 PM.

academic ladder, the hierarchy of faculty appointments in a university through which a faculty member must advance from instructor to assistant professor, to associate professor, and, finally, to professor.

acalculia /a′kalko͞o′lyə/, a type of aphasia characterized by the inability to solve simple mathematic calculations.

acampsia /əkamp′sē·ə/, a condition in which a joint becomes rigid. See also **ankylosis.**

acantha /əkan′thə/, a spine or a spinous projection. –**acanthoid,** *adj.*

acantho-, a combining form meaning 'thorny or spiky': *acanthesthesia, acanthoid, acantholysis.*

acanthocyte /əkan′thəsīt′/, an abnormal red blood cell with spurlike projections giving it a thorny appearance. Large numbers are present in abetalipoproteinemia; fewer occur in cirrhosis and in certain malabsorption syndromes. Compare **burr cell.** See also **abetalipoproteinemia, acanthocytosis.**

acanthocytosis /akan′thōsītō′sis/, the abnormal presence of acanthocytes in the circulating blood system, most commonly associated with abetalipoproteinemia in which as many as 80% of the erythrocytes are acanthocytes. See also **abetalipoproteinemia, elliptocytosis.**

acanthoid. See **acantha.**

acanthoma /ak′anthō′mə/, any benign or malignant tumor arising from the prickle-cell layer of the epidermis.

acanthoma adenoides cysticum. See **trichoepithelioma.**

acanthoma verrucosa seborrheica. See **seborrheic keratosis.**

acanthosis /ak′ənthō′sis/, an abnormal thickening of the prickle-cell layer of the skin, as in eczema and psoriasis. See also **acanthosis nigricans, epidermis.** –**acanthotic,** *adj.*

acanthosis nigricans /nē′grikanz′/, a skin disease characterized by hyperpigmented, warty lesions of the axillae and perianal body folds. There are benign and malignant forms, the latter associated with cancers of the GI tract. See also **acanthosis.**

acarbia /akär′bē·ə/, **1.** a decrease in the bicarbonate level in the blood. **2.** any condition that lowers the bicarbonate level in the blood.

acardia /akär′dē·ə/, a rare congenital anomaly in which the heart is absent. It is sometimes seen in a conjoined twin whose survival until birth depended on the circulatory system of its twin. –**acardiac,** *adj.*

acardius acephalus, an acardiac fetus that lacks a head and most of the upper part of the body.

acardius acormus, an acardiac fetus that has a grossly defective trunk.

acardius amorphus, an acardiac fetus with a rudimentary body that does not resemble the normal form. Also called **acardius anceps.**

acariasis /ak′ərī′əsis/, any disease caused by an acarid, as scrub typhus, which is transmitted by trombiculid mites.

acarid /ak′ərid/, one of the many mites that are members of the order Acarina, which includes a great number of parasitic and free-living organisms. Most are yet undescribed, but several types are of medical interest because they infect humans. The kinds associated with disease are those acting as intermediate hosts of pathogenic agents, those that directly cause skin or tissue damage, and those that cause loss of blood or tissue fluids. Important as vectors of scrub typhus and other rickettsial agents are the six-legged larvae of trombiculid mites, which are parasitic of humans, many other mammals, and birds. See **chiggers, scabies.**

acaro-, a combining form meaning 'pertaining to mites': *acarodermatitis, acaroid, acarophobia.*

acc, Acc, abbreviation for **accommodation.**

accelerated hypertension. See **malignant hypertension.**

accelerated idiojunctional rhythm /id′ē•ō-/, an automatic junctional rhythm at a rate exceeding the normal firing rate of the junction but slower than 100 per minute (60 to 100 per minute) and without retrograde conduction to the atria. It is caused by enhanced automaticity, which is commonly secondary to digitalis toxicity.

accelerated idioventricular rhythm (AIVR), an automatic ectopic ventricular rhythm, faster than the normal rate of the His-Purkinje system but slower than 100 per minute (50 to 100 per minute) and without retrograde conduction to the atria. Many examples are associated with acute myocardial infarction but are regarded as benign.

accelerated junctional rhythm, an ectopic junctional heart rhythm with a rate that exceeds the normal firing rate of junctional tissue, with or without retrograde atrial conduction.

acceleration, an increase in the speed or velocity of an object or reaction. Compare **deceleration.** **–accelerator,** *n.*

acceleration phase, (in obstetrics) the first period of active labor, characterized by an increased rate of dilatation of the cervical os as charted on a Friedman curve.

acceptable daily intake (ADI), the maximum amount of any substance that can be safely ingested by a human. Ingestion in excess of this amount may cause toxic effects.

acceptor, **1.** an organism that receives from another person or organism living tissue, as transfused blood or a transplanted organ. **2.** a substance or compound that combines with a part of another substance or compound. Compare **donor.**

access cavity, a coronal opening in a tooth, required for effective cleaning, shaping, and filling of the pulp space.

accessory, **1.** a supplement employed chiefly for convenience or for safety, as the electric elevator mechanisms for hospital beds. **2.** a structure that serves one of the main anatomic systems, as the accessory sex organs in men and women; the accessory organs of the skin; the hair; the nails; and the skin glands.

accessory chromosome, an unpaired X or Y sex chromosome. Also called **monosome.**

accessory muscle, a relatively rare anatomic duplication of a muscle that may appear anywhere in the muscular system. The most common sign associated with an accessory muscle is the appearance of a soft-tissue mass. Differential diagnosis without surgical intervention and exploration is difficult because of the similar appearance of some tumors or soft-tissue masses, as ganglia. The appearance of the soft-tissue mass associated with an accessory muscle may be transient, or it may be constant, depending on the location of the accessory muscle in relation to motion. In many individuals with accessory muscles, specific treatment is not indicated unless the accessory muscle interferes with normal function.

accessory nerve, either of a pair of cranial nerves essential for speech, swallowing, and certain movements of the head and shoulders. Each nerve has a cranial and a spinal portion, communicates with certain cervical nerves, and connects to the nucleus ambiguus of the brain. Also called **eleventh nerve, nervus accessorius, spinal accessory nerve.**

accessory pancreatic duct, a small duct opening into the pancreatic duct or duodenum near the mouth of the common bile duct.

accessory pathway, an extramuscular tract between atrium and ventricle. It may become a clinical problem when paroxysmal supraventricular tachycardia develops as a result of AV reentry, or when combined with atrial fibrillation.

accessory root canal, a lateral branching of the pulp canal in a tooth, usually occurring in the apical third of the root.

accessory phrenic nerve, the nerve that joins the phrenic nerve at the root of the neck or in the thorax, forming a loop around the subclavian vein. It may arise from the nerve to the subclavius or from the fifth cervical nerve. Resection of the phrenic nerve to immobilize the diaphragm may be only partially successful if the accessory phrenic nerve is not also resected. Compare **phrenic nerve.**

accessory sinus of the nose. See **paranasal sinus.**

accessory tooth, a supernumerary tooth that does not resemble a normal tooth in size, shape, or position.

access time, the amount of time required for a computer to retrieve a word from its memory component.

ACCH, abbreviation for **Association for the Care of Children's Health.**

accidental hemorrhage. See **abruptio placentae.**

acclimate /əklī′mit, ak′limāt/, to adjust physiologically to a different climate, especially to changes in altitude and in temperature. Also **acclimatize** /əklī′mətīz′/. **–acclimation, acclimatization,** *n.*

accommodation (A, acc, Acc), **1.** the state or process of adapting or adjusting one thing or set of things to another. **2.** the continuous process or effort of the individual to adapt or adjust to his surroundings to maintain a state of homeostasis, both physiologically and psychologically. **3.** the adjustment of the eye to variations in distance. See also **accommodation reflex.** **4.** (in sociology) the reciprocal reconciliation of conflicts between individuals or groups concerning habits and customs, usually through a process of compromise, arbitration, or negotiation. Also called **adjustment.** Compare **adaptation.**

accommodation reflex, an adjustment of the eyes for near vision, consisting of pupillary constriction, convergence of the eyes, and increased convexity of the lens. Also called **ciliary reflex.** See also **light reflex.**

accomplishment quotient, a numerical evaluation of a person's achievement age compared with mental age, expressed as a ratio multiplied by 100. See also **achievement quotient, intelligence quotient.**

accountability, being accountable or responsible for the moral and legal requirements of proper patient care.

accreditation, a process whereby a professional association or nongovernmental agency grants recognition to a school or institution for demonstrated ability in a special area of practice or training, as the accreditation of hospitals by the Joint Commission of Accreditation for Hospitals or of nursing schools by the National League for Nursing. Compare **certification, licensure.**

accrementition, growth or increase of size by the addition of similar tissue or material, as in cellular division, simple fission, budding, or gemmation.

accretio cordis /əkrē′shē•ō/, an abnormal condition in which there is an adhesion of the pericardium to a structure around the heart.

accretion /əkrē′shən/, **1.** growth or increase by the addition of material of the same nature that is already present. **2.** the adherence or growing together of parts that are normally separated. **3.** the accumulation of foreign material, especially within a cavity. –**accrete,** *v.*, **accretive,** *adj.*

accumulator, the "scratch pad" of a computer's central processing unit (CPU). Data written there can be accessed and processed very rapidly.

accuracy, the extent to which a measurement is close to the true value.

Accurbrun, a trademark for a smooth muscle relaxant (theophylline).

Accutane, a trademark for an antiacne agent (isotretinoin).

acebutolol, a beta-adrenergic blocking agent. Also called **butanamide.**

■ INDICATIONS: It is prescribed in the treatment of hypertension, angina pectoris, cardiac arrhythmias, and other cardiovascular disorders.

■ CONTRAINDICATIONS: The drug should not be given to patients with asthma, heart failure, or peripheral vascular disease.

■ ADVERSE EFFECTS: The side effects most often reported include bradycardia, flatulence, leg pains, nausea, headache, skin rashes, dizziness, and drowsiness.

acecarbromal /as′əkärbrō′məl/, a sedative-hypnotic. Also called **acetylcarbromal.**

■ INDICATION: It is prescribed in the treatment of anxiety.

■ CONTRAINDICATIONS: Known hypersensitivity to this drug or to other bromides prohibits its use.

■ ADVERSE EFFECTS: Among the more serious adverse reactions are bromism, dizziness, skin rash, and GI disturbances.

acedia /əsē′dē•ə/, a condition of listlessness and a form of melancholy, marked by indifference and sluggish mental processes.

acelius /āsē′lē•əs/, an individual without a body cavity.

acentric /āsen′trik/, **1.** having no center. **2.** (in genetics) describing a chromosome fragment that has no centromere.

-aceous, a combining form meaning 'pertaining to or of the nature of' something specified: *coriaceous, foliaceous, testaceous.*

acephalo-, a combining form meaning 'having no head': *acephalobrachia, acephalus, acephaly.*

acephalobrachia /asef′əlōbrā′kē•ə/, a congenital anomaly in which a fetus lacks both arms and a head.

acephaly /əsef′əlē/, a congenital defect in which the head is absent or not properly developed. Also called **acephalia** /as′əfā′lē•ə/, **acephalism** /əsef′əliz′əm/. –**acephalic,** *adj.*

acet-, a combining form meaning 'vinegar': *acetify, acetoin, acetyl.*

acetabulum /as′ətab′yələm/, *pl.* **acetabula,** the large, cup-shaped, articular cavity at the juncture of the ilium, the ischium, and the pubis, containing the ball-shaped head of the femur.

acetaldehyde, a colorless, volatile liquid with a pungent odor produced by the oxidation of ethyl alcohol. In the human body, acetaldehyde is produced in the liver by the action of alcohol dehydrogenase and other enzymes. It is used commercially in the manufacture of acetic acid and various aromas and flavors. Exposure to high levels of acetaldehyde can result in headache, corneal injury, rhinitis, and respiratory disorders.

acetaminophen /əset′əmin′əfin/, an analgesic and antipyretic drug used in many nonprescription pain relievers.

■ INDICATIONS: It is often prescribed for mild to moderate pain and fever.

■ CONTRAINDICATION: Known hypersensitivity to acetaminophen prohibits its use.

■ ADVERSE EFFECTS: Among the most serious adverse reactions are anaphylaxis and hemolytic anemia. Overdosage can result in fatal hepatic necrosis.

acetanilide, an analgesic drug with antipyretic and antirheumatic properties, derived from aniline. Because the use of acetanilide has been associated with an increased risk of methemoglobinemia, it has been generally replaced by acetaminophen. See **acetaminophen.**

acetate kinase, an enzyme that catalyzes the transfer of a phosphate group from adenosine triphosphate to acetate. Also called **acetokinase** /as′ətōkī′nās, əsē′tō-/.

acetazolamide /as′ətəzō′ləmīd/, a carbonic anhydrase inhibitor.

■ INDICATIONS: It is prescribed for edema, glaucoma, and epilepsy (primarily petit mal).

■ CONTRAINDICATIONS: Hyponatremia, hypocalcemia, severe liver or kidney disease or dysfunction, Addison's disease, or known hypersensitivity to this drug prohibits its use.

■ ADVERSE EFFECTS: Among the most serious adverse reactions are anorexia and depression, particularly in the elderly; acidosis; hyperuricemia; and crystalluria. GI disturbances and lethargy are common.

Acetest, a trademark for a product used to test for the presence of abnormal quantities of acetone in the urine of patients with diabetes mellitus or other metabolic disorders. A large quantity of acetone causes a rapid change in the color of the Acetest tablet. See also **acidosis, ketone bodies.**

acetic acid /əsē′tik, əset′ik/, a clear, colorless, pungent liquid that is miscible with water, alcohol, glycerin, and ether and that constitutes 3% to 5% of vinegar. Acetic acid is produced commercially by the destructive distillation of wood or from methyl alcohol, or it may be converted from ethyl alcohol by the action of many aerobic bacteria. Various concentrations of acetic acid are used in the manufacture of plastics, dyes, insecticides, cellulose acetate, photographic chemicals, and pharmaceutic preparations, including vaginal jellies and antimicrobial solutions for the treatment of superficial infections of the external auditory canal. Also called **ethanoic acid.**

acetic fermentation, the production of acetic acid or vinegar from a weak alcoholic solution.

acetoacetic acid /as′ətō·əsē′tik, əsē′tō-/, a colorless, oily ketone body produced by the metabolism of lipids and pyruvates. It is excreted in trace amounts in normal urine and in elevated levels in diabetes mellitus, especially in ketoacidosis. Acetoacetic acid is also increased during starvation as a result of incomplete oxidation of fatty acids. Soluble in water, alcohol, and ether, acetoacetic acid decomposes at temperatures below 100° C to acetone and carbon dioxide. Also called **acetone carboxylic acid** /kär′boksil′ik/, **acetylacetic acid** /əsē′tiləsē′tik, as′ətil-/, **diacetic acid** /dī·əsē′tik/.

acetohexamide, a sulfonylurea oral antidiabetic.

■ INDICATION: It is prescribed in the treatment of non-insulin-dependent diabetes mellitus.

■ CONTRAINDICATIONS: Unstable diabetes, severe liver or kidney dysfunction, or known hypersensitivity to this drug or to other sulfanylureas prohibits its use.

■ ADVERSE EFFECTS: Among the most serious adverse reactions are blood dyscrasias, hypoglycemia, and allergic reactions. GI disturbances are common.

acetokinase. See **acetate kinase.**

acetol kinase, an enzyme that catalyzes the transfer of a phosphate group from adenosine triphosphate to hydroxyacetone.

acetone /as′ətōn/, a colorless, aromatic, volatile liquid ketone body found in small amounts in normal urine and in larger quantities in the urine of diabetics. Commercially prepared acetone is used to clean the skin before injections, but prolonged exposure to the compound can be irritating. It also has many varied industrial uses.

acetone bodies. See **ketone bodies.**

acetone carboxylic acid. See **acetoacetic acid.**

acetophenazine maleate, a major phenothiazine tranquilizer.

■ INDICATION: It is prescribed in the treatment of psychotic disorders.

■ CONTRAINDICATIONS: Parkinson's disease, the concurrent administration of central nervous system depressants, liver or renal dysfunction, severe hypotension, or known hypersensitivity to any phenothiazine prohibits its use.

■ ADVERSE EFFECTS: Among the more serious adverse effects are hypotension, liver toxicity, a variety of extrapyramidal reactions, blood dyscrasias, and hypersensitivity reactions.

acetophenetidin. See **phenacetin.**

acetpyrogall, a topical irritant used as a caustic and keratolytic agent. Also called **pyrogallol triacetate.**

acetylacetic acid. See **acetoacetic acid.**

acetylcarbromal. See **acecarbromal.**

acetylcholine (ACh) /as′ətilkō′lēn, əsē′til-/, a neurotransmitter substance widely distributed in body tissues, with a primary function of mediating synaptic activity of the nervous system. Its active phase is transient because it is rapidly destroyed by acetylcholinesterase. Acetylcholine activity also can be blocked by atropine at junctions of nerve fibers with glands and smooth muscle tissue. However, atropine does not inhibit acetylcholine effects on autonomic ganglia. It is a stimulant of the vagus and parasympathetic nervous system and functions as a vasodilator and cardiac depressant. Acetylcholine is used therapeutically as an adjunct to eye surgery and has limited benefits in certain circulatory disorders. See **acetylcholinesterase, atropine.**

acetylcholine chloride, a miotic.

■ INDICATIONS: It is prescribed to cause rapid miosis during cataract or other ocular surgery and to reverse the effects of cycloplegic and mydriatic medications.

■ CONTRAINDICATION: There are no known contraindications.

■ ADVERSE EFFECTS: Systemic effects of acetylcholine may occur, and opacities of the lens of the eye may be caused by a hypertonic solution of the drug.

acetylcholinesterase, an enzyme that inactivates the neurotransmitter acetylcholine by hydrolyzing the substance to choline and acetate. The action reduces or prevents excessive firing of neurons at neuromuscular junctions. However, acetylcholinesterase activity can be blocked by many chemicals, including morphine and organophosphate pesticides.

acetylcoenzyme A /əsē′tilkō·en′zīm, as′ətil-/, a molecule that is formed in the course of several important metabolic processes. The formation of acetylcoenzyme A is the critical intermediate step between anaerobic glycolysis and the Krebs' citric acid cycle. Also called **acetyl-CoA.** See **Krebs' citric acid cycle.**

acetylcysteine, a mucolytic.

■ INDICATIONS: It is prescribed in the treatment of chronic pulmonary disease, acute bronchopulmonary disease, atelectasis resulting from mucous obstruction.

■ CONTRAINDICATION: Known sensitivity to this drug prohibits its use.

■ ADVERSE EFFECTS: Among the most serious adverse reactions are stomatitis, nausea, rhinorrhea, and bronchospasm.

acetylsalicylic acid. See **aspirin.**

acetyltransferase, any of several enzymes that transfer acetyl groups from one compound to another. See also **acetylcoenzyme A.**

ACG, abbreviation for **apexcardiography.**

ACh, abbreviation for **acetylcholine.**

achalasia /ak′əlā′zhə/, an abnormal condition characterized by the inability of a muscle to relax, particularly the cardiac sphincter of the stomach. Compare **corkscrew esophagus.** See also **dysphagia.**

Achard-Thiers syndrome /ash′ärtērz′/, a hormonal disorder seen in postmenopausal women with diabetes, characterized by growth of body hair in a masculine distribution. Treatment includes mechanic removal or bleaching of excess hair and hormonal therapy to correct endocrine imbalances related to systemic disease. See also **hirsutism, hypertrichosis.**

ache, **1.** a pain characterized by persistence, dullness, and, usually, moderate intensity. An ache may be localized, as a stomach ache, headache, or bone ache, or general, as the myalgia that accompanies a viral infection or a persistent fever. **2.** to suffer from a dull, persistent pain of moderate intensity.

achievement age, the level of a person's educational development as measured by an achievement test and compared with the normal score for chronologic age. Compare **mental age.** See also **developmental age.**

achievement motivation, an intrapsychic drive that initiates behavior directed toward the attainment of a particular goal. Compare **physiologic motivation, social motivation.**

achievement quotient (AQ), a numeric expression of a person's achievement age, determined by various achievement tests, divided by the chronologic age and expressed as a multiple of 100. Compare **intelligence quotient.** See also **accomplishment quotient.**

achievement test, a standardized test for the measurement and comparison of knowledge or proficiency in various fields of vocational or academic study. Compare **aptitude test, intelligence test, personality test, psychologic test.**

Achilles tendon. See **tendo calcaneus.**

Achilles tendon reflex /əkil′ēz/, a deep tendon reflex consisting of plantar flexion of the foot when a sharp tap is given directly to the tendon of the gastrocnemius muscle at the back of the ankle. This reflex is often absent in diabetics and people with peripheral neuropathies. A sluggish return of the flexed foot may be seen in patients with hypothyroidism. A hyperactive reflex may be caused by hyperthyroidism or by pyramidal tract disease. Also called **ankle reflex, calcaneal tendon reflex.** See also **deep tendon reflex.**

achlorhydria /ā′klôrhī′drē•ə/, an abnormal condition characterized by the absence of hydrochloric acid in the gastric juice. The ability to produce gastric juice with a pH of less than 6 is tested when the subject is stimulated with an intramuscular injection of pentagastrin. Achlorhydria occurs most commonly in atrophy of the gastric mucosa, pernicious anemia, and gastric carcinoma; it is also found in severe iron deficiency anemia. Achlorhydria in a patient with symptoms of gastric ulcer almost always indicates that the lesion is malignant. Protein digestion is severely impaired in patients with achlorhydria, but overall digestion in the alimentary tract is relatively normal, because trypsin and other enzymes of the pancreas and small intestine are not affected. See also **achylia, pernicious anemia.** **–achlorhydric,** *adj.*

acholia, **1.** the absence or decrease of bile secretion. **2.** any condition that suppresses the flow of bile into the small intestine. **–acholic,** *adj.*

acholuria, the absence or lack of pigments in the urine.

achondroplasia /ākon′drōplā′zhə/, a disorder of the growth of cartilage in the epiphyses of the long bones and skull that results in premature ossification, permanent limitation of skeletal development, and dwarfism typified by protruding forehead, and short, thick arms and legs on a normal trunk. Onset is in fetal life. Familial achondroplasia is inherited as an autosomal dominant gene; the chance is 50% that an offspring of an affected parent will be affected. The majority of affected individuals die during gestation or the first year of life. The minority that survive have relatively normal longevity. There is no treatment other than orthopedic surgery. Antenatal diagnosis is possible. Also called **chondrodystrophy, fetal rickets.**

achondroplastic dwarf, the most common type of dwarf, characterized by disproportionately short limbs, a normal-sized trunk, large head with a depressed nasal bridge and small face, stubby trident hands, and lordosis. The condition results from an inherited defect in bone-forming tissue and is often associated with other defects or abnormalities, although there is usually no involvement of the central nervous system and intelligence is normal. See also **achondroplasia.**

achromatic vision. See **color blindness.**

achromocyte /ākrō′məsīt/, a sickle-shaped, hypochromic erythrocyte, perhaps the result of a ruptured red blood cell that lost hemoglobin. Also called **achromatocyte** /ā′krōmat′əsīt/.

Achromycin V, a trademark for an antibiotic (tetracycline hydrochloride).

achylia /ākī′lē•ə/, an absence or severe deficiency of hydrochloric acid and pepsinogen in the stomach. This condition may also occur in the pancreas, when the exocrine portion of that gland fails to produce digestive enzymes. Also called **achylosis.** See also **achlorhydria.**

achylous /əkī′ləs/, **1.** of or pertaining to a lack of gastric juice or other digestive secretions. **2.** of or pertaining to a lack of chyle.

acicular /əsik′yələr/, needle-shaped, as certain leaves and crystals.

acid, **1.** a compound that yields hydrogen ions when dissociated in solution. Acids turn blue litmus red, have a sour taste, and react with bases to form salts. Acids have chemical properties essentially opposite to those of bases.

See also **alkali.** **2.** *slang.* lysergic acid diethylamide (LSD). See also **lysergide.**

acid-, a combining form meaning 'sour, acid': *acidemia, acidophil, aciduric.*

-acid, **1.** a combining form meaning an 'acid': *diacid, monacid, sulfacid.* **2.** a combining form meaning 'pertaining to acid': *subacid, semiacid, superacid.*

acid-base balance, a condition existing when the net rate at which the body produces acids or bases equals the net rate at which acids or bases are excreted. The result of acid-base balance is a stable concentration of hydrogen ions in body fluids. See also **acid, base.**

acid-base metabolism, the metabolic processes that maintain the balance of acids and bases essential in regulating the composition of body fluids. Acids release hydrogen ions, and bases accept them; the number of hydrogen ions present in a solution governs whether it is acid, alkali, or neutral. Hydrogen ions are measured on a pH scale of 1 to 14, with a reading of 7 being neutral. Above 7, the solution is alkaline; below 7, it is acid. Blood is slightly alkaline, ranging from 7.35 to 7.45. Metabolic buffer systems within the body maintain this ratio, and, when it is upset, either acidosis or alkalosis results. Acidosis may be caused by diarrhea, vomiting, uremia, diabetes mellitus, and the action of certain drugs. Alkalosis may be caused by overingestion of alkaline drugs, loss of chloride in gastric vomitus, and the action of certain diuretic drugs. See also **acid-base balance, acidosis, alkalosis, pH.**

acid bath, a bath taken in water containing a mineral acid to help reduce excessive sweating.

acid burn, damage to tissue caused by exposure to a strong acid. The severity of the burn is determined by the kind of acid and the duration and extent of exposure. Emergency treatment includes washing the affected area with large amounts of water. Compare **alkali burn.**

acid dust, an accumulation of highly acidic particles of dust. Such substances accumulate in the atmosphere and account for much of the smog hanging over large metropolitan areas. Many respiratory illnesses, as lung cancer and asthma, may be aggravated or caused by such dust. See also **acid rain.**

-acidemia, a combining form meaning an 'increased hydrogen-ion concentration in the blood': *lactacidemia, lipacedemia, oxybutyricacidemia.*

acid-fast bacillus (AFB), a type of bacillus that resists decolorizing by acid after accepting a stain. Examples include *Mycobacterium tuberculosis* and *M. leprae.*

acid-fast stain, a method of staining used in bacteriology in which a smear on a slide is treated with carbolfuchsin stain, decolorized with acid alcohol, and counterstained with methylene blue to identify acid-fast bacteria. Acid-fast organisms resist decolorization and appear red or yellow against a dark background when viewed under a microscope. The stain may be performed on any clinical specimen but is most commonly used in examining sputum for *Mycobacterium tuberculosis,* an acid-fast bacillus. See also **Ziehl-Neelsen stain.**

acid flush, a runoff of precipitation with a high acid content, as may occur during thaws in various parts of the world. Acid flushes may pollute rivers and reservoirs, killing fish and endangering the health of adjacent populations. See also **acid rain.**

acidify, **1.** to make a substance acid, as through the addition of an acid. **2.** to become acid. Compare **alkalize.**

acid mist, mist containing a high concentration of acid or particles of any toxic chemical, as carbon tetrachloride or silicon tetrachloride. Such chemicals are often used by industry and stored in tanks that may leak their contents into residential areas, becoming especially dangerous if the toxic substance mixes with fog. Inhalation of acid mists may irritate the mucous membranes, the eyes, and the respiratory tract and seriously upset the chemistry of the body. See also **acid rain.**

acidophil /as′idōfil, əsid′əfil/, **1.** a cell or cell constituent with an affinity for acid dyes. **2.** an organism that thrives in an acid medium. –**acidophilic,** *adj.*

acidophilic adenoma, a tumor of the pituitary gland characterized by cells that can be stained red with an acid dye. Gigantism and acromegaly are caused by an acidophilic adenoma. Also called **eosinophilic adenoma.**

acidophilus milk /as′idof′ələs/, milk inoculated with cultures of *Lactobacillus acidophilus,* used in various enteric disorders to change the bacterial flora of the GI tract.

acidosis, an abnormal increase in hydrogen ion concentration in the body resulting from an accumulation of an acid or the loss of a base. The various forms of acidosis are named for the cause of the condition; for example, renal tubular acidosis results from failure of the kidney to secrete hydrogen ions or reabsorb bicarbonate ions, respiratory acidosis results from respiratory retention of CO_2, and diabetic acidosis results from an accumulation of ketones associated with poorly controlled diabetes mellitus. Treatment depends on diagnosis of the underlying pathology and concurrent correction of the acid-base imbalance. Compare **alkalosis.**

acid-perfusion test, a test to demonstrate sensitivity of the esophagus to acid, a condition suggestive of reflux esophagitis. A weak hydrochloric acid solution and normal saline are dripped alternately into the esophagus via a nasal-esophageal tube without telling the patient which solution is being infused. A positive response is pain with acid but not with saline. An alternative method is to compare acid barium swallows with neutral barium swallows. If acid sensitivity is present, diffuse spasm of the esophagus may be seen by fluoroscopy when acid barium is infused and no spasm with neutral barium. Also called **Bernstein test.**

acid phosphatase, an enzyme found in the kidneys, serum, semen, and prostate gland. It is elevated in serum in cancers of the prostate and in trauma. Normal concentrations in serum are 0 to 1.1 Bodanski units/ml. See also **alkaline phosphatase.**

acid poisoning, a toxic condition caused by the ingestion of a toxic acid agent such as hydrochloric, nitric, phosphoric, or sulfuric acids, some of which are ingredients in cleaning compounds. Emergency treatment includes giving copious amounts of water, milk, or beaten eggs to dilute the acid. Vomiting is not induced, and mild solutions of alkali are not given. The victim is transported immediately to the hospital for observation of any corrosive damage to the esophagus or stomach, for metabolic abnormality, and for mechanic removal of the acid by gastric intubation and lavage. Compare **alkali poisoning.**

acid rain, the precipitation of moisture, as rain, with high acidity caused by release into the atmosphere of pollutants from industry, motor vehicle exhausts, and other sources. Acid precipitation with a pH of 5.6 or less is blamed by various authorities for numerous human health problems, fish kills, and the destruction of timber. Also called **acid precipitation, acid snow.**

acid therapy, a method for removing warts, which employs plaster patches impregnated with acid, as 40% salicylic acid, or with acid drops, as 5% to 16.7% salicylic and lactic acids in flexible collodion. The application is made every 12 to 24 hours for 2 to 4 weeks. Acid therapy is not usually recommended for body areas that perspire heavily or that are likely to become wet or for exposed body parts where the patches would detract from the patient's appearance.

Acidulin, a trademark for a gastric acidifier (glutamic acid hydrochloride).

acidulous /əsid′yələs/, slightly acidic or sour.

aciduria, the presence of acid in the urine. The condition may be caused by a diet rich in meat proteins or certain fruits, the introduction of a medication for the treatment of a urinary tract disorder, an inborn error of metabolism, or ketoacidosis.

acinar adenocarcinoma. See **acinic cell adenocarcinoma.**

Acinetobacter /as′inē′təbak′tər/, a genus of nonmotile, aerobic bacteria of the family Neisseriaceae that often occurs in clinical specimens. The *Acinetobacter* contains gram-negative or gram-variable cocci and does not produce spores. This bacterium grows on regular media without serum and is oxidase negative and catalase positive.

acinic cell adenocarcinoma, an uncommon, low-grade malignant neoplasm that develops in the secreting cells of racemose glands, especially the salivary glands. The tumor consists of cells with clear or slightly granular cytoplasm and small eccentric dark nuclei. Also called **acinar adenocarcinoma, acinous adenocarcinoma** /as′inəs/.

acinitis, any inflammation of the tiny, grape-shaped portions of certain glands.

acinous adenocarcinoma. See **acinic cell adenocarcinoma.**

acinus /as′inəs/, *pl.* **acini, 1.** also called **alveolus.** any small saclike structure, particularly one found in a gland. **2.** a subdivision of the lung consisting of the tissue distal to a terminal bronchiole.

ACMC, abbreviation for **Association of Canadian Medical Colleges.**

acmesthesia /ak′misthē′zhə/, a sensation of a pinprick or of a sharp point touching the skin.

acne /ak′nē/, an inflammatory, papulopustular skin eruption occurring usually in or near the sebaceous glands on the face, neck, shoulders, and upper back. Its cause is unknown but involves bacterial breakdown of sebum into fatty acids irritating to surrounding subcutaneous tissue. Treatment includes topical and oral antibiotics, topical vitamin A derivatives, benzyl benzoate, and dermabrasion. Kinds of acne include **acne conglobata, acne vulgaris, chloracne,** and **rosacea.** See also **comedo.**

acne artificialis, an eruption in the skin caused by an external irritant, such as tar, or ingestion of halogen compounds.

acne cachecticorum, an eruption or irritation of the skin that may occur in patients who are very weak and debilitated. It is characterized by soft, mildly infiltrated pustular lesions.

acne conglobata /kong′glōbā′tə/, a severe form of acne with abscess, cyst, scar, and keloid formation. Acne conglobata may affect the lower back, buttocks, and thighs, as well as the face and chest. Also called **cystic acne.**

acneform /ak′nifôrm/, resembling acne. Also **acneiform** /aknē′əfôrm/.

acneform drug eruption, any one of various skin reactions to a drug, characterized by papules and pustules erupting in acne, with or without comedones.

acnegenic /ak′nijen′ik/, causing or producing acne.

acne indurata, a pathologic skin condition characterized by extensive papular lesions that often produce severe scars. Also called **chronic acne vulgaris.**

acne keratosa, a skin condition characterized by hard conic plugs that usually appear at the corners of the mouth and inflame surrounding tissue.

acne necrotica miliaris, a rare, chronic type of folliculitis of the scalp, occurring mostly in adults and characterized by tiny pustules.

acne neonatorum, a skin condition of infants caused by sebaceous gland hyperplasia and characterized by the formation of comedones, nodules, and cysts on the nose, cheeks, and forehead.

acne papulosa, a common pathologic skin condition that develops small papular lesions that usually do not become inflamed. It is considered a papular form of acne vulgaris.

acne rosacea. See **rosacea.**

acne vulgaris, a common form of acne seen predominantly in adolescents and young adults. Acne vulgaris is probably an effect of androgenic hormones (which stimulate the production of sebum) and *Propionibacterium acnes* in the hair follicle.

ACNM, abbreviation for **American College of Nurse-Midwives.**

ACOG, abbreviation for **American College of Obstetricians and Gynecologists.**

acognosia /ak′og•nō′zhə/, a knowledge of remedies.

acoria /akôr′ē•ə/, a condition characterized by constant hunger, even when the appetite is small.

acorn-tipped catheter, a flexible catheter with an acorn-shaped tip used in various diagnostic procedures, especially in urology.

acou-, acu-, a combining form meaning 'pertaining to hearing': *acouesthesia, acoulalian, acouophonia.*

-acousia, -acusia, -acusis, - akusis a combining form meaning a '(specified) condition of the hearing': *amblyacousia, bradyacousia, dysacousia.*

acousma /əkōōz′mə/, *pl.* **acousmas, acousmata,** a hallucinatory impression of strange sounds.

acoustic, of or pertaining to sound or hearing. Also **acoustical.**

-acoustic, -acoustical, **1.** a combining form meaning 'pertaining to the hearing organs': *entacoustic, otacoustic.* **2.** a combining form meaning 'pertaining to amplified sound waves': *micracoustic, microcoustic, stethacoustic.*

acoustic microscope, a microscope in which the object being viewed is scanned with sound waves and its image reconstructed with light waves. Acoustic microscopes produce excellent resolution of the objects being studied and allow very close examination of cells and tissues without staining or damaging the specimen.

acoustic nerve, either of a pair of cranial nerves essential to the sense of hearing, having two distinct sets of fibers called the cochlear nerves and the vestibular nerves, and connecting to three areas in the brain. Also called **eighth nerve.**

acoustic neuroma, a benign tumor that develops from the eighth cranial (acoustic) nerve and grows within the auditory canal. Depending on the location and size of the lesion, tinnitus, increasing deafness, headache, facial numbness, papilledema, dizziness, and an unsteady gait may result. Paresis and difficulty in speaking and swallowing may occur in the later stage. It may be unilateral or bilateral. Also called **acoustic neurilemoma, acoustic neurinoma, acoustic neurofibroma.**

acoustic trauma, a gradual loss of hearing caused by exposure to loud noise over an extended period of time or a sudden loss of hearing, partial or complete, caused by an explosion, a severe blow to the head, or other accident. Hearing loss may be temporary or permanent.

acoustooptics /əkōōs′tō•op′tiks/, a field of physics that studies the generation of light waves by ultrahigh-frequency sound waves. Knowledge gained by such study is applied chiefly in the transmission of information by acoustooptic devices.

ACP, **1.** abbreviation for **American College of Pathologists. 2.** abbreviation for **American College of Physicians. 3.** abbreviation for **American College of Prosthodontists.**

acquired, of or pertaining to a characteristic, condition, or disease originating after birth and caused not by hereditary or developmental factors but by a reaction to environmental influences outside of the organism. Compare **congenital, familial, hereditary.**

acquired immune deficiency syndrome (AIDS) /ādz/, a disease involving a defect in cell-mediated immunity that has a long incubation period, follows a protracted and debilitating course, is manifested by various opportunistic infections, and has a poor prognosis. The disorder is found primarily in homosexual men and intravenous drug users and to a lesser degree in female sex partners of bisexual men and children of those with the disease. The causative agent is believed to be a retrovirus, identified as HTLV-3 (Human T-cell Lymphotropic Virus) transmitted through sexual contact or exposure to contaminated blood or possibly close personal contact. Initial symptoms include extreme fatigue, intermittent fever, night sweats, chills, lymphadenopathy, enlarged spleen, anorexia and consequent weight loss, severe diarrhea, apathy, and depression. As the disease progresses, there is a general failure to thrive, anergy, and any number and kind of recurring infections, most commonly *Pneumocystis carinii* pneumonia, meningitis, or encephalitis caused by aspergillosis, candidiasis, crytococcosis, cytomegalovirus, toxoplasmosis, or herpes simplex. Most patients with the disorder are susceptible to malignant neoplasms, especially Kaposi's sarcoma, Burkitt's lymphoma, and non-Hodgkin's lymphoma, that cause as well as result from immunodeficiency. Treatment consists primarily of combined chemotherapy to counteract the opportunistic diseases. Interferon and other immunomodulators have been used, with little success, to correct the underlying immune defect. The fatality rate is 90% in those diagnosed more than 2 years. See **HTLV, retrovirus.**

acquired immunity, any form of immunity that is not innate and is obtained during life. It may be natural or artificial and actively or passively induced. **Naturally acquired immunity** is obtained by the development of antibodies resulting from an attack of infectious disease or by the transmission of antibodies from the mother through the placenta to the fetus or to the infant through the colostrum. **Artificially acquired immunity** is obtained by vaccination or by the injection of antiserum. Compare **natural immunity.** See also **active immunity, passive immunity.**

acquired reflex. See **conditioned reflex.**

ACR, abbreviation for **American College of Radiologists.**

acrid, sharp or pungent, bitter and unpleasant to the smell or taste.

acridine /ak′ridēn/, a dibenzopyridine compound used in the synthesis of dyes and drugs. Its derivatives include fluorescent yellow dyes and the antiseptic agents acriflavine hydrochloride, acriflavine base, and proflavine.

acro-, a combining form meaning 'pertaining to the extremities': *acroagnosis, acroataxia, acrocyanosis.*

acrocentric /ak′rōsen′trik/, pertaining to a chromosome in which the centromere is located near one of the ends so that the arms of the chromatids are extremely uneven. Compare **metacentric, submetacentric, telocentric.**

acrocephalosyndactylism. See **Apert's syndrome.**

acrocephaly. See **oxycephaly.**

acrochordon /ak′rōkôr′don/, a benign, pedunculated skin tag commonly occurring on the eyelids or neck or in the axilla or groin.

acrocyanosis /ak′rōsī′ənō′sis/, a condition characterized by cyanotic discoloration, coldness, and sweating of the extremities, especially the hands, caused by arterial spasm that is usually precipitated by cold or by emotional stress. Warming induces vasodilatation, and the blue discoloration becomes mottled with red. Abnormal sympathetic nerve activity or overreaction to certain stimuli may be responsible for the vasospasm that typically occurs in Raynaud's disease and is also seen in rheumatoid arthritis, in scleroderma, and in workers who operate pneumatic air hammers. Acrocyanosis may be treated with antiadrenergic drugs, and attacks may be prevented by not smoking and by avoiding exposure to cold. A kind of acrocyanosis is **peripheral acrocyanosis of the newborn.** Acrocyanosis is also called **Raynaud's phenomenon, Raynaud's sign.**

acrodermatitis, any eruption of the skin of the hands and feet caused by a parasitic mite, which is a member of the order Acarina.

acrodermatitis enteropathica /en′tərōpath′ikə/, a rare, chronic disease of infants characterized by vesicles and bullae of the skin and mucous membranes, alopecia, diarrhea, and failure to thrive. It may be lethal if not treated. Zinc sulfate is usually prescribed.

acrodynia /ak′rōdin′ē·ə/, a disease that occurs in infants and young children: Symptoms include edema, pruritus, generalized skin rash, with pink coloration of the extremities and scarlet coloration of the cheeks and nose, profuse sweating, digestive disturbances, photophobia, polyneuritis, extreme irritability alternating with periods of listlessness and apathy, and failure to thrive. The cause is unknown, although the condition is usually associated with ingestion of or contact with mercury and often with inflammatory changes of obscure origin in the central nervous system. Also called **dermatopolyneuritis, erythredema polyneuropathy, Feer's disease, pink disease, Swift's disease.**

acromegalic eunuchoidism, a rare disorder characterized by genital atrophy and the development of female secondary sex characteristics, occurring in men with advanced acromegaly caused by a chromophobe adenoma in the anterior pituitary gland. Initially, the gonadal function of the anterior lobe may be stimulated, but with the growth of the tumor the patient may become impotent; lose facial, axillary, and pubic hair; and develop a soft skin and a feminine distribution of fat. Also called **retrograde infantilism.**

acromegaly /ak′rəmeg′əlē/, a chronic metabolic condition characterized by a gradual, marked enlargement and elongation of the bones of the face, jaw, and extremities. The condition, which afflicts middle-aged persons, is caused by the overproduction of growth hormone and is treated by x-ray or surgery, often involving partial resection of the pituitary gland. Also called **acromegalia.** Compare **gigantism.** See also **adenohypophysis, growth hormone.** –**acromegalic** /-məgal′ik/, *adj.*

acromioclavicular articulation, the gliding joint between the acromial end of the clavicle and the medial margin of the acromion of the scapula. The joint has six ligaments.

acromion /əkrō′mē·ən/, the lateral extension of the spine of the scapula, forming the highest point of the shoulder and connecting with the clavicle at a small oval surface in the middle of the spine. It gives attachment to the deltoideus and trapezius. Also called **acromion process.** Compare **coracoid process.** –**acromial,** *adj.*

acronym, a word formed by the initial letters or syllables of other words, for example, *CAT* /kat/, which is the acronym for *C*omputerized *A*xial *T*omography. Most acronyms are composed of the initial capital letters of their full forms. Acronyms differ from other abbreviations in that they are pronounced and treated as words grammatically. –**acronymic,** *adj.* Compare **letter-word.**

acroparesthesia /ak′rōpar′isthē′zhə/, **1.** an extreme sensitivity at the tips of the extremities of the body, caused by compression of the nerves in the affected area or by polyneuritis. **2.** a disease characterized by tingling, numbness, and stiffness in the extremities, especially in the fingers, the hands, and the forearms. It sometimes produces pain, skin pallor, or mild cyanosis. The disease occurs in a simple form, which may produce acrocyanosis, and in an angiospastic form, which may produce gangrene.

acrophobia, a pathologic fear or dread of high places that results in extreme anxiety. The obsessive phenomenon is most frequently seen in persons who are overconscientious, shy, pedantic, punctilious, or painstakingly addicted to orderliness and symmetry. Therapy is planned to attempt to overcome or eliminate the phobic reaction. See also **obsession, phobia.**

acrosomal cap, acrosomal head cap. See **acrosome.**

acrosomal reaction, the pattern of various chemical changes that occur in the anterior of the head of the spermatozoon in response to contact with the ovum and that lead to the penetration by the sperm and fertilization of the ovum.

acrosome /ak′rəsōm′/, the caplike structure surrounding the anterior end of the nucleus of a spermatozoon. It is derived from the Golgi apparatus within the cytoplasm and contains enzymes that function in the penetration of the ovum during fertilization. Also called **acrosomal cap, acrosomal head cap.** See also **acrosomal reaction.** –**acrosomal,** *adj.*

acrotic /əkrot′ik/, **1.** of or pertaining to the surface or to the skin glands. **2.** of or pertaining to the absence or the weakness of a pulse.

acrylic resin base, (in dentistry) a denture base made of acrylic resin. Compare **denture base.**

acrylic resin dental cement, a dental cement for restoring or repairing damaged teeth. In powder form it contains polymethyl methacrylate, which acts as filler, plasticizer, and polymerization initiator. In liquid form it contains methyl methacrylate with an inhibitor and an activator.

ACSM, abbreviation for **American College of Sports Medicine.**

act-. a combining form meaning 'to do, drive, act': *action, activate, actor.*

ACTH, abbreviation for **adrenocorticotropic hormone.**

Acthar, a trademark for adrenocorticotropic hormone (corticotropin).

Actidil, a trademark for an antihistamine (triprolidine hydrochloride), used for the symptomatic relief of allergic conditions.

Actifed, a trademark for a fixed-combination drug containing an adrenergic bronchodilator and vasoconstrictor (pseudoephedrine hydrochloride) and an antihistamine (triprolidine hydrochloride).

actigraph /ak′tigraf′/, any instrument that records changes in the activity of a substance or an organism and produces a graphic record of the process, as an electrocardiograph machine, which produces a record of cardiac activity.

actin, a protein found in muscle fibers that acts with myosin to bring about contraction and relaxation. Also called **actinin.** See also **myosin.**

actin-. See **actino-.**

acting out, the expression of intrapsychic conflict or painful emotion through overt behavior that is usually neurotic, defensive, and unconscious and that may be destructive or dangerous. In controlled situations, like psychodrama, Gestalt therapy, or play therapy, such behavior may be therapeutic in itself and may also serve to reveal to the patient the underlying conflict governing his behavior. See also **transference.**

actinic /aktin′ik/, of or pertaining to radiation, as sunlight or x-rays.

actinic dermatitis, a skin inflammation or rash resulting from exposure to sunlight, x-ray, or atomic particle radiation. Chronic or recurrent actinic dermatitis can predispose to skin cancer. See also **actinic keratosis.**

actinic keratosis, a slowly developing, localized thickening of the outer layers of the skin as a result of chronic, excessive exposure to the sun. Treatment of this potentially malignant lesion includes surgical excision, cryotherapy, and topical chemotherapy. Also called **senile keratosis, senile wart, solar keratosis.**

actinium (Ac), a rare, radioactive metallic element. Its atomic number is 89; its atomic weight is 227. It occurs in some ores of uranium.

actino-, actin-, a combining form meaning 'pertaining to a ray or to radiation': *actinocardiogram, actinocutitis, actinogen.*

Actinomyces /ak′tinōmī′sēz/, a genus of anaerobic, gram-positive bacteria. Several species that may cause disease in humans, such as *Actinomyces israelii,* are normally present in the mouth and throat. See also **actinomycosis.**

actinomycin D. See **dactinomycin.**

actinomycosis /ak′tinōmīkō′sis/, a chronic, systemic disease characterized by deep, lumpy abscesses that extrude a thin, granular pus through multiple sinuses. The disease occurs worldwide but is seen most frequently in those who live in rural areas. It is not spread from person to person or from animal to humans. The various species of *Actinomyces* are species specific. The causative organism in humans is *A. israelii,* a normal inhabitant of the bowel and mouth. Disease occurs after tissue damage, usually in the presence of another infectious organism. It is diagnosed by microscopic identification of sulfur granules, pathognomonic of *Actinomyces,* in the exudate. There are four principal forms of actinomycosis. **Cervicofacial actinomycosis** occurs with the spread of the bacterium into the subcutaneous tissues of the mouth, throat, and neck, as a result of dental or tonsillar infection. The process begins with a hard swelling over the angle of the lower jaw and neck. The swelling becomes indurated, and sinus tracts form, draining the pus to the skin. Remarkably little pain accompanies these abscesses, even when they are so deep as to involve the bone of the jaw. **Thoracic actinomycosis** may represent proliferation of the organism from cervicofacial abscesses into the esophagus, or it may result from inhalation of the bacterium into the bronchi. The infection may spread through the lungs, reaching the pleura, or through the esophagus into the mediastinum. Ribs, heart, and the great vessels may then be affected. Fever, cough, draining sinuses, weight loss, night sweats, and, rarely, pleural effusion are characteristic of this form of the disease. **Abdominal actinomycosis** usually follows an acute inflammatory process in the stomach or intestines, as appendicitis, diverticulum of the large bowel, or a perforation of the stomach. A large mass may be palpated, and sinus tracts may be found in the groin or other area that drains exudate from abscesses deep in the abdomen. Generalized actinomycosis may involve the skin, brain, liver, and urogenital system. A pelvic form of abdominal actinomycosis occurs after insertion of an intrauterine contraceptive device. All forms of actinomycosis are treated with at least 6 weeks of daily injections of penicillin in large doses. Surgical excision or incision and drainage of deep or large abscesses may be necessary. Abdominal actinomycosis can be cured in 40% of cases, thoracic actinomycosis in 80%, and cervicofacial actinomycosis in 90%.

action alternatives, (in nursing) any of several possible actions or courses of action chosen by a nurse as part of a goal-oriented nursing care plan and performed to resolve a problem or to modify the effects a particular problem has on a patient.

action current. See **action potential.**

action level, the level of concentration at which an undesirable or toxic component of a food is considered dangerous enough to public health to warrant government prohibition of the sale of that food. The United States Food and Drug Administration tests foods for action levels.

action potential, an electric impulse consisting of a self-propagating series of polarizations and depolarizations, transmitted across the cell membranes of a nerve fiber during the transmission of a nerve impulse and across the cell membranes of a muscle cell during contraction or other activity of the cell. Also called **action current.**

activated charcoal, a general-purpose antidote and a powerful pharmaceutic adsorbent.

■ INDICATIONS: It is prescribed in the treatment of acute poisoning and to control flatulence.

■ CONTRAINDICATIONS: There are no known contraindications, but activated charcoal is ineffective in poisoning caused by a strong acid or alkali or by cyanide.

■ ADVERSE EFFECTS: There are no known adverse effects.

activated 7-dehydrocholesterol. See **vitamin D_3.**

activated partial thromboplastin time (APTT), a timed blood test that determines the efficacy of various clotting factors, used in the diagnosis of coagulation disorders. The normal value in venous blood is 32 to 51 seconds.

activation energy, the energy required to convert reactants to activated or transition-state species that will spontaneously proceed to products.

activation factor. See **factor XII.**

activator, **1.** a substance, force, or device that stimulates activity in another substance or structure, especially a substance that activates an enzyme. **2.** a substance that stimulates the development of an anatomic structure in the embryo. **3.** an internal secretion of the pancreas. **4.** an apparatus for making substances radioactive, as a cyclotron or neutron generator. **5.** (in dentistry) a removable orthodontic appliance that functions as a passive transmitter and stimulator of the perioral muscles.

active algolagnia. See **sadism.**

active assisted exercise, the movement of the body or any of its parts primarily through the individual's own efforts but accompanied by the aid of a therapist or some other device, as an exercise machine. See also **exercise, passive exercise.**

active euthanasia. See **euthanasia.**

active exercise, repetitive movement of a part of the body as a result of voluntary contraction and relaxation of the controlling muscles. Compare **passive exercise.** See also **aerobic exercise, anaerobic exercise.**

active immunity, a form of long-term, acquired immunity that protects the body against a new infection, as the result of antibodies that develop naturally after an initial infection or artificially after a vaccination. Compare **passive immunity.** See also **immune response.**

active movement, muscular action at a joint as a result of voluntary effort without outside help. Compare **passive movement.**

active play, any activity from which one derives amusement, entertainment, enjoyment, or satisfaction by taking a participatory rather than a passive role. Children of all age groups engage in various forms of active play, from the exploration of objects and toys by the infant and toddler to the formal games, sports, and hobbies of the older child. Compare **passive play.**

active resistance exercise, the movement or exertion of the body or any of its parts performed totally through the individual's own efforts against a resisting force. See also **progressive resistance exercise.**

active site, the place on the surface of an enzyme where its catalytic action occurs.

active specific immunotherapy, a therapy in which a cancer patient is injected with irradiated tumor cells. The injected cells stimulate the production of antibodies that resist the tumor cells.

active transport, the movement of materials across the membrane of a cell by means of chemical activity that allows the cell to admit larger molecules than would otherwise be able to enter. Expediting active transport are carrier molecules within the cell that bind themselves to incoming molecules, rotate around them, and disconnect, setting the incoming molecule free inside the cell wall. The entry of large molecules in the process of active transport disturbs the equilibrium of the internal environment of the cell, which compensates for the imbalance by releasing materials through its membrane. Active transport is the means by which the cell absorbs glucose and other substances needed to sustain life and health. Certain enzymes play a role in active transport, providing a chemical "pump" that helps move substances through the cell membrane. Compare **osmosis, passive transport.**

active treatment. See **treatment.**

activities of daily living (ADL), the activities usually performed in the course of a normal day in the client's life, as eating, dressing, washing, or brushing the teeth. The ability to perform the activities of daily living may be compromised by a variety of causes, including chronic illnesses and accidents. The limitation imposed may be temporary or permanent; rehabilitation may involve relearning the skills or learning new ways to accomplish an activity. Nursing has a significant role in helping a client to maintain or regain his ability to perform the necessary activities of daily living, thus remaining independent to the greatest degree possible. An ADL checklist is often used before discharge from the hospital. If any activities cannot be adequately performed, arrangements are made with an outside agency, as a visiting nurse service, or with family members to provide the necessary assistance to the client. Follow-up with physical therapy on an outpatient basis may be useful in maintaining or increasing the client's ability to perform the activities.

activity, the action of an enzyme on an amount of substrate that is converted to product per unit time under defined conditions.

activity coefficient, a proportionality constant, γ, relating activity, α, to concentration, expressed in the equation, $\alpha = \gamma c$.

activity intolerance, a nursing diagnosis accepted by the Fifth National Conference on the Classification of Nursing Diagnoses. The cause of the condition may be generalized weakness, a sedentary life-style, imbalance between oxygen supply and demand, or bed rest or immobility. The defining characteristics of the condition include verbal report of fatigue or weakness, abnormal heart rate or blood pressure response to activity, exertional discomfort or dyspnea, and electrocardiographic changes reflecting arrhythmias or ischemia. See also **nursing diagnosis.**

actual cautery, the application of heat, rather than a chemical substance, in the destruction of tissue.

actual charge, the amount actually charged or billed by a medical practitioner for a service. The actual charge may not be the same as that paid for the service by an insurance plan.

actual damages. See **damages.**

actualize, the act of fulfilling a potential, as by a person who may develop capabilities through experience and education.

acu-, **1.** a combining form meaning 'pertaining to a needle': *aculosure, aculeate, acupressure.* **2.** also **acou-.** a combining form meaning 'pertaining to hearing': *acuesthesia.*

acuity, the clearness or sharpness of perception, as visual acuity.

acuminate wart. See **condyloma acuminatum.**

acupressure /ak′yəpresh′ər/, a therapeutic technique of applying digital pressure in a specified way on designated points on the body to relieve pain, produce anesthesia, or regulate a body function.

acupuncture /ak′yəpunk′tshər/, a method of producing analgesia or altering the function of a system of the body by inserting fine, wire-thin needles into the skin at specific sites on the body along a series of lines, or channels, called meridians. The needles are twirled or energized electrically or warmed. Acupuncture originated in the Far East and has gained increasing attention in the West since the early 1970s. Research seeks to determine the usefulness of acupuncture and to understand the mechanisms by which it produces analgesia or alters sensory function. Some studies indicate that the analgesic effect of this technique is reversed by naloxone, suggesting that the release of enkephalin is significantly involved. See also **moxibustion.** **–acupuncturist,** *n.*

acupuncture point, one of many discrete points on the skin along the several meridians, or chains of points of the body. Stimulation of any of the various points may induce an increase or decrease in function or sensation in an area or system of the body. The meridians are named and the points numbered to allow specific location of the points to be stimulated in acupuncture, acupressure, or moxibustion.

-acusis. See **-acousia.**

acute, **1.** (of a disease or disease symptoms) beginning abruptly with marked intensity or sharpness, then subsiding after a relatively short period of time. **2.** sharp or severe. Compare **chronic.**

acute abdomen, an abnormal condition characterized by the acute onset of severe pain within the abdominal cavity. An acute abdomen requires immediate evaluation and diagnosis, because it may indicate a condition that calls for surgical intervention. Information about the onset, duration, character, location, and symptoms associated with the pain is critical in making an accurate diagnosis. The patient is asked what decreases or increases the pain; constant, increasing pain is associated with appendicitis and diverticulitis, whereas intermittent pain is more likely indicative of a bowel obstruction, ureteral calculi, or gallstones. Appendicitis may often be differentiated from a perforated ulcer by the slower development of pain. Although sometimes misleading because of referral, radiation, or reflection of pain, the patient's report of the location of the pain may serve to identify a specific organ or system. Factors in the patient's history that are useful in the diagnosis and management of an acute abdomen include changes in bowel habits, weight loss, bloody stool, diarrhea, and clay-colored stool. Also called **surgical abdomen.** See also **abdominal pain.**

acute alcoholism, drunkenness or intoxication resulting from excessive consumption of alcoholic beverages. The syndrome is temporary and is characterized by depression of the higher nerve centers causing impaired motor control, stupor, lack of coordination, and often nausea, dehydration, headache, and other physical symptoms. Compare **chronic alcoholism.** See also **alcoholism.**

acute bacterial arthritis. See **septic arthritis.**

acute care, a pattern of health care in which a patient is treated for an acute episode of illness, for the sequelae of an accident or other trauma, or during recovery from surgery. Acute care is usually given in a hospital by specialized personnel using complex and sophisticated technical equipment and materials, and it may involve intensive care. This pattern of care is often necessary for only a short time, unlike chronic care.

acute cervicitis. See **cervicitis.**

acute childhood leukemia, a progressive, malignant disease of the blood-forming tissues that is characterized by the uncontrolled proliferation of immature leukocytes and their precursors, particularly in the bone marrow, spleen, and lymph nodes. It is the most frequent cancer in children, with a peak onset occurring between 2 and 5 years of age.

■ OBSERVATIONS: Acute leukemia is classified according to cell type: **acute lymphoid leukemia (ALL)** includes lymphatic, lymphocytic, lymphoblastic, and lymphoblastoid types; **acute nonlymphoid leukemia (ANLL)** includes granulocytic, myelocytic, monocytic, myelogenous, monoblastic, and monomyeloblastic types (the myelocytic and monocytic series are abbreviated **AML**). ALL is predominantly a disease of childhood, whereas AML occurs in all age groups. The traditional classification of leukemia into chronic and acute types is based on duration or expected course of the illness and the relative maturity of the leukemic cells. Although this classification is still used, particularly to differentiate the childhood, or acute, from the adult, or chronic, forms of the disease, it is no longer valid as a prognostic indication. The exact cause of the disease is unknown, although various factors are implicated, including genetic defects, immune deficiency, viruses, and carcinogenic environmental factors, primarily ionizing radiation. In acute leukemia, large immature leukocytes accumulate rapidly and infiltrate other tissues of the body, especially the reticuloendothelial system, causing decreased production of erythrocytes and platelets. Neutropenia, anemia, an increased susceptibility to infection and hemorrhage, and weakening of the bones with a tendency to fracture also occur. Initial symptoms of the disease include fever, pallor, fatigue, anorexia, secondary infections (usually of the mouth, throat, or lungs), bone and joint pain, subdermal or submucosal hemorrhage, and enlargement of the spleen, liver, and lymph nodes. Onset may be abrupt or follow a gradual, progressive course. Involvement of the central nervous system may lead to leukemic meningitis. Characteristically, a peripheral blood smear reveals many immature leukocytes. The diagnosis is confirmed by bone marrow aspiration or biopsy and examination, which show a highly elevated number of lymphoblasts with almost complete absence of erythrocytes, granulocytes, and megakaryocytes. The prognosis is poor in untreated cases, and death occurs usually within 6 months after the onset of symptoms. Survival rates have dramatically increased in recent years with the use of antileukemic agents in combination regimens. Remission of 5 years or longer occurs in 50% to 70% of children with ALL, with 20% to 30% achieving complete remission. For children with AML, the prognosis is poorer, and the remission rate is far less.

■ INTERVENTION: Treatment of acute leukemia consists of a three-stage process involving the use of chemotherapeutic agents and irradiation. In the first, or remission induction phase, complete destruction of all leukemic cells is achieved within a 4- to 6-week period using a combination drug-therapy regimen. The main drugs used in ALL are the corticosteroids, usually three daily oral doses of prednisone; vincristine, administered intravenously once a week; and l-asparaginase, given intramuscularly three times a week for a total of nine doses. Allopurinol, a xanthine-oxidase inhibitor, is usually administered to inhibit uric acid production. Other drugs used in various combination regimens in sequential cycles include methotrexate, 6-mercaptopurine, cyclophosphamide, cytosine arabinoside, hydroxyurea, daunorubicin, and doxorubicin. In children with AML the primary drugs for induction remission are 6-thioguanine, daunomycin, cytosine arabinoside, 5-azacytidine, vincristine, and prednisone. The child is usually hospitalized for part or all of the treatment because of the many side effects of the drugs and the high risk of complications, especially infection and hemorrhage. If severe hemorrhaging occurs and does not respond to local treatment, platelet transfusions may be necessary, and in cases of severe anemia, especially during induction therapy, whole blood or packed red cells may be needed to raise hemoglobin levels. The second stage of treatment involves prophylactic maintenance to prevent leukemic infiltration of the central nervous system. Because chemotherapy drugs do not cross the blood-brain barrier, therapy usually consists of daily high-dose cranial irradiation for about 2 weeks after induction remission and weekly or twice-weekly doses of intrathecal methotrexate, for a total of five or six injections, although in some cases only the drug is given. In small children the irradiation is limited to the cranium to prevent retardation of linear growth, but older children may receive craniospinal radiation. Therapy to maintain remission usually begins after the child is discharged from the hospital and consists of various regimens of drugs in combination. A common schedule includes daily oral doses of 6-mercaptopurine and weekly doses of oral methotrexate, intermittent short-term therapy with prednisone and vincristine, and periodic doses of intrathecal methotrexate for prophylaxis against spread to the central nervous system. Complete blood counts are done weekly or monthly, and bone marrow examinations are performed every 3 to 4 months to detect myelosuppression and drug toxicity. Maintenance therapy is discontinued after a period of 2 to 3 years if initial remission is maintained. Continuous treatment beyond 3 years is not advised, as the adverse affects of the medications increase with prolonged use. Relapse occurs in as many as 20% of treated children. If relapse occurs, the child begins the treatment cycle again, usually with prednisone, vincristine, and a combination of other drugs not previously tried. With each relapse the prognosis becomes poorer. Other treatments for prolonging remission include immunotherapy using periodic inoculation with BCG vaccine or bone marrow transplant, which has been successful in inducing long-term remissions in about 10% to 20% of the cases, especially those with AML or severe, terminal ALL.

■ NURSING CONSIDERATIONS: Nursing care for the child with acute leukemia involves intensive physical and emotional support during all phases of the disease, its diagnosis, and treatment. Foremost is the preparation of the child and parents for the various diagnostic and therapeutic procedures, including venipuncture, bone-marrow aspiration or biopsy, lumbar puncture, and x-ray treatment. Specific medical and nursing management depends on the particular regimen of drug therapy, although most of the chemotherapeutic agents used in treatment cause myelosuppression that may lead to secondary complications of infection, hemorrhage, and anemia. Overwhelming infection is a major problem and one of the most frequent causes of death. Severe neutropenia indicates increased risk of infection. It may occur during immunosuppressive therapy or after prolonged antibiotic therapy. The most common infectious organisms are viruses, especially varicella, herpes zoster, herpes simplex, measles, mumps, rubella, and poliomyelitis, both gram-positive and gram-negative bacteria, including *Staphylococcus aureus, S. epidermidis,* group-A β-hemolytic *Streptococcus, Pseudomonas aeruginosa, Escherichia coli, Proteus,* and *Klebsiella,* and various parasites and fungi, especially *Pneumocystis carinii* and *Candida albicans.* To prevent infection, the nurse isolates the child as much as possible, screens visitors for active infection, institutes strict aseptic procedures, monitors temperature closely, evaluates possible sites of infection (as needle punctures), encourages adequate nutrition, and helps the child to avoid exertion or fatigue, and, at discharge, teaches the child and parents the necessity for avoiding all known sources of infection, primarily the common childhood communicable diseases. Preventive measures to control infection also help decrease the tendency toward hemorrhage. Special attention is given to skin care, oral hygiene, cleanliness of the perineal area, and restriction of activities that could result in accidental injury. A major nursing consideration is the management of the many side effects resulting from drug toxicity and irradiation, including nausea and vomiting, anorexia, oral and rectal ulceration, alopecia, hemorrhagic cystitis, and peripheral neuropathy, including weakness and numbing of the extremities and severe jaw pain. Although corticosteroid treatment increases usually the appetite and produces a euphoric sense of well-being in the child, it also causes moon face, which is reversed with cessation of the steroid therapy. During maintenance therapy, the nurse continues to provide emotional support and guidance, specifically teaching parents which side effects are normal reactions to drugs and which indicate toxicity and require medical attention. In terminal stages of the disease, relief of discomfort and pain become the primary focus. Effective measures include careful physical handling of the child, frequent position changes, avoidance of pressure on painful areas, and control of annoying environmental factors, as excessive light and noise. Nonsalicylate analgesics are used as needed, depending on the severity of pain. See also **acute lymphocytic leukemia, acute myelocytic leukemia, leukemia.**

acute cholecystitis. See **cholecystitis.**

acute delirium, an episode of delirium that is sudden, severe, and transient. See also **delirium.**

acute disease, a disease characterized by a relatively short duration of symptoms that are usually severe. An episode of acute disease results in recovery to a state comparable to the patient's state of health and activity before the disease, in passage into a chronic phase, or in death. See also **chronic disease.**

acute epiglottitis, a severe, rapidly progressing bacterial infection of the upper respiratory tract that occurs in young children, primarily between 2 and 7 years of age. It is characterized by sore throat, croupy stridor, and an inflamed epiglottis, which may cause sudden respiratory obstruction and be quickly fatal. The infection is generally caused by *Haemophilus influenzae,* type B, although streptococci may occasionally be the causative agent. Transmission occurs by infection with airborne particles or contact with infected secretions. The diagnosis is made by bacteriologic identification of *H. influenzae,* type B, in a specimen taken from the upper respiratory tract or in the blood. An x-ray film of the neck from the side shows an enlarged epiglottis and distention of the hypopharynx, which distinguishes the condition from croup. Direct visualization of the inflamed, cherry-red epiglottis by depression of the tongue or indirect laryngoscopy is also diagnostic but may produce total acute obstruction and is attempted only by trained personnel with equipment to establish an airway or to provide respiratory resuscitation, if necessary. Compare **croup.**

■ OBSERVATIONS: The onset of the infection is abrupt and it progresses rapidly. The first signs—sore throat, hoarseness, fever, and dysphagia—may be followed by an inability to swallow, drooling, varying degrees of dyspnea, inspiratory stridor, and marked irritability and apprehension. Difficulty in breathing may progress to severe respiratory distress in minutes or hours. Suprasternal, supraclavicular, intercostal, and subcostal inspiratory retractions may be visible. The hypoxic child appears frightened and anxious; the color of the skin ranges from pallor to cyanosis.

■ INTERVENTION: Establishment of an airway is urgent, either by endotracheal intubation or by tracheostomy. Humidity and oxygen are provided, and airway secretions are drained or suctioned. Intravenous fluids are usually required, and antibiotic therapy is initiated immediately, usually with penicillin, ampicillin, or chloramphenicol. Sedatives are contraindicated because of their depressant effect on the respiratory system, and steroids, antihistamines, and adrenergic drugs are not usually of any therapeutic value.

■ NURSING CONSIDERATIONS: The nurse may assist intubation or tracheostomy once the diagnosis is confirmed. Intensive nursing care is required for a child with acute epiglottitis. Frequent changing of clothing and bed linen may be necessary to prevent chilling. The most acute phase of the condition passes within 24 to 48 hours, and intubation is rarely needed beyond 3 to 4 days. As the child responds to therapy, breathing becomes easier, and there is usually rapid recovery so that bed rest and quiet activity to relieve boredom become primary nursing concerns. The infection may spread, causing such complications as otitis media, pneumonia, and bronchiolitis. Complications of the tracheostomy may also develop, including infection, atelectasis, cannula occlusion, tracheal bleeding, granulation, and stenosis, and delayed healing of the stoma. Also called **acute epiglottiditis.**

acute febrile polyneuritis. See **Guillain-Barré syndrome.**

acute gastritis. See **gastritis.**

acute glaucoma. See **glaucoma.**

acute glomerulonephritis. See **postinfectious glomerulonephritis.**

acute hallucinatory paranoia, a form of paranoia in which hallucinations are combined with the systematized delusions. Also called **paranoia hallucinatoria.**

acute hallucinosis. See **alcoholic hallucinosis.**

acute hemorrhagic conjunctivitis, a highly contagious eye disease usually caused by enterovirus type 70 and found primarily in densely populated humid areas, particularly the developing countries or places with a high immigration or refugee population. Clinical features include sudden onset of ocular pain, itching, redness, photophobia, edema of the eyelid, and profuse watery discharge. Spontaneous improvement occurs within 2 to 4 days and is complete by 7 to 10 days. Treatment consists of hygienic measures and ophthalmic preparations.

acute hemorrhagic leukoencephalitis. See **acute necrotizing hemorrhagic encephalopathy.**

acute idiopathic polyneuritis. See **Guillain-Barré syndrome.**

acute idiopathic thrombocytopenic purpura. See **idiopathic thrombocytopenic purpura.**

acute intermittent porphyria (AIP), a genetically transmitted metabolic disorder characterized by acute attacks of neurologic dysfunction that can be started by either environmental or endogenous factors. Women are affected more frequently than men, and attacks often are precipitated by female sex hormones. Other precipitating factors include starvation or crash dieting, bacterial or viral infections, and a wide range of pharmaceutic products. Any part of the nervous system can be affected, and a common effect is mild to severe abdominal pain associated with autonomic neuropathy. Other effects can include peripheral neuropathy, hyponatremia, and organic brain dysfunction marked by seizures, coma, hallucinations, and respiratory paralysis. A frequent diagnostic factor is a high level of porphyrin precursors in the urine, which usually increase during periods of acute attacks. Treatment is generaly symptomatic, with emphasis on pain control and education of the patient about environmental factors, particularly medications, that are known to cause an onset of symptoms. A high-carbohydrate diet is reported to reduce the risk of acute attacks because glucose tends to block the induction of hepatic gamma-aminolevulinic acid (ALA) synthetase, an enzyme involved in the porphyrias. See also **porphyria.**

acute interstitial nephritis. See **interstitial nephritis.**

acute laryngotracheobronchitis. See **croup.**

acute lymphoblastic leukemia. See **acute lymphocytic leukemia.**

acute lymphocytic leukemia (ALL), a progressive, malignant disease characterized by large numbers of immature cells, closely resembling lymphoblasts in the bone marrow, the circulating blood, the lymph nodes, the spleen, the liver, and other organs. The number of normal blood cells is reduced. About 80% of the 2250 cases a year in the United States occur in children, with the greatest number diagnosed between 2 and 5 years of age. The risk of the disease is greatly increased for people with Down's syndrome and for siblings of leukemia patients. The disease has a sudden onset and rapid progression marked by fever, pallor, anorexia, fatigue, anemia, hemorrhage, bone pain, splenomegaly, and recurrent infection. Blood and bone marrow studies are used for diagnosis and for determining the type of proliferating lymphocyte, which may be B cells, T cells (that usually respond poorly to therapy), or null cells (as are found in most cases). Treatment includes intensive combination chemotherapy, therapy for secondary infections and hyperuricemia, irradiation, and intrathecal methotrexate.

acute mastitis. See **mastitis.**

acute mountain sickness. See **altitude sickness.**

acute myelocytic leukemia (AML), a malignant neoplasm of blood-forming tissues characterized by the uncontrolled proliferation of immature granular leukocytes that usually have azurophilic Auer rods in their cytoplasm. The typical symptoms, appearing abruptly or, more often, gradually, are spongy bleeding gums, anemia, fatigue, fever, dyspnea, moderate splenomegaly, joint and bone pains, and repeated infections. Chloromas (greenish granulocytic sarcomas) may develop in bone or soft tissue. AML may occur at any age, but it most frequently affects adolescents and young adults. The risk of the disease is increased among people who have been exposed to massive doses of radiation and among individuals with certain blood dyscrasias, as polycythemia vera, primary thrombocytopenia, and refractory anemia. Variants of AML, in which only one cell line proliferates, are erythroid, eosinophilic, basophilic, monocytic, and megakaryocytic leukemias. The diagnosis is based on differential blood count and bone biopsies. Chemotherapy with various combinations of drugs, including cyclophosphamide, cytosine arabinoside, daunorubicin, methotrexate, prednisone, and vincristine sulfate, is the primary form of treatment. Allopurinol is frequently administered before chemotherapy to reduce the risk of urate crystalluria and ureteral obstruction. Repeated transfusions of red cells and platelets may be required. Radiotherapy, immunotherapy, and marrow transplantation are also used, but long remissions resulting from any form of treatment are rare, and death may be caused by an infection, a hemorrhage, or an obstruction produced by leukocytes in a blood vessel. Also called **acute granulocytic leukemia (AGL), acute nonlymphocytic leukemia (ANLL), acute myelogenous leukemia, myeloid leukemia, splenomedullary leukemia, splenomyelogenous leukemia.** See also **acute childhood leukemia, chronic myelocytic leukemia.**

acute necrotizing gingivitis, a fusospirochetal infection characterized by necrotic, foul-smelling ulcers of the gums and throat, fever, and enlarged lymph nodes in the neck. It is usually associated with poor oral hygiene and is most common in conditions in which there is crowding and malnutrition. Treatment includes peroxide mouthwashes, antibiotics, analgesics, and dental care. Also called **trench mouth, Vincent's angina, Vincent's infection.**

acute necrotizing hemorrhagic encephalopathy, a degenerative disease of the brain, characterized by marked edema, numerous minute hemorrhages, necrosis of blood vessel walls, especially those of small veins, demyelination of nerve fibers, and infiltration of the meninges with neutrophils, lymphocytes, and histiocytes. Typical signs are severe headache, fever, and vomiting; convulsions may occur, and the patient may rapidly lose consciousness. Treatment consists of decompression by withdrawing cerebrospinal fluid and administration of large doses of steroids, but the disease is frequently fatal in 1 to 6 days. This kind of encephalopathy is thought to be caused by an immunologic mechanism, but the disease often resembles acute bacterial meningitis or herpes simplex encephalitis. Also called **acute hemorrhagic leukoencephalitis.**

acute necrotizing ulcerative gingivitis (ANUG), a distinct, recurring periodontal disease that primarily affects the interdental papillae, causing necrosis and ulceration.

acute nonlymphocytic leukemia. See **acute myelocytic leukemia.**

acute pain, severe pain, as may follow surgery or trauma or accompany myocardial infarction or other conditions and diseases. Acute pain occurring in the first 24 to 48 hours after surgery is often difficult to relieve, even with drugs. Some studies show that patients over 50 years of age need less analgesia to relieve acute pain than do younger patients. Another study indicates that 23% of surgical patients, except for orthopedic patients, do not require analgesia. Acute pain in individuals with orthopedic problems originates from the periosteum, the joint surfaces, and the arterial walls. Muscle pain associated with bone surgery results from muscle ischemia rather than muscle tension. Acute abdominal pain often causes the individual involved to lie on one side and draw up the legs in the fetal position. Compare **chronic pain.** See also **pain intervention.**

acute paranoid disorder, a psychopathologic condition characterized by a persecutory delusional system of rapid onset, quick development, and short duration, usually lasting less than 6 months. The disorder, which rarely becomes chronic, is most commonly seen in persons who have experienced drastic changes in their environment, such as immigrants, refugees, prisoners, military inductees, and, in a less severe form, those leaving home for the first time.

acute promyelocytic leukemia, a malignancy of the blood-forming tissues, characterized by severe bleeding, scattered bruises, a low fibrinogen level and platelet count, and the proliferation in bone marrow of promyelocytes and blast cells with distinctive Auer rods. Management of the disease requires replacement of coagulation factors and the administration of cytotoxic antileukemia drugs. See **leukemia.**

acute psychosis, one of a group of disorders in which the ability to process information is diminished and disordered. The cause of the particular disorder may be a known physiologic abnormality. In other cases the physiologic abnormality may not be recognized, but the defect in function is clearly present. Delirium and acute brain syndrome are associated with known pathophysiology in the brain and are characterized by disorientation, disturbance of memory, and lapses in consciousness. Acute functional psychosis is associated with unknown pathophysiology and varying signs and symptoms that progress from insomnia and agitation to paranoid or grandiose delusions, mania, emotional lability, and hallucinations. An acute psychosis of any kind requires prompt diagnosis and treatment. The impaired judgment, confusion, and turmoil suffered has disastrous effects on all aspects of the patient's life. Antipsychotic medication and psychotherapy often bring about remission.

acute pyelonephritis. See **pyelonephritis.**

acute pyogenic arthritis, an acute bacterial infection affecting one or more joints, caused by trauma or a penetrating wound and occurring most frequently in children. Typical signs are pain, redness, and swelling in the affected joint, muscular spasms in the area, chills, fever, diaphoresis, and leukocytosis. Treatment consists of immobilization of the joint, the intravenous administration of an antibiotic, analgesia, and sedation. If required, the joint may be irrigated with normal saline and an antibiotic. Hospitalization is usually required.

acute radial nerve palsy, a type of mononeuropathy characterized by damage to the radial nerve and consequent weakening of the muscles of the forearm. It may be caused by excessive compression of the radial nerve against a hard surface in individuals insensitized by the intake of alcohol or sedatives. It may also be caused by the repeated compression of the nerve by various weights, as the weight of the head of a bed partner. Time and the withdrawal of causative compression usually assure full recovery.

acute radiation exposure, exposure of short duration to intense ionizing radiation, usually occurring as the result of an accident in an industrial installation, a nuclear power plant, or a vehicle transporting radioactive material or from proximity to a detonated atom bomb. Exposure of the whole body to approximately 10,000 rad (100 gray) causes neurologic and cardiovascular breakdown and is fatal within 24 hours. A dose between 500 and 1200 rad (5 and 12 gray) destroys GI mucosa, produces bloody diarrhea, and may cause death in several days. Death may occur weeks after exposure to a dose of 200 to 500 rad (2 and 5 gray) because of the destructive effect on blood-forming organs, but 600 rad (6 gray) is generally considered the fatal dose. See also **radiation exposure.**

acute respiratory distress syndrome (ARDS), a respiratory emergency characterized by respiratory insufficiency and failure usually after aspiration of a foreign body, cardiopulmonary bypass surgery, gram-negative sepsis, multiple blood transfusions, oxygen toxicity, trauma, pneumonia or other respiratory infection. It may also occur in such diseases as Guillain-Barré syndrome, muscular dystrophy, myasthenia gravis, emphysema, asthma, or poliomyelitis. Also called **adult respiratory distress syndrome, congestive atelectasis, pump lung, shock lung, wet lung.** See also **chronic obstructive pulmonary disease.**

■ OBSERVATIONS: The symptoms and signs of ARDS include shortness of breath, rapid breathing, flail chest, inadequate oxygenation of the arterial blood, increase in arterial Pco_2 and a decrease in the arterial pH. The changes that occur within the lungs include damage to the membranes of the capillaries, hemorrhage, capillary leaking, interstitial edema, impairment in gas exchange, and ventilation-perfusion abnormalities. These sequelae lead to decreased compliance and increased dyspnea.

■ INTERVENTION: The patient with ARDS usually requires mechanic ventilation, often using positive-end-expiratory-pressure (PEEP). Treatment is directed toward establishing an airway, administering oxygen, improving the underlying condition, and removing the cause. Particular care in administering oxygen is necessary in patients with chronic obstructive lung disease who have elevated levels of Pco_2, because a sudden or marked decrease in the Pco_2 may result in decreased respiratory effort. These patients also receive intermittent-positive-pressure breathing (IPPB) therapy every few hours, modified to administer low-flow oxygen to aid in ventilation and to reduce co_2 levels. Also used in management are suctioning of the respiratory passages as necessary, and ultrasonic mist therapy, postural drainage, and cupping and vibration. When ventilation cannot be maintained and there is evidence of a rising Pco_2, mechanic ventilation with a respirator is necessary. Positive-end-expiratory-pressure is widely used in the treatment of ARDS. Sedatives are given with caution because they depress respiration.

■ NURSING CONSIDERATIONS: The patient with ARDS requires constant and meticulous nursing care, reassurance, and observation for changes in respiratory function and adequacy including signs of hypercapnia, especially confusion, skin flushing, and behavior changes that include aggressiveness. Increasing hypoxia may be recognized by tachycardia, elevated blood pressure, and increased peripheral resistance; fulminant respiratory failure is accompanied by falling blood pressure and cyanosis. If PEEP is being used, the nurse is careful to see that there is not a sudden disappearance of breath sounds accompanied by signs of respiratory distress—an indication that pneumothorax is present. Care is taken when weaning patients from the ventilator, and intermittent mandatory ventilation (IMV) may be used. Adequate humidification, respiratory therapy, sterile suction techniques, hourly hyperinflation, and position changes are continued as necessary. Weight is taken frequently, x-ray films of the chest are taken and evaluated, and bacteriologic cultures of secretions are analyzed in the laboratory. Throughout treatment, ventilation is carefully monitored using blood gas studies and spirometry.

acute rheumatic arthritis, arthritis that occurs during the acute phase of rheumatic fever.

acute rhinitis. See **rhinitis.**

acute schizophrenia, a form of schizophrenia that is characterized by the sudden onset of personality disorganization with symptoms that include confusion, emotional turmoil, fear, depression, dreamlike dissociation, and bizarre behavior. Episodes appear suddenly in persons whose previous behavior has been relatively normal and are usually of short duration. Recurrent episodes are common, and in some instances a more chronic type of the disorder may develop. Also called **undifferentiated schizophrenia.** See also **schizophrenia, schizophreniform disorder.**

acute toxicity, the harmful effect of a toxic agent that manifests itself in seconds, minutes, hours, or days after entering the patient.

acute transverse myelitis, an abnormal condition characterized by inflammation of the entire thickness of the spinal cord, affecting both the sensory and the motor nerves. It is the most destructive form of myelitis and can develop rapidly, accompanied by necrosis and neurologic disorder that commonly persist after recovery. Patients who develop spastic reflexes soon after the onset of this disease are more likely to recover. This disorder may develop from a variety of causes, as acute multiple sclerosis, measles, pneumonia, and the ingestion of certain toxic agents, as carbon monoxide, lead, and arsenic. Such poisonous substances can destroy the entire circumference of the spinal cord, including the myelin sheaths, the axis cylinders, and the neurons, and can also cause hemorrhage and necrosis.

■ OBSERVATIONS: Acute transverse myelitis starts very quickly with sensory and motor dysfunctions below the level of the spinal cord damage. Within 2 days of onset, one or both legs of the affected patients may suffer flaccid paralysis after the advent of pain and sensory loss. Resulting severe spinal cord damage may cause shock with associated hypotension and hypothermia. Sphincter function and reflex losses are also common signs. Diagnosis is commonly based on the rapid onset of paraplegia, but it must rule out spinal cord tumor and identify any associated underlying infection.

■ INTERVENTION: There is no effective treatment, and the prognosis for complete recovery is poor. Any underlying infection is identified and treated accordingly. Some patients with myelitis induced by multiple sclerosis or by various infections have received steroid treatments, but the results of such therapy are inconclusive.

■ NURSING CONSIDERATIONS: Proper nursing care of the patient with acute transverse myelitis involves frequent assessment of vital signs and constant vigilance for any signs of spinal shock, as hypotension and profuse sweating. Foley catheters must be meticulously maintained to avoid urinary tract infections, and proper skin care is needed to prevent infections and decubitus ulcers. To prevent contractures nurses commonly assist the patient with range-of-motion exercises and assure that the patient is properly aligned. Also important, especially for the patients who develop paraplegia, are physical therapy, bowel and bladder training, and consistent instruction and encouragement throughout the rehabilitation period.

ACVD, abbreviation for *atherosclerotic cardiovascular disease*.

-acy, a combining form meaning a 'state or quality of': *anthropocracy, lunacy, physiocracy*.

acyclovir, an antiviral (acycloguanosine).
■ INDICATIONS: It is prescribed topically in an ointment for the treatment of herpes simplex keratitis and both topically and systemically in other types of herpes infections, including genital herpes. Acyclovir appears to act selectively by inhibiting the functions of herpesvirus DNA molecules, but the drug has no demonstrated activity against other types of viral infections.
■ CONTRAINDICATION: Known senstivity to this drug prohibits its use.
■ ADVERSE EFFECTS: Used topically, irritation or pruritus may occur; used systemically, diaphoresis, headache, and nausea may occur. When it is administered intravenously in the treatment of immunosuppressed patients, there may be pain at the site of the injection.

acyesis /ā′sī•ē′sis/, **1.** the absence of pregnancy. **2.** a condition of sterility in women.

ad-, ac-, af-, ag-, ap-, as-, at-, a combining form meaning 'to, toward, addition to, or intensification': *adneural, adoral, adrenal*.

-ad, a combining form meaning 'toward (a specified terminus)': *anteriad, iniad, obeliad*.

A/D, abbreviation for **analog-to-digital.**

ADA, **1.** abbreviation for **American Dental Association.** **2.** abbreviation for **American Diabetes Association.** **3.** abbreviation for **American Dietetic Association.**

adactyly /ādak′tilē/, a congenital defect in which one or more digits of the hand or foot are missing.

Adalat, a trademark for a calcium channel blocker (nifepidine).

adamantinoma, adamantoblastoma. See **ameloblastoma.**

Adam's apple, *informal*. the bulge at the front of the neck produced by the thyroid cartilage of the larynx. Also called **laryngeal prominence.**

Adams-Stokes syndrome, a condition characterized by sudden recurrent episodes of loss of consciousness because of incomplete heart block. Seizures may accompany the episodes. Also called **Stokes-Adams syndrome.** See also **infranodal block.**

adaptation, a change or response to stress of any kind, as inflammation of the nasal mucosa in infectious rhinitis or an increase in crying in a frightened child. Adaptation may be normal, self-protective, and developmental, as a child learning to talk; it may be all encompassing, creating further stress, as polycythemia, naturally occurring at high altitudes, which provides more oxygen-carrying red blood cells but which may also lead to thrombosis, venous congestion, or edema. The degree and nature of adaptation shown by a patient is evaluated regularly by the nurse. It is a measure of the effectiveness of nursing care, the course of the disease, and the ability of the patient to cope with stress. Compare **accommodation.** See also **dark adaptation, light adaptation, stress.**

adaptation model, (in nursing) a conceptual framework that focuses on the patient as an adaptive system, one in which nursing intervention is required when a deficit develops in the patient's ability to cope with the internal and external demands of the environment. These demands are classified in four groups: physiologic needs, the need for a positive self-concept, the need to perform social roles, and the need to balance dependence and independence. The nurse assesses the patient's maladaptive response and identifies the kind of demand that is causing the problem. Nursing care is planned to promote adaptive responses to cope successfully with the current stress on the patient's well-being. This model is frequently used as a conceptual framework for programs of nursing education.

adaptation syndrome. See **general adaptation syndrome.**

adaptor RNA. See **transfer RNA.**

Addams, Jane (1860–1935), an American social reformer. In 1889 she founded Hull House in Chicago, one of the first social settlements in the United States, where volunteers from many disciplines, including nursing, lived and continued working in their professions. She was at the center of most of the social reforms of her time and was an inspiration to those in the nursing profession who were striving to establish high educational standards and better working conditions. She was co-recipient of the Nobel peace prize in 1931.

addiction, compulsive, uncontrollable dependence on a substance, habit, or practice to such a degree that cessation causes severe emotional, mental, or physiologic reactions. Compare **habituation.**

Addis count, a method for counting red blood cells, white blood cells, epithelial cells, casts, and protein content in a sedimented 12-hour urine sample. Results are expressed as the number of each formed element excreted per 24 hours. The count is useful for diagnosing and managing kidney disease, because there should be none or nearly none of these components in the urine.

addisonian anemia. See **pernicious anemia.**

addisonian crisis, Addison's crisis. See **adrenal crisis.**

Addison's disease, a life-threatening condition caused by partial or complete failure of adrenocortical function, often resulting from autoimmune processes, infection (especially tubercular or fungal), neoplasm, or hemorrhage in the gland. All three general functions of the adrenal cortex are lost: glucocorticoid, mineralocorticoid, and androgenic. Also called **addisonism, Addison's syndrome.** See also **adrenal crisis, hypoadrenalism.**

■ OBSERVATIONS: The disease is characterized by weakness, decreased endurance, increased pigmentation of the skin and mucous membranes, anorexia, dehydration, weight loss, GI disturbances, anxiety, depression and other emotional distress, and decreased tolerance to cold. The onset is usually gradual, occurring over a period of weeks or months. Laboratory tests show abnormally low blood concentrations of sodium and glucose, a greater than normal level of serum potassium, and a decreased urinary output of certain steroids. The diagnosis is established if, after stimulation with adrenocorticosteroids, the amount of cortisol in the plasma and steroid in the urine fails to increase.

■ INTERVENTION: Treatment includes replacement therapy with glucocorticoid and mineralocorticoid drugs, an adequate intake of fluids, control of sodium and potassium balance, and a diet high in carbohydrate and protein. The person's requirements for glucocorticoid, mineralocorticoid, and salt are increased by stress, as in infection, trauma, and surgical procedures. Follow-up care includes frequent monitoring of sugar in the blood or urine, urinary acetone, and continued administration of corticoid drugs.

■ NURSING CONSIDERATIONS: The complications of Addison's disease include high fever, psychotic behavior, and adrenal crisis (addisonian crisis). Under careful management, the patient's resistance to infection, capacity for work, and general well-being may be maintained. Nurses administer steroid and other drugs, observe the patient for signs of abnormal sodium and potassium levels, monitor body weight and fluid intake and output, and encourage an adequate intake of nutrients. The patient needs protection against stress while in the hospital and instruction in the importance of avoiding stress at home. The significance of emotional distress, the value of wearing a medical-alert bracelet or tag, the signs of impending crisis, the use of a prepared kit for emergencies, and the importance of scrupulous attention to drug and diet regimens are emphasized before discharge. Discharge teaching also emphasizes the need to take cortisone after meals or with milk to avoid gastric irritation and the development of ulcers.

Addison's keloid. See **morphea.**

Addison's syndrome. See **Addison's disease.**

add-on, a system or circuit that can be attached to a computer to increase its memory or performance.

address, the numbered location of one byte of data in the internal memory of a computer.

adduction, movement of a limb toward the axis of the body. Compare **abduction.**

adductor /əduk′tər/, a muscle that acts to draw a part toward the axis or midline of the body. Compare **abductor, tensor.**

adductor brevis, a somewhat triangular muscle in the thigh and one of the five medial femoral muscles. Arising from the inferior ramus of the pubis between the gracilis and the obturator externus, it passes downward, backward, and to the side to insert into the line leading from the lesser trochanter to the linea aspera of the femur. It is innervated by a branch of the obturator nerve, which contains fibers from the third and fourth lumbar nerves, and it acts to adduct and rotate the thigh medially and to flex the leg. Compare **adductor longus, adductor magnus, gracilis, pectineus.**

adductor canal, a triangular channel beneath the sartorius muscle and between the adductor longus and vastus medialis through which the femoral vessels and the saphenous nerve pass. Also called **Hunter's canal, subsartorial canal.**

adductor longus, the most superficial of the three adductor muscles of the thigh and one of five medial femoral muscles. A triangular muscle that arises from the anterior surface of the pubis, it spreads to form a broad fleshy belly, passing downward, backward, and to the side to insert into the linea aspera of the femur, between the vastus medialis and the adductor magnus. It is innervated by a branch of the obturator nerve, which contains fibers from the third and fourth lumbar nerves, and it functions to adduct and flex the thigh. Compare **adductor brevis, adductor magnus, gracilis, pectineus.**

adductor magnus, the long, heavy triangular muscle of the medial aspect of the thigh. It arises from the inferior rami of the ischium and pubis and the inferior margin of the ischial tuberosity. The fibers of the muscle insert into the rough surface of the greater trochanter, into the linea aspera via a broad aponeurosis, and into the distal third of the femur via a rounded, thick tendon. The muscle is innervated by the obturator nerve, which contains fibers of the third and fourth lumbar nerves, and by a branch of the sciatic nerve. The adductor magnus acts to adduct the thigh. The proximal portion acts to rotate the thigh medially and to flex it on the hip; the distal portion acts to extend the thigh and rotate it laterally.

aden-. See **adeno-.**

adenalgia /ad′ənal′jə/, a condition characterized by pain in any of the glands. Also called **adenodynia** /ad′ənōdin′ē·ə/.

adenectomy /ad′ənek′təmē/, the surgical removal of any gland.

Aden fever. See **dengue.**

-adenia, a combining form meaning '(condition of the) glands': *anadenia, heteradenia, poradenia.*

adenine /ad′ənin/, a purine-base component of the nucleic acids, DNA and RNA, and a constituent of cyclic AMP and the adenosine portion of AMP, ADP, and ATP. See **ATP, DNA, RNA.**

adenine arabinoside. See **vidarabine.**

adenine-D-ribose. See **adenosine.**

adenitis /ad′ənī′tis/, an inflammatory condition of a lymph node or gland. Acute adenitis of the cervical lymph nodes manifests itself as a sore throat and stiff neck, simulating mumps if severe. It is usually a sign of secondary infection related to an oral, pharyngeal, or ear infection. Scarlet fever may cause an acute suppurative cervical adenitis as may infectious mononucleosis. Swelling of the lymph nodes in the back of the neck is often the result of a scalp infection, insect bite, or infestation by head lice. Inflammation of the lymph nodes of the mesenteric portion of the peritoneum often produces pain and other symptoms similar to those of appendicitis. Mesenteric adenitis may be mistaken for appendicitis, but, characteristically, mesenteric adenitis is preceded by a respiratory infection, the pain is less localized and less constant than in appendicitis, and it does not increase in severity. Generalized adenitis is a secondary symptom of syphilis. Therapy requires treatment of the primary infection by the administration of antimicrobial agents, application of warm compresses, and, in rare cases, incision and drainage. Also called **lymphadenitis.** Compare **acinitis.**

adeno-, aden-, a combining form meaning 'pertaining to a gland': *adenocarcinoma, adenocellulitis, adenofibrosis.*

adenoacanthoma /ad'ənō•ak'anthō'mə/, a neoplasm that may be malignant or benign, derived from glandular tissue with squamous differentiation shown by some of the cells.

adenoameloblastoma /ad'ənō•amel'ōblastō'mə/, *pl.* **adenoameloblastomas, adenoameloblastomata,** a benign tumor of the maxilla composed of ducts lined with columnar or cuboidal epithelial cells. It develops in tissue that normally gives rise to the teeth, and it is most often seen in young people.

adenoassociated virus (AAV) /ad'ənō-/, a defective virus that can reproduce only in the presence of adenoviruses. It is not yet known what role, if any, these organisms have in causing disease.

adenocarcinoma /ad'ənōkärsinō'mə/, *pl.* **adenocarcinomas, adenocarcinomata,** any one of a large group of malignant, epithelial cell tumors of the glands. Specific tumors are diagnosed and named by cytologic identification of the tissue affected; for example, an adenocarcinoma of the uterine cervix is characterized by tumor cells resembling the glandular epithelium of the cervix. –**adenocarcinomatous,** *adj.*

adenocarcinoma in situ, a localized growth of abnormal glandular tissue that may become malignant. It is most common in the endometrium and in the large intestine.

adenocarcinoma of the kidney. See **renal cell carcinoma.**

adenocele /ad'ənōsēl'/, a cystic, glandular tumor.

adenochondroma /ad'ənōkondrō'mə/, *pl.* **adenochondromas, adenochondromata,** a neoplasm of cells derived from glandular and cartilaginous tissues, as a mixed tumor of the salivary glands. Also called **chondroadenoma.**

adenocyst /ad'ənōsist'/, a benign epithelial tumor in which the cells form glandular structures and cysts. Also called **adenosystoma.** A kind of adenocyst is **papillary adenocystoma lymphomatosum.**

adenocystic carcinoma, a malignant neoplasm composed of cords of uniform small epithelial cells arranged in a sievelike pattern around cystic spaces that often contain mucus. The tumor occurs most frequently in the salivary glands, breast, mucous glands of the upper and lower respiratory tract, and, occasionally, in vestibular glands of the vulva. Although it grows slowly, it is malignant and tends to spread along the nerves, causing neurologic damage. Facial paralysis often results from adenocystic carcinoma of the salivary gland. Blood-borne metastases in bones and in the liver have been reported. Also called **adenoid cystic carcinoma, adenomyoepithelioma, cribriform carcinoma, cylindroma, cylindromatous carcinoma.**

adenodynia. See **adenalgia.**

adenoepithelioma /ad'ənō•ep'ithē'lē•ō'mə/, *pl.* **adenoepitheliomas, adenoepitheliomata,** a neoplasm consisting of glandular and epithelial components.

adenofibroma /ad'ənōfībrō'mə/, *pl.* **adenofibromas, adenofibromata,** a tumor of the connective tissues that contains glandular elements. A kind of adenofibroma is **adenofibroma edematodes.**

adenofibroma edematodes, a neoplasm consisting of glandular elements and connective tissue in which there is marked edema, as in a nasal polyp.

adenohypophysis /ad'ənōhīpof'isis/, the anterior lobe of the pituitary gland. It secretes growth hormone, thyrotropin, adrenocorticotropic hormone, melanocyte stimulating hormone, follicle stimulating hormone, luteinizing hormone, prolactin, beta lipotropin molecules, and endorphins. Releasing hormones from the hypothalamus regulate secretion by the anterior pituitary. Adenohypophyseal hormones control activities of the thyroid, gonads, adrenal cortex, breast, and other endocrine glands. Also called **anterior pituitary.**

adenoid /ad'ənoid/, **1.** having a glandular appearance, particularly lymphoid. **2.** adenoids, hypertrophy of the pharyngeal tonsil. See **pharyngeal tonsil.** –**adenoidal,** *adj.*

adenoidal speech, an abnormal manner of speaking caused by hypertrophy of the adenoidal tissue that normally exists in the nasopharynx of children. It is often characterized by a muted, nasal quality and may be corrected by a natural reduction of the swollen tissues or by surgical excision of the adenoids.

adenoid cystic carcinoma. See **adenocystic carcinoma.**

adenoidectomy /ad'ənoidek'təmē/, removal of the lymphoid tissue in the nasopharynx. The surgical procedure may be performed because the adenoids are enlarged, causing obstruction, or chronically infected, and normal adenoids may be excised as a prophylactic measure during tonsillectomy. Preoperative procedures include a partial thromboplastin time test and for black patients a sickle cell preparation test. The operation is performed with general anesthesia in children, but local anesthesia may be used in adults. After removal of the adenoids, bleeding is stemmed with pressure; in some cases vessels may be ligated with sutures, or an electrocoagulation current may be used. Postoperatively, the patient is observed for signs of hemorrhage, and the pulse is checked every 15 minutes for the first hour and every 30 minutes for several hours thereafter. See also **tonsillectomy.**

adenoid hyperplasia, a condition in which enlarged adenoid glands cause partial respiratory obstruction, especially in children. Enlarged adenoids, often in association with enlarged tonsils, are a frequent cause of recurrent otitis media, sinusitis, and conduction deafness. Severe nasopharyngeal obstruction can result in alveolar hypoventilation and pulmonary hypertension with congestive heart failure. Treatment is usually surgical removal of the adenoids.

adenoleiomyofibroma /ad′ənōlī′ōmī′ōfībrō′mə/, *pl.* **adenoleiomyofibromas, adenoleiomyofibromata,** a glandular tumor with smooth muscle, connective tissue and epithelial elements.

adenolipoma /ad′ənōlipō′mə/, *pl.* **adenolipomas, adenolipomata,** a neoplasm consisting of elements of glandular and fatty tissue.

adenolipomatosis /ad′ənōlipōmətō′sis/, a condition characterized by the growth of numerous adenolipomas in the groin, axilla, and neck.

adenolymphoma. See **papillary adenocystoma lymphomatosum.**

adenoma /ad′ənō′mə/, *pl.* **adenomas, adenomata,** a tumor of glandular epithelium in which the cells of the tumor are arranged in a recognizable glandular structure. An adenoma may cause excess secretion by the affected gland, as acidophilic pituitary adenoma resulting in an excess of growth hormone. Kinds of adenomas include **acidophilic adenoma, basophilic adenoma, fibroadenoma,** and **insulinoma.** **–adenomatous,** *adj.*

-adenoma, a combining form meaning a 'tumor composed of glandular tissue or glandlike in structure': *sarcoadenoma, splenadenoma, syringadenoma.*

adenoma sebaceum /sebā′sē·əm/, an abnormal skin condition consisting of multiple, wartlike, yellowish-red, waxy papules on the face, composed chiefly of fibrovascular tissue. The lesions are not true adenomas but fibromas and part of the complex known as tuberous sclerosis. See **Bourneville's disease, tuberous sclerosis.**

adenomatoid /ad′ənō′mətoid/, resembling a glandular tumor.

adenomatosis /ad′ənōmətō′sis/, an abnormal condition in which hyperplasia or tumor development affects two or more glands, usually the thyroid, adrenals, or pituitary.

adenomatous goiter /ad′ənō′mətəs/, an enlargement of the thyroid gland because of an adenoma or numerous colloid nodules.

adenomyoepithelioma. See **adenocystic carcinoma.**

adenomyofibroma /ad′ənōmī′ōfībrō′mə/, *pl.* **adenomyofibromas, adenomyofibromata,** a fibrous tumor that contains glandular and muscular components.

adenomyoma /ad′ənōmī·ō′mə/, *pl.* **adenomyomas, adenomyomata,** a tumor of the endometrium of the uterus characterized by a mass of smooth muscle containing endometrial tissue and glands. It usually causes dysmenorrhea.

adenomyomatosis /ad′ənōmī′ōmətō′sis/, an abnormal condition characterized by the formation of benign nodules resembling adenomyomas, found in the uterus or in parauterine tissue.

adenomyosarcoma /ad′ənōmī′ōsärkō′mə/, *pl.* **adenomyosarcomas, adenomyosarcomata,** a malignant tumor of soft tissue containing glandular elements and striated muscle. A kind of adenomyosarcoma is **Wilms' tumor.**

adenomyosis /ad′ənōmī·ō′sis/, **1.** a benign neoplastic condition characterized by tumors composed of glandular tissue and smooth muscle cells. **2.** a malignant neoplastic condition characterized by the invasive growth of uterine mucosa in the wall of the uterus or the oviducts. Also called **endometriosis.**

adenopathy /ad′ənop′əthē/, an enlargement of any gland, especially a lymphatic gland. **–adenopathic,** *adj.*

adenosarcoma /ad′ənōsärkō′mə/, *pl.* **adenosarcomas, adenosarcomata,** a malignant glandular tumor of the soft tissues of the body.

adenosarcorhabdomyoma /ad′ənōsär′kōrab′dōmī-ō′mə/, *pl.* **adenosarcorhabdomyomas, adenosarcorhabdomyomata,** a tumor composed of glandular, connective tissue, and striated muscle elements.

adenosine /əden′əsin, -sēn/, a compound derived from nucleic acid, composed of adenine and a sugar, D-ribose. Adenosine is the major molecular component of the nucleotides adenosine monophosphate, adenosine diphosphate, and adenosine triphosphate, and of the nucleic acids deoxyribonucleic acid and ribonucleic acid. Also called **adenine-D-ribose.** See also **adenosine phosphate.**

adenosine deaminase /dē·am′inās,/ an enzyme that catalyzes the conversion of adenosine to the nucleoside inosine through the removal of an amino group. See also **adenosine.**

adenosine diphosphate, a product of the hydrolysis of adenosine triphosphate.

adenosine hydrolase, an enzyme that catalyzes the conversion of adenosine into adenine and ribose.

adenosine kinase, an enzyme in the liver and kidney that catalyzes the transfer of a phosphate group from adenosine triphosphate to produce adenosine phosphate.

adenosine monophosphate (AMP), an ester, composed of adenine, D-ribose, and phosphoric acid, that affects energy release in work done by a muscle. Also called **adenylic acid.**

adenosine phosphate, a compound consisting of the nucleotide adenosine attached through its ribose group to one, two, or three phosphoric acid molecules. Kinds of adenosine phosphate, all of which are interconvertible, are **adenosine diphosphate, adenosine monophosphate,** and **adenosine triphosphate.**

adenosine 3′:5′-cyclic phosphate. See **cyclic adenosine monophosphate.**

adenosine triphosphatase (ATPase), an enzyme in skeletal muscle that catalyzes the hydrolysis of adenosine triphosphate to adenosine diphosphate and inorganic phosphate. Among various enzymes in this group associated with cell membranes and intracellular structures, mitochondrial ATPase is involved in obtaining energy for cellular metabolism, and myosin ATPase is involved in muscle contraction.

adenosine triphosphate (ATP), a compound consisting of the nucleotide adenosine attached through its ribose group to three phosphoric acid molecules. It serves to store energy in muscles, which is released when it is hydrolized to adenosine diphosphate.

adenosis /ad′ənō′sis/, **1.** a disease in any gland, especially a lymphatic gland. **2.** an abnormal development or enlargement of glandular tissue.

adenovirus /ad′ənōvī′rəs/, any one of the 33 medium-sized viruses of the Adenoviridae family, pathogenic to humans, that cause conjunctivitis, upper respiratory infection, or GI infection. After the acute and symptomatic period of illness, the virus may persist in a latent stage in the tonsils, adenoids, and other lymphoid tissue. Compare **rhinovirus.** **–adenoviral,** *adj.*

adenylate /əden′ilāt/, a salt or ester of adenylic acid.

adenylate kinase, an enzyme in skeletal muscle that makes possible the reaction ATP + AMP = 2ADP. Also called **myokinase.**

adenylic acid. See **adenosine monophosphate.**

adequate and well-controlled studies, clinical and laboratory studies that the sponsors of a new drug are required by law to conduct to demonstrate the truth of the claims made for its effectiveness.

adermia /ədur′mē·ə/, a congenital or acquired skin defect or the absence of skin.

ADH, abbreviation for **antidiuretic hormone.**

adhere, to stick together or become fastened together, as two surfaces.

adherence, **1.** the quality of clinging or being closely attached. **2.** the process in which a person follows rules, guidelines, or standards, especially as a patient follows prescription and recommendations for a regimen of care.

adhesion /adhē′zhən/, a band of scar tissue that binds together two anatomic surfaces that are normally separate from each other. Adhesions are most commonly found in the abdomen where they form after abdominal surgery, inflammation, or injury. A loop of intestine may adhere to unhealed areas and cause an intestinal obstruction if scar tissue develops and constricts the lumen of the bowel, blocking the intestinal flow. The condition is characterized by abdominal pain, nausea and vomiting, distention, and an increase in pulse rate without a rise in temperature. Nasogastric intubation and suction may relieve the blockage. If not, surgery may be necessary. See also **adhesiotomy, intestinal obstruction.**

adhesiotomy /adhē′sē·ot′əmē/, the surgical dividing or separating of adhesions, usually performed to relieve an intestinal obstruction. See also **abdominal surgery.**

adhesive absorbent dressing, an absorbent dressing on an adhesive backing.

adhesive pericarditis, a condition characterized by adhesions between the visceral and the parietal layers of the pericardium or by adhesions between the pericardium and the mediastinum, diaphragm, or chest wall. Adhesions between the pericardial layers may completely obstruct the pericardial cavity. Adhesive pericarditis may seriously impair normal movements of the heart.

adhesive peritonitis, an inflammation of the peritoneum, characterized by adhesions between adjacent serous surfaces. This condition may be marked by exudations of serum, fibrin, cells, and pus, accompanied by abdominal pain and tenderness, vomiting, constipation, and fever.

adhesive plaster, a strong fabric material covered on one side with an adhesive. Often water-repellent, it may be used to hold bandages and dressings in place, to immobilize a part, or to exert pressure. Also called **adhesive tape.**

adhesive pleurisy, inflammation of the pleura with exudation, causing obliteration of the pleural space through the fusion of the visceral pleural layer covering the lungs and the parietal layer lining the walls of the thoracic cavity.

adhesive skin traction, one of two kinds of skin traction in which the therapeutic pull of traction weights is applied with adhesive straps that stick to the skin over the body structure involved, especially a fractured bone. Adhesive skin traction is used only when continuous traction is desired and skin care for the affected area presents no serious problem. The adhesive straps used to secure the traction system to the body area involved spread the pull over a wide plot of skin, decreasing the vulnerability of the patient to skin breakdown. Compare **nonadhesive skin traction.**

ADI, abbreviation for **acceptable daily intake.**

adiathermance /a′dī·əthur′məns/, the quality of being unaffected by radiated heat.

adient /ad′ē·ənt/, characterized by a tendency to move toward rather than away from stimuli. Compare **abient.** **–adience,** *n.*

Adie's pupil /ā′dēz/, an abnormal condition of the eyes marked by one pupil that reacts much more slowly to light changes or accommodation or convergence than the pupil of the other eye. There is no specific therapy for the condition, which is considered a pupillary muscle problem. Also called **tonic pupil.**

Adie's syndrome, the condition of Adie's pupil accompanied by depressed or absent tendon reflexes, particularly the ankle and knee-jerk reflexes. Also called **Adie-Holmes syndrome, Weill's syndrome.** See **Adie's pupil.**

adip-. See **adipo-.**

adipectomy. See **lipectomy.**

adiphenine hydrochloride /ədif′ənin/, an anticholinergic with smooth muscle relaxant properties that has been used for spastic disorders of the GI and genitourinary tract.

adipic /ədip′ik/, of or pertaining to fatty tissue.

adipo-, adip-, a combining form meaning 'pertaining to fat': *adipocele, adipogenesis, adipokinin.*

adipocele /ad′ipōsēl′/, a hernia containing fat or fatty tissue. Also called **lipocele.**

adipofibroma /ad′ipōfībrō′mə/, *pl.* **adipofibromas, adipofibromata,** a fibrous neoplasm of the connective tissue in which there are fatty components.

adiponecrosis /ad′ipōnikrō′sis/, a necrosis of fatty tissue in the body. **–adiponecrotic,** *adj.*

adiponecrosis subcutanea neonatorum, an abnormal dermatologic condition of the newborn characterized by patchy areas of hardened subcutaneous fatty tissue and a bluish-red discoloration of the overlying skin. The lesions, often a result of manipulation during delivery, spontaneously resolve within a period of days to several weeks without scarring. Also called **pseudosclerema, subcutaneous fat necrosis.**

adipose /ad′ipōs/, fatty. Adipose tissue is composed of fat cells arranged in lobules. See also **fat, fatty acid, lipoma.**

adipose tumor. See **lipoma.**

adiposogenital dystrophy /ad′ipō′sōjen′itəl/, a disorder occurring in adolescent boys, characterized by genital hypoplasia and feminine secondary sex characteristics, including female distribution of fat. It is caused by hypothalamic malfunction or by a tumor in the anterior pituitary gland. A subnormal body temperature, low blood pressure, and reduced blood glucose are frequently associated with the disorder. Diabetes insipidus often occurs because of hyposecretion of antidiuretic hormone, and involvement of the hypothalamic satiety center may induce overeating and result in pronounced obesity. If a tumor is present, there may be drowsiness and symptoms of increased intracranial pressure. Treatment may include the administration of testosterone and a weight reduction program, excision or radiologic ablation of a tumor, and replacement of hormones, as necessary. Also called **adiposogenital syndrome, Fröhlich's syndrome.**

adipsia, absence of thirst.

aditus /ad′itəs/, an approach or an entry.

adjunct, (in health care) an additional substance, treatment, or procedure used for increasing the efficacy or safety of the primary substance, treatment, or procedure or to facilitate its performance. **–adjunctive,** *adj.*

adjunctive psychotherapy, a form of psychotherapy that concentrates on improving a person's general mental and physical outlook without trying to resolve basic emotional problems. Some kinds of adjunctive psychotherapy are **music therapy, occupational therapy, physical therapy,** and **recreational therapy.**

adjunct to anesthesia, one of a number of drugs of five different classes. Each class of drug has a use in anesthetic procedures, as well as a therapeutic indication in other aspects of health care. Adjuncts to anesthesia are used as premedications, as intravenous supplements to hypnotic or analgesic medications, and as neuromuscular blocking agents, analeptics, and therapeutic gases. Premedications are given to reduce anxiety, sedate the patient, reduce salivation and secretions of the respiratory passages, and prevent bradycardia. Strong analgesics, sedatives and hypnotics, phenothiazenes, anticholinergics, and antianxiety agents are also sometimes prescribed as premedications. Intravenous hypnotic and analgesic supplements given to augment the effects of nitrous oxide include morphine, meperidine, diazepam, fentanyl, and droperidol. Neuromuscular blocking agents are given to produce and sustain relaxation of the skeletal muscles during the surgical procedure. These agents are of two kinds: depolarizing or nondepolarizing. Depolarizing agents (including succinylcholine) act by depolarizing the postsynaptic membranes, rendering them refractory to stimulation and producing muscle paralysis. Nondepolarizing agents (including tubocurarine, metocurine, gallamine, and pancuronium) act by competing with acetylcholine for receptor sites on the postjunctional receptor sites, producing paralysis of the muscles. The use of these agents usually requires assisted or controlled respiration by an anesthetist or anesthesiologist and a careful evaluation of the recovery of neuromuscular transmission in the postoperative period. Analeptics may be administered to stimulate the function of the central nervous system in ventilatory insufficiency caused by drug overdose, drowning, electric shock, carbon monoxide poisoning, or other conditions resulting in hypoxemia. The effects of these agents are transitory and may paradoxically result in further depression; therefore, they are not usually recommended. Therapeutic gases include carbon dioxide and oxygen and various general anesthetics. Carbon dioxide and oxygen are given to maintain normal respiratory metabolism and function and as vehicles to carry anesthetic gases.

adjustable orthodontic band, a thin metal ring, usually made of stainless steel, equipped with an adjusting screw to allow alteration in size, fitted to a tooth and serving for the attachment of orthodontic appliances. See also **orthodontic band.**

adjusted death rate. See **standardized death rate.**

adjustment. See **accommodation.**

adjustment reaction, a temporary disorder of varying severity that occurs as an acute reaction to overwhelming stress in persons of any age who have no apparent underlying mental disorders. Symptoms include anxiety, withdrawal, depression, brooding, temper outbursts, crying spells, attention-getting behavior, enuresis, loss of appetite, aches, pains, and muscle spasms. It can result from such situations as separation of an infant from its mother, the birth of a sibling, loss or change of a job, death of a loved one, or forced retirement. Symptoms usually recede and eventually disappear as stress diminishes. See also **neurotic disorder.**

adjuvant therapy /ad′jəvənt/, the treatment of a disease with substances that enhance the action of drugs, especially drugs that promote the production of antibodies.

ADL, abbreviation for **activities of daily living.**

ad lib, an abbreviation of the Latin phrase *ad libitum,* meaning to be taken as desired and sometimes used in pharmaceutic prescriptions.

administration of parenteral fluids, the intravenous infusion of various solutions to maintain adequate hydration, restore blood volume, reestablish lost electrolytes, or provide partial nutrition. See **parenteral.**

■ METHOD: Fluid is administered parenterally through a closed system consisting of a bottle of sterile solution, a catheter, and an attached intracatheter or scalp vein needle that is inserted into a peripheral vein and securely taped to the patient's arm or leg. The fluid is infused slowly. Five percent dextrose in distilled water may be used to maintain volume or restore blood volume; ascorbic acid and B vitamins are often added to the solution. Five percent dextrose in saline solution plus potassium chloride may be infused to reestablish electrolyte balance, but potassium is contraindicated in renal failure and untreated adrenal insufficiency. A one-sixth molar lactate solution may be administered if sodium is deficient, and an ammonium chloride solution may be administered when replacement of chloride is required. Distilled water containing 10% to 20% glucose or fructose may be used to supply carbohydrate, but, because these solutions are hypertonic, additional hydration is needed for proper excretion. Low molecular weight dextran is frequently used as a plasma volume expander in treating shock, but it increases bleeding time and is contraindicated in pregnancy and severe renal disease. During parenteral fluid administration, the venipuncture site is observed every 1 to 2 hours for signs of redness, swelling, warmth, and leakage; for the security and comfort of the tape; and for the position of the patient's extremity. The flow rate, the level, color, and clarity of the fluid, the label, and the patency of the tubing are checked, and the patient is monitored for signs of dehydration, fever, and signs of circulatory overload, as headache, tachycardia, elevated blood pressure, dyspnea, engorged neck veins, and pulmonary edema.

■ NURSING ORDERS: Depending on the service, the nurse may select the necessary equipment, prepare the venipuncture site, check the labels of fluid bottles for content, and perform the venipuncture. During the administration of fluid, the nurse keeps the system closed, watches the flow rate, records the amount of solution given, and observes the venipuncture site and the patient's general condition. If there are any signs of increased blood volume, the nurse reduces the flow of the infusion until further orders are obtained. The nurse changes the dressing daily and ensures that the patient understands the importance of keeping the extremity still, of not disturbing the tubing, and of reporting pain or swelling.

■ OUTCOME CRITERIA: Parenteral fluid therapy is usually uneventful, but infants, elderly patients with circulatory or renal impairment, and burn patients, whose plasma may shift suddenly from interstitial tissue, causing increased blood volume, require special attention.

adnexa, *sing.* **adnexus,** tissue or structures in the body that are next to or near another, related structure. The ovaries and the uterine tubes are adnexa of the uterus. – **adnexal,** *adj.*

adnexitis, an inflammation of the adnexal organs of the uterus, such as the ovaries or the fallopian tubes.

adolescence, **1.** the period in development between the onset of puberty and adulthood. It usually begins between 11 and 13 years of age, with the appearance of secondary sex characteristics, and spans the teen years, terminating at 18 to 20 years of age with the acquisition of completely developed adult form. During this period the individual undergoes extensive physical, psychologic, emotional, and personality changes. **2.** the state or quality of being adolescent or youthful. See also **postpuberty, prepuberty, psychosexual development, psychosocial development, pubarche.**

adolescent, **1.** of, pertaining to, or characteristic of adolescence. **2.** one in the state or process of adolescence; a teenager.

adolescent vertebral epiphysitis. See **Scheuermann's disease.**

ADP, abbreviation for **adenosine diphosphate.**

adrenal cortex, the greater portion of the adrenal or suprarenal gland, fused with the gland's medulla and producing mineralocorticoids, androgens, and glucocorticoids, hormones essential to homeostasis. The outer cortex is normally a deep yellow; the inner part, dark red or brown. It is recognizable in the embryo during the sixth week as a groove in the coelom at the base of the mesentery near the cranial end of the mesonephros.

adrenal cortical carcinoma, a malignant neoplasm of the adrenal cortex that may cause adrenogenital syndrome or Cushing's syndrome. Such tumors vary in size, occur at any age, and are more common in females than in males. Metastases frequently spread the cancer to the lungs, liver, and other organs. See also **adrenogenital syndrome, Cushing's syndrome.**

adrenal crisis, an acute, life-threatening state of profound adrenocortical insufficiency in which immediate therapy is required. It is characterized by glucocorticoid deficiency, a drop in extracellular fluid volume, and hyperkalemia. Also called **addisonian crisis, adrenergic crisis.** See also **Addison's disease, adrenal cortex.**

■ OBSERVATIONS: Typically, the patient appears to be in shock or coma with a low blood pressure, severe prostration, and loss of vasomotor tone. The person's medical history may include Addison's disease or reveal symptoms indicating its presence. Laboratory tests show hyperkalemia and hyponatremia.

■ INTERVENTION: An intravenous isotonic solution of sodium chloride containing a water-soluble glucocorticoid is administered rapidly. Vasopressor agents may be necessary to combat hypotension. If the patient is vomiting, a nasogastric tube is usually inserted. Total bed rest and the monitoring of blood pressure, temperature, and other vital signs are mandatory. After the first critical hours, the patient is followed as for Addison's disease, and steroid dosage is tapered to maintenance levels. In all cases the precipitating cause is sought. Infection and a failure to increase the maintenance dose are common causes of crisis in people who have Addison's disease. ■ NURSING CONSIDERATIONS: Nursing care during adrenal crisis includes eliminating all forms of stimuli, especially loud noises or bright lights. The patient is not moved unless absolutely necessary and is not allowed to perform self-care activities. If the condition is identified and treated promptly, the prognosis is good. Discharge instructions include a reminder to the patient to seek medical attention in any stressful situation, whether physiologic or psychologic, to prevent a recurrence of the crisis.

adrenalectomy /ədrē'nəlek'təmē/, the surgical removal of one or both adrenal glands or the resection of a portion of one or both glands, performed to reduce the excessive secretion of adrenal hormones when an adrenal tumor or a malignancy of the breast or prostate is present. The incision is made under the twelfth rib in the rear flank area with the patient under a general anesthetic. Preoperative laboratory tests include electrolytes, fasting blood glucose, and glucose tolerance. Corticosteroid drugs are given, and frequent blood-pressure measurements are recorded. Before surgery a nasogastric tube is inserted and a venous cutdown is done. Postoperative care focuses on monitoring vital signs and maintaining blood pressure with an IV solution containing a vasopressor and corticosteroids. An abrupt drop in blood pressure, increasing weakness, and a rise in temperature are signs of acute corticosteroid insufficiency. Blood electrolyte levels are checked frequently, and fluid intake and output are carefully recorded. Steroids are given by mouth a few days after surgery. When oral steroids can be tolerated, the dosage is tapered to a maintenance level; if both glands are removed, the maintenance dosage continues for life. Stress and fatigue must be avoided. See also **Addison's disease, Cushing's syndrome.**

adrenal gland, either of two secretory organs perched atop the kidneys. Each consists of two parts having independent functions: the cortex and the medulla. The adrenal cortex, in response to adrenocorticotropic hormone secreted by the anterior pituitary, secretes cortisol and androgens. Adrenal androgens serve as precursors that are converted by the liver to testosterone and estrogens. Renin from the kidney controls adrenal cortical production of aldosterone. The adrenal medulla manufactures the catecholamines epinephrine and norepinephrine.

Adrenalin, a trademark for an adrenergic (epinephrine).

adrenaline. See **epinephrine.**

adrenalize /ədrē'nəlīz/, to stimulate or excite.

adrenal medulla, the inner portion of the adrenal gland. Adrenal medulla cells secrete epinephrine and norepinephrine. See **adrenal cortex.**

adrenal virilism, the development in a female of male secondary sexual characteristics resulting from excessive production of androgenic hormones or to tumors of the ovary, as arrhenoblastoma, hilus cell tumor, or gynandroblastoma. See also **virilization.**

adrenarche /ad'rinär'kē/, the intensified activity in the adrenal cortex that occurs at about 8 years of age and increases the elaboration of various hormones, especially androgens.

adrenergic /ad'rinur'jik/, of or pertaining to sympathetic nerve fibers of the autonomic nervous system that use as neurotransmitters epinephrine or epinephrine-like substances. Compare **cholinergic.** See **sympathomimetic.**

adrenergic blocking agent. See **antiadrenergic.**

adrenergic drug. See **sympathomimetic.**

adrenergic fibers, nerve fibers of the autonomic nervous system that release the neurotransmitter norepinephrine and, in some areas, dopamine. Most postganglionic sympathetic fibers are of this type.

adrenergic receptor, a site in a sympathetic effector cell that reacts to adrenergic stimulation. Two types of adrenergic receptors are recognized: alpha-adrenergic receptors and beta-adrenergic receptors. In general, stimulation of alpha receptors is excitatory of the function of the host organ or tissue, and stimulation of the beta-receptors is inhibitory.

-adrenia, a combining form meaning '(degree or condition of) adrenal activity': *anadrenia, dysadrenia, hypadrenia.*

adrenocorticotropic /ədrē'nōkôr'tikōtrop'ik/, of or pertaining to stimulation of the adrenal cortex. Also **adrenocorticotrophic** /-trof'ik/.

adrenocorticotropic hormone (ACTH), a hormone of the anterior pituitary gland that stimulates the growth of the adrenal gland cortex and the secretion of corticosteroids. ACTH secretion, regulated by corticotropin releasing factor (CRF) from the hypothalamus, increases in response to a low level of circulating cortisol and to stress, fever, acute hypoglycemia, and major surgery. Under normal conditions there is a diurnal rhythm in ACTH secretion with an increase beginning after the first few hours of sleep and reaching a peak at the time a person awakens. ACTH stimulates the formation of cyclic adenosine monophosphate (AMP), which is thought to activate the enzyme system that catalyzes the conversion of cholesterol to pregnenolone, the precursor of all steroidal hormones. A purified preparation of ACTH in gelatin is widely used in the treatment of rheumatoid arthritis, acquired hemolytic anemia, intractable allergic states, various dermatologic diseases, and many other disorders. Also called **adrenocorticotrophic hormone, corticotropin.**

adrenodoxin /ədrē'nōdok'sin/, a protein, produced by the adrenal glands, that participates in the transfer of electrons within animal cells.

adrenogenitalism /ədrē'nōjen'itəliz'əm/, a condition characterized by hypersecretion of adrenocortical androgens, resulting in somatic masculinization. Excessive production of the hormone may be caused by a virilizing adrenal tumor, congenital adrenal hyperplasia, or an inborn deficiency of enzymes required to transform endogenous androgenic steroids to glucocorticoids. Girls born with adrenogenitalism may be pseudohermaphroditic with clitoral enlargement and labial fusion in infancy and later hirsutism, low vocal pitch, acne, amenorrhea, and masculine distribution of hair and development of muscles. Boys with congenital adrenogenitalism show precocious development of the penis and prostate and of pubic and axillary hair, but their testes remain small and immature because negative feedback from the high level of adrenal androgens prevents the normal pubertal increase in pituitary gonadotropin. Children with the disorder are unusually tall, but their epiphyses close prematurely and as adults they are abnormally short. Virilizing tumors are more common or more frequently diagnosed in women. They usually occur between 30 and 40 years of age but may arise later, after the menopause. Signs of the tumor in women include hirsutism, amenorrhea, oily skin, ovarian changes, muscular hypertrophy, and atrophy of the uterus and breasts. Treatment may involve tumor resection, administration of cortisol, and plastic surgical procedures. Electrolytic epilation may be indicated. Also called **adrenal virilism, adrenogenital syndrome.** See also **pseudohermaphroditism.**

adrenoleukodystrophy (ALD), a rare, hereditary childhood metabolic disease that is transmitted as a recessive sex-linked trait and that affects only boys. It is characterized by adrenal atrophy and widespread cerebral demyelination, producing progressive mental deterioration, aphasia, apraxia, and eventual blindness. Prognosis is poor, with death occurring usually in 1 to 5 years. ALD was formerly classified under Schilder's disease.

Adriamycin. See **doxorubicin hydrochloride.**

adromia /ədrō'mē·ə/, the absence of the conductive capacity of any nerve that normally innervates a muscle.

ADT, abbreviation for *Accepted Dental Therapeutics,* a journal published by the Council on Dental Therapeutics of the American Dental Association.

adult, **1.** one who is fully developed and matured and who has attained the intellectual capacity and the emotional and psychologic stability characteristic of a mature person. **2.** a person who has reached full legal age. Compare **child.**

adult celiac disease. See **celiac disease.**

adult day-care center, a facility for the supervised care of older adults, providing such activities as meals and socialization, during specified day hours, with the participants returning to their homes each evening.

adulteration, the debasement or dilution of the purity of any substance, process, or activity by the addition of extraneous material.

adult hemoglobin. See **hemoglobin A.**

adulthood, the phase of development characterized by physical and mental maturity.

adult nurse practioner, a registered nurse who has received additional education and training in the primary health care of adults. The additional education may be obtained through a master's degree program or a nondegree continuing education certificate program.

adult-onset diabetes. See **non-insulin-dependent diabetes.**

adult polycystic disease. See **polycystic kidney disease.**

adult respiratory distress syndrome. See **acute respiratory distress syndrome.**

adult rickets, a disease affecting adults that resembles rickets. See also **osteomalacia, rickets.**

advanced life support. See **Emergency Medical Technician-Advanced Life Support.**

adventitious /ad'ventish'əs/, of or pertaining to an accidental condition or an arbitrary action.

adventitious bursa, an abnormal bursa that develops as a response to friction or pressure.

adverse drug effect, a harmful, unintended reaction to a drug administered at normal dosage.

adynamia /ad'inā'mē·ə/, lack of physical and emotional drive because of a pathologic condition. A kind of adynamia is **adynamia episodica hereditaria.** See also **asthenia.** **–adynamic,** *adj.*

adynamia episodica hereditaria, a condition seen in infancy, characterized by muscle weakness and episodes of flaccid paralysis. It is inherited as an autosomal dominant trait. Also called **hyperkalemic periodic paralysis.**

adynamic fever, an elevated temperature with a feeble pulse, nervous depression, and a cool, moist skin. Also called **asthenic fever.**

adynamic ileus. See **ileus.**

Aedes /ā·ē'dēz/, a genus of mosquito, prevalent in tropical and subtropical regions. Several species are capable of transmitting pathogenic organisms to humans, including dengue, equine enephalitis, St. Louis encephalitis, tularemia, and yellow fever.

aer-. See **aero-.**

aerate /er'āt/, to charge a substance or a structure with air, carbon dioxide, or oxygen.

aero-, aer-, a combining form meaning 'pertaining to air or to gas': *aerobe, aerocystography, aerodontalgia.*

Aerobacter aerogenes. See ***Enterobacter cloacae.***

aerobe /er'ōb/, a microorganism that lives and grows in the presence of free oxygen. Kinds of aerobe are **facultative aerobe** and **obligate aerobe.** Compare **anaerobe, microaerophile.**

aerobic /erō'bik/, **1.** of or pertaining to the presence of air or oxygen. **2.** able to live and function in the presence of free oxygen. **3.** requiring oxygen for the maintenance of life. **4.** of or pertaining to aerobic exercise.

aerobic exercise, any physical exercise that requires additional effort by the heart and lungs to meet the increased demand by the skeletal muscles for oxygen.

The exercise generally requires heavier breathing than passive muscular activity and results in increased heart and lung efficiency with a minimum of wasted energy. Examples of aerobic exercise include running, jogging, swimming, and vigorous dancing or cycling. Also called **aerobics.** See also **active exercise, passive exercise.**

aerobic glycolysis. See **glycolysis.**

aerobics. See **aerobic exercise.**

aerodontalgia /er′ōdontal′jə/, a painful sensation in the teeth because of decreased atmospheric pressure, as may occur at high altitudes.

aeroembolism. See **embolism.**

aerophagy /erof′əjē/, the swallowing of air, usually followed by belching, gastric distress, and flatulence. Also called **aerophagia** /er′ōfā′jē·ə/.

aerosinusitis /er′ōsī′nəsī′tis/, inflammation, edema, or hemorrhage of the frontal sinuses, caused by expansion of air within the sinuses when barometric pressure is decreased, as in aircraft at high altitudes. Also called **barosinusitis.**

aerosol /er′əsol′/, **1.** nebulized particles suspended in a gas or air. **2.** a pressurized gas containing a finely nebulized medication for inhalation therapy. **3.** a pressurized gas containing a nebulized chemical agent for sterilizing the air of a room.

Aerosporin, a trademark for an antibiotic (polymyxin B sulfate).

aerotitis /er′ətī′tis/, an inflammation of the ear caused by changes in atmospheric pressure. Also called **barotitis.**

aerotitis media, inflammation or bleeding in the middle ear caused by a difference between the air pressure in the middle ear and that of the atmosphere, as occurs in sudden changes in altitude, in diving, or in hyperbaric chambers. Symptoms are pain, tinnitus, diminished hearing, and vertigo. Also called **barotitis media.**

Æsculapius /es′kyo͞olā′pē·əs/, the ancient Greek god of medicine. According to legend, Æsculapius, the son of Apollo, was trained by the centaur Chiron in the art of healing, becoming so proficient that he not only cured sick patients but also brought the dead back to life. Because Zeus feared that Æsculapius could help humans escape death altogether, he killed the healer with a bolt of lightning. Later, Æsculapius was raised to the stature of a god and was worshiped also by the Romans, who believed he could prevent pestilence. Serpents were regarded as sacred by Æsculapius, and he is symbolized in modern medicine by a staff with a serpent entwined about it.

-aesthesia, -esthesia, a combining form meaning '(condition of) feeling, perception, or sensation': *allaesthesia, cinaesthesia, hypercrysaesthesia*.

-aesthetic. See **-esthetic.**

AF, abbreviation for **atrial fibrillation.**

af-. See **ad-.**

AFB, abbreviation for **acid-fast bacillus.**

afebrile /āfē′bril, āfeb′ril/, without fever.

affect, an outward manifestation of a person's feelings or emotions. **–affective,** *adj.*

affective disorder. See **major affective disorder.**

affective melancholia, *obsolete*. the depressive phase of bipolar disorder. See also **depression.**

affect memory, a particular emotional feeling that recurs whenever a significant experience is recalled.

afferent /af′ərənt/, proceeding toward a center, as applied to arteries, veins, lymphatics, and nerves. Compare **efferent.**

affidavit /af′idā′vit/, a written statement that is sworn to before a notary public or an officer of the court.

affiliated hospital, a hospital that is associated to some degree with a medical school or health program.

affinity, the measure of the binding strength of the antibody-antigen reaction.

affirmative defense, (in law) a denial of guilt or wrongdoing based on new evidence rather than on simple denial of a charge, as a plea of immunity according to a good samaritan law. The defendant bears the burden of proof in an affirmative defense.

afibrinogenemia /afī′brinōjenē′mē·ə/, a rare, hematologic disorder characterized by a relative lack or absence of fibrinogen in the blood. It may be the result of a primary, congenital blood dyscrasia, or it may be acquired, as in disseminated intravascular coagulation.

aflatoxins, a group of carcinogenic and toxic factors produced by *Aspergillus flavus* food molds. The mucotoxins have been found to cause liver necrosis and liver cancer in laboratory animals and are believed to be responsible for a high incidence of liver cancer among people in tropic regions of Africa and Asia who may consume moldy grains, peanuts, or other *Aspergillus* contaminated foods. See ***Aspergillus***.

AFP, an abbreviation for **alpha fetoprotein.**

Afrazine, a trademark for a decongestant (oxymetazoline hydrochloride).

African lymphoma. See **Burkitt's lymphoma.**

African sleeping sickness. See **African trypanosomiasis.**

African tick fever. See **relapsing fever.**

African trypanosomiasis, a disease caused by the parasites *Trypanosoma brucei gambiense* or *Trypanosoma brucei rhodesiense,* transmitted to humans by the bite of the tsetse fly. African trypanosomiasis occurs only in the tropical areas of Africa, where tsetse flies are found. The disease progresses through three phases: localized, at the site of invasion of the organism; systemic, marked by fever, chills, headache, anemia, edema of the hands and feet, and enlargement of the lymph glands; and neurologic, marked by symptoms of central nervous system involvement, including lethargy, sleepiness, headache, convulsions, and coma. The disease is fatal unless treated, though it may be years before the patient reaches the neurologic phase. Antimicrobial medication specific for the treatment of trypanosomiasis is available in the United States only from the Centers for Disease Control. Kinds of African trypanosomiasis are **Gambian try-**

panosomiasis and **Rhodesian trypanosomiasis.** Also called **African sleeping sickness, sleeping sickness.** See also **trypanosomiasis, tsetse fly.**

Afrin, a trademark for an adrenergic vasoconstrictor (oxymetazoline hydrochloride), used as a decongestant.

afterbirth, the placenta, the amnion and the chorion, and some amniotic fluid, blood, and blood clots expelled from the uterus after childbirth.

aftercare, health care offered a patient after discharge from a hospital or other medical facility. The patient may require a certain amount of medical or nursing attention for a health problem that no longer demands inpatient status.

afterdepolarization, a slow channel depolarization that follows in the wake of an action potential. It is thought to be responsible for atrial and ventricular ectopic beats, especially in the setting of digitalis toxicity.

afterload, the load, or resistance, against which the left ventricle must eject its volume of blood during contraction. The resistance is produced by the volume of blood already in the vascular system and the vessel walls. About 90% of the oxygen required by the heart muscle is consumed in the afterload effort.

afterloading, (in radiotherapy) a technique in which an unloaded applicator or needle is placed within the patient at the time of an operative procedure and subsequently loaded with the radioactive source under controlled conditions in which health care personnel are protected against exposure to radiation. A kind of afterloading is **remote afterloading.**

afterpains, contractions of the uterus common during the first days postpartum. They tend to be strongest in nursing mothers and multiparas, resolve spontaneously, and may require analgesia. The nurse may reassure the mother that afterpains are normal and prove that the uterus is contracting as it should.

Ag, symbol for **silver.**

ag-. See **ad-.**

AGA, abbreviation for **appropriate for gestational age.**

agalactia, the failure of the mother to secrete enough milk to breast-feed an infant after childbirth.

agamete /āgam′ēt/, **1.** any of the unicellular organisms that reproduce asexually by multiple fission, such as bacteria and protozoa. **2.** any asexual reproductive cell, as a spore or merozoite, that forms a new organism without fusion with another cell.

agametic /āgəmē′tik/, asexual; without recognizable sex organs or gametes. Also **agamous** /ag′əməs/.

agamic /āgam′ik/, reproducing asexually, without the union of gametes; asexual.

agammaglobulinemia /agam′əglob′yo͞olinē′mē·ə/, a rare disorder characterized by the absence of the serum immunoglobulin, gamma globulin, associated with an increased susceptibility to infection. The condition may be transient, congenital, or acquired. The transient form is common in infancy before 6 weeks of age when the infant becomes able to synthesize the immunoglobulin. The congenital form is rare, sex-linked, and results in decreased production of antibodies. The acquired form usually occurs in association with a malignant disease such as leukemia, myeloma, or lymphoma. See also **Bruton's agammaglobulinemia, immune gamma globulin.**

agamogenesis /əgam′ōjen′əsis/, asexual reproduction, as by budding or simple fission of cells; parthenogenesis. Also called **agamocytogeny** /əgam′ōsītoj′ənē/, **agamogony** /ag′əmog′ənē/. **–agamocytogenic, agamogenetic, agamogenic, agamogonic** *adj.*

agamont. See **schizont.**

agamous. See **agametic.**

aganglionic megacolon. See **Hirschsprung's disease.**

agar-agar /a′gära′gär/, a dried hydrophilic, colloidal product obtained from certain species of red algae. Because it is unaffected by bacterial enzymes, it is widely used as the basic ingredient in solid culture media in bacteriology. Agar-agar is also used as a suspending medium, as an emulsifying agent, and as a bulk laxative. Also called **agar.**

agency, (in law) a relationship between two parties in which one authorizes the other to act in his behalf as his agent. It usually implies a contractual arrangement between two parties managed by a third party, the agent.

agenesia corticalis, the failure of the cortical cells of the brain, especially the pyramidal cells, to develop in the embryo, resulting in infantile cerebral paralysis and severe mental retardation.

agenesis /ājen′əsis/, **1.** congenital absence of an organ or part, usually caused by a lack of primordial tissue and failure of development in the embryo. **2.** impotence or sterility. Also called **agenesia** /ā′jinē′zhə/. Compare **dysgenesis.** **–agenic,** *adj.*

agenetic fracture, a spontaneous fracture caused by an imperfect osteogenesis.

ageniocephaly /ājen′ē·ōsef′əlē/, a form of otocephaly in which the brain, cranial vault, and sense organs are intact but the lower jaw is malformed. Also called **ageniocephalia** /ājen′ē·ōsəfā′lē·ə/. **–ageniocephalic, ageniocephalous,** *adj.*

agenitalism /ājen′itəliz′əm/, a condition caused by the lack of sex hormones and the absence or malfunction of the ovaries or testes.

agenosomia /əjen′əsō′mē·ə/, a congenital malformation characterized by the absence or defective formation of the genitals and protrusion of the intestines through an incompletely developed abdominal wall.

agenosomus /əjen′əsō′məs/, a fetus with agenosomia.

agent, (in law) a party authorized to act on behalf of another and to give the other an account of such actions.

Agent Orange, a U.S. military code name for a mixture of two herbicides, 2,4-D and 2,4,5-T, used as a defoliant in Southeast Asia during the 1960s war in Vietnam. The herbicides were unintentionally contaminated with the highly toxic chemical dioxin, a cause of cancer and birth defects in animals and of chloracne and porphyria cutanea tarda in humans. See **dioxin.**

age of majority, the age at which a person is considered to be an adult in the eyes of the law.

agglutination /əgloo͞′tinā′shən/, the aggregation or clumping together of cells as a result of their interaction with specific antibodies called agglutinins, commonly used in blood typing and in identifying or estimating the strength of immunoglobulins or immune sera. See also **agglutinin, blood typing, precipitin.**

agglutination-inhibition test, a serologic technique useful in testing for certain unknown soluble antigens. The unknown antigen is mixed with a known agglutinin. If there is a reaction, the agglutinin can no longer agglutinate the cells or particles that carry its corresponding antigen, and the unknown antigen is thus identified. One type of pregnancy test is based on agglutination inhibition.

agglutinin /əgloo͞′tinin/, a specific kind of antibody whose interaction with antigens is manifested as agglutination. Usually multivalent, agglutinins act on insoluble antigens in stable suspension to form a cross-linking lattice that may clump or precipitate. Compare **precipitin.** See also **agglutination, blood typing, hemagglutination.**

agglutinin absorption, the removal from immune serum of antibody by treatment with homologous antigen, followed by centrifugation and separation of the antigen-antibody complex.

agglutinogen /ag′loo͞tin′əjin/, any antigenic substance that causes agglutination by the production of agglutinin.

aggregate anaphylaxis, an exaggerated reaction of hypersensitivity rapidly induced by the injection of an antigen that forms a soluble antigen-antibody complex.

aggression, a forceful, self-assertive action or attitude that is expressed physically, verbally, or symbolically. It may arise from innate drives or occur as a defensive mechanism and is manifested by either constructive or destructive acts directed toward oneself or against others. Kinds of aggression are **constructive aggression, destructive aggression,** and **inward aggression.**

aggressive personality, a personality with behavior patterns characterized by irritability, tantrums, destructiveness, or violence in response to frustration.

aging, the process of growing old, resulting in part from a failure of body cells to function normally or to produce new body cells to replace those that are dead or malfunctioning. Normal cell function may be lost through infectious disease, malnutrition, exposure to environmental hazards, or genetic influences. Among body cells that exhibit early signs of aging are those that normally cease dividing after reaching maturity. See also **assessment of the aging patient, senile.**

agitated, describing a condition of psychomotor excitement characterized by purposeless, restless activity. Pacing, crying, and laughing without apparent cause are often seen and may serve to release nervous tension associated with anxiety, fear, or other mental stress. **–agitate,** *v.*, **agitation,** *n.*

agitated depression, a form of depression characterized by severe anxiety accompanied by continuous physical restlessness. See also **depression.**

agitographia /aj′itōgraf′ē·ə/, a condition characterized by abnormally rapid writing in which words or parts of words are unconsciously omitted. The condition is commonly associated with agitophasia.

agitophasia /aj′itōfā′zhə/, a condition characterized by abnormally rapid speech in which words, sounds, or syllables are unconsciously omitted, slurred, or distorted. The condition is commonly associated with agitographia. Also called **agitolalia.**

agnathia /ag·nath′ē·ə/, a developmental defect characterized by total or partial absence of the lower jaw. It is usually accompanied by the union or approximation of the ears. Also called **agnathy** /ag′nəthē/. Compare **synotia.** See also **otocephaly.** **–agnathous,** *adj.*

agnathocephalus /ag·nath′əsef′ələs/, a fetus with agnathocephaly.

agnathocephaly /ag·nath′əsef′əlē/, a congenital malformation characterized by the absence of the lower jaw, defective formation of the mouth, and placement of the eyes low on the face with fusion or approximation of the zygomas and the ears. Also called **agnathocephalia.** See also **otocephaly.** **–agnathocephalic, agnathocephalous,** *adj.*

agnathus /ag·nath′əs/, a fetus with agnathia.

agnathy. See **agnathia.**

agnogenic myeloid metaplasia. See **myeloid metaplasia.**

agnosia /ag·nō′zhə/, total or partial loss of the ability to recognize familiar objects or persons through sensory stimuli as a result of organic brain damage. The condition may affect any of the senses and is classified accordingly as auditory, visual, olfactory, gustatory, or tactile agnosia. Also called **agnosis.** See also **autotopagnosia.**

-agnosia, -agnosis a combining form meaning '(condition of the) loss of the faculty to perceive': *autotopagnosia, fingeragnosia, paragnosia.*

-agogue, -agog, a combining form meaning an 'agent promoting the expulsion of a (specified) substance': *lymphagogue, succagogue, uragogue.*

agonal respiration /ag′ənəl/, a type of breathing that usually follows a pattern of gasping succeeded by apnea. It generally indicates the onset of respiratory arrest.

agonal thrombus, an aggregation of blood platelets, fibrin, clotting factors, and cellular elements that forms in the heart in the process of dying.

agonist /ag′ənist/, **1.** a contracting muscle whose contraction is opposed by another muscle (an antagonist). **2.** a drug or other substance having a specific cellular affinity that produces a predictable response.

agoraphobia /ag′ərə-/, an anxiety disorder characterized by a fear of being in an open, crowded, or public place, as a field, tunnel, bridge, congested street, or busy department store, where escape may be difficult or help not available in case of sudden incapacitation. The obsessive phenomenon is observed more often in women than in men and generally can be traced to some sudden loss or separation occurring in childhood. Treatment consists of psychotherapy to uncover the cause of the phobic reaction followed by behavior therapy, specifically the systemic desensitization and flooding techniques for reducing the anxiety and altering the behavioral response. If untreated, fear and avoidance behavior dominate life, and the person refuses to leave home.

-agra, a combining form meaning a 'pain or painful seizure': *cardiagra, podagra, trachelagra.*

agranular endoplasmic reticulum. See **endoplasmic reticulum.**

agranulocyte /āgran′yo͞olōsīt′/, any leukocyte that does not contain cytoplasmic granules, as a monocyte or lymphocyte. Compare **granulocyte.** See also **leukocyte.**

agranulocytosis /āgran′yo͞olōsītō′sis/, an abnormal condition of the blood, characterized by a severe reduction in the number of granulocytes (basophils, eosinophils, and neutrophils), resulting in fever, prostration, and bleeding ulcers of the rectum, mouth, and vagina. It is an acute disease and may be an adverse reaction to a medication or the result of radiation therapy.

agraphia /āgraf′ē·ə/, an abnormal neurologic condition characterized by loss of the ability to write, resulting from injury to the language center in the cerebral cortex. Compare **dysgraphia.** –**agraphic,** *adj.*

A:G ratio, the ratio of protein albumin to globulin in the blood serum. On the basis of differential solubility with neutral salt solution the normal values are 3.5 to 5 g/dl for albumin and 2.5 to 4 g/dl for globulin.

agrypnia. See **insomnia.**

agrypnotic /ag′ripnot′ik/, **1.** insomniac. **2.** a drug or other substance that prevents sleep.

AHA, abbreviation for **American Hospital Association.**

"aha" reaction /ähä′/, (in psychology) a sudden realization or inspiration, experienced especially during creative thinking. Some psychologists associate great scientific discoveries and artistic inspirations with this reaction, which is not necessarily related to intelligence. The term has apparently replaced **"aha" experience,** formerly used by psychologists, especially those of the Gestalt school, to label experiences in which an individual utters "Aha!" during a moment of revelation.

AHF, abbreviation for **antihemophilic factor.**

AHH, abbreviation for **aryl hydrocarbon hydroxylase.**

AI, abbreviation for **artificial intelligence.**

AID, abbreviation for **artificial insemination-donor.**

AIDS /ādz/, abbreviation for **acquired immune deficiency syndrome.**

AIH, abbreviation for **artificial insemination-husband.**

air, the colorless, odorless gaseous mixture constituting the earth's atmosphere. It consists of 78% nitrogen, 21% oxygen, almost 1% argon, small amounts of carbon dioxide, hydrogen, and ozone, traces of helium, krypton, neon, and xenon, and varying amounts of water vapor.

air bath, the exposure of the naked body to warm air for therapeutic purposes. Also called **balneum pneumaticum** /bal′nē·əm no͞omat′ikəm/.

Airbron, a trademark for a mucolytic (acetylcysteine).

air cells of the nose. See **nasal sinus.**

air conditioner lung. See **humidifier lung.**

air embolism, the abnormal presence of air in the cardiovascular system, resulting in obstruction of the flow of blood through the vessel. Air may be inadvertently introduced by injection, during intravenous therapy or surgery, or traumatically, as by a puncture wound. See also **decompression sickness, embolus, gas embolism.**

air encephalography. See **encephalography.**

airplane splint, a splint used for immobilizing a fractured humerus during healing. The splint holds the arm in an abducted position at shoulder level, with the elbow bent. It extends to the waist and may be made of wire or leather, or it may be supported by a plaster body.

air pump, a pump that forces air in or out of a cavity or chamber.

air sickness. See **motion sickness.**

air thermometer, a thermometer using air as its expansible medium. See also **thermometer.**

airway, any tubular passage for the movement of air into and out of the lungs, as the trachea and bronchi, a respiratory anesthesia device, or an oropharyngeal tube used for mouth-to-mouth resuscitation.

airway clearance, ineffective, a nursing diagnosis accepted by the Fourth National Conference on the Classification of Nursing Diagnoses. The origin of the problem is decreased energy or fatigue, infection, obstruction, or secretions of the tracheobronchial tree, perceptual or cognitive impairment, or trauma. The defining characteristics of the condition include abnormal breath sounds, change in the rate or depth of respiration, tachypnea, cough, cyanosis, dyspnea, and fever. See also **nursing diagnosis.**

airway obstruction, an abnormal condition of the respiratory system characterized by a mechanic impediment to the delivery or to the absorption of oxygen in the lungs, as in bronchospasm, choking, croup, laryngospasm, chronic obstructive lung disease, goiter, tumor, or pneumothorax.

■ OBSERVATIONS: If the obstruction is minor, as in sinusitis or pharyngitis, the person is able to breathe, but not normally. If the obstruction is acute, the person may grasp the neck, gasp, become cyanotic, and lose consciousness.

■ INTERVENTION: Acute airway obstruction requires rapid intervention to save the person's life. A bolus of food, a collection of mucus, or a foreign body may be removed manually, by suction, or with the Heimlich maneuver. Obstruction of the airway caused by inflammatory or allergic reaction may be treated with bronchodilating drugs, corticosteroids, intubation, and the administration of oxygen. An emergency tracheotomy may be required if the obstruction cannot be mechanically removed or pharmacologically reduced within a few minutes.

■ NURSING CONSIDERATIONS: The patient is usually very apprehensive and may physically resist assistance. The cause of the obstruction is identified, if possible. Medical assistance is summoned, and the most highly trained person available begins emergency care, including removing the obstruction, if possible; administering oxygen; and performing cardiopulmonary resuscitation, if necessary. See also **aspiration, cardiopulmonary resuscitation, Heimlich maneuver.**

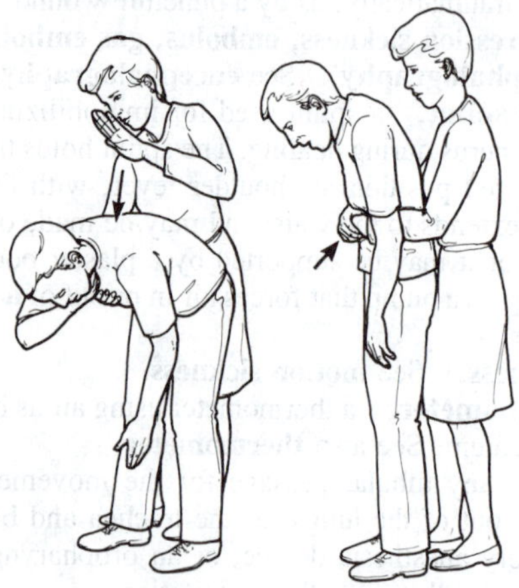

Airway obstruction: back blows and chest thrusts

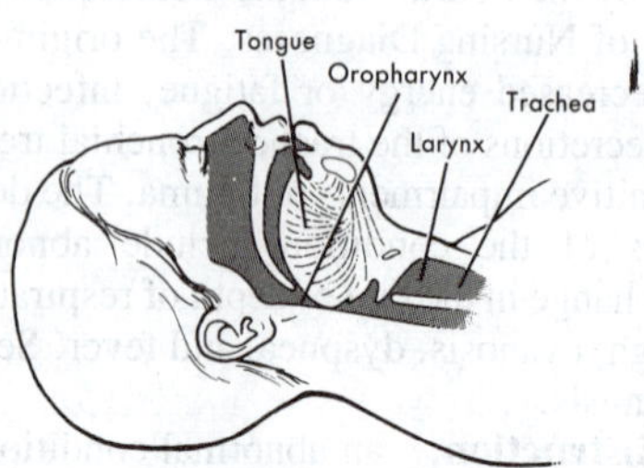

Airway obstruction by tongue

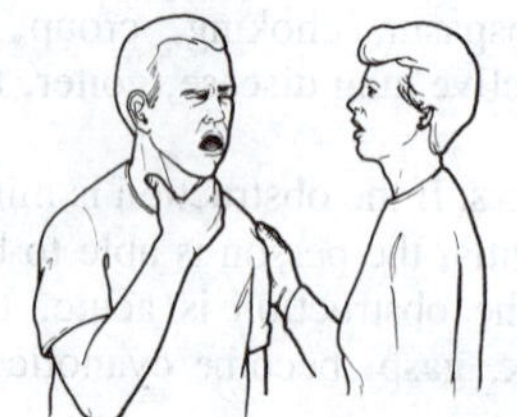

Airway obstruction: Victim gives international choking sign; rescuer asks if victim can speak

akathisia /ak′əthē′zhə/, an abnormal condition characterized by restlessness and agitation, as seen in tardive dyskinesia. **–akathisiac,** *adj.*

akinesia /ā′kinē′zhə, ā′kīnē′zhə/, an abnormal state of motor and psychic hypoactivity or muscular paralysis. **akinetic,** *adj.*

akinetic apraxia, the inability to perform a spontaneous movement. See also **apraxia.**

akinetic mutism, a state in which a person is unable or refuses to move or to make sounds, resulting from neurologic or psychologic disturbance.

Akineton, a trademark for an anticholinergic (biperiden hydrochloride or biperiden lactate), used as an antiparkinsonian.

-akusis. See **-acousia.**

Al, symbol for **aluminum.**

-al, a combining form designating a compound containing a member of the aldehyde group: *benzal, chloral, ethanal.*

-al, -ale, a combining form meaning 'pertaining to or characterized by': *appendiceal, calcyeal, meningeal.*

ala /ā′lə/, *pl.* **alae, 1.** any winglike structure. **2.** the axilla.

Ala, abbreviation for **alanine.**

ala auris, the auricle of the ear.

ala cerebelli /ser′əbel′ī/, the ala of the central lobule of the cerebellum.

ala cinerea /sinir′ē·ə/, the triangular area on the floor of the fourth ventricle of the brain from which the autonomic fibers of the vagus nerve arise.

ala nasi /nā′sī/, the outer flaring cartilaginous wall of each nostril.

alanine (Ala), a nonessential amino acid found in many proteins in the body. It is degraded in the liver to produce pyruvate and glutamate. See also **amino acid, protein.**

alanine aminotransferase (ALT), an enzyme normally present in the serum and tissues of the body, especially the tissues of the liver. This enzyme catalyzes the transfer of an amino group from l-alanine to alpha-ketoglutarate, forming pyruvate and l-glutamate. The reaction is reversible. The enzyme is released into the serum because of tissue injury and may increase in persons with acute liver damage. Also called **glutamic-pyruvic transaminase.** Compare **aspartate aminotransferase.**

Al-Anon, an international organization that offers guidance and counseling for the relatives, friends, and associates of alcoholics. See also **Alcoholics Anonymous.**

ala of the ethmoid, a small projection on each side of the crista galli of the ethmoid bone. Each ala fits into a corresponding depression of the frontal bone.

ala of the ilium, the upper flaring portion of the iliac bone.

ala of the sacrum, the flat extension of bone on each side of the sacrum.

alar ligament, one of a pair of ligaments that connects the axis to the occipital bone and limits rotation of the cranium. Also called **check ligament, odontoid ligament.** Compare **membrana tectoria.**

alarm reaction, the first stage of the general adaptation syndrome, characterized by the mobilization of the various defense mechanisms of the body or the mind to cope with a stressful situation of a physical or emotional nature. See also **stress.**

alastrim /al′əstrim/, a mild form of smallpox, thought to be caused by a weak strain of *Poxvirus variolae*. Unlike smallpox, alastrim is rarely fatal. Also called **Cuban itch, milkpox, variola minor.** See also **smallpox.**

Alateen, an international organization that offers guidance and counseling for the children of alcoholics. See also **Alcoholics Anonymous.**

ala vomeris /vō′məris/, an extension of bone on each side of the upper border of the vomer.

alb-, a combining form meaning 'white': *albedo, albugo, albumin.*

alba /al′bə/, literally, "white," as in *linea alba.*

Albers-Schönberg disease. See **osteopetrosis.**

albinism /al′biniz′əm/, an abnormal congenital condition characterized by partial or total lack of melanin pigment in the body. Total albinos have pale skin that does not tan, white hair, pink eyes, nystagmus, astigmatism, and photophobia. Albinos are prone to severe sunburn, actinic dermatitis, and skin cancer. Compare **piebald, vitiligo.**

Albright's syndrome /ôl′brīts/, a disorder characterized by fibrous dysplasia of bone, isolated brown macules on the skin, and endocrine dysfunction. It causes precocious puberty in girls but not in boys. The osseous lesions are reddish-gray, gritty fibromas containing areas of coarse fiber that may be confined to one bone or occur in several, frequently causing deformities. Hyperthyroidism is present in some cases. Treatment may involve osteotomy, curettage, and bone grafts. Also called **Albright-McCune-Sternberg syndrome, osteitis fibrosa disseminata.**

Albucid, a trademark for a topical antibacterial (sulfacetamide).

albumin /albyo͞o′min/, a water-soluble, heat-coagulable protein containing carbon, hydrogen, oxygen, nitrogen, and sulfur. Various albumins are found in practically all animal tissues and in many plant tissues. Determination of the levels and kinds of albumin in urine, blood, and other body tissues is the basis of a number of laboratory diagnostic tests.

albumin A, a blood serum constituent that gathers in cancer cells but is deficient in circulation in cancer patients.

albumin (human), a plasma-volume expander.

■ INDICATIONS: It is prescribed in the treatment of hypoproteinemia, hyperbilirubinemia, and hypovolemic shock.

■ CONTRAINDICATIONS: Severe anemia or cardiac failure prohibits its use.

■ ADVERSE EFFECTS: Among the most serious adverse reactions are chills, hypotension, fever, and urticaria.

albuminuria. See **proteinuria.**

-albuminuria, a combining form meaning a '(specified) condition characterized by excess serum proteins in the urine': *noctalbuminuria, nyctalbuminuria, pseudalbuminuria.*

albuterol, an adrenergic used a a bronchodilator.

■ INDICATION: It is prescribed in the treatment of bronchospasm in patients with reversible obstructive airway disease.

■ CONTRAINDICATION: Known sensitivity to this drug prohibits its use.

■ ADVERSE EFFECTS: Among the most serious adverse reactions are tachycardia, insomnia, dizziness, and hypertension.

Alcaine, a trademark for a local anesthetic agent (proparacaine).

Alcock's canal, a canal formed by the obturator internus muscle and the obturator fascia through which the pudendal nerve and vessels pass. Also called **pudendal canal.**

alcohol, **1.** (USP) a preparation containing at least 92.3% and not more than 93.8% by weight of ethyl alcohol, used as a topical antiseptic and solvent. **2.** a clear, colorless, volatile liquid that is miscible with water, chloroform, or ether, obtained by the fermentation of carbohydrates with yeast. **3.** a compound derived from a hydrocarbon by replacing one or more hydrogen atoms with an equal number of hydroxyl (OH) groups. Depending on the number of hydroxyl radicals, alcohols are classified as monohydric, dihydric, trihydric. Some kinds of alcohol are **rubbing alcohol, sugar alcohol,** and **unsaturated alcohol.**

alcohol bath, a procedure for decreasing an elevated body temperature. A tepid solution of 25% to 50% alcohol in water is sponged lightly on each limb, then on the trunk, turning the person only once from supine to prone position and then back again. Some sources recommend the placement of a hot-water bottle at the feet and a cold compress on the head to accelerate heat loss through vasodilatation, to promote the comfort of the patient during the procedure, and to reduce the temperature of the circulation to the brain. As the alcohol evaporates quickly, the bed is less likely to get wet, the patient does not need to be dried, and, for an equal result, the solution does not need to be as cold as a plain bath with cold water.

alcoholic cirrhosis. See **cirrhosis.**

alcoholic fermentation, the conversion of carbohydrates to ethyl alcohol.

alcoholic hallucinosis, a form of alcoholic psychosis characterized primarily by auditory hallucinations, abject fear, and delusions of persecution. The condition develops in acute alcoholism as withdrawal symptoms shortly after stopping or reducing the intake of alcohol. Also called **acute hallucinosis.** See also **alcoholic psychosis, hallucinosis.**

alcoholic hepatitis, acute toxic liver injury associated with excess ethanol consumption. This is characterized by necrosis, polymorphonuclear inflammation, and in many instances Mallory bodies.

alcoholic ketoacidosis, the fall in blood pH (acidosis) sometimes seen in alcoholics and associated with a rise in serum ketone bodies (acetone, beta-hydroxybutyric acid, and acetoacetic acid).

alcoholic-nutritional cerebellar degeneration, a sudden, severe incoordination in the lower extremity, characteristic of poorly nourished alcoholics. The patient walks, if at all, with an ataxic or wide-based gait. It is important to distinguish between this condition and cerebellar tumors, multiple sclerosis, and other neurologic disorders that have similar motor impairments. Treatment consists of improved nutrition, abstinence from alcohol, and physical therapy. Also called **cerebellar cortical degeneration.** See also **alcoholism.**

alcoholic paranoia, paranoia associated with chronic alcoholism.

alcoholic psychosis, any of a group of severe mental disorders, such as pathologic intoxication, delirium tremens, Korsakoff's psychosis, and acute hallucinosis, characterized by brain damage or dysfunction that results from the excessive use of alcohol.

Alcoholics Anonymous (AA), an international nonprofit organization, founded in 1935, consisting of abstinent alcoholics whose purpose is to help other alcoholics stop drinking and maintain sobriety through group support, shared experiences, and faith in a power greater than themselves. The AA program, which emphasizes both medical and religious resources for help in overcoming alcoholism, consists of attending meetings and coping with abstinence "one day at a time." Meetings are held at convenient times in factories, schools, churches, hospitals, and many other institutions and community buildings. Similar groups who work with the children, relatives, friends, and associates of alcoholics are **Al-Anon** and **Alateen.**

alcoholic trance, a state of automatism resulting from ethanol intoxication.

alcoholism, the extreme dependence on excessive amounts of alcohol, associated with a cumulative pattern of deviant behaviors. Alcoholism is a chronic illness with a slow, insidious onset, which may occur at any age. The cause is unknown, but cultural and psychosocial factors are suspect, and families of alcoholics have a higher incidence of alcoholism. Frequent intoxication has cumulative destructive effects on an individual's family and social life, working life, and physical health. The most frequent medical consequences of alcoholism are central nervous system depression and cirrhosis of the liver. The severity of each of these is increased in the absence of food intake. Alcoholic patients also may suffer from alcoholic gastritis, peripheral neuropathies, auditory hallucinations, and cardiac problems. Abrupt withdrawal of alcohol in addiction causes weakness, sweating, and hyperreflexia. The severe form of alcohol withdrawal is called delirium tremens. Extreme caution should be used in administering drugs to the alcoholic patient because of the possibility of additive central nervous system depression. The treatment of alcoholism consists of psychotherapy (especially group therapy, by organizations like Alcoholics Anonymous), electroshock treatments, or drugs such as disulfiram that cause an aversion to alcohol. See also **acute alcoholism, chronic alcoholism, delirium tremens.**

alcohol poisoning, poisoning caused by the ingestion of any of several alcohols, of which ethyl, isopropyl, and methyl are the most common. Ethyl alcohol (grain alcohol) is found in whiskies, brandy, gin, and other beverages. Ordinarily, it is lethal only if large quantities are ingested in a brief period. Isopropyl alcohol is more toxic: Ingestion of eight ounces may result in respiratory or circulatory failure. Methyl alcohol (wood alcohol) is extremely poisonous: In addition to nausea, vomiting, and abdominal pain, it may cause blindness, and death may follow the consumption of only 2 ounces. Treatment for alcohol poisoning includes gastric lavage, intravenous administration of sodium bicarbonate and dextrose, bed rest, the oral or intravenous administration of ethanol oxygen, and, if necessary, hemodialysis.

alcohol withdrawal syndrome, the clinical symptoms associated with cessation of alcohol consumption. These may include tremor, hallucinations, autonomic nervous system dysfunction, and seizures.

ALD, abbreviation for **adrenoleukodystrophy.**

Aldactazide, a trademark for a fixed-combination drug containing two diuretics (hydrochlorothiazide and spironolactone).

Aldactone, a trademark for a diuretic (spironolactone).

Aldase, a trademark for an enzyme (hyaluronidase), used as an adjunct to anesthesia.

aldehyde /al′dəhīd′/, any of a large category of organic compounds derived from a corresponding alcohol by the removal of two hydrogen atoms, as in the conversion of ethyl alcohol to acetaldehyde. Each aldehyde is characterized by a carbonyl (-CHO) group in its empiric formula and can be converted into a corresponding acid by the addition of one oxygen atom, as in the conversion of acetaldehyde to acetic acid.

aldolase /al′dəlās/, an enzyme found in muscle tissue that catalyzes the step in anaerobic glycolysis involving the breakdown of fructose 1,6-diphosphate to glyceraldehyde 3-phosphate. The enzyme can also catalyze the reverse reaction. See also **glycolysis.**

Aldomet, a trademark for an antihypertensive (methyldopa).

Aldoril, a trademark for a fixed-combination drug containing a diuretic (hydrochlorothiazide) and an antihypertensive (methyldopa).

aldose, the chemical form of monosaccharides in which the carbonyl group is an aldehyde.

aldosterone /al′dōstərōn′, aldos′tərōn/, a steroid hormone produced by the adrenal cortex to regulate sodium and potassium balance in the blood.

aldosteronism /al′dōstərō′nizəm, aldos′-/, a condition characterized by hypersecretion of aldosterone, occurring as a primary disease of the adrenal cortex or, more often, as a secondary disorder in response to various extra-adrenal pathologic processes. Primary aldosteronism, also called **Conn's syndrome,** may be caused by adrenal hyperplasia or by an aldosterone-secreting tumor. Secondary aldosteronism is associated with increased plasma renin activity and may be induced by the nephrotic syndrome, hepatic cirrhosis, idiopathic edema, congestive heart failure, trauma, burns, or other kinds of stress. Hypersecretion of aldosterone promotes sodium retention and potassium excretion, leading to increased blood volume and blood pressure, alkalosis, muscular weakness, tetany, paresthesias, nephropathy, ventricular arrhythmias, and other cardiac abnormalities. The electrolyte imbalance in aldosteronism usually causes polydipsia and polyuria. Treatment of primary aldosteronism caused by a tumor may include surgical resection and chemotherapy with the adrenal cytotoxic agent mitotane. Spironolactone, an aldosterone antagonist, is frequently used to treat symptoms of aldosteronism. Also called **hyperaldosteronism.**

aldosteronoma /al′dōstir′ənō′mə/, *pl.* **aldosteronomas, aldosteronomata,** an aldosterone-secreting adenoma of the adrenal cortex that is usually small and occurs more frequently in the left than the right adrenal gland, causing hyperaldosteronism with salt retention, expansion of the extracellular fluid volume, and increased blood pressure.

Aleppo boil. See **oriental sore.**

aleukemic leukemia /ā′lo͞okē′mik/, a type of leukemia in which the total leukocyte count remains within normal limits and few abnormal forms appear in the peripheral blood. Diagnosis requires tissue examination, usually of the bone marrow. Also called **subleukemic leukemia.** See also **leukemia.**

aleukemic myelosis. See **myeloid metaplasia.**

aleukia /ālo͞o′kē·ə/, a marked reduction in or the complete absence of white blood cells or blood platelets. Compare **leukopenia, thrombocytopenia.** See also **aplastic anemia.**

aleukocythemic leukemia. See **aleukemic leukemia.**

Alevaire, a trademark for a respiratory tract detergent (tyloxapol).

alexia /əlek′sē·ə/, an abnormal neurologic condition characterized by an inability to comprehend written words. Compare **dyslexia.** –**alexic,** *adj.*

alg-. See **algesi-.**

alga /al′gə/, *pl.* **algae** /al′jī, al′jē/, any of a large group of nonmotile, or motile, marine plants containing chlorophyll. Many genera and species of algae are found worldwide in fresh water, in salt water, and on land. All belong to the phylum Thallophyta. –**algal,** *adj.*

algesi-, alg-, alge-, algo-, a combining form meaning 'pertaining to pain': *algesia, algesiogenic, algesthenia.*

-algesia, a combining form meaning '(condition of) sensitivity to pain': *asphalgesia, haphalgesia, hyperthermalalgesia.*

-algesic, a combining form meaning 'pertaining to sensitivity to pain': *analgesic, hypalgesic, paralgesic.*

-algia, -algy a combining form meaning 'pain, painful condition': *epigastralgia, sacralgia, uteralgia.*

-algic, a combining form meaning 'related to pain': *cardialgic, ophthalmalgic, tibialgic.*

algid malaria, a form of malaria caused by the protozoan *Plasmodium falciparum,* characterized by coldness of the skin, profound weakness, and severe diarrhea. See also **falciparum malaria, malaria.**

algo-. See **algesi-.**

ALGOL /al′gôl/, abbreviation for *algorithmic language,* a type of computer language.

algolagnia /al′gōlag′nē·ə/, a form of sexual perversion characterized by sadism or masochism. See also **sadism, sadomasochism.**

algologist, **1.** a person who specializes in the study of or the treatment of pain. **2.** also called **phycologist.** a person who specializes in the study of algae.

algology, **1.** the branch of medicine that is concerned with the study of pain. **2.** also called **phycology.** the branch of science that is concerned with algae.

algophobia, an anxiety disorder characterized by an abnormal, pervasive fear of experiencing pain or of witnessing pain in others.

algorithm /al′gərith′əm/, **1.** a step-by-step procedure for the solution of a problem by computer, using specific mathematic or logical operations. Compare **heuristic.** **2.** an explicit protocol with well-defined rules to be followed in solving a health care problem.

alienation, the act or state of being estranged or isolated. See also **depersonalization.**

alienist, *obsolete.* a psychiatrist, especially one who specializes in giving legal evidence concerning the mental competence of persons appearing before a court of law.

alimentary bolus. See **bolus,** def. 1.

alimentary canal. See **digestive tube.**

alimentation. nourishment. See also **feeding.**

aliphatic /al′ifat′ik/, pertaining to fat or oil, specifically to those hydrocarbon compounds that open chains of carbon atoms, as the fatty acids, rather than ring structures.

aliphatic acid, an acid of a nonaromatic hydrocarbon characterized by an open carbon chain.

-alis, a combining form meaning 'pertaining to' something specified: *corticalis, rhomboidalis, vesicalis.*

alkalemia, a condition of increased pH of the blood.

alkali /al′kəlī/, a compound with the chemical characteristics of a base. Alkalis combine with fatty acids to form soaps, turn red litmus blue, and enter into reactions that form water-soluble carbonates. See also **acid, base.** –**alkaline,** *adj.* **alkalinity,** *n.*

alkali burn, tissue damage caused by exposure to an alkaline compound like lye. Treatment includes washing the area with copious amounts of water to remove the chemical and applying vinegar or other mildly acidic substance diluted with water to neutralize any remaining alkali and to decrease the discomfort. The victim should be immediately taken to a medical facility if the tissue damage is more than slight and superficial. Compare **acid burn.**

-alkaline, a combining form meaning 'of or referring to alkali': *silicoalkaline, subalkaline, vegetoalkaline.*

alkaline-ash, residue in the urine having a pH of higher than 7.

alkaline-ash producing foods, foods that may be ingested in order to produce an alkaline pH in the urine, thereby reducing the incidence of acidic urinary calculi, or that may be avoided in order to reduce the incidence of alkaline calculi. Some of the foods that result in alkaline ash are milk, cream, buttermilk, fruit (except prunes, plums, and cranberries), vegetables (except corn and lentils), almonds, chestnuts, coconuts, and olives.

alkaline bath, a bath taken in water containing sodium bicarbonate, used especially for skin disorders.

alkaline phosphatase, an enzyme present in bone, the kidneys, the intestine, plasma, and teeth. It may be elevated in the serum in some diseases of the bone and liver and in some other illnesses. The normal concentrations of this enzyme in the serum of adults are 1.5 to 4.5 Bodansky units; in children, 5 to 14 Bodansky units. See **Bodansky units.**

alkalinize /al′kəlinīz/, **1.** to make a substance alkaline, as through the addition of a base. **2.** to become alkaline. Also **alkalize** /al′kəlīz/. Compare **acidify.**

alkali poisoning, a toxic condition caused by the ingestion of an alkaline agent like liquid ammonia, lye, and some detergent powders. Emergency treatment includes giving copious amounts of water or milk to dilute the alkali. Vomiting is not induced, and mild acids are not administered. The victim is transported immediately to the hospital for observation of any corrosive damage to the esophagus or of any metabolic abnormality and for mechanic removal of the alkali by gastric intubation and lavage. Compare **acid poisoning.**

alkaloid /al′kəloid/, any of a large group of organic compounds produced by plants, including many pharmacologically active substances, such as atropine, caffeine, cocaine, morphine, nicotine, and quinine. The term also may be applied to synthetic chemicals, such as procaine, that are similar to the alkaloid substances found in leaves, stems, seeds, or other plant parts.

alkalosis /al′kəlō′sis/, an abnormal condition of body fluids, characterized by a tendency toward a pH level greater than 7.44, as from an excess of alkaline bicarbonate or a deficiency of acid. Respiratory alkalosis may be caused by hyperventilation, resulting in an excess loss of carbon dioxide and a carbonic acid deficit. Metabolic acidosis may result from an excess intake or retention of bicarbonate, loss of gastric acid in vomiting, potassium depletion, or any stimulus that increases the rate of sodium-hydrogen exchange. Alkalosis is said to be compensated if an adaptive mechanism, as a buffer system, carbon dioxide retention, or bicarbonate excretion, prevents a shift in pH. Treatment of uncompensated alkalosis involves correction of dehydration and various ionic deficits to restore the normal acid-base balance in which the ratio of carbonic acid to bicarbonate is 20:1. Compare **acidosis.**

alkaptonuria /alkap′tōno͝or′ē·ə/, a rare inherited disorder resulting from the incomplete metabolism of tyrosine, an amino acid, in which abnormal amounts of glycosuric acid are excreted, staining the urine dark. In this disorder, which is transmitted by an autosomal recessive gene, a key metabolic enzyme is absent from the body. Usually, the condition does not cause symptoms until middle age, at which point ochronosis, a type of arthritis, may develop. See also **ochronosis.** **–alkaptonuric,** *adj.*

alkene, an unsaturated aliphatic hydrocarbon containing one double bond in the carbon chain, as ethylene. Also called **olefin.**

Alkeran, a trademark for an antineoplastic (melphalan).

alkyl /al′kil/, a hydrocarbon molecule from which one of the hydrogen atoms has been removed, producing an alkyl radical.

alkylamine /al′kiləmīn′/, an amine in which an alkyl group replaces one to three of the hydrogen atoms that are attached to the nitrogen atom, as methylamine.

alkylating agent /al′kilā′ting/, any substance that contains an alkyl radical and is therefore capable of replacing a free hydrogen atom in an organic compound. Because this type of chemical reaction results in interference with mitosis and cell division, especially in rapidly proliferating tissue, such agents are particularly useful in the treatment of cancer. The types of alkylating agents applicable to medicine are the alkyl sulfonates, the ethylenimines, the nitrogen mustards, the nitrosoureas, and the triagenes. The most widely used agent is cyclophosphamide, which is also the only one not active in vitro.

alkylation, a chemical reaction in which a hydrogen atom in an organic compound is replaced by an alkyl radical from an alkylating agent. When such organic reactions occur with a biologically significant cellular constituent, as DNA, they result in interference with mitosis and cell division.

ALL, abbreviation for **acute lymphocytic leukemia.** See also **acute childhood leukemia.**

all-. See **allo-.**

allanto-, a combining form meaning 'pertaining to a sausage or to the allantois': *allantochorion, allantoid, allantotoxicon.*

allantoidoangiopagus /al′əntoidō·an′jē·op′əgəs/, conjoined monozygotic twin fetuses of unequal size that are united by the vessels of the umbilical cord. Also called **omphaloangiopagus.** See also **omphalosite.** **–allantoidoangiopagous,** *adj.*

allantoin /əlan′tō•in/, a chemical compound (5-ureido-hydantoin), $C_4H_6N_4O_3$, that occurs as a white crystallizable substance found in many plants and in the allantoic and amniotic fluids and fetal urine of primates. It is also present in the urine of mammals other than the primates as a product of purine metabolism. The substance, which can be produced synthetically by the oxidation of uric acid, was once used to promote tissue growth in the treatment of suppurating wounds and ulcers.

allantois /əlan′tois/, a tubular extension of the yolk sac endoderm that extends with the allantoic vessels into the body stalk of the embryo. In human embryos, allantoic vessels become the umbilical vessels and the chorionic villi. See also **body stalk, umbilical cord.** **–allantoic** /al′əntō′ik/, *adj.*

allele /əlēl′/, **1.** one of two or more alternative forms of a gene that occupy corresponding loci on homologous chromosomes. **2.** also called **allelomorph** /əlēl′əmôrf′/. one of two or more contrasting characteristics transmitted by alternative genes.

allelo-, a combining form meaning 'pertaining to another': *allelocatalysis, allelomorph, allelotaxis.*

allelomorph. See **allele.**

Allen correction, multichromatic analysis of reaction to correct for background absorbance.

Allen test, a test for the patency of the radial artery after insertion of an indwelling monitoring catheter. The patient's hand is formed into a fist while the nurse compresses the ulnar artery. Compression of the ulnar artery is continued while the fist is opened. If blood perfusion through the radial artery is adequate, the hand should flush and resume normal pinkish coloration.

allergen /al′ərjin/, a substance that can produce a hypersensitive reaction in the body but is not necessarily intrinsically harmful. Some common allergens are pollen, animal dander, house dust, feathers, and various foods. Some studies indicate that one of every six Americans is hypersensitive to one or more allergens. The bodies of normal individuals develop a natural or acquired immunity to allergens, but in less fortunate individuals the immune system may be overly sensitive to foreign substances and to others produced naturally by the body. The body normally protects itself against allergens or antigens by the complex chemical reactions of the humoral immune and the cell-mediated immune systems. Methods to identify specific allergens affecting individuals continue to improve. The most common method involves a skin test in which several allergens can be examined simultaneously. **–allergenic,** *adj.*

allergic, **1.** of or pertaining to allergy. **2.** having an allergy.

allergic alveolitis. See **diffuse hypersensitivity pneumonia.**

allergic asthma, a form of asthma caused by the exposure of the bronchial mucosa to an inhaled airborne antigen. This allergen causes the production of antibodies that bind to mast cells in the bronchial tree. The mast cells then release histamine, which stimulates contraction of bronchial smooth muscle and causes mucosal edema. Psychologic factors may provoke asthma attacks in bronchi already sensitized by allergens. Hyposensitization treatments are more effective for pollen sensitivity than for house dust, animal hair, molds, and insects. Often, a diurnal pattern of histamine release is seen, causing variable degrees of bronchospasm at different times of the day. Also called **extrinsic asthma.** Compare **intrinsic asthma.** See also **asthma, asthma in children, asthmatic eosinophilia, status asthmaticus.**

allergic bronchopulmonary aspergillosis, a form of aspergillosis that occurs in asthmatics when the fungus *Aspergillus fumigatus,* growing within the bronchial lumen, causes a type I or type III hypersensitivity reaction. The characteristics of the condition are similar to those of asthma, including dyspnea and wheezing. Chest examination and pulmonary function tests may reveal airway obstruction. Serologic tests usually reveal precipitating antibodies to *A. fumigatus.* Bacteriologic and microscopic examination of sputum may reveal *A. fumigatus* in addition to Charcot-Leyden crystals. Eosinophilia is usually also present. Compare **aspergillosis.**

allergic conjunctivitis, an abnormal condition characterized by hyperemia of the conjunctiva caused by an allergy. Common allergens that cause this condition are pollen, grass, topical medications, air pollutants, occupational irritants, and smoke. It is bilateral and usually starts before puberty and lasts about 10 years, commonly recurring in a seasonal pattern.

■ OBSERVATIONS: The common signs of allergic conjunctivitis are tearing and pain, accompanied by discharge and conjunctival hyperemia. Eosinophils predominate in stained blood smears, and diagnosis is commonly based on cultures and sensitivity tests to identify the causative allergen.

■ INTERVENTION: Treatment of allergic conjunctivitis commonly includes the administration of vasoconstrictor eyedrops, as epinephrine, cold compresses to relieve itching, and oral histamines.

■ NURSING CONSIDERATIONS: Warm compresses and ointments or eyedrops may be administered.

allergic coryza, acute rhinitis caused by exposure to any allergen to which the person is hypersensitive.

allergic cutaneous angiitis. See **allergic vasculitis.**

allergic interstitial pneumonitis. See **diffuse hypersensitivity pneumonia.**

allergic reaction, a hypersensitive response to an allergen to which an organism has previously been exposed and to which the organism has developed antibodies. Subsequent exposure causes the release of histamine and a variety of symptoms including urticaria, eczema, dyspnea, bronchospasm, diarrhea, rhinitis, sinusitis, laryngospasm, and anaphylaxis. Eosinophilia is usually present, revealed in a differential white blood cell count.

allergic rhinitis, inflammation of the nasal passages, usually associated with watery nasal discharge and itching of the nose and eyes, because of a localized sensitivity reaction to house dust, animal dander, or an antigen, commonly pollen. The condition may be seasonal, as in hay fever, or perennial, as in allergy to dust or animals. Treatment includes the local, systemic, or topical administration of antihistamines, avoidance of the antigen, and hyposensitization by injections of diluted antigen in gradually increasing amounts.

allergic vasculitis, an inflammatory condition of the blood vessels that is induced by an allergen. Disseminated intravascular inflammation sometimes occurs in patients treated with iodides, penicillin, sulfonamides, and thioureas. Allergic cutaneous vasculitis is characterized by itching, malaise, and a slight fever and by the presence of papules, vesicles, urticarial wheals, or small ulcers on the skin.

allergy, a hypersensitive reaction to intrinsically harmless antigens, most of which are environmental. Studies show that one of every six Americans has a severe allergy and that more than 20 million Americans have allergic reactions to airborne or inhaled allergens, as cigarette smoke, house dust, and pollens. Allergic rhinitis, which is associated with airborne allergens, affects predominantly young children and adolescents but occurs in all age groups. Allergies are classified according to types I, II, III, and IV hypersensitivity. Types I, II, and III involve different immunoglobulin antibodies and their interaction with different antigens. Type IV allergy is associated with contact dermatitis and T cells, which react directly with the antigen and cause local inflammation. Allergies are divided into those that produce immediate or antibody-mediated reactions and those that produce delayed or cell-mediated reactions. Immediate allergic reactions involve types I, II, and III hypersensitivity and antigen-antibody reactions that activate certain enzymes, creating an imbalance between these enzymes and their inhibitors. Immediate allergic reactions also release certain substances into the circulation, as histamine, bradykinin, acetylcholine, gamma globulin G, and leukotaxine. Delayed allergic reactions are caused by antigens but do not seem to depend on antibodies. Depending on the type of hypersensitivity involved, some common symptoms of allergy are bronchial congestion, conjunctivitis, edema, fever, urticaria, and vomiting. Severe allergic reactions, as anaphylaxis, can cause systemic shock and death. Symptoms of limited duration, as those associated with hay fever, serum sickness, bee stings, and urticaria, can be suppressed by glucocorticoids administered as supplements to primary therapy. The effect of such steroids may be considerably delayed. Severe allergic reactions, as anaphylaxis and angioneurotic edema of the glottis, commonly require immediate therapy with epinephrine administered subcutaneously. When allergic reactions are life threatening, steroids, as dexamethasone sodium phosphate, may be administered intravenously. For milder diseases, as serum sickness and hay fever, antihistamines are usually administered. See also **allergy testing, immunoglobulins.**

allergy testing, any one of the various procedures used in identifying the specific allergens that afflict the patients involved. Such tests are helpful in prescribing treatment to prevent allergic reactions or to reduce their severity. Skin testing is the most common kind of procedure for allergy testing and commonly exposes the patient to small quantities of the suspected allergens. Positive reactions usually occur within 20 minutes and are commonly manifested as varying degrees of erythema. Factors considered in performing allergy tests include the medical history of the patient, the allergy history, the environment, and the diet. Individuals to be tested are usually instructed to discontinue the use of any antihistamines at least 24 hours before the test, because these drugs can interfere with normal test responses. The most common kinds of allergy testing include the intradermal, scratch, patch, conjunctival, and use tests.

allied health personnel. See **paramedical personnel.**

alligator forceps, **1.** a forceps with heavy teeth and a double clamp, employed in orthopedic surgery. **2.** a forceps with long, thin, angular handles and interlocking teeth.

allo-, all-, a combining form meaning 'differing from the normal, reversal, or referring to another': *allobiosis, allochezia, allopathy.*

allodiploid /al′ōdip′loid/, **1.** also **allodiploidic.** of or pertaining to an individual, organism, strain, or cell that has two genetically distinct sets of chromosomes derived from different ancestral species, as occurs in hybridization. **2.** such an individual, organism, strain, or cell. See also **autopolyploid.**

allodiploidy /al′ōdip′loidē/, the state or condition of having two genetically distinct sets of chromosomes derived from different ancestral species.

alloeroticism, alloerotism. See **heteroeroticism.**

allogamy. See **cross fertilization.**

allogenic /al′ōjen′ik/, **1.** (in genetics) denoting an individual or cell type that is from the same species but genetically distinct. **2.** (in transplantation biology) denoting tissues that are from the same species but antigenically distinct; homologous. Compare **syngeneic, xenogeneic.**

allograft, the transfer of tissue between two genetically dissimilar individuals of the same species, as a tissue transplant between two humans who are not identical twins. Also called **homograft.** Compare **autograft, isograft, xenograft.** See also **graft.**

allohexaploid, allohexaploidic. See **allopolyploid.**

allometric growth, the increase in size of different organs or parts of an organism at various rates. Also called **heterauxesis** /het′ərôksē′sis/. Compare **isometric growth.** See also **allometry.**

allometron, a quantitative change in the proportional relationship of the parts of an organism as a result of the evolutionary process.

allometry /əlom′itrē/, the measurement and study of the changes in proportions of the various parts of an organism in relation to the growth of the whole or within a series of related organisms. See also **allometric growth.** –**allometric,** *adj.*

allopathic physician /al′ōpath′ik/, a physician who treats disease and injury with active interventions, as medical and surgical treatment, intended to bring about effects opposite from those produced by the disease or injury. Almost all practicing physicians in the United States are allopathic. Compare **chiropractic, homeopathy.**

allopathy /əlop′əthē/, a system of medical therapy in which a disease or an abnormal condition is treated by creating an environment that is antagonistic to the disease or condition; for example, an antibiotic toxic to a pathogenic organism is given in an infection, or an iron supplement may be given to increase the synthesis of hemoglobin in iron deficiency anemia.

allopentaploid, allopentaploidic. See **allopolyploid.**

alloplastic maneuver, (in psychology) a process that is part of adaptation, involving an adjustment or change in the external environment. Compare **autoplastic maneuver.**

alloploid, alloploidic. See **allodiploid, allopolyploid.**

alloploidy. See **allodiploidy, allopolyploidy.**

allopolyploid /al′əpol′iploid/, **1.** also **allopolyploidic.** of or pertaining to an individual, organism, strain, or cell that has more than two genetically distinct sets of chromosomes derived from two or more different ancestral species, as occurs in hybridization. They are referred to as allotriploid, allotetraploid, allopentaploid, allohexaploid, and so on, depending on the number of multiples of haploid sets of chromosomes they contain. **2.** such an individual, organism, strain, or cell. See also **mosaic.** Compare **autopolyploid.**

allopolyploidy /al′əpol′iploi′dē/, the state or condition of having more than two genetically distinct sets of chromosomes from two or more ancestral species. See **mosaic.** Compare **autopolyploidy.**

allopurinol /al′əpyŏŏr′ənôl/, a xanthine oxidase inhibitor.

■ INDICATIONS: It is prescribed in the treatment of gout and other hyperuricemic conditions.

■ CONTRAINDICATIONS: It is not prescribed for children (except those with hyperuricemia secondary to malignancy), for lactating mothers, or for people suffering an acute attack of gout. Known hypersensitivity to this drug prohibits its use.

■ ADVERSE EFFECTS: Among the most serious adverse reactions to this drug are blood dyscrasias and severe rashes and other allergic reactions. GI and ophthalmologic disturbances also may occur.

allorhythmia /al′ōrith′mē·ə/, any arrhythmia that tends to be repetitive.

all-or-none law, **1.** the principle in neurophysiology that if a stimulus is strong enough to trigger a nerve impulse, the entire impulse is discharged. A weak stimulus will not produce a weak reaction. **2.** the principle that the heart muscle, under any stimulus above a threshold level, will either respond with a maximum strength contraction or not at all. Also called **Bowditch's law.**

allosteric sites, the sites, other than the active site or sites, of an enzyme that bind regulatory molecules.

allotetraploid, allotetraploidic. See **allopolyploid.**

allotrio-, a combining form meaning 'strange or foreign': *allotriodontia, allotriogeustia, allotriophagy.*

allotriploid, allotriploidic. See **allopolyploid.**

allowable charge, the maximum amount that a third party, usually an insurance company, will pay to reimburse a provider for a specific service.

allowable costs, components of an institution's costs that are reimbursable as determined by a payment formula. In general, costs of services not considered to be reasonable or necessary to the proper provision of health services are excluded from allowable costs.

allowable error, the amount of error that can be tolerated without invalidating the medical usefulness of the analytical result. Allowable error is defined as having a 95% limit of analytic error; only one sample in 20 can have an error greater than this limit.

alloxan, an oxidation product of uric acid that is found in the human intestine in diarrhea. Because it can destroy the insulin-secreting islet cells of the pancreas, alloxan may cause diabetes.

alloy /al′oi/, a mixture of two or more metals or of substances with metallic properties. Most alloys are formed by mixing molten metals that dissolve in each other. A number of alloys have medical applications, as those used for prostheses and in dental amalgams. See **amalgam.**

aloe /al′ō/, the inspissated juice of various species of *Aloe* plants, formerly used as a cathartic but generally discontinued because it often causes severe intestinal cramps.

alopecia /al′əpē′shə/, partial or complete lack of hair resulting from normal aging, endocrine disorder, drug reaction, anticancer medication, or skin disease. Kinds of alopecia include **alopecia areata, alopecia totalis,** and **alopecia universalis.** See also **baldness.**

alopecia areata /er′ē·ā′tə/, a disease of unknown cause in which there are well-defined bald patches, usually round or oval, on the head and other hairy parts of the body. The condition is usually self-limited and clears

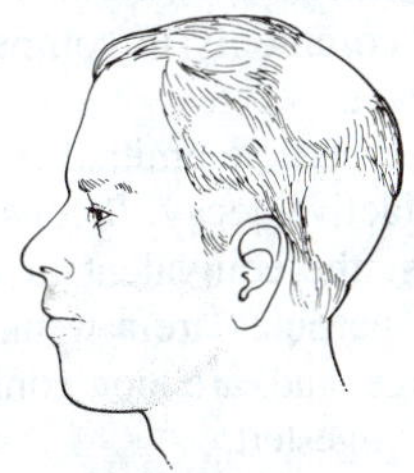

Alopecia areata

completely within 6 to 12 months without treatment. Recurrences are common. Compare **alopecia totalis, alopecia universalis.**

alopecia totalis, an uncommon condition characterized by the loss of all the hair on the scalp. The cause is unknown, and the baldness is usually permanent. No treatment is known. Compare **alopecia areata, alopecia universalis.**

alopecia universalis, a total loss of hair on all parts of the body, occasionally an extension of alopecia areata. Compare **alopecia areata, alopecia totalis.**

alpha (α), the first letter of the Greek alphabet, often used in chemical nomenclature to distinguish one variation in a chemical compound from others.

alpha-adrenergic blocking agent. See **antiadrenergic.**

alpha-adrenergic receptor. See **alpha receptor.**

alpha-aminoisovalerianic acid. See **valine.**

Alphadrol, a trademark for a glucocorticoid (fluprednisolone).

alpha fetoprotein (AFP), a protein normally synthesized by the liver, yolk sac, and GI tract of a human fetus, but which may be found elevated in the sera of adults having certain malignancies. AFP measurements in amniotic fluid are used for early diagnosis of fetal neural defects, as spina bifida and anencephaly. Elevated serum levels may be present in ataxia-telangiectasia, hereditary tyrosinemia, cirrhosis, alcoholic hepatitis, and viral hepatitis. Although not a specific marker for malignancies, AFP may be used to monitor effectiveness of surgical and chemotherapeutic management of hepatomas and germ cell neoplasms.

alpha-galactosidase, a form of the enzyme that catalyzes the conversion of alpha-D-galactoside to D-galactose.

alpha hemolysis, the development of a greenish zone around a bacterial colony growing on blood-agar medium, characteristic of pneumococci and certain streptococci and caused by the partial decomposition of hemoglobin. Compare **beta hemolysis.**

alpha-hydroxypropionic acid. See **lactic acid.**

Alphalin, a trademark for vitamin A.

alpha-methyldopa. See **methyldopa.**

alphanumeric, pertaining to a system of characters in which information is coded in combinations of letters and numerals. The characters, which also may include punctuation, are used commonly in computer programing to code signals or data.

alpha particle, a particle emitted from an atom during one kind of radioiactive decay. It consists of two protons and two neutrons, the equivalent of a helium nucleus. Ordinarily, alpha particles are a weak form of radiation with a short range and are not considered hazardous unless inhaled or ingested.

alpha receptor, any one of the postulated adrenergic components of receptor tissues that responds to norepinephrine and to various blocking agents. The activation of the alpha receptors causes such physiologic responses as increased peripheral vascular resistance, dilatation of the pupils, and contraction of pilomotor muscles. Also called **alpha-adrenergic receptor.** Compare **beta receptor.**

alpha rhythm. See **alpha wave.**

alpha state, a condition of relaxed, peaceful wakefulness devoid of concentration and sensory stimulation. It is characterized by the alpha rhythm of brain wave activity, as recorded by an electroencephalograph, and is accompanied by feelings of tranquillity and a lack of tension and anxiety. Biofeedback training and meditation techniques are used as means of achieving the state.

Alpha Tau Delta /al′fə tou′ del′tə/, a national fraternity for professional nurses.

alpha-tocopherol. See **vitamin E.**

alphavirus, any of a group of very small togaviruses consisting of a single molecule of single-stranded DNA within a lipoprotein capsule. Many alphaviruses multiply in the cytoplasm of cells of arthropods and are transmitted to humans through insect bites, such as equine encephalitis. See **encephalitis, togavirus.**

alpha wave, one of the four types of brain waves, characterized by a relatively high voltage or amplitude and a frequency of 8 to 13 Hz. Alpha waves are the "relaxed waves" of the brain and constitute the majority of waves recorded by electroencephalograms registering the activity of the parietal and the occipital lobes and the posterior parts of the temporal lobes when the individual is awake but nonattentive and relaxed, with the eyes closed. Opening and closing the eyes affects the patterns of the alpha waves and the beta waves. Also called **alpha rhythm.** Compare **beta wave, delta wave, theta wave.**

alprazolam, an antianxiety agent.

■ INDICATIONS: It is prescribed in the treatment of anxiety disorders or the short-term relief of the symptoms of anxiety.

■ CONTRAINDICATIONS: Acute narrow-angle glaucoma or known sensitivity to this drug or other benzodiazepines prohibits its use.

■ ADVERSE EFFECTS: Among the most serious adverse reactions are drowsiness and lightheadness.

ALS, 1. abbreviation for **advanced life support.** See **Emergency Medical Technician-Advanced Life Support. 2.** abbreviation for **amyotrophic lateral sclerosis. 3.** abbreviation for **antilymphocyte serum.**

ALT, abbreviation for **alanine aminotransferase.**

altered state of consciousness (ASC), any state of awareness that differs from the normal awareness of a conscious person. Altered states of consciousness have been achieved, especially in Eastern cultures, by many individuals using various techniques, as long fasting, deep breathing, whirling, and chanting. Researchers now recognize that such practices can affect the chemistry of the body and help induce the desired state. Experiments suggest that telepathy, mystical experiences, clairvoyance, and other altered states of consciousness may be subconscious capabilities in most individuals and can be used to improve health and help fight disease.

alternate generation, a type of reproduction in which a sexual generation alternates with one or more asexual generations, as in many plants and lower animals. Also called **alternation of generations.**

alternating current (AC), an electric current that reverses direction, according to a consistent sinusoidal pattern. Compare **direct current.** See also **current.**

alternating pulse, See **pulsus alternans.**

alternation of generations. See **alternate generation.**

alternative inheritance, the acquisition of all genetic traits and conditions from one parent, as in self-pollinating plants and self-fertilizing animals.

alt.h., abbreviation for the Latin prescription term *alternis horis,* meaning "every other hour."

altitude sickness, a syndrome associated with the relatively low concentrations of oxygen in the atmosphere at altitudes encountered during mountain climbing or travel in unpressurized aircraft. The acute symptoms may include dizziness, headache, irritability, breathlessness, and euphoria. Older people and those affected by pulmonary or cardiac disorders may suffer pulmonary edema, heart failure, or prostration, requiring emergency treatment and removal to lower altitudes. A chronic form of altitude sickness is characterized by an increased production of red blood cells, resulting in blood that is thick and difficult to move through the circulatory system. Also called **acute mountain sickness.** See **polycythemia.**

alum, a topical astringent, used primarily in lotions and douches. Common potassium is applied topically as a 0.5% to 5% solution.

alum bath, a bath taken in water containing alum, used primarily for skin disorders.

aluminum (Al), a widely used metallic element and the third most abundant of all the elements. Its atomic number is 13; its atomic weight is 26.97. It occurs in the ores feldspar, mica, and kaolin but most abundantly in bauxite. Aluminum is commonly obtained by purifying bauxite to produce alumina, which is reduced to aluminum. It is light and durable and used extensively in the manufacture of aircraft components, prosthetic devices, and dental appliances. It is also a component of many antacids, antiseptics, astringents, and styptics. Aluminum salts, as aluminum hydroxychloride, can cause allergic reactions in susceptible individuals. Aluminum hydroxychloride is the most commonly used agent in antiperspirants and is also effective as a deodorant.

aluminum acetate solution. See **Burow's solution.**

Alupent, a trademark for a beta-adrenergic bronchodilator (metaproterenol sulfate).

alve-, a combining form meaning 'trough, channel, cavity': *alvei, alveolate, alveolus.*

alveolar adenocarcinoma /alvē′ələr/, a neoplasm in which the tumor cells form alveoli.

alveolar canal, any of the canals of the maxilla through which the posterior superior alveolar blood vessels and the nerves to the upper teeth pass. Also called **dental canal.**

alveolar cell carcinoma, a malignant pulmonary neoplasm that arises in a bronchiole and spreads along alveolar surfaces. The tumor consists of cuboidal or nonciliated columnar epithelial cells with abundant eosinophilic cytoplasm that may contain droplets of mucus. This form of lung cancer, which occurs less frequently than bronchogenic squamous cell carcinoma or oat cell carcinoma, is characterized clinically by a severe cough and copious sputum. Also called **bronchiolar carcinoma.**

alveolar duct, any of the air passages in the lung that branch out from the respiratory bronchioles. From the ducts arise the alveolar sacs.

alveolar fiber, any one of the many white collagenous fibers of the peridontal ligament that extend from the alveolar bone to the intermediate plexus where their terminations mix with those of the cemental fibers.

alveolar fistula. See **dental fistula.**

alveolar process, the portion of the maxilla or the mandible that forms the dental arch and serves as a bony investment for the teeth. Its cortical covering is continuous with the compact bone of the body of the maxilla or the mandible, and is continuous with the spongiosa of the body of the jaws. See also **alveolar ridge.**

alveolar ridge, the bony ridge of the maxilla or the mandible that contains the alveoli of the teeth. See also **alveolar process.**

alveolar soft part sarcoma, a tumor in subcutaneous or fibromuscular tissue, consisting of numerous large round or polygonal cells in a netlike matrix of connective tissue.

alveolectomy /al′vē•əlek′təmē/, the excision of a portion of the alveolar process for aiding the extraction of a tooth or teeth, the modification of the alveolar contour after tooth extraction, or the preparation of the mouth for dentures.

alveoli /alvē′əlī/, small outpouchings of walls of alveolar space through which gas exchange takes place between alveolar air and pulmonary capillary blood.

alveolitis /al′vē•əlī′tis/, an allergic pulmonary reaction to the inhalation of antigenic substances characterized by acute episodes of dyspnea, cough, sweating, fever, weakness, and pain in the joints and muscles lasting from 12 to 18 hours. Recurrent episodes may lead to chronic obstructive lung disease with weight loss, increasing exertional dyspnea, and interstitial fibrosis. X-ray films of the lungs may show cellular thickening of alveolar septa and ill-defined generalized infiltrates. Kinds of alveolitis include **bagassosis, farmer's lung,** and **pigeon breeder's disease.**

alveolo-, a combining form meaning 'pertaining to an alveolus': *alveoloclasia, alveolodontal, alveoloplasty.*

alveolus /alvē′ələs/, *pl.* **alveoli,** a small saclike structure. Often used interchangeably with **acinus.** See also **alveoli, dental alveolus, pulmonary alveolus.** **–alveolar,** *adj.*

alymphocytosis /alim′fōsītō′sis/, an abnormal reduction in the total number of lymphocytes circulating in the blood. It is similar to lymphocytopenia but usually implies a more severe reduction. Compare **aplastic anemia, lymphocytopenia.** See also **leukocyte, lymphocyte.**

Alysine, a trademark for an analgesic, antipyretic, and antirheumatic (sodium salicylate).

Alzheimer's disease /älts′hīmərz/, presenile dementia, characterized by confusion, memory failure, disorientation, restlessness, agnosia, speech disturbances, inability to carry out purposeful movements, and hallucinosis. The patient may become hypomanic, refuse food, and lose sphincter control without local impairment. The disease usually begins in later middle life with slight defects in memory and behavior and occurs with equal frequency in men and women. Typical pathologic features are miliary plaques in the cortex and fibrillary degeneration within pyramidal ganglion cells. Treatment can only be palliative, but maintaining proper nutrition may delay the progression of the disease,which usually lasts about 7 years. Also called **senile dementia-Alzheimer type (SDAT).**

Am, symbol for **americium.**

AMA, abbreviation for **American Medical Association.**

amalgam /əmal′gəm/, **1.** a mixture or combination. **2.** an alloy of mercury and another metal or metals.

amalgam carrier, (in dentistry) an instrument for carrying plastic amalgam for inserting into a prepared tooth cavity or mold.

amalgam carver, a dental instrument for shaping plastic amalgams used in some tooth cavity fillings.

amalgam condenser, (in dentistry) an instrument used for compacting plastic amalgam in filling teeth.

amalgam core, a rigid base for the retention of a cast crown restoration, used in the replacement of a damaged tooth crown. The core may be retained by undercuts, slots, pins, or the pulp chamber of an endodontically treated tooth. Compare **cast core, composite core.** See also **core.**

Amanita, a genus of mushrooms. Some species, as *Amanita phalloides,* are poisonous, causing hallucinations, GI upset, and pain that may be followed by liver, kidney, and central nervous system damage.

amantadine hydrochloride /əman′tədēn/, an antiviral and antiparkinsonian drug.

■ INDICATIONS: It is prescribed in the prophylaxis and early treatment of influenza virus A_2, and for symptomatic treatment of parkinsonian symptoms.

■ CONTRAINDICATIONS: It is used with caution in patients with congestive heart failure and during pregnancy and lactation. Known hypersensitivity to this drug prohibits its use.

■ ADVERSE EFFECTS: Among the most serious adverse reactions are central nervous system effects and livedo reticularis. Nervousness, blurred vision, and slurred speech also may occur.

amasesis /am′əsē′sis/, the inability to chew food, caused by paralysis of the muscles of mastication, impaired teeth, poorly fitted dentures, or a psychiatric problem.

amastia /əmas′tē·ə/, absence of the breasts in women caused by a congenital defect, an endocrine disorder resulting in faulty development, lack of development of secondary sex characteristics, or a bilateral mastectomy. Also called **amazia.**

amaurosis /am′ôrō′sis/, blindness, especially lack of vision resulting from an extraocular cause, as disease of the optic nerve or brain, diabetes, renal disease, or systemic poisoning produced by excessive use of alcohol or tobacco, rather than from damage to the eye itself. Unilateral or, more rarely, bilateral amaurosis may follow an emotional shock and may continue for days or months. Amaurosis may accompany an attack of acute gastritis. One kind of congenital amaurosis is transmitted as an autosomal recessive trait. **–amaurotic,** *adj.*

amaurosis congenita of Leber. See **Leber's congenital amaurosis.**

amaurosis fugax /fo͞o′gaks/, transient episodic blindness. Compare **amaurosis.**

amaurosis partialis fugax, transitory partial blindness, usually caused by vascular insufficiency of the retina or optic nerve as a result of carotid artery disease.

amaurotic familial idiocy. See **Tay-Sachs disease.**

amazia. See **amastia.**

amb-. See **ambi-.**

ambenonium chloride /am′binō′nē·əm/, a cholinergic.

■ INDICATION: It is prescribed in the treatment of myasthenia gravis.

■ CONTRAINDICATIONS: Intestinal and urinary obstructions or known hypersensitivity to this drug prohibits its use.

■ ADVERSE EFFECTS: Among the more serious adverse reactions are increased bronchial secretions, muscle cramps, and nausea.

Ambenyl, a trademark for a fixed-combination drug containing a narcotic analgesic-antitussive (codeine sulfate), two antihistamines (bromodiphenhydramine hydrochloride and diphenhydramine hydrochloride), an expectorant (potassium guaiacolsulfonate), and ammonium chloride.

amber mutation, (in molecular genetics) a genetic alteration in which a polypeptide chain terminates prematurely, because the triplet of nucleotides that normally code for the next amino acid in the chain becomes UAG, the uracil-adenine-guanine sequence that signals the end of the chain. Also called **nonsense mutation, ochre mutation.**

ambi-, ambo-, amb-, a combining form meaning 'on both sides' or 'both': *ambidexterity, ambilateral, ambiversion.*

ambient air standard, the maximum tolerable concentration of any air pollutant, as lead, nitrogen dioxide, sodium hydroxide, or sulfuric dioxide. Federal authorities in the United States have indicated that Los Angeles, Chicago, Salt Lake City, and metropolitan New York City may not meet the ambient air standard for nitrogen dioxide and that those cities and many others throughout the world have an atmosphere polluted by various toxic chemicals that are dangerous to breathe. Research and medical evidence show the strong correlation between many diseases and toxic chemicals, but little is known about the precise effects and movement of airborne pollutants.

ambiguous genitalia, external genitalia that are not normal and morphologically typical of either sex, as occurs in pseudohermaphroditism.

ambilhar. See **niridazole.**

ambiopia. See **diplopia.**

ambivalence /ambiv'ələns/, **1.** a state in which a person experiences conflicting feelings, attitudes, drives, desires, or emotions, as love and hate, tenderness and cruelty, pleasure and pain. To some degree, ambivalence is normal. Treatment in severe, debilitating cases consists of psychotherapy appropriate to the underlying cause. **2.** uncertainty and fluctuation caused by an inability to make a choice between opposites. **3.** a continuous oscillation or fluctuation. –**ambivalent,** *adj.*

ambivert /am'bivurt'/, a person who possesses some of the characteristics of both introversion and extroversion.

amblyopia /am'blē·ō'pē·ə/, reduced vision in an eye that appears to be structurally normal when examined with an ophthalmoscope. Kinds of amblyopia are **alcoholic amblyopia, suppression amblyopia, tobacco amblyopia,** and **toxic amblyopia.**

ambo-. See **ambi-.**

Ambodryl, a trademark for an antihistamine (bromodiphenhydramine hydrochloride).

Ambu-bag, a trademark for a breathing bag used to assist respiratory ventilation.

ambulance, an emergency vehicle usually used for the transport of patients to a medical facility in cases of accident, trauma, or sudden, severe illness.

ambulatory, able to walk, hence describing a patient who is not confined to bed, or designating a health service for people who are not hospitalized.

ambulatory automatism, aimless wandering or moving about or performance of mechanic acts without conscious awareness of the behavior. See also **fugue, poriomania.**

ambulatory care, health services provided on an outpatient basis to those who visit a hospital or other health care facility and depart after treatment on the same day.

ambulatory surgery center, a medical facility designed and equipped to handle relatively minor surgery cases, as cataracts, herniorrhaphy, and meniscectomy, which do not require overnight hospitalization. Only patients who are in good health, usually children, are admitted for treatment at ambulatory surgery centers. The centers may be part of a community general hospital or independent medical facilities with prearranged hospital backup. The centers are staffed with the same health professionals as conventional surgery departments of general hospitals.

amcinonide, a topical corticosteroid.

■ INDICATION: It is used as an antiinflammatory agent.

■ CONTRAINDICATIONS: Viral and fungal diseases of the skin, circulation impairment, or known hypersensitivity to steroids prohibit its use.

■ ADVERSE REACTIONS: Among the most serious adverse reactions are various skin reactions. Systemic side effects may occur from prolonged or excessive application.

ameba /əmē'bə/, a microscopic, single-celled, parasitic organism. Several species may be parasitic in humans, including *Entamoeba coli* and *E. histolytica*. Also spelled **amoeba.** See also **amebiasis.** –**amebic,** *adj.*

-ameba, -amoeba, a combining form meaning a '(specified) protozoan': *caudameba, Dientameba, Entameba.*

amebiasis /am'ēbī'əsis/, an infection of the intestine or liver by species of pathogenic amebas, particularly *Entamoeba histolytica,* acquired by ingesting food or water contaminated with infected feces. Mild amebiasis may be asymptomatic; severe infection may cause profuse diarrhea, acute abdominal pain, jaundice, anorexia, and weight loss. It is most serious in infants, the elderly, and debilitated people. Metronidazole is often effective in curing the infection. Also spelled **amoebiasis.** See also **ameba, amebic abscess, amebic dysentery, hepatic amebiasis.**

amebic abscess, a collection of pus formed by disintegrated tissue in a cavity, usually in the liver, caused by the protozoan parasite *Entamoeba histolytica*. Cysts of the organism, ingested in fecally contaminated food or water, pass along the digestive tract into the intestine, where active trophozoites of the parasite are released. The trophozoites enter the intestinal mucosa, causing ulceration, nausea, vomiting, abdominal pain, and severe diarrhea, and they may invade the liver and produce an abscess. Oral metronidazole and chloroquine hydrochloride administered orally or intramuscularly are used in treating hepatic amebic abscesses. See also **amebiasis.**

amebic dysentery, an inflammation of the intestine caused by infestation with *Entamoeba histolytica* and characterized by frequent, loose stools flecked with blood and mucus. Intestinal amebiasis is often accompanied by symptoms of liver involvement. Also called **intestinal amebiasis.** See also **amebiasis, hepatic amebiasis.**

amelanic melanoma /am'ilan'ik/, a melanoma that lacks melanin.

amelanotic /am'ilənot'ik/, of or pertaining to tissue that is unpigmented because it lacks melanin.

amelia /əmē'lyə/, **1.** a birth defect, marked by the absence of one or more limbs. The term may be modified to indicate the number of legs or arms missing at birth, as **tetramelia** for the absence of all four limbs. **2.** a psychologic trait of apathy or indifference associated with certain forms of psychosis.

amelification /əmel′ifikā′shən/, the differentiation of ameloblasts, or enamel cells, into the enamel of the teeth.

ameloblast /am′ilōblast′/, an epithelial cell from which tooth enamel is formed. **–ameloblastic** /-blas′tik/, *adj.*

ameloblastic fibroma, an odontogenic neoplasm in which there is a simultaneous proliferation of mesenchymal and epithelial tissues but no development of dentin or enamel.

ameloblastic hemangioma, a highly vascular tumor of cells covering the dental papilla. See also **hemangioma.**

ameloblastic odontoma, an odontogenic tumor characterized by an ameloblastoma within an odontoma. Compare **composite odontoma, compound odontoma.**

ameloblastic sarcoma, a malignant odontogenic tumor, characterized by the proliferation of epithelial and mesenchymal tissue without the formation of dentin or enamel.

ameloblastoma /am′əlōblastō′mə/, a highly destructive, malignant, rapidly growing tumor of the jaw. Also called **adamantinoma, adamantoblastoma, epithelioma adamantinum.**

amelodentinal /am′əlōden′tinəl/, pertaining to both the enamel and dentin of the teeth.

amelogenesis /am′əlōjen′əsis/, the formation of the enamel of the teeth. **–amelogenic,** *adj.*

amelogenesis imperfecta, a hereditary dental defect characterized by a brown coloration of the teeth and resulting from either severe hypocalcification or hypoplasia of the enamel. The condition, which is inherited as an autosomal dominant trait, is classified according to severity as agenesis, in which there is complete lack of enamel; enamel hypoplasia, in which defective matrix formation causes the enamel to be normal in quality of hardness but deficient in quantity; or enamel hypocalcification, in which defective maturation of the ameloblasts results in the normal quantity of enamel, though it is soft and undercalcified in context. Also called **hereditary brown enamel, hereditary enamel hypoplasia.** Compare **dentinogenesis imperfecta.** See also **enamel hypocalcification, enamel hypoplasia.**

amenorrhea /ā′menərē′ə/, the absence of menstruation. Amenorrhea is normal before sexual maturity, during pregnancy, after menopause, and during the intermenstrual phase of the monthly hormonal cycle but is otherwise caused by dysfunction of the hypothalamus, pituitary gland, ovary, or uterus, by the congenital absence or surgical removal of both ovaries or the uterus, or by medication. **Primary amenorrhea** is the failure of menstrual cycles to begin. **Secondary amenorrhea** is the cessation of menstrual cycles once established. See also **hypothalamic amenorrhea, postpill amenorrhea. –amenorrheic.** *adj.*

amentia /āmen′shə/, **1.** an obsolete term for congenital mental retardation. See **mental retardation. 2.** also called **confusional insanity.** a state of mind characterized by apathy and disorientation, bordering on stupor, as in Stearns' alcoholic amentia.

Americaine, a trademark for a local anesthetic (benzocaine).

American Academy of Allergy and Immunology (AAAI), a national organization of physicians specializing in the diagnosis and treatment of allergies and immune system disorders.

American Academy of Nursing (AAN), the honorary organization of the American Nurses' Association, created to recognize superior achievement in nursing in order to promote advances and excellence in nursing practice and education. A person who is elected to membership is given the title of Fellow of the American Academy of Nursing and may use the abbreviation FAAN as an honorific.

American Academy of Physical Medicine and Rehabilitation (AAPMR), a national association of professional health care workers concerned with the diagnosis of physical impairment and the development of therapies and devices to improve physical function.

American Academy of Physicians' Assistants (AAPA), a national organization of physicians' assistants or associates.

American Association for Respiratory Therapy (AART), a national organization of nurses and other health workers in the field of respiratory therapy.

American Association of Colleges of Nursing (AACN), an organization of baccalaureate and graduate schools of nursing that was established to deal with various issues of nursing education.

American Association of Critical Care Nurses (AACN), a national organization of nurses who work in critical care units.

American Association of Industrial Nurses (AAIN), a national professional association of nurses working in industry and concerned with issues in occupational health.

American Association of Medical Colleges (AAMC), a national organization of faculty members and deans of medical schools.

American Association of Nephrology Nurses and Technicians (AANNT), an organization of nurses and technicians working in the fields of dialysis and renal diseases.

American Association of Neurological Nurses (AANN), a national organization of nurses working in the field of neurology.

American Association of of Neuroscience Nurses (AANN), a national organization of nurses working with neurologically impaired patients. The organization is affiliated with the American Association of Neurological Surgeons.

American Association of Nurse Anesthetists (AANA), a professional association of certified registered nurse anesthetists. The AANA is the accrediting agency for schools of nurse anesthetists. See also **nurse anesthetist.**

American Association of Oral and Maxillofacial Surgeons (AAOMS), a national organization of oral surgeons specializing in the diagnosis and treatment of the jaws, mouth, and teeth.

American Association of Pathologists and Bacteriologists (AAPB), a national professional organization of specialists in pathology and bacteriology.

American Association of University Professors (AAUP), a national organization of faculty members of institutions of higher learning. The AAUP represents faculty in matters of academic freedom, appointment policies, and procedures and serves as the bargaining agent for the faculties of some universities.

American College of Obstetricians and Gynecologists (ACOG), the national organization of obstetricians and gynecologists. It is concerned with the education of physicians in the specialty standards of practice, the continued education and well-being of its members, and the board certification of eligible members as fellows of the organization.

American College of Physicians (ACP), a national professional organization of physicians.

American College of Prosthodontists, an organization of dentists who specialize in restoration of dental or oral structures, as dentures, crowns, and bridges, and in the diagnosis and treatment of temporomandibular joint and maxillofacial disorders.

American College of Radiologists (ACR), a national professional organization of physicians who specialize in radiology.

American College of Surgeons (ACS), a national professional organization of physicians who specialize in surgery.

American Hospital Association (AHA), a national organization of individuals, institutions, and organizations that works to promote the improvement of health services for all people. The AHA publishes several journals and newsletters.

American Journal of Nursing, the professional journal of the American Nurses' Association (ANA). It contains articles of general and specialized clinical interest to nurses and is the principal resource regarding the profession in the United States.

American leishmaniasis, a group of mucocutaneous infections caused by various species of *Leishmania,* characterized by disfiguring ulcerative lesions of the nose, mouth, and throat. These infections are most prevalent in forested areas of southern Mexico and in Central and South America. Illness may be prolonged, rendering patients susceptible to serious secondary infections. Kinds of American leishmaniasis are **chiclero's ulcer, espundia, forest yaws,** and **uta.** Also called **mucocutaneous leishmaniasis, New World leishmaniasis.** See also **leishmaniasis.**

American Medical Association (AMA), a professional association whose membership is made up of approximately half of the total licensed physicians in the United States, including practitioners in all recognized medical specialties, as well as general primary care physicians. The AMA is governed by a Board of Trustees and House of Delegates who represent various state and local medical associations and government agencies such as the Public Health Service and medical departments of the Army, Navy, and Air Force. The AMA maintains directories of all qualified physicians (including nonmembers) in the United States, including graduates of foreign medical colleges, evaluates prescription and nonprescription drugs, advises congressional and state legislators regarding proposed health care laws, and publishes a variety of journals that report on scientific and socioeconomic developments in the field of medicine. See also **British Medical Association (BMA).**

American mountain fever. See **Colorado tick fever.**

American Nurses' Association (ANA), the national professional association of registered nurses in the United States. It was founded in 1896 to improve standards of health and the availability of health care given in order to foster high standards for nursing, to promote the professional development of nurses, and to advance the economic and general welfare of nurses. The ANA is made up of 53 constituent associations from 50 states, the District of Columbia, Guam, and the Virgin Islands, representing more than 900 district associations. National conventions are held biennially in even-numbered years. Members may join one or more of the five Divisions on Nursing Practice: Community Health, Gerontological, Maternal and Child Health, Medical-Surgical, and Psychiatric and Mental Health Nursing. These Divisions are coordinated by the Congress for Nursing Practice. The Congress evaluates changes in the scope of practice, monitors scientific and educational developments, encourages research, and develops statements that describe ANA policies regarding legislation affecting nursing practice. Other commissions within the Association include the Commission on Nursing Education, the Commission on Nursing Services, the Commission on Nursing Research, and the Economic and General Welfare Commission (E and GW), which functions at the local, state, and national level. The programs of the E and GW Commission are intended to ensure fair compensation for nurses, working conditions that are conducive to high quality nursing care, and a pool of qualified nurses adequate for the health care needs of the country. In addition, the ANA is politically active on the federal level in all issues relevant to nursing. Statistical services enable the Association to fulfill its role as the most authoritative source of data on nursing in the United States. The publications of the ANA include the *American Nurse,* a newspaper, the *Publications List,* and *The American Journal of Nursing,* the professional journal of the Association.

American Psychiatric Association (APA), a national professional psychiatric society concerned with the development of standards for psychiatric facilities, the formulation of mental health programs, the dissemination of data, and the promotion of psychiatric education and research. It publishes the *Diagnostic and Statistical Manual of Mental Disorders.*

American Red Cross, one of more than 120 national organizations that seek to reduce human suffering through various health, safety, and disaster relief programs in affiliation with the International Committee of the Red Cross. The Committee and all Red Cross organizations evolved from the Geneva Convention of 1864, following the example and urging of Swiss humanitarian Jean Henri Dunant, who aided wounded French and Austrian soldiers at the Battle of Solferino in 1859. The American Red Cross has more than 130 million members in about 3100 chapters throughout the United States. Volunteers comprise the entire staffs of about 1700 chapters. Other chapters maintain small paid staffs and some professionals but depend largely on volunteers. The American Red Cross blood program collects and distributes more blood than any other single agency in the United States and coordinates distribution of blood and blood products to the U.S. Defense Department on request or during national emergencies. The organization annually collects about four million blood donations and gives blood to more than 4000 hospitals. American Red Cross nursing and health programs include courses in the home on parenthood, prenatal and postnatal care, hygiene, and venereal disease. Nursing students are enrolled for service in American Red Cross community programs and during disasters. Four area offices at Alexandria, Virginia, Atlanta, Georgia, St. Louis, Missouri, and San Francisco, California, supervise and assist 70 divisions of the American Red Cross and direct field staff members assigned to military installations. National headquarters of the organization is at 17th and D Streets, NW, Washington, DC 20006. The President of the United States is honorary chairman of the organization, for which a 50-member board of governors, all volunteers, develops policy. The symbol of the American Red Cross, like that of most other Red Cross societies throughout the world, is a red cross on a field of white; in Switzerland it is a white cross on a red field, in Muslim countries, a red crescent, and in Israel, a red star of David.

American Registry of Radiologic Technologists (ARRT), a national professional organization of technicians specializing in radiology.

American trypanosomiasis. See **Chagas' disease.**

American Type Culture Collection (ATCC), a nonprofit, nongovernmental organization that is concerned with the preservation of specimens of cellular and microbiologic cultures and with the distribution of the cultures to research centers and laboratories in the academic, scientific, and medical communities.

americium (Am), a synthetic radioactive element of the actinide group. Its atomic number is 95; its atomic weight is 243.

Ameslan /am′islan/, abbreviation for *American Sign Language,* a method of communication with the deaf that relies primarily on the position, shape, and motion of the hands and fingers for the transmission of concepts and messages.

Ames test, a method for testing substances for possible carcinogenicity by exposing a strain of *Salmonella* bacteria to a sample of the substance. The rate of mutations observed is interpreted as an indication of the carcinogenic potential of the substance tested. Also called **mutagenicity test.**

amethocaine hydrochloride. See **tetracaine hydrochloride.**

amethopterin. See **methotrexate.**

ametropia /am′itrō′pē·ə/, a condition characterized by an optic defect involving an error of refraction, as astigmatism, hyperopia, or myopia. –**ametropic,** *adj.*

Amicar, a trademark for a hemostatic (aminocaproic acid).

amide-compound local anesthetic, any of more than two dozen compounds that are safe, versatile, and effective local anesthetics. If hypersensitivity to a drug in this group precludes its use, one of the ester-compound local anesthetics may provide analgesia without adverse effect. Some kinds of amide-compound local anesthetics are **bupivacaine, dibucaine, etiodocaine, lidocaine, mepivacaine,** and **prilocaine.**

amido-, a combining form meaning 'the presence of the radical NH_2 along with the radical CO': *amidoacetal, amidobenzene, amidopyrine.*

amidobenzene. See **aniline.**

Amigen, a trademark for a nutritional replacement or supplement (protein hydrolysate injection), used in parenteral alimentation.

amikacin sulfate, an aminoglycoside antibiotic.

▪ INDICATIONS: It is prescribed in the treatment of various severe infections that are resistant to other antibiotics.

▪ CONTRAINDICATIONS: Concurrent use of certain diuretics or known hypersensitivity to this or other aminoglycosides prohibits its use. The drug is used with caution in patients who have impaired renal function or myasthenia gravis.

▪ ADVERSE EFFECTS: Among the more serious adverse reactions are nephrotoxicity, auditory and vestibular ototoxicity, and neuromuscular blockade. GI disturbances, pain at the site of injection, and hypersensitivity reactions may occur.

Amikin, a trademark for an antibiotic (amikacin sulfate).

amiloride hydrochloride, a diuretic and hypertensive agent.

▪ INDICATIONS: It is prescribed as adjunctive therapy in the treatment of congestive heart failure or hypertension. It is often given with a thiazide medication.

▪ CONTRAINDICATIONS: Concurrent use of potassium-conserving agents, hyperkalemia, impaired renal function, or known hypersensitivity to this drug prohibits its use.

■ ADVERSE EFFECTS: Among the most serious adverse reactions are headache, diarrhea, nausea and vomiting, anorexia, hyperkalemia, dizziness, encephalopathy, impotence, muscle cramps, photosensitivity, irregular heart rhythm, mental confusion, and paresthesia.

amine /am′in, əmēn′/, (in chemistry) any organic compound that contains nitrogen.

amine pump, *informal.* an active transport system in the presynaptic nerve endings that takes up released amine neurotransmitters. Adverse reactions to some drugs, notably tricyclic antidepressants, block this function, resulting in a high concentration of norepinephrine in cardiac tissue and resultant tachycardia and arrhythmia. See also **monoamine oxidase inhibitor.**

aminoacetic acid. See **glycine.**

amino acid, an organic chemical compound composed of one or more basic amino groups and one or more acidic carboxyl groups. Twenty of the more than 100 amino acids that occur in nature are the building blocks of peptides, polypeptides, and proteins. The eight essential amino acids are isoleucine, leucine, lysine, methionine, phenylalanine, threonine, tryptophan, and valine. Arginine and histidine are essential in infants. Cysteine and tyrosine are quasi-essential because they may be synthesized from methionine and phenylalanine, respectively. The main nonessential amino acids are alanine, asparagine, aspartic acid, glutamine, glutamic acid, glycine, proline, and serine. From their structures, the amino acids can be classified as neutral, basic, or acidic, each group being transported across cell membranes by different carrier mechanisms. Arginine, histidine, and lysine are basic amino acids, aspartic acid and glutamic acid are acidic, and the remainder are neutral.

aminoaciduria /amē′nō•as′idŏŏr′ē•ə/, the abnormal presence of amino acids in the urine that usually indicates an inborn metabolic defect, as in cystinuria.

aminobenzene. See **aniline.**

aminobenzoic acid, a metabolic product of the catabolism of the amino acid tryptophan. Also called **anthranilicacid.** See also **para-aminobenzoic acid (PABA).**

aminocaproic acid /əmē′nōkəprō′ik, am′inō-/, a hemostatic.

■ INDICATION: It is prescribed to stop excessive bleeding that results from hyperfibrinolysis.

■ CONTRAINDICATION: Active intravascular coagulation prohibits its use.

■ ADVERSE EFFECTS: Among the most serious adverse reactions are thrombosis and hypotension. Inhibition of ejaculation, nasal congestion, diarrhea, and various allergic reactions also may occur.

Aminodur, a trademark for a bronchodilator (aminophylline).

aminoglycoside antibiotic. See **antibiotic.**

amino oxidase. See **monoamine oxidase.**

aminophylline /am′ənōfil′in, əmē′nō-/, a bronchodilator.

■ INDICATIONS: It is prescribed in the treatment of bronchial asthma, emphysema, and bronchitis.

■ CONTRAINDICATIONS: Known hypersensitivity to this drug or other xanthine medication prohibits its use. It is used with caution in patients who have peptic ulcer and those in whom cardiac stimulation would be harmful.

■ ADVERSE EFFECTS: Among the more serious adverse reactions are GI disturbances, central nervous system stimulation, palpitations, tachycardia, and nervousness.

aminosalicylic acid. See **paraaminosalicylic acid.**

aminosuccinic acid. See **aspartic acid.**

aminotransferase, an enzyme that catalyzes the transfer of an amino group from an alpha-amino acid to an alpha-keto acid, with pyridoxal phosphate and pyridoxamine phosphate acting as coenzymes. Aspartate amino transferase (AST), normally present in serum and various tissues, especially in the heart and liver, is released by damaged cells, and, as a result, a high serum level of AST may be diagnostic in myocardial infarction or hepatic disease. Alanine aminotransferase (ALT), a normal constituent of serum and various tissues, especially in the liver, is released by injured tissue and may be present in high concentrations in the sera of patients with acute liver disease. Also called **transaminase.**

amitosis /am′ətō′sis/, direct cell division in which there is simple fission of the nucleus and cytoplasm. It does not involve the complex stages of chromatin separation of the chromosomes that occur in mitosis. –**amitotic,** *adj.*

amitriptyline, a tricyclic antidepressant.

■ INDICATION: It is prescribed in the treatment of depression.

■ CONTRAINDICATIONS: Concomitant administration of monoamine oxidase inhibitors, recent myocardial infarction, or known hypersensitivity to this drug or to other tricyclic medication prohibits its use. It is used with caution in patients having a seizure disorder or in those with cardiovascular disease.

■ ADVERSE EFFECTS: Among the more serious adverse reactions are sedation and a variety of GI cardiovascular, and neurologic reactions. This drug interacts with many other drugs.

AML, abbreviation for **acute myelocytic leukemia.**

ammoni-, a combining form meaning 'pertaining to ammonium': *ammoniemia, ammonirrhea, ammoniuria.*

ammonia, a colorless aromatic gas consisting of nitrogen and hydrogen, produced by the decomposition of nitrogenous organic matter. Some of its many uses are as an aromatic stimulant, a detergent, and an emulsifier.

ammoniacal fermentation, the production of ammonia and carbon dioxide from urea by the enzyme urease.

Ammon's horn. See **hippocampus major.**

amnesia, a loss of memory caused by brain damage or by severe emotional trauma. Kinds of amnesia are **anterograde amnesia, hysteric amnesia, posttraumatic amnesia,** and **retrograde amnesia.**

amnestic apraxia, the inability to carry out a movement in response to a request because of a lack of ability to remember the request rather than to a loss of motor function. See also **apraxia.**

amnio-, a combining form meaning 'pertaining to the amnion': *amniogenesis, amnioma, amniorrhexis*.

amniocentesis /am′nē•ōsentē′sis/, an obstetric procedure in which a small amount of amniotic fluid is removed for laboratory analysis. It is usually performed between the sixteenth and twentieth weeks of gestation to aid in the diagnosis of fetal abnormalities.

■ METHOD: With the use of ultrasound scanning techniques the position of the fetus and the location of the placenta are determined. The skin on the mother's abdomen is aseptically prepared, and a local anesthetic is usually injected. A needle attached to a syringe is introduced into a part of the uterus where there is the least chance of perforating the placenta or scratching the fetus. Between 20 and 25 ml of amniotic fluid is aspirated. Amniocentesis is performed to diagnose various genetic defects, including chromosomal abnormalities, neural tube defects, and Tay-Sachs disease. It is also performed to discover the sex of the fetus if certain sex-linked genetic defects are suspected. Later in pregnancy, amniocentesis may be performed to assess fetal maturity by testing the lecithin-sphingomyelin (L/S) ratio in the laboratory before therapeutic termination of pregnancy. The fluid may be tested for the concentration of creatinine, another indicator of fetal maturity. When postmaturity is suspected, amniocentesis is performed to examine the amniotic fluid for meconium.

■ NURSING ORDERS: Proof of informed consent is required to be signed by the woman before amniocentesis. Specifically stated in the consent form are the reason for performing the procedure and the facts that fluid is to be removed after needle puncture of the uterus, that ultrasound imaging techniques are usual adjuncts, that the procedure may fail to give the results intended, and that spontaneous abortion, nausea, abdominal pain, or fetal injury may occur. The woman is reassured that complications and failure are rare; she is given emotional support before, during, and after the procedure. In testing for genetic abnormalities 3 or more weeks is usually necessary for tissue culture before a diagnosis may be made; this waiting period is extremely stressful for the mother. The woman is warned to report any signs of infection or of the onset of labor. Rh immune globulin is often given to pregnant women who are Rh negative.

■ OUTCOME CRITERIA: Spontaneous abortion occurs in approximately 1% of women undergoing amniocentesis. Perforation of the placenta or a blood vessel in the umbilical cord or placenta may cause hemorrhage or isoimmunization and hemolytic disease of the fetus, possibly leading to fetal death. Maternal and fetal infection with attendant morbidity or mortality may occur, but it is rare. Premature rupture of the membranes, premature labor, or trauma to the fetus or umbilical cord may occur. The procedure is not usually performed for genetic diagnosis unless the mother plans to terminate the pregnancy if the procedure indicates the presence of a genetic disease or abnormality.

amnion /am′nē•on/, a membrane, continuous with and covering the fetal side of the placenta, that forms the outer surface of the umbilical cord and becomes the outermost layer of the skin of the developing fetus. Compare **chorion.**

amniotic fluid /am′nē•ot′ik/, a liquid produced by the fetal membranes and the fetus. It surrounds the fetus throughout pregnancy, usually totaling about 1000 ml at term. In addition to providing the fetus with physical protection, the amniotic fluid is a medium of active chemical exchange. It is secreted and resorbed by cells lining the amniotic sac at a rate of 500 ml/hr at term, and is swallowed, metabolized, and excreted as fetal urine at a rate of 50 ml/hr. Its chemical constituents are those of maternal and fetal plasma in different concentrations. Its pH is close to neutral. Amniotic fluid itself is clear, though desquamated fetal cells and lipids give it a cloudy appearance.

amniotic sac, a thin-walled bag that contains the fetus and amniotic fluid during pregnancy, having a capacity of 4 to 5 L at term. The wall of the sac extends from the margin of the placenta. The amnion, chorion, and decidua that make up the wall are each a few cell layers thick. They are closely applied — though not fused — to each other and to the wall of the uterus. The intact sac and its fluid provide for the equilibration of hydrostatic pressure within the uterus and, during labor, effect the uniform transmission of the force of uterine contractions to the cervix for dilatation. See also **amnion, chorion, decidua.**

amobarbital, a barbiturate sedative-hypnotic.

■ INDICATIONS: It is prescribed for the relief of anxiety and insomnia and as an anticonvulsant.

■ CONTRAINDICATIONS: Porphyria or known hypersensitivity to barbiturates prohibits its use.

■ ADVERSE EFFECTS: Among the most serious adverse reactions are respiratory and circulatory depression, drug hangover, and various allergic reactions. It is also involved in many drug interactions.

amoeba. See **ameba.**

-amoeba. See **-ameba.**

amoebiasis. See **amebiasis.**

amoebic dysentery. See **amebic dysentery.**

amorph /ā′môrf, əmôrf′/, **1.** inactive gene; a mutant allele that has little or no effect on the expression of a trait. Compare **antimorph, hypermorph, hypomorph. 2.** abbreviation for **amorphous,** as amorph IZS (amorphous insulin zinc suspension).

amorphic, (in genetics) of or pertaining to a gene that is inactive or nearly inactive so that it has no determinable effect.

amorphous crystals, shapeless, ill-defined crystals, usually phosphates.

amoxapine, an antidepressant similar to the tricyclics.

■ INDICATION: It is prescribed in the treatment of mental depression.
■ CONTRAINDICATIONS: It is used with caution in conditions where anticholinergics are contraindicated, in seizure disorders, and in patients with cardiovascular disorders. Concomitant administration of monoamine oxidase inhibitors, recent myocardial infarction, or known hypersensitivity to this drug prohibits its use.
■ ADVERSE EFFECTS: Among the most serious adverse reactions are sedation and anticholinergic side effects. A variety of GI, cardiovascular, and neurologic reactions may also occur. It is involved in many potential drug interactions.

amoxicillin, a semisynthetic oral penicillin antibiotic similar to ampicillin.
■ INDICATIONS: It is prescribed in the treatment of several infections that are caused by a susceptible gram-negative or gram-positive organism.
■ CONTRAINDICATION: Known hypersensitivity to any penicillin prohibits its use.
■ ADVERSE EFFECTS: Among the most serious adverse reactions are anaphylaxis, nausea, and diarrhea. Various allergic reactions and rashes are common.

Amoxil, a trademark for an antibiotic (amoxicillin).

AMP, abbreviation for **adenosine monophosphate.**

ampere (A) /am′pēr/, a unit of measurement of the amount of electric current. An ampere, according to the meter-kilogram-second (MKS) system, is the amount of current passed through a resistance of 1 ohm by an electrical potential of 1 volt. The standard international ampere is the amount of current that deposits 0.001118 g of silver per second when passed, according to certain specifications, through a silver nitrate solution. See also **ohm, volt, watt.**

amperometry, the measurement of current at a single applied potential.

amph-. See **amphi-.**

amphetamines, a group of nervous system stimulants, including amphetamine and its chemical congeners dextroamphetamine and methamphetamine, that are subject to abuse because of their ability to produce wakefulness and euphoria. Abuse leads to compulsive behavior, paranoia, hallucinations, and suicidal tendencies. They have several street names, as **black beauties, lid poppers, pep pills,** and **speed,** the last being the injectable form of methamphetamine. See also **amphetamine sulfate, dextroamphetamine sulfate, methamphetamine sulfate.**

amphetamine sulfate, a central nervous system stimulant.
■ INDICATIONS: It is prescribed for narcolepsy, attention deficit disorder, or obesity.
■ CONTRAINDICATIONS: Drug abuse, hypertension, glaucoma, hyperthyroidism, arteriosclerosis, cardiovascular disease, concomitant use of monoamine oxidase, or known hypersensitivity to this drug prohibits its use.
■ ADVERSE EFFECTS: Among the most serious adverse reactions are various manifestations of central nervous system excitation, hypertension, arrhythmias and other cardiovascular effects, nausea, anorexia, and drug dependence.

amphi-, amph-, a combining form meaning 'on both sides': *amphiarthrosis, amphiaster, amphibious.*

amphiarthrosis. See **cartilaginous joint.**

amphigenesis. See **amphigony.**

amphigenetic /am′fijənet′ik/, **1.** produced by the union of gametes from both sexes. **2.** bisexual; having both testicular and ovarian tissue.

amphigenous inheritance /amfij′ənəs/, the acquisition of genetic traits and conditions from both parents. Also called **biparental inheritance, duplex inheritance.**

amphigonadism /am′figō′nədiz′əm/, true hermaphroditism; having both testicular and ovarian tissue. –**amphigonadic,** *adj.*

amphigony /amfig′ənē/, sexual reproduction. Also called **amphigenesis.** –**amphigonic** /am′figon′ik/, *adj.*

amphikaryon /am′fiker′ē·on/, a nucleus containing the diploid number of chromosomes. –**amphikaryotic,** *adj.*

amphimixis /am′fimik′sis/, **1.** the union of germ cells in reproduction so that both maternal and paternal hereditary characteristics are derived; interbreeding. **2.** (in psychoanalysis) the union and integration of oral, anal, and genital libidinal impulses in the development of heterosexuality.

amphipathic, pertaining to a molecule having two sides with characteristically different properties, as a detergent, which has both a polar (hydrophilic) end and a nonpolar (hydrophobic) end but is long enough so that each end demonstrates its own solubility characteristics.

ampho-, a combining form meaning 'both': *amphochromophil, amphodiplopia, amphogenic.*

amphoric breath sound, an abnormal, resonant, hollow blowing sound heard with a stethoscope. It indicates a cavity opening into the bronchus, or a pneumothorax.

amphoteric, a substance that can have a positive, zero, or negative charge, depending on conditions.

amphotericin B /am′fəter′əsin/, an antifungal medication.
■ INDICATIONS: It is prescribed for topical or systemic use in the treatment of fungal infections.
■ CONTRAINDICATION: Known hypersensitivity to this drug prohibits its use.
■ ADVERSE EFFECTS: Among the most serious adverse reactions are, when used systemically, thrombophlebitis, blood dyscrasias, nephrotoxicity, nausea, and fever. With topical use, local hypersensitivity reactions are the most common adverse reactions.

ampicillin /am′pəsil′in/, a semisynthetic penicillin.
■ INDICATIONS: It is prescribed in the treatment of a variety of infections caused by a broad spectrum of sensitive gram-negative and gram-positive organisms.

■ CONTRAINDICATION: Known hypersensitivity to any penicillin prohibits its use.

■ ADVERSE EFFECTS: Among the most serious adverse reactions are anaphylaxis, nausea, and diarrhea. Fever, rashes, other allergic reactions, and suprainfection also may occur.

amplification, **1.** (in molecular genetics) a process in which the amount of plasmid DNA is increased in proportion to the amount of bacterial DNA by treatment with certain substances, including chloramphenicol. **2.** the replication in bulk of an entire gene library. **–amplify,** *v.*

amplitude, width or breadth of range or extent, as amplitude of accommodation or amplitude of convergence.

amplitude of accommodation (AA), the total accommodative power of the eye, determined by the difference between the refractive power for farthest vision and that for nearest vision.

amplitude of convergence, the difference in the power needed to turn the eyes from their far point to their near point of convergence. Also called **fusional amplitude, vergence ability.**

ampule /am′pyo͞ol/, a small, sterile glass or plastic container that usually contains a single dose of a solution to be administered parenterally. Also spelled **ampoule.**

ampulla /ampo͞ol′ə/, a rounded, saclike dilatation of a duct, canal, or any tubular structure, as the lacrimal duct, semicircular canal, uterine tube, rectum, or vas deferans.

ampulla of Vater. See **hepatopancreatic ampulla.**

ampullary aneurism. See **saccular aneurism.**

ampullary tubal pregnancy /ampo͞ol′ərē, am′pəler′ē/, a kind of tubal pregnancy in which implantation occurs in the ampulla of one of the fallopian tubes. See also **tubal pregnancy.**

amputation, the surgical removal of a part of the body or a limb or part of a limb, performed to treat recurrent infections or gangrene in peripheral vascular disease, to remove malignant tumors, and in severe trauma. With the patient under general anesthesia, the part is removed and a shaped flap is cut from muscular and cutaneous tissue to cover the end of the bone, with a section left open for drainage if infection is present. Preoperative care includes an assessment of circulation in the affected part and the shaving and cleansing of the area. Postoperatively, the stump is elevated on a pillow, and, if necessary, protected with plastic from urinary and fecal contamination. Vital signs are monitored carefully. If a soft dressing is used, it is watched for excessive bleeding. The stump is moved frequently to prevent circulatory complications and tissue necrosis. If the dressing is rigid (a cast), it must remain in place for 8 to 14 days. Should the cast come off inadvertently, the stump must be wrapped tightly at once with elastic compression bandage and plans must be made to replace the cast. With the cast on, the patient who has had part of a leg removed can stand briefly after 24 hours and bear some weight on the prosthesis. Medication may relieve incisional and phantom limb pain. Kinds of amputation include **closed amputation, congenital amputation, open amputation, primary amputation,** and **secondary amputation.**

amputation neuroma, a form of traumatic neuroma that may develop near the stump after the amputation of an extremity.

amputee, a person who has had one or more extremities traumatically, congenitally, or surgically removed. See also **congenital amputation.**

Amsler grid, a checkerboard grid of intersecting dark horizontal and vertical lines with one dark spot in the middle. To discover a visual field defect, the person simply covers or closes one eye and looks at the spot with the other. A visual field defect is perceived as a defect, distortion, blank, or other fault in the grid. The person may record the defects directly on a paper copy of the grid that may be kept as a permanent record.

Amsterdam dwarf, a person affected with de Lange's syndrome, in which short stature and severe mental retardation are associated with many other abnormalities.

amyelinic neuroma, a tumor that contains only nonmyelinated nerve fibers.

amygdalin /əmig′dəlin/, a naturally occurring cyaniogenic glycoside obtained from bitter almonds and apricot pits. It has been promoted as a potential cancer remedy under the trademark of Laetrile. Also called **vitamin B_{17}.**

amyl-. See **amylo-.**

amyl alcohol, a colorless, oily liquid that is only slightly soluble in water but can be mixed with ethyl alcohol, chloroform, or ether.

amyl alcohol tertiary. See **amylene hydrate.**

amylase /am′ilās/, an enzyme that catalyzes the hydrolysis of starch into smaller carbohydrate molecules. Alpha-amylase, found in saliva, pancreatic juice, malt, certain bacteria, and molds, catalyzes the hydrolysis of starches to dextrins, maltose, and maltotriose. Beta-amylase, found in grains, vegetables, and malt, is involved in the hydrolysis of starch to maltose. See also **enzyme.**

amylene hydrate, a clear, colorless liquid with a camphorlike odor, miscible with alcohol, chloroform, ether, or glycerin and used as a solvent and a hypnotic.

amylic fermentation /əmil′ik/, the formation of amyl alcohol from sugar.

amyl nitrite, a vasodilator.

■ INDICATION: It is prescribed to relieve the vasospasm of angina pectoris.

■ CONTRAINDICATIONS: Known hypersensitivity to this drug or to other nitrites prohibits its use.

■ ADVERSE EFFECTS: Among the more serious adverse reactions are hypotension, allergic reactions, nausea, headache, and dizziness.

amylo-, amyl-, a combining form meaning 'pertaining to starch': *amyloclast, amylodextrin, amyloid.*

amylobarbitone. See **amobarbital.**

amyloidosis /am′iloidō′sis/, a disease in which a waxy, starchlike, glycoprotein (amyloid) accumulates in tissues and organs, impairing their function. There are two major forms of the condition. **Primary amyloidosis** usually occurs with multiple myeloma. Patients with **secondary amyloidosis** usually suffer from another chronic infectious or inflammatory disease, as tuberculosis, osteomyelitis, rheumatoid arthritis, or Crohn's disease. The cause of both types of amyloidosis is unknown. Almost all organs are affected, most often the heart, lungs, tongue, and intestines in primary amyloidosis, and the kidneys, liver, and spleen in the secondary type. Diagnosis is made through biopsy of the suspected organ. There is no known cure for amyloidosis, and treatment in the secondary type is aimed at alleviating the underlying chronic disease. Patients with renal amyloidosis are frequently candidates for kidney dialysis and transplantation.

amylopectinosis. See **Andersen's disease.**

amyotonia /ā′mī•ōtō′nē•ə/, an abnormal condition of skeletal muscle, characterized by a lack of tone, weakness, and wasting, usually the result of motor neuron disease. **–amyotonic,** *adj.*

amyotonia congenita. See **Oppenheim's disease.**

amyotrophic lateral sclerosis (ALS) /ā′mī•ōtrof′ik/, a degenerative disease of the motor neurons, characterized by atrophy of the muscles of the hands, forearms, and legs spreading to involve most of the body. It results from degeneration of the motor neurons of the anterior horns and corticospinal tracts, beginning in middle age and progressing rapidly, causing death within 2 to 5 years. There is no known treatment. Also called **Lou Gehrig's disease.** See also **Aran-Duchenne muscular atrophy.**

Amytal, a trademark for a barbiturate sedative-hypnotic (amobarbital).

an-, **1.** a combining form meaning 'upward, backward, excessive, or again': *anelectrotonic, anion, anode*. **2.** also **ana-.** a combining form meaning 'not': *anaerogenic, analgesia, anaphia*.

ana (āa, āā, ĀĀ), (in prescriptions) "so much of each," indication of the amount of each ingredient to be compounded. Usually written as an abreviation.

ANA, abbreviation for **American Nurses' Association.**

ana-. See **an-.**

anabolic steroid, any one of several compounds derived from testosterone or prepared synthetically to promote general body growth, to oppose the effects of endogenous estrogen, or to promote masculinizing effects. All such compounds cause a mixed androgenic-anabolic effect. Anabolic steroids are prescribed in the treatment of aplastic anemia, red-cell aplasia, and hemolytic anemia and in anemias associated with renal failure, myeloid metaplasia, and leukemia. Some common compounds used in such therapies are calusterone, methandriol, and nandrolone. Anabolic steroids used in the palliation of carcinoma of the breast in women carry the risk of causing masculinization. The earliest symptoms of such undesirable effects are acne, the growth of facial hair, and the hoarsening or deepening of the voice. Continued use of these compounds in women may also produce prominent musculature, excessive body hair, and hypertrophy of the clitoris.

anabolism /ənab′əliz′əm/, constructive metabolism characterized by the conversion of simple substances into the more complex compounds of living matter. Compare **catabolism. –anabolic** /an′əbol′ik/, *adj.*

anacatadidymus /an′əkat′ədid′iməs/, conjoined twins that are fused in the middle but separated above and below.

anaclisis /an′əklī′sis/, **1.** a condition, normal in childhood but pathologic in adulthood, in which a person is emotionally dependent on other people. **2.** a condition in which a person consciously or unconsciously chooses a love object because of a resemblance to the mother, father, or other person who was an important source of comfort and protection in infancy. **–anaclitic** /an′əklit′ik/, *adj.*

anaclitic depression, a syndrome occurring in infants, usually after sudden separation from the mothering person. Symptoms include apprehension, withdrawal, incessant crying, refusal to eat, sleep disturbances, and, eventually, stupor leading to severe impairment of the infant's physical, social, and intellectual development. If the mothering figure or a substitute is made available within 1 to 3 months, the infant recovers quickly with no long-term effects. See also **hospitalism.**

anacrotic pulse /an′əkrot′ik/, (on a sphygmographic tracing) a pulse characterized by one transient drop in amplitude on the curve of the primary elevation. It is seen in valvular aortic stenosis.

anadicrotic pulse /an′ədīkrot′ik/, (on a sphygmographic tracing) a pulse characterized by two transient drops in amplitude on the curve of primary elevation.

anadidymus /an′ədid′iməs/, conjoined twins that are united at the pelvis and lower extremities but are separated in the upper half. Also called **duplicatus anterior.** Compare **catadidymus.**

anadipsia /an′ədip′sē•ə/, extreme thirst, often occurring in the manic phase of manic-depressive psychosis. The condition is the result of dehydration caused by the excessive perspiration, continuous urination, and relentless physical activity produced by the intense excitement characteristic of the manic phase.

Anadrol, a trademark for an androgen (oxymetholone), used as an anabolic agent.

anaerobe /aner′ōb/, a microorganism that grows and lives in the complete or almost complete absence of oxygen. An example is *Clostridium botulinum*. Anaerobes are widely distributed in nature and in the body. Some kinds of anaerobes are **facultative anaerobe** and **obligate anaerobe.** Compare **aerobe, microaerophile.** See also **anaerobic infection.**

anaerobic /an′ərō′bik/, **1.** pertaining to the absence of air or oxygen. **2.** able to grow and function without air or oxygen.

anaerobic exercise, muscular exertion sufficient to result in metabolic acidosis because of accumulation of lactic acid as a product of muscle metabolism. Compare **aerobic exercise.** See also **active exercise, passive exercise.**

anaerobic glycolysis. See **glycolysis.**

anaerobic infection, an infection caused by an anaerobic organism, usually occurring in deep puncture wounds that exclude air or in tissue that has diminished oxygen-reduction potential as a result of trauma, necrosis, or overgrowth of bacteria. Kinds of anaerobic infection are **gangrene** and **tetanus.** See also ***Clostridium.***

anaerobic myositis. See **gas gangrene.**

anal /ā′nəl/, of or pertaining to the anus.

anal agenesis. See **imperforate anus.**

anal canal, the final portion of the alimentary tract, about 4 cm long, between the rectal ampulla and the anus.

anal character, (in psychoanalysis) a kind of personality exhibiting patterns of behavior originating in the anal phase of infancy, characterized by extreme orderliness, obstinacy, perfectionism, cleanliness, punctuality, and miserliness, or their extreme opposites. See also **anal eroticism, anal stage, psychosexual development.**

anal crypt, the depression between rectal columns that encloses networks of veins that, when inflamed and swollen, are called hemorrhoids.

analeptic. See **central nervous system stimulant.**

anal eroticism, (in psychoanalysis) libidinal fixation at or regression to the anal stage of psychosexual development, often reflected in such personality traits as miserliness, stubbornness, and overscrupulousness. Also called **anal erotism.** Compare **oral eroticism.** See also **anal character.**

anal fissure, a linear ulceration or laceration of the skin of the anus.

anal fistula, an abnormal opening on the cutaneous surface near the anus, usually resulting from a local crypt abscess and also common in Crohn's disease. A perianal fistula may or may not communicate with the rectum. Also called **fistula in ano.**

analgesia /an′əljē′zē·ə/, a lack of pain without loss of consciousness.

analgesia algera. See **anesthesia dolorosa.**

analgesic /an′əljē′zik/, **1.** relieving pain. **2.** a drug that relieves pain. The narcotic analgesics act on the central nervous system and alter the patient's perception; they are more often used for severe pain. The nonnarcotic analgesics act at the site of the pain, do not produce tolerance or dependence, and do not alter the patient's perception; they are used for mild to moderate pain. Compare **anodyne.** See also **pain intervention.**

analgesic cocktail, *informal.* an individualized mixture of drugs used for pain relief in specific syndromes. See also **lytic cocktail.**

anal membrane. See **cloacal membrane.**

anal membrane atresia. See **imperforate anus.**

analog /an′əlog/, **1.** a substance, tissue, or organ that is similar in appearance or function to another but differing in origin or development, as the eye of a fly and the eye of a human. **2.** a drug or other chemical compound that resembles another in structure or constituents but has different effects. Also spelled **analogue.** Compare **homolog.**

analog computer, a computer that processes information as a physical quantity, such as voltage, amperage, weight, or length and presents results of calculations that can be continuously varied and measured. Compare **digital computer, hybrid computer.**

analog signal, a continuous electric signal representing a specific condition, as temperature or ECG waveforms.

analog-to-digital converter, a device for converting analog information, such as temperature or ECG waveforms, into digital form for processing by a digital computer. Also called **A/D converter.**

anal reflex, a superficial neurologic reflex obtained by stroking the skin or mucosa of the region around the anus, which normally results in a contraction of the external anal sphincter. This reflex may be lost in disease of the pyramidal tract above the upper lumbar spine level. See also **superficial reflex.**

anal sadism, (in psychoanalysis) a sadistic form of anal eroticism, manifested by such behavior as aggressiveness and selfishness. Compare **oral sadism.**

anal stage, (in psychoanalysis) the pregenital period in psychosexual development, occurring between 1 and 3 years of age, when preoccupation with the function of the bowel and the sensations associated with the anus are the predominant source of pleasurable stimulation. It is regarded as an important determinant of ultimate personality type. Adult patterns of behavior associated with fixation on this stage include either extreme neatness, orderliness, cleanliness, perfectionism, and punctuality, or their extreme opposites. Also called **anal phase.** See also **anal character, psychosexual development.**

anal stenosis. See **imperforate anus.**

analysand /ənal′isand′/, a person undergoing psychoanalysis.

analysis, the separation of substances into their constituent parts and the determination of the nature, properties, and composition of compounds. In chemistry, **qualitative analysis** is the determination of the elements present in a substance; **quantitative analysis** is the determination of how much of each element is present in a substance. Analysis is also an informal term for **psychoanalysis.** – **analytic,** *adj.* **analyze,** *v.*

analysis of variance (ANOVA), a series of statistic procedures for determining the differences, attributable to chance alone, among two or more groups of scores.

analyst, **1.** a psychoanalyst. **2.** a person who analyzes the chemical, physical, or other properties of a substance or product.

analyte, any substance that is measured. The term is usually applied to a component of a biologic section.

analytic psychology, **1.** the system in which phenomena, such as sensations and feelings, are analyzed and classified by introspective rather than by experimental methods. Compare **experimental psychology. 2.** also called **Jungian psychology.** a system of analyzing the psyche according to the concepts developed by Carl Gustav Jung. It differs from the psychoanalysis of Sigmund Freud in stressing a "racial" or collective unconscious and a mystic, religious factor in the development of the personal unconscious and in minimizing the importance of sexual influence on early emotional and psychologic development.

analyzing, (in five-step nursing process) a category of nursing behavior in which the health care needs of the client are identified and the goals of care are selected. The nurse interprets data, identifies problems involving the client, the client's family, and significant others, establishes priorities among goals, integrates the information, and projects the expected outcomes of nursing activities. Although analyzing follows assessing and precedes planning in the five steps of the nursing process, in practice, analyzing is integral to effective nursing practice at all steps of the process. See also **assessing, evaluating, implementing, nursing process, planning.**

anamnesis /an′amnē′sis/, **1.** remembrance of the past. **2.** the accumulated data concerning a medical or psychiatric patient and the patient's background, including family, previous environment, experiences, and, particularly, recollections, for use in analyzing his condition. Compare **catamnesis.**

anaphase /an′əfāz/, the third of four stages of nuclear division in mitosis and in each of the two divisions of meiosis. In mitosis and the second meiotic division the centromeres divide, and the two chromatids, which are arranged along the equatorial plane of the spindle, separate and move to the opposite poles of the cell, forming daughter chromosomes. In the first meiotic division the pairs of homologous chromosomes separate from each other and move intact to the opposite poles of the spindle. See also **interphase, meiosis, metaphase, mitosis, prophase, telophase.**

anaphylactic hypersensitivity /an′əfilak′tik/, an IgE- or IgG-dependent, immediate-acting humoral hypersensitivity response to an exogenous antigen. An intradermal skin test produces a wheal and flare reaction and edema within 30 minutes. Histamine, kinins, and other substances are released from mast cells, causing vasodilatation and muscle contraction. Systemic anaphylaxis, atopic allergies, hayfever, and insect-sting reactions are all anaphylactic hypersensitivity reactions. Also called **type I hypersensitivity.** Compare **cell-mediated immune response, cytotoxic hypersensitivity, immune complex hypersensitivity.** See also **anaphylactic shock, immunoglobulins.**

anaphylactic shock, a severe and sometimes fatal systemic hypersensitivity reaction to a sensitizing substance, as a drug, vaccine, certain food, serum, allergen extract, insect venom, or chemical. This condition may occur within seconds from the time of exposure to the sensitizing factor and is commonly marked by respiratory distress and vascular collapse. The more quickly any systemic atopic reaction occurs in the individual after exposure, the more severe the associated shock is likely to be. The involved allergen enters the systemic circulation and triggers an incomplete humoral response that allows the allergen to combine with IgE and cause the release of histamine. Also entering into the reaction are IgG and IgM, which cause the release of complement fractions, further stimulating histamine action.

■ OBSERVATIONS: Anaphylactic shock can occur within seconds or minutes after exposure to an allergen. The first symptoms are intense anxiety, weakness, sweating, and shortness of breath. Other symptoms may include hypotension, shock, arrhythmia, respiratory congestion, laryngeal edema, nausea, and diarrhea.

■ INTERVENTION: If the patient is conscious and normotensive, treatment requires the immediate injection of epinephrine intramuscularly or subcutaneously with vigorous massage of the injection site to assure faster distribution of the drug. If the patient is unconscious, epinephrine is administered intravenously. The airway is maintained, and the patient is carefully monitored for signs of laryngeal edema, which may require the insertion of an endotracheal tube or a tracheotomy and oxygen therapy. The signs of laryngeal edema include stridor, hoarseness, and dyspnea. Cardiopulmonary resuscitation may be required for cardiac arrest; it often involves closed-chest heart massage, assisted ventilation, and the administration of sodium bicarbonate.

■ NURSING CONSIDERATIONS: Nursing care of patients experiencing anaphylactic shock requires the performance of appropriate emergency treatment and the close monitoring of the patient for hypotension and decreased circulatory volume; volume expanders, as plasma, saline, and albumin, are often ordered. After the emergency other medications, as subcutaneous epinephrine, corticosteroids, and diphenhydramine IV, are administered as prescribed; blood pressure, central venous pressure, and urinary output are monitored. Patients with food allergies that produce anaphylactic shock are instructed to avoid offending allergens; patients with insect sting allergies are instructed to carry emergency anaphylactic kits when outdoors. Such kits contain epinephrine, antihistamine, and tourniquets.

anaphylactoid purpura. See **Henoch-Schönlein purpura.**

anaphylaxis /an′əfilak′sis/, an exaggerated hypersensitivity reaction to a previously encountered antigen. The response, which is mediated by antibodies of the IgE class of immunoglobulins, causes the release of histamine, kinin, and substances that affect smooth muscle. The reaction may be a localized wheal and flare of generalized itching, hyperemia, angioneurotic edema, and in severe cases vascular collapse, bronchospasm, and shock. The severity of symptoms depends on the original sensitizing dose of the antigen, the amount and distribution of antibodies, and the route of entry and size of the dose of antigen producing anaphylaxis. Insect stings, contrast media containing iodide, aspirin, antitoxins prepared with animal serum, and allergens used in testing and desensitizing patients who are hypersensitive produce anaphylaxis in some individuals. Penicillin injection is the most common cause of anaphylactic shock. Kinds of anaphylaxis are **aggregate anaphylaxis, antiserum anaphylaxis, cutaneous anaphylaxis, cytotoxic anaphylaxis, indirect anaphylaxis,** and **inverse anaphylaxis.** **–anaphylactic, anaphylactoid,** *adj.*

anaplasia /an′əplā′zhə/, a change in the structure of cells and in their orientation to each other characterized by a loss of differentiation and reversion to a more primitive form. Anaplasia is characteristic of malignancy. Compare **metastasis.** **–anaplastic,** *adj.*

anaplastic astrocytoma. See **glioblastoma multiforme.**

Anapolon, a trademark for an androgen (oxymetholone).

anarthria /anär′thrē·ə/, a loss of control of the muscles of speech, resulting in the inability to utter words. The condition is usually caused by damage to a central or peripheral motor nerve.

anasarca /an′əsär′kə/, generalized, massive edema. Anasarca is often observed in edema associated with renal disease when fluid retention continues for an extended period of time. See also **edema.** **–anasarcous,** *adj.*

anastomosis /ənas′tōmō′sis/, *pl.* **anastomoses,** a surgical joining of two ducts or blood vessels to allow flow from one to the other. It may be performed to bypass an aneurysm or a vascular or arterial occlusion. With the patient under general anesthesia, a section of his saphenous vein or a synthetic prosthesis of Dacron, Teflon, or Orlon is grafted to the prepared vessels. Postoperative nursing care includes preventing tissue injury and wound infection by the use of a bed cradle over the incision and padded rails. An adequate airway is maintained, oxygen is given if necessary, and vital signs are closely monitored. The systolic blood pressure is kept at about 20 mm Hg above normal to maintain blood flow through the graft. Lack of blood flow may allow the graft to close, a major complication that requires exploratory surgery and sometimes amputation. Distal pulses on both legs are evaluated and their locations marked. Capillary filling time and the color and temperature of the skin are checked. Prophylactic antibiotic therapy may be started. Urinary output is monitored to be certain it is more than 30 ml for 2 consecutive hours. The patient is turned and frequently encouraged to cough and breathe deeply. Kinds of anastomoses are **end-to-end anastomosis, side-to-side anastomosis.** See also **aneurysm, bypass.**

anastomosis at elbow joint, a convergence of blood vessels at the elbow joint, consisting of various veins and portions of the brachial and deep brachial arteries and their branches.

anatomic crown, the portion of the dentin of a tooth, covered by dental enamal. Compare **artificial crown, clinical crown, complete crown, dowel crown, partial crown.**

anatomic curve, the curvature of the different segments of the vertebral column. In the lateral contour of the back, the cervical curve appears concave, the thoracic curve appears convex, and the lumbar curve appears concave.

anatomic dead space, an area in the trachea, bronchi, and air passages containing air that does not reach the alveoli during respiration. As a general rule, the volume of air in the anatomic dead space in milliliters is approximately equal to the weight in pounds of the involved individual. Certain lung disorders, as emphysema, increase the amount of anatomic dead space. Compare **physiologic dead space.**

anatomic height of contour, a line that encircles and designates the greatest convexity of a tooth. Compare **surveyed height of contour.** See also **height of contour.**

anatomic impotence. See **impotence.**

anatomic position, a position of the body in which a person stands erect, facing directly forward, feet pointed forward slightly apart, arms hanging down at the sides with palms facing forward. This is the standard neutral position of reference used to describe sites or motions of various parts of the body.

anatomic snuffbox, a small, cuplike depression on the back of the hand near the wrist formed by the tendons reaching toward the thumb and index finger as the thumb is abducted, the wrist flexed, and the digits extended.

anatomy, **1.** the study, classification, and description of structures and organs of the body. Kinds of anatomy are **applied anatomy, comparative anatomy, descriptive anatomy, gross anatomy, microscopic anatomy,** and **surface anatomy.** **2.** the structure of an organism. **3.** a text on anatomy. **4.** *archaic.* dissection of a body. Compare **physiology.**

Anavar, a trademark for an androgen (oxandrolone), used as an anabolic agent.

-ance. See **-ency.**

Ancobon, a trademark for an antifungal (flucytosine).

anconeus, one of seven superficial muscles of the posterior forearm. A small triangular muscle, it originates on the dorsal surface of the lateral condyle and inserts in the olecranon process of the ulna. It is innervated by a branch of the radial nerve, which contains fibers from the seventh and eight cervical nerves, and it functions to extend the forearm.

ancrod /ang′krod/, the venom of the Malayan pit viper, used to remove fibrinogen from the circulation, thus preventing clotting of the blood.

-ancy. See **-ency.**

ancylo-, anchylo-, ankylo-, a combining form meaning 'bent or in the form of a loop': *ancylostomatic, ancylostomiasis, ancylostomo-anemia.*

Ancylostoma /ang′kilos′təmə/, a genus of nematode that is an intestinal parasite and causes hookworm disease. See also ***Necator.***

ancylostomiasis /an′səlos′təmī′əsis/, hookworm disease, more specifically that caused by *Ancylostoma duo-*

denale, A. braziliensis, or *A. canium*. Infection by *A. duodenale* is generally more harmful and less responsive to treatment than that by *Necator americanus,* which is the hookworm most often found in the southern United States. Clinical manifestations and treatment are similar for all types of hookworms. Infection may be prevented by eliminating fecal pollution of soil and by wearing shoes. See also **hookworm.**

Andersen's disease, a rare glycogen storage disease characterized by a genetic deficiency of branching enzyme (amylo-1:4, 1:6 transglucosidase), causing the deposition in tissues of abnormal glycogen with long inner and outer chains. Infants with the disease are normal at birth but fail to thrive and soon show hepatomegaly, splenomegaly, and hypotonic muscles, associated with the progressive development of liver cirrhosis or heart failure of unknown mechanisms. Diagnosis is by enzyme assays of white blood cells and fibroblasts. There is no specific therapy for the disease, which is usually fatal in the first few years of life. Also called **amylopectinosis, glycogen storage disease type IV.**

andr-. See **andro-.**

andreioma, andreoblastoma. See **arrhenoblastoma.**

Andresen removable orthodontic appliance, an activator-type of orthodontic device intended to function as a passive transmitter and stimulator of forces of the perioral muscles by inducing or directing oral forces for the improvement of tooth position and jaw relationship.

andro-, andr-, a combining form meaning 'pertaining to man or to the male': *androcyte, androgen, androgone*.

androgamone /an'drōgam'ōn/, a gamone secreted by the male gamete.

androgen /an'drəjin/, any steroid hormone that increases male characteristics. Natural hormones, as testosterone and its esters and analogs, are primarily used as substitutional therapy during the male climacteric. Androgens may be administered orally or parenterally. –**androgenic,** *adj.*

androgynous /androj'inəs/, **1.** (of a man or woman) having some characteristics of both sexes. Social role, behavior, personality, and appearance are reflections of individuality and are not determined by gender. **2.** hermaphroditic. Compare **gynandrous.** –**androgyny,** *n.*

android pelvis, a type of pelvis in which the structure is characteristic of the male. It is not uncommon in women. The bones are thick and heavy, and the inlet is heart-shaped. The sacrum inclines anteriorly, the side walls are convergent, and the pubic arch is small. The diameters of the midplane and the outlet are smaller than in the normal gynecoid pelvis, and vaginal delivery is likely to be difficult unless the overall pelvis is large and the fetus small.

androma. See **arrhenoblastoma.**

androsterone /andros'tərōn/, originally believed to be the principal male sex hormone, it is used less frequently since the discovery of testosterone. The greater potency of several other male sex hormones has relegated androsterone largely to historic biochemical interest. See also **testosterone.**

-ane, a combining form designating hydrocarbons of the paraffin series: *butane, lindane, xylane*.

anecdotal, pertaining to medical knowledge based on isolated observations and not yet verified by controlled scientific studies.

Anectine, a trademark for a skeletal muscle relaxant (succinylcholine chloride), used as an adjunct to anesthesia.

anemia, a disorder characterized by a decrease in hemoglobin in the blood to levels below the normal range, decreased red cell production or increased red cell destruction, or blood loss. A separate and distinct morphologic classification system describes anemia by the hemoglobin content of the red cells (normochromic or hypochromic) and by differences in red cell size (macrocytic, normocytic, or microcytic). See also **hemolytic anemia, hypoplastic anemia, iron deficiency anemia, iron metabolism.**

■ OBSERVATIONS: Depending on its severity, anemia may be accompanied by some or all of a number of clinical findings that stem directly from the diminished oxygen-carrying capacity of the blood. These include fatigue, exertional dyspnea, dizziness, headache, insomnia, and pallor, especially of the mucous membranes. Anorexia and dyspepsia, palpitations, tachycardia, cardiac dilatation and systolic murmurs also occur. Understanding the pathophysiology of the anemia is a prerequisite for rational therapy, including the recognition that iron deficiency is, by far, the most common causative factor. Specific tests are first directed at this kind of anemia. Additional laboratory studies may be required to establish the presence of the less common forms.

■ INTERVENTION: The therapeutic response to anemia is highly variable and depends on the specific causative factors involved. Moderate to severe anemia, with hemoglobin levels that are below 7 to 8 g/dl, may call for transfusion of one or more units of blood, especially if the condition is acute and accompanied by specific clinical signs. Depending on the kind of anemia, treatment includes providing supplements of the deficient component, eliminating the cause of the blood loss, or alleviating the hemolytic component. The latter may involve the administration of adrenal corticosteroids or, possibly, splenectomy. Appropriate laboratory tests and other examinations are usually repeated at intervals to monitor the response, the need for continued therapy, and the extent of return to normal levels.

■ NURSING CONSIDERATIONS: The nurse emphasizes to the patient the importance of adequate diet to supply blood-building components. The patient's need for rest is stressed, especially in the face of cardiac and respiratory symptoms. The time needed for recovery and the need for repeated blood tests to evaluate the progress of therapy are outlined. The patient is also cautioned, where applicable, to be alert for signs of increasing anemia or resumption of blood loss. When transfusions are given, the nurse is alert for indications of a transfusion reaction.

-anemia, -anaemia, -nemia a combining form meaning '(condition of) red blood cell deficiency or its remedy': *achylanemia, melanemia, sulfanemia.*

anemia of pregnancy, a condition of pregnancy characterized by a reduction in the concentration of hemoglobin in the blood. It may be physiologic or pathologic. In physiologic anemia of pregnancy, the reduction in concentration results from dilution because the plasma volume expands more than the red blood cell volume. The hematocrit in pregnancy normally drops several points below the level it was before pregnancy. In pathologic anemia of pregnancy, the oxygen-carrying capacity of the blood is deficient because of disordered erythrocyte production or excessive loss of erythrocytes through destruction or bleeding. Pathologic anemia is a common complication of pregnancy occurring in approximately one half of all pregnancies. Disordered production of erythrocytes may result from nutritional deficiency of iron, folic acid, or vitamin B_{12}, or from chronic disease, malignancy, chronic malnutrition, or exposure to toxins. Destruction of erythrocytes may result from inflammation, chronic infection, sepsis, autoimmune disorders, microangiopathy, or a hematologic disease in which the red cells are abnormal. Excessive loss of erythrocytes through bleeding may result from abortion, bleeding hemorrhoids, intestinal parasites, as hookworm, placental abnormalities, as placenta previa and premature separation, or postpartum uterine atony.

anemic anoxia, a condition characterized by a deficiency of oxygen in body tissues, resulting from a decrease in the number of erythrocytes in the blood or in the amount of hemoglobin.

anemo-, a combining form meaning 'pertaining to the wind': *anemopathy, anemophobia, anemotropism.*

anencephaly /an′ensef′əlē/, congenital absence of the brain and spinal cord in which the cranium does not close and the vertebral canal remains a groove. Transmitted genetically, anencephaly is not compatible with life. It can be detected early in gestation by amniotic fluid tap and analysis or by ultrasonography. See also **neural tube defect.**

anergic stupor, a kind of dementia characterized by quietness, listlessness, and nonresistance.

anergy, **1.** lack of activity. **2.** an immunodeficient condition characterized by a lack of or diminished reaction to an antigen or group of antigens. This state may be seen in advanced tuberculosis and other serious infections, acquired immune deficiency syndrome, and some malignancies. **–anergic,** *adj.*

aneroid /an′əroid/, not containing a liquid, used especially to describe a device in contrast to one performing a similar function that does contain liquid, as aneroid sphygmomanometer, which does not contain a column of liquid mercury.

Anestacon, a trademark for an endourethral local anesthetic solution (2% lidocaine hydrochloride).

anesthesia, the absence of normal sensation, especially sensitivity to pain, as induced by an anesthetic substance or by hypnosis or as occurs with traumatic or pathophysiologic damage to nerve tissue. Anesthesia induced for medical or surgical purposes may be topical, local, regional, or general and is named for the anesthetic agent used, the method or procedure followed, the area or organ anesthetized, or the age or class of patient served. See also **general anesthesia, Guedel's signs, local anesthesia, regional anesthesia, topical anesthesia,** and see specific anesthetic agents.

anesthesia dolorosa, a severe tactile or spontaneous, paradoxical pain in an anesthetized area. Also called **analgesia algera.**

anesthesia machine, an apparatus for administering inhalant anesthetic agents. Although there are many different models, all have the following features: an accommodation for a source of gas; a meter to measure the flow of gas; vessels for volatilizing and mixing the anesthetic agents and the carrier gases; and a system for delivery of the gas to the patient.

anesthesia patients, classification of, the system by which the American Society of Anesthesiologists classifies anesthesia patients in five categories by anesthetic risk factors. Class I includes patients who are generally healthy, without serious organic, physiologic, biochemical, or psychiatric problems, and for whom anesthesia is required only for a local condition, as an inguinal hernia or fibroid uterus. Class II includes patients who have mild to moderate systemic problems, whether involving or extraneous to the condition requiring anesthesia, as anemia, mild diabetes, essential hypertension, extreme obesity, or chronic bronchitis. Class III includes patients who have severe systemic disturbances or disease, whether or not related to the procedure requiring surgical anesthesia. Class IV includes patients who are suffering from a life-threatening, but not necessarily terminal, condition that may or may not be related to the intended surgical procedure. Class V includes the moribund patient who has little chance of survival, as a person in shock with a burst abdominal aneurysm or a massive pulmonary embolus. The letter E is added to the roman numeral to indicate an emergency procedure, as a patient scheduled for an elective herniorrhaphy who becomes an emergency case when his hernia becomes an obstruction.

anesthesia screen, a metal inverted U-shaped frame that attaches to the sides of an operating table, 12 to 18 inches above a patient's upper chest. It is covered with a sheet to prevent contamination of an operative site on the chest or abdomen by airborne infection from the patient or the anesthetist and to provide a wide sterile field for the surgeon.

anesthesiologist /an′əsthē′zē·ol′əjist/, a physician trained in the administration of anesthetics and in the provision of respiratory and cardiovascular support during anesthetic procedures. Compare **nurse anesthetist.**

anesthesiology, the branch of medicine that is concerned with the relief of pain and with the administration of medication to relieve pain during surgery. It is a specialty requiring competency in general medicine, a broad understanding of surgical procedures, a wide knowledge of clinical pharmacology, biochemistry, cardiology, and respiratory physiology. See also **anesthesiologist, nurse anesthetist.**

anesthetist /ənes′thətist/, **1.** a person who administers anesthesia. **2.** an anesthesiologist. See also **nurse anesthetist.**

anetoderma /an′ətōdur′mə/, an idiopathic, patchy atrophy and looseness of skin for which there is no known effective treatment.

aneuploid /an′yo͞oploid/, **1.** of or pertaining to an individual, organism, strain, or cell that has a chromosome number that is not an exact multiple of the normal, basic haploid number characteristic of the species. Variation occurs through individual chromosomes rather than an entire set so that there are more or less than the normal diploid number found in the somatic cell. **2.** such an individual, organism, strain, or cell. Also **aneuploidic** /-ploi′dik/. Compare **euploid.** See also **monosomy, trisomy.**

aneuploidy /an′yo͞oploi′dē/, any variation in chromosome number that involves individual chromosomes rather than entire sets. There may be fewer chromosomes, as in Turner's syndrome, or more chromosomes, as in Down's syndrome. Such individuals have various abnormal physiologic and morphologic traits. Compare **euploidy.** See also **monosomy, trisomy.**

aneurysm /an′yo͞oriz′əm/, a localized dilatation of the wall of a blood vessel, usually caused by atherosclerosis and hypertension, or, less frequently, by trauma, infection, or a congenital weakness in the vessel wall. Aneurysms are most prominent and significant in the aorta but also occur in peripheral vessels and are fairly common in the lower extremities of older people, especially in the popliteal arteries. An arterial aneurysm may be a saccular distention affecting only part of the circumference of the vessel, it may be a fusiform or cylindroid dilatation of a section of the vessel, or it may be a longitudinal dissection between layers of the vascular wall. A sign of an arterial aneurysm is a pulsating swelling that produces a blowing murmur on auscultation with a stethoscope. An aneurysm may rupture, causing hemorrhage, or thrombi may form in the dilated pouch and give rise to emboli that may obstruct smaller vessels. Kinds of aneurysms include **aortic aneurysm, bacterial aneurysm, berry aneurysm, cerebral aneurysm, compound aneurysm, dissecting aneurysm, fusiform aneurysm, mycotic aneurysm, racemose aneurysm, Rasmussen's aneurysm, saccular aneurysm, varicose aneurysm,** and **ventricular aneurysm.** **–aneurysmal,** *adj.*

aneurysm needle, a needle equipped with a handle, used to ligate aneurysms.

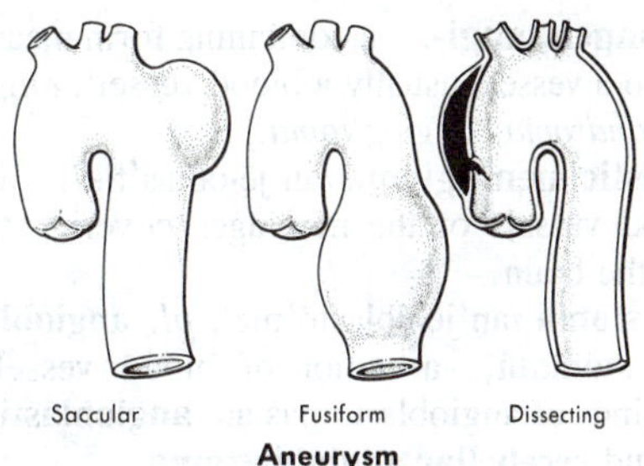

Aneurysm

ANF, abbreviation for **American Nurses' Foundation.**

anger, an emotional reaction characterized by extreme displeasure, rage, indignation, or hostility. It is considered to be of pathologic origin when such a response does not realistically reflect a person's actual circumstances. However, expressions of anger vary widely from individual to individual.

angi-. See **angio-.**

angiitis /anjē·ī′tis/, an inflammatory condition of a vessel, chiefly a blood or lymph vessel. A kind of angiitis is **consecutive angiitis.** See also **vasculitis.**

angina /anjī′nə, an′jinə/, **1.** a spasmodic, cramplike choking feeling. **2.** a term now used primarily to denote the paroxysmal thoracic pain and choking feeling caused by anoxia of the myocardium (angina pectoris). **3.** a descriptive feature of various diseases characterized by a feeling of choking, suffocation, or crushing pressure and pain. Kinds of angina are **intestinal angina, Ludwig's angina, Prinzmetal's angina,** and **streptococcal angina.** **–anginal,** *adj.*

-angina, a combining form meaning 'severe ulceration, usually of the mouth or throat': *herpangina, juxtangina, monocytangina.*

angina decubitus, a condition characterized by periodic attacks of angina pectoris that occur when the person is lying down.

angina dyspeptica, a painful condition caused by gaseous distention of the stomach that mimics angina pectoris.

angina epiglottidea, a painful condition caused by inflammation of the epiglottis.

angina pectoris, a paroxysmal thoracic pain caused most often by myocardial anoxia as a result of atherosclerosis of the coronary arteries. The pain usually radiates down the inner aspect of the left arm and is frequently accompanied by a feeling of suffocation and impending death. Attacks of angina pectoris are often related to exertion, emotional stress, and exposure to intense cold. The pain may be relieved by rest and vasodilatation of the coronary arteries by medication, as with nitroglycerin.

angina sine dolore /sē′nə dolôr′ə, sī′nē/, a painless episode of coronary insufficiency.

angina trachealis. See **croup.**

angio-, angei-, angi-, a combining form meaning 'pertaining to a vessel, usually a blood vessel': *angioblastic, angiochondroma, angioglioma*.

angioblastic meningioma /an′jē•ōblas′tik/, a tumor of the blood vessels of the meninges covering the spinal cord or the brain.

angioblastoma /an′jē•ōblastō′mə/, *pl.* **angioblastomas, angioblastomata,** a tumor of blood vessels in the brain. Kinds of angioblastomas are **angioblastic meningioma** and **cerebellar angioblastoma.**

angiocardiogram /an′jē•ōkär′dē•ōgram′/, a radiograph of the heart and the vessels of the heart. A radiopaque substance is injected forcibly into a vein in the antecubital space or directly into the heart, and x-ray films are taken as the radiopaque contrast medium passes through the heart and its vessels. Nausea and vomiting are common untoward reactions; urticaria, shortness of breath, or anaphylaxis may also occur. An antihistamine and oxygen are kept close at hand during the procedure. Angiocardiograms are performed by a member of the radiology department. See also **angiography.**

angiocatheter /an′jē•ōkath′ətər/, a hollow, flexible tube inserted into a blood vessel to withdraw or instill fluids.

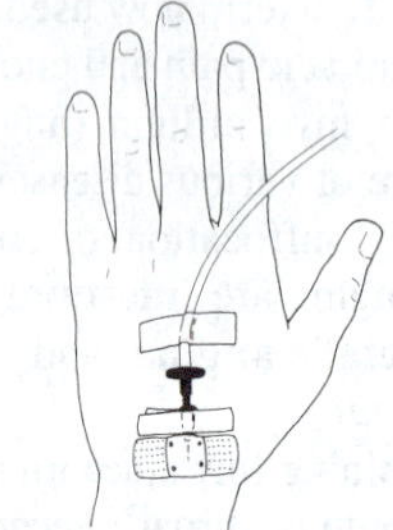

Angiocatheter securing method

angiochondroma /an′jē•ōkondrō′mə/, *pl.* **angiochondromas, angiochondromata,** a cartilaginous tumor characterized by an excessive formation of blood vessels.

angioedema. See **angioneurotic edema.**

angioendothelioma. See **hemangioendothelioma.**

angiofibroma /an′jē•ōfībrō′mə/, *pl.* **angiofibromas, angiofibromata,** an angioma containing fibrous tissue. Also called **fibroangioma, telangiectatic fibroma.**

angiogenesis /an′jē•ōjen′əsis/, the ability to evoke blood vessel formation, a common property of malignant tissue. The presence of angiogenesis in breast tissue is regarded as a precursor of histologic evidence of breast cancer.

angioglioma /an′jē•ōglē•ō′mə/, *pl.* **angiogliomas, angiogliomatas,** a highly vascular tumor composed of neuroglia.

angiography /an′jē•og′rəfē/, the x-ray visualization of the internal anatomy of the heart and blood vessels after the intravascular introduction of radiopaque contrast medium. The procedure is used as a diagnostic aid in myocardial infarction, vascular occlusion, calcified atherosclerotic plaques, cerebrovascular accident, portal hypertension, renal neoplasms, renal artery stenosis as a causative factor in hypertension, pulmonary emboli, and congenital and acquired lesions of pulmonary vessels. The contrast medium may be injected into an artery or vein or introduced into a catheter inserted in a peripheral artery and threaded through the vessel to a visceral site. Because the iodine in the contrast medium may result in a marked allergic reaction in some patients, testing for hypersensitivity is indicated before the radiopaque substance is used. After the procedure the patient is monitored for signs of bleeding, and bed rest for a number of hours is indicated. **–angiographic,** *adj.*

angiohemophilia. See **von Willebrand's disease.**

angiokeratoma /an′jē•ōker′ətō′mə/, *pl.* **angiokeratomas, angiokeratomata,** a vascular, horny neoplasm on the skin, characterized by clumps of dilated blood vessels, clusters of warts, and thickening of the epidermis, especially the scrotum and the dorsal aspect of the fingers and toes.

angiokeratoma circumscriptum, a rare skin disorder characterized by discrete papules and nodules in small patches on the legs or on the trunk.

angiokeratoma corporis diffusum, an uncommon familial disease in which phospholipids are stored in many parts of the body, especially the blood vessels, causing vasomotor, urinary, and cutaneous disorders and, in some cases, muscular abnormalities. Characteristic signs of the disease are edema, hypertension, and cardiomegaly, especially enlargement of the left ventricle; diffuse nodularity of the skin; albumin, erythrocytes, leukocytes, and casts in the urine; and vacuoles in muscle bundles. Also called **Fabry's disease, Fabry's syndrome.**

angiolipoma /an′jē•ōlipō′mə/, *pl.* **angiolipomas, angiolipomata,** a benign neoplasm containing blood vessels and tissue. Also called **lipoma cavernosum, telangiectatic lipoma.**

angioma /an′jē•ō′mə/, *pl.* **angiomas, angiomata,** any benign tumor made up primarily of blood vessels (hemangioma) or lymph vessels (lymphangioma). Most angiomas are congenital; some, like cavernous hemangiomas, disappear spontaneously.

-angioma, a combining form meaning a 'tumor composed chiefly of blood and lymph vessels': *fibroangioma, glomangioma, telangioma*.

angioma arteriale racemosum /ärtir′ē•ā′lē ras′əmō′səm/, a vascular neoplasm characterized initially by the intertwining of many small, newly formed, dilated blood vessels. Subsequently, normal blood vessels become affected.

angioma cavernosum. See **cavernous hemangioma.**

angioma cutis, a nevus composed of a network of dilated blood vessels.

angioma lymphaticum. See **lymphangioma.**

angioma serpiginosum, a cutaneous disease characterized by rings of tiny vascular points appearing as red dots. Also called **Hutchinson's disease.**

angiomatosis /an'jē·ōmətō'sis/, a condition characterized by the presence of numerous vascular tumors. A kind of angiomatosis is **Osler-Weber-Rendu syndrome.**

angiomyoma, *pl.* **angiomyomas, angiomyomata,** a tumor composed of vascular and muscular tissue elements.

angiomyoneuroma. See **glomangioma.**

angiomyosarcoma /an'jē·ōmī'ōsärkō'mə/, *pl.* **angiomyosarcomas, angiomyosarcomata,** a tumor containing vascular, muscular, and connective tissue elements.

angioneuroma. See **glomangioma.**

angioneurotic anuria, an abnormal condition characterized by an almost complete absence of urination caused by destruction of tissue in the renal cortex.

angioneurotic edema, an acute, painless, dermal, subcutaneous or submucosal swelling of short duration involving the face, neck, lips, larynx, hands, feet, genitalia, or viscera. It may result from food or drug allergy, infection, or emotional stress, or it may be hereditary. Treatment depends on the cause. For severe forms, subcutaneous injections of epinephrine, intubation, or tracheotomy may be necessary to prevent respiratory obstruction. Prevention depends on the identification and avoidance of causative factors. Also called **angioedema** /an'jē·ōdē'mə/. See also **anaphylaxis, serum sickness, urticaria.**

angiosarcoma /an'jē·ōsärkō'mə/, a rare, malignant tumor consisting of endothelial and fibroblastic tissue that proliferates and eventually surrounds vascular channels. The condition usually occurs in older persons, but recently it has been associated with exposure to vinyl chloride and arsenic. Also called **hemangiosarcoma, malignant hemangioendothelioma.** Compare **angioma.**

angiospasm, a sudden, transient constriction of a blood vessel. Also called **vasospasm.** See also **vasoconstriction.**

angiotensin /an'jē·ōten'sin/, a polypeptide occurring in the blood causing vasoconstriction, increased blood pressure, and the release of aldosterone from the adrenal cortex. Angiotensin is formed by the action of renin on angiotensinogen, an alpha-2-globulin that is produced in the liver and constantly circulates in the blood. Renin, elaborated by juxtaglomerular cells in the kidney in response to decreased blood volume and serum sodium, acts as an enzyme in the conversion of angiotensinogen to angiotensin I, which is rapidly hydrolyzed to form the active compound angiotensin II. The vasoconstrictive action of angiotensin II decreases the glomerular filtration rate, and the concomitant action of aldosterone promotes sodium retention, with the result that blood volume and sodium reabsorption increase. Plasma angiotensin increases during the luteal phase of the menstrual cycle and is probably responsible for an elevated level of aldosterone during that period. Angiotensin is inactivated by peptidases, called angiotensinases, in plasma and tissues.

angiotensinogen, a serum globulin produced in the liver that is the precursor of angiotensin.

angle, **1.** the space or the shape formed at the intersection of two lines, planes, or borders. The divergence of the lines, planes, or borders may be measured in degrees of a circle. **2.** (in anatomy and physiology) the geometric relationships between the surfaces of body structures and the positions affected by movement.

angle board, (in dentistry) a device used for facilitating the establishment of reproducible angular relationships between a patient's head, the x-ray beam, and the x-ray film.

angle-closure glaucoma. See **glaucoma.**

angle former, (in dentistry) one of a series of paired cutting instruments having cutting edges at an angle other than a right angle in relation to the axis of the blade. Compare **bayonet angle former.**

angle of mandible, the angular relationship between the body and the ramus of the mandible. Also called **gonial angle.**

Angle's classification, a classification of the various types of malocclusion, established by Edward Hartley Angle, American orthodontist (1855–1930). This system has since been modified and includes three main classes of occlusion, each class having several types or division. Classification is based on the relation of different teeth in the upper and lower jaws, as the maxillary and the mandibular molars.

angstrom (Å) /ang'strəm/, a unit of measure of length equal to 0.1 millimicron (1/10,000,000 meter). Also called **angstrom unit.**

angular movement, one of the four basic kinds of movement allowed by the various joints of the skeleton in which the angle between two adjoining bones is decreased, as in flexion, or increased, as in extension. Compare **circumduction, gliding, rotation.**

angular stomatitis, inflammation at the corner of the mouth.

angular vein, one of a pair of veins of the face, formed by the junction of the frontal and the supraorbital veins. At the root of the nose each angular vein receives the flow of venous blood from the infraorbital, the superior palpebral, the inferior palpebral, and the external nasal veins, becoming the first part of one of the two facial veins.

angulated fracture, a fracture in which the fragments of bone are angulated.

angulation, **1.** an angular shape or formation. **2.** the discipline of precisely measuring angles, as in mechanic drafting and surveying. **3.** (in radiography) the direction of the primary beam of radiation in relation to the object being radiographed and the film used to record its image. See also **horizontal angulation, vertical angulation.**

anhedonia /an'hēdō'nē·ə/, the inability to feel pleasure or happiness from experiences that are ordinarily pleasurable. –**anhedonic,** *adj.*

anhidrosis /an′hidrō′sis, an′hī-/, an abnormal condition characterized by inadequate perspiration.

anhidrotic /an′hidrot′ik, an′hī-/, **1.** of or pertaining to anhidrosis. **2.** an agent that reduces or suppresses sweating.

anhydride, a chemical compound, especially an acid, derived by the removal of water from a substance. –**anhydrous,** *adj.*

Anhydron, a trademark for a diuretic and antihypertensive (cyclothiazide).

-an, -ian, a combining form meaning 'belonging to, characteristic of, similar to': *amphibian, protozoan, salpingian.*

anicteric hepatitis /an′ikter′ik/, a mild form of hepatitis in which there is no jaundice (icterus), usually seen in infants and young children. Symptoms include anorexia, GI disturbances, and slight fever. AST and ALT are elevated. The infection may be mistaken for flu or go unnoticed. Compare **hepatitis.** See also **jaundice.**

anidean /anid′ē•ən/, formless; shapeless; denoting an undifferentiated mass, as an anideus. Also **anidian, anidous** /an′idəs./

anideus /anid′ē•əs/, an anomalous, rudimentary conceptus consisting of a simple rounded mass with little indication of the body parts. A kind of anideus is **embryonic anideus.** Also called **fetus anideus.**

aniline /an′ilēn/, an oily, colorless poisonous liquid with a strong odor and burning taste, formerly extracted from the indigo plant and now made synthetically using nitrobenzene in the manufacture of aniline dyes. Industrial workers exposed to aniline are at risk of developing methemoglobinemia and bone marrow depression. Also called **amidobenzene, aminobenzene.**

anilinparasulfonic acid. See **sulfanilic acid.**

anima /an′imə/, **1.** the soul or life. **2.** the active ingredient in a drug. **3.** (in Jungian psychology) a person's true, inner, unconscious being or personality, as distinguished from overt personality, or persona. **4.** (in analytic psychology) the female component of the male personality. Compare **animus.**

animal pole, the active, formative part of the ovum protoplasm that contains the nucleus and bulk of the cytoplasm and where the polar bodies form. In mammals it is also the site where the inner cell mass gives rise to the ectoderm. Also called **germinal pole.** Compare **vegetal pole.**

animal starch. See **glycogen.**

animus /an′iməs/, **1.** the active or rational soul; the animating principle of life. **2.** the male component of the female personality. **3.** (in psychiatry) a deep-seated antagonism that is usually controlled but may erupt with virulence under stress. Compare **anima.**

anion /an′ī·ən/, **1.** a negatively charged ion that is attracted to the positive electrode (anode) in electrolysis. **2.** a negatively charged atom, molecule, or radical. Compare **cation.**

anion exchange resin, any one of the simple organic polymers with high molecular weights that exchange anions with other ions in solution. Anion exchange resins are used as antacids in treating ulcers. Compare **cation exchange resin.**

anion gap, the difference between the concentrations of serum cations and anions, determined by measuring the concentrations of sodium cations and chloride and bicarbonate anions. It is helpful in the diagnosis and treatment of acidosis, and it is estimated by subtracting the sum of sodium and bicarbonate concentrations in the plasma from that of sodium. It is normally about 8 to 14 mEq/L and represents the negative charges contributed to plasma by unmeasured ions or ions other than those of chloride and bicarbonate, mainly phosphate, sulfate, organic acids, and plasma proteins. Anions other than chloride and bicarbonate normally constitute about 12 mEq/L of the total anion concentration in plasma. Acidosis can develop with or without an associated anion increase. An increase in the anion gap often suggests diabetic ketoacidosis, drug poisoning, renal failure, or lactic acidosis and usually warrants further laboratory tests.

anise /an′is/, the fruit of the *Pimpinella anisum* plant. Extract of anise is used in the preparation of carminatives and expectorants.

aniseikonia /an′īsīkō′nē•ə/, an abnormal ocular condition in which each eye perceives the same image as being of a different form and size.

aniso-, a combining form meaning 'unequal or dissimilar': *anisochromia, anisodont, anisognathous.*

anisocytosis /anī′sōsītō′sis/, an abnormal condition of the blood characterized by red blood cells of variable and abnormal size. Compare **poikilocytosis.** See also **anisopoikilocytosis, macrocytosis, microcytosis.**

anisogamete, a gamete that differs considerably in size and structure from the one with which it unites, as the macrogamete and microgamete of certain sporozoa. Compare **heterogamete, isogamete.** –**anisogametic,** *adj.*

anisogamy /an′īsog′əmē/, sexual conjugation of gametes that are of unequal size and structure, as in certain thallophytes and sporozoa. Compare **heterogamy, isogamy.** –**anisogamous,** *adj.*

anisognathic, /an′īsōnath′ik/, of or pertaining to an abnormal condition in which the maxillary and the mandibular arches or jaws are of significantly different sizes in the same individual.

anisokaryosis /anī′sōker′ē•ō′sis/, significant variation in the size of the nucleus of cells of the same general type. –**anisokaryotic,** *adj.*

anisometropia /anī′sōmetrō′pē•ə/, an abnormal ocular condition characterized by a difference in the refractive powers of the eyes.

anisopoikilocytosis /anī′sōpoi′kilōsītō′sis/, an abnormal condition of the blood characterized by red blood cells of variable and abnormal size and shape. See also **anisocytosis, erythrocyte, morphology, poikilocytosis.**

anisotropine, an anticholinergic drug.

■ INDICATION: It is prescribed as adjunctive therapy in the treatment of peptic ulcer.

■ CONTRAINDICATIONS: Glaucoma, obstructive uropathy, obstructive conditions of the GI tract, paralytic ileus, intestinal atony, unstable cardiovascular status in acute hemorrhage, severe ulcerative colitis or toxic megacolon complicating ulcerative colitis, or myasthenia gravis prohibits its use.

■ ADVERSE EFFECTS: Among the most serious adverse reactions are blurred vision, tachycardia, mydriasis, cycloplegia, impotence, mental confusion, urinary retention, constipation, allergic reactions, and urticaria.

ankle, **1.** the joint of the tibia, the talus, and the fibula. **2.** the part of the leg where this joint is located.

ankle bandage, a figure-of-eight bandage looped under the sole of the foot and around the ankle. The heel may be covered or left exposed, although covering is preferable because it prevents "window edema."

ankle bone. See **talus.**

ankle reflex. See **Achilles tendon reflex.**

ankylo-. See **ancylo-.**

ankyloglossia, an oral defect, characterized by an abnormally short lingual frenum that limits tongue movement and impairs the speech. It may be surgically corrected by a frenotomy. Also called **tongue-tie.**

ankylosing spondylitis /ang'kilō'sing/, a chronic inflammatory disease of unknown origin, first affecting the spine and adjacent structures, and commonly progressing to eventual fusion (ankylosis) of the involved joints. In extreme cases the patient develops a forward flexion of the spine, called a "poker spine" or "bamboo spine." The disease affects primarily males under 30 years of age, and generally burns itself out after a course of 20 years. There is a strong hereditary tendency. In addition to the spine, the joints of the hip, shoulder, neck, ribs, and jaw are often involved. When the costovertebral joints are involved, the patient may have difficulty in expanding the rib cage while breathing. Ankylosing spondylitis is a systemic disease, often affecting the eyes and the heart. Many patients with the disease also have inflammatory bowel disease. The aim of treatment is to reduce pain and inflammation in the involved joints, usually with nonsteroidal antiinflammatory drugs. Physical therapy aids in keeping the spine as erect as possible to prevent flexion contractures. In advanced cases surgery may be performed to straighten a badly deformed spine. Compare **rheumatoid arthritis.** See also **ankylosis.** Also called **Marie-Strümpell disease.**

ankylosis /ang'kilō'sis/, **1.** fixation of a joint, often in an abnormal position, usually resulting from destruction of articular cartilage and subchondral bone, as occurs in rheumatoid arthritis. **2.** also called **arthrodesis, fusion.** surgically induced fixation of a joint to relieve pain or provide support.

anlage /on'lägə/, (in embryology) the undifferentiated layer of cells from which a particular organ, tissue, or structure develops; primordium rudiment. See also **blastema.**

ANLL. abbreviation for **acute nonlymphocytic leukemia.** See **acute myelocytic leukemia.**

annular. See **anular.**

annular ligament. See **anular ligament.**

anodmia. See **anosmia.**

anodontia /an'ōdon'tē·ə/, a congenital defect in which some or all of the teeth are missing.

anodyne /an'ədīn/, a drug that relieves or lessens pain. Compare **analgesic.**

anomalo-, a combining form meaning 'uneven or irregular': *anomalopia, anomaloscope, anomalotrophy.*

anomaly /ənom'əlē/, **1.** deviation from what is regarded as normal. **2.** congenital malformation, as the absence of a limb or the presence of an extra finger. –**anomalous,** *adj.*

anomia /ənō'mē·ə/, a form of aphasia characterized by the inability to name objects, caused by a lesion in the temporal lobe of the brain.

anomie /an'əmē/, a state of apathy, alienation, anxiety, personal disorientation, and distress, resulting from the loss of social norms and goals previously valued. Also spelled **anomy.**

anoopsia /an'ō·op'sē·ə/, a strabismus in which one or both eyes are deviated upward. Also called **hypertropia.**

Anopheles /ənof'əlēz/, a genus of mosquito, many species of which transmit malaria-causing parasites to humans. See also **malaria, *Plasmodium*.**

anopia /anō'pē·ə/, blindness resulting from a defect in or the absence of one or both eyes.

-anopia, -anopsia, **1.** a combining form meaning '(condition involving) nonuse or arrested development of the eye': *hemianopia, hesperanopia, quadrantanopsia.* **2.** a combining form meaning '(condition of) defective color vision': *cyanopia, deuteranopia, tritanopia.*

anoplasty, a restorative operation on the anus.

-anopsia. See **-anopia.**

anorchia /anôr'kē·ə/, congenital absence of one or both testes. Also called **anorchism.**

anorectal /an'ōrek'təl, ā'nō-/, of or pertaining to the anal and rectal portions of the large intestine.

anorectic /an'ōrek'tik/, **1.** of or pertaining to anorexia. **2.** lacking appetite. **3.** causing a loss of appetite, as anorexiant drug. Also **anorectous, anorexiant.**

anorexia /an'ōrek'sē·ə/, lack or loss of appetite, resulting in the inability to eat. The condition may result from poorly prepared or unattractive food or surroundings, unfavorable company, or various psychologic causes. Compare **pseudoanorexia.** See also **anorexia nervosa.** –**anorexic, anorectic,** *adj.*

anorexia nervosa, a psychoneurotic disorder characterized by a prolonged refusal to eat, resulting in emaciation, amenorrhea, emotional disturbance concerning body image, and an abnormal fear of becoming obese. The condition is seen primarily in adolescents, predominantly in girls, and is usually associated with emotional stress or conflict, such as anxiety, irritation, anger, and fear, which may accompany a major change in the person's life. Treatment consists of measures to improve nourishment, followed by therapy to overcome the underlying emotional conflicts.

anosmia /anoz′mē•ə/, loss or impairment of the sense of smell, commonly occurring as a temporary condition resulting from a head cold or respiratory infection or when intranasal swelling or other obstruction prevents odors from reaching the olfactory region. It becomes a permanent condition when the olfactory neuroepithelium or any part of the olfactory nerve is destroyed as a result of intracranial trauma, neoplasms, or disease, as atrophic rhinitis or the chronic rhinitis associated with the granulomatous diseases. In some instances, the condition may be caused by psychologic factors, as a phobia or fear associated with a particular smell. Kinds of anosmia are **anosmia gustatoria** and **preferential anosmia.** Also called **anodmia, anosphrasia, olfactory anesthesia.** Compare **hyperosmia.** –**anosmatic, anosmic,** *adj.*

anosmia gustatoria, the inability to smell foods.

anosognosia /an′əsog•nō′zhə/, an abnormal condition characterized by a real or feigned inability to perceive a defect, especially paralysis, on one side of the body, possibly attributable to a lesion in the right parietal lobe of the brain.

anosphrasia, anosphresia. See **anosmia.**

ANOVA, abbreviation for **analysis of variance.**

anovular menstruation, menstrual bleeding that occurs even though ovulation has not taken place. The ovum either remains within the follicle and undergoes degeneration or in rare cases becomes impregnated, resulting in an ovarian pregnancy.

anovulation /an′ovyo͞olā′shən/, failure of the ovaries to produce, mature, or release eggs, as a result of ovarian immaturity or postmaturity; of altered ovarian function, as in pregnancy and lactation; of primary ovarian dysfunction, as in ovarian dysgenesis; or of disturbance of the interaction of the hypothalamus, pituitary gland, and ovary, caused by stress or disease. Hormonal contraceptives prevent conception by suppressing ovulation. Anovulation may be an adverse side effect of medications prescribed in the treatment of other disorders. –**anovulatory** /anov′yo͞olətôr′ē/, *adj.*

anoxia /anok′sē•ə/, an abnormal condition characterized by a lack of oxygen. Anoxia may be local or systemic and may be the result of an inadequate supply of oxygen to the respiratory system or of an inability of the blood to carry oxygen to the tissues, as in anemic anoxia, or of the tissues to absorb the oxygen from the circulation, as in histotoxic anoxia. Kinds of anoxia include **cerebral anoxia** and **stagnant anoxia.** See also **hypoxemia, hypoxia.** –**anoxic,** *adj.*

-ans, a combining form meaning '-ing': *aberrans, penetrans, proliferans.*

ansa /an′sə/, *pl.* **ansae,** (in anatomy) a looplike structure resembling a curved handle of a vase.

ansa cervicalis, one of three loops of nerves in the cervical plexus, branches of which innervate the infrahyoid muscles. It has a superior root, which connects with the hypoglossal nerve and contains fibers of the first and the second cervical nerves, and an inferior root, which connects with the second and the third cervical nerves. Also called **ansa hypoglossi.**

answer, (in law) the response of a defendant to the complaint of a plaintiff. The answer contains a denial of the plaintiff's allegations and may also contain an affirmative defense or a counterclaim. It is the principal pleading on the part of the defense and is prepared in writing, usually by the defense attorney, and submitted to the court.

ant-. See **anti-.**

Antabuse, a trademark for an alcohol abuse deterrent (disulfiram).

antacid /antas′id/, **1.** opposing acidity. **2.** a drug or dietary substance that buffers, neutralizes, or absorbs hydrochloric acid in the stomach. Most antacids are not absorbed systemically. Antacids containing aluminum and calcium are constipating; those containing magnesium have a laxative effect.

antagonist, **1.** one who contends with or is opposed to another. **2.** (in physiology) any agent, such as a drug or muscle, that exerts an opposite action to that of another or competes for the same receptor sites. Kinds of antagonists include **antimetabolite, associated antagonist, direct antagonist,** and **narcotic antagonist.** Compare **agonist. 3.** (in dentistry) a tooth in the upper jaw that articulates during mastication or occlusion with a tooth in the lower jaw. –**antagonistic,** *adj.,* **antagonize,** *v.*

ante-, a combining form meaning 'before in time or in place': *anteflexion, antenatal, antepartal.*

antecardium. See **epigastric region.**

antecubital, in front of the elbow; at the bend of the elbow.

anteflexion, an abnormal position of an organ in which the organ is tilted acutely forward, folded over on itself.

antegonial notch, a depression or concavity commonly present at the junction of the ramus and the mandible, near the attachment of the anterior margin of the masseter.

antenatal. See **prenatal.**

antenatal diagnosis. See **prenatal diagnosis.**

Antepar, a trademark for an anthelmintic (piperazine citrate).

antepartal care, care of a pregnant woman during the time in the maternity cycle that begins with conception and ends with the onset of labor. See also **intrapartal care, prenatal nutrition, postpartal care.**

■ METHOD: A medical, surgical, gynecologic, obstetric, social, and family history is taken with particular emphasis on the discovery of familial or transmissable diseases. A physical examination is performed, including observation and evaluation of the skin, thyroid gland, heart, breasts, abdomen, lungs, and pelvic organs. The vaginal part of the pelvic examination may include a Pap smear and tests for *Neisseria gonorrhoeae, Candida albicans,* and *Trichomonas vaginalis.* Blood pressure, weight, urinalysis for sugar and protein, measurement of the height

Commonly used antacids

Trade name	Dosage form	Drug composition					Sodium content†
		Calcium carbonate	*Aluminum hydroxide*	*Magnesium oxide or hydroxide*	*Magnesium trisilicate*	*Other*	
Alka-2 Chewable Antacid	Chewable tablet	500 mg	—	—	—	—	0.5 mg
Alka-Seltzer Effervescent Antacid	Tablet	—		—	—	Sodium bicarbonate Citric acid Potassium bicarbonate	95.8 mg 832 mg 312 mg
Amphojel	Tablet Suspension	—	300 or 600 mg/tablet 320 mg/5 ml	—	—	—	1.4 or 1.8 mg/tablet 6.9 mg/5 ml
Di-Gel	Tablet Suspension	—	Codried with magnesium carbonate, 282 mg/tablet	85 mg/tablet 87 mg/5 ml	—	Simethicone, 25 mg/tablet or 5 ml	10.6 mg/tablet 8.5 mg/5 ml
Gelusil	Tablet Suspension	—	200 mg/tablet or 5 ml	—	—	Mint flavor Simethicone, 25 mg/tablet or 5 ml	0.8 mg/tablet 0.7 mg/5 ml
Maalox	Suspension	—	225 mg/5 ml	200 mg/5 ml	—	—	2.5 mg/5 ml
Maalox #1	Tablet	—	200 mg	200 mg	—	—	0.84 mg
Maalox #2	Tablet	—	400 mg	400 mg	—	—	1.95 mg
Maalox Plus	Tablet Suspension	—	Dried gel, 200 mg/tablet 225 mg/5 ml	200 mg/tablet or 5 ml (hydroxide)	—	Simethicone, 25 mg/tablet or 5 ml	0.84 mg/tablet 2.5 mg/5 ml
Marblen	Tablet Suspension	NS*	NS*	—	NS*	Magnesium carbonate Peach or apricot flavor	NS* 18 mg/fl. oz.
Mylanta	Tablet Suspension	—	200 mg/tablet or 5 ml	200 mg/tablet or 5 ml (hydroxide)	—	Simethicone, 20 mg/tablet or 5 ml 150 mg sucrose	0.79 mg/tablet 11.7 mg/15 ml
Mylanta-II	Tablet Suspension	—	400 mg/tablet or 5 ml	400 mg/tablet or 5 ml (hydroxide)	—	Simethicone, 30 mg/tablet or 5 ml 105 mg sucrose	1.3 mg/tablet 1.14 mg/5 ml
Phillips' Milk of Magnesia	Suspension Tablet	—	—	—	—	Peppermint oil, 1.166 mg/30 ml or tablet	—
Riopan	Tablet Chewable tablet Suspension	—	—	—	—	Magaldrate, 400 mg/tablet or 5 ml	0.1 mg/tablet or 5 ml
Rolaids	Tablet	—	—	—	—	Dihydroxyaluminum sodium carbonate, 334 mg	53 mg
Tums	Tablet	500 mg	—	—	—	Peppermint oil	2.7 mg
WinGel	Tablet Suspension	—	180 mg/tablet or 5 ml	160 mg/tablet or 5 ml	—		2.5 mg/tablet or 5 ml

*Quantity not specified.
†If no amount is given, it should not be assumed that the product contains no sodium.
Adapted from Handbook of nonprescription drugs, ed. 7, Washington, D. C., 1982, American Pharmaceutical Association.

of the fundus and auscultation of the fetal heart are routinely performed at monthly intervals or even more frequently. Laboratory tests are performed to determine blood type and Rh factor, hematocrit, and hemoglobin. A serologic test for syphilis is performed, and various diagnostic studies may be done to discover *Chlamydia,* genital herpes, or other viral infections. Amniocentesis may be performed if certain fetal abnormalities are suspected.

■ NURSING ORDERS: The parents are encouraged to discuss their concerns about the pregnancy, to understand the physiologic processes, to report decreased fetal activity, to take a preparation-for-labor class, and to plan for the infant's needs.

■ OUTCOME CRITERIA: The basic goal of prenatal care is a healthy mother, who is ready emotionally and physically to give birth to a healthy baby. Increasingly, that goal has come to include the mother's and father's satisfaction with the birth itself and a minimal use of obstetric intervention. Information, emotional support, good nutrition, and careful observation help most mothers achieve healthy, happy intrapartal and postpartal periods of the maternity cycle.

anterior (A), **1.** the front of a structure. **2.** of or pertaining to a surface or part situated toward the front or facing forward. Compare **posterior.** See also **ventral.**

anterior asynclitism. See **asynclitism.**

anterior atlantoaxial ligament, one of five ligaments connecting the atlas to the axis. It is fixed to the inferior border of the anterior arch of the atlas and to the ventral surface of the body of the axis. Compare **posterior atlantoaxial ligament.**

anterior atlantooccipital membrane, one of two broad, densely woven fibrous sheets that form part of the atlantooccipital joint between the atlas and the occipital bone. It is continuous with two articular capsules and strengthened ventrally by a strong, rounded cord connecting the base of the occipital bone to the anterior arch of the atlas. Also called **anterior atlantooccipital ligament.** Compare **posterior atlantooccipital membrane.**

anterior cardiac vein, one of several small vessels that return deoxygenated blood from the ventral portion of the myocardium of the right ventricle to the right atrium. In some individuals, the right marginal vein opens into the right atrium and in those instances is regarded as one of the anterior cardiac veins. See also **coronary sinus.**

anterior common ligament. See **anterior longitudinal ligament.**

anterior crural nerve. See **femoral nerve.**

anterior cutaneous nerve, one of a pair of cutaneous branches of the cervical plexus. It arises from the second and the third cervical nerves, bends around the middle of the sternocleidomastoideus, crosses the muscle obliquely, passes beneath the platysma, and divides into the ascending and the descending branches. The ascending branches pass upward, pierce the platysma, and are distributed to the cranial, the ventral, and the lateral parts of the neck. The descending branches are distributed to the skin of the ventral and the lateral parts of the neck as far down as the sternum.

anterior determinants of cusp, (in dentistry) the characteristics of the anterior teeth that determine the cusp elevations and the fossa depressions in restoration of the postcanine teeth. Some such determinants are occlusion, alignment overlaps, and the capacity to disclude conjointly with condylar trajectories.

anterior fontanel. See **fontanel.**

anterior guide, (in dentistry) the portion of an articulator that is contacted by the incisal guide pin to maintain the selected separation of the upper and lower members of the articulator. The guide influences the changing relationships of mounted casts in eccentric movements. Compare **condylar guide, incisal guide.** See also **condylar guide inclination.**

anterior longitudinal ligament, the broad, strong ligament attached to the ventral surfaces of the vertebral bodies. It extends from the occipital bone and the anterior tubercle of the atlas to the sacrum. Also called **anterior common ligament.** Compare **posterior longitudinal ligament.**

anterior mediastinal node, a node in one of the three groups of thoracic visceral nodes of the lymphatic system that drains lymph from the nodes of the thymus, pericardium, and sternum. They are located ventral to the brachiocephalic veins and to the arterial trunks from the aortic arch. The efferents of the nodes form the right and the left bronchomediastinal trunks. Compare **posterior mediastinal node.** See also **lymph, lymphatic system, lymph node.**

anterior mediastinum, a caudal portion of the mediastinum in the middle of the thorax, bounded ventrally by the body of the sternum and parts of the fourth through the seventh ribs and dorsally by the parietal pericardium, extending downward as far as the diaphragm. It contains a few lymph nodes and a few vessels and a thin layer of subserous fascia, which is separated from the endothoracic fascia by a fascial cleft. Compare **middle mediastinum, posterior mediastinum, superior mediastinum.**

anterior nares, the ends of the nostrils that open anteriorly into the nasal cavity and allow the inhalation and the exhalation of air. Each is an oval opening that measures about 1.5 cm anteroposteriorly and about 1 cm in diameter. The anterior nares connect with the nasal fossae. Also called **nostrils.** Compare **posterior nares.**

anterior neuropore, the opening of the embryonic neural tube in the anterior portion of the forebrain. It closes at the 20 somite stage, which indicates the end of horizon XI in the numerical anatomic charting of human embryonic development. Compare **posterior neuropore.** See also **horizon.**

anterior pituitary. See **adenohypophysis.**

anterior tibial artery, one of the two divisions of the popliteal artery, arising in back of the knee, dividing into six branches, and supplying various muscles of the leg and foot. Its six branches are the posterior tibial recurrent, fibular, anterior tibial recurrent, muscular, anterior medial malleolar, and anterior lateral malleolar. Compare **posterior tibial artery.**

anterior tibial node, one of the small lymph glands of the lower limb, lying on the interosseous membrane near the proximal portion of the anterior tibial vessels. Compare **inguinal node, popliteal node.**

anterior tooth, any one of the incisors or canine teeth. Compare **posterior tooth.**

anterocclusion /an′tərōklo͞o′shən/, (in dentistry) a malocclusion in which the mandibular teeth are anterior to their normal position relative to the teeth in the maxillary arch. Compare **anteversion.**

anterograde amnesia, the inability to recall events of long ago with normal recall of recent events. Compare **anterograde memory, retrograde amnesia.**

anterograde memory, the ability to recall events of long ago but not those of recent occurrence. Compare **anterograde amnesia.** Also called **senile memory.**

anteroposterior /an′tərōpostir′ē·ər/, from the front to the back of the body, commonly associated with the direction of the roentgenographic beam.

anteversion, **1.** an abnormal position of an organ in which the organ is tilted forward on its axis, away from the midline. **2.** (in dentistry) the tipping or the tilting of teeth or other mandibular structures more anteriorly than normal. Compare **anterocclusion.**

anthelmintic /ant′helmin′tik/, **1.** of or pertaining to a substance that destroys or prevents the development of parasitic worms, as filariae, flukes, hookworms, pinworms, roundworms, schistosomes, tapeworms, trichinae, and whipworms. **2.** an anthelmintic drug. An anthelmintic may interfere with the parasites' carbohydrate metabolism, inhibit their respiratory enzymes, block their neuromuscular action, or render them susceptible to destruction by the host's macrophages. Among a number of drugs used in treating specific helmintic infections are piperazine, pyrantel pamoate, pyrvinium pamoate, mebendazole, niclosamide, hexylresorcinol, diethylcarbamazine, and thiabendazole.

-anthema, a combining form meaning a '(specified) type of eruption, rash': *eisanthema, enanthema, exanthema.*

anthraco-, a combining form meaning 'pertaining to a carbuncle or to carbon dioxide': *anthracoid, anthraconecrosis, anthracosis.*

anthracosis /an′thrəkō′sis/, a chronic lung disease occurring in coal miners, characterized by the deposit of coal dust in the lungs and the formation of black nodules on the bronchioles and resulting in focal emphysema. The condition is aggravated by cigarette smoking. There is no specific treatment; most cases are asymptomatic, and the progress of the condition may be halted by the prevention of further exposure to coal dust. Also called **black lung, coalworker's pneumoconiosis, miner's pneumoconiosis.** See also **inorganic dust.**

anthracosis linguae. See **parasitic glossitis.**

anthralin /an′thrəlin/, a topical antipsoriatic.

■ INDICATIONS: It is prescribed in the treatment of psoriasis and chronic dermatitis.

■ CONTRAINDICATIONS: Renal dysfunction or known hypersensitivity to this drug prohibits its use. It is not applied to acute psoriatic eruptions or near the eyes.

■ ADVERSE EFFECTS: The most serious adverse reaction is nephrotoxicity resulting from systemic absorption.

anthranilic acid. See **aminobenzoic acid.**

anthrax /an′thraks/, a disease affecting primarily farm animals (cattle, goats, pigs, sheep, and horses), caused by the bacterium *Bacillus anthracis.* Anthrax in animals is usually fatal. Humans most often acquire it when a break in the skin comes into direct contact with infected animals and their hides, but they may also contract a pulmonary form of anthrax by inhaling the spores of the bacterium. The cutaneous form begins with a reddish-brown lesion that ulcerates and then forms a dark scab. The signs and symptoms that follow include internal hemorrhage, muscle pain, headache, fever, nausea, and vomiting. The pulmonary form, called woolsorter's disease, is often fatal unless treated early. Treatment for both forms is penicillin G or tetracycline. A vaccine is available for veterinarians and for others for whom anthrax is an occupational hazard. Also called **malignant pustule.**

anthropo-, a combining form meaning 'pertaining to man or to a human being': *anthropocentric, anthropocracy, anthropoid.*

anthropoid pelvis, a type of pelvis in which the inlet is oval; the anteroposterior diameter is much greater than the transverse, and, because of the posterior inclination of the sacrum, the posterior portion of the space in the true pelvis is much greater than the anterior portion. The side walls are somewhat convergent, and the ischial spines are prominent. If the pelvis is large, vaginal delivery is not compromised, but the occiput posterior position of the fetus is favored. This type of pelvis is present in 40% of nonwhite women and in more than 25% of white women.

anthropometry /an′thrəpom′ətrē/, the science of measuring the human body as to height, weight, and size of component parts, including measurement of skinfolds, to study and compare the relative proportions under normal and abnormal conditions. Also called **anthropometric measurement.** **–anthropometric,** *adj.*

anti-, ant-, a combining form meaning 'against or over against': *antialexin, antibiosis, antichlorotic.*

antiadrenergic /an′ti·ad′rənur′jik/, **1.** of or pertaining to the blocking of the effects of impulses transmitted by the adrenergic postganglionic fibers of the sympathetic nervous system. **2.** an antiadrenergic agent. Drugs that block the response to norepinephrine by alpha-adrenergic receptors reduce the tone of smooth muscle in peripheral blood vessels, causing increased peripheral circulation and decreased blood pressure. Alpha-blocking agents include ergotamine derivatives, used in treating migraine; phenoxybenzamine and phentolamine, administered for

Anthropometric measurements

Test	Gender	Normal values	Values showing malnutrition
Tricep skinfold (TSF)	Male	11-12.5 mm	7.5-11 mm
	Female	15-16.5 mm	10-15 mm
Mid upper arm circumference (MUAC)	Male	26-29 cm	20-26 cm
	Female	26-28.5 cm	20-26 cm
Arm muscle circumference (AMC)	Male	23-25 cm	16-23 cm
	Female	20-23 cm	14-20 cm

AMC = MUAC − 0.314 = TSF

Raynaud's disease, pheochromocytoma, and diabetic gangrene; and tolazoline hydrochloride, administered to patients with spastic vascular disease. Agents that block beta-adrenergic receptors decrease the rate and force of heart contractions among other effects. Propranolol and its congeners are beta-blocking agents. Also called **sympatholytic.** Compare **adrenergic.**

antianemic, **1.** of or pertaining to a substance or procedure that counteracts or prevents a deficiency of erythrocytes. **2.** an agent used to treat or to prevent anemia. Whole blood is transfused in the treatment of anemia resulting from acute blood loss, and packed red cells are usually administered when the deficiency is caused by chronic blood loss. Transfusions of blood components are used in the treatment of aplastic anemia. Iron deficiency anemia, the most common form of anemia, is usually treated with oral preparations of ferrous sulfate, fumerate, or gluconate, but a parenteral preparation is indicated for people who are unable to absorb iron from the GI tract or for those who develop nausea and diarrhea when taking iron orally. Cyanocobalamin is administered parenterally in the treatment of pernicious anemia. Folic acid is prescribed to correct a deficiency of that vitamin in the anemias accompanying general malnutrition or alcoholic cirrhosis and to treat the common anemia of infants who are on a milk diet exclusively. A combination of folic acid and vitamin B_{12} is prescribed for people who are anemic as a result of an inadequate dietary intake of both vitamins.

antiantibody, an immunoglobulin formed as the result of the administration of an antibody that acts as an immunogen. The antiantibody then interacts with the antibody. See also **antibody, immune gamma globulin.**

antianxiety agent. See **sedative-hypnotic.**

antiarrhythmic, **1.** of or pertaining to a procedure or substance that prevents, alleviates, or corrects an abnormal cardiac rhythm. **2.** an agent used to treat a cardiac arrhythmia. A defibrillator that delivers a precordial electric shock is often used to restore a normal rhythm to rapid, irregular atrial or ventricular contractions. A pacemaker may be implanted in a patient with an extremely slow heart rate or other arrhythmia. The electrode catheter of an external pacemaker may be threaded through a vein to the heart in cases of ventricular standstill or complete heart block. Two of the major antiarrhythmic drugs are lidocaine, which increases the threshhold of electric stimulation in the ventricles during diastole, and a combination of disopyramide, procainamide, and quinidine, which decreases the excitability of the myocardium and prolongs the refractory period. The beta-adrenergic blocking agent propranolol may be used in treating arrhythmias. Isoproterenol is indicated for complete heart block and ventricular arrhythmias requiring an increased force of cardiac contractions to establish a normal rhythm. Atropine may be used in the treatment of bradycardia, a sedative in the treatment of tachycardia, and digitalis in the treatment of atrial fibrillation. Verapamil and other calcium antagonists control arrhythmias by inhibiting calcium ion influx across the cell membrane of cardiac muscle, thus slowing atrioventricular conduction and prolonging the effective refractory period within the atrioventricular node. See also **arrhythmia.**

antibacterial, **1.** of or pertaining to a substance that kills bacteria or inhibits their growth or replication. **2.** an antibacterial agent. Antibiotics synthesized chemically or derived from various microorganisms exert their bactericidal or bacteriostatic effect by interfering with the production of the bacterial cell wall, by interfering with protein synthesis, nucleic acid synthesis, or cell membrane integrity, or by inhibiting critical biosynthetic pathways in the bacteria.

antiberiberi factor. See **thiamine.**

antibiotic, **1.** of or pertaining to the ability to destroy or interfere with the development of a living organism. **2.** an antimicrobial agent, derived from cultures of a microorganism or produced semisynthetically, used to treat infections. The penicillins, derived from species of the fungus *Penicillium* or manufactured semisynthetically, consist of a thiazolidine ring fused to a beta-lactam ring connected to side chains; these agents exert their action by inhibiting mucopeptide synthesis in bacterial cell walls during multiplication of the organisms. Penicillin G and V are widely used in treating many gram-positive coccal infections but are inactivated by the enzyme penicillinase produced by strains of staphylococci; cloxacillin, dicloxacillin, methicillin, nafcillin, and oxacillin are penicillinase-resistant penicillins. Broad-spectrum penicillins effective against gram-negative organisms are ampicillin, carbenicillin, and hetacillin. Hypersensitivity reactions, as rash, fever, bronchospasm, vasculitis, and anaphylaxis, are relatively common side effects of penicillin therapy. Aminoglycoside antibiotics, composed of amino sugars in glycoside linkage, interfere with the synthesis of bacterial proteins and are used primarily for the treatment of infections caused by gram-negative organisms. The aminoglycosides include gentamicin derived from *Micromonospora,* semisynthetic amikacin, kanamycin, neomycin, streptomycin, and tobramycin. These agents commonly cause nephrotoxic and ototoxic reactions as well as GI disturbances. Macrolide antibiotics, consisting of a large lactone ring and deoxamino sugar, interfere in protein synthesis of susceptible bacteria during multiplication without affecting nucleic acid synthesis. Oleandomycin, which is added to feed to improve the growth of poultry and swine, and broad-spectrum erythromycin, used to treat various gram-positive and gram-negative infections and intestinal amebiasis, are macrolides derived from species of *Streptomyces*. Erythromycin may cause mild allergic reactions and GI discomfort, but nausea, vomiting, and diarrhea occur infrequently with the usual oral dose. Polypeptide antibiotics derived from species of *Streptomyces* or certain soil bacilli vary in their spectra; most of these agents are nephrotoxic and ototoxic. Bacitracin and vancomycin are polypeptides used to treat severe staphylococcal infections; capreomycin and vancomycin are antituberculosis agents; and gramicidin is included in ointments for topical infections. Among polypeptide antibiotics effective against gram-negative organisms, colistin and neomycin are administered for diarrhea caused by enteropathogenic *Escherichia coli*; polymyxin B, although neurotoxic, is the drug of choice for acute *Pseudomonas* infections. Antifungals, including amphotericin B, ketoconazole, and nystatin, apparently bind to sterols in fungus cell membranes and change their permeability; griseofulvin grossly distorts terminal hyphae of fungi. Amphotericin B is effective against many kinds of fungi; it may cause fever, vomiting, diarrhea, generalized pains, anemia, renal dysfunction, and other adverse effects when administered intravenously. Ketoconazole is effective against candidiasis, coccidioidomycosis, and histoplasmosis and has fewer side effects and greater ease of administration than amphotericin B. Oral griseofulvin is used to treat various fungal infections of the skin and nails and may cause hypersensitivity reactions, GI disturbances, fatigue, and insomnia. Nystatin is applied locally for the treatment of oral and vaginal candidiasis; candicidin is also used for vaginal candidiasis. The tetracyclines, including the prototype derived from *Streptomyces,* chlortetracycline, demeclocycline, doxycycline, minocycline, and oxytetracycline, are active against a wide range of gram-positive and gram-negative organisms and some rickettsiae. Antibiotics in this group are primarily bacteriostatic and are thought to exert their effect by inhibiting protein synthesis in the organisms. Tetracycline therapy may cause GI irritation, photosensitivity, renal toxicity, and hepatic toxicity, and administration of a drug of this group during the last half of pregnancy, during infancy, or before 8 years of age may result in permanent discoloration of the teeth. The cephalosporins, derived from the soil fungus *Cephalosporium* or produced semisynthetically, inhibit bacterial cell wall synthesis, resist the action of penicillinase, and are used in treating infections of the respiratory tract, urinary tract, middle ear, and bones, as well as septicemia caused by a wide range of gram-positive and gram-negative organisms. The group includes cefadroxil, cefamandole, cefazolin, cephalexin, cephaloglycin, cephaloridine, cephalothin, cephapirin, and cephradine. Treatment with a cephalosporin may cause nausea, vomiting, diarrhea, enterocolitis, or an allergic reaction, as rash, angioneurotic edema, or exfoliative dermatitis; use of antibiotics in this group is contraindicated in patients who have shown hypersensitivity to a penicillin. Chloramphenicol, a broad-spectrum antibiotic initially derived from *Streptomyces venezuelae,* inhibits protein synthesis in bacteria by interfering with the transfer of activated amino acids from soluble RNA to ribosomes. Because the drug may cause life-threatening blood dyscrasias, its use is reserved for the treatment of acute typhoid fever, serious gram-negative infections (including *Haemophilus influenzae* meningitis,) and rickettsial diseases.

Mode of action of antibiotics

Mode of action	*Representative antibiotics*
Inhibition of bacterial cell wall synthesis	Penicillins Cephalosporins Bacitracins
Alteration of membrane permeability	Polymyxin B Amphotericin B Nystatin
Inhibition of microbial DNA translation and transcription	Erythromycin Tetracyclines Streptomycin Lincomycin Kanamycin Chloramphenicol
Inhibition of essential metabolite synthesis	Para-aminosalicylic acid Sulfonamides

antibiotic sensitivity tests, a laboratory method for determining the susceptibility of bacterial infections to therapy with antibiotics. After the infecting organism has been recovered from a clinical specimen, it is cultured and tested against several antibiotic drugs, often in two groups, gram-positive and gram-negative. If the growth of the organism is inhibited by the action of the drug, it is reported as sensitive to that antibiotic. If the organism is not susceptible to the antibiotic in question, it is reported as resistant to that drug. See also **Gram's stain.**

antibody (Ab), an immunoglobulin, essential to the immune system, produced by lymphoid tissue in response to bacteria, viruses, or other antigenic substances. An antibody is specific to an antigen. Each class of antibody is named for its action. Among the many antibodies are agglutinins, bacteriolysins, opsonins, precipitin. See also **antiantibody, antigen determinant, plasma protein, T cell.**

antibody absorption, the process of removing or tying up undesired antibodies in an antiserum reagent by allowing it to react with undesired antigens.

antibody instructive theory, a theory that each antigenic contact in the life of an individual develops a new antibody, as when an immunoglobulin-covered B cell comes in contact with an antigen and subsequently produces plasma cells and memory cells. The theory maintains that the random contact of B cells with antigens induces the reticuloendothelial system to instruct memory cells to produce antibodies against antigens at any time. Compare **antibody specific theory.**

antibody specific theory, (in immunology) a theory of antibody formation proposed by F.M. Burnet, stating that preprogramed, or precommitted, clones of lymphoid cells that are produced in the fetus are capable of interacting with a limited number of antigenic determinants with which the host may come in contact. Any precommitted immunocompetent cells that encounter the specific antigen in utero are destroyed or suppressed so that entire clones are eliminated or inactivated. This in effect removes the cells programed to become endogenous autoantigens and prevents the development of autoimmume diseases, leaving intact those cells capable of reacting with exogenous antigens. The theory holds that the body contains an enormous number of diverse clones of cells, each genetically programed to synthesize a different antibody. This theory further maintains that any antigen entering the body selects the specific clone programed to synthesize the antibody for that antigen and stimulates the cells of the clone to proliferate and produce more of the same antibody. Also called **clonal selection theory.** Compare **antibody instructive theory.** See also **autoimmunity.**

antibromic. See **deodorant.**

anticholinergic, **1.** of or pertaining to a blockade of acetylcholine receptors that results in the inhibition of the transmission of parasympathetic nerve impulses. **2.** an anticholinergic agent that functions by competing with the neurotransmitter acetylcholine for its receptor sites at synaptic junctions. Anticholinergic drugs reduce spasms of smooth muscle in the bladder, bronchi, and intestine; relax the iris sphincter; decrease gastric, bronchial, and salivary secretions; decrease perspiration; and accelerate impulse conduction through the myocardium by blocking vagal impulses. Many anticholinergic agents reduce parkinsonian symptoms; atropine in large doses stimulates the central nervous system and in small doses acts as a depressant. Among numerous cholinergic blocking agents are anisotropine methylbromide, belladonna, glycopyrrolate, hyoscyamine sulfate, methixene hydrochloride, and scopolamine. Various members of the group are used to treat spastic disorders of the GI tract, to reduce salivary and bronchial secretions preoperatively, or to dilate the pupil. Also called **parasympatholytic.** Compare **cholinergic.**

anticholinergic agent. See **anticholinergic.**

anticholinesterase /an'tikol'ənes'tərās/, a drug that inhibits or inactivates the action of acetylcholinesterase. Drugs of this class cause acetylcholine to accumulate at the junctions of various cholinergic nerve fibers and their effector sites or organs, allowing potentially continuous stimulation of cholinergic fibers throughout the central and peripheral nervous systems. Anticholinesterase drugs include neostigmine, edrophonium, and pyridostigmine. Neostignine and pyridostigmine are prescribed in the treatment of myasthenia gravis; edrophonium in the diagnosis of myasthenia gravis and the treatment of overdosage of curariform drugs. Many agricultural insecticides have been developed from anticholinesterases; these are the highly toxic chemicals called organophosphates. Nerve gases developed as potential chemical warfare agents contain potent, irreversible forms of anticholinesterase.

anticipatory guidance /antis'əpətôr'ē/, the psychologic preparation of a patient to help relieve fear and anxiety of an event expected to be stressful, as the preparation of a child for surgery by explaining what will happen and what it will feel like and the showing of equipment or the part of the hospital where the child will be. It is also used to prepare parents for normal growth and development.

anticoagulant, **1.** of or pertaining to a substance that prevents or delays coagulation of the blood. **2.** an anticoagulant drug. Heparin, obtained from the liver and lungs of domestic animals, is a potent anticoagulant that interferes with the formation of thromboplastin, with the conversion of prothrombin to thrombin, and with the formation of fibrin from fibrinogen. Synthetic coumarin and phenindione derivatives administered orally are vitamin K antagonists that prevent coagulation by inhibiting the formation of certain clotting factors.

anticodon /an'tikō'don/, (in genetics) a sequence of three nucleotides in transfer RNA that pairs complementarily with a specific codon of messenger RNA during protein synthesis to specify a particular amino acid in the polypeptide chain. See also **genetic code, transcription, translation.**

anticonvulsant, **1.** of or pertaining to a substance or procedure that prevents or reduces the severity of epileptic or other convulsive seizures. **2.** an anticonvulsant drug. Hydantoin derivatives, especially sodium diphenylhydantoin, apparently exert their anticonvulsant effect by stabilizing the cell membrane and decreasing intracellular sodium, with the result that the excitability of the epileptogenic focus is reduced. Diphenylhydantoin prevents the spread of excessive discharges in cerebral motor areas and suppresses dysrhythmias originating in the thalamus, frontal lobes, and other brain areas. Phenacemide and primidone are also used in treating grand mal epilepsy, and succinic acid derivatives, valproic acid, paramethadione, and various barbiturates are among the drugs prescribed to limit or prevent petit mal seizures. Many of these agents have a potential for producing fetal malformations when administered to pregnant women.

antidepressant, **1.** of or pertaining to a substance or a measure that prevents or relieves depression. **2.** an antidepressant agent. Tricyclic antidepressant agents, as amitryptyline and imipramine hydrochloride, block reuptake of amine neurotransmitters, but the exact mechanism of the antidepressant action of these drugs is unknown. Monoamine oxidase (MAO) inhibitors, as isocarboxazid, pargyline hydrochloride, phenelzine sulfate, and tranylcypromine, increase the concentration of epinephrine, norepinephrine, and serotonin in storage sites in the nervous system, and it is theorized that this increased level of monoamines in the brainstem is responsible for the drugs' antidepressant effect. MAO inhibitors also have antihypertensive action. See also **antipsychotic.**

antidiuretic, **1.** of or pertaining to the suppression of urine formation. **2.** an antidiuretic agent. Antidiuretic hormone (vasopressin), produced in hypothalamic nuclei and stored in the posterior lobe of the pituitary gland, suppresses urine formation by stimulating the resorption of water in distal tubules and collecting ducts in the kidneys. **–antidiuresis,** *n.*

antidiuretic hormone (ADH), a hormone that decreases the production of urine by increasing the reabsorption of water by the renal tubules. ADH is secreted by cells of the hypothalamus and stored in the posterior lobe of the pituitary gland. It is released in response to a decrease in blood volume or an increased concentration of sodium or other substances in plasma, or by pain, stress, or the action of certain drugs. ADH can cause contraction of smooth muscle in the GI tract and blood vessels, especially capillaries, arterioles, and venules. Acetylcholine, methacholine, nicotine, large doses of barbiturates, anesthetics, epinephrine, and norepinephrine stimulate ADH release; ethanol and phenytoin inhibit production of the hormone. Synthetic ADH is used in the treatment of diabetes insipidus. Also called **vasopressin.**

antidote /an′tidōt/, a drug or other substance that opposes the action of a poison. An antidote may be mechanic, acting to coat the stomach and prevent absorption; or chemical, acting to make the toxin inert; or physiologic, acting to oppose the action of the poison, as a sedative given to a person who has ingested a large amount of a stimulant.

antidromic conduction /an′tidrom′ik/, the conduction of a neural impulse backward from a receptor in the midportion of an axon. It is an unnatural phenomenon and may be produced experimentally. Because synaptic junctions allow conduction in one direction only, any backward, antidromic impulses that occur fail to pass the synapse, dying at that point. Compare **orthodromic conduction.**

antiembolism hose, elasticized stockings worn to prevent the formation of emboli and thrombi, especially in patients after surgery or those restricted to bed. Return flow of the venous circulation is promoted, preventing venous stasis and dilatation of the veins, conditions that predispose to varicosities and thromboembolic disorders.

antiemetic, **1.** of or pertaining to a substance or procedure that prevents or alleviates nausea and vomiting. **2.** an antiemetic drug or agent. Belladonna derivatives, bromides, barbiturates and other sedatives, and substances that protect the stomach lining, as lime water or mild gastric astringents, have weak antiemetic properties. Chlorpromazine and other phenothiazines are the most effective antiemetic agents. In motion sickness scopolamine and antihistamines provide relief. Marijuana may alleviate the nausea induced by certain antineoplastic drugs in cancer patients.

antiepileptic. See **anticonvulsant.**

antifebrile. See **antipyretic.**

antifungal, **1.** of or pertaining to a substance that kills fungi or inhibits their growth or reproduction. **2.** an antifungal, antibiotic drug. Amphotericin B and ketoconazole, both effective against a broad spectrum of fungi, probably act by binding to sterols in the fungal cell membrane and changing the membrane's permeability. Griseofulvin, another broad-spectrum antifungal agent, binds to the host's new keratin and renders it resistant to further fungal invasion. Miconazole inhibits the growth of common dermatophytes, including yeastlike *Candida albicans,* and nystatin is effective against yeast and yeastlike fungi.

antigen /an′tijən/, a substance, usually a protein, that causes the formation of an antibody and reacts specifically with that antibody.

antigen-antibody reaction, a process of the immune system in which immunoglobulin-coated B cells recognize an intruder or antigen and stimulate antibody production to protect the body against infection. The T cells of the body assist in the antigen-antibody reaction, but the B cells play the key role. Antigen-antibody reactions activate the complement system of the body, amplifying the humoral immunity response of the B cells and causing lysis of the antigenic cells. Antigen-antibody reactions involve the binding of antigens to antibodies to form antigen-antibody complexes that may render the toxic antigen harmless, agglutinize antigens on the surface of microorganisms, or activate the complement system by exposing the complement-binding sites on the antibody molecule. Complement protein immediately binds to these sites and triggers the activity of the other complement proteins to produce cytolysis of the antigen cells. The antigen-antibody reaction may start immediately with antigen contact, or it may start as much as 48 hours later. Antigen-antibody reactions are essential to the immune response of the body and are precipitated by contact of antigenic protein molecules with antibody protein molecules. The antigen-antibody reactions occur and antigen-antibody complexes are formed when unique areas on the surfaces of antigen molecules fit precisely into appropriate concave combining sites on the surfaces of antibody molecules. Various amounts of IgM, IgG, IgA, IgE, and IgD are normally present during any antigenic challenge. Antigen-antibody reactions normally produce immunity, but they can also produce allergy, autoimmunity, and fetomaternal hematologic incompatibility. In immediate allergic reactions, antigens provoke the production of specific antibodies that may circulate freely in the serum or may become attached to specific cells. Antigen-antibody reaction in the immediate allergic response activates certain enzymes and causes an imbalance between these enzymes and their inhibitors. Simultaneously released into the circulation are certain pharmacologically active substances, as acetylcholine, bradykinin, histamine, gamma globulin G, and leukotaxine. Autoimmunity makes it impossible for the immune system to distinguish between self and a foreign substance. There are several theories that seek to explain why the body reacts to autoimmune diseases by producing antibodies that attack not only the invading organisms but the cells of the body as well. They are the forbidden clone theory, the sequestered antigens theory, and the immune complex activity theory. The antigen-antibody reactions associated with autoimmunity are still not well understood. In erythroblastosis fetalis, an antigen-antibody reaction stems from the incompatibility of the fetal and the maternal blood and produces a maternal antibody that acts against fetal red cells. ABO incompatibility involves the antigen-antibody reaction between maternal antibodies and fetal blood cells when maternal and fetal blood groups differ. See also **serum sickness.**

antigen determinant, a small area on the surface of an antigen molecule that fits a combining site of an antibody molecule and binds the antigen in the formation of an antigen-antibody complex. Antigen determinants commonly consist of a sequence of amino acids that decrees the shape of these reactive areas. Also called **epitope.** See also **antibody.**

antigenicity /an′tijənis′ətē/, the quality of causing the production of antibodies. The degree of antigenicity depends on the kind and amount of the particular substance, the condition of the host, and the degree to which the host is sensitive to the antigen and able to produce antibodies.

antigerminal pole. See **vegetal pole.**

antiglobulin /an′tiglob′yo͞olin/, an antibody against human globulin, occurring naturally or prepared in laboratory animals. Specific antiglobulins are used in the detection of specific antibodies, as in blood typing. See also **antiglobulin test, precipitin.**

antiglobulin test, a test for the presence of antibodies that coat and damage red blood cells as a result of any of several diseases or conditions. The test can detect Rh antibodies in maternal blood and is used to anticipate hemolytic disease of the newborn. It is also used to diagnose and screen for autoimmune hemolytic anemias and to determine the compatibility of blood types. When exposed to a sample of the patient's serum, the antiglobulin serum will cause agglutination if human globulin antibody or its complement is present. Also called **Coombs' test.** See also **autoimmune disease, erythroblastosis fetalis.**

antihemophilic C factor. See **factor XI.**

antihemophilic factor (AHF), blood factor VIII, a systemic hemostatic.

■ INDICATION: It is prescribed in the treatment of hemophilia A, a deficiency of factor VIII.

■ CONTRAINDICATION: There are no known contraindications.

■ ADVERSE EFFECTS: The most serious adverse reaction is hepatitis, because the factor is obtained from pools of human plasma. Various allergic reactions may also occur.

antihistamine, any substance capable of reducing the physiologic and pharmacologic effects of histamine, including a wide variety of drugs that block histamine receptors. Many such drugs are readily available as nonprescriptive medicines for the management of allergies. Toxicity resulting from the overuse of antihistamines and their accidental ingestion by children is common and sometimes fatal. These substances do not stop the release of histamine, and the ways in which they act on the central nervous system (CNS) are not completely understood. The antihistamines are divided into H_1 and H_2 blockers depending on the responses to histamine they prevent. The H_1 blocking drugs, as the alkylamines, ethanolamines, ethylenediamines, and piperazines, are effective in the symptomatic treatment of acute exudative allergies, as pollinosis and urticaria. The H_2 blocking drugs, as cimetidine, are effective in the control of gastric secretions and are often used in the treatment of duodenal ulcers. Antihistamines can both stimulate and depress the CNS. The side effects of H_1 blockers may include sedation, nausea, constipation, and dryness of the throat and respiratory tract. About 25% of the individuals who use antihistamines experience some bothersome reaction. – **antihistaminic,** *adj.*

antihypertensive, **1.** of or pertaining to a substance or procedure that reduces high blood pressure. **2.** an antihypertensive agent. Various drugs achieve their antihypertensive effect by depleting tissue stores of catecholamines in peripheral sites, by stimulating pressor receptors in the carotid sinus and heart, by blocking autonomic nerve impulses that constrict blood vessels, by stimulating central inhibitory alpha-adrenergic receptors, or by direct vasodilatation. Thiazides and other diuretic agents reduce blood pressure by decreasing blood volume. Among the numerous drugs used to treat hypertension are rauwolfia and veratrum alkaloids, diazoxide, guanethidine, methyldopa, pargyline hydrochloride, and trimethaphan camsylate.

antiinfection vitamin. See **vitamin A.**

antiinflammatory, **1.** of or pertaining to a substance or procedure that counteracts or reduces inflammation. **2.** an antiinflammatory drug or agent. Betamethasone, prednisolone, prednisone, and other synthetic glucocorticoids are used extensively in treating inflammation. The basis of the antiinflammatory effect of salicylates and nonsteroidal antiinflammatory agents, as phenylbutazone, indomethacin, appears to involve inhibition of prostaglandin biosynthesis.

antilipidemic /an′tilip′idē′mik/, **1.** of or pertaining to a regimen, diet, or agent that reduces the amount of lipids in the serum. **2.** a drug used to reduce the amount of lipids in the serum. Antilipidemic diets and drugs are prescribed to reduce the risk of atherosclerotic cardiovascular disease (ACVD) based on two facts: Atheromatous plaques contain free cholesterol, and lower serum cholesterol levels and less coronary heart disease are found in populations consuming a low-fat diet than in those on a high-fat diet. Although it has not been proven that food intake affects the development of ACVD, a prudent low-fat diet with polyunsaturates replacing saturated fats is considered a valuable preventive measure by many cardiologists. A number of pharmacologic agents are used to reduce serum lipids, but it is not established whether drug-induced lowering of serum cholesterol or triglyceride levels has a beneficial effect, no effect, or a detrimental effect on ACVD morbidity or mortality. Clofibrate reduces very low density lipoproteins in serum; the drug may reduce the risk of a second, nonfatal myocardial infarction, but it increases the risk of cholelithiasis, cardiac arrhythmias, intermittent claudication, and thromboembolism. Cholestyramine exerts its antilipidemic action by combining with bile acids in the intestine to form an insoluble complex which is excreted in the feces; it may reduce serum cholesterol markedly, but it prevents the absorption of essential fat-soluble vitamins and may be associated with several serious side effects. Colestipol also binds and removes bile acids from the intestine; sitosterol may interfere with intestinal absorption of cholesterol, but the exact mechanism of its action and that of antilipidemic probucol are unknown. Dextrothyroxine lowers serum lipid levels by stimulating hepatic catabolism and excretion of cholesterol and its metabolites. See also **hyperlipidemia.**

Antilirium, a trademark for an anticholinergic drug inhibitor (physostigmine salicylate).

antilymphocyte serum (ALS), a serum prescribed as an immunosuppressive agent for the reduction of rejection reactions in organ transplant and as an adjunct in chemotherapy for malignant neoplasms. Its effects have been promising in some cases of leukemia and in kidney transplant. It is associated with some adverse effects, as serious serum sickness, generalized infection, anaphylaxis, and antigen-antibody-induced glomerulonephritis.

antimalarial, **1.** of or pertaining to a substance that destroys or suppresses the development of malaria plasmodia or to a procedure that exterminates the mosquito vectors of the disease, as spraying insecticides or draining swamps. **2.** an antimalarial drug that destroys or prevents the development of plasmodia in human hosts. Chloroquine hydrochloride and hydroxychloroquine sulfate are effective against *Plasmodium vivax, P. malariae,* and certain strains of *P. falciparum*. Patients with drug-resistant *P. falciparum* are often treated with a combination of quinine, pyrimethamine, and sulfadoxine. See also **malaria.**

antimetabolite, a drug or other substance that is an antagonist or that resembles a normal human metabolite and interferes with its function in the body, usually by competing for the metabolite's receptors or enzymes. Among the antimetabolites used as antineoplastic agents are the folic acid analog methotrexate and the pyrimidine analogs fluorouracil and floxuridine. Antineoplastic mercaptopurine, an analog of the nucleotide adenine and the purine base hypoxanthine, is a metabolic anatagonist of both compounds. Thioguanine, another member of a large series of purine analogs, interferes with nucleic acid synthesis. Cytarabine, used in the treatment of acute myelocytic leukemia, is a synthetic nucleoside that resembles cytidine and kills cells actively synthesizing DNA, apparently by inhibiting the enzyme DNA polymerase.

antimicrobial, **1.** of or pertaining to a substance that kills microorganisms or inhibits their growth or replication. **2.** an agent that kills or inhibits the growth or replication of microorganisms.

Antiminth, a trademark for an anthelmintic (pyrantel pamoate).

antimitochondrial antibody, an antibody that acts specifically against mitochondria. These antibodies are not normally present in the blood of healthy people. A laboratory test for the presence of the antibodies in the blood is a valuable diagnostic aid in liver disease, because a biopsy of the liver may not yield affected tissue. Low titers may occur in chronic hepatitis, drug-induced hepatotoxicity, and various other diseases. High titers are virtually diagnostic of primary biliary cirrhosis.

anti-Monson curve. See **reverse curve.**

antimony /an′təmō′nē/, a bluish, crystalline metallic element occurring in nature, both free and as salts. Various antimony compounds are used in the treatment of filariasis, leishmaniasis, lymphogranuloma, schistosomiasis, and trypanosomiasis and as an emetic.

antimony poisoning, poisoning caused by the ingestion or inhalation of antimony or antimony compounds, characterized by vomiting, sweating, diarrhea, and a metallic taste in the mouth. Irritation of the skin or mucous membrane may result from external exposure. Severe poisoning resembles arsenic poisoning. Dimercaprol is used for chelation. Antimony and antimony compounds are common ingredients of many substances used in medicine and industry.

antimony potassium tartrate, an antischistosomal.

■ INDICATION: It is prescribed in the treatment of infection caused by *Schistosoma japonicum*.

■ CONTRAINDICATIONS: Anemia, severe hepatic, renal, or cardiac insufficiency, or known hypersensitivity to this drug prohibits its use.

■ ADVERSE EFFECTS: Among the most serious adverse reactions are circulatory collapse from too rapid injection and coughing and vomiting during and after injection. Potentially serious allergic reactions and blood dyscrasias are occasionally observed. Also called **tartar emetic.**

antimorph, a mutant gene that inhibits or antagonizes the normal influence of its allele in the expression of a trait. Compare **amorph, hypermorph, hypomorph.**

antimuscarinic, inhibiting the stimulation of the postganglionic parasympathetic receptor.

antimutagen /an′timyo͞o′təjən/, **1.** any substance that reduces the rate of spontaneous mutations or counteracts or reverses the action of a mutagen. **2.** any technique that protects cells against the effects of mutagenic agents. **–antimutagenic,** *adj.*

antineoplastic, **1.** of or pertaining to a substance, procedure, or measure that prevents the proliferation of malignant cells. **2.** a chemotherapeutic agent that controls or kills cancer cells. Drugs used in the treatment of cancer are cytotoxic but are generally more damaging to dividing cells than to resting cells. Cycle-specific antineoplastic agents are more effective in killing proliferating cells than in killing resting cells, and phase-specific agents are most active during a specific phase of the cell cycle. Most anticancer drugs prevent the proliferation of cells by inhibiting the synthesis of DNA by various mechanisms. Alkylating agents, as nitrogen mustard derivatives, ethylenimine derivatives, and alkyl sulfonates, interfere with DNA replication by causing cross-linking of DNA strands and abnormal pairing of nucleotides. Antimetabolites exert their action by interfering with the formation of compounds required for cell division. The folic acid analog and 5-fluorouracil, a pyrimidine analog, inhibit enzymes required for the formation of the essential DNA constituent thymidine. Hypoxanthine analog 6-mercaptopurine and 6-thioguanine, an analog of guanine, interfere with the biosynthesis of purine. Vinblastine and vincristine, alkaloids derived from the periwinkle plant, disrupt cell division by interfering with the formation of the mitotic spindle. Antineoplastic antibiotics, as doxorubicin, daunomycin, and mitomycin, block or inhibit DNA synthesis, while dactinomycin and mithramycin interfere with RNA synthesis. Cytotoxic chemotherapeutic agents may be administered orally, intravenously, or by infusion. All have untoward and unpleasant side effects and are potentially immunosuppresive and dangerous. Estrogens and androgens, although not considered antineoplastic agents, frequently cause tumor regression when administered in high doses to patients with hormone-dependent cancers. See also **alkylating agent, antimetabolite.**

antineoplastic antibiotic, a chemical substance derived from a microorganism or a synthetic analog of the substance, used in cancer chemotherapy. Dactinomycin, employed in the treatment of Wilms' tumor, testicular carcinoma, choriocarcinoma, rhabdomyosarcoma, and some other sarcomas, exerts its antineoplastic effect by interfering with RNA synthesis. Mithramycin, with a similar mechanism of action, is also administered for testicular cancer and for trophoblastic neoplasms. Doxorubicin, a broad-spectrum agent that is especially useful in treating breast carcinoma, lymphomas, sarcomas, and acute leukemia, and closely related daunomycin, which is also effective in acute leukemias, block the biosynthesis of RNA. Mitomycin C, prescribed for gastric, breast, cervical, and head and neck carcinomas, cross links strands of DNA. Bleomycin, used in the treatment of squamous cell carcinomas of the head and neck, testicular carcinoma, and lymphomas, damages DNA and prevents its repair. Antineoplastic antibiotics depress bone marrow and usually cause nausea and vomiting; several cause alopecia. Doxorubicin and daunomycin may be cardiotoxic, and mitomycin and bleomycin may produce pulmonary changes.

antineoplastic hormone, a chemical substance produced by an endocrine gland or a synthetic analog of the naturally occurring compound, used to control certain disseminated cancers. Hormonal therapy is designed to counteract the effect of an endogenous hormone required for the growth of the tumor. The estrogens diethylstilbestrol (DES) and ethinyl estradiol are employed in palliative treatment of a prostatic carcinoma that is nonresectable or unresponsive to radiotherapy. An androgen, as testosterone propionate, testolactone, or fluoxymesterone, may be administered postoperatively to control disseminated breast cancer in women whose tumors are estrogen-dependent. The antiestrogen tamoxifen produces responses in many patients with advanced estrogen-dependent breast cancer. Paradoxically, large doses of estrogen, frequently used to control disseminated breast cancer in postmenopausal women, apparently check the growth of tumors by inhibiting the secretion of estrogen by the adrenal gland. Some progestins produce a favorable response in women with disseminated endometrial carcinoma and, occasionally, in patients with prostatic or renal cancers. These progestins include megestrol acetate, medroxyprogesterone acetate, and 17-alpha-hydroxyprogesterone caproate.

antineuritic vitamin. See **thiamine.**

antinuclear antibody, an antibody directed at components of cellular nuclei, as DNA, found in patients with various diseases, as systemic lupus erythematosus.

antiparallel, (in molecular genetics) the condition in which molecules, as strands of DNA, are parallel but point in opposite directions.

antiparasitic, **1.** of or pertaining to a substance or procedure that kills parasites or inhibits their growth or reproduction. **2.** an antiparasitic drug including amebicides, anthelmintics, antimalarials, schistosomicides, trichomonacides, and trypanosomicides.

antiparkinsonian, of or pertaining to a substance or procedure used to treat parkinsonism. Drugs for this neurological disorder are of two kinds: those that compensate for the lack of dopamine in the corpus striatum of parkinsonism patients, and anticholinergic agents that counteract the activity of the abundant acetylcholine in the striatum. Synthetic levodopa, a dopamine precursor that crosses the blood-brain barrier, is administered to patients to reduce the rigidity, sluggishness, dysphagia, drooling, and instability characteristic of the disease, but the drug does not alter the relentless course of the disorder. Centrally active cholinergic blockers, notably benztropine, biperiden, procyclidine, and trihexyphenidyl, may relieve tremors and rigidity and improve mobility. The antiviral agent amantadine is often effective in the treatment of parkinsonism; the mechanism of its action is not established, but it apparently causes an increased release of dopamine in the brain. Therapeutic approaches to the relief of the symptoms of parkinsonism include alcohol injection, cautery, cryosurgery, and surgical excision performed to destroy the globus pallidus (reducing rigidity) and parts of the thalamus (reducing tremor). Extrapyramidal symptoms similar to idiopathic parkinsonism are frequently induced by antipsychotic drugs. See also **tardive dyskinesia.**

antiperistaltic, **1.** of or pertaining to a substance that inhibits or diminishes peristalsis. **2.** an antiperistaltic agent. Narcotics, as paregoric, diphenoxylate, and loperamide hydrochloride, are antiperistaltic agents used to provide symptomatic relief in diarrhea. Anticholinergic (parasympatholytic) drugs reduce spasms of intestinal smooth muscle and are frequently prescribed to decrease excessive GI motility.

antipernicious anemia factor. See **cyanocobalamin.**

antipruritic, **1.** of or pertaining to a substance or procedure that tends to relieve or prevent itching. **2.** an antipruritic drug. Topical anesthetics, corticosteroids, and antihistamines are used as antipruritic agents.

antipsychotic, **1.** of or pertaining to a substance or procedure that counteracts or diminishes symptoms of a psychosis. **2.** an antipsychotic drug. Phenothiazine derivatives are the most frequently prescribed antipsychotics for use in the treatment of schizophrenia and other major affective disorders. They apparently act by enhancing the filtering mechanisms of the reticular formation in the brainstem. Common side effects of phenothiazines are a dry mouth, blurred vision, and extrapyramidal reactions requiring treatment with antiparkinsonian agents. See also **antidepressant, neuroleptic, tranquilizer.**

antipyretic, **1.** of or pertaining to a substance or procedure that reduces fever. **2.** an antipyretic agent. Such drugs usually lower the thermodetection set point of the hypothalamic heat regulatory center, with resulting vasodilatation and sweating. Widely used antipyretic agents are acetaminophen, administered orally or through rectal suppositories, aspirin, and other salicylates. A tepid alcohol sponge bath or lukewarm tub bath may decrease an elevated temperature, and hypothermia produced by a cooling blanket is sometimes used for patients with a prolonged, high fever. Also called **antifebrile, antithermic, febrifuge.**

antipyretic bath, a bath in which tepid water is used to reduce the temperature of the body.

antiscorbutic vitamin. See **ascorbic acid.**

antisense, (in molecular genetics) a strand of DNA containing the same sequence of nucleotides as messenger RNA (mRNA). See **sense strand.**

antisepsis, destruction of microorganisms to prevent infection.

antiseptic, **1.** tending to inhibit the growth and reproduction of microorganisms. **2.** a substance that tends to inhibit the growth and reproduction of microorganisms.

antiseptic dressing, a dressing treated with an antiseptic, germicide, or bacteriostat, applied to a wound or an incision to prevent or treat infection.

antiseptic gauze, gauze permeated with an antiseptic solution, sometimes packaged in individual, sealed packets.

antiserum, *pl.* **antisera, antiserums,** serum of an animal or human containing antibodies against a specific disease, used to confer passive immunity to that disease. Antisera do not provoke the production of antibodies. There are two types of antiserum. Antitoxin is an antiserum that neutralizes the toxin produced by specific bacteria, but it does not kill the bacteria. Antimicrobial serum acts to destroy bacteria by making them more susceptible to the leukocytic action. Polyvalent antiserum acts on more than one strain of bacteria; univalent antiserum acts on only one strain. Antibiotic drugs have largely replaced antimicrobial antisera. Caution is always to be used in giving antiserum of any kind, as hepatitis or hypersensitivity reactions can occur. Also called **immune serum.** Compare **vaccine.**

antiserum anaphylaxis, an exaggerated reaction of hypersensitivity in a normal person caused by the injection of serum from a sensitized individual. Also called **passive anaphylaxis.**

antisocial personality, a person who exhibits attitudes and overt behavior contrary to the customs, standards, and moral principles accepted by society. Also called **psychopathic personality, sociopathic personality.** See also **antisocial personality disorder.**

antisocial personality disorder, a condition characterized by repetitive behavioral patterns that lack moral and ethical standards and bring a person into continuous conflict with society. Symptoms include aggressiveness, callousness, impulsiveness, irresponsibility, hostility, a low frustration level, a marked emotional immaturity, and poor judgment. A person who has this disorder neglects the rights of others, is incapable of loyalty to others or to social values, is unable to feel guilt or to learn from experience, is impervious to punishment, and tends to rationalize his behavior or to blame it on others. The disorder is usually recognized before adulthood and often persists throughout life. Adverse environmental influences, biologic deficiencies, and unconscious conflicts resulting from aberrant family relationships may contribute to the development of the disorder. Most individuals with this condition manage to function in society despite frequent bouts with authorities, but many are referred by courts to prisons. Also called **antisocial reaction.** See also **psychopathic.**

antisocial reaction. See **antisocial personality disorder.**

antistreptolysin-O test (ASOT, ASLT) /an'tistrep'-təlī'sinō'/, a streptococcal antibody test for finding and measuring serum antibodies to streptolysin-O, an exotoxin produced by most group A and some group C and G streptococci. The test is often used as an aid in the diagnosis of rheumatic fever. A low titer of antistreptolysin-O antibody is present in most people, since streptococcal infection is common. Elevated or increasing titers indicate a recent infection. See also **Lancefield's classification.**

antithermic. See **antipyretic.**

antithyroid drug, any one of several preparations that can inhibit the synthesis of thyroid hormones and are commonly used in the treatment of hyperthyroidism. The major antithyroid drugs are thioamides, as propylthiouracil, methimazole, and carbimazole. In the body such substances interfere with the incorporation of iodine into the tyrosyl residues of thyroglobulin required for the production of the hormones thyroxine and triiodothyronine. These drugs are often used to control hyperthyroidism during an anticipated remission and before a thyroidectomy. Such substances cross the placenta, can cause fetal hypothyroidism and goiter, and are contraindicated for mothers who breast-feed their children.

antitoxin, a subgroup of antisera usually prepared from the serum of horses immunized against a particular toxin-producing organism, as botulism antitoxin given therapeutically in botulism and tetanus and diphtheria antitoxin given prophylactically to prevent those infections.

antitrust, (in law) against the operation, establishment, or maintenance of a monopoly in the manufacture, production, or sale of a commodity, providing of a service, or practice of a profession.

antitussive /an′titus′iv/, **1.** against a cough. **2.** any of a large group of narcotic and nonnarcotic drugs that act on the central and peripheral nervous systems to suppress the cough reflex. Because the cough reflex is necessary for clearing the upper respiratory tract of obstructive secretions, antitussives should not be used with a productive cough. Codeine and hydrocodone are potent narcotic antitussives. Dextromethorphan is an equally effective antitussive with no dependence liability. Antitussives are administered orally, usually in a syrup with a mucolytic or expectorant and alcohol, or, sometimes, in a capsule with an antihistaminic and a mild analgesic.

antivenin /an′tiven′in/, a suspension of venom-neutralizing antibodies prepared from the serum of immunized horses. Antivenin confers passive immunity and is given as a part of emergency first aid for various snake and insect bites.

Antivert, a trademark for an antihistamine (meclizine hydrochloride).

antiviral, destructive to viruses.

antivitamin, a substance that inactivates a vitamin.

antixerophthalmic vitamin. See **vitamin A.**

antr-. See **antro-.**

antral gastritis, an abnormal narrowing of the antrum, or distal portion of the stomach. The narrowing is not a true gastritis, but a radiographic finding that may represent gastric ulcer or tumor.

antro-, antr-, a combining form meaning 'pertaining to an antrum or sinus': *antrocele, antrodynia, antrophore*.

antrum cardiacum, a constricted passage from the esophagus to the stomach, lying just inside the opening formed by the cardiac sphincter.

Anturane, a trademark for a uricosuric (sulfinpyrazone).

anular, describing a ring-shaped lesion surrounding a clear, normal, unaffected disk of skin.

anular ligament, a ligament that encircles the head of the radius and holds it in the radial notch of the skin. Distal to the notch, the anular ligament forms a complete fibrous ring.

anuresis. See **anuria.**

anuria /ənŏŏr′ē•ə/, the inability to urinate, the cessation of urine production, or a urinary output of less than 100 to 250 ml per day. Anuria may be caused by kidney failure or dysfunction, a decline in blood pressure below that required to maintain filtration pressure in the kidney, or an obstruction in the urinary passages. A rapid decline in urinary output, leading ultimately to anuria and uremia, occurs in acute renal failure. Although patients can live up to 2 weeks with anuria, death may occur within 24 hours of the total loss of urinary function. Uremia develops in anuria as the amount of waste products and potassium in the bloodstream increases because the kidneys cannot excrete them. The failure of the kidney to excrete hydrogen ions leads to acidosis, and the cells of the body then tend to release more potassium than usual. Fever, trauma, and infection, to which the uremic patient is particularly susceptible, tend to cause rapid catabolism of body tissue that further increases serum potassium levels. Symptoms of high potassium levels include extreme muscle weakness, numbness, and cardiac arrhythmia. Heart failure may suddenly occur. Management of anuria includes limitation of potassium and protein intake, medication to increase the rectal excretion of potassium, dialysis, regulation of fluid intake, and careful monitoring of blood chemistry and fluid balance. Protection of the patient from infection and from injury is critical. Kinds of anuria include **angioneurotic anuria, calculus anuria, obstructive anuria, postrenal anuria, prerenal anuria,** and **renal anuria.** Also called **anuresis** /an′yŏŏrē′sis/. **–anuric, anuretic,** *adj*. Compare **oliguria.**

anus /ā′nəs/, the opening at the terminal end of the anal canal.

anxietas /angzī′ətas/, a state of anxiety, nervous restlessness, or apprehension, often accompanied by a feeling of oppression in the epigastrium. Kinds of anxietas are **anxietas presenilis** and **restless legs syndrome.**

anxietas presenilis, a state of extreme anxiety associated with the climacteric period of life.

anxietas tibiarum. See **restless legs syndrome.**

anxiety, a nursing diagnosis accepted by the Fifth National conference on the Classification of Nursing Diagnoses. As a symptom, anxiety is a state or feeling of apprehension, uneasiness, agitation, uncertainty, and fear resulting from the anticipation of some threat or danger, usually of intrapsychic rather than external origin, whose source is generally unknown or unrecognized. The cause of the problem is complex and may involve an unconscious conflict about essential values and goals of life; a threat to self-concept; a threat of death; a threat to or change in health status, socioeconomic status, role functioning, environment, or interactive patterns; situational and maturational crises; problems involving interpersonal relationships; or unmet needs. The defining characteristics of the condition may be subjective or objective. The subjective characteristics include increased tension, apprehension, painful and persistent increased helplessness, feelings of uncertainty and inadequacy, fear, feelings of overexcitedness, distress, jitteriness, and worry. Objective characteristics include cardiovascular excitation, superficial vasoconstricition, pupil dilatation, restlessness, insomnia, glancing about, poor eye contact, trembling and extraneous movements, facial tension, quivering voice, continuous focus on the self, increased persperation, and expressed concern regarding change in life events. Kinds of anxiety include **castration anxiety, free-floating anxiety, separation anxiety,** and **situational anxiety.** See also **nursing diagnosis.**

anxiety attack, an acute, psychobiologic reaction manifested by intense anxiety and panic. Symptoms vary according to the individual and the intensity of the attack but typically include palpitations, shortness of breath, dizziness, faintness, profuse sweating, pallor of the face and extremities, GI discomfort, and a vague feeling of imminent death. Attacks usually occur suddenly, last from a few seconds to an hour or longer, and vary in frequency from several times a day to once a month. Treatment consists of reassurance, administration of a sedative, if necessary, and appropriate psychotherapy to identify the stresses perceived as threatening. See also **anxiety, anxiety neurosis.**

anxiety complex. See **castration anxiety.**

anxiety neurosis, a neurotic disorder characterized by persistent anxiety. The symptoms range from mild, chronic tenseness, with feelings of timidity, fatigue, apprehension, and indecisiveness, to more intense states of restlessness and irritability that may lead to aggressive acts or indecisiveness. In extreme cases, the overwhelming emotional discomfort is accompanied by physical reactions, including tremor, sustained muscle tension, tachycardia, dyspnea, hypertension, increased respiration, and profuse perspiration. Other physical signs include changes in skin color, nausea, vomiting, diarrhea, restlessness, immobilization, insomnia, and changes in appetite, all occurring without underlying organic cause. The symptoms of anxiety may be controlled with medication, such as tranquilizers, but psychotherapy is the preferred treatment and sometimes cures the neurosis. Also called **anxiety reaction, anxiety state.** See also **anxiety, anxiety attack.**

AORN, abbreviation for **Association of Operating Room Nurses.**

aorta /ā·ôr′tə/, the main trunk of the systemic arterial circulation, comprised of four parts: the ascending aorta, the arch of the aorta, the thoracic portion of the descending aorta, and the abdominal portion of the descending aorta. It starts at the aortic opening of the left ventricle, where it has a diameter of about 3 cm, rises a short distance toward the neck, bends to the left and dorsally over the root of the left lung, descends within the thorax on the left side of the vertebral column, and passes through the aortic hiatus of the diaphragm into the abdominal cavity. Opposite the caudal border of the fourth lumbar vertebra, it narrows to about 1.75 cm in diameter and branches into the two common iliac arteries.

aortic aneurysm, a localized dilatation of the wall of the aorta caused by atherosclerosis, hypertension, or, less frequently, syphilis. The lesion may be a saccular distention, a fusiform or cylindroid swelling of a length of the vessel, or a longitudinal dissection between the outer and middle layers of the vessel wall. Syphilitic aneurysms almost always occur in the thoracic aorta and usually involve the aortic arch, while more common atherosclerotic aneurysms are usually in the abdominal section of the great vessel below the renal arteries and above the bifurcation of the aorta. These lesions often contain atheromatous ulcers covered by thrombi that may discharge

Signs of anxiety

Appearance

↑ Muscle tension (rigidity)
Skin blanches, pales
↑ Perspiration, clammy skin
Fatigue
↑ Small motor activity (e.g., restlessness, tremor)

Behavior

↓ Attention span
↓ Ability to follow directions
↑ Acting out
↑ Somatizing
↑ Immobility

Conversation

↑ Number of questions
Constant seeking of reassurance
Frequent shifting of topics of conversation
Describes fears with sense of helplessness
Avoids focusing on feelings
Focuses on equipment or procedures

Physiologic signs mediated through autonomic nervous system

↑ Heart rate
↑ Rate or depth of respirations
Rapid extreme shifts in body temperature, blood pressure, menstrual flow
Diarrhea
Urinary urgency
Dryness of mouth
↓ Appetite
↑ Perspiration
Dilation of pupils

Signs of anxiety are dependent on the degree of anxiety. Mild anxiety heightens the use of capacities, whereas severe and panic states severely paralyze or overwork capacities.

emboli, causing obstruction of smaller vessels. A bulging abdominal aortic aneurysm may impinge on a ureter, vertebra, or other adjacent structure, causing pain. A pulsatile mass may be detected in a routine examination, but in many cases the first sign is life-threatening hemorrhage, resulting from rupture of the lesion. A diagnosis of an unruptured aneurysm may be made using x-ray films of the abdomen, which show a ring of calcification around the dilatation, or with an angiogram. The noninvasive technique of ultrasound is used to define the size and location of abdominal aortic aneurysms, being particularly useful in following the progress of aneurysms too small to require surgery. Treatment of small chronic aneurysms includes the use of antihypertensive drugs to reduce pressure on the weak area of the vessel, analgesics to relieve pain, and agents to reduce the force of cardiac contraction. Acute or large aneurysms are resected, and the segment of the aorta is replaced with synthetic prostheses. Cardiopulmonary bypass is required during surgical repair of an aneurysm of the ascending, transverse, or descending aorta but not for an abdominal aneurysm. Common postoperative complications are renal failure and ileus. See also **dissecting aneurysm.**

aortic arch. See **arch of the aorta.**

aortic arch syndrome, any of a group of occlusive conditions of the aortic arch producing a variety of symptoms related to obstruction of the large branch arteries, including the innominate, left common carotid, or left subclavian. Such conditions as atherosclerosis, Takayasu's arteritis, and syphilis may cause aortic arch syndrome. The symptoms include syncope, temporary blindness, hemiplegia, aphasia, and memory loss.

aortic body reflex, a normal chemical reflex initiated by a decrease in oxygen concentration in the blood and, to a lesser degree, by increased carbon dioxide and hydrogen ion concentrations that act on chemoreceptors in the wall of the arch of the aorta and result in nerve impulses that cause the respiratory center in the medulla to increase respiratory activity. See also **carotid body reflex.**

aortic regurgitation, the flow of blood from the aorta back into the left ventricle. Also called **aortic insufficiency.**

aortic stenosis, a cardiac anomaly characterized by a narrowing or stricture of the aortic valve because of congenital malformation or of fusion of the cusps, as may result from rheumatic fever. Aortic stenosis obstructs the flow of blood from the left ventricle into the aorta, causing decreased cardiac output and pulmonary vascular congestion. Clinical manifestations include faint peripheral pulses, exercise intolerance, anginal pain, and a systolic murmur. Diagnosis is confirmed by cardiac catheterization and echocardiography. Surgical repair is usually indicated, followed by frequent examinations, because recurrence of the stenosis and bacterial endocarditis are relatively common sequelae. Children with aortic stenosis are usually restricted from strenuous, competitive sports activities. See also **congenital cardiac anomaly, valvular disease, valvular heart disease.**

aortic valve, a valve in the heart between the left ventricle and the aorta. It is composed of three semilunar cusps that close in diastole to prevent blood from flowing back into the left ventricle from the aorta. The three cusps are separated by sinuses that resemble tiny buckets when they are filled with blood. These cup-shaped flaps grow from the lining of the aorta and, in systole, open to allow oxygenated blood to flow from the left ventricle into the aorta and on to the peripheral circulation. The right coronary artery arises from the sinus between the right posterior cusp of the valve and the aortic wall; the left coronary artery arises from the sinus of the left posterior cusp. The anterior cusp is the third flap of the valve. Compare **mitral valve, pulmonary valve, tricuspid valve.**

aortitis /ā′ôrtī′tis/, an inflammatory condition of the aorta, occurring most frequently in tertiary syphilis and occasionally in rheumatic fever. Kinds of aortitis are **rheumatic aortitis** and **syphilitic aortitis.**

aortography /ā•ôrtog′rəfē/, a radiographic process in which the aorta and its branches are injected with any of various contrast media for visualization. –**aortographic,** *adj.*

aortopulmonary fenestration, a congenital anomaly characterized by an abnormal fenestration in the ascending aorta and the pulmonary artery cephalad to the semilunar valve, allowing oxygenated and unoxygenated blood to mix, resulting in a decrease in the oxygen available in the peripheral circulation.

aosmic. See **anosmia.**

ap-, **1.** also **apo-.** a combining form meaning 'separation or derivation from': *apeidosis, apenteric.* **2.** See **ad-.**

APA, **1.** abbreviation for **American Psychiatric Association.** **2.** abbreviation for **American Psychological Association.**

apathy /ap′əthē/, an absence or suppression of emotion, feeling, concern, or passion; an indifference to things found generally to be exciting or moving. The condition is commonly seen in patients with neurasthenic neurosis and schizophrenia. –**apathetic,** *adj.*

apatite, an inorganic mineral composed of calcium and phosphate that is found in the bones and teeth.

APC, abbreviation for **aspirin, phenacetin, caffeine.**

APD, abbreviation for **adult polycystic disease.** See **polycystic kidney disease.**

apepsia nervosa. See **anorexia nervosa.**

aperient /əpir′ē•ənt/, a mild laxative.

aperitive /əper′itiv/, a stimulant of the appetite. Also called **aperitif** /əper′itif/.

Apert's syndrome /operz′/, a rare condition characterized by an abnormal craniofacial appearance in combination with partial or complete syndactyly of the hands and the feet. The specific cause of Apert's syndrome is not known, but the condition appears to be the result of a primary germ plasm defect. Characteristic features of this condition include premature synostosis of the cranial bones, with resultant growth disturbances. Some signs of Apert's syndrome are a peaked and vertically elongated head, widespread and bulging eyes, and a high, arched posterior palate with bony defects of the maxilla and the mandible. The degree of syndactyly varies greatly and may be complete, with the apparent fusion of all the digits externally. The treatment of Apert's syndrome usually includes an osteotomy of the cranial bones to prevent increased intracranial pressure. The syndactyly may be surgically corrected, the specific procedure depending on the severity of the deformity. Also called **acrocephalosyndactylism.**

aperture, an opening or hole in an object or anatomic structure. See specific apertures.

aperture of frontal sinus, an external opening of the frontal sinus into the nasal cavity.

aperture of glottis, an opening between the true vocal cords and the arytenoid cartilages.

aperture of larynx, an opening between the pharynx and larynx.

aperture of sphenoid sinus, a round opening between the sphenoid sinus and nasal cavity, situated just above the superior nasal concha.

apex /ā′peks/, *pl.* **apices** /ā′pisēz/, the top, the end, or the tip of a structure, as the apex of the heart or the apices of the teeth.

apex beat, a pulsation of the left ventricle of the heart, palpable and sometimes visible at the fifth intercostal space, approximately 9 cm to the left of the midline.

apexcardiogram, a graphic representation of the pulsations of the chest over the heart in the region of the cardiac apex.

apex cordis, the pointed lower border of the heart. It is directed downward, forward, to the left, and usually located at the level of the fifth intercostal space.

apexification, (in dentistry) the process of induced tooth root development, or apical closure of the root by the deposit of hard tissue.

apexigraph /āpek′sigraf′/, (in dentistry) a device used for determining the position of the apex of a tooth root.

apex pulmonis /pəlmō′nis/, the rounded upper border of each lung, projecting above the clavicle into the root of the neck.

Apgar score /ap′gär/, the evaluation of an infant's physical condition, usually performed 1 minute, and, again, 5 minutes after birth, based on a rating of five factors that reflect the infant's ability to adjust to extrauterine life. A pediatrician, Virginia Apgar, M.D., developed the system for the rapid identification of infants requiring immediate intervention or transfer to an intensive care nursery.

■ METHOD: The infant's heart rate, respiratory effort, muscle tone, reflex irritability, and color are scored from a low value of 0 to a normal value of 2. The five scores are combined, and the totals at 1 minute and 5 minutes are noted; for example, Apgar 9/10 is a score of 9 at 1 minute and 10 at 5 minutes. See table below.

■ NURSING ORDERS: A low 1-minute score requires immediate intervention, including the administration of oxygen, the clearing of the nasopharynx, and usually transfer to an intensive care nursery. A baby with a low score that persists at 5 minutes requires expert care, which may include assisted ventilation, umbilical catheterization, cardiac massage, blood gas evaluation, medication to correct acid-base deficit, or medication to reverse the effects of maternal medication.

■ OUTCOME CRITERIA: A score of 0 to 3 represents severe distress, a score of 4 to 7 indicates moderate distress, and a score of 7 to 10 indicates an absence of difficulty in adjusting to extrauterine life. The 5-minute total score is normally higher than the 1-minute score. Because a normal, vigorous, healthy newborn almost always has bluish hands and feet at 1 minute, the first score will include a 1 rather than a perfect 2; but at 5 minutes the blueness may have passed, and a score of 2 may be given. A 5-minute score of 0 to 1 correlates with a 50% neonatal mortality rate; infants that survive exhibit three times as many neurologic abnormalities at 1 year of age as do children with a 5-minute score of 7 or more.

APHA, abbreviation for **American Public Health Association.**

aphagia /əfā′jē·ə/, a condition characterized by the loss of the ability to swallow as a result of organic or psychologic causes. A kind of aphagia is **aphagia algera.** See also **dysphagia.**

aphagia algera, a condition characterized by the refusal to eat or swallow because doing so causes pain.

aphakia /əfā′kē·ə/, (in ophthalmology) a condition in which part or all of the crystalline lens of the eye is absent, usually because it has been surgically removed, as in the treatment of cataracts. Also called **aphacia** /əfā′shə/. –**aphakic, aphacic,** *adj.*

aphasia /əfā′zhə/, an abnormal neurologic condition in which language function is defective or absent because of an injury to certain areas of the cerebral cortex. The deficiency may be sensory or receptive, in which language is not understood, or expressive or motor, in which words cannot be formed or expressed. Sensory aphasia may be complete or partial, affecting specific language functions, as in dyslexia or alexia. Expressive aphasia may be complete, as in dysphasia, in which speech is impaired, or as in agraphia, in which writing is affected, or it may be partial, diminishing either or both functions. Most commonly, the condition is a mixture of incomplete expressive and receptive aphasia. It may occur after severe head trauma, prolonged hypoxia, or cardiovascular accident. It is sometimes transient, as when the swelling in the brain that follows a stroke or injury subsides and language returns. Intensive speech therapy and effort by the patient and the patient's family have many times been successful in restoring language function. See also **Broca's area.**

apheresis, a procedure in which blood is temporarily withdrawn, one or more components are selectively removed, and the remainder of the blood is reinfused into the donor. The process is used in treating various disease conditions in the donor and for obtaining blood elements for treating other patients or for research purposes. Also called **pheresis.** See also **leukapheresis, plasmapheresis, plateletpheresis.**

-aphia, -haphia, a combining form meaning a 'condition of the sense of touch': *araphia, hyperaphia, paraphia.*

aphonia /āfō′nē·ə/, a condition characterized by loss of the ability to produce normal speech sounds because of overuse of the vocal cords, organic disease, or psychologic causes, such as hysteria. Kinds of aphonia include **aphonia clericorum, aphonia paralytica, aphonia paranoica,** and **spastic aphonia.** See also **speech dysfunction.** –**aphonic, aphonous,** *adj.*

aphonia clericorum, a condition characterized by a loss of the voice from overuse.

aphonia paralytica /par′əlit′ikə/, a condition characterized by a loss of the voice because of paralysis or disease of the laryngeal nerves.

aphonia paranoica, an inability to speak that lacks an organic basis and that is characteristic of some forms of mental illness.

aphonic speech /āfon′ik/, abnormal speech in which vocalizations are whispered.

-aphrodisia, a combining form meaning a '(specified) condition of sexual arousal': *anaphrodisia, hypaphrodisia.*

aphronia /əfrō′nē·ə/, (in psychiatry) a condition characterized by an impaired ability to make common-sense decisions. –**aphronic,** *n., adj.*

aphthous fever. See **foot-and-mouth disease.**

aphthous stomatitis /af′thəs/, a recurring condition characterized by the eruption of painful ulcers (commonly called canker sores) on the mucous membranes of the mouth. The cause is unknown, but there is evidence to suggest that aphthous stomatitis is an immune reaction. See also **canker sore.**

APIC, abbreviation for **Association for Practitioners of Infection Control.**

apical /ap′ikəl, ā′pi-/, **1.** of or pertaining to the summit or apex. **2.** of or pertaining to the end of a tooth root.

apical curettage, (in dentistry) the surgical removal of the apex or the apical portion of a tooth root. Also called **root amputation, root resection.** Compare **root curettage, subgingival curettage.**

apical fiber, any one of the many fibers of the periodontal ligament that radiate apically from tooth to bone.

apical odontoid ligament, a ligament connecting the axis to the occipital bone. It extends from the process of the axis to the anterior margin of the foramen magnum and lies between the two alar ligaments, blending with the anterior atlantooccipital membrane. It is considered a rudimentary intervertebral disk and contains traces of the embryonic notochord.

apical pulse, the heartbeat as taken with the bell or disk of a stethoscope placed on the apex, or pointed extremety, of the heart.

APKD, abbreviation for **adult polycystic disease.** See also **polycystic kidney disease.**

aplasia /əplā′zhə/, **1.** a developmental failure resulting in the absence of an organ or tissue. **2.** in hematology, a failure of the normal process of cell generation and development. See also **aplastic anemia, hyperplasia.**

aplasia cutis congenita, the congenital absence of a localized area of skin. The defect occurs predominantly on the scalp, less frequently on the limbs and trunk, and is usually covered by a thin, translucent membrane or scar tissue, or it may be raw and ulcerated. The conditon is genetically transmitted, although the mode of inheritance is not known.

aplastic, **1.** pertaining to the absence or defective development of a tissue or organ. **2.** failure of a tissue to produce normal daughter cells by mitosis. See also **aplastic anemia.**

aplastic anemia, a deficiency of all of the formed elements of the blood, representing a failure of the cell-generating capacity of the bone marrow. It may be caused by neoplastic disease of the bone marrow or, more commonly, by destruction of the bone marrow by exposure to toxic chemicals, ionizing radiation, or some antibiotics or other medications. Rarely, an idiopathic form of the disease occurs. Compare **alymphocytosis, hemolytic anemia, hypoplastic anemia.** See also **aleukia, leukopenia.**

Infant evaluation at birth—Apgar scoring system

	0	*1*	*2*
Heart rate	Absent	Slow (below 100 beats/minute)	Over 100 beats/minute
Respiratory effort	Absent	Slow or irregular	Good crying
Muscle tone	Limp	Some flexion of extremities	Active motion
Response to catheter in nostril (tested after oropharynx is clear)	No response	Grimace	Cough or sneeze
Color	Blue or pale	Body pink, extremities blue	Completely pink

apnea /apnē′ə, ap′nē•ə/, an absence of spontaneous respiration. Kinds of apnea include **cardiac apnea, deglutition apnea, periodic apnea of the newborn, primary apnea, reflex apnea,** and **secondary apnea.** **–apneic,** *adj.*

apneustic breathing, a pattern of respirations characterized by a prolonged inspiratory phase followed by expiration apnea. The rate of apneustic breathing is usually around 1.5 cycles per minute.

apo-, ap-, a combining form meaning 'separation or derivation from': *apobiosis, apocarteresis, aponeurosis.*

apocrine gland, one of the large, deep exocrine glands located in the axillary, anal, genital, and mammary areas of the body. The apocrine glands become funtional only after puberty, and they secrete sweat that has a strong, characteristic odor. Compare **eccrine gland.** See also **exocrine gland.**

apodial symmelia. See **sirenomelia.**

apoenzyme, an enzyme without any associated cofactors or with less than the entire amount of cofactors or prosthetic groups.

apolipoprotein, the protein component of lipoprotein complexes.

apomorphine hydrochloride, an emetic.

■ INDICATION: It is prescribed to induce vomiting.

■ CONTRAINDICATIONS: Impending shock, narcosis, extreme inebriation from drugs or alcohol, or known hypersensitivity to this drug or other morphine derivatives prohibits its use. The drug is used with caution in debilitated patients or in those having cardiac decompensation.

■ ADVERSE EFFECTS: Among the more serious reactions are central nervous system depression, respiratory depression, and circulatory failure. Euphoria and tremors may occur.

aponeurosis /ap′ōnŏŏrō′sis/, *pl.* **aponeuroses,** a strong sheet of fibrous connective tissue that serves as a tendon to attach muscles to bone or as fascia to bind muscles together.

aponeurosis of the obliquus externus abdominis, the strong membrane that covers the entire ventral surface of the abdomen and lies superficial to the rectus abdominis. Fibers from both sides of the aponeurosis interlace in the midline to form the linea alba. The upper part of the aponeurosis serves as the inferior origin of the pectoralis major; the lower part ends in the inguinal ligament.

apophyseal fracture /ap′əfiz′ē•əl/, a fracture that separates an apophysis of a bone from the main osseous tissue at a point of strong tendinous attachment.

apophysitis /əpof′əsī′tis/, a condition characterized by the inflammation of an outgrowth or swelling, expecially a bony outgrowth that is not separated from the bone. Apophysitis occurs most frequently as a disorder of the foot caused by disease of the epiphysis of the quadrangular bone at the back of the tarsus.

apoplexy /ap′əplek′sē/, **1.** *obsolete.* a cerebrovascular accident, resulting in paralysis. **2.** a hemorrhage within an organ. **–apoplectic,** *adj.*

apoprotein, a polypeptide chain not yet complexed to its specific prosthetic group.

apothecaries' measure /əpoth′əker′ēz/, a system of graduated liquid volumes originally based on the minim, formerly equal to one drop of water but now standardized to 0.06 ml; 60 minims equal 1 fluid dram, 8 fluid drams equal 1 fluid ounce, 16 fluid ounces equal 1 pint, 2 pints equal 1 quart, 4 quarts equal 1 gallon. See also **apothecaries' weight, metric system.**

apothecaries' weight, a system of graduated amounts arranged in order of heaviness and based upon the grain, formerly equal to the weight of a plump grain of wheat but now standardized to 65 mg; 20 grains equal one scruple, 3 scruples equal one dram, 8 drams equal one ounce, 12 ounces equal one pound. Compare **avoirdupois weight.** See also **apothecaries' measure, metric system.**

apoxesis. See **apical curettage.**

apparatus, a device or a system composed of different parts that act together to perform some special function, as the attachment apparatus or tissues that support the teeth.

apparent death. See **death.**

appellant /əpel′ənt/, (in law) a party that brings an appeal to an appellate court. Having lost the case in a lower court, the appellant requests the court to reconsider the case.

appellate court /əpel′it/, a court of law that has the power to review the decision of a lower court. It does not make a new determination of the facts of the case; it reviews only the way in which the law was applied in the case.

appellee /ap′əlē′/, (in law) a party in an appeal that won the case in a lower court. The appellee argues that the decision of the lower court should not be modified by the appellate court.

appendage, an accessory structure attached to another part or organ. Also called **appendix.**

appendectomy /ap′əndek′təmē/, the surgical removal of the vermiform appendix through an incision in the right lower quadrant of the abdomen. The operation is performed in acute appendicitis to remove an inflammed appendix before it ruptures and prophylactically at the time of other abdominal surgery. Unless the appendix has burst and peritonitis is present or suspected, postoperative care and nursing considerations are the same as for any other abdominal operation. If the appendix has burst, a drain may be left in the incision, dressing changes are more frequent, and appropriate antibiotics are prescribed; ileus may be present and pain may be acute. Intravenous fluids, electrolytes, sedatives, and narcotic analgesics are usually given. See also **abdominal surgery, peritonitis.**

appendiceal /ap′endish′əl/, of or pertaining to the vermiform appendix. Also **appendicial, appendical** /əpen′dikəl/.

appendicitis /əpen′disī′tis/, inflammation of the vermiform appendix, usually acute, which if undiagnosed leads rapidly to perforation and peritonitis. The most common symptom is constant pain in the right lower quadrant of the abdomen around McBurney's point, which the patient describes as having begun as intermittent pain in midabdomen. To decrease the pain, the patient keeps his knees bent to avoid tension of abdominal muscles. Appendicitis is characterized by vomiting, a low-grade fever of 99° to 102°, an elevated white blood count, rebound tenderness, a rigid abdomen, and decreased or absent bowel sounds. The inflammation is caused by an obstruction as a hard mass of feces or a foreign body, in the lumen of the appendix, fibrous disease of the bowel wall, an adhesion, or a parasitic infestation. Treatment is appendectomy, within 24 to 48 hours of the first symptoms because delay usually results in rupture and peritonitis as fecal matter is released into the peritoneal cavity. The fever rises sharply once peritonitis begins, and the patient may have sudden relief from pain followed by increased, diffuse pain. The nurse is alert to the other indications of peritonitis: increasing abdominal distention, tachycardia, rapid shallow breathing, and restlessness. If peritonitis is suspected, intravenous antibiotic therapy, fluids, and electrolytes are given. Appendicitis is most apt to occur in teenagers and young adults and is more frequent in males. A kind of appendicitis is **chronic appendicitis.** See also **McBurney's point, peritonitis.**

appendix, *pl.* **appendixes, appendices,** **1.** an accessory part of a main structure. Also called **appendage. 2.** See **vermiform appendix.**

appendix dyspepsia, an abnormal condition characterized by the impairment of the digestive function associated with chronic appendicitis. See also **dyspepsia.**

appendix epididymidis /ep′ididim′idis/, a cystic structure sometimes found on the head of the epididymis. It represents a remnant of the mesonephros.

appendix epiploica, *pl.* **appendices epiploicae,** one of the fat pads, 2 to 10 cm long, scattered through the peritoneum along the colon and the upper part of the rectum, especially along the transverse and the sigmoid parts of the colon.

appendix vermiformis. See **vermiform appendix.**

apperception, **1.** mental perception or recognition. **2.** (in psychology) a conscious process of understanding or perceiving in terms of a person's previous knowledge, experiences, emotions, and memories. **–apperceptive,** *adj.*

appliance, a device or instrument designed for a specific purpose, as a dental orthodontic device.

application, a computer procedure or problem to be processed, as payroll, inventory, data about patients, scheduling of procedures and activities, pharmacy requisition and control, recording of nursing notes, or care planning.

application software, a computer program written to perform specific tasks or process particular kinds of information, as payroll, inventory, or classification systems.

applied anatomy, the study of the structure and morphology of the organs of the body as it relates to the diagnosis and treatment of disease. Kinds of applied anatomy are **pathological anatomy, radiological anatomy,** and **surgical anatomy.** Also called **practical anatomy.** See also **comparative anatomy.**

applied chemistry, the application of the study of chemical elements and compounds to industry and the arts.

applied psychology, **1.** the interpretation of historic, literary, medical, or other data according to psychologic principles. **2.** any branch of psychology that emphasizes practical rather than theoretic approaches and objectives, as clinical psychology, child psychology, industrial psychology, and educational psychology.

applied science. See **science.**

appositional growth, an increase in size by the addition of new tissue or similar material at the periphery of a particular part or structure, as in the addition of new layers in bone and tooth formation. Compare **interstitial growth.**

approach-approach conflict, a conflict resulting from the simultaneous presence of two or more incompatible impulses, desires, or goals, each of which is desirable. Also called **double-approach conflict.** See also **conflict.**

approach-avoidance conflict, a conflict resulting from the presence of a single goal or desire that is both desirable and undesirable. See also **conflict.**

appropriate for gestational age (AGA) infant, a newborn infant whose size, growth, and maturation are normal for gestational age, whether delivered prematurely, at term, or later than term. Such infants, if born at term, fall within the average range of size and weight on intrauterine growth curves, measuring from 48 to 53 cm in length and weighing between 2700 and 4000 g.

apractognosia. See **constructional apraxia.**

apraxia /əprak′sē·ə/, an impairment in the ability to perform purposeful acts or to manipulate objects. The condition is primarily neurologic but occurs in several forms. **Ideational apraxia** is characterized by impairment caused by a loss of the perception of the use of an object. **Motor apraxia** is characterized by an inability to use an object or perform a task without any loss of perception of the use of the object or the goal of the task. **Amnestic apraxia** is characterized by an inability to perform the function because of an inability to remember the command to perform it. **–apraxic,** *adj.*

Apresoline Hydrochloride, a trademark for an antihypertensive (hydralazine hydrochloride).

aprosody /āpros′odē/, a speech defect characterized by the absence of the normal variations in pitch, intonation, and rhythm of word formation.

aprosopia /ā′prəsō′pē·ə/, a congenital anomaly characterized by the absence of part or all of the facial structures. The condition is usually associated with other malformations.

aptitude, a natural ability, tendency, talent, or capability to learn, understand, or acquire a particular skill; mental alertness.

aptitude test, any of a variety of standardized tests for measuring an individual's ability to learn certain skills. Compare **achievement test, intelligence test, personality test, psychologic test.**

AQ, abbreviation for **achievement quotient.**

aqua amnii. See **amniotic fluid.**

Aquamephyton, a trademark for vitamin K (phytonadione).

aqueduct of Sylvius. See **cerebral aqueduct.**

aqueous /ā′kwē·əs, ak′wē·əs/, **1.** watery or waterlike. **2.** a medication prepared with water. See also **aqueous humor.**

aqueous humor, the clear, watery fluid circulating in the anterior and posterior chambers of the eye. It is produced by the ciliary processes and is reabsorbed into the venous system at the iridocorneal angle by means of the sinus venosus, or canal of Schlemm.

Ar, symbol for **argon.**

AR, abbreviation for **assisted respiration.**

Ara-A. See **vidarabine.**

arabinosylcytosine. See **cytarabine.**

arachidonic acid /ar′əkidon′ik/, an essential fatty acid that is a component of lecithin and a basic material for the biosynthesis of some prostaglandins.

arachno-, arachn-, a combining form meaning 'pertaining to the arachnoid membrane or to a spider': *arachnoidal, arachnoidea, arachnolysin.*

arachnodactyly /ərak′nōdak′tilē/, a congenital condition of having long, thin, spiderlike fingers and toes, which is seen in Marfan's syndrome.

arachnoid /ərak′noid/, a delicate, fibrous structure resembling a cobweb or spiderweb, as the arachnoid membrane. See also **arachnoid membrane. –arachnoidal,** *adj.*

arachnoidea encephali /ar′aknoi′dē·ə ensef′əlē/, the arachnoid membrane surrounding the brain. Also called **arachnoid of the brain, cranial arachnoid.**

arachnoidea spinalis, a continuation of the arachnoid membrane of the brain, extending along the spinal cord as far as the cauda equina with sheaths that cover the various spinal nerves as they pass outward to the intervertebral foramina. Also called **arachnoid of the spinal cord, spinal arachnoid.**

arachnoid membrane, a thin, delicate membrane enclosing the brain and the spinal cord, interposed between the pia mater and the dura mater. The subarachnoid space lies between the arachnoid membrane and the pia, and the subdural space lies between the arachnoid membrane and the dura. Also called **arachnoid.**

arachnoid of the brain. See **arachnoidea encephali.**

arachnoid of the spinal cord. See **arachnoidea spinalis.**

Aramine, a trademark for an adrenergic (metaraminol bitartrate).

Aran-Duchenne muscular atrophy /aran′do͞oshen′/, a form of amyotrophic lateral sclerosis affecting the hands, arms, shoulders, and legs at the onset before becoming more generalized. Also called **progressive spinal muscular atrophy.**

arbitrator, an impartial person appointed to resolve a dispute between parties. The arbiter listens to the evidence as presented by the parties in an informal hearing and attempts to arrive at a resolution acceptable to both parties. **–arbitration,** *n.*

arbovirus /är′bōvī′rəs/, any one of more than 300 arthropod-borne viruses that cause infections characterized by a combination of two or more of the following: fever, rash, encephalitis, and bleeding into the viscera or skin. Dengue, yellow fever, and equine encephalitis are three common arboviral infections. Treatment is symptomatic for all arbovirus infections. Vaccines have been developed to prevent infection from some arboviruses.

arch, any anatomic structure that is curved or has a bowlike appearance. Also called **arcus.**

arch-. See **archi-.**

arch bar, any one of various types of wires, bars or splints that conform to the arch of the teeth, used in the treatment of fractures of the jaws and in the stabilization of injured teeth.

arche-. See **archi-.**

archenteric canal. See **neurenteric canal.**

archenteron, *pl.* **archentera,** the primitive digestive cavity formed by the invagination into the gastrula in the embryonic development of many animals. It corresponds to the tubular cavity in the vertebrates that connects the amniotic cavity with the yolk sac. Also called **archigaster, coelenteron, gastrocoele, primitive gut.** See also **gastrula. –archenteric,** *adj.*

archetype /är′kətīp′/, **1.** an original model or pattern from which a thing or group of things is made or evolves. **2.** (in analytic psychology) an inherited primordial idea or mode of thought derived from the experiences of the human race and present in the unconscious of the individual in the form of drives, moods, and concepts. See also **anima. –archetypal, archetypic, archetypical,** *adj.*

archi- arch-, arche-, a combining form meaning 'first, beginning, or original': *archiblastoma, archenteron, archicyte.*

archiblastoma /är′kiblastō′mə/, *pl.* **archiblastomas, archiblastomata,** a tumor composed of cells derived from the layer of tissue surrounding the germinal vesicle.

archigaster. See **archenteron.**

archinephric canal, archinephric duct. See **pronephric duct.**

archinephron. See **pronephros.**

archistome. See **blastopore.**

architecture, the basic structure of a computer, including the memory, central processing unit, and input/output units.

arch length, the length of a dental arch, usually measured through the points of contact between adjoining teeth. See also **available arch length.**

arch length deficiency, the difference in any dental arch between the required length to accommodate all the natural teeth and the actual space available.

archo-, a combining form meaning 'pertaining to the rectum or anus': *archocele, archoptoma, archostenosis.*

arch of the aorta, one of the four portions of the aorta, giving rise to three arterial branches called the innominate, left common carotid, and left subclavian arteries. The arch rises at the level of the cranial border of the second sternocostal articulation of the right side, passes to the left in front of the trachea, bends dorsally, and becomes part of the descending aorta. Also called **aortic arch.**

arch width, the width of a dental arch, which varies in all diameters between the left and right opposite teeth and is determined by direct measurement between the canines, the first molars, and the second premolars. The intercanine, interpremolar, and intermolar distances may be cited as the arch width.

arch wire, an orthodontic wire fastened to two or more teeth through fixed attachments, used to cause or guide tooth movement. See also **full arch wire, sectional arch wire.**

arcing spring contraceptive diaphragm /är′king/, a kind of contraceptive diaphragm in which the flexible metal spring that forms the rim is a combination of a flexible coil spring and a flat band spring made of stainless steel. The rubber dome is approximately 4 cm deep, and the diameter of the rubber-covered rim is between 5.5 and 10 cm. Ten sizes, in increments of 0.5 cm, allow the clinician to fit the diaphragm to each individual woman. The kind of spring and the size of the rim in millimeters are stamped on the rim, as, for example, 75 mm arcing spring. This kind of diaphragm is prescribed for a woman whose vaginal musculature is relaxed and does not afford strong support, as in first degree cystocele, rectocele, or uterine prolapse; if the uterus is in an abnormal position, the arcing spring may offer better protection than the coil or flat spring, being stronger and better able to prevent the diaphragm from slipping out of the fornices of the vagina, thereby leaving the cervix exposed. Many women who have had a vaginal delivery are fitted with an arcing spring diaphragm, as some loss of vaginal muscle tone commonly occurs. An unusually long or short vagina or a vagina of unusual contour may often be well fitted with an arcing spring diaphragm. It is the most commonly prescribed kind of diaphragm and, while heavier than the other kinds, is usually found to be comfortable to use. Compare **coil spring contraceptive diaphragm, flat spring contraceptive diaphragm.** See also **contraceptive diaphragm fitting.**

arcus. See **arch.**

arcus senilis, an opaque ring, gray to white in color, that surrounds the periphery of the cornea. The condition is caused by deposits of fat granules in the cornea or hyaline degeneration and occurs primarily in older persons. Also called **gerontoxon.**

ARDS, 1. abbreviation for **acute respiratory distress syndrome. 2.** abbreviation for **adult respiratory distress syndrome.**

area, (in anatomy) a limited anatomic space that contains a specific structure of the body or within which certain physiologic functions predominate, as the aortic area and the association areas of the cerebral cortex.

areflexia /ā′rēflek′sē·ə/, a neurologic condition characterized by the absence of the reflexes.

Arenavirus /er′inəvī′rəs/, a genus of viruses usually transmitted to humans by oral or cutaneous contact with the excreta of wild rodents. Individual arenaviruses are identified with specific geographic areas, as **Bolivian hemorrhagic fever,** in one river valley in Bolivia, **Lassa fever,** in Nigeria, Liberia, and Sierra Leone, and **Argentine hemorrhagic fever,** in two agricultural provinces in Argentina. Arenavirus infections are characterized by slow onset, fever, muscle pain, rash, petechiae, hemorrhage, delirium, hypotension, and ulcers of the mouth. Treatment is supportive; there is no specific antimicrobial agent or vaccine. Fluid and electrolyte balance, rest, and adequate nutrition are the goals of treatment.

areola /erē′ōlə/, *pl.* **areolae, 1.** a small space or a cavity within a tissue. **2.** a circular area of a different color surrounding a central feature, as the discoloration about a pustule or vesicle. **3.** the part of the iris around the pupil.

areola mammae /mam′ē/, the pigmented, circular area surrounding the nipple of each breast. Also called **areola papillaris.**

areolar gland /erē′ələr/, one of the large sebaceous glands in the areolae encircling the nipples on the breasts of women. The areolar glands secrete a lipoid fluid that lubricates and protects the nipple during nursing and contain smooth muscle bundles that cause the nipples to become erect when stimulated. Also called **gland of Montgomery.**

areolar tissue, a kind of connective tissue having little tensile strength and consisting of loosely woven fibers and areolae. Also called **fibroareolar tissue.** Compare **fibrous tissue.**

Arfonad, a trademark for a ganglion blocking agent antihypertensive (trimethaphan camsylate).

Arg, abbreviation for **arginine.**

argentaffin cell /är′jentaf′in/, a cell containing serotonin-secreting granules that stain readily with silver and chromium parts. Such cells occur in most regions of the GI tract and are especially abundant in the crypts of Lieberkühn. Also called **enterochromaffin cell, Kulchitsky's cell.** See also **carcinoid, carcinoid syndrome.**

argentaffinoma /är′jentaf′inō′mə/, *pl.* **argentaffinomas, argentaffinomata,** a carcinoid tumor arising most often from argentaffin cells in epithelium of the crypts of Lieberkühn in the GI tract. The neoplasm, which occurs chiefly in middle-aged or elderly persons, may be a nodule or plaque in the early stage and a growth encircling the bowel in the later stage. Highly vascular tumors formed of silver-staining argentaffin cells may also develop in the bronchi.

argentaffinoma syndrome. See **carcinoid syndrome.**

Argentine hemorrhagic fever, an infectious disease caused by an arenavirus transmitted to humans by the ingestion of food contaminated by the excreta of infected rodents and by personal contact. Initially, it is characterized by chills, fever, headache, myalgia, anorexia, nausea, vomiting, and a general feeling of malaise. As the disease progresses, the victim may develop a high fever, dehydration, hypotension, flushed skin, abnormally slow heartbeat, bleeding from the gums and internal tissues, hematuria, and hematemesis. There may be involvement of the central nervous system, shock, and pulmonary edema. There is no specific treatment for the disease other than hydration, rest, warmth, and adequate nutrition. Rarely, intravenous fluids and dialysis are necessary. Usually, the prognosis is complete recovery. See also **Arenavirus, Bolivian hemorrhagic fever, Lassa fever.**

arginase, an enzyme that catalyzes the hydrolysis of arginine during the urea cycle, producing urea and ornithine. The enzyme is found primarily in the liver but also occurs in the mammary gland, testes, and kidney.

arginine (Arg), an amino acid produced by the digestion or hydrolysis of proteins, formed during the urea cycle by the transfer of a nitrogen atom from aspartate to citrulline. It can also be prepared synthetically. Certain compounds made from arginine, especially arginine glutamate and arginine hydrochloride, are used intravenously in the management of conditions in which there is an excess of ammonia in the blood because of liver dysfunction. See also **urea cycle.**

argininemia /är′jininē′mē·ə/, an autosomal recessive disorder characterized by an increased amount of arginine in the blood caused by a deficiency of arginase. Without arginase, ammonia cannot be metabolized into urea. Partial deficiency may result in hyperammonemia, metabolic alkalosis, convulsions, hepatomegaly, mental retardation, and growth failure; total deficiency is fatal.

argon (Ar), a colorless, odorless, chemically inactive gas and one of the six rare gases in the atmosphere. Its atomic weight is 39.95; its atomic number is 18. It forms no compounds.

Argyll Robertson pupil, a pupil that constricts on accommodation but not in response to light. It is most often seen with miosis and in advanced neurosyphilis.

arhythmia. See **arrhythmia.**

ariboflavinosis /ārī′bōflā′vinō′sis/, a condition caused by deficiency of vitamin B_2 in the diet and characterized by lesions at the corners of the mouth, on the lips, and around the nose and eyes, by seborrheic dermatitis, and by various visual disorders. See also **riboflavin.**

Aristocort, a trademark for a glucocorticoid (triamcinolone).

arithmetic mean. See **mean,** def. 2.

Arkansas stone, a fine-grained stone of novaculite, used for making hones with which surgical instruments may be sharpened.

Arlidin, a trademark for a peripheral vasodilator (nylidrin hydrochloride).

arm, **1.** a portion of the upper limb of the body between the shoulder and the elbow. The bone of the arm is the humerus. The muscles of the arm are the coracobrachialis, the biceps brachii, the brachialis, and the triceps brachii. Investing these structures is the brachial fascia. The arm is innervated by various nerves, as the ulnar nerve and the radial nerve, and is nourished by various arteries, as the brachial artery and the radial collateral artery. **2.** *nontechnical.* the arm and the forearm. See also **shoulder joint.**

arm bone. See **humerus.**

arm cylinder cast, an orthopedic device of plaster of paris or fiberglass, used for immobilizing the upper limb from the wrist to the upper arm. It is most often applied to aid the healing of a dislocated elbow, for postoperative immobilization or positioning of the elbow, or in the correction or the maintenance of a correction of a deformity of the elbow.

armpit. See **axilla.**

Arnold-Chiari malformation /är′nəldkē·är′ē/, a congenital herniation of the brainstem and lower cerebellum through the foramen magnum into the cervical vertebral canal, often associated with meningocele and spina bifida. See also **neural tube defect.**

aroma, any agreeable odor or pleasing fragrance, especially of food, drink. spices, or medication.

aromatic alcohol, a fatty alcohol in which part of the hydrogen of the alcohol radical is replaced by a phenyl hydrocarbon.

aromatic bath, a medicated bath in which aromatic substances or essential oils are added to the water.

arrest, to inhibit, restrain, or stop, as to arrest the course of a disease. See also **cardiac arrest.**

arrested dental caries, dental caries in which the area of decay has stopped progressing and infection is not present but in which the demineralized area in the tooth remains as a cavity.

arrested development, the cessation of one or more phases of the developmental process in utero before normal completion, resulting in congenital anomalies. Also called **developmental arrest.**

arrheno-, a combining form meaning 'male': *arrhenoblastoma, arrhenogenic, arrhenoplasm.*

arrhenoblastoma /erē′nōblastō′mə/, an ovarian neoplasm whose cells mimic those in testicular tubules and secrete male sex hormone, causing virilization in females. Also called **andreioma, andreoblastoma, androma, arrhenoma, Sertoli-Leydig cell tumor.**

arrhenogenic /erē′nōjen′ik/, producing only male offspring.

arrhenokaryon /erē'nōker'ē•on/, an organism that is produced from an egg that has only paternal chromosomes.

arrhenoma. See **arrhenoblastoma.**

arrhythmia /ərith'mē•ə, ərith'mē•ə/, any deviation from the normal pattern of the heartbeat. Kinds of arrhythmias include **atrial fibrillation, atrial flutter, heart block, premature atrial contraction,** and **sinus arrhythmia.** Also spelled **arhythmia.** Compare **dysrhythmia.** See also **antiarrhythmia.** **–arrhythmic, arrhythmical,** *adj.*

ARRT, abbreviation for **American Registry of Radiologic Technologists.**

arsenic (As) /är'sənik/, an element that occurs throughout the earth's crust in metal arsenides, arsenious sulfides, and arsenious oxides. Its atomic number is 33; its atomic weight is 74.91. The arsenic atom occurs in the elemental form and in trivalent and pentavalent oxidation states. This element has been used for centuries as a therapeutic agent and as a poison and continues to have limited use in some trypanocidal drugs, as melarsoprol and tryparsamide. The introduction of nonarsenic trypanosomicides with less dangerous side effects in the treatment of trypanosomiasis has greatly reduced its use. Arsenic is usually not mined in raw form but recovered as a by-product from the smelting of copper, lead, zinc, and other ores. Such processes release arsenic into the environment as does the leaching of large amounts of the element from the soil by mineral springs and the effluent from geothermal power plants. It is a component of coal, released during combustion. The environmental distribution of arsenic assures its concentration in the food chain. Many compounds containing arsenic are used as pesticides, herbicides, and feed additives for poultry and livestock. Fruit, vegetables, fish, and shellfish contain significant concentrations of arsenic. The average daily human consumption of this element is about 900 μg, most of which is ingested in food and water. The average concentration in the human adult is about 20 mg, an amount stored mainly in the liver, the kidney, the GI tract, and the lungs. Small concentrations lodge in the muscles and neural tissue. Trivalent arsenics, as inorganic arsenite, inhibit many enzymes and are poorly absorbed from the GI tract. The mechanisms for the biotransformation of arsenics in humans are not well understood. Most arsenics are slowly excreted from the body, which accounts for the toxicity of the element. Most arsenic in the body is excreted in the urine and the feces. The pentavalent forms of arsenics are rapidly excreted and cause much less toxicity than the trivalent forms. Chronic exposure to inorganic arsenics, especially the trivalent compounds, may cause severe damage to the GI lining, kidneys, central nervous system, bone marrow, liver, and blood system. Small doses of inorganic arsenic cause mild vasodilatation; larger doses induce capillary dilatation, cardiac disorders, and diminished blood volume. Various studies show a strong connection between the intensity and duration of exposure to arsenic and lung cancer in metal workers. Federal restrictions on arsenic levels in food and occupational environments have greatly reduced the incidence of both acute and chronic arsenic poisoning. **–arsenic** /ärsen'ik/, *adj.*

arsenic poisoning, poisoning caused by the ingestion or inhalation of arsenic or a substance containing arsenic, an ingredient in some pesticides, herbicides, dyes, and medicinal solutions. Small amounts absorbed over a period of time may result in chronic poisoning, producing nausea, headache, coloration and scaling of the skin, hyperkeratoses, anorexia, and white lines across the fingernails. Ingestion of large amounts of arsenic results in severe GI pain, diarrhea, vomiting, and swelling of the extremities. Renal failure and shock may occur, and death may result. Determination of the presence of arsenic in the urine, hair, or fingernails is diagnostic. Treatment includes gastric lavage with water and administration of dimercaprol, intravenous fluid therapy, and other supportive treatment as indicated for anemia, renal failure, or shock.

arsenic stomatitis, an abnormal oral condition associated with arsenic poisoning, characterized by dry, red, and painful oral mucosa, ulceration, purpura, and movility of teeth. Compare **Atabrine stomatitis, bismuth stomatitis.** See also **arsenic poisoning.**

Artane, a trademark for an anticholinergic (trihexyphenidyl hydrochloride).

arteri-. See **arterio-.**

arteria alveolaris inferior. See **inferior alveolar artery.**

arterial, of or pertaining to an artery.

arterial blood gas, the oxygen and carbon dioxide in arterial blood, measured by various methods to assess the adequacy of ventilation and oxygenation, and the acid base status. The oxygen content of arterial blood, normally 15 to 22 volumes percent, is decreased in chronic obstructive lung disease, flail chest, kyphoscoliosis, neuromuscular impairment, obesity, hypoventilation, and postoperative respiratory complications. Oxygen saturation of hemoglobin is normally 95% or higher. The partial pressure of oxygen (PaO_2), normally 80 to 100 mm Hg, is increased in polycythemia and hyperventilation and decreased in anemias, cardiac decompensation, chronic obstructive pulmonary disease, and certain neuromuscular disorders. The carbon dioxide content, normally 46%, is increased in emphysema and aldosteronism and by severe vomiting; it is decreased in starvation, acute renal failure, diabetic acidosis, and severe diarrhea. Partial pressure of carbon dioxide ($PaCO_2$), normally 38 to 42 mm Hg, may be higher in emphysema, obstructive lung disease, and reduced function of the respiratory center and lower in pregnancy and in the presence of pulmonary emboli and anxiety. The normal pH of arterial blood is 7.4.

arterial circle of Willis, the anastomosis at the base of the brain, formed by the anterior and the posterior cerebral arteries and branches of the internal carotid and the basilar arteries. The three arterial trunks, which supply each cerebral hemisphere, arise from the arterial circle of Willis. The trunks are the anterior, giving rise to the two anterior cerebral arteries, anterolateral, giving rise to the two middle cerebral arteries, and posterior, giving rise to the two posterior cerebral arteries.

arterial insufficiency, inadequate blood flow in arteries caused by occlusive atherosclerotic plaques or emboli, by damaged, diseased, or intrinsically weak vessels, by arteriovenous fistulas, by aneurysms, by hypercoagulability states, or by heavy use of tobacco. Signs of arterial inadequacy include pale, cyanotic, or mottled skin over the affected area, absent or decreased sensations, tingling, diminished sense of temperature, muscle pains, as intermittent claudication in the calf before continuous exercise, reduced or absent peripheral pulses, and, in advanced disease, atrophy of muscles of the involved extremity. Arterial insufficiency may be diagnosed by checking and comparing peripheral pulses in contralateral extremities, by angiography, by ultrasound using a Doppler device, and by skin temperature tests. Normally immersion of an extremity in hot water increases the skin temperature of the opposite limb, but this usually does not occur in arterial disease; immersion of the patient's hand in ice water raises the blood pressure about 45 mm Hg and the pulse pressure 20 mm Hg, whereas in the normal individual the blood pressure increases only 25 mm Hg and the pulse pressure does not change. Treatment of arterial insufficiency may include a diet low in saturated fats, moderate exercise, sleeping on a firm mattress, the use of a vasodilator, and, if indicated, surgical repair of an aneurysm or arteriovenous fistula. Smoking, prolonged standing, and sitting with the knees bent are discouraged.

arterial insufficiency of lower extremities, a condition characterized by hardening, thickening, and loss of elasticity of the walls of peripheral arteries causing decreased circulation, sensation, and function. Symptoms include sharp, cramping pain during exercise or rest at night, numbness, skin changes ranging from pallor to ulceration, and loss of hair on the legs. Pedal and popliteal pulses may be diminished or absent. Laboratory studies usually show elevated plasma lipids. See **intermittent claudication.**

arterial pressure, the stress exerted by the circulating blood on the walls of the arteries. The amount of arterial pressure in an individual is the product of the cardiac output and the systemic vascular resistance. A number of extrinsic and intrinsic factors serve to regulate and to maintain a reasonably constant arterial pressure. Extrinsic factors include neurologic stimulation, catecholamines, and prostaglandins and other hormones. Intrinsic factors include chemoreceptors and pressure sensitive receptors in the arterial walls that act to cause vasoconstriction or vasodilatation. Arterial blood pressure is commonly measured with a sphygmomanometer and stethoscope. Stress, hypervolemia, hypovolemia, and various drugs may alter the arterial pressure. See also **afterload blood pressure.**

arterial wall, the fibrous enclosure of the many vessels that carry oxygenated blood from the heart to structures throughout the body, and of the pulmonary arteries that carry venous blood from the heart to the lungs. The arteries, like the veins, are cylindric tubes enclosed by layers of different kinds of tissue. The inner layer is composed of a membrane of endothelium, a subendothelial layer of delicate connective tissue, and an internal elastic membrane. The endothelium of the inner layer is composed of a single layer of simple squamous cells and is continuous with the endothelium of the capillaries and the endocardium of the heart. The middle layer of tissue around each artery comprises most of the arterial wall and is composed of circular sheets of smooth muscle cells and elastic tissue. The outer layer consists of areolar connective tissue with a fine network of collagenous and elastic fibers. Most of the arteries in the body are of medium size, with a diameter of about 4 mm. The muscular coat is well developed, and nerves from the sympathetic system control the flow of blood into the areas served by the artery. The middle layer in smaller arteries is almost entirely muscular and in larger arteries is more elastic. The thickness of the outer layer varies with the location of the artery. In protected areas, as the abdominal and cranial cavities, the outer layer of associated arteries is very thin, but in more exposed locations, as in the limbs, it is much thicker. Larger arteries have a thick inner layer, which in older people may contain atherosclerotic plaques of cholesterol and calcium salts or other pathologic deposits.

arterio-, arteri-, a combining form meaning 'pertaining to an artery': *arteriosclerosis, arteriovenous, arteritis.*

arteriogram /ärtir′ē•əgram′/, an x-ray film of an artery injected with a radiopaque medium. See also **arteriography.**

arteriography /ärtir′ē•og′rəfē/, a method of radiologic visualization of arteries performed after a radiopaque contrast medium is introduced into the bloodstream or into a specific vessel by injection or through a catheter. See also **angiography.** –**arteriographic,** *adj.*

arteriole /ärtir′ē•ōl/, one of the blood vessels of the smallest branch of the arterial circulation. Blood flowing from the heart is pumped through the arteries to the arterioles to the capillaries into the veins and returned to the heart. The muscular wall of the arterioles constricts and dilates in response to neurochemical stimuli; thus, arterioles play a significant role in peripheral vascular resistance and in regulation of blood pressure. Also called **arteriola.** See also **artery.**

arteriosclerosis, a common arterial disorder characterized by thickening, loss of elasticity, and calcification of arterial walls, resulting in a decreased blood supply, especially to the cerebrum and lower extremities. The condition often develops with aging and in hypertension, nephrosclerosis, scleroderma, diabetes, and hyperlipidemia. Typical signs include intermittent claudication, changes in skin temperature and color, altered peripheral pulses, bruits over an involved artery, headache, dizziness, and memory defects. The use of vasodilators and exercise to stimulate collateral circulation may relieve symptoms of arteriosclerosis, but there is no specific treatment for the disorder. Preventive measures include therapy of predisposing diseases, continued activity in later life, adequate rest, and avoidance of stress. Kinds of arteriosclerosis are **atherosclerosis** and **Mönckeberg's arteriosclerosis.**

arteriovenous /ärtir′ē•ōvē′nəs/, of or pertaining to arteries and veins.

arteriovenous angioma of the brain, a congenital tumor consisting of a tangle of coiled, usually dilated arteries and veins, islets of sclerosed brain tissue, and, occasionally, cartilaginous cells. The lesion, which may be distinguished by an intracranial bruit, generally arises in the vascular system of the pia mater and may grow to project deeply into the brain, causing seizures and progressive hemiparesis.

arteriovenous fistula, an abnormal communication between an artery and vein occurring congenitally or resulting from trauma, infection, arterial aneurysm, or a malignancy. A continuous murmur and palpable thrill may be detected over the fistula and may be obliterated by compressing the feeding artery; this maneuver may slow the heart beat (Branham's sign). Chronic arteriovenous fistulas may give rise to varicosities, cutaneous ulcers, and cardiac enlargement. A congenital fistula may result in a cavernous hemangioma. If an arteriovenous fistula is limited in size and is in an accessible location, it can be treated by surgical excision. An arteriovenous fistula is often created surgically to provide access to the bloodstream of patients receiving hemodialysis.

arteritis /är′tərī′tis/, an inflammatory condition of the inner layers or the outer coat of one or more arteries, occurring as a clinical entity or accompanying another disorder, as rheumatoid arthritis, rheumatic fever, polymyositis, or systemic lupus erythematosus. Kinds of arteritis include **infantile arteritis, rheumatic arteritis, Takayasu's arteritis,** and **temporal arteritis.** See also **endarteritis, periarteritis.**

arteritis umbilicalis, a septic inflammation of the umbilical artery in newborn infants, usually by the bacteria of the species *Clostridium tetani*.

artery, one of the large blood vessels carrying blood in a direction away from the heart. The wall of an artery has three layers: the **tunica adventitia,** the outer coat; the **tunica media,** the middle coat; and the **tunica intima,** the inner coat. See also **arteriole.**

artery forceps, any forceps used for grasping, compressing, and holding the end of an artery during ligation. Generally self-locking, its handles are scissorlike. Also called **hemostatic forceps.**

arthr-, arthro-, a combining form meaning 'pertaining to a joint': *arthralgia, arthrocentesis*.

arthralgia /ärthral′jə/, any pain that affects a joint. – **arthralgic,** *adj*.

-arthria, a combining form meaning a '(specified) condition involving the ability to articulate': *anarthria, dysarthria, pararthria*.

-arthritic, -arthritical, a combining form meaning 'pertaining to an arthritic condition': *antarthritic, antiarthritic, postarthritic*.

arthritis /ärthrī′tis/, any inflammatory condition of the joints, characterized by pain and swelling. See also osteoarthritis, rheumatoid arthritis.

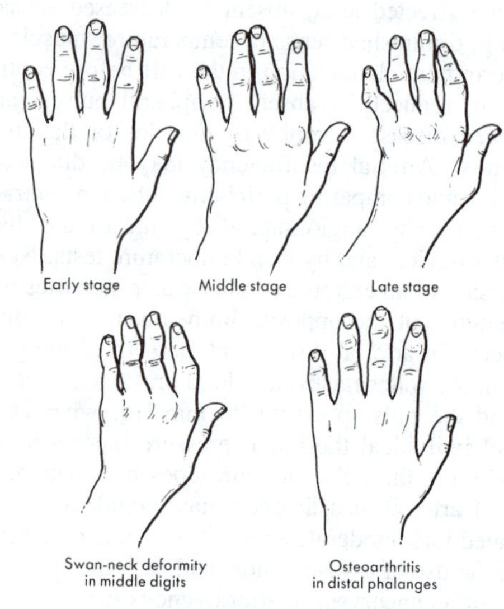

Arthritic deformities

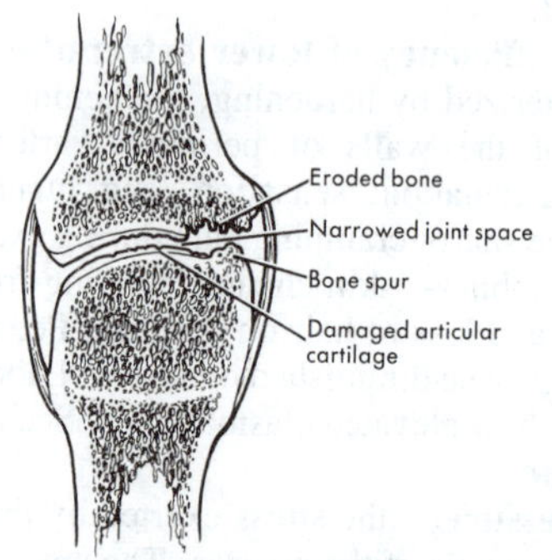

Arthritis: joint changes

arthritis deformans. See **rheumatoid arthritis.**

arthrocentesis /är′thrōsintē′sis/, the puncture of a joint with a needle and the withdrawal of fluid, performed to obtain samples of synovial fluid for diagnostic purposes. A local anesthetic is usually administered; meticulous asepsis is observed in the procedure. Normal synovial fluid is a clear, straw-colored, slightly viscous liquid that forms a white, viscous clot when mixed with glacial acetic acid; but if inflammation is present, as in rheumatoid arthritis, the fluid is watery and turbid, and its mixture with glacial acetic acid results in a flocculent, easily broken clot. The number of leukocytes, especially polymorphonuclear cells, and the protein content are increased and the glucose level is decreased if inflammation is present. Synovial fluid samples are also cultured and examined microscopically to diagnose a septic process, as bacterial arthritis.

arthrodesis. See **ankylosis,** def. 2.

arthrodia. See **gliding joint.**

arthrogryposis multiplex congenita, fibrous stiffness of one or more joints, present at birth, often associated with incomplete development of the muscles that move the involved joints and degenerative changes of the motor neurons that innervate those muscles. The cause of the condition, which is uncommon, is unknown. Physiotherapy to loosen the joints is the only treatment.

arthropathy /ärthrop′əthē/, any disease or abnormal condition affecting a joint. **–arthropathic,** *adj.*

arthroplasty /är′thrəplast′ē/, the surgical reconstruction or replacement of a painful, degenerated joint, to restore mobility to a joint in osteoarthritis or rheumatoid arthritis or to correct a congenital deformity. Under general anesthesia one of two procedures is used: Either the bones of the joint are reshaped and soft tissue or a metal disk is placed between the reshaped ends, or all or part of the joint is replaced with a metal or plastic prosthesis. Preoperative care includes the typing and crossmatching of blood. Postoperatively, the patient is immediately placed in traction to immobilize the affected limb. Exercise to increase muscle strength and range of motion is allowed in a slow, progressive schedule. Frequent checks of distal circulation are necessary if a cast is in place. The nurse watches for signs of surgical shock, thrombophlebitis, pulmonary embolism, or fat embolism. Antibiotics are usually given to prevent infection, which is the most common cause of failure of the surgery. See also **osteoarthritis.**

arthropod /är′thrəpod′/, a member of the Arthropoda, a large phylum of animal life that includes crabs and lobsters as well as mites, ticks, spiders, and insects. Arthropods generally are distinguished by a jointed exoskeleton (shell) and paired, jointed legs; they bite, sting, cause allergic reactions, and carry viruses and other disease agents.

arthroscopy /ärthros′kəpē/, the examination of the interior of a joint, performed by inserting a specially designed endoscope through a small incision. The procedure, used chiefly in knee problems, permits biopsy of cartilage or synovium, the diagnosis of a torn meniscus, and, in some instances, the removal of loose bodies in the joint space. **–arthroscopic,** *adj.*

Arthus reaction /ärto͞os′/, a rare, severe, immediate hypersensitivity reaction to a foreign substance, which is usually not irritating but in certain individuals is antigenic. An acute local inflammatory reaction, marked by edema, hemorrhage, and necrosis, occurs at the site of injection. A sterile abscess may form that is slow to heal and may become secondarily infected. Also called **Arthus phenomenon.** See also **serum sickness.**

articul-, a combining form meaning 'pertaining to a joint': *articular, articulatio.*

articular capsule, an envelope of tissue that surrounds a freely moving joint, composed of an external layer of white fibrous tissue and an internal synovial membrane. See also **fibrous capsule.**

articular cartilage. See **cartilage.**

articular disk, the platelike end of certain bones in movable joints, developed from unabsorbed mesoderm and sometimes closely associated with surrounding muscles or with cartilage.

articular fracture, a fracture involving the articular surfaces of a joint.

articulatio cubiti. See **elbow joint.**

articulatio ellipsoidea. See **condyloid joint.**

articulatio genus. See **knee joint.**

articulation. See **joint.**

articulation of the pelvis, any one of the connections between the bones of the pelvis, involving four groups of ligaments. The first group connects the sacrum and the ilium; the second, the sacrum and the ischium; the third, the sacrum and the coccyx; and the fourth, the two pubic bones.

articulatio plana. See **gliding joint.**

articulatio sellaris. See **saddle joint.**

articulator, (in dentistry) a mechanic device used in the fabrication and testing of dentures. It represents the temperomandibular joints and jaw members to which maxillary and mandibular casts may be attached. Some articulators are adjustable, allowing movement of attached casts into various eccentric relationships.

artifact, anything extraneous, irrelevant, or unwanted, as a substance, structure, or piece of data or information. In radiologic imaging, spurious electronic signals may appear as an artifact in an image with as much strength as the signals produced by the real objects, thereby confusing the radiologist and the results of any examination.

artifactual modification, a change in protein structure caused by in vitro manipulation.

artificial classification cavity, any cavity that may be classified in one of six groups, the first five of which are those proposed by G.V. Black. Class 1: cavities associated with structural tooth defects, as pits and fissures; Class 2: cavities in the proximal surfaces of premolars and molars; Class 3: cavities in the proximal surfaces of the canines and incisors that do not involve removal and restoration of the incisal angle; Class 4: cavities in the proximal surfaces of canines and molars that require the removal and restoration of the incisal angle; Class 5: cavities, except pit cavities, in the gingival third of the labial, buccal, or lingual surfaces of the teeth; Class 6: (not included in Black's classification) cavities on the incisal edges and cusp tips of the teeth.

artificial crown, a dental prosthesis that restores part or all of the coronal portion of a natural tooth. Compare anatomic crown, clinical crown, complete crown, domel crown, partial crown.**

artificial fever, an elevated body temperature produced by artificial means, as the injection of malarial parasites or of a vaccine known to produce fever symptoms, or by applying heat to the body. An artificial fever may be prescribed for a patient to arrest a disease that is sensitive to elevated body temperatures. Also called **fever therapy.**

artificial heart, a mechanic device of molded polyurethane, consisting of two ventricles implanted in the body and powered by an air compressor located outside the body. Mechanic hearts have been tested on animals since 1957, and the first artificial heart for humans was implanted in December 1982 in a retired dentist at the University of Utah Medical Center in Salt Lake City. The mechanic heart was attached to the atria and major blood vessels of the patient's normal heart with Dacron fittings. The first artificial heart for humans kept the patient alive for 112 days. Also called **Jarvik-7.**

artificial insemination, the introduction of semen into the vagina or uterus by mechanic or instrumental means rather than by sexual intercourse. The procedure is planned to coincide with the expected time of ovulation so that fertilization can occur. Kinds of artificial insemination are **artificial insemination-donor** and **artificial insemination-husband.** Also called **artificial impregnation.** See also **menstrual cycle.**

artificial insemination-donor (AID), artificial insemination in which the semen specimen is provided by an anonymous donor. The procedure is used primarily in cases where the husband is sterile. Also called **heterologous insemination.** Compare **artificial insemination-husband.**

artificial insemination-husband (AIH), artificial insemination in which the semen specimen is provided by the husband. The procedure is used primarily in cases of impotency or when the husband is incapable of sexual intercourse because of some physical disability. Also called **homologous insemination.** Compare **artificial insemination-donor.**

artificial intelligence (AI), the capability of a device, as an industrial robot, to perform functions previously thought to require human intelligence. Computer technology produces many instruments and systems that mimic and surpass some human capabilities, as speed of counting, correlating, sensing, and deducing.

artificial kidney, a device used to rid blood, circulated outside of the body, of substances commonly excreted in urine. It usually consists of a set of tubes or catheters for passing the blood between the person and a membrane unit for hemodialysis and a dialysate supply system. Also called **kidney machine.** See also **hemodialysis, peritoneal dialysis.**

artificial limb. See **prosthesis.**

artificial lung. See **Drinker respirator.**

artificially acquired immunity. See **acquired immunity.**

artificial pacemaker. See **pacemaker.**

artificial respiration, the process of maintaining respiration by manual or mechanic means when normal breathing has stopped. Effective ventilation of the lungs may fail because of bronchial obstruction by swelling, a foreign body, increased secretions, neuromuscular weakness, status asthmaticus, exhaustion, pharmacologic depression, or trauma to the chest wall. Before attempting to administer artificial respiration, the airway is tested and any obstruction removed; the pulse is palpated, and the need for cardiopulmonary resuscitation is evaluated. See also **cardiopulmonary resuscitation (CPR), resuscitation, ventilator.**

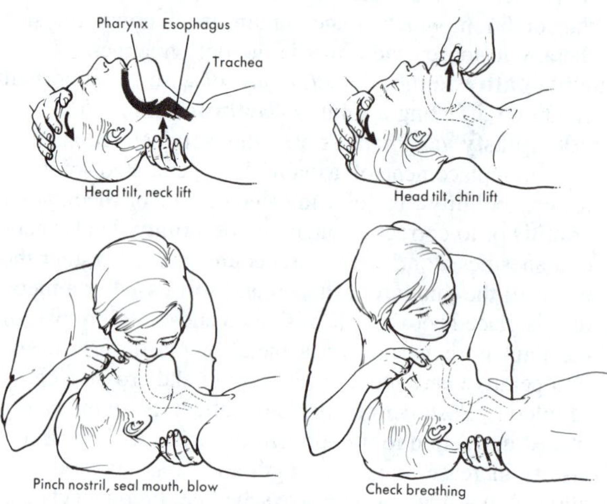

Artificial respiration

artificial selection, the process by which the genotypes of successive plant and animal generations are determined through controlled breeding. Compare **natural selection.**

artificial stone, a calcined gypsum derivative similar to but stronger than plaster of paris, used for making dental casts and dies.

aryl hydrocarbon hydroxylase (AHH), an enzyme that converts carcinogenic chemicals in tobacco smoke and in polluted air into active carcinogens within the lungs. Aryl hydrocarbon hydroxylase is the subject of numerous studies to determine why some smokers develop cancer and others do not. Experimental blood tests indicate that the level of aryl hydrocarbon hydroxylase may be a factor in hereditary predisposition of a cigarette smoker to cancer.

As, symbol for **arsenic.**

as-. See **ad.**

ASA, **1.** abbreviation for **American Society of Anesthesiologists. 2.** abbreviation for **aspirin** (acetylsalicylic acid).

asbestosis, a chronic lung disease caused by the inhalation of asbestos fibers that results in the development of alveolar, interstitial, and pleural fibrosis. Asbestos miners and workers are most frequently affected, but the disease sometimes occurs in other people who have been exposed to asbestos building materials. Chest x-ray films show the characteristic small linear opacities distributed throughout the lungs. The disease is progressive: Shortness of breath develops, eventually, into respiratory failure. Cigarette smoking and continuous exposure to asbestos aggravate the condition. Fatal mesothelial tumors sometimes occur. There is no treatment. See also **chronic obstructive pulmonary disease, inorganic dust.**

ASC, abbreviation for **altered state of consciousness.**

ascariasis /as′kərī′əsis/, an infection caused by a parasitic worm, *Ascaris lumbricoides,* that migrates through the lungs in its larval stage. The eggs are passed in human feces, contaminating the soil and allowing transmission to the mouths of others through hands, water, or food. After hatching in the small intestine, the larvae travel through the wall of the intestine, whence they are carried by the lymphatics and blood to the lungs. Early respiratory symptoms of coughing, wheezing, and fever are caused by the passage through the respiratory tract. The larvae are swallowed, they mature in the jejunum, where they release eggs, and the cycle is repeated. Intestinal infection may result in abdominal cramps and obstruction. In children, migration of the adult worms into the liver, gallbladder, or peritoneal cavity may cause death. The infective eggs are readily identified in the feces. Piperazine citrate, pyrantel pamoate, and mebendazole are effective treatments. The disease can be prevented by educating people, especially children, about good sanitation habits and handwashing.

Ascaris /as′kəris/, a genus of large parasitic intestinal roundworms, as *Ascaris lumbricoides,* a cause of ascariasis, found throughout temperate and tropic regions.

ascending aorta, one of the four main sections of the aorta, branching into the right and left coronary arteries, rising from the semilunar valve of the heart, curving to the right near the cranial border of the second right costal cartilage, and lying about 6 cm deep to the dorsal surface of the sternum. It is about 5 cm long and has three small aortic sinuses at its origin, opposite the aortic valve.

ascending colon, the segment of the colon that extends from the cecum in the lower right side of the abdomen to the transverse colon at the hepatic flexure on the right side, usually at the level of the umbilicus.

ascending current. See **centripetal current.**

ascending oblique muscle. See **obliquus internus abdominis.**

ascending pharyngeal artery, one of the smallest arteries that branch from the external carotid artery, deep in the neck, supplying various organs and muscles of the head, as the tympanic cavity, the longi capitis, and the colli. It divides into five branches, the pharyngeal, palatine, prevertebral, inferior tympanic, and posterior meningeal.

ascending urography. See **urography.**

Ascheim-Zondek (AZ) test /ash′hīmtson′dek/, an obsolete biologic test for pregnancy.

ascites /əsī′tēz/, an abnormal intraperitoneal accumulation of a fluid containing large amounts of protein and electrolytes. Ascites may be detectable when more than 500 ml of fluid has accumulated. The condition may be accompanied by general abdominal swelling, hemodilution, edema, or a decrease in urinary output. Identification of ascites is made through auscultation, percussion, and palpation. Ascites is a complication of cirrhosis, congestive heart failure, nephrosis, malignant neoplastic disease, peritonitis, or various fungal and parasitic diseases. Ascites is treated with dietary therapy and diuretic drugs; abdominal paracentesis may be performed to relieve pain and improve respiratory and visceral function by relieving the pressure of the accumulated fluid. By lowering pressure within the portal system, paracentesis is therapeutic in ascites accompanied by bleeding. See also **paracentesis.** **–ascitic,** *adj.*

ascites adiposus. See **chylous ascites.**

ascites praecox, an abnormal accumulation of fluid within the peritoneal cavity preceding the development of generalized edema associated with pericarditis. See also **ascites.**

ascorbemia /as′kôrbē′mē·ə/, the presence of ascorbic acid in the blood in amounts greater than normal, usually reflecting only an excess of ascorbic acid in the diet.

ascorbic acid /əskôr′bik/, a water-soluble, white crystalline vitamin present in citrus fruits, tomatoes, berries, potatoes, and fresh, green, leafy vegetables, such as broccoli, brussels sprouts, collards, turnip greens, parsley, sweet peppers, and cabbage. It is essential for the formation of collagen and fibrous tissue for normal intercellular matrices in teeth, bone, cartilage, connective tissue, and skin, and for the structural integrity of capillary walls. It also aids in fighting bacterial infections and interacts with other nutrients. Signs of deficiency are bleeding gums, tendency to bruising, swollen or painful joints, nosebleeds, anemia, lowered resistance to infections, and slow healing of wounds and fractures. Severe deficiency results in scurvy. An excess of ascorbic acid may cause a burning sensation during urination, diarrhea, skin rash, and nausea and may disturb the absorption and metabolism of cyanocobalamin. Tests for glycosuria, uric acid, and iron may be inaccurate when large amounts of the vitamin are being administered. Also called **antiscorbutic vitamin, cevitamic acid, vitamin C.** See also **ascorbemia, bioflavonoid, citric acid, infantile scurvy, scurvy.**

ascorburia /as′kôrbyo͝or′ē·ə/, the presence of ascorbic acid in the urine in amounts greater than normal, usually reflecting only an excess of ascorbic acid in the diet.

ASD, abbreviation for **atrial septal defect.**

-ase, a combining form used in naming enzymes: *lipase, oxidase, protease.*

Asellacrin, a trademark for a growth stimulant (somatotropin).

Asendin, a trademark for an antidepressant (amoxapine).

asepsis /āsep′sis/, **1.** the absence of germs. **2. medical asepsis,** the removal or destruction of disease organisms or infected material. **3. surgical asepsis,** protection against infection before, during, or before surgery by the use of sterile technique. **–aseptic,** *adj.*

aseptic body image, an awareness by operating room personnel of body, hair, makeup, clothing, jewelry, and placement with regard for maintenance of a sterile environment. The body image also includes an awareness of changing proximities between sterile and contaminated areas as a field becomes progressively contaminated.

aseptic conscience, a nurse's awareness that develops from a knowledge of basic operating room techniques and the importance of enforcing sterile procedures.

aseptic fever, a fever not associated with infection. Mechanic trauma, as in a crushing injury, can cause fever even when no pathogenic microorganism is present. Although the exact mechanism is not understood, fever in such cases is believed to result from the breakdown of leukocytes or from the absorption of avascular tissue.

aseptic gauze, **1.** sterile gauze prepared and packed for surgical use. **2.** any gauze that is free of microorganisms.

aseptic meningitis, an inflammation of the meninges that is caused by one of a number of viruses, including coxsackieviruses, nonparalytic polio viruses, echoviruses, and mumps. The disease is especially common in children during the late summer and early fall. In about one third of the cases no pathogen can be demonstrated, but analysis of cerebrospinal fluid reveals increased numbers of white blood cells, normal glucose concentration, and no bacteria. Symptoms vary depending upon the causative agent and may include fever, headache, stiff neck and back, nausea, and skin rash. No specific treatment is available. Supportive therapy is directed toward maintaining hydration and controlling the fever. Complete recovery, without complication or residual effect, is usual.

Asepto syringe, a trademark for a bulb-fitted, blunt-tipped syringe used primarily for irrigation of wounds.

asexual /āsek′sho͞o·əl/, **1.** not sexual. **2.** of or pertaining to an organism that has no sexual organs. **3.** of or pertaining to a process that is not sexual. **–asexuality,** *n.*

asexual dwarf, an adult dwarf whose genital organs are underdeveloped.

asexual generation, any type of reproduction that occurs without the union of male and female gametes, as fission, budding, sporulation, or parthenogenesis. Also called **direct generation, nonsexual generation.**

asexualization /āsek′sho͞o·əlīzā′shən/, the process of making one incapable of reproduction; sterilization of an individual or animal by castration, vasectomy, removal of the ovaries, or other means.

asexual reproduction, a type of reproduction found in plants and lower animals in which new organisms are formed without the union of gametes, as occurs in budding, fission, and spore formation. Compare **sexual generation.**

Asherman syndrome, secondary amenorrhea in a hormonally normal woman, caused by obliteration of the endometrial cavity by adhesions that form as a result of curettage or infection. It is diagnosed by hysterography and may be treated by secondary curettage (to remove adhesions), followed by placement in the uterus of a device to prevent reformation of adhesions during healing.

asialorrhea. See **hyposalivation.**

Asian flu. See **influenza.**

-asis, a combining form meaning an 'action, process, or result of': *basis, metabasis, oxydasis.*

ASLT, abbreviation for **antistreptolysin-O test.**

Asn, abbreviation for **asparagine.**

ASOT, abbreviation for **antistreptolysin-O test.**

asparaginase /aspar′əjinās/, an enzyme that catalyzes the hydrolysis of asparagine to asparaginic acid and ammonia. Asparaginase is used as a chemotherapeutic agent in the treatment of acute lymphoblastic leukemia.

asparagine (Asn) /aspar′əjin/, a nonessential amino acid found in many proteins in the body. It is easily hydrolyzed to aspartic acid and has diuretic properties. See also **amino acid, protein.**

aspartame, a white, almost odorless crystalline powder with an intensely sweet taste that is used as an artificial sweetener. It is approximately 180 times as sweet as the same amount of sucrose and is used to enhance the flavor of cold or uncooked foods. Aspartame tends to lose its sweetness in the presence of heat and moisture. Excessive use of aspartame should be avoided by patients with phenylketonuria (PKU) because the substance hydrolyzes to form aspartylphenylalanine.

aspartate aminotransferase (AST) /aspär′tāt/, an enzyme normally present in body serum and in certain body tissues, especially those of the heart and liver. This enzyme affects the intermolecular transfer of an amino group from aspartic acid to alpha-ketoglutaric acid, forming glutamic acid and oxaloacetic acid. The reaction is reversible. The enzyme is released into the serum because of tissue injury and thus may increase as a result of myocardial infarction and liver damage. Also called **glutamic oxaloacetic transaminase, serum glutamic oxaloacetic transaminase.** Compare **alanine aminotransferase.**

aspartate kinase, an enzyme that catalyzes the transfer of a phosphate group from adenosine triphosphate to aspartate to produce phosphoaspartate.

aspartate transaminase. See **aspartate aminotransferase.**

aspartic acid (Asp) /aspär′tik/, a nonessential amino acid present in sugar cane, beet molasses, and the breakdown products of many proteins. Pure aspartic acid is a water-soluble, colorless crystalline substance. In the Krebs' citric acid cycle, aspartic acid and oxaloacetic acid are interconvertible. Aspartic acid is used in culture media, dietary supplements, detergents, fungicides, and germicides. Also called **aminosuccinic acid.** See also **amino acid, protein.**

aspergillic acid /as′pərjil′ik/, an antibiotic substance derived from *Aspergillus flavus,* an aflatoxin-producing mold found on corn, grain, and peanuts. See **aflatoxin.**

aspergillosis /as′pərjilō′sis/, an infection caused by a fungus of the genus *Aspergillus,* most commonly affecting the ear but capable of causing inflammatory, granulomatous lesions on or in any organ. The infection is relatively uncommon and typically occurs in a person already weakened by some other disorder. Topical fungicides can be used on the skin; amphotericin B is used to treat systemic aspergillosis, especially if it has spread to the lungs. The prognosis, as for most systemic fungal infections, is poor. Compare **allergic bronchopulmonary aspergillosis.**

Aspergillus /as′pərjil′əs/, a genus of fungi that is a common contaminant in the laboratory and a cause of nosocomial infection. The fungus has hyphae and spores, lives in the soil, is ubiquitous, and proliferates rapidly. Inhalation of the spores of the two pathogenic species, *Aspergillus fumigatus* and *A. flavus,* is common, but infection is rare.

aspermia /āspur′mē·ə/, lack of formation or ejaculation of semen.

asphyxia /asfik′sē·ə/, severe hypoxia leading to hypoxemia and hypercapnea, loss of consciousness, and, if not corrected, death. Some of the more common causes of asphyxia are drowning, electric shock, aspiration of vomitus, lodging of a foreign body in the respiratory tract, inhalation of toxic gas or smoke, and poisoning. Artificial ventilation and oxygen are promptly administered to avoid damage to the brain. The underlying cause is then treated. See **artificial respiration.** –**asphyxiate,** *v.,* **asphyxiated,** *adj.*

aspirating needle, a long hollow needle used to remove fluid from a cavity, vessel, or structure of the body.

aspiration, **1.** the act of taking a breath, inhaling. **2.** the act of withdrawing a fluid, as mucus or serum, from the body by a suction device. See also **aspiration pneumonia.** –**aspirate,** *n.*

aspiration biopsy, the removal of living tissue for microscopic examination by suction through a fine needle attached to a syringe. The procedure is used primarily to obtain cells from a lesion containing fluid or when fluid is formed in a serous cavity. See also **cytology, needle biopsy.**

aspiration biopsy cytology (ABC), a microscopic examination of cells obtained directly from living body tissue by aspiration through a fine needle. It is used primarily as a diagnostic procedure, generally as a technique for detecting nuclear and cytoplasmic changes in cancerous tissue. Compare **exfoliative cytology.**

aspiration of vomitus, the inhalation of regurgitated gastric contents into the pulmonary system. See also **aspiration, aspiration pneumonia.**

aspiration pneumonia, an inflammatory condition of the lungs and bronchi caused by the inhalation of foreign material or vomitus containing acid gastric contents. Compare **bronchopneumonia.** See also **pneumonia.**

■ OBSERVATIONS: Aspiration pneumonia most often occurs during anesthesia or recovery from anesthesia or during a seizure of acute alcoholic intoxication or other condition characterized by vomiting and a decreased level of consciousness.

■ INTERVENTION: Treatment requires prompt suctioning of the bronchi and the administration, under pressure, of 100% oxygen. Continued artificial ventilation may be required. Corticosteroids are usually given to diminish inflammation. The sputum is cultured regularly, and any bacterial infection thus diagnosed is treated with an appropriate antibiotic. As long as oxygen is required, frequent analyses of the levels of gases in the blood are performed.

■ NURSING CONSIDERATIONS: The pulse rate and quality of respirations, level of consciousness, and the color of the skin are carefully monitored. Infection and respiratory failure are frequent complications. Aspiration pneumonia may be avoided by correctly positioning unconscious patients with the head low and turned to the side and by paying careful attention to the maintenance of an adequate airway. An oral airway is left in place until the patient's conditon improves, and secretions are removed by suction as necessary.

aspirator, any instrument that removes a substance from body cavities by suction, as a bulb syringe, piston pump, or hypodermic syringe.

aspirin, an analgesic, antipyretic, and antirheumatic.

■ INDICATIONS: It is prescribed to reduce fever and for the relief of pain and inflammation.

■ CONTRAINDICATIONS: Bleeding disorders, peptic ulcer, pregnancy, the concomitant use of anticoagulants, or known hypersensitivity to salicylates prohibits its use.

■ ADVERSE EFFECTS: Among the most serious adverse reactions are GI effects (ulcers, occult bleeding). Sustained treatment with large doses can cause clotting defects, liver toxicity, and renal toxicities. Reye's syndrome has been associated with aspirin use in children. An asthmatic-like and other allergic reactions are occasionally seen. Tinnitus and dyspepsia are the most common adverse effect.

aspirin poisoning. See **salicylate poisoning.**

Assam fever. See **kala-azar.**

assault, **1.** an unlawful act that places another person, without that persons's consent, in fear of immediate bodily harm or battery. The act must be apparently possible, thus causing well founded apprehension in the victim of the assault. **2.** the act of committing an assault. **3.** to threaten a person with bodily harm or injury.

assembly language, a symbolic language used for computer programing. Assembly language usually has a one on one relationship with machine language and may consist of a mnemonic code for assembling machine language computer instructions. See also **machine language.**

assertive training, a technique used in behavior therapy to help individuals become more self-assertive and self-confident in interpersonal relationships. It focuses on the direct, honest statement of feelings and beliefs, both positive and negative. The technique is learned by role playing in a therapeutic setting, usually in a group, followed by practice in actual situations. Also called **assertion training.**

assessing, (in five-step nursing process) a category of nursing behavior that includes the gathering, verifying, and communicating of information relative to the client. The nurse collects information from verbal interactions with the patient, the patient's family and significant others; examines standard data sources for information; systematically checks for symptoms and signs; determines the patient's ability to perform self-care activities; assesses the patient's environment; and identifies reactions of the staff (including the nurse who is performing the assessment) to the patient and to the patient's family and significant others. To verify the data, the nurse confirms the observations and perceptions by gathering additional information; discusses the orders and decisions made by other members of the staff with them, when indicated; and personally evaluates and checks the patient's condition. The nurse reports the information that has been gathered and verified. Although assessing is the first of the five steps of the nursing process, preceding analyzing, in practice assessing is integral to effective nursing practice at all steps of the process. See also **analyzing, evaluating, implementing, nursing process, planning.**

assessment, (in medicine and nursing) **1.** an evaluation or appraisal of a condition. **2.** the process of making such an evaluation. **3.** (in a problem oriented medical record) an examiner's evaluation of the disease or condition based on the patient's subjective report of the symptoms and course of the illness or condition and the examiner's objective findings, including data obtained through laboratory tests, physical examination, and medical history. See also **nursing assessment, problem oriented medical record.** **–assess,** *v.*

assessment of the aging patient, an evaluation of the changes characteristic of advancing years exhibited by an elderly person.

■ METHOD: The patient is measured, weighed, examined, observed, and questioned about physical, functional, and behavioral changes; height normally diminishes 0.5 inches with aging, and weight steadily decreases in men over 65 years of age but increases in women. The skin is examined for dryness, wrinkles, sagging, thinning over the back of the hands, areas of vitiligo, keratoses, warts, skin tags, and senile telangiectases, and the hair for depigmentation, lack of luster, and thinning or loss on the scalp and in the axillary and the pubic areas. Observations are made of enlargement of the nose and ears relative to face size, dryness of the eyes, discoloration of the sclera and iris, an opaque ring near the edge of the cornea (arcus senilis), decreased size of the pupil, and diminished peripheral vision. Tests are performed to determine if there is hearing loss, especially of high-frequency tones, decreased tidal volume, diminished peripheral perfusion, or deviation of the trachea, especially if scoliosis is present. Examination may reveal gum recession, loss of teeth and taste perception, diminished salivation, a decreased resting heart rate and cardiac output, and an easily palpable arterial pulse. The elderly patient may show decreased muscle mass, osteoarthritic joints, Heberden's or Bouchard's nodes at finger joints, contracture of lateral fingers, osteoporosis, a broad based stance, and slow voluntary movements. The sense of position, of smell, and of touch and the sensitivity to heat and cold may be diminished, and deep tendon reflexes may be decreased. Signs of aging that may be found in women are pendulous, flaccid breasts; vaginal narrowing and shortening and diminished lubrication, causing painful coitus; and effects of long-term estrogen therapy, as uterine bleeding, mastalgia, weight gain, fluid retention, and hypertension. Signs of aging in men include decrease in the size and firmness of the testes and in the amount and viscosity of seminal fluid, an increased diameter of the penis, and prostatic hypertrophy; libido and a sense of satisfaction usually do not diminish.

■ NURSING ORDERS: The nurse faces the patient during the evaluation, establishes eye contact, repeats questions if necessary, avoids shouting, and addresses the person by name. If the patient's visual perception and tactile sense are diminished, the nurse uses color contrasts and items of marked textural differences in the assessment.

■ OUTCOME CRITERIA: Aging does not progress at a uniform rate, and its effects may vary widely from one individual to the next, but, in many cases, changes considered normal in elderly patients are disease processes that may respond to treatment. A careful assessment distinguishes the effects of pathology from those of aging and elucidates the care needed by the patient.

assimilation, **1.** the process of incorporating nutritive material into living tissue; the end stage of the nutrition process, after digestion and absorption or occurring simultaneously with absorption. **2.** (in psychology) the incorporation of new experiences into a person's pattern of consciousness. Compare **apperception.** **3.** (in sociology) the process in which a person or a group of people of a different ethnic background become absorbed into a new culture. **–assimilate,** *v.*

assisted breech, an obstetric operation in which a baby being born feet or buttocks first is permitted to deliver spontaneously as far as its umbilicus and is then extracted. Also called **partial breech extraction.** Compare **breech extraction.**

assisted ventilation. See **IPPB.**

associate degree in nursing, an academic degree awarded on satisfactory completion of a 2-year course of study, usually at a community or junior college. The recipient is eligible to take the national licensing examination to become a registered nurse. An associate degree in nursing is not available in Canada.

associate nurse, *U.S.* **1.** (in primary nursing) a nurse who is responsible for implementing a primary nurse's care plans. **2.** in some states, a registered nurse who holds a diploma from a hospital school of nursing or an associate degree from a 2-year academic school of nursing.

associated antagonist, one of a pair of muscles or group of muscles that pull in opposite directions but whose combined action results in moving a part in one direction.

association, **1.** a connection, union, joining, or combination of things. **2.** (in psychology) the connection of remembered feelings, emotions, sensations, thoughts, or perceptions with particular persons, things, or ideas. Kinds of association are **association of ideas, clang association, controlled association, dream association,** and **free association.**

association area, any part of the cerebral cortex involved in the integration of sensory information. Also called **association cortex.**

Association for Practitioners of Infection Control (APIC), a national professional organization of nurses who work in the field of infection control.

Association for the Care of Children's Health (ACCH), an international, interdisciplinary organization concerned with the psychosocial needs of children and their families in health care settings. A quarterly journal and a bimonthly newsletter are available to members. There are affiliate organizations throughout the United States and Canada.

Association of Canadian Medical Colleges (ACMC), a Canadian organization of the deans and faculty members of the nation's 16 medical schools. It is concerned with all aspects of the education of physicians and acts as the liaison between the member schools and other professional organizations and governmental agencies. The official languages of the ACMC are French and English.

association of ideas, a mental connection established between similar or simultaneously occurring ideas, feelings, or perceptions.

Association of Operating Room Nurses (AORN), a national organization of operating room nurses.

association test, a technique used in psychiatric diagnosis and in educational and psychologic evaluation in which a person is asked to respond to a stimulus word with the first word that comes to mind. The time taken to respond and the associations offered are compared with pretested responses and are classified and enumerated for diagnostic significance. Also called **word association test.**

associative play, a form of play in which a group of children participate in similar or identical activities without formal organization, group direction, group interaction, or a definite goal. The children may borrow or lend toys or pieces of play equipment, and they may imitate others in the group, but each child acts independently, as on a playground or among a group riding tricycles or bicycles. Compare **cooperative play.** See also **parallel play, solitary play.**

AST, abbreviation for **aspartate aminotransferase.**

astatine (At), a very unstable, radioactive element that occurs naturally in tiny amounts. Its atomic number is 85; its atomic weight is 210.

-aster, a combining form meaning 'star-shaped': *cytaster, diaster, oleaster.*

astereognosis /əstir′ē•og•nō′sis/, a neurologic disorder characterized by an inability to identify objects by touch.

asterixis /as′tərik′sis/, a hand-flapping tremor, often accompanying metabolic disorders. The tremor is usually induced by extending the arm and dorsiflexing the wrist. Asterixis is seen frequently in hepatic coma. Also called **flapping tremor, liver flap.**

asteroid body, an irregular star-shaped structure that develops in the giant cells in certain diseases, including sarcoidosis, actinomycosis, and nocardiosis.

asthenia /asthē′nē•ə/, **1.** the lack or loss of strength or energy; weakness; debility. **2.** (in psychiatry) lack of dynamic force in the personality. Kinds of asthenia include **asthenia gravis hypophyseogenea, myalgic asthenia, neurocirculatory asthenia,** and **tropic anhidrotic asthenia.** See also **adynamia.** **–asthenic,** *adj.*

-asthenia, a combining form meaning '(condition of) depleted vitality': *gangliasthenia, neurasthenia phlebasthenia.*

asthenic fever. See **adynamic fever.**

asthenic habitus, a body structure characterized by a slender build with long limbs, an angular profile, and prominent muscles or bones. Compare **athletic habitus, pyknic.** See also **ectomorph.**

asthenic personality, a personality characterized by low energy, lack of enthusiasm, and oversensitivity to physical and emotional strain. A person who has this kind of personality may be easily fatigued and self-pitying, and he may place the burden of his physical and emotional difficulties on others.

asthenopia, a condition in which the eyes tire easily because of weakness of the ocular or ciliary muscles. Symptoms include pain in or around the eyes, headache, dimness of vision, dizziness, and slight nausea.

asthma /az′mə/, a respiratory disorder characterized by recurring episodes of paroxysmal dyspnea, wheezing on expiration, coughing, and viscous mucoid bronchial secretions. The episodes may be precipitated by inhalation of allergens or pollutants, infection, vigorous exercise, or emotional stress. Treatment includes elimination of the causative agent, hyposensitization, aerosol or oral bronchodilators, and short-term use of corticosteroids. Beta-adrenergic drugs, barbiturates, and narcotics are contraindicated. Repeated attacks often result in emphysema and permanent obstructive lung disease. Also called **bronchial asthma.** See also **allergic asthma, asthma in**

children, intrinsic asthma, organic dust, status asthmaticus.

-asthma, a combining form meaning '(condition of) labored breathing': *acetonasthma, cardiasthma, corasthma.*

asthma crystal. See **Charcot-Leyden crystal.**

asthma in children, an obstructive respiratory condition characterized by recurring attacks of paroxysmal dyspnea, wheezing, prolonged expiration, and an irritative cough that is a common, chronic illness in childhood. Onset usually occurs between 3 and 8 years of age. Asthmatic attacks are caused by constriction of the large and small airways, resulting from bronchial smooth muscle spasm, edema or inflammation of the bronchial wall, or excessive production of mucus. It is a complex disorder involving biochemical, immunologic, infectious, endocrinologic, and psychologic factors. Asthma in children is usually extrinsic, that is, most attacks are associated with an allergenic hypersensitivity to a foreign substance, as airborne pollen, mold, house dust, certain foods, animal hair and skin, feathers, insects, smoke, and various chemicals or drugs. In infants, especially those born into a family with a history of allergic reactions, food allergy is a common precipitating factor. In some instances, episodes are triggered by nonallergenic factors, as infection or inflammation, bronchial compression from external pressure, obstruction by a foreign body, physical stress resulting from fatigue or exercise, exposure to cold air, or psychologic stress. Such cases are classified as nonallergic, or intrinsic, asthma. A few cases may be caused by an inherited or acquired defect of adrenergic and cholinergic control of airway diameter. There is a strong hereditary factor associated with the disease. As many as 75% of children with asthma have a family history of the disorder, and the child usually has other allergic manifestations, as hay fever, eczema, or urticaria. The disease occurs twice as often in boys as in girls before puberty, but both boys and girls are affected equally during adolescence.

■ OBSERVATIONS: The condition is often confused with acute middle and lower respiratory tract infections, congenital stridor, obstruction of the bronchi or trachea, bronchial or tracheal compression, and cystic fibrosis. The diagnosis is generally determined by observation during a physical examination, a medical history confirming a presence of allergic reactions and familial allergic disease, and, to a lesser degree, laboratory tests and x-ray studies, which primarily eliminate identification of other diseases. A unique diagnostic feature is the presence of large numbers of eosinophils and their crystalloid degenerative fragments, called Charcot-Leyden crystals, in the sputum. Pulmonary function tests are valuable for assessing the degree of airway obstruction and the volume of gas exchange. Asthmatic episodes vary greatly in frequency, duration, and degree of symptoms, ranging from occasional periods of wheezing, mild coughing, and slight dypsnea to severe attacks that can lead to total airway obstruction and respiratory tract failure. An attack may begin gradually or abruptly and is often preceded by an upper respiratory infection. In general, episodes caused by infection have a gradual onset and are of long duration, whereas those resulting from allergenic factors are acute and subside quickly if the causative agent is removed. Typically, an attack begins with shortness of breath, paroxysms of wheezing, and a hacking, nonproductive cough. As secretions increase, the expiratory phase becomes prolonged, the cough gets deeper and more rattling, and a large quantity of thick, tenacious, mucoid sputum is produced as the attack subsides. The child appears apprehensive, speaks in a panting manner, and may assume a bent-over position to facilitate breathing. The prolonged expiratory phase is not as noticeable in infants and young children. In severe spasm or obstruction the respirations become shallow and irregular. A sudden increase in the rate of respiration, repeated hacking, and nonproductive coughing are indicative of lack of air movement with impending ventilatory failure and asphyxia. Children with chronic asthma develop a barrel chest from the continuous hyperventilated state and usually carry their shoulders in an elevated position to make better use of the accessory muscles of respiration.

■ INTERVENTION: An acute asthmatic attack is a medical emergency and requires immediate relief of bronchial obstruction with bronchodilating drugs, reduction of mucosal edema, and removal of excess bronchial secretions. The major drugs used to relieve bronchospasm are the beta-adrenergic agents, including epinephrine, isoproterenol, ephedrine, isoetharine, metaproterenol, terbutaline, and salbutamol; the methylxanthines, including theophylline and aminophylline; corticosteroids; expectorants; sedatives; and antibiotics for cases in which infection is the triggering mechanism. Rarely, an acute attack does not respond to any of these measures, resulting in status asthmaticus. Hospitalization is required. The child is usually in a state of dehydration and acidosis with hypoxia and hypercapnia. Management consists of intravenous fluids; humidified oxygen given by tent, face mask, or cannula; administration of sodium bicarbonate or tromethamine to keep pH at acceptable levels; and use of bronchodilators to alleviate bronchospasm and of antibiotics to reduce risk of infection. Children with mild, intermittent episodes of asthma are treated with bronchodilators in aerosol sprays, which provide quick relief and are effective in controlling an attack at the outset; oral administration is preferred for younger children. Those with persistent chronic asthma receive daily oral doses of a bronchodilator, often theophylline, usually in combination with an expectorant and corticosteroids. Bronchospasm induced by exercise can be treated prophylactically with cromolyn sodium, which inhibits the release of histamine in the lungs. Long-range management and treatment consist of physical training and exercises to induce physical and mental relaxation, improve posture, strengthen respiratory musculature, and develop better breathing patterns. Hyposensitization is recommended when an allergen is known and cannot be avoided. Prog-

nosis for children with asthma varies considerably; many children lose their symptoms at puberty. Prognosis depends on the number and severity of symptoms, emotional factors, and the family history of allergy.
■ NURSING CONSIDERATIONS: The primary focus of nursing care for children with acute asthma is to relieve symptoms of respiratory distress by initiating intravenous infusion and oxygen therapy, correcting acidosis, and administering bronchodilators and corticosteroids. The nurse implements measures to promote physical comfort, induce rest, and reduce fatigue and anxiety. It is especially important to reassure the child and parents concerning procedures, equipment, and prognosis. The nurse also plays an important role in the long-term support of children with chronic asthma, primarily in teaching the child and parents about the disease and how to cope with the condition. Once an allergen is determined, the home environment may be modified to reduce contact with the causative agents. The nurse teaches the child and parents how to use prescribed medications, especially nebulizers and aerosol devices, how to detect early signs of an attack so that it can be controlled with medication, how to determine any adverse effects of the drugs, especially the dangers of overuse, and how to implement physical exercise and play activities as therapeutic measures, especially those that promote proper breathing techniques. Children with emotional problems require special attention; psychologic stresses often trigger asthmatic attacks, and psychotherapy or behavior therapy is often necessary.

-asthmatic /azmat′ik/, a combining form meaning 'pertaining to asthma, its symptoms, or its treatment': *antiasthmatic, nonasthmatic, postasthmatic*.

asthmatic eosinophilia, a form of eosinophilic pneumonia, characterized by allergic bronchospasm, by expectoration of bronchial casts containing eosinophils and mycelium, and by cough and fever. The condition usually occurs in the fourth or fifth decade of life, and is twice as common in women as in men. It is a result of hypersensitivity to *Aspergillus fumigatus* or *Candida albicans*. Untreated, the condition may result in pleural effusion, pericarditis, ascites, encephalitis, hepatomegaly, and respiratory failure. Treatment is similar to that for asthma and includes administration of corticosteroids and antibiotics. Desensitization to the allergen is not usually effective. See also **allergic asthma, eosinophilic pneumonia.**

Astiban, a trademark for an investigational parasiticide (sodium stibocaptate), available only from the Centers for Disease Control.

astigmatism /əstig′mətiz′əm/, an abnormal condition of the eye in which the light rays cannot be focused clearly in a point on the retina because the spheric curve of the cornea is not equal in all meridians. Vision is blurred, and use of the eyes causes discomfort. The person cannot accommodate to correct the problem. The condition usually may be corrected with contact lenses or with eyeglasses ground to neutralize the defect.

astragalus. See **talus.**

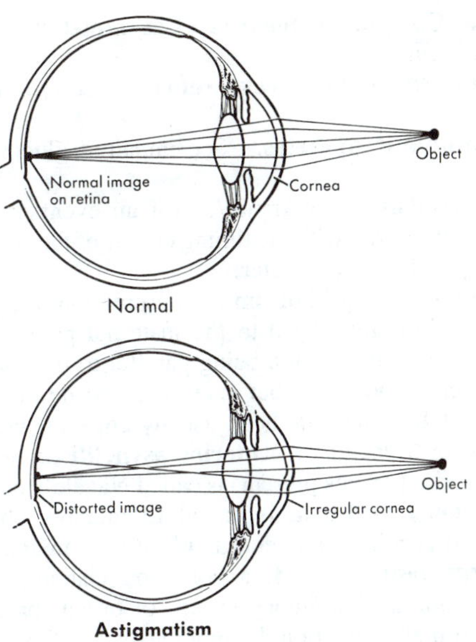

Astigmatism

astringent /əstrin′jənt/, **1.** a substance that causes contraction of tissues upon application, usually used locally. **2.** having the quality of an astringent. **–astringency,** *n.*

astringent bath, a bath in which alum, tannic acid, or another astringent is added to the water.

astro-, a combining form meaning 'pertaining to a star, or star-shaped': *astroblastoma, astrocytoma, astrophorous*.

astroblastoma /as′trōblastō′mə/, *pl.* **astroblastomas, astroblastomata,** a malignant neoplasm of the brain and spinal cord. Cells of an astroblastoma lie around blood vessels or, in some cases, around connective tissue septa.

astrocyte /as′trōsīt′/, a large, star-shaped cell found in certain tissues of the nervous system.

astrocytoma /as′trōsītō′mə/, *pl.* **astrocytomas, astrocytomata,** a primary tumor of the brain composed of astrocytes and characterized by slow growth, cyst formation, invasion of surrounding structures, and, often, the development of a highly malignant glioblastoma within the tumor mass. Complete surgical resection of an astrocytoma may be possible early in the development of the tumor. Also called **astrocytic glioma.**

astrocytosis /as′trōsītō′sis/, an increase in the number of neuroglial cells with fibrous or protoplasmic processes frequently observed in an irregular area adjacent to degenerative lesions, as abscesses, certain brain neoplasms, and encephalomalacia. Astrocytosis represents a reparative process, and in some cases it may be diffuse in a fairly large region.

asymmetric /ā′simet′rik, as′imet′rik/, (of the body or parts of the body) unequal in size or shape; different in placement or arrangement about an axis. Also **asymmet-**

rical. Compare **symmetric.** –**asymmetry** /āsim′itrē, asim′-/, *n.*

asymmetric tonic neck reflex. See **tonic neck reflex.**

asymptomatic diabetes. See impaired glucose tolerance.

asynchronous /āsing′krənəs/, (of an event or device) not synchronized with the timing circuit of the cental processing unit of a computer.

asynclitism /āsing′klitiz′əm/, presentation of a parietal aspect of the fetal head to the maternal pelvic inlet in labor, the sagittal suture being parallel to the transverse diameter of the pelvis but anterior or posterior to it. In normal labor, the fetal head usually engages with some degree of asynclitism. **Anterior asynclitism,** in which the anterior parietes present, is called Nägele's obliquity. **Posterior asynclitism** is called Litzmann's obliquity. See also **cardinal movements of labor, engagement.**

asynergy /āsin′ərjē/, **1.** a condition characterized by faulty coordination among groups of organs or muscles that normally function harmoniously. **2.** the state of muscle antagonism found in cerebellar disease. See also **ataxia, cerebellum.**

asyntaxia /ā′sintak′sē•ə/, any interference with the orderly sequence of growth and differentiation of the fetus during embryonic development, resulting in one or more congenital anomalies. A kind of asyntaxia is **asyntaxia dorsalis.** See also **developmental anomaly.**

asyntaxia dorsalis, failure of the neural tube to close during embryonic development. See also **neural tube defect.**

asystole /āsis′təlē/, the absence of a heartbeat, as distinguished from fibrillation, in which electric activity persists but contraction ceases. Cardiotoxic asystole is characterized by a brief period of cardiac arrest caused by an acceleration in the heart rate. Asystole requires immediate cardiopulmonary resuscitation with cardiac massage and adequate ventilation. If these measures fail to initiate heart contractions, a discharge with a defibrillator may be administered and, if that is ineffective, an intracardiac injection of epinephrine may be given (taking care to avoid direct myocardial injection), or 5 to 10 ml of 1% calcium chloride may be injected into the ventricular cavity. Also called **cardiac arrest, cardiac standstill.** –**asystolic** /ā′sistol′ik/, *adj.*

At, symbol for **astatine.**

at-. See **ad-.**

Atabrine Hydrochloride, a trademark for an antimalarial (quinacrine hydrochloride).

Atabrine stomatitis, an abnormal oral condition that may be associated with the use of Atabrine, characterized by oral changes simulating lichen planus. Compare **arsenic stomatitis, bismuth stomatitis.**

Atarax, a trademark for an antianxiety, antiemetic, and anticholinergic (hydroxyzine hydrochloride).

atavism /at′əviz′əm/, the appearance in an individual of traits or characteristics more like those of a grandparent or earlier ancestor than of the parents. Atavistic data may offer clues to an examining physician of genetic or familial health factors. –**atavistic,** *adj.*

ataxia /ətak′sē•ə/, an abnormal condition characterized by impaired ability to coordinate movement. A staggering gait and postural imbalance are caused by a lesion in the spinal cord or cerebellum, which might be the sequela of birth trauma, congenital disorder, infection, degenerative disorder, neoplasm, toxic substance, or head injury. See also **hereditary ataxia.**

ataxia-telangiectasia, a rare genetic disease involving immunoglobulin metabolism that is transmitted as an autosomal recessive trait. The onset usually occurs in infancy and progresses slowly with increasing cerebellar degeneration and recurrent sinopulmonary infections. Telangiectasias are most prominent on the ears, facial skin, and bulbar conjunctiva. There is an increased risk of malignancy, especially leukemia. Also called **Louis-Bar syndrome.**

ataxic aphasia. See **motor aphasia.**

ataxic breathing, a type of breathing associated with a lesion in the medullary respiratory centers and characterized by a series of inspirations and expirations.

ataxic speech, abnormal speech characterized by faulty formation of the sounds because of neuromuscular dysfunction.

ATCC, abbreviation for **American Type Culture Collection.**

-ate, **1.** a combining form meaning 'acted upon or being in a (specified) state': *degenerate, disparate, enucleate.* **2.** a combining form meaning 'possessing': *caudate, cuspidate, longipedate.* **3.** a combining form meaning a 'chemical compound derived from a (specified) source': *silicate, sulfate, opiate.* **4.** a combining form meaning an 'acid compound': *acetate, oxalate, phosphate.*

atelectasis /at′ilek′təsis/, an abnormal condition characterized by the collapse of lung tissue, preventing the respiratory exchange of carbon dioxide and oxygen. Symptoms include diminished breath sounds, a mediastinal shift toward the side of the collapse, fever, and increasing dyspnea. The condition may be caused by obstruction of the major airways and bronchioles, by pressure on the lung from fluid or air in the pleural space, or by pressure from a tumor outside the lung. As the remaining portions of the lung eventually hyperinflate, oxygen saturation of the blood is often nearly normal. Loss of functional lung tissue may secondarily cause increased heart rate, blood pressure, and respiratory rate. The retained secretions are rich in nutrients for the growth of bacteria, a condition often leading to stasis pneumonia in critically ill patients. See also **postoperative atelectasis, primary atelectasis.**

atelectatic rale /at′iləktat′ik/, an abnormal intermittent crackling sound heard during auscultation of the chest. It usually disappears after the individual being examined coughs or breathes deeply several times.

ateliotic dwarf /at′əlē•ot′ik/, a dwarf whose skeleton is incompletely formed, resulting from the nonunion of the epiphyses and diaphyses during bone development.

atelo-, a combining form meaning 'imperfect or incomplete': *atelocardia, ateloglossia, atelopodia.*

atenolol, a beta-blocker.

■ INDICATION: It is prescribed for the treatment of hypertension.

■ CONTRAINDICATIONS: Sinus bradycardia, second- or third-degree atrioventricular block, cardiogenic shock, or cardiac failure prohibits its use.

■ ADVERSE EFFECTS: Among the more serious adverse reactions are bradycardia, dizziness, and nausea.

Atensine, a trademark for a sedative and tranquilizer (diazepam).

atheroma /ath′ərō′mə/, *pl.* **atheromas, atheromata,** an abnormal mass of fat or lipids, as in a sebaceous cyst or in deposits in an arterial wall. **–atheromatous,** *adj.*

atheromatosis /ath′ərōmətō′sis/, the development of many atheromas.

atherosclerosis /ath′ərōsklərō′sis/, a common arterial disorder characterized by yellowish plaques of cholesterol, lipids, and cellular debris in the inner layers of the walls of large and medium-sized arteries. With the formation of the plaques, the vessel walls become thick, fibrotic, and calcified, and the lumen narrows, resulting in reduced circulation in organs and areas normally supplied by the artery. Atheromatous lesions are major causes of coronary heart disease, angina pectoris, myocardial infarction, and other cardiac disorders. The pathogenesis of atherosclerosis is not clear; it may be induced by injury to arterial endothelium, the proliferation of smooth muscle in vessel walls, or the accumulation of lipids in hyperlipidemia caused by dietary excesses, faulty carbohydrate metabolism, or a genetic defect, as in hyperlipidemia type II. Atherosclerosis usually occurs with aging and is often associated with obesity, hypertension, and diabetes. Segments of arteries obstructed or severely damaged by atheromatous lesions may be replaced by patch grafts or bypassed, as in coronary bypass surgery, or the lesion may be removed from the vessel in an endarterectomy. Antilipidemic agents do not reverse atherosclerosis, but a diet low in cholesterol, calories, and saturated fats, adequate exercise, and the avoidance of smoking and stress may help prevent the disorder. See also **arteriosclerosis.**

athetosis /ath′ətō′sis/, a neuromuscular condition characterized by slow, writhing, continuous, and involuntary movement of the extremities, as seen in some forms of cerebral palsy and in motor disorders resulting from lesions in the basal ganglia.

athiaminosis /athī′əminō′sis/, a condition resulting from lack of thiamine in the diet. See also **beriberi, thiamine.**

athlete's foot. See **tinea.**

athlete's heart, the typical, normal but enlarged heart of an athlete trained for endurance, characterized by a slow rate of contractions, an increased pumping capacity, and greater than average ability to deliver oxygen to skeletal muscles. Also called **athletic heart syndrome (AHS).**

athletic habitus, a physique characterized by a well-proportioned, muscular body with broad shoulders, thick neck, deep chest, and flat abdomen. Compare **asthenic habitus, pyknic.** See also **mesomorph.**

athletic heart syndrome. See **athlete's heart.**

Athrombin-K, a trademark for an anticoagulant (warfarin).

Ativan, a trademark for an antianxiety agent (lorazepam), used as an adjunct to anesthesia.

atlantooccipital joint /-oksip′itəl/, one of a pair of condyloid joints formed by the articulation of the atlas of the vertebral column with the occipital bone of the skull. It includes two articular capsules, two membranes, and two lateral ligaments. The atlantooccipital joint permits nodding and lateral movements of the head.

atlas, the first cervical vertebra, articulating with the occipital bone and the axis.

atmo-, a combining form meaning 'pertaining to steam or vapor': *atmocausis, atmolysis, atmotherapy.*

atmosphere, **1.** the natural body of air, composed of approximately 20% oxygen, 78% nitrogen, and 2% carbon dioxide and other gases, that covers the surface of the earth. **2.** an envelope of gas, which may or may not duplicate the natural atmosphere in chemical components. **3.** a unit of gas pressure that is usually defined as being equivalent to the average pressure of the earth's atmosphere at sea level, or about 14.7 pounds per square inch. **–atmospheric,** *adj.*

atmospheric pressure, the pressure exerted by the weight of the atmosphere. The atmospheric pressure at sea level is approximately 15 pounds per square inch. With increasing altitude the pressure decreases: At 30,000 feet, approximately the height of Mt. Everest, the air pressure is 4.3 pounds per square inch. Also called **barometric pressure.**

atom, **1.** (in physics) the smallest division of an element that exhibits all the properties and characteristics of the element. It comprises neutrons, electrons, and protons. The number of protons in the nucleus of every atom of any given element is the same and is called its atomic number. **2.** *nontechnical.* the amount of any substance that is so small further division is not possible. **3.** *informal.* a minute amount of any substance. **–atomic,** *adj.*

atomic number, the number of protons, or positive charges, in the nucleus of an atom of a particular element. The atomic number equals the number of electrons, and their number and arrangement determine the chemical characteristics of the atom, with the exception of its atomic weight and radioactivity. See also **atom, electron, proton.**

atomic weight (A), the relative average mass of an atom based on the mass of carbon 12 isotope.

atomize. See **nebulize.**

atomizer, a device for reducing a liquid and ejecting it as a fine spray or vapor.

atonia /ātō′nē·ə/, an abnormal lack of muscle tone.

atonia constipation, constipation caused by the failure of the colon to respond to the normal stimuli for evacuation. It may occur in elderly or bedridden patients or after prolonged dependence on laxatives. To prevent impaction of fecal material in the colon and rectum, a moderately irritant oral laxative or a mild suppository may be recommended. Patients are encouraged to develop regular, unhurried bowel habits and may be given a diet rich in fruits and vegetables. If fecal impaction develops, it may be removed by means of a mild enema or manual disimpaction, with the use of anesthetic agents. Also called **colon stasis, lazy colon.** See also **fecalith, inactive colon.**

atonic /əton′ik/, **1.** weak. **2.** lacking normal tone, as in the case of a muscle that is flaccid. **3.** lacking vigor, as an atonic ulcer, which heals slowly. **–atony** /at′onē/, *n.*

atonic bladder. See **flaccid bladder.**

atonic impotence. See **impotence.**

atony. See **atonic.**

atopic /ātop′ik/, of or pertaining to a hereditary tendency to develop immediate allergic reactions, as asthma, atopic dermatitis, or vasomotor rhinitis, because of the presence of an antibody (atopic reagin) in the skin and sometimes the bloodstream. **–atopy** /at′opē/, *n.*

atopic asthma. See **allergic asthma.**

atopic dermatitis, an intensely pruritic, often excoriated, maculopapular inflammation commonly found on the face and antecubital and popliteal areas of allergy-prone individuals. Although it may occur at any age, it is most common in infants and clears completely in half the cases by 18 months of age. Treatment includes discovery and avoidance of allergens, topical and parenteral corticosteroids, tar ointments, antihistamines, and wet compresses of Burow's solution. Also called **atopic eczema, infantile eczema.** Compare **contact dermatitis.** See also **atopic.**

atopic reagin. See **reagin.**

atopy. See **atopic.**

atoxic. See **nontoxic.**

ATP, abbreviation for **adenosine triphosphate.**

ATPase, abbreviation for **adenosine triphosphatase.**

ATPD, abbreviation for *ambient temperature, ambient pressure, dry.*

ATPS, abbreviation for *ambient temperature, ambient pressure, saturated* (with water vapor).

atresia /ətrē′zhə/, the absence of a normal body opening, duct, or canal, as the anus, vagina, or external ear canal. **–atresic, atretic,** *adj.*

-atresia, a combining form meaning a 'condition of occlusion': *gynatresia, hedratresia, urethratresia.*

atresic teratism /ətrē′sik/, a congenital anomaly in which any of the normal openings of the body, as the mouth, nares, anus, or vagina, fail to form.

atreto-, a combining form meaning 'closed, or imperforate': *atretoblepharia, atretolemia, atretorrhinia.*

atrial appendix. See **auricle.**

atrial failure /ā′trē·əl/, an abnormal condition characterized by the failure of the atrium to fill adequately and distend the associated ventricle. The atria provide a pumping function and a reservoir function for the heart and normally contribute 15% to 20% of ventricular filling. Tachycardia commonly increases this proportion. In normal individuals or in patients with mild heart disease, loss of the atrial pumping function may not change cardiac output at rest but may decrease the output during exercise. Atrial failure is commonly caused by mechanic abnormalities, fibrillation, or dysdynamic myocardial failure. Heart failure caused by atrial failure may occur with the onset of atrial fibrillation in patients who have compensated heart disease. Such individuals may develop congestive heart failure even when under treatment with digitalis to control the ventricular response rate. Atrial fibrillation rarely produces heart failure in people with otherwise normal hearts.

atrial fibrillation, a condition characterized by rapid, random contractions of the atria, causing irregular ventricular beats at the rate of 130 to 150 a minute. The atria may discharge more than 350 impulses a minute, but some do not pass the atrioventricular junction. The ventricles cannot contract in response to all the stimuli that are received, and ventricular contractions become disordered. The arrhythmia occurs most frequently in rheumatic heart disease, mitral stenosis, and atrial infarction. The rapid pulsations result in a decreased cardiac output, and the disorganized contractions of the atria promote thrombus formation in the upper chambers. Treatment consists of the administration of digitalis or of quinidine or the use of electric shock to restore a normal sinus rhythm.

atrial flutter, a condition characterized by rapid, regular contractions of the atria, approximately 300 beats per minute. The ventricles cannot respond to the stimuli and contract at a submultiple of the atrial rate, usually about 150 beats per minute. The arrhythmia occurs in rheumatic heart disease, inflammation of the atria, myocardial infarction, or arteriosclerotic heart disease. If quinidine or digitalis is ineffective, carotid sinus massage or electric shock may restore a normal sinus rhythm. Compare **atrial fibrillation.**

atrial gallop, an abnormal cardiac rhythm in which a low-pitched, extra sound is heard late in diastole on auscultation of the heart. It indicates increased resistance to ventricular filling and is frequently heard in hypertensive cardiovascular disease, coronary artery disease, and aortic stenosis. Also called **S_4.** See also **gallop, heart sound.**

atrial myxoma, a benign, pedunculated gelatinous tumor that originates in the interatrial septum of the heart. It may cause palpitations, disseminated neuritis, nausea, weight loss, fatigue, dyspnea, fever, and, occasionally, sudden loss of consciousness because of obstruction of the flow of blood through the heart.

atrial septal defect (ASD), a congenital cardiac anomaly characterized by an abnormal opening between the two atria. The severity of the condition depends on the size and location of the defect, which depend on the stage at which embryonic development of the septum structures was arrested. The defects are classified as ostium secundum defect, in which the aperture in the septum secundum, or second septum, of the fetal heart fails to close; ostium primum defect, in which there is inadequate development of the endocardial cushions of the first septum of the heart; and sinus venosus defect, in which the superior portion of the atrium fails to develop. Atrial septal defects cause an increased flow of oxygenated blood into the right side of the heart, which is usually well tolerated, since the blood is delivered under much lower pressure than in ventricular septal defect. Clinical manifestations include right atrial and ventricular enlargement, a characteristic harsh, scratchy systolic murmur, and a fixed splitting of the second heart sound, which does not vary with respiration. X-ray films and electrocardiograms generally show right atrial and ventricular enlargement, although definitive diagnosis is made by cardiac catheterization. Surgical closure is indicated in most cases, but unless the defect is severe, it is usually postponed until later childhood to prevent complications during early adulthood, as atrial arrhythmias, bacterial endocarditis, and congestive heart failure. Also called **atrioseptal defect.** See also **endocardial cushion defect.**

atrio-, a combining form meaning 'pertaining to the atrium of the heart': *atriocommissuropexy, atrionector, atrioseptopexy.*

atrioseptal defect. See **atrial septal defect.**

atrioventricular (AV) block /ā′trē·ōventrik′yələr/, the slowed conduction or stoppage of the cardiac excitatory impulse, occurring at the atrioventricular node, bundle of His, or its branches. Kinds of AV block include first-degree block, with prolonged AV conduction, second-degree block, with partial AV block, and third-degree block, with complete atrioventricular block. An overdose of digitalis, degenerative or inflammatory cardiac disease, or acute myocardial infarction may precipitate the condition. AV block is a common indication for the insertion of a cardiac pacemaker. See also **heart block, intraatrial block, intraventricular heart block, sinoatrial block.**

atrioventricular bundle. See **bundle of His.**

atrioventricular (AV) node, an area of specialized cardiac muscle that receives the cardiac impulse from the sinoatrial (SA) node and conducts it to the atrioventricular bundle of His and thence to the walls of the ventricles. The AV node is located in the septal wall of the right atrium.

atrioventricular septum, a small portion of membrane that separates the atria from the ventricles of the heart.

atrioventricular valve, a valve in the heart through which blood flows from the atria to the ventricles. The valve between the left atrium and left ventricle is the mitral valve; the right atrioventricular valve is the tricuspid valve. Also called **cuspid valve.**

at risk, the state of an individual or population being vulnerable to a particular disease or injury. The factors determining risk may be environmental or physiologic. An example of an environmental factor is exposure to harmful substances or organisms. An example of a physiologic factor is genetic predisposition to a disease.

atrium /ā′trē·əm/, *pl.* **atria,** a chamber or cavity, such as the right and left atria of the heart or the nasal cavity.

atrium of the heart, one of the two upper chambers of the heart. The right atrium receives deoxygenated blood from the superior vena cava, the inferior vena cava, and the coronary sinus. The left atrium receives oxygenated blood from the pulmonary veins. Blood is emptied into the ventricles from the atria during diastole.

Atromid-S, a trademark for an antihyperlipidemic (clofibrate).

-atrophia, -trophy, **1.** a combining form meaning a 'condition of malnutrition': *metatrophia, metratrophia, pantatrophia.* **2.** a combining form meaning a 'progressive decline of a body part': *dermatrophia, neuratrophia, splenatrophia.*

atrophic arthritis. See **rheumatoid arthritis.**

atrophic catarrh, an abnormal condition characterized by inflammation and discharge from the mucous membranes of the nose, accompanied by the loss of mucosal and submucosal tissue. Compare **hypertrophic catarrh.** See also **catarrh.**

atrophic fracture, a spontaneous fracture caused by atrophy, as in the bones of an elderly person.

atrophic gastritis, a chronic inflammation of the stomach, associated with degeneration of the gastric mucosa. Seen in elderly patients and in persons with pernicious anemia, atrophic gastritis may cause epigastric pain. Even though less acid is being produced by the stomach, antacids are helpful in relieving discomfort. See also **pernicious anemia.**

atrophoderma, the wasting away or decrease in size of the skin. The atrophy may affect the entire body surface or only localized areas. The condition, often associated with aging, may occur as a primary or secondary symptom of various diseases.

atrophy /at′rəfē/, a wasting or diminution of size or physiologic activity of a part of the body because of disease or other influences. A skeletal muscle may undergo atrophy because of lack of physical exercise or as a result of neurologic or musculoskeletal disease. Cells of the brain and central nervous system may atrophy in old age because of restricted blood flow to those areas. See also **aging.** **–atrophic,** *adj.*, **atrophy,** *v.*

atropine sulfate, an antispasmodic and anticholinergic.

■ INDICATIONS: It is prescribed in the treatment of GI hypermotility, inflammation of the iris or the uvea, cardiac dysrhythmias, parkinsonism, and certain kinds of poisoning and as an adjunct to anesthesia.

■ CONTRAINDICATIONS: GI obstruction, glaucoma, hepatitis, liver or kidney dysfunction, porphyria, or known hypersensitivity to this drug or other anticholinergics prohibits its use.

■ ADVERSE EFFECTS: Among the more serious adverse reactions are tachycardia, angina, loss of taste, nausea, diarrhea, skin rash, blurred vision, and eye pain. Dry mouth and constipation are common effects.

attachment, 1. the state or quality of being affixed or attached. 2. (in psychiatry) a mode of behavior in which one individual relates in an affiliative or dependent manner to another; a feeling of affection or loyalty that binds one person to another. Such relationships develop at critical periods during life, and any failure to form these attachments, because of lack of the opportunity or the inability to relate, can lead to personality deviation disorders or maladaptive behavior. **3.** See **bonding. 4.** (in dentistry) any device, as a retainer or artificial crown, used to secure a partial denture to a natural tooth in the mouth.

attachment apparatus, the combination of tissues that invest and support the teeth, as the cementum, the periodontal ligamanet, and the alveolar bone. See also **masticatory system.**

attending physician, the physician who is responsible for a particular, usually private, patient. In a university setting, an attending physician often also has teaching responsibilities and holds a faculty appointment. Also called *(informal)* **attending.**

attention deficit disorder, a syndrome affecting children, adolescents, and, rarely, adults characterized by learning and behavior disabilities. The symptoms may be mild or severe and are associated with functional deviations of the central nervous system without signs of major neurologic or psychiatric disturbance. The people affected are usually of normal or above average intelligence. Symptoms include impairment in perception, conceptualization, language, memory, and motor skills, decreased attention span, increased impulsivity and emotional lability, and usually, but not always, hyperactivity. The condition is 10 times more prevalent in boys than in girls and may result from genetic factors, biochemical irregularities, or perinatal or postnatal injury or disease. There is no known cure, and symptoms often subside or disappear with time. Medication with methylphenidate, pemoline, or the dextroamphetamines is frequently prescribed for children with hyperactive symptoms, and some form of psychotherapeutic counseling is often recommended. Some treatments include abstinence from certain foods and food additives. Also called **hyperactivity, hyperkinesis, minimal brain dysfunction.** See also **learning disability.**

attentuation, the process of reduction, as the attentuation of an x-ray beam by reducing its intensity or the weakening of the degree of virulence of a disease organism.

Attenuvax, a trademark for an active immunizing agent (live measles virus vaccine).

attic, the. See **epitympanic recess.**

attitudinal reflex, any reflex initiated by a change in position of the head or by a change in position of the head with respect to the position of the body. Kinds of attitudinal reflexes include **tonic neck reflex** and **tonic labyrinthine reflex.** Also called **statotonic reflex.**

attraction, a tendency of the teeth or other maxillary or mandibular structures to elevate above their normal position.

attrition, the process of wearing away or wearing down by friction.

-ature, a noun-forming combining form: *armature, ligature, tubulature.*

Au, symbol for **gold.**

audioanalgesia, the use of music to enhance relaxation and to distract a patient's mind from pain, as during dentistry. The procedure has also been tried experimentally during labor.

audio device, any computer device that accepts sound (voice recognition) or generates sound (music or speech synthesizers).

audiogram /ô′dē·əgram′/, a chart showing the acuteness of hearing of an individual as indicated by the ability to hear sounds and to distinguish different speech sounds. See also **audiometry.**

audiology, a field of research devoted to the study of hearing, especially impaired hearing that cannot be corrected by medical means. **–audiologic,** *adj.*

audiometer /ô′dē·om′ətər/, an electric device for testing the hearing and for measuring bone and air conduction. Earphones are placed over the ears; the ear not being tested receives a masking noise from the machine while the ear being tested is stimulated by a series of tones, from very low to very high frequencies at various decibels of intensity. The patient signals when a tone is heard, and the results are noted on an audiogram.

audiometry /ô′dē·om′ətrē/, the testing of the acuity of the sense of hearing. Various audiometric tests determine the lowest intensity of sound at which an individual can perceive an auditory stimulus (hearing threshold), hear different frequencies, and distinguish different speech sounds. Pure tone audiometry assesses the person's ability to hear frequencies, usually ranging from 125 to 8000 hertz (Hz), and can indicate if a hearing loss is caused by a middle ear problem or by one in the inner ear or the auditory nerve. In this test the subject sits in a soundproof booth and signals when sounds are first heard through earphones. The sound will be of a given frequency, because the operator will have been slowly increasing the decibel level. Speech audiometry tests the ability to repeat selected words. Impedance audiometry is an objective method of assessing the conductive mechanism of the middle ear by measuring muscle responses to sound with a probe inserted in the ear canal. Cortical audiometry indicates auditory acuity by measuring and averaging electric potentials evoked from the cortex of the brain by pure tones. Localization audiometry is a method for measuring the individual's ability to locate the source of a pure tone received binaurally in a sound field. **–audiometric,** *adj.*

auditory ossicles, the incus, the malleus, and the stapes, small bones in the middle ear that articulate with each other and the tympanic membrane. Sound waves are transmitted through them as the tympanic membrane vibrates.

auditory system assessment, an evaluation of the patient's ears and hearing and an investigation of present and past diseases or conditions that may be responsible for an auditory impairment.

■ METHOD: In an interview with the patient, oral or written questions are used to determine if the individual has earaches, decreased or absent hearing in one or both ears, vertigo, or a feeling of fullness, itching, or the heart pulsating in the ears. The person is asked if there is a ringing or buzzing in the ears or a popping noise when yawning or swallowing, if the voice echoes, if the ears drain a clear, yellow, red, or dark substance, and if the person uses oils, cotton swabs, or hairpins to clean the ears. Observations are recorded of the patient's general appearance, blood pressure, pulse, temperature, and respirations, the ability to hear or to lip-read or use a hearing aid. The person's startle reflex, tolerance of loud sounds, allergies, use of medication, especially of eardrops, streptomycin, salicylates, and quinine, and the color, character, and amount of ear drainage are carefully noted. The presence of otitis media, otosclerosis, acoustic nerve tumor, labyrinthitis, Ménière's disease, diabetes mellitus, arteriosclerosis, hypertension, mastoiditis, or a cerebral tumor, head contusion, or skull fracture is investigated. It is determined if the patient previously underwent stapes mobilization, suffered from otitis media, head trauma, or syphilis, or if the person is exposed to a high decibel level on the job or to recreational ear hazards, as in swimming. Diagnostic procedures indicated by the history may include an audiogram, audiometric test, a mastoid x-ray film, otologic examination, Rinne and Weber tuning-fork tests, and microbiologic studies for potential pathogens in smears of ear drainage.

■ NURSING ORDERS: The nurse conducts the interview, makes the observations, and collects the pertinent background information and the results of the diagnostic procedures.

■ OUTCOME CRITERIA: A thorough assessment of the patient's auditory system is essential in establishing the diagnosis of an ear disorder.

auditory tube. See **eustachian tube.**

Auer rod /ou′ər/, an abnormal, needle-shaped or round, pink-staining inclusion in the cytoplasm of myeloblasts and promyelocytes in acute myelogenous or myelomonocytic leukemia. These inclusions contain enzymes such as acid phosphatase, peroxidase, and esterase and may represent abnormal derivatives of cytoplasmic granules. The finding of Auer rods in stained smears of blood may help differentiate acute myelogenous leukemia from acute lymphoblastic leukemia. Also called **Auer body.**

aur-, a combining form meaning 'pertaining to the ear': *auralgan, auricle, auricular.*

aura /ôr′ə/, **1.** *pl.* **aurae** /ôr′ē/, a sensation, as of light or warmth, that may precede an attack of migraine or an epileptic seizure. **2.** *pl.* **auras,** an emanation of light or color surrounding a person as seen in Kirlian photography and studied in current nursing research in healing techniques.

aural[1] /ôr′əl/, of or pertaining to the ear or hearing. **–aurally,** *adv.*

aural[2], of or pertaining to an aura.

aural forceps, a dressing forceps with fine, bent tips, used in aural surgery.

Aureomycin, a trademark for a tetracycline antibiotic (chlortetracycline hydrochloride).

auricle /ôr′ikəl/, **1.** also called **pinna.** the external ear. **2.** the left or right cardiac atrium, so named because of its earlike shape.

auricular, 1. of or pertaining to the auricle of the ear. **2.** otic.

auricularis anterior, one of three extrinsic muscles of the ear. Arising from the anterior portion of the fascia in the temporal area and inserting into a projection in front of the helix, it is innervated by the temporal branch of the facial nerve and functions to move the auricula forward and upward. Some people can voluntarily contract the auricularis anterior to move the ears. Compare **auricularis posterior, auricularis superior.**

auricularis posterior, one of three extrinsic muscles of the ear. Arising from the mastoid area of the temporal bone by short aponeurotic fibers and inserting into the lower part of the cranial surface of the concha, it is innervated by the posterior auricular branch of the facial nerve and serves to draw the auricula backward. Compare **auricularis anterior, auricularis superior.**

auricularis superior, a thin, fan-shaped muscle that is one of three extrinsic muscles of the ear. It arises in the fascia of the temporal area and converges to insert with a thin, flattened tendon into the cranial surface of the auricula. It is innervated by a temporal branch of the facial nerve and acts to draw the auricula upward. Compare **auricularis anterior, auricularis posterior.**

auriculin, a hormonelike substance with diuretic activity produced in the atria of the heart.

auriculoventriculostomy /ôrik′yo͞olōventrik′yo͞olos′təmē/, a surgical procedure that directs cerebrospinal fluid into the general circulation in the treatment of hydrocephalus, usually in the newborn. In this procedure, a polyethylene tube is passed from the lateral ventricle through a burr hole in the parietal skull area under the scalp and into the jugular vein for the discharge of cerebrospinal fluid into the superior vena cava or the right atrium. The insertion of the tube into these structures that have one-way valves is to avoid reflux of the blood into the ventricles and to continue the drain of excess cerebrospinal fluid when ventricular pressure increases. This procedure is performed to correct the communicating and the obstructive forms of hydrocephalus. Also called **ventriculoatrial shunt, ventriculoatriostomy.**

auriosis. See **chrysiasis.**

aurothioglucose /ôr'ōthī'ōglo͞o'kōs/, an organic gold antiarthritic used in chrysotherapy.

■ INDICATION: It is prescribed for adjunctive treatment of adult and juvenile rheumatoid arthritis.

■ CONTRAINDICATIONS: Severe uncontrolled diabetes, renal or hepatic dysfunction, a history of infectious hepatitis, hypertension, heart failure, systemic lupus erythematosus, agranulocytosis, hemorrhagic diathesis, pregnancy, or known hypersensitivity to this drug prohibits its use.

■ ADVERSE EFFECTS: Among the most serious adverse effects are kidney and renal damage and various allergic reactions. Dermatitis and lesions of mucous membranes are common.

auscultation /ôs'kəltā'shən/, the act of listening for sounds within the body to evaluate the condition of the heart, lungs, pleura, intestines, or other organs or to detect the fetal heart sound. Auscultation may be performed directly, but most commonly a stethoscope is used to determine the frequency, intensity, duration, and quality of the sounds. During auscultation of the chest the patient usually sits upright and is instructed to breathe slowly and deeply through the mouth. The anterior and posterior surfaces of the thorax are auscultated from apex to base with comparisons made between the right and left sides; when the posterior chest is examined, the patient is asked to bring the shoulders forward so that a greater surface of the lung can be auscultated. The heart and abdomen may be auscultated with the patient supine or sitting upright. **–auscultate,** *v.*

auscultatory percussion. See **auscultation, percussion.**

Australia antigen, hepatitis B surface antigen (HBsAG), found in the serum of a person who has acute or chronic serum hepatitis or who is a carrier for that virus. Extremely dilute concentrations of the antigen can cause the disease. Medical personnel must take adequate precautions to avoid autoinoculation, especially in dialysis units, blood banks, and laboratories. Blood banks routinely screen for Australia antigen to avoid causing active hepatitis infection in a transfusion recipient. See also **hepatitis.**

Australian lift, a type of shoulder lift used to move a patient who is unable to assume a sitting position on a bed or other surface. The lift is executed by two persons, one on each side of the patient, who place their shoulder nearest the patient under the patient's axillae. At the same time, the two lifters grasp each other's hand under the patient's thighs and make coordinated movements needed to lift the patient onto or from a bed or wheelchair.

Australian Q fever. See **Q fever.**

autacoid /ô'təkoid/, any of a group of substances, as hormones, that are produced in one organ and are transported via blood or lymph as a means to control a physiologic process in another part of the body.

autism, a mental disorder characterized by extreme withdrawal and an abnormal absorption in fantasy, accompanied by delusion, hallucination, and an inability to communicate verbally or to otherwise relate to people. Schizophrenic children are often autistic. See also **infantile autism. –autistic,** *adj.*

auto-, a combining form meaning 'pertaining to self': *autoblast, autocatharsis, autoclasis.*

autoantibody /ô'tō•an'tibod'ē/, an immunoglobulin that reacts against a normal constituent in a person's body, as nuclear material in the patient with systemic lupus erythematosus. There are several mechanisms that may trigger the production of autoantibodies. An antigen formed during fetal development and then sequestered may be released as a result of infection or trauma and elicit the synthesis of autoantibodies, as occurs in autoimmune thyroiditis, sympathetic uveitis, and aspermia. Antibodies produced against certain streptococcal antigens during infection may cross-react with myocardial tissue, causing rheumatic heart disease, or with glomerular basement membrane, causing glomerulonephritis. Normal body proteins may be converted to autoantigens by chemicals, infectious organisms, or therapeutic drugs. Autoantibodies are found against gastric parietal cells in pernicious anemia, against platelets in autoimmune thrombocytopenia, and against antigens on the surface of erythrocytes in autoimmune hemolytic anemia.

autoantigen /ô'tō•an'tijin/, an endogenous body constituent that stimulates the production of autoantibody and a resulting autoimmune reaction against one or more tissues of the person in whom the abnormal reaction occurs. See also **autoantibody.**

autochthonous idea /ôtok'thənəs/, an idea that originates in the unconscious and arises spontaneously in the mind, independent of the conscious train of thought.

autodiploid /ô'tōdip'loid/, **1.** also **autodiploidic.** of or pertaining to an individual, organism, strain, or cell containing two genetically identical or nearly identical chromosome sets that are derived from the same ancestral species and result from the duplication of the haploid set. **2.** such an individual, organism, strain, or cell. Compare **allodiploid.** See also **autopolyploid.**

autodiploidy /ô'tōdip'loidē/, the state or condition of having two genetically identical or nearly identical chromosome sets from the same ancestral species. Such a state enables cell division to occur in a normal manner. Compare **allodiploidy.**

autoeroticism, **1.** sensual, usually sexual, gratification of the self, usually obtained through the stimulus of one's own body without the participation of another person and derived from such acts as stroking, masturbation, and fantasy, or from other oral, anal, or visual sources of stimulation. **2.** sexual feeling or desire occurring without any external stimulus. **3.** (in Freudian psychoanalytic theory) an early phase of psychosexual development, occurring in the oral and the anal stages. Also called

autoerotism. Compare **heteroeroticism.** **–autoerotic,** *adj.*

autoerythrocyte sensitization /ô′tō·ərith′rəsīt/, an unusual disorder characterized by the spontaneous appearance of painful, hemorrhagic spots on the anterior aspects of the arms and legs, resulting from hypersensitivity to the patient's own red blood cells. Autoimmune hemolytic anemia, an extreme example of hypersensitivity to antigens on the surface of the patient's erythrocytes, may cause fulminant hemolysis, fever, abdominal pain, hyperbilirubinemia, thrombosis, and shock. Psychoneurotic disorders may be associated with the disorder. Also called **Gardner-Diamond syndrome.**

autoerythrocyte sensitization syndrome. See **Gardner-Diamond syndrome.**

autogenesis /ô′tōjen′əsis/, **1.** abiogenesis. **2.** self-produced condition; a condition originating from within the organism. Also called **autogeny** /ôtoj′ənē/. Compare **heterogenesis, homogenesis.** **–autogenetic, autogenic,** *adj.*

autogenous /ôtoj′ənəs/, **1.** self-generating. **2.** originating from within the organism, as a toxin or vaccine.

autogeny. See **autogenesis.**

autograft, surgical transplantation of any tissue from one part of the body to another location in the same individual. Autografts are commonly used to replace skin lost in severe burns. Compare **allograft, isograft, xenograft.** See also **graft.**

autographism. See **dermatographia.**

autohexaploid, autohexaploidic. See **autopolyploid.**

autoimmune disease, one of a large group of diseases characterized by the subversion or alteration of the function of the immune system of the body. Antigens normally present in the internal cells stimulate the development of antibodies, and the antibodies, unable to distinguish antigens of the internal cells from external antigens, act against the internal cell to cause localized and systemic reactions. These reactions affect the epithelial and the connective tissues of the body, causing a variety of diseases that can be divided into two general categories: the collagen diseases (including systemic lupus erythematosus, dermatomyositis, periarteritis nodosa, scleroderma, and rheumatoid arthritis) and the autoimmune hemolytic disorders (including idiopathic thrombocytopenic purpura, acquired hemolytic anemia, and autoimmune leukopenia). The precise pathophysiologic processes and the origin of these diseases are unknown.

■ OBSERVATIONS: The manifestations and clinical characteristics depend on the specific disease and on the organ or systems affected. See specific diseases.

■ INTERVENTION: Therapy includes corticosteroid, anti-inflammatory, and immunosuppressive drugs. The symptoms are treated specifically, as a transfusion for hemorrhage, analgesics for pain, and physical therapy for the prevention of contracture. Diet may be regulated for specific needs; for example, iron might be increased to treat anemia in a person with thrombocytopenic purpura, or calories might be reduced in a weight-loss diet for a person with rheumatoid arthritis. Surgical treatment may be corrective or preventive, as a hip replacement in rheumatoid arthritis or a splenectomy in thrombocytopenic purpura.

■ NURSING CONSIDERATIONS: Many of these diseases are characterized by periods of crisis and periods of remission. During a crisis, the patient may be hospitalized and require extensive nursing care, with relief from pain, applications of heat or cold, range of motion exercises, or assistance in movement and ambulation. The nurse observes for signs of hemorrhage, puts side rails or a trapeze in place if necessary, protects the person from infection, and prevents chilling or overheating. Because the patient is in particular need of emotional support, the nurse helps the person verbalize feelings of anger and frustration, recognize limitations, focus on strengths, set realistic goals, and understand the disease process. It is important also to teach the patient and the family the side effects of the drugs being prescribed and how the drugs are to be taken.

autoimmunity, an abnormal characteristic or condition in which the body reacts against constituents of its own tissues. Autoimmunity may result in hypersensitivity and autoimmune disease. It is not yet fully understood, but there are several common theories to explain autoimmunity, as the forbidden clone theory and the sequestered antigens theory. See also **antibody specific theory.**

automatic behavior. See **automatism.**

automatic bladder. See **spastic bladder.**

automatic infiltration detector, a temperature-sensitive device that activates an alarm and automatically stops an intravenous infusion when infiltration of the intravenous fluid occurs. The device detects any cooling of the skin at the intravenous site, a common sign of infiltration. The detector is usually secured to the skin with tape and attaches by a small cable to the fluid-monitoring circuit of an intravenous pump.

automatic mallet condenser. See **mechanic condenser.**

automation, use of a machine designed to follow repeatedly and automatically a predetermined sequence of individual operations.

automatism /ôtom′ətiz′əm/, **1.** (in physiology) involuntary function of an organ system independent of apparent external stimuli, as the beating of the heart, or dependent on external stimuli but not consciously controlled, as the dilatation of the pupil of the eye. **2.** (in philosophy) the theory that the body acts as a machine and that the mind, whose processes depend solely on brain activity, is a noncontrolling adjunct of the body. **3.** (in psychology) mechanic, repetitive, and undirected behavior that is not consciously controlled, as seen in psychomotor epilepsy, hysteric states, and such acts as sleepwalking. Kinds of automatism include **ambulatory automatism, command automatism,** and **immediate posttraumatic automatism.** Also called **automatic behavior.**

autonomic /ô′tənom′ik/, **1.** having the ability to function independently without outside influence. **2.** of or pertaining to the autonomic nervous system.

autonomic drug, any of a large group of drugs that mimic or modify the function of the autonomic nervous system.

autonomic dysreflexia, a dysreflexia that is the result of impaired function of the autonomic nervous system caused by simultaneous sympathetic and parasympathetic activity. It occurs in quadriplegics and some paraplegics, with symptoms of hypertension, bradycardia, pallor below and flushing above the cord lesions, convulsions, and cardiomegaly. There is the possibility of a cerebrovascular accident and death occurring during an attack.

autonomic nervous system, the part of the nervous system that regulates involuntary vital function, including the activity of the cardiac muscle, the smooth muscle, and the glands. It has two divisions: The **sympathetic nervous system** accelerates heart rate, constricts blood vessels, and raises blood pressure; the **parasympathetic nervous system** slows heart rate, increases intestinal peristalsis and gland activity, and relaxes sphincters.

autonomic neuropathy, self-controlling, functionally independent disturbances in the peripheral nervous system.

autonomic reflex, any of a large number of normal reflexes governing and regulating the functions of the viscera. Autonomic reflexes control such activities of the body as blood pressure, heart rate, peristalsis, sweating, and urination.

autonomous bladder. See **flaccid bladder.**

autonomy /ôton′əmē/, the quality of having the ability or tendency to function independently. **–autonomous,** *adj.*

autopagnosia /ô′tōpəg·nō′zhə/, an inability to recognize and identify the parts of one's own body. It is associated generally with lesions of the dominant hemisphere of the patient and is manifested during a neurologic examination when the patient is unable to perform a task such as touching the right ear with the left thumb.

autopentaploid, autopentaploidic. See **autopolyploid.**

autoplastic maneuver, (in psychology) a process that is part of adaptation, involving an adjustment within the self. Compare **alloplastic maneuver.**

autopolyploid /ô′tōpol′iploid/, **1.** also **autopolyploidic.** of or pertaining to an individual, organism, strain, or cell that has more than two genetically identical or nearly identical sets of chromosomes that are derived from the same ancestral species. They result from the duplication of the haploid chromosome set and are referred to as autotriploid, autotetraploid, autopentaploid, autohexaploid, and so on, depending on the number of multiples of the haploid chromosomes they contain. **2.** such an individual, organism, strain, or cell. Compare **allopolyploid.** See also **allodiploid.**

autopolyploidy /ô′tōpol′iploi′dē/, the state or condition of having more than two identical or nearly identical sets of chromosomes. Compare **allopolyploid.**

autopsy /ô′topsē/, a postmortem examination performed to confirm or determine the cause of death. Also called **necropsy** /nek′ropsē/, **thanotopsy** /than′ətop′sē/. **–autopsic, autopsical,** *adj.*, **autopsist,** *n.*

autopsy pathology, the study of disease by the examination of the body after death by a pathologist. The organs and tissues are first described by their appearance at the time of dissection, then by their appearance in the microscopic examination or laboratory analysis of small representative samples of tissue taken for their diagnostic value.

autoserous treatment /ô′təsir′əs/, therapy of an infectious disease by inoculating the patient with the patient's own serum.

autosite /ô′təsīt/, the larger, more normally formed member of unequal or asymmetric, conjoined twins on whom the other smaller fetus depends for various physiologic functions and for nutrition and growth. Compare **parasitic fetus. –autositic.** *adj.*

autosomal /ô′təsō′məl/, **1.** pertaining to or characteristic of an autosome. **2.** pertaining to any condition transmitted by an autosome.

autosomal dominant inheritance, a pattern of inheritance in which the transmission of a dominant gene on an autosome causes a characteristic to be expressed. Males and females are affected with equal frequency. Affected individuals have an affected parent unless the condition is the result of a fresh mutation. Half of the children of a heterozygous affected parent are affected. All of the children of a homozygous affected parent are affected. Normal children of an affected parent do not carry the trait. Traits can be traced vertically through previous generations. A family history may be illustrated by drawing a pedigree. The first case, the propositus, appears suddenly in the pedigree, usually as a mutation. Achondroplasia, osteogenesis imperfecta, polydactyly, and Marfan's syndrome are autosomal dominant disorders. Compare **autosomal recessive inheritance.** See also **dominance.**

autosomal inheritance, a pattern of inheritance in which the transmission of traits depends on the presence or absence of certain genes on the autosomes. The pattern may be dominant or recessive, and males and females are affected with equal frequency. The majority of hereditary disorders are the result of a defective gene on an autosome. Kinds of autosomal inheritance are **autosomal dominant inheritance** and **autosomal recessive inheritance.** See also **inheritance.**

autosomal recessive inheritance, a pattern of inheritance in which the transmission of a recessive gene on an autosome results in a carrier state if the person is heterozygous for the trait and in the affected state if the person is homozygous for the trait. Males and females are affected with equal frequency. Affected individuals have unaffected parents who are heterozygous for the trait. One fourth of the children of two unaffected heterozygous parents are affected. All of the children of two homozygous affected parents are affected. The children of a couple in which one parent has the trait and the other does not are all carriers who show no effect of the trait. There is usually no family history of the trait; it becomes manifest when two unaffected parents who are heterozygous for a particular recessive gene have a child who is homozygous for the trait. Cystic fibrosis, phenylketonuria, and galactosemia are examples of autosomal recessive inheritance. Compare **autosomal dominant inheritance.** See also **recessive.**

autosome /ô′təsōm/, any chromosome that is not a sex chromosome and that appears as a homologous pair in the somatic cell. Humans have 22 pairs of autosomes, which are involved in transmitting all genetic traits and conditions other than those that are sex-linked. Also called **euchromosome** /yo͞o′krəsōm/. Compare **sex chromosome.**

autosplenectomy /ô′tōsplinek′təmē/, a progressive shrinking of the spleen that may occur in sickle cell anemia. The spleen is replaced by fibrous tissue and becomes nonfunctional.

autosuggestion, an idea, thought, attitude, or belief suggested to oneself, often as a formula or incantation, as a means of controlling one's behavior. Compare **suggestion.**

autotetraploid, autotetraploidic. See **autopolyploid.**

autotopagnosia /ô′tōtop′əg·nō′zhə/, the inability to recognize or localize the various parts of the body because of organic brain damage. Also called **body-image agnosia.** See also **agnosia, proprioception.**

autotriploid, autotriploidic. See **autopolyploid.**

autumn fever. See **leptospirosis.**

auxanology /ôks′ənol′əjē/, the scientific study of growth and development. **–auxanologic,** *adj.*

auxesis /ôksē′sis/, *pl.* **auxeses,** an increase in size or volume because of cell expansion rather than of an increase in the number of cells or tissue elements; hypertrophy. Also called **auxetic growth.** Compare **merisis.** **–auxetic,** *adj., n.*

auxilliary enzyme, in a coupled assay system, an enzyme that links the enzyme being measured with an indicator enzyme.

auxiliary storage, a storage device for adding to the main storage of the computer, employing such media as floppy disks, hard disks, cassette tapes, magnetic tapes, or cartridge tapes.

auxo-, a combining form meaning 'pertaining to growth, to acceleration, or to stimulation': *auxochrome, auxocyte, auxotonic.*

AV, abbreviation for *arteriovenous, atrioventricular, auricularventricular.*

available arch length, the length or space in a dental arch that is available for all the natural teeth of an individual. See also **arch length.**

avantin. See **isopropyl alcohol.**

avascular /āvas′kyo͝olər/, **1.** (of a tissue area) not receiving a sufficient supply of blood. The reduced flow may be the result of blockage by a blood clot or the deliberate stoppage of flow during surgery or of measures taken to control a hemorrhage. **2.** (of a kind of tissue) not having blood vessels.

Aventyl Hydrochloride, a trademark for an antidepressant (nortriptyline hydrochloride).

aversion therapy, a form of behavior therapy in which punishment or unpleasant or painful stimuli, such as electric shock or drugs that induce nausea, are used in the suppression of undesirable behavior. The procedure is used in treating such conditions as drug abuse, alcoholism, gambling, overeating, smoking, and various sexual deviations. Also called **aversive conditioning.** See also **behavior therapy.**

aversive stimulus, a stimulus, as electric shock, that causes psychic or physical pain. See also **aversion therapy.**

avidin, a glycoprotein in raw egg white with strong affinity for biotin.

avidity, a measure of the binding strength of antibodies to multiple antigenic determinants on natural antigens.

avitaminosis /āvī′təminō′sis/, a condition resulting from a deficiency of or the lack of absorption or use of one or more essential vitamins in the diet. Also called **hypovitaminosis.** Compare **hypervitaminosis.** See also specific vitamins.

Avloclor, a trademark for an antimalarial (chloroquine).

Avlosulfon, a trademark for a leprostatic antibacterial (dapsone).

AV nicking, a vascular abnormality on the retina of the eye, visible on ophthalmologic examination, in which a vein is compressed by an arteriovenous crossing. The vein appears "nicked," because of constriction or spasm. It is a sign of hypertension, arteriosclerosis, and other vascular conditions.

Avogadro's law /av′ōgad′rōz/, a law in physics stating that equal volumes of all gases at a given temperature and pressure contain the identical number of molecules.

avoidance, (in psychiatry) a conscious or unconscious defense mechanism, physical or psychologic, by which an individual tries to avoid or escape from unpleasant stimuli, conflicts, or feelings, as anxiety, fear, pain, or danger.

avoidance-avoidance conflict, a conflict resulting from the confrontation of two or more alternative goals or desires that are equally aversive and undesirable. Also called **double-avoidant conflict.** See also **conflict.**

avoidance conditioning, the establishment of certain patterns of behavior to avoid unpleasant or painful stimuli.

avoirdupois weight /av′ərdəpoiz′/, the English system of weights in which there are 7000 grains, 256 drams, or 16 ounces to 1 pound. One ounce in this system equals 28.35 g, and 1 pound equals 453.59 g. Compare **apothecaries' weight.** See also **metric system.**

avulsed teeth /əvulst/, teeth that have been forcibly displaced from their normal position. In some cases they can be surgically reimplanted, but this procedure is not often successful. Also spelled **evulsed teeth.** See also **avulsion.**

avulsion, the separation, by tearing, of any part of the body from the whole, as an umbilical cord torn in the process of delivering the placenta. **–avulse,** *v.*

avulsion fracture, a fracture caused by the tearing away of a fragment of bone where a strong ligamentous or tendinous attachment forcibly pulls the fragment away from osseous tissue.

awake anesthesia, an anesthetic procedure in which analgesia and anesthesia are accomplished without loss of consciousness and the concomitant need for life support equipment, personnel, and expertise. Dental procedures, surgery on a limb or an extremity, and certain kinds of head surgery are ordinarily performed using awake anesthesia. Awake anesthesia is not as complete as general anesthesia, and muscle relaxation may not be very deep. Various combinations of sedatives, tranquilizers, and low concentrations of anesthetic gas may be used. Also called **conscious sedation.**

AWOL /ā′wôl/, abbreviation for **absent without leave.**

ax-, axio-, axon-, a combining form meaning 'pertaining to an axis': *axial, axofugal, axon.*

axial (A), **1.** pertaining to or situated on the axis of a structure or part of the body. **2.** (in dentistry) relating to the long axis of a tooth.

axial current, the central part of the blood current.

axial gradient, **1.** the variation in metabolic rate in different parts of the body. **2.** the development toward the body axis or its parts in relation to the metabolic rate in the various parts.

axial illumination. See **illumination.**

axial neuritis. See **parenchymatous neuritis.**

axial spillway, a groove that crosses a cusp ridge or a marginal ridge and extends onto an axial surface of a tooth. Compare **interdental spillway, occlusal spillway.**

axilla /aksil′ə/, *pl.* **axillae,** a pyramid-shaped space forming the underside of the shoulder between the upper part of the arm and the side of the chest. Also called **armpit.**

axillary anesthesia. See **brachial plexus anesthesia.**

axillary artery /ak′səler′ē/, one of a pair of continuations of the subclavian arteries that starts at the outer border of the first rib and ends at the distal border of the teres major, where it becomes the brachial artery. It has three parts and six branches, supplying various chest and arm muscles, as the pectorals, deltoid, and subclavius. The six branches are the highest thoracic, thoracoacromial, lateral thoracic, subscapular, posterior humeral circumflex, and anterior humeral circumflex.

axillary nerve, one of the last two branches of the posterior cord of the brachial plexus before the posterior cord becomes the radial nerve. The axillary nerve passes over the insertion of the subscapularis, crosses the teres minor, and leaves the axilla, accompanied by the posterior humeral circumflex artery. It passes through the quadrilateral space bounded by the neck of the humerus, the two teres muscles, and the long head of the triceps and divides into a posterior branch and an anterior branch. The posterior branch innervates the teres minor, part of the deltoideus, and part of the skin overlying the deltoideus; the anterior branch winds around the neck of the humerus and innervates the deltoideus. Some fibers of the nerve also supply the capsule of the shoulder joint.

axillary node, one of the lymph glands of the axilla that help fight infections in the chest, armpit, neck, and arm and drain lymph from those areas. The 20 to 30 axillary nodes are divided into the lateral group, the anterior group, the posterior group, the central group, and the medial group. The lateral group is associated with lymphatic vessels that drain the whole arm, the anterior group with vessels that drain the thoracic muscles, the posterior group with vessels that drain the dorsal muscles of the neck and the muscles of the thoracic wall, the central group with vessels that drain the lymph from the nodes of the three preceding groups, and the medial group with afferent vessels that drain lymph from the breast and efferent vessels that form the subclavian lymphatic trunk. See also **lymphatic system, lymph node.**

axillary vein, one of a pair of veins of the upper limb that begins at the junction of the basilic and the brachial veins near the distal border of the teres major and becomes the subclavian vein at the outer border of the first rib. It receives deoxygenated blood from the venous tributaries that correspond to the branches of the axillary artery and near its termination, from the cephalic vein. It contains a pair of valves at the distal border of the subscapularis. Compare **subclavian vein.**

axio-. See **ax-.**

axis, *pl.* **axes** /ak′sēz/, **1.** (in anatomy) a line that passes through the center of the body, or a part of the body, as the frontal axis, binauricular axis, and basifacial axis. **2.** the second cervical vertebra about which the atlas rotates, allowing the head to be turned, extended, and flexed. Also called **epistropheus, odontoid vertebra.**

axis artery, one of a pair of extensions of the subclavian arteries, running into and supplying the upper limb, continuing into the forearm as the palmar interosseous artery. Each artery is divided into subclavian, axillary, and brachial portions, developing radial and ulnar arteries from the brachial section.

axis cylinder. See **axon.**

axis traction, **1.** the process of pulling a baby's head with obstetric forceps in a direction in line with the path of least resistance, following the curve of Carus through the mother's birth canal. **2.** *informal.* any mechanic device attached to obstetric forceps to facilitate pulling in the proper direction.

axoaxonic synapse /ak′sō•akson′ik/, a type of synapse in which the axon of one neuron comes in contact with the axon of another neuron.

axodendritic synapse /ak′sōdendrit′ik/, a type of synapse in which the axon of one neuron comes in contact with the dendrites of another neuron.

axodendrosomatic synapse /ak′sōden′drōsōmat′ik/, a type of synapse in which the axon of one neuron comes in contact with both the dendrites and the cell body of another neuron.

axon /ak′son/, the cylindric extension of a nerve cell that conducts impulses away from the neuron cell body. Axons may be bare or sheathed in myelin. Also called **axone** /ak′sōn/, **axis cylinder.** Compare **dendrite.**

axon-. See **ax-.**

axon flare, vasodilatation, reddening, and increased sensitivity of skin surrounding an injured area, caused by an axon reflex. Axon flare or reflex is considered part of a triple response in which injury or stroking of the skin results in local reddening, the release of histamine or a histamine-like substance, a surrounding flare, and wheal formation. A pinprick in the involved area causes more intense pain than a similar stimulus before injury.

axoplasmic flow /ak′sōplaz′mik/, the continuous pulsing, undulating movement of the cytoplasm between the cell body of a neuron, where protein synthesis occurs, and the axon fiber to supply it with the substances vital for the maintenance of activity and for repair. The nerve fiber depends totally on the cell body for metabolites, and any interruption in the axoplasmic flow caused by disease or trauma results in the degeneration of the unsupplied areas of the axon.

axosomatic synapse /ak′sōsōmat′ik/, a type of synapse in which the axon of one neuron comes in contact with the cell body of another neuron.

azathioprine, an immunosuppressive.

■ INDICATIONS: It is prescribed to prevent organ rejection after transplantation and in the treatment of lupus erythematosus and other systemic inflammatory diseases.

■ CONTRAINDICATION: Known hypersensitivity to this drug prohibits its use.

■ ADVERSE EFFECTS: Among the most serious adverse reactions are bone marrow depression and hepatotoxicity. Nausea and fever are common.

Azlin, a trademark for an antibiotic (azlocillin).

azlocillin sodium, a semisynthetic penicillin antibiotic.

■ INDICATIONS: It is prescribed for lower respiratory tract, urinary tract, skin, and bone and joint infections and bacterial septicemia caused by susceptible strains of microorganisms, mainly *Pseudomonas aeroginosa.*

■ CONTRAINDICATION: Hypersensitivity to any of the penicillins prohibits its use.

■ ADVERSE EFFECTS: The most serious adverse reactions are anaphylactic reactions, convulsive seisures, epigastric pain, reduction in blood elements, and elevation in hepatic and renal parameters.

azo-, a combining form meaning 'containing nitrogen': *azocarmine, azoimide, azorubin.*

azoospermia /āzō′əspur′mē·ə/, lack of spermatozoa in the semen. It may be caused by testicular dysfunction or by blockage of the tubules of the epididymis, or it may be induced by vasectomy. Infertility but not impotence is associated with azoospermia. Compare **oligospermia.**

azotemia /az′ōtē′mē·ə/, the retention in the blood of excessive amounts of nitrogenous compounds. This toxic condition is caused by failure of the kidneys to remove urea from the blood and is characteristic of uremia. See also **uremia.** **–azotemic,** *adj.*

AZ test. See **Ascheim-Zondek test.**

azul, azula. See **pinta.**

Azulfidine, a trademark for an antibacterial (sulfasalazine).

azygos. See **azygous.**

azygospore, a spore that is produced directly from a gamete that does not undergo conjugation, as in certain algae and fungi. Also called **azygosperm.**

azygous /az′əgəs/, occurring as a single entity or part, as any unpaired anatomic structure; not part of a pair. Also **azygos.** **–azygos** /az′əgos′/, *n.*

azygous vein, one of the seven veins of the thorax. Beginning opposite the first or second lumbar vertebra, it rises through the aortic hiatus in the diaphragm and passes to the right of the vertebral column to the fourth thoracic vertebra, then arches ventrally over the root of the right lung, and ends in the superior vena cava. It receives numerous veins, as the hemiazygous veins, several esophageal veins, and the right bronchial vein. Compare **internal thoracic vein, left brachiocephalic vein, right brachiocephalic vein,**

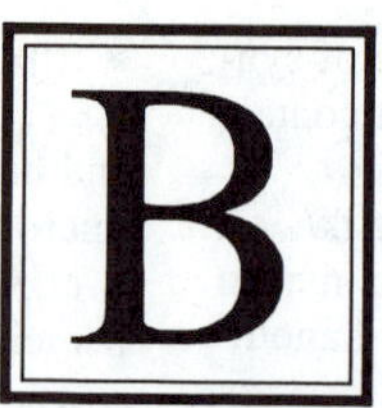

B, symbol for **boron.**
Ba, symbol for **barium.**
BA, abbreviation for **Bachelor of Arts.**
Babcock's operation, the extirpation of a varicosed saphenous vein by inserting an acorn-tipped sound, tying the vein to the sound, and drawing it out. Also called **subcutaneous stripping.**

babesiosis /bəbē′sē•ō′sis/, an infection caused by protozoa of the genus *Babesia*. The infective organism is introduced into the host through the bite of ticks of the species *Ixodes dammini*. Symptoms include headache, fever, nausea and vomiting, myalgia, and hemolysis. Also called **babesiasis.**

Babinski's reflex /bəbin′skēz/, dorsiflexion of the big toe with extension and fanning of the other toes elicited by firmly stroking the lateral aspect of the sole of the foot. The reflex is normal in newborn infants and abnormal in children and adults, in whom it may indicate a lesion in the pyramidal tract. Also called **Babinski's sign.**

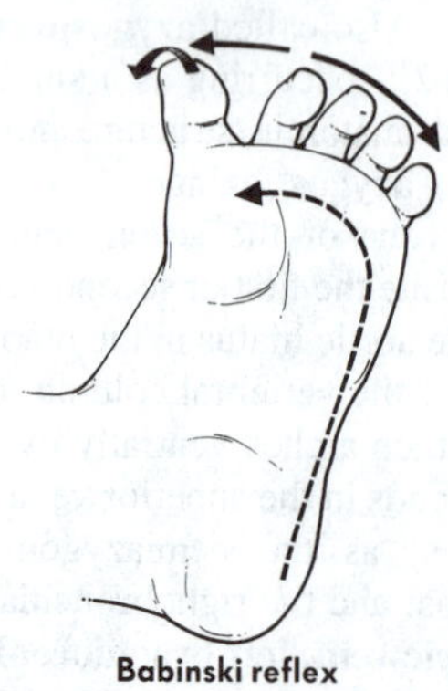
Babinski reflex

baby, 1. an infant or young child, especially one who is not yet able to walk or talk. 2. to treat gently or with special care.

Baby Jane Doe regulations, rules established in 1984 by the U.S. Health and Human Services Department requiring state governments to investigate complaints about parental decisions involving the treatment of handicapped infants. The rules also allowed the federal government to have access to children's medical records and required hospitals to post notices urging doctors and nurses to report any suspected cases of infants denied proper medical care. The controversial regulations have been held illegal by a federal court. The popular name for the federal rules was taken from the name "Jane Doe" given an infant born in New York with an open spinal column and other defects who became the object of a campaign to force lifesaving surgery for the child over the objections of the parents. Also called **Baby Doe rules.**

baby talk, 1. the speech patterns and sounds of young children learning to talk, characterized by mispronunciation, imperfect syntax, repetition, and phonetic modifications, as lisping or stuttering. See also **lallation.** 2. the intentionally oversimplified manner of speech, imitative of young children learning to talk, used by adults in addressing children or pets. 3. the speech patterns characteristic of regressive stages of various mental disorders, especially schizophrenia.

bacampicillin hydrochloride, a semisynthetic penicillin.

■ INDICATIONS: It is prescribed in the treatment of respiratory tract, urinary tract, skin, and gonococcal infections.

■ CONTRAINDICATIONS: Known sensitivity to this drug or other penicillin antibiotics prohibits its use.

■ ADVERSE EFFECTS: Among the most serious adverse reactions are hypersensitivity reactions, gastritis, enterocolitis, and transient blood disorders.

Bachelor of Science in Nursing (BSN), an academic degree awarded on satisfactory completion of a 4-year course of study in an institution of higher learning. The recipient is eligible to take the national certifying examination to become a registered nurse. A BSN degree is prerequisite to advancement in most systems and institutions that employ nurses. Compare **associate degree in nursing, diploma program in nursing.**

bacill-, a combining form meaning 'pertaining to any rod-shaped bacterium': *bacillemia, bacillicidal, bacillosis.*

Bacillaceae /bas′əlā′si•ē/, a family of *Schizomycetes* of the order *Eubacteriales,* consisting of gram-positive, rod-shaped cells that can produce cylindric, ellipsoid, or spheric endospores situated terminally, subterminally, or centrally. These cells are chemoheterotropic and mostly saprophytic, commonly appearing in soil. Some are parasitic on insects and animals and are pathogenic. The family includes the genus *Bacillus,* which is aerobic, and the genus *Clostridium,* which is facultatively anaerobic.

bacillary dysentery. See **shigellosis.**

bacille Calmette-Guérin (BCG) /kalmet′gāraN′/, an attenuated strain of tubercle bacilli, used in many countries as a vaccine against tuberculosis, most often administered intradermally, using a multiple-puncture disk. It appears to prevent the more serious forms of tuberculosis and to give some protection to persons living in areas where tuberculosis is prevalent. BCG is also administered to stimulate the immune response in people who have certain kinds of malignancy. It induces a positive tuberculin reaction and may mask early, active infection by removing the diagnostic sign of conversion from the negative to the positive skin reaction. See also **tuberculin test, tuberculosis.**

bacilliform /bəsil′ifôrm/, rod-shaped, like a bacillus.

bacilluria /bas′əlo͝or′ē•ə/, the presence of bacilli in the urine.

Bacillus, a genus of aerobic, gram-positive spore-producing bacteria in the family Bacillaceae, order Eubacteriales, including 33 species, three of which are pathogenic and the rest saprophytic soil forms. Many microorganisms formerly classified as *Bacillus* are now classified in other genera. See also **Bacillaceae.**

Bacillus anthracis, a species of gram-positive, facultative anaerobe that causes anthrax. The spores of this organism, if inhaled, can cause a pulmonary form of anthrax; spores can live for many years in animal products, as hides and wool, and in soil. See also **anthrax, wool-sorter's disease.**

bacillus Calmette-Guérin vaccine. See **BCG vaccine.**

bacitracin /bas′itrā′sin/, an antibacterial.

■ INDICATION: It is prescribed for skin infections sensitive to bacitracin.

■ CONTRAINDICATION: Known hypersensitivity to this drug prohibits its use.

■ ADVERSE EFFECTS: Among the more serious adverse reactions are nephrotoxicity and skin rash.

back, the posterior portion of the trunk of the body between the neck and the pelvis. The back is divided by a middle furrow that lies over the tips of the spinous processes of the vertebrae. The upper cervical vertebrae cannot be felt in this furrow, but the seventh cervical vertebra is easily distinguished just above the more prominent first thoracic vertebra. The skeletal portion of the back includes the thoracic and the lumbar vertebrae and both scapulas. The root of the spine of the scapula is on a level in the back with the spine of the third thoracic vertebra, and the inferior angle of the scapula is on a level with the spine of the seventh thoracic vertebra. The superficial muscles of the back are large and include the trapezius, the rhomboideus major, and the latissimus. The deep muscles of the back are the erector spinae iliocostalis, interspinales, intertransversarii, longissimus, multifidi, rotatores, splenius, semispinales, spinales, transversocostal, and transversospinal. The nerves that innervate the various muscles of the back include some branches of the dorsal primary divisions of the spinal nerves, the lateral branches of the dorsal primary division of the middle and the lower cervical nerves, some branches of the primary division of the spinal nerves, and some branches of the ventral primary divisions of the spinal nerves. The back may be affected by various orthopedic diseases and disorders of the spine, as ankylosing spondylitis, hemivertebra, kyphosis, Pott's disease, scoliosis, and spasmodic torticollis. The back may also be affected by trauma, as fractures, spinal dislocations, and ruptured intervertebral disks. Lower back problems are common.

backache, pain in the lumbar, lumbosacral, or cervical regions of the back, varying in sharpness and intensity. Causes may include muscle strain or other muscular disorders or pressure on the root of a nerve, as the sciatic nerve, caused turn by a variety of factors, including a ruptured vertebral disk. Treatment may include heat, ultrasound, and devices to provide support for the affected area while in bed or while standing or sitting, bed rest, surgical intervention, and medications to relieve pain and relax spasm of the muscle of the affected area.

back-action condenser, (in dentistry) an instrument for compacting amalgams that has a U-shaped shank to develop the condensing force from a pulling motion rather than the more common pushing motions.

backcross, **1.** (in genetics) the cross of a first filial generation hybrid with one of the parents or with a genotype that is identical to the parental strain. **2.** the organism or strain produced by such a cross.

background radiation, naturally occurring radiation emitted by materials in the soil, ground waters, and building material, radioactive substances in the body, especially potassium 40 (^{40}K), and cosmic rays from outer space. The average person is exposed each year to 44 millirads (mrad) of cosmic radiation, 44 mrads from external terrestrial radiation, and 18 mrads from naturally occurring internal radioactive sources.

back pressure, pressure that builds in a vessel or a cavity as fluid is accumulated. The pressure increases and extends backward if the normal mechanism for egress or passage of the fluid is not restored. See also **backward failure.**

backup, a duplicate computer, data file, equipment, or procedure for use in the event of failure of storage media or of components.

backscatter radiation. See **scattered radiation.**

backward failure, cardiac failure marked by elevated venous pressure and diminished arterial pressure, most commonly beginning as left ventricular failure that results in decreased output. Backward failure develops when the ventricle cannot empty and the blood backs up in the pulmonary veins and the lungs, causing pulmonary edema.

baclofen, an antispastic agent.

■ INDICATION: It is prescribed for the alleviation of spasticity.

■ CONTRAINDICATION: Known hypersensitivity to this drug prohibits is use.

■ ADVERSE EFFECTS: Among the more serious adverse reactions are confusion, hypotension, dyspnea, impotence, nausea, and transient drowsiness.

bacter-. See **bacterio-.**

bacteremia /bak′tirē′mē•ə/, the presence of bacteria in the blood. Undocumented bacteremias occur frequently and usually abate spontaneously. Bacteremia is demonstrated by blood culture. Antibiotic treatment, if given, is specific for the organism found and appropriate to the locus of infection. Compare **septicemia.** See also **septic shock.** –**bacteremic,** *adj.*

bacteremic shock. See **septic shock.**

bacteria /baktir′ē•ə/, *sing.* **bacterium,** any of the small unicellular microorganisms of the class Schizomycetes. The genera vary morphologically, being spheric (cocci), rod-shaped (bacilli), spiral (spirochetes), or comma-shaped (vibrios). The nature, severity, and outcome of any infection caused by a bacterium are characteristic of that species.

-bacteria, a combining form meaning 'genus of microscopic plants forming the class Schizomycetes': *lysobacteria, nitrobacteria, streptobacteria.*

bacterial aneurysm, a localized dilatation in the wall of a blood vessel caused by the growth of bacteria, often following septicemia or bacteremia and usually occurring in periperal vessels. See also **mycotic aneurysm.**

bacterial endocarditis, an acute or subacute bacterial infection of the endocardium or the heart valves or both. The condition is characterized by heart murmur, prolonged fever, bacteremia, splenomegaly, and embolism. The acute variety progresses rapidly and is usually caused by staphylococci or pneumococci. The subacute variety is usually caused by lodging of *Streptococcus viridans* in valves of the heart damaged by rheumatic fever. Prompt treatment of both types with antibiotics, as penicillin, cephalosporin, or gentamicin given intravenously is essential to prevent destruction of the valves and cardiac failure. See also **endocarditis, subacute bacterial endocarditis.**

bacterial food poisoning, a toxic condition resulting from the ingestion of food contaminated by certain bacteria. Acute infectious gastroenteritis caused by various species of *Salmonella* is characterized by fever, chills, nausea, vomiting, diarrhea, and general discomfort beginning 8 to 48 hours after ingestion and continuing for several days. Similar symptoms caused by *Staphylococcus,* usually *S. aureus,* appear much sooner and rarely last more than a few hours. Food poisoning caused by the neurotoxin of *Clostridium botulinum* is characterized by GI symptoms, disturbances of vision, weakness or paralysis of muscles, and, in severe cases, respiratory failure. See also **botulism.**

bacterial kinase, **1.** a kinase of bacterial origin. **2.** a bacterial enzyme that activates plasminogen, the precursor of plasmin.

bacterial meningitis. See **meningitis.**

bacterial plaque, a film comprised of microorganisms that attaches to the teeth and often causes caries and infections of the gums. Mucin secreted by the salivary glands is also a component of plaque; it varies in thickness and consistency depending on individual metabolism, dental hygiene, diet, and environmental factors. Also called **dental plaque.**

bacterial protein, a protein produced by a bacterium.

bactericidal /baktir′isī′dəl/, destructive to bacteria. Compare **bacteriostatic.**

bactericidin, an antibody that kills bacteria in the presence of complement.

bacterio-, bacter-, a combining form meaning 'pertaining to any bacterial microorganism': *bacteriogenic, bacteriophytoma, bacteriosis.*

bacteriologist, a specialist in bacteriology.

bacteriology, the scientific study of bacteria. –**bacteriologic, bacteriological,** *adj.*

bacteriolysin /baktir′ē•əlī′sin/, an antibody that causes the breakdown of a particular species of bacterial cell. Complement is usually also necessary for this reaction. See also **bacteriolysis.**

bacteriolysis /baktir′ē•ol′əsis/, the breakdown of bacteria intracellularly or extracellularly. See also **bacteriolysin.** –**bacteriolytic,** *adj.*

bacteriophage /baktir′ē•əfāj′/, any virus that causes lysis of host bacteria, including the blue-green "algae." Bacteriophages resemble other viruses in that each is composed of either ribonucleic acid or deoxyribonucleic acid. They vary in structure from simple fibrous bodies to complex forms with contractile "tails." Bacteriophages associated with temperate bacteria may be genetically intimate with the host and are named after the bacterial strain for which they are specific, as coliphage and corynebacteriophage. –**bacteriophagic,** *adj.,* **bacteriophagy** /-of′əjē/, *n.*

bacteriophage typing, the process of identifying a species of bacteria according to the type of virus that attacks it.

bacteriostatic /baktir′ē•əstat′ik/, tending to restrain the development or the reproduction of bacteria. Compare **bactericidal.**

bacteriuria /baktir′ēyŏŏr′ē•ə/, the presence of bacteria in the urine. The presence of more than 100,000 pathogenic bacteria per milliliter of urine is usually considered significant and diagnostic of urinary tract infection. See also **urinary tract infection.**

bacteroid /bak′təroid/, **1.** of, pertaining to, or resembling bacteria. **2.** a structure that resembles a bacterium. Also **bacterioid** /baktir′ē•oid/. –**bacteroidal, bacterioidal,** *adj.*

Bacteroides /bak′təroi′dēz/, a genus of obligate anaerobic bacilli normally found in the colon, mouth, genital tract, and upper respiratory system. Severe infection may result from the invasion of the bacillus through a break in the mucous membrane into the venous circulation, where thrombosis and bacteremia may occur. Foul-smelling abcesses, gas, and putrefaction are characteristic of infection with this organism. Of the 30 species, *Bacteroides fragilis* is the most common and most virulent.

Bacterial pathogens

Organism	*Disease clinical manifestation*	*Reservoir*	*Method of transmission*
Acinetobacter calcoaceticus	Wound infections, bacteremia, urinary tract infections, pneumonia	Water, humans, and animals	Endogenous (colonizes GI tract or mucous membranes); contaminated solutions; usually nosocomial
Actinomyces israelii	Actinomycosis cervicofacial and pulmonary abscesses	Humans	Endogenous (commensal of buccal cavity)
Aeromonas hydrophila	Wound infections, bacteremia, diarrhea by toxogenic strains	Water, soil, GI tract	Contact with soil, water, occasionally endogenous
Bacillus anthracis	Anthrax-malignant pustule; wool sorter's disease (pneumonia)	Infected animals (sheep, goats, cattle); contaminated soil, hides	Contact with contaminated soil or animal products; inhalation
Bacillus cereus	Food poisoning	Soil, grain	Ingestion of toxin (associated with fried rice), soil contact, trauma
Bacteroides species	Wound infections, abscesses, bacteremia	Humans, animals	Endogenous (commensals of GI tract and mucous membranes)
Bordetella bronchiseptica	Wound and respiratory infections	Respiratory tract of animals (dogs, cats, rabbit)	Bite; aerosol
Bordetella parapertussis	Pertussis-like cough	Humans	Droplet infection
Bordetella pertussis	Whooping cough; pertussis	Humans	Droplet infection
Borrelia recurrentis	Epidemic relapsing fever	Humans	Louse vector
Borrelia species	Relapsing fever	Rodents (humans)	Arthropod vector, usually tick
Branhamella catarrhalis (Neisseria catarrhalis)	Otitis, sinusitus, bronchitis	Humans	Endogenous (commensal of respiratory tract)
Brucella abortus	Brucellosis undulant fever	Dogs	Animal contact; airborne, ingestion
Brucella canis	Brucellosis undulant fever	Dogs	Contact with infected animals
Brucella melitensis	Brucellosis undulant fever	Goats, sheep	Contact with infected animals or products; ingestion of contaminated foods
Brucella suis	Brucellosis undulant fever	Swine	Contact with infected animals or products; aerosol, ingestion
Campylobacter jejuni	Diarrhea, enteritis	Humans, fowl, dogs, cats, or other animals	Contact with infected animals or ingestion of contaminated foods
Campylobacter fetus subspecies *fetus* (*C. intestinalis*)	Bacteremia and localized infections	Humans	Endogenous (GI tract) opportunistic infections in immunocompromised host
Citrobacter species	Urinary tract, wound infections, bacteremia	Humans	Endogenous (GI tract)
Clostridium botulinum	Botulism, wound botulism (rare)	GI tract or animals, soil	Ingestion of food containing preformed toxin; production of toxin by organisms growing in wound
Clostridium difficile	Pseudomembranous colitis	Humans (animals, soil?)	Endogenous in GI tract; increased numbers of toxin-producing organisms in gut usually following antibiotic therapy
Clostridium novyi (and other *Clostridium* species)	Gas gangrene, wound infections (usually with other organisms)	Humans, animals, soil	Endogenous (GI tract) or soil contact
Clostridium perfringens	Gas gangrene, wound infections	Humans, animals, soil	Endogenous (GI tract) or soil contact
	Food poisoning		Ingestion of food in which toxin-producing organisms have grown
Clostridium tetani	Tetanus	Soil, GI tract of animals, humans	Trauma and soil contact
Corynebacterium diphtheriae	Diphtheria	Humans (upper respiratory tract)	Droplet or aerosol spread
Corynebacterium species	Infections of prosthetic devices and catheters	Humans	Endogenous (commensals of skin and mucous membranes)
Enterobacter species	Urinary tract, wound infections, bacteremia	Humans (vegetable matter)	Endogenous (GI tract), contaminated solutions or equipment
Erysipelothrix rhusiopathiae	Erysipeloid (wound infection)	Animals (swine)	Contact with infected animals

By Mickelsen, Patricia, Ph.D., Associated Director, Clinical Microbiology Laboratory, Stanford University Hospital, Stanford University Medical Center, Stanford, CA, 1984.

Continued.

Bacterial pathogens—cont'd

Organism	*Disease clinical manifestation*	*Reservoir*	*Method of transmission*
Escherichia coli	Urinary tract, genital, wound infections; peritonitis, meningitis, bacteremia	Humans	Endogenous (GI tract)
	Diarrhea	Humans	Feces-borne; infestion of foods, water contaminated with toxigenic or invasive strains
Francisella tularensis	Tularemia	Rabbits, rodents, lagomorphs, squirrels	Contact with infected animals or products, contaminated food or water, inhalation, arthropod vectors
Fusobacterium species	Wound infections, abscesses	Humans (animals)	Endogenous (commensals of mucous membrane) and endogenous in female genital tract (sexual transmission?)
Haemophilus ducreyi	Chancroid (soft chancre)	Humans	Sexual contact
Haemophilus influenzae	Respiratory tract infections, otitis, meningitis, epilottitis, conjunctivitis, bacteremia	Humans	Endogenous (commensal of respiratory tract); droplet spread
Haemophilus vaginalis (Gardnerella vaginalis)	Probably not etiologic agent but associated with anaerobes in nonspecific vaginitis; postpartum bacteremia	Humans	
Klebsiella pneumoniae	Pneumonia; urinary tract, wound, infections; bacteremia	Humans (vegetable matter)	Endogenous (commensal of GI tract)
Legionella micdadei	Pittsburgh pneumonia	Water	Inhalation of aerosols
Legionella pneumophila	Legionnaires disease, Pontiac fever pneumonia	Water	Inhalation of aerosols
Leptospira interrogans	Leptospirosis		Shed in urine of infected animals; contact with infected animals, contaminated products, food, or water
Listeria monocytogenes	Meningitis, bacteremia	Humans (soil, vegetable matter)	Probably endogenous (GI tract)
Morganella morganii (Proteus morganii)	Urinary tract, wound infections	Humans (animals)	Endogenous (GI tract commensal)
Mycobacterium avium, M. intracellularis	Pulmonary or disseminated infections	Soil, water	Inhalation; opportunistic in compromised hosts
Mycobacterium bovis	Pulmonary, GI or disseminated infection	Cattle or vaccine strain: bacillcus Calmette-Guérin (BCG)	Contact with infected animals or contaminated milk; opportunistic infection after vaccination with BCG
Mycobacterium kansasii	Pulmonary infections	Soil	Inhalation; opportunistic in compromised hosts
Mycobacterium leprae	Leprosy	Humans, armadillo, rodents	Contact with infected individuals
Mycobacterium marinum	Swimming pool granuloma	Water	Water contact, broken skin, or trauma
Mycobacterium tuberculosis	Tuberculosis	Humans	Inhalation of aerosols, generated by coughing
Neisseria gonorrhoeae	gonorrhea, pelvic inflammatory disease, neonatal opthalmia	Humans	Sexual contact, contact during parturition
Neisseria meningitidis	Epidemic and sporatic meningitis, bacteremia, pneumonia	Humans	Endogenous (commensal of upper respiratory tract); droplet spread
Nocardia asteroides	Pulmonary infections, mycetoma	Soil	Inhalation (compromised hosts); soil contact with trauma
Pasteurella multocida	Cellulitis, abscesses, adenitis; osteomyelitis, meningitis; chronic respiratory tract infections	Mouth flora of cats (dogs)	Contact with animals, animal bites, scratches
Peptostreptococcus	Abscesses, wound infection	Humans	Endogenous (GI tract and mucous membranes)
Propionibacterium acnes	Infection of prosthetic devices	Humans	Endogenous (commensal skin flora)
Proteus species *(P. mirabilis, P. vulgaris)*	Urinary tract, wound infections; bacteremia	Humans	Endogenous (commensal of GI tract)
Providencia species *(P. stuartii, P. rettgeri)*	Urinary tract, wound infections; bacteremia	Humans	Endogenous (commensal of GI tract); usually nosocomial

Continued.

Bactrim, a trademark for a fixed-combination drug containing two antibacterials (sulfamethoxazole and trimethoprim).

BAEP, abbreviation for **brainstem auditory-evoked potential.**

bag, a flexible or dilatable sac or pouch designed to contain gas, fluid, or semisolid material such as crushed ice. An Ambu bag or breathing bag is used to control the flow of respiratory gases entering the lungs of a patient. Several types of bags are used in medical or surgical procedures to dilate the anus, vagina, or other body openings.

bagasse /bəgas′/, the crushed fibers or the residue of sugar cane.

bagassosis /bag′əsō′sis/, a self-limited lung disease caused by an allergic response to bagasse, the fungi-laden, dusty debris left after the syrup has been extracted from sugar cane. It is characterized by fever, dyspnea, and malaise. Treatment may include corticosteroid drugs taken by mouth. To prevent a recurrence of the condition, the antigen should be avoided. See also **diffuse hypersensitivity pneumonia, organic dust.**

bagging, *informal.* the artificial respiration performed with a ventilator or respirator bag, as an Ambu bag or Hope resuscitator. The bag is squeezed to deliver air to the patient's lungs as the mask is held over the mouth. During general anesthesia the anesthetist may also use this technique to correct the respiratory pattern of an unconscious patient.

bag of waters. the membranous sac of amniotic fluid surrounding the fetus in the uterus of a pregnant woman. See **amnion.**

Bain Breathing Circuit, a continuous-flow anesthetic system that does not require a soda-lime absorber.

Bainbridge reflex, a cardiac reflex consisting of an increased pulse rate, resulting from stimulation of stretch receptors in the wall of the left atrium. It may be produced by the infusion of large amounts of intravenous fluids.

BAL, abbreviation for **British antilewisite.** See **dimercaprol.**

Organism	*Disease clinical manifestation*	*Reservoir*	*Method of transmission*
Pseudomonas aeruginosa	Otitis, urinary tract, eye, wound and burn infections; pneumonia, bacteremia	Water, soil, plants	Endogenous (colonizes GI tract and mucous membranes); exogenous (contaminated solutions or equipment); usually nosocomial
Pseudomonas mallei	Glanders	Horses	Contact with infected animals; wound infection, droplet infection
Pseudomonas pseudomallei	Melioidosis	Soil	Ingestion, inhalation; soil contact with broken skin
Pseudomonas species (*P. cepacia, P. fluorescens, P. maltophilia*)	Urinary tract, wound infections; bacteremia	Water, soil, plants	Endogenous (colonizes GI tract and mucous membranes); infect compromised hosts; exogenous (contaminated solutions and equipment)
Salmonella choleraesuis (many serotypes)	Diarrhea, enteric fever	Animals, humans, reptiles, fowl	Ingestion of contaminated food or water
Salmonella enteritidis (many serotypes)	Diarrhea, enteric fever	Animals, reptiles, humans, fowl	Ingestion of contaminated food or water
Salmonella typhosa	Typhoid	Humans	Ingestion (fecal contamination of water, foods)
Serovar canicola		Animals; contact with dog, other animals	
Serovar icterohaemorrhagiae		Rats, other animals	
Serovar pomona		Swine, other animals	
Serratia species (*S. marcescens, S. liquefaciens*)	Urinary tract, wound infections; bacteremia	Humans (vegetable matter)	Endogenous (colonizes GI tract and mucous membranes); usually nosocomial
Shigella species (*S. boydii, S. dysenteriae, S. flexneri, S. sonnei*)	Shigellosis-bacillary dysentery	Humans	Fecal-oral transmission via hands, fomites, food
Spirillum minor	Rat-bite fever	Rats, mice (rodent-ingesting animals)	Bites
Staphylococcus	Boils, furuncles, wound infections, osteomyelitis, endocarditis, pneumonia, infection of prosthetic devices, bacteremia, meningitis	Humans	Endogenous (commensal of mucous membranes and skin)

Continued.

balance, **1.** an instrument for weighing. **2.** a normal state of physiologic equilibrium. **3.** a state of mental or emotional equilibrium. **4.** to bring into equilibrium.

balanced anesthesia, *informal*. one of a number of variable techniques of general anesthesia in which no single anesthetic agent or preset proportion of the combination of agents is used; rather, an individualized mixture of anesthetics is prescribed according to the needs of a particular patient for a particular operation. One type of balanced anesthesia may combine a local or regional anesthetic with general anesthesic agents; another may combine a muscle relaxant, an analgesic, oxygen, an anesthetic gas, and a sedative.

balanced articulation, the simultaneous contacting of the upper and lower teeth as they glide over each other when the mandible is moved from centric relation to various eccentric relations. See also **balanced occlusion.**

balanced diet, a diet containing all of the essential nutrients that cannot be synthesized in adequate quantities by the body, in amounts adequate for growth, energy needs, nitrogen equilibrium, repair of wear, and maintenance of normal health.

balanced occlusion, **1.** an occlusion of the teeth that presents a harmonious relation of the occluding surfaces in centric and eccentric positions within the functional range of mandibular positions and tooth size. **2.** the simultaneous contacting of the upper and lower teeth on both sides and in the anterior and posterior occlusal areas of the jaws. An appropriate dental prosthesis develops such an occlusion to prevent the denture base from tipping or rotating in relation to the supporting structures. This term is primarily associated with the mouth but may also be used in relation to testing the occlusion of denture casts with an articulator.

balanced polymorphism, the recurrence in a population of an equalized mixture of homozygotes and heterozygotes for specific genetic traits, which are maintained from generation to generation by the forces of natural selection. Compare **genetic polymorphism.**

balanced suspension, a system of splints, ropes, slings, pulleys, and weights for suspending the lower

Bacterial pathogens—cont'd

Organism	*Disease clinical manifestation*	*Reservoir*	*Method of transmission*
	Food poisoning		Ingestion of toxin produced by staphylococci growing in contaminated food
	Toxic shock syndrome		Toxin production by colonizing organisms
Staphylococcus epidermidis	Infections of prosthetic devices, catheters	Humans	Endogenous (commensal of mucous membranes and skin); usually nosocomial
Staphylococcus saprophyticus	Urinary tract infections	Humans	Endogenous
Streptobacillus moniliformis	Rat-bite fever, Haverhill fever	Rats, mice (cats)	Bite, ingestion of contaminated food or water
Streptococcus agalactiae (Group B)	Neonatal bacteremia, meningitis; postpartum bacteremia; urinary tract infections	Humans	Endogenous (urogenital and GI tracts)
Streptococcus faecalis (Group D—enterococcus)	Urinary tract, wound infections; endocarditis	Humans	Endogenous (commensal of GI tract)
Streptococcus pneumoniae	Pneumonia, otitis, sinusitis, eye infections, bacteremia, meningitis	Humans	Endogenous (commensal of upper respiratory tract); droplet spread
Streptococcus pyogenes (Group A)	Pharyngitis, impetigo, wound infections, erysipelas, puerperal infections	Humans	Colonizes upper respiratory tract; droplet from infected individual or carrier
	Rheumatic fever Glomerulonephritis		Segquelae of *S. pyogenes* infection
Streptococci viridans or *alpha hemolytic* (includes: *S. sanguis, S. MG-intermedius, S. mitis)*	Endocarditis, visceral abscesses	Humans	Endogenous (commensals of respiratory tract and mucous membranes)
Treponema pallidum	Syphilis	Humans	Sexual contact
Vibrio cholerae	Cholera	Humans	Contaminated food and water
Vibrio parahaemolyticus	Gastroenteritis	Shellfish	Ingestion of contaminated food
Vibrio vulnificus	Wound infections, septicemia	Marine waters	Sea water associated injury; ingestion
Yersinia enterocolitica	Gastroenteritis, mesenteric lymphadenitis	Farm animals	Infestion of contaminated food or water
Yersinia pestis	Bubonic or pneumonic plague	Rats, rodents	Fleas; droplet infection

extremities of the body, used as an aid to healing and recuperation from fractures or from surgical operations.

balanced traction, a system of balanced suspension that supplements traction in the treatment of fractures of the lower extremities or after various operations affecting the lower parts of the body.

balanced translocation, the transfer of segments between nonhomologous chromosomes in such a way that there are changes in the configuration and total number of chromosomes, but each cell or gamete contains no more or no less than the normal amount of diploid or haploid genetic material. Usually the long arm of an acrocentric chromosome is transferred to another chromosome, and the small fragment containing the centromere is lost, leaving only 45 chromosomes. A person with balanced translocation is phenotypically normal but may produce children with trisomies. Compare **reciprocal translocation, robertsonian translocation.**

balancing side, (in dentistry) the side of the mouth opposite the working side of a dentition or denture.

balanic /bəlan′ik/, of or pertaining to the glans penis or the glans clitoridis.

balanitis /bal′ənī′tis/, inflammation of the glans penis.

balanitis xerotica obliterans /zirot′ikə oblit′ərans/, a chronic skin disease of the penis, characterized by a white, indurated area surrounding the meatus. Local antibacterial and antiinflammatory agents are used to treat it.

balano-, a combining form meaning 'pertaining to the glans penis': *balanocele, balanoplasty, balanoposthitis.*

balanoplasty /bal′ənōplas′tē/, an operation involving plastic surgery of the glans penis.

balanoposthitis /bal′ənōposthī′tis/, a generalized inflammation of the glans penis and prepuce, characterized by soreness, irritation, and discharge, occurring as a complication of bacterial or fungal infection. Smear and culture can determine the causative agent—often a common venereal disease—whereupon specific antimicrobial therapy can be instituted. Circumcision may be considered in severe cases. To relieve discomfort, the inflamed area can be irrigated with a warm saline solution several times a day.

balanopreputial /bal′ənōpripyo͞o′shəl/, of or pertaining to the glans penis and the prepuce.

balanorrhagia /bal′ənōrā′jē•ə/, balanitis in which pus is discharged copiously from the penis.

balantidiasis /bal′əntidī′əsis/, an infection caused by ingestion of cysts of the protozoan *Balantidium coli.* In some cases the organism is a harmless inhabitant of the large intestine, but infection with *B. coli* usually causes diarrhea. Infrequently the infection progresses, and the protozoan invades the intestinal wall and produces ulcers or abscesses, which may cause dysentery and death. The diagnosis is made by the identification of cysts and trophozoites in the stool or in the exudate from intestinal ulcers. Metronidazole is usually prescribed to treat the infection.

Balantidium coli /bal′əntid′ē•əm/, the largest and the only ciliated protozoan species that is pathogenic to humans, causing balantidiasis. The organism is seen in two life stages: the motile trophozoite and the encysted cercaria. It is a normal inhabitant of the domestic hog and is transmitted to humans by the ingestion of cysts excreted by the hog.

baldness, absence of hair, especially from the scalp. See also **alopecia.**

BAL in Oil, a trademark for a heavy metal antagonist (dimercaprol).

Balkan frame, an overhead, rectangular frame, attached to the bed of an orthopedic patient, for use in attaching splints, suspending or changing the position of immobilized limbs, and for continuous traction involving weights and pulleys.

ball, a relatively spheric mass, as one of the chondrin balls imbedded in hyaline cartilage.

ball-and-socket joint, a synovial joint in which the globular head of an articulating bone is received into a cuplike cavity, allowing the distal bone to move around an indefinite number of axes with a common center, as in hip and shoulder joints. Also called **enarthrosis, spheroidea.** Compare **condyloid joint, pivot joint, saddle joint.**

ballism, an abnormal neuromuscular condition characterized by uncoordinated swinging of the limbs and jerky movements. Ballism is associated with extrapyramidal disorders, as Sydenham's chorea.

ballismus, an abnormal condition characterized by violent flailing motions of the arms and, occasionally, the head, resulting from injury to the subthalamic nucleus. **Hemiballismus** is a unilateral form of the condition. The term may be used interchangeably with **ballism.**

ballistocardiogram /bəlis′tōkär′′dē•əgram′/, a record of the motion of the body—toward the head and toward the feet—caused by the thrust of the heart during systolic ejection of the blood into the aorta and the pulmonary arteries. The patient is placed on a special table, a ballistocardiograph, that is so delicately balanced that vibrations of the body can be recorded by a machine attached to the table. The ballistocardiogram is a sensitive tool that is useful in measuring cardiac output and the force of contraction of the heart.

balloon septostomy. See **Rashkind procedure.**

balloon-tip catheter, a catheter bearing a nonporous inflatable sac around its distal end. After insertion of the catheter the sac can be inflated with air or sterile water, introduced via injection into a special port at the proximal end of the catheter. The inflated sac serves to secure the catheter in the correct position. Kinds of balloon-tip catheters include **Foley catheter, Swan-Ganz catheter.**

ballottable head, a fetal head that has not descended and has become fixed in the maternal bony pelvis.

ballottement /bä′lôtmäN′, bəlot′ment/, a technique of palpating an organ or floating structure by bouncing it gently and feeling it rebound. Ballottement of a fetus within a uterus is an objective sign of pregnancy. In late

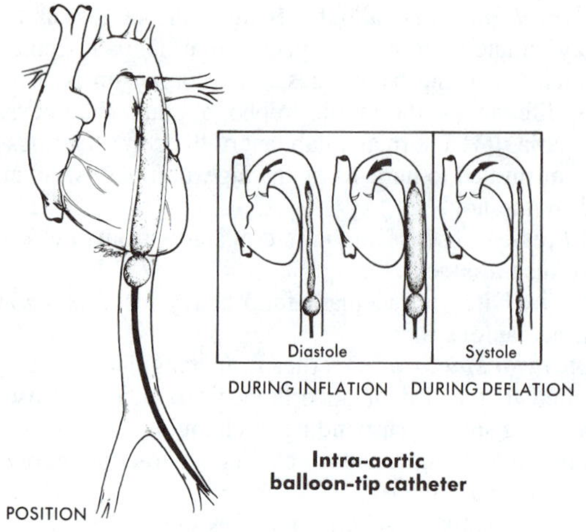

Intra-aortic balloon-tip catheter

pregnancy a fetal head that can be ballotted is said to be **floating** or **unengaged,** as differentiated from a fixed or an engaged head, which cannot be easily dislodged from the pelvis.

ball thrombus, a relatively round, coagulated mass of blood, containing platelets, fibrin, and cellular fragments, that may obstruct a blood vessel or an orifice, usually the mitral valve of the heart.

ball-valve action, the intermittent opening and closing of an orifice by a buoyant, ball-shaped mass, which acts as a valve. Some kinds of objects that may act in this manner are kidney stones, gallstones, and blood clots.

balm, **1.** also called **balsam.** a healing or a soothing substance, as any of various medicinal ointments. **2.** an aromatic plant of the genus *Melissa* that relieves pain.

balneology /bal′nē•ol′əjē/, a field of medicine that deals with the chemical compositions of various mineral waters and their healing characteristics, especially in baths. –**balneologic,** *adj.*

balneotherapy /bal′nē•ōther′əpē/, a use of baths in the treatment of many diseases and conditions.

balneum pneumaticum. See **air bath.**

balsam, any of a variety of resinous saps, generally from evergreens, usually containing benzoic or cinnamic acid. Balsam is sometimes used in rectal suppositories and dermatologic agents as a counterirritant.

bamboo spine, the characteristically rigid spine of advanced ankylosing spondylitis. Also called **poker spine.** See also **ankylosing spondylitis.**

band, **1.** (in anatomy) a bundle of fibers, as seen in striated muscle, that encircles a structure or binds one part of the body to another. **2.** (in dentistry) a strip of metal that fits around a tooth and serves as an attachment for orthodontic components. **3.** also called **stab form.** *informal.* the immature form of a segmented granulocyte characterized by a sausage-shaped nucleus. It is the only immature leukocyte normally found in the peripheral circulation. Bands represent 3% to 5% of the total white cell volume. An increase in the relative number of bands indicates bacterial infection or acute stress to the bone marrow.

band adapter, an instrument for aiding in the fitting of an orthodontic band to a tooth.

bandage, **1.** a strip or roll of cloth or other material that may be wound around a part of the body in a variety of ways to secure a dressing, maintain pressure over a compress, or immobilize a limb or other part of the body. **2.** to apply a bandage.

bandage shears, a sturdy pair of scissors used to cut through bandages. The blades of most bandage shears are angled to the shaft of the instrument, and the lower blade has a rounded blunt protuberance to facilitate insertion under the bandage without harming the patient's skin.

band cell, any one of the developing granular leukocytes in circulating blood, characterized by a curved or indented nucleus. Band cells are intermediate leukocytic forms between metamyelocytes and adult leukocytes with segmented nuclei.

banding, (in genetics) any of several techniques of staining chromosomes with fluorescent stains or chemical dyes that produce a series of lateral light and dark areas whose intensity and position are characteristic for each chromosome. Banding patterns are identified according to the staining technique used, as C-banding, G-banding, Q-banding, and R-banding. Also called **chromosome banding.**

Bandl's ring. See **pathologic retraction ring.**

band pusher, an instrument used for adapting metal orthodontic bands to the teeth.

band remover, an instrument used for removing orthodontic bands from the teeth.

Bangkok hemorrhagic fever. See **dengue.**

bank blood, anticoagulated, preserved blood collected from donors in units of 500 ml and stored under refrigeration for future use. Dated and identified as to blood type, it is stored for a usual maximum period of 21 days. Bank blood may be used directly after crossmatching against the recipient's blood or for the extraction and preparation of any of its components. See also **packed cells, pooled plasma, whole blood.**

Banocide, a trademark for an anthelmintic (diethylcarbamazine citrate).

Banthine, a trademark for an anticholinergic (methantheline bromide), used as an antispasmodic.

Banting treatment, a therapeutic regimen for obesity, consisting of a low-carbohydrate, high-protein diet. Also called **Banting diet.**

Banti's syndrome /ban′tēz/, a serious, progressive disorder involving several organ systems, characterized by portal hypertension, splenomegaly, anemia, leukopenia, GI tract bleeding, and cirrhosis of the liver. Obstruction of the blood vessels that lie between the intestines and the liver leads to venous congestion, an enlarged spleen, and abnormal destruction of red and white blood cells. Early symptoms are weakness, fatigue, and anemia. Surgical removal of the spleen and creation of a portacaval shunt to improve portal circulation are sometimes necessary. Since the syndrome is often a complication of alcoholic cirrhosis of the liver, medical treatment includes prescribing improved nutrition, vitamins, abstinence from alcohol, and rest. Also called **Banti's disease.** See also **cirrhosis, portacaval shunt, portal hypertension.**

BAO, abbreviation for **basal acid output.**

bar-. See **baro-.**

baralyme (BL) /ber′əlīm/, a mixture of calcium and barium compounds used to absorb exhaled carbon dioxide in an anesthesia rebreathing system.

Bárány's syndrome. See **caloric test.**

barber's itch. See **sycosis barbae.**

barbiturate /bärbich′o͞orāt, -ərit/, a derivative of barbituric acid that acts as a sedative or hypnotic. These derivatives are in widespread use and act by depressing the respiratory rate, blood pressure, temperature, and central nervous system. They may become addictive. Among the more common derivatives are amobarbital, butabarbital, pentobarbital, phenobarbital, secobarbital, and thiopental.

-barbituric, a combining form given to compounds derived from barbituric acid: *dibromobarbituric, isobarbituric, phenylethylbarbituric.*

barbiturism /bärbich′əriz′əm/, **1.** acute or chronic poisoning by any of the derivatives of barbituric acid. Ingestion of such preparations in excess of therapeutic quantities may be fatal or may produce physiologic, pathologic, and psychologic changes, as depressed respiration, cyanosis, disorientation, and coma. **2.** addiction to a barbiturate.

Bard-Pic syndrome /bärd′pik′/, a condition characterized by progressive jaundice, enlarged gallbladder, and cachexia, associated with advanced pancreatic cancer.

Bard's sign, the increased oscillations of the eyeball in organic nystagmus when the patient tries to visually follow a target moved from side to side across the line of sight. Such oscillations usually cease during the same test if the patient has congenital nystagmus.

bar graph, a graph in which frequencies are represented by bars extending from the ordinate or the abscissa, allowing the distribution of the entire sample to be seen at once.

bariatrics /ber′ē•at′riks/, the field of medicine that focuses on the treatment and the control of obesity and diseases associated with obesity.

barium (Ba) /ber′ē•əm/, a pale yellow, metallic element classified with the alkaline earths. Its atomic number is 56; its atomic weight is 137.36. The acid-soluble salts of barium are poisonous. Barium carbonate, formerly used in medicine, is now used to prepare the cardiac stimulant, barium chloride; fine, milky barium sulfate is used as a contrast medium in roentgenography of the digestive tract.

barium enema, a rectal infusion of barium sulfate, a radiopaque contrast medium, which is retained in the lower intestinal tract during roentgenographic studies for diagnosing obstruction, tumors, or other abnormalities, as ulcerative colitis. For the procedure to be most effective, the colon must be free of all fecal material, accomplished by a minimum residue diet for 2 days, a cathartic the night before, and a cleansing enema or suppository on the morning of the study. The patient takes only liquids the previous night and has no breakfast before the examination. After the x-ray studies are made, the barium is removed by a cleansing enema. The procedure is used therapeutically in children to reduce nonstrangulated intussusception. Also called **contrast enema.**

barium meal, the ingestion of barium sulfate, a radiopaque contrast medium, for the radiographic examination of the esophagus, stomach, and intestinal tract in the diagnosis of such conditions as dysphagia, peptic ulcer, and fistulas. The movement of the barium through the GI tract is followed by fluoroscopy, x-ray studies, or both. Before the test, the patient receives nothing by mouth for at least 8 hours. Also called **barium swallow.** See also **GI series.**

barium sulfate, a radiopaque medium used as a diagnostic aid in roentgenology.

■ INDICATION: It is prescribed for x-ray examination of the GI tract.

■ CONTRAINDICATION: Known hypersensitivity to this drug prohibits its use.

■ ADVERSE EFFECTS: Among the more serious complications is severe constipation.

barium swallow. See **barium meal.**

Barlow's disease. See **infantile scurvy.**

Barlow's syndrome, an abnormal cardiac condition characterized by an apical systolic murmur, a systolic click, and an electrocardiogram indicating inferior ischemia. These signs are associated with mitral regurgitation caused by prolapse of the mitral valve. Also called **electrocardiographic-auscultatory syndrome.**

baro-, bar-, a combining form meaning 'pertaining to pressure': *baresthesia, barognosis, barospirator.*

barognosis, *pl.* **barognoses,** the ability to perceive and evaluate weight, especially that held in the hand.

barograph /ber′əgraf′/, an instrument that continuously monitors barometric pressure and provides a record on paper of pressure changes.

barometer /bərom′ətər/, an instrument for measuring atmospheric pressure, commonly consisting of a slender tube filled with mercury, sealed at one end, and inverted into a reservoir of mercury. At sea level the normal height of mercury in the tube is 760 mm. At higher elevations the mercury column height (barometric pressure) is less. Fluctuations in barometric pressure may occur preceding major changes in the weather, making a barometer useful in weather forecasting. **–barometric,** *adj.*

barometric pressure. See **atmospheric pressure.**

baroreceptor /ber′ōrisep′tər/, one of the pressure-sensitive nerve endings in the walls of the atria of the heart, the vena cava, the aortic arch, and the carotid sinus. Baroreceptors stimulate central reflex mechanisms that allow physiologic adjustment and adaptation to changes in blood pressure via vasodilatation or vasoconstriction. Baroreceptors are essential for homeostasis.

barosinusitis. See **aerosinusitis.**

Barosperse, a trademark for a radiopaque medium (barium sulfate).

barotitis. See **aerotitis.**

barotitis media. See **aerotitis media.**

barotrauma /ber′ōtrô′mə, -trou′mə/, physical injury sustained as a result of exposure to increased environmental pressure, as barotitis media or rupture of the lungs or paranasal sinuses, as may occur among deep-sea divers or caisson workers. Compare **decompression sickness.**

Barr body. See **sex chromatin.**

barrel chest, a large, rounded thorax, considered normal in some stocky individuals and certain others who live in high-altitude areas and consequently develop increased vital capacities. Barrel chest, however, may also be a sign of pulmonary emphysema.

Barr-Epstein virus. See **Epstein-Barr virus.**

Barré's pyramidal sign /bäräz′/, the inability of a hemiplegic to maintain a flexed position on the side of the lesion when placed in a prone attitude with the lower limbs flexed 90 degrees at the knees: The leg on the side of the lesion extends.

Barrett's syndrome, a disorder of the lower esophagus marked by a benign ulcerlike lesion in columnar epithelium, resulting most often from chronic irritation of the esophagus by gastric reflux of acidic digestive juices. Major symptoms include dysphagia and heartburn. Symptoms may be relieved by eating frequent small meals, avoiding foods that produce gas, taking antacid medication, and elevating the head of the bed to prevent passive reflux when lying down. Also called **Barrett's esophagus, Barrett's ulcer.**

barrier, **1.** a wall or other obstacle that can restrain or block the passage of substances. Barrier methods of contraception, as the condom or cervical diaphragm, prevent the passage of spermatazoa into the uterus. Membranes and cell walls of body tissues function as screenlike barriers to permit the movement of water or certain other molecules from one side to the other while preventing the passage of other substances. Barriers in kidney tissues adjust automatically to regulate the retention or excretion of water and other substances according to the needs of organ systems elsewhere in the body. See also **barrier nursing.** **2.** something nonphysical that obstructs or separates, as barriers to communication or compliance.

barrier nursing, nursing care of a patient in isolation, performed to prevent the spread of infection by creating an aseptic barrier around the patient. Gown, mask, and gloves are worn by staff or visitors entering the room; the number of staff entering the room is kept to a minimum, and visitors are limited. Contaminated substances are handled according to strict protocols. Specific techniques vary with the indication for isolation. A patient with an infection may be isolated to prevent others from contracting the infection; a patient who is extremely susceptible to infection may be isolated for protection against possible infection from others. Also called **isolation technique.**

bartholinitis /bär′təlinī′tis/, an inflammatory condition of one or both Bartholin's glands, caused by bacterial infection. Usually, the causative microorganism is a species of *Streptococcus* or *Staphylococcus* or a strain of gonococci. The condition is characterized by swelling of one or both glands, pain, and the development of an abscess in the infected gland. A fistula may develop from the gland to the vagina, anus, or perineum. Treatment includes local application of heat, often by soaking in hot water, antibiotics, or, if necessary, incision of the gland and drainage of the purulent material or excision of the entire gland and its duct.

Bartholin's cyst /bär′təlinz/, a cyst that arises from one of the vestibular glands or from its ducts, filling with clear fluid that replaces the suppurative exudate characteristic of chronic inflammation.

Bartholin's duct, the major duct of the sublingual gland.

Bartholin's gland, one of two small, mucus-secreting glands located on the posterior and lateral aspect of the vestibule of the vagina. Also called **greater vestibular glands.**

Barton, Clara (1821–1912), an American philanthropist, humanitarian, and founder of the American National Red Cross. During the Civil War, she was a volunteer nurse, often on the battlefield, and at its end she organized a bureau of records to help in the search for missing men. When the Franco-Prussian War erupted, she assisted in the organization of military hospitals in Europe in association with the International Red Cross. This experience led to her advocacy of an American Red Cross organization, of which she became the first president.

Bartonella /bär′tənel′ə/, a genus of small, gram-negative flagellated pleomorphic coccobacilli. Members of the genus are intracellular parasites that infect red blood cells and the epithelial cells of the lymph nodes, liver, and spleen. They are transmitted at night by the bite of a sandfly of the genus *Phlebotomus*. The only known species of *Bartonella* is *B. bacilliformis*, the organism that causes bartonellosis. Because of its distinctive appearance, it is easily identified on microscopic examination of a smear of blood stained with Wright's stain.

bartonellosis /bär′tənəlō′sis/, an acute infection caused by *Bartonella bacilliformis*, transmitted by the bite of a sandfly. It is characterized by fever, severe anemia, bone pain, and, several weeks after the first symptoms are observed, by multiple nodular or verrucose skin lesions. The disease is endemic in the valleys of the Andes in Peru, Colombia, and Ecuador. The treatment usually includes chloramphenicol, penicillin, streptomycin, or tetracycline. Untreated, the infection is often fatal. Also called **Carrión's disease, Oroya fever, verruga peruana.**

Barton forceps. See **obstetric forceps.**

Barton's fracture, a fracture of the distal articular surface of the radius, which may be accompanied by the dorsal dislocation of the carpus on the radius.

Bartter's syndrome /bär′tərz/, a rare hereditary disorder, characterized by hyperplasia of the juxtaglomerular apparatus and secondary hyperaldosteronism. Renin and angiotensin levels may be elevated, but blood pressure usually remains normal. Early signs in childhood are abnormal physical growth and mental retardation, often accompanied by chronic hypokalemia and alkalosis.

bary-, a combining form meaning 'heavy or difficult': *baryecoia, baryencephalia, baryphonia*.

basal, of or pertaining to the fundamental or the basic, as basal anesthesia, which produces the first stage of unconsciousness, and the basal metabolic rate, which indicates the lowest metabolic rate.

basal acid output (BAO), the minimum volume of gastric fluid produced by an individual in a given period of time, used in the diagnosis of various diseases of the stomach and intestines.

basal anesthesia, **1.** a state of unconsciousness just short of complete surgical anesthesia in depth, in which the patient does not respond to words but still reacts to pinprick or other noxious stimuli. **2.** narcosis produced by injection or infusion of potent sedatives alone, without added narcotics or anesthetic agents. **3.** also called **narcoanesthesia.** any form of anesthesia in which the patient is completely unconscious, in contrast to awake anesthesia.

basal arch. See **apical arch.**

basal body temperature, the temperature of the body taken in the morning, orally or rectally, after at least 8 hours of sleep and before doing anything else, including getting out of bed, smoking a cigarette, moving around, talking, eating, or drinking.

basal-body-temperature method of family planning, a natural method of family planning that relies on the identification of the fertile period of the menstrual cycle by noting the progesterone-mediated rise in basal body temperature of 0.5° to 1° F that occurs with ovulation. The rate and pattern of the increase varies greatly from woman to woman, and somewhat from cycle to cycle in any one woman. Several cycles are observed, and careful records are kept in which the woman takes her temperature at the same time every morning, before doing anything else. It may be taken orally or rectally but should be done the same way every day. Talking, getting up, smoking a cigarette, eating, or even moving about in bed may change the temperature. Many other factors may also change the reading, including infection, stress, a bad night's sleep, medication, or environmental temperature. If any of these are present, the woman notes them on her record. The fertile period is considered to continue until the temperature is above the baseline for 5 days; the rise occurs slowly during all 5 days or increases rapidly, reaching a plateau at which it remains for 3 or 4 days. The days after that period are considered "safe" unfertile days. Abstinence is required from 6 days before the earliest day that ovulation was noted to occur during the preceding 6 months until the fifth day after the rise in temperature in the current cycle. Another way of calculating the possible beginning of the fertile days is to subtract 19 days from the shortest complete menstrual cycle of the preceding 6 months. The basal body temperature method is more effective when used with the ovulation method than is either method used alone. The combination of these methods is called the symptothermal method of family planning. Compare **calendar method of family planning, ovulation method of family planning.**

basal bone, **1.** (in prosthodontics) the osseous tissue of the mandible and the maxillae, except for the rami and the processes, which provides support for artificial dentures. **2.** (in orthodontics) the fixed osseous structure that limits the movement of teeth in the creation of a stable occlusion.

basal cell, any one of the cells in the base layer of stratified epithelium.

basal cell acanthoma. See **basal cell papilloma.**

basal cell carcinoma, a malignant, epithelial cell tumor that begins as a papule and enlarges peripherally, developing a central crater that erodes, crusts, and bleeds. Metastasis is rare, but local invasion destroys underlying and adjacent tissue. In 90% of cases, the lesion is seen between the hairline and the upper lip. The primary cause of the cancer is excessive exposure to the sun or to x-rays. Treatment is eradication of the lesion, often by electrodesiccation or cryotherapy. Also called **basal cell epithelioma, basaloma, carcinoma basocellulare, hair matrix carcinoma.** See also **rodent ulcer.**

basal cell papilloma, a benign, epidermal neoplasm characterized by multiple yellow or brown raised oval lesions that usually develop in middle age. Also called **basal cell acanthoma, seborrheic keratosis, seborrheic wart.**

basal ganglia, the islands of gray matter within each cerebral hemisphere, the most important being the caudate nucleus, the putamen, and the pallidium. The basal ganglia are surrounded by the rings of the limbic system and lie between the thalamus of the diencephalon and the white matter of the hemisphere.

basal lamina, a thin, noncellular layer of ground substance lying just under epithelial surfaces. Constituting the uppermost layer of the basement membrane, it can be examined with an electron microscope. Also called **basement lamina.**

basal layer. See **stratum basale.**

basal membrane, a sheet of tissue that forms the outer layer of the choroid and lies just under the pigmented layer of the retina. It is composed of elastic fibers and a thin homogenous layer.

basal metabolic rate (BMR), the amount of energy used in a unit of time by a fasting, resting subject to maintain vital functions. The rate, determined by the amount of oxygen used, is expressed in calories consumed per hour per square meter of body surface area or per kilogram of body weight.

basal metabolism, the amount of energy needed to maintain essential basic body functions, as respiration, circulation, temperature, peristalsis, and muscle tone, measured when the subject is awake and at complete rest, has not eaten for 14 to 18 hours, and is in a comfortable, warm environment. It is expressed as a basal metabolic rate, according to large calories per hour per square meter of body surface.

basaloid carcinoma, a rare, malignant neoplasm of the anal canal containing areas that resemble basal cell carcinoma of the skin, though a basaloid carcinoma is the more rapidly invasive and malignant of the two. The tumor may spread to the skin of the perineum.

basaloma. See **basal cell carcinoma.**

basal seat, (in dentistry) the oral tissues and structures that support a denture. See also **basal seat outline.**

basal seat area, the portion of the oral structures that is available to support a denture. Also called **denture-bearing area, stress-bearing area.**

basal seat outline, (in dentistry) a profile on the mucous membrane or on a cast of the entire oral area to be covered by a denture. See also **basal seat.**

basal temperature. See **basal body temperature.**

base, **1.** a chemical compound that combines with an acid to form a salt. Compare **alkali. 2.** a molecule or radical that takes up or accepts protons. **3.** the major ingredient of a compounded material, particularly one that is used as a medication. Petroleum jelly is frequently used as a base for ointments.

base analogue, an analogue of one of the purine or the pyrimidine bases normally found in ribonucleic acid or deoxyribonucleic acid.

Basedow's goiter /bä′sədōz/, an enlargement of the thyroid gland, characterized by the hypersecretion of thyroid hormone after iodine therapy.

baseline fetal heart rate, the fetal heart rate pattern between uterine contractions. An electronic fetal monitor is used to detect abnormally rapid or slow rates (less than 120 or more than 160 per minute) during labor.

basement lamina. See **basal lamina.**

basement membrane, the fragile, noncellular layer of tissue that secures the overlying layers of stratified epithelium. It is the deepest layer, may contain reticular fibers, and can be selectively stained with silver stains.

base of the heart, the portion of the heart opposite the apex, directed to the right side of the body. It forms the upper border of the heart, lies just below the second rib, and involves primarily the left atrium, part of the right atrium, and the proximal portions of the great vessels. Passing between the base of the heart and the bodies of the fifth to the eighth thoracic vertebrae are the descending aorta, the esophagus, and the thoracic duct.

base of the skull, the floor of the skull, containing the anterior, middle, and posterior cranial fossae and numerous foramina, as the optic foramen, foramen ovale, foramen lacerum, and foramen magnum.

base pair, a pair of nucleotides in a nucleic acid. One of the pair must be a purine, the other a pyrimidine. Base pairing finds guanine paired with cytosine and adenine paired with thymine.

base pairing, (in molecular genetics) the association in nucleic acids of the purine bases adenine and guanine with the pyrimidine bases cytosine, thymine, and uracil. In DNA, adenine always pairs with thymine, and guanine always pairs with cytosine. In RNA, adenine invariably pairs with uracil, and guanine invariably pairs with cytosine.

baseplate, a temporary form that represents the base of a denture, used for making records of maxillomandibular relationships, arranging artificial teeth, or for trial placement in the mouth to assure a precise fit of a denture. Also called **record base, temporary base.** See also **stabilized base, wax base.**

base ratio, the ratio of molar quantities of the bases in ribonucleic and deoxyribonucleic acids.

bas-fond /bäfôN′/, the bottom or fundus of any structure, especially the fundus of the urinary bladder.

basi-, basio-, a combining form meaning 'pertaining to a foundation or a base': *basicranial, basilaris, basiotribe.*

-basia, a combining form meaning 'ability to walk': *abasia, brachybasia, dysbasia.*

BASIC /bā′sik/, abbreviation for *b*eginner's *a*ll-purpose *s*ymbolic *i*nstruction *c*ode, a computer programing language considered the easiest form of programing language to learn.

-basic, a combining form meaning 'relating to or containing alkaline compounds': *ammonobasic, polybasic, tribasic.*

basic amino acid, an amino acid that has a positive electric charge in solution. The basic amino acids are arginine, histidine, and lysine.

basic group identity, (in psychiatry) the shared social characteristics, such as world view, language, and value and ideologic system, that evolve from membership in an ethnic group.

basic health services, the minimum degree of health care considered to be necessary to maintain adequate health and protection from disease.

basifacial, pertaining to the lower portion of the face.

basilar, of or pertaining to a base or a basal area.

basilar artery, the single arterial trunk formed by the junction of the two vertebral arteries at the base of the skull, extending from the inferior to the superior border of the pons, dividing into the left and right cerebral arteries, and supplying the internal ear and parts of the brain through the five branches of each artery. The branches are the pontine, labyrinthine, anterior inferior cerebellar, superior cerebellar, and posterior cerebral.

basilar artery insufficiency syndrome, the composite of clinical indicators associated with insufficient blood flow through the basilar artery, a condition that may be caused by arterial occlusion. Some of the common signs of this syndrome are dizziness, blindness, numbness, depression, dysarthria, dysphagia, and weakness on one side of the body.

basilar membrane, the cellular structure that forms the floor of the cochlear duct and is supported by bony and fibrous projections from the cochlear wall. It provides a fibrous base for the spiral organ of Corti.

basilar plexus, the venous network interlaced between the layers of the dura mater over the basilar portion of the occipital bone. It connects the two petrosal sinuses and communicates with the anterior vertebral venous plexus.

basilar sulcus, the sulcus that cradles the basilar artery, in the midline of the pons.

basilic vein /bəsil′ik/, one of the four superficial veins of the arm, beginning in the ulnar part of the dorsal venous network and running proximally on the posterior surface of the ulnar side of the forearm. It veers toward the anterior surface of the forearm distal to the elbow and is joined by the median cubital vein, then ascends obliquely between the biceps brachii and the pronator teres and crosses the brachial artery. It then runs proximally along the medial border of the biceps brachii, pierces the deep fascia, and ascends to join the brachial vein to form the axillary vein. Compare **dorsal digital vein, median antebrachial vein.**

basiloma /bas′ilō′mə/, *pl.* **basilomas, basilomata,** a carcinoma composed of basal cells. A kind of basiloma is **basiloma terebrans.** Also called **basaloma.**

basiloma terebrans /ter′əbrənz/, a basal cell epithelioma that is invasive.

basio-. See **basi-.**

basioccipital, of or pertaining to the basilar process of the occipital bone.

basion, the midpoint on the anterior margin of the foramen magnum of the occipital bone, opposite the opisthion in the middle of the posterior margin.

basis pedunculi cerebri. See **crus cerebri.**

basket cell, a degenerated leukocyte seen on a blood smear during laboratory examination.

basophil /bā′səfil/, a granulocytic white blood cell characterized by a segmented nucleus that contains granules that stain blue when exposed to a basic dye. Basophils represent 1% or less of the total white blood cell count. The relative number of basophils increases in myeloproliferative diseases and decreases in severe allergic reactions. Compare **eosinophil, neutrophil.** See also **agranulocyte, differential white blood cell count, granulocyte, leukocyte, polymorphonuclear leukocyte.**

basophilic adenoma, a tumor of the pituitary gland composed of cells that can be stained with basic dyes. Cushing's syndrome is often caused by a basophilic adenoma. Compare **acidophilic adenoma, chromophobic adenoma.**

basophilic leukemia, an acute or chronic malignant neoplasm of blood-forming tissues, characterized by large numbers of immature basophilic granulocytes in peripheral circulation and in tissues. See also **acute myelocytic leukemia.**

basophilic stippling, the abnormal presence of punctate, basophilic granules in the red blood cells, observed under the microscope on a gram-stained smear of the blood. Stippling is characteristic of lead poisoning. See also **basophil, lead poisoning.**

basosquamous cell carcinoma /bā′sōskwā′məs/, a malignant epidermal tumor composed of basal and squamous cells.

Bassen-Kornzweig syndrome. See **abetalipoproteinemia.**

batch processing, a processing mode used with some large computers in which only one user is serviced at a time and groups of similar transactions are accumulated to be processed simultaneously.

bath, (in the hospital) a cleansing procedure performed daily by or for almost all patients to help prevent infection, preserve the unbroken condition of the skin, stimulate circulation, promote oxygen intake, maintain muscle tone and joint mobility, and provide comfort.

■ METHOD: The bath may be a bed or tub bath, a shower, or a partial bath, depending on the patient's condition and preference and the room temperature. The bath period may be used to instruct the patient on hygienic measures. Observations are made of the general cleanliness and odor of the patient's body, the color, dryness, turgor, and elasticity of the skin, the condition of the hair, hands, feet, fingernails and toenails. Any discoloration, abrasion, rash, discharge, perineal or rectal irritation, clubbing of the digits, hair loss, or evidence of lice is carefully noted. Mild soap and water are used for the bath, and a lanolin-based lotion is used for the afterbath massage. The patient's hair is combed daily and shampooed as desired; finger- and toenails are cleaned and trimmed whenever required. Petroleum jelly or other suitable lubricant and a thin layer of cornstarch are applied to the perineal and perianal areas if indicated.

■ NURSING ORDERS: The nurse gives the bed bath in a setting that provides privacy for the patient. Firm, gentle strokes are used to wash, dry, and massage the person; vigorous rubbing is avoided. The partial bath is given with the patient seated in or on the side of the bed, or in a chair. Self-help is encouraged, and the procedure is completed as soon as possible to avoid chilling. In preparation for a tub bath, the nurse checks the safety strips in the bottom of the tub and the temperature of the water, and assists the patient into the tub. Precautions are taken to avoid chilling, and on completion of the bath the nurse may help the patient out of the tub. In preparation for a shower, the nurse explains the operation of the dials regulating the water temperature, provides a bath mat, and cautions the patient not to become chilled.

■ OUTCOME CRITERIA: A daily bath helps prevent decubiti, provides an opportunity to assess external signs of disease and effects of therapy, and improves the patient's sense of well-being and self-esteem.

bathesthesia /bath′əsthē′zhə/, a deep sensibility, as that associated with organs or structures beneath the surface of the body, as muscles and joints. Also called **bathyesthesia** /bath'ē·əsthē'zhə/.

bathmic evolution. See **orthogenic evolution.**

bathy-, batho-, a combining form meaning 'pertaining to depth, deep': *bathycentesis, bathypnea, bathomorphic.*

bathycardia /bath'əkär'dē·ə/, an abnormal but nonpathologic condition characterized by an unusually low position of the heart in the chest.

Batten's disease, a progressive childhood encephalopathy with disturbed metabolism of polyunsaturated fatty acids.

battered woman syndrome (BWS), repeated episodes of physical assault on a woman by the man with whom she lives, often resulting in serious physical and psychologic damage to the woman. Such violence tends to follow a predictable pattern. The violent episodes usually follow verbal argument and accusation and are accompanied by verbal abuse. Almost any subject—housekeeping, money, childrearing—may begin the episode. Over time, the violent episodes escalate in frequency and severity. Once a month becomes once a week; a shove becomes a punch. Most battered women report that they thought that the assaults would stop; but, unfortunately, study shows that the longer the women stay in the relationship the more likely they are to be seriously injured. Less and less provocation seems to be enough to trigger an attack once the syndrome has begun. The use of alcohol increases the severity of the assault; a man who usually shoves or slaps his partner is more likely to punch or kick her if he is drunk. Other drugs do not have this effect. The man is more likely to be abusive as the drug is wearing off. Battering occurs in cycles of violence. The first phase is characterized by the man acting increasingly irritable, edgy, and tense. Verbal abuse, insults, and criticism increase, and shoves or slaps begin. The second phase is the time of the acute, violent activity. As the tension mounts, the woman becomes unable to placate the man, and she may argue or defend herself. The man uses this as the justification for his anger and assaults her, often saying that he is "teaching her a lesson." The third stage is characterized by apology and remorse on the part of the man, with promises of change. The calm continues until tension builds again. The battered woman syndrome occurs at all socioeconomic levels, and one half to three quarters of female assault victims are the victims of an attack by a lover or husband. It is estimated that in the United States between one and two million women a year are beaten by their husbands. Men who grew up in homes in which the father abused the mother are more likely to beat their wives than are men who lived in nonviolent homes. Personal and cultural attitudes also affect the incidence of wife battering. Aggressive behavior is a normal part of male socialization in most cultures; physical aggression may be condoned as a means of resolving a conflict. In some studies, personality profiles obtained by psychologic testing revealed the typical battered woman to be reserved, withdrawn, depressed, and anxious, with low self-esteem. The parents of such women encouraged compliance, were not physically affectionate, and socially restricted their daughters' independence, preventing the widening of social contact that normally occurs in adolescence. Victims of the battered woman syndrome are often afraid to leave the man and the situation. Nurses are in an excellent position to offer assistance to battered women in several ways, because encouraging a woman to talk about the battering and the injuries may help her to admit what she may have been too embarrassed to reveal even to her parents. A realistic appraisal of the situation is then possible; the woman often wants to hear that the nurse thinks the battering will not recur, but the nurse can tell her only that the usual pattern is for the abuse to continue and to become more severe. The woman may be referred to the social service department or given directions for contacting special community agencies, as a battered women's shelter or a hotline to a counseling service. Caring for and counseling a battered woman often require great patience because she is usually ambivalent about her situation and may be confused to the point of believing that she deserves the assaults she has suffered. Records are maintained to document the extent of the problem, including the form of abuse reported, the injuries sustained, and a summary of similar incidents and previous admissions.

battery, **1.** a complex of two or more electrolytic cells connected together to form a single source providing direct current or voltage. **2.** a series or a combination of tests to determine the cause of a particular illness or the degree of proficiency in a particular skill or discipline. **3.** the unlawful use of force upon a person. See **assault.**

Battey bacillus /bat'ē/, any of a group of atypical mycobacteria, including *Mycobacteria avium* and *M. intracellulare,* that cause a chronic pulmonary disease resembling tuberculosis. These organisms are resistant to most of the common bacteriostatic and antibiotic medications. Surgical resection of involved lung tissue may be necessary and may improve the outcome in serious cases. Rest, good nutrition, and general supportive care are usually recommended. Compare **tuberculosis.**

battledore placenta /bat'əldôr'/, a placenta to which the umbilical cord is attached at the periphery.

Battle's sign, a small hemorrhagic spot behind the ear that appears in cases may indicate a fracture of a bone of the lower skull.

batyl alcohol, an alcohol found in fish liver oil that is used to treat bracken poisoning in cattle.

baud, binary units per second, used as a measure of the speed with which a computer device transmits information.

Baudelocque's diameter. See **external conjugate.**

Baudelocque's method, (in obstetrics) a maneuver used to convert a face presentation to a vertex presentation. The operator flexes the fetal head vaginally and applies counterpressure to the back of the head abdominally while an assistant rotates the fetus in the direction of flexion until the vertex is fixed in the pelvis.

Baynton's bandage /bān′tənz/, a spiral adhesive wrap applied to the leg over a dressing, used in the treatment of indolent ulcers of the leg.

bayonet angle former, a hoe-shaped paired cutting instrument for accenting angles in a Class 3 tooth cavity. The cutting edge of this device is at an angle to the axis of the blade that is parallel to the axis of the shaft. Compare **angle former.**

bayonet condenser, (in dentistry) an instrument for compacting restorative material. It has an offset nib device and a shank with right angle bends for varying the line of force, used primarily in condensing direct filling gold. There are many variations in angles, length, and nib diameter.

Baypen, a trademark for a semisynthetic penicillin antibiotic (mezlocillin).

BBB, abbreviation for **blood-brain barrier.**

B cell, a type of lymphocyte that originates in the bone marrow. A precursor of the plasma cell upon suitable antigenic stimulation, it is one of the two lymphocytes that play a major role in the body's immunologic response. Compare **T cell.** See also **plasma cell.**

BCG, abbreviation for **bacille Calmette-Guérin.**

BCG vaccine, an active immunizing agent prepared from bacille Calmette-Guérin.

■ INDICATION: It is prescribed most commonly for immunization against tuberculosis.

■ CONTRAINDICATIONS: Hypogammaglobulinemia, immunosuppression, or concomitant use of corticosteroids or isoniazid prohibits its use. It is not given after a vaccination for smallpox, nor is it given to patients with a positive tuberculin reaction or a burn.

■ ADVERSE EFFECTS: Among the most serious adverse reactions are anaphylaxis and disseminated pulmonary tuberculosis. Pain, inflammation, and granuloma may develop at site of injection.

BCNU. See **carmustine.**

B complex vitamins, a large group of water soluble substances that includes **vitamin B_1 (thiamine), vitamin B_2 (riboflavin), vitamin B_3 (niacin), vitamin B_6 (pyridoxine), vitamin B_{12} (cyanocobalamin), biotin, choline, carnitine, folic acid, inositol,** and **paraaminobenzoic acid.** The B complex vitamins are essential in converting carbohydrates into glucose to provide energy, for metabolism of fats and proteins, for normal functioning of the nervous system, for maintenance of muscle tone in the GI tract, and for the health of skin, hair, eyes, mouth, and liver. They are found in brewer's yeast, liver, whole grain cereals, nuts, eggs, meats, fish, and vegetables and are produced by the intestinal bacteria. Maintaining milk-free diets or taking antibiotics may destroy these bacteria. Symptoms of vitamin B deficiency include nervousness, depression, insomnia, neuritis, anemia, alopecia, acne or other skin disorders, and hypercholesterolemia. See also specific vitamins.

b.d. See **b.i.d.**

Be, symbol for **beryllium.**

beaded, **1.** of or having a resemblance to a row of beads. **2.** of or pertaining to bacterial colonies that develop along the inoculation line in various stab cultures. **3.** of or pertaining to stained bacteria that develop more deeply stained beadlike granules.

beaker cell. See **goblet cell.**

beam, a bedframe fitting for pulleys and weights, used in the treatment of patients requiring weight traction. See **Balkan frame.**

BEAM /bēm, bē′ē′ā′em′/, abbreviation for **brain electric activity map.**

bean, the pod-enclosed flattened seed of numerous leguminous plants. Beans used in pharmocologic preparations are alphabetized by specific name.

Becker's muscular dystrophy, a chronic degenerative disease of the muscles, characterized by progressive weakness. It occurs in childhood between 8 and 20 years of age. It occurs less frequently, progresses more slowly, and has a better prognosis than the more common pseudohypertrophic form of muscular dystrophy. The pathophysiology of the disease is not understood; it is transmitted genetically as an autosomal recessive trait. Also called **benign pseudohypertrophic muscular dystrophy.** Compare **Duchenne's muscular dystrophy.**

Beck I operation, a surgical procedure to provide collateral circulation to the heart. The operation roughens the surface of the epicardium and the parietal lining of the pericardium, applies an irritant, as powdered asbestos, to these surfaces, partially closes the coronary sinus at its entrance to the right atrium, and grafts the parietal pericardium and the mediastinal fat to the myocardium. Compare **Beck II operation.**

Beck II operation, an operation in two stages that provides collateral circulation to the heart. In the first stage, a venous graft is placed between the aorta and the coronary sinus to shunt arterial blood. In the second stage of the procedure, executed 2 to 3 weeks after the first stage, the coronary sinus is partially closed to raise pressure within the sinus and force oxygenated blood from the aorta to flow into the coronary vessels. Compare **Beck I operation.**

Beck's Diagnostic Inventory (BDI), a system of classifying a total of 18 criteria of depressive illness. It was developed by A.T. Beck in the 1970s as a diagnostic and therapeutic tool for the treatment of childhood affective disorders. The DBI is similar to the 21-criteria DSM-III diagnostic system of the 1980s except that the DSM-III scale includes loss of interest, restlessness, and sulkiness, which are missing from the BDI, while the Beck inventory lists somatic complaints and loneliness, which are criteria not included in the DSM-III inventory. Also called **Beck depression inventory (BDI).** See also **DSM-III.**

Beck's triad, a combination of three symptoms that characterize cardiac compression: high venous pressure, low arterial pressure, and a small, quiet heart.

Beckwith's syndrome, an hereditary disorder of unknown cause associated with neonatal hypoglycemia and hyperinsulinism. Clinical manifestations include gigantism, macroglossia, omphalocele or umbilical hernia, visceromegaly, hyperplasia of the kidney and pancreas, extreme enlargement of the cells of the adrenal cortex, and often various other abnormalities. Treatment consists of adequate glucose, diazoxide, and glucocorticoid therapy. Subtotal pancreatectomy is often necessary in cases of beta cell hyperplasia, nesidioblastosis, or beta cell tumor of the pancreas.

Beckwith-Wiedemann syndrome. See **EMG syndrome.**

beclomethasone dipropionate, a glucocorticoid.

■ INDICATION: It is prescribed in an inhaler in the treatment of bronchial asthma.

■ CONTRAINDICATIONS: Status asthmaticus, acute asthma, or known hypersensitivity to this drug prohibits its use.

■ ADVERSE EFFECTS: Among the more serious adverse reactions of systemic administration are the symptoms of adrenal insufficiency. Hoarseness, sore throat, and fungal infections of the oropharynx and larynx may occur.

becquerel (Bq), the SI unit of radioactivity, equal to one radioactive decay per second. See **curie.**

bed, (in anatomy) a supporting matrix of tissue, as the nail beds of modified epidermis over which the fingernails and the toenails move as they grow.

bedbug, a blood-sucking arthropod of either the species *Cimex lectularius* or the species *C. hemipterus* that feeds on humans and other animals. The bedbug can be removed after covering it with petrolatum. The bite, which causes itching, pain, and redness, can be treated with a lotion or cream containing a corticosteroid or other topical antiinflammatory or analgesic preparation.

Bednar's aphthae /bed′närz/, the small, yellowish, slightly elevated ulcerated patches that occur on the posterior portion of the hard palate of infants who place infected objects in their mouths. It is also associated with marasmus. Compare **Epstein's pearls, thrush.**

bedside manner, the behavior of a nurse or doctor as perceived by a patient.

bedsore. See **decubitus ulcer.**

Bee cell pessary. See **pessary.**

beef tapeworm. See ***Taenia saginata.***

beef tapeworm infection, an infection caused by the tapeworm *Taenia saginata,* transmitted to humans when they eat contaminated beef. The adult worm can live for years in the intestine of humans without causing any symptoms. The infection is rarely found in North America and Western Europe where beef is carefully inspected before being made available and is often thoroughly cooked before eating, but it is commonly found in other parts of the world. See **tapeworm infection.**

bee sting, an injury caused by the venom of bees, usually accompanied by pain and swelling. The stinger of the honeybee usually remains implanted and should be removed. Pain may be alleviated by application of an ice pack or a paste of sodium bicarbonate and water. Serious reactions may result from multiple stings, stings on some areas of the head, or the injection of venom directly into the circulatory system. In a hypersensitive person, a single bee sting may result in death because of anaphylactic shock and bronchospasm. Hypersensitive individuals are encouraged to carry emergency treatment supplies with them when the possibility of bee sting exists. Compare **wasp.**

behavior, **1.** the manner in which a person acts or performs. **2.** any or all of the activities of a person, including physical actions, which are observed directly, and mental activity, which is inferred and interpreted. Kinds of behavior include **abnormal behavior, automatic behavior, invariable behavior,** and **variable behavior.**

behavioral objective, a goal in therapy or research that concerns an act or a specific behavior or pattern of behaviors.

behavioral reflex. See **conditioned response.**

behavioral science, any of the various interrelated disciplines, as psychiatry, psychology, sociology, and anthropology, that observes and studies human activity, including psychologic and emotional development, interpersonal relationships, values, and mores.

behavior disorder, any of a group of antisocial behavior patterns occurring primarily in children and adolescents, as overaggressiveness, overactivity, destructiveness, cruelty, truancy, lying, disobedience, perverse sexual activity, criminality, alcoholism, and drug addiction. The most common motivating force for such reactions is hostility, which is manifested either overtly or covertly and is precipitated by a disturbed relationship between the child and his parents, an unstable home situation, and, in some cases, organic brain dysfunction. Behavior disorders may be symptomatic of other neuroses or psychoses, as childhood schizophrenia. Treatment may include psychotherapy, milieu therapy, medication, and family counseling. See also **antisocial personality disorder.**

behaviorism, a school of psychology founded by John B. Watson that studies and interprets behavior by observing measurable responses to stimuli without reference to consciousness, mental states, or subjective phenomena, as ideas and emotions. See also **neobehaviorism.**

behaviorist, a disciple of the school of behaviorism.

behavioristic psychology. See **behaviorism.**

behavior modification. See **behavior therapy.**

behavior systems model, a conceptual framework describing factors that may affect the stability of a person's behavior. The model examines systems of behavior, not the behavior of an individual at any particular time. In one model, behavior is defined as an integrated response to stimuli. Several subsystems of behavior form man's eight microsystems, which are: ingestion, elimination, dependency, sex, achievement, affiliation, aggression, and restoration. Each subsystem comprises several structural components called "imperatives," which are goal, set, choice, action, and support. The goal of nursing care is to attain, maintain, or restore balance of the subsystems of behavior for the stability of the patient.

behavior therapy, a kind of psychotherapy that attempts to modify observable, maladjusted patterns of behavior by the substitution of a new response or set of responses to a given stimulus. The treatment techniques involve the methods, concepts, and procedures derived from experimental psychology and include assertiveness training, aversion therapy, contingency management, flooding, modeling, operant conditioning, and systemic desensitization. Also called **behavior modification.** See also **biofeedback.**

Behçet's disease, a rare and severe illness of unknown cause, mostly affecting young males and characterized by severe uveitis and retinal vasculitis. Some other signs are optic atrophy and aphthalike lesions of the mouth and the genitals, indicating diffuse vasculitis. Also called **Behçet's syndrome.**

Behla's bodies. See **Plimmer's bodies.**

BEI, abbreviation for **butanol extractable iodine.**

bejel /bej′əl/, a nonvenereal form of syphilis prevalent among children in the Middle East and North Africa, caused by the spirochete *Treponema pallidum II*. It is transmitted by person to person contact and by the sharing of drinking and eating utensils. The primary lesion is usually on or near the mouth, appearing as a mucous patch, followed by the development of pimplelike sores on the trunk, arms, and legs. Chronic ulceration of the nose and soft palate occurs in the advanced stages of the infection. Destructive changes in the tissues of the heart, central nervous system, and mouth, often associated with the venereal form of syphilis, rarely develop. Intramuscular injection of penicillin is effective in curing the infection, but if extensive tissue destruction has occurred, scar tissue forms and may be permanently disfiguring.

Békésy audiometry /bek′əsē/, a method of testing hearing in which the subject presses a signal button while listening to a pure tone that is progressively diminished in intensity and releases the button when the sound no longer is heard. Continuous and interrupted tones are used in the test.

bel, a unit that expresses intensity of sound. It is the logarithm (to the base 10) of the ratio of the power of any specific sound to the power of a reference sound. The most common reference sound has a power of 10^{-16} watts per cm^2, or the approximate minimum intensity of sound at 1000 cycles per second, that is perceptible to the human ear. An increase of 1 bel approximately doubles the intensity or loudness of most sounds.

belching. See **eructation.**

belladonna, the dried leaves, roots, and flowering or fruiting tops of *Atropa belladonna*, a common perennial called deadly nightshade, containing the alkaloids hyoscine and hyoscyamine. Hyoscyamine is a source of atropine.

bellows murmur, a blowing sound, as air moving in and out of a bellows.

Bell's law, an axiom stating that the ventral spinal roots are motor and the dorsal spinal roots are sensory. Also called **Bell-Magendie law, Magendie's law.**

Bell's mania, *obsolete*. a mood disorder characterized by acute delirium. See also **delirium, mania.**

Bell's palsy, a paralysis of the facial nerve, resulting from trauma to the nerve, compression of the nerve by a tumor, or, possibly, an unknown infection. Any or all branches of the nerve may be affected. The person may not be able to open an eye or close the mouth. The condition may be unilateral or bilateral, transient or permanent. Plastic surgery may reduce the deformity.

Bell's phenomenon, a sign of peripheral facial paralysis, manifested by the upward and outward rolling of the eyeball when the affected individual tries to close the eyelid.

belly. See **abdomen.**

belly button. See **umbilicus.**

belonephobia /bel′ənəfō′bē·ə/, a morbid fear of sharp-pointed objects, especially needles and pins.

Benadon, a trademark for vitamin B_6.

Benadryl, a trademark for an antihistaminic (diphenhydramine hydrochloride).

Bence Jones protein /bens/, a protein found almost exclusively in the urine of patients with multiple myeloma. The protein constitutes the light chain component of myeloma globulin; it coagulates at temperatures of 45° to 55° C and redissolves completely or partially on boiling. See also **multiple myeloma, protein.**

bench research, *informal*. (in medicine) any research done in a controlled laboratory setting using other than human subjects.

Bendectin, a trademark for a fixed-combination drug containing an antihistamine (doxylamine succinate) and a vitamin (pyridoxine hydrochloride), used for treating nausea in pregnancy.

bending fracture, a fracture indirectly caused by the bending of an extremity, as of the foot or of the big toe.

bendrofluazide. See **bendroflumethiazide.**

bendroflumethiazide /ben′drōflo͞o′məthī′əzīd/, a diuretic and antihypertensive.

■ INDICATIONS: It is prescribed in the treatment of hypertension and edema.

■ CONTRAINDICATIONS: Anuria or known hypersensitivity to this drug, to other thiazide medication, or to sulfonamide derivatives prohibits its use.

■ ADVERSE EFFECTS: Among the more serious adverse reactions are hypokalemia, hyperglycemia, hyperuricemia, and various hypersensitivity reactions.

bends. See **decompression sickness.**

Benedict's qualitative test, a test for sugar in the urine based on the reduction by glucose of cupric ions to a colored cuprous oxide precipitate when it is placed in an alkaline solution. Eight drops, or 0.5 ml, of urine are added to 5 ml of Benedict's solution; the mixture is heated in boiling water for 5 minutes and then cooled. Formation of an orange or red precipitate indicates more than

2% sugar (called 4+), yellow indicates 1% to 2% sugar (called 3+), olive green indicates 0.5% to 1% sugar (called 2+), and green indicates less than 0.5% sugar (called 1+). Also called **Benedict's method.**

Benemid, a trademark for a uricosuric (probenecid).

benign, (of a tumor) noncancerous and therefore not an immediate threat, even though treatment eventually may be required for health or cosmetic reasons. See **benign neoplasm.** Compare **malignant.**

benign hypertension, a misnomer implying an innocent elevation of blood pressure. Because any sustained elevation of blood pressure may adversely affect health, it is incorrect to refer to the condition as "benign." See also **essential hypertension.**

benign intracranial hypertension. See **pseudotumor cerebri.**

benign juvenile melanoma, a benign, pink or fuchsia raised papule with a scaly surface, usually on a cheek and occurring most commonly in children between 9 and 13 years of age. It may be mistaken for a malignant melanoma. Also called **compound melanocytoma, spindle cell nevus, Spitz nevus.**

benign mesenchymoma, a benign neoplasm that has two or more definitely recognizable mesenchymal elements in addition to fibrous tissue.

benign neoplasm, a tumor, characteristically localized, that has a fibrous capsule, limited potential for growth, a regular shape, and cells that are well differentiated. A benign neoplasm does not invade surrounding tissue or metastasize to distant sites. It causes harm only by pressure and does not usually recur after surgical excision. Some kinds of benign neoplasms are **adenoma, fibroma, hemangioma,** and **lipoma.** See also **malignant neoplasm.**

benign prostatic hypertrophy, enlargement of the prostate gland, common among men after the age of 50. The condition is not malignant or inflammatory but is usually progressive and may lead to obstruction of the urethra and to interference with the flow of urine, possibly causing frequency of urination, the need to urinate during the night, pain, and urinary tract infections. Treatment consists of conservative measures: regular sexual release, hot baths, prostatic massage, avoidance of alcohol or excessive fluid intake, and voiding on the urge to do so. Surgical resection of the enlarged prostate is sometimes necessary. Compare **prostatitis.** See also **prostatectomy.**

benign pseudohypertrophic muscular dystrophy. See **Becker's muscular dystrophy.**

benign stupor, a state of apathy or lethargy, as occurs in severe depression.

benign thrombocytosis. See **thrombocytosis.**

benign tumor, a neoplasm that does not invade other tissues or metastasize in other sites. A benign tumor is usually well encapsulated, and its cells exhibit less anaplase than those of a malignant growth. Some benign tumors must be excised to prevent damage or death, because the tumor may grow to occupy space needed by an organ or tissue.

Bennett angle, (in dentistry) the angle formed by the sagittal plane and the path of the advancing condyle during lateral mandibular movement, as viewed in the horizontal plane.

Bennet's small corpuscle. See **Drysdale's corpuscle.**

Bennett's fracture, a fracture that runs obliquely through the base of the first metacarpal bone and into the carpometacarpal joint, detaching the greater part of the articular facet. Bennett's fracture may be associated with dorsal subluxation or with dislocation of the first metacarpal.

Benoquin, a trademark for a depigmenting agent (monobenzone).

benoxinate hydrochloride, a topical anesthetic.

▪ INDICATIONS: It is used for ophthalmologic anesthesia in surgical procedures, in removing sutures or foreign objects from the eye, and in tonometry.

▪ CONTRAINDICATION: Known hypersensitivity to this drug prohibits its use.

▪ ADVERSE EFFECTS: Among the more serious adverse reactions are slight pain when first instilled, corneal damage with excessive or prolonged use, and hypersensitivity reactions.

Benoxl, a trademark for a topical antiseptic (benzoyl peroxide), used in the treatment of acne.

bent fracture, an incomplete greenstick fracture.

bentonite, colloidal, hydrated aluminum silicate, that, when added to water, swells to approximately 12 times its dry size. It is used as a bulk laxative and as a base for skin care preparations.

Bentyl, a trademark for an anticholinergic antispasmodic (dicyclomine hydrochloride).

benzalkonium chloride, a disinfectant and fungicide prepared in an aqueous solution in various strengths.

benzathine penicillin G. See **penicillin G benzathine.**

Benzedrex, a trademark for an adrenergic vasoconstrictor (propylhexedrine).

Benzedrine, a trademark for a central nervous system stimulant (amphetamine sulfate).

benzene poisoning, a toxic condition caused by ingestion of benzene, the inhalation of benzene fumes, or exposure to benzene-related products such as toluene or xylene, characterized by nausea, headache, dizziness, and incoordination. In acute cases, respiratory failure or ventricular fibrillation may cause death. Chronic exposure may result in aplastic anemia or a form of leukemia. Benzene poisoning by inhalation is treated with ventilatory assistance and oxygen; poisoning by ingestion is treated with gastric intubation, removal of the poison, and lavage. See also **nitrobenzene poisoning.**

benzethonium chloride /ben′zəthō′nē•əm/, a topical antiinfective used for disinfecting the skin and for treating some infections of the eye, nose, and throat. It is also used as a preservative in some pharmaceutic preparations.

benzhexol hydrochloride. See **trihexyphenidyl hydrochloride.**

benzocaine, a local anesthetic agent derived from aminobenzoic acid, used in many over the counter compounds for pruritus and pain. Benzocaine has a low incidence of toxicity, but sensitization to it may occur with prolonged or frequent use. Topical application of benzocaine may cause methemoglobinemia in infants and small children. A minimum of 5% benzocaine is required in a compound to be effective.

benzodiazepine derivative /ben′zōdī•az′əpin/, one of a group of psychotropic agents, including the tranquilizers chlordiazepoxide, diazepam, oxazepam, and chlorazepate, prescribed to alleviate anxiety, and the hypnotics flurazepam and nitrazepam, prescribed in the treatment of insomnia. Some of the drugs have further clinical application: Diazepam is often prescribed to relieve spasm of the muscles and to increase the seizure threshold. Tolerance and physical dependence occur with prolonged high dosage. Withdrawal symptoms, including seizures, and acute psychosis, may follow abrupt discontinuation. Adverse reactions to the benzodiazepines include drowsiness, ataxia, and a paradoxical increase in aggression and hostility; these reactions are not commonly seen in association with the usual recommended dosage.

benzoic acid /benzō′ik/, a keratolytic agent, usually used with salicylic acid as an ointment in the treatment of athlete's foot and ringworm of the scalp. It has little antifungal action but makes deep infections accessible to more potent preparation. Mild irritation may occur at the site of application.

benzonatate /benzō′nənāt/, a nonopiate antitussive.

■ INDICATION: It is prescribed to suppress the cough reflex.

■ CONTRAINDICATION: Known hypersensitivity to this drug prohibits its use.

■ ADVERSE EFFECTS: A serious reaction may be convulsions. Vertigo, headache, constipation, and hypersensitivity reactions, usually mild, sometimes occur.

benzoyl peroxide, an antibacterial, keratolytic, drying agent.

■ INDICATION: It is prescribed in the treatment of acne.

■ CONTRAINDICATIONS: Known hypersensitivity to this drug prohibits its use. It is not used in the eye, on inflamed skin, or on mucous membranes.

■ ADVERSE EFFECTS: Among the more serious adverse reactions are excessive drying and allergic contact sensitization.

benzphetamine hydrochloride, a sympathomimetic used as an anorexic agent.

■ INDICATION: It is prescribed to decrease the appetite in the treatment of obesity.

■ CONTRAINDICATIONS: Arteriosclerosis, cardiovascular disease, hypertension, glaucoma, hyperthyroidism, or known hypersensitivity to this or other sympathomimetic drugs prohibits its use.

■ ADVERSE EFFECTS: Among the more serious adverse reactions are restlessness, insomnia, tachycardia, increased blood pressure, and dry mouth.

benzquinamide /benzkwin′əmīd/, an antiemetic.

■ INDICATIONS: It is prescribed in the treatment of postoperative nausea and vomiting.

■ CONTRAINDICATIONS: Severe hypertension, severe cardiovascular disease, or known hypersensitivity to this drug prohibits its use. It is not usually administered to children or to pregnant women.

■ ADVERSE EFFECTS: Among the most serious adverse reactions are sudden increase in blood pressure and cardiac arrhythmia. Drowsiness, chills, and shivering are commonly noted.

benzthiazide, a diuretic and antihypertensive.

■ INDICATIONS: It is prescribed in the treatment of hypertension and edema.

■ CONTRAINDICATIONS: Anuria or known hypersensitivity to this drug, to other thiazide medication, or to sulfonamide derivatives prohibits its use.

■ ADVERSE EFFECTS: Among the more serious adverse effects are hypokalemia, hyperglycemia, hyperuricemia, and hypersensitivity reactions.

benztropine mesylate, an anticholinergic and antihistaminic agent.

■ INDICATIONS: It is prescribed as adjunctive therapy in the treatment of all forms of parkinsonism.

■ CONTRAINDICATIONS: Known sensitivity to this drug prohibitis its use, and it is not administered to children under 3 years of age.

■ ADVERSE EFFECTS: Among the most serious adverse reactions are blurred vision, xerostoma, nausea and vomiting, constipation, depression, and skin rash.

benzyl alcohol, a clear, colorless, oily liquid, derived from certain balsams, used as a topical anesthetic and as a bacteriostatic agent in solutions for injection. Also called **phenyl carbinol, phenyl methanol.**

benzyl benzoate, a clear, oily liquid with a pleasant, aromatic odor. It is used as an agent to destroy lice and scabies, as a solvent, and as a flavor for gum.

benzyl carbonol. See **phenylethyl alcohol.**

benzylpenicillin. See **penicillin G.**

Berger rhythm, Berger wave. See **alpha wave.**

Bergonié-Tréboneau law /ber′gônē′trā′bônō′/, (in radiotherapy) a rule stating that the radiosensitivity of tissue depends on the number of undifferentiated cells, their mitotic activity, and the length of time they are actively proliferating.

beriberi /ber′ēber′ē/, a disease of the peripheral nerves caused by a deficiency of or an inability to assimilate thiamine. It is frequently the result of a diet limited to polished white rice, and it occurs in endemic form in eastern and southern Asia. Rare cases in the United States are associated with stressful conditions, as hypothyroidism, infections, pregnancy, lactation, and chronic alcoholism. Symptoms are fatigue, diarrhea, appetite and weight loss, disturbed nerve function causing paralysis and wasting of limbs, edema, and heart failure. Kinds of beriberi include alcoholic beriberi, atrophic beriberi, cardiac beriberi, and cerebral beriberi. Administration of thiamine prevents and cures most cases of the disease. Also called **athiaminosis, kakke disease.** See also **thiamine.**

berkelium (Bk), an artificial radioactive transuranic element. Its atomic number is 97; its atomic weight is 247.

Berlock dermatitis, an abnormal skin condition, characterized by hyperpigmentation and skin lesions, caused by a unique reaction to psoralen-type photosynthesizers, commonly used in perfumes, colognes, and pomades, as oil of bergamot. This condition affects mostly women and children and may result from the use of products containing psoralens and from exposure to ultraviolet light. Although only about 5% of the radiation of the sun is ultraviolet light and much of that is absorbed by oxygen and ozone, the level of ultraviolet radiation reaching the earth, especially on a sunny day, is sufficient to cause the lesion to appear. Also spelled **Berloque dermatitis.**

■ OBSERVATIONS: Berlock dermatitis commonly produces an acute erythematous reaction, as that associated with sunburn. The area affected becomes hyperpigmented and surrounded by darker pigmentation. Areas of the neck where perfume containing oil of bergamot is applied become often affected by pendantlike lesions. Diagnosis is based on the appearance of such signs and on patient history which may include recent exposure to psoralens.

■ INTERVENTION: Treatment of Berlock dermatitis seeks to identify and eliminate the cause of the condition. Topical steroids may be administered to relieve discomfort.

■ NURSING CONSIDERATIONS: Patients with Berlock dermatitis benefit from advice about the complications of prolonged exposure to sunlight and ultraviolet light. They also appreciate the justifiable reassurance that the lesions will vanish within a few months.

Bernard-Soulier syndrome /bernär′sōōlyā′/, a coagulation disorder characterized by an absence of or a deficiency in the ability of the platelets to aggregate because of the relative lack of an essential glycoprotein in the membranes of the platelets. On microscopic examination the platelets appear large and dispersed. The use of aspirin may provoke hemorrhage in people who have this condition. After trauma and surgery, loss of blood may be greater than normal and transfusion may be required.

Bernoulli's principle /bərnōō′lēz/, (in physics) a principle stating that the sum of the velocity and the kinetic energy of a fluid flowing through a tube is constant. The greater the velocity the less the lateral pressure on the wall of the tube. Thus, if an artery is narrowed by an atherosclerotic plaque, the flow of blood through the constriction increases in velocity and decreases in lateral pressure. Also called **Bernoulli's law.**

Bernstein test. See **acid perfusion test.**

berry aneurysm, a small, saccular dilatation of the wall of a cerebral artery, occurring most frequently at the junctures of vessels in the circle of Willis. A berry aneurysm may be the result of a congenital developmental defect and may rupture without warning, causing intracranial hemorrhage.

berylliosis /bəril′ē·ō′sis/, poisoning that results from the inhalation of dusts or vapors containing beryllium or beryllium compounds. It is characterized by granulomas throughout the body and by diffuse pulmonary fibrosis, resulting in a dry cough, shortness of breath, and chest pain. Symptoms may not appear for several years after exposure. See also **inorganic dust.**

beryllium (Be), a steel-gray, light weight metallic element. Its atomic number is 4; its atomic weight is 9.012. Beryllium occurs naturally as beryl and is used in metallic alloys and in fluorescent powders. Inhalation of beryllium fumes or particles may cause the formation of granulomas in the lungs, skin, and subcutaneous tissues. See also **berylliosis.**

bestiality, **1.** a brutal or animal-like character or nature. **2.** conduct or behavior characterized by beastlike appetites or instincts. **3.** also called **zooerastia** /zōō·əras′tē·ə/. sexual relations between a human being and an animal. **4.** sodomy. See also **zoophilia.**

beta (β), the second letter of the Greek alphabet, employed as a combining form with chemical names to distinguish one of two or more isomers or to indicate the position of substituted atoms in certain compounds. Compare **alpha.**

beta-adrenergic blocking agent. See **antiadrenergic.**

beta-adrenergic receptor. See **beta receptor.**

beta-adrenergic stimulating agent. See **adrenergic.**

beta-carotene, an ultraviolet screening agent.

■ INDICATION: It is prescribed to ameliorate photosensitivity in patients with erythropoetic protoporphyria.

■ CONTRAINDICATIONS: It is used with caution in patients with impaired renal or hepatic function. Known hypersensitivity to this drug prohibits its use.

■ ADVERSE EFFECTS: No serious adverse reactions have been observed. Diarrhea may occur.

beta cells, **1.** insulin-producing cells situated in the islets of Langerhans. They contain granules that are soluble in alcohol and tend to be concentrated in the central portion of each islet. The insulin-producing function of the beta cells tends to accelerate the movement of glucose, amino acids, and fatty acids out of the blood and into the cellular cytoplasm, countering glucagon function of alpha cells. **2.** the basophilic cells of the anterior lobe of the pituitary gland.

beta decay, a type of radioactivity that results in the emission of beta particles, as electrons or positrons. See **beta particle.**

Betadine, a trademark for a topical antiinfective (povidone-iodine).

beta fetoprotein, a protein found in fetal liver and in some adults with liver disease. It is now known to be identical with normal liver ferritin. See also **alpha fetoprotein, ferritin, fetoprotein.**

beta-galactosidase. See **lactase.**

beta hemolysis, the development of a clear zone around a bacterial colony growing on blood agar medium, characteristic of certain pathogenic bacteria. Compare **alpha hemolysis.**

beta-hemolytic streptococci, the pyogenic streptococci of groups A, B, C, E, F, G, H, K, L, M, and O that cause hemolysis of red blood cells in blood agar in the laboratory. These organisms cause most of the acute streptococcal infections seen in humans, including rheumatic fever, scarlet fever, many cases of pneumonia and septicemia, and streptococcal sore throat. Penicillin is usually prescribed to treat these infections when they are suspected, even before the results of the bacteriologic culture are available, because it is known that these organisms as a group are sensitive to the effects of penicillin, and because the sequelae of untreated streptococcal infection may include glomerulonephritis and rheumatic fever.

beta-ketobutyric acid. See **acetoacetic acid.**

Betalin S, a trademark for vitamin B_1 (thiamine hydrochloride).

Betaloc, a trademark for an antiadrenergic (metoprolol tartrate).

betamethasone, a glucocorticoid.
■ INDICATION: It is prescribed as a topical antiinflammatory agent.
■ CONTRAINDICATIONS: Systemic fungal infections, dermatologic viral and fungal infections, impaired circulation, or known hypersensitivity to this drug prohibits its use.
■ ADVERSE EFFECTS: Among the more serious adverse reactions associated with prolonged use of the drug are GI, endocrine, neurologic, and fluid and electrolyte disturbances.

Betapar, a trademark for a glucocorticoid (meprednisone).

beta particle, an electron or positron emitted from the nucleus of an atom during radioactive decay of the atom. Beta particles have a range of 10 meters in air and 1 mm in soft tissue. Also called **beta rays.**

beta receptor, any one of the postulated adrenergic components of receptor tissues that responds to epinephrine and such blocking agents as propranolol. Activation of beta receptors causes various physiologic reactions, as relaxation of the bronchial muscles and an increase in the rate and force of cardiac contraction. Also called **beta-adrenergic receptor.** Compare **alpha receptor.**

beta rhythm. See **beta wave.**

betatron /bā′tətron/, a cyclic accelerator that produces high-energy electrons for radiotherapy treatment. The magnetic field of the betatron deflects electrons into a circular orbit, and an increasing magnetic orbital flux produces an induced circumferential electric field that accelerates the electrons.

beta wave, one of the four types of brain waves, characterized by relatively low voltage and a frequency of more than 13 Hz. Beta waves are the "busy waves" of the brain, recorded by electroencephalograph from the frontal and the central areas of the cerebrum when the patient is awake and alert with eyes open. Also called **beta rhythm.** Compare **alpha wave, delta wave, theta wave.**

bethanechol chloride /bethan′əkol/, a cholinergic.
■ INDICATIONS: It is prescribed in the treatment of fecal and urinary retention and neurogenic atony of the bladder.
■ CONTRAINDICATIONS: Uncertain strength of the bladder, obstruction of the GI or urinary tract, hyperthyroidism, peptic ulcer, bronchial asthma, cardiovascular disease, epilepsy, Parkinson's disease, hypotension, or known hypersensitivity to this drug prohibits its use. It is not given during pregnancy.
■ ADVERSE EFFECTS: Among the more serious adverse reactions are flushing, headache, GI distress, diarrhea, excessive salivation, sweating, and hypotension.

Betnelan, a trademark for a glucocorticoid (betamethasone).

bevel, **1.** any angle, other than a right angle, between two planes or surfaces. **2.** (in dentistry) any angle other than 90 degrees between a tooth cut and a cavity wall in the preparation of a tooth cavity. Compare **cavosurface bevel, contra bevel.**

bezoar /bē′zôr/, a hard ball of hair and vegetable fiber that may develop within the intestines of humans but more often is found in the stomachs of ruminants. In some societies it was formerly considered a useful medicine and possessed of certain magical properties. It is apparently still used as a therapeutic and mystical device by some, especially in the Far East.

B/F, a symbol for *black female,* often used in the initial identifying statement in a patient record.

B-galactosidase. See **lactase.**

bhang /bang/, an Asian Indian hallucinogenic, composed of dried leaves and the young stems of uncultivated *Cannabis sativa*. It is usually ingested as a boiled mixture with milk, sugar, or water; it produces euphoria. It also may be smoked or chewed. Also spelled **bang.** See also **cannabis.**

Bi, symbol for **bismuth.**

bi-, a combining form meaning 'twice, two': *biarticular, bicapsular, bicaudal*. See also **bio-, bis-.**

-bia, a combining form meaning 'creature possessing a mode of life': *aerobia, coenobia, Euphorbia*.

bias, **1.** an oblique or a diagonal line. **2.** a prejudiced or subjective attitude. **3.** (in statistics) the systematic distortion of a statistic caused by a particular sampling process. **4.** (in electronics) a voltage applied to an electronic device, as a vacuum tube or a transistor, to control operating limits.

bicarbonate of soda. See **sodium bicarbonate.**

bicarbonate precursor, an injection of sodium lactate used in the treatment of metabolic acidosis. It is metabolized in the body to sodium bicarbonate.

biceps brachii, the long fusiform muscle of the upper arm on the anterior surface of the humerus, arising in two heads from the scapula. The short head arises in a thick flat tendon from the corocoid process, the long head arises in the glenoid cavity. Both parts of the muscle converge in a flattened tendon that inserts into the radius of the forearm. The biceps brachii is innervated by branches of the musculocutaneous nerve, containing fibers from the fifth and the sixth cervical nerves. It flexes the arm and the forearm and supinates the hand. The long head draws the humerus toward the glenoid fossa, strengthening the shoulder joint. Also called **biceps, biceps flexor cubiti.** Compare **brachialis, triceps brachii.**

biceps femoris, one of the posterior femoral muscles. It has two heads at its origin. The long head arises from the tuberosity of the ischium and from the inferior part of the sacrotuberous ligament; the short head arises from the linea aspera and from the lateral intermuscular septum. The fibers passing from both heads join in a tendon that inserts into the lateral side of the fibula, and by a few fibers, into the lateral condyle of the tibia. The tendon of insertion forms the lateral hamstring. The long head of the muscle is innervated by branches of the sciatic nerve containing fibers from the first three sacral nerves. The short head is innervated by a branch of the peroneal nerve containing fibers from the fifth lumbar and first two sacral nerves. The biceps femoris flexes the leg and rotates it laterally and extends the thigh and tends to rotate it laterally. Also called **hamstring muscle.**

biceps flexor cubiti. See **biceps brachii.**

biceps reflex, a contraction of a biceps muscle produced when the tendon is tapped with a percussor in testing deep tendon reflexes. See also **deep tendon reflex.**

Bickerdyke /bik′ərdīk/, **Mary Ann** (1817–1901), an American nurse who, after taking a short course in homeopathy, cared for the sick and wounded on the battlefields during the Civil War. She insisted on cleanliness, good food, and the best of medical care for her patients. At night, she searched the battlefield with a lantern looking for survivors.

biconcave, concave on both sides, especially as applied to a lens. **–biconcavity,** *n.*

biconvex, convex on both sides, especially as applied to a lens. **–biconvexity,** *n.*

bicornate, having two horns or processes.

bicornate uterus, an abnormal uterus that may be either a single or a double organ with two horns, or branches. The anomaly is believed to result from an embryonic development error and is associated with a high incidence of premature labor, spontaneous abortion, and infertility.

bicuspid /bīkus′pid/, **1.** having two cusps or points. **2.** also called **premolar tooth.** one of the two teeth between the molars and canines of the upper and lower jaw.

bicuspid valve. See **mitral valve.**

b.i.d., (in prescriptions) abbreviation for *bis in die* /dē′ā/, a Latin phrase meaning "twice a day." The times of administration are commonly 9 AM and 7 PM.

bidactyly /bīdak′tilē/, an abnormal condition in which the second, third, and fourth digits on the same hand are missing and only the first and fifth are represented. Also called **lobster claw deformity.** **–bidactylous,** *adj.*

bidermoma /bī′dərō′mə/, *pl.* **bidermomas, bidermomata,** a teratoid neoplasm composed of cells and tissues originating in two germ layers.

bidet /bidā′/, a fixture resembling a toilet bowl, with a rim to sit on and usually equipped with plumbing implements, for cleaning the genital and rectal areas of the body.

bidirectional printer, a computer driven printer that prints characters as the printing head moves in either direction.

biduotertian fever, a form of malaria characterized by overlapping paroxysms of chills, fever, and other symptoms, caused by infection with two strains of *Plasmodium,* each having its own cycle of symptoms, as in quartan and tertian malaria. Compare **double quartan fever.** See also **malaria.**

bifid, split into two parts.

bifocal, **1.** of or pertaining to the characteristic of having two foci. **2.** (of a lens) having two areas of different focal lengths.

bifurcation, a splitting into two branches, as the trachea, which branches into the two bronchi at about the level of the fifth thoracic vertebra.

Bigelow's lithotrite /big′əlōz/, a long-jawed lithotrite, passed through the urethra, for crushing a calculus in the bladder. See **lithoplax.**

bigeminal pulse, an abnormal pulse in which two beats in close succession are followed by a pause during which no pulse is felt. See also **trigeminal pulse, trigeminy.**

bigeminy /bījem′inē/, **1.** an association in pairs. **2.** a cardiac arrhythmia characterized by two beats in rapid succession followed by a longer interval. The arrhythmia is usually related to premature ventricular beats. **–bigeminal,** *adj.*

bilabe /bī′lāb/, a narrow forceps used to remove small calculi from the bladder.

bilaminar, pertaining to or having two layers, as the basal lamina and the reticular lamina that constitute the basement membrane of the epithelium.

bilaminar blastoderm, the stage of embryonic development before mesoderm formation in which only the ectoderm and entoderm primary germ layers have formed. Compare **trilaminar blastoderm.**

bilateral, **1.** having two sides. **2.** occurring or appearing on two sides. A patient with bilateral hearing loss may have partial or total deafness in both ears. **3.** having two layers.

bilateral long-leg spica cast, an orthopedic device of plaster of paris, fiberglass, or other casting material that encases and immobilizes the trunk cranially as far as the nipple line and both legs caudally as far as the toes. A horizontal crossbar to improve immobilization connects the parts of the cast encasing both legs at ankle level. It is used to aid the healing of fractures of the hip, the femur, the acetabulum, or the pelvis and for the correction or the maintenance of the correction of a hip deformity. Compare **one-and-a-half spica cast, unilateral long-leg spica cast.**

bile, a bitter, yellow-green secretion of the liver. Stored in the gallbladder, bile receives its color from the presence of bile pigments, as bilirubin. Bile passes from the gallbladder through the common bile duct in response to the presence of a fatty meal in the duodenum. Bile emulsifies these fats, preparing them for further digestion and absorption in the small intestine. Any interference in the flow of bile will result in the presence of unabsorbed fat in the feces and in jaundice. Also called **gall.** See also **biliary obstruction, jaundice.** –**biliary,** *adj.*

bile acid, a steroid acid of the bile, produced during the metabolism of cholesterol. On hydrolysis bile acid yields glycine and cholic acid.

bile solubility test, a bacteriologic test used in the differential diagnosis of pneumococcal and streptococcal infection. A broth culture of each organism is placed into two tubes. Ox bile is added to one and salt to the other. Pneumococci dissolve in ox bile, resulting in a clear solution; streptococci do not dissolve, resulting in a cloudy solution. The tube with salt is used for comparative purposes.

Bilharzia. See ***Schistosoma.***

bilharziasis. See **schistosomiasis.**

bili-, a combining form meaning 'pertaining to the bile': *biliary, bilidigestive, bilifuscin.*

biliary /bil′ē·er′ē/, of or pertaining to bile or to the gallbladder and its ducts, which transport bile. These are often called the **biliary tract** or the **biliary system.** Also **bilious.** See also **bile, biliary calculus.**

biliary atresia, congenital absence or underdevelopment of one or more of the biliary structures, causing jaundice and early liver damage. As the condition worsens, the child may show retarded growth and develop portal hypertension. Surgery can correct the defective ducts in only a small percentage of cases. Most infants die in early childhood from biliary cirrhosis. It is essential for the physician to distinguish between this condition and neonatal hepatitis, which is treatable. See also **biliary cirrhosis.**

biliary calculus, a stone formed in the biliary tract, consisting of bile pigments and calcium salts. Biliary calculi may cause jaundice, right upper quadrant pain, obstruction, and inflammation of the gallbladder. If stones cannot pass spontaneously into the duodenum, intravenous cholangiography will reveal their location, and they can be surgically removed. Also called **choledocholithiasis, gallstones.** See also **cholangitis, cholecystitis, cholelithiasis.**

biliary cirrhosis, an inflammatory condition in which the flow of bile through the ductules of the liver is obstructed. Biliary cirrhosis most commonly affects women in their middle years, and its cause is unknown. It is characterized by abdominal pain, jaundice, steatorrhea, and enlargement of the liver and spleen. The disease is slowly progressive and in its end stages closely resembles cirrhosis of the liver. There is no specific medical or surgical treatment. Care must be taken to rule out obstruction of the biliary structures outside the liver, because the latter condition can be treated successfully. Compare **biliary calculus, biliary obstruction.**

biliary colic, a type of smooth muscle or visceral pain specifically associated with the passing of stones through the bile ducts. Also called **cholecystalgia.** See also **biliary calculi.**

biliary duct, a duct through which bile passes from the liver to the duodenum.

biliary fistula, an abnormal passage from the gallbladder, a bile duct, or the liver to an internal organ or the surface of the body. Biliary fistulae opening into the colon, duodenum, hepatic duct, peritoneal cavity, pleural space, or skin are complications in cholelithiasis; a gallstone entering the duodenum may become impacted, usually in the ileocecal valve, and cause intestinal obstruction.

biliary obstruction, blockage of the common or cystic bile duct, usually caused by one or more gallstones. It impedes bile drainage and produces an inflammatory reaction. Uncommon causes of biliary obstruction include choledochal cysts, pancreatic and duodenal tumors, Crohn's disease, pancreatitis, echinococcosis, ascariasis, and sclerosing cholangitis. Stones, consisting chiefly of cholesterol, bile pigment, and calcium, may form in the gallbladder and in the hepatic duct in persons of either sex at any age but are more common in middle-aged women. Increased amounts of serum cholesterol in the blood, as occurs in obesity, diabetes, hypothyroidism, biliary stasis, and inflammation of the biliary system, promote the formation of gallstones. Cholelithiasis may be asymptomatic until a stone lodges in a biliary duct, but the patient usually has a prior history of indigestion and discomfort after eating fatty foods.

■ OBSERVATIONS: Biliary obstruction is characterized by severe epigastric pain, often radiating to the back and shoulder, nausea, vomiting, and profuse diaphoresis. The dehydrated patient may have chills, fever, jaundice, clay-colored stools, dark, concentrated urine, an electrolyte imbalance, and a tendency to bleed because the absence of bile prevents the synthesis and absorption of fat-soluble vitamin K.

■ INTERVENTION: The patient is placed in bed in a semi-Fowler's position and is usually administered intermittent nasogastric suctioning, parenteral fluids with electrolytes and fat-soluble vitamins, and medication for pain. Antibiotics, anticholinergic and antispasmodic drugs, and a cholecystogram or ultrasound scan may be ordered. The blood pressure, temperature, pulse, and respirations are noted, and the patient is helped to turn, cough, and deep breathe every 2 to 4 hours. The intake and output of fluids are measured, and the color and character of urine and stools are noted. When the nasogastric tube is removed, the patient initially receives a low-fat liquid diet and progresses to a soft or normal diet, as tolerated; up to 2500 ml of fluids a day are forced, unless contraindicated. Cholecystectomy is usually the definitive treatment, but, in most cases, surgery is delayed until the patient's condition is stabilized and any prothrombin deficiency (caused by vitamin K malabsorption) is corrected.

■ NURSING CONSIDERATIONS: The patient may experience intense pain as obstruction causes biliary colic. Instruction is given on the importance of adhering to a low-fat diet and reporting recurrence of symptoms if discharge occurs before surgery. Cholecystectomy usually requires several days of intensive nursing care and support. See **cholecystectomy.**

biliary tract cancer, a relatively rare malignancy in an extrahepatic bile duct, occurring slightly more often in men than in women, characterized by progressive jaundice, pruritus, weight loss, and, in the later stages, severe pain. Transhepatic cholangiography and x-ray examination after the introduction of a contrast medium into the common bile duct and pancreatic duct are used to identify and determine the site of the lesion. Results of laboratory studies indicative of extrahepatic biliary obstruction include greater than normal levels of serum alkaline phosphatase and bilirubin in the blood. If the tumor is in the ampulla of Vater, occult blood may be found in the stool. The tumor is an adenocarcinoma; it may be papillary or flat and ulcerated. It is generally inoperable if it is located in the hepatic or common bile duct, but periampullary lesions may be treated by pancreatoduodenectomy. In cases of an inoperable tumor, various surgical procedures may be performed palliatively to improve the flow of bile. Preoperative, postoperative, and palliative irradiation are also used. With the exception of a rare remission induced by 5-fluorouracil, chemotherapy is not effective in treating these lesions.

bilingulate /bīling'gyəlit/, having two tongues or two tonguelike structures.

bilious /bil'yəs/, **1.** of or pertaining to bile. **2.** characterized by an excessive secretion of bile. **3.** characterized by a disorder affecting the bile.

bilirubin /bil'iroo͞'bin/, the orange-yellow pigment of bile, formed principally by the breakdown of hemoglobin in red blood cells after termination of their normal lifespan. Water-insoluble, unconjugated bilirubin normally travels in the bloodstream to the liver, where it is converted to a water-soluble, conjugated form and excreted into the bile. In a healthy person, about 250 mg of bilirubin are produced daily, and the majority of that is eventually excreted from the body in the stool. The characteristic yellow pallor of jaundice is caused by the accumulation of bilirubin in the blood and in the tissues of the skin. Testing for bilirubin in the blood provides valuable information for diagnosis and evaluation of liver disease, biliary obstruction, and hemolytic anemia. See also **jaundice, van den Bergh test.**

bilirubinuria, the presence of bilirubin in urine.

biliuria /bil'iyoo͝r'ē·ə/, the presence of bile in the urine.

biliverdin /bil'ivur'din/, a greenish bile pigment formed in the breakdown of hemoglobin and converted to bilirubin. See also **bile, bilirubin.**

Billings method, a method of estimating ovulation time by changes in the cervical mucus that occur during the menstrual cycle.

Billroth's operation I, the surgical removal of the pylorus in the treatment of gastric cancer. The proximal end of the duodenum is anastomosed to the stomach.

Billroth's operation II, the surgical removal of the pylorus and duodenum. The cut end of the stomach is anastomosed to the jejunum through the transverse mesocolon.

bilobate, having two lobes.

bilobulate, having two lobules. Also **bilobular.**

bilocular, **1.** divided into two cells. **2.** containing two cells. Also **biloculate.**

Bilticide, a trademark for a trematocide (praziquantel).

bimanual, of or pertaining to the functioning of both hands.

bimaxillary, of or pertaining to the right and left maxilla.

bimodal distribution, the distribution of quantitative data around two separate modes. It is suggestive of two separate normally distributed populations from which the data are drawn.

binangle, a surgical instrument that has a shank with two offsetting angles to keep the cutting edge of the instrument within 3 mm of the shaft axis.

binary fission /bī'nərē/, direct division of a cell or nucleus into two equal parts. It is the common form of asexual reproduction of bacteria, protozoa, and other lower forms of life. Also called **simple fission.** Compare **multiple fission.**

binary number, a number represented in the binary system, and usually represented by 0s and 1s. See **binary system.**

binary system, a number system based on the number two, used in digital computers. Each digit, represented by a zero or one, represents a power of two. Thus, the decimal number 47 (actually representing $4 \times 10^2 + 7 \times 10^0$) is expressed in binary notation as 101111 (that is, $1 \times 2^5 + 0 \times 2^4 + 1 \times 2^3 + 1 \times 2^2 + 1 \times 2^1 + 1 \times 2^0$).

binaural stethoscope /bīnôr'əl/, a stethoscope having two earpieces.

bind, **1.** to bandage or wrap in a band. **2.** to join together with a band or with a ligature. **3.** (in chemistry) to combine or unite molecules by employing reactive groups within the molecules or by using a binding chemical. Binding is especially associated with chemical bonds that are fairly easily broken, as in the bonds between toxins and antitoxins.

Binet age /binā'/, the mental age of an individual, especially a child, as determined by the Binet-Simon tests, which are evaluated on the basis of tested intelligence of the "normal" individual at any given age. The Binet age corresponding to "profoundly retarded" is 1 to 2 years; to "severely retarded," 3 to 7 years; and to "mildly retarded," 8 to 12 years.

binocular, **1.** pertaining to both eyes, especially regarding vision. **2.** a microscope, telescope, or field glass that can accommodate viewing by both eyes.

binocular fixation, the process of having both eyes directed at the same object at the same time. This is essential to having good depth perception.

binocular ophthalmoscope, an ophthalmoscope having two eyepieces through which stereoscopic examination of the eye may be made.

binocular parallax /par′əlaks/, the difference in the angles formed by the sight lines to two objects situated at different distances from the eyes. Binocular parallax is a major factor in depth perception. Also called **stereoscopic parallax.**

binocular perception, the visual ability to judge depth or distance by virtue of having two eyes.

binocular vision, the use of both eyes simultaneously so that the images perceived by each eye are combined to appear as a single image. Compare **diplopia.**

binomial, containing two names or terms.

binovular, developing from two distinct ova, as in dizygotic twins. Also **diovular.** Compare **uniovular.**

binovular twins. See **dizygotic twins.**

bio-, bi-, a combining form meaning 'pertaining to life': *bioassay, biogenesis, biolysis.*

bioactive, of or pertaining to a substance that has an effect on or causes a reaction in living tissue.

bioactivity, any response from or reaction in living tissue.

bioassay /bī′ō·as′ā, -əsā′/, the laboratory determination of the concentration of a drug or other substance in a specimen by comparing its effect on an organism, an animal, or an isolated tissue with that of a standard preparation. Also called **biologic assay.**

bioavailability, the degree of activity or amount of an administered drug or other substance that becomes available for activity in the target tissue.

biochemical genetics. See **molecular genetics.**

biochemistry, the chemistry of living organisms and life processes. Also called **biologic chemistry, physiologic chemistry.**

biochromatic analysis, the spectrophotometric monitoring of a reaction at two wavelengths. It is used to correct for background color.

bioelectricity, electric current that is generated by living tissues, such as nerves and muscles. The electric potentials of human tissues, recorded by electrocardiograph, electroencephalograph, and similar sensitive devices, are used in diagnosing the condition of various vital organs.

bioenergetics, a system of exercises based on the concept that natural healing will be enhanced by bringing into harmony the patient's body rhythms and the natural environment.

bioequivalent /bī′ō·ikwiv′ələnt/, **1.** (in pharmacology) of or pertaining to a drug that has the same effect on the body as another drug, usually one nearly identical in its chemical formulation. **2.** a bioequivalent drug. **–bioequivalence,** *n.*

biofeedback, a process providing a person with visual or auditory information about the autonomic physiologic functions of his or her body, as blood pressure, muscle tension, and brain wave activity, usually through use of instrumentation. By trial and error, the person learns to consciously control these processes, which were previously regarded as involuntary. Biofeedback may be used clinically to treat many conditions, as hypertension, insomnia, and migraine headache.

bioflavonoid /bī′ōflā′vənoid/, a generic term for any of a group of colored flavones found in many fruits and essential for the absorption and metabolism of ascorbic acid. The bioflavonoids are needed for the maintenance of collagen and of the capillary walls and may aid in protection against infection. The components are citrin, hesperidin, rutin, flavones, and flavonoids. Rich sources include lemons, grapes, plums, grapefruit, black currants, apricots, buckwheat, cherries, blackberries, and rose hips. Deficiency can result in a tendency to bleed or bruise easily. The bioflavonoids are completely nontoxic. Also called **vitamin P.** See also **ascorbic acid.**

biogenesis /bī′ōjen′əsis/, **1.** also called **biogeny** /bī·oj′ənē/. the doctrine that living material can originate only from preexisting life and not from inanimate matter. **2.** the origin of life and living organisms; ontogeny and phylogeny. **–biogenetic,** *adj.*

biogenetic law. See **recapitulation theory.**

biogenic /bī′ōjen′ik/, **1.** produced by the action of a living organism, as fermentation. **2.** essential to life and the maintenance of health, as food, water, and proper rest.

biogenic amine, one of a large group of naturally occurring biologically active compounds most of which act as neurotransmitters. The most dominant, norepinephrine, is involved in such physiologic functions as emotional reactions, memory, sleep, and arousal from sleep. Other biochemicals of the group include three catecholamines: histamine, serotonin, and dopamine. These substances are active in regulating blood pressure, elimination, body temperature, and many other centrally mediated body functions.

biogenous /bī·oj′ənəs/, **1.** biogenetic. **2.** biogenic.

biogeny. See **biogenesis.**

biologic, **1.** pertaining to living organisms and their products. **2.** any preparation made from living organisms or the products of living organisms and used as diagnostic, preventive, or therapeutic agents. Kinds of biologics are **antigens, antitoxins, serums,** and **vaccines.** Also called **biological.**

biologic assay. See **bioassay.**

biologic half-life, the time required for the body to eliminate one half of an administered dosage of any substance by regular physiologic processes. The time required is approximately the same for both the stable and radioactive isotopes of a specific element. Also called **metabolic half-life.** See also **effective half-life, half-life.**

biologic plausibility, a method of reasoning used to establish a cause and effect relationship between a biologic factor and a particular disease.

biologic psychiatry, a school of psychiatric thought that stresses the physical, chemical, and neurologic causes of and treatments for mental and emotional disorders.

biologic vector. See **vector.**

biology, the scientific study of plants and animals. Some branches of biology are **biometry, ecology, molecular biology,** and **paleontology.**

biome /bī′ōm/, the total group of biologic communities existing in and characteristic of a given geographic region, as a desert, woodland, or marsh. A biome includes all plants, animals, and microorganisms of a particular region.

biomechanics, the study of mechanic laws and their application to living organisms, especially the human body and its locomotor system. –**biomechanic, biomechanical,** *adj.*

biomedical engineering, a system of techniques in which knowledge of biologic processes is applied to solve practical medical problems and to answer questions in biomedical research.

bionics /bī·on′iks/, the science of applying electronic principles and devices, as computers and solid state miniaturized circuitry, to medical problems, as artificial pacemakers used to correct abnormal heart rhythms. –**bionic,** *adj.*

biophore /bī′əfôr′/, according to German biologist A.F.L. Weismann, the basic hereditary unit contained in the germ plasm from which all living cells develop and all inherited characteristics are transmitted. Compare **gemmule.**

biopsy, **1.** the removal of a small piece of living tissue from an organ or other part of the body for microscopic examination to confirm or establish a diagnosis, estimate prognosis, or follow the course of a disease. **2.** the tissue excised for examination. **3.** *informal.* to excise tissue for examination. Kinds of biopsy include **aspiration biopsy, needle biopsy, punch biopsy,** and **surface biopsy.** –**bioptic,** *adj.*

biopsychic, of or pertaining to psychic factors as they relate to living organisms.

biopsychology. See **psychobiology.**

biopsychosocial, of or pertaining to the complex of biologic, psychologic, and social aspects of life.

biorhythm, any cyclic, biologic event or phenomenon, as the sleep cycle, the menstrual cycle, or the respiratory cycle. –**biorhythmic,** *adj.*

-biosis, a combining form meaning 'life': *macrobiosis, necrobiosis, otobiosis.*

biostatistics, numeric data on births, deaths, diseases, injuries, and other factors affecting the general health and condition of human populations. Also called **vital statistics.**

biosynthesis, any one of thousands of chemical reactions continually occurring throughout the body in which molecules form more complex biomolecules, especially the carbohydrates, the lipids, the proteins, the nucleotides, and the nucleic acids. Biosynthetic reactions constitute the anabolism of the body. –**biosynthetic,** *adj.*

biotaxis /bī′ōtak′sis/, the ability of living cells to develop into certain forms and arrangements. See also **cytoclesis.** –**biotactic,** *adj.*

biotaxy /bī′ōtak′sē/, **1.** biotaxis. **2.** the systematic classification of living organisms according to their anatomic characteristics; taxonomy.

biotechnology, **1.** the study of the relationships between humans or other living organisms and machinery, as the health effects of word processor equipment on office workers or the ability of airplane pilots to perform tasks when traveling at supersonic speeds. **2.** the industrial application of the results of biologic research, particularly in fields such as recombinant DNA or gene splicing, which permits the production of synthetic hormones or enzymes by combining genetic material from different species. See **recombinant DNA.**

-biotic, **1.** a combining form meaning 'pertaining to life': *anabiotic, catabiotic, microbiotic.* **2.** a combining form meaning 'possessing a (specified) mode of life': *endobiotic, parabiotic, photobiotic.*

biotin /bī′ətin/, a colorless, crystalline, water-soluble B complex vitamin that acts as a coenzyme in fatty acid production and in the oxidation of fatty acids and carbohydrates. It also aids in the use of protein, folic acid, pantothenic acid, and vitamin B_{12}. Rich sources are egg yolk, beef liver, kidney, unpolished rice, brewer's yeast, peanuts, cauliflower, and mushrooms. Because biotin is synthesized by intestinal bacteria, naturally occurring deficiency disease is unknown, although it can be induced by large quantities of raw egg whites in the diet. Symptoms include scaly dermatitis, grayish pallor, extreme lassitude, anorexia, muscle pains, insomnia, some precordial distress, and slight anemia. Also called **vitamin H.**

biotin deficiency syndrome, an abnormal condition caused by a deficiency of biotin, characterized by dermatitis, hyperesthesia, muscle pain, anorexia, slight anemia, and changes in electrocardiographic activity of the heart. The average daily requirement of biotin for an adult is 100 to 200 μg; the average American diet provides 100 to 300 μg of the vitamin. Authorities have observed spontaneous deficiency of biotin in some individuals who have eaten raw eggs over a long period of time. Some authorities consider seborrheic dermatitis in infants a form of biotin deficiency. Some common sources of biotin are egg yolks, liver, and yeast.

biotope, a specific biologic habitat or site.

biotransformation, the chemical changes a substance undergoes in the body, as by the action of enzymes. See also **metabolic.**

Biot's respiration /bē•ōz′/, an abnormal respiratory pattern, characterized by irregular breathing with periods of apnea. The breathing may be slow and deep or rapid and shallow and is often accompanied by sighing. Biot's respiration is symptomatic of meningitis or increased intracranial pressure.

biparental inheritance. See **amphigenous inheritance.**

biparietal /bīpərī′ətəl/, of or pertaining to the two parietal bones of the head, as the biparietal diameter.

biparietal diameter, the distance between the protuberances of the two parietal bones of the skull.

bipartite, having two parts.

biped, **1.** having two feet. **2.** any animal with only two feet.

bipedal, capable of locomotion on two feet.

bipenniform /bīpen′ifôrm′/, (of bodily structure) having the bilateral symmetry of a feather, as the pattern formed by the fasciculi that converge on both sides of a muscle tendon in the rectus femoris. Compare **multipenniform, penniform, radiate.**

biperiden, a synthetic anticholinergic agent.

■ INDICATIONS: It is prescribed in the treatment of Parkinson's disease and drug-induced extrapyramidal disorders. Biperiden hydrochloride is administered orally, and biperiden lactate is administered intramuscularly or intravenously.

■ CONTRAINDICATIONS: Narrow-angle glaucoma, asthma, obstruction of the genitourinary or GI tract, or known hypersensitivity to this drug prohibits its use.

■ ADVERSE EFFECTS: Among the more serious adverse reactions are blurred vision, central nervous system effects, tachycardia, dry mouth, decreased sweating, and hypersensitivity reactions.

biphasic /bīfā′zik/, having two phases, parts, aspects, or stages.

Biphetamine, a trademark for a fixed-combination drug containing two central stimulants (amphetamine and dextroamphetamine), formerly prescribed as an anorexiant.

bipolar, **1.** having two poles, as in certain electrotherapeutic treatments using two poles or in certain bacterial staining that affects only the two poles of the microorganism under study. **2.** (of a nerve cell) having an afferent and an efferent process.

bipolar disorder, a major affective disorder characterized by episodes of mania and depression. One or the other phase may be predominant at any given time, one phase may appear alternately with the other, or elements of both phases may be present simultaneously. Characteristics of the manic phase are excessive emotional displays, excitement, euphoria, hyperactivity accompanied by elation, boisterousness, impaired ability to concentrate, decreased need for sleep, and seemingly unbounded energy, often accompanied by delusions of grandeur. In the depressive phase, marked apathy and underactivity are accompanied by feelings of profound sadness, loneliness, guilt, and lowered self-esteem. Causes of the disorder are multiple and complex, often involving biologic, psychologic, interpersonal, and social and cultural factors. Treatment includes antidepressants, tranquilizers and antianxiety drugs, or the use of electroconvulsive therapy for persons who present an immediate and serious risk of suicide, followed by long-term psychotherapy. Careful nursing observation is important during depression, particularly during the recovery from depression, because of the possibility of suicide.

bipolar lead /lēd/, **1.** an electrocardiographic conductor having two electrodes placed on different body regions, with each electrode contributing significantly to the record. **2.** *informal.* a tracing produced by such a lead on an electrocardiograph.

bipotentiality, the characteristic of acting or reacting according to either of two potentials.

bird breeder's lung. See **pigeon breeder's lung.**

bird face retrognathism, an abnormal facial profile with an undeveloped mandible, which may be caused by interference of condylar growth associated with trauma or condylar infection. Compare **prognathism.**

bird headed dwarf, a person affected with Seckel's syndrome, a congenital disorder characterized by a proportionate shortness of stature; a proportionately small head with hypoplasia of the jaws, large eyes, and a beaklike protrusion of the nose; mental retardation; and various other skeletal, cutaneous, and genital defects. Also called **nanocephalic dwarf.**

birth, **1.** the event of being born, the coming of a new person out of its mother into the world. Kinds of birth are **breech birth, live birth,** and **stillbirth.** See also **effacement, labor.** **2.** the child-bearing event, the bringing forth by a mother of a baby. **3.** a medical event, the delivery of a fetus by an obstetric attendant.

birth canal, *informal.* the passage that extends from the inlet of the true pelvis to the vaginal orifice through which an infant passes during vaginal birth. See also **clinical pelvimetry.**

birth control. See **contraception.**

birth defect. See **congenital anomaly.**

birthing chair, a chair used in labor and delivery to promote the comfort of the mother and the efficiency of parturition. The chair may be specially designed, having many technic features, or it may be a simple three-legged stool with a high, slanted back and a circular seat with a large central hole in it. The newer birthing chairs allow the woman to sit straight up or to recline. The chair has a lower section that may be removed or folded out of the way. Lights, mirrors, and basins may be attached for the attendant's convenience. The upright position appears to shorten the time in labor, particularly the second or expulsive stage of labor, probably because of gravity and increased participation of the mother. The chair is not suitable for use with anesthesia.

birth injury, trauma suffered by a baby while being born. Some kinds of birth injury are **Bell's palsy, cerebral palsy,** and **Erb's palsy.**

birthmark. See **nevus.**

birth rate, the proportion of the number of births in a specific area during a given period to the total population of that area, usually expressed as the number of births per 1000 of population. Compare **crude birth rate, refined birth rate, true birth rate.**

birth trauma, **1.** any physical injury suffered by an infant during the process of delivery. **2.** the supposed psychic shock, according to some psychiatric theories, that an infant suffers during delivery.

birth weight, the measured heaviness of a baby when born, usually about 3500 g (7.5 pounds). In the United States, 97% of newborns weigh between 2500 g (5.5 pounds) and 4500 g (10 pounds). Babies weighing less than 2500 g at term are considered **small for gestational age.** Babies weighing more than 4500 g are considered **large for gestational age** and are often infants of mothers with diabetes.

bis-, bi-, a combining form meaning 'twice, two': *bisacromial, bisaxillary, bisferious.*

bisacodyl /bisak′ōdil/, a cathartic.

■ INDICATIONS: It is prescribed in the treatment of acute or chronic constipation, to empty the bowel pre- or postoperatively or before diagnostic radiographic procedures.

■ CONTRAINDICATIONS: Abdominal pain, nausea, vomiting, rectal fissures, ulcerated hemorrhoids, or known hypersensitivity to this drug prohibits its use.

■ ADVERSE EFFECTS: Among the more serious adverse reactions are colic, abdominal pain, and diarrhea.

bisect, to divide into two equal lengths or parts.

bisexual /bīsek′sho͞o•əl/, **1.** hermaphroditic; having gonads of both sexes. **2.** possessing physical or psychologic characteristics of both sexes. **3.** engaging in both heterosexual and homosexual activity. **4.** desiring sexual contact with persons of both sexes.

bisexual libido, (in psychoanalysis) the tendency in a person to seek sexual gratification with people of either sex.

bishydroxycoumarin. See **dicumarol.**

bis in die (b.d., b.i.d.) /dē′ā/, a Latin phrase, used in prescriptions, meaning "twice a day." It is more commonly used in its abbreviated form.

bismuth (Bi), a reddish, crystalline, trivalent metallic element. Its atomic number is 83; its atomic weight is 209. It is combined with various other elements, as oxygen, to produce numerous salts used in the manufacture of many pharmaceutic substances.

bismuth gingivitis, a symptom of metallic poisoning caused by bismuth administered in the treatment of systemic disease. It is characterized by a dark bluish line along the gingival margin. See also **gingivitis.**

bismuth stomatitis, an abnormal oral condition caused by systemic use of bismuth compounds over prolonged periods, characterized by a blue-black line on the inner aspect of the gingival sulcus or pigmentation of the buccal mucosa, a sore tongue, metallic taste, and a burning sensation in the mouth. Compare **arsenic stomatitis, Atabrine stomatitis.**

bit /bit/, abbreviation for *bi*nary digi*t*, a single digit of a binary number. See also **byte.**

bite, **1.** the act of cutting, tearing, holding, or gripping with the teeth. **2.** the lingual portion of an artificial tooth between its shoulder and incisal edge. **3.** an occlusal record or relationship. Compare **closed bite, open bite.**

bite block. See **occlusion rim.**

bitegage /bīt′gāj′/, a prosthetic dental device that helps attain proper occlusion of the teeth rooted in the maxilla and the mandible.

biteguard, a resin appliance that covers the occlusal and incisal surfaces of the teeth. It is designed to stabilize the teeth and provide a platform for the excursive glides of the mandible. Also called **night guard.** Compare **biteplane.**

biteguard splint, a device, usually made of resin, for covering the occlusal and incisal surfaces of the teeth and for protecting them from traumatic occlusal forces during immobilization and stabilization processes. See also **Gunning's splint.**

bitelock /bīt′lok′/, a dental device for retaining the occlusion rims in the same relation outside the mouth as inside the mouth.

bitemporal, of or pertaining to both temples or both temporal bones.

biteplane /bīt′plān/, a removable dental appliance for covering the occlusal surfaces of the teeth and to prevent their articulation.

biteplate, a device used in dentistry as a diagnostic or a therapeutic aid for prosthodontics or for orthodontics. It is fabricated of wire and plastic and worn in the palate. It may also be used to correct temperomandibular joint problems or as a splint in restoring the full mouth.

bite wing film, a type of dental x-ray film that has a central tab or wing on which the teeth close to maintain film position during radiographic examination. Also called **interproximal film.**

bite wing radiograph, a kind of dental radiograph that reveals approximately the coronal portions of maxillary and mandibular teeth and portions of the interdental septa on the same film. Compare **occlusal radiograph.**

bithionol (TBP) /bithī′ənôl/, a pale gray powder, soluble in acetone, alcohol, or ether, used as a local antiseptic and administered orally in the treatment of infestations of the giant liver fluke (*Fasciola gigantica hepatica*) and of the lung fluke (*Paragonimus westermani*) that cause parasitic hemoptysis in Asiatic countries.

Bithynia /bəthin′ē•ə/, a genus of snails, species of which act as intermediate hosts to *Opisthorchis.*

biting in childhood, a natural behavior trait and reflex action in infants, acquired at about 5 to 6 months of age in response to the introduction of solid foods in the diet and the beginning of the teething process. The activity represents a significant modality in the psychosocial development of the child, because it is the first aggressive action the infant learns, and through it the infant learns to control the environment. The behavior also confronts the infant with one of the first inner conflicts, because biting can produce both pleasing and displeasing results. Biting during breast feeding causes withdrawal of the nipple and anxiety in the mother, yet it also serves as a means of soothing teething discomfort. Infants continue to use biting as a mechanism for exploring their surroundings. Toddlers and older children often use biting for expressing aggression toward their parents and other children, especially during play or as a means of gaining attention. Most children normally outgrow the tendency unless severe maladaptive or emotional problems are present. See also **psychosexual development, psychosocial development.**

Bitot's spots /bitōz′/, white or gray triangular deposits on the bulbar conjunctiva adjacent to the lateral margin of the cornea, a clinical sign of vitamin A deficiency. Also called **Bitot's patches.**

bitrochanteric lipodystrophy, an abnormal and excessive deposition of fat on the buttocks and the outer aspect of the upper thighs, occurring most commonly in women. See also **lipodystrophy.**

bitterling test, a Japanese test for pregnancy in which a female bitterling fish is immersed in 1 L of fresh water containing 10 ml of the urine of the woman being tested. If the woman is pregnant, the long oviduct of the bitterling grows from its belly.

biuret test, a method for detecting urea and other soluble proteins in serum. In alkaline solution, copper sulfate ions react with the peptide bonds of proteins to produce a purple color, called the biuret reaction. The amount of serum protein in a sample solution is estimated by comparing its color with that of a standard solution whose protein concentration is known.

bivalent /bīvā′lənt/, **1.** also **divalent.** (in genetics) a pair of synapsed homologous chromosomes that are attached to each other by chiasmata during the early first meiotic prophase of gametogenesis. The structure serves as the basis for the tetrads from which gametes are produced during the two meiotic divisions. **2.** See **valence,** def. 1. **–bivalence,** *n.*

bivalent chromosome, a pair of synapsed homologous chromosomes during the early stages of gametogenesis. See also **bivalent.**

bivalve cast, an orthopedic cast used for immobilizing a section of the body for the healing of one or more broken bones or for correction or the maintenance of correction of an orthopedic deformity. The cast is cut in half to monitor and detect pressure under the cast, especially with a patient who has decreased sensation or who has no sensation in the portion of the body surrounded by the cast. An area of the skin that is subjected to prolonged pressure from a cast may become infected, and early signs of pressure are almost impossible to detect. If dangerous pressure areas are detected, "windows" are often cut out of the cast over the pressure areas to relieve the problem.

bizarre leiomyoma. See **epithelioid leiomyoma.**

Bk, symbol for **berkelium.**

BL, abbreviation for **baralyme.**

black beauties, *slang.* amphetamines.

black damp. See **damp.**

Black Death, *informal.* bubonic plague, especially the epidemic in the fourteenth century that killed over 25,000,000 people in Europe. See also **bubonic plague, plague, *Yersinia pestis.***

black fever. See **kala-azar.**

black hairy tongue. See **parasitic glossitis.**

blackhead. See **comedo.**

black light. See **Wood's light.**

black lung. See **anthracosis.**

black lung disease. See **pneumoconiosis.**

blackout, *informal.* a temporary loss of vision or consciousness resulting from cerebral ischemia.

black plague. See **bubonic plague.**

black spots film fault, a defect in a radiograph, seen as dark spots thoughout the image area. It is caused by dust particles or developer on the x-ray film before development or by outdated film.

black tongue. See **parasitic glossitis.**

blackwater fever, a serious complication of chronic falciparum malaria, characterized by jaundice, hemoglobinuria, acute renal failure, and the passage of bloody dark red or black urine because of massive intravascular hemolysis. Death occurs in 20% to 30% of all cases; mortality is particularly high among Europeans. See also **falciparum malaria, malaria, *Plasmodium.***

Blackwell, Elizabeth (1821–1910), a British-born American physician, the first woman to receive a medical degree. She established the New York Infirmary, a 40 bed hospital staffed entirely by women, with which Marie Zakrzewski was associated for a time. At the infirmary, she began training nurses in a 4 month course. Her influence helped others establish nursing schools to improve patient care.

black widow spider, a poisonous arachnid found in many parts of the world. The venom injected with its bite causes perspiration, abdominal cramps, nausea, headaches, and dizziness of various levels of intensity. Small children, old people, or persons with heart conditions are most severely affected and may require hospitalization and the administration of an antivenin.

black widow spider antivenin, a passive immunizing agent.

■ INDICATION: It is prescribed in the treatment of black widow spider bite.

■ CONTRAINDICATIONS: Known hypersensitivity to this drug or to horse serum prohibits its use.

■ ADVERSE EFFECTS: Among the more serious adverse effects are allergic reactions.

bladder, **1.** a membranous sac serving as a receptacle for secretions. **2.** the urinary bladder.

bladder cancer, the most common malignancy of the urinary tract. It is characterized by a tumor or by multiple growths that tend to recur in a more aggressive form. Malignant neoplasia of the bladder occurs 2.3 times more often in men than in women, is more prevalent in urban than in rural areas, and may be increasing in incidence. The risk for developing bladder cancer is increased with cigarette smoking and exposure to carcinogens, as aniline dyes, and with the use of beta-naphthylamine, mixtures of aromatic hydrocarbons, or benzidine and its salts, used in chemical, paint, plastics, rubber, textile, petroleum, and wood industries and in medical laboratories. Other predisposing factors are chronic urinary tract infections, calculous disease, and schistosomiasis; in Egypt, where *Schistosoma haematobium* infestations are extremely common, the bladder is the most frequent site of cancer. Early symptoms of a bladder cancer include hematuria, frequent urination, dysuria, and cystitis. Urinalysis, excretory urography, cystoscopy, or transurethral biopsy are performed for diagnosis. The majority of bladder malignancies are transitional cell carcinomas; a small percentage are squamous cell carcinomas or adenocarcinomas. Superficial or multiple lesions may be treated by fulguration or open loop resection. A segmental resection is usually performed if the tumor is at the dome or in a lateral wall of the bladder, but total cystectomy may be performed for an invasive lesion of the trigone. In patients requiring cystectomy, a conduit is constructed to divert urine to the colon, to a rectal bladder, or to an abdominal stoma. External radiation may be administered preoperatively or as palliation for inoperable lesions. Internal radiation, the introduction of radioisotopes via a balloon of a catheter, or the implantation of radon seeds may be used in treating small localized tumors on the bladder wall. Medications that are often used as palliatives are 5-fluorouracil and adriamycin. See also **cystectomy.**

bladder flap, *informal.* the vesicouterine fold of peritoneum that is incised during low cervical cesarean section so that the bladder can be separated from the uterus to expose the lower uterine segment for incision. The flap is reapproximated with sutures during closure to cover the uterine incision. See also **cesarean section.**

bladder stone. See **vesicle calculus.**

Blakemore-Sengstaken tube. See **Sengstaken-Blakemore tube.**

Blalock-Taussig procedure /blā′loktô′sig/, surgical construction of a shunt as a temporary measure to overcome congenital pulmonary stenosis and atrial septal defect, as in an infant born with tetralogy of Fallot. Preoperatively, a cardiac catheterization is done to identify the defect or defects, and the levels of arterial blood gases are analyzed. Hypothermia anesthesia and a cardiac bypass machine are used. The subclavian artery is joined end to end with the pulmonary artery, directing blood from the systemic circulation to the lungs. Thrombosis of the shunt is the major postoperative complication. Nursing care includes giving humidified oxygen by nasotracheal tube, monitoring fluids and electrolytes, maintaining the IV, and giving nasogastric feedings. Restlessness may signal a lack of oxygen or a low cardiac output. Permanent surgical correction is performed in early childhood. See also **heart surgery.**

blanch, **1.** to cause to become pale, as a spider angiomata may be blanched using digital pressure. **2.** to whiten or bleach a surface or substance. **3.** to become white or pale, as from vasoconstriction accompanying fear or anger.

bland, mild or having a soothing effect.

bland diet, a diet that is mechanically, chemically, physiologically, and, sometimes, thermally nonirritating. It is often prescribed in the treatment of peptic ulcer, ulcerative colitis, gallbladder disease, diverticulosis and diverticulitis, gastritis, idiopathic spastic constipation, and mucous colitis and after abdominal surgery. The diet may include eggs, meat, poultry, fish, and enriched fine cereals; milk is usually an important ingredient. A bland diet may be planned that includes or excludes any specific foods. Spicy or highly seasoned foods, carbonated beverages, raw fruits and vegetables, and rich desserts are avoided. See also **sippy diet.**

blanket bath, the procedure of wrapping the patient in a wet pack and then in blankets.

-blast, a combining form meaning an 'embryonic state of development': *leucoblast, megaloblast, osteoblast.*

blast cell, any immature cell, as an erythroblast, a lymphoblast, or a neuroblast.

blastema /blastē′mə/, *pl.* **blastemas, blastemata,** **1.** any mass of living protoplasm capable of growth and differentiation, specifically the primordial undifferentiated cellular material from which a particular organ or tissue develops. **2.** in certain animals, a group of cells capable of regenerating a lost or damaged part or of giving rise to a complete organism in asexual reproduction. **3.** the budding or sprouting area of a plant. See also **anlage.** – **blastemal, blastematic, blastemic,** *adj.*

-blastema, a combining form meaning a 'mass of living substance': *epiblastema, scleroblastema, scytoblastema.*

blastid, the site in the fertilized ovum where the pronuclei fuse and the nucleus forms. Also called **blastide.**

blastin, any substance that provides nourishment for or stimulates the growth or proliferation of cells, as allantoin.

blasto-, a combining form meaning 'pertaining to an early embryonic or developing stage': *blastocele, blastocytoma, blastomatosis.*

blastocoele /blas′təsēl′/, the fluid-filled cavity of the blastocyst in mammals and the blastula or discoblastula of lower animals. The cavity increases the surface area of the developing embryo for better absorption of nutrients and oxygen. Also spelled **blastocoel, blastocele.** Also called **cleavage cavity, segmentation cavity, subgerminal cavity.**

blastocyst /blas′təsist/, the embryonic form that follows the morula in human development. It is a spheric mass of cells having a central, fluid-filled cavity (blastocele) surrounded by two layers of cells. The outer layer (trophoblast) later forms the placenta; the inner layer (embryoblast) later forms the embryo. Implantation in the wall of the uterus usually occurs at this stage, on approximately the eighth day after fertilization.

blastocyte /blas′təsīt/, an undifferentiated embryonic cell before germ layer formation. **–blastocytic,** *adj.*

blastocytoma. See **blastoma.**

blastoderm /blas′tədurm′/, the layer of cells forming the wall of the blastocyst in mammals and the blastula in lower animals during the early stages of embryonic development. It is produced by the cleavage of the fertilized ovum and gives rise to the primary germ layers, the ectoderm, mesoderm, and endoderm from which the embryo and all of its membranes are derived. In animals in which the ovum contains a large amount of yolk and undergoes partial cleavage, the cells form a small caplike structure, or cellular disk, above the yolk mass. Kinds of blastoderm are **bilaminar blastoderm, embryonic blastoderm, extraembryonic blastoderm,** and **trilaminar blastoderm.** Also called **germinal membrane.** **–blastodermal, blastodermic,** *adj.*

blastodisk, the disklike nonyolk area of the protoplasm surrounding the animal pole where cleavage occurs in a fertilized ovum containing a large amount of yolk, as in birds and reptiles. As cleavage continues, the blastomeres form a convex structure, the blastula, which eventually develops into the embryo. Also spelled **blastodisc.**

blastogenesis /blas′tōjen′əsis/, **1.** asexual reproduction by budding. **2.** the theory of the transmission of hereditary characteristics by the germ plasm, as opposed to the theory of pangenesis. **3.** the early development of the embryo during cleavage and formation of the germ layers. **4.** the process of transforming small lymphocytes in tissue culture into large blastlike cells by exposure to phytohemagglutin or other substances, often for the purpose of inducing mitosis. **–blastogenetic,** *adj.*

blastogenic, **1.** originating in the germ plasm. **2.** initiating tissue proliferation. **3.** relating to or characterized by blastogenesis.

blastogeny /blastoj′ənē/, the early stages in ontogeny; the germ plasm history of an organism or species, which traces the history of the inherited characteristics.

blastokinin /blas′təkī′nin/, a globulin, secreted by the uterus in many mammals, that may stimulate and regulate the implantation process of the blastocyst in the uterine wall. Also called **uteroglobulin.**

blastolysis /blastol′isis/, destruction of a germ cell or blastoderm. **–blastolytic,** *adj.*

blastoma /blastō′mə/, *pl.* **blastomas, blastomata,** a neoplasm of embryonic tissue developing from the blastema of an organ or tissue. A blastoma derived from a number of scattered cells is pluricentric, and one arising from a single cell or group of cells is unicentric. Also called **blastocytoma.** **–blastomatous,** *adj.*

blastomatosis /blast′tōmətō′sis/, the development of many tumors derived from embryonic tissue.

blastomere /blas′təmēr/, one of a pair of cells that develops in the first mitotic division of the segmentation nucleus of a fertilized ovum. The two blastomeres divide and subdivide to form the morula in the first several days of pregnancy. **–blastomeric,** *adj.*

blastomerotomy, the destruction or the separation of blastomeres, either caused naturally or induced artificially. Also called **blastotomy.** **–blastomerotomic,** *adj.*

Blastomyces /blas′tōmī′sēz/, a genus of yeastlike fungus, usually including the species *Blastomyces dermatitidis,* which causes North American blastomycosis, and *Paracoccidioides brasiliensis,* which causes South American blastomycosis.

blastomycosis /blas′tōmīkō′sis/, an infectious disease caused by a yeastlike fungus, *Blastomyces dermatitidis,* that usually affects only the skin but may invade the lungs, kidneys, central nervous system, and bones. The disease is most common in young men living in North America, particularly the southeastern United States, but outbreaks have occurred in Africa and Latin America. Skin infections often begin as small papules on the hand, face, neck, or other exposed areas where there has been a cut, bruise, or other injury and spread gradually and irregularly into surrounding areas. When the lungs are involved, x-ray films of the chest show tumors resembling cancer. The person usually has a cough, dyspnea, chest pain, chills, and a fever with heavy sweating. Diagnosis is made by identification of the disease organism in a culture of specimens from lesions. Treatment usually involves the administration of a fungicidal antibiotic, amphotericin B. Recovery usually begins within the first week of treatment. Also called **Gilchrist's disease.** See also **fungus, mycosis.**

blastopore /blas′təpôr/, (in embryology) the invagination into a blastula that occurs in the process of the blastula becoming a gastrula.

blastoporic canal. See **neurenteric canal.**

blastosphere. See **blastula.**

blastotomy. See **blastomerotomy.**

blastula, an early stage of the process through which a zygote develops into an embryo, characterized by a fluid-filled sphere formed by a single layer of cells. The spheric layer of cells is called a blastoderm, and the fluid-filled cavity is the blastocoele. The blastula develops from the morula stage and is usually the form in which the embryo becomes implanted in the wall of the uterus. Also called **blastosphere.**

-blastula, a combining form meaning an 'early embryonic stage in the development of a fertilized egg': *coeloblastula, diblastula, steroblastula.*

blastulation, the transformation of the morula into a blastocyst or blastula by the development of a central cavity, the blastocoele.

BLB mask, abbreviation for **Boothby-Lovelace-Bulbulian mask.**

bleb /bleb/, an accumulation of fluid under the skin, usually associated with lesions that are smaller than normal blisters. **–blebby,** *adj.*

bleed, 1. to lose blood from the blood vessels of the body. The blood may flow externally, through an orifice or a break in the skin, or it may flow internally, into a cavity, an organ, or the spaces between the tissues. The color, quantity, and source of the blood are noted. **2.** to cause blood to flow from a vein or an artery.

bleeder, *informal.* **1.** a person who has hemophilia or any other vascular or hematologic condition associated with a tendency to hemorrhage. **2.** a bleeding blood vessel, especially one cut during a surgical procedure.

bleeding, the release of blood from the vascular system as a result of damage to or inadequacy of one or more blood vessels. See also **blood clotting.**

bleeding diasthesis, a predisposition to abnormal blood clotting.

bleeding time, the time required for blood to stop flowing from a tiny wound. A test of bleeding time is the Ivy method, in which a blood pressure cuff on the upper arm is inflated to 40 mm of mercury and a small wound is made with a scalpel and a template on the volar surface of the arm. Prolonged bleeding times are most often the result of uremia, a disorder of platelet function, or the ingestion of aspirin or other antiinflammatory medications. Normal Ivy bleeding time is from 2 to 6 minutes. See also **hemostasis.**

blending inheritance, the apparent fusion in the offspring of distinct, dissimilar characteristics of the parents, usually of a quantitative nature, as height, with segregation of the specific traits failing to appear in successive generations. This premendelian concept of inheritance is now explained in terms of multiple pairs of genes that have a cumulative effect. See also **polygene.**

blenno-, blenn-, a combining form meaning 'pertaining to mucus': *blennemesis, blennostasis, blennothorax.*

blennorrhea /blen′ərē′ə/, **1.** excessive discharge of mucus. See also **swimming pool conjuntivitis. 2.** *obsolete.* gonorrhea. Also called **blennorrhagia.**

Blenoxane, a trademark for an antineoplastic (bleomycin sulfate).

bleomycin sulfate, an antineoplastic antibiotic.

■ INDICATIONS: It is prescribed in the treatment of a variety of neoplasms.

■ CONTRAINDICATION: Hypersensitivity to this drug prohibits its use.

■ ADVERSE EFFECTS: Among the most serious adverse reactions are pneumonitis, pulmonary fibrosis, and a syndrome of hyperpyrexia and circulatory collapse. Rashes and skin reactions commonly occur.

blephar-. See **blepharo-.**

blepharal /blef′ərəl/, of or pertaining to the eyelids.

-blepharia, a combining form meaning '(condition of the) eyelid': *ablepharia, atretoblepharia, macroblepharia.*

blepharitis /blef′ərī′tis/, an inflammatory condition of the lash follicles and meibomian glands of the eyelids, characterized by swelling, redness, and crusts of dried mucus on the lids. **Ulcerative blepharitis** is caused by bacterial infection. **Nonulcerative blepharitis** may be caused by psoriasis, seborrhea, or an allergic response.

blepharo-, blephar-, a combining form meaning 'pertaining to the eyelid or eyelash': *blepharochalasis, blepharal, blepharelosis.*

blepharoadenoma /blef′ərō·ad′inō′mə/, *pl.* **blepharoadenomas, blepharoadenomata,** a glandular epithelial tumor of the eyelid.

blepharoatheroma /blef′ərō·ath′ərō′mə/, *pl.* **blepharoatheromas, blepharoatheromata,** a tumor of the eyelid.

blepharoncus /blef′əron′kəs/, a neoplasm of the eyelid.

blepharoplegia /blef′əroplē′jē·ə/, paralysis of the eyelid.

plepharospasm, a spasm of the eyelid.

-blepsia, -blepsy a combining form meaning '(condition of) sight': *acyanoblepsia, chionablepsia, hemiablepsia.*

blight, any disease of plants caused by fungus.

blighted ovum, a fertilized ovum that fails to develop. On x-ray or ultrasonic visualization it appears to be a fluid-filled cyst attached to the wall of the uterus. It may be empty, or it may contain amorphous parts. Many first trimester spontaneous abortions represent the expulsion of a blighted ovum. Suction curettage may be necessary if the blighted ovum is retained.

blind fistula, an abnormal passage with only one open end; the opening may be on the body surface or on or within an internal organ or structure. Also called **incomplete fistula.**

blind intubation. See **intubation.**

blind loop, a redundant segment of intestine. Bacterial overgrowth occurs and may lead to malabsorption, obstruction, and necrosis. Blind loops may be created inadvertently by surgical procedures, as side to side ileotransverse colostomy.

blindness, the inability to see.

blind operation, any surgical procedure performed by using the sense of touch and knowledge of surgical anatomy without making a significant cutaneous or membranous incision to provide a view of the structure or organ involved. Compare **open operation.**

blind spot, 1. a normal gap in the visual field occurring when an image is focused on the space in the retina occupied by the optic disc. **2.** an abnormal gap in the visual field because of a lesion on the retina or in the optic pathways or because of hemorrhage or choroiditis, often perceived as light spots or flashes.

blister, a vesicle or bulla.

bloat, a swelling or filling with gas, as the distention of the abdomen from swallowing air or from intestinal gas.

Blocadren, a trademark for a beta-adrenergic receptor blocking agent (timolol maleate).

block anesthesia. See **conduction anesthesia.**

blocking, **1.** preventing the transmission of an impulse as by an antiadrenergic agent or by the injection of an anesthetic. **2.** interrupting an intracellular biosynthetic process, as by the injection of actinomycin D or the action of an antivitamin. **3.** being unable to remember or involuntarily interrupting a train of thought or speech, usually because of emotional or mental conflict. **4.** repressing an idea or emotion to keep it from obtruding into the consciousness.

blocking antibody, an antibody that fails to cross-link and cause agglutination. When such antibodies are present in high concentration, they tend to interfere with the action of other antibodies by occupying all the antigenic sites. See also **antigen-antibody reaction, hapten.**

blood, the liquid pumped by the heart through all the arteries, veins, and capillaries. It consists of a clear yellow fluid, called plasma, and the formed elements, a series of different cell types, all with varying functions. The major function of the blood is to transport oxygen and nutrients to the cells and to remove from the cells carbon dioxide and other waste products for detoxification and elimination. The normal adult has a total blood volume of 7% to 8% of body weight. This is approximately equivalent to 70 ml/kg of body weight for men and about 65 ml/kg for women. It moves at a speed of about 30 cm/second, with a complete circulation time of 20 seconds. Compare **lymph.** See also **blood cell, erythrocyte, leukocyte, plasma, platelet.**

blood agar, a culture medium consisting of blood and nutrient agar, used in bacteriology to cultivate certain microorganisms, including *Staphylococcus epidermidis, Diplococcus pneumoniae,* and *Clostridium perfringens.*

blood bank, an organizational unit responsible for collecting, processing, and storing blood to be used for transfusion and other purposes. It is usually a subdivision of a laboratory in a hospital and is often charged with the responsibility for all serologic testing. See also **bank blood, component therapy, transfusion.**

blood-brain barrier (BBB), an anatomic-physiologic feature of the brain thought to consist of walls of capillaries in the central nervous system and surrounding glial membranes. The barrier separates the parenchyma of the central nervous system from blood. The blood-brain barrier functions in preventing or slowing the passage of various chemical compounds, radioactive ions, and disease-causing organisms, as viruses, from the blood into the central nervous system.

blood buffers, a system of buffers, composed primarily of dissolved carbon dioxide and bicarbonate ions, which functions in maintaining the proper pH of the blood. See also **buffer, pH.**

blood cell, any one of the formed elements of the blood, including red cells (erythrocytes), white cells (leukocytes), and platelets (thrombocytes). Together they normally constitute about 50% of the total volume of the blood. See also **erythrocyte, leukocyte, platelet.**

blood clot, a semisolid, gelatinous mass, the end result of the clotting process in blood. It ordinarily consists of red cells, white cells, and platelets enmeshed in an insoluble fibrin network. Compare **embolus, thrombus.** See also **blood clotting, fibrinogen.**

blood clotting, the conversion of blood from a free flowing liquid to a semisolid gel. Although it can occur within the intact blood vessel, the process usually starts with tissue damage and exposure of the blood to air. Within seconds of injury to the vessel wall, platelets clump at the site. If normal amounts of calcium, platelets, and tissue factors are present, prothrombin will be converted to thrombin. Thrombin then acts as a catalyst for the conversion of fibrinogen to a mesh of insoluble fibrin, in which all the formed elements are immobilized. Also called **blood coagulation.** Compare **hemostasis.** See also **anticoagulant, coagulation,** table.

blood count, See **complete blood count.**

blood culture medium, a liquid enrichment medium for the growth of bacteria in the diagnosis of blood infections. It contains a suspension of brain tissue in meat broth with dextrose, peptone, and citrate and has a pH of 7.4.

blood donor, anyone who donates his or her blood to a blood bank or directly to another person. See also **blood bank, transfusion.**

blood dyscrasia, a pathologic condition in which any of the constituents of the blood are abnormal or are present in abnormal quantity, as in leukemia or hemophilia.

blood fluke, a parasitic flatworm of the class Trematoda, genus *Schistosoma,* including the species *S. haematobium, S. japonicum,* and *S. mansoni.* See also ***Schistosoma,*** **schistosomiasis.**

blood gas, gas dissolved in the liquid part of the blood. Blood gases include oxygen, carbon dioxide, and nitrogen. (Figure, page 146)

blood gas determination, an analysis of the pH of the blood and the concentration and pressure of oxygen, carbon dioxide, and hydrogen ion in the blood. It can be performed rapidly as an emergency procedure to assess acid base balance and ventilatory status. Blood gas determination is often important in the evaluation of cardiac failure, hemorrhage, kidney failure, drug overdose, shock, uncontrolled diabetes mellitus, or any other condition of severe stress. The blood for examination is drawn from a vein or artery as ordered, placed in ice, and immediately transported for analysis. See also **acid base balance, acidosis, alkalosis, oxygenation,** $\mathbf{P_{CO_2}}$**, pH,** $\mathbf{P_{O_2}}$**.**

blood glucose. See **blood sugar.**

blood group, the classification of blood based on the presence or absence of genetically determined antigens on the surface of the red cell. Several different grouping systems have been described. These include ABO, Auberger, Diego, Dombrock, Duffy, high-frequency, I, Kell, Kidd, Lewis, low-frequency, Lutheran, MNS, P, Rh, Sutter, and Xg. Their relative importance depends on

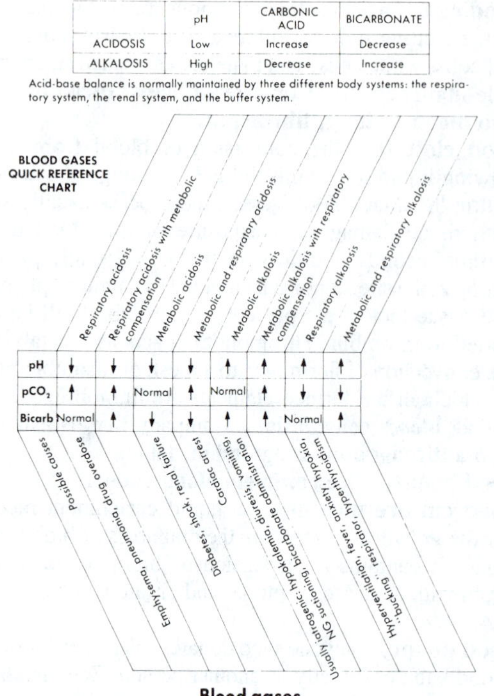

	pH	CARBONIC ACID	BICARBONATE
ACIDOSIS	Low	Increase	Decrease
ALKALOSIS	High	Decrease	Increase

Acid-base balance is normally maintained by three different body systems: the respiratory system, the renal system, and the buffer system.

Blood gases

their clinical significance in transfusion therapy, organ transplantation, disputed paternity cases, maternal-fetal compatibility, and genetic studies. See also **ABO blood groups.**

blood island, one of the clusters of mesodermal cells that proliferate on the outer surface of the embryonic yolk sac and give it a lumpy appearance. The outermost cells flatten into primitive endothelium; the inner cells develop primitive blood plasma and elaborate hemoglobin within their cytoplasm.

blood lavage, the removal of toxic elements from the blood by the injection of serum into the veins.

blood osmotality, the osmotic pressure of blood. The normal values in serum are 280 to 295 mOsm/L.

blood patch. See **epidural blood patch.**

blood pH, the hydrogen ion concentration of the blood, or a measure of its acidity or alkalinity. The normal pH values for arterial whole blood are 7.38 to 7.44; for venous whole blood, 7.36 to 7.41; for venous serum or plasma, 7.35 to 7.45.

blood plasma, the liquid portion of the blood, free of its formed elements and particles. Plasma represents approximately 50% of the total volume of blood and contains glucose, proteins, amino acids, and other nutritive materials, urea and other excretory products, as well as hormones, enzymes, vitamins, and minerals. Compare **serum.** See also **blood, plasma protein, pooled plasma.**

blood poisoning. See **septicemia.**

blood pressure (BP), the pressure exerted by the circulating volume of blood on the walls of the arteries, the veins, and the chambers of the heart. Overall blood pressure is maintained by the complex interaction of the homeostatic mechanisms of the body, moderated by the volume of the blood, the lumen of the arteries and arterioles, and the force of the cardiac contraction. The pressure in the aorta and the large arteries of a healthy young adult is approximately 120 mm Hg during systole and 70 mm Hg in diastole. The pulse pressure is approximately 50 mm Hg. See also **hypertension, hypotension.**

■ METHOD: The blood pressure is most often measured by auscultation, using an aneroid or mercury sphygmomanometer, a stethoscope, and a blood pressure cuff. The cuff is placed around the upper arm and inflated to a pressure greater than the systolic pressure, occluding the artery. The diaphragm of the stethoscope is placed over the brachial artery in the antecubital space, and the pressure in the cuff is slowly released. No sound is heard until the cuff pressure falls to less than the systolic pressure in the artery; at that point a pulse is heard. As the cuff pressure continues to fall slowly, the pulse continues; first becoming louder, then dull and muffled. These sounds, called the sounds of Korotkoff, are produced by turbulence of the blood flowing through a vessel that is partially occluded as the arterial pressure falls to the low pressure of diastole. When the cuff pressure is less than the diastolic pressure, no pulse is heard. Thus the cuff pressure at which the first sound is heard is the systolic blood pressure indicative of the pressure in the large arteries during systole; the cuff pressure at which the sounds stop is the diastolic blood pressure, indicative of the pressure on the arteries during diastole. Other methods include the use of palpation in place of auscultation to determine the systolic pressure: The pressure at which a pulse is first palpated in the antecubital space is noted; with the use of a calibrated strain gauge or a mercury manometer attached to an oscillograph, the arterial pressure may be monitored directly through a cannula placed in the artery. A Doppler instrument translates changes in ultrasound frequency caused by blood movement within the artery to audible sound by means of a transducer in the cuff. The flush method is used when pressure is difficult to obtain and reflects mean blood pressure. The cuff is applied, and complete capillary emptying is performed, usually with an elastic bandage. The cuff is inflated, the elastic bandage is removed, and the earliest discernible flush is observed as the cuff is deflated.

■ NURSING ORDERS: The intervals at which the patient's blood pressure is to be taken are specified. The pressure in both arms is taken the first time the procedure is performed; persistent major difference between the two readings is indicative of the presence of a vascular occlusion. The blood pressure may be taken using the thigh and the popliteal space, but to obtain an accurate reading, the leg should be at the level of the heart. A larger cuff is used when taking the blood pressure of an obese person and for all people when using the thigh location.

■ OUTCOME CRITERIA: Any factor that increases peripheral resistance or cardiac output affects the blood pressure. Strong emotion, for example, tends to do both; therefore, it is important to try to secure a blood pressure reading when the person is at rest. Increased peripheral resistance usually increases the diastolic pressure, and increased cardiac output tends to increase the systolic pressure. Blood pressure increases with age, primarily because of the decreased distensibility of the veins. As a person grows older, an increase in systolic pressure precedes an increase in diastolic pressure.

Classification of blood pressure

Diastolic blood pressure (mm Hg)	Category*
<85	Normal blood pressure
85 to 89	High normal blood pressure
90 to 104	Mild hypertension
105 to 114	Moderate hypertension
≥115	Severe hypertension
Systolic blood pressure (mm Hg) when DBP <90 mm Hg	**Category**
<140	Normal blood pressure
140 to 159	Borderline isolated systolic hypertension
≥160	Isolated systolic hypertension

*A classification of borderline isolated systolic hypertension (SBP 140 to 159 mm Hg) or isolated systolic hypertension (SBP ≥ 160 mm Hg) takes precedence over a classification of high normal blood pressure (DBP 85 to 89 mm Hg) when both occur in the same individual. A classification of high normal blood pressure (DBP 85 to 89 mm Hg) takes precedence over a classification of normal blood pressure (SBP <140 mm Hg) when both occur in the same person.
From The 1984 Report of the Joint National Committee on Detection, Evaluation, and Treatment of High Blood Pressure, U.S. Dept. of Health and Human Services, Public Health Service, NIH Publication No. 84-1088, Bethesda, MD, June 1984, National Institutes of Health.

blood pump, **1.** a pump for regulating the flow of blood into a blood vessel during transfusion. **2.** a component of a heart-lung machine that pumps the blood through the machine for oxygenation and then through the peripheral circulatory system of the body. See also **oxygenation.**

blood serum. See **serum.**

blood substitute, a substance used as a replacement for circulating blood or for extending its volume. Plasma, human serum albumin, packed red cells, platelets, leukocytes, and concentrates of clotting factors are often administered in place of whole blood transfusions in the treatment of various disorders. Substances that are sometimes used in solution to expand blood volume include dextran, hetastarch, albumin solutions, or plasma protein fraction. Perfluorocarbon emulsions that are being tested as blood substitutes are able to carry oxygen to tissues, have a long shelf life without refrigeration, and do not induce antigen-antibody reactions. See also **synthetic blood.**

blood sugar, **1.** one of a group of closely related substances, as glucose, fructose, and galactose, that are normal constituents of the blood and are essential for cellular metabolism. **2.** *nontechnical.* the concentration of glucose in the blood, represented in milligrams of glucose per deciliter of blood. Also called **blood glucose.** See also **hyperglycemia, hypoglycemia.**

blood test, **1.** any test that determines something about the characteristics or properties of the blood. **2.** *informal.* a serologic test for syphilis.

blood transfusion, the administration of whole blood or a component, as packed red cells, to replace blood lost through trauma, surgery, or disease.

■ METHOD: Blood for transfusion is obtained from a healthy donor or donors whose ABO blood group and antigenic subgroups match those of the recipient and who have an adequate hemoglobin level (above 13.5 g/100 ml for men and above 12.5 g/100 ml for women). Each 500 ml of blood collected from a donor is stored in a plastic bag containing citrate-dextrose or citrate-phosphate. A unit can be stored under refrigeration for only 3 weeks; at that time, the leukocytes, platelets, and 20% to 30% of the red cells are nonviable, and the levels of clotting factors V and VIII are low. The blood is removed from the refrigerator no more than 30 minutes before transfusion and is checked according to hospital policy. The necessary equipment is assembled, the blood tubing is flushed with normal saline solution, and the patient's venipuncture site is prepared. During transfusion the position of the extremity is checked, and the venipuncture site is observed for signs of erythema, swelling, or leakage. The procedure is stopped if there is evidence of a systemic reaction. An acute hemolytic reaction, characterized by chills, fever, headache, back pain, decreased blood pressure, hematuria, and nausea, may occur if the recipient's and donor's blood groups are not exactly matched. Circulatory overload may cause shortness of breath, lung congestion, and frothy sputum. A pyrogenic reaction caused by bacteria or an antigen on the leukocytes or platelets of the transfused blood may result in fever, chills, and palpitations. An allergic reaction to serum protein in transfused blood may be characterized by urticaria, laryngeal edema, and asthmatic wheezing. After a transfusion has been completed, pressure is applied to the venipuncture site and a bandage or dressing is applied. The patient is observed for 1 hour to make certain that a reaction does not occur.

■ NURSING ORDERS: The nurse prepares the required equipment and venipuncture site, observes the patient during and after transfusion, and instructs the patient to report any symptoms associated with the procedure.

■ OUTCOME CRITERIA: All possible measures are taken to prevent the reactions that occur in an estimated 2% to 3% of transfused patients. Acute hemolytic reactions can be fatal; delayed hemolysis, characterized by jaundice and anemia, may occur weeks or months after transfusion. Air embolism may occur if blood is administered under air pressure after hemorrhaging; massive replacement may cause hyperkalemia, thrombocytopenia, ammonia, and citrate toxicity. Viral hepatitis and cytomegalovirus disease may be transmitted by transfused blood. But in most cases transfusion is an uneventful procedure.

blood typing, identification of genetically determined antigens on the surface of the red blood cell, used to determine a person's blood group. Usually a blood bank prodecure, it is the first step in testing donor's and recipient's blood to be used in transfusion and is followed by crossmatching. See also **ABO blood groups, blood group, Rh factor, transfusion reaction.**

blood urea nitrogen (BUN), the amount of nitrogenous substance present in the blood as urea. BUN is a rough indicator of kidney function. It is elevated in kidney failure, shock, GI bleeding, diabetes mellitus, and some tumors. BUN levels are decreased in liver disease, malnutrition, and normal pregnancy. See also **azotemia.**

blood vessel, any one of the network of tubes that carries blood. Kinds of blood vessels are **arteries, arterioles, capillaries, veins,** and **venules.**

blood warming coil, a device constructed of coiled plastic tubing, used for the warming of reserve blood before massive transfusions, as those often required for patients who develop extensive GI bleeding. Administration of cold blood in such transfusions may cause the patient to go into shock. The blood warming coil is a prepackaged, sterile single use device. Aseptic technique is used to remove the coil from its wrapper. The coil is immersed in water warmed to 99° F (37.6° C), and blood from the transfusion bag is allowed to flow through the coil until warm enough to administer. The coil is equipped with clamps for control of the blood flow to the primary transfusion line. During prolonged transfusions the blood warming coil is replaced every 24 hours. Compare **electric blood warmer.**

bloody show. See **vaginal bleeding.**

Bloom's syndrome, a rare genetic disease occuring mainly in Ashkenazi Jews. It is transmitted as an autosomal recessive trait and is characterized by growth retardation, telangiectatic erythema of the face and arms, sensitivity to sunlight, and an increased risk of leukemia.

blow-out fracture, a fracture of the floor of the orbit caused by a blow that suddenly increases the intraocular pressure.

blue baby, an infant born with cyanosis caused by a congenital heart lesion, as transposition of the great vessels, by tetralogy of Fallot, or by incomplete expansion of the lungs (congenital atelectasis). Tetralogy of Fallot is the most common congenital cyanotic cardiac lesion. Congenital cyanotic heart lesions are diagnosed by cardiac catheterization, angiography, or echocardiography and are corrected surgically, preferably in early childhood. See also **congenital atelectasis, congenital cardiac anomaly, tetralogy of Fallot, transposition of the great vessels.**

blue bloater. See **chronic bronchitis.**

blue fever, *informal.* Rocky Mountain spotted fever, so named for the dark cyanotic discoloration of the skin after the initial rickettsial infection. See also **rickettsiosis, Rocky Mountain spotted fever, typhus.**

blue nevus, a sharply circumscribed, usually benign, steel blue skin nodule with a diameter between 2 and 7 mm. It is found on the face or upper extremities, grows very slowly, and persists throughout life. Nodular blue nevi found on the buttocks or in the sacrococcygeal region occasionally become malignant. Any sudden change in the size of such a lesion demands surgical attention and biopsy. The dark color is caused by large, densely packed melanocytes deep in the dermis of the nevus. Compare **melanoma.**

blue phlebitis. See **phlegmasia cerulea dolens.**

blue spot, **1.** also called **macula cerulea.** one of a number of small grayish blue spots that may appear near the armpits or around the groins of individuals infested with lice, as in pediculosis corporis and pediculosis pubis. These spots are usually less than 1 cm in diameter and are caused by a substance in the saliva of lice that converts bilirubin to biliverdin. **2.** one of a number of dark blue or mulberry hued round or oval spots that may appear as a congenital condition in the sacral regions of certain children under 4 or 5 years of age. They usually disappear spontaneously as the affected individual matures. Also called **mongolian spot.**

blunt dissection, a dissection performed by separating tissues along natural lines of cleavage, without cutting.

blunthook, **1.** a sturdy hook-shaped bar used in obstetrics for traction between the abdomen and the thigh in cases of difficult breech deliveries. **2.** a hook-shaped device with a blunt end used in embryotomy.

blurred film fault, a defect in a photograph or radiograph that appears as an indistinct or blurred image. It is caused by film movement during exposure, bent film during exposure, double exposure, or film emulsion flow during processing in excessively warm solutions.

blush, a brief, diffuse erythema of the face and neck, commonly the result of dilatation of superficial small blood vessels in response to heat or sudden emotion.

B lymphocyte. See **B cell.**

B/M, symbol for black male, often used in the initial identifying statement in a patient record.

BMA, abbreviation for **British Medical Association.**

B-mode, brightness modulation, an imaging technique used in ultrasound scanning in which bright dots on an oscilloscope screen represents echos, and the intensity of the brightness indicates the strength of the echo.

BMR, abbreviation for **basal metabolic rate.**

BOA, abbreviation for **born out of asepsis.**

board certification, a process in which an individual is tested in a medical specialty or subspecialty. Physicians are approved to practice after successfully completing requirements of specialty or subspecialty boards. The various medical professional organizations provide board certification examinations. Successful candidates are called "fellows," as Fellow of the American College of Surgeons (FACS), Fellow of the American College of Obstetrics and Gynecology (FACOG). Board certification is required to attain the privilege of professional practice in a hospital, including the admission of patients, the use of hospital resources, or the performance of certain diagnostic tests or surgery.

board certified, denoting a physician who has passed the certification examination administered by a medical specialty board and has been certified as a specialist in a particular field of medicine. The professional is then called a ''fellow'' of the specialty organization.

board of health, an administrative body acting on a municipal, county, state, provincial, or national level. The functions, powers, and responsibilities of boards of health vary with the locales. Each board is generally concerned with the recognition of the health needs of the people and the coordination of projects and resources to meet and identify these needs. Among the tasks of most boards of health are prevention of disease, health education, and implementation of laws pertaining to health.

Boas' test /bō′az/, **1.** also called **resorcinol test.** a test for hydrochloric acid in the contents of the stomach, in which a glass rod dipped in a specially prepared reagent is touched to a drop of filtered stomach liquid. A scarlet streak forms along the rod in the presence of hydrochloric acid. The reagent, which is warmed before the rod is dipped, contains 5 g of resorcinol and 5 g of sugar dissolved in 100 ml of dilute alcohol. **2.** a test for free hydrochloric acid in the contents of the stomach in which filtered stomach fluid is boiled with a special reagent, containing five parts of resorcinol, three parts of cane sugar, and 92 parts of 94% alcohol. Free hydrochloric acid produces a transient rosy mirror. **3.** a test for lactic acid in a sample of gastric juice that depends on the oxidation of the lactic acid to aldehyde and formic acid by the action of sulfuric acid and manganese. The test detects the aldehyde by the addition of Nessler's reagent or by the formation of iodoform with the addition of iodine solution. **4.** also called **chlorophyll test.** a test for gastric motility in which a fasting patient drinks 400 ml of water that has been tinted green by the addition of 20 drops of chlorophyll solution. After 30 minutes, the contents of the stomach are aspirated and the amount of tinted water that has passed through the stomach is determined.

Bodansky unit, the quantity of phosphotase in 100 ml of serum to liberate 1 mg of phosphorous as phosphate ion from sodium betaglycerophosphate in 1 hour at 37° C. It is used to express the measure of certain enzymes, as acid phosphatase in the body.

body, **1.** the whole structure of an individual with all the organs. **2.** a cadaver or a corpse. **3.** the largest or the main part of any organ, as the body of the tibia or the body of the vastus lateralis. Also called **corpus, soma.**

body fluid, a fluid contained in the three fluid compartments of the body: the blood plasma of the circulating blood, the interstitial fluid between the cells, and the cell fluid within the cells. Blood plasma and interstitial fluid make up the extracellular fluid; the cell fluid is the intracellular fluid. The chemical constituents of the fluids vary greatly; for example, sodium is present in large amounts in both compartments of the extracellular fluid but is nearly absent in the intracellular fluid; protein is present in the blood plasma and cell fluid but not in the interstitial fluid.

body image, a person's subjective concept of his or her physical appearance. The mental representation, which may be realistic or unrealistic, is constructed from self-observation, the reactions of others, and a complex interaction of attitudes, emotions, memories, fantasies, and experiences, both conscious and unconscious. A marked inability to conceptualize one's personal body characteristics may be caused by organic brain damage, as in autotopagnosia, by a physical disability, as the loss of a limb, or by psychologic and emotional disturbances, as in anorexia nervosa.

body image agnosia. See **autotopagnosia.**

body jacket, an orthopedic cast that encases the trunk of the body but does not extend over the cervical area; it may be equipped with shoulder straps. It is used to help immobilize the trunk for the healing of spinal injuries and scoliosis and for postoperative positioning and immobilization after spinal surgery. Compare **Risser cast.**

body language, a set of nonverbal signals, including body movements, postures, gestures, spatial positions, facial expressions, and bodily adornment, that give expression to various physical, mental, and emotional states. See also **kinesics.**

body mechanics, the field of physiology that studies muscular actions and the function of muscles in maintaining the posture of the body.

body movement, motion of all or part of the body, especially at a joint or joints. Some kinds of body movements are **abduction, adduction, extension, flexion,** and **rotation.**

body odor, a fetid smell associated with stale perspiration. Freshly secreted perspiration is odorless, but after exposure to the atmosphere and bacterial activity at the surface of the skin, chemical changes occur to produce the odor. Common body odor usually can be eliminated by bathing with soap and water. Body odors also can be the result of discharges from a variety of skin conditions, including cancer, fungus, hemorrhoids, leukemia, and ulcers. See also **bromhidrosis.**

body of Retzius /ret′sē·əs/, any one of the masses of protoplasm containing pigment granules at the lower end of a hair cell of the organ of Corti in the internal ear.

body position, attitude or posture of the body. Some kinds of body position are **anatomic position, decubitus, Fowler's position, prone, supine,** and **Trendelenburg position.**

body righting reflex, any one of the neuromuscular responses to restore the body to its normal upright position when it has been displaced. The righting reflexes involve complicated mechanisms and processes associated with the structures of the internal ear, as the utricle, the saccule, the macula, and the semicircular canals. Also involved in the righting mechanism are receptors for the vestibular branch of the eighth cranial nerve. Any change in the position of the head produces a change in the pressure on the gelatinous membrane of the macula and causes tiny otoliths within the membrane to pull on hair cells, stimulating adjacent receptors of the vestibular nerve. The fibers of the nerve transmit impulses to the brain, producing a sense of position of the head by a sensation of change in the gravitational pull, activating muscles that tend to restore the body to its optimum position. Also activating righting reflexes are proprioceptors in muscles and tendons and visual nerve impulses. Interruption of the impulses associated with body righting reflexes may disturb equilibrium and cause nausea and vomiting.

body stalk, the elongated part of the embryo that is connected to the chorion. The stalk first extends from the posterior end of the embryo to the chorion but later moves to the midventral region and forms the lengthening umbilical cord. As the embryo develops and the amnion expands, the umbilical cord comes to enclose the body stalk and the yolk sac. See also **allantois.**

body surface area. See **surface area.**

body systems model, (in nursing education) a conceptual framework in which illness is studied in relation to the functional systems of the body, as the circulatory, nervous, GI, and reproductive. In this model, nursing care is directed toward manipulating the patient's environment in such a way that the signs and symptoms of the health problem are alleviated. As the body systems model focuses on the disease rather than the patient, current educational programs tend to integrate it with other concepts that allow the nurse to approach the patient in a more holistic framework, recognizing the complexity of the external and internal agents that contribute to illness and to health.

body temperature, the level of heat produced and sustained by the body processes. Variations and changes in body temperature are major indicators of disease and other abnormalities. Heat is generated within the body through metabolism of food and lost from the body surface through radiation, convection, and evaporation of perspiration. Heat production and loss are regulated and controlled in the hypothalamus and brainstem. Fever is usually a function of an increase in the generation of heat, but some abnormal conditions, as congestive heart failure, produce slight elevations of body temperature through impairment of the heat loss function. Contributing to the failure to dissipate heat are reduced activity of the heart, lower rate of blood flow to the skin, and the insulating effect of edema. Diseases of the hypothalamus or interference with the other regulatory centers may produce abnormally low body temperatures. Normal adult body temperature, as measured orally, is 98.6° F. Oral temperatures ranging from 96.5° F to 99° F are consistent with good health, depending on the physical activity of the person, the ambient temperature, and the particular, normal body temperature for that person. Axillary temperature is usually 1° F lower than the oral temperature. Rectal temperatures may be 0.5° to 1° F higher than oral readings. Body temperature appears to vary 1° to 2° F throughout the day, with lows recorded early in the morning and peaks between 6 PM and 10 PM. This diurnal variation may increase in range during a fever. While adult body temperature, normal and abnormal, tends to vary within a relatively narrow range, the temperatures of children respond more dramatically and rapidly to disease, changes in ambient temperature, and levels of physical activity.

Boeck's sarcoid. See **sarcoidosis.**

boil, a skin abscess. See **furuncle.**

boiling point, the temperature at which a substance passes from the liquid to the gaseous state at a particular atmospheric pressure. See also **evaporation.**

bole, any of a variety of soft, friable clays of various colors although usually red from iron oxide. They consist of hydrous silicate of aluminum, are used as pigments, and were once commonly used as absorbents and astringents.

Bolivian hemorrhagic fever, an infectious disease caused by an arenavirus, generally transmitted from infected rodents to humans through contamination of food by rodent urine, though direct transmission between people has also been observed. After an incubation period of from 1 to 2 weeks, the patient experiences chills, fever, headache, muscle ache, anorexia, nausea, and vomiting. As the disease progresses, hypotension, dehydration, bradycardia, pulmonary edema, and internal hemorrhages may occur. The mortality may reach 30%; pulmonary edema is the most common cause of death. There is no specific therapy. Peritoneal dialysis is sometimes performed. Also called **Machupo.** See also **arenavirus, Argentine hemorrhagic fever, Lassa fever.**

bolus, **1.** also called **alimentary bolus.** a round mass, specifically a masticated lump of food ready to be swallowed. **2.** a large round preparation of medicinal material for oral ingestion, usually soft and not prepackaged. **3.** a dose of a medication or a contrast material, radioactive isotope, or other pharmaceutic preparation injected all at once intravenously. **4.** in radiotherapy, material used to fill in irregular body surfaces in order to get a better dose distribution for hyperthermia or to increase the dose to the skin when high-energy photon beams are used.

Bombay phenotype, a rare genetic trait involving the phenotypic expression of the ABO blood groups. The gene for the H antigen, which in the usual dominant form of HH or Hh is responsible for the precursor necessary for the production of the A and B antigens, is homozygous recessive in individuals with this trait so that the expression of the A, B, and H antigens is suppressed. Cells of such individuals are phenotypically of blood type O even though they are genotype AB, and the serum contains anti-A, anti-B, and anti-H antigens. In such cases the offspring from two phenotypic O blood type parents may be blood type AB. The phenomenon is an example of the intricate interaction of linked genes in which one gene on a chromosome controls the expression or suppression of another gene that is not its allele. The trait is named for the city in which it was first reported. See also **ABO blood groups.**

bonding, the attachment process that occurs between an infant and the parents, especially the mother, and is significant in the formation of affectionate ties that later influence both the physical and psychologic development of the child. The process is reciprocal and is usually initiated immediately after birth by placing the nude infant on the mother's abdomen so that both the parents and child can see and touch one another and begin to interact. The newborn is in an alert, reactive state for about 30 minutes to 1 hour after birth and displays such behavior as crying, sucking, clinging, grasping, and following with the eyes, which in turn stimulates the expression of the parenting instincts. Especially important in initiating bonding is eye to eye contact, fondling of the infant, soothing talk, and other affectionate behavior that begins to create positive emotional ties. Another essential element is the amount of contact that occurs between parents and the newborn, especially crucial with premature and high risk infants. New concepts in normal delivery procedures, especially the trend toward more natural childbirth, allowing the father to participate and even to assist in the delivery, and the parental involvement in the care of premature and ill newborns help to facilitate stronger parent-infant relationships. Specific behavioral traits are common for each parent during the early attachment process. Mothers are more concerned with physically touching and holding the infant, whereas fathers are more intent on forming a sense of absorption, preoccupation, and visual interest in the child—what has been called paternal engrossment. By about the second to third week of life, there is a definite reciprocal pattern of interacting behavior, involving an attention and nonattention cycle, during each encounter of parents and child. At the peak of the attention phase, the infant reaches out toward the parent and is very attentive. This is followed in a short time by deceleration of excitement in the infant and a turning away from the parent. This nonattentive phase prevents the infant from being overwhelmed by excessive stimuli, and no amount of visual or verbal attempt will regain his attention. Recognition of these cycles and especially the fact that the nonattention phase is not a form of rejection help both the mother and father to develop competence in parenting. Assessment of the attachment process is an important function of the nurse and requires skill in terms of observation and interviewing. The nurse observes the mother's reactions, especially while feeding, bathing, and comforting her infant, for potential signs of inadequate or delayed mothering. Perhaps the most important actions for forming positive parent-child attachment are eye contact in the en face position and embracing the infant close to the body. Many variables determine the development of attachment and parenting, including the parents' fantasies about the child, the conditions surrounding the pregnancy, what arrangements have been made concerning changes in life-style with the addition of a dependent family member, and what type of parenting the mother and father received as children. Because bonding is always a reciprocal process, the nurse can also instruct parents on ways of encouraging various developmental behavior, especially during the first year of life, which, in turn, enhances the responsiveness of the infant and creates a closer attachment. Parents who are aware of the child's expected level of performance promote trust and security in the child. Such awareness and especially early contact between parents and child, primarily during the neonatal period, reduce the later risk of neglect or child abuse. Although bonding is considered primarily an emotional response, it is theorized that there may be some biochemical and hormonal interaction in the mother that may stimulate the response, but studies are still inconclusive. Also called **maternal-child attachment.** See also **maternal deprivation syndrome, maternal-infant bonding.**

bond specificity, the nature of enzyme action that causes the disruption of only certain bonds between atoms.

bone, **1.** the dense, hard, and slightly elastic connective tissue, comprising the 206 bones of the human skeleton. It is composed of compact osseous tissue surrounding spongy cancelous tissue permeated by many blood vessels and nerves and enclosed in membranous periosteum. Long bones contain yellow marrow in longitudinal cavities and red marrow in their articular ends. Red marrow also fills the cavities of the flat and the short bones, the bodies of the vertebrae, the cranial diploe, the sternum, and the ribs. Blood cells are produced in active red marrow. Osteocytes form bone tissue in concentric rings around an intricate haversian system of interconnecting canals that accommodates blood vessels, lymphatic vessels, and nerve fibers. **2.** any single element of the skel-

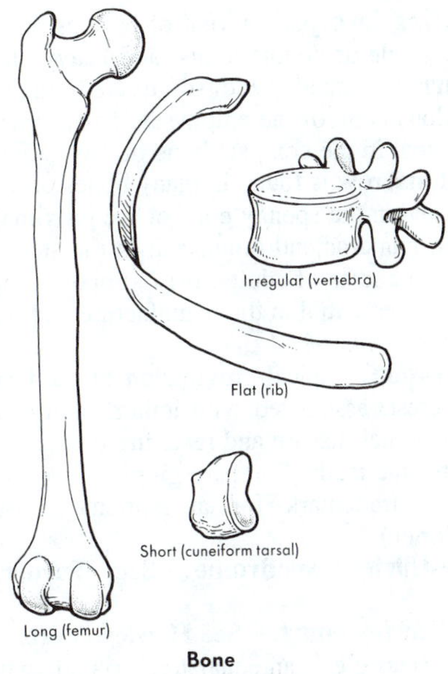

Bone

eton, as a rib, the sternum, or the femur. See also **connective tissue.**

bone cancer, a skeletal malignancy occurring as a primary sarcomatous tumor in an area of rapid growth or, more frequently, as a metastasis from cancer elsewhere in the body. Primary bone tumors are comparatively rare; the incidence peaks during adolescence, then decreases, and rises slowly after the age of 35. In adults bone cancer is strongly linked to exposure to ionizing radiation, especially in applying paints containing radium to watch dials. Paget's disease, hyperparathyroidism, chronic osteomyelitis, old bone infarcts, and fracture callosities increase the risk of bone tumors, but most osseous malignancies are metastatic lesions found most often in the spine or pelvis and less often in sites away from the trunk. Bone cancers progress rapidly but are often difficult to detect; pain that increases at night may be the only symptom. X-ray films, radioisotopic scans, arteriography, and biopsies are diagnostic; alkaline phosphatase levels are elevated in osteoblastic tumors, and serum calcium and urinary calcium are increased in highly destructive lesions; but in other bone lesions, blood studies are often equivocal. The most common osseous malignancies are osteosarcomas, followed by chrondrosarcomas, fibrosarcomas, and Ewing's sarcoma. Surgical treatment consists of local resection of slow-growing tumors or amputation, including the joint above the tumor, if the lesion is particularly virulent and fast-growing. Radiotherapy may be administered preoperatively or as the primary form of treatment of radiosensitive tumors, as Ewing's sarcoma, reticulum cell sarcoma, and multiple myeloma. Chemotherapy, using a combination of adriamycin, cyclophosphamide, vincristine, and actinomycin D, is often effective in curing Ewing's tumors. The use of interferon and other forms of immunotherapy has been experimental.

bone cutting forceps, a kind of forceps that has long handles, single or double joints, and heavy blades.

bone marrow, specialized, soft tissue filling the spaces in cancelous bone of the epiphyses. Fatty, **yellow marrow** is found in the compact bone of most adult epiphyses. **Red marrow** is found in many bones of infants and children and in the spongy bone of the proximal epiphyses of the humerus and femur and in the sternum, ribs, and vertical bodies of adults. It is composed of myeloid tissue and is essential in the manufacture and maturation of red blood cells.

bone recession, apical progression of the level of the alveolar crest, associated with inflammatory or dystrophic periodontal disease and resulting in decreased bone support for the teeth. Compare **gingival recession.**

Bonine, a trademark for an antiemetic (meclizine hydrochloride).

Bonnevie-Ullrich syndrome. See **Turner's syndrome.**

Bonwitt-Hawley chart. See **Hawley chart.**

Bonwitt's triangle, an equalateral triangle with 4 inch (10 cm) sides formed by lines from the contact points of the lower central incisors (or the median line of the residual ridge of the mandible) to the condyle on either side and from one condyle to the other. Compare **Tweed triangle.**

booster injection, the administration of an antigen, as a vaccine or toxoid, usually in a smaller amount than the original immunization, given to maintain the immune response at an appropriate level.

Boothby-Lovelace-Bulbulian (BLB) mask, an apparatus for the administration of oxygen, consisting of a mask fitted with an inspiratory-expiratory valve and a rebreathing bag.

boracic acid. See **boric acid.**

borate, any salt of boric acid. Borate salts and boric acid, although formerly used as mild antiseptic irrigant solutions, especially for ophthalmic conditions, are highly poisonous when taken internally or absorbed through a cut, abrasion, or other wound in the skin. Because of the potential for fatal poisoning, such solutions are rarely used now. See also **boric acid.**

borax bath, a medicated bath in which borax and glycerin are added to the water.

borborygmus /bôr′bərig′məs/, *pl.* **borborygmi,** an audible abdominal sound produced by hyperactive intestinal peristalsis. Borborygmi are rumbling, gurgling, and tinkling noises heard in auscultation. Although increased intestinal activity may be noted in cases of gastroenteritis and diarrhea, true borborygmi are more intense and episodic. Borborygmi accompanied by vomiting, distension, and intestinal cramps suggest a mechanic obstruction of the small intestine.

borderline schizophrenia. See **latent schizophrenia.**

Bordetella /bôr′ditel′ə/, a genus of gram-negative coccobacilli, some species of which are pathogens of the respiratory tract of humans, including *Bordetella bronchiseptica, B. parapertussis,* and *B. pertussis.* See also **parapertussis, pertussis.**

boric acid /bôr′ik/, a white, odorless powder or crystalline substance used as a buffer and formerly employed as a topical antiseptic and eye wash. Also called **boracic acid, orthoboric acid.**

Bornholm disease. See **epidemic pleurodynia.**

born out of asepsis (BOA), (in a hospital) denoting a newborn infant that was not delivered in the usual place in an obstetric unit. Depending on the policy of the institution, a BOA-designated infant may have been born on the way to the hospital or in the hospital, on the way to the delivery suite or in a labor room.

■ OBSERVATIONS: Initial assessment on the admitting unit includes evaluation of respiration, quality of cry, skin color, apical pulse rate, muscle tone, reflexes, temperature, condition of umbilical cord or cord stump, ability to suck, presence of meconium, congenital defect, skin eruption, or signs of sepsis, including jaundice, anorexia, vomiting, diahrrea, irritability or lethargy, high-pitched cry, and hypothermia or hyperthermia.

■ INTERVENTION: The usual steps in caring for a newborn are performed. Head and chest circumferences are measured, weight is taken, the baby is placed in a warmer until the axillary temperature is 36.5° C. Vitamin K and silver nitrate are usually given, and a bath is given when the body temperature is over 36.5° C and stable. In many hospitals BOA infants are placed in a special nursery, isolated from other infants to prevent contagion should the BOA baby be infected.

■ NURSING CONSIDERATIONS: Daily care for the newborn BOA is the same as that given to other newborns, but, in addition, close observation for signs of sepsis is made. The parents are involved in the care of the infant as soon as is possible, and the usual instructions are given for care of the baby at home after discharge.

boron (B), a nonmetallic element, similar to aluminum. Its atomic number is 5; its atomic weight is 10.8. Elemental boron occurs in the form of dark crystals and as a greenish yellow amorphous mass. Certain concentrations of this element are toxic to plant and animal life, but plants need traces of boron for normal growth. It is the characteristic element of boric acid, which is used chiefly as a dusting powder and ointment for minor skin disorders. Boric acid in solution was formerly extensively employed as an antiinfective and eyewash, but the high incidence of toxic reactions and fatalities associated with these preparations has greatly reduced their use.

Borrelia /bərel′ē·ə/, a genus of coarse, unevenly coiled, helical spirochetes, several species of which cause tick-borne and louseborne relapsing fever. The organism is spread to offspring from generation to generation. This does not occur in lice. Many animals serve as reservoirs and hosts for *Borrelia*. The spirochete may be identified by microscopic examination of a smear of blood stained with Wright's stain; it is also easily inoculated onto culture media for bacterial culture and identification.

Bostock's catarrh, an obsolete term for **hay fever.**

Boston exanthem, an epidemic disease characterized by scattered, pale red maculopapules on the face, chest, and back, occasionally accompanied by small ulcerations on the tonsils and soft palate. There is little or no adenopathy, and the rash disappears spontaneously in 2 or 3 weeks. It is caused by echovirus 16 and requires no treatment. Compare **herpangina.**

bottle feeding, feeding an infant or young child from a bottle with a rubber nipple on the end, sometimes called artificial feeding because it is done as a substitute for or supplement to breast feeding.

■ METHOD: The infant is held on one arm close to the body of the mother or nurse during feeding. The bottle is held at an angle to assure that the nipple is always filled with liquid so that the infant does not ingest air while feeding. For a newborn infant, rest periods may be given every several minutes. Once or twice in the course of the feeding and again at the end the infant is encouraged to burp by being held upright on the mother's or nurse's shoulder or on its stomach on the feeder's lap. Gentle rubbing or patting on the back and pressure on the stomach often helps to induce burping.

■ NURSING ORDERS: The formula contains protein, fats, carbohydrates, vitamins, and minerals in amounts similar to those in breast milk. The formula may be warmed before feeding by immersing the bottle in warm water for several minutes (although this is not necessary), and the size of the nipple hole is adjusted to the needs of the infant. Smaller infants need larger nipple holes, which require less sucking. Premature, or weak infants, may be fed using a special, long soft nipple through which it is very easy for the infant to feed.

■ OUTCOME CRITERIA: Bottle feeding is used as a substitute for breast feeding when the mother is unable to breast-feed or chooses not to. Bottle feeding can also be substituted for breast feeding occasionally, once lactation has been established. Bottle feeding is recommended if the mother has active tuberculosis or other active, acute contagious disease, if she has a serious chronic disease, as cancer or cardiac disease, or if she has recently undergone extensive surgery. Severe mastitis, narcotic addiction, or concurrent use of medication that is secreted in the breast milk usually requires the mother to bottle-feed.

bottle mouth syndrome. See **nursing bottle caries.**

botulism /boch′əliz′əm/, an often fatal form of food poisoning caused by an endotoxin produced by the bacillus *Clostridium botulinum*. The toxin is ingested in food contaminated by *C. botulinum,* although it is not necessary for the live bacillus to be present if the toxin has been produced. In rare instances, the toxin may be introduced into the human body through a wound contaminated by the organism. Botulism differs from most other types of food poisoning in that it develops without gastric distress and may not occur for from 18 hours up to 1 week after the contaminated food has been ingested. Botulism is characterized by a period of lassitude and fatigue followed by visual disturbances, as double vision, difficulty in focusing the eyes, and loss of ability of the pupil to accommodate to light. Muscles may become weak, and the victim often develops dysphagia. Nausea and vomiting occur in less than half the cases. Hospitalization is required, and antitoxins are administered. Sedatives are given, mainly to relieve anxiety. Approximately two thirds of the cases of botulism are fatal, usually as a result of delayed diagnosis and respiratory complications. For those who survive, recovery is slow. Most botulism occurs after eating improperly canned or cooked foods. See also ***Clostridium.***

bouba. See **yaws.**

Bouchard's node /bo͞oshärz′/, an abnormal cartilaginous or bony enlargement of a proximal interphalangeal joint of a finger, usually occurring in degenerative diseases of the joints. Compare **Heberden's node.**

bougie /bo͞o′zhē, bo͞ozhē′/, a thin, cylindric instrument made of rubber, waxed silk, or other flexible material for insertion into canals of the body in order to dilate, examine, or measure them.

-boulia. See **-bulia.**

boulimia. See **bulimia.**

bounding pulse, a pulse that, on palpation, feels full and springlike because of an increased thrust of cardiac contraction or an increased volume of circulating blood within the elastic structures of the vascular system.

bouquet fever. See **dengue.**

Bourneville's disease. See **tuberous sclerosis.**

boutonneuse fever /bo͞o′təno͞oz′/, an infectious disease caused by *Rickettsia conorii,* transmitted to humans through the bite of a tick. The onset of the disease is characterized by a lesion called a tache noire /täshnô·är′/, or black spot, at the site of the infection, fever lasting from a few days to 2 weeks, and a papular erythematous rash that spreads over the body to include the skin of the palms and soles. Treatment usually involves administration of antibiotics. There is no prophylactic medication available, and prevention depends primarily on avoiding ticks. The disease is similar to Rocky Mountain spotted fever and to other rickettsial diseases. It is prevalent in parts of Europe, Asia, Africa, and the Middle East. See also **rickettsiosis, Rocky Mountain spotted fever.**

Bowditch's law. See **all-or-none law.**

bowel. See **intestine.**

bowel elimination, alteration in: constipation, a nursing diagnosis accepted by the Fourth National Conference on the Classification of Nursing Diagnoses. The cause of the condition, developed at the Fifth National Conference, is less than adequate intake and bulk, less than adequate physical activity, a side effect of medications, chronic use of medications and enemas, GI obstructive lesions, neuromuscular or musculoskeletal impairment, weak abdominal musculature, pain on defecation, diagnostic procedures, lack of privacy for personal habits, pregnancy, or emotional stature. The defining characteristics include decreased frequency of elimination; a hard, formed stool; a palpable rectal mass; straining at stool; decreased bowel sounds; reported feeling of abdominal or rectal fullness or pressure; less than useful amount of stool; and nausea. Abdominal pain, appetite impairment, back pain, headache, and interference with daily living may also be present. See also **nursing diagnosis.**

bowel elimination, alteration in: diarrhea, a nursing diagnosis accepted by the Fourth National Conference on the Classification of Nursing Diagnoses. The cause of the condition, developed at the Fifth National Conference, includes stress and anxiety; dietary intake; the side effects of medications; inflammation, irritation, or malabsorption of the bowel; and the effects of toxins, contaminants, or radiation. The defining characteristics include abdominal pain, cramping, increased frequency of elimination, increased frequency of bowel sounds, loose or liquid stools, urgency of defecation, and a change in the color of the feces. See also **nursing diagnosis.**

bowel elimination, alteration in: incontinence, a nursing diagnosis accepted by the Fourth National Conference on the Classification of Nursing Diagnoses. The cause of the condition, developed at the Fifth National Conference, is neuromuscular or musculoskeletal impairment; depression, severe anxiety, or perceptive or cognitive impairment; multiple life changes; inadequate relaxation; little or no exercise; poor nutrition; work-related tensions; no vacations; unmet expectations; unrealistic perceptions; and inadequate support systems or coping methods. The defining characteristic of the problem is the involuntary passage of stool. See also **nursing diagnosis.**

bowel training, a method of establishing regular evacuation by reflex conditioning, used in the treatment of fecal incontinence, impaction, chronic diarrhea, and autonomic hyperreflexia. In patients with autonomic hyperreflexia, distention of the rectum and bladder causes paroxysmal hypertension, restlessness, chills, diaphoresis, headache, elevated temperature, and bradycardia.

■ METHOD: The patient's previous bowel habits are ascertained, and the necessity of developing a program to induce an evacuation at the same time each day or every other day is explained. Exercises to strengthen abdominal muscles, as pushing up, bearing down, and contracting the musculature, are demonstrated. A bedside commode is provided, and privacy is ensured. The patient is instructed to recognize and respond promptly to signals indicating a full bowel, as goose pimples, perspiration, piloerection on arms or legs, and to develop cues to stimulate the urge to defecate, as drinking coffee, massaging the abdomen, pressing the inner thigh, or stroking the anus. Fluids to 3000 ml daily are encouraged; prune juice, orange juice, and coffee are included in the daily diet, and the importance of having well balanced meals that include bulk and roughage and of avoiding constipating foods, as bananas, beans, and cabbage, is discussed. Depending on the patient and the problem, the training program may involve drinking 4 to 10 ounces of prune juice each night or 12 hours before the time set for evacuation, drinking warm water, coffee, or milk 30 minutes before the set time, and inserting a lubricated glycerine suppository before the set time. The patient is told that no formed stools for 3 days, semiliquid feces, restlessness, and discomfort are signs of impending impaction and that the condition may be treated with a laxative suppository or with a tap water or oil retention enema. The importance of reporting symptoms of autonomic hyperreflexia to the physician is stressed. The possibility that emotional stress or illness may cause accidental incontinence after the program is established is discussed.

■ NURSING ORDERS: The nurse provides instruction and encourages the patient to establish a program of regular evacuation.

■ OUTCOME CRITERIA: Reflex conditioning is often an effective method of developing regular bowel habits in incontinent patients, especially those who are highly motivated and are given good instruction and understanding support. Young persons with spinal cord lesions are able to develop automatic defecation when adequately trained, but some elderly incontinent people may not be able to learn the program.

Bowen's disease, Bowen's precancerous dermatosis. See **intraepidermal carcinoma.**

bowleg. See **genu varum.**

Bowman's capsule /bō′mənz/, the cup-shaped end of a renal tubule containing a glomerulus. Also called **glomerular capsule.**

box bath. See **cabinet bath.**

boxer's fracture, a fracture of one or more metacarpal bones, usually the fourth or the fifth, caused by punching a hard object. Such a fracture is often distal, angulated, and impacted.

boxing, (in dentistry) the forming of vertical walls, most commonly made of wax, to produce the desired shape and size of the base of a cast.

Boyle's law, (in physics) a law stating that the product of the volume and pressure of a gas compressed at a constant temperature remains constant.

BP, abbreviation for **blood pressure.**

Br, symbol for **bromine.**

brace, an orthopedic device, sometimes jointed, to support and hold any movable part of the body in the correct position to allow function, as a leg brace that permits walking and standing. Compare **splint.**

brachi-, a combining form meaning 'pertaining to the arm': *brachialgia, brachiation, brachiocyllosis.*

-brachia, a combining form meaning an 'anatomic condition involving an arm': *acephalobrachia, diantebrachia, monobrachia.*

brachial /brā′kē·əl/, of or pertaining to the arm.

brachial artery, the principal artery of the upper arm that is the continuation of the axillary artery. It has three branches and terminates at the bifurcation of its main trunk into the radial artery and the ulnar artery.

brachialis /brā′kē·al′is/, a muscle of the upper arm, covering the anterior part of the elbow joint and the distal half of the humerus. It arises from the anterior surface of the humerus and inserts, by a thick tendon, into the tuberosity of the coronoid process of the ulna. It is innervated by a branch of the musculocutaneous nerve, containing fibers from the fifth and the sixth cervical nerves, and functions to flex the forearm. Compare **biceps brachii, triceps brachii.**

brachial plexus, a network of nerves in the neck, passing under the clavicle and into the axilla, originating in the fifth, sixth, seventh, and eighth cervical and first two thoracic spinal nerves and innervating the muscles and skin of the chest, shoulders, and arms.

brachial plexus anesthesia, an anesthetic block of the region innervated by the anterior divisions of the last four cervical and first two thoracic nerves. The plexus extends from the transverse processes to the apex of the axilla, where the terminal nerves are formed. Because of the anatomy of the area, many approaches are possible, the axillary being most common; supraclavicular and interscalene are also used. Perivascular axillary block has the least incidence of complications, it being limited to minimal extravasation of blood. Other approaches may result in Horner's syndrome, phrenic nerve palsy, pneumothorax, recurrent laryngeal paralysis, sensory deficits, paresthesias, or hematomas. See also **regional anesthesia.**

brachial plexus paralysis. See **Erb's palsy.**

brachial pulse, the pulse of the brachial artery, palpated in the antecubital space.

brachiocephalic, of or relating to the arm and head.

brachiocephalic arteritis. See **Takayasu's arteritis.**

brachiocephalic artery, brachiocephalic trunk. See **innominate artery.**

brachiocephalic vein. See **innominate vein.**

brachioradialis /brā′kē·ôrā′dē·al′is/, the most superficial muscle on the radial side of the forearm. It arises from the lateral supracondylar ridge of the humerus and from the lateral intermuscular septum and inserts, by a flat tendon, into the styloid process of the radius. It is innervated by a branch of the radial nerve, which contains fibers from the fifth and the sixth cervical nerves, and it functions to flex the forearm.

brachioradialis reflex, a deep tendon reflex, elicited by striking the lateral surface of the forearm proximal to the distal head of the radius, characterized by normal slight elbow flexion and forearm supination. It is accentuated by disease of the pyramidal tract above the level of the fifth cervical vertebra. See also **deep tendon reflex.**

-brachium, a combining form meaning 'arm or armlike growth': *antibrachium, prebrachium, pontibrachium.*

brachy-, a combining form meaning 'short': *brachycheilia, brachygnathia, brachyskelous.*

brachycephaly /brak′isef′əlē/, a congenital malformation of the skull in which premature closure of the coronal suture results in excessive lateral growth of the head, giving it a short, broad appearance with a cephalic index of between 81 and 85. Also called **brachycephalia, brachycephalism.** See also **craniostenosis.** –**brachycephalic, brachycephalous,** *adj.*

brachytherapy, the use of radioactive materials in the treatment of malignant neoplasms by placing the radioactive sources in contact with or implanted into the tissues to be treated. Compare **teletherapy.**

Bradford frame, a rectangular orthopedic frame made of pipes to which heavy movable straps of canvas are attached, running from side to side to support a patient in a prone or supine position. The straps can be removed to permit the patient to urinate or defecate while remaining immobile.

Bradford solid frame, a rectangular orthopedic device of metal covered with canvas to aid in immobilization, especially of children in traction. The Bradford solid frame provides support for the entire body and is especially appropriate for patients who are under 5 years of age, hyperactive, or mentally retarded. The main purpose of the device is to assist in maintaining proper immobilization, positioning, and alignment by controlling movement. To facilitate nursing care, the Bradford solid frame is not placed directly on a bed but elevated at both ends by plywood blocks or by other suitable devices. It is most often used with Bryant traction but never with balanced suspension traction, cervical traction, cervical tongs, or certain other kinds of traction.

Bradford split frame, a rectangular orthopedic device of metal covered with two separate pieces of canvas fastened at both ends of the frame. Used especially in pediatrics to aid in the immobilization of children in traction, it is divided in the middle by a large opening designed to accommodate the excretory functions of an incontinent patient in a hip spica cast. The division also allows for the upper and lower extremities of the patient to be elevated separately and for the maintenance of a clean and dry cast. When the purpose of the frame is to provide elevation only, the head end of the frame is elevated to help assure a clean and dry cast by the flow of excretory matter by gravity. The frame is equipped with three webbing straps to prevent the patient from sliding on the frame. Two straps are anchored at the upper end of the frame around the metal portion, one strap on each side. Both straps are then passed under the canvas cover to the opening in the middle of the frame. If the cast encasing the patient is a short-leg hip spica, the straps are secured around the thigh section of the cast. If the cast extends to the toes of one or both legs, the straps are wrapped around the portion of the frame at the opening in the middle and then secured around the thigh section. The third strap is placed around the waist of the patient and around the frame. For an incontinent child, a plastic funnel leading into the bedpan is positioned below the opening in the frame.

Bradley method, a method of psychophysical preparation for childbirth developed by Robert Bradley, M.D., comprising education about the physiology of childbirth, exercise and nutrition during pregnancy, and techniques of breathing and relaxation for control and comfort during labor and delivery. The father is extensively involved in the classes and acts as the mother's "coach" during labor. The first stage of labor is divided into two parts. During the latent phase the woman is encouraged to carry on her normal activities until she feels the need to concentrate on the contractions. During the active phase the uterine cervix dilates from about 5 cm to 10 cm, the contractions occur every 1.5 to 3 minutes and last from 40 to 90 seconds, the interval between contractions tends to decrease, and the length and intensity of the contractions tend to increase. The father helps the mother to relax by repeating reminders to relax the various parts of her body, by massaging and touching her as he has learned she finds relaxing, and by arranging and rearranging pillows to support her in a "lounge chair" position. During contractions, she breathes deeply and slowly—in through the nose and out through the mouth. Her abdominal wall lifts with each inhalation and falls with each exhalation. She may close her eyes and try to visualize the baby's head pressing against the cervix, causing it to dilate. She is encouraged by the close support of the father, the midwife or obstetrician, and the nurse. During the second stage of labor, the uterine cervix is fully dilated, the contractions are strong and expulsive, occurring every 1.5 to 2 minutes and lasting 60 to 90 seconds. The mother, feeling the urge to bear down and push, allows her knees to fall away from each other without forcibly drawing her thighs against her abdomen as in other methods. She breathes in and out deeply once or twice, waiting for the contraction to build in strength, then she bears down while holding her breath. She pushes as hard as necessary to relieve the pressure or urgency of the contraction. The father may count seconds for her so that she can push for 10 or for 15 seconds, as necessary. He also checks to see that her legs and buttocks are relaxed, and he reminds her to keep her perineum relaxed, to concentrate, and to "let the baby out." As the baby is born, with the mother still in a semisitting position, the infant is placed on her abdomen and then nursed as soon as it wants. The mother is given a glass of orange juice and often walks back to her room with the father and the baby. Among the advantages of the method are its simplicity, the involvement of the father, and the realistic approach to the efforts and discomfort of labor. Also called **husband-coached childbirth.** Compare **Lamaze method, Read method.**

brady-, a combining form meaning 'slow, dull': *bradyacusia, bradydiastalsis, bradyphagia.*

bradycardia /brad′ikär′dē·ə/, an abnormal circulatory condition in which the myocardium contracts steadily but at a rate of less than 60 contractions a minute. The heart normally slows during sleep, and in some physically fit people the pulse may be quite slow. Pathologic bradycardia may be symptomatic of a brain tumor, digitalis toxicity, or vagotonus. Cardiac output is decreased, causing faintness, dizziness, chest pain, and eventually syncope and circulatory collapse. Treatment may include administration of atropine, implantation of a pacemaker, or reduction of digitalis dosage.

bradycardia-tachycardia syndrome, a heart disorder characterized by a heart rate that alternates between abnormally slow and abnormally rapid rhythms.

bradykinesia /brad′ikinē′zhə, -kīnē′zhə/, an abnormal condition characterized by slowness of all voluntary movement and speech, as caused by parkinsonism, other extrapyramidal disorders, and certain tranquilizers.

bradykinin, a peptide of nonprotein origin containing nine amino acid residues. It is produced from α_2-globulin by kallikrein, and it is a potent vasodilator.

bradypnea /brad′ipnē′ə/, an abnormally slow rate of breathing. Also called **oligopnea.** Compare **hypopnea.** See also **respiratory rate.**

Bragg curve, in radiation therapy, the path followed by ionizing particles used in a treatment. Because certain particles reach a peak of potential near the end of their path, the Bragg curve can be used to direct the radiation so that it reaches deep seated tumors while significantly sparing the normal overlying tissues.

Braille /brāl, brä′yə/, a system of printing for the blind consisting of raised dots or points that can be read by touch.

brain, the portion of the central nervous system contained within the cranium. It consists of the cerebrum, cerebellum, pons, medulla, and midbrain. Specialized cells in its mass of convoluted, soft, gray or white tissue coordinate and regulate the functions of the central nervous system.

brain concussion, a violent jarring, or shaking, or other blunt, nonpenetrating injury to the brain caused by a sudden change in momentum of the head. Characteristically, after a mild concussion there may be a transient loss of consciousness followed, on awakening, by a headache. Severe concussion may cause prolonged unconsciousness and disruption of certain vital functions of the brainstem, as respiration and vasomotor stability. The treatment for a person recovering from a concussion consists principally of observation for signs of intracranial bleeding. Also called **concussion.**

brain death, an irreversible form of unconsciousness characterized by a complete loss of brain function while the heart continues to beat. The legal definition of this condition varies from state to state. The usual clinical criteria for brain death include the absence of reflex activity, movements, and respiration. The pupils are dilated and fixed. Because hypothermia, anesthesia, poisoning, or drug intoxication may cause deep physiologic depression that resembles brain death, a diagnosis of brain death requires that the electric activity of the brain be evaluated and shown to be absent on two electroencephalograms performed 12 to 24 hours apart. Also called **irreversible coma.** Compare **coma, sleep, stupor.**

brain electric activity map (BEAM), a topographic map of the brain created by a computer that is able to respond to the electric potentials evoked in the brain by a flash of light. Potentials recorded at 4-millisecond intervals are converted into a many-colored map of the brain showing them to be positive or negative. The waves may be observed traveling through the brain. If the wave is disordered, blocked, too small, or too large, there may be a tumor or other lesion causing the abnormal pattern.

brain fever, *informal.* any inflammation of the brain or meninges. See also **encephalitis.**

brain scan, a diagnostic procedure employing radioisotope imaging techniques to localize and identify intracranial masses, lesions, tumors, or infarcts. Radioisotopes are injected intravenously to circulate to the brain where they accumulate in abnormal tissue. The radioisotopes are traced and photographed by a scintillator, or scanner, and the size and location of the abnormality are determined. The nature and rate of accumulation of radioisotopes in pathologic tissue in some cases are diagnostic of a particular lesion. A brain scan, which is painless, requires no special preparation other than injection of the isotopes and an explanation of the procedure. Compare **CAT scan.** See also **isotope, radioisotope.**

brainstem, the portion of the brain comprising the medulla oblongata, the pons, and the mesencephalon. It performs motor, sensory, and reflex functions and contains the corticospinal and the reticulospinal tracts. The 12 pairs of cranial nerves from the brain arise mostly from the brainstem. Compare **medulla oblongata, mesencephalon, pons.**

brainstem auditory evoked potential (BAEP), the most reliable evoked potential for predicting nerve damage during surgery in the auditory nerve region. A clicking sound is made, and the EEG waves from the auditory area of the patient's brain are observed. Cessation or absence of electric activity may indicate damage or destruction.

brain tumor, a neoplasm of the intracranial portion of the central nervous system that is usually invasive but does not spread beyond the cerebrospinal axis. Brain tumors, which are not rare, cause significant morbidity and mortality, but increasing numbers are successfully treated. Intracranial tumors in children are usually the result of a developmental defect. In adults 20% to 40% of malignancies in the brain are metastatic lesions from cancers in the breast, lung, GI tract, kidney, or any site of a malignant melanoma. The origin of primary brain tumors is not known, but the risk is increased in individuals exposed to vinyl chloride, in the siblings of cancer patients, and in recipients of renal transplant being treated with immunosuppressant medication. During pregnancy a meningioma may suddenly develop or increase in size, suggesting that this tumor is stimulated by hormonal factors. Symptoms of a brain tumor are often those of increased intracranial pressure, as headache, nausea, vomiting, papilledema, lethargy, and disorientation. Various localizing signs also occur, as loss of vision in the eye on the side of an occipital neoplasm. Diagnostic measures include visual field and funduscopic examinations, skull x-ray examinations, electroencephalography, cerebral angiography, brain scanning, computerized axial tomography, and spinal fluid studies. Lumbar puncture may not be performed if increased intracranial pressure is obvious. A broad spectrum of tumors may be found in the brain, but gliomas, chiefly astrocytomas, are the most common malignancies. Rapidly growing medulloblastomas often occur in children. Benign meningiomas are the only intracranial neoplasms more common in women than in men. Craniopharyngiomas, generally found in children and young adults, are benign but impinge on critical structures and are difficult to remove. Schwannomas most often arise from the eighth cranial nerve and cause deafness; but they are generally benign. Surgery is the initial treatment for most primary tumors of the brain. Radiotherapy is indicated for inoperable lesions, medulloblastomas, and tumors with multiple foci, and as postoperative treatment of residual tumor tissue. Beams of neutrons and high energy pi-mesons currently show promise in the treatment of highly malignant brain lesions. The blood-brain barrier impedes the effect of some antineoplastic agents, but responses are obtained in some cases treated with procarbazine and various nitrosoureas administered alone or with vincristine. Compare **spinal cord tumor.**

bran bath, a bath in which bran has been boiled in the water, used for the relief of skin irritation.
branched chain ketoaciduria. See **maple syrup urine disease.**
branched tubular gland, one of the many multicellular glands with one excretory duct from two or more tube-shaped secretory branches, as some of the gastric glands.
branchial fistula, a congenital, abnormal passage from the pharynx to the external surface of the neck, resulting from the failure of a branchial cleft to close during fetal development. Introduction of a sound into a branchial fistula may cause pallor and arrhythmic pounding of the heart. Also called **cervical fistula.**
branching canal. See **collateral pulp canal.**
brand name. See **trademark.**
brassfounder's ague. See **metal fume fever.**
brassy eye. See **chalkitis.**
Braun's canal. See **neurenteric canal.**
Braxton Hicks contraction /brak′stənhiks′/, irregular tightening of the pregnant uterus that begins in the first trimester and increases in frequency, duration, and intensity as pregnancy progresses. Contractility of uterine muscle increases in pregnancy. Near term, strong Braxton Hicks contractions are often difficult to distinguish from the contractions of true labor. See also **false labor.** Also called **Braxton Hicks sign.**
Brazelton assessment, a system for assessing the interactional behavior of newborns with a series of 27 reaction tests, including response to inanimate objects, to a pinprick, to light, and to the sound of a rattle or bell.
Brazilian trypanosomiasis. See **Chagas' disease.**
breach of contract, the failure to perform as promised or agreed in a contract. The breach may be complete or partial and may occur by repudiation, by failure to recognize the contract, or by prevention or hindrance of performance.
breach of duty, **1.** the failure to perform an act required by law. **2.** the performance of an act in an unlawful way.
breakbone fever. See **dengue.**
breakthrough bleeding, the escape of uterine blood between menstrual periods, a side effect experienced by some women using oral contraceptives.
breast, **1.** the anterior aspect of the surface of the chest. **2.** a mammary gland.
breast cancer, a malignant neoplastic disease of breast tissue, the most common malignancy in women in the United States. The incidence increases exponentially with age from the third to the fifth decade and reaches a second peak at age 65, suggesting that breast cancer in premenopausal women may be related to ovarian hormonal function and in postmenopausal patients to adrenal function. Based on the great prevalence of breast cancer in affluent countries, especially in high socioeconomic groups, it is thought that a high fat diet may be a causative factor, but the relationship is unproven and the origin is unknown. Risk factors include a family history of breast cancer, nulliparity, exposure to ionizing radiation, early menarche, late menopause, obesity, diabetes, hypertension, chronic cystic disease of the breast, and, possibly, postmenopausal estrogen therapy. Women who are over 40 years of age when they bear their first child and patients with malignancies in other body sites also have an increased risk of developing breast cancer. Initial symptoms, detected in most cases by self-examination, include a small painless lump, thick or dimpled skin, or nipple retraction. As the lesion progresses, there may be nipple discharge, pain, ulceration, and enlarged axillary glands. The diagnosis may be established by a careful physical examination, mammography, and cytologic examination of tumor cells obtained by biopsy. Infiltrating ductal carcinomas are found in about 75% of cases, and infiltrating lobular, infiltrating medullary, colloid, comedo, or papillary carcinomas in the others. Tumors are more common in the left than in the right breast and in the upper and outer quadrant than in the other quadrants. Metastasis through the lymphatic system to axillary lymph nodes and to bone, lung, brain, and liver is common, but there is evidence that primary carcinomas of the breast may exist in multiple sites and that tumor cells may enter the bloodstream directly without passing through lymph nodes. Surgical treatment, depending on the assessment of the tumor, may be a radical, modified radical, or simple mastectomy, with dissection of axillary nodes, or a lumpectomy. Postoperative radiotherapy, chemotherapy, or both are usually prescribed. Chemotherapeutic agents frequently administered in various combinations are cyclophosphamide, methotrexate, 5-fluorouracil, phenylalanine mustard (L-PAM), thio-TEPA, doxorubicin, vincristine, and prednisone. The presence of estrogen receptors in breast tumors is considered an indication for ovarian ablation, adrenalectomy, or hypophysectomy or for the administration of androgens or antiestrogens in order to reduce the amount of endogenous estrogen. Implantation of a prosthesis after mastectomy is gaining currency but is painful initially and is not universally approved. Less than 1% of breast cancers occur in men, but those with Klinefelter's syndrome are at 60 times greater risk. In men, the tumor may be successfully treated with surgical excision and with combination chemotherapy, orchiectomy, adrenalectomy, or hypophysectomy. The prognosis is generally less favorable in women. See also **lumpectomy, mastectomy, scirrhous carcinoma.**
breast examination, a process in which the breasts and their accessory structures are observed and palpated in assessing the presence of changes or abnormalities that could indicate malignant disease. See also **self-breast examination.**
■ METHOD: The breasts are observed with the patient sitting with her arms at her sides, sitting with her arms over her head, back straight, then leaning forward, and, finally, sitting upright, as she contracts the pectoral muscles. The breasts are observed for symmetry of shape and size and for surface characteristics, including moles or nevi,

hyperpigmentation, retraction or dimpling, edema, abnormal distribution of hair, focal vascularity, or lesions. With the patient still sitting, the axillary nodes and the supraclavicular and subclavicular areas are palpated. With the patient lying down on her back, each breast is shifted medially, and the glandular area in each is palpated with the flat of the fingers of a hand in concentric circles or in a pattern like the spokes of a wheel, from the periphery inward. The areolar areas, the nipples, and the axillary tail of Spence in the upper outer quadrant extending toward the axilla are then palpated.

■ NURSING ORDERS: The patient should be taught how to perform a self-breast examination and encouraged to do it monthly. Many women find it helpful to check their breasts every time they shower for the first few months after being taught the procedure to practice and to become very familiar with their own breasts.

■ OUTCOME CRITERIA: Early diagnosis greatly improves the rate of cure in cancer of the breast. The breast examination thoroughly performed serves as a valuable means of screening women to discover those who require further diagnostic examination by xeroradiography, mammography, biopsy, or, less frequently, thermoradiography.

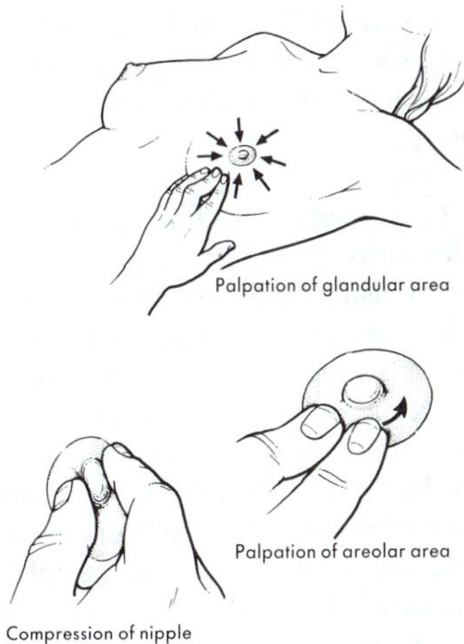

Breast palpation

breast feeding, 1. suckling or nursing, as giving a baby milk from the breast. Breast feeding encourages postpartum uterine involution and slows the natural return of the menses, providing a measure of contraception. 2. taking milk from the breast. See also **breast milk, lactation.**

breast milk, human milk, the ideal food for most babies. The nurse should counsel mothers that it is easily digested, clean, and warm, that it confers some immunities (bronchiolitis and gastroenteritis are rare in breast-fed babies), and promotes emotional bonding between mother and baby. Infants fed breast milk are less likely to become obese or to develop dental malocclusions. See also **breast feeding.**

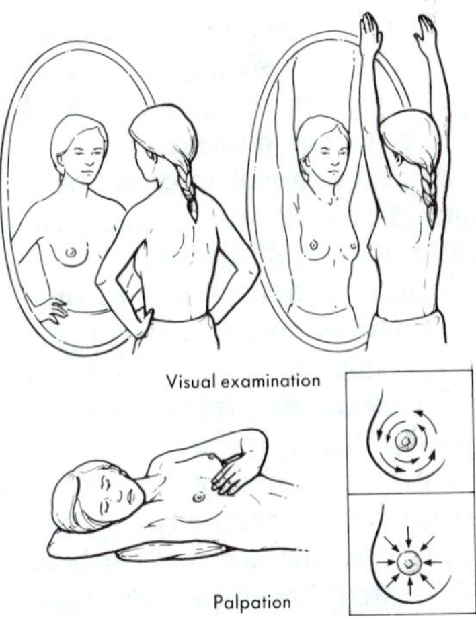

Breast self-examination

breast milk jaundice, jaundice and hyperbilirubinemia in breast-fed infants that occur in the first weeks of life as a result of a metabolite in the mother's milk that inhibits the infant's ability to conjugate bilirubin to protein for excretion. See also **hyperbilirubinemia of the newborn.**

■ OBSERVATIONS: Breast milk jaundice usually occurs after the fifth day of life and peaks toward the end of the second or third week. Serum bilirubin levels usually exceed 5 mg/100 ml but rarely reach dangerous levels of 20 mg/100 ml, at which point kernicterus may develop. The infant seems normal and healthy, but the skin, the whites of the eyes, and the serum are jaundiced.

■ INTERVENTION: If serum bilirubin exceeds acceptable levels, breast feeding may be interrupted until there is a decrease to the normal range, usually a period of 1 to 3 days. During this interval, the infant is bottle-fed with a supplemental formula and the mother uses a breast pump or manual devices to maintain lactation without becoming engorged. Phototherapy may be used to accelerate excretion of bilirubin through the skin.

■ NURSING CONSIDERATIONS: The primary concern of the nurse is to observe for signs of increasing jaundice, to monitor serum bilirubin levels, and, usually, to reassure the mother that her child is well and that the jaundice resolves slowly but completely in time.

breast pump, a device for withdrawing milk from the breast.

breast self-examination. See **self-breast examination.**

breathing. See **respiration.**

breathing pattern: ineffective, a nursing diagnosis accepted by the Fourth National Conference on the Classification of Nursing Diagnoses. The cause of the condition includes neuromuscular impairment, pain, musculoskeletal impairment, impairment of perception or cognition, anxiety, decreased energy, and fatigue. The defining characteristics of the problem include dyspnea, shortness of breath, tachypnea, fremitus, abnormal concentrations of arterial blood gases, cyanosis, cough, nasal flaring, change in depth of respiration, pursed lip breathing or prolonged expiratory phase, increased anteroposterior diameter of the chest, use of accessory muscles of breathing, and altered excursion of the chest wall with respiration. See also **nursing diagnosis.**

breathing tube, a device inserted into the trachea through the mouth or nose to assure a patent airway for adequate respiration during artificial or assisted ventilation. See also **extubation, intubation.**

breathlessness. See **dyspnea.**

breath sound, the sound of air and carbon dioxide passing in and out of the respiratory system as heard with a stethoscope. Vesicular and tracheal breath sounds are normal. Decreased breath sounds may indicate an obstruction of an airway, collapse of a portion or all of a lung, thickening of the pleurae of the lungs, emphysema, or other chronic obstructive lung disease.

Breckinridge, Mary (1881–1965), an American nurse, who founded the Frontier Nursing Service, in Kentucky. The Service was designed to improve the obstetric care of women living in the remote mountainous area. The nurses in the Service had training in midwifery and reached their patients on horseback and on foot, often encountering personal danger. The Service began training midwives and stimulated the increase of other midwifery schools.

breech birth, parturition in which the baby emerges feet, knees, or buttocks first. Breech birth is often hazardous: The body may deliver easily, but the aftercoming head may become trapped by an incompletely dilated cervix because babies' heads are usually larger than their bodies. See also **assisted breech, breech presentation, complete breech, footling breech, frank breech, version and extraction.**

breech extraction, an obstetric operation in which a baby being born feet or buttocks first is grasped before any part of the trunk is born and delivered by traction. Compare **assisted breech.**

breech presentation, intrauterine position of the fetus in which the buttocks or feet present, occurring in approximately 3% of labors. Kinds of breech presentation are **complete breech, footling breech,** and **frank breech.** Compare **vertex presentation.** See also **breech birth.**

bregma /breg′mə/, the junction of the coronal and sagittal sutures on the top of the skull. **–bregmatic,** *adj.*

Brenner tumor, an uncommon, benign ovarian neoplasm consisting of nests or cords of epithelial cells containing glycogen that are enclosed in fibrous connective tissue. The tumor may be solid or cystic and is sometimes difficult to distinguish from certain granulosa-theca cell neoplasms.

brepho-, a combining form meaning 'pertaining to an embryo, fetus, or newborn infant': *brephoplastic, brephopolysarcia, brephotrophic.*

Brethine, a trademark for a bronchodilator (terbutaline sulfate).

bretylium tosylate /britil′ē·əm/, an antiarrhythmic agent.

■ INDICATION: It is prescribed in the treatment of life-threatening ventricular arrhythmias when other measures have not been effective.

■ CONTRAINDICATION: Known hypersensitivity to this drug prohibits its use.

■ ADVERSE EFFECTS: Among the more serious adverse reactions are hypotension, nausea and vomiting, anginal pain, and nasal stuffiness.

Bretylol, a trademark for an adrenergic blocking agent (bretylium tosylate), used as an antiarrhythmic agent.

brevi-, a combining form meaning 'short': *brevicollis, breviflexor, breviradiate.*

Brevital Sodium, a trademark for a barbiturate (methohexital sodium), used as a general anesthetic.

brewer's yeast, a preparation containing the dried pulverized cells of a yeast, as *Saccharomyces cerevisiae,* that is used as a leavening agent and as a dietary supplement. It is one of the best sources of the B complex vitamins and of many minerals and is also a high grade of protein. Brewer's yeast may protect against toxicity of large doses of vitamin D, is used to prevent constipation, and is a good source of enzyme-producing agent.

Bricanyl, a trademark for a beta-adrenergic drug (terbutaline sulfate).

bridge of Varolius. See **pons.**

bridging, 1. a nursing technique of positioning a patient so that bony prominences are free of pressure on the mattress by using pads, bolsters of foam rubber, or pillows to distribute body weight over a larger surface. **2.** a nursing technique for supporting a part of the body, as the testicles in treating orchitis using a Bellevue bridge made of a towel or other material.

brief psychotherapy, (in psychiatry) treatment directed toward the active resolution of personality or behavioral problems rather than toward the speculative analysis of the unconscious. It usually concentrates on a specific problem or symptom and is limited to a specified number of sessions with the therapist.

Bright's disease, an obsolete term for a kidney disease, especially glomerulonephritis.

Brill-Symmers disease. See **giant follicular lymphoma.**

Brill-Zinsser disease /bril′zin′sər/, a mild form of typhus that recurs in a person who appears to have completely recovered from a severe case of the disease. Some rickettsiae remain in the body after the symptoms of the disease abate, causing the recurrence of symptoms, especially when stress, illness, or malnutrition weaken the person. Treatment with antibiotics may eradicate the organism. See also **epidemic typhus, murine typhus, rickettsiosis, typhus.**

brim, the edge of the upper border of the true pelvis, or the pelvic inlet. See also **pelvis.**

Brinnell hardness test, a means of determining the surface hardness of a material by measuring the amount of resistance to the impact of a steel ball. The test result is recorded as the Brinnell hardness number (BHN); the higher the number, the harder the material. The BHN is generally indicative of abrasion resistance, and the associated test is commonly used to measure this quality in various materials used in dental restorations, as amalgams, cements, and porcelains. Compare **Knoop hardness test.**

Briquet's syndrome. See **somatization disorder.**

Brissaud's dwarf /brisōz′/, a person affected with infantile myxedema in which short stature is associated with hypothyroidism.

British antilewisite. See **dimercaprol.**

British Medical Association (BMA), a national professional organization of physicians in the United Kingdom.

British Pharmacopoeia (BP), the official British reference work setting forth standards of strength and purity of medications and containing directions for their preparation to ensure that the same prescription written by different doctors and filled by different pharmacists will contain exactly the same ingredients in the same proportions. The first *British Pharmacopoeia* was published in 1864 by the General Medical Council; it superseded the *London Pharmacopoeia,* which had been published since 1618. See also **British Medical Association, *United States Pharmacopeia (USP).***

brittle bones. See **osteogenesis imperfecta.**

brittle diabetes. See **insulin-independent diabetes mellitus.**

broad beta disease, a familial type of hyperlipoproteinemia in which a lipoprotein, high in cholesterol and triglycerides, accumulates in the blood. The condition, which affects males in their 20s and females in their 30s and 40s, is characterized by yellowish nodules (xanthomas) on the elbows and knees, peripheral vascular disease, and elevated serum cholesterol levels. People with this disease are at risk of developing early coronary disease. Therapy includes dietary measures to reduce weight and serum lipids. See also **hyperlipidemia, hyperlipoproteinemia.**

broad ligament, a folded sheet of peritoneum draped over the uterine tubes, the uterus, and the ovaries. It extends from the sides of the uterus to the sidewalls of the pelvis, dividing the pelvis from side to side and creating the vesicouterine fossa and pouch in front of the uterus and the rectouterine fossa and pouch behind it. Also called **ligamentum latum uteri.** See also **cardinal ligament.**

Broca's area /brō′kəz/, an area, involved in speech production, situated on the inferior frontal gyrus of the brain. See also **aphasia.**

Broca's plane, a plane that extends from the tip of the interalveolar septum between the upper central incisors to the lowest point of the occipital condyle.

Brodie's abscess, a form of osteomyelitis consisting of an indolent staphylococcal infection of bone, usually in the metaphysis of a long bone of a child, characterized by a necrotic cavity surrounded by dense granulation tissue. See also **osteomyelitis.** Also called **circumscribed abscess of bone.**

Brodmann's areas /brod′manz, brōt′mons/, the 47 different areas of the cerebral cortex that are associated with specific neurologic functions and distinguished by different cellular components. Compare **motor area.** See also **cerebral cortex.**

brom-, bromo-, a combining form meaning 'odor, stench': *bromacetone, bromhidrosis, bromoacetophenon.*

bromhidrosis /brō′midrō′sis/, an abnormal condition in which the apocrine sweat has an unpleasant odor. The odor is usually caused by bacterial decomposition of perspiration on the skin. Treatment includes frequent bathing, changing of socks and underclothes, and the use of deodorants, antibacterial soaps, and dusting powders. Also called **body odor.**

bromide /brō′mīd/, a compound in which the negative element is bromine, especially a salt of hydrobromic acid. Bromides, once widely prescribed as sedatives, are now seldom used for that purpose because they may cause serious mental disturbances as side effects.

bromine (Br), a toxic, red-brown, liquid element of the halogen group. Its atomic number is 35; its atomic weight is 79.909. Bromine is used in industry, in photography, in the manufacture of organic chemicals and fuels, and in medications. Bromine gives off a red vapor that is extremely irritating to the eyes and the respiratory tract. Liquid bromine is irritating to the skin; bromates used as neutralizers in cold wave products are toxic if ingested. Bromides are binary compounds of bromine; they have been used as sedatives, hypnotics, and analgesics and are still used in some nonprescription, over the counter preparations. Prolonged use of these products may cause brominism, a toxic condition characterized by acneiform eruptions, headache, loss of libido, drowsiness, and fatigue. See also **bromide.**

bromo-. See **brom-.**

bromocriptine, a dopamine receptor agonist.

■ INDICATIONS: It is prescribed for the treatment of amenorrhea and galactorrhea associated with hyperprolactinemia, female infertility, and Parkinson's disease.

■ CONTRAINDICATION: Sensitivity to any ergot alkaloid prohibits its use.

■ ADVERSE EFFECTS: Among the more severe adverse reactions are palpitations, hypotension, bradycardia, hallucinations, syncope, nausea, ataxia, dyspnea, dysphagia, confusion, and asthenia.

bromoderma /brō′mōdur′mə/, an acneiform, bullous, or nodular skin rash, occurring as a hypersensitivity reaction to ingested bromides.

brompheniramine maleate /brom′fənir′əmin/, an antihistamine.

■ INDICATIONS: It is prescribed in the treatment of a variety of hypersensitivity reactions, including rhinitis, skin reactions, and itching.

■ CONTRAINDICATIONS: Asthma or known hypersensitivity to this drug prohibits its use. It is not given to newborn infants, lactating mothers, or other people for whom anticholinergic medications are contraindicated.

■ ADVERSE EFFECTS: Drowsiness, skin rash, hypersensitivity reactions, dry mouth, and tachycardia commonly occur.

Brompton's cocktail, an analgesic solution containing alcohol, morphine or heroin, cocaine, and, in some cases, a phenothiazine. Formulations vary, and recently cocaine has generally been eliminated from the mixture. The cocktail is administered in the control of pain in the terminally ill patient. Given frequently at the lowest effective dose, it may relieve pain for many months. It was developed at the Brompton Hospital in England. Also called **Brompton's mixture.**

Bromsulphalein (BSP) test /bromsul'falin/, a trademark for sulfobromophthalein, a dye prepared for use in a highly sensitive, nonspecific test that measures the ability of liver cells to remove the sulfobromophthalein from the blood. Forty-five minutes after intravenous injection, more than 95% of the dye is normally cleared from the blood. The test is rarely indicated in current clinical practice because it may cause severe allergic reactions and because it cannot indicate a specific dysfunction of the liver. See also **sulfobromophthalein.**

bronch-, a combining form meaning 'pertaining to the bronchus': *bronchiectasis, bronchiotetany, bronchodilatation.*

bronchial asthma. See **asthma.**

bronchial breath sound, an abnormal sound heard with a stethoscope over the lungs, indicating consolidation because of pneumonia or compression. Expiration and inspiration produce loud, high-pitched sounds of equal duration.

bronchial fremitus, a vibration that can be palpated or auscultated on the chest wall over a bronchus congested by secretions that rattle as the air passes during respiration.

bronchial hyperreactivity, an abnormal respiratory condition characterized by reflex bronchospasm in response to histamine or a cholinergic drug. It is a universal feature of asthma and is used in the differential diagnosis of asthma and heart disease. An asthmatic person experiences episodes of bronchospasm in response to the cholinergic effect of endogenous histamine and to exposure via inhalation of histamine or a cholinergic drug such as methacholine in testing for asthma.

bronchial tree, an anatomic complex of the bronchi and the bronchial tubes. The bronchi branch from the trachea, and the bronchial tubes branch from the bronchi. The right bronchus is wider and shorter than the left bronchus, and it diverges less abruptly from the trachea. The right bronchus branches into three subsidiary bronchi, one passing to each of the three lobes that comprise the right lung. The left bronchus is smaller in diameter but about twice as long as the right bronchus and passes inferior to the pulmonary artery before branching into the bronchi for the inferior and the superior lobes of the left lung.

bronchiectasis /brong'kē•ek'təsis/, an abnormal condition of the bronchial tree, characterized by irreversible dilatation and destruction of the bronchial walls. The condition is sometimes congenital but is more often a result of bronchial infection or of obstruction by a tumor or an aspirated foreign body. Symptoms of bronchiectasis include a constant cough productive of copious purulent sputum, hemoptysis, chronic sinusitis, clubbing of fingers, and persistent moist, coarse rales. Some of the complications of bronchiectasis are pneumonia, lung abscess, empyema, brain abscess, and amyloidosis. Treatment includes frequent postural drainage, antibiotics, and, rarely, surgical resection of the affected part of the lungs.

bronchiolar. See **bronchiole.**

bronchiolar carcinoma. See **alveolar cell carcinoma.**

bronchiole /brong'kē•ōl/, a small airway of the respiratory system extending from the bronchi into the lobes of the lung. There are two divisions of bronchioles: The terminal bronchioles pass inspired air from the bronchi to the respiratory bronchioles and expired waste gases from the respiratory bronchioles to the bronchi. The respiratory bronchioles function similarly, allowing the exchange of air and waste gases between the alveolar ducts and the terminal bronchioles. –**bronchiolar,** *adj.*

bronchiolitis /brong'kē•ōlī'tis/, an acute viral infection of the lower respiratory tract that occurs primarily in infants under 18 months of age, characterized by expiratory wheezing, respiratory distress, inflammation, and obstruction at the level of the bronchioles. The most common causative agents are the respiratory syncytial viruses (RSV) and the parainfluenza viruses. *Mycoplasma pneumoniae,* the rhinoviruses, enteroviruses, and measles virus are less common causative agents. Transmission occurs by infection with airborne particles or by contact with infected secretions. The diagnosis consists of evidence of hyperinflation of the lungs through percussion or chest x-ray examination.

■ OBSERVATIONS: The condition typically begins as an upper respiratory tract infection with serous nasal discharge and, often, low-grade fever. Increasing respiratory distress follows, characterized by tachypnea, tachycardia, intercostal and subcostal retractions, a paroxysmal cough, an expiratory wheeze, and, often, an elevated temperature. The chest may appear barrel-shaped; x-ray films show hyperinflated lungs and a depressed diaphragm. Respiration becomes more shallow, causing increased alveolar oxygen tension and leading to respiratory acidosis. Complete obstruction and absorption of trapped air may lead to atelectasis and respiratory failure. Blood gas determinations indicate the degree of oxygen saturation and carbon dioxide retention.

■ INTERVENTION: Routine treatment includes humidity and oxygen via a mist tent, vaporizer, or Croupette, generally combined with oxygen; an adequate fluid intake, usually given intravenously because of tachypnea, weakness, and fatigue; suctioning of the airways to remove secretions; and rest. Endotracheal intubation is indicated when carbon dioxide retention occurs, when bronchial secretions do not loosen and clear, or when oxygen therapy does not alleviate hypoxia. Such medications as antibiotics, bronchodilators, corticosteroids, cough suppressants, and expectorants are not routinely used. Sedatives are contraindicated because of the suppressant effect they exert on the respiratory tract. The infection typically runs its course in 7 to 10 days, with good prognosis. A major complication is bacterial infection, most commonly after prolonged use of a mist tent. The disorder is often confused with asthma: A family history of allergy, the presence of other allergic manifestations, and improvement with epinephrine injection is usually indicative of asthma, not bronchiolitis. Cystic fibrosis, pertussis, the bronchopneumonias, and foreign body obstruction of the trachea are other disorders that may be confused with bronchiolitis.

■ NURSING CONSIDERATIONS: The focus of nursing care is to promote rest and to conserve the child's energy by reducing anxiety and apprehension; to increase the ease of breathing with humidity and oxygen as needed; to aid in changing position for comfort; and to induce drainage of secretions or to suction when necessary. Fever is usually controlled by the cool atmosphere of the mist tent and by administering antipyretics as needed. Frequent changing of clothing and bed linen is often necessary in a mist environment to reduce chilling. Vital signs and chest and breath sounds are continuously monitored to detect early signs of respiratory distress. Children with bacterial infections are isolated to prevent cross-contamination.

bronchitis /brongkī′tis/, an acute or chronic inflammation of the mucous membranes of the tracheobronchial tree. **Acute bronchitis** is characterized by a productive cough, fever, hypertrophy of mucus-secreting structures, and back pain. Caused by the spread of upper respiratory viral infections to the bronchi, it is often observed with or after childhood infections like measles, whooping cough, diphtheria, and typhoid fever. Treatment includes bedrest, aspirin, expectorants, and appropriate antibiotic therapy. **Chronic bronchitis** is distinguished by an excessive secretion of mucus in the bronchi with a productive cough for at least 3 consecutive months in at least 2 successive years. Additional symptoms are frequent chest infections, cyanosis, hypoxemia, hypercapnia, and a marked tendency for the development of cor pulmonale and respiratory failure. Predisposing factors for chronic bronchitis include cigarette smoking, air pollution, chronic infections, and abnormal physical development of the bronchi that distorts the structures sufficiently to interfere with bronchial drainage. Most common in adults, it is often a complication of cystic fibrosis in children. Treatment includes the cessation of cigarette smoking, avoidance of airway irritants, the use of expectorants, and postural drainage. Currently, prophylactic antibiotics, steroids, and desensitization therapy are not recommended. See also **chronic obstructive pulmonary disease (COPD), respiratory syncytial virus.**

bronchodilator, a substance, especially a drug, that relaxes contractions of the smooth muscle of the bronchioles to improve ventilation to the lungs. Pharmacologic bronchodilators are prescribed to improve aeration in asthma, bronchiectasis, bronchitis, and emphysema. Commonly used bronchodilators include corticosteroids, ephedrine, isoproterenol hydrochloride, theophylline, and various derivatives and combinations of these drugs. Beclomethasone dipropionate and triamcinolone are available in aerosol form. The adverse effects vary, depending on the particular class of the bronchodilating drug. In general, bronchodilators are given with caution to people with impaired cardiac function. Nervousness, irritability, gastritis, or palpitations of the heart may occur.

bronchofibroscopy. See **fiberoptic bronchoscopy.**

bronchogenic carcinoma, one of the more than 90% of malignant lung tumors that originate in bronchi. Lesions, usually associated with cigarette smoking, may cause coughing and wheezing, fatigue, chest tightness, aching joints, and, in the late stages, bloody sputum, clubbing of the fingers, weight loss, and pleural effusion. Diagnosis is made by bronchoscopy, sputum cytology, lymph node biopsy, radioisotope scanning procedures, or exploratory surgery. About 45% of the tumors are squamous cell or epidermoid carcinomas, 33% are oat cell carcinomas, and 15% to 20% are adenocarcinomas. Surgery is the most effective treatment, but approximately 50% of cases are advanced and inoperable when first seen. Palliative treatment includes radiotherapy and chemotherapy.

bronchography /brongkog′rəfē/, an x-ray examination of the bronchi after they have been coated with a radiopaque substance.

bronchopneumonia, an acute inflammation of the lungs and bronchioles, characterized by chills, fever, high pulse and respiratory rates, bronchial breathing, cough with purulent bloody sputum, severe chest pain, and abdominal distension. The disease is usually a result of the spread of bacterial infection from the upper respiratory tract to the lower respiratory tract, caused by *Mycoplasma pneumoniae, Staphylococcus pyogenes,* or *Streptococcus pneumoniae*. Atypical forms of bronchopneumonia may occur in viral and rickettsial infections. The most common cause in infancy is the respiratory syncytial virus. The condition results in pleural effusion, empyema, lung abscess, peripheral thrombophlebitis, respiratory failure, congestive heart failure, and jaundice. Treatment includes an antibiotic, often penicillin or ampicillin, oxygen therapy, supportive measures to keep the bronchi clear of secretions, and relief of pleural pain. Compare **aspiration pneumonia, eosinophilic pneumo-**

nia, interstitial pneumonia. See also **lobar pneumonia, respiratory syncytial virus.**

bronchopulmonary, of or pertaining to the bronchi and the lungs of the respiratory system.

bronchoscope /brong′kəskōp′/, a curved, flexible tube for visual examination of the bronchi. It contains fibers that carry light down the tube and project an enlarged image up the tube to the viewer. The bronchoscope is used to examine the bronchi, to secure a specimen for biopsy or culture, or to aspirate a foreign body from the respiratory tract. See also **fiberoptic bronchoscopy.** –**bronchoscopic,** *adj.*

bronchoscopy /brongkos′kəpē/, the visual examination of the tracheobronchial tree, using the standard rigid, tubular metal bronchoscope or the narrower, flexible fiberoptic bronchoscope. The patient is in a fasting state and is usually sedated before the examination, which is routinely performed under topical anesthesia. In addition to visualization, the procedure can be used for suctioning, for obtaining a biopsy and fluid or sputum for examination, for removal of foreign bodies, and for diagnosing such conditions as localized atelectasis, bronchial obstruction, lung abscess, and tracheal extubation. See also **bronchoscope.**

bronchospasm, an abnormal contraction of the smooth muscle of the bronchi, resulting in an acute narrowing and obstruction of the respiratory airway. A cough with generalized wheezing usually indicates this condition. Bronchospasm is a chief characteristic of asthma and bronchitis. Treatment includes the use of active bronchodilators, catecholamines, corticosteroids, or methylxanthines, and preventive drugs, as cromolyn sodium. See also **asthma, bronchitis.**

bronchus /brong′kəs/, *pl.* **bronchi,** any one of several large air passages in the lungs through which pass inspired air and exhaled waste gases. Each bronchus has a wall consisting of three layers. The outermost is made of dense fibrous tissue, reinforced with cartilage. The middle layer is a network of smooth muscle. The innermost layer consists of ciliated mucous membrane. Kinds of bronchi are **lobar bronchus, primary bronchus, secondary bronchus,** and **segmental bronchus.** See also **arteriole, bronchiole.** –**bronchial,** *adj.*

Bronkephrine, a trademark for a sympathomimetic bronchodilator (ethylnorepinephrine hydrochloride).

Bronkodyl, a trademark for a smooth muscle relaxant (theophylline).

Bronkosol, a trademark for a bronchodilator (isoetharine hydrochloride), used for temporary relief of bronchial asthma, acute paroxysms, and bronchial spasms of bronchitis and emphysema.

brown fat, a type of fat present in newborn infants and rarely found in adults. Brown fat is a unique source of heat energy for the infant because it has greater thermogenic activity than ordinary fat. Brown fat deposits occur around the kidneys, neck, and upper chest area.

Brown-Séquard's treatment. See **organotherapy.**

Brown-Séquard syndrome /broun′sākär′/, a traumatic neurologic disorder resulting from compression of one side of the spinal cord, above the tenth thoracic vertebrae, characterized by spastic paralysis on the injured side of the body, loss of postural sense, and loss of the senses of pain and heat on the other side of the body.

brown spider, a poisonous insect, also known as the brown recluse or violin spider, found in both North and South America. The venom from its bite usually creates a blister surrounded by concentric white and red circles. This so-called "bull's eye" appearance is helpful in distinguishing it from other spider bites. The wound ordinarily ulcerates and sometimes becomes infected. Pain, nausea, fever, and chills are common, but the reaction is usually self-limited. Antivenin is not available in the United States, but corticosteroids may be administered.

Brucella abortus. See **abortus fever.**

brucellosis /bro͞o′səlō′sis/, a disease caused by any of several species of the gram-negative coccobacillus *Brucella.* Brucellosis is most prevalent in rural areas among farmers, veterinarians, meat packers, slaughterhouse workers, and livestock producers. It is primarily a disease of animals (including cattle, pigs, and goats), and humans usually acquire it by ingesting contaminated milk or milk products or through a break in the skin. It is characterized by fever, chills, sweating, malaise, and weakness. The fever often comes in waves, rising in the evening and subsiding during the day, occurring at intervals separated by periods of remission. Other signs and symptoms may include anorexia and weight loss, headache, muscle and joint pain, and an enlarged spleen. In some victims, the disease is acute; more often, it is chronic, recurring over a period of months or years. Although brucellosis itself is rarely fatal, treatment is important because serious complications such as pneumonia, meningitis, and encephalitis can develop. Tetracycline plus streptomycin is the treatment of choice; bed rest is also important. Also called **Cyprus fever, Gibraltar fever, Malta fever, Mediterranean fever, rock fever, undulant fever.** See also **abortus fever.**

Bruch's disease. See **Marseilles fever.**

Brudzinski's sign /bro͞odzin′skēz/, an involuntary flexion of the arm, hip, and knee when the neck is passively flexed, seen in patients with meningitis.

bruise. See **contusion, ecchymosis.**

bruit /bro͞o′ē/, an abnormal sound or murmur heard while auscultating an organ or gland, as the liver or thyroid. The specific character of the bruit, its location, and the time of its occurrence in a cycle of other sounds are all of diagnostic importance.

Brushfield's spots, pinpoint, white or light yellow spots on the iris of a child with Down's syndrome. Occasionally, they are seen in normal infants, but their absence may help rule out Down's syndrome.

Bruton's agammaglobulinemia, a sex-linked, inherited condition characterized by the absence of gamma globulin in the blood. Patients with this syndrome are deficient in antibodies and susceptible to repeated infections. Compare **agammaglobulinemia.** See also **gamma globulin.**

bruxism /bruk′sizəm/, the compulsive, unconscious grinding of the teeth, especially during sleep or as a mechanism for the release of tension during periods of extreme stress in the waking hours. Also called **bruxomania.**

bry-, a combining form meaning 'full of life': *bryocyte, bryocytole, bryocytic.*

Bryant's traction, an orthopedic mechanism used only with infants to immobilize both lower extremities in the treatment of a fractured femur or in the correction of the congenital dislocation of the hip. This mechanism consists of a traction frame supporting weights, connected by ropes that run through pulleys to traction foot plates worn by the infant. The traction pull elevates the lower extremities to a vertical position with the patient supine, the trunk and the lower extremities forming a right angle. The weight applied to the traction mechanism is usually less than 35 pounds. Compare **Buck's traction.**

BSA, **1.** abbreviation for **body surface area.** See **surface area.** **2.** abbreviation for **bovine serum albumin.**

BSE, abbreviation for **breast self-examination.** See **self-breast examination.**

BSN, abbreviation for **Bachelor of Science in Nursing.**

BSP, abbreviation for **Bromsulphalein.**

BT, abbreviation for **bleeding time.**

BTPD, abbreviation for *body temperature, ambient pressure, dry.*

BTPS, abbreviation for *body temperature, ambient pressure, saturated* (with water vapor).

bubbling rale, an abnormal chest sound characteristic of moisture moving in the lungs. Compare **amphoric breath sound, atelectatic rale, dry rale.**

bubble oxygenator, a heart-lung device that oxygenates the blood while it is diverted outside the patient's body.

bubo /byōō′bō/, *pl.* **buboes,** a greatly enlarged, inflamed lymph node usually in the axilla or groin, associated with such diseases as chancroid, lymphogranuloma venereum, bubonic plague, and syphilis. Treatment includes specific antibiotic therapy, application of moist heat, and, sometimes, incision and drainage.

bubonic plague, the most common form of plague, characterized by painful buboes in the axilla, groin, or neck, fever often rising to 106° F, prostration with a rapid, thready pulse, hypotension, delirium, and bleeding into the skin from the superficial blood vessels. The symptoms are caused by an endotoxin released by a bacillus, *Yersinia pestis,* usually introduced into the body by the bite of a rat flea that has bitten an infected rat. Inoculation with plague vaccine confers partial immunity; infection provides lifetime immunity. Treatment includes antibiotics, supportive nursing care, surgical drainage of buboes, isolation, and stringent precautions against spread of the disease. Conditions favor a plague epidemic when a large infected rodent population lives with a large nonimmune human population in a damp, warm climate. Improved sanitary conditions and the eradication of rats and other rodent reservoirs of *Y. pestis* may prevent outbreaks of the disease. Killing the infected rodents, which may include squirrels and rabbits, and not the fleas allows a continued threat of human infection. Also called **Black Death, black plague.** Compare **pneumonic plague, septicemic plague.** See also **bubo.**

bucca-. See **bucco-.**

buccal /buk′əl/, of or pertaining to the inside of the cheek, the surface of a tooth, or the gum next to the cheek.

buccal administration of medication, oral administration of a drug, usually in the form of a tablet, by placing it between the cheek and the teeth or gum until it dissolves.

buccal bar, an orthodontic appliance auxillary that consists of a rigid metal wire extending anteriorly from the buccal side of a molar band anteriorly. See also **arch bar, labial bar, lingual bar.**

buccal contour, the shape of the buccal side of a posterior tooth, usually characterized by a slight occlusocervical convexity with its largest prominence at the gingival third of the clinical buccal surface.

buccal fat pad, a fat pad in the cheek under the subcutaneous layer of the skin, over the buccinator. It is particularly prominent in infants and is often called a sucking pad.

buccal flange, the portion of a denture flange that occupies the buccal vestible of the mouth and extends distally from the buccal notch. Compare **labial flange, lingual flange.** See also **flange.**

buccal notch, a depression in a denture flange that accomodates the buccal frenum. Compare **labial notch.**

buccal splint, any material, usually plaster, placed on the buccal surfaces of fixed partial denture units to hold the units in position for assembly.

bucci-. See **bucco-.**

buccinator /buk′sinā′tər/, the main muscle of the cheek, one of the 12 muscles of the mouth. It arises from the maxilla above and the mandible below, inserting in the lips; its superficial surface is covered by the buccopharyngeal fascia and the buccal fat pad. Its deep part is pierced by the duct of the parotid gland opposite the second molar tooth. The buccinator, innervated by buccal branches of the facial nerve, compresses the cheek, acting as an important accessory muscle of mastication by holding food under the teeth.

bucco-, bucca-, bucci-, a combining form meaning 'pertaining to the cheek': *buccocervical, buccodistal, buccogingival.*

buccopharyngeal /buk′ōfərin′jē·əl/, of or pertaining to the cheek and the pharynx or to the mouth and the pharynx.

bucket handle fracture, a fracture that produces a tear in a semilunar cartilage along the medial side of the knee joint.

bucking, *informal.* **1.** gagging on an endotracheal tube. **2.** involuntarily resisting insufflation by a positive pressure respirator.

buck knife, a periodontal surgical knife with a spear-shaped cutting point, used for interdental incision associated with a gingivectomy.

Buck's skin traction, an orthopedic procedure that applies traction to the lower extremity, with the hips and the knees extended. It is used to help in the treatment of hip and knee contractures, in postoperative positioning and immobilization, and in disease processes of the hip and the knee. This type of traction may be unilateral, involving one leg, or bilateral, involving both legs.

Buck's traction, one of the most common orthopedic mechanisms by which pull is exerted on the lower extremity with a system of ropes, weights, and pulleys. Buck's traction, which may be unilateral or bilateral, is used to immobilize, position, and align the lower extremity in the treatment of contractures and diseases of the hip and knee. The mechanism commonly consists of a metal bar extending from a frame at the foot of the patient's bed, supporting traction weights connected by a rope passing through a pulley to a cast or a splint around the affected body structure. Compare **Bryant traction.**

Bucky diaphragm, (in radiology) a device consisting of a moving grid that limits the amount of scattered radiation and thus obtains finer x-ray film contrast and detail.

Budd-Chiari syndrome /bud′kē·är′ē/, a disorder of hepatic circulation, marked by venous obstruction, that leads to liver enlargement, ascites, extensive development of collateral vessels, and severe portal hypertension. Also called **Chiari's syndrome, Rokitansky's disease.**

budding, a type of asexual reproduction in which the cell produces a budlike projection containing chromatin that eventually separates from the parent and develops into an independent organism. It is a common form of reproduction in the lower animals and plants, as sponges, yeasts, and molds.

Buerger's disease. See **thromboangiitis obliterans.**

buffer, a substance or group of substances that tends to control the hydrogen ion concentration in a solution by absorbing hydrogen ions when a base is added to the system and releasing hydrogen ions upon the addition of an acid. Buffers minimize significant changes of pH in a chemical system. Among the functions carried out by buffer systems in the body are maintenance of the acid-base balance of the blood and maintenance of the proper pH in kidney tubules. See also **blood buffers, pH.**

buffy coat transfusion. See **granulocyte transfusion.**

bug, an error in a computer program (software bug) or a design flaw in computer hardware (hardware bug), usually resulting in the inability to make a computer process data correctly.

bulbar paralysis, a degenerative neurologic condition characterized by progressive paralysis of the lips, tongue, mouth, pharynx, and larynx. The condition occurs most commonly in people over 50 years of age, in multiple sclerosis, and in amyotrophic lateral sclerosis.

bulbourethral gland, one of two small glands located on each side of the prostate, draining to the urethra. Bulbourethral glands secrete a fluid component of the seminal fluid. Also called **Cowper's gland.**

bulb syringe, a blunt-tipped, flexible syringe usually made of rubber or plastic. Bulb syringes are used primarily for irrigating external orifices, as the auditory canal.

bulbus oculi. See **eye.**

-bulia, -boulia, a combining form meaning '(condition of the) will': *abulia, parabulia, hyperbulia.*

bulimia /byo͞olim′ē·ə/, an insatiable craving for food, often resulting in episodes of continous eating followed by periods of depression and self-deprivation. Also spelled **boulimia.** –**bulemic,** *n., adj.*

bulk. See **dietary fiber.**

bulk cathartic, a cathartic that acts by softening and increasing the mass of fecal material in the bowel. Bulk cathartics contain a hydrophilic agent such as methylcellulose or psyllium seed.

bulla /bo͝ol′ə, bul′ə/, *pl.* **bullae,** a thin-walled blister of the skin or mucous membranes greater than one centimeter in diameter containing clear, serous fluid. Compare **vesicle.** –**bullous,** *adj.*

bulldog forceps, short, spring forceps for clamping an artery or vein for hemostasis. The jaws may be padded to avoid injury to vascular tissue.

bullet forceps, a kind of forceps that has thin, curved, serrated blades designed for extracting a foreign object, as a bullet, from the base of a puncture wound.

bullous myringitis, an inflammatory condition of the ear, characterized by fluid-filled vesicles on the tympanic membrane and the sudden onset of severe pain in the ear. The condition often occurs with bacterial otitis media. Treatment includes the administration of antibiotics, analgesics, and surgical draining of the vesicles. See also **otitis media.**

bumetanide, a diuretic.

■ INDICATIONS: It is prescribed in the treatment of edema caused by cardiac, hepatic, or renal disease.

■ CONTRAINDICATIONS: Anuria, electrolyte depletion, or known sensitivity to this drug prohibits its use.

■ ADVERSE EFFECTS: Among the most serious adverse reactions are hypokalemia, hyperuricemia, azotemia.

Bumex, a trademark for a diuretic (bumetanide).

Buminate, a trademark for a blood volume expander (human albumin).

BUN, abbreviation for **blood urea nitrogen.**

-bund, a combining form meaning 'prone to' something specified: *furibund, moribund.*

bundle branch block, an abnormality in the conduction of the cardiac impulse through the fibers of the bundle of His. If many fibers are affected, the heart rate is reduced; the pacemaker function is relegated to the ventricles and peripheral perfusion is impaired. The condition may occur after myocardial infarction, in ischemic heart disease, or in certain degenerative neurologic diseases. An artificial pacemaker may be used to maintain adequate cardiac function. Compare **infranodal block, intraventricular block.** See also **atrioventricular block, heart block, intraatrial block, sinoatrial block.**

bundle of His /his/, a band of fibers in the myocardium through which the cardiac impulse is transmitted from the atrioventricular (AV) node to the ventricles. The bundle of His begins at the AV node, follows the membranous septum of the heart and divides to form the left bundle branch and the right bundle branch. The right bundle branch continues toward the apex and spreads throughout the right ventricle. The left bundle branch penetrates the fibrous septum and spreads throughout the left ventricle. The ends of both bundle branches within the ventricles are composed of Purkinje fibers. Also called **atrioventricular bundle, His bundle.**

bunion /bun′yən/, an abnormal enlargement of the joint at the base of the great toe. It is caused by inflammation of the bursa, usually as a result of chronic irritation and pressure from poorly fitted shoes. It is characterized by soreness, swelling, thickening of the skin, and lateral displacement of the great toe.

bunionectomy, excision of a bunion.

bunionette /bun′yənet′/, an abnormal enlargement and inflamation of the joint at the base of the small toe. Also called **tailor's bunion.**

Bunyamwera arbovirus, one of a group of arthropod-borne viruses that infect humans, carried by mosquitoes from rodent hosts causing California encephalitis, Rift Valley fever, and other diseases characterized by headache, weakness, low-grade fever, myalgia, and a rash. Convalescence is prolonged. Outbreaks have occurred in North America, South America, Africa, and Europe.

buphthalmos. See **congenital glaucoma.**

bupivacaine hydrochloride /byo͞opiv′əkān/, a local anesthetic.

■ INDICATIONS: It is prescribed for caudal, epidural, peripheral, or sympathetic anesthetic block.

■ CONTRAINDICATIONS: Known hypersensitivity to this drug or to any of the amide class of local anesthetics prohibits its use.

■ ADVERSE EFFECTS: Among the more serious adverse reactions are central nervous system disturbances, cardiovascular depression, respiratory arrest, cardiac arrest, and hypersensitivity reactions. The adverse effects vary depending on the condition of the patient, the dosage, and the route of administration.

buret, a laboratory utensil used to deliver a wide range of volumes accurately. Also spelled **burette.**

Burkitt's lymphoma /bur′kits/, a malignant neoplasm composed of undifferentiated lymphoreticular cells that form a large osteolytic lesion in the jaw or, in children, an abdominal mass. The tumor, which is seen chiefly in Central Africa, is characteristically a gray-white mass with a branlike consistency, sometimes containing areas of hemorrhage and necrosis. Central nervous system involvement often occurs, and other organs may be affected. The Epstein-Barr virus (EBV), a herpesvirus, may be the cause of this lymphoma. Chemotherapy usually results in rapid shrinking of the osteolytic lesion and complete cure of the disease. Also called **African lymphoma, Burkitt's tumor.**

burn, any injury to tissues of the body caused by heat, electricity, chemicals, radiation, or gases in which the extent of the injury is determined by the amount of exposure of the cell to the agent and to the nature of the agent. The treatment of burns includes pain relief, careful asepsis, prevention of infection, maintenance of the balance in the body of fluids and electrolytes, and good nutrition. Severe burns of any origin may cause shock, which is treated before the wound. See also **chemical burn, electrocution, thermal burn.**

burn center, a health care facility that is designed to care for patients who have been severely burned. A network of burn centers has been established throughout the United States and Canada, which provide sophisticated advanced techniques of care for burn victims.

burnout, a popular term for the condition of having mental or physical energy depletion after a period of chronic, unrelieved job-related stress characterized sometimes by physical illness. The health professional loses concern or respect for patients, and often develops cynical, dehumanized perceptions of people, labeling them in a derogatory manner. Causes of burnout peculiar to the nursing profession often include stressful, even dangerous, work environments; lack of support; lack of respectful relationships within the health care team; low pay scales, compared with physician's salaries; shift changes and long work hours; understaffing of hospitals; pressure from the responsibility of providing continuous high levels of care over long periods of time; and frustration and disillusionment resulting from the difference between job realities and job expectations.

burn therapy, the management of a patient burned by flames, a hot liquid, or explosive, chemical, or electric current. Partial thickness burns may be first degree, involving only the epidermis, or second degree, involving the epidermis and corium, whereas full thickness or third degree burns involve all skin layers. Second degree burns covering more than 30% of the body and third degree burns on the face and extremities, or more than 10% of the body surface, are critical. In the first 48 hours of a severe burn, vascular fluid, sodium chloride, and protein rapidly pass into the affected area causing local edema, blister formation, hypovolemia, hypoproteinemia, hyponatremia, hyperkalemia, hypotension, and oliguria. The initial hypovolemic stage is followed by a shift of fluid in the opposite direction resulting in diuresis, increased blood volume, and decreased serum electrolytes. Potential complications in serious burns include circulatory collapse, renal damage, gastric atony, paralytic ileus, infections, septic shock, pneumonia, and stress ulcer (Curling's ulcer), characterized by hematemesis and peritonitis.

■ **METHOD**: The extent of the burn, its cause, and time of occurrence and the patient's age, weight, allergies, and any preexisting illness are recorded. If respiratory distress is present, endotracheal intubation or tracheostomy may be performed. Specimens are obtained for urinalysis, blood type, blood urea nitrogen level, hematocrit, prothrombin time, electrolyte levels, blood gases, and cultures of nasal, throat, wound, and stool organisms. Parenteral fluids and electrolytes, antibiotics, tetanus prophylaxis, and pain medication are administered as ordered; large doses of analgesics and sedatives are avoided when possible to prevent depressing respiration and the masking of symptoms. An indwelling urinary catheter is inserted, and a nasogastric tube and catheter for monitoring central venous pressure may be indicated. Local treatment of the burn may be by the closed method or the more frequently used open method in which the injured area is cleaned and exposed to air and the patient is kept warm by a blanket or linen over a bed cradle or by a heater or lamp. In the closed method, a germicidal or bacteriostatic cream, ointment, or solution is applied to the burn, and the wound is covered with a dressing. A porcine heterograft may be used to cover the wound temporarily; this technique prevents loss of fluid and reduces the risk of infection, but the graft dries in 1 or 2 days and may pull and cause pain. Newly developed artificial skin holds great promise for treating severe burns. During the acute stage of a burn, the patient's blood pressure, pulse, respiration, and cerebrovascular pressure are checked every 30 to 60 minutes, and the rectal temperature every 2 to 4 hours. Oral hygiene, assistance in turning, coughing, and deep breathing are provided every 2 hours, and the patient's sensorium is evaluated hourly. If oral fluids are ordered, juices and carbonated drinks are offered, but plain water and ice chips are avoided. Fluid intake and output are measured hourly; if a child excretes less than 1 ml/kg of urine or an adult less than 0.5 ml/kg, a diuretic or an increase in intravenous infusion of fluid may be necessary. Blood transfusions, steroid therapy, and antipyretics may be ordered; aspirin is contraindicated. Excessive chilling and exposure to upper respiratory and wound infections are carefully avoided. Burned extremities are elevated, and contractures are prevented by using firm supports to keep affected areas properly aligned, as by using a footboard to keep the feet at a 90 degree angle to the ankles in burns of the lower extremities or by having the patient grasp a ball when the back of the hand is burned. In burns of the arm, axilla, or chest, the arm of the affected side is supported at a 90 degree angle to the body slightly above shoulder height. Linear incision of the eschar on the wound may be required if the constricting crust interferes with circulation or respiration. The patient is weighed daily at the same time on the same scale, and, after the initial acute period, an adequate intake of a high-calorie, high-protein diet is encouraged; to stimulate appetite, the patient is offered frequent small meals of preferred foods and beverages that are high in

Depth of burn		Detailed classification	Pain and pinprick sensitivity	Appearance	Healing time	End result of healing	Treatment
1°		Erythema only, no loss of epidermis	Hyperalgesia	Erythema		Normal skin	Allow to heal by natural processes Protect from further injury and infection
2°	Partial skin loss	Superficial, no loss of dermis	Hyperalgesia or normal		6-10 days		
		Intermediate, healing from hair follicles	Normal to hypo-algesia	Erythema to opaque, white blisters are characteristic	7-14 days	Normal to slightly pitted and/or poorly pigmented	
		Deep, healing from sweat glands	Hypoalgesia to analgesia		14-21 days	Hairless and depigmented Texture normal to pitted or flat and shiny	Elective skin grafting may save time and give better end result
3°	Whole skin loss	Deep dermal, occassionally heal from scattered epithelium	Analgesia	White opaque to charred, coagulated; subcutaneous veins may be visible	More than 21 days	Poor texture Hypertrophic Scar frequent	
		Whole skin loss, healing from edges only			Never if area is large	Hypertrophic scar and chronic granulations unless grafted	Skin grafting mandatory
4°	Deep tissue loss	Deep structure loss	May be some algesia				

Burn classification

potassium. Vitamins may be required. Tranquilizers may be given before wound care, but narcotics for pain usually are not needed after the acute phase. The patient is encouraged to stand for a few minutes every hour or every second hour and is generally able to walk in 7 to 10 days, but convalescence may be prolonged. Burned patients often are frightened, withdrawn, and disoriented initially, but after a few days they may become angry, depressed, or rebellious and in need of emotional support to help them cooperate with their treatment and rehabilitation. Extensive plastic surgery and repeated skin grafts may be required to restore function and the physical appearance of burn patients.

■ NURSING ORDERS: The burned patient requires intensive, prolonged care to avoid complications and prevent disfiguring contractures. The nurse administers parenteral fluids, medication, and wound care, closely monitors the patient, limits physical discomfort, provides emotional support and diversion, and encourages the family to visit regularly and to become involved in the patient's care.

■ OUTCOME CRITERIA: The outcome for the severely burned patient depends greatly on the detailed, near-constant care required during the acute phase of treatment. Scarring may cause residual dysfunction and discouragement. Encouragement to participate fully in physical therapy and to continue treatments may be helpful. Although protection from infection is essential, the nurse does not isolate the patient unless necessary.

Burow's solution /byŏŏr′ōz/, a liquid preparation containing aluminum sulfate, acetic acid, precipitated calcium carbonate, and water, used as a topical astringent, antiseptic, and antipyretic for a wide variety of skin disorders. Also called **aluminum acetate solution.**

burp, *informal.* **1.** to belch, or eructate. **2.** a belch, or eructation.

burr cell, a form of mature erythrocyte in which the cells or cell fragments have spicules, or tiny projections, on the surface. Compare **acanthocyte.**

burrowing flea. See ***Tunga penetrans.***

bursa /bur′sə/, *pl.* **bursae, 1.** a fibrous sac between certain tendons and the bones beneath them. Lined with a synovial membrane that secretes synovial fluid, the bursa acts as a small cushion that allows the tendon as it contracts and relaxes to move over the bone. See also **adventitious bursa, bursa of Achilles, olecranon bursa, prepatellar bursa. 2.** a sac or closed cavity. See also **omental bursa, pharyngeal bursa.**

bursa of Achilles, bursa separating the tendon of Achilles and the calcaneus.

bursitis /bursī′tis/, an inflammation of the bursa, the connective tissue structure surrounding a joint. Bursitis may be precipitated by arthritis, infection, injury, or excessive or traumatic exercise or effort. The chief symptom is severe pain of the affected joint, particularly on movement. The goals of treatment for bursitis include the control of pain and the maintenance of joint motion. A frequent measure used for the relief of acute pain is an intrabursal injection of an adrenocorticosteroid, followed by procaine infusion. Other commonly used treatments are analgesics, antiinflammatory agents, cold, and immobilization of the inflamed site. After the inflammatory process has subsided, heat may be helpful. In chronic cases surgery may be required to remove calcium deposits. Some kinds of bursitis are **housemaid's knee, miner's elbow,** and **weaver's bottom.** See also **rheumatism.**

bursting fracture, any fracture that disperses multiple bone fragments, usually at or near the end of a bone.

bus, a group of wires in a computer in which each separate wire carries the electric current representing one bit. Buses interconnect the parts of the computer that communicate with each other.

Buschke's disease. See **cryptococcosis.**

busulfan, an alkylating agent.

■ INDICATION: It is prescribed in the treatment of chronic myelocytic leukemia.

■ CONTRAINDICATIONS: Radiation, depressed neutrophil or platelet counts, concurrent administration of neoplastic medication, or known hypersensitivity to this drug prohibits its use.

■ ADVERSE REACTIONS: Among the more serious adverse reactions are alveolar hyperplasia (busulfan lung), depression of the bone marrow and severe nausea and diarrhea. Amenorrhea commonly occurs.

butabarbital sodium /byo͞o′təbär′bitôl/, a sedative.

■ INDICATIONS: It is prescribed for the relief of anxiety, nervous tension, and insomnia.

■ CONTRAINDICATIONS: Porphyria, seizure disorders, or known hypersensitivity to this drug prohibits its use.

■ ADVERSE EFFECTS: Among the more serious adverse reactions are jaundice, skin rash, and paradoxical excitement.

butamben picrate, a local anesthetic for the temporary relief of pain from minor burns.

butanoic acid. See **butyric acid.**

butanol. See **butyl alcohol.**

butanol-extractable iodine (BEI) /byo͞o′tənôl/, iodine that can be separated from plasma proteins by a solvent, as butanol, and measured for analyzing thyroid function. The normal concentrations of butanol-extractable iodine in serum are 3.5 to 6.5 mcg/dl. Concentration values are inaccurate if the patient has ingested any iodine compound just before a butanol-extractable iodine test. See also **thyroxine assays.**

butaperazine maleate, an antipsychotic.

■ INDICATIONS: It is prescribed in the treatment of schizophrenia and chronic brain syndrome.

■ CONTRAINDICATIONS: Bone marrow depression, the concomitant use of an antiadrenergic, or known hypersensitivity to this drug or to other phenothiazines prohibits its use. It is not given to children under 12 years of age.

■ ADVERSE EFFECTS: Among the more serious adverse reactions are skin rash, leukopenia, tardue dyskinesia, and jaundice.

Butazolidin, a trademark for an antirheumatic (phenylbutazone).

Butesin Picrate, a trademark for a local anesthetic (butamben picrate).

Butisol Sodium, a trademark for a sedative (butabarbital sodium).

butorphanol tartrate /byo͞otôr′fənôl/, a parenteral narcotic of the phenanthrene family, given for surgical premedication and as an analgesic component of balanced anesthesia. Because it provides almost immediate relief from pain when given intravenously and begins to take effect within 10 minutes when given intramuscularly (with peak analgesic activity within 30 to 60 minutes), it is useful for the relief of moderate to severe pain associated with surgical procedures. Butorphanol tartrate is not given to patients known to be sensitive to phenanthrenes or to persons dependent on narcotics, because it may provoke withdrawal symptoms. Toxicity may result from the use of butorphanol with other narcotics.

butterfly bandage, a narrow adhesive strip with broader winglike ends used to approximate the edges of a superficial wound and to hold the sides together as they heal. It is used in place of a suture in certain cases. Also called **butterfly.**

butterfly fracture, a bone break in which the center fragment contained by two cracks forms a triangle.

butterfly rash, an erythematous, scaling eruption of both cheeks joined by a narrow band of rash across the nose. It is seen in lupus erythematosus, rosacea, and seborrheic dermatitis.

buttermilk, **1.** the slightly sour tasting liquid residue remaining after the solids in cream have been churned into butter. It is nearly fat free and, except for a relatively low content of vitamin A, is nutritionally comparable to whole milk. **2.** cultured milk made by the addition of certain organisms to fat-free milk.

buttock. See **nates.**

buttonhole, a small slitlike hole in the wall of a structure or a cavity of the body.

buttonhole fracture, any fracture caused by the perforation of a bone by a bullet.

button suture, a technique in suturing in which the ends of the suture material are passed through buttons on the surface of the skin and tied. It is used to prevent the suture from cutting through the skin.

butyl /byo͞o′til/, a hydrocarbon radical (C_4H_9), the compounds of which are obtained from petroleum. Butyl compounds, some of which are toxic and irritating, are used in a variety of industrial and medical applications, including anesthesia.

butyl alcohol, a clear, toxic liquid used as an organic solvent. It is one of four isomers, the others being isobutyl, secondary butyl, and tertiary butyl alcohol. Also called **butanol.**

butyr-, a combining form meaning 'pertaining to butter': *butyraceous, butyric, butyrinase.*

butyric acid /byo͞otir′ik/, a fatty acid occurring in rancid butter, feces, urine, perspiration, and, in trace amounts, in the spleen and blood. Butyric acid is used in the preparation of flavorings, emulsifying agents, and pharmaceutics. Also called **butanoic acid, propylformic acid.**

butyric fermentation, the conversion to butyric acid of carbohydrates.

butyrophenone /byo͞o′tərōfē′nōn/, one of a small group of major tranquilizers used in treating psychosis, to decrease the choreic symptoms of Huntington's chorea and the tics and coprolalia of Gilles de la Tourette's syndrome, and as an adjunct in neuroleptanesthesia. Principal butyrophenones are pimozide, fluspirilene, haloperidol, and droperidol. Butyrophenones are pharmacologically and clinically similar to the phenothiazines.

BWS, abbreviation for **battered woman syndrome.**

bypass, any one of various surgical procedures to divert the flow of blood or other natural fluids from normal anatomic courses. A bypass may be either temporary or permanent. Bypass surgery is commonly performed in the treatment of cardiac and GI disorders.

byssinosis /bis′inō′sis/, an occupational respiratory disease characterized by shortness of breath, cough, and wheezing. The condition is an allergic reaction to dust or fungi in cotton, flax, and hemp fibers. The symptoms are typically more pronounced on Mondays when the workers return after a weekend break and are reversible in the early stages. Prolonged exposure of many years results in chronic airway obstruction, bronchitis, and emphysema with fibrosis, leading to respiratory failure, pulmonary hypertension, and cor pulmonale. Treatment is symptomatic for the irreversible changes of emphysema and chronic bronchitis. Compare **pneumoconiosis.** See also **organic dust**

byte /bīt/, the number of bits required to encode one character of information (letter, number, or symbol) in a computer system. See also **bit.**

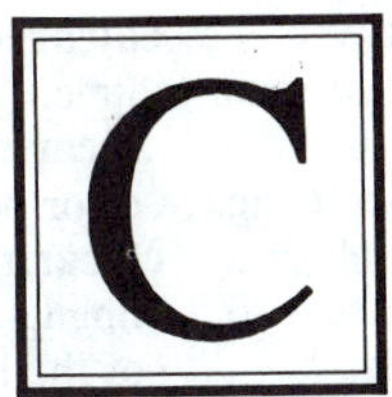

c, **1.** symbol for **capillary blood.** **2.** abbreviation for **curie.**

C, symbol for concentration of gas in the blood.

Ca, symbol for **calcium.**

cabinet bath, a bath in which the patient is enclosed in a cabinet, except for the head, heated by hot air or radiant heat. Also called **box bath.**

Cabot rings /kab′ot/, threadlike figures, often appearing as loops or rings, observed in red blood cells of patients with severe anemia. The inclusions are seen after blood cells are treated with a blue stain. Also called **Cabot bodies.**

Cabot's splint, a metal splint worn behind the thigh and leg for support.

cac-. See **caco-.**

cacao, **1.** cocoa. **2.** the substance *Theobroma cacao.* **3.** the seeds of *Theobroma cacao.*

cacesthesia /kak′əsthē′zhə/, any morbid feeling or disordered sensibility. **–cacesthetic,** *adj.*

cachet /käshā′/, any lenticular edible capsule that encloses a dose of medicine.

cachexia /kəkek′sē·ə/, general ill health and malnutrition, marked by weakness and emaciation, usually associated with serious disease, as tuberculosis or cancer. Also called **cachexy** /kəkek′sē/. **–cachectic,** *adj.*

cachinnation /kak′ənā′shən/, an excessive laughter for no apparent reason, often part of the behavioral pattern in schizophrenia. **–cachinnate,** *v.*

caco-, cac-, a combining form meaning 'ill, bad': *cacodontia, cacogeusia, cacosmia.*

cacodemonomania /kak′ōdē′mənōmā′nē·ə/, an abnormal mental condition in which the patient claims to be possessed by an evil spirit.

cacophony /kəkof′ənē/, *pl.* **cacophonies,** a harsh or discordant sound or a mixture of confused, different sounds. **–cacophonic, cacophonous,** *adj.*

cacosmia, the perception of foul odors or stench when none exists. In most instances the condition results from psychologic factors, as in olfactory hallucinations that occur during certain psychoses, although it may be caused by a brain lesion. Also spelled **kakosmia.**

cadaver, a dead body used for dissection and study.

cadmium (Cd), a metallic, bluish-white element that resembles tin. Its atomic number is 48; its atomic weight is 112.40. Cadmium has many uses in industry and was formerly used in medications. Such medications have been replaced by less toxic drugs. Cadmium bromide, used in engraving, lithography, and photography, can cause severe GI symptoms if swallowed. Cadmium may also cause poisoning by inhalation of fumes from metal-plating processes or by the ingestion of acidic foods prepared and stored in cadmium-lined containers, as lemonade in certain metal cans.

cadmium poisoning, poisoning resulting from the inhalation of cadmium in fumes created by welding, smelting, or other industrial processes involving solder. The effects may include vomiting, dyspnea, headache, prostration, pulmonary edema, and, possibly, years later, cancer. Treatment for acute poisoning includes intravenous fluids and hyperbaric oxygen.

caduceus /kədo͞o′sē·əs/, the wand of the god Hermes or Mercury, used as the symbol for the U.S. Army Medical Corps. It is represented as a staff with two serpents coiled around it and is often confused with the staff of Æsculapius, a rod with one snake entwined about it.

caenogenesis. See **cenogenesis.**

Caesarean hysterectomy. See **cesarean hysterectomy.**

Caesarean section. See **cesarean section.**

café-au-lait spot /kaf′ā·ōlā′/, a pale tan macule the color of coffee with milk. Several café-au-lait spots developing simultaneously are associated with neurofibromatosis, but occasional café-au-lait spots occur normally. See also **neurofibromatosis.**

Cafergot, a trademark for a fixed-combination drug containing caffeine and ergotamine, commonly administered in the treatment of migraine headaches.

caffeine /kafēn′, kaf′ē·in/, a central nervous system stimulant.

■ INDICATIONS: It is prescribed to counteract migraine, drowsiness, and mental fatigue.

■ CONTRAINDICATIONS: It is used with caution in patients with heart disease and peptic ulcer. Known hypersensitivity to this drug prohibits its use.

■ ADVERSE EFFECTS: Among the most serious adverse reactions are tachycardia and diuresis. GI distress, restlessness, and insomnia are common.

caffeinism, a toxic condition caused by the chronic ingestion of excessive amounts of caffeine. Symptoms include restlessness, anxiety, general depression, tachycardia, tremors, nausea, diuresis, and insomnia. In cases of caffeine poisoning, death may occur from cardiovascular and respiratory collapse. See also **xanthine derivative.**

CAH, abbreviation for **chronic active hepatitis.**

CAI, abbreviation for **computer-assisted instruction.**

-caine, a combining form usually indicating a synthetic alkaloid anesthetic: *isocaine, metycaine, neurocaine.*

caisson disease. See **decompression sickness.**
caked, formed into a compact mass or crust, as the scab of coagulated blood on a healing wound.
caked breast, an accumulation of milk in the secreting ducts of the breast after child delivery, causing all or a part of the breast to become hardened and the tissues to become engorged. Also called **lactation mastitis.**
calabar swelling /kal′əbär/, an abnormal condition characterized by fugitive, swollen lumps of subcutaneous tissue caused by a parasitic, filarial worm endemic to central and west Africa. The swollen areas migrate with the worm through the body at a speed of about one cm per minute and may become as large as a small egg. At times the worm may move under the conjunctiva of the eye and may live in the anterior chamber of the eye. Treatment includes the oral administration of diethylcarbamazine, which destroys the adult worms and their offspring. Antihistamines and other medications may be given. A kind of calabar swelling is *Loa loa*. See also **loiasis.**
Caladryl, a trademark for a topical, fixed-combination drug containing a protectant (calamine) and an antihistaminic (diphenhydramine hydrochloride).
calamine /kal′əmīn/, a pink, odorless, powdered concoction used as a protectant or as an astringent and sometimes prepared as a lotion. It is composed of zinc oxide with 0.5% ferric oxide.
Calan, a trademark for a slow channel blocker or calcium ion antagonist (verapamil).
calc-, **1.** a combining form meaning 'pertaining to lime or limestone': *calcarea, calcariuria, calciosis*. **2.** a combining form meaning 'pertaining to the heel': *calcaneum, calcaneocavus, calcanodynia*.
calcaneal /kalkā′nē·əl/, of or pertaining to the calcaneus at the back of the tarsus.
calcaneal spurs, abnormal, often painful, bony outgrowths on the lower surface of the calcaneus, resulting from chronic traumatic pressure on the heel.
calcaneal tendon. See **Achilles tendon.**
calcaneal tendon reflex. See **Achilles tendon reflex.**
calcaneal tuberosity, a transverse elevation on the plantar surface of the calcaneus to which are attached the abductor digiti minimi, the long plantar ligament, and various other muscles, including the abductor hallucis and the flexor digitorum brevis.
calcaneodynia /kalkā′nē·ōdin′ē·ə/, a painful condition of the heel.
calcaneum. See **calcaneus.**
calcaneus /kalkā′nē·əs/, the heel bone. The largest of the tarsal bones, it articulates proximally with the talus and distally with the cuboid. **–calcaneal, calcanean,** *adj.*
calcar /kal′kär/, *pl.* **calcaria,** a spur or a structure that resembles a spur.
calcar avis, a projection on the medial wall of the posterior horn of the lateral ventricle of the brain. It is associated with the lateral extension of the calcarine fissure. Also called **hippocampus minor.**
calcareous /kalker′ē·əs/, of or pertaining to calcium or lime.
calcarine /kal′kərīn/, **1.** having the shape of a spur. **2.** of or pertaining to the calcar.
calcarine fissure, a fissure between the cuneus and the lingual gyrus on the medial surface of the occipital lobe of the brain. Also called **calcarine sulcus.**
calcifediol, a physiologic form of vitamin D.
■ INDICATION: It is prescribed in the treatment of metabolic bone disease associated with chronic renal failure.
■ CONTRAINDICATIONS: Hypercalcemia, vitamin D toxicity, or known hypersensitivity to this drug prohibits its use.
■ ADVERSE EFFECTS: Among the most serious adverse reactions are renal toxicity and those reactions associated with hypercalcemia, as soft tissue calcification and GI and central nervous system disturbances.
calciferol /kalsif′ərôl/, a fat-soluble, crystalline, unsaturated alcohol produced by ultraviolet irradiation of ergosterol and used as a dietary supplement in the prophylaxis and treatment of rickets, osteomalacia, and other hypocalcemic disorders. It occurs naturally in milk and fish-liver oils. Also called **ergocalciferol, oleovitamin D_2, vitamin D_2.** See also **rickets, viosterol.**
calcific aortic disease, an abnormal condition characterized by small deposits of calcium in the aorta.
calcification, the accumulation of calcium salts in tissues. Normally, about 99% of all the calcium entering the human body is deposited in the bones and teeth; the remaining 1% is dissolved in body fluids, as the blood. Disorders affecting the delicate balance between calcium and other minerals, parathyroid hormone, and vitamin D can result in calcium deposits in arteries, kidneys, lung alveoli, and other tissues, interfering with usual organ functions. See also **calcitonin, calcium, calculus.**
calcified fetus. See **lithopedion.**
calcifying epithelial odontogenic tumor, an uncommon tumor that develops in odontogenic epithelium, characterized by focal areas of calcification. It has the same age, sex, and size distribution as the ameloblastoma. Also called **Pindorg tumor.**
Calcimar, a trademark for calcitonin.
calcination, (in dentistry) a process of removing water by heat, used in the manufacture of plaster and stone from gypsum. Compare **calcification.**
calcinosis /kal′sənō′sis/, a condition characterized by abnormal deposits of calcium salts in various tissues of the body. The deposits appear as nodules or plaques and may occur in the skin, connective tissue, muscles, or intervertebral disks. Usually the nodules occur secondary to a preexisting inflammatory degenerative or neoplastic dermatosis, primarily scleroderma, and dermatomyositis.
calcitonin /kal′sitō′nin/, a hormone produced in parafollicular cells of the thyroid that participates in regulating the blood level of calcium and stimulates bone mineralization. A synthetic preparation of the hormone is

used in the treatment of certain bone disorders. Calcitonin acts to reduce the blood level of calcium and to inhibit bone resorption, while parathyroid hormone acts to increase blood calcium and bone resorption. Calcitonin has a short-term effect in enhancing bone formation and causes transient decreases in the volume and acidity of gastric juice and in the volume of amylase and trypsin in pancreatic juice. The hormone also promotes the excretion of phosphate, sodium, and calcium by decreasing their reabsorption in kidney tubules. The secretion of calcitonin is regulated by the amount of calcium in plasma, and an infusion of calcium may increase the concentration of the circulating hormone two- to threefold. Men usually have a higher level of plasma calcitonin than women.

calcitriol /kalsit′rē•ôl/, a regulator of calcium metabolism.

■ INDICATION: It is prescribed in the management of hypocalcemia occurring in patients undergoing chronic renal dialysis.

■ CONTRAINDICATIONS: Hypercalcemia, evidence of vitamin D toxicity, or known sensitivity to this drug prohibits its use.

■ ADVERSE EFFECTS: Among the more serious adverse reactions are renal toxicity and those associated with hypercalcemia, as soft tissue calcification, and GI and central nervous system disturbances.

calcium (Ca), an alkaline earth metal element. Its atomic number is 20; its atomic weight is 40. Its metallic form is a white, flammable solid, somewhat harder than lead. Calcium is commonly produced by the electrolysis or by the thermal dissociation of calcium chloride. Calcium carbonate is the most common calcium compound, which, when treated with hydrochloric acid, forms calcium chloride. Calcium also occurs as a component of the natural compound gypsum, which forms plaster of paris when heated. It is also a component of calcium cyanamid, a fertilizer and progenitor of other nitrogen compounds. Calcium is the fifth most abundant element in the human body and occurs mainly in the bone. The body requires calcium ions for the transmission of nerve impulses, muscle contraction, blood coagulation, cardiac functions, and other processes. It is a component of extracellular fluid and of soft tissue cells. The average daily human intake of calcium varies from 200 to 2500 mg. In the United States dairy products are the major dietary sources of this element. The daily dietary allowances recommended by the Federal Food and Nutrition Board vary from 360 mg for infants to 1200 mg for women 15 to 18 years of age. More than 90% of the calcium in the body is stored in the skeleton, which constantly exchanges its supplies with the calcium of the interstitial fluids. The endocrine system controls the concentration of ionized calcium in the plasma. Only a fraction of this amount is ionized and diffusable; the rest is bound to proteins, especially albumin. It is the ionized, diffusable portion of calcium that figures in the physiologic changes associated with hypocalcemia. About one third of the calcium ingested by humans is absorbed, primarily in the small bowel. Vitamin D, calcitonin, and parathyroid hormone are essential in the metabolism of calcium. The degree of cell permeability varies inversely with calcium ion concentration. Abnormally high levels of ionized calcium in the extracellular fluid can produce muscle weakness, lethargy, and coma. A relatively small decrease from the normal level of this element can produce tetanic seizures.

calcium channel blocker, a drug that inhibits the flow of calcium ions across the membranes of smooth muscle cells. By reducing the calcium flow, smooth muscle tone is relaxed and the risk of muscle spasms is diminished. Calcium channel blockers are used primarily in the treatment of heart diseases marked by coronary artery spasms. Also called **calcium antagonist, calcium blocker.**

calcium chloride, a concentrated solution of the chloride salt of calcium used to replenish calcium in the blood.

■ INDICATIONS: It is prescribed for hypocalcemic tetany and as an antidote for magnesium poisoning or an overdose of magnesium sulfate.

■ CONTRAINDICATIONS: Renal insufficiency, ventricular fibrillation, hypercalcemia, or known hypersensitivity to this drug prohibits its use.

■ ADVERSE EFFECTS: Among the more serious adverse reactions is hypercalcemia.

■ CAUTION: Calcium chloride is never injected into tissue.

calcium pump, a theoretical, energy-requiring mechanism for transmitting calcium ions across a cell membrane from a region of low calcium ion concentration to one of higher concentration. Compare **sodium pump.**

calculus /kal′kyələs/, *pl.* **calculi** /kal′kyəlī/, an abnormal stone formed in body tissues by an accumulation of mineral salts. Calculi are usually found within hollow organs or ducts and can cause obstruction and inflammation. Kinds of calculi include **biliary calculus** and **urinary calculus.** Also called **stone.** See also **gallstone.**

calculus anuria, the cessation of urine production caused by renal calculi.

Calderol, a trademark for a calcium regulator (calcifediol).

Caldwell-Moloy pelvic classification /kôl′dwelməloi′/, a system for classifying the structure of the bony pelvis of the female. The types in this system are android, anthropoid, gynecoid, and platypelloid. The sacrum, sidewalls, sacrosciatic notch, ischial spines, pubic arch, and ischial tuberosities are the anatomic points of reference used to determine pelvic type. The classification system requires that a mixed pelvis be named for the character of its posterior section with the name of the type characterized by the anterior portion following a hyphen, as in a gynecoid-android pelvis. See also **pelvic classification.**

calefacient /kal′əfā′shənt/, **1.** making or tending to make anything warm or hot. **2.** an agent that imparts a sense of warmth when applied, as a hot-water bottle or a hot compress.

calendar method of family planning. See **rhythm method.**

calf, *pl.* **calves,** the fleshy mass at the back of the leg below the knee, composed chiefly of the gastrocnemius muscle.

calf bone. See **fibula.**

caliber, the diameter of a tube or a canal, as any of the blood vessels. Also spelled **calibre.**

California encephalitis, a common, acute viral infection that affects the central nervous system. Epidemics occur mainly in the Midwest, on the Eastern seaboard, and in Texas and Louisiana. The virus was first isolated in California. The infection generally follows one of two clinical courses. The mild form is characterized by headache, malaise, GI symptoms, and a fever that may reach 104° F. The more severe form may be marked by a sudden onset of fever, vomiting, headaches, lethargy, and signs of neurologic involvement, as loss of reflexes, disorientation, seizure, loss of consciousness, and flaccid paralysis. Recovery usually begins in 1 week. Mortality is very low, but a significant number of patients have neurologic sequelae for 1 year or more. Treatment usually involves administration of anticonvulsant and sedative medications. See also **arbovirus, encephalitis.**

californium (Cf), an artificial element in the actinide group. Its atomic number is 98; its atomic weight is 251. Californium 252 isotope is a potent source of neutrons.

calipers, an instrument with two hinged, adjustable, curved legs, used to measure the thickness or the diameter of a convex body or solid.

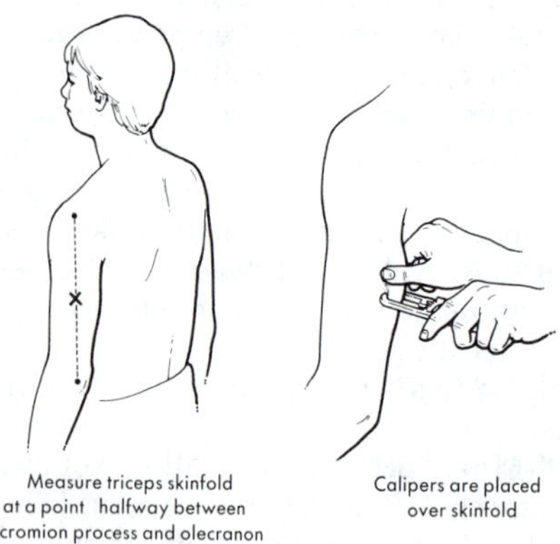

Measure triceps skinfold at a point halfway between acromion process and olecranon
Calipers are placed over skinfold

Calipers

caliper splint, a splint for the leg consisting of two metal rods running from the back of a band around the thigh or from a cushioned ring around the lower portion of the pelvis. The rods are attached to a metal plate under the shoe below the arch of the foot.

Calliphoridae /kal′əfôr′ədē/, a family of medium-sized to large flies that belong to the order Diptera, serve as pathogenic vectors, and may cause intestinal or nasopharyngeal myiasis in humans. These flies include the genera *Auchmeromyia, Calliphora, Cordylobia, Cochliomyia, Chrysomyia, Lucilia, Phaenicia,* and *Phormia.*

callomania, an abnormal psychologic condition characterized by delusions of personal beauty.

callosal fissure, a groove following the convex aspect of the corpus callosum.

callosity. See **callus.**

calloso marginal fissure /kəlō′sō/, a long, irregular groove on the medial surface of a cerebral hemisphere. It divides the cingulate gyrus from the medial frontal gyrus and from the paracentral lobule. Also called **cingulate sulcus.**

callus, **1.** also called **callosity.** a common, usually painless thickening of the epidermis at locations of external pressure or friction. Compare **corn. 2.** bony deposit formed between and around the broken ends of a fractured bone during healing. –**callous,** *adj.*

calmodulin, a calcium-binding protein that mediates a variety of biochemical and physiologic processes, including the contraction of muscles and the release of norepinephrine. Depending on its form and function, calmodulin may act independently of, in concert with, or antagonistically to reactions involving cyclic adenosinemonophosphate.

calor /kal′ôr/, heat, as that generated by inflammation of tissues or that from the normal metabolic processes of the body.

calor-, a combining form meaning 'pertaining to heat': *calorie, calorifacient, calorization.*

caloric, of or pertaining to heat or calories.

caloric test, a procedure for determining if the ear is diseased or normal. The test alternately irrigates the ear with hot water and cold water. If the ear is normal, the hot water irrigation produces a rotatory nystagmus toward the irrigated side. Cold water irrigation produces a rotatory nystagamus away from the irrigated side. If the ear is diseased, irrigation produces no nystagmus. Also called **Barany's test.**

calorie, **1.** also called **gram calorie, small calorie (cal.).** the amount of heat required to raise 1 g of water 1° C at atmospheric pressure. **2.** also called **great calorie, kilocalorie, kilogram calorie, large calorie (Cal.).** a quantity of heat equal to 1000 small calories. **3.** a unit, equal to the large calorie, used to denote the heat expenditure of an organism and the fuel or energy value of food. –**caloric,** *adj.*

calorific /kal′ərif′ik/, pertaining to the production of heat.

calorigenic /kəlôr′ijen′ik/, of or pertaining to a substance or process that produces heat or energy or that increases the consumption of oxygen.

calorimeter /kal′ərim′ətər/, a device used for measuring quantities of heat generated by friction, by chemical reaction, or by the human body. –**calorimetric,** *adj.*

calorimetry /kal′ərim′ətrē/, the measurement of the amounts of heat radiated and the amounts of heat absorbed. Compare **direct calorimetry, indirect calorimetry.** –**calorimetric,** *adj.*

calusterone /kəlo͞o′stərōn/, an antineoplastic androgen.
■ INDICATION: It is prescribed in the treatment of cancer of the breast.
■ CONTRAINDICATIONS: Cardiac and renal disease, hypercalcemia, or known sensitivity to the drug prohibits its use. It is not given to pregnant or lactating women.
■ ADVERSE EFFECTS: Among the more severe adverse reactions are fluid retention and hypercalcemia. Masculinization with clitoral enlargement, hirsutism, acne, alopecia, and erythrocytemia also occur.

calvaria /kalver′ē·ə/, the skull cap or superior portion of the skull, which varies greatly in shape from individual to individual. In some persons, the calvaria is relatively oval, in others it is more circular. It is traversed by the coronal suture between the frontal and the parietal bones, by the sagittal suture in the midline between the two parietal bones, and by the upper part of the lambdoidal suture between the parietal bones and the occipital bone. The inner surface of the calvaria is indented to accept the convolutions of the cerebrum and furrowed for the branches of the meningeal vessels. It also contains the superior sagittal sinus, affords attachment at its margins for the falx cerebri, and posteriorly, in some individuals, it accommodates the openings of the parietal foramina. The soft spots in the skull of an infant are situated on the surface of the calvaria at the junction of the sagittal and the coronal sutures and at the junction of the sagittal and lambdoid sutures. See also **bregma.**

calvities /kalvish′i·ēz/, the condition of baldness. –**calvous,** *adj.*

calyx /kā′liks/, *pl.* **calyces** /kal′isēz/, **calyxes, 1.** a cup-shaped organ. **2.** a renal calyx. **3.** the wall of an ovarian follicle after expulsion of the ovum at ovulation. Also spelled **calix.**

cambium layer, 1. the loose, inner cellular layer of the periosteum that develops during ossification. **2.** a cellular layer of formative tissue that lies between the wood and the bark in plants.

camera, (in anatomy) any cavity or chamber, as those of the eye or the heart.

camphor, a colorless or white crystalline substance with a penetrating odor and pungent taste, occurring naturally in certain plants, especially *Cinnamomum camphora.* Also called **camphora, gum camphor.**

camphor bath, an air bath in which the air is filled with camphor vapor.

camphor salicylate, a crystalline substance formed by the fusion of 84 parts of camphor and 65 parts of salicylic acid, previously used in skin ointments and administered internally for diarrhea.

camptodactyly /kamp′tədak′təlē/, the permanent flexion of one or more fingers. –**campodactylic,** *adj.*

camptomelia /kamp′təmē′lyə/, a congenital anomaly characterized by bending of one or more limbs causing permanent bowing or curving of the affected area. –**camptomelic,** *adj.*

Campylobacter, a genus of bacteria found in the family Spirillaceae. The organisms consist of gram-negative, non-spore-forming, spirally curved, motile rods that have a single polar flagellum at either or both ends of the cell and move in a characteristic coil-like motion. The organisms require little or no oxygen for growth. The type species is *C. fetus,* which consists of several subspecies that cause human infections as well as abortion and infertility in cattle. Also called ***Vibrio fetus.***

Canadian Association of University Schools of Nursing (CAUSN), a national Canadian organization of nursing schools affiliated with institutions of higher learning.

Canadian Association of University Teachers (CAUT), a national Canadian organization representing the interests of all who teach in the universities of the provinces and territories of Canada. The official languages of the CAUT are French and English.

Canadian crutch, a wooden or a metal device that helps a disabled patient stand or walk. It consists of two uprights with a crosspiece to accommodate the hand and a concave crosspiece that fits the armpit for support.

Canadian Journal of Public Health (CJPH), the official publication of the Canadian Public Health Association.

Canadian Medical Association Journal (CMAJ), the official publication of the Canadian Medical Association.

Canadian Nurses' Association (CNA), the official national organization for the professional registered nurses of Canada who are members of the 10 provincial nurses' associations and the Northwest Territory's association. The CNA, a federation of these 11 associations, is supported by contributions of the 140,000 members of the regional associations. The chief objective of the CNA is to promote conditions conducive to the good health of the people and to good patient care. It is concerned with the quality and quantity of nurses available, the standards of preparation for nurses, the social and economic welfare of nurses, the advancement of competence and expertise within the profession, the promotion of unity and understanding among the members, and the representation of the organized profession of nurses nationally and internationally. A board of 23 elected volunteers and a permanent staff working at CNA House in Ottawa manage the affairs of the organization. Among the services provided are a research and advisory unit that studies trends in nursing and health and prepares briefs, when necessary; a library containing reference works, the archives of the CNA, and up-to-date lists of educational programs in nursing; an information service that collects and disseminates information about nursing and publishes *The Canadian Nurse* and *L'Infirmière Canadienne;* a labor relations service; a testing service; a governmental liaison service; and an international service that facilitates a working relationship with various organizations, as the World Health Organization and the Pan American Health

Organization. All services are provided in the two official languages, English and French.

Canadian Nurses' Association Testing Service (CNATS), the organizational affiliate of the Canadian Nurses' Association that is concerned with testing the graduates of approved schools of nursing to qualify them as registered nurses.

Canadian Nurses' Foundation (CNF), a national Canadian foundation organized to support scholarship in nursing. The CNF awards financial support to nurses undertaking graduate studies in nursing and to nurses planning research in nursing.

Canadian Nurses' Respiratory Society (CNRS), an organization of nurses working with or interested in alleviating the problems of respiratory disease. The CNRS is an affiliate of the Canadian Nurses' Association, and it is a section of the Canadian Lung Association.

Canadian Orthopedic Nurses' Association (CONA), a national Canadian organization concerned with the nursing care of orthopedic patients and the continuing education of nurses working in orthopedics. Membership includes orthopedic nurses and other professionals concerned with orthopedics.

Canadian Public Health Association (CPHA), a national Canadian organization concerned with issues in public health and epidemiology. Membership is open to professionals and to others interested in these issues.

canal, **1.** (in anatomy) a narrow tube or channel. Some kinds of canals are **adducto canal, Alcock's canal,** and **alveolar canal. 2.** (in dentistry) one of the accessory root canals and collateral pulp canals in the teeth.

canaliculus /kan'əlik'yələs/, *pl.* **canaliculi,** a very small tube or channel, like the tiny haversian canaliculi throughout bone tissue.

canalization, the formation of canals or of passages through any tissue.

canal of Schlemm /shlem/, a tiny vein at the angle of the anterior chamber of the eye that connects with the pectinate villi, draining the aqueous humor and funneling it into the bloodstream. Also called **Schlemm's canal.**

cancellous /kan'siləs/, (of tissue) latticelike, porous, spongy. Cancellous tissue is normally present in the interior of many bones, where the spaces are usually filled with marrow.

cancer, **1.** a neoplasm characterized by the uncontrolled growth of anaplastic cells that tend to invade surrounding tissue and to metastasize to distant body sites. **2.** any of a large group of malignant neoplastic diseases characterized by the presence of malignant cells. Each cancer is distinguished by the nature, site, or clinical course of the lesion. The basic origin of cancer is undetermined, but many potential causes are recognized. More than 80% of cases of cancer are attributed to cigarette smoking, exposure to carcinogenic chemicals, ionizing radiation, and ultraviolet rays; overexposure to the sun is the major cause of skin cancer. Many viruses induce malignant tumors in animals, and viral particles are detected in some human tumors; but there is no clear evidence that any microorganism causes human cancer. The high incidence of various kinds of cancer in certain families suggests that genetic susceptibility is an important factor. An excess rate of malignant tumors in organ transplant recipients after immunosuppressive therapy indicates that the immune system plays a major role in controlling the proliferation of anaplastic cells. The basic defect may be a biochemical anomaly that triggers abnormal cell growth and glucose metabolism and in which certain vital proteins and respiratory enzymes are reduced. The incidence of different kinds of cancer varies markedly with sex, age, ethnic group, and geographic location. The age-adjusted death rate for oral cancer is almost 10 times higher in Hong Kong than in Denmark, and that for prostate cancer is more than 10 times greater in Sweden than in Japan, but leukemia mortality is similar throughout the world. In the United States, cancer is second only to heart disease as a cause of mortality and is a leading cause of death in children between 3 and 14 years of age. The most common sites for the development of malignant tumors are the lung, breast, colon, uterus, oral cavity, and bone marrow. Surgery remains the major form of treatment, but irradiation is widely used as preoperative, postoperative, or primary therapy; chemotherapy, with single or multiple antineoplastic agents, is often highly effective. Many malignant lesions are curable if detected in the early stage. Depending on the site, the warning signal may be a change in bowel or bladder habits, a nonhealing sore, unusual bleeding or discharge, a thickening or lump in the breast or elsewhere, indigestion or dysphagia, an obvious change in a wart or mole, or a nagging cough or persistent hoarseness.

cancer bodies. See **Russell's bodies.**

cancericidal /kan'sərisī'dəl/, of or pertaining to a substance or procedure capable of destroying cancer cells.

cancer in situ. See **carcinoma in situ.**

cancer of the small intestine, a neoplastic disease of the duodenum, jejunum, or ileum. Its characteristics vary, depending on the kind of tumor and the site, but may include abdominal pain, vomiting, weight loss, diarrhea, intermittent bowel obstruction, GI bleeding, or a mass deep in the right abdomen. Diagnosis is made with barium x-ray examination, but such studies may be inconclusive until lesions are large. Adenocarcinomas, the most common tumors, occur more frequently in the duodenum or upper jejunum and form polypoid or constricting napkin-ring growths. Lymphomas, found most often in the lower small intestine, may impair bowel motility by invading nerves and in some cases are associated with a malabsorption syndrome. Less common tumors of the small intestine are carcinoids, usually found in the ileum, and sarcomas, usually seen in the jejunum and ileum. A leiomyosarcoma may sometimes form a large extraluminal mass but does not metastasize, unlike other cancers of the small intestine. Surgery, including a wide resection of mesenteric lymph nodes, is indicated for adenocarcinomas. Irradiation is not effective in ablation of these tumors but is recommended post-

Cancer's seven warning signals

Adults	*Children*
Change in bowel or bladder habit	Marked change in bowel or bladder habits; nausea and vomiting for no apparent cause
Unusual bleeding or discharge	Bloody discharge of any sort: blood in urine, spontaneous nosebleed or other type hemorrhage, failure to stop bleeding in the usual time
Thickening or lump in breast or elsewhere	Swellings, lumps, or masses anywhere in the body
Obvious change in wart or mole	Any change in the size or appearance of outward growths, such as moles or birthmarks
Nagging cough or hoarseness	Unexplained stumbling in a child
A sore that does not heal	A generally run-down condition
Indigestion or difficulty in swallowing	Pains or the persistent crying of a baby or child, for which no reason can be found

From American Cancer Society: cancer facts and figures (1982), New York, 1982, American Cancer Society.

operatively for lymphomas to treat metastatic lesions in mesenteric lymph nodes, the liver, and spleen. Resection of carcinoids is advised to prevent bowel obstruction even if metastatic disease is present, and some patients with these lesions may respond to chemotherapeutic agents, as cyclophosphamide, 5-fluorouracil, methotrexate, and streptozocin. Cancer of the small intestine, which is uncommon considering the great length and surface area of that organ, occurs slightly more often in men than in women.

cancer staging, a system for describing the extent of a malignant tumor and its metastases, used to plan appropriate treatment and predict prognosis. Staging involves a careful physical examination, diagnostic procedures, and, ultimately, surgical exploration. The standardized system developed by the American Joint Committee for Cancer Staging and End Results Reporting uses the letter T to represent the tumor, N for the regional lymph node involvement, M for distant metastases, and numeric subscripts in each category to indicate the degree of dissemination. According to this system $T_1N_0M_0$ designates a small, localized tumor; $T_2N_1M_0$ is a larger primary tumor that has extended to regional nodes; and $T_4N_3M_3$ is a very large lesion involving regional nodes and distant sites. The Ann Arbor System classifies Hodgkin's disease as Stages I to IV according to the number and location of involved lymph nodes in relation to the diaphragm and the involvement of extralymphatic organs or tissues, based on numerous diagnostic procedures and by a staging laparotomy. Other systems may be used for staging breast carcinoma, colorectal cancer, and cutaneous melanoma.

TNM cancer staging classification system

T† subclasses	Tx—tumor cannot be adequately assessed
	T0—no evidence of primary tumor
	TIS—carcinoma in situ
	T1, T2, T3, T4—progressive increase in tumor size and involvement
N‡ subclasses	Nx—regional lymph nodes cannot be assessed clinically
	N0—regional lymph nodes demonstrably abnormal
	N1, N2, N3, N4—increasing degrees of demonstrable abnormality of regional lymph nodes
M§ subclasses	Mx—not assessed
	M0—no (known) distant metastasis
	M1—distant metastasis present, specify site(s)
Histopathology	G1—well-differentiated grade
	G2—moderately well-differentiated grade
	G3, G4—poorly to very poorly differentiated grade

From American Joint Committee for Cancer Staging and End Results Reporting: Manual for staging of cancer, 1977, Chicago, 1977, American Joint Committee.
†T = Primary tumor.
‡N = Regional lymph nodes.
§M = Distant metastasis.

cancer-ulcer, a carcinomatous ulceration.

cancr-, chancr-, a combining form meaning 'pertaining to cancer': *cancriform, cancroid, cancrology*.

cancriform /kang′krifôrm′/, of or pertaining to a lesion resembling a cancer.

cancroid, **1.** of or pertaining to a lesion resembling a cancer. **2.** a moderately malignant skin cancer.

candela. See **candle.**

candicidin /kan′dəsī′din/, a topical antifungal agent.
■ INDICATIONS: It is prescribed in the treatment of vaginitis caused by *Candida albicans* or by other species of *Candida*.
■ CONTRAINDICATION: Known hypersensitivity to this drug prohibits its use.
■ ADVERSE EFFECTS: Among the most serious adverse reactions are irritation of the vulvar and perivulvar area. Allergic reactions occur rarely.

Candida /kan′didə/, a genus of yeastlike fungi including the common pathogen, *Candida albicans*.

Candida albicans /al′bəkanz/, a common, budding, yeastlike, microscopic fungal organism normally present in the mucous membranes of the mouth, intestinal tract, and vagina and on the skin of healthy people. Under certain circumstances, it may cause superficial infections of the mouth or vagina and, less commonly, serious invasive systemic infection and toxic reaction. See also **candidiasis.**

candidiasis /kan′didī′əsis/, any infection caused by a species of *Candida*, usually *Candida albicans*, characterized by pruritus, a white exudate, peeling, and easy bleeding. Diaper rash, intertrigo, vaginitis, and thrush are common topical manifestations of candidiasis. Endocarditis, other inflammatory conditions of the heart and liver, and infection of the kidney, spleen, and lungs sometimes occur in debilitated patients. Treatment includes the oral and topical administration of antifungal drugs, as nystatin, clotrimazole, and, rarely, amphotericin B. Also called **candidosis.**

Candiru fever /kan′diro͞o′/, an arbovirus infection transmitted to humans by the bite of a sandfly, characterized by an acute fever, headache, and muscle aches. Recovery occurs, without treatment, within a few days. It occurs mainly in the forests of Brazil. See also **arbovirus, phlebotomus fever, sandfly fever.**

candle, (in optics) the basic unit of measurement for luminous intensity, equal to 1/60 of the luminous intensity of a square centimeter of a black body heated to 1773.5° C or the solidification temperature of platinum, adopted in 1948 as the international standard of luminous intensity. Also called **candela** /kandē′lə/.

candy-striper, *informal.* a hospital volunteer, named for the striped pink and white uniforms traditionally worn by the young people who perform this service.

cane-cutter's cramp. See **heat cramp.**

canefield fever. See **field fever.**

canine fossa /kā′nīn/, (in dentistry) either of the wide depressions on the external surface of each maxilla, superolateral to the canine tooth socket. It is the origin of the levator anguli oris muscle. Also called **maxillary fossa.**

canine tooth, any one of the four teeth, two in each jaw, situated immediately lateral to the incisor teeth in the human dental arches. The canine teeth are larger and stronger than the incisors, and they project beyond the level of the other teeth in both arches. Their roots sink deeply into the bones, causing marked prominences on the alveolar arch. The upper canine teeth, or eye teeth, are larger and longer than the lower ones and have a distinct basal ridge. The lower canine teeth, or stomach teeth, are situated nearer the middle line than the upper ones, and their summits correspond to the intervals between the upper canines and the incisors. The crowns of the canines are very large and conic and taper to blunted points or cusps. The canines erupt as deciduous teeth about 16 to 20 months after birth. The eruption of the permanent canines occurs during the eleventh or the twelfth year of life.

canker, an ulcer or sore, especially in the mouth. Also called **aphthous stomatitis.**

canker sore, an ulcerous lesion of the mouth, characteristic of aphthous stomatitis. See also **aphthous stomatitis.**

cannabis /kan′əbis/, a psychoactive drug derived from the flowering tops of hemp plants. It has no currently acceptable clinical use in the United States but has been employed in the treatment of glaucoma and as an antiemetic in some cancer patients to counter the nausea and vomiting associated with chemotherapy. Cannabis is controlled under Schedule I of the Comprehensive Drug Abuse Prevention and Control Act of 1970 and may be legally obtained for research and special medical applications authorized by the Drug Enforcement Administration of the U.S. Department of Justice. The common hemp from which cannabis is obtained is an herbaceous annual of which *Cannabis sativa* is the sole species. The two subspecies are *indica* and *americana*. All parts of the plant contain psychoactive substances or cannabinoids, the highest concentrations of which are in the resin of the flowering tops of the plant. *Cannabis sativa* grows in many parts of the world, and cannabis is used in different psychoactive ways among various populations. The cannabinoids synthesized by the hemp plant include cannabinol, cannabidiol, cannabinolic acid, cannabigerol, cannabicyclol, and several isomers of tetrahydrocannabinol (THC). THC is believed to cause the most characteristic psychologic effects, which include alterations of mood, memory, motor coordination, cognitive ability, and self-perception. Most users of cannabis smoke marijuana cigarettes containing dried and chopped leaves of the hemp plant. Other users ingest the drug. The effects vary, depending on the dosage, the type of administration, and the experience of the user. In marijuana illicitly obtained and used in the United States the concentration of THC varies widely from 0.5% to 6%, and its absorption into the bloodstream depends on the smoking technique of the user and the destruction of cannabinoids by pyrolysis. Oral doses of 20 mg of THC or the smoking of a cigarette containing 2% of THC most commonly produces euphoria in the user and changes in mood and sense of time. Oral doses of cannabis equivalent to several cigarettes impair short-term memory and the capacity to complete tasks requiring multiple steps to reach a specific goal. Low doses of cannabis seldom impair the ability to perform simple motor tasks but commonly hinder more complex actions, as driving and flying, which involve complex sensory perception, concentration, and information processing. Cannabis may also enhance the nondominant senses of touch, taste, and smell. Higher doses in some persons can produce delusions, paranoid feelings, anxiety, and panic. This drug also increases the heart rate and systolic blood pressure. Pharmacologic effects of smoking marijuana occur within minutes after smoking begins and produce peak plasma concentrations of THC within 10 to 30 minutes. The effects of one cigarette rarely last more than 2 or 3 hours. Marijuana is about three times more powerful when smoked than when taken orally. The smoking of marijuana has increased throughout the world since the 1960s, and in 1977 approximately 60% of young adults polled in the United States reported some experience with the drug. Studies indicate that it is used by many individuals in all socioeconomic and ethnic groups. Research indicates that some cannabinoids may be therapeutic as anticonvulsants and helpful in reducing intraocular pressure associated with glaucoma. Also called **bhang, ganja, grass, hashish, marijuana, pot, reefer, tea, weed.**

cannabism, a condition associated with excessive or extended use of cannabis drugs. It is characterized by anxiety, disorientation, hallucinations, memory defects, and paranoia.

cannon wave, a powerful "a" wave in the jugular pulse, characteristic of a complete heart block and of premature ventricular beats of the heart. Cannon waves are caused by the contraction of the right atrium of the heart immediately after contraction of the right ventricle has closed the tricuspid valve.

cannula /kan′yələ/, *pl.* **cannulas, cannulae,** a flexible tube containing a stiff, pointed trocar that may be inserted into the body, guided by the trocar. As the trocar is removed, a body fluid may be passed through the cannula to the outside. **–cannular, cannulate,** *adj.*

cannulation, the insertion of a cannula into a body duct or cavity, as into the trachea, bladder, or a blood vessel. Also called **cannulization. –cannulate, cannulize,** *v.*

cantharis /kan′thäris/, *pl.* **cantharides** /kanther′idēz/, the dried insects *Cantharis vesicatoria* containing cantharidin, formerly used as a topical vesicant. Also called **Spanish fly.**

cantho-, a combining form meaning 'pertaining to the canthus': *cantholysis, canthorraphy, canthotomy.*

canthus /kan′thəs/, *pl.* **canthi,** the angle at the medial and the lateral margins of the eyelids. The medial canthus opens into a small space containing the opening to a lacrimal duct. Also called **palpebral commissure. –canthic,** *adj.*

Cantil, a trademark for an anticholinergic antispasmodic (mepenzolate bromide).

cap, abbreviation for Latin *capiat,* "let him or her take," used in prescriptions.

CAP, **1.** abbreviation for **College of American Pathologists. 2.** (in molecular genetics) abbreviation for **catabolic activator protein.** CAP participates in initiating the transcription of RNA in organisms without a true nucleus, as bacteria.

capacity factor, the ratio of the elution volume of a substance to the void volume in the column.

Capastat, a trademark for an antibiotic (capreomycin).

capeline bandage /kap′əlin/, a caplike covering used for protecting the head, shoulder, or a stump. Also called **Hippocrates' bandage.**

capillaritis, an abnormal condition characterized by a progressive pigmentary disorder of the skin without inflammation but with dilatation. It does not involve any systemic problems and runs a benign self-limiting course.

capillarity. See **capillary action.**

capillary /kap′iler′ē/, one of the tiny blood vessels (about 0.008 mm in diameter) joining arterioles and venules. Through their walls, which consist of a single layer of endothelial cells, blood and tissue cells exchange various substances.

capillary action, the action involving molecular adhesion by which the surface of a liquid in a tube is either elevated or depressed, depending on the cohesiveness of the liquid molecules. The more cohesive the molecules the more elevated will be the surface of the liquid. Less cohesive liquid molecules will adhere to the surfaces of the tube in which they are contained and depress the surface of the liquid. Also called **capillarity.**

capillary angioma. See **cherry angioma.**

capillary bed, a capillary network.

capillary flames. See **telangiectatic nevus.**

capillary fracture, any thin hairlike fracture.

capillary hemangioma, a blood-filled birthmark or benign tumor consisting of closely packed, small blood vessels. Commonly found in infants, it first grows, then spontaneously disappears in early childhood without treatment. Surgical removal will not usually be attempted unless frequent trauma and bleeding are present. Also called **hemangioma simplex, port-wine stain, strawberry hemangioma, strawberry mark, nevus vascularis.** Compare **cavernous hemangioma, nevus flammeus.**

capillary pulse. See **Quincke's pulse.**

capillovenous, of or pertaining to the venous capillaries.

capillus /kəpil′əs/, *pl.* **capilli,** one of the hairs of the body, especially one of the hairs of the scalp.

capit-, a combining form meaning 'pertaining to the head': *capitate, capitopedal, capitular.*

capitate, having the shape of a head.

capitate bone, one of the largest carpal bones, located at the center of the wrist and presenting a rounded head that fits the concavity of the scaphoid and the lunate bones. Various ligaments are attached to the rough dorsal and palmar surfaces. The capitate articulates with the scaphoid and lunate proximally, the second, third, and fourth metacarpals distally, the trapezoid on the radial side, and the hamate on the ulnar side. Also called **os capitatum, os magnum.**

capitulum /kəpich′ələm/, *pl.* **capitula,** a small, rounded prominence on a bone where it articulates with another bone.

capitulum humeri /hyo͞o′mərī, ho͞o′mərē/, a rounded eminence at the distal end of the humerus. It articulates with the radius.

-capnia, a combining form meaning '(condition of) carbon dioxide content in the blood': *acapnia, eucapnia, hypocapnia.*

capnograph /kap′nəgraf′/, an instrument used in anesthesia, respiratory physiology, and respiratory therapy to produce a tracing, or capnogram, which shows the proportion of carbon dioxide in expired air.

Capoten, a trademark for an angiotensin-converting enzyme (captopril).

capreomycin /kap′rē·ōmī′sin/, an antibiotic.

■ INDICATIONS: It is prescribed in the treatment of pulmonary infections caused by capreomycin-susceptible strains of *Mycobacterium tuberculosis* when the primary agents are ineffective or cannot be used.

■ CONTRAINDICATIONS: Known sensitivity to this drug prohibits its use. It must be used with caution in patients with preexisting renal or auditory impairment.

■ ADVERSE EFFECTS: Among the most serious adverse reactions are nephrotoxicity, hearing loss, tinnitus, vertigo, leukocytosis, leukopenia, urticaria, and skin rash.

capric acid /kap′rik/, a white, crystalline substance with a rancid odor, occurring as a glyceride in natural oils. Capric acid is used in the production of perfumes, flavors, wetting agents, and food additives. Also called **decanoic acid, decoic acid.**

caps-, kaps-, a combining form meaning 'capsule or container': *capsitis, capsulation, capsuloplasty.*

capsid /kap′sid/, the layer of protein enveloping a virion. A capsid is composed of structural units, called capsomeres, and its symmetry may be cubic or helical.

capsula. See **capsule.**

capsular swelling test. See **quellung reaction.**

capsule, 1. a small, soluble container, usually made of gelatin, used for enclosing a dose of medication for swallowing. Compare **tablet. 2.** a membranous shell surrounding certain microorganisms, as the pneumococcus bacterium. **3.** a well-defined anatomic structure that encloses an organ or part, as the capsule of the adrenal gland. Also called **capsula** (*pl.* **capsuli**).

capsulectomy /kap′səlek′təmē/, the surgical excision of a capsule, usually the capsule of a joint or the capsule of the lens of the eye.

capsule of Tenon. See **fascia bulbi.**

capsule of the kidney, the fatty enclosure of the kidney, consisting of adipose tissue continuous at the hilus with the fat of the renal sinus. This investment of perirenal fat covers the fibrous capsule and helps protect the organ from bumps and shocks. Compare **Bowman's capsule.**

capsule of the lens. See **lens capsule.**

capsuloma /kap′səlō′mə/, *pl.* **capsulomas, capsulomata,** a neoplasm of the renal capsule or the subcapsular area.

capsulotomy /kap′səlot′əmē/, an incision into the capsule of the eye, as in an operation to remove a cataract.

captain-of-the-ship doctrine, the medicolegal principle that the physician is ultimately responsible for all patient-care activities and thus may be held accountable and may be sued for negligence or malpractice when the act at issue is performed by an employee or other person under the physician's control, even if not ordered by the physician.

captopril, an angiotensin-converting enzyme inhibitor.

■ INDICATION: It is prescribed for the treatment of severe hypertension.

■ CONTRAINDICATION: Known sensitivity to this drug prohibits its use.

■ ADVERSE EFFECTS: Among the most serious adverse reactions are proteinurea, renal failure, neutropenia, agranulocytosis, angioneurotic edema, hypotension, angina, myocardial infarction, Raynaud's disease, congestive heart failure.

caput /kā′pət, kap′ət/, *pl.* **capita** /cap′itə/, **1.** the head. **2.** the enlarged or prominent extremity of an organ or part. Kinds of capita include **caput costae, caput epididymis, caput femoris, caput fibulae, caput humeri, caput mallei, caput mandibulae, caput ossis metacarpalis, caput phalangis, caput radii, caput stapedis,** and **caput succedaneum.**

caput costae, the head of a rib; it articulates with a vertebral body.

caput epididymidis, the head of the epididymis.

caput femoris, the head of the femur; it fits into the acetabulum.

caput fibulae, the head of the fibula; it articulates with the lateral condyle of the tibia.

caput humeri, the head of the humerus; it fits into the glenoid cavity of the scapula.

caput mallei, the head of the malleus.

caput mandibulae, the articular process of the ramus of the mandible.

caput ossis metacarpalis, the metacarpal head; it articulates with the proximal phalanx of the same digit.

caput phalangis, the articular head at the distal end of the proximal and middle phalanges.

caput radii, the head of the radius; it articulates with the capitulum of the humerus.

caput stapedis, the head of the stapes.

caput succedaneum, a localized pitting edema in the scalp of a fetus that may overlie sutures of the skull. It is usually formed during labor as a result of the circular pressure of the cervix on the fetal occiput. On vaginal examination the swelling may be mistaken for unruptured membranes. If the caput enlarges appreciably during labor, it may give an erroneous impression of fetal descent on successive examinations. At birth the baby's head may appear markedly deformed, but the swelling begins to resolve immediately and is usually gone in a few days. Compare **cephalhematoma, molding.**

caramiphen edisylate, an antitussive.

■ INDICATION: It is prescribed in the treatment of coughs.

■ CONTRAINDICATION: Known sensitivity to this drug prohibits its use.

■ ADVERSE EFFECTS: Among the most serious adverse reactions are dizziness, GI upset, nausea, and drowsiness.

carapace /kar′əpās/, a horny shield or shell covering the dorsal surface of an animal, as a turtle.

carate. See **pinta.**

carbachol /kär′bəkôl/, a parasympathomimetic agent.

■ INDICATIONS: It is prescribed in the treatment of glaucoma, for use in ocular surgery, and to oppose the action of cycloplegic and mydriatic medication.

■ CONTRAINDICATIONS: Corneal abrasion, acute iritis, or known hypersensitivity to this drug prohibits its use.

■ ADVERSE EFFECTS: Among the more serious adverse reactions are accommodative spasm and conjunctival hyperemia.

carbamate kinase, a liver enzyme that catalyzes the transfer of a phosphate group from adenosine triphosphate, associated with ammonia and carbon dioxide, to form adenosine diphosphate and carbamoylphosphate.

carbamazepine /kär′bəmaz′əpin/, an analgesic and anticonvulsant.

■ INDICATIONS: It is prescribed in the treatment of trigeminal neuralgia and certain seizure disorders.

■ CONTRAINDICATIONS: Concomitant use of monoamine oxidase inhibitors, a history of bone marrow depression, or known hypersensitivity to this drug or to any of the tricyclic antidepressants prohibits its use.

■ ADVERSE EFFECTS: Among the more serious adverse reactions are life-threatening blood dyscrasias, drowsiness, dizziness, ataxia, and nausea. Dermatologic and hypersensitivity reactions may occur.

carbamide peroxide, a topical antiinfective and cerumenolytic.

■ INDICATIONS: It is prescribed in the treatment of canker sores and other minor inflammatory conditions of the gums and mouth and to soften impacted earwax.

■ CONTRAINDICATION: Perforated eardrum prohibits its use.

■ ADVERSE EFFECTS: The most serious adverse reaction is local irritation.

carbenicillin disodium /kär′bənəsil′in/, a semisynthetic penicillin antibiotic.

■ INDICATIONS: It is prescribed in the treatment of certain infections.

■ CONTRAINDICATIONS: Known hypersensitivity to this drug or to other penicillins prohibits its use.

■ ADVERSE EFFECTS: Among the more serious adverse effects are hypersensitivity reactions, neurologic disturbances, and clotting defects. The high sodium content (5.5-6.5 mEq/g) may aggravate fluid and electrolyte imbalance in people affected with kidney, heart, or liver disease.

carbidopa, a decarboxylase inhibitor.

■ INDICATION: It is prescribed in combination with levodopa in the treatment of idiopathic Parkinson's disease.

■ CONTRAINDICATIONS: Glaucoma, hypertension, the use of a monoamine oxidase inhibitor within the past 14 days, or known hypersensitivity to this drug prohibits its use.

■ ADVERSE EFFECTS: Among the most serious adverse reactions are GI bleeding, cardiac irregularity, hemolytic anemia, tardive dyskinesia, mental depression, blurred vision, and activation of malignant melanoma.

carbinoxamine maleate /kär′bənok′səmēn/, an antihistamine.

■ INDICATIONS: It is prescribed in the treatment of a variety of hypersensitivity reactions, including rhinitis, skin reactions, and itching.

■ CONTRAINDICATIONS: Asthma or known hypersensitivity to this drug prohibits its use. It should not be administered to newborn infants or lactating mothers.

■ ADVERSE EFFECTS: Among the more serious adverse reactions are tachycardia and other side effects of anticholinergic medications. Drowsiness, skin rash, hypersensitivity reactions, and dry mouth commonly occur.

carbo-, carbon-, a combining form meaning 'carbon, charcoal': *carbonate, carboneol, carbonometry*.

Carbocaine Hydrochloride, a trademark for a local anesthetic (mepivacaine hydrochloride).

carbocyclic. See **closed-chain.**

carbohydrate, any of a group of organic compounds, the most important being sugar, starch, cellulose, and gum. They are classified according to molecular structure as mono-, di-, tri-, poly-, and heterosaccharides. Carbohydrates constitute the main source of energy for all body functions and are necessary for the metabolism of other nutrients. They are synthesized by all green plants and in the body are either absorbed immediately or stored in the form of glycogen. Cereals, vegetables, fruits, rice, potatoes, legumes, and flour products are the major sources of carbohydrates. They can also be manufactured in the body from some amino acids and the glycerol component of fats. Symptoms of deficiency include fatigue, depression, breakdown of essential body protein, and electrolyte imbalance. Excessive consumption of carbohydrates is associated with tooth decay, obesity, diabetes mellitus, and cardiovascular disease.

carbohydrate metabolism, the sum of the anabolic and catabolic processes of the body involved in the synthesis and breakdown of carbohydrates, principally galactose, fructose, and glucose. Some of the processes are glycogenesis, glyconeogenesis, and glycolysis. Energy-rich phosphate bonds are produced in many metabolic reactions requiring carbohydrates.

carbolated camphor, a mixture of 1.5 parts camphor with 1 part each of alcohol and phenol, used as an antiseptic dressing for wounds.

carbol-fuchsin solution /kär′bolfo͝ok′sin/, a preparation used in the treatment of superficial fungal infections. It contains boric acid, phenol, resorcinol, fuchsin, acetone, and alcohol in water. Also called **Castellani's paint.**

carbol-fuchsin stain, a solution of dilute phenol and basic fuchsin used on microorganisms and cell nuclei for microscopic examination. Also called **Ziehl's stain.**

carbolic acid /kärbol′ik/, a poisonous, colorless to pale pink crystalline compound obtained from coal tar distillation and converted to a clear liquid with a strong odor and burning taste by the addition of 10% water. Low concentrations of carbolic acid are used in antiseptic preparations. Also called **hydroxybenzene, oxybenzene, phenic acid, phenol, phenylic acid, phenylic alcohol.**

carbolic acid poisoning. See **phenol poisoning.**

carbon (C), a nonmetallic, chiefly tetravalent element. Its atomic number is 6; its atomic weight is 12.011. Carbon occurs in pure form in diamond and graphite and is a component of all living tissue. Most of the study of organic chemistry focuses on the vast number of carbon compounds. Carbon occurs in impure form in charcoal, coke, and soot, and in the atmosphere as carbon dioxide. Carbon is essential to the chemistry of the body, participating in many metabolic processes and acting as a component of carbohydrates, amino acids, triglycerides, deoxyribonucleic and ribonucleic acids, and many other compounds. Carbon dioxide produced in glycolysis is important in the acid-base balance of the body and in controlling respiration. Carbon is a component of carbon monoxide, which can be lethal if inhaled, and of many hydrocarbons, the fumes of which can cause death from respiratory failure. Brief incidental exposures to low concentrations of solvent vapors that contain carbon, as gasoline, lighter fluids, aerosol sprays, and spot removers, may be relatively harmless, but exposures to concentrations of hydrocarbon vapors often found in the home and in manufacturing environments may be dangerous. Many occupational pulmonary diseases, as coal worker's pneumoconiosis, black lung disease, and byssinosis, are caused by chronic inhalation of dusts containing carbon compounds. See also **carbon 11, carbon 14.**

carbon-. See **carbo-.**

carbon 11, a radioisotope of carbon with a half-life of 20 minutes. It is produced by a cyclotron and emits positrons. Compare **carbon 14.**

carbon 14, a beta-emitter with a half-life of 5760 years. It occurs naturally, arising from cosmic rays, and is used as a tracer in studying various aspects of metabolism and in dating relics that contain natural carbonaceous materials. Compare **carbon 11.**

carbon arc lamp, an electric lamp producing a strong white light of adjustable intensity from an arc of current between carbon electrodes.

carbon cycle, the steps by which carbon in the form of carbon dioxide is extracted from and returned to the atmosphere by living organisms, especially human beings. The process starts with the photosynthetic production of carbohydrates by plants, progresses through the consumption of carbohydrates by animals and human beings, and ends with the exhalation of carbon dioxide by those same animals and human beings, and also with the release of carbon dioxide during the decomposition of dead plants and animals. Various chemical processes intervene between the ingestion of carbohydrates and the release of carbon dioxide. Carbohydrate metabolism starts with the movement of glucose through cell membranes and subsequently involves glycolysis, the processes of the citric acid cycle, electron transport, and oxidative phosphorylation. See also **Krebs' citric acid cycle.**

carbon damp. See **damp.**

carbon dioxide (CO_2), a colorless, odorless gas produced by the oxidation of carbon. Carbon dioxide, as a product of cell respiration, is carried by the blood to the lungs and is exhaled. The acid-base balance of body fluids and tissues is affected by the level of carbon dioxide and its carbonate compounds. Solid carbon dioxide (dry ice) is used in the treatment of some skin conditions.

carbon dioxide bath, a bath taken in water that is saturated with carbon dioxide. See also **Nauheim bath.**

carbon dioxide tension, the partial pressure of carbon dioxide gas, expressed as $Paco_2$, which is proportional to its percentage in the blood or lungs. It is expressed quantitatively in millimeters of mercury. Alveolar $Paco_2$ directly reflects adequate pulmonary gas exchange in relation to blood flow. A high rate of ventilation causes a lower alveolar $Paco_2$, a lower rate of breathing leads to higher amounts of alveolar and blood carbon dioxide. The $Paco_2$ is measured by glass electrodes in samples of arterial blood. Normal values for arterial and alveolar carbon dioxide tension are between 37 and 43 mm Hg. Higher levels occur in conditions of slow blood flow or increased metabolic rate. Below normal values are caused by hyperventilation, respiratory alkalosis, or rapid rates of blood flow. See also **carbon dioxide, hypercapnia, hyperventilation, hypoventilation.**

carbonic anhydrase, an enzyme that catalyzes the union of carbon dioxide and water to form carbonic acid. It also reverses the action.

carbon monoxide, a colorless, odorless, poisonous gas produced by the combustion of carbon or organic fuels in a limited oxygen supply, as in the cylinders of an internal combustion engine. Carbon monoxide combines irreversibly with hemoglobin, preventing the formation of oxyhemoglobin and reducing the oxygen supply to the tissues. Prolonged exposure to high levels of carbon monoxide results in asphyxiation.

carbon monoxide poisoning, a toxic condition in which carbon monoxide gas has been inhaled and absorbed by erythrocytes in the pulmonary circulation, displacing oxygen from the red blood cells and decreasing the capacity of the blood to carry oxygen to the cells of the body. Characteristically, headache, dyspnea, drowsiness, confusion, cherry-pink skin, unconsciousness, and apnea occur in sequence as the level of carbon monoxide in the blood increases. The most common source of carbon monoxide in cases of poisoning is exhaust fumes from an automobile. Treatment includes removal of the victim from the toxic environment, resuscitation, and administration of oxygen.

carbon tetrachloride, a colorless, volatile, toxic liquid used as a solvent and in fire extinguishers. Ingestion of the liquid or inhalation of the fumes usually results in headaches, nausea, depression, abdominal pain, and convulsions. In poisoning by inhalation, ventilatory assistance and oxygen may be necessary. In poisoning by ingestion, removal of the poison and gastric lavage are the usual treatments. Carbon tetrachloride is particularly toxic to the kidneys and liver; permanent damage to these organs may result.

carboprost tromethamine, an oxytocic prostaglandin.

■ INDICATION: It is prescribed to induce abortion during the second trimester.

■ CONTRAINDICATIONS: Acute pelvic inflammatory disease and known hypersensitivity to this drug prohibits its use. It should be used with caution in patients who have cardiac, pulmonary, hepatic, or renal disease, asthma, jaundice, diabetes, or epilepsy, and in those who have had uterine surgery.

■ ADVERSE EFFECTS: Among the more serious adverse reactions are fever, vomiting, and diarrhea. Cervical trauma may occur.

carboxyhemoglobin /kärbok′sēhē′məglō′bin, -hem′-/, a compound produced by the exposure of hemoglobin to carbon monoxide. Carbon monoxide from the environment is inhaled into the lungs, absorbed through the alveoli, and bound to hemoglobin in the blood, blocking the sites for oxygen transport. Oxygen levels decrease, and, when the decrease is excessive, hypoxia and anoxia result. See also **carbon monoxide poisoning, oxyhemoglobin.**

carboxyl /kärbok′sil/, a monovalent radical COOH characteristic of organic acids. The hydrogen of the radical can be replaced by metals to form salts.

carbuncle /kär′bungkəl/, a large staphylococcal infection containing purulent matter in deep, interconnecting, subcutaneous pockets. Eventually pus discharges to the skin surface through openings. Common sites for carbuncles are the back of the neck and the buttocks. Diabetes mellitus and hypogammaglobulinemia may be associated diseases. Treatment may include the use of antibiotics, hot compresses, and surgical drainage. Compare **furuncle.**

carbunculosis, an abnormal condition characterized by a cluster of deep painful abscesses that drain through multiple openings onto the skin surface, usually around hair follicles. Carbunculosis is a form of folliculitis, most commonly caused by the coagulase-positive *Staphylococcus aureus*. The lesions caused by this condition may result in fever and malaise.

■ OBSERVATIONS: Carbunculosis commonly follows persistent *S. aureus* infection and furunculosis. Diagnosis is based on obvious skin lesions, a patient history of previous furunculosis, and *S. aureus* in wound culture.

■ INTERVENTION: Treatment of carbunculosis requires the administration of systemic antibiotics. The prognosis depends on the severity of the infection and the physical condition of the patient.

■ NURSING CONSIDERATIONS: Nursing care for this disorder is mainly supportive and educative to impress the patient with the importance of meticulous personal and family hygiene. The nurse explains that reducing the intake of sugars and fats is important and cautions the patient never to squeeze a carbuncle or furuncle because it may rupture into the surrounding area. The patient is also instructed not to share towels and washcloths with other family members because this may spread the bacteria. Also stressed is the importance of boiling towels and washcloths before reusing them and the need for daily changes of boiled clothes and bedsheets. The patient is additionally encouraged to change dressings frequently and to discard them in paper bags. Because carbunculosis often follows furunculosis, a disorder associated with diabetes, the patient should have a thorough physical examination.

carcin-, a combining form meaning 'pertaining to cancer': *carcinelcosis, carcinogen, carcinolytic*.

carcinectomy /kär′sinek′təmē/, the excision of a cancer.

carcinoembryonic antigen (CEA), an antigen present in very small quantities in adult tissue. A greater than normal amount is suggestive of cancer. Tests for its presence aid in screening, in evaluating recurrent or disseminated disease, and in gauging the success of surgical ablation of malignant tumors.

carcinogen /kärsin′əjin/, a substance or agent that causes the development or increases the incidence of cancer.

carcinogenesis /kär′sinəjen′əsis/, the process of initiating and promoting cancer. Compare **oncogenesis, sarcomagenesis, tumorigenesis.**

carcinogenic /kär′sinəjen′ik/, of or pertaining to the ability to cause the development of a cancer. Also called **cancerigenic, cancerogenic.**

carcinoid /kär′sinoid/, a small yellow tumor derived from argentaffin cells in the GI mucosa that secrete serotonin, other catecholamines, and similar compounds. Carcinoid tumors spread slowly locally but may later metastasize widely. Their secretions often cause systemic symptoms. Also called **argentaffinoma, Kulchitsky-cell carcinoma.** See also **argentaffin cell, carcinoid syndrome.**

carcinoid syndrome, the systemic effects of serotonin-secreting carcinoid tumors manifested by flushing, diarrhea, cramps, skin lesions resembling pellagra, labored breathing, palpitations, and valvular heart disease, especially of the pulmonary valve. Treatment includes surgical excision of the tumor, if feasible, administration of alpha-adrenergic blocking agents to produce vasodilatation, and medication to counteract bronchospasm. Also called **argentaffinoma syndrome.** See also **carcinoid.**

carcinolysis /kär′sinol′isis/, the destruction of cancer cells, as by the action of an antineoplastic drug. **–carcinolytic,** *adj.*

carcinoma /kär′sinō′mə/, *pl.* **carcinomas, carcinomata,** a malignant epithelial neoplasm that tends to invade surrounding tissue and to metastasize to distant regions of the body. It develops most frequently in the skin, large intestine, lungs, stomach, prostate gland, cervix, or breast. The tumor is characteristically firm, irregular, and nodular, with a well-defined border in some places. It usually cannot be clearly dissected and excised without removing normal surrounding tissue. Macroscopically, it is whitish with diffuse, dark hemorrhagic patches, and it has yellow areas of necrosis in the center. Microscopically, the tumor cells are characterized by anaplasia, abnormal size and shape, disproportionately large nuclei, and clumps of nuclear chromatin. **–carcinomatous,** *adj.*

-carcinoma, a combining form meaning a 'malignant tumor composed of epithelial cells, with a tendency to metastasize': *ophthalmocarcinoma, osteocarcinoma, phlebocarcinoma.*

carcinoma basocellulare. See **basal cell carcinoma.**

carcinoma cutaneum. See **basal cell carcinoma, squamous carcinoma.**

carcinoma en cuirasse /äN′kēräs′/, a rare neoplasm accompanying advanced breast cancer and characterized by progressive extensive fibrosis and rigidity of the skin of the chest, neck, back, and, occasionally, abdomen. Another type, an extraperitoneal extension of gelatinous carcinoma of the rectum, encases the abdominal cavity in a rigid shell.

carcinoma fibrosum. See **scirrhous carcinoma.**

carcinoma gigantocellulare. See **giant cell carcinoma.**

carcinoma in situ, a premalignant neoplasm that has not invaded the basement membrane but shows cytologic characteristics of invasive cancer. Such neoplastic changes in stratified squamous or glandular epithelium are frequently seen on the uterine cervix and also occur in the anus, bronchi, buccal mucosa, esophagus, eye, lip, penis, uterine endometrium, vagina, and lesions of senile keratosis. Cervical carcinoma in situ is treated successfully by various methods, including cryosurgery, electrocautery, and simple hysterectomy. Lesions of this kind in pregnant women sometimes regress in the months after delivery. Also called **cancer in situ, intraepithelial carcinoma, preinvasive carcinoma.** See also **erythroplasia of Queyrat.**

carcinoma lenticulare /len′ticŏŏlär′ə/, a form of carcinoma tuberosum or scirrhous skin cancer characterized by the development of many small, relatively flat nodules that often coalesce to form larger areas resembling a fungous infection.

carcinoma medullare, carcinoma molle. See **medullary carcinoma.**

carcinoma mucocellulare. See **Krukenberg's tumor.**

carcinoma scroti, an epithelial cell carcinoma of the scrotum.

carcinoma simplex, an undifferentiated epithelial tumor in which the stroma and neoplastic epithelial cells do not have a definite microscopic pattern.

carcinoma spongiosum, a carcinoma that is soft and spongy with small and large cavities in it. See also **medullary carcinoma.**

carcinoma telangiectaticum, a neoplasm of the capillaries of the skin causing dilatation of the vessels and red spots on the skin that blanch with pressure.

carcinomatoid /kär′sinō′mətoid/, resembling a carcinoma.

carcinomatosis, an abnormal condition characterized by the extensive spread of carcinoma throughout the body.

carcinomatous, pertaining to carcinoma. Also **carcinous.**

carcinoma tuberosum. See **tuberous carcinoma.**

carcinoma villosum. See **villous carcinoma.**

carcinomectomy. See **carcinectomy.**

carcinophilia /kär′sinōfil′yə/, the property in which there is an affinity for carcinomatous tissue. **–carcinophilic,** *adj.*

carcinosarcoma /kär′sinōsärkō′mə/, *pl.* **carcinosarcomas, carsinosarcomata,** a malignant neoplasm composed of carcinomatous and sarcomatous cells. Tumors of this type may occur in the esophagus, thyroid gland, and uterus.

carcinosis /kär′sinō′sis/, *pl.* **carcinoses,** a condition characterized by the development of many carcinomas throughout the body. Kinds of carcinoses are **carcinosis pleurae, miliary carcinosis, pulmonary carcinosis.** Also called **carcinomatosis.**

carcinosis pleurae /plo͞o′rē/, a secondary malignancy of the pleura in which nodules develop throughout the membranes.

carcinostatic /kär′sinōstat′ik/, of or pertaining to the tendency to slow or halt the growth of a carcinoma.

carcinous /kär′sinəs/, carcinomatous.

card-, cardio-, a combining form meaning 'heart': *cardioclasis, cardiography, cardiomegaly.*

cardia, **1.** the opening between the esophagus and the cardiac portion of the stomach. **2.** the portion of the stomach surrounding the esophagogastric connection, characterized by the absence of acid cells. **3.** an obsolete term formerly and vaguely used to describe the heart and the region around the heart. **–cardiac,** *adj.*

cardia-. See **cardio-.**

-cardia, a combining form meaning a 'type of heart action or location': *araiocardia, brachycardia, miocardia.*

cardiac, **1.** of or pertaining to the heart. **2.** pertaining to a person with heart disease. **3.** of or pertaining to the proximal part of the stomach.

-cardiac, **1.** a combining form meaning 'to characterize types and locations of heart ailments': *gravidocardiac, intracardiac, precardiac.* **2.** a combining form meaning 'to identify heart ailment patients': *diplocardiac, hemicardiac, phrenopericardiac.*

cardiac aneurysm. See **ventricular aneurysm.**

cardiac apnea, abnormal, temporary absence of respiration, as in Cheynes-Stokes respiration.

cardiac arrest, a sudden cessation of cardiac output and effective circulation, usually precipitated by ventricular fibrillation and, in some instances, by ventricular asystole. When cardiac arrest occurs, delivery of oxygen and removal of carbon dioxide stop, tissue cell metabolism becomes anaerobic, and metabolic and repiratory acidosis ensue. Immediate initiation of cardiopulmonary resuscitation is required to prevent heart, lung, kidney, and brain damage. Also called **cardiopulmonary arrest.** See also **cardiac standstill, cardiopulmonary resuscitation.**

cardiac arrhythmia, an abnormal rate or rhythm of atrial or ventricular myocardial contraction. The condition may be caused by a defect in the ability of the sinoatrial node to maintain its pacemaker function, or by a failure of the bundle of His, the bundle branches, or the Purkinje network to conduct the contractile impulse. Increased metabolic demand, as in exercise or fever, or altered metabolic function, as in acidosis, alkalosis, hypokalemia, or hypocalcemia, results in an arrhythmia if the capacity of the heart to adjust to the particular stress is exceeded. Kinds of arrhythmia include **bradycardia, extrasystole, heart block, premature atrial contraction, premature ventricular contraction, tachycardia.** (Table, pages 186-188)

cardiac asthma, an attack of asthma associated with heart disease, as ventricular failure, and characterized by predominant pulmonary congestion with some bronchoconstriction.

cardiac catheter, a long, fine catheter designed to be passed into the heart through a blood vessel. Used for diagnosis, it allows the determination of blood pressure and the rate of flow in the vessels and chambers of the heart and the identification of abnormal anatomy. Medication may be instilled directly into a coronary vessel, often with visualization by tomography.

cardiac catheterization, a diagnostic procedure in which a catheter is introduced into a large vein or artery, usually of an arm or a leg, and threaded through the circulatory system to the heart.

■ METHOD: A sterile radiopaque catheter 100 to 125 cm in length is passed through an incision into the vein, through the vein to the superior vena cava, and into the right atrium (or through an artery leading to the left ventricle) and other structures to be studied. The course of the catheter is followed with fluoroscopy, and radiographs may be taken. An electrocardiogram is monitored on an oscilloscope. As the catheter tip passes through the chambers and vessels of the heart, the pressure of the flow of blood is monitored, and samples of the blood are taken to study the oxygen content.

■ NURSING ORDERS: Cardiac catheterization takes from 1 to 3 hours, and the patient has to lie still during the entire procedure. It is not painful, but, because it is anxiety producing, the patient needs explanation and emotional support. A young child may need a sedative in order to lie still. An antiobiotic is often given the day before. The pulse on the operative side and the blood pressure on the other side of the body are monitored every 15 minutes for 1 hour and every half hour thereafter. In left heart catheterization, peripheral pulses are also monitored. The temperature may be elevated for several hours, and there may be pain at the site of the incision. The nurse observes the site for bleeding and for signs of infection, thrombophlebitis, and cardiac arrhythmia. Cardiac catheterization is often performed by a special team in a special laboratory. By offering information and counseling, a member of the team may be of great help to the patient and the nursing staff before and after the procedure.

■ OUTCOME CRITERIA: Many conditions may be accurately identified and assessed using cardiac catheterization, including congenital heart disease, tricuspid stenosis, and valvular incompetence. Among the risks of the procedure are local infection, cardiac arrhythmia, and thrombophlebitis.

cardiac compression. See **cardiac tamponade.**

cardiac conduction defect, any impairment of the electrical pathways and the specialized muscular fibers that conduct action impulses to contract the atria and the ventricles. Conduction defects may develop in the sinus node, the atrioventricular node, the bundle of His, the left or the right fiber bundles, or the Purkinje fibers. Defective transmission of cardiac impulses along the conduction routes may be caused by ischemic coronary disease or by an occlusion, a lesion, or other pathologic factor. See also **heart block.**

cardiac cycle, the cycle of events during which an electrical impulse is conducted through special fibers over the muscle of the myocardium, from the sinoatrial (SA) node to the atrioventricular (AV) node, to the bundle of His and the bundle branches, and to the Purkinje fibers, causing contraction of the atria followed by contraction of the ventricles. Contraction occurs with depolarization of the muscle fibers; recovery requires repolarization. Deoxygenated blood enters the right atrium of the heart from the superior vena cava and is pumped through the tricuspid valve into the right ventricle. With ventricular contraction, the blood is pumped through the pulmonary valve into the pulmonary artery and the lungs for oxygenation. Oxygen-rich blood is returned to the heart through the branches of the pulmonary veins to the left atrium and is then passed through the mitral valve into the left ventricle. With ventricular contraction, the blood is pumped through the aortic semilunar valve into the aorta for peripheral circulation. The contractions of the left and the right atria are nearly simultaneous; they precede the nearly simultaneous contractions of the ventricles. The atria begin to repolarize during ventricular depolarization. On electrocardiogram the cycle is shown as a series of waves, called P, Q, R, S, and T waves, that includes the QRS complex and two segments that connect the waves, the PR segment and the ST segment. Structural, chemical, or electric abnormalities may cause a large variety of anomalies in electric conduction, muscular contraction, and blood flow in the heart. The ECG may reflect these abnormalities by changes in the shape and duration of the waves and segments of the ECG that represent phases of the cardiac cycle. See also specific waves and specific segments.

cardiac failure. See **heart failure.**

cardiac impulse, the movement of the thorax, caused by the beating of the heart. It is readily palpable and easily recorded.

cardiac index, a measure of the cardiac output of a patient per square meter of body surface area. It is obtained by dividing the cardiac output in liters per minute by the body surface area.

Comparison of basic cardiac arrhythmias

Arrhythmia	*Description*	*Etiology*	*Symptoms/consequences*	*Treatment*
Sinus tachycardia	P waves present followed by QRS Rhythm regular Heart rate 100 to 150	Increased metabolic demands Decreased oxygen delivery; CHF, shock, hemorrhage, anemia	May produce palpitations Prolonged episodes may lead to decreased cardiac output	None Treat underlying cause Occasionally sedatives

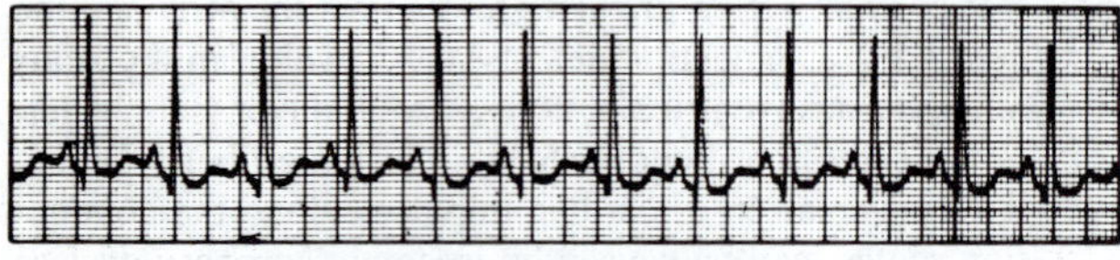

Rate of sinus node is 110; conduction is normal

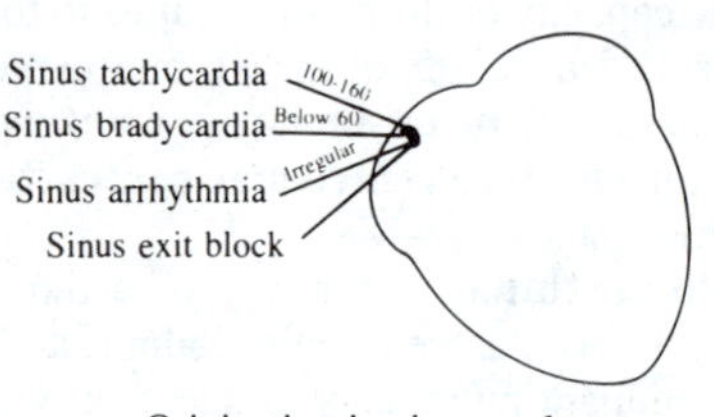

Originating in sinus node

Arrhythmia	*Description*	*Etiology*	*Symptoms/consequences*	*Treatment*
Sinus bradycardia	P waves present Rhythm regular Heart rate less than 60	Physical fitness Parasympathetic stimulation Sleep Increased intracranial pressure Digitalis excess	Very low rates may cause decreased cardiac output; light-headedness, faintness, chest pain	None or atropine if cardiac output is decreased Pacemaker

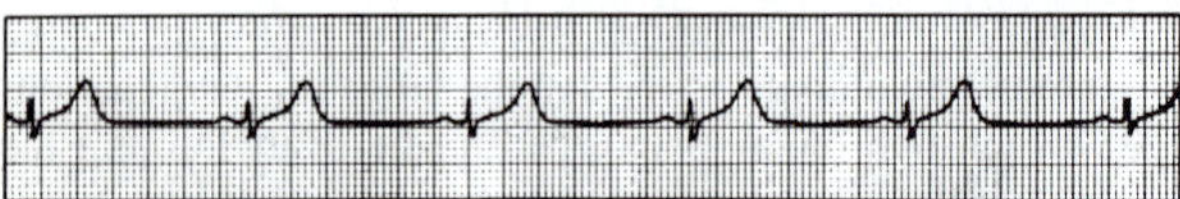

Rate is 48; Rhythm is regular and conduction is normal

Arrhythmia	*Description*	*Etiology*	*Symptoms/consequences*	*Treatment*
Complete heart block	No conduction in presence of slow ventricular rhythm and plentiful P waves P waves have no relation to QRS Heart rate approx. 20 to 45	Digitalis toxicity Infectious disease Coronary artery disease Myocardial infarction	Very low rates may cause decreased cardiac output; light-headedness, faintness, chest pain	Depends on clinical setting Pacemaker Isoproterenol to increase heart rate

II

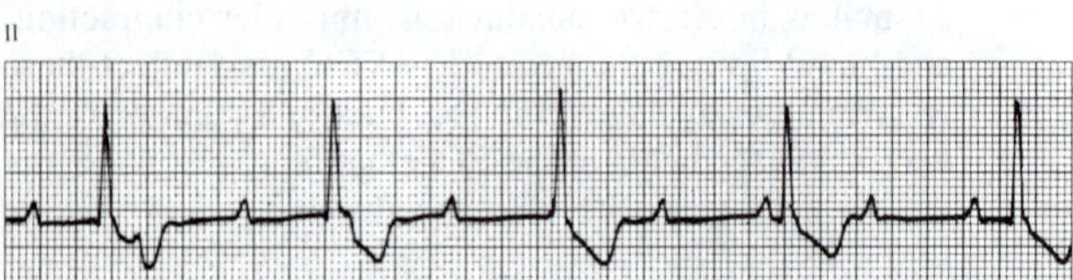

P waves are clearly seen and occur regularly at rate of 72. Ventricles are beating independently under control of junctional pacemaker rate of 46

Arrhythmia	Description	Etiology	Symptoms/consequences	Treatment
Atrial fibrillation	Rapid, irregular atrial waves Ventricular rhythm irregularly irregular Heart rate varies, may be increased to 150 to 170/min	Rheumatic heart disease Mitral and tricuspid valvular disease Atrial infarction	Pulse deficit Decreased cardiac output if rate is rapid Promotes thrombus formation in atria	Verapamil Digitalis Quinidine Cardioversion

Disorganized electrical activity

Atrial fibrillation with controlled ventricular response and coarse fibrillatory line

Arrhythmia	Description	Etiology	Symptoms/consequences	Treatment
Premature atrial beats	Early P wave followed by normal QRS Rhythm irregular	Stress, ischemia, atrial enlargement, caffeine, nicotine Chronic rheumatic valvular disease Electrolyte imbalance Hypoxia Digitalis toxicity Thyrotoxicosis Anxiety	May produce palpitations Frequent episodes may decrease cardiac output Is sign of chamber irritability	Potassium Magnesium Oxygen Reassurance Sedation Quinidine

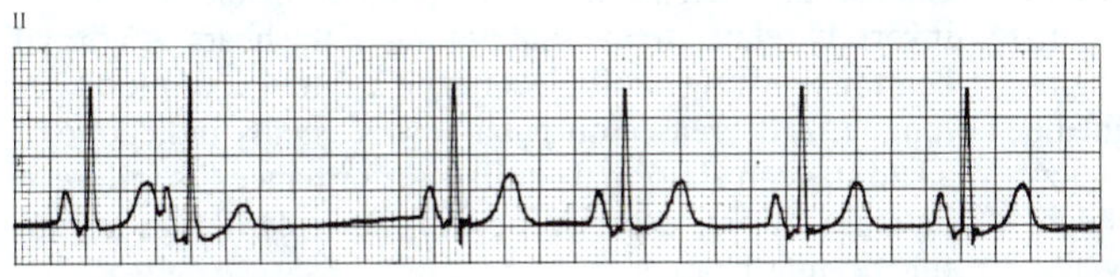

Atrial premature beats

Arrhythmia	Description	Etiology	Symptoms/consequences	Treatment
Premature ventricular beats	Early wide bizarre QRS, not associated with a P wave Rhythm irregular	Cardiac disease Myocardial infarction Stress May be benign Electrolyte imbalance Drug toxicity (digitalis, quinidine) Hypoxemia, hypercapnia	Same as premature atrial beats (PAB)	Lidocaine Procainamide (Pronestyl) Oxygen Sodium bicarbonate Potassium Magnesium Treat CHF None

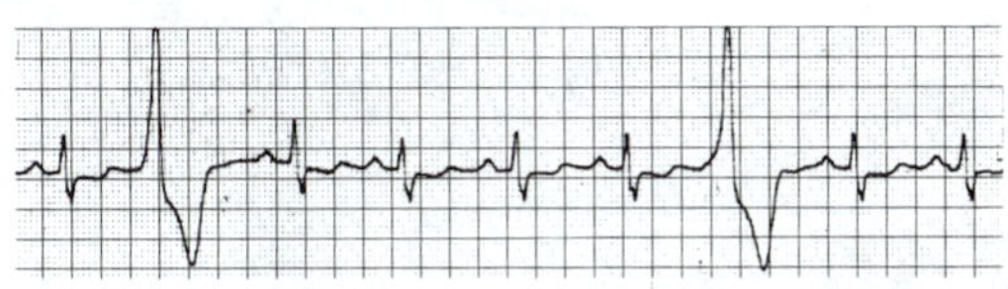

Ventricular premature beats

Continued.

cardiac insufficiency, the inability of the heart to perform its normal functions properly.

cardiac massage, repeated, rhythmic compression of the heart applied directly, during surgery, or through the intact chest wall in an effort to maintain circulation after cardiac arrest or ventricular fibrillation. Also called **heart massage.** See also **cardiopulmonary resuscitation.**

cardiac monitor, a device for the continuous observation of cardiac function. It may include electrocardiograph and oscilloscope readings, recording devices, and a visual or audible record of heart function and rhythm. An alarm system may be set to alert staff of variation from a certain rate.

cardiac monitoring, a continuous check on the functioning of the heart with an electronic instrument that provides an electrocardiographic reading on an oscilloscope. Each ventricular contraction of the heart is indicated by either a flashing light or an audible sound. The indicator is often integrated with an alarm system that is triggered by a pulse rate above or below predetermined limits. The procedure is performed most often in an intensive care unit, although devices are available for patients who are ambulatory. See also **electrocardiography.**

cardiac murmur, an abnormal sound heard during auscultory examination of the heart, caused by the flow of blood into a chamber or through a valve or by a valve opening or closing. A murmur is classified by the time of its occurence during the cardiac cycle, the duration, and the intensity of the sound on a scale of I to V. For example, a moderately loud murmur that begins at the beginning of systole and ends just as systole ends might be described as a grade III/V pansystolic murmur. Also noted is the part of the heart over which the murmur is heard and any parts to which it radiates. In general, many systolic murmurs are benign and of no significance, but some signal cardiac pathophysiology. Most diastolic murmurs are pathologic. Also called **heart murmur.**

cardiac muscle, a special striated muscle of the myocardium, containing dark intercalated disks at the junctions of abutting fibers. Cardiac muscle is an exception among involuntary muscles, which are characteristically smooth. Its contractile fibrillae resemble those of skeletal muscle but are only one third as large in diameter, are richer in sarcoplasm, and contain centrally located instead of peripheral nuclei. Studies with the electron microscope indicate that the intercalated disks in cardiac muscle represent cell boundaries. The connective tissue of cardiac muscle is sparser than that of skeletal muscle.

cardiac output, the volume of blood expelled by the ventricles of the heart, equal to the amount of blood ejected at each beat (the stroke output), multiplied by the number of beats in the period of time used in the computation. Cardiac output is commonly measured by the thermodilution technique in which a Swan-Ganz catheter with a thermistor electrode at the tip is inserted in the pulmonary artery, and a certain amount of a cold solution is injected through the lumen of the catheter into the right atrium. The thermistor determines the temperature of the solution when it reaches the pulmonary artery, and the output is calculated on the basis of the temperature change; the increase in the temperature of the solution is inversely related to the functioning of the heart. A normal heart in a resting adult ejects from 2.5 to 4 L of blood per minute. A decreased output at rest is usually indicative of a late stage in abnormal cardiac performance; its failure to increase during exercise occurs much earlier in a malfunctioning heart.

Comparison of basic cardiac arrhythmias—cont'd

Arrhythmia	*Description*	*Etiology*	*Symptoms/consequences*	*Treatment*
Ventricular fibrillation	Chaotic electric activity No recognizable QRS complex	Myocardial infarction Electrocution Freshwater drowning Drug toxicity	No cardiac output Absent pulse or respiration Cardiac arrest	Defibrillation Epinephrine Sodium bicarbonate
Ventricular standstill	Can only be distinguished from ventricular fibrillation by ECG P waves *may* be present No QRS "straight line"	Myocardial infarction Chronic diseases of conducting system	Same as ventricular fibrillation	CPR Pacemaker Intracardiac epinephrine

Chaotic ventricular activity is reflected in erratic ECG pattern

Disorganized electrical activity

cardiac output, alteration in: decreased, a nursing diagnosis accepted by the Fourth National Conference on the Classification of Nursing Diagnoses. The origin of the condition is to be developed at a later conference. The defining characteristics include variations in blood pressure, arrhythmias, fatigue, jugular vein distention, color changes of the skin and mucous membranes, oliguria, decreased peripheral pulses, cold and clammy skin, rales, dyspnea, orthopnea, and restlessness. Other characteristics that frequently occur are change in mental status, shortness of breath, syncope, vertigo, edema, cough, frothy sputum, cardiac gallop, and weakness. See also **nursing diagnosis.**

cardiac pacemaker. See **pacemaker.**

cardiac plexus, one of several nerve complexes situated close to the arch of the aorta. The cardiac plexuses contain sympathetic and parasympathetic nerve fibers that leave the plexuses, accompany the right and the left coronary arteries, and enter the heart. Some of the fibers from the plexuses terminate in the sinoatrial node; others terminate in the atrioventricular node and in the atrial myocardium.

cardiac radionuclide imaging, the noninvasive examination of the heart, using a radiopharmaceutic, as thallium 201, and a detection device, as a gamma camera, positron camera, or rectilinear scanner. The main clinical applications of cardiac radionuclide imaging are the gated cardiac blood pool scan, myocardial imaging, and the detection of myocardial necrosis.

cardiac reserve, the potential capacity of the heart to function well beyond its basal level, responding to the demands of various physiologic and psychologic changes.

cardiac resuscitation. See **cardiopulmonary resuscitation.**

cardiac sphincter, a ring of muscle fibers at the juncture of the esophagus and stomach.

cardiac standstill, the complete cessation of ventricular contractions and ejection of blood by the heart. Cardiac standstill requires immediate cardiopulmonary resuscitation, intravenous or intracardiac administration of epinephrine or isoproterenol, or stimulation of the heart with an electric current. It may be caused by severe generalized anoxia or local myocardial oxygen deficiency. See also **cardiac arrest.**

cardiac stimulant, a pharmacologic agent that increases the action of the heart. Cardiac glycosides, as digitalis, digitoxin, digoxin, deslanoside, lanatoside, acetyldigitoxin, and ouabain, increase the force of myocardial contractions and decrease the heart rate and conduction velocity, allowing more time for the ventricles to relax and become filled with blood. These glycosides, which are composed of a steroid nucleus, a lactone ring, and a sugar, are used in the treatment of congestive heart failure, atrial flutter and fibrillation, paroxysmal atrial tachycardia, and cardiogenic shock. Toxic signs and symptoms, resulting from an overdose or the cumulative effect of slowly eliminated digitalis preparations, include anorexia, nausea, vomiting, diarrhea, abdominal pain, headache, muscle weakness, confusion, drowsiness, irritability, visual disturbances, bradycardia or tachycardia, ectopic heart beats, bigeminy, and a pulse deficit. Epinephrine, a potent vasopressor and cardiac stimulant, is sometimes used to restore heart rhythm in cardiac arrest but is not employed in treating heart failure or cardiogenic shock. Isoproterenol hydrochloride, which is related to epinephrine, may be used in treating heart block. Dobutamine hydrochloride and dopamine are employed in the short-term treatment of cardiac decompensation resulting from depressed contractility.

cardiac tamponade, compression of the heart produced by the accumulation in the pericardial sac of fluid or of blood resulting from the rupture of a blood vessel of the myocardium, as by a penetrating wound. Also called **cardiac compression.**

■ OBSERVATIONS: Signs of cardiac tamponade may include distended neck veins, hypotension, decreased heart sounds, tachypnea, peripheral pulses that are weak or absent or that fall sharply during inspiration (pulsus paradoxus), elevated cerebrovascular pressure, reduced left atrial pressure, and a pericardial friction rub. The patient, who is usually anxious and restless, may sit upright or lean forward, and the skin may be pale, dusky, or cyanotic. The electrocardiogram generally shows decreased cardiac voltage, and the chest x-ray film may reveal an enlarged heart shadow (''water bottle'' heart).

■ INTERVENTION: The patient is maintained on bed rest; the head of the bed is elevated 45 degrees, and a defibrillator and emergency drugs are kept at the bedside. Blood pressure, respiration, apical pulse, and cerebrovascular, atrial, and pulmonary wedge pressures are checked every 15 to 30 minutes. Auscultation for pulsus paradoxus is performed and peripheral pulses are checked every 30 minutes. A 12-lead electrocardiogram is usually ordered, and, when possible, the patient is placed on a cardiac monitor and the rhythm strip is checked every hour. Cardiotonic and antiarrhythmic drugs and measures for controlling pain are administered as ordered. Aspiration of the fluid or blood in the pericardial sac (pericardiocentesis) is performed for diagnosis and for therapy. If surgery is indicated, the patient is prepared for the procedure, and the bleeding vessel or vessels are ligated.

■ NURSING CONSIDERATIONS: The patient with life-threatening cardiac tamponade is usually cared for in an intensive care unit. A drain may be in place in the pericardial sac. Coughing and deep breathing are painful, and recovery may be lengthy and difficult. The patient requires extensive physical and emotional care.

cardiac valve. See **heart valve.**

Cardilate, a trademark for an antianginal (erythrityl tetranitrate).

cardinal frontal plane, the plane that divides the body into front and back portions. Also called **vertical plane.**

cardinal horizontal plane. See **transverse plane.**

cardinal ligament, a sheet of subserous fascia extending across the female pelvic floor as a continuation of the broad ligament. It is embedded in the adipose tissue on each side of the vagina and is formed by the fasciae of the vagina and the cervix converging at the lateral borders of these organs. The ligament forms ventral and dorsal extensions at the lateral portion of the pelvic diaphragm. The ventral extension joins the tissue supporting the bladder. The dorsal extension blends with the uterosacral ligaments. The vaginal arteries course across the pelvis in close association with the cardinal ligament. See also **broad ligament.**

cardinal movements of labor, the typical sequence of positions assumed by the fetus as it descends through the pelvis during labor and delivery, usually designated as engagement, flexion, descent, internal rotation, extension, and external rotation or restitution. The birth canal is a curved cylinder; the head must enter it in a downward, transverse direction but exit it in a more forward, anteroposterior direction. In a vertex presentation, engagement of the head in the pelvic inlet requires flexion of the head with chin on chest. After descent, the head must undergo extension to turn forward and be born under the symphysis. The pelvic inlet is heart-shaped, and the fetal head enters it facing obliquely; but the pelvic outlet is diamond-shaped, and the head usually exits it facing posteriorly and must undergo internal rotation to do so. After delivery of the head, the shoulders remain for a time in the oblique plane and the head undergoes external rotation or restitution to allow the widest diameter of the shoulders to be delivered from the longer anteroposterior diameter of the pelvic outlet. See illustration at **labor.**

cardinal position of gaze, (in ophthalmology) one of six positions to which the normal eye may be turned. Each position requires the function of a specific ocular muscle and a cranial nerve. The positions and the corresponding muscles and nerves are as follows:
1) Straight nasal: medial rectus and the third cranial nerve.
2) Up nasal: inferior oblique and the third cranial nerve.
3) Down nasal: superior oblique and the fourth cranial nerve.
4) Straight temporal: lateral rectus and the sixth cranial nerve.
5) Up temporal: superior rectus and the third cranial nerve.
6) Down temporal: inferior rectus and the third cranial nerve.

cardinal sagittal plane. See **median plane.**

cardinal symptom. See **symptom.**

cardio-, cardia-, a combining form meaning 'pertaining to the heart': *cardiocele, cardiocirrhosis, cardiodynia.*

cardiocirculatory /kär′dē•ōsur′kyo͝olətôr′ē/, of or pertaining to the heart and the circulation.

cardiogenic shock /kär′dē•ōjen′ik/, an abnormal condition often characterized by low cardiac output in association with acute myocardial infarction and congestive heart failure. This condition is difficult to diagnose because of complex hemodynamic variations in affected individuals. Although low cardiac output is a common sign of this disorder, cardiogenic shock may also occur in association with normal or higher than normal output. Fast determination of blood volume is important to proper therapy. Cardiogenic shock is fatal in about 80% of cases, and immediate therapy is necessary to save affected individuals. Depending on the signs, therapy may include the administration of fluids, diuretics, or vasoactive drugs and the application of various devices, as pacing catheters. A variety of surgical procedures may be part of the therapy but are not usually employed. Compare **hypovolemic shock.** See also **electric shock, shock.**

cardiogram, an electronically recorded tracing of cardiac activity.

cardiography /kär′dē•og′rəfē/, the technique of graphically recording the movements of the heart by means of a cardiograph.

cardiologist, a physician specializing in the diagnosis and treatment of disorders of the heart.

cardiology, the study of the anatomy, normal functions, and disorders of the heart.

cardiolysis /kär′dē•ol′isis/, an operation that separates the heart and the pericardium from the sternal periosteum in a procedure to correct adhesive mediastinopericarditis. The operation resects the ribs and the sternum over the pericardium.

cardiomegaly /kär′dē•ōmeg′əlē/, hypertrophy of the heart caused most frequently by pulmonary hypertension and also occurring in arteriovenous fistula, congenital aortic stenosis, ventricular septal defect, patent ductus arteriosus, and Paget's disease. In athletes an enlarged, well-functioning heart is a normal finding. See also **athlete's heart.**

cardiomyopathy /kär′dē•ōmī•op′əthē/, any disease that affects the myocardium, as alcoholic cardiomyopathy.

cardioplegia, **1.** paralysis of the heart. **2.** the arrest of myocardial contractions by injection of chemicals, hypothermia, or electrical stimuli for the purpose of performing surgery on the heart. See also **cardiac standstill.**

cardiopulmonary, of or pertaining to the heart and the lungs.

cardiopulmonary arrest. See **cardiac arrest.**

cardiopulmonary bypass, a procedure used in heart surgery in which the blood is diverted from the heart and lungs by means of a pump oxygenator and returned directly to the aorta.

cardiopulmonary resuscitation (CPR), a basic emergency procedure for life support, consisting of artificial respiration and manual external cardiac massage. It is used in cases of cardiac arrest to establish effective circulation and ventilation in order to prevent irreversible cerebral damage resulting from anoxia. External cardiac massage compresses the heart between the lower sternum and the thoracic vertebral column. During compressions, blood is forced into systemic and pulmonary circulation, and venous blood refills the heart when the compression is released. Mouth-to-mouth breathing or a mechanic form of ventilation is used concomitantly with CPR to oxygenate the blood being pumped through the circulatory system. (Table, pages 192-193)

■ METHOD: Basic cardiopulmonary resuscitation requires no adjunctive equipment, although mechanic devices can be used. It can be done by one or two rescuers and involves three interrelated actions: opening the airway, restoring breathing, and restoring circulation. For an adult, the procedure is performed in the following manner:

1) The victim is placed on a hard flat surface, as a CPR board, a backboard, or, if necessary, the floor. Resuscitation efforts are not delayed while the rescuer is waiting for such a support.

2) The victim is examined closely. If unresponsive, the victim is tapped on the shoulder, or the ear is pinched. The rescuer asks loudly, "Can you hear me? Are you all right?" If there is no response, it is assumed the victim is unconscious.

3) The rescuer establishes and maintains an open airway. In the supine position, relaxed muscles allow the tongue to drop back in the throat, blocking the airway. This can be easily relieved by tilting the head. One hand is placed beneath the victim's neck and the other on the forehead, the one lifting the neck while the other applies pressure on the forehead. This extends the neck and lifts the tongue from the back of the throat. In a case of suspected cervical spine injury, the neck is not hyperextended. Instead, the lower jaw is lifted by placing the fingers behind the angles of the victim's jaw in front of the earlobes and displacing it upward. If available, an oropharyngeal airway is inserted; if not, the head is held in position, either tilted back or with jaw lifted, throughout the resuscitation procedure.

4) The rescuer evaluates the need for artificial respiration by looking, listening, and feeling for signs of air exchange or respiratory effort. If there is no spontaneous exchange and if there is no stoma (artificial airway device) over the larynx, regular artificial respiration is begun immediately. If there is a stoma, mouth-to-stoma respiration is initiated.

5) To begin artificial respiration, the rescuer rotates the hand that has been placed on the victim's forehead and, using the thumb and index finger of this hand, pinches the nostrils closed. A tight seal is made with the rescuer's mouth around the mouth of the victim, and four breaths, each of increasing strength and volume, are given. The rescuer's mouth is removed, and the victim is allowed to exhale passively. The rescuer watches the chest fall and then breathes in another series of breaths. The cycle is repeated every 5 seconds as long as respiratory deficiency exists. If indicated, mouth-to-nose respiration may be used. If the chest does not expand, the head is repositioned and ventilation is again attempted. A second unsuccessful attempt indicates an obstructed airway. See also **Heimlich maneuver.**

6) The rescuer takes the pulse and checks for cardiac arrest. If the pulse is absent or inadequate, the carotid artery is palpated for 5 seconds immediately after the four initial breaths are given. Absence or questionable pressure of the pulse at that time indicates the need to begin external cardiac compression.

7) To start external massage, the rescuer takes a position facing the side of the victim. To find the correct location for the hands (the landmark position), the chest is uncovered and the xiphoid process is identified. With the middle finger on the notch and the index finger next to it, the heel of the other hand is placed on the sternum, directly adjacent to the fingers marking the xiphoid. With the fingers extended upward and away from the ribs, the first hand is placed on top of the second and the fingers are interlocked. With arms straight, the rescuer rocks back and forth from the hip joints, exerting sufficient downward pressure with the forward swing of the body to depress the victim's sternum from 1.5 to 2 inches. It is extremely important to be positioned properly to avoid depressing the xiphoid process and the possibility of causing severe internal injury. After each compression, a rest is allowed for a time equal to the time of compression, but the hands are not moved from their position on the chest. The cycle is repeated using a ratio of 15 compressions to two breaths at the rate of 80 compressions a minute. The proper rhythm may be achieved by counting "one and two and three," up to 15. If two rescuers are available, CPR is performed with one rescuer giving compressions and the other giving breaths, at a 5:1 ratio at a rate of 60 compressions a minute. The proper rhythm can be determined by counting "one-one thousand, two-one thousand," up to "five-one thousand." Effectiveness of CPR is checked frequently by palpating the carotid artery for the return of a spontaneous heartbeat and by watching for "pinking" of the skin, constriction of the pupils, and a return of respiration. If the rescuer doing compressions becomes tired, a switch may be made by changing the counting rhythm to "switch-one thousand, two-one thousand," up to "five-one thousand." At the end of that cycle, the rescuer giving compressions moves to the victim's head and checks the pulse. The rescuer who has been at the head, after giving a breath, moves to the victim's side, and checks the pulse for 5 seconds. If the pulse is absent or its pressure is inadequate, the rescuer at the head says, "No pulse. Continue CPR."

The technique for infants up to 1 year of age and for children up to 8 years of age is like that for adults, with the following exceptions. In infants, the neck is not hyperextended because soft cartilage and neck tissues may occlude the airway if the head is tilted too far; placing a hand beneath the shoulders of an infant provides adequate tilt. The rescuer's mouth covers the infant's mouth and nose, and the infant's pulse is checked on the

Emergency cardiopulmonary resuscitation (CPR)

Findings	*CPR basic sequence*	*ABCD's of action*
1. No response	1. Call for help Stimulate or arouse	
2. Absence of respirations Cyanosis Dilated pupils Limp extremities	2. Open airway a. Head tilt, neck lift; or b. Head tilt, chin lift c. Back blows (if airway obstructed) d. Chest thrusts (if airway obstructed)	A - Open airway 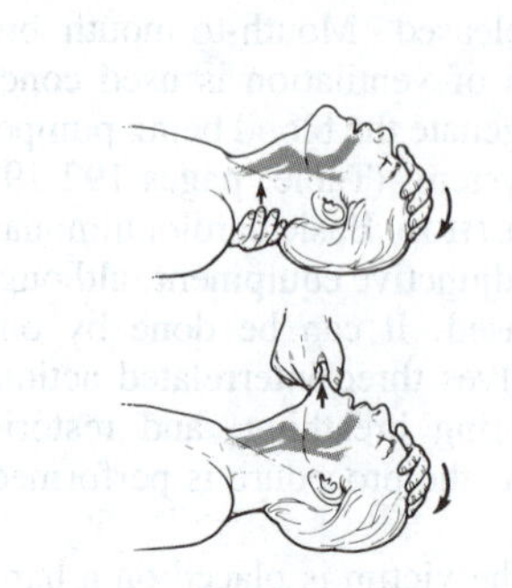
3. Respirations still absent	3. Initiate artificial respiration a. Pinch nostrils & make a seal with rescuer's mouth; four quick breaths - only enough to make chest rise and fall	B - Restore breathing 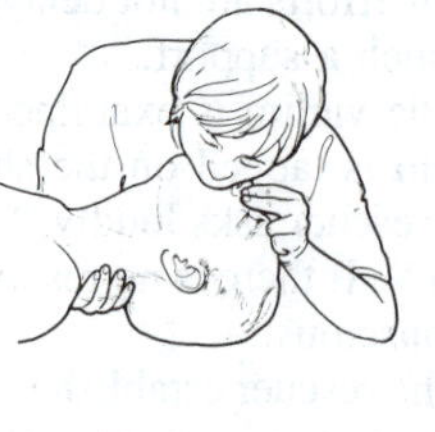
4. Pulse—not palpable	4. a. Palpate brachial artery in infants, carotid artery in children & adults b. Initiate external cardiac compressions & continue rescue breathing	C - Restore circulation 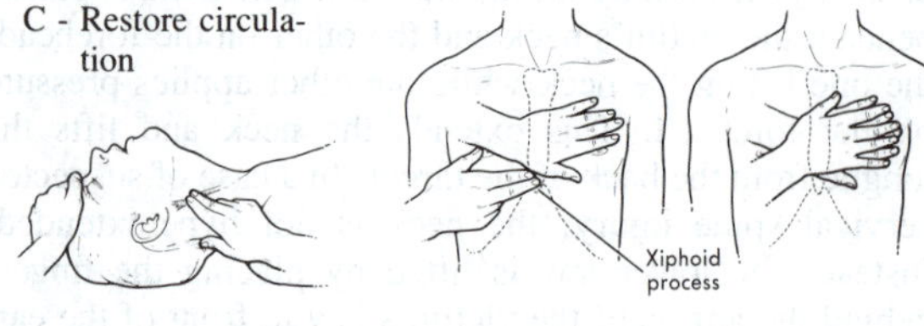
5. ECG ventricular fibrillation; ventricular tachycardia; asystole; Electromechanical Dissociation (EMD)	5. Drug therapy; defibrillation	D - Provide definitive treatment 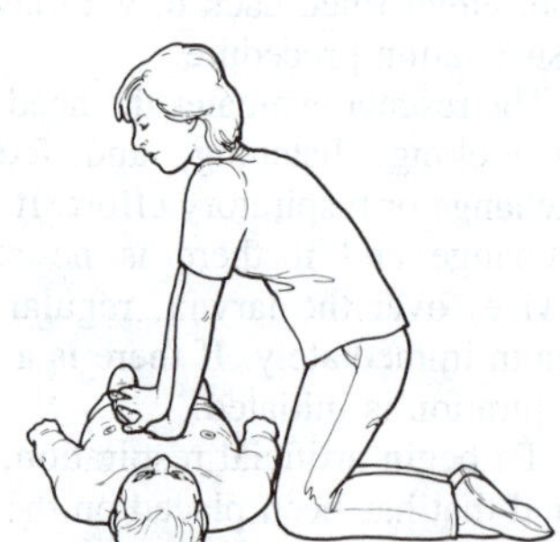

Victim *must* be supported on hard surface; gastric emptying (decompression) is recommended only if the abdomen is so tense that ventilation is ineffective; effective CPR is accompanied by improvement in skin color, pupillary constriction, spontaneous movement, and some gasping respirations; effectiveness should be evaluated after 1 minute, and periodically thereafter (every 1 to 3 minutes)

Adapted from the Supplement to Journal of the American Medical Association, August 1, 1980.

Age	Procedures: Consideration	
Infants (less than 1 year)	Breathing point	Mouth *and* nose
	Pressure point	Midsternum—on line with nipples
	Hands	Tips of 2 or 3 fingers
	Compression distance	½ to 1 inch (1.3 to 2.5 cm)
	Compression/ventilation C/V ratio	5/1 100C/20V/minute; use only slight hyperextension of neck; mouth or mask covers nose and mouth; use only small breaths from cheeks
Children (1 through 8 years)	Breathing point	Mouth
	Pressure point	Slightly below midsternum
	Hands	Heel of one hand
	Compression distance	1 to 1½ inches (2.5 to 3.8 cm)
	Compression/ventilation C/V ratio	5/1 80C/15V/minute
Older children and adults	Breathing point	Mouth
	Pressure point	Lower half of sternum
	Hands	Both
	Compression distance	1½ to 2 inches (4 to 5 cm)
	Compression/ventilation C/V ratio	Alone—15/2 2 Rescuers—5/1 60C/12V/minute

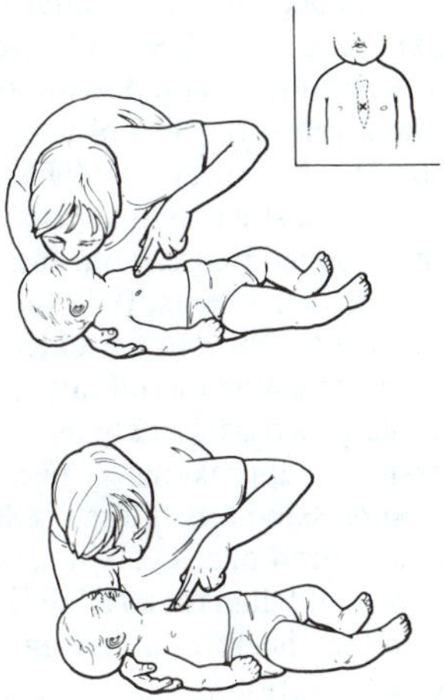

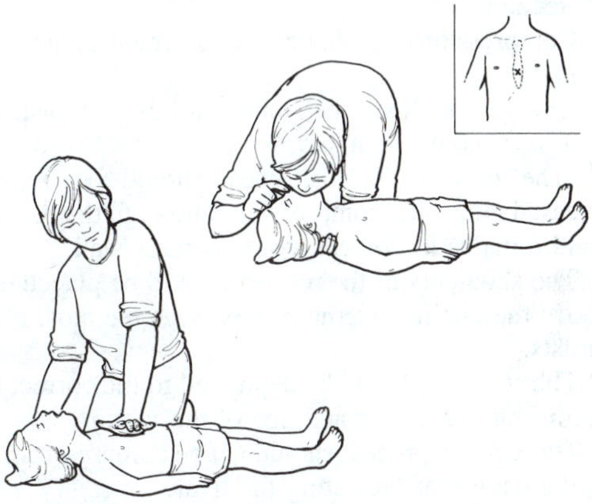

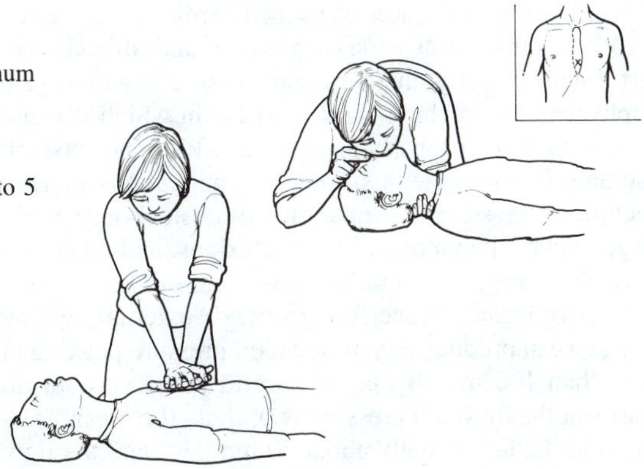

brachial artery. For small infants, both thumbs are placed on the midsternum while joining the fingers behind the infant's back. It is best applied from the superior direction with the operator at the infant's head. For an older infant, pressure is applied with two fingers on the midsternum, exerting a sharp downward thrust. For children older than 5 years, the heel of one hand is used. Because the ventricles of the heart in infants and small children lie higher in the chest cavity than they do in adults, external pressure is applied midsternum and only to a depth of 0.5 to 0.75 inches for infants, 0.75 to 1 inch for young children, and 1.5 to 2 inches for older children. The rate of cardiac compression for infants is 100 a minute, with breaths interposed as quickly as possible after each five compressions—approximately one every 3 seconds. The rate of compression for children is 80 a minute, with ventilations delivered once every 4 seconds. Less air is necessary for a child than for an adult. For an infant, only the air held in the cheeks is puffed in.

■ OUTCOME CRITERIA: To provide adequate basic life support, these rules for correct performance should be followed:

1) CPR should not be interrupted for more than 5 seconds, except for endotracheal intubation or for moving a victim. In these cases, the interruption should not exceed 15 seconds.

2) Compressions should be smooth, regular, and uninterrupted.

3) The victim should be stabilized before transportation to a more convenient site.

4) The pressure on the chest should be completely released after each compression, although the palm of the hand remains in contact with the chest wall.

5) The shoulders of the rescuer should be placed directly above the victim's sternum to provide the most effective thrusts.

6) The sternum should be depressed to the correct degree according to the size and age of the victim.

7) The xiphoid process should not be compressed because of the danger of lacerating the liver.

8) Gastric distension should not be relieved unless it becomes so severe that it interferes with ventilation.

CPR is used only in cases of sudden cardiac arrest. Even if CPR is initiated as soon as possible and all steps are performed correctly, there are some cases, as with severe emphysema or crushing chest injuries, in which it is not successful. Even properly performed, CPR may cause rib fractures in some victims. Other complications include fracture of the sternum, separation of costochondral cartilage, hepatic hematoma, lung contusions, and fat embolism. The danger of complications is minimized by correct performance. Properly performed, external cardiac massage can produce a systolic blood pressure peaking at more than 100 mm Hg in the carotid arteries. With no heartbeat the diastolic pressure is 0; thus, the mean pressure with CPR is usually about 40 mm Hg, and the flow of arterial blood is approximately 25% to 35% of the normal flow. These figures point out the need for immediate action and for continuous effort to effect a rescue; they also indicate that CPR can be effective and can save lives if properly given in a carefully monitored fashion. CPR is an interim measure used until advanced life support action and definitive measures can be taken. Once initiated, it is continued until one of the following occurs: Spontaneous circulation and respiration are restored; resuscitation efforts are transferred to someone who can continue life-support procedures, either basic or advanced; a physician assumes responsibility for the victim; the victim is handed over to the care of a medical facility; or the rescuer is physically unable to continue.

■ NURSING ORDERS: Cardiopulmonary resuscitation is considered an emergency procedure, and knowledge of the principles, procedures, requirements, and complications of this maneuver is essential. In the hospital, there are additional tasks to perform to implement CPR. Primarily, the nurse evaluates the extent of the emergency and the indications for initiating lifesaving measures. The nurse is also prepared to undertake immediate action should it be necessary to do so before the medical team arrives. If not immediately involved in performing CPR, the nurse prepares for the initiation of definitive therapy by readying equipment, including an electrocardiograph, a defibrillator, a tracheostomy set, oxygen, and a suction machine. Epinephrine for direct injection into the heart, sodium bicarbonate to combat acidosis, and calcium chloride to stimulate cardiac contraction are also prepared for injection and properly labeled. While resuscitation proceeds, efforts are made to start an intravenous infusion, and ECG electrodes are applied to the patient. In the hospital, the decision to terminate resuscitation efforts is made by a physician.

cardiorrhaphy /kär′dē•ôr′əfē/, an operation in which the heart muscle is sutured.

cardioscope, an obsolete device for inspecting and manipulating the internal structures of the heart.

cardiospasm /kär′dē•ōspaz′əm/, a form of achalasia characterized by a failure of the cardia at the distal end of the esophagus to relax, causing dysphagia and regurgitation, and sometimes requiring surgical division of the muscle.

cardiotachometer /kär′dē•ōtəkom′ətər/, an instrument that continuously monitors and records the heartbeat.

cardiotomy /kär′dē•ot′əmē/, **1.** an operation in which the heart is incised. **2.** an operation in which the cardiac end of the stomach or cardiac orifice is incised.

cardiotonic /kär′dē•ōton′ik/, **1.** of or pertaining to a substance that tends to increase the efficiency of contractions of the heart muscle. **2.** a pharmacologic agent that increases the force of myocardial contractions. Cardiac glycosides, derived from certain plant alkaloids, exert a tonic effect by altering the transport of electrolytes across the myocardial membrane, causing an increased influx of sodium and calcium and an increased efflux of potassium. Digitalis, digitoxin, and digoxin, widely used cardiac glycosides obtained from leaves of a species of foxglove, increase the force of myocardial contractions, extend the refractory period of the atrioventricular node, and, to a lesser degree, affect the sinoatrial node and the heart's conduction system. Other cardiac glycosides are ouabain and strophanthin, obtained from species of *Strophanthus;* scillaridin, derived from squill; and bufotalin, obtained from the skin and saliva of a European toad.

cardiotoxic, having a toxic or injurious effect on the heart.

cardiovascular /kär′dē•ōvas′kyələr/, of or pertaining to the heart and blood vessels.

cardiovascular assessment, an evaluation of the condition, function, and abnormalities of the heart and circulatory system.

▪ METHOD: The patient is asked to describe the onset, duration, location, and characteristics of any pain present and the occurrence of weakness, fatigue, shortness of breath, fever, coughing, wheezing, and palpitations. Questions are asked regarding episodes of fainting, indigestion, nausea, edema of extremities, cyanosis, and changes in vision, and whether the hands and feet ever feel numb or cold. The person's general appearance, color, assumed position, rate and rhythm of arterial pulses, the presence of pulsus paradoxus or pulsus alternans, and the distention, pulsation, and pressure of neck veins are observed. Blood pressure, temperature, rate, and character of respirations are checked, and the precordium is examined for the point of maximal impulse, symmetry, the cardiac border, pulsations, and evidence of lifts or bulges. Auscultation of the chest is performed to determine the intensity, pitch, duration, timbre, origin, and frequency of heart sounds and murmurs and to identify the location and character of breath sounds, including rales, rhonchi, and rubs. Color, temperature, turgor, and dryness or sweating of the skin are noted, and the appearance of the extremities, capillary filling time, nails, and lesions are described. The patient's level of consciousness, reflexes, neurologic signs, and responses to pain are recorded, along with data on concurrent hypertension, obesity, diabetes, and any pulmonary and renal conditions. Information is obtained on any previous cardiovascular surgery and illnesses, as rheumatic fever, myocardial infarction, angina, congenital heart disease, occlusive vascular disease, and lung and kidney disorders. Pertinent background data include the patient's response to stress, methods of coping, relationships, occupation, environment, sleep pattern, exercise levels, leisure activities, and use of alcohol and tobacco. Other factors considered in the evaluation are the patient's history of medication with digitalis preparations, antihypertensives, diuretics, aspirin, sleeping pills, and over-the-counter cold and influenza remedies and family history of heart disease, hypertension, diabetes, obesity, vascular disorders, stroke, and renal disease. Diagnostic aids used are electrocardiogram, chest x-ray film, echocardiogram, radionuclide imaging, coronary arteriogram, cardiac catheterization, and arterial and pulmonary wedge pressure readings. Appropriate laboratory studies include a complete blood count, hemoglobin and hematocrit determinations, electrolyte and clotting profiles, and assays of serum cholesterol, triglycerides, serum glutamic oxaloacetic transaminase (SGOT), serum glutamic pyruvic transaminase (SGPT), creatine phosphokinase (CP), and lactic acid dehydrogenase (LAD).

▪ NURSING ORDERS: The nurse usually obtains the patient's history, records the external observations, checks the blood pressure, temperature, respiration, and pulse, auscultates the chest, and assembles the pertinent background information and the reports on diagnostic tests. In a coronary care unit the nurse may have a greatly expanded role, interpreting the data on an electrocardiographic tracing and adjusting medications.

▪ OUTCOME CRITERIA: An accurate and complete assessment of cardiovascular function is an essential adjunct to a complete physical examination and is vital to the diagnosis and proper continuing care of a patient who has cardiovascular disease.

cardiovascular disease, any one of numerous abnormal conditions characterized by dysfunction of the heart and blood vessels. Some common kinds of cardiovascular disease are **atherosclerosis, cor pulmonale, rheumatic heart disease, syphilitic heart disease,** and **systemic hypertension.** In the United States cardiovascular disease is second to cancer as the leading cause of death, accounting for about 50% of all deaths from disease annually. More than a quarter of a million persons under 65 years of age in the United States die each year from this disorder; about half of such deaths are attributed to atherosclerosis. The prevalent kinds of cardiovascular disease are the rheumatic, the syphilitic, and the traumatic varieties.

cardiovascular system, the network of structures, including the heart and the blood vessels, that pump and convey the blood throughout the body. The system includes thousands of miles of vessels, capillaries, and venules and is vital to maintaining homeostasis. Numerous control mechanisms of the system assure that the blood is delivered to the structures where it is most needed and at the proper rate. The system delivers nutrients and other essential materials to the fluids surrounding the cells and removes waste products, which are conveyed to excretory organs, as the kidneys and the intestine. The cardiovascular system functions in close association with the respiratory system, transporting oxygen inhaled into the lungs and conveying carbon dioxide to the lungs for expiration. Sympathetic and parasympathetic impulses from the medulla and cardiac baroreceptors sensitive to changes in pressure control the function of the heart, which pumps oxygenated blood carried by the arteries and receives deoxygenated blood from the veins. Cardiovascular diseases affect a large number of individuals throughout the world, and half a million Americans die each year from coronary diseases. A variety of factors, as diet, exercise, and stress, affect the cardiovascular system.

cardioversion, the restoration of the heart's normal sinus rhythm by delivery of a synchronized electric shock through two metal paddles placed on the patient's chest. Cardioversion is used in the treatment of atrial fibrillation and in ventricular, nodal, and atrial arrhythmias.

■ METHOD: The synchronized electric voltage is delivered by placing one of the insulated electrode paddles, covered with a thick layer of conductive paste, below the angle of the patient's left scapula; the other paddle is placed over the right parasternal area of the third intercostal space. The instrument is automatically preset to deliver an electric discharge during the interval in which the normal cardiac impulse spreads through the bundle of His and its branches to initiate contraction (the QRS complex). The instrument is set initially to deliver 5 to 10 watts per second, but if the normal rhythm does not resume, successive shocks of up to 400 watts per second are delivered. To prepare the patient for cardioversion, the physician's explanation of the procedure is reinforced, a signed informed consent is obtained, and diuretics and digitalis preparations are withheld for 24 to 72 hours as ordered. The patient's serum potassium level is checked for possible hypokalemia and a 12-lead electrocardiogram and rhythm strip are obtained. Nothing is given orally for 6 to 8 hours before the procedure. Parenteral fluids are maintained, and oxygen, delivered by mask or cannula, may be ordered. The patient voids and receives a sedative about an hour before cardioversion; dentures are removed. An emergency cart with cardiac drugs and airway equipment is placed at the bedside, and conductive gel, paste, or saline pads are applied to the electrode paddles. During and after cardioversion, observations are made of the patient's level of consciousness, pulse, respirations, and blood pressure; also noted are electrocardiographic changes, as return to sinus rhythm, atrial fibrillation, premature ventricular contractions, ventricular tachycardia, or cardiac standstill. Any signs of pulmonary embolus are noted. After the procedure, the patient is maintained in a supine position in bed. The blood pressure, respirations, and apical pulse are checked every 15 minutes for 1 hour, then every 4 hours. Cardiac activity is monitored, and oxygen is administered as ordered. The patient's skin areas exposed to the electrodes' gel or saline pads are washed with plain water, and a lanolin-based lotion is applied.

■ NURSING ORDERS: The nurse prepares the patient for cardioversion, assembles the necessary emergency equipment, and checks the vital signs during and after the procedure.

■ OUTCOME CRITERIA: Cardioversion is usually an effective method for restoring the heart's normal sinus rhythm.

carditis /kärdī′tis/, an inflammatory condition of the muscles of the heart, usually resulting from infection. In most cases more than one layer of muscles is involved. Chest pain, cardiac arrhythmia, circulatory failure, and damage to the structures of the heart may occur. Kinds of carditis are **endocarditis, myocarditis,** and **pericarditis.**

Cardizem, a trademark for a slow channel blocker or calcium antagonist (diltiazem).

career ladder, (in nursing education) a pathway for upward mobility that begins with a course of study in practical nursing or a program that grants an associate degree in nursing. On completion of this basic level, the candidate may continue up the ladder, taking a baccalaureate program in nursing. After this, the person may continue on to a masters and a doctoral program.

care of the sick, (in public health nursing) the care of sick patients in their homes, as distinguished from health supervision. Public health nursing agencies are reimbursed for the nursing services rendered by the nurses according to the kind of service rendered, as a sick visit or a health supervision visit. Compare **health supervision.**

care plan. See **nursing care plan.**

caries /ker′ēz/, an abnormal condition of a tooth or a bone characterized by decay, disintegration, and destruction of the structure. Kinds of caries include **dental caries, radiation caries,** and **spinal caries.**

carina /kərē′nə/, *pl.* **carinae,** any structure shaped like a ridge or keel, as the carina of the trachea, which projects from the lowest tracheal cartilage.

cariogenic /ker′ē·ōjen′ik/, tending to produce caries.

carisoprodol, a skeletal muscle relaxant.

■ INDICATION: It is prescribed for the relief of muscle spasm.

■ CONTRAINDICATIONS: Porphyria or known hypersensitivity to this drug or to chemically similar drugs prohibits its use.

■ ADVERSE EFFECTS: Among the more serious adverse reactions are ataxia, drowsiness, pronounced weakness, visual disturbances, mental confusion, and allergic reactions.

carmalum. See **carmine dy.**

carminative /kärmin′ətiv/, **1.** of or pertaining to a substance that relieves flatulence and abdominal distention. **2.** a carminative agent that relieves gaseous distention and painful spasms, especially after meals. Volatile oils of anise, bitter almond, cinnamon, fennel, peppermint, spearmint, and wintergreen, which have a soothing effect passing through the stomach, were formerly used as carminatives, but they are rarely used in modern medicine except as flavoring agents.

carmine dye /kär′min/, a red coloring substance, produced by the addition of alum to an extract of cochineal, used for staining specimens in histology. Also called **carmalum.**

carmustine /kärmus′tin/, a lipid-soluble nitrosourea, 1,3-bis(2-chloroethyl)-1-nitrosourea,used as a single antineoplastic agent or with other approved chemotherapeutic agents in the treatment of brain tumors, multiple myeloma, Hodgkin's disease, and non-Hodgkin's lymphomas. Also called **BCNU.**

carneous /kär′nē·əs/, having the quality of flesh.

carnitine /kär′nitin/, a substance found in skeletal and cardiac muscle and certain other tissues that functions as a carrier of fatty acids across the membranes of the mitochondria. It is used therapeutically in treating angina and certain deficiency diseases, particularly endocardial fibroelastosis. It has actions that closely resemble those of amino acids and B vitamins.

carnivore, an animal belonging to the order *Carnivora,* classified as a flesheater, with appropriate teeth and a characteristically simple stomach and a short intestine for such a diet. –**carnivorous,** *adj.*

carotene /kar′ətin/, a red or orange hydrocarbon found in carrots, sweet potatoes, milk fat, egg yolk, and leafy vegetables, as beet greens, spinach, and broccoli. Carotene is a provitamin and in the body is converted into vitamin A. An inability to utilize carotene results in vitamin A deficiency. Also spelled **carotin, carrotene, carrotine.** See also **vitamin A.**

carotenemia /kar′ətinē′mē·ə/, the presence of high levels of carotene in the blood resulting in an abnormal yellow appearance of the plasma and skin. The conjunctivae are not discolored. Also called **pseudojaundice.** Compare **bilirubinemia.** See also **jaundice, icterus.**

carotenoid /kərot′ənoid/, any of a group of red, yellow, or orange highly unsaturated pigments that are found in some animal tissue and in foods, as carrots, sweet potatoes, and leafy green vegetables. Many of these substances, as carotene, are necessary for the formation of vitamin A in the body, while others, including lycopene and xanthophyll, show no vitamin A activity. Also spelled **carotinoid.**

carotenosis. See **carotenemia.**

carotid /kərot′id/, of or pertaining to the carotid artery. See also **carotid body, carotid sinus, common carotid artery.**

carotid body, a small structure containing neural tissue at the bifurcation of the carotid arteries. It monitors the oxygen content of the blood and assists in regulating respiration.

carotid-body reflex, a normal chemical reflex initiated by a decrease in oxygen concentration in the blood and, to a lesser degree, by increased carbon dioxide and hydrogen ion concentrations that act on chemoreceptors at the bifurcation of the common carotid arteries and result in nerve impulses that cause the respiratory center in the medulla to increase respiratory activity. See also **aortic-body reflex.**

carotid body tumor, a benign, round, firm growth that develops at the bifurcation of the common carotid artery. The tumor usually has no effect but it sometimes may cause dizziness, nausea, and vomiting, especially if it impedes the flow of blood because pressure is increased in the vascular system. It may be surgically excised in some cases.

carotid plexus, any one of three nerve plexuses associated with the carotid arteries. Compare **common carotid plexus, external carotid plexus, internal carotid plexus.**

carotid pulse, the pulse of the carotid artery, palpated by gently pressing a finger in the groove between the larynx and the sternocleidomastoid muscle in the neck.

carotid sinus, a dilatation of the arterial wall at the bifurcation of the common carotid artery. It contains sensory nerve endings from the vagus nerve that respond to changes in blood pressure.

carotid sinus reflex, the decrease in the heart rate as a reflex reaction from pressure on or within the carotid artery at the level of its bifurcation. This reflex starts in the sinus of the internal carotid artery. See also **carotid sinus syndrome.**

carotid sinus syndrome, a temporary loss of consciousness that sometimes accompanies convulsive seizures because of the intensity of the carotid sinus reflex when pressure builds in one or both carotid sinuses.

carotodynia /kərot′ōdin′ē·ə/, a tenderness along the length of the common carotid artery.

-carp, a combining form meaning 'fruit': *archicarp, ascocarp, pericarp.*

carpal /kär′pəl/, of or pertaining to the carpus, or wrist.

-carpal, a combining form referring to the wrist: *extracarpal, radiocarpal, trapeziometacarpal.*

carpal tunnel, a conduit for the median nerve and the flexor tendons, formed by the carpal bones and the flexor retinaculum.

carpal tunnel syndrome, a common painful disorder of the wrist and hand, induced by compression on the median nerve between the inelastic carpal ligament and other structures within the carpal tunnel. The syndrome is seen more often in women, especially in pregnant and in menopausal women. Symptoms may result from trauma, synovitis, or tumor, or may develop with rheumatoid arthritis, amyloidosis, agromegaly, or diabetes. The median nerve innervates the palm and the radial side of the hand; compression of the nerve causes weakness, pain with opposition of the thumb, and burning, tingling, or aching, sometimes radiating to the forearm and to the shoulder joint. Weakness and atrophy of muscles may increase from lack of use, impairing thumb and finger dexterity. Pain may be intermittent or constant and is often most intense at night. Symptomatic treatment usually relieves mild symptoms of recent onset, but if the pain becomes disabling, the injection of corticosteroids often brings dramatic relief. Surgical division of the volar carpal ligament to relieve nerve pressure is usually curative. Nursing treatment includes emotional support, nocturnal splinting of the hand and forearm, elevation of the arm to relieve the swelling of soft tissue, and encouragement of mild wrist and finger movements to prevent atrophy of muscles.

carphenazine maleate, a phenothiazine antipsychotic agent.

■ INDICATION: It is prescribed in the treatment of psychotic disorders.

■ CONTRAINDICATIONS: Parkinson's disease, concurrent administration of central nervous system depressants, liver or renal dysfunction, severe hypotension, or known hypersensitivity to this drug or to phenothiazine medication prohibits its use.

■ ADVERSE EFFECTS: Among the more serious adverse effects are hypotension, liver toxicity, a variety of extrapyramidal reactions, blood dyscrasias, and hypersensitivity reactions.

carpopedal spasm, a spasm of the hand, or thumbs, or foot, or toes that sometimes accompanies tetany.

carpus /kär′pəs/, the wrist, made up of eight bones arranged in two rows. The proximal row consists of the scaphoid, lunate, triangular, and pisiform. The distal row consists of the trapezium, trapezoid, capitate, and hamate.

Carrel-Lindbergh pump. See **Lindbergh pump.**

carrier, **1.** a person or animal who harbors and spreads an organism causing disease in others but who does not become ill. **2.** one whose chromosomes carry a recessive gene.

Carrión's disease. See **bartonellosis.**

carry-over, contamination of a specimen by the previous one.

car sickness. See **motion sickness.**

cartilage, a nonvascular supporting connective tissue composed of various cells and fibers, found chiefly in the joints, the thorax, and various rigid tubes, as the larynx, trachea, nose, and ear. Temporary cartilage, as that comprising most of the fetal skeleton at an early stage, is later replaced by bone. Permanent cartilage remains unossified, except in certain diseases and, sometimes, in advanced age. Kinds of permanent cartilage are **hyaline cartilage, white fibrocartilage,** and **yellow cartilage.** **–cartilaginous,** *adj.*

cartilage-hair hypoplasia, a genetic disorder, inherited as an autosomal recessive trait, characterized by dwarfism caused by hypoplasia of the cartilage, multiple skeletal abnormalities, and excessively sparse, short, fine, brittle hair that is usually light colored. The condition is found primarily among Amish people in the United States and Canada.

cartilaginous joint, a slightly movable joint in which cartilage unites bony surfaces. Two types of articulation involving cartilaginous joints are synchondrosis and symphysis. Also called **amphiarthrosis, junctura cartilaginea.** Compare **fibrous joint, synovial joint.**

CARTOS /kär′tos/, abbreviation for *computer-aided reconstruction by tracing of serial sections,* a technique in which serial, hand-drawn copies of electron micrographs are programed on a computer for display on a television screen. The image can be manipulated for study of all dimensions of the structure.

caruncle /kär′ungkəl/, a small, fleshy projection, as one of the lacrimal caruncles at the inner canthus of the eye or the hymenal caruncles that are the hymenal remnants. Also called **caruncula.**

carunculae hymenales, remnants of a ruptured hymen that appear as irregular projections of normal skin around the introitus to the vagina. Also called **hymenal tags.**

caryo-, karyo-, a combining form meaning 'pertaining to a nucleus': *caryokinesis, caryophyllus.*

cascade, any process that develops in stages, with each stage dependent on the preceding one, often producing a cumulative effect.

cascara sagrada /kasker′ə səgrä′də/, a stimulant cathartic prepared from the bark of the *Rhamnus purshianus* tree.

■ INDICATION: It is prescribed for constipation.

■ CONTRAINDICATIONS: Symptoms of appendicitis, intestinal obstruction or perforation, fecal impaction, or known hypersensitivity to this drug prohibits its use. It is not given to lactating mothers.

■ ADVERSE EFFECTS: Among the more serious adverse reactions are rectal bleeding, muscle cramps, dizziness, and laxative dependence.

caseation /kā′sē·ā′shən/, a form of tissue necrosis in which there is loss of cellular outline and the appearance is that of crumbly cheese. It is typical of tuberculosis. See also **caseous.** **–caseate,** *v.*

caseation necrosis, necrosis that transforms tissue into a dry cheeselike mass.

case fatality rate, the number of registered deaths caused by any specific disease, expressed as a percentage of the total number of reported cases of a specific disease.

case nursing, a health care system in which one nurse is assigned to a single patient for delivery of total nursing care.

caseous /kā′sē·əs/, cheeselike; describing the mixture of fat and protein that appear in some body tissues undergoing necrosis.

caseous fermentation, the coagulation of soluble casein through the action of rennin.

cassette, a device used in radiography for holding a sheet of x-ray film and a set of screens. A cassette also may have a grid to absorb scattered radiation.

cast, **1.** a stiff, solid dressing formed with plaster of paris or other material around a limb or other body part to immobilize it during healing. **2.** a mold of a part or all of a patient's teeth and internal jaw area for fitting prostheses or dentures. **3.** a tiny structure formed by deposits of mineral or other substances on the walls of renal tubules, bronchioles, or other organs. Casts often appear in samples of urine or blood collected for laboratory examination. **4.** the deviation of an eye from the normal parallel lines of vision, as in strabismus.

cast core, a metal casting, employing a post in the root canal for retaining an artificial tooth crown. Compare **amalgam core, composite core.** See also **core.**

Castellani's paint. See **carbol-fuchsin solution.**

castor oil, an oil derived from *Ricinus communis,* used as a stimulant cathartic.

■ INDICATIONS: It is prescribed for constipation and for a cleansing preparation of the bowel or colon before examination.

■ CONTRAINDICATIONS: Symptoms of appendicitis, intestinal obstruction or perforation, and fecal impaction prohibit its use. It is not to be used during menstruation or pregnancy.

■ ADVERSE EFFECTS: Among the most serious adverse reactions are rectal bleeding and laxative dependence. Nausea, abdominal cramps, and dizziness also may occur.

castration, the surgical excision of one or both testicles or ovaries, performed most frequently to reduce the production and secretion of certain hormones that may stimulate the proliferation of malignant cells in women with breast cancer or in men with cancer of the prostate. The patient must be informed that bilateral excision of the gonads causes sterility. See also **oophorectomy, orchiectomy.**

castration anxiety, **1.** the fantasized fear of injury or loss of the genital organs, often as the reaction to a repressed feeling of punishment for forbidden sexual desires. It may also be caused by some apparently threatening everyday occurrence, such as a humiliating experience, loss of a job, or loss of authority. **2.** a general threat to the masculinity or femininity of a person or an unrealistic fear of bodily injury or loss of power. Also called **anxiety complex.** See also **anxiety neurosis.**

castration complex. See **castration anxiety.**

casuistics, the recording and the study of the cases of any disease.

CAT /kat/, abbreviation for **computerized axial tomography.**

cata-, cat-, a combining form meaning 'down, under, against, with': *catabasis, catabolic, catacausis.*

catabasis /kətab′əsis/, *pl.* **catabases,** the phase in which a disease declines. **–catabatic,** *adj.*

catabiosis, the normal aging of cells. **–catabiotic,** *adj.*

catabolic activator protein. See **CAP.**

catabolism /kətab′əliz′əm/, a complex, metabolic process in which energy is liberated for use in work, energy storage, or heat production by the destruction of complex substances by living cells to form simple compounds. Carbon dioxide and water are produced as well as energy. Compare **anabolism.** **–catabolic,** *adj.*

catacrotism /kətak′rətiz′əm/, an anomaly of the pulse, characterized by one or more small additional waves in the descending limb of the pulse tracing. **–catacrotic,** *adj.*

catagen. See **hair.**

catalase, a heme enzyme, found in almost all biologic cells, that catalyzes the decomposition of hydrogen peroxide to water and oxygen.

catalepsy /kat′əlep′sē/, an abnormal state characterized by a trancelike level of consciousness and postural rigidity. It occurs in hypnosis and in certain organic and psychologic disorders, as schizophrenia, epilepsy, and hysteria.

catalysis /kətal′əsis/, an increase in the rate of any chemical reaction, caused by a chemical material that is neither part of the process itself nor consumed or affected by the reaction. Compare **negative catalysis.** See also **catalyst.** **–catalytic,** *adj.*

catalyst /kat′əlist/, a substance that influences the rate of a chemical reaction without being permanently altered by the process. Most catalysts, including enzymes in living organisms, accelerate chemical reactions; negative catalysts retard such reactions. See also **enzyme.**

-catalytic, -catalytical, a combining form meaning 'pertaining to a chemical reaction caused by an agent unchanged by the reaction': *allelocatalytic, autocatalytic, photocatalytic.*

catamenia. See **menses.**

catamnesis /kat′amnē′sis/, the medical history of a patient from the onset of an illness. Compare **anamnesis.**

cataphylaxis /kat′əfəlak′sis/, **1.** the migration of leukocytes and antibodies to the site of an infection. **2.** the deterioration of the natural defense system of the body. **–cataphylactic,** *adj.*

cataplexy /kat′əplek′sē/, a condition characterized by sudden muscular weakness and hypotonia, caused by emotions, as anger, fear or surprise, often associated with narcolepsy. **–cataplectic,** *adj.*

Catapres, a trademark for an antihypertensive (clonidine hydrochloride).

cataract, an abnormal progressive condition of the lens of the eye, characterized by loss of transparency. A gray-white opacity can be seen within the lens, behind the pupil. Most cataracts are caused by degenerative changes, occurring most often after 50 years of age. The tendency to develop cataracts is inherited. Trauma, as a puncture wound, may result in cataract formation; less often, exposure to such poisons as dinitrophenol or naphthalene causes them. **Congenital cataracts** are usually hereditary but may be caused by viral infection during the first trimester of gestation. If cataracts are untreated, sight is eventually lost. At first vision is blurred; then, bright lights glare diffusely, and distortion and double vision may develop. Uncomplicated cataracts of old age (**senile cataracts**) are usually treated with excision of the lens and prescription of special contact lenses or glasses. The soft cataracts of children and young adults may either be incised and drained or fragmented by ultrasound, followed by irrigation and aspiration of the fragments through a minute incision.

catarrh, *obsolete.* inflammation of the mucous membranes with discharge, especially inflammation of the air passages of the nose and the trachea. **–catarrhal, catarrhous,** *adj.*

catarrhal dysentery. See **sprue.**

catastrophic care, a pattern of medical and nursing care that involves intensive, highly technical life-support care of an acutely ill or severely traumatized patient.

catastrophic health insurance, health insurance that awards benefits to pay for the cost of severe or lengthy disability or illness. Benefits on some policies are not paid until a specified minimum amount, paid by the insured, is exceeded. Most policies have a limit in total benefits paid, and payment for certain kinds of services may either be precluded or limited to a maximum indemnity.

catastrophic reaction, the uncoordinated response to a drastic shock or a sudden threatening condition, as often occurs in the victims of car crashes and disasters.

catatonia /kat′ətō′nē•ə/, a state or condition characterized by conspicuous motor disturbance, manifested usually as immobility with extreme muscular rigidity or, less commonly, as excessive, impulsive activity. See also **catatonic schizophrenia.** –**catatonic,** *adj.*

catatonic schizophrenia, a form of schizophrenia characterized by alternating periods of extreme withdrawal and extreme excitement. During the withdrawal stage stupor, muscular rigidity, mutism, blocking, negativism, and catalepsy (cerea flexibilitas) may be seen; during the period of excitement, purposeless and impulsive activity may range from mild agitation to violence. Either phase may last for a period of hours, days, or weeks, and the change to the alternate phase is usually abrupt and rapid. Treatment may include tranquilizers, an antidepressant or antianxiety drug, followed by long-term psychotherapy. See also **catatonia.**

cat-bite fever. See **cat-scratch fever.**

catchment area, the specific geographic area for which a particular institution, especially a mental health center, is responsible.

catch-up growth, an acceleration of the growth rate following a period of growth retardation caused by a secondary deficiency, as acute malnutrition or severe illness. The phenomenon, which is routinely seen in premature infants, involves rapid increase in weight, length, and head circumference and continues until the normal individual growth pattern is resumed. The severity, duration, and the developmental timing at which the deficiency occurs may result in some growth inadequacy or permanent deficit, especially in such tissue as the brain.

cat-cry syndrome, a rare, congenital disorder recognized at birth by a kittenlike cry caused by a laryngeal anomaly. The condition is associated with a defect in chromosome 5. Other characteristics include low birth weight, microcephaly, "moon face," wide-set eyes, strabismus, and low-set misshaped ears. Infants are hypotonic; heart defects and mental and physical retardation are common. Also called **cri-du-chat syndrome** /crēdo͞oshä′/, **chromosome 5p– syndrome.**

catecholamine /kat′əkəlam′in/, any one of a group of sympathomimetic compounds composed of a catechol molecule and the aliphatic portion of an amine. Some catecholamines are produced naturally by the body and function as key neurologic chemicals. Catecholamines are also synthesized as drugs used in the treatment of various disorders, as anaphylaxis, asthma, cardiac failure, and hypertension. Some important endogenous catecholamines are dopamine, epinephrine, and norepinephrine. Norepinephrine mediates a host of physiologic and metabolic responses that follow the stimulation of the sympathetic nerves. In response to stress, the adrenal medulla is stimulated, causing the elevation of epinephrine and norepinephrine concentrations in the circulation. Epinephrine dilates blood vessels to the skeletal muscles. Norepinephrine slightly constricts these blood vessels. Both compounds stimulate the myocardium. Dopamine is found primarily in the basal ganglia of the central nervous system (CNS), but dopaminergic nerve endings and specific receptors for this compound have been found in other CNS areas. The major functions of catecholamines and drugs that mimic their actions include the peripheral excitation of certain muscles, peripheral inhibition of certain muscles, cardiac excitation, metabolic actions, endocrine actions, and CNS actions. Differences in the actions of the catecholamines depend on alpha and beta receptors in nerve terminals throughout the body. The brain contains separate neuronal systems that use dopamine, epinephrine, and norepinephrine. More than half of the catecholamine content of the CNS is dopamine, large quantities of which are found in the basal ganglia, the central nucleus of the amygdala, the median eminence, the olfactory tubercle, and the restricted fields of the frontal cortex. The hypothalamus and certain zones of the limbic system contain relatively large amounts of norepinephrine, which is also found in lesser amounts in other brain areas. Neurons in the CNS that contain epinephrine are situated primarily in the medullary reticular formation. Norepinephrine is converted to epinephrine in the adrenal medulla. Catecholamines act directly on sympathetic effector cells by binding to receptors in cellular plasma membranes. Sympathomimetic drugs influence biochemical reactions and functional responses in all the tissues they effect.

cat-eye syndrome, a rare, congenital autosomal anomaly, marked by the presence of an extra, small chromosome 22 and pupils that resemble the vertical pupils of a cat. Anal atresia, heart abnormalities, and severe mental retardation are common.

categoric data, (in research) any data that are classified by name rather than by number, as race, religion, ethnicity, or marital status.

catgut, a nonabsorbable suture material, prepared from the intestines of sheep, used to close surgical wounds. Compare **chromic.**

catharsis /kəthär′sis/, **1.** a cleansing or purging. –**cathartic,** *n.* **2.** the therapeutic release of pent-up feelings and emotions by open discussion of ideas and thoughts. **3.** also called **psychocatharsis.** the process of bringing repressed ideas and feelings into the consciousness by the technique of free association, often in conjunction with hypnosis and the use of hypnotic drugs. See also **abreaction.**

cathartic /kəthär′tik/, **1.** of or pertaining to a substance that causes evacuation of the bowel. **2.** also called **coprogogue.** a cathartic agent that promotes bowel evacuation by stimulating peristalsis, increasing the fluidity or bulk of intestinal contents, softening the feces, or lubricating the intestinal wall. The term *cathartic* implies a fluid evacuation; this is in contrast to *laxative,* which implies the elimination of a soft, formed stool. Cathartics that increase peristalsis, usually by irritating intestinal mucosa, include certain plant substances, as aloe, colocynth, croton oil, podophyllum senna, phenolphthalein, bisacodyl, and dehydrocholic acid. Saline cathartics, as sodium sulfate, magnesium sulfate, and magnesium hydroxide, dilute the intestinal contents by retaining water through osmotic forces. Suppositories containing sodium biphosphate, sodium acid pyrophosphate, and sodium bicarbonate induce defecation when the salts react to form carbon dioxide and the expanding gas stimulates peristalsis. See also **laxative.** –**catharsis,** *n.*

-cathartic, a combining form meaning 'pertaining to cleaning': *cephalocathartic, emetocathartic, hematocathartic.*

catheter /kath′ətər/, a hollow, flexible tube that can be inserted into a vessel or cavity of the body to withdraw or to instill fluids. Most catheters are made of soft plastic or rubber and may be used for treatment or diagnosis. Kinds of catheters include **acorn-tipped catheter, Foley catheter,** and **intrauterine catheter.**

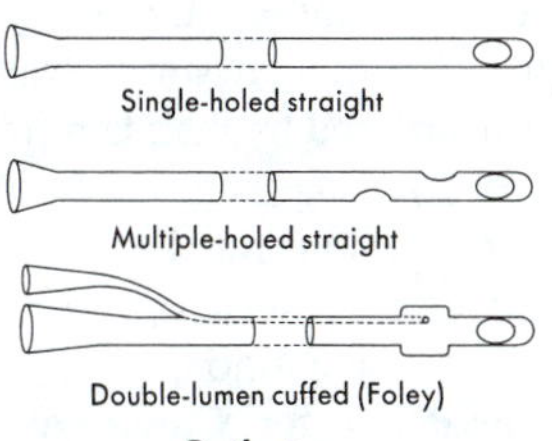

Catheters

catheterization, the introduction of a catheter into a body cavity or organ to inject or remove a fluid. The most common procedure is the insertion of a catheter into the bladder through the urethra for the relief of urinary retention and for emptying the bladder completely before surgery. It is also used when a urine specimen may otherwise be contaminated, as when a woman is menstruating. Self-catheterization is taught to those patients with neurogenic bladder. Sterile, aseptic techniques are necessary to prevent infection; trauma is also to be avoided, particularly to the male urethra and when the procedure is performed on children, who are frightened by the technique and cannot cooperate. For indwelling catheters, attention is given to maintaining continuous free drainage and to the increased possibility of infection. Frequent washing of the area surrounding the urinary meatus reduces the risk of infection and eliminates unpleasant odors and irritation. Kinds of catheterization are **cardiac catheterization, hepatic vein catheterization,** and **laryngeal catheterization.** See also **female catheterization, Foley catheter, male catheterization.** –**catheterize,** *v.*

cathexis /kəthek′sis/, the conscious or unconscious attachment of emotional feeling and importance to a specific idea, person, or object. –**cathectic,** *adj.*

cathode, the electrode at which reduction occurs.

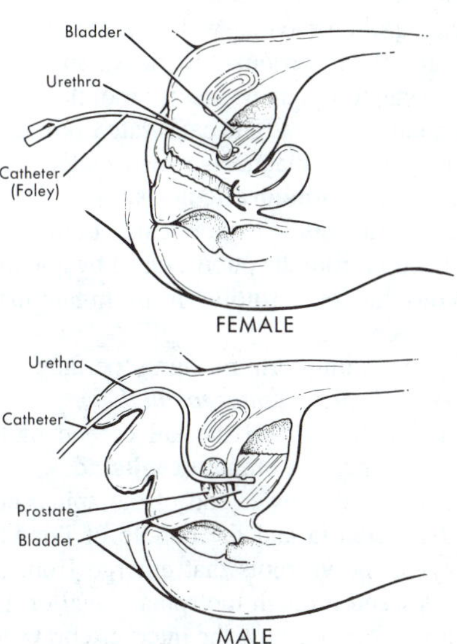

Catheterization (urethral)

cathode ray, a stream of electrons emitted by the negative electrode of a gaseous discharge device when the cathode is bombarded by positive ions, as in a cathode ray tube, an oscilloscope, or a television picture tube. The ray itself is usually focused by a series of electromagnets that control its direction and position on a screen coated with a phosphor to create a visible pattern.

cathode ray oscilloscope, an instrument that produces a visual representation of electric variations by means of the fluorescent screen of a cathode ray tube. Oscilloscopes have many applications in medicine and in nursing, as the displaying of patients' brain waves and heart beats for monitoring and diagnostic purposes.

cathode ray tube (CRT), a vacuum tube that focuses a beam of electrons onto a spot on a screen coated with a phosphor, creating a visible image of information on the face of the tube. The CRT provides a means for representing graphically data processed by a computer.

cation /kat′ī·on/, a positively charged ion that in solution is attracted to the negative electrode. Compare **anion.**

cation-exchange resin, any one of various insoluble organic polymers with high molecular weights that exchange their cations for other ions in solution. Cation-exchange resins are used especially to restrict intestinal sodium absorption in patients with edema. Compare **anion-exchange resin.**

catling, a long, sharp, double-edged knife used in amputation. Also called **catlin.**

catoptric /kətop′trik/, of or pertaining to a reflected image or reflected light, as from a mirror.

CAT scan. See **computerized axial tomography.**

cat scratch fever, a disease that results from the scratch or bite of a healthy cat. Inflammation and pustules are found on the scratched skin, and lymph nodes in the neck, head, groin, or axilla swell 2 weeks later. Although patients are seldom seriously ill, fever and malaise may occur and symptoms can persist for months. Tetracycline may aid rapid recovery. The cat scratch skin test is available to help in the diagnosis. Also called **cat scratch disease, benign lymphoreticulosis.**

cat's eye amaurosis, a monocular blindness, with a bright reflection from the pupil caused by a white mass in the vitreous humor resulting from inflammation or a malignant lesion.

caud-, a combining form meaning 'pertaining to a tail': *caudal, caudalward, caudocephalad.*

caudad /kô′dad/, toward the tail or end of the body, away from the head. Compare **cephalad.**

cauda equina, the lower end of the spinal cord at the first lumbar vertebra and the bundle of lumbar, sacral, and coccygeal nerve roots that emerge from the spinal cord and descend through the spinal canal of the sacrum and coccyx before reaching the intervertebral foramina of their particular vertebrae. The cauda equina looks like a horse's tail.

caudal, signifying a position toward the distal end of the spine.

caudal anesthesia, the injection of a local anesthetic agent into the caudal portion of the spinal canal through the sacrum. It is performed in labor and in such procedures as culdoscopy and anorectal and genitourinary surgery. Caudal anesthesia has largely been replaced by epidural anesthesia because of the difficulty of controlling the level of anesthesia, the need for large volumes (10 to 15 ml) of anesthetic solution, a high 5% to 10% rate of failure, frequent neurologic complications, arterial hypotension, and, in obstetrics, reduced force of labor. Other complications of caudal anesthesia include maternal infection and inadvertent injection into the fetus. See also **regional anesthesia.**

caudate, having a tail.

caudate process, a small elevation of tissue that extends obliquely from the lower extremity of the caudate lobe of the liver to the visceral surface of the right lobe. It separates the fossa for the gallbladder from the beginning of the fossa for the inferior vena cava.

caul, the intact amniotic sac surrounding the fetus at birth. The sac usually ruptures or is ruptured during the course of labor or delivery; when it remains intact, it must be torn or cut to allow the baby to breathe. In the past, pieces of the caul were sold to sailors as a good luck token that would protect the bearer from death by drowning.

cauliflower ear, a thickened, deformed ear caused by repeated trauma, as that suffered by boxers. Plastic surgery may be a means of restoring the normal appearance of the ear.

caumesthesia /kô′məsthē′zhə/, an abnormal condition in which a patient has a low temperature but experiences a sense of intense heat. **–caumesthetic,** *adj.*

causalgia /kôzal′jə/, a severe sensation of burning pain, often in an extremity, sometimes with local erythema of the skin. It is the result of injury to a peripheral sensory nerve.

causal hypothesis, (in research) a hypothesis that predicts a cause-and-effect relationship among the variables to be studied.

causal hypothesis testing study, (in nursing research) an experimental design used in testing a hypothesis that predicts a cause-and-effect relationship within the data to be studied.

causality, (in research) a relationship between one phenomenon or event (A) and another (B) in which A precedes and causes B and the direction of influence and the nature of the effect are predictable and reproducible and may be empirically observed. Causality is difficult to prove; some social scientists contend that it is impossible to prove a causal relationship.

causal treatment. See **treatment.**

causation, (in law) the existence of a reasonable connection between the misfeasance, malfeasance, or nonfeasance of the defendant and the injury or damage suffered by the plaintiff. In a lawsuit in which negligence is alleged the harm suffered by the plaintiff must be proven to result directly from the negligence of the defendant; causation must be demonstrated.

cause, any process, substance, or organism that produces an effect or condition.

CAUSN, abbreviation for **Canadian Association of University Schools of Nursing.**

caustic, **1.** any substance that is destructive to living tissue, as silver nitrate, nitric acid, or sulfuric acid. **2.** exerting a burning or corrosive effect.

CAUT, abbreviation for **Canadian Association of University Teachers.**

cautery /kô′tərē/, **1.** a device or agent that scars and burns the skin, as in the coagulation of tissue by heat or caustic substances. **2.** a destructive effect produced by a cauterizing agent.

cautery knife, a surgical knife that cuts tissue and cauterizes it to prevent bleeding. The knife is connected to an electric source that generates the heat necessary for cauterization.

cav-, a combining form meaning 'hollow': *cavascope, cavernome, cavity.*

cavalry bone. See **rider's bone.**

Cavell /kəvel′/, **Edith,** (1865–1915), an English nurse who trained at London Hospital. In 1907 she became the head of a nurses' training school in Brussels, with the task of raising nursing standards to match those of Britain. By 1912, the school offered a 3-year intensive course and was associated with four hospitals in Brussels. After the Germans occupied Belgium in World War I, she nursed or sheltered more than 200 fleeing soldiers and helped them reach Holland; to her, this was an extension of her nursing: helping those in need. She was arrested by the Germans, tried, and shot on October 12, 1915. Her execution, which she met with courage and fortitude, brought her widespread fame.

cavernoma. See **cavernous hemangioma.**

cavernous, containing cavities or hollow spaces. See also **cavernous hemangioma.**

cavernous angioma. See **cavernous hemangioma.**

cavernous body of the clitoris, cavernous body of the penis. See **corpus cavernosum.**

cavernous hemangioma, a benign, congenital tumor consisting of large, blood-filled, cystic spaces. The scalp, face, and neck are the most common sites, but these tumors have been found in the liver and other organs. Superficial cavernous hemangiomas are friable and easily infected if the skin is broken. Treatment includes observation, irradiation, sclerosing solutions, and surgery. Also called **angioma cavernosum, cavernoma.** Compare **capillary hemangioma, nevus flammeus.**

cavernous lymphangioma. See **lymphangioma cavernosum.**

cavernous rale, an abnormal hollow, metallic sound heard during auscultation of the thorax. It is caused by contraction and expansion of a pulmonary cavity during respiration and indicates a pathologic condition.

cavernous sinus, one of a pair of irregularly shaped, bilateral venous channels between the sphenoid bone of the skull and the dura mater. It is one of the five anterior inferior venous sinuses that drain the blood from the dura mater into the internal jugular vein. Like the other anterior inferior sinuses, the cavernous sinus has no valves. Coursing through the sinus are the oculomotor nerve, the trochlear nerve, the abducent nerve, the ophthalmic and the maxillary divisions of the trigeminal nerve, and the internal carotid artery. The cavernous sinus receives the superior and the inferior ophthalmic veins, some of the cerebral veins, and the sphenoparietal sinus, and joins the cavernous sinus from the opposite side through the intercavernous sinuses. The cavernous sinus drains into the inferior petrosal sinus, thence into the internal jugular vein.

cavernous sinus syndrome, an abnormal condition characterized by edema of the conjunctiva, the upper eyelid, and the root of the nose and by paralysis of the third, the fourth, and the sixth nerves. It is caused by a thrombosis of the cavernous sinus.

cavernous sinus thrombosis, a syndrome, usually secondary to infections near the eye or nose, characterized by orbital edema, venous congestion of the eye, and palsy of the nerves supplying the extraocular muscles. The infection may spread to involve the cerebrospinal fluid and meninges. Treatment is with antibiotics and, sometimes, with anticoagulants. Prevention includes avoidance of squeezing pimples and other skin lesions in the area of the nose and central face.

cavitary, **1.** denoting the presence of one or more cavities. **2.** any entozoon having a body cavity or an alimentary canal.

cavitate, the act of rapidly forming and collapsing vapor pockets or bubbles in a flowing fluid with low pressure areas, often causing damage to surrounding structures.

cavitation, **1.** the formation of cavities within the body, as those formed in the lung by tuberculosis. **2.** any cavity within the body, as the pleural cavities.

cavity, **1.** a hollow space within a larger structure, as the peritoneal cavity or the oral cavity. **2.** *nontechnical.* a space in a tooth formed by dental caries.

cavity classification, the taxonomy of carious lesions according to the tooth surfaces on which they occur, as labial, buccal, or occlusal; type of surface, as pitted or smooth; numeric designation of cavity type according to the classification proposed by G.V. Black. See also **artificial classification cavity.**

cavogram /kav′əgram′/, an angiogram of the inferior or superior vena cava.

cavosurface angle, (in dentistry) the angle formed by the junction of the wall of a prepared cavity with the external surface of the tooth.

cavosurface bevel, the incline of the cavosurface angle of a prepared tooth cavity wall relative to the enamel wall. Compare **bevel, contra bevel.**

cavum /kā′vəm/, *pl.* **cava,** **1.** any hollow or cavity. **2.** the inferior or superior vena cava.

Cb, symbol for **columbium.**

CBC, abbreviation for **complete blood count.**

CBF, abbreviation for *cerebral blood flow.*

CBS, abbreviation for **chronic brain syndrome.**

CCK, abbreviation for **cholecystokinin.**

CCU, abbreviation for **coronary care unit.**

Cd, symbol for **cadmium.**

CDC, abbreviation for **Centers for Disease Control.**

CDE, the major symbols used in one system for the nomenclature of the Rh system, in which D is the same as Rh_0, the major determining factor of Rh positivity.

Ce, symbol for **cerium.**

CEA, abbreviation for **carcinoembryonic antigen.**

ceasmic /sē·az′mik/, pertaining to or characterized by a persistent embryonic fissure or abnormal cleavage of parts.

ceasmic teratism, a congenital anomaly, caused by developmental arrest, in which parts of the body that should be fused remain in their fissured embryonic state, as in cleft palate.

cec-, a combining form meaning 'pertaining to a cecum': *cecitis, cecectomy, cecoplication.*

cecal /sē′kəl/, **1.** of or pertaining to the cecum. **2.** of or pertaining to the optic disc or the blind spot in the retina. Also spelled **caecal.**

cecal appendix. See **vermiform appendix.**

Ceclor, a trademark for a cephalosporin antibiotic (cefaclor).

cecocolostomy /sē′kōkəlos′təmē/, **1.** a surgical operation that creates an anastomosis between the cecum and the colon. **2.** the anastomosis produced by this operation.

cecofixation. See **cecopexy.**

cecoileostomy /sē′kō•il′ē•os′təmē/, a surgical operation that connects the ileum with the cecum. Also called **ileocecostomy** /il′ē•ōsēkos′təmē/.

cecopexy /sē′kōpek′sē/, a surgical operation that fixes or suspends the cecum to correct its excessive mobility. Also called **cecofixation.**

cecostomy /sēkos′təmē/, the surgical construction of an opening into the cecum, performed as a temporary measure to relieve intestinal obstruction in a patient who cannot tolerate major surgery. Twenty-four hours before surgery, if time permits, a low residue diet is given, with only clear liquids allowed. Cleansing enemas and antibiotics are prescribed to reduce the number of bacteria in the bowel. IV fluids and electrolytes are given, and a nasointestinal tube is inserted. With the patient under local anesthesia, a tube is inserted into the cecum to allow drainage of feces. The procedure may also be done to decompress the large bowel and prevent distention until peristalsis is restored after intestinal surgery. Postoperatively, the tube is connected to a drainage bottle. The nurse irrigates the cecostomy tube with saline solution as necessary, allowing the solution to flow in and out by gravity, if possible. Frequent changes of dressings are needed to keep the skin clean and dry. An ileostomy bag may be used. When edema and inflammation have subsided, the obstruction (usually cancer) is resected, the healthy sections of bowel reconnected, and the cecostomy closed. See also **abdominal surgery, intestinal obstruction.**

cecum /sē′kəm/, a cul-de-sac constituting the first part of the large intestine.

Cedilanid-D, a trademark for a cardiotonic (deslanoside).

CeeNU, a trademark for an antineoplastic (lomustine).

cefaclor, a cephalosporin antibiotic.

■ INDICATIONS: It is prescribed in the treatment of certain infections.

■ CONTRAINDICATIONS: Known hypersensitivity to cephalosporins prohibits its use. It is administered with caution to patients who have a history of allergy to penicillin.

■ ADVERSE EFFECTS: Among the most serious adverse reactions are hypersensitivity reactions and severe diarrhea, nausea, and vomiting.

cefadroxil monohydrate, a cephalosporin antibiotic.

■ INDICATIONS: It is prescribed in the treatment of certain bacterial infections.

■ CONTRAINDICATIONS: Known hypersensitivity to cephalosporins prohibits its use. It is administered with caution to patients with a history of allergy to penicillins.

■ ADVERSE EFFECTS: Among the most serious adverse reactions are hypersensitivity reactions and severe diarrhea, nausea, and vomiting.

Cefadyl, a trademark for an antibiotic (cephapirin).

cefamandole naffate, a cephalosporin antibiotic.

■ INDICATIONS: It is prescribed in the treatment of certain bacterial infections.

■ CONTRAINDICATIONS: Known hypersensitivity to cephalosporins prohibits its use. It is administered with caution to patients who have a history of allergy to penicillin.

■ ADVERSE EFFECTS: Among the most serious adverse reactions are various hypersensitivity reactions, phlebitis, suprainfection, and pain on intramuscular injection.

cefazolin sodium, a cephalosporin antibacterial.

■ INDICATIONS: It is prescribed in the treatment of a variety of infections.

■ CONTRAINDICATIONS: Known hypersensitivity to this drug or to any cephalosporin medication prohibits its use. It is used with caution in patients who are allergic to penicillin.

■ ADVERSE EFFECTS: Among the more serious adverse reactions are pain at the site of injection and hypersensitivity reactions.

Cefizox, a trademark for a cephalosporin antibiotic (ceftizoxime).

Cefobid, a trademark for a cephalosporin antibiotic (cefoperazone).

cefoperazone sodium, a cephalosporin antibiotic.

■ INDICATIONS: It is prescribed in the treatment of respiratory tract, intraabdominal, skin, and female genital tract infections and bacterial septicemia.

■ CONTRAINDICATIONS: Hypersensitvity to the cephalosporins or known sensitivity to this drug prohibits its use.

■ ADVERSE EFFECTS: Among the most serious adverse reactions are pruritus, urticaria, transient eosinophilia, neutropenia, and injection site reactions.

cefotaxime sodium, a cephalosporin antibiotic.

■ INDICATIONS: It is prescribed for lower respiratory tract, genitourinary, gynecologic, intraabdominal, skin, bone and joint, and central nervous system infections and bacterial septicemia caused by susceptible strains of microorganisms.

■ CONTRAINDICATIONS: Hypersensitivity to the cephalosporins or known hypersensitivity to this drug prohibits its use.

■ ADVERSE EFFECTS: The most serious adverse reactions are pruritus, colitis, fungal infections, and injection site reactions.

cefoxitin sodium, a cephalosporin antibiotic.

■ INDICATIONS: It is prescribed in the treatment of certain bacterial infections.

■ CONTRAINDICATIONS: Known hypersensitivity to cephalosporins prohibits its use. It is administered with caution to patients who have a history of allergy to penicillin.

■ ADVERSE EFFECTS: Among the most serious adverse

reactions are various hypersensitivity reactions, phlebitis, suprainfection, and pain on intramuscular injection.

ceftizoxime sodium, a cephalosporin antibiotic.

■ INDICATIONS: It is prescribed in the treatment of several bacterial infections.

■ CONTRAINDICATIONS: Known sensitivity to this drug prohibits its use. It is administered with caution to patients who are allergic to penicillin.

■ ADVERSE EFFECTS: Among the most serious adverse reactions are hypersensitivity reactions, neutropenia, leukopenia, thrombocytopenia, and pain at the injection site.

cefuroxime sodium, a cephalosporin antibiotic.

■ INDICATIONS: It is prescribed in the treatment of lower respiratory tract, urinary tract, skin, and gonococcal infections, bacterial septicemia, meningitis, and for the prevention of postoperative infections.

■ CONTRAINDICATIONS: Hypersensitivity to the cephalosporins or known sensitivity to this drug prohibits its use.

■ ADVERSE EFFECTS: Among the most serious adverse reactions are pruritus, urticaria, transient eosinophilia, neutropenia, leukopenia, and injection site reactions.

cel-, coel-, **1.** a combining form meaning 'a cavity of the body': *celarium, celoschisis, celozoic*. **2.** a combining form meaning 'a swelling or tumor, hernia': *celectome, celology, celosomia*.

-cele, a combining form meaning a 'tumor or swelling': *hematoscheocele, oodeocele, tracheocele*.

-cele, -coel, -coele a combining form meaning a 'cavity': *paracele, orchidocele, syringocele*.

Celestone, a trademark for a glucocorticoid (betamethasone).

celiac artery, a thick visceral branch of the abdominal aorta, arising caudal to the diaphragm, usually dividing into the left gastric, the common hepatic, and the splenic arteries.

celiac disease, an inborn error of metabolism characterized by the inability to hydrolyze peptides contained in gluten. The disease affects adults and young children, who suffer from abdominal distention, vomiting, diarrhea, muscle wasting, and extreme lethargy. A characteristic sign is a pale, foul-smelling stool that floats on water because of its high fat content. There may be a secondary lactose intolerance, and it may become necessary to eliminate all milk products from the diet. Most patients respond well to a high-protein, high-calorie, gluten-free diet. Rice and corn are good substitutes for wheat, and any vitamin or mineral deficiencies can be corrected with oral preparations. Prognosis for full recovery is excellent. Failure to respond generally indicates misdiagnosis. Also called **celiac sprue, gluten-induced enteropathy, nontropical sprue.** Compare **malabsorption syndrome.**

celiac plexus. See **solar plexus.**

celiac rickets, arrested growth and osseous deformities resulting from malabsorption of fat and calcium. See also **celiac disease, rickets.**

celio-, a combining form meaning 'pertaining to the abdomen': *celioma, celiopathy, celiorrhaphy*.

celiocolpotomy /sē'lē·ōkəlpot'əmē/, an incision into the abdomen through the vagina.

celioma /sēlē·ō'mə/, *pl.* **celiomas, celiomata,** an abdominal neoplasm, especially a mesothelial tumor of the peritoneum.

celioscope. See **laparoscope.**

celiothelioma /sē'lē·ōthē'lē·ō'mə/, *pl.* **celiotheliomas, celiotheliomata,** a mesothelioma of the abdomen.

cell, the fundamental unit of all living tissue. Eukaryotic cells consist of a nucleus, cytoplasm, and organelles surrounded by a cytoplasmic membrane. Within the nucleus are the nucleolus (containing RNA) and chromatin granules (containing protein and DNA) which develop into chromosomes, the determinants of hereditary characteristics. Organelles within the cytoplasm include the endoplasmic reticulum, ribosomes, the Golgi complex, mitochondria, lysosomes, and the centrosome. Prokaryotic cells are similar, but lack a nucleus. The specialized nature of body tissue reflects the specialized structure and function of its constituent cells. See also **cell theory.**

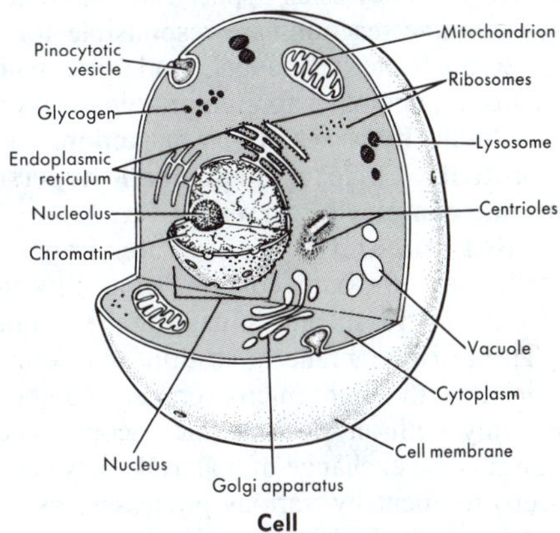

Cell

cella /sel'ə/, *pl.* **cellae,** an enclosed space.

cell biology, the science that deals with the structures, living processes, and functions of cells, especially human cells.

cell body, the part of a cell that contains the nucleus and surrounding cytoplasm exclusive of any projections or processes, as the axon and dendrites of a neuron or the tail of a spermatozoon. This enlarged area is concerned more with the metabolism of the cell than with a specific function.

cell death, **1.** terminal failure of a cell to maintain the essential life functions. **2.** the point in the process of dying at which vital functions have ceased at the cellular level.

cell division, the continuous process by which a cell divides in four stages; prophase, metaphase, anaphase, and telophase. Preliminary to prophase, the centrosome of the cell divides into two parts, which become oriented at opposite poles of the nucleus. During the prophase, previously dispersed chromatin condenses into chromomeres strung along a threadlike chromonema composed of deoxyribonucleic acid. The chromonema then condenses into compact chromosomes. During metaphase, the chromosomes become oriented in the equatorial plane with a clear area directed toward the two centrosomes. Each chromosome meanwhile has doubled into chromatids attached to each other at the centromere. Each centromere divides during late metaphase and early anaphase. In telophase, the chromosomes form a compact mass, lose their individuality, and disperse into the chromatin of the intermitotic nucleus. Cell division does not occur in discrete steps; each phase is part of a continuous process that may require hours to complete. The cycle of cell division includes an interphase period during which new DNA, RNA, and protein molecules are synthesized before the start of the next prophase. Also called **mitosis.** Compare **meiosis.**

cell line, a colony of animal cells developed as a subculture from a primary culture.

cell-mediated immune response, a delayed type IV hypersensitivity reaction, mediated primarily by sensitized T cell lymphocytes as opposed to antibodies. Cell-mediated immune reactions are responsible for defense against certain bacterial, fungal, and viral pathogens, malignant cells, and other foreign protein or tissue. Also called **cellular hypersensitivity reaction, type IV hypersensitivity.** Compare **anaphylactic hypersensitivity, immune complex hypersensitivity.**

cell-mediated immunity. See **cellular immunity.**

cell membrane, the outer covering of a cell, often having projecting microvilli and containing the cellular cytoplasm. The cell membrane is so thin and delicate it is barely visible with a light microscope and can be studied in detail only with an electron microscope. The membrane controls the exchange of materials between the cell and its environment by various processes, as osmosis, phagocytosis, pinocytosis, and secretion. Also called **plasma membrane.**

cell theory, the proposition that cells are the basic units of all living substance and that cellular function is the essential process of life.

cellular hypersensitivity reaction. See **cell-mediated immune response.**

cellular immunity, the mechanism of acquired immunity characterized by the dominant role of small T cell lymphocytes. Cellular immunity is involved in resistance to infectious diseases caused by viruses and some bacteria, in delayed hypersensitivity reactions, some aspects of resistance to cancer, certain autoimmune diseases, graft rejection, and certain allergies. Also called **cell-mediated immunity.** Compare **humoral immunity.**

cellular infiltration, the migration and grouping of cells within tissues throughout the body.

cellulitis, an infection of the skin characterized most commonly by local heat, redness, pain, and swelling, and occasionally by fever, malaise, chills, and headache. Abscess and tissue destruction usually follow if antibiotics are not taken. Damaged skin, poor circulation, and diabetes mellitus favor the development of cellulitis. Treatment in addition to appropriate antibiotics includes warm soaks and avoidance of pressure to the affected areas.

cellulose /sel′yo͞olōs/, a colorless, insoluble, nondigestible, transparent solid carbohydrate that is the primary constituent of the skeletal substances of the cell walls of plants. In the diet it provides the bulk necessary for proper GI functioning. Rich sources are fruits, as apples and bananas, and legumes, bran, and green vegetables, especially celery. See also **dietary fiber.**

cell wall, the structure that covers and protects the cell membrane in some kinds of cells, as certain bacteria and all plant cells. The cell walls of plant cells are composed of cellulose.

celom. See **coelom.**

Celontin, a trademark for an anticonvulsant (methsuximide).

celosomia /sē′ləsō′mē·ə/, a congenital malformation characterized by a fissure or absence of the sternum and ribs and protrusion of the viscera.

celosomus /sē′ləsō′məs/, a fetus with celosomia.

celothelioma. See **mesothelioma.**

Celsius (C) /sel′sē·əs/, denoting a temperature scale in which 0° is the freezing point of water and 100° is the boiling point of water at sea level. Also called **centigrade.** Compare **Fahrenheit.**

cement, **1.** a sticky or mucilaginous substance that helps neighboring tissue cells stick together. **2.** any of a variety of dental materials used to fill cavities or to hold bridgework or other dental prostheses in place. **3.** a material used in the fixation of a prosthetic joint in adjacent bone, as methyl mathacrylate.

cemental fiber, any one of the many fibers of the periodontal membrane that extend from the cementum to the intermediate plexus, where their terminations are mixed with those of the alveolar fibers.

cement base, (in dentistry) a layer of insulated dental cement, sometimes medicated, pressed into the bottom of a prepared cavity to protect the pulp, to reduce the bulk of metallic restoration, or eliminate undercuts in a tapered preparation.

cementifying fibroma, **1.** an intrabony lesion that is not associated with the teeth, composed of fibrous connective tissue enclosing foci of calcified material resembling cementum. **2.** a rare odontogenic tumor composed of varying amounts of fibrous connective tissue resembling cementum. **3.** a central lesion of the jaws.

cementoblastoma /simen′tōblastō′mə/, *pl.* **cementoblastomas, cementoblastomata,** an odontogenic fibrous tumor consisting of cells developing into cementoblasts but containing only a small amount of calcified tissue.

cementoma /sē′mentō′mə/, *pl.* **cementomas, cementomata,** an accumulation of cementum existing free at the apex of a tooth, probably caused by trauma rather than neoplastic growth.

cementopathia, an abnormal condition of the teeth caused by necrotic cementum and insufficient cementogenesis. Cementopathia is implicated in periodontitis and periodontosis.

cementum, the bonelike connective tissue that covers the roots of the teeth and helps to support them.

cen, abbreviation for **centromere.**

cen-, a combining form meaning 'common': *cenadelphus, cenesthesia, cenesthopathia.*

cenesthesia /sē′nesthē′zhə/, the general sense of existing, derived as the aggregate of all the various stimuli and reactions throughout the body at any specific moment to produce a feeling of health or of illness. Also called **cenesthesis, coenesthesis.**

ceno-, a combining form meaning 'new': *cenogenesis, cenophobia, cenopsychic.*

cenogenesis, the development of structural characteristics that are absent in earlier forms of a species, as an adaptive response to environmental conditions. Also spelled **coenogenesis, caenogenesis, kenogenesis.** Compare **palingenesis.** **–cenogenetic, coenogenetic, caenogenetic,** *adj.*

cenophobia. See **kenophobia.**

censor, **1.** a person who monitors or evaluates books, newspapers, plays, works of art, speech, or other means of expression in order to suppress certain kinds of information. **2.** (in psychoanalysis) a psychic suppression that allows unconscious thoughts to rise to consciousness only if they are heavily disguised.

cente-, a combining form meaning 'puncture': *centesis.*

center, **1.** the middle point of the body or geometric entity, equidistant from points on the periphery. **2.** a group of neurons with a common function, as the accelerating center in the brain that controls the heartbeat. Also spelled *(chiefly British)* **centre.**

Centers for Disease Control (CDC), a federal agency of the U.S. government that provides facilities and services for the investigation, identification, prevention, and control of disease. It is concerned with all aspects of the epidemiology and the laboratory diagnosis of disease. Immunization programs, quarantine regulations and programs, laboratory standards, and community surveillance for disease are among the activities of the CDC, which is located in Atlanta. Many state and local health workers and scientists receive training in specific techniques there. Formerly, the Communicable Disease Center, it was concerned only with communicable diseases; today its interests include environmental health, smoking, malnutrition, poisoning, and issues in occupational health.

centesis /sentē′sis/, a perforation or a puncture, as a paracentesis, abdominocentesis, or thoracocentesis.

centi-, a combining form meaning 'a hundred or a hundredth': *centibar, centiliter, centipoise.*

centigrade. See **Celsius.**

centimeter (cm) /sen′timē′tər/, the metric unit of measurement equal to one hundredth of a meter, or 0.3937 inches.

centimeter-gram-second system (cgs, CGS), the internationally accepted scientific system of expressing length, mass, and time in basic units of centimeters, grams, and seconds. The CGS system is gradually being replaced by the Système International d'Unités (SI) or the International System of Units based on the meter, kilogram, and second.

centipede bite, a wound produced by the poison claws and the first body segment of a centipede, an elongate arthropod with many pairs of legs. The bite of a few species, including *Scolopendra morsitans* in the southern United States, may cause painful local inflammation, fever, headache, vomiting, and dizziness.

central, pertaining to or situated at a center.

central amaurosis, blindness caused by a disease of the central nervous system.

central canal of spinal cord, the conduit that runs the entire length of the spinal cord and contains most of the 140 ml of cerebrospinal fluid in the body of the average individual. The central canal of the spinal cord lies in the center of the cord between the ventral and the dorsal gray commissures and extends cranialward into the medulla oblongata where it opens into the fourth ventricle of the brain. Caudalward, the canal runs into the filum terminale after forming a triangular, fusiform dilatation about 10 mm long in the conus medullaris. Cerebrospinal fluid flows into the canal from the fourth ventricle of the brain, into the subarachnoid space around the spinal cord, and into the subarachnoid space around the brain. Subarachnoid hemorrhage may form blood clots that block drainage of the cerebrospinal fluid from the subarachnoid space. Lumbar puncture, often performed to obtain samples of cerebrospinal fluid for diagnostic purposes, draws fluid from the subarachnoid space around the spinal cord and not from the central canal. See also **lumbar puncture.**

central chondrosarcoma, a malignant cartilaginous tumor that forms inside a bone. Also called **enchondrosarcoma.**

central fissure. See **central sulcus.**

central implantation. See **superficial implantation.**

central lobe, one of the lobes constituting each of the cerebral hemispheres, lying hidden in the depths of the lateral sulcus. The central lobe can be seen only if the lips of the sulcus are parted or cut away. The lips of the lateral sulcus are parts of the frontal, the parietal, and the temporal lobes and are separated by the rami of the lateral sulcus, thus constituting the frontal, the parietal, and the temporal opercula. With the opercula cut away, the insula appears as a triangular area with the limen insulae as the apex. Also called **island of Reil.** Compare **frontal lobe, occipital lobe, parietal lobe, temporal lobe.**

central nervous system (CNS), one of the two main divisions of the nervous system of the body, consisting of the brain and the spinal cord. The central nervous system processes information to and from the peripheral nervous system and is the main network of coordination and control for the entire body. The brain controls many functions and sensations, as sleep, sexual activity, muscular movement, hunger, thirst, memory, and the emotions. The spinal cord extends various types of nerve fibers from the brain and acts as a switching and relay terminal for the peripheral nervous system. The 12 pairs of cranial nerves emerge directly from the brain. Sensory nerves and motor nerves of the peripheral system leave the spinal cord separately between the vertebrae but unite to form 31 pairs of spinal nerves containing sensory fibers and motor fibers. More than 10 billion neurons constitute but one tenth of the brain cells, the other cells consisting of neuroglia. The neurons and the neuroglia form the soft, jellylike substance of the brain, which is supported and protected by the skull. Flowing through various cavities of the central nervous system, as the ventricles of the brain, the subarachnoid spaces of the brain and spinal cord, and the central canal of the spinal cord is the cerebrospinal fluid. This fluid helps to protect surrounding structures and affects the rate of respiration through changes in its content of carbon dioxide. The brain and the spinal cord are composed of gray matter and white matter. The gray matter contains primarily nerve cells and associated processes; the white matter consists of bundles of predominantly myelinated nerve fibers. The central nervous system develops from the embryonic neural tube, which first appears as the neural fold in the third week of pregnancy. The cavity of the neural tube is retained after birth in the ventricles of the brain and in the central canal of the spinal cord. Compare **peripheral nervous system.** See also **brain, spinal cord.**

central nervous system depressant, any drug that decreases the function of the central nervous system, as alcohol, barbiturates, and hypnotics. Such drugs can produce tolerance, physical dependence, and compulsive drug use. The compulsive use of barbiturates, benzodiazepines, and related drugs varies greatly and is believed to exceed that of the opiates. Depressants, especially the benzodiazepines, are the most widely prescribed drugs throughout the world. These substances depress excitable tissue throughout the central nervous system by stabilizing neuronal membranes, decreasing the amount of transmitter released by the nerve impulse, and generally depressing postsynaptic responsiveness and ion movement. The central nervous system is more affected by alcohol than any other body system, with effects generally proportional to the concentration of alcohol in the blood. Central nervous system depressants elevate the seizure threshold and can produce physical dependence in a relatively short period of time. All depressants are subject to abuse, particularly through the use of illicitly procured depressants. The most abused depressants are the short-acting barbiturates, especially pentobarbital, secobarbital, glutethimide, methyprylon, and methaqualone. These substances have popular street names on the illicit market, as "reds" (secobarbital) and "yellows" (pentobarbital). Sudden withdrawal of general central nervous system depressants that have been used in high doses for prolonged periods can be fatal to some individuals. Withdrawal treatment commonly involves the substitution of pentobarbital administered orally to produce a stabilization level followed by gradual reduction in dosage for a period of 10 days to 3 weeks.

central nervous system stimulant, a substance that quickens the activity of the central nervous system by increasing the rate of neuronal discharge or by blocking an inhibitory neurotransmitter. Many natural and synthetic compounds stimulate the central nervous system but only a few are used therapeutically. Caffeine, a potent central nervous system stimulant, is used to help restore mental alertness and overcome respiratory depression, but it may cause nausea, nervousness, tinnitus, tremor, tachycardia, extra systoles, diuresis, and visual disturbances. Amphetamines, sympathomimetic amines with central nervous system stimulating activity, are employed in treating narcolepsy and obesity, but these drugs have a high potential for abuse and may cause dizziness, restlessness, tachycardia, increased blood pressure, headache, mouth dryness, an unpleasant taste, GI symptoms, and urticaria. Various amphetamines, especially methylphenidate, and deanol acetamidobenzoate, a precursor of acetylcholine, are prescribed for the hyperkinetic child syndrome because central nervous system stimulants may act as depressants on children. Doxapram, ethamivan, and nikethamide are used to stimulate the respiratory center and restore consciousness after anesthesia or in the treatment of acute sedative-hypnotic intoxication. Flurothyl is employed in convulsive therapy in psychiatry. Also called **analeptic.**

central nervous system syndrome (CNS syndrome), a constellation of neurologic and emotional signs and symptoms that results from a massive whole-body dosage of radiation. The syndrome includes hysteria and disorientation, increasing during the last 24 to 48 hours before death.

central nervous system tumor, a neoplasm of the brain or spinal cord that characteristically does not spread beyond the cerebrospinal axis, although it may be highly invasive locally and have widespread effects on body functions. Intracranial neoplasms are about four times more common than those arising in the spinal cord. From 20% to 40% of brain tumors are metastatic lesions from primary cancer in the breast, lung, GI tract, kidney, or a site of melanoma. See also **brain tumor, spinal cord tumor.**

central neuritis. See **parenchymatous neuritis.**

central neurogenic hyperventilation (CNHV), a pattern of breathing marked by rapid and regular respirations at a rate of about 25 per minute. Increasing regularity, rather than rate, is an important diagnostic sign as it indicates an increasing depth of coma.

central placenta previa, placenta previa in which the placenta is implanted in the lower segment of the uterus and completely covers the internal os of the uterine cer-

vix. In labor, as the cervix dilates, the placenta is gradually separated from the underlying blood vessels in the uterine lining, resulting in bleeding that usually begins slowly, is painless, and progresses to hemorrhage that is life-threatening to the mother and the baby. Cesarean section is usually performed to save the mother and the baby. The condition may be discovered before any bleeding occurs by ultrasound visualization or by digital palpation in the normal course of prenatal care. See also **placenta previa.**

central processing unit (cpu, CPU), a component of a computer that controls the encoding and execution of instructions, consisting mainly of an arithmetic unit, which performs arithmetic functions, and an internal memory, which controls the sequencing of operations. Also called **processor.**

central ray (CR), the portion of the x-ray beam that is directed toward the center of the film or of the object being radiographed.

central scotoma, an area of blindness or site of depressed vision involving the macula of the retina.

central stimulant. See **central nervous system stimulant.**

central sulcus, a cleft separating the frontal from the parietal lobes of brain. Also called **central fissure, fissure of Rolando.**

central venous pressure (CVP) monitor, a device for measuring and recording the venous blood pressure by means of an indwelling catheter and a pressure manometer. It is used to evaluate the right ventricular function, the right atrial filling pressure, and the capacity of the blood vessels.

central venous return, the blood from the venous system that flows into the right atrium through the vena cava.

central vision, vision that results from images falling on the macula of the retina.

Centrax, a trademark for an antianxiety agent (prazepam).

centrencephalic /sen′trensifal′ik/, of, pertaining to, or involving the center of the encephalon.

centri-. See **centro-.**

centrifugal /sentrif′o͞ogəl/, **1.** denoting a force that is directed outward, away from a central point or axis, as the force that keeps the moon in its orbit around the earth. **2.** a direction away from the head.

centrifugal analyzer, equipment that uses centrifugal force to mix the sample aliquot with reagent and a spinning rotor to pass the reaction mixture through a detector.

centrifugal current, an electric current in the body with the positive pole near the nerve center and the negative pole at the periphery. Also called **descending current.**

centrifuge /sen′trifyo͞oj′/, a device for separating components of different densities contained in liquid by spinning them at high speeds. Centrifugal force causes the heavier components to move to one part of the container, leaving the lighter substances in another. –**centrifugal,** *adj.*, **centrifuge,** *v.*

centrilobular /sen′trəlob′yələr/, pertaining to, or situated at the center of a lobule.

centriole /sen′trē·ōl′/, an intracellular organelle, usually as a component of the centrosome. Often occurring in pairs, centrioles are associated with cell division and can be closely studied only with an electron microscope; under light microscope the centrioles appear as tiny dots. They are actually tiny cylinders positioned at right angles to each other, with walls consisting of nine bundles of fine tubules, three tubules to a bundle. The centriole measures approximately 150 nm by 300 nm to 500 nm. Numerous centrioles occur in some large cells, as the giant cells in bone marrow. The precise function of centrioles is still a mystery, but they appear to aid in the formation of the spindle that develops during mitosis.

centripetal /sentrip′ətəl/, **1.** denoting an afferent direction, as that of a sensory nerve impulse traveling toward the brain. **2.** denoting the direction of a force pulling an object toward an axis of rotation or constraining an object to a specific curved path.

centripetal current, an electric current passing through the body from a peripheral positive electrode to a negative pole near the nerve center. Also called **ascending current.**

centro-, centri-, a combining form meaning 'center': *centrocecal, centrocinesia, centrosclerosis.*

centromere /sen′trəmir/, the specialized, constricted region of the chromosome that joins the two chromatids to each other and attaches to the spindle fiber in mitosis and meiosis. During cell division the centromeres split longitudinally, half going to each of the new daughter chromosomes. The position of the centromere is constant for a specific chromosome and is identified accordingly as acrocentric, metacentric, submetacentric, or telocentric. Also called **kinetochore, kinomere, primary constriction.** –**centromeric,** *adj.*

centrosome, a self-propagating cytoplasmic organelle present in animal cells and in those of some lower plants. The structure, which consists of the centrosphere and the centrioles, is located near the nucleus and functions as the dynamic center of the cell, especially during mitosis. Also called **cytocentrum, microcentrum, paranuclear body.**

centrosphere, the differentiated, condensed area of cytoplasm surrounding the centrioles in the centrosome of the cell.

centrum, *pl.* **centra,** any kind of center, especially one related to a structure of the body, as the centrum semiovale of a cerebral hemisphere.

CEO, C.E.O., abbreviation for **Chief Executive Officer.**

cephal-. See **cephalo.**

cephalad /sef′əlad/, toward the head, away from the end, or tail. Compare **caudad.**

cephalalgia /sef′əlal′jə/, headache, often combined with another word to indicate a specific type of headache, as histamine cephalalgia. See also **histamine headache.**

cephalexin /sef′əlek′sin/, a cephalosporin antibacterial.

■ INDICATIONS: It is prescribed orally in the treatment of certain infections.

■ CONTRAINDICATIONS: Known hypersensitivity to this drug or to any cephalosporin medication prohibits its use. It is used with caution in patients who are allergic to penicillin.

■ ADVERSE EFFECTS: Nausea, diarrhea, and hypersensitivity reactions may occur.

cephalhematoma /sef′əlhē′mətō′mə, -hem′ətō′mə/, swelling caused by subcutaneous bleeding and accumulation of blood. It may begin to form in the scalp of a fetus during labor and enlarge slowly in the first few days after birth. It is usually a result of trauma, often from forceps. Large cephalhematomas may become infected, require surgical drainage, and take several months to resolve. Compare **caput succedaneum, molding.**

-cephalia, a combining form meaning '(condition of the) head': *hemicephalia, megacephalia, notancephalia.*

cephalic /sifal′ik/, of or pertaining to the head.

-cephalic, a combining form meaning 'relating to the head': *holocephalic, megalocephalic, postcephalic.*

cephalic presentation, a classification of fetal position in which the head of the fetus is at the uterine cervix. Cephalic presentation is usually further qualified by an indication of the part of the head presenting, as the occiput, bregma, or mentum.

cephalic vein, one of the four superficial veins of the upper limb. It begins in the dorsal venous network of the hand and winds upward to end in the axillary vein just caudal to the clavicle. It receives deoxygenated blood from the dorsal and the palmar surfaces of the forearm. Just distal to the antecubital fossa, it has a wide anastomosis with the median cubital vein. In the proximal third of the arm it passes between the pectoralis major and the deltoideus where it is accompanied by the thoracoacromial artery. Compare **basilic vein, dorsal digital vein, median antebrachial vein.**

cephalo-, cephal-, a combining form meaning 'pertaining to the head': *cephalocaudal, cephalocentesis, cephalogenesis.*

cephalomelus /sef′əlom′ələs/, a deformed individual with a structure resembling an arm or a leg protruding from the head.

cephalometry /sef′əlom′ətrē/, scientific measurement of the head, as that performed in dentistry to determine appropriate orthodontic procedures for correcting malocclusions and other abnormal conditions. **–cephalometric,** *adj.*

cephalopagus. See **craniopagus.**

cephalopelvic disproportion (CPD), an obstetric condition in which a baby's head is too large or a mother's birth canal too small to permit normal labor or birth. In **relative CPD,** the size of the baby's head is within normal limits but larger than average or the size of the mother's birth canal is within normal limits but smaller than average, or both; relative CPD is often overcome by molding of the head, the forces of labor, or by the use of forceps to effect delivery. In **absolute CPD,** the baby's head is markedly or abnormally enlarged or the mother's birth canal is markedly or abnormally contracted, making vaginal delivery impossible. See also **clinical pelvimetry, x-ray pelvimetry.**

cephaloridine, a cephalosporin antibiotic.

■ INDICATIONS: It is prescribed in the treatment of a variety of infections.

■ CONTRAINDICATIONS: Concurrent administration of medications causing nephrotoxicity or known hypersensitivity to this drug or to cephalosporin medication prohibits its use. It is used with caution in patients who are allergic to penicillin.

■ ADVERSE EFFECTS: Among the more serious adverse reactions are nephrotoxicity, pain at the site of injection, and hypersensitivity reactions.

cephalosporin /sef′əlōspôr′in/, a semisynthetic derivative of an antibiotic originally derived from the microorganism *Cephalosporium acremonium.* Cephalosporins are similar in structure to penicillins except for a beta-lactam-dihydrothiazine ring in place of beta-lactam-thiazolidin in penicillin.

cephalothin sodium /sef′əlōthin/, a cephalosporin antibacterial.

■ INDICATIONS: It is prescribed in the treatment of a variety of infections.

■ CONTRAINDICATIONS: Known hypersensitivity to this drug or to any cephalosporin medication prohibits its use. It is used with caution in patients who are allergic to penicillin.

■ ADVERSE EFFECTS: Among the more serious adverse reactions are pain at the site of injection and hypersensitivity reactions.

cephalothoracoiliopagus. See **synadelphus.**

cephalothoracopagus /sef′əlōthôr′əkop′əgəs/, a conjoined twin fetal monster united at the head, neck, and thorax.

-cephaly, -cephalia, a combining form meaning a '(specified) condition of the head': *macrencephaly, platycephaly, trochocephaly.*

cephapirin, an antibiotic.

■ INDICATIONS: It is prescribed in the treatment of infections caused by cephapirin-susceptible strains of a wide variety of microorganisms causing septicemia, endocarditis, osteomyelitis, and infections of the respiratory tract, urinary tract, and skin.

■ CONTRAINDICATION: Known sensitivity to cephalosporin antibiotics prohibits its use.

■ ADVERSE EFFECTS: Among the most serious adverse reactions are neutropenia, leukopenia, anemia, and allergic reactions.

cephradine, a cephalosporin antibacterial.

■ INDICATIONS: It is prescribed in the treatment of certain bacterial infections.

■ CONTRAINDICATIONS: Known hypersensitivity to this drug or to any cephalosporin medication prohibits its use. It is used with caution in patients who are allergic to penicillin.

■ ADVERSE EFFECTS: Nausea, diarrhea, and hypersensitivity reactions may occur.

cer-, a combining form meaning 'wax': *ceraceous, cerate, cerumen.*

ceramics, (in dentistry) the technology of making dental restorations from fused porcelain and other glasses.

cerato-, kerato-, a combining form meaning 'pertaining to the cornea or to horny tissue': *ceratocricoid, ceratohyal, ceratopharyngeus.*

cercaria /sərker′ē·ə/, *pl.* **cercariae,** a minute, wormlike early developmental form of trematode. It develops in a freshwater snail, is released into the water, and swims toward the sun, rising to the surface of the water in the warmest part of the day. Cercariae enter the body of the next host by ingestion, by direct invasion through the skin, or through a cut or other break in the skin. Some cercariae of the genera *Schistosoma, Chlonorchis, Paragonimus, Fasciolopsis,* and *Fasciola* are known to infect humans. They encyst and complete their development in various organs of the body. Each species tends to migrate to one organ, as *Fasciola hepatica,* which grows to become a liver fluke. See also **fluke, schistosomiasis.**

cerclage /serkläzh′/, **1.** an orthopedic procedure in which the ends of an oblique bone fracture or the chips of a broken patella are bound together with a wire loop or a metal band to hold the bone fragments in position until healed. **2.** a procedure in which a taut silicone band is applied around the sclera to restore contact between the retina and the choroid when the retina is detached. **3.** an obstetric procedure in which a nonabsorbable suture is used for holding the cervix closed to prevent spontaneous abortion in a woman who has an incompetent cervix. The band is usually released when the pregnancy is at full term to allow labor to begin. See also **incompetent cervix.**

cerea flexibilitas /sirē′ə flek′sibil′itas/, a cataleptic state, frequently observed in catatonic schizophrenia, in which the limbs retain for an indefinite period of time the positions in which they are placed. Also called **flexibilitas cerea, waxy flexibility.** See also **catalepsy.**

cerebellar /ser′əbel′ər/, of or pertaining to the cerebellum.

cerebellar angioblastoma, a tumor in the cerebellum composed of a mass of blood vessels. It may be cystic and is frequently associated with von Hippel-Lindau disease.

cerebellar cortex, the superficial gray matter of the cerebellum covering the white substance in the medullary core and consisting of two layers, an external molecular layer and an internal granule cell layer. The layers are separated by an incomplete stratum of Purkinje cells. Also called **cortical substance of cerebellum.**

cerebellar cortical degeneration. See **alcoholic nutritional cerebellar degeneration.**

cerebellar speech, abnormal speech seen in diseases of the cerebellum. It is characterized by slow, jerky, and slurred articulation that may be intermittent and explosive or monotonous and unvaried in pitch.

cerebellopontine /ser′əbel′ōpon′tīn/, leading from the cerebellum to the pons varolii.

cerebellospinal /ser′əbel′ōspī′nəl/, leading from the cerebellum to the spinal cord.

cerebellum /ser′əbel′əm/, *pl.* **cerebellums, cerebella,** the part of the brain located in the posterior cranial fossa behind the brainstem. It consists of two lateral cerebellar hemispheres, or lobes, and a middle section called the vermis. Three pairs of peduncles link it with the brainstem. Its functions are concerned with coordinating voluntary muscular activity.

cerebr-, a combining form meaning 'pertaining to the cerebrum': *cerebralgia, cerebrocardiac, cerebropathy.*

cerebral, of or pertaining to the cerebrum.

-cerebral, a combining form referring to the brain: *craniocerebral, medicerebral, postcerebral.*

cerebral aneurysm, an abnormal localized dilatation of a cerebral artery, most commonly the result of congenital weakness of the media or muscle layer of the vessel wall. Cerebral aneurysms may also be caused by infection, as subacute bacterial endocarditis or syphilis, and by neoplasms, arteriosclerosis, and trauma. The most frequent sites are the middle cerebral, internal carotid, basilar, and anterior cerebral arteries, especially at bifurcations of vessels. Cerebral aneurysms may occur in infancy or old age and may be fusiform dilatations of the entire circumference of an artery or saccular outcroppings of the side of a vessel, which may be as small as a pinhead or as large as an orange but are usually the size of a pea.

■ OBSERVATIONS: Depending on its size and site, a cerebral aneurysm may cause headache, drowsiness, confusion, vertigo, facial weakness and pain, tinnitus, visual impairment, neck stiffness, and monoplegia or hemiplegia. Because about half the cases of cerebral aneurysm rupture, the patient is closely monitored for signs of subarachnoid hemorrhage and increased intracranial pressure. Few aneurysms rupture that are less than 1 cm in diameter.

■ INTERVENTION: The patient is placed in a bed, in which the head is raised at a 45-degree angle, and is maintained in a quiet, darkened environment. Antifibrinolytic, analgesic, anticonvulsant, antiemetic, or antihypertensive medication, steroids, and parenteral fluids may be administered as ordered. The pulse, blood pressure, respiration, and neurologic status of the patient are checked frequently. Any sudden change in blood pressure or pupillary response is reported promptly. An icebag may be applied to relieve headache, and hypothermia or cooling measures may be indicated to reduce blood flow to the brain and decrease the risk of rupture of the aneurysm. The patient is turned gently every 2 to 4 hours and may need to be fed. Passive range of motion exercises to the extremities are performed to maintain function. A lumbar puncture, which can reveal rupture of the aneurysm if there is blood in the cerebrospinal fluid, and an angiogram, to show the site of the lesion, may be ordered; the contrast medium for angiography can be injected into the carotid artery, but placement in a femoral artery is preferred because there is less risk of dislodging a carotid plaque. Surgery, if indicated, involves a craniotomy and the application of a silver clip to the neck of the aneurysm or the use of an electric current to produce thrombosis. If the base of the aneurysm is too large to be ligated, a coating containing methyl methacrylate may be applied to support the weakened artery. When craniotomy is contraindicated, the neurosurgeon may apply a special clamp to a common carotid artery to reduce blood flow to the site of the aneurysm if collateral vessels can supply enough blood to maintain vital brain functions.

■ NURSING CONSIDERATIONS: The patient with a cerebral aneurysm requires intensive care and as little stress as possible. The nurse limits the number of visitors and the length of visits but involves the family in the patient's care and instructions. The patient is almost certain to be anxious about the possibility of rupture of the aneurysm and resultant neurologic problems. This concern may be anticipated by the nurse in order to help the patient express the fear and adapt to the situation.

cerebral angiography, an x-ray procedure for visualizing the vascular system of the brain by injecting a radiopaque contrast material into a carotid, subclavian, brachial, or femoral artery and taking x-rays at specific intervals in a series.

cerebral anoxia, a condition in which oxygen is deficient in brain tissue. This state, which is caused by circulatory failure, can exist for no more than 4 to 6 minutes before the onset of irreversible brain damage.

cerebral aqueduct, the narrow conduit, between the third and the fourth ventricles in the midbrain, that conveys the cerebrospinal fluid. Also called **aqueduct of Sylvius.**

cerebral cortex, a thin layer of gray matter on the surface of the cerebral hemisphere, folded into gyri with about two thirds of its area buried in fissures. It integrates higher mental functions, general movement, visceral functions, perception, and behavioral reactions. It has been classified many different ways, with reference according to supposed phylogenetic and ontogenetic differences, structure, cell, and fiber layers, and function areas. Research has described more than 200 areas on the basis of differences in myelinated fiber patterns and has defined 47 separate function areas with different cell designs. The precentral cortex or motor area has received special attention because its stimulation with electrodes causes voluntary muscle contractions. A motor speech area in the frontal operculum is better developed in the left hemisphere of right-handed persons, and its destruction causes motor aphasia or speech defects despite healthy, intact vocal organs. The surgical operation of lobotomy isolates the frontal area from the rest of the brain, especially the thalamus, and has been used in the treatment of severe psychoses. Stimulation of the frontal area affects circulation, respiration, pupillary reaction, and other visceral activity. Also called **pallium.**

cerebral dominance, the specialization of each of the two cerebral hemispheres in the integration and control of different functions. In 90% of the population, the left cerebral hemisphere specializes in or dominates the ability to speak and write and the ability to understand spoken and written words. The areas that control these activities are situated in the frontal, parietal, and temporal lobes of the left hemisphere. In the other 10% of the population, either the right hemisphere or both hemispheres dominate the speech and writing abilities. The right cerebral hemisphere dominates the integration of certain sounds other than those associated with speaking, as sounds of coughing, laughter, crying, and melodies. The right cerebral hemisphere perceives tactual stimuli and visual spatial relationships better than the left cerebral hemisphere. See also **Brodmann's areas.**

cerebral embolism, a cerebrovascular accident caused by an embolus that blocks the flow of blood through the vessels of the cerebrum, resulting in tissue ischemia distal to the occlusion. See also **cerebrovascular accident.**

cerebral gigantism, an abnormal condition characterized by excessive weight and size at birth, accelerated growth during the first 4 or 5 years after birth without any increase in the level of growth hormone, and then reversion to normal growth. Some typical signs of this condition are prognathism, antimongoloid slant, dolichocephalic skull, moderate mental retardation, and impaired coordination. Also called **Sotos' syndrome.**

cerebral hemiplegia, paralysis of one side of the body caused by a lesion in the brain.

cerebral hemisphere, one of the halves of the cerebrum. The two cerebral hemispheres are divided by a deep longitudinal fissure and are connected medially at the bottom of the fissure by the corpus callosum. Prominent grooves, subdividing each hemisphere into four major lobes, are the central sulcus, the lateral fissure, and the parietooccipital fissure. Each hemisphere also has a fifth major lobe deep in the brain. The central fissure separates the frontal lobe from the parietal lobe. The lateral fissure separates the temporal lobe, which lies below the fissure, from the frontal and parietal lobes, which lie above it. The parietooccipital fissure separates the occipital lobe from the two parietal lobes. The hemispheres consist of external gray substance, internal white substance, and internal gray substance and are covered by cerebral cortexes at the surface.

cerebral hemorrhage, a hemorrhage from a blood vessel in the brain. Three criteria used to classify cerebral hemorrhages are location (subarachnoid, extradural, subdural), the kind of vessel involved (arterial, venous, capillary), and origin (traumatic, degenerative). Each kind of cerebral hemorrhage has its own clinical characteristics. Most cerebral hemorrhages occur in the region of the basal ganglia and are caused by the rupture of a sclerotic artery as a result of hypertension. Other causes of rupture include congenital aneurysm, cerebrovascular infarction, and head trauma.

■ OBSERVATIONS: Bleeding may lead to displacement or destruction of brain tissue and to medullary anemia. Extensive hemorrhage is usually fatal. Recovery from the condition, which occurs more often in men than in women, may be complete. Depending on the extent and the location of the damaged tissue, residual effects may include aphasia, diminished mental function, or disturbance of the function of a special sense.

■ INTERVENTION: Lumbar puncture may reveal blood in the spinal fluid. A CAT scan may be performed to locate the lesion and to differentiate the hemorrhage from an embolus or thrombus, or cerebral angiography may be utilized for these purposes. Surgery is often necessary to stop the bleeding to prevent death from medullary anemia or from greatly increased intracranial pressure. The person is kept immobile, with the body in a position that assures adequate blood flow to and from the head. Physical therapy and speech therapy may be necessary during convalescence.

■ NURSING CONSIDERATIONS: Initially, bedside care is directed toward the prevention of recurrence and of the sequelae of prolonged immobility. Special care is taken in the positioning of the head of the patient to avoid flexion of the head or the neck, which might impair circulation to the brain. Fastidious skin care to prevent decubiti and emotional support are required to keep the person comfortable and calm. During convalescence the nurse may be called on to assist the patient in developing self-help capabilities. See also **subarachnoid hemorrhage.**

cerebral localization, **1.** the determination of various areas in the cerebral cortex associated with specific functions, as the 47 areas of Brodmann. **2.** the diagnosis of a cerebral condition, as a brain lesion, by determining the area of the brain affected, a determination made by analysis of the signs manifested by the patient and of electroencephalograms.

cerebral nerve. See **cranial nerve.**

cerebral palsy, a motor function disorder caused by a permanent, nonprogressive brain defect or lesion present at birth or shortly thereafter. The neurologic deficit may result in spastic hemiplegia, monoplegia, diplegia, or quadriplegia, athetosis or ataxia, seizures, paresthesia, varying degrees of mental retardation, and impaired speech, vision, and hearing. The disorder is usually associated with premature or abnormal birth and intrapartum asphyxia, causing damage to the nervous system. Abnormalities in breathing, sucking, swallowing, and responsiveness are usually apparent soon after birth, but the characteristic stiff, awkward movements of the infant's limbs may be overlooked for several months. Walking is usually delayed, and, when attempted, the child manifests a typical scissors gait. The arms may be affected only slightly, but the fingers are often spastic. Deep-tendon reflexes are exaggerated, and there may be slurred speech, delay in acquiring sphincter control, and athetotic movements of the face and hands. Early identification of the disorder facilitates the handling of palsied infants and the initiation of an exercise and training program. Treatment is individualized and may include the use of braces, surgical correction of deformities, speech therapy, and various indicated drugs, as muscle relaxants and anticonvulsants. Also called **congenital cerebral diplegia, Little's disease.**

cerebral tabes. See **general paresis.**

cerebral thrombosis, a clotting of blood in any cerebral vessel, as the middle cerebral artery or the ascending parietal artery.

cerebriform carcinoma. See **medullary carcinoma.**

cerebritis /ser′əbrī′tis/, *obsolete.* **1.** any inflammation of the cerebrum or brain. **2.** bacterial meningitis.

cerebrocerebellar atrophy, a deterioration of the cerebellum caused by certain abiotrophic diseases.

cerebroid /ser′əbroid/, resembling the substance of the brain.

cerebroma /ser′əbrō′mə/, *pl.* **cerebromas, cerebromata,** any unusual mass of brain tissue.

cerebromedullary tube. See **neural tube.**

cerebropathia psychia toxemia. See **Korsakoff's psychosis.**

cerebroretinal angiomatosis /ser′əbrōret′ənəl, sərē′brō-/, a hereditary disease characterized by congenital, tumorlike vascular nodules in the retina and cerebellum. Similar spinal cord lesions, cysts of the pancreas, kidneys, and other viscera, seizures, and mental retardation may be present. Also called **Lindau-von Hippel disease, retinocerebral angiomatosis, von Hippel-Lindau disease.**

cerebroside /ser′əbrōsīd′/, any of a group of glycolipids found in the brain and other tissue of the nervous system, especially the myelin sheath.

cerebrospinal /ser′əbrōspī′nəl, sərē′brō-/, pertaining to or involving the brain and the spinal cord.

cerebrospinal fluid (CSF), the fluid that flows through and protects the four ventricles of the brain, the subarachnoid space, and the spinal canal. It is composed mainly of secretions of the choroid plexi in the lateral ventricles and in the third and the fourth ventricles of the brain. Openings in the roof of the fourth ventricle allow the fluid to flow into the subarachnoid spaces around the brain and the spinal cord. The flow of fluid is from the blood in the choroid plexi, through the ventricles, the central canal, the subarachnoid spaces, and back into the blood. The volume of CSF in the average adult is about 140 ml, including about 23 ml in the ventricles and 117 ml in the subarachnoid spaces of the brain and the spinal cord. Changes in the carbon dioxide content of CSF affect the respiratory center in the medulla, helping to control breathing. A brain tumor may press against the cerebral aqueduct and shut off the flow of the fluid from the third to the fourth ventricle, resulting in an accumulation of fluid in the lateral and the third ventricles, called internal hydrocephalus. Other blockages of the flow of CSF, as those caused by blood clots, result in serious complications. Certain illnesses and various diagnoses may require microscopic examination and chemical analysis of CSF. Samples of the fluid may be removed by lumbar puncture between the third and the fourth lumbar vertebrae.

cerebrovascular /ser'əbrōvas'kyələr, sərē'brō-/, of or pertaining to the vascular system and blood supply of the brain.

cerebrovascular accident (CVA), an abnormal condition of the blood vessels of the brain characterized by occlusion by an embolus or cerebrovascular hemorrhage, resulting in ischemia of the brain tissues normally perfused by the damaged vessels. The sequelae of a cerebrovascular accident depend on the location and extent of ischemia. Paralysis, weakness, speech defect, aphasia, or death may occur. Symptoms remit somewhat after the first few days as brain swelling subsides. Physical therapy and speech therapy may restore much lost function.

cerebrum /ser'əbrəm, sərē'brəm/, *pl.* **cerebrums, cerebra,** the largest and uppermost section of the brain, divided by a central sulcus into the left and the right cerebral hemispheres. At the bottom of the groove, the hemispheres are connected by the corpus callosum. The internal structures of the hemispheres merge with those of the diencephalon and further communicate with the brain stem through the cerebral peduncles. Each cerebral hemisphere is composed of the extensive outer cerebral cortex with its gray substance, the underlying semiovale with its white substance, the internal basal ganglia, and certain centrally and medially located structures comprising the rhinencephalon. The surface of the cerebrum is convoluted and lobed, each lobe bearing the name of the bone under which it lies. The cerebrum performs sensory functions, motor functions, and less easily defined integration functions associated with various mental activities. It generates a variety of electric waves that may be recorded on an electroencephalogram to localize areas of brain dysfunction, to identify altered states of consciousness, or to establish brain death. Some of the other processes that are controlled or affected by the cerebrum are memory, speech, writing, and emotional response. See also **cerebral cortex.** –**cerebral,** *adj.*

cerium (Ce), a ductile, gray rare-earth element. Its atomic number is 58; its atomic weight is 140.13. A compound of cerium, cerium oxalate, is used as a sedative, an antiemetic, and an antitussive.

ceroid /sir'oid/, a golden, waxy pigment appearing in the cirrhotic livers of some individuals, in the GI tract, in the nervous system, and in the muscles. It is an insoluble, acid-fast, sudanophilic pigment.

ceroma /sirō'mə/, *pl.* **ceromas, ceromata,** a neoplasm that has undergone waxy degeneration.

certificate-of-need or -necessity, a statement or certificate issued by a governmental agency to the effect that a proposed construction or modification of a health facility will be needed at the time of its completion. The certificate is issued to the individual or group intending to build or modify the facility.

certification, **1.** a process in which an individual, an institution, or an educational program is evaluated and recognized as meeting certain predetermined standards. Certification is usually made by a nongovernmental agency. The purpose of certification is to assure that the standards met are those necessary for safe and ethical practice of the profession or service. **2.** (in nursing) a process in which the professional organization or association verifies the fact that a person who is licensed to practice has met the standards for specialty practice specified by the profession. The purpose of certification is to assure other professionals and the public that the person has mastered the skills necessary to practice a particular specialty and has acquired the standard body of knowledge common to that specialty.

certification for excellence, (in nursing) certification that recognizes professional achievement, advanced training, and superior performance in a special or subspecial field of practice.

certification in nursing, one of two processes in which a professional organization formally recognizes the right of a nurse to practice a subspecialty of nursing. One process, certification for excellence, bases recognition on professional achievement, advanced training, and superior performance. The second process, entry level certification, bases recognition on advanced training in a program approved by the certifying organization. Criteria vary according to the particular requirements of the professional organization but always require current licensure as a registered nurse and usually include an examination and certain educational or practice requirements. Submission and evaluation of documented clinical practice and a statement of a philosophy of practice may also be required by some professional organizations.

certified dental assistant, a person who has successfully completed the education, training, and testing of the Certification Board of the American Dental Assistant Association.

certified milk, raw milk that is obtained, handled, and marketed in compliance with state health laws. The milk must be produced by disease-free cows, which are regularly inspected by a veterinarian and are milked by sterilized equipment in hygienic surroundings, contain less than a specified low bacterial count, and be not older than 36 hours when delivered.

Certified Nurse-Midwife (CNM), (according to the American College of Nurse-Midwives) "an individual educated in the two disciplines of nursing and midwifery, who possesses evidence of certification according to the requirements of the American College of Nurse-Midwives. Nurse-midwifery practice is the independent management of care of essentially normal newborns and women, antepartally, intrapartally, postpartally, and/or gynecologically, occurring within a health care system which provides for medical consultation, collaborative management, or referral and is in accord with the qualifications, standards, and functions for the practice of nurse-midwifery as defined by the American College of Nurse-Midwives." See also **midwife.**

certified registered nurse anesthetist. See **nurse anesthetist.**

certify, **1.** to guarantee formally that certain requirements have been met based on expert knowledge of significant, pertinent facts. **2.** to attest, by a legal process, that someone is insane. **3.** to attest to the fact of someone's death in writing, usually on a form as required by local authority. **4.** to declare that a person has satisified certain requirements for membership or acceptance into a professional or other group. See also **board certification.** –**certification,** *n.*, **certifiable,** *adj.*

Cerubidine, a trademark for an antineoplastic (daunorubicin hydrochloride).

cerulean /sirōō′lē·ən/, sky-blue in color.

ceruloplasmin /sirōō′lōplaz′min/, a glycoprotein in plasma that transports 96% of the plasma copper.

cerumen /sirōō′mən/, a yellowish or brownish waxy secretion produced by vestigial apocrine sweat glands in the external ear canal. Also called **earwax.**

ceruminosis /sirōō′minō′sis/, excessive buildup of cerumen or earwax in the external auditory canal. It can cause discomfort, symptoms of hearing loss, and irritation leading to the development of infection. Removal of excess cerumen is accomplished by the local use of a wax softening agent followed by careful flushing with an ear syringe. A cerumen spoon is sometimes used to scoop out hard collections of old wax.

ceruminous gland /sirōō′minəs/, one of a number of tiny structures in the external ear canal, believed to be modified sweat glands. They secrete a waxy cerumen instead of watery sweat.

cervic-, a combining form meaning 'pertaining to the neck': *cervicectomy, cervicitis, cervicobrachial.*

cervical /sur′vikəl/, **1.** of or pertaining to the neck or the region of the neck. **2.** of or pertaining to the constricted area of a necklike structure, as the neck of a tooth or the cervix of the uterus.

cervical abortion, spontaneous expulsion of a cervical pregnancy.

cervical adenitis, an abnormal condition characterized by enlarged, tender lymph nodes of the neck. It often occurs in association with acute infections of the throat.

cervical canal, the canal within the uterine cervix, which protrudes into the vagina. The uterine end of the canal is closed at the internal os and, in the nullipara, at the distal end by the external os. The canal is a passageway through which the menstrual flow escapes and, vastly dilated and effaced by labor, through which the infant must come to be delivered vaginally. Various diagnostic and therapeutic procedures require dilatation of the muscular cervix surrounding the canal, including endometrial biopsy, suction or surgical curettage, or radium implantation. Pelvic inflammatory disease is the result of the entry of pathogenic bacteria into the uterus through the cervical canal. Sperm must travel upward through the canal to reach the uterus and fallopian tubes. The mucus that is secreted by endocervical glands changes in appearance and consistency through the menstrual cycle. For the first few days after menstruation little mucus is secreted. As ovulation approaches, increasing amounts of sticky, cloudy-white or yellowish secretions are seen. Around the time of ovulation, the volume of mucus increases, and it becomes clear, slippery, and elastic, resembling the uncooked white of an egg. After ovulation the mucus becomes cloudy, thick, sticky, and progressively less profuse until menstruation supervenes to begin the cycle again.

cervical cancer, a neoplasm of the uterine cervix that can be detected in the early, curable stage by the Papanicolaou (Pap) test. Factors associated with the development of cervical cancer are coitus at an early age, many sexual partners, genital herpesvirus infections, multiparity, and poor obstetric and gynecologic care. Early cervical neoplasia is usually asymptomatic, but there may be a watery vaginal discharge or occasional spotting of blood; advanced lesions may cause a dark, foul-smelling vaginal discharge, leakage from bladder or rectal fistulas, anorexia, weight loss, and back and leg pains. Pap smears of cervical cells are highly important in screening, but definitive diagnoses are based on colposcopic examination and cytologic study of specimens obtained by biopsy. Suitable sites for biopsy may be indicated by applying 3% acetic acid to the cervix to accentuate characteristic changes in neoplastic epithelium or by using Schiller's test in which an iodine solution stains normal cervical cells dark brown and does not stain the nonglycogen-producing cells of malignant epithelium. Cervical dysplasia may regress, persist, or progress to clinical disease, but carcinoma in situ is considered to be a precursor of invasive carcinoma. About 90% of cervical tumors are squamous cell carcinomas, fewer than 10% are adenocarcinomas, and others are mixtures of these kinds, or, in rare cases, sarcomas. Tumors on the surface of the cervix may be huge, polypoid masses while endophytic lesions tend to be small and hard; ulcerative lesions may cause extensive erosion. Cervical cancer invades the tissues of adjacent organs and may metastasize through lymphatic channels to distant sites, including the lungs, bone, liver, brain, and paraaortic nodes. Treatment depends on the kind and the extent of the malignancy, the age of the woman, and her general health. Also considered are her wishes in regard to maintaining her reproductive function. Carcinoma in situ may be treated by excisional conization or cryosurgery. Invasive tumors may be treated with radiotherapy or vaginal or abdominal hysterectomy.

cervical cap, a contraceptive device consisting of a small rubber cup fitted over the uterine cervix to prevent spermatozoa from entering the cervical canal. In some studies, its contraceptive effectiveness equals or exceeds that of the diaphragm. It may be more comfortable than the diaphragm and may be left safely on the cervix for days or weeks and remain effective. Accurate initial fitting by a trained person is necessary. Practice by the user may be required to manipulate the cap into proper position on the cervix. The cap has become a popular contraceptive in Great Britain and Europe among women who require nonsystemic, noninvasive means of preventing conception.

cervical disk syndrome, an abnormal condition characterized by compression or irritation of the cervical nerve roots in or near the intervertebral foramina before the roots divide into the anterior and the posterior rami. Cervical disk syndrome may be caused by ruptured intervertebral disks, degenerative cervical disk disease, or cervical injuries. The form caused by ruptured cervical intervertebral disks or by degenerative disease may produce varying degrees of malalignment, causing nerve root compression. Most cervical disk syndromes are caused by injuries that involve hyperextension, which results in compression of the anatomic structures. Flexion injuries in the cervical area do not result in nerve compression. Edema usually occurs in all cases of cervical disk syndrome. Pain, the most common symptom, usually emanates from the cervical area but may radiate down the arm to the fingers and increase with cervical motion. The pain may increase sharply with coughing, sneezing, or any radical movement. Other signs and symptoms associated with cervical disk syndrome may be paresthesia, headache, blurred vision, decreased skeletal function, and weakened hand grip. Physical examination may reveal varying degrees of muscular atrophy, sensory abnormalities, muscular weakness, and decreased reflexes. Radiographic examination may show a loss of normal lordosis associated with the cervical vertebrae and may also reveal some minor malalignment of the vertebrae. Nonsurgical intervention, which is usually a successful treatment, may include immobilization of the cervical vertebrae to decrease irritation and to provide rest for the traumatized area. Other treatment may include special exercises, heat therapy, and intermittent traction. Mild analgesics are usually successful in controlling the pain associated with cervical disk syndrome, especially when employed with immobilization. Surgery is usually recommended only when signs and symptoms persist despite nonsurgical treatment. The prognosis for this condition is usually good, but recurrence of symptoms is common. Also called **cervical root syndrome.** See also **ruptured intervertebral disk, whiplash injury.**

cervical endometritis, an inflammation of the inner lining of the cervix uteri. See also **endometritis.**

cervical erosion, a condition in which the squamous epithelium of the cervix is abraded as a result of irritation caused by infection or trauma, as childbirth, and is replaced by columnar epithelium. Early treatment is desirable to avoid possible malignancy later and consists of cauterization and douches.

cervical fistula, an abnormal passage from the cervix to the vagina or bladder that may be caused by a malignant lesion, radiotherapy, surgical trauma, or injury during childbirth. A cervical fistula communicating with the bladder permits leakage of urine, causing irritation, odor, and embarrassment. When surgical repair is not possible, the patient is advised to take sitz baths, use a deodorizing douche or powder, as sodium borate, and wear plastic pants or a protective apron. See also **branchial fistula.**

cervical mucus method of family planning. See **ovulation method of family planning.**

cervical os. See **external cervical os, internal cervical os.**

cervical plexus, the network of nerves formed by the ventral primary divisions of the first four cervical nerves. Each nerve, except the first, divides into the superior branch and the inferior branch, and both branches unite to form three loops. The plexus is located opposite the cranial aspect of the first four cervical vertebrae, ventrolateral to the levator scapulae and the scalenus medius, and deep to the sternocleidomastoideus. It communicates with certain cranial nerves and numerous muscular and cutaneous branches.

cervical plexus anesthesia, nerve block at any point below the mastoid process from C_2 to the second cervical vertebra transverse process of the sixth cervical vertebra. This method is used for operations on the area between the jaw and clavicle. Complications may include Horner's syndrome, inadvertent stellate ganglion or brachial plexus block, vertebral artery bleeding, subarachnoid or peridural penetration, phrenic nerve block or palsy, or laryngeal nerve block, manifested by sudden hoarseness.

cervical polyp, an outgrowth of columnar epithelial tissue of the endocervical canal, usually attached to the wall of the canal by a slender pedicle. Often there are no symptoms, but multiple or abraded polyps may cause bleeding, especially with contact during coitus. Polyps are most common in women over 40 years of age. The cause is not known. Treatment of a symptomatic polyp is removal by simple torsion, turning the polyp on its stalk while pulling gently until it tears off. Scant bleeding and prompt healing usually follow. The polyp is removed and sent to the laboratory for pathologic evaluation and histologic examination. Squamous metaplasia is a common finding; malignancy is rare. A Pap smear and endometrial biopsy may be performed at the same visit if other pathology is suspected.

cervical smear, a small amount of the secretions and superficial cells of the cervix, secured with a sterile applicator or special small wooden or plastic spatula from the external os of the uterine cervix. For a Pap smear, it is obtained from the squamocolumnar junction of the uterine cervix and from the vaginal vault and endocervical canal. The specimen is spread on a specially labeled glass slide and sent for cytologic examination by a special laboratory. For bacteriologic culture and identification, only the applicator is used; the specimen is spread on a glass slide and stained and examined under a microscope or placed in or on a culture medium and sent to a bacteriologic laboratory for culture and identification.

cervical tenaculum. See **tenaculum.**

cervical triangle, one of two triangular areas formed in the neck by the oblique course of the sternocleidomastoideus. The anterior triangle is bounded by the midline of the throat anteriorly, the sternocleidomastoideus laterally, and the body of the mandible superiorly. The posterior triangle is bounded by the clavicle inferiorly and by the borders of the sternocleidomastoideus and the trapezius superiorly.

cervical vertebra, one of the first seven segments of the vertebral column. They differ from the thoracic and the lumbar vertebrae by the presence of a foramen in each transverse process. The first, second, and seventh cervical vertebrae present exceptional features. The bodies of the four remaining cervical vertebrae are small, oval, and broader than the other three in transverse diameter and contain large, triangular foramina within their tranverse processes. Their spinous processes are short and bifid. The first cervical vertebra has no body, supports the head, and contains a smooth, oval facet for articulation with the dens of the second cervical vertebra. The dens extends from the cranial portion of the body of the second cervical vertebra, which has a very large, strong spinous process with a bifid extremity. The seventh cervical vertebra has a very long, prominent spinous process that is nearly horizontal in direction and is often used as a palpable reference for locating the other cervical spines. Compare **coccygeal vertebra, lumbar vertebra, sacral vertebra, thoracic vertebra.** See also **vertebra.**

cervicitis /sur'visī'tis/, acute or chronic inflammation of the uterine cervix. **Acute cervicitis** is infection of the cervix marked by redness, edema, and bleeding on contact. Symptoms do not always occur but may include any or all of the following: copious, foul-smelling discharge from the vagina, pelvic pressure or pain, scant bleeding with intercourse, and itching or burning of the external genitalia. The principal causative organisms are: *Trichomonas vaginalis, Candida albicans,* and *Haemophilus vaginalis*. Diagnosis is by microscopic examination, confirmed, in some cases, by culture and Pap smear. Specific antimicrobial medication may be effective. Acute cervicitis tends to be a recurrent problem because of reexposure to the germ, undertreatment, or predisposing factors such as multiple sexual partners or poor nutritional status. **Chronic cervicitis** is a persistent inflammation of the cervix usually occurring among women in their reproductive years. Symptoms include a thick, irritating, malodorous discharge that may, in severe cases, be accompanied by significant pelvic pain. The cervix looks congested and enlarged, nabothian cysts are often present, and there are signs of eversion of the cervix and often old lacerations from childbirth. A Pap smear should be performed before treatment. Antibiotic treatment is seldom effective. The symptoms of mild chronic cervicitis may abate with topical treatment, but the underlying inflammatory condition will not change. The most effective treatments are hot or cold cautery. See also ***Candida albicans,* cautery, cervical cancer, cervical polyp, condylomatum accuminatum, nabothian cyst.**

cervico-, a combining form meaning 'neck': *cervicodynia, cervicolabial, cervicotomy.*

cervicodynia /sur'vikōdin'ē·ə/, pain in the neck. Also called **trachelodynia.**

cervicofacial actinomycosis. See **actinomycosis.**

cervicolabial /sur'vikōlā'bē·əl/, pertaining to or situated in the labial area of the neck of an incisor or a canine tooth.

cervicouterine /sur'vikōyo͞o'tərin/, pertaining to or situated at the cervix of the uterus.

cervicovesical /sur'vikōves'ikəl/, of or pertaining to the cervix of the uterus and the bladder.

cervix /sur'viks/, the part of the uterus that protrudes into the cavity of the vagina. The cervix is divided into the supravaginal portion and the vaginal portion. The supravaginal portion is separated ventrally from the bladder by the parametrium, which attaches to the sides of the cervix and contains the uterine arteries. The vaginal portion of the cervix projects into the cavity of the vagina and contains the cervical canal and the internal and external os of the canal. The mucous membrane lining the endocervix is broken by numerous oblique ridges, deep glandular follicles, little cysts, and papillae. See also **effacement.**

ceryl alcohol /sē'ril/, a fatty alcohol present in many waxes. Also called **hexacosanol.**

cesarean hysterectomy, a surgical operation in which the uterus is removed at the time of cesarean section. It is performed most often for complications of cesarean section, usually intractable hemorrhage. Less often it is done to treat preexisting gynecologic disease, as an intraepithelial cervical neoplasia. It is rarely done electively for sterilization because the danger of hemorrhage is greater when both procedures are performed simultaneously.

cesarean section, a surgical procedure in which the abdomen and uterus are incised and a baby is delivered transabdominally. It is performed when abnormal maternal or fetal conditions exist that are judged likely to make vaginal delivery hazardous. Approximately 15% of births in the United States are by cesarean section; the operation is performed less frequently in other countries. The maternal mortality is 0.1% to 0.2%. Maternal indications for the operation include hemorrhage from placenta previa or abruptio placenta, severe preeclampsia, and dysfunctional labor. Delivery by cesarean section at a prior parturition is no longer considered an absolute indication for repeating it in future deliveries. Cesarean birth is less traumatic for babies than difficult midforceps delivery. Fetal indications for the operation include fetal distress, cephalopelvic disproportion, and abnormal presentation, as breech and transverse lie. The incision in the skin of the abdomen may be horizontal or vertical, regardless of the kind of internal incision into the uterus. Because she must begin mothering while she is recovering from major surgery, the mother requires special care that provides for both her postoperative medical needs and her need to nurture her new baby, who may also be ill or recovering during the crucial neonatal period. See also **classical**

cesarean section, extraperitoneal cesarean section, low cervical cesarean section.

cesium (Cs) /sē′zē·əm/, an alkali metal element. Its atomic number is 55; its atomic weight is 132.9. Like other alkali metals cesium emits electrons when exposed to visible light and is used in photoelectric cells and in television cameras.

cesium 137, a radioactive material with a half-life of 30.2 years that is used in radiotherapy as a sealed source of gamma rays intended for application to various malignancies that are treated by brachytherapy. Cesium has replaced radium for such applications. See also **brachytherapy.**

cesspool fever, *informal.* typhoid fever.

cestode. See **tapeworm.**

cestode infection, cestodiasis. See **tapeworm infection.**

cestoid /ses′toid/, **1.** resembling a tapeworm. **2.** a tapeworm of the Cestoda subclass.

Cetacaine, a trademark for a fixed-combination, anesthetic spray, containing several local anesthetics (benzocaine, butyl aminobenzoate, tetracaine), applied to mucous membranes.

cetyl alcohol /sē′til/, a fatty alcohol, derived from spermaceti, used as an emulsifier and stiffening agent in creams and ointments. Also called **hexadecanol, palmityl alcohol.**

cetylpyridinium chloride, an antiinfective used as a preservative in pharmaceutic preparations and as a topical cleanser.

■ INDICATIONS: It is prescribed prophylactically to prevent infection of the skin or mucous membranes.

■ CONTRAINDICATIONS: Known hypersensitivity to this drug is the only contraindication.

■ NOTE: It is inactivated by soap, serum, and tissue fluids; therefore, the surface of the skin must be clean and well rinsed.

CEU, abbreviation for **continuing education unit.**

Ce-Vi-Sol, a trademark for vitamin C (ascorbic acid).

cevitamic acid. See **ascorbic acid.**

Cf, symbol for **californium.**

CF test, abbreviation for **complement-fixation test.**

cgs, CGS, abbreviation for **centimeter-gram-second system.**

Ch[1], symbol for **Christchurch chromosome.**

Chaddock reflex, an abnormal reflex, induced by firmly stroking the ulnar surface of the forearm, characterized by flexion of the wrist and extension of the fingers in fanlike position. It is seen on the affected side in hemiplegia. Compare **Gordon reflex, Oppenheim reflex.** See also **Babinski's reflex.**

Chaddock's sign, a variation of Babinski's reflex, elicited by firmly stroking the side of the foot just distal to the lateral malleolus, characterized by extension of the great toe and fanning of the other toes. It is seen in pyramidal tract disease.

chadless paper tape, chad paper tape. See **paper tape punch.**

Chadwick's sign /chad′wiks/, the bluish coloration of the vulva and vagina that develops after the sixth week of pregnancy as a normal result of local venous congestion. It is an early sign of pregnancy.

chafe, an irritation of the skin by friction, as when rough material rubs against an unprotected area of the body.

chafing, superficial irritation of the skin by friction.

Chagas-Cruz disease. See **Chagas' disease.**

Chagas' disease /chag′əs/, a parasitic disease caused by *Trypanosoma cruzi* or by *Schizotrypanum cruzi,* transmitted to humans by the bite of bloodsucking insects. It may occur in acute or chronic form. The acute form, which is common in children and rare in adults, is marked by a lesion at the site of the bite, fever, weakness, enlarged spleen and lymph nodes, edema of the face and legs, and tachycardia. This form resolves within 4 months unless complications, as encephalitis, develop. The chronic form may be manifested by cardiomyopathy or by dilatation of the esophagus or colon. Often, infections are asymptomatic. Also called **African sleeping sickness, African trypanosomiasis, Brazilian trypanosomiasis, Chagas-Cruz disease, Cruz trypanosomiasis, South American trypanosomiasis.** See also **trypanosomiasis.**

Chagres fever /chag′ris/, a phlebotomus arbovirus infection transmitted to humans through the bite of a sandfly. The disease is rarely fatal and is characterized by fever, headache, and muscle pains of the chest or abdomen. There may be nausea and vomiting, giddiness, weakness, photophobia, and pain on moving the eyes. The infection subsides within a week. Supportive treatment includes analgesics, bed rest, and adequate fluid intake. The disease is most common in Central America. Also called **Panama fever.**

chain, **1.** a length of several units linked together in a linear pattern, as a polypeptide chain of amino acids or a chain of atoms forming a chemical molecule. **2.** a group of individual bacteria linked together, as streptococci formed by a chain of cocci. **3.** the serial relationship of certain structures essential to function, as the chain of ossicles in the middle ear. Each of the small bones moves successively in response to vibration of the tympanic membrane, thus transmitting the auditory stimulus to the oval window. See also **chain ligature.**

chain ligature, an interlocking ligature that ties off a pedicle at several places by passing a long thread through the pedicle at different points.

chain reaction, **1.** (in chemistry) a reaction that produces a compound needed for the reaction to continue, as each product that is produced in the chain reaction of glycolysis which is essential for each succeeding reaction and the total catabolism of glucose. **2.** (in physics) a reaction that perpetuates itself by the proliferating fission of nuclei and the release of atomic particles that cause more nuclear fissions.

chain reflex, a series of reflexes, each stimulated by the preceding one.

chain printer, a character printer for computers in which the die for each character is on a separate link of a continuous chain that is passed over the area to be printed. As the desired character passes in front of the desired position where it is to be printed, a hammer strikes the die and the pattern is impressed on the paper through an inked ribbon.

chain-stitch suture, a continuous surgical stitch in which each loop of the suture is secured by the next loop.

chalasia /kəlā′zhə/, abnormal relaxation or incompetence of the cardiac sphincter of the stomach, resulting in reflux of the gastric contents into the esophagus with subsequent regurgitation. Conservative treatment in infancy includes feeding several small meals a day to avoid distention of the stomach and holding the baby upright while giving the feeding. The symptoms and treatment are similar to those of a hiatal hernia. See also **gastroesophageal reflux.**

chalazion /kəlā′zion/, a small, localized swelling of the eyelid resulting from obstruction and retained secretions of the meibomian glands. A nonmalignant condition, it often requires surgery for correction. Compare **hordeolum, sty.**

chalice cell. See **goblet cell.**

chalkitis /kalkī′tis/, an abnormal condition characterized by inflammation of the eyes, caused by rubbing the eyes with the hands after touching or handling brass. Also called **brassy eye.**

chalone /kā′lōn/, any one of numerous polypeptide inhibitors that is elaborated by a tissue and functions like a hormone on specific target organs.

chamaeprosopy /kam′əpros′əpē/, a facial appearance characterized by a low brow and a broad face with a facial index of 90 or less. **–chamaeprosopic,** *adj.*

chamber, **1.** a hollow but not necessarily an empty space or cavity in an organ, as in the anterior and posterior chambers of the eye or the atrial and ventricular chambers of the heart. **2.** a room or closed space used for research or therapeutic purposes, as a decompression chamber or hyperbaric oxygen chamber.

Chamberlain's line, a line that extends from the posterior of the hard palate to the dorsum of the foramen magnum.

Chamberlen forceps, one of the earliest kinds of obstetric forceps, introduced in the seventeenth century.

CHAMPUS, abbreviation for **Civilian Health and Medical Programs for Uniformed Services.**

chancr-. See **cancr-.**

chancre /shang′kər/, **1.** also called **venereal sore.** a skin lesion, usually of primary syphilis, that begins at the site of infection as a papule and develops into a red, bloodless, painless ulcer with a scooped-out appearance. It heals without treatment and leaves no scar. Two or more chancres may develop at the same time, occurring usually in the genital area but sometimes on the hands, face, or other body surface. The chancre teams with *Treponema pallidum* spirochetes and is highly contagious. **2.** a papular lesion or ulcerated area of the skin that marks the point of infection of a nonsyphilitic disease, as tuberculosis. Compare **chancroid.** See also **syphilis.**

chancroid /shang′kroid/, a highly contagious, sexually transmitted disease caused by infection with a bacillus, *Haemophilus ducreyi.* It characteristically begins as a papule, usually on the skin of the external genitalia; it then grows and ulcerates, other papules form, and, if untreated, the bacillus spreads, causing buboes in the groin. An intradermal skin test is more reliable than smear and culture techniques in diagnosing this condition. Sulfonamide drugs are prescribed to treat chancroid. Because the lesion resembles syphilis and lymphogranuloma venereum, the diagnosis must be made before treatment in order to avoid obscuring simultaneous infections. Compare **chancre.**

change of life, *informal.* the female climacteric; menopause.

channel, a passageway or groove that conveys fluid, as the central channels that connect the arterioles with the venules.

channel ulcer, a rare type of peptic ulcer found in the pyloric canal between the stomach and the duodenum. See also **peptic ulcer.**

chaotic atrial tachycardia, a form of atrial tachycardia marked by an abnormal electrocardiogram tracing in which the P wave, representing contraction of the atria, is irregular in time and variable in shape.

chapped, pertaining to skin that is roughened, cracked, or reddened by exposure to cold or excessive surface evaporation. Stinging or burning sensations often accompany the disorder. Prevention is by protection against exposure to cold and wind. Treatment includes the avoidance of frequent washing, the replacement of soaps and detergents with superfatted soaps, and the application of emollients. Compare **frostbite.** **–chap,** *v.*

character, **1.** the integrated composite of traits and behavioral tendencies that enable a person to react in a relatively consistent way to the customs and mores of society. Character, as contrasted with personality, implies volition and morality. Compare **personality.** **2.** any letter, number, symbol, or punctuation mark, usually composed of eight bits or one byte, that can be transmitted as output by a computer. See also **bit.**

character analysis, a systematic investigation of the personality of an individual with special attention to psychologic defenses and motivations, usually undertaken to improve behavior.

character disorder, a chronic, habitual, maladaptive, and socially unacceptable pattern of behavior and emotional response. The condition is usually accompanied by minimal feelings of anxiety. Also called **character neurosis.** See also **antisocial personality disorder.**

characteristic curve, (in radiotherapy) a plot of the amount of blackening that a film or film-screen combination will achieve as a function of differing levels of radiation exposure.

character neurosis. See **character disorder.**

character printer, a printer for computers that prints a fully formed character, as a letter, number, or symbol, with each impression stroke. Compare **dot-matrix printer.**

charcoal. See **activated charcoal.**

Charcot-Bouchard aneurysm /shärkō′bo͝oshär′/, a small, round aneurysm of a small artery of the cerebral cortex or basal ganglia, which some authorities believe is the cause of massive cerebral hemorrhage. Charcot-Bouchard aneurysms often occur in individuals with very high blood pressure.

Charcot-Leyden crystal /shärkō′lī′dən/, any one of the crystalline structures shaped like narrow, double pyramids found in the sputum of individuals suffering from bronchial asthma. They are also found in the feces of dysentery patients. The Charcot-Leyden crystals are protein compounds and occur in association with the fragmentation of eosinophils. Also called **asthma crystal, leukocytic crystal.**

Charcot-Marie-Tooth atrophy /shärkō′mərē′to͞oth′/, a progressive hereditary disorder characterized by degeneration of the peroneal muscles of the fibula, resulting in clubfoot, foot drop, and ataxia.

Charcot's fever /shärkōz′/, a syndrome characterized by a recurrent fever, jaundice, and abdominal pain in the right upper quadrant occurring with inflammation of the bile ducts. It is caused by the intermittent impaction of a stone in the ducts.

Charcot's joint, See **neuropathic joint disease.**

charlatan, a totally unqualified individual posing as an expert, especially an individual pretending to be a physician. Also called **quack.** **–charlatanical,** *adj.*

Charles' law. See **Gay-Lussac's law.**

charley horse, a painful condition of the quadricep or hamstring muscles characterized by soreness and stiffness. It is the result of a strain, tear, or bruise of the muscle and is often associated with athletic activity. Compare **cramp.**

chart, **1.** *informal.* a patient record. **2.** to note data in a patient record, usually at prescribed intervals.

charta /kär′tə/, *pl.* **chartae,** a piece of paper, especially one treated with medicine, as for external application, or with a chemical for a special purpose, as litmus paper.

chauffeur's fracture, any fracture of the radial styloid, produced by a twisting or a snapping type injury.

Chaussier's areola /shôsyāz′/, an areola of indurated tissue surrounding a malignant pustule.

CHC, abbreviation for *community health center.*

check ligament. See **alar ligament.**

check-up, a thorough study or examination of the health of an individual.

Chediak-Higashi syndrome /ched′ē•ak•higä′shē/, a congenital, autosomal disorder, characterized by partial albinism, photophobia, massive leukocytic inclusions, psychomotor abnormalities, recurrent infections, and early death. Antenatal diagnosis can be made by amniocentesis and tissue culture. Treatment includes antibiotics and transfusions.

cheek, a fleshy prominence, especially the fleshy protuberances on both sides of the face between the eye and the jaw and the ear and the nose and mouth. Also called **bucca.**

cheekbone. See **zygomatic bone.**

cheesewasher's lung, a lung disease caused by an allergic reaction to the mold of cheese. Avoidance of the causative agent assures prevention of the condition. No treatment is necessary.

cheil-. See **cheilo-.**

-cheilia, -chilia, a combining form meaning '(condition of the) lips': *atelocheilia, dicheilia, xerocheilia.*

cheilitis /kīlī′tis/, an abnormal condition of the lips characterized by inflammation and cracking of the skin. There are several forms including those caused by excessive exposure to sunlight, allergic sensitivity to cosmetics, and vitamin deficiency. Compare **cheilosis.**

cheilo-, cheil-, a combining form meaning 'pertaining to the lip': *cheiloangioscopy, cheilocarcinoma, cheiloplasty.*

cheilocarcinoma /kī′lōkär′sinō′mə/, *pl.* **cheilocarcinomas, cheilocarcinomata,** a malignant epithelial tumor of the lip.

cheiloplasty /kī′ləplas′tē/, surgical correction of a defect of the lip.

cheilorraphy /kīlôr′əfē/, a surgical procedure that sutures the lip, as in the repair of a congenitally cleft lip or a lacerated lip.

cheilosis /kīlō′sis/, a disorder of the lips and mouth characterized by scales and fissures, resulting from a deficiency of riboflavin in the diet.

cheir-. See **cheiro-.**

cheiralgia /kəral′jə/, a pain in the hand, especially the pain associated with arthritis. **–cheiralgic,** *adj.*

-cheiria. See **-chiria.**

cheiro-, cheir-, chir-, chiro-, a combining form meaning 'pertaining to the hand': *cheiragra, cheiromegaly, cheiroplasty.*

cheiromegaly /kī′rōmeg′əlē/, an abnormal condition characterized by excessively large hands. **–cheiromegalic,** *adj.*

cheiroplasty /kī′rōplas′tē/, an operation involving plastic surgery of the hand. **–cheiroplastic,** *adj.*

chelate /kē′lāt/, **1.** (of a metal ion and two or more polar groups of a single molecule) to form a bond, thus creating a ringlike complex. **2.** (in medicine) any coordination compound composed of a central metal ion and an organic molecule with multiple bonds, arranged in ring formations, used especially in chemotherapeutic treatments for metal poisoning. **3.** of or pertaining to chelation.

chelating agent, a substance that promotes chelation. Chelating agents are used in the treatment of metal poisoning. See also **chelation.**

chelation /kēlā′shən/, a chemical reaction in which there is a combination with a metal to form a ring-shaped molecular complex in which the metal is firmly bound and sequestered. See also **chelating agent.**

cheloid. See **keloid.**

cheloidosis. See **keloidosis.**

chemical, **1.** a substance composed of chemical elements or a substance produced by or used in chemical processes. **2.** pertaining to chemistry.

chemical action, any process in which natural elements and compounds react with each other to produce a chemical change or a different compound, as hydrogen and oxygen, which combine to produce water.

chemical agent, any chemical power, active principle, or substance that can produce an effect in the body by interacting with various body substances, as aspirin, which produces an analgesic effect.

chemical antidote, any substance that reacts chemically with a poison to form a compound that is harmless. There are few true antidotes, and treatment of poisoning depends largely on eliminating the toxic agent before it can be absorbed by the body.

chemical burn, tissue damage caused by exposure to a strong acid or alkali, as phenol, creosol, mustard gas, or phosphorus. Emergency treatment includes washing the surface with copious amounts of water to remove the chemical and, if the damage is more than slight and superficial, immediate transport to a medical facility. See also **acid burn, acid poisoning, alkali burn, alkali poisoning.**

chemical cauterization, the corroding or burning of living tissue by a caustic chemical substance, as potassium hydroxide. Also called **chemocautery.**

chemical diabetes. See **impaired glucose tolerance.**

chemical equivalent, a drug or chemical containing similar amounts of the same ingredients as another drug or chemical.

chemical gastritis, inflammation of the stomach caused by the ingestion of a chemical compound. Treatment is determined by the substance ingested. Gastric lavage is often advisable, but neither lavage nor emetics should be administered in cases involving the most corrosive poisons. Compare **corrosive gastritis, erosive gastritis.**

chemical name, the exact designation of the chemical structure of a drug as determined by the rules of accepted systems of chemical nomenclature. For example, N,N-bis-(2-chloroethyl)-N′-(3-hydroxypropyl) phosphordiamidic acid cyclic acid monohydrate is the chemical name of cyclophosphamide, a drug used in cancer chemotherapy.

chemical shift, the slight departure in the nuclear magnetic resonance spectrum of an element, as hydrogen, when it is a constituent in a complex biomolecule, from the spectrum for a sample containing that element in pure form. Detecting chemical shift is an important step in identifying molecular structure.

chemical warfare, the waging of war with poisonous chemicals and gases.

cheminosis /kem′ənō′sis/, any disease caused by a chemical substance.

chemistry, the science dealing with the elements, their compounds, and the chemical structure and interactions of matter. Kinds of chemistry include **inorganic chemistry** and **organic chemistry.**

chemistry, normal values, the amounts of various substances in the normal human body, determined by testing a large sample of people presumed to be healthy. Normal values are expressed in ranges of numbers, and ranges vary from laboratory to laboratory. For example, a normal concentration of a substance in the blood might be expressed as 5 to 20 mg/dl. Although variations from normal values may be highly significant tools in the diagnoses of certain diseases, in all cases an abnormal result must be cautiously interpreted. See also specific tests.

chemo-, a combining form meaning 'pertaining to a chemical or to chemistry': *chemoantigen, chemobiotic, chemokinesis.*

chemocautery. See **chemical cauterization.**

chemodifferentiation /kē′mō-, kem′ō-/, a stage in embryonic development that precedes and controls specialization and differentiation of the cells into rudimentary organs.

chemonucleolysis /kē′mōno͞o′klē·ol′isis, kem′-/, a method of dissolving the nucleus pulposus of an intervertebral disk by the injection of a chemolytic agent, as the enzyme chymopapain. The procedure is used primarily in the treatment of a herniated disk and other intervertebral disk lesions.

chemoreceptor, a sensory nerve cell activated by chemical stimuli, as a chemoreceptor in the carotid that is sensitive to the PCO_2 in the blood, signaling the respiratory center in the brain to increase or decrease respiration.

chemoreflex, any reflex initiated by the stimulation of chemical receptors, as the carotid and aortic bodies, which respond to changes in carbon dioxide, hydrogen ion, and oxygen concentrations in the blood. See also **chemoreceptor.**

chemosis /kimō′sis/, an abnormal edematous swelling of the mucous membrane covering the eyeball and lining the eyelids that is usually the result of local trauma or infection. Chemosis may also occur in acute conjunctivitis. An obstruction of normal lymph flow, as might occur from growth of a tumor within the eye socket, may less commonly be found to be the cause of chemosis. Systemic disorders, as angioneurotic edema, anemia, and Bright's disease, may also cause the condition. Also called **conjunctival edema.**

chemostat /kē′məstat′/, a device that assures a steady rate of cell division in bacterial populations by maintaining a constant environment.

chemosurgery, the destruction of malignant, infected, or gangrenous tissue by the application of chemicals. The technique is used successfully to remove skin cancers.

chemotaxis, a response involving movement that is positive (toward) or negative (away from) to a chemical stimulus.

chemotherapeutic index. See **therapeutic index.**

chemotherapy, the treatment of infections and other diseases with chemical agents. The term has been applied over the centuries to a variety of therapies, including the treatment of malaria with herbs and the use of mercury for syphilis. In modern usage, chemotherapy usually refers to the use of chemicals to destroy cancer cells on a selective basis. The cytotoxic agents used in cancer treatments generally function in the same manner as ionizing radiation; they do not kill the cancer cells directly but instead impair their ability to replicate. Most of the nearly 40 anticancer drugs commonly used act by interfering with DNA and RNA activities associated with cell division. Chemotherapeutic agents are often used in combination with radiation treatments for their synergistic effect. A cytotoxic agent, for example, may be used to render a tumor cell more sensitive to the effects of radiation. Thus, by making the cancer cell more vulnerable to the effects of ionizing radiation, the cancer can be controlled with smaller doses of radiation than would be possible with radiation alone.

chemotherapy (unsealed radioactive), the oral or parenteral administration of a radioisotope, as iodine 131 (^{131}I) for the treatment of hyperthyroidism or thyroid cancer, phosphorus 32 (^{32}P) for leukemia or polycythemia vera, or gold 198 (^{198}Au) for lung cancer or peritoneal ascites resulting from widely disseminated carcinoma.

■ METHOD: Before unsealed radioactive chemotherapy is administered, the patient receives an explanation of the procedure and of the need for isolation during the half-life of the radioisotope (8.1 days for ^{131}I, 14 days for ^{32}P, and 2.7 days for ^{198}Au). The room in which the patient is isolated adjoins a private bathroom and is equipped with convenient furniture, a freshly made bed placed next to the building's outer wall, a functioning phone and television set, adequate lighting, reading and hobby materials, and containers for contaminated linen, dressings, and excreta. Radioactive tags are posted on the door. The patient's chart and individual radioactive badges, kept at the door, are worn by each staff member entering the room to record the amount of radiation exposure; pregnant staff members are not assigned to the patient's care. Urine excreted by a patient treated with ^{131}I is collected directly or via an indwelling catheter, in a lead-lined container, which is sent to the laboratory for assay of the radioisotope. Feces, sputum, and vomitus are placed in the toilet and decontaminated with a dropperful of a saturated solution of potassium iodide before the bowl is flushed. If excreta spills on the skin, the area is rinsed in running water for 2 minutes and washed in soap and water for an additional 3 minutes. If the bed or another surface in the room is contaminated with excreta, the radiation control officer is notified and the area is monitored before being cleaned. Dressings and bed linen are handled with rubber or plastic gloves; contaminated linens are placed in a hamper and trash in plastic bags, and they are not removed from the room until monitored with a Geiger-Müller counter. The staff member limits exposure by repositioning the debilitated patient with a turn sheet, by bathing only the soiled body areas, and by preparing and cutting food on the diet tray before entering the room. The patient treated with ^{131}I is observed for evidence of neck tenderness, changes in exophthalmia, a transient productive cough, hypoparathyroidism, hypothyroidism, and hyperthyroidism. Special precautions are required in caring for the patient treated with radioactive gold, which emits gamma and beta rays. After purple liquid ^{198}Au is injected into the body cavity, the patient is turned with a sheet every 15 minutes for 2 hours so that the radionuclide can spread. Dressings and cleansing tissues contaminated by the purple seepage from wounds are burned immediately; linen in contact with wounds is placed in special containers. The patient injected with ^{198}Au is usually terminally ill, and, if death occurs, a tag is placed on the body to alert the mortician to the presence of the radionuclide.

■ NURSING ORDERS: The nurse wears a radiation badge when entering the patient's room and limits exposure by performing planned procedures efficiently. Routine nursing functions are kept to a minimum, especially if the patient is ambulatory, but emotional support is provided in brief hourly visits at the door and via the intercommunication system. The nurse anticipates and fulfills the isolated patient's requests as promptly as possible, arranges diversional activities, and assures the patient that when a certain period of time has passed the patient will no longer be a source of radioactivity.

■ OUTCOME CRITERIA: Radioactive iodine usually counteracts hyperthyroidism and is frequently used in conjunction with surgery in the treatment of thyroid cancer. Radioactive phosphorus often controls polycythemia vera, but other agents are generally more effective in leukemia therapy. Radioactive gold is usually administered as a last resort in advanced lung cancer or peritoneal ascites resulting from malignant disease.

chenodeoxycholic acid, a secondary bile acid. It is used in vivo to dissolve cholesterol gallstones, particularly in the elderly and poor-risk patients. See also **ursodeoxycholic acid.**

cherry angioma, a small, bright red, clearly circumscribed vascular tumor on the skin. It occurs most often on the trunk but may be found anywhere on the body. The lesion is very common; more than 85% of people over 45 years of age have several cherry angiomas. Also called **capillary angioma, capillary hemangioma, De Morgan's spots, senile angioma.**

cherry red spot, an abnormal red circular area of the choroid, seen through the fovea centralis of the eye and surrounded by a contrasting white edema. It is associated with cases of infantile cerebral sphingolipidosis and sometimes appears in the late infantile form of amaurotic familial idiocy. Also called **Tay's spot.**

cherubism /cher′əbiz′əm/, an abnormal hereditary condition characterized by progressive bilateral swelling at the angle of the mandible, especially in children. In some cases of cherubism, the entire jaw swells and the eyes turn up, enhancing the cherubic facial appearance. The condition tends to regress during adult life.

chest. See **thorax.**

chest lead /lēd/, **1.** an electrocardiographic conductor in which the exploring electrode is placed on the chest or precordium. The indifferent electrode is placed on the patient's back for a CB (chest back) lead, on the front of the chest for a CF (chest front) lead, on the left arm for a CL (chest left) lead, and on the right arm for a CR (chest right) lead. **2.** *informal.* the tracing produced by such a lead on an electrocardiograph.

chest pain, a physical complaint that requires immediate diagnosis and evaluation. Chest pain may be symptomatic of cardiac disease, as angina pectoris, myocardial infarction, or pericarditis, or of disease of the lungs, as pleurisy, pneumonia, or pulmonary embolism or infarction. The source of chest pain may also be musculoskeletal, GI, or psychogenic. Over 90% of severe chest pain is caused by coronary disease, spinal root compression, or psychologic disturbance. Because of its association with serious, life-threatening heart disease, chest pain causes extreme anxiety, which tends to mask other symptoms that would aid in diagnosis and treatment; reassuring the person being examined assists in proper diagnosis. Evaluation of chest pain requires determining the quality of the pain—dull, sharp, or crushing—locating the site of the pain—in the center or side of the chest—and determining how long the pain has persisted, how it has developed, and whether or not it has occurred in the past. The patient is asked to describe the spread of pain to other parts of the body and to identify factors, as exertion, emotional distress, movement, or deep breathing, that aggravate or relieve the pain. Specific cardiovascular conditions associated with chest pain are myocardial infarction, angina pectoris, pericarditis, and a dissecting aneurysm of the thoracic aorta. Musculoskeletal conditions include rib fractures, swelling of the rib cartilage, and muscle strain. GI conditions associated with chest pain include esophagitis, peptic ulcers, hiatus hernia, and pancreatitis.

chest physiotherapy. See **chest wall percussion.**

chest tube, a catheter inserted through the thorax into the chest cavity for removing air or fluid. It is commonly used after chest surgery and lung collapse.

chest wall percussion. See **percussion.**

Cheyne-Stokes respiration (CSR) /chān′stōks′/, an abnormal pattern of respiration, characterized by alternating periods of apnea and deep, rapid breathing. The respiratory cycle begins with slow, shallow breaths that gradually increase to abnormal depth and rapidity. Respiration gradually subsides as breathing slows and becomes shallower, climaxing in a 10- to 20-second period without respiration before the cycle is repeated. Each cyclic episode may last from 45 seconds to 3 minutes. The immediate cause of CSR is a complex alteration in the functioning of the respiratory center in the brain. Changes in blood gases, especially an increase in carbon dioxide, may be the proximal cause. Alternatively, a direct reduction in the sensitivity of the respiratory center may occur in the presence of normal concentrations of blood gases, as seen in cerebral vascular disease, in tumors of the brainstem, or as a result of severe head injury. The most common cause of an alteration in the blood chemistry that might induce CSR is congestive heart failure, especially in elderly patients with degenerative arterial disease. Bronchopneumonia or other respiratory diseases in elderly people may likewise induce Cheyne-Stokes breathing, and CSR may occur in an otherwise healthy person through hyperventilation or exposure to high altitudes. This pattern of breathing may also be induced by an overdose of a narcotic or hypnotic drug, and it occurs more frequently during sleep. Compare **Biot's respiration.**

-chezia, -chesia, a combining form meaning '(condition of) defecation, especially involving the discharge of foreign substances': *dyschezia, hematochezia, pyochezia.*

CHF, abbreviation for **congestive heart failure.**

Chiari-Frommel syndrome /kē·är′ēfrom′əl/, a hormonal disorder that occurs after a pregnancy in which weaning does not spontaneously end lactation. The syndrome is usually the result of a decrease in pituitary gonadotropins and an excess of pituitary prolactin and may be accompanied by amenorrhea. Treatment includes observation, hormonal therapy, and investigation to confirm or rule out pituitary tumor.

Chiari's syndrome. See **Budd-Chiari syndrome.**

chiasm /kī′azəm/, **1.** the crossing of two lines or tracts, as the crossing of the optic nerves at the optic chiasm. **2.** (in genetics) the crossing of two chromatids in the prophase of meiosis. **–chiasmal, chiasmic,** *adj.*

chiasma /kī·az′mə/, *pl.* **chiasmata,** (in genetics), the visible point of connection between homologous chromosomes during the first meiotic division in gametogenesis. The X-shaped configurations form during the late prophase stage and provide the means by which exchange of genetic material occurs. See also **crossing over.** **–chiasmatic, chiasmic.** *adj.*

chiasmatypy. See **crossing over.**

chiasmic. See **chiasm, chiasma.**

chickenpox, an acute, highly contagious viral disease caused by a herpesvirus, varicella zoster virus (VZV). It occurs primarily in young children and is characterized by crops of pruritic vesicular eruptions on the skin. The disease is transmitted by direct contact with skin lesions or, more commonly, by droplets spread from the respiratory tract of infected persons, usually in the prodromal period or the early stages of the rash. The vesicular fluid and the scabs are infectious until entirely dry. Indirect transmission through uninfected persons or objects is rare. The diagnosis is usually made by physical examination and by the characteristic appearance of the disease. The virus may be identified by culture of the vesicle fluid. Also called **varicella.**

■ OBSERVATIONS: The incubation period averages 2 to 3 weeks, followed by slight fever, mild headache, malaise, and anorexia occurring about 24 to 36 hours before the rash begins. The prodromal period is usually mild in children but may be severe in adults. The rash, which is highly pruritic, begins as macules and progresses in a day or two to papules and, finally, to vesicles surrounding an erythematous base and containing clear fluid. Within 24 to 48 hours the vesicles turn cloudy and become umbilicated, are easily broken, and become encrusted. The lesions, which erupt in crops so that all three stages are present simultaneously, appear first on the back and chest and then spread to the face, neck, and limbs; they occur only rarely on the soles and palms. In severe cases, laryngeal or tracheal vesicles in the pharynx, larynx, and trachea may cause dyspnea and dysphagia. Prolonged fever, lymphadenopathy, and extreme irritability from pruritis are other symptoms. The symptoms last from a few days to 2 weeks.

■ INTERVENTION: Routine treatment consists of bed rest; antipyretics to reduce fever; applications of topical antipruritics, as wet compresses, calamine lotion, or a paste made from baking soda and water; or oral antihistamines, given for the relief of itching. Infected vesicles may be treated with neomycin-bacitracin, and systemic antibiotics may be given if the secondary bacterial infection is extensive. People who are susceptible and at risk for severe disease when exposed to the infection may be passively protected with zoster immune globulin (ZIG), varicella-zoster immune globulin (VZIG), immune serum globulin (ISG), or zoster immune plasma (ZIP). A preparation of the virus for active immunization is not yet available. Babies born to women who develop chickenpox within 5 days of delivery are especially likely to get a severe case of the disease. One attack of the disease confers permanent immunity, although recurring episodes of

Differential diagnosis of chest pain

Cause	*Onset of pain*	*Characteristic of pain*	*Location of pain*
Acute myocardial infarction	Sudden onset; lasts more than 30 minutes to 1 hour	Pressure, burning, aching, tightness, choking	Across chest; may radiate to jaws and neck and down arms and back
Angina	Sudden onset; lasts only a few minutes	Aches, squeezing, choking, heaviness, burning	Substernal: may radiate to jaws and neck and down arms and back
Dissecting aortic aneurysm	Sudden onset	Excruciating, tearing	Center of chest: radiates into back; may radiate to abdomen
Pericarditis	Sudden onset or may be variable	Sharp, knifelike	Restrosternal: may radiate up neck and down left arm
Pneumothorax	Sudden onset	Tearing, pleuritic	Lateral side of chest
Pulmonary embolus	Sudden onset	Crushing (but not always)	Lateral side of onset
Hiatal hernia	Sudden onset	Sharp, severe	Lower chest: upper abdomen
Gastrointestinal disturbance or cholecystitis, reflux esophagitis	Sudden onset	Gripping, burning	Lower substernal and upper abdomen
Degenerative disk (cervical or thoracic spine) disease	Sudden onset	Sharp, severe	Substernal: may radiate to neck, jaw, arms, and shoulders
Degenerative or inflammatory lesions of shoulder, ribs, scalenus anterior	Sudden onset	Sharp, severe	Substernal: radiates to shoulder
Hyperventilation	Sudden onset	Vague	Vague
Pleurisy	Gradual onset	Sharp, knifelike	Unilateral side of chest, usually can isolate the area
Costochondritis	Variable	Sharp, tearing	Pain in area of cartilage between ribs

herpes zoster occur, especially in elderly or debilitated people, resulting from reactivation of the virus. Herpes zoster virus (HZV), like all herpesviruses, lies dormant in certain sensory nerve roots after primary infection.
■ NURSING CONSIDERATIONS: Chickenpox in childhood is usually benign. Few cases require hospitalization. It may be serious or fatal in immunocompromised people, as those receiving chemotherapy or radiotherapy for malignant disease, in those who have undergone organ transplantation, in those with congenital or acquired defects in cell-mediated immunity, or in those receiving high doses of steroids. Common complications are secondary bacterial infections, as abscesses, cellulitis, pneumonia, and sepsis, and hemorrhagic varicella (tiny hemorrhages that may occur in the vesicles or surrounding skin). Less common complications are encephalitis, Reye's syndrome, thrombocytopenia, and hepatitis.

chiclero's ulcer /chikler′ōz/, a kind of American leishmaniasis caused by *Leishmania mexicana*. It is endemic among the workers in the Yucatan and Central America who harvest chicle from the forest. The disease is characterized by cutaneous ulcers on the head that usually heal spontaneously by six months, except for those on the pinna of the ear, which may last for years and cause scarring and deformities. See also **American leishmaniasis, leishmaniasis.**

chief cell, **1.** also called **zymogenic cell.** any one of the columnar epithelial cells or the cuboidal epithelial cells that line the gastric glands and secrete pepsinogen and intrinsic factor, which is needed for the absorption of vitamin B_{12} and the normal development of red blood cells. Anemia is caused by the absence of intrinsic factor. **2.** any one of the epithelioid cells with pale-staining cytoplasm and a large nucleus containing a prominent nucleolus. Cords of such cells form the main substance of the pineal body. **3.** also called **principal cell.** any one of the polyhedral epithelial cells, within the parathyroid glands, which contain pale, clear cytoplasm and a vesicular nucleus.

History	*Pain worsened by*	*Pain relieved by*	*Other*
40 to 70 years of age; may or may not have history of angina	Movement, anxiety	Nothing; no movement, stillness, position, or breath holding; only relieved by medication (morphine sulfate)	Shortness of breath, diaphoresis, weakness, anxiety
May have history of angina; circumstances precipitating; pain characteristic; response to nitroglycerin	Lying down, eating, effort, cold weather, smoking, stress, anger, worry, hunger	Rest, nitroglycerin	Unstable angina appears even at rest
Nothing specific except that pain is usually worse at onset			Blood pressure difference between right and left arms, murmur of aortic regurgitation
Short history of upper respiratory infection or fever	Deep breathing, trunk movement, maybe swallowing	Sitting-up, leaning forward	Friction rub, paradoxic pulse over 10 mm Hg
None	Breathing		Dyspnea, increased pulse, decreased breath sounds, deviated trachea
Sometimes, phlebitis	Breathing		Cyanosis, dyspnea, cough with hemoptysis
May have none	Heavy meal, bending, lying down	Bland diet, walking, antacids, semi-Fowler position	
May have none	Eating, lying down	Antacids	
May have none	Movement of neck or spine, lifting, straining	Rest, decreased movement	Pain usually on outer aspect of arm, thumb, or index finger
May have none	Movement of arm or shoulder	Elevation and arm support to shoulder, postural exercises	
Hyperventilation, anxiety, stress, emotional upset	Increased respiratory rate	Slowing of respiratory rate	Be *sure* hyperventilation is from nonmedical cause!
May have history of viral infection, pneumonia, TB	Inspiratory effort, deep breathing, coughing	Analgesics, regional anesthesia	Dyspnea, may hear friction rub
Variable	Inspiratory effort, deep breathing, coughing	Analgesics, regional anesthesia	

chief complaint, a subjective statement made by a patient describing the patient's most significant or serious symptoms or signs of illness or dysfunction.

Chief Executive Officer (CEO, C.E.O.), the most senior official of an organization or institution.

chief resident, a senior resident physician who acts temporarily as the clinical and administrative director of the house staff in a department of the hospital. The period of duty varies depending on the size of the department, the length of the residency, and the number of house staff members.

chief surgeon, a surgeon appointed or elected head of the surgeons on the staff of a health care facility.

chigger /chig′ər/, the larva of *Trombicula* mites found in tall grass and weeds. It sticks to the skin and causes irritation and severe itching. Also called **harvest mite, red mite.**

chigoe /chig′ō/, a flea found in tropic and subtropic America and Africa. The pregnant female flea burrows into the skin of the feet, causing an inflammatory condition that may lead to spontaneous amputation of a toe. Also called **burrowing flea, jigger, sand flea.** See also **chigger.**

chikungunya encephalitis /chik′ən•gun′yə/, an arbovirus infection characterized by a high fever that begins abruptly, muscle aches, a rash, and pain in the joints. It is transmitted by the bite of a mosquito and occurs mainly in Africa, Asia, and on some of the Pacific islands, including Guam. The fever may last for a week, then rise again after a remission of several days. Pain in the joints may continue after other symptoms have ceased. Supportive nursing care and symptomatic relief are the only treatments.

chilblain /chil′blān/, redness and swelling of the skin because of excessive exposure to cold. Burning, itching, blistering, and ulceration, similar to a thermal burn, may occur. Treatment includes protection against cold and injury, gentle warming, and avoidance of tobacco. Also called **pernio.** Compare **frostbite.**

child, **1.** a person of either sex between the time of birth and adolescence. **2.** an unborn or recently born human being; fetus, neonate, infant. **3.** an offspring or descendant; a son or daughter or a member of a particular tribe or clan. **4.** one who is like a child or immature.

child abuse, the physical, sexual, or emotional maltreatment of a child. It may be overt or covert and often results in permanent physical or psychiatric injury, mental impairment, or, sometimes, death. Child abuse occurs predominantly with children less than 3 years of age and is the result of multiple and complex factors involving both the parents and the child, compounded by various stressful environmental circumstances, as poor socioeconomic conditions, inadequate physical and emotional support within the family, and any major life change or crisis, especially those crises arising from marital strife. Parents at high risk for abuse are characterized as having unsatisfied needs, difficulty in forming adequate interpersonal relationships, unrealistic expectations of the child, and a lack of nuturing experience, often involving neglect or abuse in their own childhoods. Predisposing factors among children include the temperament, personality, and activity level of the child, order of birth in the family, sensitivity to parental needs, and a need for special physical or emotional care resulting from illness, premature birth, or congenital or genetic abnormalities. Identification of abused children or potential child abusers is a major concern for all health care workers. Obvious physical marks on a child's body, as burns, welts, or bruises, and signs of emotional distress, including symptoms of failure to thrive, are common indications of some degree of neglect or abuse. Often, x-ray film to detect healed or new fractures of the extremities or diagnostic tests to identify sexual molestation are necessary. If abuse is suspected, the nurse is required to make the necessary report. Special counseling services or support groups, as Parents Anonymous, exist to help families in which a child is abused. The nurse can play a significant role in preventing abuse by promoting a positive parent-child relationship, especially in the neonatal period, by teaching parents proper child care and disciplinary techniques, and by explaining normal child development and behavior so that parents can formulate realistic guidelines for discipline. Compare **child neglect.** See also **battered child syndrome.**

Guidelines for identifying potential child abusers

One or both parents were often abused as children. Studies indicate over 90% of abusive parents were abused children.
Parents tend to be lonely adults, attracted to each other as they search for loving parent figures.
Extreme personal and social isolation. These parents lack group and community integration and most often lack family support.
Unstable marital relationship. Parents lack positive feedback and support.
Low self-esteem.
Parent-child role reversal. The parents want the infant to meet their unfulfilled needs for mothering.
Unrealistic expectations of infants. Parents expect children to act older.
Parents unable to reach out and ask for help.

Special traits that make a child vulnerable to abuse

Usually young child, under 3 years of age.
Something different about child (i.e., pregnancy or delivery uncomfortable, child unwanted, premature birth).
Child is extremely irritable or cries often.
Birth order. Most often the first or last child is abused.

childbearing period, the reproductive period in a woman's life, from puberty to menopause. It is the time during which she is physiologically able to conceive children.

childbed fever. See **puerperal fever.**

childbirth. See **birth.**

childbirth center, a health facility where prenatal care and delivery services are made available to low-risk pregnant women by a team of nurse-midwives, obstetricians, pediatricians, and ancillary health professionals.

child development, the various stages of physical, social, and psychologic growth that occur from birth through adulthood. See also **adolescence, development, growth, infant, neonatal period, psychosexual development, psychosocial development, toddler.**

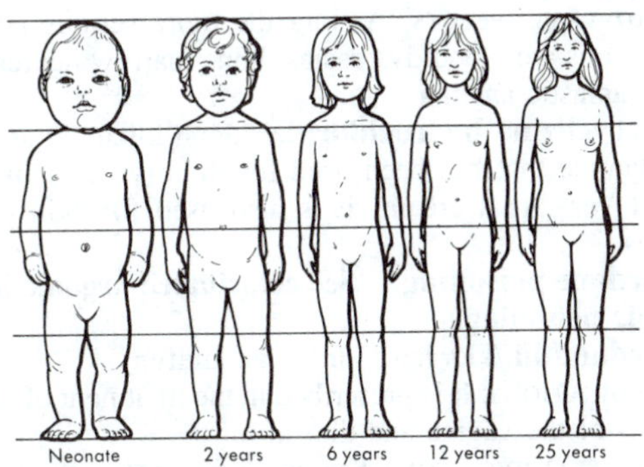

Child development and proportion

childhood, **1.** the period in human development that extends from birth until the onset of puberty. **2.** the state or quality of being a child. See also **development, growth.**

childhood polycystic disease. See **polycystic kidney disease.**

childhood schizophrenia, a form of schizophrenia, occurring before the onset of puberty, resulting from organic brain damage or from environmental conditions. It is characterized by autistic withdrawal into fantasy, obsessional attachments, failure to communicate verbally, repetitive gestures, emotional unresponsiveness, and a severely impaired sense of identity. Two kinds of childhood schizophrenia are **early infantile autism** and **symbiotic infantile psychotic syndrome.**

child neglect, the failure by parents or guardians to provide for the basic needs of a child by physical or emotional deprivation that interferes with normal growth and development or that places the child in jeopardy. Compare **child abuse.** See also **failure to thrive, maternal deprivation syndrome.**

child psychology, the study of the mental, emotional, and behavioral development of infants and children.

child welfare, any service sponsored by the community or special organizations that provide for the physical, social, or psychologic care of children in need of it.

-chilia. See **-cheilia.**

chill, **1.** the sensation of cold caused by exposure to a cold environment. **2.** an attack of shivering with pallor and a feeling of coldness, often occurring at the beginning of an infection and accompanied by a rapid rise in temperature.

Chilomastix /kī′lōmas′tiks/, a genus of flagellate protozoa, as *Chilomastix mesnili,* a nonpathogenic intestinal parasite of humans.

chimera /kimir′ə, kīmir′ə/, an organism carrying cell populations derived from two or more different zygotes of the same or of different species. It may be a natural phenomenon, as in a bone marrow graft. Compare **mosaic.**

chimney-sweeps' cancer. See **scrotal cancer.**

Chinese restaurant syndrome, a syndrome consisting of tingling and burning sensations of the skin, facial pressure, headache, and chest pain that occurs immediately after eating food containing monosodium glutamate, frequently used in Chinese cooking.

chip, **1.** a relatively small piece of a bone or tooth. **2.** to break off or cut away a small piece.

chip fracture, any small fragmental fracture, usually one involving a bony process near a joint.

chir-. See **cheiro-.**

chirality. See **handedness.**

-chiria, -cheiria, **1.** a combining form meaning a '(specified) condition involving hands': *acephalochiria, atelochiria, dichiria.* **2.** a combining form meaning a '(specified) condition involving stimulus and its perception': *allochiria, dyschiria, synchiria.*

chiro-. See **cheiro-.**

chiropodist /kirop′ədist, shir-/, a health professional trained to diagnose and treat diseases and other disorders of the feet. A chiropodist may be awarded a degree of D.S.C. (Doctor of Surgical Chiropody) or Pod.D. (Doctor of Podiatry) after completing at least 2 years of premedical studies followed by 4 years of study in an accredited college of podiatry. Internship is optional, but a graduate must pass an examination and receive a state license before being allowed to practice. After a refresher course, a D.S.C. or a Pod.D. may be granted the postgraduate degree D.P.M. (Doctor of Podiatric Medicine). Also called **podiatrist.**

chiropody /kirop′ədē, shir-/, the study of minor disorders of the feet and the practice of treating these disorders. Practitioners trained in chiropody are licensed to practice by the various states but do not hold a medical degree or license.

chiropractic /kī′rōprak′tik/, a system of therapy based on the theory that the state of a person's health is determined in general by the condition of his nervous system. In most cases treatment provided by chiropractors involves the mechanic manipulation of the spinal column. Some practitioners employ radiology for diagnosis and use physiotherapy and diet in addition to spinal manipulation. Chiropractic does not employ drugs or surgery, the primary basis of treatment used by medical physicians. A chiropractor is awarded the degree of Doctor of Chiropractic, or D.C., after completing at least 2 years of premedical studies followed by 4 years of training in an approved chiropractic school. Compare **allopathic.**

-chirurgia. See **-surgery.**

chisel fracture, any fracture in which there is an oblique detachment of a bone fragment from the head of the radius.

chi square (χ^2) /kī/, (in statistics) a statistic test for an association between observed data and expected data represented by frequencies. The test yields a statement of the probability of the obtained distribution having occurred by chance alone.

Chlamydia /kləmid′ē•ə/, **1.** a microorganism of the genus *Chlamydia*. **2.** a genus of microorganisms that live as intracellular parasites, have a number of properties in common with gram-negative bacteria, and are currently classified as specialized bacteria. Two species of *Chlamydia* have been recognized; both are pathogenic to humans. ***Chlamydia trachomatis,*** an organism that lives in the conjunctiva of the eye and the epithelium of the urethra and cervix, is responsible for inclusion conjunctivitis, lymphogranuloma venereum, and trachoma. It is one of the most common sexually transmitted diseases in North America and a frequent cause of sterility. ***Chlamydia psittaci*** is an organism that infects birds and causes a type of pneumonia in humans. See also **psittacosis.** – **chlamydial,** *adj*.

chloasma /klō•az′mə/, tan or brown pigmentation, particularly of the forehead, cheeks, and nose, commonly associated with pregnancy or the use of oral contraceptives. The hyperpigmentation may be permanent or may disappear only to recur with subsequent pregnancies or use of oral contraceptives. Also called **mask of pregnancy, melasma.**

chlor-, a combining form meaning 'green': *chloremia, chlorephidrosis, chlorine*.

chloracne /klôrak′nē/, a skin condition characterized by small, black follicular plugs and papules on exposed surfaces, especially on the arms, face, and neck of workers in contact with chlorinated compounds, as cutting oils, paints, varnishes, and lacquers. Avoidance of contact with chlorinated compounds or the use of protective garments prevents the condition.

chloral camphor, a mixture of equal parts of camphor and chloral hydrate, used externally as a sedative.

chloral hydrate, a sedative and hypnotic.

■ INDICATIONS: It is prescribed for the relief of insomnia, anxiety, or tension.

■ CONTRAINDICATIONS: Liver or kidney dysfunction or known hypersensitivity to this drug prohibits its use.

■ ADVERSE EFFECTS: Among the more serious adverse reactions are GI disturbances, skin rash, paradoxic excitement, and hypotension.

chlorambucil, an alkylating agent.

■ INDICATIONS: It is prescribed in the treatment of a variety of malignant neoplastic diseases, including chronic lymphocytic leukemia and Hodgkin's disease.

■ CONTRAINDICATIONS: Bone marrow depression or known hypersensitivity to this drug prohibits its use. It is not given during the first trimester of pregnancy or within 28 days of chemotherapy or radiation therapy.

■ ADVERSE EFFECTS: Among the more serious adverse reactions are bone marrow depression, GI disturbance, skin rash, and hepatotoxicity.

chloramphenicol, an antibacterial and antirickettsial.

■ INDICATIONS: It is prescribed in the treatment of a wide variety of serious infections.

■ CONTRAINDICATIONS: Mild or unidentified infections, pregnancy, lactation, or known hypersensitivity to this drug prohibits its use.

■ ADVERSE EFFECTS: Among the more serious adverse reactions are blood dyscrasias, bone marrow depression, and aplastic anemia.

chlorcyclizine hydrochloride /klôrsī′klizin/, an antihistamine that has been used for rhinitis, sinusitis, and hayfever. As a cream, it is also used for skin conditions.

chlordane poisoning. See **chlorinated organic insecticide poisoning.**

chlordantoin /klôrdan′tō•in/, an antifungal.

■ INDICATIONS: It is prescribed in the treatment of candidiasis of the vagina and the skin.

■ CONTRAINDICATION: Known hypersensitivity to this drug prohibits its use.

■ ADVERSE EFFECTS: Among the more serious adverse reactions are irritation and allergic reactions.

chlordiazepoxide /klôr′dī•az′əpok′sīd/, a minor tranquilizer.

■ INDICATIONS: It is prescribed in the treatment of anxiety and nervous tension and alcohol withdrawal symptoms.

■ CONTRAINDICATIONS: Psychosis, acute narrow-angle glaucoma, or known hypersensitivity to this drug prohibits its use.

■ ADVERSE EFFECTS: Among the more serious adverse reactions are withdrawal symptoms occurring on discontinuation of treatment. Drowsiness and fatigue commonly occur.

chlorhexidine, an antimicrobial agent used as a surgical scrub, hand rinse, and topical antiseptic.

-chloric, a combining form meaning 'referring to or containing chlorine': *hydrochloric, hyperchloric, perchloric*.

chloride /klôr′īd/, a compound in which the negative element is chlorine. Chlorides are salts of hydrochloric acid, the most common being sodium chloride (table salt).

chloride shift, an exchange of chloride ions in red blood cells in peripheral tissues in response to P_{CO_2} of blood. The shift reverses in the lungs.

chlorinated organic insecticide poisoning, poisoning resulting from the inhalation, ingestion, or absorption of DDT and other insecticides containing chlorophenothane, as heptachlor, dieldrin, and chlordane. It is characterized by vomiting, weakness, malaise, convulsions, tremors, ventricular fibrillation, respiratory failure, and pulmonary edema. Treatment includes control of the neurologic and neuromuscular symptoms with phenobarbitol and gastric lavage, instillation of a demulcent and absorbent such as sodium sulfate or charcoal in the stomach, parenteral fluids, and supportive therapy as indicated by monitoring vital functions. Also called **DDT poisoning.**

chlorine (Cl) /klôr′ēn/, a yellowish-green, gaseous element of the halogen group. Its atomic number is 17; its atomic weight is 35.453. It has a strong, distinctive odor, is irritating to the respiratory tract, and is poisonous if ingested or inhaled. It occurs in nature chiefly as a component of sodium chloride in sea water and in salt deposits. It is used as a bleach and as a disinfectant to purify water for drinking or for use in swimming pools. Chlorine compounds in general use include many solvents, cleaning fluids, and chloroform. Most of the solvents and cleaning fluids containing chlorine are toxic when inhaled or ingested. Chloroform was formerly in general use as an anesthetic.

chlormezanone, an antianxiety agent.

▪ INDICATIONS: It is prescribed for mild anxiety and for nervous tension.

▪ CONTRAINDICATION: Known hypersensitivity to this drug prohibits its use.

▪ ADVERSE EFFECTS: Among the most serious adverse reactions are hypersensitivity and sedation. Dizziness, nausea, and rashes often occur.

chloroform /klôr′əfôrm′/, a nonflammable, volatile liquid that was the first inhalation anesthetic to be discovered. Because of ease of administration—often just a medicine dropper and a handkerchief face mask—it is still the principal general anesthetic in many underdeveloped countries, where anesthesia equipment for the newer agents is not available. Chloroform is a dangerous anesthetic drug: A difference of only 10% in drug-plasma levels can result in hypotension, myocardial and respiratory depression, cardiogenic shock, ventricular fibrillation, coma, and death. Delayed poisoning, even weeks after apparently complete recovery, can occur, and serious ocular damage is frequently reported.

chloroformism, **1.** the habit of inhaling chloroform for its narcotic effect. **2.** the anesthetic effect of chloroform.

chloroguanide hydrochloride /klôr′əgwan′īd/, an antimalarial.

▪ INDICATIONS: It is prescribed in the prophylaxis of malaria, particularly in cases caused by *Plasmodium falciparum.*

▪ CONTRAINDICATIONS: Hypersensitivity to the drug prohibits its use. It is prescribed with caution during pregnancy, especially in the first trimester.

▪ ADVERSE EFFECTS: Among the more serious adverse reactions are megaloblastic anemia, anorexia, and weight loss, usually occurring with prolonged prophylactic use.

chloroleukemia /klôr′ōlo͞okē′mē•ə/, a kind of myelogenous leukemia in which specific tumor masses are not seen at autopsy but body fluids and organs are green. See also **myelogenous leukemia.**

chlorolymphosarcoma /klôr′ōlim′fōsärkō′mə/, *pl.* **chlorolymphosarcomas, chlorolymphosarcomata,** a greenish neoplasm of myeloid tissue occurring in patients with myelogenous leukemia. The mononuclear cells in the peripheral blood are believed to be lymphocytes rather than myeloblasts, as found with chloroma.

chloroma /klôrō′mə/, *pl.* **chloromas, chloromata,** a malignant, greenish neoplasm of myeloid tissue occurring anywhere in the body in patients with myelogenous leukemia. The green pigment, primarily myeloperoxidase (verdoperoxidase), has no definite metabolic function. The tumor tissue fluoresces bright red under ultraviolet light. Also called **granulocytic sarcoma, green cancer.**

Chloromycetin, a trademark for an antibacterial and antirickettsial (chloramphenicol).

chloromyeloma. See **chloroma.**

chlorophyll /klôr′əfil/, a plant pigment capable of absorbing light and converting it to energy for the oxidation and reduction involved in the photosynthesis of carbohydrates. Chlorophylls a and b are found in green plants; chlorophyll c occurs in brown algae, and chlorophyll d occurs in red algae. See also **photosynthesis.**

chlorophyll test. See **Boas' test.**

chloroprocaine /klôr′ōprō′kān/, a local anesthetic with a chemical structure similar to procaine.

chloroquine /klôr′əkwīn′/, an antimalarial.

▪ INDICATIONS: It is prescribed in the treatment of malaria, extraintestinal amebiasis, rheumatoid arthritis, some forms of lupus erythematosus, and photoallergic reactions.

▪ CONTRAINDICATIONS: Retinal or visual field changes, porphyria, or known hypersensitivity to this drug prohibits its use.

▪ ADVERSE EFFECTS: Among the more serious adverse reactions are GI disturbances, headache, visual disturbances, and pruritus.

chlorosis /klôrō′sis/, *archaic.* an iron deficiency anemia of young women characterized by hypochromic, microcytic erythrocytes and a small reduction in the total number of erythrocytes. See also **anemia.**

chlorothiazide, a diuretic and antihypertensive.

▪ INDICATIONS: It is prescribed in the treatment of hypertension and edema.

▪ CONTRAINDICATIONS: Anuria or known hypersensitivity to thiazide medication or to sulfonamide derivatives prohibits its use.

▪ ADVERSE EFFECTS: Among the more serious adverse reactions are hypokalemia, hyperglycemia, and hyperuricemia. Hypersensitivity reactions may occur.

chlorotrianisene, an estrogen.

▪ INDICATIONS: It is prescribed in the treatment of postpartum breast engorgement, menopausal symptoms, and prostatic cancer.

▪ CONTRAINDICATIONS: Liver dysfunction, thromboembolic disorders, unusual vaginal bleeding, known or suspected pregnancy, suspected estrogen-dependent neoplastic disease, or known hypersensitivity to this drug prohibits its use.

■ ADVERSE EFFECTS: Among the more serious adverse reactions are GI distress, breakthrough bleeding, and, in men, gynecomastia, decreased libido, and impotence.

chlorpheniramine maleate, an antihistamine.

■ INDICATIONS: It is prescribed in the treatment of a variety of hypersensitivity reactions, including rhinitis, skin rash, and pruritus.

■ CONTRAINDICATIONS: Asthma or known hypersensitivity to this drug prohibits its use. It is not given to newborn infants or nursing mothers.

■ ADVERSE EFFECTS: Among the more serious adverse reactions are skin rash, hypersensitivity reactions, and tachycardia. Drowsiness and dry mouth commonly occur.

chlorpromazine /klôrprō′məzēn/, a phenothiazine tranquilizer and antiemetic.

■ INDICATIONS: It is prescribed in the treatment of psychotic disorders, severe nausea and vomiting, and intractable hiccups.

■ CONTRAINDICATIONS: Parkinson's disease, concurrent administration of central nervous system depressants, liver or renal dysfunction, severe hypotension, or known hypersensitivity to this drug or to other phenothiazine medication prohibits its use.

■ ADVERSE EFFECTS: Among the more serious adverse effects are hypotension, liver toxicity, a variety of extrapyramidal reactions, blood dyscrasias, and hypersensitivity reactions.

chlorpropamide, an oral antidiabetic.

■ INDICATION: It is prescribed in the treatment of mild, stable non-insulin-dependent diabetes mellitus.

■ CONTRAINDICATIONS: Liver or kidney dysfunction or known hypersensitivity to this drug prohibits its use.

■ ADVERSE EFFECTS: Among the most serious adverse reactions are hematologic derangements and jaundice. GI distress and rashes are common adverse effects.

chlorprothixene /klôr′prōthik′sēn/, a thioxanthine antipsychotic agent.

■ INDICATIONS: It is prescribed in the treatment of psychotic disorders.

■ CONTRAINDICATIONS: Parkinson's disease, concurrent administration of central nervous system depressants, liver or renal dysfunction, severe hypotension, or known hypersensitivitity to this drug prohibits its use.

■ ADVERSE EFFECTS: Among the more serious adverse effects are hypotension, liver toxicity, a variety of extrapyramidal reactions, blood dycrasias, and hypersensitivity reactions.

chlortetracycline hydrochloride, an antibiotic.

■ INDICATIONS: It is prescribed in the treatment of a variety of infections.

■ CONTRAINDICATIONS: Renal or liver dysfunction, pregnancy, early childhood, or known hypersensitivity to this drug or to other tetracycline medication prohibits its use.

■ ADVERSE EFFECTS: Among the more serious adverse effects are GI disturbances, phototoxicity, potentially serious suprainfections, and hypersensitivity reactions. Discoloration of teeth may occur in children exposed to this drug in utero or before 8 years of age.

chlorthalidone, a diuretic and antihypertensive.

■ INDICATIONS: It is prescribed in the treatment of high blood pressure and edema.

■ CONTRAINDICATIONS: Anuria or known hypersensitivity to this drug, to other thiazide medication, or to sulfonamide derivatives prohibits its use.

■ ADVERSE EFFECTS: Among the more serious adverse reactions are hypokalemia, hyperglycemia, hyperuricemia, and hypersensitivity reactions.

Chlor-Trimeton, a trademark for an antihistamine (chlorpheniramine maleate).

chlorzoxazone /klôrzok′səzōn/, a skeletal muscle relaxant.

■ INDICATION: It is prescribed for the relief of muscle spasm.

■ CONTRAINDICATION: Known hypersensitivity to this drug is the only contraindication.

■ ADVERSE EFFECTS: Among the more serious adverse reactions are jaundice and GI bleeding.

choana /kō′ənə/, *pl.* **choanae, 1.** a funnel-shaped channel. **2.** See **posterior nares.**

choanal atresia /kō′ənəl/, a congenital anomaly in which a bony or membranous occlusion blocks the passageway between the nose and pharynx. The condition, which is caused by the failure of the nasopharyngeal septum to rupture during embryonic development, can result in serious ventilation problems in the neonate, and providing an oral airway or endotracheal intubation may be necessary. The defect is usually repaired surgically shortly after birth.

choke, to interrupt respiration by compression or obstruction of larynx or trachea.

choke damp. See **damp.**

choked disc. *informal.* papilledema.

chokes, a respiratory condition, occurring in decompression sickness, characterized by shortness of breath, substernal pain, and a nonproductive cough caused by bubbles of gas in the blood vessels of the lungs.

choking, the condition in which a respiratory passage is blocked by constriction of the neck, an obstruction in the trachea, or swelling of the larynx. It is characterized by sudden coughing and a red face that rapidly becomes cyanotic. The person cannot breathe and clutches his throat. Emergency treatment requires removal of the obstruction and resuscitation if necessary. See also **Heimlich maneuver.**

chol-. See **chole-.**

cholangeostomy /kōlan′jē·os′təmē/, a surgical operation to form an opening in a bile duct.

cholangiogram /kōlan′jē·əgram′/, an x-ray film of the bile ducts produced after injection of a radiopaque contrast medium. A cholangiogram is routinely performed as a part of biliary tract surgery, before or after the procedure. A postoperative radiogram may be made after injecting an iodinated contrast medium through an indwelling T-tube. The medium also may be introduced directly into the biliary system or intravenously. See also **cholangiography, cholecystography.**

cholangiography /kōlan′jē•og′rəfē/, a special roentgenographic test procedure for outlining the major bile ducts by the intravenous injection or the direct instillation of a radiopaque contrast material.

■ METHOD: For intravenous cholangiography the contrast agent is given slowly by vein, and x-ray films are taken of the region of the gallbladder. If the gallbladder has not been removed, a fatty meal may then be given and further x-ray films taken to show contraction of the gallbladder. Operative and postoperative cholangiography employ the injection of contrast material into the common bile duct via a drainage T-tube inserted during surgery, the purpose being to discover any small, residual gallstones. In percutaneous transhepatic cholangiography the contrast material is injected through a long needle or needle-catheter, which is introduced directly through the skin into the substance of the liver. Endoscopic retrograde cholangiography is accomplished by cannulating the ampulla of Vater through a flexible fiberoptic duodenoscope and instilling radiopaque material directly into the common bile duct.

■ NURSING ORDERS: Intravenous cholangiography cannot be used in the presence of severe liver disease or jaundice, because the dye will not be concentrated and excreted into the bile. The patient fasts and fluids are restricted overnight. An early morning cleansing enema is given, usually followed by a sedative. The patient is warned about a brief period of a burning sensation that occurs as the dye is injected. For percutaneous transhepatic cholangiography, sedative premedication is often ordered and a local anesthetic injected at the site of needle puncture. Appropriate evaluation for bleeding tendencies must be carried out before percutaneous transhepatic cholangiography. Bile peritonitis is occasionally a complication of T-tube or percutaneous cholangiography, and close nursing observation is essential after the test is completed. For endoscopic retrograde cholangiography, nothing is given by mouth after midnight, an explanation is given to the patient, dentures are removed, and, to permit administration of medications, intravenous infusion is begun. The endoscope is passed with the patient in the left lateral position; then the patient is turned to the prone position, the ampulla is cannulated, the dye is injected, and films are taken. Vital signs are observed and the patient is given a light meal in 2 to 4 hours after the procedure.

■ OUTCOME CRITERIA: The resulting cholangiograms from any of these procedures are examined for unobstructed outlining of the biliary system. Calculi may be noted as shadows within the opaque medium. See also **cholecystography.**

cholangiohepatoma /kōlan′jē•ōhep′ətō′mə/, *pl.* **cholangiohepatomas, cholangiohepatomata,** a neoplasm in which there is an abnormal mixture of liver cord cells and bile ducts.

cholangiolitis /kōlan′jē•əlī′tis/, an abnormal condition characterized by inflammation of the fine tubules of the bile duct system, which may cause cholangiolitic cirrhosis. **–cholangiolitic,** *adj*.

cholangioma /kōlan′jē•ō′mə/, *pl.* **cholangiomas, cholangiomata,** a neoplasm of the bile ducts.

cholangitis /kō′lanjī′tis/, inflammation of the bile ducts, caused either by bacterial invasion or by obstruction of the ducts by calculi or a tumor. The condition is characterized by severe right upper quadrant pain, jaundice (if an obstruction is present), and intermittent fever. Blood tests reveal an elevated level of serum bilirubin. Diagnosis is made by oral cholecystogram or intravenous cholangiogram. Treatment is with antibiotics for infection and with surgery for acute obstruction. See also **biliary calculus.**

chole-, chol-, cholo-, a combining form meaning 'pertaining to the bile': *cholecystectomy, cholelithotomy, cholesterase*.

cholecalciferol. See **vitamin D_3.**

cholecystectomy /kō′lisistek′təmē/, the surgical removal of the gallbladder, performed to treat cholelithiasis and cholecystitis. Surgery may be delayed while the acute inflammation is treated. A cholecystogram is done to confirm the diagnosis, and an electrocardiogram and tests of hepatic function may be ordered. The prothrombin level is evaluated, and, if it is low, vitamin K is given. Under general anesthesia, the gallbladder is excised and the cystic duct ligated; the common duct is searched, and any stones found are removed. A T-tube is left in place to ensure adequate bile drainage; a Penrose drain may be left in a separate stab wound to prevent the formation of an abcess. The most common complication is a disruption of the hepatic or other ducts of the biliary system, requiring surgical correction. Wound infection, hemorrhage, bile leakage, and jaundice may also occur. A nasogastric tube is left in place postoperatively until bowel function has returned and food can be tolerated. See also **cholecystitis, cholelithiasis.**

cholecystitis /kō′lisistī′tis/, acute or chronic inflammation of the gallbladder. **Acute cholecystitis** is usually caused by a gallstone that cannot pass through the cystic duct. Pain is felt in the right upper quadrant of the abdomen, accompanied by nausea, vomiting, eructation, and flatulence. Diagnosis is usually made with oral cholecystogram, useful in ruling out acute appendicitis, intestinal obstruction, peptic ulcer, and other upper abdominal disorders. Surgery is the preferred mode of treatment. **Chronic cholecystitis,** the more common type, has an insidious onset. Pain, often felt at night, may follow a fatty meal. Complications include biliary calculi, pancreatitis, and carcinoma of the gallbladder. Again, surgery is the preferred treatment. See also **biliary calculus, cholecystectomy, cholelithiasis.**

cholecystogram /kō′lisis′təgram′/, an x-ray film of the gallbladder, made after the ingestion or injection of a radiopaque substance, usually a contrast material containing iodine.

cholecystography /kō′lisistog′rəfē/, an x-ray examination of the gallbladder. At least 12 hours before the study the patient has a fat-free meal and ingests a contrast material containing iodine, usually in the form of tablets; it may also be given intravenously. The iodine, which is opaque to x-rays, is excreted by the liver into the bile in the gallbladder. After the procedure, the patient consumes a fatty meal or cholecystokinin, which stimulates the gallbladder to contract, expelling bile and contrast material into the bile duct. Additional x-ray films are taken about 1 hour later. The test is useful in the diagnosis of cholecystitis, cholelithiasis, tumors, and the differential diagnosis of a mass in the upper right quadrant of the stomach.

cholecystokinin /kol′isis′təkī′nin/, a hormone, produced by the mucosa of the upper intestine, that stimulates contraction of the gallbladder and the secretion of pancreatic enzymes.

choledocholithiasis. See **biliary calculus.**

choledocholithotomy /kōled′ōkō′lithot′əmē/, a surgical operation to make an incision in the common bile duct to remove a stone.

Choledyl, a trademark for a theophylline derivative (oxtriphylline), used as a bronchodilator.

cholelithiasis /kō′lilithī′əsis/, the presence of gallstones in the gallbladder. The condition affects about 20% of the population over 40 years of age and is more prevalent in women and in persons with cirrhosis of the liver. Many patients complain of unlocalized abdominal discomfort, eructation, and intolerance to certain foods. Other patients will have no symptoms at all. In patients with severe attacks of biliary pain associated with cholelithiasis, cholecystectomy is recommended to prevent such complications as cholecystitis, cholangitis, and pancreatitis. See also **biliary calculus, cholecystitis.**

cholelithic dyspepsia /kō′lilith′ik/, an abnormal condition characterized by sudden attacks of indigestion associated with the dysfunction of the gallbladder. See also **dyspepsia.**

cholelithotomy /kō′lilithot′əmē/, a surgical operation to remove gallstones through an incision in the gallbladder.

cholera /kol′ərə/, an acute bacterial infection of the small intestine, characterized by severe diarrhea and vomiting, muscular cramps, dehydration, and depletion of electrolytes. The disease is spread by water and food that have been contaminated by feces of persons previously infected. The symptoms are caused by toxic substances produced by the infecting organism, *Vibrio cholerae*. The profuse, watery diarrhea, as much as a liter an hour, depletes the body of fluids and minerals. Complications include circulatory collapse, cyanosis, destruction of kidney tissue, and metabolic acidosis. Mortality is as high as 50% if the infection remains untreated. Treatment includes the administration of antibiotics that destroy the infecting bacteria and the restoration of normal amounts of fluids and electrolytes with intravenous solutions. A cholera vaccine is available for people traveling to areas where the infection is endemic. Other preventive measures include drinking only boiled or bottled water and eating only cooked foods. See also ***Vibrio cholerae, Vibrio gastroenteritis.***

choleragen /kol′ərəjin/, an exotoxin, produced by the cholera vibrio, that stimulates the secretion of electrolyte and water into the small intestine in Asiatic cholera, draining the fluids of the body and weakening the patient.

cholera vaccine, an active immunizing agent.

■ INDICATION: It is prescribed as an immunization against cholera.

■ CONTRAINDICATIONS: Immunosuppression, acute infection, concomitant administration of corticosteroids, or known hypersensitivity to this drug prohibits its use.

■ ADVERSE EFFECTS: The most serious adverse reaction is anaphylaxis.

choleretic /kō′ləret′ik/, **1.** stimulating the production of bile either by cholepoiesis or by hydrocholeresis. **2.** a choleretic agent.

choleric /kol′ərik, kəler′ik/, having a hot temper or an irascible nature.

cholestasis /kō′listā′sis/, interruption in the flow of bile through any part of the biliary system, from liver to duodenum. It is essential for the physician to discover whether the cause is within the liver (intrahepatic) or outside it (extrahepatic). Intrahepatic causes include hepatitis, drug and alcohol use, metastatic carcinoma, and pregnancy. Extrahepatic causes may be an obstructing calculus or tumor in the common bile duct or carcinoma of the pancreas. Symptoms of both types of cholestasis include jaundice, pale and fatty stools, dark urine, and intense itching over the skin. If liver disease is suspected, liver biopsy can confirm the suspicion, and attempts can be made to treat the underlying disorder. Extrahepatic cholestasis usually requires surgery. See also **cholestatic hepatitis, hyperbilirubinemia of the newborn.** **–cholestatic,** *adj.*

cholestatic hepatitis /kō′listat′ik/, inflammation of the liver caused by hepatitis infection that produces interruption of the flow of bile in the intrahepatic ducts. Signs are persistent jaundice, itching, and elevated alkaline phosphatase. These signs usually abate when the hepatitis remits. See also **cholestasis, hepatitis.**

cholesteatoma /kōles′tē•ətō′mə/, a cystic mass composed of epithelial cells and cholesterol that is found in the middle ear and occurs as a congenital defect or as a serious complication of chronic otitis media. The mass may occlude the middle ear, or enzymes produced by it may destroy the adjacent bones, including the ossicles. Surgery is required to remove a cholesteatoma. See also **otitis media.**

cholesterase /kəles′tərās′/, an enzyme in the blood and other tissues that forms cholesterol and fatty acids by hydrolyzing cholesterol esters.

cholesteremia. See **cholesterolemia.**

cholesterol /kəles′tərôl/, a fat-soluble crystalline steroid alcohol found in animal fats and oils, and egg yolk, and widely distributed in the body, especially in the bile, blood, brain tissue, liver, kidneys, adrenal glands, and myelin sheaths of nerve fibers. It facilitates the absorption and transport of fatty acids and acts as the precursor for the synthesis of vitamin D at the surface of the skin as well as for the synthesis of the various steroid hormones, including cortisol, cortisone, and aldosterone in the adrenal glands and of the sex hormones progesterone, estrogen, and testosterone. It sometimes crystallizes in the gallbladder to form gallstones. Cholesterol is found almost exclusively in foods of animal origin and is continuously synthesized in the body, primarily in the liver and the adrenal cortex. Increased levels of serum cholesterol may be associated with the pathogenesis of atherosclerosis. Also called **cholesterin.** See also **high-density lipoprotein, low-density lipoprotein, vitamin D.**

cholesterolemia, **1.** the presence of excessive amounts of cholesterol in the blood. **2.** the abnormal condition of having excessive amounts of cholesterol in the blood. Also called **cholesteremia.**

cholesteroleresis /kəles′tərôler′isis/, the increased elimination of cholesterol in the bile.

cholesterol metabolism, the sum of the anabolic and catabolic processes in the synthesis and degradation of cholesterol in the body. Ingested cholesterol is quickly absorbed. It is also synthesized in the liver and can be synthesized by most other tissues of the body. As more cholesterol is ingested, less is synthesized. Cholesterol is removed from the body by conversion in the liver and excretion in the bile.

cholesterolopoiesis /kəles′tərôlōpō·ē′sis/, the elaboration of cholesterol by the liver.

cholesterolosis /kəles′tərəlō′sis/, an abnormal condition, found in about 5% of patients with chronic cholecystitis, in which there are deposits of cholesterol within large macrophages in the submucosa of the gallbladder. This produces a spotty appearance, sometimes referred to as a strawberry gallbladder. Cholesterolosis is often associated with gallstones and may be asymptomatic or accompanied by biliary colic. See also **cholecystitis.**

cholestyramine resin, an ion-exchange resin and antihyperlipoproteinemic agent.

■ INDICATIONS: It is prescribed for hyperlipoproteinemia and for pruritus resulting from partial biliary obstruction.

■ CONTRAINDICATIONS: Complete biliary obstruction or known hypersensitivity to this drug prohibits its use.

■ ADVERSE EFFECTS: Among the more serious adverse reactions are fecal impaction, GI disturbances, and depletion of vitamins A, D, and K. Constipation is common.

-cholia, -choly, a combining form meaning '(condition of the) bile': *albuminocholia, syncholia, uricocholia.*

choline /kō′lēn/, one of the B complex vitamins, essential for the metabolism of fats in the body. It is a primary component of acetylcholine, the neurotransmitter, and functions with inositol as a basic constituent of lecithin. It prevents the deposition of fats in the liver and facilitates the movement of fats into the cells. The richest sources of choline are liver, kidneys, brains, wheat germ, brewer's yeast, and egg yolk. Deficiency leads to hepatic cirrhosis, resulting in bleeding stomach ulcers and impaired kidney function, hypertension, high blood levels of cholesterol, and atherosclerosis and arteriosclerosis. See also **inositol, lecithin.**

cholinergic, **1.** of or pertaining to nerve fibers that elaborate acetylcholine at the myoneural junctions. **2.** the tendency to transmit or to be stimulated by or to stimulate the elaboration of acetylcholine. Compare **adrenergic, anticholinergic.**

cholinergic blocking agent, any agent that blocks the action of acetylcholine and substances similar to acetylcholine. Such agents, in effect, block the action of cholinergic nerves that transmit impulses by the release of acetylcholine at their synapses.

cholinergic crisis, a pronounced muscular weakness and respiratory paralysis caused by excessive acetylcholine, often apparent in patients suffering from myasthenia gravis as a result of overmedication with anticholinesterase drugs.

cholinergic nerve, a nerve that releases the neurotransmitter acetylcholine at its synapse. The cholinergic nerves include all the preganglionic sympathetic and the preganglionic parasympathetic nerves, the postganglionic parasympathetic nerves, the somatic motor nerves to skeletal muscles, and some nerves to sweat glands and to certain blood vessels.

cholinergic stimulant. See **cholinergic.**

cholinergic urticaria, an abnormal and usually transient vascular reaction of the skin, often associated with sweating in susceptible individuals subjected to stress, strong exertion, or hot weather. The condition is characterized by small, pale, itchy papules surrounded by reddish areas; it is caused by the action of acetylcholine on mast cells.

cholinesterase /kō′lines′tərās/, an enzyme that acts as a catalyst in the hydrolysis of acetylcholine to choline and acetate.

choliopancreatography, the x-ray visualization of the bile and pancreatic ducts.

cholo-. See **chole-.**

Cholografin, a trademark for a diagnostic dye (iodipamide), used in radiology.

Choloxin, a trademark for an antihyperlipoproteinemic (dextrothyroxine sodium).

-choly. See **-cholia.**

chondr-. See **chondro-.**

chondral /kon′drəl/, of or pertaining to cartilage.

chondrectomy /kondrek′təmē/, the surgical excision of a cartilage.

chondri-. See **chondro-.**

-chondria, **1.** a combining form meaning a 'condition involving granules in cell composition': *lipochondria, mitochondria, plastochondria.* **2.** a combining form meaning an 'abnormal preoccupation with worry about disease': *hypochondria*.

chondriocont /kon′drē•ōkont′/, a threadlike or rod-shaped mitochondrion.

chondriome /kon′drē•ōm/, the total mitochondria content of a cell, taken as a unit. Also called **chondrioma.**

chondriomite /kon′drē•ōmīt′/, a single granular mitochondrion or a group of such organelles appearing in a chain formation.

chondriosome. See **mitochondrion.**

chondritis /kondrī′tis/, any inflammatory condition affecting the joints.

chondro-, chondr-, chondri-, a combining form meaning 'pertaining to cartilage': *chondroblast, chondroclast, chondrocostal*.

chondroadenoma. See **adenochondroma.**

chondroangioma /kon′drō•an′jē•ō′mə/, *pl.* **chondroangiomas, chondroangiomata,** a benign, mesenchymal tumor containing vascular and cartilaginous elements.

chondroblast /kon′drōblast/, any one of the cells that develops from the mesenchyma and forms cartilage. Also called **chondroplast.**

chondroblastoma /kon′drōblastō′mə/, *pl.* **chondroblastomas, chondroblastomata,** a benign tumor, derived from precursors of cartilage cells, that develops most frequently in epiphyses of the femur and humerus, especially in young men. The lesions may contain scattered areas of calcification and necrosis. Also called **Codman's tumor.**

chondrocalcinosis /kon′drōkal′sinō′sis/, an arthritic disease in which calcium deposits are found in the peripheral joints. Chondrocalcinosis, which resembles gout, is often found in patients over 50 years of age who have osteoarthritis or diabetes mellitus. Aspiration of synovial fluid from the affected joints reveals crystals of calcium salts. Inflammation and pain may be relieved by intraarticular injections of hydrocortisone and by antiinflammatory medications. Prognosis for recovery is excellent. Also called **pseudogout.** Compare **gout, gouty arthritis.**

chondrocarcinoma /kon′drōkär′sinō′mə/, *pl.* **chondrocarcinoma, chondrocarcinomata,** a malignant epithelial tumor in which there is cartilaginous metaplasia.

chondroclast /kon′drōklast′/, a giant multinucleated cell associated with the resorption of cartilage. **–chondroclastic,** *adj.*

chondrocostal /kon′drōkos′təl/, of or pertaining to the ribs and the costal cartilages.

chondrocyte /kon′drəsīt/, any one of the polymorphic cells that form the cartilage of the body. Each contains a nucleus, a relatively large amount of clear cytoplasm, and the common organelles. **–chondrocytic,** *adj.*

chondrodystrophia calcificans congenita, an inherited defect characterized by many small opacities in the epiphyses of the long bones. This sign is present on x-ray films of the newborn. Dwarfism, contractures, cataracts, mental retardation, and short stubby fingers develop as the infant grows into childhood. Also called **chondrodystrophia fetalis calcificans, Conradi's disease.**

chondrodystrophy /kon′drōdis′trəfē/, a group of disorders in which there is abnormal conversion of cartilage to bone, particularly in the epiphyses of the long bones. Patients are dwarfed, with normal trunks and shortened extremities. See also **achondroplasia.**

chondroendothelioma /kon′drō•en′dōthē′lē•ō′mə/, *pl.* **chondroendotheliomas, chondroendotheliomata,** a benign mesenchymal tumor containing cartilaginous and endothelial components.

chondrofibroma /kon′drōfībrō′mə/, *pl.* **chondrofibromas, chondrofibromata,** a fibrous tumor containing cartilaginous components.

chondrogenesis /kon′drōjen′əsis/, the development of cartilage. **–chondrogenetic,** *adj.*

chondroid /kon′droid/, resembling cartilage.

chondrolipoma /kon′drōlipō′mə/, *pl.* **chondrolipomas, chondrolipomata,** a benign mesenchymal tumor containing fatty and cartilaginous components.

chondroma /kondrō′mə/, *pl.* **chondromas, chondromata,** a benign, fairly common tumor of cartilage cells that grows slowly within cartilage (enchondroma) or on the surface (ecchondroma). Kinds of chondromas are **joint chondroma** and **synovial chondroma.** See also **ecchondroma, enchondroma. –chondromatous,** *adj.*

-chondroma, a combining form meaning a 'benign cartilaginous tumor': *hyaloenchondroma, osteochondroma*.

chondromalacia /kon′drōməlā′shə/, a softening of cartilage. **Chondromalacia fetalis** is a lethal congenital form of the condition in which the stillborn infant is born with soft and pliable limbs. **Chondromalacia patellae** occurs in young adults after knee injury and is characterized by swelling and pain and by degenerative changes, which are revealed on examination by x-ray.

chondroma sarcomatosum. See **chondrosarcoma.**

chondromatosis /kon′drōmətō′sis/, a condition characterized by the presence of many cartilaginous tumors. A kind of chondromatosis is **synovial chondromatosis.**

chondromere /kon′drōmir/, a cartilaginous, embryonic vertebra and its costal component.

chondromyoma /kon′drōmī•ō′mə/, *pl.* **chondromyomas, chondromyomata,** a benign mesenchymal tumor containing myomatous and cartilaginous tissue.

chondromyxofibroma /kon′drōmik′sōfībrō′mə/, a benign tumor that develops from cartilage-forming connective tissue. The lesion, typically a firm, grayish-white, somewhat rubbery mass, tends to occur in the knee and small bones of the foot and may be confused with chondrosarcoma. Also called **chondromyxoid fibroma.**

chondromyxoid /kon′drōmik′soid/, composed of cartilaginous and myxoid elements.

chondromyxoid fibroma. See **chondromyxofibroma.**

chondrophyte /kon′drōfīt′/, an abnormal mass of cartilage. **–chondrophytic,** *adj.*

chondroplast. See **chondroblast.**

chondroplasty /kon′drōplas′tē/, the surgical repair of cartilage.

chondrosarcoma /kon′drōsärkō′mə/, *pl.* **chondrosarcomas, chondrosarcomata,** a malignant neoplasm of cartilaginous cells or their precursors that occurs most frequently on long bones, the pelvic girdle, and the scapula. The characteristic tumor is a large, smooth, lobulated growth composed of nodules of hyaline cartilage that may show slight to marked calcification. Kinds of chondrosarcomas are **central chondrosarcoma** and **mesenchymal chondrosarcoma.** Also called **chondroma sarcomatosum.** **–chondrosarcomatous,** *adj.*

chondrosarcomatosis /kon′drōsär′kōmətō′sis/, a condition characterized by multiple, malignant cartilaginous tumors.

chondrosis /kondrō′sis/, **1.** the development of the cartilage of the body. **2.** a cartilaginous tumor.

chondrotomy /kondrot′əmē/, a surgical procedure for dividing a cartilage.

chord-, a combining form meaning 'string, cord': *chordoblastoma, chordoma, chordotomy.*

chordae tendineae, *sing.* **chorda tendinea,** the strands of tendon that anchor the cusps of the mitral and the tricuspid valves to the papillary muscles of the ventricles of the heart, preventing prolaspe of the valves into the atria during ventricular contraction. Also called **chordae tendineae cordis, tendinous cords.**

chordal canal. See **notochordal canal.**

chorda spinalis. See **spinal cord.**

chorda umbilicalis. See **umbilical cord.**

chordee /kôr′dē, kôr′dā/, a congenital defect of the genitourinary tract resulting in a ventral curvature of the penis, caused by a fibrous band of tissue instead of normal skin along the corpus spongiosum. The condition is often associated with hypospadias and is surgically corrected in early childhood. The goals of surgery are to improve the appearance of the genitalia cosmetically for psychologic reasons, to construct an organ that allows the boy to void in a standing position, and to produce a sexually adequate organ.

chordencephalon /kôrd′ensef′əlon/, the portion of the central nervous system that develops in the early weeks of pregnancy from the neural tube and includes the mesencephalon, the rhombencephalon, and the spinal cord. The chordencephalon is segmented and divided into the alar and the basal plates. The alar plate becomes the sensory portion of the gray substance of the spinal cord; the basal plate becomes the motor portion of the gray substance. **–chordencephalic,** *adj.*

chorditis /kôrdī′tis/, **1.** inflammation of a spermatic cord. **2.** inflammation of the vocal cords or of the vocal folds.

chordoid /kôr′doid/, resembling the notocord or notochordal tissue.

chordoma /kôrdō′mə/, *pl.* **chordomas, chordomata,** a rare, congenital tumor of the brain developing from the fetal notochord. It is usually located in the midline, behind the sella, and is slow growing but highly invasive. Surgical removal is rarely possible.

chordotomy /kôrdot′əmē/, an operation in which the anterolateral tracts of the spinal cord are surgically divided to relieve pain.

chorea /kôrē′ə/, a condition characterized by involuntary, purposeless, rapid motions, as flexing and extending the fingers, raising and lowering the shoulders, or grimacing. In some forms the person is also irritable, emotionally unstable, weak, restless, and fretful. See also **chorea gravidarum, Huntington's chorea, Sydenham's chorea.** **–choreic** /kôrā′ik/, *adj.*

-chorea, a combining form meaning a '(specified) nervous disorder': *hemichorea, monochorea, orthochorea.*

chorea gravidarum, a form of chorea occurring during a first pregnancy subsequent to an episode of Sydenham's chorea in childhood. Similar symptoms may develop in a woman taking oral contraceptives.

chorea minor. See **Sydenham's chorea.**

choreiform /kərē′əfôrm′/, resembling the rapid jerky movements associated with chorea.

chorio-, a combining form meaning 'pertaining to the protective fetal membrane': *chorioblastosis, choriocele, chorioma.*

chorioadenoma /kərē′ō·ad′inō′mə/, *pl.* **chorioadenomas, chorioadenomata,** an epithelial cell tumor of the outermost fetal membrane that is intermediate in the malignant development of a hydatid mole to invasive choriocarcinoma.

chorioadenoma destruens, an invasive hydatidiform mole in which the chorionic villi of the mole penetrate into the myometrium and parametrium of the uterus and metastasize to distant parts of the body, most commonly to the lungs. Also called **invasive mole, malignant mole, metastasizing mole.**

chorioallantoic graft, the grafting of tissue onto the chorioallantoic membrane of the egg of a hen to improve the environment for embryonic growth.

chorioamnionic /kôr′ē·ō·am′nē·ot′ik/, of or pertaining to the chorion and the amnion.

chorioamnionitis, an inflammatory reaction in the amniotic membranes caused by organisms in the amniotic fluid. The membranes become infiltrated with polymorphonuclear leukocytes.

choriocarcinoma /kôr′ē·ōkär′sinō′mə/, *pl.* **choriocarcinomas, choriocarcinomata,** an epithelial malignancy of fetal origin that develops from the chorionic portion of the products of conception, usually from a hydatidiform mole. Less frequently it develops after an abortion, during a normal or ectopic pregnancy, or from a genital or extragenital teratoma. The primary tumor usually appears in the uterus as a soft, dark red, crumbling mass. It may invade and destroy the uterine wall and metastasize through lymph or blood vessels, forming secondary hemorrhagic and necrotic tumors in the vaginal wall, vulva, lymph nodes, lungs, liver, and brain. The urine often contains much more chorionic gonadotropin than is expected in pregnancy. The hormone level returns to normal when the tumor is completely removed. This form of cancer, which is more common in older than in younger women, responds to chemotherapy with cytotoxic drugs, as methotrexate. Rarely, a choriocarcinoma may arise in a teratoma of the testis, mediastinum, or pineal gland, and chemotherapy is usually not effective in treating these tumors. Also called **chorioblastoma, chorioepithelioma, chorionic carcinoma, chorionic epithelioma.**

choriocele /kôr′ē•əsēl′/, a hernia or protrusion of the tissue of the choroid layer of the eye.

chorioepithelioma. See **choriocarcinoma.**

choriogenesis /kôr′ē•ōjen′əsis/, the development of the chorion, which is first evident in the first month of pregnancy, after the trophoblast anchors to the uterine tissue and extends primary villi into the intervillous space. The chorion at first contains fluid and loose filaments of extraembryonic mesoderm. As pregnancy proceeds, the amnion grows into the chorionic space and obliterates it. The chorion continues to expand to accommodate the fetus and serves as the outer barrier between the fetus and the uterus. –**choriogenetic,** *adj.*

choriomeningitis. See **lymphocytic choriomeningitis.**

chorion /kôr′ē•on/, (in biology) the outermost extraembryonic membrane composed of trophoblast lined with mesoderm. It develops villi about 2 weeks after fertilization and is vascularized by allantoic vessels 1 week later. It gives rise to the placenta and persists until birth as the outer of the two layers of membrane containing the amniotic fluid and the fetus. Compare **amnion.** See also **amniotic sac.**

-chorion, a combining form meaning a 'membrane': *allantochorion, omphalochorion, prochorion.*

chorionic carcinoma, chorionic epithelioma. See **choriocarcinoma.**

chorionic gonadotropin (CG), a chemical component of the urine of pregnant women or pregnant mares. This glycoprotein hormone is secreted by the placental trophoblastic cells. It is composed of two subunits, alpha and beta human chorionic gonadotropin. The alpha subunit is nearly identical to similar subunits of the follicle-stimulating, luteinizing, and thyroid-stimulating hormones. The specific hormonal effects of chorionic gonadotropin are activated by the beta portion. They include stimulation of the corpus luteum to secrete estrogen and progesterone and to decrease lymphocyte activation, both important factors in preparing the uterus to accept the fetus immunologically. Chorionic gonadotropin is also administered in the treatment of some cases of cryptorchidism and male hypogonadism, and to induce ovulation in some infertile women. Also called **human chorionic gonadotropin (HCG).** See also **gonadotropin.**

chorionic plate, the part of the fetal placenta that gives rise to chorionic villi, which attach to the uterus during the early stage of formation of the placenta.

chorionic villi, tiny vascular fibrils on the surface of the chorion that infiltrate the maternal blood sinuses of the endometrium and help form the placenta. They are also a source of the HCG hormone of pregnancy.

chorioretinitis /kôr′ē•ōret′inī′tis/, an inflammatory condition of the choroid and retina of the eye, usually as a result of parasitic or bacterial infection. It is characterized by blurred vision, photophobia, and distorted images.

chorioretinopathy /kôr′ē•ōret′ənop′əthē/, a noninflammatory process caused by disease that involves the choroid and the retina. Also called **choroidoretinitis.**

choroid /kôr′oid/, a thin, highly vascular membrane covering the posterior five sixths of the eye between the retina and sclera.

choroidal malignant melanoma, a tumor of the choroid coat that grows into the vitreous humor, causing detachment and degeneration of the overlying retina. Typically mound shaped or mushroom shaped, the neoplasm may break through the sclera and present under the conjunctiva.

choroiditis /kôr′oidī′tis/, an inflammatory condition of the choroid membrane of the eye. See also **chorioretinitis.**

choroidocyclitis /kôroi′dōsiklī′tis/, an abnormal condition characterized by inflammation of the choroid and the ciliary processes.

choroidoretinitis. See **chorioretinopathy.**

choroid plexectomy /pleksek′təmē/, a surgical procedure for the reduction of cerebrospinal fluid production in the ventricles of the brain in hydrocephalus, usually in the newborn. The procedure involves transcortical entry of the lateral ventricles to coagulate or to excise the choroid plexuses and seeks to correct a communicating type of hydrocephalus.

choroid plexus, any one of the tangled masses of tiny blood vessels contained within the third, the lateral, and the fourth ventricles of the brain. The choroid plexus of the third ventricle is part of the roof of the anterior commissure of the third ventricle, lying above the interventricular foramen. The choroid plexus of the lateral ventricle is continuous with the choroid plexus of the third ventricle, extending from the interventricular foramen, through the body of the ventricle, to the rostral end of the inferior horn. The choroid plexus of the fourth ventricle, on each side, is an elongated tuft of blood vessels extending through the roof of the ventricle.

Christchurch chromosome (Ch^1), an abnormally small acrocentric chromosome of the G group, involving any members of chromosome pairs 21 or 22, in which the short arms are missing or partially deleted. The aberration is associated with chronic lymphocytic leukemia but has also been found in patients with various other defects. See also **Philadelphia chromosome.**

Christmas disease. See **hemophilia B.**

Christmas factor. See **factor IX.**

-chroia, a combining form meaning '(condition of) coloration': *cacochroia, cyanochroia, xanthochroia.*

chrom-. See **chromo-.**

chromaffin /krō′məfin/, having an affinity for strong staining with chromium salts, especially strong staining of the cells of the adrenal, the coccygeal, and the carotid glands, certain cells of the adrenal medulla, and the cells of the paraganglions. Also **chromaphil** /krō′məfil/.

chromaffin body. See **paraganglion.**

chromaffin cell, any one of the special cells comprising the paraganglia and connected to the ganglia of the celiac, the renal, the suprarenal, the aortic, and the hypogastric plexuses. Chromaffin cells are also sometimes found in association with other sympathetic plexuses. The chromaffin cells of the adrenal medulla secrete two catecholamines, epinephrine and norepinephrine, which affect smooth muscle, cardiac muscle, and glands in the same way as sympathetic stimulation, increasing and prolonging sympathetic effects. The chromaffin cells of the adrenal medulla are especially active in response to stress and the associated reception of nerve impulses from the hypothalamus. These impulses synapse with the chromaffin cells in the adrenal medulla and stimulate them to increase hormonal production, about 80% of which is epinephrine, the rest being norepinephrine.

chromaffinoma. See **pheochromocytoma.**

chromaphil. See **chromaffin.**

-chromasia, **1.** a combining form meaning '(condition of) color (as of cells, skin)': *allochromasia, hyperchromasia, oligochromasia.* **2.** a combining form meaning '(condition of the) stainability of tissues': *amblychromasia, anisochromasia, anochromasia.*

chromatic, **1.** of or pertaining to color. **2.** stainable by a dye. **3.** of or pertaining to chromatin. Also **chromatinic.**

-chromatic, a combining form meaning the 'staining properties of tissues and microorganisms': *lithochromatic, orthochromatic, panchromatic.*

chromatic dispersion, the splitting of light into its various component wavelengths or frequencies, as with a prism, to separate and study the different colors.

chromatid /krō′mətid/, one of the two identical threadlike filaments of a chromosome. It results from the self-replication of the chromosome during interphase, is held together by a common centromere, and, during anaphase of mitosis and meiosis, divides longitudinally to form daughter chromosomes.

chromatin /krō′mətin/, the material within the cell nucleus from which the chromosomes are formed. It consists of fine, threadlike strands of deoxyribonucleic acid attached to a protein base, usually histone; it is readily stained with basic dyes; and it occurs in two different forms, euchromatin and heterochromatin, which are distinguishable during the phases of the cell cycle by variant degrees of staining depending on the amount of dispersion or coiling that occurs. During cell division, portions of the chromatin condense and coil to form the chromosomes. A kind of chromatin is **sex chromatin.** Chromatin is also called **chromoplasm, karyotin.** See also **chromatid, euchromatin, heterochromatin.** **–chromatinic,** *adj.*

chromatin-negative, pertaining to or descriptive of the nuclei of cells that lack sex chromatin, specifically characteristic of the normal male, but also occurring in certain chromosomal abnormalities.

chromatin nucleolus. See **karyosome.**

chromatin-positive, pertaining to or descriptive of the nuclei of cells that contain sex chromatin, specifically characteristic of the normal female, but occurring also in certain chromosomal abnormalities.

chromatism /krō′mətiz′əm/, **1.** an abnormal condition characterized by hallucinations in which the affected individual sees colored lights. **2.** abnormal pigmentation.

chromato-, chromat-, **1.** a combining form meaning 'pertaining to color': *chromatism, chromatogram, chromatopsia.* **2.** See **chromo-.**

chromatogram /krōmat′əgram′/, **1.** the record produced by the separation of gaseous substances or dissolved chemical substances moving through a column of absorbent material that filters out the various absorbates in different layers. **2.** any graphic record produced by any chromatographic method.

chromatography /krō′mətog′rəfē/, any one of several processes for separating and analyzing various gaseous or dissolved chemical materials according to differences in their absorbency with respect to a specific substance and according to their different pigments. Some kinds of chromatography are **column chromatography, displacement chromatography, gas chromatography, ion-exchange chromatography,** and **paper chromatography.** **–chromatographic,** *adj.*

chromatopsia /krō′mətop′sē·ə/, **1.** an abnormal condition characterized by a visual defect that makes colorless objects appear tinged with color. **2.** a form of color blindness characterized by the imperfect perception of various colors. It may be caused by a deficiency in one or more of the retinal cones or from defective nerve circuits that convey color-associated impulses to the cerebral cortex. The most common defect in color sense is the inability to distinguish red from green, a defect evident in about 10% of men and 1% of women. Everyone is color-blind in very dim light because the color-discriminating cones of the retina are insufficiently stimulated to function. In very dim light only the retinal rods, which have the capacity to distinguish black from white, are sufficiently stimulated to function. Some color-blind persons may not be able to see red and green or blue and yellow; others cannot perceive any color, seeing everything as gray. Very few individuals are color-blind to blue. Compare **chromesthesia.**

-chrome, a combining form distinguishing 'chromium alloys': *hallachrome, nichrome, nicochrome.*

-chrome, -chromatic, a combining form meaning a 'coloring substance within a cell or chemical compound': *cytochrome, hemochrome, serochrome.*

-chromemia, a combining form meaning '(condition of the) hemoglobin in the blood': *hyperchromemia, lipochromemia, polychromemia.*

chromesthesia /krō′misthē′zhə/, **1.** the color sense that depends on the mixture of wavelengths in the light that enters the eye and the response of the different types of retinal cones associated with color vision. According to one theory of color vision, one type of cone responds to green light, a second type to red light, a third to blue light. The human eye can distinguish hundreds of different colors which are combinations of the basic light wavelengths for red, green, and blue. Some of the retinal cones can be stimulated by the whole visual spectrum, and variable stimulation of all the cones can produce all the color sensations known to humans. Changes in the pigments within the cones affect color vision, and defects in the cones cause various kinds of color blindness. **2.** an abnormal condition characterized by the confusion of other senses, as taste and smell, with imagined sensations of color. Compare **chromatopsia.**

chromhidrosis /krō′midrō′sis/, a rare, functional disorder in which apocrine sweat glands secrete colored sweat. The sweat may be yellow, blue, green, or black and often also fluoresces. A known cause is occupational exposure to copper, catechols, or ferrous oxide. Industrial nurses should be aware of this benign condition.

-chromia, a combining form meaning a 'state or condition of pigmentation': *metachromia, normochromia, orthochromia.*

-chromic, -chromatic, **1.** a combining form meaning the '(specified) number of colors seen by the eye': *bichromic, hexachromic, tetrachromic.* **2.** a combining form meaning a '(specified) color of the blood indicating the hemoglobin content': *hypochromic, normochromic.* **3.** a combining form meaning the 'staining ability of bacteria and tissues': *bathochromic, hemochromic, perchromic.* **4.** a combining form meaning a '(specified) skin color as indicative of disease': *heterochromic, pleiochromic, xanthochromic.*

chromic myopia, a kind of color blindness characterized by the ability to distinguish colors only of those objects that are close to the eye.

chromium (Cr), a hard, brittle, metallic element. Its atomic number is 24; its atomic weight is 51.9. It does not occur naturally in pure form but exists in combination with iron and oxygen in chromite, a mineral found chiefly in Africa, Albania, Russia, and Turkey. Chromium strongly resists corrosion and is used extensively to plate other metals and harden steel and, in combination with other elements, to form colored compounds. Stainless steels are more than 10% chromium and strongly resist rusting. Traces of chromium occur in plants and animals, and there is evidence this element may be important in human nutrition, especially in carbohydrate metabolism. Some experts estimate that the safe and adequate daily intake of chromium ranges from 0.1 to 0.2 mg, depending on the age of the individual. Workers in chromite mines are susceptible to pneumoconiosis caused by the inhalation of chromite dust particles that lodge in the lung. Chromium 51 isotope is used in blood studies.

chromo-, chrom-, chromato-, a combining form meaning 'pertaining to color': *chromocrinia, chromocyte, chromotrichia.*

chromobacteriosis /krō′məbaktir′ē·ō′sis/, an extremely rare, usually fatal systemic infection caused by a gram-negative bacillus *Chromobacterium violaceum,* found in fresh water in tropic and subtropic regions, which enters the body through a break in the skin. The disease is characterized by sepsis, multiple liver abscesses, and severe prostration. Early diagnosis, surgical drainage of abscesses, and the administration of chloramphenicol markedly improve the chance of survival.

chromoblastomycosis /krō′mōblas′tōmīkō′sis/, an infectious skin disease caused by any of a variety of fungi and characterized by the appearance of pruritic, warty nodules that develop in a cut or other break in the skin. What may first appear as a small dull-red lesion gradually develops into a large ulcerated growth. Over a period of weeks or months, additional warty growths may appear elsewhere on the skin along the path of lymphatic drainage. Treatment includes surgical excision and, in some cases, topical application of antibiotics. Also called **chromomycosis, verrucous dermatitis.** See also **mycosis,** and see specific fungal infections.

chromocenter. See **karyosome.**

chromogen, a substance that absorbs light, producing color.

chromolipid, chromolipoid. See **lipochrome.**

chromomere /krō′əmir/, any of the series of beadlike structures that lie along the chromonema of a chromosome during the early stages of cell division. The position of each chromomere is relatively constant for each chromosome and probably reflects the coiling pattern of the DNA molecule for the particular chromosome. Also called **idiomere.** See also **granulomere.**

chromomycosis. See **chromoblastomycosis.**

chromonema /krō′mənē′mə/, *pl.* **chromonemata,** the coiled filament along which the chromomeres lie that forms the central part of the chromatid of the chromosome during cell division. Also called **chromoneme** /krō′mənēm/. See also **chromosome.** **–chromonemal, chromonematic, chromonemic,** *adj.*

chromophilic /krō′məfil′ik/, denoting a cell, tissue, or microorganism that is easily stained, particularly certain leukocytes. Compare **chromophobic.**

chromophobe adenoma. See **chromophobic adenoma.**

chromophobia /krō′mə-/, **1.** the resistance of certain cells and tissues to stains. **2.** a morbid aversion to colors. **–chromophobe,** *n.*

chromophobic /krō′məfō′bik/, denoting a cell, tissue, or microorganism that is not easily stained, particularly certain cells of the anterior lobe of the pituitary gland. Compare **chromophilic.**

chromophobic adenoma, a tumor of the pituitary gland composed of cells that do not stain with acid or basic dyes. Diabetes insipidus and other conditions resulting from deficiency of one or more pituitary hormones are associated with this tumor. Also called **chromophobe adenoma.**

chromoplasm. See **chromatin.**

chromosomal aberration, any change in the structure or number of any of the chromosomes for a given species, which can result in anomalies of varying severity. In humans, a number of physical disabilities and disorders are directly associated with chromosomal defects of both the autosomes and the sex chromosomes, including Down's syndrome, Turner's syndrome, and Kleinfelter's syndrome. The incidence for most of the chromosomal disorders is significantly higher than that for the single gene disorders. See also specific trisomy syndromes.

chromosomal nomenclature, a standard nomenclature that serves to identify the complement of chromosomes in an individual according to the number of chromosomes, sex, and the deletion or addition of a specific chromosome or part of a chromosome. Complement in a normal female is recorded as 46,XX, and for a normal male, 46,XY. The morphologically paired autosomes are separated into 7 groups and numbered from 1 to 22, with 1 through 3 being designated group A; 4 and 5, group B; 6 through 12, group C; 13 through 15, group D; 16 through 18, group E; 19 and 20, group F; and 21 and 22, group G. The chromosomes are arranged according to decreasing length, followed by the sex chromosome complement, in the usual karyotype representation. Chromosomal aberrations are designated by indicating the total chromosomal number, sex complement, and the group or specific chromosome in which the addition or deletion occurs. For example, 47,XY,G+ indicates a male with an extra chromosome in the G group; 47,XX,21+ shows a female with an extra chromosome 21, or Down's syndrome. The short arm of a chromosome is designated "p," the long arm is "q," and a translocation is "t".

chromosome /krō'məsōm/, any one of the threadlike structures in the nucleus of a cell that function in the transmission of genetic information. Each consists of a double strand of the nucleoprotein deoxyribonucleic acid (DNA), which is coiled in a helix formation and attached to a protein base, usually a histone. The genes, which contain the genetic material that controls the inheritance of traits, are arranged in a linear pattern along the entire length of each DNA strand. Chromosomes are readily stainable with basic dyes and can be seen easily during cell division when they are compactly coiled and in their most condensed state. During interphase, the chromosomes disperse into chromatin and undergo self-replication, forming identical chromatids that separate during mitosis so that each new cell receives a full set of chromosomes. Each species has a characteristic number of chromosomes in the somatic cell, which in humans is 46 and includes 22 homologous pairs of autosomes and one pair of sex chromosomes, with one member of each pair being derived from each parent. Kinds of chromosomes include **accessory chromosome, Christchurch chromosome, daughter chromosome, gametic chromosome, giant chromosome, homologous chromosomes, Philadelphia chromosome, sex chromosome, somatic chromosome, W chromosome,** and **Z chromosome.** See also **centromere, chromatid, chromatin, Denver classification, gene, karyotype, mitosis. –chromosomal,** *adj.*

chromosome banding. See **banding.**

chromosome coil, the spiral formed by the coiling of two or more chromonemata of the chromatid within the chromosome.

chromosome complement, the normal number of chromosomes found in the somatic cell of any given species. In humans it is 46, consisting of 22 pairs of homologous autosomes and one pair of sex chromosomes.

chromosome 5p– syndrome. See **cat-cry syndrome.**

chromosome mapping. See **mapping.**

chromosome puff, a band of accumulated chromatic material located at a specific site on a giant chromosome. It is indicative of gene activity, specifically DNA and RNA synthesis, for the particular locus. Such bands appear at certain chromosomal locations within a given tissue at specific developmental stages in insects and are significant for studying the mode of genetic transmission.

chromosome walking, the process by which overlapping molecular clones that span large chromosomal intervals are isolated.

chromotrope /krō'mətrōp/, **1.** a component of tissue that stains metachromatically with metachromatic dyes. **2.** any one of several dyes differentiated by numeric suffixes. **–chromotropic,** *adj.*

chron-. See **chrono-.**

-chronia, -chrone, 1. a combining form meaning '(condition of) processes with respect to time': *isochronia, heterochronia, synchronia.* **2.** a combining form meaning '(condition of) chronaxy between muscle and nerve': *isochronia.* **3.** a combining form meaning the 'time of formation of a part or tissue': *heterochronia, synchronia.*

chronic /kron'ik/, (of a disease or disorder) developing slowly and persisting for a long period of time, often for the remainder of the lifetime of the individual. Glaucoma is an example of a disease that may develop gradually and insidiously, although it may also occur as an acute disorder marked by sudden severe pain, requiring emergency treatment. Compare **acute.**

chronic alcoholic delirium. See **Korsakoff's psychosis.**

chronic alcoholism, a pathologic condition resulting from the habitual use of alcohol in excessive amounts. The syndrome involves complex cultural, psychologic, social, and physiologic factors and usually impairs an individual's health and ability to function normally in society. Symptoms of the disease include anorexia, diarrhea, weight loss, neurologic and psychiatric disturbances (most notably depression), and fatty deterioration of the liver, sometimes leading to cirrhosis. Treatment depends on the severity of the disease and its resulting complications; hospitalization may be necessary. Nutritional therapy, use of tranquilizers in the detoxification process, use of disulfiram as an aid to continued abstinence, and psychotherapy are all methods of treatment. Alcoholism often goes unrecognized in patients admitted to the hospital for care after an accident or for esophagitis, gastritis, peripheral neuropathy, anemia, or depression, all of which are secondary effects of their alcoholism. If alcoholism is not diagnosed and treated, the patient may not recover. The nurse usually spends more time with a patient than the physician does and is in a better position to discover the condition and to observe signs of withdrawal; the nurse should inform the physician responsible so that detoxification, sedation, and other treatment can be instituted. If the patient is to undergo an operation, it is imperative that the anesthesiologist be notified of the alcoholism, which can affect sensitivity to anesthetics. Alcoholism is a family disease, and the nurse can be instrumental in guiding the patient's family to seek treatment. Long-term support for the alcoholic and his family is offered by such organizations as Alcoholics Anonymous, Al-Anon, and Alateen, and rehabilitation facilities for alcoholism. Compare **acute alcoholism.** See also **alcoholism.**

chronic appendicitis, **1.** a type of appendicitis characterized by thickening or scarring of the vermiform appendix, caused by previous inflammation. **2.** an obsolete term for chronic pain in the appendiceal area without any evidence of inflammation.

chronic brain syndrome (CBS), an abnormal condition that is caused by impairment of the cerebral tissue function, characterized by loss of memory and disorientation. It may occur in dementia paralytica, cerebral arteriosclerosis, brain trauma, and Huntington's chorea.

chronic bronchitis, a very common debilitating respiratory disease, characterized by greatly increased production of mucus by the glands of the trachea and bronchi and resulting in a cough with expectoration for at least 3 months of the year for more than 2 consecutive years. ■ OBSERVATIONS: The condition has a strong association with smoking and occupational and environmental pollutants. Formerly seen almost exclusively in males, the disease is becoming more common in women who smoke. Productive cough, often with wheezing, is a universal feature, followed by progressive dyspnea on exertion, repeated purulent respiratory infections, airway narrowing and obstruction, and often respiratory failure. Cor pulmonale with right ventricular heart failure is a common result. Some patients develop secondary polycythemia caused by chronic hypoxemia. Acute attacks of respiratory distress with rapid, labored respirations, prolonged expiratory phase, prominent cough, and cyanosis

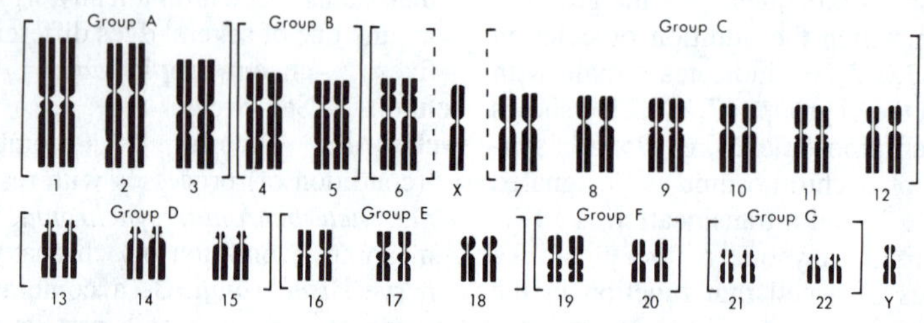

HUMAN CHROMOSOMAL PAIRS

Analysis of human chromosomes

Description of chromosomes					*Number of chromosomes in all body (somatic) cells*	
Size	*Position of centromere*	*Group*	*Autosomes*	*Sex chromosomes*	*Male*	*Female*
Large	Metacentric or submetacentric	A	1, 2, 3		6	6
Large	Submetacentric	B	4, 5		4	4
Medium	Metacentric and submetacentric	C	6, 7, 8, 9, 10, 11, 12	X	15	16
Medium	Acrocentric (subterminal)	D	13, 14, 15		6	6
Small	Metacentric and submetacentric	E	16, 17, 18		6	6
Smallest	Metacentric	F	19, 20			
Small	Acrocentric (subterminal)	G	21, 22	Y	5	4
				TOTAL	46	46

has resulted in these patients being called "blue bloaters." Common laboratory findings include elevated hematocrit, hypoxemia with or without respiratory acidosis, abnormal liver function caused by right-sided heart failure and hepatic congestion, pathogenic bacteria in the sputum, abnormal pulmonary function tests, and often chest x-ray signs of increased bronchial markings and emphysema.

■ INTERVENTION: Broad-spectrum antibiotics, as ampicillin or erythromycin, are usually prescribed during acute exacerbations of symptoms. Bronchodilators, as theophylline or metaproterenol, as well as sympathomimetic drugs, such as terbutaline, are prescribed to prevent worsening of the condition. Heart failure is managed with sodium restriction, diuretics, and sometimes digitalis.

■ NURSING CONSIDERATIONS: A major effort should be made to have the patient discontinue smoking and avoid exposure to toxic inhalants, as hair sprays, aerosol insecticides, and occupational irritants and poisons. Patients with chronic bronchitis should be immunized against influenza and pneumococcal infections. The use of low-flow oxygen in the home may require patient education and monitoring. Exercise, especially walking, chest physiotherapy, and postural drainage are often indicated, and nurses may give instruction to patients and their families in these therapeutic programs. See also **asthma, chronic obstructive pulmonary disease, cor pulmonale, emphysema, respiratory failure.**

chronic care, a pattern of medical and nursing care that focuses on long-term care of people with chronic diseases or conditions, either at home or in a medical facility. It includes care specific to the problem, as well as other measures to encourage self-care, to promote health, and to prevent loss of function.

chronic carrier, an individual who acts as host to pathogenic organisms for an extended period of time without displaying any signs of disease.

chronic cervicitis. See **cervicitis.**

chronic cholecystitis. See **cholecystitis.**

chronic chorea. See **Huntington's chorea.**

chronic cystic mastitis. See **fibrocystic disease.**

chronic disease, a disease that persists over a long period of time as compared with the course of an acute disease. The symptoms of chronic disease are usually less severe than those of the acute phase of the same disease. Chronic disease may result in complete or partial disability.

chronic gastritis. See **gastritis.**

chronic glaucoma. See **glaucoma.**

chronic glomerulonephritis, a noninfectious disease of the glomerulus of the kidney characterized by proteinuria, hematuria, edema, and decreased production of urine. Of unknown cause, it is asymptomatic for years: The symptoms develop slowly, but the disease progresses to kidney failure. Transplantation and dialysis are the only treatments available. See also **postinfectious glomerulonephritis, subacute glomerulonephritis, uremia.**

chronic idiopathic thrombocytopenic purpura. See **idiopathic thrombocytopenic purpura.**

chronic intestinal ischemia. See **intestinal angina.**

chronic interstitial nephritis. See **interstitial nephritis.**

chronic lingual papillitis, an inflammatory disorder of the tongue, sometimes extending to the buccal mucosa and palate, characterized by irregularly scattered red patches, thinning of the lingual papillae, severe burning pain, and shedding of epidermal tissue. The disorder affects middle-aged individuals, especially women, and occurs in attacks alternating with remissions lasting weeks or months. Also called **Moeller's glossitis.**

chronic lymphocytic leukemia (CLL), a neoplasm of blood-forming tissues, characterized by a proliferation of small, long-lived lymphocytes, chiefly B cells, in bone marrow, blood liver, and lymphoid organs. CLL is rare under 35 years of age, increases in frequency with age, and is more common in men than in women. The disease has an insidious onset and progresses to cause malaise, easy fatigability, anorexia, weight loss, nocturnal sweating, lymphadenopathy, and hepatosplenomegaly. Most patients can continue normal activities for years; 25% die of unrelated diseases. No treatment is curative, but remissions may be induced by chemotherapy with chlorambucil and glucocorticoids or by thymic, splenic, or total body irradiation.

chronic mastitis. See **mastitis.**

chronic mucocutaneous candidiasis, an abnormal condition and rare form of candidiasis, characterized by lesions of the skin, viral infections, and recurrent respiratory tract infections. This disease usually occurs during the first year of life but can develop as late as the 20s. It affects both men and women and is associated with an inherited defect of the cell-mediated immune system and apparently allows autoantibodies to develop against target organs. The humoral immune system functions normally in this disease. The onset of infections associated with the disease may precede endocrinopathy.

■ OBSERVATIONS: Chronic mucocutaneous candidiasis may affect the skin, the mucous membranes, the nails, and the vagina, usually causing large, circular lesions. Associated viral infections may lead to endocrinopathy and hepatitis. Infections of the mouth, nose, and palate may cause problems with speech and eating. Tetany and hypocalcemia are the most common symptoms associated with the endocrinopathy and are usually confined to the involved organ. Other complications associated with chronic mucocutaneous candidiasis may include diabetes, Addison's disease, hypothyroidism, and pernicious anemia. Some patients also develop psychiatric problems because of disfigurements and extensive endocrinal disorders. Diagnosis of this disease usually includes laboratory tests, which commonly show a normal T-cell count and normal immunologic responses to antigens other than *Candida albicans*. The endocrinopathy associated with this disease may include nonimmunologic aberrations, as hypocalcemia, abnormal hepatic function, hyperglycemia, iron deficiency, and abnormal vitamin B_{12} absorption. Other immunodeficiency diseases associated with chronic *Candida* infection must be excluded by diagnosis. Such immunodeficiency diseases as Di-George's syndrome, ataxiatelangiectasia, and severe combined immunodeficiency disease all cause serious immunologic defects. Required after diagnosis of chronic mucocutaneous candidiasis are evaluations of numerous functions of the patient, as adrenal, gonadal, pancreatic, parathyroid, pituitary, and thyroid functions. Chronic mucocutaneous candidiasis is progressive and usually leads to endocrinopathy.

■ INTERVENTION: Chronic mucocutaneous candidiasis resists treatment with topical antifungal agents, miconazole, and nystatin. Endocrinopathies associated with the disease must be treated individually by hormone replacement; some success in this regard has been reported with experimental injections of thymosin and levamisole. Most success in treating severe cases has been with transfer factor from a *Candida*-positive donor, with intravenous amphotericin B. Some success may also be possible against systemic infection with amphotericin B, but that agent is highly nephrotoxic. Some patients respond fairly well to fetal thymus transplants. Plastic surgery may also be part of the treatment to aid patients in coping with disfigurements caused by the disease. Treatment may also include iron replacement orally or intramuscularly.

■ NURSING CONSIDERATIONS: Patients with chronic mucocutaneous candidiasis must be closely monitored for signs of other associated diseases, as Addison's disease, diabetes, hepatitis, and pernicious anemia. Patients suffering psychologically from disfigurements associated with the disease often respond positively to the counsel, encouragement, and kindness of the nursing staff. If amphotericin B is involved in the treatment, the patient must be carefully monitored for renal function, because amphotericin B is nephrotoxic. Patients benefit from calm explanations about the progressive manifestations of the disease and the importance of regular endocrinologic checkups.

chronic myelocytic leukemia (CML), a malignant neoplasm of blood-forming tissues, characterized by a proliferation of granular leukocytes and, often, of megakaryocytes. The disease occurs most frequently in mature adults and begins insidiously. Its progress is marked by malaise, fatigue, heat intolerance, bleeding gums, purpura, skin lesions, weight loss, hyperuricemia, abdominal discomfort, and massive splenomegaly. Differential blood count and bone-marrow biopsies are performed to aid in the diagnosis. The alkaline phosphatase activity of the leukocytes is low, and the Philadelphia chromosome is present in myeloblasts in most patients with CML. Therapy with an oral alkylating agent is usual, but advanced CML is refractory to chemotherapy. Also called **chronic granulocytic leukemia (CGL), chronic myelogenous leukemia (CML), chronic myeloid leukemia, splenomedullary leukemia, splenomyelogenous leukemia.**

chronic obstructive pulmonary disease (COPD), a progressive and irreversible condition characterized by diminished inspiratory and expiratory capacity of the lungs. The person complains of dyspnea with physical exertion, of difficulty in inhaling or exhaling deeply, and sometimes of a chronic cough. The condition may result from chronic bronchitis, pulmonary emphysema, asthma, or chronic bronchiolitis and is aggravated by cigarette smoking and air pollution. Also called **chronic obstructive lung disease.**

chronic (open-angle) glaucoma. See **glaucoma.**

chronic pain, pain that continues or recurs over a prolonged period, caused by various diseases or abnormal conditions, as rheumatoid arthritis. Chronic pain is often less intense than the acute pain. The person with chronic pain does not display increased pulse and rapid respiration because these autonomic reactions to pain cannot be sustained for long periods. A characteristic of many persons with chronic pain is their impulse to control their surroundings. They cannot control their disease so they seek to control other people and their environment and are often labeled "uncooperative" or "manipulative." Others with chronic pain may withdraw from their environment and concentrate solely on their affliction, totally ignoring their family, their friends, and external stimuli. Some of the factors that can complicate the treatment of persons with chronic pain are scarring, continuing psychologic stress, and medication. Compare **acute pain.** See also **pain intervention, pain mechanism.**

chronic pyelonephritis. See **pyelonephritis.**

chronic tuberculous mastitis, a rare infection of the breast resulting from extension of tuberculosis of underlying ribs. The condition is also characterized by multiple sinus tracts and the presence of tuberculosis elsewhere in the body.

chrono-, chron-, a combining form meaning 'pertaining to time': *chronognosis, chronophobia, chronotropism.*

chronograph, a device that records small intervals of time, as a stopwatch. **–chronographic,** *adj.*

chronologic, **1.** arranged in time sequence. **2.** of or pertaining to chronology. Also **chronological.**

chronologic age, the age of an individual expressed as a period of time that has elapsed since birth, as the age of an infant, which is expressed in hours, days, or months, and the age of children and adults, expressed in years.

chronotropism /krənot′rəpiz′əm/, the act or process of affecting the regularity of a periodic function, especially interference with the rate of heartbeat. **–chronotropic,** *adj.*

chrysiasis /krəsī′əsis/, an abnormal condition characterized by the deposition of gold in the tissues of the body. Also called **auriosis.**

chrysotherapy /kris′ōther′əpē/, the treatment of any disease with gold salts. **–chrysotherapeutic,** *adj.*

Churg-Strauss syndrome /churg′strous′/, an allergic disorder marked by granulomatosis, usually of the lungs, and often involving the circulatory system.

Chvostek's sign /khvôsh′teks/, an abnormal spasm of the facial muscles elicited by light taps on the facial nerve in patients who are hypocalcemic. It is a sign of tetany.

Chvostek-Weiss sign. See **Chvostek's sign.**

chyl-. See **chylo-.**

chyle /kīl/, the cloudy liquid products of digestion taken up by the small intestine. Consisting mainly of emulsified fats, chyle passes through fingerlike projections in the small intestine, called lacteals, and into the lymphatic system for transport to the venous circulation at the thoracic duct in the neck. Also called **chylus.** **–chylous,** *adj.*

chyli-. See **chylo-.**

-chylia, a combining form meaning '(condition of the) digestive juices': *dyschylia, euchylia, polychylia.*

chyliform ascites. See **chylous ascites.**

chylo-, chyl-, chyli-, a combining form meaning 'pertaining to chyle': *chylocyst, chylophonic, chylosis.*

chyloid /kī′loid/, resembling the chyle that fills the lacteals of the small intestine during the digestion of fatty foods.

chylomicron /kī′lōmī′kron/, minute droplets of the lipoproteins measuring less than 0.5 μm in diameter. Chylomicrons consist of about 90% triglycerides with small amounts of cholesterol, phospholipids, and protein. They are synthesized in the GI tract and carry dietary glycerides from the intestinal mucosa via the thoracic duct into the plasma and ultimately to sites of utilization in the tissues. The remnant chylomicron particles are removed by the liver.

chylosus ascites. See **chylous ascites.**

chylothorax /kī′lōthôr′aks/, a condition marked by the effusion of chyle from the thoracic duct into the pleural space. The cause is usually a traumatic injury to the neck or a tumor that invades the thoracic duct. Treatment is directed at repairing damage to the duct.

chylous ascites, an abnormal condition characterized by an accumulation of chyle in the peritoneal cavity. Chylous ascites results from an obstruction of the thoracic duct that may be caused by a tumor or by a destructive lesion resulting in rupture of a lymph vessel. Also called **ascites adiposus, chylosus ascites, chyliform ascites, fatty ascites, milky ascites.** See also **ascites.**

chyluria /kīlŏŏr′ē·ə/, a condition characterized by the milky appearance of the urine because of the presence of chyle.

chylus. See **chyle.**

chyme /kīm/, the viscous, semifluid contents of the stomach present during digestion of a meal. Chyme then passes through the pylorus into the duodenum, where further digestion occurs.

-chymia, -chymy, a combining form meaning '(condition of) partly digested food in the duodenum': *achymia, ischochymia, oligochymia.*

chymopapain, a proteolytic enzyme isolated from the fruit of *Carica papaya* and related to papain. It is used in the treatment of prolapsed intervertebral or herniated disks.

chymosin. See **rennin.**

chymotrypsin /kī′mōtrip′sin/, **1.** a proteolytic enzyme, produced by the pancreas, that catalyzes the hydrolysis of casein and gelatin. **2.** a yellow crystalline powder prepared from an extract of ox pancreas, used in treating digestive disorders in which the enzyme is

Physical signs in COPD

Stage	*Signs*
Early	Examination may be negative or show only slight prolongation of forced expiration (which can be timed while auscultating over the trachea—normally 3 seconds or less), slight diminution of breath sounds at the apices or bases, scattered rhonchi or wheezes, especially on expiration, often best heard over the hila anteriorly (the rhonchi often clear after cough)
Moderate	Above signs are usually present and more pronounced, often with decreased rib expansion, use of the accessory muscles of respiration, retraction of the supraclavicular fossae in inspiration, generalized hyperresonance, decreased area of cardiac dullness, diminished heart sounds at base, increased anteroposterior distance of the chest†
Advanced	Examination usually shows the above findings to a greater degree, and often shows evidence of weight loss, depression of the liver, hyperpnea and tachycardia with mild exertion, low and relatively immobile diaphragm, contraction of abdominal muscles on inspiration, inaudible heart sounds except in the xiphoid area, cyanosis
Cor pulmonale	Increased intensity and splitting of pulmonic second sound, right-sided diastolic gallop, left parasternal heave (right ventricular overactivity), early systolic pulmonary ejection click with or without systolic ejection murmur
	With failure: distended neck veins, functional tricuspid insufficiency, V waves and hepatojugular reflux, hepatomegaly, peripheral edema

From American Lung Association: Chronic obstructive pulmonary disease, ed. 5, New York, 1977, The Association.
†Physicians may put misplaced confidence in relating the shape of the thorax to the presence or absence of obstructive lung disease. It has been shown that the classic ''barrel chest'' with poor rib separation may be caused solely or largely by dorsal kyphosis. In such patients ventilatory function may nonetheless be normal because of good diaphragmatic motion.

present in less than normal amounts or is totally lacking.

chymotrypsinogen /kī′mōtripsin′əjən/, a substance, produced in the pancreas, that is the zymogen precursor to the enzyme chymotrypsin. It is converted to chymotrypsin by trypsin.

-chymy. See **-chymia.**

Ci, abbreviation for **curie.**

C.I., abbreviation for **color index.**

***C.I.*,** abbreviation for **Colour Index.**

cibophobia /sē′bə-/, an abnormal or morbid aversion to food or to eating.

cicatricial entropion. See **cicatrix, entropion.**

cicatricial stenosis, the narrowing of a duct or tube because of the formation of scar tissue.

cicatrix /sik′ətriks, sikā′triks/, *pl.* **cicatrices** /sik′ətrī′sēz/, scar tissue that is avascular, pale, contracted, and firm after the earlier phase of skin healing characterized by redness and softness. **–cicatricial** /sik′ətrish′əl/, *adj.* **–cicatrize,** *v.*

ciclopirox, an antifungal agent.

■ INDICATIONS: It is prescribed in the treatment of tinea and candidiasis.

■ CONTRAINDICATION: Known sensitivity to this drug prohibits its use.

■ ADVERSE EFFECTS: Among the most serious adverse reactions are hypersensitivity of the skin.

ciclosporin. See **cyclosporine.**

cicutism /sik′yōōtiz′əm/, poisoning caused by water hemlock, resulting in cyanosis, dilated pupils, convulsions, and coma.

CID, abbreviation for **cytomegalic inclusion disease.**

-cide, -cid, a combining form meaning 'killing': *amebicide, herbicide, protozoacide.*

cigarette drain, a surgical drain fashioned from a section of gauze or surgical sponge drawn into a tube of gutta-percha.

ciguatera poisoning /sē′gwəter′ə/, a nonbacterial food poisoning that results from eating fish contaminated with the ciguatera toxin. Any of over 300 varieties of fish from the Caribbean or South Pacific have been implicated. The toxin is believed to block acetylcholinesterase activity. Characteristics of ciguatera poisoning are vomiting, diarrhea, tingling or numbness of extremities and the skin around the mouth, itching, muscle weakness, and pain. Cold liquids feel hot to the surfaces of the mouth and throat. No specific treatment has been developed.

cili-, **1.** a combining form meaning 'pertaining to an eyelid': *ciliectomy, cilioretinal, cilioscleral.* **2.** a combining form meaning 'pertaining to an eyelash': *ciliary, cilium.* **3.** a combining form meaning 'pertaining to a minute vibratile': *ciliated, ciliogenesis.*

cilia /sil′ē•ə/, *sing.* **cilium,** **1.** the eyelids or eyelashes. **2.** small, hairlike processes on the outer surfaces of some cells, aiding metabolism by producing motion, eddies, or current in a fluid. **–ciliary,** *adj.*

ciliary body, the thickened part of the vascular tunic of the eye that joins the iris with the anterior portion of the choroid. It is composed of the ciliary crown, ciliary processes and folds, ciliary orbiculus, ciliary muscle, and a basal lamina.

ciliary canal, the spaces of the iridocorneal angle.

ciliary gland, one of the numerous tiny, modified sweat glands arranged in several rows near the free margins of the eyelids. The apertures of the glands lie near the attachments of the eyelashes. Acute localized bacterial infection of one or more of the ciliary glands causes external sties. Also called **gland of Zeiss.** Compare **tarsal gland.**

ciliary margin, the peripheral border of the iris, continuous with the ciliary body.

ciliary movement, the waving motion of the hairlike processes projecting from the epithelium of the respiratory tract and from certain microorganisms.

ciliary muscle, a semitransparent, circular band of smooth muscle fibers attached to the choroid of the eye, the chief agent in adjusting the eye to view near objects. It draws the ciliary process centripetally, relaxing the suspensory ligament of the crystalline lens and allowing the lens to become more convex. It consists of meridional fibers and circular fibers and is thickest anteriorly. The circular fibers close to the circumference of the iris are well developed in hypermetropic eyes but are rudimentary or absent in myopic eyes.

ciliary process, any one of about 80 tiny fleshy projections on the posterior surface of the iris, forming a frill around the margin of the crystalline lens of the eye. The larger ciliary processes are about 2.5 mm long and are more regularly arranged than the smaller ones. The processes comprise one of the two zones of the ciliary body of the eye and are formed by infolding of the various layers of the choroid. They are attached anteriorly to the orbicularis ciliaris and posteriorly to the suspensory ligament of the crystalline lens. See also **ciliary body.**

ciliary reflex. See **accommodation reflex.**

ciliary ring, a small grooved band of tissue, about 4 mm wide, that forms the posterior part of the ciliary body of the eye. It extends from the ora serrata of the retina to the ciliary processes and is thicker near the ciliary processes, because of the thickness of the ciliary muscle.

ciliary zone, an outer circular area on the anterior surface of the iris, separated from the inner circular area by the angular line. The ciliary zone contains the stroma of the iris. Also called **zonula ciliaris.**

Ciliata /sil′ē•ā′tə/, a class of protozoa of the subphylum Ciliophora, characterized by cilia throughout the life cycle. The class includes the subclasses Euciliata and Protociliata. The only significant ciliate in humans is the intestinal parasite *Balantidium coli*, which causes dysentery.

ciliate /sil′ē•it/, of or having cilia, as certain epithelial cells of the body or protozoa of the class Ciliata.

ciliated epithelium, any epithelial tissue that projects cilia from its surface, as portions of the epithelium in the respiratory tract.

ciliospinal reflex /sil′ē·ōspī′nəl/, a normal brainstem reflex initiated by scratching or pinching the skin of the back of the neck, resulting in dilatation of the pupil. Also called **pupillary skin reflex.**

cimetidine, a histamine H_2-receptor antagonist.

■ INDICATIONS: It is prescribed to inhibit the production and secretion of acid in the stomach in the treatment of duodenal ulcer, pancreatitis, and hypersecretory conditions.

■ CONTRAINDICATION: Known hypersensitivity to this drug prohibits its use.

■ ADVERSE EFFECTS: Among the more serious adverse reactions are diarrhea, dizziness, rash, confusion (usually in elderly patients given large doses), and gynecomastia.

Cimex lectularius. See **bedbug.**

Cinchocaine, a trademark for a local anesthetic (dibucaine hydrochloride).

cinchona /singkō′nə, sinchō′nə/, the dried bark of the stem or root of species of *Cinchona,* containing the alkaloids quinine and quinidine.

cinchonism /sin′kōniz′əm/, a condition resulting from excessive ingestion of cinchona bark or its alkaloid derivatives. Cinchonism is characterized by deafness, headache, ringing in the ears, and signs of cerebral congestion. See also **quinine.**

cine-, kine-, kinesio-, a combining form meaning 'pertaining to movement': *cineangiogram, cinefluorography, cineradiography.*

cineangiocardiogram /sin′ē·an′jē·ōkär′dē·əgram′/, a radiograph of the cardiovascular system obtained by special instruments that employ a combination of x-ray, fluoroscopic, and motion-picture techniques.

cineangiocardiography /sin′ē·an′jē·ōkär′dē·og′rəfē/, the filming of fluorescent images of the cardiovascular system combining use of fluoroscopic, x-ray, and motion-picture techniques. See also **cineradiography.**

cineangiogram /sin′ē·an′jē·əgram′/, a movie film record of a blood vessel or of a portion of the cardiovascular system, obtained by injecting a patient with a nontoxic radiopaque medium and filming the action of the vessels through which it courses.

cineangiograph /sin′ē·an′jē·əgraf′/, a special movie camera for recording fluorescent images of the cardiovascular system.

cinefluorography. See **cineradiography.**

cinematics. See **kinematics.**

cineradiography /sin′irā′dē·og′rəfē/, the filming with a movie camera of the images that appear on a fluorescent screen, especially those images of body structures that have been injected with a nontoxic, radiopaque medium, for diagnostic purposes. Cineradiography incorporates the techniques of cinematography, fluoroscopy, and radiography as a diagnostic technique. Also called **cinefluorography, cineroentgenofluorography.** See also **cineangiocardiography.**

-cinesis, -cinesia, See **-kinesis.**

cingulate /sing′gyəlit/, **1.** having a zone or a girdle, usually with transverse markings. **2.** of or pertaining to a cingulum.

cingulate sulcus. See **callosomarginal fissure.**

cingulectomy /sing′gyo͞olek′təmē/, the surgical excision of a portion of the cingulate gyrus in the frontal lobe of the brain and the immediately surrounding tissue.

cingulotomy /sing′gyo͞olot′əmē/, a procedure in brain surgery to alleviate intractable pain by producing lesions in the tissue of the cingulate gyrus of the frontal lobe. The operation interrupts the fibers of the white matter in the gyrus by the stereotactic application of heat or cold.

cinnamon, the aromatic inner bark of several species of *Cinnamomum,* a tree native to the East Indies and China. Saigon cinnamon is commonly used as a carminative, an aromatic stimulant, or a spice. **–cinnamic,** *adj.*

CIPM, abbreviation for **Comité International des Poids et Mesures.**

circadian rhythm /sərkā′dē·ən, sur′kədē′ən/, a pattern based on a 24-hour cycle, especially the repetition of certain physiologic phenomena, as sleeping and eating.

circinate /sur′sināt/, having a ring-shaped outline or formation; annular.

circle, (in anatomy) a circular or nearly circular structure of the body, as the circle of Willis and circle of Zinn. **–circular,** *adj.*

circle of Carus. See **curve of Carus.**

circle of Willis, a vascular network at the base of the brain, formed by the interconnection of the internal carotid, anterior cerebral, posterior cerebral, anterior communicating, and posterior communicating arteries.

Circolectric (COL) bed, a trademark for an electronically controlled bed that can be vertically rotated 210 degrees and permits vertical alteration of the position of the bed patient from prone to supine. This type of bed is used especially in orthopedics and in the treatment of patients with severe burns. The bed consists of a strong aluminum circular frame supporting an anterior and a posterior straight frame within the exterior aluminum circle. The patient is "sandwiched" and secured between the two straight frames during rotation, the anterior frame covering the patient's chest and abdomen and the posterior frame covering the patient's back. The COL bed is equipped with an electric motor operated by a toggle switch with "up" and "down" positions and by a lever button. Moving the switch to the "up" position and depressing the lever button rotates the circular bed frame clockwise, thus changing the vertical orientation of the patient. Moving the toggle switch to the "down" position and depressing the lever button rotates the circular frame counterclockwise. Release of the lever button stops rotation. If electric power fails, the COL bed can be operated by a hand crank inserted into the control box. The anterior frame of the COL bed is secured to the posterior mattress by tightening the nut on the stud at each end of the frame. The stud at the head end is tightened first. The anterior frame footboard is adjusted gently against the patient's feet and the nut tightened on the foot-end stud.

The forehead support is moved to just above brow level, and the chin support is moved to just below the level of the upper lip. The distance between the frames is adjusted by pulling the adjusting knobs on the anterior support bar and lowering the anterior frame until it rests on the patient's chest. Many orthopedists caution about the use of the COL bed for patients with unstable spines and the dangers of vertical turning of the bed in the management of such patients. Another disadvantage of the COL bed can be the development of "Circolectric feet," when a patient without protective sensations may get decubiti from the pressure of the footboard against the feet and from the posterior mattress resting on the heels when the patient is prone. These pressure complications can be prevented if the attending staff takes proper precautions to eliminate the pressure on the dorsum of the feet by releasing the footplate after turning the patient prone and by repositioning the footplate before turning the patient supine. An additional hazard of the COL bed is the height of the frame and the absence of any high-low electric adjustment mechanism. Patients that are elderly, post-anesthesia, or heavily sedated may be injured by falling from the bed unless they are properly secured with safety belts. The COL bed has many safety features, including caster locks to stabilize the mechanism when it is being operated and permanent stops to prevent the bed from rotating beyond 210 degrees. The bed also has two stops that may be engaged by levers to prevent the bed from rotating past the sitting position and from rotating past the standing position. Some of the greatest advantages of the COL bed are its versatility in changing bed-patient position, the accommodation for patient transfer to walkers, and the capability for gradually orienting the cardiovascular patient to a vertical position before walking. The COL bed also permits greater patient comfort during position changes essential to postoperative treatment for orthopedic surgery, controlled weight-bearing for patients after hip surgery, and easy mobilization of elderly patients who may be at lesser risk in a COL bed than they would be with 5 to 7 days of bedrest in a regular hospital bed. Compare **Foster bed, hyperextension bed, Stryker wedge frame.**

circuit, a course or pathway, particularly one through which an electric current passes. Current passes through a closed or continuous circuit and stops if the circuit is open, interrupted, or broken. See also **volt.**

circular bandage, a bandage wrapped around an injured part, usually a limb.

circular fiber, any one of the many fibers in the free gingiva that encircle the teeth. Compare **alveolar fiber, apical fiber.**

circular fold, one of the numerous annular projections in the small intestine. They vary in size and frequency in the duodenum, the jejunum, and the ileum, and are formed by mucous and submucous tissue. Most of the folds make less than a full turn around the inside circumference of the intestine, but others spiral through the lumen, making as many as three turns. Also called **plica circularis, valve of Kerkring.**

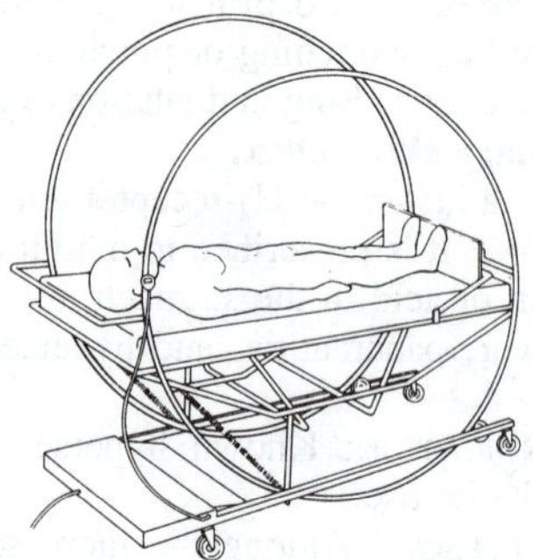

CircOlectric bed

circulation, movement of an object or substance through a circular course so that it returns to its starting point, such as the circulation of blood through the circuitous network of arteries and veins.

circulation time, normal, the time required for blood to flow from one part of the body to another. Timing a particle of blood involves injecting a traceable dye or radioisotope into a vein and timing its reappearance in an artery at the point of injection. Alternatively, a tastable substance such as saccharin can be injected, and the time it takes to travel to the tongue can be noted.

circulatory failure, failure of the cardiovascular system to supply the cells of the body with a volume of blood adequate to meet the metabolic demands of the cells. The condition results from abnormal function of the myocardium, as in myocardial infarction; from an inadequate circulatory volume of blood, as with hemorrhage; or from collapse of the peripheral vascular system, as in gram-negative septicemia. See also **shock.**

circulatory system, the network of channels through which the nutrient fluids of the body circulate. See also **Color Atlas of Human Anatomy.**

circulus arteriosus minor, the small artery encircling the outer circumference of the iris. Also called **circulus arteriosis iridus.**

circum-, a combining form meaning 'around': *circumanal, circumgemmal, circumvascular.*

circumanal /sur′kəmā′nəl/, of or pertaining to the area surrounding the anus.

circumcision, a surgical procedure in which the prepuce of the penis or, rarely, the prepuce of the clitoris is excised. Circumcision is widely performed on newborn boys despite the demonstrable lack of medical benefit and the small but significant risk of serious or lethal complications, as hemorrhage, urethral injury, or postoperative infection. These problems occur as often as the penile diseases of uncircumcised adults that circumcision is intended to prevent. The operation is performed on newborns without anesthesia, using one of several kinds of clamp. Circumcision is sometimes performed on adult males in the treatment of phymosis and balanitis. Ritual circumcision is required by the religions of approximately one sixth of the population of the world.

circumduction /sur′kəmduk′shən/, **1.** the circular movement of a limb or of the eye. **2.** the motion of the head of a bone within an articulating cavity, as the hip joint. The bone circumscribes a conic space, the apex of which is in the cavity and the base of which is described by the distal end of the bone. Circumduction is one of the four basic kinds of motion allowed by various joints of the skeleton and is a combination of abduction, adduction, extension, and flexion. Compare **angular movement, gliding, rotation.** See also **joint.**

circumferential fibrocartilage, a structure made of fibrocartilage, in which fibrocartilaginous rims surround the margins of various articular cavities, as the glenoid labra of the hip and the shoulder. The rims deepen such cavities and protect their edges. Compare **connecting fibrocartilage, interarticular fibrocartilage, stratiform cartilage.**

circumferential implantation. See **superficial implantation.**

circumoral /sur′kəmôr′əl/, of or pertaining to the area of the face around the mouth.

circumscribed scleroderma. See **morphea.**

circum-speech, (in psychiatry) behavioral characteristics associated with conversation. The characteristics include body language, maintenance of personal space between individuals, handsweeps, head nods, and task-oriented activities such as walking or knitting while carrying on a conversation.

circumstantiality, (in psychiatry) a speech pattern in which a patient has difficulty in separating relevant from irrelevant information while describing an event. The patient may not only include every detail but present the details in a sequential order with the result that the main thread of thought becomes lost as one association leads to another. Very often the person may need to have questions repeated because the main point of answers become lost in the confusion of unnecessary detail. Circumstantiality may be a sign of chronic brain dysfunction. Compare **flight of ideas.**

circumvallate papilla. See **papilla.**

circus movement, **1.** an unusual and involuntary rolling or somersaulting, because of injured neurologic mechanisms that control body posture, as the cerebral pedicles or the vestibular apparatus. **2.** an unusual circular gait caused by injury to the brain or to basal nerve centers. **3.** a mechanism associated with the excitatory wave of the atrium of the heart and atrial flutter or fibrillation. The wave travels a circular path characterized by a gap between the refractory and the excitatory tissue, usually resulting in conduction of only a fraction of the impulses to the ventricle.

cirrhosis /sirō′sis/, a chronic degenerative disease of the liver in which the lobes are covered with fibrous tissue, the parenchyma degenerates, and the lobules are infiltrated with fat. Gluconeogenesis, detoxification of drugs and alcohol, bilirubin metabolism, vitamin absorption, GI function, hormonal metabolism, and other functions of the liver deteriorate. Blood flow through the liver is obstructed, causing back pressure and leading to portal hypertension and esophageal varices. Eventually, unless the cause of the disease is removed, hepatic coma, GI hemorrhage, and kidney failure usually occur. Cirrhosis is most commonly the result of chronic alcohol abuse but can be the result of nutritional deprivation or hepatitis or other infection. The symptoms of cirrhosis are the same regardless of the cause: nausea, flatulence, anorexia, weight loss, ascites, light-colored stools, weakness, abdominal pain, varicosities, and spider angiomas. Diagnosis is made definitively by biopsy, but x-ray and physical examinations and several blood tests of liver function are serially performed to monitor the course of the disease. Treatment usually includes a balanced diet, as rich in protein as can be tolerated, vitamins (especially folic acid), rest, and total abstinence from alcohol. The liver has remarkable ability to regenerate, but recovery may be very slow. Kinds of cirrhosis are **biliary cirrhosis, fatty cirrhosis,** and **posthepatic cirrhosis.** See also **hepatic coma.** **–cirrhotic,** *adj.*

cirsoid aneurysm. See **racemose aneurysm.**

cis configuration /sis/, **1.** the presence of the dominant alleles of two or more pairs of genes on one chromosome and the recessive alleles on the homologous chromosome. **2.** the presence of the mutant genes of a pair of pseudoalleles on one chromosome and the wild-type genes on the homologous chromosome. Compare **coupling, transconfiguration.** **3.** (in chemistry) a form of isomerism in which two substituent groups are on the same side of a double bond. Also called **cis arrangement, cis position.**

cisplatin, an antineoplastic.

■ INDICATIONS: It is prescribed in the treatment of a wide variety of neoplasms, as metastatic testicular, prostatic, and ovarian tumors.

■ CONTRAINDICATIONS: Preexisting renal dysfunction, myelosuppression, hearing impairment, or known hypersensitivity to this drug or other drugs containing platinum prohibits its use.

■ ADVERSE EFFECTS: Among the most serious adverse reactions are nephrotoxicity, ototoxicity, myelosuppression, severe nausea, anorexia, vomiting, and allergic reactions.

cisterna /sistur′nə/, *pl.* **cisternae,** a cavity that serves as a reservoir for lymph or other body fluids. Kinds of cisternae include **cisterna chyli** and **cisterna subarachnoidea.**

cisterna chyli, a dilatation at the beginning of the thoracic duct, situated ventral to the body of the second lumbar vertebra, on the right side of and dorsal to the aorta. It receives the two lumbar lymphatic trunks and the intestinal lymphatic trunk.

cisternal puncture, the insertion of a needle into the cerebellomedullary cistern to withdraw cerebrospinal fluid for examination. The puncture is made between the atlas and the occipital bone.

cisterna subarachnoidea, any one of many small subarachnoid spaces that serve as reservoirs for cerebrospinal fluid.

cistron /sis′tron/, a fragment or portion of DNA that codes for a specific polypeptide. It is the smallest unit functioning as a transmitter of genetic information. In modern molecular genetics the cistron is essentially synonymous with the gene. **–cistronic,** *adj.*

cisvestitism /sisves′titiz′əm/, the practice of wearing attire appropriate to the sex of the individual involved but not suitable to the age, occupation, or status of the wearer, as when a male bookkeeper impersonates a male police officer by wearing a police uniform.

Citanest Hydrochloride, a trademark for a local anesthetic (prilocaine hydrochloride).

citrate /sit′rāt, sī′trāt/, **1.** any salt or ester of citric acid. **2.** the act of treating with a citrate or citric acid. **–citration,** *n.*

citric acid /sit′rik/, a white, crystalline, organic acid soluble in water and alcohol. It is extracted from citrus fruits, especially lemons and limes, or obtained by fermentation of sugars and is used as a flavoring agent in foods, carbonated beverages, and certain pharmaceutic products, especially laxatives. It is also used as a preventive of scurvy. See also **ascorbic acid, infantile scurvy, scurvy.**

citrin /sit′rin/, a crystalline flavonoid concentrate that is used as a source of bioflavonoid.

citrovorum factor. See **folinic acid.**

citrulline, an amino acid that is produced from ornithine during the urea cycle and is subsequently transformed to arginine by the transfer of a nitrogen atom from aspartate.

Civilian Health and Medical Programs for Uniformed Services (CHAMPUS), a health care insurance system for military dependents and members of the military services when certain kinds of care are not available through the usual military medical service. CHAMPUS is the first, and one of the few, federal third-party reimbursement systems that pay for care rendered by nurse-midwives and nurse practitioners.

CJPH, abbreviation for ***Canadian Journal of Public Health.***

Cl, symbol for **chlorine.**

Claforan, a trademark for an antibiotic (cefotaxime sodium).

claims-made policy, a professional liability-insurance policy that covers the holder for the period in which a claim of malpractice is made. The alleged act of malpractice may have occurred at some previous time, but the policy insures the holder when the claim is made. Compare **occurrence policy.**

clairvoyance /klervoi′əns/, the alleged power or ability to perceive or to be aware of objects or events without the use of the physical senses. Also called **clairsentience.** See also **extrasensory perception, parapsychology, telepathy.**

clairvoyant /klervoi′ənt/, **1.** pertaining to or characterized by clairvoyance. **2.** one who allegedly possesses the powers of clairvoyance.

clamp, an instrument with serrated tips and locking handles, used for gripping, holding, joining, supporting, or compressing an organ or vessel. In surgery, clamps generally are used for hemostasis.

clamp forceps. See **pedicle clamp.**

clang association, the mental connection between dissociated ideas made because of similarity in the sounds of the words used to describe the ideas. The phenomenon occurs frequently in the manic phase of bipolar disorder. Also spelled **klang association.**

clapping, (in massage) the procedure of making percussive movements on the body of a patient by lowering the cupped palms alternately in a series of rapid, stimulating blows. In this procedure the movement of the hands is from the wrist. Clapping stimulates the circulation and refreshes the skin and is often done to improve the comfort of bedridden patients, especially during the administration of a bed bath.

clarify, (in chemistry) to clear a turbid liquid by allowing any suspended matter to settle, by adding a substance that precipitates any suspended matter, or by heating. **–clarification,** *n.*

Clark's rule, a method of calculating the approximate pediatric dosage of a drug for a child using this formula: weight in pounds/150 × adult dose. See also **pediatric dosage.**

clas-, a combining form meaning 'a piece broken off': *clasmatocyte, clasmatodendrosis, clasmatosis.*

-clasia, a combining form meaning a '(specified) condition involving crushing or breaking up': *aortoclasia, colloidoclasia, osteoclasia.*

clasmocytic lymphoma. See **histiocytic malignant lymphoma.**

clasp, **1.** (in dentistry) a sleevelike fitting that is fastened over a tooth to hold a partial denture in place. **2.** (in surgery) any device for holding tissues together, especially bones.

clasp-knife reflex, an abnormal sign in which a spastic limb resists passive motion and then suddenly gives way, similar to the blade of a jackknife. It is an indication of damage to the pyramidal tract.

clasp torsion, the twisting of a dental retentive clasp arm on its long axis.

classic apraxia. See **ideomotor apraxia.**

classic cesarean section, a method for surgically delivering a baby through a vertical midline incision of the upper segment of the uterus. For many practitioners this is the fastest method of cesarean delivery, but it is attended with a weaker scar, and because the upper segment is thicker and more vascular, there is more bleeding during surgery than from the low cervical cesarean section. Compare **extraperitoneal cesarean section.** See also **cesarean section.**

classic conditioning, a form of learning in which a previously neutral stimulus comes to elicit a given response through associative training. Also called **respondent conditioning.** See also **conditioned reflex.**

classic tomography, a method that moves the x-ray source and the x-ray plate during an exposure to produce an image in which all but a particular plane is blurred out. This enables an approximate isolation of the image of a detail, which might otherwise be obscured by overlying or underlying structures. See also **computerized axial tomography.**

classic typhus. See **epidemic typhus.**

classification, (in research) a process in data collection and analysis in which data are grouped according to previously determined characteristics. –**classify,** *v.*

classification schemes, systems of organizing data or information, usually involving categories of items with similar characteristics. An example is the *International Classification of Diseases (ICD)* compiled by the World Health Organization (WHO), in which basic disease categories are assigned a three-digit code with optional digits for specific disease entities. An example is candidiasis, which is assigned the basic three-digit code 112. Candidiasis of the mouth is 112.0, of the skin and nails, 112.3. A fifth digit is assigned to specified sites, such as 112.81 for candidal endocarditis and 112.82 for candidal otitis externa. Other classification schemes include that of the North American Nursing Diagnoses Association (NANDA) and the *Diagnostic and Statistical Manual of Mental Disorders (DSM),* prepared by the American Psychiatric Association. See also **nursing diagnosis.**

-clast, a combining form meaning 'something that breaks': *angioclast, cranioclast, myeloclast.*

-clastic, a combining form meaning 'causing disintegration': *hemoclastic, histoclastic, lipoclastic.*

claudication, a weakness of the legs accompanied by cramplike pains in the calves caused by poor circulation of the blood to the leg muscles. The condition is commonly associated with atherosclerosis and may be marked by a lameness or limping. Intermittent claudication is a form of the disorder that is manifested only at certain times, usually after an extended period of walking, and is relieved by a period of rest.

claustrophobia /klôs′trə-/, a morbid fear of being in or becoming trapped in enclosed or narrow places. The phenomenon is observed more often in women than in men and can generally be traced to some traumatic situation involving enclosed spaces, usually occurring in childhood. Treatment consists of psychotherapy to uncover the cause of the phobic reaction, followed by behavior therapy, specifically systematic desensitization or flooding technique.

claustrum /klôs′trəm/, *pl.* **claustra,** **1.** a barrier, as a membrane that partially closes an aperture. **2.** a thin sheet of gray matter, composed chiefly of spindle cells, situated lateral to the external capsule of the brain and separating the internal capsule from white matter of the insula. Also called **claustrum of insula.**

clavicle /klav′ikəl/, a long, curved, horizontal bone just above the first rib, forming the ventral portion of the shoulder girdle. It articulates medially with the sternum and laterally with the acromion of the scapula and accommodates the attachment of numerous muscles. It starts to ossify before any other bone in the body and does not totally unite with the sternum until about the twenty-fifth year. It is shorter, thinner, less curved, and smoother in the female than in the male and is thicker, more curved, and more prominently ridged for muscle attachment in persons performing consistent, strenuous manual labor.

clavicular notch /kləvik′yələr/, one of a pair of oval depressions at the superior end of the sternum. Each clavicular notch is situated on one side of the sternum and articulates with the clavicle from the same side.

clavus. See **corn.**

clawfoot. See **pes cavus.**

clawhand, a hand fixed in a position of acute flexion. Also called **main en griffe** /menäNgrif′/.

claw-type traction frame, an orthopedic apparatus that holds various pieces of traction equipment, as the pulleys, the ropes, and the weights by which traction is applied to various parts of the body or by which various parts of the body are suspended. It consists of two metal uprights, one at the head of the bed and the other at the foot. Both the uprights are secured by claw-type attachments and support an overhead metal bar secured by metal clamps. Compare **Balkan frame, IV-type traction frame.**

clearance, the removal of a substance from the blood via the kidneys. Kidney function can be tested by measuring the amount of a specific substance excreted in the urine in a given length of time.

clear cell, **1.** a type of cell found in the parathyroid gland that does not take on a color with the ordinary tissue stains used for microscopic examination. **2.** the principal cell of most renal cell carcinomas and, occasionally, of ovarian and parathyroid tumors. **3.** a specific type of epidermal cell, probably of neural origin, that has a dark-staining nucleus but clear cytoplasm with hematoxylin and eosin stain.

clear cell carcinoma, **1.** a malignant tumor of the tubular epithelium of the kidney. Characteristically the malignant cells contain abundant clear cytoplasm. See also **renal cell carcinoma.** **2.** an uncommon ovarian neoplasm characterized by cells with clear cytoplasm.

clear cell carcinoma of the kidney. See **renal cell carcinoma.**

clear-liquid diet, a diet that supplies fluids and provides minimal residue. It consists primarily of dissolved sugar and flavored liquids, as ginger ale, sweetened tea or coffee, fat-free broth, plain gelatin desserts, and strained fruit juices. The diet is nutritionally inadequate and is usually prescribed for a limited amount of time, as 1 day, postoperatively.

cleavage, **1.** the series of repeated mitotic cell divisions occurring in the ovum immediately after fertilization to form a mass of cells that transforms the single-celled zygote into a multicellular embryo capable of growth and differentiation. At this initial stage, as the zygote remains uniform in size, the cleavage cells, or blastomeres, become smaller with each division. **2.** the act or process of cleaving or splitting, primarily the splitting of a complex molecule into two or more simpler molecules. Kinds of cleavage include **determinate cleavage, equal cleavage, indeterminate cleavage, partial cleavage, total cleavage,** and **unequal cleavage.**

cleavage cavity. See **blastocoele.**

cleavage cell. See **blastomere.**

cleavage fracture, any fracture that splits cartilage with the avulsion of a small piece of bone from the distal portion of the lateral condyle of the humerus.

cleavage line, any one of a number of linear striations in the skin that delineate the general structural pattern and tension of the subcutaneous fibrous tissue. They correspond closely to the crease lines on the surface of the skin and are present in all areas of the body but are visible only in certain sites, as the palms of the hands and soles of the feet. The lines follow a characteristic pattern for each region of the body, although they vary with body configuration; they are consistent in persons of the same build regardless of age. In general, the lines run obliquely, lying in the direction in which the skin stretches the least, perpendicular to the direction of the greatest stretch. Incisions made parallel to these lines heal with much less scarring than those made perpendicular to them. To a certain degree, cleavage lines determine the direction and arrangement of lesions in skin diseases. Also called **Langer's line.**

cleavage nucleus. See **segmentation nucleus.**

cleavage plane, **1.** the area in a fertilized ovum where cleavage takes place; the axis along which any cell division occurs. **2.** any plane within the body where organs or structures can be separated with minimal damage to surrounding tissue.

cleft, **1.** divided. **2.** a fissure, especially one that originates in the embryo, as the branchial cleft or the facial cleft.

cleft foot, an abnormal condition in which the division between third and fourth toes extends into the metatarsum of the foot.

cleft lip, a congenital anomaly consisting of one or more clefts in the upper lip resulting from the failure in the embryo of the maxillary and median nasal processes to close. Treatment is surgical repair in infancy. Also called **harelip.** See also **cleft palate.**

cleft-lip repair, the surgical correction of a unilateral or bilateral congenital interruption of the upper lip, usually resulting from the embryologic failure of the median nasal and maxillary processes to unite.

■ METHOD: A cleft lip may sometimes be repaired during the infant's first 48 hours of life, but some surgeons follow a "rule of 10s" and perform the operation when the child is 10 weeks old, weighs 10 or more pounds, and has a hemoglobin of at least 10 g per 100 ml. Preoperatively, elbow restraints, used to prevent the infant from touching

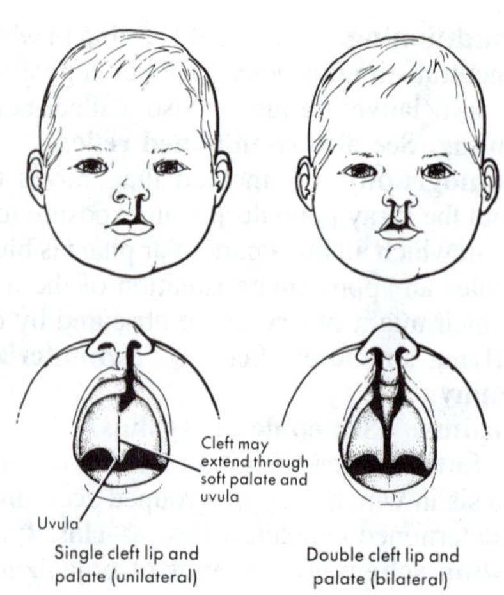

Cleft lip and palate

the incision, are prepared in the proper size and are sent to the operating room with the patient. Postoperatively, the infant is maintained with ventilatory support as necessary until respirations are normal and is observed for respiratory stridor or obstruction, excessive bleeding, separation of the incision, and redness under the elbow restraints. The wire bow applied to the infant's upper lip and taped to the cheeks to prevent tension on the sutures is kept in place; if it becomes loose, it is reapplied with tincture of benzoin. The infant is given clear liquids and juices through an Asepto syringe or special feeding unit; parenteral fluids are administered until the oral intake is adequate; milk products, solids, and a nipple or pacifier are not allowed. The diet and manner of feeding may vary, but the infant is fed while held with the head up or is placed in a cardiac chair and burped after the intake of each ounce of food. The intake and output of fluids are measured. The elbow restraints are worn at all times except when range-of-motion exercises are performed, one arm at a time, while skin care is administered to that limb.

■ NURSING ORDERS: The nurse administers preoperative and postoperative care and prepares for the infant's discharge by ensuring that the parents understand the proper diet and feeding schedule and technique, by emphasizing the importance of using elbow restraints, and by explaining the importance of maintaining motion and skin integrity of the arms, of avoiding injury to the surgical area, and of reporting symptoms of infection, including separation of the incision, excessive swelling, redness, bleeding, and drainage.

■ OUTCOME CRITERIA: Modern surgical techniques permit remarkable repair of cleft lips, but in some cases a second operation is required to eliminate the scar.

cleft palate, a congenital defect characterized by a fissure in the midline of the palate, resulting from the failure of the two sides to fuse during embryonic development. The fissure may be complete, extending through both the hard and soft palates into the nasal cavities, or it may show any degree of incomplete or partial cleft. The condition, which occurs approximately once in every 2500 live births and affects females more than males, is often associated with a cleft in the upper lip. Together, these abnormalities are the most common of the craniofacial malformations, accounting for half of the total number of defects. Feeding is best accomplished with special feeding devices. Surgical repair of the defect is usually not begun until the first or second year of life and is usually performed in steps. Care of the child requires a team approach that includes a plastic surgeon, orthodontist, dentist, nurse, speech and hearing therapists, and social workers. Long-term postoperative problems, including speech impairment and hearing loss, improper tooth development and alignment, chronic respiratory and ear infections, and varying levels of emotional and social maladjustment, may be largely prevented by modern techniques and reconstructive surgery. See also **cleft lip.**

cleft-palate repair, the surgical correction of a congenital fissure in the midline of the partition separating the oral and nasal cavities. Palatine clefts range from a simple separation in the uvula to an extensive fissure involving the soft and hard palate and extending forward unilaterally or bilaterally through the alveolar ridge. A cleft lip often accompanies a cleft palate. Repair of a cleft palate is usually undertaken in the child's second year.

■ METHOD: Before surgery, properly sized elbow restraints to prevent the child from touching the mouth are prepared and sent to the operating room with the patient. Postoperatively, the youngster is kept in a moist oxygen-rich environment using a Croupette or other tent device until respirations are normal and is observed for signs of airway obstruction or excessive bleeding. Parenteral fluids are administered until the oral intake is adequate. Clear liquids and juices are given by cup only; straws, nipples, pacifiers, utensils, or toys may not be put in the mouth. Milk products and solids are contraindicated, but the kind of feeding ordered may vary. The child is fed in a high chair when possible, and a bib is used to accommodate drooling. Only circumoral mouth care is administered; the teeth are not brushed. The intake and output of fluids are measured. The elbow restraints are worn continuously, except when daily range-of-motion exercises are performed and skin care is administered, to one arm at a time. With improvement, the child is permitted to walk as tolerated.

■ NURSING ORDERS: Before discharge, the nurse ensures that the parents understand the required diet and the need to feed by cup only, to use elbow restraints, to maintain the motion and skin integrity of the arms, and to avoid injury to the mouth. The nurse reminds the parents to administer the required medication in the proper dosage and on schedule and to report symptoms of incision infection, as drainage, mouth odor, or bleeding.

■ OUTCOME CRITERIA: Depending on the extent and nature of a cleft palate, it may be repaired in one or in several operations. Some experts believe that early repair of a defect in the bony palate can lead to structural malrelations and advise delaying the operation until the child is between 5 and 7 years of age and has achieved more bone growth. Successful repair often greatly improves the child's oronasopharyngeal physiology, speech, and appearance.

cleft uvula, an abnormal congenital condition in which the uvula is split into halves because of the failure of the posterior palatine folds to unite.

cleido-, cleid-, a combining form meaning 'pertaining to the clavicle': *cleidocostal, cleidocranial, cleidomastoid.*

cleidocranial dysostosis /klē′dōkrā′nē•əl/, a rare, abnormal hereditary condition characterized by defective ossification of the cranial bones and by the complete or partial absence of the clavicles. It is transmitted as an autosomal dominant trait. The defective ossification of the cranial bones delays the closing of the cranial sutures and results in large fontanels. The complete or partial absence of the clavicles allows the shoulders to be brought together. This condition also involves dental and vertebral anomalies. Also called **cleidocranial dysplasia.** See also **dysostosis.**

cleidocranial dystrophia. See **cleidocranial dysostosis.**

clemastine, an antihistaminic agent.

■ INDICATIONS: It is prescribed in the treatment of symptoms of allergic rhinitis, as sneezing, rhinorrhea, pruritus, or lacrimation.

■ CONTRAINDICATIONS: Use by nursing mothers or those undergoing monamine oxidase inhibitor therapy or having known sensitivity to this drug or other antihistamines is contraindicated.

■ ADVERSE EFFECTS: Among the most serious adverse reactions are hypersensitivity reactions, skin rash, and tachycardia. Transient drowsiness commonly occurs.

Cleocin, a trademark for an antibacterial (clindamycin).

cleptomania. See **kleptomania.**

click, (in cardiology) an extra heart sound that occurs during systole. See also **ejection click, systolic click.**

client, **1.** a person who is recipient of a professional service. **2.** a recipient of health care regardless of the state of health. **3.** a recipient of health care who is not ill or hospitalized. **4.** a patient.

client-centered therapy, a nondirective method of group or individual psychotherapy, originated by Carl Rogers, in which the role of the therapist is to listen to and then reflect or restate without judgment or interpretation the words of the client. The goal of the therapy is personal growth achieved by the client's increased awareness and understanding of his attitudes, feelings, and behavior.

client interview. See **patient interview.**

climacteric. See **menopause.**

climacteric melancholia. See **involutional melancholia.**

climate, a composite of the prevailing weather conditions that characterizes any particular geographic region. Various phenomena constitute climate, as air pressure, temperature, precipitation, sunshine, and humidity—all health factors considered in the diagnosis and treatment of certain illnesses, especially those affecting respiration. **–climatic,** *adj*.

clindamycin hydrochloride, an antibacterial.

■ INDICATIONS: It is prescribed in the treatment of certain serious infections.

■ CONTRAINDICATION: Hypersensitivity to this drug or to lincomycin prohibits its use.

■ ADVERSE EFFECTS: Among the more serious adverse reactions are colitis, severe GI disturbances, and hypersensitivity reactions.

clinic, **1.** a department in a hospital where persons not requiring hospitalization may receive medical care. Formerly it was called a dispensary. **2.** a group practice of doctors, as the Mayo Clinic. **3.** a meeting place for doctors and medical students where instruction can be given at the bedside of a patient or in a similar setting. **4.** a seminar or other scientific medical meeting. **5.** a detailed published report of the diagnosis and treatment of a health care problem.

-clinic, a combining form meaning 'places set aside for medical treatment': *policlinic, polyclinic, psychoclinic*.

clinical, **1.** of or pertaining to a clinic. **2.** of or pertaining to direct, bedside medical care. **3.** of or pertaining to materials or equipment used in the care of a sick person.

clinical crown, **1.** the portion of a tooth that is covered by enamel and visible in the mouth. **2.** the portion of a tooth that is occlusal to the deepest part of the gingival crevice. Compare **anatomic crown, artificial crown, complete crown, partial crown.**

clinical-crown/clinical-root ratio, the proportion between the length of the portion of the teeth lying coronal to the epithelial attachment and the length of the portion of the root lying apical to the epithelial attachment. The clinical-crown/clinical-root ratio is useful in the diagnosis and prognosis of periodontal disease.

clinical cytogenetics, the branch of genetics that studies the relationship between chromosomal abnormalities and pathologic conditions.

clinical diagnosis, a diagnosis made on the basis of knowledge obtained by medical history and physical examination alone, without benefit of laboratory tests or x-rays films.

clinical disease, a stage in the history of a pathologic condition that begins with anatomic or physiologic changes that are sufficient to produce recognizable signs and symptoms of a disease.

clinical genetics, a branch of genetics that studies inherited disorders and investigates the possible genetic factors that may influence the occurrence of any pathologic condition. Also called **medical genetics.**

clinical horizon, the imaginary line above which detectable signs and symptoms of a disease first begin to appear. Compare **subclinical.**

clinical laboratory, a laboratory in which tests directly related to the care of patients are performed. Such laboratories use material obtained from patients for testing, as compared with research laboratories, where animal and other sources of test material are also used.

clinical nurse specialist (CNS), a registered nurse who holds a master-of-science degree in nursing (M.S.N.) and who has acquired advanced knowledge and clinical skills in a specific area of nursing and health care. The CNS, as a practitioner, assumes a leadership role in the distribution of clinical care to a specific patient population while interacting within the total health care system. The unique functions of the CNS are based on clinical expertise and judgment and include caring for patients, delegating responsibility, teaching other staff members, and influencing and effecting change with respect to the needs of the patient and family and the total health care system.

clinical-pathologic conference, a teaching conference in which a case is presented to a clinician who then demonstrates the process of reasoning that leads to his diagnosis. A pathologist then presents an anatomic diagnosis, based on the study of tissue removed at surgery or obtained in autopsy. Often the students will have been asked to suggest a diagnosis based on the same information presented to the clinician. A discussion usually follows that serves to demonstrate the origin of errors present in any of the diagnoses offered. The pathologist's diagnosis is usually the definitive one. The clinical-pathological conference is the model for the long series called "case-reports" in the *New England Journal of Medicine* and is a part of the curricula of most medical schools.

clinical pathology, the laboratory study of disease by a pathologist using techniques appropriate to the specimen being studied. Among the many branches of clinical pathology are hematology, bacteriology, chemistry, and serology.

clinical pelvimetry, a process used to assess the size of the birth canal by means of the systematic vaginal palpation of specific bony landmarks in the pelvis and an estimation of the distances between them. Internal pelvic diameters are not accessible to direct measurement; they must be inferred. Clinical pelvimetry is usually performedby a midwife or an obstetrician during the first prenatal examination of a pregnant woman. Findings are commonly recorded in terms such as "adequate,""borderline," or "inadequate," rather than in centimeters or inches. Compare **x-ray pelvimetry.** See also **birth canal, cephalopelvic disproportion, contraction, dystocia.**

clinical psychology, the branch of psychology concerned with the diagnosis, treatment, and prevention of personality and behavioral disorders.

clinical research center, an organization, often associated with a medical school or a teaching hospital, that studies, analyzes, correlates, and describes medical cases. Such centers usually have extensive laboratory facilities and specialized staffs of physicians and medical technicians. Clinical research centers often offer free or very inexpensive diagnoses and treatment for patients participating in various research programs and often produce significant new medical information distributed through articles, journals, reports, seminars, and lectures. Funding for such facilities may come from minimal fees for various medical services and from grants.

clinical specialist, a physician or nurse having advanced training in a particular field of practice, as a nurse-midwife, pediatrician, or radiologist.

clinical thermometry, a method for determining temperature in heated tissue.

clinical trials, organized studies to provide large bodies of clinical data for statistically valid evaluation of treatment.

Clinitest, a trademark for reagent tablets used to test for the presence of reducing sugars, as glucose, in the urine. The tablets contain copper sulfate, and the procedure is a modified version of Benedict's test.

clino-, a combining form meaning 'to bend or make lie down': *clinodactyl, clinostatic, clinostatism.*

clinocephaly /klī′nōsef′əlē/, a congenital anomaly of the head in which the upper surface of the skull is saddle-shaped or concave. Also called **clinocephalism.** **–clinocephalic, clinocephalous,** *adj.*

clinodactyly /klī′nōdak′təlē/, a congenital anomaly characterized by abnormal lateral or medial bending of one or more fingers or toes. Also called **clinodactylism.** **–clinodactylic, clinodactylous,** *adj.*

Clinoril, a trademark for an antiinflammatory (sulindac).

-clinous, a combining form meaning 'pertaining to ancestry': *matriclinous, matroclinous, patroclinous.*

clioquinol. See **iodochlorhydroxyquin.**

clip, a surgical device used for grasping the skin to align the edges of a wound and to stop bleeding, especially of the smaller blood vessels. It is also used in radiography for localization.

clipped speech. See **scamping speech.**

Clistin, a trademark for an antihistamine (carbinoxamine maleate).

clitoris /klit′əris/, the vaginal erectile structure homologous to the corpora cavernosa of the penis. It consists of two corpora cavernosa within a dense layer of fibrous membrane, joined along their inner surfaces by an incomplete fibrous septum. It is situated beneath the anterior commissure, partially hidden between the anterior extremities of the labia minora.

CLL, abbreviation for **chronic lymphocytic leukemia.**

cloaca /klō·ā′kə/, *pl.* **cloacae,** **1.** (in embryology) the end of the hindgut before the developmental division into the rectum, the bladder, and the primitive genital structures. **2.** (in pathology) an opening into the sheath of tissue around a necrotic bone.

cloacal membrane, a thin sheath that separates the internal and external portions of the cloaca in the developing embryo. It is formed from endoderm and ectoderm and closes the fetal anus during early prenatal development; it later ruptures and is absorbed so that the anal canal becomes continuous with the rectum. Also called **anal membrane.**

cloacal septum. See **urorectal septum.**

clocortolone pivalate, a topical corticosteroid.
■ INDICATION: It is used topically as an antiinflammatory agent.
■ CONTRAINDICATIONS: Viral and fungal diseases of the skin or local impairment of circulation prohibits its use.
■ ADVERSE REACTIONS: Among the more serious adverse reactions are various systemic side effects that may occur from prolonged or excessive application. Local irritation of the skin may occur.

Cloderm, a trademark for a glucocorticoid (clocortolone pivalate).

clofibrate /klō′fəbrāt/, an antihyperlipoproteinemic.
■ INDICATIONS: It is prescribed in the treatment of high blood levels of cholesterol, triglycerides, or both.
■ CONTRAINDICATIONS: Liver or kidney dysfunction, pregnancy, lactation, biliary cirrhosis, or known hypersensitivity to this drug prohibits its use.
■ ADVERSE EFFECTS: Among the more serious adverse reactions are nausea, diarrhea, weight gain, and a syndrome resembling influenza. This drug interacts with many other drugs.

Clomid, a trademark for a nonsteroidal fertility drug (clomiphene citrate).

clomiphene citrate /klō′məfēn/, a nonsteroidal antiestrogen that acts to stimulate ovulation.
■ INDICATIONS: It is prescribed principally in the treatment of anovulation and oligoovulation in women.
■ CONTRAINDICATIONS: Abnormal vaginal bleeding, liver dysfunction, or known hypersensitivity to this drug prohibits its use.
■ ADVERSE EFFECTS: Among the more serious adverse reactions are enlargement of the ovaries, blurred vision, gastric upset, rashes, and abdominal pain.

clomiphene stimulation test, a test used to evaluate gonadal function in males who show signs of abnormal pubertal development. Clomiphene, a nonsteroid analog of estrogen, stimulates the hypothalamic-pituitary system to raise FSH and LH levels of the blood. Failure to respond to clomiphene indicates hypothalamic-pituitary disease, possibly a pituitary tumor. See also **clomiphene citrate, gonadotropins.**

clonal selection theory. See **antibody specific theory.**

clonazepam /klōnaz′əpam/, an anticonvulsant.
■ INDICATIONS: It is prescribed in the prevention of seizures in petit mal epilepsy and other convulsive disorders.

■ CONTRAINDICATIONS: Liver disease, acute narrow-angle glaucoma, or known hypersensitivity to this drug or to other benzodiazepine drugs prohibits its use. It is not given during lactation.

■ ADVERSE EFFECTS: Among the more serious adverse reactions are anemia, coma, palpitations, mental and respiratory depression, muscle weakness, and shortness of breath.

clone, a group of genetically identical cells or organisms derived from a single common cell or organism through mitosis.

-clonia, a combining form meaning '(condition involving) spasms': *logoclonia, myoclonia, polyclonia.*

clonidine hydrochloride /klō′nədēn/, an antihypertensive.

■ INDICATIONS: It is prescribed for the reduction of high blood pressure.

■ CONTRAINDICATIONS: Known hypersensitivity to this drug prohibits its use.

■ ADVERSE EFFECTS: Among the more serious adverse reactions are a withdrawal syndrome occurring on discontinuation of the medication, characterized by tachycardia, a rapid increase in blood pressure, and anxiety. Drowsiness and dry mouth commonly occur.

Clonopin, a trademark for an anticonvulsant (clonazepam).

Clonorchis sinensis /klōnôr′kis sinen′sis/, the Chinese or Oriental liver fluke, a form of tapeworm that is acquired by humans who eat raw or imperfectly cooked fish that is the intermediate host of the parasite. The fluke exists in a dormant stage as a cercaria, encysted in the skin of a fish and unable to continue its life cycle until ingested by a warmblooded animal in which the larvae mature and produce eggs. The eggs are excreted in the feces of the host to enter water where the new generation evolves first in aquatic snails and then in fish. In human hosts, the liver fluke lives in the bile ducts and gallbladder, causing chronic liver disease with enlargement of the liver, diarrhea, edema, and, eventually, death. Also called ***Opisthorchis sinensis.***

clonus /klō′nəs/, an abnormal pattern of neuromuscular activity, characterized by rapidly alternating involuntary contraction and relaxation of skeletal muscle. Compare **tonus.** –**clonic,** *adj.*

C-loop, a surgically formed loop of bowel with a C-shape.

clorazepate dipotassium, a minor tranquilizer.

■ INDICATIONS: It is prescribed in the treatment of anxiety, nervous tension, and alcohol withdrawal.

■ CONTRAINDICATIONS: Psychosis, acute narrow-angle glaucoma, or known hypersensitivity to this drug prohibits its use.

■ ADVERSE EFFECTS: Among the more serious adverse reactions are withdrawal symptoms occurring on discontinuation of treatment. Drowsiness and fatigue commonly occur.

closed amputation, a kind of amputation in which one or two broad flaps of muscular and cutaneous tissue are retained to form a cover over the end of the bone. It is performed only when no infection is present. A rigid dressing may be applied and the patient may be fitted for a prosthesis immediately after surgery. Compare **open amputation.**

closed-angle glaucoma. See **glaucoma.**

closed bite, **1.** an abnormal overbite. **2.** a decrease in the occlusal vertical dimension produced by various factors, as tooth abrasion and insufficient eruption of supportive posterior teeth. Compare **open bite.**

closed-chain, (in organic chemistry) of or pertaining to a compound in which the carbon atoms are bonded together to form a closed ring. Also called **carbocyclic.**

closed drainage. See **drainage.**

closed-wound suction, any one of several techniques for draining potentially harmful fluids, as blood, pus, serosanguineous fluid, and tissue secretions from surgical wounds. Such fluids interfere with the healing of wounds and often promote infection. Postoperative drainage aids the healing process by removing dead spaces where extravascular fluids collect and helps draw healing tissues together. Many surgical authorities prefer closed-wound suction to other wound-drainage methods, as pressure bandages and wicks, because it minimizes danger of infection. Closed-wound suction is often an important part of postoperative treatment and may be accomplished with a variety of reliable devices that create a gentle negative pressure to drain away undesirable exudates. The uses of closed-wound suction are as varied as the different surgical procedures. The technique is used as an aid to many operations, as mastectomies, augmentations, plastic and reconstructive procedures, and urologic and urogenital procedures. Closed-wound suction devices usually consist of disposable transparent containers attached to suction tubes and portable suction pumps. After thoroughly irrigating the wound to remove blood clots and debris, the surgeon inserts the perforated wound tubing into the wound and brings it out through healthy tissue, approximately 5 cm from the incision line. When silicone tubing is used, the tube is passed through a stab wound made adjacent to the surgical wound. With the drainage tubing brought out away from the incision line, the closed-wound suction system remains completely closed. Air cannot infiltrate the wound and cause contamination. When the suction tube has been inserted, the wound is closed and a light dressing is applied. Since the tubing drains most fluids, the dressing usually does not require frequent changing. Closed-wound suction usually continues postoperatively for 2 or 3 days or until the wound stops exuding fluid. The surgeon then removes the suction tubing, and all drainage components of the suction device are discarded. The transparent tubing and reservoir are checked regularly while the suction is functioning as a precaution against clogging and to monitor the volume of exudate drawn from the wound. In some individuals closed-wound suction systems can also accommodate antibiotic drips, which are connected to accessory tubing placed within the wound beside the suction tube. Closed-wound suction also allows irrigation of the wound with special flow controls to permit a periodic change in the flow direction of solutions.

clostridial /klostrid′ē•əl/, of or pertaining to anaerobic spore-forming bacteria of the genus *Clostridium*.

clostridial myonecrosis. See **myonecrosis.**

***Clostridium*,** a genus of spore-forming, anaerobic bacteria of the Bacillaceae family: *Clostridium novyi, C. septicum, and C. bifermentans* are involved in gas gangrene; *C. botulinum* causes botulism; *C. perfringens* causes food poisoning, cellulitis, and wound infections; *C. tetani* is the cause of tetanus.

closure /klō′zhər/, the surgical closing of a wound by suture. See also **flask closure, velopharyngeal closure.**

clot. See **blood clot.**

clotrimazole, an antifungal.

■ INDICATIONS: It is prescribed in the treatment of a variety of superficial fungal infections and for candidal vulvovaginitis.

■ CONTRAINDICATIONS: Known hypersensitivity to this drug prohibits its use. It is not prescribed for ophthalmic use; contact with eyes is avoided.

■ ADVERSE EFFECTS: The most serious adverse reactions are severe hypersensitivity reactions of the skin.

clotting. See **blood clotting.**

clotting time, the time required for blood to form a clot, tested by collecting 4 ml of blood in a glass tube and examining it for clot formation. The first appearance of a clot is noted and timed. This simple test has been used to diagnose hemophilias, but it does not detect mild coagulation disorders. Its chief application is in monitoring anticoagulant therapy. Also called **coagulation time.**

cloud baby, a newborn who appears well and healthy but is a carrier of infectious bacterial or viral organisms. The infant may contaminate the surrounding environment with airborne droplets from the respiratory tract forming clouds of the organisms. A cloud baby may be the source of a nursery epidemic, especially one caused by a staphylococcal organism.

clove, the dried flower bud of *Eugenia caryophyllata*. It contains the lactone caryophyllin and a volatile oil used as a dental analgesic, a germicide, and a salve. Clove is also used as a spice and a carminative against nausea, vomiting, and flatulence.

cloverleaf nail, a surgical nail shaped in cross section like a cloverleaf, used especially in the repair of fractures of the femur.

cloverleaf skull deformity, a congenital defect characterized by a trilobed skull resulting from the premature closure of multiple cranial sutures during embryonic development. The condition is associated with hydrocephalus, facial anomalies, and skeletal deformities. Also called **kleeblattschädel deformity syndrome** /klā′blochā′dəl/.

cloxacillin sodium, an antibacterial.

■ INDICATIONS: It is prescribed in the treatment of certain serious infections, primarily those caused by penicillin-resistant strains of staphylococci.

■ CONTRAINDICATION: Known hypersensitivity to this drug or to any penicillin prohibits its use.

■ ADVERSE EFFECTS: Among the more serious adverse reactions are GI discomfort, rash, and hypersensitivity reactions.

clubbing, an abnormal enlargement of the distal phalanges, usually associated with cyanotic heart disease or advanced chronic pulmonary disease but sometimes occurring with biliary cirrhosis, colitis, chronic dysentery, and thyrotoxicosis. The mechanism whereby diminished oxygen tension in the blood causes clubbing is not understood. Clubbing occurs in all the digits but is most easily seen in the fingers. Advanced clubbing is obvious, but early clubbing is difficult to diagnose. Clubbing is present if the transverse diameter of the base of the fingernail is greater than the transverse diameter of the most distal joint of the digit. The affected phalange is full, fleshy, and quite vascular; the skin may be excoriated.

clubfoot, a congenital deformity of the foot, sometimes resulting from intrauterine constriction and characterized by unilateral or bilateral deviation of the metatarsal bones of the forefoot. Ninety-five percent of clubfoot deformities are **equinovarus,** characterized by medial deviation and plantar flexion of the forefoot, but a few are **calcaneovalgus,** or **calcaneovarus,** characterized by lateral deviation and dorsiflexion either outward from or inward toward the midline of the body. Treatment depends on the extent and rigidity of the deformity. Splints and casts in infancy may produce complete correction; surgery in several steps may be necessary to achieve normal function. See also **Denis Browne splint, talipes.**

club hair, a hair in the resting, or final, stage of the growth cycle. See also **hair.**

cluster analysis, (in statistics) a complex technique of data analysis of numeric scale scores that produces clusters of variables related to one another. The technique is performed with a computer.

cluster breathing, a breathing pattern in which a closely grouped series of respirations is followed by apnea. The activity is associated with a lesion in the lower pontine region of the brainstem.

cluster headache. See **histamine headache.**

cluttering, a speech defect characterized by a rapid, confused, nervous delivery with uneven rhythmic patterns and the omission or transposition of various letters or syllables. The condition is commonly associated with other language disorders, as difficulty in learning to speak, read, and spell, and with various personality and behavior problems.

Cm, symbol for **curium.**

***CMAJ*,** abbreviation for ***Canadian Medical Association Journal*.**

CMHC, abbreviation for **community mental health center.**

CMI, abbreviation for **computer-managed instruction.**

CML, abbreviation for **chronic myelocytic.**

CMRNG, abbreviation for **chromosomally mediated resistant *Neisseria gonorrhea.***

CMV, abbreviation for **cytomegalovirus.**

CNA, abbreviation for **Canadian Nurses' Association.**

CNATS, abbreviation for **Canadian Nurses' Association Testing Service.**

-cnemia, a combining form meaning '(condition of the) leg below the knee': *bucnemia, cacocnemia, microcnemia.*

CNF, abbreviation for **Canadian Nurses' Foundation.**

CNM, abbreviation for **Certified Nurse-Midwife.**

CNP, abbreviation for **community nurse practitioner.**

CNRS, abbreviation for **Canadian Nurses' Respiratory Society.**

CNS, **1.** abbreviation for **central nervous system.** **2.** abbreviation for **clinical nurse specialist.**

CNS syndrome. See **central nervous system syndrome.**

Co, symbol for **cobalt.**

co-, col-, com-, con-, cor-, a combining form meaning 'together, with': *coadaptation, coagulate, coarctate.*

CO_2, symbol for **carbon dioxide.**

coagulase /kō•ag′yəlās/, an enzyme produced by bacteria, particularly the *Staphylococcus aureus,* that promotes the formation of thrombi.

coagulation /kō•ag′yəlā′shən/, **1.** the process of transforming a liquid into a solid, especially of the blood. See also **blood clotting.** **2.** (in colloid chemistry) the transforming of the liquid dispersion medium into a gelatinous mass. **3.** the hardening of tissue by some physical means, as by electrocoagulation or photocoagulation.

coagulation current, an electric current delivered by a needle ball or other variously shaped points that coagulates tissue. See also **electrocautery, electrocoagulation.**

coagulation factor, one of 13 factors in the blood, the interactions of which are responsible for the process of blood clotting. The factors, using standardized numeric nomenclature, are factor I, fibrinogen; factor II, prothrombin; factor III, tissue thromboplastin; factor IV, calcium ions; factors V and VI, proaccelerin or labile factors; factor VII, proconvertin or stable factor; factor VIII, antihemophilic globulin; factor IX, plasma thromboplastin component (PTC); factor X, Stuart factor; factor XI, plasma thromboplastin antecedent (PTA); factor XII, Hageman factor or glass factor; factor XIII, fibrin stabilizing factor or Laki-Lorand factor. See also **blood clotting, coagulation, fibrinogen, hemophilia A, hemophilia B, hemophilia C, prothrombin, thromboplastin,** and see **factor IV** through **factor XIII.**

coagulation necrosis. See **necrosis.**

coagulation time. See **clotting time.**

coagulopathy /kō•ag′yəlop′əthē/, a pathologic condition affecting the ability of the blood to coagulate.

coal tar, a topical antieczematic.

■ INDICATIONS: It is prescribed in the treatment of chronic skin diseases, as eczema and psoriasis.

■ CONTRAINDICATIONS: Known hypersensitivity to this drug prohibits its use.

■ ADVERSE EFFECTS: Among the most serious adverse effects are skin irritation and local hypersensitivity reactions.

coal worker's pneumoconiosis. See **anthracosis.**

coaptation splint /kō′aptā′shən/, a small splint fitted to a fractured limb to prevent overriding of the fragments of bone. A longer splint usually covers the small one to provide for more support and fixation of the entire limb.

coarct /kō•ärkt′/, the act of narrowing or constricting, especially the lumen of a blood vessel.

coarctation /kō′ärktā′shən/, a stricture or contraction of the walls of a vessel as the aorta.

coarctation of the aorta, a congenital cardiac anomaly characterized by a localized narrowing of the aorta, which results in increased pressure proximal to the defect and decreased pressure distal to it. Symptoms of the condition are directly related to the pressure changes created by the constriction. The most common site of coarctation is just beyond the origin of the left subclavian artery from the aorta, resulting in high blood pressure in the upper extremities and head and low blood pressure in the lower extremities. Clinical manifestations include dizziness, headaches, fainting, epistaxis, reduced or absent femoral pulses, and muscle cramps in the legs from tissue anoxia during increased exercise. Diagnosis is based on characteristic pressure changes in the upper and lower body and specific radiologic findings, including notching of the lower ribs, left ventricular hypertrophy, and dilatation of the aorta proximal to the stricture. A murmur may or may not be present. Surgical repair is recommended for minor defects because of the high incidence of untreated complications, including aortic rupture, hypertension, infective endocarditis, subarachnoid hemorrhage, and congestive heart failure.

coarse, (in physiology) involving a wide range of movements, as those associated with tremors and other involuntary movements of the skeletal muscle.

coarse fremitus, a rough, loud, tremulous vibration of the chest wall noted on palpation of the chest during a physical examination as the person inhales and exhales. It is most common in pulmonary conditions characterized by consolidation.

coat, **1.** a membrane that covers the outside of an organ or part. **2.** one of the layers of a wall of an organ or part, especially a canal or a vessel.

cobalamin /kōbôl′əmin/, a generic term for a chemical portion of the vitamin B_{12} group. See also **cyanocobalamin.**

cobalt (Co), a metallic element that occurs in the minerals cobaltite, smaltite, and linnaeite. Its atomic number is 27; its atomic weight is 58.9. Extensive deposits of cobalt minerals are found in Ontario, Canada. Pure cobalt is obtained by reducing the oxide with alumium or with carbon. It is used in special alloys, as Alnico. Cobalt is a component of vitamin B_{12}, is found in most common foods, and is readily absorbed by the GI tract. Research has established that this element is common in the human diet, but the precise daily intake requirement is not known, and cobalt deficiency in humans is not known. The administration of cobalt in the form of cobaltous chloride has been successful in some patients with certain types of anemia because of the capacity of cobalt to produce polycythemia. Accidental intoxication by cobaltous chloride, especially in children, may produce cyanosis, coma, and death. Certain amounts of cobalt stimulate the production of erythropoietin, but the exact mechanisms of this process are not completely understood. Large doses of cobalt depress erythrocyte production. It is believed that in stimulating the production of erythropoietin cobalt inhibits enzymes involved in oxidative metabolism and that erythropoietin increases as the result of tissue hypoxia. The only disease for which some experts still advocate the use of cobalt is normochromic, normocytic anemia associated with renal failure. The radioisotope ^{60}Co emits gamma rays and is often used as an encapsulated radiation source in the treatment of cancer.

cobalt 60 (^{60}Co), (in radiotherapy) a radioactive isotope of the silver-white metallic element cobalt with a mass number of 60 and a half-life of 5.2 years. ^{60}Co emits high-energy gamma rays and is the most frequently used radioisotope in radiotherapy. In ^{60}Co machines, the high-energy radioactive source is stored in a position well shielded by lead or uranium.

COBOL /kō′bol/, abbreviation for *common business oriented language,* a high-level compiler computer language for programing.

coca, a species of South American shrubs, native to Bolivia and Peru and cultivated in Indonesia. The leaves are dried and then chewed for their stimulant effect by some of the people of the region. It is a natural source of cocaine. See also **ecgonine.**

cocaine hydrochloride, a white crystalline powder used as a local anesthetic. It was originally derived from coca leaves but can also be prepared synthetically.

■ INDICATIONS: In solution the drug is an effective topical anesthetic commonly used in the examination and treatment of the eye, ear, nose, and throat. The vasoconstrictive action of the drug slows bleeding and limits absorption. Prolonged or frequent use may damage the mucous membranes.

■ CONTRAINDICATIONS: Cocaine is incompatible with all alkaloid precipitants, mercurials, and silver nitrate. Central nervous system overstimulation may result from use with monoamine oxidase inhibitors, amphetamines, or guanethidine. Combination with epinephrine or norepinephrine can lead to cardiac arrhythmias or ventricular fibrillation. Cocaine is not given to patients with severe cardiovascular disease, thyrotoxicosis, hypotension, or hypertension.

■ ADVERSE REACTIONS: Among the most serious adverse reactions are excitement, depression, euphoria, restlessness, tremors, vertigo, nausea, vomiting, hypotension, hypertension, abdominal cramps, exophthalmia, mydriasis, peripheral vascular collapse, tachypnea, tachycardia, chills, fever, coma, or death from respiratory failure.

■ NOTE: Cocaine hydrochloride solution should be freshly made; it deteriorates rapidly on standing and cannot be heat-sterilized. Cocaine is a Schedule II drug under the Controlled Substances Act.

cocarcinogen, an agent that, by itself, does not transform a normal cell into a cancerous state but in concert with another can effect the transformation.

cocci-, cocco-, a combining form meaning 'seed or berry; pertaining to a spherical bacterial cell': *coccobacillus, coccogenous, coccoid.*

coccidioidomycosis /koksid′ē•oi′dōmīkō′sis/, an infectious fungal disease caused by the inhalation of spores of the bacterium *Coccidioides immitis,* which is carried on windborne dust particles. The disease is endemic in hot, dry regions of the southwestern United States and Central and South America. Primary infection is characterized by symptoms resembling those of the common cold or influenza. Secondary infection, occurring after a period of remission and lasting from weeks to years, is marked by low-grade fever, anorexia and weight loss, cyanosis, dyspnea, hemoptysis, focal skin lesions resembling erythema nodosum, and arthritic pain in the bones and joints. The diagnosis is made by learning that the patient was living in or visiting an endemic area and by identifying *C. immitis* in sputum, exudate, or tissue. Treatment usually consists of bed rest and the administration of antibiotics. Also called **desert fever, desert rheumatism, San Joaquin fever, valley fever.**

coccidiosis /kok′sidē•ō′sis/, a parasitic disease of tropic and subtropic regions caused by the ingestion of oocysts of the protozoa *Isospora belli* or *I. hominis*. Symptoms include fever, malaise, abdominal discomfort, and watery diarrhea. The infection is usually self-limited, lasting 1 to 2 weeks, but occasionally it persists, resulting in malabsorption syndrome and, rarely, death. No specific therapy has been found. Compare **coccidioidomycosis.**

cocco-. See **cocci-.**

coccus /kok′əs/, *pl.* **cocci,** a bacterium that is round, spheric, or oval, as gonococcus, pneumococcus, staphylococcus, streptococcus. –**coccal,** *adj.*

-coccus, a combining form meaning a 'berry-shaped organism': *dermococcus, enterococcus, pneumonococcus.*

coccyg-, coccygo-, a combining form meaning 'coccyx': *coccygeal, coccygectomy, coccygodynia.*

coccygeal vertebra, one of the four segments of the vertebral column that fuse to form the adult coccyx. They are considered rudimentary vertebrae and have no pedicles, laminae, or spinous processes. Compare **cervical vertebra, lumbar vertebra, sacral vertebra, thoracic vertebra.** See also **coccyx, vertebra.**

coccygeus /koksij′ē·əs/, one of two muscles in the pelvic diaphragm. Stretching across the pelvic cavity like a hammock, it is a triangular sheet of muscle and tendinous fibers, dorsal to the levator ani, arising from the spine of the ischium and from the sacrospinous ligament. It inserts into the coccyx and into the sacrum, it is innervated by branches of the pudendal plexus, which contain fibers from the fourth and the fifth sacral nerves, and it acts to draw the coccyx ventrally, helping to support the pelvic floor. Compare **levator ani.**

coccygodynia /kok′sigōdin′ē·ə/, a pain in the coccygeal area of the body.

coccyx /kok′siks/, *pl.* **coccyges** /koksī′jēz, kok′sijēz/, the beaklike bone joined to the sacrum by a disk of fibrocartilage at the base of the vertebral column. It is formed by the union of three to five rudimentary vertebrae. The pieces of the coccyx fuse together in men at an earlier period in life than in women. In men and in women, the coccyx becomes fused with the sacrum by the sixth decade of life. The coccyx is freely movable on the sacrum during pregnancy. **–coccygeal** /koksij′ē·əl/, *adj.*

cochineal /koch′inēl′/, a red dye prepared from the dried female insects of the species *Coccus cacti* containing young larvae. During the preparation of the dye the larvae are extracted with an aqueous solution of alum, and the resulting dye has been used in coloring medicines.

cochlea /kok′lē·ə/, a conic bony structure of the inner ear, perforated by numerous apertures for passage of the cochlear division of the acoustic nerve. Part of a complex tubular network called the osseous labyrinth, it is a spiral tunnel about 30 mm long with two full and three quarter-turns, resembling a tiny snail shell. **–cochlear** /kok′lē·ər/, *adj.*

cochlear canal, a bony spiral tunnel within the cochlea of the internal ear. It narrows gradually in diameter as it rises to the apex of the cochlea. It contains one opening that communicates with the tympanic cavity, a second that connects with the vestibule, and a third that leads to a tiny canal opening on the inferior surface of the temporal bone.

cochlear duct. See **cochlear canal.**

cockscomb papilloma, a benign, small red lesion that may project from the uterine cervix during pregnancy; it regresses after delivery.

cocktail, *informal.* an unofficial mixture of drugs, usually in solution, combined to achieve a specific purpose. See also **Brompton's cocktail.**

Coco-Quinine, a trademark for an antimalarial (quinine sulfate).

code, **1.** (in law) a published body of statutes, as a civil code. **2.** a collection of standards and rules of behavior, as a dress code. **3.** a symbolic means of representing information for communication or transfer, as a genetic code. **4.** a system of notation that allows information to be transmitted rapidly, as Morse code, or in secrecy, as a cryptographic code. **5.** *informal.* a discreet signal used to summon a special team to resuscitate a patient, as in "code zero, 3 west" announced over a public address system to bring the team to the west wing of the third floor without alarming patients or visitors. See also **no-code.** **6.** to enter data by use of a given programing language into a computer. Compare **decode, encode.**

codeine, a narcotic analgesic and antitussive.

■ INDICATIONS: It is used to treat mild to moderate pain, to treat diarrhea, and as an antitussive.

■ CONTRAINDICATIONS: Known hypersensitivity to this drug prohibits its use.

■ ADVERSE EFFECTS: Among the most serious adverse reactions are constipation, nausea, drowsiness, and allergic reactions. High doses are associated with respiratory and circulatory depression. The drug is potentially addictive.

codeine phosphate, a narcotic analgesic and antitussive.

■ INDICATIONS: It is prescribed to suppress cough and to relieve pain.

■ CONTRAINDICATION: Known hypersensitivity to opiates is the only contraindication.

■ ADVERSE EFFECTS: Among the more serious adverse reactions are depression of the central nervous system, paradoxical excitement, and drug dependence.

code of ethics, a statement encompassing the set of rules by which practitioners of a profession are expected to conform. See also **Hippocratic Oath.**

code team, a specially trained and equipped team of physicians, nurses, and technicians that is available to provide cardiopulmonary resuscitation when summoned by a code set by the institution. A code team usually includes a physician, registered nurse, respiratory therapist, and pharmacist. The members may work in any department or unit of the hospital. A schedule is made that ensures a full team on duty at all times.

coding, the process of organizing information into categories, which are assigned codes for the purposes of sorting, storing, and retrieving the data.

cod-liver oil, a pale-yellow, fatty oil extracted from the fresh livers of the codfish and other related species. It is a rich source of vitamins A and D, useful in the treatment of nutritional deficiency of those vitamins or of conditions resulting from abnormal absorption of calcium and phosphorus. The oil must be stored in a cool, dark place, or it becomes rancid. See also **osteomalacia, rickets, tetany.**

Codman's tumor. See **chondroblastoma.**

codominant, of or pertaining to the alleles or to the trait resulting from the full expression of both alleles of a pair in a heterozygote, as the AB or MNS blood group antigens. **–codominance,** *n.*

codominant inheritance, the transmission of a trait or condition in which both alleles of a pair are given full expression in a heterozygote, as in the AB or MNS blood group antigens and the leukocyte antigens.

codon /kō′don/, a unit of three adjacent nucleotides along a DNA or messenger RNA molecule that designates a specific amino acid in the polypeptide chain during protein synthesis. Each codon consists of a specific section of the DNA molecule so that the order of the codons along the molecule determines the sequence of the amino acids in each protein. See also **genetic code.**

coefficient, a mathematic relationship between factors that can be used to measure or evaluate a characteristic under specified conditions. An example is the **oxygen-utilization coefficient,** which measures the amount of oxygen in a patient's venous blood in terms of the proportion of oxygen in his arterial blood.

coel-, a combining form meaning 'pertaining to the colon': *colalgia, colauxe, colectasia*. See also **cel-.**

-coel, -coele. See **-cele²**.

coelenteron, *pl.* **coelentera,** the digestive cavity of those animals having only two germ layers, as the hydra and jellyfish. See also **archenteron.**

coelom, the body cavity of the developing embryo. It is situated between the layers of mesoderm and in mammals gives rise to the pericardial, pleural, and peritoneal cavities. A kind of coelom is **extraembryonic coelom.** Also spelled **coelome, celom.** Also called **coeloma** (*pl.* **coelomata**), **somatic cavity.** –**coelomic, celomic,** *adj.*

coelosomy, a congenital anomaly characterized by the protrusion of the viscera from the body cavity.

coenesthesia, coenesthesis, coenogenesis. See **cenesthesia.**

coenzyme /kō•en′zīm/, a nonprotein substance that combines with an apoenzyme to form a complete enzyme or holoenzyme. Coenzymes include some of the vitamins, as B_1 and B_2, and have smaller molecules than enzymes. Coenzymes are dialyzable and heat-stable and usually dissociate easily from the protein portions of the enzymes with which they combine. See also **acetylcoenzyme A.**

coffee, the dried and roasted ripe seeds of *Coffea arabica, C. liberica,* and *C. robusta* trees that may have originated in Africa but now grow in almost all tropic areas. Coffee contains the alkaloid caffeine and is the basis for a stimulating drink that has been used in treating the common headache, chronic asthma, and narcotic poisoning.

coffee-and- . . . , (in psychiatric nursing) a method of treatment for chronically ill psychiatric outpatients. Patients meet on a regular schedule, with professional staff, in a quasi-social environment for mutual support and encouragement of the patients. Coffee and something to eat may be served.

coffee-ground vomitus, dark brown vomitus the color and consistency of coffee grounds, composed of gastric juices and old blood and indicative of slow upper GI bleeding. Compare **hematemesis.**

coffee worker's lung, a respiratory condition caused by an allergic reaction to the dust of the coffee bean. See also **organic dust.**

Cogentin, a trademark for an antiparkinsonian (benztropine mesylate).

cognition, the mental process characterized by knowing, thinking, learning, and judging. Compare **conation.** –**cognitive,** *adj.*

cognitive development, the developmental process by which an infant becomes an intelligent person, acquiring, with growth, knowledge and the ability to think, learn, reason, and abstract. Jean Piaget demonstrated the orderly sequence of this process from early infancy through childhood. See also **psychosexual development, psychosocial development.**

cognitive dissonance, a state of tension resulting from a discrepancy in a person's emotional and intellectual frame of reference for interpreting and coping with his environment. It usually occurs when new information contradicts existing assumptions or knowledge.

cognitive function, an intellectual process by which one becomes aware of, perceives, or comprehends ideas. It involves all aspects of perception, thinking, reasoning, and remembering. Compare **conation.**

cognitive learning, learning that is concerned with acquisition of problem-solving abilities and with intelligence and conscious thought.

cognitive psychology, the study of the development of thought, language, and intelligence in infants and children.

cognitive therapy, any of the various methods of treating mental and emotional disorders that help a person change attitudes, perceptions, and patterns of thinking. Therapeutic approaches include behavior therapy, existential therapy, Gestalt therapy, and transactional analysis.

cogwheel rigidity, an abnormal rigor in muscle tissue, characterized by jerky movements when the muscle is passively stretched. Some authorities believe cogwheel rigidity masks a muscular tremor that is not evident until the affected muscle is manipulated.

cohere, to stick together, as similar molecules of a common substance.

coherence, **1.** the property of sticking together, as the molecules within a common substance. **2.** (in psychology) the logical pattern of expression and thought evident in the speech of a normal, stable individual. –**coherent,** *adj.*

cohesive termini, (in molecular genetics) the complementary single-stranded ends projecting from a double-stranded DNA segment that can be joined to introduced fragments. Also called **sticky ends.**

cohort, (in statistics) a collection or sampling of individuals who share a common characteristic, as members of the same age or the same sex.

cohort study, (in research) a study concerning a specific subpopulation, as the children born between December and May in 1975 and the children born in the same months in 1955. See also **prospective study.**

coil. See **intrauterine device.**

coiled tubular gland, one of the many multicellular glands that contain a coiled, tube-shaped secretory portion, as the sweat glands.

coil-spring contraceptive diaphragm, a kind of contraceptive diaphragm in which the flexible metal spring that forms the rim is a coiled, circular spring. The rubber dome of the diaphragm is approximately 3.8 cm deep, and the diameter of the rubber-covered rim is from 5.5 to 10 cm. Ten sizes, in increments of 0.5 cm, allow the clinician to fit the diaphragm to the individual woman. The kind of spring and the size of the rim in millimeters is stamped on the rim, as, for example, a 75 mm coil spring. This kind of diaphragm is prescribed for a woman whose vaginal musculature offers good support, whose uterus is not acutely retroflexed or anteflexed, and whose vagina, neither very long nor very short, has a deeper than usual arch behind the symphysis pubis. The coil-spring diaphragm is lighter than an arcing spring, and, if it is well fitted and conforms to the woman's vaginal contour, it is effective and comfortable to use. Compare **arcing-spring contraceptive diaphragm, flat-spring contraceptive diaphragm.** See also **contraceptive-diaphragm fitting.**

coincidence counting, (in radiotherapy) the detection of two photons that arrive at separate counters simultaneously as the result of annihilation of a positron (created during a radioactive decay) and an electron. As an imaging technique, the coincidence counting of two photons greatly reduces the significance of any background radiation.

coitus /kō′itəs/, the sexual union of two people of opposite sex in which the penis is introduced into the vagina, typically resulting in mutual excitation and usually orgasm. Also called **coition, copulation, sexual intercourse.** **–coital,** *adj.*

coitus interruptus. See **withdrawal method.**

col-, a combining form meaning 'pertaining to the colon': *colalgia, colauxe, colectasia.* See also **co-.**

Colace, a trademark for a stool softener (docusate sodium sulfosuccinate).

colation, the act of filtering or straining, as urine is often strained for medical examination.

COL bed. See **Circolectric (COL) bed.**

colchicine /kol′chəsēn/, a gout suppressant.

■ INDICATIONS: It is prescribed in the treatment of acute gout and prophylaxis of recurrent gouty arthritis.

■ CONTRAINDICATIONS: Ulcer, ulcerative colitis, or known hypersensitivity to this drug prohibits its use. The drug is highly toxic and is not given to elderly, debilitated patients or to those people who have chronic renal, hepatic, cardiovascular, or GI disease.

■ ADVERSE EFFECTS: Among the most serious adverse reactions are severe GI distress including diarrhea with blood, bone marrow depression, peripheral neuritis, liver dysfunction, and alopecia.

cold, **1.** the absence of heat. **2.** also called **common cold.** a contagious viral infection of the upper respiratory tract, usually caused by a strain of rhinovirus. It is characterized by rhinitis, tearing, low-grade fever, and malaise and is treated symptomatically with rest, mild analgesia, decongestants, and an increased intake of fluids.

cold abscess, a site of infection that does not show common signs of heat, redness, and swelling.

cold agglutinin, a nonspecific antibody, found on the surface of red blood cells in certain diseases, that may cause clumping of the cells at temperatures below 4° C and may cause hemolysis. The phenomenon does not occur at body temperature. Mycoplasma pneumonia, infectious mononucleosis, and many lymphoproliferative disorders are associated with cold agglutinins.

cold bath, a bath in which the water temperature is approximately 50° F (10° C) to 65° F (18° C), used primarily to reduce body temperature.

cold-blooded, unable to regulate body heat, as fishes, reptiles, and amphibians that have internal temperatures that are close to the temperatures of the environments in which they live. Also called **poikilothermic.** Compare **warm-blooded.**

cold cautery. See **cryocautery.**

cold caloric irrigation, a procedure for testing the integrity of brainstem function. It is carried out by irrigating the external auditory canal of the patient with a cold saline solution while the head is flexed at approximately 30 degrees, after checking the patency of the ear canal. The stimulus results in jerky but regular eye movements in a normal patient. Absence of the reaction may be a sign of a lesion at the pontine level of the brainstem.

cold hemoglobinuria. See **hemoglobinuria.**

cold injury, any of several abnormal and often serious physical conditions caused by exposure to cold temperatures. See also **chilblain, frostbite, hypothermia, immersion foot.**

cold-pressor test, a test for the tendency to develop essential hypertension. One hand of the individual is immersed in ice water for about 60 seconds. An excessive rise in the blood pressure or an unusual delay in the return of normal blood pressure when the hand is removed from the water is believed to indicate that the individual is at risk for hypertension.

cold-sensitive mutation, a genetic alteration resulting in a gene that functions at a high temperature and not at a low temperature.

cold sore. See **herpes simplex.**

colectomy /kəlek′təmē/, surgical excision of part or all of the colon, performed to treat cancer of the colon or severe chronic ulcerative colitis. For several days before surgery, a low-residue diet is prescribed. Antibiotics and cleansing enemas are given to reduce the number of bacteria in the bowel. Parenteral fluids and electrolytes are given, and a nasointestinal tube is passed. The colon is removed under general anesthesia. The nurse gives postoperative care as for any abdominal surgery. The nasointestinal tube is connected to suction and remains in place until bowel sounds are heard. See also **abdominal surgery.**

Colestid, a trademark for an antihyperlipoproteinemic (colestipol hydrochloride).

colestipol hydrochloride, an antihyperlipoproteinemic that acts by sequestering bile acids in the intestine, thus reducing plasma levels of cholesterol.

▪ INDICATIONS: It is prescribed in the treatment of hypercholesterolemia and xanthoma.

▪ CONTRAINDICATIONS: Biliary obstruction or known hypersensitivity to this drug prohibits its use.

▪ ADVERSE EFFECTS: Among the more serious adverse reactions are skin rash, fecal impaction, and a deficiency of vitamins A, D, and K.

colic /kol′ik/, **1.** sharp visceral pain resulting from torsion, obstruction, or smooth muscle spasm of a hollow or tubular organ, as a ureter or the intestines. Kinds of colic include **biliary colic, infantile colic,** and **renal colic. 2.** of or pertaining to the colon. **–colicky,** *adj.*

colicinogen /kol′isin′əjən/, an episome in some strains of *Escherichia coli* that induces secretion of a colicin, a protein lethal to other strains of the bacterium. Specific colicins attach to specific receptors on the cell membrane and impair the synthesis of macromolecules or the production of energy. Also called **colicinogenic factor.**

coliform /kol′ifôrm/, **1.** of or pertaining to the colon-aerogenes group, or the *Escherichia coli* species of microorganisms, constituting most of the intestinal flora in humans and other animals. **2.** having the characteristic of a sieve or cribriform structure, as some of the porous bones of the skull.

colistimethate sodium, an antibacterial. Also called **colistin sulfomethate sodium.**

▪ INDICATIONS: It is prescribed in the treatment of GI infections caused by certain gram-negative microorganisms and as a topical medication.

▪ CONTRAINDICATIONS: Known hypersensitivity to this drug or to polymyxin B prohibits its use.

▪ ADVERSE EFFECTS: Among the more serious adverse reactions are nephrotoxicity and neurotoxicity, including neuromuscular blockade.

colistin sulfate, an antibacterial.

▪ INDICATIONS: It is prescribed topically in the treatment of infections of the outer ear and systemically for serious gram-negative infections and for the treatment of gastroenteritis caused by *Escherichia coli* infections.

▪ CONTRAINDICATION: Known hypersensitivity to this drug prohibits its use.

▪ ADVERSE EFFECTS: Among the more serious systemic reactions are respiratory arrest, renal toxicity, and neuromuscular blockade.

colitis, an inflammatory condition of the large intestine, either one of the episodic, functional, irritable bowel syndromes or one of the more serious chronic, progressive, inflammatory bowel diseases. Irritable bowel syndrome is characterized by bouts of colicky pain and diarrhea or constipation, often resulting from emotional stress. Treatment includes stress reduction and adherence to a diet that may include bland foods and less roughage than in a usual diet. Because individuals with colitis may be irritated by different substances, the diet is individualized to avoid known irritants. Kinds of irritable bowel syndrome are **spastic colon** and **mucous colitis.** Inflammatory bowel disease is characterized by abscess formation, severe diarrhea, bleeding, and ulceration of the mucosa of the intestine. Weight loss and pain are significant. Steroids, fluids, electrolytes, antibiotics, and careful attention to diet are the usual modes of therapy. Most of the diseases of this group are of unknown origin. Kinds of inflammatory bowel disease include **Crohn's disease** and **ulcerative colitis. –colitic,** *adj.*

collagen /kol′əjən/, a protein consisting of bundles of tiny reticular fibrils, which combine to form the white glistening inelastic fibers of the tendons, the ligaments, and the fascia. **–collagenous** /kəlaj′ənəs/, *adj.*

collagenase ointment, a medication used in the treatment of decubitus ulcers, burns, and other epidermal lesions. It is an enzyme preparation derived from the fermentation of *Clostridium histolyticum.*

collagen disease, any one of the various abnormal conditions characterized by extensive disruption of the connective tissue, as inflammation and fibrinoid degeneration. Some collagen diseases are polyarteritis nodosa, disseminated lupus erythematosus, rheumatic fever, rheumatoid coronary arteritis, and ankylosing spondylitis. Such disorders may also cause coronary problems, which are often controlled with glucocorticoids.

collagenoblast /kəlaj′ənōblast′/, a cell that differentiates from a fibroblast and functions in the formation of collagen. It can also transform into cartilage and bone tissue by metaplasia.

collagenous fiber, any one of the tough, white fibers that constitute much of the intercellular substance and the connective tissue of the body. Collagenous fibers contain collagen; they are often arranged in bundles that strengthen the tissues in which they are imbedded.

collagen vascular disease, any of a group of acquired disorders that have in common diffuse immunologic and inflammatory changes in small blood vessels and connective tissue. The cause of most of these diseases is unknown. Hereditary factors and deficiencies, environmental antigens, infections, allergies, and antigen-antibody complexes in various combinations are probably involved. Common features of most of these entities include arthritis, skin lesions, iritis and episcleritis, pericarditis, pleuritis, subcutaneous nodules, myocarditis, vasculitis, and nephritis. Often associated are also Coombs test-positive hemolytic anemia, thrombocytopenia, leukopenia, B and T cell abnormalities, antinuclear antibodies, cryoglobulins, rheumatoid factors, false-positive serologic tests for syphilis, alterations in serum complement, and immunologic abnormalities. The diseases usually included in this category are mixed connective tissue disease, necrotizing vasculitis, polyarteritis nodosa, polymyositis, relapsing polychondritis, rheumatic fever, rheumatoid arthritis, scleroderma, and systemic lupus erythematosus. Also called **connective tissue disease.**

collapse, **1.** *nontechnical.* a state of extreme depression or a condition of complete exhaustion because of physical or psychosomatic problems. **2.** an abnormal condition characterized by shock. **3.** the abnormal sagging of an organ or the obliteration of its cavity.

collar, any structure that encircles another, usually around its neck, as the periosteal bone collars that form around the diaphyses of young bones.

collarbone. See **clavicle.**

collateral, **1.** secondary or accessory. **2.** (in anatomy) a small branch, as any one of the arterioles or venules in the body.

collateral fissure, a fissure separating the subcalcarine and the subcollateral gyri of the cerebral hemisphere.

collateral pulp canal, (in dentistry) a branch of the pulp canal that emerges from the root at a place other than the apex. Also called **branching canal.** Compare **accessory root canal.**

collecting tubule, any one of the many relatively large straight tubules of the kidney that funnel urine into the renal pelvis. The collecting tubules drain the urine from the distal convoluted tubules in the renal cortex and descend into the renal medulla before connecting with each other at various intervals along the path to the renal pelvis. The collecting tubules play an important role in maintaining the fluid balance of the body by allowing water to osmose through their membranes into the interstitial fluid in the renal medulla. Antidiuretic hormone in the blood makes the collecting tubules permeable to water. If no antidiuretic hormone is present in the blood, the membranes of the collecting tubules are practically impermeable to water. See also **Bowman's capsule, kidney.**

collective unconscious, (in analytic psychology) that portion of the unconscious common to all mankind. Also called **racial unconscious.** See also **analytic psychology.**

collector, (in medicine) a device with various modifications, used for collecting secretions from the bronchi and esophagus for bacteriologic and cytologic examination.

college, **1.** an organization of individuals with common professional training and interests, as the American College of Nurse-Midwives, the American College of Cardiology, or the American College of Surgeons. **2.** an institution of higher learning.

College of American Pathologists (CAP), a national professional organization of physicians who specialize in pathology.

Colles' fascia /kol′ēz/, the deep layer of the subcutaneous fascia of the perineum, constituting a distinctive structure in the urogenital region of the body. It is a strong, smooth sheet of tissue containing elastic fibers that give it a characteristic yellow tint. Ventrally, it is continuous with the deep layer of the subcutaneous abdominal fascia and fills a groove between the scrotum and the thigh or between the labium and the thigh; medially, it joins the superficial layer of the subcutaneous perineal fascia to form the dartos tunic of the scrotum or to form the thick fascial sheath of the labium; laterally, it firmly adheres to the ischiopubic ramus; and dorsally, it dips toward the ischiorectal fossa and attaches firmly to deep perineal fascia. In the anal region of the perineum, Colles' fascia adheres to both the superficial layer and the deep layer of the subcutaneous fascia.

Colles' fracture, a fracture of the radius at the epiphysis within 1 inch of the joint of the wrist, easily recognized by the dorsal and lateral position of the hand that it causes.

colligative /kol′igā′tiv/, (in physical chemistry) of or pertaining to those properties of matter that depend on the concentration of particles, as molecules and ions, rather than the chemical properties of any substance. One such colligative property is the pressure of a specific volume of gas.

collimator /kol′imā′tər/, a device for limiting particles of radiation to parallel paths, used to restrict the beam of a radiotherapy machine to a specified area.

colliquation /kol′ikwā′shən/, the degeneration of a tissue of the body to a liquid state, usually associated with necrotic tissue.

colliquative /kol′ikwā′tiv/, characterized by the profuse discharge of fluid, as in suppurating wounds and structures of the body that are infected.

collision tumor, a tumor formed as two separate growths, developing close to each other, join. See also **carcinoma.**

collodion /kəlō′dē·ən/, a clear or a slightly opaque, highly inflammable liquid composed of pyroxylin, ether, and alcohol. It dries to a strong, transparent film that is used as a surgical dressing.

collodion baby, an infant whose skin at birth is covered with a scaly, parchmentlike membrane. See also **harlequin fetus, lamellar exfoliation of the newborn.**

colloid /kol′oid/, a state or division of matter in which large molecules or aggregates of molecules that do not precipitate, and that measure between 1 and 100 nm, are dispersed in another medium. In a suspension colloid the particles are insoluble and the medium may be solid, liquid, or gas. In an emulsion colloid the particles are usually water and the medium is any of several complex hydrophilic, organic substances that become evenly dispersed among the particles of water. Compare **solution, suspension.**

colloid bath, a bath taken in water that contains such substances as bran, gelatin, and starch, used to relieve irritation and inflammation. See also **emollient bath.**

colloid carcinoma, a former term for mucinous carcinoma.

colloid chemistry, the science dealing with the composition and nature of chemical colloids.

colloid goiter, a greatly enlarged, soft thyroid gland in which the follicles are distended with colloid.

colloid osmotic pressure, an abnormal condition of the kidney caused by the pressure of concentrations of large particles, such as protein molecules, that will not pass through a membrane. Also called **oncotic pressure.**

colo-, colon-, a combining form meaning 'pertaining to the colon': *colocolic, colodyspepsia, colitis.*

coloboma /kol'əbō'mə/, *pl.* **colobomas, colobomata,** a congenital or pathologic defect in the ocular tissue of the body, usually affecting the iris, ciliary body, or choroid by forming a cleft that extends inferiorly. Colobomas are usually the result of the failure of part of the fetal fissure to close. **–colobomatous,** *adj.*

-coloboma, a combining form meaning the 'absence or defect of an ocular tissue affecting function, especially of the iris': *blepharocoloboma, iridocoloboma, pseudocoloboma.*

colon /kō'lən/, the portion of the large intestine extending from the cecum to the rectum. It has four segments: ascending colon, transverse colon, descending colon, and sigmoid colon. **–colonic** /kəlon'ik/, *adj.*

colon-. See **colo-.**

-colon, a combining form meaning the 'part of the large intestine between the cecum and rectum': *cecocolon, megacolon, paracolon.*

colonic. See **colon.**

-colonic, a combining form meaning 'relating to the colon': *pericolonic, rectocolonic, vesicocolonic.*

colonic fistula, an abnormal passage from the colon to the surface of the body or an internal organ or structure. In regional enteritis, chronic inflammation may lead to the formation of a fistula between two adjacent loops of bowel. An external opening from the colon to the surface of the abdomen may be created surgically after the removal of a malignant or severely ulcerated segment of the bowel. See also **colostomy.**

colon stasis. See **atonia constipation.**

colony, **1.** (in bacteriology) a mass of microorganisms in a culture that originates from a single cell. Some kinds of colonies, according to different configurations, are smooth colonies, rough colonies, and dwarf colonies. **2.** (in cell biology) a mass of cells in a culture or in certain experimental tissues, as a spleen colony.

colony counter, a device used for counting colonies of bacteria growing in a culture and usually consisting of an illuminated, transparent plate that is divided into sections of known area. Petri dishes containing colonies of bacteria are placed over the plate, and the colonies are counted according to the number within the areas viewed.

-color, a combining form meaning 'hue or hues': *cuticolor, tricolor, versicolor.*

Colorado tick fever, a relatively mild, self-limited arbovirus infection transmitted to humans by the bite of a tick. It is most prevalent in the spring and summer months throughout the Rocky Mountains, particularly in Colorado. Symptoms, occurring in two phases separated by a period of remission, include chills, fever, headache, pain in the eyes, legs, and back, and sensitivity to light. Treatment is supportive; analgesics can be given for headache and other pains. Also called **American mountain fever, mountain fever, mountain tick fever. Compare Rocky Mountain spotted fever.**

color blindness, an abnormal condition characterized by an inability to clearly distinguish colors of the spectrum. In most cases it is not a blindness but a weakness in perceiving them distinctly. There are two forms of color blindness. **Daltonism** is the most common form and is characterized by an inability to distinguish reds from greens. It is an inherited, sex-linked disorder. **Total color blindness,** or **achromatic vision,** is characterized by an inability to perceive any color at all. Only white, gray, and black are seen. It may be the result of a defect in or the absence of the cones in the retina.

color dysnomia /disnō'mē·ə/, an inability to name colors despite an ability to match and distinguish them. It may be caused by expressive dysphasis.

colorectal cancer /kō'lərek'təl/, a malignant neoplastic disease of the large intestine, characterized by melena, a change in bowel habits, and the passing of blood. Malignant tumors of the large bowel usually occur after the age of 50, are slightly more frequent in women than in men, and are almost as common as lung cancer in the United States. The high incidence of colorectal cancer in the western world, as contrasted with the low incidence in Japan and rural Africa, suggests that a diet high in refined carbohydrates and beef and low in roughage may be a causative factor. The risk of large bowel cancer is increased in chronic ulcerative colitis, in diverticulosis, in villous adenomas, and especially in familial polyposis of the colon. People who have inhaled asbestos fibers or who have been irradiated are more likely than others to develop colorectal cancer. In the vermiform appendix, carcinoid is the most common tumor. Most lesions of the large bowel are adenocarcinomas; one half arise in the rectum, one fifth in the sigmoid colon, approximately one sixth in the cecum and ascending colon, and the rest in other sites. Rectal tumors may cause pain, bleeding, and a feeling of incomplete evacuation; they may metastasize slowly through lymphatic channels and veins, and, occasionally, prolapse through the anus. Typical napkin ring tumors in the sigmoid and descending colon constrict the intestinal lumen, causing partial obstruction and the production of flat or pencil-shaped stools. Malignant lesions in the ascending colon are usually large growths that may be palpable on physical examination; they generally cause severe anemia, nausea, and alternating constipation and diarrhea. The diagnosis of colorectal cancer is based on digital rectal examination, testing for blood in the stool, proctosigmoidoscopic examination of the sigmoid, and x-ray studies of the GI tract after a barium enema. Suspicious polyps may be removed for histologic study, often through a sigmoidoscope or colposcope or by a laparotomy. Surgical treatment of colorectal cancer may involve a wide resection of the lesion, the surrounding colon, and the attached tissues, with an end-to-end anastomosis of the remaining intestinal segments whenever possible. Tumors of the lower two thirds of the rectum usually require removal of the entire rectum by abdominoperineal resection and the creation of a permanent colostomy. Transanal electric coagulation is currently being studied and tried in the treatment of certain rectal cancers. Irradiation may be administered preoperatively and postoperatively as palliative therapy for inoperable tumors or as the sole method of treating certain rectal cancers. Chemotherapy with 5-fluorouracil infused intraluminally in the bowel at surgery and intravenously after surgery may be used as adjunctive treatment. Combinations of 5-fluorouracil, the nitrosourea lomustine, and vincristine may offer palliation of the symptoms of the disease.

colorimetry /kol′ərim′ətrē/, **1.** measurement of the intensity of color in a fluid or substance. See also **spectrophotometry. 2.** measurement of color in the blood by using of a colorimeter to determine hemoglobin concentration. The technique is useful only for gross screening purposes, because it is not exact and interpretation is subjective. –**colorimetric,** *adj.*

color index (C.I.), the ratio between the concentration of hemoglobin and the number of red blood cells in any given sample of blood. The color index is computed by dividing the concentration of hemoglobin, expressed as a percentage of normal concentration, by the approximate number of red blood cells, expressed as a percentage of a normal concentration of 5 million red cells per cubic millimeter. The average color index is about 0.85. Compare ***Colour Index.***

color vision, a recognition of color as the result of changes in the pigments of the cones in the retina that react to varying intensities of red, green, and blue light. The exact mechanisms of color vision are not completely understood, but some experts believe they depend on three specialized types of cones, each type responding to red, green, or blue light. Some retinal cones respond to the entire visual spectrum. See also **color blindness.**

colostomate /kəlos′təmāt/, a person who has undergone a colostomy.

colostomy /kəlos′təmē/, surgical creation of an artificial anus on the abdominal wall by incising the colon and bringing it out to the surface, performed for cancer of the colon and benign obstructive tumors, and severe abdominal wounds. A colostomy may be single-barreled, with one opening, or double-barreled, with distal and proximal loops open onto the abdomen. The latter is performed when the lower bowel is completely blocked or in paraplegia to simplify daily management. A temporary colostomy may be done to divert feces, after surgery, as in the repair of Hirschsprung's disease, from an inflamed area; it is repaired when the colon has healed or the inflammation subsides. Preoperative nursing care focuses on teaching the patient what to expect after surgery. A high-calorie, low-residue diet is given; an antibiotic, usually neomycin, is prescribed to reduce the bacterial count in the bowel, and enemas are given until returns are clear. The surgery is done under general anesthesia. Immediate postoperative care is the same as for abdominal surgery. The color of the stoma is checked: a dark blue-black color (rather than bright red) indicates a circulation block, and the surgeon is notified. Saline irrigations are begun on the fourth or fifth day. A type of colostomy is **loop colostomy.** Compare **enterostomy.**

colostomy irrigation, a procedure used by colostomates to clear the bowel of fecal matter and to help establish an evacuation schedule.

■ METHOD: Daily irrigation may be ordered beginning 7 to 10 days after the operation, and the patient is involved in assisting in the procedure as soon as possible. In preparation for self-care, the technique is explained in a step-by-step manner and irrigation is carried out with the equipment the patient will use at home. In the hospital the procedure is performed as the patient sits in bed in a semi- or high-Fowler's position or on a commode, if ambulatory; at home the individual will probably find a toilet more convenient. A catheter, lubricated with petroleum jelly, is gently inserted in the stoma to a depth of about 3 inches; the catheter tip is advanced only as far as it will go easily and is never forced. If it is not accepted, the stoma is usually dilated by gently inserting and rotating a gloved, lubricated finger approximating the size of the opening. An irrigating bag containing 500 to 1000 ml of warm solution is held 12 to 18 inches above the stoma, and the fluid is allowed to flow slowly into the colon. If

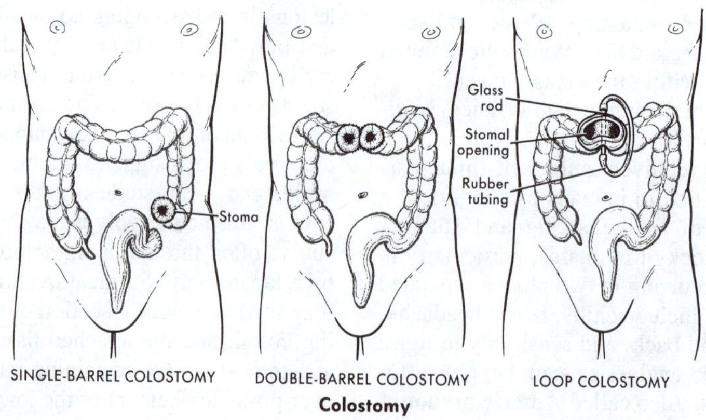

Colostomy

the patient complains of cramps, the catheter is clamped for a few minutes before the flow is resumed. The fluid is retained for several minutes and then drained through outlet tubing into a basin or commode. From 30 to 45 minutes is allowed for draining; if the return is slow, the patient is asked to lean forward or move from side to side; the abdomen may be massaged. The character and amount of the return flow is noted. A dehydrated patient may retain some fluid.

■ NURSING ORDERS: The nurse performs and teaches colostomy irrigation and ensures that the patient knows how to carry out the procedure correctly and where to purchase the necessary equipment. The person is urged to report any symptoms of obstruction or prolapse of the stoma. A public health nurse is available in many areas for home visits if help is needed.

■ OUTCOME CRITERIA: Many colostomates establish a regular schedule of evacuation with irrigation, but the procedure may be unsatisfactory for patients with a liquid or semisoft fecal stream, for patients who, before the operation, had a tendency to develop diarrhea under stress, or for patients with irregular bowel habits.

colostrum /kəlos′trəm/, the fluid secreted by the breast during pregnancy and the first days postpartum before lactation begins, consisting of immunologically active substances and white blood cells, water, protein, fat, and carbohydrate in a thin, yellow, serous fluid.

Colour Index (C.I.), a publication of dyers, colorists, and textile chemists that specifies all the standard industrial pigments and stains according to five-digit numbers associated with chemical coloring materials. For example, methylene blue is assigned number 52015. Compare **color index.**

colpectomy, the surgical excision of the vagina.

colpo-, colp-, kolpo-, kysth-, kystho-, a combining form meaning 'pertaining to the vagina': *colpocele, colpocystitis, colpodynia.*

colpohysterectomy, vaginal hysterectomy. See also **hysterectomy.**

colporrhaphy, a surgical procedure in which the vagina is sutured, as for the purpose of narrowing the vagina.

colpotomy, any surgical incision into the wall of the vagina.

columbium, former name for **niobium.**

column chromatography, the process of separating and analyzing a group of substances according to the differences in their absorption affinities for a given absorbent as evidenced by pigments deposited during filtration through the same absorbent contained in a glass cylinder or tube. The substances are dissolved in a liquid that is passed through the absorbent. The absorbates move down the column at different rates and leave behind a band of pigments that is subsequently washed with a pure solvent to "develop" discrete pigmented bands that constitute a chromatograph. The cylinder of absorbent is then pushed from the tube, and the individual bands are either separated with a knife or further diluted with the pure solvent and collected in the bottom of the tube for analysis. Effective column chromatography depends on the selection of the appropriate absorbent and solvent and a flow rate that is slow enough to allow complete diffusion of the absorbates from the solvent to the absorbent and the retardation of the absorbates according to their different affinities for the absorbent. Compare **gas chromatography, ion-exchange chromatography.**

Coly-Mycin M, a trademark for a parenteral antibacterial (colistimethate sodium).

Coly-Mycin S, a trademark for an oral antibacterial (colistin sulfate).

com-. See **co-.**

coma, a state of profound unconsciousness, characterized by the absence of spontaneous eye movements, response to painful stimuli, and vocalization. The person cannot be aroused. Coma may be the result of trauma, space-occupying brain tumor, hematoma, toxic condition, acute infectious disease with encephalitis, vascular disease, poisoning, diabetic acidosis, or intoxication. See also **Glasgow Coma Scale, unconscious.**

-coma, **1.** a combining form meaning '(condition of) profound unconsciousness': *narcoma, semicoma.* **2.** a combining form meaning '(condition of) torpor': *agrypnocoma.*

combat fatigue, any of a variety of psychoneurotic disorders, usually temporary but sometimes leading to permanent neurosis, resulting from exhaustion, the stress of combat, or the cumulative emotions and psychologic strain of warfare or similar situations. It is characterized by anxiety, depression, irritability, memory and sleep disorders, and various related symptoms. Also called **combat neurosis, war neurosis.** See also **posttraumatic stress disorder, shell shock.**

Combid, a trademark for a GI fixed-combination drug containing an anticholinergic (isopropamide iodide) and a phenothiazine antipsychotic (prochlorperazine).

combined anesthesia. See **balanced anesthesia.**

combined system disease, a disorder of the nervous system caused by a deficiency of vitamin B_{12} that results in pernicious anemia and degeneration of the spinal cord and peripheral nerves, marked by increased difficulty in walking, a feeling of vibration in the legs, and a loss of sense of position. Also known as **subacute combined degeneration of the spinal cord.** See also **pernicious anemia, vitamin B_{12}.**

combining form, a component of a word, often derived from Latin or Greek. It may be a root, a prefix, or a suffix, or all three. For example, in the words *arthralgia, encephalitis, hepatomegaly,* and *oliguria,* the combining forms are *arthr-, -algia, en-, -cephal-, -itis, hepato-, -megaly, olig-,* and *-uria.*

comedo /kom′idō/, *pl.* **comedones** /komidō′nēz/, blackhead, the basic lesion of acne vulgaris, caused by an accumulation of keratin and sebum within the opening of a hair follicle. It is dark because of the effect of oxygen on sebum, not because of the presence of dirt. Compare **milium.**

comedocarcinoma /kom′idōkär′sinō′mə/, *pl.* **comedocarcinomas, comedocarcinomata,** a malignant intraductal neoplasm of the breast, in which the central cells degenerate and may be easily expressed from the cut surface of the tumor. As the growth is confined in the mammary ducts, the prognosis is better than in cases of invasive breast lesions.

COMDU, abbreviation for **cardiac monitor and diagnostic unit.**

comfort, alteration in: pain, a nursing diagnosis accepted by the Fourth National Conference on the Classification of Nursing Diagnoses. The origin of the condition includes injury by biologic, chemical, physical, or psychologic agents. The defining characteristic is the verbal or nonverbal communication by the client of the presence of pain, including behavior that is self-protective; a narrowed focus that is indicated by an altered time perception, withdrawal from social contact, or impaired thought processes; distraction behavior, marked by moaning, crying, pacing, restlessness, or the seeking out of other people or activities; a facial mask of pain, recognized by eyes that appear dull and lusterless, a ''beaten'' look, fixed or scattered facial movements or grimace; alteration in muscle tone, ranging from listlessness to rigidity; and autonomic responses to increasing pain, including diaphoresis, changes in blood pressure and pulse rate, pupillary dilatation, and an increased or decreased rate of respiration. See also **nursing diagnosis.**

comfort measure, any action taken to promote comfort of the patient, as a back rub, a change in position, or the prewarming of a stethoscope or a bedpan.

Comité International des Poids et Mesures (CIPM) /kômitā′ aNternäsyōnäl′ dā pô•ä′ ā mesYr′/, a group of scientists that meet periodically to define the international (SI) units of physical quantities, as the volume of a liter, the length of a meter, or the precise amount of time in a minute. See also **SI units.**

-comma, a combining form meaning a 'piece of a structure': *inocomma, myocomma, osteocomma.*

command, an order given to the computer to execute a specific instruction, as a code that evokes a particular program or performs a particular function.

command automatism, a condition characterized by an abnormal mechanical responsiveness to commands, usually followed without critical judgment, as may be seen in hypnosis and certain psychotic states.

command hallucination, a psychotic condition in which the patient hears and obeys voices that command him to perform certain acts. The hallucinations may influence the individual to engage in behavior that is dangerous to himself or to others.

commensal /kəmen′səl/, (of two different organisms) living together in an arrangement that is not harmful to either and may be beneficial to both. Some bacteria in the digestive tract of humans aid in the processing of food and produce B vitamins needed for normal health while causing no harm. Compare **parasite, synergist.**

comminuted fracture, a fracture in which there are several breaks in the bone, creating numerous fragments.

commissurotomy /kom′ishŏŏrot′əmē/, the surgical division of a fibrous band or ring connecting corresponding parts of a body structure. A commissurotomy is commonly performed to separate the thickened, adherent leaves of a stenosed mitral valve.

commitment, 1. the placement or confinement of an individual in a specialized hospital or other institutional facility. See also **institutionalize. 2.** the legal procedure of admitting a mentally ill person to an institution for psychiatric treatment. The process varies from state to state but usually involves judicial or court action based on medical evidence certifying that the person is mentally ill. See also **certification. 3.** a pledge or contract to fulfill some obligation or agreement, used especially in some forms of psychotherapy or marriage counseling.

common bile duct, the duct formed by the juncture of the cystic duct and hepatic duct.

common carotid artery, one of the major arteries supplying blood to the head and neck. The left common carotid is a branch of the brachiocephalic trunk. Each divides into an external common carotid and an internal common carotid. Branches of the external carotid supply the face, scalp, and most of the neck and throat tissues. The internal common carotids supply the brain and other tissues generally accessible from within the skull, as the eyes.

common carotid plexus, a network of nerves on the common carotid artery, supplying sympathetic fibers to the head and the neck, with branches that accompany the cranial blood vessels. The common carotid plexus is formed by the internal and external carotid plexuses and by the cervical ganglia of the sympathetic system. Compare **external carotid plexus, internal carotid plexus.**

common cold. See **cold.**

common hepatic artery, the visceral branch of the celiac trunk of the abdominal aorta, passing to the pyloris and dividing into five branches, the gastroduodenal, right gastric, right hepatic, left hepatic, and middle hepatic.

common iliac artery, a division of the abdominal aorta, starting to the left of the fourth lumbar vertebra, passing caudally about 5 cm, and dividing into external and internal iliac arteries. The right common iliac artery is somewhat longer than the left.

common iliac node, a node in one of the seven groups of parietal lymph nodes serving the abdomen and the pelvis. The nodes are arranged in clusters of about five nodes lying along the dorsal aspect of the common iliac artery. They drain the internal and the external iliac nodes and pass their efferents to the lateral aortic nodes. Compare **external iliac node, internal iliac node, iliac circumflex node.** See also **lymph, lymphatic system, lymph node.**

common iliac vein, one of the two veins that are the sources of the inferior vena cava, formed by the union of the internal and the external iliac veins, ventral to the sacroiliac articulation. The right common iliac vein runs almost vertically, ascends dorsal and lateral to its corresponding artery, and is shorter than the left common iliac vein. The left common iliac vein ascends more obliquely, at first to the medial side of the corresponding artery and then dorsal to the right common iliac vein. Each common iliac vein receives the iliolumbar and, in some individuals, the lateral sacral veins. The left common iliac vein also receives the middle sacral vein. Neither of the common iliacs contains valves. Compare **external iliac vein, internal iliac vein.**

communicable, contagious; transmissible by direct or indirect means, as a communicable disease.

communicable disease, any disease transmitted from one person or animal to another directly, by contact with excreta or other discharges from the body; or indirectly, via substances or inanimate objects, as contaminated drinking glasses, toys, or water; or via vectors, as flies, mosquitoes, ticks, or other insects. To control a communicable disease, it is important to identify the organism, prevent its spread to the environment, protect others against contamination, and treat the infected person. Many communicable diseases, by law, must be reported to the local health department. Kinds of communicable diseases include those caused by bacteria, chlamydia, fungi, parasites, rickettsiae, and viruses. Also called **contagious disease.** See also **infectious disease.**

Communicable Disease Center, former name of the **Centers for Disease Control.**

communicating hydrocephalus. See **hydrocephalus.**

communication, any process in which a message containing information is transferred, especially from one person to another, via any of a number of media. Communication may be verbal or nonverbal; it may occur directly, as in a face-to-face conversation or with the observation of a gesture; or it may occur remotely, spanning space and time, as in writing and reading or in making or playing back a recording. Communication is basic to all nursing and contributes to the development of all therapeutic relationships. See also **kinesics.**

communication channels, (in communication theory) any gesture, action, sound, written word, or visual image used in transmitting messages.

communication, impaired verbal, a nursing diagnosis accepted by the Fourth National Conference on the Classification of Nursing Diagnoses. The origin of the condition includes decreased circulation to the brain; a physical barrier to speech, as a brain tumor, laryngectomy, tracheostomy, or intubation; an anatomic deficit, as a cleft palate; a psychologic barrier, as a psychosis or lack of stimuli; a cultural difference; or a developmental or age-related factor. The defining characteristics of the condition include slurring, stuttering, difficulty in forming words or sentences, difficulty in expressing thoughts verbally, inappropriate verbalization, dyspnea, and disorientation. The critical defining characteristics, one of which must be present for the diagnosis to be made, are an inability to speak the dominant language of the culture, a difficulty in speaking or verbalizing, or the absence of speech. See also **nursing diagnosis.**

communication theme, (in psychiatry) a recurrent concept or idea that ties together components of communication. Kinds of communication themes include **content theme,** in which a single concept links varied topics of discussion; **mood theme,** in which the underlying idea is the emotion communicated by the individual; and **interaction theme,** in which a particular idea best describes the dynamics between communicating participants.

communication theory, a theory that describes a model of a system of communication consisting of a source of information (the sender), a transmitter, a communication channel, a source of noise (interference), a receiver, and a purpose for the message.

community health nursing, a field of nursing that is a blend of primary health care and nursing practice with public health nursing. The community health nurse conducts a continuing and comprehensive practice that is preventive, curative, and rehabilitative. The philosophy of care is based on the belief that care directed to the individual, the family, and the group contributes to the health care of the population as a whole. The community health nurse is not restricted to the care of a particular age or diagnostic group. Participation of all consumers of health care is encouraged in the development of community activities that contribute to the promotion, education, and maintenance of good health. These activities require comprehensive health programs that pay special attention to social and ecologic influences and specific populations at risk.

community medicine, a branch of medicine that is concerned with the health of the members of a community, municipality, or region. The emphasis in community medicine is on the early diagnosis of disease, the recognition of environmental and occupational hazards to good health, and the prevention of disease in the community.

community mental health center (CMHC), a community-based center that provides comprehensive mental health services, including ambulatory and inpatient care. The specific services to be provided are defined in an act of Congress, the Community Mental Health Centers Act; these requirements have been updated periodically. The costs of consultation and educational services, instruction, development, and initial operation of the facility are provided by the federal government. The organization, management, and operation of CMHCs are specified by the Act. Consumer representation in each of these areas is required.

community nurse practitioner (CNP), a nurse who has completed a postbaccalaureate program in community nursing.

community psychiatry, the branch of psychiatry concerned with the development of an adequate and coordinated program of mental health care for residents of specified catchment areas. See also **community mental health center.**

companionship, (in psychiatric nursing) the assignment of a staff member or of another patient to stay with a disturbed patient to provide support and to protect the patient from self-harm or the harming of others. In constant companionship, the disturbed patient is accompanied in all activities until the companion is convinced the patient has regained control.

comparative anatomy, the study of the morphology and function of all living animals. A comparison of the forms indicates a progression on a scale from the simplest to the most highly specialized animals. The adult stage of animals that are lower in the scale resembles the immature stages of many animals that are higher in the scale. See also **applied anatomy, ontogeny, phylogeny.**

comparative embryology, the study of the similarities and differences among various organisms during the embryologic period of development.

comparative method, the analytic method to which the test method is compared in the comparison-of-methods experiment. This term makes no inference about the quality of the comparative method.

comparative physiology, the study of the similarities and differences of the vital processes found in various species of living organisms to determine fundamental physiologic relationships between members of the animal and plant kingdoms.

comparative psychology, **1.** the study of human behavior as it relates to or differs from animal behavior. **2.** the study of the psychologic and behavioral differences among various peoples.

compartment syndrome, a pathologic condition caused by the progressive development of arterial compression and reduced blood supply. It can result in a permanent contracture deformity of the hand or foot, with or without a fracture. See also **Volkmann's contracture.**

compatibility, **1.** the quality or state of existing together in harmony; congruity. **2.** the orderly, efficient integration of the elements of one system with those of another. **3.** the formation of a stable chemical or biochemical system, specifically in medication, so that two or more drugs can be administered at the same time without producing undesired side effects or without canceling or changing the therapeutic effects of the others. **4.** (in immunology) the degree to which the body's defense system will tolerate the presence of foreign material, as transfused blood, grafted tissue, or transplanted organs, without an immune reaction. Usually, complete compatibility exists between identical twins. **5.** (in blood grouping or crossmatching) the lack of reaction between blood groups so that there is no agglutination when the red blood cells of one sample are mixed with the serum of another sample; no reaction from transfused blood. – **compatible,** *adj.*

Compazine, a trademark for a phenothiazine (prochlorperazine), used as an antiemetic and antipsychotic.

compendium /kəmpen'dē·əm/, *pl.* **compendia,** a collected body of information on the standards of strength, purity, and quality of drugs. The official compendia in the United States are the *United States Pharmacopoeia,* the *Homeopathic Pharmacopoeia of the United States,* the *National Formulary,* and their supplements. See also **formulary.**

compensated gluteal gait, one of the more common abnormal gaits associated with a weakness of the gluteus medius. It is a variation of the Trendelenburg gait and involves the dropping of the pelvis on the unaffected side of the body during the walking cycle between the moment of heelstrike on the affected side and the moment of heelstrike on the unaffected side. The compensated gluteal gait is also characterized by the dropping of the entire trunk downward and sideways over the affected hip and a short step on the unaffected side. In a compensated gait, the trunk is forcibly thrown laterally during the weight-bearing or stance phase in the movement of the affected lower limb. This lateral movement is the result of an attempt to shift a significant portion of body weight above and outside the center of rotation of the affected hip. During this movement, the erector spinae and the quadratus lumborum of the involved side function to lift the whole weight of the pelvis and the opposite lower extremity off the ground to allow the uninvolved leg to clear during its swing phase. Also called **gluteal gait.**

compensated heart failure, an abnormal cardiac condition in which heart failure is compensated for by such mechanisms as increased sympathetic adrenergic stimulation of the heart, fluid retention with increased venous return, increased end-diastolic ventricular volume and fiber length, and hypertrophy. Compensation may be aided by the administration of digitalis glycosides, with associated improved myocardial function, or by diuresis. However, diuretics may relieve only the symptoms of pulmonary and peripheral congestion, whereas the ventricular function remains severely abnormal. See also **heart failure.**

compensating current, an electric current that neutralizes the intensity of a muscle current.

compensating curve, the curvature of alignment of the occlusal surfaces of the teeth, developed to compensate for the paths of the condyles as the mandible moves from centric to eccentric positions. It is used to maintain posterior tooth contacts on the molar teeth and to provide balancing contacts on dentures associated with a protruding mandible. The compensating curve corresponds to the curve of Spee of natural teeth. See also **alignment.**

compensation, **1.** the process of counterbalancing any defect in bodily structure or function. **2.** (in cardiology) the process of maintaining an adequate blood flow through such normal cardiac and circulatory mechanisms as tachycardia, fluid retention with increased venous return, and hypertrophy. Failure of the heart to compensate and to provide the required cardiac output indicates a diseased heart muscle. See also **compensated heart failure.** **3.** (in psychiatry) a complex defense mechanism that allows one to avoid the unpleasant or painful emotional stimuli that result from a feeling of inferiority or inadequacy. This is accomplished by any of several patterns of behavior, for example, one in which an extraordinary effort is spent in overcoming a handicap, one in which the quality lacking is scorned (''sour grapes''), one in which hard work and excellent performance in one field are substituted for a lack of ability in another, or one in which a fantasy of excellence, achievement, or perfection replaces awareness of a weakness or failure. A kind of compensation is **dosage compensation.** See also **overcompensation.**

compensation neurosis, an unconscious process by which one prolongs the symptoms resulting from an injury or disease in order to receive secondary gains, especially money. Compare **malingering.**

compensator, a device used in radiotherapy to correct for irregularities in body surfaces by providing a differential attenuation of the beam before it reaches the patient. The result is a more uniform distribution of radiation dose in the tumor. Compensators are generally mounted on the collimator system of a teletherapy unit.

compensatory hypertrophy, an increase in the size or the function of an organ or part to counterbalance a structural or functional defect. See also **compensated heart failure.**

competence, **1.** (in embryology) the total capacity of an embryonic cell to react to determinative stimuli in various ways of differentiation. **2.** the ability of bacteria to take up donor DNA molecules.

competitive antagonist. See **antimetabolite.**

competitive-binding assay, an analytic procedure based on the reversible binding of a ligand to a binding protein. In proportion to its concentration, the ligand competes with a labeled derivative for binding to the limited number of available binding sites.

competitive identification, the unconscious modeling of one's personality on that of another as a means of outdoing or bettering the other person. See also **identification.**

competitive inhibitor, an inhibitor of an enzyme reaction that competes with the substrate by binding at the active site.

compiler, a computer program that converts high-level language into machine code in order to convert a symbolic text representation of a program into a set of numbers that the computer can interpret.

complaint, **1.** (in law) a pleading by a plaintiff made under oath to initiate a suit. It is a statement of the formal charge and the cause for action against the defendant. For a minor offense, the defendant is tried on the basis of the complaint. A more serious felony prosecution requires an indictment with evidence presented by a state's attorney. **2.** *informal.* any ailment, problem, or symptom identified by the client, patient, member of the person's family, or other knowledgeable person. The chief complaint is often the reason that the person has sought health care.

complement, one of 11 complex, enzymatic serum proteins. In an antigen-antibody reaction, complement causes lysis. Complement is also involved in other physiologic reactions, including anaphylaxis and phagocytosis. See also **antibody, antigen, antigen-antibody reaction, immune gamma globulin.**

complement abnormality, an unusual condition characterized by deficiencies or by dysfunctions of any of the nine functional components of the enzymatic proteins of blood serum. The components are labeled C1 through C9. Intensive research currently seeks to determine the relationship between complement abnormalities or deficiencies and numerous disorders. Theoretically, any of the nine complement components may be lacking. The most common abnormalities are C2 and C3 deficiencies and C5 familial dysfunction. Patients with complement deficiencies or with complement dysfunctions may be more susceptible to infections and to collagen vascular diseases. Some patients with lupus erythematosus or dermatomyositis have displayed complement abnormalities. Studies indicate that primary complement deficiencies may be inherited. Secondary complementary deficiencies may stem from immunologic reactions, as drug-induced serum disease, which depletes complement. Complement deficiencies may be associated with other illnesses, as acute streptococcal glomerulonephritis and acute systemic lupus erythematosus.

■ OBSERVATIONS: Increased susceptibility to systemic bacterial infection is associated with C2 and C3 deficiencies and with C5 familial dysfunction. Chronic renal failure and lupus erythematosus may also be associated with C2 deficiency. Signs of C5 dysfunction are malaise, diarrhea, and seborrheic dermatitis. It is difficult and often expensive to diagnose complement abnormalities, but some indications are ECG conduction abnormalities, detection of complement and immunoglobulin in the walls of blood vessels in glomerulonephritis, cerebrospinal fluid pleocytosis, increased erythrocyte sedimentation rate, and the presence in urine of RBCs, RBC casts, and protein.

■ INTERVENTION: Replacement of complement-fixing antibodies and the control of infection and associated illnesses are part of the standard treatment of complement abnormalities. The patient with complement deficiency or dysfunction commonly receives transfusions of fresh plasma to replace antibodies. Bone marrow transplants and injections of gamma globulin may also be employed, but bone marrow transplant carries the risk of a fatal graft-versus-host reaction. Complement abnormalities may usually be temporarily corrected by replacement therapy, but no permanent cure is yet available.

■ NURSING CONSIDERATIONS: Authorities recommend careful monitoring of patients with complement abnormalities, especially patients who receive gamma globulin injections. The gamma globulin is injected into a large muscle mass and massaged well after each injection.

More than one site is usually selected if the dosage is more than 1.5 ml. If frequent doses are ordered, the injection sites are rotated. With plasma infusions, careful matching of leukocytes for HLA cell types is important to prevent graft-versus-host reaction and other undesirable responses. Bone marrow transplants require close monitoring for transfusion reactions and are usually followed by instructions to the patient for scrupulous hygiene, prompt treatment of the smallest wound, and avoidance of crowds or persons with active infections. Renal infections require meticulous monitoring of intake and output, tests for serum electrolytes and acid-base balance, and observation for symptoms of renal failure. Neurologic damage resulting from infection is cause for special alertness to detect early signs of ataxia or slight changes in mental activity.

complemental inheritance, the acquisition or expression of a trait or condition from the presence of two independent pairs of nonallelic genes. Both of the genes must be present for the characteristic to appear in the phenotype.

complementary feeding, a supplemental feeding given an infant that is still hungry after breast feeding.

complementary gene, either member of two or more nonallelic gene pairs that interact to produce an effect not expressed in the absence of any of the pairs. Also called **reciprocal gene.**

complement cascade, a biochemical process involving the C1 to C9 complement components in which one complement interacts with another in a specific sequence called a complement pathway. The reaction sequence is C1, 4, 2, 3, 5, 6, 7, 8, 9 (the first complements being out of numerical sequence for historical reasons). The cascade effect leads to an accumulation of fluid in a cell and finally lysis of the membrane, causing the cell to rupture.

complement fixation, an immunologic reaction in which an antigen combines with an antibody and its complement, causing the complement factor to become inactive or "fixed." The complement-fixation reaction can be tested in the laboratory by exposing the patient's serum to antigen, complement, and specially sensitized red blood cells. Complement-fixation tests are widely used to detect antibodies for infectious diseases, especially syphilis and viral illnesses. See also **complement, immune system, immunity, Wassermann test.**

complement-fixation test (C-F test), any serologic test in which complement fixation is detected, indicating the presence of a particular antigen. Specific C-F tests are used to aid in the diagnosis of amebiasis, Rocky Mountain spotted fever, trypanosomiasis, and typhus. The Wassermann test is a C-F test for syphilis.

complete abortion, termination of pregnancy in which the conceptus is expelled or removed in its entirety. Because no products of conception remain in the uterus, surgical evacuation is not necessary. Compare **incomplete abortion.**

complete blood count (CBC), a determination of the number of red and white blood cells per cubic millimeter of blood. A complete blood count is one of the most routinely performed tests in a clinical laboratory and one of the most valuable screening and diagnostic techniques. The count can be performed manually by staining a smear of blood on a slide and counting the different types of cells under a microscope. Most laboratories use an electronic counter for reporting numbers of red and white blood cells. Platelets are more difficult to count automatically, and many laboratories continue to do this manually. Examining a stained slide of blood yields useful information about red-cell morphology. Each type of white cell can be represented as a percentage of the total number of white cells observed. This is called a differential count. Many electronic blood counters also automatically determine hemoglobin or hematocrit and include this value in the complete blood count. See also **differential white blood cell count, erythrocyte, hematocrit, hemoglobin, leukocyte.**

complete breech, a fetal presentation in which the nates present with the legs folded on the thighs and the thighs on the abdomen. The position of the fetus is the same as in a normal vertex presentation but upside down. Compare **frank breech.** See also **breech birth.**

complete fistula, an abnormal passage from an internal organ or structure to the surface of the body or to another internal organ or structure.

complete fracture, a bone break that completely disrupts the continuity of osseous tissue across the entire width of the bone involved.

complete health history, a health history that includes a history of the present illness, a health history, social history, occupational history, sexual history, and a family health history. See also **health history.**

complete rachischisis, a rare congenital fissure of the entire vertebral column and spinal cord, resulting from the failure of the embryonic neural tube to close. The condition is characterized by flaccid paralysis and impaired sensations. It is often accompanied by other birth defects, as cleft palate, harelip, and hydrocephalus, and is frequently fatal. Also called **rachischisis totalis, holorachischisis.** See also **spina bifida.**

complete response (CR), the total disappearance of a tumor.

complex, **1.** a group of items, as chemical molecules, that are related in structure or function as are the iron and protein portions of hemoglobin or the cobalt and protein portions of vitamin B_{12}. **2.** a combination of signs and symptoms of disease that forms a syndrome. **3.** (in psychology) a group of associated ideas with strong emotional overtones affecting a person's attitudes.

complex cavity, a cavity that involves more than one surface of a tooth. Compare **gingival cavity.**

complex fracture, a closed fracture in which the soft tissue surrounding the bone is severely damaged.

complex odontoma. See **composite odontoma.**

complex protein, a protein that contains a simple protein and at least one molecule of another substance, as a glycoprotein, nucleoprotein, or hemoglobin.

complex sugars, sugar molecules that can be hydrolyzed or digested to yield two molecules of the same or different simple sugars, as sucrose, lactose, and maltose. Also called **disaccharides.**

compliance, fulfillment by the patient of the care-giver's prescribed course of treatment.

component, a significant part of a larger unit.

component drip set, a device used for delivering intravenous fluids, especially whole blood. It includes plastic tubing and a combination drip-chamber and filter. Compare **component syringe set, microaggregate recipient set, straight-line blood set, Y-set.**

component syringe set, a device used for delivering intravenous fluids. It includes plastic tubing, two slide clamps, a Y-connector, and a syringe. The component syringe set may be used in various procedures, as in the transfusion of platelets and in the transfusion of cryoprecipitates. In such transfusions the component syringe set is used primarily to avoid clogging the intravenous line. Compare **component drip set, microaggregate recipient set, straight-line blood set, Y-set.**

component therapy, a kind of transfusion in which specific blood components are administered instead of whole blood. Packed red cells or platelet-rich plasma suspensions may be transfused in larger quantities than would be possible if whole blood were used. More sophisticated processing provides fibrinogen or antihemophilic globulin solutions for administration in therapeutic amounts in excess of what might be given with conventional blood transfusion therapy. Compare **plasmaphoresis.** See also **packed cells, pooled plasma.**

composite core, a buildup of composite resin, designed and installed to retain an artificial tooth crown. See also **core.** Compare **amalgam core, cast core.**

composite odontoma, an odontogenic tumor composed of abnormally arranged calcified enamel and dentin. Also called **complex odontoma.**

compound, **1.** (in chemistry) a substance composed of two or more different elements, chemically combined in definite proportions, that cannot be separated by physical means. **2.** any substance composed of two or more different ingredients. **3.** to make a substance by combining ingredients, as a pharmaceutic. **4.** denoting an injury characterized by multiple factors, as a compound fracture.

compound aneurysm, a localized dilatation of an arterial wall in which some of the layers are distended and others are ruptured or dissected. Also called **mixed aneurysm.**

compound fracture, a fracture in which the broken end or ends of the bone have torn through the skin. Also called **open fracture.**

compound melanocytoma. See **benign juvenile melanoma.**

compound monster, a fetus in which some of the parts or organs are duplicated but not fully developed.

compound tubuloalveolar gland, one of the many multicellular glands with more than one secretory duct that contains both tube-shaped and sac-shaped portions, as the salivary glands.

comprehensive care. See **holistic health care.**

Comprehensive Health Manpower Act of 1971, legislation passed by the U.S. Congress providing educational funding for nurse-practitioner (NP) and physician-assistant (PA) programs. See also **Nurse Training Act of 1971.**

Comprehensive Health Planning (CHP) and Public Health Services Amendments, legislation passed by the U.S. Congress in 1966 that emphasized regional planning and established for the first time the concept that each person has a "right to health care."

compress, a soft pad, usually made of cloth, used to apply heat, cold, or medications to the surface of a body area. A compress also may be applied over a wound to help control bleeding. Compare **dressing.**

compression, the act of pressing, squeezing, or otherwise applying pressure to an organ, tissue, or body area. An intracranial tumor or hemorrhage may cause compression of brain tissue. Kinds of pathologic compression include **compression fracture,** in which bone surfaces are forced against each other, causing a break, and **compression paralysis,** marked by paralysis of a body area caused by pressure on a nerve.

compression fracture, a bone break, especially in a short bone, that disrupts osseous tissue and collapses the affected bone. The bodies of vertebrae are often sites of compression fractures.

compression neuropathy, any of several disorders involving damage to sensory nerve roots or peripheral nerves, caused by mechanic pressure or localized trauma and characterized by paresthesia, weakness, or paralysis. The carpal, peroneal, radial, and ulnar nerves are most commonly involved. Compare **neuritis.** See also **paresthesia, pressure palsy.**

compressor naris, the transverse part of the nasalis muscle that serves to depress the cartilage of the nose and to draw the ala toward the septum. Compare **dilatator naris.**

compromised host, a person who is less-than-normally able to resist infection, because of immunosuppressive therapy, immunologic defect, severe anemia, or concurrent disease or condition, including metastatic malignancy, cachexia, or severe malnutrition.

Compton scatter, the principal interaction process of photons with tissue in the diagnostic and therapeutic radiology energy range. In this process, the incoming photon transfers energy to an electron in the material and is deflected with reduced energy into a path that generally leads to additional interactions.

compulsion, an irresistible, repetitive, irrational impulse to perform an act that is usually contrary to one's ordinary judgments or standards yet results in overt anxiety if it is not completed. The impulse is usually the result of an obsession. A kind of compulsion is **repetition compulsion.** Compare **phobia.** See also **obsession.** –**compulsive,** *adj.*

compulsive idea, a recurring, irrational idea that persists in the mind, usually resulting in an irresistible urge to perform some inappropriate act. Also called **imperative idea.**

compulsive personality, a type of character structure in which there is a pattern of chronic and obsessive adherence to rigid standards of conduct. The person is usually excessively conscientious and inhibited, is extremely inflexible, has an extraordinary capacity for work, and lacks a normal ability to relax and to relate to other people. The compulsive person is likely to follow repetitive patterns of behavior, as snapping the fingers, crossing the legs, tapping the foot, or refusing to walk on cracks in the sidewalk, and often leads an impoverished emotional life, being dominated by a need for order, cleanliness, punctuality, rules, and systems. See also **compulsive personality disorder, obsessive-compulsive neurosis.**

compulsive personality disorder, a condition in which an irrational preoccupation with order, rules, ritual, and detail interferes with everyday functioning and normal behavior. The disorder is characterized by an excessive devotion to work, a pathologic adherence to a definite set of rules or system of behavior, and a persistent, compulsive following of specific rituals. The person cannot make decisions when faced with unexpected situations and cannot take pleasure in the normal activities of daily life. Psychotherapy is the usual treatment and may include behavior therapy with desensitization and flooding in order to reduce maladaptive anxiety. See also **compulsive personality, obsessive-compulsive neurosis.**

compulsive polydipsia, a neurotic, compelling urge to drink excessive amounts of liquid. The condition is psychogenic; it is not caused by any organic dysfunction or physical deprivation. Extreme cases can result in death from water intoxication and electrolyte imbalance. See also **polydipsia.**

compulsive ritual, a series of acts a person feels must be carried out even though he recognizes the behavior to be useless and inappropriate. Failure to complete the acts results in extreme tension or anxiety. See also **obsessive-compulsive neurosis.**

computer, an electronic device for processing and storing large amounts of information very quickly. See also **analog computer, digital computer, main-frame computer, microcomputer, minicomputer.**

computer-assisted instruction (CAI), a teaching process employing a computer in the presentation of instructional materials, often in such a way as to require the student to interact with it. Also called **computer-assisted learning (CAL).**

computerized axial tomography (CAT), (in radiology) a technique in which an EMI scanner, comprising an x-ray tube, two scintillation detectors, a line printer, a teletyper, and a computer-and-magnetic disk unit, is used to attain a series of detailed visualizations of the tissues, especially of brain, at any depth desired. The procedure is painless, noninvasive, and requires no special preparation. The head is scanned in two planes simultaneously at various angles. The computer calculates tissue absorption, displays a printout of the numeric values, and produces a visualization of the tissues that demonstrates the densities of the various intracranial structures. Tumor masses, infarctions, bone displacement, and accumulations of fluid may be detected. Also called **computerized transverse axial tomography.** See also **computerized tomography.**

computerized tomography (CT), a tomographic method that employs a narrowly collimated beam of x-rays to image the body in cross-sectional slices. (*Tomos* comes from the Greek word for slice.) An array of detectors, positioned at several angles, records those x-rays that pass through the body. The term, computerized tomography, may also apply to forms of tomography using positrons or ultrasound for imaging instead of x-rays, and it is sometimes used interchangeably with **computerized axial tomography.**

computer-managed instruction (CMI), a system in which a computer is employed to direct an entire instructional process, including CAI, as well as traditional forms of instruction that do not use the computer.

con-. See **co-.**

CONA, abbreviation for **Canadian Orthopedic Nurses' Association.**

conation, the mental process characterized by desire, impulse, volition, and striving. Compare **cognition.** –**conative,** *adj.*

concanavalin A, a hemagglutinin, isolated from the meal of the jack bean, that reacts with polyglucosans in the blood of mammals causing agglutination. It has been used in immunology to stimulate T cell production.

concealed accessory pathway, (in cardiology) an extramuscular tract between the atria and ventricles that conducts only in a retrograde direction. It often results in evidence of the Wolff-Parkinson-White syndrome.

concealed bigeminy, (in cardiology) a bigeminal cardiac arrhythmia that may not be revealed on an electrocardiogram except through the appearance of odd numbers of P waves between manifest extrasystoles. See also **bigeminy.**

concealed junctional extrasystole, a junctional impulse that arises in and discharges the atrioventricular junction but fails to reach either atria or ventricles.

concentrate, **1.** to decrease the bulk of a liquid and increase its strength per unit of volume by the removal of inactive ingredients through evaporation or other means. **2.** a substance, particularly a liquid, that has been strengthened and reduced in volume through such means.

concentration gradient, a gradient that exists across a membrane separating a high concentration of a particular ion from a low concentration of the same ion.

concentric, describing two or more circles that have a common center.

concentric fibroma, a fibrous tumor surrounding the uterine cavity.

concept, a construct or abstract idea or thought that originates and is held within the mind. **–conceptual,** *adj.*

conception, **1.** the beginning of pregnancy, usually taken to be the instant that a spermatozoon enters an ovum and forms a viable zygote. **2.** the act or process of fertilization. **3.** the act or process of creating an idea or notion. **4.** the idea or notion created; a general impression resulting from the interpretation of a symbol or set of symbols.

conceptional age, in fetal development, the number of weeks since conception. Because the exact time of conception is difficult to determine, conceptional age is assumed to be 2 weeks less than gestational age.

conception control. See **contraception.**

conceptive, **1.** able to become pregnant. **2.** pertaining to or characteristic of the mental process of forming ideas or impressions.

conceptual framework, a group of concepts that are broadly defined and systematically organized to provide a focus, a rationale, and a tool for the integration and interpretation of information. Usually expressed abstractly using word models, a conceptual framework is the basis for many theories, as communication theory and general systems theory.

conceptus, the product of conception; the fertilized ovum and its enclosing membranes at all stages of intrauterine development, from the time of implantation to birth. See also **embryo, fetus.**

concomitant, designating one or more of two or more things, occurring simultaneously, that may or may not be interrelated or produced as a result of the others; accompanying.

concordance, (in genetics) the expression of one or more specific traits in both members of a pair of twins. Compare **discordance.** **–concordant,** *adj.*

concrete thinking, a stage in the development of the cognitive thought processes in the child. During this phase, thought becomes increasingly logical and coherent so that the child is able to classify, sort, order, and organize facts while still being incapable of generalizing or dealing in abstractions. Problem solving is accomplished in a concrete, systematic fashion based on what is perceived, keeping to the literal meaning of words, as the word "horse" applying to a particular animal and not to horses in general. In Piaget's classification, this stage occurs between 7 and 11 years of age, is preceded by syncretic thinking, and is followed by abstract thinking.

concretion. See **calculus.**

concurrent disinfection, the daily handling and disposal of contaminated material or equipment.

concurrent nursing audit. See **nursing audit.**

concurrent sterilization, a method of preparing an infant-feeding formula in which all ingredients and equipment are sterilized before mixing the formula.

concurrent validity, validity of a test or a measurement tool that is established by concurrently applying a previously validated tool or test to the same phenomena, or data base, and comparing the results. Concurrent validity is achieved if the results are the same or similar at a statistically significant level. See also **validity.**

concussion, **1.** a violent jarring or shaking, as caused by a blow or an explosion. **2.** *informal.* **brain concussion.**

condensed milk, a thick liquid prepared by the evaporation of half of the water content of cow's milk and the addition of sugar. The final product contains 40% to 50% sugar and is used to prepare desserts and confectionery.

condenser, (in dentistry) an instrument for compacting restorative material into a prepared tooth cavity. It has a working end, or nib, with a flat or serrated face.

condition, **1.** a state of being, specifically in reference to physical and mental health or well-being. **2.** anything that is essential for or that restricts or modifies the appearance or occurrence of something else. **3.** to train the body or mind, usually through specific exercises and repeated exposure to a particular state or thing. **4.** (in psychology) to subject a person or animal to conditioning or associative learning so that a specific stimulus will always elicit a particular response. See also **classical conditioning.**

conditioned avoidance response, a learned reaction that is performed either consciously or unconsciously to avoid an unpleasant or painful stimulus or to prevent such stimuli from occurring.

conditioned escape response, a learned reaction that is performed either consciously or unconsciously to stop or to escape from an aversive stimulus.

conditioned reflex, a reflex developed gradually by training in association with a specific, repeated external stimulus. An example of a conditioned reflex is Pavlov's experiment in which a dog salivates at the ringing of a bell if over a period of time every feeding is preceded by the bell-ringing stimulus.

conditioned response, an automatic reaction to a stimulus that does not normally elicit such response but which has been learned through training. Such responses can be physical or psychologic and are produced by repeated association of some physiologic function or behavioral pattern with an unrelated stimulus or event. In Pavlov's classic experiments, dogs learned to associate the ringing of a bell with feeding time so that they would salivate at the sound of the bell regardless of whether or not food was given to them. Also called **acquired reflex, behavior reflex, conditioned reflex, trained reflex.** Compare **unconditioned response.** See also **classical conditioning.**

conditioning, a form of learning based on the development of a response or set of responses to a stimulus or series of stimuli. Kinds of conditioning are **classical conditioning, instrumental conditioning,** and **operant conditioning.**

condom, a soft, flexible sheath that covers the penis and prevents semen from entering the vagina in sexual intercourse, used to avoid the transmittal of an infection and to prevent conception. Condoms are made of plastic, rubber, or skin. Also called **prophylactic,** *(informal)* **rubber.**

conduction, **1.** (in physics) a process in which heat is transferred from one substance to another because of a difference in temperature; a process in which energy is transmitted through a conductor. **2.** (in physiology) the process by which a nerve impulse is transmitted.

conduction anesthesia, a loss of sensation, especially pain, in a region of the body, produced by injecting a local anesthetic along the course of a nerve or nerves to inhibit the conduction of impulses to and from the area supplied by that nerve or nerves. Also called **block anesthesia, nerve block anesthesia.**

conduction aphasia, a dissociative speech phenomenon in which there is no difficulty in comprehending words seen or heard and in which there is no dysarthria, yet the patient has problems in self-expression. The patient may substitute words similar in sound or meaning for the correct ones but is unable to repeat from dictation, to spell, and to read aloud. The patient is alert and aware of the deficit. A common cause is an embolus in a branch of the middle cerebral artery. The nurse should try to reduce tension and frustration in the patient, encourage socialization, find the best means of communication for the patient, use simple language and direct questions requiring simple answers, and help the family to understand the problem and deal with it. See also **aphasia.**

conductive hearing loss, a form of hearing loss in which sound is inadequately conducted through the external or middle ear to the sensorineural apparatus of the inner ear. Sensitivity to sound is diminished, but clarity (interpretation of the sound) is not changed. If volume is increased to compensate for the loss, hearing is normal. Compare **sensorineural hearing loss.**

condylar fracture /kon′dilər/, any fracture of the round end of a hinge joint, usually occurring at the distal end of the humerus or at the distal end of the femur, frequently detaching a small bone fragment that includes the condyle.

condylar guide, a mechanic device on a dental articulator, designed to guide articular movement similar to that produced by the paths of the condyles in the temporomandibular joints. Compare **anterior guide, incisal guide.** See also **condylar guide inclination.**

condyle /kon′dīl/, a rounded projection at the end of a bone that anchors muscle ligaments and articulates with adjacent bones.

-condyle, -condylus, a combining form meaning a 'knucklelike projection on a bone': *entepicondyle, epicondyle, entocondyle.*

condyloid joint, a synovial joint in which a condyle is received into an elliptic cavity, as the wrist joint. A condyloid joint permits no axial rotation but allows flexion, extension, adduction, abduction, and circumduction. Also called **articulatio ellipsoidea.** Compare **ball-and-socket joint, pivot joint, saddle joint.**

condyloma /kon′dilō′mə/, *pl.* **condylomata,** a wartlike growth on the anus, vulva, or glans penis.

condyloma acuminatum, *pl.* **condylomata acuminata,** a soft, wartlike or papillomatous growth common on warm and moist skin and the mucous membrane of the genitalia. It is caused by a virus and is transmitted by sexual contact. Also called **acuminate wart, venereal wart.**

condyloma latum, *pl.* **condylomata lata,** a flat, moist, papular growth that appears in secondary syphilis in the coronal sulcus of the perineum or on the glans penis.

-condylus. See **-condyle.**

cone, **1.** a photoreceptor cell in the retina of the eye that enables a person to visualize colors. There are three kinds of retinal cones, one for each of the colors, blue, green, and red; other colors are seen by stimulation of more than one type of cone. **2.** a cone-shaped device attached to radiologic equipment to focus x-rays on a small target of tissue. See also **cone biopsy.** **–conic, conical,** *adj.*

cone biopsy, surgical removal of a cone-shaped segment of the cervix, including both epithelial and endocervical tissue. General anesthesia is used. The cone of tissue is excised and examined microscopically to establish a precise diagnosis, usually to confirm or evaluate a positive Papanicolaou test. Postoperatively, hemorrhage sometimes occurs. If bleeding occurs 7 to 10 days later, suturing is required. See also **biopsy, cone.**

cone of light, **1.** a triangular reflection observed during an ear examination when the light of an otoscope is focused on the image of the malleus. **2.** the group of light rays entering the pupil of the eye and forming an image on the retina.

confabulation, the fabrication of experiences or situations, often recounted in a detailed and plausible way to fill in and cover up gaps in the memory. The phenomenon occurs principally as a defense mechanism and is most commonly seen in alcoholics, especially those who have Korsakoff's psychosis, and persons with head injuries or lead poisoning. Also called **fabrication.**

configuration, the hardware, software, and peripherals assembled to work as a computer unit in a specific situation.

configurationism. See **Gestalt psychology.**

confinement, **1.** a state of being held or restrained within a specific place in order to hinder or minimize activity. **2.** the final phase of pregnancy during which labor and childbirth occur; parturition. See also **puerperium.**

conflict, **1.** a mental struggle, either conscious or unconscious, resulting from the simultaneous presence of opposing or incompatible thoughts, ideas, goals, or emotional forces, such as impulses, desires, or drives. **2.** a painful state of consciousness caused by the arousal of such opposing forces and the inability to resolve them; a kind of stress found to a certain degree in every person. **3.** (in psychoanalysis) the unconscious emotional struggle between the demands of the id and those of the ego and superego or between the demands of the ego and the restrictions imposed by society. Kinds of conflict include **approach-approach conflict, approach-avoidance conflict, avoidance-avoidance conflict, extrapsychic conflict,** and **intrapsychic conflict.**

confluence of the sinuses, the wide junction of the superior sagittal, the straight, and the occipital sinuses with the two large transverse sinuses of the dura mater. The right tranverse sinus usually receives most of the blood from the superior sagittal sinus, and the left transverse sinus receives the blood from the straight sinus. The confluence is one of six posterior superior sinuses of the dura matter, draining blood from the section and an inner bulging granular section.

confusion, a mental state characterized by disorientation regarding time, place, or person, causing bewilderment, perplexity, lack of orderly thought, and inability to choose or act decisively. It is usually symptomatic of an organic mental disorder, but it may accompany severe emotional stress and various psychologic disorders. –**confusional,** *adj.*

confusional insanity. See **amentia.**

congener /kon′jənər/, one of two or more things that are similar or closely related in structure, function, or origin. Examples of congeners are muscles that function identically, chemical compounds similar in composition and effect, or species from the same genus of plants or animals. –**congenerous** /kənjen′ərəs/, *adj.*

congenital, present at birth, as a congenital anomaly or defect.

congenital absence of sacrum and lumbar vertebrae, an abnormal condition present at birth and characterized by varying degrees of deformity, ranging from the absence of the lower segment of the coccyx to the absence of the entire sacrum and all lumbar vertebrae. Congenital absence of the sacrum and the lumbar vertebrae is relatively rare. Lesser degrees of this anomaly may present so few signs that marked deformities are not present, and the condition may not be diagnosed unless accidentally found on radiographic examination. More severe forms display gross deformities and neurologic deficits. Signs and symptoms of the more severe kinds include short stature, flattened buttocks, muscle paralysis to varying degrees, muscle atrophy in the lower extremities, foot deformities, contractures of the hips and the knees, and varying degrees of loss of sensation, especially sensation distal to the knees. The treatment varies greatly for the congenital absence of the sacrum and the lumbar vertebrae and depends on severity. Surgical intervention may be reconstructive or may involve disarticulation procedures at various spinal levels and subsequent fusion of the remaining vertebrae. Depending on the severity, many patients with this anomaly may be surgically provided with enough stability to sit and to walk with assistance. The most severe forms are usually fatal.

congenital adrenal hyperplasia. See **adrenogenital syndrome.**

congenital amputation, the absence of a fetal limb or part at birth, previously attributed to amputation by constricting bands in utero but now regarded as a developmental defect. See also **amputee.**

congenital anomaly, any abnormality present at birth, particularly a structural one, which may be inherited genetically, acquired during gestation, or inflicted during parturition. Also called **birth defect.**

congenital cardiac anomaly, any structural or functional abnormality or defect of the heart or great vessels existing from birth. Congenital heart disease is a major cause of neonatal distress and is the most common cause of death in the newborn other than problems related to prematurity. The incidence of congenital cardiovascular anomalies is 8 to 10 per 1000 live births, with the mortality rate greatest in the neonatal period. Approximately 90% of all deaths from congenital heart disease occur during the first year of life. Congenital heart defects may result from genetic causes, primarily single-gene mutations and chromosomal aberrations, or from environmental factors, as maternal infection or exposure to radiation or noxious substances during pregnancy. Most defects are probably caused by some interaction between genetic and environmental factors that results in arrested embryonic development. Congenital heart anomalies are classified broadly according to the resulting alteration in circulation as acyanotic, in which no unoxygenated blood mixes in the circulatory system, or cyanotic, in which unoxygenated blood enters the system. The general effects of cardiac malformations on cardiovascular functioning are increased cardiac workload, involving either systolic or diastolic overloading, increased pulmonary vascular resistance, inadequate systemic cardiac output, and decreased oxygen saturation from the shunting of unoxygenated blood directly into the circulatory system. The general physical symptoms of these pathophysiologic alterations are growth retardation, decreased exercise tolerance, recurrent respiratory infections, dyspnea, tachypnea, tachycardia, cyanosis, tissue hypoxia, and murmurs, all of which vary in severity depending on the type and degree of the defect. Kinds of congenital cardiac anomalies include **atrial septal defect, coarctation of the aorta, tetralogy of Fallot, transposition of the great vessels, tricuspid atresia,** and **ventricular septal defect.** See also **aortic stenosis, patent ductus arteriosus, pulmonic stenosis, valvular stenosis.**

congenital cloaca. See **persistent cloaca.**

congenital condition. See **congenital anomaly.**

congenital dermal sinus, a channel present at birth, extending from the surface of the body and passing between the bodies of two adjacent lumbar vertebrae to the spinal canal.

congenital dislocation of the hip, a congenital orthopedic defect in which the head of the femur does not articulate with the acetabulum, because of an abnormal shallowness of the acetabulum. Treatment consists of maintaining continuous abduction of the thigh so that the head of the femur presses into the center of the shallow cavity causing it to deepen. Also called **congenital dysplasia of the hip, congenital subluxation of the hip.** See also **Frejka splint.**

congenital facial diplegia. See **Möbius' syndrome.**

congenital glaucoma, a rare form of glaucoma affecting infants and young children, resulting from a congenital closure of the iridocorneal angle by a membrane that obstructs the flow of aqueous humor and increases the intraorbital pressure. The condition is progressive, usually bilateral, and may damage the optic nerve. It may be corrected surgically. Also called **buphthalmos, hydrophthalmos.**

congenital goiter, an enlargement of the thyroid gland at birth. It may be caused by a deficiency of enzymes required for the production of thyroxine.

congenital heart disease. See **congenital cardiac anomaly.**

congenital hypoplastic anemia. See **Diamond-Blackfan syndrome.**

congenital megacolon. See **Hirschsprung's disease.**

congenital nonspherocytic hemolytic anemia, a large group of blood disorders made up of a number of

Typical murmurs associated with common congenital heart anomalies

Sounds heard	*Characteristics and location*	*May indicate*
Pansystolic murmur	Maximum in the 4th, 5th, and 6th intercostal spaces at left sternal border; high, harsh murmur heard throughout systole; may be associated with palpable thrill	Ventricular septal defect (blood passes from left to right ventricle)
	Heard in the apical area	Endocardial cushion defect
Split S_2 on expiration Systolic ejection murmur	Split is heard in 2nd, 3rd, or 4th intercostal space; murmur maximum in 2nd and 3rd left intercostal spaces	Atrial septal defect (oxygenated and unoxygenated blood mix)
Loud aortic closure sound Systolic murmur	Aortic sound heard at 2nd left intercostal space; murmur heard if ventricular septal defect is present	Transposition of the great arteries

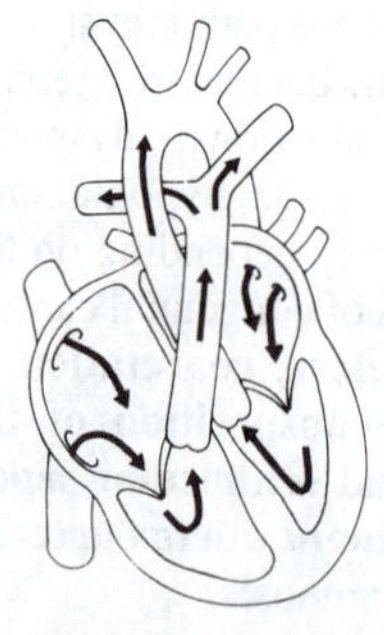
NORMAL HEART

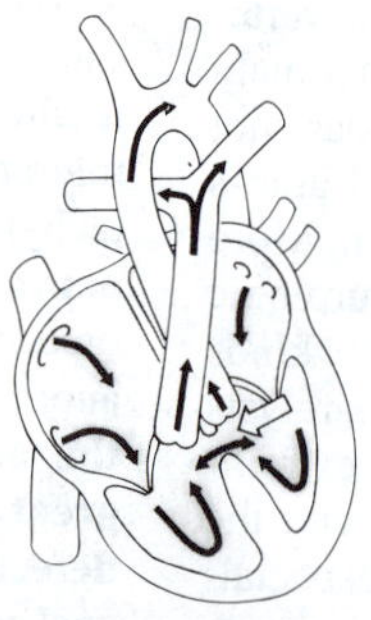
VENTRICULAR SEPTAL DEFECT

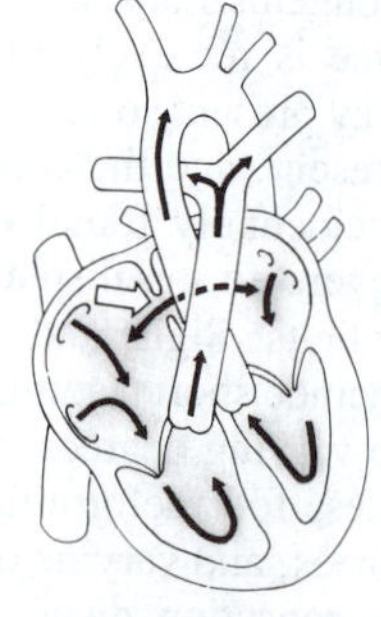
ATRIAL SEPTAL DEFECT

Adapted from Shor, V.Z.: Congenital cardiac defects assessment and case finding, Am. J. Nurs. **78**:259, Feb. 1978.
The preceding murmurs and abnormal heart sounds are generally, but not always, associated with the indentified congenital defects. In the presence of multiple defects, various combinations of these sounds may be heard.

similar inherited diseases, each with a deficiency of one of the enzymes of red-cell glycolysis. Most are associated with varying degrees of hemolysis, but all are less severe than and are to be differentiated from the more serious disorder associated with spherocytosis. Compare **hemolytic anemia, spherocytic anemia.** See also **elliptocytosis, heme, sickle cell anemia.**

congenital oculofacial paralysis. See **Möbius' syndrome.**

congenital polycystic disease. See **polycystic kidney disease.**

congenital pulmonary arteriovenous fistula, a direct connection between the arterial and venous systems of the lung present at birth that results in a right-to-left shunt and permits unoxygenated blood to enter systemic circulation. The anomaly is probably caused by faulty development of the network of vessels covering the embryonic lungs and is often accompanied by hereditary hemorrhagic telangiectasis (Rendu-Osler-Weber disease). The fistula may be single or multiple and may occur in any part of the lung; if it is in an accessible site, surgical correction is the method of treatment.

congenital scoliosis, an abnormal condition present at birth, characterized by a lateral curvature of the spine, resulting from specific congenital rib and vertebral anomalies. The etiologic and the pathologic characteristics of congenital scoliosis are divided into six categories. Category I is associated with partial unilateral failure of the

Sounds heard	*Characteristics and location*	*May indicate*
Single S_2 Systolic murmur	Murmur maximal in 2nd and 3rd intercostal spaces at left sternal border	Tetralogy of Fallot (*1,* narrowing of pulmonary artery or valve; *2,* ventricular septal defect; *3,* overriding aorta; *4,* hypertrophied right ventricle)
Continuous murmur	Maximum in 2nd left intercostal space; envelops S_2 with late systolic accentuation; terminates in late or middiastole; radiates to 1st intercostal space and beneath left clavicle	Patent ducus arteriosus (blood tends to bypass lungs)
Systolic ejection click	Loudest to left of sternum; sometimes heard at apex	Aortic stenosis
	Loudest during expiration; heard at base of the heart	Pulmonary stenosis
	Heard at both base and apex of the heart; associated with systolic or continuous murmur between scapulae	Coarctation of the aorta (aortic lumen is narrowed)

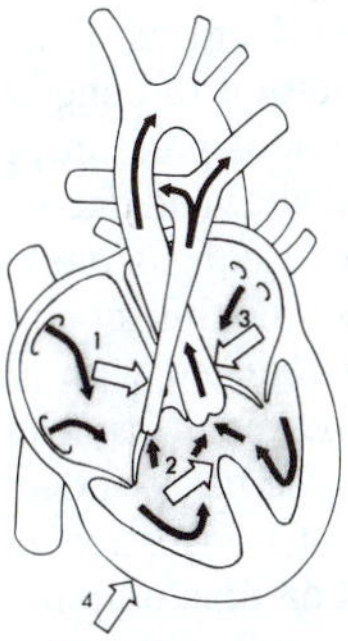

TETRALOGY OF FALLOT

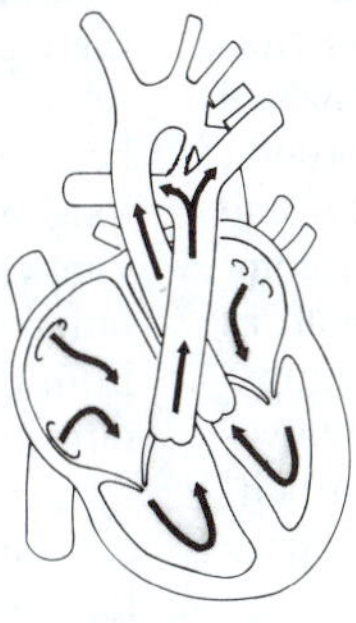

PATENT DUCUS ARTERIOSUS

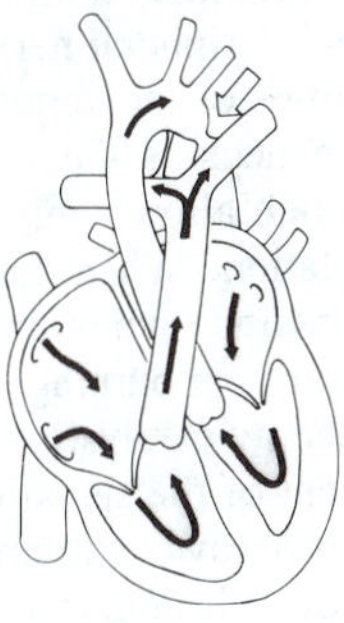

COARCTATION OF THE AORTA

formation of a vertebra. Category II is associated with complete unilateral failure of the formation of a vertebra. Category III is associated with bilateral failure of segmentation with the absence of disk space. Category IV is associated with the unilateral failure of segmentation with the unsegmented bar. Category V is associated with the fusion of ribs. Category VI is associated with any condition not covered in the other categories. Category IV scoliosis seems to progress more rapidly and cause the greatest degree of deformity. The degree of obvious deformity caused by congenital scoliosis depends on the cause of the disease. The deformity increases with growth and age, usually progressing slowly during periods of slow growth of the trunk of the body. Diagnosis of the specific congenital anomaly may be confirmed by radiographic examination. The specific rate of progression of many congenital curvatures cannot be predicted. There may be little correlation between the rate of progression and the severity of the curvature at the time of diagnosis. Treatment of congenital scoliosis may be surgical or nonsurgical. Some kinds of nonsurgical treatment techniques are exercise programs and the use of orthotic devices, as scoliosis splints, a Milwaukee brace, a Risser localizer, or a turnbuckle cast. Surgical intervention in this disease may involve an anterior or a posterior spinal fusion. In a few individuals with this disease, additional surgical procedures, as spinal osteotomy or halo traction, may be required. See also **scoliosis.**

congenital short neck syndrome, a rare congenital malformation of the cervical spine in which the cervical vertebrae are fused, usually in pairs, into one mass of bone, resulting in decreased neck motion and decreased cervical length, sometimes with neurologic involvement. The posterior portion of the laminar arches in the cervical area is not fully developed, resulting in spina bifida in the cervical region, usually involving the lower cervical vertebrae and, in some cases, one or more of the upper thoracic vertebrae. Congenital short neck syndrome is often associated with a cervical rib or with hemivertebrae. Neurologic complications, as nerve-root compression and peripheral nerve symptoms, are secondary to deformities of the vertebral bodies. The extreme shortness of the neck is the most common sign of this deformity, which allows only limited motion, lateral bending, and rotation. When the deformity involves nerve-root compression, symptoms of peripheral nerve involvement, as pain or a burning sensation, may be evident, accompanied by paralysis, hyperesthesia, or paresthesia. Involvement of the spinal cord may present signs of abnormalities of lower extremities with associated signs of an upper motor lesion. Congenital short neck syndrome may require no treatment. Mild associated symptoms may be alleviated with traction, cast application, or cervical collars. Surgery may be required to relieve neurologic manifestations. Also called **Klippel-Feil syndrome** /klipel′fel′, klip′əlfīl′/.

congenital subluxation of the hip. See **congenital dislocation of the hip.**

congestion, abnormal accumulation of fluid in an organ or body area. The fluid is often blood, but it may be bile or mucus.

congestive atelectasis, severe pulmonary congestion characterized by diffuse injury to alveolar-capillary membranes, resulting in hemorrhagic edema, stiffness of the lungs, difficult ventilation, and respiratory failure. Fulminating sepsis, especially when gram-negative organisms are involved, is the most common cause, but congestive atelectasis may occur after trauma, near drowning, aspiration of gastric acid, paraquat ingestion, inhalation of corrosive chemicals, as chlorine, ammonia, or phosgene, or the use of certain drugs, including barbiturates, chlordiazepoxide, heroin, methadone, propoxyphene, and salicylates. This serious pulmonary disorder may also be caused by diabetic ketoacidosis, fungal infections, high altitudes, pancreatitis, tuberculosis, and uremia. Management of congestive atelectasis consists of treatment of the underlying cause, frequent changes of the patient's position to promote drainage, careful dehydration, assistance with ventilation, and the use of bronchodilators and steroids. Also called **adult respiratory distress syndrome, hemorrhagic lung, pump lung, stiff lung, wet lung.**

congestive heart failure (CHF), an abnormal condition characterized by circulatory congestion caused by cardiac disorders, especially myocardial infarction of the ventricles. This condition usually develops chronically in association with the retention of sodium and water by the kidneys. Humoral agents that significantly affect such retention include renin, angiotensin, aldosterone, vasopressin, estrogen, and norepinephrine. Acute congestive heart failure may develop after myocardial infarction of the left ventricle and cause a significant shift of blood from the systemic to the pulmonary circulation before the typical retention of sodium and water occurs. Pulmonary congestion in this situation may be caused by mechanic obstruction at the left mitral valve or by ventricular failure, impairing the ventilatory function of the lungs. Ischemia may also affect the respiratory muscles, producing chest pains difficult to distinguish from the pains of myocardial infarction. Common symptoms of congestive heart failure include dyspnea, high venous pressure, prolonged circulation time, peripheral edema, and decreased vital capacity. Confirming diagnosis of congestive heart failure often depends on distinguishing this condition from the congested systemic state associated with rapid infusions, severe anemia, and chronic renal insufficiency. Such distinction is often made on the basis of cardiac catheterization, which, in the case of congestive heart failure, reveals an insufficient rise in cardiac output during exercise and a significant rise in cardiac output after the administration of digitalis. Treatment of this condition includes prolonged rest and the administration of oxygen, digitalis, and diuretics. The nurse keeps the patient in as quiet a room as possible and endeavors to reduce the patient's fear and anxiety, which can exacerbate the condition. Signs of the results of prolonged bed rest, as mental depression, thrombophlebitis, hypostatic pneumonia, renal caluli, and pulmonary embolism, should be watched for. After the patient becomes ambulatory, the nurse observes for distended neck veins, edema, dyspnea, and weight gain. When the patient leaves the hospital, the nurse also advises the patient and family on care and exercise programs. See also **heart failure.**

Congolese red fever. See **murine typhus.**

-conia, a combining form meaning 'small particles in the (specified) fluid or part of the body': *chondroconia, otoconia, statoconia.*

conic papilla. See **papilla.**

conjoined manipulation, the use of both hands in obstetric and gynecologic procedures, with one positioned in the vagina and the other on the abdomen.

conjoined tendon. See **inguinal falx.**

conjoined twins, two fetuses developed from the same ovum who are physically united at birth. The defect ranges from a superficial anatomic union of varying extent between equally or nearly equally formed fetuses to one in which only a part of the body is duplicated or in which a small, incompletely developed fetus, or parasite, is attached to a more fully formed one, the autosite. Conjoined twins result when separation of the blastomeres in early embryonic development does not occur until a late cleavage phase and is incomplete, causing the fused condition. Viability depends on the extent of the fusion and the degree of development of the fetuses. See also **Siamese twins.**

conjugated estrogen, a mixture of sodium salts of estrogen sulfates, chiefly those of estrone, equilin, and 17-alpha-dihydroequilin, blended to approximate the average composition of estrogenic substances in the urine of pregnant mares. Conjugated estrogens may be prescribed to relieve postmenopausal vasomotor symptoms, as hot flushes, for the treatment of atrophic vaginitis, female hypogonadism, primary ovarian failure, and palliation in advanced prostatic carcinoma and metastatic breast cancer in selected patients. The drug, in conjunction with other therapeutic measures, may also retard the progress of postmenopausal osteoporosis. Continued use of estrogens increases the risk of endometrial carcinoma, gallbladder disease, and thromboembolic disorders; because of the danger of damage to the fetus, all female sex hormones are contraindicated during pregnancy. Among the adverse effects of conjugated estrogens are breakthrough bleeding, breast tenderness, nausea, headache, water retention, and acneiform skin eruptions.

conjugated protein, a compound that contains a protein molecule united to a nonprotein substance.

conjugation, (in genetics) a form of sexual reproduction in unicellular organisms in which the gametes temporarily fuse so that genetic material can transfer from the donor male to the recipient female, where it is incorporated, recombined, and then passed on to the progeny through replication.

conjugon /kon′jo͞ogon/, an episome that induces bacterial conjugation.

conjunctiva /kon′jungktī′və/, the mucous membrane lining the inner surfaces of the eyelids and anterior part of the sclera. The **palpebral conjunctiva** lines the inner surface of the eyelids and is thick, opaque, and highly vascular. The **bulbar conjunctiva** is loosely connected, thin, and transparent, covering the sclera of the anterior third of the eye.

conjunctival edema. See **chemosis.**

conjunctival fornix. See **inferior conjunctival fornix, superior conjunctival fornix.**

conjunctival reflex, a protective mechanism for the eye in which the eyelids close whenever the conjunctiva is touched. Compare **corneal reflex.**

conjunctival test, a procedure used to identify offending allergens by instilling the eye with a dilute solution of the allergenic extract. A positive reaction in the allergic patient causes tearing and redness of the conjunctiva within 5 to 15 minutes. See also **allergy testing.**

conjunctivitis /kənjungk′tivī′tis/, inflammation of the conjunctiva, caused by bacterial or viral infection, allergy, or environmental factors. Red eyes, a thick discharge, sticky eyelids in the morning, and inflammation without pain are characteristic. The cause may be found by microscopic examination or bacteriologic culture of a specimen of the discharge. Choice of treatment depends on the causative agent and may include antibacterial agents, antibiotics, or corticosteroids. Also called **pinkeye.** See also **choroiditis, uveitis.**

connecting fibrocartilage, a disk of fibrocartilage found between many joints, especially those with limited mobility, as the spinal vertebrae. Each disk is composed of concentric rings of fibrous tissue separated by cartilaginous laminae. The disk swells outward if it is compressed by the vertebrae above or below. Compare **circumferential fibrocartilage, interarticular fibrocartilage, stratiform fibrocartilage.**

connective tissue, tissue that supports and binds other body tissue and parts. It derives from the mesoderm of the embryo and is dense, containing large numbers of cells and large amounts of intercellular material. The intercellular material is composed of fibers in a matrix or ground substance that may be liquid, gelatinous, or solid, as in bone and cartilage. Connective tissue fibers may be collagenous or elastic. The matrix or ground material surrounding fibers and cells is not composed of living material, as protoplasm, but is nonetheless a dynamic substance, varying with the general condition of the body, susceptible to its own special diseases, and transporting materials for metabolism, nutrition, and waste elimination. The most common cell in connective tissue is the histiocyte or microphage. Mast cells, plasma cells, and white blood cells are also found in connective tissue throughout different parts of the body. Red blood cells are not usually found in connective tissue unless blood vessels have been injured. Kinds of connective tissue are **bone, cartilage,** and **fibrous connective tissue.**

connective tissue disease. See **collagen vascular disease.**

Conn's syndrome. See **primary aldosteronism.**
Conor's disease. See **Marseilles fever.**
Conradi's disease. See **chondrodystrophia calcificans congenita.**
consanguinity, a hereditary or "blood" relationship between persons, by having a common parent or ancestor.
conscience, **1.** the moral, self-critical sense of what is right and wrong. **2.** (in psychoanalysis) the superego.
conscious, **1.** (in neurology) capable of responding to sensory stimuli; awake, alert; aware of one's external environment. **2.** (in psychiatry) that part of the psyche or mental functioning in which thoughts, ideas, emotions, and other mental content are in complete awareness. Compare **preconscious, unconscious.**
conscious sedation. See **awake anesthesia.**
consecutive angiitis, an inflammatory condition of blood or lymph vessels resulting from a similar process in surrounding tissues.
consensual light reflex, a normally present crossed reflex in which light directed at one eye causes the opposite pupil to contract. See also **light reflex.**
consensual reaction to light, the constriction of the pupil of one eye when the other eye is illuminated. Stimulation of either optic nerve causes constriction of both pupils. In monocular blindness the pupil of the blind eye reacts consensually with stimulation of the seeing eye but does not cause constriction of the pupil of either eye. Compare **direct reaction to light.** See also **light reflex.**
consensus sequence, (in molecular genetics) a sequence in a strand of RNA nucleotides that is used as a site for the insertion of a splice of an RNA sequence from another source into the segment.
conservation of energy, (in physics) a law stating that in any closed system the total amount of energy is constant.
conservation of matter, (in physics) a law stating that matter can neither be created nor destroyed and that the amount of matter in the universe is finite. Also called **conservation of mass.** See also **conservation of energy.**
conservation principles of nursing, a conceptual framework for nursing that is directed toward maintaining the wholeness or integrity of the patient when the normal ability to cope is disturbed or exceeded by stress. Nursing intervention is determined by the patient's need to conserve energy and to maintain structural, personal, and social integrity. The patient is perceived as a person whose wholeness is threatened by stress. Subjective and objective indicators of stress are assessed by the nurse, the stimuli for the stress are identified, and the level of integrity in each area is evaluated. The nurse acts as a "conservationist."
conservative treatment. See **treatment.**
consolidation, **1.** the combining of separate parts into a single whole. **2.** a state of solidification. **3.** (in medicine) the process of becoming solid, as when the lungs become firm and inelastic in pneumonia.
constipation, difficulty in passing stools or an incomplete or infrequent passage of hard stools. There are many causes, both organic and functional. Among the organic causes are intestinal obstruction, diverticulitis, and tumors. Functional impairment of the colon may occur in elderly or bedridden patients who fail to respond to the urge to defecate. For constipation that is not organically caused, the nurse can encourage a liberal diet of fruits, vegetables, and plenty of water. The patient should be encouraged to exercise moderately, if possible, and to develop regular, unhurried bowel habits. See also **atonia constipation.** **–constipated,** *adj.*
constitutional psychology, the study of the relationship of individual psychologic makeup to body morphology and organic functioning.
constitutional symptom. See **symptom.**
constriction ring, a band of contracted uterine muscle that forms a stricture around part of the fetus during labor, usually after premature rupture of the membranes and sometimes impeding labor. The uterine wall is thickened in the zone of the ring and is not prone to rupture. Compare **pathologic retraction ring.**
constructional apraxia, a form of apraxia characterized by the inability to copy drawings or to manipulate objects to form patterns or designs.
constructive aggression, an act of self-assertiveness in response to a threatening action for purposes of self-protection and preservation. See also **aggression.**
construct validity, validity of a test or a measurement tool that is established by demonstrating its ability to identify the variables that it proposes to identify. See also **validity.**
consumption, an obsolete term for tuberculosis.
contact, **1.** the touching or bringing together of two surfaces, as those of upper and lower teeth. The term is often used attributively, as in contact dermatitis and contact lens. **2.** the bringing together either directly or indirectly, as through the handling of food or clothing, of two individuals so as to allow the transmission of an infectious organism from one to the other. **3.** a person who has been exposed to an infectious disease.
contact dermatitis, skin rash resulting from exposure to a primary irritant or to a sensitizing antigen. In the first, or nonallergic, type, a primary irritant, as an alkaline detergent or an acid, causes a lesion similar to a thermal burn. Emergency treatment is to drench liberally and immediately with water. In the second, or allergic, type, sensitizing antigens, on first exposure, result in an immunologic change in certain lymphocytes. Subsequent exposure to the antigen causes the lymphocytes to release irritating chemicals leading to inflammation, edema, and vesiculation. Poison ivy and nickel dermatitis are common examples of this delayed hypersensitivity reaction. The diagnosis can be aided by patch testing with suspected antigens. Treatment includes avoidance of the irritant or sensitizer, topical corticosteroid preparations, and

soothing or drying lotions. In severe cases, systemic corticosteroids may be used. Also called **dermatitis venenata.** Compare **atopic dermatitis.** See also **delayed hypersensitivity.**

contact factor. See **factor XII.**

contact lens, a small, curved, glass or plastic lens shaped to fit the person's eye and to correct refraction. Contact lenses float on the precorneal tear film and must be inserted, removed, cleaned, and stored as directed to avoid damage or infection to the eyes.

contagious, communicable, as a disease that may be transmitted by direct or indirect contact. **–contagion,** *n.*

contagious disease. See **communicable disease.**

content validity, validity of a test or a measurement as a result of the use of previously tested items or concepts within the tool. See also **validity.**

context, (in communications theory) the setting, meaning, and language of a message. If a message is interpreted without strict regard for these limits, it will be taken out of context.

continent ileostomy, an ileostomy that drains into a surgically created pouch or reservoir in the abdomen. Involuntary discharge of intestinal contents is prevented by a nipple valve created from the ileum.

■ METHOD: After surgery, the pouch is kept relatively empty by means of a catheter placed in it at surgery. It is removed a week or two afterward, depending on the status of intestinal function and wound healing. Once the indwelling catheter is removed, the pouch is drained by periodically inserting a catheter through the stoma into the pouch through the valve. The length of time allowed to elapse between catheterizations is gradually lengthened as the capacity of the pouch increases to between 500 and 1000 ml. Six months after surgery, drainage may be necessary only 3 or 4 times a day. The patient learns to recognize a feeling of fullness that indicates the need for drainage. When the patient is seated on the toilet, the dressing over the stoma is removed, and the tip of a French size 28 to 32 catheter is lubricated and inserted into the stoma. The distal end of the catheter is in a receptacle or in the toilet, at least 30 cm below the stoma. The lubricated tip of the catheter is advanced carefully through the stoma. Resistance is usually felt at a depth of about 5 cm where the valve covers the opening to the pouch. Flow usually begins when the tip of the catheter has passed the valve, at a distance of approximately 7.5 cm from the stoma. Drainage may take up to 15 minutes to complete.

■ NURSING ORDERS: After surgery, the patient is usually instructed to add foods one at a time. High-fiber foods and those that cause gas formation are particularily likely to be problematic. Thick secretions may be thinned by the injection of a little water into the pouch through the catheter. The stoma may be covered with a 3-inch square cut from a disposable diaper. It is important to teach the patient to avoid irritation of the skin around the stoma. Nonallergenic tape may be used to hold the pad in place. After healing, if there is no danger of a blow to the abdomen, a pad is often not necessary. After surgery, activity is resumed as the patient is able. There is no reason for activity to be curtailed once healing is complete and the person feels well.

■ OUTCOME CRITERIA: The patient may expect to be able to care for the stoma and to manage the drainage of the pouch before discharge from the hospital. A continent ileostomy has several advantages, including the avoidance of unpleasant odors, and the convenience of not having to use a colostomy or ileostomy bag.

contingency contracting, a formal agreement between a psychotherapist and a patient undergoing behavior therapy regarding the consequences of certain actions by both parties.

contingency management, any of a group of techniques used in behavior therapy that attempts to modify a behavioral response by controlling the consequences of that response. Kinds of contingency management include **contingency contracting, shaping,** and **token economy.**

continuing education, (in nursing) formal, organized, educational programs designed to promote the knowledge, skills, and professional attitudes of nurses. The programs are usually short-term and specific; a certificate may be offered for completion of a course, and a number of continuing education units (C.E.U.s) may be conferred. Continuing education is required for relicensure in many states. It is not to be confused with academic, degree-granting programs, as advanced education or postgraduate education.

continuing education unit (C.E.U.), a point awarded to a professional person by a professional organization for having attended an educational program relevant to the goals of the organization. A value is established for the course and that number of points is given. Many states require professionals in the various fields of medicine and nursing to obtain a specific number of C.E.U.s annually for relicensure.

continuous anesthesia, a method for maintaining regional nerve block in anesthesia for surgical operations or labor in which an anesthetic solution drips either at intervals or at a low rate of flow. Barbiturates or other central nervous system depressant drugs are used. The procedure is named according to the area infiltrated: continuous spinal, caudal, epidural, peridural, or lumbar. Also called **fractional anesthesia.**

continuous bath. See **continuous tub bath.**

continuous fever, a fever that persists steadily for a prolonged period of time. Compare **intermittent fever.**

continuous positive airway pressure (CPAP), (in respiratory therapy) ventilation assisted by a flow of air delivered at a constant pressure throughout the respiratory cycle. It is performed for patients who can initiate their own respirations but who are not able to maintain adequate arterial oxygen levels without assistance. CPAP may be given through a ventilator and endotracheal tube, through a nasal cannula, or into a hood over the patient's head. Respiratory distress syndrome in the newborn is often treated with CPAP. Also called **continuous positive pressure breathing.** Compare **positive end expiratory pressure.**

continuous positive pressure ventilation (CPPV), positive end-expiratory pressure applied to the airway during mechanic ventilation. See **continuous positive airway pressure.**

continuous tremor, fine, rhythmic, purposeless movements that persist during rest but sometimes disappear briefly during voluntary movements. The pill-rolling movements and trembling seen in Parkinson's disease are typical continuous tremors. Compare **intention tremor.** See also **tremor.**

continuous tub bath, a therapeutic bath, usually prescribed in the treatment of some dermatologic conditions, in which the patient lies supported in a medicated solution of tepid water.

■ METHOD: The bath is prepared as for a medicated tub bath. The patient is immersed in the water, and a towel saturated with the solution is placed over the torso. The patient may wear a loin cloth, and a harness is fitted comfortably around the chest and under the shoulders and head to hold the head safely out of the water as the patient sleeps or dozes. A pillow or folded towel is placed over the wide supporting straps under the head and neck to add to the patient's comfort. A board is placed on top of the tub from the patient's shoulders to the end of the tub, and a sheet is draped over it. A bell for calling for assistance, a container of drinking water with a flexible straw, and any other materials that may be needed are placed on the board.

■ NURSING ORDERS: The method and the reason for the treatment are explained to the patient. Privacy is maintained; close supervision by a nurse is available throughout the treatment. The procedure is psychologically trying and may be physically unpleasant for the patient. Psychosocial support and attention to making the patient as comfortable as possible improves the patient's tolerance for the procedure.

■ OUTCOME CRITERIA: The patient is observed for any febrile reaction, rapid or weak pulse, faintness, or increased severity of symptoms, as itching, burning, or pain. The solution is changed completely every 4 hours, the linen is changed twice a day, and the harness is changed once a day.

continuum /kəntin′yo͞o·əm/, *pl.* **continua,** **1.** a continuous series or whole. **2.** (in mathematics) a system of real numbers.

contra-, a combining form meaning 'against': *contraception, contralateral, contraparetic.*

contra bevel, **1.** also called **reverse bevel.** (in dentistry) the angle between a cutting blade and the base of the periodontal pocket when the blade is held so that it separates the sulcular epithelium from the external epithelium of the gingiva. **2.** (in dentistry) an external bevel of a tooth preparation extending onto a buccal or lingual cusp from an intracoronal restoration.

contraception, a process or technique for the prevention of pregnancy by means of a medication, device, or method that blocks or alters one or more of the processes of reproduction in such a way that sexual union can occur without impregnation. Kinds of contraception include **cervical cap, condom, contraceptive diaphragm, intrauterine device, natural family-planning method, oral contraceptive, spermatocide,** and **sterilization.** Also called **birth control, conception control, family planning.** See also **planned parenthood.**

contraceptive diaphragm, a contraceptive device consisting of a hemisphere of thin rubber bonded to a flexible ring, inserted in the vagina together with spermaticidal jelly or cream. Fitted between the pubic symphysis and the posterior fornix of the vagina, the diaphragm cups the cervix in a pool of spermatocide so that spermatozoa cannot enter the uterus, thus preventing conception. The rate of failure of the diaphragm method of contraception is approximately 5 to 10 unplanned pregnancies in 100 women using the method properly for 1 year. The principal advantages of the diaphragm are that it has no systemic effects and that it needs to be used only during coitus. The most often reported disadvantages are that it is messy, that it is uncomfortable for some people, and that insertion may interfere with spontaneity or continuity in making love. Diaphragms are manufactured in seven standard sizes from 60 mm to 90 mm in diameter. Kinds of diaphragms are **arcing spring, coil spring,** and **flat spring.** Also called **diaphragm.**

contraceptive diaphragm fitting, a procedure, performed in an office or clinic, in which a contraceptive diaphragm is selected according to the clinical assessment of certain anatomic factors specific to the woman being fitted, including the size of the vagina, the position of the uterus, the depth of the arch behind the symphysis pubis, and the degree of support afforded by the muscles surrounding the vagina. See also **arcing-spring contraceptive diaphragm, coil-spring contraceptive diaphragm, flat-spring contraceptive diaphragm.**

■ METHOD: A vaginal and pelvic examination is performed to determine the appropriate kind of diaphragm and to estimate the size of the vagina. Fitting rings, which are available in various sizes and styles, or sets of actual diaphragms may be used for the fitting. With experience the clinician becomes able to choose a size with which to begin the fitting that is close to the best size for the woman being fitted. The ring or the rim of the diaphragm is lubricated, the rim is drawn together, and the diaphragm is inserted (domeside down) and directed upward toward the sacrum. As it enters the vagina, the posterior aspect of the rim is directed into the posterior fornix of the vagina, behind the cervix; the anterior rim is placed in the arch above and behind the symphysis. A digital examination is done to check that the cervix is covered; through the rubber dome it feels like a nose or a great toe with a dimple or depression in its center. When, by trial and error, the correct size has been determined, the woman is instructed in the technique of inserting it herself and checking its placement. A model may be used before she tries self-insertion. She is shown how to apply the correct amount of contraceptive cream or jelly in the dome and around the rim and how to place her hands on the diaphragm for easiest insertion. The device is inserted while squatting or standing with one foot on a low stool or chair. After she has inserted the diaphragm in her vagina, the clinician checks its placement. The woman may then remove and replace the diaphragm for practice.

■ NURSING ORDERS: Careful and thorough instruction in the correct use of the contraceptive diaphragm is essential to its acceptance and use and, therefore, to its effectiveness in preventing pregnancy. Adequate time must be allowed for a diaphragm fitting. The woman is shown how to examine the dome regularly for holes, tears, or weak spots and how to use the spermicidal cream or jelly. She is told to leave the diaphragm in place for at least 6 to 8 hours after coitus and never to have sexual intercourse without it, because pregnancy has been know to occur at all times during the menstrual cycle in women who have

Contraceptives in common use, their modes of action, and female/male involvement

Contraceptive	*Woman*	*Man*	*Mode of action*	*Involvement time* — *Periodic*	*Involvement time* — *Daily*
Natural family planning Rhythm/calendar	X		Couple cooperation: abstinence during fertile periods	Mathematic formula calculated once every month	
BBT	X		Couple cooperation: abstinence during fertile periods	Ovulation determined from daily record of BBT	X
Cervical mucus	X		Couple cooperation: abstinence during fertile periods	Ovulation determined from daily record of cervical mucus characteristics	X
Symptothermal	X	Assists	Couple cooperation: abstinence during fertile periods	Combination of BBT, cervical mucus observation, and record of secondary symptoms by couple	X
Oral contraceptives	X		Suppress ovulation by inhibiting hypothalamus and pituitary	Ingestion of OC at same time each day; physical examination by physician every 6 mo	X
IUDs (unmedicated)	X		Prevent implantation within uterus	Inserted into uterus by trained person; placement checked often; IUD changed every 2-3 yr, prn	
Mechanical barriers Diaphragms	X		Prevent sperm migration into uterus	Inserted into vagina over cervix before intercourse	
Condoms		X	Prevent sperm migration into uterus	Applied to penis before intercourse	
Chemical barriers: foams, gels, suppositories*	X	X	Destroy sperm or make them immobile within vaginal vault	Inserted into vagina before each intercourse; applied with diaphragm or condom	
Fertility awareness	X	X	Family planning method combined with a barrier method of contraception		
Vaginal sponge	X		Releases spermicide Blocks cervical opening Absorbs semen	Inserted into upper vagina before intercourse; can be left in place to provide protection for 24 hr	

*Chemicals may be combined with other forms of contraception to enhance their effectiveness (e.g., Cu-7 IUD; spermicide with diaphragm or condom).

had coitus only once during the cycle. A new fitting is necessary if the woman gains or loses more than 20 pounds or of she has an abortion or a vaginal delivery. If the woman has not been sexually active before the fitting, the fit is reevaluated after 1 or 2 months of sexual activity has passed. After use, the diaphragm is washed and dried, powdered with a powder that does not contain perfume or talc, and stored in a dry container, preferably the plastic case in which it was dispensed. The prescription may be written with instructions to the pharmacist to allow one replacement of the diaphragm, in case of its loss or destruction.

■ OUTCOME CRITERIA: The diaphragm method of contraception is subject to great variation in effectiveness, largely because of inconsistent or incorrect use of the device by the woman. After a woman has used it for several years, the pregnancy rate may be as low as two to three pregnancies per 100 woman-years. The pregnancy rate may be much greater, regardless of the perfect and consistent practice of the user, if the woman has a second- or third-degree uterine prolapse, a second- or third-degree cystocele, or an acute displacement of the uterus (severe anteversion, anteflexion, retroversion, or retroflexion), or if the diaphragm is too small or the wrong kind, allowing spermatozoa to reach the cervix from around and under a loose-fitting rim. Hypersensitivity to the spermicidal cream or jelly used in conjunction with the diaphragm sometimes occurs; another product containing different ingredients may not cause an allergic reaction. The method usually causes no other major adverse reactions.

contraceptive effectiveness, the effectiveness of a method of contraception in preventing pregnancy. For clinical purposes, it combines the theoretic effectiveness of the device, medication, or method and the use effectiveness. It is sometimes represented as a percentage but more accurately as the number of pregnancies per 100 woman-years. The average pregnancy rate for a couple that is sexually active without the use of contraceptives is equivalent to 90 pregnancies per 100 woman-years. A contraceptive method that results in a pregnancy rate of less than 10 pregnancies per 100 woman-years is considered highly effective. See also **pregnancy rate, woman-year.**

contraceptive method, any act, device, or medication for avoiding conception or a viable pregnancy. See also **cervical cap, condom, diaphragm, intrauterine device, natural family-planning method, oral contraceptive, spermatocide, sterilization.**

contract, **1.** an agreement or a promise that meets certain legal requirements, including competence of both or all parties to the contract, proper lawful subject matter, mutuality of agreement, mutuality of obligation, and consideration (the giving of something of value in payment for the obligation undertaken). **2.** to make such an agreement or promise. –**contractual,** *adj.*

contractile ring dysphagia, an abnormal condition characterized by difficulty in swallowing because of an overreactive interior esophageal sphincteric mechanism that induces painful sticking sensations under the lower sternum. Compare **dysphagia lusoria, vallecular dysphagia.**

contractility, (in cardiology) the force of a heart contraction when preload and afterload are constant.

contraction, **1.** a reduction in size, especially of muscle fibers. **2.** an abnormal shrinkage. **3.** (in labor) a rhythmic tightening of the musculature of the upper uterine segment that begins mildly and becomes very strong late in labor, occurring as frequently as every 2 minutes, and lasting over 1 minute. Contractions decrease the size of the uterus and squeeze the fetus through the birth canal. **4.** abnormal smallness of the birth canal or part of it, a cause of dystocia. **Inlet contraction** exists if the anteroposterior diameter is 10 cm or less or if the transverse diameter is 11.5 cm or less. **Midpelvic contraction** exists if the sum of the measurements in centimeters of the interspinous diameter (normally 10.5 cm) and the posterior sagittal diameter (normally 5 cm) is 13.5 cm or less. **Outlet contraction** exists if the intertuberous diameter is 8 cm or less. See also **clinical pelvimetry, dystocia, x-ray.**

contracture, an abnormal, usually permanent condition of a joint, characterized by flexion and fixation and caused by atrophy and shortening of muscle fibers or by loss of the normal elasticity of the skin, as from the formation of extensive scar tissue over a joint. See also **Volkmann's contracture.**

contraindication, a factor that prohibits the administration of a drug or the performance of a procedure in the care of a specific patient; for example, pregnancy is a contraindication for the prescription of tetracycline, immunosuppression is a contraindication for vaccination, and complete placenta previa is a contraindication for vaginal delivery.

contralateral, affecting or originating in the opposite side of a point or reference, as a point on a body.

contrast, a measure of the differences between two adjacent areas in an image. Contrast may be based on differences in optic density or differences in radiation transmission, or other parameters. Contrast plays an important role in the ability of a radiologist to perceive image detail.

contrast bath, a bath in which the patient alternately immerses a part of the body, usually the hands or feet, in hot and cold water for a specified period of time. The procedure is used to increase the blood flow to a particular area.

contrast enema. See **barium enema.**

contrast medium, a radiopaque substance injected into the body to facilitate roentgen imaging of internal structures that otherwise are difficult to visualize on x-ray films.

contribution, (in law) a right of a defendant who has been required to pay a judgment to demand that others who are equally liable for the plaintiff's injuries contribute a share of the payment.

control, to exercise restraint or maintain influence over a situation, as in self-control, the conscious limitation or suppression of impulses.

control gene, (in molecular genetics) a gene, as the operator gene or regulator gene, that controls the transcription of the amino-acid sequence in the structural gene by either inducing or repressing protein synthesis.

control group. See **group.**

controlled association, **1.** a direct connection of relevant ideas as the result of a specific stimulus. **2.** a process of bringing repressed ideas into the consciousness in response to words spoken by a psychoanalyst. Also called **word association.**

controlled hypotension. See **deliberate hypotension.**

controlled ventilation, the use of an intermittent positive pressure breathing unit or other respirator that has an automatic cycling device that replaces spontaneous respiration. Some units measure expired volume, nebulize medication or fluids in the air, exert negative pressure at the end of the expiration, or have a variety of alarms.

control of hemorrhage, the limitation of the flow of blood from a break in the wall of a blood vessel.

■ METHOD: Some of the methods for controlling hemorrhage are direct pressure, use of a tourniquet, or application of pressure on pressure points proximal to the wound. Direct pressure with a thick compress is applied in such a way that the edges of the wound are brought together. A tourniquet is applied proximal to the site of bleeding only in the most drastic emergency, for the limb may then have to be sacrificed because of tissue anoxia stemming from the use of the tourniquet. Pressure is applied to a pressure point by using firm manual pressure over the main artery supplying the wound. Points used to obtain the pulse may be used as pressure points to stop hemorrhage. See also **tourniquet.**

■ NURSING ORDERS: The flow of blood to an area is limited by restricting activity, elevating the part, and applying pressure. Specific treatment depends on the cause of the hemorrhage and the condition of the patient. In addition to intravenous infusion equipment and fluids, the nurse may anticipate the need for vasopressor drugs, ventilatory assistance, central venous pressure monitoring equipment, and materials for obtaining and recording the blood pressure and urinary output. If signs of shock are present, the patient may be placed supine at a 45-degree angle to the pelvis, with the knees straight and the pelvis slightly higher than the chest. The head may be supported with a pillow. If Trendelenburg's position is used, a pillow is placed under the left shoulder to maximize filling of the right atrium of the heart and to maintain an open airway. The person may be given oxygen, and the central venous pressure may be measured to determine the need for replacement of fluid volume. Sudden, severe hemorrhage with signs of shock usually is treated with intravenous infusion of fluids and a transfusion of blood. The application of additional warmth to the skin is not recommended, because heat increases the metabolism and the need for oxygen.

■ OUTCOME CRITERIA: Signs of continued bleeding, tachycardia, cold sweat, decreasing blood pressure, and anxiety on the part of the patient alert the nurse to the probability that bleeding has begun again or that replacement fluids administered after the hemorrhage are not adequate. The person is kept calm and quiet; if the fluid balance is promptly restored, recovery is usual. Excessive loss of blood leads to anoxia of all the tissues of the body, including the brain and vital organs, and causes death.

control process, a system of establishing standards, objectives, and methods, and measuring actual performance, comparing results, reinforcing strengths, and taking necessary corrective action.

control unit, a part of the central processing unit that controls the sequence of operations within a computer.

contusion, an injury that does not break the skin, caused by a blow to the body and characterized by swelling, discoloration, and pain. The immediate application of cold may limit the development of a contusion. Also called **bruise.** Compare **ecchymosis.**

convalescence, the period of recovery after an illness, injury, or surgery.

convalescent home. See **extended care facility.**

convection, (in physics) the transfer of heat through a gas or liquid by the circulation of heated particles.

convergent evolution, the development of similar structures or functions within widely differing phylogenetic species in response to similar environmental conditions.

convergent strabismus. See **esotropia.**

conversion, **1.** changing from one form to another, transmutation. **2.** (in obstetrics) the correction of a fetal position during labor. **3.** (in psychiatry) an unconscious defense mechanism by which emotional conflicts ordinarily resulting in anxiety are repressed and transformed into symbolic physical symptoms having no organic basis. Loss of sensation, paralysis, pain, or other dysfunction of the nervous system are the most common somatic expressions of conversion.

conversion disorder, a kind of hysteric neurosis in which emotional conflicts are repressed and converted into sensory, motor, or visceral symptoms having no underlying organic cause, as blindness, anesthesia, hypesthesia, hyperesthesia, paresthesia, involuntary muscular movements (as tics or tremors), paralysis, aphonia, mutism, hallucinations, catalepsy, choking sensations, and respiratory difficulties. The person who has conversion disorder is usually indifferent to the symptoms yet firmly believes the condition exists. Causal factors include a conscious or unconscious desire to escape from or avoid some unpleasant situation or responsibility or to obtain sympathy or some other secondary gain. Treatment usually consists of psychotherapy. Also called **conversion hysteria, conversion reaction.**

convulsion, a sudden, violent involuntary contraction of a group of muscles that may be paroxysmal and episodic, as in a seizure disorder, or transient and acute, as after a head concussion. A convulsion may be clonic or tonic, focal, unilateral, or bilateral.

Cooley's anemia. See **thalassemia.**

cooling, reducing body temperature by the application of a hypothermia blanket, cold moist dressings, ice packs, or an alcohol bath. Subnormal body temperature may be induced to reduce metabolic function before some kinds of surgery. Very high fevers of any origen may be treated in part by reduction of the fever with cooling techniques. See also **alcohol bath, hypothermia, hypothermia blanket.**

cooling rate, the rate at which temperature decreases with time (°C/minute) immediately after the completion of hyperthermia treatment.

Coombs' test. See **antiglobulin test.**

cooperative play, any organized play among a group of children in which activities are planned for the purpose of achieving some goal. It usually occurs among older children. Compare **associative play, parallel play, solitary play.**

coordinated reflex, a sequence of muscular actions occurring in a purposeful, orderly progression, as the act of swallowing.

coping, a process by which a person deals with stress, solves problems, and makes decisions. The process has two components, cognitive and noncognitive. The cognitive component includes the thought and learning necessary to identify the source of the stress. The cognitive components are automatic and focus on relieving the discomfort. Many defense mechanisms fall into this category. While sometimes useful, noncognitive measures may fail to relieve the stress because the response may be inappropriate, may have the wrong effect, and, as it replaces cognitive coping measures, may prevent the person from learning more about the cause and a better solution for the problem.

coping ability, the degree to which an individual is able to adapt to any stress encountered in the activities of daily life, whether of a physical or psychologic nature, through the use of both conscious and unconscious mechanisms. Abnormal behavior patterns result when such demands or problems cannot be adequately met.

coping, family: potential for growth, a nursing diagnosis accepted by the Fourth National Conference on the Classification of Nursing Diagnoses. The cause of the problem is the need for self-actualization that occurs when a person's basic needs have been satisfied and the adaptive tasks required by the client's health problem have been mastered. The defining characteristics of the family's potential for growth in this area are the family's expressed wish to discuss the impact of the situation on the client's own life and values, interest in meeting with others in similar situations, and choice of healthful options available to the client. See also **nursing diagnosis.**

coping, ineffective family: compromised, a nursing diagnosis accepted by the Fourth National Conference on the Classification of Nursing Diagnoses. The diagnosis refers to a lack or absence of emotional and psychologic support for the client that is usually available from a family member or other supportive person, a deficiency that causes further difficulty for the client in coping with the current health problem. The cause of the situation may be inadequate or faulty understanding of the health problem by the supportive person, or it may result from temporary preoccupation with emotional conflicts on the part of the supportive person. Illness or health problems may cause changes in roles, resulting in temporary disorganization of the network of family and friends, who may become exhausted by the demands of filling the needs of the client. Many situational crises may interrupt or prevent adequate expression of support for the client, and the client may be able to give little support in return. The defining characteristics of ineffective compromised family coping include expression by the client that support is lacking or expression by the supportive person that fear, anticipatory grief, anxiety, or other reaction is interfering with the ability to give support to the client. A frank statement of an inadequate understanding of the health problem from the client or supportive person may be made. Objectively, the nurse may observe that the support given is inadequate, that the communication between the parties is limited and unsatisfactory, or that the supportive person offers help that is disproportionate to the need. See also **nursing diagnosis.**

coping, ineffective family: disabling, a nursing diagnosis accepted by the Fourth National Conference on the Classification of Nursing Diagnoses. The diagnosis refers to the detrimental attitudes and behavior of a family, a family member, or other person who is important to the client. The cause of the problem is often the disablement of the significant person by grief, anxiety, guilt, hostility, or despair. The defining characteristics of this kind of ineffective family coping include neglect in the care of the client, intolerance, rejection or abandonment, adoption of the symptoms of the client, disregard of the client's needs, and marked distortion of reality in regard to the client's health problem. See also **nursing diagnosis.**

coping, ineffective individual, a nursing diagnosis accepted by the Fourth National Conference on the Classification of Nursing Diagnoses. The cause of the problem includes situational crises, maturational or developmental crises, or personal vulnerability. The defining characteristics include an inability to meet the expectations of a role, an inability to meet one's basic needs, or an alteration in ability to participate in society. The critical defining characteristics, one of which must be present for the diagnosis to be made, are an inability to ask for help, an inability to solve problems, and verbalization of the inability to cope. Other characteristics that may be present are destructive behavior, inappropriate or excessive use of defense mechanisms, a change in patterns of communication, verbal manipulation, and a greater-than-expected incidence of accidents and illness. See also **nursing diagnosis.**

copper (Cu), a malleable, reddish-brown, metallic element. Its atomic number is 29; its atomic weight is 63.54. Copper occurs in a pure state in nature and in many ores. It is a component of several important enzymes in the body and is essential to good health. Copper deficiency in the body is rare because only 2 to 5 mg daily, easily obtained from a variety of foods, is sufficient for a proper balance. Copper accumulates in individuals with Wilson's disease, primary biliary cirrhosis, and, occasionally, chronic extrahepatic biliary tract obstruction. Copper is an excellent conductor of heat and electricity and a valuable component of numerous alloys, and it may be compounded with arsenic to form insecticides. Copper-sulfate solution is commonly used to test for reducing agents, as glucose, in the urine. See also **ceruloplasmin, hepatolenticular degeneration.**

copperhead, a poisonous pit viper found mainly in the southeastern United States. A similar snake of a different genus is found in Australia. The reddish-brown, darkly banded snake is responsible for nearly 40% of the snake bites in the United States; few bites are fatal. Pain, swelling, fang marks, and a bruise are usually present. Immediate treatment includes placing a constricting band above the bite that is tight enough to prevent lymphatic and superficial venous flow from the wound to the general circulation but that is not tight enough to stop deep arterial and venous flow to the limb. The fang marks are incised, the venom is drained, and free bleeding is allowed. The victim should be taken to a medical facility and given antivenin if necessary. The medication is usually needed only for children and older people. See also **coral snake, cottonmouth, rattlesnake.**

Copper Kettle, a trademark for a kind of vaporizer used in the circuits of an anesthesia machine to mix the carrier gas and the volatile anesthetic liquid to form an anesthetizing vapor.

copro-, copr-, kopr-, kopra-, a combining form meaning 'pertaining to feces': *coprolalia, coprolith.*

coprogogue. See **cathartic.**

coprolalia /kop′rōlā′lyə/, the excessive use of obscene language.

coproporphyria /kop′rōpôrfir′ē·ə/, a rare, hereditary, metabolic disorder in which large quantities of nitrogenous substances, called porphyrins, are excreted in the urine. Attacks, with varying GI and neurologic symptoms, may be precipitated by certain drugs, including barbiturates, sulfonamides, and steroids. Patients are often helped by a high-carbohydrate diet. See also **acute intermittent porphyria, coproporphyrin, porphyria.**

coproporphyrin /kop′rōpôr′firin/, any of the nitrogenous organic substances normally excreted in the feces that are products of the breakdown of bilirubin from hemoglobin decomposition.

copulation. See **coitus.**

cor, **1.** the heart. **2.** relating to the heart.

cor-. See **co-.**

coracoid process, the thick, curved extension of the superior border of the scapula, to which the pectoralis minor is attached. Compare **acromion.**

coral snake, a poisonous snake with transverse red, black, and yellow bands that is native to the southern United States. Bites are rare; pain is not always present, but neuromuscular and respiratory effects may be severe. Coral snake antivenin and oxygen are the usual emergency treatments.

Coramine, a trademark for a respiratory stimulant (nikethamide).

cord, any long, rounded, flexible structure. The body contains many different cords, as the spermatic, vocal, spinal, nerve, umbilical, and hepatic cords. Cords serve many different purposes, depending on location, kind of enclosed cells, and body parts or tissue involved. – **cordal,** *adj.*

corditis /kôrdī′tis/, an abnormal inflammation of the spermatic cord, accompanied by pain in the testis, often caused by an infection originating in the urethra or by tumor, hydrocele, or varicocele. Injury to the groin often causes hematoma of the cord. Inflammatory conditions of the testis may lead to swelling and tenderness.

Cordran, a trademark for a glucocorticoid (flurandrenolide).

core, **1.** a kind of main computer memory. **2.** (in dentistry) a section of a mold, usually of plaster, made over assembled parts of a dental restoration to record and maintain their relationships so that the parts can be reassembled in their original position. Also called **laboratory core.**

core-, coro-, a combining form meaning 'pertaining to the pupil of the eye': *coreclisis, corectasis, corectopia.*

core gender identity. See **gender identity.**

Corgard, a trademark for a beta-adrenergic blocking agent (nadolol).

-coria, **1.** a combining form meaning '(condition of the) sense of satiety': *acoria, hypercoria, saccharacoria.* **2.** a combining form meaning '(condition of the) pupil': *anisocoria, diplocoria, platycoria.*

Cori's disease /kôr′ēz/, a rare type of glycogen storage disease, in which a missing enzyme results in abnormally large deposits of glycogen in the liver, skeletal muscles, and heart. Signs are an enlarged liver, hypoglycemia, acidosis, and, occasionally, stunted growth. Symptoms can be controlled by giving the patient frequent, small meals rich in carbohydrate and protein. Also called **Forbes' disease, glycogenosis, glycogen storage disease, type III.** See also **glycogen storage disease.**

corium /kôr′ē·əm/, the layer of skin, just below the epidermis, consisting of papillary and reticular layers and containing blood and lymphatic vessels, nerves and nerve endings, glands, and hair follicles.

corkscrew esophagus, a neurogenic disorder in which normal peristaltic contractions of the esophagus are replaced by spastic movements occurring spontaneously or with swallowing or gastric acid reflux. Difficulty in swallowing, weight loss, severe pain over the upper chest, and a characteristic corkscrew image on x-ray pictures are the symptoms usually present. Management may include the use of antispasmodic drugs, avoidance of cold fluids, surgical dilatation, or myotomy. Compare **achalasia.** See also **dysphagia.**

cork worker's lung, a lung disease caused by an allergic reaction to cork dust. Also called **suberosis.** See also **organic dust.**

-cormia, -cormy, a combining form meaning an 'abnormal development of the trunk of the body': *camptocormia, nanocormia, schistocormia.*

corn, a horny mass of condensed epithelial cells overlying a bony prominence. Corns result from chronic friction and pressure. The conic shape of the corn compresses the underlying dermis, making it thin and tender. Corns can become soft and macerated by perspiration. Treatment includes relief of the mechanic pressure and surgical paring or chemical peeling of the excess keratin. Also called **clavus.** Compare **callus.**

cornea /kôr′nē•ə/, the convex, transparent, anterior part of the eye, comprising one sixth of the outermost tunic of the eye bulb. It is a fibrous structure with five layers: the anterior corneal epithelium, continuous with that of the conjunctiva; the anterior limiting layer (Bowman's membrane); the substantia propria; the posterior limiting layer (Descemet's membrane); and the endothelium of the anterior chamber (keratoderma). It is dense, uniform in thickness, and nonvascular, and it projects like a dome beyond the sclera, which forms the other five sixths of the eye's outermost tunic. The degree of corneal curvature varies in different individuals and in the same person at different ages, the curvature being more pronounced in youth than in advanced age.

-cornea, a combining form meaning 'condition of the cornea': *entocornea, mesocornea, microcornea.*

corneal abrasion, the rubbing off of the outer layers of the cornea.

corneal grafting, transplantation of corneal tissue from one human eye to another, performed to improve vision in corneal scarring or distortion or to remove a perforating ulcer. Preoperative preparation includes constricting the pupil with a miotic drug, as pilocarpine. Under local anesthesia the affected area is excised; an identical section of clear cornea is cut from the donor eye and sutured in place, using an operating microscope. Cataract surgery may be performed at the same time. Postoperatively, the eye is covered with a protective metal shield, and the patient is cautioned to avoid coughing, sneezing, sudden movement, or lifting. The dressing is changed daily, and antibiotics are instilled. A complication that may occur after several weeks is a clouding over of the graft, because of the body's rejection of foreign tissue. Corticosteroid drugs administered immediately postoperatively may prevent the reaction. Healing is slow, and the sutures are usually left in place for 1 year. Also called **keratoplasty.**

corneal loupe, (in ophthalmology) a loupe designed especially for examining the cornea.

corneal reflex, a protective mechanism for the eye in which the eyelids close when the cornea is touched. This reflex is mediated by the ophthalmic division of the fifth cranial nerve and may be used as a test of integrity of that nerve branch. People who wear contact lenses may have a diminished or absent corneal reflex. Compare **conjunctival reflex.**

cornification, thickening of the skin by a buildup of dead, keratinized epithelial cells.

corn pad, a device that helps relieve the pressure and the pain of a corn by transferring the pressure to surrounding, unaffected areas. Corn pads are constructed of pliable fabric and fashioned in various ways to accommodate different conditions. Some common kinds of corn pads are the foam toe cap, the foam toe sleeve, the soft corn shield, and the hard corn shield.

cornual pregnancy, an ectopic pregnancy that implants in the portion of the fallopian tube that is within the horn of the uterus. Also called **interstitial pregnancy.** See also **ectopic pregnancy.**

coro-. See **core-.**

corona /kərō′nə/, **1.** a crown. **2.** a crownlike projection or encircling structure, as a process extending from a bone. **–coronal, coronoid,** *adj.*

coronal plane. See **frontal plane.**

coronal suture, the serrated transverse suture between the frontal bone and the parietal bone on each side of the skull.

corona radiata, *pl.* **coronae radiatae, 1.** a network of fibers that weaves through the internal capsule of the cerebral cortex and intermingles with the fibers of the corpus callosum. **2.** an aggregate of cells that surrounds the zona pellucida of the ovum.

coronary /kôr′əner′ē/, **1.** (in anatomy) of or pertaining to encircling structures, as the coronary arteries; of or pertaining to the heart. **2.** *nontechnical.* myocardial infarction or occlusion.

coronary arteriovenous fistula, an unusual congenital abnormality characterized by a direct communication between a coronary artery, usually the right, and the right atrium or ventricle, the coronary sinus, or the vena cava. There may be a left-to-right shunt of small magnitude causing no symptoms, but a large shunt may result in growth failure, limited exercise tolerance, dyspnea, and anginal pain. Possible complications with a large shunt are bacterial endocarditis, rupture of an aneurysmal fistula, thrombus formation causing occlusion or distal embolization, and, in rare cases, pulmonary hypertension and congestive heart failure. A loud continuous murmur heard at the lower or midsternal border of the heart suggests a coronary arteriovenous fistula; the diagnosis may be confirmed by coronary arteriography or aortography. Closure of the fistulous tract is a safe surgical procedure with excellent long-term results.

coronary artery, one of a pair of arteries that branch from the aorta, including the left and the right coronary arteries. As these vessels and their branches supply the heart, any dysfunction or disease that affects them can cause serious, sometimes fatal complications. Coronary arterial anastomoses occur throughout the heart and are especially numerous within the interventricular and interatrial septums, at the apex of the heart, at the crux, over the anterior surface of the right ventricle, and between the sinus-node artery and the other atrial arteries. These anastomoses are more numerous and larger in the epicardium than in the endocardium, and they provide important collateral circulation in the recovery of patients who suffer coronary occlusions. The branches of the coronary arteries are affected by many different disorders, as embolic, neoplastic, inflammatory, and noninflammatory diseases.

coronary artery disease, any one of the abnormal conditions that may affect the arteries of the heart and produce various pathologic effects, especially the reduced flow of oxygen and nutrients to the myocardium. Any of the coronary artery diseases, as coronary atherosclerosis, coronary arteritis, or fibromuscular hyperplasia of the coronary arteries, may produce the common characteristic symptom of angina pectoris, which, however, may also be associated with cardiomyopathy, in which the coronary arteries are normal. The most common kind of coronary artery disease is coronary atherosclerosis, which has increased dramatically in the last 50 years and is now the leading cause of death in the Western world. Epidemiologic studies show marked regional differences in the incidence and prevalence of coronary atherosclerosis. The disease is not necessarily part of the aging process. It affects more men than women and occurs more often in whites, the middle-aged or elderly, and individuals from affluent countries. Coronary atherosclerosis affects more premenopausal women today than in the past, possibly because of the pathologic effects of increased cigarette smoking by women, stressful sedentary jobs, and the use of oral contraceptives. Studies over the last 30 years confirm that coronary atherosclerosis occurs most frequently in populations with regular diets high in calories, total fat, saturated fat, cholesterol, and refined carbohydrates. The risk of developing coronary atherosclerosis and the risk of death from the disease is two to six times greater among cigarette smokers than nonsmokers and appears to be proportional to the number of cigarettes smoked per day. Significantly less risk is associated with pipe and cigar smoking. Hypertension is also a prime risk factor in atherosclerosis. Some studies show the combination of cigarette smoking and cholesterol level above 275 mg/dl increases the coronary risk 14 to 16 times. Some studies also have implicated other factors as possibly contributing to the risk of atherosclerosis. They include coffee intake, alcohol intake, deficiencies of vitamins C and E, water hardness, hypoxia, carbon monoxide, social overcrowding, heredity, climate, and viruses. Atherosclerosis develops with the formation of fatty fibrous plaques that narrow the lumen of the coronary arteries and may lead to thrombosis and myocardial infarction. Although no single cause of atherosclerosis has been found, the development of the disease is closely associated with the plasma lipids and the lipoproteins that transport the plasma lipids from one tissue to another. The plasma lipids, composed chiefly of cholesterol, triglycerides, phospholipids, and free fatty acids are insoluble in water. The major classes of lipoproteins are chylomicra, very-low-density lipoproteins, low-density lipoproteins, high-density lipoproteins, and the free fatty acid-albumin complex.

■ OBSERVATIONS: Angina pectoris, the classic symptom of coronary artery disease, results from infarction and myocardial ischemia. Angina is usually described as a crushing substernal pain that radiates to the left arm, neck, jaw, and shoulder blade. In affected individuals, angina commonly follows physical exertion, emotional excitement, or exposure to cold. Angina may be stable, unstable, or decubitus. The frequency and the duration of stable angina are predictable, and this type of pain may be relieved with nitrates and rest. Unstable angina occurs more often and lasts longer than stable angina. Decubitis angina may recur even when the affected individual is resting. Prolonged, intense angina commonly indicates myocardial infarction with possible fatal coronary obstruction spasms, and arrythmias. Diagnosis of coronary artery disease is usually based on patient history, especially a history with characteristic risk factors. Other diagnostic procedures are ECG during angina, treadmill or bicycle exercise tests, coronary angiography, and myocardial perfusion imaging.

■ INTERVENTION: Treatment of the patient with coronary artery disease concentrates on reducing myocardial oxygen demand or on increasing oxygen supply. Therapy commonly includes the administration of nitrates, as nitroglycerin, isosorbide dinitrate, or propranolol, a beta-adrenergic blocker. Coronary-artery-bypass surgery may use vein grafts to obviate obstructive lesions. Angioplasty to relieve occlusion by compressing fatty deposits in coronary arteries with no calcification may also be performed. The prevalence of coronary artery disease highlights the importance of preventive measures, as the reduction of caloric intake for the obese patient; reduction of salt, fats, and cholesterol; regular exercise; abstention from smoking; and reduction of stress. Other preventive measures include the control of hypertension, reduction of elevated serum cholesterol and triglyceride levels, and reduction of dangers of blood clots and platelet aggregation. Hypertension may be controlled with diuretics or with sympathetic blocking agents, as propranolol. Serum cholesterol and triglyceride levels may be reduced with hypolipidemic drugs, as clofibrate. Clinical trials with various antithrombotic drugs seek to reduce the danger of blood clots from platelet aggregation. Further studies may determine the efficacy of aspirin in the prevention of platelet plugs as the predominant form of arterial thrombi. Aspirin inhibits the aggregation of platelets but may not retard their adherence to the walls of blood vessels.

■ NURSING CONSIDERATIONS: Nursing care of the patient with coronary artery disease involves monitoring of blood pressure and heart rate, taking of ECGs during anginal episodes, and administration of nitrates, as nitroglycerin. Meticulous maintenance of pulmonary artery catheters and of IV and endotracheal tubes often associated with treatment is important. Nurses are especially alert to signs of ischemia and arrhythmias and, before the patient is discharged, stress the importance of following the prescribed regimens of diet, medication, and exercise.

coronary artery fistula, a congenital anomaly characterized by an abnormal communication between a coronary artery and the right side of the heart or the pulmonary artery.

coronary autoregulation, the process of coronary artery vasodilatation in response to myocardia ischemia.

coronary bypass, open-heart surgery in which a prosthesis or a section of a blood vessel is grafted onto one of the coronary arteries and connected to the ascending aorta, bypassing a narrowing or blockage in a coronary artery. The operation is performed in coronary artery disease to improve the blood supply to the heart muscle, to reduce the workload of the heart, and to relieve anginal pain. Coronary arteriography pinpoints the areas of obstruction preoperatively. Under general anesthesia and with the use of a heart-lung machine, one end of a 15 to 20 cm prosthesis or a segment of saphenous vein from the patient's leg is grafted to the ascending aorta, and the other end is sutured to the clogged coronary artery at a point distal to the stoppage. The internal mammary artery may also be used as graft tissue. Usually, double or triple grafts are done for multiple areas of blockage. Postoperatively, close observation in a coronary intensive care unit or surgical recovery unit is essential to ensure adequate ventilation and cardiac output. The systolic blood pressure is not allowed to drop more than 10 mm Hg below the preoperative baseline, nor is it allowed to rise significantly, as hypertension can rupture a graft site. Arrhythmias occur frequently and are treated with lidocaine, procainamide, or digitalis, given intravenously, or by electrical cardioversion. The patient is usually discharged within 10 to 14 days. Nearly 20% of cases are associated with thrombosis within the first year after surgery, making the surgery controversial.

coronary care nursing, the nursing care provided in a hospital in a coronary care unit. Nursing in this setting requires technical knowledge, judgment, and skills as well as an ability to give emotional support to patients and their families during the acute stage of cardiac dysfunction.

coronary care unit (CCU), a specially equipped hospital area designed for the treatment of patients with sudden, life-threatening cardiac conditions, as acute coronary thrombosis. Such units contain resuscitation and monitoring equipment and are staffed by personnel especially trained and skilled in recognizing and immediately responding to cardiac emergencies with cardiopulmonary resuscitation techniques, the administration of antiarrhythmic drugs, and other appropriate therapeutic measures. See also **intensive care unit.**

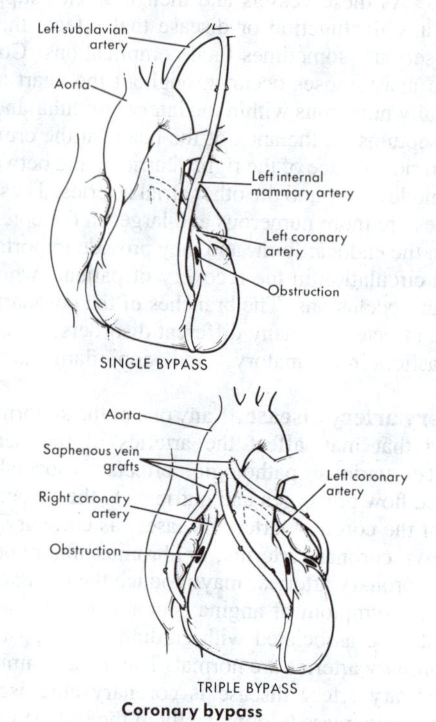

Coronary bypass

coronary occlusion, an obstruction of any one of the coronary arteries, usually caused by progressive atherosclerosis and sometimes complicated by thrombosis. Coronary occlusions are rarely caused by embolisms, arteritis, or dissecting aneurysms. More often, an obstruction of a coronary artery develops gradually from the accumulation of fatty, fibrous plaques that narrow the arterial lumen, reduce the blood flow, and lead to myocardial infarction. In certain heart diseases arterial spasms may narrow the lumen of a coronary artery, blocking blood flow, and causing the characteristic signs of myocardial infarction, as crushing substernal pain that radiates to the arms, jaw, and neck. Atherosclerosis, which commonly develops in high-flow, high-pressure arteries, is associated with numerous factors, including family history, hypertension, obesity, smoking, diabetes mellitus, stress, sedentary occupations, and high serum cholesterol and triglyceride levels. Occlusions that lead to myocardial infarction are common, and mortality is high when treatment is delayed. Almost half the sudden deaths caused by myocardial infarction occur before the affected individual is hospitalized, often within 1 hour of the onset of symptoms. If treatment begins immediately after the onset of symptoms, the prognosis significantly improves. Occlusion of the circumflex branch of the left coronary artery causes a lateral wall infarction. Occlusion of the anterior descending branch of the left coronary artery causes an infarction of the anterior heart wall. Occlusion of the right coronary artery or one of its branches causes a posterior wall infarction. Many patients who suffer coronary occlusions recover because of fast treatment and collateral circulation provided by extensive arterial anastomoses of the heart. The reasons why the arterial anastomoses function for collateral circulation in some patients with occlusions and not in others are apparently associated with individual differences in arterial pressure and configurations of the arterial anastomoses. In normal hearts, the coronary anastomoses are usually straight or gently curving; in hearts with coronary occlusion, the arterial anastomoses are twisted and tortuous. Occlusions of the sinus-node artery and the main coronary artery proximal to the origin of the sinus-node branch commonly cause infarctions of the atrium and the sinus node and lead to atrial arrhythmias. Coronary occlusions that produce posterior myocardial infarction cut off the blood supply to the atrioventricular node, resulting in characteristic signs, as fainting and syncope during angina. Treatment of coronary occlusion and associated myocardial infarction often includes the administration of lidocaine or other antiarrhythmic drugs, nitroglycerin to relieve pain, oxygen, and bed rest and the implantation of a temporary pacemaker. See also **coronary artery disease.**

coronary sinus, the wide venous channel, about 2.25 cm long, situated in the coronary sulcus and covered by muscular fibers from the left atrium. It drains five coronary veins through a single semilunar valve. They are the great cardiac vein, the small cardiac vein, the middle cardiac vein, the posterior vein of the left ventricle, and the oblique vein of the left atrium.

coronary thrombosis, a development of a thrombus that blocks a coronary artery, often causing myocardial infarction and death. Coronary thromboses commonly develop in segments of arteries with atherosclerotic lesions, thus supporting the opinion of many authorities that atherosclerosis favors the development of thrombi.

coronary vein, one of the veins of the heart that drains blood from the capillary beds of the myocardium through the coronary sinus into the right atrium. A few small coronary veins that collect blood from a small area in the right ventricle drain directly into the right atrium.

coronavirus /kôr′ənəvī′rəs/, a member of a family of viruses that includes several types capable of causing acute respiratory illnesses.

coroner /kôr′ənər/, a public official who investigates the causes and circumstances of a death occurring within a specific legal jurisdiction or territory, especially a death that may have resulted from unnatural causes. Also called **medical examiner.**

coronoid fossa, a small depression in the distal, dorsal surface of the humerus that receives the coronoid process of the ulna when the forearm is flexed.

coronoid process of mandible, a prominence on the anterior surface of the ramus of the mandible to which each temporal muscle attaches.

coronoid process of ulna, a wide, flaring projection of the proximal end of the ulna. The proximal surface of the process forms the lower part of the trochlear notch.

corpor-, a combining form meaning 'pertaining to the body': *corpora, corporeal, corporic.*

cor pulmonale /kôr po͝ol′mənal′ē/, an abnormal cardiac condition characterized by hypertrophy of the right ventricle of the heart as a result of hypertension of the pulmonary circulation. Pulmonary hypertension associated with this condition is caused by some disorder of the pulmonary parenchyma or of the pulmonary vascular system between the origin of the left pulmonary artery and the entry of the pulmonary veins into the left atrium. Chronic cor pulmonale commonly increases the size of the right ventricle of the heart, because the right ventricle cannot accommodate an increase in pressure as easily as the left ventricle. In some patients, however, the disease also increases the size of the left ventricle. Some of the diseases associated with cor pulmonale include cystic fibrosis, myasthenia gravis, myopathies, and pulmonary arteritis. Approximately 85% of patients with cor pulmonale have chronic obstructive pulmonary disease; 25% of patients with emphysema eventually develop cor pulmonale. Pulmonary capillary destruction and pulmonary vasoconstriction decrease the cross-sectional area of the pulmonary vascular bed, increasing pulmonary vascular resistance and causing pulmonary hypertension. The right ventricle dilates and hypertrophies to compensate for the extra work required in forcing blood through the lungs. To compensate for the low oxygen content associated with cor pulmonale, the bone marrow produces more red blood cells, causing erythrocytosis. Right ventricular failure results when blood viscosity increases and further aggravates pulmonary hypertension, increasing the hemodynamic load on the right ventricle. Cor pulmonale accounts for about 25% of all types of heart failure and is most prevalent in populations where the incidence of cigarette smoking and chronic obstructive pulmonary disease is high. The disease affects middle-aged and elderly men more than women. Cor pulmonale in children may be a complication of cystic fibrosis, hemosiderosis, scleroderma, neurologic diseases affecting respiratory muscles, or disorders of the respiratory control center.

■ OBSERVATIONS: Some of the early signs of cor pulmonale include chronic cough, exertional dyspnea, fatigue, wheezing, and weakness. As the disease progresses, dyspnea may become more severe, and other signs, as tachypnea, orthopnea, and edema, may emerge. Signs of this condition and right ventricular failure may include dependent edema, distended neck veins, hepatojugular reflux, and tachycardia. A weak pulse and hypotension may result from decreased cardiac output, and chest examination may reveal various signs, depending on the cause of the condition. In chronic obstructive pulmonary disease, auscultation may reveal rales, rhonchi, and diminished breath sounds. When cor pulmonale is secondary to obstruction of the upper airway or to damage of central nervous system respiratory centers, auscultation may reveal a right ventricular lift, a gallop rhythm, and a systolic pulmonic click. A pansystolic murmur, which intensifies on inspiration, may indicate tricuspid insufficiency. The patient with cor pulmonale may also experience fluctuating levels of drowsiness and consciousness. Diagnosis of the condition may be confirmed by measurements of pulmonary-artery pressure by pulmonary-artery catheterization. Systolic pressures of the right ventricle and the pulmonary arteries are usually more than 30 mm Hg in cor pulmonale, and the diastolic pressure of the pulmonary arteries is usually more than 15 mm Hg. Other diagnostic indicators commonly associated with this condition are an echocardiograph or an angiograph indicating right ventricular enlargement, a chest x-ray films showing large pulmonary arteries, and arterial oxygen pressure of less than 70 mm Hg and not more than 90 mm Hg. The ECG with cor pulmonale frequently shows arrhythmias, as ventricular and premature atrial contractions, and may also show right bundle branch block, right axis deviation, pronounced P waves and inverted T wave in the right precordial leads, and hypertrophy of the right ventricle. The hematocrit in cor pulmonale is often greater than 50%.

■ INTERVENTION: The treatment of cor pulmonale seeks to reduce hypoxia, increase exercise tolerance, and correct the functional defect whenever possible. The prognosis is usually poor, because cor pulmonale commonly develops as the result of chronic obstructive pulmonary disease and other irreversible conditions. Treatment includes bed rest, the administration of digitalis glycoside, antibiotics to fight any respiratory infection, oxygen therapy, low-salt diet, restricted fluid intake, diuretics, and anticoagulants. Oxygen may be administered by mask or by cannula in concentrations from 24% to 40%, depending on arterial oxygen pressure. A tracheotomy may be performed to open an obstructed upper airway, and mechanic ventilation may be used in acute cases. A phlebotomy may be performed to reduce red cell mass.

■ NURSING CONSIDERATIONS: Nursing care in the treatment of cor pulmonale commonly requires careful diet planning with frequent small meals, because the patient may tire easily during regular feedings. The nurse often helps to prevent edema by limiting the daily fluid intake of the patient to between 1000 and 2000 ml. It is important to monitor closely the serum potassium levels of the patient receiving diuretics, because low-serum potassium levels can increase the risk of arrhythmias associated with digitalis. Digitalis toxicity is often a danger and may be indicated by anorexia, nausea, vomiting, and the observance by the patient of yellow halos surrounding visual images. Nurses commonly instruct the patient to check the radial pulse before ingesting any digitalis glycoside and to report any changes in pulse rate. The frequent repositioning of bed patients with cor pulmonale helps to prevent atelectasis. The nursing responsibility also usually includes respiratory care, including oxygen therapy, the periodic measuring of arterial blood gases, and monitoring for signs of respiratory failure, pulse rate changes, labored respirations, and exertional fatigue levels. Before the patient is discharged from the hospital, nurses instruct the patient on personal maintenance, especially the detection of pitting edema of the extremities. The cor pulmonale patient being discharged can also benefit from instructions about breathing exercises, the importance of reporting early signs of infection, the dangers of mingling with crowds, especially during the flu season, and the danger of using nonprescribed medications, especially sedatives, which can depress the ventilatory drive.

corpus. See **body.**

corpus cavernosum /kôr′pəs/, a type of spongy erectile tissue within the penis or clitoris. The tissue becomes engorged with blood during sexual excitement.

corpuscle /kôr′pəsəl/, **1.** any cell of the body. **2.** a red or white blood cell. Also called **corpuscule.** –**corpuscular,** *adj.*

corpuscular radiation, the radiation associated with subatomic particles, as electrons, protons, neutrons, or alpha particles, that travel in streams at various velocities. All these particles have definite masses and have radiation properties very different from electromagnetic radiations, which have no mass and travel in wave forms at the speed of light. See also **background radiation, leakage radiation, scattered radiation.**

corpus luteum, *pl.* **corpora lutea,** an anatomic structure on the surface of the ovary, consisting of a spheroid of yellowish tissue 1 to 2 cm in diameter that grows within the ruptured ovarian follicle after ovulation. The pleated wall of the collapsed follicle is made up of several layers of granulosa cells that grow toward the center of the cavity to form the structure. During the reproductive years of a woman's life, a corpus luteum forms after every ovulation. It acts as a short-lived endocrine organ that secretes progesterone, which serves to maintain the decidual layer of the endometrium in the richly vascular state necessary for implantation and pregnancy. If conception occurs, the corpus luteum grows and secretes increasing amounts of progesterone. It reaches its maximum function and size (2 to 3 cm) at 10 to 12 weeks of gestation. It persists, slowly diminishing in size and function, until 6 months after the onset of gestation. During the 2 weeks before menstruation, the corpus luteum secretes progesterone in decreasing amounts, atrophies, undergoes fibrotic degeneration, and becomes a pale spot (corpus albicans) on the surface of the ovary.

corpus vitreum. See **vitreous humor.**

corrective exercise, a program of physical therapy to restore normal function to diseased, defective, or injured parts of the body. Also called **therapeutic exercise.** See also **exercise, osteopathy.**

correlation, (in statistics) a relationship between variables that may be negative (inverse), positive, or curvilinear. Correlation is measured and expressed using numeric scales.

correlative differentiation, (in embryology) specialization or diversification of cells or tissues caused by an inductor or other external factor. Also called **dependent differentiation.**

Corrigan's pulse, a bounding pulse in which a great surge is felt followed by a sudden and complete absence of force or fullness in the artery. This kind of pulse occurs in excited emotional states, in various abnormal cardiac conditions, including patent ductus arteriosus, and as a result of systemic arteriosclerosis.

corrosion of surgical instruments, the rusting of surgical instruments or the gradual wearing away of their polished surfaces because of oxidation and the action of contaminants. Though minimized by the use of stainless steel alloys in the fabrication of the instruments, corrosion persists as a problem, even when cleaning procedures seem more than adequate. It usually occurs because of inadequate cleaning and drying of surgical instruments after use, the use of sterilizing solutions that eat into the surface, overexposure to such solutions, or a faulty autoclave. Cleanliness is the single most important factor in preventing corrosion. Any foreign material, either organic or inorganic, on the surface of stainless steel is likely to promote corrosion, and microscopic examinations often reveal foreign material and chlorides from cleaning solutions scattered over the surface of cleaned and sterilized instruments. A good soap, with rubbing, is required, and a soft brush is often needed. Instruments must then be rinsed and dried. They must be disassembled after use and thoroughly cleaned and dried before they are reassembled. Assembled instruments will corrode if they are stored with trapped moisture. An efficient method of removing corrosive products from inaccessible places on an instrument is to soak it in a mixture of equal parts of ethyl alcohol and aqueous ammonia. After soaking in this solution for about 12 hours, corrosive products may be rinsed or lightly brushed away. Polishing in the manufacturing process of surgical instruments is one of the steps that reduces corrosion. Box locks often corrode because they are more inaccessible than other parts of surgical instruments and their intersurfaces are not polished. Certain quaternary ammonium chlorides are effective cold sterilizing agents because they are both potent germicides and powerful detergents. The chloride ions in such compounds are corrosive. Corrosion during autoclaving will occur if the autoclave is not functioning properly, if corrosive materials are in contact with the instruments, or if tap water instead of distilled water is used to generate steam. Also, autoclaves in which a lot of corrosion occurs may have leaking valves. The bleaches and detergents remaining in laundered cloths and wrappings for autoclaving instruments may also cause corrosion; their chemical activity is increased by high autoclave temperatures. The more chromium in the stainless steel alloys of which surgical instruments are made, the more resistant the instruments are to corrosion. Carbon, which hardens such alloys, also reduces their resistance to corrosion. Most corrosion of surgical instruments is superficial and may be removed by soaking in a solution of ammonia and alcohol or by repolishing by the manufacturer.

corrosive, **1.** eating away a substance or tissue, especially by chemical action. **2.** an agent or substance that eats away a substance or tissue. **–corrode,** *v.*, **corrosion,** *n.*

corrosive gastritis, an acute inflammatory condition of the stomach caused by the ingestion of an acid, alkali, or other corrosive chemical in which the lining of the stomach is eaten away by the corrosive substance. The amount of tissue destruction and recommended treatment depend on the nature of the corrosive agent and the extent of exposure. Compare **chemical gastritis, erosive gastritis.** See also **acid poisoning, alkali poisoning.**

corrugator supercilii, one of the three muscles of the eyelid. Arising from the medial end of the supercilliary arch and inserting into the skin above the orbital arch, it is innervated by temporal and zygomatic branches of the facial nerve and functions to draw the eyebrow downward and inward, as if to frown. Also called **corrugator.** Compare **levator palpebrae superioris, orbicularis oculi.**

Cortef, a trademark for a glucocorticoid (cortisol).

Cortef Acetate, a trademark for a glucocorticoid (cortisol acetate).

Cortef Fluid, a trademark for a glucocorticoid (cortisol cypionate).

cortex, *pl.* **cortices** /kôr′tisēz/, the outer layer of a body organ or other structure, as distinguished from the internal substance.

cortic-, a combining form meaning 'pertaining to the cortex or bark': *corticipetal, corticobulbar, corticothalamic.*

cortical apraxia. See **motor apraxia.**

cortical audiometry. See **audiometry.**

cortical blindness, blindness that results from a lesion in the visual center of the cerebral cortex of the brain.

cortical fracture, any fracture that involves the cortex of the bone.

cortical substance of cerebellum. See **cerebellar cortex.**

corticosteroid /kôr′tikōstir′oid/, any one of the natural or the synthetic hormones associated with the adrenal cortex, which influences or controls key processes of the body, as carbohydrate and protein metabolism, electrolyte and water balance, and the functions of the cardiovascular system, the skeletal muscle, the kidneys, and other organs. The corticosteroids synthesized by the adrenal glands include the glucocorticoids and the mineralocorticoids. The principal glucocorticoids are cortisol and corticosterone. The only physiologically important mineralocorticoid in humans is aldosterone. The glucocorticoids tend to cause the cells of the body to shift from carbohydrate catabolism to fat catabolism, to accelerate the breakdown of proteins to amino acids, and to help maintain normal blood pressure. The secretion of these hormones increases during stress, especially that produced by anxiety and severe injury. Chronic overproduction of these substances is associated with various disorders, as Cushing's syndrome. A high blood level of glucocorticoids markedly increases the number of eosinophils and decreases the size of lymphatic tissues, especially the thymus and the lymph nodes. The decrease in lymphocytes retards antibody formation and affects the immune system of the body. Aldosterone is the most powerful of the natural mineralocorticoids in the regulation of electrolyte balance, especially in the balance of sodium and potassium. Cortisol induces sodium retention and potassium excretion but not as effectively as aldosterone. The effects of the corticosteroids on the cardiovascular system, which are not precisely understood, are most evident in hypocorticism when the reduction in blood volume, accompanied by increased viscosity, may cause hypotension and cardiovascular collapse. The absence of corticosteroids increases capillary permeability, decreases the vasomotor response of the small vessels, and reduces cardiac size and output. The skeletal muscles require adequate amounts of the corticosteroids to function normally; excessive amounts cause them to function abnormally. Cortisol and its synthetic analogs can prevent or reduce inflammation by inhibiting edema, leukocytic migration, disposition of collagen, and other complications associated with inflammatory processes. The antiinflammatory powers of synthetic hormones can be dangerous, however, because they mask the disease process and prevent accurate observation of its progress. Pharmacologic doses of glucocorticosteroids retard bone growth of children and inhibit cell division in various developing structures, as the gastric mucosa, liver, lung, and brain. Glucocorticoids are absorbed from sites of local application, as synovial spaces, the conjunctival sac, and the skin. When large areas of the skin are involved or when the administration is prolonged, absorption may cause systemic effects, including adrenocortical suppression. Corticosteroids may be administered orally, parenterally, or topically. Toxic effects may result from the too rapid withdrawal of such drugs after prolonged therapy or from the continued use of large doses. Toxic effects associated with prolonged corticosteroid therapy include fluid and electrolyte imbalance, hyperglycemia and glycosuria, increased susceptibility to infections, myopathy, arrested growth, ecchymoses, Cushing's syndrome, acne, and behavioral disturbances. The increased susceptibility to infection associated with corticosteroids is not specific for any particular pathogen, and those patients who develop infections while undergoing corticosteroid therapy are usually treated concomitantly with appropriate antibacterial agents. Peptic ulceration occurs in some patients undergoing corticosteroid therapy, and some patients receiving large doses of these drugs develop myopathy, characterized by weakness of the proximal musculature of the arms and the legs and of associated shoulder and pelvic muscles. Corticosteroid therapy may also produce behavioral changes, as schizophrenia, suicidal tendencies, nervousness, and insomnia.

corticotropin. See **adrenocorticotropic hormone.**

cortisol, a steroid hormone occurring naturally in the body and produced synthetically for pharmacologic use. Also called **hydrocortisone.**

■ INDICATION: It is prescribed as an antiinflammatory agent.

■ CONTRAINDICATIONS: Fungal infections or known hypersensitivity to this drug prohibits its systemic use. Viral or fungal infections of the skin, impaired circulation, or known hypersensitivity to this drug prohibits its topical use.

■ ADVERSE EFFECTS: Among the more serious adverse reactions to the systemic administration of this drug are GI, endocrine, neurologic, fluid, and electrolyte disturbances. A variety of hypersensitivity reactions may occur from topical administration of this drug.

cortisone, a glucocorticoid produced in the liver and also made synthetically.

■ INDICATION: It is prescribed as an antiinflammatory agent.

■ CONTRAINDICATIONS: Fungal infections or known hypersensitivity to this drug prohibits its systemic use. Viral or fungal infections of the skin, impaired circulation, or known hypersensitivity to this drug prohibits its topical use.

■ ADVERSE EFFECTS: Among the more serious adverse reactions to the systemic administration of the drug are GI, endocrine, neurologic, fluid, and electrolyte disturbances. A variety of skin reactions may occur from topical administration of this drug.

Corti's organ /kôr′tēz/, a small, spiral structure within the cochlea of the internal ear, containing hair cells in contact with the acoustic nerve. Also called **spiral organ of Corti.**

Cortisporin, a trademark for a topical fixed-combination drug containing a glucocorticoid (hydrocortisone) and three antibacterials (neomycin sulfate, polymyxin B sulfate, and gramicidin).

Corynebacterium /kôr′inēbaktir′ē·əm/, a common genus of rod-shaped, curved bacilli having many species. The most common pathogenic species are *Corynebacterium acnes,* commonly found in acne lesions, and *C. diphtheriae,* the cause of diphtheria. See also ***Propionibacterium.***

coryza. See **rhinitis.**

coryza spasmodica. See **hay fever.**

Cosmegen, a trademark for an antineoplastic (dactinomycin).

cosmetic surgery, reconstruction of cutaneous or underlying tissues, usually about the face and neck, performed to correct a structural defect or to remove a scar, birthmark, or some normal evidence of aging. A local anesthetic is usually sufficient. Kinds of cosmetic surgery include **rhinoplasty, rhytidoplasty.** Compare **plastic surgery.**

cosmic radiation, high-energy particles with great penetrating power originating in outer space and reaching the earth as normal background radiation. The rays consist partly of high-energy atomic nuclei.

cost-. See **costi-.**

costal, **1.** of or pertaining to a rib. **2.** situated near a rib or on a side close to a rib.

costal cartilage. See **cartilage.**

cost analysis, an analysis of the disbursements of a given activity, agency, department, or program.

COSTAR /kō′stär/, abbreviation for *COmputer STored Ambulatory Record* system, an on-line interactive computerized information system, accessible via a minicomputer, for the public health field.

cost-benefit ratio, a ratio that represents the relationship of the cost of an activity to the benefit of its outcome or product.

cost cap, *informal.* a limit on the amount of money that an agency, department, or institution may spend.

cost center, a department, division, or other subunit of an institution established within its accounting system so that the income and expenses of the subunit can be separated from the income or expenses of other centers and monitored for cost and benefit.

cost control, the process of monitoring and regulating of the expenditure of funds by an agency or institution. Budgets, reports, and cost-accounting procedures are performed to achieve cost control.

cost effectiveness, the extent to which an activity is thought to be as valuable as it is expensive, as a public-assistance program that gives vouchers for nutritious foods in pregnancy being be cost-effective if it were to prevent the costly incidence of perinatal morbidity.

Costen's syndrome. See **temporomandibular joint pain-dysfunction syndrome.**

costi-, cost-, costo-, a combining form meaning 'pertaining to a rib': *costicartillage, costicervical, costifluous.*

costochondral /kos′təkon′drəl/, of or pertaining to a rib and its cartilage.

costotransverse articulation, any one of 20 gliding joints between the ribs and associated vertebrae, except for the eleventh and twelfth ribs. The five ligaments that associate with each costotransverse joint are the articular capsule, the superior costotransverse ligament, the posterior costotransverse ligament, the ligament of the neck of the rib, and the ligament of the tubercle of the rib.

costovertebral, of or relating to a rib and the vertebral column.

costovertebral angle (CVA), one of two angles that outline a space over the kidneys. The angle is formed by the lateral and downward curve of the lowest rib and the vertical column of the spine itself. CVA tenderness to percussion is a common finding in pyelonephritis and other infections of the kidney and adjacent structures.

Cotazym, a trademark for an enzyme (pancrelipase).

cot death. See **sudden infant death syndrome.**

cotton-mill fever. See **byssinosis.**

cottonmouth, a poisonous pit viper commonly found near water and swamps of the southeastern part of the United States. The symptoms of the bite of a cottonmouth are rapid swelling, severe pain, skin discoloration at bite marks, and weakness. Antivenin and oxygen are the usual treatments. Also called **water moccasin.**

Cotton's fracture, a trimalleolar fracture involving medial, lateral, and posterior malleoli.

cotyledon, one of the visible segments on the maternal surface of the placenta. A typical placenta may have 15 to 28 cotyledons, each consisting of fetal vessels, chorionic villi, and intervillous space.

cotyloid cavity. See **acetabulum.**

cough, a sudden, audible expulsion of air from the lungs. Coughing is preceded by inspiration, the glottis is partially closed, and the accessory muscles of expiration contract to expel the air forcibly from the respiratory passages. Coughing is an essential protective response that serves to clear the lungs, bronchi, or trachea of irritants and secretions or to prevent aspiration of foreign material into the lungs. It is a common symptom of diseases of the chest and larynx. Chronic coughing may be indicative of tuberculosis, lung cancer, bronchiectasis, or bronchitis. Otitis media, subdiaphragmatic irritation, congestive heart failure, and mitral valve disease may be associated with episodes of severe chronic coughing. Coughing is a reflex action that may be induced voluntarily and, to some extent, voluntarily inhibited. The cough-reflex center is located in the medulla of the brain. It responds to stimulation transmitted by the glossopharyngeal or vagus nerve. The reflex is initiated by chemical or mechanic irritation of the pharynx, larynx, or tracheobronchial tree. Because the function of coughing is to clear the respiratory tract of secretions, it is important that the cough bring out accumulated debris. Where it does not, because of weakness or inhibition of the force of the cough caused by pain, instruction and assistance in effective coughing and deep-breathing exercises are required. Persons with chronic coughs may obtain symptomatic relief through environmental controls that reduce irritants in the air and provide humidification. Medication may be supplied to dilate the bronchi, liquefy secretions, and increase expectoration. Rest, increased fluid intake, and adequate nutrition are necessary. Antitussive medications are sometimes prescribed in the treatment of a cough in the absence of mucus or congestion.

cough fracture, any fracture of a rib, usually the fifth or the seventh rib, caused by violent coughing.

coulomb /ko͞o′lōm/, the SI unit of electricity equal to the quantity of charge transferred in 1 second across a conductor in which there is a constant current of 1 ampere, or 1 ampere-second.

Coulomb's law, (in physics) a law stating that the force of attraction or repulsion between two electrically charged bodies is directly proportional to the strength of the electric charges and inversely proportional to the square of the distance between them.

Coulter counter /kōl′tər/, a trademark for an electric device that rapidly identifies, sorts, and counts the various kinds of cells present in a small specimen of blood.

Coumadin, a trademark for an anticoagulant (warfarin sodium).

coumarin /ko͞o′mərin/, an anticoagulant.

■ INDICATIONS: It is prescribed for prophylaxis and treatment of thrombosis and embolism.

■ CONTRAINDICATIONS: Known hypersensitivity to the drug prohibits its use. It is not used in situations where there is a risk of hemorrhage.

■ ADVERSE EFFECTS: The most serious adverse reaction is hemorrhage. Many other drugs interact with this drug to increase or decrease its effect.

count, a computation of the number of objects or elements present per unit of measurement. Kinds of counts include **Addis count, bacteria count, blood count,** and **platelet count.**

counterclaim, (in law) a claim made by a defendant establishing a cause for action in his favor against the plaintiff. The purpose of a counterclaim is to oppose or detract from the plaintiff's claim or complaint.

counterpulsation **1.** the action of a circulatory-assist pumping device synchronized counter to the normal action of the heart. **2.** the process of increasing the intraaortic pressure in diastole by inflation of an intraaortic balloon and deflation of the balloon immediately preceding the next systole.

countershock, (in cardiology) a high-intensity, short-duration electric shock applied to the area of the heart, resulting in total cardiac depolarization. See also **cardioversion, defibrillation.**

countertraction, a force that counteracts the pull of traction, especially in orthopedics, as the force of body weight resulting from the pull of gravity. Orthopedic countertraction may also be obtained by altering the angle of the body force in relation to the pull of traction, as by elevating the foot of the bed with shock blocks to attain Trendelenburg's position. The magnitude of countertraction depends on the amount of force needed to counteract the pull of the traction and is usually developed gradually by methodically changing the position of a patient and by adding or by removing weights from weight hangers.

countertransference, the conscious or unconscious emotional response of a psychotherapist or psychoanalyst to a patient. See also **transference.**

countertransport, the simultaneous transport of two different substances across the same membrane, each in the opposite direction.

coup /ko͞o/, any blow or stroke or the effects of such a blow to the body, usually used with a French word identifying a type of stroke: **1. coup de sabre** /ko͞odəsäb′r(ə)/, a wound resembling a sword cut. **2. coup de soleil.** See **sunstroke. 3. coup sur coup** /ko͞osYrko͞o′/, administration of a drug in small amounts over a short period of time rather than in a single larger dose. **4. contre coup** /kôNtrəko͞o′/, an injury most often associated with a blow to the skull in which the force of the impact is transmitted through the skull bones to the opposite side of the head where the bruise, fracture, or other sign of injury appears.

coupling, **1.** the act of coming together, joining, or pairing. **2.** (in genetics) the situation in linked inheritance in which the nonalleles of two or more mutant genes are located on the same chromosome and are close enough so that they are likely to be inherited together. **3.** (in radiation therapy) the efficiency of transfer of power from an applicator to the treatment site. Compare **repulsion.** See also **cis configuration.**

coupling interval, the interval between the dominant heartbeat and a coupled extrasystole.

courseware, software programs for use in instruction.

Courvoisier's law /ko͝orvô•äzē•äz′/ a statement that the gallbladder is smaller than usual if a gallstone blocks the common bile duct but is dilated if the common bile duct is blocked as a result of a cause other than a gallstone, as cancer of the pancreas.

Couvelaire uterus /ko͞o′vəler′/, a hemorrhagic process in uterine musculature that may accompany severe abruptio placenta. Extravasated blood effuses between the muscle fibrils and under the uterine peritoneum. The uterus takes on a purplish color and does not contract well. Also called **uteroplacental apoplexy.** See also **abruptio placenta.**

Cowling's rule, a method of calculating the approximate pediatric dosage of a drug for a child using this formula: (age at next birthday/24) × adult dose. See also **pediatric dosage.**

Cowper's gland /kou′pərz/, either of two round, pea-sized glands embedded in the urethral sphincter of the male. Normally yellow in color, they consist of several lobes with ducts that join and form a single excretory duct. Also called **bulbourethral gland.** Compare **Bartholin's gland.**

cowpox, a mild infectious disease characterized by a pustular rash, caused by the vaccinia virus transmitted to humans from infected cattle. Cowpox infection usually confers immunity to smallpox, because of the similarity of the variola and vaccinia viruses. See also **smallpox, vaccinia, variola.**

coxa /kok′sə/, *pl.* **coxae,** the hip joint; the head of the femur and the acetabulum of the innominate bone.

coxa adducta, coxa flexa. See **coxa vara.**

coxal articulation, the ball-and-socket joint of the hip, formed by the articulation of the head of the femur into the cup-shaped cavity of the acetabulum. It involves seven ligaments and permits very extensive movements, as flexion, extension, adduction, abduction, circumduction, and rotation. Also called **hip joint.** Compare **shoulder joint.**

coxa magna, an abnormal widening of the head and neck of the femur.

coxa plana. See **Perthes' disease.**

coxa valga, a hip deformity in which the angle formed by the axis of the head and neck of the femur and the axis of its shaft is significantly increased.

coxa vara, a hip deformity in which the angle formed by the axis of the head and neck of the femur and the axis of its shaft is decreased. Also called **coxa adducta, coxa flexa.**

coxa vara luxans, a fissure or crack in the neck of the femur with dislocation of the head, caused by coxa vara.

coxsackievirus /koksak′ē-/, any of 30 serologically different enteroviruses associated with a variety of symptoms and primarily affecting children during warm weather. The coxsackieviruses resemble the virus responsible for poliomyelitis, particularly in size; both are picornaviruses. Among the diseases associated with coxsackievirus infections are herpangina, hand, foot, and mouth disease, epidemic pleurodynia, myocarditis, pericarditis, aseptic meninigitis, and several exanthems. There is no known preventive measure except isolation of infected persons, and the treatment is generally directed toward relief of symptoms. See also **viral infection.**

CPAP, abbreviation for **continuous positive airway pressure.**

CPD, **1.** abbreviation for **cephalopelvic disproportion.** **2.** abbreviation for **childhood polycystic disease.** See **polycystic kidney disease.** **3.** abbreviation for **congenital polycystic disease.** See **polycystic kidney disease.**

CPHA, abbreviation for the **Canadian Public Health Association.**

CPK, abbreviation for *creatinine phosphokinase*. See **Duchenne's muscular dystrophy.**

CPPB, abbreviation for **continuous positive pressure breathing.**

CPPV, abbreviation for **continuous positive pressure ventilation.**

CPR, abbreviation for **cardiopulmonary resuscitation.**

CPRAM, abbreviation for *controlled partial rebreathing anesthesia method*.

CPT, abbreviation for **current procedural terminology.**

cpu, CPU, abbreviation for **central processing unit** of a computer.

Cr, symbol for **chromium.**

CR, abbreviation for *controlled respiration*.

crab louse, a species of body louse, *Phthirus pubis,* that infests the hairs of the genital area and is often transmitted between persons by venereal contact. Also called ***Pediculus pubis, (informal)* crab.** See also **pediculosis.**

cradle cap, a common seborrheic dermatitis of infants consisting of thick, yellow, greasy scales on the scalp. Treatment includes oil or ointment to soften the scales, and frequent shampoos.

cramp, **1.** a spasmodic and often painful contraction of one or more muscles. **2.** a pain resembling a muscular cramp. Kinds of cramps include **cane-cutter's cramp, fireman's cramp, miner's cramp, stoker's cramp,** and **writer's cramp.** See also **charley horse, dysmenorrhea, heat cramp, wryneck.**

-crania, a combining form meaning '(condition of the) skull or head': *diastematocrania, hemicrania, platycrania.*

cranial arachnoid. See **arachnoidea encephali.**

cranial arteritis. See **temporal arteritis.**

cranial nerves, the 12 pairs of nerves emerging from the cranial cavity through various openings in the skull. Beginning with the most anterior, they are designated by Roman numerals and named (I) olfactory, (II) optic, (III) oculomotor, (IV) trochlear, (V) trigeminal, (VI) abducens, (VII) facial, (VIII) acoustic, (IX) glossopharyngeal, (X) vagal, (XI) accessory, (XII) hypoglossal. The cranial nerves are attached to the base of the brain and carry impulses for such functions as smell, vision, ocular movement, pupil contraction, muscular sensibility, general sensibility, mastication, facial expression, glandular secretion, taste, cutaneous sensibility, hearing, equilibrium, swallowing, phonation, tongue movement, head movement, and shoulder movement. Certain cranial nerves, particularly V, VII, and VIII, contain two or more distinct functional components considered as independent nerves by some authorities. In this category the masticatory nerve would be separated from the trigeminal (V), the glossopalatine from the facial (VII), and the equilibrium from the acoustic (VIII), making 15 pairs in all. Some anatomists also classify the terminal nerve as the first cranial. Also called **cerebral nerves.** See also the specific nerves. (Figure, page 298)

cranio-, a combining form meaning 'pertaining to the skull or cranium': *craniobuccal, craniognomy, craniosacral.*

craniocele. See **encephalocele.**

craniodidymus /krā′nē·ōdid′iməs/, a two-headed fetal monster in which the bodies are fused.

craniofacial dysostosis, an abnormal hereditary condition characterized by acrocephaly, exophthalmos, hypertelorism, strabismus, parrot-beaked nose, and hypoplastic maxilla with relative mandibular prognathism. This condition is transmitted as an autosomal dominant trait. See also **dysostosis.**

craniohypophyseal xanthoma /krā′nē·ōhī′pōfiz′ē·əl/, a condition in which cholesterol deposits are formed around the hypophyses of the bones, as in Hand-Schüller-Christian disease.

craniopagus /krā′nē·op′əgəs/, conjoined twins that are united at the heads. Fusion can occur at the frontal, occipital, or parietal regions. Also called **cephalopagus.**

craniopharyngeal /krā′nē·ōfərin′jē·əl/, of or pertaining to the cranium and the pharynx.

craniopharyngioma /krā′nē·ōfərin′jē·ō′mə/, *pl.* **craniopharyngiomas, craniopharyngiomata,** a congenital pituitary tumor, appearing most often in children and adolescents, that arises in cells derived from Rathke's pouch or the hypophyseal stalk. The lesion, a solid or cystic body ranging in size from 1 to 8 cm, may expand into the third ventricle or the temporal lobe, frequently becoming calcified. The tumor may interfere with pituitary function, damage the optic chiasm, disrupt hypothalamic control of the autonomic nervous system, and result in hydrocephalus. Increased intracranial pressure, severe headaches, vomiting, stunted growth, defective vision, irritability, somnolence, and infantile genitalia are often associated with the lesion in children. Development of the tumor after puberty usually results in amenorrhea in women and loss of libido and potency in men. Also called **ameloblastoma, craniopharyngeal duct tumor, pituitary adamantinoma, Rathke's pouch tumor.**

craniostenosis /krā′nē•ōstənō′sis/, a congenital deformity of the skull resulting from premature closure of the sutures between the cranial bones. The severity of the malformation depends on which sutures close, the point in the developmental process the closure occurred, and the success or failure of the other sutures to compensate by expansion. Impaired brain growth may or may not be involved. The most common form of the condition is permanent closure of the sagittal suture with anteroposterior elongation of the skull. Surgery is generally indicated when multiple sutures are fused to relieve cerebral pressure and may be performed for cosmetic reasons. See also **brachycephaly, oxycephaly, plagiocephaly, scaphocephaly.** –**craniostenotic,** *adj.*

craniostosis /krā′nē•ostō′sis/, premature ossification of the sutures of the skull, often associated with other skeletal defects. The sutures close before or soon after birth. If no surgical correction is made, the growth of the skull is inhibited, the head is deformed, and the eyes and brain are often damaged. Also called **craniosynostosis.**

craniotabes /krā′nē•ōtā′bēz/, benign, congenital thinness of the top and back of the skull of a newborn, common because the rate of brain growth exceeds the rate of calcification of the skull during the last month of gestation. The bones feel brittle when pressed by an examiner's fingers. The condition disappears with normal nutrition and growth but may persist in infants who develop rickets.

craniotomy /kran′ē•ot′əmē/, any surgical opening into the skull, performed to relieve intracranial pressure, to control bleeding, or to remove a tumor. X-ray films of the skull are taken preoperatively, and a CAT scan or an electroencephalogram is done to establish the diagnosis. The entire head is shaved and cleansed. Parenteral corticosteroids are given to reduce cerebral edema; mannitol and urea are administered to promote diuresis and decrease intracranial pressure. Narcotics are not given, because they depress cerebral function. Neuroleptic drugs that sedate but do not narcotize the patient may be combined with local anesthesia, or general anesthesia may be given. A semicircular skin incision is made just above the hairline, a series of burr holes are made and connected with a cut, and the flap of bone is removed. The meninges are incised, and the brain is exposed. The flap may be replaced after surgery or left off temporarily to prevent the buildup of pressure from the cerebral edema. Postoperatively, if the cerebral area is involved, the head of the patient's bed is elevated to 45 degrees to

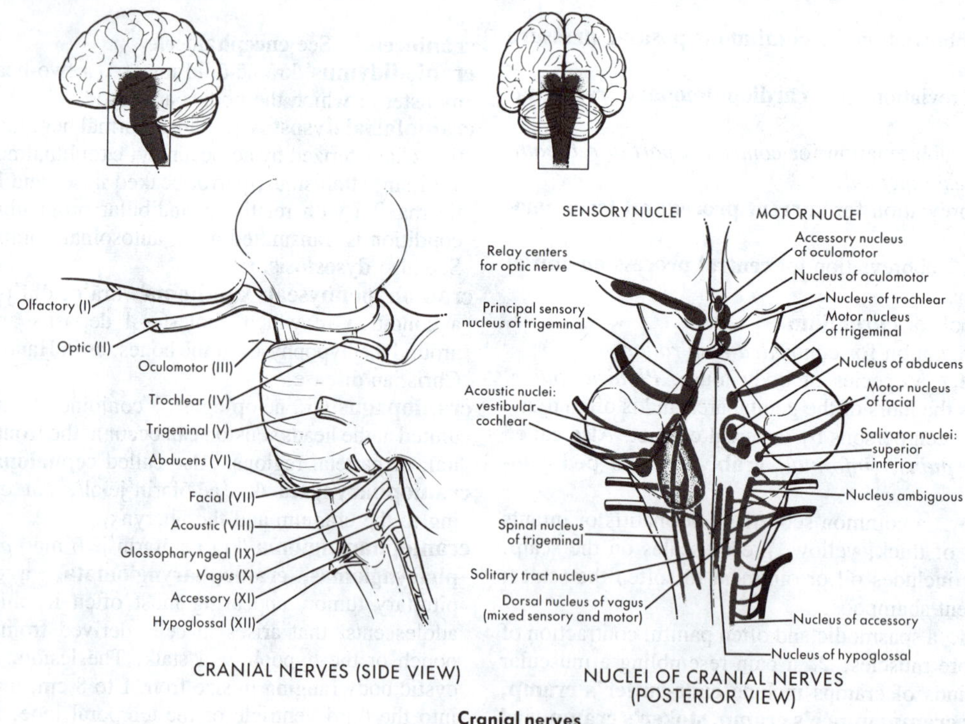

Cranial nerves

reduce the risk of hemorrhage and edema; if the cerebellum or brainstem is affected, the patient is kept flat. The dressing is checked frequently for yellowish drainage of cerebrospinal fluid. Any moist areas are reinforced with sterile materials to avoid infection. Frequent observation of neurologic signs, including the level of consciousness, speech, and strength, is essential.

cranium /krā′nē·əm/, the bony skull that holds the brain. It is composed of eight bones: frontal, occipital, sphenoid, and ethmoid bones, and paired temporal and parietal bones. **–cranial,** *adj.*

-cranium, a combining form meaning 'referring to the skull': *chondrocranium, desmocranium, endocranium.*

crankcase-spool catheter, a special, elastic catheter stored within a plastic spool to facilitate its insertion, especially for hyperalimentation. Most experts recommend the indirect method of venipuncture for insertion of this kind of catheter, usually into a peripheral vein that connects with the subclavian vein. When fully inserted, the crankcase-spool catheter is usually lodged in the subclavian vein. The catheter is highly flexible, and each revolution of the crankcase spool feeds about 5 inches of the catheter into the vein involved. When the crankcase-spool catheter is fully inserted, an x-ray exposure is made of the insertion area to confirm its correct placement. The venipuncture site for insertion is prepared, dressed, and taped in the same manner as any other venipuncture site. The crankcase-spool catheter is less irritating than a regular catheter, allows greater limb movement, and minimizes the risk of thrombosis. It may, however, cause complications, as occlusion, phlebitis, infection, and catheter sensitivity. Occlusion of the vein, a common risk, is usually countered by flushing the vein with dilute streptokinase. If the patient develops phlebitis and receives proper treatment, the catheter may be left in place. Infection, usually evidenced by purulent drainage at the insertion site, is accompanied by an elevated white blood cell count. In cases of such infection the attending physician may order an antibiotic or the removal of the catheter. Catheter sensitivity, evidenced by fever and phlebitis, may require removal of the catheter.

crash, a malfunction of computer hardware or software.

crash cart, a cart carrying emergency equipment, as analgesics, antiseptics, suction devices, sutures, scalpels, surgical needles, sponges, swabs, retractors, hemostats, forceps, trachea tubes, and often a defibrillator. Hospital emergency rooms and intensive care units usually have several crash carts equipped according to prescribed specifications. Efficient, effective emergency care often depends on the careful provisioning of crash carts and the precise knowledge of their layouts.

-crasia, **1.** a combining form meaning '(condition of a) mixture, good or bad': *eucrasia, orthocrasia, spermacrasia.* **2.** a combining form meaning a '(specified) condition involving loss of control': *copracrasia, uracrasia.*

-cratia, a combining form meaning '(condition of) incontinence': *scatacratia, scoracratia, uracratia.*

cravat bandage /krəvat′/, a triangular bandage, folded lengthwise. It may be used as a circular, figure-of-eight, or spiral bandage to control bleeding or to tie splints in place.

crawling reflex. See **symmetric tonic neck reflex.**

C-reactive protein (CRP), a protein not normally detected in the serum but present in many acute inflammatory conditions and with necrosis. CRP appears in the serum before the erythrocyte-sedimentation rate begins to rise, often within 24 to 48 hours of the onset of inflammation. After a myocardial infarction, it is present in 24 hours, begins to fall 3 days later, and is absent after 2 weeks. Acute rheumatic fever is monitored with serial estimations of CRP, as the serum level of the protein is the most sensitive indicator of rheumatic activity. Bacterial infections and widespread neoplastic disease are also associated with C-reactive protein in the serum. CRP disappears when an inflammatory process is suppressed by salicylates and steroids, or both. Also called **serum C-reactive protein.**

cream, **1.** the portion of milk rich in butterfat. **2.** any fluid mixture of thick consistency. Creams are often used as a method of applying medication to the surface of the body. Compare **ointment.**

crease, an indentation or margin formed by a doubling back of tissue, as the folds or creases on the palm of the hand and sole of the foot.

creat-, a combining form meaning 'pertaining to flesh': *creaton, creatorrhea, creatotoxism.*

creatine /krē′ətēn, -tin/, an important nitrogenous compound produced by metabolic processes in the body. Combined with phosphorus, it forms high-energy phosphate. In normal metabolic reactions the phosphorus is yielded to combine with a molecule of adenosine diphosphate to produce a molecule of the very-high-energy molecule adenosine triphosphate. See also **creatinine.**

creatine kinase, an enzyme in muscle, brain, and other tissues that catalyzes the transfer of a phosphate group from adenosine triphosphate to creatine, producing adenosine diphosphate and phosphocreatine.

creatinine /krē·at′inēn, -nin/, a substance formed from the metabolism of creatine, commonly found in blood, urine, and muscle tissue. See also **creatine.**

creatinine phosphokinase. See **Duchenne's muscular dystrophy.**

creatinism /krē·at′iniz′əm/, a condition caused by a congenital absence of the thyroid gland or its secretions.

Crede's prophylaxis, the instillation of a 1% silver-nitrate solution into the conjunctiva of newborn infants to prevent ophthalmia neonatorum

creeping eruption, a skin lesion characterized by irregular, wandering red lines made by the burrowing larvae of hookworms and certain roundworms. Infestation occurs when people walk barefoot where these parasites are known to be endemic. Antiparasitic treatment is specific to the organism. Also called **larva migrans.**

cremaster /krimas′tər/, a thin, muscular layer spreading out over the spermatic cord in a series of loops. It is a continuation of the obliquus internus. The muscle arises from the inguinal ligament and inserts into the crest of the pubis and into the sheath of the rectus abdominis. It is innervated by the genital branch of the genitofemoral nerve and functions to draw the testis up toward the superficial inguinal ring in response to cold or to stimulation of the nerve.

cremasteric reflex /krē′məster′ik/, a superficial neural reflex elicited by stroking the skin of the upper inner aspect of the thigh in a male. This normally results in a brisk retraction of the testis on the side of the stimulus. The reflex is lost in diseases of the pyramidal tract above the level of the first lumbar vertebra. See also **superficial reflex.**

crenation /krinā′shən/, the formation of notches or leaflike, scalloped edges on an object. Red blood cells exposed to a hypertonic saline solution acquire a notched, shriveled surface because of the osmotic effect of the solution. They are then called crenated red blood cells. **–crenate, crenated,** *adj.*

creosote poisoning. See **phenol poisoning.**

crepitus /krep′itəs/, **1.** flatulence or the noisy discharge of fetid gas from the intestine through the anus. **2.** a sound that resembles the crackling noise heard when rubbing hair between the fingers or throwing salt on an open fire. Crepitus is associated with gas gangrene, the rubbing of bone fragments, or the rales of a consolidated area of the lung in pneumonia. Also called **crepitation.**

cresc-, a combining form meaning 'to grow': *crescograph.*

crescendo angina, a form of anginal discomfort associated with ischemic electrocardiographic changes, marked by increased frequency, provocation, intensity, or character.

cresol /krē′sol/, a colorless to yellow-brown liquid obtained from coal tar. It is similar to phenol but is not as poisonous. It is used as an antiseptic and disinfectant.

CREST syndrome /krest/, abbreviation for **calcinosis, Raynaud's phenomenon, esophageal dysfunction, sclerodactyly,** and **telangiectasis,** which may occur for varying periods of time in patients with scleroderma.

cretin dwarf /krē′tən/, a person in whom short stature is caused by infantile hypothyroidism and severe deficiency of thyroid hormone. Also called **hypothyroid dwarf.** See also **cretinism.**

cretinism /krē′təniz′əm/, a condition characterized by severe congenital hypothyroidism and often associated with other endocrine abnormalities. Typical signs of cretinism include dwarfism, mental deficiency, puffy facial features, dry skin, a large tongue, umbilical hernia, and muscular incoordination. The disorder occurs usually in areas where the diet is deficient in iodine and where goiter is endemic. Early treatment with thyroid hormone generally promotes normal physical growth but may not prevent mental retardation. The use of iodized salt dramatically reduces the incidence of cretinism in a population. The condition is rare in the United States, but in some areas, including parts of Ecuador, the Himalayas, and Zaire, more than 5% of the people are cretins. See also **familial cretinism. –cretinoid, cretinous,** *adj.,* **cretin,** *n.*

Creutzfeldt-Jakob disease /kroits′feltyä′kôp/, a rare, fatal encephalopathy caused by an as yet unidentified slow virus. The disease occurs in middle age, and symptoms are progressive dementia, dysarthria, muscle wasting, and various involuntary movements, as myoclonus and athetosis. Deterioration is obvious week to week. Death ensues, usually within a year. Transmission between humans is unusual, but the disease has been observed years after exposure to needles, instruments, and electrodes previously used in the treatment of a patient with the disease. Isolation is not necessary. Special care in disposal or sterilization of potentially infective items is always necessary. Also called **Jakob-Creutzfeldt disease, spastic pseudoparalysis, spastic pseudosclerosis.**

crib death. See **sudden infant death syndrome.**

cribriform carcinoma. See **adenocystic carcinoma.**

crico-, a combining form meaning 'ring': *cricoderma, cricoid, cricoidectomy.*

cricoid /krī′koid/, **1.** having a ring shape. **2.** a ring-shaped cartilage connected to the thyroid cartilage by the cricothyroid ligament at the level of the sixth cervical vertebra.

cricoid pressure, a technique to reduce the risk of the aspiration of stomach contents during induction of general anesthesia. The cricoid cartilage is pushed against the esophagus to prevent passive regurgitation. The technique cannot, however, stop vomiting that has begun. Cricoid pressure is applied before intubation, immediately after injection of the anesthetic drug or muscle relaxant.

cricopharyngeal /krī′kōfərin′jē·əl/, of or pertaining to the cricoid cartilage and the pharynx.

cricopharyngeal incoordination, a defect in the normal swallowing reflex. The cricopharyngeus muscle ordinarily serves as a sphincter to keep the top of the esophagus closed except when the person is swallowing, vomiting, or belching. The trachea remains open for breathing, but air normally does not enter the esophagus during respiration. In swallowing, the reverse effect occurs and the larynx is closed while food slides past it into the esophagus, which is located immediately behind the larynx. When the somewhat complex series of neuromuscular actions is not properly coordinated as a result of disease or injury, the patient may choke, swallow air, regurgitate fluid into the nose, or experience discomfort in swallowing food. See also **dysphagia.**

cricothyrotomy /krī′kōthīrot′əmē/, an emergency incision into the larynx, performed to open the airway in a person who is choking. A small vertical midline cut is made just below the Adam's apple and above the cricoid cartilage. The incision is opened further with a transverse cut through the cricothyroid membrane, and the wound is spread open with a knife handle or other dilator. The new opening must be held open with a tube that is open at both ends to allow air to move in and out. The cartridge end of a ballpoint pen will suffice until a tracheostomy can be done. Compare **tracheostomy.**

cri-du-chat syndrome. See **cat-cry syndrome.**

Crigler-Najjar syndrome /krig′lərnaj′är/, a congenital, familial, autosomal anomaly, in which glucuronyl transferase, an enzyme, is deficient or absent. The condition is characterized by nonhemolytic jaundice, an accumulation of unconjugated bilirubin in the blood, and severe disorders of the central nervous system. See also **hyperbilirubinemia of the newborn.**

Crimean-Congo hemorrhagic fever /krīmē′ən/, an arbovirus infection transmitted to humans through the bite of a tick, characterized by fever, dizziness, muscle ache, vomiting, headache, and other neurologic symptoms. After several days, in severe cases, bleeding from the skin and mucous membranes, particularly from the mouth and nose, bloody sputum or vomit, and blood-tinged feces may be seen. Transfusion may be necessary to replace lost blood; otherwise, treatment is symptomatic and supportive. There is no specific medication or therapy available for prevention or cure. It occurs mainly in the U.S.S.R., Asia, and Africa; agricultural workers are most often afflicted. See also **hemorrhagic fever, Omsk hemorrhagic fever.**

criminal abortion, the intentional termination of pregnancy under any condition prohibited by law. See also **induced abortion.**

criminal psychology, the study of the mental processes, motivational patterns, and behavior of criminals.

crin-, a combining form meaning 'to separate': *crinin, crinogenic.*

-crinia, a combining form meaning '(condition of) endocrine secretion': *hemocrinia, hypercrinia, neurocrinia.*

-crisia, **1.** a combining form meaning a 'diagnosis': *acrisia, urocrisia.* **2.** a combining form meaning a '(specified) condition of endocrine secretion': *hypercrisia, hyperendocrisia, hypocrisia.*

crisis, **1.** a turning point for better or worse in the course of a disease, usually indicated by a marked change in the intensity of signs and symptoms. A crisis may be celiac, marked by an attack of watery diarrhea and vomiting leading, in turn, to dehydration; hepatic, characterized by intense pain in the region of the liver; or ocular, manifested by eye pain, a flow of tears, and sensitivity to light. **2.** a turning point in events affecting the emotional state of a person, as death or divorce. See also **crisis intervention.**

crisis intervention, (in psychiatry) therapeutic intervention to help resolve a particular and immediate problem. No attempt is made at in-depth analysis. The goal is to restore in the person the level of functioning that existed before the current crisis.

crisis-intervention unit, a group trained in emergency medical treatment and in various methods for rendering psychiatric therapeutic assistance to a person or group of persons during a period of crisis, especially instances involving suicide attempts or drug abuse. Such networks are found within community hospitals, health care centers, or as specialized self-contained units, as suicide-prevention centers, and operate 24 hours a day. The primary objective of such crisis assistance is to help the person cope with the immediate problem and to offer guidance and support for long-term therapy.

crisis theory, a conceptual framework for defining and explaining the phenomena that occur when a person faces a problem that appears to be insoluble. The theory is the basis of crisis therapy.

crisscross inheritance, the acquisition of genetic characteristics or conditions from the parent of the opposite sex.

crista supraventricularis /kris′tə so͞o′prəven′trik′-yəler′is/, the muscular ridge on the interior dorsal wall of the right ventricle of the heart. It defines the limit of the arterial cone and extends toward the pulmonary trunk from the ventral cusp of the atrioventricular ring. Compare **moderator band.**

critical care. See **intensive care.**

critical organs, tissues that are the most sensitive to irradiation, as the gonads, lymphoid organs, and intestine. The skin, cornea, oral cavity, esophagus, vagina, cervix, and optic lens are the next most sensitive organs to irradiation.

CRNA, abbreviation for **certified registered nurse anesthetist.** See also **nurse anesthetist.**

Crohn's disease, a chronic inflammatory bowel disease of unknown origin, usually affecting the ileum, the colon, or both structures. Diseased segments may be separated by normal bowel segments. Also called **regional enteritis.** Compare **ulcerative colitis.** See also **colitis, ileitis.**

■ OBSERVATIONS: Crohn's disease is characterized by frequent attacks of diarrhea, severe abdominal pain, nausea, fever, chills, weakness, anorexia, and weight loss. Children with the disease often suffer retarded physical growth. The diagnosis of Crohn's disease is based on clinical signs, x-ray studies using a contrast medium, and endoscopy. The disease is easily confused with ulcerative colitis, which is also an inflammatory bowel disease affecting the colon and rectum.

■ INTERVENTION: Corticosteroids, antibiotics, and antiinflammatory agents are used to control symptoms and to attempt to induce remission. In patients who are malnourished because of the disease, intravenous hyperalimentation is used to ensure adequate intake of nutrients and to rest the bowel. Surgical removal of the diseased segment of the bowel provides some relief, but recurrence after surgery is likely.

■ NURSING CONSIDERATIONS: In many cases the inflammation extends to other areas of the bowel or to the stomach, duodenum, or mouth. Other complications are arthritis, ankylosing spondylitis, kidney and liver disease, and skin and eye disorders. The formation of fistulas from the diseased bowel to the anus, vagina, skin surface, or to other loops of bowel are common. Persons with Crohn's disease are hospitalized frequently and often become depressed because of the relentless, painful character of the disease. Continued support and encouragement are essential in helping the patient maintain a hopeful outlook.

Comparison of Crohn's disease and ulcerative colitis

	Crohn's disease	*Ulcerative colitis*
General appearance	Usually normal	May feel and look ill
Age	Bimodal: 20-30 yr and 40-50 yr	Mostly young adults
Area affected	Mainly terminal ileum, cecum, and ascending colon (right side)	Colon only, primarily the descending colon (left side)
Extent of involvement	Segmental areas of involvement	Continuous, diffuse areas of involvement
Inflammation	Mostly submucosal	Mostly mucosal
Mucosal appearance	Cobblestone effect; granulomas	Ulcerations
Cancer potential	Normal incidence	Increased incidence
Character of stools	No blood; may have some fat; three to four semisoft per day	Blood present; no fat; frequent liquid stools
Reasons for surgery	Fistulas; intestinal obstruction	Poor response to medical therapy; hemorrhage; perforation
Complications	Fistulas; perianal disease; strictures; vitamin and iron dificiencies; fistulas to other organs	Pseudopolyps; hemorrhage; toxic megacolon; cachexia; perforation less often, causes peritonitis

cromoglycic acid. See **cromolyn sodium.**

cromolyn sodium, an antiasthmatic that acts by decreasing allergic bronchospasm resulting from an inhaled allergen.

■ INDICATION: It is prophylactically prescribed in the treatment of bronchial asthma. The drug has no effect after an attack has begun.

■ CONTRAINDICATION: Known hypersensitivity to this drug prohibits its use.

■ ADVERSE EFFECTS: Bronchospasm, wheezing, nasal congestion, pharyngeal irritation, and other hypersensitivity reactions may occur.

Cronkhite-Canada syndrome, an abnormal familial condition characterized by GI polyposis accompanied by ectodermal defects, as nail atrophy, alopecia, and excessive skin pigmentation. In some individuals it is also accompanied by protein-losing enteropathy, malabsorption, and deficiency of blood calcium, potassium, and magnesium.

cross, (in genetics) any method of crossbreeding or any individual, organism, or strain produced from crossbreeding. Kinds of crosses include **dihybrid cross, monohybrid cross, polyhybrid cross,** and **trihybrid cross.**

cross-bite tooth, any of the posterior teeth that allow the modified buccal cusps of the upper teeth to be positioned in the central fossae of the lower teeth.

crossbreeding, the production of offspring by the mating of plants and animals from different varieties, strains, or species; hybridization. See also **inbreeding.** **–crossbred,** *adj.*

crossed grid, (in radiography) an assembly of two parallel x-ray grids that may be rotated at right angles to each other. See also **grid.**

crossed reflex, any neural reflex in which stimulation of one side of the body results in a response on the other side, as the consensual light reflex.

cross-eye. See **esophoria.**

cross fertilization, 1. (in zoology), the union of gametes from different species or varieties to form hybrids. **2.** (in botany) the fertilization of the flower of one plant by the pollen from a different plant, as opposed to self-fertilization. Also called **allogamy.**

crossing over, the exchange of sections of chromatids between homologous pairs of chromosomes during the prophase stage of the first meiotic division. The process occurs through the formation of chiasmata and results in the recombination of genes. Also called **chiasmatypy.**

crossmatching of blood, a procedure used by blood banks to determine compatibility of a donor's blood with that of a recipient after the specimens have been matched for major blood type. Serum from the donor's blood is mixed with red cells from the recipient's blood, and cells from the donor are mixed with serum from the recipient. If agglutination occurs, an antigenic substance is present and the bloods are not compatible. If no agglutination occurs, the donor's blood may safely be transfused to the recipient. Compare **blood typing.** See also **ABO blood groups, Rh factor, transfusion, transfusion reaction.**

crossover, the result of the recombination of genes on homologous pairs of chromosomes during meiosis. See also **crossing over.**

cross-sectional, (in statistics) pertaining to the comparative data of two groups of persons at one point in time.

cross-sectional anatomy, the study of the relationship of the structures of the body by the examination of cross sections of the tissue or organ. Compare **surface anatomy.**

cross-sequential, (in statistics) pertaining to data that compare several cohorts at different points in time.

crotamiton, a scabicide.

■ INDICATIONS: It is prescribed in treating scabies and other pruritic skin diseases.

■ CONTRAINDICATIONS: Known hypersensitivity to this drug prohibits its use. It is not applied near the eyes or on the mouth or raw skin.

■ ADVERSE EFFECTS: Among the most serious adverse reactions are irritation and allergic reactions of the skin.

croup /kro͞op/, an acute viral infection of the upper and lower respiratory tract that occurs primarily in infants and young children 3 months to 3 years of age after an upper respiratory tract infection. It is characterized by hoarseness, fever, a distinctive harsh, brassy cough, persistent stridor during inspiration, and varying degrees of respiratory distress resulting from obstruction of the larynx. The most common causative agents are the parainfluenza viruses, especially type 1, followed by the respiratory syncytial viruses (RSV) and influenza A and B viruses. Also called **acute laryngotracheobronchitis (LTB), angina trachealis, exudative angina, laryngostasis.** Compare **acute epiglottitis.** **–croupous, croupy,** *adj.*

■ OBSERVATIONS: Transmission occurs by infection with airborne particles or by contact with infected secretions. Leukocytosis with an increased proportion of polymorphonuclear cells may be present at first, followed by leukopenia and lymphocytosis. A lateral neck x-ray film shows subepiglottic narrowing and a normal-sized epiglottis, which differentiate the condition from acute epiglottitis. Onset of the acute stage is rapid, usually occurs at night, and may be preciptated by exposure to cold air. The child becomes irritable, develops stridor, dyspnea, tachypnea, the characteristic barking cough, and, in severe cases, cyanosis or pallor. The child's condition often improves in the morning, but it may worsen at night.

■ INTERVENTION: Routine treatment consists of bed rest, adequate fluid intake, and the alleviation of airway obstruction to ensure adequate respiratory exchange. Children with mild infections are usually managed at home with supportive measures, as vaporizers, humidifiers, or steam from hot running water in an enclosed bathroom to reduce the spasm of the laryngeal muscles and to free secretions. Hospitalization is indicated for children with high temperatures, progressive stridor and respiratory distress, and hypoxia, cyanosis, or pallor. Endotracheal intubation and tracheostomy may be necessary. Humidity and oxygen are usually prescribed. The vital signs are continuously monitored; a change in pulse and respiration may be early signs of hypoxia and impending airway obstruction. Arterial blood gas analysis is performed. Fluids are often given intravenously to reduce physical exertion and the possibility of vomiting, with its attendant increased risk of aspiration. Corticosteroids or other drugs, as expectorants, bronchodilators, and antihistamines, are rarely used, and sedatives are contraindicated, because they exert a depressant effect on the respiratory tract. Nebulized racemic epinephrine, administered diluted with water by a face-mask aerosol, may provide temporary relief in the acute phase in some children.

■ NURSING CONSIDERATIONS: The primary focus of nursing care is to ease breathing by providing humidity and to maintain continuous monitoring and surveillance for signs of respiratory distress and impending airway obstruction, with intubation and tracheostomy equipment kept readily available. To conserve the child's energy and to reduce apprehension, the nurse encourages rest, disturbs the child as little as possible, remains in constant attendance, provides comfort with a familiar toy or other device, and encourages parental involvement whenever possible. Fever is usually reduced by the cool atmosphere of the mist tent; antipyretics are given as needed. To prevent chilling, frequent changes of clothing and bed linen are often necessary in the humid environment. The nurse also explains the condition to the parents and discusses appropriate care after discharge, including continued use of humidity and ensurance of adequate hydration and proper nutrition. In most children the condition is relatively mild and runs its course in 3 to 7 days. The infection may spread to other areas of the respiratory tract and may cause complications, as bronchiolitis, pneumonia, and otitis media. The most serious complication is laryngeal obstruction, which may cause death. If a tracheostomy is required, as may happen with a small percentage of children, other complications, as infection, atelectasis, cannula occlusion, tracheal bleeding, granulation, stenosis, and delayed healing of the stoma, may develop.

Croupette /kro͞opet′/, a trademark for a device that provides cool humidification with the administration of oxygen or of compressed air, used especially in the treatment of pediatric patients. The Croupette consists of a nebulizer with attached tubing that connects with a canopy to enclose the patient and contain the humidifying mist. The environment of the patient may be cooled by adding ice to the ice compartment or by using a Croupette with its own refrigeration unit. This device is especially used with pediatric patients from 1 month to 10 years of age to relieve hypoxia, liquefy secretions, and cool the environment of the patient. It is also often used in the treatment of the croup, bronchiolitis, cystic fibrosis, asthma, laryngitis, postoperative dehydration, and hyperpyrexia. The oxygen concentration obtainable is approximately 21% to 60%. Nursing care associated with this device usually involves assembling the unit, ensuring proper water level in the nebulizer, and adjusting the oxygen flow rate. The flow rate may be adjusted from 6 L to 10 L per minute or according to equipment specifications. Explaining the equipment and the humidifying treatment also helps reassure the patient. Precautions in using the Croupette with a patient receiving periodic therapy involve ensuring that the flow of oxygen or compressed air is turned on when the canopy is placed over the patient and that the patient is carefully monitored throughout the therapy period. Some of the advantages of the Croupette are its capability for providing a cool, moist environment, its adaptability for the delivery of oxygen or the delivery of compressed air, and the ease of canopy installation. Croupette canopies are disposable. Some of the limitations associated with the device are that some Croupette units have awkward, bulky frames; nebulizer water reservoirs are usually small and require constant refilling; periodic refills of ice are required; and excess humidity may wet the bed linen and the patient.

crown, **1.** the upper part of an organ or structure, as the top of the head. **2.** the portion of a human tooth that is covered by enamel.

crowning, (in obstetrics) the phase at the end of labor in which the fetal head is seen at the introitus of the vagina. The labia are stretched in a crown around the head just before delivery.

crown/root ratio, the relation of the clinical crown to the clinical root of a tooth.

CRP, abbreviation for **C-reactive protein.**

CRT, abbreviation for **cathode-ray tube.**

crucial bandage. See **T bandage.**

cruciate ligament of the atlas, a crosslike ligament attaching the atlas to the base of the occipital bone above and the posterior surface of the body of the axis below.

crude birth rate, the number of births per 1000 people in a population during 1 year. Compare **birth rate, refined birth rate, true birth rate.**

crur-, a combining form meaning 'pertaining to the leg': *crura, crural, crureus.*

crura anthelicis /kro͝or′ə anthel′isis/, the two ridges on the external ear marking the superior termination of the anthelix and bounding the triangular fossa. Also called **crura of anthelix.**

crureus. See **vastus intermedius.**

crus /krus/, *pl.* **crura** /kro͝or′ə/, **1.** the leg, from knee to foot. **2.** a structure resembling a leg, as crura anthelicis.

crus cerebri /ser′əbrī, -brē/, the ventral part of the cerebral peduncle, composed of the descending fiber tracts passing from the cerebral cortex to form the longitudinal fascicles of the pons. Also called **basis pedunculi cerebri.**

crush syndrome, **1.** a severe, life-threatening condition caused by extensive crushing trauma, characterized by destruction of muscle and bone tissue, hemorrhage, and fluid loss resulting in hypovolemic shock, hematuria, renal failure, and coma. Massive supportive therapy, with fluids, electrolytes, antibiotics, analgesia, oxygen, and intensive care with close monitoring of all vital functions are usually necessary. **2.** a severe complication of heroin-induced coma characterized by edema, vascular occlusion, and lymphatic obstruction.

crust, a solidified, hard outer layer formed by the drying of a bodily exudate, common in such dermatologic conditions as eczema, impetigo, seborrhea, and favus, and during the healing of burns and lesions; a scab.

crutch, a wooden or metal staff, the most common kind of which reaches from the ground almost to the axilla, to aid a person in walking. A padded, curved surface at the top fits under the arm; a grip in the form of a crossbar is held in the hand at the level of the palms to support the body. It is important that the person be taught how to use the crutches safely and how to achieve a stable and acceptable gait. Kinds of crutches include **axillary crutches, forearm crutches.**

Crutchfield tongs, an instrument inserted into the skull to hyperextend the head and neck of patients with fractured cervical vertebrae.

■ METHOD: The tongs are inserted into small bur holes drilled in each parietal region of the skull; the surrounding skin is sutured and covered with a collodion dressing. A weight of from 10 to 20 pounds is suspended from a rope extending from the center of the tongs, over a pulley attached to head of the bed allowing the weights to hang freely. The insertion sites of the tongs are inspected and cleaned every 1 to 2 hours; any formed crusts are removed with hydrogen peroxide twice a day or as required. The patient is turned and assisted in deep breathing every other hour and is given scalp and skin care every 2 to 4 hours. The bed linen is kept dry and smooth, an air mattress or sheepskin is used, and back rubs are administered to prevent decubiti, especially of the scapulae, coccyx, and heels. Passive range-of-motion exercises of all extremities are performed. Sandbags may be used to prevent the patient from sliding to the head of the bed, and the call bell is placed within easy reach. The immobilized patient receives food that is easy to swallow and is fed with care to prevent aspiration into the trachea; suction apparatus is kept at the bedside as an emergency measure.

■ NURSING ORDERS: The nurse maintains the patient's body alignment, checks the weight and traction apparatus, administers meticulous skin care, feeds the patient, and provides for other care as necessary.

■ OUTCOME CRITERIA: A patient may be immobilized by Crutchfield tongs for weeks before surgery is performed; during an operation on the cervical spine and cord, the tongs may be left in place for proper alignment.

crutch gait, a gait achieved by a person on crutches by alternately bearing weight on one or both legs and on the crutches. The gait selected and learned is determined by physical and functional abilities of the patient and on the diagnosis. In a three-point gait, weight is borne on the noninvolved leg, then on both crutches, then on the noninvolved leg. Touchdown and progression to full-weight bearing on the involved leg are usual. Four-point gait gives stability but requires bearing weight on both legs. Each leg is used alternately with each crutch. Two-point gait characteristically uses each crutch with the opposing leg. The swing-to and swing-through gaits are often used by paraplegic patients with weight-supporting braces on the legs. Weight is borne on the supported legs; the crutches are placed one stride in front of the person who then swings to that point or through the crutches to a spot in front of them.

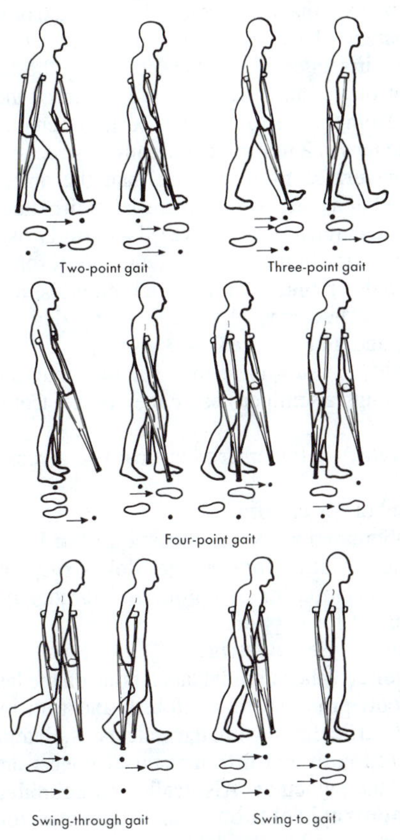

Crutch gaits

Cruz trypanosomiasis. See **Chagas' disease.**

cry, **1.** a sudden, loud, voluntary, or automatic vocalization in response to pain, fear, or a startle reflex. **2.** weeping, because of pain or as an emotional response to depression or grief. **3.** See **cri-du-chat syndrome.**

cryo-, cry-, crymo-, a combining form meaning 'pertaining to cold': *cryocautery, cryophilia, cryotolerant.*

cryoanesthesia /krī'ō·an'isthē'zhə/, the freezing of a part to achieve adequate deadening of neural sensitivity to pain during brief minor surgical procedures.

cryocautery /krī'ōkô'tərē/, the application of any substance, as solid carbon dioxide, that destroys tissue by freezing. Also called **cold cautery.**

cryogen /krī'əjən/, a chemical that induces freezing, used to destroy diseased tissue without injury to adjacent structures. Cell death is caused by dehydration after cell membranes rupture. Kinds of cryogens include **carbon dioxide, freon, liquid nitrogen,** and **nitrous oxide.** –**cryogenic,** *adj.*

cryoglobulin /krī'ōglob'yo͞olin/, an abnormal plasma protein that precipitates and coalesces at low temperatures and dissolves and disperses at body temperature.

cryoglobulinemia /krī'ōglob'yo͞olinē'mē·ə/, an abnormal condition in which cryoglobulins are present in the blood. Cryoglobulins may be found associated with multiple myeloma and angioneurotic edema.

cryonics /krī·on'iks/, the techniques in which cold is applied for a variety of therapeutic goals, including brief local anesthesia, destruction of superficial skin lesions, and preservation of cells, tissue, organs, or the entire body. –**cryonic,** *adj.*

cryoprecipitate. **1.** any precipitate formed upon cooling a solution. **2.** a preparation rich in factor VIII needed to restore normal coagulation in hemophilia. It is collected from fresh human plasma that has been frozen and thawed.

cryostat, a device used in surgical pathology that consists of a special microtome used for freezing and slicing sections of tissue for study by a surgical pathologist.

cryosurgery, use of subfreezing temperature to destroy tissue, as in the destruction of the ganglion of nerve cells in the thalamus in the treatment of Parkinson's disease, in the destruction of the pituitary gland to halt the progress of some kinds of metastatic cancer, and in the treatment of various cancers and lesions of the skin. The process is also used in ophthalmology to cause the edges of a detached retina to heal and to remove cataracts. The coolant is circulated through a metal probe, chilling it to as low as −160° C, depending on the chemical used. The moist tissues adhere to the cold metal of the probe and freeze. Cells are dehydrated as their membranes burst; they are eventually discarded or absorbed by the body. No specific postoperative nursing care is required.

cryotherapy /krī·ōther'əpē/, a treatment using cold as a destructive medium. Cutaneous tags, warts, condylomata acuminatum, actinic keratosis, and dermatofibromas are some of the common skin disorders amenable to cryotherapy. Solid carbon dioxide or liquid nitrogen are applied briefly with a sterile cotton-tipped applicator. A blister forms, followed by necrosis. The procedure may be repeated.

crypt, a blind pit or tube on a free surface. Some kinds of crypts are **anal crypt, dental crypt,** and **synovial crypt.**

crypt-. See **crypto-.**

cryptitis /kriptī'tis/, an inflammation of a crypt, usually a perianal crypt, often accompanied by pain, pruritus, and spasm of the sphincter. Treatment may include hot compresses, sitz baths, antibiotics, or excision.

crypto-, crypt-, krypto-, a combining form meaning 'hidden': *cryptocephalus, cryptocrystalline, cryptodidymus.*

cryptocephalus /krip'tōsef'ələs/, a malformed fetus that has a small, underdeveloped head. –**cryptocephalic, cryptocephalous,** *adj.,* **cryptocephaly,** *n.*

cryptococcosis /krip'tōkokō'sis/, an infectious disease caused by a fungus, *Cryptococcus neoformans,* which spreads through the lungs to the brain and central nervous system, skin, skeletal system, and urinary tract. The disease occurs in all parts of the world, but in North America it is most likely to afflict middle-aged men in the southeastern states. It is characterized by the development of nodules or tumors filled with a gelatinous material in visceral and subcutaneous tissues. Initial symptoms may include coughing or other respiratory effects because the lungs are a primary site of infection. After the fungus spreads to the meninges, neurologic symptoms may develop, including headache, blurred vision, and difficulty in speaking. The diagnosis is made by isolation and identification of the fungus in specimens of sputum, pus, or tissue biopsy. Amphotericin B and flucytosine may be administered to control the infection. Also called **Buschke's disease, European blastomycosis, torulosis.** See also ***Cryptococcus,*** and see specific fungal infections.

Cryptococcus, a genus of yeastlike fungi that reproduces by budding rather than by producing spores. Many nonpathogenic species of *Cryptococcus* are commonly found in the soil and on the skin and mucous membranes of people who are well. Certain pathogenic species exist; *C. neoformans* is the most important. See also **fungus, yeast.**

Cryptococcus neoformans, a species of yeastlike fungus that causes cryptococcosis, a potentially fatal infection that can affect the lungs, skin, and brain.

cryptodidymus /krip′tōdid′əməs/, conjoined twins in which one fetus is small, underdeveloped, and concealed within the body of the other, more fully formed autosite.

crypt of iris, any one of the small pits in the iris along its free margin encircled by the circulus arteriosus minor. Also called **crypt of Fuchs.**

cryptomenorrhea /krip′tōmenôrē′ə/, an abnormal condition in which the products of menstruation are retained within the vagina because of an imperforate hymen, or, less often, within the uterus because of an occlusion of the cervical canal. Cryptomenorrhea is usually accompanied by subjective symptoms of menstruation with scant or absent flow and sometimes by severe pain. If the flow is completely obstructed, uterotubal reflux of menstrual flow into the pelvic cavity may cause peritonitis, pain, adhesions, and endometriosis. **–cryptomenorrheal,** *adj.*

cryptophthalmos /krip′təfthal′məs/, a developmental anomaly characterized by complete fusion of the eyelids, usually with defective formation or lack of the eyes.

cryptorchidism /kriptôr′kidiz′əm/, failure of one or both of the testicles to descend into the scrotum. If spontaneous descent does not occur by the age of 1 year, hormonal injections may be given. If not successful, surgery, called orchipexy, will likely be performed before the boy is 5 years of age. Also called **undescended testis.**

crystal, a solid inorganic substance, the atoms or molecules of which are arranged in a regular, repeating three-dimensional pattern, which determines the shape of a crystal. **–crystalline,** *adj.*

crystalline lens /kris′təlin, -līn/, a transparent structure of the eye, enclosed in a capsule, situated between the iris and the vitreous humor, and slightly overlapped at its margin by the ciliary processes. The capsule of the lens is a transparent, elastic membrane that touches the free border of the iris anteriorly and is secured by the suspensory ligament of the lens. The circumference of the capsule recedes from the iris to form the posterior chamber of the eye. The lens is a transparent biconvex structure with the posterior surface more convex than the anterior. It is composed of a soft, cortical material, a firm nucleus, and concentric laminae and is covered anteriorly by transparent epithelium. In the fetus the lens is very soft and has a slightly reddish tint; in the adult it is colorless and firm; in old age it becomes flattened, more dense, slightly opaque, and amber-tinted. See also **eye.**

crystalloid, a substance in a solution that can be diffused through a semipermeable membrane. Compare **colloid.**

Crystodigin, a trademark for a cardiac glycoside (digitoxin).

Cs, symbol for **cesium.**

CSF, abbreviation for **cerebrospinal fluid.**

CSR, abbreviation for **Cheyne-Stokes respiration.**

CT, abbreviation for **computerized tomography.**

Cu, symbol for **copper.**

Cuban itch. See **alastrim.**

cuboid bone, the cuboidal tarsal bone on the lateral side of the foot, proximal to the fourth and fifth metatarsal bones. It articulates with the calcaneus, lateral cuneiform, and fourth and fifth metatarsal bones, and, occasionally, the navicular. Also called **os cuboideum.**

cuffed endotracheal tube, an endotracheal tube with a balloon at one end that may be inflated to tighten the fit of the tube in the lumen of the airway. The balloon forms a cuff that prevents gastric contents from passing into the lungs and gas from leaking back from the lungs. Hard or soft cuffs are in use. The pressure of a cuffed tube often causes sore throat after general anesthesia. In patients with tracheitis, arteriosclerosis, or general debility, overinflation of the cuff can cause contusion, hemorrhage, mucosal sloughing, or rupture.

cul-de-sac /kul′dəsak, kYdesok′/, *pl.* **culs-de-sac, cul-de-sacs,** a blind pouch or cecum, as the conjunctival cul-de-sac and the dural cul-de-sac.

cul-de-sac of Douglas, a pouch formed by the caudal portion of the parietal peritoneum. Also called **pouch of Douglas, rectouterine excavation, rectouterine pouch.**

Cullen's sign, the appearance of faint, irregularly formed hemorrhagic patches on the skin around the umbilicus. The discolored skin is blue-black and becomes greenish-brown or yellow. Cullen's sign may appear 1 to 2 days after the onset of anorexia and the severe, poorly localized abdominal pains that are characteristic of acute pancreatitis. Cullen's sign is also present in massive upper GI hemorrhage and ruptured ectopic pregnancy. Compare **Grey Turner's sign.** See also **pancreatitis.**

culture-bound, pertaining to a health condition that is specific to a particular culture, as a belief in the effects of certain kinds prayer or the "evil eye."
culture medium. See **medium.**
culture procedure, (in bacteriology) any of several techniques for growing colonies of microorganisms to identify a pathogen and to determine which antibiotics are effective in combating the infection caused by the organism. Usually, a specimen is secured and a small amount is placed in or on one or more culture media, because different organisms are nourished by different nutrients and grow best at specific but different pH levels. The environment in which the media are held during observation is maintained at body temperature, and the ambient oxygen level is adjusted to achieve an aerobic or anaerobic state. All procedures are aseptic and all equipment is sterile to avoid accidental contamination of the media. As colonies appear in or on the media, small amounts of each (there are often several) are spread on other media to allow examination of a pure specimen of the microorganisms.
culture shock, the psychologic effect of a drastic change in the cultural environment of an individual. The person may exhibit feelings of helplessness, discomfort, and disorientation in attempting to adapt to a different cultural group with dissimilar practices, values, and beliefs.
cumulative, increasing by incremental steps with an eventual total that may exceed the expected result.
cumulative action, **1.** the increased activity of a therapeutic measure or agent when administered repeatedly, as the cumulative action of a regular exercise program. **2.** the increased activity demonstrated by a drug when repeated doses accumulate in the body and exert a greater biologic effect than the initial dose.
cumulative dose, the total dose that accumulates from repeated exposure to radiation or a radiopharmaceutic product.
cumulative gene. See **polygene.**
cune-, a combining form meaning 'pertaining to a wedge': *cuneate, cuneiform, cuneus.*
cuneate /kyo͞o′nē·āt/, (of tissue) wedge-shaped, used especially in describing cells of the nervous system.
cuneiform /kyo͞onē′əfôrm′/, (of bone and cartilage) wedge-shaped.
cuneiform bone. See **triangular bone.**
cup arthroplasty of the hip joint, the surgical replacement of the head of the femur by a metal or plastic mold to relieve pain and increase motion in arthritis or to correct a deformity. The damaged or diseased bone is removed under general anesthesia, and the acetabulum and the head of the femur are reshaped. A metal Vitallium cup is inserted between the two and becomes the articulating surface of the femur. Postoperatively, the patient's leg is suspended in traction to hold it in a position of abduction and internal rotation to keep the disk in place in the acetabulum. Continued abduction is necessary for 6 weeks. Possible complications include infection, thrombophlebitis, pulmonary embolism, and fat embolism. The patient receives extensive physical therapy; crutches are necessary to avoid bearing of full weight for 6 months, and an exercise program must be followed for several years. Compare **hip replacement.** See also **arthroplasty, knee replacement, osteoarthritis, plastic surgery.**
cupping and vibrating, the procedures to help remove mucus and fluid from the lungs by the use of the clinical nursing techniques of manual percussion and vibration to dislodge and mobilize the secretions.
■ METHOD: Cupping is performed by the rhythmic percussion of the affected segments of the lungs or bronchi by the cupped hands of the nurse. Cupping is begun gently and is increased in forcefulness as the patient tolerates increased percussion. Vibration is done by placing the nurse's hands over the affected area and tensing and contracting the muscles of the hand, arm, and, mainly, shoulder, as if having a shaking chill. The movements are transmitted to the patient's chest, which increases the turbulence and velocity of exhaled air in the small bronchi. See also **postural drainage.**
■ NURSING ORDERS: Cupping is never performed over breast tissue, over the spine, or below the ribs because it causes discomfort and can cause damage to soft tissue. After head-down postural drainage with cupping and vibrating, the patient is helped to a position favorable for effective coughing and asked to breathe deeply at least three times and to cough at least twice.
■ OUTCOME CRITERIA: Thick, tenacious mucus is difficult to evacuate from the bronchi, the bronchioles, and the alveoli. As an adjunct to postural drainage, cupping and vibrating may greatly facilitate the clearing of the passages. The patient can breathe more deeply and with less effort, and the danger of pneumonia or atelectasis is reduced.
cupric /kyo͞o′prik/, of or pertaining to copper in its divalent form, as cupric sulfate.
Cuprimine, a trademark for a chelating agent (D-penicillamine), used in treating poisoning by heavy metals.
cupulolithiasis /kyo͞o′pyo͝olōlithī′əsis/, a severe, long-lasting vertigo brought on by movement of the head to certain positions. There are many possible causes, among them otitis media, ear surgery, or injury to the inner ear. In addition to extreme dizziness, signs are nausea, vomiting, and ataxia. There is no treatment except avoidance of the offending head positions. Also called **postural vertigo.**
curare /kyo͝orä′rē/, a substance derived from tropic plants of the genus *Stryknos*. It is a potent muscle relaxant that acts by preventing transmission of neural impulses across the myoneural junctions. Large dosage can cause complete paralysis, but action is usually reversible with anticholinergics. Pharmacologic preparations of the substance are used as adjuncts to general anesthesia. The use of curare or other neuromuscular blocking agents requires respiratory and ventilatory assistance by a qualified anes-

thetist or anesthesiologist. See also **tubocurarine chloride.**

curariform /kyo͞orä′rifôrm′/, **1.** chemically similar to curare. **2.** having the effect of curare.

curative treatment. See **treatment.**

cure, **1.** restoration to health of a person afflicted with a disease or other disorder. **2.** the favorable outcome of the treatment of a disease or other disorder. **3.** a course of therapy, a medication, a therapeutic measure, or another remedy used in treatment of a medical problem, as faith healing, fasting, rest cure, or work cure.

curet /kyo͞oret′/, **1.** a surgical instrument shaped like a spoon or scoop for scraping and removing material or tissue from an organ, cavity, or surface. A curet may be blunt or sharp and is designed in a shape and size appropriate to its use. **2.** to remove tissue or debris with such a device. Kinds of curets include **Hartmann's curet.**

curettage /kyo͝or′ətäzh′/, scraping of material from the wall of a cavity or other surface, performed to remove tumors or other abnormal tissue or to obtain tissue for microscopic examination. Curettage also refers to clearing unwanted material from fistulas and areas of chronic infection. It may be performed with a blunt or a sharp curet or by suction.

curie (c, Ci) /kyo͝or′ē/, a unit of radioactivity used before adoption of the becquerel (Bq) as the SI unit. It is equal to 3.70×10^{10} Bq.

curium (Cm), a radioactive metallic element. Its atomic number is 96; its atomic weight is 247. Curium is an artificial element produced by bombarding plutonium with helium ions in a cyclotron. Numerous isotopes of curium are produced by bombarding lighter transuranium elements. Curium is so radioactive that it glows in the dark.

Curling's ulcer, a duodenal ulcer that develops in people who have severe burns on the surface of the body. Also called **Curling's stress ulcer.** See also **milk therapy.**

current, **1.** a flowing or streaming movement. **2.** a flow of electrons along a conductor in a closed circuit; an electric current. **3.** certain physiologic electric activity and characteristics of blood circulation. Physiologic currents include abnerval current, action current, axial current, centrifugal current, centripetal current, compensating current, demarcation current, and electrotonic current. See also **alternating current, direct current, volt, watt.**

-current, a combining form meaning 'running, flowing, happening': *concurrent, excurrent, intercurrent.*

current of injury. See **demarcation current.**

Current Procedural Terminology (CPT), a system developed by the American Medical Association for standardizing the terminology and coding used to describe medical services and procedures.

curriculum vitae (CV) /kərik′ələm wē′tī, vē′tē/, *pl.* **curricula vitae,** a summary of educational and professional experiences, including activities and honors, to be used in seeking employment, for biographic citations on professional meeting programs, or for related purposes. Also called **résumé, resume** /rā′zəmā/.

Curschmann spiral /ko͝orsh′mon/, one of the coiled fibrils of mucus occasionally found in the sputum of persons with bronchial asthma.

curvature myopia, a type of nearsightedness caused by refractive errors associated with an excessive curvature of the cornea.

curve, (in statistics) a straight or curved line used as a graphic method of demonstrating the distribution of data collected in a study or survey.

curve of Carus, the normal axis of the pelvic outlet. Also called **circle of Carus.**

curve of occlusion, **1.** a curved occlusal surface that simultaneously contacts the major portion of the incisal and occlusal prominances of the existing teeth. **2.** the curve of dentition on which lie the occlusal surfaces of the teeth. See also **alignment, reverse curve.**

curve of Spee, **1.** the anatomic curvature of the occlusal alignment of the teeth, beginning at the tip of the lower canine, following the buccal cusps of the natural premolars and molars, and continuing to the anterior border of the ramus. **2.** the curve of the occlusal surfaces of the arches in vertical dimension, produced by a downward dipping of the mandibular premolars, with a corresponding adjustment of the upper premolars. See also **alignment.**

curvilinear trend, (in statistics) a trend in which a graphic representation of the data yields a curved line. The value of the independent variable may be expressed as a polynomial coefficient, by a more complete mathematic expression, as a logistic curve, or by a smoothing process, as a moving average.

cushingoid /ko͝osh′ingoid/, having the habitus and facies characteristic of Cushing's disease: fat pads on the upper back and face, striae on the limbs and trunk, and excess hair on the face.

Cushing's disease /ko͝osh′ingz/, a metabolic disorder characterized by the abnormally increased secretion of adrenocortical steroids caused by increased amounts of adrenocorticotropic hormone (ACTH) secreted by the pituitary, as by a pituitary adenoma. Excess adrenocortical hormones result in accumulations of fat on the chest, upper back, and face and in edema, hyperglycemia, increased gluconeogenesis, muscle weakness, purplish striae on the skin, decreased immunity to infection, osteoporosis with susceptibility to fracture of bones, acne, and facial hirsutism. Hyperglycemia resulting from Cushing's disease does not usually respond to treatment; diabetes mellitus may become a chronic condition. Therapy is aimed at removal or destruction of ACTH secreting tissue, most commonly by surgical or radiologic procedures. If this is not possible, the adrenal glands are totally or subtotally removed and pharmacologic preparations of adrenal steroids are administered. Also called **hyperadrenalism.** Compare **Cushing's syndrome.**

Cushing's syndrome, a metabolic disorder resulting from the chronic and excessive production of cortisol by the adrenal cortex or by the administration of glucocorticoids in large doses for several weeks or longer. When occurring spontaneously, the syndrome represents a failure in the body's ability to regulate the secretion of cortisol or adrenocorticotropic hormone (ACTH). (Normally cortisol is produced only in response to ACTH, and ACTH is not secreted in the presence of high levels of cortisol.) The most common cause of the syndrome is a pituitary tumor that causes an increased secretion of ACTH. Also called **hyperadrenocorticism.** See also **Addison's disease, Cushing's disease, Nelson's syndrome.**

■ OBSERVATIONS: Characteristically, the patient with Cushing's syndrome has a decreased glucose tolerance, central obesity, round "moon" face, supraclavicular fat pads, a pendulous, striae-covered pad of fat on the chest and abdomen, oligomenorrhea or decreased testosterone levels, muscular atrophy, edema, hypokalemia, and some degree of emotional change. The skin may be abnormally pigmented and fragile; minor infections may become systemic and long-lasting. Children with the disorder may stop growing. Occasionally, hypertension, kidney stones, and psychosis occur.

■ INTERVENTION: The objective of all treatment is reduction of the secretion of cortisol. The source of the excess ACTH is discovered by a series of tests that challenge the function of the adrenal and pituitary glands. Once known, the cause is treated. If the excess ACTH is caused by an adenoma of the anterior pituitary, x-ray irradiation or surgical excision of the tumor corrects the condition. If the condition is the result of medication, decreasing or changing the medication may alleviate the symptoms.

■ NURSING CONSIDERATIONS: In caring for children, the nurse normally observes height and weight, because rapidly developing obesity and failure to grow are suggestive of Cushing's syndrome. The patient with the syndrome may usually be reassured that treatment is largely successful and that the appearance may be expected to return to normal. Some of the medications used for some forms of the condition may cause nausea and anorexia, somnolence, and lethargy, and the patient is informed of this. Nursing care of the hospitalized patient with Cushing's syndrome is similar to that of Addison's disease, Cushing's disease, and other endocrinologic disorders; weight and electrolyte and fluid balance are monitored, an adequate, balanced diet is urged, and emotional changes are observed with a goal of maintaining emotional equilibrium.

cusp, **1.** a sharp projection or a rounded eminence that rises from the chewing surface of a tooth, as the two pyramidal cusps that arise from the premolars. **2.** any one of the small flaps on the valves of the heart, as the ventral, dorsal, and medial cusps attached to the right atrioventricular valve.

cuspid valve. See **atrioventricular valve.**

cuspless tooth, a tooth without cuspal prominences on its masticatory surface.

custodial care, services and care of a nonmedical nature provided on a long-term basis, usually for convalescent and chronically ill individuals. Kinds of custodial care include **board, room,** and **personal assistance.**

cut, (in molecular genetics) a fissure or split in a double strand of DNA in contrast to a nick in a single strand. See also **nick.**

cut-, a combining form meaning 'pertaining to the skin': *cutaneous, cuticle, cuticularization.*

cutaneous /kyo͞otā′nē·əs/, of or pertaining to the skin.

cutaneous absorption, the taking up of substances through the skin.

cutaneous anaphylaxis, a localized, exaggerated reaction of hypersensitivity in the form of a wheal and flare caused by an antigen injected into the skin of a sensitized individual, generally used as a test of sensitivity to various allergens. Passive cutaneous anaphylaxis, the response to an intradermally injected antibody, is used in studies of antibodies that induce immediate reactions of hypersensitivity.

cutaneous emphysema. See **subcutaneous emphysema.**

cutaneous horn, a hard, skin-colored projection of the epidermis, usually on the head or face. The lesion may be precancerous and is usually excised.

cutaneous larva migrans, a skin condition caused by a hookworm, *Ancylostoma braziliense,* a parasite of cats and dogs. Its ova are deposited in the ground with the feces of infected animals, develop into larvae, and invade the skin of people, particularly bare feet, but any skin may be involved. The larvae rarely develop into adult hookworms in the human body, but as the larvae migrate through the epidermis, a trail of inflammation follows the burrow causing severe pruritus. Secondary infections often occur if the skin has been broken by scratching. Topical application of a solution of thiabendazole usually eradicates the larvae. Also called **creeping eruption.**

cutaneous leishmaniasis. See **oriental sore.**

cutaneous lupus erythematosus. See **discoid lupus erythematosus.**

cutaneous membrane. See **skin.**

cutaneous papilloma, a small brown or flesh-colored outgrowth of skin, occurring most frequently on the neck of an older person. Also called **cutaneous tag, skin tag.**

cutdown, an incision into a vein with insertion of a polyethylene catheter for intravenous infusion. It is performed when an infusion cannot be started by venipuncture and in hyperalimentation therapy, when highly concentrated solutions are given via catheter into the superior vena cava. The skin is cleansed before the procedure; the incision is sutured, and a sterile dressing is applied at its conclusion. See also **hyperalimentation, venipuncture.**

cuticle /kyo͞o′təkəl/, **1.** epidermis. **2.** the sheath of a hair follicle. **3.** the thin edge of cornified epithelium at the base of a nail.

cutis. See **skin.**

cutis laxa /kyo͞o′təs/, abnormally loose, relaxed skin resulting from an absence of elastic fibers in the body, usually a hereditary condition.

cutis marmorata. See **livedo.**

cuvette /kyo͞ovet′/, a small transparent tube or container with specific optical properties that is used in laboratory research and analyses, as photometric evaluations, colorimetric determinations, and turbidity studies. The chemical composition of the container determines the vessel's use, as Pyrex glass for examining materials in the visible spectrum and one containing silica for those in the ultraviolet range.

CVA, 1. abbreviation for **cerebrovascular accident. 2.** abbreviation for **costovertebral angle.**

CVP monitor. See **central venous pressure monitor.**

cyan-. See **cyano-.**

cyanide poisoning, poisoning resulting from the ingestion or inhalation of cyanide from such substances as bitter almond oil, wild cherry syrup, prussic acid, hydrocyanic acid, or potassium or sodium cyanide. Characterized by tachycardia, drowsiness, convulsion, and headache, cyanide poisoning may result in death within 1 to 15 minutes. Treatment includes gastric lavage, amyl-nitrite inhalation, oxygen, and sodium thiosulfate.

cyano-, cyan-, a combining form meaning 'blue': *cyanochroia, cyanocrystallin, cyanodermia.*

cyanocobalamin /sī′ənōkōbal′əmin/, a red, crystalline, water-soluble substance with activity similar to that of vitamin B_{12}. It is involved in the metabolism of protein, fats, and carbohydrates, normal blood formation, and neural function. It is the first substance containing cobalt that is found to be vital to life. It cannot be produced synthetically but can be obtained from cultures of *Streptomyces griseus*. Rich dietary sources are liver, kidney, meats, fish, and dairy products. Deficiency is usually caused by the absence of intrinsic factor, which is necessary for the absorption of cyanocobalamin from the GI tract and which results in pernicious anemia and brain damage. Symptoms of deficiency include nervousness, neuritis, numbness and tingling in the hands and feet, poor muscular coordination, unpleasant body odor, and menstrual disturbances. Cyanocobalamin is used in the prophylaxis and treatment of pernicious anemia, tropic and nontropic sprue, and other macrocytic and megaloblastic anemias. It is nontoxic, even when administered in amounts greater than those recommended for therapeutic purposes. Also called **antipernicious anemia factor, extrinsic factor, LLD factor, vitamin B_{12}.** See also **intrinsic factor, pernicious anemia.**

cyanomethemoglobin /sī′ənōmethē′məglō′bin/, a hemoglobin derivative formed during nitrite therapy for cyanide poisoning.

cyanosis /sī′ənō′sis/, bluish discoloration of the skin and mucous membranes caused by an excess of deoxygenated hemoglobin in the blood or a structural defect in the hemoglobin molecule, as in methemoglobin. **–cyanotic,** *adj.*

Cyantin, a trademark for a urinary antibacterial (nitrofurantoin).

cycl-. See **cyclo-.**

cyclacillin, a penicillin antibiotic.

■ INDICATIONS: It is prescribed in the treatment of certain bacterial infections.

■ CONTRAINDICATION: Known hypersensitivity to penicillins prohibits its use.

■ ADVERSE EFFECTS: Among the most serious adverse reactions are hypersensitivity reactions and severe diarrhea and nausea. Skin rash may also occur.

Cyclaine, a trademark for a local anesthetic (hexylcaine hydrochloride).

cyclamate /sī′kləmāt/, an artificial, nonnutritive sweetener formerly used in the form of calcium or sodium salt. It was withdrawn from the market in the United States because of evidence that it caused cancer in laboratory animals.

cyclandelate /sīklan′dəlāt/, a vasodilator.

■ INDICATIONS: It is prescribed in the treatment of muscular ischemia and peripheral vascular obstruction or spasm.

■ CONTRAINDICATIONS: Pregnancy or known hypersensitivity to this drug prohibits its use.

■ ADVERSE EFFECTS: Tachycardia, GI distress, and flushing may occur.

Cyclapen-W, a trademark for a penicillin antibiotic (cyclacillin).

cycle. See **menstrual cycle.**

cyclencephaly /sīk′lənsef′əlē/, a developmental anomaly characterized by the fusion of the two cerebral hemispheres. **–cyclencephalic, cyclencephalous,** *adj.,* **cyclencephalus,** *n.*

cyclic adenosine monophosphate, a cyclic nucleotide formed from adenosine triphosphate by the action of adenyl cyclase. This cyclic compound, known as the "second messenger," participates in the action of catecholomines, vasopressin, adrenocorticotropic hormone, and many other hormones. Also called **cyclic AMP, adenosine 3′:5′-cyclic phosphate.**

cyclitis /siklī′tis/, inflammation of the ciliary body causing redness of the sclera adjacent to the cornea of the eye.

cyclizine hydrochloride, an antihistamine.

■ INDICATION: It is prescribed in the treatment or prevention of motion sickness.

■ CONTRAINDICATIONS: Asthma or known hypersensitivity to this drug prohibits its use. It is not given to newborn infants or nursing mothers.

■ ADVERSE EFFECTS: Among the more serious adverse reactions are skin rash, hypersensitivity reactions, and tachycardia. Drowsiness and dry mouth commonly occur.

cyclo-, cycl-, a combining form meaning 'round, recurring'; often with reference to the eye: *cyclodialysis, cycloid, cyclops.*

cyclobenzaprine hydrochloride, a muscle relaxant.

■ INDICATION: It is prescribed in the short-term treatment of muscle spasm.

■ CONTRAINDICATIONS: Hyperthyroidism, cardiac arrhythmia, cardiac failure, concomitant use of a monoamine oxidase inhibitor, or known hypersensitivity to this drug prohibits its use. It is used with caution in conditions in which anticholinergics are contraindicated.

■ ADVERSE EFFECTS: The most serious adverse effects are hypersensitivity reactions. Drowsiness, dry mouth, and dizziness commonly occur.

cyclocephalic, cyclocephalous, cyclocephaly. See **cyclopia.**

Cyclocort, a trademark for a glucocorticoid (amcinonide).

Cyclogyl, a trademark for an ophthalmic anticholinergic (cyclopentolate hydrochloride).

cyclomethycaine sulfate, a local anesthetic agent for use on nontraumatized mucus membranes before clinical examination or instrumentation.

Cyclopar, a trademark for a broad-spectrum antibiotic (tetracycline).

cyclopentolate hydrochloride, an ophthalmic anticholinergic.

■ INDICATIONS: It is prescribed to provide mydriasis and cycloplegia for diagnostic procedures in ophthalmology.

■ CONTRAINDICATIONS: Narrow-angle glaucoma or known hypersensitivity to this drug prohibits its use.

■ ADVERSE EFFECTS: Among the most serious adverse reactions are psychic disturbances and systemic anticholinergic effects, particularly in children. Local irritation and burning may also occur.

cyclophosphamide, an alkylating agent.

■ INDICATIONS: It is prescribed in the treatment of a variety of neoplasms and as an immunosuppressant in organ transplants.

■ CONTRAINDICATIONS: This drug is teratogenic in animals. It is not used during pregnancy; adequate methods of contraception should be considered for both males and females taking the drug. It is used with caution with impaired renal or hepatic function or with various blood disorders.

■ ADVERSE EFFECTS: Among the more serious adverse reactions are anorexia, vomiting, alopecia, leukopenia, and potentially serious hemorrhagic cystitis.

cyclopia /sīklō′pē·ə/, a developmental anomaly characterized by fusion of the orbits into a single cavity containing one eye. The condition is usually combined with various other head and facial defects. Also called **cyclocephaly** (*adj.* **cyclocephalic, cyclocephalous**), **synophthalmia.** **–cyclops,** *n.*

cycloplegia /sī′kləplē′jə/, paralysis of the ciliary muscles, as induced by certain ophthalmic drugs to allow examination of the eye. See also **cycloplegic.**

cycloplegic /sī′kləplē′jik/, **1.** of or pertaining to a drug or treatment that causes paralysis of the ciliary muscles of the eye. **2.** one of a group of anticholinergic drugs used to paralyze the ciliary muscles of the eye for ophthalmologic examination or surgery. Any of the cycloplegics may cause adverse effects in persons sensitive to anticholinergics.

cyclopropane /sī′klōprō′pān/, a highly flammable and explosive potent anesthetic gas that gives good analgesia and skeletal muscle relaxation, with low toxicity, minimal adverse effects, and rapid induction and emergence. It has been largely replaced by the nonflammable halogenated hydrocarbons and is now used for anesthesia only when characteristics of other anesthetic agents contraindicate their use in a specific patient. Also called **trimethylene.**

cycloserine /sī′klōser′ēn/, an antibiotic.

■ INDICATIONS: It is prescribed in the treatment of active pulmonary and extrapulmonary tuberculosis.

■ CONTRAINDICATIONS: Epilepsy, depression, severe anxiety, psychosis, severe renal insufficiency, excessive concurrent use of alcohol, or known hypersensitivity to this drug prohibits its use.

■ ADVERSE EFFECTS: Among the most serious reactions are central nervous system toxicity, including tremor, drowsiness, convulsions, and psychotic changes.

Cyclospasmol, a trademark for a vasodilator (cyclandelate).

cyclosporine, a fungal metabolite that has immunosuppressive properties. It is used in research as an immunosuppressive agent in transplant surgery. Also spelled **ciclosporin.**

cyclothiazide, a diuretic and antihypertensive.

■ INDICATIONS: It is prescribed in the treatment of hypertension and edema.

■ CONTRAINDICATIONS: Anemia or known hypersensitivity to this drug, to other thiazide medication, or to sulfonamide derivatives prohibits its use.

■ ADVERSE EFFECTS: Among the more serious adverse effects are hypokalemia, hyperglycemia, hyperuricemia, and hypersensitivity reactions.

cyclothymic disorder, a mild form of bipolar disorder.

cyclothymic personality, **1.** a personality characterized by extreme swings in mood from elation to depression. **2.** a person who has this disorder, which is also called **bipolar disorder.**

cyclotron /sī′klətron/, a device used to accelerate charged particles or ions. The particles bombard special targets where they create radioactive species to be used as radiopharmaceutics or to make neutrons that can be used for radiotherapy.

cycrimine hydrochloride, an anticholinergic.

■ INDICATION: It is prescribed in the treatment of Parkinson's disease.

■ CONTRAINDICATIONS: Narrow-angle glaucoma, asthma, obstruction of the genitourinary or GI tract, severe ulcerative colitis, or known hypersensitivity to this drug prohibits its use.

■ ADVERSE EFFECTS: Among the more serious adverse reactions are blurred vision, central nervous system effects, tachycardia, dry mouth, decreased sweating, and hypersensitivity reactions.

Cylert, a trademark for a central nervous system stimulant (pemoline).

cylindroma /sil′indrō′mə/, *pl.* **cylindromas, cylindromata,** **1.** See **adenocystic carcinoma.** **2.** also called **cylindromatous spiradenoma, trichobasalioma hyalinicum.** a benign neoplasm of the skin, usually of the scalp or face, developing from a hair follicle or sweat gland.

cylindromatous carcinoma. See **adenocystic carcinoma.**

cylindromatous spiradenoma. See **cylindroma.**

cyno-, cyn-, a combining form meaning 'pertaining to dogs, doglike': *cynobax, cynocephalic, cynophobia.*

cyproheptadine hydrochloride, an antihistamine.

■ INDICATIONS: It is prescribed in the treatment of a variety of hypersensitivity reactions, including rhinitis, skin rash, and pruritus.

■ CONTRAINDICATIONS: Asthma or known hypersensitivity to this drug prohibits its use. It is not given to newborn infants or lactating mothers.

■ ADVERSE EFFECTS: Among the more serious adverse reactions are skin rash, hypersensitivity reactions, and tachycardia. Drowsiness and dry mouth commonly occur.

Cyprus fever. See **brucellosis.**

Cys, abbreviation for **cysteine.**

cyst, a closed sac in or under the skin lined with epithelium and containing fluid or semisolid material, as a **sebaceous cyst.**

cyst-. See **cysto-.**

-cyst, -cystis, a combining form meaning a 'pouch or bladder': *enterocyst, microcyst, zoocyst.*

cystadenoma /sis′tədinō′mə/, *pl.* **cystadenomas, cystadenomata,** **1.** an adenoma associated with a cystoma. **2.** an adenoma containing multiple cystic structures. The cysts may be serous, containing serum, or pseudomucinous, containing clear serous fluid or thick, viscid fluid.

cystectomy /sistek′təmē/, a surgical procedure in which all or a part of the bladder is removed, as may be required in treating cancer of the bladder.

cysteine (Cys) /sis′tēn/, a nonessential amino acid found in many proteins in the body, including keratin. It is a metabolic precursor of cystine and an important source of sulfur for various body functions.

cysti-. See **cysto-.**

cystic acne. See **acne conglobata.**

cystic carcinoma, a malignant neoplasm containing cysts or cystlike spaces. Tumors of this kind occur in the breast and ovary.

cystic duct, the duct through which bile from the gallbladder passes into the common bile duct.

cysticercosis /sis′tisərkō′sis/, an infection and infestation by the larval stage of the pork tapeworm *Taenia solium* or the beef tapeworm *T. saginata.* The eggs are ingested and hatch in the intestine; the larvae invade the subcutaneous tissue, brain, eye, muscle, heart, liver, lung, and peritoneum. They attach themselves with two rows of hooklets, grow, mature, and become covered with a dense, fibrous capsule. The invasive, early phase of the infection is characterized by fever, malaise, muscle pain, and eosinophilia. Years later, epilepsy and personality change may appear if the brain is affected, and calcification and destruction of local structures are apparent in other infested areas of the body. Prophylaxis depends on avoiding ingestion of inadequately cooked, infected pork or beef.

cystic fibroma, a fibrous tumor in which cystic degeneration has occurred.

cystic fibrosis, an inherited disorder of the exocrine glands, causing those glands to produce abnormally thick secretions of mucus, elevation of sweat electrolytes, increased organic and enzymatic constituents of saliva, and overactivity of the autonomic nervous system. The glands most affected are those in the pancreas, the respiratory system, and the sweat glands. Cystic fibrosis is usually recognized in infancy or early childhood, occurring chiefly among whites. When present in infancy, the ealiest manifestation is meconium ileus, an obstruction of the small bowel by viscid stool. Other early signs are a chronic cough, frequent, foul-smelling stools, and persistent upper respiratory infections. The most reliable diagnostic tool is the sweat test, which shows elevations of both sodium and chloride. Because there is no known cure, treatment is directed at the prevention of respiratory infections, which are the most frequent cause of death. Mucolytic agents, bronchodilators, and mist tents are used to help liquefy the thick, tenacious mucus. Physical therapy measures, as postural drainage and breathing exercises, can also dislodge secretions. Broad spectrum antibiotics may be used prophylactically. The nurse's role is vital in instructing the family in health promotion and in all the aspects of care needed by the child. Particular attention is paid to teaching the child and family the use of pancreatic enzymes, equipment, food selection, prevention of infection, and techniques of expectorating sputum. The nurse can provide emotional support for the family and counsel them on community resources. Life expectancy in cystic fibrosis has improved markedly over the past several decades, and with early diagnosis and treatment, most patients can be expected to reach adulthood. Also called **fibrocystic disease of the pancreas, mucoviscidosis.**

cystic goiter, an enlargement of the thyroid gland containing cysts resulting from mucoid or colloid degeneration.

cystic lymphangioma, a cystic growth formed by lymph vessels; usually congenital, it most frequently occurs in the neck, axilla, or groin of children. Also called **cystic hygroma, lymphangioma cysticum.**

cystic mole. See **hydatid mole.**

cystic myxoma, a tumor of the connective tissue that has undergone cystic degeneration.

cystic neuroma, a neoplasm of nerve tissue that has degenerated and become cystic. Also called **false neuroma.**

cystic tumor, a tumor with cavities or sacs containing a semisolid or a liquid material.

cystido-. See **cysto-.**

cystine /sis′tin/, a nonessential amino acid found in many proteins in the body, including keratin and insulin. Cystine is a product of the oxidation of two cysteine molecules.

cystinosis /sis′tinō′sis/, a congenital disease characterized by glucosuria, proteinuria, cystine deposits in the liver, spleen, bone marrow, and cornea, rickets, excessive amounts of phosphates in the urine, and retardation of growth. Also called **cystine storage disease, Fanconi's syndrome.** See also **cystine.**

cystinuria /sis′tino͝or′ē·ə/, **1.** abnormal presence in the urine of the amino acid cystine. **2.** an inherited defect of the renal tubules, characterized by excessive urinary excretion of cystine and several other amino acids. The disorder is caused by an autosomal recessive trait that impairs cystine reabsorption by the kidney tubules. In high concentration, cystine tends to precipitate in the urinary tract and form kidney or bladder stones. Treatment attempts to prevent the formation of stones or to dissolve them by increasing the volume of urine flow, decreasing the pH of the urine, and increasing the solubility of cystine. In addition to a large fluid intake, sodium bicarbonate, acetazolamide, and, in refractory cases, D-penicillamine are sometimes prescribed.

-cystis. See **-cyst.**

cystitis /sistī′tis/, an inflammatory condition of the urinary bladder and ureters, characterized by pain, by urgency and frequency of urination, and by hematuria. It may be caused by a bacterial infection, calculus, or tumor. Depending on the diagnosis, treatment may include antibiotics, increased fluid intake, bed rest, medications to control bladder wall spasms, and, when necessary, surgery.

-cystitis, a combining form meaning an 'inflammation of the bladder or cyst': *epicystitis, gonecystitis, pericystitis.*

cysto-, cyst-, cysti-, cystido-, a combining form meaning 'pertaining to the bladder, or to a cyst or sac': *cystocele, cystodynia, cystomyoma.*

cystocele /sis′təsēl′/, protrusion of the urinary bladder through the wall of the vagina, in hernia. Compare **rectocele.**

cystogram /sis′təgram′/, a graphic record, usually a series of x-ray films, obtained as a part of any excretory urographic procedure, as in retrograde pyelography or retrograde cystoscopy.

cystolith. See **vesicle calculus.**

cystoma /sistō′mə/, *pl.* **cystomas, cystomata,** any tumor or growth containing cysts, especially one in or near the ovary.

-cystoma, a combining form meaning a 'cystic tumor': *enterocystoma, hydrocystoma, inocystoma.*

cystometry /sistom′ətrē/, the study of bladder function by use of a **cystometer** /sistom′ətər/, an instrument that measures capacity in relation to changing pressure. The urologic procedure, **cystometography** /sis′tōmətog′rəfē/, measures the amount of pressure exerted on the bladder at varying degrees of capacity. The results of the measurements are traced graphically on a **cystometogram** /sis′tōmet′əgram′/.

cystoscope /sis′təskōp′/, an instrument for examining and treating lesions of the urinary bladder, ureter, and kidney. It consists of an outer sheath with a lighting system, a viewing obturator, and a passage for catheters and operative devices.

cystoscopic urography. See **retrograde cystoscopy.**

cystoscopy /sistos′kəpē/, the direct visualization of the urinary tract by means of a cystoscope inserted in the urethra. For the examination the bladder is distended with air or water and the patient is in a fasting state; the procedure is usually performed under sedation or anesthesia with the patient in the lithotomy position. In addition to visualization, cystoscopy is used for obtaining biopsies of tumors or other growths and for the removal of polyps. After the examination, the patient is observed for the common complications of trauma and signs of urinary infection. See also **cystoscope.** –**cystoscopic,** *adj.*

Cystospaz, a trademark for an anticholinergic (hyoscyamine).

cyt-, cyto-, a combining form meaning 'cell or cytoplasm': *cytochrome, cytogenesis, cytosome.*

Cytadren, a trademark for an inhibitor of adrenocorticosteroid biosynthesis (aminoglutethimide).

cytarabine, an antineoplastic agent. Also called **arabinosylcitosine, cytosine arabinoside.**

■ INDICATIONS: It is prescribed in the treatment of acute and chronic myelocytic leukemia, acute lymphocytic leukemia, and erythroleukemia.

■ CONTRAINDICATION: Known hypersensitivity to this drug prohibits its use.

■ ADVERSE EFFECTS: The most serious adverse reactions are bone marrow depression, stomatitis, phlebitis, liver toxicity, and fever. GI disturbances may occur.

-cyte, a combining form meaning a 'cell' of a specified type: *gliacyte, hemacyte, plasmacyte.*

-cythemia, -cythaemia, a combining form meaning a 'condition involving cells in the blood': *achroiocythemia, rhestocythemia, thrombocythemia.*

cyto-. See **cyt-.**

cytoarchitectonic /sī′tō-/, pertaining to the cellular arrangement within a tissue or structure.

cytoarchitecture, the typical pattern of cellular arrangement within a particular tissue or organ, as in the cerebral cortex. –**cytoarchitectural,** *adj.*

cytobiotaxis. See **cytoclesis.**

cytoblast /sī′təblast′/, *obsolete.* the nucleus of a cell.

cytocentrum. See **centrosome.**

cytocerastic. See **cytokerastic.**

cytochemism /sī′tōkem′izəm/, the chemical activity within the living cell, specifically the various reactions to and affinity for chemical substances.

cytochemistry, the study of the various chemicals within a living cell and their actions and functions.

cytocide, any substance that is destructive to cells. –**cytocidal,** *adj.*

cytoclesis /sī′tōklē′sis/, the influence exerted by one cell on the action of other cells; the vital principle of all living tissue. Also called **cytobiotaxis.** –**cytocletic, cytobiotactic,** *adj.*

cytoctony /sītok′tənē/, the destruction of cells, specifically the killing of cells in culture by viruses.

cytode /sī′tōd/, the simplest type of cell, consisting of a protoplasmic mass without a nucleus, as a bacterium.

cytodieresis /sī′tōdī·er′isis/, *pl.* **cytodiereses,** cell division, especially the phenomena involving the division of the cytoplasm. See also **meiosis, mitosis.** –**cytodieretic,** *adj.*

cytodifferentiation, **1.** a process by which embryonic cells acquire biochemical and morphologic properties essential for specialization and diversification. **2.** the total and gradual transformation from an undifferentiated to a fully differentiated state.

cytogene /sī′təjēn/, a particle within the cytoplasm of a cell that is self-replicating, derived from the genes in the nucleus, and capable of transmitting hereditary information.

cytogenesis /sī′tōjen′əsis/, the origin, development, and differentiation of cells. –**cytogenetic, cytogenic,** *adj.*

cytogeneticist /sī′tōjənet′isist/, one who specializes in cytogenetics.

cytogenetics /sī′tōjənet′iks/, the branch of genetics that studies the cellular constituents concerned with heredity, primarily the structure, function, and origin of the chromosomes. One kind of cytogenetics is **clinical cytogenetics.** –**cytogenetic,** *adj.*

cytogenic gland, a glandular organ that secretes living cells, specifically the testes and ovary.

cytogenic reproduction, the formation of a new organism from a unicellular germ cell, either sexually through the fusion of gametes to form a zygote or asexually by means of spores.

cytogeny /sītoj′ənē/, **1.** cytogenetics. **2.** the origin and development of the cell. –**cytogenic, cytogenous,** *adj.*

cytogony /sītog′ənē/, cytogenic reproduction.

cytohistogenesis /sī′tōhis′tōjen′əsis/, the structural development and formation of cells. –**cytohistogenetic,** *adj.*

cytohyaloplasm. See **hyaloplasm.**

cytoid /sī′toid/, like or resembling a cell.

cytoid body, a small white spot on the retina of each eye that is seen by using an ophthalmoscope in examining the eyes of a patient affected with systemic lupus erythematosus.

cytokerastic /sī′tōkəras′tik/, pertaining to or characteristic of cellular development from a lower to a higher form or from a simple to more complex arrangement. Also **cytocerastic** /-səras′tik/.

cytokinesis /sī′tōkinē′sis, -kīnē′sis/, the division of the cytoplasm, exclusive of nuclear division, that occurs during the final stages of mitosis and meiosis to form daughter cells; the sum total of all the changes that occur in the cytoplasm during mitosis, meiosis, and fertilization. –**cytokinetic,** *adj.*

cytologic map /sī′tō-/, the graphic representation of the location of genes on a chromosome, based on correlating genetic recombination testcrossing results with the structural analysis of chromosomes that have undergone such changes as deletions or translocations as detected by banding techniques.

cytologist /sītol′əjist/, one who specializes in the study of cells, specifically one who uses cytologic techniques in the differential diagnosis of neoplasms.

cytology /sītol′əjē/, the study of cells, including their formation, origin, structure, function, biochemical activities, and pathology. Kinds of cytology are **aspiration biopsy cytology** and **exfoliative cytology.** –**cytologic, cytological,** *adj.*

cytolymph. See **hyaloplasm.**

cytolysin /sītol′isin/, an antibody that dissolves antigenic cells. Kinds of cytolysin are **bacteriolysin** and **hemolysin.**

cytolysis /sītol′isis/, *pl.* **cytolyses,** the destruction or breakdown of the living cell, primarily by the disintegration of the outer membrane. A kind of cytolysis is **immune cytolysis.** –**cytolytic,** *adj.*

cytomegalic inclusion disease (CID) /sī′tōmegal′ik/, an infection caused by the cytomegalovirus, a "salivary gland" virus related to the herpesviruses. It is primarily a congenitally acquired disease of newborn infants and is characterized by microcephaly, retarded growth, hepatosplenomegaly, hemolytic anemia, and pathologic fracture of long bones. See also **cytomegalovirus (CMV) disease, TORCH syndrome.**

cytomegalovirus (CMV) /sī′tōmeg′əlōvī′rəs/, a member of a group of large species-specific herpes-type viruses with a wide variety of disease effects. It causes serious illness in newborns and in people being treated with immunosuppressive drugs and therapy, especially after an organ transplant. See also **cytomegalic inclusion disease, TORCH syndrome.**

cytomegalovirus (CMV) disease, a viral infection caused by the cytomegalovirus, characterized by malaise, fever, lymphadinopathy, pneumonia, hepatosplenomegaly, and superinfection with various bacteria and fungi as a result of the depression of immune response characteristic of herpesviruses. See also **cytomegalic inclusion disease.**

Cytomel, a trademark for a thyroid hormone (liothyronine sodium).

cytometer /sītom′ətər/, a device for counting and measuring the number of cells within a given amount of fluid, as blood, urine, or cerebrospinal fluid.

cytometry /sītom′ətrē/, the counting and measuring of cells, specifically blood cells. **–cytometric,** *adj.*

cytomitome /sī′təmī′tōm/, the fibrillary network within the cytoplasm of a cell, as contrasted with that in the nucleoplasm. See also **karyomitome.**

cytomorphology, the study of the various forms of cells and the structures contained within them. **–cytomorphologic, cytomorphological,** *adj.*, **cytomorphologist,** *n.*

cytomorphosis /sī′tōmôr′fəsis/, *pl.* **cytomorphoses,** the various changes that occur within a cell during the course of its life cycle, from the earliest undifferentiated stage until destruction.

cyton /sī′tən/, the cell body of a neuron or that portion containing the nucleus and its surrounding cytoplasm from which the axon and dendrites are formed. Also called **cytone** /sī′tōn/.

cytophoresis /sī′tōfôr′əsis/, **1.** a therapeutic technique that uses the principle of centrifugation to remove red or white blood cells or platelets from patients with certain blood disorders. **2.** a laboratory procedure for separating specific components, as white blood cells or platelets, from donor blood by centrifugation.

cytophotometer /sī′tōfətom′ətər/, an instrument for measuring light density through stained portions of cytoplasm, used for locating and identifying chemical substances within cells.

cytophotometry /sī′tōfətom′ətrē/, the identification of chemical substances within cells, using a cytophotometer. Also called **microfluorometry. –cytophotometric,** *adj.*

cytophysiology, the study of the biochemical processes involved in the functioning of an individual cell, as contrasted with the functioning of organs or tissues. **–cytophysiologic, cytophysiological,** *adj.*, **cytophysiologist,** *n.*

cytoplasm /sī′təplaz′əm/, all of the substance of a cell other than the nucleus. See also **cell, nucleus.**

cytoplasmic bridge. See **intercellular bridge.**

cytoplasmic inheritance /sī′tōplaz′mik/, the acquisition of traits or conditions controlled by self-replicating substances within the cytoplasm, as mitochondria or chloroplasts, rather than by the genes on the chromosomes in the nucleus. The phenomenon occurs in plants and lower animals but has not yet been demonstrated in humans.

Cytosar-U, a trademark for an antineoplastic (cytarabine).

cytosine /sī′təsin/, a major pyrimidine base found in nucleotides and a fundamental constituent of DNA and RNA. In free or uncombined form it occurs in trace amounts in most cells, usually as products of the enzymatic hydrolysis of nucleic acids and nucleotides. Upon hydrolysis, it is converted to urea and ammonia. See also **thymine, uracil.**

cytosine arabinoside. See **cytarabine.**

cytoskeleton, the cytoplasmic elements, including the tonofibrils, keratin, and other microfibrils, that function as a supportive system within a cell, especially an epithelial cell.

cytotoxic anaphylaxis, an exaggerated reaction of hypersensitivity to an injection of antibodies specific for antigenic substances that occur normally on the surfaces of body cells.

cytotoxic drug, any pharmacologic compound that inhibits the proliferation of cells within the body. Such compounds, as the alkylating agents and the antimetabolites, are designed to destroy abnormal cells selectively, while sparing as many normal cells as possible; they are commonly used in chemotherapy. Cytotoxic agents have a potential for producing teratogenesis, mutagenesis, and carcinogenesis.

cytotoxic hypersensitivity, an IgG or an IgM complement-dependent, immediate-acting hypersensitive humoral response to foreign cells or to alterations of surface antigens on the cells. Direct and immediate destruction of cells occurs, as seen in hemolytic disease of the newborn and in severe transfusion reactions. Also called **type II hypersensitivity.** Compare **anaphylactic hypersensitivity, immune complex hypersensitivity.** See also **immune gamma globulin.**

cytotoxin /sī′tōtok′sin/, a substance that has a toxic effect on certain cells. An antibody may act as a cytotoxin. **–cytotoxic,** *adj.*

cytotrophoblast /sī′tōtrof′əblast′/, the inner layer of cells of the trophoblast of the early mammalian embryo that gives rise to the outer surface and villi of the chorion. Also called **Langhans' layer.** Compare **syncytiotrophoblast. –cytotrophoblastic,** *adj.*

Cytoxan, a trademark for an antineoplastic (cyclophosphamide).

D, **1.** symbol for **dead space gas.** **2.** symbol for **diffusing capacity.** **3.** abbreviation for **diopter.** **4.** abbreviation for *dexter,* meaning "right."

DA, abbreviation for **developmental age.**

D & C, abbreviation for **dilatation and curettage.**

dacarbazine, an alkylating agent used as an antineoplastic.

■ INDICATIONS: It is prescribed primarily in the treatment of malignant melanoma, sarcoma, and Hodgkin's disease.

■ CONTRAINDICATION: Known hypersensitivity to this drug prohibits its use.

■ ADVERSE EFFECTS: Among the more serious adverse reactions are bone marrow depression, GI symptoms, kidney and liver impairment, alopecia, and fever.

D/A converter. See **digital-to-analog converter.**

Dacriose, a trademark for an isotonic ophthalmic irrigating solution containing boric acid, sodium carbonate, potassium chloride, benzalkonium chloride, and EDTA.

dacryo-, dacry-, a combining form meaning 'pertaining to tears': *dacryocele, dacryolin, dacryorrhea.*

dacryocyst /dak′re·ōsist′/, a lacrimal sac at the medial angle of the eye, a normal anatomic feature.

dacryocystectomy /dak′rē·ōsistek′təmē/, partial or total excision of the lacrimal sac.

dacryocystitis /dak′rē·ōsistī′tis/, an infection of the lacrimal sac caused by obstruction of the nasolacrimal duct, characterized by tearing and discharge from the eye. In the acute phase, the sac becomes inflamed and painful. The disorder is nearly always unilateral and usually occurs in infants. Systemic administration of antibiotics is usual; local, topical treatment is seldom effective; and, rarely, a dacryocystorhinostomy may be required. Compare **dacryostenosis.**

dacryocystorhinostomy /dak′rē·ōsis′tôrīnos′təmē/, a surgical procedure for restoring drainage into the nose from the lacrimal sac when the nasolacrimal duct is obstructed.

dacryostenosis /dak′rē·ōstinō′sis/, an abnormal stricture of the nasolacrimal duct, occurring either as a congenital condition or as a result of infection or trauma. Dacryocystorhinostomy may be required to correct this condition. Compare **dacryocystitis.**

Dactil, a trademark for an anticholinergic (piperidolate hydrochloride).

dactinomycin, an antibiotic used as an antineoplastic agent.

■ INDICATIONS: It is prescribed in the treatment of a variety of malignant neoplastic diseases, including Wilms' tumor and rhabdomyosarcoma in children.

■ CONTRAINDICATIONS: Herpes zoster infection or known hypersensitivity to this drug prohibits its use.

■ ADVERSE EFFECTS: Among the more serious adverse reactions are bone marrow depression, severe GI disturbances, proctitis, alopecia, and ulcers of the mouth.

dactyl /dak′til/, a digit (finger or toe). **–dactylic,** *adj.*

dactyl-. See **dactylo-.**

-dactyl, a combining form meaning 'digit (finger or toe)': *hermodactyl, pachydactyl, pentadactyl.*

-dactylia, -dactyly, a combining form meaning '(condition of the) fingers or toes': *ankylodactylia, heptadactylia, oligodactylia.*

dactylo-, dactyl-, a combining form meaning 'pertaining to a finger or toe': *dactylophasia, dactylospasm, dactylosymphysis.*

-dactyly. See **-dactylia.**

daisy-wheel printer, a character printer for computers in which the character dies are on a number of narrow, flexible "fingers" projecting from a central hub, resembling a daisy. The wheel spins in front of the position for printing, and as the desired character appears, it is struck by a hammer and the pattern is impressed on the paper through an inked ribbon. Compare **dot-matrix printer.**

Dakin's solution, an antiseptic solution containing boric acid and 0.4% to 0.5% of sodium hypochlorite.

Dalmane, a trademark for a sedative-hypnotic (flurazepam hydrochloride).

daltonism /dôl′təniz′əm/, *informal.* a form of red-green color blindness. It is genetically transmitted as a sex-linked autosomal recessive trait. Also called **protanopia.**

Dalton's law of partial pressures /dôl′tənz/, (in physics) a law stating that the sum of the pressure exerted by a mixture of gases is equal to the total of the partial pressures that could be exerted by the gases if they were separated. See also **Avogadro's law, Boyle's law, Gay-Lussac's law.**

damages, (in law) a sum of money awarded to a plaintiff by a court as compensation for any loss, detriment, or injury to the plaintiff's person, property, or rights caused by the malfeasance or negligence of the defendant. **Actual damages** are awarded to reimburse the plaintiff for the loss or injury sustained. **Nominal damages** are awarded to show that a legal wrong has been committed although no recoverable loss can be determined. **Punitive damag-**

es exceed the actual cost of injury or damage and are awarded when the defendant has acted maliciously or in reckless disregard of the plaintiff's rights.

damp, a potentially lethal atmosphere in caves and mines. **Black damp** or **choke damp** is caused by absorption of the available oxygen by coal seams. **Fire damp** is composed of methane and other explosive hydrocarbon gases. **White damp** is another name for carbon monoxide.

damping, (in cardiology) pertaining to a diminishing of the amplitude of a series of waves or oscillations and eventual arrest of any fluctuations.

danazol, a synthetic androgen that acts to suppress the output of gonadotropins from the pituitary.

■ INDICATION: It is prescribed in the treatment of endometriosis.

■ CONTRAINDICATIONS: Genital bleeding, cardiac, liver, or kidney dysfunction, or known hypersensitivity to this drug prohibits its use. It is not used in pregnancy or during lactation.

■ ADVERSE EFFECTS: Among the most serious adverse reactions are muscle spasms, nausea, weight gain, acne, edema, oily skin, voice changes, and other androgenic effects.

dance reflex, a normal response in the neonate to simulate walking by a reciprocal flexion and extension of the legs when held in an erect position with the soles touching a hard surface. The reflex disappears by about 3 to 4 weeks of age and is replaced by controlled, deliberate movement. Also called **step reflex, stepping reflex.**

D & C, abbreviation for **dilatation and curettage.**

dander, dry scales shed from the skin or hair of animals or feathers of birds that may cause an allergic reaction in some individuals.

dandruff, an excessive amount of scaly material composed of dead, keratinized epithelium shed from the scalp that may be a mild form of seborrheic dermatitis. Treatment with a keratolytic shampoo is usually recommended to soften and remove the scales.

dandy fever. See **dengue fever.**

Dandy-Walker cyst, a cystic malformation of the fourth ventricle of the brain, resulting from hydrocephalus. Diagnosis of the defect is made with CAT scan, with x-ray films, and less commonly with a ventriculogram. See also **hydrocephalus, shunt.**

Danocrine, a trademark for an anterior pituitary suppressant (danazol).

danthron, a stimulant laxative.

■ INDICATIONS: It is prescribed in the treatment of constipation or for bowel evacuation before radiologic or surgical procedures.

■ CONTRAINDICATIONS: Abdominal pain, nausea, vomiting, or other signs and symptoms of appendicitis prohibit its use. It is not recommended for nursing mothers.

■ ADVERSE EFFECTS: Among the most serious adverse reactions are dizziness, palpitations, stomach cramps, and excessive bowel activity.

Dantrium, a trademark for a skeletal muscle relaxant (dantrolene sodium), used as an adjunct to anesthesia.

dantrolene sodium, a skeletal muscle relaxant.

■ INDICATIONS: It is prescribed in the treatment of muscle spasticity resulting from injury to the spinal cord or cerebrum. It is not indicated in treatment of spasm from rheumatic disorders.

■ CONTRAINDICATIONS: Liver dysfunction or known hypersensitivity to this drug prohibits its use.

■ ADVERSE EFFECTS: The most serious adverse reaction is potentially fatal hepatotoxicity. Common reactions include confusion, drowsiness, diarrhea, dizziness, fatigue, and muscular weakness. Side effects may continue for several days.

dapsone (DADPS), a bacteriostatic sulfone derivative.

■ INDICATIONS: It is prescribed in the treatment of lepromatous leprosy and dermatitis herpetiformis.

■ CONTRAINDICATIONS: Pregnancy or known hypersensitivity to this drug prohibits its use.

■ ADVERSE EFFECTS: Among the more serious adverse reactions are hemolysis (particularly in people who have glucose-6-phosphate dehydrogenase deficiency), lepra reactions, methemoglobinemia, neuropathy, nausea, anorexia, and skin rash.

Daraprim, a trademark for an antimalarial (pyrimethamine).

Darbid, a trademark for an anticholinergic (isopropamide iodide).

Darenthin, a trademark for bretylium tosylate.

Daricon, a trademark for an anticholinergic (oxyphencyclimine hydrochloride).

Darier's disease. See **keratosis follicularis.**

dark-adapted eye, an eye in which the pupil has dilated, making it more sensitive to dim light.

darkfield microscopy, examination with a darkfield microscope, in which the specimen is illuminated by a peripheral light source. Organisms in specimens that have been prepared for use with a darkfield microscope appear to glow against a dark background. The technique is used primarily to identify the syphilis spirochete. Also called **darkfield illumination, ultramicroscopy.**

dark-film fault, a defect in a photograph or radiograph, which appears as an excessively darkened image and image area. It is caused by overexposure of the film to light or radiation, film fog from excessive development, accidental exposure to light, or an unsafe darkroom light.

Darvocet-N, a trademark for a fixed-combination drug containing an analgesic-antipyretic (acetaminophen) and an analgesic (propoxyphene napsylate).

Darvon, a trademark for an analgesic (propoxyphene hydrochloride).

Darvon Compound, a trademark for a fixed-combination drug containing an analgesic (propoxyphene hydrochloride) and APC (aspirin, phenacetin, and caffeine).

Darvon-N, a trademark for an analgesic (propoxyphene napsylate).

darwinian theory, the theory postulated by Charles Darwin that organic evolution results from the process of natural selection of those variants of plants and animals best suited to survive in their environmental surroundings. Also called **darwinism.** Compare **lamarckism.** – **darwinian,** *adj., n.*

D.A.S.E., abbreviation for **Denver Articulation Screening Examination.**

data, *sing.* **datum,** **1.** pieces of information, especially those that are part of a collection of information to be used in an analysis of a problem, as the diagnosis of a health problem. **2.** information stored and processed by a computer.

data analysis, (in research) the phase of a study that includes classifying, coding, and tabulating information needed to perform statistic or qualitative analyses according to the research design and appropriate to the data. Data analysis follows data collection and precedes interpretation or application of the data.

data base, a large store or bank of information, especially in a form that can be processed by computer.

data base management systems (DBMS), a set of computer programs written to aid a user in the storage and retrieval of large amounts of related information.

data collection, (in research) the phase of a study that includes the gathering of information and identification of sampling units as directed by the research design. Data collection precedes data analysis.

data processing, the techniques and practices involved in the manipulation of information by a computer.

dataset, **1.** a modem. **2.** files of data for processing by computer.

datum. See **data.**

daughter chromosome, either of the paired chromatids that during the anaphase stage of mitosis separate and migrate to opposite ends of the cell before division. Each contains the complete genetic information of the original chromosome and was formed during interphase by the duplication of the DNA molecule.

daughter element, an element that results from the radioactive decay of a parent element. An example is technetium 99, which is the daughter element created by the decay of an atom of molybdenum 99.

daughter product. See **decay product.**

daunorubicin hydrochloride, an anthracycline antibiotic antineoplastic agent.

■ INDICATIONS: It is prescribed in the treatment of cancer, particularly the leukemias and neuroblastoma.

■ CONTRAINDICATIONS: Preexisting drug-induced bone marrow depression or known hypersensitivity to this drug prohibits its use. It is not given to patients who have previously received a complete course of treatment with daunorubicin or doxorubicin.

■ ADVERSE EFFECTS: Among the most serious adverse reactions are bone marrow depression and cardiotoxicity. GI disturbances, stomatitis, and alopecia are common.

DAVA, a trademark for an antineoplastic agent (vindesine sulfate).

Davidson regimen, a method of treating chronic constipation in children, of developing regular bowel habits, and of identifying those with functional bowel disease or obstructive disorders. If necessary, the fecal impactions are removed by a series of hypertonic phosphate enemas. The child is then given mineral oil in increasing doses, until four or five loose bowel movements occur daily. The condition usually subsides within 2 to 3 weeks unless Hirschsprung's disease or another obstructive disorder is present. Some children, especially those under 2 years of age, require supplemental, fat-soluble vitamins to maintain proper nutrition. The regimen may be continued in children older than 3 years as a training procedure for developing regular bowel habits. The child is placed on a potty-chair at a specific time each day for 5 to 15 minutes, and, as regular habits develop, the mineral oil is gradually withdrawn over a period of several weeks. See also **toilet training.**

day blindness. See **hemeralopia.**

day care, a specialized program or facility that provides care for preschool children, usually within a group framework, either as a substitute for or extension of home care, particularly for single parents or for parents who are both employed outside the home. Day care groups vary in size and function and range from casual neighborhood parent-supervised play groups to formal nursery schools or organized centers run by trained personnel. Most day care programs incorporate a daily schedule of quiet play, outdoor activities, group games and projects, creative or educational play, and snack and rest periods. Group participation provides extensive opportunity for social, educational, and physical development, enables the child to learn how to cope with frustration, dissatisfaction, anger, and fear, especially fear of being separated from the parents, and may offer excellent preparation for entrance into elementary school.

day health care services, the provision of hospitals, nursing homes, or other facilities for health-related services to adult patients who are ambulatory or can be transported and who regularly use such services for a certain number of daytime hours but do not require continuous inpatient care.

day hospital, a psychiatric facility that offers a therapeutic program during daytime hours for formerly institutionalized patients.

day patient. See **inpatient.**

day sight. See **nyctalopia.**

dB, abbreviation for **decibel.**

DC, abbreviation for **direct current.**

D & C, abbreviation for **dilatation and curettage.**

DD, abbreviation for **developmental disability.**

DDAVP, a trademark for an antidiuretic (desmopressin acetate).

D.D.S., abbreviation for *Doctor of Dental Surgery.*

DDST, abbreviation for **Denver Developmental Screening Test.**

DDT (dichlorodiphenyltrichloroethane), a nondegradable water-insoluble chlorinated hydrocarbon once used worldwide as a major insecticide, especially in agriculture. In recent years, knowledge of its adverse impact on the environment has led to restrictions in its use. In addition, because tolerance in formerly susceptible organisms develops rapidly, DDT has been largely replaced by organophosphate insecticides in the United States, where DDT was banned by the FDA in 1971. It is still used as a pediculocide where epidemic-scale delousing is justified, as in barracks and refugee camps. Its value as a scabicide is marginal, since scabies and crab lice quickly become resistant to it. See also **scabicide.**

DDT poisoning. See **chlorinated organic insecticide poisoning.**

de-, a combining form meaning 'down or from': *deaquation, decartation, dedentition.*

DEA, **1.** abbreviation for **Drug Enforcement Administration.** **2.** abbreviation for **Drug Enforcement Agency.**

dead-end host, any animal from which a parasite cannot escape to continue its life cycle. Humans are dead-end hosts for trichinosis, because the larvae encyst in muscle and human flesh is unlikely to be a source of food for other animals susceptible to this parasite. Compare **definitive host, intermediate host, reservoir host.**

dead space, a cavity that remains after the incomplete closure of a surgical or traumatic wound, leaving an area in which blood can collect and delay healing. See also **anatomic dead space, physiologic dead space.**

deaf, **1.** unable to hear; hard of hearing. **2.** people who are unable to hear or who suffer hearing impairment. – **deafness,** *n.*

deaf-mute, a person who is unable to hear or to speak because of disability of the brain or the organs of hearing and speech.

deafness, a condition characterized by a partial or complete loss of hearing. In assessing deafness, the patient's ears are examined for drainage, crusts, accumulation of cerumen, or structural abnormality. It is determined if the deafness is conductive or sensory, temporary or permanent, and congenital or acquired in childhood, adolescence, or adulthood. The effect of aging, when applicable, is evaluated, and a psychosocial assessment is conducted to ascertain if the individual is well adjusted to deafness or reacts to the handicap with fear, anxiety, frustration, depression, anger, or hostility. In all cases the degree of loss and the kind of impairment causing the loss are determined. See also **conductive hearing loss, sensorineural hearing loss.**

■ OBSERVATIONS: Many conditions and diseases may result in deafness. More than 6 million people in the United States have some degree of bilateral hearing loss, and more than 50% of those people are over 65 years old. The person with a slight hearing loss may be initially unaware of the problem and then, as the impairment increases, may tend to hide or deny it. Recognition, diagnosis, and early treatment may help prevent further impairment and prevent frustration, embarrassment, and danger for the person. An older person with a hearing impairment usually has a sensorineural loss as well as a conductive hearing loss. High sounds are hard to hear, and discernment of such letter sounds as /s/ and /f/ becomes difficult. Speaking clearly and slowly, allowing the person to lip-read, is helpful, as are visual cues clear with enunciation; shouting is not. A severe or sudden hearing loss usually drives the person to seek help. If the loss is sudden, confusion, fear, and even panic are common. The person's speech becomes loud and slurred. There is new danger because the person cannot hear horns, whistles, or sirens and has not developed a way to cope with the impairment safely. The congenitally deaf person needs special speech and language training before reaching school age. Most affected children also have a disturbance of visual perception and are more dependent and less mature emotionally and socially; also reading and writing are learned with more difficulty.

■ INTERVENTION: The treatment of deafness depends on the cause. Merely removing impacted cerumen from the external auditory canal may significantly improve hearing. Hearing aids, amplification of sound, or lip reading may be useful. Speech therapy is useful in teaching a person to speak or helping a person to retain the ability to speak.

■ NURSING CONSIDERATIONS: Caring for a deaf person who is hospitalized for treatment of another problem requires certain adjustments in communication between nurse and patient. To communicate with the deaf patient who lip-reads, staff members speak slowly, enunciate distinctly, use simple phrases, and rephrase any statements that are not understood; the speaker avoids shouting, chewing gum, or covering or obscuring the mouth in other ways while speaking. If the patient uses a hearing aid, its placement and operation are checked before the speaker begins to talk; the voice is modulated to a pitch that is comfortable for the patient, and the speaker stands or sits where the lips are visible to the deaf individual. If the patient uses sign language, an interpreter or another means of communication is sought; when a pad and pencil are used, a frequent practice with the newly deaf, the messages are written clearly in short, simple phrases, and adequate time is allowed for the patient to understand and answer. Because hospitalization increases the stress imposed by deafness and because persons with impaired hearing are acutely aware of movement and changes in light, the patient is maintained in a calm, nonstressful, and safe environment. The bed is located so that the patient can see the door. The call bell is placed within reach and is answered promptly and in person; if the patient's eyes are closed when he is approached, a gentle pat on the arm is used to arouse him without causing undue alarm. The patient is encouraged to express himself, to communicate with friends and relatives, and to participate in planning his own care. When possible, pictures are used to explain procedures or treatment. In addition to physical care, the nurse provides emotional support in frequent visits and communication with the deaf patient and suggests diversions, as working puzzles, playing cards, knitting, sewing, or various hobbies. In preparing the newly deaf patient for discharge, the nurse points out the availability of lip-reading or sign-language classes, of organizations for the deaf, and of amplifiers and flashing lights for telephones and doorbells. The importance of a safe environment, of continuing the prescribed regimen of care of the ears, and of keeping outpatient appointments are stressed. If the patient is to wear a hearing aid, the nurse may assist in demonstrating its use and care.

deaminase /dē•am′inās/, an enzyme that catalyses the hydrolysis of the NH_2 bond in amino compounds. The enzymes are usually named according to the substrate, as **adenosine deaminase, guanine deaminase,** or **guanosine deaminase.**

deamination /dē′aminā′shən/, the removal, usually by hydrolysis, of the NH_2 radical from an amino compound. Also called **deaminization.**

dean, the chief executive and educational officer of a unit of a university, school, or college.

Deaner, a trademark for a psychostimulant (deanol).

deanol, a psychostimulant.

■ INDICATIONS: It is prescribed in the treatment of learning problems and hyperkinetic-behavior problems.

■ CONTRAINDICATIONS: There are no known absolute contraindications, but it should be used with caution in patients with grand mal epilepsy.

■ ADVERSE EFFECTS: Among the most serious adverse reactions are insomnia, mild overstimulation, and pruritus.

death, **1. apparent death,** the cessation of life as indicated by the absence of heartbeat or respiration. **2. legal death,** the total absence of activity in the brain and central nervous system, the cardiovascular system, and the respiratory system as observed and declared by a physician. See also **cell death, emotional care of the dying patient, fetal death, stages of dying, sudden infant death syndrome.**

death trance, a state in which a person appears to be dead.

debility, feebleness, weakness, or loss of strength. See also **asthenia.**

debride /dibrēd′/, to remove dirt, foreign objects, damaged tissue, and cellular debris from a wound or a burn to prevent infection and to promote healing. In treating a wound, debridement is the first step in cleansing it; debridement also allows thorough examination of the extent of the injury. In treating a burn, debridement of the eschar may be performed in a hydrotherapy bath. – **debridement** /debrēdmäN′/, *n.*

Debrox, a trademark for a topical antiinfective (carbamide peroxide).

debug, to find and correct errors in a computer program or hardware.

dec-, **1.** a combining form meaning 'ten': *decagram, decaliter, decipara.* **2.** a combining form meaning 'tenth': *decigram, deciliter, decinormal.*

Decadron, a trademark for a glucocorticoid (dexamethasone).

Deca-Durabolin, a trademark for an androgen (nandrolone decanoate), used as an anabolic agent.

decalcification, loss of calcium salts from the teeth and bones caused by malnutrition, malabsorption, or other dietary or physiologic factors. It may result, particularly in older people, from a diet that lacks adequate calcium. Malabsorption may be caused by a lack of vitamin D necessary for the absorption of calcium from the intestine, by an excess of dietary fats that can combine with calcium to form an indigestible soaplike compound, by the presence of oxalic acid that can combine with calcium to form a relatively insoluble calcium oxalate salt, or by a relative lack of acid in the digestive tract that can decrease the solubility of calcium. Other factors include the parathyroid hormone control of the calcium level in the bloodstream, the ratio of calcium to phosphorus in the blood, and the relative activity of osteoblast cells that form calcium deposits in the bones and teeth and osteoclast cells that absorb calcium from bones and teeth. Bone tissue tends to be maintained in quantities no greater than needed to meet current physical stress. Therefore inactive and, particularly, bedridden people lose calcium from their bones; osteoclastic activity exceeds osteoblastic activity, and decalcification occurs. See also **calcium, mineral.**

decamethonium bromide /dek′əmithō′nē•əm/, a skeletal muscle relaxant.

■ INDICATIONS: It is prescribed as an adjunct to anesthesia to induce skeletal muscle relaxation and to lessen skeletal muscle contractions in convulsions.

■ CONTRAINDICATIONS: Severe renal disease, myotonia, shock, or known hypersensitivity to this drug or to other bromides prohibits its use. It is not recommended for use in surgery lasting more than 20 minutes.

■ ADVERSE EFFECTS: Among the more serious adverse reactions are ventricular arrhythmias, increased arterial pressure, and cardiac arrest.

decanoic acid. See **capric acid.**

Decapryn, a trademark for an antihistaminic (doxylamine succinate).

decay product, (in radiology) a stable or radioactive nuclide formed directly from the radioactive disintegration of a radionuclide or as a result of successive transformation in a radioactive series. Also called **daughter product.**

deceleration, a decrease in the speed or velocity of an object or reaction. Compare **acceleration.**

deceleration phase, (in obstetrics) the latter part of active labor characterized by a decreased rate of dilatation of the cervical os on a Friedman curve.

decerebrate posture /dēser′əbrāt/, the position of a patient, who is usually comatose, in which the arms are extended and internally rotated and the legs are extended with the feet in forced plantar flexion. The posture is usually observed in patients afflicted by compression of the brainstem at a low level. Also called **decerebrate rigidity.** See also **tonic labyrinthine reflex.**

decibel (dB), a unit of measure of the intensity of sound. A decibel is one tenth of 1 bel; an increase of 1 bel is perceived as an approximate doubling of loudness, based on a sound-pressure reference level of 0.0002 dyn/cc.

decidua /disij′o͞o•ə/, the epithelial tissue of the endometrium lining the uterus. It envelops the conceptus during gestation and is shed in the puerperium. It is also shed periodically during menstruation. Kinds of decidua are **decidua basalis, decidua capsularis,** and **decidua vera.** See also **amniotic sac.**

decidua basalis, the decidua of the endometrium in the uterus that lies beneath the implanted ovum. Also called **decidua serotina.**

decidua capsularis, the decidua of the endometrium of the uterus covering the implanted ovum. Also called **decidua reflexa.**

decidual endometritis /disij′o͞o•əl/, an inflammation or infection of any portion of the decidua during pregnancy. See also **endometritis.**

decidua menstrualis, the endometrium shed during menstruation.

decidua parietalis. See **decidua vera.**

decidua reflexa. See **decidua capsularis.**

decidua serotina. See **decidua basalis.**

decidua vera, the decidua of the endometrium lining the uterus except for those areas beneath and above the implanted and developing ovum called, respectively, the decidua basalis and the decidua capsularis. Also called **decidua parietalis.**

deciduous dentition. See **deciduous tooth.**

deciduous tooth /disij′o͞o•əs/, any one of the set of 20 teeth that appear normally during infancy, consisting of four incisors, two canines, and four molars in each jaw. Deciduous teeth start developing at about the sixth week of fetal life as a thickening of the epithelium along the line of the future jaw. During the seventh week, the epithelium splits longitudinally into the labial strand and the lingual strand. The labial strand forms the labiodental lamina. The lingual strand becomes the dental lamina, which develops ten enlargements in each jaw. The enlargements appear about the ninth week and correspond to the future deciduous teeth. In most individuals the first deciduous tooth erupts through the gum about 6 months after birth. Thereafter, one or more deciduous teeth erupt about every month until all 20 have appeared. The deciduous teeth are usually shed between the ages of 6 and 13, although the timing varies greatly from person to person. Also called **milk tooth, deciduous dentition, first dentition, primary dentition.** Compare **permanent tooth.** See also **predeciduous dentition, teething, tooth.**

Declomycin, a trademark for an antibacterial (demeclocycline hydrochloride).

decode, to interpret coded information into a form usable by people.

decoded message, (in communication theory) a message as translated by a receiver. If it is correctly interpreted within the context of the message as sent by the sender, the decoded message is the same as the encoded message; if it is not understood and interpreted as sent, it is not the same as the encoded message.

decoic acid. See **capric acid.**

decompensation, the failure of a system, as cardiac decompensation in heart failure.

decomposition, the dissolution of a substance into simpler chemical forms.

decompression sickness, a painful, sometimes fatal syndrome caused by the formation of nitrogen bubbles in the tissues of divers, caisson workers, and aviators who move too rapidly from environments of higher to those of lower atmospheric pressures. Nitrogen breathed in air under pressure dissolves in tissue fluids. When ambient pressure is reduced too rapidly, nitrogen comes out of solution faster than it can be circulated to the lungs for expiration. Gaseous nitrogen then accumulates in the joint spaces and peripheral circulation, impairing tissue oxygenation. Disorientation, severe pain, and syncope follow. Treatment is by rapid return of the patient to an environment of higher pressure followed by gradual decompression. Death is more often caused by accident during syncope rather than by decompression sickness itself. Also called **bends, caisson disease.** Compare **barotrauma.**

decongestant, **1.** of or pertaining to a substance or procedure that eliminates or reduces congestion or swelling. **2.** a decongestant drug. Antihistaminic agents, as chlorpheniramine maleate, and adrenergic drugs, as epinephrine, ephedrine, and phenylpropanolamine hydrochloride, that cause bronchodilatation or vasoconstriction of nasal mucosa are used as decongestants. Respiratory tract congestion caused by bacterial infection is usually treated with an antibiotic, and nasal congestion produced by the common cold may be relieved by the inhalation of plain or mentholated steam.

decorticate posture /dēkôr′tikāt/, the position of a comatose patient in which the upper extremities are flexed at the elbows and at the wrists. The legs also may be flexed. The decorticate posture indicates a lesion in a mesencephalic region of the brain. In some instances the posture may be produced by application of a painful stimulation to a comatose patient.

decortication /dēkôr′tikā′shən/, (in medicine) the removal of the cortical tissue of an organ or structure, as the kidney, the brain, and the lung. **–decorticate,** *v., adj.*

decremental conduction, (in cardiology) conduction that slows progressively as the effectiveness of the propagating impulse gradually decreases.

decubitus /dikyo͞o′bitəs/, a recumbent or horizontal position, as lateral decubitus, which is lying on one side. See also **decubitus care, decubitus ulcer.**

decubitus care, the management and prevention of decubitus ulcers that occur most frequently on the sacrum, elbows, heels, outer ankles, inner knees, hips, shoulder blades, and ear rims of immobilized patients, especially those who are obese, elderly, or suffering from infections, injuries, or a poor nutritional state.

■ METHOD: Decubiti may be prevented by repositioning the immobile patient every 2 hours, keeping the skin dry, and inspecting pressure areas every 4 to 6 hours for signs of redness. Bed linen is kept dry and wrinkle-free; a sheet is used to lift the patient, who is moved frequently from the bed but is not allowed to sit in one place for more than 30 minutes. A high-protein diet, vitamins, and iron may be ordered for vulnerable patients, and a prophylactic measure is daily skin care, in which all areas are washed, rinsed, and dried thoroughly and lotion is gently rubbed on bony prominences. A thin layer of cornstarch or a noncaking powder is applied to areas showing excessive perspiration, and the perineal and perianal areas are washed with soap and water after each defecation and urination. Preventive devices include air mattresses, flotation mattresses, sheepskins, silicone pads, foam cushions for wheelchairs, and heel and elbow guards. Stage I decubiti, characterized by redness that is not relieved by circulatory stimulation or removal of pressure, and Stage II lesions, involving excoriation, vesiculation, or breaks in the skin, are treated similarly. The area is cleaned every 8 hours as indicated with mild soap and water, dilute hydrogen peroxide, or normal saline solution and is blotted dry. To increase circulation, the area is massaged gently and exposed every 2 to 4 hours for 15 minutes to air, sunlight, or a heat lamp. Magnesium aluminum hydroxide gel, karaya powder, A & D ointment, tincture of benzoin, or povidone-iodine may be applied to the area, but if there is no improvement within 48 hours, a different kind of dressing is tried. Pressure and irritation to excoriated areas are avoided at all times. Stage III decubiti, in which there is full-thickness skin loss, and Stage IV pressure ulcers, which characteristically invade fascia, connective tissue, muscle, or bone, require more extensive treatment. The patient is turned every 1 to 2 hours, and the lesion is irrigated with hydrogen peroxide and water every 6 to 8 hours. The affected area is exposed to air for 15 to 30 minutes every 2 to 4 hours and to a heat lamp for 15 minutes every 4 to 6 hours. The ulcer may be incised, debrided, and covered with a nonadhering dressing secured by nonallergenic tape. Proteolytic enzyme preparations, antibiotics, magnesium aluminum hydroxide gel, gold-leaf flakes, or povidone-iodine may be applied to the wound, and granulated sugar dressings may be used after removal of necrotic tissue, although they are contraindicated in diabetic patients.

■ NURSING ORDERS: The nurse plays a major role in the prevention of decubiti and in their treatment if they occur, turning the patient at frequent intervals, applying the ordered medications and dressings to the lesions, and, in the administration of daily skin care, avoiding vigorous rubbing. The nurse conducts active or passive exercises with massage to the patient's extremities and, when indicated, prepares for incision and debridement of advanced ulcers.

■ OUTCOME CRITERIA: Decubiti are often resistant to treatment, and large areas of ulceration can be life-threatening, especially in a debilitated patient. Prompt and continued care of early lesions can prevent invasion of underlying tissue and promote healing. The nurse may elicit the cooperation and participation of the patient in a nursing care plan that includes all preventive measures. The importance of frequent change of position, dryness, cleanliness, and good nutrition are emphasized.

decubitus ulcer, an inflammation, sore, or ulcer in the skin over a bony prominence. It results from ischemic hypoxia of the tissues because of prolonged pressure on the part. Decubitus ulcers are most often seen in aged, debilitated, immobilized, or cachectic patients. The sores are graded by stages of severity: Stage I: The skin is red; with massage and relief of pressure, the color of the skin does not return to normal. Stage II: The skin is blistered, peeling, or cracked, although damage is still superficial. Stage III: The skin is broken; a full thickness of skin is lost, subcutaneous tissue may also be damaged, and a serous or bloody drainage may be seen. Stage IV: A deep, craterlike ulcer has formed. The full thickness of skin and the subcutaneous tissues are destroyed. Fascia, connective tissue, bone, or muscle underlying the ulcer are exposed and may be damaged. Prevention of decubitus ulcers is a cardinal aspect of nursing care; treatment is planned specific to the location and the extent of the condition.

decussate /dəcus′āt/, to cross in the form of an "X," as certain nerve fibers from the retina cross at the optic chiasm. –**decussation,** *n.*

deduction, a system of reasoning that leads from a known principle to an unknown, or from the general to the specific. Deductive reasoning is used to test diagnostic hypotheses.

deemed status, a status conferred on a hospital by a professional standards review organization (PSRO) in formal recognition that the hospital's review, continued-stay review, and medical care evaluation programs meet certain effectiveness criteria.

deep brachial artery, a branch of each of the brachial arteries, arising at the distal border of the teres major, passing deeply into the arm between the long and lateral heads of the triceps brachii, and supplying the humerus and the muscles of the upper arm. It has five branches: ascending, radial collateral, middle collateral, muscular, and nutrient. Also called **superior profunda artery.**

deep breathing and coughing exercises, the exercises taught to a person to improve aeration or to maintain respiratory function, especially after prolonged inactivity or after general anesthesia. Incisional pain after surgery in the chest or abdomen often inhibits normal respiratory excursion. See also **cupping and vibrating, postural drainage.**

■ METHOD: The person is assisted to a comfortable position, supine or sitting up. An analgesic is given before the exercises if pain is present. Inhalation through the nose and exhalation through the mouth are encouraged. After a deep inhalation, with the incision supported, the patient is asked to cough. If pain prevents the person from producing a deep, effective cough, a series of short barklike coughs may be encouraged.

■ NURSING ORDERS: The use of simple nursing techniques and patience and encouragement significantly improve the effectiveness of the exercises. Positioning increases comfort, allows the abdominal contents to fall away from the diaphragm, and encourages full expansion of the chest wall on inspiration. If an incision is present, it may be supported with the hands or with a book or pillow held against the abdomen. The person is often reluctant to breathe deeply or to cough; adequate analgesia, encouragement, and a patient explanation to the person of the benefits may overcome that resistance. Various devices are available for use in respiratory exercises, as those used in atelectasis to strengthen the muscles used in expiration and to empty the air sacs of retained gas. Postural drainage is commonly performed concurrently with coughing and deep-breathing exercises.

■ OUTCOME CRITERIA: When shallow breathing has replaced deep breathing, secretions tend to dry in the respiratory passages, causing damage to the mucous membranes lining the passages. Coughing and deep breathing serve to clear the dried or thick and viscid mucus, to allow moisturized air to enter the bronchi, bronchioles, and alveoli, and to expand the lungs and increase the exchange of gases, thereby improving ventilation.

deep coma. See **coma.**

deep fascia, the most extensive of three kinds of fascia comprising an intricate series of connective sheets and bands that hold the muscles and other structures in place throughout the body, wrapping the muscles in gray, feltlike membranes. The deep fasciae comprise a continuous system, splitting and fusing in an elaborate network attached to the skeleton and divided into the outer investing layer, the internal investing layer, and the intermediate membranes. Compare **subcutaneous fascia, subserous fascia.**

deep palmar arch, the termination of the radial artery, joining the deep palmar branch of the ulnar artery in the palm of the hand.

deep sensation, the awareness or perception of pain, pressure, or tension in the deep layers of the skin, the muscles, tendons, or joints. Such sensations are conveyed to the brain via the spinal column. Compare **superficial sensation.**

deep temporal artery, one of the branches of the maxillary artery on each side of the head. It branches into the anterior portion and the posterior portion, both rising between the temporalis and the pericranium to supply the temporalis and to anastomose with the middle temporal artery. The anterior branch communicates with the lacrimal artery by small branches that pierce the zygomatic bone and the great wing of the sphenoid. Compare **middle temporal artery, superficial temporal artery.**

deep tendon reflex (DTR), a brisk contraction of a muscle in response to a sudden stretch induced by a sharp tap by a finger or rubber hammer on the tendon of insertion of the muscle. Absence of the reflex may have been caused by damage to the muscle, the peripheral nerve, nerve roots, or the spinal cord at that level. A hyperactive reflex may indicate disease of the pyramidal tract above the level of the reflex arc being tested. Generalized hyperactivity of DTRs may be caused by hyperthyroidism. Kinds of DTRs include **Achilles tendon reflex, biceps reflex, brachioradialis reflex, patellar reflex,** and **triceps reflex.** Also called **myotatic reflex, tendon reflex.** See also **hung-up reflex.**

deep vein, one of the many systemic veins that accompany the arteries, usually enclosed in a sheath that wraps both the vein and the associated artery. The larger arteries, as the axillary, the femoral, the popliteal, and the subclavian, are usually accompanied by only one deep vein. The deep veins accompanying the smaller arteries, as the brachial, the peroneal, and the radial, occur usually in pairs, one vein on each side of the artery. Various structures, as the skull, the vertebral column, and the liver, are served by less closely associated arteries and veins. Compare **superficial vein.**

deep x-ray therapy, the treatment of internal neoplasms, as Wilms' tumor of the kidney, Hodgkin's disease, and other cancers, with ionizing radiation from an external source. The dose delivered is determined according to the radiosensitivity, size, pathologic grade and differentiation of the tumor, the tolerance of normal surrounding tissue to irradiation, and the condition of the patient. Deep x-ray therapy frequently causes nausea, malaise, diarrhea, and skin reactions, as blanching, erythema, itching, burning, oozing, or desquamation, but with modern techniques the ray is beamed directly to the site, reducing side scatter, and the skin can be spared. Because tumor cells are hypoxic and are more effectively eradicated when they are well oxygenated, the patient may breathe hyperbaric oxygen or atmospheric oxygen with 5% carbon dioxide during deep x-ray therapy.

deerfly fever. See **tularemia.**

defamation, any communication, written or spoken, that is untrue and that injures the good name or reputation of another or that in any way brings that person into disrepute.

default judgment, (in law) a judgment rendered against a defendant because of the defendant's failure to appear in court or to answer the plaintiff's claim within the proper time.

defecation /def′ikā′shən/, the elimination of feces from the digestive tract through the rectum. See also **constipation, diarrhea, feces.** **–defecate** /def′ikāt/, *v.*

defecation reflex. See **rectal reflex.**

defendant, (in law) the party that is named in a plaintiff's complaint and against whom the plaintiff's allegations are made. The defendant must respond to the allegations.

defense mechanism, an unconscious, intrapsychic reaction that offers protection to the self from a stressful situation. Kinds of defense mechanisms include **compensation, conversion, dissociation, displacement,** and **sublimation.** Also called **ego-defense mechanism.**

deferent duct. See **vas deferens.**

deferoxamine mesylate, a chelating agent.

■ INDICATIONS: It is prescribed in the treatment of acute iron intoxication and chronic iron overload.

■ CONTRAINDICATIONS: Renal disease or anuria prohibits its use.

■ ADVERSE EFFECTS: Among the most serious adverse reactions are hypotension, tachycardia, dysuria, visual difficulties, and allergic-type reactions.

defervescence /di′fərves′əns/, the diminishing or disappearance of a fever. –**defervescent,** *adj.*

defibrillate /difī′brilāt, difib′-/, to stop fibrillation of the atria or the ventricles of the heart, usually by delivering an electric shock to the myocardium through the chest wall by the use of a defibrillator. See also **defibrillation.**

defibrillation /difī′brilā′shən/, the termination of ventricular fibrillation, by delivering a direct electric countershock to the patient's precordium.

■ METHOD: Defibrillation by electric countershock is a common emergency measure generally performed by a physician or specially trained nurse or paramedic. The electrode paddles of the defibrillator are covered with a conductive jelly or applied over wet saline sponges. One paddle is placed to the right of the upper sternum below the clavicle, and the other is applied to the midaxillary line of the left lower rib cage. In another method, one paddle is placed over the upper precordium, and the other is applied beneath the patient's chest. The defibrillator, usually a condenser-discharge system, is set to deliver between 200 and 400 W seconds. Respiratory support is suspended during the shock but is promptly resumed. If one or two shocks fail to cause defibrillation, cardiopulmonary resuscitation (CPR) may be conducted until another shock is attempted. Before the procedure, the patient's level of consciousness, pulse, respirations, and electrocardiogram are observed. After defibrillation, the patient's level of consciousness, irritation or sloughing of the exposed skin of the chest, and electrocardiographic signs of the return of sinus rhythm, continued fibrillation, and the development of cardiac standstill are investigated. Blood pressure, apical pulse, and respirations are checked every 5 to 10 minutes for 4 hours, and then every 30 to 60 minutes. CPR is initiated if no pulse is present. Cardiac activity is monitored; arterial blood gases may be determined, and oxygen with assisted ventilation may be ordered. Parenteral fluids are maintained, and the patient's skin, which may be irritated by the shock, receives care by application of a lanolin-based lotion.

■ NURSING ORDERS: The nurse performs all the required procedures before and after defibrillation and makes certain that all equipment surrounding the patient is grounded.

■ OUTCOME CRITERIA: Successful defibrillation by electrical countershock can reverse life-threatening cardiac arrythmias, especially ventricular fibrillation.

defibrillator /difī′brilā′tər, difib′-/, a device that delivers an electric shock at a preset voltage to the myocardium through the chest wall. It is used for restoring the normal cardiac rhythm and rate when the heart has stopped beating or is fibrillating.

deficiency disease, a condition resulting from the lack of one or more essential nutrients in the diet, from metabolic dysfunction, or from impaired digestion or absorption, excessive excretion, or increased biologic requirements. Compare **malnutrition.** See also **avitaminosis.**

definitive /difin′ətiv/, **1.** final; clearly established without doubt or question. **2.** (in embryology) fully formed in the final differentiation of a tissue, structure, or organ. Compare **primitive. 3.** (in parasitology) of or pertaining to the host in which the parasite undergoes the sexual phase of its reproductive cycle.

definitive host, any animal in which the reproductive stages of a parasite develop. The female *Anopheles* mosquito is the definitive host for malaria. Humans are definitive hosts for pinworms, schistosomes, and tapeworms. Also called **primary host.** Compare **dead-end host, intermediate host, reservoir host.** See also **host.**

definitive treatment, any therapy generally accepted as a specific cure of a disease. Compare **expectant treatment, palliative treatment, supportive treatment.**

deformity, a condition of being distorted, disfigured, flawed, malformed, or misshapen, which may affect the body in general or any part of it and may be the result of disease, injury, or birth defect, as Arnold-Chiari deformity, in which a part of the brain protrudes through the base of the skull into the spinal canal, and seal-fin deformity, characterized by a deviation of the fingers as an effect of rheumatoid arthritis.

degeneration, the gradual deterioration of normal cells and body functions.

degenerative chorea. See **Huntington's chorea.**

degenerative disease /dijen′ərətiv/, any disease in which there is deterioration of structure or function of tissue. Some kinds of degenerative disease are **arteriosclerosis, cancer,** and **osteoarthritis.**

degenerative joint disease. See **osteoarthritis.**

degloving, the exposure of the bony mandibular anterior or posterior regions by oral surgery.

deglutition /di′glo͞otish′ən/, swallowing.

deglutition apnea, the normal absence of respiration during swallowing.

degradation, the reduction of a chemical compound to a compound less complex, usually by splitting off one or more groups or subgroups of atoms, as deamination.

dehiscence /dihis′əns/, the separation of a surgical incision or rupture of a wound closure.

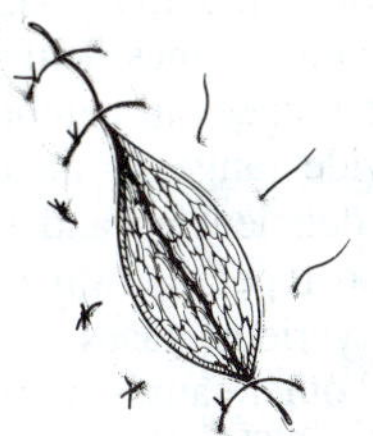
Wound dehiscence

dehydrate /dihī′drāt/, **1.** to remove or lose water from a substance. **2.** to lose excessive water from the body. –**dehydration,** *n.*

dehydrated alcohol, a clear, colorless, highly hygroscopic liquid with a burning taste, containing at least 99.5% ethyl alcohol by volume. Also called **absolute alcohol.**

dehydration, **1.** excessive loss of water from the body tissues. Dehydration is accompanied by a disturbance in the balance of essential electrolytes, particularly sodium, potassium, and chloride. Dehydration may follow prolonged fever, diarrhea, vomiting, acidosis, and any condition in which there is rapid depletion of body fluids. It is of particular concern among infants and young children, because their electrolyte balance is normally precarious. Signs of dehydration include poor skin turgor, flushed dry skin, coated tongue, oliguria, irritability, and confusion. Normal fluid volume and balanced electrolyte values are the primary goals of therapy. **2.** rendering a substance free from water.

dehydration fever, a fever that frequently occurs in newborns, thought to be caused by dehydration. Also called **inanition fever.** Compare **inanition, starvation.**

dehydration of gingivae, the drying of gingival tissue, often the result of mouth breathing, which lowers the resistance of the gingival tissue to infection.

deinstitutionalization, the practice of discharging certain long-term mentally ill patients into the local community.

déjà vu /dāzhävY′, -vē′, -vo͞o′/, the sensation or illusion that one is encountering a set of circumstances or a place that was previously experienced. The phenomenon, which is normal in everyone but occurs more frequently or continuously in certain emotional and organic disorders, results from some unconscious emotional connection with the present experience. Compare **jamais vu, paramnesia.**

Dejerine-Sottas disease /dezh′ərinsot′əz/, a rare, congenital spinocerebellar disorder characterized by the development of palpable thickenings along peripheral nerves, degeneration of the peripheral nervous system, pain, paresthesia, ataxia, diminished sensation, and deep tendon reflexes. Diagnosis is made by a histologic examination of a peripheral nerve. There is no specific treatment. Also called **progressive interstitial hypertrophic neuropathy.**

del, (in cytogenetics) abbreviation for **deletion.**

Deladumone, a trademark for a fixed-combination drug containing an androgen (testosterone enanthate), an estrogen (estradiol valerate), and chlorobutanol.

Delalutin, a trademark for a progestin (hydroxyprogesterone caproate).

de Lange's syndrome. See **Amsterdam dwarf.**

Delano, Jane A. (1862–1919), an American nurse who organized the American Red Cross Nursing Service, an organization formed to supply nurses to the military forces. In 1891 she became the director of the Nurses' Training School of the University of Pennsylvania and was later appointed the director of the Bellevue Hospital Training School for Nurses in New York, where she had

Physical signs of dehydration

	Isotonic (loss of water and salt)	*Hypotonic (loss of salt in excess of water)*	*Hypertonic (loss of water in excess of salt)*
Skin			
Color	Gray	Gray	Gray
Temperature	Cold	Cold	Cold or hot
Turgor	Poor	Very poor	Fair
Feel	Dry	Clammy	Thickened
Mucous membranes	Dry	Slightly moist	Parched
Tearing and salivation	Absent	Absent	Absent
Eyeball	Sunken and soft	Sunken and soft	Sunken
Fontanel	Sunken	Sunken	Sunken
Body temperature	Subnormal or elevated	Subnormal	Subnormal or elevated
Pulse	Rapid	Very rapid	Moderately rapid
Respirations	Rapid	Rapid	Rapid
Behavior	Irritable to lethargic	Lethargic to comatose; convulsions	Marked lethargy with extreme hyperirritability on stimulation

been trained. On a trip to survey nursing conditions in Europe, she died after surgery for a mastoid infection at Base Hospital, Savenay, France, in March 1919.

Delatestryl, a trademark for an androgen (testosterone enanthate).

delayed dentition. See **retarded dentition.**

delayed echolalia, a phenomenon, commonly seen in schizophrenia, involving the meaningless, automatic repetition of overheard words and phrases. It occurs hours, days, or even weeks after the original stimulus.

delayed hypersensitivity reaction. See **cell-mediated immune response.**

delayed postpartum hemorrhage, hemorrhage occurring later than 24 hours after delivery. It is most often caused by retained fragments of the placenta, a laceration of the cervix or vagina that was not discovered or that was not completely sutured, or by subinvolution of the placental site within the uterus. Characteristics of delayed postpartum hemorrhage are heavy bleeding and signs of impending shock and anemia. The cause is diagnosed and treated. A laceration is closed with suture, retained fragments of placenta are removed, infection is treated with antibiotics, or the uterus is caused to contract by the administration of ergotrate or oxytocin. See also **postpartum hemorrhage.**

delayed sensation, a feeling or impression that is not experienced immediately after a stimulus. See also **sensation,** def. 1.

Delestrogen, a trademark for an estrogen (estradiol valerate).

deletion (del), (in cytogenetics) the loss of a piece of a chromosome because it has broken away from the genetic material.

deletion syndrome, any of a group of congenital autosomal anomalies that result from the loss of chromosomal genetic material, because of breakage of a chromatid during cell division, as the cat-cry syndrome, which results from the absence of the short arm of chromosome 5.

Delhi boil. See **oriental sore.**

deliberate hypotension, an anesthetic process in which a short-acting hypotensive agent such as sodium nitroprusside or trimethaphan camsylate is given to reduce blood pressure and thus bleeding during surgery. The procedure facilitates surgery by making vessels and tissues more visible and reducing blood loss.

delinquency, **1.** negligence or failure to fulfill a duty or obligation. **2.** an offense, fault, misdemeanor, or misdeed; a tendency to commit such acts. See also **juvenile delinquency.**

delinquent, **1.** characterized by neglect of duty or violation of law. **2.** one whose behavior is characterized by persistent antisocial, illegal, violent, or criminal acts; a juvenile delinquent.

délire de toucher /dālir′dətōōshā′/, an abnormal desire or irresistable urge to touch or handle objects.

delirium /dilir′ē·əm/, **1.** a state of frenzied excitement or wild enthusiasm. **2.** an acute organic mental disorder characterized by confusion, disorientation, restlessness, clouding of the consciousness, incoherence, fear, anxiety, excitement, and often illusions, hallucinations, usually of visual origin, and at times delusions. The condition is caused by disturbances in cerebral functions that may result from a wide range of metabolic disorders, including nutritional deficiencies and endocrine imbalances; postpartum or postoperative stress; the ingestion of toxic substances, as various gases, metals, or drugs, including alcohol; and other causes of physical and mental shock or exhaustion. The symptoms are usually of short duration and reversible with treatment of the underlying cause, although in extreme cases, where the toxic condition is exceedingly severe or prolonged, permanent brain damage may occur. Bed rest in a quiet environment is essential. The delirious patient must be protected from accidents and self-injury. In prolonged cases, dehydration and vitamin deficiency may occur. Sedatives or tranquilizing drugs are often used to relieve excitability. Kinds of delirium include **acute delirium, delirium tremens, exhaustion delirium, senile delirium,** and **traumatic delirium.** Compare **dementia.** **–delirious,** *adj.*

delirium tremens (DTs), an acute and sometimes fatal psychotic reaction caused by excessive intake of alcoholic beverages over a long period of time. The reaction may follow a prolonged alcoholic binge without an adequate intake of food, occur during a period of abstinence, be precipitated by a head injury or infection, or result from the partial or total withdrawal of alcohol after prolonged drinking. Initial symptoms include loss of appetite, insomnia, and general restlessness, followed by agitation, excitement, disorientation, mental confusion, vivid and often frightening hallucinations, acute fear and anxiety, illusions and delusions, coarse tremors of the hands, feet, legs, and tongue, fever, increased heart rate, extreme perspiration, GI distress, and precordial pain. The episode, which usually constitutes a medical emergency, typically lasts from 3 to 6 days and is generally followed by a deep sleep. Treatment includes a quiet, nonstimulating environment in which the person is watched closely and protected from self-injury, not only during the period of delirium but, more important, during convalescence, when depression and remorse often lead to attempted suicide. Extreme fatigue, pneumonia, respiratory infections, and heart failure are common complications, as are severe dehydration and nutritional deficiencies. Dietary supplements are often given; tube feeding and intravenous fluids may be needed. Sedatives and tranquilizing agents are useful for quieting the person. Compare **alcoholic hallucinosis, Stearns' alcoholic amentia.** See also **Korsakoff's psychosis.**

delivery, (in obstetrics) the birth of a child; parturition.

delivery room, a unit of a hospital utilized for obstetric delivery and infant resuscitation.

Delta-Cortef, a trademark for a glucocorticoid (prednisolone).

Delta Dental Plan, a dental fee and payment plan of the Delta Dental Plans Association for providing prepaid dental care to the public on a group basis. The association is organized and guided by state dental societies throughout the United States.

delta-1-testolactone. See **testolactone.**

delta-9-tetrahydrocannabinol (THC), a pharmacologically active ingredient of cannabis that has been used in treating some cases of nausea and vomiting associated with cancer chemotherapy. See **cannabis.**

delta optical density analysis, a technique used to diagnose anemia in a fetus by measuring the proportion of bilirubin decomposition products in the aminiotic fluid. The method involves spectrographic examination of a fluid sample. It measures the bilirubin and bilirubin-products concentration according to the wavelengths of light absorbed by the hemolytic products, as the bilirubin products alter the normal color of the amniotic fluid. The data are sometimes expressed in terms of δOD_{450}, the number representing the wavelength in nm at which maximum absorption of light by bilirubin occurs. If the delta optical density analysis indicates the fetus is moderately to severely anemic, immediate delivery is usually recommended when the gestational age permits. Otherwise, intrauterine fetal blood transfusions may be recommended.

delta wave, **1.** also called **delta rhythm.** the slowest of the four types of brain waves, characterized by a frequency of 4 Hz and a relatively high voltage. Delta waves are "deep-sleep waves" associated with a dreamless state from which an individual is not easily aroused. Compare **alpha wave, beta wave, theta wave.** **2.** (in cardiology) a slurring of the QRS portion of an ECG tracing caused by preexcitation.

deltoid, **1.** triangular. **2.** of or pertaining to the deltoid muscle that covers the shoulder.

deltoid muscle, a large, thick triangular muscle that covers the shoulder joint and abducts, flexes, extends, and rotates the arm. It arises from various surfaces on the clavicle, acromion, and scapula and inserts, with a thick tendon, into the humerus. Also called **deltoideus.**

delusion, a persistent, aberrant belief or perception held inviolable by a person even though it is illogical, unique, and probably wrong. Kinds of delusion include **delusion of being controlled, delusion of grandeur, delusion of persecution, nihilistic delusion,** and **somatic delusion.** Compare **illusion.**

delusion of being controlled, the false belief that one's feelings, beliefs, thoughts, and acts are governed by some external force, as seen in various forms of schizophrenia. See also **delusion.**

delusion of grandeur, the gross exaggeration of one's importance, wealth, power, or talents, as seen in such disorders as megalomania, general paresis, and paranoid schizophrenia. See also **delusion.**

delusion of persecution, a morbid belief that one is being mistreated and harassed by unidentified enemies, as seen in paranoia and paranoid schizophrenia. See also **delusion.**

delusion of reference. See **idea of reference.**

delusion stupor, the state of lethargy and unresponsiveness observed in catatonic schizophrenia.

demarcation current, an electric current that flows from an uninjured to an injured end of a muscle. Also called **current of injury.**

Demazin, a trademark for a respiratory, fixed-combination drug containing an adrenergic (phenylephrine hydrochloride) and an antihistaminic (chlorpheniramine maleate).

deme /dēm/, a small, closely related, interbreeding population of organisms or individuals, usually occupying a circumscribed area. Also called **genetic population.**

demecarium bromide, an ophthalmic anticholinesterase agent.

■ INDICATION: It is prescribed in the treatment of open-angle glaucoma.

■ CONTRAINDICATIONS: Active uveal inflammation, narrow-angle glaucoma, glaucoma associated with iridocyclitis, bronchial asthma, peptic ulcer, epilepsy, recent myocardial infarction, or known hypersensitivity to this drug prohibits its use.

■ ADVERSE EFFECTS: Among the most serious adverse reactions are symptoms associated with systemic absorption of anticholinesterase agents (including certain insecticides), as bradycardia and diarrhea. Eye irritation, hypotension, headache, formation of cysts, and lens opacities also may occur.

demeclocycline hydrochloride, a tetracycline antibiotic.

■ INDICATIONS: It is prescribed in the treatment of a variety of infections, including infections in which use of penicillin is contraindicated.

■ CONTRAINDICATIONS: Renal or liver dysfunction, pregnancy, early childhood, or known hypersensitivity to this drug or to other tetracycline medication prohibits its use.

■ ADVERSE EFFECTS: Among the more serious adverse effects are blood disorders, GI disturbances, phototoxicity, potentially serious suprainfections, and hypersensitivity reactions. Discoloration of teeth may occur in children exposed to the drug in utero or before 8 years of age.

dementia /dimen'shə/, a progressive, organic mental disorder characterized by chronic personality disintegration, confusion, disorientation, stupor, deterioration of intellectual capacity and function, and impairment of control of memory, judgment, and impulses. Dementia caused by drug intoxication, hyperthyroidism, pernicious anemia, paresis, subdural hematoma, benign brain tumor, hydrocephalus, insulin shock, and tumor of islet cells of the pancreas can be reversed by treating the condition; Alzheimer's disease, Pick's disease, Huntington's disease, and traumatic injuries to the brain are not amenable to treatment. Kinds of dementia include **Alzheimer's disease, dementia paralytica, Pick's disease,**

secondary dementia, senile dementia, and **toxic dementia.**

dementia paralytica. See **general paresis.**

dementia praecox /prē′koks/, an absolete term for schizophrenia, especially developing in adolescence or early adulthood. See also **schizophrenia.**

Demerol, a trademark for a narcotic analgesic (meperidine).

Demerol Hydrochloride, a trademark for a narcotic analgesic (meperidine hydrochloride).

-demic, a combining form meaning 'relating to disease in a (specified) region': *interedemic, philodemic, prosodemic.*

demigauntlet bandage /dem′igônt′lit/, a glovelike bandage covering only the hand and leaving the fingers free. See also **gauntlet bandage.**

demineralization, a decrease in the amount of minerals or inorganic salts in tissues, as occurs in certain diseases.

demography /dəmog′rəfē/, the study of human populations, particularly the size, distribution, and characteristics of members of population groups. Demography is applied in studies of health problems involving ethnic groups, populations of a specific geographic region, religious groups with special dietary restrictions, as Mormons (Church of Jesus Christ of Latter-Day Saints) or Seventh-Day Adventists, and members of population groups that may represent a typical cross-section of the entire nation, as in the continuing study of residents of Framingham, Massachusetts, by the National Institutes of Health. Compare **epidemiology.**

De Morgan's spots. See **cherry angioma.**

Demser, a trademark for an antihypertensive (metyrosine).

demulcent /dimul′sənt/, **1.** any of several oily substances used for soothing and reducing irritation of surfaces that have been abraded or irritated. **2.** soothing, as a counterirritant or balm.

Demulen, a trademark for an oral contraceptive containing an estrogen (ethinyl estradiol) and a progestogen (ethynodiol diacetate).

demyelination /dimī′əlinā′shən/, the process of destruction or removal of the myelin sheath from a nerve or nerve fiber.

denatured alcohol, ethyl alcohol made unfit for ingestion by the addition of acetone or methanol, used as a solvent and in chemical processes.

dendr-, a combining form meaning 'pertaining to a tree or branches': *dendriceptor, dendroid, dendrophobia.*

-dendria, a combining form meaning the 'twiglike branching of nerve fibers': *oligodendria, telodendria, zoodendria.*

dendrite /den′drīt/, a branching process that extends from the cell body of a neuron. Each neuron usually possesses several dendrites, which receive impulses that are conducted to the cell body. The number of dendrites varies with the functions of a neuron. Compare **axon.**

dendritic /dendrit′ik/, **1.** treelike, with branches that spread toward or into neighboring tissues, as dendritic keratitis. **2.** of or pertaining to a dendrite.

dendritic keratitis, a serious herpes virus infection of the eye, characterized by an ulceration of the surface of the cornea resembling a tree with knobs at the ends of the branches. Photophobia, the sensation of a foreign body in the eye, pain, and conjunctivitis are usual. Treatment includes application of idoxuridine (IDU), chemical debridement with an iodine tincture, or surgical removal of the involved layer of corneal tissue cells. Untreated dendritic keratitis may result in permanent scarring of the cornea with impaired vision or blindness.

dendrodendritic synapse, a type of synapse in which a dendrite of one neuron comes in contact with a dendrite of another neuron. Compare **axodendritic synapse.**

-dendron, a combining form meaning a 'treelike formation': *neurodendron, telodendron, toxicodendron.*

dengue fever /deng′gē, den′gā/, an acute arbovirus infection transmitted to humans by the *Aedes* mosquito and occurring in tropic and subtropic regions. The disease usually produces a triad of symptoms: fever, rash, and severe head, back, and muscle pain. Manifestations of dengue usually occur in two phases, separated by a day of remission. In the first attack, the patient experiences fever, extreme weakness, headache, sore throat, muscle pains, and edema of the hands and feet. The second attack is marked by a return of fever and by a bright-red scarlatinaform rash. Dengue is a self-limited illness, though it may take patients several weeks to recover. Treatment is symptomatic; analgesics may be given to relieve headache and other pains. Also called **Aden fever, bouquet fever, breakbone fever, dandy fever, solar fever.** See also ***Aedes*, arbovirus.**

dengue hemorrhagic fever shock syndrome (DHFS), a grave form of dengue fever characterized by shock with collapse or prostration; cold, clammy extremities; a weak, thready pulse; respiratory distress; and all of the symptoms of dengue fever. Hemorrhage, bruises, small reddish spots indicating bleeding from skin capillaries, and bloody vomit, urine, and feces may occur and precede circulatory collapse. Treatment includes fluid and electrolyte replacement and fresh blood, plasma, or platelet transfusions as needed. Oxygen and sedatives may be administered. See also **breakbone fever, dandy fever, dengue fever.**

denial, 1. refusal or restriction of something requested, claimed, or needed, often resulting in physical or emotional deficiency. **2.** an unconscious defense mechanism in which emotional conflict and anxiety are avoided by refusing to acknowledge those thoughts, feelings, desires, impulses, or external facts that are consciously intolerable.

Denis Browne splint, a splint for the correction of talipes equinovarus (clubfoot), composed of a curved bar attached to the soles of a pair of high-top shoes. The splint is equipped with wing nuts, allowing abduction of each foot to be individualized. The splint is commonly applied nightly in late infancy after casting and manipulation have effectively reduced the deformity.

Denman's spontaneous evolution, a natural, unassisted turning of the fetus from the transverse presentation. The head rotates back and, as the breech descends, the shoulder ascends in the pelvis. The back of the fetus is generally posterior. Also called **Denman's method, Denman's spontaneous version.**

dens, *pl.* **dentes** /den′tēz/, a tooth or toothlike structure or process. See also **dentition, tooth.**

dens deciduus. See **deciduous tooth.**

dense fibrous tissue, a fibrous connective tissue consisting of compact, strong, inelastic bundles of parallel collagenous fibers that have a glistening white color. Organized dense fibrous tissue comprises the tendons, the aponeuroses, and the ligaments; unorganized dense fibrous tissue comprises the fascial membranes, the dermis of the skin, the periosteum, and the capsules of organs. Compare **loose fibrous tissue.**

dens in dente /den′tə/, an anomaly of the teeth, found chiefly in the maxillary lateral incisors and characterized by invagination of the enamel. This condition results in a radiographic image suggestive of a tooth within a tooth. Also called **dens invaginatus, gestant odontoma.**

densitometer /den′sitom′ətər/, a device that uses a photoelectric cell to detect differences in the density of light transmitted through a liquid, as in spectrophotometric analysis of biologic substances.

density, the amount of mass of a substance in a given volume. The greater the mass in a given volume, the greater the density. See also **mass, volume.**

density gradient, the variation of the concentration of a solute in a confined solution.

dens serotinus. See **wisdom tooth.**

dent-, denta-. See **dento-.**

dental, of or pertaining to a tooth or teeth.

dental alveolus /alvē′ələs/, a tooth socket in the mandible or maxilla.

dental amalgam, an alloy of silver, tin, and mercury with small amounts of copper and sometimes zinc, used for filling tooth cavities.

dental anesthesia, any of several anesthetic procedures used in dental surgery. Injectable local anesthetics have largely replaced the use of inhalational general anesthesics, especially of nitrous oxide.

dental anomaly, an aberration in which one or more teeth deviate from the normal in form, function, or position.

dental arch, the curving shape formed by the arrangement of a normal set of teeth.

dental assistant, a person who assists a dentist in the performance of generalized tasks, including chairside assistance, clerical work, reception, and some radiography and dental laboratory work.

dental biomechanics, the field of biomechanics that deals with the biologic effects of dental restoration on oral structures.

dental calculus, a salivary deposit of calcium phosphate and calcium carbonate with organic matter on the teeth or a dental prosthesis. See also **subgingival calculus, supragingival calculus.**

dental canal. See **alveolar canal.**

dental caries, an abnormal destructive condition in a tooth, caused by the complex interaction of food, especially starches and sugars, with bacteria that form dental plaque. This material adheres to the surfaces of the teeth and provides the medium for the growth of bacteria and the production of organic acids that cause breaks in the enamel sheath of the tooth. Enzymes produced by the bacteria then attack the protein component of the tooth. This process, if untreated, ultimately leads to the formation of deep cavities and bacterial infection of the pulp chamber and nerves. Dental caries may be prevented by avoidance of sugar in the diet, regular brushing and removal of food particles from the surfaces and interstices of the teeth, fluoridation of drinking water, and the topical application of fluorides to the teeth. Removal of plaque by a dental hygienist is performed to eliminate the source of decay as well as to prevent infection and destruction of the peridontal tissues. Treatment of dental caries includes removal of the decayed material and the refilling of the cavity with an amalgam of silver or another restorative material. If the lesion has reached the nerve of the tooth, it may be necessary to remove the nerve tissue to alleviate pain, to prevent the spread of infection to the rest of the body, and to allow the continued use of the natural tooth. Alternatively, the entire tooth may be extracted. The development of dental caries in a debilitated patient is a concern because of the danger that infections of the teeth or gums might spread to the rest of the body. In addition, missing, decayed, or painful teeth inhibit mastication and lead to dietary changes, which may in turn cause nutritional and digestive disorders. Kinds of dental caries include **active caries, arrested caries, primary caries,** and **secondary caries.**

dental crypt, the space occupied by a developing tooth.

dental engine, an apparatus consisting of a hand instrument to which various rotating tools or drills can be fitted. It is driven by an electric motor via a continuous cordlike belt.

dental erosion, the chemical or mechanicochemical destruction of a tooth substance that causes variously shaped concavities at the cementoenamel junctions of teeth. The surfaces of these depressions, unlike those of carious cavities, are hard and smooth.

dental extracting forceps, a type of forceps used for grasping teeth in extractions.

dental filling. See **filling.**

dental fistula, an abnormal passage from the apical periodontal area of a tooth to the surface of oral mucous membrane, permitting the discharge of inflammatory or suppurative material. Also called **alveolar fistula.**

dental floss, a waxed or unwaxed thread used to clean tooth surfaces and spaces between the teeth.

dental granuloma, a disorder characterized by a mass of granulation tissue which is surrounded by a fibrous capsule attached to the apex of a pulp-involved tooth. On x-ray film it appears as a well-defined radiolucency.

dental hygienist, a person with special training to provide dental services under the supervision of a dentist. Services supplied by a dental hygienist include dental prophylaxis, radiography, application of medications, and provision of dental education at chairside and in the community.

dental plaque. See **bacterial plaque.**

dental review committee, a group of dentists and administrative personnel that reviews questionable dental claims and practices and suggests dental care policies.

dental root cyst. See **periodontal cyst.**

dental sealants, plastic films that are applied to the chewing surfaces of teeth to seal pits and grooves where food and bacteria usually become trapped. The procedure generally involves isolation of the teeth to be treated, beginning with the molars, to ensure that saliva contamination will not interfere with the process. The tooth surfaces are cleaned with a special brush and cleansing agent, then dried and etched with a phosphoric-acid solution. Fluoride is applied to the enamel after the acid has been washed away, followed by application of a resin sealant. Dental sealants reportedly reduce the incidence of cavities in children's teeth by 50%.

dental stone. See **artificial stone.**

dental technician, a person who makes dental prostheses and orthodontic appliances as prescribed by a dentist. Kinds of dental prostheses made by dental technicians include full dentures, partial dentures, crowns, bridgework, and other dental restorations.

-dentate, a combining form meaning 'possessing teeth': *edentate, multidentate, tridentate.*

dentate fracture /den′tāt/, any fracture that causes serrated bone ends that fit together like the teeth of gears.

denti-, dentia-. See **dento-.**

denticle, a calcified body in the pulp chamber of a tooth. Also called **endolith, pulp stone.** Compare **true denticle, false denticle.**

dentifrice /den′tifris/, a pharmaceutic compound used with a toothbrush for cleaning and polishing the teeth. It typically contains a mild abrasive, a detergent, flavoring agent, and a binder. Other common ingredients are various medications to prevent dental caries and deodorants.

dentigerous cyst /dentij′ərəs/, one of three kinds of follicular cyst, consisting of an epithelium-lined sac, filled with fluid or viscous material that surrounds the crown of an unerupted tooth or odontoma. Compare **primordial cyst, multilocular cyst.**

dentin /den′tin/, the chief material of teeth, surrounding the pulp and situated inside of the enamel and cementum. Harder and denser than bone, it consists of solid organic substratum infiltrated with lime salts. Also spelled **dentine.**

dentin eburnation, a change in carious teeth in which softened and decalcified dentin develops a hard, brown, polished appearance.

dentin globule, a small spheric body in peripheral dentin, created by early calcification.

dentinoenamel /den′tinō·inam′əl/, pertaining to both the dentin and the enamel of the teeth.

dentinoenamal junction, the interface of enamel and dentin of a tooth crown, generally conforming to the shape of the crown. Also called **dentoenamal junction.**

dentinogenesis /den′tinōjen′əsis/, the formation of the dentin of the teeth. **–dentinogenic,** *adj.*

dentinogenesis imperfecta, hereditary dysplasia of dentin of deciduous and permanent teeth in which brown, opalescent dentin overgrows and obliterates the pulp cavity. The teeth have short roots and wear rapidly. Early restorative dentistry is indicated. The condition is often associated with osteogenesis imperfecta and other congenital mesodermal dysplasias.

dentist, a person who is qualified by training and licensed by the state to practice dentistry. Training requires a minimum of 2 years, preferably 4, in an undergraduate college and a satisfactory score on a Dental Aptitude Test (DAT), followed by 3 to 4 years at an approved dental college. After completing dental college, a dentist is awarded a degree of either Doctor of Dental Surgery (D.D.S.) or Doctor of Dental Medicine (D.M.D.), which are equivalent degrees. Dental internships and residencies are not required for general practice, although written and practical examinations must be passed to obtain a state license. In various states, licensing requirements can be met by providing a certificate from the National Board of Dental Examiners in place of a written test and by taking the practical examination before a Regional Dental Examining Board rather than appearing before a state board. See also **dentistry.**

dentistry, the art of practicing the prevention and treatment of diseases and disorders of the teeth and surrounding structures of the oral cavity. Responsibilities include the repair and restoration of teeth and replacement of missing teeth, as well as the detection of signs of diseases, as tumors, that would require treatment by a physician. In addition to the general practice of dentistry, there are eight recognized specialties, each requiring additional training after graduation from a dental college: **endodontics, oral pathology, oral surgery, orthodontics, pedodontics, periodontics, prosthodontics,** and **public health dentistry.**

dentition, **1.** the development and eruption of the teeth. See also **teething.** **2.** the arrangement, number, and kind of teeth as they appear in the dental arch of the mouth. **3.** the character of the teeth of an individual or species as determined by their form and arrangement. Kinds of dentition include **artificial dentition, deciduous dentition, mixed dentition, natural dentition, permanent dentition, precocious dentition, predeciduous dentition,** and **retarded dentition.**

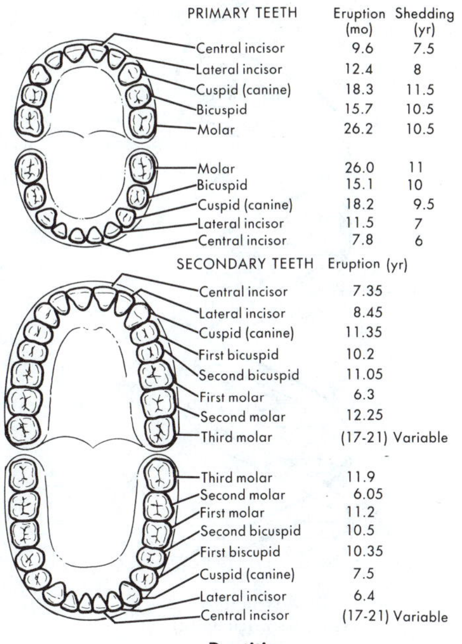

Dentition

dento-, dent-, denta-, denti-, dentia-, a combining form meaning 'pertaining to a tooth or the teeth': *dentography, dentoidin, dentonomy.*

dentoalveolar abscess /den′tō•alvē′ələr/, the formation and accumulation of pus in a tooth socket or the jawbone around the base of a tooth. The pus results from a bacterial infection that is usually secondary to an infection or injury to the tooth or alveolar tissues. Also called **periapical abscess.**

dentoalveolar cyst. See **periodontal cyst.**

dentoenamal junction. See **dentinoenamal junction.**

dentofacial, of or pertaining to an oral or gnathic structure.

dentofacial anomaly, an abnormality in which an oral or gnathic structure deviates from the normal in form, function, or position.

dentogenesis imperfecta /den′tōjen′əsis/, **1.** a genetic disturbance of the dentin, characterized by early calcification of the pulp chambers, marked attrition, and an opalescent hue to the teeth. **2.** a localized form of mesodermal dysplasia affecting the dentin of the teeth. It may be hereditary and associated with osteogenesis imperfecta. **3.** also called **hereditary opalescent dentin.** a genetic condition that produces defective dentin but normal tooth enamel.

dentogingival fiber /den′tōjinjī′vəl/, any one of the many fibers that spread like a fan, emerge from the supraalveolar portion of the cementum, and terminate in the free gingiva.

dentogingival junction, the junction between the gingival attachment, a nonkeratinized epithelium, and the surface of the teeth.

dentoperiosteal fiber /den′tōper′ē•os′tē•əl/, any one of the many fibers that emerge from the supraalveolar part of the cementum of a tooth and extend apically beyond the alveolar crest into the mucoperiosteum of the attached gingiva.

dentulous dental arch, a dental arch that contains natural teeth.

denture /den′chər/, an artificial tooth or a set of artificial teeth not permanently fixed or implanted. Compare **fixed bridgework.**

denture base, 1. the portion of a denture that fits the oral mucosa of the basal seat and supports artificial teeth. **2.** the part of a denture that covers the soft tissue of the mouth, commonly made of resin or a combination of resins and metal.

denture flask, a sectional metal case in which plaster of paris or artificial stone is molded to process dentures or other resin restorations.

denture packing, the laboratory procedure of filling and compressing a denture-base material into a mold in a flask.

denturist, a person who performs the same type of work as a dental technician but without a dentist's prescription, providing dental prostheses directly to clients. In the United States, the practice is limited to certain states. See also **dental technician.**

Denver Articulation Screening Examination (DASE), a test for evaluating the clarity of pronunciation in children between 2½ and 6 years of age. Each child's performance may be compared with a standardized norm for the age.

Denver classification, the system of identifying and classifying human chromosomes according to the criteria established at the Denver (1960), London (1963), and Chicago (1966) conferences of cytogeneticists. It is based on chromosome size and position of the centromere as determined during mitotic metaphase and is divided into seven major groups, designated A through G, which are arranged according to decreasing length. See also **chromosome, karyotype.**

Denver Developmental Screening Test (DDST), a test for evaluating development in children from 1 month to 6 years of age. The developmental level of motor, social, and language skills may be discovered by comparing the child's performance with the average performance of other children. The score, or the developmental age, is expressed as a ratio in which the child's age is the denominator and the age at which the norm possesses skills equal to those of the child being tested is the numerator.

deodorant, 1. destroying or masking odors. **2.** a substance that destroys or masks odors. Underarm deodorants are available as sprays, creams, solid gels, and liquids containing an antiperspirant, as aluminum chloride, aluminum hydroxyl, aluminum sulfate, or aluminum zirconyl hydroxychloride. These aluminum salts form an obstructive hydroxide gel in sweat ducts. Aluminum salts may produce an allergic reaction in some individuals, and hydrolyzed aluminum chloride can cause local tissue necrosis. Some underarm deodorants contain antibacterial agents or fragrances. Vaginal deodorant sprays contain a fatty ester emollient, a masking fragrance, and an antimicrobial agent, as benzethonium chloride, chlorhexidine hydrochloride, or triacetin, and are often associated with allergic reactions. Room and breath deodorants contain masking agents, as various mints, pine, eucalyptus, lemon, lavender, rosemary, sassafras, or thyme. Ozone masks odors by decreasing olfactory sensitivity. Chlorophyll has a deodorizing action that is enhanced by croconic acid. Also called **antibromic.**

deodorized alcohol, a liquid, free of organic impurities, containing 92.5% absolute alcohol.

deontologism /dē′ontol′əgiz′əm/, a doctrine of ethics that states that moral duty or obligation is binding; also, that what makes acts right are nonconsequential characteristics such as fidelity, veracity, justice, and honesty. Compare **natural law, utilitarianism.**

deoxy-, desoxy-, a combining form meaning 'deoxidized or a reduction product of': *deoxygenation, desoxymorphine, desoxyribose.*

deoxyribonucleic acid (DNA) /dē•ok′sirī′bōnōōklē′ik/, a large nucleic acid molecule, found principally in the chromosomes of the nucleus of a cell, that is the carrier of genetic information. The genetic information is coded in the sequence of the nitrogenous, molecular subunits that are constituents of the deoxyribonucleic acid molecule. Also called **desoxyribonucleic acid.** See also **nucleic acid, ribonucleic acid.**

Depakene, a trademark for an anticonvulsant (valproic acid).

dependence, **1.** the state of being dependent. **2.** the total psychophysical state of one addicted to drugs or alcohol who must receive an increasing amount of the substance to prevent the onset of abstinence symptoms.

dependency needs, the sum of the physical and emotional requirements of an infant for survival, including mothering (or ''fathering''), love, affection, shelter, protection, food, and warmth. Reliance on others to satisfy these needs decreases with age and maturity; continuance in later years, in overt or latent form, is indicative of a pathologic emotional disorder. These needs may increase under stress, as during physical illness, in which case they do not reflect a psychopathologic condition. Compare **emotional need.**

dependent, of or pertaining to a condition of being reliant on someone or something else for help, support, favor, and other need, as a child is dependent on a parent, a narcotics addict is dependent on a drug, or one variable is dependent on another variable. **–depend,** *v.*

dependent differentiation. See **correlative differentiation.**

dependent personality, behavior characterized by excessive or compulsive needs for attention, acceptance, and approval from other people to maintain security and self-esteem.

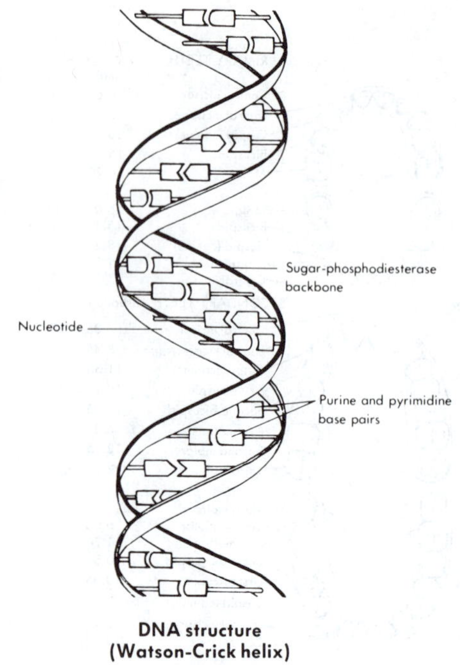

DNA structure (Watson-Crick helix)

dependent variable, (in research) a factor that is measured to learn the effect of one or more independent variables; for example, in a study of the effect of preoperative nursing intervention on postoperative vomiting, vomiting is the dependent variable measured to determine the effect of the nursing intervention. Compare **independent variable.**

depersonalization, a feeling of strangeness or unreality concerning oneself or the environment, often resulting from anxiety. In severe cases, it may lead to a neurotic reaction. See also **alienation, depersonalization disorder.**

depersonalization disorder, an emotional disturbance characterized by depersonalization feelings in which a dreamlike atmosphere pervades the consciousness. The body may not feel like one's own, and dramatic and important events may be watched with equanimity. The reaction is commonly seen in various forms of schizophrenia and in severe depression.

depilation /dep′ilā′shən/, the removal or extraction of hair from the body, either temporarily, by mechanic or chemical means or permanently, by electrolysis, which destroys the hair follicle. Also called **epilation.** **–depilate,** *v.*

depilatory /dipil′ətôrē/, **1.** of or pertaining to a substance or procedure that removes hair. **2.** a depilatory agent.

depolarization, the reduction of a membrane potential to a less negative value. The positive current responsible for the buildup of positive ions on the inside of the cell is called a depolarizing current. It occurs relatively slowly, as during phase 4 of pacemaker cells or because of injury to nonpacemaker cells, or it occurs very rapidly, as during phase 0 of the action potential. Rapid depolarization of the cell permits calcium to enter the cell so that contraction can take place. See also **action potential.**

deposition, (in law) a sworn pretrial testimony given by a witness in response to oral or written questions and cross-examination. The deposition is transcribed and may be used for further pretrial investigation. It may also be presented at the trial if the witness cannot be present. Compare **discovery, interrogatories.**

depot, **1.** any area of the body in which drugs or other substances, as fat, are stored and from which they can be distributed. **2.** (of a drug) injected or implanted to be slowly absorbed into the circulation.

depressant, **1.** (of a drug) tending to decrease the function or activity of a system of the body. **2.** such a drug; for example, a cardiac depressant or a respiratory depressant.

depressed fracture, any fracture of the skull in which fragments are depressed below the normal surface of the skull.

depression, **1.** a depressed area, hollow, or fossa; downward or inward displacement. **2.** a decrease of vital functional activity. **3.** a mood disturbance characterized by feelings of sadness, despair, and discouragement resulting from and normally proportionate to some personal loss or tragedy. **4.** an abnormal emotional state characterized by exaggerated feelings of sadness, melancholy, dejection, worthlessness, emptiness, and hopelessness that are inappropriate and out of proportion to reality. The overt manifestations, which are extremely variable, range from a slight lack of motivation and inability to concentrate to severe physiologic alterations of body functions and may represent symptoms of a variety of mental and physical conditions, a syndrome of related symptoms associated with a particular disease, or a specific mental illness. The condition is neurotic when the precipitating cause is an intrapsychic conflict or a traumatic situation or event that is identifiable, even though the person is unable to explain the overreaction to it. The condition is psychotic when there is severe physical and mental functional impairment because of some unidentifiable intrapsychic conflict; it is often accompanied by hallucinations, delusions, and confusion concerning time, place, and identity. Depression may be expressed in a wide spectrum of affective, physiologic, cognitive, and behavioral manifestations. The varied behaviors represent the complex actions, reactions, and interactions of the depressed person to stimuli that may be either internal or external. Because the origin of depression can be genetic, pharmacologic, endocrinal, infectious, nutritional, neoplastic, or neurologic, the behavioral effects can appear as aggression or withdrawal, anorexia or overeating, anger or apathy or any of a myriad of responses. Kinds of depression include **agitated depression, anaclitic depression, endogenous depression, involutional melancholia, reactive depression,** and **retarded depression.** See also **bipolar disorder.** –**depressive,** *adj.*

depressor, any agent that reduces activity when applied to nerves and muscles. See also **depressant.**

depressor septi, one of the three muscles of the nose. Arising from the maxilla and inserting into the septum and the posterior aspect of the ala, it lies between the mucous membrane and the muscular structure of the lip and is a direct antagonist of the other muscles of the nose. It is innervated by buccal branches of the facial nerve and serves to draw the ala down, constricting the nostril. Compare **nasalis, procerus.**

deprivation, the loss of something considered valuable or necessary by taking it away or denying access to it. In experimental psychology, animal or human subjects may be deprived of something desired or expected for study of their reactions.

depth dose, (in radiotherapy) the relationship between dose at any depth from a beam of radiation compared with the dose at the entrance from that beam.

depth electroencephalography. See **electroencephalography.**

depth perception, the ability to judge depth or the relative distance of objects in space and to orient one's position in relation to them. Binocular vision is essential to this ability.

depth psychology, any approach to psychology that emphasizes the study of personality and behavior in relation to unconscious motivation. See also **psychoanalysis.**

de Quervain's fracture /də kərvänz′/, fracture of the navicular bone of the hand, with dislocation of the lunate bone.

de Quervain's thyroiditis, an inflammatory condition of the thyroid, characterized by swelling and tenderness of the gland, fever, dysphagia, fatigue, and severe pain in the neck, ears, and jaw. The disorder often occurs after a viral infection of the upper respiratory tract and tends to remit spontaneously and to recur several times. The diagnosis may be made by a radiologic scan showing depressed uptake of radioactive iodine in involved areas. Occasionally, a needle biopsy of the thyroid is performed. Treatment may include antiinflammatory medication, as aspirin or thyroid hormone, if the condition continues for more than a few days. Corticosteroids are prescribed for prolonged or severe cases. Also called **giant cell thyroiditis, granulomatous thyroiditis, subacute thyroiditis.**

der, (in cytogenetics) abbreviation for **derivative chromosome.**

der-, a combining form meaning 'pertaining to the neck': *deradelphus, deradenitis, deranencephalia.*

derby hat fracture. See **dishpan fracture.**

dereflection, a technique of logotherapeutic psychology that is directed toward taking a person's mind off a certain goal through a positive redirection to another goal, with emphasis on assets and abilities rather than the problems at hand. Dereflection results often in accomplishment of the original goal.

derivative, anything that is derived or obtained from another substance or object; for example, organs and tissues are derivatives of the primordial germ cells.

derived protein, a metabolic product of protein hydrolysis, as proteose, peptone, or peptide.

-derm, a combining form meaning a 'skin': *angioderm, mucoderm, paraderm.*

-derma, **1.** a combining form meaning a '(specified) skin or covering': *chrysderma, micoderma, sarcoderma.* **2.** a combining form meaning a 'skin ailment or skin of a specified type': *rhinoderma, syphiloderma, vaselinoderma.*

derma-. See **dermato-.**

dermabrasion /dur′məbrā′zhən/, a treatment for the removal of scars on the skin by the use of revolving wire brushes or sandpaper. An aerosol spray is used to freeze the skin for this procedure. Dermabrasion is used to reduce facial scars of severe acne and to remove pigment from undesired tattoos.

dermat-. See **dermato-.**

dermatitis /dur′mətī′tis/, an inflammatory condition of the skin, characterized by erythema and pain or pruritus. Various cutaneous eruptions occur and may be unique to a particular allergen, disease, or infection. The condition may be chronic or acute; treatment is specific to the cause. Some kinds of dermatitis are **actinic dermatitis, contact dermatitis, rhus dermatitis,** and **seborrheic dermatitis.**

dermatitis exfoliativa neonatorum. See **Ritter's disease.**

dermatitis herpetiformis, a chronic, severely pruritic skin disease with symmetrically located groups of red, papulovesicular, vesicular, bullous, or urticarial lesions that leave hyperpigmented spots. It is occasionally associated with a malignancy of an internal organ or with celiac disease, patch, or IgA immunotherapy. Treatment may include a diet free of gluten and the administration of sulfone, dapsone, sulfapyridine, or antipruritic drugs.

dermatitis medicamentosa. See **drug eruption.**

dermatitis venenata. See **contact dermatitis.**

dermato-, derma-, dermat-, dermo-, a combining form meaning 'pertaining to the skin': *dermatobiasis, dermatocele, dermatocyst.*

dermatofibroma /dur′mətōfībrō′mə/, *pl.* **dermatofibromas, dermatofibromata,** a cutaneous nodule that is painless, round, firm, gray or red, and elevated. It is most commonly found on the extremities, requires no treatment, and is sometimes associated with systemic lupus erythematosus. Also called **fibrous histiocytoma.**

dermatoglyphics /dur′mətōglif′iks/, the study of the skin ridge patterns on fingers, toes, palms of hands, and soles of feet. The patterns are used as a basis of identification and also have diagnostic value because of associations between certain patterns and chromosomal anomalies.

dermatographia /dur′mətōgraf′ē·ə/, an abnormal skin condition characterized by wheals that develop from tracing on the skin with the fingernail or a blunted instrument. This condition makes the skin especially susceptible to irritation and may be associated with urticaria. Also called **autographism, dermatographism, Ebbecke's reaction.**

dermatologist, a physician specializing in disorders of the skin.

dermatology, the study of the skin, including the anatomy, physiology, and pathology of the skin and the diagnosis and treatment of skin disorders.

dermatome /dur′mətōm/, **1.** (in embryology) the mesodermal layer in the early developing embryo that gives rise to the dermal layers of the skin. **2.** (in surgery) an instrument used to cut thin slices of skin for grafting. **3.** an area on the surface of a body innervated by afferent fibers from one spinal root.

dermatomycosis /dur′mətōmīkō′sis/, a superficial, fungal infection of the skin, characteristically found on parts that are moist and protected by clothing, as the groin or feet. It is caused by a dermatophyte. See also **dermatophytosis.** –**dermatomycotic,** *adj.*

dermatomyositis /dur′mətōmī·ōsī′tis/, a disease of the connective tissues, characterized by pruritic or eczematous inflammation of the skin and tenderness and weakness of the muscles. Muscle tissue is destroyed, and loss is often so severe that the person may become unable to walk or to perform simple tasks. Swelling of the eyelids and face and loss of weight are common manifestations. The cause is unknown, but in 15% of cases the condition develops with an internal malignancy. Viral infection and antibacterial medication are also associated with an increased incidence of dermatomyositis.

Dermatophagoides farinae, a ubiquitous species of household dust mite responsible for allergic reactions in sensitive individuals. Protection against the microscopically small mite includes use of insecticides, vacuum cleaning, and control of the temperature and humidity. The mites thrive on skin scales, hair, pet foods, carpets, and bedding, in addition to ordinary house dust.

dermatophyte /dur′mətōfīt′, dərmat′əfīt/, any of several fungi that cause parasitic skin disease in humans. See also **dermatophytid,** and see specific fungal infections.

dermatophytid /dur′mətof′itid, dur′mətōfī′tid/, an allergic skin reaction characterized by small vesicles and associated with dermatomycosis. The lesions result from sensitization to the infection elsewhere on the skin and do not contain fungi. See also **dermatomycosis, dermatophyte.**

dermatophytosis /dur′mətō′fītō′sis/, a superficial fungus infection of the skin, caused by *Microsporum, Epidermophyton,* or *Trichophyton* species of dermatophyte. On the trunk and upper extremities it is commonly called ''ringworm'' infection and is characterized by round or oval, scaly patches with slightly raised borders and clearing centers. On the feet small vesicles, cracking, itching, scaling, and often secondary bacterial infections occur and are commonly called "athlete's foot." Treatment includes topical antifungal agents, as tolnaftate, clotrimazole, and undecylenic acid, and oral griseofulvin. Fingernails and toenails respond poorly to topical treatment. See also **tinea.**

dermatopolyneuritis. See **acrodynia.**

dermatosis /dur′mətō′sis/, any disorder of the skin, especially if not associated with inflammation. Compare **dermatitis.**

dermatosis papulosa nigra, a common abnormal skin condition in blacks consisting of multiple, tiny, benign, skin-colored or hyperpigmented papules on the cheeks. The lesions are permanent and increase in number with age.

-dermia, -derma, a combining form meaning a '(specified) skin condition': *allergodermia, carotenodermia, toxidermia.*

-dermic, **1.** a combining form meaning 'related to the skin': *diadermic, epidermic, intradermic.* **2.** a combining form meaning 'related to the variety of skin': *leptodermic, pachydermic, sarcodermic.* **3.** a combining form meaning 'related to skin ailments': *leukodermic, toxicodermic, xerodermic.* **4.** a combining form meaning 'related to a cell division process': *blastodermic, ectodermic, endodermic.*

dermis. See **corium.**

-dermis, a combining form meaning 'tissue or skin': *hypodermis, endepidermis, osteodermis.*

dermo-. See **dermato-.**

dermographism. See **dermatographia.**

dermoid /dur′moid/, **1.** of or pertaining to the skin. **2.** *informal.* a dermoid cyst.

dermoid cyst, a tumor, derived from embryonal tissues. It consists of a fibrous wall lined with epithelium and a cavity containing fatty material, and frequently hair, teeth, bits of bone, and cartilage. More than 10% of all ovarian tumors are dermoid cysts. They are usually benign, but they may cause granulomatous peritonitis if they rupture. Kinds of dermoid cysts are **implantation dermoid cyst, inclusion dermoid cyst, thyroid dermoid cyst,** and **tubal dermoid cyst.** Also called **organoid tumor, teratoid tumor.**

-dermoma, a combining form meaning a 'tumor of the skin layers': *epidermoma, monodermoma, tridermoma.*

DES, abbreviation for **diethylstilbestrol.**

descending aorta, the main portion of the aorta, consisting of the thoracic aorta and the abdominal aorta, that continues from the aortic arch into the trunk of the body and supplies many parts, as the esophagus, lymph glands, ribs, and stomach.

descending colon, the segment of the colon that extends from the end of the transverse colon at the splenic flexure on the left side of the abdomen down to the beginning of the sigmoid colon in the pelvis.

descending current. See **centrifugal current.**

descending oblique muscle. See **obliquus externus abdominis.**

descending urography. See **intravenous pyelography.**

descensus, the process of falling or descending; prolapse.

descriptive anatomy, the study of the morphology and structure of the body by systems, as the vascular system and the nervous system. Each system is composed of similar tissues that are essential to a particular function.

descriptive embryology, the study of the changes that occur in cells, tissues, and organs during the progressive stages of prenatal development.

descriptive epidemiology, the first stage of epidemiological investigation. It focuses on describing disease distribution by characteristics relating to time, place, and person.

descriptive psychiatry, the study of external, readily observable behavior. Compare **dynamic psychiatry.**

Desenex, a trademark for a fixed-combination topical drug containing two antifungals (undecylenic acid and zinc undecylenate).

desensitization. See **systemic desensitization.**

desensitize, **1.** (in immunology) to render an individual insensitive to any of the various antigens. **2.** (in psychiatry) to relieve an emotionally disturbed person of the stress of phobias and neuroses by encouraging discussion of the anxieties and the stressful experiences that cause the emotional problems involved. **3.** (in dentistry) to remove or reduce the painful response of vital, exposed dentin to irritating substances and temperature changes.

deserpidine /disur′pədēn/, a rauwolfia alkaloid used as an antihypertensive.

■ INDICATIONS: It is prescribed for mild hypertension and for mild anxiety.

■ CONTRAINDICATIONS: Mental depression, peptic ulcer, ulcerative colitis, or known hypersensitivity to this drug prohibits its use. It interacts with monoamine oxydase inhibitors, which can increase hypertension and excitability.

■ ADVERSE EFFECTS: Among the more serious adverse reactions are orthostatic hypotension, potentially severe mental depression, and lethargy.

desert fever. See **coccidioidomycosis.**

desert rheumatism, a form of coccidioidomycosis characterized by pain in the bones and joints.

Desferal Mesylate, a trademark for a chelating agent (deferoxamine mesylate).

desiccant /des′ikənt/, any agent or procedure that promotes drying or causes a substance to dry up. Also called **exsiccant.**

desiccate /des′ikāt/, **1.** to dry thoroughly. **2.** to preserve by drying, especially food. Also **exsiccate.**

desipramine hydrochloride, a tricyclic antidepressant.

■ INDICATION: It is prescribed in the treatment of mental depression.

■ CONTRAINDICATIONS: Concomitant administration of monoamine oxidase inhibitors, heart block, recent myocardial infarction, or known hypersensitivity to this drug or to tricyclic medication prohibits its use. It is used with caution in patients who have seizure disorders or cardiovascular disease.

■ ADVERSE EFFECTS: Among the more serious adverse reactions are sedation as well as GI, cardiovascular, and neurologic reactions. This drug interacts with many other drugs.

deslanoside /dislan′əsīd/, a cardiotonic.

■ INDICATIONS: It is prescribed for congestive heart failure and certain arrhythmias.

■ CONTRAINDICATIONS: Ventricular fibrillation, tachycardia, or known hypersensitivity to this drug prohibits its use.

■ ADVERSE EFFECTS: The most serious reactions are various cardiac arrhythmias.

-desma, a combining form meaning 'something bridging or connecting': *cytodesma, mesodesma, plasmodesma.*

desmo-, a combining form meaning 'pertaining to a ligament': *desmoma, desmorrhexis, desmotomy.*

desmocyte. See **fibroblast.**

desmoid tumor, a neoplasm in skeletal muscle and fascia that may occur in the head, neck, upper arm, abdomen, or lower extremities. The tumor is usually a firm, circumscribed, rubbery mass. Injury may be a factor in the development of this lesion, which is often regarded as overproliferation of scar tissue.

desmopressin acetate, an antidiuretic analog of vasopressin.

■ INDICATION: It is prescribed in the treatment of diabetes insipidus.

■ CONTRAINDICATION: Known hypersensitivity to this drug prohibits its use.

■ ADVERSE EFFECTS: Among the most serious adverse reactions are hyponatremia and water intoxication. Mild effects, as headache, cramps, and nasal congestion, also may occur.

desmosis, any disease of the connective tissue.

desmosome /des′məsōm/, a small, circular, dense area within the intercellular bridge that forms the site of adhesion between certain epithelial cells, especially the stratified epithelium of the epidermis. Also called **macula adherens.**

desonide, a topical corticosteroid.

■ INDICATION: It is prescribed topically as an antiinflammatory agent.

■ CONTRAINDICATIONS: Viral and fungal diseases of the skin, impaired circulation, or known hypersensitivity to this drug or to steroid medication prohibits its use.

■ ADVERSE EFFECTS: Among the more serious adverse reactions, usually occurring after prolonged or excessive application, are striae, hypopigmentation or local irritation of the skin, and various systemic effects.

desoximetasone, a topical corticosteroid.

■ INDICATION: It is prescribed topically as an antiinflammatory agent.

■ CONTRAINDICATIONS: Viral and fungal diseases of the skin, impaired circulation, or known hypersensitivity to this drug or to other steroid medication prohibits its use. Caution should be used in applying occlusive dressings over topical steroid medications.

■ ADVERSE EFFECTS: Among the more serious adverse reactions, usually occurring after prolonged or excessive application, are striae, hypopigmentation, or local irritation of the skin and various systemic effects.

desoxy-. See **deoxy-.**

desoxycorticosterone acetate /desok′sikôr′təkōstē′-rōn/, a mineralocorticoid hormone.

■ INDICATIONS: It is prescribed in replacement therapy, in congenital adrenal hyperplasia, and in chronic primary adrenocortical insufficiency to prevent the excess loss of salt from the body.

■ CONTRAINDICATIONS: Hypertension, congestive heart failure, or known hypersensitivity to this drug prohibits its use.

■ ADVERSE EFFECTS: Among the more serious adverse reactions are excessive sodium and water retention and potassium loss, hypertension, edema, and heart failure.

Desoxyn, a trademark for a central nervous system stimulant (methamphetamine hydrochloride).

desoxyribonucleic acid. See **deoxyribonucleic acid.**

desquamation /des′kwəmā′shən/, a normal process in which the cornified layer of the epidermis is sloughed in fine scales. Certain conditions, injuries, and medications accelerate desquamation and may cause peeling and the loss of deeper layers of the skin. Also called **exfoliation.** –**desquamate,** *v.*, **desquamative** /deskwam′ətiv/, *adj.*

desquamative gingivitis, a gingival inflammation, characterized by peeling of the surface epithelium. It is a clinical rather than a pathologic condition and is most frequently associated with menopause. It may also be associated with any biologic stress. Compare **eruptive gingivitis.**

destructive aggression, an act of hostility unnecessary for self-protection or preservation that is directed toward an external object or person. See also **aggression.**

Desyrel, a trademark for an antidepressant (trazodone).

detached retina. See **retinal detachment.**

detergent, **1.** a cleansing agent. **2.** cleansing. See also **surfactant.**

determinant evolution, the theory that evolution progresses according to a predetermined course. See also **orthogenesis.**

determinants of occlusion, (in dentistry) the classifiable factors that influence proper closure of the teeth. The common fixed factors are the intercondylar distance, anatomy, mandibular centricity, and relationship of the jaws. The common changeable factors are tooth shapes, tooth positions, and vertical dimensions of occlusion, cusp height, and fossa depth.

determinate cleavage, mitotic division of the fertilized ovum into blastomeres that are each destined to form a specific part of the embryo. If such cells are isolated, they are incapable of giving rise to an individual, complete embryo. Damage to or destruction of any of these cells results in a malformed organism. Also called **mosaic cleavage.** Compare **indeterminate cleavage.** See also **mosaic development.**

detoxification service, a hospital service providing treatment to diminish or remove from a patient's body the toxic effects of chemical substances, as alcohol or drugs, usually as an initial step in the treatment of a chemical-dependent person. The service may also be used to remove poisonous substances to which a person may have been exposed. See also **alcoholism, drug addiction.**

detrusor urinae muscle /ditro͞o′zər/, a complex of longitudinal fibers that form the external layer of the muscular coat of the bladder. These fibers arise from the posterior surface of the pubis, traverse the inferior surface of the bladder, descend along the fundus, and attach to the prostate in men and to the front of the vagina in women. Along the sides of the bladder the fibers pass obliquely and intersect. The detrusor muscle is supplied by branches from the internal iliac artery and is innervated by medullated fibers from the third and fourth sacral nerves and by nonmedullated fibers from the hypogastric plexus.

deuterium (^{2}H), a radioactive isotope of the hydrogen atom, used as a tracer. Also called **heavy hydrogen.** See also **tritium.**

deutero-, deuto-, a combining form meaning 'second': *deuteroalbumose, deuteroconidium, deuteroelastose.*

deuteroplasm. See **deutoplasm.**

deuto-. See **deutero-.**

deutoplasm /do͞o′təplaz′əm/, the inactive elements of the protoplasm, primarily the stored nutritive material contained in the yolk. Also called **deuteroplasm.**

DEV, abbreviation for **duck embryo vaccine.** See also **rabies vaccine.**

development, **1.** the gradual process of change and differentiation from a simple to a more advanced level of complexity. In humans the physical, mental, and emotional capacities that allow complex adaptation to the environment and function within society are acquired through growth, maturation, and learning. Kinds of development include **arrested development, mosaic development, psychomotor development, psychosexual development, psychosocial development,** and **regulative development.** **2.** (in biology) the series of events that occur within an organism from the time of fertilization of the ovum to the adult stage. **–developmental,** *adj.*

developmental age (DA), an expression of a child's developmental progress stated in age and determined by standardized measurements, as of body size and dimensions, by social and psychologic functioning, by observations of motor skills, and by the giving of mental and aptitude tests. Compare **achievement age, developmental quotient, mental age.**

developmental agraphia, a deficiency in a child's ability to learn to form letters and to write. Other learning is normal, and the child usually has no musculoskeletal or neurologic problems.

developmental anatomy, the study of the differentiation and the growth of an organism from one cell to birth. Also called **embryology.**

developmental anomaly, any congenital defect that results from the interference with the normal growth and differentiation of the fetus. Such defects can arise at any stage of embryonic development, vary greatly in type and severity, and are caused by a wide variety of determining factors, including genetic mutations, chromosomal aberrations, teratogenic agents, and environmental factors. Developmental anomalies are classified either according to the organ system affected, as congenital heart defects, or according to the way in which the defect occurred, as developmental failure or arrest, failure to atrophy or subdivide, fusion, splitting, incorrect migration, and misplacement. Most developmental defects are apparent at birth, especially any structural malformation, but some, especially those involving the organ systems, do not become evident until days, weeks, or even years later.

developmental arrest. See **arrested development.**

developmental crisis, severe, usually transient, stress that occurs when a person is unable to complete the tasks of a psychosocial stage of development and is therefore unable to move on to the next stage. See also **psychosocial development.**

developmental disability (DD), a pathologic condition that starts developing before 18 years of age. Most developmental disabilities persist throughout the life of the individual, although many can be effectively treated. See also **congenital condition.**

developmental groove, a fine recessed line in the enamel of a tooth that marks the union of the lobes of the crown in its development.

developmental guidance, (in dentistry) the comprehensive dentofacial orthopedic control over the growth of the jaws and the eruption of the teeth. It may require precisely timed active appliance therapy and supervisory examinations, including radiography and other diagnostic records, at various developmental stages. The control may be needed throughout the entire growth and maturation of the face, beginning at the earliest detection of a developing malformation.

developmental horizon, any one of 25 stages in the development of the human embryo from the one-cell stage at conception to the morphologically and physiologically complex organism at the end of the seventh week of gestation.

developmental idiocy, *obsolete.* Severe mental retardation resulting from arrest of brain development.

developmental model, **1.** a conceptual framework devised to be used as a guide in making a diagnosis, in understanding a developmental process, and in forming a prognosis for continued development. It has five components. The "identifiable state" describes the stage, level, phase, or period of the condition or process; the "shift in state" identifies qualities of change as progressive, sudden, abrupt, or recurrent; and the "form of progression" describes patterns of development as linear, spiral, or oscillating. The "force" that triggers the change or the step in development may be self-actualization or any form of stress. Development is ultimately constrained by the fifth component, "potentiality," the genetic and environmental potential for growth. **2.** (in nursing) a conceptual framework describing four stages, or processes, of development in the patient during therapy. In the first stage, called orientation, the patient begins a relationship with the nurse or other therapist and begins to clarify the problem with the help of the therapist. In the second stage, called identification, the patient develops a sense of closeness and attachment to the therapist. During this period the patient and the therapist work comfortably together. In the third stage, called exploitation, the patient makes full use of the nursing services offered, begins to assume some control of the interactions, and becomes more independent. During the last stage, called resolution, the therapeutic relationship is terminated; the patient is independent and no longer needs the nurse or therapist. With this model the nurse therapist may plan nursing interventions appropriate to the developmental level of the patient. The developmental model is one of the earliest nursing models to be developed. It views the person as a psychobiologic being whose needs are expressed in behavior and as one who is unique and capable of learning and changing. Health is viewed as a forward movement of personality development and other ongoing processes, reflected by the person's creative, constructive, and productive community living. Thus, the focus of nursing is to promote this forward movement by assisting the patient in self-repair and self-renewal.

developmental physiology, the study of the physiologic processes as they relate to embryonic development.

developmental quotient (DQ), the numeric expression of a child's developmental level as measured by dividing the developmental age by the chronologic age and multiplying by 100. Compare **intelligence quotient.** See also **developmental age.**

developmental task, a physical or cognitive skill that a person must accomplish during a particular age period to continue developing, as walking, which precedes the development of a sense of autonomy in the toddler period. The nurse may also outline developmental tasks for families.

developmental theory of aging, a concept based on the premise that traits and characteristics developed early in life tend to continue into the later years.

deviance /dē′vē·əns/, behavior that is contrary to the accepted standards of a community or culture.

deviate /dē′vē·it/, **1.** a person or an act that varies from that which is considered standard, as a social or sexual deviate, or that which is within a statistic norm. **2.** to vary from that which is considered standard or within a statistic norm. –**deviant,** *adj.*, **deviation,** *n.*

deviated septum, a shifted medial partition of the nasal cavity, a condition affecting many adults. The nasal septum more commonly shifts to the left during normal growth, but this deflection may be aggravated by a blow to the nose or by other trauma. A severe deflection of the septum may significantly obstruct the nasal passages and result in infection, sinusitis, shortness of breath, headache, or recurring nosebleeds. Severe septal deviation may be corrected by various surgical procedures, as rhinoplasty or septoplasty. Postoperative care in such cases usually includes various measures, as the maintenance of nasal packing, the administration of sedatives, and the placement of ice packs around the affected area to reduce swelling.

deviation from normal, a quality, characteristic, symptom, or clinical finding that is different from what is commonly regarded as normal, as an elevated temperature, multiple gestation, or an extra digit.

device, an item other than a drug that has application in the healing arts. The term is sometimes restricted to items used directly by, on, or in the patient and not surgical instruments or other equipment used for diagnosis and treatment. Devices include orthopedic appliances, crutches, artificial heart valves, pacemakers, prostheses, wheelchairs, cervical collars, hearing aids, and eye glasses.

devil's grip. See **epidemic pleurodynia.**

devital tooth. See **pulpless tooth.**

dexamethasone, a glucocorticoid.

■ INDICATIONS: It is prescribed in the treatment of a variety of inflammatory conditions.

■ CONTRAINDICATIONS: Systemic fungal infections or known hypersensitivity to this drug prohibits its use.

■ ADVERSE EFFECTS: Among the more serious adverse reactions are GI, endocrine, neurologic, fluid, and electrolyte disturbances.

dexchlorpheniramine maleate, an antihistamine.

■ INDICATIONS: It is prescribed in the treatment of a variety of hypersensitivity reactions, including rhinitis, skin rash, and pruritus.

■ CONTRAINDICATIONS: Asthma or known hypersensitivity to this drug prohibits its use. It should not be given to newborn infants or lactating mothers.

■ ADVERSE EFFECTS: Drowsiness, skin rash, hypersensitivity reactions, dry mouth, and tachycardia may occur.

Dexedrine, a trademark for a central nervous system stimulant (dextroamphetamine sulfate).

dextrality. See **right-handedness.**

dextran fermentation /dek′strən/, the conversion of dextrose to dextran by the action of *Leuconostoc mesenteroides* dextran (LMD) bacteria.

dextran preparation, any of a group of solutions containing polysaccharides, water, and, in some preparations, electrolytes. These solutions are used as plasma-volume extenders in cases of hypovolemia from hemorrhage, dehydration, or another cause and are available for intravenous administration in several concentrations.

dextro-, dextr-, a combining form meaning 'right': *dextrocardia, dextrocerebral, dextrogastria.*

dextroamphetamine sulfate, a central nervous system stimulant.

■ INDICATIONS: It is prescribed in the treatment of narcolepsy and in the treatment of hyperkinetic disorders in children. It has also been prescribed as an anorexiant in treating exogenous obesity.

■ CONTRAINDICATIONS: Cardiovascular disease, glaucoma, hypertension, hyperthyroidism, agitation, history of drug abuse, concomitant administration of a monoamine oxidase inhibitor within 14 days, or known hypersensitivity to this drug prohibits its use.

■ ADVERSE EFFECTS: Among the more serious adverse reactions are various manifestations of central nervous system excitation, increased blood pressure, arrhythmias and other cardiovascular effects, nausea, anorexia, and drug dependence.

dextromethorphan hydrobromide, an antitussive derived from morphine, but lacking narcotic effects.

■ INDICATION: It is prescribed for the suppression of nonproductive cough.

■ CONTRAINDICATIONS: Use of a monoamine oxidase inhibitor within the past 14 days or known hypersensitivity to this drug prohibits its use.

■ ADVERSE EFFECTS: The most serious adverse reaction is respiratory depression resulting from large doses.

dextrose /dek'strōs/, a glucose available in various solutions for intravenous administration.

■ INDICATIONS: It is prescribed to provide calories and fluid and to correct hypoglycemia.

■ CONTRAINDICATIONS: Diabetic coma, intracranial or intraspinal hemorrhage, or delirium tremens prohibits its use.

■ ADVERSE EFFECTS: Among the more serious adverse reactions are hyperglycemia, glycosuria, and phlebitis.

dextrose and sodium chloride injection, a fluid, nutrient, and electrolyte replenisher. It is available for parenteral use in a variety of concentrations.

dextrothyroxine sodium, an antihyperlipidemic.

■ INDICATION: It is prescribed in the treatment of hyperlipidemia.

■ CONTRAINDICATIONS: Known organic heart disease, hypertension, advanced liver or kidney disease, pregnancy, and a history of iodism prohibits its use. It is also prohibited for lactating mothers.

■ ADVERSE EFFECTS: Among the most serious adverse reactions are angina pectoris, supraventricular tachycardia, cardiomegaly, myocardial infarction, insomnia, alopecia, hyperthermia, diuresis, dizziness, paresthesia, gallstones, and psychic changes.

D.H.E.-45, a trademark for an alpha-adrenergic blocking agent (dihydroergotamine mesylate).

DHFS, abbreviation for **dengue hemorrhagic fever shock syndrome.**

dhobie itch /dō'bē/, a form of contact dermatitis associated with the use of laundry marking fluids. See also **jock itch, jockstrap itch.**

di-, **1.** a combining form meaning 'two, twice': *diacid, diamide, dimorphic.* **2.** also **dia-.** a combining form meaning 'apart, through': *diuresia, diactinism.* **3.** a combining form meaning 'apart, away from': *diffraction, discission, divergent.*

diabetes /dī'əbē'tēz/, **1.** a clinical condition characterized by the excessive excretion of urine. The excess may be caused by a deficiency of antidiuretic hormone (ADH), as in diabetes insipidus, or it may be the result of the hyperglycemia occurring in diabetes mellitus. **2.** diabetes mellitus. See also **diabetic.**

diabetes insipidus /insip'idəs/, a metabolic disorder, characterized by extreme polyuria and polydipsia, caused by deficient production or secretion of the antidiuretic hormone (ADH) or an inability of the kidney tubules to respond to ADH. Rarely, the symptoms are self-induced by an excessive water intake. The condition may be acquired, familial, idiopathic, or nephrogenic.

■ OBSERVATIONS: The onset may be dramatic and sudden, and urinary output may exceed 10 L in 24 hours. The patient is usually well and comfortable except for the annoyance of frequent urination and a constant need to drink. A person with diabetes insipidus who is unconscious because of trauma or surgery continues to produce massive quantities of urine. If fluids are not administered in adequate amounts, the patient becomes severely dehydrated and hypernatremic.

■ INTERVENTION: In mild cases, no treatment is necessary. Vasopressin in an intramuscular injection or spray is effective. Oral hypoglycemic agents improve the response of the kidneys to the decreased amount of available ADH in some cases, and thiazide diuretics, by inducing a state of salt depletion, sometimes decrease the diuresis of water by as much as 50%.

■ NURSING CONSIDERATIONS: Infants and small children are particularly vulnerable to serious circulatory disturbances when dehydrated; therefore, exceedingly careful monitoring is essential in cases where the condition is suspected, especially after head surgery or trauma.

diabetes mellitus (DM) /məlī'təs/, a complex disorder of carbohydrate, fat, and protein metabolism that is primarily a result of a relative or complete lack of insulin secretion by the beta cells of the pancreas or of defects of the insulin receptors. The disease is often familial but may be acquired, such as in Cushing's syndrome, as a result of the administration of excessive glucocorticoid. The various forms of diabetes have been organized into a series of categories developed by the National Diabetes Data Group of the National Institutes of Health. Type I diabetes in this classification scheme includes patients dependent upon insulin to prevent ketosis. The category is also known as the insulin-dependent diabetes mellitus (IDDM) subclass. This group was previously called juvenile-onset diabetes, brittle diabetes, or ketosis-prone diabetes. Patients with Type II, or non-insulin-dependent diabetes mellitus (NIDDM), are those previously designated as having maturity-onset diabetes, adult-onset diabetes, ketosis-resistant diabetes, or stable diabetes. Type II patients are further subdivided into obese NIDDM and nonobese NIDDM groups. Those with gestational diabetes (GDM), usually identified as Type III, are in a separate subclass composed of women who developed glucose intolerance in association with pregnancy. Type IV, also identified as Other Types of Diabetes, includes patients whose diabetes is associated with a pancreatic disease, hormonal changes, adverse effects of drugs, or genetic or other anomalies. A fifth subclass, the impaired glucose tolerance (IGT) group, includes persons whose plasma glucose levels are abnormal although not sufficiently beyond the normal range to be diagnosed as diabetic. Kinds of diabetes mellitus are **gestational diabetes, insulin-dependent diabetes,** and **non-insulin-dependent diabetes.** See also **impaired glucose tolerance, potential abnormality of glucose tolerance, previous abnormality of glucose tolerance.**

■ OBSERVATIONS: The onset of diabetes mellitus is sudden in children and usually insidious in non-insulin-dependent diabetes mellitus (type II). Characteristically, the course is progressive and includes polyuria, polydipsia, weight loss, polyphagia, hyperglycemia, and glycosuria. The eyes, kidneys, nervous system, skin, and circulatory system may be affected, infections are common, and atherosclerosis often develops. In childhood and in the Type I, advanced stage of the disease, when no endogenous insulin is being secreted, ketoacidosis is a constant danger. The diagnosis is confirmed by glucose-tolerance tests, history, and urinalysis.

■ INTERVENTION: The goal of treatment is to maintain insulin-glucose homeostasis. Mild early or late onset of the disease may be controlled by diet alone. In more severe diabetes, insulin is administered to keep blood-glucose levels below the point where ketoacidosis is likely. Good control of diabetes may decrease the severity of the symptoms and the progression of the disease. The kind and amount of insulin given varies with the person's condition. Stress of any kind may require an adjustment in the dosage. See also **diabetic foot and leg care.**

■ NURSING CONSIDERATIONS: Diabetic patients need extensive teaching and emotional support. The nurse may help the person to accept the diagnosis, to understand the disease, and to learn self-administration of the medication. The person is also taught the need for continued medical supervision and dietary restriction, how to test the urine for sugar and interpret the results, and how to recognize the signs of impending coma: restlessness, thirst, hot dry skin, rapid pulse, fruity odor to the breath, and nausea. The patient also learns to recognize the signs of hypoglycemia and impending insulin shock: headache, nervousness, diaphoresis, thready pulse, and slurred speech. Certain safety precautions are emphasized; the patient should avoid infection, carry a supply of glucose at all times, wear a medical alert tag, and use sterile technique in giving self-medication.

diabetes, other types. See **other types of diabetes.**

diabetic /dī'əbet'ik/, **1.** of or pertaining to diabetes. **2.** affected with diabetes. **3.** a person who has diabetes mellitus.

diabetic amaurosis, blindness associated with diabetes, caused by a proliferative, hemorrhagic form of retinopathy that is characterized by capillary microaneurysms and hard or waxy exudates. Cataracts are also common in non-insulin-dependent diabetes, and, in insulin-dependent diabetes, snowflake cataract may progress until the entire lens is milky white.

diabetic coma, a life-threatening condition occurring in diabetic patients, caused by inadequate treatment, by failure to take prescribed insulin, or, most frequently, by infection, surgery, trauma, or other stress that increases the body's need for insulin. Without insulin to metabolize glucose, fats are burned for energy, resulting in ketosis and acidosis. The body's effort to counteract acidosis depletes the alkali reserve, causes a loss of sodium, chloride, potassium, and water, increases respiration (Kussmaul breathing) and urinary excretion, and leads to dehydration and generalized hypoxia. Warning signs of diabetic coma include a dull headache, fatigue, inordinate thirst, epigastric pain, nausea, vomiting, parched lips, a flushed face, and sunken eyes. The temperature usually rises and then falls; the systolic blood pressure drops, and circulatory collapse may occur. Immediate treatment consists of administering insulin and replacing electrolytes and fluids to correct the acidosis and dehydration. Nonketotic coma may occur in patients with poorly controlled diabetes and high levels of blood glucose but no acetone in the urine. The plasma hyperosmolarity causes water to leave cells, and the dehydration of cerebral cells results in coma.

diabetic diet, a diet prescribed in the treatment of diabetes mellitus, usually containing limited amounts of sugar or readily available carbohydrates and increased amounts of proteins, complex carbohydrates, and unsaturated fats. Dietary regulation depends on the severity of the disease and on the type and extent of insulin therapy. The diet should be designed to prevent wide fluctuation in the amount of glucose in the blood in order to preserve pancreatic function and to prevent chronic diabetic complications. See also **diabetes mellitus, insulin.**

diabetic foot and leg care, the special attention given to prevent the circulatory disorders and infections that frequently occur in the lower extremities of diabetic patients.

■ METHOD: The patient's legs and feet are examined daily for signs of dry, scaly, red, itching, or cracked skin, blisters, corns, calluses, abrasions, infection, blueness and swelling around varicosities, and thickened, discolored nails. The feet are bathed daily in tepid water with mild or superfatted soap and are dried gently but thoroughly with a soft towel. A lanolin-based lotion is then applied, starting with the distal end of the toes; excess lotion is removed with a dry towel; vigorous rubbing and the use of alcohol preparations are avoided. The toenails are cut straight across above the level of soft tissue after the feet are soaked for 3 to 5 minutes in tepid water. The feet are also soaked in tepid water for several minutes before hardened areas are treated by applying soft soap and rubbing the area with a washcloth; calluses and corns are removed, and thickened, deformed nails are cut by a podiatrist.

■ NURSING ORDERS: The nurse provides foot and leg care while the diabetic patient is hospitalized. Before discharge, the patient is instructed to examine and bathe the feet daily according to the recommended method, to report abnormalities, to keep the feet dry at all times, to wear cotton socks or stockings with cotton feet, and to place clean lamb's wool or cotton between the toes if they perspire. The patient is cautioned to avoid foot or leg trauma, walking barefoot, scratching insect bites, using a hot-water bottle or heating pad on the lower extremities, getting sunburned, wearing constricting garments, remaining in the same position for long periods, sitting at more than a right-angle bend, and crossing the knees. The diabetic individual is advised to alternate the wearing of two pairs of rubber-soled, well-fitted shoes wide enough to prevent pressure and rubbing, to air each pair of shoes between use, and to break in new shoes gradually. The patient is urged to walk to tolerance daily, to plan exercise periods after meals, to bend and straighten the knees and rotate the ankles occasionally when sitting, and, when standing, to shift weight from time to time and walk in place.

■ OUTCOME CRITERIA: Meticulous care of the feet and legs can prevent serious complications to which diabetic patients are subject, including local infection, skin ulcers, cellulitis, and gangrene.

diabetic ketoacidosis, an acute, life-threatening complication of uncontrolled diabetes mellitus in which urinary loss of water, potassium, ammonium, and sodium results in hypovolemia, electrolyte imbalance, extremely high blood-glucose levels, and the breakdown of free fatty acids causing acidosis, often with coma. Compare **insulin shock.**

■ OBSERVATIONS: The person appears flushed, has hot, dry skin, is restless, uncomfortable, agitated, diaphoretic, and has a fruity odor to the breath. Coma, confusion, and nausea are often noted. Diabetics who have no endogenous insulin are the most often affected, although the insulin concentration may be normal but inappropriately low for the degree of hyperglycemia. Untreated, the condition invariably proceeds to coma and death.

■ INTERVENTION: Intravenous insulin and hypotonic saline solution are administered immediately. Nasogastric intubation and bladder catheterization are usual. Blood glucose and ketone levels are determined hourly, and electrolyte and acid-base balance are monitored frequently. Bicarbonate or potassium may be given in dosages dependent on the degree of acidosis. Plasma or a plasma expander may be necessary to prevent or correct shock resulting from hypovolemia.

■ NURSING CONSIDERATIONS: The cause for the episode of ketoacidosis is sought. The most common precipitating factors are infection, GI upset, alcohol consumption, and the patient's failure to take insulin. In childhood, diabetes characteristically begins suddenly and progresses rapidly; therefore, the diagnosis of insulin-dependent diabetes is usually made when the child is brought to the hospital in diabetic ketoacidosis. The care of a patient in the hospital after an episode of ketoacidosis is the same as for diabetes mellitus.

diabetic retinopathy, a disorder of retinal blood vessels characterized by capillary microaneurysms, hemorrhage, exudates, and the formation of new vessels and

Classification of diabetes mellitus and descriptive characteristics for each type

Class	*Clinical and associated factors and former terminology*
Type I: insulin-dependent diabetes mellitus (IDDM)	Patients dependent on insulin to prevent ketosis; onset usually in youth but may occur in adults; associated with certain HLA types, islet cell antibodies are frequently present; formerly called juvenile-onset diabetes, ketosis-prone diabetes, brittle diabetes
Type II: noninsulin-dependent diabetes mellitus (NIDDM)	Patients not dependent on insulin to preserve life, although they may be treated with insulin (even if treated with insulin, they are still classified as NIDDM); ketosis resistant except in very special circumstances such as presence of infection; not HLA related; onset usually after 40 years of age but may occur in youth; serum insulin levels may be depressed, normal, or elevated; 60% to 90% of diabetics in this class are obese; formerly called maturity-onset diabetes, adult-onset diabetes, ketosis-resistant diabetes, and stable diabetes; class may be subdivided into two classes: (1) obese type II, and (2) nonobese type II
Type III: gestational diabetes mellitus (GDM)	Glucose intolerance occurs during pregnancy; group does not include known diabetics who become pregnant; after delivery, glucose intolerance may remain but not be serious enough to be treated or the patient may have characteristics of type I or type II diabetes, or glucose intolerance may disappear; patient is reclassified after delivery, formerly called gestational diabetes
Type IV: other types, includes diabetes mellitus associated with pancreatic disease, other hormonal abnormalities, drugs	Patients in this class must have diabetes mellitus and one of the other diseases, syndromes, or casual factors; formerly called secondary diabetes

connective tissue. The disorder occurs most frequently in patients with long-standing, poorly controlled diabetes. Repeated hemorrhage may result in permanent opacity of the vitreous humor, and blindness may eventually set in. Photocoagulation of damaged retinal blood vessels by a laser beam may be performed to prevent hemorrhage from the vessels. Rarely, cloudy vitreous humor is surgically removed by vitrectomy.

diabetic treatment, therapy of diabetes mellitus by means of a low carbohydrate diet, insulin injections, or oral hypoglycemic agents, as chlorpropamide, acetohexamide, tolbutamide, and tolazamide.

diabetic xanthoma, an eruption of yellow papules or plaques on the skin in uncontrolled diabetes mellitus. The lesion disappears as the metabolic functions are stabilized and the disease is brought under control.

diabetogenic state, a health condition manifested by signs and symptoms of diabetes.

Diabinese, a trademark for an oral antidiabetic (chlorpropamide).

diacetic acid. See **acetoacetic acid.**

diacondylar fracture /dī′əkon′dilər/, any fracture that runs across the line of a condyle.

Diagnex blue test, a trademark for a test for the presence of hydrochloric acid in gastric secretions. Diagnex blue tablets, which contain the dye azuresin, are taken by mouth. If the urine appears blue, it can be inferred that the stomach is secreting hydrochloric acid. See also **gastric analysis.**

diagnosis, *pl.* **diagnoses, 1.** identification of a disease or condition by a scientific evaluation of physical signs, symptoms, history, laboratory tests, and procedures. Kinds of diagnoses are **clinical diagnosis, differential diagnosis, laboratory diagnosis, nursing diagnosis,** and **physical diagnosis. 2.** the art of naming a disease or condition. –**diagnostic,** *adj.*, **diagnose,** *v.*

diagnosis-related group (DRG), a designation in a system that classifies patients by age, diagnosis, and surgical procedure, producing 300 different categories used in predicting the use of hospital resources, including length of stay. The system is being tested for use in anticipating the cost of reimbursement to hospitals by studying the population served to improve the cash flow to the hospital. It is performed using grouped data about how much each particular DRG may be expected to cost in hospital services.

diagnostic, pertaining to a diagnosis.

Diagnostic and Statistical Manual of Mental Disorders (DSM), a manual, published by the American Psychiatric Association, listing the official diagnostic classifications of mental disorders. The *DSM* recommends the use of a multiaxial evaluation system as a holistic diagnostic approach. It consists of five axes, each of which refers to a different class of information, including both mental and physical data. Axes I and II include all of the mental disorders, classified broadly as clinical syndromes and personality disorders; axis III contains physical disorders and conditions; and axes IV and V provide a coded outline of supplemental information on, for example, psychosocial stressors and adaptive functioning, which may be useful for planning individual treatment and predicting its outcome. Each of the classifications of the mental disorders contains a code that provides a reference to the WHO *International Classification of Diseases (ICD)* and offers such useful diagnostic criteria as essential and associated features of the disorder, age at onset, course, impairment, complications, predisposing factors, prevalence, sex ratio, familial patterns, and differential diagnoses.

diagnostic anesthesia, a procedure in which analgesia is induced to a depth adequate to comfortably permit performance of moderately painful diagnostic procedures of short duration. Awake anesthesia is often used for this purpose. See also **awake anesthesia.**

diagnostician, a person skilled and trained in making diagnoses.

diagnostic position of gaze. See **cardinal position of gaze.**

diagnostic radiology, medical imaging using external sources of radiation.

diagnostic radiopharmaceutic, a radioactive drug administered to a patient as a diagnostic tracer to differentiate normal from abnormal anatomic structures or biochemical or physiologic functions. Most diagnostic radioactive tracers indicate their position within the body by emitting gamma rays. By monitoring the emissions with a collimated external gamma-ray detector, the concentration of the tracer in different organs can be inferred and low-resolution images of the organs can be obtained. Tracers prepared with tritium, carbon 14, or phosphorus 32, which do not emit gamma rays, are used diagnostically by analyzing the concentration of the isotope in a metabolic end product in the patient's blood, urine, breath, or, in some cases, biopsy samples. When glucose containing ^{14}C is administered, the subsequent monitoring of $^{14}CO_2$ in the patient's breath can indicate the absorption of the compound, its metabolism, and elimination as a metabolic end product.

diagnostic services, services related to the diagnosis made by a physician but which may be performed also by nurses or other health professionals.

diakinesis /dī′əkinē′sis, dī′əkī-/, the final stage in the first meiotic prophase in gametogenesis in which the chromosomes achieve maximum contraction and are ready to separate. The chiasmata and nucleolus disappear, the nuclear membrane degenerates, and the spindle fibers form in preparation for the formation of dyads. See also **diplotene, leptotene, pachytene, zygotene.**

dialogue, a complex form of computer-assisted instruction in which the student is actively engaged in "true conversation" with a computer. A less formally structured mode, it does not present textual material as a basis for questioning the student.

Dialose, a trademark for a GI, fixed-combination drug containing a stool softener (docusate sodium sulfosuccinate) and a laxative (sodium carboxymethylcellulose).

dialysate /dī·al′isāt/, a solution used in dialysis.

dialysis /dī·al′isis/, **1.** the process of separating colloids and crystalline substances in solution by the difference in their rate of diffusion through a semipermeable membrane. **2.** a medical procedure for the removal of certain elements from the blood or lymph by virtue of the difference in their rates of diffusion through an external semipermeable membrane or, in the case of peritoneal dialysis, through the peritoneum. Dialysis may be used to remove poisons and excessive amounts of drugs, to correct serious electrolyte and acid-base imbalances, and to remove urea, uric acid, and creatinine in patients with chronic end-stage renal disease. Dialysis involves diffusion of particles from an area of high to lower concentration, osmosis of fluid across the membrane from an area of lesser to greater concentration of particles, and the ultrafiltration or movement of the fluid across the membrane as a result of an artificially created pressure differential. See also **hemodialysis, peritoneal dialysis.**

dialysis disequilibrium syndrome, a disorder caused by a rapid change in extracellular fluid composition during dialysis. The syndrome may be marked by cerebral or neurologic disturbances, cardiac arrhythmias, and pulmonary edema.

dialysis fluid, the solution that flows on the opposite side of a semipermeable membrane to blood.

dialyzer /dī′əlī′zər/, **1.** a machine used in dialysis. **2.** a semipermeable membrane or porous diaphragm in a dialysis machine. See also **hemodialysis, peritoneal dialysis.**

Diamond-Blackfan syndrome, a rare congenital disorder evident in the first 3 months of life, characterized by severe anemia, very low reticulocyte count, but normal numbers of platelets and white cells. It is caused by a deficiency of erythrocyte precursors. Also called **congenital hypoplastic anemia.** See also **anemia.**

diamond stone, (in dentistry) any of the rotary devices that contain diamond chips as an abrasive.

Diamox, a trademark for a carbonic anhydrase inhibitor (acetazolamide), used as an adjunct in anticonvulsant therapy for certain seizure disorders and to reduce intraocular pressure in glaucoma.

Dianabol, a trademark for an androgen (methandrostenolone), used as an anabolic agent.

Dianeal, a trademark for a peritoneal dialysis solution containing dextrose and a number of electrolytes.

diapedesis /dī′əpidē′sis/, the passage of red or white blood corpuscles through the walls of the vessels that contain them without damage to the vessels.

diaper rash, a maculopapular and occasionally excoriated eruption in the diaper area of infants caused by irritation from feces, moisture, heat, or ammonia produced by the bacterial decomposition of urine. Secondary infection by *Candida albicans* is common. Principles of treatment include frequent diaper changes, dryness, cleanliness, coolness, and ventilation of the affected area. Specific topical antimicrobial medication may be prescribed for secondary infection. Also called **diaper dermatitis.**

diaper restraint, a therapeutic device used especially in orthopedics for countertraction with lower extremity traction when other methods of countertraction are not effective. Diaper restraints are commonly used in treating children with orthopedic diseases and abnormalities and are designed to fit over the pelvic area like a diaper, with rings incorporated at each of four corners. A webbing strap is threaded through the rings and attached to the top side of the bedspring frame. Diaper restraints applied to incontinent patients are usually checked every half hour as a precaution against urinary tract infections that can develop from urinary wastes accumulating within such restraints. Diaper restraints are used with Russell traction and with split Russell traction if additional countertraction is required but are not usually used with other kinds of traction. Compare **jacket restraint, sling restraint.**

diaphanoscopy /dī·af′ənos′kəpē/, examination of an internal structure with a **diaphanoscope,** an instrument that transilluminates body tissues. It is sometimes used in the diagnosis of breast tumors.

diaphoresis /dī′əfərē′sis/, the secretion of sweat, especially the profuse secretion associated with an elevated body temperature, physical exertion, exposure to heat, and mental or emotional stress. Sweating is centrally controlled by the sympathetic nervous system and is primarily a thermoregulatory mechanism, but the sweat glands on the palms and soles respond to emotional stimuli and do not participate in thermal sweating. The rate of sweating is generally not affected by water deficiency, but it may be reduced by severe dehydration and diminishes when salt intake exceeds salt loss. Also called **sweating.** See also **sudorific.**

diaphoretic. See **sudorific.**

diaphragm /dī′əfram/, **1.** (in anatomy) a dome-shaped musculofibrous partition that separates the thoracic and the abdominal cavities. The convex cranial surface of the diaphragm forms the floor of the thoracic cavity, and the concave surface forms the roof of the abdominal cavity. This partition is pierced by various openings through which pass the aorta, esophagus, and vena cava. The diaphragm aids respiration by moving up and down. During inspiration it moves down and increases the volume of the thoracic cavity; during expiration it moves up, decreasing the volume. During deep inspiration and expiration the range of diaphragmatic movement in the adult is about 30 mm on the right side and about 28 mm on the left side. The height of this structure also varies with the degree of distension of the stomach and the intestines and with the size of the liver. It is innervated by the phrenic nerve from the cervical plexus. **2.** *informal.* a contraceptive diaphragm. **3.** (in optics) an opening that controls the amount of light passing through an optical network. **4.** a thin, membranous partition, as that employed in dialysis. **5.** (in radiography) a metal plate with a small opening that limits the diameter of the radiographic beam. –**diaphragmatic,** *adj.*

diaphragmatic hernia, the protrusion of part of the stomach through an opening in the diaphragm, most commonly an abnormally enlarged esophageal hiatus. In some cases the intestines may also herniate into the chest. The enlargement of the normal opening for the esophagus may be caused by trauma, congenital weakness, increased abdominal pressure, or relaxation of ligaments of skeletal muscles, and permits part of the stomach to slide into the thorax. A sliding hiatus hernia, one of the most common pathologic conditions of the upper GI tract, may occur at any age but is most frequent in elderly and middle-aged people. A kind of diaphragmatic hernia is **hiatus hernia.**

■ OBSERVATIONS: Symptoms of diaphragmatic hernia vary but usually include heartburn after meals, when in a supine position, and on exertion, especially when bending forward. There may be regurgitation of food, dysphagia, abdominal distention after eating, belching, rumbling in the intestines, rapid breathing, and a dull epigastric pain radiating to the shoulder. The similarity of some of the symptoms to those of myocardial infarction may make the patient fearful and anxious. The continued reflux of gastric juice into the esophagus may lead to ulceration with bleeding and the formation of fibrous tissue. Gastric contents regurgitated during sleep may be aspirated into the lungs. Rarely, a part of the stomach or other viscera becomes incarcerated in the chest.

■ INTERVENTION: The patient is placed in bed in a semi-Fowler's position and raised to a high Fowler's position during and after small, frequent meals of a bland diet. The individual is encouraged to chew slowly and thoroughly, to drink one or two glasses of water with a meal (unless contraindicated), and to avoid smoking. The blood pressure, pulse, respirations, and temperature are monitored. Medication for pain, an antacid, as aluminum hydroxide gel, and diagnostic endoscopy and x-ray films may be ordered; to facilitate visualization of the hernia, the patient may be placed in a Trendelenburg position during studies of barium swallowing. If symptoms are severe and persistent and if they are unrelieved by conservative measures, the hernia may be repaired surgically.

■ NURSING CONSIDERATIONS: Diaphragmatic hernias are very common, especially among older people who are in the hospital for other indications. The recurrence of the symptoms of diaphragmatic hernia may often be prevented by instructing the patient, before discharge, to have frequent, small bland meals, not to recline after eating, to lose weight (if indicated), not to smoke, and to avoid constipation. Serious complications and severe discomfort may usually be avoided by the patient if the instructions are observed.

diaphragmatic node, a node in one of three groups of thoracic parietal lymph nodes, situated on the thoracic side of the diaphragm and consisting of the anterior set, the middle set, and the posterior set. The anterior set includes about three nodes dorsal to the base of the xiphoid process and one or two nodes on either side near the junction of the seventh rib. The nodes dorsal to the xiphoid process receive afferent lymphatic vessels from the convex surface of the liver. The afferents of the nodes near the seventh rib drain the ventral side of the diaphragm. The efferents of the anterior set pass to the sternal nodes. The middle set of about three nodes on each side is close to the diaphragmatic entry of the phrenic nerves. Some of the nodes of the middle set on the right side lie within the pericardium. The afferents of the middle set drain parts of the diaphragm and the liver. The efferents of the middle set pass to the posterior mediastinal nodes. The posterior set of diaphragmatic nodes consists of a few nodes on the crura of the diaphragm, connecting with the lumbar nodes and the posterior mediastinal nodes. Compare **intercostal node, sternal node.** See also **lymphatic system, lymph node.**

diaphragm pessary. See **pessary.**

diaphragm stethoscope, an instrument for auscultation of bodily sounds. Originally designed by René Laënnec, it consists of a vibrating disk, or diaphragm, which transmits sound waves through tubing to two earpieces. Also called **binaural stethoscope.** See also **stethoscope.**

diaphyseal aclasis /dī′əfiz′ē·əl ak′ləsis/, a relatively rare abnormal condition that affects the skeletal system. Characterized by multiple exostoses or bony protrusions, it is hereditary, being transmitted as a dominant trait. Approximately half of the children of an individual with diaphyseal aclasis display varying degrees of its symptoms. The characteristic exostoses are radiographically and microscopically similar to osteochondromas. Evident involvement is diffuse, with the long bones usually affected more severely and more frequently than the short bones. Depending on the specific area involved, various angular or rotational deformities may result. Diaphyseal aclasis is usually bilateral and occurs more frequently in boys than in girls. Although this disease is hereditary, its signs and symptoms are not usually evident until the affected individual is 2 years of age or older. Children of a parent who has the disease are often routinely examined for symptoms. The major signs of the disease are the noticeable protrusions in the areas of the exostoses. Pain is not usually associated with the exostoses and, if present, is usually minimal. Deformities of the extremities may be evident, depending on the severity and the location of the exostoses. Radiographic examination reveals a broadened metaphyseal area, and the specific lesion is exhibited by abnormal continuity and decreased density. Asymptomatic lesions characteristic of diaphyseal aclasis usually require little or no treatment other than continued observation. The lesions located near the joints that interfere with joint motion or impair neurovascular function may be surgically excised. Angular and rotational deformities caused by the lesions may require surgical correction to facilitate improved function. Inequalities in the length of lower extremities resulting from unilateral involvement may require epiphysiodesis. A relatively small number of these lesions may become malignant. One form of the disorder, dyschondroplasia, results in dwarfism. Also called **hereditary deforming chondroplasia, multiple cartilaginous exostoses.**

diaphysis /dī•af′isis/, the shaft of a long bone, consisting of a tube of compact bone enclosing the medullary cavity.

Diapid, a trademark for a pituitary antidiuretic hormone (lypressin).

diarrhea, the frequent passage of loose, watery stools, generally the result of increased motility in the colon. The stool may also contain mucus, pus, blood, or excessive amounts of fat. Diarrhea is usually a symptom of some underlying disorder. Conditions in which diarrhea is an important symptom are dysenteric diseases, malabsorption syndrome, lactose intolerance, irritable bowel syndrome, GI tumors, and inflammatory bowel disease. In addition to stool frequency, patients may complain of abdominal cramps and generalized weakness. Untreated, diarrhea may lead to rapid dehydration and electrolyte imbalance and should be treated symptomatically until proper diagnosis can be made. Antidiarrheal preparations, as diphenoxylate and paregoric, are helpful. If diarrhea is accompanied by vomiting, intravenous fluids may be necessary to prevent fluid depletion. See also **dehydration.** **–diarrheal, diarrheic,** *adj.*

diarthrosis. See **synovial joint.**

Diasone Sodium Enterab, a trademark for a leprostatic antibacterial (sulfoxone sodium).

diastasis /dī•as′təsis/, the forcible separation of two parts that normally are joined together, as the separation of parts of a bone at an epiphysis or the separation of two bones that lack a synovial joint.

diastasis recti abdominis, the separation of the two rectus muscles along the median line of the abdominal wall. In a newborn infant, the condition is the result of incomplete development. In an adult woman, the abnormality is often caused by repeated pregnancies or a multiple birth, as the delivery of triplets.

diastatic fermentation /dī′əstat′ik/, the conversion of starch to glucose by the enzyme ptyalin.

diastole /dī•as′təlē/, **1.** the period of time between contractions of the atria or the ventricles during which blood enters the relaxed chambers from the systemic circulation and the lungs. Ventricular diastole begins with the onset of the second heart sound and ends with the first heart sound. **2.** phase 4 of the action potential (from the end of phase 3 to the beginning of phase 0). Compare **systole.** **–diastolic** /dī′əstol′ik/, *adj.*

-diastole, a combining form referring to 'types and locations of the lower blood pressure measurement': *adiastole, hyperdiastole, prediastole.*

diastolic augmentation, an increase in arterial diastolic pressure caused by the counterpulsation of a circulatory assist device, as an intraaortic balloon pump. Counterpulsation is produced because the mechanic device pumps when the heart is in diastole and relaxes when the heart is in systole.

diastolic blood pressure, the minimum level of blood pressure measured between contractions of the heart. Diastolic pressures for an individual may vary with age, sex, body weight, emotional state, and such other factors as the time of day and whether the patient has just finished a meal.

diastolic filling pressure, the blood pressure in the ventricle during diastole.

diastrophic dwarf /dī′əstrof′ik/, a person in whom short stature is caused by osteochondrodysplasia and is associated with various deformities of the bones and joints, including scoliosis, clubfoot, micromelia, hand defects, multiple joint contractures and subluxations, ear deformities, and cleft palate. The condition may be genetically related and transmitted as an autosomal recessive trait.

diathermy /dī′əthur′mē/, the production of heat in body tissues for therapeutic purposes by high-frequency currents that are insufficiently intense to destroy tissues or to impair their vitality. Diathermy is used in treating chronic arthritis, bursitis, fractures, gynecologic diseases, sinusitis, and other conditions.

diathesis /dī•əthē′sis/, *pl.* **diatheses,** an inherited physical constitution predisposing to certain diseases or conditions, many of which are believed associated with the Y chromosome, because males appear to be more susceptible than females. A diasthesis may be bilious, indicating a familial tendency to develop GI distress, or gouty, indicating a predisposition to the accumulation of urates in the tissues, particularly in mature males.

diazepam, a sedative and tranquilizer.

■ INDICATIONS: It is prescribed in the treatment of anxiety, nervous tension, and muscle spasm, and as an anticonvulsant.

■ CONTRAINDICATIONS: Acute narrow-angle glaucoma, psychosis, or known hypersensitivity to this drug or to any benzodiazepine medication prohibits its use.

■ ADVERSE EFFECTS: Among the more serious adverse reactions are withdrawal symptoms resulting from discontinuation of treatment. Hypotonia, respiratory depression, drowsiness, and fatigue commonly occur.

diazoxide /dī′əzok′sīd/, a vasodilator used as an antihypertensive.

■ INDICATIONS: It is prescribed for the emergency reduction of blood pressure in malignant hypertension when drastic reduction of the diastolic blood pressure is required and in some cases of hypoglycemia.

■ CONTRAINDICATIONS: Compensatory hypertension or known hypersensitivity to this drug or other thiazides prohibits its use. Caution is advised in heart disease, pregnancy, and impaired kidney function.

■ ADVERSE EFFECTS: Among the more serious adverse reactions are tachycardia, sodium and water retention, hyperglycemia, and severe hypotension.

■ NOTE: This drug is for intravenous use in hospitalized patients only. Severe hypotension may result.

Dibenzyline, a trademark for an alpha-adrenergic blocker (phenoxybenzamine hydrochloride).

dibromodulcitol. See **mitolactol.**

dibucaine, a topical anesthetic ointment.

dic, (in cytogenetics) abbreviation for *dicentric*.

DIC, abbreviation for **disseminated intravascular coagulation.**

dicalcium phosphate and calcium gluconate with vitamin D, a source of calcium and phosphorus.

■ INDICATIONS: It is prescribed for hypocalcemia, especially in pregnancy and lactation.

■ CONTRAINDICATIONS: Hypoparathyroidism or known hypersensitivity to any of the ingredients of this drug prohibits its use.

■ ADVERSE EFFECTS: There are no known adverse reactions.

dicephaly /dīsef′əlē/, a developmental anomaly in which the fetus has two heads. –**dicephalous, dicephalic,** *adj.*, **dicephalus,** *n.*

dichlorodiphenyltrichloroethane. See **DDT.**

dichlorphenamide /dī′klôrfen′əmīd/, a carbonic anhydrase inhibitor.

■ INDICATION: It is prescribed in the treatment of chronic glaucoma.

■ CONTRAINDICATIONS: Liver and adrenocortical insufficiency, kidney failure, hyperchloremic acidosis, depressed sodium or potassium levels, pulmonary obstruction, Addison's disease, known or suspected pregnancy, or known hypersensitivity to this drug prohibits its use.

■ ADVERSE EFFECTS: Among the more serious adverse reactions are anorexia, GI disturbances, acidosis, ureteral calculus formation, and aplastic anemia.

dichorial twins, dichorionic twins. See **dizygotic twins.**

dichotomy /dīkot′əmē/, a division or separation into two equal parts.

dichotomy planning, the preparation for ongoing and future needs for health care resources of patients as they move along the health/illness continuum.

Dick test, a skin test for determining sensitivity to an erythrotoxin produced by the group A streptococci that cause scarlet fever. A skin-test dose of the toxin is injected intradermally. An area of inflammation 1 cm in diameter indicates that the person is not immune, has no antitoxin, and therefore is susceptible to the toxin. Larger doses may then be given to induce immunity. Compare **Shultz-Charlton phenomenon.**

dicloxacillin sodium /dī′kloksəsil′in/, an antibacterial.

■ INDICATIONS: It is prescribed in the treatment of staphylococcal infections, especially those caused by penicillinase-producing strains of staphylococci.

■ CONTRAINDICATIONS: Known hypersensitivity to this drug or to any penicillin medication prohibits its use.

■ ADVERSE EFFECTS: The most serious adverse effect is hypersensitivity reaction. Other side effects include nausea, diarrhea, and epigastric distress.

Dicodid, a trademark for an antitussive (hydrocodone bitartrate).

dicumarol, an anticoagulant.

■ INDICATIONS: It is prescribed for the prophylaxis and treatment of thrombosis and embolism.

■ CONTRAINDICATIONS: Risk of hemorrhage, peptic ulcer, ulcerative colitis, or known hypersensitivity to this drug prohibits its use.

■ ADVERSE EFFECTS: Among the more serious adverse reactions are GI disturbances, nausea, and diarrhea.

dicyclomine hydrochloride, an anticholinergic.

■ INDICATION: It is prescribed as an adjunct to ulcer therapy.

■ CONTRAINDICATIONS: Narrow-angle glaucoma, asthma, obstruction of the genitourinary or GI tract, ulcerative colitis, or known hypersensitivity to this drug prohibits its use.

■ ADVERSE EFFECTS: Among the more serious adverse reactions are blurred vision, central nervous system effects, tachycardia, dry mouth, decreased sweating, and hypersensitivity reactions.

Didrex, a trademark for an anorexiant (benzphetamine hydrochloride).

Didronel, a trademark for a calcium regulator (etidronate disodium).

didym-, a combining form meaning 'pertaining to a testis': *didymalgia, didymitis, didymodynia.*

-didymus, **1.** a combining form meaning a 'pair of twins joined at a (specified) part of the body': *gastrodidymus, thoracodidymus, vertebrodidymus.* **2.** a combining form meaning a 'fetal monster with supernumerary organ(s)': *atlodidymus, opodidymus, pygodidymus.*

diecious /dī·ē′shəs/, an animal or plant that is sexually distinct, having either male or female reproductive organs. Also spelled **dioecious.**

diencephalon /dī′ənsef′əlon/, the division of the brain between the telencephalon and the mesencephalon. It consists of the hypothalamus, thalamus, metathalamus, and the epithalamus and includes most of the third ventricle.

diener /dē′nər/, an individual (German, for "man-servant") who maintains the hospital laboratory or equipment and facilities. The morgue diener may also assist the pathologist in performing autopsies.

dienestrol /dī′ines′trôl/, an estrogen.

■ INDICATIONS: It is prescribed in the treatment of atrophic vaginitis and kraurosis vulvae.

■ CONTRAINDICATIONS: Pregnancy, known or suspected cancer of the breast, thrombophlebitis, unusual vaginal bleeding, or known hypersensitivity to this drug prohibits its use.

■ ADVERSE EFFECTS: Among the more serious adverse reactions are increased risk of cancer, thrombophlebitis, hepatic adenoma, embolism, and gallbladder disease.

diet, **1.** food and drink considered with regard to their nutritional qualities, composition, and effects on health. **2.** nutrients prescribed, regulated, or restricted as to kind and amount for therapeutic or other purposes. **3.** the customary allowance of food and drink regularly provided or consumed. Compare **nutrition.** See also specific diets. –**dietetic,** *adj.*

dietary allowances, the recommended allowances of essential nutrients formulated by the Food and Nutrition

Board of the National Research Council to serve as a guide for planning the diet to maintain good nutrition in healthy individuals. In general the recommended allowances exceed average nutritional requirements and are lower than the amounts needed in disease or deficiency states. See also **recommended dietary allowances (RDA), minimum daily requirments (MDR).**

dietary fiber, a generic term for nondigestible chemical substances found in plant cell walls and surrounding cellular material, each with a different effect on the various GI functions, as colon transit time, water absorption, and lipid metabolism. The main dietary fiber components are cellulose, lignin, hemicellulose, pectin, and gums. Foods high in dietary fiber are fruits; green leafy vegetables, as lettuce, spinach, celery, and cabbage; root vegetables, as carrots, turnips, and potatoes; and whole-grain cereals and breads. Also called **bulk, roughage.**

dietetic assistant, a person who assists in providing food-service supervison and nutritional-care services under the guidance of a registered or consultant dietitian or administrator. A dietetic assistant is usually required to complete a training program approved by the American Dietetic Association in order to be qualified.

dietetic food, **1.** a specially prepared low-calorie food, often containing artificial sweeteners. **2.** a food prepared for any specific dietary need or restriction, as salt-free or vegetarian foods. See also **dietetics.**

dietetics /dī′itet′iks/, the science of applying nutritional principles to the planning and preparation of foods and regulation of the diet in relation to both health and disease.

dietetic technician, a person qualified by an associate degree program approved by the American Dietetic Association who may assist in providing food service management or nutritional-care services under the supervision of a dietitian or administrator.

diethylcarbamazine citrate /dī·eth′əlkärbam′əzēn/, an anthelmintic.

■ INDICATIONS: It is prescribed in the treatment of ascariasis, filariasis, onchocerciasis, loiasis, and tropic eosinophilia.

■ CONTRAINDICATIONS: Hypertension, severe heart, kidney, or liver impairment, or known hypersensitivity to this drug prohibits its use.

■ ADVERSE EFFECTS: Among the most serious adverse reactions are tachycardia, breathing difficulties, hypotension, and severe allergic reactions caused by the death of parasites.

diethyl ether. See **ether.**

diethylpropion hydrochloride, an appetite depressant.

■ INDICATION: It is prescribed in the treatment of exogenous obesity.

■ CONTRAINDICATIONS: Arteriosclerosis, hyperthyroidism, glaucoma, history of drug dependence, hypertension, concomitant administration of a monoamine oxidase inhibitor within 14 days, or known hypersensitivity to this drug prohibits its use.

■ ADVERSE EFFECTS: Among the more serious adverse reactions are restlessness and insomnia, increased blood pressure, arrhythmias, cardiovascular effects, nausea, dry mouth, and drug dependence.

diethylstilbestrol (DES), a synthetic hormone with estrogenic properties. Also called **stilbestrol.**

diethylstilbestrol diphosphate, an antineoplastic agent.

■ INDICATION: It is prescribed for inoperable, progressing prostatic cancer.

■ CONTRAINDICATIONS: Present or previous conditions of markedly impaired liver, thrombophlebitis, thromboembolic disorders, or cerebral apoplexy prohibits its use.

■ ADVERSE EFFECTS: The most serious adverse reactions are thrombophlebitis, pulmonary embolism, cerebral thrombosis, cholestatic jaundice, mental depression, erythema nodosum and erythema multiforme, changes in libido, and dizziness.

dietitian, a person who meets all the requirements for active membership in the American Dietetic Association after completing special educational training in the nutritional care of groups and individuals. A registered dietitian is one who has successfully completed an examination and maintains continuing education requirements of the Commission on Dietetic Registration.

Dietl's crisis /dē′təlz/, a sudden, excruciating pain in the kidney, caused by distention of the renal pelvis, by the rapid ingestion of very large amounts of liquid, or by a kinking of a ureter that produces temporary occlusion of the flow of urine from the kidney. The pain may be accompanied by nausea, vomiting, hematuria, and general collapse. See also **hydronephrosis.**

differential diagnosis, the distinguishing between two or more diseases with similar symptoms by systematically comparing their signs and symptoms. See also **diagnosis.**

differential growth, a comparison of the various increases in size or the different rates of growth of dissimilar organisms, tissues, or structures.

differential white blood cell count, an examination and enumeration of the distribution of leukocytes in a stained blood smear. The different kinds of white cells are counted and reported as percentages of the total examined. Compare **complete blood count.** See also **hematocrit, hemoglobin, leukocyte, red cell indices.**

differentiation, **1.** (in embryology) a process in development in which unspecialized cells or tissues are systemically modified and altered to achieve specific and characteristic physical forms, physiologic functions, and chemical properties. Kinds of differentiation are **correlative differentiation, functional differentiation, invisible differentiation,** and **self-differentiation. 2.** progressive diversification leading to complexity. **3.** the acquisition of functions and forms different from those of the original. **4.** the distinguishing of one thing or disease from another, as in differential diagnosis. **–differentiate,** *v.*

diffraction, the bending and scattering of wavelengths of light or other radiation, as the radiation that passes around obstacles in its path. X-ray diffraction is used in the study of the internal structure of cells. The x-rays are diffracted by cell parts into patterns that are indicative of chemical and physical structure. See also **refraction.**

diffuse, becoming widely spread, as through a membrane or fluid.

diffuse fibrosing alveolitis. See **interstitial pneumonia.**

diffuse goiter, an enlargement of all parts of the thyroid gland.

diffuse hypersensitivity pneumonia, an immunologically mediated inflammatory reaction in the lungs induced by exposure to an allergen derived from a fungus, bird excreta, piscine, porcine, or bovine proteins, wood dust, or fur, or by an adverse reaction to a drug, as chlorpropamide, hydrochlorothiazide, mecamylamine, mephenesin, methotrexate, nitrofurantoin, para-aminosalicylic acid, or penicillin. The disorder is characterized by cough, fever, dyspnea, malaise, pulmonary edema, and infiltration of the alveoli with eosinophils and large mononuclear cells. Also called **allergic alveolitis, allergic interstitial pneumonitis, extrinsic allergic pneumonia.** See also **bagassosis, P.I.E.**

diffuse lipoma, diffuse lipomatosis. See **multiple lipomatosis.**

diffusion, the process in which solid, particulate matter in a fluid moves from an area of higher concentration to an area of lower concentration, resulting in an even distribution of the particles in the fluid.

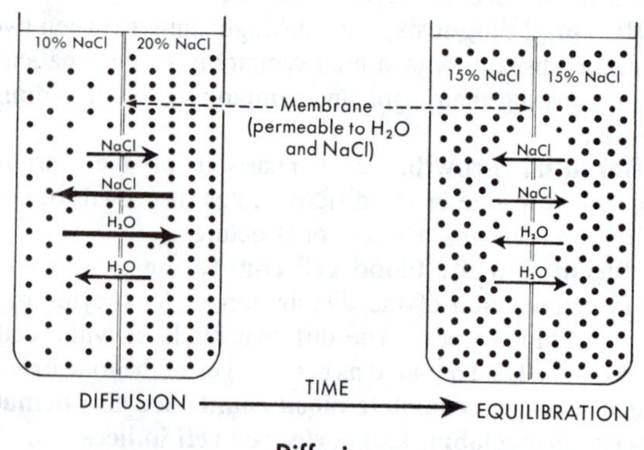

Diffusion

diffusion of gases, a natural process, essential in respiration, in which molecules of a gas pass from an area of high concentration to one of a lower concentration.

diflorasone diacetate, a topical corticosteroid.

■ INDICATION: It is prescribed topically as an antiinflammatory agent.

■ CONTRAINDICATIONS: Viral and fungal diseases of the skin, impaired circulation, or known hypersensitivity to this drug or to other steroidal medication prohibits its use.

■ ADVERSE EFFECTS: Among the more serious adverse reactions, usually occurring after prolonged or excessive application, are striae, hypopigmentation, local irritation of the skin, and various systemic effects.

diflunisal, a nonsteroidal antiinflammatory agent.

■ INDICATIONS: It is prescribed for mild to moderate pain and inflammation in osteoarthritis and other musculoskeletal disorders.

■ CONTRAINDICATIONS: Hypersensitivity to aspirin and other nonsteroidal antiinflammatory drugs or known sensitivity to this drug prohibits its use.

■ ADVERSE EFFECTS: The most serious adverse reactions are GI pain, diarrhea, peptic ulcer, anorexia, and edema.

digastricus /dīgas′trikəs/, one of four suprahyoid muscles having two parts, an anterior belly and a posterior belly. The anterior belly originates in the lower border of the mandible and inserts in the body and great cornu of the hyoid bone. It is innervated by fibers of the mandibular branch of the trigeminal nerve. It acts to open the jaw and to draw the hyoid bone forward. The posterior belly originates in the mastoid notch of the temporal bone and inserts in the body and great cornu of the hyoid bone. It is innervated by fibers of the mandibular branch of the facial nerve and acts to draw back and to raise the hyoid bone. Also called **digastric muscle.** Compare **geniohyoideus, mylohyoideus, stylohyoideus.**

DiGeorge's syndrome /dijôrj′əz/, a congenital disorder characterized by severe immunodeficiency and structural abnormalities, including hypertelorism, notched, low-set ears, small mouth, downward slanting eyes, cardiovascular defects, and the absence of the thymus and parathyroid glands. Death, often from infection, usually occurs before 2 years of age. Rarely, transplantation of a human fetal thymus is performed. Also called **thymic parathyroid aplasia.**

digest, **1.** to soften by heat and moisture. **2.** to break into smaller parts and simpler compounds by mastication, hydrolysis, and the action of intestinal secretions and enzymes, especially in the way the body digests food for the absorption of nutrients required in metabolism. The small intestine digests food by enzymatic actions that produce absorbable amino acids, emulsified fat particles, and monosaccharides. **3.** any material that results from digestion or hydrolysis.

digestion, the conversion of food into absorbable substances in the GI tract. Digestion is accomplished through the mechanic and chemical breakdown of food into smaller and smaller molecules, with the help of glands located both inside and outside the gut. **–digestive,** *adj.*

digestive fever, a slight rise in body temperature that normally accompanies the digestive process.

digestive gland, any one of the many structures that secretes reactive agents involved in the breaking down of food into the constituent absorbable substances needed for metabolism. Some kinds of digestive glands are the salivary glands, gastric glands, intestinal glands, liver, and pancreas. Some important secretions produced by different digestive glands are hydrochloric acid, bile, mucus, and various enzymes.

digestive system, the organs, structures, and accessory glands of the digestive tube of the body through which food passes from the mouth to the esophagus, stomach, and intestines. The accessory glands secrete the digestive enzymes, used by the digestive system to break down food substances in preparation for absorption into the bloodstream before carrying the waste to the intestines for excretion. See also **Color Atlas of Human Anatomy.**

digestive tract, a musculomembranous tube, about 9 m long, extending from the mouth to the anus and lined with mucous membrane. Its various portions are the mouth, pharynx, esophagus, stomach, small intestine, and large intestine. The tube, which is part of the digestive system of the body, includes numerous accessory organs. Also called **alimentary canal, digestive tube.** See also **digestive system.**

digit-, a combining form meaning 'pertaining to a finger or toe': *digitate, digitigrade, digitoplantar*.

digital, **1.** of or pertaining to a digit, that is, a finger or toe. **2.** resembling a finger or toe. See also **digitate. 3.** the characterization or measurement of a signal in terms of a series of numbers rather than in terms of some continuously varying value.

digital computer, a computer that processes information in numeric form. Compare **analog computer, hybrid computer.**

digitalis, a cardiotonic.

■ INDICATIONS: It is prescribed in the treatment of congestive heart failure and certain cardiac arrhythmias.

■ CONTRAINDICATIONS: Ventricular fibrillation, ventricular tachycardia, or known hypersensitivity to this drug prohibits its use.

■ ADVERSE EFFECTS: The most serious reactions are various cardiac arrhythmias.

digitalis glycoside. See **glycoside.**

digitalis therapy, the administration of a digitalis preparation to a person with a heart disorder to increase the force of myocardial contractions, produce a slower, more regular apical rate, and slow the transmission of impulses through the conduction system. Digitalis may be used in treating many cardiac disorders, including atrial fibrillation, atrial septal defect, coarctation of the aorta, congenital heart block, congestive heart failure, endocardial fibroelastosis, great vessel transposition, malformation of the tricuspid valve, myocarditis, paroxysmal atrial tachycardia, and patent ductus arteriosus.

■ METHOD: The completeness of the orders is ensured regarding the name of the digitalis preparation, the dosage in milligrams, the route and intervals of administration, and the pulse rate under which the drug is to be withheld. The dosage volume of the drug is carefully calculated by two people: two registered nurses, an RN and pharmacist, or an RN and physician. If the drug is to be given orally, the best method of ensuring that a child receives the full dose is determined: whether by spoon, nipple, or dropper. It is administered before feeding and is never mixed with the formula or food. Before each administration, the person's resting apical pulse is checked for rate and rhythm for a full minute; if the rate is slower than desired, if it is irregular or shows a rapid rise or fall, if there are any signs of toxicity, as anorexia, nausea, vomiting, or if there are visual disturbances, the drug is withheld and the problem is reported.

■ NURSING ORDERS: The nurse participates in calculating the dosage volume ordered, administers the drug, and observes for and reports any undesirable effects. Once the dosage is stabilized and before discharge, the nurse ensures that the patient understands the proper method, time, and purpose of administering the drug, as well as the need and the time to give the complete dose, when to withhold medication, and how to recognize and report signs of toxicity to the drug.

■ OUTCOME CRITERIA: In addition to promoting more forceful myocardial contractions and a slower, more regular apical beat, digitalis therapy can reduce venous pressure, improve pulmonary and systemic circulation, increase urinary output, reduce edema, and stop paroxysmal atrial tachycardia and atrial fibrillation.

digitalization, the administration of digitalis in doses sufficient to achieve maximum pharmacologic effects without also producing toxic symptoms.

digital radiography (DR), any method of x-ray image formation that uses a computer to store and manipulate data.

digital subtraction angiography (DSA), a method by which x-ray images of blood vessels filled with contrast material are digitized and then subtracted from images stored before the administration of contrast. Thus, the background is eliminated and only the vessels appear.

digital-to-analog converter, a device for converting digital information into analog form for representation as a continuous method of interpreting data, as from an ohmmeter or thermometer. Also called **D/A converter.**

digitate /dij′itāt/, having fingers or fingerlike projections. See also **digital.**

digitate wart, a fingerlike, horny projection that arises from a pea-shaped base and occurs on the scalp or near the hairline. Like other kinds of warts, it is a benign viral infection of the skin and the adjacent mucous membrane. It may disappear spontaneously as the host develops an immune response, or it may require treatment, as by electrodesiccation and curettage.

digitoxin, a cardiac glycoside obtained from leaves of *Digitalis purpurea*.

■ INDICATIONS: It is prescribed in the treatment of congestive heart failure and certain cardiac arrhythmias.

■ CONTRAINDICATIONS: Ventricular fibrillation, ventricular tachycardia, or known hypersensitivity to this drug prohibits its use.

■ ADVERSE EFFECTS: The most serious adverse reactions are cardiac arrhythmia and heart block.

digoxin /dijok′sin/, a cardiac glycoside obtained from leaves of *Digitalis lanata*.

■ INDICATIONS: It is prescribed in the treatment of congestive heart failure and certain cardiac arrhythmias.

■ CONTRAINDICATIONS: Ventricular fibrillation, ventricular tachycardia, or known hypersensitivity to this drug prohibits its use.

■ ADVERSE EFFECTS: The most serious adverse reactions are cardiac arrhythmia and heart block.

diGuglielmo's disease, diGuglielmo's syndrome. See **erythroleukemia.**

dihybrid /dī′hī′brid/, (in genetics) pertaining to or describing a person, organism, or strain that is heterozygous for two specific traits, that is the offspring of parents differing in two specific gene pairs, or that is heterozygous for two particular traits or gene loci under consideration.

dihybrid cross, (in genetics) the mating of two individuals, organisms, or strains that have different gene pairs that determine two specific traits or in which two particular characteristics or gene loci are being followed.

dihydric alcohol, an alcohol containing two hydroxyl groups.

dihydroergotamine mesylate, an alpha-adrenergic blocking agent.

■ INDICATIONS: It is prescribed for migraine and for vascular headache.

■ CONTRAINDICATIONS: Cardiovascular disease, hypertension, liver or kidney dysfunction, sepsis, pregnancy, or known hypersensitivity to this drug prohibits its use.

■ ADVERSE EFFECTS: Among the more serious adverse reactions are gangrene and the toxicity of the ergot alkaloids.

dihydrotachysterol /dīhī′drōtəkis′tərol/, a rapid-acting form of vitamin D.

■ INDICATIONS: It is prescribed in the treatment of hypocalcemia resulting from hypoparathyroidism and pseudohypoparathyroidism.

■ CONTRAINDICATIONS: Hypercalcemia, hypocalcemia with kidney insufficiency, hyperphosphatemia, or known hypersensitivity to this drug or to vitamin D prohibits its use. Caution is advised for lactating mothers.

■ ADVERSE EFFECTS: The most serious adverse reaction is hypercalcemia. With overdosage, calcification of soft tissues, including those of the heart, or cardiovascular or kidney failure may occur.

diiodohydroxyquin. See **iodoquinol.**

Dilantin, a trademark for an anticonvulsant (phenytoin).

dilatation /dil′ətā′shən/, **1.** normal physiologic increase in the diameter of a body opening, blood vessel, or tube, as the widening of the pupil of the eye in response to decreased light or the widening of the opening of the uterine cervix during labor. See also **effacement, station. 2.** artificial increase in the diameter of such an opening either by medication, as in the use of cycloplegic eyedrops to open the pupil wide for examination of the retina, or by instrumentation as in the use of a dilator to open the uterine cervix to facilitate curettage. **3.** the diameter of the opening of the cervix in labor as measured on vaginal examination, expressed in centimeters or finger breadths, one finger breadth being approximately 2 cm. At full dilatation the diameter of the cervical opening is 10 cm. Also called **dilation** /dīlā′shən/. **–dilatate, dilate** /dī′lāt/, *v.*, **dilatator, dilator,** *n.*

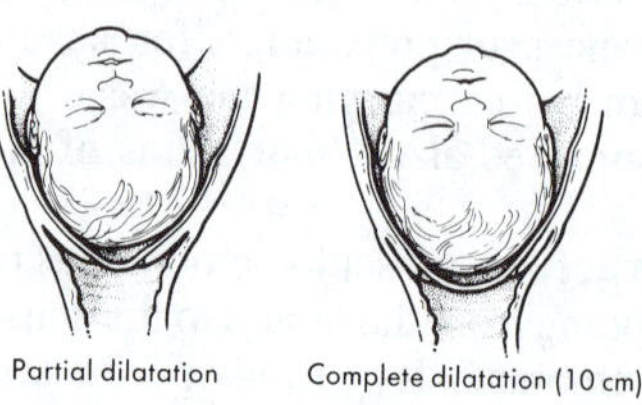

Cervical dilatation

dilatation and curettage (D & C), dilatation of the uterine cervix and scraping of the endometrium of the uterus, performed to diagnose disease of the uterus, to correct heavy or prolonged vaginal bleeding, or to empty uterine contents of the products of conception. It is also done to remove tumors, to rule out carcinoma of the uterus, to remove retained placental fragments postpartum or after an incomplete abortion, and to find the cause of infertility. Under a light, general anesthesia the cervix is dilated with a series of dilators of increasing size to allow the insertion of a curet into the uterus. Vaginal packing may sometimes be inserted to slow bleeding but is not usually recommended. It may be left in place for 24 hours. A sterile perineal pad is applied. Postoperative care requires emotional support appropriate to the clinical situation and close observation for hemorrhage, infection, or dysuria. See also **abortion.**

dilatator naris, the alar portion of the nasalis muscle that dilates the nostril. Compare **compressor naris.**

dilatator pupillae, a muscle that contracts the iris of the eye and dilates the pupil. It is composed of radiating fibers that converge from the circumference of the iris toward the center and blend with fibers of the sphincter pupillae near the margin of the pupil. The dilatator pupillae is innervated by nerve fibers from the sympathetic system. Compare **sphincter pupillae.**

dilate, dilator. See **dilatation.**

Dilaudid Hydrochloride, a trademark for a narcotic analgesic (hydromorphone hydrochloride).

Dilor, a trademark for a bronchodilator (dyphylline).

diltiazem, a slow channel blocker or calcium antagonist.

■ INDICATIONS: It is prescribed for the treatment of vasospastic and effort-associated angina.

■ CONTRAINDICATIONS: Sick sinus syndrome, second- or third-degree atrioventricular block, or hypotension prohibits its use.

■ ADVERSE EFFECTS: Among the more serious adverse reactions are edema, arrhythmia, bradycardia, hypotension, syncope, rash, headache, and dizziness.

dimenhydrinate /dim′ənhī′drināt/, an antihistamine. ▪ INDICATIONS: It is prescribed in the treatment of nausea and motion sickness. ▪ CONTRAINDICATIONS: Asthma or known hypersensitivity to this drug prohibits its use. It is not given to newborn infants or lactating mothers. ▪ ADVERSE EFFECTS: Among the more serious adverse reactions are skin rash, hypersensitivity reactions, and tachycardia. Drowsiness and dry mouth are common.

dimer /dī′mər/, a compound formed by the union of two radicals or two molecules of a simpler compound, as a polymer formed from two or more molecules of a monomer.

dimercaprol /dī′mərkap′rol/, a heavy-metal antagonist. Previously called **British antilewisite (BAL).** ▪ INDICATIONS: It is prescribed in the treatment of Wilson's disease and in the treatment of acute arsenic, mercury, or gold poisoning, as from an overdosage with mercurial diuretics, arsenics, or gold salts or from an accidental ingestion of mercury, gold, or arsenic. ▪ CONTRAINDICATIONS: Hepatic or renal insufficiency, poisoning with cadmium, iron, or selenium, or known hypersensitivity to the drug prohibits its use. ▪ ADVERSE EFFECTS: Among the most serious adverse reactions are nephrotoxicity, acidosis, convulsions, and abnormal cardiovascular functions. Mild reactions include pain at the injection site, nausea, excessive salivation, and parasthesia.

Dimetane, a trademark for an antihistamine (brompheniramine maleate).

Dimetapp, a trademark for a fixed-combination drug containing two decongestants (phenylephrine hydrochloride and phenylpropanolamine hydrochloride) and an antihistamine (brompheniramine maleate).

dimethindene maleate /dīmeth′indēn/, an antihistamine. ▪ INDICATIONS: It is prescribed in the treatment of a variety of hypersensitivity reactions, including rhinitis, skin reactions, and itching. ▪ CONTRAINDICATIONS: The drug is not given to newborn infants or to lactating mothers. Asthma or known hypersensitivity to this drug prohibits its use. ▪ ADVERSE EFFECTS: Drowsiness, skin rash, hypersensitivity reactions, dry mouth, and tachycardia commonly occur.

dimethoxymethylamphetamine (DOM), a psychedelic agent.

dimethyl carbinol. See **isopropyl alcohol.**

dimethyl sulfoxide (DMSO), an antiinflammatory agent. ▪ INDICATIONS: It is prescribed in the treatment of interstitial cystitis and is being investigated as a topical antiinflammatory agent in orthopedic sports injuries. ▪ CONTRAINDICATION: Known hypersensitivity to this drug prohibits its use. ▪ ADVERSE EFFECTS: Among the most serious adverse reactions are GI disturbances, photophobia, disturbance of color vision, and headache. A garliclike body odor and taste in the mouth may occur. When applied to the skin, it can cause local irritations.

dimethyl tubocurarine iodide. See **metocurine iodide.**

Dimitri's disease. See **Sturge-Weber syndrome.**

dinoprost /dī′nəprōst/, a prostaglandin abortifacient. ▪ INDICATION: It is prescribed to terminate a pregnancy during the second trimester. ▪ CONTRAINDICATIONS: Acute pelvic inflammatory disease or known hypersensitivity to this drug prohibits its use. ▪ ADVERSE EFFECTS: Among the more serious adverse reactions are cardiac arrhythmias, vomiting, and bronchospasm.

dinoprostone /dī′nōpros′tōn/, a naturally occurring form of prostaglandin E_2 (PGE_2) administered in a vaginal suppository as an oxytocic agent. ▪ INDICATIONS: It is prescribed to cause termination of pregnancy from 12 to 20 weeks of gestation, to evacuate the uterus after fetal death up to 28 weeks of gestation, in missed abortion, and in nonmetastatic gestational trophoblastic disease. ▪ CONTRAINDICATIONS: Acute inflammatory disease, concurrent administration of oxytocin, or known hypersensitivity to this drug prohibits its use. It is used with caution in patients who have cardiac, pulmonary, hepatic, or renal disease, asthma, diabetes, or epilepsy or in patients who have had uterine surgery. ▪ ADVERSE EFFECTS: Among the more serious reactions are wheezing, dyspnea, fever, vomiting, and diarrhea. Trauma to the cervix and to the lower uterine segment has occurred after administration of the drug because of forceful expulsion of the uterine contents before full dilatation of the cervix.

dioctyl calcium sulfosuccinate, dioctyl sodium sulfosuccinate. See **docusate.**

dioecious. See **diecious.**

Dionysian, the personal attitude of one who is uninhibited, mystic, sensual, emotional, and irrational and who may seek to escape from the boundaries imposed by the limits of one's senses.

Diothane, a trademark for a local anesthetic (diperodon monohydrate).

diovular. See **binovular.**

diovulatory, routinely releasing two ova during each ovarian cycle. Compare **monovulatory.**

dioxin /dī·ok′sin/, a contaminant of the herbicide 2,4,5-trichlorophenoxyacetic acid (2,4,5-T), widely used throughout the world in forestry, on grassland, against woody shrubs and trees on industrial sites, and for rice and sugar-cane weed control. Because of its toxicity, it is no longer manufactured in the United States. Exposure to dioxin is associated with chloracne and porphyria cutanea tarda (PCT). Dioxin was a contaminant of the jungle defoliant Agent Orange sprayed by the United States military aircraft over areas of southeast Asia from 1965 to 1970. Also called **TCDD (2,3,7,8-tetrachlorodibenzo-para-dioxin).**

dioxybenzone, an ultraviolet screen.

■ INDICATION: It is prescribed to prevent burning from exposure to the sun.

■ CONTRAINDICATIONS: Known hypersensitivity to this drug prohibits its use. It should not come into contact with the eyes.

■ ADVERSE EFFECTS: The only known adverse reaction is skin rash.

dioxyline phosphate, a synthetic antispasmodic and vasodilator. Also called **dimoxyline phosphate.**

■ INDICATIONS: It is prescribed for the relief of angina pectoris and for spasm of blood vessels in arms, legs, or lungs.

■ CONTRAINDICATION: Known hypersensitivity to this drug prohibits its use.

■ ADVERSE EFFECTS: Among the most serious adverse reactions are nausea, dizziness, and flushing, which occur rarely.

Dipaxin, a trademark for an anticoagulant (diphenadione).

diphemanil methylsulfate /dīfē′mənil/, an anticholinergic.

■ INDICATION: It is prescribed as an adjunct to ulcer therapy.

■ CONTRAINDICATIONS: Narrow-angle glaucoma, asthma, obstruction of the genitourinary or GI tract, ulcerative colitis, or known hypersensitivity to this drug prohibits its use.

■ ADVERSE EFFECTS: Among the more serious adverse reactions are blurred vision, central nervous system effects, tachycardia, dry mouth, decreased sweating, and hypersensitivity reactions.

diphenadione /dī′fənad′ē·ōn/, an anticoagulant.

■ INDICATIONS: It is prescribed in the treatment of thrombosis and embolism.

■ CONTRAINDICATIONS: Hemorrhage or known hypersensitivity to this drug prohibits its use.

■ ADVERSE EFFECTS: The most serious adverse reaction is hemorrhage. This drug interacts with many other drugs.

diphenhydramine hydrochloride, an antihistamine.

■ INDICATIONS: It is prescribed in the treatment of a variety of hypersensitivity reactions, including rhinitis, skin rash, and pruritus, and in the treatment of motion sickness.

■ CONTRAINDICATIONS: Asthma or known hypersensitivity to this drug prohibits its use. It is not given to newborn infants or lactating mothers.

■ ADVERSE EFFECTS: Among the more serious adverse reactions are skin rash, hypersensitivity reactions, and tachycardia. Drowsiness and dry mouth commonly occur.

diphenidol, an antiemetic, antivertigo agent.

■ INDICATIONS: It is prescribed in the treatment of vertigo and to control nausea and vomiting.

■ CONTRAINDICATIONS: Anuria or known sensitivity to this drug prohibits its use.

■ ADVERSE EFFECTS: Among the most serious adverse reactions are transient hypotension, hallucinations, disorientation, and mental confusion.

diphenoxylate hydrochloride, an antidiarrheal.

■ INDICATIONS: It is prescribed in the treatment of diarrhea and intestinal cramping.

■ CONTRAINDICATIONS: Liver disease, antibiotic-associated diarrhea, or known hypersensitivity to this drug prohibits its use. It is not given to children under 2 years of age.

■ ADVERSE EFFECTS: Among the more serious adverse reactions are abdominal discomfort, intestinal obstruction, skin rash, and nausea.

diphenylhydantoin. See **phenytoin.**

diphenylpyraline hydrochloride /dī′fenəlpī′rəlēn/, an antihistamine.

■ INDICATIONS: It is prescribed in the treatment of a variety of hypersensitivity reactions, including rhinitis, skin rash, and pruritus.

■ CONTRAINDICATIONS: Asthma or known hypersensitivity to this drug prohibits its use. It is not given to newborn infants or lactating mothers.

■ ADVERSE EFFECTS: Among the more serious adverse reactions are skin rash, hypersensitivity reactions, and tachycardia. Drowsiness and dry mouth commonly occur.

diphtheria /difthir′ē·ə, dipthir′ē·ə/, an acute, contagious disease caused by the bacterium *Corynebacterium diphtheriae,* characterized by the production of a systemic toxin and a false membrane lining of the mucous membrane of the throat. The toxin is particularly damaging to the tissues of the heart and central nervous system, and the dense pseudomembrane in the throat may interfere with eating, drinking, and breathing. The membrane may occur in other body tissues. Lymph glands in the neck swell, and the neck becomes edematous. Untreated, the disease is often fatal, causing heart and kidney failure. Patients are usually hospitalized in isolation rooms. Treatment of the isolated patient may include administration of diphtheria antitoxin, antibiotics, bed rest, fluids, and an adequate diet. Tracheostomy is sometimes necessary. Recovery is slow, but it is usually complete. Immunization against diphtheria is available to all children in the United States and is usually given in conjunction with pertussis and tetanus immunization early in infancy. See also **Schick test.**

diphtheria and tetanus toxoids (DT), an active immunizing agent.

■ INDICATIONS: It is prescribed for immunization against diphtheria and tetanus.

■ CONTRAINDICATIONS: Immunosuppression, acute infection, or concomitant use of corticosteroids prohibits its use.

■ ADVERSE EFFECTS: The most serious adverse reaction is anaphylaxis.

diphtheria and tetanus toxoids and pertussis vaccine (DTP), an active immunizing agent.

■ INDICATIONS: It is prescribed for the routine immunization of children under 6 years of age against diphtheria, tetanus, and pertussis.

■ CONTRAINDICATIONS: Immunosuppressive therapy, active infection, or neurologic disorders prohibit its use.

■ ADVERSE EFFECT: The most serious adverse reaction is anaphylaxis.

diphtheroid /dif′thəroid′/, **1.** of or pertaining to diphtheria. **2.** resembling the bacillus *Corynebacterium diphtheriae*.

Diphyllobothrium /dəfil′ōboth′rē·əm/, a genus of large, parasitic, intestinal flatworms having a scolex with two slitlike grooves. The species that most often infects humans is *Diphyllobothrium latum,* a giant freshwater fish tapeworm of North America and Europe. See also **tapeworm infection.**

dipivefrin, an ophthalmic adrenergic.

■ INDICATION: It is prescribed in the treatment of open-angle glaucoma.

■ CONTRAINDICATIONS: Narrow-angle glaucoma or known hypersensitivity to this drug prohibits its use.

■ ADVERSE EFFECTS: Among the most serious adverse effects are reactive hyperemia, conjunctivitis, allergic reactions, and macular edema. Systemic reactions, as tachycardia, are possible.

diplegia /dīplē′jē·ə/, bilateral paralysis of both sides of any part of the body or of like parts on the opposite sides of the body. A kind of diplegia is **facial diplegia.** Compare **hemiplegia.** **–diplegic,** *adj.*

diplo-, a combining form meaning 'double': *diplobacilli, diplococcus, diplokaryon.*

diplococcus /dip′lōkok′əs/, *pl.* **diplococci** /-kok′sī/, a coccus that occurs in pairs.

diploë /dip′lō·ē/, the loose tissue filled with red bone marrow between the two tables of the cranial bones.

diploid /dip′loid/, of or pertaining to an individual, organism, strain, or cell that has two complete sets of homologous chromosomes, such as is normally found in the somatic cells and the primordial germ cells before maturation. In humans the normal diploid number is 46. Compare **haploid, tetraploid, triploid.** **–diploidic,** *adj.*

diploidy /dip′loidē/, the state or condition of having two complete sets of homologous chromosomes.

diplokaryon /dip′lōker′ē·on/, a nucleus that contains twice the diploid number of chromosomes.

diploma program in nursing, an educational program that trains nurses in a hospital setting, usually in 2 or 3 years. The recipient of a diploma is eligible to take the national certifying examination to become a registered nurse. In Canada, diploma programs are generally conducted in junior or community colleges, as well as in some hospital schools in the Atlantic provinces.

diplomate /dip′ləmāt/, an individual who has earned a diploma or certificate, especially a physician who has been certified by a specialty board. See also **board certified.**

diplonema /dip′lənē′mə/, the looplike formation of the chromosomes in the diplotene stage of the first meiotic prophase of gametogenesis.

diplopagus /diplop′əgəs/, conjoined twins that are more or less equally developed, although one or several internal organs may be shared.

diplopia /diplō′pē·ə/, double vision caused by defective function of the extraocular muscles or a disorder of the nerves that innervate the muscles. A transient episode of diplopia is usually of no clinical significance, indicating only a brief relaxation of the fusion mechanism of the central nervous system that maintains ocular straightness. Also called **ambiopia.** Compare **binocular vision.**

-diplopia, a combining form meaning '(condition of) double vision': *amphodiplopia, amphoterodiplopia, monodiplopia.*

diplosomatia /dip′lōsōmā′shə/, a congenital anomaly in which fully formed twins are joined at one or more areas of their bodies. Also called **diplosomia.**

diplotene /dip′lətēn/, the fourth stage in the first meiotic prophase in gametogenesis in which the tetrads exhibit chiasmata between the chromatids of the paired homologous chromosomes and genetic crossing-over occurs. The chromosomes then begin to repel each other and separate longitudinally, forming loops. See also **diakinesis, leptotene, pachytene, zygotene.**

dipodia /dīpō′dē·ə/, a developmental anomaly characterized by the duplication of one or both feet.

diprosopus /dīpros′əpəs, dī′prəsō′pəs/, a malformed fetus that has a double face showing varying degrees of development.

-dipsia, -dipsy, a combining form meaning '(condition of) thirst': *hydroadipsia, oligodipsia, polydipsia.*

dipsomania, an uncontrollable, often periodic craving for and indulgence in alcoholic beverages; alcoholism.

-dipsy. See **-dipsia.**

dipus /dī′pəs/, conjoined twins that have only two feet.

dipygus /dīpī′gəs, dip′əgəs/, a malformed fetus that has a double pelvis, one of which is usually not fully developed.

dipyridamole, a coronary vasodilator.

■ INDICATION: It is prescribed for the long-term treatment of angina.

■ CONTRAINDICATIONS: The drug should be used with caution in hypotension and anticoagulant therapy.

■ ADVERSE EFFECTS: The adverse reactions are mild and transient, as headache, dizziness, rash, nausea, and flushing.

dipyrone /dī′pīrōn/, an analgesic, antipyretic, and antiinflammatory that was formerly used for pain and fever. Its use has been discontinued, except in rare cases of intractable fever, because the drug may cause fatal agranulocytosis.

direct antagonist, one of a pair or a group of muscles that pull in opposite directions and whose combined action keeps the part from moving.

direct calorimetry, the measurement of the amount of heat directly generated by any oxidation reaction, especially one involving a living organism. Compare **indirect calorimetry.**

direct causal association, a cause-and-effect relationship between a causative factor and a disease with no other factors intervening in the process.

direct contact, mutual touching of two individuals or organisms. Many communicable diseases may be spread by the direct contact between an infected and a healthy person. Some kinds of diseases that may be spread by direct contact are gonorrhea, impetigo, staphylococcal skin infections, and syphilis. Other infections are transmitted by insect or animal vectors, droplets, or contaminated food.

direct current, an electric current that flows in one direction only and is substantially constant in value. Compare **alternating current.**

direct fracture, any fracture occurring at a specific point of injury that is a direct result of that injury.

direct generation. See **asexual generation.**

direct gold, any form of pure gold that may be compacted directly into a prepared tooth cavity to form a restoration.

direct illumination. See **illumination.**

directive therapy, a psychotherapeutic approach in which the psychotherapist directs the course of therapy by intervening to ask questions and offer interpretations. Compare **nondirective therapy.** See also **psychoanalysis.**

direct lead, **1.** an electrocardiographic conductor in which the exploring electrode is placed directly on the surface of the exposed heart. **2.** *informal.* a tracing produced by such a lead on an electrocardiograph.

direct patient care, (in nursing) care of a patient provided in person by a member of the staff. Direct patient care may involve any aspects of the health care of a patient, including treatments, counseling, self-care, patient education, and administration of medication.

direct percussion. See **percussion.**

direct provider reimbursement, a method of direct payment for health care services, as fee-for-service.

direct reaction to light, the constriction of a pupil receiving increased illumination, as by a flashlight during an ophthalmologic examination. Compare **consensual reaction to light.**

direct relationship. See **positive relationship.**

direct retainer, a clasp, attachment, or assembly fastened to an abutment tooth for the purpose of maintaining a removable restoration in its planned position in relation to oral structures.

dis-, **1.** a combining form meaning 'reversal or separation': *disacidify, dischronation, disinfect.* **2.** a combining form meaning 'duplication': *disdiaclast, dissogeny, districhiasis.*

disability, the loss, absence, or impairment of physical or mental fitness that is observable and measurable. Compare **handicap.**

disadvantaged, **1.** any group of people who lack money, education, literacy, or another status advantage. **2.** a euphemism for "poor."

disaster-preparedness plan, a formal plan of action, usually prepared in written form, for coordinating the response of a hospital staff in the event of a disaster within the hospital or the surrounding community.

disc. See **disk.**

discharge, **1.** also **evacuate, excrete, secrete.** to release a substance or object. **2.** to release a patient from a hospital. **3.** to release an electric charge, which may be manifested by a spark or surge of electricity, from a storage battery, condenser, or other source. **4.** to release a burst of energy from or through a neuron. **5.** a release of emotions, often accompanied by a wide range of voluntary and involuntary reflexes, weeping, rage, or other emotional displays, called **affective discharge** in psychology. **6.** also called **evacuate, excretion, secretion.** a substance or object discharged.

discharge abstract, items of information compiled from medical records of patients discharged from a hospital, organized and recorded in a uniform format to provide data for statistic studies, reports, or research.

discharge coordinator, an individual who arranges with community agencies and institutions for the continuing care of patients after their discharge from a hospital.

discharge planning, a schedule of events often planned by a multidisciplinary team leading to the return of a patient from hospital confinement to a normal life at home.

discharge summary, a clinical report prepared by a physician or other health professional at the conclusion of a hospital stay or series of treatments, outlining the patient's chief complaint, the diagnostic findings, the therapy administered and the patient's response to it, and recommendations on discharge.

disciform keratitis, an inflammatory condition of the eye that often follows an attack of dendritic keratitis and is believed to be an immunologic response to an ocular herpes simplex infection. The condition is characterized by disclike opacities in the cornea, usually with inflammation of the iris. See also **herpesvirus simplex.**

disclosing solution, a topically applied dye, used in aqueous solution to stain and reveal plaque and other deposits on teeth.

disco-, a combining form meaning 'pertaining to a disk, disk-shaped': *discophorous, discopathy, discoplacenta.*

discoblastula, a blastula formed from the partial cleavage that occurs in a fertilized ovum containing a large amount of yolk. It develops from the blastodisc and consists of a cellular cap, or blastoderm, separated from the uncleaved yolk mass by a small cavity, the blastocele.

discocyte /dis′kəsīt/, a mature, normal, erythrocyte, exhibiting one of its many steady-state configurations. It is a biconcave disk without a nucleus.

discoid lupus erythematosus (DLE), a chronic, recurrent disease, primarily of the skin, characterized by red macules that are covered with scales and extend into follicles. The lesions are typically distributed in a butterfly pattern covering the cheeks and bridge of the nose but may also occur on other parts of the body. On healing, the lesions atrophy and leave hyperpigmented or hypopigmented scars, and, if hairy areas are involved, alopecia may result. The cause of the disease is not established, but there is evidence that it may be an autoimmune disorder, and some cases seem to be induced by certain drugs. It is at least five times more common in women than in men and occurs most frequently in the third and fourth decades of life. Treatment includes the use of a sunscreen lotion or ointment when exposure to sunlight cannot be avoided, the application of steroids to the lesions, and systemic antimalarial drugs, as hydroxychloroquine; systemic corticosteroid agents may be used in severe cases. Also called **cutaneous lupus erythematosus.** See also **systemic lupus erythematosus.**

discoid meniscus, an abnormal condition characterized by a discoid rather than semilunar shape of the cartilaginous meniscus of the knee. The lateral meniscus is most often affected, although the medial meniscus may also become involved. The condition is a developmental anomaly, asymptomatic in the infant or in the young child, and occurs most frequently in children between 6 and 8 years of age. Common complaints are that a "clicking" occurs in the knee joint or that the knee joint gives way. These characteristics are often associated with an injury to the knee but occur also without any history of trauma. Examination demonstrates the "clicking," usually when the knee is moved from flexion to extension, during the last 15 to 20 degrees. Surgical excision of the meniscus is seldom warranted in treating this benign condition.

discordance, (in genetics) the expression of one or more specific traits in only one member of a pair of twins. Compare **concordance.** **–discordant,** *adj.*

discovery, (in law) a pretrial procedure allowing one party to examine vital witnesses and documents held exclusively by the adverse party. Discovery is limited to materials, facts, and other resources that could not otherwise be reasonably expected to be discovered and that are necessary to the preparation of the case for trial. Also called **pretrial discovery.** Compare **deposition, interrogatories.**

discus. See **disk.**

discus interpubicus. See **interpubic disk.**

discus nervi optici. See **optic disc.**

disease, **1.** a condition of abnormal vital function involving any structure, part, or system of an organism. **2.** a specific illness or disorder characterized by a recognizable set of signs and symptoms, attributable to heredity, infection, diet, or environment. Compare **condition, diathesis.**

disease prevention, activities designed to protect patients or other members of the public from actual or potential health threats and their harmful consequences.

disengagement, **1.** an obstetrical manipulation in which the presenting part of the baby is dislodged from the maternal pelvis as part of an operative delivery. See also **Kielland rotation, version and extraction.** **2.** the release or detachment of oneself from other persons or responsibilities.

disengagement theory, a concept that as individuals grow older they tend to withdraw from society.

dishpan fracture, a fracture that depresses the skull. Also called **derby hat fracture.**

disinfectant, a chemical that can be applied to objects to destroy microorganisms.

disinfection, the process of killing pathogenic organisms or of rendering them inert.

disjunction, (in genetics) the separation of the paired homologous chromosomes during the anaphase stage of the first meiotic division or of the chromatids of a chromosome during anaphase of mitosis and the second meiotic division. Compare **nondisjunction.**

disk, **1.** also spelled (chiefly in ophthalmology) **disc.** a flat, circular platelike structure, as an articular disk or an optic disc. **2.** *informal.* an intervertebral disk. Also called *(Latin)* **discus.**

disk drive, a computer device containing a disk that spins at high speeds, equipped with a head that allows electric impulses to be written onto and read from the electromagnetic surface.

diskette, a flexible plastic, oxide-coated disk, contained in a special square jacket, for use in a computer disk drive. Also called **floppy disk, flexible disk, floppy.**

dislocation, the displacement of any part of the body from its normal position, particularly a bone from its normal articulation with a joint. See also **subluxation.** **–dislocate,** *v.*

dismiss, (in law) to discharge or dispose of an action, suit, or motion trial. **–dismissal,** *n.*

disodium edetate. See **edetate disodium.**

Disophrol, a trademark for a respiratory, fixed-combination drug containing an antihistamine (dexbrompheniramine maleate) and an adrenergic bronchodilator (pseudoephedrine sulfate).

disopyramide phosphate /dī′sōpir′əmīd/, a cardiac depressant.

▪ INDICATIONS: It is prescribed in the treatment of premature ventricular contractions and ventricular tachycardia.

▪ CONTRAINDICATIONS: Heart failure, preexisting second- or third-degree heart block in the absence of a pacemaker, sick sinus syndrome, or known hypersensitivity to this drug prohibits its use.

▪ ADVERSE EFFECTS: Among the more serious adverse reactions are severe hypotension, precipitation of heart failure, and aggravation of heart block. Urinary retention, dry mouth, and constipation commonly occur.

disorganized schizophrenia, a form of schizophrenia characterized by an earlier age of onset, usually at puberty, and a more severe disintegration of the personality than occurs in other forms of the disease. Symptoms include inappropriate laughter and silliness; peculiar mannerisms, like grimaces; talking and gesturing to oneself; regressive, bizarre, and often obscene behavior; extreme social withdrawal; and fantastic and unsystematized hallucinations and delusions, which are usually of a sexual, religious, persecutory, or hypochondriacal nature. Also called **hebephrenia, hebephrenic schizophrenia.** See also **schizophrenia.**

disorient, to cause to lose awareness or perception of space, time, or personal identity and relationships.

disorientation, a state of mental confusion characterized by inadequate or incorrect perceptions of place, time, or identity. Disorientation may occur in organic mental disorders, in drug and alcohol intoxication, and, less commonly, after severe stress.

dispersing agent, a chemical additive used in pharmaceutics to cause the even distribution of the ingredients throughout the product, as in dermatologic emulsions containing both oil and water. Dispersing agents commonly used in skin creams, lotions, and ointments include glyceryl monostearate, sodium lauryl sulfate, and polyethylene glycol derivatives, as polysorbate 80 and polyoxyl 40 stearate. A dispersing agent may cause an allergic reaction or adverse effect in a hypersensitive person.

dispersion medium. See **medium.**

displaced fracture, a traumatic bone break in which two ends of a fractured bone are separated from each other. The ends of broken bones in displaced fractures often pierce surrounding skin, as in an open fracture, or may be contained within the skin, as in a closed fracture.

displacement, **1.** the state of being displaced or the act of displacing. **2.** (in chemistry) a reaction in which an atom, molecule, or radical is removed from combination and replaced by another. **3.** (in physics) the displacing in space of one mass by another, as the weight or volume of a fluid being displaced by a floating or submerged body. **4.** (in psychiatry) an unconscious defense mechanism for avoiding emotional conflict and anxiety by transferring emotions, ideas, or wishes from one object to a substitute that is less anxiety-producing. Compare **sublimation.** See also **percolation.**

dissect, to cut apart tissues for visual or microscopic study using a scalpel, a probe, or scissors. Compare **bisect.** **–dissection,** *n.*

dissecting aneurysm, a localized dilatation of an artery, most commonly the aorta, characterized by a longitudinal dissection between the outer and middle layers of the vascular wall. Aortic dissecting aneurysms occur most frequently in men between the ages of 40 and 60 and are, in more than 90% of cases, preceded by hypertension. Blood entering a tear in the intimal lining of the vessel causes a separation of weakened elastic and fibromuscular elements in the medial layer and leads to the formation of cystic spaces filled with ground substance. Dissecting aneurysms in the thoracic aorta may extend into blood vessels of the neck. Rupture of a dissecting aneurysm may be fatal in less than 1 hour. Treatment consists of resection and replacement of the excised section of aorta with a synthetic prosthesis. See also **aortic aneurysm.**

disseminated intravascular coagulation (DIC), a grave coagulopathy resulting from the overstimulation of the body's clotting and anticlotting processes in response to disease or injury, as septicemia, acute hypotension, poisonous snake bites, neoplasms, obstetric emergencies, severe trauma, or extensive surgery and hemorrhage. The primary disorder initiates generalized intravascular clotting which, in turn, overstimulates fibrinolytic mechanisms; as a result the initial hypercoagulability is succeeded by a deficiency in clotting factors with hypocoagulability and hemorrhaging.

■ OBSERVATIONS: Widespread purpura on the chest and abdomen, reflecting fibrin deposits in capillaries, is a common first sign of DIC and is often followed by the appearance of hemorrhagic bullae, acral cyanosis, and focal gangrene in the skin and mucous membranes. There may be hemorrhages from incisions, catheter or injection sites, GI bleeding, hematuria, pulmonary edema, pulmonary embolism, progressive hypotension, tachycardia, an absence of peripheral pulses, restlessness, convulsions, or coma. Laboratory studies show generally a marked deficiency of blood platelets, low levels of fibrinogen and other clotting factors, prolonged prothrombin and partial thromboplastin times, and abnormal erythrocyte morphology.

■ INTERVENTION: Treatment of the primary disorder is essential in the management of DIC. Heparin may be infused intravenously to prevent clot formation, but, because it may increase bleeding, it is not always used for surgical patients with DIC. Transfusions of whole blood, plasma, platelets, and other blood products are administered to replace depleted factors. Patients are maintained in a quiet, nonstressful environment and are protected from trauma and bleeding. The side rails of the bed are padded, foam or cotton swabs are used for mouth care, and, whenever possible, the use of tape or any invasive procedure that might cause bleeding is avoided.

■ NURSING CONSIDERATIONS: The care of a patient with life-threatening DIC is a challenge requiring monitoring of vital signs, observation for evidence of bleeding, extremely gentle handling, and the giving of considerable emotional support.

disseminated lupus erythematosus. See **systemic lupus erythematosus.**

disseminated multiple sclerosis. See **multiple sclerosis.**

dissent, (in law) a statement written by a judge who disagrees with the decision of the majority of the court. The dissent explicitly states the reasons for the dissenting judge's contrary opinion. **–dissenting,** *adj.*

dissimilar twins. See **dizygotic twins.**

dissociation, **1.** the act of separating into parts or sections. **2.** an unconscious defense mechanism by which an idea, thought, emotion, or other mental process is separated from the consciousness and thereby loses emotional significance. See also **dissociative disorder, dissociative reaction.** –**dissociative** /disō′shē•ətiv/, *adj.*

dissociative anesthesia, an anesthetic procedure characterized by analgesia and amnesia without loss of respiratory function or pharyngeal and laryngeal reflexes. This form of anesthesia may be used to provide analgesia during brief, superficial operative procedures or diagnostic processes. It is especially useful for people who are sensitive to general or local anesthetics or for those who, for other reasons, may not be safely anesthetized with inhalant gases. Because the most commonly used drug is a hallucinogenic (ketamine hydrochloride), emergence may be accompanied by delirium, excitement, and confusion.

dissociative disorder, a type of hysteric neurosis in which emotional conflicts are so repressed that a separation or split in the personality occurs, resulting in an altered state of consciousness or a confusion in identity. Symptoms include amnesia, somnambulism, fugue, dream state, or multiple personality. The disorder is caused by an inability to cope with severe stress or conflict and usually occurs suddenly, after a situation catastrophic to the person. Treatment may include hypnosis, especially when amnesia is the primary symptom, psychotherapy, and antianxiety medication. Also called **dissociative reaction.** Compare **conversion disorder.** See also **dissociation.**

distal /dis′təl/, **1.** away from or being the farthest from a point of origin. **2.** away from or being the farthest from the midline or a central point, as a distal phalanx. Compare **proximal.**

distal muscular dystrophy, a rare form of muscular dystrophy, usually affecting adults, characterized by moderate weakness and by wasting that begins in the arms and legs and then extends gradually to the proximal and facial muscles. Also called **Gowers' muscular dystrophy.**

distal phalanx, any one of the small distal bones in the third row of phalanges of the hand or the foot. Each one at the end of the finger has a convex dorsal surface and a flat palmar surface, with a rough elevation at the end of the palmar surface that supports a fingernail and its sensitive pulp. Each distal phalanx of the toes is smaller and more flattened than that of a finger; it also has a rough elevation to support the toenail and its pulp. Also called **ungual phalanx.**

distal radioulnar articulation, the pivotlike articulation of the head of the ulna and the ulnar notch on the lower end of the radius, involving two ligaments. The joint allows rotation of the distal end of the radius around an axis that passes through the center of the head of the ulna. Also called **inferior radioulnar joint.** Compare **proximal radioulnar articulation.**

distal renal tubular acidosis (distal RTA), an abnormal condition characterized by excessive acid accumulation and bicarbonate excretion. It is caused by the inability of the distal tubules of the kidney to secrete hydrogen ions, thus decreasing the excretion of titratable acids and ammonium and increasing the urinary loss of potassium and bicarbonate. This condition may result in hypercalciuria and the formation of kidney stones. Treatment is as for renal tubular acidosis. **Primary distal RTA** occurs mostly in females, adolescents, older children, and young adults. It may occur sporadically or as the result of hereditary defects. **Secondary distal RTA** is associated with numerous disorders, as cirrhosis of the liver, malnutrition, starvation, and various genetic problems. Compare **proximal renal tubular acidosis.**

distance regulation, behavior that is related to the control of personal space. Most humans establish a quantum of space between themselves and others that offers security from either psychologic or physical threat while not creating a feeling of isolation. The amount of social distance thus maintained varies with different individuals and in different cultures. A wild animal generally maintains a flight distance, the minimum it will allow between itself and a potential enemy before fleeing. Animals of the same species also maintain a personal distance from each other.

distension, the state of being distended or swollen.

distraction techniques, procedures that prevent or lessen the perception of pain by focusing attention on sensations unrelated to pain.

distress of the human spirit. See **spiritual distress.**

distributed processing, a combination of local and remote computers in a network connected to a central computer to distribute the processing and thereby reduce the load on the central computer.

distributive analysis and synthesis, the system of psychotherapy used by the psychobiologic school of psychiatry. It involves an extensive and systematic investigation and analysis of a person's total past experiences to discover the emotional factors underlying personality problems and how they can be synthesized into constructive behavioral patterns.

distributive care, a pattern of health care that is concerned with environment, heredity, living conditions, life-style, and early detection of pathologic effects. The system is usually directed toward continuous care of persons not confined to hospitals or other health care facilities.

district, **1.** (in hospital nursing) a group of patients in an area of the unit for whom a head nurse or primary nurse is responsible, usually a subdivision of a ward unit. Patients are customarily assigned to a district on the basis of certain shared needs for nursing care. **2.** the area of a city or town assigned to a public health nurse.

district nurse. See **public health nurse.**

disulfiram, an alcohol-use deterrent.

■ INDICATIONS: It is prescribed as a deterrent to drinking alcohol in the treatment of chronic alcoholism. It causes severe intestinal cramping, diaphoresis, and nausea if alcohol is ingested.

■ CONTRAINDICATIONS: Alcoholic intoxication, recent or concomitant administration of metronidazole, paraldehyde, or alcohol, severe myocardial disease, coronary occlusion, psychosis, or known hypersensitivity to this drug prohibits its use.

■ ADVERSE EFFECTS: The most serious adverse reactions occur after alcohol is ingested, including optic neuritis, psychotic reaction, and polyneuritis. Drowsiness, headache, and skin rash may occur. This drug interacts with several other drugs.

disuse phenomena, the physical and the psychologic changes, usually degenerative, that result from the lack of use of a part of the body or a body system. Disuse phenomena are associated with confinement and immobility, especially in orthopedics. Individuals under treatment for fractures and other orthopedic disorders must often be confined to beds and immobilized in traction for long periods. Such patients are often deprived of interaction with the world around them and lose motivations, expectations, and even acquired abilities because of lack of practice. Some studies have shown that young, healthy individuals confined to bed rest for even 3 hours experience disturbances of time sense and memory. Other individuals in similar circumstances have experienced tactile, auditory, and visual hallucinations. Such disorientation is compounded by pain and therapeutic narcotic drugs commonly associated with the treatment of many illnesses and abnormal conditions. In hospital environments often requiring patients to drastically reduce physical and social movement during treatment and recuperation, many patients become egocentric, expecting other people to direct all their time and energy toward them. Unable to interact with the normal world outside the hospital, many patients become less efficient in remembering, problem solving, and learning. The physical changes often induced by continued bed rest constitute problems affecting many key areas and systems of the body, as the skin, the musculoskeletal system, the GI tract, the cardiovascular system, and the respiratory system. The skin of the patient on prolonged bed rest is commonly subjected to abnormal conditions, as pressure exerted by the bed, moisture, friction, and inadequate nutrition. Pressure exerted on the skin by the bed is slightly higher than capillary hydrostatic pressure, often causing problems in blood circulation and inadequate airing of the skin surface. Any pressure that causes collapse of the superficial capillaries will lead to ischemia and eventual tissue necrosis. Of particular interest to the orthopedic nurse is the phenomenon, accompanying disuse, that may prevent the neurologically impaired patient from feeling pain. This phenomenon may be the first sign of ischemia followed by a rapid breakdown of the skin. Some indications of skin ischemia are redness, pain, edema, and skin breakdown. Elderly patients are often more susceptible to skin breakdown because of possible poor nutrition, more restricted mobility, and generally poor skin condition. Younger patients may also develop ischemia if they are not sufficiently mobile. Tissue ischemia can occur in any individual in 1 or 2 hours. One of the biggest problems associated with extended bed rest or limited activity of a part of the body is disuse atrophy, which may affect the bones and muscles. The normal stress applied to these structures is important to their health and function. Unused muscles lose size and strength, often wasting away until they are unable to perform their vital functions of support and contraction. Another disuse phenomenon is contracture, which may result from constant flexion or extension of a body part by the patient on prolonged bed rest. Contractures are usually caused by flexion, because patients flex knees and hips whenever possible to relax muscles, especially when cold or in pain. The amputee often flexes the remaining portion of the affected limb for comfort or to reduce edema. Continued flexion in such circumstances may produce stiffness in the affected joint which, if not manipulated, may become permanently impaired. Prevention of contractures involves manipulation and various range-of-motion exercises, when possible. Constipation is a disuse phenomenon commonly developing from the weakening of abdominal muscles required for normal evacuation of the bowel. This problem is often compounded by the horizontal position of the bed patient, dietary changes, and the administration of narcotics and anesthetic agents, which slow peristalsis. The immobilized patient may experience bone demineralization because of a restricted diet and decreased motility. Calcium and phosphorus are dependent on vitamin D for absorption from the gut and movement into the bones, and some nutritional experts describe calcium loss as a natural disuse phenomenon of bed rest. Muscle action is required to maintain the blood flow to the bones, and the immobilized patient may not be capable of sufficient muscular activity to assure such blood flow, with its attendant delivery of critical nutrients. The peak loss of calcium from the bones occurs in the fifth and the sixth weeks of bed rest. Disuse osteoporosis develops as the result of an imbalance between osteoblasts and osteoclasts; both types of cells proliferate during bed rest, but osteoclasts at a greater rate. Degeneration of bone matrix apparently occurs before osteoclastic resorption, causing the breakdown of the bony matrix and the resultant loss of minerals. The dangers of osteoporosis are pathologic fracture and softening of bones, which can lead to deformity and pain in joints from calcium deposits. Calcium released from the bone enters the bloodstream and is deposited in the joints or carried to the kidneys for excretion in the urine. When the kidney cannot process the calcium fast enough, kidney stones develop, blocking the ureters and causing kidney damage, with glomerular degeneration, and acute pain. The pooling of respiratory secretions is another disuse phenomenon caused by the immobility and the horizontal position of the bed-rest patient. When the individual lies down, secretions in the lungs tend to accumulate in the bronchioles unevenly, wetting the dependent side of the bronchioles and drying the other surfaces. The diameter of the bronchioles also decreases when the individual is supine, and a thicker coating of mucus develops, creating a ripe medium for bacterial growth. Hypostatic pneumonia may result if the mucus is not removed. Prolonged bed rest also encourages certain cardiovascular problems, as venous stasis in the pelvis and the lower extremities, dehydration, and clot formation. Dehydration increases the risk of clot formation by increasing the viscosity of the blood. Some common therapeutic measures to deal with disuse phenomena are the improvement of diet and nutrition, proper positioning and regular movement of the bed-rest patient, meticulous hygiene, scrupulous skin care, and positive social interaction with the patient. See also **hypostatic pneumonia.**

Ditropan, a trademark for an antispasmodic (oxybutynin chloride).

Diucardin, a trademark for an antihypertensive and diuretic (hydroflumethiazide).

Diupres, a trademark for a fixed-combination drug containing a diuretic (chlorothiazide) and an antihypertensive (reserpine).

diuresis /dī'yo͞orē'sis/, increased formation and secretion of urine. Diuresis occurs in conditions such as diabetes mellitus and diabetes insipidus. It is normal in the first 48 hours postpartum. Coffee, tea, certain foods, diuretic drugs, and some steroids cause diuresis.

diuretic /dī'yo͞oret'ik/, **1.** (of a drug or other substance) tending to promote the formation and excretion of urine. **2.** a drug that promotes the formation and excretion of urine. The more than 50 diuretic drugs available in the United States and Canada are classified by chemical structure and pharmacologic activity into these groups: aldosterone antagonists, carbonic anhydrase inhibitors, loop diuretics, mercurials, osmotics, potassium-sparing diuretics, and thiazides. A diuretic medication may contain drugs from one or more of these groups. Diuretics are prescribed to reduce the volume of extracellular fluid in the treatment of many disorders, including hypertension, congestive heart failure, and edema. The particular drug to be prescribed is selected according to the action desired and the physical status of the patient. Hypersensitivity to sulfonamides prohibits use of this class of drug, and diabetes mellitus may be aggravated by thiazide medications; thus, the presence of a particular condition may prohibit the use of a particular agent. Several adverse reactions are common to all diuretics, including hypovolemia and electrolyte imbalance. Mercurial diuretics are rarely used because of the nephrotoxicity, and carbonic anhydrase inhibitors have only a weak diuretic activity. Mannitol and urea osmotics are used primarily in emergency situations, as in the treatment of cerebral edema, rather than as hypertensive or cardiovascular medications.

Diuril, a trademark for a diuretic (chlorothiazide).

diurnal variation, the range of the output or excretion rate of a substance in a specimen being collected for laboratory analysis over a 24-hour period.

divalent. See **bivalent.**

diversional activity deficit, a nursing diagnosis accepted by the Fourth National Conference on the Classification of Nursing Diagnoses. The causes of the situation include a lack of diversion in the environment, long-term hospitalization, or frequent or prolonged treatment. The defining characteristics of the diagnosis include statements from the client that there is nothing to do or that everything is boring, but the usual diversions or hobbies pursued at home are not undertaken. See also **nursing diagnosis.**

diverticulitis /dī'vurtik'yo͞olī'tis/, inflammation of one or more diverticula. The penetration of fecal matter through the thin-walled diverticula causes inflammation and abcess formation in the tissues surrounding the colon. With repeated inflammation, the lumen of the colon narrows and may become obstructed. During periods of inflammation, the patient will experience crampy pain, particularly over the sigmoid colon, fever, and leukocytosis. Barium enemas and proctoscopy are performed to rule out carcinoma of the colon, which exhibits some of the same symptoms. Conservative treatment includes bed rest, intravenous fluids, antibiotics, and nothing taken by mouth. In acute cases, bowel resection of the affected part greatly reduces mortality and morbidity. Compare **diverticulosis.**

diverticulosis /dī'vurtik'yo͞olō'sis/, the presence of pouchlike herniations through the muscular layer of the colon, particularly the sigmoid colon. Diverticulosis affects increasing numbers of people over 50 years of age and may be the result of the modern, highly refined, low-residue diet. Most patients with this condition have few symptoms except for occasional bleeding from the rectum. The physician must exercise care in ruling out other reasons for bleeding, as carcinoma and inflammatory bowel disease. Barium enemas and proctoscopic examination are used in establishing diagnosis. An increase in the dietary fiber can aid in propelling the feces through the colon. Hemorrhage from bleeding diverticula can become quite severe, and the patient may require surgery. Diverticulosis may lead to diverticulitis. See also **diverticulitis.**

diverticulum /dī'vurtik'yo͞oləm/, *pl.* **diverticula,** a pouchlike herniation through the muscular wall of a tubular organ. A diverticulum may be present in the stomach, in the small intestine, or, most commonly, the colon. See also **diverticulitis, diverticulosis, Meckel's diverticulum.** **–diverticular,** *adj.*

diving goiter, a large movable thyroid gland located at times above the sternal notch and at other times below the notch. Also called **plunging goiter, wandering goiter.**

division, **1.** an administrative subunit in a hospital, as a division of medical nursing or a division of surgical nursing. **2.** (in public health nursing) an area that encompasses several geographic districts. **3.** the separation of something into two or more parts or sections. A kind of division is **cell division.**

Dix, Dorothea Lynde (1802–87), an American humanitarian who achieved fame as a social reformer, primarily for her work in improving prison conditions and care of the mentally ill. During her lifetime, she helped to establish mental institutions in 30 states and in Canada. During the Civil War, she was appointed superintendent of army nurses for government hospitals.

dizygotic /dī′zīgot′ik/, of or pertaining to twins from two fertilized ova. Compare **monozygotic.** See also **twinning.**

dizygotic twins, two offspring born of the same pregnancy and developed from two ova that were released from the ovary simultaneously and fertilized at the same time. They may be of the same or opposite sex, differ both physically and in genetic constitution, and have two separate and distinct placentas and membranes, both amnion and chorion. The frequency of dizygotic twinning varies according to ethnic origin, the highest incidence being in the black race, the lowest in Orientals, with the white races being intermediate; maternal age, the highest rate occurring when the mother is 35 to 39 years of age; and heredity, showing an increase in the female genetic line rather than the male, although fathers may transmit the disposition toward double ovulation to their daughters. In general, the overall ratio is two-thirds dizygotic twinning to one-third monozygotic. Also called **binovular twins, dissimilar twins, false twins, fraternal twins, heterologous twins.** Compare **monozygotic twins.**

dizziness, a sensation of faintness or an inability to maintain normal balance in a standing or seated position, sometimes associated with giddiness, mental confusion, nausea, and weakness. A patient who experiences dizziness should be carefully lowered to a safe position on a bed, chair, or floor because of the danger of injury from falling. Compare **syncope.** See also **vertigo.**

DLE, abbreviation for **discoid lupus erythematosus.**

DM, abbreviation for **diabetes mellitus.**

D.M.D., abbreviation for *Doctor of Dental Medicine.*

DMSO, abbreviation for **dimethyl sulfoxide.**

DNA, abbreviation for **deoxyribonucleic acid.**

DNA chimera /kīmē′rə/, (in molecular genetics) a recombinant molecule of DNA composed of segments from more than one source.

DNA ligase, an enzyme that can repair breaks in a strand of DNA by synthesizing a bond between adjoining nucleotides. Under some circumstances the enzyme can join together loose ends of DNA strands, and in some cases it can repair breaks in RNA.

DNA polymerase, (in molecular genetics) an enzyme that catalyzes the assembly of deoxyribonucleoside triphosphates into DNA, with single-stranded DNA serving as the template. The enzyme is often found in tumor cells. Also called **DNA nucleotidyltransferase.**

DNCB, abbreviation for **dinitrochlorobenzene.**

DNR, abbreviation for *do not resuscitate.* See **no-code.**

D.O., abbreviation for *Doctor of Osteopathy.* See **physician.**

Dobie's globule /dō′bēz/, a very small stainable body in the transparent disk of a striated muscle fiber. Also called **Krause's line, Z disk.**

dobutamine hydrochloride, a beta-adrenergic stimulating agent.

■ INDICATIONS: It is prescribed to increase cardiac output in severe chronic congestive heart failure and as an adjunct in cardiac surgery.

■ CONTRAINDICATIONS: Idiopathic hypertrophic subaortic stenosis or known hypersensitivity to this drug prohibits its use. It is not recommended for use in pregnancy.

■ ADVERSE EFFECTS: Among the most serious adverse reactions are cardiovascular effects, including tachycardia, hypertension, arrythmias, and precipitation of angina. Nausea, vomiting, and headache may also occur.

Dobutrex, a trademark for a synthetic catecholamine (dobutamine hydrochloride), which stimulates beta-adrenergic receptors.

Dock, Lavinia Lloyd (1858–1956), an American public health nurse. A graduate of the Bellevue Hospital Training School for Nurses in New York in 1886, she started a visiting-nurse service in Norwalk, Connecticut, and then joined the New York City Mission before becoming an assistant to Isabel Hampton Robb at Johns Hopkins Hospital in Baltimore. She returned to public health nursing when she joined the Henry Street Settlement in New York to work with Lillian Wald. She advocated an international public health movement and the improvement of education for nurses. With M. Adelaide Nutting, she wrote *History of Nursing,* a classic in nursing literature.

doctoral program in nursing, an educational program of study that offers preparation for a doctoral degree in the field of nursing designed to prepare nurses for advanced practice and research. Upon successful completion of the course of study, the degree Ph.D. or Ed.D in nursing or D.S.N. (Doctor of Science in Nursing) is awarded. Higher standards of professional practice and the desire for scholarly achievement have caused nurses to work toward advanced educational degrees. Many nurses obtain a doctoral degree in fields ancillary to nursing, as the social or biologic sciences, education, and the humanities.

Doctor of Medicine, Doctor of Osteopathy. See **physician.**

documentation, written material associated with a computer or a program. Kinds of documentation include **user documentation,** an instruction manual that provides enough information for the individual to use the system; **system documentation,** a complete description of the hardware and the software that make up a system; and **program documentation,** a general and specific description of what a program does and how it does it.

docusate /dok′yo͞osāt/, a stool softener. Also called **dioctyl calcium sulfosuccinate, dioctyl sodium sulfosuccinate.**

■ INDICATION: It is prescribed in the treatment of constipation.

■ CONTRAINDICATIONS: Signs or symptoms of appendicitis, concomitant administration of mineral oil, or known hypersensitivity to the drug prohibits its use.

■ ADVERSE EFFECTS: No serious adverse reactions are known.

δOD, abbreviation for **delta optic density.**

Doederlein's bacillus, a gram-positive bacterium present in normal vaginal secretions.

Doehle bodies, blue inclusions in the cytoplasm of some leukocytes in May-Hegglin anomaly and in blood smears from patients with acute infections.

Döhle-Heller disease. See **syphilitic aortitis.**

Dolene, a trademark for an analgesic (propoxyphene hydrochloride).

dolicho-, a combining form meaning 'long': *dolichocephaly, dolichocolon, dolichomorphic*.

dolichocephaly. See **scaphocephaly.**

doll's-eye reflex, a normal response in newborns to keep the eyes stationary as the head is moved to the right or left. The reflex disappears as ocular fixation develops.

Dolobid, a trademark for an antiinflammatory agent (diflunisal).

Dolophine Hydrochloride, a trademark for a narcotic analgesic (methadone hydrochloride).

DOM, abbreviation for **dimethoxymethylamphetamine.**

dome fracture, any fracture of the acetabulum, specifically involving a weight-bearing surface.

dominance, (in genetics) a basic principle stating that not all genes determining a given trait operate with equal vigor. If two genes at a given locus produce a different effect, as eye color, they compete for expression. The gene that is manifest is dominant; it masks the effect of the other gene, which is recessive. See also **autosomal-dominant inheritance, independent assortment, recessive, segregation.** **–dominant,** *adj.*

dominant gene, one that produces a phenotypic effect regardless of whether its allele is the same or different. Compare **recessive gene.**

Donath-Landsteiner syndrome, a rare blood disorder, marked by hemolysis minutes or hours after exposure to cold. Systemic symptoms include the passage of dark urine, severe pain in the back and legs, headache, vomiting, diarrhea, and moderate reticulocytosis. There may be temporary hepatosplenomegaly and mild hyperbilirubinemia following the onset of an attack. The condition may occur with congenital or acquired syphilis, in which case antisyphilitic treatment may be curative. Also called **paroxysmal cold hemoglobinuria.**

Don Juan, a seductive and sexually promiscuous man.

Donnatal, a trademark for a GI fixed-combination drug containing a sedative (phenobarbital) and three anticholinergics (hyoscyamine sulfate, atropine sulfate, and hyoscine hydrobromide), used to decrease the motility of the GI tract.

donor, **1.** a human or other organism that gives living tissue to be used in another body, for example, blood for transfusion or a kidney for transplantation. **2.** a substance or compound that gives part of itself to another substance. Compare **acceptor.** See also **universal donor.**

Donovan bodies, encapsulated gram-negative rods of the species *Calymmatobacterium granulomatis,* present in the cytoplasm of mononuclear phagocytes obtained from the lesions of granuloma inguinale. They may be seen under the microscope in a Wright-stained smear of infected tissue. See also **granuloma inguinale.**

dopamine hydrochloride /dō′pəmin/, a sympathomimetic catecholamine.

■ INDICATIONS: It is prescribed in the treatment of shock, hypotension, and low cardiac output.

■ CONTRAINDICATIONS: Pheochromocytoma, tachyarrhythmias, ventricular fibrillation, or known hypersensitivity to this drug prohibits its use.

■ ADVERSE EFFECTS: Among the more serious adverse reactions are arrhythmias, hypotension, hypertension, and tachycardia.

dopaminergic /dō′pəminur′jik/, having the effect of dopamine.

Dopar, a trademark for an antiparkinsonian (levodopa).

dope, *slang.* morphine, heroin, or another narcotic, or marijuana or another substance illicitly bought, or sold, and often self-administered for sedative, hypnotic, euphoric, or other mood-altering purpose.

Doppler effect /dop′lər/, the apparent change in frequency of sound or light waves emitted by a source as it moves away from or toward an observer. The frequency increases as the source moves toward the observer and decreases as it moves away, as the rising pitch of the whistle of an approaching train and the falling pitch of a departing train. The Doppler effect is also observed in electromagnetic radiation, as light and radio waves. See also **electromagnetic radiation, ultrasonography, wavelength.**

Doppler scanning, a technique used in ultrasound imaging to monitor the behavior of a moving structure, as flowing blood or a beating heart. The frequency of ultrasonic waves reflected from a moving surface is slightly different from that of the incident waves. The detected frequency shift yields information about the moving structure. Fetal heart detectors work on this principle.

Dopram, a trademark for a respiratory stimulant (doxapram hydrochloride).

Dorantamin, a trademark for an antihistamine (pyrilamine maleate).

Dorbane, a trademark for a laxative (danthron).

Dorbantyl, a trademark for a fixed-combination drug containing a stool softener (dioctyl sodium sulfosuccinate) and a laxative (danthron).

Doriden, a trademark for a sedative (glutethimide).

dorsal /dôr′səl/, pertaining to the back or posterior. Compare **ventral.** See also **dorsiflect.** **–dorsum,** *n.*

-dorsal, a combining form meaning 'the back of something' or 'the back': *predorsal, thoracodorsal, ventrodorsal.*

dorsal carpal ligament. See **retinaculum extensorum manus.**

dorsal digital vein, one of the communicating veins along the sides of the fingers. The veins from the adjacent sides of the fingers unite to form three dorsal metacarpal veins, which end in a dorsal venous network on the back of the hand. Compare **basilic vein, cephalic vein, median antebrachial vein.**

dorsal interventricular artery, the arterial branch of the right coronary artery, branching to supply both ventricles. It runs down the dorsal sulcus two thirds of the way to the apex of the heart. Also called **right interventricular artery.**

dorsalis pedis artery, the continuation of the anterior tibial artery, starting at the ankle joint, dividing into five branches, and supplying various muscles of the foot and toes. Its branches are the lateral tarsal, medial tarsal, arcuate, first dorsal metatarsal, and deep plantar.

dorsalis pedis pulse, the pulse of the dorsalis pedis artery, palpable between the first and second metatarsal bones on the top of the foot. It can be felt in approximately 90% of people.

dorsal lip, the marginal fold of the blastopore during gastrulation in the early stages of embryonic development of many animals. It marks the dorsal limit of the developing embryo, constitutes the primary organizer, gives rise to neural tissue, and corresponds to the primitive node in humans and higher animals.

dorsal scapular nerve, one of a pair of supraclavicular branches from the roots of the brachial plexus. It arises from the fifth cervical nerve near the intervertebral foramen, pierces the scalenus medius, and runs dorsally and caudally to the vertebral border of the scapula. It supplies the rhomboideus major and the rhomboideus minor and sends a branch to the levator.

dorsi-. See **dorso-.**

dorsiflect /dôr′siflekt/, to bend or flex backward as in the upward bending of the fingers, wrist, foot, or toes.

dorsiflexion /dôr′siflek′shən/, flexion toward the back, as accomplished by a muscle. See also **dorsiflexor.**

dorsiflexor /dôr′siflek′sər/, a muscle causing backward flexion of a part of the body, as the hand or foot.

dorsiflexor gait, an abnormal gait caused by the weakness of the dorsiflexors of the ankle. It is characterized by footdrop during the entire gait cycle and excessive knee and hip flexion to allow clearance of the involved extremity during the swing phase. The sole of the affected foot also slaps forcibly against the ground at the moment of heelstrike because of the inability of the dorsiflexor to decelerate the body weight as the heel strikes the ground. Compare **Trendelenburg gait.**

dorso-, dorsi-, a combining form meaning 'pertaining to a dorsum or to the back': *dorsocephalad, dorsomesial, dorsoscapular.*

dorsosacral position. See **lithotomy position.**

dosage, the regimen governing the size, frequency, and number of doses of a therapeutic agent to be administered to a patient.

dosage compensation, (in genetics) the mechanism that counterbalances the number of X-linked gene doses in the sex chromosomes so that they are equal in both the male, which has one X chromosome, and the female, which has two. In mammals this is accomplished by genetic activation of only one of the X chromosomes in the somatic cells of females. See also **Lyon hypothesis.**

dose, the amount of a drug or other substance to be administered at one time. See also **absorbed dose.**

dose equivalent, a quantity used in radiation-safety work that equates on a unified scale the amount of radiation dose and the physical damages that it might produce. It is the product of the dose (in rad or gray) and modifying factors that are specific to the type and energy of the radiation delivering that dose. The unit of dose equivalent is the sievert (Sv) or the rem.

dose fractionation. See **fractionation,** def. 5.

dose rate, (in radiotherapy) the amount of delivered radiation absorbed per unit of time.

dose ratemeter, (in radiotherapy) an instrument for measuring the dose rate of radiation.

dose threshold, (in radiotherapy) the minimum amount of absorbed radiation that produces a detectable degree of a given effect.

dose to skin, (in radiotherapy) the amount of absorbed radiation at the center of the irradiation field on the skin. It is the sum of the dose in the air and the scatter from body parts.

dosimeter /dōsim′ətər/, an instrument to detect and measure accumulated radiation exposure. A pencil-sized ionization chamber with a self-reading electrometer is used to monitor exposure to personnel.

dot-matrix printer, a printer that imprints a character by creating it from a pattern of dots, each of which is produced by actuating selected wires in a set so that their ends strike the paper through an inked ribbon. Compare **character printer, daisy-wheel printer.**

double-approach conflict. See **approach-approach conflict.**

double-avoidant conflict. See **avoidance-avoidance conflict.**

double-blind study, an experiment designed to test the effect of a treatment or substance using groups of experimental and control subjects in which neither the subjects nor the investigators know which treatment or substance is being administered to which group. In a double-blind test of a new drug, the substance may be identified to the investigators by only a code. The purpose of a double-blind study is to eliminate the risk of prejudgment by the participants, which could distort the results. A double-blind study may be augmented by a **cross-over experiment**, in which experimental subjects unknowingly become control subjects, and vice versa, at some point in the study. See also **placebo.**

double fracture, a fracture consisting of breaks or cracks in two places in a bone, resulting in more than two bone segments.

double gel diffusion. See **immunodiffusion.**

double innervation, innervation of effector organs by fibers of the sympathetic and parasympathetic divisions of the autonomic nervous system. The pelvic viscera, bronchioles, heart, eyes, and digestive system are all doubly innervated. The fibers of the two divisions operate at cross-purposes to achieve a state of balance and to maintain the homeostatic condition of the body. The mode of action of each division varies: in some structures one division is stimulating and the other inhibiting; in others, separate fibers from each division act to stimulate and inhibit complementary function.

double monster, a fetus that has developed from a single ovum but has two heads, trunks, and multiple limbs. Also called **twin monster.**

double quartan fever, a form of malaria in which paroxysms of fever occur in a repeating pattern of 2 consecutive days followed by 1 day of remission. The pattern is usually the result of concurrent infections by two species of the genus *Plasmodium,* one causing paroxysms every 72 hours and the other every 48 hours. Compare **biduotertian fever.**

double setup, a nursing procedure in which an obstetric operating room is prepared for both vaginal delivery and cesarean section. The circulating and scrub nurses lay out the equipment required for both procedures, possibly including a vacuum aspirator, forceps, and cesarean-section packs. The scrub nurse remains scrubbed until the infant is delivered but does not participate unless a cesarean section is performed.

double tachycardia, the simultaneous but independent firing of two rapid heart contraction impulses, one controlling the atria and one the ventricles.

double vision. See **diplopia.**

douche /do͞osh/, **1.** a procedure in which a liter or more of a solution of a medication or cleansing agent in warm water is introduced into the vagina under low pressure. The woman often performs the procedure herself. Sitting on a toilet seat or semisitting in a bathtub, she introduces the douche tip into the vagina and releases a clamp on the tubing connected to the douche bag, which is suspended 2 feet above the introitus. She allows the solution to flow in, while holding the lips of the vagina closed to retain the fluid. As the accumulation of fluid distends the vagina, she clamps the tubing and, after a few minutes, allows the fluid to flow out. The process is repeated until the entire quantity of solution in the douche bag has been used. Douching may be recommended in the treatment of various pelvic and vaginal infections. **2.** to perform a douche.

doughnut pessary. See **pessary.**

Douglas' cul-de-sac, a rectouterine pouch or recess formed by a fold of peritoneum that extends between the rectum and the uterus. Also called **excavatio rectouterina.**

down, (of a computer) one that is not operating as a result of malfunction or maintenance or for other reasons.

Downey cells, lymphocytes identified in one system of classification of the blood cells of patients with infectious mononucleosis. The cells are designated as Downey I, II, or III lymphocytes.

Down's syndrome, a congenital condition characterized by varying degrees of mental retardation and multiple defects. It is the most common chromosomal abnormality of a generalized syndrome and is caused by the presence of an extra chromosome 21 in the G group or, in a small percentage of cases, by the translocation of chromosomes 14 or 15 in the D group and chromosomes 21 or 22. Also called **mongolism, mongoloid idiocy, trisomy G syndrome, trisomy 21.**

■ OBSERVATIONS: Down's syndrome occurs in approximately 1 in 600 to 650 live births and is associated with advanced maternal age, particularly over 35 years of age. The incidence is as high as 1 in 80 for offspring of women older than 40 years. In those cases caused by translocation, which is a genetic aberration that is hereditary rather than a chromosomal aberration caused by nondisjunction during cell division, the incidence is not associated with maternal age, and the risk is low, about 1 in 5 if the mother is the carrier and 1 in 20 if the father is the carrier. The condition, which can be diagnosed prenatally by amniocentesis, also occurs as a mosaic variant, in which there is a mixture of trisomy 21 and normal cells. Such patients have fewer physical defects and less-severe retardation depending on the degree of mosaicism. Infants with the syndrome are small and hypotonic, with characteristic microcephaly, brachycephaly, a flattened occiput, and typical facies with a mongoloid slant to the eyes, depressed nasal bridge, low-set ears, and a large, protruding tongue that is furrowed and lacks the central fissure. The hands are short and broad with a transverse palmar or simian crease; the fingers are stubby and show clinodactyly, primarily of the fifth finger. The feet are broad and stubby with a wide space between the first and second toes and a prominent plantar crease. Other anomalies associated with the disorder are bowel defects, congenital heart disease (primarily septal defects), chronic respiratory infections, visual problems, abnormalities in tooth development, and susceptibility to acute leukemia. The most significant feature of the syndrome is mental retardation, which varies considerably, although the average IQ is in the range of 50 to 60, so that the child is generally trainable and in most instances can be reared at home. Those more severely affected are often institutionalized. The mortality rate is high within the first few years, especially in children with cardiac anomalies. Those who survive tend to be shorter than average and stocky in build, they show delayed or incomplete sexual development, and they can live to middle or old age, although adults with Down's syndrome are prone to respiratory infections, pneumonia, and lung disease.

■ INTERVENTION: Care for the child with Down's syndrome involves several short- and long-term goals, depending on the severity of physical defects and the degree of mental impairment. Of immediate importance is the prevention of physical problems associated with the disorder, as respiratory infections, inadequate nutrition and feeding difficulties because of the large protruding tongue, skin breakdown caused by the characteristic dry, cracked dermal condition, and positioning difficulties caused by the hypotonicity of muscles and hyperextensibility of the joints. Long-term intervention centers on carefully planned programs to promote optimal development, both in motor and mental skills. Since the developmental potential of a child with Down's syndrome is greatest during infancy, a stimulation program of exercise based on the child's ability and potential is mandatory for teaching gross motor skills.

■ NURSING CONSIDERATIONS: The primary role of the nurse is to offer support to the parents, to teach them how to provide adequate care, and to plan both short- and long-term programs that will realize the full physical and mental potential of the child. The nurse helps the parents to learn the child's limitations and to function within that range, periodically assesses the child's developmental progress, and advises parents on the various community programs and vocational classes that are available. Of utmost importance is that all family members understand that the child has the same basic needs as other children, as play, discipline, and social interaction. The nurse also functions in the genetic counseling of high-risk women and encourages those at risk to consider amniocentesis in the event of pregnancy.

down-time, a period during which a computer system is inoperable, for maintenance, as a result of malfunction, or for other reasons.

doxapram hydrochloride, a respiratory stimulant.

■ INDICATIONS: It is prescribed to improve respiratory function after anesthesia, in drug-induced central nervous system depression, and for chronic pulmonary disease associated with acute hypercapnia.

■ CONTRAINDICATIONS: Seizure disorder, pulmonary disease, coronary artery disease, hypertension, or known hypersensitivity to this drug prohibits its use.

■ ADVERSE EFFECTS: Among the more serious adverse reactions are convulsions, bronchospasm, cardiovascular symptoms, and phlebitis.

doxepin hydrochloride /dok′səpin/, a tricyclic antidepressant.

■ INDICATION: It is prescribed in the treatment of depression.

■ CONTRAINDICATIONS: Concomitant administration of monoamine oxidase inhibitors, recent myocardial infarction, seizure disorders, or known hypersensitivity to tricyclic medication prohibits its use.

■ ADVERSE EFFECTS: Among the more serious adverse reactions are GI, cardiovascular, and neurologic disturbances. Sedation, dry mouth, and many drug interactions may occur.

doxorubicin hydrochloride, an anthracycline antibiotic.

■ INDICATIONS: It is prescribed in the treatment of a variety of malignant neoplastic diseases.

■ CONTRAINDICATIONS: Myelosuppression, heart disease, concurrent administration of daunorubicin, or known hypersensitivity to this drug prohibits its use.

■ ADVERSE EFFECTS: Among the more serious adverse reactions are myelosuppression and cardiomyopathy. Stomatitis, GI disturbances, and alopecia commonly occur.

doxycycline, a tetracycline antibacterial.

■ INDICATIONS: It is prescribed in the treatment of a variety of infections.

■ CONTRAINDICATIONS: Renal or liver dysfunction or known hypersensitivity to this drug or to other tetracycline medication prohibits its use. It is not given during pregnancy or to children under 8 years of age.

■ ADVERSE EFFECTS: Among the more serious adverse reactions are GI disturbances, phototoxicity, potentially serious suprainfections, and hypersensitivity reactions. Discoloration of teeth may occur in children exposed to the drug in utero or under 8 years of age.

doxylamine succinate /dok′silam′ēn/, an antihistamine.

■ INDICATIONS: It is prescribed for the treatment of acute allergic symptoms produced by the release of histamine.

■ CONTRAINDICATIONS: Known hypersensitivity to this drug prohibits its use. It is not recommended for use during pregnancy or lactation and is not given to children under 6 years of age.

■ ADVERSE EFFECTS: Among the more serious reactions are sedation, ataxia, tachycardia, hemolytic anemia, and thrombocytopenia.

dp/dt, (in cardiology) the rate of pressure change per unit of time.

DPT vaccine, abbreviation for **diphtheria, tetanus toxoids, and pertussis vaccine.**

DQ, abbreviation for **developmental quotient.**

dracunculiasis /drakun′kyo͝olī′əsis/, a parasitic infection caused by infestation by the nematode *Dracunculus medinensis*. It is characterized by ulcerative skin lesions on the legs and feet that are produced by gravid female worms. People are infected by drinking contaminated water or eating contaminated shellfish. It is common in densely populated tropic and subtropic areas of the world. Also called **dracontiasis, guinea worm infection.**

Dracunculus medinensis /drakun′kyo͝oləs/, a parasitic nematode of the Mediterranean area that causes dracunculiasis. An American species is *Dracunculus insignis*. Also called **fiery serpent.**

drainage, the removal of fluids from a body cavity, wound, or other source of discharge by one or more methods. **Closed drainage** is a system of tubing and other apparatus attached to the body to remove fluid in an airtight circuit that prevents environmental contaminants from entering the wound or cavity. **Open drainage** is drainage in which discharge passes through an open-ended tube into a receptacle. **Suction drainage** utilizes a pump or other mechanic device to assist in extracting a fluid. **Tidal drainage** is drainage in which a body area is washed out by alternately flooding and then emptying it with the aid of gravity, a technique that may be used in treating a urinary bladder disorder. See also **postural drainage.**

drainage tube, a heavy-gauge catheter used for the evacuation of air or a fluid from a cavity or wound in the body. The tube may be attached to a suction device or simply allow flow by gravity into a receptacle.

Draize test, a controversial method of testing the toxicity of pharmaceutic and other products to be used by humans by placing a small amount of the substance in the eyes of rabbits. The eye-irritancy potential of a substance is considered a measure of the possible effect the product could have on similar human tissues. The Draize in vivo test is recognized by the U.S. Food and Drug Administration as a reliable method of predicting the risk of new products to human eyesight, although alternative testing methods are being sought.

dram, a unit of mass equivalent to an apothecaries' measure of 60 grains or ⅛ ounce and to 1/16 ounce or 27.34 grains avoirdupois.

Dramamine, a trademark for an antihistamine (dimenhydrinate), used as an antiemetic.

dramatic play, an imitative activity in which a child fantasizes and acts out various domestic and social roles and situations, as rocking a doll, pretending to be a doctor or nurse, or teaching school. It is the predominant form of play among preschool children.

drape, a sheet of fabric or paper, usually the size of a small bed sheet, for covering all or a part of a person's body during a physical examination or treatment. –**drape,** *v.*

drawing, *informal.* a vague sensation of muscle tension.

dream, **1.** a sequence of ideas, thoughts, emotions, or images that pass through the mind during the rapid-eye-movement stage of sleep. **2.** the sleeping state in which this process occurs. **3.** a visionary creation of the imagination experienced during wakefulness. **4.** (in psychoanalysis) the expression of thoughts, emotions, memories, or impulses repressed from the consciousness. **5.** (in analytic psychology) the wishes, emotions, and impulses that reflect the personal unconscious and the archetypes that originate in the collective unconscious. See also **dream analysis, dream state.**

dream analysis, a process of gaining access to the unconscious mind by means of examining the content of dreams, usually through the method of free association.

dream association, a relationship of thoughts or emotions discovered or experienced when a dream is remembered or analyzed. See also **dream analysis.**

dream state, a condition of altered consciousness in which a person does not recognize the environment and reacts in a manner opposed to his or her usual behavior, as by flight or an act of violence. The state is seen in epilepsy and certain neuroses. See also **automatism, fugue.**

drepanocytic anemia, sickle cell anemia.

dress code, the standards set by an institution for the dress of the members of the institution.

dressing, a clean or sterile covering applied directly to wounded or diseased tissue for absorption of secretions, for protection from trauma, for administration of medications, to keep the wound clean, or to stop bleeding. Kinds of dressings include **absorbent dressing, antiseptic dressing, occlusive dressing, pressure dressing,** and **wet dressing.**

dressing forceps, a kind of forceps that has narrow blades and blunt or notched teeth, designed for dressing wounds, removing drainage tubes, or extracting fragments of necrotic tissue.

Dressler's syndrome /dres′lərz/, an autoimmune disorder that may occur several days after acute coronary infarction, characterized by fever, pericarditis, pleurisy, pleural effusions, and joint pain. It results from the body's immunologic response to a damaged myocardium and pericardium. Treatment usually includes intensive aspirin therapy and, in severe cases, corticosteroids. A similar syndrome may occur after cardiac surgery.

DRG, abbreviation for **diagnosis-related group.**

drift, **1. antigenic drift,** a change that occurs in a strain of virus so that variations appear periodically with alterations in antigenic qualities. **2. genetic drift,** random variations in gene frequency of a population from one generation to the next.

drifting tooth, any one of the teeth that migrate from normal position in the associated dental arch. This anomaly may result from the loss of proximal support, loss of functional antagonists, occlusal traumatic tooth relationships, inflammatory and retrograde changes in the attachment apparatus, or oral habits, as thumb-sucking and bruxism.

drill and practice, a form of computer-assisted instruction in which the computer is used as a means for practice and provides little or no information.

Drinker respirator, an airtight respirator consisting of a metal tank that encloses the entire body, except for the head. Used for long-term therapy, it alternates positive and negative air pressure within the tank, providing artificial respiration by contracting and expanding the walls of the chest. Also called **artificial lung, iron lung.**

drip, **1.** the process of a liquid or moisture forming and falling in drops. Kinds of drip are **nasal drip** and **postnasal drip.** **2.** the slow but continuous infusion of a liquid into the body, as into the stomach or a vein. **3.** to infuse a liquid continuously into the body.

drip system, (in intravenous therapy) an apparatus for delivering specific volumes of intravenous solutions within predetermined periods of time and at a specific flow rate. See also **macrodrip, microdrip.**

Drisdol, a trademark for vitamin D_2 (ergocalciferol).

drive, an electromechanic device that holds a secondary-storage medium and allows for the transfer of data to and from the computer, as a disk drive or tape drive.

Drixoral, a trademark for a fixed-combination drug containing an antihistamine (dexbrompheniramine maleate) and a vasoconstrictor and bronchodilator (pseudoephedrine sulfate), used for the relief of congestion of the upper respiratory tract.

drocode. See **dihydrocodeine.**

Drolban, a trademark for a synthetic androgen (dromostanolone propionate), which is used in cancer therapy.

-drome, a combining form meaning 'that which runs' in a specified way: *dermadrome, heterodrome, syndrome.*

dromo-, a combining form meaning 'pertaining to running or conduction': *dromonania, dromophobic, dromotropic.*

dromostanolone propionate, a synthetic androgen.

■ INDICATION: It is prescribed for female breast cancer.

■ CONTRAINDICATIONS: It is not used for male breast cancer or in premenopausal women.

■ ADVERSE EFFECTS: Among the more serious adverse reactions are masculinization, edema, and hypercalcemia.

droperidol /drəper′ədol/, an antipsychotic, sedative drug of the butyrophenone group, used most commonly with a narcotic analgesic (fentanyl) in neuroleptanesthesia.

drop foot, a condition in which the foot is plantarflexed and cannot voluntarily be dorsiflexed. It is usually caused by damage to the peroneal nerve.

droplet infection, an infection acquired by the inhalation of pathogenic microorganisms suspended in particles of liquid exhaled, sneezed, or coughed by another infected person or animal. Some diseases spread by droplets are chickenpox, common cold, influenza, measles, and mumps.

dropped foot. See **footdrop.**

dropsy. See **hydrops.**

Drosophila /drōsof′ilə/, a genus of fly, including *Drosophila melanogaster,* the Mediterranean fruit fly, useful in genetic experiments because of the large chromosomes found in its salivary glands and its sensitivity to environmental effects, as exposure to radiation.

drowning, asphyxiation because of submersion in a liquid. See also **near drowning.**

drug, **1.** also called **medicine.** any substance taken by mouth, injected into a muscle, the skin, a blood vessel, or a cavity of the body, or applied topically to treat or prevent a disease or condition. **2.** *informal.* a narcotic substance.

drug abuse, the use of a drug for a nontherapeutic effect, especially one for which it was not prescribed or intended. Some of the most commonly abused drugs are alcohol, amphetamines, barbiturates, cocaine, methaqualone, and opium alkaloids. Drug abuse may lead to organ damage, addiction, and disturbed patterns of behavior. Some illicit drugs, as heroin, lysergic acid diethylamide (LSD), and phencylidine hydrochloride (PCP), have no recognized therapeutic effect in humans. Use of these drugs often incurs criminal penalty in addition to the potential for physical, social, and psychologic harm. See also **drug addiction.**

drug action, the means by which a drug exerts a desired effect. Drugs are usually classified by their actions; for example, a vasodilator, prescribed to decrease the blood pressure, acts by dilating the blood vessels.

drug addiction, a condition characterized by an overwhelming desire to continue taking a drug to which one has become habituated through repeated consumption because it produces a particular effect, usually an alteration of mental activity, attitude, or outlook. Addiction is usually accompanied by a compulsion to obtain the drug, a tendency to increase the dose, a psychologic or physical dependence, and detrimental consequences for the individual and society. Common addictive drugs are barbiturates, alcohol, and morphine and other narcotics, especially heroin, which has slightly greater euphorigenic properties than other opium derivatives. See also **alcoholism, drug abuse.**

drug administration, the giving by a nurse or other authorized person of a single dose of a drug to a patient.

drug allergy, hypersensitivity to a pharmacologic agent, manifested by reactions ranging from a mild rash to anaphylactic shock, depending on the individual, the allergen, and the dose. Allergic responses are frequently produced by contrast media containing iodine, aspirin, phenylbutazone, novobiocin, penicillin, and other antibiotics, but they may be caused by any drug.

drug dependence, a psychologic craving for or a physiologic reliance on a chemical agent, resulting from habituation, abuse, or addiction. See also **drug abuse, drug addiction.**

drug dispensing, the preparation, packaging, labeling, record keeping, and transfer of a prescription drug to a patient or an intermediary, such as a nurse, who is responsible for administration of the drug.

drug-drug interaction, a modification of the effect of a drug when administered with another drug. The effect may be an increase or a decrease in the action of either substance, or it may be an adverse effect that is not normally associated with either drug. The particular interaction may be the result of a chemical-physical incompatibility of the two drugs or a change in the rate of absorption or the quantity absorbed in the body, the binding ability of either drug, or an alteration in the ability of receptor sites and cell membranes to bind either drug.

Drug Enforcement Agency (DEA), an agency of the Drug Enforcement Administration of the federal government, empowered to enforce regulations regarding the import or export of narcotic drugs and certain other substances or the traffic of these substances across state lines.

drug eruption, any skin lesion or rash caused by a drug taken internally. Also called **dermatitis medicamentosa.** See also **fixed drug eruption.**

drug fever, a fever caused by the pharmacologic action of a medication, its thermoregulatory action, a local complication of parenteral administration, or, most commonly, an immunologic reaction mediated by drug-induced antibodies. The onset of fever occurs usually between 7 and 10 days after the medication is begun; a return to normal is seen within 2 days of the discontinuance of the drug. The correct diagnosis of drug fever and the discontinuance of the medication are important to prevent further adverse reactions and to avoid possibly dangerous and expensive diagnostic and therapeutic interventions. See also **Jarisch-Herxheimer reaction.**

drug monograph, a statement that specifies the kinds and amounts of ingredients a drug or class of drugs may contain, the directions for the drug's use, the conditions in which it may be used, and contraindications for its use.

dry catarrh, a dry cough, accompanied by almost no expectoration that occurs in severe coughing spells. It is associated with asthma and emphysema in older people.

dry dressing, a plain dressing containing no medication, applied directly to an incision or a wound to prevent contamination or trauma or to absorb secretions.

dry gangrene. See **gangrene.**

dry labor, *informal.* labor in which the amniotic fluid has already escaped.

dry rale, an abnormal chest sound produced by air passing through a constricted bronchial tube. Compare **amphoric breath sound, atelectatic rale, bubbling rale.**

Drysdale's corpuscle /drīz′dālz/, one of a number of transparent cells in the fluid of some ovarian cysts. Also called **Bennet's small corpuscle.**

dry skin, epidermis lacking moisture or sebum, often characterized by a pattern of fine lines, scaling, and itching. Causes include too frequent bathing, low humidity, decreased production of sebum in aging skin, and ichthyosis. Treatment includes decreased frequency of bathing, increased humidity, bath oils, emollients such as lanolin and glycerine, and hydrophilic ointments. Also called **xerosis** /zērō′sis/.

dry tooth socket, an inflamed condition of a tooth socket (alveolus) after extraction. Normally, a blood clot forms over the alveolar bone at the base of the tooth socket after an extraction. If the clot fails to form properly or becomes dislodged, the bone tissue is exposed to the environment and can become infected, a usually painful condition requiring analgesics and sedatives in addition to treatment to cure the infection.

Dryvax, a trademark for an active immunizing agent (smallpox vaccine).

DSM*,** abbreviation for ***Diagnostic and Statistical Manual of Mental Disorders.

D.S.N., abbreviation for *Doctor of Science in Nursing.*

DSR, abbreviation for **dynamic spatial reconstructor.**

DT, abbreviation for **diphtheria and tetanus toxoids.**

dTc, abbreviation for **d-tubocurarine.**

DTIC-Dome, a trademark for an antineoplastic (dacarbazine).

DTR, abbreviation for **deep tendon reflex.**

DTs, abbreviation for **delirium tremens.**

DUB, **1.** abbreviaiton for **dysfunctional uterine bleeding.** **2.** a genetically determined human blood factor that is associated with immunity to certain diseases.

Dubin-Johnson syndrome /do͞o′binjon′sən/, a rare, chronic, hereditary hyperbilirubinemia, characterized by nonhemolytic jaundice, abnormal liver pigmentation, and abnormal function of the gallbladder. It is caused by an inability of the liver to excrete several organic anions. See also **hyperbilirubinemia of the newborn, Rotor syndrome.**

Dubowitz assessment, a system of estimating the gestational age of a newborn child according to such factors as posture, ankle dorsiflexion, and arm and leg recoil.

Duchenne-Erb paralysis. See **Erb's palsy.**

Duchenne's disease /do͞oshenz′/, a series of three different neurologic conditions: **spinal muscular atrophy, bulbar paralysis,** and **tabes dorsalis.** See also **muscular dystrophy.**

Duchenne's muscular dystrophy, an abnormal congenital condition characterized by progressive symmetric wasting of the leg and pelvic muscles. This disease affects predominantly males and accounts for 50% of all muscular dystrophy diseases. It is an X-linked recessive disease that appears insidiously between 3 and 5 years of age and spreads from the leg and pelvic muscles to the involuntary muscles. Associated muscle weakness produces a waddling gait and pronounced lordosis. Muscles rapidly deteriorate, and calf muscles become firm and enlarged from fatty deposits. Affected children develop contractures, have difficulty climbing stairs, often stumble and fall, and display wing scapulae when they raise their arms. Such persons are usually confined to wheelchairs by 12 years of age, and progressive weakening of cardiac muscle causes tachycardia and pulmonary problems. There is no correlation between the degree of muscular dystrophy and the severity of cardiac problems, but the electrocardiogram is abnormal in 40% to 90% of the affected patients. The characteristic clinical finding is tachycardia persisting during sleep and often associated with arrhythmia and with cardiac enlargement. Certain distinctive electrocardiographic abnormalities, as tall R waves in the right precordial leads and deep Q waves in the limb leads, may be present in affected family members and also in asymptomatic maternal carriers. The patients affected may also have cardiac murmurs, faint heart sounds, and chest pain and may suffer arrhythmias or infections that produce overt heart failure. Such complications, especially in the later stages of this disease, can cause sudden death. Duchenne's muscular dystrophy usually results in death within 10 to 15 years of the onset of symptoms. Also called **pseudohypertrophic muscular dystrophy.**

■ OBSERVATIONS: Abnormal cardiac signs may precede recognition of Duchenne's muscular dystrophy and may aid diagnosis based on other abnormalities of gait and voluntary movement. Typical medical and family history may also suggest the disease. Confirming diagnosis is usually aided by a muscle biopsy showing fat and connective tissue deposits. Electromyography is often used to help rule out neurogenic muscle atrophy by demonstrating viable muscle innervation. Laboratory results that indicate the disease include increased urinary creatinine excretion and increased serum levels of creatinine phosphokinase (CPK), lactic dehydrogenase (LDH), and transaminase. The CPK level often rises before muscular weakness becomes severe.

■ INTERVENTION: There is no successful treatment of the disease. Orthopedic appliances, exercise, physical therapy, and surgery to correct contractures can help preserve mobility. Doctors and nurses often caution family members who are carriers about the risk of transmitting this disease. No form of muscular dystrophy can be detected by amniocentesis, but this procedure can determine the sex of the fetus and is often recommended for carriers who are pregnant.

■ NURSING CONSIDERATIONS: Nursing care involves the psychologic support of the patient and the family and the encouragement of the patient to avoid long periods of bed rest and inactivity to assure maximum physical activity. Splints, braces, grab bars, and overhead slings help the patient exercise. A wheelchair helps preserve mobility. Other devices that can increase comfort and help prevent footdrop include footboards, high-topped sneakers, and foot cradles. Nurses encourage the patient to maintain peer relationships and often encourage the parents to keep the child in school as long as possible. Nurses provide emotional support for the parents and the patient in coping with continuing changes in the patient's body, and they commonly refer parents to the Muscular Dystrophy Association for futher support and assistance.

duck embryo vaccine. See **rabies vaccine.**

duck walk. See **metatarsus valgus.**

duct, a narrow tubular structure, especially one through which material is secreted or excreted.

duct carcinoma, a neoplasm developed from the epithelium of ducts, especially in the breast or pancreas.

ductless gland, a gland lacking an excretory duct, as an endocrine gland, which secretes hormones into blood or lymph.

duct of Rivinus /rivē′nəs/, one of the minor sublingual ducts. Compare **Bartholin's duct.**

duct of Wirsung. See **pancreatic duct.**

ductus /duk′təs/, *pl.* **ductus** /duk′to͞os/, a duct.

ductus arteriosus, a vascular channel in the fetus that joins the pulmonary artery directly to the descending aorta.

ductus deferens. See **vas deferens.**

ductus epididymidis, a tube into which the efferent ductules of the testes empty.

ductus venosus, the vascular channel in the fetus passing through the liver and joining the umbilical vein with the inferior vena cava. Before birth, it carries highly oxygenated blood from the placenta to the fetal circulation. It closes shortly after birth as pulmonary circulation is established and as the vessels in the umbilical cord collapse and become occluded. See also **ductus arteriosus, foramen ovale.**

Duke diet. See **rice diet.**

Dulcolax, a trademark for a laxative (bisacodyl).

dumb terminal, a computer terminal that serves as an input or output device only and is incapable of performing any data-processing functions by itself. Compare **intelligent terminal.**

dumdum fever. See **kala-azar.**

dump, **1.** to preserve the contents of one computer memory by transferring it into another memory. **2.** to print out the contents of a computer memory or other computer-storage medium. **3.** the printout resulting from such an operation.

dumping syndrome, the combination of profuse sweating, nausea, dizziness, and weakness experienced by patients who have had a subtotal gastrectomy. Symptoms are felt soon after eating, when the contents of the stomach empty too rapidly into the duodenum. A high-protein, high-calorie diet, with small meals taken frequently, should prevent discomfort and ensure adequate nutrition. See also **gastrectomy.**

Duncan's mechanism, a technique for delivery of the placenta with the maternal rather than the fetal surface presenting.

Dunlop skeletal traction, an orthopedic mechanism that helps immobilize the upper limb in the treatment of the contracture or the supracondylar fracture of the elbow. The mechanism employs a system of traction weights, pulleys, and ropes. The system is attached to the bone involved with a pin or wire; it may be further secured by adhesive or nonadhesive skin-traction components. Dunlop skeletal traction is usually applied unilaterally but may also be applied bilaterally. Compare **Dunlop skin traction.**

Dunlop skin traction, an orthopedic mechanism that helps immobilize the upper limb in the treatment of contracture and supracondylar fracture of the elbow. The mechanism employs a system of traction weights, pulleys, and ropes, usually applied unilaterally but sometimes bilaterally. Dunlop skin traction may be applied as adhesive skin traction or nonadhesive skin traction. Compare **Dunlop skeletal traction.**

duodenal /do͞o′ədē′nəl/, of or pertaining to the duodenum.

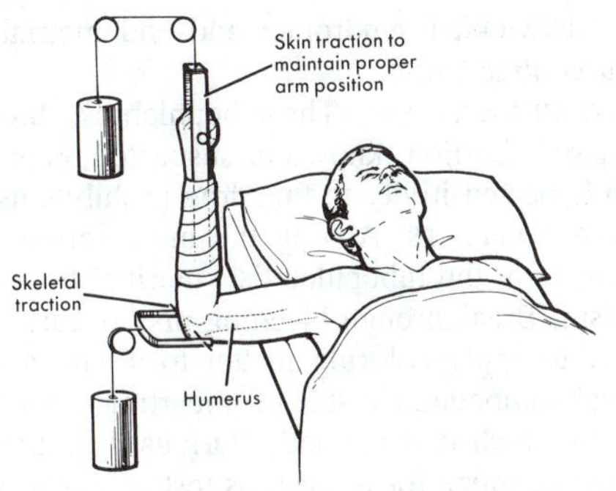

Dunlop skeletal traction

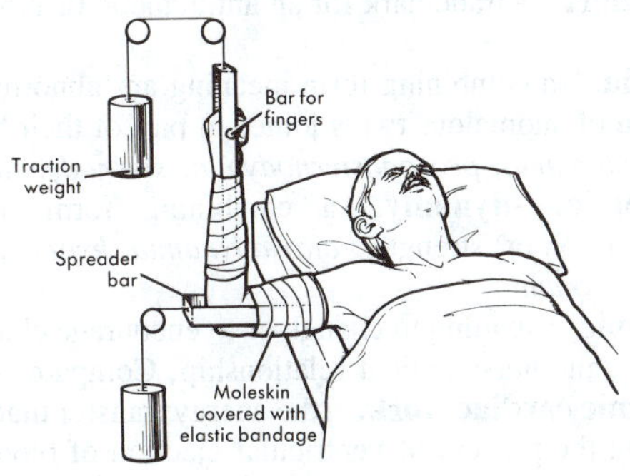

Dunlop skin traction

duodenal ulcer, an ulcer in the duodenum, the most common type of peptic ulcer. See also **peptic ulcer.**

duodeno-, a combining form meaning 'pertaining to the duodenum': *duodenocolic, duodenohepatic, duodenostomy.*

duodenoscope /do͞o′ədē′nəskōp′/, an endoscopic instrument, usually fiberoptic, for the visual examination of the duodenum.

duodenoscopy /do͞o′ədənos′kəpē/, the visual examination of the duodenum by means of an endoscope.

duodenum /do͞o′ədē′nəm, do͞o•od′inəm/, *pl.* **duodena, duodenums,** the shortest, widest, and most fixed portion of the small intestine, taking an almost circular course from the pyloric valve of the stomach so that its termination is close to its starting point. It is about 25 cm long and is divided into superior, descending, horizontal, and ascending portions. The superior portion is about 6 cm long and extends from the pylorus to the neck of the gallbladder. The descending portion is about 8 cm long and extends from the neck of the gallbladder at the level of the first lumbar vertebra to the cranial border of the fourth lumbar vertebra. The horizontal portion is about 7 cm long and passes from right to left, from the level of the fourth lumbar vertebra to the diaphragm. The ascending portion is about 4 cm long and rises on the left side of the aorta to the level of the second lumbar vertebra, turning ventrally to become the jejunum at the duodenojejunal flexure. Compare **jejunum, ileum.**

dup, (in cytogenetics) abbreviation for **duplication.**

duplex inheritance. See **amphigenous inheritance.**

duplex transmission, the passage of a neural impulse in both directions along a nerve fiber.

Dupuytren's contracture /dYpY•itraNs′, dēpē•itranz′/, a progressive, painless thickening and tightening of subcutaneous tissue of the palm, causing the fourth and fifth fingers to bend into the palm and resist extension. Tendons and nerves are not involved. Although the condition begins in one hand, both will become symmetrically affected. Of unknown cause, it is most frequent in middle-aged males. Early surgical removal of the excess fibrous tissue under general anesthesia will restore full use of the hand. An incision is made into the palm, and the thickened tissue is excised carefully to avoid injury to adjacent ligaments.

Dupuytren's fracture. See **Galeazzi's fracture.**

Durabolin, a trademark for an anabolic steroid (nandrolone phenpropionate).

dura mater /do͝o′rə mā′tər, dyo͝o′rə/, the outermost and most fibrous of the three membranes surrounding the brain and spinal cord. The **dura mater encephali** covers the brain, and the **dura mater spinalis** covers the cord. See also **meninges.**

Duranest, a trademark for a local anesthetic (etidocaine hydrochloride).

duress, (in law) an action compelling another person to do what otherwise would not be done voluntarily. A consent form signed under duress is not valid.

dust, any fine, particulate, dry matter. Kinds of dust are **inorganic dust** and **organic dust.**

dust fever. See **brucellosis.**

Dutton's relapsing fever, an infection caused by a spirochete, *Borrelia duttonii,* which is transmitted by a soft tick, *Ornithodoros moubata,* found in human dwellings in tropic Africa. The spirochete enters the lesion through the tick bite, characteristically producing a high fever, chills, rapid heartbeat, headache, joint and muscle pain, vomiting, and neurologic disorders. The symptoms recur in a pattern of remissions and peaks of fever and other effects. The infection is spread through the community as ticks bite infected people, thereby acquiring the spirochete for inoculation in others. Treatment with tetracycline is usually effective in curing the infection. Also called **African relapsing fever, Dutton's disease.** See also **relapsing fever.**

duty, (in law) an obligation owed by one party to another. Duty may be established by statute or other legal process, as by contract or oath supported by statute, or it may be voluntarily undertaken. Every person has a duty of care to all other people to avoid causing harm or injury by negligence.

Duverney's fracture /do͞o′vərnāz′/, fracture of the ilium just below the anterior superior spine.

dv/dt, (in cardiology) the rate of change of voltage with respect to time.

dwarf, **1.** also called **nanus.** an abnormally short, undersized person, especially one whose bodily parts are not proportional. Kinds of dwarfs include **achondroplastic dwarf, Amsterdam dwarf, asexual dwarf, ateliotic dwarf, bird-headed dwarf, Brissaud's dwarf, cretin dwarf, diastrophic dwarf, phocomelic dwarf, pituitary dwarf, primordial dwarf, rachitic dwarf, renal dwarf, Russell dwarf, sexual dwarf, Silver dwarf,** and **thanatophoric dwarf. 2.** to prevent or retard normal growth.

dwarfism, the abnormal underdevelopment of the body, characterized predominantly by extreme shortness of stature, although the condition is associated with numerous other defects and may involve varying degrees of mental retardation. Dwarfism has multiple causes, including genetic defects, endocrine dysfunction involving either the pituitary or thyroid glands, chronic diseases, as rickets, renal failure, and intestinal malabsorption defects, and psychosocial stress, as in the maternal deprivation syndrome. See also **dwarf.**

dwindles, *informal.* a condition of physical deterioration involving several systems of the body, usually in an elderly person.

Dwyer cable instrumentation, one of the two most common surgical methods for correcting the spinal curvature associated with scoliosis. The Dwyer cable method uses a mechanic device that assists in obtaining the curvature correction. The device is inserted to assist in maintaining the corrected curvature while the fusion heals; it is not usually removed unless there is postoperative indication of displacement or a pattern of associated symptoms. Dwyer cable instrumentation involves surgical intervention through the pulmonary cavity and the rib cage and is accompanied by a relatively greater surgical risk than a posterior approach. It is often inadequate to correct the spinal curvature involved and must frequently be followed several weeks later by a posterior spinal fusion.

Dy, symbol for **dysprosium.**

dyad /dī′ad/, (in genetics) one of the paired homologous chromosomes, consisting of two chromatids, which result from the division of a tetrad in the first meiotic division of gametogenesis. **–dyadic,** *adj.*

dyadic interpersonal communication, a process in which two people interact face to face as senders and receivers, as in a conversation.

Dyazide, a trademark for a fixed-combination drug containing two diuretic agents (triamterene and hydrochlorothiazide).

Dyclone, a trademark for a local anesthetic (dyclonine hydrochloride).

dyclonine hydrochloride, a local anesthetic, with bactericidal and fungicidal properties, for oral pain, pruritis, insect bites, and minor skin burns and injuries.

dydrogesterone /dī′drəjes′tərōn/, a synthetic oral progestin.

■ INDICATIONS: It may be prescribed in the treatment of abnormal uterine bleeding, menopausal vasomotor symptoms, pickwickian syndrome, and endometrial cancer, and for contraception.

■ CONTRAINDICATIONS: Thrombophlebitis, breast cancer, missed abortion, known or suspected pregnancy, or known hypersensitivity to this drug prohibits its use.

■ ADVERSE EFFECTS: Among the more serious adverse reactions are thrombophlebitis, uterine fibroma, and embolism. Breakthrough bleeding may occur.

dye, **1.** to apply coloring matter to a substance. **2.** a chemical compound capable of imparting color to a substance to which it is applied. Various dyes are used in medicine as stains for tissues, as test reagents, as therapeutic agents, and to color pharmaceutic preparations.

Dymelor, a trademark for an antidiabetic (acetohexamide).

-dymia, a combining form meaning an 'abnormal condition of anomalous twins joined at part of their bodies': *cephalodymia, prosoposternodymia, sternodymia.*

-dynamia, -dynamy, a combining form meaning '(condition of) strength': *ataxiadynamia, hyperdynamia, plastodynamia.*

dynamic, tending to change or to encourage change, as a dynamic nurse-patient relationship. Compare **static.**

dynamic cardiac work, the energy transfer that occurs during the process of ventricular ejection of blood.

dynamic nurse-patient relationship, a conceptual framework in which the interpersonal aspects of the nurse-patient relationship are analyzed. The relationship is affected by many factors. Elements in the process include the behavior of the patient, the reaction of the nurse, and the actions of the nurse that are intended to aid the patient. Also examined are the means for validating nurses' perceptions and interpretations and for evaluating the effects of the nursing actions taken.

dynamic psychiatry, the study of motivational, emotional, and biologic factors as determinants of human behavior.

dynamic response, the accuracy with which a physiologic monitoring system, as an electrocardiograph, will simulate the actual event being recorded.

dynamic spatial reconstructor (DSR), a kind of roentgenographic machine used in research permitting moving three-dimensional images of human organs to be examined visually and from any direction.

dynamo-, a combining form meaning 'pertaining to power or strength': *dynamogenesis, dynamometer, dynamophore.*

dynamometer /dī′nəmom′ətər/, a device for measuring the amount of energy expended in the contraction of a muscle or a group of muscles, as a squeeze dynamometer, which measures the force of the hand when squeezing the device.

-dynamy. See **-dynamia.**

Dynapen, a trademark for an antibacterial (dicloxacillin sodium).

dyphylline, a bronchodilator.

■ INDICATIONS: It is prescribed in the treatment of

bronchospasm in acute bronchial asthma, bronchitis, and emphysema.

■ CONTRAINDICATIONS: It is used with caution in patients with peptic ulcer or cardiovascular disease. Known hypersensitivity to this or to other xanthines prohibits its use.

■ ADVERSE EFFECTS: Among the more serious adverse reactions are GI distress, dizziness, tachycardia, headache, and palpitations.

Dyrenium, a trademark for a diuretic (triamterene).

dys-, a combining form meaning 'bad, painful, disordered': *dysadrenia, dysbolism, dysmnesia.*

dysadrenia, abnormal adrenal function characterized by decreased production of hormones, as in hypoadrenalism or hypoadrenocorticism, or by increased secretion of the products of the gland, as in hyperadrenalism or hyperadrenocorticism. Also called **dysadrenalism.**

dysarthria /disär′thrē·ə/, difficult, poorly articulated speech, resulting from interference in the control over the muscles of speech, usually because of damage to a central or peripheral motor nerve.

dyscholia /diskō′lē·ə/, any abnormal condition of the bile, either regarding the quantity secreted or the condition of the constituents.

dyschondroplasia. See **enchondromatosis.**

dyschroic film fault, a defect in a radiograph that appears as a pinkish coloration when the film is viewed by transmitted light and as a green coloration when the film is viewed by reflected light. It is usually caused by incomplete fixation of the film or an overused fixing solution with a depleted acid concentration.

dyscrasia /diskrā′zhə/, an abnormal blood or bone marrow condition, as leukemia, aplastic anemia, or Rh incompatibility.

dyscrasic fracture /diskraz′ik/, any fracture caused by the weakening of a specific bone as a result of a debilitating disease.

dysentery /dis′inter′ē/, an inflammation of the intestine, especially of the colon, that may be caused by chemical irritants, bacteria, protozoa, or parasites. It is characterized by frequent and bloody stools, abdominal pain, and tenesmus. Dysentery is common in underdeveloped areas of the world and in times of disaster and social disorganization when sanitary living conditions, clean food, and safe water are not available. See also **amebic dysentery, shigellosis.**

dysfunctional, (of a body organ or system) unable to function normally. –**dysfunction,** *n.*

dysfunctional uterine bleeding (DUB), uterine bleeding as a result of endocrine imbalance rather than a pathologic condition.

dysgenesis /disjen′əsis/, **1.** also called **dysgenesia.** defective or abnormal formation of an organ or part, primarily during embryonic development. **2.** impairment or loss of the ability to procreate. A kind of dysgenesis is **gonadal dysgenesis.** Compare **agenesis.** –**dysgenic,** *adj.*

dysgenics /disjen′iks/, the study of those factors or situations that are genetically detrimental to the future of a race or species. Compare **eugenics.**

dysgenitalism /disjen′itəliz′əm/, any condition involving the abnormal development of the genital organs.

dysgerminoma, *pl.* **dysgerminomas, dysgerminomata,** a rare malignant tumor of the ovary, believed to arise from the undifferentiated germ cells of the embryonic gonad. It is found in young women and is histologically identical to seminoma. Also called **embryoma of the ovary, ovarian seminoma.**

dysgnathic anomaly /disnath′ik/, (in dentistry) an abnormality that extends beyond the teeth, affecting the maxilla, the mandible, or both.

dysgraphia /disgraf′ē·ə/, an impairment of the ability to write, caused by a pathologic disorder. Compare **agraphia.** See also **learning disability.** –**dysgraphic,** *adj.*

dyshidrosis /dis′hidrō′sis, dis′hī-/, a condition in which abnormal sweating occurs. Kinds of dyshidrosis are **hyperhidrosis** and **miliaria.** Also called **pompholyx.** Compare **anhidrosis.** –**dyshidrotic,** *adj.*

dyskeratosis /dis′kerətō′sis/, an abnormal or premature keratinization of epithelial cells.

dyskinesia /dis′kinē′zhə/, an impairment of the ability to execute voluntary movements. –**dyskinetic** /-et′ik/, *adj.*

dyslexia /dislek′sē·ə/, an impairment of the ability to read, as a result of a variety of pathologic conditions, some of which are associated with the central nervous system. Dyslexic persons often reverse letters and words, cannot adequately distinguish the letter sequences in written words, and have difficulty determining left from right. Some reading experts doubt that dyslexia is a pathologic disorder and believe the condition represents a combination of reading problems, each of which should be isolated by specific tests. The problems cited by these authorities are poor vision, impaired hearing, emotional immaturity, lack of physical development, psychic stress, and inadequate reading instruction. Compare **alexia.** –**dyslexic,** *adj.*

dysmaturity, **1.** the failure of an organism to develop, ripen, or otherwise achieve maturity in structure or function. **2.** the condition of a fetus or newborn being abnormally small or large for its age of gestation. Kinds of dysmaturity are **small for gestational age** and **large for gestational age.** Compare **postmature, premature.** –**dysmature,** *adj.*

dysmelia /dismē′lyə/, an abnormal congenital condition characterized by missing or shortened extremities of the body and associated with abnormalities of the spine in some individuals. It is caused by abnormal metabolism during the development of the embryonic limbs. See also **phocomelia.**

dysmenorrhea /dis′menərē′ə/, pain associated with menstruation. Primary dysmenorrhea is menstrual pain that results from factors intrinsic to the uterus and the process of menstruation. It is extremely common, occurring at least occasionally in almost all women. If the painful episode is mild and brief, it is considered functional and normal and requires no treatment. In approximately 10% of women, dysmenorrhea is sufficiently severe to cause episodes of partial or total disability. The cause in most cases is poorly understood; various anatomic, neurohormonal, and psychosomatic abnormalities have been suggested. Pain occurs typically in the lower abdomen or back and is crampy, coming in successive waves—apparently in conjunction with intense uterine contractions and slight cervical dilatation. Pain usually begins just before, or at the onset of, menstrual flow and lasts from a few hours to 1 day or more; but it may persist through the entire period in a few women. Pain is frequently associated with nausea, vomiting, and frequent bowel movements with intestinal cramping. Dizziness, fainting, pallor, and obvious distress may also be observed. Treatment with an antiprostaglandin provides relief for many women if begun 1 to 3 days premenstrually and continued through the first day of the menses. Oral contraceptive steroids are also effective for many women and are taken through the full monthly cycle. Potent analgesics or narcotics may be required by a few women. Secondary dysmenorrhea is menstrual pain that occurs secondary to specific pelvic abnormalities, as endometriosis, adenomyosis, chronic pelvic infection, chronic pelvic congestion, or degenerating fibroid tumors. Typically, the pain begins earlier in the cycle and lasts longer than the pain of primary dysmenorrhea. Painful bowel or bladder function may accompany the condition, depending on the location of the specific lesions. Diagnosis of the chief cause is made by pelvic examination, ultrasonography, laparoscopy, or laparotomy. Treatment, most often surgical, is directed at the specific organic disease involved.

dysmetria /dismē′trē•ə/, an abnormal condition that prevents the affected individual from properly measuring distances associated with muscular acts and from controlling muscular action. See also **hypermetria, hypometria.**

dysmorphophobia /dis′môrfō-/, **1.** a fundamental delusion of body image. **2.** the morbid fear of deformity.

dysostosis /dis′ostō′sis/, an abnormal condition characterized by defective ossification, especially by defects in the normal ossification of fetal cartilages. Kinds of dysostoses include **cleidocranial dysostosis, craniofacial dysostosis, mandibulofacial dysostosis, metaphyseal dysostosis,** and **Nager's acrofacial dysostosis.**

dyspareunia /dis′pərо͞o′nē•ə/, an abnormal condition of women, in which sexual intercourse is accompanied by pain. The pain may result from abnormal conditions of the genitalia, dysfunctional psychophysiologic reaction to sexual union, forcible coition, or incomplete sexual arousal. See also **vaginismus.**

Dyspas, a trademark for an anticholinergic (dicyclomine hydrochloride).

dyspepsia /dispep′sē•ə/, a vague feeling of epigastric discomfort, felt after eating. There is an uncomfortable feeling of fullness, heartburn, bloating, and nausea. Dyspepsia is not a distinct condition, but it may be a sign of underlying intestinal disorder, as peptic ulcer, gallbladder disease, or chronic appendicitis. **–dyspeptic,** *adj.*

dysphagia /disfā′jē•ə/, difficulty in swallowing, commonly associated with obstructive or motor disorders of the esophagus. Patients with obstructive disorders like esophageal tumor or lower esophageal ring are unable to swallow solids but can tolerate liquids. Persons with motor disorders, as achalasia, are unable to swallow solids or liquids. Diagnosis of the underlying condition is made through barium studies, the observed clinical signs, and evaluation of the patient's symptoms. See also **achalasia, aphagia, corkscrew esophagus.**

dysphagia lusoria, an abnormal condition, characterized by difficulty in swallowing, caused by the compression of the esophagus from an anomalous right subclavian artery that arises from the descending aorta and courses behind or in front of the esophagus. Compare **contractile ring dysphagia, vallecular dysphagia.**

dysphasia /disfā′zhə/, an impairment of speech, not as severe as aphasia, usually the result of an injury to the speech area in the cerebral cortex of the brain. It may follow a stroke or brain tumor and may be accompanied by other language disorders, as dysgraphia. Compare **dysarthria.**

-dysplasia, a combining form meaning '(condition of) abnormal development': *chondrodysplasia, epidermodysplasia, osteomyelodysplasia.*

dyspnea /dispnē′ə/, a shortness of breath or a difficulty in breathing that may be caused by certain heart conditions, strenuous exercise, or anxiety. Compare **hyperpnea. –dyspneal, dyspneic,** *adj.*

dyspraxia /disprak′sē•ə/, a partial loss of the ability to perform skilled, coordinated movements in the absence of any associated defect in motor or sensory functions. See also **apraxia.**

dysprosium (Dy), a rare-earth metallic element. Its atomic number is 66; its atomic weight is 162.50. Radioactive isotopes of dysprosium are used in radioisotope scanning, particularly in studies of the bones and joints.

dysproteinemia /disprō′tēnē′mē•ə/, an abnormality of the protein content of the blood, usually involving the immunoglobulins.

dysraphia /disrā′fē•ə/, failure of a raphe to fuse completely, as in incomplete closure of the neural tube. Also called **status dysraphicus.**

dysreflexia /dis′riflek′sē•ə/, an abnormal neuromuscular condition characterized by abnormal motor response to stimuli that normally produce a specific response. **–dysreflexic,** *adj.*

dysrhythmia /disrith′mē•ə/, any disturbance or abnormality in a normal rhythmic pattern, specifically, irregularity in the brain waves or cadence of speech. Compare **arrhythmia.**

dyssebacea /disibā′shē•ə/, a skin condition characterized by red, scaly, greasy patches on the nose, eyelids, scrotum, and labia. It results from a deficiency of vitamin B_2 and is most commonly associated with chronic alcoholism, liver disease, chronic diarrhea, and protein malnutrition. Also called *(informal)* **shark skin.**

dystocia /distō′shə/, pathologic or difficult labor, which may be caused by an obstruction or constriction of the birth passage or an abnormal size, shape, position, or condition of the fetus. See also **clinical pelvimetry, fetal contraction, presentation, x-ray pelvimetry.**

dystonia musculorum deformans /distō′nē·ə/, a rare abnormal condition characterized by intense, irregular torsion muscle spasms that contort the body. The muscles of the trunk, shoulder, and pelvis are commonly involved. This disease appears in several forms, generally classified as autosomal recessive or autosomal dominant. The cause of this disorder is not known; a biochemical dysfunction is suspected. The autosomal recessive form appears most often in Ashkenazic Jews and starts between 5 and 15 years of age, causing abnormalities of movement and speech. Muscle power and tone appear normal, but convulsive spasms make the involved muscles relatively useless. The autosomal recessive form of the disease commonly begins with intermittent spasmodic inversion of the foot, so that the affected individual has difficulty in placing the heel on the ground when walking and develops an odd, bowing gait. Lordosis and torsion of pelvis appear as the proximal muscles become more involved. Torticollis is often an early sign if the muscles of the neck and shoulder girdle are involved. The autosomal dominant form of the disease appears in early adult life, generally affects the axial musculature, and progresses more slowly than the autosomal recessive form. Some muscle-relaxing drugs, as the benzodiazepines, have been helpful in treating both forms of the condition. Mild cases have been successfully controlled for long periods with treatments that combine the use of muscle-relaxing drugs and psychotherapy. Some patients with this disease have also responded well for long periods to stereotactic thalamotomy, which, however, carries the risk of producing speech disorders.

dystrophic calcification, the pathologic accumulation of calcium salts in necrotic or degenerated tissues. Compare **metastatic calcification.**

dystrophy /dis′trəfē/, any abnormal condition caused by defective nutrition, often applied to a developmental change in muscles that does not involve the nervous system, as fatty degeneration associated with increased size but decreased strength. Also called **dystrophia.** **–dystrophic** /distrof′ik/, *adj.*

dysuria /disyŏŏr′ē·ə/, painful urination, usually the result of a bacterial infection or obstructive condition in the urinary tract. The patient complains of a burning sensation when passing urine, and laboratory examination may reveal the presence of blood, bacteria, or white blood cells. Dysuria is a symptom of such conditions as cystitis, urethritis, prostatitis, urinary tract tumors, and some gynecologic disorders. Compare **hematuria, pyuria.**

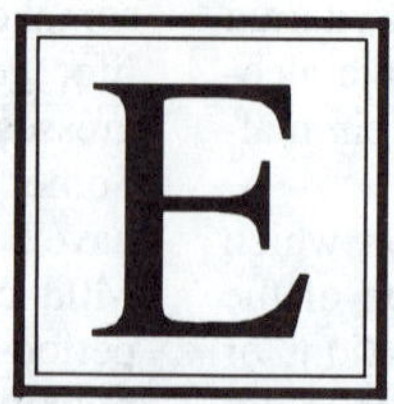

E, symbol for **expired gas.**

e-, a combining form meaning 'out from': *ebonation, egesta, emollient.*

E and GW, abbreviation for **Economic and General Welfare.**

ear, the organ of hearing, consisting of the internal, middle, and external ear. The external ear includes the skin-covered cartilaginous auricle visible on either side of the head and the portion of the external auditory canal that is outside the skull. Together they form a funnel that directs sound waves toward the eardrum, or tympanic membrane, which marks the boundary between the external ear and the air-filled middle ear. The middle ear contains three very small bones, the malleus, incus, and stapes, which transmit vibrations caused by sound waves reaching the tympanic membrane to the oval window of the inner ear. The leverage of the ossicles, or middle-ear bones, increases the intensity of sound vibrations by more than 25 dB. Because the inner ear is filled with fluid, the increased intensity helps compensate for the loss of signal normally caused by sound-wave reflection of the fluid. The inner ear contains two separate organs: the vestibular apparatus, which provides the sense of balance, and the organ of Corti, which receives vibrations from the middle ear and translates them into nerve impulses, which are again interpreted by brain cells as specific sounds.

earache, a pain in the ear, sensed as sharp, dull, burning, intermittent, or constant. The cause is not necessarily a disease of the ear, because infections and other disorders of the nose, oral cavity, larynx, and temporomandibular joint can produce referred pain in the ear. Also called **otalgia, otodynia.**

eardrop instillation, the instillation of a medicated solution into the external auditory canal of the ear. The patient is asked to turn the head to the side so that the ear being treated faces upward. The orifice is exposed, and the drops of medicine are directed toward the internal wall of the canal. The pinna is pulled up and back in a person over 3 years of age and down and back in a child younger than 2 or 3 years of age.

eardrops, a topical, liquid form of medication for the local treatment of various conditions of the ear, as inflammation or infection of the lining of the external auditory canal or impacted cerumen.

eardrum. See **tympanic membrane.**

Early and Periodic Screening Diagnosis and Treatment (EPSDT), a section of the Medicaid program that requires all states to maintain a program to determine the physical and mental defects of persons under 21 who are covered by the program and to provide short- and long-range treatment. See also **Medicaid.**

earth bath, the covering of a part of the body with warm sand or earth.

earwax. See **cerumen.**

East African Sleeping Sickness. See **Rhodesian trypanosomiasis.**

eastern equine encephalitis. See **equine encephalitis.**

Eaton agent pneumonia. See **mycoplasma pneumonia.**

Ebbecke's reaction. See **dermatographia.**

EBP, abbreviation for **epidural blood patch.**

EBV, abbreviation for **Epstein-Barr virus.**

ec-, a combining form meaning 'out of ': *ecbolic, eccephalosis, ecchondroma.*

eccentric implantation, (in embryology) the embedding of the blastocyst within a fold or recess of the uterine wall, which then closes off from the main cavity.

eccentricity, behavior that is regarded as odd or peculiar for a particular culture or community although not unusual enough to be considered pathologic.

eccentric jaw relation, (in dentistry) any jaw relation other than centric relation.

ecchondroma /ek′əndrō′mə/, a benign cartilaginous tumor that develops on the surface of a cartilage or under the periosteum of bone.

ecchondrosis. See **ecchondroma.**

ecchymosis /ek′imō′sis/, *pl.* **ecchymoses,** discoloration of an area of the skin or mucous membrane caused by the extravasation of blood into the subcutaneous tissues as a result of trauma to the underlying blood vessels or by fragility of the vessel walls. Also called **bruise.** Compare **contusion, petechiae.**

eccrine /ek′rin/, of or pertaining to a sweat gland that secretes outwardly through a duct to the surface of the skin. See also **exocrine.**

eccrine gland, one of two kinds of sweat glands in the corium of the skin. Such glands are unbranched, coiled, and tubular, and they are distributed throughout the dermal covering of the body. They promote cooling by evaporation of their secretion, which is clear, has a faint odor, and contains water, sodium chloride, and traces of albumin, urea, and other compounds. Compare **apocrine gland.**

eccyesis. See **ectopic pregnancy.**

ECF, 1. abbreviation for **extended care facility.** 2. abbreviation for **extracellular fluid.**

ECG, **1.** abbreviation for **electrocardiogram.** **2.** abbreviation for **electrocardiograph.**

-echia, a combining form meaning a 'condition of holding': *asynechia, blepharosynechia, synechia.*

echino-, a combining form meaning 'pertaining to spines, or spiny': *echinochroma, echinosis, echinostomiasis.*

echinococcosis /ekī'nōkokō'sis/, an infestation, usually of the liver, caused by the larval stage of a tapeworm of the genus *Echinococcus.* Dogs are the principal hosts of the adult worm; sheep, cattle, rodents, and deer are the natural intermediate hosts for the larvae. Humans, especially children, can become infested with larvae by ingesting eggs shed in the stool of infected dogs. The disease is most common in countries where domestic animals are raised with the help of dogs. Clinical manifestations and prognosis vary, depending upon the tissue invaded and the extent of infestation. Diagnosis is made by skin tests for sensitivity, serologic tests, radiologic evidence of cyst formation, and identification of larval cysts in infected tissue. Surgical excision of the cysts is the only treatment available. The disease can be prevented by avoiding contact with infected dogs, deworming pet animals, and preventing dogs from eating carcasses of infected intermediate hosts. Also called **hydatid disease, hydatidosis.** See also **cysticercosis, tapeworm infection.**

Echinococcus /ekī'nōkok'əs/, a genus of small tapeworms that infects primarily canines. See also **echinococcosis, hydatid cyst.**

echinocyte. See **burr cell.**

echo, *informal.* echoradiography.

echo beat, a reciprocal heart beat, or one that results from the return of an impulse to an atrium or ventricle to reactivate a contraction.

echocardiography /ek'ōkär'dē·og'rəfē/, a diagnostic procedure for studying the structure and motion of the heart. Ultrasonic waves directed through the heart are reflected backward, or echoed, when they pass from one type of tissue to another, as from cardiac muscle to blood. The sound waves are transmitted from and received by a transducer and are recorded on a strip chart. Major diagnostic uses include the detection of atrial tumors and pericardial effusion, the measurement of the ventricular septa and the ventricular chambers, and the determination of mitral valve motion abnormalities and congenital lesions. Also called **ultrasonic cardiography.** See also **phonocardiograph, ultrasonography.**

echoencephalogram /ek'ō·ensef'ələgram'/, a recording produced by an echoencephalograph.

echoencephalography /ek'ō·ensef'əlog'rəfē/, the use of ultrasound to study the intracranial structures of the brain. The technique is useful for showing ventricular dilatation and a major shift of midline structures as a result of an expanding lesion. See also **ultrasonography.** –**echoencephalographic,** *adj.*

echography. See **ultrasonography.**

echolalia /ek'ōlā'lyə/, **1.** also called **echophrasia, echo speech.** (in psychiatry) the automatic and meaningless repetition of another's words or phrases, especially as seen in schizophrenia. A kind of echolalia is **delayed echolalia. 2.** (in pediatrics) a baby's imitation or repetition of sounds or words produced by others. It occurs normally in early childhood development. –**echolalic,** *adj.*

echopraxia /ek'ōprak'sē·ə/, imitation or repetition of the body movements of another person, a behavior exhibited by some schizophrenic patients.

echoradiography /ek'ōrā'dē·og'rəfē/, a diagnostic procedure using ultrasonography and various devices for the visualization of internal structures of the body.

echo speech. See **echolalia.**

echothiophate iodide, an anticholinesterase used for ophthalmic purposes.

■ INDICATIONS: It is prescribed for chronic open-angle glaucoma and accommodative esotropia.

■ CONTRAINDICATIONS: Uveal inflammation, most types of angle-closure glaucoma, or known hypersensitivity to this drug prohibits its use.

■ ADVERSE EFFECTS: Among the more serious adverse reactions are retinal detachment, nonreversible cataract, lens opacity, activation of iritis or uveitis, and iris cysts.

echovirus /ek'ōvī'rəs/, a picornavirus associated with many clinical syndromes but not identified as the causative organism of any specific disease. There are many echoviruses; most are harmless. Bacterial or viral disease may be complicated by echovirus infection, as seen in aseptic meningitis accompanying some severe bacterial and viral infections.

eclampsia /iklamp'sē·ə/, the gravest form of toxemia of pregnancy, characterized by grand mal convulsion, coma, hypertension, proteinuria, and edema. The symptoms of impending convulsion often include anxiety, epigastric pain, headache, and blurred vision. The nurse is alert to persistently and extremely high blood pressure and to increasingly hyperactive deep-tendon reflexes, or clonus. Convulsions may be prevented by bed rest in a quiet, dimly lit room and parenteral administration of magnesium sulfate. The nurse attentively monitors the mother's general condition, blood pressure, and urine excretion, and the baby's heart rate. Treatment of a convulsion must include maintenance of the mother's airway, protection against self-injury, and administration of medication to check the convulsion and decrease the blood pressure. Once this is accomplished, delivery is indicated. Convulsions rarely occur in the puerperium. Complications of eclampsia include cerebral hemorrhage, pulmonary edema, renal failure, necrosis of the liver, abruptio placentae, hypofibrinogenemia, hemolysis, and retinal hemorrhages, sometimes with temporary blindness. Maternal mortality in eclampsia is 10%; fetal mortality is 25%. Eclampsia occurs in 0.2% of pregnancies. The cause is not known.

Eclipse, a trademark for a topical, fixed-combination drug containing an ultraviolet sunscreen (padimate).

-ecoia, a combining form meaning '(condition of the) sense of hearing': *bradyecoia, dysecoia, oxyecoia.*

ecologic chemistry, the study of chemical compounds synthesized by plants that influence ecology because of their toxic effects.

ecologic fallacy, a false assumption that the presence of a pathogenic factor and a disease in a population can be accepted as proof that the agent is the cause of the disease in a particular individual.

ecology, the study of the interaction between living organisms and the various influences of their environment.

econazole, an antifungal agent.

■ INDICATIONS: It is prescribed in the treatment of tinea and candidiasis.

■ CONTRAINDICATION: Known sensitivity to this drug prohibits its use.

■ ADVERSE EFFECTS: Among the most serious adverse reactions are local irritation and hypersensitivity of the skin.

Econochlor, a trademark for an antibacterial and antirickettsial (chloramphenicol).

Economic and General Welfare (E and GW), a unit of the American Nurses' Association that works to upgrade the salaries, benefits, and working conditions of nurses.

Econopred, a trademark for a glucocorticoid (prednisolone acetate).

ecosystem, the sum total of all living and nonliving things that support a chain of life events within a particular area.

ecstasy, an emotional state characterized by exultation, rapturous delight, or frenzy. Compare **euphoria, mania.** –**ecstatic,** *adj.*

ECT, abbreviation for **electroconvulsive therapy.**

-ectasia, -ectasis, -ectasy, a combining form meaning '(condition of) dilatation, extension, or distension of an organ': *esophagectasia, lymphectasia, pharyngectasia.*

ecthyma /ek'thimə/, a deep, burrowing form of impetigo characterized by large pustules, crusts, and ulcerations surrounded by erythema. Staphylococci and streptococci are the offending bacteria, and the skin of the legs is most frequently affected. Treatment includes vigorous cleanliness, compresses of cool Burow's solution to soften and remove crusts, and penicillin or erythromycin given systemically. Compare **folliculitis, impetigo.**

ecto-, a combining form meaning 'outside': *ectoblast, ectocolon, ectodermal.*

ectoderm, the outermost of the three primary cell layers of an embryo. The ectoderm gives rise to the nervous system; the organs of special sense, as the eyes and ears; the epidermis and epidermal tissue, as fingernails, hair, and skin glands; and the mucous membranes of the mouth and anus. See also **embryo, endoderm, mesoderm.** –**ectodermal, ectodermic,** *adj.*

ectodermal cloaca, a part of the cloaca in the developing embryo that lies external to the cloacal membrane and eventually gives rise to the anus and anal canal. Compare **endodermal cloaca.**

ectomorph /ek'təmôrf'/, a person whose physique is characterized by slenderness, fragility, and a predominance of structures derived from the ectoderm. Compare **endomorph, mesomorph.** See also **asthenic habitus.**

-ectomy, a combining form meaning the 'surgical removal' of something specified: *lobectomy, thrombectomy, thyroidectomy.*

ectoparasite /ek'tōper'əsīt/, (in medical parasitology) an organism that lives on the outside of the body of the host, as a louse.

-ectopia, a combining form meaning a 'condition in which a (specified) organ or part is out of its normal place': *corectopia, osteectopia, tarsectopia.*

ectopic /ektop'ik/, **1.** (of an object or organ) situated in an unusual place, away from its normal location; for example, an ectopic pregnancy is a pregnancy that occurs outside the uterus. **2.** (of an event) occurring at the wrong time, as a premature heart beat or premature ventricular contraction.

ectopic myelopoiesis. See **extramedullary myelopoiesis.**

ectopic pregnancy, an abnormal pregnancy in which the conceptus implants outside the uterine cavity. Kinds of ectopic pregnancy are **abdominal pregnancy, ovarian pregnancy,** and **tubal pregnancy.** Also called **eccyesis** /ek'sī•ē'sis/.

ectopic teratism, a congenital anomaly in which one or more parts are misplaced, as dextrocardia, palatine teeth, and transposition of the great vessels.

ectotoxin. See **exotoxin.**

ectrodactyly /ek'trōdak'təlē/, a congenital anomaly characterized by the absence of part or all of one or more of the fingers or toes. Also called **ectrodactylia, ectrodactylism.**

ectrogenic teratism, a congenital anomaly caused by developmental failure in which one or more parts or organs are missing.

ectrogeny /ektroj'ənē/, the congenital absence or defect of any organ or part of the body. –**ectrogenic,** *adj.*

ectromelia /ek'trōmē'lyə/, the congenital absence or incomplete development of the long bones of one or more of the limbs. Kinds of ectromelia are **amelia, hemimelia,** and **phocomelia.** –**ectromelic,** *adj.,* **ectromelus,** *n.*

ectropion /ektrō'pē•on/, eversion, most commonly of the eyelid, exposing the conjunctival membrane lining the eyelid and part of the eyeball. The condition may involve only the lower eyelid or both eyelids. The cause may be paralysis of the facial nerve or, in an older person, atrophy of the eyelid tissues. Compare **entropion.**

ectrosyndactyly /ek'trōsindak'təlē/, a congenital anomaly characterized by the absence of some but not all of the digits, with those that are formed being webbed so as to appear fused. Also called **ectrosyndactylia.**

ECU, abbreviation for **extended care unit.**

eczema /ek′simə/, superficial dermatitis of unknown cause. In the early stage it may be pruritic, erythematous, papulovesicular, edematous, and weeping. Later it becomes crusted, scaly, thickened, and lichenified. Eczema is not a distinct disease entity. See also **atopic dermatitis, nummular dermatitis.** –**eczematous,** *adj.*

eczema herpeticum, a generalized vesiculopustular skin disease caused by herpes simplex virus or vaccinia virus infection of a preexisting rash like atopic dermatitis. Hospitalization is advisable because fatalities have occurred with this condition. Also called **Kaposi's varicelliform eruption.**

eczema marginatum. See **tinea cruris.**

eczematous conjunctivitis, conjunctival and corneal inflammation associated with multiple, tiny, ulcerated vesicles. The cause is believed to be a delayed hypersensitivity to bacterial protein. If untreated, the condition may lead to ingrowth of small blood vessels in the cornea, eventually obscuring vision. Treatment usually includes topical instillation of corticosteroids.

ED, abbreviation for **effective dose.**

ED50, symbol for **median effective dose.**

edaphon /ed′əfon/, the composite of organisms that live in the soil. –**edaphic,** *adj.*

EDB, abbreviation for **ethylene dibromide.**

EDC, abbreviation for **expected date of confinement.**

Edecrin, a trademark for a diuretic (ethacrynic acid).

Edecrin Sodium, a trademark for a diuretic (ethacrynate sodium).

edema /idē′mə/, the abnormal accumulation of fluid in interstitial spaces of tissues, as in the pericardial sac, intrapleural space, peritoneal cavity, or joint capsules. Edema may be caused by increased capillary fluid pressure, venous obstruction, as occurs in varicosities, thrombophlebitis, or pressure from casts, tight bandages, or garters, congestive heart failure, overloading with parenteral fluids, renal failure, hepatic cirrhosis, hyperaldosteronism, as in Cushing's syndrome, corticosteroid therapy, and inflammatory reactions. Edema may also occur because of loss of serum protein in burns, draining wounds, fistulas, hemorrhage, nephrotic syndrome, or chronic diarrhea; in malnutrition, especially kwashiorkor; in allergic reactions; and in blockage of lymphatic vessels caused by malignant diseases, filariasis, or other disorders. Treatment of edema is directed to correction of the basic cause. Potassium-sparing diuretics may be administered to promote excretion of sodium and water, and care should be exercised in protecting edematous parts of the body from prolonged pressure, injury, and temperature extremes. In the evaluation of tissue turgor, the nurse evaluates edema according to position change, specific location, and response to pressure, as in pitting edema in which pressing the fingers into the edematous area causes a temporary indentation. When a limb is edematous because of venous stasis, elevating the extremity and applying an elastic stocking or sleeve facilitates venous return. See also **anasarca, lymphedema.** –**edematous, edematose,** *adj.* (Table, page 378)

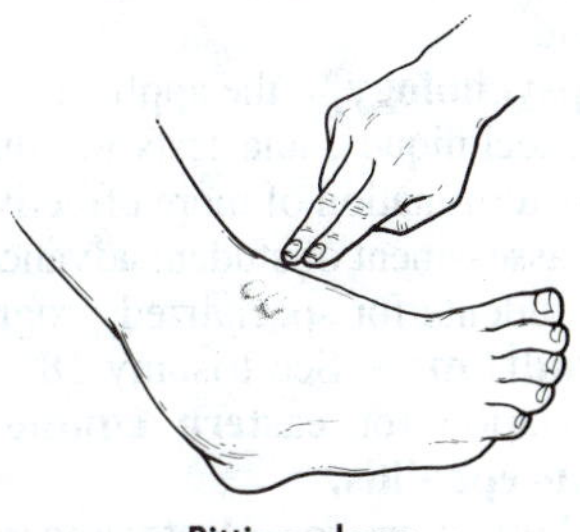

Pitting edema

-edema, a combining form meaning 'swelling resulting from an excessive accumulation of serous fluid in the tissues of the body in (specified) locations': *cephaledema, dactyledema, papilledema.*

edetate (EDTA) /ed′ətāt/, one of several salts of edetic acid, including calcium disodium edetate and edetate disodium, used as a chelating agent in treating poisoning with heavy metals.

edetate disodium, a parenteral chelating agent.

■ INDICATIONS: It is prescribed for hypercalcemic crisis, for ventricular arrhythmia and heart block resulting from digitalis toxicity, and for lead poisoning.

■ CONTRAINDICATIONS: Hypocalcemia, kidney disease, or known hypersensitivity to this drug prohibits its use.

■ ADVERSE EFFECTS: Among the more serious adverse reactions are hypocalcemia, thrombophlebitis, kidney damage, and hemorrhage associated with hypocoagulability.

edetic acid (EDTA) /idet′ik/, a chelating agent.

EDG, abbreviation for **electrodynogram.**

edgewise fixed orthodontic appliance, an orthodontic appliance, characterized by tooth attachment brackets with a rectangular slot that engages a round or a rectangular arch wire. It is used to correct or improve malocclusion.

EDNA, abbreviation for **Emergency Department Nurses' Association.**

edrophonium chloride, a cholinesterase inhibitor that acts as an antidote to curare and is an aid in the diagnosis of myasthenia gravis.

■ INDICATIONS: It is prescribed in the treatment of curare toxicity, in the diagnosis of suspected myasthenia gravis, and to terminate paroxysmal supraventricular tachycardia.

■ CONTRAINDICATIONS: Obstruction of the GI or urinary tract, hypotension, bradycardia, or known hypersensitivity to this drug prohibits its use.

■ ADVERSE EFFECTS: Among the most serious adverse reactions are respiratory paralysis, hypotension, bradycardia, and bronchospasm.

Edsall's disease, a cramping condition that is the result of excessive exposure to heat. Also called **heat cramp.**

EDTA, **1.** abbreviation for **edetate. 2.** abbreviation for **edetic acid.**

educational psychology, the application of psychologic principles, techniques, and tests to educational problems, as the determination of more effective instructional methods, the assessment of student advancement, and the selection of students for specialized programs.

Edwards' syndrome. See trisomy 18.

EEE, abbreviation for **eastern equine encephalitis.** See **equine encephalitis.**

EEG, **1.** abbreviation for **electroencephalogram. 2.** abbreviation for **electroencephalography.**

EEOC, abbreviation for **Equal Employment Opportunity Commission.**

ef-. See **ex-.**

effacement, the shortening of the vaginal portion of the cervix and thinning of its walls as it is stretched and dilated by the fetus during labor. When the cervix is fully effaced, the constrictive neck of the uterus is obliterated, the cervix being then continuous with the lower uterine segment. The extent of effacement, determined by vaginal examination, is expressed as a percentage of full effacement. See also **birth, cervix, dilatation, station.**

effective compliance, the ratio of tidal volume to peak airway pressure.

effective dose (ED), the dosage of a drug that may be expected to cause a specific intensity of effect in the people to whom it is given.

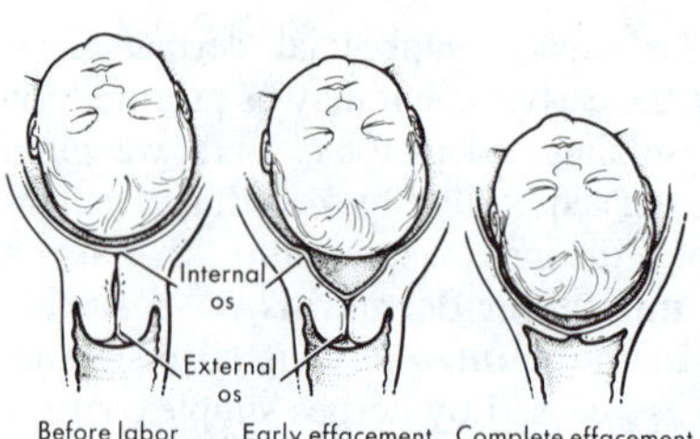

Cervical effacement

effective half-life (ehl), (in radiotherapy) the time required for a radioactive element in an animal body to be diminished 50% as a result of the combined action of radioactive decay and biologic elimination. The effective half-life is equal to the product of the biologic half-life (*bhl*) and the radioactive half-life (*rhl*) divided by the product of the biologic half-life plus the radioactive half-life $ehl = (bhl \times rhl)/(bhl + rhl)$. See also **biologic half-life.**

effective refractory period, the period after the firing of an impulse during which a fiber may respond at the cellular level to a stimulus but the response will not be propagated.

efferent /ef′ərənt/, directed away from a center, as certain arteries, veins, nerves, and lymphatics. Compare **afferent.**

efferent duct, any duct through which a gland releases its secretions.

Cause of edema

Etiologic factors	*Associated conditions*
Increased capillary permeability	Inflammatory reactions Burns Trauma Allergic reactions
Increased capillary hydrostatic pressure Na$^+$ retention and increased blood volume	Congestive heart failure Trauma and stress Renal failure Refeeding edema Adrenocortical hormone secretion Drugs; estrogen, phenylbutazone
Venous obstruction	Local obstruction Hepatic obstruction Pulmonary edema
Decreased plasma oncotic pressure Decreased synthesis of plasma proteins	Liver disease Malnutrition
Increased loss of plasma proteins	Nephrotic syndrome Burns Protein losing enteropathy
Increased interstitial pressure (plasma protein lost to interstitium)	Lymphatic obstruction Increased capillary permeability

efficacy /ef′əkəsē/, (of a drug or treatment) the maximum ability of a drug or treatment to produce a result, regardless of dosage. Narcotics have a nearly identical efficacy but require various dosages to obtain the effect.

effleurage /ef′ləräzh′/, a technique in massage in which long, light, or firm strokes are used, usually over the spine and back. Fingertip effleurage is a light technique performed with the tips of the fingers in a circular pattern over one part of the body or in long strokes over the back or an extremity. Fingertip effleurage of the abdomen is a technique commonly used in the Lamaze method of natural childbirth. Compare **pétrissage, rolling effleurage.**

effort syndrome, an abnormal condition characterized by chest pain, dizziness, fatigue, and palpitations. This condition is often associated with soldiers in combat but occurs also in other individuals. The symptoms of effort syndrome often mimic angina pectoris but are more closely connected to anxiety states. Some indications that pain and other symptoms are related to effort syndrome rather than angina pectoris include cold, moist hands, sighing respiration, and chest pain after, rather than during, exercise. In some patients effort syndrome may be directly and obviously related to psychologic problems, but angina may also be associated with anxiety, and positive diagnosis may require an exercise electrocardiogram. Other chest pains that mimic effort syndrome and angina may be caused by musculoskeletal problems, as inflammation of the costochondral junctions, fractured ribs, and cervical spondylosis. Also called **neurocirculatory asthenia.**

effraction, a breaking open or weakening.

effusion, **1.** the escape of fluid from blood vessels because of rupture or seepage, usually into a body cavity. The condition is usually associated with a circulatory or renal disorder and is often an early sign of congestive heart disease. The term may be associated with an affected body area, as pleural effusion. See also **edema, transudate.** **2.** the outward spread of a bacterial growth.

EFM, abbreviation for **electronic fetal monitor.**

Efudex, a trademark for an antineoplastic (fluorouracil).

egest /ijest′/, to discharge or evacuate a substance from the body, especially to evacuate unabsorbed residue of foods from the intestines. **–egesta,** *n. pl.,* **egestive,** *adj.*

ego /ē′gō, eg′ō/, **1.** the conscious sense of the self; those elements of a person, such as thinking, feeling, willing, and emotions, that distinguish the person as an individual. **2.** (in psychoanalysis) the part of the psyche that experiences and maintains conscious contact with reality and which tempers the primitive drives of the id and the demands of the superego with the social and physical needs of society. It represents the rational element of the personality, is the seat of such mental processes as perception and memory, and develops defense mechanisms against anxiety. See also **id, superego.**

ego-alien. See **ego-dystonic.**

ego analysis, (in psychoanalysis) the intensive study of the ego, especially the defense mechanisms.

ego boundary, (in psychiatry) a sense or awareness that there is a distinction between the self and others. In some psychoses the person does not have an ego boundary and cannot differentiate personal perceptions and feelings from other people's perceptions and feelings.

egocentric, **1.** regarding the self as the center, object, and norm of all experience and having little regard for the needs, interests, ideas, and attitudes of others. **2.** a person possessing these characteristics.

ego-defense mechanism. See **defense mechanism.**

ego-dystonic /ē′gōdiston′ik/, describing the elements of a person's behavior, thoughts, impulses, drives, and attitudes that are at variance with the standards of the ego and inconsistent with the total personality. Also called **ego-alien, self-alien.** Compare **ego-syntonic.**

ego-dystonic homosexuality, a psychosexual disorder in which there is a persistent desire to change sexual orientation from homosexuality to heterosexuality. See also **homosexual.**

ego ideal, the image of the self to which a person aspires both consciously and unconsciously and against which he measures himself and his performance. It is usually based on a positive identification with the significant and influential figures of the early childhood years. See also **identification.**

egoism /ē′gō•iz′əm, eg′-/, **1.** an overvaluation of the importance of the self, expressed as a willingness to gain an advantage at the expense of others. See also **egotism.** **2.** the belief that individual self-interest is, or ought to be, the basic motive for all conscious behavior.

egoist /ē′gō•ist, eg′-/, **1.** a person who seeks to satisfy his own interests at the expense of others. **2.** a person who believes in or follows the concept that all conscious action is justifiably motivated by self-interest. **–egoistic, egoistical,** *adj.*

ego libido, (in psychoanalysis) concentration of the libido on the self; self-love, narcissism.

egomania, a pathologic preoccupation with the self and an exaggerated sense of one's own importance.

ego strength, (in psychotherapy) the ability to maintain the ego by a cluster of traits that together contribute to good mental health. The traits usually considered important include tolerance of the pain of loss, disappointment, shame, or guilt; forgiveness of those who have caused an injury, with feelings of compassion rather than anger and retaliation; acceptance of substitutes and the ability to defer gratification; persistence and perseverance in the pursuit of goals; openness, flexibility, and creativity in learning to adapt; and vitality and power in the activities of life. The psychiatric prognosis for a client correlates positively with ego strength.

ego-syntonic /ē′gōsinton′ik/, those elements of a person's behavior, thoughts, impulses, drives, and attitudes that agree with the standards of the ego and are consistent with the total personality. Compare **ego-dystonic.**

egotism /ē′gətiz′əm, eg′-/, the overvaluation of the importance of the self and undervaluation or contempt of others. See also **egoism.** –**egotistic, egotistical,** *adj.*

egotist /ē′gətist, eg′-/, one who places too much importance on the self and is boastful, egocentric, and arrogant.

egress /ē′gres/, the act of emerging or moving forward.

Egyptian ophthalmia. See **trachoma.**

EHD, abbreviation for **electrohemodynamics.**

Ehlers-Danlos syndrome /ā′lərzdan′ləs/, a hereditary disorder of connective tissue, marked by hyperplasticity of skin, tissue fragility, and hypermotility of joints. Minor trauma may cause a gaping wound with little bleeding. Sprains, joint dislocations, and synovial effusions are common; life expectancy is usually normal. Nursing management includes emotional support of the patient and the family, with emphasis on avoiding trauma in childhood.

eidetic /īdet′ik/, **1.** pertaining to or characterized by the ability to visualize and reproduce accurately the image of objects or events previously seen or imagined. **2.** a person possessing such ability.

eidetic image, an unusually vivid, elaborate, and apparently exact mental image resulting from a visual experience and occurring as a fantasy, dream, or memory. See also **image.**

eighth nerve. See **acoustic nerve.**

einsteinium (Es) /īnstī′nē·əm/, a synthetic transuranic metallic element. Its atomic number is 99; its atomic weight is 254. Einsteinium was first found in the debris from a hydrogen-bomb explosion. It decays rapidly into berkelium.

ejaculate /ijak′yəlit/, the semen discharged in a single emission. See also **ejaculation.** –**ejaculate** /ijak′yəlāt/, *v.*

ejaculation, the sudden emission of semen from the male urethra, usually occurring during copulation, masturbation, and nocturnal emission. It is a reflex action in two phases: First, sperm, seminal fluid, and prostatic and bulbourethral gland secretions are moved into the urethra; second, strong spasmodic peristaltic contractions force ejaculation. The sensation of ejaculation is commonly also called orgasm. The fluid volume of the ejaculate is usually between 2 and 5 ml; each milliliter usually contains 50 million to 150 million spermatozoa. –**ejaculatory** /ijak′yələtôr′ē/, *adj.*

ejaculatory duct, the passage through which semen enters the urethra.

ejection clicks, sharp clicking sounds from the heart, which may be caused by the sudden swelling of a pulmonary artery, the abrupt dilatation of the aorta, or the forceful opening of the aortic cusps. Ejection clicks, often heard during examinations of individuals with septal defects and in cases of patent ductus arteriosis, are associated with high pulmonary resistance and hypertension, but are common and of no clinical significance in pregnant women and in many other healthy people. See also **ejection sounds.**

ejection fraction (EF), the proportion of blood that is ejected during each ventricular contraction compared with the total ventricular volume. The EF is an index of left ventricular function, and the normal fraction is 65%.

ejection murmur. See **systolic murmur.**

ejection sounds, sharp clicking sounds heard early in systole, coinciding with the onset of either right or left ventricular systolic ejection and reflecting either dilatation of the pulmonary artery or aorta or the presence of valvular abnormalities. The term "systolic click" is reserved for the nonejection sounds heard in mid or late systole. Aortic ejection sounds are commonly heard in the presence of aortic valvular stenosis, aortic insufficiency, coarctation of the aorta, and hypertension with aortic dilatation. Pulmonary ejection sounds are heard in mild to moderate pulmonary stenosis, in pulmonary hypertension, and in cases of dilatation of the pulmonary artery. See also **ejection clicks.**

Ekbom syndrome. See **restless legs syndrome.**

EKG, abbreviation for **electrocardiogram.**

elaborate, (in endocrinology) a process by which a gland synthesizes a complex substance from simpler substances and secretes it, usually under the stimulation of a tropic hormone from the pituitary gland. This process, regulated by a negative feedback system, serves to maintain homeostasis in body function. –**elaboration,** *n.*

Elase, a trademark for a topical, fixed-combination drug containing enzymes (fibrinolysin and desoxyribonuclease).

Elase with Chloromycetin, a trademark for a topical, fixed-combination drug containing two lytic enzymes and an antibacterial (chloramphenicol).

elastance, **1.** the quality of recoiling or returning to an original form after the removal of pressure. **2.** the degree to which an air-filled or fluid-filled organ, as a lung, bladder, or blood vessel, can return to its original dimensions when a distending or compressing force is removed. **3.** the measurement of the unit volume of change in such an organ per unit of decreased pressure change. **4.** the reciprocal of compliance.

elastic bandage, a bandage of elasticized fabric that provides support and allows movement.

elastic-band fixation, a method of treatment of fractures of the jaw using rubber bands to connect metal splints or wires that are attached to the maxilla and mandible. The rubber bands produce traction and bring the teeth into occlusion and proper alignment while the fracture is healing. Rubber bands are safer than rigid wires in the event of vomiting. See also **maxillomandibular fixation, nasomandibular fixation.**

elastic bougie, a flexible bougie that can be passed through angular or winding channels.

elastic cartilage. See **yellow cartilage.**

elasticity, the ability of tissue to regain its original shape and size after being stretched, squeezed, or otherwise deformed. Muscle tissue is generally regarded as elastic because it is able to change size and shape and return to its original condition.

elastin /ilas′tin/, a protein that forms the principal substance of yellow elastic tissue fibers.

elation, an emotional reaction characterized by euphoria, excitement, extreme joyfulness, optimism, and self-satisfaction. It is considered to be of pathologic origin when such a response does not realistically reflect a person's actual circumstances. Thus an elated mood may be characteristic of a manic state.

Elavil, a trademark for an antidepressant (amitriptyline hydrochloride).

elbow, the bend of the arm at the joint that connects the arm and forearm. It is a common site of inflammation and injuries, as those incurred during participation in various sports. See also **elbow joint.**

elbow bone. See **ulna.**

elbow joint, the hinged articulation of the humerus, the ulna, and the radius. It is covered by a protective capsule associated with three ligaments and an extensive synovial membrane. The elbow joint allows flexion and extension of the forearm and accommodates the radioulnar articulation. Also called **articulatio cubiti.**

elbow reflex. See **triceps reflex.**

Eldesine, a trademark for an antineoplastic agent (vindesine sulfate).

Eldopaque, a trademark for a dermatologic bleaching agent (hydroquinone).

elective, of or pertaining to a procedure that is performed by choice but which is not essential, as elective surgery.

elective abortion, induced termination of a pregnancy, usually before the fetus has developed enough to live if born, deemed necessary by the woman carrying it and performed at her request. Commonly (but incorrectly) called **therapeutic abortion.** See also **induced abortion, therapeutic abortion.**

elective induction of labor. See **induction of labor.**

electrically stimulated osteogenesis, a bone regeneration process induced by surgically implanted electrodes conveying electric current, especially at nonunion fracture sites. The process is effective because of the different electrical potentials within bone tissue. Viable nonstressed bone is electronegative in the metaphyseal regions and over a fracture callus and electropositive in the diaphyses and other less active regions. Electric stimulation of fractures can accelerate osteogenesis, forming bone more quickly in the area of a surgically inserted negative electrode. The precise mechanisms by which electricity induces osteogenesis are not understood, but research shows that when cathodes are implanted at a fracture site and an electric potential of less than 1 volt is applied, oxygen is consumed at the cathode, and hydroxyl ions are produced, decreasing the oxygen tension of the local tissue and increasing the alkalinity. Low tissue-oxygen tension encourages bone formation, which follows a predominantly anaerobic metabolic pathway. Studies of bone-forming junctions demonstrate that an alkaline pH exists in the zone of hypertrophic cells of the bone growth plate when calcification starts. Electrically stimulated osteogenesis can be achieved with a device that stimulates the fracture site electrically by means of several surgically implanted cathodes. Cathode pins are connected to an external power supply that delivers 20 μamp to each pin. The cathodes are inserted and positioned in the fracture space with the aid of image intensification or other radiographic techniques. Other methods for applying electric current to fractured bone involve open surgical procedures and the implantation of electrodes. The percutaneous technique involving the insertion of cathode pins is performed with a local anesthetic and usually involves less postoperative pain than open surgery methods. The number and the position of the cathodes in the percutaneous technique vary, depending on the bone involved. Generally two cathodes are used for nonunion fractures of small bones, as the medial malleolus or the carpal navicular. Three or more cathodes are used in the clavicle and the bones of the forearm. Four cathodes are used in the treatment of large bones, as the tibia, the femur, and the humerus. Cathodes are generally inserted from opposite directions into the nonunion site. If four cathodes are used, two are placed above and two below the fracture site, the exposed tips of the cathodes resting directly in the nonunion space. Patients who receive such treatment are routinely released from the hospital the day after the procedure, and the stimulation of their fractures continues during the healing period from a portable power supply strapped to the skin over the fracture site. The osteogenesis is radiographically monitored, and after about 12 weeks the cathode pins are removed and the affected portion of the limb involved is placed in a weight-bearing cast. Use of the cathode-pin method of electrically stimulated osteogenesis is contraindicated in the treatment of pathologic fractures associated with benign or malignant tumors and in the treatment of congenital conditions, as congenital pseudarthrosis and osteogenesis imperfecta. The cathode-pin method is also contraindicated in the presence of active systemic infections, clinically active osteomyelitis, proven patient sensitivity to the nickel or chromium from which the pins are made, or synovial pseudarthrosis, unless the fluid-filled cavity at the nonunion site is excised before the cathode pins are inserted. The success rate of treatment with the percutaneous method of electrically stimulated osteogenesis is significantly reduced in nonunions in which the gap is wider than one half the diameter of the bone involved.

electric blood warmer, an electric device for heating blood before infusions, especially massive transfusions in which cold blood might put the patient into shock. The electric blood warmer includes a receptacle containing an electric heater and space for the insertion of a disposable blood-warming bag composed of parallel plastic tubes. The warmer is also equipped with a temperature indicator, which shows when the heating bag reaches the proper temperature of 99° F (37.6° C). An intravenous Y-set is commonly employed in transfusions involving the electric blood warmer. The tubing of the warming bag is primed with normal saline solution. One lead of the warming bag is connected to the primed Y-set; the other lead is connected to the patient. Once the system is primed with normal saline solution, the line conveying the solution is clamped off, and blood is allowed to flow through the warming bag and into the vein of the patient. During transfusion, the electric blood warmer is attached to an IV pole or placed on a bedside table at mattress level. The warming bag must be discarded after one use.

electric burns, the tissue damage resulting from heat of up to 5000° C generated by an electric current. The point of contact on the skin is burned, and the muscle and subcutaneous tissues may be damaged. If the burn is severe, circulatory and respiratory failure may occur and are treated before the burn. Artificial ventilation and cardiac resuscitation are performed as the person is rapidly transported to a medical facility.

electric cautery. See **electrocautery.**

electric potential gradient, the net difference in electric charge across the membrane of a cell.

electric shock, a traumatic physical state caused by the passage of electric current through the body. It usually involves accidental contact with exposed parts of electric circuits in home appliances and domestic power supplies but may also result from lightning or contact with high-voltage wires. About 1000 persons in the United States die from electric shock each year. The damage electricity does in passing through the body depends on the intensity of the electric current, the type of current, and the duration and the frequency of current flow. Alternating current (AC), direct current (DC), and mixed current cause different kinds and degrees of damage in passing through body tissues. High-frequency current produces more heat than low-frequency current and can cause burns, coagulation, and necrosis of affected body parts. Low-frequency current can burn tissues if the area of contact is small and concentrated. Severe electric shock commonly causes unconsciousness, respiratory paralysis, muscle contractions, bone fractures, and cardiac disorders. Even small electric currents passing through the heart can cause fibrillation. Treatment of electric shock commonly involves such measures as cardiopulmonary resuscitation, defibrillation, and the intravenous administration of electrolytes to help stabilize vital functions. See also **cardiogenic shock, hypovolemic shock.**

electric shock therapy. See **electroconvulsive therapy.**

electric spinal orthosis, an electric device that helps control curvature of the spine by stimulating back muscles. The portable, battery-powered machine does not correct scoliosis, but prevents worsening of the condition.

electro-, a combining form meaning 'pertaining to electricity': *electrobiology, electrocatalysis, electrolepsy.*

electroanalytic chemistry, the branch of chemistry concerned with the analysis of compounds using electric current to produce characteristic, observable change in the substance being studied. See also **chemistry.**

electrocardiogram (ECG, EKG), a graphic record produced by an electrocardiograph.

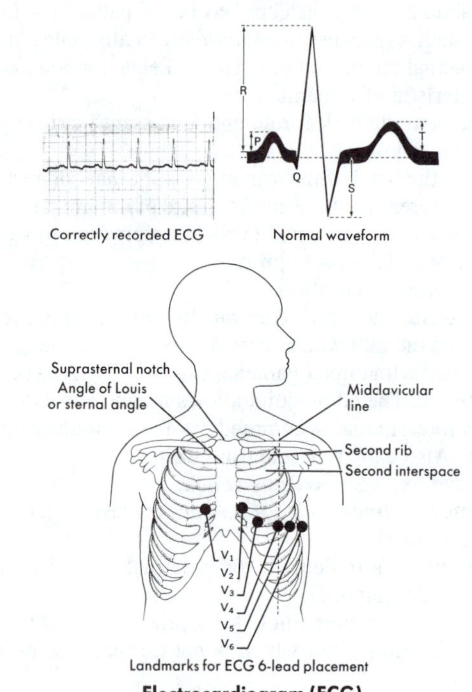

Electrocardiogram (ECG)

electrocardiograph (ECG), a device used for recording the electric activity of the myocardium to detect abnormal transmission of the cardiac impulse through the conductive tissues of the muscle. Electrocardiography allows diagnosis of specific cardiac abnormalities. Leads are affixed to certain anatomic points on the patient's chest, usually with an adhesive gel that promotes transmission of the electric impulse to the recording device. The patient is positioned supine on an examining table and asked to lie quietly during the test. **–electrocardiographic,** *adj.*

electrocardiographic-auscultatory syndrome. See **Barlow's syndrome.**

electrocardiograph lead /lēd/, **1.** an electrode placed on part of the body and connected to an electrocardiograph. **2.** a record, made by the electrocardiograph, that varies depending on the site of the electrode. Electrocardiography is generally performed with the use of three peripheral leads and six leads placed on the precordium. The peripheral or extremity leads are designated I, II, and III, and the chest leads are designated V_1, V_2, V_3, V_4, V_5, and V_6 to indicate the points on the precordium on which the electrodes are placed.

electrocautery /ilek'trōkô'tərē/, the application of a needle or snare heated by electric current for the destruction of tissue, as for the removal of warts or polyps. Also called **electric cautery, galvanic cautery, galvanocautery.** See also **diathermy.**

electrocoagulation /ilek'trōko•ag'yo͞olā'shən/, a therapeutic, destructive form of electrosurgery in which tissue is hardened by the passage of high-frequency current from an electric cautery device. Also called **surgical diathermy.** Compare **electrodesiccation.**

electroconvulsive therapy (ECT), the induction of a brief convulsion by passing an electric current through the brain for the treatment of affective disorders, especially in patients resistant to psychoactive-drug therapy. The patient is placed in a comfortable supine position with the limbs lightly restrained and with a padded tongue depressor between the back teeth, after premedication with succinylcholine to prevent fractures. Conductive paste is applied to the skin on both sides of the forehead where the electrodes are placed, and a 70 to 130 volt current is delivered for 0.1 to 0.5 seconds. The patient loses consciousness and undergoes tonic contractions for approximately 10 seconds, followed by a somewhat longer period of clonic convulsions accompanied by apnea; on awakening the individual has no memory of the shock. ECT is usually administered three times a week for 2 months and is used primarily for the treatment of acute depression. Also called **electric shock therapy, electroshock therapy.**

electrocution, death caused by the passage of electric current through the body. See also **electric shock.**

electrode /ilek'trōd/, **1.** a contact for the induction or detection of electric activity. **2.** a medium for conducting an electric current from the body to physiologic monitoring equipment.

electrodermal audiometry, a method of testing hearing in which a harmless electric shock is used to condition the subject to a pure tone; thereafter the tone, coupled with the anticipation of a shock, elicits a brief electrodermal response, which is recorded, and the lowest intensity of the sound producing the skin response is considered the subject's hearing threshold.

electrodesiccation /ilek'trōdes'ikā'shən/, a technique in electrosurgery in which tissue is destroyed by burning with an electric spark. It is used primarily for eliminating small superficial growths but may be used with curettage for eradicating abnormal tissue deeper in the skin, in which case layers of skin may be burned, then successively scraped away. The procedure is performed under local anesthesia.

electrodynograph (EDG) /ilek'trōdin'əgraf'/, an electronic device used to measure pressures exerted in biologic activity, as the pressures exerted by the human foot in walking, running, jogging, or climbing stairs.

electroencephalogram (EEG) /ilek'trō•ensef'ələgram'/, a graphic chart on which is traced the electric potential produced by the brain cells, as detected by electrodes placed on the scalp. The resulting brain waves are called alpha, beta, delta, and theta rhythms, according to the frequencies they produce, which range from 2 to 12 cps with an amplitude of up to 100 μV. Variations in brain-wave activity correlate with neurologic conditions, psychologic states, and level of consciousness. See also **encephalography.**

electroencephalograph /ilek'trō•ensef'ələgraf'/, an instrument for receiving and recording the electric potential produced by the brain cells. It consists of a vacuum-tube amplifier that magnifies the electric currents received through electrodes placed on the scalp and electromagnetically records the patterns on a graphic chart. See also **electroencephalography.**

electroencephalographic technologist, a person trained in the management of an electroencephalographic laboratory. The technologist may supervise electroencephalographic technicians who are generally responsible for the operation and maintenance of the equipment.

electroencephalography (EEG) /ilek'trō•ensef'əlog'rəfē/, the process of recording brain-wave activity. Electrodes are attached to various areas of the patient's head with collodion. During the procedure the patient remains quiet, with eyes closed, and refrains from talking or moving, although, in certain cases, prescribed activities may be requested, especially hyperventilation. The test is used to diagnose seizure disorders, brainstem disorders, focal lesions, and impaired consciousness. During neurosurgery, the electrodes can be applied directly to the surface of the brain (intracranial electroencephalography) or placed within the brain tissue (depth electroencephalography) to detect lesions or tumors. See also **electroencephalogram.** **–electroencephalographic,** *adj.*

electrogram /ilek'trōgram'/, a unipolar or bipolar record of electric activity of the heart as recorded from electrodes within the cardiac chambers or on the epicardium. Examples are atrial electrogram (AEG), ventricular electrogram (VEG), and His bundle electrogram (HBE).

electrohemodynamics (EHD) /ilek'trōhē'mōdīnam'iks/, a technique for noninvasively measuring the mechanic properties and hemodynamic characteristics of the vascular system, including arterial blood pressure, electric impedance, blood flow, and resistance to blood flow.

electrohydraulic heart, a type of artificial heart in which the ventricles are driven by the alternate pumping of a fluid rather than by compressed air. The device is powered by a compact electric motor, which can be implanted in a patient's chest along with the hydraulic pump. Also called **Jarvik-7 artificial heart.** See also **artificial heart.**

electroimmunodiffusion. See **immunodiffusion.**

electrolysis /il'ektrol'isis/, a process in which electric energy causes a chemical change in a conducting medium, usually a solution or a molten substance. Electrodes, usually pieces of metal, induce the flow of electric energy through the medium. Electrons enter the solution through the cathode and leave the solution through the anode. Negatively charged ions, or anions, are attracted to the anode; positively charged ions, or cations, are attracted to the cathode. Various conducting mediums are used, as solutions of copper, zinc, nickel, lead, and silver. Electric energy passing through such solutions causes deposition of pure metal at the cathode. Passing electric energy through solutions of alkali and alkaline-earth salts liberates hydrogen at the cathode. A metal anode causes metal ions to flow from the anode into the solution as the electric current passes through the medium. An inert electrode, as one of platinum, may liberate oxygen at the anode in an aqueous medium. A halogen salt solution liberates free bromine, chlorine, or iodine. Fluorine, which has a high oxidation potential, is not liberated by electrolysis. **–electrolytic,** *adj.*

electrolyte /ilek′trōlīt/, an element or compound that, when melted or dissolved in water or other solvent, dissociates into ions and is able to conduct an electric current. Electrolytes differ in their concentrations in blood plasma, interstitial fluid, and cell fluid and affect the movement of substances between those compartments. Proper quantities of principal electrolytes and balance among them are critical to normal metabolism and function. For example, calcium (Ca^{++}) is necessary for the relaxation of skeletal muscle and contraction of cardiac muscle; potassium (K^+) is required for the contraction of skeletal muscle and relaxation of cardiac muscle. Sodium (Na^+) is essential in maintaining fluid balance. Certain diseases, conditions, and medications may lead to a deficiency of one or more electrolytes and to an imbalance among them, as certain diuretics and a low-sodium diet prescribed in hypertension may cause hypokalemic shock resulting from a loss of potassium. Diarrhea may cause a loss of many electrolytes, leading to hypovolemia and shock, especially in infants. Careful and regular monitoring of electrolytes and intravenous replacement of fluid and electrolytes are part of the acute care in many illnesses. **–electrolytic,** *adj.*

Normal electrolyte content of body fluids*

Electrolytes (anions and cations)	*Extracellular*		*Intracellular (mEq/L)*
	Intravascular (mEq/L)	*Interstitial (mEq/L)*	
Sodium (Na^+)	142	146	15
Potassium (K^+)	5	5	150
Calcium (Ca^{++})	5	3	2
Magnesium (Mg^{++})	2	1	27
Chloride (Cl^-)	102	114	1
Bicarbonate (HCO_3^-)	27	30	10
Protein ($Prot^-$)	16	1	63
Phosphate ($HPO_4^=$)	2	2	100
Sulfate ($SO_4^=$)	1	1	20
Organic acids	5	8	0

*Note that the electrolyte level of the intravascular and interstitial fluids (extracellular) is approximately the same and that sodium and chloride contents are markedly higher in these fluids, whereas potassium, phosphate, and protein contents are markedly higher in intracellular fluid.

electrolyte balance, the equilibrium between electrolytes in the body.

electrolyte solution, any solution containing electrolytes prepared for oral, parenteral, or rectal administration for the replacement or supplementation of ions necessary for homeostasis. The loss of potassium ion (K^+) by vomiting, by diarrhea, or by the action of certain medications, including diuretics and corticosteroids, may be corrected by administering a solution high in potassium. Other electrolyte solutions containing combinations of calcium, sodium, phosphate, chloride, or magnesium may be given to treat acid-base disturbance, as seen in chronic renal dysfunction or diabetic ketoacidosis. The solutions are available in a wide range of balanced formulas for replacement or maintenance, and most include various trace minerals.

electromagnetic induction, the production in tissue of electric fields and associated eddy currents by magnetic fields generated by coils carrying an electric current.

electromagnetic radiation, every kind of electric and magnetic radiation, regarded as a continuous spectrum of energy that includes energy with the shortest wavelength (gamma rays, with a wavelength of 0.0011 Å) to that with the longest wavelength (long radio waves, with a wavelength of more than 1 million kilometers). The visible part of the electromagnetic spectrum is between 3800 and 7600 Å. Ultraviolet radiation occurs beyond the short-wave (violet) end of the visible spectrum, having a wavelength of less than 4000 Å; x-rays have a much shorter wavelength (from 0.05 to a few hundred Å). Infrared radiation occurs just beyond the longer wave end of the visible spectrum, having a wavelength of 7000 Å or more.

electromagnetic tape. See **mag tape.**

electromallet condenser, an electromechanic device for compacting direct filling gold in prepared tooth cavities. The frequency of the blows delivered by this instrument may be varied from 200 to 3600 strokes per minute. The intensity of the blows is electrically controlled. Also called **McShirley's electromallet.**

electromyogram (EMG) /ilek′trōmī′əgram′/, a record of the intrinsic electric activity in a skeletal muscle. Such data help in diagnosing neuromuscular problems and are obtained by applying surface electrodes or by inserting a needle electrode into the muscle and observing electric activity with an oscilloscope and a loudspeaker. Some electromyograms show abnormalities, as spontaneous electric potentials within the muscle under study, and help pinpoint lesions of motor nerves. Electromyograms also measure electric potentials induced by voluntary muscular contraction. See also **electroneuromyography.**

electron, **1.** a negatively charged elementary particle that has a specific charge, mass, and spin. The number of electrons circling the nucleus of an atom is equal to the atomic number of the substance. Electrons may be shared or exchanged by two atoms; after the exchange the atom becomes an ion. **2.** a negative beta particle emitted from a radioactive substance. See also **atom, element, ion, neutron, proton.**

electronarcosis /ilek′trōnärkō′sis/, general anesthesia without the use of anesthetic gases or drugs. Narcosis is produced by passing an electric current through the brain, but adequate control and prevention of undesirable side effects, especially convulsions, remain a problem. The procedure is experimental. Compare **electrosleep therapy.**

electron capture, a radioactive decay process in which a nucleus with an excess of electrons brings one of them into the nucleus, creating a neutron out of a proton, thus decreasing the atomic number of the atom by 1. The resulting atom is often unstable and gives off a gamma ray to achieve stability.

electroneuromyography /ilek′trōnŏŏr′ōmī·og′rəfē/, a procedure for testing and recording neuromuscular activity by the electric stimulation of nerves. The procedure involves the insertion of needle electrodes into any skeletal muscle being studied, applying electric current to the electrodes, and observing and recording neuromuscular functions by means of instruments, as a cathode-ray oscilloscope and an appropriate recording device. The procedure helps in studying neuromuscular conduction, the extent of nerve lesions, and reflex responses. See also **electromyogram.**

electronic fetal monitor (EFM), a device that allows observation of the fetal heart rate and the maternal uterine contractions. It may be applied externally, in which case the fetal heart is detected by an ultrasound transducer on the abdomen and the uterine contractions by a pressure sensor applied to the abdomen. Internal monitoring of the fetal heart rate is accomplished via an electrode clipped to the fetal scalp; the amplitude, frequency, and duration of the uterine contractions are detected by the use of an intrauterine catheter.

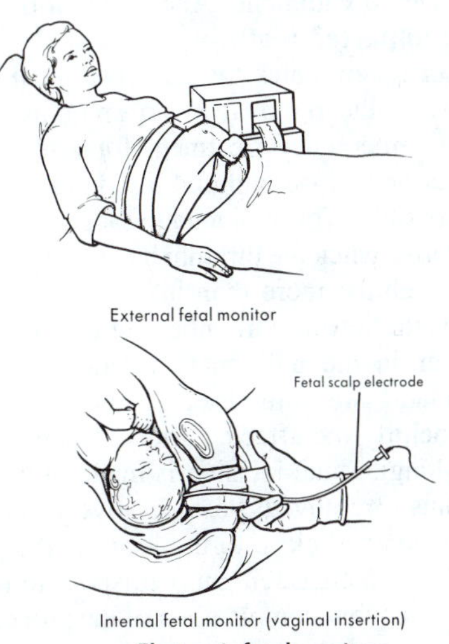

Electronic fetal monitors

electronic thermometer, a thermometer that registers temperature rapidly by electronic means.

electron microscope, an instrument, similar to an optic microscope, that scans cell surfaces with a beam of electrons, instead of visible light, creating an image that can be photographed or viewed on a fluorescent screen. Compare **scanning electron microscope.** See also **electron microscopy.**

electron microscopy, a technique, using an electron microscope, in which a beam of electrons is focused by an electromagnetic lens and directed onto an extremely thin specimen. The electrons emerging are focused and directed by a second lens onto a fluorescent screen. The magnified image produced is 1000 times greater than with an optic microscope, and well resolved, but it is two-dimensional because of the thinness of the specimen. Also called **transmission electron microscopy.** Compare **scanning electron microscopy, transmission scanning electron microscopy.**

electron scanning microscope. See **scanning electron microscope.**

electron volt (eV), a unit of energy equal to the energy acquired by an electron in falling through a potential difference of one volt. One eV equals 1.6×10^{-12} erg or 1.6×10^{-19} J.

electronystagmography /ilek′trōnis′tagmog′rəfē/, a method of assessing and recording eye movements by measuring the electric activity of the extraocular muscles. See also **electroencephalogram, nystagmus.**

electrophoresis /ilek′trōfərē′sis/, the movement of charged suspended particles through a liquid medium in response to changes in an electric field. Charged particles of a given substance migrate in a predictable direction and at a characteristic speed. The pattern of migration can be recorded in bands on an **electrophoretogram** ilek′trōfəret′ōgram. The technique is widely used to separate and identify serum proteins and other substances. **–electrophoretic,** *adj.*

electroresection, a technique for the removal of bladder tumors by the insertion of an electric wire through the urethra. The electric wire is guided to the site with the aid of an optic probe. The electric lead is not energized until it is properly located in the tumor to be destroyed. The procedure is performed after administration of an anesthetic.

electroshock therapy. See **electroconvulsive therapy.**

electrosleep therapy, a technique designed to induce sleep, especially in psychiatric patients, by administering a low-amplitude pulsating current to the brain. The cathode is placed supraorbitally, and the anode is placed over the mastoid process. The current, which is discharged for 15 to 20 minutes, produces a tingling sensation, but does not always induce sleep. The procedure is repeated from five to 30 times. Electrosleep therapy is said to be beneficial for patients with anxiety, depression, gastric distress, insomnia, personality disorders, and schizophrenia, but double-blind studies have yielded conflicting results. Compare **electronarcosis.**

electrostatic imaging, techniques for producing radiographic images in which the ionic charge liberated during the irradiation process is converted to a visible image using electronic read-out devices or by the use of liquid or powder ''toner'' to convert a latent charge image into a visible one.

electrosurgery, surgery performed with various electric instruments that operate on high-frequency electric current. Kinds of electrosurgery include **electrocoagulation, electrodesiccation.**

electrotonic current, a current induced in a nerve sheath by an action potential within the nerve or an adjacent nerve.

eleidin /əlē′ədin/, a transparent protein substance, resembling keratin, found in the stratum lucidum of the epidermis.

element, one of more than 100 primary, simple substances that cannot be broken down by chemical means into any other substance. Each atom of any element contains a specific number of electrons orbiting the nucleus. The nucleus contains a variable number of neutrons. A **stable element** contains an equal number of neutrons and electrons and does not easily give up neutrons. A **radioactive element** does not contain a balanced number of electrons and neutrons, giving off neutrons readily. See also **atom, compound, molecule.**

element 104, a synthetic, radioactive element, the twelfth transuranic element, and the first transactinide element. Proposed names are rutherfordium (Rf) and kurchatovium (Ku).

element 105, a synthetic element, and the thirteenth transuranic element. A proposed name is hahnium (Ha).

element 106, a synthetic element, with a half-life of 0.9 seconds. It was first synthesized in 1974 by scientists working independently in the United States and the U.S.S.R.

element 107, an element reportedly synthesized in 1976 by Soviet scientists who bombarded isotopes of bismuth with heavy nuclei of chromium 54. The finding was not confirmed by scientists of other nations.

eleo-, a combining form meaning 'pertaining to oil': *eleoma, eleomyenchysis, eleopten.*

elephantiasis /el′əfəntī′əsis/, the end-stage lesion of filariasis, characterized by tremendous swelling, usually of the external genitalia and the legs. The overlying skin becomes dark, thick, and coarse. Elephantiasis results from filariasis that has lasted for many years. See also **filariasis.**

elephantoid fever. See **elephantiasis, filariasis.**

eleventh nerve. See **accessory nerve.**

elimination diet, a procedure for identifying a food or foods to which a person is allergic by successively omitting from the diet certain foods in order to detect those responsible for the symptoms.

elixir /ilik′sər/, a clear liquid containing water, alcohol, sweeteners, or flavors, used primarily as a vehicle for the oral administration of a drug.

Elixophyllin, a trademark for a smooth muscle relaxant (theophylline), used as a bronchodilator.

Elliot forceps. See **obstetric forceps.**

Elliot's position, a supine posture assumed by the patient on the operating table, with a support placed under the lower costal margin to elevate the chest. The position is used in gallbladder surgery.

elliptocyte, an oval-shaped red blood cell. See also **elliptocytosis.**

elliptocytosis /ilip′tōsītō′sis/, a mild abnormal condition of the blood that is characterized by increased numbers of elliptocytes or oval erythrocytes. Less than 15% of the red cells appear in this form in normal blood; modest increases occur in a variety of anemias, including a rare congenital disorder, hereditary elliptocytosis, which may or may not be associated with a mild hemolytic anemia. Also called **ovalocytosis.** Compare **spherocytosis.** See also **acanthocytosis, congenital nonspherocytic hemolytic anemia, sickle cell anemia, spherocytic anemia.**

elope, *informal.* to leave a locked psychiatric institution without notice or permission.

Elspar, a trademark for an antineoplastic (asparaginase).

em-, a combining form meaning 'in, on': *embolism, empasma, emphysis.*

emaciation /imā′shi•ā′shən/, excessive leanness caused by disease or lack of nutrition.

Embden-Meyerhof pathway /emb′denmī′ərhof/, a sequence of enzymatic reactions in the anaerobic conversion of glucose to lactic acid, producing energy in the form of adenosine triphosphate.

embedded tooth, an unerupted tooth, usually completely covered with bone. Also called **imbedded tooth.** Compare **impacted tooth.**

embolectomy /em′bəlek′təmē/, a surgical incision into an artery for the removal of an embolus or clot, performed as emergency treatment for arterial embolism. The operation is done within 4 to 6 hours of the onset of pain, if possible. Thrombi tend to lodge at the juncture of major arteries when the thrombi have broken away from a thrombophlebitis; more than half lodge in the aorta, in arteries of the lower extremities, in the common carotid arteries, or in the pulmonary arteries. Preoperatively, anticoagulants are administered, and an arteriogram is done to identify the affected artery. Under general anesthesia, a longitudinal incision is made in the artery, and the embolus is removed. Postoperatively, the blood pressure is maintained close to the level of the preoperative baseline, as a decrease might predispose to new clot formation. A frequent complication of the procedure is hemorrhage from small arteries that may have been clogged with the embolus but overlooked while tying larger bleeding vessels.

embolism /em′bəliz′əm/, an abnormal circulatory condition in which an embolus travels through the bloodstream and becomes lodged in a blood vessel. The symptoms vary with the degree of occlusion that the embolism causes, the character of the embolus, and the size, nature, and location of the occluded vessel. Kinds of embolism include **air embolism** and **fat embolism.**

embolized atheroma, an embolized fat particle lodged in a blood vessel.

embolotherapy, a technique of blocking a blood vessel with a balloon catheter. It is used for treating bleeding ulcers and blood vessel defects and, during surgery, to stop blood flow to a tumor.

embolus /em′bələs/, *pl.* **emboli,** a foreign object, a quantity of air or gas, a bit of tissue or tumor, or a piece of a thrombus that circulates in the bloodstream until it becomes lodged in a vessel. Kinds of emboli include **air embolus** and **fat embolus.** **–embolic, emboloid,** *adj.*

embryatrics. See **fetology.**

embryectomy /em′brē•ek′təmē/, the surgical removal of an embryo, most commonly in an ectopic pregnancy.

embryo /em′brē•ō/, **1.** any organism in the earliest stages of development. **2.** in humans, the stage of prenatal development between the time of implantation of the fertilized ovum about 2 weeks after conception until the end of the seventh or eighth week. The period is characterized by rapid growth, differentiation of the major organ systems, and development of the main external features. Compare **fetus, zygote.** **–embryonal, embryonoid, embryonic,** *adj.*

embryo-, a combining form meaning a 'fetus': *embryoctony, embryology.*

embryoctony /em′brē•ok′tənē/, the intentional destruction of the living embryo or fetus in utero. Also called **feticide.** See also **abortion.**

embryogenesis /em′brē•ōjen′əsis/, the process in sexual reproduction in which an embryo forms from the fertilization of an ovum. Also called **embryogeny** /em′brē•oj′ənē/. See also **heterogenesis, homogenesis.** **–embryogenetic, embryogenic.** *adj.*

embryologic development, the various intrauterine stages and processes involved in the growth and differentiation of the conceptus from the time of fertilization of the ovum until the eighth week of gestation. The stages are related to the biologic status of the unborn child and are divided into two distinct periods. The first is embryogenesis, or the formation of the embryo, which occurs during the 10 days to 2 weeks after fertilization until implantation. The second period, organogenesis, involves the differentiation of the various cells, tissues, and organ systems and the development of the main external features of the embryo; it occurs from approximately the end of the second week to the eighth week of intrauterine life. The fetal stage follows these stages, beginning at about the ninth week of gestation. The entire process of the growth and development of the embryo and fetus is loosely called prenatal development. Embryogenesis is initiated shortly after fertilization by the formation of the zygote from the fusion of the pronuclei of the spermatozoon and the ovum. The zygote then divides by cleavage to form blastomeres, which eventually cluster into a solid mass of cells, called the morula, that are uniform in size, shape, and physiologic capabilities. With continued division the cells become unequal in size and shape, and fluid accumulates between them to produce the blastocyst. This hollow ball of cells consists of an outer layer, the trophoblast, and a localized inner cluster, the inner cell mass, which protrudes into the cavity. The inner cell mass contains two formative layers that differentiate into the primary germ layers and develop into the embryo. The trophoblastic cells contain the enzymes and other substances necessary for the implantation of the blastocyst onto the uterine wall and the formation of the extraembryonic structures, as the chorion and the placenta. By the time of implantation and the beginning of organogenesis, the endoderm, ectoderm, and mesoderm germ layers have differentiated into the embryonic disk and have formed the amniotic cavity and yolk sac cavity. During this stage, the embryo develops rapidly, changing from a flat, disklike shape into an elongated, cylindric, curved mass that contains the primitive structures, which will subsequently differentiate into all the organs and cavities of the body. By the fourth week of development, the primitive body includes the neural tube, which will develop into the brain, spinal cord, and other neural tissue of the central nervous system; the notochord, which will be replaced by the vertebral column; the somites, which will segment into skeletal and muscle tissue; the nephrotomes, which will form the urogenital system; the gut, which will differentiate into the digestive and respiratory systems; the coelom, which will subdivide into separate cavities for the heart, lungs, and abdominal viscera; and the primitive heart and tiny spaces within the mesoderm that will become the vessels of the circulatory and lymphatic systems. At 8 weeks of development, major differentiation of all the organs has occurred, and the main external features, as the eyes, ears, nose, mouth, and digits, are recognizable. The embryo is now remarkably humanlike in appearance and at this stage is called a fetus. For the remaining 7 months of intrauterine life, the primary changes in the fetus are growth, further tissue differentiation, elaboration of structural detail, and specialization of organs and systems. See also **prenatal development.**

embryologist /em′brē•ol′əjist/, one who specializes in the study of embryology.

embryology /em′brē•ol′əjē/, the study of the origin, growth, development, and function of an organism from fertilization to birth. Kinds of embryology include **comparative embryology, descriptive embryology,** and **experimental embryology.** **–embryologic, embryological,** *adj.*

embryoma /em'brē·ō'mə/, *pl.* **embryomas, embryomata,** a tumor arising from embryonic cells or tissues.

embryoma of the ovary. See **dysgerminoma**

embryomorph /embrē'əmôrf'/, any structure that resembles an embryo, especially a mass of tissue that may represent an aborted conceptus. –**embryomorphous,** *adj.*

embryonal adenomyosarcoma, embroyonal adenosarcoma. See **Wilms' tumor.**

embryonal carcinoma, an extremely malignant neoplasm derived from germinal cells, which usually develops in gonads, especially the testes. The tumor, a firm, nodular mass with many hemorrhagic areas, is characterized histologically by large, undifferentiated cells with indistinct borders, eosinophilic cytoplasm, and prominent nucleoli in pleomorphic nuclei. Bodies resembling a 1- or 2-week-old embryo are occasionally seen in these tumors. The neoplasm is relatively resistant to radiation therapy, and, early in its development, it metastasizes by way of lymph channels. Surgery and chemotherapy are usually included in the treatment. See also **choriocarcinoma.**

embryonal leukemia. See **stem cell leukemia.**

embryonate /em'brē-ənāt'/, **1.** impregnated; containing an embryo. **2.** of, pertaining to, or resembling an embryo.

embryonic abortion, **1.** termination of pregnancy before the twentieth week of gestation. **2.** expelled products of conception before the twentieth week. Compare **fetal abortion.**

embryonic anideus, a blastoderm in which the axial elongation of the primitive streak and primitive groove fail to develop.

embryonic blastoderm, the area of the blastoderm that gives rise to the primitive streak from which the embryonic body develops. Compare **extraembryonic blastoderm.**

embryonic competence, the ability of an embryonic cell to react normally to the stimulation of an inductor allowing continued, normal growth or differentiation of the embryo.

embryonic disk, the thickened plate from which the embryo develops in the second week of pregnancy. Scattered cells from the border of the disk migrate to the space between the trophoblast and yolk sac and become the embryonic mesoderm. The disk develops from the ectoderm and endoderm. Also called **gastrodisk, germ disk.**

embryonic layer, one of the three layers of cells in the embryo, the endoderm, the mesoderm, and the ectoderm. From these layers of cells arise all of the structures and organs and parts of the body. The endoderm is the first to develop, followed by the ectoderm. During the third week of gestation, the mesoderm arises between the ectoderm and the endoderm.

embryonic rest, a portion of embryonic tissue that remains in the adult organism. Such tissue may act as organ-specific indicators in certain types of cancer and can assist in the prediction of metastases and provide an objective therapeutic monitor. Also called **epithelial rest, fetal rest.**

embryonic stage, (in embryology) the interval of time from the end of the germinal stage, at 10 days of gestation, to the eighth week.

embryoniform /em'brē·on'ifôrm'/, resembling an embryo.

embryopathy /em'brē-op'əthē/, any anomaly occurring in the embryo or fetus as a result of interference with normal intrauterine development. A kind of embryopathy is **rubella embryopathy.**

embryoplastic /em'brē·ōplas'tik/, of or pertaining to the formation of an embryo, usually with reference to cells.

embryotome /em'brē·ətōm'/, an instrument used in embryotomy.

embryotomy /em'brē·ot'əmē/, **1.** the dismemberment or mutilation of a fetus for removal from the uterus when normal delivery is not possible. **2.** the dissection of an embryo for examination and analysis.

embryotoxon. See **arcus juvenilis.**

embryotroph /em'brē-ətrof'/, the liquefied uterine nutritive material, composed of glandular secretions and degenerative tissue, that nourishes the mammalian embryo until placental circulation is established. Also called **embryotrophe** /-trōf'/, **histotroph, histotrophic nutrition.** Compare **hemotroph.**

embryotrophy /em'brē·ot'trəfē/, the nourishment of the embryo. See also **embryotroph, hemotroph.** –**embryotrophic,** *adj.*

embryulcia /em'brē·ul'sē·ə/, the surgical extraction of the embryo or fetus from the uterus.

Emcyt, a trademark for an antineoplastic agent (estramustine phosphate sodium).

emergence, a stage in the process of recovery from general anesthesia that includes spontaneous respiration, voluntary swallowing, and consciousness. See also **postoperative care.**

emergency, a serious situation that arises suddenly and threatens the life or welfare of a person or a group of people, as a natural disaster or a medical crisis.

emergency childbirth, a birth that occurs accidentally or precipitously in or out of the hospital, without standard obstetric preparations and procedures. Signs and symptoms of impending delivery include increased bloody show, frequent strong contractions, a desire on the part of the mother to bear down forcibly or her report that she feels as though she is going to defecate, visible bulging of the bag of waters, or crowning of the baby's head at the vaginal introitus.

■ METHOD: If time permits, equipment is readied, but the delivery is not delayed for such preparations. Useful equipment includes sterile gloves, towels, bulb syringe, receiving blankets, scissors, two Kelly clamps, cord clamp or tie, and a basin for the placenta. The mother's vital signs are taken, and her baby's heart tones are listened to if time permits and if equipment is available. The mother is reassured that emergency deliveries are usually simple and that all procedures and events will be explained. Despite her compelling urge to push and to deliver quickly, the mother is encouraged to ease the baby out slowly by not pushing and by blowing air forcibly out through pursed lips as she feels the strength of the urge building. As the head emerges, it is supported but allowed to rotate naturally. A check is made immediately to determine whether or not the umbilical cord is wound around the neck. If it is, a gentle attempt is made to slip it over the baby's head; if it is too tight, it is immediately clamped with two Kelly clamps placed 2 or 3 inches apart, cut between the clamps, and unwound from the neck. If the baby does not deliver immediately, mucus and fluid in the nose and the mouth are sucked out with a bulb syringe. The shoulders are delivered one at a time by guiding the head downward to deliver the anterior (upper) shoulder under the symphysis pubis, and then upward to deliver the posterior (lower) shoulder over the perineum. The rest of the baby is quickly born. If the membranes of the amniotic sac are intact, the sac is snipped or torn behind the baby's neck and peeled away from the face so that the baby can breathe. If necessary, the nares, nasopharynx, and mouth may be suctioned with the bulb syringe, taking care not to slow the heart rate by stimulating the vagus nerve with the tip of the syringe on the back of the throat. The baby is kept warm and held with the head lower than the chest; it may be laid skin-to-skin on the mother's abdomen. The baby may thus be positioned, observed, and warmed in one place as the nurse or other helper covers mother and baby with a dry blanket or towel and continues to provide emergency care as necessary through the third stage of labor. There is no urgent need to cut the cord or to deliver the placenta. When it is desired, the cord may be cut by clamping it in two places several inches from the baby and cutting it between the clamps with sterile scissors. The cord clamp may be put on later. If possible, an Apgar score is assigned first at 5 minutes of age, then at 10. The placenta is ready to be delivered when the cord is seen to advance a few inches, the uterus becomes firmer and rises in the abdomen, and a small gush of bright red blood is seen coming from the vagina. The mother may help expel it by bearing down. The placenta is lifted out of the vagina slowly, with care, so that all of the membranes are brought out with it. The placenta and membranes are kept for further evaluation. The uterus is massaged to ensure that it is well contracted, and the baby is put to breast if the mother wishes. The uterus is frequently palpated, and it is massaged when necessary. The baby is kept with the mother and observed for warmth, color, activity, and respiration. After delivery of the placenta, the perianal area is rinsed with warm sterile water and dried with a clean towel or cloth, and an ice pack and a sanitary pad or small towel are applied in such a way that the mother can hold them in place by bringing her legs together.

■ OUTCOME CRITERIA: Almost all births are normal and do not constitute true medical emergencies. If a mother is healthy and is not bleeding, if her vital signs are normal, and if the baby's heart tones are normal, there is no immediate cause for alarm, even if the birth is imminent. Emergency care is directed toward ensuring that the baby breathes well and is kept warm, that the mother is protected from hemorrhage, and that her privacy is maintained. The nurse is likely to be the person who must initially evaluate the situation and decide whether to attempt to transfer or transport the mother or to prepare for emergency delivery. If a mother says the baby is coming, the attendant is advised to believe her and to act accordingly. Throughout the delivery and the third stage of labor, the nurse works to help the mother to feel calm, confident, and well cared for.

emergency department, (in a health care facility) a section of an institution that is staffed and equipped to provide rapid and varied emergency care, especially for those stricken with sudden and acute illness or those who are the victims of severe trauma.

Emergency Department Nurses' Association (EDNA), a national professional organization of emergency department nurses that defines and promotes emergency nursing practice. The Association, which was founded in 1970 and has more than 11,000 members, has written and implemented the Standards of Emergency Nursing Practice. The Association offers a certification examination and awards the designation Certified Emergency Nurse (CEN) to nurses who successfully complete it. EDNA publishes the *Journal of Emergency Nursing (JEN)* and *Continuing Education Core Curriculum of Emergency Nursing Practice*. The Association, which has its headquarters in Chicago, works closely with its members and with related associations to define practice and to prepare professionals to practice in the area of emergency care.

emergency doctrine, (in law) a doctrine that assumes a person's consent to medical treatment when the person is in imminent danger and unable to give informed consent to treatment. Emergency doctrine assumes that the person would consent if able to do so.

Emergency Medical Service (EMS), a national network of services coordinated to provide aid and medical assistance from primary response to definitive care, involving personnel trained in the rescue, stabilization, transportation, and advanced treatment of traumatic or medical emergencies. Linked by a communications system that operates on both a local and regional level, EMS is a tiered system of care, which is usually initiated by citizen action in the form of a telephone call to an emergency number. Subsequent stages include the first medical responder, ambulance personnel, medium and heavy rescue equipment, and paramedic units, if necessary, continuing in the hospital with emergency room nurses, emergency room physicians, specialists, and critical care nurses and physicians. See also **Emergency Medical Technician, Emergency Medical Technician-Advanced Life Support, Emergency Medical Technician-Intermediate, Emergency Medical Technician-**

Intravenous, Emergency Medical Technician-Paramedic.

Emergency Medical Technician (EMT), a person trained in and responsible for the administration of specialized emergency care and the transportation to a medical facility of victims of acute illness or injury. In addition to basic life-support skills, the EMT is trained in extrication and disentanglement, operation of emergency vehicles, basic anatomy, basic assessment of injury or illness, triage, care for specific injuries and illnesses, environmental emergencies, childbirth, and transport of the patient. EMTs undergo ongoing training in new procedures and must qualify for national recertification every 2 years. See also **Emergency Medical Service.**

Emergency Medical Technician-Advanced Life Support (EMT-ALS), a third-level EMT. The EMT-ALS is locally certified in all the skills of the basic-level EMT and EMT-IV. Additionally, the EMT-ALS may administer certain medications following the orders of the hospital physician, with whom radio contact is maintained. An EMT-ALS is also trained in the use of advanced life-support systems, including electric defibrillation equipment. See also **Emergency Medical Service.**

Emergency Medical Technician-Intermediate (EMT-I), a second-level emergency medical technician nationally certified as both an EMT-ALS and an EMT-IV. See also **Emergency Medical Service**

Emergency Medical Technician-Intravenous (EMT-IV), a second-level emergency medical technician. The EMT-IV is trained and locally certified in intravenous therapy, endotracheal intubation, and the use of other antishock techniques. See also **Emergency Medical Service.**

Emergency Medical Technician-Paramedic (EMT-P), an advanced-level emergency medical technician. The EMT-P is nationally certified in all the skills of EMTs of other levels, with additional training in pharmacology and the administration of emergency drugs. See also **Emergency Medical Service.**

emergency medicine, a branch of medicine concerned with the diagnosis and treatment of conditions resulting from trauma or sudden illness. The patient's condition is stabilized, and care of the patient is transferred to the primary physician or to a specialist. Emergency medicine requires a broad interdisciplinary training in the physiology and pathology of all of the systems of the body.

emergency nurse practitioner, a registered nurse with additional education through a master's degree program or through a nondegree certificate program approved for preparing nursing personnel to deliver primary care in an emergency room setting.

emergency nursing, nursing care provided to prevent imminent severe damage or death or to avert serious injury. Activities that exemplify emergency nursing are basic life support, cardiopulmonary resuscitation, and control of hemorrhage.

emergency room (ER, E.R.), a hospital area specially designed to receive and initially treat patients suffering from sudden trauma or medical problems, as accidental hemorrhage, poisoning, fracture, heart attack, and respiratory failure.

emergency theory, (in physiology) a theory stating that when a person is faced with an emergency, the adrenal medulla is stimulated by the sympathetic nervous system to release epinephrine, which increases heart rate, raises blood pressure, reduces blood flow to viscera, and mobilizes blood glucose, preparing the body for flight from danger or for the fight to survive. See also **flight-or-fight reaction.**

emergent evolution, the theory that evolution occurs in a series of major changes at certain critical stages and results from the total rearrangement of existing elements so that completely new and unpredictable characteristics appear within the species. See also **saltatory evolution.**

emesis. See **vomit,** def. 2.

Emete-con, a trademark for an antiemetic (benzquinamide hydrochloride), used after anesthesia.

emetic /imetʹik/, **1.** of or pertaining to a substance that causes vomiting. **2.** an emetic agent. Apomorphine hydrochloride, acting through the central nervous system, induces vomiting 10 to 15 minutes after parenteral administration. Syrup of ipecac is used in the emergency treatment of drug overdosage and in certain cases of poisoning, but it can be cardiotoxic if it is absorbed and not vomited.

-emetic, -emetical, a combining form meaning 'pertaining to vomiting': *antiemetic, hematemetic, hyperemetic.*

emetine hydrochloride /emʹətēn/, a potent, parenteral antiamebic.

■ INDICATIONS: It is prescribed in the treatment of acute fulminating amebic dysentery, amebic abscesses, and amebic hepatitis.

■ CONTRAINDICATIONS: Previous emetine therapy within 6 to 8 weeks, heart disease, polyneuropathy, kidney disease, or known hypersensitivity to this drug prohibits its use.

■ ADVERSE EFFECTS: Among the more serious adverse reactions are cardiovascular irregularities, hypotension, and neuromuscular effects.

Emetrol, a trademark for a fixed-combination drug containing fructose, glucose, and orthophosphoric acid, used to treat nausea and vomiting.

EMG, 1. abbreviation for **electromyogram. 2.** abbreviation for **exophthalmos, macroglossia, and gigantism.**

EMG syndrome, a hereditary disorder transmitted as an autosomal recessive trait. Clinical manifestations include exophthalmos, macroglossia, and gigantism, often accompanied by visceromegaly, dysplasia of the renal medulla, and enlargement of the cells of the adrenal cortex. Also called **Beckwith-Wiedemann syndrome, exophthalmos-macroglossia-gigantism syndrome.**

-emia, -aemia, -hemia, -haemia, 1. a combining form meaning a '(specified) blood condition': *hypoki-*

nemia, panhyperemia, pyknemia. **2.** a combining form meaning a 'blood condition involving a (specified) substance': *calcemia, iodemia, melitemia.*

emissary veins /em'əser'ē/, the small vessels in the skull that connect the sinuses of the dura with the veins on the exterior of the skull through a series of anastomoses. The major emissary veins are the mastoid emissary vein, the parietal emissary vein, the internal carotid plexus, the rete canalis hypoglossi, the condyloid emissary vein, the rete foraminis ovalis, and the small veins passing through the foramen lacerum to connect the cavernous sinus with the pterygoid plexus. Also included in the emissary group is a vein passing through the foramen cecum, connecting the superior sagittal sinus with the veins of the nasal cavity.

emission computed tomography (ECT), a form of tomography in which the emitted decay products, as positrons or gamma rays, of an ingested radioactive pharmaceutic are recorded in detectors outside the body. Computer reconstruction of the data yields a cross-sectional image of the body.

Emivan, a trademark for an analeptic agent (ethamivan).

emmetropia /em'ətrō'pē·ə/, a state of normal vision characterized by the proper relationship between the refractive system of the eyeball and its axial length. This correlation ensures that light rays entering the eye parallel to the optic axis are focused exactly on the retina. Compare **amblyopia, hyperopia, myopia.** **–emmetropic,** *adj.*

emollient /imol'yənt/, a substance that softens tissue, particularly the skin and mucous membranes.

emollient bath, a bath taken in water containing an emollient, as bran, to relieve irritation and inflammation. See also **colloid bath.**

emotion, the affective aspect of consciousness as compared with volition and cognition. Physiologic alterations often occur with a marked change of emotion regardless of whether the feelings are conscious or unconscious, expressed or unexpressed. See also **emotional need, emotional response.**

emotional abuse, the debasement of a person's feelings so that he perceives himself as inept, uncared for, and worthless.

emotional amalgam, an unconscious effort to deny or counteract anxiety.

emotional care of the dying patient, the compassionate, consistent support offered to help the terminally ill patient and the family cope with impending death. See also **stages of dying.**

■ METHOD: The professional person providing emotional support for the terminally ill encourages the expression of personal feelings, anxieties, and experiences regarding death, and empathizes with the patient and the family. The patient needs gentle, realistic care, but not all questions require answers, and the decision to tell the prognosis rests with the physician and family. To avoid conflicting statements, it is essential to know what the physician, other professionals, and family members tell the patient about the outcome. Effective support in terminal illness involves a nonjudgmental approach to the patient's relatives, an understanding of their problems, and efforts to assist them in the grieving process. The patient needs relief from pain, tender care, and continued attention through all the stages of dying: characteristically, a period of denial, followed by anger, bargaining, depression, and, finally, acceptance. When the patient denies the prognosis and refuses to follow directions, the nursing staff does not interfere with or support the denial mechanism but spends time with the sick person and encourages self-care. During the stage of anger, often manifested by refusal of care and food and by abusive language and negative criticism of the staff, the patient is not allowed to indulge in physically harmful behavior but is encouraged to verbalize the anger. In the period in which the patient tries to make bargains, as "If I could live until . . . ," it is recognized that time is needed to accept death and that the person may appreciate discussing the importance of various events and people in earlier life. When depression, marked by apathy, insomnia, inability to concentrate, poor appetite, and weariness, sets in, efforts to cheer the patient or interrupt crying are inappropriate; the patient may want only the most beloved person to be present. In the final stage of acceptance, the patient usually experiences less pain and discomfort, seems peaceful and lacking in emotional affect, and appreciates care from people who are close and familiar.

■ NURSING ORDERS: The nurse has the major role in providing emotional care for the hospitalized, terminally ill patient and may help the family arrange for home care when it is possible and desirable for the person to die at home. The nurse may teach methods of care required at home, may assist the family in realizing the patient's need to live as normally and as long as possible, and may refer the family to the social service department and to community resources for assistance.

■ OUTCOME CRITERIA: Sensitive emotional support appropriate to the stage of dying may help the person to move more rapidly through the usual stages of acceptance of dying. The family usually goes through similar stages; therefore, support and counseling by an experienced person may greatly enhance the quality of life of the patient and the patient's family.

emotional illness. See **mental disorder.**

emotional need, a psychologic or mental requirement of intrapsychic origin, usually centering on such basic feelings as love, fear, anger, sorrow, anxiety, frustration, and depression and involving the understanding, empathy, and support of one person for another. Such needs normally occur in everyone but usually are increased during periods of excessive stress or physical and mental illness and during various stages of life, as infancy, early childhood, and old age. If these needs are not routinely met by appropriate, socially accepted means, they can precipitate psychopathologic conditions. Appropriate measures common in nursing for anticipating and satisfying the emotional needs of patients in stress include physical closeness, especially remaining with the person during periods when the feeling is acute; empathic listening as the patient discusses the feeling; encouragement to talk; and planning activities that provide a constructive outlet for the feeling or the situation causing it. Compare **dependency needs.** See also **emotion.**

emotional response, a reaction to a particular intrapsychic feeling or feelings, accompanied by physiologic changes that may or may not be outwardly manifest but that motivate or precipitate some action or behavioral response. See also **emotion.**

emotional support, the sensitive, understanding approach that helps patients accept and deal with their illnesses, communicate their anxieties and fears, derive comfort from a gentle, sympathetic, caring person, and increase their ability to care for themselves.

■ METHOD: Essential in providing emotional support is recognizing and respecting the individuality, personal preferences, and human needs of each patient. Understanding the sick and appreciating the psychologic effects on the patient of the transition from health to illness are also important. The patient is encouraged to verbalize feelings and concerns, and the attentive listener avoids interjecting clichés, as "Don't worry," "Take it easy," or "Everything will be all right." The nurse and other workers realize that the patient may express some fears but may act out others through anger, hostility, silence, or assumed joviality. Efforts to change the patient, negative criticism, a judgmental attitude, and facial expressions that may indicate rejection are carefully avoided. Opportunities to listen to the troubled patient and provide compassionate and realistic counseling and care are sought.

■ NURSING ORDERS: The nurse establishes means of communication, provides an atmosphere that invites the patient to discuss the worrisome feelings, and presents a caring attitude. This is especially important when the illness damages the person's body image or self-concept. Care is administered by the nurse in a quiet, unhurried manner with the realization that a gentle touch is important and that the patient has a right to be informed of all procedures and their rationale.

■ OUTCOME CRITERIA: Emotional support frequently improves the patient's psychologic and physical state, often enabling the patient to accept the illness, to adjust with less anxiety, and to cope with the changes required.

empathy /em′pəthē/, the ability to recognize and to some extent share the emotions and states of mind of another and to understand the meaning and significance of that person's behavior. It is an essential quality for effective psychotherapy. Compare **sympathy.** **–empathic,** *adj.*, **empathize,** *v.*

emphysema /em′fəsē′mə/, an abnormal condition of the pulmonary system, characterized by overinflation and destructive changes of alveolar walls, resulting in a loss of lung elasticity and decreased gases. When emphysema occurs early in life, it is usually related to a rare genetic deficiency of serum alpha-1-antitrypsin, which inactivates the enzymes leukocyte collagenase and elastase. Acute emphysema may be caused by the rupture of alveoli by severe respiratory efforts, as in acute bronchopneumonia, suffocation, and whooping cough, and occasionally during labor. Chronic emphysema usually accompanies chronic bronchitis, a major cause of which is cigarette smoking. Emphysema is also seen after asthma or tuberculosis, conditions in which the lungs are overstretched until the elastic fibers of the alveolar walls are destroyed. In old age, the alveolar membranes atrophy and may collapse, resulting in large air-filled spaces with decreased total surface area of the pulmonary membranes.

■ OBSERVATIONS: The person may have shortness of breath, dyspnea, cough, cyanosis, orthopnea, unequal chest expansion, tachypnea, tachycardia, and an elevated temperature. Anxiety, carbon dioxide narcosis with a decreased pH, increased Pco_2, restlessness, confusion, weakness, anorexia, congestive heart failure, pulmonary edema, and respiratory failure are common in advanced cases.

■ INTERVENTION: The airway is kept open, and a low concentration of oxygen with humidification may be given for a prescribed number of minutes every hour. Bronchodilators, antibiotics, expectorants, and corticosteroids may be prescribed. Sedation is to be avoided, because most sedatives depress respiratory function. Postural drainage, cupping and vibration, and IPPB may improve pulmonary function.

■ NURSING CONSIDERATIONS: The patient is taught breathing exercises and encouraged to drink between 2000 and 3000 ml of fluids daily. Activity is encouraged to the limit of the patient's tolerance. Fatigue, constipation, and upper respiratory tract infection and irritation are to be avoided. A respirator and oxygen equipment may be prescribed for the patient's use at home. The patient is taught the adverse role that smoking plays in the disease and is encouraged to stop smoking.

empiric /empir′ik/, of or pertaining to a method of treating disease based on observations and experience without an understanding of the cause or mechanism of the disorder or the way the employed therapeutic agent or procedure effects improvement or cure. The empiric treatment of a new disease may be based on observations and experience gained in the management of analogous disorders. **–empirical,** *adj.*

empiricism, a form of therapy based on personal experience and the experience of other practitioners. **–empiricist,** *n.*

empiric treatment. See **treatment.**

Empirin, a trademark for a fixed-combination drug containing two analgesic-antipyretics (aspirin and phenacetin) and a central nervous system stimulant (caffeine).

emprosthotonos /em'prosthot'ənəs/, a position of the body characterized by a forward, rigid flexure of the body at the waist. The position is the result of a prolonged, involuntary, muscle spasm that is most commonly associated with tetanus infection or strychnine poisoning.

empty sella syndrome, an abnormal enlargement of the sella turcica in which no pituitary tumor is present; the gland may be smaller than normal, or it may be absent. Signs and symptoms of hormonal imbalance may be present, but some patients show no evidence of hypopituitarism or of any other endocrine abnormality. The condition is especially frequent in overweight, middle-aged, multiparous women. The diagnosis may be made by computerized axial tomography scan, skull x-ray study, or pneumoencephalography.

empyema /em'pī·ē'mə, em'pē·ē'mə/, an accumulation of pus in a body cavity, especially the pleural space, as a result of bacterial infection, as pleurisy or tuberculosis. It is usually removed by surgical incision, aspiration, and drainage. Antibiotics are administered to correct the cause of the underlying infection.

-empyema, a combining form meaning an 'accumulation of pus, especially thoracic': *arthroempyema, pneumoempyema, typhloempyema.*

EMS, abbreviation for **Emergency Medical Service.**

EMT, abbreviation for **Emergency Medical Technician.**

EMT-ALS, abbreviation for **Emergency Medical Technician-Advanced Life Support.**

EMT-I, abbreviation for **Emergency Medical Technician-Intermediate.**

EMT-IV, abbreviation for **Emergency Medical Technician-Intravenous.**

EMT-P, abbreviation for **Emergency Medical Technician-Paramedic.**

emulsify, to disperse a liquid into another liquid, making a colloidal suspension. Soaps and detergents emulsify by surrounding small globules of fat, preventing them from settling out. Bile acts as an emulsifying agent in the digestive tract by dispersing ingested fats into small globules. –**emulsification,** *n.*

emulsion, **1.** a system consisting of two immiscible liquids, one of which is dispersed in the other in the form of small droplets. **2.** (in photography) a composition sensitive to actinic rays of light, consisting of one or more silver halides suspended in gelatin applied in a thin layer to film.

E-Mycin, a trademark for an antibiotic (erythromycin).

en-, em- a combining form meaning 'in, on': *enanthema, encelialgia, enostosis.*

enamel, a hard white substance that covers the dentin of the crown of a tooth.

enamel hypocalcification, a hereditary dental defect in which the enamel of the teeth is soft and undercalcified in context yet normal in quantity, caused by defective maturation of the ameloblasts. The teeth are chalky in consistency, the surfaces wear down rapidly, and a yellow-to-brown stain appears as the underlying dentin is exposed. The condition affects both deciduous and permanent teeth. Compare **enamel hypoplasia.** See also **amelogenesis imperfecta.**

enamel hypoplasia, a developmental dental defect in which the enamel of the teeth is hard in context but thin and deficient in amount, caused by defective enamel matrix formation with a deficiency in the cementing substance. There is lack of contact between teeth, rapid breakdown of occlusive surfaces, and a yellowish brown stain that appears where the dentin is exposed. The condition, which affects both the deciduous and permanent teeth, is transmitted genetically or caused by environmental factors, as vitamin deficiency, fluorosis, exanthematous diseases, congenital syphilis, or injury or trauma to the mouth. Administration of tetracyclines during the second half of pregnancy or during tooth development in the child can also cause the condition. Compare **enamel hypocalcification.** See also **ameliogenesis imperfecta.**

enanthema /en'anthē'mə/, an eruptive lesion from the surface of a mucous membrane. Also called **enanthem** /ənan'thəm/.

Enarax, a trademark for a fixed-combination gastric antisecretory agent containing an anticholinergic (oxyphencyclimine hydrochloride) and a tranquilizer (hydroxyzine hydrochloride).

enarthrosis. See **ball-and-socket joint.**

encapsulated, (of arteries, muscles, nerves, and other body parts) enclosed in fibrous or membranous sheaths. See also **fascia bulbi, synovial sheath.**

-ence. See **-ency.**

-encephalia, -encephaly, a combining form meaning '(condition of the) brain': *amyelencephalia, rhinencephalia, synencephalia.*

encephalitis /ensef'əlī'tis/, *pl.* **encephalitides** /-tidēz/, an inflammatory condition of the brain. The cause is usually an arbovirus infection transmitted by the bite of an infected mosquito, but it may be the result of lead or other poisoning or of hemorrhage. **Postinfectious encephalitis** occurs as a complication of another infection, as chickenpox, influenza, or measles, or after smallpox vaccination. The condition is characterized by headache, neck pain, fever, nausea, and vomiting. Neurologic disturbances may occur, including seizures, personality change, irritability, lethargy, paralysis, weakness, and coma. The outcome depends on the cause, the age and condition of the person, and the extent of inflammation. Severe inflammation with destruction of nerve tissue may result in a seizure disorder, loss of a special sense or other permanent neurologic problem, or death. Usually, the inflammation involves the spinal cord and brain; hence, in most cases, a more accurate term is *encephalomyelitis.* Compare **meningitis.** See also **encephalomyelitis, equine encephalitis.**

encephalitis lethargica. See **epidemic encephalitis.**

encephalitis periaxialis diffusa. See **Schilder's disease.**

encephalocele /ensef′ələsēl′/, protrusion of the brain through a congenital defect in the skull; hernia of the brain. See also **neural tube defect.**

encephalodysplasia, any congenital anomaly of the brain.

encephalogram /ensef′ələgram′/, a radiograph of the brain made during encephalography.

encephalography /ensef′əlog′rəfē/, radiographic delineation of the structures of the brain containing fluid after the cerebrospinal fluid is withdrawn and replaced by a gas, as air, helium, or oxygen. The procedure is used mainly for indicating the site of cerebrospinal fluid obstruction in hydrocephalus or the structural abnormalities of the posterior fossa. Because of the risks involved, it is used only when computerized tomography is not definitive. Kinds of encephalography are **pneumoencephalography** and **ventriculography.** Also called **air encephalography.** Compare **echoencephalography, electroencephalography.** **–encephalographic,** *adj.*

encephaloid carcinoma. See **medullary carcinoma.**

encephalomeningocele. See **meningoencephalocele.**

encephalomyelitis /ensef′əlōmī′əlī′tis/, an inflammatory condition of the brain and spinal cord characterized by fever, headache, stiff neck, back pain, and vomiting. Depending on the cause, the age and condition of the person, and the extent of the inflammation and irritation to the central nervous system, seizures, paralysis, personality changes, a decreased level of consciousness, coma, or death may occur. Sequelae, as seizure disorders or decreased mental ability, may occur after severe inflammation that causes extensive damage to the cells and tissues of the nervous system. See also **encephalitis, equine encephalitis.**

encephalomyocarditis /ensef′əlōmī′ōkärdī′tis/, an infectious disease of the central nervous system and heart tissue caused by a group of small RNA picornaviruses. Rodents are a major reservoir of the infection. Human illness ranges from asymptomatic infection to severe encephalomyelitis. Symptoms are generally similar to those of poliomyelitis. Myocarditis is not a feature of infection in humans, and most victims recover promptly without sequelae. Treatment is supportive. See also **picornavirus.**

encephalopathy /ensef′əlop′əthē/, any abnormal condition of the structure or function of tissues of the brain, especially chronic, destructive, or degenerative conditions, as Wernicke's encephalopathy or Schilder's disease.

encephalotrigeminal angiomatosis. See **Sturge-Weber syndrome.**

-encephaly. See **-encephalia.**

enchondroma /en′kəndrō′mə/, *pl.* **enchondromas, enchondromata,** a benign, slowly growing tumor of cartilage cells that arises in the extremity of the shaft of tubular bones, usually in the hands or feet. The growth of the neoplasm, by cell proliferation and the accession of small satellite tumors, may distend the bone. Also called **enchondrosis, true chondroma.**

enchondromatosis /en′kəndrō′mətō′sis/, a congenital disorder characterized by the proliferation of cartilage within the extremity of the shafts of several bones, causing thinning of the cortex and distortion in length. Also called **dyschondroplasia, multiple enchondromatosis, Ollier's disease, skeletal enchondromatosis.** See also **Maffucci's syndrome.**

enchondromatous myxoma, a tumor of the connective tissue, characterized by the presence of cartilage between the cells of connective tissue. See also **myxoma.**

enchondrosarcoma. See **central chondrosarcoma.**

enchondrosis. See **enchondroma.**

enchylema. See **hyaloplasm.**

-enchyma, a combining form meaning the 'liquid that nourishes tissue, or tissue itself': *karyenchyma, mesenchyma, sclerenchyma.*

encode, 1. to translate a message, signal, or stimulus into a code. **2.** to rewrite, manually or automatically, as by a computer program, information into a form that can be interpreted by a computer.

encoded message, (in communication theory) a message as transmitted by a sender to a receiver.

encopresis /en′kōprē′sis/, fecal incontinence. **–encopretic,** *adj.*

encounter, (in psychotherapy) the interaction between a patient and a psychotherapist, as occurs in existential therapy, or among several members of a small group, as in encounter or sensitivity training groups, in which emotional change and personal growth are brought about by the expression of strong feelings by the participants.

encounter group, (in psychology) a small group of people who meet to increase self-awareness, promote personal growth, and improve interpersonal communication. Members focus on becoming aware of their feelings and on developing the ability to express those feelings openly, honestly, and clearly. See also **group therapy, psychotherapy, sensitivity training group.**

enculturation, the process of learning the concepts, values, and behavioral standards of a particular culture.

-ency, -ance, -ancy, -ence, 1. a combining form meaning a 'quality or state': *deficiency, dependency.* **2.** a combining form meaning a 'person or thing in a state': *latency.* **3.** a combining form meaning an 'instance of a quality or state': *emergency.*

encyst /ensist′/, to form a cyst or capsule. See also **cyst.** **–encysted,** *adj.*

end /ē′en′dē′, end/, (in cytogenetics) abbreviation for **endoreduplication.**

end-. See **endo-.**

Endameba. See ***Entamoeba.***

endamebiasis. See **amebiasis.**

Endamoeba. See ***Entamoeba.***

endamoebiasis. See **amebiasis.**

endarterectomy /en′därtərek′təmē/, a surgical procedure that excises tunica intima, or core, of an artery that has become thickened by atherosclerosis.

endarteritis /en′därtərī′tis/, an inflammatory disorder of the inner layer of one or more arteries, which may become partially or completely occluded.

endarteritis obliterans, an inflammatory condition of the lining of the arterial walls in which the intima proliferates, narrowing the lumen of the vessels and occluding the smaller vessels.

end bud, a mass of undifferentiated cells produced from the remnants of the primitive node and the primitive streak at the caudal end of the developing embryo after the formation of the somites is completed. In lower animals it gives rise to the tail or any other caudal appendage and part of the trunk; in humans it forms the caudal portion of the trunk. Also called **tail bud.**

end bulbs of Krause. See **Krause's corpuscles.**

endemic /endem′ik/, (of a disease or microorganism) indigenous to a geographic area or population. See also **epidemic, pandemic.**

endemic goiter, an enlargement of the thyroid gland caused by the dietary intake of inadequate amounts of dietary iodine. Iodine deprivation leads to diminished production and secretion of thyroid hormone by the gland. The pituitary gland, operating on a negative feedback system, senses the deficiency and secretes increased amounts of thyroid-stimulating hormone, causing hyperplasia and hypertrophy of the thyroid gland. The goiter may grow during the winter months and shrink during the summer months when more iodine-bearing fresh vegetables are eaten. Initially, the goiter is diffuse; later, it becomes multinodular. Endemic goiter occurs occasionally in adolescents at puberty and widely in population groups in geographic areas in which limited amounts of iodine are present in the soil, water, and food. The use of iodized salt is a prophylactic treatment. Dessicated thyroid given orally may prevent further growth of adult goiters and may reduce the size of diffuse goiters. A large goiter may cause dysphagia, dyspnea, tracheal deviation, and cosmetic problems.

endemic typhus. See **murine typhus.**

endo-, end-, ento-, a combining form meaning 'inward, within': *endobiotic, endocranial, endognathion.*

endobronchial anesthesia, a procedure, rarely performed, in which anesthetic gas is administered into the bronchi.

endocardial cushion defect, any cardiac defect resulting from the failure of the endocardial cushions in the embryonic heart to fuse and form the atrial septum. See also **atrial septal defect, congenital cardiac anomaly.**

endocardial cushions, a pair of thickened tissue sections in the embryonic atrial canal. During embryonic development, they meet and fuse to form a septum that divides the canal into two channels that eventually become the atrioventricular orifices.

endocardial fibroelastosis /fī′brō•ē′lastō′sis/, an abnormal condition characterized by hypertrophy of the wall of the left ventricle and the development of a thick, fibroelastic endocardium. This condition often increases the ventricular capacity but sometimes decreases it. Some studies have incriminated the mumps virus in endocardial fibroelastosis, while other investigations refute such a connection.

endocarditis /en′dōkärdī′tis/, an abnormal condition that affects the endocardium and the heart valves and is characterized by lesions caused by a variety of diseases. The kinds of endocarditis are bacterial endocarditis, nonbacterial thrombotic endocarditis, and Libman-Sacks endocarditis. Untreated, all types of endocarditis are rapidly lethal, but they are often successfully treated by various antibacterial and surgical measures. With adequate treatment about 65% to 80% of the patients with endocarditis survive. See also **bacterial endocarditis, subacute bacterial endocarditis.**

endocardium /en′dōkär′dē•əm/, *pl.* **endocardia,** the lining of the heart chambers, containing small blood vessels and a few bundles of smooth muscle. It is continuous with the endothelium of the great blood vessels. Compare **epicardium, myocardium.**

endocervical, pertaining to the interior of the cervix and uterus.

endocervicitis /en′dōsur′visī′tis/, an abnormal condition characterized by inflammation of the epithelium and glands of the canal of the uterine cervix. See also **cervicitis.**

endocervix /en′dōsur′viks/, **1.** the membrane lining the canal of the uterine cervix. **2.** the opening of the cervix into the uterine cavity.

endocrine fracture /en′dōkrīn, -krēn/, any fracture that results from weakness of a specific bone because of an endocrine disorder, as hyperparathyroidism.

endocrine system, the network of ductless glands and other structures that elaborate and secrete hormones directly into the bloodstream, affecting the function of specific target organs. Glands of the endocrine system include the thyroid and the parathyroid, the anterior pituitary, the posterior pituitary, the pancreas, the suprarenal glands, and the gonads. The pineal gland is also considered an endocrine gland because it is ductless, although its precise endocrine function is not established. The thymus gland, once considered an endocrine gland, is now classified in the lymphatic system. Various other organs have some endocrinologic function. Secretions from the endocrine glands affect various processes throughout the body, as metabolism, growth, and secretions from other organs. Compare **exocrine.** See also the Color Atlas of Human Anatomy.

endocrinologist /en′dōkrinol′əjist/, a physician who specializes in endocrinology.

endocrinology, the study of the anatomy, physiology, and pathology of the endocrine system and of the treatment of endocrine problems.

endoderm /en′dədurm/, (in embryology) the innermost of the cell layers that develop from the embryonic disk of the inner cell mass of the blastocyst. From the endoderm arises the epithelium of the trachea, bronchi, lungs, GI tract, liver, pancreas, urinary bladder and canal, pharynx, thyroid, tympanic cavity, tonsils, and parathyroid glands. The endoderm thus comprises the lining of the cavities and passages of the body and the covering for most of the internal organs. Compare **ectoderm, mesoderm.**

endodermal cloaca, a part of the cloaca in the developing embryo that lies internal to the cloacal membrane and gives rise to the bladder and urogenital ducts. Compare **ectodermal cloaca.** See also **urogenital sinus.**

endogenous /endoj′ənəs/, **1.** growing within the body. **2.** originating from within the body or produced from internal causes, as a disease caused by the structural or functional failure of an organ or system. Compare **exogenous.** –**endogenic,** *adj.*

endogenous depression, a major affective disorder characterized by a persistent dysphoric mood, anxiety, irritability, fear, brooding, appetite and sleep disturbances, weight loss, psychomotor agitation or retardation, decreased energy, feelings of worthlessness or guilt, difficulty in concentrating or thinking, occasional delusions and hallucinations, and thoughts of death or suicide. The disorder, which occurs in children, adolescents, and adults, may develop over a period of days, weeks, or months; episodes may occur in clusters or singly, separated by several years of normality. The causes of the disorder are multiple and complex and may involve biologic, psychologic, interpersonal, and sociocultural factors that lead to some unidentifiable intrapsychic conflict. Treatment includes the use of antidepressants and electroconvulsive therapy, followed by long-term psychotherapy. In severe cases, proper nursing care is needed for adequate nutrition, appropriate balance of fluid intake and output, good personal hygiene, and protection of the patient from self-injury. Also called **major depressive episode.** See also **bipolar disorder, depression.**

endogenous infection, an infection caused by the reactivation of previously dormant organisms, as in coccidioidomycosis, histoplasmosis, and tuberculosis. Compare **germinal infection, mixed infection, retrograde infection, secondary infection.**

endogenous obesity, obesity resulting from dysfunction of the endocrine or metabolic systems. Compare **exogenous obesity.** See also **obesity.**

endolith. See **denticle.**

endolymph /en′dəlimf/, the fluid in the membranous labyrinth of the internal ear. Compare **perilymph.**

endolymphatic duct, a labyrinthine passage joining an endolymphatic sac with a utricle and saccule.

endolymphatic hydrops, an obsolete term for **Ménière's disease.**

endometrial /en′dōmē′trē·əl/, **1.** of or pertaining to endometrium. **2.** of or pertaining to the uterine cavity.

endometrial cancer, a maligant neoplastic disease of the endometrium of the uterus most often occurring in the fifth or sixth decade of life. Some of the factors associated with an increased incidence of the disease are a medical history of infertility, anovulation, administration of exogenous estrogen, uterine polyps, and a combination of diabetes, hypertension, and obesity. Abnormal vaginal bleeding, especially in a postmenopausal woman, is the cardinal symptom. There also may be lower abdominal and low back pain; a large, boggy uterus is often a sign of advanced disease. Less than half the patients with endometrial cancer have a positive Papanicolaou (Pap) test of the cervix and vagina, because the tumor cells rarely exfoliate in early stages of the lesion. A Pap test of cells removed from the endometrium obtained from jet washings of the uterine cavity provides more accurate data. Vacuum curettage is also used to extract endometrial cells for study, but the diagnostic technique most frequently recommended is a dilatation and curettage in which each section of the uterus is examined and curetted for biopsy specimens. Adenocarcinomas constitute roughly 90% of all endometrial tumors; mixed carcinomas, sarcomas, and benign adenoacanthomas comprise the rest. Endometrial lesions may spread to the cervix, but rarely invade the vagina. They metastasize to the broad ligaments, fallopian tubes, and ovaries so frequently that bilateral salpingo-oophorectomy with abdominal hysterectomy is the usual treatment. Radiotherapy is usually administered preoperatively and postoperatively. High doses of a progestogen may be administered for palliation in advanced or inoperable cases.

endometrial hyperplasia, an abnormal condition characterized by overgrowth of the endometrium resulting from sustained stimulation by estrogen (of endogenous or exogenous origin) that is not opposed by progesterone. Estrogens act as growth hormone for the endometrium. Through a complex intercellular mechanism, endometrial cells bind estrogens preferentially and undergo changes characteristic of the proliferative phase of the menstrual cycle. If estrogen stimulation continues for 3 to 6 months without periodic cessation or counteractive progesterone stimulation, as occurs in anovulatory or perimenopausal women or in women receiving replacement estrogen without added progestogen, the endometrium becomes abnormally thickened and glandularized. Unremitting estrogen stimulation eventually causes cystic or adenomatous endometrial hyperplasia, the latter a premalignant lesion that undergoes malignant degeneration in approximately 25% of women having it. The causative relationship between estrogen and endometrial hyperplasia is well established; there is implication but not proof that estrogen also provokes the change from hyperplasia to neoplasia and malignancy. Endometrial hyperplasia often results in abnormal uterine bleeding; such bleeding, particularly in older women, constitutes an indication for biopsy or curettage of the endometrium to establish histopathologic diagnosis and to rule out malignancy. A functioning estrogen-secreting tumor is suspected if the woman is not taking estrogen medication. Progestogen therapy is effective in reversing the abnormal histopathologic changes of endometrial hyperplasia; if hyperplasia is adenomatous, hysterectomy is commonly performed.

endometrial polyp, a pedunculated overgrowth of endometrium, usually benign. Polyps are a common cause of vaginal bleeding in perimenopausal women and are often associated with other uterine abnormalities, as endometrial hyperplasia or fibroids. They may occur singly or in clusters and are usually 1 cm or less in diameter, but they may become much larger and prolapse through the cervix. Treatment for the condition includes surgical dilatation and curettage.

endometriosis /en′dōmē′trē•ō′sis/, an abnormal gynecologic condition characterized by ectopic growth and function of endometrial tissue. Precise incidence of the disease is unknown, but evidence of it is found in approximately 15% of women who undergo pelvic laparotomy for other indications. Women of higher socioeconomic status and women who defer pregnancy are more likely to contract the disease. The average age of women found to have endometriosis is 37 years. The disease is uncommon among black women. Pregnancy has a definite but inconsistent influence in preventing or ameliorating the disease. The causes of endometriosis are unknown; evidence suggests that the ectopic endometrium of endometriosis develops from vestigial tissue of the wolffian or müllerian ducts; other evidence strongly suggests that fragments of endometrium from the lining of the uterus are regurgitated during menstruation backward through the fallopian tubes into the peritoneal cavity, where they attach, grow, and function. Fragments of this tissue, which is microscopically similar to or identical with endometrium, having glands or glandlike structures, stroma, and areas of hemorrhage, may be found in the wall of the uterus or on its surface, in or on the tubes, ovaries, rectosigmoid, or pelvic peritoneum, or, occasionally, in remote extrapelvic areas. Foci of endometriosis have been found in surgical scars, the umbilicus, the bowel, the lung, the eye, and the brain. When endometriosis occurs in a critical location, it may result in grave dysfunction of the organ involved or, rarely, in death; intestinal obstruction is a common complication. The lesions of pelvic endometriosis are typically small cystic structures a few millimeters in diameter that appear individually or in clusters as black nodules on the visceral and parietal peritoneum. Ovarian endometrial cysts, however, commonly grow to several centimeters in diameter. The endometrial tissue of endometriosis in both large and small lesions functions cyclically and undergoes periodic menstrual breakdown that results in bleeding within cysts, stretching of the cyst wall, and pain. Ovarian endometrial cysts containing menstruum that has become a thick, dark-brown liquid are called "chocolate cysts." The most characteristic symptom of endometriosis is pain, particularly dysmenorrhea and dyspareunia, but also dysuria, painful defecation, and suprapubic soreness. Pain is not always present, however, and its absence does not rule out the presence of the disease. Other common symptoms include premenstrual vaginal staining of blood, hypermenorrhea, and infertility. On pelvic examination, tender nodularity of the uterosacral ligaments is commonly found. Diagnosis is made by biopsy of tissue obtained from lesions found on culdoscopy, laparoscopy, or laparotomy. Some of the measures that have been recommended to prevent endometrial regurgitation include avoidance by examiners of forceful manipulation of the pelvic organs, particularly during a woman's menstruation, anteversion of retroverted uteri to provide better menstrual drainage, correction of cervical obstruction, and avoidance by women of prolonged deferral of pregnancy. Treatment of endometriosis in its milder forms may consist only of medication with analgesics and expectant follow-up, because many women will outgrow mild endometriosis or become pregnant. When the disease is more extensive, the treatment is hormonal or surgical and is directed at reducing the size and number of lesions, relieving symptoms, and correcting infertility, if present. Prolonged suppression of ovulation may produce a hormonal milieu similar to pregnancy and result in partial or total regression of lesions; this condition of "pseudopregnancy" may be brought about with danazol, with estrogen and progestogen separately or in combination, or, less often, with androgen. Among women with endometriosis and infertility who undergo prolonged hormonal therapy, approximately 40% become pregnant after treatment. Conservative surgery to preserve reproductive function entails excision or ablation of individual lesions, restoration of normal uterine and adnexal position, freeing of adhesions, and obliteration of the cul-de-sac, a most common site of endometrial implantation. Advanced endometriosis often requires surgery, including total abdominal hysterectomy and bilateral salpingo-oophorectomy to remove large lesions and to terminate cyclic ovarian stimulation on which endometrial growth depends so that retained lesions atrophy and heal.

endometritis /en′dōmitrī′tis/, an inflammatory condition of the endometrium, usually caused by bacterial infection, commonly gonococci or hemolytic streptococci. It is characterized by fever, abdominal pain, malodorous discharge, and enlargement of the uterus. It occurs most frequently after childbirth or abortion and in women fitted with an intrauterine contraceptive device. The diagnosis may be made by physical examination, history, laboratory analysis revealing an elevated white blood cell count, ultrasound, and bacteriologic identification of the pathogen. Treatment includes antibiotics, rest, analgesia, an adequate intake of fluids, and, if necessary, surgical drainage of a suppurating abscess, hysterectomy, or salpingo-oophorectomy. Endometritis may be mild and self-limited, chronic or acute, and unilateral or bilateral. It may result in sterility because of scar formation occluding the passage of the fallopian tubes. Septic abortion and puerperal fever are forms of endometritis that caused many deaths before antibiotics and asepsis became commonly available. A kind of endometritis is **decidua endometritis.** See also **pelvic inflammatory disease.**

endometritis dessicans, *obsolete.* endometritis characterized by ulceration and shedding of the endometrium of the uterus.

endometrium /en′dōmē′trē•əm/, the mucous membrane lining of the uterus, consisting of the stratum compactum, the stratum spongiosum, and the stratum basale.

The endometrium changes in thickness and structure with the menstrual cycle. The stratum compactum and the stratum spongiosum comprise the pars functionalis and are shed with each menstrual flow. The pars functionalis is known as the decidua during pregnancy, when it underlies the placenta. Compare **parametrium.**

endomorph /en′dəmôrf′/, a person whose body build is characterized by a soft, round physique with a large trunk and thighs, tapering extremities, an accumulation of fat throughout the body, and a predominance of structures derived from the endoderm. Compare **ectomorph, mesomorph.** See also **pyknic.**

endoparasite /en′dōper′əsīt/, (in medical parasitology) an organism that lives within the body of the host, as a tapeworm.

endophthalmitis /endof′thalmī′tis/, an inflammatory condition of the internal eye in which the eye becomes red, swollen, painful, and, sometimes, filled with pus. This condition may blur the vision and cause vomiting, fever, and headache. Endophthalmitis may result from bacterial or fungal infection, trauma, allergy, drug or chemical toxicity, or vascular disease. Depending on the cause, therapy requires surgical intervention or the administration of an antibiotic, atropine, or a corticosteroid. Also called **endophthalmia.**

endophthalmitis phacoanaphylactica /fak′ō•an′əfilak′təkə/, an abnormal condition characterized by an acute autoimmune reaction of the eye. It is caused by hypersensitivity of the eye to the protein of the crystalline lens and commonly occurs after trauma to the crystalline lens or after a cataract operation. Associated symptoms include swelling and inflammation of the eye, severe pain, and blurred vision. The substance of the lens is invaded by polymorphonuclear cells and mononuclear phagocytes. Sensitization of one eye often follows the extracapsular removal of the lens of the eye on the opposite side. Accurate diagnosis must differentiate between this condition and infectious endophthalmitis. Therapy is supportive and commonly includes the administration of corticosteroids and atropine. Refractory cases may require surgical removal of the lens. Compare **uveitis.**

endophytic /en′dōfit′ik/, of or pertaining to the tendency to grow inward, as an endophytic tumor that grows on the inside of an organ or structure.

endoplasmic reticulum, an extensive network of membrane-enclosed tubules in the cytoplasm of cells. The ultramicroscopic organelle, which can be seen only with an electron microscope, is classified as granular or rough-surfaced when ribosomes are attached to the surface of the membrane and agranular or smooth-surfaced when ribosomes are absent. The structure functions in the synthesis of proteins and lipids and in the transport of these metabolites within the cell.

endorphin /endôr′fin/, any one of the neuropeptides composed of many amino acids, elaborated by the pituitary gland and acting on the central and the peripheral nervous systems to reduce pain. Endorphins isolated by researchers are alpha-endorphin, beta-endorphin, and gamma-endorphin, all chemicals producing pharmacologic effects similar to morphine. Beta-endorphin has been isolated in the brain and in the GI tract and seems to be the most potent of the endorphins. Beta-endorphin is composed of 31 amino acids that are identical to part of the sequence of 91 amino acids of the hormone beta-lipoprotein, also produced by the pituitary gland. Behavioral tests indicate that beta-endorphin is a powerful analgesic in humans and animals. Brain-stimulated analgesia in humans releases beta-endorphin into the cerebrospinal fluid. Compare **enkephalin.**

endorsement, a statement of recognition of the license of a health practitioner in one state by another state. An endorsement relieves the health practitioner of the necessity of going through the full licensing procedure of the state in which practice is to be undertaken.

endoscope, an illuminated optic instrument for the visualization of the interior of a body cavity or organ. Instruments are available in varying lengths, and the fiberopticendoscope has great flexibility, reaching previously inaccessible areas. Although the endoscope is generally introduced through a natural opening in the body, it may also be inserted through an incision. Other instruments for viewing specific areas of the body include the bronchoscope, cystoscope, gastroscope, laparoscope, otoscope, and vaginoscope. See also **fiberoptics.** **–endoscopic,** *adj.*

endoscopic retrograde cholangiography, (in radiology) a diagnostic procedure for outlining the common bile duct. A flexible fiberoptic duodenoscope is placed in the common bile duct. A radiopaque substance is instilled directly into the duct, and serial x-ray films are taken. See also **cholangiography.**

endoscopy /endos′kəpē/, the visualization of the interior of organs and cavities of the body with an endoscope. The procedure is indicated for the diagnosis of gastric ulcers with atypical radiologic features, to locate the source of upper GI bleeding, to establish the presence and extent of varices in the lower esophagus and stomach in patients with liver disease, and to detect any abnormalities of the lower colon. For examination of the upper GI tract, the stomach of the patient is lavaged with ice water through a large-bore gastric tube, with the patient placed on the side to reduce the chance of aspiration. For examination of the lower colon, fecal material is removed by enema, laxative, or suppository. The patient is placed in the knee-chest position for the procedure and afterward is observed by the nurse for abdominal pain or rectal bleeding. Aseptic rather than sterile techniques are routinely followed. Endoscopy can also be used to obtain samples for cytologic and histologic examination and to follow the course of a disease, as the assessment of the healing of gastric and duodenal ulcers. See also **bronchoscopy, cystoscopy, gastroscopy, laparoscopy.**

endostomy therapist. See **enterostomal therapist.**

endothelial myeloma /en′dōthē′lē•əl/, a malignant myeloma that develops in the bone marrow, occurring most frequently in the long bones. Pain, fever, and leukocytosis are characteristically present. Also called **Ewing's tumor.**

-endothelioma, a combining form meaning 'a tumor of endothelial tissue': *hemendothelioma, lymphendothelioma.*

endothelium /en'dōthē'lē•əm/, the layer of squamous epithelial cells that lines the heart, the blood and the lymph vessels, and the serous cavities of the body. It is highly vascular, heals quickly, and is derived from the mesoderm.

endotoxin /en'dōtok'sin/, a toxin contained in the cell walls of some microorganisms, especially gram-negative bacteria, that is released when the bacterium dies and is broken down in the body. Fever, chills, shock, leukopenia, and a variety of other symptoms result, depending on the particular organism and the condition of the infected person. Compare **exotoxin.**

endotracheal /en'dōtrā'kē•əl/, within or through the trachea.

endotracheal anesthesia, inhalation anesthesia that is achieved by the passage of an anesthetic gas or mixture of gases through an endotracheal tube into the respiratory tract. General anesthesia is usually obtained by endotracheal anesthesia.

endotracheal intubation, the management of the patient with an airway catheter inserted through the mouth or nose into the trachea. An endotracheal tube may be used to maintain a patent airway, to prevent aspiration of material from the digestive tract in the unconscious or paralyzed patient, to permit suctioning of tracheobronchial secretions, or to administer positive-pressure ventilation that cannot be given effectively by a mask. Endotracheal tubes may be made of rubber or plastic and usually have an inflatable cuff to maintain a closed system with the ventilator.

■ METHOD: The endotracheal tube is inserted via the mouth or nose through the larynx into the trachea; if the oral route is used, a bite block may be required to keep the patient from biting and obstructing the tube. Breath sounds are auscultated immediately after insertion and every 1 or 2 hours thereafter to make certain the tube is properly positioned and is not obstructing one of the mainstem bronchi. Once the tube is correctly positioned, it is taped securely in place and checked for patency and slippage every 15 to 60 minutes. The trachea is suctioned every hour and irrigated with normal saline solution, if so ordered. The patient is usually on intermittent positive-pressure breathing (IPPB) or a volume respirator with the cuff of the endotracheal tube inflated; if the patient can breathe independently, the trachea and mouth are suctioned, the cuff is deflated, and the respiratory rate and quality are checked hourly. The patient is turned every 1 to 2 hours, with the blood pressure and pulse checked every 2 to 4 hours. Parenteral fluids are administered as ordered; nothing is given orally; the intake and output of fluids are measured and recorded. The patient's level of consciousness is determined hourly, and if he is sufficiently conscious, a method of communication is established.

■ NURSING ORDERS: The nurse monitors the position and patency of the endotracheal tube, performs the necessary suctioning, inflates and deflates the cuff at appropriate times, and administers IPPB or support with the volume respirator. The nurse checks the vital signs at the ordered intervals and provides emotional support as well as physical care for the patient, who is usually acutely ill, unable to communicate, and suffering from the discomfort of an endotracheal tube.

■ OUTCOME CRITERIA: Meticulous care of the patient with an endotracheal tube can result in the survival of a critically ill person.

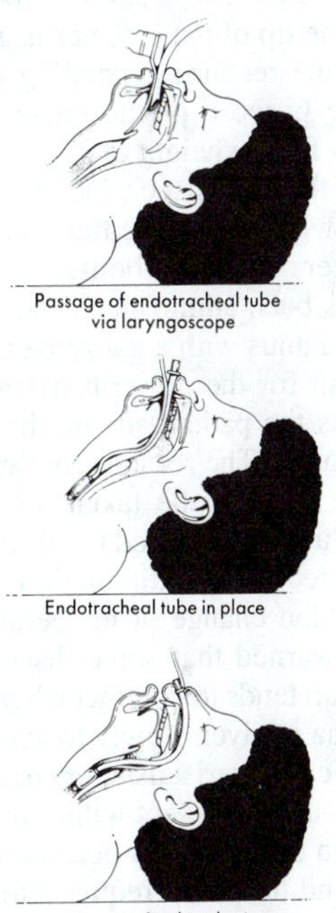

Passage of endotracheal tube via laryngoscope
Endotracheal tube in place
Nasotracheal intubation

Endotracheal intubation

endotracheal tube, a large-bore catheter inserted through the mouth or nose and into the trachea to a point above the bifurcation of the trachea proximal to the bronchi. It is used for delivering oxygen under pressure when ventilation must be totally controlled and in general anesthetic procedures. See also **endotracheal intubation.**

endoxin /endok'sin/, an endogenous analog of digoxin, occurring naturally in humans. It is a hormone that may regulate the excretion of salt.

Endrate, a trademark for a chelating agent (edetate disodium).

Enduron, a trademark for a diuretic and antihypertensive (methyclothiazide).

Enduronyl, a trademark for a cardiovascular, fixed-combination drug containing a diuretic (methyclothiazide) and an antihypertensive (deserpidine).

-ene, a combining form naming hydrocarbons: *ethidene, somnifene, xanthene.*

enema, a procedure in which a solution is introduced into the rectum for cleansing or therapeutic purposes. Enemas may be commercially packed disposable units or reusable equipment prepared just before use.

■ METHOD: The equipment is assembled; if reusable equipment is to be used, an 18-to-20 French gauge catheter, a 2- to 3-foot length of tubing, an enema can, the solution, a clamp, and a thermometer are collected and brought to the bedside. If a disposable set is to be used, no other equipment is necessary. The patient is positioned in the left lateral knee-chest or dorsal position. After air is expelled from the tubing, the tip of the catheter is lubricated. (Disposable units usually have prelubricated tips.) The patient is asked to bear down, as if to defecate, and the tip of the catheter is gently inserted 7.5 to 10 cm into the rectum, depending on the size of the patient and the purpose of the enema. The solution is allowed to flow from a height of 45 cm above the level of the hips, or, with some disposable enemas, the container is squeezed slowly to force the fluid into the rectum. The tip of the catheter or squeeze-bottle is withdrawn when all the solution has been administered, and light pressure is applied over the anus with a gauze pad. The fluid is held in by the patient for the prescribed length of time. It is then expelled as the patient sits on the toilet.

■ NURSING ORDERS: The reasons for performing the procedure and the steps to be taken are explained to the patient. The solution is warmed to 99° F (37.8° C) to 105° F (40.6° C) to reduce the stimulation of intestinal peristalsis by a sudden change of temperature in the colon. The patient is warned that some discomfort may occur because the colon tends to contract when distended by the fluid. The enema is given slowly to avoid sudden distention that would cause peristalsis, or spasm, and increased discomfort. A call bell is kept within reach of the patient during expulsion of the enema because the discomfort of the procedure and the effort required to expel the enema may cause faintness. The color, consistency, and amount of material evacuated are evaluated. If reusable equipment is used, it is rinsed in cold water before being washed with warm soapy water and sterilized.

■ OUTCOME CRITERIA: Careful observation of the patient during the procedure, slow and gentle administration of the enema, evaluation of the results of the procedure, and a thorough explanation to the patient of all aspects of the procedure are important to achieve the desired effect of the enema.

energy, the capacity to do work or to perform vigorous activity. Compare **anergy.** –**energetic,** *adj.*

energy-protein malnutrition, a condition resulting from a diet deficient in both calories and proteins. Also called **protein-calorie malnutrition.** See also **marasmic kwashiorkor, marasmus.**

energy subtraction, subtraction of two digitized x-ray images that were produced by x-rays whose energies were different.

enervation, **1.** the reduction or lack of nervous energy; weakness; lassitude; languor. **2.** removal of a complete nerve or of a section of nerve.

en face /äNfäs′/, "face-to-face"; a position in which the mother's face and the infant's face are approximately 8 inches apart and on the same plane, as when the mother holds the infant up in front of her face or when she nurses the child. Studies of maternal and infant bonding have shown that mothers seek eye-to-eye contact, and that they will instinctively move the baby to an en face position. In addition, infants have been shown to prefer a human face over other visual stimuli and to be best able to focus at a distance of 8 to 10 inches.

enflurane /en′flo͞orān/, a nonflammable anesthetic gas belonging to the ether family, used for induction and maintenance of general anesthesia in cases in which ethers are the drugs of choice. A halogenated volatile liquid, enflurane is administered through vaporizers specially calibrated for delivery via nitrous oxide or an oxygen-nitrous oxide mixture, permitting close control of dosage. Because excitement may occur on induction, a hypnotic dose of short-acting barbiturate is sometimes used for premedication. Adverse reactions may include seizure activity, muscle fasciculation, hypotension, cardiac arrhythmia, shivering, and elevated white blood cell count. Nausea and vomiting on emergence from anesthesia sometimes occur.

engagement, **1.** fixation of the presenting part of the fetus in the maternal pelvis. The lowest part of the presenting part is at or below the level of the ischial spines. **2.** fixation of the fetal head in the maternal pelvis with the biparietal diameter of the head level with the ischial spines.

English position. See **lateral recumbent position.**

engorgement, distention or vascular congestion of body tissues, as the swelling of breast tissue caused by an increased flow of blood and lymph preceding true lactation.

engrossment. See **bonding.**

Enisyl, a trademark for an amino acid (lysine hydrochloride).

enkephalin /enkef′əlin/, one of two pain-relieving pentapeptides produced in the body. Researchers have isolated enkephalins in the pituitary gland, brain, and GI tract. The enkephalins are methionine-enkephalin and isoleucine-enkephalin, each composed of five amino acids, four of which are identical in both compounds. It is believed that these two neuropeptides can depress neurons throughout the central nervous system. Axon terminals that release enkephalins are concentrated in the posterior horn of the gray matter of the spinal cord, in the central part of the thalamus, and in the amygdala of the limbic system of the cerebrum. Enkephalins inhibit neurotransmitters in the pathway for pain perception, thereby reducing the emotional as well as the physical impact of pain. Although it is not known exactly how these two neuropeptides function, many experts believe that the enkephalins are natural pain killers and that they may be involved, with other neuropeptides, in the development of psychopathologic behavior in some cases. Compare **endorphin.**

enomania. See **oinomania.**

enophthalmos /en'əfthal'məs/, backward displacement of the eye in the bony socket, caused by traumatic injury or developmental defect. Ptosis may cause a false impression of enophthalmos. –**enophthalmic,** *adj.*

Enovid, a trademark for an oral contraceptive containing an estrogen (mestranol) and a progestin (norethynodrel).

ensiform process. See **xiphoid process.**

Ensure, a trademark for a lactose-free nutritional supplement containing protein, carbohydrate, fat, vitamins and minerals.

Entameba. See ***Entamoeba.***

entamebiasis. See **amebiasis.**

Entamoeba /en'təmē'bə/, a genus of intestinal amebic parasites of which several species are pathogenic to humans. Also spelled ***Entameba.*** See also ***Entamoeba histolytica.***

Entamoeba histolytica, a pathogenic species of ameba that causes amebic dysentery and hepatic amebiasis in humans. See also **amebiasis, amebic dysentery, hepatic amebiasis.**

entamoebiasis. See **amebiasis.**

enter-. See **entero-.**

enteric coating, a coating added to oral medications that are designed to be absorbed from the intestinal tract. The coating resists the effects of stomach juices, which can interact with or destroy certain drugs.

enteric fever. See **typhoid fever.**

enteric infection, a disease of the intestine caused by any infection. Symptoms similar to those caused by pathogens may be produced by chemical toxins in ingested foods and by allergic reactions to certain food substances. Among bacteria commonly involved in enteric infections are *Escherichia coli, Vibrio cholerae,* and several species of *Salmonella, Shigella,* and anaerobic streptococci. Enteric infections are characterized by diarrhea, abdominal discomfort, nausea and vomiting, and anorexia. There may be a significant loss of fluid and electrolytes as a result of severe vomiting and diarrhea. Nothing is offered by mouth until vomiting has ceased. At that time, a clear fluid diet may be given. In severe cases, an IV solution containing glucose, saline, and electrolytes may be administered. Medication for sedation and relief of abdominal cramps may be prescribed. Antibiotics may be recommended, depending upon the specific microorganism causing the infection.

entericoid fever, a typhoidlike febrile disease characterized by intestinal inflammation and dysfunction. See also **enteric infection, typhoid fever.**

enteritis /en'tərī'tis/, inflammation of the mucosal lining of the small intestine, resulting from a variety of causes—bacterial, viral, functional, and inflammatory. Involvement of small and large intestine is called **enterocolitis.** Compare **gastroenteritis.**

entero-, enter-, a combining form meaning 'pertaining to the intestines': *enteric, enterobiliary, enteroptosis.*

Enterobacter cloacae /en'tirōbak'tər klō·ā'kē, klō·ā'sē/, a common species of bacterium found in human and animal feces, dairy products, sewage, soil, and water. It is rarely the cause of disease. Also called ***Aerobacter aerogenes*** /eroj'inēz/, ***Enterobacter aerogenes.***

Enterobacteriaceae /en'tirōbaktir'ē·ā'si·ē/, a family of aerobic and anaerobic bacteria that includes both normal and pathogenic enteric microorganisms. Among the significant genera of the family are ***Escherichia, Klebsiella, Proteus,*** and ***Salmonella.***

enterobacterial, of or pertaining to a species of bacterium found in the digestive tract.

enterobiasis /en'tirōbī'əsis/, a parasitic infestation with *Enterobius vermicularis,* the common pinworm. The worms infect the large intestine, and the females deposit eggs in the perianal area, causing pruritus and insomnia. Reinfection commonly occurs by transfer of eggs to the mouth by contaminated fingers. Airborne transmission is possible, as eggs remain viable for two or three days in contaminated bedclothes. To make the diagnosis, the sticky side of an adhesive cellophane tape swab is pressed against the perianal skin and examined for eggs under a microscope. Therapy for the whole family may be necessary. Effective anthelmintics include piperazine, pyrantel pamoate, pyrvinium pamoate, and thiabendazole. Personal hygiene, including handwashing, is the best preventive measure. There appears to be little benefit from disinfection procedures for the home. Also called **oxyuriasis.**

Enterobius vermicularis, a common parasitic nematode that resembles a white thread between 0.5 and 1 cm long. Also called **pinworm, seatworm, threadworm.**

enterochromaffin cell. See **argentaffin cell.**

enterococcus, *pl.* **enterococci,** any *Streptococcus* that inhabits the intestinal tract.

enterocolitis, an inflammation involving both the large and small intestines.

enterokinase /en'tirōkī'nās/, an intestinal juice enzyme that activates the proteolytic enzyme in pancreatic juice by converting trypsinogen to trypsin.

enterolith /en'tərōlith'/, a stone or concretion found within the intestine. See also **calculus.**

enterolithiasis /en'tərōlithī'əsis/, the presence of enteroliths in the intestine.

enterostomal therapist, a registered nurse who is qualified by training in an accredited program in enterostomal therapy to provide wound drainage services to patients. Also called **endostomy therapist.**

enterostomy /en'təros'təmē/, a surgical procedure that produces an artificial anus or fistula in the intestine by incision through the abdominal wall. Compare **colostomy.**

enterovirus, a virus that multiplies primarily in the intestinal tract. Kinds of enteroviruses are **coxsackievirus, echovirus,** and **poliovirus.** –**enteroviral,** *adj.*

ento-. See **endo-.**

entoderm. See **endoderm.**

Entozyme, a trademark for a GI fixed-combination drug containing bile salts and the digestive enzymes (pancreatin and pepsin).

entrainment, a phenomenon observed in the microanalysis of sound films in which the speaker moves several parts of the body and the listener responds to the sounds by moving in ways that are coordinated with the rhythm of the sounds. Infants have been observed to move in time to the rhythms of adult speech but not to random noises or disconnected words or vowels. Entrainment is thought to be an essential factor in the process of maternal-infant bonding.

entrance block, (in cardiology) a theoretic zone surrounding the heart's natural pacemaker focus, protecting it from discharge by an extraneous impulse that might trigger ectopic ventricular contractions.

entropion, turning inward or turning toward, usually a condition in which the eyelid turns inward toward the eye. **Cicatricial entropion** can occur in either the upper or lower eyelid as a result of scar tissue formation. **Spastic entropion** results from an inflammation or other factor that affects tissue tone. An inflammation of the eyelid may be the result of an infectious disease or irritation from an inverted eyelash. Compare **ectropion.** See also **blepharitis.**

entropy /en′trəpē/, the tendency of a system to go from a state of order to a state of disorder, expressed in physics as a measure of the part of the heat or energy in a thermodynamic system that is not available to perform work. Living organisms tend to go from a state of disorder to a state of order in their development and thus appear to reverse entropy. However, maintaining a living system requires the expenditure of energy, leaving less energy available for work, with the result that the entropy of the system and its surroundings increases.

ENT specialist, a physician who specializes in the treatment of the eye, nose, and throat. See also **otolaryngologist.**

enucleation, **1.** removal of an organ or tumor in one piece. **2.** removal of the eyeball, performed for malignancy, severe infection, or extensive trauma or to control pain in glaucoma. Local or general anesthesia is used. The optic nerve and muscle attachments are cut; if possible, the surrounding layer of fascia is left with the muscles. A ball-shaped implant of silicone, plastic, or tantalum is inserted, and the muscles are sutured around it, providing a permanent stump to give support and motion to an artificial eye. Postoperatively, pressure dressings are kept in place for 1 or 2 days to prevent hemorrhage. Other possible complications include thrombosis of nearby blood vessels, which may lead to infection, including meningitis.

Enuclene, a trademark for an ophthalmic, fixed-combination drug containing a detergent (tyloxapol) and a preservative (benzalkonium chloride).

enuresis /en′yo͝orē′sis/, incontinence of urine, especially in bed at night.

environment, all of the many factors, as physical and psychologic, that influence or affect the life and survival of a person. See also **biome, climate.** –**environmental,** *adj.*

environmental carcinogen, any of many natural or synthetic substances that can cause cancer. Such agents, or oncogens, may be divided into chemical agents, physical agents, and certain hormones and viruses. Some environmental carcinogens are arsenic, asbestos, uranium, vinyl chloride, ionizing radiation, ultraviolet rays, x-rays, and various coal tar derivatives. Carcinogenic effects of chemicals may be delayed as long as 30 years. Other carcinogens produce more immediate effects. Some studies indicate that the carcinogens in cigarette smoke are involved in 80% of all lung cancers. Most carcinogens are unreactive or secondary carcinogens but are converted to primary carcinogens in the body. Research indicates that numerous factors, as heredity, affect the susceptibilities of different individuals to cancer-causing agents.

environmental health, the total of various aspects of substances, forces, and conditions in and about a community that affect the health and well-being of the population.

environmental services, a housekeeping function of a hospital or other health care facility. It has the responsibility for laundry, liquid and solid waste control, safe disposal of materials contaminated by radiation or pathogenic organisms, and general maintenance of safety and sanitation.

Enzactin, a trademark for a topical antifungal (triacetin).

enzygotic twins. See **monozygotic twins.**

enzyme, a protein produced by living cells that catalyzes chemical reactions in organic matter. Most enzymes are produced in minute quantities and catalyze reactions that take place within the cells. Digestive enzymes, however, are produced in relatively large quantities and act outside the cells in the lumen of the digestive tube.

eosin /ē′əsin/, a group of red, acidic xanthine dyes often used in combination with a blue-purple, basic dye, as hematoxylin, to stain tissue slides in the laboratory.

eosinophil /ē′əsin′əfil/, a granulocytic, bilobed leukocyte somewhat larger than a neutrophil characterized by the large number of coarse, refractile, cytoplasmic granules that stain intensely with the acid dye, eosin. Eosinophils constitute 1% to 3% of the white blood cells of the body. They increase in number with allergy and some infections and decrease when steroid medications are being administered. Compare **basophil, neutrophil.** –**eosinophilic,** *adj.*

eosinophilia /ē′əsin′ōfil′ē·ə/, an increase in the number of eosinophils in the blood, accompanying many inflammatory conditions. Substantial increases are considered a reflection of an allergic response.

eosinophilic /ē′əsin′əfil′ik/, **1.** the tendency of a cell, tissue, or organism to be readily stained by the dye eosin. **2.** of or pertaining to an eosinophilic leukocyte.

eosinophilic adenoma. See **acidophilic adenoma.**

eosinophilic enteropathy, a rare form of food allergy that is characterized by nausea, crampy abdominal pain, diarrhea, urticaria, an elevated eosinophil count in the blood, and eosinophilic infiltrates in the intestine. Diagnosis is made by an elimination diet; symptoms usually disappear when the offending food is removed from the diet.

eosinophilic granuloma, a growth characterized by numerous eosinophils and histiocytes, occurring as a single or multiple lesion in bone. Eosinophilic granulomas may also develop in the lung and occur most frequently in children and adolescents.

eosinophilic leukemia, a malignant neoplasm of leukocytes in which eosinophils are the predominant cells. It resembles chronic myelocytic leukemia but may have an acute course even though there are no blast forms in the peripheral blood.

eosinophilic pneumonia, inflammation of the lungs, characterized by infiltration of the alveoli with eosinophils and large mononuclear cells, pulmonary edema, fever, night sweats, cough, dyspnea, and weight loss. The disease may be caused by a hypersensitivity reaction to spores of fungi, plant fibers, wood dust, bird droppings, porcine or bovine or piscine proteins, *Bacillus subtilis* enzyme in detergents, or certain drugs. Treatment consists of removal of the offending allergen and symptomatic and supportive therapy. Compare **bronchopneumonia.** See also **asthmatic eosinophilia.**

-eous, a combining form meaning 'like' or 'composed of' or 'relating to' something specified: *anedeous, cutaneous, osseous.*

EP, abbreviaiton for **evoked potential.**

ep-. See **epi-.**

ependyma /ipen′dimə/, a layer of ciliated epithelium that lines the central canal of the spinal cord and the ventricles of the brain.

ependymal glioma, a large, vascular, fairly solid glioma in the fourth ventricle.

ependymoblastoma /ipen′dimōblastō′mə/, a malignant neoplasm composed of primitive cells of the ependyma. Also called **malignant ependymoma.**

ependymoma /ipen′dimō′mə/, a neoplasm composed of differentiated cells of the ependyma. The tumor, which is usually a benign, pale, firm, encapsulated, somewhat nodular mass, commonly arises from the roof of the fourth ventricle and usually grows slowly. It may extend to the spinal cord. Primary lesions may also develop in the spinal cord. Also called **ependymocytoma.**

ephapse /ef′aps/, a point of lateral contact between nerve fibers across which impulses may be transmitted directly through the membranes of the cells rather than across a synapse. Compare **synapse.** **–ephaptic,** *adj.*

ephaptic transmission /ifap′tik/, the passage of a neural impulse from one nerve fiber, axon, or dendrite to another through the membranes. The mechanism may be a factor in epileptic seizures. Compare **synaptic transmission.**

ephedrine, an adrenergic bronchodilator.

■ INDICATIONS: It is prescribed in the treatment of asthma and bronchitis and is used topically as a nasal decongestant.

■ CONTRAINDICATIONS: Concomitant administration of monoamine oxidase inhibitors, hypertension, cardiac artery disease, cardiac arrhythmia, or known hypersensitivity to this drug prohibits its use.

■ ADVERSE EFFECTS: Among the more serious adverse reactions are nervousness, insomnia, anorexia, and increased blood pressure.

ephemeral fever, any febrile condition lasting only 24 to 48 hours that is uncomplicated and of unknown origin.

epi-, ep-, a combining form meaning 'on, upon': *epicanthus, epicostal, epidural.*

epiblast, the primordial outer layer of the blastocyst or blastula, before differentiation of the germ layers, that gives rise to the ectoderm and contains cells capable of forming the endoderm and mesoderm. See also **ectoderm.** **–epiblastic,** *adj.*

epicanthus /ep′ikan′thəs/, a vertical fold of skin over the angle of the inner canthus of the eye. It may be slight or marked, covering the canthus and the caruncle. It is normal in Oriental people and is of no clinical significance. Some infants with Down's syndrome have the folds. Also called **epicanthal fold, epicanthic fold.** **–epicanthal, epicanthic,** *adj.*

epicardium /ep′ikär′dē·əm/, one of the three layers of tissue that form the wall of the heart. It is composed of a single sheet of squamous epithelial cells overlying delicate connective tissue. The epicardium is the visceral portion of the serous pericardium and folds back upon itself to form the parietal portion of the serous pericardium. Compare **myocardium.** **–epicardial,** *adj.*

epicondylar fracture, any fracture that involves the medial or the lateral epicondyle of a specific bone, as the humerus.

epicondyle /ep′ikon′dəl/, a projection on the surface of a bone above its condyle. **–epicondylar,** *adj.*

epicondylitis /ep′ikon′dili′tis/, a painful and sometimes disabling inflammation of the muscle and surrounding tissues of the elbow, caused by repeated strain on the forearm near the lateral epicondyle of the humerus, as from violent extension or supination of the wrist against a resisting force. The strain may result from activities, as tennis or golf, twisting a screwdriver, or carrying a heavy load with the arm extended. Treatment usually includes rest, injection of procaine with or without hydrocortisone, and, in some cases, surgery to release part of the muscle from the epicondyle. See also **lateral humeral epicondylitis.**

epicranial aponeurosis, a fibrous membrane that covers the cranium between the occipital and frontal muscles of the scalp. Also called **galea aponeurotica.**

epicranium, the complete scalp, including the integument, the muscular sheets, and the aponeuroses. Compare **epicranius.** **–epicranial,** *adj.*

epicranius, the broad, muscular, and tendinous layer of tissue covering the top and the sides of the skull from the occipital bone to the eyebrows. It consists of broad, thin muscular bellies, connected by an extensive aponeurosis. Innervation of the epicranius by branches of the facial nerves can draw back the scalp, raise the eyebrows, and move the ears. Compare **epicranium.** See also **epicranial aponeurosis, occipitofrontalis, temperoparietalis.**

epidemic, **1.** affecting a significantly large number of people at the same time. **2.** a disease that spreads rapidly through a demographic segment of the human population, as everyone in a given geographic area, a military base, or similar population unit, or everyone of a certain age or sex, as the children or women of a region. **3.** a widespread disease that tends to occur periodically. Compare **endemic, epizootic, pandemic.**

epidemic encephalitis, any diffuse inflammation of the brain occurring in epidemic form. Two kinds of epidemic encephalitis are **Japanese encephalitis** and **St. Louis encephalitis.** See also **encephalitis.**

epidemic hemoglobinuria. See **hemoglobinuria.**

epidemic hemorrhagic fever, a severe viral infection marked by fever and bleeding. The disorder develops rapidly, characterized initially by fever and muscle ache, possibly followed by hemorrhage, peripheral vascular collapse, hypovolemic shock, and acute kidney failure. The arbovirus or other pathogen is believed transmitted by mosquitoes, ticks, or mites. The pathophysiology of the hemorrhagic effect is uncertain, although it is assumed the disease organism causes the development of lesions in the lining of the capillaries. Among the various forms of epidemic hemorrhagic fevers are **Argentine hemorrhagic fever, Bolivian hemorrhagic fever, dengue hemorrhagic fever, Lassa fever,** and **yellow fever.** See also specific viral infections.

epidemic myalgia, a disease caused by coxsackie B virus, characterized by sudden, acute chest or epigastric pain and fever lasting a few days, followed by complete, spontaneous recovery. Also called **devil's grip, epidemic myositis, epidemic pleurodynia.**

epidemic myositis. See **epidemic myalgia, epidemic pleurodynia.**

epidemic parotitis. See **mumps.**

epidemic pleurodynia, an infection caused by a coxsackievirus, affecting mainly children. It is characterized by severe intermittent pain in the abdomen or lower chest, fever, headache, sore throat, malaise, and extreme myalgia. The symptoms may continue for weeks or subside after a few days and recur for a period of weeks. Treatment is symptomatic; complete recovery is usual. Also called **Bornholm disease, devil's grip, epidemic myositis.**

epidemic typhus, an acute, severe rickettsial infection characterized by prolonged high fever, headache, and a dark maculopapular rash that covers most of the body. The causative organism, *Rickettsia prowazekii,* is transmitted indirectly as a result of the bite of the human body louse; the pathogen is contained in feces of the louse and enters the body tissues as the bite is scratched. An intense headache and a fever reaching 40° C (104° F) begin after an incubation period of 10 days to 2 weeks. The rash follows. Complications may include vascular collapse, renal failure, pneumonia, or gangrene. Mortality is high among older patients. Treatment may include chloramphenicol or tetracycline, aspirin, and supportive, symptomatic care. Also called **classic typhus, European typhus, jail fever, louse-borne typhus.** Compare **murine typhus.** See also **Brill-Zinsser disease, rickettsia, typhus.**

epidemiologist, a physician or medical scientist who studies the incidence, prevalence, spread, prevention, and control of disease in a community or a specific group of individuals. In a hospital, a physician may be assigned as a staff epidemiologist with responsibility for directing infection control programs within the facility.

epidemiology, the study of the occurrence, distribution, and causes of disease in humankind. **–epidemiologic,** *adj.,* **epidemiologist,** *n.*

epiderm-, epidermo-, a combining form meaning 'of or pertaining to the epidermis': *epidermoid, epidermolysis, epidermolytic.*

epidermis /ep′idur′mis/, the superficial, avascular layers of the skin, made up of an outer, dead, cornified portion and a deeper, living, cellular portion. Epidermal cells gradually move outward to the skin surface, undergoing change as they migrate, until they are desquamated as cornified flakes. Cells in various transitional stages make up the basal cell layer, the prickle cell layer, the granular layer, the clear cell layer, and the cornified layer. Altogether, these layers are between 0.5 and 1.1 mm in thickness. Also called **cuticle. –epidermal, epidermoid,** *adj.*

epidermoid carcinoma, a malignant neoplasm in which the tumor cells tend to differentiate in the manner of epidermal cells, then form horny cells called prickle cells.

epidermoid cyst, a common, benign, variable, subcutaneous swelling lined by keratinizing epithelium and filled with a cheesy material composed of sebum and epithelial debris. The cyst is movable but attached to the skin by the remains of the duct of a sebaceous gland. Frequently, epidermoid cysts become infected. Treatment is surgical excision. Also called **sebaceous cyst, wen.** Compare **pilar cyst.**

epidermolysis bullosa /ep′idərmol′isis/, a group of rare, hereditary skin diseases in which vesicles and bullae develop, usually at sites of trauma. Severe forms may also involve mucous membranes and may leave scars and contractures on healing. Basal cell and squamous cell carcinomas sometimes develop in the scar tissue. Treatment is symptomatic.

epidermophytosis, a fungus infection of the skin.

epididymis /ep′idid′imis/, *pl.* **epidiymides,** one of a pair of long, tightly coiled ducts that carry sperm from the seminiferous tubules of the testes to the vas deferens.

epididymitis /ep'idid'imī'tis/, acute or chronic inflammation of the epididymis. It may result from venereal disease, urinary tract infection, prostatitis, or prostatectomy. Symptoms include fever and chills, pain in the groin, and tender, swollen epididymis. Treatment includes bed rest, scrotal support, and antibiotics, as appropriate.

epididymoorchitis /ep'idid'imō•ôrkī'tis/, inflammation of the epididymis and of the testis. See also **epididymitis, orchitis.**

epidural /ep'ido͞or'əl/, outside the dura mater.

epidural anesthesia, the process of achieving regional anesthesia of the pelvic, abdominal, genital, or other area by the injection of a local anesthetic into the epidural space of the spinal column.

epidural blood patch, a patch repairing a tear or a hole in the dura mater around the spinal cord. The tear is usually the result of needle puncture during spinal anesthesia or lumbar puncture. Spinal fluid leaks through the hole, resulting in a spinal headache. To form a seal, 10 to 15 ml of the patient's blood is injected into the epidural space. A clot forms, covering the hole and preventing further loss of fluid. The technique is used to treat persistent or severe spinal headache.

epidural space, the space immediately surrounding the dura mater of the brain or spinal cord, beneath the periosteum of the cranium and the spinal column.

Epifrin, a trademark for an adrenergic (epinephrine hydrochloride).

epigastric node, a node in one of the seven groups of parietal lymph nodes serving the abdomen and the pelvis, comprising about four nodes along the caudal portion of the inferior epigastric vessels. See also **lymph, lymphatic system, lymph node.**

epigastric region, the part of the abdomen in the upper zone between the right and left hypochondriac regions. Also called **antecardium, epigastrium.** See also **abdominal regions.**

epigastric sensation, a weak, sinking feeling of undefined nature that is usually localized in the pit of the stomach but may occur throughout the abdominal region. See also **sensation,** def.1.

epigastrium. See **epigastric region.**

epigenesis /ep'ijen'əsis/, (in embryology) a theory of development in which the organism grows from a simple to more complex form through the progressive differentiation of an undifferentiated cellular unit. Compare **preformation.** –**epigenesist,** *n.* **epigenetic,** *adj.*

epiglottiditis. See **epiglottitis.**

epiglottis /ep'iglot'is/, the cartilaginous structure that overhangs the larynx like a lid and prevents food from entering the larynx and the trachea while swallowing.

epiglottitis /ep'iglotī'tis/, an inflammation of the epiglottis. Acute epiglottitis is a severe form of the condition, affecting primarily children. It is characterized by fever, sore throat, stridor, croupy cough, and an erythematous, swollen epiglottis. The child may become cyanotic and require an emergency tracheostomy to maintain respiration. The causative organism is usually *Haemophilus influenzae,* type B. Antibiotics, rest, oxygen, and supportive care are usually included in treatment. Also called **epiglottiditis.** See also **acute epiglottitis.**

epilating forceps /ep'ilā'ting/, a kind of small spring forceps, used for removing unwanted hair.

epilation. See **depilation.**

epilepsy, a group of neurologic disorders characterized by recurrent episodes of convulsive seizures, sensory disturbances, abnormal behavior, loss of consciousness, or all of these. Common to all types of epilepsy is an uncontrolled electric discharge from the nerve cells of the cerebral cortex. Although most epilepsy is of unknown cause, it may sometimes be associated with cerebral trauma, intracranial infection, brain tumor, vascular disturbances, intoxication, or chemical imbalance. See also **focal seizure, grand mal seizure, petit mal seizure, psychomotor seizure.**

■ OBSERVATIONS: The frequency of attacks may range from several times a day to intervals of several years. In predisposed individuals, seizures may occur during sleep or after physical stimulation, as by a flickering light or sudden loud sound. Emotional disturbances also may be significant trigger factors. Some seizures are preceded by an aura, but others have no warning symptoms. Most epileptic attacks are brief. They may be localized or general, with or without clonic movements, and are often followed by drowsiness or confusion. Diagnosis is made by observation of the pattern of seizures and abnormalities on an electroencephalogram. Diagnosis is also aided by a system of classification of the criteria that characterize the different types of epileptic seizures. One major category in the classification scheme encompasses the partial seizures, which often begin focally then "march," or spread, to other brain areas. A second major category includes the generalized seizures, which usually begin deep in the brain and may involve both consciousness and motor functions.

■ INTERVENTION: The kind of epilepsy determines the selection of preventive medication. Correctable lesions and metabolic causes are eliminated when possible. During an attack the patient should be protected from injury without being severely restrained.

■ NURSING CONSIDERATIONS: A nurse observing an epileptic attack, in addition to protecting the patient from injury, should carefully note and accurately describe the sequence of seizure activity. The patient and family must be fully informed and counseled about the disorder, the importance of regularly taking prescribed medication and never discontinuing treatment without professional advice, toxic effects of medication, wearing a medical identification tag, and continuing to live as normal a life as possible. Nurses also have a responsibility to help improve the public's attitude toward epilepsy and to correct misunderstanding that limits educational and occupational opportunities for patients with this diagnosis. See also **anticonvulsant, aura, central nervous system stimulant, clonus, ictus, tonic.** –**epileptic,** *adj., n.*

International classification of epileptic seizures

Generalized seizures
  Tonic-clonic (grand mal)
  Absence (petit mal)
  Infantile spasms
  Other (myoclonic seizures, akinetic seizures, undetermined)
Partial seizures
  Simple partial seizures (e.g., disturbances in movement only)
  Complex partial seizures (psychomotor, other)
  Secondarily generalized seizures

From The Office of Scientific and Health Reports, National Institute of Neurological and Communicative Disorders and Stroke: Epilepsy: hope through research, NIH Publication No. 81-156, Bethesda, MD, July 1981, National Institutes of Health.

epileptic mania, *obsolete.* a mood disorder characterized by attacks of violence that occur immediately before, after, or in place of an epileptic seizure. See also **epilepsy, mania.**

epileptic stupor, the state of unawareness and unresponsiveness after an epileptic seizure.

epiloia. See **tuberous sclerosis.**

epimysium /ep′imiz′ē·əm/, a fibrous sheath that enfolds a muscle and extends between the bundles of muscle fibers, as the perimysium. It is sturdy in some areas but more delicate in others, as those areas where the muscle moves freely under a strong sheet of fascia. The epimysium may also fuse with fascia that attaches a muscle to a bone.

Epinal, a trademark for an adrenergic (epinephryl borate).

epinephrine /ep′ənef′rin/, an adrenal hormone and synthetic adrenergic vasoconstrictor.

■ INDICATIONS: It is prescribed in the treatment of anaphylaxis, acute bronchial spasm, and nasal congestion and to increase the effectiveness of a local anesthetic.

■ CONTRAINDICATION: Known hypersensitivity to this drug prohibits its use.

■ ADVERSE EFFECTS: Among the most serious adverse reactions are arrhythmias, increases in blood pressure, and rebound congestion (when used as a decongestant).

epinephryl borate, an adrenergic.

■ INDICATIONS: It is prescribed in the treatment of primary open-angle glaucoma.

■ CONTRAINDICATIONS: Narrow-angle glaucoma, aphakia, or known hypersensitivity to this drug prohibits its use. It should not be given before peripheral iridectomy and should not be administered to eyes that are capable of angle closure.

■ ADVERSE EFFECTS: Among the more serious adverse reactions are tachycardia, hypertension, headache, blurred vision, and allergic reaction.

epiphora. See **tearing.**

epiphyseal fracture, a fracture involving the epiphyseal growth plate of a long bone, resulting in separation or in fragmentation of the plate. Also called **Salter fracture.**

epiphysis /ipif′isis/, *pl.* **epiphyses,** the head of a long bone that is separated from the shaft of the bone by the epiphyseal plate until the bone stops growing, the plate is obliterated, and the shaft and the head become united. Compare **diaphysis.** –**epiphyseal** /ipif′əsē′əl/, *adj.*

epiphysis cerebri. See **pineal body.**

epiploic foramen, a passage between the peritoneal cavity and the omental bursa. It is lined with peritoneum and is approximately 3 cm in diameter.

epipygus. See **pygomelus.**

episcleritis /ep′isklərī′tis/, inflammation of the outermost layers of the sclera and of the tissues overlying the posterior portions of this tough, white outer coat of the eyeball.

episiotomy /epē′zē·ot′əmē/, a surgical procedure, usually required for forceps delivery, in which an incision is made in a woman's perineum to enlarge her vaginal opening for delivery, performed most often electively to prevent tearing of the perineum, to hasten or facilitate delivery of the baby, or to prevent stretching of perineal muscles and connective tissue thought to predispose to subsequent abnormalities of pelvic outlet relaxation, as cystocele, rectocele, and uterine prolapse; its prophylactic efficacy is debated. The incision into the vaginal and perineal tissue is closed with absorbable sutures that need not be removed. Deep incisions require closure in two or more layers. Immediate complications include hemorrhage and extension of the incision along the vaginal sulcus or into the anal sphincter or rectum. Delayed complications include hematoma and abscess. Application of cold packs to the perineum for several hours immediately postpartum minimizes swelling. Alternating applications later of heat and cold and warm sitz baths reduce discomfort, but sitz baths longer than 10 minutes soften tissue and prolong healing. A mediolateral episiotomy is an episiotomy cut at an angle of approximately 45 degrees with the midline. Although it affords wide exposure for delivery, it is painful postpartum and is prone to hematoma and infection. A median or midline episiotomy is an incision in the perineum in the midline; although less painful postpartum, it affords less exposure for delivery and may extend into or through the anal sphincter and into the rectum.

episode, an incident or event that stands out from the continuity of everyday life, as an episode of illness or a traumatic episode in the course of a child's development. **episodic,** *adj.*

episode of hospital care, the services provided by a hospital in the continuous course of care for a patient with a medical problem or other health condition. It may cover a sequence from emergency through inpatient to outpatient services.

episodic care, a pattern of medical and nursing care in which care is given to a person for a particular problem, without an ongoing relationship being established between the person and health care professionals. Emergency rooms provide episodic care.

episodic health history, an abbreviated form of the health history that is focused on the factors relevant to an illness or complaint that has been previously noted, as in a follow-up visit after a treatment or surgical procedure, or in the regular periodic visits for a chronic illness or condition. The current health status of the person is noted with an account of his health since the last visit as it pertains to the particular condition. An episodic health history is a partial history that serves to bring the data base up to date. In the patient's chart it may precede the progress notes made for the current visit.

episome /ep′isōm/, (in bacterial genetics) an extrachromosomal replicating unit that exists autonomously or functions with a chromosome. See also **colicinogen, conjugon, F factor, R factor.**

epispadias /ep′ispā′dē·əs/, a congenital defect in which the urethra opens on the dorsum of the penis at some point proximal to the glans. Treatment is directed at correcting or managing urinary incontinence, which occurs because the urinary sphincters are defective, and at permitting sexual function. The corresponding defect in women, fissure of the upper wall of the urethra, is quite rare. Compare **hypospadias.**

epistasis /epis′təsis/, (in genetics) a type of interaction between genes at different loci on a chromosome in which one is able to mask or suppress the expression of the other. The epistatic effect, which is nonallelic and therefore the opposite of the dominance relationship, may be caused by the presence of homozygous recessives at one gene pair, as occurs in the Bombay phenotype, or by the presence of a dominant allele that counteracts the expression of another dominant gene. Compare **dominance.** –**epistatic,** *adj.*

epistaxis /ep′istak′sis/, bleeding from the nose caused by local irritation of mucous membranes, violent sneezing, fragility of the mucous membrane or of the arterial walls, chronic infection, trauma, hypertension, leukemia, vitamin K deficiency, or, most often, picking of the nose. Also called **nosebleed.**

■ OBSERVATIONS: Epistaxis may result from rupture of tiny vessels in the anterior nasal septum; this occurs most frequently in early childhood and adolescence. In adults, it occurs more commonly in men than in women, may be severe in elderly persons, may be accompanied by respiratory distress, apprehension, restlessness, vertigo, and nausea, and may lead to syncope.

■ INTERVENTION: The patient suffering epistaxis is instructed to breathe through the mouth, to sit quietly with the head tilted slightly forward to prevent blood from entering the pharynx, and to avoid swallowing blood. The bleeding may be controlled by pinching the nose firmly with the fingers, by inserting a cotton ball soaked in a topical vasoconstrictor and applying pressure to the skin on both sides of the nose, occluding the blood supply to the nostrils, or by placing an ice compress over the nose. If bleeding continues, the clots may be removed by suction. The nasal mucosa may be anesthetized with topical lidocaine, cauterized with a silver nitrate stick or an electric cautery, and then sprayed with epinephrine. Severe bleeding, especially from the posterior nasal septum, may be treated by inserting packing, which generally is left in place for 1 to 3 days. During that period the patient is kept in high Fowler's position, the placement of the packing is checked frequently, and a sedative, antibiotics, vitamins C and K, and a cool, nonirritating liquid diet may be ordered. Persistent or recurrent profuse epistaxis may be treated by ligating an artery supplying the nose, as the external carotid, ethmoid, or internal maxillary.

■ NURSING CONSIDERATIONS: The nurse administers first aid and ordered medication; assists in cauterization and nasal packing; checks the patient's blood pressure, pulse, and respiration every half hour until bleeding subsides; and then continues to check them every 4 hours. The nurse limits the patient's activity, avoids serving milk and hot liquids, encourages expectoration rather than swallowing of blood, and reports symptoms of respiratory distress, vertigo, and any bleeding. Before the patient is discharged, the nurse provides instruction on the prevention of epistaxis by using a vaporizer and applying petroleum jelly with a cotton swab gently to the mucous membrane lining the nostrils.

epistropheus. See **axis.**

epithalamus /ep′ithal′əməs/, one of the portions of the diencephalon. It includes the trigonum habenulae, the pineal body, and the posterior commissure. Compare **hypothalamus, metathalamus, subthalamus, thalamus.** –**epithalamic,** *adj.*

epithelial peg, any of the papillary projections of the epithelius that penetrate the underlying stroma of connecting tissue and normally develop in mucous membranes and dermal tissues. Also called **rete peg** /rē′tē/.

epithelial rest. See **embryonic rest.**

epitheliofibril. See **tonofibril.**

epithelioid leiomyoma /ep′ithē′lē·oid/, an uncommon neoplasm of smooth muscle in which the cells are polygonal in shape. It usually develops in the stomach. Also called **bizarre leiomyoma, leiomyoblastoma.**

epithelioma, **1.** a neoplasm derived from the epithelium. **2.** *obsolete.* any carcinoma.

-epithelioma, a combining form meaning a 'tumor of epithelial tissue': *inoepithelioma, periepithelioma, trichoepithelioma.*

epithelioma adamantinum. See **ameloblastoma.**

epithelioma adenoides cysticum. See **trichoepithelioma.**

epithelium, the covering of the internal and the external organs of the body, including the lining of vessels. It consists of cells bound together by connective material and varies in the number of layers and the kinds of cells. Epithelium in different parts of the body is made of simple squamous cells, simple cuboidal cells, and stratified columnar cells. The stratified squamous epithelium of the epidermis is comprised of five different cellular layers. **epithelial,** *adj*.

epitope /ep′itōp/, an antigenic determinant that causes a specific reaction by an immunoglobulin. It consists of a group of amino acids on the surface of the antigen. See also **antibody.**

Epitrate, a trademark for an ophthalmic adrenergic (epinephrine bitartrate).

epitympanic recess, one of two areas of the tympanic cavity, the other being the tympanic cavity proper. The recess is cranial to the tympanic membrane and contains the upper half of the malleus and greater part of the incus. Also called **the attic.**

epizootic /ep′izō•ot′ik/, a disease or condition that occurs at about the same time in many of the animals of a species in a geographic area.

EPO, abbreviation for **erythropoietin.**

eponychium. See **cuticle,** def. 3.

epoophorectomy /ep′ō•of′ərek′təmē/, surgical removal of the epoophoron.

epoophoron /ep′ō•of′əron/, a structure that is situated in the mesosalpinx between the ovary and the uterine tube. It is composed of a few short tubules. The ends of the tubules converge in one direction toward the ovary and, in the opposite direction, open into a rudimentary duct. The epoophoron is a persistent portion of the embryonic mesonephric duct. Also called **parovarium.**

Eppy, a trademark for an adrenergic (epinephryl borate).

Eprolin, a trademark for vitamin E (alpha tocopherol).

EPSDT, abbreviation for **Early and Periodic Screening Diagnosis and Treatment.**

Epsom salt. See **magnesium sulfate.**

Epstein-Barr virus (EBV) /ep′stīnbär′/, the herpesvirus that causes infectious mononucleosis.

Epstein's pearls, small, white, pearl-like epithelial cysts that occur on both sides of the midline of the hard palate of the newborn baby. They are normal and usually disappear within a few weeks. Compare **Bednar's aphthae, thrush.**

epulis /epyo͞o′lis/, *pl.* **epulides,** any tumor or growth on the gingiva.

Equagesic, a trademark for a central nervous system, fixed-combination drug containing analgesics (aspirin and ethoheptazine citrate) and a sedative (meprobamate).

equal cleavage, mitotic division of the fertilized ovum into blastomeres of identical size, as occurs in humans and most mammals. Compare **unequal cleavage.**

Equal Employment Opportunity Commission (EEOC), a commission appointed by the President of the United States to administer the Civil Rights Act of 1964, particularly to investigate complaints of discrimination in employment in businesses engaged in interstate commerce. Discrimination based on race, color, creed, or national origin is forbidden, but certain kinds of employers and certain conditions of employment allow exceptions to the act. Women and men must both be considered for a position that both can perform, and men and women must be paid equal wages for equal work.

Equanil, a trademark for a sedative (meprobamate).

Equanitrate, a trademark for a cardiovascular, fixed-combination drug containing a vasodilator (pentaerythritol tetranitrate) and a sedative (meprobamate).

equatorial plate, the platelike configuration formed by the chromosomes at the center of the spindle during the metaphase stage of mitosis and meiosis.

equilibration, the balancing and integrating of new experiences with those of the past in the psychologic development of an individual.

equilibrium, **1.** a state of balance or rest resulting from the equal action of opposing forces, as calcium and phosphorus in the body. **2.** (in psychiatry) a state of mental or emotional balance. **3.** (in radiotherapy) a point at which the rate of production of a daughter element is equal to the rate of decay of the parent element and the activites of parent and daughter are identical.

equine encephalitis /ē′kwīn, ek′win/, an arbovirus infection, characterized by inflammation of the nerve tissues of the brain and spinal cord, with high fever, headache, nausea, vomiting, myalgia and neurologic symptoms, as visual disturbances, tremor, lethargy, and disorientation. The virus is transmitted by the bite of an infected mosquito. Horses are the primary host of the particular viruses that cause the infection; humans are secondary hosts. **Eastern equine encephalitis (EEE)** is a severe form of the infection. It occurs along the eastern seaboard of the United States and lasts longer and causes more deaths and residual morbidity than **western equine encephalitis (WEE),** which occurs throughout the United States and results in a mild, brief illness, as does **Venezuelan equine encephalitis (VEE),** which is common in Central and South America, Florida, and Texas. See also **encephalitis, encephalomyelitis.**

Er, symbol for **erbium.**

ER,E.R., abbreviation for **emergency room.**

Erb-Duchenne paralysis. See **Erb's palsy.**

erbium (Er), a rare-earth, metallic element. Its atomic number is 68; its atomic weight is 167.26.

Erb's muscular dystrophy, a form of muscular dystrophy that first affects the shoulder girdle and later often involves the pelvic girdle. It is a progressively crippling disease with onset in childhood or adolescence and is usually inherited as an autosomal recessive trait. It affects both sexes. In males, differential diagnosis between Erb's muscular dystrophy and Duchenne's muscular dystrophy may be difficult.

Erb's palsy, a kind of paralysis caused by traumatic injury to the upper brachial plexus. It occurs most commonly in childbirth from forcible traction during delivery, with injury to one or more cervical nerve roots. The signs of Erb's palsy include loss of sensation in the arm and paralysis and atrophy of the deltoid, the biceps, and the brachialis muscles. The arm on the affected side hangs loosely with the elbow extended and the forearm pronated. Treatment initially requires that the arm and shoulder be immobilized to allow the swelling and inflammation of the associated neuritis to resolve. Physical therapy and splinting may be necessary to improve function of the muscles and to prevent flexion contracture of the elbow. Also called **Erb-Duchenne paralysis.**

erectile /irek′til, -tīl/, capable of being erected or raised to an erect position. The term is usually applied in the description of spongy tissue of the penis or clitoris that becomes turgid and erectile when filled with blood. It also may be used when referring to the epidermal tissue involved in the appearance of "goose bumps" (horripilation) in response to fear, anger, cold, or other stimuli.

erectile myxoma, an angioma that contains areas of myxomatous tissue.

erection, the condition of hardness, swelling, and elevation observed in the penis and to a lesser degree in the clitoris, usually caused by sexual arousal but also occurring during sleep or as a result of physical stimulation. It occurs as additional blood enters the organ and blood pressure increases and is influenced by psychic and nerve stimulation. It is needed to enable the penis to enter the vagina and to emit semen. See also **ejaculation, nocturnal emission, priapism.**

erector spinae. See **sacrospinalis.**

erethistic idiocy /er′ithis′tik/, *obsolete.* severe mental retardation associated with continuous, purposeless activity and restlessness.

-ergasia, a combining form meaning 'interfunctioning of the mind and body': *cacergasia, dysgasia, orthergasia.*

ergastoplasm, a network of cytoplasmic structures that show basophilic staining properties; granular endoplasmic reticulum. See **endoplasmic reticulum.**

-ergic, -ergetic, a combining form meaning an 'effect of activity': *allergic, pathergic, telergic.*

ergo-, a combining form meaning 'pertaining to work': *ergodermatosis, ergomaniac, ergotropy.*

ergocalciferol. See **calciferol.**

ergoloid mesylates, an adrenergic with psychotropic actions.

■ INDICATIONS: It is prescribed in the treatment of symptomatic decline in mental capacity for an unknown cause, as in senile dementia.

■ CONTRAINDICATIONS: Psychosis or known sensitivity to this drug prohibits its use.

■ ADVERSE EFFECTS: Among the most serious adverse reactions are sublingual irritation, transient nausea, and gastric disturbance.

Ergomar, a trademark for an ergot alkaloid (ergotamine tartrate) used to treat migraine.

ergonomics, a scientific discipline devoted to the study and analysis of human work, especially as it is affected by individual anatomy, psychology, and other human factors. –**ergonomic,** *adj.*

ergonovine maleate /ur′gōnō′vēn/, an oxytocic ergot alkaloid. Also called **ergometrine maleate.**

■ INDICATIONS: It is prescribed to contract the uterus in the treatment or prevention of postpartum or postabortion hemorrhage.

■ CONTRAINDICATIONS: Pregnancy, peripheral vascular disease, elevated blood pressure, or known hypersensitivity to this drug prohibits its use.

■ ADVERSE EFFECTS: Among the more serious adverse effects are hypertension, nausea, headache, blurred vision, and hypersensitivity reactions. Fetal death may occur if the drug is given in pregnancy.

ergosome. See **polysome.**

ergosterol /ərgos′tərôl/, an unsaturated hydrocarbon of the vitamin D group isolated from yeast, mushrooms, ergot, and other fungi. When treated with ultraviolet irradiation it is converted into vitamin D_2. See also **calciferol, viosterol, vitamin D.**

ergot /ur′gət/, (in pharmacology) the food storage body of a fungus, *Claviceps purpurea,* which commonly infects rye and other cereal grasses. It contains ergot alkaloids.

ergot alkaloid, one of a large group of alkaloids derived from a common fungus, *Claviceps purpurea,* that grows on rye and other grains throughout the temperate areas of the world. The alkaloids are divided into three groups; the amino acid alkaloids, typified by ergotamine; the dihydrogenated amino acid alkaloids, as dihydroergotamine; and the amine alkaloids, as ergonovine. Ergotamine and dihydroergotamine are not as effective oxytocics as ergonovine; therefore, ergonovine, given orally or intravenously, is currently used in obstetrics to treat or prevent postpartum uterine atony and to complete an incomplete or missed abortion. Ergotamine is prescribed to relieve migraine headache. It acts by reducing the amplitude of arterial pulsations in the external carotid branches of the cranial arteries. Dihydroergotamine was formerly used to enhance cerebral blood flow in elderly patients to improve mental function but is no longer thought to be a useful or effective drug for that purpose. Contraindications to the use of any of the ergot alkaloids include peripheral vascular disease, coronary artery disease, hypertension, renal or hepatic dysfunction, and sepsis. Pregnancy prohibits use of the drugs because contractions of the uterus and decreased blood flow to the fetus may result, causing fetal death. Ergot poisoning may occur with prolonged or excessive use of the drug or by accidental ingestion of contaminated grain. Signs of toxicity are thirst, diarrhea, dizziness, chest pain, abnormal and variable rate of cardiac contraction, nausea and vomiting, digital paresthesia, severe cramping, and seizures. Tissue anoxia and gangrene of the extremities may occur, as a result of prolonged vasoconstriction, if poisoning is severe.

ergotamine tartrate /ərgot′əmēn/, a vasoconstrictor and oxytocic.

■ INDICATIONS: It is prescribed in the treatment of migraine and postpartum uterine atony.

■ CONTRAINDICATIONS: Pregnancy, peripheral vascular

disease, infectious disease, or known hypersensitivity to this drug prohibits its use.

■ ADVERSE EFFECTS: Among the more serious adverse reactions are vomiting, diarrhea, thirst, tingling of fingers and toes, and increased blood pressure. Fetal death may occur if the drug is administered to a woman during pregnancy.

ergotherapy, the use of physical activity and exercise in the treatment of disease. By extension, the therapy includes any procedure that increases the blood supply to a diseased or injured part, as massage or various types of hot baths. **–ergotherapeutic,** *adj.*

Ergotrate Maleate, a trademark for an ergot alkaloid (ergonovine maleate), used as an oxytocic.

-ergy, **1.** a combining form meaning an 'action': *abioenergy, leukergy, synergy.* **2.** a combining form meaning an 'effect or result': *allergy, anabolergy, pathergy.*

Eros, a Freudian term for the drive or instinct for survival, including self-preservation and survival of the species through reproduction.

erosion, the wearing away or gradual destruction of a surface, such as a mucosal or epidermal surface as a result of inflammation, injury, or other effects, usually marked by the appearance of an ulcer. See also **necrosis.**

erosive gastritis, an inflammatory condition characterized by multiple erosions of the mucous membrane lining the stomach. Nausea, anorexia, pain, and gastric hemorrhage may occur. Treatment includes removal of the irritating substance, and supportive care includes intravenous fluids, electrolytes, and, if necessary, blood transfusion. See also **chemical gastritis, corrosive gastritis.**

erosive osteoarthritis. See **Kellgren's syndrome.**

-erotic, a combining form meaning 'pertaining to sexual love or desire': *anterotic, homoerotic, hysteroerotic.*

eroticism, **1.** sexual impulse or desire. **2.** the arousal or attempt to arouse the sexual instinct through suggestive or symbolic means. **3.** the expression of sexual instinct or desire. **4.** an abnormally persistent sexual drive. Also called **erotism.** See also **anal eroticism, oral eroticism.**

eroto-, a combining form meaning 'pertaining to love or sexual desire': *erotogenic, erotopath, erotophobia.*

erotomania, *obsolete.* a psychopathologic state characterized by preoccupation with sexuality and sexual behavior.

erotomaniac, *obsolete.* a person displaying characteristics of erotomania.

error, (in research) a defect in the design of a study, in the development of measurements or instruments, or in the interpretation of the findings.

error message, a brief statement delivered by a computer via a peripheral device, as a CRT or printer, that something has been done incorrectly.

ERT, abbreviation for **external radiation therapy.**

erucic acid, a fatty acid that has been associated with heart disease. It is present in rapeseed oil and is used in some countries as a vegetable oil for salad dressings, margarines, and mayonnaise.

eructation, the act of bringing up air from the stomach with a characteristic sound. Also called **belching.**

eruption, the rapid development of a skin lesion, especially of a viral exanthem or of the rash commonly accompanying a drug reaction.

eruptive fever, any disease characterized by fever and a rash.

eruptive gingivitis, a gingival inflammation that may occur concurrently with the eruption of the permanent teeth. Compare **desquamative gingivitis.**

eruptive xanthoma, a skin disorder associated with elevated triglyceride levels in the blood. Erythematous or pale raised papules suddenly appear in large numbers on the trunk, legs, arms, and buttocks.

ERV, abbreviation for **expiratory reserve volume.**

Erypar, a trademark for an antibacterial (erythromycin stearate).

erysipelas /er′isip′ələs/, an infectious skin disease characterized by redness, swelling, vesicles, bullae, fever, pain, and lymphadenopathy. It is caused by a species of group A, beta-hemolytic streptococci. Treatment includes antibiotics, analgesics, and packs or dressings applied locally to the lesions.

erysipeloid /er′isip′əloid/, an infection of the hands characterized by blue-red nodules or patches and, occasionally, by erythema. It is acquired by handling meat or fish infected with *Erysipelothrix rhusiopathiae.* The disease is self-limited, lasting about 3 weeks, but will respond to penicillin. Also called **fish-handler's disease.** Compare **erysipelas.**

erythema /er′ithē′mə/, redness or inflammation of the skin or mucous membranes that is the result of dilatation and congestion of superficial capillaries. Examples of erythema are nervous blushes and mild sunburn. See also **erythroderma, rubor.** **–erythematous,** *adj.*

erythema chronicum migrans, a skin lesion that begins as a small papule and spreads peripherally, extending by a raised, red margin and clearing in the center. It may be associated with **Lyme arthritis,** which is caused by the bite of a small tick.

erythema infectiosum, an acute, benign infectious disease, mainly of children, characterized by fever and an erythematous rash beginning on the cheeks and appearing later on the arms, thighs, buttocks, and trunk. As the rash progresses, earlier lesions fade. Sunlight aggravates the eruption, which usually lasts about 10 days. For a period of time the rash may reappear whenever the skin is irritated. Its cause is unknown, no treatment is necessary, and prognosis is excellent. The isolation of patients is not required. Also called **fifth disease.**

erythema marginatum, a variant of **erythema multiforme** seen in acute rheumatic fever, characterized by transient, disk-shaped, nonpruritic, reddened macules that fade in the center, leaving raised margins.

erythema multiforme /mul'tifôr'mē, mo͝ol'tēfôr'mā/, a hypersensitivity syndrome characterized by polymorphous eruption of skin and mucous membranes. Macules, papules, nodules, vesicles or bullae, and target, or bull's-eye-shaped, lesions are seen. Erythema multiforme has been associated with many infections, collagen diseases, drug sensitivities, allergies, and pregnancy. Definitive and preventive treatment depends on finding the specific cause, but topical or systemic corticosteroids are helpful in most cases. A severe form of this condition is known as **Stevens-Johnson syndrome.**

erythema neonatorum, a common skin condition of neonates characterized by a pink papular rash frequently superimposed with vesicles or pustules. The rash appears within 24 to 48 hours after birth, covers the thorax, abdomen, back, and diaper area, and disappears spontaneously after several days. A smear of the papules shows eosinophils rather than neutrophils to differentiate the condition from neonatal pustular melanosis. Also called **toxic erythema of the newborn,** *(informal)* **flea bites.**

erythema nodosum, a hypersensitivity vasculitis characterized by bilateral, reddened, tender, subcutaneous nodules on the shins and, occasionally, on other parts of the body. The nodules last for several days or weeks, never ulcerate, and are often associated with mild fever, malaise, and pains in muscles and joints. This condition may be seen with streptococcal infections, tuberculosis, sarcoidosis, drug sensitivity, ulcerative colitis, and pregnancy. The prognosis is good, given appropriate treatment of the underlying disease. A course of corticosteroids is usually effective in diminishing the symptoms of this condition.

erythema perstans, a persistent local redness of the skin, often caused by a fixed-combination drug eruption.

erythrasma /er'ithraz'mə/, a bacterial skin infection of the axillary or inguinal regions, characterized by irregular, reddish brown, raised patches. An asymptomatic disease, it is more common in diabetics and responds quickly to oral erythromycin. Compare **intertrigo, tinea cruris.**

erythredema polyneuropathy. See **acrodynia.**

erythremia /er'ithrē'mē·ə/, an abnormal increase in the number of red blood cells.

erythrityl tetranitrate, a coronary vasodilator.

▪ INDICATIONS: It is prescribed in the treatment of angina pectoris.

▪ CONTRAINDICATIONS: It is used with caution when glaucoma is present. Known hypersensitivity to this drug prohibits its use.

▪ ADVERSE EFFECTS: Among the most serious adverse reactions are hypotension, allergic reactions, headache, and flushing.

erythro-, a combining form meaning 'red': *erythroblast, erythroclast, erythrocyte.*

erythroblastosis fetalis, a type of hemolytic anemia that occurs in newborns as a result of maternal-fetal blood group incompatibility, specifically involving the Rh factor and the ABO blood groups. The condition is caused by an antigen-antibody reaction in the bloodstream of the infant resulting from the placental transmission of maternally formed antibodies against the incompatible antigens of the fetal blood. In Rh factor incompatibility, the hemolytic reaction occurs only when the mother is Rh negative and the infant is Rh positive. The isoimmunization process rarely occurs with the first pregnancy, but there is increased risk with each succeeding pregnancy. However, maternal sensitization to the Rh factor can be prevented by injection of a high-titer anti-Rh gamma globulin preparation after delivery or abortion of an Rh positive fetus. No sensitization may occur in situations in which a strong placental barrier prevents transfer of fetal blood into the maternal circulation. In about 10% to 15% of sensitized mothers, there is no hemolytic reaction in the newborn. Clinical manifestations of the condition include severe anemia, jaundice, and enlargement of the liver and spleen, which, without intervention, can lead to hypoxia, cardiac failure, generalized edema, respiratory distress, and death. Prenatal diagnosis of the disease is confirmed through amniocentesis and analysis of bilirubin levels in amniotic fluid. Higher than normal levels result from the breakdown of hemoglobin from the lysed erythrocytes. Treatment consists of intrauterine transfusion when placental bilirubin levels progressively increase or immediate exchange transfusions after birth. Hemolytic reactions involving the ABO blood groups have similar manifestations but are generally less severe. See also **hydrops fetalis, hyperbilirubinemia of the newborn, Rh factor.**

Erythrocin, a trademark for an antibacterial (erythromycin).

erythrocyte /erith'rəsīt'/, a biconcave disk about 7 micrometers in diameter that contains hemoglobin confined within a lipoid membrane. The major cellular element of the circulating blood, its principal function is to transport oxygen. The number of cells per cubic millimeter of blood is usually maintained between 4.5 and 5.5 million in men and between 4.2 and 4.8 million in women. It varies with age, activity, and environmental conditions. For example, an increase to a level of 8 million/cu mm can normally occur at over 10,000 feet above sea level. An erythrocyte normally lives for 110 to 120 days, at which time it is removed from the bloodstream and broken down by the reticuloendothelial system. New erythrocytes are produced at a rate of slightly more than 1% a day; thus, a constant level is usually maintained. With acute blood loss, hemolytic anemia, or chronic oxygen deprivation, erythrocyte production may increase greatly. Erythrocytes originate in the marrow of the long bones. Maturation proceeds from a stem cell (promegaloblast) through the pronormoblast stage to the normoblast, the last stage before the mature adult cell develops. Kinds of erythrocyte include **burr cell, discocyte, macrocyte, meniscocyte,** and **spherocyte.** Also called **red blood cell, red cell, red corpuscle.** Compare **normoblast, reticulocyte.** See also **anisopoikilocytosis, erythropoiesis, hemoglobin, red cell indices.**

erythrocyte sedimentation rate (ESR), the rate at which red blood cells settle out in a tube of unclotted blood, expressed in millimeters per hour. Blood is collected in an anticoagulant and allowed to form a sediment in a calibrated glass column. At the end of 1 hour, the laboratory technician measures the distance the erythrocytes have fallen in the tube. Elevated sedimentation rates are not specific for any disorder but indicate the presence of inflammation. Inflammation causes an alteration of the blood proteins, which makes the red blood cells aggregate, becoming heavier than normal. The speed with which they fall to the bottom of the tube corresponds to the degree of inflammation. Serial evaluations of erythrocyte sedimentation rate are useful in monitoring the course of inflammatory activity in rheumatic diseases and, when performed with a white blood cell count, can indicate infection. Certain noninflammatory conditions, as pregnancy, are also characterized by high sedimentation rates. Two methods are used. The Wintrobe ESR is performed in a 10 cm Wintrobe tube, and the Westergren ESR is performed in a 200 mm Westergren tube. Values are higher for women in both methods and vary according to the method used. Also called *(informal)* **sed. rate.** See also **inflammation.**

erythrocythemia /erith′rōsīthē′mē•ə/, an increase in the number of erythrocytes circulating in the blood.

erythrocytosis /erith′rōsītō′sis/, an abnormal increase in the number of circulating red cells. See also **polycythemia.**

erythroderma /erith′rōdur′mə/, any dermatosis associated with abnormal redness of the skin. Compare **erythema, rubor.**

erythroleukemia, a malignant blood disorder characterized by a proliferation of erythropoietic elements in bone marrow, erythroblasts with bizarre lobulated nuclei, and abnormal myeloblasts in peripheral blood. The disease may have an acute or chronic course. Also called **diGuglielmo's disease** /di′gōōlyel′mōs/, **diGuglielmo's syndrome, erythromyeloblastic leukemia.**

erythromelalgia /erith′rōmilal′jə/, a rare disorder characterized by a paroxysmal dilatation of the peripheral blood vessels. It occurs bilaterally, usually in the extremities, and is associated with burning, redness of the skin, and pain. –**erythromelalgic,** *adj.*

erythromycin /erith′rōmī′sin/, an antibacterial antibiotic.

■ INDICATIONS: It is prescribed in the treatment of many bacterial and mycoplasmic infections, particularly infections that cannot be treated by penicillins.

■ CONTRAINDICATIONS: Liver disease or known hypersensitivity to this drug prohibits its use.

■ ADVERSE EFFECTS: Among the more serious adverse effects are cholestatic hepatitis and hypersensitivity reactions.

erythromyeloblastic leukemia. See **erythroleukemia.**

erythrophobia, **1.** an anxiety disorder characterized by an irrational fear of blushing or of displaying embarrassment. **2.** a neurotic symptom manifested by blushing at the slightest provocation. **3.** a morbid fear of or aversion to the color red. –**erythrophobic,** *adj.*

erythroplasia of Queyrat /erith′rōplā′zhə/, a premalignant lesion on the glans or corona of the penis. It is a well-circumscribed reddish patch on the skin. It is usually excised surgically. See also **carcinoma in situ.**

erythropoiesis /erith′rōpō•ē′sis/, the process of erythrocyte production involving the maturation of a nucleated precursor into a hemoglobin-filled, nucleus-free erythrocyte that is regulated by erythropoietin, a hormone produced by the kidney. See also **erthrocyte, erythropoietin, hemoglobin, leukopoiesis.** –**erythropoietic,** *adj.*

erythropoietic porphyria. See **porphyria.**

erythropoietin (EPO) /erith′rōpō•ē′tin/, a glycoprotein hormone synthesized mainly in the kidneys and released into the bloodstream in response to anoxia. The hormone acts to stimulate and to regulate the production of erythrocytes and is thus able to increase the oxygen-carrying capacity of the blood. See also **erythropoiesis.**

Es, symbol for **einsteinium.**

escape beat, an automatic beat of the heart that occurs after an interval longer than the duration of the dominant heart beat cycle. Escape beats function as safety mechanisms, and anything that produces a pause in the prevailing heart cycle may allow an escape to occur. Some kinds of pauses in which escape beats occur are caused by sinoatrial (SA) block, atrioventricular (AV) block, extra systole, and the completion of a paroxysm of tachycardia. In the presence of atrial fibrillation, nodal escape beats present a unique diagnostic problem because fibrillation obviates any dominant heart beat cycle. In the electrocardiogram, the nodal escape beat commonly presents a QRS-T contour similar to that of the sinus beats but sometimes varies slightly from the dominant beats. Ventricular escape beats are associated with the late rather than the early occurrence of the usual ventricular beat patterns.

-escent, **1.** a combining form meaning 'beginning to be': *alkalescent, convalescent, turgescent.* **2.** a combining form meaning 'emitting or reflecting light': *incandescent, iridescent, opalescent.*

eschar /es′kär/, a scab or dry crust resulting from a thermal or chemical burn, infection, or excoriating skin disease. –**escharotic,** *adj.*

escharonodulaire, escarronodulaire. See **Marseilles fever.**

Escherichia coli /eshirī′kē•ə kō′lī/, a species of coliform bacteria of the family Enterobacteriaceae, normally present in the intestines and common in water, milk, and soil. *Escherichia coli* is the most frequent cause of urinary tract infection and is a serious pathogen in wounds. *E. coli* septicemia may rapidly result in shock and death because of the action of an endotoxin released from the bacteria.

escutcheon, the shieldlike pattern of distribution of pubic hair.

eserine, eserine sulfate. See **physostigmine.**

Esidrix, a trademark for a diuretic (hydrochlorothiazide).

-esis, a combining form meaning an 'action, process, or result of': *enuresis, oxydesis, synthesis.*

Eskalith, a trademark for an antidepressant (lithium carbonate).

Eskatrol, a trademark for a fixed-combination drug containing a central nervous system stimulant (dextroamphetamine sulfate) and a tranquilizer (prochlorperazine maleate), used as an appetite suppressant.

Esmarch's bandage /es′märks/, a broad, flat, elastic bandage wrapped around an elevated limb to force blood out of the limb. It is used before certain surgical procedures to create a blood-free field.

ESO, abbreviation for **electrical spinal orthosis.**

eso-, a combining form meaning 'within': *esocataphoria, esogastritis, esotropia.*

esophageal cancer /əsof′əjē′əl, es′ofā′jē·əl/, a malignant neoplastic disease of the esophagus that occurs three times more frequently in men than in women and more often in Asia and Africa than in North America. Risk factors associated with the disease are heavy consumption of alcohol, smoking, betel-nut chewing, Plummer-Vinson syndrome, hiatus hernia, and achalasia. Aflatoxin in moldy grain and peanuts or a dietary deficiency, especially of molybdenum, may be involved. Esophageal cancer does not often cause any symptoms in the early stages but in later stages causes painful dysphagia, anorexia, weight loss, regurgitation, cervical adenopathy, and, in some cases, a persistent cough. Left vocal cord paralysis and hemoptysis indicate an advanced state of the disease. The tumor may spread locally to invade the trachea, bronchi, pericardium, great blood vessels, and thoracic vertebrae or may metastasize to lymph nodes, the lungs, and the liver. Diagnostic measures include fluoroscopic observation of the esophagus as the patient swallows barium, fiberoptic esophagoscopy, and biopsy and cytologic examination of the primary lesion and regional nodes. Most esophageal tumors are poorly differentiated squamous cell carcinomas; adenocarcinomas occur less frequently and are usually found in the lower third of the esophagus as extensions of gastric cancer. Surgical treatment may require total or partial esophagectomy with the resected segment replaced by a Dacron graft or a section of the colon. If only the lower third of the esophagus is removed, the proximal end may be anastomosed to the stomach. A catheter inserted into the stomach through an incision or a nasogastric tube may be used to feed patients who have inoperable esophageal cancer. Radiotherapy may eradicate early local tumors and may effectively palliate the symptoms of advanced lesion. Methotrexate given before irradiation may increase the chances of survival. See also **esophagectomy.**

esophageal dysfunction, any disturbance, impairment, or abnormality that interferes with the normal functioning of the esophagus, as dysphagia, esophagitis, or sphincter incompetence. The condition is one of the primary symptoms of scleroderma.

esophageal lead, **1.** an electrocardiographic conductor in which the exploring electrode is placed within the lumen of the esophagus. It is used to detect sizable atrial deflections as an aid in identifying cardiac arrhythmias. **2.** *informal.* a tracing produced by such a lead on an electrocardiograph.

esophageal varices, a complex of longitudinal, tortuous veins at the lower end of the esophagus, enlarged and swollen as the result of portal hypertension. These vessels are especially susceptible to ulceration and hemorrhage.

esophagectomy /esof′əjek′təmē/, a surgical procedure in which all or part of the esophagus is removed, as may be required to treat severe, recurrent, bleeding esophageal varices.

esophagitis /esof′əjī′tis/, inflammation of the mucosal lining of the esophagus, caused by infection, irritation from a nasogastric tube, or, most commonly, backflow of gastric juice from the stomach. See also **gastroesophageal reflux.**

esophagoscopy /esof′əgos′kəpē/, examination of the esophagus with an endoscope.

esophagus /esof′əgəs/, the muscular canal, about 24 cm long, extending from the pharynx to the stomach. It begins in the neck at the inferior border of the cricoid cartilage, opposite the sixth cervical vertebra, and descends to the cardiac sphincter of the stomach in a vertical path with two slight curves. It is the narrowest part of the digestive tube and is most constricted at its commencement and at the point where it passes through the diaphragm. The esophagus is composed of a fibrous coat, a muscular coat, and a submucous coat and is lined with mucous membrane. Also called **gullet.** **–esophageal,** *adj.*

esophoria /es′əfôr′ē·ə/, deviation of the visual axis of one eye toward that of the other eye in the absence of visual stimuli for fusion. Also called **cross-eye.** Compare **esotropia.** **–esophoric,** *adj.*

esotropia /es′ətrō′pē·ə/, a kind of strabismus characterized by an inward deviation of one eye relative to the other eye. Also called **convergent strabismus, internal strabismus.** Compare **esophoria, exotropia.** See also **strabismus.** **–esotropic,** *adj.*

ESP, abbreviation for **extrasensory perception.**

espundia /espun′dē·ə/, a cutaneous form of American leishmaniasis most common in Brazil, caused by *Leishmania brasiliensis.* The primary lesion often disappears spontaneously followed by mucocutaneous lesions that destroy the mucosal surface of the nose, pharynx, and larynx. If the condition is left untreated, secondary bacterial infections that are potentially fatal may occur.

ESR, abbreviation for **erythrocyte sedimentation rate.**

essential amino acid, an organic compound not synthesized in the body that is essential for nitrogen equilibrium in adults and optimal growth in infants and children.

Adults require isoleucine, leucine, lysine, methionine, phenylalanine, threonine, tryptophan, and valine. Infants need these eight amino acids plus arginine and histidine. Cysteine and tyrosine, limited substitutes respectively for methionine and phenylalanine, are considered quasi-essential. See also **amino acid.**

essential fatty acid, a polyunsaturated acid, as linoleic, linolenic, and arachidonic, essential in the diet for the proper growth, maintenance, and functioning of the body. It is a precursor of the prostaglandins and has an important role in fat transport and metabolism and in maintaining the function and integrity of cellular membranes. It is also necessary for the normal functioning of the reproductive and endocrine systems and for the breaking up of cholesterol deposits on arterial walls. The best dietary sources are natural vegetable oils, as safflower, soy, and corn oils; margarines blended with vegetable oils; wheat germ; edible seeds, as pumpkin, sesame, and sunflower; poultry fat; and fish oils, especially cod-liver oil. A deficiency of essential fatty acids causes changes in cell structure and enzyme function resulting in decreased growth and other disorders. Symptoms include brittle and lusterless hair, nail problems, dandruff, allergic conditions, and dermatoses, especially eczema in infants. Excessive amounts may reduce the level of vitamin E in the tissues and cause other metabolic disturbances as well as abnormal weight gain.

essential fever, any fever of unknown origin.

essential hypertension, an elevated systemic arterial pressure for which no cause can be found and which is often the only significant clinical finding. Elevated blood pressure is always considered a risk, and individuals with elevated pressures are at risk for cardiovascular disease. In examining patients with essential hypertension, clinicians consider the normal complex mechanisms that control pressure, as the arterial baroreflex, body fluid regulators, the renin-angiotensin system, and vascular autoregulation. These mechanisms are closely integrated, and it is not precisely clear how their impairment affects normotension and hypertension. Also called **primary hypertension.** See also **benign hypertension, malignant hypertension.**

essential nutrient, the carbohydrates, proteins, fats, minerals, and vitamins necessary for growth, normal function, and body maintenance. These substances are supplied by food, because some are not synthesized by the body in the quantities required for normal health.

essential thrombocythemia. See **thrombocytosis.**

essential tremor, an involuntary fine shaking of the hand, the head, and the face, especially during routine movements of the body. It is a familial disorder inherited as an autosomal dominant trait and appears during adolescence or in middle age, slowly progressing as a more pronounced disorder. The precise cause of this condition is not known, but it is believed to involve the central nervous system. Essential tremor is aggravated by activity and emotion and can be reduced in some patients by the administration of alcohol and mild sedatives, as propranolol and diazepam. Also called **familial tremor.** Compare **parkinsonism.**

EST, abbreviation for **electric shock therapy.**

established name, the name assigned to a drug by the U.S. Adopted Names Council. The established name, generally shorter than the chemical name, is the name by which the drug is known to health practitioners. Also called **generic name.** See also **chemical name, trademark.**

Estar, a trademark for a coal tar preparation used to treat eczema and psoriasis.

ester /es′tər/, a class of chemical compounds formed by the bonding of an alcohol and one or more organic acids. Fats are esters, formed by the bonding of fatty acids with the alcohol glycerol.

esterase, any enzyme that splits esters.

ester-compound local anesthetic, any one of four potent local anesthetics slightly different in chemical structure from the amide group of local anesthetics. Tetracaine is the most commonly used. Kinds of ester-compound local anesthetics are **chloroprocaine, cocaine hydrochloride,** and **procaine hydrochloride.**

esterified estrogen, an ester of natural estrogen.

■ INDICATIONS: It is prescribed in the treatment of menstrual irregularities, contraception, and menopausal symptoms.

■ CONTRAINDICATIONS: Pregnancy, known or suspected breast cancer, thrombophlebitis, vaginal bleeding of unknown origin, or known hypersensitivity to this drug prohibit its use.

■ ADVERSE EFFECTS: Among the more serious adverse reactions are gallbladder disease, thromboembolic disease, and a possible increase in risk of cancer.

esthesio-, a combining form meaning 'pertaining to feeling or to the perceptive faculties': *esthesiogenic, esthesioneure, esthesioscopy.*

-esthetic, -esthetical, -aesthetic, -aesthetical, a combining form meaning 'pertaining to a person's consciousness of something': *cenesthetic, photoesthetic, somatesthetic.*

Estinyl, a trademark for an estrogen (ethinyl estradiol).

Estrace, a trademark for an estrogen (estradiol).

estradiol /es′trədī′ôl/, the most potent naturally occurring human estrogen, also found in hog ovaries and in the urine of pregnant mares. Various esters of estradiol administered intramuscularly or orally are used as estrogens. See also **estrogen.**

Estradurin, a trademark for an antineoplastic estrogen (polyestradiol phosphate).

estramustine phosphate sodium, an antineoplastic agent.

■ INDICATIONS: It is prescribed for metastatic or progressive carcinoma of the prostate.

■ CONTRAINDICATIONS: Thromboembolytic disorders or known hypersensitivity to this drug prohibits its use.

■ ADVERSE EFFECTS: The most serious adverse reactions are cerebrovascular accident, myocardial infarction, thrombophlebitis, pulmonary emboli, and congestive heart failure.

estrangement, a psychologic effect caused by the required separation of a mother from her newborn child when the infant is ill, premature, or has a congenital defect, thereby diverting the mother from establishment of a normal relationship with her child.

Estratab, a trademark for esterified estrogens.

Estraval, a trademark for an estrogen (estradiol valerate).

estriol /es'trē•ôl/, a relatively weak, naturally occurring human estrogen found in high concentrations in urine. See also **estrogen.**

estrogen /es'trojən/, one of a group of hormonal steroid compounds that promote the development of female secondary sex characteristics. Human estrogen is elaborated in the ovaries, adrenal cortices, testes, and fetoplacental unit. During the menstrual cycle estrogen renders the female genital tract suitable for fertilization, implantation, and nutrition of the early embryo. Pharmaceutic preparations of estrogen are used in oral contraceptives, to palliate postmenopausal breast cancer and prostatic cancer, to inhibit lactation, and to treat threatened abortion, osteoporosis, and ovarian disease. Estrogen is also prescribed to relieve discomforts of menopause, but its long-term, continued use increases the risk of endometrial carcinoma. Kinds of estrogen are **conjugated estrogen, esterified estrogen, estradiol, estriol,** and **estrone.** –**estrogenic,** *adj.*

estrone /es'trōn/, a relatively potent estrogen.

■ INDICATIONS: It is prescribed in the treatment of menstrual cycle irregularities, prostatic cancer, and menopausal vasomotor symptoms, and to prevent pregnancy.

■ CONTRAINDICATIONS: Thrombophlebitis, abnormal genital bleeding, known or suspected pregnancy, or known hypersensitivity to this drug prohibits its use.

■ ADVERSE EFFECTS: Among the more serious adverse reactions are thrombophlebitis, embolism, and hypercalcemia.

Estronol, a trademark for an estrogen (estrone).

estropipate, an estrogen.

■ INDICATIONS: It is prescribed in the treatment of vasomotor symptoms of menopause, atrophic vaginitis, kraurosis vulvae, female hypogonadism, female castration, and primary ovarian failure.

■ CONTRAINDICATIONS: Known or suspected cancer of the breast or estrogen-dependent neoplasia, pregnancy, thrombophlebitis or thromboembolic disorders, undiagnosed abnormal genital bleeding, or complications from previous administration of estrogen prohibits its use.

■ ADVERSE EFFECTS: Among the most serious adverse reactions are a possible increased risk of cancer, gallbladder disease, and thromboembolic disorders.

estrus, the cyclic period of sexual activity in mammals other than primates.

ethacrynate sodium. See **ethacrynic acid.**

ethacrynic acid, a potent diuretic.

■ INDICATIONS: It is prescribed to relieve the effects of severe edema and hypertension.

■ CONTRAINDICATIONS: Pregnancy, anuria, or known hypersensitivity to this drug prohibits its use. It is not given to infants.

■ ADVERSE EFFECTS: Among the more serious adverse reactions are tetany, muscle weakness, cramps, and excessive diuresis. Hearing loss or deafness may occur.

ethambutol hydrochloride, a tuberculostatic antibiotic.

■ INDICATION: It is prescribed in the treatment of pulmonary tuberculosis.

■ CONTRAINDICATIONS: Optic neuritis or known hypersensitivity to this drug prohibits its use. It is not recommended for small children.

■ ADVERSE EFFECTS: Among the most serious adverse reactions are diminished visual acuity and allergic reactions, as rashes.

Ethamide, a trademark for a carbonic anhydrase inhibitor (ethoxzolamide).

ethanoic acid. See **acetic acid.**

ethanol, ethyl alcohol. See also **alcohol.**

ethaverine hydrochloride, a smooth muscle relaxant.

■ INDICATIONS: It is prescribed to relieve spasm of the GI or genitourinary tract, arterial vasospasm, and cerebral insufficiency.

■ CONTRAINDICATIONS: Liver disease, atrioventricular dissociation, or known hypersensitivity to this drug prohibits its use. It is used with caution in patients who have glaucoma.

■ ADVERSE EFFECTS: Among the more serious adverse reactions are hypotension, abdominal distress, cardiac arrhythmia, and headache.

ethchlorvynol /ethklôr'vənôl/, a sedative and hypnotic.

■ INDICATIONS: It is prescribed in the treatment of insomnia.

■ CONTRAINDICATIONS: Porphyria or known hypersensitivity to this drug prohibits its use.

■ ADVERSE EFFECTS: Among the most serious adverse effects are allergic reactions, nausea, dizziness, aftertaste, and drug hangover.

ethene. See **ethylene.**

ether, a nonhalogenated, volatile liquid used as a general anesthetic. Because it provides excellent analgesia and profound muscle relaxation, adjuncts to anesthesia, as narcotic analgesics and neuromuscular blocking agents, are often unnecessary. Ether has little depressant effect on the respiratory and cardiovascular systems but may cause hyperglycemia, decreased excretion of urine, decreased intestinal tone and motility, and transient abnormalities in the function of the liver. It has an irritating, pungent odor, is highly flammable and explosive, and frequently causes postoperative nausea and vomiting.

ethical drug, a drug available only by prescription and advertised only to physicians and other health professionals. Also called **prescription drug.** Compare **over the counter.**

ethics, the science or study of moral values or principles, including ideals of autonomy, beneficence, and justice.

Code for nurses

1. The nurse provides services with respect for human dignity and the uniqueness of the client unrestricted by considerations of social or economic status, personal attributes, or the nature of health problems.
2. The nurse safeguards the client's right to privacy by judiciously protecting information of a confidential nature.
3. The nurse acts to safeguard the client and the public when health care and safety are affected by the incompetent, unethical, or illegal practice of any person.
4. The nurse assumes responsibility and accountability for individual nursing judgments and actions.
5. The nurse maintains competence in nursing.
6. The nurse exercises informed judgment and uses individual competence and qualification as criteria in seeking consultation, accepting responsibilities, and delegating nursing activities to others.
7. The nurse participates in activities that contribute to the ongoing development of the profession's body of knowledge.
8. The nurse participates in the profession's efforts to implement and improve standards of nursing.
9. The nurse participates in the professional's efforts to establish and maintain conditions of employment conducive to high quality nursing care.
10. The nurse participates in the profession's efforts to protect the public from misinformation and misrepresentation and to maintain the integrity of nursing.
11. The nurse collaborates with members of the health professions and other citizens in promoting community and national efforts to meet the health needs of the public.

From Code for Nurses With Interpretive Statements, Kansas City, MO, American Nurses' Association, 1976.

ethinamate /ethin′əmāt/, a sedative.

■ INDICATION: It is prescribed in the treatment of insomnia.

■ CONTRAINDICATIONS: Known hypersensitivity to this drug prohibits its use. It is not recommended for pregnant women, for people under 15 years of age, or for persons with a history of drug abuse.

■ ADVERSE EFFECTS: Among the more serious adverse reactions are thrombocytopenic purpura, physical and psychologic dependence, and skin rash.

ethinyl estradiol /eth′inil/, an estrogen.

■ INDICATIONS: It is prescribed in the treatment of postmenopausal breast cancer, menstrual cycle irregularities and prostatic cancer, and hypogonadism, for contraception, and to relieve menopausal vasomotor symptoms.

■ CONTRAINDICATIONS: Thrombophlebitis, abnormal genital bleeding, known or suspected pregnancy, or known hypersensitivity to this drug prohibits its use.

■ ADVERSE EFFECTS: Among the more serious adverse reactions are thrombophlebitis, embolism, and hypercalcemia.

ethionamide /eth′ē·ənam′īd/, a tuberculostatic antibacterial.

■ INDICATION: It is prescribed for tuberculosis.

■ CONTRAINDICATIONS: Existing liver damage or known hypersensitivity to this drug prohibits its use.

■ ADVERSE EFFECTS: Among the more serious adverse reactions are skin rash, jaundice, and mental depression. GI side effects are common.

ethmoidal air cell /ethmoi′dəl/, one of the numerous, small thin-walled cavities in the ethmoid bone of the skull, rimmed by the frontal maxilla, lacrimal, sphenoidal, and palatine bones. The cavities are lined with mucous membrane continuous with that of the nasal cavity and lie between the upper part of the nasal cavities and the orbits. They are divided bilaterally into anterior, middle, and posterior cavities. The anterior and the middle cavities open into the middle meatus of the nose; the posterior cavities open into the superior meatus. The ethmoidal air cells start to develop at birth. Compare **frontal sinus, maxillary sinus, sphenoidal sinus.**

ethmoid bone, the very light and spongy bone at the base of the cranium, forming most of the walls of the superior part of the nasal cavity and consisting of four parts: a horizontal plate, a perpendicular plate, and two lateral labyrinths.

ethnocentrism, **1.** a belief in the inherent superiority of the "race" or group to which one belongs. **2.** a proclivity to consider other ethnic groups in terms of one's own racial origins.

Ethobral, a trademark for a sedative-hypnotic, fixed-combination drug containing three barbiturates (phenobarbital, butabarbital sodium, and secobarbital sodium).

Ethocaine, a trademark for a local anesthetic (procaine hydrochloride).

ethoheptazine citrate, a nonnarcotic analgesic.

■ INDICATION: It is prescribed to relieve mild to moderate pain.

■ CONTRAINDICATION: Known hypersensitivity to this drug prohibits its use.

■ ADVERSE EFFECTS: Among the most common adverse reactions are GI distress and dizziness.

ethology, **1.** (in zoology) the scientific study of the behavioral patterns of animals, specifically in their native habitat. **2.** (in psychology) the empiric study of human behavior, primarily social customs, manners, and mores. –**ethologic, ethological,** *adj.*, **ethologist,** *n.*

ethopropazine hydrochloride, a phenothiazine anticholinergic agent.

■ INDICATIONS: It is prescribed in the treatment of extrapyramidal parkinsonism and other nervous system disorders.

■ CONTRAINDICATIONS: Narrow-angle glaucoma, asthma, obstruction of the genitourinary or GI tract, severe ulcerative colitis, or known hypersensitivity to this drug or to phenothiazine medication prohibits its use.

■ ADVERSE EFFECTS: Among the more serious adverse effects are blurred vision, central nervous system effects, tachycardia, dry mouth, decreased sweating, and hypersensitivity reactions.

ethosuximide, an anticonvulsant.

■ INDICATION: It is prescribed in the treatment of petit mal epilepsy.

■ CONTRAINDICATIONS: Known hypersensitivity to this drug or to any succinimide medication prohibits its use.

■ ADVERSE EFFECTS: Among the more serious adverse reactions are blood dyscrasias, GI disturbance, hematopoietic complications, and systemic lupus erythematosus.

ethotoin /ethō′tō•in/, an anticonvulsant.

■ INDICATIONS: It is prescribed in the treatment of grand mal and psychomotor seizures.

■ CONTRAINDICATIONS: Liver disease, hematologic disorders, or known hypersensitivity to this drug or to any hydantoin prohibits its use. It is not recommended for use during pregnancy or lactation.

■ ADVERSE EFFECTS: Among the more serious adverse reactions are blood disorders, nausea, fatigue, skin rash, and chest pain.

ethoxzolamide, a carbonic anhydrase inhibitor.

■ INDICATIONS: It is prescribed primarily in the treatment of certain types of glaucoma and congestive heart failure.

■ CONTRAINDICATIONS: Liver or kidney dysfunction, hyponatremia, hypokalemia, or known hypersensitivity to this drug prohibits its use.

■ ADVERSE EFFECTS: Among the most serious adverse reactions are bone marrow depression, kidney stones, and crystalluria. Fever and skin rash may also occur.

Ethrane, a trademark for an inhalational general anesthetic (enflurane).

Ethril, a trademark for an antibacterial (erythromycin stearate).

ethyl alcohol. See **alcohol.**

ethyl aminobenzoate. See **benzocaine.**

ethyl chloride, a topical anesthetic for short operations.

■ INDICATIONS: It is prescribed in the treatment of skin irritations and in minor skin surgery.

■ CONTRAINDICATIONS: Known hypersensitivity to this drug prohibits its use. It is not used on broken skin or on mucous membrane.

■ ADVERSE EFFECTS: Among the more serious adverse reactions are pain, muscle spasm, and, from excessive use, frostbite.

■ NOTE: It is highly flammable.

ethylene /eth′əlēn/, a colorless, flammable gas that is lighter than air and has a slightly sweet odor and taste. It was previously used as a general anesthetic, being slightly more potent than nitrous oxide. Also called **ethene, olefiant gas.**

ethylenediamine /eth′əlēndi•am′ēn/, a clear, thick liquid having the odor of ammonia. It is used as a solvent, an emulsifier, and a stabilizer with aminophylline injections.

ethylene dibromide (EDB), a volatile liquid used as an insecticide and gasoline additive. Because it has been found to be a cause of cancer in animals, the Environmental Protection Agency has restricted the use of EDB to control insect pests in grains and fruits intended for human use.

ethylene oxide, a gas used to sterilize surgical instruments and other supplies.

ethylestrenol, an anabolic steroid.

ethylnorepinephrine hydrochloride /eth′ilnôrep′inef′rin/, a bronchodilator.

■ INDICATION: It is prescribed in the treatment of bronchial asthma.

■ CONTRAINDICATIONS: Known hypersensitivity to this drug or to other sympathomimetic medication prohibits its use.

■ ADVERSE EFFECTS: Among the more serious adverse reactions are increased or decreased blood pressure, palpitations, and an increase in heart rate.

ethyl oxide, a colorless highly volatile liquid solvent similar to diethyl ether. It is widely used in various pharmaceutic processes.

ethynodiol diacetate /eth′inōdī′ôl/, a synthetic progestin derivative.

ethynodiol diacetate and ethinyl estradiol, an oral contraceptive.

■ INDICATION: It is prescribed for contraception.

■ CONTRAINDICATIONS: Thrombophlebitis, cardiovascular disease, breast or reproductive organ cancer, or known hypersensitivity to either ingredient prohibits its use.

■ ADVERSE EFFECTS: Among the more serious adverse reactions are thrombophlebitis, uterine fibroma, gallbladder disease, embolism, and hepatic lesions.

ethynodiol diacetate and mestranol, an oral contraceptive.

■ INDICATION: It is prescribed for contraception.

■ CONTRAINDICATIONS: Thrombophlebitis, cardiovascular disease, breast or reproductive organ cancer, or known hypersensitivity to either ingredient prohibits its use.

■ ADVERSE EFFECTS: Among the more serious adverse reactions are thrombophlebitis, uterine fibroma, gallbladder disease, embolism, and hepatic lesions.

-etic, a combining form used as the equivalent of *-ic* in forming adjectives: *enuretic, genetic, kinetic.*

etidronate disodium /etid′rənāt/, a regulator of calcium metabolism. Also called **sodium etidronate.**

■ INDICATIONS: It is prescribed in the treatment of Paget's disease, for heterotopic ossification caused by injury to the spinal cord, and after total hip replacement.

■ CONTRAINDICATIONS: There are no known contraindications.

■ ADVERSE EFFECTS: Among the more serious adverse reactions are bone pain at both Pagetic sites and previously asymptomatic sites, GI disturbances, and elevated serum phosphate concentrations.

etiology /ē′tē·ol′əjē/, **1.** the study of all factors that may be involved in the development of a disease, including susceptibility of the patient, the nature of the disease agent, and the way in which the patient's body is invaded by the agent. **2.** the cause of a disease. Compare **pathogenesis.** –**etiologic,** *adj.*

etomidate /etom′idāt/, a hypnotic and short-acting, investigational nonbarbiturate intravenous induction agent for general anesthesia. It is reported to have minimal adverse cardiovascular and respiratory effects, thus providing a greater margin of safety in patients at risk because of heart disease.

Etrafon, a trademark for a central nervous system fixed-combination drug containing a tranquilizer (perphenazine) and an antidepressant (amitriptyline hydrochloride).

Eu, symbol for **europium.**

eu-, a combining form meaning 'well, easily, good': *euangiotic, eucrasia, euthyroid.*

eucaryon. See **eukaryon.**

eucaryosis. See **eukaryosis.**

eucatropine hydrochloride /yo͞okat′rəpin/, an ophthalmic anticholinergic.

■ INDICATION: It is prescribed for dilating the pupil in an ophthalmoscopic examination of the eye.

■ CONTRAINDICATIONS: Known hypersensitivity to this drug or to other anticholinergics prohibits its use.

■ ADVERSE EFFECTS: Among the most serious adverse reactions are tachycardia and severe constipation. Dry mouth, heat intolerance, and other effects associated with systemic absorption of an anticholinergic agent may also occur.

eucholia /yo͞okō′lyə/, the normal state of the bile as to the quantity secreted and the condition of the constituents.

euchromatin /yo͞okrō′mətin/, that portion of chromosome material that is active in gene expression during cell division. It stains most deeply during mitosis when it is in a coiled, condensed state, and during each division of the cell it passes through a continuous cycle of condensation and dispersion. Compare **heterochromatin.** See also **chromatin.** –**euchromatic,** *adj.*

euchromosome. See **autosome.**

eugamy /yo͞o′gəmē/, the union of those gametes that contain the same haploid number of chromosomes. –**eugamic,** *adj.*

eugenics /yo͞ojen′iks/, the study of methods for controlling the characteristics of future human populations through selective breeding.

euglobulin, a "true" globulin (a protein insoluble in distilled water). This is one of a number of different properties used to classify proteins. Compare **albumin, cryoglobulin.** See also **plasma protein, electrophoresis.**

eugnathic anomaly /yo͞onath′ik/, (in dentistry) an abnormality of the teeth and their alveolar supports. Compare **dysgnathic anomaly.**

eukaryocyte /yo͞oker′ē·ōsīt′/, a cell with a true nucleus, found in all higher organisms and in some microorganisms, as amebae, plasmodia, and trypanosomes. Also spelled **eucaryocyte.** Compare **prokaryocyte.** –**eukaryotic,** *adj.*

eukaryon /yo͞oker′ē·on/, **1.** a nucleus that is highly complex, organized, and surrounded by a nuclear membrane, usually characteristic of higher organisms. **2.** an organism containing such a nucleus. Also spelled **eucaryon.** Compare **prokaryon.**

eukaryosis, the state of having a highly complex, organized nucleus containing organelles surrounded by a nuclear membrane, such as is characteristic of all organisms except bacteria, viruses, and blue-green algae. Also spelled **eucaryosis.** Compare **prokaryosis.**

eukaryote /yo͞oker′ē·ot/, an organism having cells that contain a true nucleus. Also spelled **eucaryote.** –**eukaryotic, eucaryotic,** *adj.*

eunuch /yo͞o′nək/, a male whose testicles have been destroyed or removed. If this occurs before puberty, secondary sex characteristics fail to develop and symptoms such as a feminine voice and absence of facial hair can stem from the absence of male hormones. See also **secondary sex characteristic.**

eunuchoidism /yo͞o′nəkoidiz′əm/, deficiency of the function of male hormone or of its formation by the testes. The deficiency leads to sterility and to abnormal tallness, small testes, and deficient development of secondary sexual characteristics, libido, and potency.

euphoretic /yo͞o′fəret′ik/, **1.** (of a substance or event) tending to produce a condition of euphoria. **2.** a substance tending to produce euphoria, as LSD, mescaline, marijuana, and other hallucinogenic drugs.

euphoria /yo͞ofôr′ē·ə/, **1.** a feeling or state of well-being or elation. **2.** an exaggerated or abnormal sense of physical and emotional well-being not based on reality or truth, disproportionate to its cause, and inappropriate to the situation, as commonly seen in the manic stage of bipolar disorder, in some forms of schizophrenia, in organic mental disorders, and in toxic and drug-induced states. Compare **ecstasy.**

euploid /yo͞o′ploid/, **1.** of or pertaining to an individual, organism, strain, or cell with a chromosome number that is an exact multiple of the normal, basic haploid number characteristic of the species, as diploid, triploid, tetraploid, or polyploid. Variation occurs through entire sets rather than individual chromosomes, so that there is a balanced number of chromosomes. **2.** such an individual, organism, strain, or cell. Compare **aneuploid.**

euploidy /yo͞o′ploidē/, the state or condition of having a variation in chromosome number that is an exact multiple of the characteristic haploid number. Compare **aneuploidy.**

Eurax, a trademark for a scabicide (crotamiton).

European blastomycosis. See **cryptococcosis.**

European typhus. See **epidemic typhus.**
europium (Eu), a rare-earth, metallic element. Its atomic number is 63; its atomic weight is 151.96.
eury-, a combining form meaning 'wide, broad': *eurycephalic, eurygnathic, euryopia.*
eustachian tube /yo͞ostā'shən/, a tube, lined with mucous membrane, that joins the nasopharynx and the tympanic cavity, allowing equalization of the air pressure in the inner ear with atmospheric pressure. Also called **auditory tube.**
eustress /yo͞o'stres/, **1.** a positive form of stress. **2.** a balance between selfishness and altruism through which an individual develops the drive and energy to care for others.
euthanasia /yo͞o'thənā'zhə/, deliberately bringing about the death of a person who is suffering from an incurable disease or condition, actively, as by administering a lethal drug, or passively, by allowing the person to die by withholding treatment. Legal authorities, church leaders, philosophers, and commentators on ethics and morality usually treat passive euthanasia differently from active euthanasia. Also called **mercy killing.**
euthenics, the science that deals with improvement of the human species through the control of environmental factors, as pollution, malnutrition, disease, and drug abuse. Compare **eugenics.**
Euthroid, a trademark for a thyroid hormone preparation (liotrix; a combination of levothyroxine sodium and liothryonine sodium).
euthymism /yo͞othī'mizm/, the characteristic of normal mood responses.
Eutonyl, a trademark for a monoamine oxidase inhibitor (pargyline hydrochloride).
Eutron, a trademark for a fixed-combination drug containing a diuretic (methyclothiazide) and a monoamine oxidase inhibitor (pargyline hydrochloride), used as an antihypertensive.
evacuate, **1.** to discharge or to remove a substance from a cavity, space, organ, or tract of the body. **2.** a substance discharged or removed from the body. – **evacuation,** *n.*
evaluating, (in five-step nursing process) a category of nursing behavior in which a determination is made and recorded regarding the extent to which the established goals of care have been met. To make this judgment, the nurse estimates the degree of success in meeting the goals, evaluates the implementation of nursing measures, investigates the client's compliance with therapy, and records the client's response to therapy. The nurse evaluates effects of the measures used, the need for change in goals of care, the accuracy of the implementation of nursing measures, and the need for change in the client's environment or in the equipment or procedures used. The impact of the care or treatment on the client, the client's family, and the staff is evaluated, the accuracy of tests and measurements is checked, and the client's and the family's understanding of the information given them is evaluated. The client's expressed and observed response to care is recorded. Although evaluating is the final step of the five-step nursing process, after implementing, evaluating is, in practice, integral to effective nursing practice at all steps of the process. See also **analyzing, assessing, implementing, nursing process, planning.**
evaporated milk, homogenized whole milk from which 50% to 60% of the water content has been evaporated. It is fortified with vitamin D, canned, and sterilized. When it is diluted with an equal amount of water, its nutritional value is comparable to that of fresh whole milk.
evaporation, the change of a substance from a solid or liquid state to a gaseous state. The process of evaporation is hastened by an increase in temperature and a decrease in atmospheric pressure. See also **boiling point.** – **evaporate,** *v.*
event-related potential (ERP), a type of brain wave that is associated with a response to a specific stimulus, as a particular wave pattern observed when a patient hears a clicking sound. See also **evoked potential.**
Evex, a trademark for a type of esterified estrogen (sodium estrone sulfate).
evisceration, **1.** the removal of the viscera from the abdominal cavity; disembowelment. **2.** the removal of the contents from an organ or an organ from its cavity. **3.** the protrusion of an internal organ through a wound or surgical incision, especially in the abdominal wall. – **eviscerate,** *v.*

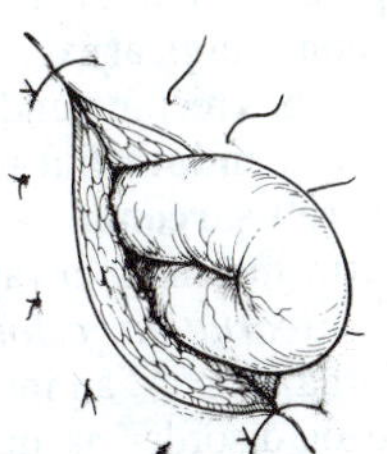

Wound evisceration

evocation, (in embryology) a specific morphogenetic change within a developing embryo that occurs as a result of the action of a single evocator. See also **induction.**
evocator, a specific chemical substance or hormone that is emitted from the organizer part of the embryonic tissue and acts as a morphogenetic stimulus in the developing embryo.
evoked potential (EP), a tracing of a brain wave measured on the surface of the head at various places. The EP, unlike the waves seen on an electroencephalogram, is elicited by a specific stimulus. The stimulus may originate in the visual, auditory, or somatosensory areas normally evoked by the stimulus of the nervous system. The activity and function of the system may be monitored during surgery, while the patient is unconscious. The surgeon is thus able to avoid damage to the nerves during

operative procedures. Evoked potentials are also used to diagnose multiple sclerosis and various disorders of hearing and of sight. Kinds of evoked potentials include **brainstem auditory evoked potential, somatosensory evoked potential,** and **visual evoked potential.** See also **brain electric activity map.**

evolution, **1.** a gradual, orderly, and continuous process of change and development from one condition or state to another. It encompasses all aspects of life, including physical, psychologic, sociologic, cultural, and intellectual development, and involves a progressive advancement from a simple to a more complex form or state through the processes of modification, differentiation, and growth. **2.** (in genetics) the theory of the origin and propagation of all plant and animal species, including humans, and their development from lower to more complex forms through the natural selection of variants produced through genetic mutations, hybridization, and inbreeding. Kinds of evolution are **convergent evolution, determinant evolution, emergent evolution, organic evolution, orthogenic evolution,** and **saltatory evolution.** **–evolutionist,** *n.*

evulsed tooth. See **avulsed tooth.**

Ewing's sarcoma, a malignant tumor developing from bone marrow, usually in long bones or the pelvis. It occurs most frequently in adolescent boys and is characterized by pain, swelling, fever, and leukocytosis. The tumor, a soft, crumbly grayish mass that may invade surrounding soft tissues, is difficult to distinguish histologically from a neuroblastoma or a reticulum cell sarcoma. Radiotherapy often produces a dramatic initial response, but relapses are common. Surgical excision, often requiring amputation, may be recommended. Also called **Ewing's tumor.** See also **endothelial myeloma, neuroblastoma, reticulum cell sarcoma.**

ex-, a combining form meaning 'away from, outside, without': *exacrinous, excoriation, exfoliato.*

exacerbation /igzas′ərbā′shən/, an increase in the seriousness of a disease or disorder as marked by greater intensity in the signs or symptoms of the patient being treated.

exanthema /ig′zanthē′mə/, a skin eruption or rash that may have specific diagnostic features of an infectious disease. Chickenpox, measles, roseola infantum, and rubella are usually characterized by a particular type of exanthema. Also called **exanthem.** Compare **enanthema.** **–exanthematous,** *adj.*

exanthem subitum. See **roseola infantum.**

excess mortality, a premature death or one that occurs before the average life expectancy for a person of a particular demographic category.

exchange transfusion in the newborn, the introduction of whole blood in exchange for 75% to 85% of an infant's circulating blood that is repeatedly withdrawn in small amounts and replaced with equal amounts of donor blood. The procedure is performed to improve the oxygen-carrying capacity of the blood in the treatment of erythroblastosis neonatorum by removing Rh and ABO antibodies, sensitized erythrocytes producing hemolysis, and accumulated bilirubin.

■ METHOD: A radiant heat warmer, pacifier, and cardiac and respiratory monitors are prepared, and resuscitative equipment and drugs, including oxygen, a mask, a bag, suction apparatus, glucose, calcium, and sodium bicarbonate, are made readily available. The results of laboratory studies of the infant's bilirubin, hemoglobin, and calcium levels, hematocrit, blood culture, and random blood glucose test and the donor blood culture are checked. The donor blood is checked to make certain that it is not more than 48 hours old; if fresh whole blood is not used, stored blood is mixed in amounts as ordered with frozen plasma or plasmanate. Before exchange transfusion, nothing is administered by mouth for 3 to 4 hours, or the contents of the infant's stomach are aspirated. The baby's extremities are restrained; the blood is warmed as ordered, and the physician is assisted with the insertion of an umbilical venous line, if one is not in place. The physician may administer albumin with the donor blood. The procedure may be carried out under phototherapy lights, and, unless contraindicated, the infant's parents may be in attendance. During the procedure the young patient is observed for bradycardia with less than 100 beats a minute, cyanosis, hypothermia, vomiting, aspiration, apnea, an air embolus, abdominal distention, or cardiac arrest. The respiratory and cardiac rates are checked every 5 minutes, the axillary temperature every 15 to 30 minutes. The integrity of all blood tubing connections is inspected periodically. The amount of blood withdrawn and infused is recorded, and the physician is notified when each 100 ml of blood has been exchanged. A repetition of laboratory studies is requested as ordered for the last amount of blood removed from the infant. After the procedure, the infant is observed for signs of tachycardia or bradycardia, tachypnea or bradypnea, hypothermia, lethargy, jitteriness, increasing jaundice, cyanosis, edema, dark urine, bleeding from the cord, convulsions, or complications, as hemorrhage, hypocalcemia, heart failure, hypoglycemia, sepsis, acidosis, hyperkalemia, thrombus formation, or shock. The infant is maintained in a neutral thermal environment and is handled gently and minimally for the next 2 to 4 hours. The cardiac and respiratory rates are monitored every 15 minutes for 4 hours, then every 30 to 60 minutes for 24 to 48 hours or as ordered. The axillary temperature is checked every 1 to 3 hours for 48 hours, and the cord is observed for bleeding every 5 to 15 minutes for 1 to 2 hours after the procedure. Feeding, by gavage or a bottle having a soft nipple with a large enough hole to ensure adequate intake, is initiated 4 to 6 hours after the transfusion, as ordered; the infant is fed slowly and repositioned after each feeding. Intake and output of fluids are measured, and ongoing care is provided as for all high-risk infants.

■ NURSING ORDERS: The nurse prepares the equipment and infant for the exchange transfusion, assists the physician in the insertion of the umbilical venous line, and

monitors the baby during and after the procedure. The nurse offers the parents an explanation of the reason for the procedure and encourages them to participate in the infant's care as much as possible.
■ OUTCOME CRITERIA: An exchange transfusion is usually administered only to a high-risk infant, but the procedure often effectively counteracts the hemolytic anemia and hyperbilirubinemia associated with erythroblastosis neonatorum.

excise /iksīz′/, to remove completely, as in the surgical excision of the palatine tonsils. Compare **resect.**

excision, **1.** the process of excising or amputating. **2.** (in molecular genetics) the process by which a genetic element is removed from a strand of DNA.

excitability, the property of a cell that enables it to react to irritation or stimulation, as the reaction of a nerve or myocardial cell to an adequate stimulus.

exciting eye, (in sympathetic ophthalmia) the eye that is primarily affected by an injury or infection in a bilateral disorder. Also called **inciting eye.**

excoriation /ekskôr′ē·ā′shən/, an injury to the surface of the skin or other part of the body caused by scratching or abrasion.

excreta /ekskrē′tə/, any waste matter discharged from the body.

excrete, to evacuate a waste substance from the body, often via a normal secretion; for example, a drug may be excreted in breast milk.

excretion, the process of eliminating, shedding, or getting rid of substances by body organs or tissues, as part of a natural metabolic activity. Excretion usually begins at the cellular level where water, carbon dioxide, and other waste products of cellular life are emptied into the capillaries. The epidermis excretes dead skin cells by shedding them daily.

excretory /eks′krətôr′ē/, relating to the process of excretion, often used in combination with a term to identify an object or procedure associated with excretion, as in **excretory urography.**

excretory duct, a duct that is conductive but not secretory.

excretory urography. See **intravenous pyelography.**

execute, (of a computer) to follow a set of instructions to complete a program or specified function.

executive physical, a physical examination including extensive laboratory, x-ray, and other tests that is provided periodically to management level personnel at employer expense. Such examinations may be detailed, expensive, and overly complete.

exercise, **1.** the performance of any physical activity for the purpose of conditioning the body, improving health, or maintaining fitness or as a means of therapy for correcting a deformity or restoring the organs and bodily functions to a state of health. **2.** any action, skill, or maneuver that exerts the muscles and is performed repeatedly in order to develop or strengthen the body or any of its parts. **3.** to use a muscle or part of the body in a repetitive way to maintain or develop its strength. The nurse constantly assesses the patient's needs and provides the proper type and amount of exercise, taking into account the patient's physical or mental limitations. Exercise has a beneficial effect on each of the body systems, although in excess it can lead to the breakdown of tissue and cause injury. Kinds of exercise are **active assisted exercise, active exercise, active resistance exercise, aerobic exercise, anaerobic exercise, corrective exercise, isometric exercise, isotonic exercise, muscle-setting exercise, passive exercise, progressive resistance exercise, range of motion exercise,** and **underwater exercise.**

exercise electrocardiogram (exercise ECG), a stress test that is important in the diagnosis of coronary artery disease. An exercise electrocardiogram is recorded as a person walks on a treadmill or pedals a stationary bicycle for a given length of time at a specific rate of speed. Abnormal changes in cardiac function that were absent during rest may appear with exercise.

exfoliation, peeling and sloughing off of tissue cells. This is a normal process that may be exaggerated in certain skin diseases or after a severe sunburn. See also **desquamation, exfoliative dermatitis. –exfoliative,** *adj.*

exfoliative cytology, the microscopic examination of desquamated cells for diagnostic purposes. The cells are obtained from lesions, sputum, secretions, urine, and other material by aspiration, scraping, a smear, or washings of the tissue. Compare **aspiration biopsy cytology.**

exfoliative dermatitis, any inflammatory skin disorder in which there is excessive peeling or shedding of skin. The cause is unknown in about half of the cases. Known causes include drug reactions, scarlet fever, leukemia, lymphoma, and generalized dermatitis. Treatment is individualized, but care is essential to prevent secondary infection, to avoid further irritation, and to maintain fluid balance.

exhalation. See **expiration.**

exhale, to breathe out or to let out with the breath. –**exhalation,** *n.*

exhaustion delirium, a delirium that may result from prolonged physical or emotional stress, fatigue, or shock associated with severe metabolic or nutritional problems. See also **delirium.**

exhibitionism, **1.** the flaunting of oneself or one's abilities in order to attract attention. **2.** (in psychiatry) a psychosexual disorder occurring in men in which the repetitive act of exposing the genitals to unsuspecting women or girls in socially unacceptable situations is the preferred means of achieving sexual excitement and gratification. See also **paraphilia, scopophilia. –exhibitionist,** *n.*

existential humanistic psychotherapy. See **humanistic existential therapy.**

existential psychiatry, a school of psychiatry based on the philosophy of existentialism that emphasizes an analytic, holistic approach in which mental disorders are viewed as deviations within the total structure of an individual's existence rather than as caused by any biologically or culturally related factors.

existential therapy, a kind of psychotherapy that emphasizes the development of a sense of self-direction through choice, awareness, and acceptance of individual responsibility.

exit block, (in cardiology) the failure of an expected impulse to emerge from its focus of origin and cause a contraction.

exit dose, (in radiotherapy) the amount of radiation at the side of the body opposite the surface to which the beam is directed.

Exna, a trademark for a diuretic and antihypertensive (benzthiazide).

exo-, a combining form meaning 'outside, outward': *exocataphoria, exohysteropexy, exotoxin*.

exocoelom. See **extraembryonic coelom.**

exocrine /ek′səkrin/, of or pertaining to the process of secreting outwardly through a duct to the surface of an organ or tissue or into a vessel, as a gland that secretes through a duct. Compare **endocrine system.** See also **eccrine.**

exocrine gland, any one of the two kinds of multicellular glands that open on the surface of the skin through ducts in the epithelium, as the sweat glands and the sebaceous glands. Exocrine glands include simple glands having only one duct and compound glands having more than one duct. See also **apocrine gland.**

exogenous /igzoj′ənəs/, **1.** growing outside the body, **2.** originating outside the body or an organ of the body or produced from external causes, as a disease caused by a bacterial or viral agent foreign to the body. Compare **endogenous.** **–exogenic,** *adj.*

exogenous depression. See **reactive depression.**

exogenous hyperlipemia. See **Type I hyperlipidemia.**

exogenous obesity, obesity caused by a caloric intake greater than needed to meet the metabolic needs of the body. Compare **endogenous obesity.** See also **obesity.**

exon /ek′son/, (in molecular genetics) the part of a DNA molecule that produces the code for the final messenger RNA.

exonuclease /ek′sōnōō′klē•ās/, (in molecular genetics) a nuclease that digests DNA or RNA from the ends of the strands.

exophoria /ek′səfôr′ē•ə/, deviation of the visual axis of one eye away from that of the other eye, occurring in the absence of visual stimuli for fusion. Compare **exotropia.** **–exophoric,** *adj.*

exophthalmia /ek′softhal′mē•ə/, an abnormal condition characterized by a marked protrusion of the eyeballs (**exophthalmos, exophthalmus**), usually resulting from the increased volume of the orbital contents caused by a tumor; swelling associated with cerebral, intraocular, or intraorbital edema or hemorrhage; paralysis of or trauma to the extraocular muscles; or cavernous sinus thrombosis. It may also be caused by endocrine disorders, as hyperthyroidism and Graves' disease, by varicose veins within the orbit, or by injury to orbital bones. Visual acuity may be impaired in exophthalmia; keratitis, ulceration, infection, and blindness may also occur. Treatment depends on the underlying cause. The outcome depends on the cause and the stage at which the condition is detected and treatment is begun. Acute advanced exophthalmia is often irreversible. Also called **proptosis, protrusio bulbi.** **–exophthalmic,** *adj.*

exophthalmic goiter, exophthalmos occurring in association with goiter, as in Graves' disease.

exophthalmometer /ek′səfthalmom′ətər/, an instrument used for measuring the degree of forward displacement of the eye in exophthalmos. The device allows measurement of the distance from the center of the cornea to the lateral orbital rim. This distance is rarely more than 18 mm.

exophthalmos. See **exophthalmia.**

exophthalmos-macroglossia-gigantism syndrome. See **EMG syndrome.**

exophthalmus. See **exophthalmia.**

exophytic /ek′səfit′ik/, of or pertaining to the tendency to grow outward, as an exophytic tumor that grows on the surface or exterior portion of an organ or structure.

exophytic carcinoma, a malignant, epithelial neoplasm that resembles a papilloma or wart.

exostosis /ek′səstō′sis/, an abnormal, benign growth on the surface of a bone. **–exostosed, exostotic,** *adj.*

exotoxin /ek′sətok′sin/, a toxin that is secreted or excreted by a living microorganism. Compare **endotoxin.**

exotropia /ek′sətrō′pē•ə/, strabismus characterized by the outward deviation of one eye relative to the other. Compare **esotropia, exophoria.** See also **strabismus.** **–exotropic,** *adj.*

expanded role, the role of a nurse beyond the traditional limits of nursing practice legislation. Common roles are primary nurse and nurse practitioner, necessitating legal coverage through the establishment of standardized procedures or amendments or changes in nursing practice acts.

expectant treatment, applying therapeutic measures to relieve symptoms as they arise in the course of a disease rather than treating the cause of the illness itself. Some kinds of expectant treatment are amputations for gangrene in a patient with diabetes, coronary bypass procedures in a patient with generalized atherosclerosis, and transplantation of tendons in a patient with severe rheumatoid arthritis. Compare **definitive treatment, palliative treatment, treatment.**

expectation, (in nursing) **1.** anticipation by the staff of a patient's behavior based on a knowledge and understanding of the person's abilities and problems. **2.** anticipation of the performance of the nursing staff, as role expectation.

expectation of life, the probable number of years a person will live after a given age, as determined by the mortality rate in a specific geographic area. It may be individually qualified by the person's condition or race, sex, age, or other demographic factor. Also called **life expectancy.**

expected date of confinement (EDC), the predicted date of a pregnant woman's delivery. Pregnancy lasts approximately 266 days or 38 weeks from the day of fertilization but is considered clinically to last 280 days, or 40 weeks, or 10 lunar months, or 9⅓ calendar months from the first day of the last menstrual period (LMP). The EDC is usually calculated on the basis of 9⅓ calendar months, but if a woman is certain that coitus occurred only once during the month and if she knows the date on which it occurred, the EDC may be calculated as 38 weeks from that date. In the absence of a special calendar or device for calculating the EDC, it is arrived at by counting back 3 months from the first day of the LMP and then adding 7 days and 1 year; thus, if the first day of a woman's LMP was July 18, 1985, one counts back 3 months to April 18, 1985, then adds 7 days and 1 year to arrive at an EDC of April 25, 1986. Because calendar months differ in length, this calculation may give a date that is a few days more or less than 280 days from the first day of the LMP, but it provides a very close approximation, and a trivial error will not be of clinical significance because of the variability of the actual durations of normal pregnancies. The expectant mother is advised that the EDC is only an estimate and that the chances are that she will give birth within 2 weeks before or, more commonly, after the calculated date. Also called **expected date of confinement.**

expectorant, **1.** of or pertaining to a substance that promotes the ejection of mucus or other exudates from the lung, bronchi, and trachea. **2.** an agent that promotes expectoration by reducing the viscosity of pulmonary secretions or by decreasing the tenacity with which exudates adhere to the lower respiratory tract. Expectorant drugs include acetylcysteine, guaifenesin, terpin hydrate, and tyloxapol. Also called **mucolytic.** –**expectorate,** *v.*

expectoration, the ejection of mucus, sputum, or fluids from the trachea and lungs by coughing or spitting.

experience rating, a rating system used by an insurance company to set the premium to be paid by the insured, based on the risk to the insurance company of providing the insurance. Experience rating may lead to very high malpractice premiums in some medical specialties, for the insurance company calculates the premium on the basis of settlements made in related malpractice cases during a specified period. Experience rating is also used to set annual membership health maintenance fees in organizations in which the cost of providing the services in a previous accounting period is used to determine the premiums for the next fiscal year.

experimental design, (in research) a study design used to test cause-and-effect relationships between variables. The classic experimental design specifies an experimental group and a control group. The independent variable is administered to the experimental group and not to the control group, and both groups are measured on the same dependent variable. Subsequent experimental designs have used more groups and more measurements over longer periods of time.

experimental embryology, the study and analysis through experimental techniques of the factors, mechanisms, and relationships that determine and influence prenatal development.

experimental epidemiology, a stage of epidemiologic investigation that uses an experimental model for studies to confirm a causal relationship suggested by observational studies.

experimental group. See **group.**

experimental medicine, a branch of the practice of medicine in which new drugs or treatments are evaluated for safety and efficacy in a clinical laboratory setting by using animals or, in certain cases, human subjects.

experimental physiology, a branch of the study of physiology in which the functions of various body systems are evaluated in a clinical laboratory setting by using animals or, in some cases, human subjects.

experimental psychology, the study of mental processes and phenomena by observation in a controlled environment using various tests, manipulations, and experiments. Compare **analytic psychology.**

experimental variable. See **independent variable.**

expertise, pertaining to special skills or knowledge acquired by a person through education, training, or experience.

expert witness, a person who has special knowledge of a subject about which a court requests testimony. Special knowledge may be acquired by experience, education, observation, or study but is not possessed by the average person. An expert witness gives expert testimony or expert evidence. This evidence often serves to educate the court and the jury in the subject under consideration.

expiration, **1.** also called **exhalation.** breathing out, normally a passive process, depending on the elastic qualities of lung tissue and the thorax. Compare **inspiration.** **2.** termination or death. –**expire,** *v.*

expiratory reserve volume (ERV), the maximum volume of gas that can be expired from the resting expiratory level. See also **vital capacity.**

expired gas (E), any gas exhaled from the lungs.

explosive personality, behavior characterized by episodes of uncontrolled rage and physical abusiveness in reaction to relatively minor stressors.

explosive speech, abnormal speech characterized by slow, jerky articulation interspersed with the sudden loud enunciation of words, often seen in brain disorders.

exposure, (in radiotherapy) a measure of the ionization of air produced by a beam of radiation. Exposure is defined in coulomb per kilogram of air, but there is no special unit in the SI system for this concept. An older unit, the roentgen (R), was defined as 2.58×10^{-4} C/kg.

expression, 1. the indication of a physical or emotional state through facial appearance or vocal intonation. 2. the act of pressing or squeezing to expel something, as milk from the breast after pregnancy or the fetus from the uterus by exerting pressure on the abdominal wall. 3. (in genetics) the detectable effect or appearance in the phenotype of a particular trait or condition. See also **expressivity.** **–express,** *v.*

expressive aphasia. See **motor aphasia.**

expressivity, (in genetics) the variability with which basic patterns of inheritance are modified, both in degree and in variety, by the effect of a given gene in people of the same genotype. Polydactyly may be expressed as extra toes in one generation and extra fingers in another.

expulsive stage of labor, the second stage of labor, during which the mother's uterine contractions are accompanied by a bearing-down reflex. It begins after full dilatation of the cervix and continues to the complete delivery of the infant.

exsanguination, a loss of blood.

exsiccant. See **desiccant.**

exsiccate. See **desiccate.**

extended care facility, an institution devoted to providing medical, nursing, or custodial care for an individual over a prolonged period of time, as during the course of a chronic disease or during the rehabilitation phase after an acute illness. Kinds of extended care facilities are **intermediate care facility** and **skilled nursing facility.** Also called **convalescent home, nursing home.**

extended family, a family group consisting of the biologic parents, their children, the grandparents, and other family members. The extended family is the basic family group in many societies. Among its characteristics are increased exchange of information from experienced older members to less experienced younger ones, care of the older family members in the home by the younger ones, and care by the older people for the children of the younger members. Compare **nuclear family.**

extended insulin-zinc suspension, a long-acting insulin that is slowly absorbed and slow to act.

Extendryl, a trademark for a fixed-combination nasal decongestant drug containing an adrenergic (phenylephrine hydrochloride), an antihistaminic (chlorpheniramine maleate), and an anticholinergic (methscopolamine nitrate).

extension, a movement allowed by certain joints of the skeleton that increases the angle between two adjoining bones, as extending the leg, which increases the angle between the femur and the tibia. Compare **flexion.**

extensor carpi radialis brevis, one of the muscles of the posterior forearm. Lying beneath the extensor carpi radialis longus, it arises from the lateral epicondyle of the humerus, from the radial collateral ligament of the elbow joint, and from various intermuscular septa. It inserts into the dorsal surface of the third metacarpal bone. The muscle is innervated by a branch of the radial nerve that contains fibers from the sixth and the seventh cervical nerves, and it functions to extend the hand.

extensor carpi radialis longus, one of the seven superficial muscles of the posterior forearm. Lying above the extensor carpi radialis brevis, it arises from the lateral supracondylar ridge of the humerus, from the lateral intermuscular septum, and from the common tendon of the extensor muscles of the forearm. It inserts into the dorsal surface of the second metacarpal bone. The muscle is innervated by a branch of the radial nerve that contains fibers from the sixth and seventh cervical nerves, and it serves to extend and flex the hand radially.

extensor carpi ulnaris, one of the muscles of the lateral forearm. It arises from the lateral epicondyle of the humerus and inserts by a tendon into the ulnar side of the fifth metacarpal bone. It is innervated by a branch of the deep radial nerve, containing fibers of the sixth, seventh, and eighth cervical nerves, and functions to extend and adduct the hand.

extensor digiti minimi, an extensor muscle of the posterior forearm. Located on the medial side of the extensor digitorum, it is a slender muscle that arises from the common extensor tendon and joins the expansion of the extensor digitorum tendon on the back of the first phalanx of the little finger. It is innervated by a branch of the deep radial nerve that contains fibers from the sixth, seventh, and eighth cervical nerves, and it functions to extend the little finger.

extensor digitorum, the principal muscle of the medial digits of the posterior forearm. Arising from the lateral epicondyle of the humerus, the intermuscular septa between it and adjacent muscles, and the antebrachial fascia, it divides distally into four tendons that pass through the extensor retinaculum and diverge on the back of the hand, inserting into the second and the third phalanges of the fingers. The muscle is innervated by a branch of the deep radial nerve that contains fibers from the sixth, seventh, and eighth cervical nerves, and it functions to extend the phalanges and, by continued action, the wrist. Also called **extensor digitorum communis.**

extensor digitorum longus, a penniform muscle located at the lateral part of the anterior leg. It is one of three anterior crural muscles and arises from the lateral condyle of the tibia, the anterior surface of the fibula, the deep surface of the fascia, and from intermuscular septa. Its distal tendon passes under the extensor retinacula and divides into four slips that insert into the second and third phalanges of the four lesser toes. The muscle is innervated by branches of the deep peroneal nerve containing fibers from the fourth and the fifth lumbar and first sacral nerves. It extends the proximal phalanges of the four small toes and dorsally flexes and pronates the foot.

extensor retinaculum of the hand. See **retinaculum extensorum manus.**

extern, a medical or dental student who lives outside the institution but provides medical or dental care to patients as an extracurricular activity under the professional supervision of hospital staff members. Compare **intern.**

external, **1.** being on the outside or exterior of the body or an organ. **2.** acting from the outside, as an external influence or exogenous factor. **3.** pertaining to the outward or visible appearance. Compare **internal.**

external abdominal region. See **lateral region.**

external absorption, the taking up of substances through the mucous membranes or the skin.

external acoustic meatus, the canal of the external ear, comprised of bone and cartilage, extending from the auricle to the tympanic membrane. Also called **external auditory canal.**

external aperture of aqueduct of vestibule, an external opening for the small canal extending from the vestibule of the inner ear, located on the internal surface of the petrous part of the temporal bone lateral to the opening for the internal acoustic passage.

external aperture of canaliculus of cochlea, an external opening of the cochlear channel on the margin of the jugular opening in the temporal bone.

external aperture of tympanic canaliculus, the lower opening of the tympanic channel on the inferior surface of the petrous part of the temporal bone.

external auditory canal. See **external acoustic meatus.**

external carotid artery, one of a pair of arteries with eight major temporal or maxillary branches, rising from the common carotid arteries and supplying various parts and tissues of the head and neck.

external carotid plexus, a network of nerves around the external carotid artery, formed by the external carotid nerves from the superior cervical ganglion and supplying sympathetic fibers associated with branches of the external carotid artery. Compare **common carotid plexus, internal carotid plexus.**

external cervical os, an external opening of the uterus that leads into the cavity of the cervix. This opening, bounded by the ventral lip and the dorsal lip, is in the center of the rounded extremity of the cervix that projects into the cavity of the vagina. Compare **internal cervical os.**

external conjugate, the distance measured with obstetric calipers from the depression below the lowest lumbar vertebra posteriorly to the upper border of the symphysis anteriorly (usually about 21 cm). Also called **Baudelocque's diameter.**

external counterpulsation, (in cardiology) a noninvasive technique for providing counterpulsation by encasing the legs of a patient in a rigid case housing a water-filled bladder. The legs are pressurized by the bladder during diastole to produce counterpulsation, using an electrocardiogram to control the timing.

external cuneiform bone. See **lateral cuneiform bone.**

external ear, the outer structure of the ear, consisting of the auricle and the external acoustic meatus. Sound waves are funneled through the external ear to the middle ear. Compare **internal ear, middle ear.**

external fertilization, the union of male and female gametes outside of the bodies from which they originated, as occurs in fish and frogs.

external fistula, an abnormal passage between an internal organ or structure and the cutaneous surface of the body.

external iliac artery, a division of the common iliac artery descending into the thigh and becoming the femoral artery. The external iliac supplies the lower limb and is larger than the internal iliac, except in the fetus, where it is smaller. Compare **internal iliac artery.**

external iliac node, a node in one of the seven groups of parietal nodes serving the lymphatic system in the abdomen and the pelvis. About 10 external iliac nodes, arranged in three groups, lie along the external iliac vessels. Their afferents drain lymph from numerous abdominal and pelvic structures, as the deep abdominal wall, the adductor region of the thigh, the prostate, and the vagina. Compare **common iliac node, iliac circumflex node, internal iliac node.** See also **lymph, lymphatic system, lymph node.**

external iliac vein, one of a pair of veins in the lower body that join the internal iliac vein to form the two common iliac veins. Each external iliac vein begins under the inguinal ligament, ascends along the brim of the lesser pelvis, and ends opposite the sacroiliac articulation by joining the internal iliac vein. In many individuals it contains at least one valve and sometimes two. It receives the inferior epigastric vein, the deep iliac circumflex vein, and the pubic veins. Compare **internal iliac vein.**

external jugular vein, one of a pair of large vessels in the neck that receive most of the blood from the exterior of the cranium and the deep tissues of the face. Each external jugular vein is formed by the junction of the retromandibular vein with the posterior auricular vein and arises in the parotid gland on a level with the angle of the mandible. It runs perpendicularly down the neck and joins the subclavian vein lateral or ventral to the scalenus anterior. It contains two pairs of valves, the inferior pair at the junction with the subclavian vein and the superior pair, usually about 4 cm above the clavicle. A sinus lies between the two sets of valves. Compare **internal jugular vein.**

external oblique muscle. See **obliquus externus abdominis.**

external perimysium. See **epimysium.**

external pin fixation, a method of holding together the fragments of a fractured bone by employing transfixing metal pins through the fragments and a compression device attached to the pins outside the skin surface. Nursing care includes regular cleansing of the skin around the pins and, often, the application of antibiotic solutions or ointments. The pins are removed at a later procedure when the fracture is healed. Compare **internal fixation.**

external pterygoid muscle. See **pterygoideus lateralis.**

external radiation therapy (ERT), the therapeutic application of ionizing radiation from an external beam of a kilovoltage x-ray machine, a megavoltage cobalt 60 machine, or a supervoltage linear accelerator, cyclotron, or betatron. ERT is used most frequently in the treatment of cancer but also in the therapy of keloids and some dermatologic conditions and in counteracting the body's physiologic rejection of transplanted organs.

external rotation, turning outwardly or away from the midline of the body, as when a leg is externally rotated with the toes turned outward or away from the body's midline.

external shunt, a device for the passage of a body fluid from one compartment of the body to another, consisting of a tube or catheter or a series of such containers that passes over the surface of the body from one compartment or cavity to another. See also **hemodialysis, hydrocephalus.**

external version, an obstetric procedure in which a fetus is turned, usually from a breech to a vertex presentation, by external manipulation of the fetus through the wall of the abdomen. Compare **version and extraction.**

exteroceptive, pertaining to stimuli that originate from outside of the body or to the sensory receptors that they activate. Compare **interoceptive, proprioception.**

exteroceptor, any sensory nerve ending, as those located in the skin, mucous membranes, or sense organs, that responds to stimuli originating from outside of the body, as touch, pressure, or sound. Compare **interoceptor, proprioceptor.** See also **chemoreceptor.**

extra-, a combining form meaning 'outside of, beyond, in addition to': *extrabronchial, extradural, extramarginal.*

extrabuccal feeding, the administration of nutrients by means other than the mouth. Also called **extraoral feeding.** See also **gavage, intravenous feeding.**

extracapsular fracture, any fracture that occurs near a joint but does not directly involve the joint capsule. This type of fracture is extremely common in the hip.

extracellular, occurring outside a cell or cell tissue or in cavities or spaces between cell layers or groups of cells. See also **cell, edema, interstitial.**

extracellular fluid (ECF), the portion of the body fluid comprising the interstitial fluid and blood plasma. The adult body contains about 11.2 L of interstitial fluid, constituting about 16% of body weight, and about 2.8 L of plasma, constituting about 4% of body weight. Plasma and interstitial fluid are very similar chemically and, in conjunction with intracellular fluid, help control the movement of water and electrolytes throughout the body. Some of the important ionized components of extracellular fluid are protein, magnesium, potassium, chlorine, calcium, and certain sulfates.

extracoronal retainer, **1.** a kind of dental retainer that incorporates a cast restoration lying largely external to the coronal portion of a tooth and complements the contour of the tooth crown. The retention or resistance to displacement is developed between the inner surfaces of the casting and the external walls of the prepared tooth. An extracoronal crown may be a complete or partial crown. **2.** a direct clasp type retainer that engages an abutment tooth on its external surface, used for the retention and stabilization of a removable partial denture. **3.** a manufactured direct retainer, the protruding portion of which is attached to the external surface of a cast crown on an abutment tooth.

extracorporeal, something that is outside the body, as extracorporeal circulation in which venous blood is diverted outside the body to a heart-lung machine and returned to the body through a femoral or other artery.

extracorporeal technician. See **perfusion technologist.**

extract, to remove a tooth from the oral cavity by means of elevators, or forceps, or both. **–extraction,** *n.*

extradural /ek′trədo͞or′əl/, outside the dura mater.

extradural anesthesia, anesthetic nerve block achieved by the injection of a local anesthetic solution into the space in the spinal canal outside the dura mater of the spinal cord, as in epidural, caudal, or paravertebral anesthesia.

extradural hemorrhage, a hemorrhage of an area surrounding but outside of the dura of the brain or spinal cord.

extraembryonic blastoderm, the area of the blastoderm outside the embryo that gives rise to the membranes that surround the embryo during gestation. Compare **embryonic blastoderm.** See also **allantois, amnion, chorion, yolk sac.**

extraembryonic coelom, a cavity external to the developing embryo that forms between the mesoderm of the chorion and that covering the amniotic cavity and yolk sac. During early prenatal development, there is direct contact with the embryonic coelom at the umbilicus, but this junction is obliterated by the growth of the amnion and the closing of the body wall. Also called **exocoelom.**

extramedullary myeloma, a plasma cell tumor that occurs outside of the bone marrow, usually affecting the visceral organs or the nasopharyngeal and oral mucosa. Also called **extramedullary plasmacytoma, peripheral plasma cell myeloma, plasma cell tumor.**

extramedullary myelopoiesis, the formation and development of myeloid tissue outside of the bone marrow. Also called **ectopic myelopoiesis.**

extraocular /ek′strə•ok′yo͞olər/, outside the eye.

extraocular muscle palsy, an abnormal condition characterized by paralysis of the extrinsic muscles of the eye, as the superior, inferior, medial, and lateral rectus muscles, and the superior and the inferior oblique muscles. See also **strabismus.**

extraoral anchorage, an orthodontic anchorage outside the mouth, typically linking dental attachments to a wire bow or to hooks extending between the lips and attached by elastic to a cap, a neck strap, or another extraoral device.

extraoral feeding. See **extrabuccal feeding.**

extraoral orthodontic appliance, a device secured to a portion of the face, the neck, or the back of the head to deliver traction force to the teeth or jaws for changing the relative postitions of dentitions.

extraperitoneal, occurring or located outside the peritoneal cavity.

extraperitoneal cesarean section, a method for surgically delivering a baby through an incision in the lower uterine segment without entering the peritoneal cavity. The uterus is approached through the paravesicle space. This procedure is performed most often to avoid spread of infection from the uterus into the peritoneal cavity. It is somewhat slower to perform than the low cervical or classical cesarean operations. Compare **classical cesarean section, low cervical cesarean section.** See also **cesarean section.**

extrapsychic conflict, an emotional conflict usually occurring when one's inner needs and desires do not coincide with the restrictions of the environment or society. Compare **intrapsychic conflict.** See also **conflict.**

extrapyramidal /ek'strəpiram'ədəl/, **1.** of or pertaining to the tissues and structures outside the cerebrospinal pyramidal tracts of the brain that are associated with movement of the body, excluding motor neurons, the motor cortex, and the corticospinal and corticobulbar tracts. **2.** of or pertaining to the function of these tissues and structures.

extrapyramidal disease, any of a large group of conditions characterized by involuntary movement, changes in muscle tone, and abnormal posture, as in tardive dyskinesia, chorea, athetosis, and Parkinson's disease.

extrapyramidal reaction, a response to a treatment or a drug characterized by the signs of extrapyramidal disease. The reaction may persist or regress after discontinuation of the treatment or drug.

extrapyramidal side effects, side effects caused by drugs that block dopamine receptor sites in the extrapyramidal system tract.

extrapyramidal system, the part of the nervous system that includes the basal ganglia, substantia nigra, subthalamic nucleus, part of the midbrain, and the motor neurons of the spine. See also **extrapyramidal tracts.**

extrapyramidal tracts, the tracts of motor nerves from the brain to the anterior horns of the spinal cord, except for the fibers of the pyramidal tracts. Within the brain, extrapyramidal tracts comprise various relays of motoneurons between motor areas of the cerebral cortex, the basal ganglia, the thalamus, the cerebellum, and the brainstem. The extrapyramidal tracts are functional rather than anatomic units, comprising the nuclei and the fibers and excluding the pyramidal tracts. They especially control and coordinate the postural, static, supporting, and locomotor mechanisms and cause contractions of muscle groups in sequence or simultaneously. The extrapyramidal tracts include the corpus striatum, the subthalamic nucleus, the substantia nigra, and the red nucleus, together with their interconnections with the reticular formation, the cerebellum, and the cerebrum. Compare **pyramidal tract.**

extrasensory perception (ESP), alleged awareness or knowledge acquired without using the physical senses. See also **clairvoyance, parapsychology, telepathy.**

extrasystole /ek'strəsis'təlē/, cardiac contraction that is abnormal in timing or in origin of impulse with respect to the fundamental rhythm of the heart.

extrauterine /ek'strəyōō'tərin/, occurring or located outside the uterus, as an ectopic pregnancy.

extravasation /ikstrav'əsā'shən/, a passage or escape into the tissues, usually of blood, serum, or lymph. Compare **bleeding.** See also **exudate, transudate.** –**extravasate,** *v.*

extraventricular hydrocephalus. See **hydrocephalus.**

extraversion. See **extroversion.**

extrinsic allergic alveolitis, an inflammatory form of interstitial pneumonia that results from an immunologic reaction in a hypersensitive person. The reaction may be provoked by a variety of inhaled organic dusts, often those containing fungal spores. The disease can be prevented by avoiding contact with the causative agents. Extrinsic allergic alveolitis is a disease in which classification is based solely on the character of the immune response rather than on its clinical manifestations. A wide variety of symptoms may occur, including asthma, fever, chills, malaise, and muscle aches, which usually develop 4 to 6 hours after exposure. On laboratory examination of the blood, leukocytosis is commonly found. Recovery is usually spontaneous. In an acute attack, corticosteroids may be given to diminish the inflammatory response. Kinds of extrinsic allergic alveolitis include **bagassosis, farmer's lung, humidifier lung, mushroom worker's lung,** and **suberosis.** Also called **hypersensitivity pneumonitis.** See also **Arthus reaction.**

extrinsic allergic pneumonia. See **diffuse hypersensitivity pneumonia.**

extrinsic asthma. See **allergic asthma.**

extrinsic factor. See **cyanocobalamin.**

extroversion, **1.** the tendency to direct one's interests and energies toward external values or things outside the self. **2.** the state of being totally or primarily concerned with what is outside the self. Also spelled **extraversion.** Compare **introversion.**

extrovert, **1.** a person whose interests are directed away from the self and concerned primarily with external reality and the physical environment rather than with inner feelings and thoughts. This person is usually highly sociable, outgoing, impulsive, and emotionally expressive. **2.** a person characterized by extroversion. Also spelled **extravert.** Compare **introvert.**

extrusion reflex, a normal response in infants to force the tongue outward when touched or depressed. The reflex begins to disappear by about 3 or 4 months of age. Before it fades, food must be placed well back in the mouth to be retained and swallowed. Constant protrusion of a large tongue may be a sign of Down's syndrome.

extubation, the process of withdrawing a tube from an orifice or cavity of the body. **–extubate,** *v.*

exuberant callus. See **heterotopic ossification.**

exudate /eks′yōōdāt/, fluid, cells, or other substances that have been slowly exuded, or discharged, from cells or blood vessels through small pores or breaks in cell membranes. Perspiration, pus, and serum are sometimes identified as exudates.

exudative /igzōō′dətiv/, relating to the exudation or oozing of fluid and other materials from cells and tissues, usually as a result of inflammation or injury.

exudative angina. See **croup.**

exudative enteropathy, diarrhea seen in diseases characterized by inflammation or destruction of intestinal mucosa. Crohn's disease, ulcerative colitis, tuberculosis, and some lymphomas cause an increase of plasma, blood, mucus, and protein to accumulate in the intestine, adding to fecal bulk and frequency. See also **diarrhea.**

eye, one of a pair of organs of sight, contained in a bony orbit at the front of the skull, embedded in orbital fat, and innervated by one of a pair of optic nerves from the forebrain. Associated with the eye are certain accessory structures, as the muscles, the fasciae, the eyebrow, the eyelids, the conjunctiva, and the lacrimal gland. The bulb of the eye is composed of segments of two spheres with nearly parallel axes that constitute the outside tunic and one of three fibrous layers enclosing two internal cavities separated by the crystalline lens. The smaller cavity anterior to the lens is divided by the iris into two chambers, both filled with aqueous humor. The posterior chamber is larger than the anterior chamber and contains the jellylike vitreous body that is divided by the hyaloid canal. The outside tunic of the bulb consists of the transparent cornea anteriorly, constituting one fifth of the tunic, and the opaque sclera posteriorly, constituting five sixths of the tunic. The intermediate vascular, pigmented tunic consists of the choroid, the ciliary body, and the iris. The internal tunic of nervous tissue is the retina. Light waves passing through the lens strike a layer of rods and cones in the retina creating impulses that are transmitted by the optic nerve to the brain. The transverse and the anteroposterior diameters of the eye bulb are slightly greater than the vertical diameter; the bulb in women is usually smaller than the bulb in men. Also called **bulbus oculi, eyeball.**

eyebrow, **1.** the supraorbital arch of the frontal bone that separates the orbit of the eye from the forehead. **2.** the arch of hairs growing along the ridge formed by the supraorbital arch of the frontal bone.

eyeground, the fundus of the eye. See also **funduscopy.**

eyelash, one of many cilia growing in double or triple rows along the border of the eyelids in front of a row of ciliary glands that are in front of a row of meibomian glands.

eyelid, a movable fold of thin skin over the eye, with eyelashes and ciliary and meibomian glands along its margin. It consists of loose connective tissue containing a thin plate of fibrous tissue lined with mucous membrane. The orbicularis oculi muscle and the oculomotor nerve control the opening and closing of the eyelid. The upper and lower eyelids are separated by the palpebral fissure. Also called **palpebra** /pal′pəbrə/.

eye memory. See **visual memory.**

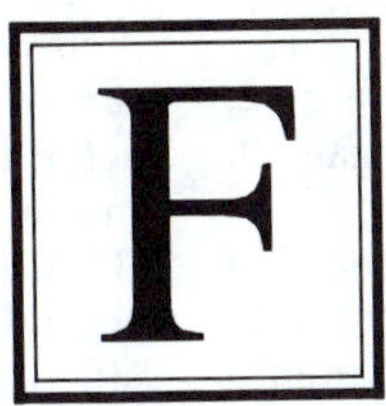

f, **1.** symbol for *breaths per unit time*. **2.** symbol for *respiratory frequency*.

F, **1.** abbreviation for **farad.** **2.** symbol for **fluorine.**

F_1, (in genetics) the symbol for the first filial generation; the heterozygous offspring produced by the mating of two unrelated individuals or by the crossing of a homozygous dominant strain with a homozygous recessive.

F_2, (in genetics) the symbol for the second filial generation; the offspring produced by mating two members of the F_1 generation or, broadly, by crossing any two heterozygous strains.

FAAN, abbreviation for **Fellow of the American Academy of Nursing.**

fabrication. See **confabulation.**

Fabry's disease, Fabry's syndrome. See **angiokeratoma corporis diffusum.**

F.A.C.C.P., abbreviation for **Fellow of the American College of Chest Physicians.**

face, **1.** the front of the head from the chin to the brow, including the skin and muscles and structures of the forehead, eyes, nose, mouth, cheeks, and jaw. **2.** the visage. **3.** to direct the face toward something. See also **en face.** **–facial,** *adj*.

face-bow, a device resembling a caliper, used for measuring the relationship of the maxillae to the temporomandibular joints required for the fabrication of denture casts.

facet, (in dentistry) a flattened, highly polished wear pattern on a tooth.

face validity, the apparent validity of a test or measurement device as it is to be used in a particular study. See also **validity.**

facial angle, an anthropomorphic expression of the degree of protrusion of the lower face, assessed by measuring the inclination of the facial plane relative to the horizontal reference plane.

facial artery, one of a pair of tortuous arteries that arise from the external carotid arteries, divide into four cervical and five facial branches, and supply various organs and tissues in the head. The cervical branches of the facial artery are the ascending palatine, tonsillar, glandular, and submental. The facial branches are the inferior labial, superior labial, lateral nasal, angular, and muscular.

facial diplegia, a rare neuromuscular condition characterized by bilateral paralysis of various muscles of the face. See also **Möbius' syndrome.**

facial hemiplegia, paralysis of the muscles of one side of the face, with the rest of the body not being affected.

facial muscle, one of numerous muscles of the face, seldom remaining distinct over its entire length because of a tendency to merge with a neighboring muscle at its termination or its attachment. The five groups of facial muscles include the muscles of the scalp, the extrinsic muscles of the ear, the muscles of the nose, the muscles of the eyelid, and the muscles of the mouth. The platysma is one of the facial group but is described with the muscles of the neck. Also called **muscle of expression.**

facial nerve, either of a pair of mixed sensory and motor cranial nerves that arises from the brainstem at the base of the pons and divides just in front of the ear into its six branches, innervating the scalp, forehead, eyelids, muscles of facial expression, cheeks, and jaw. Also called **seventh nerve.**

facial paralysis, an abnormal condition characterized by the partial or the total loss of the functions of the facial muscles or the loss of sensation in the face. It may be caused by disease or by trauma. The degree of paralysis depends on the nerves affected. Brain injury above the facial nucleus usually does not block the innervation of the brow and the forehead muscles. Injury to the nucleus of the facial nerve or injury to its peripheral neurons paralyzes all the ipsilateral facial muscles. See also **Bell's palsy.**

facial perception, the ability to judge the distance and direction of objects through the sensation felt in the skin of the face. The phenomenon is commonly experienced by those who are blind and is rarely experienced in the dark by those with sight. Also called **facial vision.**

facial vein, one of a pair of superficial veins that drain deoxygenated blood from the superficial structures of the face. Each facial vein starts as the angular vein at the union of the frontal and the supraorbital veins and accompanies the facial artery, passing deep to the zygomaticus major and the zygomaticus minor, following the border of the masseter, curving around the mandible into the neck, and communicating with the anterior jugular vein and the external jugular vein to empty into the internal jugular vein. The facial vein anastomoses with the cavernous sinus through various veins, as the angular, the supraorbital, and the superior ophthalmic. Because the vein has no valves that prevent the backflow of blood, infections of the skin near the nose and mouth may cause meningitis: Blood-borne organisms can reach the cavernous sinus through the anastomoses.

facial vision. See **facial perception.**
facies /fā′shē·ēs/, *pl.* **facies** /fā′shē·ēs/, **1.** the face. **2.** the surface of any body structure, part, or organ. **3.** facial expression or appearance.
facilitation, **1.** the enhancement or reinforcement of any action or function so that it is carried out with increased ease. Compare **inhibition.** See also **summation.** **2.** (in neurology) the phenomenon whereby two or more afferent impulses that individually are not strong enough to elicit a response in a neuron can collectively produce a reflex discharge greater than the sum of the separate responses. **3.** also called **law of facilitation.** (in neurology) the process of lowering the threshold action potential of a neuron by the repeated passage of an impulse along the same pathway.
facio-, a combining form meaning 'pertaining to the face': *faciocervical, faciolingual, facioplegia.*
facitis /fasī′tis/, an abnormal, benign growth resembling a tumor that develops in the subcutaneous oral tissues, usually in the cheek. Commonly growing rapidly and then regressing, it consists of young fibroblasts and many capillaries and may be mistaken for fibrosarcoma.
F.A.C.O.G., abbreviation for *Fellow of the American College of Obstetricians and Gynecologists.*
F.A.C.S. abbreviation for **Fellow of the American College of Surgeons.**
-faction, a combining form meaning a 'process of making': *bilifaction, chylifaction, liquefaction.*
factitial /fakti′shəl/, artificial or self-induced, as a factitial dermatitis.
factitial dermatitis, a skin rash caused by the patient, usually for secondary gain or as a manifestation of psychiatric illness.
-factive, -fying, a combining form meaning 'making': *liquefactive, stupefactive, vasofactive.*
factor I. See **fibrinogen.**
factor II. See **prothrombin.**
factor III. See **thromboplastin.**
factor IV, a designation for calcium as an element in the process of the coagulation of blood.
factor V, an unstable procoagulant that occurs in normal plasma but is deficient in the blood of parahemophiliacs. It is needed to convert prothrombin rapidly to thrombin. Some research indicates that during coagulation, factor V changes from an inactive agent to an active prothrombin accelerator. Also called **proaccelerin.**
factor VI, a hypothetic chemical agent that some suggest is derived from proaccelerin, or factor V, in the process of blood coagulation.
factor VII, a blood procoagulant present in the blood plasma and synthesized in the liver in the presence of vitamin K. Also called **proconvertin.**
factor VIII, a coagulation factor present in normal plasma but deficient in the blood of persons with hemophilia A. It is a macromolecular complex composed of two separate entities, one of which, when deficient, results in hemophilia A, and the other, when deficient, results in Von Willebrand's disease. See also **antihemophilic factor.**
factor IX, a coagulation factor present in normal plasma but deficient in the blood of persons with hemophilia B. Also called **Christmas factor.**
factor IX complex, a hemostatic containing factors II, VII, IX, and X.

■ INDICATION: It is prescribed in the treatment of hemophilia B. It is a vitamin K-dependent protein sythesized in the liver.

■ CONTRAINDICATION: Liver disease with intravascular coagulation and fibrinolysis is the only contraindication.

■ ADVERSE EFFECTS: Among the more serious adverse reactions are hepatitis, intravascular coagulation, circulatory collapse, and hypersensitivity reaction.

factor X, a coagulation factor that occurs in normal plasma but is deficient in some inherited defects in coagulation. Factor X and prothrombin are closely related; both are synthesized in the liver in the presence of vitamin K. Also called **Stuart-Power factor.**
factor XI, a coagulation factor present in normal plasma. Deficiency results in hemophilia C.
factor XII, a coagulation factor present in normal plasma. It triggers the formation of bradykinin and associated enzymatic reactions. It is required for rapid coagulation in vitro but is apparently not needed for hemostasis in vivo. It can be activated in the laboratory by contact with negatively charged surfaces, which can develop on glass and kaolin or on biologic material, as collagen. Also called **activation factor, contact factor, glass factor, Hageman factor.**
factor XIII, a coagulation factor present in normal plasma that acts with calcium to produce an insoluble fibrin clot. Also called **fibrinase, fibrin stabilizing factor.**
Factorate, a trademark for human antihemophilic factor VIII.
factor-searching study, (in nursing research) a study design that produces a qualitative, narrative description including categories or classifications of phenomena. It may be used to describe various aspects of nursing practice, characteristics of a population, or both. Factor searching is often a preliminary step in a study at a higher level of inquiry.
facultative /fak′əltā′tiv/, not obligatory; having the ability to adapt to more than one condition, as a facultative anaerobe.
facultative aerobe, an organism able to grow under anaerobic conditions but that develops most rapidly in an aerobic environment. Compare **obligate aerobe.** See also **aerobe.**
facultative anaerobe, an organism able to grow under aerobic conditions but that develops most rapidly in an anaerobic environment. Compare **obligate anaerobe.** See also **anaerobe, anaerobic infection.**
facultative parasite. See **parasite.**
faculty, **1.** any normal physiologic function or natural ability of a living organism, as the digestive faculty or the

ability to perceive and distinguish sensory stimuli. **2.** an ability to do something specific, as learn languages or remember names. **3.** any mental ability or power, as memory or thought. **4.** a department in an institution of learning or the people who teach in a department of such an institution.

faculty practice plan, a system in a medical school by which faculty members are able to increase the income to their department or themselves by practicing their specialty of medicine in a departmental practice in a school-controlled organization. Nursing school faculties are beginning to use the same device for retrieval of incomes from service.

Faget's sign /fazhāz'/, a falling pulse rate associated with a constant temperature, or a constant pulse associated with a rising temperature. It is an unusual sign found in yellow fever. Also called **Faget's law.**

fagicladosporic acid /faj'iklad'ōspôr'ik/, a toxin produced by *Cladosporium epiphyllum,* a member of a genus of fungi that cause "black spot" in stored meat, tinea negra, and black degeneration of the brain.

Fahrenheit /fer'ənhīt/, a scale for the measurement of temperature in which the boiling point of water is 212° and the freezing point of water is 32° at sea level. Compare **Celsius.**

failed forceps, an attempted mid-forceps operation that is abandoned because there is a greater degree of resistance to rotation or traction than anticipated, as a result of cephalopelvic disproportion. Cesarean section is performed to deliver the infant. Compare **trial forceps.** See also **cephalopelvic disproportion.**

failure to thrive, the abnormal retardation of the growth and development of an infant resulting from conditions that interfere with normal metabolism, appetite, and activity. Causative factors include chromosomal abnormalities, as in Turner's syndrome and the various trisomies; major organ system defects that lead to deficiency or malfunction; systemic disease or acute illness; physical deprivation, primarily malnutrition; and various psychosocial factors, as seen in severe cases of maternal deprivation syndrome. Metabolic disturbances of short duration, as occur during acute illness, have usually no long-term effects on development and are usually followed by a period of rapid growth. Prolonged nutritional deficiency may cause permanent and irreversible retardation of physical, mental, or social development.

faint, *nontechnical.* **1.** to lose consciousness, as in a syncopal attack. **2.** a syncopal attack. See also **syncope.**

faith healing, alleged healing through the power to cause a cure or recovery from an illness or injury without the aid of conventional medical treatment because the healer is believed to have been given that power by a supernatural force.

falciform body. See **sporozoite.**

falciparum malaria /falsip'ərəm/, the most severe form of malaria, caused by the protozoan *Plasmodium falciparum,* characterized by extremely grave systemic symptoms, mental confusion, enlarged spleen, edema, GI symptoms, and anemia. Falciparum malaria does not last as long as other forms of malaria; if treatment is begun promptly, the disease may be mild and the recovery uneventful. Relapses are uncommon, but death may result from dehydration and anemia. The usual treatment is chloroquine, but patients known to have contracted malaria in an area that harbors drug-resistant *P. falciparum* are often treated with a combination of quinine, pyrimethamine, and one of the sulfones or sulfonamides. Compare **quartan malaria, tertian malaria.** See also **algid malaria, blackwater fever, malaria.**

fallopian tube /fəlō'pē·ən/, one of a pair of ducts opening at one end into the uterus and at the other end into the peritoneal cavity, over the ovary. Each tube serves as the passage through which an ovum is carried to the uterus and through which spermatozoa move out toward the ovary. The tube lies in the upper border of the broad ligament (the mesosalpinx). Each tube has four parts: the fimbriae, the infundibulum, the ampulla, and the isthmus. The fimbriae drape in fingerlike projections from the infundibulum over the ovary. Just proximal to the infundibulum is the ampulla, the widest portion of the tube. The ampulla is connected to the fundus of the uterus by the isthmus. Also called **oviduct, uterine tube.**

Fallot's syndrome. See **tetralogy of Fallot.**

fallout, the deposition of radioactive debris after a nuclear explosion. The debris from an atmospheric explosion of an atomic bomb may travel thousands of miles in the atmosphere and be deposited over a large geographic area.

false anorexia. See **pseudoanorexia.**

false imprisonment, (in law) the intentional, unjustified, nonconsensual detention or confinement of a person for any length of time.

false labor. See **Braxton Hicks contractions.**

false negative, an incorrect result of a diagnostic test or procedure that falsely indicates the absence of a finding, condition, or disease. The rate of occurrence of false negative results varies with the diagnostic accuracy and the specificity of the test or procedure. As the accuracy and specificity of a test increase, the rate of false negatives decreases. Certain tests are known to yield false negative results at a certain rate; in all tests, a small number will occur by chance alone. False negative results are more common than false positive results, because the person conducting the test is more likely to fail to observe a finding than to imagine seeing something that does not exist. Compare **false positive.**

false neuroma, **1.** a neoplasm that does not contain nerve elements. **2.** a cystic neuroma.

false nucleolus. See **karyosome.**

false positive, a test result that wrongly indicates the presence of a disease or other condition the test is designed to reveal. Compare **false negative.**

false pregnancy. See **pseudocyesis.**

false rib. See **rib.**

false suture, an immovable fibrous joint in which rough articulating surfaces form the connection between certain bones of the skull. Two kinds of false sutures are **sutura plana** and **sutura squamosa.** Compare **true suture.**

false twins. See **dizygotic twins.**

false vocal cord, either of two thick folds of mucous membrane in the larynx separating the ventricle from the vestibule. Each fold encloses a narrow band of fibrous tissue (the ventricular ligament). Compare **vocal cord.**

falx /falks, fôlks/, *pl.* **falces** /fal′sēz, fôl′sēz/, **1.** a sickle-shaped structure. **2.** sickle-shaped.

falx cerebelli, a small sickle-shaped process of the dura mater attached to the occipital bone above and projecting into the posterior cerebellar notch between the two cerebellar hemispheres.

falx cerebri, a sickle-shaped fold of dura mater membrane extending into and following along the longitudinal fissure of the two hemispheres of the cerebrum.

falx inguinalis, transverse and internal oblique muscles.

falx ligamentosa, the broad ligament of the liver.

familial, pertaining to a characteristic, condition, or disease that is present in some families and not others or that occurs in more family members than would be expected by chance. It is usually but not always hereditary. Compare **acquired, congenital, hereditary.**

familial cretinism, a rare genetic disorder caused by an inborn error of metabolism resulting from an enzyme deficiency that interferes with thyroid hormone biosynthesis. Clinical manifestations include lethargy, stunted growth, and mental retardation. The condition, which is transmitted as an autosomal recessive trait, is treated by early administration of thyroid hormone, if possible in utero, to reduce the abnormalities of mental development. See also **cretinism.**

familial hypercholesterolemia, an inherited disorder transmitted as a dominant trait and characterized by a high level of serum cholesterol, tendinous xanthomas, and early evidence of atherosclerosis, especially of the coronary arteries. Affected individuals at 50 years of age have three to 10 times greater risk of ischemic heart disease than the general population. Cholesterol levels are elevated at birth, increase with age, and average 250 to 500 mg/dl in heterozygous adults and 500 to 1000 mg/dl in adults who are homozygous for the gene. Xanthomas begin to appear at 20 years of age and occur most frequently on the Achilles tendon, extensor tendons of the hands, elbows, and tibial tuberosities. In Type IIa familial hypercholesterolemia, only low-density lipoprotein (LDL) is elevated, while in Type IIb, LDL and very low-density lipoprotein (VLDL) are increased. The disorder occurs in whites, blacks, and Orientals, and the prevalence of the gene in the United States is 1:1000. Treatment includes a low-cholesterol and low-saturated-fat diet. Cholestyramine may be given to patients with Type IIa familial hypercholesterolemia but not to those with Type IIb. Also called **hypercholesterolemic xanthomatosis, type II hyperlipoproteinemia.**

familial iminoglycinuria. See **iminoglycinuria.**

familial juvenile nephronophthisis. See **medullary cystic disease.**

familial lipoprotein lipase deficiency. See **hyperchylomicronemia.**

familial osteochondrodystrophy. See **Morquio's disease.**

familial polyposis, an abnormal condition characterized by multiple polyps in the colon and rectum. The disease, which has high malignancy potential, is inherited as a heterozygous, autosomal dominant trait. Total proctocolectomy eliminates the risk of cancer, which, if untreated, occurs before 40 years of age. Genetic counseling is advised. A kind of familial polyposis is **Gardner's syndrome.** See also **polyposis.**

familial spinal muscular atrophy. See **Werdnig-Hoffmann disease.**

familial tremor. See **essential tremor.**

family, **1.** a group of people related by heredity, as parents, children, and siblings. The term sometimes is broadened to include persons living in the same household or those related by marriage. **2.** a group of persons having a common surname, as the Anderson family. **3.** a category of animals or plants situated on a taxonomic scale between order and genus. Humans are members of the genus *Homo sapiens,* which is a part of the hominid family which, in turn, is a division of the primate order of mammals. See also **genetics, heredity.** **–familial,** *adj.*

family-centered care, primary health care that includes an assessment of the health of an entire family, identification of actual or potential factors that might influence the health of its members, and implementation of actions needed to maintain or improve the health of the unit and its members.

family-centered maternity care, a system for the delivery of safe, high-quality health care adapted to the physical and psychosocial needs of the patient, the patient's family, and the newly born offspring.

family-centered nursing care, nursing care directed toward improving the potential health of a family or any of its members by assessing individual and family health needs and strengths, by identifying problems influencing the health care of the family as a whole and those influencing the individual members, by using family resources, by teaching and counseling, and by evaluating progress toward stated goals.

family ganging, an unethical medical practice in which the patient is encouraged or required to involve the entire family in a program of health care even if the other family members do not require such care. The practice enables the health care facility to obtain third-party compensation for all family members. Family ganging is often practiced in so-called Medicaid mills. See also **Medicaid.**

family health, (in a health history) an account of the health of the members of the immediate family. Hereditary and familial diseases are especially noted. The age and health of each person, the ages at death, and the causes of death are charted. The family health history is obtained from the patient or family in the initial interview and becomes a part of the permanent record.

family history, an essential portion of a patient's medical history in which the patient is asked about the health of the other members of the family in a series of specific questions, as "Has anyone in your family had tuberculosis? diabetes mellitus? breast cancer?," to discover any diseases to which the patient may be particularly vulnerable. Other questions, as those concerning the age, sex, relationships of others in the household, and the marital history of the patient, may also be asked if the information has not already been secured.

family medicine, the branch of medicine that is concerned with the diagnosis and treatment of health problems in people of either sex and any age. Practitioners of family medicine are often called family practice physicians, family physicians, or, formerly, general practitioners. They often act as the primary health care providers, referring complicated problems to a specialist.

family nurse practitioner (FNP), a nurse practitioner possessing skills necessary for the detection and management of acute self-limiting conditions and management of chronic stable conditions. An FNP provides primary, ambulatory care for families in collaboration with primary care physicians. The FNP meets the needs of health and specified illness care by providing direct care and by guiding or counseling the family as required. Consultation, copractice, and referral to associated physicians occur in the course of the FNP's practice.

family physician, **1.** a medical practitioner of the specialty of family medicine. **2.** a general practitioner. **3.** a family practice physician. See also **family medicine.**

family planning. See **contraception.**

family practice physician, a practitioner of family medicine, usually one who has completed a residency program in the specialty. See also **family medicine.**

family process, alteration in, a nursing diagnosis accepted by the Fifth National Conference on the Classification of Nursing Diagnoses. The origin of the problem is a situational or developmental change or crisis within the family network. The defining characteristics include the inability of the family system to meet the physical, emotional, spiritual, or security needs of its members; the inability of family members to communicate adequately, to express or accept a wide range of feelings, or to relate to each other for mutual growth and maturation; the parents' disrespect for each other's views on child-rearing practices; family rigidity in function and roles and its uninvolvement in community activities; the inability of the family to accept or receive appropriate help, to adapt to change, or to deal with traumatic experience constructively; disrespect for individuality and autonomy; failure to accomplish current or past developmental tasks; ineffective decision-making processes; inappropriate or poorly communicated family rules, rituals, or symbols; and unexamined family myths. See also **nursing diagnosis.**

family therapy, (in psychiatry) a therapeutic approach to the care of any one of the members of a family. The entire immediate family may meet together, usually with a male and a female therapist, in order to discover the dynamics of the situation, especially as it affects the disturbed, symptomatic family member.

famine fever. See **relapsing fever.**

FANCAP, *U.S.* a mnemonic device, for helping student nurses learn to assess, provide, and evaluate direct patient care. It stands for fluids, aeration, nutrition, communication, activity, and pain. Occasionally a variant, FANCAS, is substituted for FANCAP in which case the 'S' stands for stimulation.

Fanconi's anemia, a rare, usually congenital disorder, characterized by aplastic anemia in childhood or early adult life, bone abnormalities, chromatin breaks, and developmental anomalies. Also called **congenital pancytopenia, pancytopenia-dysmelia.**

Fanconi's syndrome, a group of disorders including renal tubular function, glycosuria, phosphaturia, and bicarbonate wasting. The condition is often marked by osteomalacia, acidosis, and hypokalemia. Two main types of the syndrome have been differentiated. Idiopathic Fanconi's syndrome is inherited and usually appears in early middle age. Acquired Fanconi's syndrome is usually the result of toxicity from various sources, including the ingestion of outdated tetracycline. Because of numerous variations of the syndrome, it is believed that different alleles are responsible for the different recessively inherited factors expressed as signs and symptoms of the group of disorders.

Fansidar, a trademark for a fixed-combination antimalarial agent (pyrimethamine and sulfadoxine).

fantasy, **1.** the unrestrained free play of the imagination; fancy. **2.** a mental image, usually distorted or grotesque in nature, often the result of the action of drugs or a disease of the central nervous system. **3.** the mental process of transforming undesirable experiences into imagined events or into a sequence of ideas in order to fulfill an unconscious wish, need, or desire or to give expression to unconscious conflicts, as a daydream.

farad (F) /fer′əd/, a unit of capacitance that increases the potential difference between the plates of a capacitor by 1 volt with a charge of 1 coulomb.

Farber test, a microscopic examination of newborn meconium for lanugo and squamous cells. The fetus normally swallows amniotic fluid containing these large proteins, which then pass through the digestive system to be excreted, usually after birth, in the first stools. The absence of hair or skin cells is suggestive of intestinal obstruction or atresia and requires further evaluation.

Far Eastern hemorrhagic fever, a form of epidemic hemorrhagic fever, indigenous to Asia, that is transmitted by a virus carried by an Asian rodent. The infection is characterized by chills, fever, headache, abdominal pain, nausea, vomiting, anorexia, and extreme thirst. Hypotensive shock may occur as the fever subsides. Thirst continues into the second week, oliguria develops, and the blood pressure returns to normal. Blood urea nitrogen levels increase hyperphosphatemia and hypercalcemia, and other complications occur. Diuresis follows the oliguric phase, resulting in an output of as much as 8 L a day of urine and in electrolyte imbalance. Mortality may be as high as 33%. There is no specific treatment.

farmer's lung, a respiratory disorder caused by the inhalation of actinomycetes or other organic dusts from moldy hay. It is a form of hypersensitivity pneumonitis, affecting individuals who have developed antibodies to the mold spores. It is characterized by coughing, dyspnea, cyanosis, tachycardia, nausea, chills, and fever. Treatment may include cromolyn sodium and a corticosteroid.

farsightedness. See **hyperopia.**

FAS, abbreviation for **fetal alcohol syndrome.**

fasci-, a combining form meaning 'pertaining to a band or bundle of fibrous tissue': *fasciagram, fascicular, fasciitis.*

fascia /fash′ē·ə/, *pl.* **fasciae,** the fibrous connective tissue of the body that may be separated from other specifically organized structures, as the tendons, the aponeuroses, and the ligaments. It varies in thickness and density and in the amounts of fat, collagenous fiber, elastic fiber, and tissue fluid it contains. Kinds of fasciae are **deep fascia, subcutaneous fascia,** and **subserous fascia.** **–fascial,** *adj.*

fascia bulbi, a thin membranous socket that envelops the eyeball from the optic nerve to the ciliary region and allows the eyeball to move freely. The fascia bulbi has a smooth inner surface, pierced by vessels and nerves, and fuses with the sheath of the optic nerve and with the sclera. The lower part of the membrane thickens into the suspensory ligament, which attaches to the zygomatic arch and the lacrimal bones. Also called **Tenon's capsule.**

fascial cleft, a place of cleavage between two contiguous fascial surfaces, as the deep fasciae and the subcutaneous fasciae. A fascial cleft is rich in fluid but poor in traversing fibers; thus, two fascial surfaces may move or be separated from each other easily. Compare **fascial compartment, fascial membrane lamination.**

fascial compartment, a part of the body that is walled off by fascial membranes, usually containing a muscle or group of muscles or an organ, as the heart is contained by the mediastinum. Compare **fascial cleft, fascial membrane lamination.**

fascial membrane lamination, a pad of connective tissue that contains fat and an occasional blood vessel or a lymph node. It is found where a fascial membrane splits into two sheets, as at the division of the outer cervical fascia above the sternum. Compare **fascial cleft, fascial compartment.**

fascia thoracolumbalis, the extensive subdivision of the vertebral fascia that sheaths the sacrospinalis muscle. It spreads caudally to become the glistening, white lumbar aponeurosis and the origin of the latissimus dorsi. Medially it attaches to the sacrum, laterally to the ribs and the intercostal fascia, and cranially to the ligamentum nuchae. Also called **lumbodorsal fascia.**

fascicle. See **fasciculus.**

fascicular neuroma, a neoplasm composed of myelinated nerve fibers. Also called **medullated neuroma.**

fasciculation /fasik′yo͞olā′shən/, a localized, uncoordinated, uncontrollable twitching of a single muscle group innervated by a single motor nerve fiber or filament that may be palpated and seen under the skin. It results from a variety of drugs as a side effect with normal dosage or from an overdose, or it may be symptomatic of a number of disorders, including dietary deficiency, cerebral palsy, fever, neuralgia, polio, rheumatic heart disease, sodium deficiency, tic, or uremia. Fasciculation of the heart muscle is known as fibrillation. **–fascicular,** *adj.*, **fasciculate,** *v.*

fasciculus /fəsik′yələs/, *pl.* **fasciculi,** a small bundle of muscle, tendon, or nerve fibers. The arrangement of fasciculi in a muscle is correlated with the power of the muscle and its range of motion. The patterns of muscular fasciculi are penniform, bipenniform, multipenniform, and radiated. **–fascicular,** *adj.*

fascioliasis /fas′ē·ōlī′əsis/, infection with the liver fluke *Fasciola hepatica,* characterized by epigastric pain, fever, jaundice, eosinophilia, urticaria, and diarrhea, with fibrosis of the liver a consequence of prolonged infection. It is acquired by ingestion of encysted forms of the fluke found on aquatic plants, as raw watercress. The disease is prevalent in many parts of the world, including southern and western United States. Bithionol, given orally, is the usual treatment.

fasciolopsiasis /fas′ē·ōlopsī′əsis/, an intestinal infection, prevalent in the Far East, characterized by abdominal pain, diarrhea, constipation, eosinophilia, ascites, and, sometimes, edema; caused by the fluke *Fasciolopsis buski.* The disease is usually acquired by eating contaminated water plants, as raw water chestnuts. It is easily treated with anthelmintics, as piperazine.

fascioscapulohumeral dystrophy /fas′ē·ōskap′yo͞olōhyo͞o′mərəl/, an abnormal congenital condition and one of the main types of muscular dystrophy. It is characterized by progressive symmetric wasting of the skeletal muscles, especially the muscles of the face, the shoulders, and the upper arms, without any associated neural or sensory disorders. This disease is not usually fatal but spreads to all the voluntary muscles and commonly produces a pendulous lower lip and the absence of the nasolabial fold. It is an autosomal dominant disease that may be transmitted to males and females. Compare **Duchenne's muscular dystrophy.**

■ OBSERVATIONS: Fascioscapulohumeral dystrophy usually occurs before 10 years of age but may also develop during adolescence. Early symptoms include the inability to pucker the lips, abnormal facial movements when laughing or crying, facial flattening, winging of the scapulae, inability to raise the arms over the head, and, in infants, the inability to suckle. Diagnosis of this disease is based on the typical family and medical history and associated characteristic signs of abnormality. Confirming diagnosis is based on muscle biopsy showing abnormal deposits of fat and connective tissue. Electromyography may show attenuated electric activity, an inconclusive sign when considered alone but helpful in ruling out neurogenic muscle atrophy.

■ INTERVENTION: No known treatment can halt the progression of this disease and associated muscle impairment. Some measures that may help preserve mobility are physical therapy, surgery, and the use of orthopedic appliances.

■ NURSING CONSIDERATIONS: Nurses usually help preserve the mobility of the patient by assisting with therapeutic exercises. Encouragement and instruction can help the patient and the family deal with long-term care and adjustment. The individual with a dystrophy disorder often becomes constipated because activity is increasingly limited. High-protein, high-fiber diets and the use of stool softeners can help avoid constipation. Nurses often counsel family members who are carriers of the disease about the dangers of transmitting the disorder and refer patients who must learn new job skills to the appropriate agencies. Information about social services and financial assistance for patients and families is available from the Muscular Dystrophy Association, Inc.

fasciotomy /fas′ē•ot′əmē/, a surgical incision into an area of fascia.

fast, **1.** resistant to change, especially to the action of a specific drug or chemical, as a staining agent. **2.** to abstain from all or certain foods. See also **fasting.**

fast-acting insulin, one of a group of insulin preparations in which the onset of action is rapid, approximately 1 hour, and the duration of the action is relatively brief, approximately 6 to 14 hours. Kinds of fast-acting insulins include **insulin injection** and **prompt insulin zinc suspension.**

fastigium /fastij′ē•əm/, **1.** the highest point in the course of a fever, or the most symptomatic point in the course of an illness. **2.** the angle at the top of the roof of the fourth ventricle in the brain.

Fastin, a trademark for an anorexiant (phentermine hydrochloride).

fasting, the act of abstaining from food for a specific period of time, usually for therapeutic or religious purposes.

fat, **1.** a substance composed of lipids or fatty acids and occurring in various forms or consistencies ranging from oil to tallow. **2.** a type of body tissue composed of cells containing stored fat (depot fat). Stored fat is usually identified as white fat, which is found in large cellular vesicles, or brown fat, which consists of lipid droplets. Stored fat contains more than twice as many calories per gram as sugars and serves as a source of quickly mobilized body energy. In addition, stored fat helps cushion and insulate vital organs. See also **adipose, obesity.**

fat cell lipoma. See **hibernoma.**

fat embolism, a serious circulatory condition characterized by the blocking of an artery by an embolus of fat that entered the circulatory system after the fracture of a long bone or, less commonly, after traumatic injury to adipose tissue or to a fatty liver. A systemic condition may occur after extensive trauma, because lipid metabolism is altered by the injury and causes release of free fatty acids resulting in vasculitis with obstruction of many small pulmonary and cerebral arteries. Fat embolism usually occurs suddenly 12 to 36 hours after the injury and is characterized by severe chest pain, pallor, dyspnea, tachycardia, delirium, prostration, and, in some cases, coma. Anemia and thrombocytopenia are common. Classic signs of systemic fat embolism are petechial hemorrhages on the neck, shoulders, axillae, and conjunctivae, appearing 2 or 3 days after the injury. There is no specific therapy for systemic fat embolism; the patient is placed in a high Fowler's position and given oxygen, digitalis, corticosteroids, blood transfusion, respiratory assistance, and other supportive care.

FA test. See **fluorescent antibody test.**

father complex, *nontechnical.* a repressed desire for an incestuous relationship with one's father. See also **Oedipus complex.**

father fixation, an arrest in psychosexual development characterized by an abnormally persistent, close, and often paralyzing emotional attachment to one's father. Compare **mother fixation.** See also **Freudian fixation.**

fatigue, **1.** a state of exhaustion or a loss of strength or endurance, as may follow strenuous physical activity. **2.** loss of ability of tissues to respond to stimuli that normally evoke muscular contraction or other activity. Muscle cells generally require a refractory or recovery period after activity, during which time cells restore their energy supplies and excrete metabolic waste products. **3.** a sense of weariness or tiredness. **4.** an emotional state associated with extreme or extended exposure to psychic pressure, as in battle or combat fatigue.

fatigue fever, a benign episode of fever and muscle pain after overexertion. The symptoms are caused by an accumulation of the metabolic waste products of muscle contractions and may persist for several days.

fatigue fracture, any fracture that results from excessive physical activity and not from any specific injury, as commonly occurs in the metatarsal bones of runners.

fat metabolism, the biochemical process by which fats are broken down and elaborated by the cells of the body. Fats provide more food energy than carbohydrates; the catabolism of 1 g of fat provides 9 kg of heat as compared with 4.1 kcal yielded in the catabolism of 1 g of carbohydrate. Fat catabolism involves a series of chemical reactions, the last stages of which are similar to the final reactions of carbohydrate catabolism. Before the final reactions in fat catabolism can occur, fats must be hydrolyzed into fatty acids and glycerol. Conversion of glycerol provides a compound that can enter the citric acid cycle. Catabolism of fatty acids continues by beta-oxidation to produce acetyl-CoA, which also enters the citric acid cycle. The body synthesizes fats from fatty acids and glycerol or from compounds derived from excess glucose or from amino acids. Fat anabolism also includes the synthesis of complex compounds, as phospholipid, an important component of cell membranes. The body can synthesize only saturated fatty acids. Essential unsaturated fatty acids can be supplied only by the diet. Certain hormones, as insulin, growth hormone, adrenocorticotropic horomone, and the glucocorticoids, control fat metabolism. Fat catabolism is inversely related to the rate of carbohydrate catabolism, and in some conditions, as diabetes mellitus, the secretion of these hormones increases to counter a decrease in carbohydrate catabolism.

fatty acid, any of several organic acids produced by the hydrolysis of neutral fats. In a living cell a fatty acid usually occurs in combination with another molecule rather than in a free state. Essential fatty acids are unsaturated molecules that cannot be produced by the body and must therefore be included in the diet. Kinds of essential fatty acids are **arachidonic** and **linoleic.** See also **saturated fatty acid, unsaturated fatty acid.**

fatty alcohol, a hydroxide of a hydrocarbon from the paraffin series.

fatty ascites. See **chylous ascites.**

fatty cirrhosis. See **cirrhosis.**

fatty liver, an accumulation of triglycerides in the liver. The causes include alcoholic cirrhosis, IV administration of drugs such as tetracycline and corticosteroids, and exposure to toxic substances, as carbon tetrachloride and yellow phosphorus. Fatty liver is also seen in kwashiorkor and is a rare complication of unknown origin in late pregnancy. The symptoms are anorexia, hepatomegaly, and abdominal discomfort; fat cells can be seen under the microscope after liver biopsy. The condition is usually reversible after the underlying condition is corrected or the offending drug is withdrawn. See also **cirrhosis.**

fauces /fô′sēz/, the opening of the mouth into the pharynx. The anterior pillars of the fauces form the glossopalatine arch, and the posterior pillars form the pharyngopalatine arch.

faulty restoration, any dental restoration that contains flaws, as overhanging or incomplete tooth fillings, incorrect anatomy of occlusal and marginal ridge areas, and faulty clasps. Such faults may mar individual tooth restorations and fixed or removable partial dentures, which may cause inflammatory and dystrophic diseases of the teeth and periodontium. See also **restoration.**

favism /fā′vizəm/, an acute hemolytic anemia caused by ingestion of the beans or inhalation of the pollen from the *Vicia faba* (fava) plant. Sensitive individuals show a deficiency of glucose-6-phosphate dehydrogenase, usually the result of a hereditary biochemical abnormality of the erythrocytes. Symptoms include dizziness, headache, vomiting, fever, jaundice, eosinophilia, and often diarrhea. The condition is found primarily in persons of southern Italian extraction and is treated by blood transfusion and avoidance of fava beans and pollen. See also **glucose-6-phosphate dehydrogenase deficiency.**

favus /fā′vəs/, a fungal infection of the scalp, more common in children than adults. It is caused by *Trichophyton* fungi. Favus is characterized by thick, yellow crusts with suppuration, a distinct "mousy" odor, permanent scars, and alopecia. Rarely seen in North America, it is common in the Middle East and Africa.

F.C.A.P., abbreviation for **Fellow of the College of American Pathologists.**

F.D.A., abbreviation for **Food and Drug Administration.**

Fe, symbol for **iron.**

fear, a nursing diagnosis accepted by the Fourth National Conference on the Classification of Nursing Diagnoses. As a symptom, fear is a feeling of dread related to an identifiable source that the client is able to validate. The etiology of the problem, developed at the Fifth National Conference, results from natural or innate origins, as a sudden noise, loss of physical support, pain, heights, or other environmental stimuli; from a learned or conditioned response; separation from a support system in a potentially threatening situation, as hospitalization; knowledge defect or unfamiliarity; language barrier; sensory impairment; phobia or phobic stimulus. The defining characteristics may be subjective or objective. Subjective characteristics include increased tension, apprehension, impulsiveness, terror, panic, and decreased self-assurance. Objective characteristics are increased alertness and concentration on the source of fear; a wide-eyed, aggressive attack mode of behavior or withdrawal from the source of fear; and cardiovascular excitation, superficial vasoconstriction, and pupil dilatation. See also **nursing diagnosis.**

fear-tension-pain syndrome, a concept formulated by Grantly Dick-Read, M.D., to explain the pain commonly expected and reported in childbirth. The concept proposes that mistaken cultural attitudes induce anxiety before labor and cause fear in labor. This fear causes muscular and psychologic tension that interferes with the natural processes of dilatation and delivery, resulting in pain. He advocated education, exercise, and warm emotional and physical support in labor to counteract the syndrome, coining the term "natural childbirth" for a labor or delivery in which the well-trained woman joyfully, comfortably, and with a calm, cooperative attitude, participates in the natural experience. Elements of his method of psychophysical preparation for childbirth are incorporated into most other methods of natural childbirth. See also **Bradley method, Lamaze method.**

febri-, a combining form meaning 'pertaining to a fever': *febricant, febrifugal, febriphobia.*

febrifuge. See **antipyretic.**

febrile /fē′bril, feb′ril/, pertaining to or characterized by an elevated body temperature, as a febrile reaction to an infectious agent. –**febrility,** *n.*

-febrile, a combining form meaning 'pertaining to fever': *afebrile, nonfebrile, subfebrile.*

fecal fistula, an abnormal passage from the colon to the external surface of the body, discharging feces. Fistulas of this kind are usually created surgically in operations involving the removal of malignant or severely ulcerated bowel segments. See also **colostomy.**

fecal impaction, an accumulation of hardened or inspissated feces in the rectum or sigmoid colon that the individual is unable to move. Diarrhea may be a sign of fecal impaction since only liquid material is able to pass the obstruction. Occasionally, fecal impaction may cause urinary incontinence because of pressure on the bladder. Treatment includes oil and cleansing enemas and manual breaking up and removal of the stool by a gloved finger. Persons who are dehydrated, nutritionally depleted, on long periods of bedrest, receiving constipating medications such as iron or opiates, or undergoing barium x-ray studies are at risk of developing fecal impaction. Prevention includes adequate bulk food, fluids, exercise, regular bowel habits, privacy for defecation, and occasional stool softeners or laxatives. See also **constipation, obstipation.**

fecalith /fē′kəlith/, a hard, impacted mass of feces in the colon. To allow evacuation, an oil retention enema is usually administered; if ineffective, manual removal can be performed. See also **atonia constipation, constipation.**

fecal softener, a drug that lowers the surface tension of the fecal mass, allowing the intestinal fluids to penetrate and soften the stool. Also called **stool softener.**

feces /fē′sēz/, waste or excrement from the digestive tract that is formed in the intestine and expelled through the rectum. Feces consist of water, food residue, bacteria, and secretions of the intestines and liver. Gross examination of feces for color, odor, quantity, and consistency and microscopic examination for the presence of blood, fat, mucus, or parasites are common diagnostic procedures. Also called **stool.** See also **defecation.** –**fecal,** *adj*.

fecundation /fē′kəndā′shən, fek′-/, impregnation or fertilization; the act of fertilizing. See also **artificial insemination.** –**fecundate,** *v*.

fecundity /fikun′ditē/, the ability to produce offspring, especially in large numbers and rapidly; fertility. –**fecund,** *adj*.

Federal Register, a document published by the U.S. government each working day to inform the public of executive regulations, presidential orders, hearings and meetings schedules of various federal agencies, and related matters. The *Federal Register* contains announcements of the Food and Drug Administration, the Environmental Protection Agency, and other government bureaus that regulate matters of health and safety.

Federal Tort Claims Act, a statute passed in 1946 that allows the federal government to be sued for the wrongful action or negligence of its employees. The act, for most purposes, eliminates the doctrine of governmental immunity, which formerly prohibited the bringing of a suit against the federal government.

Federal Trade Commission (FTC), an agency in the executive branch of the federal government created to promote trade and to prevent practices that restrain free enterprise and competition. In the area of health care, the Commission successfully challenged the American Medical Association's ban on physician advertising. The FTC held that competition among physicians and the free choice of the consumer were impaired by the antiadvertising policy.

Federation Licensing Examination (FLEX), the standardized licensing examination for state licensure of physicians. Developed by the Federation of State Medical Boards of the United States, the examination is based on National Board of Medical Examiners test materials.

Fede's disease. See **Riga-Fede disease.**

feeblemindedness. See **mental retardation.**

feedback, (in communication theory) information produced by a receiver and perceived by a sender that informs the sender about the receiver's reaction to the message. Feedback is a cyclic part of the process of communication that regulates and modifies the content of messages.

feeding, the act or process of taking or giving food or nourishment. Kinds of feeding include **breastfeeding** and **forced feeding.** See also **alimentation, parenteral nutrition.**

fee-for-service, **1.** a charge made for a professional activity, as for a physical examination, the fitting of a contraceptive diaphragm, or the monitoring of a person's blood pressure. **2.** a system for the payment of professional services in which the practitioner is paid for the particular service rendered, rather than receiving a salary for providing professional services as needed during scheduled hours of work or time on call.

feel life, *nontechnical*. to experience quickening.

Feer's disease. See **acrodynia.**

fee screen system, a method of establishing payment for physician services based on the usual, customary, or reasonable charge according to a regional evaluation. It allows physicians to establish their own reimbursement level for units of service.

Fehling's solution /fā′lingz/, a solution containing cupric sulfate with sodium hydroxide and potassium sodium tartrate, used for testing for the presence of glucose and other reducing substances in the urine. Also called **Fehling's reagent.**

Feldene, a trademark for an antiinflammatory agent (piroxicam).

feldspar, a crystalline mineral of aluminum silicate with potassium, sodium, barium, and calcium. It melts over a range of 1100° F to 2000° F (593.5° C to 1093° C) and is an important component of dental porcelain.

Fellow of the American Academy of Nursing (FAAN), a member of the American Academy of Nursing.

Fellow of the American College of Chest Physicians (F.A.C.C.P.), a physician who is a board-certified member of the American College of Chest Physicians.

Fellow of the American College of Surgeons (F.A.C.S.), a member of the American College of Surgeons, recognized by that professional organization as being qualified by education, training, and experience to practice surgery.

Fellow of the College of American Pathologists (F.C.A.P.), a physician who is a member of the **College of American Pathologists.**

fellowship, a grant given to a person for study or training or to allow payment for work on a special project, but not for study toward a degree. It provides a salary and, in some cases, the miscellaneous expenses involved in the study, training, or project.

felon, a suppurative abscess on the distal phalanx of a finger.

felonious assault. See **assault, felony.**

felony, (in criminal law) a crime declared by statute to be more serious than a misdemeanor and deserving of a more severe penalty. Conviction usually requires imprisonment in a penitentiary for longer than 1 year. Crimes of murder, rape, burglary, and arson are tried as felonies in most cases. Compare **misdemeanor.**

Felty's syndrome /fel′tēz/, hypersplenism occurring with adult rheumatoid arthritis, characterized by splenomegaly, leukopenia, and frequent infections. The cause of the syndrome is unknown. Surgical resection of the spleen offers temporary improvement in about one half of the cases. See also **hypersplenism.**

female, **1.** of or pertaining to the sex that becomes pregnant and bears children; feminine. **2.** a female person.

female catheterization, a procedure for removing urine by means of a urinary catheter introduced through the urinary meatus and urethra into the bladder. The procedure is performed to relieve distention if voluntary micturition is not possible (as after trauma or surgery), as a preparation for and during anesthesia, if a specimen of urine from the bladder is required, or if medication is to be instilled into the bladder. A straight catheter or a retention catheter with a balloon may be used. A French size 12 to 16 is usually selected for straight drainage. See also **catheterization, male catheterization.**

■ METHOD: The necessary sterile equipment is obtained, including cotton swabs, a bowl for collecting the urine, a disposable catheter, a sponge stick for holding the swabs, a disinfectant for washing the urinary meatus and the perineal area adjacent to it, gloves, a lubricant for the catheter tip, and a drape. Often, a preassembled kit of disposable sterile equipment is available, leaving only the separately packaged catheter to be selected. The patient is positioned on her back, with the knees flexed and the legs abducted, and is then draped. A bright light is directed at the perineum. The nurse then scrubs the hands, dries them well, and opens the catheterization kit or tray carefully, not touching the inside of the wrapper or the contents. Sterile gloves are put on, and the tray is lifted and placed between the patient's legs. The small sterile drape in the kit is placed over the patient so that the window in it allows access to the urinary meatus. With the thumb and the forefinger, the labia are separated and the tissues are retracted, exposing the meatus. The area is cleansed from the front to the back using one pledget or swab for each stroke. Each pledget is discarded before beginning another stroke; three or more strokes are used, and the location of the meatus is verified while the area is cleaned. The labia are separated, the catheter is picked up approximately 4 cm from its tip, the tip is lubricated, and the end is placed in the basin. While the patient's attention is diverted, the catheter is inserted approximately 7.5 cm until the urine begins to flow. When the urine stops flowing, the bladder is gently massaged to empty it completely, and the catheter is slowly withdrawn. A sterile sponge is gently pressed to the meatus to remove any lubricant and to dry the area. The urine is measured, and the odor, color, and any abnormal precipitate are noted. A specimen for bacteriologic culture and antibiotic sensitivity is often secured, labeled, and sent to the laboratory.

■ NURSING ORDERS: Catheterization is usually ordered by a physician for an individual patient, or the conditions under which a catheterization is to be performed are stated in written standing orders. Catheterization is needlessly dreaded by many patients; careful explanation may allay the fears. Having the woman take a deep breath may cause the meatus to open slightly, revealing its presence, and asking her to bear down slightly may minimize the momentary discomfort that commonly accompanies the insertion of the catheter into the bladder. Voluntary micturition is almost always preferable, and the nurse encourages the woman to try to void spontaneously. Signs of infection are carefully observed. If a woman is to be catheterized more than twice, an indwelling catheter is usually preferred to a third catheterization.

■ OUTCOME CRITERIA: Catheterization predisposes the urinary tract to infection, and traumatic catheterization further increases the risk. Care, gentleness, and asepsis are essential. If the bladder is distended with urine, the first 1000 ml may be withdrawn, the catheter clamped, and the physician consulted, as withdrawing more than that amount at once may cause damage to the bladder, chills, and shock. Certain conditions, including radical vulvectomy, postoperative swelling, or structural anomalies, may obscure the urinary meatus. The indication for catheterization, the age of the patient, and the condition and size of the urethra affect the choice of catheter style and size.

female dietary allowance. See **dietary allowances.**

female reproductive system assessment, an evaluation of a patient's genital tract and breasts and an investigation of past and present disorders that may be factors in the individual's current gynecologic condition. See also **pelvic examination.**

■ METHOD: The patient is interviewed to determine if she has lower abdominal pain, cramps, vaginal bleeding, itching, swelling, redness, or a discharge that is mucoid, watery, frothy, or thick in consistency and white, yellow, greenish, bloody, or brown in color. She is asked if she experiences pain on intercourse and pain or burning on urination. Observations are recorded of her general appearance, vital signs, weight, breast symmetry, texture, and lumps or bumps, nipple color, and the presence of a serous, bloody, or purulent nipple discharge. The abdomen is examined for contour, symmetry, stretch marks, scars, lesions, and visible pulsations and peristaltic waves, and is auscultated for bowel sounds in each quadrant. Carefully noted are edema or redness of the external genitalia, cervix, and perineum, lumps or lesions on the labia majora, the size of the urethral orifice, the presence or absence of the hymenal ring, hymenal tags, perineal scars or excoriation, and a bloody, purulent, or odoriferous discharge. The normal mucoid secretion is distinguished from the thick, white, cheesy discharge typical of candidosis, the frothy, yellow-green, watery liquid characteristic of trichomoniasis, and the thick, yellow-green or brown, and bloody drainage typical of upper genital tract infection. The patient's age at onset of menses, the duration, spacing, and regularity of cycles, the amount and character of the flow, the date of the last menstrual period, and associated symptoms, as pain and menorrhagia, are investigated. The complications and outcome of each of the patient's pregnancies, the kind of delivery, the incidence and outcome of any abortion, and the date of menopause and associated symptoms, as hot flushes and dry vaginal mucosa, are explored. It is determined if the patient suffers from a venereal disease, constipation, hemorrhoids, hypothyroidism or hyperthyroidism, polycystic ovary syndrome, hypertension, or blood dyscrasias or has a history of gynecologic or other major abdominal surgery or a serious illness, especially one related to the endocrine system. The patient's smoking habits, sexual activity, use of oral contraceptives or an intrauterine device, her experience with estrogen therapy, and family history of gynecologic diseases and deaths are reported in the assessment. Diagnostic procedures indicated by the history may include a manual examination, Pap test, basal body temperature determination, culture of vaginal discharge, punch biopsy, endometrial biopsy, dilatation and curettage, cold-knife conization, laparoscopy, ultrasound study, and tubal insufflation. Laboratory studies that may be performed include determinations of levels of human chorionic gonadotropin, serum luteinizing and follicle-stimulating hormones, 17-ketosteroids, and corticosteroids, tests for venereal diseases, and thyroid function tests, as the basal metabolic rate and protein-bound iodine level.

■ NURSING ORDERS: The nurse conducts the interview, records observations of the patient, and collects the pertinent background information and the results of the diagnostic procedures and laboratory studies.

■ OUTCOME CRITERIA: A careful assessment of the patient's reproductive system is essential in establishing the diagnosis.

female sexual dysfunction, impaired or inadequate ability of a woman to engage in or enjoy satisfactory sexual intercourse and orgasm. Symptoms, usually psychologic in origin, include dyspareunia, vaginismus, persistent inability to reach orgasm, and inhibition in sexual arousal, so that congestion and vaginal lubrication are minimal or absent. Causes include anxiety, fear, negative emotions associated with sexual arousal and intercourse, and interpersonal problems. Treatment is focused on eliminating physical problems and sexual anxieties and on enhancing erotic sensitivities. Compare **male sexual dysfunction.** See also **sexual dysfunction.**

feminization, **1.** the normal development or induction of female sex characteristics. **2.** the induction of female sex characteristics in a genotypic male. Testicular feminization may be caused by the inability of target tissues to respond to endogenous or administered androgen; some cases seem related to an absent or inadequate conversion of testosterone to dihydrotestosterone, which presumably is the active form of the androgen. Testicular feminization in males with an X and Y chromosome and a female phenotype may be caused by fetal hypogonadism and is often familial. Individuals with this defect usually have undescended or labial testes, a short, blind vaginal pouch, no uterus, well-developed breasts, sparse or absent axillary and pubic hair, normal plasma levels of testosterone and follicle-stimulating hormone, and increased concentrations of estradiol and luteinizing hormone. Treatment consists of orchiectomy because of the risk of cancer in gonads of these patients. Feminization may also be caused by adrenocortical estrogen-secreting tumor, by failure of the liver to inactivate endogenous estrogens, as in advanced alcoholism, or by the administration of estrogen therapy for androgen-dependent neoplasms. Some testicular tumors may produce feminizing symptoms, and gynecomastia may be caused by Klinefelter's syndrome and by certain drugs, as reserpine, digitalis, meprobamate, and cimetidine. Compare **virilization.** See also **pseudohermaphroditism.**

feminizing adrenal tumor, a rare neoplasm of the adrenal cortex, characterized in males by gynecomastia, hypertension, diffuse pigmentation, a high level of estrogen in urine, and loss of potency. Testicular atrophy frequently occurs, but the prostate and penis are usually normal in size. The tumor may be large enough to palpate or to be diagnosed by intravenous urography or arteriography. In most cases it is a carcinoma. Treatment includes surgical resection and chemotherapy with mitotane. In women, these tumors, which are extremely rare, are associated with precocious puberty.

Feminone, a trademark for an estrogen (ethinyl estradiol).

Femogen, a trademark for esterified estrogens.

femoral /fem′ərəl/, of or pertaining to the femur or the thigh.

femoral artery, an extension of the external iliac artery into the lower limb, starting just distal to the inguinal ligament and ending at the junction of the middle and lower thirds of the thigh. It divides into seven branches and supplies various parts of the lower limb and trunk, as the groin and its organs. Its branches are the superficial epigastric, superficial iliac circumflex, superficial external pudendal, deep external pudendal, muscular, profundis femoris, and descending genicular.

femoral hernia, a hernia in which a loop of intestine descends through the femoral canal into the groin. Surgical repair, herniorrhaphy, is the usual treatment. See also **hernia.**

femoral nerve, the largest of the seven branches from the lumbar plexus and the main nerve of the anterior part of the thigh. It arises from the dorsal parts of the ventral primary divisions of the second, third, and fourth lumbar nerves, passes through the lateral, distal fibers of the psoas major, and descends between the psoas major and the iliacus under the cover of the transversalis fascia. Lateral to the femoral artery, it passes under the inguinal ligament, enters the thigh, and breaks into the muscular branches, the anterior cutaneous branches, the intermediate cutaneous nerve, the medial cutaneous nerve, the nerve to the pectineus, the nerve to the sartorius, the saphenous nerve, the branches to the quadriceps femoris, the articular branch to the hip joint, and the articular branches to the knee joint. Also called **anterior crural nerve.**

femoral pulse, the pulse of the femoral artery, palpated in the groin.

femoral torsion, an extreme lateral or a medial twisting rotation of the femur on its longitudinal axis, as may occur because of the action of the gluteal muscles. Compare **tibial torsion.**

femoral vein, a large vein in the thigh originating in the popliteal vein and accompanying the femoral artery in the proximal two thirds of the thigh. Its distal portion lies lateral to the artery; its proximal portion deeper to the artery. About 4 cm below the inguinal ligament it is joined by the deep femoral vein. Near its termination it is joined by the great saphenous vein. It receives tributaries from the branches of the deep femoral artery and receives the medial and the lateral femoral circumflex veins. At the inguinal ligament it becomes the external iliac vein. The femoral vein has four valves.

femur /fē′mər/, *pl.* **femora, femurs,** the thigh bone, which extends from the pelvis to the knee. It is largely cylindric and is the longest and strongest bone in the body. It has a large, round head that fits the acetabulum of the hip, and it displays a large neck and several prominences and ridges for muscle attachments. In an erect posture it inclines medially, bringing the knee joint near the line of gravity of the body. The degree of this inclination is usually greater in a woman than in a man. Also called **thigh bone.**

fenestra /fines′trə/, *pl.* **fenestrae,** an aperture, especially in a bandage or cast, that is often cut out to relieve pressure or to administer regular skin care.

fenestration, **1.** a surgical procedure in which an opening is created in order to gain access to the cavity within an organ or a bone. **2.** an opening created surgically in a bone or organ of the body. Also called **window.** – **fenestrate,** *v.*

fenfluramine hydrochloride /fenflŏŏr′əmēn/, a sympathomimetic anorectic agent.

■ INDICATION: It is prescribed to decrease the appetite in exogenous obesity.

■ CONTRAINDICATIONS: Glaucoma, alcoholism, severe hypertension, use of a monoamine oxidase inhibitor within 14 days, or known hypersensitivity to this drug or to other sympathomimetic medication prohibits its use.

■ ADVERSE EFFECTS: Among the more serious adverse reactions are drug dependence, diarrhea, mental confusion, and depression.

fenoprofen calcium, a nonsteroidal antiinflammatory agent and analgesic.

■ INDICATIONS: It is prescribed in the treatment of arthritis and other painful inflammatory conditions.

■ CONTRAINDICATIONS: Renal dysfunction, upper GI disease, or known hypersensitivity to this drug, to aspirin, or to nonsteroidal antiinflammatory medication prohibits its use.

■ ADVERSE EFFECTS: Among the more serious adverse reactions are GI disturbances, gastric or duodenal ulceration, dizziness, skin rash, and tinnitus. The drug interacts with many other drugs.

fentanyl, a potent, narcotic analgesic, used most commonly with the sedative and antipsychotic drug droperidol as an adjunct in anesthesia.

fentanyl citrate /fen′tənil/, a narcotic analgesic.

■ INDICATIONS: It is prescribed as an adjunct to general anesthesia, as a preoperative and postoperative analgesic, and as a component in neuroleptanesthesia and analgesia.

■ CONTRAINDICATIONS: Myasthenia gravis, use of a monoamine oxidase inhibitor within 14 days, or known hypersensitivity to this drug prohibits its use.

■ ADVERSE EFFECTS: Among the more serious adverse reactions are drug dependence, hypotension, pruritus, respiratory depression, and laryngospasm.

fentanyl citrate and droperidol, a parenteral anesthetic.

■ INDICATION: It is given to induce neuroleptanesthesia for various brief surgical or diagnostic procedures.

■ CONTRAINDICATIONS: Use of monoamine oxidase inhibitors within 14 days or known hypersensitivity to either ingredient prohibits its use. It is used with caution in elderly and poor-risk patients, in patients with head injury or brain tumor, and in children younger than 2 years of age.

■ ADVERSE EFFECTS: Among the more serious adverse reactions are hypotension, respiratory depression, laryngospasm, and drug dependence.

Feosol, a trademark for a hematinic (ferrous sulfate).

-fer, a combining form meaning 'something that carries something': *parasitifer, sonifer, vaccinifer.*

Fergon, a trademark for a hematinic (ferrous gluconate).

Ferguson's reflex, a contraction of the uterus after the cervix is stimulated. The reflex is an important function of labor.

fermentation, a chemical change that is brought about in a substance by the action of an enzyme or microorganism, especially the anaerobic conversion of foodstuffs to certain products. Kinds of fermentation are **acetic fermentation, alcoholic fermentation, ammoniacal fermentation, amylic fermentation, butyric fermentation, caseous fermentation, dextran fermentation, diastatic fermentation, lactic acid fermentation, propionic fermentation, storing fermentation,** and **viscous fermentation.**

fermentative dyspepsia /fərmen′tətiv/, an abnormal condition characterized by impaired digestion associated with the fermentation of digested food. See also **dyspepsia.**

fermium (Fm), a synthetic transuranic metallic element. Its atomic number is 100; its atomic weight is 257. Fermium was first detected in the debris from a hydrogen bomb explosion and later produced in a reactor. Ten isotopes of fermium have been identified.

ferning test, a technique used to determine the presence of estrogen in the uterine cervical mucus. When it is used as a test for ovulation, high levels of estrogen cause the cervical mucus to dry on a slide in a fernlike pattern. When it is used in pregnancy testing, the fern pattern does not appear because of the high levels of progesterone present along with the estrogen.

-ferous, a combining form meaning 'producing or carrying' something specified: *lactiferous, sebiferous, tubiferous.*

ferr-, ferri-. See **ferro-.**

ferritin /fur′itin/, an iron compound found in the intestinal mucosa, the spleen, and the liver. It contains over 20% iron and is essential for hematopoiesis.

ferro-, ferr-, ferri-, a combining form meaning 'pertaining to iron': *ferrocyanide, ferropectic, ferrosilicon.*

ferrous sulfate, a hematinic agent.

■ INDICATION: It is prescribed in the treatment of iron deficiency anemia.

■ CONTRAINDICATIONS: There are no known contraindications.

■ ADVERSE EFFECTS: Among the most serious adverse reactions are diarrhea and constipation.

fertile, **1.** capable of reproducing or bearing offspring. **2.** of a gamete, capable of inducing fertilization or being fertilized. **3.** prolific; fruitful; not sterile. **–fertility,** *n.,* **fertilize,** *v.*

fertile eunuch syndrome, a hypogonadotropic hormonal disorder occurring only in males in which the quantity of testosterone and follicle stimulating hormone is inadequate for the inducement of spermatogenesis and the development of secondary sexual characteristics. If supplemental hormones are not prescribed, the affected person acquires the appearance of a eunuch.

fertile period, the time in the menstrual cycle during which fertilization may occur. Spermatozoa can survive for 48 to 72 hours; the ovum lives for 24 hours. Thus, the fertile period begins 2 to 3 days before ovulation and lasts for 2 to 3 days afterward. To increase the contraceptive effectiveness of natural family-planning methods, some allowance is made for the possibility of longer survival of the spermatozoa and the ovum, extending the length of the fertile period to 7 or 8 days. The fertile period may be identified by observation of the changes in the quantity and character of cervical mucus or of changes in the basal body temperature, or it may be deduced from a calendar record of six or more menstrual cycles, applying the fact that ovulation usually occurs 14 days before menstruation.

fertility factor. See **F factor.**

fertilization, the union of male and female gametes to form a zygote from which the embryo develops. The process takes place in the fallopian tube of the female when a spermatozoon, carried in the seminal fluid discharged during coitus, comes in contact with and penetrates the ovum. Rapid chemical changes in the membrane of the ovum prevent the entrance of additional spermatozoa. Penetration by the spermatozoon stimulates the completion of the second meiotic division and formation of the pronucleus in the ovum. Fusion and synapsis of the male and female pronuclei restore the diploid number of chromosomes to the germ cell, resulting in the determination of the sex of the zygote and of the characteristics inherited from each parent, and stimulate the initiation of development through cleavage. Kinds of fertilization include **cross-fertilization, external fertilization,** and **internal fertilization.** See also **oogenesis, spermatogenesis.**

fertilization age. See **fetal age.**

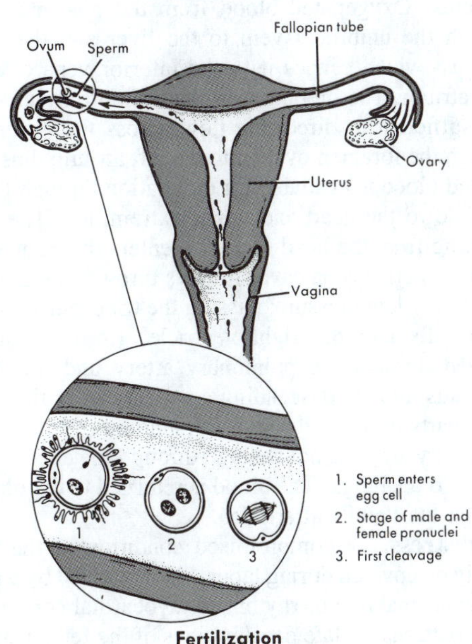

Fertilization

fertilization membrane, a viscous membrane surrounding the fertilized ovum that prevents the penetration of additional spermatozoa. It is formed by granules from the cytoplasm of the fertilized ovum adhering to the vitelline membrane.

fertilizin /fərtil′izin/, a glycoprotein found on the plasma membrane of the ovum in various species. It was once thought that the specific agglutinizing receptor groups of the substance were complementary to antifertilizin, a substance extracted from the sperm, and were responsible for binding the spermatozoon to the ovum during the early stage of fertilization, but the theory has since been discarded. See also **acrosomal reaction.**

Festal, a trademark for a GI fixed-combination drug containing a group of digestive enzymes and bile constituents.

festoon, a carving in the base material of a denture that simulates the contours of the natural gingival tissues.

fetal abortion, termination of pregnancy after the twentieth week of gestation but before the fetus has developed enough to live outside of the uterus. Compare **embryonic abortion.**

fetal advocate, a person who regards the health and well-being of the fetus as a matter of top priority.

fetal age, the age of the conceptus computed from the time elapsed since fertilization. Also called **fertilization age.** Compare **gestational age.**

fetal attitude, the relationship of the fetal parts to each other, as in the "military" attitude, in which the fetal head is not flexed and the chin on chest is as usual but is held straight up. Compare **fetal position, fetal presentation.**

fetal bradycardia, an abnormally slow fetal heart rate, usually below 100 beats per minute.

fetal circulation, the pathway of blood circulation in the fetus. Oxygenated blood from the placenta travels through the umbilical vein to the liver and the ductus venosus, which carries it to the inferior vena cava and right atrium. The blood enters the right atrium at a pressure sufficient to direct the flow across the atrium and through the foramen ovale into the left atrium; thus, oxygenated blood is available for circulation through the left ventricle to the head and upper extremities. The blood returning from the head and arms enters the right atrium via the superior vena cava. It flows through the atrium at a relatively low pressure; passing the tricuspid valve, the blood falls into the right ventricle, from which it is pumped through the pulmonary artery and the ductus arteriosus into the descending aorta for circulation to the lower parts of the body. A small amount of blood in the pulmonary artery is not shunted through the ductus and is carried to the lungs. The blood is returned to the placenta through the umbilical arteries.

fetal distress, a compromised condition of the fetus, usually discovered during labor, characterized by a markedly abnormal rate or rhythm of myocardial contraction. Some patterns, as late decelerations of the fetal heart rate

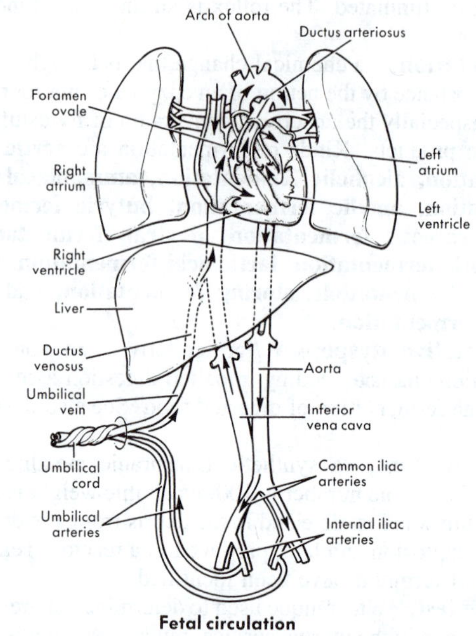

Fetal circulation

seen on records of electronic fetal monitoring, are indicative of fetal distress. If possible, the cause of the situation is identified and corrected and the acid-base balance of the fetal blood is tested. Labor is allowed to continue if the pH is within normal range and if the abnormal pattern does not recur or persist. Cesarean section may be necessary if the fetus is markedly alkalotic or acidotic or if the cause of the problem cannot be corrected. If possible, the baby is stabilized before being delivered by giving the mother oxygen, increased fluids, or a narcotic antagonist, a vasopressor, or an agent to relax the uterus. A pediatrician is required to attend the birth of a distressed baby to manage resuscitation and care immediately after delivery.

fetal heart rate (FHR), the number of heartbeats in the fetus occurring in a given unit of time. The FHR varies in cycles of fetal rest and activity and is affected by many factors, including maternal fever, uterine contractions, maternal-fetal hypotension, and many drugs. The normal FHR is more than 100 beats per minute and less than 160 beats per minute. In labor the FHR is monitored with a fetoscope or an electronic fetal monitor to detect abnormal alterations in the rate, especially recurrent decelerations that continue past the end of uterine contractions.

fetal heart tones (fht), the pulsations of the fetal heart heard through the maternal abdomen in pregnancy. The rate, usually between 120 and 160 beats per minute, tends to increase briefly with or just after fetal movement.

fetal hemoglobin, hemoglobin F, the major hemoglobin present in the blood of a fetus and neonate. Hemoglobin F is present in only trace amounts in the blood of normal adults.

fetal hydantoin syndrome (FHS), a complex of birth defects associated with prenatal maternal ingestion of hydantoin derivatives. Symptoms of FHS include microcephaly, hypoplasia or absence of nails on the fingers or toes, abnormal facies, mental and physical retardation, and cardiac defects. The syndrome occurs to some degree in 10% to 40% of infants born of mothers for whom this anticonvulsant has been prescribed. Hydantoin sometimes appears to be associated with hemorrhage and, more rarely, with neural crest tumors in the newborn.

fetal hydrops. See **hydrops fetalis.**

fetal lie, the relationship of the long axis of the fetus to the long axis of the mother. See also **fetal presentation.**

fetal lipoma. See **hibernoma.**

fetal monitor. See **electronic fetal monitor.**

fetal position, the relationship of the part of the fetus that presents in the pelvis to four quadrants of the maternal pelvis identified by initial L (left), R (right), A (anterior), and P (posterior). The presenting part is also identified by initial O (occiput), M (mentum), and S (sacrum). If a fetus presents with the occiput directed to the posterior aspect of the mother's right side, the fetal position is right occiput posterior (ROP). Compare **fetal attitude, fetal presentation.**

fetal presentation, the part of the fetus that first appears in the pelvis. Cephalic presentations include vertex, brow, and chin; breech presentations include frank breech, complete breech, and single or double footling breech. Shoulder presentations are rare and require cesarean section or turning before vaginal delivery. Compound presentation involves the entry of more than one part in the true pelvis; most commonly a hand next to the head. See also **fetal attitude, fetal lie, fetal position.**

fetal rest. See **embryonic rest.**

fetal rickets. See **achondroplasia.**

fetal stage, (in embryology) the interval of time from the end of the embryonic stage, at the end of the seventh week of gestation, to birth, 38 to 42 weeks after the first day of the last menstrual period.

fetal tachycardia, a fetal heart rate that continues at 160 or more beats per minute for more than 10 minutes.

feti-, feto-, foeti-, foeto-, a combining form meaning 'fetus or fetal': *feticide, fetochorionic, fetoscope.*

feticide. See **embryoctony.**

fetish, **1.** any object or idea given unreasonable or excessive attention or reverence. **2.** (in psychology) any inanimate object or any part of the body not of a sexual nature that arouses erotic feelings or fixation. The erotic symbology is unique to the fetishist and results from unconscious associations. **–fetishism,** *n.*

fetishist, a person who believes in or receives erotic gratification from fetishes.

feto-. See **feti-.**

fetochorionic /fē′tōkôr′ē·on′ik/, of or pertaining to the fetus and the chorion.

fetography /fētog′rəfē/, roentgenography of the fetus in utero. See also **fetometry.**

fetology /fētol′əjē/, the branch of medicine that is concerned with the fetus in utero, including the diagnosis of abnormalities, congenital anomalies, the prevention of teratogenic influences, and the treatment of certain disorders. Also called **embryatrics.**

fetometry /fētom′ətrē/, the measurement of the size of the fetus, especially the diameter of the head and circumference of the trunk. A kind of fetometry is **roentgen fetometry.**

fetoplacental, of or pertaining to the fetus and the placenta.

fetoprotein, an antigen that occurs naturally in fetuses and occasionally in adults as the result of certain diseases. Leukemia, hepatoma, sarcoma, and other neoplasms are associated with **beta fetoprotein** in the blood of adults. An increased amount of **alpha fetoprotein** in the fetus is diagnostic for neural tube defects.

fetor hepaticus, foul-smelling breath associated with severe liver disease. Also called **liver breath.**

fetoscope /fē′təskōp′/, a stethoscope for auscultating the fetal heartbeat through the mother's abdomen.

fetoscopy /fētos′kəpē/, a procedure in which a fetus may be directly observed in utero, using a fetoscope introduced through a small incision in the abdomen under local anesthesia. Photographs of the fetus may be taken, and amniotic fluid, fetal cells, or blood may be sampled for prenatal diagnosis of many congenital anomalies or genetic defects.

fetotoxic, pertaining to anything that is poisonous to a fetus.

fetus /fē′təs/, the unborn offspring of a viviparous animal after it has attained the particular form of the species, more specifically, the human child in utero after the embryonic period and the beginning of the development of the major structural features, usually from the eighth week after fertilization until birth. Kinds of fetuses include **acardius, anideus, lithopedion, mummified fetus, parasitic fetus,** and **sirenomelia.** Also spelled **foetus.** Compare **embryo.** See also **prenatal development.** **–fetal, foetal,** *adj.*

fetus acardiacus, fetus acardius. See **acardius.**

fetus amorphus, a shapeless conceptus in which there are no formed or recognizable parts.

fetus anideus. See **anideus.**

fetus in fetu, a fetal anomaly in which a small, imperfectly formed twin, incapable of independent existence, is contained within the body of the normal twin, the autosite.

fetus papyraceus, a twin fetus that has died in utero early in development and has been pressed flat against the uterine wall by the living fetus. Also called **paper-doll fetus, papyraceous fetus.**

fetus sanguinolentis /sang′gwinəlen′tis/, a darkly colored, partly macerated fetus that has died in utero.

FEV, abbreviation for **forced expiratory volume.**

fever, an abnormal elevation of the temperature of the body above 37° C (98.6° F) because of disease. Fever results from an imbalance between the elimination and the production of heat. Exercise, anxiety, and dehydration may increase the temperature of healthy people. Infection, neurologic disease, malignancy, pernicious anemia, thromboembolic disease, paroxysmal tachycardia, congestive heart failure, crushing injury, severe trauma, and many drugs may cause the development of fever. No single theory explains the mechanism whereby the temperature is increased. Fever has no recognized function in conditions other than infection. It increases metabolic activity by 7% per degree Celsius, requiring a greater intake of food. Convulsions may occur in children whose fevers tend to rise abruptly, and delirium is seen with high fevers in adults and in children. Very high temperatures, as in heatstroke, may be fatal. The course of a fever varies with the cause and the condition of the patient and with the treatment given. The onset may be abrupt or gradual, and the period of maximum elevation, called the stadium or fastigium, may last for a few days or up to 3 weeks. The fever may resolve suddenly, by crisis, or gradually, by lysis. Certain diseases and conditions are associated with fevers that begin, rise, and fall in such characteristic curves that diagnosis may be made by studying a graphic record of the course of the fever. Kinds of hyperthermia include **habitual fever, intermittent fever,** and **relapsing fever.** See also **fever treatment, hyperpyrexia.**

fever blister, a cold sore caused by herpesvirus I or II. Also called **herpes simplex.**

fever therapy. See **artificial fever.**

fever treatment, the care and management of a person with an elevated temperature.

■ METHOD: The patient is observed for symptoms of fever, as tachycardia; a full, bounding pulse or a weak, thready pulse; rapid breathing; hot, dry, hyperemic skin; chills; headache; diaphoresis; restlessness; delirium; dehydration; tremors; convulsions; and coma. Treatment may include the administration of antibiotic, antipyretic, and sedative drugs. If the temperature is extremely high, an alcohol sponge bath, cooling tub bath, cold wet sheet, ice packs, or hypothermia may be ordered. The patient's temperature is checked every 2 to 4 hours. Antipyretic and sedative therapy is continued as ordered and, if necessary, cooling measures are reinstituted; the room temperature is reduced, and air currents are increased by a fan. Increased amounts of fluids are given orally or parenterally, physical activity is reduced, and the skin is exposed to air.

■ NURSING ORDERS: The nurse observes and records the symptoms accompanying fever, administers the ordered medication and cooling measures, reassures the patient, and explains the importance of therapy and of drinking adequate fluids.

■ OUTCOME CRITERIA: Antipyretic drugs and cooling measures usually reduce the temperature, but the patient may require additional fluids and treatment for the underlying cause of the fever.

F factor, (in bacterial genetics) an episome present in conjugating male bacteria but absent in females. Also called **F element, fertility factor, sex factor.**

FHR, abbreviation for **fetal heart rate.**

FHS, abbreviation for **fetal hydantoin syndrome.**

fht, abbreviation for **fetal heart tones.**

fiberoptic bronchoscopy, the visual examination of the tracheobronchial tree through a fiberoptic bronchoscope. Also called **bronchofibroscopy.** See also **bronchoscopy, fiberoptics.**

fiberoptic duodenoscope, an instrument for visualizing the interior of the duodenum, consisting of an eyepiece, a flexible tube incorporating bundles of coated glass or plastic fibers with special optic properties, and a terminal light. When the duodenoscope is introduced into the patient's mouth and threaded through the upper digestive tract to the duodenum, the light illuminates the internal structures and any lesions present, and the fiberoptic bundles transmit the image to the observer's eyepiece.

fiberoptics, the technical process by which an internal organ or cavity can be viewed, using glass or plastic fibers to transmit light through a specially designed tube and reflect a magnified image. **–fiberoptic,** *adj.*

fiberscope, a flexible fiberoptic instrument having an inner shaft coated with light-conveying glass or plastic fibers for visualization of internal structures. Fiberscopes are specially designed for the examination of particular organs and cavities of the body and are used in bronchoscopy, endoscopy, and gastroscopy.

fibril /fī′bril/, a small filamentous structure that often is a component of a cell, as in a mitotic spindle.

fibrillation /fī′brilā′shən/, involuntary recurrent contraction of a single muscle fiber or of an isolated bundle of nerve fibers. Fibrillation of a chamber of the heart results in inefficient random contraction of that chamber and disruption of the normal sinus rhythm of the heart. Fibrillation is usually described by the part that is contracting abnormally, as atrial fibrillation or ventricular fibrillation.

fibrin /fī′brin/, a stringy, insoluble protein that is a product of the action of thrombin on fibrinogen in the clotting process. It is responsible for the semisolid character of a blood clot. Compare **fibrinogen.** See also **blood clotting, coagulation, fibrinolysis, thrombin.**

fibrinase. See **factor XIII.**

Fibrindex, a trademark for a local hemostatic (thrombin).

fibrinogen /fībrin′əjən/, a plasma protein essential to the blood clotting process that is converted into fibrin by thrombin in the presence of calcium ions. Compare **fibrin.** See also **afibrinogenemia, blood clotting, fibrinolysis, thrombin.**

fibrinogenopenia, a condition in which there is a deficiency of fibrinogen in the blood.

fibrinokinase /fī'brinōkī'nās/, a non-water-soluble enzyme in animal tissue that activates plasminogen. Also called **tissue activator, tissue kinase.**

fibrinolysin /fī'brinol'isin/, a proteolytic enzyme that dissolves fibrin. It is formed from plasminogen in the blood plasma. Also called **plasmin.** See also **fibrinolysis.**

fibrinolysis /fī'brinol'isis/, the continual process of fibrin decomposition by fibrinolysin that is the normal mechanism for the removal of small fibrin clots. It is stimulated by anoxia, inflammatory reactions, and other kinds of stress. **–fibrinolytic,** *adj.*

fibrinopeptide /fī'brinōpep'tīd/, a product of the action of thrombin on fibrinogen. The enzymatic cleavage responsible for the release of this protein fragment produces fibrin as well as the fibrinopeptides A and B. The latter consist of short peptides derived from the N-terminal ends of the alpha and beta chains of the fibrinogen molecule. See also **fibrinogen, thrombin.**

fibrin-stabilizing factor. See **factor XIII.**

fibro-, a combining form meaning 'pertaining to fiber': *fibroadipose, fibroblast, fibroelastosis.*

fibroadenoma /fī'brō·ad'inō'mə/, *pl.* **fibroadenomas, fibroadenomata,** a benign tumor composed of dense epithelial and fibroblastic tissue. A fibroadenoma of the breast is nontender, encapsulated, round, movable, and firm. It occurs most frequently in women under 25 years of age and is caused by greater than usual amounts of estrogen. Surgical excision under local anesthesia and cytologic examination of the mass are usually performed to be sure it is not cancerous.

fibroangioma. See **angiofibroma.**

fibroareolar tissue. See **areolar tissue.**

fibroblast, a flat, elongated undifferentiated cell in the connective tissue that gives rise to various precursor cells, as the chondroblast, collagenoblast, and osteoblast, that form the fibrous, binding, and supporting tissue of the body. Also called **desmocyte, fibrocyte. –fibroblastic,** *adj.*

fibroblastoma, *pl.* **fibroblastomas, fibroblastomata,** a tumor derived from a fibroblast, now differentiated as a fibroma or a fibrosarcoma.

fibrocarcinoma. See **scirrhous carcinoma.**

fibrocartilage, cartilage that consists of a dense matrix of white collagenous fibers. Of the three kinds of cartilage in the body, fibrocartilage has the greatest tensile strength. Fibrocartilaginous disks between the vertebrae help to cushion the jolts to which the vertebral column is continually subjected. See also **elastic cartilage, hyaline cartilage. –fibrocartilaginous,** *adj.*

fibrocartilaginous joint. See **symphysis.**

fibrocystic disease, **1.** (of the breast) the presence of single or multiple cysts in the breasts. The cysts are benign and fairly common, yet must be considered potentially malignant and observed carefully for growth or change. Women with fibrocystic disease of the breast are at greater than usual risk of developing breast cancer later in life. The cysts can be aspirated and a biopsy performed. In most cases no treatment is required. The nurse must vigorously counsel women who have fibrocystic disease to examine their own breasts frequently. A woman is shown any cysts present, palpation is taught, and the importance of any change is emphasized. Reassurance should also be given that the condition is very common and generally not associated with cancer. Also called **chronic cystic mastitis. 2.** See **cystic fibrosis.**

fibrocyte. See **fibroblast.**

fibroelastic tissue. See **fibrous tissue.**

fibroepithelial papilloma, a benign epithelial tumor containing extensive fibrous tissue. Also called **fibropapilloma.**

fibroepithelioma /fī'brō·ep'ithē'lē·ō'mə/, *pl.* **fibroepitheliomas, fibroepitheliomata,** a neoplasm consisting of fibrous and epithelial components. A kind of fibroepithelioma is **premalignant fibroepithelioma.**

fibroid /fī'broid/, **1.** having fibers. **2.** *informal.* a fibroma or myoma, particularly of the uterus.

fibroid tumor. See **fibroma.**

fibroma /fībrō'mə/, *pl.* **fibromas, fibromata,** a benign neoplasm consisting largely of fibrous or fully developed connective tissue. See also specific fibromas.

-fibroma, a combining form meaning a 'benign tumor made up of fibrous tissue': *neurofibroma, hemangiofibroma, lymphangiofibroma.*

fibroma cavernosum, a tumor containing large vascular spaces, an excessive amount of fibrous tissue, and blood or lymph vessels.

fibroma cutis, a fibrous tumor of the skin.

fibroma durum. See **hard fibroma.**

fibroma molle. See **soft fibroma.**

fibroma mucinosum, a fibrous tumor in which there is mucoid material with degeneration.

fibroma myxomatodes. See **myxofibroma.**

fibroma pendulum, a pendulous fibrous tumor of the skin.

fibroma sarcomatosum. See **fibrosarcoma.**

fibroma thecocellulare xanthomatodes. See **theca cell tumor.**

fibromatosis, a gingival enlargement believed to be hereditary, manifesting in the permanent dentition and characterized by a firm hyperplastic tissue that covers the surfaces of the teeth. Differentiation between this condition and diphenylhydantoin hyperplasia is based on a history of drug ingestion.

fibromyoma uteri. See **leiomyoma uteri.**

fibromyositis /fī'brōmī'əsī'tis/, any one of a large number of disorders in which the common element is stiffness and joint or muscle pain, accompanied by localized inflammation of the muscle tissues and of the fibrous connective tissues. The condition may develop after climatic change, infection, or physical or emotional trauma. Fibromyositis may recur and become chronic. Treatment includes rest, heat, massage, salicylates, and, in severe cases, intraarticular injections of a corticosteroid and procaine. Kinds of fibromyositis include **lumbago, pleurodynia,** and **torticollis.** See also **rheumatism.**

fibropapilloma. See **fibroepithelial papilloma.**

fibrosarcoma, *pl.* **fibrosarcomas, fibrosarcomata,** a sarcoma that contains connective tissue. It develops suddenly from small nodules on the skin; metastases often occur before the nodules begin to change.

fibrosing alveolitis /fī′brōsing/, a severe form of alveolitis characterized by dyspnea and hypoxia, occurring in advanced rheumatoid arthritis and other autoimmune diseases. X-ray films show thickening of the alveolar septa and diffuse pulmonary infiltrates. See also **alveolitis.**

fibrosis /fībrō′sis/, **1.** a proliferation of fibrous connective tissue. The process occurs normally in the formation of scar tissue to replace normal tissue lost through injury or infection. **2.** an abnormal condition in which fibrous connective tissue spreads over or replaces normal smooth muscle or other normal organ tissue. Fibrosis is most common in the heart, lung, peritoneum, and kidney. See also **cystic fibrosis, fibrositis.**

fibrositis /fī′brəsī′tis/, an inflammation of fibrous connective tissue, usually characterized by a poorly defined set of symptoms, including pain and stiffness of the neck, shoulder, and trunk. Fibrositis usually develops in middle age. There are no objectively measurable signs on radiologic examination. The person is often tense, and the origin of the condition may be psychogenic. Salicylates, sedatives, tranquilizers, muscle relaxants, and intraarticular injection of a local anesthetic may be prescribed in treatment. Compare **fibromyositis, myositis.**

fibrous, consisting mainly of fibers or fiber-containing materials, as fibrous connective tissue. See also **fibrosis.**

-fibrous, a combining form meaning 'composed of fibrous tissue': *cellulofibrous, fibrofibrous, interfibrous.*

fibrous capsule, **1.** the external layer of an articular capsule. It surrounds the articulation of two adjoining bones. **2.** the external, tough membranous envelope surrounding some visceral organs, as the liver. Compare **synovial membrane.**

fibrous dysplasia, an abnormal condition characterized by the fibrous displacement of the osseous tissue within the bones affected. The specific cause of fibrous dysplasia is unknown, but indications are that the disease is of developmental or congenital origin. The distinct kinds of fibrous dysplasia are monostotic fibrous dysplasia, polyostotic fibrous dysplasia, and polyostotic fibrous dysplasia with associated endocrine disorders. Any bone may be affected with monostotic fibrous dysplasia. The polyostotic type usually displays a segmental distribution of the involved bones, all of which show varying degrees of the characteristic fibrous replacement of the osseous tissue. The onset of fibrous dysplasia is usually during childhood, progressing beyond puberty and through adulthood. The onset of symptoms is usually during childhood although diagnosis may be delayed until adolescence or even early adulthood if symptoms are minimal. The initial signs may be a limp, a pain, or a fracture on the affected side. Girls affected may have an early onset of menses and breast development and early epiphyseal closure. Albright's syndrome is usually diagnosed on the basis of a triad of symptoms, including the polyostotic type of fibrous dysplasia, café-au-lait patches on the skin, and precocious puberty. Pathologic fractures are frequently associated with this process, and angulation deformities may follow. The involved extremity may be shortened, and the classic ''shepherd's crook'' deformity is common. Radiographic examination usually reveals a well-circumscribed lesion occupying all or a portion of the shaft of the long bone involved. Pathologic fractures in patients with fibrous dysplasia usually heal with conservative treatment, but residual deformities often remain. When symptoms are mild and limited, this disease usually progresses slowly. Radiation therapy is not employed because it may provoke malignant degeneration. Biopsies are commonly performed if pain increases or if alterations are seen on radiographic examination.

fibrous goiter, an enlargement of the thyroid gland, characterized by hyperplasia of the capsule and connective tissue.

fibrous gold. See **gold foil.**

fibrous histiocytoma. See **dermatofibroma.**

fibrous joint, any one of many immovable joints, as those of the skull segments, in which a fibrous tissue or a hyaline cartilage connects the bones. The three kinds of articulation associated with fibrous joints are syndesmosis, sutura, and gomphosis. Also called **junctura fibrosa, synarthrosis.** Compare **cartilaginous joint, synovial joint.**

fibrous thyroiditis, a disorder characterized by slowly progressive fibrosis of an enlarged thyroid with replacement of normal thyroid tissue by dense fibrous tissue. The gland eventually becomes fixed to the adjacent muscles, nerves, blood vessels, and trachea by means of this fibrous tissue. The disease occurs more frequently in women than in men and usually arises after the age of 40. Symptoms include a choking sensation, dyspnea, dysphagia, and hypothyroidism, but in some patients the gland functions normally. Treatment includes surgical excision and thyroid hormone administered postoperatively, as required. Also called **ligneous thyroiditis, Riedel's struma, Riedel's thyroiditis.**

fibrous tissue, the fibrous connective tissue of the body, consisting of closely woven elastic fibers and fluid-filled areolae. Also called **fibroelastic tissue.** Compare **areolar tissue.**

fibula /fib′yo͞olə/, the bone of the leg, lateral to and smaller than the tibia. In proportion to its length, it is the most slender of the long bones and presents three borders and three surfaces, attaching to various muscles, including the peronei longus and brevis and the soleus longus. Also called **calf bone.**

Fick principle, a method for making indirect measurements, based on the law of conservation of mass. It is used specifically to determine cardiac output, in which the amount of oxygen uptake of each unit of blood as it passes through the lungs is equal to the oxygen concentration difference between arterial and mixed venous blood. Cardiac output is calculated by measuring the uptake of oxygen for a given period of time, noted as milliliters per minute, then dividing that ratio by the difference in oxygen saturation of arterial and mixed venous blood samples in milliliters per 100 ml of blood, and multiplying the total by 100.

Fick's law, **1.** (in chemistry and physics) an observed law stating that the rate at which one substance diffuses through another is directly proportional to the concentration gradient of the diffusing substance. **2.** (in medicine) an observed law stating that the rate of diffusion across a membrane is directly proportional to the concentration gradient of the substance on the two sides of the membrane and inversely related to the thickness of the membrane.

field fever, a form of leptospirosis caused by *Leptospira grippotyphosa,* affecting primarily agricultural workers. It is characterized by fever, abdominal pain, diarrhea, vomiting, stupor, and conjunctivitis. Also called **canefield fever, harvest fever.** See also **leptospirosis.**

fiery serpent, an informal term for *Dracunculus medinesis.* See also **dracunculiasis.**

fifth disease. See **erythema infectiosum.**

fifth nerve. See **trigeminal nerve.**

FIGLU, abbreviation for **formiminoglutamic acid.**

figure-ground relationship, a perceptual field that is divided into a figure, which is the object of focus, and a diffuse background.

figure-of-eight bandage, a bandage with successive laps crossing over and around each other like the figure eight. See also **bandage.**

fila-, a combining form meaning 'pertaining to a thread, or threadlike': *filaceous, filamentous, filaria.*

filament, a fine threadlike fiber. Filaments are found in most tissues and cells of the body and serve various morphologic or physiologic functions.

filariasis /fil′ərī′əsis/, a disease caused by the presence of filariae or microfilariae in the tissues of the body. Filarial worms are round, long, and threadlike and are common in most tropic and subtropic regions of the world. They tend to infest the lymph glands and channels after entering the body as microscopic larvae through the bite of a mosquito or other insect. The infection is characterized by occlusion of the lymphatic vessels, with swelling and pain of the limb distal to the blockage. After many years, the limb may become greatly swollen and the skin coarse and tough. Treatment is by oral administration of diethylcarbamazine. The most effective means of preventing infestation is mosquito control. See also **elephantiasis.**

filial generation, the offspring produced from a given mating or cross in a genetic sequence. See also $\mathbf{F_1}$, $\mathbf{F_2}$.

filiform bougie, an extremely thin bougie for passage through a narrow stricture, as a sinus tract.

filiform catheter, a catheter with a slender, threadlike tip that allows the wider portion of the instrument to be passed through canals that are constricted or irregular because of an obstruction or an angulation in the canal. It may bypass obstructions or dilate strictures.

filiform papilla. See **papilla.**

filling factor, a measure of the geometric relationship of a radiofrequency coil used in NMR imaging and the body. This relationship affects the efficiency of irradiating the body and detecting NMR signals, and thereby affects the signal-to-noise ratio and, ultimately, image quality. Achieving a high filling factor requires fitting the coil closely to the body, thus potentially decreasing patient comfort.

film, **1.** a thin sheet or layer of any material, as a coating of oil on a metal part. **2.** (in photography and radiography) a thin, flexible, transparent sheet of cellulose acetate or similar material coated with a light-sensitive emulsion, used to record images, as of organs, structures, and tissues that may be involved in disease and diagnoses.

film badge, a photographic film packet, sensitive to ionizing radiation, used for estimating the exposure of personnel working with x-rays and other radioactive sources.

film fault, a defect in a photograph or radiograph, usually caused by a chemical, physical, or electric error in its production.

film on teeth, a collection of mucinous deposits adhering to the teeth, which contains microorganisms, desquamated tissue elements, blood cellular elements, and other debris. See also **plaque.**

filtered back projection, a mathematic technique used in NMR imaging and computed tomography to create images from a set of multiple projection profiles.

filtration, the addition of sheets of metal into a beam of x-rays, altering the energy spectrum and thus the imaging characteristics and penetrating ability of the radiation. Filtration is generally provided by aluminum or copper at low to medium energies, and by tin, copper, and aluminum for higher energy beams.

fimbria, any structure that forms a border or edge or that resembles a fringe. Kinds of fimbria are **fimbria hippocampi, fimbria ovarica,** and **fimbriae tubae.** See also **pilus,** def. 2.

fimbriae tubae, the branched, fingerlike projections at the distal end of each of the fallopian tubes. The projections are connected to the ovary and have epithelial cells with cilia that serve to move the ovum toward the uterus.

fimbria hippocampi, a band of efferent fibers formed by the alveus hippocampi that is continuous with the posterior pillar of the fornix.

fimbrial tubal pregnancy, a kind of tubal pregnancy in which implantation occurs in the fimbriated distal end of one of the fallopian tubes. See also **tubal pregnancy.**

fimbria ovarica, the longest of the fimbriae tubae. It extends from the infundibulum to the ovary. Also called **fimbriated extremity.**

fineness, (in dentistry) a means of grading alloys relative to gold content. The fineness of an alloy is designated in parts per thousand of pure gold, which is 1000 fine. Gold alloys and pure gold may be used in dental restorations, as in some tooth crowns and prepared tooth cavity fillings.

finger, any of the digits of the hand. The fingers of the hand are composed of a metacarpal bone and three bony phalanges. Some anatomists regard the thumb as a finger, since its metacarpal bone ossifies in the same way as a phalanx. Other anatomists regard the thumb as being composed of a metacarpal bone and two phalanges. The digits of the hand are anatomically numbered 1 to 5, starting with the thumb.

finger percussion. See **percussion.**

Finnish bath. See **Russian bath.**

FiO_2, the percentage of inspired oxygen a patient is receiving, usually expressed as a fraction.

Fiorinal, a trademark for a group of fixed-combination drugs containing a sedative-hypnotic (butalbital), an analgesic, antipyretic, and antiinflammatory (aspirin), an analgesic (phenacetin), and a central nervous system stimulant (caffeine).

fire damp. See **damp.**

fireman's cramp. See **heat cramp.**

firmware, computer routines, instructions, and programs that are unalterable and are permanently fixed on a **Read Only Memory (ROM)** chip. See also **hardware, software, wetware.**

first aid, the immediate care that is given to an injured or ill person before to treatment by medically trained personnel. Attention is directed first to the most critical problems: evaluation of the patency of the airway, the presence of bleeding, and the adequacy of cardiac function. The patient is kept warm and as comfortable as possible. The conscious patient is reassured and is queried for significant details of his medical history, as diabetes, a known heart condition, or allergic reactions to drugs; if the patient is unconscious, a medical identification card, bracelet, or necklace is sought. The patient is moved as little as possible, particularly if there is a possibility of fracture. If there is vomiting, the patient's head is moved to a position for the vomitus to exit easily to avoid aspiration. See also **cardiopulmonary resuscitation, control of hemorrhage, emergency medicine, emergency nursing.**

first cuneiform. See **medial cuneiform bone.**

first dentition. See **deciduous dentition.**

first-dollar coverage, an insurance plan under which the third-party payer assumes liability for covered services as soon as the first dollar of expense for such services is incurred, without requiring the insured to pay a deductible.

first filial generation. See **F_1.**

first intention. See **intention.**

first metacarpal bone, the metacarpal bone of the thumb.

first nerve. See **olfactory nerve.**

first-state cementoma. See **periapical fibroma.**

fish tapeworm infection, an infection caused by the tapeworm *Diphyllobothrium latum* that is transmitted to humans when they eat contaminated raw or undercooked freshwater fish. Fish tapeworm infection is common in temperate zones throughout the world and is found in the Great Lakes region of the United States. See also ***diphyllobothrium*, tapeworm infection.**

fiss-, a combining form meaning 'pertaining to a split or cleft': *fissile, fissiparous, fissula.*

fission, **1.** the act or process of splitting or breaking up into parts. **2.** a type of asexual reproduction common in bacteria, protozoa, and other lower forms of life in which the cell divides into two or more equal components, each of which eventually develops into a complete organism. Kinds of fission are **binary fission** and **multiple fission.** **3.** also called **nuclear fission.** (in physics) the splitting of the nucleus of an atom and subsequent release of energy.

fissiparous /fisip'ərəs/, reproduced by fission.

fissural angioma /fish'ərəl/, a tumor composed of a cluster of dilated blood vessels found in an embryonal fissure, especially on a lip, the face, or the neck.

fissure /fish'ər/, **1.** a cleft or a groove on the surface of an organ, often marking division of the organ into parts, as the lobes of the lung. **2.** a cracklike lesion of the skin, as an anal fissure. **3.** a lineal fault on a bony surface occurring during the development of a part, as a fissure in the enamel of a tooth. A fissure is usually deeper than a sulcus but, in the terminology of anatomy, *fissure* and *sulcus* are often used interchangeably. Also called **fissura.** Compare **sulcus.** **–fissured,** *adj.*

fissure fracture, any fracture in which a crack extends into the cortex of the bone but not through the entire bone.

fissure of Bichat. See **transverse fissure.**

fissure of Rolando. See **central sulcus.**

fissure of Sylvius. See **lateral cerebral sulcus.**

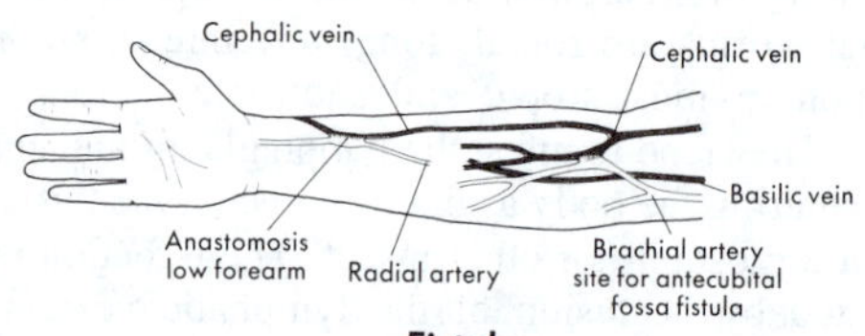

Fistula

fistula /fis'cho͝olə, -chələ/, *pl.* **fistulas, fistulae,** an abnormal passage from an internal organ to the body surface or between two internal organs, as a hepatopleural or pulmonoperitoneal fistula, caused by a congenital defect, injury, infection, the spreading of a malignant lesion, radiotherapy of a cancerous growth, or trauma during childbirth. Fistulas may occur in many sites from the gingiva to the anus and may be created for therapeutic purposes or to obtain body secretions for physiologic studies. An arteriovenous fistula is commonly created to gain access to the patient's bloodstream for the administration of hemodialysis. Anal fistulas resulting from rupture or drainage of abscesses may be treated by fistulectomy or fistulotomy, and fistulas between the vagina and bladder, urethra, ureter, or rectum may be repaired surgically, but the results are not always successful. **–fistulous, fistular, fistulate,** *adj.*

fistula in ano. See **anal fistula.**

fit, **1.** *nontechnical.* a paroxysm or seizure. **2.** the sudden onset of an episode of symptoms, as a fit of coughing. **3.** the manner in which one surface is aligned to another, as the fit of a denture to the gingiva and jaw.

Fitzgerald treatment. See **zone therapy.**

five-day fever, *informal.* trench fever.

five-step nursing process, a nursing process comprising five broad categories of nursing behaviors: assessing, analyzing, planning, implementing, and evaluating. The nurse gathers information about the client, identifies the specific needs of the client, develops a plan of care with the client to answer these needs, implements the plan of care, and evaluates the effects of the implementation. The nurse involves the client, the client's family, and significant others in each step of the process to the greatest extent possible and compensates for and acknowledges the factors that might influence the provision of care by the nurse and staff. Implicit in the nursing process is a therapeutic and personal relationship between the nurse, the client, the client's family, and significant others. See also **nursing process.**

five-year survival, a benchmark in the evaluation of response to therapy for cancer patients. The raw data are corrected for expected deaths from other causes by actuarial methods.

fixating eye, (in strabismus) the normal eye that can be focused. Compare **squinting eye.**

fixation, (in psychoanalysis) an arrest at a particular stage of psychosexual development, as anal fixation. **–fixate,** *v.*, **fixated,** *adj.*

fixation muscle, a muscle that acts to hold a part of the body in appropriate position. Compare **antagonist, prime mover, synergist.**

fixative, **1.** any substance used to bind, glue, or stabilize. **2.** any substance used to preserve gross or histologic specimens of tissue for later examination.

fixed bridgework, a dental device incorporating artificial teeth permanently attached in the upper or the lower jaw.

fixed-combination drug, any of a group of multiple-ingredient preparations that provides concomitant administration of specific amounts of two or more drugs.

fixed coupling, a precise distance between a normal and ectopic beat that is duplicated each time the ectopic beat occurs.

fixed dressing, a dressing usually made of gauze impregnated with a hardening agent, as plaster of paris, sodium silicate, starch, or dextrin, applied to support or immobilize a part of the body. The dressing is soaked in water, applied to the part to be immobilized, and allowed to harden. See also **cast.**

fixed drug eruption, a circumscribed skin lesion either persisting or recurring in the same location, caused by continuing or repeated exposure to a sensitizing drug.

fixed idea, **1.** a persistent, obsessional thought or notion. **2.** in certain mental disorders, especially obsessive-compulsive neurosis, a delusional idea that dominates mental activity and persists despite contrary evidence or rational refutation. Also called **idée fixe** /idā′fiks′/.

fixed orthodontic appliance, a prosthetic device cemented to the teeth or attached by adhesive material, for changing the relative positions of dentitions.

fixed phagocyte. See **phagocyte.**

flaccid /flak′sid/, weak, soft, and flabby; lacking normal muscle tone, as flaccid muscles. **–flaccidity, flaccidness,** *n.*

flaccid bladder, a form of neurogenic bladder caused by interruption of the reflex arc associated with the voiding reflex in the spinal cord. It is marked by continual filling and occasional overfilling of the bladder, absence of bladder sensation, and inability to urinate voluntarily. It is most often produced by trauma. The bladder can be emptied by pressure to the area. Also called **atonic bladder, autonomous bladder, nonreflex bladder.** Compare **spastic bladder.**

flaccid paralysis, an abnormal condition characterized by the weakening or the loss of muscle tone. It may be caused by disease or by trauma affecting the nerves associated with the involved muscles. Compare **spastic paralysis.**

flagell-, a combining form meaning 'pertaining to a whiplike process, tapping': *flagellation, flagelliform, flagellospore.*

flagella, hairlike projections that extend from some unicellular organisms and aid in their movement.

flagellant, a person who receives sexual gratification from the practice of flagellation.

flagellate /flaj′əlāt′, -lit/, a microorganism that propels itself by waving whiplike filaments or cilia behind its body, as *Trypanosoma, Leishmania, Trichomonas,* and *Giardia.* See also **protozoa.**

flagellation, **1.** the act of whipping, beating, or flogging. **2.** a type of massage administered by tapping the body with the fingers. See also **massage.** **3.** a type of sexual deviation in which a person is erotically gratified by being whipped or by whipping another. See also **masochism, sadism.** **4.** the arrangement of flagella on an organism; exflagellation.

Flagyl, a trademark for an antiprotozoal (metronidazole).

flail chest, a thorax in which multiple rib fractures cause instability in part of the chest wall and paradoxical breathing, with the lung underlying the injured area contracting on inspiration and bulging on expiration. The condition, if uncorrected, leads to hypoxia.

■ OBSERVATIONS: Flail chest is characterized by sharp pain, uneven chest expansion, shallow, rapid respirations, and decreased breath sounds. Tachycardia and cyanosis may be present, and potential complications are atelectasis, pneumothorax, hemothorax, cardiac tamponade, shock, and respiratory arrest.

■ INTERVENTION: The treatment of choice is internal stabilization of the chest wall through the use of a volume-controlled ventilator with a cuffed tracheostomy tube or endotracheal tube. If the patient breathes against the automatic ventilator, a sedative and muscle relaxant may be ordered to achieve ventilatory control. Chest tubes may be required to remove air or fluid preventing expansion of the affected lung, and a nasogastric tube may be ordered to provide food and fluids. The patient's blood pressure, pulse, respirations, and breath sounds are checked every 1 to 2 hours, the rectal temperature every 2 to 4 hours, and arterial blood gases are determined as ordered. Traction is less frequently used in treating flail chest but may be applied by attaching a steel wire to the ribs or sternum under local anesthesia and connecting the wire to a rope, pulley, and weight.

■ NURSING CONSIDERATIONS: The patient with flail chest usually requires a long period of care involving frequent repositioning, scrupulous attention to the patency and cleanliness of the tracheostomy or endotracheal tube, skin care, oral hygiene, and emotional support. The nurse performs passive range-of-motion exercises to the extremities, explains the various procedures, and provides a pad and pencil or a magic slate so that the patient is able to communicate.

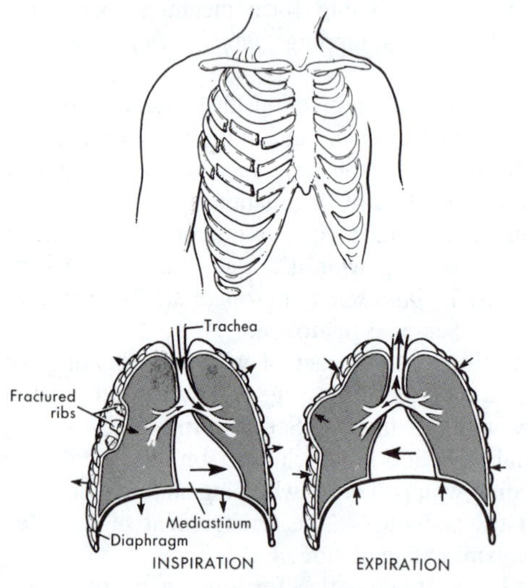

Flail chest

flame photometry, measurement of the wavelength of light rays emitted by excited metallic electrons exposed to the heat energy of a flame, used to identify characteristics in clinical specimens of body fluids. The intensity of the emitted light is proportional to the concentration of atoms in the fluid, and a quantitative analysis can be made on that basis. In the clinical laboratory, flame photometry is used to measure sodium, potassium, and lithium levels.

flange, **1.** the part of a denture base that extends from the cervical ends of the teeth to the border of the denture. **2.** a prosthesis with a lateral vertical extension designed to direct a resected mandible into centric occlusion.

flapping tremor. See **asterixis.**

flare, **1.** a red blush on the skin at the periphery of an urticarial lesion seen in immediate hypersensitivity reactions. **2.** an expanding skin flush, spreading from an infective lesion or extending from the principal site of a reaction to an irritant. **3.** the sudden intensification of a disease.

flaring of nostrils, a widening of the nostrils during inspiration, a sign of air hunger or respiratory distress.

flask closure, (in dentistry) the joining of two halves of a flask that encloses and forms a denture base. Compare **closure, velopharyngeal closure.**

Flatau-Schilder disease. See **Schilder's disease.**

flat electroencephalogram, a graphic chart on which no tracings were recorded during electroencephalography, indicating a lack of brain-wave activity. Flat readings are indicative of death except in cases of profound hypothermia and central nervous system depression. Also called **isoelectric electroencephalogram.**

flatfoot. See **pes planus.**

flat spring contraceptive diaphragm, a kind of contraceptive diaphragm in which the flexible metal spring that forms the rim is a thin, light, flat band made of stainless steel. The rubber dome is approximately 1.5 inches deep, and the diameter of the rubber-covered rim is between 5.5 and 10 cm. Ten sizes, in increments of 5 mm, allow the clinician to fit the diaphragm to each individual woman. The kind of spring and the size of the rim in millimeters is stamped on the rim, as, for example, 75 mm flat spring. This kind of diaphragm is prescribed for a woman whose vaginal musculature provides good support, whose uterus is in the normal position and not acutely retroflexed or anteflexed, and whose vagina, neither very long nor very short, has a shallow arch behind the symphysis pubis. The flat spring diaphragm offers protection equal to the other kinds of diaphragm if it is appropriate for the woman and is correctly fitted. It is preferred by many women because it is very light and comfortable to use. Compare **arcing spring contraceptive diaphragm, coil spring contraceptive diaphragm.** See also **contraceptive diaphragm fitting.**

flatulence, the presence of an excessive amount of air or gas in the stomach and intestinal tract, causing distension of the organs and in some cases mild to moderate pain.

flatus /flā'təs/, air or gas in the intestine that is passed through the rectum. See also **aerophagia.**

flat wart. See **verruca plana.**

flav-, a combining form meaning 'yellow': *flavescens, flavin, flavism.*

flavone /flā′vōn/, a colorless, crystalline, flavonoid derivative and component of bioflavonoid that increases capillary resistance.

flavoxate hydrochloride, a smooth muscle relaxant.
■ INDICATION: It is prescribed for spastic conditions of the urinary tract.
■ CONTRAINDICATIONS: GI hemorrhage or obstruction, urinary tract obstruction, or known hypersensitivity to this drug prohibits its use.
■ ADVERSE EFFECTS: Among the more serious adverse reactions are nervousness, nausea, abdominal pain, fever, and tachycardia.

Flaxedil, a trademark for a neuromuscular blocking agent (gallamine triethiodide), used as an adjunct to general anesthesia.

flea, a wingless, bloodsucking insect of the order Siphonaptera, some species of which transmit arboviruses to humans by acting as host or vector to the organism.

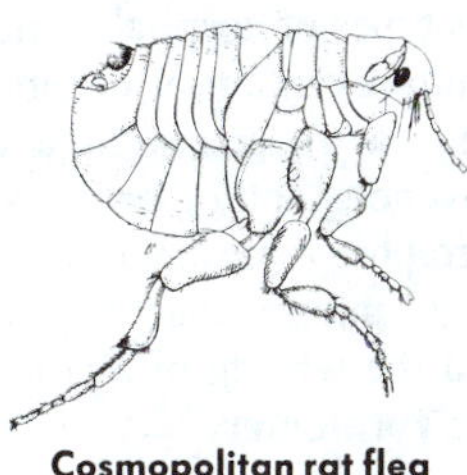

Cosmopolitan rat flea

flea bite, a small puncture wound produced by a bloodsucking flea. Certain species of fleas transmit plague, murine typhus, and probably tularemia.

flea bites, *informal.* erythema toxicum neonatorum.

flea-borne typhus. See **murine typhus.**

-flect, a combining form meaning 'to bend': *anteflect, circumflect.*

Fleet Theophylline, a trademark for a smooth muscle relaxant (theophylline ethanolamine), administered rectally as a bronchodilator.

FLEX, abbreviation for **Federation Licensing Examination.**

Flexeril, a trademark for a muscle relaxant (cyclobenzaprine hydrochloride).

flexibilitas cerea. See **cerea flexibilitas.**

Flexical, a trademark for a nutritional supplement containing protein, carbohydrate, and fat.

flexion /flek′shən/, a movement allowed by certain joints of the skeleton that decreases the angle between two adjoining bones, as bending the elbow, which decreases the angle between the humerus and the ulna. Compare **extension.**

flexor carpi radialis, a slender, superficial muscle of the forearm that lies on the ulnar side of the pronator teres. It arises from the medial epicondyle, the fascia of the forearm, and several intermuscular septa, and it inserts by a long tendon into the base of the second metacarpal bone. Fibers of the muscle extend to the base of the third metacarpal bone. The flexor carpi radialis is innervated by a branch of the median nerve that contains fibers from the sixth and the seventh cervical nerves, and it functions to flex and to help abduct the hand. Compare **flexor carpi ulnaris, palmaris longus.**

flexor carpi ulnaris, a superficial muscle lying along the ulnar side of the forearm that arises in a humeral and an ulnar head and inserts in a long tendon into the pisiform bone, extending by ligaments to the hamate and the fifth metacarpal bones. It is innervated by a branch of the ulnar nerve, which contains fibers from the eighth cervical and the first thoracic nerves. The flexor carpi ulnaris functions to flex and adduct the hand. Compare **flexor carpi radialis, palmaris longus.**

flexor digitorum superficialis, the largest superficial muscle of the forearm, lying on the ulnar side under the palmaris longus, arising by a humeral, an ulnar, and a radial head. The humeral head originates in the medial epicondyle of the humerus, in the ulnar collateral ligament of the elbow joint, and in various intermuscular septa; the ulnar head originates in the medial side of the coronoid process; the radial head originates in the oblique line of the radius. The muscle separates into a superficial layer and a deep layer and inserts by four tendons into the second phalanx of the fingers. The flexor digitorum superficialis is innervated by branches of the median nerve that contains fibers from the seventh and the eighth cervical and the first thoracic nerves. The muscle flexes the second phalanx of each finger and, by continued action, the hand. Also called **flexor digitorum sublimis.** Compare **flexor carpi radialis, flexor carpi ulnaris, palmaris longus, pronator teres.**

flexor retinaculum of the hand. See **retinaculum flexorum manus.**

flextime, a system of staffing that allows the individualization of work schedules. A person working days might choose to work from 7 to 3, 9 to 5, or other hours. Full staffing must be maintained, but within the group flextime can be arranged. Use of the system tends to improve morale and decrease turnover. Also called **flexitime.**

flight into health, an abnormal but common reaction to an unpleasant physical sensation or symptom in which the person denies the reality of the feeling or observation, insisting that there is nothing wrong. See also **illness experience.**

flight of ideas, (in psychiatry) a continuous stream of talk in which the patient switches rapidly from one topic to another, each subject being incoherent and not related to the preceding one or stimulated by some environmental circumstance. The condition is frequently a symptom of acute manic states and schizophrenia. Compare **circumstantiality.**

flight-or-fight reaction, **1.** (in physiology) the reaction of the body to stress, in which the sympathetic nervous system and the adrenal medulla act to increase the cardiac output, dilate the pupils of the eyes, increase the rate of the heartbeat, constrict the blood vessels of the skin, increase the glucose and fatty acids in the circulation, and induce an alert, aroused mental state. **2.** (in psychiatry) a person's reaction to stress by either fleeing from a situation or remaining and attempting to deal with it.

flip angle, in NMR imaging, the amount of rotation of the macroscopic magnetization vector produced by a radiofrequency pulse with respect to the direction of the static magnetic field.

floater, one or more spots that appear to drift in front of the eye, caused by a shadow cast on the retina by vitreous debris. Most floaters are benign and represent remnants of a network of blood vessels that existed prenatally in the vitreous cavity. The sudden onset of several floaters may indicate serious disease. Hemorrhage into the vitreous humor may cause a large number of big and little shadows and a red discoloration of vision. The cause is often traumatic injury, but spontaneous intraocular hemorrhage is seen in severe diabetes mellitus, hypertension, or increased intracranial pressure. Cancer, detachment of the retina, occlusion of a retinal vein, and other purely ocular diseases may also cause hemorrhage into the vitreous cavity. Inflammation of the retina resulting from chorioretinitis may cause entry of inflammatory cells into the vitreous humor. Inflammatory debris may adhere to the vitreous framework in netlike masses that are very disruptive of normal vision. Retinal detachment also causes a sudden appearance of lightninglike floaters and a diminished field of vision as a shower of red cells and pigment is released into the vitreous humor. Careful ophthalmologic examination through a well-dilated pupil is recommended for all people who experience a sudden occurrence of floaters, because each of the pathologic causes can be treated in the early stages and loss of vision can usually be avoided. The technical term for floaters is **muscae volitantes.**

floating head, unengaged fetal head. See also **ballottement, engagement.**

floating kidney, a kidney that is not securely fixed in the usual anatomic location because of congenital malplacement or traumatic injury. Compare **ptotic kidney.**

floating rib. See **rib.**

float nurse, a nurse who is available for assignment to duty on an ad hoc basis, usually to assist in times of unusually heavy work loads or to assume the duties of absent nursing personnel. A float nurse is recruited from a group of nurses called a float pool.

flocculant /flok′yo͝olənt/, an agent or substance that causes flocculation.

flocculation test /flok′yo͝olā′shən/, a serologic test in which a positive result depends on the degree of flocculent precipitation produced in the material being tested. Many tests for syphilis, including the VDRL slide test, are flocculation tests.

flocculent /flok′yo͝olənt/, clumped or tufted, as a cloud, or covered with a woolly, fuzzy surface. **–flocculate,** *v.*, **flocculation, floccule,** *n.*

flood fever. See **typhus.**

flooding, a technique used in behavior therapy for the reduction of anxiety associated with various phobias. Exposure to a stimulus that usually provokes anxiety desensitizes a person to that stimulus, thereby reducing fear and anxiety. Also called **implosive therapy.** Compare **systemic desensitization.**

floppy, floppy disk. See **diskette.**

floppy infant syndrome, a general term for juvenile spinal muscular atrophies, including Werdnig-Hoffmann disease and Wohlfart-Kugelberg-Welander disease.

Florinef Acetate, a trademark for an adrenocortical steroid (fludrocortisone acetate).

Florone, a trademark for an antiinflammatory agent (diflorasone diacetate).

Floropryl, a trademark for an inhibitor of cholinesterase (isoflurophate), used ophthalmically.

flotation therapy, a state of semiweightlessness produced by various types of hospital equipment and used in the treatment and prevention of decubitus ulcers.

Flo-Trol clamp, a trademark of a triggerlike off-on control for intravenous and other infusion lines.

flow chart, a graphic representation of a computer program sequence, an intermediate step between algorithm development and the writing of a computer program.

flowmeter. See **rotameter.**

flow sheet, (in a patient record) a graphic summary of several changing factors, especially the patient's vital signs or weight and the treatments and medications given. In labor, the flow sheet displays the progress of labor, including the centimeters of cervical dilatation, cervical effacement, the position of the baby's head, the baby's heart rate, the frequency of contractions, the mother's temperature and blood pressure, and any medications given or procedures performed.

floxuridine /floksyo͝or′ədēn/, an antineoplastic agent.

▪ INDICATIONS: It is prescribed in the treatment of malignant neoplastic disease of the brain, breast, liver, and gallbladder.

▪ CONTRAINDICATIONS: Bone marrow depression, infection, poor nutritional state, or known hypersensitivity to this drug prohibits its use.

▪ ADVERSE EFFECTS: Among the more serious adverse reactions are severe depression of the bone marrow and acute GI disturbances, including nausea, vomiting, diarrhea, and stomatitis. Alopecia and dermatitis commonly occur.

flu, *informal.* **1.** influenza. **2.** any viral infection, especially of the respiratory or intestinal system.

Fluax, a trademark for an active immunizing agent (influenza whole virus vaccine).

flucytosine /flo͞osī′təsēn/, an antifungal.

▪ INDICATION: It is prescribed in the treatment of certain serious fungal infections.

■ CONTRAINDICATIONS: Known hypersensitivity to this drug prohibits its use. Close monitoring is required when administering this drug to patients with renal disorders or bone marrow depression.
■ ADVERSE EFFECTS: Among the more serious adverse reactions are GI disturbances, including enterocolitis, abnormal liver function, hepatomegaly, and bone marrow depression.

fludrocortisone acetate /flo͞o′drōkôr′təsōn/, a mineralocorticosteroid.
■ INDICATIONS: It is prescribed in the treatment of Addison's disease and in salt-losing adrenogenital syndrome. It is not used as a glucocorticoid.
■ CONTRAINDICATIONS: Systemic fungal infections or known hypersensitivity to this drug prohibits its use.
■ ADVERSE EFFECTS: Among the more serious adverse reactions are salt and water retention. This drug has the potential for the adverse effects of glucocorticoids, including peptic ulcer, hyperglycemia, mental disturbances, and adrenal failure.

-fluent, a combining form meaning 'flowing': *diffluent, ossifluent*.

fluid, **1.** a substance, as a liquid or gas, that is able to flow and to adjust its shape to that of a container because it is composed of molecules that are able to change positions with respect to each other without separating from the total mass. **2.** a body fluid, either intracellular or extracellular, that is involved in the transport of electrolytes and other vital chemicals to, through, and from tissue cells. See also **blood, lymph, cerebrospinal fluid.**

fluid dram. See **dram,** def. 2.

fluid ounce, a measure of liquid volume in the apothecaries' system, which is equal to 8 fluidrams or 29.57 ml. See also **apothecaries' measure, metric system.**

fluid volume, alteration in: excess, a nursing diagnosis accepted by the Fifth National Conference of the Classification of Nursing Diagnoses. The cause of the problem is a compromised regulatory mechanism of the homeostatic mechanisms that regulate the retention and excretion of body fluids or an excess fluid or sodium intake. The defining characteristics of the condition include edema, effusion, weight gain, shortness of breath, third heart sound, pulmonary congestion changes in respiratory pattern and abnormal breath sounds, decreased hemoglobin and hematocrit, blood pressure changes, an alteration in electrolyte balance, and restlessness, anxiety, and other changes in mental status. See also **nursing diagnosis.**

fluid volume deficit, actual, **1.** a nursing diagnosis accepted by the Fourth National Conference on the Classification of Nursing Diagnoses. The cause of the condition is a failure of the body's homeostatic mechanisms that regulate the retention and excretion of body fluids. The defining characteristics of the problem are dilute urine, increased output of urine, and a sudden loss of body weight. Several other characteristics may be observed, including hypotension, increased pulse rate, decreased turgor, increased body temperature, hemoconcentration, weakness, and thirst. **2.** a nursing diagnosis accepted by the Fourth National Conference on the Classification of Nursing Diagnoses. The cause of the condition is the active loss of excessive amounts of body fluid. The defining characteristics of the condition are decreased output of urine, high specific gravity of the urine, output of urine that is greater than the intake of fluid into the body, a sudden loss of weight, hemoconcentration, and increased serum levels of sodium. Other characteristics that may be observed are increased thirst, alteration in the mental state, dryness of skin and mucous membranes, elevated temperature, and an increased pulse rate. See also **nursing diagnosis.**

fluid volume deficit, potential, a nursing diagnosis accepted by the Fifth National Conference on the Classification of Nursing Diagnoses. The cause of the problem is advanced age; excessive weight; extreme loss of fluid through normal routes, as in diarrhea, or abnormal routes, as indwelling tubes; the lack of intake of fluids, as in physical immobility; increased fluid needs, as in hypermetabolic states; and the use of diuretics or other medications affecting the retention and excretion of body fluids. The defining characteristics of the condition include increased fluid output, urinary frequency, thirst, and any alteration in fluid intake. See also **nursing diagnosis.**

fluke, a parasitic flatworm of the class Trematoda, including the genus *Schistosoma*. See also **schistosomiasis.**

flumethasone pivalate, a topical glucocorticoid.
■ INDICATION: It is prescribed as a topical antiinflammatory agent.
■ CONTRAINDICATIONS: Viral and fungal diseases of the skin, impaired circulation, or known hypersensitivity to this drug or to steroid medication prohibits its use.
■ ADVERSE EFFECTS: Among the more serious adverse reactions, usually occurring after prolonged and excessive application, are striae, hypopigmentation, local irritation of the skin, and various systemic effects.

fluocinolone acetonide, a topical glucocorticoid.
■ INDICATION: It is prescribed as an antiinflammatory agent.
■ CONTRAINDICATIONS: Impaired circulation, viral and fungal diseases of the skin, or known hypersensitivity to this drug or to other steroid medication prohibits its use.
■ ADVERSE EFFECTS: Among the more serious adverse reactions are systemic side effects resulting from prolonged use or excessive application. Various hypersensitivity reactions may occur.

fluocinonide /flo͞o′ōsin′ənīd/, a synthetic corticosteroid.
■ INDICATION: It is prescribed to reduce inflammation.
■ CONTRAINDICATIONS: Viral and fungal diseases of the skin, tuberculosis of the skin, or known hypersensitivity to this drug prohibits its use.
■ ADVERSE EFFECTS: Among the more serious adverse

reactions are secondary infections, striae, miliaria, and contact dermatitis.

Fluonid, a trademark for a glucocorticoid (fluocinolone acetonide).

fluorescence /flo͞ores′əns/, the emission of light of one wavelength (usually ultraviolet) when exposed to light of a different, usually shorter, wavelength, a property possessed by certain substances. Fluorescent substances that simultaneously absorb and emit light appear luminous. –**fluoresce,** *v.*, **fluorescent,** *adj.*

fluorescent antibody test (FA test), a test in which a fluorescent dye is used to stain an antibody for identification of clinical specimens. Fluorescent dyes conjugate with immunoglobulins without altering the antibody-antigen reaction, making the dyed organisms glow visibly when examined under a fluorescent microscope. The fluorescent antibody technique can be used to identify *Mycobacterium tuberculosis* and is used in the most common serologic screening test for syphilis. Kinds of fluorescent antibody tests include the **FTA-ABS test.** Also called **immunofluorescence test.**

fluorescent microscopy, examination with a fluorescent microscope equipped with a source of ultraviolet light rays, used to study specimens, as tissues or microorganisms, that have been stained with fluorescent dye. Also called **ultraviolet microscopy.** See also **fluorescent antibody test.**

Fluorescent Treponemal Antibody Absorption Test (FTA-ABS test), a serologic test for syphilis. See also **fluorescent antibody test.**

fluoridation /flôr′idā′shən/, the process of adding fluoride, especially to a public water supply, to reduce tooth decay. See also **fluoride.**

fluoride, a salt of hydrofluoric acid introduced into drinking water and applied directly to the teeth to prevent tooth decay.

Fluori-Methane, a trademark for a local anesthetic (fluoromethane vapocoolant spray).

fluorine (F) /flo͞o′ərēn/, an element of the halogen family and the most reactive of the nonmetals. Its atomic number is 9; its atomic weight is 19. It occurs in nature only as a component of substances as fluorspar, cryolite, and phosphate rocks. It can be prepared by the electrolytic decomposition of hydrogen fluoride and in its pure form is a pale-yellow, flammable, toxic gas 1.6 times heavier than air. It is also a component of very stable fluorocarbons used in the manufacture of resins and plastics. As a component of fluorides it is widely distributed throughout the soils of the earth, enters plants, is ingested by humans, and is absorbed from the GI tract. Fluorides in the atmosphere and industrial dust are absorbed by the lungs and the skin. Relatively soluble compounds, as sodium fluoride, are almost completely absorbed by humans. The relatively insoluble compounds, as cryolite, are poorly absorbed. Small amounts of sodium fluoride are added to the water supply of many communities to harden tooth enamel and decrease dental caries. Excessive amounts of fluoride can mottle tooth enamel and cause osteosclerosis. Acute fluoride poisoning and death can result from the accidental ingestion of insecticides and rodenticides containing fluoride salts.

fluoroacetic acid /flo͞or′ō•asē′tik, -aset′ik/, a colorless, water-soluble, highly toxic compound that blocks the Krebs' citric acid cycle, causing convulsions and ventricular fibrillation. It is derived from a South African tree and is used in some potent pesticides.

fluorometholone, a topical glucocorticoid.

■ INDICATION: It is prescribed as an antiinflammatory agent.

■ CONTRAINDICATIONS: Impaired circulation, viral and fungal diseases of the skin, or known hypersensitivity to this drug or to steroid medication prohibits its use.

■ ADVERSE EFFECTS: Among the more serious adverse reactions are systemic side effects resulting from prolonged use or excessive application. Various hypersensitivity reactions may occur.

fluorometry /flo͞orom′ətrē/, measurement of fluorescence emitted by compounds when exposed to ultraviolet or other intense radiant energy. The atoms of certain substances produce fluorescence of a characteristic color and wavelength, enabling identification and quantification of several clinically significant compounds in biologic specimens. Fluorometry is used to measure urinary estrogens, triglycerides, catecholamines, and other substances. Although it is a highly sensitive method of analysis, test interference by other compounds, especially drugs, may limit its usefulness in some situations. –**fluorometric,** *adj.*

Fluoroplex, a trademark for a topical preparation of antineoplastic (fluorouracil).

fluoroscope /flo͞or′əskōp′/, a device used for the immediate projection of an x-ray image on a fluorescent screen for visual examination. –**fluoroscopic,** *adj.*

fluoroscopy /flo͞oros′kəpē/, a technique in radiology for visually examining a part of the body or the function of an organ using a fluoroscope. The technique offers immediate, serial images that are invaluable in many clinical situations, as in intrauterine fetal transfusion and cardiac catheterization.

fluorosis /flo͞orō′sis/, the condition that results from excessive, prolonged ingestion of fluorine. Unusually high concentration of fluorine in the drinking water typically causes mottled discoloration and pitting of the enamel of the permanent and deciduous teeth in children whose teeth developed while maternal intake of fluorinated water was high. Severe chronic fluorine poisoning will lead to osteosclerosis and other pathologic bone and joint changes in adults. See also **fluoridation, fluoride.**

fluorouracil /flo͞o′ərōyo͞or′əsil/, an antineoplastic.

■ INDICATIONS: It is prescribed in the treatment of malignant neoplastic disease of the skin and internal organs.

■ CONTRAINDICATIONS: Bone marrow depression, infection, poor nutritional status, or known hypersensitivity to this drug prohibits its use.

■ ADVERSE EFFECTS: Among the more serious adverse reactions are severe depression of the bone marrow and acute GI disturbances, including nausea, vomiting, diarrhea, and stomatitis. Alopecia and dermatitis commonly occur.

Fluothane, a trademark for an inhalational general anesthetic (halothane).

fluoxymesterone /flo͞o·ok′simes′tərōn/, an androgenic and anabolic steroid.

■ INDICATIONS: It is prescribed in the treatment of testosterone deficiency, breast cancer in females, and delayed puberty in males.

■ CONTRAINDICATIONS: Male breast or prostate cancer, liver disease, known or suspected pregnancy, or known hypersensitivity to this drug prohibits its use.

■ ADVERSE EFFECTS: Among the more serious adverse reactions are anaphylaxis, hypercalcemia, and jaundice.

fluphenazine hydrochloride, a phenothiazine tranquilizer.

■ INDICATION: It is prescribed in the treatment of psychotic disorders.

■ CONTRAINDICATIONS: Parkinson's disease, concurrent administration of central nervous system depressants, liver or renal dysfunction, severe hypotension, or known hypersensitivity to this drug or to other phenothiazine medication prohibits its use.

■ ADVERSE EFFECTS: Among the more serious adverse effects are hypotension, liver toxicity, a variety of extrapyramidal reactions, blood dyscrasias, and hypersensitivity reactions.

fluprednisolone /flo͞o′prednis′əlōn/, a glucocorticoid.

■ INDICATIONS: It is prescribed in the treatment of inflammatory and hypersensitivity reactions.

■ CONTRAINDICATIONS: Systemic fungal infection or known hypersensitivity to this drug prohibits its use.

■ ADVERSE EFFECTS: Among the more serious adverse reactions are GI, endocrine, neurologic, and fluid and electrolyte disturbances.

flurandrenolide, a topical glucocorticoid.

■ INDICATION: It is prescribed as an antiinflammatory agent.

■ CONTRAINDICATIONS: Impaired circulation, viral and fungal diseases of the skin, or known hypersensitivity to this drug or to steroid medication prohibits its use.

■ ADVERSE EFFECTS: Among the more serious adverse reactions are systemic side effects resulting from prolonged use or excessive application. Various hypersensitivity reactions may occur.

flurandrenolone. See **flurandrenolide.**

flurazepam hydrochloride /flo͝oraz′əpam/, a benzodiazepine minor tranquilizer.

■ INDICATION: It is prescribed in the treatment of insomnia.

■ CONTRAINDICATION: Known hypersensitivity to this drug prohibits its use.

■ ADVERSE EFFECTS: Among the most serious adverse reactions are possible physical and psychologic dependence. Dizziness and drug hangover may also occur.

Fluress, a trademark for a topical ophthalmic fixed-combination drug containing a dye (fluorescein sodium) and a topical anesthetic (benoxinate hydrochloride).

flush, **1.** a blush or sudden reddening of the face and neck. **2.** a sudden, subjective feeling of heat. **3.** a prolonged reddening of the face such as may be seen with fever, certain drugs, or hyperthyroidism. **4.** a sudden, rapid flow of water or other liquid.

flush device, a device for the accurate transmission of a pressure wave from a catheter to a transducer in an IV line.

fly, a two-winged insect of the order Diptera, some species of which transmit arboviruses to humans.

Fm, symbol for **fermium.**

FMET, abbreviation for **formylmethionine.**

FMG, abbreviation for **foreign medical graduate.**

FML, a trademark for an ophthalmic glucocorticoid agent (fluorometholone).

FNP, abbreviation for **family nurse practitioner.**

foam bath, a bath taken in water containing a saporin substance that covers the surface of the liquid and through which air or oxygen is blown to form the foam.

focal illumination. See **illumination.**

focal motor seizure. See **motor seizure.**

focal seizure, a transitory disturbance in motor, sensory, or autonomic function resulting from abnormal neuronal discharges in a localized part of the brain, most frequently motor or sensory areas adjacent to the central sulcus. Focal motor seizures commonly begin as spasmodic movements in the hand, face, or foot and may spread progressively to other muscles to end in a generalized convulsion. Abnormal neuronal discharges arising in the motor area controlling mastication and salivation may be manifested by chewing, lip-smacking, swallowing movements, and by profuse salivation. Seizures originating in the eye-turning area of the brain may begin with a forced turning of the head and eyes away from the side of the focus or lesion. Abnormal electric activity in the sensory strip of the cortex may be evident initially as a numb, prickling, tingling, or crawling feeling, and the neuronal discharge may spread to motor areas. Focal seizures may be caused by localized anoxia or a small lesion in the brain. Also called **jacksonian seizure.** See also **epilepsy, motor seizure.**

focal spot, the area on the anode of an x-ray tube or the target of an accelerator that is struck by electrons and from which the resulting x-rays are emitted. The shape and size of a focal spot will influence the resolution of a diagnostic image.

focus, a specific location, as the site of an infection or the point at which an electrochemical impulse originates.

focused grid, (in radiography) an x-ray grid that has lead foils placed at an angle so that they all point toward a focus at a specific distance.

foeti-, foeto-. See **feti-.**

foetus. See **fetus.**

fogged film fault, a defect in a photograph or radiograph, which appears as a foggy image or image area. It is usually caused by stray light or radiation, use of expired film, or an unsafe darkroom light.

foil assistant. See **foil holder.**

foil carrier. See **foil passer.**

foil holder, an instrument used for holding a foil pellet in place while it is being condensed or for retaining a bulk of gold while additions are being made to it for various dental restorations. Also called **foil assistant.** Compare **foil passer.**

foil passer, a pointed or forked instrument for carrying pellets of gold foil through an annealing flame or from the annealing tray to a prepared tooth cavity. Also called **foil carrier.** Compare **foil holder.**

foil pellet, a loosely rolled piece of gold foil, used for making various dental restorations, as a permanent tooth cavity filling or tooth crown. Pellets are prepared, as needed, from a piece of gold cut from foil that usually comes in 4 inch (10 cm) square sections. See also **gold foil.**

folacin. See **folic acid.**

folate /fō′lāt/, **1.** a salt of folic acid. **2.** any of a group of substances found in some foods and in mammalian cells that act as coenzymes and promote the chemical transfer of single carbon units from one molecule to another.

Foley catheter /fō′lē/, a rubber catheter with a balloon tip to be filled with air or a sterile liquid after it has been placed in the bladder. This kind of catheter is used when continuous drainage of the bladder is desired, as in surgery, or when repeated urinary catheterization would be necessary if an indwelling catheter were not used. Sterile technique is used in placing the catheter. See also **catheterization.**

folic acid /fō′lik, fol′ik/, a yellow, crystalline, water-soluble vitamin of the B complex group essential for cell growth and reproduction. It functions as a coenzyme with vitamins B_{12} and C in the breakdown and utilization of proteins and in the formation of nucleic acids and heme in hemoglobin. It also increases the appetite and stimulates the production of hydrochloric acid in the digestive tract. The vitamin is stored in the liver and may by synthesized by the bacterial flora of the GI tract. Deficiency of the vitamin results in poor growth, graying hair, glossitis, stomatitis, GI lesions, and diarrhea, and it may lead to megaloblastic anemia. Deficiency is caused by inadequate dietary intake of the vitamin, malabsorption, or metabolic abnormalities. Need for folic acid is increased in pregnancy, in infancy, and by stress. Rich dietary sources include spinach and other green leafy vegetables, liver, kidney, asparagus, lima beans, nuts, and whole-grain cereals. It is both heat and light labile, and considerable loss of the vitamin occurs when it has been stored for a long period. The vitamin, which is nontoxic, is effective in treating the specific deficiency states and may be beneficial in alleviating menstrual problems and leg ulcers. Also called **folacin, pteroylglutamic acid, vitamin B_9.**

folie /fōlē′/, a mental disorder; any of a variety of psychopathologic reactions. Kinds of folie include **folie à deux, folie circulaire, folie du doute, folie du pourquoi, folie gemellaire, folie musculaire,** and **folie raisonnante.**

folie à deux. See **shared paranoid disorder.**

folie circulaire. See **bipolar disorder.**

folie du doute /dYdo͞ot′/, an extreme obsessive-compulsive reaction characterized by persistent doubting, vacillation, repetition of a particular act or behavior, and pathologic indecisiveness to the point of being unable to make even the most trifling decision.

folie du pourquoi /dYpo͞orkwô·ä′/, a psychopathologic condition characterized by the persistent tendency to ask questions, usually concerning unrelated topics.

folie gemellaire /zhemeler′/, a psychotic condition occurring simultaneously in twins, sometimes in those not living together or closely associated at the time.

folie musculaire /mYskYler′/, severe chorea.

folie raisonnante /rezônäNt′/, a delusional form of any psychosis marked by an apparent logical thought process but lacking common sense.

folinic acid /fōlin′ik/, an active form of folic acid. Folinic acid is used in the treatment of megaloblastic anemias not caused by vitamin B_{12} deficiency and to counteract the toxic effects of antineoplastic folic acid antagonists, as methotrexate. Also called **citrovorum factor, leucovorin.**

follicle, a pouchlike depression, as the dental follicles that enclose the teeth before eruption or the hair follicles within the epidermis. **–follicular,** *adj.*

follicle stimulating hormone (FSH), a gonadotropin, secreted by the anterior pituitary gland, that stimulates the growth and maturation of graafian follicles in the ovary and promotes spermatogenesis in the male. FSH-releasing factor produced in the median eminence of the hypothalamus controls the release of FSH by the pituitary. Increasing amounts of FSH are secreted in the post-menstrual or resting phase of the menstrual cycle, causing a primordial follicle to develop into a mature Graafian follicle containing a mature ovum. The Graafian follicle produces estrogen, which reaches a high level before ovulation and suppresses release of FSH. In males, FSH maintains the integrity of the seminiferous tubules and influences all the stages of spermatogenesis. FSH may be given in treating some conditions. One form is derived from the urine of postmenopausal women. Also called **menotropins.**

follicular adenocarcinoma, a neoplasm characterized by a follicular arrangement of cells that are usually derived from the thyroid gland. It is not especially malignant, but it has a greater tendency to metastasize distantly to the lungs and bones than the more common papillary adenocarcinoma of the thyroid. Surgery is the preferred treatment; if complete excision of the primary tumor is not feasible, radioiodine therapy is indicated. See also **medullary carcinoma, papillary adenocarcinoma.**

follicular cyst, an odontogenic cyst that arises from the epithelium of a tooth bud and dental lamina. The kinds of follicular cysts are dentigerous, primordial, and multilocular.

follicular goiter, an enlargement of the thyroid gland characterized by proliferation of the follicles and epithelial tissue.

folliculitis /fōlik′yo͞olī′tis/, inflammation of hair follicles, as in sycosis barbae.

folliculoma. See **granulosa cell tumor.**

Follutein, a trademark for a placental hormone (human chorionic gonadotropin).

fomentation, **1.** a topical treatment of pain or inflammation with a warm, moist application. **2.** a substance or poultice that is used as a warm, moist application.

fomite, nonliving material, as bed linens, which may convey pathogenic organisms.

Fone's method, a toothbrushing technique that employs large, sweeping, scrubbing circles over occluded teeth, with the toothbrush held at right angles to the tooth surfaces. With the jaws parted, the palatal and lingual surfaces of the teeth are scrubbed in smaller circles. Occlusal surfaces of the teeth are scrubbed in an anteroposterior direction.

fontanel /fon′tənel′/, a space covered by tough membranes between the bones of an infant's cranium. The anterior fontanel, roughly diamond-shaped, remains palpable until about 2 years of age. The posterior fontanel, triangular in shape, closes about 2 months after birth. Increased intracranial pressure may cause a fontanel to become tense or bulge. A fontanel may be soft and depressed in the presence of dehydration. Also spelled **fontanelle.**

food, **1.** any substance, usually of plant or animal origin, consisting of carbohydrates, proteins, fats, and such supplementary elements as minerals and vitamins, that is ingested or otherwise taken into the body and assimilated to provide energy and to promote the growth, repair, and maintenance essential for sustaining life. **2.** nourishment in solid form as contrasted with liquid form. **3.** a particular kind of solid nourishment, such as breakfast food or snack food.

food allergy, a hypersensitive state resulting from the ingestion of a specific food antigen. Symptoms of sensitivity to specific foods can include allergic rhinitis, bronchial asthma, urticaria, angioneurotic edema, dermatitis, pruritus, headache, labyrinthitis and conjunctivitis, nausea, vomiting, diarrhea, pylorospasm, colic, spastic constipation, mucous colitis, and perianal eczema. Food allergens are predominantly protein in nature. The most common foods causing allergic reactions are wheat, milk, eggs, fish and other sea foods, chocolate, corn, nuts, strawberries, chicken, pork, legumes, tomatoes, cucumbers, garlic, and citrus fruits. Foods that are rarely allergenic are rice, lamb, gelatin, peaches, pears, carrots, lettuce, artichokes, sesame oil, and apples. Diagnosis of a specific food allergy is obtained by a detailed food history, food diary, elimination diet, or cutaneous tests.

Food and Drug Administration (F.D.A.), a federal agency responsible for the enforcement of federal regulations regarding the manufacture and distribution of food, drugs, and cosmetics as protection against the sale of impure or dangerous substances.

food exchange list, a grouping of foods in which the carbohydrate, fat, and protein values are equal for the items listed. The list is used for meal planning in various diseases and deficiency states and was compiled by a joint committee of The American Dietetic Association, The American Diabetes Association, and the National Institutes of Health. The six groups of foods included on the list are milk, vegetables, fruits, bread, meat, and fats. Starchy vegetables are listed as bread exchanges; fish and cheese are meat exchanges.

food poisoning, any of a large group of toxic processes resulting from the ingestion of a food contaminated by toxic substances or by bacteria containing toxins. Kinds of food poisoning include **bacterial food poisoning, ciguatera poisoning, Minamato disease, mushroom poisoning,** and **shellfish poisoning.** See also **botulism, ergot alkaloid, phalloidine poisoning, toadstool poisoning.**

food service administrator, a member of a hospital staff who is responsible for the planning and management of the food service system of the facility.

food service department, the department of a hospital or similar health facility that is responsible for food preparation and services to patients and personnel. It also provides nutritional care to patients.

foot, the distal extremity of the leg, consisting of the tarsus, the metatarsus, and the phalanges.

foot-and-mouth disease, an acute, extremely contagious, rhinovirus infection of cloven-hooved animals. It is characterized by the development of ulcers on the skin around the mouth, on the mucous membrane in the mouth, and on the udders. Horses are immune. Uncommonly, the virus is transmitted to humans by direct contact with infected animals or their secretions or with contaminated milk. Symptoms and signs in humans include headache, fever, malaise, and vesicles on tongue, oral mucous membranes, hands, and feet. Generalized pruritus and painful ulcerations may occur; however, the temperature soon falls, the lesions subside in about a week, and total healing without scars is complete by 2 or 3 weeks. Treatment is symptomatic. See also **picornavirus.**

footdrop, an abnormal neuromuscular condition of the lower leg and foot, characterized by an inability to dorsiflect, or invert, the foot because of damage to the peroneal nerve.

-footed, a combining form meaning 'having feet' of a specified sort or number: *clubfooted, flatfooted, fourfooted.*

footling breech, an intrauterine position of the fetus in which one or both feet are folded under the buttocks at the inlet of the maternal pelvis, one foot presenting in a single footling breech, both feet in a double footling breech. Compare **frank breech.** See also **breech birth.**

foot-pound, a unit for the measurement of work or energy. One foot-pound is the amount of work required to move 1 pound a distance of 1 foot in the same direction as that of the applied force.

for-, a combining form meaning 'pertaining to an opening': *foramen, foramina, foration.*

foramen /fôrā′mən/, *pl.* **foramina,** an opening or aperture in a membranous structure or bone, as the apical dental foramen and the carotid foramen.

foramen magnum, a passage in the occipital bone through which the spinal cord enters the spinal column.

foramen of Monro /monrō′/, a passage between the lateral and third ventricles of the brain.

foramen ovale /ōvā′lē, ōvä′lā/, an opening in the septum between the right and the left atria in the fetal heart. This opening provides a bypass for blood that would otherwise flow to the fetal lungs. Most of the blood from the inferior vena cava in the fetus flows through the foramen ovale into the left atrium. After birth, the foramen ovale functionally closes when the newborn takes the first breath and full circulation through the lungs begins. Complete closure of this opening takes about 9 months, and the foramen ovale eventually becomes the fossa ovale in the wall of the right atrial septum. See also **ductus arteriosus.**

Forane, a trademark for a general anesthetic (isoflurane).

Forbes-Albright syndrome, an endocrine disease characterized by amenorrhea, prolactinemia, and galactorrhea, caused by an adenoma of the anterior pituitary. Diagnosis is made by x-ray film of the anterior pituitary and a blood test for prolactin. Surgical resection of the adenoma is usually indicated. See also **galactorrhea, pituitary gland.**

Forbes' disease. See **Cori's disease.**

forbidden clone theory, a theory, associated with autoimmunity, based on the clonal evolution theory that at birth all the cells of the body that might react against the body have been eliminated, leaving only the cells that will react against foreign substances. The forbidden clone theory postulates that certain clone cells that can react against the body persist after birth and can be activated by a viral infection or by some metabolic change, especially if the viral organism is structurally similar to a body cell. The theory holds that the regular cells of the immune system attack only the virus, but the clone cells attack the tissues of the body. Compare **sequestered antigens theory.**

force, energy applied in such a way that it initiates motion, changes the speed or direction of motion, or alters the size or shape of an object.

forced expiratory volume (FEV), the volume of air that can be forcibly expelled in 1 second after full inspiration. Compare **vital capacity.** See also **expiratory reserve volume.**

forced feeding, the administration of food by force, as nasal feeding, to persons who cannot or will not eat.

forceps, *pl.* **forceps,** a pair of any of a large variety and number of surgical instruments, all of which have two handles or sides, each attached to a blade. The handles may be joined at one end, as a pair of tweezers, or the two sides may be separate to be conjoined in use, as obstetric forceps. Forceps are used to grasp, handle, compress, pull, or join tissue, equipment, or supplies. See specific forceps.

forceps delivery, an obstetric operation in which instruments are used to deliver a baby. It is performed to overcome dystocia, to quickly deliver a baby experiencing fetal distress, or, most often, to shorten normal labor. Local or regional anesthesia is usual, as is episiotomy. Prerequisites to forceps delivery include full dilatation of the cervix, engagement of the fetal head, and certain knowledge of the position of the head. The blades of the forceps are introduced into the vagina one at a time and applied symmetrically to opposite sides of the baby's head; the handles of the forceps are brought together so that the head is held firmly between the blades; the head is rotated, if necessary, to the occiput anterior or occiput posterior position; and traction is applied so as to draw the head from the birth passage. When the head has been delivered, the forceps are removed and the delivery is completed manually. Forceps produce marks on a baby's head and face; unless application has been imperfect, the marks are usually superficial and disappear in few days. Because cesarean section is performed more often now than formerly, traumatic forceps deliveries are uncommon. Kinds of forceps delivery are **high forceps, low forceps,** and **mid forceps.** Compare **failed forceps, forceps rotation, trial forceps.** See also **obstetric forceps.**

forceps rotation, an obstetric operation in which forceps are used to turn a baby's head that is arrested in transverse or posterior position in the birth canal. It may be performed to facilitate spontaneous birth or as the first step in a forceps delivery. Kinds of forceps rotation are **Kielland rotation** and **Scanzoni rotation.** Compare **forceps delivery, manual rotation.** See also **obstetric forceps.**

forceps tenaculum. See **tenaculum.**

fore-, a combining form meaning 'front or before': *forearm, foregut, forewaters.*

forebrain. See **prosencephalon.**

foregut, the cephalic portion of the embryonic alimentary canal. It consists of endodermal tissue and gives rise to the pharynx, esophagus, stomach, liver, pancreas, most of the small intestine, and the respiratory ducts. Compare **hindgut, midgut.**

foreign body, any object or substance found in the body in an organ or tissue in which it does not belong under normal circumstances, as a bolus of food in the trachea or a particle of dust in the eye.

foreign body obstruction, a disturbance in normal function or a pathologic condition caused by an object lodged in a body orifice, passage, or organ. Most cases occur in children who suddenly inhale or swallow a foreign object or insert it in a body opening. In adults, large boluses of hastily eaten food frequently lodge in the esophagus, causing coughing, choking, and, if the airway is obstructed, asphyxia. Forceful blows to the victim's back between the shoulder blades or the Heimlich maneuver may dislodge the bolus. Esophageal foreign bodies usually produce an immediate reaction, but occasionally children have a long asymptomatic period before signs of obstruction or infection are evident. Laryngeal foreign bodies usually cause hoarseness, wheezing, and dyspnea; a sharp object, as a chicken bone, may perforate the larynx and produce swelling and infection. Objects may be removed from the larynx, using a grasping forceps through a direct laryngoscope, with the patient under local or general anesthesia in the Trendelenburg position. A foreign body in the trachea may cause wheezing, an audible slap, coughing, and dyspnea; a small object may become lodged in a bronchus, producing coughing, which is often followed by an asymptomatic period before signs of obstruction and inflammation appear; vegetable foreign bodies produce earlier, more severe inflammatory symptoms than other objects. A bronchoscope with suitable forceps and general anesthesia are usually employed in removing bronchial foreign bodies, but thoracotomy may be required if the object is in the periphery of a lung. Objects that children sometimes insert in their nostrils may cause local obstruction, mild discomfort, or infection and may be removed by forceps or nasal suction. Needles and hairpins ingested by children often pass through the esophagus and stomach without incident but may become lodged at the turn of the duodenum and require removal by a magnetized nasogastric tube or by laparotomy; laxatives are contraindicated, and if tenderness, rigidity, pain, nausea, or vomiting ensues, immediate surgery is necessary. Coins, marbles, and closed safety pins usually pass through the digestive tract without creating problems; but hairballs, vegetable fibers, or shellac concretions, sometimes found in the stomach of emotionally disturbed or retarded patients, may cause anorexia, nausea, and vomiting. Hairballs may be fragmented, using an endoscope, and removed by lavage; surgery may be required. Urethral inflammation and hematuria, sometimes caused by the introduction of a foreign body into the urethra during self-exploration, may be treated symptomatically.

foreign medical graduate (FMG), a physician trained in and graduated from a medical school outside the United States and Canada. United States citizens graduated from medical schools outside the United States and Canada are also classified as FMGs.

forensic medicine, a branch of medicine that deals with the legal aspects of health care.

forensic dentistry, the branch of dentistry that deals with the legal aspects of professional dental practices and treatment.

forensic psychiatry, the branch of psychiatry that deals with legal issues and problems relating to mental disorders, especially the determination of insanity for legal purposes.

foreskin, a loose fold of skin that covers the end of the penis or clitoris. Its removal constitutes circumcision. The nurse observes for any interference with urination in infants. Also called **prepuce.**

forest yaws, a cutaneous form of American leishmaniasis, common in South and Central America, caused by *Leishmania guyanensis*. The disease is chronic, with multiple deep skin ulcers that occasionally spread to the nasal mucosa. Also called **pian bois.**

forewaters, the amniotic fluid between the presenting part and the intact membranes.

Forhistal Maleate, a trademark for an antihistaminic (dimethindene maleate).

-form, -forme, a combining form meaning 'having a (specified) shape or form': *linguiform, toruliform.*

formaldehyde /fərmal′dəhīd/, a toxic, colorless, foul-smelling gas that is soluble in water and used in that form as a disinfectant, fixative, or preservative.

formalin /fôr′məlin/, a clear solution of formaldehyde in water. A 37% solution is used for fixing and preserving biologic specimens for pathologic and histologic examination.

Formatrix, a trademark for a hormonal fixed-combination drug containing conjugated estrogens, an androgen (methyltestosterone), and vitamin C (ascorbic acid).

formic acid /fôr′mik/, a colorless, pungent liquid found in nature in nettles, in ants, and in other insects. It is prepared commercially from oxalic acid and glycerin and from the oxidation of formaldehyde. Formerly used as a vesicant, it currently has no therapeutic applications.

formiminoglutamic acid (FIGLU) /fôrmim′inōgloo͞tam′ik/, a compound formed in the metabolism of histidine, occurring in urine in elevated levels in folic acid deficiency. Increased excretion of FIGLU may indicate folic acid deficiency.

formol. See **formaldehyde.**

formula, a simplified statement, generally using numerals and other symbols, expressing the constituents of a chemical compound, a method for preparing a substance, or a procedure for achieving a desired value or result. –**formulaic,** *adj.*

formulary, a listing of drugs intended to include a large enough range of drugs and sufficient information about them to enable health practitioners to prescribe treatment that is medically appropriate. Hospitals maintain formularies that list all drugs commonly stocked in the hospital pharmacy. Third-party organizations, as insurance companies, usually maintain formularies listing drugs for which the company will pay in settlement of claims. See also **compendium,** ***United States Pharmacopeia.***

formulation, **1.** a pharmacologic substance prepared according to a formula. **2.** a systematic and precise statement of a problem, a theory, or a method of analysis in research.

formylmethionine (FMET) /fôr′milməthī′ənēn/, (in molecular genetics) the first amino acid in a protein sequence.

fornication, (in law) sexual intercourse between two people who are not married to each other. The specific legal definition varies from jurisdiction to jurisdiction. In some, both persons are unmarried; in some, one is unmarried; in some, the charge is adultery rather than fornication if the woman is married, regardless of the man's marital status.

fornix /fôr′niks/, *pl.* **fornices** /fôr′nisēz/, an archlike structure or space, as the fornix cerebri, the superior or inferior conjunctival fornices, or the vaginal fornices.

fornix cerebri, an archlike body of nerve fibers that lies beneath the corpus callosum of the cranium and serves as the efferent pathway from the hipppocampus.

fornix vaginae. See **vaginal fornix.**

Fort Bragg fever. See **pretibial fever.**

fortified milk, pasturized milk enriched with one or more nutrients, usually vitamin D, which has been standardized at 400 International Units per quart **(fortified vitamin D milk).**

FORTRAN /fôr′tran/, abbreviation for *FORmula TRANslator,* a high-level, compiler computer language developed to optimize mathematic computation.

fossa /fos′ə/, *pl.* **fossae,** a hollow or depression, especially on the surface of the end of a bone, as the olecranon fossa or the coronoid fossa.

Foster bed, a special bed used in the care and treatment of severely injured patients, especially those with spinal injuries. It consists of two Bradford frames mounted on a castered base and secured with locking bars to the head and foot assemblies. The assembly at each end is attached to a rotary bearing mechanism, permitting horizontal turning of the patient without moving the spine. The patient can be rotated to supine and prone positions while maintaining proper immobilization and alignment of injured body structures. The Foster bed has a horizontal turning frame that permits hyperextension and traction at each end of the frame, and either end of the bed can be elevated to provide countertraction. It can be used in posttraumatic management of patients with spinal instability, with or without cord damage, and in the management of the postoperative patient with multilevel spinal fusion when weight-bearing or ambulation is contraindicated. The Foster bed is also used in many scoliosis centers for halo-femoral traction, preparatory to spinal procedures with Harrington rods and Dwyer instrumentation. This preoperative technique permits stretching of the paravertebral soft tissues on the concavity of the spinal curve before operative correction and fusion. The bed also allows techniques for maintaining continuous cervical traction in flexion for selected patients with unstable cervical neck problems. An outrigger attachment for the bed maintains a constant angle with the patient in the supine or prone position. The bed, which allows clockwise and counterclockwise rotation around its long axis, is equipped with a convenient storage rack at the base of the bed. The weight of each frame is approximately 20 pounds, and the bed can be turned by one person, although hospital and nursing officials recommend that two trained hospital staff members perform each turning to ensure the safety of the patient and the welfare of the nursing staff. Also, two safety straps are required to guard against slippage and to decrease the margin of human error. A pillow is placed over the patient's lower legs to prevent slippage in turning. The length of the canvas on the Foster bed must be adjusted to correspond to the size of the patient, so that correct ankle posture can be maintained when the patient is prone. The relative position of the patient on the posterior frame must correspond so that when the bedpan section is released, the buttocks of the patient will not sag and compromise the alignment of the lumbosacral spine. The anatomic landmark in this adjustment is the level of the trochanters, which should be even with the bottom edge of the torso canvas to prevent hyperextension of the lumbosacral spine. The turn sheet is placed under the patient's torso to adjust movement up and down the frame, without endangering proper alignment. Other safety precautions in caring for a patient confined to a Foster bed include the placement of IV and catheter tubing at the head and the foot of the frame before rotating the patient. A Foster bed patient with thoracotomy tubing must be rotated toward the chest tube side. A Foster bed patient recovering from anesthesia or heavy sedation is usually secured with a safety strap at thigh level to help prevent turning or falling. The prone position with the use of a reading board permits self-feeding by the patient and participation in personal hygiene. Massage of the patient's forehead and chin areas toughens the skin and increases the patient's tolerance of the prone position. Foster bed patients sometimes display claustrophobia on being "sandwiched" between Foster frames, and skillful techniques to minimize the "sandwiching" time are needed to ensure the greatest possible tranquillity of the patient. Frequent sensory stimulation with patient-staff interaction, discussions and games, and prism glasses that allow the patient to read and watch TV increase the person's comfort and tolerance of prolonged immobility. Compare **Circolectric bed, hyperextension bed, Stryker wedge frame.**

foulage. See **pétrissage.**

foundation, **1.** a charitable organization usually established to allocate private funds to worthy projects or to provide other services. **2.** (in dentistry) any device or material added to a remaining tooth structure to enhance the stability and retention of an overlying cast restoration, as a pin retainer, amalgam, or a casting.

fourchette /fo͞orshet′/, a tense band of mucous membranes at the posterior angle of the vagina connecting the posterior ends of the labia minora.

four-forty (4-40), a work schedule in which a person works four 10-hour days each week rather than five 8-hour days.

four-handed dentistry, a technique of chairside operating in which four hands simultaneously perform tasks directly associated with dental work being accomplished in the oral cavity of a patient.

Fourier transform (FT), (in medical physics) a mathematic procedure that separates out the frequency components of a signal from its amplitudes as a function of time, or vice versa.

Fourier transform imaging, (in medical physics) NMR imaging techniques in which at least one dimension is phase encoded by applying variable gradient pulses along that dimension before ''reading out'' the NMR signal with a gradient magnetic field perpendicular to the variable gradient. The Fourier transform is then used to reconstruct an image from the set of encoded NMR signals.

four-tailed bandage, a narrow piece of cloth with two ties on each end for wrapping a joint, as an elbow or knee, or a prominence, as the nose or chin.

fourth nerve. See **trochlear nerve.**

Fowler's position, the posture assumed by the patient when the head of the bed is raised 18 or 20 inches and the individual's knees are elevated.

Fox's knife. See **Goldman-Fox knife.**

Fr, symbol for **francium.**

fract-, a combining form meaning 'pertaining to a breaking': *fractional, fractography, fracture.*

fractional anesthesia. See **continuous anesthesia.**

fractional dilatation and curettage, a diagnostic technique in which each section of the uterus is examined and curetted to obtain specimens of the endometrium from all parts of the uterus. It is often performed under regional anesthesia in the diagnosis of endometrial cancer.

fractionation, **1.** (in neurology) a mechanism within the neural arch of the vertebrae whereby only a portion of the efferent nerves innervating a muscle reacts to a stimulus, even when the reflex requirement is maximal, so that there is a reserve of neurons to respond to additional stimuli. Through this phenomenon muscle tension is maintained. **2.** (in chemistry) the separation of a substance into its basic constituents, by using such procedures as fractional distillation or crystallization. **3.** (in bacteriology) the process of isolating a pure culture by successive culturing of a small portion of a colony of bacteria. **4.** (in histology) the process of isolating the different components of living cells by centrifugation. **5.** also called **dose fractionation, fractionation radiation.** (in radiology) the process of administering a dose of radiation in smaller units over a period of time to minimize tissue damage rather than in a single large dose.

fracture, a traumatic injury to a bone in which the continuity of the tissue of the bone is broken. A fracture is classified by the bone involved, the part of that bone, and the nature of the break, as a comminuted fracture of the head of the tibia. Kinds of fracture include **butterfly fracture, comminuted fracture, complete fracture, compression fracture, displaced fracture, impacted fracture, incomplete fracture, segmental fracture, spiral fracture,** and **undisplaced fracture.**

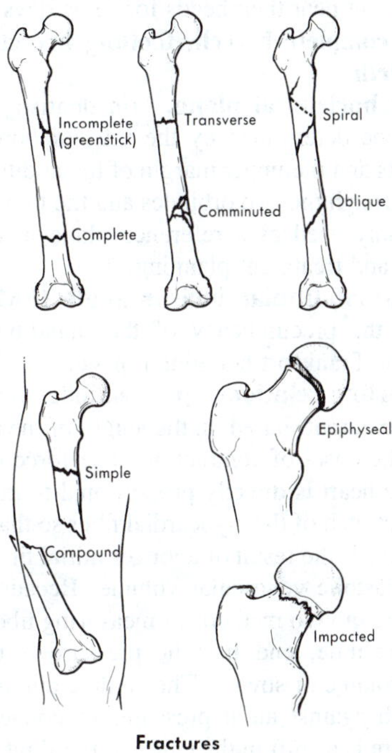

Fractures

fracture-dislocation, a fracture involving the bony structures of any joint, with associated dislocation of the same joint.

fragilitas ossium. See **osteogenesis imperfecta.**

fragmented fracture, a fracture that results in multiple bone fragments.

frambesia. See **yaws.**

frame of reference, the personal guidelines of an individual, taken as a whole. An individual frame of reference reflects the person's social status, cultural norms, and concepts.

Franceschetti's syndrome /fran′chesket′ēz/, a complete form of mandibulofacial dysostosis. See also **Treacher Collins' syndrome.**

franchise dentistry, the practice of dentistry under a trade name, which has been purchased from another dentist or dental practice. Under a franchise license agreement the franchiser may use the trade name, the associated marketing products, and treatment techniques for a sum of money, in accordance with the franchise rules and regulations.

francium (Fr), a metallic element of the alkali metal group. Its atomic number is 87; its atomic weight is 223. Formed from the decay of actinium, all of its 20 isotopes are radioactive and short-lived.

frank, obvious or clinically evident, as the unequivocal presence of a condition or a disease.

frank breech, an intrauterine position of the fetus in which the buttocks present at the maternal pelvic inlet, the legs are straight up in front of the body, and the feet are at the shoulders. Babies born in this position tend to hold their feet near their heads for some days after birth. Compare **complete breech, footling breech.** See also **breech birth.**

Frankfort horizontal plane, (in dentistry) a craniometric plane determined by the inferior borders of the bony orbits and the upper margin of the auditory meatus, passing through the two orbitales and the two tragions. It is commonly used as a reference plane in orthodontic diagnosis and treatment planning.

Frankfort-mandibular incisor angle (FMTA), (in dentistry) the precumbency of the mandibular incisor tooth to the Frankfort horizontal plane.

Frank-Starling relationship, an index for determining cardiac output, based on the length of the myocardial fibers at the onset of contraction. The force exerted per beat of the heart is directly proportional to the length or degree of stretch of the myocardial fiber so that improved performance is the result of a longer initial fiber length or a larger diastolic ventricular volume. Because there are no adequate in vivo methods of measuring fiber length or diastolic volume, end-diastolic pressure is used as an index of volume or stretch. The cardiac output is plotted on a graph against atrial pressure. In congestive heart failure there is a shift in the curve to the right and downward. Also called **Frank-Starling mechanism.**

fraternal twins. See **dizygotic twins.**

fraud, (in law) the act of intentionally misleading or deceiving another person by any means so as to cause him legal injury, usually the loss of something valuable or the surrender of a legal right.

FRC, abbreviation for **functional residual capacity.**

FreAmine II, a trademark for a nutritional supplement containing protein, amino acids, and electrolytes.

freckle, a brown or tan macule on the skin, usually resulting from exposure to sunlight. There is an inherited tendency to freckling, most frequently seen in persons with red hair. Freckles are harmless in themselves, but people who freckle easily should avoid excessive sun exposure or use protective sunscreen lotions because such individuals have a tendency to develop more serious actinic skin changes. Compare **lentigo.**

Fredet-Ramstedt's operation. See **pyloromyotomy.**

free-air chamber, a device used as a primary standard for calibrating x-ray exposure. It is used in national calibration laboratories throughout the world.

free association, **1.** the spontaneous, consciously unrestricted association of ideas, feelings, or mental images. **2.** spontaneous verbalization of thoughts and emotions entering the consciousness during psychoanalysis.

free clinic, a clinic or health program, usually located in a neighborhood setting, that provides health care for ambulatory patients at nominal or no cost.

free-floating anxiety, a generalized, persistent, pervasive fear that is not attributable to any specific object, event, or source. See also **anxiety, anxiety neurosis.**

free gingiva, the unattached coronal portion of the gingiva that encircles a tooth and forms a gingival sulcus.

free gingival groove, a shallow line or depression on the gingival surface at the junction of the free and attached gingivae.

free phagocyte. See **phagocyte.**

free-radical theory of aging, a concept of aging based on the premise that the main causative factor is an imbalance between the production and elimination of free chemical radicals in the body tissues.

free thyroxine, the amount of the unbound, active thyroid hormone, thyroxine (T_4), circulating in the blood, measured by special laboratory procedures. See also **free thyroxine index.**

free thyroxine index, the amount of unbound, physiologically active thyroxine (T_4) in serum, determined by direct assay or, more frequently, calculated on the basis of an in vitro uptake test. In this test the uptake (by resin or charcoal) of labeled triiodothyronine (T_3) is measured; because T_3 is less strongly bound by serum, it is used rather than T_4. The free T_4 index is then obtained by multiplying the T_3 uptake by the total concentration of T_4 in serum.

freeway space, the interocclusal distance or separation between the occlusal surfaces of the teeth when the mandible is in its rest position.

Freiberg's infarction, an abnormal orthopedic condition characterized by osteochondritis or aseptic necrosis of bone tissue, most commonly affecting the head of the second metatarsal.

Frei test /frī/, a test performed to confirm a diagnosis of lymphogranuloma venereum. Killed antigen, originally derived from infected patients, is injected intradermally in one forearm, and a control material is injected into the other arm. If a red, thickened papule develops at the site of injection of antigen, the test is positive. See also ***Chlamydia.***

Frejka splint /frā′kə/, a corrective device consisting of a pillow that is belted between the legs of a baby born with dislocated hips to maintain abduction and articulation of the head of the femur with the acetabulum. See also **congenital dysplasia of the hips.**

fremitus /frem′itəs/, a tremulous vibration of the chest wall that can be auscultated or palpated during physical examination. Kinds of fremitus include **bronchial fremitus, coarse fremitus, tactile fremitus,** and **vocal fremitus.**

frenectomy /frənek′təmē/, a surgical procedure for excising a frenum or frenulum, as the excision of the lingual frenum from its attachment into the mucoperiosteal covering of the alveolar process to correct ankyloglossia. Compare **frenotomy.**

frenotomy /frənot′əmē/, a surgical procedure for repairing a defective frenum, as the cutting or lengthening of the lingual frenum to correct ankyloglossia. Compare **frenectomy.**

frenulum linguae. See **lingual frenum.**

frenum /frē′nəm/, *pl.* **frenums, frena,** a restraining portion or structure. Also called **frenulum.**

Freon, the trademark for a hydrocarbon gas commonly used as a refrigerant and propellant.

frequency, **1.** the number of repetitions of any phenomenon within a fixed period of time, as the number of heart beats per minute. **2.** (in biometry) the proportion of the number of persons having a discrete characteristic to the total number of persons being studied. **3.** (in electronics) the number of cycles of a periodic quantity, as alternating current, that occur in a period of 1 second. Electromagnetic frequencies, formerly expressed in cycles per second (cps), are now expressed in hertz (Hz).

freudian /froi′dē•ən/, **1.** of or pertaining to Sigmund Freud (1856–1939), his theories and doctrines, which stress the formative years of childhood as the basis for later psychoneurotic disorders, primarily through the unconscious repression of instinctual drives and sexual desires, and his system of psychoanalysis for treating such disturbances. **2.** anything that is easily interpreted according to the theories of Freud or in psychoanalytic terms. **3.** of or pertaining to the school of psychiatry based on Freud's teachings. **4.** one who adheres to Freud's school of psychiatry. See also **psychoanalysis.**

freudian fixation, an arrest in psychosexual development characterized by a firm emotional attachment to another person or object. Some kinds of freudian fixation are **father fixation** and **mother fixation.**

freudianism, the school of psychiatry based on the psychoanalytic theories and psychotherapeutic methods of treating psychoneurotic disorders developed by Sigmund Freud and his followers. Also called **freudism.** See also **psychoanalysis.**

Fricke dosimeter, a chemical radiation dosimeter that uses the change of concentration of ferric ions in a solution subject to irradiation to quantify the amount of dose delivered to the sample.

friction, **1.** the act of rubbing one object against another. See also **attrition.** **2.** a type of massage in which deeper tissues are stroked or rubbed, usually through strong circular movements of the hand. See also **massage.**

friction burn, tissue injury caused by abrasion of the skin. See also **abrasion.**

friction rub, a dry, grating sound heard with a stethoscope during auscultation. It is a normal finding when heard over the liver and splenic areas. A pericardial friction rub auscultated over the pericardial area is suggestive of pericarditis; a pleural friction rub over the lungs may be present in heart or lung disease.

Friedländer's bacillus /frēd′lendərz/, a bacterium of the species *Klebsiella pneumonia,* which is associated with infection of the respiratory tract, especially lobar pneumonia.

Friedman curve /frēd′mən/, a graph depicting the progress of labor, prepared by labor attendants to facilitate detection of dysfunctional labor. Observations of cervical dilatation and fetal descent are plotted on the vertical axis against time on the horizontal axis. The labor curve is divided into latent and active phases, with the latter subdivided into latent, acceleration, maximum slope, and deceleration phases.

Friedman's test, a modification of the Aschheim-Zondek pregnancy test. A sample of urine from a woman is injected into a mature, unmated female rabbit. If, days later, the rabbit ovaries contain fresh corpora lutea or hemorrhaging corpora, the test is positive as a sign that the woman is pregnant.

Friedreich's ataxia /frēd′rīshs/, an abnormal condition characterized by muscular weakness, loss of muscular control, weakness of the lower extremities, and an abnormal gait. Friedreich's ataxia, which may be hereditary, exhibits both dominant and recessive inheritance patterns. The primary pathologic feature of the disease is pronounced sclerosis of the posterior columns of the spinal cord with possible involvement of the spinocerebellar tracts and the corticospinal tracts. Friedreich's ataxia usually affects individuals between 5 and 20 years of age. The highest incidence of onset is at puberty. The characteristically ataxic gait may progress to severe disability. Over a period of years a child affected by Friedrich's ataxia may also develop ataxia of the upper extremities and have difficulty performing simple maneuvers, as writing or handling silverware while eating. The characteristic gait of this disease is caused by a cavus deformity, or clawfoot. The gait and the stance of the affected individual are unsteady. A positive Romberg's sign may be evident, and Babinski's sign is present with absent or decreased deep reflexes. The condition may also cause slurred speech, head tremors, tachycardia, and cardiac failure. Thoracic scoliosis is present in approximately 80% to 90% of the patients afflicted. All the signs and symptoms are progressive. There is no curative treatment for Friedreich's ataxia. Orthoses may be useful to varying degrees in the prevention of associated deformities and the maintenance of an ambulatory status. Correction of the foot deformity allows the patient to remain ambulatory as long as possible and is preferred when the lack of progression of the disease process is demonstrated, thereby reducing the potential for recurrence. Spinal fusion may correct the associated scoliosis. Death in the progression of this disease is usually the result of myocardial failure.

frigid, **1.** lacking warmth of feeling; unemotional; unimaginative; without passion or ardor and stiff or formal in manner. **2.** a woman who is unresponsive to sexual advances or stimuli, abnormally indifferent or averse to sexual intercourse, or unable to have an orgasm during sexual intercourse. Compare **impotence.** See also **orgasm.** **–frigidity,** *n.*

frit, a partially or wholly fused porcelain from which dental porcelain powders are made.

Fröhlich's syndrome. See **adiposogenital dystrophy.**

frôlement /frôlmäN′/, **1.** the rustling type of sound often heard on auscultating the chest in diseases of the pericardium. **2.** a kind of massage that uses a light brushing stroke with the hand. See also **massage.**

front-, a combining form meaning 'pertaining to the forehead, or front': *frontad, frontalis, frontonasal.*

frontal lobe, the largest of five lobes constituting each of the two cerebral hemispheres. It lies beneath the frontal bone, occupies part of the lateral, the medial, and the inferior surfaces of each hemisphere, and extends posteriorly to the central sulcus and inferiorly to the lateral fissure. The frontal lobe significantly influences personality and is associated with the higher mental activities, as planning, judgment, and conceptualizing. Research indicates that the right frontal and the right temporal lobes are associated with the nonverbal, specialized activities of the right cerebral hemisphere and that the left frontal and the left temporal lobes are associated with the verbal activities of the left cerebral hemisphere. The lateral surface of each frontal lobe contains the precentral, the superior, and the inferior sulci, which divide the lobe into the precentral, the superior, the middle, and the inferior frontal gyri. The left inferior frontal gyrus constitutes Broca's speech area and, in most individuals, is more convoluted than the right inferior frontal gyrus. An H-shaped orbital sulcus on the inferior surface of the frontal lobe divides its inferior surface into the medial, the anterior, the lateral, and the posterior orbital gyri. The olfactory sulcus on the inferior surface contains the olfactory tract and separates the gyrus rectus from the medial orbital gyrus. The medial surface of the frontal lobe is limited posteriorly by an imaginary line that extends downward and anteriorly to the corpus callosum from the intersection of the central sulcus with the superior margin of the lobe. The medial surface of the frontal lobe includes the superior frontal gyrus and part of the cingulate gyrus. The superior frontal gyrus extends posteriorly as the paracentral lobule into the parietal lobe of the hemisphere. Compare **central lobe, occipital lobe, parietal lobe, temporal lobe.**

frontal lobe syndrome, behavioral and personality changes observed after a neoplastic or traumatic frontal lobe lesion. The patient may become sociopathic, boastful, hypomanic, uninhibited, exhibitionistic, and subject to outbursts of irritability or violence; but in other cases the person may become depressed, apathetic, lacking in initiative, negligent about personal appearance, and inclined to perseverate. Partial frontal lobectomy or leukotomy was formerly performed by some psychosurgeons to reduce drive in extremely disturbed psychotic patients, but the results were highly questionable.

frontal plane, any one of the vertical planes passing through the body from the head to the feet, perpendicular to the sagittal planes, dividing the body into front and back portions. Also called **coronal plane.** Compare **median plane, sagittal plane, transverse plane.**

frontal sinus, one of a pair of small cavities in the frontal bone of the skull that communicates with the nasal cavity. The frontal sinuses, which are rarely symmetric, are situated behind the superciliary arches. Each sinus measures approximately 3 cm in height, 2.5 cm in width, and 2.5 cm in depth and is lined with a mucous membrane that is continuous with that of the nasal cavity. A large frontal sinus may project over most of the orbit. Each sinus opens into the anterior part of the middle meatus through the frontonasal duct. The frontal sinuses are absent at birth, well developed between the seventh and eighth years, and reach their full size after puberty. Compare **ethmoidal air cell, maxillary sinus, sphenoidal sinus.**

frontal vein, one of a pair of superficial veins of the face, arising in the plexus of the forehead. Each frontal vein communicates with the frontal tributaries of the superficial temporal vein and lies near the vein of the opposite side as it courses toward the root of the nose. The two frontal veins communicate by a transverse vessel before joining the supraorbital veins. Compare **angular vein, facial vein.**

frontocortical aphasia. See **motor aphasia.**

frostbite, traumatic effect of extreme cold on skin and subcutaneous tissues that is first recognized by distinct pallor of exposed skin surfaces, particularly the nose, ears, fingers, and toes. Vasoconstriction and damage to blood vessels impair local circulation and result in anoxia, edema, vesiculation, and necrosis. Gentle warming is appropriate first aid treatment; rubbing of the affected part is avoided. Later, therapy is similar to treatment of thermal burns. Iatrogenic frostbite is the result of excessive use of ethyl chloride sprays for local anesthesia for the relief of muscle and tendon strains. Compare **chilblain, immersion foot.**

frottage /frôtäzh′/, sexual gratification obtained by rubbing (especially one's genital area) against the clothing of another person, as can occur in a crowd.

frotteur /frôtœr′/, a person who obtains sexual gratification by the practice of frottage.

frozen section method, (in surgical pathology) a method used in preparing a selected portion of tissue for pathologic examination. The tissue is moistened and, fixed or unfixed, is rapidly frozen and cut by a microtome in a cryostat. This method is very rapid, allowing the pathologist to examine the specimen during a surgical procedure.

fructokinase /fruk′tōkī′nās/, an enzyme that catalyzes the transfer of a phosphate group from adenosine triphosphate to D-fructose.

fructose /fruk′tōs, fro͝ok′-/, a yellowish-to-white, crystalline, water-soluble levorotatory ketose monosaccharide that is sweeter than sucrose and found in honey, several fruits, and combined in many disaccharides and polysaccharides. It is used as a preservative and in solution as an intravenous nutrient. In the absence of insulin it is metabolized or converted in the body to glycogen. Also called **fruit sugar, levulose.**

fructosuria /frŏŏk′tōsŏŏr′ē·ə/, presence of the sugar, fructose, in the urine. This usually harmless and asymptomatic condition is caused by the hereditary absence of the enzyme fructokinase, which normally helps metabolize fructose. Essential fructosuria is associated with symptoms of diabetes. Also called **levulosuria.**

fruit sugar. See **fructose.**

FSH, abbreviation for **follicle stimulating hormone.**

FTA-ABS test. See **Fluorescent Treponemal Antibody Absorption Test.**

FTC, abbreviation for **Federal Trade Commission.**

fuchsin bodies. See **Russell's bodies.**

FUDR, a trademark for an antiviral and antineoplastic (floxuridine).

fugue /fyōōg/, a state of dissociative reaction characterized by amnesia and physical flight from an intolerable situation. During the episode, the person appears normal and acts as though consciously aware of what may be very complex activities and behavior, but after the episode, the person has no recollection of the actions or behavior. The condition may last for only a few days or weeks, or it may continue for several years, during which the person wanders away from the customary environment, enters a new occupation, and undertakes an entirely different way of life. The syndrome appears to be caused by an inability to cope with a severe conflict or with a chronically stressful life situation. A form of fugue also occurs briefly after an epileptic seizure. See also **ambulatory automatism, automatism.**

fulcrum /fŏŏl′krəm, ful′-/, the stable point or the position on which a lever, as the ulna and the femur, turns in moving an object. Numerous common movements of the body, as raising the arm and walking, are combinations of lever actions involving fulcrums. The muscles of the body provide the forces that move the numerous bones acting as levers.

fulfillment, a perception of harmony in life that results when an individual has found meaning and leads a purposeful life.

fulguration. See **electrodesiccation.**

full-arch wire, a wire that is attached to the teeth and extends from the molar region of one side of a dental arch to the other. It is used to cause or guide orthodontic tooth movement. Compare **sectional arch wire.**

full bath, a bath in which the patient's body is immersed in water up to the neck.

full diet. See **regular diet.**

full-liquid diet, a diet consisting of only liquids and foods that liquefy at body temperature. It includes milk, milk drinks, carbonated beverages, coffee, tea, strained fruit juices, broth, strained cream soup, raw eggs, cream, melted butter or margarine, strained precooked infant cereals in milk, thin custards, gelatin desserts, ice cream, sherbet, strained vegetables in soup, honey, syrups, sugar, and dry skim milk dissolved in liquids. The diet is prescribed after surgery, in some acute infections of short duration, in the treatment of acute GI disorders, and for patients too ill to chew. See also **liquid diet.**

fulminating /ful′minā′ting/, (of a disease or condition) rapid, sudden, severe, as an infection, fever, or hemorrhage. Also **fulminant. –fulminate,** *v.*

Fulvicin, a trademark for an antifungal (griseofulvin).

fumagillin, fumigacin. See **helvolic acid.**

function, 1. an act, process, or series of processes that serve a purpose. **2.** to perform an activity or to work properly and normally.

functional contracture. See **hypertonic contracture.**

functional differentiation, (in embryology) the specialization or diversification as a result of the particular function of a cell or tissue.

functional disease, 1. a disease that affects function or performance. **2.** a condition marked by signs or symptoms of an organic disease or disorder although careful examination fails to reveal any evidence of structural or physiologic abnormalities. The symptoms of a functional disorder are as real as those of an organic disease. Headache, impotence, certain heart murmurs, and constipation may be symptoms of organic disease or of functional disease.

functional dyspepsia, an abnormal condition characterized by impaired digestion caused by an atonic or a neurologic problem. See also **dyspepsia.**

functional imaging, (in nuclear medicine) a diagnostic procedure in which a sequence of radiographic or scintillation camera images of the distribution of an administered radioactive tracer delineates one or more physiologic processes in the body.

functional impotence. See **impotence.**

functional nursing, a centralized system of nursing care that is task and activity oriented, using auxiliary health workers trained in a variety of skills. Each person is assigned specific functions that are carried out for all patients in a given unit.

functional occlusal harmony, an occlusal relationship of opposing teeth in all functional ranges and movements that provides the maximum masticatory efficiency without pathogenic force on the supporting oral structures.

functional psychosis, a severe emotional disorder characterized by personality derangement and the loss of ability to function in reality, but without evidence that the disorder is related to the physical processes of the brain.

functional refractory period, (in cardiology) the shortest interval at which a tissue is capable of conducting consecutive impulses, as measured by the time intervening between the arrival of an initial impulse and the earliest subsequent premature impulse at the distal end of the same conducting tissue.

functional residual capacity, the volume of gas in the lungs at the end of a normal expiration. The functional residual capacity is equal to the residual volume plus the expiratory reserve volume.

fundal height, the height of the fundus, measured in centimeters from the top of the symphysis pubis to the highest point in the midline at the top of the uterus. Fundal height is measured at each prenatal visit with large, blunt calipers or with a tape measure. From the twentieth to the thirty-second weeks of pregnancy, the height in centimeters is equal to the gestation in weeks. Two measurements 2 weeks apart showing a deviation of more than 2 cm may indicate that the fetus is large or small for dates, that the estimated gestation is in error, or that the woman is carrying a multiple pregnancy.

fundamental needs of humans, (in nursing education) the 14 basic needs of human beings as described in a curriculum for basic nursing. The needs are respiration; nutrition; elimination; mobility, including posture and locomotion; sleep and rest; clothing; maintenance of normal body temperature; cleanliness; safety; communication; worship, according to the person's faith; work that is satisfying to the person; recreation; and learning and discovery. Recognition and identification of a need precede and serve as the basis for a nurse's plan for care, taking into consideration that the need and the ability to cope with the need vary according to age, temperament, social and cultural status, and physical and intellectual ability.

fundamentals of nursing, the basic principles and practices of nursing as taught in educational programs for nurses. In a course called "the fundamentals of nursing," traditionally required in the first semester of the program, the student attends classes and gives care to selected patients. The emphasis of this phase of training is the acquisition by the student of the basic skills of nursing. Currently, nursing educators emphasize the importance of knowledge and understanding of the fundamental needs of humans as well as competence in the basic skills as prerequisites to providing comprehensive nursing care.

fundus /fun′dəs/, *pl.* **fundi** /fun′dī/, the base or the deepest part of an organ; the portion farthest from the mouth of an organ, as the fundus of the uterus or the fundus of an eye.

funduscope. See **ophthalmoscope.**

funduscopy /fundus′kəpē/, the examination and study of the fundus of the eye by means of an ophthalmoscope. –**fundoscopic, funduscopic,** *adj.*

fundus microscopy, examination of the base of the interior of the eye using an instrument that combines an ophthalmoscope and a lens with high magnifying power for observing minute structures in the cornea and iris.

fundus reflex. See **light reflex.**

fungal infection, any inflammatory condition caused by a fungus. Most fungal infections are superficial and mild, though persistent and difficult to eradicate. Some, particularly in older, debilitated, or immunosuppressed people, may become systemic and life-threatening. Some kinds of fungal infections are **aspergillosis, blastomycosis, candidiasis, coccidioidomycosis,** and **histoplasmosis.**

fungemia /funjē′mē·ə/, the presence of fungi in the blood. Compare **bacteremia, parasitemia, viremia.**

fungicide /fun′jisīd/, a drug that kills fungi. See also **antifungal,** def. 2. –**fungicidal,** *adj.*

fungiform papilla. See **papilla.**

Fungizone, a trademark for an antifungal (amphotericin B).

fungus /fung′gəs/, *pl.* **fungi** /fun′jī/, a simple parasitic plant that, lacking chlorophyll, is unable to make its own food and is dependent on other life forms. A simple fungus reproduces by budding; multicellular fungi reproduce by spore formation. Of the 100,000 identified species of fungi, 100 are common in humans and 10 are pathogenic. See also **fungal infection.** –**fungal, fungous,** *adj.*

funiculitis /fənik′yo͞olī′tis/, any abnormal inflammatory condition of a cordlike structure of the body, as the spinal cord or spermatic cord.

funiculus /fənik′yələs/, a division of the white matter of the spinal cord, consisting of fasciculi or fiber tracts.

funiculus umbilicalis. See **umbilical cord.**

funnel feeding, a technique in which liquids may be given orally to a patient who cannot move the lips or masticate, as may occur after surgery at the mouth or lips. A rubber tube attached to a funnel is placed in the mouth, usually at one corner, and a liquid is poured slowly through the funnel and tube into the mouth near the back of the tongue. The patient quickly learns to control the flow with sucking action and the position of the tongue. If the method is used for a weak or young infant, a rubber bulb or a large syringe may be used instead of a funnel. The bulb or syringe is compressed gently, slowly, and continuously to control the rate of flow and prevent choking.

Furacin, a trademark for a topical antiinfective (nitrofurazone).

Furadantin, a trademark for an antibacterial (nitrofurantoin).

furazolidone, an antiinfective and antiprotozoal.

■ INDICATIONS: It is prescribed for certain bacterial or protozoal infections of the GI tract.

■ CONTRAINDICATIONS: Known hypersensitivity to this drug prohibits its use. It is not given to children under 1 month of age, and it is not used with drugs that are contraindicated with monoamine oxidase inhibitors.

■ ADVERSE EFFECTS: Among the more serious adverse reactions are hemolytic anemia and fever; skin rash and abdominal pain sometimes occur.

furcation, the region of division of the root portion of a tooth.

furosemide /fyərō′səmid/, a diuretic.

■ INDICATIONS: It is prescribed in the treatment of hypertension, renal failure, and edema.

■ CONTRAINDICATIONS: Anuria, pregnancy, lactation, electrolyte depletion, or known hypersensitivity to this drug prohibits its use.

■ ADVERSE EFFECTS: Among the more serious adverse reactions are fluid and electrolyte imbalance.

Fungal pathogens

Organism	Disease clinical manifestation	Reservoir	Method of transmission
Absidia species	Zygomycosis (mucormycosis) infections of nose, ear, sinuses, eye, CNS; lungs, GI tract	Organic debris, soil	Inhalation; trauma
Acremonium species (cephalosporium)	Mycotic keratitis; mycetoma	Organic debris, soil	Trauma
Aspergillus species (A. flavus, A. fumigatus, A. niger)	Aspergillosis; pneumonia or disseminated infections; keratitis; fungus ball; allergic aspergillosis	Ubiquitous	Inhalation; trauma
Blastomyces dermatidis	North American blastomycosis (lungs, disseminates to skin, bone)	Unknown (endemic to central and central eastern U.S.A.); possibly dogs, mice	Inhalation
Candida albicans	Mucocutaneous candidiasis (thrush); infections of mucous membranes, nails skin, catheters, urinary tract; fungemia, endocarditis, bronchitis	Humans, ubiquitous	Endogenous (GI tract, mucous membranes)
Candida species (C. stellatoidea C. tropicalis)	Infections of mucous membranes, catheters, urinary tract, fungemia, endocarditis	Humans, ubiquitous	Endogenous (GI tract, skin)
Cladosporium species (C. bantianum, C. carrionii)	Chromoblastomycosis (granulomas of skin, brain abscess)	Soil, woody plant material	Trauma
Coccidioides immitis	Coccidioidomycosis (San Joaquin Valley fever); pulmonary, cutaneous, or disseminated infections	Soil (endemic to areas of southwestern U.S.A. and South America)	Inhalation; trauma
Cryptococcus neoformans	Cryptococcosis (meningitis, lung, bone, skin lesions)	Pigeon droppings and nesting areas	Inhalation
Curvularia species	Phaeohyphomycosis (localized abscesses); keratitis, endocarditis	Ubiquitous	Trauma
Epidermophyton floccosum	Tinea cruris, tinea pedis, tinea corpons, tinea nanus	Humans	Contact
Exophiala jeanselmei	Mycetoma (localized subcutaneous infections)	Soil	Trauma
Exophiala werneckii (cladosporium werneckii)	Tinea nigra (superficial skin infection)	Soil, plant material	Contact
Fonsecaea species (F. compactum, F. pedrosoi)	Chromoblastomycosis (granulomas of skin, brain abscess)	Soil, woody plant material	Trauma
Fusarium species	Mycotic keratitis	Soil, plant material	Trauma
Geotrichum candidum	Geotrichosis (lung infections)	Milk products, soil	Inhalation; endogenous to humans (GI tract)
Histoplasma capsulatum	Histoplasmosis (pulmonary, mucocutaneous, disseminated)	Bird droppings, bat droppings (endemic to Mississippi Valley)	Inhalation
Loboa loboi	Lobomycosis (keloidal blastomycosis)	Unknown (a South American disease)	Trauma (?)
Madurella species (M. grisea, M. mycetomatis)	Mycetoma	Soil	Trauma
Malassezia furfur	Tinea versicolor (superficial infection of skin)	Humans	Contact
Microsporum audounii	Tinea capitis, tinea corporis	Humans, fomites	Contact
Microsporum canis	Tinea capitis, tinea corporis	Animals (dogs)	Contact with infected animals
Mucor species	Zygomycosis (mucormycosis); infections of nose, sinuses, eye, CNS; lungs, GI tract	Soil, organic debris	Inhalation; contact, trauma
Paracoccidioides brasiliensis	Paracoccidioidomycosis (South American blastomycosis); skin especially, lips, nose, mouth; lymph nodes, lung, bone	Woody plants (soil ?) (endemic to Brazil)	Inhalation; contact possibly requiring broken skin (?)
Phialophora verrucosa	Chromoblastomycosis	Soil, woody plant material	Trauma
Piedraia hortae	Black piedra (hair infection)	Ubiquitous	?
Pseud Allescheria boydii	Mycetoma; systemic infections	Soil	Trauma; inhalation
Rhizopus species	Zygomycosis (mucormycosis) infections of nose, sinuses, eye, CNS; lungs, GI tract	Organic debris, soil	Inhalation; contact, trauma
Scorpulariopsis species	Onychomycosis (nail infection)	Organic debris, soil	Contact, trauma?

Continued.

Fungal pathogens—cont'd

Organism	*Disease clinical manifestation*	*Reservoir*	*Method of transmission*
Sporothrix schenckii	Sporotrichosis (lymphocutaneous, pulmonary, and disseminated infections)	Plant material, wood, soil	Contact (broken skin or splinters)
Torulopsis glabrata	Urinary tract infections, peritonitis, catheter infections	Humans	Endogenous (GI tract)
Trichophyton mentagrophytes	Tinea pedis (athelete's foot), tinea corporis, tinea barbae	Humans, animals	Contact with infected individual
Trichophyton rubrum	Tinea corporis, tinea barbae, tinea pedis	Humans	Contact with infected individual
Trichophyton tonsurans	Tinea capitis, tinea corporis, tinea unquium	Humans	Contact with infected individual
Trichosporon beigelii	White piedra (hair infection)	Ubiquitous	?

By Mickelsen, Patricia, Ph.D., Associate Director, Clinical Microbiology Laboratory, and McClenny, Nancy, M.T. (ASCP), Mycology Supervisor, Stanford University Hospital, Stanford University Medical Center, Stanford, CA, 1984.

Furoxone, a trademark for an antiinfective antiprotozoal (furazolidone).

furuncle /fyo͝or′ungkəl/, a localized, suppurative staphylococcal skin infection originating in a gland or hair follicle, characterized by pain, redness, and swelling. Necrosis deep in the center of the inflamed area forms a core of dead tissue that will be spontaneously extruded, eventually resorbed, or surgically removed. To prevent spread of infection, it is important to avoid irritating or squeezing the lesion. Treatment may include antibiotics, local moist heat, and, when there is definite fluctuation and the hard white core is evident, incision and drainage. Also called **boil.** **–furunculous,** *adj.*

furunculosis /fyo͝orung′kyo͝olō′sis/, an acute skin disease characterized by boils or successive crops of boils that are caused by staphylococci or streptococci.

-fuse, a combining form meaning 'to pour or flow': *diffuse, effuse, perfuse.*

fusiform, a structure that is tapered at both ends.

fusiform aneurysm, a localized dilatation of an artery in which the entire circumference of the vessel is distended, creating an elongated tubular or spindlelike swelling. Also called **Richet's aneurysm.** Compare **saccular aneurysm.**

fusimotor /fyo͞o′zimō′tər/, pertaining to the motor nerve fibers, or gamma efferent fibers, that innervate the intrafusal fibers of the muscle spindle.

fusion, **1.** the bringing together into a single entity, as in optic fusion. **2.** also called **ankylosis.** the act of uniting two or more bones of a joint. **3.** the surgical joining together of two or more spinal vertebrae, performed to stabilize a segment of the spinal column after severe trauma, a herniated disk, or degenerative disease. Under general anesthesia, the cartilage pads are removed from between the posterior portions of the involved vertebrae. Bone chips are cut from one of the patient's iliac crests and inserted in place of the cartilage, fusing the articulating surfaces into one segment of bone. Postoperative nursing care focuses on strict limitations of motion for the graft site until bony healing occurs. The patient's bed is completely flat; a Stryker frame may be used. In a standard bed, the patient is log-rolled from side to side to avoid twisting the trunk. The nurse observes the dressing for any drainage of spinal fluid. Ambulation takes place before sitting.

fusion beat, (in cardiology) a QRS complex that is the result of a collision of impulses within the atria or ventricles as a result of simultaneous activation of those chambers by two foci, usually the sinus node and a ventricular ectopic beat, but sometimes the sinus node and an atrial ectopic beat. The more common ventricular fusion beat has the same clinical significance as other late diastolic ventricular ectopic beats. The shape of the fusion complex varies even when the same focus is involved because the amount of tissue involved with each focus may vary slightly each time. The PR interval may be normal if the ventricular ectopic focus discharges after the sinus impulse enters the ventricle, or it may be shorter than normal if that impulse discharges before the sinus impulse can enter the ventricles. Some arrhythmias in which fusion beats are commonly noted are parasystole and accelerated idioventricular rhythm.

fusospirochetal disease /fyo͞o′zōspī′rōkē′təl/, any infection characterized by ulcerative lesions in which both a fusiform bacillus and a spirochete are found, as trench mouth or Vincent's angina.

f waves, (in cardiology) waves that represent fibrillation or flutter.

-fy, a combining form meaning 'to make into' something specified: *acidify, decalcify, salify.*

-fying. See **-factive.**

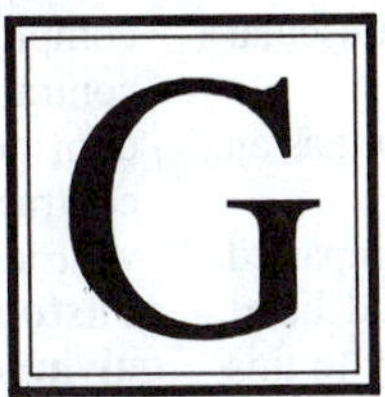

g, abbreviation for **gram.**
Ga, symbol for **gallium.**
GA, abbreviation for **general anesthesia.**
GABA, abbreviation for **gamma-aminobutyric acid.**
gadolinium (Gd), a rare earth metallic element. Its atomic number is 64; its atomic weight is 157.25.
gag reflex, a normal neural reflex elicited by touching the soft palate or posterior pharynx, the response being elevation of the palate, retraction of the tongue, and contraction of the pharyngeal muscles. The reflex is used as a test of the integrity of the vagus and glossopharyngeal nerves. Also called **pharyngeal reflex.**
gait, the manner or style of walking, including rhythm, cadence, and speed.
gait determinant, one of a number of the kinetic anatomic factors that govern the locomotion of an individual in the process of walking. Some authorities have defined pelvic rotation, pelvic tilt, knee and hip flexion, knee and ankle interaction, and lateral pelvic displacement as the main determinants of gait. Such descriptions are often important in analyzing and correcting pathologic gaits of individuals afflicted by orthopedic diseases, deformities, or abnormal bone conditions.
galact-, galacta-. See **galacto-.**
-galactia, a combining form meaning a 'condition involving secretion of milk': *cacogalactia, dysgalactia, oligogalactia.*
galacto-, galact-, galacta-, a combining form meaning 'pertaining to milk': *galactochloral, galactogen, galactorrhea.*
galactokinase /gəlak'tōkī'nās/, an enzyme that functions in the metabolism of glycogen. Galactokinase catalyzes a metabolic step involving the transfer of a high-energy phosphate group from a donor molecule to a molecule of galactose producing a molecule of D-galactose-1-phosphate.
galactokinase deficiency, an inherited disorder of carbohydrate metabolism in which the enzyme galactokinase is deficient or absent. As a result, dietary galactose is not metabolized, galactose accumulates in the blood, and cataracts may develop rapidly. Food containing galactose, as milk and certain milk products, must be eliminated from the diet. Compare **lactase deficiency.**
galactophorous duct, a passage for milk in the lobes of the breast.
galactorrhea /gəlak'tərē'ə/,, lactation not associated with childbirth or nursing. The condition is sometimes a symptom of a pituitary gland tumor. See also **Forbes-Albright syndrome.**
galactose /gəlak'tōs/, a simple sugar found in the dextrorotatory form in lactose (milk sugar), nerve cell membranes, sugar beets, gums, and seaweed and, in the levorotatory form, in flaxseed mucilage. Prepared galactose, a white crystalline substance, is less sweet and less soluble in water than glucose but is similar in other properties.
galactosemia /gəlak'tōsē'mē•ə/, an inherited, autosomal recessive disorder of galactose metabolism, characterized by a deficiency of the enzyme galactose-1-phosphate uridyl transferase. Shortly after birth, an intolerance to milk is evident. Hepatosplenomegaly, cataracts, and mental retardation develop. Greater than normal amounts of galactose are present in the blood, the galactose tolerance test indicates an abnormality, and the red cells show deficient galactose-1-phosphate uridyl transferase activity. Because the elimination of galactose from the diet results in the rapid amelioration of all symptoms except mental retardation, early diagnosis and prompt therapy are essential. Compare **diabetes mellitus, glycogen storage disease.** See also **galactose, inborn error of metabolism.**
galactosyl ceramide lipidosis, a rare, fatal, inherited disorder of lipid metabolism, present at birth. Infants become paralyzed, blind, deaf, and increasingly retarded, and eventually die of bulbar paralysis. There is no known treatment for the disorder, but it can be detected in pregnancy by amniocentesis. Also called **globoid leukodystrophy, Krabbe's disease.** Compare **Tay-Sachs disease.**
Galant reflex /gəlant'/, a normal response in the neonate to move the hips toward the stimulated side when the back is stroked along the spinal cord. The reflex disappears by about 4 weeks of age. Absence of the reflex may indicate spinal cord lesion. Also called **trunk incurvation reflex.**
galea aponeurotica. See **epicranial aponeurosis.**
Galeazzi's fracture /gal'ē•at'sēz/, a fracture of the distal radius accompanied by dislocation of the radioulnar joint. Also called **Dupuytren's fracture.**
Galen's bandage /gā'lənz/, a bandage for the head, consisting of a strip of cloth with each end divided into three pieces. The center of the cloth is placed on top of the head; the two strips in front are joined at the back of the neck; the two strips at the back are pulled up and fastened on the forehead; the remaining middle strips are fastened under the chin.
gall. See **bile.**

gallamine triethiodide, a curare-like neuromuscular blocking agent.

■ INDICATION: It is prescribed as a muscle relaxant as an adjunct to anesthesia.

■ CONTRAINDICATIONS: Myasthenia gravis, impaired kidney function, use in patients where increased heart rate may be hazardous, or known hypersensitivity to this drug or to iodine prohibits its use.

■ ADVERSE EFFECTS: Among the most serious adverse reactions are risks associated with skeletal muscle relaxation, as respiratory depression and apnea, and tachycardia. Allergic reactions may also occur.

gallbladder, a pear-shaped excretory sac lodged in a fossa on the visceral surface of the right lobe of the liver. It serves as a reservoir for bile. About 8 cm long and 2.5 cm wide at its thickest part, it holds about 32 cc of bile. During digestion of fats, the gallbladder contracts, ejecting bile through the common bile duct into the duodenum. The gallbladder is divided into a fundus, body, and neck and is covered by the peritoneum. Obstruction of the biliary system by gallstones may lead to jaundice and pain; it is a common condition in overweight, middle-aged women and may require surgical excision.

gallbladder cancer, a malignant neoplasm of the bile reservoir, characterized by anorexia, nausea, vomiting, weight loss, progressively severe right upper quadrant pain, and, eventually, jaundice. Tumors of the gallbladder are predominantly adenocarcinomas; often associated with biliary calculi, they are three to four times more common in women than in men and rarely occur before 40 years of age. Physical examination reveals an enlarged gallbladder in about one half of the cases. X-ray film may aid in making a diagnosis, but obstruction of the biliary duct by the cancer or the inability of the gallbladder to concentrate the radiopaque dye often prevents visualization of the lesion, and the diagnosis is usually made during a laparotomy. Complete removal of the gallbladder may be curative, but partial hepatectomy may be required because the liver is often a site of early metastases. Surgery is contraindicated if there are distant metastases, as frequently occur in the lungs, bone, and adrenal glands. Radiotherapy may be palliative; chemotherapy is usually ineffective.

gallium (Ga), a metallic element. Its atomic number is 31; its atomic weight is 69.72. The melting point of gallium is 29.8° C (88.6° F); it will melt if held in the hand. Because of its high boiling point (1983° C; 3602° F), it is used in high-temperature thermometers. Radioisotopes of gallium are used in total body scanning procedures. Many of its compounds are poisonous.

gallop, a pathologic third or fourth heart sound, which at certain heart rates sometimes mimics the gait of a horse. The third heart sound (S3) may normally be heard in healthy children and young adults, but is called a ventricular gallop when it is pathologic and, as such, may be the first sign of cardiac decompensation. An S3 gallop occurs early in diastole and is caused by the sudden deceleration of the diastolic filling wave as a result of a noncompliant ventricular wall. An S4 gallop follows atrial contraction and precedes the first heart sound. It is seldom normal and is related to either left or right atrial contraction and the resultant distension of a noncompliant ventricle just before systole.

gallstone. See **biliary calculus.**

galvanic cautery, galvanocautery. See **electrocautery.**

gam-. See **gamo-.**

Gambian trypanosomiasis, a usually chronic form of African trypanosomiasis, caused by the parasite *Trypanosoma brucei gambiense*. An infected individual may have relatively mild symptoms for months or years before developing the neurologic symptoms of the terminal stage. Also called **West African sleeping sickness.** Compare **Rhodesian trypanosomiasis.** See also **African trypanosomiasis.**

Gamene, a trademark for a pediculicide and scabicide (gamma-benzene hexachloride).

gamet-, See **gameto-.**

gamete /gam′ēt/, **1.** a mature male or female germ cell that is capable of functioning in fertilization or conjugation and contains the haploid number of chromosomes of the somatic cell. **2.** the ovum or spermatozoon. See also **meiosis.** **–gametic,** *adj.*

gametic chromosome, any of the chromosomes contained in the haploid cell, specifically the spermatozoon or ovum, as contrasted to those in the diploid, or somatic cell.

gameto-, gamet-, a combining form meaning 'reproductive cell': **gametocyte, gametophore, gametogenesis.**

gametocide /gəmē′tōsīd/, any agent that is destructive to gametes or gametocytes, specifically to the malarial gametocytes. **–gametocidal,** *adj.*

gametocyte /gəmē′təsīt/, (in genetics) any cell capable of dividing into or in the process of developing into a gamete, specifically an oocyte or spermatocyte.

gametogenesis /gam′itōjen′əsis/, the origin and maturation of gametes, which occurs through the process of meiosis. See also **oogenesis, spermatogenesis.** **–gametogenic, gametogenous,** *adj.*

gamma-aminobutyric acid (GABA), an amino acid with neurotransmitter activity found in the brain and also in the heart, lungs, kidneys, and certain plants.

gamma-benzene hexachloride. See **lindane.**

gamma camera, a device that uses the emission of light from a crystal struck by gamma rays to produce an image of the distribution of radioactive material in a body organ. The light is detected by an array of light-sensitive electronic tubes and is converted to electric signals for further processing. The gamma camera is a workhorse of nuclear medicine departments, where it is used to produce scans of patients who have been injected with small amounts of radioactive materials.

gamma efferent fiber, any of the motor nerve fibers that transmit impulses from the central nervous system to the intrafusal fibers of the muscle spindle. The gamma efferent fibers are responsible for deep tendon reflexes, spasticity, and rigidity but not for the degree of contractile response. They function in regulating the sensitivity of the spindle and the total tension of the muscle. See also **primary afferent fiber.**

gamma globulin. See **immune gamma globulin.**

gamma radiation, a very high frequency electromagnetic emission of photons from certain radioactive elements in the course of nuclear transition or from nuclear reactions. Gamma radiation is more penetrating than alpha radiation and beta radiation but has less ionizing power and is not deflected in electric and magnetic fields. The wavelengths of gamma rays emitted by radioactive substances are characteristic of the radioisotopes involved and range from about 4×10^{-10} to 5×10^{-13} m. High-voltage generators can produce x-rays of a wavelength much shorter than that of most gamma rays. The depth to which gamma rays penetrate depends on their wavelengths and energy. Gamma radiation and other forms of radiation can injure, distort, or destroy body cells and tissue, especially cell nuclei, but controlled radiation is used in the diagnosis and treatment of various diseases. Gamma radiation can penetrate thousands of meters of air and several centimeters of soft tissue and bone. Sixty percent of a dose of gamma radiation that enters the body tissue normally exits the same tissue. Radiation is an important form of therapy in the treatment of skin cancer and malignancies deep within the body. The ionizing effect of radiation affects all the cells of the body, but young, growing, and dividing cells are most susceptible. Radiation therapy tends to destroy the nuclei of rapidly dividing cancer cells by bombarding the nuclei with selective doses of radiation that spare normal slower dividing tissue. Any cell is vulnerable to injury if radiated while dividing, and the injury to the cells and tissue from radiation is basically the same, regardless of the type of radiant energy. There is no practical application of radiation in routine sterilization, but both heat and gamma radiation are employed to sterilize spacecraft. Body cells especially sensitive to radiation include lymphoid cells, bone marrow cells, cells that line the alimentary tract, and cells of the testes and the ovaries. Exposure of the entire body to sizable doses of radiation can cause acute radiation sickness. See also **ultraviolet radiation.**

gamma ray, an electromagnetic radiation of short wavelength emitted by the nucleus of an atom during a nuclear reaction. Composed of high-energy photons, gamma rays lack mass and an electric charge and travel at the speed of light. They are usually associated with alpha particles and beta rays (electrons ejected at high velocities from radioactive substances).

gammopathy /gamop′əthē/, an abnormal condition characterized by the presence of markedly increased levels of gamma globulin in the blood. Two different types of hypergammaglobulinemia can be distinguished. **Monoclonal gammopathy** is commonly associated with an electrophoretic pattern showing one sharp, homogenous electrophoretic band in the gamma globulin region. This reflects the presence of excessive amounts of one type of immunoglobulin secreted by a single clone of B cells. **Polyclonal gammopathy** reflects the presence of a diffuse hypergammaglobulinemia in which all immunoglobulin classes are proportionally increased. See also **Bence Jones protein, multiple myeloma.**

gamo-, gam-, a combining form meaning 'pertaining to marriage or sexual union': *gamobium, gamont, gamophagia.*

gamogenesis /gam′ōjen′əsis/, sexual reproduction through the fusion of gametes. **–gamogenetic,** *adj.*

gamone /gam′ōn/, a chemical substance secreted by the ova and spermatozoa that supposedly attracts the gametes of the opposite sex to facilitate union. Kinds of gamones are **androgamone** and **gynogamone.**

gampsodactyly. See **pes cavus.**

Gamulin R, a trademark for a passive immunizing agent, Rh_o(D), immune human globulin.

-gamy, **1.** a combining form meaning a '(specified) type of marriage': *endogamy, monogamy, pedogamy.* **2.** a combining form meaning 'possession of organs for reproduction': *cleistogamy, dichogamy, homogamy.* **3.** a combining form meaning a 'union for propagation': *hologamy, macrogamy, syngamy.*

gangli-. See **ganglio-.**

ganglia. See **ganglion.**

ganglio-, gangli-, a combining form meaning 'pertaining to a ganglion': *gangliocytoma, ganglioneuroma, ganglioplexus.*

ganglion /gang′glē•on/, *pl.* **ganglia,** **1.** a knot, or knotlike mass. **2.** one of the nerve cells, chiefly collected in groups outside the central nervous system. Individual cells and very small groups abound in association with alimentary organs. The two types of ganglia in the body are the sensory ganglia on the dorsal roots of spinal nerves and on the sensory roots of the trigeminal, facial, glossopharyngeal, and vagus nerves and the autonomic ganglia of the sympathetic and parasympathetic systems.

ganglionar neuroma, a tumor composed of nerve cells. Also called **ganglionated neuroma, ganglionic neuroma.**

ganglionic blocking agent, any one of a group of drugs prescribed to produce controlled hypotension, as required in certain surgical procedures or in emergency management of hypertensive crisis. The drugs act by occupying receptor sites on sympathetic and parasympathetic nerve endings of autonomic ganglia, preventing response of these nerves to the action of acetylcholine liberated by the presynaptic nerve endings. Trimethaphan and mecamylamine are the most commonly prescribed ganglionic blocking agents. They are used with great caution in treating patients who are affected with coronary, cerebrovascular, or renal insufficiency or who have a history of severe allergy. Adverse reactions to the drugs include sudden marked hypotension, paralytic ileus, urinary retention, constipation, visual disturbances, heartburn, and nausea.

ganglionic crest. See **neural crest.**

ganglionic glioma, a tumor composed of glial cells and ganglion cells that are nearly mature. See also **neuroblastoma.**

ganglionic neuroma. See **ganglionar neuroma.**

ganglionic ridge. See **neural crest.**

ganglioside, a glycolipid found in the brain and other nervous system tissues. Gangliosides are members of a group of galactose-containing cerebrosides with a basic composition of ceramide-glucose-galactose-N-acetyl neuraminic acid. Accumulation of gangliosides because of an inborn error of metabolism results in gangliosidosis or Tay-Sachs disease.

gangliosidosis type I. See **Tay-Sachs disease.**

gangliosidosis type II. See **Sandhoff's disease.**

gangrene, necrosis or death of tissue, usually the result of ischemia (loss of blood supply), bacterial invasion, and subsequent putrefaction. The extremities are most often affected, but it can occur in the intestines and gallbladder. Internally, gangrene may be a complication of strangulated hernia, appendicitis, cholecystitis, or thrombosis of the mesenteric arteries to the gut. **Dry gangrene** is a late complication of diabetes mellitus that is already complicated by arteriosclerosis in which the affected extremity becomes cold, dry, and shriveled and eventually turns black. **Moist gangrene** may follow a crushing injury or an obstruction of blood flow by an embolism, tight bandages, or tourniquet. This form of gangrene has an offensive odor, spreads rapidly, and may result in death in a few days. In all types of gangrene, surgical debridement is necessary to remove the necrotic tissue before healing can progress. Cleanliness and the maintenance of good circulation are nursing considerations essential in preventing this condition. See also **gas gangrene, open amputation.** **–gangrenous,** *adj.*

gangrenous necrosis. See **necrosis.**

gangrenous stomatitis. See **noma.**

ganja. See **cannabis.**

Gantanol, a trademark for an antibacterial (sulfamethoxazole).

Gantrisin, a trademark for an antibacterial (sulfisoxazole).

Ganzfeld effect, a visual field that is patternless, as a whitewashed surface, producing a sensation of an inability to see.

gap, (in molecular genetics) a short, missing segment in one strand of double-stranded DNA.

gap phenomenon, (in cardiology) a condition in which a premature stimulus encounters a block where an earlier or later stimulus could be conducted.

Garamycin, a trademark for an antibacterial (gentamicin sulfate).

Gardner, Mary Sewell (1871–1961), an American public health nurse who wrote the classic *Public Health Nurse*. She directed the Providence, Rhode Island, District Nursing Association and was instrumental in the development of the National Organization for Public Health Nursing and of public health nursing in the American Red Cross.

Gardner-Diamond syndrome, a condition resulting from autoerythrocyte sensitization, marked by large, painful, transient ecchymoses that appear without apparent cause but often accompany emotional upsets, various collagen disorders, and abnormalities of protein metabolism. Treatment includes topical and systemic corticosteroids. Also called **autoerythrocyte sensitization syndrome.**

Gardner's syndrome, familial polyposis of the large bowel, with fibrous dysplasia of the skull, extra teeth, osteomas, fibromas, and epidermal cysts. The condition is inherited as a dominant trait, and malignancies occur more often than usual in families having this syndrome.

gargle, **1.** to hold and agitate a liquid at the back of the throat by tilting the head backward and forcing air through the solution. The procedure is used for cleansing or medicating the mouth and oropharynx. **2.** a solution used to rinse the mouth and oropharynx.

gargoylism. See **Hurler's syndrome.**

Gartner's duct, one of two vestigial, closed ducts, each one parallel to a uterine tube.

gas, an aeriform fluid possessing complete molecular mobility and the property of indefinite expansion. A gas has no definite shape and its volume is determined by temperature and pressure. Compare **liquid, solid.**

gas chromatography, the separation and analysis of different substances according to their different affinities for a standard absorbent. In the process a gaseous mixture of the substances is passed through a glass cylinder containing the absorbent, which may be dampened with a nonvolatile liquid solvent for one or more of the gaseous components. As the mixture passes through the absorbent, each substance is absorbed to a different extent and leaves a characteristic pigment. The bands of different colors left when all the gaseous mixture has moved through the absorbent constitute a chromatograph for analysis. Compare **column chromatography, ion-exchange chromatography.**

gas embolism, an occlusion of one or more small blood vessels, especially in the muscles, tendons, and joints, caused by expanding bubbles of gases. Gas emboli can rupture tissue and blood vessels, causing decompression sickness and death. This phenomenon commonly affects deep-sea divers who rise too quickly to the surface without adequate decompression. Gas emboli are most dangerous in the central nervous system because of associated neurologic changes, as syncope, paralysis, and aphasia. Such emboli are extremely painful. The prevention and treatment of gas emboli involve gradual decompression of atmospheric gases, especially nitrogen, that are dissolved in the blood. See also **air embolism, decompression sickness, embolism.**

gas exchange, impaired, a nursing diagnosis accepted by the Fourth National Conference on the Classification of Nursing Diagnoses. The cause of the condition is an imbalance in ventilatory perfusion. The defining characteristics are confusion, restlessness, irritability, somnolence, hypercapnea, and hypoxia. See also **nursing diagnosis.**

gas gangrene, necrosis accompanied by gas bubbles in soft tissue after surgery or trauma. It is caused by anaerobic organisms, as various species of *Clostridium,* particularly *C. perfringens.* Symptoms include pain, swelling, and tenderness of the wound area, moderate fever, tachycardia, and hypotension. The skin around the wound becomes necrotic and ruptures, revealing necrotic muscle. A characteristic finding is toxic delirium. If untreated, gas gangrene is rapidly fatal. Prompt treatment, including excision of gangrenous tissue and administration of penicillin G intravenously, saves 80% of patients. The disease is prevented by proper wound care. Also called **anaerobic myositis.**

gasoline poisoning. See **petroleum distillate poisoning.**

gas-scavenging system, the equipment and procedures used to eliminate anesthetic gases that escape into the atmosphere of the operating room. See also **trace gas.**

gaster-, gastr-. See **gastro-.**

gastrectomy, surgical excision of all or, more commonly, part of the stomach, performed to remove a chronic peptic ulcer, to stop hemorrhage in a perforating ulcer, or to remove a malignancy. Preoperatively, a GI series is done and a nasogastric tube is introduced. Under general anesthesia, one half to two thirds of the stomach is removed, including the ulcer and a large area of acid-secreting mucosa. A gastroenterostomy is then done, joining the remainder of the stomach to the jejunum or duodenum. If a malignant tumor is found, the chest cavity is opened and the entire stomach is removed, along with the omentum and, usually, the spleen; the jejunum is anastomosed to the esophagus. Postoperatively, the nurse observes the drainage from the nasogastric suction tube for bright red blood, indicative of hemorrhage. The nurse encourages the patient to breathe deeply and to cough. With the return of peristalsis, water is given orally, and, if tolerated without pain or nausea, the tube is removed. A temperature elevation or dyspnea may indicate a leakage of the oral liquids from the incision into the abdomen. Complications of gastrectomy include fullness and discomfort after meals, a marginal ulcer formed when gastric acids come into contact with the mucous membrane of the anastomosis of the jejunum, and painful contractions and vomiting of bile from a blockage of pancreatic juices and bile in the distal end of the duodenum. The diet gradually progresses to six small, bland meals a day, with 120 ml of fluid hourly between meals. See also **dumping syndrome, gastroenterostomy, nasogastric tube, peptic ulcer.**

-gastria, a combining form meaning '(condition of) possessing a stomach or stomachs': *atretogastria, macrogastria, megalogastria.*

gastric, of or pertaining to the stomach.

-gastric, a combining form meaning a 'type of stomach or number of stomachs': *endogastric, paragastric, trigastric.*

gastric analysis, examination of the contents of the stomach, primarily to determine the quantity of acid present and incidentally to ascertain the presence of blood, bile, bacteria, and abnormal cells. A sample of gastric secretion is obtained via a nasogastric tube. The technique used varies according to the information desired. The total absence of hydrochloric acid is diagnostic of pernicious anemia. Patients with gastric ulcer and gastric cancer may secrete less acid than normal, whereas patients with duodenal ulcers secrete more. The composition and volume of the secretions may also provide diagnostic information. See also **Diagnex Blue test.**

gastric antacid. See **antacid.**

gastric atrophy. See **atrophic gastritis.**

gastric cancer, a malignancy of the stomach that is declining in incidence in North America and western Europe. Dietary factors, as nitrates, smoked and salted fish and meats, and moldy foods containing aflatoxin are thought to cause gastric cancer, but the etiology remains unknown. The incidence is higher in men than in women and peaks in the 50- to 59-year-old age group. The risk is increased in workers exposed to asbestos and in patients with pernicious anemia. Gastric ulcers may become malignant, and those that do may have originated as ulcerating cancerous lesions. Symptoms of gastric cancer are vague epigastric discomfort, anorexia, weight loss, and unexplained iron deficiency anemia; but many cases are asymptomatic in the early stages, and metastatic enlargement of the left supraclavicular lymph node may be the first manifestation of a stomach lesion. Diagnostic measures include a test for occult blood in the stool, gastric analysis, x-ray films of the upper GI tract afterbarium ingestion, examination of gastric mucosa with a flexible endoscope, biopsy, and cytologic studies of exfoliated tumor cells. Approximately 97% of stomach tumors are adenocarcinomas that may be ulcerating, polypoid, diffuse and fibrous, or superficial spreading lesions; lymphomas and leiomyosarcomas account for less than 3%. Radical subtotal gastrectomy with excision of contiguous involved tissues and reconstruction by anastomosing the remainder of the stomach to the duodenum or jejunum is usually recommended. Total gastrectomy is associated with high morbidity and mortality, and it usually leads to pernicious anemia. Radiotherapy and chemotherapy are usually not effective, but postoperative irradiation is recommended to control microscopic residual tumor; combinations of antineoplastic antimetabolites are used in treating advanced, metastatic gastric cancer.

gastric dyspepsia, pain or discomfort localized in the stomach. See also **dyspepsia.**

gastric fistula, an abnormal passage into the stomach, communicating most frequently with an opening on the external surface of the abdomen. A gastric fistula may be created surgically to provide tube feeding for patients with severe esophageal disorders.

gastric intubation, a procedure in which a Levin tube or other small-caliber catheter is passed through the nose into the esophagus and stomach for the introduction into the stomach of liquid formulas to provide nutrition for unconscious patients or for premature or sick newborn infants. Medication or a contrast medium may be instilled for treatment or for radiologic examination. Gastric intubation is most often performed to remove the contents of the stomach to prevent postoperative gastric distention, to prevent aspiration of gastric contents during general anesthesia, or to remove a poisonous substance and wash the stomach. See also **gastric lavage, Levin tube.**

gastric juice, digestive secretions of the gastric glands in the stomach, consisting chiefly of pepsin, hydrochloric acid, rennin, lipase, and mucin. The pH is strongly acid (0.9 to 1.5). Achlorhydria (a deficiency of hydrochloric acid in gastric juice) is present in pernicious anemia and stomach cancer. Excessive secretion of gastric juice may lead to mucosal irritation and to peptic ulcer. See also **achlorhydria, gastric analysis, gastric ulcer.**

gastric lavage, the washing out of the stomach with sterile water or a saline solution. The procedure is performed before and after surgery to remove irritants or toxic substances and before such examinations as endoscopy or gastroscopy. See also **irrigation.**

gastric motility, the spontaneous peristaltic movements of the stomach that aid in digestion, moving food through the stomach and out through the pyloric sphincter into the duodenum. Excess gastric motility causes pain that is usually treated with antispasmodic medication. Less than normal motility is common in labor, after general anesthesia, and as a side effect of some sedative hypnotics.

gastric node, a node in one of three groups of lymph glands associated with the abdominal and pelvic viscera supplied by branches of the celiac artery. The gastric nodes accompany the left gastric artery and are divided into the superior and inferior gastric nodes. Compare **hepatic node, pancreaticolienal node.**

gastric ulcer, a circumscribed erosion of the mucosal layer of the stomach that may penetrate the muscle layer and perforate the stomach wall. It tends to recur with stress and is characterized by episodes of burning epigastric pain, belching, and nausea, especially when the stomach is empty or after eating certain foods. Characteristically, antacid medication or milk quickly relieves the pain. Treatment includes medication to decrease the acidity and motility of the stomach and to relieve symptomatic stress. If perforation and hemorrhage occur, surgical resection of part of the stomach may be necessary. Also called **peptic ulcer.**

gastrin /gas′trin/, a polypeptide hormone, secreted by the pylorus, that stimulates the flow of gastric juice and contributes to the stimulus causing bile and pancreatic enzymes secretion.

gastritis /gastrī′tis/, an inflammation of the lining of the stomach that occurs in two forms. **Acute gastritis** may be caused by severe burns, major surgery, aspirin, or other antiinflammatory agents, corticosteroids, drugs, or food allergens or by the presence of viral, bacterial, or chemical toxins. The symptoms—anorexia, nausea, vomiting, and discomfort after eating—usually abate after the causative agent has been removed. **Chronic gastritis** is usually a sign of underlying disease, as peptic ulcer, stomach cancer, Zollinger-Ellison syndrome, or pernicious anemia. Differential diagnosis is by endoscopy with biopsy. Kinds of gastritis include **antral gastritis, atrophic gastritis, hemorrhagic gastritis,** and **hypertrophic gastritis.** Compare **peptic ulcer.**

gastro-, gaster-, gastr-, a combining form meaning 'pertaining to the stomach or abdomen': *gastroadynamia, gastrocolitis, gastrophrenic.*

gastrocnemius /gas′troknē′mē•əs/, the most superficial muscle in the posterior part of the leg. It arises by a lateral head and a medial head and forms the greater part of the calf. The lateral head arises from the lateral condyle of the femur and the capsule of the knee. The medial head arises from the medial condyle of the femur and from the capsule of the knee. The fibers of both heads insert into a broad aponeurosis that narrows distally to join the tendon of the soleus as part of the tendo calcaneus. Compare **soleus, plantaris.**

gastrocnemius gait, an abnormal gait associated with a weakness of the gastrocnemius. It is characterized by the dropping of the pelvis on the affected side at the last moment of the stance phase in the walking cycle, accompanied by the lagging or the slowness of forward pelvic movement.

gastrocoele. See **archenteron.**

gastrocolic omentum. See **greater omentum.**

gastrocolic reflex, a mass peristaltic movement of the colon that often occurs when food enters the stomach. When an infant is fed, this reflex may result in a bowel movement.

gastrodidymus, conjoined, equally developed twins united at the abdominal region. Also called **omphalodidymus.**

gastrodisciasis /gas′trōdiskī′əsis/, an infection of trematodes of the genus *Gastrodiscoides,* which are digestive tract parasites. The species *G. hominis,* a reddish-orange fluke averaging 1 cm in length, is endemic in the hog populations of Southeast Asia and is transmitted to humans.

gastrodisk. See **embryonic disk.**

gastroenteritis /gas′trō•en′tərī′tis/, inflammation of the stomach and intestines accompanying numerous GI disorders. Symptoms are anorexia, nausea, vomiting, abdominal discomfort, and diarrhea. The condition may be attributed to bacterial enterotoxins, bacterial or viral invasion, chemical toxins, or miscellaneous conditions, as lactose intolerance. The onset may be slow, but more often it is abrupt and violent, with rapid loss of fluids and electrolytes from persistent vomiting and diarrhea. Hypokalemia and hyponatremia, acidosis, or alkalosis may develop. Treatment is supportive, employing bed rest, sedation, intravenous replacement of electrolytes, and antispasmodic medication to control vomiting and diarrhea. With a precise diagnosis, medication and treatment can be specific and curative, as an antitoxin that might be prescribed for gastroenteritis resulting from a bacterial endotoxin. After the acute phase, water may be given by mouth. If it produces no vomiting or diarrhea, clear fluids may be added, followed, if tolerated, by a bland diet.

gastroenterologist /gas'trō•en'tərol'əjist/, a physician who specializes in gastroenterology.

gastroenterology /gas'trō•en'tərol'əjē/, the study of diseases affecting the GI tract, including the stomach, intestines, gallbladder, and bile duct.

gastroenterostomy /gas'trō•en'təros'təmē/, surgical formation of an artificial opening between the stomach and the small intestine, usually at the jejunum. The operation is performed with a gastrectomy, to route food from the remainder of the stomach into the small intestine, or by itself, for perforating ulcer of the duodenum. A GI series is done preoperatively, and a nasogastric tube is inserted. Under general anesthesia, the jejunum is pulled up and anastomosed with the stomach. A new opening is then made for food to pass from the stomach directly into the jejunum. Pancreatic juices and bile are still secreted into the duodenum and pass through its distal end to the jejunum. Postoperatively, drainage from the nasogastric suction tube is observed for bright red bleeding, indicative of hemorrhage. Deep breathing and coughing are encouraged. The nasogastric tube is removed when peristalsis returns and when water given orally does not cause pain or nausea. Temperature elevation or dyspnea may indicate a leakage of the fluids from the incision around the anastomosis. The diet is gradually increased to six small, bland meals a day, with 120 ml of fluids hourly between meals. Compare **gastrectomy.**

gastroesophageal /gas'trō•isof'əjē'əl/, of or pertaining to the stomach and the esophagus.

gastroesophageal hemorrhage. See **Mallory-Weiss syndrome.**

gastroesophageal reflux, a backflow of contents of the stomach into the esophagus that is often the result of incompetence of the lower esophageal sphincter. Gastric juices are acid and therefore produce burning pain in the esophagus. Repeated episodes of reflux may cause esophagitis, peptic esophageal stricture, or esophageal ulcer. In uncomplicated cases, treatment consists of elevation of the head of the bed, avoidance of acid-stimulating foods, and regular administration of antacids. In complicated cases, surgical repair may provide relief. See also **chalasia, esophagitis, heartburn, hiatus hernia.**

gastrogavage. See **gastrostomy feeding.**

gastrohepatic omentum. See **lesser omentum.**

gastrointestinal (GI) /gas'trō•intes'tinəl/, of or pertaining to the organs of the GI tract, from mouth to anus.

gastrointestinal allergy, an immediate reaction of hypersensitivity after the ingestion of certain foods or drugs. GI allergy differs from food allergy, which can affect organ systems other than the digestive system. Characteristic symptoms include itching and swelling of the mouth and oral passages, nausea, vomiting, diarrhea (sometimes containing blood), severe abdominal pain, and, if severe, anaphylactic shock. Treatment includes identification and removal of the allergen. In an acute attack epinephrine may be administered as a stimulant, and muscle relaxants may be given to reduce intestinal spasms causing abdominal pain. In childhood, GI allergy is most often caused by hypersensitivity to cow's milk and is characterized by diarrhea and colicky pain, sometimes with vomiting, eczema, respiratory distress, and thrombocytopenia. See also **lactose intolerance.**

gastrointestinal bleeding, any bleeding from the GI tract. The most common underlying conditions are peptic ulcer, esophageal varices, diverticulitis, ulcerative colitis, and carcinoma of the stomach and colon. Vomiting of bright red blood or the passage of coffee ground vomitus indicates upper GI bleeding, usually from the esophagus, stomach, or upper duodenum. Aspiration of the gastric contents, lavage, and endoscopy are performed to determine the site and rate of bleeding. Tarry, black stools indicate a bleeding source in the upper GI tract; bright red blood from the rectum usually indicates bleeding in the distal colon. GI bleeding is treated as a potential emergency. Patients may require transfusions or fluid replacement and are watched carefully for signs of shock and hypovolemia. In all patients, blood loss is evaluated and ability to coagulate is tested. See also **coffee ground vomitus, hematochezia, melena.**

gastrointestinal obstruction, any obstruction of the passage of intestinal contents, caused by mechanic blockage or failure of motility. Mechanic blockage may be caused by adhesions resulting from surgery or inflammatory bowel disease, an incarcerated hernia, fecal impaction, tumor, intussusception, or volvulus. Failure of motility may follow anesthesia, abdominal surgery, or occlusion of any of the mesenteric arteries to the gut. Symptoms vary with the cause of obstruction but generally include vomiting, abdominal pain, and increasing abdominal distention. Dehydration and prostration may follow. Characteristically, borborygmus is diminished or absent and abdominal guarding is prominent. A barium enema may be performed, but barium is never given by mouth in such cases because it would increase the volume of the obstruction. The objective of therapy is to remove the obstruction as quickly and safely as possible. A tube is inserted into the stomach or small intestine to aspirate contents and relieve distention. During these procedures, the patient is monitored for proper fluid and electrolyte balance. Surgical intervention may be necessary. The nurse helps the patient to understand that medication for pain can aggravate the condition by further decreasing motility of the GI tract and that it may not be prescribed in the acute period, before the location and extent of the obstruction is discovered.

gastrointestinal system assessment, an evaluation of the patient's digestive system and symptoms.

■ METHOD: Discussion of symptoms is encouraged, and the patient is asked if there is or has been pain or tenderness in the oral cavity, gums, tongue, lips, or abdomen, and if there have been instances of dysphagia, belching, heartburn, anorexia, nausea, vomiting, constipation, diarrhea, or painful defecation. Information is elicited concerning any changes in eating, bowel habits, the color, character, and frequency of stools and urine, the use of laxatives or enemas, and the occurrence of fatigue, hemorrhoids, and edema of the extremities. The patient's general appearance, weight, and temperature are noted; the blood pressure, pulse, and respirations are checked in the supine, sitting, and standing positions, and the urinary output and color are determined. The presence of allergies, stomatitis, halitosis, and the condition of the tongue, gums, oral mucosa, and teeth are recorded. The abdomen is examined for distention, rigidity, ascites, symmetry, hepatomegaly, keloid tissue, visible peristalsis, bowel sounds, masses, and the presence of an ostomy. The perianal area is inspected for its general condition, color, odor, and hemorrhoids, the sclera for signs of jaundice, and the skin for pruritis, spider angioma, purpura, palmar erythema, peripheral edema, jaundice, and distended, tortuous blood vessels. Relevant to the assessment are the patient's concurrent endocrine, cardiovascular, and neurologic disorders, severe burns, psychologic problems, carcinoma, alcohol or drug abuse, and previous GI surgery and illnesses, as hepatitis, liver cirrhosis, or pancreatitis. The patient's personality type, attitude toward work, use of tobacco, antacids, laxatives, anticholinergics, steroids, antidiarrheals, antiemetics, sedatives, tranquilizers, barbiturates, antihypertensives, antibiotics, and aspirin are investigated. The family history, especially of GI disease, carcinoma, and diabetes, is an important aspect of the evaluation. Diagnostic aids include a complete blood count, stool examination, prothrombin time, and determinations of levels of alkaline phosphatase, serum and urine bilirubin, serum glutamic oxaloacetic transaminase (SGOT), serum glutamic pyruvic transaminase (SGPT), lactic acid dehydrogenase (LDH), blood urea nitrogen, and serum lipase, cholinesterase, calcium, albumin, and glucose. Additional laboratory studies for the evaluation are the total protein level, a serum electrolyte profile, serum carotene, delta-xylose tolerance, galactose tolerance, hippuric acid, and bromosulphalein tests, the albumin-globulin ratio, serum flocculation and thymol turbidity tests, urobilinogen level, the polyvinylpyrrolidone (PVP) test for protein loss, Sulkowitch's test for calcium in urine, and Schilling's test for GI absorption of vitamin B_{12}. Procedures that may be required for the diagnosis include upper GI, small bowel, and gallbladder series, esophageal and gastric endoscopy and biopsy, scans of the liver and pancreas, biopsies of the liver, colon, or rectum, gastric analysis, sigmoidoscopy, abdominal x-ray films, fluoroscopy, percutaneous transhepatic cholangiography, splenoportography, and digital rectal examinations.

■ NURSING ORDERS: The nurse conducts the interview, records observations of the patient, and assembles the results of the diagnostic laboratory studies and procedures.

■ OUTCOME CRITERIA: A well-conducted assessment of the patient's GI system is a valuable contribution to the diagnosis and plan of treatment.

gastropore. See **blastopore.**

gastroschisis /gastros′kəsis/, a congenital defect characterized by incomplete closure of the abdominal wall with protrusion of the viscera. Compare **omphalocele.**

gastroscope, a fiberoptic instrument for examining the interior of the stomach. See also **fiberoptics.** **–gastroscopy,** *n.*, **gastroscopic,** *adj.*

gastroscopy /gastros′kəpē/, the visual inspection of the interior of the stomach by means of a gastroscope inserted through the esophagus. The flexible fiberoptic gastroscope has increased the visualization of the prepyloric antrum, but the fundus is still not visible. See also **endoscopy, fiberoptics.** **–gastroscopic,** *adj.*

gastrostomy /gastros′təmē/, surgical creation of an artificial opening into the stomach through the abdominal wall, performed to feed a patient who has cancer of the esophagus or tracheoesophageal fistula or one who is expected to be unconscious for a prolonged period. Under local anesthesia, the anterior wall of the stomach is drawn forward and sutured to the abdominal wall. A Foley catheter or other tube or a special prosthesis is then inserted into an incision in the stomach, and the opening is tightly sutured to prevent leakage of the contents of the stomach. The device is clamped, and opened when food is instilled. Postoperatively, glucose in water may be given; then a warm, blended formula is given every 4 hours. The skin is kept clean and dry around the site. Skin irritation indicates a leakage of gastric secretions and digestive enzymes. After 2 weeks the tube is withdrawn after feeding and reinserted before the next meal.

gastrostomy feeding, the introduction of a nutrient solution through a tube that has been surgically inserted into the stomach through the abdominal wall. Also called **gastrogavage.**

gastrothoracopagus /gas′trōthôr′əkop′əgəs/, conjoined twins that are united at the thorax and abdomen.

gastrula /gas′tro͞olə/, the early embryonic stage formed by the invagination of the blastula. The cup-shaped gastrula consists of an outer layer of ectoderm and an inner layer of mesentoderm that subsequently differentiates into the mesoderm and endoderm. See also **blastula, embryonic layer.**

-gastrula, a combining form meaning an 'embryonic stage after the blastula': *amphigastrula, discogastrula, paragastrula.*

gastrulation, the development of the gastrula in lower animals and the formation of the three germ layers in the embryo of humans and higher animals. It is characterized by an extensive series of coordinated morphogenetic movements within the blastula or blastocyst by which the primitive body plan of the organism is established and by which the areas that later differentiate into various structures and organs are in their proper position for development.

gatch bed, a bed that has an adjustable joint, allowing the knees to be flexed and the legs supported.

gate, a simple electronic circuit, a fundamental building block of a computer.

gate theory of pain. See **pain mechanism.**

gating mechanism, (in cardiology) the increasing duration of an action potential from the AV node to a point in the distal Purkinje system, beyond which it again decreases.

Gaucher's disease /gôshāz′/, a rare, familial disorder of fat metabolism, caused by an enzyme deficiency, characterized by widespread reticulum cell hyperplasia in the liver, spleen, lymph nodes, and bone marrow. Beginning in infancy or early childhood, splenomegaly, hepatomegaly, and abnormal bone growth develop. Diagnosis is made through biopsy of the liver, spleen, or bone marrow. Mortality is high, but children who survive adolescence may live for many years. Also called **glucosyl cerebroside lipidosis.**

gauntlet bandage /gônt′lət/, a glovelike bandage covering the hand and the fingers. See also **demigauntlet bandage.**

gauze, a transparent fabric of open weave and differing degrees of fineness, most often cotton muslin, used in surgical procedures and for bandages and dressings. It may be sterilized and permeated by an antiseptic or lotion. Kinds of gauze include **absorbable gauze, absorbent gauze,** and **petrolatum gauze.** See also **bandage.**

gavage /gäväzh′/, the process of feeding a patient through a nasogastric tube. See also **gastronomy feeding.**

gavage feeding of the newborn, a procedure in which a tube passed through the nose or mouth into the stomach is used to feed a newborn infant with weak sucking, uncoordinated sucking and swallowing, respiratory distress, tachypnea, or repeated apneic spells.

■ METHOD: After the gastric tube is inserted, its placement is checked by instilling air and auscultating the stomach for air sounds or by immersing the proximal end of the tube in water (which bubbles if the distal end is misplaced in the infant's respiratory tract). During feeding, the infant is held in a low Fowler's position, preferably by the mother, and is restrained only if necessary. The feeding syringe is held 6 to 8 inches above the infant's head, and the flow is initiated by pressure on the plunger. As the formula is slowly instilled, the baby is stroked and is offered a pacifier to promote gravity flow, exert a calming effect, and reinforce the relationship between sucking and feeding. If the infant gags, spits, chokes, regurgitates, vomits, or becomes cyanotic, the rate of flow of formula is reduced and the feeding may be stopped. To prevent air from entering the stomach when the feeding is completed, the tube is pinched closed as it is withdrawn. The infant is burped gently by patting or rubbing the back and then positioned on the right side in the crib; postural drainage and percussion are avoided for at least 1 hour after feeding. The time, amount, and kind of feeding and the size of tube used are entered in the nursing care plan; if the amount of residual formula left in the infant's stomach at the time of the next feeding exceeds the quantity specified, the next feeding may be delayed or omitted.

■ NURSING ORDERS: The nurse administers intermittent gavage feeding to the infant, offers an explanation to the parents of the need for the procedure, and points out that nipple feedings may be instituted when the infant sucks on the gavage tube or pacifier, actively seeks nourishment, shows good suck and swallow coordination, gains weight, and has a respiratory rate of less than 60 breaths per minute.

■ OUTCOME CRITERIA: Intermittent gavage feedings can enable the high-risk infant to survive.

gay, **1.** any person who is homosexual. **2.** of or pertaining to homosexuality.

Gay-Lussac's law /gā′ləsaks′/, (in physics) a law stating that the volume of a specific mass of a gas will increase as the temperature is increased at a constant rate, determined by the volume of the gas at 0° C if the pressure remains constant. Also called **Charles' law.**

Gay Nurses' Alliance (GNA), a national organization of homosexual nurses.

gaze palsy, a partial or complete inability to move the eyes to all directions of gaze. A gaze palsy is often named for the absent direction of gaze, as a right lateral gaze palsy.

GBIA. See **Guthrie bacterial inhibition assay test.**

g.c., *informal.* abbreviation for **gonococcus.**

Gd, symbol for **gadolinium.**

GDM, abbreviation for **gestational diabetes mellitus.**

Ge, symbol for **germanium.**

Geiger-Müller (GM) counter /gī′gərmil′ər/, an electronic device that indicates the level of radioactivity of any substance by counting the number of subatomic particles, as electrons, emitted by a substance. It cannot identify the type or energy of a particle. The counter detects ionizing particles with a Geiger-Müller tube. As ionizing particles cross the tube, they ionize the gas within the tube and cause an electric discharge. Also called **Geiger counter.**

gel, a colloid that is firm even though it contains a large amount of liquid, used in many medicines as a demulcent, a vehicle for other drugs, an antacid, or an astringent, depending on the drug from which it is derived.

gelat-, a combining form meaning 'to freeze, congeal': *gelatigenous, gelatinoid, gelatum.*

gelatin film, absorbable, a hemostatic.

■ INDICATIONS: It is used to attain hemostasis during surgery, particularly neurologic, thoracic, and ophthalmic procedures.

■ CONTRAINDICATIONS: Infection or gross contamination of the surgical wound prohibits its use.

■ ADVERSE EFFECTS: There are no known adverse reactions.

gelatiniform carcinoma. See **mucinous carcinoma.**

gelatinous carcinoma, a former term for **mucinous carcinoma.**

gelatin sponge, an absorbable local hemostatic.

■ INDICATIONS: It is prescribed to control bleeding in various surgical procedures and in the treatment of decubitus ulcers to promote healing and hemostasis.

■ CONTRAINDICATIONS: Frank infection, extensive and abnormal bleeding, postpartum bleeding, or menorrhagia prohibits its use.

■ ADVERSE EFFECTS: There are no known adverse reactions.

gel diffusion. See **immunodiffusion.**

Gelfilm, a trademark for an absorbable, hemostatic gelatin film.

Gelfoam, a trademark for an absorbable hemostatic gelatin sponge.

Gellhorn pessary. See **pessary.**

Gelusil, a trademark for a GI, fixed-combination drug containing an antiflatulent (simethicone) and antacids (aluminum and magnesium hydroxide).

gemellary /jem′əler′ē/, of or pertaining to twins.

gemellipara /jem′əlip′ərə/, a woman who has given birth to twins.

gemellology /jem′əlol′əjē/, the study of twins and the phenomenon of twinning.

gemfibrozil, an antihyperlipidemic agent.

■ INDICATION: It is prescribed for hyperlipidemia.

■ CONTRAINDICATIONS: Renal or hepatic dysfunction, gallbladder disease, or known hypersensitivity to this drug prohibits its use.

■ ADVERSE EFFECTS: Among the adverse reactions are abdominal or epigastric pain, urticaria, dizziness, and anemia.

gemin-, a combining form meaning 'pertaining to a twin, or double': *geminate, gemini, geminous.*

gemma /jem′ə/, *pl.* **gemmae,** 1. a budlike projection produced by lower forms of life during the budding process of asexual reproduction. 2. any budlike or bulblike structure, as a taste bud or end bulb. –**gemmaceous,** *adj.*

gemmate /jem′āt/, 1. having buds or gemmae. 2. to reproduce by budding.

gemmation /jemā′shən/, the process of cell reproduction by budding. Also called **gemmulation.**

gemmiferous /jemif′ərəs/, having buds or gemmae; gemmiparous.

gemmiform /jem′ifôrm′/, resembling a bud or gemma.

gemmipara /jemip′ərə/, an animal that produces gemmae or reproduces by budding, such as the hydra. –**gemmiparous,** *adj.*

gemmulation. See **gemmation.**

gemmule /jem′yo͞ol/, 1. the small, asexual reproductive structure produced by the parent during budding that eventually develops into an independent organism. 2. (according to the early theory of pangenesis) any of the submicroscopic particles containing hereditary elements that are produced by each somatic cell of the parent, are transmitted through the bloodstream to the gametes, and, after fertilization, give rise to cells and tissues that have the exact characteristics as those from which they originated. Compare **biophore.**

Gemonil, a trademark for an anticonvulsant (metharbital).

gen-, a combining form meaning 'to become or produce': *generic, genesiology, genus.*

-gen, -gene, 1. a combining form meaning 'that which generates': *aerogen, proteinogen, venogen.* 2. a combining form meaning 'that which is generated': *immunogen, ionogen, nitrogen.*

Genapax Tampon, a trademark for an antiinfective tampon (gentian violet).

gender, 1. the classification of the sex of a person into male, female, or intersexual. 2. the particular sex of a person. See also **sex.**

gender identity, the sense or awareness of knowing to which sex one belongs. The process begins in infancy, continues throughout childhood, and is reinforced during adolescence. Also called **core gender identity.**

gender identity disorder, a condition characterized by a persistent feeling of discomfort or inappropriateness concerning one's anatomic sex. The disorder typically begins in childhood with gender identity problems and is manifested in adolescence or adulthood as asexuality, homosexuality, transvestism, or transsexualism.

gender role, the expression of a person's gender identity; the image that a person presents to both himself or herself and others demonstrating maleness or femaleness.

gene, the biologic unit of genetic material and inheritance. Since the time the concept of the gene was introduced with mendelian genetics, it has undergone considerable modification and change and is still evolving as techniques for studying the molecular components of the cell are refined. The gene is now considered to be a particular nucleic acid sequence within a DNA molecule that occupies a precise locus on a chromosome and is capable of self-replication by coding for a specific polypeptide chain. In diploid organisms, which include humans and other mammals, genes occur as paired alleles and function in numerous capacities, primarily as structural and regulative components in controlling the differentiation of the cells and tissues of the body. Kinds of genes include **complementary genes, dominant gene, lethal gene, mutant gene, operator gene, pleiotropic gene, recessive gene, regulator gene, structural gene, sublethal gene, supplementary genes,** and **wild-type gene.** See also **chromosome, cistron, DNA, operon.**

-gene. See **-gen.**

gene library, (in molecular genetics) a collection of all of the genetic information of a specific species, obtained from cloned fragments.

general adaptation syndrome (GAS), the defense response of the body or the psyche to injury or prolonged stress, as described by Hans Selye (1907–1982). It consists of an initial stage of shock or alarm reaction, followed by a phase of increasing resistance or adaptation, using the various defense mechanisms of the body or mind, and culminating in either a state of adjustment and healing or of exhaustion and disintegration. Also called **adaptation syndrome.** See also **posttraumatic stress disorder, stress.**

general anesthesia, the absence of sensation and consciousness as induced by various anesthetic agents, given primarily by inhalation or intravenous injection. Four kinds of nerve blocks attained by general anesthesia are sensory, voluntary motor, reflex motor, and mental. There are several levels of mental block: calmness, sedation, hypnosis, narcosis, and complete, potentially lethal depression of all vital regulatory functions of the medulla in the brain. The kind of anesthesia selected and the dose and route by which it is given depend on the indication for anesthesia. The depth of anesthesia is planned to allow the surgical procedure to be performed without the patient's experiencing pain or having any recall of the procedure. Endotracheal intubation and respiratory support are often necessary. General anesthesia may be administered only by a physician or a Certified Registered Nurse Anesthetist. See also **anesthesia, Guedel's signs, local anesthesia, regional anesthesia.**

generalization, the process of reducing or bringing under a general rule or statement, as classifying items under general categories.

generalized anaphylaxis, a severe reagin-mediated reaction to an allergen characterized by itching, edema, wheezing respirations, apprehension, cyanosis, dyspnea, pupillary dilatation, a rapid, weak pulse, and falling blood pressure that may rapidly result in shock and death. Systemic anaphylaxis, the most extreme form of hypersensitivity, may be caused by insect stings, proteins in animal sera, food, or certain drugs; parenterally administered penicillin and contrast media containing iodide are frequent causes of anaphylactic shock, especially in individuals with a history of allergies. An anaphylactic reaction is mediated by reaginic antibodies (IgE) that form in response to an initial sensitizing dose of an allergen and render the individual hypersensitive to the allergen by binding it to mast cells and basophils. A subsequent challenging dose of the allergen, causing the cells to degranulate and release histamine, bradykinin, and other vasoactive amines, produces anaphylaxis; the severity of the reaction depends on several factors, including the amount and route of entrance of the sensitizing and challenging doses of the allergen. Treatment of generalized anaphylaxis consists of an immediate subcutaneous or intramuscular injection of 1:1000 epinephrine hydrochloride, the administration of an antihistamine, as tripelennamine or diphenhydramine, and isoproterenol or aminophylline to relieve bronchial spasm. A vasopressor may be given to increase blood pressure, and a corticosteroid to suppress the immune response. The patient's legs are elevated to counteract shock; oxygen may be administered by a positive pressure mask, and, if tracheal edema is present, an endotracheal tube may be inserted or a tracheostomy performed. See also **reagin-mediated disorder.**

generally recognized as effective (GRAE), one of the statutory criteria that must be met by a drug before it can be approved as a "new drug." Meeting these criteria relieves the manufacturer of the necessity of obtaining premarket approval as required by the Federal Food, Drug, and Cosmetic Act. To be recognized as effective, the drug must be, according to the Act, considered safe and effective by "experts qualified by scientific training and experience."

general paresis, an organic mental disorder resulting from chronic syphilitic infection, characterized by degeneration of the cortical neurons; progressive dementia, tremor, and speech disturbances; muscular weakness; and, ultimately, generalized paralysis. It is often accompanied by periods of exultation and delusions of grandeur. Treatment usually consists of large doses of penicillin without which the outcome is almost invariably progressive deterioration and death. Also called **cerebral tabes, dementia paralytica,** *(obsolete)* **general paralysis of the insane, paretic dementia, syphilitic meningoencephalitis.**

general practitioner (GP), a family practice physician. See also **family medicine.**

generation, **1.** the act or process of reproduction; procreation. **2.** a group of contemporary individuals, animals, or plants that are the same number of life cycles from a common ancestor. **3.** the period of time between the birth of one individual or organism and the birth of its offspring. Kinds of generation include **alternate generation, asexual generation, filial generation, parental generation, sexual generation,** and **spontaneous generation.**

generative, pertaining to activity that generates new physical or mental growth, as creative problem solving.

generic, **1.** of or pertaining to a genus. **2.** of or pertaining to a substance, product, or drug that is not protected by trademark. **3.** of or pertaining to the name of a kind of drug that is also the description of the drug, as penicillin or tetracycline.

generic equivalent, a drug product sold under its generic name, identical in chemical composition to one or more others sold under a trademark but not, necessarily, equivalent in therapeutic effect.

generic name, the official, established nonproprietary name assigned to a drug. A given drug is licensed under its generic name, and all manufacturers of the drug list it by its generic name. However, a drug is usually marketed under a trademark chosen by the manufacturer. See also **chemical name, established name, trademark.**

generic nursing program, a program to prepare people with no previous professional nursing experience for entry into the field of nursing. The term is now usually used to distinguish baccalaureate programs from master's programs or practitioner programs.

-genesia, **1.** a combining form meaning a '(specified) condition concerning information': *agenesia, morphogenesia, paragenesia.* **2.** also **-genesis.** a combining form meaning 'the production or procreation of something (specified)': *algogenesia, palingenesia, syngenesia.*

genesis, **1.** the origin, generation, or developmental evolution of anything. **2.** the act of producing or procreating.

-genesis. See **-genesia.**

gene splicing, (in molecular genetics) the process by which a segment of DNA is attached to or inserted in a strand of DNA from another source. In recombinant DNA technology genetic material from humans and other mammals is spliced into bacterial plasmids.

genetic, **1.** pertaining to reproduction, birth, or origin. **2.** pertaining to genetics or heredity. **3.** pertaining to or produced by a gene; inherited.

-genetic, -genic, -genous, -geneous, **1.** a combining form meaning 'pertaining to generation by (specified) agents': *gamogenetic, mitogenetic, spermatogenetic.* **2.** a combining form meaning 'generating': *glycogenetic, ovigenetic, ureagenetic.* **3.** a combining form meaning 'pertaining to something generated by a (specified) agent': *biogenetic, ideogenetic, phylogenetic.*

genetic affinity, relationship by direct descent.

genetic code, the information carried by the DNA molecules that determines the specific amino acids and their arrangement in the polypeptide chain of each protein synthesized by the cell. The code represents the sequence of nucleotides along the DNA molecule of each chromosome, and, during transcription, this arrangement is synthesized in messenger RNA and carried from the nucleus to the cytoplasm of the cell where it is translated into protein at the site of the ribosomes. A unit of three consecutive nucleotides, or a codon, codes for each amino acid of the protein molecule. Any change in the code results in the incorrect arrangement of the amino acids in the protein, causing a mutation. See also **anticodon, transcription, translation.**

genetic colonization, the process by which a parasite introduces into its host genetic information that induces the host to synthesize products solely for the use of the parasite.

genetic counseling, the process of determining the occurrence or risk of occurrence of a genetic disorder within a family and of providing appropriate information and advice about the courses of action that are available, whether care of a child already affected, prenatal diagnosis, termination of a pregnancy, sterilization, or artificial insemination is involved. Effective genetic counseling requires an accurate diagnosis of the condition, sometimes necessitating special biochemical or cytogenetic tests, because many of the some 2000 known inherited disorders have similar clinical manifestations but totally different modes of inheritance; a careful, detailed family history, recorded in the form of a pedigree chart; and an understanding of genetic principles, especially a knowledge of the risks related to multifactorial inheritance. The most efficient counseling services consist of a group of specialists, including physicians, geneticists, psychologists, biochemists, cytologists, nurses, and social workers. It is especially important that nurses be alert to those situations in which persons may need genetic counseling, become familiar with facilities in the area that provide genetic counseling services, and help couples arrive at tentative decisions regarding future family planning or the care of a child with a genetic disorder. See also **genetic screening, prenatal diagnosis.**

genetic death, **1.** the failure of an organism to survive as a result of its genetic makeup. **2.** the removal of a gene or genotype from the gene pool of a population or a given familial descent because of sterility, failure of the individual or organism to reproduce, or death before sexual maturity.

genetic disorder. See **inherited disorder.**

genetic drift, the chance fluctuations in gene frequencies within a population. The smaller the population, the greater the tendency for variation within each generation, so that eventually small, isolated inbreeding groups become genetically quite different from the ancestors from which they derived. Also called **drift, random genetic drift.**

genetic engineering, the process of producing recombinant DNA so that the genotype and phenotype of organisms can be altered and controlled. Enzymes are used to break the DNA molecule into fragments so that genes from another organism can be inserted and the nucleotides rearranged in any desired sequence. Through genetic engineering, such human proteins as the growth hormone, insulin, and interferon have been produced in bacteria by using the recombinant DNA technique. At present, genetic engineering represents a powerful tool for medical research and is possible only in microorganisms; but in the future, the technique may be applicable to higher organisms, with the possibility of controlling and eliminating genetic disorders and malformations in humans.

genetic equilibrium, the state within a population at which the frequency of genes and genotypes does not change from generation to generation. The condition routinely occurs in a large interbreeding population in which mating is random and there are no or relatively few mutations. See also **Hardy-Weinberg equilibrium principle.**

genetic homeostasis, the maintenance of genetic variability within a population through adaptation to varied or changing environments and conditions of life as a result of shifts or resistance to shifts in gene frequencies.

genetic immunity. See **natural immunity.**

genetic isolate, a group of plants, animals, or individuals that are genetically separated by geographic, racial, social, cultural, or any other barriers that prevent them from interbreeding with those outside of the group. Depending on the size of the group and the amount of inbreeding that occurs, genetic isolates generally show an increased incidence of otherwise rare, inherited defects. See also **deme.**

geneticist, one who specializes in the study or application of genetics.

genetic load, the average number of accumulated detrimental genes per individual within a population, including those caused by mutation and selection within a recent generation and those inherited from ancestors. Genetic load is measured according to lethal equivalents.

genetic map, the graphic representation of the linear arrangement of genes on a chromosome and the relative distance between them, as expressed in map or morgan units. Also called **linkage map.**

genetic marker, any specific gene that produces a readily recognizable genetic trait that can be used in family and population studies or in linkage analysis. Also called **gene marker, marker gene.**

genetic polymorphism, the recurrence within a population of two or more discontinuous genetic variants of a specific trait in such proportions that they cannot be maintained simply by mutation, as the sickle cell trait, the Rh factor, and the blood groups. Compare **balanced polymorphism.**

genetic population. See **deme.**

genetics, **1.** the science that studies the principles and mechanics of heredity, specifically the means by which traits are passed from parents to offspring and the causes of the similarities and differences between related organisms. **2.** the total genetic makeup of a particular individual, family, group, or condition. Kinds of genetics are **clinical genetics, molecular genetics,** and **population genetics.** See also **cytogenetics, Mendel's laws.**

genetic screening, the process of investigating a specific population of persons for the purpose of detecting the presence of disease, either incipient or overt, as the generalized screening of all newborn infants for phenylketonuria, of identifying those who possess defective genes, of gaining information concerning the incidence of a disorder in the population, and of providing reproductive information, specifically to those at risk, as the close relatives of persons affected with inborn errors of metabolism or those in certain ethnic groups who have a high incidence of a particular disease, specifically sickle cell anemia in blacks and Tay-Sachs disease in Ashkenazic Jews. When accompanied by education and counseling, mass screening programs can be effective in the management of genetic disorders. See also **genetic counseling.** (Table, page 482)

Genga's bandage. See **Theden's bandage.**

-genia, a combining form meaning '(condition or development of the) jaw': *microgenia, opisthogenia, progenia.*

-genic, **1.** a combining form meaning 'causing, forming, producing': *collagenic, hemorrhagenic, phosphagenic.* **2.** a combining form meaning 'produced by or formed from': *bacillogenic, coccigenic, pituitarigenic.* **3.** a combining form meaning 'related to a gene': *intragenic, polygenic, trigenic.*

geniculate neuralgia, a severe, debilitating, inflammatory condition of the geniculate ganglion of the facial nerve, characterized by pain, loss of the sense of taste, facial paralysis, and a decrease in salivation and lacrimation. It sometimes follows herpes zoster infection. See also **Ramsay Hunt's syndrome.**

geniculate zoster. See **herpes zoster.**

geniohyoideus /jē′nē·ōhī·oi′dē·əs/, one of the four suprahyoid muscles, arising from the symphysis menti of the lower jaw and inserting into the body of the hyoid bone. A narrow muscle, it is innervated by a branch of the first cervical nerve, and it acts to draw the hyoid bone and the tongue forward. Also called **geniohyoid muscle.** Compare **digastricus, mylohyoideus, stylohyoideus.**

genital herpes. See **herpes genitalis, herpes simplex.**

genital reflex. See **sexual reflex.**

genitals, the reproductive organs. Also called **genitalia.** **–genital,** *adj.*

genital stage, (in psychoanalysis) the final period in psychosexual development, beginning with adolescence and continuing through the adult years when the genitals are the predominant source of pleasurable stimulation. The most significant feature of this stage is direction of sexual interest not just toward self-satisfaction but toward the establishment of a stable and meaningful heterosexual relationship. See also **psychosexual development.**

genitourinary (GU), referring to the genital and urinary systems of the body, either the organ structures or functions or both. Also called **urogenital.**

genitourinary system. See **urogenital system.**

genome /jē′nōm/, the complete set of genes in the chromosomes of each cell of a particular organism.

genontopia. See **senopia.**

genotype /jē′nōtīp′/, **1.** the complete genetic constitution of an organism or group, as determined by the particular combination and location of the genes on the chromosomes. **2.** the alleles situated at one or more sites on homologous chromosomes. The genetic information carried by a pair of alleles determines a specific characteristic or trait, usually designated by a letter or symbol, as AA when the alleles are identical and Aa when they are different. **3.** a group or class of organisms having the same genetic makeup; the type species of a genus. Compare **phenotype.** **–genotypic,** *adj.*

-genous, a combining form meaning 'producing or produced by': *tetanigenous, thyroigenous, tuberculigenous.*

Gensoul's disease. See **Ludwig's angina.**

gentamicin sulfate /jen′təmī′sin/, an aminoglycoside antibiotic.

■ INDICATION: It is prescribed to relieve the effects of severe infections caused by organisms sensitive to gentamicin.

■ CONTRAINDICATIONS: Concomitant administration of other potentially ototoxic drugs or known hypersensitivity to this drug or to other aminoglycoside medications prohibits its use. It is used with caution in patients having impaired renal function.

■ ADVERSE EFFECTS: Among the more serious adverse reactions are nephrotoxicity, auditory or vestibular ototoxicity, impairment of neuromuscular transmission, and hypersensitivity reactions.

gentian violet /jen′shən/, an antibacterial antiinfective, antifungal, and anthelmintic.

■ INDICATIONS: It is prescribed in the treatment of pinworms, superficial infections of the skin, and vaginal infections.

■ CONTRAINDICATIONS: Known hypersensitivity to this drug prohibits its use. It is not applied to ulcerative lesions of the face.

■ ADVERSE EFFECTS: Among the most serious adverse reactions are permanent discoloration of the skin after topical exposure to the drug. GI distress and purple vomitus may occur after oral administration.

gentiotannic acid /jen′shē·ətan′ik/, a form of tannic acid once used as an astringent and in the treatment of burns but no longer recommended because the compound is hepatotoxic.

Gentran 40, a trademark for a plasma volume extender (dextran 40).

Gentran 75, a trademark for a plasma volume extender (dextran 75).

genu /jē′nōō/, the knee or any angular structure resembling the flexed knee.

genuine issue, (in law) an issue that is upheld by substantial evidence. It is a real issue, not a false one or one that is subject to interpretation.

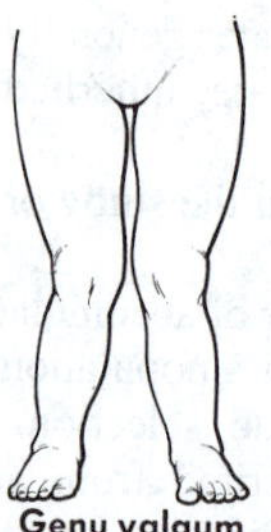

Genu valgum

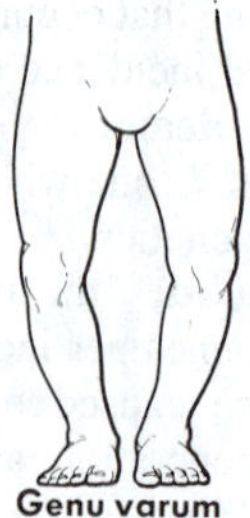

Genu varum

genupectoral position, knee-chest position. To assume the genupectoral position, the person kneels so that the weight of the body is supported by the knees and chest, with the abdomen raised. The head is turned to one side and the arms are flexed so that the upper part of the body can be supported in part by the elbows.

genus /jē′nəs/, *pl.* **genera** /jen′ərə/, a subdivision of a family of animals or plants. A genus usually is composed of several closely related species, but the genus *Homo sapiens* has only one species, humans. See also **family.**

genu valgum, a deformity in which the legs are curved inward so that the knees are close together, knocking as the person walks, with the ankles widely separated. Also called **knock-knee.**

genu varum, a deformity in which one or both legs are bent outward at the knee. Also called **bowleg.** Compare **genu valgum.**

-geny, a combining form meaning 'production, generation, origin': *homogeny, hylogeny, morphogeny.*

Genetic diseases

Disorders of carbohydrate metabolism
Diabetes mellitus
Pentosuria
Glycogen storage diseases
Galactosemia

Disorders of lipid metabolism
Familial lipoprotein deficiency
Familial lecithin-cholesterol acyl-transferase (L-CAT) deficiency
Tay-Sachs disease
Gaucher's disease

Disorders of protein metabolism
Familial goiter
Phenylketonuria
Albinism
Alkaptonuria
Tyrosinosis

Disorders of purine and pyrimidine metabolism
Gout
Lesch-Nyhan syndrome

Disorders of metal metabolism
Wilson's disease
Hemochromatosis

Disorders of connective tissue, bone, and muscle
Familial periodic paralysis
Muscular dystrophies
Mucopolysaccharidoses

Disorders of the hematopoietic system and blood
Sickle cell anemia
Glucose 6-phosphate dehydrogenase deficiency
Thalassemias
Hereditary spherocytosis

Disorders of exocrine glands
Cystic fibrosis

geo-, a combining form meaning 'pertaining to the earth, or soil': *geobiology, geophagia, geotropism.*

Geocillin, a trademark for an antibacterial (carbenicillin indanyl sodium).

geographic tongue, a disorder in which small white or yellowish plaques develop on the tongue, gradually enlarge, and desquamate in the center, leaving denuded red patches surrounded by thickened white borders that converge, forming figures with scalloped outlines. The disorder, which may persist for months or years, causes a burning or itching sensation, is aggravated by food, and is often associated with digestive problems, especially in children. Also called **benign migratory glossitis.**

geometric mean. See **mean,** def. 3.

Geopen, a trademark for an antibacterial (carbenicillin disodium).

geotrichosis /jē′ōtrikō′sis/, an abnormal condition associated with the fungus *Geotrichum candidum,* which may cause oral, bronchial, pharyngeal, and intestinal disorders. *Geotrichum candidum,* normally found in healthy individuals, the soil, and in dairy products, is not necessarily pathogenic. Geotrichosis most commonly occurs in immunosuppressed individuals and in diabetics. Bronchopulmonary complications associated with this disorder may produce a cough with thick, bloody sputum. Geotrichosis has been associated with allergic asthmatic reactions similar to allergic aspergillosis and a type of intestinal disorder characterized by abdominal pain, diarrhea, and rectal bleeding. Oral lesions that may occur with this disorder are commonly treated with a solution of gentian violet; associated abdominal lesions are treated with the oral administration of gentian violet capsules; associated pulmonary lesions are treated with the oral administration of potassium iodide.

geriatric day care, an ambulatory health care facility for elderly people. It usually offers a broad range of professional and community services to maximize functional independence for the patients.

geriatrician /jer′ē·ətrish′ən/, a medical specialist in the field of geriatrics.

geriatric nurse practitioner, a registered nurse with additional education and training through a master's degree program in nursing or a nondegree certificate program that prepares the nurse to deliver primary health care to elderly adults.

geriatrics /jer′ē·at′riks/, the branch of medicine dealing with the physiology of aging and the diagnosis and treatment of diseases affecting the aged.

germ, **1.** any microorganism, especially one that is pathogenic. **2.** a unit of living matter able to develop into a self-sufficient organism, as a seed, spore, or egg. **3.** (in embryology) the first stage in development, as a spermatozoon or other germ cell.

germanium (Ge), a metallic element with some nonmetallic properties. Its atomic number is 32; its atomic weight is 72.59.

German measles. See **rubella.**

germ cell, **1.** a sexual reproductive cell in any stage of development, from the primordial embryonic form to the mature gamete. **2.** an ovum or spermatozoon or any of their preceding forms. **3.** any cell undergoing gametogenesis. Also called **gonoblast, gonocyte.** Compare **somatic cell.**

germ disk. See **embryonic disk.**

germicide, a drug that kills pathogenic microorganisms. See also **antibacterial,** def. 2, **antifungal,** def. 2, **antiviral,** def. 2. **–germicidal,** *adj.*

germinal /jur′minəl/, pertaining to or characteristic of a germ cell or to the early stages of development.

germinal disk. See **embryonic disk.**

germinal epithelium, **1.** the epithelial layer covering the genital ridge from which the gonads are derived in early embryonic development. **2.** the epithelial covering of the ovary, formerly thought to be the site of the formation of the oogonia. See also **oogenesis.**

germinal infection, an infection transmitted to a child by the ovum or sperm of a parent. Compare **endogenous infection, mixed infection, retrograde infection, secondary infection.**

germinal membrane. See **blastoderm.**

germinal nucleus. See **pronucleus.**

germinal pole. See **animal pole.**

germinal spot, the nucleolus of a mature oocyte, before fertilization. See also **oogenesis, ovum.**

germinal stage, (in embryology) the interval of time from fertilization to implantation during which the ovum undergoes cell division several times, travels to the uterus, and, in the form of a blastocyst, begins to implant itself in the endometrium. The germinal stage is over at about 10 days of gestation.

germinal vesicle, the nucleus of a mature oocyte before fertilization. Much larger than the nucleus of other cells, it initiates the completion of meiotic division after fertilization. See also **oogenesis, ovum.**

germination, **1.** the initial growth and development of an organism from the time of fertilization to the formation of the embryo. **2.** the sprouting of a spore or the seed of a plant. **–germinate,** *v.*

germ layer, one of the three primordial cell layers formed during gastrulation in the early stages of embryonic development from which the entire range of body tissue is derived. Each layer has the potentiality for forming different cellular types that differentiate into the various structures and organs of the body. See also **ectoderm, endoderm, mesoderm.**

germ nucleus. See **pronucleus.**

germ plasm, **1.** the protoplasm of the germ cells containing the basic reproductive and hereditary material; the sum total of the DNA in a particular cell or organism. The substance was first named by August Weismann (1834–1914) to indicate the material that originates in the germ cell, produces new organisms, transmits hereditary characteristics, and passes in direct continuity to germ cells of succeeding generations. **2.** *nontechnical.* germ cells in any stage of development together with the tissues from which they originated. Compare **somatoplasm.** See also **weismannism.**

germ-plasm theory. See **weismannism.**

gero-, geronto-, a combining form meaning 'pertaining to old age or the aged': *gerocomia, gerodontology, geromarasmus.*

-gerontic, -gerontal, a combining form meaning 'pertaining to old age': *parageronitc, phylogerontic, ungerontic.*

geronto-. See **gero-.**

gerontology, the study of all aspects of the aging process, including the clinical, psychologic, economic, and sociologic problems encountered by the elderly and their consequences for both the individual and society.

gerontoxon. See **arcus senilis.**

geropsychiatry, the study and treatment of mental illness in elderly persons.

-gerous, a combining form meaning 'bearing or characterized by' something specified: *calcigerous, ovigerous, setigerous.*

Gestalt /gəshtält′/, *pl.* **Gestalts, Gestalten** /gəshtäl′tən/, a single physical, psychologic, or symbolic configuration, pattern, or experience consisting of a number of elements that has an effect as a whole different from that of the sum of its parts.

Gestalt psychology, a school of psychology, originating in Germany, that maintains that a psychologic phenomenon is perceived as a total configuration or pattern, rising from the relationships among its constituent elements, rather than as discrete elements possessing attributes of their own, and that the pattern, or Gestalt, cannot be derived from the summation of its constituents. Thus, learning is regarded as resulting from insight, defined as a process or reorganization, rather than from association or trial and error, and behavior is seen as an integrated response to a unitary situation rather than as a series of reflexes and sensations. Also called **configurationism, Gestaltism.** See also **Gestalt.**

Gestalt therapy, a form of psychotherapy that stresses the unity of self-awareness, behavior, and experience. It incorporates elements of psychoanalytic, behavioristic, and humanistic existential therapy. See **Gestalt psychology.**

gestant anomaly. See **odontoma.**

gestate, 1. to carry a developing fetus in the womb. **2.** to grow and develop slowly toward maturity, as a fetus in the womb.

gestation, in viviparous animals, the period of time from the fertilization of the ovum until birth. Gestation varies with the species; in humans the average duration is 266 days or approximately 280 days from the onset of the last menstrual period. See also **pregnancy.**

gestational age, the age of a fetus or a newborn, usually expressed in weeks dating from the first day of the mother's last menstrual period.

gestational diabetes mellitus (GDM), a disorder characterized by an impaired ability to metabolize carbohydrate, usually caused by a deficiency of insulin, occurring in pregnancy and disappearing after delivery but, in some cases, returning years later. There is evidence that placental lactogen and considerable destruction of insulin by the placenta play a role in precipitating gestational diabetes. Treatment consists of insulin injections, a high-protein diet, and an adequate intake of calcium and iron, but no attempt is made to keep the patient's urine free of sugar. See also **diabetes mellitus.**

-geusia, -geustia, a combining form meaning, '(condition of the) sense of taste': *glycogeusia, hemiageusia, parageusia.*

GH, abbreviation for **growth hormone.**

ghost cells, red blood cells that have lost their hemoglobin so that only the cell membranes are observed in microscopic examinations of urine samples. The hemoglobin is destroyed by the presence of urine. Also called **shadow cells.**

GHRF, abbreviation for **growth hormone releasing factor.**

GI, abbreviation for **gastrointestinal.**

giant cell arteritis. See **temporal arteritis.**

giant cell carcinoma, a malignant epithelial neoplasm characteristically containing numerous very large anaplastic cells. A small percentage of adenocarcinomas of the lung and some liver tumors also contain such cells. Also called **carcinoma gigantocellulare.**

giant cell interstitial pneumonia. See **interstitial pneumonia.**

giant cell myeloma, a bone tumor of multinucleated giant cells that resembles osteoclasts scattered in a matrix of spindle cells. Myelomas of this kind may be benign or malignant and may cause pain, functional disability, and, in some cases, pathologic fractures. Also called **giant cell tumor of bone.**

giant cell thyroiditis. See **de Quervain's thyroiditis.**

giant cell tumor of bone. See **giant cell myeloma.**

giant chromosome, any of the excessively large chromosomes found in insects and the lower animals, specifically the lampbrush chromosome and polytene chromosome.

giant follicular lymphoma, a nodular, well-differentiated, lymphocytic, malignant lymphoma in which many nodules distort the normal structure of a lymph node. Also called **Brill-Symmers disease, giant follicular lymphadenopathy, Symmers' disease.**

giant hypertrophic gastritis, a rare disease characterized by large folds of nodular gastric rugae that may cover the wall of the stomach, causing anorexia, nausea, vomiting, and abdominal distress. X-ray or endoscopic examination or surgery may be necessary for diagnosis. The nurse usually recommends periodic reexamination because the disease is associated with an incidence of stomach cancer that is greater than normal.

Giardia /jē·är′dē·ə/, a common genus of the flagellate protozoans. Many species of *Giardia* normally inhabit the digestive tract causing inflammation in association with other factors that produce rapid proliferation of the organism. See also **giardiasis.**

giardiasis /jē·ärdī′əsis/, an inflammatory, intestinal condition caused by overgrowth of the protozoan *Giardia lamblia*. The source of infection is usually untreated water contaminated with *G. lamblia* cysts. Also called **traveler's diarrhea.**

gibbus /gib′əs, jib′əs/, **1.** a hump, swelling, or enlargement on a body surface, usually confined to one side. **2.** a convex spinal curvature that may occur after the collapse of a vertebral body as may result from a fracture or tuberculosis of the spine.

Gibraltar fever. See **brucellosis.**

Gibson walking splint, a kind of Thomas splint that allows a patient to be ambulatory.

Giemsa's stain /gē·em′zəz/, an azure dye used as a stain in the microscopic examination of the blood for certain protozoan parasites, viral inclusion bodies, and rickettsia, and, more routinely, in the preparation of a smear for a differential white cell count.

gigantic acid, an antibiotic substance derived from *Aspergillus giganteus,* a species of mold.

gigantism /jigan′tizəm/, an abnormal condition characterized by excessive size and stature, caused most frequently by hypersecretion of growth hormone (GH) and occurring to a lesser degree in hypogonadism and in certain genetic disorders. Gigantism with normal body proportions and normal sexual development usually results from hypersecretion of GH in early childhood. Hypogonadism, by delaying puberty and closure of the epiphyses, may lead to gigantism. Excessive linear growth often occurs in males with more than one Y chromosome, and it may accompany Klinefelter's syndrome, Marfan's syndrome, and some cases of generalized lipodystrophy. Children with cerebral gigantism are mentally retarded and have a large head and extremities and a clumsy gait. They grow rapidly during their first few years and then at a normal rate. Appropriate gonadal hormones may be administered to control abnormal growth of children with hypogonadism. The treatment of acromegalic gigantism is usually irradiation, but hypophysectomy may be indicated. See also **acromegaly, eunuchoidism.**

giganto-, a combining form meaning 'huge': *gigantoblast, gigantochromoblast, gigantocyte.*

Gilbert's syndrome, a benign, hereditary condition characterized by hyperbilirubinemia and jaundice. No treatment is required. See also **hyperbilirubinemia of the newborn.**

Gilchrist's disease. See **blastomycosis.**

Gilles de la Tourette's syndrome /zhēl′dəlätŏŏrets′/, an abnormal condition characterized by facial grimaces, tics, and involuntary arm and shoulder movements. In adolescence, the condition worsens; the child may grunt, snort, and shout involuntarily. Coprolalia often develops, to the consternation of the person and the people around the person afflicted. In adulthood the condition usually does not worsen; it comes and goes. Recently, treatment with dopamine antagonists has been found to be very effective, demonstrating an organic cause for this syndrome.

Gillies' operation /gil′ēz/, a surgical procedure for reducing fractures of the zygoma and zygomatic arch by making an incision in the temporal hairline.

gingiva /jinjī′və/, *pl.* **gingivae,** the gum of the mouth, a mucous membrane with supporting fibrous tissue that overlies the crowns of unerupted teeth and encircles the necks of those that have erupted. **–gingival,** *adj.*

gingival blanching, the lightening of gingival color, usually temporary, caused by the stretching of gingival tissue with decreased blood supply.

gingival blood supply, the vascular supply to the gingivae, arising from blood vessels that pass on the gingival side of the outer periosteum of bone and anastomose with blood vessels of the periodontal membrane and intraalveolar blood vessels.

gingival cavity, a cavity that occurs in the gingival third of the clinical crown of the tooth.

gingival color, the color of healthy or diseased gingival tissues. It varies with the thickness and degree of keratinization of the epithelium, blood supply, pigmentation, and alterations produced by gingival diseases.

gingival consistency, the combination of visual and tactile characteristics of healthy gingival tissue. The visual characteristic varies from the look of smooth velvet to that of a finely or coarsely grained orange peel. The tactile consistency of healthy gingival tissue is firm and resilient. Compare **gingival color.**

gingival corium, the most stable connective tissue of the gingiva, lying between the periosteum and the lamina propria mucosae.

gingival crater, a depression in the gingival tissue, especially in the area of the former apex of interdental papilla. It is commonly caused by necrotizing ulcerative gingivitis and food impaction against the tissue subjacent to the contact areas of adjacent teeth.

gingival crevice, a normal fissure between the free gingiva and the tooth enamel.

gingival discoloration, a change in the normal coloration the gingivae, associated with inflammation, reduced blood supply, abnormal pigmentation and other problems.

gingival festoon, the distinct rounding and enlargement of the margins of the gingival tissue found in early gingival involvement. Compare **festoon, McCall's festoon.**

gingival hormonal enlargement, the enlargement of the gingivae associated with hormonal imbalance during pregnancy, puberty, and hormonal therapy.

gingival hyperplasia, overgrowth of the soft tissue of the gums, often seen in patients treated with phenytoin for epileptic seizures.

gingival massage, the massage of gingival tissues for cleansing purposes, improving tissue tone and blood circulation, and for keratinization of the surface epithelium

gingival mat, the gingival connective tissue composed of coarse, broad collagen fibers that attach the gingivae to the teeth and hold the free gingivae in close approximation to the teeth.

gingival papilla. See **papilla.**

gingival physiology, the function of the gingivae as supportive and protective investments of the teeth and subjacent tissues. The gingival fiber apparatus serves as a barrier to apical migration of the epithelial attachment and binds the gingival tissues to the teeth. Normal gingival topograpy permits the free flow of food away from the occlusal surfaces and from the cervical and interproximal areas of the teeth.

gingival position, the level of the gingival margin in relation to the teeth.

gingival shrinkage, the reduction in the size of gingival tissue, especially as the result of therapeutic elimination of subgingival deposits and curettement of the soft tissue wall of the gingival pocket.

gingival stippling, a series of small depressions in the surface of healthy gingivae, producing an appearance that varies from that of smooth, undulated velvet to that of an orange peel. See also **gingival consistency.**

gingival sulcus, any of the normal spaces between the free gingivae and the teeth.

gingivectomy, surgical removal of infected and diseased gingival tissue, performed to arrest the development of pyorrhea. Under general anesthesia, all pockets around the teeth are scraped and hypertrophied tissue is removed. The exposed surface of the gum is covered with packing to prevent trauma while eating and to allow new epithelial tissue to cover and fill in the areas. Considerable bleeding and pain are associated with the procedure. Postoperatively, the patient is closely observed for signs that may indicate hemorrhage, frequent swallowing, or a rise in pulse rate. The packing is removed 1 week later. Compare **gingivoplasty.**

gingivitis /jin′jivī′tis/, a condition in which the gums are red, swollen, and bleeding. Most gingivitis is the result of poor oral hygiene and of the accumulation of bacterial plaque on the teeth, but gingivitis may be a sign of another condition, as diabetes mellitus, leukemia, or vitamin deficiency. It is common in pregnancy, usually painless, and may be acute or chronic. Frequent removal of plaque and regular visits to the dentist may be preventive. Compare **Vincent's infection.** See also **hypertrophic gingivitis.**

gingivo-, a combining form meaning 'pertaining to the gingiva': *gingivoglossitis, gingivolabial, gingivosis.*

gingivoplasty, the surgical contouring of the gingival tissues to maintain healthy gingival tissue. Compare **gingivectomy.**

gingivostomatitis /jin′jivōstō′mətī′tis/, multiple, painful ulcers on the gums and mucous membranes of the mouth, the result of a herpesvirus infection. Seen most frequently in infants and young children, the condition usually subsides after 1 week, but, in rare cases, it may progress to a systemic viral infection. See also **herpes simplex.**

ginglymus joint. See **hinge joint.**

Giordano-Giovannetti diet /jôrdä′nōjō′vənet′ē/, a low-protein, low-fat, high-carbohydrate diet with controlled potassium and sodium intake, used in chronic renal insufficiency and liver failure. Protein is given only in the form of essential amino acids so that the body will use excess blood urea nitrogen to synthesize the nonessential amino acids for the production of tissue protein. The foods included are eggs, small amounts of milk, low-protein bread, some fruits and vegetables low in potassium, as green beans, summer squash, cabbage, pears, grapefruit, and fresh or frozen blackberries, blueberries, and boysenberries. There are many modified forms of this diet depending on patient requirements and tolerance, usually varying in the amount and origin of the protein. Also called **Giovannetti diet.** See also **renal diet.**

girdle sensation. See **zonesthesia.**

Gitaligin, a trademark for a cardiotonic (gitalin).

gitalin /jit′əlin/, a combination of digitalis glycosides.

■ INDICATIONS: It is prescribed as a cardiotonic in the treatment of congestive heart failure, atrial fibrillation, and atrial tachycardia.

■ CONTRAINDICATIONS: Ventricular fibrillation, ventricular tachycardia, concomitant administration of calcium salts, or known hypersensitivity to this drug prohibits its use.

■ ADVERSE EFFECTS: The most serious adverse reactions are various cardiac arrhythmias.

glabella, a flat triangular area of bone between the two superciliary ridges of the forehead. It is sometimes used as a baseline for cephalometric measurements.

glabrous skin, smooth, hairless skin.

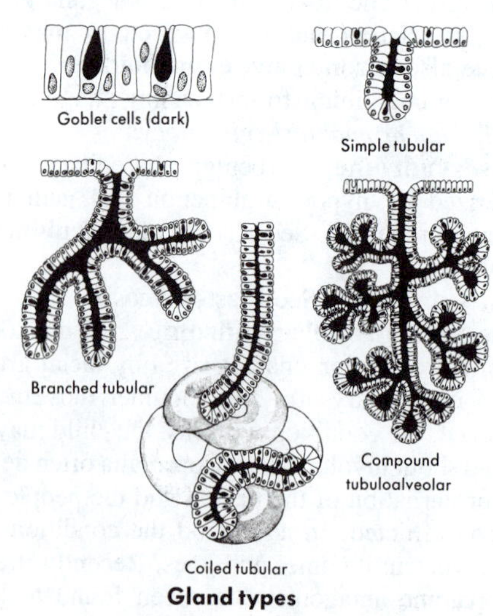

Gland types

gland, any one of many organs in the body, comprising specialized cells that secrete or excrete materials not related to their ordinary metabolism. Some glands lubricate; others, as the pituitary gland, produce hormones; hematopoietic glands, as the spleen, thyroid, and certain lymph nodes, take part in the production of blood.

glanders, an infection caused by the bacillus *Pseudomonas mallei,* transmitted to humans from horses and other domestic animals. It is characterized by purulent inflammation of the mucous membranes and the development of skin nodules that ulcerate. If untreated with antibiotics, the infection may spread to the bones, liver, central nervous system, and other tissues and cause death. It is endemic in Africa, Asia, and South America but has been eradicated in Europe and North America.

gland of Montgomery. See **areolar gland.**

glands of Zeiss. See **ciliary gland.**

glandular carcinoma. See **adenocarcinoma.**

glandular fever. See **infectious mononucleosis.**

glandula vestibularis major. See **Bartholin's gland.**

glans /glanz/, *pl.* **glandes** /glan′dēz/, **1.** a general term for a small, rounded mass, or glandlike body. **2.** erectile tissue, as on the ends of the clitoris and the penis.

glans of clitoris, the erectile tissue at the end of the clitoris, continuous with the intermediate part of the vaginal vestibular bulbs. It comprises two corpora cavernosa enclosed in a dense, fibrous membrane and connected to the pubis and ischium. Also called **glans clitoridis.**

glans penis, the conical tip of the penis that covers the end of the corpora cavernosa penis and the corpus spongiosom like a cap. The urethral orifice is normally located at the center of the distal tip of the glans penis; the corona glandis, the widest part of the glans penis, is around the base of the proximal portion. A fold of dark, thin, hairless skin forms the foreskin covering the glans penis.

Glanzmann's disease. See **thrombasthenia.**

Glasgow Coma Scale, a quick, practical, and standardized system for assessing the degree of conscious impairment in the critically ill and for predicting the duration and ultimate outcome of coma, primarily in patients with head injuries. The system involves three determinants: eye opening, verbal response, and motor response, all of which are evaluated independently according to a rank order that indicates the level of consciousness and degree of dysfunction. There are four grades of eye opening: spontaneous, which indicates that the arousal mechanisms in the brainstem are unimpaired, receives the

Glasgow coma scale

The Glasgow coma scale has been designed to quantitatively relate consciousness to motor responses, verbal responses, and eye opening. Coma is defined as no response and no eye opening. Scores of 7 or less on the Glasgow scale qualify as "coma"; all scores of 9 or more do not qualify as "coma." The examiner determines the *best* response the patient can make to a set of standardized stimuli. Higher points are assigned to responses that indicate increasing degrees of arousal.

1. **Best motor response.** (Examiner determines the *best* response with *either* arm.)
   a. *6 points.* Obeys simple commands. Raises arm on request or holds up specified number of fingers. Releasing a grip (not grasping, which can be reflexive) is also an appropriate test.
   b. *5 points.* Localizes noxious stimuli. Fails to obey commands but can move either arm toward a noxious cutaneous stimulus and eventually contacts it with the hand. The stimulus should be maximal and applied in various locations, i.e., sternum pressure, or trapezius pinch.
   c. *4 points.* Flexion withdrawal. Responds to noxious stimulus with arm flexion but does not localize it with the hand.
   d. *3 points.* Abnormal flexion. Adducts shoulder, flexes and pronates arm, flexes wrist, and makes a fist in response to a noxious stimulus (decorticate rigidity).
   e. *2 points.* Abnormal extension. Adducts and internally rotates shoulder, extends forearm, flexes wrist, and makes a fist in response to a noxious stimulus (decerebrate rigidity).
   f. *1 point.* No motor response. Exclude reasons for no response; for example, insufficient stimulus or spinal cord injury.
2. **Best verbal response.** (Examiner determines the *best* response after arousal. Noxious stimuli are employed if necessary.) Omit this test if the patient is dysphasic, has oral injuries, or is intubated. Place a check mark after other two test category scores after totaling to indicate omission of the verbal response section.
   a. *5 points.* Oriented patient. Can converse and relate who he is, where he is, and the year and month.
   b. *4 points.* Confused patient. Is not fully oriented or demonstrates confusion.
   c. *3 points.* Verbalizes. Does not engage in sustained conversation, but uses intelligible words in an exclamation (curse) or in a disorganized manner which is nonsensical.
   d. *2 points.* Vocalizes. Makes moaning or groaning sounds that are not recognizable words.
   e. *1 point.* No vocalization. Does not make any sound even in response to noxious stimulus.
3. **Eye opening.** (Examiner determines the minimum stimulus that evokes opening of one or both eyes.) If the patient cannot realistically open the eyes because of bandages or lid edema, write "E" after the total test score to indicate omission of this component.
   a. *4 points.* Eyes open spontaneously.
   b. *3 points.* Eyes open to speech. Patient opens eyes in response to command or on being called by name.
   c. *2 points.* Eyes open to noxious stimuli.
   d. *1 point.* No eye opening in response to noxious stimuli.

From Teasdale, G., and Jennett, B.: Assessment of coma and impaired consciousness: a practical scale, Lancet **2:**81-84, 1974.

highest score; opening in response to a verbal statement; opening in response to pain, which should be tested on the limbs, because facial pressure may cause eye closure; and no response. Verbal response has five grades: Orientation is indicated by the patient's awareness of who he or she is, where he or she is, and why he or she is there, as well as the month and year; confused conversation is identified by the patient's verbal responses to questions accompanied by varying degrees of confusion and disorientation; inappropriate speech is indicated by the inability to sustain conversation, the shouting of intelligible words, and swearing; incomprehensible speech is identified by verbalization using unrecognizable "words"; speechlessness is the fifth grade, in which the patient does not make any sound, even in response to a noxious stimulus. Motor responses also have five grades of dysfunction: The patient obeys commands, with care being taken not to confuse the grasp reflex or postural adjustment for a response; a localizing response is the result of a painful stimulus to more than one site causing a limb to move; flexor responses may be slow or rapid; extension responses are usually associated with adduction, internal rotation of the shoulder, and pronation of the forearm; no response indicates hypotonia, and spinal transection must be ruled out. The degree of consciousness may vary from determinant to determinant and is assessed numerically by the best response. The results are plotted on a graph to provide a visual representation of the improvement, stability, or deterioration of a patient's level of consciousness, which is crucial to predicting the eventual outcome of coma. The sum of the numeric values for each parameter can also be used as an overall objective measurement, with 14 being indicative of no impairment, 3 being compatible with brain death, and 7 usually accepted as a state of coma. The test score can also function as an indicator for certain diagnostic tests or treatments, as the need for a CAT scan, intracranial pressure monitoring, and intubation. The scale has a high degree of consistency even when used by staff of varied experience.

glass factor. See **factor XII.**

glaucoma /glôkō′mə, glou-/, an abnormal condition of elevated pressure within an eye because of obstruction of the outflow of aqueous humor. **Acute (angle-closure, closed-angle,** or **narrow-angle) glaucoma** occurs if the pupil in an eye with a narrow angle between the iris and cornea dilates markedly, causing the folded iris to block the exit of aqueous humor from the anterior chamber. **Chronic (open-angle** or **wide-angle) glaucoma** is much more common, often bilateral; it develops slowly and is genetically determined. The obstruction is believed to be within the canal of Schlemm. –**glaucomatous,** *adj.*

■ OBSERVATIONS: Acute glaucoma is accompanied by extreme ocular pain, blurred vision, a red eye, and a dilated pupil. Nausea and vomiting may occur. If untreated, acute glaucoma results in complete and permanent blindness within 2 to 5 days. Chronic glaucoma may produce no symptoms except for gradual loss of peripheral vision over a period of years. Sometimes headaches, blurred vision, and dull pain in the eye are present. Cupping of the optic discs may be noted on ophthalmoscopic examination. Halos around lights and central blindness are late manifestations. Both types have elevated intraocular pressure by tonometry.

■ INTERVENTION: Acute glaucoma is treated with eye drops to constrict the pupil and draw the iris away from the cornea, osmotic agents such as urea, mannitol, or glycerol given systemically to lower intraocular pressure, acetazolamide to reduce fluid formation, and surgical iridectomy to produce a filtration pathway for aqueous humor. Chronic glaucoma can usually be controlled with miotic eye drops such as pilocarpine. Other treatment includes carbonic anhydrase inhibitors, epinephrine eye drops, and timolol, a beta-adrenergic blocking agent.

■ NURSING CONSIDERATIONS: Persons who complain of tunnel vision or who bump into objects frequently should be referred for evaluation. Routine tonometry and ophthalmoscopic examinations are advised for all adults every 3 to 5 years. Nurses should remember that the use of mydriatic and cycloplegic eye drops, atropine-like drugs, and epinephrine in a person with a narrow anterior chamber angle is dangerous. Patients who have glaucoma are cautioned to avoid straining at defecation, to reduce excessive emotional and exertional stress, and to wear a medical identification tag. The nurse stresses the importance of regular eye examinations and the continuous use of medications prescribed for glaucoma.

Glaucon, a trademark for a mydriatic (epinephrine hydrochloride).

-glea, -gloea, a combining form meaning a 'binding gelatinous medium': *ooglea, mesoglea, zooglea.*

glia. See **neuroglia.**

gliadin /glī′ədin/, a protein substance that is obtained from wheat and rye. Its solubility in diluted alcohol distinguishes gliadin from another grain protein, glutenin.

gliding, **1.** a smooth, continuous movement. **2.** the simplest of the four basic movements allowed by various joints of the skeleton. It is common to all movable joints and allows one surface to move smoothly over an adjacent surface, regardless of shape. Gliding is the only motion allowed by most of the wrist and the ankle joints. Compare **angular movement, circumduction, rotation.**

gliding joint, a synovial joint in which articulation of contiguous bones allows only gliding movements, as in the wrist and the ankle. The ligaments or the osseous processes around each gliding joint limit movements of apposed plane surfaces or concavoconvex articulations. Also called **arthrodia, articulatio plana.** Compare **hinge joint, pivot joint.**

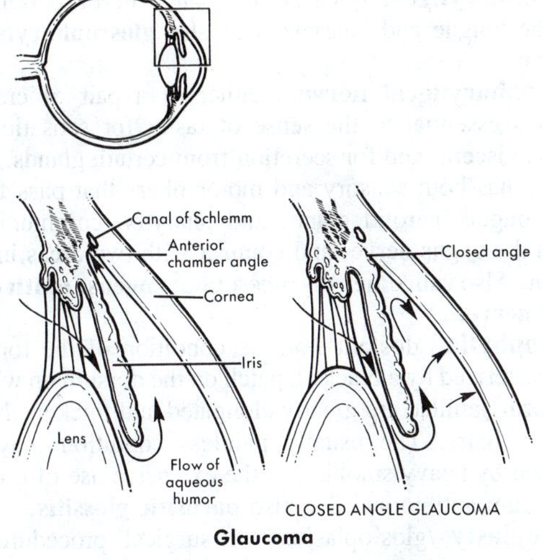

Glaucoma

glio-, a combining form meaning 'pertaining to the neuroglia, or a gluey substance': *gliococcus, gliosarcoma, gliosome.*

glioblastoma. See **spongioblastoma.**

glioblastoma multiforme, a malignant, rapidly growing, pulpy or cystic tumor of the cerebrum or, occasionally, of the spinal cord. The lesion spreads with pseudopod-like projections. It is composed of a mixture of monocytes, pyriform cells, immature and mature astrocytes, and neural ectodermal cells with fibrous or protoplasmic processes. Also called **anaplastic astrocytoma, glioma multiforme.**

glioma /glī·ō′mə/, *pl.* **gliomas, gliomata,** any of the largest group of primary tumors of the brain, composed of malignant glial cells. Kinds of gliomas are **astrocytoma, ependymoma, glioblastoma multiforme, medulloblastoma,** and **oligodendroglioma.**

-glioma, a combining form meaning a 'tumor arising from the neuroglia': *angioglioma, fibroglioma, ganglioma.*

glioma multiforme. See **gliobastoma multiforme.**

glioma retinae. See **retinoblastoma.**

glioma sarcomatosum. See **gliosarcoma.**

glioneuroma /glī′ōnŏŏrō′mə/, *pl.* **glioneuromas, glioneuromata,** a neoplasm composed of nerve cells and elements of their supporting connective tissue.

gliosarcoma /glī′ōsärkō′mə/, *pl.* **gliosarcomas, gliosarcomata,** a tumor composed of spindle-shaped cells in the delicate supporting connective tissue of nerve cells. Also called **glioma, glioblastoma, spongioblastoma, spongiocytoma.**

gliosarcoma retinae. See **retinoblastoma.**

Glisson's sling, *obsolete.* an apparatus with a collar for the neck and chin, which is attached to weights and a pulley and used for traction of the cervical spine.

glitter cells, white blood cells in which movement of granules is observed in their cytoplasm. They are seen in microscopic examination of urine samples in cases of pyelonephritis or disorders marked by low osmolality.

Gln, abbreviation for **glutamine.**

-globinuria, a combining form meaning '(condition involving) the presence of complex proteins in the urine': *hemoglobinuria, methemoglobinuria, myoglobinuria.*

globin zinc insulin injection, a form of intermediate-acting lente insulin in a mixture with zinc chloride and a protein, globin, from beef hemoglobin. It is seldom used in current diabetic treatment regimens.

globoid leukodystrophy. See **galactosyl ceramide lipidosis.**

globule /glob′yŏŏl/, a small spheric mass. Kinds of globules are **dentin globule, Dobie's globule, Marchi's globule, Margagni's globule, milk globule,** and **myelin globule.**

globulin /glob′yŏŏlin/, one of a broad category of simple proteins classified by solubility, electrophoretic mobility, and size. Compare **albumin.** See also **euglobulin, plasma protein, protein electrophoresis.**

globus hystericus, a transitory sensation of a lump in the throat that cannot be swallowed or coughed up, often accompanying emotional conflict or acute anxiety. The condition is thought to be caused by a functional disturbance of the ninth cranial nerve and spasm of the inferior constrictor muscle that encircles the lower part of the throat. The physical examination tends to be normal, as does the barium esophagram.

globus pallidus, the smaller and more medial part of the lentiform nucleus of the brain, separated from the putamen by the lateral medullary lamina and divided into external and internal portions closely connected to the stratium, thalamus, and mesencephalon.

-gloea. See **-glea.**

glomangioma /glōman′jē·ō′mə/, *pl.* **glomangiomas, glomangiomata,** a benign tumor that develops from a cluster of blood cells in the skin. Also called **angiomyoneuroma, angioneuroma.**

glomerular /glōmer′yŏŏlər/, of or pertaining to a glomerulus, especially a renal glomerulus.

glomerular capsule. See **Bowman's capsule.**

glomerular disease, any of a group of diseases in which the glomerulus of the kidney is affected. Depending on the particular disease, there may be hyperplasia, atrophy, necrosis, scarring, or deposits in the glomeruli. The symptoms may be abrupt in onset or slowly progressive. See also **glomerulonephritis.**

glomerulonephritis /glōmer′yŏŏlōnəfrī′tis/, an inflammation of the glomerulus of the kidney, characterized by proteinuria, hematuria, decreased urine production, and edema. Kinds of glomerulonephritis are **acute glomerulonephritis, chronic glomerulonephritis,** and **subacute glomerulonephritis.**

glomerulus /glōmer′yŏŏləs/, *pl.* **glomeruli, 1.** a tuft or cluster. **2.** a structure composed of blood vessels or nerve fibers, as a renal glomerulus.

glomus /glō′məs/, *pl.* **glomera** /glom′ərə/, a small group of arterioles connecting directly to veins and having a rich nerve supply.

gloss-. See **glosso-.**

-glossia, **1.** a combining form meaning the 'possession of a specified type or condition of tongue': *cacoglossia, megaloglossia, schistoglossia.* **2.** a combining form meaning the 'possession of a specified number of tongues': *aglossia, diglossia.*

glossitis /glosī′tis/, inflammation of the tongue. Acute glossitis, characterized by swelling, intense pain that may be referred to the ears, salivation, fever, and enlarged regional lymph nodes, may develop during an infectious disease or after a burn, bite, or other injury. Glossitis in which there is smooth atrophy of the surface and edges of the tongue is seen in pernicious anemia. Chronic superficial glossitis (Moeller's glossitis), in which irregular, bright red patches appear on the tip or sides of the tongue, occurs in middle-aged people, chiefly women. The condition causes pain or a burning sensation and sensitivity to hot or spicy foods; it often resists treatment. In congenital glossitis, there is a flat or slightly elevated patch or plaque anterior to the circumvallate papillae in the midline of the dorsal surface of the tongue.

glossitis parasitica. See **parasitic glossitis.**

glossitis rhomboidea mediana. See **median rhomboid glossitis.**

glosso-, gloss-, a combining form meaning 'pertaining to the tongue': *glossocele, glossodynia, glossoplegia.*

glossodynia /glos′ōdin′ē·ə/, pain in the tongue, caused by acute or chronic inflammation, an abscess, or an ulcer.

glossodynia exfoliativa, a form of chronic glossitis, characterized by pain and sensitivity to spicy foods without any evidence of a pathologic condition. It occurs primarily in middle-aged women. Also called **Moeller's glossitis.**

glossohyal /glos′ōhī′əl/, of or pertaining to the tongue and the horseshoe-shaped hyoid bone at the base of the tongue immediately above the thyroid cartilage. Also called **hyoglossal.**

glossolalia /glos′ōlā′lyə/, speech in an unknown "language," as "speaking in tongues" during a state of religious ecstasy when the message being transmitted through the speaker is believed to be a message from a celestial spirit or from God.

glossoncus /glosong′kəs/, a local swelling or general enlargement of the tongue.

glossopathy /glosop′əthē/, a pathologic condition of the tongue, as acute inflammation caused by a burn, bite, injury, or infectious disease, enlargement resulting from congenital lymphangioma, or a disorder produced by mycotic infection, a malignant lesion, or a congenital anomaly.

glossopexy /glos′əpek′sē/, an adhesion of the tongue to the lip.

glossopharyngeal /glos′ōfərin′jē·əl/, of or pertaining to the tongue and pharynx. See also **glossopharyngeal nerve.**

glossopharyngeal nerve, either of a pair of cranial nerves essential to the sense of taste, for sensation in some viscera, and for secretion from certain glands. The nerve has both sensory and motor fibers that pass from the tongue, parotid gland, and pharynx, communicate with the vagus nerve, and connect with two areas in the brain. Also called **nervus glossopharyngeus, ninth cranial nerve.**

glossophytia /glos′əfit′ē·ə/, a condition of the tongue characterized by a blackish patch on the dorsum on which filiform papillae are greatly elongated and thickened like bristly hairs. The usually painless condition may be caused by heavy smoking or the extensive use of broad-spectrum antibiotics. See also **parasitic glossitis.**

glossoplasty /glos′ōplas′tē/, a surgical procedure or plastic operation on the tongue performed to correct a congenital anomaly, repair an injury, or restore a measure of function after excision of a malignant lesion.

glossoptosis /glos′optō′sis/, the retraction or downward displacement of the tongue.

glossopyrosis /glos′ōpīrō′sis/, a burning sensation in the tongue caused by chronic inflammation, by exposure to extremely hot or spicy food, or by psychogenic glossitis.

glossorrhaphy /glosôr′əfē/, the surgical suturing of a wound in the tongue.

glossotrichia /glos′ətrik′ē·ə/, a condition of the tongue characterized by a hairlike appearance of the papillae. Also called **hairy tongue.**

glott-, a combining form meaning 'pertaining to the glottis': *glottic, glottidas, glottis.*

glottis, *pl.* **glottises, glottides,** **1.** also called **true glottis, rima glottidis.** a slitlike opening between the true vocal cords (plica vocalis). **2.** the phonation apparatus of the larynx, composed of the true vocal cords and the opening between them (rima glottidis). **–glottal, glottic,** *adj.*

Glu, abbreviation for **glutamic acid.**

glucagon /glo͞o′kəgon/, a hormone, produced by alpha cells in the islets of Langerhans, that stimulates the conversion of glycogen to glucose in the liver. Secretion of glucagon is stimulated by hypoglycemia and by the growth hormone of the anterior pituitary. A preparation of purified, crystallized glucagon is used in the treatment of certain hypoglycemic states. Also called **hyperglycemic-glycogenolytic factor.**

glucagonoma syndrome /glo͞o′kəgonō′mə/, a disease associated with a glucagon-secreting tumor of the islet cells of the pancreas, characterized by hyperglycemia, stomatitis, anemia, weight loss, and a characteristic rash.

gluco-, glyco-, a combining form meaning 'pertaining to sweetness or to glucose': *glucofuranose, glucokinetic, glucosuria.*

glucocorticoid /glo͞o′kōkôr′təkoid/, an adrenocortical steroid hormone that increases glyconeogenesis, exerts an antiinflammatory effect, and influences many body functions. The most important of the three glucocorticoids is cortisol (hydrocortisone); corticosterone is less active, and cortisone is inactive until converted to cortisol. Glucocorticoids promote the release of amino acids from muscle, mobilize fatty acids from fat stores, and increase the ability of skeletal muscles to maintain contractions and avoid fatigue. In vitro, these hormones are known to stabilize mitochondrial and lysosomal membranes, increase the production of adenosine triphosphate, promote the formation of certain liver enzymes, and decrease antibody production and the number of circulating eosinophils. A deficiency of glucocorticoids is characterized by hyperpigmentation of the skin, fasting hypoglycemia, weight loss, and apathy. An excess is associated with impaired glucose tolerance, thinning of the skin, ecchymosis, osteoporosis, poor wound healing, increased susceptibility to infection, and obesity. Glucocorticoid secretion is stimulated by the adrenocorticotropic hormone of the anterior pituitary, which in turn is regulated by the corticotropin-releasing factor of the hypothalamus. Synthetic or semisynthetic glucocorticoids, derived chiefly from cortisol, include prednisone, prednisolone, dexamethasone, methylprednisolone, triamcinolone, and betamethasone. Compare **mineralocorticoid.**

glucosan, any of a large group of anhydrous polysaccharides that on hydrolysis yield a hexose, primarily anhydrides of glucose. The glucosans include cellulose, glycogen, starch, and the dextrins.

glucose /glo͞o′kōs/, a simple sugar found in certain foods, especially fruits, and a major source of energy occurring in human and animal body fluids. Glucose, when ingested or produced by the digestive hydrolysis of double sugars and starches, is absorbed into the blood from the intestines. Excess glucose in circulation is normally polymerized and stored in the liver and muscles as glycogen, which is depolymerized to glucose and liberated as needed. The determination of blood glucose levels is an important diagnostic test in diabetes and other disorders. Prepared glucose is a syrupy sweetening agent. Pharmaceutic preparations of glucose are widely used in the treatment of many disorders. See also **dextrose, glycogen.**

glucose 1-phosphate, an intermediate compound in carbohydrate metabolism.

glucose 6-phosphate, an intermediate compound in carbohydrate metabolism.

glucose-6-phosphate dehydrogenase (G-6-PD) deficiency, an inherited disorder characterized by red cells partially or completely deficient in glucose-6-phosphate dehydrogenase, a critical enzyme in aerobic glycolysis. The gene for this enzyme is sex-linked, and the defect is fully expressed in affected males despite a heterozygous pattern of inheritance. The disorder is associated with episodes of acute hemolysis under conditions of stress or in response to certain chemicals or drugs. The anemia that results is a kind of nonspherocytic hemolytic anemia. See also **congenital nonspherocytic hemolytic anemia, favism.**

glucose tolerance test, a test of the body's ability to metabolize carbohydrates by administering a standard dose of glucose and measuring the blood and urine for glucose at regular intervals thereafter. The patient usually eats a high carbohydrate diet for the 3 days preceding the test and fasts the night before. A fasting blood glucose is obtained the next morning, and then the patient drinks a 100 g dose of glucose. Blood and urine are collected periodically for up to 6 hours. The glucose tolerance test is most often used to assist in the diagnosis of diabetes or other disorders that affect carbohydrate metabolism.

glucosuria /glo͞o′kōso͝or′ē·ə/, abnormal presence of glucose in the urine resulting from the ingestion of large amounts of carbohydrate or from a kidney disease, as nephrosis, or a metabolic disease, as diabetes mellitus. See also **glycosuria.** **–glucosuric,** *adj.*

glucosyl cerebroside lipidosis. See **Gaucher's disease.**

glue sniffing, the practice of inhaling the vapors of toluene, a volatile organic compound used as a solvent in certain glues. The glue is squeezed into a plastic bag, which is then placed over the nose and mouth. Intoxication and dizziness result. Prolonged accidental or occupational exposure or repeated recreational use may damage a variety of organ systems. Death has been reported from asphyxiation by the plastic bag.

glutamate /glo͞o′təmāt/, a salt of glutamic acid.

glutamic acid (Glu) /glo͞otam′ik/, a nonessential amino acid occurring widely in a number of proteins. Preparations of glutamic acid are used as aids for digestion. See also **amino acid, protein.**

glutamic acid hydrochloride, a gastric acidifier.

■ INDICATION: It is prescribed for hypoacidity.

■ CONTRAINDICATIONS: Hyperacidity, peptic ulcer, or known hypersensitivity to this drug prohibits its use.

■ ADVERSE EFFECTS: The most serious adverse reaction is systemic acidosis resulting from overdose.

glutamic-oxaloacetic transaminase. See **aspartate aminotransferase.**

glutamic-pyruvic transaminase. See **alanine aminotransferase.**

glutamine (Gln), a nonessential amino acid found in many proteins in the body. It functions as an amino donor for many reactions and it is also a nontoxic transport for ammonia, being easily hydrolyzed to glutamic acid and free ammonia, the latter being excreted in the urine. See also **amino acid, protein.**

glutargin, arginine glutamate. See also **arginine.**

glutathione, an enzyme whose deficiency is commonly associated with hemolytic anemia.

gluteal gait. See **Trendelenburg gait.**

gluteal tuberosity, a ridge on the lateral posterior surface of the thigh bone to which is attached the gluteus maximus.

gluten /glo͞o′tən/, the insoluble protein constituent of wheat and other grains. It is obtained from flour by washing out the starch and is used as an adhesive agent, giving to dough its tough, elastic character.

gluten enteropathy. See **celiac disease.**

glutethimide /glo͞oteth′əmīd/, a sedative.

■ INDICATION: It is prescribed in the treatment of anxiety and insomnia.

■ CONTRAINDICATION: Known hypersensitivity to this drug prohibits its use.

■ ADVERSE EFFECTS: Among the most serious adverse reactions are physical and psychologic dependence. Rashes also may occur.

Gly, abbreviation for **glycine.**

-glycemia, -glycaemia, a combining form meaning a 'condition of sugar in the blood': *dysglycemia, hepatoglycemia, hyperglycemia.*

glycerin, a sweet, colorless, oily fluid that is a pharmaceutic preparation of glycerol. Glycerin is used as a moistening agent for chapped skin, as an ingredient of suppositories for constipation, and as a sweetening agent and vehicle for drug preparations. Also spelled **glycerine.**

glycerol /glis′ərôl/, an alcohol that is a component of fats. Glycerol is soluble in ethyl alcohol and water. See also **glycerin.**

glycerol kinase, an enzyme in the liver and kidneys that catalyzes the transfer of a phosphate group from adenosin triphosphate to form adenosine diphosphate and L-glycerol-3-phosphate.

glyceryl alcohol. See **glycerin.**

glyceryl guaiacolate. See **guaifenesin.**

glyceryl triacetate. See **triacetin.**

glycine (Gly) /glī′sin/, a nonessential amino acid occurring widely as a component of animal and plant proteins. Synthetically produced glycine is used in solutions for irrigation, in the treatment of various muscle diseases, and as an antacid and dietary supplement. See also **amino acid, protein.**

glyco-. See **gluco-.**

glycobiarsol, an antiamebic containing arsenic and bismuth, formerly used to treat intestinal amebiasis.

glycocoll. See **glycine.**

glycogen /glī′kəjən/, a polysaccharide that is the major carbohydrate stored in animal cells. It is formed from glucose and stored chiefly in the liver and, to a lesser extent, in muscle cells. Glycogen is depolymerized to glucose and released into circulation as needed by the body. Also called **animal starch, hepatin, tissue dextrin.** See also **glucose.**

glycogenesis, the synthesis of glycogen from glucose.

glycogenolysis /glī′kōjenol′isis/, the breakdown of glycogen to glucose.

glycogenosis. See **glycogen storage disease.**

glycogen storage disease, any of a group of inherited disorders of glycogen metabolism. An enzyme deficiency causes glycogen to accumulate in abnormally large amounts in various parts of the body. Biopsy and chemical analysis reveal the missing enzyme. Also called **glycogenosis.**

glycogen storage disease, type I. See **von Gierke's disease.**

glycogen storage disease, type II. See **Pompe's disease.**

glycogen storage disease, type III. See **Cori's disease.**

glycogen storage disease, type IV. See **Andersen's disease.**

glycogen storage disease, type V. See **McArdle's disease.**

glycogen storage disease, type VI. See **Hers' disease.**

glycolic acid, a substance in bile, formed by glycine and cholic acid, that aids in digestion and absorption of fats. Glycolic acid is used as a food additive and an emulsifying agent.

glycolipid, a compound that consists of a lipid and a carbohydrate, usually galactose, found primarily in the tissue of the nervous system, especially the myelin sheath and the ganglion cells.

glycolysis /glīkol′isis/, a series of enzymatically catalyzed reactions, occurring within cells, by which glucose and other sugars are broken down to yield lactic acid or pyruvic acid, releasing energy in the form of adenosine triphosphate. **Aerobic glycolysis** yields pyruvic acid in the presence of adequate oxygen. **Anaerobic glycolysis** yields lactic acid. See also **aldolase, Krebs' citric acid cycle, lactic acid.**

glycoprotein, any of the large group of conjugated proteins in which the nonprotein substance is a carbohydrate. These include the mucins, the mucoids, and the chondroproteins.

glycopyrrolate /glī′kōpir′əlāt/, an anticholinergic.

■ INDICATION: It is prescribed as an adjunct to ulcer therapy.

■ CONTRAINDICATIONS: Narrow-angle glaucoma, asthma, obstruction of the genitourinary or GI tract, ulcerative colitis, or known hypersensitivity to this drug prohibits its use.

■ ADVERSE EFFECTS: Among the more serious adverse reactions are blurred vision, central nervous system effects, tachycardia, dry mouth, decreased sweating, and hypersensitivity reactions.

glycoside /glī′kəsīd/, any of several carbohydrates that yield a sugar and a nonsugar on hydrolysis. The plant *Digitalis purpurea* yields a glycoside used in the treatment of heart disease.

glycosuria /glī′kōso͝or′ē·ə/, abnormal presence of a sugar, especially glucose, in the urine. Glycosuria can result from the ingestion of large amounts of carbohydrate, or it may be the result of endocrine or renal disorders. It is a finding most routinely associated with diabetes mellitus. **–glycosuric,** *adj.*

glycosuric acid, a compound that is an intermediate product of the metabolism of tyrosine. It forms a melanin-like staining substance in the urine of people who have alkaptonuria.

glycyl alcohol. See **glycerin.**

Glysennid, a trademark for a stimulant laxative (sennosides A and B).

gm, abbreviation for **gram.** Preferred is the abbreviation *g.*

GMENAC, abbreviation for **Graduate Medical Education National Advisory Committee.**

GMP, abbreviation for **guanosine monophosphate.**

GNA, abbreviation for **Gay Nurses' Alliance.**

gnath-. See **gnatho-.**

-gnathia, a combining form meaning a 'condition of the jaw': *brachygnathia, campylognathia, retrognathia.*

gnathic /nath′ik/, of or pertaining to the jaw or cheek.

gnathion /nā′thē·on/, the lowest point in the lower border of the mandible in the median plane. It is on the bony mandibular border palpated from below and naturally lies posterior to the tegumental border of the chin. It is a common reference point in the diagnosis and orthodontic treatment of various kinds of malocclusion.

gnatho-, gnath-, a combining form meaning 'pertaining to the jaw': *gnathocephalus, gnathodynia, gnathoplasty.*

gnathodynamometer /nā′thōdī′nəmom′ətər/, an instrument used for measuring the biting pressure of the jaws of an individual. Also called **occlusometer.**

gnathodynia /nā′thōdin′ē·ə/, a pain in the jaw, as that commonly associated with an impacted wisdom tooth.

gnathology /nāthol′əjē/, a field of dental or medical study that deals with the entire masticatory apparatus, including its anatomy, histology, morphology, physiology, pathology, and therapeutics.

gnathoschisis. See **cleft palate.**

gnathostatic cast /nā′thōstat′ik/, a cast of the teeth trimmed so that its occlusal plane is in its normal oral attitude when the cast is set on a plane surface. It is used in orthodontic diagnosis based on the ganthostatic technique. See also **gnathostatics.**

gnathostatics /nā′thōstat′iks/, a technique of orthodontic diagnosis based on an analysis of the relationships between the teeth and certain reference points on the skull. See also **gnathostatic cast.**

gno-, a combining form meaning 'to know or discern': *gnosia, gnosis.*

-gnomonic, -gnomonical, a combining form meaning 'signs or experience in knowing or judging (a condition)': *pathognomonic, physiognomonic, thanatognomonic.*

-gnomy, a combining form meaning the 'science or means of judging' something specified: *craniognomy, pathognomy, physiognomy.*

-gnosia, a combining form meaning a '(condition of) perceiving or recognizing': *acognosia, hypergnosia, topognosia.*

-gnosis, a combining form meaning 'knowledge': *acrognosis, diagnosis, topognosis.*

goal, the purpose toward which an endeavor is directed, as the outcome of diagnostic, therapeutic, and educational management of a patient's health problem.

goblet cell, one of the many specialized cells that secrete mucus and form glands of the epithelium of the stomach, the intestine, and parts of the respiratory tract. Also called **beaker cell, chalice cell.** See also **gland.**

goiter, a hypertrophic thyroid gland, usually evident as a pronounced swelling in the neck. The enlargement may be associated with hyperthyroidism, hypothyroidism, or normal levels of thyroid function. The goiter may be cystic or fibrous, containing nodules or an increased number of follicles; it may surround a large blood vessel, or a part of the enlarged gland may be situated beneath the sternum or in the thoracic cavity. Treatment may include total or subtotal surgical removal, the administration of antithyroid drugs or radioiodine, or the use of thyroid hormone to block the hypothalamic-hypophyseal mechanism that releases thyroid-stimulating hormone. After thyroidectomy, maintenance therapy with thyroid hormone may be required. See specific goiters. **–goitrous,** *adj.*

gold (Au), a yellowish, soft metallic element that occurs naturally as a free metal and as the telluride $AuAgTe_4$. Its atomic number is 79; its atomic weight is 197. Gold has been highly valued since antiquity and has been and is used for currency, ornamentation, and as a dental restorative material. It is usually hardened by alloying it with small amounts of nickel or copper. Gold is highly resistive to oxidation but can be dissolved in aqua regia and aqueous potassium cyanide. Gold salts, in which gold is attached to sulfur, are often used in the treatment, or chrysotherapy, of patients with rheumatoid arthritis but cause serious toxicity in about 10% of patients and some toxicity in 25% to 50%. See also **chrysotherapy.**

gold 198, a radioactive gold antineoplastic.

■ INDICATIONS: It is prescribed for cancer of the prostate, cervix, and bladder and for the reduction of fluid accumulation secondary to a cancer.

■ CONTRAINDICATIONS: Ulcerative tumors, pregnancy, lactation, or unhealed surgical wounds prohibit its use. It is not prescribed for patients under 18 years of age.

■ ADVERSE EFFECTS: The most serious adverse reaction is radiation sickness.

gold compound, a drug containing gold salts, usually administered with other drugs in the treatment of rheumatoid arthritis. Gold is potentially toxic and is administered only under the supervision of a specialist in chrysotherapy. Toxic reactions range from mild dermatoses to lethal poisoning. Various radioisotopes of gold have been used in diagnostic radiology and in the radiologic treatment of certain malignant neoplastic diseases.

Goldent, a trademark for a direct gold restorative material which is composed of various amounts of powdered gold contained in a wrapping or envelope of gold foil for use in dentistry.

gold file, (in dentistry) an instrument designed for removing surplus gold from gold restorations. It may be designed and used as either a pull-cut or push-cut file.

gold foil, (in dentistry) pure gold that has been rolled and beaten into a very thin sheet. The thickness of different gold foils varies from 1/40,000 inch for No. 2 foil to 1/20,000 inch for No. 4 foil. The main types of gold foil are cohesive, semicohesive, and noncohesive. It is commonly compacted into a retentive tooth cavity form, using gold's property of cold welding. Also called **fibrous gold.**

gold inlay, an intracoronal cast restoration of gold alloy. Compare **inlay gold.**

gold knife, an instrument that may be contraangled, with a blade or cutting edge, used for trimming excess metal and for developing contour in foil restorations.

Goldman-Fox knife, a dental surgical instrument with a sharp cutting edge, designed for the incision and contouring of gingival tissue.

gold sodium thiomalate, an antirheumatic.

■ INDICATION: It is prescribed for rheumatoid arthritis.

■ CONTRAINDICATIONS: Severe debilitation, systemic lupus erythematosus, renal or liver disease, blood dyscrasias, Sjögren's syndrome (in rheumatoid arthritis), or known hypersensitivity to this drug or to other gold or heavy metal salts prohibits its use.

■ ADVERSE EFFECTS: Among the most serious adverse reactions are various blood dyscrasias, renal damage, and allergic reactions. Dermatitis, stomatitis, and lesions of the mucous membranes also may occur.

gold therapy. See **chrysotherapy.**

Golgi apparatus /gôl′jē/, one of many small membranous structures found in most cells, composed of various elements associated with the formation of carbohydrate side chains of glycoproteins, mucopolysaccharides, and other substances. Saccules within each structure migrate through the cell membrane and release substances associated with external and internal secretion. Also called **Golgi body, Golgi complex.**

Golgi-Mazzoni corpuscles /gôl′jēmatsō′nē/, a number of thin capsules enveloping terminal nerve fibrils in the subcutaneous tissue of the fingers. They have thicker cores than Pacini's corpuscles but are similar special sensory end organs. Also called **Krause's terminal bulbs.** Compare **Pacini's corpuscles, Ruffini's corpuscles.**

gomphosis /gomfō′sis/, *pl.* **gomphoses,** an articulation by the insertion of a conic process into a socket, as the insertion of a root of a tooth into an alveolus of the mandible or the maxilla. Gomphosis is not a connection between true bones but is considered a type of fibrous joint. Compare **sutura, syndesmosis.**

gon-. See **gono-, gony-.**

gonad /gō′nad/, a gamete-producing gland, as an ovary or a testis. –**gonadal,** *adj.*

gonadal dysgenesis, a general designation for a variety of conditions involving anomalies in the development of the gonads, as Turner's syndrome, hermaphroditism, and gonadal aplasia.

gonadotropin, a hormonal substance that stimulates the function of the testes and the ovaries. The gonadotropic follicle stimulating hormone and luteinizing hormone are produced and secreted by the anterior pituitary gland. In early pregnancy, chorionic gonadotropin is produced by the placenta. It acts to sustain the function of the corpus luteum of the ovary, forestalling menstruation and thus maintaining pregnancy. Gonadotropins are prescribed to induce ovulation in infertility that is caused by inadequate stimulation of the ovary by endogenous gonadotropic hormones. Excessive stimulation of the ovary may result in vast enlargement of the gland, maturation of many follicles, multiple pregnancy, bleeding into the abdomen, and pain. Also called **gonadotrophin.** –**gonadotropic, gonadotrophic,** *adj.*

gonial angle. See **angle of mandible.**

-gonic, a combining form meaning 'agents, processes, or results of generation, reproduction, including the sexual': *dysgonic, endergonic, exergonic.*

gonio-, a combining form meaning 'pertaining to an angle': *goniocraniometry, goniometer, gonion.*

goniometry /gō′nē·om′ətrē/, a system of testing for various labyrinthine diseases which affect the sense of balance. One test uses a plank, one end of which may be raised to any desired height. The patient stands on the plank as one end is gradually raised, and the point where the patient can no longer maintain balance is noted. –**goniometric,** *adj.*

gonioscope, an ophthalmoscope used to examine the angle of the anterior chamber of the eye and for demonstrating ocular motility and rotation.

gono-, gon-, a combining form meaning 'pertaining to semen or seed': *gonococcin, gonophore, gonotome.*

gonoblast. See **germ cell.**

gonococcal pyomyositis, an acute inflammatory condition of a muscle caused by infection with a *Neisseria gonorrhoeae,* characterized by abscess formation and pain. It is an unusual form of gonorrhea and must be differentiated from sarcoma. The diagnosis is made by the discovery of the gonocococcal diplococci within the abscess when a bacterial culture of a specimen is prepared after exploratory surgery. The patient is then usually found to be asymptomatically infected in the urogenital organs. Antibiotic treatment, most often with ampicillin, is rapidly effective in curing the infection.

gonococcus /gon′əkok′əs/, *pl.* **gonococci** /gon′əkok′sī/, a gram-negative, intracellular diplococcus of the species *Neisseria gonorrhoeae,* the cause of gonorrhea.

gonocyte. See **germ cell.**

gonorrhea /gon′ərē′ə/, a common sexually transmitted disease most often affecting the genitourinary tract and, occasionally, the pharynx, conjunctiva, or rectum. Infection results from contact with an infected person or by contact with secretions containing the causative organism *Neisseria gonorrhoeae.* –**gonorrheal, gonorrheic,** *adj.*

■ OBSERVATIONS: Urethritis, dysuria, purulent, greenish-yellow urethral or vaginal discharge, red or edematous urethral meatus, and itching, burning, or pain around the vaginal or urethral orifice are characteristic. The vagina may be massively swollen and red, and the lower abdomen may be tense and very tender. As the infection spreads, which is more common in women than in men, nausea, vomiting, fever, and tachycardia may occur as salpingitis, oophoritis, or peritonitis develops. Inflammation of the tissues surrounding the liver may also occur, causing pain in the upper right quadrant of the abdomen. Severe disseminated infection is also more common in women than in men and is characterized by signs of septicemia with polyarthritis, tender papillary lesions on the skin of the hands and feet, and inflammation of the tendons of the wrists, knees, and ankles. Gonoccocal ophthalmia involves infection of the conjunctiva and may lead to scarring and blindness. Gonorrhea is diagnosed by bacteriologic culture of the organism from a smear obtained from a specimen of exudate. In men a microscopic study of a gram-stained specimen of exudate that reveals gram-negative intracellular diplococci is diagnostic of gonorrheal infection, but this finding is not diagnostic in women.

■ INTERVENTION: Penicillin is used to treat uncomplicated gonorrhea. It is given, usually by intramuscular injection, ½ hour after an oral dose of probenecid that acts to slow the excretion of the penicillin from the body. Oral treatment with a large, one-time dose of ampicillin is also held to be effective, and erythromycin or tetracycline is sometimes used to treat the infection, most commonly in people who are sensitive to penicillin and penicillin-like drugs. The patient is tested 1 or 2 weeks after treatment to confirm eradication of the organism. The routine instillation of 1% silver nitrate in the eyes of the newborn provides effective prophylaxis against infection in the newborn period that might otherwise result from contact with the infected secretions of an asymptomatic infected mother during vaginal delivery.

■ NURSING CONSIDERATIONS: It is important that the patient's sexual contacts be treated. Before giving any antibiotic, it is ascertained that the patient does not have any known sensitivity to the drug being given and that equipment and drugs are available to treat any hypersensitivity reaction that may occur. The patient is alerted that until it is proven that the microorganism has been eradicated, transmission of the infection is possible and therefore precautions against spread are recommended. It may also be appropriate to inform the patient that use of condoms during coitus affords excellent protection against venereal infection.

gonorrheal conjunctivitis, a severe, destructive form of purulent conjunctivitis caused by the gonococcus *Neisseria gonorrhoeae*. Prompt treatment by the intravenous administration of antibiotics is required to prevent scarring of the cornea and blindness. Newborn infants receive routine prophylaxis of a topical instillation of 1% solution of silver nitrate or an antibiotic ointment, which has largely eradicated the infection in infants. See also **ophthalmia neonatorum.**

gony-, gon-, a combining form meaning 'pertaining to a knee': *gonycampsis, gonyectyposis, gonyoncus*.

-gony, a combining form meaning 'birth or origin': *amphigony, merogony, zoogony*.

Goodell's sign /go͝odelz′/, softening of the uterine cervix, a probable sign of pregnancy.

Goodpasture's syndrome, a chronic, relapsing pulmonary hemosiderosis, usually associated with glomerulonephritis and characterized by a cough with hemoptysis, dyspnea, anemia, and progressive renal failure. Mild forms of the syndrome may respond to corticosteroids or immunosuppressive drugs. Severe recurrent cases have a poor prognosis; hemodialysis and kidney transplantation are the only treatments.

Goodrich, Annie Warburton (1866–1954), an American nursing educator, instrumental in bringing nursing from an apprenticeship to a profession. She was superintendent of nurses at several New York hospitals before going to Teachers College, Columbia University, in 1914. In addition to teaching, she was associated with the Henry Street Settlement and the Nursing Department of the U. S. Army. In 1923 she became dean of the newly formed Yale School of Nursing at Yale University, bringing to nursing the same university rank as other professions.

Good Samaritan legislation, laws enacted in some states to protect physicians, dentists, and some other health professionals from liability in rendering emergency medical or dental aid, unless there is proven willful wrong or gross negligence.

gooseflesh. See **pilomotor reflex.**

Gordon's elementary body, a particle found in tissues containing eosinophils once thought to be the viral cause of Hodgkin's disease. Also called **Gordon's encephalopathic agent.**

Gordon's reflex, **1.** an abnormal variation of Babinski's reflex, elicited by compressing the calf muscles, characterized by extension of the great toe and fanning of the other toes. It is evidence of disease of the pyramidal tract. **2.** an abnormal reflex, elicited by compressing the forearm muscles, characterized by flexion of the fingers or of the thumb and index finger. It is seen in diseases of the pyramidal tract. Compare **Chaddock reflex, Oppenheim's reflex.** See also **Babinski's reflex.**

Gosselin's fracture /gôslaNz′/, a V-shaped fracture of the distal tibia, extending to the ankle.

GOT, abbreviation for **glutamic-oxaloacetic transaminase.**

goundou /go͞on′do͞o/, a condition characterized by bony exostoses of the nasal and maxillary bones, usually occurring as a late sequela of yaws in people in Africa and Latin America.

gout, a disease associated with an inborn error of uric acid metabolism that increases production or interferes with excretion of uric acid. Excess uric acid is converted to sodium urate crystals that precipitate from the blood and become deposited in joints and other tissues. Men are more often affected than women. The great toe is a common site for the accumulation of urate crystals. The condition can result in exceedingly painful swelling of a joint, accompanied by chills and fever. The symptoms are recurrent; episodes become longer each year. The disorder is disabling and, if untreated, can progress to the development of tophi and destructive joint changes. Treatment usually includes administration of colchicine, phenylbutazone, indomethacin, or glucocorticoid drugs, a diet that excludes purine-rich foods, as organ meats, and may include surgical removal of tophi. Acquired gout is a condition having the signs and symptoms of gout but occurring as a result of another disorder or treatment for a different condition. Diuretic drugs can alter the concentration of uric acid so that uric acid salts precipitate from the blood and are carried to the joints. See also **chondrocalcinosis, Lesch-Nyhan syndrome, pseudogout, tophus.**

gouty arthritis. See **gout.**

Gowers' muscular dystrophy. See **distal muscular dystrophy.**

GP, abbreviation for **general practitioner.**

GPI, *obsolete.* abbreviation for *general paralysis of the insane.* See **general paresis.**

GPT, abbreviation for **glutamic-pyruvic transaminase.** See **alanine aminotransferase.**

gr, abbreviation for **grain.**

graafian follicle /graf′ē·ən/, a mature ovarian vesicle, measuring about 10 to 12 mm in diameter, that ruptures during ovulation to release the ovum. Many primary ovarian follicles, each containing an immature ovum about 35 μ in diameter, are imbedded near the surface of the ovary, just below the tunica albuginea. Under the influence of the follicle stimulating hormone from the adenohypophysis, one ovarian follicle ripens into a graafian follicle during the proliferative phase of each menstrual cycle. The cells that form the graafian follicle are arranged in a layer three to four cells thick around a relatively large volume of follicular fluid. Within the follicle the ovum grows to about 100 μ in diameter and, when the follicle ruptures, is swept into the fimbriated opening of the uterine tube. The cavity of the follicle collapses when the ovum is released, and the remaining follicular cells greatly enlarge to become the corpus luteum. If the ovum is fertilized, the corpus luteum grows and becomes the corpus luteum of pregnancy that, at the end of 9 months, has a diameter of about 30 mm. As the ovarian follicle ripens into the graafian follicle, it produces estrogen, which stimulates the proliferation of the endometrium and the enlargement of the uterine glands. The growing corpus luteum produces progesterone, which triggers endometrial gland secretion and prepares the uterus to receive the fertilized ovum. If the ovum is not fertilized, the graafian follicle forms the corpus luteum of menstruation, which degenerates, leaving the small scarred corpus albicans.

gracile /gras′il/, long, slender, and graceful.

gracilis /gras′ilis/, the most superficial of the five medial femoral muscles. A thin, flattened muscle that is broad proximally and narrow distally, it originates in a thin aponeurosis secured on the inferior aspect of the symphysis pubis and the superior half of the pubic arch. The muscle curves around the medial condyle of the tibia and inserts into the body of the tibia, distal to the condyle. It is innervated by a branch of the obturator nerve, which contains fibers from the third and fourth lumbar nerves, and it functions to adduct the thigh and flex the leg and to assist in the medial rotation of the leg after it is flexed. Compare **adductor brevis, adductor longus, adductor magnus, pectineus.**

gradient, 1. the rate of increase or decrease of a measurable phenomenon, as temperature or pressure. **2.** a visual representation of the rate of change of a measurable phenomenon; a curve.

gradient magnetic field, a magnetic field that changes in strength in a certain given direction. Such fields are used in NMR imaging to select a region for imaging and also to encode the location of NMR signals received from the object being imaged.

gradient of approach, the inverse relationship between the distance from a positive stimulus and the tendency to approach it.

gradient of avoidance, the inverse relationship between the distance from a negative stimulus and the tendency to avoid it.

graduated bath, a bath in which the temperature of the water is slowly reduced.

graduated resistance exercise. See **progressive resistance exercise.**

graduate medical education, formal medical education pursued after receipt of M.D. or other professional degree in the medical sciences. Graduate medical education is usually obtained as an intern, resident, or fellow, or in continuing medical education programs.

Graduate Medical Education National Advisory Committee (GMENAC), a committee established by order of the Secretary of the Department of Health, Education and Welfare (now the Department of Health and Human Services) to study the personnel issues in medicine. The Committee issued its final report in September 1980. Among its conclusions were those regarding the supply of nurses in expanded roles, including nurse practitioners and nurse midwives.

Graduate Record Examination (GRE), an examination administered to graduates of institutions of higher learning. The scores are used as criteria for admission to masters and doctoral programs in many institutions and areas of specialization, including nursing. The examination tests verbal and mathematic aptitudes and abilities.

GRAE, abbreviation for **generally recognized as effective.**

graft, a tissue or an organ taken from a site or a person and inserted into a new site or person, performed to repair a defect in structure. The graft may be temporary, as an emergency skin transplant for extensive burns, or permanent, as the grafted tissue growing to become a part of the body. Skin, bone, cartilage, blood vessel, nerve, muscle, cornea, and whole organs, as the kidney or the heart, may be grafted. Preoperative care focuses on a high protein diet and vitamins to ensure optimum physical condition and on freedom from infection. Under general or local anesthesia the tissue is transferred and sutured into place. Rejection is the major complication: fever, pain in the graft area, and evidence of loss of function 4 to 15 days after the procedure are indicative of rejection. Immunosuppressive drugs are given in large doses to suppress antibody production and rejection. Even if an early reaction is blocked, late rejection may occur 1 year or more after the graft is done. Also called **transplant.** See also **allograft, autograft, isograft, skin graft, xenograft.**

graft-versus-host reaction, a rejection response of certain grafts, especially bone marrow. It involves an incompatibility resulting from a deficiency in the immune response of some patients and is commonly associated with inadequate immunosuppressive therapy. Characteristic signs may include skin lesions with edema, erythema, ulceration, scaling, and loss of hair. Such reactions may also cause lesions of the joints and the heart and hemolytic anemia with a positive Coombs' reaction. The graft-versus-host reaction is similar to the Type IV reaction in hypersensitive individuals who receive tuberculin injections. Some experts believe that it involves certain immunologically active cells that originate as the result of defective tolerance mechanisms or as the result of somatic mutation of certain host cells. Also called **homologous disease.**

grain (gr), the smallest unit of mass in avoirdupois, troy, and apothecaries' weights, being the same in all and equal to 4.79891 mg. The troy and apothecaries' ounces contain 480 grains; the avoirdupois ounce contains 437.5 grains.

grain itch, a skin condition caused by a mite that lives in grain or straw. The lesion consists of an intensely itchy, urticarial papule surmounted by a tiny vesicle.

gram (g, gm), a unit of mass in the metric system equal to $\frac{1}{1000}$ of a kilogram, 15.432 grains, and 0.0353 ounce avoirdupois. The preferred abbreviation is *g*.

-gram, -gramme, 1. a combining form meaning a 'drawing': *cephalogram, mammogram, splenogram.* **2.** a combining form meaning '1/1000 kilogram': *centigram, decagram, microgram.*

gram calorie. See **calorie.**

gram-molecular weight, the molecular weight of a substance expressed in grams. See also **mole, molecular weight.**

gram-negative, having the pink color of the counterstain used in Gram's method of staining microorganisms. This property is a primary method of characterizing organisms in microbiology. Some of the most common gram-negative pathogenic bacteria are *Bacteroides fragilis, Brucella abortus, Escherichia coli, Haemophilus influenzae, Klebsiella pneumoniae, Neisseria gonorrhoeae, Proteus vulgaris, Pseudomonas aeruginosa, Salmonella typhi, Shigella dysenteriae,* and *Yersinia pestis.*

gram-positive, retaining the violet color of the stain used in Gram's method of staining microorganisms. This property is a primary method of characterizing organisms in microbiology. Some of the most common kinds of gram-positive pathogenic bacteria are *Bacillus anthracis, Clostridium, Mycobacterium leprae, Mycobacterium tuberculosis, Staphylococcus aureus, Streptococcus pneumoniae,* and *Streptococcus pyogenes.*

Gram's stain, the method of staining microorganisms using a violet stain, followed by an iodine solution, decolorizing with an alcohol or acetone solution, and counterstaining with safranin. The retention of either the violet color of the stain or the pink color of the counterstain serves as a primary means of identifying and classifying bacteria. Also called **Gram's method.** See also **gram-negative, gram-positive.**

grand mal seizure, an epileptic seizure characterized by a generalized involuntary muscular contraction and cessation of respiration followed by tonic and clonic spasms of the muscles. Breathing resumes with noisy respirations. The teeth may be clenched, the tongue bitten, and control of the bladder lost. As this phase of the seizure passes, the person may fall into a deep sleep for 1 hour or more. Usually, the person has no recall of the seizure on awakening. A sensory warning, or aura, usually precedes each grand mal seizure. These seizures may occur singly, at intervals, or in close succession. Anticonvulsant medications are usually prescribed as prophylaxis against grand mal seizures. Compare **focal seizure, petit mal seizure, psychomotor seizure.**

grand rounds, a formal conference in which one usually expert person presents a lecture concerning a clinical issue intended to be educational for the listeners. Charts, tables, films, slides, tapes, and demonstrations are often used in presentation at grand rounds. Historically the patient was present. In some settings grand rounds may be formal teaching rounds conducted by an expert at the bedsides of selected patients.

grant, an award given to an institution, a project, or an individual usually consisting of a sum of money. A grant is given by a granting agency, the federal government, a foundation, private enterprise, or institution to provide financial support for research, service, or training. The applicant usually writes a formal application (proposal) for the grant, which is reviewed by the granting agency and compared with other proposals. The selected grantee is usually required to sign a contract with the agency, specifying the terms of the grant and the responsibilities of the grantee.

granul-, a combining form meaning 'pertaining to grains or granules': *granulase, granulocorpuscle, granulocytemia.*

granular, 1. macroscopically looking or feeling like sand. **2.** microscopically appearing to have a few or many particles within or on its surface, as a stained granular leucocyte. **–granularity,** *n.*

granular conjunctivitis. See **trachoma.**

granular endoplasmic reticulum. See **endoplasmic reticulum.**

granularity. See **granular.**

granulation tissue, any soft, pink, fleshy projections that form during the healing process in a wound not healing by first intention, consisting of many capillaries surrounded by fibrous collagen. Overgrowth of granulation tissue results in proud flesh growing above the skin. See also **pyogenic granuloma.**

granulocyte /gran′yo͞oləsīt′/, one of a group of leukocytes characterized by the presence of cytoplasmic granules. Kinds of granulocytes are **basophil, eosinophil,** and **neutrophil.** Compare **agranulocyte.**

granulocyte transfusion, the use of specially prepared leukocytes for the treatment of severe granulocytopenia and prophylactically for the prevention of serious infection in patients with leukemia or those receiving cancer chemotherapy. The procedure has the same risks as a blood transfusion. Also called **buffy coat transfusion.**

granulocytic leukemia. See **acute myelocytic leukemia, chronic myelocytic leukemia.**

granulocytic sarcoma. See **chloroma.**

granulocytopenia /gran′yo͞olōsī′tōpē′nē·ə/, an abnormal condition of the blood, characterized by a decrease in the total number of granulocytes. Also called **neutropenia.** Compare **granulocytosis.** See also **leukopenia.** –**granulocytopenic,** *adj.*

granulocytosis /gran′yo͞olōsītō′sis/, an abnormal condition of the blood, characterized by an increase in the total number of granulocytes. Compare **granulocytopenia.**

granuloma /gran′yo͞olō′mə/, *pl.* **granulomas, granulomata,** a mass of nodular granulation tissue resulting from inflammation, injury, or infection. It is composed of capillary buds and growing fibroblasts. Granulomas may resolve spontaneously, become gangrenous, spread, or remain as a focus of infection. Treatment depends on the cause and probable course of the particular granuloma.

-granuloma, a combining form meaning a 'tumorlike mass or nodule of granulation tissue': *paragranuloma, ulcerogranuloma, xanthogranuloma.*

granuloma annulare, a self-limited, chronic skin disease of unknown cause, consisting of reddish papules and nodules arranged in a ring and most commonly seen on the distal portions of the extremities in children. No treatment is necessary.

granuloma gluteale infantum, a skin condition of the neonate characterized by large, elevated bluish or brownish-red nodules on the buttocks, often occurring as a secondary reaction to the application of strong steroid salves over a period of time. The lesions routinely disappear within a couple of months after the use of the preparations is discontinued.

granuloma inguinale, a sexually transmitted disease characterized by ulcers of the skin and subcutaneous tissues of the groin and genitalia. It is caused by infection with *Calymmatobacterium granulomatis,* a small gram-negative rod-shaped bacillus. The diagnosis is made by the microscopic examination and identification of characteristic "safety-pin"-shaped bodies in the cytoplasm of phagocytes taken from a lesion and dyed with Wright's stain. Untreated, the lesions spread, deepen, multiply, and become secondarily infected. Streptomycin is usually effective in treating the infection. All persons who have or are suspected of having granuloma inguinale are also tested for syphilis, because concurrent infection is common.

granulomatosis /gran′yo͞olōmətō′sis/, a condition or disease characterized by the development of granulomas, as **berylliosis, pulmonary Wegener's granulomatosis,** or **Wegener's granulomatosis.**

granulomatous thyroiditis. See **de Quervain's thyroiditis.**

granulosa cell carcinoma. See **granulosa cell tumor.**

granulosa cell tumor, a fleshy ovarian tumor with yellow streaks that originates in cells of the primordial membrana granulosa and may grow to an extremely large size. It may be associated with the excessive production of estrogen, resulting in endometrial hyperplagia and menorrhagia.

-graph, **1.** a combining form meaning the 'product of drawing or writing': *hemophotograph, micrograph, retinograph.* **2.** a combining form meaning a 'machine for making something drawn': *clonograph, pneumograph, scopograph.*

-grapher, a combining form meaning 'one who writes about' something specified: *nosographer, syphilographer.*

-graphia, a combining form meaning a 'psychologic abnormality revealed through handwriting': *dysantigraphia, echographia, palingraphia.*

grapho-, a combining form meaning 'pertaining to writing': *graphocatharsis, graphomania, graphophobia.*

graphospasm, muscle cramping and pain in the hand and forearm resulting from prolonged writing. Also called **writer's cramp.**

-graphy, a combining form meaning a 'kind of printing': *arteriography, cardiography, dermagraphy.*

GRAS, abbreviation for *generally recognized as safe.*

grasp reflex, a pathologic reflex induced by stroking the palm or sole with the result that the fingers or toes flex in a grasping motion. The reflex occurs in diseases of the premotor cortex. In young infants the tonic grasp reflex is normal: When an examiner strokes the infant's palms, the examiner's fingers are grasped so firmly that the child can be lifted into the air.

grass. See **cannabis.**

grass-line ligature, a fine cord composed of the fibers of a grass-cloth plant, used in orthodontics for minor adjustments or movement of the teeth. Its action depends on a property of shrinkage when the ligature is wetted by saliva.

Graves' disease, a disorder characterized by pronounced hyperthyroidism usually associated with an enlarged thyroid gland and exophthalmos. The origin is unknown, but the disease is familial and may be autoimmune; antibodies to thyroglobulin or to thyroid microsomes are found in more than 60% of patients with the disorder. Graves' disease, which is five times more common in women than in men, occurs most frequently between 20 and 40 years of age and often arises after an infection or physical or emotional stress. Typical signs are nervousness, a fine tremor of the hands, weight loss, fatigue, breathlessness, palpitations, heat intolerance, increased metabolic rate, and GI motility. There may be an enlarged thymus, generalized hyperplasia of the lymph nodes, blurred or double vision, localized edema, atrial arrhythmias, and osteoporosis. The diagnosis may be established by tests that measure thyroxine and triiodothyronine levels in serum. If necessary, radioactive iodine uptake in the gland may be tested. Treatment may include subtotal thyroidectomy or prescription of antithyroid drugs, as methimazole, propylthiouracil, and iodine preparations. Radioactive iodine may be administered, but hospitalization for a few days is recommended for patients treated with a large dose. In patients with inadequately controlled Graves' disease, infection or stress may precipitate a life-threatening thyroid storm. Also called **exophthalmic goiter, thyrotoxicosis, toxic goiter.**

gravid /grav′id/, pregnant; carrying fertilized eggs or a fetus. **–gravidity, gravidness,** *n.*

gravid-, a combining form meaning 'pertaining to pregnancy, or pregnant': *gravida, graviditas, gravidocardiac.*

-gravida, a combining form meaning 'pregnant woman with (specified) quantity of pregnancies': *nonigravida, plurigravida, unigravida.*

gravida 1. See **primigravida.**

gravida 2. See **secundigravida.**

gravidity, gravidness. See **gravid.**

gravity, the heaviness or weight of an object resulting from the universal effect of the attraction between any body of matter and any planetary body. The force of the attraction depends on the relative masses of the bodies and on the distance between them.

gray (Gy), the absorption of one joule per kilogram by material exposed to ionizing radiation. One gray equals 100 rad.

gray baby syndrome. See **gray syndrome.**

gray hepatization. See **hepatization.**

gray substance, the gray tissue that makes up the inner core of the spinal column, arranged in two large lateral masses connected across the midline by a narrow commissure. Each lateral portion of the gray substance splays outward, forming the posterior and anterior horns of the spinal cord. The horns consist primarily of cell bodies of interneurons and cell bodies of motoneurons. The quantity of gray substance varies greatly at different levels of the cord, and its shape is characteristic at each level. In the thoracic region, the gray substance is small in comparison with surrounding white substance; in the cervical and the lumbar regions it is larger; and in the conus medullaris its proportion to the white substance is the greatest. Nuclei in the gray matter of the spinal cord function as centers for all spinal reflexes. Also called **gray matter.** Compare **white substance.** See also **spinal cord, spinal nerves.**

gray syndrome, a toxic condition in neonates, especially premature infants, caused by a reaction to chloramphenicol. Because the body's mechanisms for detoxification and excretion of drugs are immature, the infant has limited ability to conjugate and thus eliminate the chloramphenicol. The name of the condition comes from a characteristic ashen-gray cyanosis, which is accompanied by abdominal distention, hypothermia, vomiting, respiratory distress, and vascular collapse. The condition, which is fatal if the drug is continued, can be prevented by conservative dosages of the drug and by restricting its use in women during late pregnancy or labor (because chloramphenicol readily crosses the placental barrier) and in lactating mothers. Also called **gray baby syndrome.**

GRE, abbreviation for **Graduate Record Examination.**

great auricular nerve, one of a pair of cutaneous branches of the cervical plexus, arising from the second and the third cranial nerves. It winds around the border of the sternocleidomastoideus, perforates the deep fascia, and ascends on the surface of the muscle before dividing into the anterior branch and the posterior branch. The anterior branch is distributed to the skin of the face over the parotid gland, communicating within the gland with the facial nerve. The posterior branch supplies the skin of the mastoid process and the back of the auricula. It also communicates with the smaller occipital nerve, the auricular branch of the vagus nerve, and the posterior auricular branch of the facial nerve.

great calorie. See **calorie.**

great cardiac vein, one of the five tributaries of the coronary sinus, beginning at the apex of the heart and ascending along the anterior interventricular sulcus to the base of the ventricles. It then curves left in the coronary sulcus, reaches the back of the heart, and opens into the left part of the coronary sinus. It receives various tributaries from the left atrium, as the large left marginal vein, which ascends along the left margin of the heart. The great cardiac vein drains the blood through its tributaries from the capillaries of the myocardium. Also called **vena cordis magna.** Compare **middle cardiac vein, small cardiac vein.**

greater multangular. See **trapezium.**

greater omentum, a filmy, transparent extension of the peritoneum, draping the transverse colon and coils of the small intestine. It is attached along the greater curvature of the stomach and the first part of the duodenum, and between its two layers contains blood vessels and fat pads. Between the stomach and the colon the greater omentum forms the gastrocolic ligament, which contains the right and the left gastroepiploic blood vessels near the greater curvature of the stomach. The greater omentum is a very movable structure that spreads easily into areas of trauma, often sealing hernias and walling off infections that would otherwise cause general peritonitis, as can occur from a ruptured vermiform appendix. Also called **gastrocolic omentum.** Compare **lesser omentum.**

greater trochanter, a large projection of the femur, to which are attached various muscles, including the gluteus medius, gluteus maximus, and obturator internus. The greater trochanter projects from the angle formed by the neck and the body of the femur.

greater vestibular gland. See **Bartholin's gland.**

great saphenous vein, one of a pair of the longest veins in the body, containing 10 to 20 valves along its course through the leg and the thigh before ending in the femoral vein. It begins in the medial marginal vein of the dorsum of the foot, ascends anterior to the tibial malleolus and up the medial side of the leg in relation to the saphenous nerve. It runs posterior to the medial condyles of the tibia and the femur and passes through the hiatus saphenus just before joining the femoral vein. It contains more valves in the leg than in the thigh and receives many cutaneous veins and numerous tributaries, as those from the sole of the foot. Near the saphenous hiatus it is joined by the superficial epigastric vein, the superficial epigastric circumflex, and the superficial external pudendal veins. Compare **common iliac vein, femoral vein.**

great vessels, the large arteries and veins entering and leaving the heart. They include the aorta, the pulmonary arteries and veins, and the superior and inferior venae cavae.

green cancer. See **chloroma.**

green journal, *informal.* **1.** *American Journal of Medicine.* **2.** *American Journal of Psychiatry.* **3.** *Obstetrics and Gynecology.* Each is so named for the color of its cover. Compare **grey journal, yellow journal.**

Greenough microscope. See **stereoscopic microscope.**

greenstick fracture, an incomplete fracture in which the bone is bent but fractured only on the outer arc of the bend. Children are particularly likely to have greenstick fractures. Immobilization is usually effective, and healing is rapid. See also **fracture.**

grenade-thrower's fracture, a fracture of the humerus caused by violent muscular contraction.

Grenz rays, low-energy x-rays used for treatment of skin conditions. They have very little penetrating ability and are frequently applied by dermatologists rather than by radiotherapists.

grey journal, *informal. The American Journal of Obstetrics and Gynecology;* so named for the color of its cover. Compare **green journal, yellow journal.**

Grey Turner's sign, bruising of the skin of the loin in acute hemorrhagic pancreatitis. Also called **Turner's sign.**

grid, a device used to absorb scattered radiation produced during an x-ray examination in the body of the patient. Such scatter does not contribute to the useful information and thus constitutes a source of unwanted noise. A grid selectively absorbs radiation that is not heading along straight lines from the x-ray source to the film.

grief, a nearly universal pattern of physical and emotional responses to bereavement, separation, or loss. The physical components are similar to those of fear, hunger, rage, and pain. Stimulation of the sympathetic portion of the autonomic nervous system causes increased heart and respiratory rates, dilatation of the pupils, sweating, bristling of the hair, increased flow of blood to the muscles, and increased reserves of energy. Digestion is slowed. The emotional components proceed in stages from alarm to disbelief and denial, to anger and guilt, to finding a source of comfort, and, finally, to adjustment to the loss. The way in which a grieving person behaves is greatly affected by the culture in which the person has been raised.

grief reaction, a complex of somatic and psychologic symptoms associated with some extreme sorrow or loss, specifically the death of a loved one. Somatic symptoms include feelings of tightness in the throat and chest with choking and shortness of breath, abdominal distress, lack of muscular power, and extreme tiredness and lethargy. Psychologic reactions involve a generalized awareness of mental anguish and discomfort accompanied by feelings of guilt, anger, hostility, extreme restlessness, inability to concentrate, and the lack of capacity to initiate and maintain organized patterns of activities. Such symptoms may appear immediately after a crisis, or they may be delayed, exaggerated, or apparently absent, depending on the degree of involvement of the relationship and the physical and mental status of the person. Although both the somatic and psychologic reactions have the potential for developing into pathologic conditions, appropriate adaptive behavior and normal responses, as sobbing or talking about the dead person or tragedy, are methods of working through the acute grief and lead to successful resolution of the crisis. Most acute grief reactions are resolved within 4 to 6 weeks, although the period varies and may be much longer, especially in cases of unexpected and sudden death. Intervention by health care professionals, especially nurses, is necessary when individuals exhibit maladaptive behavioral patterns that avoid the resolution of grief and can lead to morbid reactions, including such accepted psychosomatic illnesses as asthma and ulcers. Also called **grief process.** See also **death, parental grief.**

grieving, anticipatory, a nursing diagnosis accepted by the Fourth National Conference on the Classification of Nursing Diagnoses. As a symptom, anticipatory grieving is grieving before an actual loss, as contrasted with grief in response to an actual loss. The cause of the condition, developed at the Fifth National Conference, is the perceived potential loss of a significant person in one's life, of one's physiopsychosocial well-being, or of one's personal possessions. The defining characteristics of the problem include the potential loss of something or someone important, expressions of distress, denial of potential loss, anger, guilt, or sorrow, and changes in eating habits, sleep patterns, activity level, libido, and patterns of communication. See also **nursing diagnosis.**

grieving, dysfunctional, a nursing diagnosis accepted by the Fourth National Conference on the Classification of Nursing Diagnoses. The cause of the problem is an actual or perceived loss of someone or something of great importance to the patient, thwarted grieving response to a loss, absence of anticipatory grieving, chronic fatal illness, or lack of resolution of a previous grieving response. The defining characteristics of the problem include expressions of distress or a denial of the loss; grief, anger, sadness, and weeping; changes in patterns and habits of sleeping, eating, and dreaming; and alterations in libido and activity levels. The lost person or object is idealized, past experience is relived, and concentration and purposeful work are diminished. The patient has a labile affect and seems to regress developmentally. See also **nursing diagnosis.**

griffe des orteils. See **pes cavus.**

Grifulvin, a trademark for an antifungal (griseofulvin).

grinder's asthma, a condition characterized by asthmatic symptoms caused by inhalation of fine particles produced by industrial grinding processes. See also **pneumoconiosis.**

grinder's disease. See **silicosis.**

grinding-in, a clinical corrective grinding of one or more natural or artificial teeth to improve centric and eccentric occlusions. Compare **selective grinding.**

gripes, severe and usually spasmodic pain in the abdominal region caused by an intestinal disorder. Also called **gripping.**

grippe. See **influenza.**

gripping. See **gripes.**

Grisactin, a trademark for an antifungal (griseofulvin).

griseofulvin /gris′ē·ōful′vin/, an antifungal.

■ INDICATIONS: It is prescribed in the treatment of certain infections of the skin, hair, and nails.

■ CONTRAINDICATIONS: Liver dysfunction, porphyria, or known hypersensitivity to this drug prohibits its use.

■ ADVERSE EFFECTS: The most serious adverse reactions are blood dyscrasias. Headache, GI symptoms, and rashes also may occur.

groin, each of two areas where the abdomen joins the thighs.

Grönblad-Strandberg syndrome /grōn′bladstrand′-bərg/, an autosomal recessive disorder of connective tissue characterized by premature aging and breakdown of the skin, gray or brown streaks on the retina, and hemorrhagic arterial degeneration, including retinal bleeding that causes loss of vision. Angina pectoris and hypertension are common; weak pulse, episodic claudication, and fatigue with exertion may affect the extremities. The prognosis depends on vessel involvement, but life expectancy is shortened by the condition. Treatment is symptomatic. Also called **pseudoxanthoma elasticum.**

groove, a shallow, linear depression in various structures throughout the body, as those that form channels for nerves along the bones, those in bones for the insertion of muscles, and those between certain areas of the brain.

gross, **1.** macroscopic, as *gross pathology,* from the study of tissue changes without magnification by a microscope. **2.** large or obese. Compare **microscopic.**

gross anatomy, the study of the organs or parts of the body large enough to be seen with the naked eye. Also called **macroscopic anatomy.**

ground, **1.** (in electricity) a connection between the electric circuit and the ground, which becomes a part of the circuit. **2.** (in psychology) the background of a visual field that can enhance or inhibit the ability of a patient to focus on an object. See also **figure-ground.**

ground itch, pruritic macules, papules, and vesicles secondary to penetration of the skin by hookworm larvae, prevalent in tropic and subtropic climates. It may be prevented by wearing shoes and by establishing sanitary disposal of feces. See also **hookworm.**

ground substance. See **matrix.**

group, (in research) any set of items or groups of people under study. An **experimental group** is studied to determine the effect of an event, a substance, or a technique. A **control group** serves as a standard or reference for comparison with an experimental group. A control group is similar to the experimental group in number and is identical in specified characteristics, as sex, age, annual income, parity, or other factors. Subjects meeting the study criteria are selected from a larger group at random or by a protocol that ensures nonbiased selection.

group function, (in dentistry) the simultaneous contacting of opposing teeth in a segment or a group.

group therapy, the application of psychotherapeutic techniques within a small group of emotionally disturbed persons who, usually under the leadership of a psychotherapist, discuss their problems in an attempt to promote individual psychologic growth and favorable personality change. The procedure provides opportunities for treating a greater number of people in a shorter period of time than would be possible with individual therapy, and it is used in clinics, in institutions, and in private practice. Group therapy has been found to be particularly effective in the treatment of various addictions. A kind of group therapy is **psychodrama.** See also **Gestalt therapy, psychotherapy, self-help group, transactional analysis.**

growing fractures, a fracture, usually linear, in which consecutive x-ray images show a gradual separation of the fracture edges with the passage of time. The cause often is pressure of soft tissues forcing the edges apart, as when arachnoid tissues expand through edges of a skull fracture.

growing pains, **1.** rheumatism-like pains that occur in the muscles and joints of children or adolescents as a result of fatigue, emotional problems, postural defects, and other causes that are not related to growth and that may be symptoms of various disorders. **2.** emotional and psychologic problems experienced during adolescence.

growth, **1.** an increase in the size of an organism or any of its parts, as measured in increments of weight, volume, or linear dimensions, that occurs as a result of hyperplasia or hypertrophy. **2.** the normal progressive anatomic, physiologic, psychologic, intellectual, social, and cultural development from infancy to adulthood as a result of the gradual and normal processes of accretion and assimilation. The total of the numerous changes that occur during the lifetime of an individual constitute a dynamic and complex process that involves many interrelated components, notably heredity, environment, nutrition, hygiene, and disease, all of which are subject to a variety of influences. In childhood, growth is categorized according to the approximate age at which distinctive physical changes usually appear and at which specific developmental tasks are achieved. Such stages include the prenatal period, infancy, early childhood (including the toddler and the preschool child), middle childhood, and adolescence. There are two periods of accelerated growth: the first 12 months, in which the infant triples in weight, grows approximately 50% of the height at birth, and undergoes rapid motor, cognitive, and social development; the second, in the months around puberty, when the child approaches adult height and secondary sexual characteristics emerge. Physical growth may be abnormally accelerated or slowed by a defect in the hypophyseal or pituitary gland. **3.** any abnormal localized increase of the size or number of cells, as in a tumor or neoplasm. **4.** a proliferation of cells, specifically a bacterial culture or mold. Compare **development, differentiation, maturation.**

growth failure, a lack of normal physical and psychologic development as a result of genetic, nutritional, pathologic, or psychosocial factors. See also **failure to thrive, maternal deprivation syndrome.**

growth hormone (GH), a single-chain peptide secreted by the anterior pituitary gland in response to growth hormone releasing factor (GHRF) from the hypothalamus. Growth hormone promotes protein synthesis in all cells, increases fat mobilization and use of fatty acids for energy, and decreases use of carbohydrate. Growth effects depend on the presence of thyroid hormone, insulin, and carbohydrate. Somatomedins, proteins produced chiefly in the liver, play a vital role in GH-induced skeletal growth, but the hormone cannot cause elongation of long bones after the epiphyses close, so that stature does not increase after puberty. Growth hormone accelerates the transport of specific amino acids into cells, stimulates the synthesis of messenger RNA and ribosomal RNA, influences the activity of several enzymes, increases the storage of phosphorus and potassium, and promotes a moderate retention of sodium. The secretion of GH, controlled almost exclusively by the central nervous system, occurs in bursts with more than one half of the total daily amount released during early sleep. Somatostatin, an anterior pituitary regulating hormone produced in the hypothalamus, inhibits GH secretion. A deficiency of GH causes dwarfism; an excess results in gigantism or acromegaly. Also called **somatotropic hormone, somatotropin.** See also **acromegaly, dwarfism, gigantism, somatostatin.**

growth hormone release inhibiting hormone. See **somatostatin.**

growth hormone releasing factor (GHRF), somatotropin releasing factor released by the hypothalamus. Also called **somatoliberin.**

Grünfelder's reflex /grYn′feldərz, grēn′-/, an involuntary dorsal flexion of the great toe with a fanlike spreading of the other toes, caused by continued pressure on the posterior lateral fontanel. The reflex occurs in children who have middle-ear disease.

grunting, abnormal, short audible gruntlike breaks in exhalation that often accompany severe chest pain. The grunt occurs because the glottis briefly stops the flow of air, halting the movement of the lungs and their surrounding or supporting structures. Grunting is most often heard in a person who has pneumonia, pulmonary edema, or fractured or bruised ribs. Atelectasis in the newborn also causes grunting as a result of the effort required for the baby to fill the lungs.

G-6-PD deficiency, abbreviation for **glucose-6-phosphate dehydrogenase deficiency.**

GTP, abbreviation for **guanosine triphosphate.**

GU, abbreviation for **genitourinary.**

guaiac /gwī′ak/, a wood resin, commonly used as a reagent in laboratory tests for the presence of occult blood.

guaiacol poisoning. See **phenol poisoning.**

guaiac test, a test, using guaiac as a reagent, performed on feces and urine for detecting occult blood in the intestinal and urinary tracts.

guaifenesin, glyceryl guaiacolate, a white to slightly gray powder with a bitter taste and faint odor, widely used as an expectorant. Guaifenesin increases the flow of fluid in the respiratory tract, reducing the viscosity of bronchial and tracheal secretions and facilitating their removal by the cough reflex and ciliary action.

guanabenz acetate, an antihypertensive agent.

■ INDICATION: It is prescribed for hypertension.

■ CONTRAINDICATION: Known hypersensitivity to this drug prohibits its use.

■ ADVERSE EFFECTS: Among adverse reactions are dizziness, sedation, and dry mouth.

guanadrel sulfate, an antihypertensive agent.

■ INDICATION: It is prescribed in the treatment of hypertension in patients not responding to a thiazide-type diuretic.

■ CONTRAINDICATIONS: Pheochromocytoma, monoamine oxidase antagonist inhibitors, frank congestive heart failure, or known sensitivity to this drug prohibits its use.

■ ADVERSE EFFECTS: Among the most serious adverse reactions are orthostatic hypotension and syncope.

guanase. See **guanine deaminase.**

guanethidine sulfate, an antihypertensive.

■ INDICATION: It is prescribed in the treatment of moderate and severe hypertension.

■ CONTRAINDICATIONS: Heart failure, concomitant administration of monoamine oxidase inhibitors, pheochromocytoma, or known hypersensitivity to this drug prohibits its use.

■ ADVERSE EFFECTS: Among the more serious adverse reactions are orthostatic hypotension, salt and water retention, bradycardia, diarrhea, and an inability to ejaculate.

guanine /gwan′ēn/, a major purine base found in nucleotides and a fundamental constituent of DNA and RNA. In free or uncombined form it occurs in trace amounts in most cells, usually as a product of the enzymatic hydrolysis of nucleic acids and nucleotides. On enzymatic hydrolysis, it is first converted into xanthine and finally uric acid, its end product. See also **adenine.**

guanine deaminase, an enzyme that catalyzes the hydrolysis of guanine to xanthine and ammonia. Also called **guanase** /gwan′ās/.

guanine deaminase assay, the measurement of an enzyme in the blood that commonly increases in patients with hepatitis and other types of liver disease and mononucleosis. The normal value in serum is less than 3 nm/-ml/min.

guanosine /gwan′ōsēn/, a compound derived from a nucleic acid, composed of guanine and a sugar, D-ribose. It is a major molecular component of the nucleotides guanosine mono- and triphosphate and of DNA and RNA.

guanosine monophosphate (GMP), a nucleotide that plays an important role in various metabolic reactions and in the formation of RNA from DNA templates.

guanosine triphosphate (GTP), a high-energy nucleotide, similar to adenosine triphosphate, that functions in various metabolic reactions, as the activation of fatty acids and the formation of the peptide bond in protein synthesis.

guaranine /gwərä′nin/, caffeine.

guardian ad litem /ad lī′təm/, (in law) a person who is appointed by a court to prosecute or defend a suit for an infant or an incapacitated person. A guardian ad litem is sometimes appointed when a person's life is in imminent danger and that person refuses treatment.

Guedel's signs, a system for describing the stages and planes of anesthesia during an operative procedure.

■ STAGE I (amnesia and analgesia) begins with the administration of an anesthetic and continues to the loss of consciousness. Respiration is quiet, though sometimes irregular, and reflexes are still present.

■ STAGE II (delirium or excitement) begins with the loss of consciousness and includes the onset of total anesthesia. During this stage the patient may move the limbs, chatter incoherently, hold the breath, or become violent. Vomiting, with the attendant danger of aspiration, may occur. No avoidable stimulation is allowed at this stage; the patient is brought to Stage III as quickly and smoothly as possible.

■ STAGE III (surgical anesthesia) begins with establishment of a regular pattern of breathing and total loss of consciousness and includes the period during which signs of respiratory or cardiovascular failure first appear. This stage is divided into four planes: At *plane 1* all movements cease and respiration is regular and "automatic." Eyelid reflexes are lost, but eyeball movements are marked. Pharyngeal reflexes disappear, but laryngeal and peritoneal reflexes are still present. Tonicity of the abdominal muscles can be judged by the tonicity of the extraocular muscles. At *plane 2* the eyeballs become fixed centrally, conjunctivae lose their luster, and intercostal muscle activity diminishes. Respiration remains regular, with reduced tidal volume, and does not change in quality or rate in response to incision. Intubation no longer causes laryngospasm. At *plane 3* intercostal paralysis occurs, and respiration becomes solely diaphragmatic. The pupils no longer react to light, and total muscle relaxation is achieved. At *plane 4* deep anesthesia is achieved, with the cessation of spontaneous respiration and the absence of sensation.

■ STAGE IV (premortem) signals danger. This stage is characterized by pupils that are maximally dilated and skin that is cold and ashen. Blood pressure is extremely low, often unmeasurable, and the brachial pulse is feeble or entirely absent. Cardiac arrest is imminent. Anesthetic is reduced, the lungs are manually ventilated with 100% oxygen, and the reservoir bag is continually emptied. See also **anesthesia.**

Guérin's fracture /gāraNz′/, a fracture of the maxilla. Also called **Le Fort I fracture** /ləfôr′/.

guide plane, **1.** a part of an orthodontic appliance that has an established inclined plane for changing the occlusal relation of the maxillary and mandibular teeth and for permitting their movement to normal positions. **2.** a plane that is developed on the occlusal sufaces of occlusion rims for positioning the mandible in centric relation. **3.** two or more vertically parallel surfaces of abutment teeth shaped to direct the path of placement and removal of a partial denture.

Guillain-Barré syndrome /gēyaN′bärā′/, an idiopathic, peripheral polyneuritis occurring between 1 and 3 weeks after a mild episode of fever associated with a viral infection or with immunization. Symmetric pain and weakness affect the extremities, and paralysis may develop. The neuritis may spread, ascending to the trunk and involving the face, arms, and thoracic muscles. The course of the disease is variable; some people may have minimal symptoms whereas others may have symptoms severe enough to require critical nursing care, including respiratory assistance and a Circolectric bed. The disease resolves itself completely in a few weeks or a few months. There is no treatment other than supportive care. Also called **acute febrile polyneuritis, acute idiopathic polyneuritis, infectious polyneuritis.**

guilt, a feeling caused by tension between the ego and superego when one falls below the standards set for oneself.

guilty, (in criminal law) a verdict by the court, finding that to a moral certainty it is beyond reasonable doubt that the defendant committed the crime and is responsible for the offense as charged.

Guinea worm infection. See **dracunculiasis.**

gullet. See **esophagus.**

gum, **1.** a sticky excretion from certain plants. **2.** See **gingiva.**

gumboil, an abscess of the gingiva and periosteum resulting from injury, infection, or dental decay. The gum is characteristically red, swollen, and tender. The abscess may rupture spontaneously, or it may require incision. Treatment may include antibiotics and hot mouthwashes. Also called **parulis.**

gum camphor. See **camphor.**

gumma /gum′ə/, *pl.* **gummas, gummata,** **1.** a granuloma, characteristic of tertiary syphilis, varying from 1 mm to 1 cm in diameter. It is usually encapsulated and contains a central necrotic mass surrounded by inflammatory and fibrotic zones of tissue. Infectious organisms of the genus *Treponema* may be found in a gumma. The lesion may be localized or diffuse, occurring on the trunk, legs, and face and on various internal organs, especially the liver. A ruptured gumma results in a shallow ulcer that heals slowly. **2.** a soft granulomatous lesion sometimes occurring with tuberculosis.

Gunning's splint, a maxillomandibular splint used for supporting the maxilla and the mandible in surgery of the jaws.

gunshot fracture, a fracture caused by a bullet or similar missile.

Gunther's disease /gun′thərz/, a rare congenital disorder of porphyrin metabolism that is associated with sunlight-induced skin lesions. See also **porphyria.**

gurgling rale, an abnormal coarse sound heard during auscultation, especially over large cavities or over a trachea nearly filled with secretions.

gurry /gur′ē/, *slang.* the detritus incident to physical trauma or surgery, including body fluids, secretions, and tissue.

Gurvich radiation. See **mitogenetic radiation.**

gustatory organ. See **taste bud.**

gut, **1.** intestine. **2.** *informal.* digestive tract. **3.** suture material manufactured from the intestines of sheep.

Guthrie test /guth′rē/, a screening for phenylketonuria used to detect the abnormal presence of phenylalanine metabolites in the blood. A small amount of blood is obtained and placed in a medium with a strain of *Bacillus subtilis,* a bacterium that cannot grow without phenylalanine. If phenylalanine metabolites are present, the bacteria reproduce and the test is positive, indicating that the patient has phenylketonuria. In most states, this test is done twice on all infants, once before discharge from the hospital and again at 2 weeks of age. See also **phenylketonuria.**

gutta-percha, the coagulated, rubbery sap of various tropical trees, used for temporarily sealing the dressings of prepared tooth cavities. Small cones of gutta-percha may be used to fill dental root canals. When combined with fillers and coloring materials, it may be rolled into sheets and used to make temporary bases for dentures.

gutta-percha point, any of the fine, tapered cylinders of gutta-percha that may be used to fill a root canal. The radiopacity of gutta-percha points is an asset in their use as probes for determining the depth and topography of periodontal pockets by means of radiography.

guttate psoriasis, an acute form of psoriasis consisting of teardrop-shaped, red, scaly patches measuring 3 to 10 mm all over the body. A beta-hemolytic streptococcal pharyngitis or other upper respiratory infection may precipitate this reaction in susceptible individuals. Adequate treatment is essential to prevent a more severe form of psoriasis. Compare **pustular psoriasis.** See also **psoriasis.**

GVS, a trademark for a topical antiinfective (gentian violet).

gymno-, a combining form meaning 'pertaining to nakedness': *gymnocarpus, gymnocyte, gymnospore.*

gyn, *informal.* **1.** abbreviation for **gynecologist.** **2.** abbreviation for **gynecology.**

gyn-. See **gyneco-.**

gynandrous /gīnan′drəs, jī-/, describing a man or a woman who has some of the physical characteristics usually attributed to the other sex, as a female pseudohermaphrodite. Compare **androgynous.** **–gynandry,** *n.*

gyne-. See **gyneco-.**

-gyne, -gyn, a combining form meaning '(specified) female characteristics': *androgyne, epigyne, trichogyne.*

gyneco-, gyn-, gyne-, gyno-, a combining form meaning 'pertaining to a woman or the female sex': *gynecoid, gynecomastia, gynotermon.*

gynecoid pelvis, a type of pelvis characteristic of the normal female and associated with the smallest incidence of fetopelvic disproportion. The inlet is nearly round, the sacrum is parallel to the posterior aspect of the symphysis pubis, the sidewalls are straight, and the ischial spines are blunt and do not encroach on the space in the true pelvis. It is the ideal pelvic type for childbirth.

gynecologic examination, pelvic examination.

gynecologist /gī′nəkol′əjist, jī′-, jin′-/, a physician who specializes in gynecology.

gynecology /gī′nəkol′əjē, jī′-, jin′-/, a branch of medicine concerned with the health care of women, including their sexual and reproductive function and the diseases of their reproductive organs, except diseases of the breast that require surgery. Unlike most specialities in medicine, gynecology encompasses surgical and nonsurgical expertise. It is almost always studied and practiced in conjunction with obstetrics. –**gynecologic, gynecological,** *adj.*

gynecomastia /gī′nəkōmas′tē•ə, jī′-, jin′-/, an abnormal enlargement of one or both breasts in men. The condition is usually temporary and benign. It may be caused by hormonal imbalance, tumor of the testis or pituitary, medication with estrogens or steroidal compounds, or failure of the liver to inactivate circulating estrogen, as in alcoholic cirrhosis. Less commonly, the gynecomastia may be caused by a hormone-secreting tumor of the breast, lung, or other organ. It tends to remit spontaneously, but, if marked, may be corrected surgically for cosmetic or psychologic reasons. Biopsy may be performed to rule out the presence of cancer. Malignant neoplastic gynecomastia is usually inoperable and only briefly responsive to chemotherapy. Also called **gynecomasty.**

Gyne-Lotrimin, a trademark for an antifungal (clotrimazole).

gynephobia /gī′nəfō′bē•ə, jī′-, jin′-/, an anxiety disorder characterized by a morbid fear of women or by a morbid aversion to the society of women. It is an obsessive, phobic phenomenon occurring almost entirely in men and may usually be traced to some frightening experience involving women that occurred in childhood. Treatment consists of psychotherapy to uncover the causative emotional conflict, followed by behavior therapy, specifically systemic desensitization and flooding to reduce anxiety.

Gynergen, a trademark for an ergot alkaloid (ergotamine tartrate), used to treat migraine.

Gynetone, a trademark for a hormonal fixed-combination drug containing an estrogen (ethinyl estradiol) and an androgen (methyltestosterone).

-gynic, a combining form meaning 'relating to the human female': *hologynic, monogynic, polygynic.*

gyno-. See **gyneco-.**

gynogamone /gī′nōgam′ōn/, a gamone secreted by the female gamete.

-gynous, -gynic, a combining form meaning 'pertaining to female characteristics': *androgynous.*

-gyria, a combining form meaning '(condition of the) development of the convolutions of the cerebral cortex': *oculogyria, polymicrogyria, ulegyria.*

gyri cerebri, the convolutions of the outer surface of the cerebral hemisphere, separated from each other by sulci, most of which appear during the sixth or seventh months of fetal life.

gyrus /jī′rəs/, *pl.* **gyri** /jī′rī/, one of the tortuous convolutions of the surface of the brain caused by infolding of the cortex.

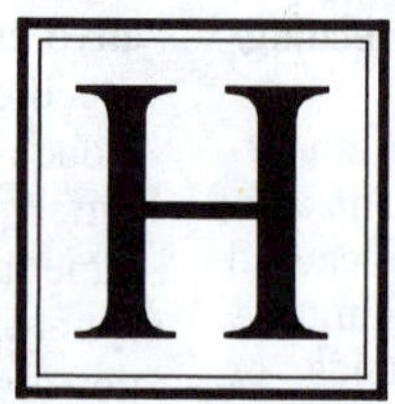

H, symbol for **hydrogen.**

^{2}H, symbol for **deuterium.**

^{3}H, symbol for **tritium.**

habit, **1.** a customary or particular practice, manner, or mode of behavior. **2.** an involuntary pattern of behavior or thought. **3.** also called **habitus.** *archaic.* appearance or physique, as pyknic habit. **4.** the habitual use of drugs or narcotics. See also **habit spasm, habit training.**

habitat, a natural environment where a species of a plant or animal, including humans, may live and grow normally.

habit spasm, an involuntary twitching or tic usually involving a small muscle group of the face, neck, or shoulders and resulting in movements as spasmodic blinking or rapid jerking of the head to the side. The movements are often generated by emotional conflicts rather than caused by any organic disorder. They may serve as a release for tension or anxiety.

habit training, the process of teaching a child how to adjust to the demands of the external world by forming certain habits, primarily those related to eating, sleeping, elimination, and dress.

habitual abortion, spontaneous termination of three successive pregnancies before the twentieth week of gestation. Habitual abortion can result from chronic infection, abnormalities of the conceptus, maternal hormonal dysfunction, or uterine abnormalities as cervical incompetence. See also **cerclage, incompetent cervix.**

habitual fever. See **habitual hyperthermia.**

habitual hyperthermia, a condition of unknown cause occurring in young females, characterized by body temperatures of 99° to 100.5° F regularly or intermittently for years, associated with fatigue, malaise, vague aches and pains, insomnia, bowel disturbances, and headaches. No organic cause can be found; the diagnosis is usually made only after a prolonged period of study and observation. No specific treatment is recommended. Reassurance and psychotherapy offer the best relief. Also called **habitual fever.**

habituation, **1.** an acquired tolerance from repeated exposure to a particular stimulus. **2.** also called **negative adaptation.** a decline and eventual elimination of a conditioned response by repetition of the conditioned stimulus. **3.** psychologic and emotional dependence on a drug, tobacco, or alcohol resulting from the repeated use of the substance but without the addictive, physiologic need to increase dosage. Compare **addiction.**

habitus /hab′itəs/, describing a person's appearance or physique, as an athletic habitus. See also **habit.**

Haeckel's law. See **recapitulation theory.**

-haemia. See **-emia.**

Haemophilus /hēmof′iləs/, a genus of gram-negative pathogenic bacteria, frequently found in the respiratory tract of humans and other animals, as *Haemophilus influenzae,* which causes influenza and one form of meningitis, *H. haemolyticus,* a hemolytic species pathogenic in the upper respiratory tract of humans, and *H. ducreyi,* which causes chancroid. *Haemophilus* species are generally sensitive to tetracyclines and sulfonamides.

Haemophilus influenzae, a small, gram-negative, nonmotile, parasitic bacterium that occurs in two forms, encapsulated and nonencapsulated, and in six types, a, b, c, d, e, and f. Almost all infections are caused by encapsulated type b organisms. *Haemophilus influenzae* is found in the throats of 30% of healthy, normal people. In children and in debilitated older people severe destructive inflammation of the larynx, trachea, and bronchi may result from infection. Subacute bacterial endocarditis and purulent meningitis may also be caused by it. Secondary infection by *H. influenzae* occurs in influenza and in many other respiratory diseases. Immunization is available by inoculation with anti-*Haemophilus influenzae* serum.

hafnium (Hf), a hard, brittle, silver-gray metallic element of the first transition group. Its atomic number is 72; its atomic weight is 178.49. Elements in this group show some nonmetallic chemical characteristics.

Hagedorn needle /hä′gedôrn/, a flat surgical needle with a cutting edge near its point and a very large eye at the other end.

Hageman factor. See **factor XII.**

hair, a filament of keratin consisting of a root and a shaft formed in a specialized follicle in the epidermis. There are three stages of hair development: **anagen,** the active growing stage; **catagen,** a short interlude between the growth and resting phases; and **telogen,** the resting, or club stage before shedding. Scalp hair grows at an average rate of 1 mm every 3 days, body and eyebrow hair at a much slower rate. Hair plucking does not stop hair growth. See also **hirsutism, lanugo.**

hair matrix carcinoma. See **basal cell carcinoma.**

hair pulling. See **trichotillomania.**

hairy-cell leukemia, an uncommon neoplasm of blood-forming tissues, characterized by pancytopenia, a massively enlarged spleen, and the presence in blood and bone marrow of reticulum cells with many fine projections on their surface. The disease occurs six times more frequently in men than in women, usually appears in the fifth decade with an insidious onset and a variable course marked by anemia, thrombocytopenia, and spontaneous bruising. A tartrate-resistant acid phosphate isoenzyme found in hairy cells may aid in the diagnosis. Splenectomy may control the cytopenia, and some cases may improve with chemotherapy using vincristine and prednisone. Also called **leukemic reticuloendotheliosis.**

hairy tongue, a dark, pigmented overgrowth of the filiform papillae of the tongue that is a benign and frequent side effect of some antibiotics. The condition gradually subsides, and no treatment is indicated. See also **glossitis.**

halcinonide, a topical glucocorticoid.

■ INDICATION: It is prescribed topically as an antiinflammatory agent.

■ CONTRAINDICATIONS: Viral and fungal diseases of the skin, impaired circulation, or known hypersensitivity to this drug or to steroid medication prohibits its use.

■ ADVERSE EFFECTS: Among the more serious adverse effects are skin reactions and systemic side effects occurring from prolonged or excessive application.

Halcion, a trademark for a hypnotic agent (triazolam).

Haldol, a trademark for a tranquilizer (haloperidol).

Haldrone, a trademark for a glucocorticoid (paramethasone acetate).

half-life (t½), **1.** the time required for a radioactive substance to lose 50% of its activity through decay. Each radionuclide has a unique half-life. **2.** the amount of time required to reduce a drug level to one half of its initial value. Usually the term refers to time necessary to reduce the plasma value to one half of its initial value, and is also applied to the disappearance of the total amount of drug from the body. Also called **radioactive half-life.** See also **biologic half-life, effective half-life.**

half-sibling, one of two or more children who have at least one parent in common; a half brother or half sister. Also called **half-sib.**

half-value layer, the amount of material required to attenuate a beam of radiation to one half of its original level. Units are given in lengths, as centimeters.

halfway house, a specialized treatment facility, usually for psychiatric patients who no longer require complete hospitalization but who need some care and time to adjust to living independently.

halisteresis, a theoretic process of bone resorption in which bone salts may be removed by humoral mechanisms and returned to body tissue fluids, leaving behind a decalcified bone matrix. See also **osteolysis.**

halitosis /hal′itō′sis/, offensive breath resulting from poor oral hygiene, dental or oral infections, the ingestion of certain foods, as garlic or alcohol, use of tobacco, or some systemic diseases, as the odor of acetone in diabetes and ammonia in liver disease.

Hallpike caloric test, a method for evaluating the function of the vestibule of the ear in patients with vertigo or hearing loss. Irrigation of the ears with cool and warm water or air mimics the stimulus of turning in the vestibular apparatus, causing nystagmus. Nystagmus can then be evaluated, and specific disorders of the vestibule may be diagnosed. See also **caloric test, nystagmus.**

hallucination, a sensory perception that does not result from an external stimulus. It can occur in any of the senses and is classified accordingly as auditory, gustatory, olfactory, tactile, or visual. Kinds of hallucinations are **hypnagogic hallucination, lilliputian hallucination,** and **stump hallucination.** **–hallucinate,** *v.*

hallucinogen /həlo͞o′sənəjen′, hal′əsin′əjən, hal′yəsin′əjən/, a substance that causes excitation of the central nervous system, characterized by hallucination, mood change, anxiety, sensory distortion, delusion, depersonalization, increased pulse, temperature, and blood pressure, and dilatation of the pupils. Psychic dependence may occur, and depressive or suicidal psychotic states may result from the ingestion of hallucinogenic substances. Some kinds of hallucinogens are **lysergine, mescaline, peyote, phencyclidine hydrochloride,** and **psilocybin.**

hallucinosis /halo͞o′sinō′sis/, a pathologic mental state in which awareness consists primarily or exclusively of hallucinations. A kind of hallucinosis is **alcoholic hallucinosis.**

hallux /hal′əks/, *pl.* **halluces** /hal′yo͞osēz/, the great toe.

hallux rigidus, a painful deformity of the great toe, limiting motion at the metatarsophalangeal joint.

hallux valgus, a deformity in which the great toe is angulated away from the midline of the body toward the other toes; in some cases the great toe rides over or under the other toes.

halo cast, an orthopedic device used to help immobilize the neck and head. It incorporates the trunk, usually with shoulder straps, and an apparatus by means of an outrigger within the cast to secure pins to a band around the skull. The halo cast is used to help the healing of cervical injuries and cervical dislocations and for postoperative positioning and immobilization after cervical surgery.

halo effect, the beneficial effect of an interview or other encounter, as may occur in the course of a research project or a health care visit. The halo effect cannot be attributed to the content of the interview or to any specific act or treatment; it is the result of indefinable interpersonal factors present in the interaction.

Halog, a trademark for a topical glucocorticoid (halcinonide).

halogenated hydrocarbon, a volatile liquid used for general anesthesia, administered in combination with nitrous oxide, oxygen, or both. Nausea, vomiting, laryngospasm, and pharyngeal irritation are less severe and frequent when this anesthesia is used. Because the secretion of mucus is reduced, premedication with atropine and scopolamine may be reduced. Kinds of halogenated hydrocarbons are **enflurane, halothane, isoflurane, methoxyflurane,** and **trichoroethylene.**

haloperidol /hal′ōper′ədôl/, a butyrophenone tranquilizer.

■ INDICATIONS: It is prescribed in the treatment of psychotic disorders and in the control of Gilles de la Tourette's syndrome.

■ CONTRAINDICATIONS: Parkinson's disease, concurrent administration of central nervous system depressants, liver or renal dysfunction, severe hypotension, or known hypersensitivity to this drug prohibits its use.

■ ADVERSE EFFECTS: Among the more serious adverse effects are hypotension and a variety of extrapyramidal and hypersensitivity reactions.

haloprogin /hā′lōprō′jin/, an antibacterial and antifungal.

■ INDICATION: It is prescribed in the treatment of susceptible fungal infections, including athlete's foot.

■ CONTRAINDICATION: Known hypersensitivity to this drug prohibits its use.

■ ADVERSE EFFECTS: Among the most serious adverse reactions are exacerbation of existing lesions, formation of vesicles, and pruritus.

Halotestin, a trademark for an androgen (fluoxymesterone).

Halotex, a trademark for an antibacterial (haloprogin).

halothane /hal′əthān/, an inhalation anesthetic.

■ INDICATION: It is prescribed for induction and maintenance of general anesthesia.

■ CONTRAINDICATION: It is not recommended for obstetric anesthesia unless uterine relaxation is required.

■ ADVERSE EFFECTS: Among the more serious adverse reactions are hepatic necrosis, cardiac arrest or arrhythmia, hypotension, nausea, and emesis.

Halsted's forceps /hal′stedz/, **1.** also called **mosquito forceps.** a small, pointed hemostatic forceps. **2.** a forceps with slender jaws for grasping arteries and other blood vessels.

hamamelis water. See **witch hazel,** def 2.

hamate bone /ham′āt/, a carpal bone that rests on the fourth and fifth metacarpal bones and projects a hooklike process, the hamulus, from its palmar surface. Its dorsal surface is rough for ligamentous attachment. The hamate bone articulates with the lunate proximally, the fourth and fifth metacarpal distally, the triangular medially, and the capitate laterally. Also called **os hamatum, unciform bone.**

Hamman-Rich syndrome. See **interstitial pneumonia.**

hammertoe, a foot digit permanently flexed at the midphalangeal joint, resulting in a clawlike appearance. The anomaly may be present in more than one digit but is most common in the second toe.

hamstring muscle, any one of three muscles at the back of the thigh; medially, the semimembranosus and the semitendinosus and laterally, the biceps femoris.

hamstring reflex, a normal deep tendon reflex elicited by tapping one of the hamstring tendons behind the knee, resulting in contraction of the tendon and flexion of the knee. The patient should be lying in the supine position with the knee and hip partially flexed and the leg supported by the examiner's hand. An accentuated hamstring reflex may result from a lesion of the pyramidal system above the level of the fourth lumbar nerve root. See also **deep tendon reflex.**

hamstring tendon, one of the three tendons from the three hamstring muscles in the back of the thigh. The one lateral and the two medial hamstring tendons connect the hamstring muscles to the knee.

hamular notch. See **pterygomaxillary notch.**

hand, the part of the upper limb distal to the forearm. It is the most flexible part of the skeleton and has a total of 27 bones, 8 forming the carpus, 5 forming the metacarpus, and 14 comprising the phalangeal section. Also called **manus.**

handblock, a device made of a wood block several inches high with a firm handle that can be gripped by a disabled patient to provide a certain amount of body support in minor ambulatory activities, as getting into or out of a bed.

hand condenser, (in dentistry) an instrument for compacting amalgams or gold foil using force applied by the operator, with or without supplementary force from a mallet of an assistant.

handedness, voluntary or involuntary preference for use of either the left or right hand. The preference is related to cerebral dominance, with left-handedness corresponding to dominance of the right side of the brain and vice versa. Also called **chirality, laterality.**

hand-foot syndrome. See **sickle cell crisis.**

handicapped, referring to a person who has a congenital or acquired mental or physical defect that interferes with normal functioning of the body system or the ability to be self-sufficient in modern society. Compare **disability.**

handpiece, a device for holding rotary instruments in a dental engine or condensing points in mechanic condensing units. It is connected by an arm, cable, belt, or tube to a power source, as a motor, or an air-pressure or water-pressure hose.

Hand-Schüller-Christian syndrome /hand′shōō′-lərkris′chən/, *obsolete.* a triad of symptoms, exopthalmos, diabetes insipidus, and bone destruction, which may occur in any of several disorders. See also **eosinophilic granuloma, Letterer-Siwe disease.**

hanging drop preparation, a technique used for the examination and identification of certain microorganisms, as spirochetes or trichomonads. The technique requires a cover slip, a microscope, and a special slide that has a central concavity. A specimen suspected of containing the microorganism is diluted with a sterile isotonic solution. A drop of this fluid mixture is placed on a glass cover slip, which is then inverted carefully and placed over the slide so that the drop is hanging from the slip into the concavity in the slide. The delicate structures and the method of movement characteristic of the species may then be viewed through the microscope. An ordinary glass slide can be prepared for hanging drop examination by making a ring of petroleum jelly on the slide and inverting a cover slip bearing the drop of solution over the ring.

hangman's fracture, a fracture of the posterior elements of the cervical vertebrae with dislocation of C2 or C3.

hangnail, a piece of partially disconnected epidermis of the cuticle or nail fold. Tearing the skin fragment causes a red, painful, easily infected sore. ("Hang" is not related to the verb but is an old English word for pain.) Early treatment is to trim the hangnail close with nail clippers. For inflamed situations an antibiotic ointment and protective bandage are used.

Hanot's disease /hanōz′/, primary biliary cirrhosis. See also **biliary cirrhosis.**

Hansen's disease. See **leprosy.**

-haphia. See **-aphia.**

haploid /hap′loid/, having only one complete set of nonhomologous chromosomes. Also called **monoploid.** –**haploidy,** *n.*

hapten /hap′tən/, a nonproteinaceous substance that acts as an antigen by combining with particular bonding sites on an antibody. Unlike a true antigen, it does not induce the formation of antibodies. A hapten bonded to a carrier protein may induce an immune response. Also called **haptene** /hap′tēn/.

haptics, the science concerned with studying the sense of touch. –**haptic,** *adj.*

haptoglobin /hap′tōglō′bin/, a plasma protein whose only known function is to bind free hemoglobin. The quantity of haptoglobin is increased in certain chronic diseases and inflammatory disorders and is decreased or absent in hemolytic anemia. Compare **transferrin.** See also **hemoglobinemia, hemoglobinuria.**

hard copy, any readable output from a computer that is produced on paper or another permanent medium.

hard data, information about a patient that is obtained by observation and measurement, including laboratory data, as opposed to information collected by interviewing the patient.

hard disk, a computer data storage medium that consists of a rigid disk with an electromagnetic coating allowing information to be transcribed on it and from it. Usually permanently mounted in a dust-proof container, a hard disk has a storage capacity approximately 10 to 100 times that of a diskette. Compare **diskette.**

hardening of the arteries, arteriosclerosis.

hard fibroma, a neoplasm composed of fibrous tissue in which there are few cells. Also called **fibroma durum.**

hard money, *informal.* (in a university, school, or agency) income from stable sources, as an endowment, tuition, or fees.

hardness of x-rays, the relative penetrating power of x-rays. In general, the shorter the wavelength, the harder the radiation. Also called **hard radiation.** Compare **soft radiation.**

hard palate, the bony portion of the roof of the mouth, continuous posteriorly with the soft palate and bounded anteriorly and laterally by the alveolar arches and the gums. The palatine process of the maxilla and the horizontal portion of the palatine bone form the bony support for the hard palate that is covered by periosteum and by the mucous membrane of the mouth. A linear raphe along its middle line ends anteriorly in a small papilla, which corresponds with the incisive canal. On each side and anterior to the raphe, the mucous membrane is thick, pale in color, and corrugated. Posteriorly the mucous membrane is thin, smooth, and darker. The hard palate is covered with squamous epithelium and furnished with numerous palatal glands lying between the mucous membrane and the surface of the bone. Compare **soft palate.**

hard radiation. See **hardness of x-rays.**

hardware, the tangible parts of a computer, as chips, boards, wires, transformers, and peripheral devices. See also **firmware, software, wetware.**

hardware bug. See **bug.**

Hardy-Weinberg equilibrium principle, the mathematic relationship between the frequency of genes and the resulting genotypes in populations. In a large interbreeding population characterized by random mating, mendelian inheritance, and the absence of migration, mutation, and selection, the ratio of individuals homozygous for a dominant gene to those heterozygous to those homozygous for a recessive gene is 1:2:1, at which point equilibrium is established; and the frequency of genes and genotypes remains relatively unchanged from generation to generation. See also **genetic equilibrium.**

harelip. See **cleft lip.**

hare's eye. See **lagophthalmos.**

harlequin color, a transient flushing of the skin on the lower side of the body with pallor of the upward side. Commonly seen in normal young infants, it disappears as the child matures.

harlequin fetus, an infant whose skin at birth is completely covered with thick, horny scales that resemble armor and are divided by deep red fissures. The condition is the most severe form of lamellar exfoliation of the newborn, and the infant is stillborn or dies within a few days of birth. Also called **ichthyosis fetus.**

Harmonyl, a trademark for an antihypertensive (deserpidine).

Harris tube, a tube used for gastric and intestinal decompression. It is a mercury weighted, single lumen tube that is passed through the nose and carried through the alimentary tract by gravity. The amount of mercury in the soft bag surrounding the tube varies from 2 to 5 ml according to the age, size, and condition of the patient. The location of the tube is followed by fluoroscopy, and its final placement is also checked. The tube is lubricated before the procedure is begun, and the patient is positioned in such a way that gravity can aid advancement of the tube through the alimentary tract.

Hartmann's curet, a curet used for the removal of adenoids. See also **curet.**

Hartnup disease, a recessive genetic metabolic disorder characterized by pellagra-like skin lesions, transient cerebellar ataxia, and hyperaminoaciduria, caused by defects in intestinal absorption and renal reabsorption of neutral amino acids. Bacterial degradation of unabsorbed amino acids in the gut leads to the absorption of breakdown products and their appearance in urine; the unavailability of tryptophan leads to a deficiency of niacin, the antipellagra vitamin. Common symptoms of the disease are dry, scaly, well-circumscribed skin lesions, glossitis, stomatitis, diarrhea, psychiatric problems, and pronounced photosensitivity; brief exposure to the sun may cause erythema, edema, and vesiculation. Treatment consists of oral nicotinamide and a diet containing proteins composed of more easily absorbed small peptides.

Harvard pump, a small pump that can be adjusted to deliver small amounts of medication in solution through an intravenous infusion set. It is commonly used to administer oxytocin in the induction or augmentation of labor. Compare **Abbot pump.**

harvest fever. See **leptospirosis.**

harvest mite. See **chigger.**

Hashimoto's disease /hä′shimō′tōz/, an autoimmune thyroid disorder, characterized by the production of antibodies in response to thyroid antigens and the replacement of normal thyroid structures with lymphocytes and lymphoid germinal centers. The disease shows a marked hereditary pattern, but it is 20 times more common in women than in men. It occurs most frequently between 30 and 50 years of age but may arise in young children. The thyroid, typically enlarged, pale yellow, and lumpy on the surface, shows dense lymphocytic infiltration, and the remaining thyroid tissue frequently contains small empty follicles. The goiter is usually asymptomatic, but occasionally patients complain of dysphagia and a feeling of local pressure. The thymus is usually enlarged, and regional lymph nodes often show hyperplasia. A definitive diagnosis can be made if a fluorescent scan shows a decrease or absence of thyroid-stable iodine and if a hemagglutination test for thyroid antigens is positive. Replacement therapy with thyroid hormone is indicated for patients with thyroid deficiency and can prevent further enlargement of the goiter. Also called **Hashimoto's struma, Hashimoto's thyroiditis, lymphocytic thyroiditis, struma lymphomatosa.**

hashish. See **cannabis.**

Haverhill fever /hā′vəril/, a febrile disease, caused by infection with *Streptobacillus moniliformis,* transmitted by the bite of a rat. The spirochete-like bacterium is normally present in rat saliva. Characteristically the wound from the bite heals, but within 10 days fever, chills, vomiting, headache, muscle and joint pain, and a rash appear. Treatment with antibiotics is effective. *S. moniliformis* is identified by laboratory analysis using fluorescent antibody screening. Also called **streptobacillary ratbite fever.**

haversian canal /havur′shən/, one of the many tiny longitudinal canals in bone tissue, averaging about 0.05 mm in diameter. Each contains blood vessels, connective tissue, nerve filaments, and, occasionally, lymphatic vessels. The canals are interconnected and part of an intricate network. See also **haversian canaliculus, haversian system, Volkmann's canal.**

haversian canaliculus, any one of the many tiny passages radiating from the lacunae of bone tissue to larger haversian canals. See also **haversian canal, haversian system.**

haversian system, a circular district of bone tissue, consisting of lamellae in the bone around a central canal. See also **haversian canal, haversian canaliculus, Volkmann's canal.**

Hawthorne effect, a general, unintentional, but usually beneficial effect on a person, a group of people, or the function of the system being studied. The Hawthorne effect is the effect of an encounter, as with an investigator or health care provider, or of a change in a program or facility, as by painting an office or changing the lighting system. The Hawthorne effect is likely to confound the results of a study or investigation, because it is usually present and difficult to identify. It was named for a study in industrial management at the Hawthorne (Illinois) facility of the Western Electric Company.

hay fever, *informal.* an acute seasonal allergic rhinitis stimulated by tree, grass, or weed pollens. Also called **pollinosis.** See also **allergic rhinitis, organic dust.**

hazard, a condition or phenomenon that increases the probability of a loss arising from some danger that may result in injury or illness. **–hazardous,** *adj.*

Hb, abbreviation for **hemoglobin.**

HB, abbreviation for **hepatitis B.**

Hb A, abbreviation for **hemoglobin A.**

Hb A_2, abbreviation for **hemoglobin A_2.**

Hb C, abbreviation for **hemoglobin C.**

HBE, abbreviation for **His bundle electrocardiogram.**

Hb F, abbreviation for **hemoglobin F.**

HBIG, abbreviation for **hepatitis B immune globulin.**

Hb S, abbreviation for **hemoglobin S.**

HBsAG, abbreviation for **hepatitis B surface antigen.** See also **Australia antigen.**

Hb S-C, abbreviation for **hemoglobin S-C.**

HCG, abbreviation for **human chorionic gonadotropin.** See also **chorionic gonadotropin.**

HCG radioreceptor assay, a urine test to detect pregnancy or missed abortion, performed by measuring human chorionic gonadotropin, a chemical found only in the urine of pregnant women or in tumors that produce HCG. The normal values are negative (within 2 hours) if the patient is not pregnant and positive (within 1 hour) if the patient is pregnant. Also called **pregnancy test.**

H deflection, (in cardiology) an indication on an electrocardiogram of His bundle activation.

HDL, abbreviation for **high-density lipoprotein.**

He, symbol for **helium.**

headache, a pain in the head from any cause. Kinds of headaches include **functional headache, migraine headache, organic headache, sinus headache,** and **tension headache.** Also called **cephalalgia.**

head and neck cancer, any malignant neoplasms of the upper aerodigestive tract, facial features, and structures in the neck, presenting as masses, ulcerations, or flat lesions that usually produce early symptoms. Tumors of the oral cavity, lips, and tongue characteristically begin as a swelling or nonhealing ulcer and are most commonly epidermoid carcinomas that occur in men over 60 years of age; predisposing factors are chronic alcoholism, heavy use of tobacco, poor oral hygiene, syphilis, and Plummer-Vinson syndrome. Nasal and paranasal sinus malignancies, most often epidermoid cancers, cause a bloody discharge, obstruction in breathing, and facial and dental pain. Nasopharyngeal tumors, predominantly squamous cell and undifferentiated carcinomas occurring most frequently in Orientals, are associated with nasal obstruction, serous otitis media, hearing loss, lymphadenopathy, and cranial nerve involvement. Oropharyngeal and tonsillar neoplasms, usually squamous cell carcinomas and less frequently lymphomas, produce dysphagia, pain, dyspnea, and trismus. Most hypopharyngeal and laryngeal tumors are carcinomas that cause hoarseness, dysphagia, dyspnea, cough, and cervical adenopathy. Salivary gland carcinomas occur most frequently in the parotid gland and may cause facial palsy. Cancer of the mandible, including extremely painful osteosarcoma and, often, painless giant cell tumor, Ewing's sarcoma, and ameloblastoma, may erode through the gingiva, producing an intraoral ulcer, and may cause pathologic fractures. Ear neoplasms involve the auricle in most cases, usually occur in persons over 50 years of age, and are most commonly squamous cell carcinomas that cause pain, deafness, and facial nerve paralysis. Cancers of the lacrimal glands, lacrimal sacs, and parathyroid glands are rare, but hypercalcemia, hypercalcinuria, kidney stones, and renal and bone diseases are associated with parathyroid carcinoma. Tumors of the eye, as malignant melanoma in patients over 50 years of age and retinoblastoma in children, are also rare. Head and neck tumors are diagnosed by clinical examination, x-ray examinations, tomograms, biopsies, arteriograms, supravital staining of lesions, and cytologic studies. Surgery and radiotherapy are the primary treatments, but their use may cause problems with swallowing and speaking; the effectiveness of chemotherapy is limited by the poor nutritional status of many patients with head or neck lesions. Plastic surgery and various prostheses are often essential in correcting deformities and restoring functions in patients who have undergone the excision or radiotherapy of a head or neck tumor. See also specific cancer.

head, eye, ear, nose, and throat (HEENT), a specialty in medicine concerned with the anatomy, physiology, and pathology of the head, eyes, ears, nose, and throat and with the diagnosis and treatment of disorders of those structures.

head injury, any traumatic damage to the head resulting from penetration of the skull or from too rapid inertial acceleration or deceleration of the brain within the skull. Blood vessels, nerves, and meninges are torn; bleeding, edema, and ischemia may result. Meningeal infection is a grave and frequent complication of fracture of the bones of the paranasal sinuses. See also **concussion.**

head kidney. See **pronephros.**

head nurse, the clinical and administrative leader of the nurses working in a given geographic division of an institution, usually a floor, ward, or unit. The responsibilities of a head nurse may include directing nursing care activities, scheduling of staff, evaluation of nursing personnel, and hiring, firing, or promoting staff nurses. The head nurse may also be responsible for budget preparation and general clinical leadership. The head nurse acts as liaison in the communication between the nursing staff and others, including physicians, institutional personnel, and nursing educators.

head process, a strand of cells that extends forward from the primitive node in the early stages of embryonic development in vertebrates. It is the precursor of the notochord and forms the primitive axis around which the embryo develops. Also called **notochordal plate.**

Heaf test /hēf/, a tuberculin skin test using a multiple puncture technique. See also **tuberculin test.**

healing, the act or process in which the normal structural and functional characteristics of health are restored to diseased, dysfunctional, or damaged tissues, organs, or systems of the body. See also **intention, wound repair.**

health, a condition of physical, mental, and social well-being and the absence of disease or other abnormal condition. It is not a static condition; constant change and adaptation to stress result in homeostasis. René Dubos, often quoted in nursing education, says, "The states of health or disease are the expressions of the success or failure experienced by the organism in its efforts to respond adaptively to environmental challenges." See also **high-level wellness, homeostasis.**

health assessment, an evaluation of the health status of an individual by performing a physical examination after obtaining a health history. Various laboratory tests may also be ordered to confirm a clinical impression or to screen for dysfunction. The depth of investigation and the frequency of the assessment varies with the condition and age of the client and the facility in which the assessment is performed. A significant part of the health assessment is counseling and education that may explain aspects of anatomy, physiology, and pathophysiology and that introduces or affirms the general tenets of a healthful way of life. The person's response to any dysfunction present is observed and noted. The techniques of the health assessment include: palpation, percussion, auscultation, and inspection, including sight, sound, and smell.

health behavior, an action taken by a person to maintain, attain, or regain good health and to prevent illness. Health behavior reflects a person's health beliefs. Some common health behaviors are exercising regularly, eating a balanced diet, and obtaining necessary inoculations.

health belief model, a conceptual framework that describes a person's health behavior as an expression of health beliefs. The model was designed to predict a person's health behavior, including the use of health services, and to justify intervention to alter maladaptive health behavior. Components of the model include the person's own perception of susceptibility to a disease or condition, the likelihood of contracting that disease or condition, the person's perception of the severity of the consequences of contracting the condition or the disease, the perceived benefits of care and barriers to preventive behavior, and the internal or external stimuli that result in appropriate health behavior by the person.

health care consumer, any actual or potential recipient of health care, as a patient in a hospital, a client in a community mental health center, or a member of a prepaid health maintenance organization.

health care industry, the complex of preventive, remedial, and therapeutic services provided by hospitals and other institutions, nurses, doctors, dentists, government agencies, voluntary agencies, noninstitutional care facilities, pharmaceutic and medical equipment manufacturers, and health insurance companies.

health care system, the complete network of agencies, facilities, and all providers of health care in a specified geographic area. Nursing services are integral to all levels and patterns of care, and nurses form the largest number of providers in a health care system.

health certificate, a statement signed by a health care provider that attests to the state of health of a person.

health consumer. See **health care consumer.**

health culture, a system that attempts to explain and treat sickness and to maintain health. Health cultures are part of the larger culture or tradition of a people. It may be a popular or folk system, or it may be a technical or scientific one.

health economics, a social system that studies the supply and demand of health care resources and the impact of health services on a population.

health education, an educational program directed to the general public that attempts to improve, maintain, and safeguard the health of the community.

health history, (in nursing and medicine) a collection of information obtained from the patient and from other sources concerning the patient's physical status and psychologic, social, and sexual functions. The history provides a data base on which a plan for management of the diagnosis, treatment, care, and follow-up of the patient may be made. The first part of the history describes the present illness (PI), including its signs and symptoms, onset and character, and any factors or behaviors that aggravate or ameliorate the symptoms. The patient's own words often serve as the best description and may be quoted. The second part of the history comprises an account of previous illnesses, conditions, allergies, transfusions, immunizations, screening tests, and hospitalizations. An occupational history, describing the patient's work and exposure to stress, toxins, radiation, or other occupational hazards, may be included. The effect of the current illness on the patient's work is also noted. A social history is taken in which the patient's social, cultural, and familial milieux are outlined, focusing on aspects that might have an effect on the current illness. In some instances a sexual history may be relevant. A review of systems may follow or be incorporated into the health history. Kinds of history include **complete health history, episodic health history,** and **interval health history.** Also called **medical history.** See also **occupational history, review of systems, sexual history.**

health maintenance, a program or procedure planned to prevent illness, to maintain maximal function, and to promote health. It is central to health care, especially to nursing care at all levels (primary, secondary, and tertiary) and in all patterns (preventive, episodic, acute, chronic, and catastrophic).

health maintenance, alterations in, a nursing diagnosis accepted by the Fifth National Conference on the Classification of Nursing Diagnoses. This diagnosis describes the condition in which the patient is unable to identify, manage, or seek help to maintain health. The causes of the problem include the lack of or significant alteration in written, verbal, or other communication skills; perceptual or cognitive impairment or the inability to make deliberate and thoughtful judgments; impairment or lack of motor skills; lack of material resources; or the inability to cope. The defining characteristics include a demonstrated lack of knowledge regarding basic health practices or the inability to take responsibility for meeting those needs, the inability to adapt to internal or external environmental change, a lack of financial or other resources or support systems, a history of the lack of health-seeking behavior, or an increased interest in improving health behavior. See also **nursing diagnosis.**

Health Maintenance Organization (HMO), a type of group health care practice that provides basic and supplemental health maintenance and treatment services to voluntary enrollees who prepay a fixed periodic fee that is set without regard to the amount or kind of services received. Some of the first HMOs, Kaiser-Permanente among them, have demonstrated that high quality medical care can often be provided at less expense by such a system than by other health care systems. In addition to diagnostic and treatment services, including hospitalization and surgery, an HMO often offers supplemental services, as dental, mental, and eye care, and prescription drugs. Federal financial support for the establishment of

HMOs was provided under Title XIII of the 1973 U.S. Public Health Service Act.

health physicist, a health scientist who directs research, training, and management of programs in which patients and health professionals are exposed to potential hazards associated with the use of diagnostic and therapeutic equipment, as radioactive materials.

health physics, the study of the effects of ionizing radiation on the body and the methods for protecting people from the undesirable effects of the radiation. Health physics is concerned with the development and evaluation of methods, techniques, materials, and procedures to be used to protect people from these untoward effects. Also called **medical physics.**

health policy, **1.** a statement of a decision regarding a goal in health care and a plan for achieving that goal; for example, to prevent an epidemic, a program for innoculating a population is developed and implemented. **2.** a field of study and practice in which the priorities and values underlying health resource allocation are determined.

health professional, any person who has completed a course of study in a field of health, such as a registered nurse, physical therapist, or physician. The person is usually licensed by a government agency or certified by a professional organization.

health provider, any individual who provides health services to health care consumers.

health-related services, services of a health facility other than medical care that may contribute directly or indirectly to the physical or mental health and well-being of patients, as personal or social services.

health resources, all materials, personnel, facilities, funds, and anything else that can be used for providing health care and services.

health risk, a disease precursor associated with a higher than average morbidity or mortality. The disease precursors may include demographic variables, certain individual behaviors, familial and individual histories, and certain physiologic changes.

health risk appraisal, a process of gathering, analyzing, and comparing an individual's prognostic characteristics of health with a standard age group, thereby predicting the likelihood that a person may develop prematurely a health problem associated with a high morbidity and mortality rate.

health screening, a program designed to evaluate the health status and potential of an individual. In the process it may be found that a person has a particular disease or condition or is at greater than normal risk of developing it. Health screening may include taking a personal and family health history and performing a physical examination or tests, laboratory tests, or radiologic examination, and may be followed by counseling, education, referral, or further testing.

health service area, a geographic region designated under the National Health Planning and Resources Development Act of 1974, covering such factors as geography, political boundaries, population, and health resources, for the effective planning and development of health services.

health supervision, health teaching, counseling, or monitoring the status of the patient's health rather than for physical care. Such supervision occurs in health care agencies, clinics, physician's offices, or the patient's home. Compare **care of the sick.**

health systems agency (HSA), an agency established under the terms of the National Health Planning and Resources Development Act of 1974. Health planning agencies are intended to provide networks of health planning and resource development services in each of several health service areas established by the Act. Health systems agencies are nonprofit and include private organizations, public regional planning bodies, or local government agencies and consumers. See also **health systems plan.**

health systems plan, a plan in which the long-range health goals of a health services area are specified. Health systems plans are prepared by health systems agencies. See also **health policy.**

hearing, the special sense that enables sound to be perceived. It is the major function of the ear. Any reduction in the ability to perceive sounds results in hearing loss, which can range from mild impairment to complete deafness. See also **deafness.**

hearing aid, an electronic device that amplifies sound for persons with impaired hearing. The device consists of a microphone, a battery power supply, an amplifier, and a receiver. The microphone receives sound waves directed toward the person with normal hearing loss, the sound waves are converted to electric impulses that are amplified with the aid of the power supply, and the receiver converts the electric impulses back into sound vibrations. The receiver is designed, according to the cause of the hearing loss, to transmit sound through the external auditory canal or through the mastoid area of the skull. See also **cochlear implants.**

heart, the muscular, cone-shaped organ, about the size of a clenched fist, that pumps blood throughout the body and beats normally about 70 times per minute by coordinated nerve impulses and muscular contractions. Enclosed in pericardium, the heart rests on the diaphragm between the lower borders of the lungs, occupying the middle of the mediastinum. It is covered ventrally by the sternum and the adjoining parts of the third to the sixth costal cartilages. The organ is about 12 cm long, 8 cm wide at its broadest part, and 6 cm thick. The weight of the heart in men averages between 280 and 340 g and in women, between 230 and 280 g. The layers of the heart, starting from the outside, are the epicardium, the myocardium, and the endocardium. The epicardium includes the visceral pericardium and a layer of fibroelastic connective tissue interspersed with fat. The myocardium is composed of layers and bundles of cardiac muscle laced by blood vessels. The endocardium is continuous with the endothelial lining of the blood vessels and is composed of squamous endothelium. The chambers of the heart include two ventricles with thick muscular walls, making up the bulk of the organ, and two atria with thin muscular walls. A septum separates the ventricles and extends between the atria, dividing the heart into the right and the left sides. The left side of the heart pumps oxygenated blood from the pulmonary veins into the aorta and on to all parts of the body. The right side of the heart pumps deoxygenated blood, received through the venae cavae, into the pulmonary arteries. The sinoatrial node in the right atrium of the heart initiates the cardiac impulse, causing the atria to contract. The atrioventricular node in the septal wall of the right atrium spreads the impulse over the bundle of His, causing the ventricles to contract. Both atria contract almost simultaneously, followed quickly by the nearly simultaneous contraction of the ventricles. The valves of the heart include the tricuspid valve between the right atrium and the right ventricle, the mitral valve between the left atrium and the left ventricle, the aortic valve at the exit of the left ventricle, and the pulmonary valve at the exit of the right ventricle. The sinoatrial node of the pulse sets the rate. Other factors affecting the pulse are emotion, exercise, hormones, temperature, pain, and stress.

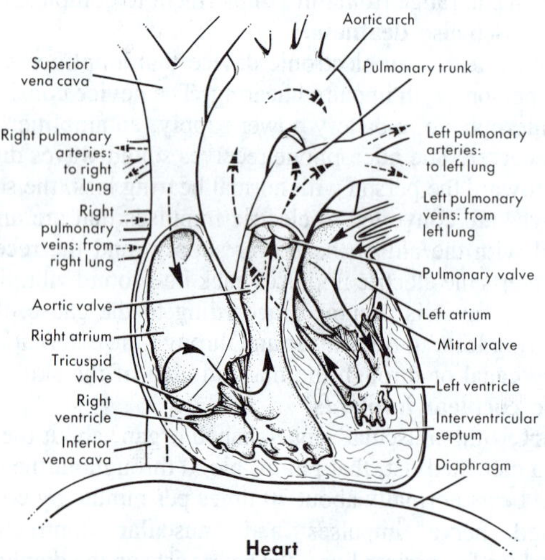

Heart

heart block, an interference with the normal conduction of electric impulses that control activity of the heart muscle. Heart block usually is further defined as to the location of the block and the type, as a first degree AV block in which all atrial impulses that should be conducted to the ventricles reach the ventricles but are delayed by a fraction of a second. The delay or block can occur in the sinoatrial node, atria, atrioventricular node, the bundle of His, the fascicles, or a combination of these. See also **atrioventricular block, bundle branch block, cardiac conduction defect, infranodal block, intraatrial block, intraventricular block, sinoatrial block.**

heartburn, a painful burning sensation in the esophagus just below the sternum. Heartburn is usually caused by the reflux of gastric contents into the esophagus but may be caused by gastric hyperacidity or peptic ulcer. Antacids relieve the symptoms but do not cure the heartburn. Also called **pyrosis.** See also **gastroesophageal reflux, hiatus hernia.**

heart failure, a condition in which the heart cannot pump enough blood in relation to the venous return and the metabolic requirements of body tissues. Extreme exertion may cause heart failure in individuals with normal hearts if there is a discrepancy between the needs of the body and the volume of blood pumped by the heart. Heart failure may be generally classified as cardiac mechanic failure, myocardial failure, and arrhythmic failure. Most forms of heart failure are caused by atrial failure or by ventricular failure, and many patients develop heart failure from more than one cause. Many of the symptoms associated with heart failure are caused by the dysfunction of organs other than the heart, especially the lungs, kidneys, and liver. Ventricular dysfunction is usually the basic disorder in congestive heart failure and often triggers compensatory mechanisms that preserve cardiac output but produce symptoms and signs, as dyspnea, orthopnea, rales, and edema. Heart failure is closely associated with many forms of heart disease and is commonly diagnosed only after the diagnosis of heart disease. Most kinds of heart disease initially affect the left side of the heart, and clinicians commonly divide associated heart failure into left-sided heart failure and right-sided heart failure. Peripheral edema occurs in connection with right-sided heart failure and dyspnea in connection with left-sided heart failure. The adjustments of the body to heart failure are divided into the acute adjustments, the subacute adjustments, and the chronic adjustments, depending on how long the adjustment takes. The acute adjustments involve numerous complex mechanisms, the most important of which increase autonomic sympathetic excitation to the heart and most of the arteries and veins. The stimulation of the peripheral arteries helps maintain arterial pressure. The stimulation of the veins helps increase venous tone and venous pressure. The increased venous pressure aids venous return, ventricular filling, and the diastolic stretching of the ventricular fibers. The subacute adjustments of the body to heart failure mainly involve those mechanisms that cause the kidneys to retain salt and water, resulting in increased blood volume. The localization of edema produced by the excess fluid and salt depends on various hydrostatic factors, as the position of the patient. The main chronic adjustment of the body to heart failure is hypertrophy of the ventricular myocardium, apparently caused by a chronic increase in the tension of the myocardial fibers. Current studies indicate that heart failure in infants and children is usually the result of congenital heart disease, but it may also be caused by myocarditis and ectopic tachycardia. The most frequent cause of congestive heart failure between birth and 1 week of age is aortic atresia.

Between 1 week and 1 month of age, the most common causes are coarctation of the aorta and transposition of the great vessels, followed in order of causative frequency by endomyocardial disease, ventricular septal defect, and patent ductus arteriosus. Between 3 and 6 months of age, endomyocardial disease is the most common cause of cardiac failure, followed in frequency by ventricular septal defect, patent ductus arteriosus, total anomalous pulmonary venous return, coarctation of the aorta, and transposition of the great vessels. From birth to 6 months of age, paroxysmal atrial tachycardia may cause acute catastrophic heart failure without other evidence of heart disease. The most common causes of heart failure between 5 and 15 years of age are acute rheumatic myocarditis, acute glomerulonephritis, and congenital heart disease, especially ventricular septal defect, atrial septal defect, and patent ductus arteriosus. Heart failure during early life is rarely caused by secundum-type atrial septal defect, congenital valve disease, or acquired valve disease. Rheumatic mitral disease and aortic valve disease frequently cause congestive heart failure in young adults. Mitral valve disease, especially mitral stenosis, is the most common cause of heart failure and affects more young women than men. Other heart diseases that may affect young adults are nonrheumatic myocardial disease and congenital heart disease. The common causes of heart failure after 40 years of age are coronary atherosclerosis with myocardial infarction, diastolic hypertension in which the pressure is usually above 110 mm Hg, valvular heart disease, pulmonary disease, and diffuse myocardial disease. Some individuals may suffer heart failure caused by a combination of congenital heart disease and acquired disease. After 50 years of age, a common cause of heart failure, especially in men, is calcific aortic stenosis. Some of the behavioral and environmental factors that may cause heart failure in asymptomatic patients with heart disease are sudden extraordinary effort, increased work load, excessive dietary intake of sodium, sudden emotional upset, and the administration of excessive volumes of intravenous fluids. Some signs of heart failure based on physical examination may be divided into those signs caused by the effects of cardiac failure on other organs and those signs of cardiac failure that are associated with the heart, the arteries, and the veins. Some of the extracardiac signs are ascites, bronchial wheezing, hydrothorax, edema, enlargement of the liver, moist rales, and splenomegaly. Some of the cardiac signs associated with heart failure are abnormalities in the jugular venous pulsation and the carotid pulse, and abnormal cardiographic tracings of the apex wave. The treatment for heart failure commonly involves the reduction of the workload of the heart, the administration of certain drugs, as digitalis, to increase myocardial contractility and cardiac output, salt-free diets, diuretics, and surgical intervention. Many patients with heart failure, especially elderly patients, become constipated and require laxatives, as mineral oil, milk of magnesia, and cascara sagrada. In acute heart failure, a complex autonomic response and local regulatory mechanisms redistribute the available blood flow, and body tissues receiving less blood than required may use anaerobic metabolism or withdraw more oxygen from each unit of available blood. The sudden onset of acute pulmonary edema associated with some cases of heart failure is a life-threatening condition requiring immediate treatment. Acute pulmonary edema may develop in patients with chronic heart failure because of atherosclerosis and old infarcts or in patients with normal hearts who develop ectopic tachycardia or pulmonary embolism. Acute pulmonary edema may sometimes be confused with bronchial asthma, and caution is required in the administration of appropriate drugs. Aminophylline and oxygen are used in therapy for both pulmonary edema and acute asthma. See also **compensated heart failure, congestive heart failure.**

heart-lung machine, an apparatus consisting of a pump and an oxygenator that takes over the functions of the heart and lungs, especially during cardiac surgery. The blood is shunted from the venous system through an oxygenator and returned to the arterial circulation.

heart massage. See **cardiac massage.**

heart murmur. See **cardiac murmur.**

heart rate, the pulse, calculated by counting the number of QRS complexes or contractions of the cardiac ventricles per unit of time. Tachycardia is a heart rate of more than 100 beats per minute; bradycardia is a heart rate of fewer than 60 beats per minute. See also **pulse.**

heart scan, a radiographic scan of the heart, performed after injecting a radioactive material into a vein, used for determining the size, shape, and location of the heart, for diagnosing pericarditis, and for viewing the chambers of the heart. See also **cardiography, echocardiogram.**

heart sound, a normal noise produced within the heart during the cardiac cycle that can be heard over the precordium and may reveal abnormalities in cardiac structure or function. Cardiac auscultation is performed systematically from apex to base of the heart or from base to apex, using a stethoscope to listen initially with the diaphragm and then with the bell of the instrument. The first heart sound (S_1), a dull, prolonged "lub," occurs with the closure of the mitral and tricuspid valves and marks the onset of ventricular systole; the mitral valve sound is loudest at the apex of the heart and that of the tricuspid valve at the left sternal border in the fourth intercostal space. The second heart sound (S_2), a short, sharp "dup," occurs with the closing of the aortic and pulmonic valves at the beginning of ventricular diastole; the aortic valve closure is heard loudest on the right sternal border, and that of the pulmonic valve is most distinct on the left sternal border over the second intercostal space. A weak, low-pitched, dull third heart sound (S_3) is sometimes heard and is thought to be caused by vibrations of the walls of the ventricles when they are suddenly distended by blood from the atria. S_3, which is heard most clearly at the apex of the heart with the bell of a stethoscope, is called a ventricular or diastolic gallop; it may be normal in children, adolescents, or very thin adults, or it may be a sign of congestive heart failure or hypertension causing left ventricular failure. A left-sided fourth heart sound (S_4), which may be heard with the stethoscope's bell at the apex of the heart during expiration, is caused by vibrations of the atria after contraction. Called an atrial or presystolic gallop, S_4 is usually a sign of pathology, as myocardial infarction or impending heart failure from another cause. Asynchronous closure of cardiac valves may result in split heart sounds. An S_1 split occurs in right bundle branch block, mitral stenosis, and tricuspid valve dysfunction associated with pulmonary hypertension. S_2 splits may occur in normal inspiration but may also indicate septal defects, pulmonic stenosis, or other mechanic problems. Brief, periodic endocardial murmurs may indicate various disorders. A murmur characteristic of incompetency of the mitral orifice is loudest at the cardiac apex, a murmur characteristic of tricuspid incompetency is loudest at the ensiform cartilage, and a murmur typical of obstruction of the pulmonic orifice is loudest at the left second intercostal space near the sternum. Systolic and diastolic murmurs that are loudest at the junction of the right second costal cartilage and sternum indicate problems in the aortic orifice, and a presystolic murmur over the body of the heart may be the result of mitral orifice obstruction. A phonocardiogram recorded simultaneously with the electrocardiogram shows the relationships between heart sounds and electric events. S_1 begins midway in the QRS complex; during this interval the mitral and tricuspid valves close, the pulmonic and aortic valves open, and ejection of blood from the right ventricle begins. Left ventricular ejection occurs between S_1 and S_2, which begins immediately after the T wave and is signaled by closure of the aortic valve, followed by closure of the pulmonic valve and opening of the tricuspid and mitral valves. S_3 occurs between the T and P wave on the ECG at the end of the rapid-filling phase of the ventricles, and S_4 begins at the peak of the P wave during vibrations of the atria.

heart surgery, any surgical procedure involving the heart, performed to correct acquired or congenital defects, to replace diseased valves, to open or bypass blocked vessels, or to graft a prosthesis or a transplant in place. Two major types of heart surgery are performed, closed and open. The closed technique is done through a small incision, without using the heart-lung machine. In the open technique the heart chambers are open and fully visible, and blood is detoured around the surgical field by the heart-lung machine. Preoperative care focuses on the correction of metabolic imbalances and cardiac and pulmonary ailments and on diagnostic and laboratory tests. General anesthesia is used, the chest cavity is opened, and the heart-lung machine is connected. Hypothermia may also be used to reduce the metabolic rate and the need of the tissues for oxygen. The heart is opened, and the defect is corrected. Postoperatively, constant observation is required in an intensive care unit for signs of hemorrhage, shock, fibrillation, arrhythmia, sudden chest pain, and pulmonary edema. The blood pressure, all pulses, respirations, and venous and pulmonary artery pressures are monitored. If the blood pressure is high enough to assure cerebral profusion, the head of the patient's bed is lifted to a semi-Fowler's position to encourage chest drainage and lung expansion. Oxygen is given via the endotracheal tube for 18 to 24 hours. The chest tube is cleared hourly to dislodge clots; urinary output and temperature are noted hourly; and intravenous infusions and blood transfusions are often given. Small doses of a narcotic will help to control pain and allow coughing and deep breathing. Antibiotics are given to prevent infection. The mortality rate is highest during the first 48 hours after surgery. Kinds of heart surgery include **Blalock-Taussig procedure, coronary bypass,** and **endarterectomy.** See also **arrhythmia, fibrillation, heart-lung machine, hypothermia, pulmonary edema.**

heart valve, one of the four structures within the heart that control the flow of blood by opening and closing with each heartbeat. The valves include two semilunar valves, the aortic and pulmonary, the mitral valve, and the tricuspid valve. The valves permit the flow of blood in only one direction, and any one of the valves may become defective permitting the backflow associated with heart murmurs. Also called **cardiac valve.** See also **heart, semilunar valve, tricuspid valve.**

heat cramp, any cramp in the arm, leg, or abdomen caused by depletion in the body of both water and salt because of heat exhaustion. It usually occurs after vigorous physical exertion in an extremely hot environment or under other conditions that cause profuse sweating and depletion of body fluids and electrolytes. Also called **cane-cutter's cramp, fireman's cramp, miner's cramp, stoker's cramp.** See also **heat exhaustion.**

heated nebulization, a method of inhalation therapy using a heating device with a nebulizer that produces a spray with a higher water content than that of a cold atomizer. The mist may be administered through a mask or in a tent. Croup in infancy is often treated with a heated nebulizer.

heat exhaustion, an abnormal condition characterized by weakness, vertigo, nausea, muscle cramps, and loss of consciousness, caused by depletion of body fluid and electrolytes resulting from exposure to intense heat or the inability to acclimatize to heat. Body temperature is near normal; blood pressure may drop but usually returns to normal as the person is placed in a recumbent position; the skin is cool, damp, and pale. The person usually recovers with rest and replacement of water and electrolytes. Compare **heat hyperpyrexia.** See also **heat cramp.**

heat hyperpyrexia, a severe and sometimes fatal condition resulting from the failure of the temperature regulating capacity of the body, caused by prolonged exposure to the sun or to high temperatures. Reduction or cessation of sweating is an early symptom. Body temperature of 105° F or higher, tachycardia, hot and dry skin, headache, confusion, unconsciousness, and convulsions may occur. Treatment includes cooling, sedation, and fluid replacement. Also called **heatstroke, siriasis, sunstroke.** See also **hyperpyrexia.** Compare **heat exhaustion.**

heat labile. See **thermolabile.**

heat rash, a finely papular or vesicular inflammation of the skin resulting from prolonged exposure to heat and high humidity. Tingling and prickling sensations are common. Prevention and treatment include cool, dry temperatures, ventilation, and absorbent powders. See also **miliaria.**

heatstroke. See **heat hyperpyrexia.**

heaves, **1.** a chronic respiratory disease of horses, similar to human pulmonary emphysema, characterized by wheezing, coughing, and dyspnea on exertion. The causes of the condition are unknown. **2.** *informal.* vomiting and retching.

heavy function, (in dentistry) an increase in the functional activities of the teeth.

heavy hydrogen. See **deuterium.**

heavy metal, a metallic element with a specific gravity five or more times that of water. The heavy metals are antimony, arsenic, bismuth, cadmium, cerium, chromium, cobalt, copper, gallium, gold, iron, lead, manganese, mercury, nickel, platinum, silver, tellurium, thallium, tin, uranium, vanadium, and zinc. Small amounts of many of these elements are common and necessary in the diet. Large amounts of any of them may cause poisoning.

heavy metal poisoning, poisoning caused by the ingestion, inhalation, or absorption of various toxic heavy metals. Kinds of heavy metal poisoning include **antimony poisoning, arsenic poisoning, cadmium poisoning, lead poisoning,** and **mercury poisoning.** See also **heavy metal.**

heavy vaginal bleeding. See **vaginal bleeding.**

hebephrenia, hebephrenic schizophrenia. See **disorganized schizophrenia.**

Heberden's node /hē′bərdənz/, an abnormal cartilaginous or bony enlargement of a distal interphalangeal joint of a finger, usually occurring in degenerative diseases of the joints. Compare **Bouchard's node.**

hebetude /heb′ito͞od′/, a state of dullness or lethargy, characteristic of some forms of schizophrenia.

heboid paranoia. See **paranoid schizophrenia.**

-hedonia, a combining form meaning '(condition of) pleasure, cheerfulness': *anhedonia, hyphedonia, parhedonia.*

-hedron, a combining form meaning a 'geometric figure with (specified) sides': *decahedron, octahedron, polyhedron.*

Hedulin, a trademark for an anticoagulant (phenindione).

heel, the posterior part of the foot, formed by the largest tarsal bone, the calcaneus.

heel-knee test, a method of assessing coordination of movements of the extremities. In the test the patient, lying prone, is asked to touch the knee of one leg with the heel of the other.

heel-shin test, a method of assessing coordination of movements of the extremities. In the test the patient, lying prone, is asked to pass the heel of one leg slowly down the shin of the other leg from the knee to the ankle.

HEENT, abbreviation for **head, eyes, ears, nose, and throat.**

Hegar's sign /hā′gärz/, a softening of the isthmus of the uterine cervix early in gestation. It is a probable sign of pregnancy.

height, the vertical measurement of a structure, organ, or other object from bottom to top, when it is placed or projected in an upright position.

height of contour, the greatest convexity of a tooth surface, viewed from a predetermined position.

Heimlich maneuver /hīm′lik/, an emergency procedure for dislodging a bolus of food or other obstruction from the trachea to prevent asphyxiation. The choking person is grasped from behind by the rescuer whose fist, thumb side in, is placed just below the victim's sternum with the other hand placed firmly over the fist. The rescuer then pulls the fist firmly and abruptly into the epigastrium forcing the obstruction up the trachea. If repeated attempts do not free the airway, an emergency tracheotomy may be necessary. See also **cardiopulmonary resuscitation.**

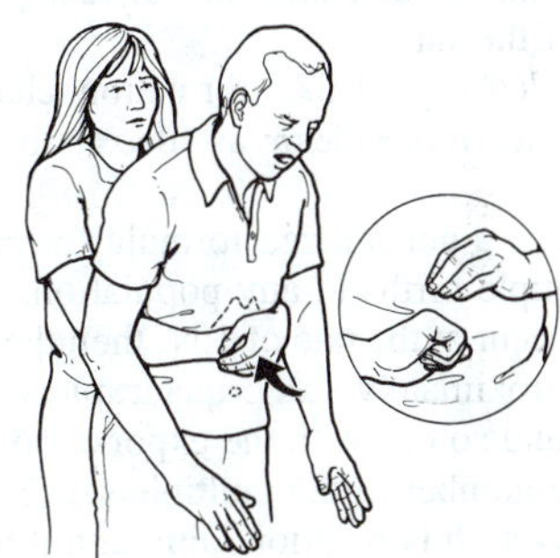

Heimlich maneuver

Heinz bodies /hīnts/, irregularly shaped bits of altered hemoglobin found in the red blood cells of persons who are hypersensitive to certain chemicals, as aniline, phenylhydrazine, and primaquine.

Helen, Sister (Helen Bowden), a nurse who received her education in England and became the first director of the newly formed Bellevue Hospital Training School for Nurses in New York, in 1873. Although she had not trained under Florence Nightingale, she set up the Bellevue school along Nightingale's principles. She was a member of the All Saints Sisterhood. After several years at Bellevue, having established one of the leading nursing schools in the United States, she went to South Africa.

Heliodorus' bandage. See **T bandage.**

helium (He), a colorless, odorless, gaseous element; the second lightest element after hydrogen. Its atomic number is 2; its atomic weight is 4. Helium is one of the rare or inert gases and does not usually combine with other elements. Most of the commercial helium in the world comes from natural gas reservoirs in Texas and Louisiana where it is recovered after natural gas has been liquefied. It is produced in nature by the decay of radioactive elements and is produced in the sun from hydrogen. It occurs in the atmosphere in the ratio of five parts per million. Helium is used industrially in arc welding, refining, and other processes. Because of its lightness and lack of flammability it is also used to lift airships and balloons. The main physiologic and medical uses of helium are in respiratory therapy and testing and the prevention of nitrogen narcosis and decompression sickness in hyperbaric environments. A mixture of 80% helium and 20% oxygen is commonly breathed by deep-sea divers to prevent gas emboli and by patients undergoing treatment to clear obstructed respiratory tracts. Problems associated with such uses involve the high velocity of acoustic transmission in helium and the high thermal conductivity of the gas. These characteristics produce voice distortions and hypothermia in persons who inhale it. Helium is one third as soluble in lipids as nitrogen, which accounts for its preferred use in hyperbaric atmospheres, as those associated with deep-sea diving. The low density of helium reduces the effort of breathing any gas mixture of which it is a component. Helium is used in pulmonary function testing to calculate the diffusing and residual capacities of the lungs.

helix, a coiled, spiral-like formation characteristic of many organic molecules, as deoxyribonucleic acid (DNA).

Hellin's law, a generalized formula for calculating the ratio of multiple births in any population, stating that if twin births occur at the rate of 1:N, then the rate of triplet births is approximately $1{:}N^2$, quadruplets $1{:}N^3$, quintuplets $1{:}N^4$, and so on, with the exponent of N being one less than the number in the multiple set. The constant N varies greatly with population, although it was originally set at 89 when the law was formulated. In general, twin births occur approximately once in every 80 pregnancies. Also called **Hellin-Zeleny law.**

helminth /hel′minth/, a worm, especially one of the pathogenic parasites of the division Metazoa fluke, including flukes, tapeworms, and roundworms.

-helminth, a combining form meaning 'worm': *nemathelminth, platyhelminth.*

helminthiasis /hel′minthī′əsis/, a parasitic infestation of the body by helminths that may be cutaneous, visceral, or intestinal. Ascariasis, bilharziasis, filariasis, hookworm, and trichinosis are common forms of the disease.

helper T cell. See **T cell.**

Helsinki accords, a declaration signed by the representatives of 35 member nations of the Conference on Security and Cooperation in Europe in Helsinki, Finland, on August 1, 1975. The declared goals of the nonbinding document comprised four principal aspects of European security: economic cooperation, humanitarian issues, contact between the East and West, and provision for a later follow-up conference (held in Belgrade in 1978). Follow-up conferences were planned in part to allow the member nations to monitor each other's performance on humanitarian issues, as the right to self-determination of all people and respect for the fundamental freedoms, including thought, conscience, and religion or belief, without regard to race, language, sex, or religion. The Helsinki accords grew from the precedent set by the judgments at the trials of the Nuremberg tribunals—that crimes against humanity are offenses subject to criminal prosecution. The principal and the practice of informed consent in health care grew from this precedent. Also called **Helsinki Declaration.** See also **Nuremberg tribunals.**

helvolic acid /helvol′ik/, an antibiotic, derived from the mold *Aspergillus fumigatus,* formerly used as an amebicide. Also called **fumagillin, fumigacin.**

hemadsorption /hē′madsôrp′shən, hem′-/, a process in which a substance or an agent, as certain viruses and bacilli, adheres to the surface of an erythrocyte. The process occurs naturally, or it may be induced for laboratory identification of bacteriologic specimens.

hemagglutination /hē′məglo͞o′tinā′shən, hem′-/, an antigen-antibody reaction resulting in the agglutination of red cells. See **ABO blood groups.**

hemagglutinin, a kind of antibody that agglutinates red blood cells. These substances are classified according to the source of cells agglutinated as **autologous** (from the same organism), **homologous** (from an organism of the same species), and **heterologous** (from an organism of a different species). Some hemagglutinins clump red cells together as they are suspended in 0.85% sodium chloride solution; others will not agglutinate red cells unless hydrophilic colloids are added or unless the red cells have been treated with a proteolytic enzyme.

hemangioblastoma /hēman′jē·ōblastō′mə/, *pl.* **hemangioblastomas, hemangioblastomata,** a brain tumor composed of a proliferation of capillaries and of disorganized clusters of capillary cells or angioblasts.

hemangioendothelioma /hēman′jē·ō·en′dōthē′lē·ō′mə/, *pl.* **hemangioendotheliomas, hemangioendotheliomata, 1.** also called **angioendothelioma.** a tumor, consisting of endothelial cells, that grows around an artery or a vein. The benign form is seen in children and is usually cured by local excision. It rarely becomes malignant. **2.** malignant hemangioendothelioma. See also **angiosarcoma.**

hemangioma /hēman′jē·ō′mə/, *pl.* **hemangiomas, hemangiomata,** a benign tumor consisting of a mass of blood vessels. Kinds of hemangiomas include **capillary hemangioma, cavernous hemangioma,** and **nevus flammeus.**

hemangioma simplex. See **capillary hemangioma.**

hemangiosarcoma. See **angiosarcoma.**

hematemesis /hē′mətem′əsis, hem′-/, vomiting of bright red blood, indicating rapid upper GI bleeding, commonly associated with esophageal varices or peptic ulcer. The rate and the source of bleeding are determined by endoscopic examination. Any blood found in the stomach is removed by nasogastric suction. Treatment requires replacement of blood by transfusion and administration of intravenous fluids for maintenance of fluid and electrolyte balance. Vasoconstrictors may sometimes be infused at the site of bleeding. Surgery may be necessary. The patient is usually very anxious and needs quiet, warmth, and reassurance. See also **gastrointestinal bleeding.**

hematochezia, the passage of red blood through the rectum. The cause is usually bleeding in the colon or rectum, but it can result from the loss of blood higher in the digestive tract, depending on the transit time. Blood passed from the stomach or small intestine generally loses its red coloration through enzymatic activity on the erythrocytes. Cancer, colitis, and ulcers are among causes of hematochezia. Compare **melena.**

hematocrit /himat′ōkrit/, a measure of the packed cell volume of red cells, expressed as a percentage of the total blood volume. The normal range is between 43% and 49% in men, and between 37% and 43% in women. See also **complete blood count, differential white blood cell count.**

hematogenic shock, a condition of shock caused by the loss of blood or plasma.

hematogenous /hēmətoj′ənəs/, originating or transported in the blood.

hematologist /hē′mətol′əjist, hem′-/, a medical specialist in the field of hematology.

hematology /hē′mətol′əjē, hem′-/, scientific medical study of blood and blood-forming tissues. **–hematologic, hematological,** *adj.*

hematoma /hē′mətō′mə, hem′-/, *pl.* **hematomas, hematomata,** a collection of extravasated blood trapped in the tissues of the skin or in an organ, resulting from trauma or incomplete hemostasis after surgery. Initially, there is frank bleeding into the space; if the space is limited, pressure slows and eventually stops the flow of blood. The blood clots, serum collects, the clot hardens, and the mass becomes palpable to the examiner and is often painful to the patient. A hematoma may be drained early in the process and bleeding arrested with pressure or, if necessary, with surgical ligation of the bleeding vessel. Considerable blood may be lost, and infection is a serious complication. Also called **blood blister.**

-hematoma, a combining form meaning a 'swelling containing blood': *cephalhematoma, episiohematoma, othematoma*.

hematomyelia, the appearance of frank blood in the fluid of the spinal cord.

hematopoiesis /hē′mətōpō•ē′sis, hem′-/, the normal formation and development of blood cells in the bone marrow. In severe anemia and other hematologic disorders, cells may be produced in organs outside the marrow (extramedullary hematopoiesis). See also **erythropoiesis. –hematopoietic,** *adj.*

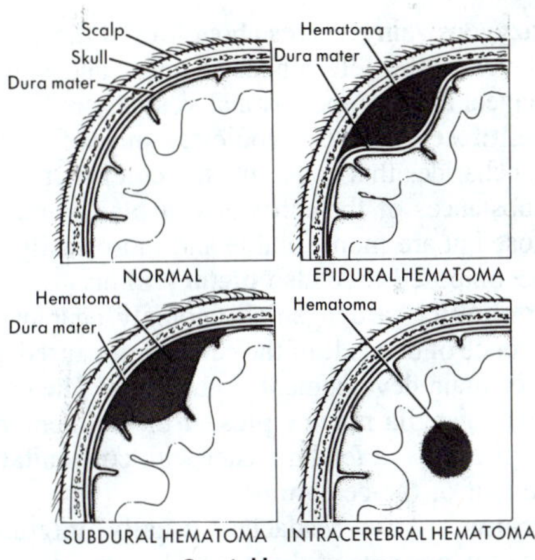

Cranial hematomas

hematoxylin-eosin, a stain commonly used to treat tissue sections on microsope slides.

hematuria /hē′mətŏŏr′ē•ə, hem′-/, abnormal presence of blood in the urine. Hematuria is symptomatic of many renal diseases and disorders of the genitourinary system. Microscopic examination of the urine, culture and sensitivity of the urine, and physical examination of the patient are usually performed. **–hematuric,** *adj.*

heme /hēm/, the pigmented, iron containing, nonprotein portion of the hemoglobin molecule. There are four heme groups in a hemoglobin molecule, each consisting of a cyclic structure of four pyrrole residues, called protoporphyrin, and an atom of iron in the center. Heme binds and carries oxygen in the red blood cells, releasing it to tissues that give off excess amounts of CO_2. See also **hemoglobin, porphobilinogen, protoporphyrin.**

hemeralopia /hem′ərəlō′pē•ə/, an abnormal visual condition in which bright light causes blurring of vision. Hemeralopia is an unpleasant side effect of certain anticonvulsant medications, including trimethadione, prescribed in treating children affected with petit mal epilepsy. Also called **day blindness, night sight. –hemeralopic,** *adj.*

-hemia. See **-emia.**

hemiacephalus, a fetal monster in which the brain and most of the cranium are lacking. See also **anencephaly.**

hemianesthesia, a loss of feeling on one side of the body.

hemianopia, defective vision or blindness in one half of the visual field.

hemiazygous vein /hem′ē•əzī′gəs/, one of the tributaries of the azygous vein of the thorax. It starts in the left ascending lumbar vein, enters the thorax through the left crus of the diaphragm, ascends on the left side of the vertebral column as high as the ninth thoracic vertebra, and passes dorsal to the aorta to enter the azygous. The hemiazygous vein receives about four of the caudal intercostal veins, the left subcostal vein, and some of the esophageal and the mediastinal veins.

hemicellulose /hem′ēsel′yo͞olōs/, any of a group of polysaccharides that constitute the chief part of the skeletal substances of the cell walls of plants and resemble cellulose but are more soluble and more easily extracted and decomposed. See also **dietary fiber.**

hemicephalia, a congenital anomaly characterized by the absence of one side of the cerebrum, caused by severe arrest of brain development in the fetus. The cerebellum and basal ganglia may be present in rudimentary form.

hemicephalus, a fetal monster with congenital absence of one half of the cerebrum.

hemicrania, **1.** a headache, usually migraine, that affects only one side of the head. **2.** a congenital anomaly characterized by the absence of one half of the skull in the fetus; incomplete anencephaly.

hemiectromelia, a congenital anomaly characterized by the incomplete development of the limbs on one side of the body. **–hemiectromelus,** *n.*

hemignathia /hem′ēnā′thē·ə/, **1.** a congenital anomaly characterized by incomplete development of the lower jaw on one side of the face. **2.** a condition of having only one jaw. **–hemignathus,** *n.*

hemihyperplasia, overdevelopment or excessive growth of one half of a specific organ or part or of all the organs and parts on one side of the body.

hemihypoplasia, partial or incomplete development of one half of a specific organ or part or of all the organs and parts on one side of the body.

hemikaryon /hem′ēker′ē·on/, a cell nucleus that contains the haploid number of chromosomes, or one half of the diploid number, as that of the gametes. Compare **amphikaryon. –hemikaryotic,** *adj.*

hemimelia, a developmental anomaly characterized by the absence or gross shortening of the lower portion of one or more of the limbs. The condition may involve either or both of the bones of the distal arm or leg and is designated according to whichever is absent or defective, as fibular, radial, tibial, or ulnar hemimelia. See also **ectromelia, phocomelia.**

hemipagus /hemip′əgəs/, conjoined symmetric twins who are united at the thorax.

hemiparesis, muscular weakness of one half of the body.

hemiplegia /hem′iplē′jə/, paralysis of one side of the body. Kinds of hemiplegia are **cerebral hemiplegia, facial hemiplegia, infantile hemiplegia,** and **spastic hemiplegia.** Also called **unilateral paralysis.** Compare **diplegia, paraplegia, quadriplegia. –hemiplegic,** *adj.*

hemisomus /hem′isō′məs/, a fetus or individual in which one side of the body is malformed, defective, or absent.

hemisphere, **1.** one half of a sphere or globe. **2.** the lateral half of the cerebrum or of the cerebellum. **–hemispherical,** *adj.*

hemiteras /hem′ēter′əs/, *pl.* **hemiterata,** any individual with a congenital malformation that is not so severe or disabling as to be classified as a monstrous or teratic condition. **–hemiteratic,** *adj.*

hemivertebra, an abnormal condition characterized by the congenital failure of a vertebra to develop completely, possibly caused by the complete failure of the growth center of one vertebral body. Usually one half of the vertebra involved is completely or partially developed and the other half is absent. One or more vertebrae may be involved, the different conditions producing varying degrees of balanced or unbalanced scoliosis. As a result of the developmental abnormality of the spine a wedge-shaped vertebra develops, and adjacent vertebral bodies expand to fit the deformity or tilt to accommodate wedge-shaped articulation. Hemivertebra may be classified according to the degree of developmental failure of involved vertebral growth centers. There may be involvement of two vertebral bodies in which growth centers on the same side fail to develop, resulting in moderate to severe unbalanced congenital scoliosis, or there may be involvement of two vertebral bodies in which growth centers fail to develop on opposite sides, creating balanced congenital scoliosis. Singular hemivertebra may pose few if any signs and symptoms. Depending on the degree of congenital scoliosis involved, any associated deformity may become more apparent with growth. Other types of hemivertebra, especially those involving unbalanced congenital scoliosis, usually progress markedly with growth and have a relatively poor prognosis unless early spinal fusion prevents further spinal curvature. No treatment may be required for the form of the condition associated with balanced congenital scoliosis.

hemizygote, an individual, organism, or cell that has only one of a pair of genes for a specific characteristic. Such traits are expressed regardless of whether the genes transmitting them are dominant or recessive, as with the X-linked genes on the single X chromosome in males, which have no alleles on the Y chromosome. **–hemizygosity,** *n.*, **hemizygous, hemizygotic,** *adj.*

hemoblastic leukemia. See **stem cell leukemia.**

hemochromatosis /hē′mōkrō′mətō′sis, hem′-/, a rare disease of iron metabolism, characterized pathologically by excess iron deposits throughout the body. Hepatomegaly, skin pigmentation, diabetes mellitus, and cardiac failure may occur. The disease most often develops in men over 40 years of age and as a complication of some hemolytic anemias requiring multiple blood transfusions. Compare **hemosiderosis.** See also **iron metabolism, siderosis, thalassemia.**

hemoconcentration, an increase in the number of red blood cells resulting either from a decrease in plasma volume or increased production of erythrocytes.

hemocytoblastic leukemia. See **stem cell leukemia.**

hemodialysis /hē′mōdī·al′isis, hem′-/, a procedure in which impurities or wastes are removed from the blood, used in treating renal insufficiency and various toxic conditions. The patient's blood is shunted from the body through a machine for diffusion and ultrafiltration and then returned to the patient's circulation. Hemodialysis requires access to the patient's bloodstream, a mechanism for the transport of the blood to and from the dialyzer, and a dialyzer. See also **arteriovenous fistula, external shunt.**

■ METHOD: Access may be achieved by an external shunt or an arteriovenous fistula. The external shunt is constructed by inserting two cannulas through the skin into a large vein and a large artery. When dialysis is not being performed, the cannulas are joined, allowing the blood to flow from artery to vein. When dialysis is being performed, the cannulas are separated, allowing the arterial blood to flow to the dialyzer and the dialyzed blood to return from the dialyzer to the circulation through the cannula in the vein. An arteriovenous fistula is created by the anastomosis of a large vein to an artery. Large-bore needles are threaded into superficial vessels enlarged by the increased flow caused by the fistula. Various dialyzers may be used. The procedure takes from 3 to 8 hours and may be necessary daily in acute situations or 2 or 3 times a week in chronic renal failure.

■ NURSING ORDERS: A decrease in the flow of blood through the shunt may result in clotting; therefore, any factor that may result in a slowing of the flow is to be avoided. Some of these factors are systemic hypotension, infection of the shunt or fistula, compression of the shunt or fistula, thrombophlebitis, and prolonged inflation of a blood pressure cuff. Infection is avoided in the area around an external shunt by placing a sterile dressing over the shunt and changing the dressing daily. Before the procedure is begun, the patient is told how long the procedure will take, what pain or discomfort may be expected, what will be felt afterward, what food or activity will be allowed during the procedure, and whether or not family or friends may be present during treatment. Headache and nausea are common, especially during the procedure and for a few hours afterward. The patient usually feels the best on the day after hemodialysis. Rest, an antiemetic, and a mild analgesic may make the procedure more comfortable. Most patients need emotional support and some physical assistance during hemodialysis. The physical status of the patient is monitored frequently throughout; blood pressure, pulse, and blood tests for electrolyte and acid-base balance are performed. Normal saline may be administered to counteract hypotension that occurs as a result of a rapid removal of fluid from the intravascular compartment. The patient is weighed before and after the treatment to determine the amount of fluid lost during the procedure. An anticoagulant is usually given to prevent coagulation of the blood in the dialyzer, cannulas, or catheters; to prevent hemorrhage, protamine sulfate may be given after the procedure to reverse the effect of the anticoagulant. Any treatment that causes tissue trauma, as dental extraction, venipuncture, or intramuscular injection, is not recommended during or immediately after dialysis.

■ OUTCOME CRITERIA: Infection and clotting of the shunt or erosion of the skin around the shunt are frequent complications of the external shunt; therefore, the method using an arteriovenous fistula is more common. The discomfort before, during, and just after dialysis, the prolonged time of relative immobility during the procedure, and the dietary restrictions necessary in renal insufficiency all place considerable stress on the patient. Adjustments in the patterns of daily life are necessary and require the assistance of professionals with experience and training in the field.

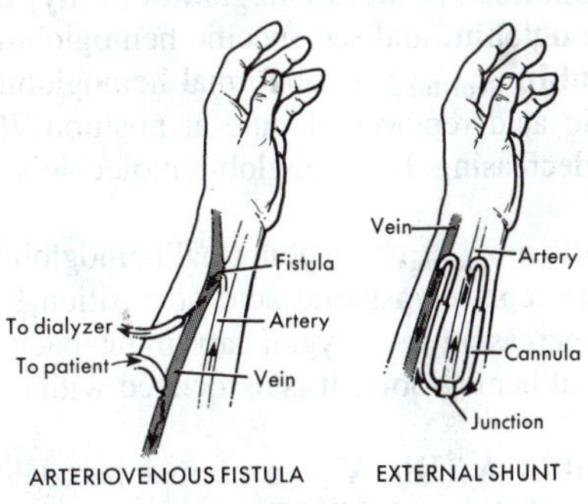

Hemodialysis

hemodialysis technician, a registered nurse who has received special training in the operation of hemodialysis equipment and treatment of patients with kidney disorders.

hemodialyzer. See **dialyzer.**

hemodynamics, the study of factors affecting the force and flow of circulating blood.

Hemofil, a trademark for human antihemophilic factor.

hemoglobin (Hb) /hē′məglō′bən/, a complex protein-iron compound in the blood that carries oxygen to the cells from the lungs and carbon dioxide away from the cells to the lungs. Each erythrocyte contains 200 to 300 molecules of hemoglobin, each molecule of hemoglobin contains several molecules of heme, and each molecule of heme can carry one molecule of oxygen. A hemoglobin molecule contains four globin polypeptide chains, designated in adults as the alpha (α), beta (β), gamma (γ), and delta (δ) chains. Each polypeptide chain is composed of several hundred amino acids, and the absence, replacement, or addition of only one amino acid modifies the properties of the hemoglobin. Different kinds of hemoglobin are identified by their specific combination of polypeptide chains, the number of chains of the different types in the molecule indicated by subscript numerals and superscript capital letters. More than 100 hemoglobins with different electrophoretic mobilities and characteristics have been identified and classified, as S, C, D, E, G, H, I, J, K, L, M, N, and O. Improved research methods may reveal many more. New hemoglobins are named for the laboratory, town, or hospital where they are discovered, as hemoglobin $_{\text{Seattle}}$ and hemoglobin $_{\text{Yakima}}$.

The normal concentrations of hemoglobin in the blood are 12 to 16 g/dl in women and 13.5 to 18 g/dl in men. In an atmosphere of high oxygen concentration, as in the lungs, hemoglobin binds with oxygen to form oxyhemoglobin. In an atmosphere of low oxygen concentration, as in the peripheral tissues of the body, oxygen is replaced by carbon dioxide to form carboxyhemoglobin. Hemoglobin releases the carboxyhemoglobin in the lungs for excretion and picks up more oxygen for transport to the cells. See also **carboxyhemoglobin, complete blood count, differential white blood cell count, erythrocyte, erythropoiesis, heme, hemoglobinopathy, hemolysin, oxyhemoglobin,** and see specific hemoglobins.

hemoglobin $_{Seattle}$, an abnormal hemoglobin in which glutamic acid replaces alanine at position 76 of the β chain, decreasing the hemoglobin molecule's affinity for oxygen.

hemoglobin $_{Yakima}$, an abnormal hemoglobin in which histadine replaces aspartic acid at position 99 in the β chain, increasing the oxygen carrying capacity over that of normal hemoglobin. It is associated with erythrocytosis.

hemoglobin A (Hb A), a normal hemoglobin. Also called **adult hemoglobin.** Compare **hemoglobin F.** See also **hemoglobinopathy, hemoglobin variant.**

hemoglobin A_2 (Hb A_2), a normal hemoglobin that occurs in small amounts in adults, characterized by the substitution of δ chains for β chains. Its concentration in the blood increases in various diseases. It normally constitutes 1.5% to 3.5% of the total hemoglobin.

hemoglobin C, an abnormal type of hemoglobin characterized by the substitution of lysine for glutamic acid at position 6 of the β chain of the hemoglobin molecule. Hemoglobin C moves slowly and reduces the plasticity of the erythrocytes.

hemoglobin C (Hb C) disease, a genetic blood disorder characterized by a moderate, chronic hemolytic anemia and associated with the presence of hemoglobin C, an abnormal form of the red cell pigment. Hemoglobin C is inherited as an autosomal codominant gene. In the heterozygous form, hemoglobin C trait, there is no anemia or increased blood hemolysis. Target cells may be seen in microscopic examination of a blood smear. Abnormal hemoglobin C is accompanied by an approximately equal amount of its normal counterpart, hemoglobin A. See also **hemoglobin C, hemoglobin S-C disease, hemoglobin variant.**

hemoglobin electrophoresis, a test to identify various abnormal hemoglobins in the blood, including certain genetic disorders, as sickle cell anemia.

hemoglobinemia /hē′mōglō′binē′mē·ə, hem′-/, presence of free hemoglobin in the blood plasma.

hemoglobin F (Hb F), the normal hemoglobin of the fetus, most of which is broken down in the first days after birth and replaced by hemoglobin A. It has an increased capacity to carry oxygen and is present in increased amounts in some pathologic conditions, including sickle cell anemia, aplastic anemia, and leukemia. Small amounts are produced throughout life.

hemoglobinopathy /hē′mōglō′binop′əthē, hem′-/, any of a group of inherited disorders characterized by variation of the structure of the hemoglobin molecule. The alteration appears as the substitution of one or more amino acids in the globin portion of the molecule at selected positions in the two alpha or two beta polypeptide chains. Although more than 100 variants have been described and identified, only hemoglobins S, C, and D are seen regularly. The abnormality may occur in the heterozygous or the homozygous form. In the heterozygous form, the normal adult pigment, hemoglobin A, and its variant both appear in the red cell; there may be little or no clinical manifestation of disease. In the homozygous form, only the variant hemoglobin is present, and the characteristic symptoms of that hemoglobinopathy appear. Mixed heterozygous forms are also known to occur. These are characterized by the absence of the normal hemoglobin A and the presence of two or three hemoglobin variants. Kinds of hemoglobinopathies include **hemoglobin C disease, hemoglobin S-C disease,** and **sickle cell anemia.** Compare **thalassemia.** See also **hemoglobin, hemoglobin A, sickle cell thalassemia, sickle cell trait.**

hemoglobin S (Hb S), an abnormal type of hemoglobin, characterized by the substitution of the amino acid valine for glutamic acid in the β chain of the hemoglobin molecule. It moves more slowly and is much less soluble than hemoglobin A. As the abnormal molecules become deoxygenated, because of decreased oxygen tension in the peripheral circulation, they tend to become sickle-shaped, to move slowly, to clump together, and to hemolyze. If the proportion of Hb S to Hb A is large, as in sickle cell anemia, local thrombosis and infarction may occur. See also **hemoglobin variant, sickle cell anemia, sickle cell crisis, sickle cell trait.**

hemoglobin S-C (Hb S-C) disease, a genetic blood disorder in which two different abnormal alleles, one for hemoglobin S and one for hemoglobin C, are inherited. The disorder is characterized by a clinical course considerably less severe than sickle cell anemia despite the absence of normal hemoglobin. See also **hemoglobin C disease, sickle cell thalassemia.**

hemoglobinuria, an abnormal presence in the urine of hemoglobin that is unattached to red blood cells. Hemoglobinuria can result from various autoimmune diseases or episodic hemolytic disorders. It can be diagnosed using a dipstick reagent that is sensitive to free hemoglobin. Kinds of hemoglobinuria include **cold hemoglobinuria, march hemoglobinuria,** and **nocturnal hemoglobinuria.**

hemoglobin variant, any type of hemoglobin other than hemoglobin A. All variants are characterized by an alteration in the sequence of amino acids in the polypeptide chains of globin contained in the hemoglobin molecule. These variations are genetically determined and, depending on the kind and extent of change, result in altered physical and chemical function of the red blood cells. See also **hemoglobin C, hemoglobinopathy, hemoglobin S, sickle cell thalassimia.**

hemogram, a written or graphic record of a differential blood count that emphasizes the size, shape, special characteristics, and numbers of the solid components of the blood. See also **complete blood count.**

hemolysin /himol′əsin/, any one of the numerous substances that lyse or dissolve red blood cells. Hemolysins are produced by strains of many kinds of bacteria, including some of the staphylococci and streptococci. They are also contained in venoms and in certain vegetables. Bacterial hemolysins are divided into those that are filterable and those that cluster around the bacterial colony on a culture medium containing red blood cells. Hemolysins appear to aid the invasive power of bacteria. See also **hemoglobin, hemolysis.**

hemolysis /himol′isis/, the breakdown of red blood cells and the release of hemoglobin. It occurs normally at the end of the life span of a red cell, but it may occur under a variety of other circumstances, including certain antigen-antibody reactions, metabolic abnormalities of the red cell that significantly shorten its life span, and mechanic trauma, as in hemodialysis, cardiac prosthesis, or exposure to snake venoms. Dilution of the blood by intravenous administration of excessive amounts of hypotonic solutions, which cause progressive swelling and eventual rupture of the erythrocyte, also results in hemolysis. See also **hemolysin, hemolytic anemia, transfusion reaction. –hemolytic,** *adj.*

hemolytic anemia, a disorder characterized by the premature destruction of red blood cells. Anemia may be minimal or absent, reflecting the ability of the bone marrow to increase production of red blood cells. The condition may occur in association with some infectious diseases, with certain inherited red cell disorders, or as a response to drugs or other toxic agents. Compare **aplastic anemia, congenital nonspherocytic hemolytic anemia, iron deficiency anemia, myelophthisic anemia, nonspherocytic anemia.** See also **anemia, hemolysis, spherocytosis.**

hemolytic jaundice, a yellowish discoloration of the skin caused by a breakdown of red blood cells, resulting in excess production of bilirubin.

hemolytic uremia syndrome, a rare kidney disorder marked by renal failure, microangiopathic hemolytic anemia, and platelet deficiency. The syndrome, the cause of which is unknown, usually occurs in infancy.

hemopericardium, an accumulation of blood within the pericardial sac surrounding the heart.

hemoperitoneum, the presence of extravasated blood in the peritoneal cavity.

hemophilia /hē′mōfē′lyə, hem′-/, a group of hereditary bleeding disorders in which there is a deficiency of one of the factors necessary for coagulation of the blood. The two most common forms of the disorder, but clinically indistinguishable entities, are hemophilia A and hemophilia B. Hemophilia A is the result of a deficiency or absence of antihemophilic factor VIII, a trace protein that acts to accelerate the conversion of prothrombin to thrombin through the formation of thromboplastin. Hemophilia B (Christmas disease) represents a deficiency of plasma thromboplastin component, another plasma protein active in the formation of thromboplastin. The clinical severity of the disorder varies markedly with the extent of the deficiency. Greater than usual loss of blood during dental procedures, epistaxis, hematoma, and hemarthrosis are common problems in hemophilia. Severe internal hemorrhage and hematuria are less common. The primary objective of nursing care is to prevent bleeding and to make the environment as safe as possible. The nurse teaches measures for controlling bleeding and for limiting local joint damage and ways that the patient can be physically active without danger of injury. The nurse also provides assistance in coping with the disorder, refers the parents for genetic counseling and to parent discussion groups, and implements home care. See **von Willebrand's disease,** and see specific blood factors. **–hemophiliac,** *n.,* **hemophilic,** *adj.*

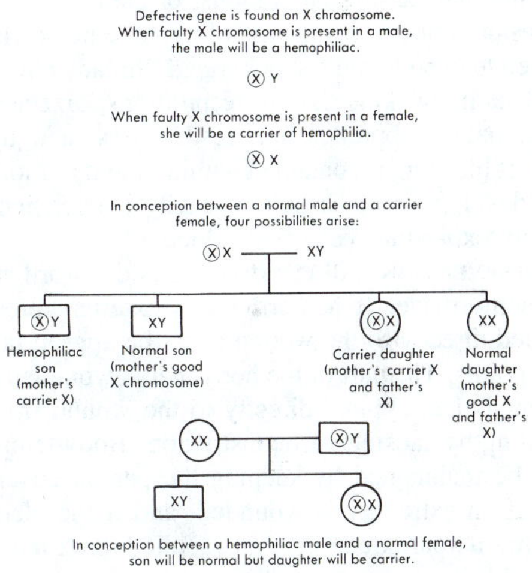

Hemophilia inheritance pattern

hemophilia A, a hereditary blood disorder, transmitted as an X-linked recessive trait, caused by a deficiency of coagulation factor VIII. Hemophilia A is considered the classic type of hemophilia in contrast to hemophilia B and hemophilia C, which may be less severe. See also **coagulation factor, hemophilia.**

hemophilia B, a hereditary blood disorder, transmitted as an X-linked recessive trait, caused by a deficiency of factor IX, the plasma thromboplastin component. The condition is clinically similar to but less severe than hemophilia A. Also called **Christmas disease.** See **coagulation factor, hemophilia.**

hemophilia C, a hereditary blood disorder, transmitted as an X-linked recessive trait, caused by a deficiency of factor XI, the plasma thromboplastin antecedent. The condition is clinically similar to but may be less severe than hemophilia A. Also called **Rosenthal's syndrome.** See also **coagulation factor, hemophilia.**

hemopoietic /hē′mōpō•et′ik, hem′-/, related to the process of formation and development of the various types of blood cells.

hemoptysis /himop′tisis/, coughing up of blood from the respiratory tract. Blood-streaked sputum often occurs in minor upper respiratory infections or in bronchitis. More profuse bleeding may indicate *Aspergillus* infection, lung abcess, tuberculosis, or bronchogenic carcinoma. X-ray examination, endoscopy, and bronchoscopy are often used to diagnose hemoptysis. Treatment of significant hemoptysis includes monitoring the patient for signs of shock, preventing asphyxiation, and localizing and stopping the bleeding. Antibiotics and antitussives may be given. The frightened patient may be calmed by quiet and warmth; sedatives and tranquilizers are not given because of their tendency to depress respiration. Compare **hematemesis.**

hemorrhage, a loss of a large amount of blood in a short period of time, either externally or internally. Hemorrhage may be arterial, venous, or capillary.

■ OBSERVATIONS: Symptoms of massive hemorrhage are related to hypovolemic shock: rapid, thready pulse; thirst; cold, clammy skin; sighing respirations; dizziness; syncope; pallor; apprehension; restlessness; and hypotension. If bleeding is contained within a cavity or joint, pain will develop as the capsule or cavity is stretched by the rapidly expanding volume of blood.

■ INTERVENTION: All effort is directed toward stopping the hemorrhage. If hemorrhage is external, pressure is applied directly to the wound or to the appropriate pressure points. The part of the body that is wounded may be elevated. Ice, applied directly to the wound, may slow bleeding by causing vasoconstriction. Body temperature may be maintained by keeping the person covered and flat. If an extremity is wounded, and if the bleeding is severe, a tourniquet may be applied proximal to the wound.

■ NURSING CONSIDERATIONS: A tourniquet is not applied if there is any other way to stanch the flow, because the risk is great that the limb will not survive the hypoxia induced by obstruction of the supply of blood. The tourniquet is not removed until surgical repair of the wound is possible. Internal bleeding requires prompt medical intervention. The patient is kept warm and quiet. **–hemorrhagic,** *adj.*

hemorrhagic diathesis, an inherited predisposition to any one of a number of abnormalities characterized by excessive bleeding. See also **Fanconi's syndrome, hemophilia, von Willebrand's disease.**

hemorrhagic disease of newborn, a bleeding disorder of neonates that is usually caused by a deficiency of vitamin K.

hemorrhagic familial angiomatosis. See **Osler-Weber-Rendu disease.**

hemorrhagic fever, an arbovirus infection, characterized by fever, chills, headache, malaise, and respiratory or GI symptoms, followed by capillary hemorrhages, and, in severe infection, oliguria, kidney failure, hypotension, and, possibly, death. Many forms of the disease occur in specific geographic areas. Some kinds of hemorrhagic fever are **Argentine hemorrhagic fever, dengue fever,** and **Far Eastern hemorrhagic fever.**

hemorrhagic gastritis, a form of acute gastritis usually caused by a toxic agent, as alcohol, aspirin or other drugs, or bacterial toxins that irritate the lining of the stomach. If bleeding is significant, vasoconstrictors and ice water lavage of the stomach may be necessary. Nausea, vomiting, and epigastric distress may persist after the irritant is removed. Treatment is symptomatic; the nurse usually includes identification of the irritant and dietary counseling for a patient with hemorrhagic gastritis.

hemorrhagic lung. See **congestive atelectasis.**

hemorrhagic scurvy. See **infantile scurvy.**

hemorrhagic shock, a state of physical collapse and prostration associated with the sudden and rapid loss of significant amounts of blood. Severe traumatic injuries often cause such blood losses, which, in turn, produce low blood pressure in affected individuals. Death occurs within a relatively short time unless transfusion quickly restores normal blood volume. Hemorrhagic shock often accompanies secondary shock. Compare **primary shock.**

hemorrhoid, a varicosity in the lower rectum or anus caused by congestion in the veins of the hemorrhoidal plexus.

■ OBSERVATIONS: Internal hemorrhoids originate above the internal sphincter of the anus. If they become large enough to protude from the anus, they become constricted and painful. Small internal hemorrhoids may bleed with defecation. External hemorrhoids appear outside the anal sphincter. They are usually not painful, and bleeding does not occur unless a hemorrhoidal vein ruptures or thromboses.

■ INTERVENTION: Treatment includes local application of a topical medication to lubricate, anesthetize, and shrink the hemorrhoid; sitz baths and cold or hot compresses are also soothing. The hemorrhoids may require sclerosing by injection, ligation, or excision by a surgical procedure. Ligation is increasingly the preferred treatment: It is simple, effective, and does not require anesthesia. The hemorrhoid is grasped with a forceps, and a rubber band is slipped over the varicosity, causing tissue necrosis and sloughing of the hemorrhoid, usually within 1 week.

■ NURSING CONSIDERATIONS: Straining to defecate, constipation, and prolonged sitting contribute to the development of hemorrhoids. The client is counseled in ways to avoid these predisposing factors. Because pregnancy is associated with an increased incidence of hemorrhoids, the pregnant woman, in particular, is advised to avoid constipation.

hemosiderin /hē′mōsid′ərin/, an iron-rich pigment that is a product of red cell hemolysis. Iron is often stored in this form.

hemosiderosis /hē′mōsid′ərō′sis, hem′-/, an increased deposition of iron in a variety of tissues, usually in the form of hemosiderin, and usually without tissue damage. It is often associated with diseases involving chronic, extensive destruction of red blood cells, as thalassemia major. Compare **hemochromatosis, sideroblastic anemia.** See also **ferritin, iron transport, siderosis, thalassemia, transferrin.**

hemostasis /himos′təsis, hē′məstā′sis/, the termination of bleeding by mechanic or chemical means or by the complex coagulation process of the body, consisting of vasoconstriction, platelet aggregation, and thrombin and fibrin synthesis. Compare **blood clotting.** See also **platelet, thrombus, vasoconstriction.**

hemostat. See **Halsted's forceps.**

hemostatic, of or pertaining to a procedure, device, or substance that arrests the flow of blood. Direct pressure, tourniquets, and surgical clamps are mechanic hemostatic measures. Cold applications are hemostatic and include the use of an ice bag on the abdomen to halt uterine bleeding and irrigation of the stomach with an iced solution to check gastric bleeding. Gelatin sponges, solutions of thrombin, and microfibrillar collagen, which causes the aggregation of platelets and the formation of clots, are used to arrest bleeding in surgical procedures. Aminocaproic acid is administered orally or intravenously in the treatment of excessive bleeding caused by systemic hyperfibrinolysis. Phytonadione (vitamin K_1) is used for the prevention and treatment of hemorrhagic disease in newborn infants and for the treatment of prothrombin deficiency induced by anticoagulants or other drugs.

hemostatic forceps. See **artery forceps.**

hemothorax /hē′mōthôr′aks, hem′-/, an accumulation of blood and fluid in the pleural cavity, between the parietal and visceral pleura, usually the result of trauma. Hemothorax may also be caused by the rupture of small blood vessels as a result of inflammation from pneumonia, tuberculosis, or tumors. Shock from hemorrhage, pain, and respiratory failure follows if emergency care is not available.

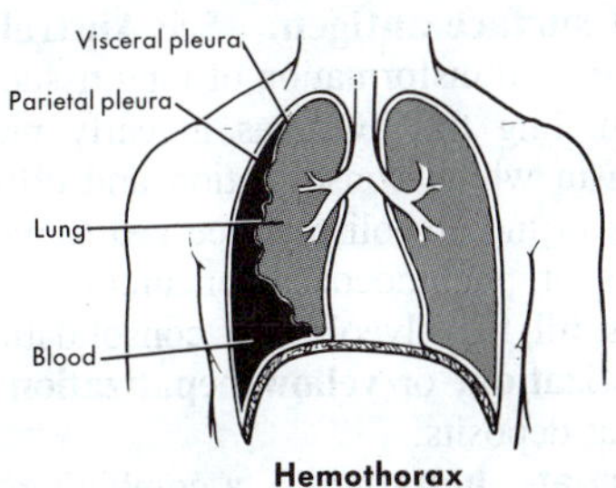

Hemothorax

hemotroph /hē′mətrof/, the total nutritive substances supplied to the embryo from the maternal circulation after the development of the placenta. Also spelled **hemotrophe.** Also called **hemotrophic nutrition.** Compare **embryotroph.** –**hemotrophic,** *adj.*

Henderson-Hasselbalch equation, the relationship between pH, the pK_a of a buffer system, and the ratio of the conjugate base and a weak acid.

Henderson, Virginia, a nursing theorist who introduced a holistic approach to nursing in 1966. It is based on the concepts that the body and mind are inseparable, no two individuals are alike, and the role of nursing is independent of the functions of the physician. The Henderson theory proposes that there are 14 components of basic nursing care that contribute to the health of a patient. The components relate to: (1) breathing, (2) eating and drinking, (3) elimination, (4) movement and posture, (5) sleep and rest, (6) clothing, (7) maintenance of body temperature, (8) cleaning and grooming the body, (9) avoiding environmental dangers and injury, (10) communication, (11) worship, (12) work, (13) play and recreation, and (14) learning and discovery.

Henle's fissure /hen′lēz/, one of many patches of connective tissue between the muscle fibers of the heart.

Henle's loop, a U-shaped portion of the renal tubule.

Henoch-Schönlein purpura /hen′ôkhshœn′līn/, a self-limited hypersensitivity vasculitis, chiefly of children, characterized by purpuric skin lesions that appear predominantly on the lower abdomen, buttocks, and legs,and usually associated with pain in the knees and ankles. Other joint involvement, GI bleeding, and hematuria are also common findings. The disease lasts up to 6 weeks and has no sequelae if renal involvement is not severe. Immunosuppressive drugs, as corticosteroids, may help the nephropathy. Also called **anaphylactoid purpura, Schönlein-Henoch purpura.**

Henry's law, (in physics) a law stating that the solubility of a gas in a liquid is proportional to the pressure of the gas if the temperature is constant and if the gas does not chemically react with the liquid.

Hensen's knot, Hensen's node. See **primitive node.**

hen worker's lung. See **pigeon breeder's lung.**

heparin /hep′ərin/, a naturally occurring mucopolysaccharide that acts in the body as an antithrombin factor to prevent intravascular clotting. It is produced by basophils and mast cells, which are found in large numbers in the connective tissue surrounding capillaries, particularly in the lungs and liver. In the form of its sodium salt, heparin is used therapeutically as an anticoagulant. See also **heparin sodium.**

heparin rebound, the phenomenon of reactivation of heparin effect occurring from 5 minutes to 5 hours after neutralization with protamine sulfate.

heparin sodium, an anticoagulant.

■ INDICATIONS: It is prescribed in the treatment and prophylaxis of a variety of thromboembolic disorders.

■ CONTRAINDICATIONS: Known hypersensitivity to this drug prohibits its use. It is given only when frequent monitoring of the coagulation status of the patient's blood is possible.

■ ADVERSE EFFECTS: The most serious adverse reaction is hemorrhage. Vasospastic disorders may occur.

hepat-. See **hepato-.**

-hepatia, a combining form meaning '(condition of the) liver or its functioning': *anhepatia, dyshepatia, hypohepatia.*

hepatic /hipat′ik/, of or pertaining to the liver.

hepatic adenoma, a rapidly growing liver tumor that may become very large and may rupture, causing a lethal internal hemorrhage. It is sometimes called a ''pill tumor'' because of its frequent association with the use of oral contraceptives.

hepatic amebiasis, enlargement and tenderness of the liver that often occurs in association with amebic dysentery. The inflammation results from infection with *Entamoeba histolytica.* See also **amebiasis, amebic dysentery, *Entamoeba histolytica.***

hepatic coma, a neuropsychiatric manifestation of extensive liver damage caused by chronic or acute liver disease. Either endogenous or exogenous waste toxic to the brain is not neutralized in the liver before being shunted back into the peripheral circulation of the blood, or substances required for cerebral function are not synthesized in the liver and, therefore, are not available to the brain. The condition is characterized by variable consciousness, lethargy, stupor, and coma; a tremor of the hands, personality change, memory loss, hyperreflexia, and hyperventilation. Respiratory alkalosis, mania convulsions, and death may occur. The outcome varies according to the pathogenesis of the condition and the treatment. Treatment in most cases includes cleansing enemas, low-protein diet, parenteral hydration with a balanced electrolyte solution, and specific treatment for the underlying cause. Also called **portal-systemic encephalopathy.** See also **cirrhosis, hepatitis.**

hepatic cord, a mass of cells, arranged in irregular radiating columns and plates, spreading outward from the central vein of the hepatic lobule. The cells are many-sided and contain one or, sometimes, two distinct nuclei. Many such cords join to form the parenchyma of the lobule. Each cell usually contains granules, some of which are protoplasmic whereas others consist of glycogen, fat, or an iron compound. Also called **hepatic cells.**

hepatic fistula, an abnormal passage from the liver to another organ or body structure.

hepatic node, a node in one of three groups of lymph glands associated with the abdominal and the pelvic viscera supplied by branches of the celiac artery. The hepatic nodes are divided into the hepatic and subpyloric groups. The hepatic group, on the stem of the hepatic artery, extends along the common bile duct, between the two layers of the lesser omentum, as far as the porta hepatis. The subpyloric group comprises about five nodes closely relating to the division of the gastroduodenal artery. Both groups receive afferents from the stomach, the duodenum, the liver, the gallbladder, and the pancreas. Their efferents join the celiac set of preaortic nodes. Compare **gastric node, pancreaticolienal node.**

hepatico-. See **hepato-.**

hepatic porphyria. See **porphyria.**

hepatic vein catheterization, the introduction of a long, fine catheter into a hepatic venule for the purpose of recording intrahepatic venous pressure. The catheter is inserted through a vein in the arm and is passed through the right atrium, the inferior vena cava, and hepatic vein into the small hepatic vessel.

hepatin. See **glycogen.**

hepatitis /hep′ətī′tis/, an inflammatory condition of the liver, characterized by jaundice, hepatomegaly, anorexia, abdominal and gastric discomfort, abnormal liver function, clay-colored stools, and dark urine. The condition may be caused by bacterial or viral infection, parasitic infestation, alcohol, drugs, toxins, or transfusion of incompatible blood. It may be mild and brief or severe, fulminant, and life-threatening. The liver usually is able to regenerate its tissue, but severe hepatitis may lead to cirrhosis and chronic liver dysfunction. Compare **anicteric hepatitis.** See also **viral hepatitis.**

hepatitis A, a form of infectious viral hepatitis caused by the hepatitis A virus, characterized by slow onset of signs and symptoms. The virus may be spread by direct contact or through fecal-contaminated food or water. The infection most often occurs in young adults and is usually followed by complete recovery. Also called **acute infective hepatitis.** See **viral hepatitis.**

hepatitis B, a form of viral hepatitis caused by the hepatitis B virus, characterized by rapid onset of acute symptoms and signs. The virus is transmitted in contaminated serum in blood transfusion or by the use of contaminated needles and instruments. The infection may be severe and result in prolonged illness, destruction of liver cells, cirrhosis, or death. Also called **serum hepatitis.** See **viral hepatitis.**

hepatitis B immune globulin (HBIG), a passive immunizing agent.

■ INDICATION: It is prescribed for postexposure prophylaxis against infection by the hepatitis B virus.

■ CONTRAINDICATIONS: Known hypersensitivity to the drug or to gamma globulin prohibits its use.

■ ADVERSE EFFECTS: Among the most serious adverse reactions are severe hypersensitivity reactions. Pain and inflammation at the site of injection also may occur.

hepatitis B surface antigen. See **Australia antigen.**

hepatization, transformation of lung tissue into a solid mass resembling the liver, as in early pneumococcal pneumonia in which consolidation and effusion of red blood cells in the alveoli produce **red hepatization.** In later stages of pneumococcal pneumonia, when white blood cells fill the alveoli, the consolidation becomes **gray hepatization,** or **yellow hepatization** when infiltrated by fat deposits.

hepato-, hepat-, hepatico-, a combining form meaning 'pertaining to the liver': *hepatobiliary, hepatocarcinogenic, hepatocellular.*

hepatocarcinoma, hepatocellular carcinoma. See **malignant hepatoma.**

hepatocyte, a parenchymal liver cell that performs all the functions ascribed to the liver.

hepatoduodenal ligament /hep′ətōdōō•ədē′nəl, -dōō•od′inəl/, the portion of the lesser omentum between the liver and the duodenum, containing the hepatic artery, the common bile duct, the portal vein, lymphatics, and the hepatic plexus of nerves. These structures are enclosed within a fibrous capsule between the two layers of the ligament. Compare **hepatogastric ligament.**

hepatogastric ligament /hep′ətōgas′trik/, the portion of the lesser omentum between the liver and the stomach. Compare **hepatoduodenal ligament.**

hepatojugular reflux /hep′ətōjug′yōōlər/, an increase in jugular venous pressure when pressure is applied for 30 to 60 seconds over the abdomen, suggestive of right-sided heart failure.

hepatolenticular degeneration /həpat′ōlentik′yōōlər/, an abnormal condition associated with defective copper metabolism in the body, characterized by decreased serum ceruloplasmin and copper levels and increased secretion of urinary copper. Individuals with this condition develop tissue deposits of copper associated with hepatic cirrhosis, deep marginal pigmentation of the cornea, and extensive degeneration of the central nervous system, especially the basal ganglions. Also called **Wilson's disease.**

hepatoma /hep′ətō′mə/, *pl.* **hepatomas, hepatomata,** a primary malignant tumor of the liver characterized by hepatomegaly, pain, hypoglycemia, weight loss, anorexia, ascites, and the presence of alpha fetoprotein in the plasma. It occurs most frequently in association with hepatitis or cirrhosis of the liver and, geographically, in those parts of the world where the mycotoxin, aflatoxin, is commonly found.

hepatomegaly /hep′ətōmeg′əlē/, abnormal enlargement of the liver that is usually a sign of liver disease. It is often discovered by percussion and palpation as part of a physical examination: the liver is easily palpable below the ribs and is tender to the touch. Hepatomegaly may be caused by hepatitis or other infection, fatty infiltration, as in alcoholism, biliary obstruction, or malignancy.

hepatopancreatic ampulla, the dilatation formed by the junction of the pancreatic and bile ducts as they open into the lumen of the duodenum. Also called **ampulla of the bile duct, ampulla of Vater.**

hepatotoxic, potentially destructive of liver cells.

hepatotoxicity /hep′ətōtoksis′itē/, the tendency of an agent, usually a drug or alcohol, to have a destructive effect on the liver.

hepta-, hept-, a combining form meaning 'seven': *heptachromic, heptadactylia, heptavalent.*

heptachlor poisoning /hep′təklôr′/, a form of chlorinated organic insecticide poisoning.

heptaploid. See **polyploid.**

herald patch. See **pityriasis rosea.**

herb bath, a medicinal bath taken in water containing a decoction of aromatic herbs.

herbicide poisoning, a poisoning caused by the ingestion, inhalation, or absorption of a substance intended for use as a weed killer or defoliant. Many of the commonly used agricultural herbicides can produce symptoms ranging from skin irritation to hypotension, liver and kidney damage, and coma or convulsions. Estimated fatal doses may be as small as 1 to 10 g. If ingested, an emetic or gastric lavage is administered. Some herbicides contain extremely toxic substances; poisoning is characterized by dysphagia, burning stomach pain, throat constriction, diarrhea, or other severe symptoms. The substance is identified, the victim is rapidly taken to a medical facility, and therapy specific to the poison is promptly instituted.

hereditability, the degree to which a given trait is controlled by inheritance.

hereditary, pertaining to a characteristic, condition, or disease transmitted from parent to offspring; inborn; inherited. Compare **acquired, congenital, familial.**

hereditary ataxia, one of a group of inherited degenerative diseases of the spinal cord, cerebellum, and, often, other parts of the nervous system, characterized by tremor, spasm, wasting of muscle, skeletal change, and sensory disturbances resulting in impaired motor activity. Kinds of hereditary ataxia include **ataxia telangiectasia** and **Friedreich's ataxia.**

hereditary brown enamel. See **amelogenesis imperfecta.**

hereditary deforming chondroplasia. See **diaphyseal aclasis.**

hereditary disorder. See **inherited disorder.**

hereditary elliptocytosis. See **elliptocytosis.**

hereditary enamel hypoplasia. See **amelogenesis imperfecta.**

hereditary essential tremor. See **essential tremor.**

hereditary hemorrhagic telangiectasia. See **Osler-Weber-Rendu disease.**

hereditary hyperuricemia. See **Lesch-Nyhan syndrome.**

hereditary multiple exostoses, a rare, familial, dyschondroplastic disease in which bony protruberances form on the shafts of the long bones and eventually develop into caps of cartilage covering the ends of the bones. The affected joints lose their mobility, and the bones stop growing. The disease begins in childhood and has no cure. Very rarely, a chondrosarcoma may develop from the cap of an exostosis. See also **Ollier's dyschondroplasia.**

hereditary opalescent dentin. See **dentinogenesis imperfecta.**

hereditary oral disease, any abnormal condition characterized by genetic defects of oral and paraoral structures, as deformed dentition, ankyloglossia, hereditary gingivofibromatosis, or cleft palate. Many hereditary oral diseases are associated with generalized defects, as Crouzon's disease, sickle cell anemia, gargoylism, familial amyloidosis, and achondroplasia.

hereditary protoporphyria. See **porphyria.**

hereditary spherocytosis. See **spherocytic anemia.**
hereditary tyrosinemia. See **tyrosinemia.**
heredity, **1.** the process by which particular traits or conditions are genetically transmitted from parents to offspring, resulting in resemblance of individuals related by descent. It involves the separation and recombination of genes during meiosis and fertilization and the further interaction of developmental influences and genetic material during embryogenesis. **2.** the total genetic constitution of an individual; the sum of the qualities inherited from ancestors and the potentialities of transmitting these qualities to offspring.
heredo-, a combining form meaning 'hereditary': *heredobiologic, heredosyphilitic, heredotrophedema.*
heredofamilial tremor. See **essential tremor.**
Hering-Breuer reflexes, inhibitory and excitatory impulses that maintain the rhythm of respiration and prevent the overdistension of alveoli. The impulses originate in stretch receptors of the bronchi and bronchioles, travel via afferent fibers of the vagus nerves to the medullary respiratory centers, and back by motor neurons to the respiratory muscles of the chest. Hering-Breuer reflexes are well developed at birth. They are stimulated by distension of the airway, increased intratracheal pressures, or pulmonary inflation. The inflation reflex stops inspiration and stimulates expiration; the deflation reflex inhibits expiration and brings on inspiration. These reflexes are hyperactive in conditions of restrictive ventilatory insufficiency.
hermaphroditism /hərmaf'rədītiz'əm/, a rare condition in which both testicular and ovarian tissue exist in the same person, the testicular tissue containing seminiferous tubules or spermatozoa and the ovarian tissue containing follicles or corpora albicantia. The condition results from a chromosomal abnormality. Also called **hermaphrodism.** Compare **pseudohermaphroditism.**
hernia, protrusion of an organ through an abnormal opening in the muscle wall of the cavity that surrounds it. A hernia may be congenital, may result from the failure of certain structures to close after birth, or may be acquired later in life because of obesity, muscular weakness, surgery, or illness. Kinds of hernia include **abdominal hernia, diaphragmatic hernia, femoral hernia, hiatus hernia, inguinal hernia,** and **umbilical hernia.** See also **herniorrhaphy.**
herniated disk, a rupture of the fibrocartilage surrounding an intervertebral disk, releasing the nucleus pulposus that cushions the vertebrae above and below. The resultant pressure on spinal nerve roots may cause considerable pain and damage the nerves. The condition most frequently occurs in the lumbar region. Also called **herniated nucleus pulposus, ruptured intervertebral disk, slipped disk.**
herniated intervertebral disk. See **herniated disk.**
herniation, a protrusion of a body organ or portion of an organ through an abnormal opening in a membrane, muscle, or other tissue. See also **hernia, hiatus.**
herniorrhaphy, the surgical repair of a hernia.
heroin, a morphinelike drug with no currently acceptable medical use in the United States. Heroin is included in Schedule I of the Comprehensive Drug Abuse Prevention and Control Act of 1970. As covered in this legislation, it may not be obtained by prescription but only for research and instructional use or for chemical analysis by application to the Drug Enforcement Administration of the Department of Justice. Heroin, like other opium alkaloids, can produce analgesia, respiratory depression, GI spasm, and physical dependence. It produces its major effects on the central nervous system (CNS) and the bowel and alters the endocrine and the autonomic nervous systems. The binding sites for heroin are widely distributed in the CNS, especially throughout the limbic system, thalamus, striatum, hypothalamus, midbrain, and spinal cord. Illicitly obtained heroin is commonly used by individuals who become addicted and have a higher death rate than nonaddicts of similar age. Some studies conducted in the United States and England have shown that the majority of heroin users are relatively young people who have been introduced to the drug by friends and first start using heroin out of curiosity but continue because of its euphoric effects. Such individuals commonly show similar patterns of behavior, social adjustment, and health impairment. Heroin use in the United States reached epidemic proportions during the 1960s and in 1971 became a major cause of death in New York City among males between 15 and 35 years of age. The problem abated somewhat during the 1970s but has apparently increased and spread from the larger cities to the smaller communities across the country. Initial street use of the drug commonly involves sniffing powdered heroin, which is absorbed through the mucous membranes of the nasopharynx and the respiratory tract. Other methods of self-administration include subcutaneous injection and intravenous injection. Heroin, which loses much of its analgesic power when taken orally, is more powerful than morphine and acts more rapidly. It is hydrolyzed to morphine by the body and becomes concentrated in the parenchymatous tissues, skeletal muscle, and brain. Heroin metabolites are detected by tests for morphine. Heroin administered intravenously is almost immediately effective and produces reactions that last from 3 to 6 hours. Many users liken the initial sensation to a sexual orgasm. Heroin addicts may spend as much as $300 daily for the drug and inject themselves every 3 to 6 hours. Repeated use of this drug produces tolerance to most of the acute narcotic effects; physical dependence develops concurrently with tolerance. Withdrawal from heroin after relatively few exposures commonly produces acute abstinence syndrome. Withdrawal signs are usually observed shortly before the next planned dose and commonly include anxiety, restlessness, irritability, and craving for another dose. Other withdrawal signs that may appear 8 to 15 hours after the last dose include lacrimation, perspiration, yawning, and restless sleep. On awakening from such sleep the severely addicted heroin user may experience withdrawal signs, as vomiting, pain in

the bones, diarrhea, convulsions, and cardiovascular collapse. Withdrawal signs usually peak at between 36 and 48 hours and gradually subside during the following 10 days. Associated anxiety and depression may persist for months in many heroin addicts under treatment. Most authorities consider such addiction a complex disease caused by heroin-induced neurochemical disturbances in combination with deep psychologic and social factors. A variety of diluents, as quinine, are used to dissolve street heroin for subcutaneous and intravenous injection. Toxic diluents in combination with unhygienic administration and other unhealthy factors are responsible for more than half the fatalities associated with the illegal use of opiates. The most frequent disorders associated with injections of adulterated heroin are tetanus, skin abscesses, cellulitis, and thrombophlebitis. Heroin-connected pulmonary complications may include pneumonia, infarction, and tuberculosis. Neurologic disorders stemming from the use of street heroin may include transverse myelitis, peripheral nerve lesions, and fibrosing chronic myopathy. Women heroin addicts who become pregnant often give birth to premature babies who are highly susceptible to toxemia. Relapses of heroin addicts during withdrawal treatment are common, and protracted abstinence signs, as altered blood pressure and pulse rate, anxiety, and depression, may persist for months. Methadone is commonly used as a substitute drug in the treatment of heroin addiction. Also being studied is the effectiveness of the synthetic methadone congener, alpha acetyl methadol (methadone alcohol), which can prolong opiate effects for 72 hours. Numerous outpatient programs staffed by former opiate users seek to provide psychologic and therapeutic support for addicts trying to break their drug habits. Some of these programs are Synanon, Daytop Village, and Phoenix House. Research and community-supported psychotherapy projects continue to seek more effective treatment methods for addicts, many of whom are successfully rehabilitated. Enforced abstinence from heroin and other opiates in penal institutions has been much less effective in rehabilitating addicts, and most authorities propose a combination of medically prescribed withdrawal psychotherapeutic procedures and rehabilitative programs as the most promising approach. Also called **diacetylmorphine.**

herpangina /hur′panjī′nə/, a viral infection, usually of young children, characterized by sore throat, headache, anorexia, and pain in the abdomen, neck, and extremities. Febrile convulsions and vomiting may occur in infants. Papules or vesicles may form in the pharynx and on the tongue, the palate, or the tonsils. The lesions evolve into shallow ulcers that heal spontaneously. The disease usually runs its course in less than 1 week. Treatment is symptomatic. The cause is often infection by a strain of coxsackievirus.

herpes genitalis, an infection caused by Type 2 herpes simplex virus (HSV2), usually transmitted by sexual contact, that causes painful vesicular eruptions on the skin and mucous membranes of the genitalia of males and females. When acquired during pregnancy, HSV2 may be transmitted through the placenta to the fetus and to the newborn by direct contact with infected tissue during birth.

■ OBSERVATIONS: In the male, herpes genitalis infections may resemble penile ulcers. A small group of vesicular lesions surrounded by erythematous tissue may occur on the glans or prepuce. The lesions erupt into superficial ulcers that often heal in 5 to 7 days, although they also may become the sites of secondary infections. The lesions are painful and are often associated with a burning sensation, urinary dysfunction, fever, malaise, and swelling of the lymph nodes in the inguinal area. The female patient may exhibit the same or similar systemic effects, and members of both sexes may complain of painful sexual intercourse. In the female, herpes genitalis lesions are likely to appear as multiple superficial eruptions on the surfaces of the cervix, vagina, or perineum. There may be a discharge from the cervix. Vaginal lesions may appear as mucous patches with grayish ulcerations. Laboratory tests from smears of fluid taken from the base of lesions show a positive Tzanck reaction with multiple nucleated giant cells that distinguishes HSV2 infections from other venereal diseases. HSV2 tends to recur.

■ INTERVENTION: Treatment of uncomplicated initial herpes genitalis is with the antibiotic ancyclovir. Untreated, an attack of the disease is generally self-limiting. Lesions may be cleansed with soap and water, where feasible, to limit the risk of secondary infections, and drying medications may be applied to lesions that rupture or ooze. Secondary infections are treated with appropriate antibiotics. Except for experimental antiviral drugs, there are no specific cures or vaccines for the control of recurrent HSV2 infections.

■ NURSING CONSIDERATIONS: The nurse exercises extreme caution in contacts with infected patients. Smears for laboratory analysis are obtained by cleansing fresh vesicles with alcohol and removing fluid from the base of lesions with a cotton swab or wooden applicator. Rubber gloves are worn and the hands washed after contact to prevent transfer of virus particles from vesicles to other skin or mucous membranes of the patient or other individuals. Transfer of the virus to the cornea or conjunctiva results in herpetic keratitis. Primary infections that develop in pregnant women may progress to viremia and a marked incidence of mortality and morbidity in the fetus. Active HSV2 lesions within 3 weeks of delivery usually require that the infant be delivered by cesarean section to avoid dangerous neonatal herpesvirus infection.

herpes gestationis, a generalized, pruritic, vesicular or bullous rash appearing in the second or third trimester of pregnancy and disappearing several weeks postpartum. The lesions often recur with succeeding pregnancies and are associated with premature birth and increased fetal mortality. The disease closely resembles erythema multiforme.

herpes labialis. See **herpes simplex.**

herpes simplex, an infection caused by a herpes simplex virus (HSV), which has an affinity for the skin and nervous system and usually produces small, transient, irritating, and sometimes painful fluid-filled blisters on the skin and mucous membranes. HSV1 (oral herpes, herpes labialis) infections tend to occur in the facial area, particularly around the mouth and nose; HSV2 (herpes genitalis) infections are usually limited to the genital region.

■ OBSERVATIONS: The initial symptoms of a herpes simplex infection usually include burning, tingling, or itching sensations about the edges of the lips or nose within 1 week or 2 after contact with an infected person. Several hours later, small red papules develop in the irritated area, followed by the eruption of small vesicles, or fever blisters, filled with fluid. Several small vesicles may merge to form a larger blister. The vesicles generally are associated with itching, pain, or similar discomfort. Other effects often include a mild fever and enlargement of the lymph nodes in the neck. Laboratory analysis of the vesicular fluid usually shows the presence of herpesvirus particles and the absence of pyogenic bacteria. Within 1 week after the onset of symptoms, thin yellow crusts form on the vesicles as healing begins. In skin areas that are moist or protected or in severe cases, healing may be delayed. HSV2 infections in adolescence are associated with an increased incidence of cervical cancer in adulthood.

■ INTERVENTION: Treatment of herpes simplex is symptomatic. The lesions may be washed gently with soap and water to reduce the risk of secondary infection. Topical applications of drying medications, as alcohol solutions, may speed healing, but they are very painful. Where secondary infections have begun, antibiotics are prescribed.

■ NURSING CONSIDERATIONS: Because herpesviruses are extremely contagious, the nurse follows all appropriate procedures in contacts with patients to avoid acquiring the infection and carrying it to other persons. Washing the hands and wearing rubber gloves while working about the mouth of a patient help prevent transmission of the virus. Once acquired, the virus tends to remain latent in the skin or tissues of the nervous system and may be reactivated by a variety of stimuli, including a febrile illness, physical or emotional stress, exposure to sunlight, or ingestion of certain foods or drugs. Topical sunscreen preparations offer some protection against exposure to the sun, and patients are advised to avoid repeated exposure to stimuli to which they are sensitive. The complications of herpetic infections may include encephalitis, herpes simplex keratitis, and gingivostomatitis. In cases involving system complications, antibiotics, blood transfusions, IV solutions, and other therapy may be required. In uncomplicated cases, the herpes attack is usually self-limiting and runs its course in 3 weeks or less.

herpesvirus /hur′pēzvī′rəs/, any of five related viruses including herpes simplex viruses 1 and 2, varicellazoster virus, Epstein-Barr virus, and cytomegalovirus.

herpesvirus hominis. See **herpes simplex.**

herpes zoster, an acute infection caused by the varicellazoster virus (VZV), affecting mainly adults and characterized by the development of painful vesicular skin eruptions that follow the underlying route of cranial or spinal nerves inflamed by the virus.

■ OBSERVATIONS: Distribution of the pain and vesicular eruptions is usually unilateral, although both sides of the body may be involved. Any sensory nerve may be affected, but the virus in most cases tends to invade the posterior root ganglia associated with thoracic and trigeminal nerves. The pain, which may be constant or intermittent, superficial or deep, usually precedes other effects and may mimic other disorders, as appendicitis or pleurisy. Early symptoms may include GI disturbances, malaise, fever, and headache. The vesicles usually evolve from small red macules along the path of a nerve, and the skin of the area is hypersensitive. All of the lesions may appear within a period of hours, but they most often develop gradually over a period of several days. The macules vesiculate and, after about 3 days, become turbid with cellular debris. Usually, at the end of the first week, the vesicules develop crusts. The symptoms may persist for 3 to 5 weeks, but in most cases they diminish after 2 weeks.

■ INTERVENTION: Treatment is primarily symptomatic and includes application of calamine lotion or similar medications to relieve itching and administration of analgesics for pain symptoms. Cool compresses may be applied to the affected skin areas. Topical corticosteroids may be prescribed for severe cases and for elderly patients who are potential candidates for a common sequela of postherpetic neuralgia. Surgical intervention to excise an affected nerve may be advised in cases of severe pain that fail to respond to more conservative treatment.

■ NURSING CONSIDERATIONS: The nurse encourages bed rest during the early stages of zoster infection, when fever and other systemic effects occur. Irritation of the vesicles may be exacerbated by contact with clothing or bed linen. The use of nonadherent dressings and of cradles to prevent direct contact of affected skin areas with irritating fabrics relieves discomfort. Older patients are most susceptible to complications, as exhaustion and postherpetic neuralgia, which may persist for several months after the skin lesions have cleared. Other complications are geniculate zoster, with involvement of the ear, face, and soft palate, and ophthalmic herpes zoster, which can result in corneal damage. An attack of herpes zoster does not confer immunity, but most patients recover without permanent effects except for occasional scarring at sites of severe vesicular lesions. Evidence indicates VZV remains latent in the body of a person once infected, and a person lacking varicella immunity can acquire chickenpox from a herpes zoster patient. Also called **shingles.** See also **herpes simplex, varicellazoster virus.**

herpes zoster oticus, a herpes zoster infection of the eighth cervical nerve ganglia and geniculate ganglion, causing severe pain in the external ear structures and pain or paralysis along the facial nerve. The disease may also result in hearing loss and vertigo. The vertigo is usually transient, but the hearing loss and facial paralysis may be permanent. There may be vesicular eruptions along the external ear canal and ear pinna. Treatment is generally symptomatic, with diazepam administered for vertigo, analgesics for pain, and corticosteroids for other symptoms.

herpes zoster virus. See **chickenpox.**

herpetiform /hərpet′ifôrm′/, having clusters of vesicles; resembling the skin lesions of some herpesvirus infections.

Herplex, a trademark for an antiviral (idoxuridine).

Hers' disease, an uncommon metabolic disorder of glycogen storage, characterized by hepatomegaly and an accumulation of abnormally large amounts of glycogen in the liver as a result of its inability to break down glycogen. The condition is inherited as an autosomal recessive trait. There is no known treatment. Also called **glycogen storage disease, type VI.** See also **glycogen storage disease.**

hertz (Hz), a unit of measurement of wave frequency equal to one cycle per second (cps).

hesperidin /hesper′idin/, a crystalline flavone glycoside found in bioflavonoid and occurring in most citrus fruits, especially in the spongy casing of oranges and lemons.

hetacillin, a penicillinase sensitive penicillin antibiotic that has no antibacterial activity until it is converted into ampicillin in the body.

■ INDICATION: It is prescribed in the treatment of certain infections.

■ CONTRAINDICATIONS: Known hypersensitivity to this drug or to any penicillin medication prohibits its use. Severe impairment of kidney function or a history of hypersensitivity reactions, as eczema, asthma, or hives, require that the drug be administered with caution.

■ ADVERSE EFFECTS: Among the more serious adverse reactions are diarrhea, GI distress, skin rash, and hypersensitivity reactions.

hetastarch, a plasma volume extender.

■ INDICATIONS: It is prescribed as an adjunct in shock and leukophoresis.

■ CONTRAINDICATIONS: Severe bleeding, severe heart or kidney dysfunction with oliguria or anuria, or known hypersensitivity to this drug prohibits its use.

■ ADVERSE EFFECTS: Among the more serious adverse reactions are influenza-like symptoms, muscle pain, edema, and anaphylaxis.

heter-. See **hetero-.**

heterauxesis. See **allometric growth.**

hetero-, heter-, a combining form meaning 'pertaining to another': *heteroalbumose, heterochronia, heterogamy.*

heteroallele /het′ərō-əlēl′/, one of a set of genes located at a specific locus on homologous chromosomes that differs from the other of the pair, resulting in a mutation. –**heteroallelic,** *adj.*

heteroblastic, developing from different germ layers or kinds of tissue rather than from a single type. Compare **homoblastic.**

heterocephalus, a malformed fetus that has two heads of unequal size. –**heterocephalous, heterocephalic,** *adj.*

heterochromatin, that portion of chromosome material that is inactive in gene expression but may function in controlling metabolic activities, transcription, and cell division. It stains most intensely during the interphase stage and usually remains in a condensed state throughout the cell cycle. It consists of two types, constitutive heterochromatin, which occurs in the centromeric region of the chromosome and is characteristic of the Y chromosome, and facultative heterochromatin, which is present in the inactivated X chromosome of the mammalian female. Compare **euchromatin.** See also **chromatin** –**heterchromatic,** *adj.*

heterochromatinization, the transformation of genetically active euchromatin into genetically inactive heterochromatin; the inactivation of one of the X chromosomes in the mammalian female during the early stages of embryogenesis. See also **Lyon hypothesis.**

heterochromosome, a sex chromosome. See also **heterotypical chromosomes.** –**heterochromosomal,** *adj.*

heterodidymus /het′ərōdid′iməs/, a conjoined twin fetus in which the parasitic elements consist of a head, neck, and thorax attached to the thoracic wall of the autosite. Also called **heterodymus.**

heteroduplex, (in molecular genetics) a DNA molecule in which the two strands are derived from different individuals, with the result that some pairs or blocks of base pairs may not match.

heteroeroticism, sexual feeling or activity directed toward another individual. Also called **alloeroticism, heteroerotism.** Compare **autoeroticism.**

heterogamete, a gamete that differs considerably in size and structure from the one with which it unites, specifically denoting those of higher organisms as opposed to those of lower plants and animals. Compare **anisogamete, isogamete.**

heterogamy /het′ərog′əmē/, **1.** sexual reproduction in which there is fusion of dissimilar gametes, usually differing in size and structure. The word is used primarily to denote the reproductive processes of higher organisms as opposed to certain lower plants and animals. Compare **anisogamy, isogamy. 2.** reproduction by the alternation of sexual and asexual generations; heterogenesis. –**heterogamous,** *adj.*

heterogeneous, **1.** consisting of dissimilar elements or parts; unlike; incongruous. **2.** not having a uniform quality throughout. Compare **homogeneous.** –**heterogeneity,** *adj.*

heterogenesis, **1.** also called **heterogeny, heterogony.** reproduction that differs in successive generations, as the alternation of sexual with asexual reproduction, so that offspring have characteristics different from those of the parents. In the asexual stage, it often involves one or more parthenogenic or hermaphroditic generations, often with various hosts, as in the case of many trematode parasites. **2.** asexual generation. **3.** abiogenesis. Compare **autogenesis, homogenesis.** See also **metagenesis.** –**heterogenetic, heterogenic,** *adj.*

heterogenous /het′əroj′ənəs/, derived or developed from another source or from two different sources.

heterogeny. See **heterogenesis.**

heterograft. See **xenograft.**

heterologous. See **xenogeneic.**

heterologous insemination. See **artificial insemination-donor.**

heterologous tumor, a neoplasm consisting of tissue different from that of its site.

heterologous twins. See **dizygotic twins.**

heterophil antibody test, a test for the presence of heterophil antibodies in the serum of patients suspected of having infectious mononucleosis, based on an agglutination reaction between heterophil antibodies in a person's serum and heterophil antigen, a normal component of sheep erythrocytes. This antibody eventually appears in the serum of more than 80% of the patients with mononucleosis, hence is highly diagnostic of the disease. See also **Epstein-Barr virus.**

heteroploid /het′əraploid′/, **1.** of or pertaining to an individual, organism, strain, or cell that has a variation in the number of whole chromosomes characteristic for the somatic cell of the species. The change may involve entire sets of chromosomes or the addition or loss of single whole chromosomes. **2.** such an individual, organism, strain, or cell. See also **aneuploid, euploid.**

heteroploidy /het′əraploi′dē/, the state or condition of having an abnormal number of chromosomes, either more or less than that characteristic of the somatic cell of the species.

heteropolymer, a compound formed from subunits that are not all the same, as a protein composed of various amino acid subunits.

heterosexual, **1.** a person whose sexual desire or preference is for people of the opposite sex. **2.** of or pertaining to sexual desire or preference for people of the opposite sex. –**heterosexuality,** *n.*

heterosexual panic, an acute attack of anxiety resulting in the frantic pursuit of heterosexual activity in response to unconscious or latent homosexual impulses. Compare **homosexual panic.**

heterosis /het′ərō′sis/, the superiority of first generation hybrid plants and animals in respect to one or more traits when compared with either of the parent strains or with corresponding inbred strains. Also called **hybrid vigor.**

heterotopic ossification, a nonmalignant overgrowth of bone, frequently occurring after a fracture, that is sometimes confused with certain bone tumors when visualized on x-ray film. Also called **exuberant callus, myositis ossificans.**

heterotypic /het′ərōtip′ik/, pertaining to or characteristic of a type differing from the usual or the normal, specifically regarding the first meiotic division of germ cells in gametogenesis as distinguished from the second or mitotic division. Also called **heterotypical.** Compare **homeotypic.**

heterotypic chromosomes, any unmatched pair of chromosomes, specifically the sex chromosomes.

heterotypic mitosis, the division of bivalent chromosomes, as occurs in the first meiotic division of germ cells in gametogenesis; a reduction division. Compare **homeotypic mitosis.**

heterozygosis /het′ərōzīgō′sis/, **1.** the formation of a zygote by the union of two gametes that have dissimilar pairs of genes. **2.** the production of hybrids through crossbreeding. –**heterozygotic,** *adj.*

heterozygous /het′ərəzī′gəs/, having two different genes at corresponding loci on homologous chromosomes. An individual who is heterozygous for a particular characteristic has inherited a gene for that characteristic from one parent and the alternative gene from the other parent. A person heterozygous for a genetic disease caused by a dominant gene, as Huntington's chorea, manifests the disorder. An individual heterozygous for a hereditary disorder produced by a recessive gene, as sickle cell anemia, is asymptomatic or exhibits reduced symptoms of the disease. The offspring of a heterozygous carrier of a genetic disorder have a 50% chance of inheriting the gene associated with the trait. Compare **homozygous.**

Hetrazan, a trademark for an anthelmintic (diethylcarbamazine citrate).

heuristic /hyo͞oris′tik/, **1.** serving to stimulate interest for further investigation. **2.** a teaching method in which the student is encouraged to learn through independent research and investigation. **3.** a method of argument that postulates what is to be proved.

hex-, hexa-, a combining form meaning 'six': *hexabasic, hexavaccine, hexhydric.*

Hexa-Betalin, a trademark for vitamin B_6 (pyridoxine hydrochloride).

hexachlorophene, a topical antiinfective and detergent.

■ INDICATIONS: It is used as an antiseptic scrub and as a disinfectant for inanimate objects.

■ CONTRAINDICATIONS: Known hypersensitivity to this drug prohibts its use. Systemic absorption can occur when used on burns, broken skin, mucous membranes, and infant skin, with hemotoxic effects.

■ ADVERSE EFFECTS: Among the more serious adverse reactions are skin rash and neurologic abnormalities.

■ NOTE: The skin should be rinsed thoroughly to prevent systemic absorption.

Hexadrol, a trademark for a glucocorticoid (dexamethasone).

hexafluorenium bromide, an inhibitor of acetylcholinesterase.
■ INDICATIONS: It is used as an adjunct to anesthesia to prolong the skeletal muscle relaxation caused by succinylcholine.
■ CONTRAINDICATIONS: Known hypersensitivity to this drug or to bromides prohibits its use.
■ ADVERSE EFFECTS: Among the more serious adverse reactions are excessive prolongation of muscle relaxation and resultant apnea, allergic reactions, and hypotension.

hexamethylenamine. See **methenamine.**

hexamethylmelamine, an experimental antineoplastic that has been used to treat bronchogenic, cervical, and ovarian carcinomas.

hexaploid. See **polyploid.**

hexenmilch. See **witch's milk.**

hexobarbital, a short-acting barbiturate.
■ INDICATIONS: It is prescribed as a hypnotic and as a short-acting sedative for insomnia.
■ CONTRAINDICATIONS: Porphyria, liver dysfunction, or known hypersensitivity to this drug prohibits its use.
■ ADVERSE EFFECTS: Among the most serious adverse reactions are respiratory depression, paradoxical excitement, porphyria, allergic reactions, and drug dependence.

hexocyclium methylsulfate, an anticholinergic.
■ INDICATION: It is prescribed as an adjunct to ulcer therapy.
■ CONTRAINDICATIONS: Narrow-angle glaucoma, asthma, obstruction of the genitourinary or GI tract, ulcerative colitis, or known hypersensitivity to this drug prohibits its use.
■ ADVERSE EFFECTS: Among the more serious adverse reactions are blurred vision, central nervous system effects, tachycardia, dry mouth, decreased sweating, and hypersensitivity reactions.

hexokinase /hek'səkī'nās/, an enzyme that catalyzes the transfer of a phosphate group from adenosine triphosphate to D-glucose.

hexose, a monosaccharide that contains six carbon atoms in the molecule. Glucose and fructose are the principal hexoses found in nature.

hexylcaine hydrochloride, a local anesthetic for use on intact mucous membranes of the respiratory, upper GI, and urinary tracts.

Hf, symbol for **hafnium.**

Hg, symbol for **mercury.**

hiatus /hī·ā'təs/, a usually normal opening in a membrane or other body tissue. **–hiatal,** *adj.*

hiatus hernia, protrusion of a portion of the stomach upward through the diaphragm. The condition occurs in about 40% of the population, and most people display few, if any, symptoms. The major difficulty in symptomatic patients is gastroesophageal reflux, the backflow of the acid contents of the stomach into the esophagus. Diagnosis is made easily on x-ray films. Surgical treatment is usually unnecessary, and efforts should be directed toward alleviating the discomfort associated with reflux. See also **diaphragmatic hernia, gastroesophageal reflux, heartburn.**

hibernoma /hī'bərnō'mə/, *pl.* **hibernomas, hibernomata,** a benign tumor, usually on the hips or the back, composed of fat cells that are partly or entirely of fetal origin. Also called **fat cell lipoma, fetal lipoma.**

hiccup, a characteristic sound that is produced by the involuntary contraction of the diaphragm, followed by rapid closure of the glottis. Hiccups have a variety of causes, including indigestion, rapid eating, certain types of surgery, and epidemic encephalitis. Most episodes of hiccups do not persist longer than a few minutes, but recurrent and prolonged attacks sometimes occur. The condition is most often seen in men. Sedatives are used in extreme cases. Also spelled **hiccough.** Also called **singultus.**

hickory stick fracture. See **greenstick fracture.**

hidradenitis. See **hydradenitis.**

hidro-, a combining form meaning 'pertaining to sweat or a sweat gland': *hidrocystoma, hidrosadenitis.*

hidrosis /hidrō'sis, hī-/, sweat production and secretion. Compare **anhidrosis, dyshidrosis, hyperhidrosis.** **–hidrotic,** *adj.*

hiero-, hier-, a combining form meaning 'pertaining to the sacrum, or to religion': *hierolisthesis, hieromania, hierotherapy.*

high blood pressure. See **hypertension.**

high-density lipoprotein (HDL), a plasma protein containing about 50% protein (apoprotein) with cholesterol and triglycerides. It may serve to stabilize very low-density lipoprotein and is involved in transporting cholesterol and other lipids from the plasma to the tissues. See also **low-density lipoprotein, very low-density lipoprotein.**

high-energy phosphate compound, a chemical compound containing a high-energy bond between phosphoric acid residues and certain organic substances. When the bond is hydrolyzed, a large amount of energy is released. Adenosine triphosphate is the most powerful and ubiquitous of the high-energy phosphate compounds found in the body. All of these compounds liberate energy to fuel muscle contraction, active transport across cell membranes, and the synthesis of many substances in the body.

highest intercostal vein, one of a pair of veins that drain the blood from the upper two or three intercostal spaces. The right vein descends and opens into the azygous vein. The left vein crosses the arch of the aorta and opens into the left brachiocephalic vein, usually receiving the left bronchial vein.

high forceps, an obstetric operation in which forceps are used to deliver a baby whose head is not engaged in the birth canal. The procedure is considered hazardous and is generally condemned. Compare **low forceps, mid forceps.** See also **forceps delivery, obstetric forceps.**

high-Fowler's position, placement of the patient in a semisitting position by raising the head of the bed more than 20 inches.

high labial arch, a labial arch wire adapted to lie gingival to the anterior tooth crowns, having auxiliary springs that extend downward in contact with the teeth to be moved.

high-level language, a computer programing language that approaches English in its syntax, as BASIC, FORTRAN, and PASCAL. See also **low-level language.**

high-level wellness, a concept of optimal health that emphasizes the integration of body, mind, and environment to maximize the function of an individual.

high-potassium diet, a diet that contains foods rich in potassium, including all leafy green vegetables, brussels sprouts, citrus fruits, bananas, dates, raisins, legumes, meats, and whole grains. It is indicated for any condition resulting in the loss of extracellular fluid, as acute diarrhea, congenital renal alkalosis, aldosteronism, hypokalemia, hypertension, and diabetic coma. It is also indicated for patients receiving thiazide or corticosteroid therapy.

high-protein diet, a diet that contains large amounts of protein, consisting largely of meats, fish, milk, legumes, and nuts. It may be indicated in protein depletion from any cause, as a preoperative preparation, in nephrotic syndromes, or in hepatic disorders. It may be contraindicated in liver failure or when function of the kidneys is so impaired that added protein could result in azotemia and acidosis.

high-risk infant, any neonate, regardless of birth weight, size, or gestational age, who, because of preconceptual, prenatal, natal, or postnatal conditions or circumstances that interfere with the normal birth process or impede adjustment to extrauterine growth and development, has a greater than average chance of morbidity or mortality, especially within the first 28 days of life. See also **neonatal period, premature infant.**

high-speed handpiece, a rotary or vibratory cutting instrument that operates at high speeds, powered by a conventional dental engine and propelled by gears, a belt drive, or turbine.

high-vitamin diet, a dietary regimen that includes a variety of foods that contain therapeutic amounts of all of the vitamins necessary for the metabolic processes of the body. It is often ordered in combination with other therapeutic diets containing larger than usual amounts of protein or calories, especially when treating severe or chronic infection, malnutrition, or vitamin deficiency.

Hill-Burton Act, a 1946 amendment to the U.S. Public Health Service Act authorizing grants to states for surveying their hospital and public health center needs and for the planning and construction of additional facilities. Subsequent amendments authorized federal funding for as much as two thirds of the cost of construction projects and broadened the scope of the legislation to include diagnostic and treatment centers, long-term treatment centers, and nursing homes and to aid in modernization of existing hospitals. Also called **Hospital Survey and Construction Act.**

Hill-Burton programs, a cluster of programs created by legislation included in the National Health Planning and Resources Development Act of 1974. The programs allow federal monetary assistance for modernization of health facilities, construction of outpatient health centers, construction of inpatient facilities in underserved areas, and the conversion of existing health care facilities for the provision of new health services.

hilus /hī′ləs/, *pl.* **hili,** a depression or pit at that part of an organ where vessels and nerves enter.

hindgut, the caudal portion of the embryonic alimentary canal. Consisting of endodermal tissue, it is formed by the development of the tail fold and eventually gives rise to part of the small and large intestines, rectum, bladder, and urogenital ducts. Compare **foregut, midgut.** See also **cloaca.**

hind kidney. See **metanephros.**

hinge axis-orbital plane, a craniofacial plane that is usually determined by marking three points on the face of the patient. Two of the points, one on each side of the face, are located on the hinge axis. The third point is located on the face at the level of the orbital rim just beneath the eye. The hinge axis-orbital plane is a reference plane for the diagnosis of various types of malocclusions and the development of associated prostheses.

hinge joint, a synovial joint providing a connection in which articular surfaces are closely molded together in a manner that permits extensive motion in one plane. The distal bone of a hinge joint seldom moves in the same plane as that of the axis of the proximal bone. The interphalangeal joints are hinge joints. Also called **ginglymus joint.** Compare **gliding joint, pivot joint.**

hip. See **coxa.**

hip bath. See **sitz bath.**

hipbone. See **innominate bone.**

hip joint. See **coxal articulation.**

hippocampal commissure, a thin, triangular layer of transverse fibers that connects the medial edges of the posterior pillars of the fornix.

hippocampal fissure, a fissure reaching from the posterior aspect of the corpus callosum to the tip of the temporal lobe.

hippocampus, *pl.* **hippocampi,** a curved convoluted elevation of the floor of the inferior horn of the lateral ventricle of the brain. It is composed of gray substance covered by a layer of white fibers, the alveus, and functions as an important component of the limbic system. Its efferent projections form the fornix of the cerebrum. Also called **Ammon's horn, hippocampus major.**

hippocampus minor. See **calcar avis.**

Hippocrates /hipok′rətēz/, a Greek physician, born about 460 BC on the island of Cos, a center for the worship of Æsculapius. Called the "Father of Medicine," Hippocrates introduced a scientific approach to healing by seeking physical causes for disease rather than magic or mythic relationships employed by members of the

...also compiled case ...lts of treatments ...ethical bedside ...ath.

...lage.

...ributed to ...he med- ...nto the ...ds as ... physician, by Æsculapius, ...ygeia, and Panacea, and I take to witness all the gods, and all the goddesses, to keep according to my ability and my judgment the following Oath:

To consider dear to me as my parents him who taught me this art; to live in common with him and if necessary to share my goods with him; to look upon his children as my own brothers, to teach them this art if they so desire without fee or written promise; to impart to my sons and the sons of the master who taught me and the disciples who have enrolled themselves and have agreed to the rules of the profession, but to these alone, the precepts and the instruction. I will prescribe regimen for the good of my patients according to my ability and my judgment and never do harm to anyone. To please no one will I prescribe a deadly drug, nor give advice which may cause his death. Nor will I give a woman a pessary to procure abortion. But I will preserve the purity of my life and my art. I will not cut for stone, even for patients in whom the disease is manifest; I will leave this operation to be performed by practitioners (specialists in this art). In every house where I come I will enter only for the good of my patients, keeping myself far from all intentional ill-doing and all seduction, and especially from the pleasures of love with women or with men, be they free or slaves. All that may come to my knowledge in the exercise of my profession or outside of my profession or in daily commerce with men, which ought not to be spread abroad, I will keep secret and will never reveal. If I keep this oath faithfully, may I enjoy my life and practice my art, respected by all men and in all times; but if I swerve from it or violate it, may the reverse be my lot. See also **Æsculapius, Hippocrates.**

hip replacement, replacement of the hip joint with an artificial ball and socket joint, performed to relieve a chronically painful and stiff hip in advanced osteoarthritis, an improperly healed fracture, or degeneration of the joint. Antibiotic therapy is begun preoperatively, and the patient is taught to walk with crutches. General anesthesia is used, the femoral head, neck, and part of the shaft are removed, and the contours of the socket are smoothed. A prosthesis of a durable, hard metal alloy or stainless steel is shaped to resemble a femur and head of a femur and is attached to the femur with screws or an acrylic cement; a metal or a plastic acetablum is implanted. Postoperatively, the patient is placed in traction. The affected leg is kept abducted and in straight alignment with pillows; external rotation of the leg must

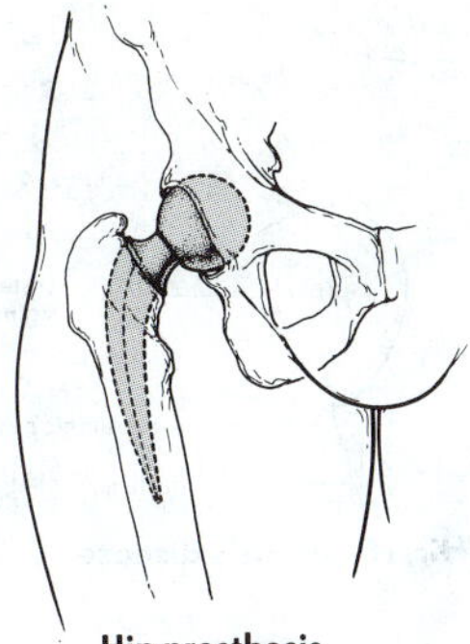

Hip prosthesis

be prevented. The nurse observes nerve function and circulation in the leg frequently during the first postoperative day. Support hose may be ordered and anticoagulant therapy begun. The most frequent complications are infection requiring removal of the new joint, or its dislocation. Ambulation begins gradually, with frequent short walks. Sitting for more than 1 hour is to be avoided, and hip flexion beyond 90 degrees may cause dislocation of the prosthesis. The patient continues an exercise program after discharge to maintain functional motion of the hip joint and to strengthen the abductor muscles.

Hiprex, a trademark for a urinary antibacterial (methenamine hippurate).

Hirschfeld-Dunlop file, a kind of periodontal file, used with a pull stroke to remove tooth calculus. Various models with different angulations are available for different tooth surfaces.

Hirschfeld's method, a toothbrushing technique in which the bristles are placed against the axial surfaces of the teeth at a slight incisal or occlusal angle and in contact with the teeth and gingivae, then vigorously rotated in very small circles.

Hirschsprung's disease /hirsh′spro͞ongz/, the congenital absence of autonomic ganglia in the smooth muscle wall of the colon, resulting in poor or absent peristalsis in the involved segment of colon, accumulation of feces, and dilatation of the bowel (megacolon). Symptoms include intermittent vomiting, diarrhea, and constipation. The abdomen may become distended to several times its normal size. The condition is usually diagnosed in infancy, but it may not be recognized until much later in childhood, when there is anorexia, lack of urge to defecate, distention of the abdomen, and poor health. Diagnosis is confirmed by barium enema; biopsy of the affected tissue shows the absence of ganglia. Surgical repair in early childhood is usually successful. A temporary colostomy is performed, and the aganglionic portion of the bowel is resected. The colostomy is almost always reversed a few months later. Also called **aganglionic megacolon, congenital megacolon.**

hirsutism /hur′so͞otiz′əm/, excessive body hair in a masculine distribution as a result of heredity, hormonal

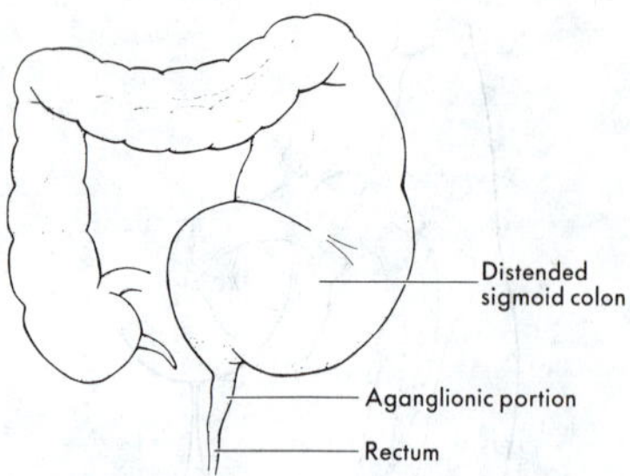

Hirschsprung's disease

dysfunction, porphyria, or medication. Treatment of the specific cause will usually stop growth of more hair. Excess hair may be removed by dermabrasion, electrolysis, chemical depilation, shaving, plucking, or rubbing with pumice. Fine facial hair may be most effectively minimized by bleaching. Also called **hypertrichosis.** –**hirsute,** *adj.*, **hirsuteness,** *n.*

hirsutoid papilloma of the penis /hur′sōōtoid/, a condition characterized by clusters of small, white papules on the coronal edge of the glans penis. Also called **papillomatosis coronae penis, pearly penile papules.**

His. See **histidine.**

His bundle. See **bundle of His.**

His bundle electrogram (HBE), (in cardiology) a direct recording of the electric activity in the bundle of His.

His-Purkinje system, the conduction system in the cardiac tissues from the bundle of His to the distal Purkinje fibers.

Hispril, a trademark for an antihistaminic (diphenylpyraline hydrochloride).

hist-. See **histo-.**

histamine /his′təmēn, -min/, a compound, found in all cells, produced by the breakdown of histidine. It is released in allergic, inflammatory reactions and causes dilatation of capillaries, decreased blood pressure, increased secretion of gastric juice, and constriction of smooth muscles of the bronchi and uterus.

histamine headache, a headache associated with the release of histamine from the body tissues and marked by symptoms of dilated carotid arteries, fluid accumulation under the eyes, tearing or lacrimation, and rhinorrhea (runny nose). Symptoms include sudden sharp pain on one side of the head, involving the facial area from the neck to the temple. Treatment includes the use of preparations of antihistamines and ergot that help constrict the arteries. Also called **cluster headache, Horton's histamine cephalalgia.** See also **cephalalgia.**

-histechia, a combining form meaning a 'tissue retaining a (specified) substance': *cholesterohistechia, glycohistechia, uratohistechia.*

histidine (His), a basic amino acid found in many proteins and a precursor of histamine. It is an essential amino acid in infants. See also **amino acid, protein.**

histiocyte. See **macrophage.**

histiocytic leukemia. See **monocytic leukemia.**

histiocytic malignant lymphoma, a lymphoid neoplasm containing undifferentiated primitive cells or differentiated reticulum cells. Also called **clasmocytic lymphoma, reticulum cell sarcoma.**

histiocytosis X /his′tē·ōsītō′sis/, *obsolete.* a cluster of conditions encompassing benign eosinophilic granuloma and several malignant lymphomatous diseases.

histiotypic growth /his′tē·ōtip′ik/, the uncontrolled proliferation of cells, as occurs in bacterial cultures and molds. Compare **organotypic growth.**

histo-, hist-, a combining form meaning 'pertaining to tissue': *histoclastic, histohematin, histonectomy.*

histocompatibility antigens, a group of genetically determined antigens on the surface of many cells. Histocompatibility antigens are the cause of most graft rejections that occur in organ transplantation. See also **isoantigen, histocompatibility locus.**

histocompatibility locus, a set of positions on a chromosome occupied by a complex of genes that govern several tissue antigens. Together, the loci and the genes comprise the human leukocyte antigen complex.

histogram /his′təgram′/, (in research) a graph showing the values of one or more variables plotted against time or against frequency of occurrence. A graph of a patient's temperature, pulse, and respiration is an example of a histogram.

histography /histog′rəfē/, the process of describing or creating visualizations of tissues and cells. –**histographer,** *n.*, **histographic,** *adj.*, **histographically,** *adv.*

histoid neoplasm, a growth that resembles the tissues in which it originates. Compare **organoid neoplasm.**

histologist /histol′əjist/, a medical scientist who specializes in the study of histology. See also **histology.**

histology /histol′əjē/, **1.** the science dealing with the microscopic identification of cells and tissue. **2.** the structure of organ tissues, including the composition of cells and their organization into various body tissues. –**histologic, histological,** *adj.*, **histologically,** *adv.*

histone /his′tōn/, any of a group of strongly basic, low molecular weight proteins that are soluble in water, insoluble in dilute ammonia, and combine with nucleic acid to form nucleoproteins. They are found in the cell nucleus, especially of glandular tissue, where they form a complex with deoxyribonucleic acid in the chromatin and function in regulating gene activity. Histones also interfere with coagulation of the blood and have been isolated from the urine of patients with leukemia and febrile conditions.

histoplasma agglutinin, an agglutinin associated with fungal lung infections.

Histoplasma capsulatum, a dimorphic fungal organism that is a single budding yeast at body temperature and a mold at room temperature. It is the causative organism in histoplasmosis, common in the Mississippi River Valley. The fungus, spread by airborne spores from soil contaminated with excreta from infected birds, acts as a parasite on the cells of the reticuloendothelial system.

histoplasmosis /his′tōplazmō′sis/, an infection caused by inhalation of spores of the fungus *Histoplasma capsulatum*. **Primary histoplasmosis** is characterized by fever, malaise, cough, and lymphadenopathy. Spontaneous recovery is usual; small calcifications remain in the lungs and affected lymph glands. **Progressive histoplasmosis,** the sometimes fatal, disseminated form of the infection, is characterized by ulcerating sores in the mouth and nose, enlargement of the spleen, liver, and lymph nodes, and severe and extensive infiltration of the lungs. Infection confers immunity; a histoplasmin skin test may be performed to identify people who may safely work with contaminated soil. The disease is most common in the Mississippi and Ohio Valleys.

history, **1.** a record of past events. **2.** a systematic account of the medical and psychosocial occurrences in a patient's life and of factors in family, ancestors, and environment that may have a bearing on the patient's condition.

history of present illness, an account obtained during the interview with the patient of the onset, duration, and character of the present illness, as well as of any acts or factors that aggravate or ameliorate the symptoms. The patient is asked what is believed to be the cause of the symptoms and whether or not a similar condition has occurred in the past.

histotoxin, any substance that is poisonous to the body tissues. It is usually generated from within the body rather than being introduced externally. **–histotoxic,** *adj.*

histotroph, histotrophe, histotrophic nutrition. See **embryotroph.**

histrionic personality, a personality characterized by behavioral patterns and attitudes that are overreactive, emotionally unstable, overly dramatic, and self-centered, exhibited as a means of attracting attention, consciously or unconsciously. Also called **hysteric personality.** See also **histrionic personality disorder.**

histrionic personality disorder, a disorder characterized by dramatic, reactive, and intensely exaggerated behavior, which is typically self-centered and results in severe disturbance in interpersonal relationships that can lead to psychosomatic disorders, depression, alcoholism, and drug dependency. Symptoms include emotional excitability, such as irrational angry outbursts or tantrums; abnormal craving for activity and excitement; overreaction to minor events; manipulative threats and gestures; egocentricity; inconsiderateness; inconsistency; and continuous demand for reassurance because of feelings of helplessness and dependency. A person having this disorder is perceived by others as vain, demanding, superficial, self-centered, and self-indulgent. The disorder is more prevalent in women than in men and is treated by various psychotherapies, depending on the individual and the severity of the condition. See also **narcissistic personality disorder.**

hives. See **urticaria.**

HLA, abbreviation for **human leukocyte antigen.**

HLA-A, abbreviation for *human leukocyte antigen A.* See **human leukocyte antigen.**

HLA-B, abbreviation for *human leukocyte antigen B.* See **human leukocyte antigen.**

HLA-D, abbreviation for *human leukocyte antigen D.* See **human leukocyte antigen.**

HLH, abbreviation for **human luteinizing hormone.**

HMO, abbreviation for **Health Maintenance Organization.**

HMS Liquifilm, a trademark for an ophthalmic preparation containing a glucocorticoid (medrysone).

Ho, symbol for **holmium.**

H_2O, symbol for **water.**

Hô, symbol for **null hypothesis.**

hod-, a combining form meaning 'pertaining to pathways': *hodology, hodoneuromere.*

Hodgkin's disease /hoj′kinz/, a malignant disorder characterized by painless, progressive enlargement of lymphoid tissue, usually first evident in cervical lymph nodes; splenomegaly; and the presence of Reed-Sternberg cells, large, atypical macrophages with multiple or hyperlobulated nuclei and prominent nucleoli. Symptoms include anorexia, weight loss, generalized pruritus, low-grade fever, night sweats, anemia, and leukocytosis. The disease is diagnosed in about 7100 Americans annually, causes approximately 1700 deaths a year, affects twice as many males as females, and usually develops between 15 and 35 years of age. The diagnosis is established by blood studies, x-ray films, lymphangiograms, lymph node biopsies, and ultrasonic and computerized tomographic scans. Total lymphoid radiotherapy, using a covering mantle to protect other organs, is the treatment of choice for early stages of the disease; combination chemotherapy is the treatment for advanced disease. Long-term remissions are achieved in more than one half of the patients treated, and 60% to 90% of those with localized disease may be cured. It is widely held that Hodgkin's disease may start as an inflammatory or infectious process and then become a neoplasm; according to another theory it may be an immune disorder. Clusters of cases have been reported, but there is no conclusive evidence of a causative infectious agent, and the cause of the disease remains an enigma.

Hoffmann's atrophy. See **Werdnig-Hoffmann disease.**

Hoffmann's reflex, an abnormal reflex elicited by sudden, forceful flicking of the nail of the index, middle, or ring finger, resulting in flexion of the thumb and of the middle and distal phalanges of one of the other fingers. It is not a very reliable sign of pyramidal tract disease above the level of the seventh or eighth cervical and first thoracic vertebrae. Also called **Hoffmann's sign.**

hol-. See **holo-.**

holandric /holan′drik/, **1.** designating genes located on the nonhomologous portion of the Y chromosome. **2.** of or pertaining to traits or conditions transmitted only through the paternal line. Compare **hologynic.**

holistic health care, a system of comprehensive or total patient care that considers the physical, emotional, social, economic, and spiritual needs of the person, the response to the illness, and the impact of the illness on the person's ability to meet self-care needs. Holistic nursing is the modern nursing practice that expresses this philosophy of care. Also called **comprehensive care.**

Hollenback condenser. See **pneumatic condenser.**

hollow cathode lamp, a lamp consisting of a metal cathode and an inert gas. When an electric current is passed through the cathode, metal is dislodged. After colliding with the gas in the lamp, it emits a line spectrum of specific wavelengths related to the metal of the cathode.

holmium (Ho), a rare earth metallic element. Its atomic number is 67; its atomic weight is 164.93.

holo-, hol-, a combining form meaning 'entire, or pertaining to the whole': *holodiastolic, holomastigote, holotonia.*

holoacardius /hō′lō·əkär′dē·əs/, a separate, grossly defective monozygotic twin fetus, usually represented by a shapeless, nonformed mass in which the heart is absent and the circulation in utero is accomplished totally by the heart of the viable twin through a vascular shunt.

holoacardius acephalus, a grossly defective separate twin fetus that lacks a heart, a head, and most of the upper portion of the body.

holoacardius acormus, a grossly defective, separate twin fetus in which the trunk is malformed and little more than the head is recognizable.

holoacardius amorphus, a malformed separate twin fetus in which there are no recognizable or formed parts.

holoblastic /hol′əblas′tik/, of or pertaining to an ovum that contains little or no yolk and undergoes total cleavage. Compare **meroblastic.**

holocephalic /hō′lōsifal′ik/, a malformed fetus in which several parts are deficient although the head is complete.

holodiastolic. See **pandiastolic.**

holoenzyme, a complete enzyme-cofactor complex that gives full catalytic activity.

hologynic /hol′ōjin′ik/, **1.** designating genes located on attached X chromosomes. **2.** of or pertaining to traits or conditions transmitted only through the maternal line. Compare **holandric.**

trisomy 13. —**holoprosencephalic, holoprosencephalous,** *adj*.

holorachischisis. See **complete rachischisis.**

holosystolic. See **pansystolic.**

Holtzman inkblot technique, a modification of the Rorschach test in which many more pictures of inkblots are used, the subject is permitted only one response to each design, and the scoring is predominantly objective rather than subjective.

Homan's sign, pain in the calf with dorsiflexion of the foot, indicating thrombophlebitis or thrombosis.

homatropine methylbromide, a quaternary anticholinergic.

■ INDICATIONS: It is prescribed as an antispasmodic and as a cycloplegic and mydriatic medication in ophthalmic procedures.

■ CONTRAINDICATIONS: Narrow-angle glaucoma, asthma, obstruction of the genitourinary or GI tract, ulcerative colitis, or known hypersensitivity to this drug prohibits its use.

■ ADVERSE EFFECTS: Among the more serious adverse reactions are blurred vision, central nervous system effects, tachycardia, dry mouth, decreased sweating, and hypersensitivity reactions.

home care, a health service provided in the patient's place of residence for the purpose of promoting, maintaining, or restoring health or minimizing the effects of illness and disability. Service may include such elements as medical, dental, and nursing care, speech and physical therapy, the homemaking services of a home health aide, or the provision of transportation. The level of care needed is determined by an assessment of the nature and extent of care needed and by the ability of the patient's family and friends to assume responsibility for the care needed. Nursing may be provided by a registered nurse, licensed practical nurse, or a home health aide. Some hospitals have home care services that include regular visits by a nurse and a physician to patients in their homes.

home health agency, an organization that provides health care in the home. Medicare certification for a home health agency is dependent on the providing of skilled nursing services and of at least one additional therapeutic service.

home maintenance management: impaired, a nursing diagnosis accepted by the Fourth National Conference on the Classification of Nursing Diagnoses. This diagnosis describes the situation in which a person is unable to maintain a safe, healthy home environment without help. The causes may include any of the following: disease or injury of a member of the family or household, disorganization of the family, inadequate finances, lack of knowledge of community or neighborhood resources, impaired or disordered emotional or cognitive function, inadequate support from others, lack of knowledge, or lack of role models competent in home maintenance. Among the defining characteristics reported by the client and other members of the household are difficulty in maintaining the home in a comfortable condition, a need for help from the outside in maintaining the home, and the existence of debt or a financial crisis. Among the defining characteristics that may be observed in the home are disorder, an offensive odor, an inappropriate temperature, lack of necessary equipment or supplies, and the presence of rodents or vermin. The critical defining characteristics, at least one of which must be present for the diagnosis to be made, are unwashed or unavailable cooking utensils, clothes, or linens; the presence of accumulations of dirt, food, waste, and refuse; exhausted or distressed family or household members; and repeated infections and infestations resulting from a lack of hygiene. See also **nursing diagnosis.**

homeo-, homoeo-, homoio-, a combining form meaning 'sameness, similarity': *homeochrome, homeomorphus, homeothermal.*

homeodynamics, the constantly changing interrelatedness of body components while maintaining an overall equilibrium.

Homeopathic Pharmacopoeia of the United States, one of the three official drug compendia specified in the Federal Food, Drug, and Cosmetic Act. See also **compendium, National Formulary, United States Pharmacopoeia.**

homeopathist /hō′mē·op′əthist/, a physician who practices homeopathy.

homeopathy /hō′mē·op′əthē/, a system of therapeutics based on the theory that "like cures like." The theory was advanced in the late eighteenth century by Dr. Samuel Hahnemann, who believed that a large amount of a particular drug may cause symptoms of a disease and moderate dosage may reduce those symptoms; thus, some disease symptoms could be treated by very small doses of medicine. In practice, homeopathists dilute drugs with milk sugar in ratios of 1 to 10 to achieve the smallest dose of a drug that seems necessary to control the symptoms in a patient and prescribe only one medication at a time. Compare **allopathy.** –**homeopathic,** *adj.*

homeostasis /hō′mē·əstā′sis/, a relative constancy in the internal environment of the body, naturally maintained by adaptive responses that promote healthy survival. Various sensing, feedback, and control mechanisms function to effect this steady state. Some of the key control mechanisms are the reticular formation in the brainstem and the endocrine glands. Some of the functions controlled by homeostatic mechanisms are the heartbeat, hematopoiesis, blood pressure, body temperature, electrolytic balance, respiration, and glandular secretion. –**homeostatic,** *adj.*

homeotypic /hō′mē·ōtip′ik/, pertaining to or characteristic of the regular or usual type, specifically applied to the second meiotic division of germ cells in gametogenesis as distinguished from the first meiotic division. Also **homeotypical.** Compare **heterotypic.**

homeotypic mitosis, the equational division of chromosomes, as occurs in the second meiotic division of germ cells in gametogenesis. Compare **heterotypic mitosis.**

Home's silver precipitation method, (in dentistry) a technique for depositing silver in enamel and dentin by the application of ammoniac silver nitrate solution and its reduction with formalin or eugenol.

homicide, the death of one human being caused by another human. Homicide is usually intentional and often violent.

hominal physiology, the study of the specific physical and chemical processes involved in the normal functioning of humans; human physiology.

homiothermal. See **warm-blooded.**

homiothermic, pertaining to the ability of warm-blooded animals to maintain a relatively stable internal temperature regardless of the temperature of the environment. This ability is not fully developed in newborn humans.

homo-, **1.** a combining form meaning 'the same': *homocentric, homodont, homolysis.* **2.** a combining form meaning 'the addition of one CH_2 group to the main compound': *homochelidonine, homocystine, homoquinine.*

homoblastic, developing from the same germ layer or a single type of tissue. Compare **heteroblastic.**

homochronous inheritance, the appearance of traits or conditions in the offspring at the same age as they appeared in the parents.

homocystinuria /hō′mōsis′tino͝or′ē·ə/, a rare biochemical abnormality characterized by the abnormal presence of homocystine, an amino acid, in the blood and urine, caused by any of several enzyme deficiencies in the metabolic pathway of methionine to cystine. Inherited as an autosomal recessive trait, the clinical signs of the disease are similar to Marfan's syndrome, including mental retardation, osteoporosis leading to skeletal abnormalities, dislocated lenses, and thromboembolism. Treatment may include a diet low in methionine and supplementation with large doses of vitamin B_6. Long-term results of treatment are not available. –**homocystinuric,** *adj.*

homoeo-. See **homeo-.**

homogeneous, **1.** consisting of similar elements or parts. **2.** having a uniform quality throughout. Compare **heterogeneous.** –**homogeneity,** *adj.*

homogenesis, reproduction by the same process in succeeding generations so that offspring are similar to the parents. Compare **heterogenesis.**

origin. Compare **homoplasty.**

homograft. See **allograft.**

homoio-. See **homeo-.**

homolateral, pertaining to the same side of the body.

homolog /hom′əlog/, **1.** any organ corresponding in function, origin, and structure to another organ, as the flippers of a seal that correspond to human hands. **2.** (in chemistry) one of a series of compounds, each formed by an added common element; for example, CO, carbon monoxide, is followed by CO_2, carbon dioxide, with the addition of an oxygen atom. Also spelled **homologue.** Compare **analog.** **–homologous,** *adj.*

homologous chromosomes, any two chromosomes in the diploid complement of the somatic cell that are identical in size, shape, and gene loci. In humans there are 22 pairs of homologous chromosomes and one pair of sex chromosomes, with one member of each pair being derived from the mother and the other from the father. Any deviation in the size, number, or genetic makeup of the chromosomes results in defects or disorders of varying severity in the affected individual.

homologous disease. See **graft-versus-host reaction.**

homologous insemination. See **artificial insemination-husband.**

homologous tumor, a neoplasm made up of cells resembling those of the tissue in which it is growing.

homonymous hemianopia, blindness or defective vision in the right or left halves of the visual fields of both eyes.

homoplasty, having a likeness in form or structure acquired through similar environmental conditions or parallel evolution rather than because of common ancestral origin. Compare **homogeny.** **–homoplastic,** *adj.*

homopolymer, a compound formed from subunits that are the same, as a carbohydrate composed of a series of glucose units.

homosexual, **1.** of, pertaining to, or denoting the same sex. **2.** a person who is sexually attracted to members of the same sex. Compare **heterosexual.** See also **lesbian.**

homosexual panic, an acute attack of anxiety based on unconscious conflicts concerning gender identity and a fear of being homosexual. Compare **heterosexual panic.**

individual who is homozygous for a particular characteristic has inherited from each parent one of two identical genes for that characteristic. A person homozygous for a genetic disease caused by a pair of recessive genes, as sickle cell anemia, manifests the disorder, and his or her offspring have a 100% chance of inheriting the gene for the disease. Compare **heterozygous.**

homunculus /hōmung′kyələs/, *pl.* **homunculi,** **1.** a dwarf in which all the body parts are proportionally developed and in which there is no deformity or abnormality. **2.** (in early embryologic theories of development, primarily preformation) a minute and complete human being contained in each of the germ cells that after fertilization grows from the microscopic to normal size; by extension, the human fetus. **3.** a small anatomic model of the human form; a manikin, specifically, one believed to have been produced by an alchemist and placed in a flask. **4.** (in psychiatry) a little man created by the imagination who possesses magical powers.

hookworm, *nontechnical.* a nematode of the genera *Ancylostoma, Necator,* or *Uncinaria.* Most hookworm infections in the Western Hemisphere are caused by the species *Necator americanus.*

hopelessness, a psychologic condition characterized by a belief that all efforts to alter one's life situation will be fruitless.

hordeolum /hôrdē′ələm/, a furuncle of the margin of the eyelid originating in the sebaceous gland of an eyelash. Treatment includes hot compresses and antibiotic ophthalmic preparations; it occasionally requires incision and drainage. Also called **sty.** Compare **chalazion.**

horizon, a specific stage of human embryonic development based on the appearance and ultimate formation of certain anatomic characteristics. The classification comprises 23 stages, each lasting 2 to 3 days, beginning with the fertilization of the ovum and ending 7 to 9 weeks later with the initiation of the fetal period of intrauterine life.

horizontal angulation, (in dentistry) the measured angle within the occlusal plane at which the primary x-ray beam is directed, relative to a reference in the vertical or sagital plane. Compare **vertical angulation.**

horizontal fissure of the right lung, a cleft that marks the separation of the upper and middle lobes of the right lung.

horizontal resorption, a pattern of bone reduction in marginal periodontitis whereby the marginal crest of the alveolar bone between adjacent teeth remains level and the bases of the periodontal pockets are supracrestal. Compare **vertical resorption.** See also **resorption.**

horizontal transmission, the spread of an infectious agent from one person or group to another, usually through contact with contaminated material, such as sputum or feces.

horm-, a combining form meaning 'to urge or stimulate': *hormesis, hormonal, hormothyrin.*

hormic psychology, (in psychology) the school that stresses the purposive, goal-oriented nature of human behavior. Also called **hormism.**

hormone, a complex chemical substance produced in one part or organ of the body that initiates or regulates the activity of an organ or a group of cells in another part of the body. Hormones secreted by the endocrine glands are carried through the bloodstream to the target organ. Secretion of these hormones is regulated by other hormones, by neurotransmitters, and by a negative feedback system in which an excess of target organ activity signals a decreased need for the stimulating hormone. This principal is integral to oral contraceptive pills. A steady supply of estrogen and progesterone in the medication causes a reduction in the secretion of the pituitary hormones that ordinarily stimulate the ovary to develop the follicle, release the egg, and secrete the estrogen and progesterone. Other hormones are released by organs for local effect, most commonly in the digestive tract.

-hormone, **1.** a combining form meaning a 'chemical substance possessing a regulatory effect' classified by source: *necrohormone, phytohormone, zoohormone.* **2.** a combining form meaning a 'chemical substance possessing a regulatory effect' classified by activity affected: *cytohormone, neurohormone, parathormone.*

Horner's syndrome, a neurologic condition characterized by miotic pupils, ptosis, and facial anhidrosis, resulting from a lesion in the spinal cord, with damage to a cervical nerve. In the case of traumatic injury, the person is carried prone or supine with as little movement as possible.

horny layer. See **stratum corneum.**

horripilation. See **pilomotor reflex.**

horse serum, immune serum prepared from the blood of a horse, especially tetanus antitoxin. Because many people are sensitive to horse serum, a skin test for sensitivity is usually performed before immunization. Tetanus immune globulin prepared from human immune serum is preferred.

horseshoe fistula, an abnormal, semicircular passage in the perianal area with both openings on the surface of the skin.

Hortega cells. See **microglia.**

Horton's arteritis. See **temporal arteritis.**

Horton's headache. See **migrainous cranial neuralgia.**

Horton's histamine cephalalgia. See **histamine headache.**

hospice /hos′pis/, a system of family-centered care designed to assist the chronically ill person to be comfortable and to maintain a satisfactory life style through the terminal phases of dying. Hospice care is multidisciplinary and includes home visits, professional medical help available on call, teaching and emotional support of the family, and physical care of the client. Some hospice programs provide care in a center, as well as in the home. See also **emotional care of the dying patient, stages of dying.**

hospital-acquired infection. See **nosocomial infection.**

hospitalism, the physical or mental effects of hospitalization or institutionalization on patients, especially infants and children in whom the condition is characterized by social regression, personality disorders, and stunted growth. See also **anaclitic depression.**

Hospital Survey and Construction Act. See **Hill-Burton Act.**

host, **1.** an organism in which another, usually parasitic, organism is nourished and harbored. A **primary** or **definitive host** is one in which the adult parasite lives and reproduces. A **secondary,** or **intermediate host** is one in which the parasite exists in its nonsexual, larval stage. A **reservoir host** is a primary animal host for organisms that are sometimes parasitic in humans and from which humans may become infected. **2.** the recipient of a transplanted organ or tissue. Compare **donor.**

hostility, the tendency of an organism to threaten harm to another or to itself. The hostility may be expressed passively and actively.

hot bath, a bath in which the temperature of the water is gradually raised to about 106° F.

hot flash, a transient sensation of warmth experienced by some women during or after menopause. Hot flashes result from autonomic vasomotor disturbances that accompany changes in the neurohormonal activity of the ovaries, hypothalamus, and pituitary. The exact causative mechanism is not known. Most menopausal women do not experience hot flashes; among those who do, the frequency, duration, and intensity of flashes vary widely. Though physically harmless, the symptom may be extremely disturbing or, rarely, disabling. Hot flashes may be alleviated by cyclic administration of exogenous estrogen. Also called **hot flush.**

hot line, a means of contacting a trained counselor or specific agency for help with a particular problem, as a rape hot line or a battered child hot line. The person needing help calls a telephone number and speaks to a counselor who remains anonymous and who offers emotional support, specific recommendations for action, and referral to other medical, social, or community services. Such services are usually maintained by volunteers who answer phones 24 hours a day, 7 days a week.

in front of the kneecap, characterized by redness and swelling. It is caused by prolonged and repetitive pressure of the knee on a hard surface.

house organ, a publication designed for distribution to the employees or members of an institution or business. A house organ may be prepared by a staff within the institution or business, or it may be prepared by an outside agency for the institution or business.

house physician, a physician on call and immediately available in a hospital or other health care facility.

house surgeon, a surgeon on call and immediately available on the premises of a hospital.

housewives' eczema, *nontechnical.* contact dermatitis of the hands caused and exacerbated by their frequent immersion in water and by the use of soaps and detergents.

Houston's valves. See **plicae transversales recti.**

Howell-Jolly bodies, spheric and granular inclusions in the erythrocytes observed on microscopic examination of stained blood smears. They are most commonly seen in people who have hemolytic or pernicious anemia, leukemia, thalassemia, or congenital absence of the spleen and in those who have had a splenectomy.

HPL, abbreviation for **human placental lactogen.**

h.s., (in prescriptions) abbreviation for *hora somni,* a Latin phrase meaning "bedtime."

HSA, abbreviation for **health systems agency.**

HSV, abbreviation for *herpes simplex virus*. See **herpes genitalis, herpes simplex.**

Hubbard tank, a large tank in which a patient may be immersed to perform underwater exercise. The mechanism provides superficial heat and is generally used for exercising the trunk and lower limbs. See also **whirlpool bath.**

Huhn's gland, an anterior lingual gland imbedded in tissues on the inferior surface and near the apex and midline of the tongue.

Humafac, a trademark for human antihemophilic factor (factor VIII).

human bite, a wound caused by the piercing of skin by human teeth. Bacteria are usually present, and serious infection often follows. The area is thoroughly washed, using an antiseptic, and rinsed well. The wound is examined frequently and appropriate antibiotic therapy instituted, if necessary.

DNA technology. The advantages of human insulin are in eliminating allergic reactions that occur with the use of animal insulins, especially in patients who are non-insulin-dependent but who require insulin on a short-term basis. See also **insulin,** def.2.

human investigations committee, a committee established in a hospital, school, or university to review applications for research involving human subjects to protect the rights of the people to be studied. Also called **human subjects review committee.**

humanistic existential therapy, a kind of psychotherapy that promotes self-awareness and personal growth by stressing current reality and by analyzing and altering specific patterns of response to help realize the potential of a person. This process may be facilitated in a group setting, where additional aspects of problems are revealed through interaction with others. Kinds of humanistic existential psychotherapy are **client-oriented therapy, existential therapy, Gestalt therapy.** Also called **existential humanistic psychotherapy.**

humanistic nursing model, a conceptual framework in which the nurse-patient relationship is analyzed as a human-to-human event rather than a nurse-to-patient interaction. The nurse makes therapeutic use of therself, understanding the effects of nursing actions. Four phases are recognized in the development of the therapeutic relationship. The encounter phase is followed by the phase in which the identities of the nurse and patient emerge. The nurse empathizes and then sympathizes with the patient. The meaning of the patient's experience is important; hope and suffering are seen as central to that experience. Self-knowledge and self-awareness on the part of the nurse are essential. Nursing intervention proceeds in five steps: observation of the need for intervention; validation of this observation; determination of the ability of the nurse to meet the necessity for referral; formulation of a plan for meeting the need; and evaluation of the degree to which the need was met.

humanistic psychology, a branch of psychology that emphasizes a person's struggle to develop and maintain an integrated, harmonious personality as the primary motivational force in human behavior. See also **self-actualization.**

human leukocyte antigen (HLA), any one of four significant genetic markers identified as specific loci on chromosome 6. They are HLA-A, HLA-B, HLA-C, and HLA-D. Each locus has several genetically determined alleles; each of these is associated with certain diseases or conditions, as HLA-B27 is usually present in people who have ankylosing spondylitis. The HLA system is used to assess tissue compatibility. White blood cells are used for testing. Perfect tissue compatibility exists only between identical twins.

human placental lactogen (HPL), a placental hormone that may be deficient in certain abnormalities of pregnancy. The normal concentrations of this hormone in serum after the fifth week of pregnancy are 0.5 mcg/ml and increase to approximately 8 mcg/ml at the time of delivery.

human subjects investigation committee. See **human investigations committee.**

Humatin, a trademark for an antiamebic (paromomycin sulfate).

humeral. See **humerus.**

humeral articulation. See **shoulder joint.**

humerus /hyo͞o′mərəs/, *pl.* **humeri,** the largest bone of the upper arm, comprising a body, a head, and a condyle. The body is almost cylindric proximally and prismatic and flattened distally, and has two borders and three surfaces. The nearly hemispheric head articulates with the glenoid cavity of the scapula and has a constriction called the surgical neck, frequently the seat of a fracture. The condyle at the distal end has several depressions into which articulate the radius and ulna. Also called **arm bone.** **–humeral,** *adj.*

humidifier lung, a type of hypersensitivity pneumonitis common among workers involved with refrigeration and air conditioning equipment. The antigens to which the hypersensitive reaction occurs are genera of the fungi *Micropolyspora* and *Thermoactinomyces*. Symptoms of the acute form of the disease include chills, cough, fever, dyspnea, anorexia, nausea, and vomiting. The chronic form of the disease is characterized by fatigue, chronic cough, weight loss, and dyspnea on exercise. Also called **air conditioner lung.** See also **pneumonitis.**

humoral immunity /hyo͞o′mərəl/, one of the two forms of immunity that respond to antigens such as bacteria and foreign tissue. Humoral immunity is the result of the development and the continuing presence of circulating antibodies carried in the immunoglobulins IgA, IgB, and IgM. Circulating antibodies are produced by the plasma cells of the reticuloendothelial system. Compare **cellular immunity.**

humoral response, one of a broad category of hypersensitivity reactions. Humoral responses are mediated by B cell lymphocytes and occur in type I, type II, and type III hypersensitivity reactions. Compare **cell-mediated immunity.**

Humorsol, a trademark for an ophthalmic anticholinesterase agent (demecarium bromide).

hung-up reflex, a deep tendon reflex in which, after a stimulus is given and the reflex action takes place, there is a slow return of the limb to its neutral position. This prolonged relaxation phase is characteristic of the reflexes in patients with hypothyroidism. See also **deep tendon reflex.**

Hunner's ulcer. See **interstitial cystitis.**

Hunter's canal. See **adductor canal.**

Hunter's syndrome, a hereditary defect in mucopolysaccharide metabolism affecting only males, characterized by dwarfism, kyphosis, gargoylism, and mental retardation. It is transmitted as an X-linked recessive trait. Females who carry the gene can be identified by biochemical tests, and known carriers may choose to abort if amniocentesis reveals a male fetus, because males born of women who carry the trait have a 50% chance of having the syndrome. Also called **MPS II.** See also **mucopolysaccharidosis.**

Huntington's chorea, a rare, abnormal hereditary condition characterized by chronic, progressive chorea and mental deterioration that terminates in dementia. An individual afflicted with the condition usually shows the first signs in the fourth decade of life and dies about 15 years later. The condition is transmitted as an autosomal trait. Also called **chronic chorea, degenerative chorea.**

Hurler's syndrome, a type of mucopolysaccharidosis, transmitted as an autosomal-recessive trait, that results in severe mental retardation. The onset of the symptoms of Hurler's syndrome occurs within the first few months of life. Characteristic signs of the disease are enlargement of the liver and the spleen, often with cardiovascular involvement. Facial characteristics of individuals affected by Hurler's syndrome include a low forehead and enlargement of the head, sometimes resulting from hydrocephalus. Corneal clouding is common, and the neck is short. Marked kyphosis is apparent at the dorsolumbar level, and the hands and the fingers are short and broad. Flexion contractures are common with this disease. Hurler's syndrome usually results in death during childhood from cardiac complications or pulmonary disorders. Also called **gargoylism, MPS I.** See also **mucopolysaccharidosis.**

Hürthle cell adenoma, a benign tumor of the thyroid gland composed of large cells with granular eosinophilic cytoplasm (Hürthle cells). Compare **Hürthle cell carcinoma.**

Hürthle cell carcinoma, a malignant neoplasm of the thyroid gland composed of Hürthle cells. Tumors of this kind, which occur more often in women than in men, are encapsulated and resemble adenomas, but they are locally invasive. See also **Hürthle cell adenoma.**

Hürthle cell tumor, a neoplasm of the thyroid gland composed of large cells with granular eosinophilic cytoplasm (Hürthle cells); it may be benign (Hürthle cell adenoma) or malignant (Hürthle cell carcinoma).

husband-coached childbirth. See **Bradley method.**

Hutchinson's disease. See **angioma serpiginosum.**

Hutchinson's freckle, a tan patch on the skin that grows slowly, becoming mottled, dark, thick, and nodular. The lesion is usually seen on one side of the face of an elderly person. Local excision is recommended because it

time through the His-Purkinje system, measured from the earliest onset of the His potential to the onset of ventricular activation as recorded on the electrocardiogram leads.

hyal-. See **hyalo-.**

hyaline cartilage, the gristly, elastic connective tissue comprised of specialized cells in a translucent, pearly-blue matrix. Hyaline cartilage thinly covers the articulating ends of bones, connects the ribs to the sternum, and supports the nose, trachea, and part of the larynx. It is covered by a membranous perichondrium, except where it coats the ends of bones, and tends to calcify in advanced age. Compare **yellow cartilage, white fibrocartilage.**

hyaline cast, a transparent cast composed of mucoprotein.

hyaline membrane disease. See **acute respiratory distress syndrome of the newborn.**

hyaline thrombus, a translucent, colorless mass consisting of hemolyzed erythrocytes.

hyalo-, hyal-, a combining form meaning 'resembling glass': *hyaloenchondroma, hyaloplasm, hyaloid.*

hyaloid artery /hī′əloid/, an embryonic blood vessel that branches to supply the vitreous body of the eye and develops part of the blood supply to the capsula vasculosa lentis. The hyaloid artery disappears from the fetus in the ninth month of pregnancy, leaving a vestigial remnant, the hyaloid canal, which persists in the adult as a narrow passage through the vitreous body from the optic disc to the posterior surface of the crystalline lens.

hyaloplasm /hī′əlōplaz′əm/, the portion of the cytoplasm that is clear and more fluid, as opposed to the granular and reticular part. Also called **cytohyaloplasm, cytolymph, enchylema, hyalotome, interfilar mass, interfibrillar mass of Flemming, paramitome, paraplasm.**

hyaluronic acid /hī′əlo͞oron′ik/, a mucopolysaccharide formed by the polymerization of acetylglucosamine and glucuronic acid, occurring in vitreous humor, synovial fluids, and various tissues. Known as the cement substance of tissues, it forms a gel in intercellular spaces.

hyaluronidase /hī′əlyo͞oron′ədās/, an enzyme that hydrolyzes hyaluronic acid.

■ INDICATIONS: It is prescribed to increase the absorption and dispersion of other parenteral drugs, for hypodermo-

hybrid computer, a computer that combines the characteristics of a digital computer and an analog computer by its capacity to accept input and provide output in either digital or analog form and to process information digitally. Compare **analog computer, digital computer.**

hybridization, **1.** the process of producing hybrids by crossbreeding. **2.** (in molecular genetics) the process of combining single-stranded nucleic acids whose base composition is identical but whose base sequence is different to form stable double-stranded duplex molecules. The technique involves the fragmentation and separation of the double-stranded molecules by heating, then recombination through cooling. The resulting hybrids can be of a DNA-DNA, DNA-RNA, or RNA-RNA nature.

hybrid subtraction, a two step subtraction method for producing digitalized x-ray images that uses at least four images. Both energy and temporal subtraction steps are used to mitigate patient motion artifacts.

hybrid vigor. See **heterosis.**

Hycodan, a trademark for a fixed-combination drug containing an anticholinergic (homatropine methylbromide) and an antitussive (hydrocodone bitartrate), used for cough relief.

Hycomine, a trademark for a fixed-combination drug containing an adrenergic (phenylpropanolamine hydrochloride) and an antitussive (hydrocodone bitartrate), used to treat coughs.

hydantoin /hīdan′tō•in/, any one of a group of anticonvulsant medications, chemically and pharmacologically similar to the barbiturates, that act to limit seizure activity and reduce the spread of the abnormal electric excitation from the focus of the seizure. A primary drug in the management of almost all forms of epilepsy, the most common hydantoin in current use is phenytoin, formerly known as diphenylhydantoin. Toxic effects of the drug include cardiovascular collapse and central nervous system depression when it is given in excessive dosage intravenously, as may occur in the emergency treatment of status epilepticus. Chronic toxicity, which is related to the dosage and the route of administration, may result in behavioral change, GI disturbance, osteomalacia, gingival hyperplasia, or megaloblastic anemia. Hypersensitivity reactions are rare but serious. Frequent observation for the blood concentrations of hydantoin are necessary. Seizures are usually controlled at a level of 10 μg/ml;

higher levels of concentration are associated with toxic effects. Phenytoin interacts with many drugs, including chloramphenicol, dicumarol, disulfiram, isoniazid, salicylates, phenylbutazone, antihistamines, and some sulfonamides. The interaction usually has the adverse effect of increasing the concentration of phenytoin in the blood, resulting in toxicity. Phenytoin is sometimes also prescribed in the treatment of trigeminal neuralgia and cardiac arrhythmias.

hydatid /hī′dətid/, a cyst or cystlike structure that usually is filled with fluid, especially the cyst formed around the developing scolex of the dog tapeworm *Echinococcus granulosus*. Humans and sheep can become hosts to the larval stage by ingesting the eggs. Hydatid cysts may be identified by palpation; they occur most commonly in the liver. An acute anaphylactoid allergic reaction may occur if the cyst ruptures. See also **hydatid cyst, hydatid mole, hydatidosis.** **–hydatidiform,** *adj.*

hydatid cyst, a cyst in the liver that contains larvae of the tapeworm *Echinococcus granulosus*, whose eggs are carried from the intestinal tract to the liver via the portal circulation. Patients are generally asymptomatic, except for hepatomegaly and a dull ache over the right upper quadrant of the abdomen. Radiologic tests are employed in diagnosis, and because no medical treatment is available, surgical removal of the cyst is indicated. Compare **hydatid mole.**

hydatid disease. See **echinococcosis.**

hydatid mole, an intrauterine neoplastic mass of grapelike enlarged chorionic villi occurring in approximately one in 1500 pregnancies in the United States and eight times more frequently in some oriental countries. Molar pregnancies are more common in older and younger women than in those between 20 and 40 years of age. The cause of the degenerative disorder is not known; it may be the result of a primary ovular defect, an intrauterine abnormality, or nutritional deficiency. Characteristic signs of the condition are extreme nausea, uterine bleeding, anemia, hyperthyroidism, an unusually large uterus for the length of pregnancy, absence of fetal heart sounds, edema, and high blood pressure. Diagnostic measures include ultrasonography, amniography, and serial bioassay of chorionic gonadotropin in the blood. In most cases the mole is discovered when abortion is threatened or in progress. Oxytocin may be used to stimulate the evacuation of a mole that is not spontaneously aborted, and curettage is usually performed several days later to be certain that no molar tissue remains in the uterus. It is important that pregnancy be avoided for at least 1 year and that assays for chorionic gonadotropin be performed to minimize the risk of developing trophoblastic choriocarcinoma. Also called **hydatidiform mole.** See also **trophoblastic disease.**

hydatidosis /hī′dətidō′sis/, infestation with the tapeworm *Echinococcus granulosus*. See also **hydatid cyst.**

Hydeltrasol, a trademark for a glucocorticoid (prednisolone sodium phosphate).

Hydeltra TBA, a trademark for a glucocorticoid (prednisolone tebutate).

Hydergine, a trademark for a fixed-combination drug containing various ergoloid mesylates.

hydr-. See **hydro-.**

hydradenitis /hī′dradənī′tis/, an infection or inflammation of the sweat glands. Also spelled **hidradenitis.**

hydralazine /hīdral′əzēn/, an antihypertensive.

■ INDICATION: It is prescribed in the treatment of hypertension.

■ CONTRAINDICATIONS: Coronary artery disease, mitral valvular rheumatic heart disease, or known sensitivity to this drug prohibits its use.

■ ADVERSE EFFECTS: Among the most serious adverse reactions are angina pectoris, palpitations, tachycardia, anorexia, tremors, blood dyscrasias, depression, nausea, and peripheral neuritis.

hydralazine hydrochloride, a vasodilator.

■ INDICATION: It is prescribed in the treatment of high blood pressure.

■ CONTRAINDICATIONS: Coronary artery disease, mitral valvular rheumatic heart disease, or known hypersensitivity to this drug prohibits its use.

■ ADVERSE EFFECTS: Among the more serious adverse reactions are headache, anorexia, tachycardia, GI disturbances, and a syndrome resembling lupus erythematosus.

hydramnios /hīdram′nē·əs/, an abnormal condition of pregnancy characterized by an excess of amniotic fluid. It occurs in less than 1% of pregnancies and is diagnosed by palpation, ultrasound, or x-ray examination. It is associated with maternal disorders, including toxemia of pregnancy and diabetes mellitus. Some fetal disorders, including anomalies of the GI tract, respiratory tract, and cardiovascular system may interfere with normal exchange of amniotic fluid, resulting in hydramnios. Fetal hydrops and multiple gestation are also associated with the condition. The incidence of premature rupture of the membranes, premature labor, and perinatal mortality are increased. Periodic amniocentesis may be necessary. Also called **hydramnion, polyhydramnios.** Compare **acute hydramnios, oligohydramnios.**

hydrargyrism. See **mercury poisoning.**

Hydrazol, a trademark for a carbonic anhydrase inhibitor (acetazolamide).

Hydrea, a trademark for an antineoplastic (hydroxyurea).

hydremic ascites, an abnormal accumulation of fluid within the peritoneal cavity accompanied by hemodilution, as in protein calorie malnutrition. See also **ascites.**

-hydria, a combining form meaning 'level of fluid in the body': *histohydria, isohydria, oligohydria*.

hydro-, hydr-, a combining form meaning 'pertaining to water or hydrogen': *hydroadipsia, hydrocele, hydropexis*.

hydroa /hīdrō′ə/, an unusual vesicular and bullous skin condition of childhood that recurs each summer after

peritoneal cavity and the scrotum to close completely during prenatal development. In some newborn infants the defect may resolve spontaneously after neonatal obliteration of the communication. Treatment for persistent hydrocele is surgery. Aspiration is only a temporary measure and may induce secondary infection. See also **inguinal hernia.**

hydrocephalus, a pathologic condition characterized by an abnormal accumulation of cerebrospinal fluid, usually under increased pressure, within the cranial vault and subsequent dilatation of the ventricles. Interference with the normal flow of cerebrospinal fluid may be caused by increased secretion of the fluid, obstruction within the ventricular system (noncommunicating or intraventricular hydrocephalus), or defective reabsorption from the cerebral subarachnoid space (communicating or extraventricular hydrocephalus), resulting from developmental anomalies, infection, trauma, or brain tumors. Also called **hydrocephaly.** **–hydrocephalic,** *adj., n.*

■ OBSERVATIONS: The condition may be congenital with rapid onset of symptoms or it may progress slowly so that neurologic manifestations do not appear until early to late childhood or even until early adulthood. In infants, the head grows at an abnormal rate with separation of the sutures, bulging fontanelles, and dilated scalp veins, the face becomes disproportionately small, and the eyes appear depressed within the sockets. Typical behavior includes irritability with lethargy and vomiting, opisthotonos, lower extremity spasticity, and failure to perform normal reflex actions. If the condition progresses, lower brainstem function is disrupted, the skull becomes enormous, the cortex is destroyed, and the infant displays somnolence, seizures, and cardiopulmonary obstruction, usually not surviving the neonatal period. At later onset, after the cranial sutures have fused and the skull has formed, symptoms are primarily neurologic and include headache, edema of the optic disc, strabismus, and loss of muscular coordination. Hydrocephalus in infants is suspected when head growth is observed to be in excess of the normal rate. In all age groups diagnosis is confirmed by such procedures as cerebrospinal fluid examination, computerized axial tomography, air encephalography, arteriography, and echoencephalography.

nutrition, proper positioning and support to prevent extra strain on the neck, and assistance with diagnostic evaluation and procedures. Postoperatively, in addition to routine care and observation to prevent complications, especially infection, the nurse gives support to the parents and teaches them how to care for a child with a functioning shunt, specifically how to recognize signs that indicate shunt malfunction or infection and how to pump the shunt.

hydrochloric acid, a compound consisting of hydrogen and chlorine. Hydrochloric acid is secreted in the stomach and is a major component of gastric juice.

hydrochlorothiazide, a diuretic and antihypertensive.

■ INDICATIONS: It is prescribed in the treatment of hypertension and edema.

■ CONTRAINDICATIONS: Anuria or known hypersensitivity to this drug, to other thiazide medication, or to sulfonamide derivatives prohibits its use.

■ ADVERSE EFFECTS: Among the more serious adverse effects are hypoglycemia, hyperglycemia, hyperuricemia, and hypersensitivity reactions.

hydrocholeretics, drugs that stimulate the production of bile with a low specific gravity, or with a minimal proportion of solid constituents.

Hydrocil, a trademark for a laxative (psyllium hydrophilic muciloid).

hydrocodone bitartrate, a narcotic antitussive.

■ INDICATION: It is prescribed in the treatment of cough.

■ CONTRAINDICATIONS: Drug dependence or known hypersensitivity to this drug prohibits its use.

■ ADVERSE EFFECTS: Among the more serious adverse reactions are drug dependence and respiratory and circulatory depression.

hydrocortisone, hydrocortisone acetate, hydrocortisone cyclopentylpropionate, hydrocortisone sodium succinate. See **cortisol.**

hydrocortisone valerate, a topical corticosteroid.

■ INDICATION: It is used topically as an antiinflammatory agent.

■ CONTRAINDICATIONS: Viral and fungal diseases of the skin that occur where circulation is impaired or known hypersensitivity to steroids prohibits its use.

■ ADVERSE REACTIONS: Among the more serious adverse reactions are various systemic side effects that may occur from prolonged or excessive use. Local irritation of the skin may occur.

Hydrocortone, a trademark for a glucocorticoid (hydrocortisone acetate).

Hydro Diuril, a trademark for a diuretic (hydrochlorothiazide).

hydroflumethiazide, a diuretic and antihypertensive.

■ INDICATIONS: It is prescribed in the treatment of hypertension and edema.

■ CONTRAINDICATIONS: Anuria or known hypersensitivity to this drug, to other thiazide medication, or to sulfonamide derivatives prohibits its use.

■ ADVERSE EFFECTS: Among the more serious adverse effects are blood disorders, hypotension, hypokalemia, hyperglycemia, hyperuricemia, and hypersensitivity reactions.

hydrogen (H), a gaseous, univalent element. Its atomic number is 1; its atomic weight is 1.008. It is the simplest and the lightest of the elements and is normally a colorless, odorless, highly inflammable diatomic gas. It occurs in pure form only sparsely in the earth and the atmosphere but is plentiful in the sun and in many other stars. Hydrogen is a component of numerous compounds, many of them produced by the body. As a component of water, hydrogen is crucial in the metabolic interaction of acids, bases, and salts within the body and in the fluid balance necessary for the body to survive. Hydrogen makes it possible for water, which serves as a host to many body functions, to dissolve the many different substances on which the body depends, as oxygen and food substances. Hydrogen makes possible the process of hydrolysis by which compounds unite with water and split into simpler compounds.

hydrogenation. See **reduction.**

hydrogen bonding, the attractive force of compounds in which a hydrogen atom covalently linked to an electronegative element, as oxygen, nitrogen, or sulfur, has a large degree of positive character relative to the electronegative atom, thereby causing the compound to possess a large dipole.

hydrogen peroxide, a topical antiinfective.

■ INDICATIONS: It is prescribed to cleanse open wounds, as a mouthwash, and to aid in the removal of cerumen in the external ear.

■ CONTRAINDICATIONS: Irritations to skin or mucous membranes or known hypersensitivity to this agent prohibits its use.

■ ADVERSE EFFECTS: There are no known adverse effects.

hydrolase, an enzyme that cleaves ester bonds by the addition of water.

Hydrolose, a trademark for a laxative (methylcellulose).

hydrolysis /hīdrol′isis/, the chemical alteration or decomposition of a compound with water.

hydrometer /hīdrom′ətər/, a device that determines the specific gravity or density of a liquid by a comparison of its weight with that of an equal volume of water. A calibrated, hollow glass device is placed in the liquid being examined, and the depth to which the device settles in the liquid is noted.

hydromorphone hydrochloride, a narcotic analgesic.

■ INDICATION: It is used to treat moderate to severe pain.

■ CONTRAINDICATIONS: It is used with caution in many conditions, including head injuries, asthma, impaired renal or hepatic function, or unstable cardiovascular status. Known hypersensitivity to this drug prohibits its use.

■ ADVERSE EFFECTS: Among the most serious adverse reactions are drowsiness, dizziness, nausea, constipation, respiratory and circulatory depression, and drug addiction.

hydronephrosis /hī′drōnefrō′sis/, distention of the pelvis and calyces of the kidney by urine that cannot flow past an obstruction in a ureter. Ureteral obstruction may be caused by a tumor, a calculus lodged in the ureter, inflammation of the prostate gland, or edema caused by a urinary tract infection. The person may experience pain in the flank and, in some cases, hematuria, pyuria, and hyperpyrexia. Intravenous pyelography, cytoscopy, or retrograde pyelography may be used in diagnosis. Surgical repair or removal of the obstruction may be necessary. Prolonged hydronephrosis will result in atrophy and eventual loss of kidney function. See also **urinary calculi.** **–hydronephrotic,** *adj.*

hydropenia, lack of water in the body tissues.

hydrophilic, pertaining to the property of attracting water molecules, possessed by polar radicals or ions. Compare **hydrophobic.**

hydrophobia, **1.** *nontechnical.* rabies. **2.** a morbid, extreme fear of water.

hydrophobic, pertaining to the property of repelling water molecules or side chains that are more soluble in organic solvents. Compare **hydrophilic.**

hydrophthalmos. See **congenital glaucoma.**

Hydropres, a trademark for a fixed-combination drug containing a diuretic (hydrochlorothiazide) and an antihypertensive (reserpine).

hydrops /hī′drops/, an abnormal accumulation of clear, watery fluid in a body tissue or cavity, as a joint, a graafian follicle, a fallopian tube, the abdomen, the middle ear, or the gallbladder. Hydrops in the entire body may occur in infants born with thalassemia or severe Rh sensitization. Formerly called **dropsy.**

hydrops fetalis, massive edema in the fetus or newborn, usually in association with severe erythroblastosis fetalis. Severe anemia and effusions of the pericardial, pleural, and peritoneal spaces also occur. The condition usually leads to death, even with immediate exchange transfusions after delivery. Also called **fetal hydrops.**

hydroquinone /hī′drōkwin′ōn/, a dermatologic bleaching agent.

■ INDICATIONS: It is prescribed to reduce pigmentation of the skin in certain skin conditions in which an excess of

phase of the inflammatory process.

hydrostatic pressure, the pressure exerted by a liquid.

hydrotherapy, the use of water in the treatment of various mental and physical disorders. Hydrotherapy may include continuous tub baths, wet sheet packs, or shower sprays.

hydrothorax, a noninflammatory accumulation of serous fluid in one or both plural cavities.

hydrotropism, the tendency of a cell or organism to turn or move in a certain direction under the influence of a water stimulus. Compare **chemotropism.**

hydrous wool fat. See **lanolin.**

hydroxyamphetamine hydrobromide, an adrenergic and mydriatic.

■ INDICATIONS: It is prescribed for dilatation of the pupil for ophthalmoscopy and as a diagnostic aid in Horner's syndrome.

■ CONTRAINDICATIONS: Narrow-angle glaucoma or known hypersensitivity to this drug prohibits its use.

■ ADVERSE EFFECTS: Among the more serious adverse reactions are increased intraocular pressure and photophobia.

hydroxyandrosterone, a sex hormone that is secreted by the testes and adrenal glands. Its normal accumulation in the urine of men after 24-hour collection is 0.1 to 8 mg; in women, 0 to 0.5 mg.

hydroxyapatite, an inorganic compound composed of calcium, phosphate, and hydroxide. It is found in the bones and teeth in a crystallized latticelike form that gives these structures rigidity.

hydroxybenzene. See carbolic acid.

hydroxychloroquine sulfate, an antiprotozoal, antirheumatic drug that is also a suppressant of lupus erythematosus and of polymorphous light eruption.

■ INDICATIONS: It is prescribed in the treatment of malaria and for the suppression of acute paroxysmal attacks of the disease, in the treatment of extraintestinal, usually hepatic, amebiasis, and in the reduction of symptoms of lupus erythematosus and rheumatoid arthritis.

■ CONTRAINDICATIONS: Concurrent use of other 4-aminoquinolones or of gold salts or a known hypersensitivity to this drug or to other 4-aminoquinolones prohibits its use. It is used with caution in people affected with alcoholism, blood dyscrasia, severe neurologic disorder, ret-

17-hydroxycorticosteroid, any of the hormones, as cortisol, secreted by adrenal glands, measured in the urine in a test for determining adrenal function and diagnosing hypoadrenalism or hyperadrenalism. The normal accumulation of this hormone in the urine of men after 24-hour collection is 5.5 to 14.5 μg; in women, 4.9 to 12.9 μg; slightly lower in children. The levels are two to four times higher in all cases after injection of 25 USP units of adrenocorticotropic hormone.

11-hydroxyetiocholanolone, a sex hormone secreted by the testes and adrenal glands. The normal accumulation in the urine of men after 24-hour collection is 0.2 to 0.6 mg; in women, 0.1 to 1 mg.

5-hydroxyindoleacetic acid, an acid produced by serotonin metabolism, measured in the blood and urine to aid in the diagnosis of certain kinds of tumors. It commonly rises above normal levels in whole blood in association with asthma, diarrhea, rapid heartbeat, and other symptoms and is elevated in the urine of patients with carcinoid syndrome. Its normal concentrations in whole blood are 0.05 to 0.20 μg/ml; in urine after 24-hour collection, 1 to 5 mg.

hydroxyl (OH) /hīdrok′sil/, a radical compound containing an oxygen atom and a hydrogen atom.

hydroxyprogesterone caproate, a progestational steroid.

■ INDICATIONS: It is prescribed in the treatment of advanced adenocarcinoma of the uterine corpus, amenorrhea, and abnormal uterine bleeding caused by hormonal imbalance in the absence of organic disease.

■ CONTRAINDICATIONS: Markedly impaired liver function, carcinoma of the breast, undiagnosed abnormal genital bleeding, near abortion, thromboembolitic disorders, or known sensitivity to this drug prohibits its use.

■ ADVERSE EFFECTS: Among the most serious adverse reactions are thrombophlebitis, pulmonary embolism, cerebrovascular accident, neuroocular lesions, anorexia, edema, hypertension, cholestatic jaundice, and depression.

hydroxyproline, an amino acid that is elevated in the urine in diseases of the bone and certain genetic disorders, as Marfan's syndrome. Its normal accumulations in urine after 24-hour collection are 10 to 75 mg.

5-hydroxytryptamine. See **serotonin.**

hydroxyurea /hīdrok′siyŏŏrē′ə/, an antineoplastic.

■ INDICATION: It is prescribed in the treatment of a variety of neoplasms.

■ CONTRAINDICATIONS: Bone marrow depression or known hypersensitivity to this drug prohibits its use. It is not to be given to women who are or might become pregnant.

■ ADVERSE EFFECTS: The most serious adverse reaction is bone marrow depression. GI disturbances and dermatitis may also occur.

hydroxyzine hydrochloride /hīdrok′səzēn/, a minor tranquilizer.

■ INDICATIONS: It is prescribed to relieve anxiety, nervous tension, hyperkinesis, and motion sickness.

■ CONTRAINDICATION: Known hypersensitivity to this drug is the only contraindication.

■ ADVERSE EFFECTS: No serious adverse reactions have been observed. Decreased mental alertness is sometimes seen.

hygroscopic humidifier, a humidifying device attached to the tubing circuit of a mechanic ventilator or anesthesia gas machine to maintain a constant rate of humidity in the patient's trachea.

Hygroton, a trademark for a diuretic (chlorthalidone).

Hylorel, a trademark for an antihypertensive (guanadrel sulfate).

hymen /hī′mən/, a fold of mucous membrane, skin, and fibrous tissue at the introitus of the vagina. It may be absent, small, thin and pliant, or, rarely, tough and dense, completely occluding the introitus. When the hymen is ruptured, small rounded elevations remain. See also **carunculae hymenales.**

hymenal tag /hī′mənəl/, normal, redundant hymenal tissue protruding from the floor of the vagina during the first weeks after birth. It eventually disappears without treatment.

Hymenolepis /hī′minol′əpis/, a genus of intestinal tapeworms infesting humans, as *Hymenolepis nana*, the dwarf tapeworm, and *H. diminuta*. Heavy infestation by *H. nana* may cause abdominal pain, bloody stools, and disorders of the nervous system, especially in children. Contaminated food spreads the disease, which is endemic in the United States. Quinacrine hydrochloride or hexylresorcinol is used to treat the infestation.

hymenotomy /hī′mənot′əmē/, the surgical incision of the hymen.

hyoglossal. See **glossohyal.**

hyoid bone /hī′oid/, a single U-shaped bone suspended from the styloid processes of the temporal bones. The body of the hyoid is square and flat, its ventral surface convex and angled cranially. Two greater wings of the bone attach to the lateral thyroid ligaments, and the body of the bone attaches to various muscles, as the hypoglossus and the sternohyoideus. The hyoid is palpable in the neck. Also called **lingual bone, os hyoideum.**

hyoscine hydrobromide. See **scopolamine hydrobromide.**

hyoscyamine /hī′əsī′əmēn/, an anticholinergic.

■ INDICATIONS: It is prescribed in the treatment of hypermotility of the GI and the lower urinary tracts.

■ CONTRAINDICATIONS: Narrow-angle glaucoma, asthma, obstruction of the genitourinary or GI tracts, severe ulcerative colitis, or known hypersensitivity to this drug prohibits its use.

■ ADVERSE EFFECTS: Among the more serious adverse reactions are blurred vision, central nervous system effects, tachycardia, dry mouth, decreased sweating, and hypersensitivity reactions.

hypalgesia, the perception of a painful stimulus to a degree that varies significantly from a normal perception of the same stimulus.

hyp-. See **hypo-.**

hyper-, a combining form meaning 'excessive, above, or beyond': *hyperacidaminuria, hyperalkalinity, hyperechema.*

Hyperab, a trademark for a passive immunizing agent (rabies immune globulin).

hyperacidity, an excessive amount of acidity, as in the stomach. See also **hyperchlorhydria.**

hyperactivity, any abnormally increased activity involving either the entire organism or a particular organ, as the heart or thyroid. Compare **hypoactivity.** See also **attention deficit disorder.**

hyperadrenalism. See **Cushing's disease.**

hyperadrenocorticism. See **Cushing's syndrome.**

hyperaldosteronism. See **aldosteronism.**

hyperalimentation, **1.** overfeeding or the ingestion or administration of a greater than optimal amount of nutrients in excess of the demands of the appetite. **2.** See **total parenteral nutrition.**

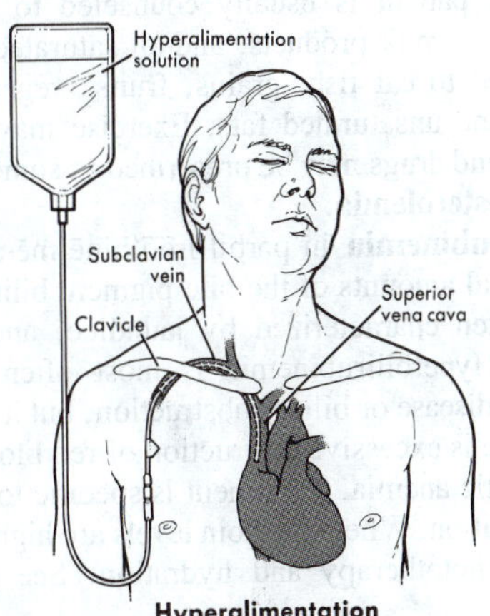

Hyperalimentation

hyperammonemia /hī′pəram′ōnē′mē·ə/, abnormally high levels of ammonia in the blood. Ammonia is produced in the intestine, absorbed into the blood, and detoxified in the liver. If there is an increased production of ammonia or a decreased ability to detoxify it, levels of ammonia in the blood may increase. Untreated, the condition leads to asterixis, vomiting, lethargy, coma, and death.

hyperbaric oxygenation, the administration of oxygen at greater than normal atmospheric pressure. The proce-

tion, acute cyanide poisoning, decompression sickness, Clostridial myonecrosis, and certain cases of blood loss or anemia in which increased oxygen transport may compensate in part for the hemoglobin deficiency. Factors limiting the usefulness of hyperbaric oxygenation include the hazards of fire and explosive decompression, pulmonary damage and neurologic toxicity at high atmospheric pressures, cardiovascular debility of the patient, and the need to interrupt treatments repeatedly because exposures at maximum atmospheric pressures must be limited to 90 minutes.

hyperbetalipoproteinemia /hī′pərbā′təlip′ōprō′tēnē′mē·ə/, type II hyperlipoproteinemia, a genetic disorder of lipid metabolism, in which there are abnormally high levels of serum cholesterol, and xanthomas appear on the tendons of the heels, knees, and fingers. There is a marked tendency to develop atherosclerosis and early myocardial infarction, especially among males. Treatment attempts to reduce blood cholesterol levels in the hope of lowering the risk of early death from heart disease. The patient is usually counseled to avoid most meats, eggs, milk products, and all saturated fats and is encouraged to eat fish, grains, fruits, vegetables, lean poultry, and unsaturated fats. Exercise may be recommended, and drugs may be prescribed in some cases. See also **cholesterolemia.**

hyperbilirubinemia /hī′pərbil′iro͞o′binē′mē·ə/, greater than normal amounts of the bile pigment bilirubin in the blood, often characterized by jaundice, anorexia, and malaise. Hyperbilirubinemia is most often associated with liver disease or biliary obstruction, but it also occurs when there is excessive destruction of red blood cells, as in hemolytic anemia. Treatment is specific to the underlying condition. When bilirubin levels are high, treatment includes phototherapy and hydration. See also **jaundice.**

hyperbilirubinemia of the newborn, an excess of bilirubin in the blood of the neonate, resulting from hepatic dysfunction. It is usually caused by a deficiency of an enzyme, resulting from physiologic immaturity, or increased hemolysis, especially from blood group incompatibility, which, in severe cases, can lead to kernicterus. Also called **neonatal hyperbilirubinemia.** See also **breast milk jaundice, cholestasis, Crigler-Najjar syndrome, Dubin-Johnson syndrome, erythroblastosis fetalis, Gilbert's syndrome, kernicterus, phototherapy in the newborn, Rotor syndrome.**

hours of life are abnormal and indicate a pathologic cause of hyperbilirubinemia. In erythroblastosis fetalis, jaundice is evident shortly after birth and bilirubin levels rise rapidly. Severely affected infants also show hepatosplenomegaly and signs of anemia, which quickly worsen, causing decreased oxygen carrying capacity that may lead to cardiac failure and shock. Early symptoms of kernicterus are lethargy, poor feeding, and vomiting, followed by severe neurologic excitation or depression, including tremors, twitching, convulsion, opisthotonos, a high-pitched cry, hypotonia, diminished deep tendon reflexes, and the absence of Moro and sucking reflexes. Brain damage generally does not occur at serum bilirubin levels below 20 mg/100 ml. Factors such as metabolic acidosis, lowered albumin levels, hypoxia, hypothermia, free fatty acids, and certain drugs, especially salicylates and sulfonamides, increase the risk at much lower levels. The mortality may reach 50%. Sequelae of kernicterus include mental retardation, minimal brain dysfunction, cerebral palsy, delayed or abnormal motor development, hearing loss, ataxia, athetosis, perceptual problems, and behavioral disorders.

■ INTERVENTION: Such preventive measures as frequent feedings during the first 6 to 12 hours of life to increase GI motility have little justification. Infants with mild jaundice require no treatment, only observation. Phototherapy is the usual treatment for severe or increasing hyperbilirubinemia. If hyperbilirubinemia is the result of increased hemolysis caused by blood group incompatibility, exchange transfusion is the standard procedure. It is usually indicated if laboratory analysis reveals a positive antiglobulin test, a hemoglobin concentration of the cord blood below 12 g/100 ml, or a bilirubin level of 20 mg/100 ml or more in a full-term infant or 15 mg/100 ml or more in a premature infant. Phototherapy may be used in conjunction with exchange transfusion, except in Rh incompatibility. If used immediately after the initial exchange transfusion, phototherapy may remove enough bilirubin from the tissues to make subsequent transfusions unnecessary. Pharmacologic management, as the use of barbiturates to stimulate protein synthesis that, in turn, increases albumin for conjugating bilirubin and promotes hepatic glucuronyl transferase synthesis, is indicated in some instances, although this form of therapy is controversial because of the known side effects of the drugs.

■ NURSING CONSIDERATIONS: An initial concern is to identify high-risk infants who may develop hyperbilirubinemia and kernicterus. The nurse may monitor the serum bilirubin levels and observe for evidence of jaundice, anemia, central nervous system irritability, and such conditions as acidosis, hypoxia, and hypothermia. In erythroblastosis fetalis, exchange transfusion may be necessary. The amounts of blood infused and withdrawn, the vital signs, and any signs of exchange reactions are noted. Resuscitative equipment is kept available. Optimal body temperature is maintained: hypothermia increases oxygen and glucose consumption, causing metabolic acidosis, and hyperthermia damages the donor's erythrocytes, causing an elevation in the amount of free potassium that may lead to infant cardiac arrest. After the procedure, a sterile dressing is applied to the catheter site.

hypercalcemia /hī′pərkalsē′mē•ə/, greater than normal amounts of calcium in the blood, most often resulting from excessive bone resorption and release of calcium, as occurs in hyperparathyroidism, metastatic tumors of bone, Paget's disease, and osteoporosis. Clinically, patients with hypercalcemia are confused and have anorexia, abdominal pain, and muscle pain and weakness. Extremely high levels of blood calcium may result in shock, kidney failure, and death. Hypercalciuria is also found in most patients with elevated blood calcium. Prednisone, diuretics, isotonic saline, and other drugs may be used in treatment. –**hypercalcemic,** *adj.*

hypercalciuria /hī′pərkal′sēyŏŏr′ē•ə/, the presence of abnormally great amounts of calcium in the urine, resulting from conditions such as sarcoid, hyperparathyroidism, or certain types of arthritis, characterized by augmented bone resorption. Immobilized patients are often hypercalciuric. Some people absorb more calcium than is normal and therefore excrete greater than normal amounts into their urine. Concentrated amounts of calcium in the urinary tract may form kidney stones. Treatment is directed toward correcting any underlying disease condition and limiting dietary intake of calcium. Also called **hypercalcinuria.** Compare **hypercalcemia.** –**hypercalciuric,** *adj.*

hypercapnia /hī′pərkap′nē•ə/, greater than normal amounts of carbon dioxide in the blood. Also called **hypercarbia.**

hyperchloremia, an excessive level of chloride in the blood.

hyperchlorhydria, the excessive secretion of hydrochloric acid by cells lining the stomach. See also **hyperacidity.**

hypercholesterolemia, a condition in which greater than normal amounts of cholesterol are present in the blood. High levels of cholesterol and other lipids may lead to the development of atherosclerosis. Hypercholesterolemia may be reduced or prevented by avoiding saturated fats, which are found in red meats, eggs, and dairy products.

hypercholesterolemic xanthomatosis. See **familial hypercholesterolemia.**

hyperchromic, having a greater density of color or pigment.

hyperchylomicronemia type I hyperlipoproteinemia, a rare congenital deficiency of an enzyme essential to fat metabolism. Fat accumulates in the blood as chylomicrons. The condition affects children and young adults, who develop xanthomas (fatty deposits) in the skin, hepatomegaly, and abdominal pain. Pancreatitis is the most significant complication. Strict limitation of dietary fat may allow the person to avoid discomfort and complications. Also called **familial lipoprotein lipase deficiency.** See also **chylomicron.**

hypercoagulability, a tendency of the blood to coagulate more rapidly than is normal.

hyperdactyly. See **polydactyly.**

hyperdiploid. See **hyperploid.**

hyperdynamic syndrome, a cluster of symptoms that signal the onset of septic shock, often including a shaking chill, rapid rise in temperature, flushing of the skin, galloping pulse, and alternating rise and fall of the blood pressure. This is a medical emergency that requires expert medical support in a hospital. Emergency measures include keeping the patient warm and elevating the feet to assist venous return. Usually, it is ordered that nothing be given by mouth and that the patient's head be turned to avoid aspiration if there is vomiting. See also **septic shock.**

hyperemesis gravidarum /hī′pərem′isis/, an abnormal condition of pregnancy characterized by protracted vomiting, weight loss, and fluid and electrolyte imbalance. If the condition is severe and intractable, brain damage, liver and kidney failure, and death may result. The cause of the condition is not known; an increase in chorionic gonadotropins or other hormones, an immunologic sensitivity to products of conception, or aggravation of preexisting emotional conflicts has been suggested, but a causal relationship has not been proven. It occurs in approximately three of every 1000 pregnancies, its incidence having diminished in recent years.

■ OBSERVATIONS: Women are frightened of and uncomfortable and embarrassed about their illness. Dehydration results in dry mucous membranes, decreased skin elasticity, a rapid pulse, and falling blood pressure. The specific gravity of the urine rises, and the volume of urine excreted falls. The hematocrit is elevated because of hemoconcentration. Loss of electrolytes in vomitus leads to metabolic acidosis with hypokalemia, hypochloremia, and hyponatremia. Severe potassium deficit alters myocardial function; the electrocardiogram may show prolonged P-R and Q-T intervals and inverted T waves. In addition to weight loss, undernourishment causes fever, ketosis, and acetonuria. Severe vitamin B deficiency may result in encephalopathy manifested by confusion and, eventually, coma. Laboratory analyses of blood indicate increased concentrations of metabolic products normally cleared from the blood by the liver and kidneys. Forceful vomiting may cause retinal hemorrhages that impair

apy are sometimes beneficial. Termination of pregnancy is curative but almost never required.

... thetic listening and supportive, nonjudgmental care are provided. The woman and her family are told often that the prognosis is excellent for both mother and baby. She is weighed regularly, and her weight is accurately recorded, for the best evidence of recovery is steady weight gain.

hyperemia /hī′pərē′mē·ə/, increased blood in part of the body, caused by increased blood flow, as in the inflammatory response, local relaxation of arterioles, or obstruction of the outflow of blood from an area. Skin overlying a hyperemic area usually becomes reddened and warm. –**hyperemic,** *adj*.

hyperextension, (of a joint) a position of maximum extension.

hyperextension bed, a bed used in pediatric orthopedics to maintain any correction achieved by suspension of a body part and to increase the range of motion of the hips after an operative muscle release procedure. The hyperextension bed may be purchased or it may be converted from a regular hospital bed. Removal of the mattress from a regular hospital bed and the addition of three half mattresses allows sufficient height to permit alternating prone and supine positions and the concomitant alternating flexion and extension of the hips. The bilateral extremities of the patient, in casts, are suspended over the lower half of the bed with rings and traction apparatus. The position of the patient's hips is alternated at 2-hour intervals; abduction and adduction can be controlled by the position of the pulleys. Restraints are required to maintain the child in position so that the horizontal, gluteal folds are even with the bottom edge of the stacked mattresses. Also called **Schwartz bed.** Compare **Circolectric bed, Foster bed, Stryker wedge frame.**

hyperextension suspension, an orthopedic procedure used in the postoperative positioning of hip muscles. The procedure uses traction equipment, including metal frames, ropes, and pulleys to relieve the weight of the lower limbs and to position properly the muscles of the hip, without applying traction to the lower limbs involved. The ropes used to suspend the lower limbs in this procedure are attached by rings to long leg casts encasing the lower limbs of the patient. Compare **balanced suspension, lower extremity suspension, upper extremity suspension.**

hyperglycemia ... a greater than normal amount of glucose in the blood. Most frequently associated with diabetes mellitus, the condition may occur in newborns, after the administration of glucocorticoid hormones, and with an excess infusion of intravenous solutions containing glucose, especially in poorly monitored, long-term hyperalimentation. Compare **hypoglycemia.**

hyperglycemic-glycogenolytic factor. See **glucagon.**

hyperglycemic-hyperosmolar nonketotic coma, a diabetic coma in which the level of ketone bodies is normal; caused by hyperosmolarity of extracellular fluid and resulting in dehydration of intracellular fluid, often a consequence of overtreatment with hyperosmolar solutions.

hyperhidrosis /hī′pərhīdrō′sis, -hidrō′sis/, excessive perspiration, often caused by heat, hyperthyroidism, strong emotion, menopause, or infection. Symptomatic therapy usually includes topical antiperspirants and may involve surgery to remove axillary sweat glands.

hyperimmune, a characteristic associated with an unusual abundance of antibodies, producing a greater than normal immunity.

hyperinsulinism, an excessive amount of insulin in the body, as may occur when a greater than required dose is administered.

hyperintention, an excessive amount of concentration on an objective, which may result in failure to accomplish the goal.

hyperkalemia /hī′pərkalē′mē·ə/, greater than normal amounts of potassium in the blood. This condition is seen frequently in acute renal failure. Early signs are nausea, diarrhea, and muscle weakness. As potassium levels increase, marked cardiac changes are observed in the ECG. Treatment of severe hyperkalemia includes the intravenous administration of sodium bicarbonate, calcium salts, and dextrose. Hemodialysis is used if these measures fail.

hyperkalemic periodic paralysis. See **adynamia episodica hereditaria.**

hyperkeratosis /hī′pərker′ətō′sis/, overgrowth of the cornified epithelial layer of the skin. See also **callus, corn.**

hyperkinesis. See **attention deficit disorder.**

hyperlipidemia, an excess of lipids in the plasma, including the glycolipids, lipoproteins, and the phospholipids. See also **antilipidemic.**

hyperlipoproteinemia /hī′pərlip′ōprō′tēnē′mē·ə/, any of a large group of inherited and acquired disorders of lipoprotein metabolism characterized by greater than normal amounts of certain protein-bound lipids and other fatty substances in the blood. The treatment includes diet to control obesity; diet may reduce lipoprotein levels in the blood. Medication and other treatment vary according to the specific metabolic defect, its cause, and its prognosis.

hypermagnesemia /hī′pərmag′nisē′mē·ə/, a greater than normal amount of magnesium in the plasma, found in people with kidney failure and in those who use a large quantity of drugs containing magnesium, as antacids. Toxic levels of magnesium cause cardiac arrhythmias and depression of deep tendon reflexes and respiration. Treatment often includes intravenous fluids, a diuretic, and hemodialysis.

hypermenorrhea. See **menorrhagia.**

hypermetria /hī′pərmē′trē·ə/, an abnormal condition, a form of dysmetria, characterized by a dysfunction of the power to control the range of muscular action, resulting in movements that overreach the intended goal of the affected individual. Compare **hypometria.**

hypermetropia, hypermetropy, See **hyperopia.**

hypermorph /hī′pərmôrf′/, **1.** a person whose arms and legs are disproportionately long in relation to the trunk, and whose sitting height is disproportionate to the standing height. **2.** (in genetics) a mutant gene that shows an increased activity in the expression of a trait. Compare **amorph, antimorph, hypomorph.**

hypernatremia /hī′pərnatrē′mē·ə/, greater than normal concentration of sodium in the blood, caused by excessive loss of water and electrolytes resulting from polyuria, diarrhea, excessive sweating, or inadequate water intake. When water loss is caused by kidney dysfunction, urine is profuse and dilute. If water loss is not through the kidneys, as in diarrhea and excessive sweating, the urine is scanty and highly concentrated. People with hypernatremia may become mentally confused, have seizures, and lapse into coma. The treatment is restoration of fluid and electrolyte balance by mouth or by IV infusion. Care must be taken to restore water balance slowly, because further electrolyte imbalances may occur. See also **diabetes insipidus.**

hyperopia /hī′pərō′pē·ə/, farsightedness, a condition resulting from an error of refraction in which rays of light entering the eye are brought into focus behind the retina. Also called **hypermetropuia, hypermetropy.** Compare **myopia.**

hyperosmia, an abnormally increased sensitivity to odors. Compare **anosmia.**

hyperosmolarity, a state or condition of abnormally increased osmolarity. **–hyperosmolar,** *adj.*

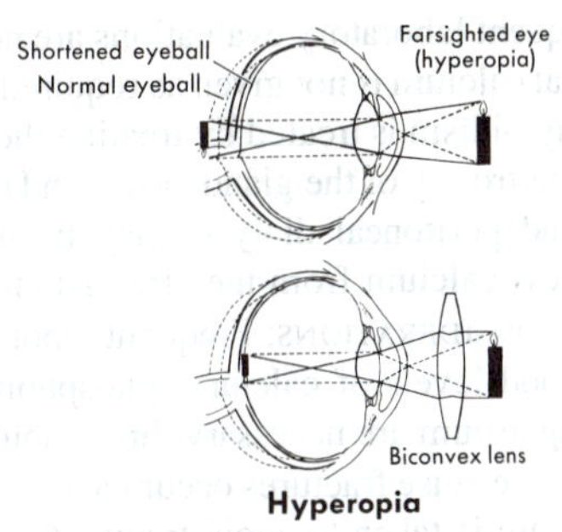

Hyperopia

hyperoxia, a condition of abnormally high oxygen tension in the blood.

hyperparathyroidism, an abnormal endocrine condition characterized by hyperactivity of any of the four parathyroid glands with excessive secretion of parathyroid hormone (PTH) that results in increased resorption of calcium from the skeletal system and increased absorption of calcium by the kidneys and GI system. The condition may be primary, originating in one or more of the parathyroid glands, or secondary, resulting from an abnormal hypocalcemia-producing condition in another part of the body causing a compensatory hyperactivity of the parathyroid glands.

■ OBSERVATIONS: Hypercalcemia in primary hyperparathyroidism results in dysfunction of most of the systems of the body. In the kidneys, tissue calcifies, calculi form, and renal failure may ensue. In the bones and joints, osteoporosis develops, causing pain and fragility; fractures, synovitis, and pseudogout often occur. In the GI tract, chronic, piercing epigastric pain may develop caused by pancreatitis. Hematemesis, anorexia, and nausea may be seen if peptic ulceration occurs. In the neuromuscular system, generalized weakness and atrophy develop if the condition is not corrected, and changes in the central nervous system result in alteration of consciousness, coma, psychosis, abnormal behavior, and disturbances of personality. Secondary hyperparathyroidism may result in many of these signs of calcium imbalance and in various abnormalities of the long bones, as in rickets. The diagnosis of primary hyperparathyroidism is made by laboratory findings of increased levels of PTH and calcium in the blood and by the characteristic appearance of the bones on x-ray films. Calcium in the blood and urine and chloride and alkaline phosphatase in the blood are present in excessive amounts; phosphorus is present in the serum in less than normal amounts.

■ INTERVENTION: Primary parathyroidism that is the result of an adenoma of one of the glands is treated by excision of the tumor; other causes of primary disease might require excision of up to one half of the glandular tissue. Dietary intake of calcium may be limited, and diuretics that promote urinary excretion of calcium and sodium may be administered. Postoperatively, calcium levels in the blood may drop rapidly to dangerously low

and percussed regularly to detect pulmonary edema in its earliest stages. Tetany is a warning sign of severe hypoglycemia; calcium gluconate is kept available for immediate use postoperatively. Walking and moving about cause pain to the patient but accelerate healing of the affected bones and are therefore encouraged.

hyperphenylalaninemia /hī′pərfen′ilal′əninē′mē·ə/, an abnormally high concentration of phenylalanine in the blood. This symptom may be the result of one of several defects in the metabolic process of breaking down phenylalanine. See also **phenylketonuria.**

hyperphoria /hī′pərfôr′ē·ə/, the tendency of an eye to deviate upward.

hyperpigmentation, unusual darkening of the skin. Causes include heredity, drugs, exposure to the sun, and adrenal insufficiency. Compare **hypopigmentation.** See also **chloasma, melanocyte stimulating hormone.**

hyperplasia /hī′pərplā′zhə/, an increase in the number of cells of a body part. Compare **hypertrophy, hypoplasia.**

hyperplastic endometritis, *obsolete*. endometritis with endometrial hyperplasia.

hyperploid /hī′pərploid/, **1.** of or pertaining to an individual, organism, strain, or cell that has one or more chromosomes in excess of the basic haploid number or of an exact multiple of the haploid number characteristic of the species. The result is unbalanced sets of chromosomes, which are referred to as hyperdiploid, hypertriploid, hypertetraploid, and so on, depending on the number of multiples of the haploid chromosomes they contain. **2.** such an individual, organism, strain, or cell. Compare **hypoploid.** See also **trisomy.**

hyperploidy /hī′pərploi′dē/, any increase in chromosome number that involves individual chromosomes rather than entire sets, resulting in more than the normal haploid number characteristic of the species, as in Down's syndrome. Compare **hypoploidy.**

hyperpnea /hī′pərpnē′ə/, a deep, rapid, or labored respiration. It occurs normally with exercise, and abnormally with pain, fever, hysteria, or any condition in which the supply of oxygen is inadequate, as cardiac disease and respiratory disease. Also spelled **hyperpnoea.** Compare

rexia, characterized by a rapid rise in temperature, tachycardia, tachypnea, sweating, rigidity, and blotchy cyanosis, occasionally occurs in patients undergoing general anesthesia. A high temperature may be reduced by sponging the body with tepid water and alcohol, by giving a tepid tub bath, by hypothermia treatment, or by administering antipyretic medication, as aspirin or acetaminophen. See also **fever.** –**hyperpyretic,** *adj.*

hyperreflection, a compulsion to devote excessive attention to oneself.

hyperreflexia, a neurologic condition characterized by increased reflex reactions.

hypersensitivity, an abnormal condition characterized by an excessive reaction to a particular stimulus. See also **allergy.** –**hypersensitive,** *adj.*

hypersensitivity pneumonitis. See **extrinsic allergic alveolitis.**

hypersensitivity reaction, an inappropriate and excessive response of the immune system to a sensitizing antigen. The antigenic stimulant is an allergen. There are several factors that determine the degree of an allergic response: the responsiveness of the host to the allergen, the amount of allergen, the kind of allergen, its route of entrance into the body, the timing of the exposures, and the site of the allergen-immune mediator reaction. Hypersensitivity reactions are classified by the components of the immune system involved in their mediation. Humoral reactions, mediated by the circulating B lymphocytes, are immediate and include three types: anaphylactic hypersensitivity, cytotoxic hypersensitivity, and immune system hypersensitivity. Cellular reactions, mediated by the T lymphocytes, are delayed, cell-mediated hypersensitivity reactions.

hypersomnia /hī′pərsom′nē·ə/, **1.** sleep of excessive depth or abnormal duration, usually caused by psychologic rather than physical factors and characterized by a state of confusion on awakening. **2.** extreme drowsiness, often associated with lethargy. **3.** a condition characterized by periods of deep, long sleep. Compare **narcolepsy.**

hyperspadias. See **epispadias.**

hypersplenism /hī′pərsplē′nizəm/, a syndrome consisting of splenomegaly and a deficiency of one or more types of blood cells. The numerous causes of this syndrome include the lymphomas, the hemolytic anemias, malaria, tuberculosis, and various connective tissue and inflammatory diseases. Patients complain of abdominal pain on the left side and often experience fullness after eating very little, because the greatly enlarged spleen is pressing against the stomach. On physical examination the enlarged spleen is felt and abnormal bruits (vascular sounds) are heard with a stethoscope over the epigastric area. Treatment of the underlying disorder may cure the syndrome. Splenectomy is usually performed only in treating the hemolytic anemias or when splenic enlargement is severe and the danger of vascular accident is significant. See also **splenectomy.**

Hyperstat, a trademark for a vasodilator (diazoxide).

hypertelorism /hī′pərtel′əriz′əm/, a developmental defect characterized by an abnormally wide space between two organs or parts. A kind of hypertelorism is **ocular hypertelorism.** Compare **hypotelorism.**

hypertension, a common, often asymptomatic disorder characterized by elevated blood pressure persistently exceeding 140/90 mm Hg. Essential hypertension, the most frequent kind, has no single identifiable cause, but the risk of the disorder is increased by obesity, a high sodium level in serum, hypercholesterolemia, and a family history of high blood pressure. Known causes of hypertension include adrenal disorders, as aldosteronism, Cushing's syndrome, and pheochromocytoma, thyrotoxicosis, toxemia of pregnancy, and chronic glomerulonephritis. The incidence of hypertension is higher in men than in women and is twice as great in blacks as in whites. Persons with mild or moderate hypertension may be asymptomatic or may experience suboccipital headaches, especially on rising, tinnitus, lightheadness, easy fatigability, and palpitations. With sustained hypertension arterial walls become thickened, inelastic, and resistant to blood flow, and, as a result, the left ventricle becomes distended and hypertrophied in its efforts to maintain normal circulation. Inadequate blood supply to the coronary arteries may cause angina or myocardial infarction. Left ventricular hypertrophy may lead to congestive heart failure. High blood pressure associated with hypersecretion of catecholamines in pheochromocytoma is often accompanied by anxiety attacks, palpitation, profuse sweating, pallor, nausea, and, in some cases, pulmonary edema. Malignant hypertension, characterized by a diastolic pressure higher than 120 mm Hg, severe headaches, blurred vision, and confusion, may result in fatal uremia, myocardial infarction, congestive heart failure, or a cerebrovascular accident. Drugs used to treat hypertension include diuretics, as furosemide and thiazide derivatives; vasodilators, as hydralazine and prazosin; sympathetic nervous system (SNS) depressants, as rauwolfia alkaloids; SNS inhibitors, as guanethidine and methyldopa; and ganglionic blocking agents, as clonidine and propranolol. Patients with high blood pressure are advised to follow a low-sodium, low-saturated fat diet, to reduce calories to control obesity, to exercise, to avoid stress, and to take adequate rest. Kinds of hypertension are **essential hypertension, malignant hypertension,** and **secondary hypertension.** See also **blood pressure.**

hypertensive crisis, a sudden severe increase in blood pressure to a level exceeding 200/120 mm Hg, occurring most frequently in untreated hypertension and in patients who have stopped taking prescribed antihypertensive medication.

■ OBSERVATIONS: Characteristic signs include severe headache, vertigo, diplopia, tinnitus, nosebleed, twitching muscles, tachycardia or other cardiac arrhythmia, distended neck veins, narrowed pulse pressure, nausea, and vomiting. The patient may be confused, irritable, or stuporous, and the condition may lead to convulsions, coma, myocardial infarction, renal failure, cardiac arrest, or stroke.

■ INTERVENTION: Treatment consists of antihypertensive drugs, administered intravenously or intramuscularly, and diuretics and may include the use of anticonvulsants, sedatives, and antiemetics, if indicated. The patient is usually placed on a cardiac monitor in a bed with the head elevated and is maintained in a quiet environment. The diet is low in calories, and sodium and fluids may be restricted. As the condition improves, the patient is permitted progressive ambulation but is carefully observed for symptoms of orthostatic hypotension, as pallor, diaphoresis, or faintness.

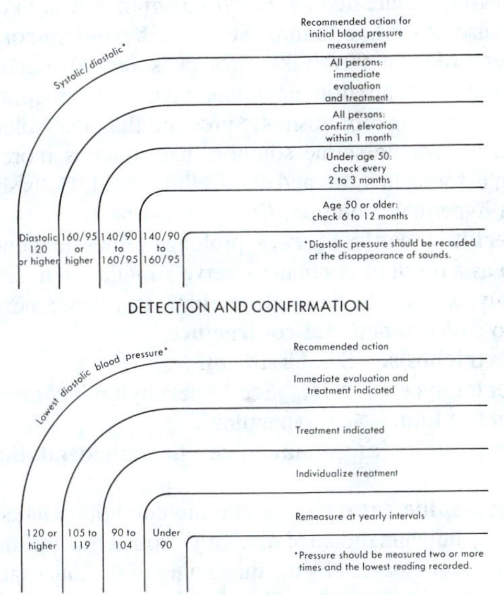

High blood pressure

■ NURSING CONSIDERATIONS: A major concern in caring for patients who have suffered a hypertensive crisis is observing and reporting of any sign of hypotension. In preparation for discharge the nurse advises the patient to recognize symptoms of any dramatic increase or decrease in blood pressure, to adhere to the prescribed diet and medication, and to avoid fatigue, heavy lifting, smoking, and stressful situations.

[illegible]

hypertetraploid. See **hyperploid.**

[illegible]

hyperthyroidism, a condition characterized by hyper- [illegible] ... roid hormones, and the metabolic processes in the body are accelerated. [illegible] constant hunger, weight loss, fatigue, heat intolerance, palpitations, and diarrhea may develop. Antithyroid drugs, as propylthiouracil or methimazole, are usually prescribed. Radioactive iodine may be prescribed in certain cases. Surgical ablation of the gland is sometimes necessary. Untreated hyperthyroidism may lead to death because of cardiac failure. See also **thyroid storm.**

hypertonic /hī′pərton′ik/, (of a solution) having a greater concentration of solute than another solution, hence exerting more osmotic pressure than that solution, as a hypertonic saline solution that contains more salt than is found in intra- and extracellular fluid. Cells shrink in a hypertonic solution. Compare **isotonic.**

hypertonic contracture, prolonged muscle contraction as a result of continuous nerve stimulation in spastic paralysis. Anesthesia or sleep eliminates this condition. Also called **functional contracture.**

hypertrichosis. See **hirsutism.**

hypertriglyceridemia. See **hyperchylomicronemia.**

hypertriploid. See **hyperploid.**

hypertrophic angioma. See **hemangioendothelioma.**

hypertrophic catarrh, a chronic condition characterized by inflammation and discharge from a mucous membrane, accompanied by the thickening of the mucosal and submucosal tissue. Compare **atrophic catarrh.** See also **catarrh.**

hypertrophic endometritis, *obsolete.* endometritis with endometrial hyperplasia.

hypertrophic gastritis, an inflammatory condition of the stomach characterized by epigastric pain, nausea, vomiting, and distention. It is differentiated from other forms of gastritis by the presence of prominent rugae (folds), enlarged glands, and nodules on the wall of the stomach. This condition often occurs with peptic ulcer, Zollinger-Ellison syndrome, or gastric hypersecretion.

hypertrophic gingivitis. See **gingivitis.**

hypertrophy /hīpur′trəfē/, an increase in the size of an organ caused by an increase in the size of the cells rather than the number of cells. Kinds of hypertrophy include **adaptive hypertrophy, compensatory hypertrophy, Marie's hypertrophy, physiologic hypertrophy,** and **unilateral hypertrophy. Compare atrophy, hyperplasia. –hypertrophic,** *adj.*

[illegible]

hyperventilation, [illegible] ... Hypocapnia and respiratory alkalosis then occur, [illegible] ... increased metabolism because of exercise, fever, hyperthyroidism, or infections; lesions of the central nervous system, as in cerebral thrombosis, encephalitis, head injuries, or meningitis; hypoxia or metabolic acidosis; hormones and drugs, as epinephrine, progesterone, salicylates; difficulties with mechanic respirators; and psychogenic factors, as acute anxiety or pain. Compare **hypoventilation.** See also **respiratory center.**

hypervitaminosis, an abnormal condition resulting from excessive intake of toxic amounts of one or more vitamins, especially over a long period of time. Serious effects may result from overdoses of vitamins A, D, E, or K, but rarely with the water-soluble B and C vitamins. Compare **avitaminosis.** See also specific vitamins.

hypervolemia, an increase in the amount of extracellular fluid, particularly in the volume of circulating blood or its components.

hypesthesia /hī′pəristhē′zhə/, an abnormal weakness of sensation in response to stimulation of the sensory nerves. Touch, pain, heat, and cold are poorly perceived. Also called **hypoesthesia. –hypesthetic,** *adj.*

hypha /hī′fə/, *pl.* **hyphae,** the threadlike structure of the mycelium in a fungus.

hyphema /hīfē′mə/, a hemorrhage into the anterior chamber of the eye, usually caused by a blunt or percussive injury. Bedrest and a sedative are indicated. The patient is treated by an ophthalmologist who evaluates the need for evacuation of the blood, the use of mydriatic or miotic medications, or a carbonic anhydrase inhibitor. Glaucoma may result from recurrent bleeding. Also called **hyphemia** /hīfē′mē·ə/.

hypnagogic hallucination, one that occurs in the period between wakefulness and sleep. See also **hallucination.**

hypnagogue /hip′nəgog/, an agent or substance that tends to induce sleep or the feeling of dreamy sleepiness, as occurs before falling asleep. See also **hypnotic. –hypnagogic,** *adj.*

hypnoanalysis, the use of hypnosis as an adjunct to other techniques in psychoanalysis.

hypnosis, a passive, trancelike state that resembles normal sleep during which perception and memory are altered, resulting in increased responsiveness to suggestion. The condition is usually induced by the monotonous repetition of words and gestures while the subject is completely relaxed. Susceptibility to hypnosis varies from person to person. Hypnosis is used in some forms of psychotherapy and psychoanalysis to gain access to the subconscious, in behavior modification programs to help a person stop overeating or smoking or to end other unwanted behavior, or in medicine to reduce pain and promote relaxation.

hypnotherapy, the use of hypnosis as an adjunct to other techniques in psychotherapy.

-hypnotic, a combining form meaning 'pertaining to hypnosis': *anhypnotic, autohypnotic, posthypnotic*.

hypnotics, a class of drugs often used as sedatives.

hypnotic trance, an artificially induced sleeplike state, as in hypnosis.

hypnotism, the study or practice of inducing hypnosis.

hypnotist, one who practices hypnotism.

hypnotize, **1.** to put into a state of hypnosis. **2.** to fascinate, entrance, or control through personal charm.

hypo-, hyp-, a combining form meaning 'beneath, deficient,' or, in chemistry, 'lacking oxygen': *hypochlorite, hypodermic, hypodontia*.

hypoacidity, a deficiency of acid.

hypoactivity, any abnormally diminished activity of the body or its organs, as decreased cardiac output, thyroid secretion, or peristalsis. Compare **hyperactivity,** def. 1.

hypoadrenalism. See **Addison's disease.**

hypoalimentation, a condition of insufficient or inadequate nourishment.

hypobetalipoproteinemia /hī′pōbā′təlip′ōprō′tēnē′mē•ə/, an inherited disorder in which there are less than normal amounts of beta-lipoprotein in the serum. Blood lipids and cholesterol are present at less than the expected levels regardless of dietary intake of fats. There are no clinical signs, and treatment is unnecessary. Compare **hyperbetalipoproteinemia.**

hypocalcemia /hī′pōkalsē′mē•ə/, a deficiency of calcium in the serum that may be caused by hypoparathyroidism, vitamin D deficiency, kidney failure, acute pancreatitis, or inadequate plasma magnesium and protein. Mild hypocalcemia is asymptomatic. Severe hypocalcemia is characterized by cardiac arrhythmias and tetany with hyperparesthesia of the hands, feet, lips, and tongue. The underlying disorder is diagnosed and treated, and calcium is given by mouth or by intravenous infusion. Hypocalcemia is also seen in dysmature newborns, in infants born of mothers with diabetes, or in normal babies delivered by normal mothers after a long or stressful labor and delivery. It is recognized by vomiting, twitching of extremities, poor muscle tone, high-pitched crying, and difficulty in breathing. See also **tetany.** **–hypocalcemic,** *adj.*

hypochloremia, a decrease in the chloride level in the blood serum, below 95 mEq/L. The condition may occur as a result of prolonged gastric suctioning.

hypochloremic alkalosis, a metabolic alkalosis resulting from increased blood bicarbonate secondary to loss of chloride from the body.

hypochlorhydria, a deficiency of hydrochloric acid in the stomach's gastric juice.

hypochlorous acid, a greenish-yellow liquid derived from an aqueous solution of lime. An unstable compound that decomposes to hydrochloric acid and water, hypochlorous acid is used as a bleaching agent and disinfectant.

hypochondria, hypochondriac neurosis. See **hypochondriasis.**

hypochondriac region, the part of the abdomen in the upper zone on both sides of the epigastric region and beneath the cartilages of the lower ribs. Also called **hypochondrium.** See also **abdominal regions.**

hypochondriasis /hī′pōkəndrī′əsis/, **1.** also called **hypochondria.** a chronic, abnormal concern about the health of the body. **2.** also called **hypochondriac neurosis.** a disorder characterized by extreme anxiety, depression, and an unrealistic interpretation of real or imagined physical symptoms as indications of a serious illness or disease despite rational medical evidence that no disorder is present. The condition is caused by some unresolved intrapsychic conflict and may involve a specific organ, as the heart, lungs, or eyes, or several body systems at various times or simultaneously. In severe cases, the distorted body-mind relationship is so strong that actual symptoms and disease may develop. Treatment usually consists of psychotherapy to uncover the underlying emotional conflict. **–hypochondriac** /hī′pōkon′drē•ak/, *adj., n.,* **hypochondriac** /hī′pōkəndrī′ak/, **hypochondriacal,** *adj.*

hypochondrium. See **hypochondriac region.**

hypochromic /hī′pōkrō′mik/, having less than normal color, usually describing a red blood cell and characterizing anemias associated with decreased synthesis of hemoglobin. Compare **normochromic.** See also **hypochromic anemia, red cell indices.**

hypochromic anemia, any of a large group of anemias characterized by a decreased concentration of hemoglobin in the red blood cells. See also **anemia, red cell indices.**

hypocytic leukemia. See **aleukemic leukemia.**

hypodermatoclysis. See **hypodermoclysis.**

hypodermic, of or pertaining to the area below the skin, as a hypodermic injection.

hypodermic needle, a short, thin, hollow needle that attaches to a syringe for injecting a drug or medication under the skin or into vessels and for withdrawing a fluid, as blood, for examination.

hypodermoclysis /hī′pōdərmok′lisis/, the injection of an isotonic or hypotonic solution into subcutaneous tissue to supply the patient with a continuous and large amount of fluid, electrolytes, and nutrients. The procedure is used to replace the loss or inadequate intake of water and salt during illness or surgery or after shock or hemorrhage and is performed only when the patient is unable to take

[illegible]

hypodiploid. See **hypoploid.**
hypoesthesia. See **hypesthesia.**
hypofibrinogenemia, a deficiency of fibrinogen, a blood clotting factor, in the blood. The condition may occur as a complication of abruptio placentae.
hypogammaglobulinemia, a less than normal concentration of gamma globulin in the blood, usually the result of increased protein catabolism or the loss of protein in the urine, as in nephrosis. The condition is associated with a decreased resistance to infection. Compare **agammaglobulinemia.**
hypogastric artery. See **internal iliac artery.**
hypogastrium. See **pubic region.**
hypogenitalism, a condition of retarded sexual development caused by a defect in male or female hormonal production in the testis or ovary.
hypogeusia, reduced taste.
hypoglossal nerve, either of a pair of cranial nerves essential for swallowing and for moving the tongue. Each nerve has four major branches, communicates with the vagus nerve, and connects to nucleus XII in the brain. Also called **nervus hypoglossus, twelfth nerve.**
hypoglycemia /hī′pōglīsē′mē·ə/, a less than normal amount of glucose in the blood, usually caused by administration of too much insulin, excessive secretion of insulin by the islet cells of the pancreas, or dietary deficiency. The condition may result in weakness, headache, hunger, visual disturbances, ataxia, anxiety, personality changes, and, if untreated, delirium, coma, and death. The treatment is the administration of glucose in orange juice by mouth if the person is conscious or in an intravenous glucose solution if the person is unconscious. Compare **diabetic coma.**

Signs and symptoms of hypoglycemia

Sympathetic nervous system activity	Central nervous system activity
Pallor	Headache
Perspiration	Blurred vision
Piloerection	Diplopia
Tachycardia	Incoherent speech
Palpitation	Emotional changes
Nervousness	Fatigue
Irritability	Numbness of lips, tongue
Weakness	Mental confusion
Trembling	Convulsions
Hunger	Coma

[illegible] formin has been recently removed from the market in the United States, primarily because of its tendency to cause lactic acidosis. The adverse reactions of any hypoglycemic agent and contraindications for its prescription depend on the class of drug and the condition of the patient.
hypoglycemic shock treatment. See **insulin shock treatment.**
hypokalemia /hī′pōkəlē′mē·ə/, a condition in which an inadequate amount of potassium, the major intracellular cation, is found in the circulating bloodstream. Hypokalemia is characterized by abnormal ECG, weakness, and flaccid paralysis and may be caused by starvation, treatment of diabetic acidosis, adrenal tumor, or diuretic therapy. Mild hypokalemia may resolve itself when the underlying disorder is corrected. Severe hypokalemia may be treated by the administration of potassium chloride, orally or parenterally, and by a diet high in potassium. Compare **hyperkalemia.** See also **electrolyte balance.**
hypokalemic alkalosis, a pathologic condition resulting from the accumulation of base or the loss of acid from the body associated with a low level of serum potassium. The retention of alkali or the loss of acid occurs primarily in extracellular fluid, but the pH of intracellular fluid may also be subnormal. See also **hypokalemia.**
hypolipemia. See **hypolipoproteinemia.**
hypolipoproteinemia /hī′pōlip′ōprō′tēnē′mē·ə/, a group of defects of lipoprotein metabolism that result in varying complexes of signs. Primary, or hereditary, hypolipoproteinemia factors include abnormal transport of triglycerides in the blood, low levels of high-density lipoproteins, high levels of low-density lipoproteins, and abnormal deposition of lipids in the body, especially in the kidneys and the liver. In some of the syndromes ocular, intestinal, and neurologic effects are also present. The condition may also be secondary to anemia, malabsorption syndromes, or malnutrition. Kinds of hypolipoproteinemias are **abetalipoproteinemia, hypobetalipoproteinemia, lecithin-cholesterol acyltransferase deficiency,** and **Tangier disease.**
hypomagnesemia /hī′pōmag′nisē′mē·ə/, an abnormally low concentration of magnesium in the blood plasma, resulting in nausea, vomiting, muscle weakness, tremors, tetany, and lethargy. Mild hypomagnesemia is usually

the result of inadequate absorption of kidney or intestine, although it is al longed parenteral feeding and during severe form is associated with malabs protein malnutrition, and parathyroid sium salts to correct the deficiency may intravenously.

hypomania, a psychopathologic state optimism, excitability, a marked hyper ativeness, heightened sexual interest, irritability, and a decreased need for sle **niac,** *n.,* **hypomanic,** *adj.*

hypometria /hī′pōmē′trē·ə/, an abnormal condition, a form of dysmetria, characterized by a dysfunction of the power to control the range of muscular action, resulting in movements that fall short of the intended goals of the affected individual. Compare **hypermetria.**

hypomorph, **1.** a person whose legs are disproportionately short in relation to the trunk and whose sitting height is greater in proportion than the person's standing height. **2.** (in genetics) a mutant allele that has a reduced effect on the expression of a trait but at a level too low to result in abnormal development. Also called **leaky gene.** Compare **amorph, antimorph, hypermorph.**

hyponatremia /hī′pōnatrē′mē·ə/, a less than normal concentration of sodium in the blood, caused by inadequate excretion of water or by excessive water in the circulating bloodstream. In a severe case, the person may develop water intoxication, with confusion and lethargy, leading to muscle excitability, convulsions, and coma. Restoration of fluid and electrolyte balance may be by intravenous infusion of a balanced solution.

hypoosmolarity, a state or condition of abnormally reduced osmolarity.

hypoparathyroidism, a condition of diminished parathyroid function, which can be caused by primary parathyroid dysfunction or by elevated serum calcium levels.

hypopharyngeal, **1.** of, pertaining to, or involving the hypopharynx. **2.** situated below the pharynx.

hypophosphatasia /hī′pōfos′fətā′zhə/, congenital absence of alkaline phosphatase, an enzyme essential to the calcification of bone tissue. Affected newborns vomit, grow slowly, and often die in infancy. Children who survive have numerous skeletal abnormalities and are dwarfs. There is no known treatment.

hypophosphatemic rickets /hī′pōfos′fətē′mik/, a rare familial disorder in which there is impaired resorption of phosphate in the kidneys and poor absorption of calcium in the small intestine, resulting in osteomalacia, retarded growth, skeletal deformities, and pain. Treatment includes the prescription of phosphate and vitamin D, to be taken by mouth.

hypophyseal cachexia. See **panhypopituitarism.**

hypophyseal dwarf. See **pituitary dwarf.**

hypophysectomy /hīpof′əsek′təmē/, surgical removal of the pituitary gland. It may be performed to slow the growth and spread of endocrine-dependent malignant

monitored for early signs of thyroid crisis, crisis, electrolyte imbalance, hemorrhage, and meningitis. –**hypophysectomize,** *v.*

hypophysis cerebri. See **pituitary gland.**

hypopigmentation, unusual lack of skin color, seen in albinism or vitiligo. Compare **hyperpigmentation.**

hypopituitarism, an abnormal condition caused by diminished activity of the pituitary gland and marked by excessive deposits of fat and persistence or acquisition of adolescent characteristics.

hypoplasia /hī′pōplā′zhə/, incomplete or underdeveloped organ or tissue, usually the result of a decrease in the number of cells. Kinds of hypoplasia are **cartilage-hair hypoplasia** and **enamel hypoplasia.** Also called **hypoplasty.** Compare **aplasia, hyperplasia.** See also **oligomeganephronia, osteogenesis imperfecta.** –**hypoplastic,** *adj.*

hypoplasia of the mesenchyme. See **osteogenesis imperfecta.**

hypoplastic anemia, a broad category of anemias characterized by decreased production of red blood cells. Compare **aplastic anemia, polycythemia.** See also **anemia.**

hypoplastic dwarf. See **primordial dwarf.**

hypoploid /hī′pəploid/, **1.** also **hypoploidic.** of or pertaining to an individual, organism, strain, or cell that has fewer than the normal haploid number or an exact multiple of the haploid number of chromosomes characteristic of the species. The result is unbalanced sets of chromosomes, which are referred to as hypodiploid, hypotriploid, hypotetraploid, and so on, depending on the number of multiples of the haploid chromosomes they contain. **2.** such an individual, organism, strain, or cell. Compare **hyperploid.** See also **monosomy.**

hypoploidy /hī′pōploi′dē/, any decrease in chromosome number that involves individual chromosomes rather than entire sets, resulting in fewer than the normal haploid number characteristic of the species, as in Turner's syndrome. Compare **hyperploidy.**

hypopnea /hīpop′nē·ə, hī′pōnē′ə/, shallow or slow respiration. In well-conditioned athletes it is normal and is accompanied by a slow pulse; otherwise, it is characteristic of damage to the brainstem, in which case it is accompanied by a rapid, weak pulse and is a grave sign. See also **respiratory rate.**

hypopotassemia, a deficiency of potassium in the blood.

hypoproteinemia /hī′pōprō′tēnē′mē·ə/, a disorder characterized by a decrease in the amount of protein in the blood to an abnormally low level, accompanied by edema, nausea, vomiting, diarrhea, and abdominal pain. It may be caused by an inadequate dietary supply of protein, by intestinal lymphangiectasia, or by renal failure. Also called **intestinal lymphangiectasia.**

hypoprothrombinemia /hī′pōprōthrom′binē′mē·ə/, an abnormal reduction in the amount of prothrombin (factor II) in the circulating blood, characterized by poor clot formation, longer bleeding time, and possible hemorrhage. The condition is usually the result of inadequate synthesis of prothrombin in the liver, most often the result of a deficiency of vitamin K caused by severe liver disease or by anticoagulant therapy with the drug dicumarol. See also **blood clotting.**

hypoptyalism /hī′pōtī′əliz′əm/, a condition in which there is a decrease in the amount of saliva secreted by the salivary glands. See also **hyposalivation, ptyalism.**

hypopyon, an accumulation of pus in the anterior chamber of an eye, appearing as a gray fluid between the cornea and the iris. It may occur as a complication of conjunctivitis, herpetic keratitis, or corneal ulcer.

hyporeflexia, a neurologic condition characterized by weakened reflex reactions.

hyposalivation, a decreased flow of saliva that may be associated with dehydration, radiation therapy of the salivary gland regions, anxiety, the use of drugs, as atropine and antihistamines, vitamin deficiency, various forms of parotitis, or various syndromes, as Plummer-Vinson syndrome. Also called **xerostomia, asialorrhea.**

hyposensitization. See **immunotherapy.**

hypospadias /hī′pəspā′dē·əs/, a congenital defect in which the urinary meatus is on the underside of the penis. Incontinence does not occur because the sphincters are not defective. The opening may be off center or anywhere along the underside of the penis or on the perineum. Surgical correction is performed as necessary for cosmetic, urologic, or reproductive indications. A corresponding defect in women is rare but recognized by the location of the urinary meatus in the vagina. Compare **epispadias.**

hypostatic pneumonia, a type of pneumomia associated with elderly or debilitated persons who remain in the same position for long periods. Gravity tends to accelerate fluid congestion in one area of the lungs, increasing the susceptibility to infection.

hypotelorism /hī′pōtel′əriz′əm/, a developmental defect characterized by an abnormally decreased distance between two organs or parts. A kind of hypotelorism is **ocular hypotelorism.** Compare **hypertelorism.**

hypotension, an abnormal condition in which the blood pressure is not adequate for normal perfusion and oxygenation of the tissues. An expanded intravascular space, a decreased intravascular volume, or a diminished cardiac thrust may be the cause.

hypotensive anesthesia. See **deliberate hypotension.**

hypotetraploid. See **hypoploid.**

hypothalamic amenorrhea, cessation of menses caused by disorders that inhibit the hypothalamus from initiating the cycle of neurohormonal interactions of the brain, pituitary, and ovary necessary for ovulation and subsequent menstruation. Examples of causes are stress, anxiety, and acute weight loss. See **amenorrhea.**

hypothalamus /hī′pōthal′əməs/, a portion of the diencephalon of the brain, forming the floor and part of the lateral wall of the third ventricle. It activates, controls, and integrates the peripheral autonomic nervous system, endocrine processes, and many somatic functions, as body temperature, sleep, and appetite. Compare **epithalamus, metathalamus, subthalamus, thalamus.** – **hypothalamic,** *adj.*

hypothenar, an eminence or fleshy elevation on the ulnar side of the palm of the hand.

hypothermia /hī′pōthur′mē·ə/, **1.** an abnormal and dangerous condition in which the temperature of the body is below 95° F (35° C), usually caused by prolonged exposure to cold. Respiration is shallow and slow, and the heart rate is faint and slow. The person is very pale and may appear to be dead. People who are very old or very young, people who have cardiovascular problems, and people who are hungry, tired, or under the influence of alcohol are most susceptible to hypothermia. Treatment includes slowly warming the person. Hospitalization is necessary for evaluating and treating any metabolic abnormalities that may result from hypothermia. **2.** the deliberate and controlled reduction of body temperature with cooling mattresses or ice as preparation for some surgical procedures.

hypothermia blanket, a covering used to conserve heat in the body of a patient suffering from hypothermia.

hypothermia therapy, the reduction of a patient's body temperature to counteract high prolonged fever caused by an infectious or neurologic disease, or, less frequently, as an adjunct to anesthesia in heart or brain surgery.

■ METHOD: Hypothermia may be produced by placing crushed ice around the patient, by immersing the body in ice water, by autotransfusing blood after it is circulated through coils submerged in a refrigerant, or, most commonly, by applying cooling blankets or vinyl pads containing coils through which cold water and alcohol are circulated by a pump. The cooling unit is placed in an open area; any kinks or twists in the tubing are removed, and the blanket is checked for leaks. The patient is wrapped in bath blankets and then covered with the cooling blanket; the patient's temperature, registered by means of a probe inserted in the rectum, is read and recorded before hypothermia is initiated, every 5 minutes until the desired reduction is achieved, and then every 15 minutes. The blood pressure, pulse, respirations, and neurologic status are checked every 5 to 10 minutes until the temperature is stabilized, then every 30 minutes for 2 hours, every 4 hours in the next 24 hours, and subsequently as required. Every 1 to 2 hours the patient is assisted in turning, coughing, and deep breathing. At similar intervals the chest is auscultated for breath sounds, and oral, nose, and skin care are administered; the skin is lubricated with oil or lotion before and during the procedure. An indwelling catheter is connected to a closed gravity drainage system, as ordered, and fluid intake and output are measured; if less than 30 ml of urine per hour is excreted, the physician is notified. If the patient's temperature is less than 90° F (32.2° C), the gag reflex is tested before any oral fluids or foods are administered. Nasooral suction is performed as indicated; body alignment is maintained, and passive or active range of motion exercises are performed every 4 hours. Because shivering increases body heat, medication for its prevention, as chlorpromazine hydrochloride, may be ordered. The patient is observed for medication reactions, decreased blood pressure, bradycardia, arrhythmias, bradypnea, respiratory failure, unequal pupils, increased intracranial pressure, changes in consciousness, intestinal ileus, and frostbite. Any changes in skin color or signs of edema and induration are reported to the physician immediately. At the termination of hypothermia, the cooling blanket is replaced by regular blankets and the patient usually warms at his or her own rate. As the patient's temperature approaches normal, the warming blankets are removed, but the temperature probe remains in place until the body temperature is stable.

■ NURSING ORDERS: The nurse administers hypothermia, carefully monitoring the patient's vital signs and any evidence of complications.

■ OUTCOME CRITERIA: Hypothermia used in the treatment of high fever associated with generalized severe infections reduces body heat by decreasing metabolism and also inhibits the multiplication of the causative pathogenic organisms. Patients with a high temperature caused by a neurologic disease may be maintained in a state of mild hypothermia (87° to 95° F or 30.6° to 35° C) for as long as 5 days. The procedure is successful if the fever is broken and complications do not occur.

hypothesis /hīpoth′isis/, (in research) a statement derived from a theory that predicts the relationship among variables representing concepts, constructs, or events. Kinds of hypotheses include **causal hypothesis, null hypothesis,** and **predictive hypothesis.**

hypothyroid dwarf. See **cretin dwarf.**

hypothyroidism, a condition characterized by decreased activity of the thyroid gland. It is caused by surgical removal of all or part of the gland, overdosage with antithyroid medication, decreased effect of thyroid releasing hormone secreted by the hypothalamus, decreased secretion of thyroid stimulating hormone by the pituitary gland, or by atrophy of the thyroid gland itself. Weight gain, sluggishness, dryness of the skin, constipation, arthritis, and slowing of the metabolic processes of the body may occur. Untreated, hypothyroidism leads to myxedema, coma, and death. Treatment is by administration of the deficient hormone. Dosage is adjusted to maintain normal levels of thyroid hormones.

hypotonic /hī′pōton′ik/, (of a solution) having a smaller concentration of solute than another solution, hence exerting less osmotic pressure than that solution, as a hypotonic saline solution that contains less salt than is found in intra- or extracellular fluid. Cells expand in a hypotonic solution.

hypotriploid. See **hypoploid.**

hypoventilation, an abnormal condition of the respiratory system, characterized by cyanosis, clubbing of the fingers, polycythemia, increased carbon dioxide arterial tension, Cheyne-Stokes breathing, and generalized decreased respiratory function. It occurs when the volume of air that enters the alveoli and takes part in gas exchanges is not adequate for the metabolic needs of the body. Hypoventilation may be caused by uneven distribution of inspired air (as in bronchitis), obesity, neuromuscular or skeletal disease affecting the thorax, decreased response of the respiratory center to carbon dioxide, and reduced functional lung tissue, as in atelectasis, emphysema, and pleural effusion. The result of hypoventilation is hypoxia, hypercapnia, pulmonary hypertension with cor pulmonale, and respiratory acidosis. Treatment includes weight reduction in cases of obesity, artificial respiration, and tracheostomy. Compare **hyperventilation.** See also **respiratory center.**

hypovitaminosis. See **avitaminosis.**

hypovolemia, an abnormally low circulating blood volume.

hypovolemic shock, a state of physical collapse and prostration caused by massive blood loss, circulatory dysfunction, and inadequate tissue perfusion. The loss of about one fifth of total blood volume in the affected individual can produce this condition. The common signs include low blood pressure, feeble pulse, clammy skin, tachycardia, rapid breathing, and reduced urinary output. The associated blood losses may stem from GI bleeding, internal hemorrhage, external hemorrhage, or excessive reduction of intravascular plasma volume and body fluids. Disorders that may cause hypovolemic shock are dehydration from excessive perspiration, severe diarrhea, protracted vomiting, intestinal obstruction, peritonitis, acute pancreatitis, and severe burns, which deplete body fluids. Associated effects may include metabolic acidosis with the accumulation of lactic acid, irreversible cerebral and renal damage, and disseminated intravascular coagulation. Treatment of hypovolemic shock focuses on prompt replacement of blood and fluid volumes, identification of bleeding sites, and the control of bleeding. Without fast aggressive treatment there is further collapse that can cause death. Compare **cardiogenic shock.** See also **electric shock, shock.**

hypoxemia /hī′poksē′mē·ə/, an abnormal deficiency of oxygen in the arterial blood. Symptoms of acute hypoxemia are cyanosis, restlessness, stupor, coma, Cheyne-

Stokes breathing, apnea, increased blood pressure, tachycardia, and an initial increase in cardiac output that later falls, resulting in hypotension and ventricular fibrillation or asystole. Chronic hypoxemia stimulates red blood cell production by the bone marrow, leading to secondary polycythemia. Hypoxemia caused by decreased alveolar oxygen tension or underventilation improves with oxygen therapy. Hypoxemia resulting from shunting of blood from the right side of the heart to the left side of the heart without exchange of gases in the lungs is treated with bronchial hygiene and positive and expiratory pressure therapy. Compare **hypoxia.** See also **anoxia, asphyxia.**

hypoxia, an inadequate, reduced tension of cellular oxygen, characterized by cyanosis, tachycardia, hypertension, peripheral vasoconstriction, dizziness, and mental confusion. Mild hypoxia stimulates the peripheral chemoreceptors to increase heart and respiratory rates. However, the central mechanisms that regulate breathing fail in severe hypoxia, leading to irregular respiration, Cheyne-Stokes breathing, apnea, and respiratory and cardiac failure. Increased sensitivity to the depressant effect on the respiratory system by certain drugs is common in chronic hypoxia, resulting in severe depression or apnea from relatively small doses of opiates. If the amounts of oxygen are not adequate for aerobic cellular metabolism, energy is provided by less efficient anaerobic pathways that produce metabolites other than carbon dioxide. The tissues most sensitive to hypoxia are the brain, heart, pulmonary vessels, and liver. Treatment may include cardiotonic and respiratory stimulant drugs, oxygen therapy, mechanic ventilation, and frequent analysis of blood gases. Compare **hypoxemia.** See also **anoxia, chemoreceptor, hyperventilation, respiratory center.**

hypsi-, a combining form meaning 'high': *hypsicephalia, hypsiconchous, hypsistaphylie.*

hypsibrachycephaly /hips′ibrakisef′əlē/, the condition of having a skull that is high with a broad forehead. See also **brachycephaly, oxycephaly. –hypsibrachycephalic,** *adj., n.*

hypsicephaly. See **oxycephaly.**

hypso-, a combining form meaning 'pertaining to height': *hypsonosus, hypsophobia, hypsotherapy.*

hyster-. See **hystero-.**

hysterectomy, surgical removal of the uterus, performed to remove fibroid tumors of the uterus or to treat chronic pelvic inflammatory disease, severe recurrent endometrial hyperplasia, uterine hemorrhage, and precancerous and cancerous conditions of the uterus. Types of hysterectomy include **total hysterectomy,** in which the uterus and cervix are removed, and **radical hysterectomy,** in which ovaries, oviducts, lymph nodes and lymph channels are removed with the uterus and cervix. Menstruation ceases after either type is performed. A vaginal douche may be given preoperatively. Under general or spinal anesthesia the uterus is excised and removed, either through the abdominal wall or, if plastic repair of vaginal structures is needed, through the vagina. One or both ovaries and oviducts may be removed at the same time. Postoperatively, the nurse will frequently observe the abdominal dressing, if present, for bleeding. Food and oral fluids are restricted to prevent abdominal distention. Toe to knee elastic stockings or bandages are reapplied twice a day to give snug, even support and to prevent circulatory stasis. The lower half of the bed is kept flat, and the patient is instructed to avoid sharply flexing the thighs or knees, because thrombophlebitis of the blood vessels of the pelvis and upper thigh is a frequent complication. Low back pain or scanty urine may indicate a ligated ureter. A kind of hysterectomy is **cesarean hysterectomy.** Compare **hysterosalpingo-oophorectomy. –hysterectomize,** *v.*

hysteria, **1.** a general state of tension or excitement in a person or a group, characterized by unmanageable fear and temporary loss of control over the emotions. **2.** *obsolete.* a psychoneurosis, now commonly called **hysteric neurosis.**

hysteric amaurosis, monocular or, more rarely, binocular blindness occurring after an emotional shock and lasting for hours, days, or months.

hysteric apepsia. See **anorexia nervosa.**

hysteric fever, an abnormal rise in body temperature without general symptoms, often seen in hysteric neurosis.

hysteric lethargy, a sleep induced by hypnosis. See also **hypnosis, lethargy.**

hysteric mania, a mood disorder characterized by symptoms of hysteria and mania.

hysteric neurosis, a form of psychoneurosis in which extreme excitability and anxiety resulting from an underlying emotional conflict are converted either into physical symptoms having no organic basis or into states of altered consciousness or identity. Kinds of hysteric neurosis are **conversion disorder** and **dissociative disorder.**

hysteric personality. See **histrionic personality.**

hysteric trance, a somnambulistic state occurring as a symptom of hysteric neurosis.

hystero-, hyster-, a combining form meaning 'pertaining to the uterus': *hysterocarcinoma, hysterocleisis, hysterolith.*

hysterogram, the radiographic record of a uterus made after the injection of a contrast medium into the uterine cavity. See also **hysterosalpingogram.**

hysterolaparotomy /his′tərōlap′ərot′əmē/, abdominal hysterectomy or hysterotomy.

hysterosalpingogram /his′tərōsalping′gōgram′/, an x-ray film of the uterus and the fallopian tubes using gas or a radiopaque substance introduced through the cervix to allow visualization of the cavity of the uterus and the passageway of the tubes. A blockage of a structure is demonstrated on the film because the radiopaque substance cannot pass to the more distal structures and escape from the ends of the tubes into the peritoneal cavity. Serial hysterosalpingograms are useful in the diagnosis of the cause of infertility.

hysterosalpingo-oophorectomy, surgical removal of one or both ovaries and oviducts along with the uterus, performed commonly to treat malignant neoplastic disease of the reproductive tract and chronic endometriosis. To avoid the severe symptoms of sudden menopause, a portion of one ovary is left, unless a malignancy is present. Under general anesthesia, the uterus, one or both oviducts, and one or both ovaries are removed. If both ovaries are removed and no malignancy is present, estrogen replacement therapy is often begun immediately. Elastic stockings or bandages are applied to the legs twice a day to prevent circulatory stasis because thrombophlebitis of the blood vessels of the pelvis or thigh is a frequent complication. The lower half of the bed is kept flat, and the patient is instructed to avoid flexing of the thighs or knees. Low back pain or scanty urine may indicate a ligated ureter. Compare **hysterectomy.**

hysteroscopy, direct visual inspection of the cervical canal and uterine cavity through a hysteroscope, performed to examine the endometrium, to secure a specimen for biopsy, to remove an intrauterine device, or to excise cervical polyps. Under spinal anesthesia, the endoscope is passed through the vagina and into the uterus, and the surrounding tissues are examined. The nurse keeps the patient flat in bed for the next 8 hours. The procedure is contraindicated in pregnancy, acute pelvic inflammatory disease, chronic upper genital tract infection, recent uterine perforation, and known or suspected cervical malignancy. **–hysteroscope,** *n.,* **hysteroscopic,** *adj.*

hysterotomy, surgical incision of the uterus, performed as a method of abortion in a pregnancy beyond the first trimester of gestation in which a saline-injection abortion was incomplete, or in which a tubal sterilization is to be done with the abortion. Under general or spinal anesthesia, the lower segment of the uterus is incised, and the products of conception are withdrawn. Postoperative care includes close observation for excessive vaginal bleeding.

Hytakerol, a trademark for a calcium regulator (dihydrotachysterol).

Hytone, a trademark for a glucocorticoid (hydrocortisone), used in a topical ointment for dermatitis.

Hz, abbreviation for **hertz.**

HZV, abbreviation for **herpes zoster virus.** See **chickenpox.**

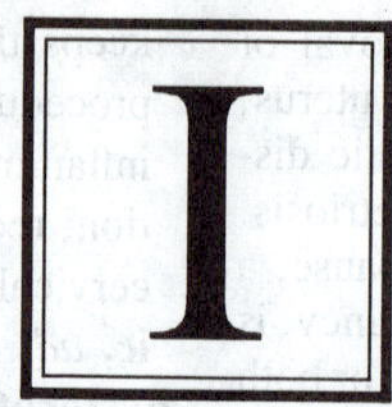

I, **1.** symbol for **inspired gas.** **2.** symbol for **iodine.**

-i, a plural-forming element used in native and later scientific Latin words: *bacilli, bronchi, plumbi*, and in scientific terms derived through Latin from Greek: *encephali, pylori, tympani*.

-ia, a combining form meaning a 'specified condition (disease)': *athrombia, phrenoblabia, pontobulbia*.

I.A.D.R., abbreviation for **International Association for Dental Research.**

-iasis, **1.** a combining form meaning a 'disease produced' by something specified: *cestodiasis, dicrocoeliasis, myiasis*. **2.** a combining form meaning a 'disease producing (specified) characteristics': *elephantiasis, leontiasis, lithiasis*.

-iatria. See **-iatry.**

-iatric, -iatrical, a combining form meaning 'relating to medical treatment': *neuropsychiatric, orthopsychiatric, pithiatric*.

-iatrist, -iatrician, a combining form meaning a 'physician': *hydriatrist, pediatrist, podiatrist*.

iatro-, a combining form meaning 'pertaining to a physician or to treatment': *iatrogenic, iatrophysics, iatrotechnics*.

iatrogenic /ī′atrōjen′ik, yat-/, caused by treatment or diagnostic procedures. An iatrogenic disorder is a condition caused by medical personnel or procedures or through exposure to the environment of a health-care facility. See also **nosocomial.** –**iatrogenesis,** *n.*

-iatry, -iatria, a combining form meaning a '(specified) type of medical treatment': *andriatry, pediatry, pithiatry*.

ibuprofen /ībyo͞o′prəfin/, a nonsteroidal antiinflammatory agent.

■ INDICATIONS: It is prescribed in the treatment of rheumatoid and osteoarthritis conditions.

■ CONTRAINDICATIONS: Renal dysfunction, disorders of the GI tract, or known hypersensitivity to this drug, to other nonsteroidal antiinflammatory drugs, or to aspirin prohibits its use.

■ ADVERSE EFFECTS: Among the more serious adverse reactions are GI disturbances, gastric or duodenal ulceration, dizziness, skin rash, and tinnitus. Ibuprofen may interact with other drugs.

IC, abbreviation for **inspiratory capacity.**

-ic, -ac, a combining form meaning 'pertaining to, similar to': *allelic, cadaveric, hypochondriac*.

ICD, abbreviation for ***International Classification of Diseases.***

ICDA, abbreviation for ***International Classification of Disease Adapted for Use in the United States.***

ICF, abbreviation for **intermediate care facility.**

ICF/MR, abbreviation for **intermediate care facility for the mentally retarded.**

ichthammol /ik′thəmôl/, a topical antiinfective used for treating certain skin diseases.

ichthyo-, a combining form meaning 'pertaining to fish': *ichthyocolla, ichthyophagy, ichthyotoxic*.

Ichthyol, a trademark for a topical antiinfective (ichthammol).

ichthyosis /ik′thē·ō′sis/, any of several inherited dermatologic conditions in which the skin is dry, hyperkeratotic, and fissured, resembling fish scales. It usually appears at or shortly after birth and may be part of one of several rare syndromes. Some types respond temporarily to bath oils, topical retinoic acid, or propylene glycol. A rare, acquired variety occurs in adult life accompanying a lymphoma or multiple myeloma. Also called **fish skin disease, xeroderma.** –**ichthyotic,** *adj.*

ichthyosis congenita, ichthyosis fetalis. See **lamellar exfoliation of the newborn.**

ichthyosis fetus. See **harlequin fetus.**

ichthyosis vulgaris, a hereditary skin disorder characterized by large, dry, dark scales that cover the face, neck, scalp, ears, back, and extensor surfaces but not the flexor surfaces of the body. The condition is transmitted as an autosomal dominant trait; not present at birth, it appears several months to 1 year after birth. Management consists of topical application of emollients and the use of keratolytic agents to facilitate removal of the scales. Also called **ichthyosis simplex.** See also **sex-linked ichthyosis.**

-ician, a combining form meaning a 'specialist in a field': *clinician, pediatrician, technician*.

ICN, abbreviation for **International Council of Nurses.**

ICP, abbreviation for **intracranial pressure.**

-ics, a combining form meaning the 'systematic formulation of a body of knowledge': *bionomics, osmics, psychics*.

I.C.S., abbreviation for **International Congress of Surgeons.**

ICSH, abbreviation for **interstitial cell-stimulating hormone.** See **luteinizing hormone.**

ictal, pertaining to a sudden, acute onset, as convulsions of an epileptic seizure.

icterus. See **jaundice.**

icterus index, a liver function test in which the blood serum is compared in intensity of color with that of potassium dichromate, normal being recorded in a numerical range of 3 to 5. When an excessive amount of bilirubin is present and jaundice becomes apparent, the index is usually 15 or higher; subnormal values are associated with various anemias.

icterus neonatorum, a jaundice condition in a newborn infant.

ictus /ik′təs/, *pl.* **ictuses, ictus,** **1.** a seizure. **2.** a cerebrovascular accident. **–ictal, ictic,** *adj.*

ICU, abbreviation for **intensive care unit.**

id, **1.** (in psychoanalysis) the part of the psyche functioning in the unconscious that is the source of instinctive energy, impulses, and drives. It is based on the pleasure principle and has strong tendencies toward self-preservation. Compare **ego, superego. 2.** the true unconscious.

ID, abbreviation for **infectious disease.**

-id, **1.** a combining form meaning a 'structural element of teeth': *protoconid, talonid, trigonid.* **2.** a combining form meaning a '(specified) body or particle': *cuspid, rhabdoid, sporid.*

IDDM, abbreviation for **insulin-dependent diabetes mellitus.**

-ide, a combining form naming binary compounds composed of a metallic and a nonmetallic element: *chloride, monoxide, sulfide.*

idea, any thought, concept, intention, or impression that exists in the mind as a result of awareness, understanding, or other mental activity. Kinds of ideas include **autochthonous idea, compulsive idea, dominant idea, fixed idea, idea of influence, idea of persecution,** and **idea of reference.**

ideal gas law, a rule that PV = nRT, with the product of pressure (P) and volume (V) equal to the product of the number of moles of gas (n), temperature (T), and a gas constant (R).

idea of influence, an obsessive delusion, often seen in paranoid disorders, that external forces or persons are controlling one's thoughts, actions, and feelings.

idea of persecution, an obsessive delusion, often seen in paranoid disorders, that one is being threatened, discriminated against, or mistreated by other persons or by external forces.

idea of reference, an obsessive delusion that the statements or actions of others refer to oneself, usually taken to be depreciatory, often seen in paranoid disorders. Also called **delusion of reference, referential idea.**

ideational apraxia, a condition in which the conceptual process is lost, often because of a lesion in the submarginal gyrus of the parietal lobe. The individual is unable to formulate a plan of movement and does not know the proper use of an object because of a lack of perception of its purpose. There is no loss of motor movement, but the reason for the movement is confused. Also called **sensory apraxia.** See also **apraxia.**

idée fixe. See **fixed idea.**

identical twins. See **monozygotic twins.**

identification, an unconscious defense mechanism by which a person patterns his personality on that of another person, assuming the person's qualities, characteristics, and actions. The process is a normal function of personality development and learning, and it contributes to the acquisition of interests and ideals. Kinds of identification are **competitive identification** and **positive identification.**

identity crisis, a period of disorientation concerning an individual's sense of self and role in society, occurring most frequently in the transition from one stage of life to the next. Identity crises are most common during adolescence, when a sudden increase in the strength of internal drives combined with greater peer pressure and parents' or society's expectations of more mature behavior often results in conflicts. The youngster may become confused about personal worth, abilities, values, goals, choice of vocation, and place in the world. The erosion of family life, social fluidity, mobility of the population, and changes in the relationships between the sexes all contribute to an increased incidence of identity crises. Although confusion regarding one's identity is usually considered an adolescent problem, it also is widespread among elderly people who lose their status in the community and their position as head of a family.

ideomotor apraxia, the inability to translate an idea into motion, resulting from some interference with the transmission of the appropriate impulses from the brain to the motor centers. There is no loss of the ability to perform an action automatically, as tying the shoelaces, but the action cannot be performed on request. The condition is often caused by diffuse cortical disease. Also called **classic apraxia, ideokinetic apraxia, limb-kinetic apraxia, transcortical apraxia.** See also **apraxia.**

ideophobia /ī′dē•ō-/, an anxiety disorder characterized by the irrational fear or distrust of ideas or reason. See also **phobia.**

idio-, a combining form meaning 'pertaining to self or to something separate': *idiocratic, idioneurosis, idioventricular.*

idiojunctional rhythm, a heart rhythm emanating from the AV junction but without retrograde conduction to the atria.

idiomere, See **chromomere.**

idiopathic /id′ē•ōpath′ik/, without a known cause.

idiopathic disease, a disease that develops without an apparent or known cause although it may have a recognizable pattern of signs and symptoms and may be curable.

idiopathic multiple pigmented hemorrhagic sarcoma. See **Kaposi's sarcoma.**

idiopathic respiratory distress syndrome. See **hyaline membrane disease.**

idiopathic scoliosis, an abnormal condition characterized by a lateral curvature of the spine. It is the most common type of scoliosis, evident in 70% of all patients with scoliosis and up to 80% of those with structural scoliosis. It may occur at any age, but three types are commonly associated with certain age groups. The infantile type affects 1- to 3-year-olds. The juvenile type affects 3- to 10-year-olds. The adolescent type affects preadolescents and adolescents. The main factors in diagnosing idiopathic scoliosis are the degree, balance, and rotational component of the curvature. The rotational component may contribute to rib cage deformities and impingement on the pulmonary and the cardiac systems. The most common type is the adolescent type. Early diagnosis is difficult because the associated curvature is often hidden by clothing, and many states have started scoliosis screening programs for the early detection of this condition. The signs commonly associated with scoliosis include unlevel shoulders, a prominent scapula, a prominent breast, a prominent flank area, an unlevel or a prominent hip, poor posture, and an obvious curvature. During diagnosis it is necessary to view the patient from the front and from the back and while the patient is bending. Other signs that may be associated with idiopathic scoliosis are occasional transient pain and fatigue and decreased pulmonary function. Radiographic films of the spine in the bending position are important in ascertaining the flexibility of the curvature and the potential of spontaneous correction. Neurologic deficits are commonly associated with severe curvature and vary according to the extent to which the curvature has impinged on the spinal cord. Some signs of such impingement are reflex, sensation, and motor alterations of the lower extremities. Nonsurgical intervention commonly employs observation, an exercise program, and a Milwaukee brace. Observation and an exercise program often suffice, the observation implemented by frequent physical examinations and radiographic monitoring of the progress of the curvature. Exercise programs are designed to promote the maximum correction possible, as indicated by the degree of flexibility shown in the initial x-ray examination. Observation and the exercise program are employed with patients who have a curvature under 15 to 20 degrees. Greater degrees of curvature usually require the use of a Milwaukee brace in addition to observation and an exercise program. The Milwaukee brace, which is usually worn 23 hours a day, is used to control the progress of the curvature. The exercise program is implemented when the adolescent is out of the brace, and additional exercises are performed while in the brace. Surgical intervention may be required if the curvature has progressed to 40 degrees or more at the time of diagnosis or if a slightly lesser degree of curvature exists with a high degree of rotational component or imbalance. Approximately 5% to 10% of patients with idiopathic scoliosis require surgical intervention, which involves fusing of the involved vertebrae to prevent progress of the deformity. Preoperative traction, as Cotrel traction and halo-femoral traction, may also be used to encourage gradual tissue alterations and to decrease postoperative complications. The patient involved may be placed in Cotrel traction for a period of 5 to 10 days preoperatively. If halo-femoral traction is used, the patient may be placed in traction 1 to 3 weeks preoperatively. Some physicians apply a preoperative cast to their patients with idiopathic scoliosis to achieve immobilization and adjustment, especially if surgery must be postponed for a considerable period after diagnosis. Common surgical intervention techniques for this condition are Harrington rod instrumentation technique and Dwyer cable instrumentation technique, the former being more common. Initial postoperative immobilization is achieved with a posterior plaster shell, a Milwaukee brace, or a windowed cast. A Stryker frame, Foster frame, or Circolectric bed may also be used. Blood replacement may be required postoperatively, and appropriate intravenous therapy is usually employed for several days. Additional postoperative immobilization by means of cast therapy is often required for 8 to 12 months or until the bony union of the fused area is absolutely assured. The usual type of cast in this application is a Risser localizer cast, applied with a degree of traction. The Risser turnbuckle cast may also be used when instrumentation has not been employed. A Milwaukee brace or a plastic body jacket may be used when less immobilization is desired.

idiopathic thrombocytopenic purpura (ITP), bleeding into the skin and other organs caused by a deficiency of platelets. **Acute ITP** is a disease of children that may follow a viral infection, lasts a few weeks to a few months, and usually has no residual effects. **Chronic ITP** is more common in adolescents and adults, begins more insidiously, and lasts longer. Antibodies to platelets are found in patients with ITP; the condition may be transmitted to the fetus if a pregnant woman develops it. Treatment includes corticosteroids and splenectomy. See also **thrombocytopenia, thrombocytopenic purpura.**

idiopathy /id′ē·op′əthē/, any primary disease that arises without an apparent cause. –**idiopathic,** *adj.*

idiosyncrasy /id′ē·ōsin′krəsē/, **1.** a physical or behavioral characteristic or manner that is unique to an individual or to a group. **2.** an individual's unique hypersensitivity to a particular drug, food, or other substance. Also called **idiocrasy** /id′ē·ok′rəsē/. See also **allergy.** –**idiosyncratic,** *adj.*

idiot, an obsolete term for a severely retarded person having an intelligence quotient of less than 20, incapable of developing beyond the mental age of 3 or 4 years. Compare **imbecile, moron.** See also **mental retardation.** –**idiocy,** *n.,* **idiotic,** *adj.*

idiot savant /idē·ō′ savänt′/, *pl.* **idiot savants, idiots savants,** an individual with severe mental retardation who is nonetheless capable of performing certain unusual mental feats, primarily those involving music, puzzle-solving, or the manipulation of numbers.

idiotype, the portion of an immunoglobulin molecule conferring unique character; most often including its binding site.

idioventricular, originating in a ventricle.

-idium, a noun-forming combining form: *coracidium, parorchidium, thrombidium.*

IDL (intermediate-density lipoprotein), a lipid-protein complex with a density between VLDL (very-low-density lipoprotein) and LDL (low-density lipoprotein). It is a product that has a relatively very short half-life and is in the blood of normal persons in very low concentrations. In a type III hyperlipoproteinemic person the IDL concentration in the blood is found to be elevated.

IDM, abbreviation for **infant of a diabetic mother.**

idoxuridine /ī′doksyo͞or′ədēn/, an ophthalmic antiviral.

■ INDICATION: It is prescribed for herpes simplex keratitis.

■ CONTRAINDICATIONS: Deep ulceration of the cornea or known hypersensitivity to this drug prohibits its use.

■ ADVERSE EFFECTS: Among the more serious adverse reactions are visual disturbances and eye discomfort.

id reaction, the autosensitization resulting from a fungal infection that causes pruritus and vesicular lesions. These secondary lesions, caused by circulating antigens, are usually distant from the primary fungal infection.

-iform, a combining form meaning 'in the form of': *amebiform, bulbiform, nucleiform.*

Ig, abbreviation for **immunoglobulin.**

IgA, abbreviation for **immunoglobulin A.**

IgA deficiency, a selective lack of immunoglobulin A, the most common type of immunoglobulin deficiency, appearing in about 1 in 400 individuals. Immunoglobulin A is a major protein antibody in the saliva and the mucous membranes of the intestines and the bronchi. It protects against bacterial and viral infections. A deficiency of immunoglobulin A is associated with autosomal dominant or with autosomal recessive inheritance, and with autoimmune abnormalities. The IgA deficiency is common in patients with rheumatoid arthritis and in patients with systemic lupus erythematosus. Many individuals with this deficiency have normal numbers of peripheral blood lymphocytes with IgA receptors and normal amounts of other immunoglobulins. Normality accompanied by IgA deficiency suggests that the B-lymphocytes of the involved patient may not secrete IgA. In some patients with this deficiency, T cells seem to depress the synthesis of IgA.

■ OBSERVATIONS: Symptoms of IgA deficiency are often lacking in patients whose humoral immune systems may be compensating for low IgA with extra amounts of IgM to assure adequate defenses. Common symptoms are respiratory allergies associated with chronic sinopulmonary infection, GI diseases, as celiac disease and regional enteritis, autoimmune diseases, as rheumatoid arthritis, systemic lupus erythematosus, and chronic hepatitis, malignant tumors, as squamous cell carcinoma of the lungs, recticulum cell sarcoma, and thymoma. The age of onset varies. Some children with IgA deficiency may begin to synthesize the immunoglobulin spontaneously when their recurrent infections wane and their conditions improve. Diagnoses of IgA-deficient patients depend on the results of tests that commonly show normal IgE and IgM levels while IgA levels are below 5 mg/dl in serum. Cell-mediated response and circulating B cells commonly appear normal, although tests may indicate autoantibodies and antibodies against IgG, IgM, and cow's milk. T cell interferon production may be decreased in some patients with IgA deficiency, increasing the chances of infection.

■ INTERVENTION: There is no known cure for selective IgA deficiency; treatment usually involves the effort to control associated diseases, as respiratory and GI infections.

■ NURSING CONSIDERATIONS: The patient with IgA deficiency should not receive gamma globulin because associated sensitization may cause anaphylaxis during administration of blood products. When the IgA deficient patient requires a blood transfusion, the risk of any harmful reaction can be reduced by using washed red blood cells. Using the crossmatched blood of an IgA-deficient donor in such a transfusion is considered a safer method and completely avoids the risk of an adverse reaction. The IgA deficiency is a lifelong condition, and patients with this disorder are commonly instructed to identify its symptoms and to seek treatment promptly.

IgD, abbreviation for **immunoglobulin D.**

IgE, abbreviation for **immunoglobulin E.**

IgG, abbreviation for **immunoglobulin G.**

IgM, abbreviation for **immunoglobulin M.**

IGT, abbreviation for **impaired glucose tolerance.**

Ikwa fever. See **trench fever.**

-il, -ile, a combining form meaning a 'substance related to another': *benzil, uracil, uramil.*

Ile, abbreviation for **isoleucine.**

ileal conduit, a method of urinary diversion through intestinal tract tissue. Ureters are implanted in a section of dissected ileum which is then sewed to an ostomy in the abdominal wall where a collecting device is attached.

ileitis /il′ē·ī′tis/, inflammation of the ileum. See also **Crohn's disease.**

ileo-, a combining form meaning 'pertaining to the ileum': *ileocecum, ileorectostomy, ileotomy.*

ileocecal valve, the valve between the ileum of the small intestine and the cecum of the large intestine. The valve consists of two flaps that project into the lumen of the large intestine, just above the vermiform appendix, allowing the contents of the intestine to pass only in a forward direction.

ileocecostomy. See **cecolieostomy.**

ileocolic node /il′ē·ōkol′ik/, a node in one of three groups of superior mesenteric lymph glands, forming a chain of approximately 15 nodes around the ileocolic (mesenteric) artery. They tend to form in two main groups, one near the duodenum, the other on the lower part of the ileocolic artery. The chain breaks into several groups where the artery divides into its terminal branches. The ileocolic nodes receive afferents from the jejunum, ileum, cecum, vermiform appendix, ascending colon, and transverse colon. Their efferents pass to the preaortic nodes. Compare **mesenteric node, mesocolic node.**

ileocystoplasty, a surgical procedure in which the bladder is reconstructed using a segment of the ileum for the bladder wall.

ileostomate /il′ē·os′təmāt/, a person who has undergone an ileostomy.

ileostomy /il′ē·os′təmē/, surgical formation of an opening of the ileum onto the surface of the abdomen, through which fecal matter is emptied. The operation is performed in advanced or recurrent ulcerative colitis, Crohn's disease, or cancer of the large bowel. A low-residue diet is given preoperatively and is reduced to fluids 24 hours before surgery to decrease intestinal residue. Intestinal antibiotics are given to decrease the bacterial count. A nasogastric or intestinal tube is passed. The diseased portion of the large bowel is removed in a permanent ileostomy; occasionally, the distal and proximal segments of bowel may be reconnected after ulcerated areas have healed. A loop of the proximal ileum is then brought out onto the abdomen and sutured in place, and a stoma is formed. A pouch may be made with part of the terminal ileum, in which the open end is woven through the rectus muscles to form a valve and then opens onto the abdomen. Postoperatively, the patient wears a temporary disposable bag to collect the semiliquid fecal matter, which begins to drain once peristalsis is restored and the tube is removed. Since the secretions contain digestive enzymes that can ulcerate the skin around the stoma, the nurse ensures that nothing leaks from the bag. The nurse instructs the patient how to apply and care for the stoma and the colostomy bag. If a pouch is present, it is irrigated or drained three or four times a day through a small irrigating catheter through the valve. Compare **colostomy.** See also **enterostomy, ostomy irrigation, stoma.**

ileum /il′ē·əm/, *pl.* **ilea,** the distal portion of the small intestine, extending from the jejunum to the cecum. It has a few small circular folds and numerous clusters of lymph nodes. It ends in the right iliac fossa, opening into the medial side of the large intestine. –**ileac, ileal,** *adj.*

ileus /il′ē·əs/, an obstruction of the intestines, as an adynamic ileus caused by immobility of the bowel, or a mechanic ileus in which the intestine is blocked by mechanic means.

-iliac, a combining form meaning 'the ilium': *occipitoiliac, subiliac, vertebroiliac.*

iliac circumflex node /il′ē·ak/, a node in one of the seven clusters of parietal lymph nodes of the abdomen. This node is one of a group found along the course of the deep iliac circumflex vessels. Compare **common iliac node, external iliac node, internal iliac node.** See also **lymph, lymphatic system, lymph node.**

iliac fascia, the portion of the endoabdominal fascia that is attached with the iliacus to the crest of the ilium and passes under the inguinal ligament into the thigh.

iliac region. See **inguinal region.**

iliacus /ilī′əkəs/, a flat, triangular muscle that covers the inner curved surface of the iliac fossa. It arises from the inner aspect of the superior iliac crest, from the anterior and the iliolumbar ligaments, and from the sacrum. It joins the psoas major to form the iliopsoas at the inguinal ligament. The iliacus is innervated by branches of the femoral nerve that contain fibers from the second and the third lumbar nerves. It acts to flex and laterally rotate the thigh. Compare **psoas major, psoas minor.**

ilio-, a combining form meaning 'of or pertaining to the ilium or flank': *iliocostal, iliolumbar, iliometer.*

iliofemoral /il′ē·ōfem′ərəl/, of or pertaining to the ilium and femur.

ilioinguinal /il′ē·ō·ing′gwinəl/, of or pertaining to the hip and inguinal regions.

iliolumbar ligament, one of a pair of ligaments forming part of the connection between the vertebral column and the pelvis. Each iliolumbar ligament attaches to a transverse process of the fifth lumbar vertebra and passes to the base of the sacrum.

iliopectineal line, a bony ridge on the inner surface of the ilium and pubic bones that divides the true and false pelvises. Also called **brim of true pelvic cavity, inlet.**

iliopsoas /il′ē·ōsō′əs/, one of the pair of muscle complexes that flexes the thigh and the lumbar vertebral column. Each complex is comprised of the psoas major, the psoas minor, and the iliacus, although the psoas minor is often absent. The psoas major is a long fusiform muscle, arising from certain lumbar vertebrae and inserting into the femur. The iliacus is a flat, triangular muscle arising from the iliac fossa and inserting into the femur and the tendon of the psoas major. The psoas minor is a long slender muscle ventral to the psoas major.

ilium /il′ē·əm/, *pl.* **ilia,** one of the three bones that make up the innominate bone. The ilium forms part of the acetabulum and provides attachment for several muscles, including the obturator internus, the gluteals, the iliacus, and the sartorius. The ilium is divided into the body, which forms less than two fifths of the acetabulum, and the ala ossis ilii, which is the large, winglike portion of the greater pelvis. The ala contains the iliac fossa and the greater sciatic notch and presents various prominences for muscle attachment, as the iliac crest, the anterior superior and the posterior superior iliac spines, and the anterior inferior and the posterior inferior iliac spines. Compare **ischium, pubis.** –**iliac,** *adj.*

illicit, pertaining to an act that is unlawful or otherwise not permitted.

illness, an abnormal process in which aspects of the social, physical, emotional, or intellectual condition and function of a person are diminished or impaired, compared with that person's previous condition.

illness experience, the process of being ill, comprised of five stages: phase I, experiencing a symptom; phase II, assuming a sick role; phase III, making contact for health care; phase IV, being dependent (a patient); and phase V, recovering or being rehabilitated. Each stage is characterized by certain decisions, behaviors, and end points. During phase I, in which a symptom is experienced, the person decides that something is wrong and tries to remedy the situation. Phase I ends with the person accepting the reality of the symptom, no longer delaying any action toward help or denying the symptom (flight into health). During phase II the person decides that the illness is real and that care is necessary. Advice, guidance, and validation are sought. This gives the person permission to act sick and to be excused temporarily from usual obligations. The outcome of this phase is acceptance of the role—or denial of its necessity. In phase III professional advice is sought; authoritative declarations identify and validate the illness and legitimize the sick role. The person usually asks for help and negotiates for treatment. Denial may still occur and the patient may ''shop'' further for medical care or may accept the illness, the medical authority, and the plan for treatment. In phase IV professional treatment is performed and accepted by the person, who is now perceived as a patient. At any time during this phase the dependent patient may develop ambivalent feelings and may decide to reject the treatment, the care giver, and the illness. More often, care is accepted with ambivalence. The patient has a particular need to be informed and to be given emotional support during this phase. During phase V, the last stage of the illness experience, the patient relinquishes the sick role. The usual tasks and roles are resumed to the greatest degree possible. Some people do not willingly give up the sick role, becoming, in their own eyes, chronically ill, or, for secondary gain, they malinger, acting sick. Most people accept the recovery and work toward rehabilitation.

illumination, the lighting up of a part of the body or of an object under a microscope for the purpose of examination. –**illuminate,** *v.*

illusion, a false interpretation of an external sensory stimulus, usually visual or auditory, as a mirage in the desert or voices on the wind. Compare **delusion, hallucination.**

Ilopan, a trademark for a precursor of coenzyme A (dexpanthenol).

Ilosone, a trademark for an antibacterial (erythromycin estolate).

Ilozyme, a trademark for a digestant (pancrelipase).

im-, a combining form in chemistry indicating the bivalent group > NH: *imadyl, imide, imperialine.*

I.M.A., abbreviation for **Industrial Medical Association.**

image, **1.** a representation or visual reproduction of the likeness of someone or something, as a painting, photograph, or sculpture. **2.** an optic representation of an object, as that produced by refraction or reflection. **3.** a person or thing that closely resembles another; semblance. **4.** a mental picture, representation, idea, or concept of an objective reality. **5.** (in psychology) a mental representation of something previously perceived and subsequently modified by other experiences resulting from intrapsychic or extrapsychic stimuli, or both. Kinds of images include **body image, eidetic image, memory image, mental image, motor image,** and **tactile image.**

image acquistion time, the time required to carry out an NMR imaging procedure comprising only the data acquisition time. The additional image reconstruction time will also be important to determine how quickly the image can be viewed. In comparing sequential plane imaging and volume imaging techniques, the equivalent image acquisition time per slice must be considered, as well as the actual image acquisition time.

image intensifier, an electronic device used to produce a fluoroscopic image with a low-radiation exposure. A beam of x-rays passing through the patient is converted in a special vacuum tube into a pattern of electrons. The electrons are accelerated and concentrated onto a small fluorescent screen where they present a bright image. This is generally displayed on a TV monitor.

imagery, (in psychiatry) the formation of mental concepts, figures, ideas; any product of the imagination. In mentally disturbed persons these images are often bizarre and delusional.

imagination, **1.** the ability to form, or the act or process of forming mental images or conscious concepts of things that are not immediately available to the senses. **2.** (in psychology) the ability to reproduce images or ideas stored in the memory by the stimulation or suggestion of associated ideas or to regroup former ideas and concepts to form new images and ideas concerned with a particular goal or problem. See also **fantasy.**

imaging, the formation of a mental picture or representation of someone or something using the imagination. See also **fantasy.**

imago /imā′gō/, (in analytic psychology) an unconscious, usually idealized mental image of a significant individual, as one's mother, in a person's early, formative years. See also **identification.**

imbalance, **1.** lack of balance between opposing muscle groups, as in the imbalance of extraocular muscles leading to strabismus. **2.** an abnormal balance of fluid and electrolytes in the body tissues. **3.** an unequal distribution of subjects in a population group, as an only girl in a large family of boys. **4.** a person with mental abilities that are remarkable in one area but deficient in others, as an idiot savant.

imbecile, *obsolete.* a moderately retarded person having an intelligence quotient of 20 to 49, incapable of developing beyond a mental age of 7 or 8 years. Compare **idiot, moron.** See also **mental retardation.** –**imbecile, imbecilic,** *adj.,* **imbecility,** *n.*

imbricate /im′brikāt/, to build a surface with overlapping layers of material. Surgeons may imbricate with layers of tissue when closing a wound or other opening in a body part. –**imbrication,** *n.*

Imferon, a trademark for an injectable hematinic (iron dextran).

imide-, imido-, a combining form indicating the presence in a chemical compound of the bivalent group > NH: *imidogen.*

imino-, a combining form indicating the presence of the bivalent group > NH attached to a nonacid radical: *iminourea*.

iminoglycinuria, a benign familial condition characterized by the abnormal urinary excretion of the amino acids glycine, proline, and hydroxyproline.

imipramine hydrochloride, a tricyclic antidepressant with a slow onset of action.

■ INDICATION: It is prescribed in the treatment of mental depression.

■ CONTRAINDICATIONS: Concomitant administration of monoamine oxidase inhibitors, recent myocardial infarction, cardiovascular disease or seizure disorder, or known hypersensitivity to this drug or to other tricyclic medication prohibits its use.

■ ADVERSE EFFECTS: Among the more serious adverse reactions are sedation, GI disturbances, and cardiovascular and neurologic reactions. It should not be withdrawn abruptly. This drug interacts with many other drugs.

immature baby, a term sometimes applied to an infant weighing less than 1134 g (2.5 lb) and who is considerably underdeveloped at birth.

immediate auscultation, a method of examining a patient by placing an ear or stethoscope on the skin directly over the body part being studied.

immediate hypersensitivity, an allergic reaction that occurs within minutes after exposure to an allergen.

immediate percussion. See **percussion.**

immediate posttraumatic automatism, a posttraumatic state in which a person acts spontaneously and automatically without having any recollection of the behavior.

immersion, the placing of a body or an object into water or other liquid so that it is completely covered by the liquid. **–immerse,** *v.*

immersion foot, an abnormal condition of the feet characterized by damage to the muscles, nerves, skin and blood vessels, caused by prolonged exposure to dampness or by prolonged immersion in cold water. See also **frostbite.**

imminent abortion. See **inevitable abortion.**

immiscible /imis′əbəl/, not capable of being mixed, as oil and water. Compare **miscible.**

immune complex hypersensitivity, an IgG or IgM complement dependent, immediate acting humoral hypersensitivity to certain soluble antigens. An intradermal skin test results in erythema and edema within 3 to 8 hours and an acute inflammatory reaction with an increase in polymorphonuclear leukocytes. It is seen in serum sickness, Arthus reaction, and glomerulonephritis. Also called **type III hypersensitivity.** Compare **anaphylactic hypersensitivity, cell-mediated immune response, cytotoxic hypersensitivity.**

immune cytolysis, cell destruction mediated by a particular antibody in conjunction with complement.

immune gamma globulin, passive immunizing agents obtained from pooled human plasma. Also called **immune globulin.** See also **immunoglobulin G.**

■ INDICATIONS: It is prescribed for immunization against measles, poliomyelitis, chickenpox, serum hepatitis following transfusion, hepatitis A, agammaglobulinemia, and hypogammaglobulinemia.

■ CONTRAINDICATION: Known hypersensitivity to gamma globulins prohibits its use.

■ ADVERSE EFFECTS: Among the more serious adverse reactions are pain and inflammation at the site of injection and allergic reactions.

immune globulin. See **immune gamma globulin.**

immune human globulin, a sterile solution of globulins that is used as a passive immunizing agent and derived from adult human blood.

immune response, a defense function of the body that produces antibodies to destroy invading antigens and malignancies. Important components of the immune system and response are immunoglobulins, lymphocytes, phagocytes, complement, properdin, the migratory inhibitory factor, and interferon. Antigens, which are largely foreign protein macromolecules, trigger the immune response during interaction with countless cells of the reticuloendothelial system of the body. The kinds of immune response are humoral immune response, involving B lymphocytes or B cells, and cell-mediated immune response, involving T lymphocytes or T cells. The B cells and the T cells derive from the hemopoietic stem cells, which originate in the embryonic yolk sac. Every normal baby is born with many different clones of B cells in the bone marrow, the lymph nodes, and the spleen. All the cells of each clone synthesize a specific antibody with a different sequence of amino acids from that of any of the other numerous clones of B cells. The receptor sites on the surface membranes of the B cells are the combining sites of immunoglobulin molecules. The classes of immunoglobulins, identified by letter names, are M, G, A, E, and D. Immunoglobulin M, the antibody that immature B cells synthesize and incorporate in their cytoplasmic membranes, is the predominant antibody produced after initial contact with an antigen. The T cells develop in the thymus gland and proliferate with antigen receptors on their surface membranes. The T cells assist in the antigen-antibody reaction of the B cells and control the cell-mediated response associated with the reduction of tissue inflammation. The cell-mediated response is also effective against fungi, viruses, and tumors and is the major reaction in the rejection of organ transplants. In transplant surgery, certain methods, as the administration of appropriate drugs and radiation, suppress transplant rejection. The T cells have little or no immunoglobulin on their surfaces and always maintain their leukocyte structure. They are divided into circulating T cells, noncirculating T cells, and memory T cells. Circulating T cells function within circulating fluids; noncirculating T cells include those that produce lymphokines and selectively migrate to inflamed tissue sites. Memory T cells recognize antigens as foreign and mobilize tissue macrophages in the presence of the migratory inhibitory factor. Humoral immune response protects the body against bacterial and viral infections through the stimulation of antibodies associated with the B cells. Plasma cells, which derive from B cells through the stimulation of antigens, secrete trillions of antibody molecules that aid the humoral immune response. Such molecules recognize microinvaders of the body as ''foreigners'' when the antigens bind to them. The antigen-antibody reaction may transform the toxic antigen into a harmless substance, or it may agglutinate antigens, allowing macrophages and other phagocytes to digest large numbers of antigens at one time. The antigen-antibody reactions of the humoral immune response also activate the complement in the blood serum, which triggers a nonspecific series of chemical reactions to amplify the humoral immune response. Activated discrete plasma proteins C1 to C3 in the complement system cause lysis of the antigenic cell and opsonize the antigen for phagocytosis. Humoral immune response may begin immediately with antigen contact or may be delayed for as long as 48 hours. The speed of humoral response is demonstrated in anaphylaxis. Other proteins associated with the immune response are properdin and interferon. Properdin provides an alternate process for activating complement. Interferon is synthesized by body cells after viral invasion acts to combat viruses and may retard the growth of cancer cells. Humoral immune response and cell-mediated immune response immunity are interdependent. The former can influence the function of T cells and the latter the function of B cells. Humoral and cell-mediated immunity can be natural or acquired. Natural immunity, or genetically inherited resistance to specific infectious organisms, can be affected by diet, mental health, environment, metabolism, and the virulence of invading pathogens.

immune serum. See **antiserum.**

immune serum globulin. See **chickenpox, immune human globulin, immunoglobulin antibody.**

immune system, a biochemical complex that protects the body against pathogenic organisms and other foreign bodies. The system incorporates the humoral immune response, which produces antibodies to react with specific antigens, and the cell-mediated response, which uses T cells to mobilize tissue macrophages in the presence of a foreign body. The immune system also protects the body from invasion by creating local barriers and inflammation. The local barriers provide chemical and mechanic defenses through the skin, the mucous membranes, and the conjunctiva. Inflammation draws polymorphonuclear leukocytes and neutrophils to the site of injury where these phagocytes engulf the invading organism. The humoral response and the cell-mediated response develop if these first-line defenses fail or are inadequate to protect the body. The humoral immune response is especially effective against bacterial and viral invasions and employs B cells that produce appropriate antibodies. The principal organs of the immune response system include the bone marrow, the thymus, and the lymphoid tissues. The system also employs peripheral organs, as the lymph nodes, the spleen, and the lymphatic vessels. The antigen-antibody reactions of the immune system activate the complement system, which removes antigens from the body. The complement system contains several discrete proteins that function to produce lysis of the antigenic cells. The humoral response may begin immediately on invasion by the antigen or may start as long as 48 hours later.

immunity, **1.** (in civil law) exemption from a duty or an obligation generally required by law, as an exemption from taxation, exemption from penalty for wrongdoing, or protection against liability. **2.** the quality of being insusceptible to or unaffected by a particular disease or condition. Kinds of immunity are **active immunity** and **passive immunity.** –**immune,** *adj.*

immunization, a process by which resistance to an infectious disease is induced or augmented.

immunoassay, a competitive-binding assay in which the binding protein is an antibody.

immunodeficient, an abnormal condition of the immune system in which cellular or humoral immunity is inadequate and resistance to infection is decreased. Kinds of immunodeficient conditions are **hypogammaglobulinemia** and **lymphoid aplasia.**

immunodiagnosis. See **serologic diagnosis.**

immunodiagnostic, pertaining to or characterizing a diagnosis based on an antigen-antibody reaction. In many cases, a tumor releases a discrete antigenic substance into the blood; detection of a particular antigen can provide an immunodiagnostic sign of the presence of the tumor associated with that antigen.

immunodiffusion, a technique for the identification and quantification of any of the immunoglobulins. It is based on the presence of a visible precipitate that results from an antigen-antibody combination under certain circumstances. **Gel diffusion** is a technique that involves evaluation of the precipitin reaction in a clear gel, seen when an antigen placed in a hole in the agarose diffuses evenly into the medium. An obvious ring forms where the antigen meets the antibody. **Electroimmunodiffusion** is a gel diffusion to which an electric field is applied, accelerating the reaction. **Double gel diffusion** is a technique that permits identification of antibodies in mixed specimens. In an agar plate, antigen is placed in one well, antibody in another. Antigen and antibody diffuse out of their wells. In mixed antigen specimens, each antigen-antibody combination forms a separate line; observation of the location, shape, and thickness of a line permits identification and quantification of the antibody.

immunoelectrodiffusion. See **immunodiffusion.**

immunoelectrophoresis, a technique that combines electrophoresis and immunodiffusion to separate and allow identification of complex proteins. The proteins in the test serum are spread out in agar and separated by electrophoresis. Wells or troughs are then cut into the agar, and aliquots of antibody are placed in the troughs and allowed to diffuse toward the separated proteins. A visible precipitin will form in a series of arcs in the agar when an antigen-antibody reaction occurs. The shape and location of each arc are specific for known proteins. Unusual arcs are representative of abnormal or unknown protein. Although the density of the precipitation corresponds to the concentration of protein in each electrophoretic band, immunoelectrophoresis does not accurately quantify the amount of protein in the test serum. –**immunoelectrophoretic,** *adj.*

immunofluorescence, a technique used for the rapid identification of an antigen by exposing it to known antibodies tagged with the fluorescent dye fluorescein and observing the characteristic antigen-antibody reaction of precipitation. As the fluorescent antibody reacts with its specific antigen, the precipitate appears luminous in the ultraviolet light projected by a fluorescent microscope. Many of the most common infectious organisms can be identified using this technique. Among them are *Candida albicans, Haemophilus influenzae, Neisseria gonorrhae, Shigella, Staphylococcus aureus,* and several viruses, including rabies virus and many enteroviruses. See also **fluorescent microscopy.** –**immunofluorescent,** *adj.*

immunofluorescence test. See **fluorescent antibody test.**

immunofluorescent microscopy. See **fluorescent microscopy, immunofluorescence.**

immunogen /imyōō′nəjən/, any agent or substance capable of provoking an immune response or producing immunity. –**immunogenic,** *adj.*

immunoglobulin, any of five structurally and antigenically distinct antibodies present in the serum and external secretions of the body. In response to specific antigens, immunoglobulins are formed in the bone marrow, spleen, and all lymphoid tissue of the body except the thymus. Kinds of immunoglobulins are **IgA, IgD, IgE, IgG,** and **IgM.** Also called **immune serum globulin.** See also **antibody, antigen, immunity.**

immunoglobulin A (IgA), one of the five classes of humoral antibodies produced by the body and one of the most prevalent. It is found in all secretions of the body and is the major antibody in the mucous membrane lining the intestines and in the bronchi, saliva, and tears. IgA combines with a protein in the mucosa and defends body surfaces against invading microorganisms. Research indicates that it protects body tissues by seeking out foreign microorganisms and triggering an antigen-antibody reaction. The normal concentrations of IgA in serum are 50 to 250 mg/dl. Compare **immunoglobulin D, immunoglobulin E, immunoglobulin G, immunoglobulin M.**

immunoglobulin D (IgD), one of the five classes of humoral antibodies produced by the body. It is a specialized protein found in small amounts in serum tissue. The precise function of IgD is not known, but it increases in quantity during allergic reactions to milk, insulin, penicillin, and various toxins. The normal concentrations of IgD in serum are 0.5 to 3 mg/dl. Compare **immunoglobulin A, immunoglobulin E, immunoglobulin G, immunoglobulin M.**

immunoglobulin E (IgE), one of the five classes of humoral antibodies produced by the body. It is concentrated in the lung, the skin, and the cells of mucous membranes. It provides the primary defense against environmental antigens and is believed to be responsive to immunoglobulin A. IgE reacts with certain antigens to release certain chemical mediators that cause Type I hypersensitivity reactions characterized by wheal and flare. The normal concentrations of IgE in serum are 0.01 to 0.04 mg/dl. Compare **immunoglobulin A, immunoglobulin D, immunoglobulin G, immunoglobulin M.**

immunoglobulin G (IgG), one of the five classes of humoral antibodies produced by the body. It is a specialized protein synthesized by the body in response to invasions by bacteria, fungi, and viruses. IgG crosses the placenta and protects against red cell antigens and white cell antigens. The normal concentrations of IgG in serum are 800 to 1600 mg/dl. Compare **immunoglobulin A, immunoglobulin D, immunoglobulin E, immunoglobulin M.**

immunoglobulin M (IgM), one of the five classes of humoral antibodies produced by the body and the largest in molecular structure. It is the first immunoglobulin the body produces when challenged by antigens and is found in circulating fluids. IgM triggers the increased production of immunoglobulin G and the complement fixation required for effective antibody response. It is the dominant antibody in ABO incompatibilities. The normal concentrations of IgM in serum are 40 to 120 mg/dl. Compare **immunoglobulin A, immunoglobulin D, immunoglobulin E, immunoglobulin G.**

immunohematology, the study of antigen-antibody reactions and their effects on blood.

immunologic tests, tests based on the principles of antigen-antibody reactions.

immunologic theory of aging, a concept based on the premise that normal cells are unrecognized as such, thereby triggering immune reactions within the individual's own body.

immunologist, a specialist in immunology.

immunology, the study of the reaction of tissues of the immune system of the body to antigenic stimulation.

immunomodulator, a substance that acts to alter the immune response by augmenting or reducing the ability of the immune system to produce specifically modified serum antibodies or sensitized cells that recognize and react with the antigen that initiated their production. Corticosteroids, cytotoxic agents, thymosin, and the immunoglobulins are among the immunomodulating substances. Some immunomodulating substances are naturally present in the body; some of these are available in various pharmacologic preparations. –**immunomodulation,** *n.*

immunopotency, the ability of an antigen to elicit an immune response.

immunosuppression, **1.** the administration of agents that significantly interfere with the ability of the immune system to respond to antigenic stimulation by inhibiting cellular and humoral immunity. Corticosteroid hormones given in large amounts, cytotoxic drugs, including antimetabolites and alkylating agents, antilymphocytic serum (ALS), and irradiation may result in immunosuppression. Immunosuppression may be deliberate, as in preparation for bone marrow or other transplantation to prevent rejection by the host of the donor tissue, or incidental, as often results from chemotherapy for the treatment of cancer. **2.** an abnormal condition of the immune system characterized by markedly inhibited ability to respond to antigenic stimuli. **–immunosuppressed,** *adj.*

immunosuppressive, **1.** of or pertaining to a substance or procedure that lessens or prevents an immune response. **2.** an immunosuppressive agent. The immunosuppressive drugs used most frequently to prevent homograft rejection are the cytotoxic purine antimetabolite azathioprine, the alkylating agent cyclophosphamide, and the adrenocorticosteroid prednisone. Methotrexate, cytarabine, dactinomycin, thioguanine, and antilymphocyte globulin are also potent immunosuppressives. The use of some of these agents is being explored for the treatment of autoimmune diseases, as systemic lupus erythematosus, and for many other disorders.

immunotherapy, a special treatment of allergic responses that administers increasingly large doses of the offending allergens to gradually develop immunity. Immunotherapy is based on the premise that low doses of the offending allergen will bind with IgG to prevent an allergic reaction by damping the action of IgE by fostering the synthesis of the blocking IgG antibody. The individual who is exposed to the offending allergen develops an amount of blocking antibody in proportion to the extent of the exposure. The blocking antibody binds to the circulating antigen and seems to decrease the allergic response, or it eliminates the allergic response by producing an immunologic tolerance toward the antigen. In immunotherapy low doses of the offending allergen are gradually increased throughout the year or during a 3- to 6-month period before the allergy season starts; it usually continues until the patient shows no significant allergic response for 2 to 5 years. Also called **hyposensitization.** **–immunotherapeutic,** *adj.*

Imodium, a trademark for an intestinal antiperistaltic (loperamide hydrochloride), used as an antidiarrheal agent.

Imovax, a trademark for a rabies virus vaccine (rabies human diploid cell vaccine).

impacted, tightly or firmly wedged in a limited amount of space. **–impact,** *v.,* **impaction,** *n.*

impacted fracture, a bone break in which the adjacent fragmented ends of the fractured bone are wedged together.

impacted tooth, a tooth so positioned against another tooth, bone, or soft tissue that its complete and normal eruption is impossible or unlikely. An impacted third molar tooth may be further described according to its position, as buccoangular, distoangular, or vertical. Compare **embedded tooth.**

impact printer, a mechanic printer that imprints computer characters on paper by striking it as a typewriter does, usually through an inked ribbon. Compare **nonimpact printer.**

impaired glucose tolerance (IGT), a condition in which fasting plasma glucose levels are higher than normal but lower than those diagnostic of diabetes mellitus. In some patients this represents a stage in the natural history of diabetes, but in a substantial number of persons IGT either does not progress or reverts to normal. See also **diabetes mellitus.**

impairment, any disorder in structure or function resulting from anatomic, physiologic, or psychologic abnormalities that interfere with normal activities.

impedance, a form of electric resistance observed in an alternating current that is analagous to the classic electric resistance that occurs in a direct current circuit. It is expressed as a ratio of voltage applied to a circuit to the current it produces, as an alternating current oscillates ahead of or behind the voltage.

impedance audiometry. See **audiometry.**

impedance plethysmography, a technique for detecting blood vessel occlusion that determines volumetric changes in the limb by measuring changes in its girth as indicated by changes in the electric impedance of mercury-containing Silastic tubes in a pressure cuff. The method is based on the principle that any circumferential rate of change in a limb segment is directly proportional to the volumetric rate of change, which in turn reflects occlusion of venous and arterial blood flow. However, the technique does not accurately indicate the presence or absence of partially obstructing thrombi in major vessels.

imperative conception, a thought or impression that appears spontaneously in the mind and cannot be eliminated, as an obsession.

imperative idea. See **compulsive idea.**

imperforate /impur′fərit/, lacking a normal opening in a body organ or passageway. An infant may be born with an imperforate anus. Compare **perforate.**

imperforate anus, any of several congenital, developmental malformations of the anorectal portion of the GI tract.

■ OBSERVATION: The most common form is anal agenesis, in which the rectal pouch ends blindly above the surface of the perineum. An anal fistula is present in 80% to 90% of cases. Other forms include anal stenosis, in which the anal aperture is small, and anal membrane atresia, in which the anal membrane covers the aperture creating an obstruction.

■ INTERVENTION: The defect is usually discovered at birth; inspection reveals an absence of the anus or the presence of a thin translucent membrane covering it. Digital and endoscopic examination allows identification of the anatomic character of the malformation. X-ray examination is performed to outline the rectal pouch. A radiopaque marker is placed at the usual site of the anus, and the infant is held upside down. Air moving through the intestines into the distal portion of the bowel or the rectum is visible on the x-ray film. Anal stenosis is treated with daily digital dilatation begun in the hospital and continued at home by the parents. An imperforate anal membrane is excised, and digital dilatation is performed daily as the skin heals. Surgical reconstruction is performed to treat anal agenesis in infants in whom the pouch is below the puborectalis of the levator ani; an anus is created surgically by an anoplasty. Anal atresia in which the pouch at the end of the bowel is high above the perineum may require a colostomy.

■ NURSING CONSIDERATIONS: Often it is the nurse who identifies the anal malformation because the thermometer cannot be inserted during the routine newborn assessment. A newborn who does not pass any stool in the first 24 hours requires further evaluation for the possibility of the defect. The passage of meconium from the vagina or urinary meatus clearly indicates the presence of anal fistula and usually occurs in association with an imperforate anus. Postoperative care in the newborn treated surgically for any of these conditions requires scrupulous perineal care.

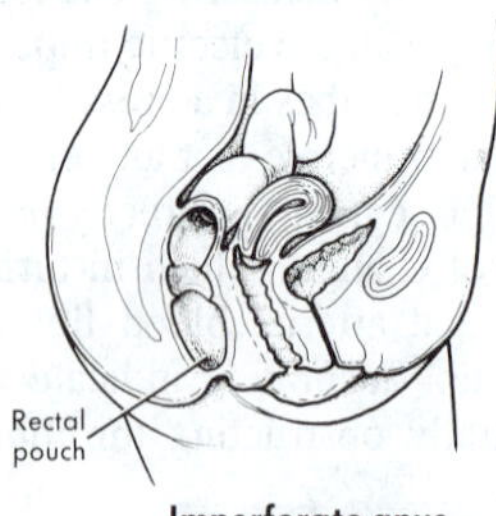

Imperforate anus

impermeable, (of a tissue, membrane, or film) preventing the passage of a substance through it.

impetigo /im′pətī′gō/, a streptococcal, a staphylococcal, or a combined infection of the skin beginning as focal erythema and progressing to pruritic vesicles, erosions, and honey-colored crusts. Lesions usually form on the face and spread locally. The disorder is highly contagious by contact with the discharge from the lesions. Acute glomerulonephritis is an occasional complication. Treatment includes thorough cleansing with antibacterial soap and water, compresses of Burow's solution, removal of crusts, and topical or oral antibiotics. Essential to prevent spread of infection are treatment of the sores, use of individual wash cloths and linens, and scrupulous hand washing. –**impetiginous,** *adj.*

implant, **1.** (in radiotherapy) an encapsulated radioactive substance embedded in tissue for therapy. Seeds containing iodine 125 may be implanted permanently in prostate and chest tumors and seeds of iridium 192 in ribbons or wire may be embedded temporarily in head and neck cancers. Sealed sources of cesium 137 or radium 226 may be implanted in the body cavity temporarily in the treatment of gynecologic malignancies; strontium 90 in sealed sources may be embedded for a brief period (usually less than 2 minutes) in the treatment of eye tumors; needles containing radium 226 may be used as temporary interstitial implants. Patients with radioactive implants are isolated from other patients whenever possible. **2.** (in surgery) material inserted or grafted into an organ or structure of the body. The implant may be of tissue, as in a blood vessel graft, or of an artificial substance, as in a hip prosthesis, a cardiac pacemaker, or a container of radioactive material.

implantation, (in embryology) the process involving the attachment, penetration, and embedding of the blastocyst in the lining of the uterine wall during the early stages of prenatal development. The degree of invasiveness required for an adequate maternal-fetal exchange varies greatly among species. In humans, the process occurs over a period of a few days, beginning about the seventh or eighth day after fertilization, and consists of the complete embedding of the conceptus within the uterine endometrium. Kinds of implantation include **eccentric implantation, interstitial implantation,** and **superficial implantation.** Also called **nidation.**

implantation dermoid cyst, a tumor derived from embryonal tissues, caused by an injury that forces part of the ectoderm into the body.

implant restoration, a single-tooth implant crown or multiple-tooth implant crown or bridge that replaces a missing tooth or teeth.

implementation, a deliberate action performed to achieve a goal, as carrying out a plan in caring for a patient. –**implement,** *v.*

implementation mechanism, the means by which innovations are transferred from the planners to the units of service.

implementing, (in five-step nursing process) a category of nursing behavior in which the actions necessary for accomplishing the health care plan are initiated and completed. Implementing includes the performance or assisting in the performance of the patient's activities of daily living; counseling and teaching the patient or the patient's family; giving care to achieve therapeutic goals and to optimize the achievement of health goals by the patient; supervising and evaluating the work of staff members; and recording and exchanging information relevant to the patient's continued health care. The patient may require assistance in performing certain activities of daily living. The nurse helps the patient to maintain optimal function, while instituting measures for the patient's comfort as necessary. The nurse helps the patient and the patient's family to recognize and manage the emotional and psychologic stress attendant on the patient's condition and facilitates the relationships of the patient, patient's family, staff, and other significant people. Correct principles, procedures, and techniques of health care are taught, and the patient is informed about the current status of health. If necessary, the patient or the patient's family is referred to a health or social resource in the community. Care is given to achieve therapeutic goals, including acting to compensate for adverse reactions; using preventive and precautionary measures and correct technique in administering care; preparing the patient for surgery, delivery, or other procedure; or initiating life-saving measures for emergency situations. Care is given to the patient in a manner and to a degree that best promotes attainment of the goals by the patient by providing an environment that is conducive to attaining the goals; by adjusting the care given according to the patient's needs; by stimulating and motivating the patient to achieve independence; by encouraging the patient to comply with and accept the regimen of care; and by compensating for the staff reactions to factors that influence the relationship with the patient and the therapy planned. Implementing follows planning and precedes evaluating in the five-step nursing process. See also **analyzing, assessing, evaluating, nursing process, planning.**

implosion, **1.** a bursting inward. **2.** a psychiatric treatment for people disabled by phobias and anxiety in which the person is desensitized to anxiety-producing stimuli by repeated intense exposure in imagination or reality, until the stimuli are no longer stressful. Also called **flooding.** –**implode,** *v.*

implosive therapy. See **flooding.**

impotence, **1.** weakness. **2.** inability of the adult male to achieve penile erection or, less commonly, to ejaculate having achieved an erection. Several forms are recognized. **Functional impotence** has a psychologic basis. **Anatomic impotence** results from physically defective genitalia. **Atonic impotence** involves disturbed neuromuscular function. Poor health, age, drugs, and fatigue can inhibit normal sexual function. Also called **impotency.** –**impotent,** *adj.*

impregnate, **1.** to inseminate and make pregnant; to fertilize. **2.** to saturate or mix with another substance. –**impregnable,** *adj.*, **impregnation,** *n.*

impression, **1.** (in dentistry and prosthetic medicine) a mold of a part of the mouth or other part of the body from which a replacement or prosthesis may be formed. **2.** (in the medical record) the examiner's diagnosis or assessment of a problem, disease, or condition. **3.** a strong sensation or effect on the mind, intellect, or feelings.

imprinting, (in ethology) a special type of learning that occurs at critical points during the early stages of development in animals. It involves behavioral patterning and social attachment, is characterized by rapid acquisition and irreversibility, and is usually species-specific, although animals exposed to members of a different species during this short period may become attached to and identify with that particular species instead of their own. The degree to which imprinting occurs in human development has not been determined. See also **bonding.**

imprisonment, (in law) the act of confining, detaining, or arresting a person or in any way restraining personal liberty and preventing free exercise of movement. Imprisonment may be in a prison or other special facility, but every confinement is an imprisonment.

impulse, **1.** (in psychology) a sudden, irresistible, often irrational inclination, urge, desire, or action resulting from a particular feeling or mental state. **2.** also called **nerve impulse, neural impulse.** (in physiology) the electrochemical process involved in neural transmission. –**impulsive,** *adj.*

impulsion, an abnormal, irrational urge to commit an unlawful or socially unacceptable act.

Imuran, a trademark for an immunosuppressive (azathioprine).

IMV, abbreviation for **intermittent mandatory ventilation.**

In, symbol for **indium.**

in-, **1.** a combining form meaning 'of or pertaining to fibers': *inaxon, inemia, initis.* **2.** a combining form meaning 'in, on': *incineration, indigitation, induced.* **3.** a combining form meaning 'not': *inaction, inassimilable, incompetence.*

-in, -ine, **1.** a combining form meaning an 'antibiotic': *bacitracin, penicillin, streptomycin.* **2.** a combining form meaning a 'pharmaceutic product': *aspirin, niacin.* **3.** a combining form meaning a 'chemical compound': *albumin, gelatin, palmitin.* **4.** a combining form meaning an 'enzyme': *emulsin, pepsin, myrosin.*

inactivation, a reversible denaturation of a protein.

inactive colon, hypotonicity of the bowel resulting in decreased contractions and propulsive movements and a delay in the normal 12-hour transit time of luminal contents from cecum to anus. Colonic inactivity may be caused by acquired or congenital megacolon, aging, anticholinergic drugs, depression, faulty habits of elimination, inadequate fluid intake, lack of exercise, a low-residue or starvation diet, neuroendocrine response to surgical stress, prolonged bed rest, or a neurologic disease, as diabetic visceral neuropathy, multiple sclerosis, parkinsonism, and spinal cord lesions. Normal motility of the colon is frequently compromised by the continued use of laxatives. Acquired megacolon, characterized by an abnormally large, inactive bowel and chronic constipation, is common in retarded children and adults with chronic mental illness. In congenital megacolon (Hirschsprung's disease) congenital absence of myenteric innervation in a distal segment of the colon results in loss of motility and causes massive dilatation of the proximal segment of the large bowel and extreme constipation. The disorder is more common in males than females and in severe cases retards growth. Treatment of colonic inactivity includes a stimulus-response training program to establish regular bowel habits, the use of stool softeners and hydrophilic colloids to increase fecal bulk, and a diet containing adequate roughage.

inadequate personality, a personality characterized by a lack of physical stamina, emotional immaturity, social instability, poor judgment, reduced motivation, ineptness—especially in interpersonal relationships—

and an inability to adapt or react effectively to new or stressful situations.

inanimate, not alive; lacking signs of life.

inanition /in′ənish′ən/, **1.** an exhausted condition resulting from lack of food and water or a defect in assimilation; starvation. **2.** a state of lethargy characterized by a loss of vitality or vigor in all aspects of social, moral, and intellectual life.

inanition fever, a temporary, mild, febrile condition of the newborn in the first few days after birth, usually caused by dehydration.

inborn, innate; acquired or occurring during intrauterine life, with reference to both normally inherited traits and developmental or genetically transmitted anomalies. See also **congenital, hereditary, inborn error of metabolism.**

inborn error of metabolism, one of many abnormal metabolic conditions caused by an inherited defect of a single enzyme or other protein. Though people with such diseases are each defective in only protein, they generally display a large number of physical signs that are characteristic of the genetic trait. The diseases are rare. Kinds of inborn errors of metabolism include **phenylketonuria, Tay-Sachs disease, Lesch-Nyhan syndrome, galactosemia,** and **glucose-6-phosphate dehydrogenase deficiency.**

■ OBSERVATIONS: Inborn errors of metabolism may be detected in the fetus in utero by the examination of squamous and blood cells obtained by amniocentesis and fetoscopy. Laboratory tests after birth often show higher than normal levels of particular metabolites in the blood and urine, as phenylpyruvic acid and phenylalanine in PKU and galactose in galactosemia. The values are higher in homozygous than in heterozygous carriers. Physical stigmata of the various defects are usually seen only in homozygous carriers.

■ INTERVENTION: Treatment for some pathologic inborn errors may be initiated by removing dietary precursors of the nondegradable metabolite in order to prevent its accumulation. Removal of dietary phenylalanine in PKU and galactose in galactosemia are effective in preventing the development of symptoms if treatment is begun early. In those cases of inborn errors of metabolism in which the nondegradable metabolite is endogenous, as in the mucopolysaccaridoses, there is no treatment available.

inborn reflex. See **unconditioned response.**

inbreeding, the production of offspring by the mating of closely related individuals, organisms, or plants; self-fertilization is the most extreme form, which normally occurs in certain plants and lower animals. The practice provides a greater chance for recessive genes for both desirable and undesirable traits to become homozygous and to be expressed phenotypically. In humans, the amount of inbreeding in a specific population is largely controlled by tradition and cultural practices. In plants and animals, inbreeding is a standard method for developing desirable genotypes and pure lines. Compare **outbreeding.**

incarcerate, to trap, imprison, or confine, as a loop of intestine in an inguinal hernia. See also **hernia.**

incest, sexual intercourse between members of the same family who are so closely related as to be legally prohibited from marrying one another by reason of their consanguinity. **–incestuous,** *adj.*

incidence, 1. the number of times an event occurs. **2.** (in epidemiology) the number of new cases in a particular period of time. Incidence is often expressed as a ratio, in which the number of cases is the numerator and the population at risk is the denominator. See also **rate.**

incidental additives, food additives caused by the use of pesticides, herbicides, or chemicals involved in food processing.

incineration, the removal or reduction of waste materials by burning.

incipient, coming into existence; at an initial stage; beginning to appear, as a symptom or disease.

incipient dental caries, a dental condition in which a lesion of tooth decay is initially detectable.

incisal angle, the degree of slope between the axis-orbital plane and the discluding surface of the maxillary incisor teeth.

incisal guide, the part of a dental articulator that maintains the incisal guide angle. Also called **anterior guide.**

incisal guide pin, a metal rod, attached to the upper member of an articulator, that touches the incisal guide table to maintain the established vertical separation of the upper and lower members of the articulator.

incision, 1. a cut produced surgically by a sharp instrument creating an opening into an organ or space in the body. **2.** the act of making an incision.

incisor, one of the eight front teeth, four in each dental arch, that first appear as milk teeth during infancy, are replaced by permanent incisors during childhood, and last until old age. The crown of the incisor is chisel shaped and has a sharp cutting edge. Its labial surface is convex, smooth, and highly polished; its lingual surface is concave and, in many individuals, is marked by an inverted V-shaped basal ridge near the gum of the upper arch. The neck of the incisor is constricted. The root is single, long, and conic. The upper incisors are larger and stronger than the lower and are directed obliquely downward and forward. Compare **canine tooth, molar, premolar.**

inclusion, 1. the act of enclosing or the condition of being enclosed. **2.** a structure within another, as inclusions in the cytoplasm of the cells.

inclusion bodies, microscopic objects of various shapes and sizes observed in the nucleus or cytoplasm of blood cells or other tissue cells, depending on the type of disease.

inclusion conjunctivitis, an acute, purulent, conjunctival infection caused by *Chlamydia* organisms. It occurs in two forms: Bilateral chemosis, redness, and purulent discharge characterize the infection in infants; the adult variety is unilateral, less severe, less purulent, and associated with preauricular lymphadenopathy. Local instillation of antibiotics is effective treatment. Also called **swimming pool conjunctivitis.**

inclusion dermoid cyst, a tumor derived from embryonal tissues, caused by the inclusion of a foreign tissue when a developmental cleft closes.

inclusiveness principle, a rule that response to various objects in the environment is proportional to the amount of stimulus provided by each object.

inclusive rate, a method of calculating inpatient hospital charges in which a fixed amount covers all services, regardless of the number or intensity of services provided.

incoherent, **1.** disordered; without logical connection; disjointed; lacking orderly continuity or relevance. **2.** unable to express one's thoughts or ideas in an orderly, intelligible manner, usually as a result of emotional stress.

incompatible, unable to coexist. A tissue transplant may be rejected because recipient and donor antibody factors are incompatible.

incompetence, lack of ability. Body organs that do not function adequately may be described as incompetent. Kinds of incompetence include **aortic incompetence, ileocecal incompetence,** and **valvular incompetence.** **–incompetent,** *adj.*

incompetent cervix, (in obstetrics) a condition characterized by dilatation of the cervical os of the uterus before term without labor or contractions of the uterus. Miscarriage or premature delivery may result. Incompetent cervix is treated prophylactically by a Shirodkar or other procedure in which the cervix is held closed by a surgically implanted suture.

incomplete abortion, termination of pregnancy in which the products of conception are not entirely expelled or removed, often causing hemorrhage that may require surgical evacuation by curettage, oxytocics, and blood replacement. Infection is also a frequent complication of incomplete abortion. Compare **complete abortion.**

incomplete fistula. See **blind fistula.**

incomplete fracture, a bone break in which the crack in the osseous tissue does not completely traverse the width of the affected bone but may angle off in one or more directions.

incontinence, the inability to control urination or defecation. Urinary incontinence may be caused by cerebral clouding in the aged, infection, lesions in the brain or spinal cord, damage to peripheral nerves of the bladder, or injury to the sphincter or perineal structures, sometimes occurring in childbirth. Treatment includes bladder retraining, the implantation of an artificial sphincter, and the use of internal or external drainage devices. Stress incontinence precipitated by coughing, straining, or heavy lifting occurs more often in women than in men, and mild cases may be treated by exercises involving tightening and relaxing perineal and gluteal muscles, or they may respond to sympathomimetic drug therapy. Severe cases may require surgery to correct the underlying anatomic defect. Fecal incontinence may result from relaxation of the anal sphincter or by central nervous system or spinal cord disorders and may be treated by a program of bowel training. A Bradford frame with an opening for a bedpan or urinal may be used for bedridden incontinent patients. See also **bowel training.** **–incontinent,** *adj.*

increment, **1.** an increase or gain. **2.** the act of growing or increasing. **3.** the amount of an increase or gain in intrauterine pressure as uterine contractions begin in labor. **–incremental,** *adj.*

increto-, a combining form meaning 'of or pertaining to internal secretions': *incretodiagnosis, incretogenous, incretology.*

incrustation, hardened exudate, scale, or scab.

incubation period, **1.** the time between exposure to a pathogenic organism and the onset of symptoms of a disease. **2.** the time required to induce the development of an embryo in an egg or to induce the development and replication of tissue cells or microorganisms being grown in culture media or other special laboratory environment. **3.** the time allowed for a chemical reaction or process to proceed.

incubator, an apparatus used to provide a controlled environment, especially a particular temperature. Other environmental components, as darkness, light, oxygen, moisture, or dryness, may also be provided, as in an incubator for the cultivation of eggs or microorganisms in a laboratory or an incubator for premature infants.

incud-, a combining form meaning 'of or pertaining to an anvil (the incus)': *incudectomy, incudiform, incudomalleal.*

incudectomy /in′kyo͞odek′təmē/, surgical removal of the incus, performed to treat conductive deafness resulting from necrosis of the tip of the incus. Local or general anesthesia is used. The defective incus is excised and replaced with a bone chip graft so that sound vibrations are again transmitted. Postoperatively, the nurse instructs the patient to change position slowly to avoid dizziness, to avoid blowing the nose and sneezing, and to report any fever, headache, dizziness or pain in the ear.

incus /ing′kəs/, *pl.* **incudes** /inko͞o′dēz/, one of the three ossicles in the middle ear, resembling an anvil. It communicates sound vibrations from the malleus to the stapes. Compare **malleus, stapes.** See also **middle ear.**

IND, abbreviation for **investigational new drug.**

indandione derivative, one of a small group of oral anticoagulants designed for long-term therapeutic use in patients who cannot tolerate other oral anticoagulants. The indandiones are difficult to control and may cause grave adverse effects, including severe renal and hepatic toxicity, agranulocytosis, and leukopenia. For this reason coumarin derivatives are preferred. Regular evaluations of prothrombin are necessary. Extreme fatigue, sore throat, chills, and fever are signs of impending toxicity and require discontinuation of the drug. Compare **coumarin.**

indentation, a notch, pit, or depression in the surface of an object, as toothmarks on the tongue or skin. –**indent,** *v.*

independence, **1.** also called **independency.** the state or quality of being independent; autonomy; free from the influence, guidance, or control of a person or a group. **2.** a lack of requirement or reliance on another for physical existence or emotional needs. –**independent,** *adj.*

independent assortment, (in genetics) a basic principle stating that the members of a pair of genes are randomly distributed in the gametes, independent of the distribution of other pairs of genes. See also **dominance, segregation.**

independent practice, (in nursing) the practice of certain aspects of professional nursing that are encompassed by applicable licensure and law and require no supervision or direction from others. Nurses in independent practice may have an office in which they see patients and charge fees for service. In all nursing settings, state practice acts define certain aspects of nursing practice that are independent and may define those that must be done only under supervision or direction of another individual, usually a physician.

independent variable, (in research) a variable that is controlled by the researcher and evaluated by its measurable effect on the dependent variable or variables; for example, in a study of the effect of nursing intervention on postoperative vomiting, nursing intervention is the independent variable evaluated by its effect on the incidence of postoperative vomiting. Also called **experimental variable, predictor variable.** Compare **dependent variable.**

Inderal, a trademark for a beta-adrenergic blocking agent (propranolol).

indeterminate cleavage, mitotic division of the fertilized ovum into blastomeres that have similar developmental potential and, if isolated, can give rise to a complete individual embryo. Also called **regulative cleavage.** Compare **determinate cleavage.** See also **regulative development.**

index case, (in epidemiology) the first case of a disease as contrasted with the appearance of subsequent cases. See also **propositus.**

Index Medicus, an index published monthly by the National Library of Medicine, which lists articles from the medical literature from throughout the world by subject and by author. An annual edition, the *Cumulative Index Medicus,* is published yearly; it contains the citations in all 12 issues of the *Index Medicus.*

index myopia, a kind of nearsightedness caused by a variation in the index of refraction of the media of the eye.

Indian Health Service, a bureau within the Department of Health and Human Services for providing public health and medical services to Native Americans in the United States.

Indian tick fever. See **Marseilles fever.**

indican, a substance (potassium indoxyl sulfate) produced in the intestine by the decomposition of tryptophan, absorbed by the intestinal wall, and excreted in the urine. It may be elevated in the urine of patients on high-protein diets or those suffering from GI disease. The normal accumulation of indican in urine after 24-hour collection is 10 to 20 mg.

indication, a reason to prescribe a medication or perform a treatment, as a bacterial infection may be an indication for the prescription of a specific antibiotic or as appendicitis is an indication for appendectomy. –**indicate,** *v.*

indicator, a tape, paper, tablet, or any other substance that is used to test for a particular reaction because it changes in a predictable visible way. Some kinds of indicators are **autoclave indicator, dipsticks,** and **litmus paper.** Also called **reagent.**

indigence /in′dijəns/, a condition of having insufficient income to pay for adequate medical care without depriving oneself or one's dependents of food, clothing, shelter, or other living essentials.

indigenous /indij′ənəs/, native to or occurring naturally in a specified area or environment, as certain species of bacteria in the human digestive tract.

indigestion. See **dyspepsia.**

indirect anaphylaxis, an exaggerated reaction of hypersensitivity to a person's own antigen that occurs because the antigen has been altered in some way.

indirect calorimetry, the measurement of the amount of heat generated in an oxidation reaction by determining the intake or consumption of oxygen or by measuring the amount of carbon dioxide or the amount of nitrogen released and translating these quantities into a heat equivalent. Compare **direct calorimetry.**

indirect division. See **mitosis.**

indirect ophthalmoscope, an ophthalmoscope with a biconvex lens that produces a reversed direct image.

indirect percussion. See **percussion.**

indirect provider reimbursement, a method of payment to an agency for health services delivered by providers, as nurses.

indirect restorative method, the technique for fabricating a restoration on a cast of the original, as the indirect construction of an inlay. After a die is made from an impression of the prepared tooth, a wax pattern is formed and inverted. The cast inlay is then fitted and finished on the die, and fused to the tooth.

indirect retainer, a portion of a removable partial denture that resists movement of a distal extension away from its tissue support by means of lever action opposite the fulcrum line of the direct retention.

indium (In), a silvery metallic element with some nonmetallic chemical properties. Its atomic number is 49; its atomic weight is 114.82. It is used in electronic semiconductors.

individual immunity, a form of natural immunity not shared by most other members of the race and species. It is rare and probably occurs as the result of the person having had an infection that went unrecognized. Compare **racial immunity, species immunity.**

individual psychology, a modified system of psychoanalysis, developed by Alfred Adler, that views maladaptive behavior and personality disorders as resulting from a conflict between the desire to dominate and feelings of inferiority. See also **inferiority complex.**

Indocin, a trademark for an antiinflammatory agent (indomethacin).

Indoklon, a trademark for an inhalation anesthetic agent (flurothyl).

indoleacetic acid /in'dōləsē'tik, -əset'ik/, a major terminal metabolite of tryptophan that is present in very small amounts in normal urine and excreted in elevated quantities by patients with carcinoid tumors.

indomethacin, a nonsteroidal antiinflammatory agent.

■ INDICATIONS: It is prescribed in the treatment of arthritis and certain other inflammatory conditions.

■ CONTRAINDICATIONS: Upper GI disease or known hypersensitivity to this drug or to aspirin prohibits its use. It is not given to children under 15 years of age or to pregnant or lactating women.

■ ADVERSE EFFECTS: The most serious adverse reaction is peptic ulcers. GI upset, dizziness, tinnitus, and rashes also may occur.

induce, to cause or stimulate the start of an activity, as an enzyme induces a metabolic activity. See also **induced fever.** –**inducer, induction,** *n.*

induced abortion, an intentional termination of pregnancy before the fetus has developed enough to live if born. Twenty to 50% of pregnancies are terminated deliberately, at the request of the mother or for medical indications—during the first trimester by curettage, or during the second trimester by induction of labor or hysterotomy. Termination of pregnancy by a trained person under proper conditions is safe. Unskilled abortions can be extremely hazardous because of the susceptibility of the uterus to infection and laceration. Puerperal sepsis and hemorrhage after criminal abortion have been leading causes of maternal death. Compare **spontaneous abortion.** See also **criminal abortion, septic abortion, therapeutic abortion.**

induced fever, a deliberate elevation of body temperature by application of heat or by inoculation with a fever-producing organism in order to kill heat-sensitive pathogens.

induced hypotension. See **deliberate hypotension.**

induced lethargy, a trancelike state produced during hypnosis. See also **hypnosis, lethargy.**

induced trance, a somnambulistic state resulting from a hysteric neurosis or hypnotism.

inducer, (in molecular genetics) a substance, usually a molecular substrate of a specific enzyme, that combines with and deactivates the active repressor produced by the regulator gene. The result of this combination is the activation of the operator gene, which was previously inactivated by the active repressor, and initiation of the transcription of the amino acid sequence in the structural gene for the eventual synthesis of protein.

induction, (in embryology) the process of stimulating and determining morphogenetic differentiation in a developing embryo through the action of chemical substances transmitted from one to another of the embryonic parts. See also **evocation.**

induction of anesthesia, all portions of the anesthetic process that occur before attaining the desired level of anesthesia, including premedication with a sedative, hypnotic, tranquilizer, or curariform adjunct to anesthesia, intubation, administration of oxygen, and administration of the anesthetic.

induction of labor, an obstetric procedure in which labor is initiated artificially by means of amniotomy or the administration of oxytocics. It is performed electively or for fetal or maternal indications. Elective induction is carried out for the convenience of the mother or the obstetrician, often to avert the possibility of delivery outside of the hospital when labor is judged to be imminent and the mother is expected to have an unusually rapid birth. Elective inductions are performed less often now than in the past. Prerequisites for elective induction are a term gestation, a fetal weight of at least 2500 g, a cervix judged ready to dilate, a vertex presentation, and engagement of the presenting part of the fetus in the pelvis. Errors in the estimation of gestational age and fetal weight may result in the delivery of an unexpectedly immature or low-birthweight infant. Indicated induction is performed when the risk of induction is judged to be less than that of continuing the pregnancy in such conditions as premature rupture of the membranes, severe maternal diabetes, and intractable preeclampsia. Surgical induction is effected by amniotomy, often with stripping of the membranes and digital stretching of the cervix; it is very often carried out in conjunction with medical induction. Medical induction is achieved through the administration of oxytocin, almost always by intravenous infusion, in a carefully controlled manner using microdrip equipment or an infusion pump. Beginning with very small amounts of oxytocin in an intravenous solution, the dosage is increased by gradual increments of the rate or concentration of infusion until effective labor is established. Oxytocin can be administered by buccal lozenge or by subcutaneous or intramuscular injection, but these methods are less controllable and are considered less safe than the intravenous method. Prostaglandins are now used to induce labor more often than formerly, particularly for therapeutic abortions in the second trimester. With intravenous oxytocin inductions, a secondary, piggyback infusion without medication is usually attached to the tubing so that an unmedicated infusion can be maintained if oxytocin is stopped. Electronic fetal and uterine monitoring is usually instituted during induction of labor to avoid hyperstimulation of the uterus and fetal distress. Ideally, induced labor mimics natural labor, but in practice this is not usually achieved. Longer and harder contractions commonly occur. In addition to unexpected fetal immaturity, complications of induction of labor include umbilical cord prolapse after amniotomy, tumultuous labor, tetanic uterine contractions, rupture of the uterus, placental abruption, fetal maternal hypotension, water intoxication, postpartum uterine atony and hemorrhage, and fetal asphyxia, hypoxia, or death. If the induction fails to produce effective labor, cesarean section is often required to prevent the adverse sequelae of the procedures used in the induction. For this reason, it is usually recommended that induction of labor not be attempted unless delivery must be accomplished to avoid severe fetal or maternal morbidity.

induction phase, the period of time during which a normal cell becomes transformed into a cancerous cell.

inductive approach, the analysis of data and examination of practice problems within their own context rather than from a predetermined theoretical basis.

inductor, (in embryology) a tissue or cell that emits a chemical substance that stimulates some morphogenetic effect in the developing embryo. See also **evocator, organizer.**

induration, hardening of a tissue, particularly the skin, because of edema, inflammation, or infiltration by a neoplasm. **–indurated,** *adj.*

Industrial Medical Association (I.M.A.), a professional organization whose members are concerned with the identification, prevention, diagnosis, and treatment of disorders associated with technology and industry.

industrial psychology, the application of psychologic principles and techniques to the problems of business and industry, including the selection of personnel, the motivation of workers, and the development of training programs.

indwelling catheter, any catheter designed to be left in place for a prolonged period. See also **self-retaining catheter.**

-ine, a combining form meaning a 'chemical substance': *chlorine, pyrroline, strychnine.*

inert, **1.** not moving or acting, as inert matter. **2.** (of a chemical substance) not taking part in a chemical reaction or acting as a catalyst, as neon or an inert gas. **3.** (of a medical ingredient) not active pharmacologically; serving only as a bulking, binding, or sweetening agent or other excipient in a medication.

inert gas, a chemically inactive gaseous element. The inert gases are argon, helium, krypton, neon, radon, and xenon. Also called **noble gas.**

inertia, **1.** the tendency of a body at rest to remain at rest unless acted on by an outside force, and the tendency of a body in motion to remain at motion in the direction in which it is moving unless acted on by an outside force. **2.** an abnormal condition characterized by a general inactivity or sluggishness, as colonic inertia or uterine inertia.

inevitable abortion, a condition of pregnancy in which spontaneous termination is imminent and cannot be prevented. It is characterized by bleeding, uterine cramping, dilatation of the cervix, and presentation of the conceptus in the cervical os. If heavy bleeding supervenes, immediate evacuation of the uterus may be required. The point at which an inevitable abortion becomes an incomplete abortion is of medicolegal interest because of the statutory difference between spontaneous and induced abortion. In clinical practice precise differentiation is seldom practicable. Compare **incomplete abortion, imminent abortion, threatened abortion.**

infant, **1.** a child who is in the earliest stage of extrauterine life, a time extending from birth to approximately 12 months of age, when the baby is able to assume an erect posture; some extend the period to 24 months of age. **2.** (in law) a person not of full legal age; a minor. **3.** of or pertaining to infancy; in an early stage of development. **–infantile,** *adj.*

infant botulism, an intoxication from neurotoxins produced by *Clostridium botulinum* that occurs in children less than 6 months of age. The condition is characterized by severe hypotonicity of all muscles, constipation, lethargy, and feeding difficulties, and it may lead to respiratory insufficiency. The botulism neurotoxin is usually found in the GI tract rather than in the blood, indicating that it is probably produced in the gut rather than ingested, although the epidemiology and pathophysiology of the syndrome are not clearly understood. Treatment is supportive, including optimal management of fluids, electrolytes, and nutrition. Ventilatory support may also be necessary. There is no evidence that antitoxin therapy is helpful, and it is usually not recommended.

infant death, the death of a live-born infant before 1 year of age.

infant feeder, a device for feeding small or weak infants who cannot suck hard enough to nurse from the breast or to get milk from a bottle. The feeder resembles a bulb syringe with a long soft nipple on the end. The bulb is squeezed slowly and gently, permitting the baby to suck and swallow without great effort and preventing the escape of fluid into the infant's trachea, where it might cause asphyxiation or aspiration pneumonia.

infant feeding. See **bottle feeding, breast feeding.**

infanticide /infan′tisīd/, **1.** the killing of an infant or young child. The act is usually a psychotic reaction often associated with severe depression, as occurs in bipolar disorder and, occasionally, in extreme postpartum disturbances. Infanticide may become a neurotic obsession among mothers who do not want the baby or who do not feel physically, mentally, or emotionally capable of caring for or coping with the infant. **2.** one who takes the life of an infant or young child. **–infanticidal,** *adj.*

infantile, **1.** of, relating to, or characteristic of infants or infancy. **2.** lacking maturity, sophistication, or reasonableness. **3.** affected with infantilism. **4.** being in a very early stage of development.

infantile arteritis, a disorder in infants and young children characterized by inflammation of many arteries in which atherosclerotic lesions are rarely present.

infantile autism, a disability characterized by abnormal emotional, social, and linguistic development in a child. It may result from organic brain dysfunction, in which case it occurs before 3 years of age, or it may be associated with childhood schizophrenia, in which case the autism occurs later, but before the onset of adolescence. The autistic child remains fixed at one of the consecutive stages through which a normal infant passes as it develops. If the condition is the result of organic brain disease, the child appears to be unable to proceed beyond the current stage of development, though there is no regression to an earlier stage. If the condition accompanies schizophrenia in later childhood, regression occurs. Treatment includes psychotherapy, often accompanied by play therapy.

infantile celiac disease. See **celiac disease.**

infantile cerebral sphingolipidosis. See **Tay-Sachs disease.**

infantile dwarf, a person whose mental and physical development is greatly retarded as a result of various causes, as genetic or developmental defects.

infantile eczema. See **atopic dermatitis.**

infantile hemiplegia, paralysis of one side of the body that may occur at birth from a cerebral hemorrhage, in utero from lack of oxygen, or during a febrile illness in infancy.

infantile paralysis. See **poliomyelitis.**

infantile pellagra. See **kwashiorkor.**

infantile scurvy, a nutritional disease caused by an inadequate dietary supply of vitamin C, most commonly occurring because cow's milk, unfortified with vitamin C, is the principal food in an infant's diet. Families are counseled to feed their children foods rich in vitamin C or to use a formula supplemented with this vitamin. Also called **Barlow's disease, hemorrhagic scurvy.** See also **ascorbic acid, citric acid, scurvy.**

infantile spinal muscular atrophy. See **Werdnig-Hoffmann disease.**

infantile uterus, a uterus that has failed to attain adult characteristics.

infantilism /in′fəntəliz′əm/, **1.** a condition in which various anatomic, physiologic, and psychologic characteristics of childhood persist in the adult. It is characterized by mental retardation, underdeveloped sexual organs, and, usually, small stature. Compare **progeria. 2.** a condition, usually of psychologic rather than organic origin, characterized by speech and voice patterns in an older child or adult that are typical of very young children.

infant mortality, the statistic rate of infant death during the first year after live birth, expressed as the number of such births per 1000 live births in a specific geographic area or institution in a given period of time. Neonatal mortality accounts for 70% of infant mortality.

infant of addicted mother, a newborn infant showing withdrawal symptoms, usually within the first 24 hours of life, most commonly caused by maternal antepartum dependence on heroin, methadone, diazepam, phenobarbital, or alcohol. See also **fetal alcohol syndrome.**

■ OBSERVATIONS: Characteristic symptoms include tremors, irritability, hyperactive reflexes, increased muscle tone, twitching, increased mucus production, nasal congestion, respiratory distress, excessive sweating, elevated temperature, vomiting, diarrhea, and dehydration. The infants cry shrilly, often sneeze, frantically suck their fists but feed poorly, and frequently yawn but have difficulty falling asleep. They are usually pale, are often born with nose and knee abrasions, and are subject to convulsions.

■ INTERVENTION: The infant is kept warm, snugly swaddled in a padded crib, and exposed to minimal visual, auditory, and tactile stimulation. The baby is handled only when necessary and is then held firmly, close to the body. Parenteral fluid therapy and drugs, as paregoric, phenobarbital, chlorpromazine, or diazepam, may be administered. Small, frequent feedings of concentrated formula are usually ordered, and before each feeding the infant's nasopharynx is suctioned. If the buttocks become excoriated because of diarrhea, a paste of zinc oxide and karaya powder is applied, and if the infant's flailing about is likely to cause abrasions, bony prominences of the body may be protected with light padding and the hands with the mitts of the infant shirt.

■ NURSING CONSIDERATIONS: These high-risk infants require special attention, and it is important for the mother to be encouraged to participate in her baby's care as soon as possible. The nurse may help to promote parent-child bonding.

infant psychiatry, the branch of psychiatry that specializes in the diagnosis, etiology, and treatment of the psychopathologic syndromes and symptoms of infants. Such conditons are associated with early pathology, tactile hypersensitivity, and homeostatic disorders and include poor infant-parent attachment, infantile autism, anaclitic depression, avoidance reaction, persistent stranger and separation anxiety, early signs of aggression, hyperactivity, cyclic vomiting, and disturbances in sleeping, eating, and elimination.

infarct /infärkt′/, a localized area of necrosis in a tissue, vessel, organ, or part resulting from tissue anoxia caused by an interruption in the blood supply to the area, or, less frequently, by circulatory stasis produced by the occlusion of a vein that ordinarily carries blood away from the area. An infarct may resemble a red swollen bruise, because of hemorrhage and an accumulation of blood in the area. Some infarcts are pale and white, caused by a lack of circulation to the area. Kinds of infarct include **anemic infarct, calcareous infarct, cicatrized infarct, hemorrhagic infarct,** and **uric acid infarct.** –**infarcted,** *adj.*

infarct extension, a myocardial infarction that has spread beyond the original area, usually as a result of the death of cells in the ischemic margin of the infarct zone.

infarction, 1. the development and formation of an infarct. **2.** an infarct. Kinds of infarction include **myocardial infarction** and **pulmonary infarction.**

infect, to transmit a pathogen that may induce development of an infectious disease in another person.

infected abortion, a spontaneous or induced termination of an immature pregnancy in which the products of conception have become infected, causing fever and requiring antibiotic therapy and evacuation of the uterus. Compare **septic abortion.**

infection, **1.** the invasion of the body by pathogenic microorganisms that reproduce and multiply, causing disease by local cellular injury, secretion of a toxin, or antigen-antibody reaction in the host. **2.** a disease caused by the invasion of the body by pathogenic microorganisms. Compare **infestation.** **–infectious,** *adj.*

infection control, the policies and procedures of a hospital or other health facility to minimize the risk of nosocomial or community-acquired infections spreading to patients or members of the staff.

infection control committee, a group of hospital health professionals composed of infection control personnel, with medical, nursing, administrative, and occasionally dietary and housekeeping department representatives, who plan and supervise infection control activities.

infection control nurse, a registered nurse who is assigned responsibility for surveillance and infection prevention and control activities.

infectious, **1.** capable of causing an infection. **2.** caused by an infection.

infectious hepatitis. See **hepatitis A.**

infectious mononucleosis, an acute herpesvirus infection caused by the Epstein-Barr virus (EBV). It is characterized by fever, sore throat, swollen lymph glands, atypical lymphocytes, splenomegaly, hepatomegaly, abnormal liver function, and bruising. The disease is usually transmitted by droplet infection but is not highly or predictably contagious. Young people are most often affected. In childhood, the disease is mild and usually unnoticed; the older the person, the more severe the symptoms are likely to be. Infection confers permanent immunity. Treatment is primarily symptomatic, with enforced bed rest to prevent serious complications of the liver or spleen, analgesics to control pain, and saline gargles for throat discomfort. Rupture of the spleen may occur, requiring immediate surgery and blood transfusion. See also **Epstein-Barr virus, viral infection.**

infectious myringitis, an inflammatory, contagious condition of the eardrum caused by viral or bacterial infection, characterized by the development of painful vesicles on the drum. Also called **bullous myringitis.**

infectious nucleic acid, DNA or, more commonly, viral RNA that is able to infect the nucleic acid of a cell and to induce the host to produce viruses.

infectious parotitis. See **mumps.**

infectious polyneuritis. See **Guillain-Barré syndrome.**

infective tubulointerstitial nephritis, an acute inflammation of the kidneys caused by an infection by *Escherichia coli* or other pyogenic pathogen. The condition is characterized by chills, fever, nausea and vomiting, flank pain, dysuria, proteinuria, and hematuria. The kidney may become enlarged, and portions of the renal cortex may be destroyed. Infection is usually the result of bacterial contamination of a urinary catheter, but it may occur in any condition characterized by urinary stasis.

infectivity, the ability of a pathogen to spread rapidly from one host to another.

inferior, **1.** situated below or lower than a given point of reference, as the feet are inferior to the legs. **2.** of poorer quality or value. Compare **superior.**

inferior alveolar artery, an artery that descends with the inferior alveolar nerve from the first or mandibular portion of the maxillary artery to the mandibular foramen on the medial surface of the ramus of the mandible. It enters the mandibular canal and runs through to the first premolar tooth where it divides into the mental and incisor branches. Also called **arteria alveolaris inferior.**

inferior aperture of minor pelvis, an irregular aperture bounded by the coccyx, the sacrotuberous ligaments, part of the ischium, the sides of the pubic arch, and the pubic symphysis.

inferior aperture of thorax, an irregular opening bounded by the twelfth thoracic vertebra, the eleventh and twelfth ribs, and the edge of the costal cartilages as they meet the sternum.

inferior conjunctival fornix, the space in the fold of conjunctiva created by the reflection of the conjunctiva covering the eyeball and the lining of the lower eyelid. Compare **superior conjunctival fornix.**

inferior gastric node, a node in one of two groups of gastric lymph glands, lying between the two layers of the lesser omentum along the pyloric half of the greater curvature of the stomach. Compare **hepatic node, superior gastric node.**

inferiority complex, **1.** a feeling of fear and resentment resulting from a sense of being physically inadequate, characterized by a variety of abnormal behaviors. **2.** (in psychoanalysis) a complex characterized by striving for unrealistic goals because of an unresolved Oedipus complex. **3.** *informal.* a feeling of being inferior.

inferior maxillary bone. See **mandible.**

inferior mesenteric node, a node in one of the three groups of visceral lymph glands serving the viscera of the abdomen and the pelvis. The inferior mesenteric nodes are associated with the branches of the inferior mesenteric artery and are divided into a group of small nodes along the branches of the left colic and sigmoid arteries, another group in the sigmoid mesocolon, and a pararectal group touching the muscular coat of the rectum. The inferior mesenteric nodes drain the descending colon, the iliac and sigmoid parts of the colon, and the upper part of the rectum. Their efferents pass to the preaortic nodes. Compare **gastric node, superior mesenteric node.**

inferior mesenteric vein, the vein in the lower body that returns the blood from the rectum, the sigmoid colon, and the descending colon. It begins in the rectum as the superior rectal vein, ascends through the lesser pelvis, and continues upward as the inferior mesenteric vein. It passes dorsal to the pancreas and opens into the lienal vein. It receives the sigmoid veins from the sigmoid colon and the iliac colon and the left colic vein from the descending colon and the left colic flexure. Compare **superior mesenteric vein.**

inferior orbital fissure, a groove in the inferolateral wall of the orbit that contains the infraorbital and zygomatic nerves and the infraorbital vessels.

inferior phrenic artery, a small, visceral branch of the abdominal aorta, arising from the aorta itself, the renal artery, or the celiac artery. It divides into the medial and lateral branches and supplies the diaphragm. A few vessels of the inferior vena cava stem from the lateral branch of the right phrenic artery. Some branches of the left phrenic artery supply the esophagus.

inferior radioulnar joint. See **distal radioulnar articulation.**

inferior sagittal sinus, one of the six venous channels of the posterior dura mater, draining blood from the brain into the internal jugular vein. It is a cylindric sinus contained in the posterior portion of the free margin of the falx cerebri, increases in size as it courses posteriorly, and ends in the straight sinus. It receives deoxygenated blood from several veins from the falx cerebri and, in some individuals, a few veins from the cerebral hemispheres. Compare **straight sinus, superior sagittal sinus, transverse sinus.**

inferior subscapular nerve /subskap′yo͞olər/, one of two small nerves on opposite sides of the back that arise from the posterior cord of the brachial plexus. It supplies the distal part of the subscapularis and ends in the teres major. Compare **superior subscapular nerve.**

inferior thyroid vein, one of the few veins that arise in the venous plexus on the thyroid gland and form a plexus ventral to the trachea, under the sternothyroideus muscle. A left vein descends from this plexus to join the left brachiocephalic trunk; a right vein descends obliquely to open into the right brachiocephalic vein at its junction with the superior vena cava. The inferior thyroid veins contain valves at their terminations and receive the esophageal, the tracheal, and the inferior laryngeal veins.

inferior ulnar collateral artery, one of a pair of branches of the deep brachial arteries, arising about 5 cm from the elbow, passing inward to form an arch with the deep brachial artery, and carrying blood to the muscles of the forearm. Compare **superior ulnar collateral artery.**

inferior vena cava, the large vein that returns deoxygenated blood to the heart from parts of the body below the diaphragm. It is formed by the junction of the two common iliac veins at the right of the fifth lumbar vertebra and ascends along the vertebral column, pierces the diaphragm and opens into the right atrium of the heart. As it passes through the diaphragm, it receives a covering of serous pericardium. The inferior vena cava contains a semilunar valve that is rudimentary in the adult but very large and important in the fetus. The vessel receives blood from the two common iliacs, the lumbar veins, and the testicular veins. Compare **superior vena cava.**

infero-, a combining form meaning 'low': *inferolateral, inferomedial, inferoposterior.*

inferolateral /in′fərōlat′ərəl/, situated below and to the side.

inferomedial, situated below and toward the center.

infertile, denoting the inability to produce offspring. This condition may be present in one or both sex partners and may be temporary and reversible. The cause may be physical, including immature sexual organs, abnormalities of the reproductive system, hormonal imbalance, and dysfunction or anomalies in other organ systems, or may result from psychologic or emotional problems. The condition is classified as primary, in which pregnancy has never occurred, and secondary, when there have been one or more pregnancies. Compare **sterile.** **–infertility.** *n.*

infest, to attack, invade, and subsist on the skin or in the internal organs of a host. Compare **infect.**

infestation, the presence of animal parasites in the environment, on the skin, or in the hair of a host.

infiltration, the process whereby a fluid passes into the tissues, as when a local anesthetic is administered.

inflammation, the protective response of the tissues of the body to irritation or injury. Inflammation may be acute or chronic; its cardinal signs are redness (rubor), heat (calor), swelling (tumor), and pain (dolor), accompanied by loss of function. The process begins with a brief increase in vascular permeability. The second stage is prolonged and consists of sustained increase in vascular permeability, exudation of fluids from the vessels, clustering of leukocytes along the vessel walls, phagocytosis of microorganisms, deposition of fibrin in the vessel, disposal of the accumulated debris by macrophages, and, finally, the migration of fibroblasts to the area and the development of new, normal cells. The severity, timing, and local character of any particular inflammatory response depend on the cause, the area affected, and the condition of the host. Histamine, kinins, and various other substances mediate the inflammatory process.

inflammatory bowel disease. See **ulcerative colitis.**

inflammatory fracture, a fracture of bone tissue weakened by inflammation.

inflatable pessary. See **pessary.**

influenza, a highly contagious infection of the respiratory tract caused by a myxovirus and transmitted by airborne droplet infection. It occurs in isolated cases, epidemics, and pandemics. Symptoms include sore throat, cough, fever, muscular pains, and weakness. The incubation period is brief (from 1 to 3 days), and the onset is usually sudden, with chills, fever, and general malaise. Treatment is symptomatic and usually involves bed rest, aspirin, and drinking of fluids. Fever and constitutional symptoms distinguish influenza from the common cold. Complete recovery in from 3 to 10 days is the rule, but bacterial pneumonia may occur among high-risk patients, as the elderly, the very young, and people who have chronic pulmonary disease. Three main strains of influenza virus have been recognized: type A, type B, and type C. New strains of the virus emerge at regular intervals and are named according to their geographic origin. **Asian flu** is a type A influenza. Yearly vaccination with the currently prevalent strain of influenza virus is recommended for elderly or debilitated persons. Also called **grippe, la grippe,** *(informal)* **flu.**

influenza-virus vaccine, an active immunizing agent.

■ INDICATION: It is prescribed for immunization against influenza.

■ CONTRAINDICATIONS: Acute infection or allergy to eggs prohibits its use.

■ ADVERSE EFFECTS: Among the more serious adverse reactions are anaphylaxis and Guillain-Barré syndrome.

information systems director, a person who directs and administers the data processing facilities of a hospital or other health facility.

informed consent, permission obtained from a patient to perform a specific test or procedure. Informed consent is required before performing most invasive procedures and before admitting a patient to a research study. The document used must be written in a language understood by the patient and be dated and signed by the patient and at least one witness. Included in the document are clear, rational statements that describe the procedure or test, the risk to the patient, the expected benefits to the patient, the natural anticipated consequences of not allowing the test or procedure, and the alternative procedures or diagnostic aids that are available. Also required is a statement that care will not be withheld if the patient does not consent; informed consent is voluntary. By law, informed consent must be obtained more than a given number of days or hours before certain procedures, including therapeutic abortion and sterilization, and must always be obtained when the patient is fully competent.

infra-, a combining form meaning 'situated, formed, or occurring beneath': *infraclavicular, infracortical, infratemporal.*

infraction fracture, a pathologic fracture characterized by a small radiolucent line and most commonly associated with a disorder of metabolism. See also **greenstick fracture.**

infranodal block /in'frənō'dəl/, a type of atrioventricular (AV) block in which an impairment of the stimulatory mechanism of the heart causes blockage of the impulse in the bundle of His or in both bundle branches after leaving the AV node. The condition is often the result of arteriosclerosis, degenerative diseases, a defect in the conduction system, or tumor; it is most often seen in older patients. Symptoms include frequent episodes of fainting and a pulse rate of between 20 and 50 beats per minute. Diagnosis is made by an electrocardiogram, which shows intraventricular conduction disturbances during sinus rhythm and distinguishes nodal from infranodal block. The usual therapy is the implantation of a pacemaker of the demand type. Compare **bundle branch block, intraventricular block.** See also **Adams-Stokes syndrome, atrioventricular block, cardiac conduction defect, heart block, intraatrial block, sinoatrial block.**

infraradian rhythm, a biorhythm that repeats in patterns greater than 24-hour periods.

infrared radiation, electromagnetic radiation in which the wavelengths are between 10^{-5} m and 10^{-4} m, or longer than those of visible light waves but shorter than those of radio waves. Infrared radiation striking the body surface is perceived as heat.

infrared therapy, treatment by exposure to various wavelengths of infrared radiation. Hot water bottles and heating pads of all kinds emit longwave infrared radiation; incandescent lights emit shortwave infrared radiation. Infrared treatment is performed to relieve pain and to stimulate circulation of blood.

infrared thermography, measurement of temperature through the detection of infrared radiation emitted from heated tissue.

infundibulum, *pl.* **infundibula,** a funnel-shaped structure or passage, as the cavity formed by the fimbriae tubae at the distal end of the fallopian tubes, the stalk that extends from the posterior lobe of the pituitary gland, or the passage connecting the middle meatus of the nose with the frontal sinus.

infusion, **1.** the introduction of a substance, as a fluid, electrolyte, nutrient, or drug, directly into a vein or interstitially by means of gravity flow. Sterile techniques are maintained, the equipment is periodically checked for mechanic difficulties, and the patient is observed for swelling at the site of injection and for cardiac or respiratory difficulties. Compare **injection, instillation, insufflation.** **2.** the substance introduced into the body by infusion. **3.** the steeping of a substance, as an herb, in order to extract its medicinal properties. **4.** the extract obtained by the steeping process. **–infuse,** *v.*

infusion pump, an apparatus designed to deliver measured amounts of a drug through injection over a period of time. Some kinds of infusion pumps can be implanted surgically.

ingrown hair, a hair that fails to follow the normal follicle channel to the surface, with the free end becoming embedded in the skin. The hair then acts like a foreign body, and inflammation and suppuration follow.

ingrown toenail, a toenail whose free distal margin grows or is pressed into the skin of the toe, causing an inflammatory reaction. Granulation tissue may develop and secondary infection is common. Treatment includes wider shoes, proper trimming of the nail, and various surgical procedures to narrow the nail or to reduce the size of the lateral nail fold.

inguinal /ing'gwinəl/, of or pertaining to the groin.

inguinal canal, the tubular passage through the lower layers of the abdominal wall that contains the spermatic cord in the male and the round ligament in the female. It is a common site for hernias.

inguinal falx, the inferior terminal portion of the common aponeurosis of the obliquus internus abdominis and the transverse abdominis. It is inserted into the crest of the pubis, just under the superficial inguinal ring, and strengthens that part of the anterior abdominal wall. The width and the strength of the inguinal falx vary. Also called **conjoined tendon.**

inguinal hernia, a hernia in which a loop of intestine enters the inguinal canal, sometimes filling, in a male, the entire scrotal sac. An inguinal hernia is usually repaired surgically to prevent the herniated segment from becoming strangulated, gangrenous, or obstructive, thereby blocking passage of waste through the bowel. Of all hernias, 75% to 80% are inguinal hernias. See also **hernia.**

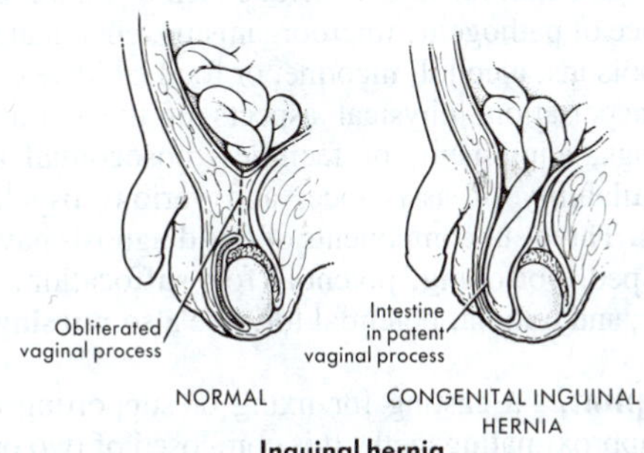

Inguinal hernia

inguinal node, one of approximately 18 nodes in the group of lymph glands in the upper femoral triangle of the thigh. These nodes are divided into the superficial inguinal nodes and the subinguinal nodes. Compare **anterior tibial node, popliteal node.**

inguinal region, the part of the abdomen surrounding the inguinal canal, in the lower zone on both sides of the pubic region. Also called **iliac region.** See also **abdominal regions.**

inguinal ring, either of the two apertures of the inguinal canal, the internal end opening into the abdominal wall and the external end opening into the aponeurosis of the obliquus externus abdominis above the pubis.

inguino-, a combining form meaning 'of or pertaining to the groin': *inguinocrural, inguinodynia, inguinoscrotal.*

INH. See **isoniazid.**

inhalation administration of medication, the administration of a drug by inhalation of the vapor released from a fragile ampoule packed in a fine mesh that is crushed for immediate administration. Amyl nitrate and ammonia act quickly and are often used in this way. The medication is absorbed into the circulation through the mucous membrane of the nasal passages. Vaporized medication is also given by inhalation. See also **inhalation therapy.**

inhalation analgesia, the occasional administration of anesthetic gas during the second stage of labor to reduce pain. Consciousness is retained to allow the woman to follow instructions and to avoid the adverse effects of general anesthesia.

inhalation anesthesia, surgical narcosis achieved by the administration of an anesthetic gas or a volatile anesthetic liquid via a carrier gas. Although general anesthesia by gas inhalation has been used to permit surgical operations for over a century, the mechanism by which these anesthetics dull the pain centers of the brain is not yet understood. Administration of an inhalation anesthetic is usually preceded by intravenous or intramuscular administration of a short-acting sedative or hypnotic drug, often a barbiturate. The procedure almost always requires endotracheal intubation. Among the principal inhalation anesthetics are nitrous oxide, cyclopropane, ethylene, halothane, enflurane, fluroxene, methoxyflurane, trichloroethylene, and isoflurane. Some other inhalation anesthetics, including chloroform, ether, and ethyl chloride, are rarely used in the United States because of adverse effects, potential toxicity, or the possibility of explosion.

inhalation therapy, a treatment in which a substance is introduced into the respiratory tract with inspired air. Oxygen, water, and various drugs may be administered using techniques of inhalation therapy. The goals of treatment are varied, as improved strength of respiratory function in a bedridden patient, bronchodilatation in an asthmatic, or liquefaction of mucus in a person with chronic obstructive lung disease.

inhale, to breathe in or to draw in with the breath. –**inhalation,** *n.*

inherent, inborn, innate; natural to an environment. Compare **indigenous.**

inherent rate, the frequency of impulse formation attributed to a given pacemaker location. The following are representative of the adult heart: SA node: 50-100/minute; AV junction: 40-60/minute; ventricle: 35-40/minute.

inheritance, **1.** the acquisition or expression of traits or conditions by transmission of genetic material from parents to offspring. **2.** the sum total of the genetic qualities or traits transmitted from parents to offspring; the total genetic makeup of the fertilized ovum. Kinds of inheritance include **alternative inheritance, amphigenous inheritance, autosomal inheritance, blending inheritance, codominant inheritance, complemental inheritance, crisscross inheritance, cytoplasmic inheritance, holandric inheritance, hologynic inheritance, homochronous inheritance, maternal inheritance, mendelism, monofactorial inheritance, multifactorial inheritance, supplemental inheritance,** and **x-linked inheritance.** –**inherited,** *adj.* **inherit,** *v.*

inherited disorder, any disease or condition that is genetically determined and involves either a single gene mutation, multifactorial inheritance, or a chromosomal aberration. Also called **genetic disorder, hereditary disorder.**

inhibiting hormone. See **hormone.**

inhibition, **1.** the act or state of inhibiting or of being inhibited, restrained, prevented, or held back. **2.** (in psychology) the unconscious restraint of a behavioral process, usually resulting from the social or cultural forces of the environment; the condition inducing such restraint. **3.** (in psychoanalysis) the process in which the superego prevents the conscious expression of an unconscious instinctual drive, thought, or urge. **4.** (in physiology) restraining, checking, or arresting the action of an organ or cell or the reducing of a physiologic activity by an antagonistic stimulation. **5.** (in chemistry) the stopping or slowing down of the rate of a chemical reaction.

inhibition assay, an immunoassay in which an excess of antigens prevents or inhibits the completion of either the initial or indicator phase of the reaction.

inhibitory, tending to stop or slow a process, as a neuron that suppresses the intensity of a nerve impulse. Compare **induce.**

inio-, a combining form meaning 'of or pertaining to the occiput': *iniodymus, iniopagus, iniops.*

inion /in′ē·on/, the most prominent point of the back of the head, where the occipital bone protrudes the farthest.

initial contact stance stage, one of the five stages in the stance phase of walking or gait, specifically associated with the moment when the foot touches the ground or floor, and the leg prepares to accept the weight of the body. The initial contact stance stage figures in the diagnoses of many abnormal orthopedic conditions and is often correlated with electromyographic studies of the muscles used in walking, as the pretibial muscle and the gluteus maximus. Compare **loading response stance stage, midstance, preswing stance stage, terminal stance.** See also **swing phase of gait.**

initial plan of care, a medical plan prepared by a physician for the care of a patient.

initiation codon /kō′don/, (in molecular genetics) the triplet of nucleotides, usually adenine-uracil-guanine (AUG) or, in some cases, guanine-uracil-guanine (GUG), that code for formylmethionine, the first amino acid in protein sequences. Also called **start codon.**

injection, **1.** the act of forcing a liquid into the body by means of a syringe. Injections are designated according to the anatomic site involved; the most common are intra-arterial, intradermal, intramuscular, intravenous, and subcutaneous. Parenteral injections are usually given for therapeutic reasons, although they may be used diagnostically. Sterile technique is maintained. Compare **infusion, instillation, insufflate.** **2.** the substance injected. **3.** redness and swelling observed in the physical examination of a part of the body, caused by dilatation of the blood vessels secondary to an inflammatory or infectious process. **–inject,** *v.*

injection technique. See **intradermal injection, intramuscular injection, intrathecal injection, intravenous injection, subcutaneous injection,** and see other specific injection techniques.

injunction, a court order that prevents a party from performing a particular act.

injury: potential for, a nursing diagnosis accepted by the Fourth National Conference on the Classification of Nursing Diagnoses. The cause of the condition may be somatic (internal) or environmental (external). The somatic factors may be biologic, chemical, physiologic, psychologic, or developmental; the environmental factors may be biologic, chemical, physiologic, psychologic, or interpersonal. The defining characteristics of a somatic potential for injury include abnormal sensory function, autoimmune condition, malnutrition, hemoglobinopathy or other abnormal hematologic condition, broken skin, developmental abnormality, or psychologic dysfunction. The defining characteristics of an environmental potential for injury include lack of immunization; presence of pathogenic microorganisms, chemical pollutants, poisons, alcohol, nicotine, or food additives; modes of transportation; physical aspects of the community, buildings, equipment, or facilities; nosocomial agents; nonavailability of assistance; and various psychologic factors. Three subcomponents of this diagnosis have been developed: poisoning, potential for; suffocation, potential for; and trauma, potential for. See also **nursing diagnosis.**

inlay splint, a casting for fixing or supporting one or more approximating teeth. It is composed of two or more inlays soldered together or a single casting for prepared cavities in approximating teeth.

inlet, a passage leading into a cavity, as the pelvic inlet that marks the brim of the pelvic cavity.

inlet contraction. See **contraction.**

in loco parentis /in lō′kō pəren′tis/, a Latin phrase meaning "in the place of the parent": the assumption by a person or institution of the parental obligations of caring for a child without adoption.

innate, **1.** existing in or belonging to a person from birth; inborn; hereditary; congenital. **2.** a natural and essential characteristic of something or someone; inherent. **3.** originating in or produced by the intellect or the mind.

innate immunity. See **natural immunity.**

inner cell mass, a cluster of cells localized around the animal pole of the blastocyst of placental mammals from which the embryo develops. See also **trophoblast.**

inner ear. See **internal ear.**

innervation, the distribution or supply of nerve fibers or nerve impulses to a part of the body.

innervation apraxia. See **motor apraxia.**

innidation. See **nidation.**

innocent, benign, innocuous, or functional; not malignant, as an innocent heart murmur.

innominate, without a name; unnamed. The term is traditionally applied to certain anatomic structures, often identified by their descriptive name, as the hipbone, brachiocephalic artery, and brachiocephalic vein.

innominate artery, one of the three arteries that branch from the arch of the aorta, running about 5 cm from the level of the cranial border of the second right costal cartilage, ascending cranially, dorsally, and obliquely to the right, and dividing into the right common carotid and the right subclavian arteries. Also called **brachicephalic artery, brachiocephalic trunk.**

innominate bone, the hipbone. It consists of the ilium, ischium, and pubis and unites with the sacrum and coccyx to form the pelvis. Also called **os coxae.**

innominate vein, a large vein on either side of the neck that is formed by the union of the internal jugular and subclavian veins. The two veins drain blood from the head, neck, and upper extremities and unite to form the superior vena cava. Also called **brachiocephalic vein.**

inoculate, to introduce a substance (inoculum) into the body to produce or to increase immunity to the disease or condition associated with the substance. It is introduced by making multiple scratches in the skin after placing a drop of the substance on the skin, by puncture of the skin with an implement bearing multiple short tines, or by intradermal, subcutaneous, or intramuscular injection.

inoculum /inok′yo͞oləm/, *pl.* **inocula,** a substance introduced into the body to cause or to increase immunity to a specific disease or condition. It may be a toxin, a live, attenuated, or killed virus or bacterium, or an immune serum. Also called **inoculant.** See also **immune system.**

inorganic, (in chemistry) a chemical compound that does not contain carbon.

inorganic acid, a compound containing no carbon that is made up of hydrogen and an electronegative element, as hydrochloric acid. Some organic acids, as carbonic acid, contain carbon dioxide.

inorganic chemistry, the study of the properties and reactions of all chemical elements and compounds other than hydrocarbons.

inorganic dust, dry, finely powdered particles of an inorganic substance, especially dust, which, when inhaled, can cause abnormal conditions of the lungs. See also **anthracosis, asbestosis, berylliosis, pneumoconiosis, silicosis.**

inorganic phosphorus, phosphorus that may be measured in the blood as phosphate ions. Its increased concentration may indicate bone, kidney, or glandular diseases; decreased concentration may be associated with alcoholism, vitamin deficiency, and other problems. Normal concentrations in the serum of adults are 1.8 to 2.6 mEq/L. See also **phosphorus.**

inosine /in′əsēn, -sīn/, a nucleoside, derived from animal tissue, especially intestines, originally used in food processing and flavoring. It has been used in the treatment of cardiac disorders and now is under investigation in studies of cancer and virology chemotherapy. See also **inosiplex.**

inosiplex, a form of inosine that acts as a stimulator of the immune system. It is currently under investigation for use in cancer therapy and in the treatment of herpesvirus and rhinovirus infections. Also called **methisoprinol.**

inositol /inō′sətōl, inos′-/, an isomer of glucose that occurs widely in plant and animal cells. Although inositol has no current therapeutic use, it may be an essential cell constituent.

inotropic, pertaining to the force or energy of muscular contractions, particularly contractions of the heart muscle. An inotropic agent increases myocardial contractility.

inpatient, **1.** a patient who has been admitted to a hospital or other health care facility for at least an overnight stay. **2.** of or pertaining to the treatment or care of such a patient or to a health care facility to which a patient may be admitted for 24-hour care. Compare **outpatient.**

inpatient care unit, a unit of a hospital organized for medical and continuous nursing services for a group of inpatients who are usually grouped according to diagnosis or other common characteristics, as maternity or surgical patients.

input device, a device that allows for the entry of commands or information for processing in a form acceptable to a computer, as a typewriter, keyboard, tape drive, disk drive, microphone, or light pen.

insanity, *informal.* a severe mental disorder or defect, as a psychosis, rather than a neurosis. It is used more in legal and social than in medical terminology and refers to those mental illnesses that are of such a serious or debilitating nature as to interfere with one's capability of functioning within the legal limits of society and from looking after one's personal affairs. When a person is classified as insane, various legal actions can ensue, as commitment to an institution, appointment of a guardian, or dissolution of a contract. See also **psychosis.**

insect bite, the bite of any parasitic or venomous arthropod as a louse, flea, mite, tick, or arachnid. Many arthropods inject venom that produces poisoning or severe local reaction, saliva that may contain viruses, or substances that produce mild irritation. The degree of irritation of an insect's bite is affected by the design and shape of its mouthparts: A horsefly, for example, makes a short lateral and coarse wound, while a tick takes hold with its backward curved teeth, making its removal difficult. Spiders inflict a sharp pinprick bite that may remain unnoticed until the injected venom has begun to produce a painful reaction. Treatment of a bite depends on the species of insect, the reaction to the bite, and the risk of sequelae from it. First aid treatment is generally symptomatic and includes ice or cold packs, careful cleaning of the wound, and antihistamines or specific antivenin as necessary.

insecticide, a chemical agent that kills insects.

insecticide poisoning. See **chlorinated organic insecticide poisoning.**

insensible perspiration, the loss of fluid from the body by evaporation, as normally occurs during respiration. A small amount of perspiration is continually excreted by the sweat glands in the skin; the portion that evaporates before it may be observed also contributes to insensible perspiration. Also called **insensible water loss.**

insertion, (in anatomy) the place of attachment, as of a muscle to the bone it moves.

insertion forceps. See **point forceps.**

in-service education, a program of instruction or training that is provided by an agency or institution for its employees. The program is held in the institution or at the agency and is intended to increase the skills and competence of the employees in a specific area. In-service education may be a part of any program of staff development.

insidious /insid′ē·əs/, of, pertaining to, or describing a development that is gradual, subtle, or imperceptible. Certain chronic diseases, as glaucoma, can develop insidiously with symptoms that are not detected by the patient until the disorder is established. Compare **acute.**

insight, **1.** the capacity of comprehending the true nature of a situation or of penetrating an underlying truth. **2.** an instance of penetrating or comprehending an underlying truth, primarily through intuitive understanding. **3.** (in psychology) a type of self-understanding encompassing both an intellectual and emotional awareness of the unconscious nature, origin, and mechanisms of one's attitudes, feelings, and behavior. It is one of the most important goals of psychotherapy and, with integration, leads to modification of maladaptive behavioral patterns. See also **integration.**

in situ /in sī′to͞o, sit′o͞o/, **1.** in the natural or usual place. **2.** describing a cancer that has not metastasized or invaded neighboring tissues, as carcinoma in situ.

insoluble, unable to be dissolved, usually in a specific solvent, as a substance that is insoluble in water.

insomnia, chronic inability to sleep or to remain asleep throughout the night; wakefulness; sleeplessness. The condition is caused by a variety of physical and psychologic factors, including emotional stress, physical pain and discomfort, disturbances in cerebral function, like toxic delirium and senile dementia, drug abuse and drug dependence, psychosomatic disorders, neuroses, psychoses, and psychologic problems that produce anxiety, irrational fears, and tensions. Treatment may include medication with sedatives, tranquilizers or hypnotics, psychotherapy, and exercise.

insomniac, **1.** a person with insomnia. **2.** pertaining to, causing, or associated with insomnia. **3.** characteristic of or occurring during a period of sleeplessness.

inspiration, the act of drawing air into the lungs in order to exchange oxygen for carbon dioxide, the end product of tissue metabolism. The major muscle of inspiration is the diaphragm, the contraction of which creates a negative pressure in the chest, causing the lungs to expand and air to flow inward. Additional muscles aiding inspiratory efforts are the external intercostals, scaleni, scapular elevators, and sternocleidomastoids. Since expiration is usually a passive process, these muscles of inspiration alone perform normal respiration. Lungs at maximal inspiration have an average total capacity of 5500 to 6000 ml of air. Compare **expiration.** See also **inspiratory reserve volume.**

inspiratory, of or pertaining to inspiration.

inspiratory capacity (IC), the maximum volume of gas that can be inhaled from the resting expiratory level. Equal to the sum of the tidal volume and the inspiratory reserve volume, it is measured with a spirometer.

inspiratory reserve volume, the maximum volume of gas that can be inspired from the end-tidal inspiratory level.

inspissate /inspis′āt/, (of a fluid) to thicken or harden through the absorption or evaporation of the liquid portion, as milk in an inspissated milk duct. **–inspissation,** *n.*

instillation, **1.** a procedure in which a fluid is slowly introduced into a cavity or passage of the body and allowed to remain for a specific length of time before being drained or withdrawn. It is performed to expose the tissues of the area to the solution, to warmth or cold, or to a drug or substance in the solution. **2.** a solution so introduced. Compare **infusion, injection, insufflate.** **–instill,** *v.*

instinctive reflex. See **unconditioned response.**

institutionalize, to place a person in an institution for psychologic or physical treatment or for the protection of the person or society. **–institutionalization,** *n.*, **institutionalized,** *adj.*

institutional licensure, a proposed procedure in which licensure for almost all health professions would be abandoned and the responsibility for assessing professional competence would fall to the health care facility where the health professional is employed. Proponents of the procedure maintain that health needs would be better and more flexibly served. Opponents maintain that knowledge, judgment, and competency are the products of a good basic education in the profession and that educators cannot teach the profession without a set of standardized expectations, as are now provided by government-controlled licensing procedures and certifying examinations. In addition, health care facilities may not have the expertise or resources necessary to evaluate the various kinds of health care providers.

institutional review board (IRB), a federally approved committee that reviews all research proposals before submission of requests for funding to federal government granting agencies.

instrument, a surgical tool or device designed to perform a specific function, as cutting, dissecting, grasping, holding, retracting, or suturing. Surgical instruments are usually made of steel and are specially treated to be durable, heat-resistant, rust-resistant, and stain-proof. Proper care of surgical instruments is essential and includes correct use, careful handling, inspection for defects, adequate and appropriate sterilization, and proper labeling, dating, and storage. Some kinds of instruments are **clamp, needle holder, retractor,** and **speculum.**

instrumental conditioning. See **operant conditioning.**

instrumentation, the use of instruments for treatment and diagnosis.

insufficiency, inability to perform a necessary function adequately. Some kinds of insufficiency are **adrenal insufficiency, aortic insufficiency, ileocecal insufficiency, pulmonary insufficiency,** and **valvular insufficiency.**

insufflate /insuf′lāt/, to blow a gas or powder into a tube, cavity, or organ to allow visual examination, to remove an obstruction, or to apply medication. See also **Rubin's test.** –**insufflation,** *n.*

insul-, a combining form meaning 'of or pertaining to an island, or island-shaped': *insula, insulin, insuloma.*

insulin, **1.** a naturally occurring hormone secreted by the beta cells of the islands of Langerhans in the pancreas in response to increased levels of glucose in the blood. The hormone acts to regulate the metabolism of glucose and the processes necessary for the intermediary metabolism of fats, carbohydrates, and proteins. Insulin lowers blood glucose levels and promotes transport and entry of glucose into the muscle cells and other tissues. Inadequate secretion of insulin results in hyperglycemia, hyperlipemia, ketonemia, and azoturia and in the characteristic signs of diabetes mellitus, including polyphagia, polydipsia, and polyuria, and, eventually, lethargy and weight loss. Uncorrected severe deficiency of insulin is incompatible with life. **2.** a pharmacologic preparation of the hormone administered in treating diabetes mellitus. The various preparations of insulin available for prescription vary in promptness, intensity, and duration of action. They are termed rapid-acting, intermediate-acting and long-acting. Most forms of insulin drugs are given by subcutaneous injection in individualized dosage schedules. Adverse reactions include hypoglycemia and insulin shock from excess dosage and hyperglycemia and diabetic ketoacidosis from inadequate dosage. Many drugs interact with insulin, among them the monoamine oxidase inhibitors, corticosteroids, salicylates, thiazide diuretics, and phenytoin. Fever, stress, infection, pregnancy, surgery, and hyperthyroidism may significantly increase insulin requirements; liver disease, hypothyroidism, vomiting, and renal disease may decrease the need for insulin. Urine or blood tests for glucose and ketones are performed to determine the need for adjustment of the dosage or of the schedule of administration. See also **human insulin.** (Table, page 590)

insulin-dependent diabetes mellitus (IDDM), an inability to metabolize carbohydrate caused by an overt insulin deficiency, occurring in children and characterized by polydipsia, polyuria, polyphagia, loss of weight, diminished strength, and marked irritability. The onset is usually rapid, but approximately one third of the patients have a remission within 3 months; this stage may continue for days or years, but diabetes then progresses quickly to a state of total dependence on insulin. Occasionally, the disease is asymptomatic and is discovered only by postprandial hyperglycemia or glucose tolerance tests. Insulin-dependent diabetes mellitus tends to be unstable and brittle, with the patients quite sensitive to insulin and physical activity and liable to develop ketoacidosis. Recent evidence suggests that insulin-dependent diabetes mellitus may be caused by environmental factors, as a virus. Previously called brittle diabetes, juvenile diabetes, juvenile-onset diabetes, JOD, juvenile-onset-type diabetes, ketosis-prone diabetes. Compare **non-insulin-dependent diabetes mellitus.** See also **diabetes mellitus.**

insulin injection, a fast-acting, regular insulin prescribed in the treatment of diabetes mellitus when the desired action is prompt, intense, and short-acting. Insulin injection prepared from zinc insulin crystals is slightly longer-acting than the amorphous noncrystalline form of this type of insulin preparation. Insulin injection is the only form of insulin suitable for intramuscular administration. Also called **regular insulin.**

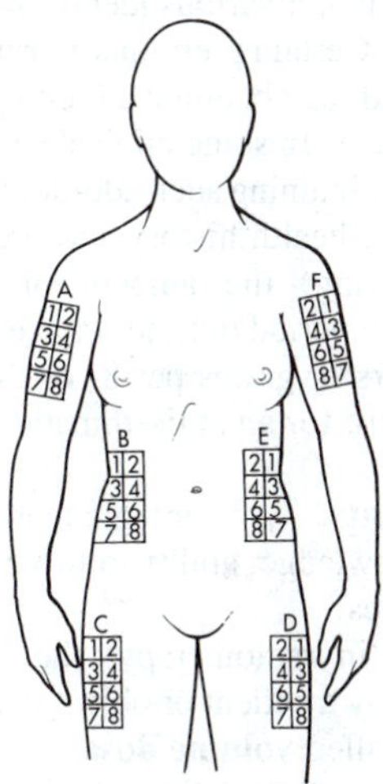

Insulin injection sites

insulin kinase, an enzyme, assumed to be present in the liver, that activates insulin.

insulinogenic, promoting the production and release of insulin by the islands of Langerhans in the pancreas.

insulinoma /in′so͞olinō′mə/, *pl.* **insulinomas, insulinomata,** a benign tumor of the insulin-secreting cells of the islands of Langerhans. Surgical resection of the tumor may be possible, thus limiting the development of hypoglycemia. Also called **insuloma, islet cell adenoma.** Compare **islet cell tumor.**

insulin reaction, the adverse effects caused by excessive levels of circulating insulin. See **hyperinsulinism.**

insulin shock, hypoglycemic shock caused by an overdose of insulin, a decreased intake of food, or excessive exercise. It is characterized by sweating, trembling, chilliness, nervousness, irritability, hunger, hallucination, numbness, and pallor. Uncorrected, it will progress to convulsions, coma, and death. Treatment requires an immediate dose of glucose. Compare **ketoacidosis.**

insulin shock treatment, the injection of large, convulsion-producing doses of insulin, administered as a therapeutic measure in psychoses, especially schizophrenia. Electroconvulsive therapy is currently administered more commonly than insulin shock and is used chiefly for manic-depressive psychosis. Also called **hypoglycemic shock treatment.**

insulin tolerance test, a test of the body's ability to use insulin, in which insulin is given and blood glucose is measured at regular intervals. Thirty minutes after the insulin is given, blood glucose is usually lower but not less than half of the fasting glucose level. Glucose levels usually return to normal after about 90 minutes. In people with hypoglycemia, the glucose levels may drop lower and be slower to return to normal.

insuloma. See **insulinoma.**

intake, **1.** the process in which a person is admitted to a clinic or hospital or is signed in for an office visit. The reason for the visit and various identifying data about the patient are noted. Certain preliminary, routine procedures may be performed, as obtaining a blood pressure reading or a urine specimen. In some clinical settings, the intake may also include obtaining such additional information as the patient's basic health history and previous source of care. **2.** (in nursing) the amount of food or fluids ingested in a given period of time. Intake is measured and noted in milliliters or grams per 8- or 24-hour period.

Intal, a trademark for an antiasthmatic (cromolyn sodium).

intangible elements, psychologic factors, such as cognitive ability, knowledge, ability to solve problems, emotions, and attitudes.

integral dose, (in radiotherapy) the total amount of energy absorbed by a patient or object during exposure to radiation. Also called **volume dose.**

integrating dose meter, (in radiotherapy) an ionization chamber, usually designed to be placed on the patient's skin, with a measuring system for determining the total radiation administered during an exposure. A device may be included to terminate the exposure when the desired value is reached.

integration, **1.** the act or process of unifying or bringing together. **2.** (in psychology) the organization of all elements of the personality into a coordinated, functional whole that is in harmony with the environment, one of the primary goals in psychotherapy. It involves the assimilation of insight and the coordination of new and old data, experiences, and emotional reactions so that an effective change can occur in behavior, thinking, or feeling. See also **insight.** **–integrate,** *v.*

integration of self, one of the components of high-level wellness. It is a prerequisite for the achievement of maturity and is characterized by the integration of mind, body, and spirit into one harmoniously functioning unit.

integument /integ′yo͞omənt/, a covering or skin. –**integumentary,** *adj.*

integumentary system, the skin and its appendages, hair, nails, and sweat and sebaceous glands. See also the Color Atlas of Human Anatomy.

integumentary system assessment, an evaluation of the general condition of a patient's integument and of factors or abnormalities that may contribute to the presence of a dermatologic disorder.

■ METHOD: The nurse askes if the patient suffers from itching, pain, rashes, blisters, or boils; if the skin usually is dry, oily, thin, rough, bumpy, or puffy; or if it feels hot or cold, peels, changes in color, or is marked with dark liver (aging) spots. Observations are made of the intactness, turgor, elasticity, temperature, cleanliness, odor, wetness or dryness, and color of the skin. Cyanosis of the lips, circumoral area, or mucous membranes, earlobes, or nailbeds; jaundice of the sclera; pale conjunctivae; the distribution of pigment; and evidence of plethora are noted. Indications of rashes, edema, needle marks, insect bites, scabies, acne, sclerema, decubiti, uremic frost on the beard or eyebrows, or pressure areas over bony prominences are recorded. The nails are examined for brittleness, lines, a convex ram's horn or concave spoon shape, and the condition of surrounding tissue, including clubbing of the fingers and toes. The existence and characteristics of maculae, papules, vesicles, pustules, bullae, hives, warts, moles, ulcers, scars, keloids, petechiae,

Action of insulin preparations

Type of insulin	*Time of onset (hr)*	*Peak of action (hr)*	*Duration of action (hr)*	*Insulin appearance*
Rapid acting				
Regular	< 1	2-4	4-6	Clear
Crystalline zinc	< 1	2-4	5-8	Clear
Semilente	< 1	4-7	12-16	Cloudy
Intermediate acting				
NPH	1-2	8-12	18-24	Cloudy
Globin zinc	2-4	6-10	12-18	Clear
Lente	1-4	8-12	18-24	Cloudy
Slow acting				
Protamine zinc	4-8	16-18	36+	Cloudy
Ultralente	4-8	16-18	36+	Cloudy

lipomas, crusts of dried exudate, flakes of dead epidermis, excoriations, blackheads, or a chancre are noted. The patient's exposure to parasites, to internal allergens in food and drugs, and to external allergens in cosmetics, soaps, topical medication, and plants, as well as a family history of allergies, is investigated. The patient's currently used medication, creams, lotions, ointments, hygienic measures, and sexual practices are ascertained. Diagnostic aids contributing to the evaluation are skin and lesion cultures, punch biopsies, skin tests for allergies, a lupus erythematosus preparation, and a blood culture.

■ NURSING ORDERS: the nurse conducts the interview to obtain subjective data on the patient's condition, makes the necessary observations, and assembles the background information and the results of the diagnostic tests.

■ OUTCOME CRITERIA: A well-conducted assessment of the patient's integument is a valuable aid in diagnosing a dermatologic disorder.

intellect, **1.** the power and ability of the mind for knowing and understanding, as contrasted with feeling or with willing. **2.** a person possessing a great capacity for thought and knowledge. –**intellectual,** *adj., n.*

intellectualization, (in psychiatry) a defense mechanism in which reasoning is used as a means of blocking a confrontation with an unconscious conflict and the emotional stress associated with it.

intelligence, **1.** the potential ability and capacity to acquire, retain, and apply experience, understanding, knowledge, reasoning, and judgment in coping with new experiences and in solving problems. **2.** the manifestation of such ability. See also **intelligence quotient.** –**intelligent,** *adj.*

intelligence quotient (IQ), a numeric expression of a person's intellectual level as measured against the statistical average of his or her age group. On several of the traditional scales it is determined by dividing the mental age, derived through psychologic testing, by the chronologic age and multiplying the result by 100. Average IQ is considered to be 100. See also **mental retardation.**

intelligence test, any of a variety of standarized tests designed to determine the mental age of an individual by measuring the relative capacity to absorb information and to solve problems. These tests are routinely used by the medical profession to diagnose and determine degrees of mental retardation and to aid in the planning of therapeutic programs for such persons. Two kinds of intelligence tests are **Stanford-Binet** and **Wechsler-Bellevue scale.** Compare **achievement test, aptitude test, personality test, psychologic test.**

intelligent terminal, a computer terminal that can function as a processing device in addition to providing input/output facilities, whether operated independently or connected to a main computer. Also called **smart terminal.**

intensifying screen, a device consisting of fluorescent material, which is placed in contact with the film in a radiographic cassette. Radiation from a therapeutic process interacts with the fluorescent phosphor, releasing light photons. These expose the film with greater efficiency than would the radiation alone. Thus patient exposure can be reduced.

intensive care, constant, complex, detailed health care as provided in various acute life-threatening conditions, as multiple trauma, severe burns, myocardial infarction, or after certain kinds of surgery. Special training is often necessary to provide intensive care. Care is most frequently given in an intensive care unit equipped with various advanced machines and devices for treating and monitoring the patient. Also called **critical care.**

intensive care unit (ICU), a hospital unit in which patients requiring close monitoring and intensive care are housed for as long as needed. An ICU contains highly technical and sophisticated monitoring devices and equipment, and the staff in the unit is educated to give critical care as needed by the patients. A large tertiary care facility usually has separate units specifically designed for the intensive care of adults, infants, children or newborns or for other groups of patients requiring a certain kind of treatment. See also **coronary care unit, neonatal care unit.**

intention, a kind of healing process: Healing by **first intention** is the primary union of the edges of a wound, progressing to complete healing without scar formation or granulation; healing by **second intention** is wound closure in which the edges are separated, granulation tissue develops to fill the gap, and, finally, epithelium grows in over the granulations, producing a scar. Healing by **third intention** is wound closure in which granulation tissue fills the gap between the edges of the wound with epithelium growing over the granulation at a slower rate and producing a larger scar than results from healing from second intention. Usually there is also suppuration.

intentional additives, substances that are deliberately added in the manufacture of food or pharmaceutic products to improve or maintain flavor, color, texture, or consistency, or to enhance or conserve nutritional value. Compare **incidental additives.**

intention tremor, fine, rhythmic, purposeless movements that tend to increase during voluntary movements. Compare **continuous tremor.** See also **tremor.**

inter-, a combining form meaning 'situated, formed, or occurring between': *interacinar, intercalary, intercartilaginous.*

interaction processes, a component of the theory of effective practice. The processes consist of a series of interactions between a nurse and a patient. The series occurs in a sequence of actions and reactions until the patient and the nurse both understand what is wanted and the desired behavior or act is achieved.

interarticular fibrocartilage, one of four kinds of fibrocartilage, consisting of flattened fibrocartilaginous plates between the articular cartilage of the most active joints, as the sternoclavicular, wrist, and knee joints. The synovial surfaces extend over the fibrocartilaginous plates and attach to surrounding ligaments. The fibrocartilaginous plates absorb shocks and increase mobility. Compare **circumferential fibrocartilage, connecting fibrocartilage, stratiform fibrocartilage.**

intercalary /intur′kəler′ē, in′tərkal′ərē/, occurring between two others, as the absence of the middle part of a bone with the proximal and the distal parts present.

intercalate /intur′kəlāt/, to insert between adjacent surfaces or structures. **–intercalation,** *n.*

intercapillary glomerulosclerosis, an abnormal condition characterized by degeneration of the renal glomeruli. It is associated with diabetes and often produces albuminuria, nephrotic edema, hypertension, and renal insufficiency. Also called **Kimmelstiel-Wilson disease.**

intercellular, between or among cells.

intercellular bridge, a structure that connects adjacent cells, occurring primarily in the epithelium and other stratified squamous epithelia. It consists of slender strands of cytoplasm that project from the surfaces of adjacent cells and merge at the desmosome. Also called **cytoplasmic bridge.**

interchange. See **reciprocal translocation.**

interconceptional gynecologic care, health care of a woman during her reproductive years, between pregnancies, and after 6 weeks after delivery. Papanicolaou testing for cervical cancer, breast and pelvic examinations, evaluation of general health, and laboratory determination of glucosuria and proteinuria and of the hematocrit or hemoglobin are common and routine aspects of interconceptional care. Testing and treatment for pelvic, vaginal, or genital infections may be required. A contraceptive method may also be discussed, taught, prescribed, or provided. Ordinarily, the basic examination is performed annually. The method of contraception may be adjusted or changed at interim visits; infections or other complaints are investigated, diagnosed, and treated as symptoms appear. Interconceptional care is increasingly given by nurse practitioners or nurse midwives who follow protocols for treatment and referral formulated in consultation with a supervising gynecologist.

intercondylar fracture /in′tərkon′dilər/, a fracture of the tissue between condyles.

intercostal, of or pertaining to the space between two ribs.

intercostal bulging, the visible bulging of the soft tissues of the intercostal spaces that occurs when increased expiratory effort is needed to exhale, as in asthma, cystic fibrosis, or obstruction of a respiratory passage by a foreign body. Compare **retraction of the chest.**

intercostal node, a node in one of three groups of thoracic parietal lymph nodes situated near the dorsal parts of the intercostal spaces and associated with lymphatic vessels that drain the posterolateral area of the chest. The efferent vessels from the nodes in the caudal four or five spaces form a descending trunk that opens into the dilated origin of the thoracic duct. The efferents from the nodes in the upper intercostal spaces on the left side connect with the thoracic duct; those on the right side end in the right lymphatic duct. Compare **diaphragmatic node, sternal node.** See also **lymphatic system, lymph node.**

intercourse, *informal.* sexual intercourse. See **coitus.**

intercristal, of or pertaining to the space between two crests.

intercurrent disease, a disease that develops in and may alter the course of another disease.

interdental canal, any one of the nutrient channels that pass upward to the teeth through the body of the mandible. Also called **nutrient canal.**

interdental gingiva, the soft supporting tissue, consisting of prominent horizontal collagen fibers, that normally fills the space between two approximating teeth.

interdental groove, a linear, vertical depression on the surface of the interdental papillae, which functions as a sluiceway for the egress of food from the interproximal areas.

interdental spillway, a sluiceway formed by the interproximal contours of adjoining teeth and their investing tissues.

interface, the connection between different elements of a computer system or between different computers.

interference, the effect of a component on the accuracy of measurement of the desired analyte.

interferent, any chemical or physical phenomena that can interfere or disrupt a reaction or process.

interfibrillar mass of Flemming, interfilar mass. See **hyaloplasm.**

interim rate, a method of third-party payment for costs of hospital services in which an amount is paid periodically pending an accounting of actual costs at the end of a designated period.

interiorization, the merging of reflex and cognitive processes as a response to the environment.

interior mesenteric artery, a visceral branch of the abdominal aorta, arising just above the division into the common iliacs and supplying the left half of the transverse colon, all of the descending and iliac colons, and most of the rectum. It has left colic, sigmoid, and superior rectal branches.

interkinesis /in′tərkinē′sis, -kīnē′sis/, the interval between the first and second nuclear divisions in meiosis. See also **interphase.**

interlobular duct, any duct connecting or draining the lobules of a gland.

interlocked twins, monozygotic twins so positioned in the uterus that the neck of one becomes entwined with that of the other during presentation so that vaginal delivery is not possible. Such interlocking occurs when one fetus is a breech presentation and the other a vertex presentation. Also called **interlocking twins.**

intermediary, a Blue Cross plan, private insurance company, or public or private agency selected by health care providers to pay claims under Medicare.

intermediate-acting insulin, a preparation of the antidiabetic principle of beef pancreas or pork pancreas modified by interaction with zinc under specific chemical conditions and having an intermediate range of action.

The action of semilente insulin begins within 1 hour of injection, reaches a peak in 6 to 10 hours, and lasts for 12 to 16 hours. Three other intermediate-acting preparations begin to act 2 to 4 hours after injection; globin zinc insulin reaches a peak in 6 to 10 hours and lasts for 18 to 24 hours; neutral protamine Hagedorn insulin (NPH) has a peak action in 8 to 12 hours and a duration of action of 28 to 32 hours, while lente insulin has a similar peak interval and a slightly shorter duration of action. See also **insulin.** Compare **long-acting insulin, short-acting insulin.**

intermediate care, a level of medical care for certain chronically ill or disabled individuals in which room and board are provided but skilled nursing care is not. Title XI of U.S. Medicaid legislation mandates standards and federal subsidies for intermediate care of the recipients of public assistance.

intermediate care facility, a health facility that provides medical-related services to persons with a variety of physical or emotional conditions requiring institutional facilities but without the degree of care provided by a hospital or skilled nursing facility. An example is a health care facility for mentally retarded persons.

intermediate cell mass. See **nephrotome.**

intermediate cuneiform bone, the smallest of the three cuneiform bones of the foot, located between the medial and the lateral cuneiform bones. It has six surfaces, is attached to various ligaments, and articulates with the navicular, medial, and lateral cuneiform bones and with the second metatarsal. Also called **middle cuneiform bone, second cuneiform bone.**

intermediate host, any animal in which the larval or intermediate stages of a parasite develop. Certain snails are intermediate hosts for liver flukes and schistosomes. Humans are intermediate hosts for malaria parasites. Also called **secondary host.** Compare **dead-end host, definitive host, reservoir host.** See also **host,** def. 1.

intermediate mesoderm. See **nephrotome.**

intermenstrual, of or pertaining to the time between menstrual periods.

intermenstrual fever, the normal, slight elevation of temperature that marks ovulation, usually occurring about 14 days before the onset of menses.

intermittent, occurring at intervals; alternating between periods of activity and inactivity, as rheumatoid arthritis, which is marked by periods of signs and symptoms followed by periods of remission.

intermittent fever, a fever that recurs in cycles of paroxysms and remissions, as in malaria. Kinds of intermittent fever include **bidoutertian malaria, double quartan malaria,** and **quartan malaria.**

intermittent mandatory ventilation (IMV), a method of respiratory therapy in which the patient is allowed to breathe independently and then, at certain prescribed intervals, a ventilation machine forces him to take a breath either under positive pressure or in a measured volume. Compare **continuous positive pressure breathing, intermittent positive pressure breathing.** See also **respiratory therapy.**

intermittent positive pressure breathing. See **IPPB.**

intermittent positive pressure breathing unit. See **IPPB unit.**

intermittent positive pressure ventilation. See **IPPB.**

intern, **1.** a physician in the first postgraduate year, learning medical practice under supervision before beginning a residency program. **2.** any immediate postgraduate trainee in a clinical program. **3.** to work as an intern. Also spelled **interne.**

internal, within or inside. **–internally,** *adv.*

internal aperture of tympanic canaliculus, the upper opening of the tympanic channel in the temporal bone, leading to the tympanum.

internal carotid artery, each of two arteries starting at the bifurcation of the common carotid arteries, opposite the cranial border of the thyroid cartilage, through which blood circulates to many structures and organs in the head. Each artery includes cervical, petrous, cavernous, and cerebral portions and divides into 11 branches. There are no branches from the cervical portion. The four branches from the petrous portion are the caroticotympanic, the artery of the pterygoid canal, the cavernous, and the hypophyseal. The five branches from the cavernous portion are the ganglionic, anterior meningeal, ophthalmic, anterior cerebral, and middle cerebral. The two branches from the cerebral portion are the posterior communicating and the anterior choroidal.

internal carotid plexus, a network of nerves on the internal carotid artery, formed by the internal carotid nerve. The internal carotid plexus supplies sympathetic fibers to the branches of the internal carotid artery, the tympanic plexus, the nerves of the cavernous sinus, and the cranial parasympathetic ganglia through which the fibers pass. Compare **common carotid plexus, external carotid plexus.**

internal cervical os, an internal opening of the uterus that corresponds to the slight constriction or isthmus of that organ about midway in its length. The internal cervical os separates the body of the uterus from the cervix. Compare **external cervical os.**

internal cuneiform bone. See **medial cuneiform bone.**

internal ear, the complex inner structure of the ear, communicating directly with the acoustic nerve, transmitting sound vibrations from the middle ear through the fluid-filled network of three semicircular canals joining at a vestibule connected to the cochlea. It has two parts: the osseous labyrinth and the membranous labyrinth. Also called **inner ear, labyrinth.** Compare **external ear, middle ear.**

internal fertilization, the union of gametes within the body of the female after insemination. See also **artificial insemination.**

internal fistula, an abnormal passage between two internal organs or structures.

internal fixation, any method of holding together the fragments of a fractured bone without the use of appliances external to the skin. After open reduction of the fracture, smooth or threaded pins, Kirschner wires, screws, plates attached by screws, or medullary nails may be used to stabilize the fragments. In some instances the device is removed at a later operation, but sometimes it may remain in the body permanently. Compare **external pin fixation.**

internal iliac artery, a division of the common iliac artery, supplying the walls of the pelvis, the pelvic viscera, the genital organs, and part of the medial thigh. The pattern of its branches is the most variable of any artery in the body. Its 10 most common branches are umbilical, inferior vesical, middle rectal, uterine, obturator, internal pudendal, iliolumbar, lateral sacral, superior gluteal, and inferior gluteal. In the fetus, the internal iliac artery is twice as large as the external iliac and is the direct continuation of the common iliac artery. After birth, the internal iliac becomes smaller than the external iliac. Also called **hypogastric artery.** Compare **external iliac artery.**

internal iliac node, a node in one of seven groups of parietal lymph nodes serving the abdomen and the pelvis. The internal iliac nodes surround the internal iliac vessels and receive lymphatic vessels corresponding to the branches of the internal iliac artery. Their afferent vessels drain lymph from the pelvic viscera, the buttocks, and dorsal portions of the thighs. Their efferents end in the common iliac nodes. Compare **external iliac node, iliac circumflex node.** See also **lymph, lymphatic system, lymph node.**

internal iliac vein, one of the pair of veins in the lower body that join the external iliac vein to form the two common iliac veins. Each internal iliac vein begins at the greater sciatic foramen, ascends dorsal to its corresponding artery, and at the pelvic brim joins the external iliac vein. It receives various tributaries, as the superior gluteal, the inferior gluteal, the internal pudendal, the obturator, the lateral sacral, the middle rectal, the dorsal veins of the penis, the vesical, the uterine, and the vaginal. Compare **external iliac vein.**

internalization, the process of adopting within the self, either unconsciously or consciously through learning and socialization, the attitudes, beliefs, values, and standards of another person or, more generally, of the society or group to which one belongs. See also **socialization.**

internal jugular vein, one of a pair of veins in the neck. Each vein collects blood from one side of the brain, the face, and the neck, and both unite with the subclavian vein to form the brachiocephalic vein. The left internal jugular vein is usually smaller than the right, and each vein contains a pair of valves located about 2.5 cm above its termination. The thoracic duct on the left side and the right lymphatic duct on the right side drain into the junction of the internal jugular and the subclavian veins. Each internal jugular vein is continuous with the transverse sinus in the posterior part of the jugular foramen at the base of the skull where, in some people, the vein forms a jugular bulb. Just above the termination is the inferior bulb. Compare **external jugular vein.**

internal mammary artery bypass, a surgical procedure to correct a coronary artery obstruction. The internal mammary artery in situ and still attached to the subclavian artery is anastomosed to the coronary artery beyond the obstruction.

internal medicine, the branch of medicine concerned with the study of the physiology and pathology of the internal organs and with the medical diagnosis and treatment of disorders of these organs.

internal oblique muscle. See **obliquus internus abdominis.**

internal os, the internal opening of the cervical canal.

internal podalic version and total breech extraction. See **version and extraction.**

internal pterygoid muscle. See **pterygoideus medialis.**

internal respiratory nerve of Bell. See **phrenic nerve.**

internal rotation, the turning of a limb toward the midline of the body.

internal standard, an element or compound added in a known amount to yield a signal against which an instrument or an analyte to be measured can be calibrated.

internal strabismus. See **esotropia.**

internal thoracic artery, one of a pair of arteries that arise from the first portions of the subclavian arteries, descend to the margin of the sternum, and divide into the musculophrenic and superior gastric arteries at the level of the sixth intercostal space, supplying the pectoral muscles, the breasts, the pericardium, and the abdominal muscles. Each artery has eight branches: pericardiophrenic, mediastinal, thymic, sternal, anterior intercostal, perforating, musculophrenic, and superior epigastric.

internal thoracic vein, one of a pair of veins that accompanies the internal thoracic artery, receiving tributaries that correspond to those of the artery. It forms a single trunk that runs up on the medial side of the artery and ends in the corresponding brachiocephalic vein. The superior phrenic vein usually opens into the internal thoracic vein.

International Association for Dental Research (I.A.D.R.), an international organization concerned with research in dentistry and the exchange of information regarding such research.

International Classification of Disease Adapted for Use in the United States (ICDA), a classification system adapted by the U.S. Public Health Service from the parent system developed by the World Health Organization. The system is used in categorizing and indexing hospital records. Each disease is listed as belonging to a major section, as infectious disease or neoplastic disease, and then further coded into major disease categories and subdivisions. The system is updated every 10 years.

International Classification of Diseases (ICD), an official list of categories of diseases, physical and mental, issued by the World Health Organization (WHO). It is used primarily for statistic purposes in the classification of morbidity and mortality data. Any nation belonging to WHO may adjust the classification to meet specific needs; for example, in the United States, the *ICD-9-CM,* a clinical modification of the 1975 revision, *ICD-9,* was adopted to provide additional data required by clinicians, research workers, epidemiologists, medical record librarians, and administrators of inpatient, outpatient, and community programs. See also ***Diagnostic and Statistical Manual of Mental Disorders.***

International Congress of Surgeons (I.C.S.), an international professional organization of surgeons.

International Council of Nurses (ICN), the oldest international health organization. It is a federation of nurses' associations from 93 nations and was one of the first health organizations to develop strict policies of nondiscrimination based on nationality, race, creed, color, politics, sex, or social status. The objectives of the ICN include promotion of national associations of nurses, improvement of standards of nursing and competence of nurses, improvement of the status of nurses within their countries, and provision of an authoritative international voice for nurses. The following ICN definition of the nurse is accepted internationally and serves as a pattern in developing nursing practice and nursing education throughout the world: "A nurse is a person who has completed a program of basic education and is qualified and authorized in her/his country to practice nursing. Basic nursing education is a formally recognized program of study which provides a broad and sound foundation for the practice of nursing and for post-basic education which develops specific competency. At the first level, the educational program prepares the nurse, through study of behavior, life, and nursing sciences and clinical experience, for effective practice and direction of nursing care and for the leadership role. The first level nurse is responsible for planning, providing, and evaluating nursing care in all settings for the promotion of health, prevention of illness, care of the sick, and rehabilitation; and functions as a member of the health team. In countries with more than one level of nursing personnel, the second level program prepares the nurse, through study of nursing theory and clinical practice, to give nursing care in co-operation with and under the supervision of a first level nurse." The ICN is active in the World Health Organization (WHO), the United Nations Educational, Scientific, and Cultural Organization (UNESCO), and other international organizations.

International Red Cross Society, an international philanthropic organization, based in Geneva, Switzerland, concerned primarily with the humane treatment and welfare of the victims of war and calamity and with the neutrality of hospitals and medical personnel in times of war. See also **American Red Cross.**

International System of Units, a system for the standardization of the measurement of certain substances, including some antibiotics, vitamins, enzymes, and hormones. An International Unit (I.U.) of substance is the amount that produces a specific biologic result. Each I.U. of a substance has the same potency and action as another unit of the same substance. See also **centimeter-gram-second system, CIPM.**

International Unit (IU, I.U.), a unit of measure in the International System of Units. See also **SI units.**

internist, a physician who specializes in internal medicine.

internuncial neuron, a connecting neuron in a neural pathway, usually serving as a link between two other neurons.

interocclusal record, a record of the positional relation of opposing teeth or jaws to each other, made on the occlusal surfaces of occlusal rims or teeth with a plastic material that hardens, as plaster of paris, wax, zinc oxide-eugenol paste, or acrylic resin.

interoceptive /in′tərōsep′tiv/, pertaining to stimuli originating from within the body regarding the functioning of the internal organs or to the receptors they activate. Compare **exteroceptive, proprioception.**

interoceptor, any sensory nerve ending located in cells in the viscera that responds to stimuli originating from within the body regarding the function of the internal organs, as digestion, excretion, and blood pressure. Compare **exteroceptor, proprioceptor.**

interparietal fissure. See **intraparietal sulcus.**

interperiosteal fracture /in′tərper′ē•os′tē•əl/, an incomplete fracture in which the periosteum is not disrupted.

interpersonal therapy, a kind of psychotherapy that views faulty communications, interactions, and interrelationships as basic factors in maladaptive behavior. A kind of interpersonal therapy is **transactional analysis.**

interphase, the metabolic stage in the cell cycle during which the cell is not dividing, the chromosomes are not individually distinguishable, and such biochemical and physiologic activities as DNA synthesis occur. The stage follows telophase of one division and extends to the beginning of prophase of the next division. See also **anaphase, interkinesis, metaphase, mitosis, prophase, telophase.**

interpolated PVC, a ventricular extrasystole sandwiched between two sinus-conducted beats.

interpolated VPB, a ventricular extrasystole that occurs between two consecutive beats of the dominant heart rhythm.

interpreter, a computer program that remains in the memory and interprets or executes higher-level language.

interproximal film. See **bite-wing film.**

interpubic disk, the fibrocartilaginous plate connecting the opposed surfaces of the pubic bones at the pubic symphysis. Varying in thickness, it is strengthened by interlacing fibers and often contains a cavity that usually appears after the tenth year of life. Also called **discus interpubicus.**

interradicular space, the area between the roots of a multirooted tooth, normally occupied by a bony septum and the periodontal membrane.

interrogatories, (in law) a series of written questions submitted to a witness or other person having information of interest to the court. The answers are transcribed and are sworn to under oath. Interrogatories are used during pretrial preparation as a means of discovery. They differ from depositions in that there is no opportunity for cross-examination. Compare **discovery, deposition.**

intersex, any individual who has anatomic characteristics of both sexes or whose external genitalia are ambiguous or inappropriate for either the normal male or female. See also **hermaphrodite, intersexuality, pseudohermaphrodite.**

intersexuality, the condition in which an individual has both male and female anatomic characteristics to varying degrees or in which the appearance of the external genitalia is ambiguous or differs from the gonadal or genetic sex. See also **hermaphroditism, pseudohermaphroditism. –intersexual,** *adj.*

■ OBSERVATIONS: Any disturbance in the normal sequence of sex determination during embryonic development, including sex chromosome aberrations, abnormal differentiation of the gonads or ductal systems, or hormonal imbalance, may result in situations in which the phenotypic sex differs from the genotypic sex. Those conditions characterized by ambiguous or inappropriate genitalia are apparent at birth, but others, as Turner's syndrome or Kleinfelter's syndrome, may not be diagnosed until later as a result of delayed development or infertility. There are conditions producing ambiguous genitalia in the newborn that require prompt evaluation and attention: the masculinized female, or female pseudohermaphrodite, of which the most common type is congenital adrenal hyperplasia, caused by an inherited deficiency in the enzymes of adrenal corticoid synthesis; the incompletely masculinized male, or male pseudohermaphrodite, produced as an inherited X-linked recessive or autosomal dominant trait and caused by a deficiency in any of the enzymes needed for testosterone biosynthesis or the unresponsiveness of genital structures to testosterone; the true hermaphrodite, which is rare; and mixed gonadal dysgenesis, in which affected infants are sex chromosomal mosaics. In cases of sexual ambiguity at birth, several diagnostic tests are performed to determine gender assignment. These include a buccal smear to determine the presence or absence of sex chromatin, which is found only in the female; gonadal biopsy; chromosomal analysis to detect chromosomal abnormalities and the precise genetic sex; endoscopic and x-ray contrast studies to show the presence, absence, or nature of internal genital structures; and biochemical tests to measure adrenocortical function.

■ INTERVENTION: Sex determination should be made as soon as possible after birth to minimize medical, social, and psychologic problems. The primary criterion for the choice of gender is the infant's anatomy rather than genetic sex, although diagnostic tests are performed to assist in gender selection. Usually, female pseudohermaphrodites are reared as females with early genital reconstruction and corticosteroid treatment throughout life. Male intersex conditions caused by developmental abnormalities are usually treated surgically to establish male genital appearance and function. In instances of ambiguous genitalia, it is most often recommended that the infant be reared as a female because the outcome of surgical and medical treatment is likely to be better.

■ NURSING CONSIDERATIONS: Gender determination of an infant whose sex is doubtful constitutes more of a psychologic and social problem rather than a medical emergency. Such situations are always highly emotional for the parents, who are often overwhelmed by feelings of guilt and shame, and a great deal of support and encouragement are needed. Of special importance is the education of the family about the abnormality, primarily what measures can be undertaken immediately and what will be involved in the long-term management of the condition. The nurse also helps the parents to set realistic goals for the child, depending on the severity of the condition and the degree of medical and surgical treatment possible.

interspinal ligament, one of many thin, narrow membranous ligaments that connect adjoining spinous processes and extend from the root of each process to the apex. The interspinal ligaments meet the ligamenta flava ventrally and the supraspinal ligament dorsally and are only slightly developed in the neck.

interspinous, of or pertaining to the space between any spinous processes.

interstitial /in′tərstish′əl/, of or pertaining to the space between tissues, as interstitial fluid.

interstitial cell-stimulating hormone (ICSH), the luteinizing hormone that also stimulates the production of testosterone by the Leydig, or interstitial, cells of the testis.

interstitial cystitis, an inflammation of the bladder, believed to be associated with an autoimmune or allergic response. The bladder wall becomes inflamed, ulcerated, and scarred, causing frequent, painful urination. Hematuria often occurs. Treatment may include distention of the bladder and cauterization of the ulcers or weekly lavage of the bladder until the inflammation clears. Both procedures are performed under anesthesia. Corticosteroids are often prescribed to control inflammation. Ulceration is rarely severe enough to require cystectomy with urinary diversion. The condition occurs most often in women of middle age and may resemble the early stages of cancer of the bladder. Cystoscopy and biopsy are required for a diagnosis. Also called **Hunner's ulcer.**

interstitial emphysema, a form of emphysema in which air or gas escapes into the interstitial tissues of the lung after a penetrating injury or as the result of a rupture in an alveolar wall. As the alveoli must be decompressed, there is danger that the pleura will be torn, resulting in a pneumothorax. The condition is diagnosed by chest x-ray films. See also **emphysema, pneumothorax.**

interstitial fluid, an extracellular fluid that fills the spaces between most of the cells of the body and provides a substantial portion of the liquid environment of the body. Formed by filtration through the blood capillaries, it is drained away as lymph. It closely resembles blood plasma in composition but contains less protein. Compare **intracellular fluid, lymph, plasma.**

interstitial growth, an increase in size by hyperplasia or hypertrophy within the interior of a part or structure that is already formed. Compare **appositional growth.**

interstitial hypertrophic neuropathy. See **Dejerine-Sottas disease.**

interstitial implantation, (in embryology) the complete embedding of the blastocyst within the endometrium of the uterine wall.

interstitial infusion. See **hypodermoclysis.**

interstitial keratitis, an uncommon inflammation within the layers of the cornea, the first symptom of which is a diffuse haziness. Blood vessels may grow into the area and cause permanent opacities. Its causes are syphilis, tuberculosis, leprosy, and vascular hypersensitivity. Treatment is specific to the infection or condition.

interstitial myositis. See **myositis.**

interstitial nephritis, inflammation of the interstitial tissue of the kidney, including the tubules. The condition may be acute or chronic. **Acute interstitial nephritis** is an immunologic, adverse reaction to certain drugs, often sulfonamide or methicillin. Acute renal failure, fever, rash, and proteinuria are characteristic of this condition. Most people regain normal function of the kidneys when the offending drug is removed. **Chronic interstitial nephritis** is a syndrome of interstitial inflammation and structural changes, sometimes associated with such conditions as ureteral obstruction, pyelonephritis, exposure of the kidney to a toxin, rejection of a transplant, and certain systemic diseases. Gradually, renal failure, nausea, vomiting, weight loss, fatigue, and anemia develop. Acidosis and hyperkalemia may follow. The nurse watches carefully for signs of electrolyte imbalance, dehydration, and hypovolemia, especially if there is frequent vomiting. Fluids and electrolytes may be replaced intravenously. Treatment includes correction of the underlying cause. If the cause is an obstruction of the urinary tract, rapid recovery may follow removal of the obstruction; in other cases hemodialysis and kidney transplantation may be necessary.

interstitial plasma cell pneumonia. See **pneumocystosis.**

interstitial pneumonia, a diffuse, chronic inflammation of the lungs beyond the terminal bronchioles, characterized by fibrosis and collagen formation in the alveolar walls and by the presence of large mononuclear cells in the alveolar spaces. The symptoms of this condition are progressive dyspnea, clubbing of the fingers, cyanosis, and fever. The disease may result from a hypersensitive reaction to busulfan, chlorambucil, hexamethonium, or methotrexate. Interstitial pneumonia may also be an autoimmune reaction, since it often accompanies celiac disease, rheumatoid arthritis, Sjögren's syndrome, and systemic sclerosis. X-ray films of the lungs show patchy shadows and mottling, as in bronchopneumonia. Later stages of the disease reveal bronchiectasis, dilatation of the bronchi, and shrinkage of the lungs. Treatment includes bed rest, oxygen therapy, and corticosteroids. Most patients die within 6 months to a few years, usually from cardiac or respiratory failure. Also called **diffuse fibrosing alveolitis, giant cell interstitial pneumonia, Hamman-Rich syndrome.** Compare **bronchopneumonia.**

interstitial pregnancy. See **ectopic pregnancy.**

interstitial therapy, radiotherapy in which needles or wires that contain radioactive material are implanted directly into tumor areas.

interstitial tubal pregnancy, a kind of tubal pregnancy in which implantation occurs in the proximal, interstitial portion of one of the fallopian tubes. See also **tubal pregnancy.**

intertransverse ligament, one of many fibrous bands connecting the transverse processes of vertebrae. In the cervical region, intertransverse ligaments consist of a few scattered fibers; in the thoracic region, they are rounded cords intimately connected with the deep muscles of the back; in the lumbar region, they are thin and membranous.

intertrigo /in'tərtrī'gō/, an erythematous irritation of opposing skin surfaces caused by friction. Common sites are the axillae, the folds beneath large or pendulous breasts, and the inner aspects of the thighs. Maceration and monilial infection may complicate the picture if the area is also warm and moist. Prevention is by weight reduction, powdering, cleansing, and antifungal topical medication when necessary. **–intertriginous,** *adj.*

intertrochanteric crest /in'tərtrō'kanter'ik/, one of a pair of ridges along the thigh bones, curving obliquely from the greater to the lesser trochanter. Immediately distal to the crest a slight ridge, the linea quadrata, receives the insertion of the quadratus femoris and a few fibers of the adductor magnus.

intertrochanteric fracture, a fracture characterized by a crack in the tissue of the proximal femur between the greater and the lesser trochanters.

intertrochanteric line, a line that runs across the anterior surface of the thigh bone from the greater to the lesser trochanter, winding around the medial surface, and ending in the linea aspera. The proximal half of the intertrochanteric line is the attachment for the iliofemoral ligament; the distal half holds the vastus medialis muscle.

intertuberous diameter, the distance between the ischial tuberosities, a factor used in determining the dimensions of the pelvic outlet.

interval health history, a kind of health history that notes the general condition of a client during the period between visits and is not limited to facts relevant to a particular condition. The interval health history provides an ongoing account of a person's health, serving to bring the data base up to date.

intervention, any act performed to prevent harm from occurring to a patient or to improve the mental, emotional, or physical function of a patient. A physiologic process may be monitored or enhanced, or a pathologic process may be arrested or controlled. See also **nursing intervention.**

intervertebral /in'tərvur'təbrəl/, of or pertaining to the space between any two vertebrae, as the fibrocartilaginous disks.

intervertebral disk, one of the fibrous disks found between adjacent spinal vertebrae, except the axis and the atlas. The disks vary in size, shape, thickness, and number depending on the location in the back and on the particular vertebrae they separate.

intervertebral fibrocartilage. See **intervertebral disk.**

intervertebral foramen, any of the passages between adjacent vertebrae through which the spinal nerves and vessels pass.

intervillous space /in'tərvil'əs/, one of many spaces between the chorionic villi of the endometrium of the gravid uterus, beneath the placenta. The intervillous spaces act as small reservoirs for oxygenated maternal blood from which the fetal circulation may take up the nutrients and gases by osmosis, hydrostatic pressure, and diffusion. The spaces form early in gestation, when the trophoblastic layer of the embryo embeds itself in the wall of the uterus.

intestinal absorption, the passage of the products of digestion from the lumen of the small intestine into the blood and lymphatic vessels in the wall of the gut. The surface area of the intestine is greatly increased by the presence of fingerlike projections, called villi, each of which contains capillaries and a lymphatic vessel, or lacteal. Most dissolved nutrients pass quickly into the capillary bed for transport through the portal circulation to the liver. Lipids enter the lymphatic channels, which eventually rejoin the venous circulation at the thoracic duct in the neck.

intestinal amebiasis. See **amebic dysentery.**

intestinal angina, chronic vascular insufficiency of the mesentery caused by atherosclerosis and resulting ischemia of the smooth muscle of the small bowel. Abdominal pain or cramping after eating, constipation, melena, malabsorption, and weight loss are characteristic of the condition. Also called **chronic intestinal ischemia.**

intestinal apoplexy, the sudden occlusion of one of the three principal arteries to the intestine by an embolism or a thrombus. This condition leads rapidly to necrosis of intestinal tissue and is often fatal. Treatment is usually surgical: The occlusion is removed, and, often, the affected portion of the bowel is resected. See also **atherosclerosis.**

intestinal dyspepsia, an abnormal condition characterized by impaired digestion associated with a problem that originates in the intestines. See also **dyspepsia.**

intestinal fistula, an abnormal passage from the intestine to an external abdominal opening or stoma, usually created surgically for the exit of feces after removal of a malignant or severely ulcerated segment of the bowel. See also **colostomy.**

intestinal infarction. See **intestinal strangulation.**

intestinal flu, a viral gastroenteritis, usually caused by infection by an enterovirus. It is characterized by abdominal cramps, diarrhea, nausea, and vomiting. Outbreaks may be sporadic or epidemic, and the disease usually is mild and self-limited. Treatment is symptomatic. Control of diarrhea may be achieved with antidiarrheal medication and a diet limited to clear fluids. See also **enteric infection, gastroenteritis.**

intestinal juices, the secretions of glands lining the intestine.

intestinal lymphangiectasia. See **hypoproteinemia.**

intestinal obstruction, any obstruction that results in failure of the contents of the intestine to pass through the lumen of the bowel. The most common cause is a mechanic blockage resulting from adhesions, impacted feces, tumor of the bowel, hernia, intussusception, volvulus, or the strictures of inflammatory bowel disease. Obstruction may also be the result of paralytic ileus. Obstruction of the small bowel may cause severe pain, vomiting of fecal matter, dehydration, and eventually a drop in blood pressure. Obstruction of the colon causes less severe pain, marked abdominal distention, and constipation. X-ray examination reveals the level of obstruction and its cause. Treatment includes the evacuation of intestinal contents by means of an intestinal tube. Surgical repair is sometimes necessary. Fluid balance and electrolyte balance are restored by carefully monitored intravenous infusion. Nonnarcotic analgesics are usually prescribed in order to avoid the decrease in intestinal motility that often accompanies the administration of narcotic analgesics. Also called *(informal)* **ileus.** See also **hernia, intussusception, volvulus.**

intestinal strangulation, the arrest of blood flow to the bowel, resulting in edema, cyanosis, and gangrene of the affected loop of bowel. This condition is usually caused by a hernia, intussusception, or volvulus. Early signs of intestinal strangulation resemble those of intestinal obstruction, but peritonitis, shock, and the presence of a tender mass in the abdomen are important in making a differential diagnosis. In addition to surgery, treatment includes the immediate correction of fluid and electrolyte imbalance. Also called **intestinal infarction.**

intestinal tonsil, one of a group of lymphatic nodules forming a single layer in the mucous membrane of the ileum opposite the mesenteric attachment. They are oval patches about 1 cm wide and extend for about 4 cm along the intestine. In most individuals they appear in the distal ileum but also appear in the jejunum of a few individuals.

Also called **Peyer's patches.** Compare **lingual tonsil, palatine tonsil, pharyngeal tonsil.**

intestine, the portion of the alimentary canal extending from the pyloric opening of the stomach to the anus. It includes the small and large intestines. **–intestinal,** *adj.*

intima /in′timə/, *pl.* **intimae,** the innermost layer of a structure, as the lining membrane of an artery, vein, lymphatic, or organ. **–intimal,** *adj.*

intoe. See **metatarsus varus.**

intolerance, a condition characterized by an inability to absorb or metabolize a nutrient or medication. Exposure to the substance may cause an adverse reaction, as in lactose intolerance. Compare **allergy, atopic.**

intoxication, **1.** the state of being poisoned by a drug or other toxic substance. **2.** the state of being inebriated because of an excessive consumption of alcohol. **3.** a state of mental or emotional hyperexcitability, usually euphoric.

intoxication amaurosis, loss of vision occurring without an apparent ophthalmic lesion, caused by a systemic poison, as alcohol or tobacco.

intra-, a combining form meaning 'situated, formed, or occurring within': *intrabronchial, intracutaneous, intramatrical.*

intraaortic balloon pump, a counterpulsation device that provides temporary cardiac assist in the management of refractory left ventricular failure, as may follow myocardial infarction or occur in preinfarction angina. The balloon is attached to a catheter inserted in the aorta and is automatically inflated during diastole and deflated during systole. See also **counterpulsation.**

intraarticular, within a joint.

intraarticular fracture, a fracture involving the articular surfaces of a joint.

intraarticular injection, the injection of a medication into a joint space, usually to reduce inflammation, as in bursitis or fibromyositis. With the same technique, fluid may be withdrawn from the joint space in abnormal, excessive accumulations of fluid in a joint, as a result of trauma or inflammation.

intraarticular ligament, a ligament that forms part of the joints between 16 of the 24 ribs, dividing the joints into two cavities, each containing a synovial membrane. Each intraarticular ligament consists of a short, flattened band of fibers inside the joint, attached by one extremity to the rib and by the other to the intervertebral disk. Intraarticular ligaments are not present in the joints of the first, tenth, eleventh, and twelfth ribs, each of which has only one synovial cavity. Compare **radiate ligament.**

intraatrial, within an atrium in the heart.

intraatrial block, delayed or abnormal conduction within the atria, identified on an electrocardiogram by a prolonged and often notched P wave. See also **atrioventricular block, heart block, intraventricular block, sinoatrial block.**

intracanalicular fibroma /in′trəkan′əlik′yo͞olər/, a tumor containing glandular epithelium and fibrous tissue, occurring in the breast.

intracanicular papilloma /in′trəkənik′yo͞olər/, a benign warty growth in certain glands, especially the breast.

intracapsular fracture /in′trəkap′so͞olər/, a fracture within the capsule of a joint.

intracardiac catheter. See **cardiac catheter.**

intracardiac lead, **1.** an electrocardiographic conductor in which the exploring electrode is placed within one of the cardiac chambers, usually by means of cardiac catheterization. **2.** *informal.* a tracing produced by such a lead on an electrocardiograph.

intracartilaginous ossification. See **ossification.**

intracatheter, a thin, flexible plastic catheter introduced and threaded into a blood vessel to infuse blood, fluid, or medication. Also called *(informal)* **intracath.**

intracavitary therapy, a kind of radiotherapy in which one or more radioactive sources are placed, usually with the help of an applicator or holding device, within a body cavity in order to irradiate the walls of the cavity or adjacent tissues.

intracellular fluid, a fluid within cell membranes throughout most of the body, containing dissolved solutes that are essential to electrolytic balance and to healthy metabolism. Also called **intracellular water (ICW).** Compare **extracellular fluid, interstitial fluid, lymph, plasma.**

intracerebral, within the tissue of the brain, inside the bony skull.

intracistronic /in′trəsistron′ik/, within a cistron.

intracoronal retainer, **1.** a retainer in which the prepared tooth cavity and its cast restoration lie largely within the body of the coronal portion of a tooth and within the contour of the tooth crown, as an inlay. The retention or resistance to displacement is developed between the casting and the internal walls of the prepared tooth cavity. **2.** a direct retainer used in the construction of removable partial dentures. It consists of a female portion within the coronal segment of the crown of an abutment and a fitted male portion attached to the denture proper.

intracranial, within the cranium.

intracranial aneurysm, any aneurysm of any of the cerebral arteries. Rupture of an intracranial aneurysm results in mortality approaching 50%, and there is a high risk of recurrence in survivors of a rupture. Characteristics of the condition include sudden severe headache, stiff neck, nausea, vomiting, and, sometimes, loss of consciousness. Some forms of intracranial aneurysm may be treated surgically. Kinds of intracranial aneurysms include **berry aneurysm, fusiform aneurysm,** and **mycotic aneurysm.**

intracranial electroencephalography. See **electroencephalography.**

intracranial pressure, pressure that occurs within the cranium.

intractable, having no relief, as a symptom or a disease that remains unrelieved by the therapeutic measures employed.

intracutaneous, within the layers of the skin.

intracystic papilloma, a benign epithelial tumor formed with a cystic adenoma.

intradermal test, a procedure used to identify suspected allergens by subcutaneously injecting the patient with small amounts of extracts of the suspected allergens. The injections are made at spaced intervals, usually in the forearm or in the scapular region. The patient is concurrently injected with the diluent alone as a control procedure. The test is positive if, within 15 to 30 minutes, the injection of extract produces a wheal surrounded by erythema and the control injection produces no symptoms. The intradermal test is started with highly diluted solutions, and, if the initial test is negative, the procedure is repeated with stronger solutions. This gradual method is used to prevent a systemic reaction, which is more of a risk with intradermal testing than with other kinds of allergy testing, as the scratch test. Intradermal testing tends to be more accurate than the scratch test and is often performed if scratch test results are negative or unclear. Intradermal testing also limits to between 20 and 30 the number of suspected allergens that can be examined simultaneously in the skin of one patient. Also called **subcutaneous test.** Compare **patch test, scratch test.** See also **conjunctival test, use test.**

intradermal injection, the introduction of a hypodermic needle into the dermis for the purpose of instilling a substance, as a serum or vaccine.

intraductal carcinoma, a frequently large neoplasm occurring most often in the breast. The lesion on cross section usually shows well differentiated tumor cells in calcified and dilated ducts of the breast.

intradural lipoma, a fatty tumor in or beneath the dura mater of the spine or sacrum that tends to infiltrate the dorsal column and roots of spinal nerves, causing pain and dysfunction.

intraepidermal carcinoma, a neoplasm of squamous epidermal cells that does not proliferate into the basal area and often occurs at many sites simultaneously. The lesions, which enlarge slowly without healing at the center, are resistant to chemotherapy and to radiation. Also called **Bowen's disease, Bowen's precancerous dermatosis, precancerous dermatitis.**

intraepithelial carcinoma. See **carcinoma in situ.**

intramembranous ossification. See **ossification.**

intramuscular injection, the introduction of a hypodermic needle into a muscle to administer a medication.

■ METHOD: The equipment is selected and the medication drawn up into the syringe. The site that has been selected is prepared by cleansing with alcohol or acetone. The sites most commonly used are the upper, outer quadrant of the gluteal area, the ventrogluteal area, the vastus lateralis of the thigh, or the deltoid muscle. The skin is stretched between the thumb and forefinger. The needle is introduced at a 90-degree angle with a quick thrust and advanced as necessary—not as far as the hub of the needle, but deep into the muscle. The plunger is withdrawn slightly to be sure that the needle has not been placed in a blood vessel. The solution is injected slowly, the needle is withdrawn, and the injection site is massaged.

■ NURSING ORDERS: If the gluteal area is chosen, the patient is asked to lie prone with ankles bent and feet curved in, so that the toes of each foot are directed toward the opposite foot to relax the gluteal muscles, thus making the injection less painful. Injection in deltoid muscles is more painful than in other sites and is avoided if possible. The ventrogluteal area and the vastus lateralis are the preferred injection sites in infants. Care is taken not to hit the femur with the tip of the needle when injecting into the vastus lateralis. Needles and syringes are always disposed of in a safe way; they are usually destroyed.

■ OUTCOME CRITERIA: Infection may result from nonaseptic technique; care is taken not to contaminate the needle before injection. Certain medications can cause tissue necrosis if injected into the subcutaneous tissues. Many medications may be given intravenously or intramuscularly, but the intravenous dose may be much smaller; inadvertent injection into a blood vessel could result in severe systemic reactions of an overdose. Often, biologicals may leave a knot in the muscle that is not painful and that subsides slowly over several weeks or months, though it may cause concern in the patient or in the parents of younger patients. The lump should not grow larger or become more painful; if it does, it may be assumed that an abscess has formed.

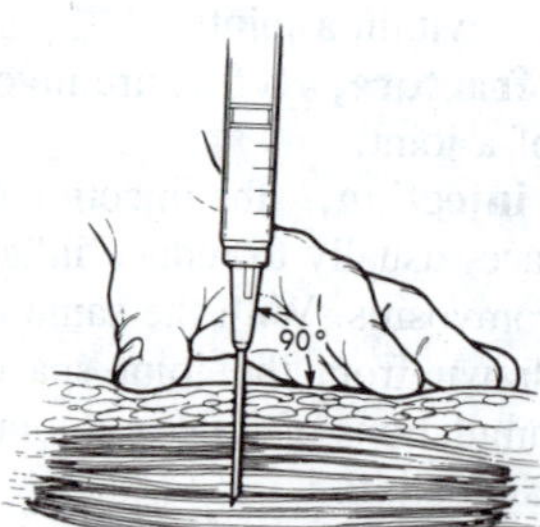

Intramuscular injection

intraocular, pertaining to structures or substances within the eyeball.

intraocular pressure, the internal pressure of the eye, regulated by resistance to the flow of aqueous humor through the fine sieve of the trabecular meshwork. Contraction or relaxation of the longitudinal muscles of the ciliary body affects the size of the apertures in the meshwork. In older persons, the trabecular meshwork may become sclerotic and obstructed, preventing the normal flow of aqueous humor from passing out at the proper rate and causing an increase in the intraocular pressure. See also **glaucoma.**

intraoperative ultrasound, a diagnostic technique that uses a portable ultrasound device to scan the spinal cord during spinal surgery. The method enables surgeons to locate and identify the size of tumors of the central nervous system that may not be detected by computerized axial tomography or other techniques. Intraoperative ultrasound can distinguish between syrinxes, or fluid filled cysts, and neoplastic growths in nervous system tissue.

intraoral orthodontic appliance, an orthodontic device placed inside the mouth to correct or alleviate malocclusion.

intraparietal sulcus, an irregular groove on the convex surface of the parietal lobe that marks the division of the inferior and superior parietal lobules. Also called **interparietal fissure.**

intrapartal care, care of a pregnant woman from the onset of labor to the completion of the third stage of labor with the expulsion of the placenta. See also **antepartal care, newborn intrapartal care, postpartal care.**

■ METHOD: The signs and symptoms of true labor are observed. Uterine contractions increase in frequency, duration, and strength. Pressure of the presenting part of the fetus causes dilatation and effacement of the cervix, producing a bloody discharge called "bloody show." A physical examination of the mother is performed, urine is measured regularly through labor and tested for ketones, protein, glucose, and specific gravity, and a microhematocrit is often done. The position, attitude, and presentation of the fetus is ascertained by abdominal palpation. The cervical effacement and dilatation and the station of the presenting part of the fetus are determined periodically by vaginal examination, using careful aseptic technique. If the amniotic sac has broken, the color, character, and quantity of the amniotic fluid is noted. The fetal heart rate is counted, and variations are noted in relation to the timing and intensity of contractions. See also **emergency childbirth.**

■ NURSING ORDERS: Emotional support and measures to increase physical comfort are provided by the nurse throughout labor and delivery. Asepsis is maintained, the progress of labor is monitored, and the well-being of the fetus and the mother are continually observed. After delivery of the infant, the mother is observed for hemorrhage; the uterine fundus may need to be massaged to cause it to contract. The placenta is weighed and examined for completeness. The episiotomy, if performed, or any laceration that occurred is usually repaired after delivery of the placenta. Depending on the mother's preference and condition and the policy of the maternity service, the infant may be placed in a warmer or on the mother's abdomen. The mother and infant are observed for a brief period in the delivery area before being transferred to the postpartum unit.

■ OUTCOME CRITERIA: During labor and delivery several danger signs alert the observer to problems. These danger signs include strong, continuous uterine contractions, marked variation of the fetal heart rate, sudden, excessive fetal movement, continuous abdominal pain with increased fundal height, vaginal bleeding, protrusion of the umbilical cord, a large amount of amniotic fluid, meconium-stained amniotic fluid, or an elevation or drop in the mother's temperature, pulse, or blood pressure. Observation for these danger signs is important in providing intrapartal care, but normal spontaneous vaginal delivery of a healthy baby from a healthy mother is the usual outcome of this period.

intrapartal period, the period spanning labor and birth.

intraperiosteal fracture /in′trəper′ē•os′tē•əl/, a fracture that does not rupture the periosteum.

intrapsychic conflict, an emotional conflict within oneself. See also **conflict.**

intrasocial idiocy, *obsolete*. a state of mental retardation in which the person is capable of undertaking some form of regular occupation.

intrathecal /in′trəthē′kəl/, of or pertaining to a structure, process, or substance within a sheath, as the cerebrospinal fluid within the theca of the spinal canal.

intrathecal injection, the introduction of a hypodermic needle into the subarachnoid space for the purpose of instilling a material for diffusion throughout the spinal fluid.

intrathoracic goiter, an enlargement of the thyroid gland that protrudes into the thoracic cavity.

intrauterine device (IUD) /in′trəyo͞o′tərin/, a contraceptive device consisting of a bent strip of radiopaque plastic with a fine monofilament tail that is inserted and left in the uterine cavity for the purpose of altering the physiology of the uterus and fallopian tubes to prevent pregnancy. The mechanism of action is not known. Insertion is performed during or just after menstruation when the cervix is slightly open and menstruation assures that a pregnancy does not exist. The tail string of the IUD is left projecting a few centimeters from the cervix. By feeling the string with her finger from time to time the wearer can be sure the device is in place. The string also provides a hold for removing the IUD. The rate of failure for the IUD method of contraception is approximately two to four unplanned pregnancies in 100 women using the device for 1 year. IUDs can cause complications, the most serious being infection. Such infections occurring in pregnancy may be overwhelming and lethal; therefore, the IUD is removed if pregnancy is suspected. Some other complications are cervicitis, perforation of the uterus, salpingitis causing sterility, ectopic pregnancy, abortion, embedding of the device in the wall of the uterus, endometritis, bleeding, pain, cramping, undetected expulsion, and irritation of the penis. Women who do not have complications using an IUD are commonly able to retain the device safely for several years, or indefinitely. Also called **intrauterine contraceptive device (IUCD),** *(informal)* **coil,** *(informal)* **loop.**

intrauterine fracture, a fracture that occurs during fetal life.

intrauterine growth curve, a line on a standardized graph representing the mean weight for gestational age through pregnancy to term. It provides a method for classifying infants according to their state of maturity and fetal development.

intrauterine growth retardation, an abnormal process in which the development and maturation of the fetus is impeded or delayed by genetic factors, maternal disease, or fetal malnutrition caused by placental insufficiency. See also **small for gestational age infant.**

intravascular coagulation test, a test for detecting internal coagulation of blood.

intravenous (IV), of or pertaining to the inside of a vein, as of a thrombus or an injection, infusion, or catheter.

intravenous alimentation. See **total parenteral nutrition.**

intravenous bolus, a relatively large dose of medication administered IV in a short period of time, usually within 1 to 30 minutes. The IV bolus is commonly used when administration of a medication is needed quickly, as in an emergency, when drugs are administered that cannot be diluted, as many cancer chemotherapeutic drugs, and when the therapeutic purpose is to achieve a peak drug level in the bloodstream of the patient. The IV bolus is not used when the medication involved must be diluted in a large-volume parenteral before entering the bloodstream or when the rapid administration of a medication, as potassium chloride, could be life-threatening. The IV bolus is normally not used for patients with decreased cardiac outputs, decreased urinary outputs, pulmonary congestion, or systemic edema. Such patients have decreased tolerances to medications, which therefore must be diluted more than usual and administered at slower rates. A wristwatch with a second hand is recommended for the timing of all IV bolus injections. The amount of medication to be delivered per minute is determined by dividing the total amount of medication to be injected by the prescribed time for delivery. The IV bolus site is prepared with an appropriate antiseptic, and the site is entered with a venipuncture needle. A winged-tip needle is used for administering an IV bolus because it is small enough to lessen the risk of collapsing the vein and causing trauma and is more stable than a syringe needle. If a primary IV line is already established, the IV bolus is administered by mixing the prescribed drug with the appropriate amount of diluent, after first determining whether the drug is compatible with the primary IV solution. Also called **intravenous push.**

intravenous cholangiography, (in diagnostic radiology) a procedure for outlining the major bile ducts. A radiopaque contrast material is injected intravenously, and serial x-ray films are taken. See also **cholangiography.**

Intravenous controller, any one of several devices that automatically deliver IV fluid at selectable flow rates, usually between 1 and 69 drops per minute. The controller is commonly equipped with a rate selector, drop sensor, drop indicator, and drop alarm. When the infusion does not flow at the prescribed rate, the drop alarm emits a visual and an audible signal. The IV controller works by gravity so that the IV container must be placed at least 30 inches above the venipuncture site. The controller cannot exert the positive pressure of a true pump and is not recommended for the delivery of highly viscous fluid or for keeping an arterial line open. Compare **intravenous peristaltic pump, intravenous piston pump, intravenous syringe pump.**

intravenous DSA (IV-DSA), a form of digital subtraction angiography in which radiopaque dye is injected into a vein, rather than an artery, in order to visualize arteries in the body.

intravenous fat emulsion, a preparation of 10% fat administered intravenously to help maintain the weight of an adult patient or the weight and growth of a younger patient. Such fat emulsions are prepared from refined soybean oil and egg-yolk phospholipids and may contain such major fatty acids as linoleic, oleic, palmitic, and linolenic acids. The IV fat emulsion is isotonic and may be administered into a peripheral vein, but it is not mixed with other solutions employed in parenteral alimentation. IV fat emulsions are often administered when hyperalimentation is not sufficient to maintain adequate treatment of a patient or when the patient needs calories but cannot tolerate the high percentage of dextrose contained in hyperalimentation solutions. Such emulsions may also be administered to patients who need more essential fatty acids than are contained in hyperalimentation solutions or to patients who need general nutritional improvement, especially postoperative patients. IV emulsions are not administered to patients suffering from disturbances of normal fat metabolism (as hyperlipemia), severe hepatic diseases, blood coagulation defects caused by decreased blood-platelet counts, pulmonary diseases, lipoid nephrosis, hepatocellular damage, or bone marrow dyscrasia, or to patients being treated with anabolic inhibitory drugs. If possible, the IV fat emulsion is usually administered during the daytime hours so that the patient may follow a normal eating pattern with rest during the night and a lower nocturnal urinary flow. Once the primary IV line has been established, IV fat emulsions are usually administered with the aid of an electronic control device to maintain an even flow rate and avoid any fatty-acid overload. The patient's fluid intake and output are regularly measured during the delivery of such an emulsion, and daily blood studies are conducted to determine the level of free-floating triglycerides. Hepatic function tests are performed if the patient receives consecutive IV fat emulsion infusions over a long period of time. Immediate adverse reactions or those that may occur up to 2 ½ hours after the onset of the infusion may include temperature rise, flushing, sweating, pressure sensations over the eyes, nausea, vomiting, headache, chest and back pains, dyspnea, and cyanosis. Delayed adverse reactions or those that may occur within 10 days of the onset of such infusions may include hepatomegaly, splenomegaly, thrombocytopenia, focal seizures, hyperlipemia, hepatic damage, jaundice, hemorrhagic diathesis, and gastroduodenal ulcer.

intravenous feeding, the administration of nutrients through a vein or veins.

intravenous infusion, **1.** a solution administered intravenously through an infusion set that includes a plastic or glass vacuum bottle or bag containing the solution and tubing connecting the bottle to a catheter or a needle in the patient's vein. **2.** the process of administering a solution intravenously. Swelling of the limb around and distal to the site of injection may indicate that the tip of the catheter or needle is in the subcutaneous tissue, and not in the vein. The fluid may be infiltrating the tissue spaces. It should be withdrawn and the limb elevated. Redness, swelling, heat, and pain around the vein at the site of injection or proximal to it may indicate thrombophlebitis. The infusion should be discontinued and the inflammatory condition treated. The infusion is usually begun again at another site. See also **venipuncture.**

intravenous infusion filter, any one of the numerous devices used in helping to ensure the purity of an IV solution. IV filters strain the IV solution to remove such contaminants as dissolved impurities (detergents, proteins, and polysaccharides), extraneous salts, microorganisms, particles, precipitates, and undissolved drug powders. Any such contaminants may complicate the IV therapy and the recovery of the patient. Some filters are built into the primary IV tubing; others must be attached. Manufacturers' instructions come with most filters to assure proper use. One of the main criteria for selecting a filter is the assurance that the filter is not too fine for the IV solution to be strained. Filters that are too fine will clog. The size of filter membranes vary from 5 μ to 0.22 m. Filters of 1 to 5 μ will remove most particulate debris but not most fungi or bacteria. Filters that are 0.45 μ or less will remove fungi and most bacteria; filters that are 0.22 μ will remove all fungi and bacteria but will also reduce the flow rate of the IV solution, which is crucial when rapid delivery is required. Aseptic techniques are essential in attaching all filters to the IV delivery system. Once attached, filters must be primed according to manufacturers' instructions. Most filters should be upright to function properly, but some filters must be inverted. See also **needle filter.**

intravenous infusion technique, the calculations for determining the delivery rate of IV fluid for the individual patient and the necessary spiking of the container and priming of the tubing before venipuncture and administration of the fluid.

■ METHOD: The rate at which solution is to be administered by IV infusion can be determined from this formula:

$$\frac{\text{total amount of solution (in ml)}}{\text{period over which delivered (in hrs)}} = \text{rate (in ml) per hr.}$$

Thus, if 1,000 ml are to be delivered in 8 hrs:

$$\frac{1000}{8} = 125 \text{ ml per hr}$$

To determine which drip system to use, the following formula is useful:

$$\frac{\text{drops per ml} \times \text{amount of solution (in ml) per hr}}{\text{60 min}} = \text{drops per min.}$$

Thus, if a macrodrip system of 15 drops per one ml is used, following the preceding example:

$$\frac{15}{60} \times 125 = 31 \text{ drops per min.}$$

Or, if a microdrip system (60 drops per ml) is used:

$$\frac{60}{60} \times 125 = 125 \text{ drops per min.}$$

The hands are washed thoroughly before assembling the container of IV solution, the IV pole, and the proper tubing with the flow clamp placed in a position directly beneath the drip chamber and clamped. If a bottle with a rubber stopper is used, the protective metal cap is removed, and, with the bottle held securely on a stable surface, the spike of the tubing is pushed firmly into the stopper. To spike an IV bottle with an indwelling vent and latex diaphragm, the metal cap and diaphragm are removed and the spike is inserted into the nonvented hole; if a hiss, indicating a vacuum, is not heard, the bottle is contaminated and should be discarded. Nonvented tubing is used with this kind of bottle. A plastic bag of IV fluid is hung on a hook for spiking; the cap is removed by pulling it smoothly to the right, and a nonvented spike is inserted into the port using one quick, even motion to prevent the escape of fluid. An IV bag with a firm, easily grasped port with a lip to prevent touch contamination may be spiked before hanging by grasping the port firmly; squeezing the bag may expel air and is carefully avoided. After the hanging bag or bottle is spiked, the drip chamber is gently squeezed until it is half full before the tubing is primed. The end of the tubing is held over a sink or wastebasket as the protective cap is removed, and the cap is kept uncontaminated for reuse. The flow clamp is released, and the tubing is allowed to fill with fluid until all air bubbles are expelled; if a backcheck valve is on the tubing, the valve is inverted during priming. The flow clamp is then closed, the protective cap is replaced, and the tubing is looped over the IV pole so that it is out of the way during venipuncture. Once the needle or intracatheter is inserted and connected to the tubing, the fluid container is hung securely from the IV pole or a hook at a height 3 feet above the insertion site. The flow clamp is opened and adjusted to deliver the proper rate of delivery of fluid by counting the number of drops entering the drip chamber in a minute. Throughout the administration of IV fluid, the rate of flow is checked periodically and any necessary readjustments of the clamp are made.

■ NURSING ORDERS: The nurse assembles the apparatus for the IV infusion, spikes the fluid container, primes the tubing, calculates the proper rate for the patient, and ensures that the rate of delivery and asepsis are maintained. The nurse carefully observes the patient for signs of circulatory overload, as a bounding pulse, engorged peripheral veins, dyspnea, cough, and pulmonary edema, indicating that the infusion rate is too rapid and requires adjustment.

■ OUTCOME CRITERIA: IV solutions administered to maintain normal body fluid levels and the electrolyte balance do not overload the circulation when delivered at the flow rate required by the individual patient.

intravenous injection, a hypodermic injection into a vein for the purpose of instilling a single dose of medication, injecting a contrast medium, or beginning an IV infusion of blood, medication, or a fluid solution, as saline or dextrose in water. See also **venipuncture.**

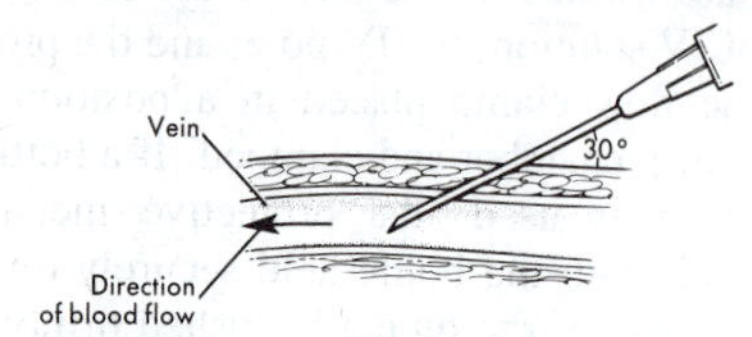

Intravenous injection (note bevel direction of needle)

intravenous peristaltic pump, any one of several devices for administering IV fluids by exerting pressure on the IV tubing rather than on the fluid itself. Most peristaltic pumps operate with normal IV tubing and deliver fluid at a selectable drop-per-minute rate. This device typically can infuse between 1 and 99 drops of IV fluid per minute and is equipped with a drop sensor, rate selector, power switch indicator lamp, and drop indicator and alarm. The drop indicator flashes whenever a drop of IV fluid passes the drop sensor. The drop alarm sounds when the infusion does not flow at the prescribed rate. Compare **intravenous controller, intravenous piston pump, intravenous syringe pump.**

intravenous piston pump, any one of several devices that accurately control the infusion of IV fluids by piston action. Most IV piston pumps can be operated by battery as well as by electric current and require special tubing. Some models are portable. IV piston pumps are commonly equipped with controls that allow selectable flow rates and indicators that display flow rates, dose limits, and cumulative fluid volumes. Such pumps commonly monitor the patient's skin for infiltration by IV fluid and are equipped with infiltration and flow alarms. The IV piston pump monitors the actual volume of IV fluid administered instead of counting drops of fluid. Hence, its accuracy is not affected by drop size, temperature, or fluid viscosity. The pump is designed to reduce the delivery rate to a keep-vein-open rate if the proper flow rate or the dose limit is exceeded. The pump also stops delivery of the IV fluid if the IV line is clogged or if infiltration is detected. Compare **intravenous controller, intravenous peristaltic pump, intravenous syringe pump.**

intravenous pump, a pump designed to regulate the rate of flow of a fluid given intravenously through an intracatheter or a scalp vein needle. See also **Abbot pump, Harvard pump.**

intravenous push. See **intravenous bolus.**

intravenous pyelography (IVP), a technique in radiology for examining the structures and evaluating the function of the urinary system. A contrast medium is injected intravenously, and serial x-ray films are taken as the medium is cleared from the blood by glomerular filtration. The renal calyces, renal pelvis, ureters, and urinary bladder are all visible on the x-ray films. Tumors, cysts, stones, and many structural and functional abnormalities may be diagnosed using this technique. A cathartic or an enema is usually given the day before the procedure, because the kidneys lie retroperitoneally and gas or fecal material in the bowel may prevent visualization of the urinary tract. The person is given nothing by mouth from midnight before the test to induce a moderate state of dehydration, thereby allowing concentration of the contrast medium in the collecting structures. The patient may also be asked to void immediately before injection of the dye to avoid dilution of the medium in the bladder. Also called **descending urography, excretory urography.**

intravenous syringe pump, any one of several devices that automatically compress a syringe plunger at a controlled rate. Such devices are used with disposable syringes that can deliver blood, medications, or nutrients by IV, arterial, or subcutaneous routes. IV syringe pumps can deliver small volumes of fluid at rates as low as 0.01 ml/hour and are often used in the treatment of infants. They are ideal for keeping arterial lines open and are usually battery-operated and portable. They are especially useful in treating ambulatory patients. Compare **intravenous controller, intravenous peristaltic pump, intravenous piston pump.**

intravenous team, a group of registered nurses and licensed practical nurses with special training who administer IV therapy under the direction of a physician.

intravenous therapy, the administration of fluids or drugs, or both, into the general circulation through a venipuncture.

intravenous urography. See **intravenous pyelography.**

intraventricular /in′trəventrik′yo͞olər/, of or pertaining to the space within a ventricle.

intraventricular block, the slowed conduction or stoppage of the cardiac excitatory impulse, occurring within the ventricles. The block can occur as a right bundle branch block, a left bundle branch block, or left anterior or posterior fascicular block. The block is identified on an electrocardiogram, when the QRS duration is greater than 100 msec. The block can be caused by coronary artery disease, valvular heart disease, ventricular hypertrophy and fibrosis, cardiomyopathy, or idiopathic degeneration of the conduction system. Prognosis is based on the underlying cardiac condition. Kinds of intraventricular block include **bundle branch block** and **infranodal block.** See also **heart block, intraatrial block, Purkinje's network, sinoatrial block.**

intraventricular hydrocephalus. See **hydrocephalus.**

intrinsic, **1.** denoting a natural or inherent part or quality. **2.** originating from or situated within an organ or tissue.

intrinsic asthma, a nonseasonal, nonallergic form of asthma, usually first occurring later in life than allergic asthma, that tends to be chronic and persistent rather than episodic. The precipitating factors include inhalation of irritating pollutants in the atmosphere, as dust particles, smoke, aerosols, strong cooking odors, paint fumes, and other volatile substances. Bronchospasm may also occur in cold, damp weather, after the sudden inhalation of cold, dry air, and after physical exercise or violent coughing or laughing. Respiratory infections, as the common cold, and psychologic factors, as anxiety, may also induce an attack. Compare **allergic asthma.** See also **asthma.**

intrinsic factor, a substance secreted by the gastric mucosa that is essential for the intestinal absorption of cyanocobalamin. Intrinsic factor forms a bond with molecules of cyanocobalamin and transports them across the membranes of the ileum. A deficiency of intrinsic factor, caused by gastrectomy, myxedema, or atrophy of the gastric mucosa, results in pernicious anemia. See also **pernicious anemia.**

intro-, a combining form meaning 'into or within': *introgastric, introjection, introspection.*

introitus /intrō′itəs/, an entrance or orifice to a cavity or a hollow tubular structure of the body, as the vaginal introitus.

introjection, an unconscious mechanism in which an individual incorporates into his own ego structure the qualities of another person.

intron /in′tron/, (in molecular genetics) a sequence of base pairs in DNA that interrupts the continuity of genetic information. Some genes contain a number of long intervening sequences.

introperative hyperthermia, hyperthermia delivered to internal sites that have been exposed by a surgical procedure. After heating the patient is "closed."

Intropin, a trademark for an adrenergic (dopamine hydrochloride).

introspection, **1.** the act of examining one's own thoughts and emotions by concentrating on the inner self. **2.** a tendency to look inward and view the inner self. –**introspective,** *adj.*

introversion, **1.** the tendency to direct one's interests, thoughts, and energies inward or toward things concerned only with the self. **2.** the state of being totally or primarily concerned with one's own intrapsychic experience. Also spelled **intraversion.** Compare **extroversion.**

introvert, **1.** a person whose interests are directed inward and who is shy, withdrawn, emotionally reserved, and self-absorbed. **2.** to turn inward or to direct one's interests and thoughts toward oneself. Compare **extrovert.** See also **egocentric.**

intubation, passage of a tube into a body aperture, specifically the insertion of a breathing tube through the mouth or nose or into the trachea to ensure a patent airway for the delivery of an anesthetic gas or oxygen. **Blind intubation** is the insertion of a breathing tube without the use of a laryngoscope. Kinds of intubation are **endotracheal intubation, nasogastric intubation.**

intussusception /in′təsəsep′shən/, prolapse of one segment of bowel into the lumen of another segment. This kind of intestinal obstruction may involve segments of the small intestine, the colon, or the terminal ileum and cecum. Intussusception occurs most often in infants and small children and is characterized by abdominal pain, vomiting, and bloody mucus in the stool. Barium enema is used to confirm the diagnosis, and surgery is usually necessary to correct the obstruction. See also **intestinal obstruction.**

inulin /in′yo͝olin/, a fructose-derived substance used as a diagnostic aid in tests of kidney function, specifically glomerular filtration. It is not metabolized or absorbed by the body but is readily filtered through the kidney.

inulin clearance, a test of the rate of filtration of a starch, inulin, in the glomerulus of the kidney. Inulin is given by mouth, and the glomerular filtration rate can be estimated from the length of time needed for the inulin to appear in the urine. The normal clearance rate of inulin in urine is 100 to 150 ml/minute.

inunction, **1.** the rubbing of a drug mixed with an oil or fatty substance into the skin, with absorption of the active ingredient. **2.** any compound so applied.

inundation fever. See **scrub typhus.**

invagination, **1.** a condition in which one part of a structure telescopes into another part, as the intestine during peristalsis. If the invagination is extensive or involves a tumor or polyps, it may cause an intestinal obstruction, and surgery is indicated. **2.** surgery for repair of a hernia by replacing the contents of the hernial sac in the abdominal cavity. General or spinal anesthesia may be used. No upper respiratory infection, chronic cough, or allergy with sneezing can be present, for it will weaken the repair. Postoperatively, the nurse checks for retention of urine. See also **hernia, intestinal obstruction, peristalsis.** –**invaginate,** *v.*

invariable behavior, behavior that results from physiologic response to a stimulus and is not modified by individual experience, as a reflex. Compare **variable behavior.**

invasion, the process by which malignant cells move into deeper tissue and through the basement membrane and gain access to blood vessels and lymphatic channels.

invasion of privacy, (in law) the violation of another person's right to be left alone and free from unwarranted publicity and intrusion.

invasive, characterized by a tendency to spread, infiltrate, and intrude.

invasive carcinoma, a malignant neoplasm composed of epithelial cells that infiltrate and destroy surrounding tissues.

invasive mole. See **chorioadenoma destruens.**

invasive thermometry, measurement of tissue temperature using probes placed directly in the tissue.

inverse anaphylaxis, an exaggerated reaction of hypersensitivity induced by an antibody rather than by an antigen. Also called **reverse anaphylaxis.**

inverse relationship. See **negative relationship.**

inverse square law, a law stating that the amount of radiation emitted is inversely proportional to the square of the distance between the source and the irradiated surface, as a person 2 feet from a patient being treated with radium is exposed to four times more radiation than he would be exposed to at 4 feet.

Inversine, a trademark for a ganglionic blocking agent (mecamylamine hydrochloride).

inversion, **1.** an abnormal condition in which an organ is turned inside out, as a uterine inversion. **2.** a chromosomal defect in which two or more segments of a chromosome break off and become separated. They rejoin the chromosome in the wrong order, causing the genes carried on one arm of the chromosome to be in a position and sequence different from those on the other arm.

invert, **1.** a homosexual. **2.** to turn something upside down or inside out.

investigational device exemption (I.D.E.), an agreement through which the federal government permits the testing of new medical devices.

investigational new drug (IND), a drug not yet approved for marketing by the Food and Drug Administration and available only for use in experiments to determine its safety and effectiveness. The use of an investigational new drug in human subjects requires approval by the Food and Drug Administration of an application that includes reports of animal toxicity tests, descriptions of proposed clinical trials, and a list of the investigators and their qualifications.

invisible differentiation, (in embryology) a fixed determination for specialization and diversification that exists in embryonic cells but is not yet visibly apparent. See also **chemodifferentiation.**

in vitro /in vē′trō/, (of a biologic reaction) occurring in laboratory apparatus. Compare **in vivo.**

in vivo /in vē′vō/, (of a biologic reaction) occurring in a living organism. Compare **in vitro.**

in vivo tracer study, (in nuclear medicine) a diagnostic procedure in which a series of radiograms of an administered radioactive tracer as it passes through a compartment in the patient's body demonstrates normal or abnormal structures or processes. A strip chart recording of an in vivo tracer study, as a radionuclide angiocardiogram, shows the passage of the tracer through the central circulation.

involucrum /in′vəlo͞o′krəm/, *pl.* **involucra,** a sheath or coating, as that encasing a sequestrum of necrotic bone.

involuntary, occurring without conscious control or direction. See also **autonomy.**

involuntary muscle. See **smooth muscle.**

involuntary nervous system. See **visceral nervous system.**

involution, **1.** a normal process characterized by a decrease in the size of an organ caused by a decrease in the size of its cells, as postpartum involution of the uterus. **2.** (in embryology) a developmental process in which a group of cells grows over the rim at the border of the organ or part and, rolling inward, rejoins the organ or part to form a tube, as in the heart or bladder.

involutional melancholia, a state of depression occurring during the climacteric. The disorder begins gradually and is characterized by pessimism, irritability, insomnia, loss of appetite, feelings of anxiety, and an increase in motor activity, ranging from mere restlessness to extreme agitation. In the rare instances where treatment is necessary, antidepressant drugs, electroconvulsive treatment, and various forms of psychotherapy may be used. Also called **climacteric melancholia, involutional depression, involutional psychosis.** See also **depression.**

inward aggression, destructive behavior that is directed against oneself. See also **aggression, masochism.**

-io, a noun-forming combining form: *abrasio, evulsio, injectio.*

iodinated ^{125}I serum albumin /ī′ədinā′tid/, a sterile, buffered isotonic solution containing radioiodinated normal human serum adjusted to provide not more than 1 mCi of radioactivity per milliliter in diagnostic tests of blood volume and cardiac output.

iodine (I), a nonmetallic element of the halogen group. Its atomic number is 53; its atomic weight is 126.90. Iodine is a bluish-black solid that becomes a violet vapor on heating without going through a liquid phase. An essential micronutrient or trace element, almost 80% of the iodine present in the body is in the thyroid gland, mostly in the form of thyroglobulin. Iodine deficiency can result in goiter or cretinism. Iodine is found in seafoods, iodized salt, and some dairy products. Radioisotopes of iodine are used in radioisotope scanning procedures and in palliative treatment of cancer of the thyroid.

iodism, a condition produced by excessive amounts of iodine in the body. It is characterized by increased lacrimation and salivation, rhinitis, weakness, and a typical skin eruption. See also **ioderma.**

iodize, to treat or impregnate with iodine or an iodide. Table salt is iodized to prevent the occurrence of goiter in areas with insufficient iodine in the drinking water or food. Iodized oil, a viscous liquid with the odor of garlic, has been used as a contrast medium in roentgenology.

iodo-, a combining form meaning 'of or pertaining to iodine': *iododerma, iodogenic, iodolography.*

iodochlorhydroxyquin /ī·ō′dōklôrhīdrok′səkwin/, an antiamebic and topical antiinfective.

■ INDICATIONS: It is prescribed in the treatment of eczema, athlete's foot, and other fungal infections.

■ CONTRAINDICATIONS: The presence of tuberculosis or viral skin conditions or known hypersensitivity to this drug or to iodine prohibits its use.

■ ADVERSE EFFECTS: The most serious adverse reaction is irritation to sensitive skin.

iododerma /ī•ō′dōdur′mə/, a skin rash caused by a hypersensitivity to ingested iodides. The lesions may be acneiform, bullous, or fungating. Treatment requires removal of iodides from the diet.

iodoform, a topical antiinfective used as an antiseptic.

iodophor, an antiseptic or disinfectant that combines iodine with another agent, as a detergent.

iodopsin /ī′ōdop′sin/, a photosensitive chemical in the cones of the retina, which reacts in association with other chemicals and plays a part in color vision. Iodopsin is more stable when exposed to bright light than rhodopsin, which is found in the rods of the retina. Color vision, a synthesis of red, green, and blue light, is induced by changes within the pigments of different types of cones during a photochemical process in which coded nerve impulses are sent to the brain. Research continues into color vision, and the exact role of iodopsin is still unknown.

iodoquinol, an amebicide.

■ INDICATION: It is prescribed in the treatment of intestinal amebiasis.

■ CONTRAINDICATIONS: Hepatic disease and known hypersensitivity to iodine or 8-hydroxyquinolines prohibits its use.

■ ADVERSE EFFECTS: Among the most serious adverse reactions are dizziness, thyroid enlargement, optic neuropathy, optic atrophy, and peripheral neuropathy.

ion /ī′ən, ī′on/, an atom or group of atoms that has acquired an electric charge through the gain or loss of an electron or electrons.

-ion, **1.** a combining form meaning an 'electrically charged particle': *anion, cation, ion.* **2.** a noun-forming combining form: *endognathion, osteopedion, parhelion.*

Ionamin, a trademark for an anoretic (phentermine).

ion exchange chromatography, the process of separating and analyzing different substances according to their affinities for chemically stable but very reactive synthetic exchangers, which are composed largely of polystyrene and cellulose. The process uses an absorbent containing ionizing groups and accommodates the exchange of ions between a solution of substances to be analyzed and the absorbent. Ion exchange chromatography is often used to separate components of nucleic acids and proteins elaborated by various structures throughout the body. Different ions deposited in the absorbent during the exchange produce bands of different colors, which constitute a chromatograph. Compare **column chromatography, gas chromatography.**

ionic strength, the sum of the concentrations of all ions in a solution, weighted by the squares of their charges.

ionization, the process in which a neutral atom or molecule gains or loses electrons and thus acquires a negative or positive electric charge. Ionization occurs when atoms or molecules dissociate in solution or when those of gases dissociate in an electric field. Ionizing radiation produces ionization in its passage through body tissue or other matter. Ionization can also cause cell death or mutation.

ionization chamber, a small cavity filled with air that has the capability of collecting the ionic charge liberated during irradiation. A measure of this charge combined with knowledge of the mass of air in the chamber is a means of determining exposure and dose.

ionize /ī′ənīz/, to separate or change into ions. See also **ion.**

ionized calcium, the ionized, unbound, noncomplexed fraction of serum calcium that is biologically active.

ionizing energy, the average energy lost by ionizing radiation in producing an ion pair in a gas. In air, the value is approximately 33.73 electron-volts (eV).

ionizing radiation, high-energy electromagnetic waves (as x-rays and gamma rays) and particulate rays (as alpha particles, beta rays, electrons, neutrons, positrons, protons, and heavy nuclei) that dissociate substances in their paths into ions. The spatial distribution of the ionization depends on the kind of radiation, its penetrating power, the location of the source, and the nature of the irradiated material. High energy x-rays penetrate deeply, most beta particles penetrate only a few millimeters, and alpha particles penetrate only a fraction of a millimeter, but they all produce intense ionization along their tracks. Ionizing radiation directly affects living organisms by killing cells or retarding their development; its indirect effects include the production of gene mutations and chromosome breaks by striking a DNA molecule in the path of a particle ray. Animal tissues containing elements with relatively high atomic weights, as calcium in bones and teeth, absorb much higher doses from a given radiation than are absorbed by soft tissue.

ion-selective electrode, a potentiometric electrode that develops a potential in the presence of one ion (or class of ions) but not in the presence of a similar concentration of other ions.

iontophoretic pilocarpine test, a sweat test used in the diagnosis of cystic fibrosis. Pilocarpine iontophoresis is employed to stimulate production of sweat, which is absorbed from the forearm in a previously weighed gauze pad. The sweat sample is then analyzed for concentrations of sodium and chloride electrolytes.

Iowa trumpet, a kind of needle guide used in performing a pudendal block. It consists of a long thin cylinder through which a needle may be passed. A ring is attached to the proximal end of the guide, allowing the operator to hold it securely.

ipecac, an emetic.

■ INDICATIONS: It is prescribed to cause emesis in certain types of poisoning and drug overdose.

■ CONTRAINDICATIONS: Known hypersensitivity to this drug prohibits its use. It is not used in unconscious patients or for poisoning by petroleum distillates, strong alkalis, acids, or strychnine.

■ ADVERSE EFFECT: The most serious adverse reaction is cardiotoxicity if vomiting does not occur and the substance is retained.

■ NOTE: If vomiting does not occur, the ipecac is recovered by gastric lavage.

ipomea /ipəmē′ə/, a resin prepared from the dried root of *Ipomoea orizabensis,* formerly used as a cathartic.

IPPB (intermittent positive pressure breathing), a form of assisted or controlled respiration produced by a ventilatory apparatus in which compressed gas is delivered under positive pressure into the person's airways until a preset pressure is reached. Passive exhalation is allowed through a valve, and the cycle begins again as the flow of gas is triggered by inhalation. Also called **(IPPV) intermittent positive pressure ventilation.**

■ METHOD: The use of the IPPB unit involves the combined efforts of the physician, the inhalation therapist or technician, and the nurse. The specific pressure and volume and the use of nebulizing or other attachments are ordered individually. The equipment is tested and is introduced to the patient by the inhalation therapist. The nurse observes that the patient closes the lips around the mouthpiece and does not allow air to escape from the nose or mouth during inspiration and that the therapy is effective.

■ NURSING ORDERS: The patient may require reassurance that the machine will automatically shut off the flow of air at the end of inspiration and encouragement to relax and allow the lungs to be completely filled by the machine. The patient is cautioned not to manipulate any of the controls.

■ OUTCOME CRITERIA: Ventilation may be greatly improved by the use of the IPPB unit. Secretions may be thinned and cleared, and the passages may be humidified, allowing greater comfort and a better exchange of gases.

IPPB unit, a pressure-cycled ventilator for providing a flow of air into the lungs at a predetermined pressure. As the pressure is attained, the flow is stopped, pressure is released, and the patient exhales. The device is used to prevent postoperative atelectasis, to promote full expansion of the lungs, to improve oxygenation, and to administer nebulized medications into the respiratory passages.

IPPV, abbreviation for **intermittent positive pressure ventilation.** See **IPPB.**

ipsilateral, pertaining to the same side of the body. Compare **contralateral.**

IQ, abbreviation for **intelligence quotient.**

Ir, symbol for **iridium.**

iralgia /iral′jə/, *obsolete.* any pain or inflammation in the iris. Also called *(obsolete)* **iridalgia. –iralgic, iridalgic,** *adj.*

IRB, abbreviation for **institutional review board.**

iridectomy, surgical removal of part of the iris of the eye, performed most often to restore drainage of the aqueous humor in glaucoma or to remove a foreign body or a malignant tumor. General anesthesia is used. An incision is made through the cornea, and the iris is grasped with forceps or a hook and drawn out through the incision. The area involved is cut away, and the elastic iris is allowed to slip back into place. Atropine and an antibiotic are instilled, and a dressing and a shield are applied. Postoperatively, the patient is observed for signs of local hemorrhage or excessive pain.

iridium (Ir), a silvery-bluish metallic element. Its atomic number is 77; its atomic weight is 192.2.

irido-, a combining form meaning 'of or pertaining to the iris, or to a colored circle': *iridocele, iridokeratitis, iridoplegia.*

iridotomy, a surgical incision into the iris of the eye, performed to relieve occlusion of the pupil, to enlarge the pupil in cataract extraction, or to treat postoperative glaucoma. Local or general anesthesia is used. An incision is made through the cornea, and a cut is made transversely across the sphincter fibers of the iris. Atropine and an antibiotic are instilled, and a dressing and shield are applied. Postoperatively, the dressing is observed for signs of drainage. Excessive pain is abnormal. See also **iridectomy, iris.**

iris, a circular, contractile disc suspended in aqueous humor between the cornea and the crystalline lens of the eye and perforated by a circular pupil. The periphery of the iris is continuous with the ciliary body and is connected to the cornea by the pectinate ligament. The iris divides the space between the lens and the cornea into an anterior and a posterior chamber. In the adult, the two chambers communicate through the pupil, but they are separated in the fetus, up to the seventh month, by the membrana pupillaris. The involuntary muscle of the iris is composed of circular fibers and radiating fibers. Dark pigment cells under the translucent tissue of the iris are variously arranged in different people to produce different colored irises. The pigment is absent in albinos. In blue eyes the pigment cells are confined to the posterior surface of the iris, but in gray eyes, brown eyes, and black eyes the pigment cells appear in the anterior layer of epithelium and in the stroma. See also **dilatator pupillae, sphincter pupillae. –iridic,** *adj.*

iritis, an inflammatory condition of the iris of the eye characterized by pain, lacrimation, photophobia, and, if severe, diminished visual acuity. On ophthalmic examination the eye looks cloudy, the iris bulges, and the pupil is contracted. The underlying cause is treated if known, but the condition is most often idiopathic. The pupil is dilated, usually with atropine, and a corticosteroid may be prescribed to reduce inflammation. If the inflammation is allowed to continue and the pupil is left constricted, permanent scarring may occur, causing an opacity over the lens and diminished vision.

iron (Fe), a common metallic element essential for the synthesis of hemoglobin. Its atomic number is 26; its atomic weight is 55.85. It is used as a hematinic in the form of its salts and complexes, as ferrocholinate, ferrous fumarate, ferrous gluconate, ferrous sulfate, and iron-dextran.

iron deficiency anemia, a microcytic, hypochromic anemia caused by inadequate supplies of iron needed to synthesize hemoglobin, characterized by pallor, fatigue, and weakness. Laboratory diagnosis includes hemoglobin, hematocrit, transferrin, and serum iron evaluation. Iron deficiency may be the result of an inadequate dietary supply of iron, of poor absorption of iron in the digestive system, or of chronic bleeding. Replacement iron can be supplied by ferrous sulfate, the oral form being preferable, if tolerated. The anemia should be corrected in 2 months, but therapy is continued for another 4 months to replace tissue stores. Compare **hemolytic anemia, hypoplastic anemia.** See also **anemia, iron metabolism, nutritional anemia, red cell indices.**

iron dextran, an injectable hematinic.

■ INDICATION: It is prescribed in the treatment of iron deficiency anemia not responsive to oral iron therapy.

■ CONTRAINDICATIONS: Early pregnancy, anemias other than iron deficiency anemia, or known hypersensitivity to this drug prohibits its use.

■ ADVERSE EFFECTS: Among the more serious adverse effects are severe hypersensitivity reactions, including fatal anaphylaxis. Inflammation or phlebitis at the site of injection, arthralgia, headache, GI distress, fever, and lesser hypersensitivity reactions may occur.

iron lung. See **Drinker respirator.**

iron metabolism, a series of processes involved in the entry of iron into the body through its absorption, its transport and storage throughout the body, its utilization for the formation of hemoglobin and other iron compounds, and its eventual excretion. Iron normally enters the body through the epithelium of the intestinal mucosa, being oxidized from ferrous to ferric iron in the process. The rate at which iron enters is modulated by this absorption mechanism. When iron stores are high, iron no longer passes through but, instead, is trapped by the mucosal cells of the intestine to be eliminated upon their death. Once iron enters the blood, it is in a closed system in which, attached to transferrin, it cycles between the plasma and the reticuloendothelial or erythropoietic system. Plasma iron is delivered to the normoblast for hemoglobin synthesis where it remains up to 4 months, trapped in the hemoglobin molecules of a mature red cell. Senescent red cells then deteriorate and break down. The iron is released from the hemoglobin by the reticuloendothelial system to reenter the transport pool for recycling. The normal iron distribution in a 70 kg adult (male) totals approximately 3.7 g with more than 65% of this in circulating hemoglobin. Another 27% is found in the storage pool as hemosiderin or ferritin. The body normally conserves iron so well that loss, usually only through the feces, is normally limited to about 1 mg/day. This amount is easily provided by a dietary intake of only 10 mg/day. Iron deficiency may follow extended intervals of inadequate iron intake (especially in women) or after excessive blood loss. Iron overload sometimes occurs in disorders in which normal regulation of absorption of iron is impaired. It is most commonly produced iatrogenically through the parenteral administration of large amounts of iron or blood for therapeutic purposes. See also **anemia, hemochromatosis, iron deficiency anemia, iron transport.**

iron-rich food, any nutrient containing a relatively large amount of iron. The best source of dietary iron is liver, with oysters, clams, heart, kidney, lean meat, and tongue as second choices. Leafy green vegetables are the best plant sources. See also **iron, iron deficiency anemia.**

iron salts poisoning, poisoning caused by overdosage of ferric or ferrous salts, characterized by vomiting, bloody diarrhea, cyanosis, and gastric and intestinal pain. Therapy includes gastric lavage, administration of an emetic, deferoxamine, and supportive therapy as indicated by the severity of the symptoms.

iron saturation, the capacity of iron to saturate transferrin, measured in the blood to detect iron excess or deficiency. The normal iron saturation capacity in serum is 20% to 55%. See also **total iron.**

iron transport, the process whereby iron is carried from its entry point into the body, the intestinal mucosa, to the various sites of utilization and storage. Transferrin binds with free iron and shuttles it to storage and utilization sites. Transferrin becomes attached to exogenous iron entering through the intestinal villi or to iron reentering the plasma from the sinusoids of the spleen. The iron is then released to the normoblasts, and the transferrin is freed for additional transport functions that may, to a small extent, involve iron stored as ferritin or hemosiderin. See also **hemosiderosis, iron metabolism, transferrin.**

irradiation, exposure to any form of radiant energy like heat, light, or x-ray. Radioactive sources of radiant energy, such as x-rays or isotopes of iodine or cobalt, are used diagnostically to examine internal body structures, using knowledge of the ways in which various tissues absorb or reflect radioactive emissions. The same or similar sources of radioactivity in larger amounts are used to destroy microorganisms or tissue cells that have become cancerous. Infrared or ultraviolet light may be used to produce heat in body tissues to relieve pain and soreness or to treat acne, psoriasis, or other skin ailments. Ultraviolet light is also used to identify certain bacteria and toxic molds. See also **radiation sickness, radioactivity, ultraviolet. –irradiate,** *v.*

irreducible, unable to be returned to the normal position or condition, as an irreducible hernia. See also **incarcerate.**

irrelevance, (in psychiatry) any response, action, or statement not pertinent to the existing situation or condition that is indicative of a neurotic or psychotic condition.

irreversible coma. See **brain death.**

irrigation, the process of washing out a body cavity or wounded area with a stream of water or other fluid. It is also used to cleanse a tube or drain inserted into the body, as an indwelling catheter. The procedure is most commonly performed with water, saline, aminoacetic acid, or antiseptic solutions on the eye, ear, throat, vagina, and urinary tract. Gentle pressure is applied in the introduction of the fluid, except in the debridement of wounds, and the solution is removed from internal cavities through suction or by drainage. See also **lavage.** **–irrigate,** *v.*

irrigator, an apparatus with a flexible tube for flushing or washing out a body cavity.

irritable bowel syndrome, abnormally increased motility of the small and large intestines, generally associated with emotional stress. Most of those affected are young adults, who complain of diarrhea and, occasionally, pain in the lower abdomen. The pain is usually relieved by moving the bowels. In diagnosing irritable bowel syndrome, other more serious conditions, as dysentery, lactose intolerance, and the inflammatory bowel diseases, must be ruled out. Because there is no organic disease present in irritable bowel syndrome, no specific treatment is necessary. Many persons benefit from the use of bulk-producing agents in the diet, because bulk tends to stabilize the water content of the stool. Antidiarrheal drugs are helpful in decreasing the frequency of stool. Although this is a functional disorder, patients experience pain and discomfort and need emotional support. Mild tranquilizers or antidepressants are sometimes given to relieve anxiety or depression. Also called **mucous colitis, spastic colon.**

irritation fibroma, a localized peripheral, tumorlike enlargement of connective tissue caused by prolonged irritation. It commonly develops on the gingivae or the buccal mucosa.

IRV, abbreviation for *inspiratory reserve volume*. See **pulmonary function test.**

ischemia /iskē′mē·ə/, decreased blood supply to a body organ or part, often marked by pain and organ dysfunction, as in ischemic heart disease. Some causes of ischemia are arterial embolism, atherosclerosis, thrombosis, and vasoconstriction. Compare **infarction.** **–ischemic,** *adj.*

ischemic contracture. See **Volkmann's contracture.**

ischemic heart disease, a pathologic condition of the myocardium caused by lack of oxygen reaching the tissue cells.

ischemic lumbago, a pain in the lower back and buttocks caused by vascular insufficiency, as in occlusion of the abdominal aorta.

ischemic pain, the unpleasant, often excruciating sensation associated with ischemia, resulting from peripheral vascular disease, from decreased blood flow caused by constricting orthopedic casts, or from insufficient blood flow caused by surgical trauma or accidental injury. Ischemic pain caused by occlusive arterial disease is often severe and may not be relieved, even with narcotics. The individual with peripheral vascular disease may experience ischemic pain only while exercising because the metabolic demands for oxygen cannot be met by the occluded flow of blood. The ischemic pain of partial arterial occlusion is not as severe as the abrupt, excruciating pain associated with a complete blocking of the artery, as by an embolism. The ischemic pain caused by the pressure of an orthopedic cast is difficult to differentiate from the acute pain caused by surgical intervention, because both types of pain may be localized rather than diffused, as is the pain caused by trauma. See also **pain intervention, pain mechanism.**

ischio-, a combining form meaning 'of or pertaining to the ischium, or to the hip': *ischioanal, ischiodidymus, ischiopagus*.

ischium /is′kē·əm/, *pl.* **ischia,** one of the three parts of the hip bone, joining the ilium and the pubis to form the acetabulum. The ischium comprises the dorsal part of the hip bone and is divided into the body of the ischium, which forms two fifths of the acetabulum, and the ramus, which joins the inferior ramus of the pubis. The spine of the ischium provides attachment for various muscles, as the gemellus superior, the coccygeus, and the levator ani. The greater sciatic notch above the spine transmits the superior and the inferior gluteal vessels and various nerves, as gluteal nerves, the sciatic nerve, and the nerves to the obturator internus and the quadratus femoris. A notch below the spine of the ischium transmits various ligaments, vessels, and nerves for other parts. The large dorsal tuberosity of the ischium provides attachment for various muscles, as the adductor longus, the semimembranosus, the biceps femoris, and the semitendinosus. Compare **ilium, pubis.**

ISG, abbreviation for **immune serum globulin.**

Ishihara color test /ish′ēhä′rə/, a test of color vision using a series of plates on which are printed round dots in a variety of colors and patterns. People with normal color vision are able to discern specific numbers or patterns on the plates; the inability to pick out a given number or shape is symptomatic of a specific deficiency in color perception.

island fever. See **scrub typhus.**

islands of Langerhans /lang′gərhanz/, clusters of cells within the pancreas that produce insulin, glucagon, and pancreatic polypeptide. They form the endocrine portion of the gland and their hormonal secretions released into the bloodstream are balanced, important regulators of sugar metabolism. The islands of Langerhans are scattered throughout the pancreas; the beta cells, which secrete insulin, usually appear in the center of each of the lobules. Alpha cells secrete glucagon, and pancreatic peptide cells secrete pancreatic peptide. The cells comprising the islands are arranged in plates interspersed by capillaries. Also called **islets of Langerhans.**

islet cell adenoma. See **insulinoma.**

islet cell antibody, an immunoglobulin that reacts with the cytoplasm of all of the cells of the pancreatic islets. These antibodies occur in about 60% to 70% of newly diagnosed insulin-dependent diabetic patients, and the presence of the antibody is transient.

islet cell tumor, any tumor of the islands of Langerhans.

islets of Langerhans. See **islands of Langerhans.**

-ism, -ismus, a combining form meaning 'condition of, practice of, theory of': *hyperthyroidism, hypopituitarism, strabismus.*

Ismelin, a trademark for an antihypertensive (guanethidine sulfate).

iso-, a combining form meaning 'equal': *isobar, isochromatic, isohydric.*

isoagglutinin /ī'sō•əglo͞o'tinin/, an antibody that causes agglutination of erythrocytes in other members of the same species that carry an isoagglutinogen on their erythrocytes. Also called **isohemagglutinin.** Compare **isoagglutinogen.** See also **ABO blood groups, antibody.**

isoagglutinogen /ī'sō•əglo͞otin'əjən/, an antigen that causes the agglutination of erythrocytes in others of the same species that carry a corresponding isoagglutinin in their serum. Also called **isohemagglutinin.** Compare **agglutinin.** See also **ABO blood groups.**

isoamyl alcohol. See **amyl alcohol.**

isoantibody, an antibody to isoantigens found in other members of the same species. See also **autoimmune disease, tissue typing.**

isoantigen /ī'sō•an'tijən/, a substance that interacts with isoantibodies in other members of the same species. Compare **autoantigen, autoimmune disease.** See also **antigen, isoagglutinogen.**

isobar /ī'səbär/, (in nuclear medicine) one of a group of nuclides having the same total number of neutrons and protons in the nucleus but so proportioned as to result in different values of the atomic number.

isobutyl alcohol /ī'sōbyo͞o'til/, a clear, colorless liquid that is miscible with ethyl alcohol or ether.

isocarboxazid, a monoamine oxidase inhibitor.

■ INDICATION: It is prescribed in the treatment of mental depression.

■ CONTRAINDICATIONS: Liver or kidney dysfunction, congestive heart failure, pheochromocytoma, concomitant use of a sympathomimetic drug or foods high in tryptophan or tyramine, or known hypersensitivity to this drug prohibits its use.

■ ADVERSE EFFECTS: Among the more serious adverse reactions are hyperactivity, cardiac arrhythmia, hypotension, vertigo, dryness of mouth, constipation, and blurred vision. Monoamine oxidase inhibitors produce many adverse drug interactions.

isodose chart, (in radiotherapy) a graphic representation of the distribution of radiation in a medium; lines are drawn through points receiving equal doses. Isodose charts are determined for x-rays traversing the body, for radium applicators used in intracavitary or interstitial treatment, and for working areas where x-rays or radionuclides are employed.

isoelectric, pertaining to the electric base line of an electrocardiogram.

isoelectric electroencephalogram. See **flat electroencephalogram.**

isoelectric focusing, the ordering and concentration of substances according to their isoelectric points.

isoelectric point, the pH at which a molecule containing many ionizable groups is electrically neutral. The number of positively charged groups equals the number of negatively charged groups.

isoenzyme, an enzyme that may appear in multiple forms, with slightly different chemical or other characteristics, and be produced in different organs, although each enzyme performs essentially the same function. The various forms are distinguishable in analysis of blood samples, which aids in the diagnosis of diseases. Isoenzymes that catalyze the same physiologic reaction may also appear in different forms in different animal species. Also called **isozyme.**

isoetharine, isoetharine hydrochloride. See **isoetharine mesylate.**

isoetharine mesylate, a beta-adrenergic bronchodilator.

■ INDICATIONS: It is prescribed in the treatment of bronchial asthma, bronchitis, and emphysema.

■ CONTRAINDICATIONS: A history of cardiac arrhythmias or known hypersensitivity to this drug or to sympathomimetic medications prohibits its use.

■ ADVERSE EFFECTS: Among the more serious adverse reactions are palpitations, tachycardia, arrhythmias, vertigo, nervousness, and headache.

isoimmunization, the development of antibodies in a species with antigens from the same species, as the development of anti-Rh antibodies in an Rh-negative person.

isoflurophate, a cholinesterase inhibitor.

■ INDICATIONS: It is prescribed in the treatment of open-angle glaucoma and esotropia.

■ CONTRAINDICATIONS: Uveal inflammation or known hypersensitivity to this drug or to other organophosphates prohibits its use.

■ ADVERSE EFFECTS: Among the more serious adverse reactions are systemic cholinergic effects, visual disturbances, a paradoxical increase in intraocular pressure, and, with long-term administration, the development of cataracts.

isofosfamide. See isophosphamide.

isogamete /ī'sōgam'ēt/, a reproductive cell of the same size and structure as the one with which it unites. Compare **anisogamete, heterogamete.** –**isogametic,** *adj.*

isogamy /īsog'əmē/, sexual reproduction in which there is fusion of gametes of the same size and structure, as in certain algae, fungi, and protozoa. Compare **anisogamy, heterogamy.** –**isogamous,** *adj.*

isogeneic. See **syngeneic.**

isogenesis, development from a common origin and according to similar processes. Also called **isogeny** /īsoj'ənē/. –**isogenetic, isogenic,** *adj.*

isograft, surgical transplantation of histocompatible tissue obtained from genetically identical individuals, as between a patient and identical twin or between animals of a highly inbred strain. Compare **allograft, autograft, xenograft.** See also **graft.**

isohemagglutinin. See **isoagglutinin.**

isohydric shift, the series of reactions in red blood cells in which CO_2 is taken up and oxygen is released without the production of excess hydrogen ions.

isolation, the separation of a seriously ill patient from others to prevent the spread of an infection or to protect the patient from irritating environmental factors. A patient undergoing radiation therapy may also be isolated to reduce the exposure of hospital personnel to effects of radioactive materials.

isolation incubator, an incubator bed regularly maintained for premature or other infants who require isolation.

Isolette, a trademark for a self-contained incubator unit that provides a controlled heat, humidity, and oxygen microenvironment for the isolation and care of premature and low birth-weight neonates. The apparatus is made of a clear plastic material and has a large door and portholes for easy access to the infant with a minimum of heat and oxygen loss. A servocontrol mechanism constantly monitors the infant's temperature and controls the heat within the unit.

isoleucine (Ile) /ī′sōlo͞o′sēn/, an amino acid, occurring in most dietary proteins, that is essential for proper growth in infants and for nitrogen balance in adults. See also **amino acid, maple syrup urine disease, protein.**

isometheptene hydrochloride, an antispasmodic and vasoconstrictor drug that is a component in some fixed-combination drugs used to treat migraine.

isometric /ī′səmet′rik/, maintaining the same length or dimension.

isometric exercise, a form of active exercise that increases muscle tension by applying pressure against stable resistance. This may be accomplished by opposing different muscles in the same individual, as by pressing the hands together or by making a limb push or pull against an immovable object. There is no joint movement and the length of the muscle remains unchanged, but muscle strength and tone are maintained or improved. Compare **isotonic exercise.** See also **exercise.**

isometric growth, an increase in size of different organs or parts of an organism at the same rate. Compare **allometric growth.**

isoniazid /ī′sənī′əzid/, a tuberculostatic antibacterial. Also called **INH (isonicotinic acid hydrazide).**

■ INDICATION: It is prescribed in the treatment of tuberculosis caused by mycobacteria sensitive to the drug.

■ CONTRAINDICATIONS: Liver disease, a previous history of a hepatotoxic reaction to isoniazid, or known hypersensitivity to this drug prohibits its use.

■ ADVERSE EFFECTS: Among the more serious adverse reactions in long-term treatment are hepatoxicity and peripheral neuropathy. Rashes, fever, and central nervous system effects commonly occur.

isopentoic acid. See **isovaleric acid.**

isophane insulin suspension, a modified form of protamine zinc insulin suspension. It is an intermediate-acting insulin that is a stable, commonly prescribed preparation. Also called **NPH insulin.**

isophosphamide, an antineoplastic that is a derivative of cyclophosphamide and used similarly to cyclophosphamide. Also called **isofosfamide.** See also **cyclophosphamide.**

isoprenaline. See **isoproterenol hydrochloride.**

isopropamide iodide, an anticholinergic.

■ INDICATION: It is prescribed as an adjunct to ulcer therapy.

■ CONTRAINDICATIONS: Narrow-angle glaucoma, asthma, obstruction of the genitourinary or GI tract, ulcerative colitis, or known hypersensitivity to this drug prohibits its use.

■ ADVERSE EFFECTS: Among the more serious adverse reactions are blurred vision, central nervous system effects, tachycardia, dry mouth, decreased sweating, and hypersensitivity reactions.

isopropanol. See **isopropyl alcohol.**

isopropylacetic acid. See **isovaleric acid.**

isopropyl alcohol /ī′sōprō′pil/, a clear, colorless, bitter aromatic liquid that is miscible with water, ether, chloroform, and ethyl alcohol. A solution of approximately 70% isopropyl alcohol in water is used as a rubbing compound. Also called **avantin, dimethyl carbinol, isopropanol.** See also **alcohol.**

isopropylaminoacetic acid. See **valine.**

isoproterenol hydrochloride /ī′sōprəter′ənol/, a beta-adrenergic stimulant.

■ INDICATIONS: It is used as a bronchodilator and as a cardiac stimulant.

■ CONTRAINDICATIONS: Cardiac arrhythmia or known hypersensitivity to this drug prohibits its use.

■ ADVERSE EFFECTS: Among the more serious adverse reactions are arrhythmias, tachycardia, hypotension, and intensification of angina.

Isoptin, a trademark for a slow channel blocker or calcium ion antagonist (verapamil).

Isopto Atropine, a trademark for an anticholinergic (atropine sulfate).

Isopto Carbachol, a trademark for a cholinergic (carbachol).

Isopto Carpine, a trademark for a cholinergic (pilocarpine hydrochloride).

Isopto Cetamide, a trademark for an antibacterial (sulfacetamide sodium).

Isopto Homatropine, a trademark for an anticholinergic (homatropine hydrobromide).

Isopto Hyoscine, a trademark for an anticholinergic (scopolamine hydrobromide).

Isordil, a trademark for an antianginal agent (isosorbide dinitrate).

Isordil with Phenobarbital, a trademark for a cardiovascular fixed-combination drug containing an antianginal agent (isosorbide dinitrate) and a sedative-hypnotic (phenobarbital).

isosmotic. See **isotonic.**

isosorbide dinitrate, an antianginal agent.
■ INDICATIONS: It is prescribed as a coronary vasodilator in the treatment of angina pectoris and congestive heart failure.
■ CONTRAINDICATION: Known hypersensitivity to this drug prohibits its use.
■ ADVERSE EFFECTS: The most serious reaction is occasional marked hypotension. Flushing, headache, and dizziness also may occur.

isotachophoresis, the ordering and concentration of substances of intermediate effective mobilities between an ion of high effective mobility and one of much lower effective mobility, followed by their migration at a uniform velocity.

isotonic /ī′səton′ik/, (of a solution) having the same concentration of solute as another solution, hence exerting the same amount of osmotic pressure as that solution, as an isotonic saline solution that contains an amount of salt equal to that found in the intra- and extracellular fluid. Also **isosmotic.** Compare **hypertonic, hypotonic.**

isotonic exercise, a form of active exercise in which the muscle contracts and causes movement. Throughout the procedure there is no significant change in the resistance so that the force of the contraction remains constant. Such exercise greatly improves joint mobility and helps to improve muscle strength and tone. Compare **isometric exercise.** See also **exercise.**

isotope /ī′sətōp/, one of two or more forms of a chemical element having almost identical properties: They have the same number of protons in the atomic nucleus and the same atomic number, but they differ in the number of their nuclear neutrons and atomic weights. Carbon (^{12}C) has six nuclear neutrons, while its isotope ^{14}C has eight. Many hundreds of radioactive isotopes are used in diagnostic and therapeutic procedures.

isotopic tracer /ī′sətop′ik/, an isotope or artificial mixture of isotopes of an element incorporated into a sample to permit observation of the course of the element, alone or in combination, through a chemical, physical, or biologic process. The observations may be made by measuring the radioactivity or the abundance of the isotope.

isotretinoin, an antiacne agent.
■ INDICATION: It is prescribed for cystic acne.
■ CONTRAINDICATIONS: Pregnancy or sensitivity to hydroxybenzoic acid esters prohibits its use.
■ ADVERSE EFFECTS: The most serious adverse reactions are epistaxis, cheilitis, conjunctivitis, paresthesia, dizziness, serum lipid, and hematologic disturbances.

isovaleric acid, a fatty acid with a pungent taste and disagreeable odor that is found in valerian and other plant products as well as in cheese. It also occurs as a metabolite of the amino acid leucine and is found in the sweat of feet and in urine in smallpox, hepatitis, and typhus. It has been used commercially in a variety of drugs, perfumes, and flavorings. Isovaleric acidemia occurs in patients who have inherited a deficiency of the enzyme isovaleryl coA dehydrogenase, resulting in abnormally high levels of isovaleric acid in the blood and urine. The condition is treated with diets that contain low-leucine foods. Also called **isopentoic acid, isopropylacetic acid.**

isovolumic contraction, (in cardiology) an early phase of systole in which the left ventricle is generating enough tension to overcome the resistance of the aortic end-diastolic pressure. See also **afterload.**

isoxsuprine hydrochloride, a peripheral vasodilator.
■ INDICATIONS: It is prescribed for the symptomatic relief of cerebrovascular insufficiency and to improve the circulation in arteriosclerosis, Raynaud's disease, and Buerger's disease.
■ CONTRAINDICATION: Known hypersensitivity to this drug is the only contraindication.
■ ADVERSE EFFECTS: Among the more serious adverse reactions are tachycardia, hypotension, and dermatitis.

-ist, a combining form meaning a 'practitioner of a science': *audiologist, pharmacist, psychosomaticist.*

isthmus /is′məs/, *pl.* **isthmuses, isthmi,** a narrow connection between two larger bodies or parts, as the isthmus of the auditory tube in the ear, which connects the bony and the cartilaginous parts of the tube.

Isuprel, a trademark for a beta-adrenergic stimulant (isoproterenol).

itch, **1.** to feel a sensation, usually on the skin, that makes one want to scratch. **2.** a tingling, annoying sensation on an area of the skin that makes one want to scratch it, as may be caused in some people by rhus dermatitis, a mosquito bite, or an allergic reaction. **3.** the pruritic condition of the skin caused by infestation with the parasitic mite *Sarcoptes scabiei.* –**itchy,** *adj.*

-ite, **1.** a combining form meaning 'compounds': *nitrite, phosphite, sulfite.* **2.** a combining form meaning a 'body part': *chondriomite, osteite, zygoite.*

ithy-, a combining form meaning 'straight': *ithylordosis, ithyokyphosis.*

-itic, a combining form meaning 'of or related to something specified': *encephalitic, nephritic, syphilitic.*

-itis, a combining form meaning an 'inflammation of a (specified) organ': *carditis, cecitis, sarcitis.*

ITP, abbreviation for **idiopathic thrombocytopenic purpura.**

IU, I.U., abbreviation for **International Unit.**

IUCD, abbreviation for **intrauterine contraceptive device.** See **intrauterine device.**

IUD, abbreviation for **intrauterine device.**

-ium, a combining form used to name metallic elements: *aluminum, radium, sodium.*

IV, **1.** abbreviation for **intravenous.** **2.** *informal.* equipment consisting of a bottle of fluid, infusion set with tubing, and an intracatheter, used in intravenous therapy. **3.** intravenous administration of fluids or medication by injection into a vein.

IVAC pump, a trademark for a portable IV pump that electronically regulates and monitors the flow of fluid. It is usually attached to the IV stand. See also **intravenous pump.**

ivory bones. See **osteopetrosis.**

IVP, abbreviation for **intravenous pyelography.**

IV push, a technique in which a bolus of medication or a large volume of IV fluid is given rapidly via IV injection or infusion. Methergine may be given in this way to cause immediate contraction of the uterus in postpartum hemorrhage. See also **intravenous injection.**

IV-type traction frame, a metal support that holds traction equipment consisting of two metal uprights, one at each end of the bed, which support an overhead metal bar. Each upright is clamped to a horizontal bar that fits into holders inserting at the corners of the bed. Compare **claw-type traction frame.** See also **traction frame.**

Ixodes /iksō′dēz/,, a genus of parasitic hard-shelled ticks associated with the transmission of a variety of arbovirus infections, as Rocky Mountain spotted fever.

ixodi-, a combining form meaning 'of or pertaining to ticks': *ixodiasis, ixodism.*

ixodid /iksod′id, iksō′did/, of or pertaining to hard ticks of the family Ixodidae.

-ize, a combining form meaning 'do, treat, cause': *anesthetize, canalize, fertilize.*

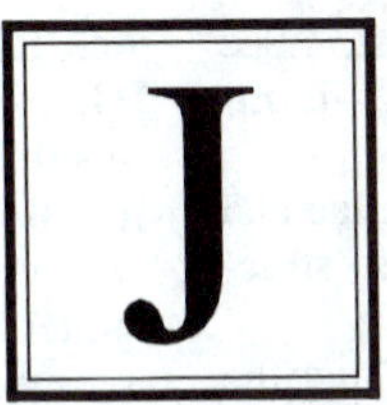

jacket, a supportive or confining therapeutic casing or garment for the torso. Some kinds of jackets are **Minerva jacket** and **Sayre's jacket.**

jacket restraint, an orthopedic device used to help immobilize the trunk of a patient in traction and to discourage the patient from sitting up in bed. The jacket restraint is attached to both sides of the bedspring frame by means of buckled webbing straps that are sewn into the side seams of the restraint. The jacket restraint may be used with most kinds of traction but is not usually used with Dunlop skin traction or Dunlop skeletal traction, Bryant traction, halo-femoral traction, or halo-pelvic traction. Compare **diaper restraint, sling restraint.**

jackknife position, an anatomic position in which the patient is placed on the back in a semisitting position, with the shoulders elevated and the thighs flexed at right angles to the abdomen. Examination and instrumentation of the male urethra is facilitated by this position.

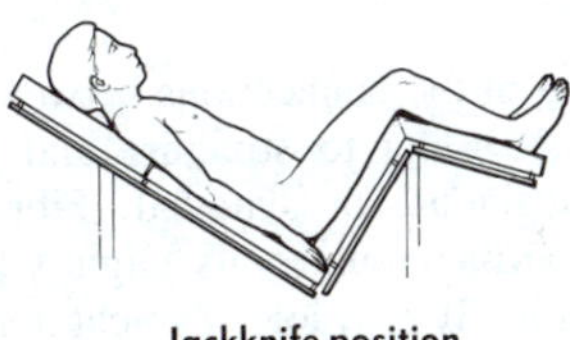

Jackknife position

Jackson crib, a removable orthodontic appliance retained in position by crib-shaped wires.

jacksonian seizure. See **focal seizure.**

Jacob's membrane, the outermost of the nine layers of the retina, composed of rods and cones interacting directly with the optic nerve.

Jacquemier's sign /zhäkmē·äz′/, a deepening of the color of the vaginal mucosa just below the urethral orifice. It may sometimes be noted after the fourth week of pregnancy, but it is not a reliable sign of pregnancy.

jail fever. See **epidemic typhus.**

Jakob-Creutzfeldt disease. See **Creutzfeldt-Jakob disease.**

JAMA /jä′mä, jam′ə, jā′ā′em′ā′/, abbreviation for *Journal of the American Medical Association.*

jamais vu /zhämävY′, -vē′, -vo͞o′/, the sensation of being a stranger when with a person one knows or when in a familiar place. The phenomenon occurs occasionally in normal people but more frequently in people who have temporal lobe epilepsy. The French phrase means literally "never seen." Compare **déjà vu.**

Janeway lesion, a small erythematous or hemorrhagic macule occurring on the palms or soles, sometimes diagnostic of subacute bacterial endocarditis.

janiceps /jan′əseps/, a conjoined, twin fetal monster in which the heads are fused, with the faces looking in opposite directions. The faces and bodies of both twins may be fully formed or one member may be only partially formed and act as a parasite on the more fully developed fetus.

Jansen's disease. See **metaphyseal dysostosis.**

Japanese encephalitis, a severe epidemic infection of brain tissue seen in East Asia and the South Pacific, including Australia and New Zealand, characterized by shaking chills, paralysis, and weight loss, and caused by a group of B arboviruses transmitted by mosquitoes. Mortality may be as high as 33%. Various neurologic and psychiatric sequelae are common. There is no specific treatment. Also called **Japanese B encephalitis.**

Japanese flood fever, Japanese river fever. See **scrub typhus.**

JAPHA /jaf′ə, jā′ā′pē′āch′ā′/, abbreviation for *Journal of the American Public Health Association.*

Jarisch-Herxheimer reaction /jä′risherks′hīmər/, a sudden transient fever and exacerbation of skin lesions observed several hours after administration of penicillin or other antibiotics in the treatment of syphilis, leptospirosis, or relapsing fever. The effect lasts less than 24 hours and requires no treatment.

Jarvik-7, an artificial heart designed by R.K. Jarvik for use in humans. The Jarvik-7 was an early model that depended on air pressure to drive the ventricles. See also **electrohydraulic heart.**

Jarotzky's treatment /jərot′skēz/, therapy of gastric ulcer using a bland diet consisting of egg whites, fresh butter, bread, milk, and noodles.

jaundice, a yellow discoloration of the skin, mucous membranes, and sclerae of the eyes, caused by greater than normal amounts of bilirubin in the blood. Persons with jaundice may also experience nausea, vomiting, and abdominal pain and may pass dark urine. Jaundice is a symptom of many disorders, including liver diseases, biliary obstruction, and the hemolytic anemias. Newborns commonly develop physiologic jaundice, which disappears after a few days. Rarer disorders causing jaundice are Crigler-Najjar syndrome and Gilbert's syndrome. Useful diagnostic procedures include a clinical evaluation of the signs and symptoms, tests of liver function, techniques for direct or indirect visualization as x-ray film, CAT scan, ultrasound, endoscopy or exploratory surgery, and biopsy. Also called **icterus** /ik′tərəs/. See also **anicteric hepatitis, hyperbilirubinemia.** –**jaundiced,** *adj*.

jaw, a common term used to describe the maxillae and the mandible and the soft tissue that covers these structures. See also **jaw relation.**

jaw reflex, an abnormal reflex elicited by tapping the chin with a rubber hammer while the mouth is half open and the jaw muscles are relaxed. A quick snapping shut of the jaw implies damage to the area of cerebral cortex governing motor activity of the fifth cranial nerve. Also called **chin reflex, jaw jerk, mandibular reflex.**

jaw relation, any relation of the mandible to the maxillae.

JCAH, abbreviation for **Joint Commission on Accreditation of Hospitals.**

J chain, the portion of IgM molecule possibly holding structure together, thus ''joining chain.''

jeco-, a combining form meaning 'of or pertaining to the liver': *jecolein, jecoral, jecorin*.

Jefferson fracture, a fracture characterized by bursting of the ring of the atlas.

jejuno-, a combining form meaning 'of or pertaining to the jejunum': *jejunocecostomy, jejunocolostomy, jejunotomy*.

jejunoileitis. See **Crohn's disease.**

jejunum /jijo͞o′nəm/, *pl.* **jejuna,** one of the three portions of the small intestine, connecting proximally with the duodenum and distally with the ileum. The jejunum has a slightly larger diameter, a deeper color, and a thicker wall than the ileum and contains heavy, circular folds that are absent in the lower part of the ileum. The jejunum also has larger villi than the ileum. Compare **ileum.** –**jejunal,** *adj*.

jellyfish sting, a wound caused by skin contact with a jellyfish, a sea animal with a bell-shaped gelatinous body and suspended numerous long tentacles containing stinging structures. In most cases a tender, red welt develops on the affected skin. In some cases, depending on the sensitivity of the person and the particular species of jellyfish, severe localized pain and nausea, weakness, excessive lacrimation, nasal discharge, muscle spasm, perspiration, and dyspnea may occur. Treatment includes carefully removing any tentacles and applying a compress of alcohol, aromatic spirits of ammonia, or Dakin's solution. Calcium gluconate may be administered to control muscle spasms.

Jendrassik's maneuver /yendrä′shiks/, (in neurology) a diagnostic procedure in which the patient hooks the flexed fingers of the two hands together and forcibly tries to pull them apart. While this tension is being exerted, the lower extremity reflexes are tested, particularly the patellar reflex.

jet lag, a condition characterized by fatigue, insomnia, and sluggish body functions caused by disruption of the normal circadian rhythm resulting from air travel across several time zones.

jigger. See **chigoe.**

jock itch. See **tinea cruris.**

JOD, abbreviation for *juvenile-onset diabetes*. See **insulin-dependent diabetes mellitus.**

Jod-Basedow phenomenon, thyrotoxicosis occurring when dietary iodine is given to a patient with endemic goiter in an area of environmental iodine deficiency. It is presumed that iodine deficiency protects some patients with endemic goiter from developing thyrotoxicosis. The phenomenon may also occur when large doses of iodine are given to patients with nontoxic multinodular goiter in areas with sufficient environmental iodine. There is a danger of inducing the phenomenon if iodine-containing drugs, as x-ray contrast media, are administered to elderly patients with nontoxic multinodular goiter.

jogger's heel, a painful condition, common among joggers and distance runners. It is characterized by bruising, bursitis, fasciitis, or calcaneal spurs, caused by repetitive and forceful strikes of the heel on the ground. Judicious selection of well-fitting running shoes and avoidance of running on hard surfaces are recommended to avoid occurrence or recurrence of the condition. Rest, heat, or corticosteroid medication or aspirin may be recommended.

Johnson's method, (in dentistry) a technique for filling root canals, in which gutta-percha cones are dissolved in a chloroform-rosin solution in the root canal to form a plastic mass. The plastic material is forced into the apex of the root canal with more added until the canal is sealed.

joint, any one of the connections between bones. Each is classified according to structure and movability as fibrous, cartilaginous, or synovial. Fibrous joints are immovable, cartilaginous joints slightly movable, and synovial joints freely movable. Typical immovable joints are those connecting most of the bones of the skull with a

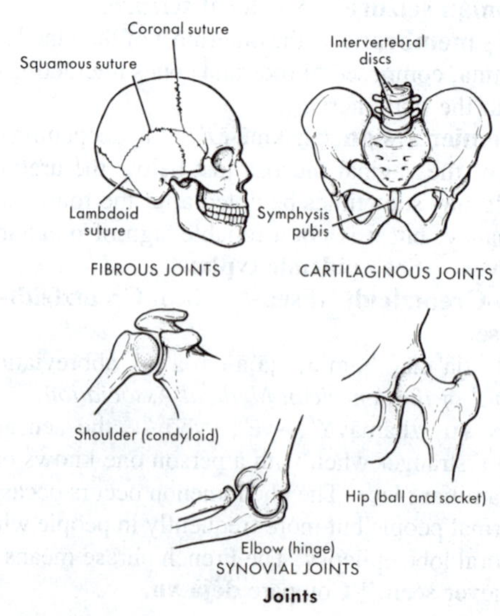

Joints

sutural ligament. Typical slightly movable joints are those connecting the vertebrae and the pubic bones. Most of the joints in the body are freely movable and allow gliding, circumduction, rotation, and angular movement. Also called **articulation.** See also **cartilaginous joint, fibrous joint, synovial joint.**

joint and several liability, (in law) a condition in which several persons share the liability for a plaintiff's injury and may be found liable individually or as a group.

joint appointment, **1.** a faculty appointment to two institutions within a university or system, as to the schools of nursing and medicine of the same university. **2.** (in academic nursing) the appointment of a member of the faculty of a university to a clinical service of an associated service institution. A psychiatric nurse might hold appointment in a university as an assistant professor and might also be a clinical nurse specialist in a service institution. The practice of joint appointments is said to have begun at Case Western Reserve University, University Hospital. See also **unification model.**

joint audit. See **nursing audit.**

joint chondroma, a cartilaginous mass that develops in the synovial membrane of a joint.

Joint Commission on Accreditation of Hospitals (JCAH), a private, nongovernmental agency that establishes guidelines for the operation of hospitals and other health care facilities, conducts accreditation programs and surveys, and encourages the attainment of high standards of institutional medical care. Members of the JCAH include representatives from the American Medical Association, American College of Physicians, and American College of Surgeons.

joint conference committee, a hospital organization composed of the governing board, administration, and medical staff representatives whose purpose is to facilitate communication between the groups.

joint fracture, a fracture of the articular surfaces of the bony structures of a joint.

jointly exhaustive categories, categories on a research instrument that are sufficiently complete to allow every possible subject, factor, or variable to be classified and assigned to a category.

joint planning, the development by two or more health care providers of a strategic plan to serve the health care needs of an area while sharing clinical or administrative services, or the sharing of data, without the sharing of assets.

joint practice, **1.** the practice of a physician and a nurse practitioner, usually private, who work as a team, sharing responsibility for a group of patients. **2.** (in inpatient nursing) the practice of making joint decisions about patient care by committees of the physicians and nurses working on a division.

Jones criteria, a standardized set of guidelines for the diagnosis of rheumatic fever, as recommended by the American Heart Association. See also **rheumatic fever.**

joule /jo͞ol/, a unit of energy or work in the MKS (meter-kilogram-second) system. It is equivalent to 10^7 ergs or 1 watt second. The unit was named for nineteenth century English physicist James P. Joule.

judgment, **1.** (in law) the final decision of the court regarding the case before it. **2.** the reason given by the court for its decision; an opinion. **3.** an award, penalty, or other sentence of law given by the court. **4.** (in psychiatry) the ability to recognize the relationships of ideas and to form correct conclusions from those data as well as from those acquired from experience.

judgment call, *slang.* a decision based on experience, especially a judgment that resolves a serious problem in which the data are inconclusive or equivocal.

jug-, a combining form meaning 'yoke': *jugal, jugum, conjugal.*

jugu-, a combining form meaning 'throat or neck': *jugular, jugulation.*

jugular foramen, one of a pair of openings between the lateral part of the occipital bone and the petrous part of the temporal bones in the skull. The foramen contains the inferior petrosal sinus, the transverse sinus, some meningeal branches of the occipital and ascending pharyngeal arteries, and the glossopharyngeal, vagus, and accessory nerves.

juice, any fluid secreted by the tissues of animals or plants. In humans, it usually refers to the secretions of the digestive glands. Kinds of juices include **gastric juice, intestinal juice,** and **pancreatic juice.**

jumentous, having a strong animal odor, especially that of a horse. It is used to describe the odor of urine during certain disease conditions.

jumping gene, (in molecular genetics) a unit of genetic information associated with a segment of DNA that can move from one position in the genome to another.

junctional extrasystole, an extrasystole arising from the atrioventricular junction. See also **atrioventricular junction.**

junctional rhythm, the cardiac rhythm originating in the atrioventricular junction.

junctional tachycardia, an automatic heart rhythm of greater than 100 beats/minute, emanating from the AV junction. The mechanism is enhanced automatically, usually caused by digitalis toxicity.

junction nevus, a hairless, flat or slightly raised, brown skin blemish arising from pigment cells at the epidermal-dermal junction. A junction nevus may be found anywhere on the surface of body. All nevi of the palms and soles and all pigmented nevi in early childhood are of this type. Malignant change may be signaled by increase in size, hardness or darkening, bleeding, or the appearance of satellite discoloration around the nevus. Junction nevi undergoing these changes and lesions found in areas subject to trauma should be removed.

junctura cartilaginea. See **cartilaginous joint.**

junctura fibrosa. See **fibrous joint.**

junctura synovialis. See **synovial joint.**

jungian psychology. See **analytic psychology.**

Junin fever. See **Argentine hemorrhagic fever.**
junk, *slang*. heroin.
justo major, *archaic*. atypically large, as a woman's bony pelvis.
juvenile, **1.** a young person; youth; child; youngster. **2.** of, pertaining to, characteristic of, or suitable for a young person; youthful. **3.** physiologically underdeveloped or immature. **4.** denoting psychologic or intellectual immaturity; childish.
juvenile alveolar rhabdomyosarcoma, a rapidly growing tumor of striated muscle with a grave prognosis, occurring in children and adolescents, chiefly in the extremities.
juvenile angiofibroma. See **nasopharyngeal angiofibroma.**
juvenile delinquency, persistent antisocial, illegal, or criminal behavior by children or adolescents to the degree that it cannot be controlled or corrected by the parents, it endangers others in the community, and it becomes the concern of a law enforcement agency. Such behavioral patterns are characterized by aggressiveness, destructiveness, hostility, and cruelty and occur more frequently in boys than in girls. Causative factors typically involve poor parent-child relationships, especially parental rejection, indifference, and apathy, and unstable family environments where disciplinary methods are lax, erratic, or overly strict, or involve harsh physical punishment. Traditional punitive treatments, primarily correctional institutions and reform schools, usually aggravate rather than remedy the situation. More progressive approaches, such as foster home placement, work and recreational programs, and various community and family counseling services, have been more successful. Behavior therapy and other forms of psychotherapy, often involving the parents as well as the child, are also used as modes of treatment and prevention. See also **antisocial personality disorder, behavior disorder.**
juvenile delinquent, a person who performs illegal acts and who has not reached an age at which treatment as an adult can be accorded under the laws of the community having jurisdiction. Also called **juvenile offender.**
juvenile diabetes. See **insulin-dependent diabetes mellitus.**
juvenile kyphosis. See **Scheuermann's disease.**
juvenile lentigo. See **lentigo.**
juvenile-onset diabetes. See **insulin-dependent diabetes mellitus.**
juvenile periodontitis, an abnormal condition that may affect the dental alveoli, expecially in the anterior and first molar regions of children and adolescents. It is characterized by severe pocketing and bone loss. Formerly called **periodontosis.**
juvenile rheumatoid arthritis, a form of rheumatoid arthritis, usually affecting the larger joints of children under 16 years of age. As bone growth in chilren is dependent on the epiphyseal plates of the distal epiphyses, skeletal development may be impaired if these structures are damaged. Treatment includes analgesia, antiinflammatory medication, and rest. The recovery rate in this juvenile form is better than in the adult forms of rheumatoid arthritis. Also called **Still's disease.**
juvenile xanthogranuloma, a skin disorder characterized by groups of yellow, red, or brown papules or nodules on the extensor surfaces of the arms and legs, and in some cases on the eyeball, meninges, and testes. The lesions typically appear in infancy or early childhood and usually disappear in a few years.
juxta-, a combining form meaning 'near': *juxtaglomerular, juxtangina, juxtaposition*.
juxtaglomerular cells, smooth muscle cells lining the glomerular end of the afferent arterioles in the kidney that are in opposition to the macula densa region of the early distal tubule. These cells synthesize and store renin and release it in response to decreased renal perfusion pressure, increased sympathetic nerve stimulation of the kidneys, or decreased sodium concentration in fluid in the distal tubule.

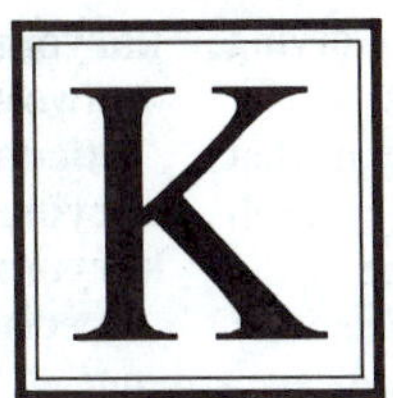

K, symbol for **potassium.**

K_m, symbol for **Michaelis-Menten constant.**

Kafocin, a trademark for an antibacterial (cephaloglycin).

Kahn test, **1.** one of the older serologic tests for syphilis. The appearance of a white precipitate in a serum sample allowed to stand overnight in a mixture with a sensitized antigen is regarded as a positive reaction. **2.** a test for the presence of cancer by measuring the proportion of albumin A in a blood sample.

kak-, a combining form meaning 'bad': *kakidrosis, kakosmia.*

kakke disease. See **beriberi.**

kakosmia. See **cacosmia.**

kala-azar /kä′lə·əzär′/, a disease caused by the protozoan *Leishmania donovani,* transmitted to humans, particularly to children, by the bite of the sand fly. Kala-azar occurs primarily in Asia, parts of Africa, several South and Central American countries, and in the Mediterranean region. The liver and spleen are the main sites of infection; signs and symptoms include anemia, hepatomegaly, splenomegaly, irregular fever, and emaciation. Patients with kala-azar are also susceptible to secondary bacterial infections. Untreated, the disease has an extremely high mortality. Treatment includes sodium antimony gluconate, blood transfusions (for anemia), bed rest, and adequate nutrition. Also called **Assam fever, black fever, dumdum fever, ponos, visceral leishmaniasis.** See also **leishmaniasis.**

kali-, a combining form meaning 'of or pertaining to potassium': *kaligenous, kalium, kalinite.*

Kallmann's syndrome, a condition characterized by the absence of the sense of smell because of agenesis of the olfactory bulbs and by secondary hypogonadism because of the lack of LHRH.

kanamycin /kan′əmī′sin/, an antibacterial substance derived from *Streptomyces kanamyceticus.*

kanamycin sulfate, an aminoglycoside antibiotic.

■ INDICATIONS: It is prescribed in the treatment of certain severe infections and those resistant to other antibiotics.

■ CONTRAINDICATIONS: Concomitant administration of ototoxic drugs or known hypersensitivity to this drug or to other aminoglycoside antibiotics prohibits its use. It is used with caution in patients having impaired renal function and in the elderly.

■ ADVERSE EFFECTS: Among the more serious adverse reactions are nephrotoxicity, vestibular and auditory ototoxicity, neuromuscular blockade, and hypersensitivity reactions.

Kantrex, a trademark for an antibacterial (kanamycin sulfate).

Kanulase, a trademark for a GI, fixed-combination drug containing various antiflatulent ingredients.

Kaochlor, a trademark for an electrolyte-replacement solution (potassium chloride).

kaodzera. See **Rhodesian trypanosomiasis.**

kaolin /kā′əlin/, an adsorbent used internally to treat diarrhea, often in combination with pectin. Kaolin in an ointment base is also used topically as an absorbent and a protective emollient.

Kaon, a trademark for the electrolyte-replacement solution (potassium chloride).

Kaopectate, a trademark for an antidiarrheal fixed-combination drug containing an adsorbent (kaolin) and an emollient (pectin).

Kaposi's sarcoma /kap′əsēz/, a malignant, multifocal neoplasm of reticuloendothelial cells that begins as soft, brownish or purple papules on the feet and slowly spreads in the skin, metastasizing to the lymph nodes and viscera. It occurs most often in men and is occasionally associated with diabetes, malignant lymphoma, or other disorders. Radiotherapy and chemotherapy are usually recommended. Also called **idiopathic multiple pigmented hemorrhagic sarcoma, multiple idiopathic hemorrhagic sarcoma.**

Kaposi's varicelliform eruption. See **eczema herpeticum.**

kaps-. See **caps-.**

karaya powder, a dried form of *Sterculia urens* or other species of *Sterculia,* used as a bulk cathartic. Like other bulk-forming agents, karaya powder reduces the intraluminal rectosigmoid pressure and helps relieve symptoms in patients with irritable bowel disease and diverticular disease of the colon. Relief of pain and other symptoms may occur progressively over several months. Because of its ability to absorb water and form an emollient intestinal mass, karaya powder also may be useful in relieving the symptoms of acute diarrhea, in modifying the effluent in the patient with an ileostomy or a colostomy, and in the care of skin surfaces around a stoma. The use of such a bulk-forming cathartic may also increase the loss of sodium, potassium, and water in such patients. With some individuals the use of karaya powder may cause allergic reactions, as urticaria, rhinitis, dermatitis, and asthma. Methylcellulose has largely replaced this drug in modern use. Externally, it is used as a drying agent for Stage I and Stage II decubitus ulcers.

Kardex. a trademark for a card-filing system that allows quick reference to the particular needs of each patient for certain aspects of nursing care. Included on the card may be a schedule of medications, level of activity allowed, ability to perform basic self-care, diet, any special problems, a schedule of treatments and procedures, and a care plan. The Kardex is updated as necessary and is usually kept at the nurses' station.

karyenchyma. See **karyolymph.**

karyo-, a combining form meaning 'of or pertaining to a nucleus': *karyochrome, karyokinesis, karyolymph.*

karyogamy /ker'ē•og'əmē/, the fusion of cell nuclei, as in conjugation and zygosis. **–karyogamic,** *adj.*

karyogenesis /ker'ē•ōjen'əsis/, the formation and development of the nucleus of a cell. **–karyogenetic,** *adj.*

karyokinesis /ker'ē•ōkinē'sis, -kīnē'sis/, the division of the nucleus and equal distribution of nuclear material during mitosis and meiosis. The process involves the four stages of prophase, metaphase, anaphase, and telophase, and it precedes the division of the cytoplasm. Also called **karyomitosis.** See also **cytokinesis. –karyokinetic,** *adj.*

karyoklasis /ker'ē•ok'ləsis/, **1.** the disintegration of the cell nucleus or nuclear membrane. **2.** the interruption of mitosis. Also spelled **karyoclasis. –karyoklastic, karyoclastic,** *adj.*

karyology /ker'ē•ol'əjē/, the branch of cytology that concentrates on the study of the cell nucleus, especially the structure and function of the chromosomes. **–karyologic, karyological,** *adj.*, **karyologist,** *n.*

karyolymph /ker'ē•əlimf'/, the clear, usually nonstaining, fluid substance of the nucleus. It consists primarily of proteinaceous, colloidal material in which the nucleolus, chromatin, linin, and various submicroscopic particles are dispersed. Also called **karyenchyma, nuclear hyaloplasm, nuclear sap, nucleochyme. –karyolymphatic,** *adj.*

karyolysis /ker'ē•ol'isis/, the dissolution of the cell nucleus. It occurs normally, both as a form of necrobiosis and during the generation of new cells through mitosis and meiosis.

karyolytic /ker'ē•əlit'ik/, **1.** of or pertaining to karyolysis. **2.** that which causes the destruction of the cell nucleus.

karyomere /ker'ē•əmir'/, **1.** a saclike structure containing an unequal portion of the nuclear material after atypical mitosis. **2.** a segment of the chromosome. See also **chromomere.**

karyometry, the measurement of the nucleus of a cell. **–karyometric,** *adj.*

karyomit /ker'ē•əmit'/, **1.** a single chromatin fibril of the network within the nucleus of a cell. **2.** a chromosome.

karyomitome /ker'ē•om'itōm/, the fibrillar chromatin network within the nucleus of a cell. Also called **karyoreticulum.**

karyomitosis. See **karyokinesis.**

karyomorphism, the shape or form of a cell nucleus, especially that of the leukocyte. **–karyomorphic,** *adj.*

karyon /ker'ē•on/, the nucleus of a cell. **–karyontic,** *adj.*

karyophage /ker'ē•ōfāj'/, an intracellular protozoan parasite that destroys the nucleus of the cell it infects. **–karyophagic, karyophagous,** *adj.*

karyoplasm. See **nucleoplasm.**

karyoplasmic ratio. See **nucleocytoplasmic ratio.**

karyopyknosis /ker'ē•ōpiknō'sis/, the state of a cell in which the nucleus has shrunk and the chromatin has condensed into solid masses, as in cornified cells of stratified squamous epithelium. **–karyopyknotic,** *adj.*

karyoreticulum. See **karyomitome.**

karyorrhexis /ker'ē•ərek'sis/, the fragmentation of chromatin and distribution of it throughout the cytoplasm as a result of nuclear disintegration. **–karyorrhectic,** *adj.*

karyosome /ker'ē•əsōm'/, a dense irregular mass of chromatin filaments in the cell nucleus. It is often seen during interphase and may be confused with the nucleolus because of similar staining properties. Also called **chromatin nucleolus, chromocenter, false nucleolus, prochromosome.**

karyospherical /ker'ē•ōsfer'ikəl/, **1.** of or pertaining to a nucleus that is spherical in shape. **2.** such a nucleus.

karyostasis /ker'ē•os'təsis/, the resting stage of the nucleus between cell division. See also **interphase. –karyostatic,** *adj.*

karyotheca /ker'ē•əthē'kə/, the membrane that encloses a cell nucleus. **–karyothecal,** *adj.*

karyotin. See **chromatin.**

karyotype /ker'ē•ətīp'/, **1.** the total morphologic characteristics of the somatic chromosome complement of an individual or species, described in terms of number, form, size, and arrangement within the nucleus, as determined by a microphotograph taken during the metaphase stage of mitosis. **2.** a diagrammatic representation of the chromosome complement of an individual or species, arranged in pairs in descending order of size and according to the position of the centromere. See also **chromosome, Denver classification. –karyotypic,** *adj.*

Kasai operation. See **portoenterostomy.**

kat-, kata-, cat-, cata-, a combining form meaning 'down, against': *katadidymus, katakinetomeric, katolysis.*

katadidymus /kat'ədid'əməs/, conjoined twins that are united in the lower portion of the body and separated at the top.

katal (K, kat), an enzyme unit in moles per second defined by the SI system: 1 K = 6.6 × 10^9 U.

Kavrin, a trademark for a smooth muscle relaxant (papaverine hydrochloride).

Kawasaki disease. See **mucocutaneous lymph node syndrome.**

KayCiel, a trademark for an electrolyte replacement solution (potassium chloride).

Kayser-Fleischer ring /kī′zərflī′shər/, a gray-green to red-gold pigmented ring at the outer margin of the cornea, pathognomonic of hepatolenticular degeneration, a rare progressive disease caused by a defect in copper metabolism and transmitted as an autosomal recessive trait. The disease is characterized by cerebral degenerative changes, liver cirrhosis, splenomegaly, involuntary movements, muscle rigidity, psychic disturbances, and dysphagia. See also **Wilson's disease.**

Kazanjian's operation, a surgical procedure for extending the vestibular sulcus to improve prosthetic foundation of edentulous ridges.

K capture, an electron capture process in which a K-shell electron is captured by the atomic nucleus.

K cell. See **null cell.**

Kedani fever. See **scrub typhus.**

kefir /kef′ər/, a slightly effervescent, acidulous beverage prepared from the milk of cows, sheep, or goats through fermentation by kefir grains, which contain yeasts and lactobacilli. It is an important source of the bacteria necessary in the GI tract to synthesize vitamin K. Also spelled **kephir.**

Keflex, a trademark for an antibacterial (cephalexin).

Keflin, a trademark for an antibiotic (cephalothin).

Kefzol, a trademark for an antibacterial (cefazolin sodium).

Kegel exercises. See **pubococcygeus exercises.**

Keith-Flack node. See **sinoatrial node.**

kel-, a combining form meaning 'of or pertaining to a tumor': *kelectome, keloid, keloplasty*.

Kellgren's syndrome /kel′grinz/, a form of osteoarthritis affecting the proximal and distal interphalangeal joints, the first metatarsophalangeal and carpometacarpal joints, the knees, and the spine. The absence of rheumatoid factor and rheumatoid nodules and the lack of systemic involvement differentiate this syndrome from rheumatoid arthritis. Also called **erosive osteoarthritis.**

Kelly clamp, a curved hemostat without teeth, used primarily in gynecologic procedures for grasping vascular tissue.

Kelly's pad, a horseshoe-shaped, inflatable rubber drainage pad used in a bed or on the operating table.

keloid /kē′loid/, overgrowth of collagenous scar tissue at the site of a wound of the skin. The new tissue is elevated, rounded, and firm, with irregular, clawlike margins. Young women and blacks are particularly susceptible to keloid formation. Most keloids flatten and become less noticeable over a period of years. Types of therapy include solid carbon dioxide, liquid nitrogen, intralesional corticosteroid injections, radiation, and surgery. Treatment may worsen the condition and should be performed only by skilled professionals. Also spelled **cheloid. –keloidal, cheloidal,** *adj.*

keloidosis /kē′loidō′sis/, habitual or multiple formation of keloids. Also spelled **cheloidosis.**

Kemadrin, a trademark for an antiparkinsonian skeletal muscle relaxant (procyclidine hydrochloride).

Kempner rice-fruit diet. See **rice diet.**

Kenacort Diacetate, a trademark for a glucocorticoid (triamcinolone diacetate).

Kenalog, a trademark for a glucocorticoid (triamcinolone acetonide).

Kennedy classification, a method of classifying edentulous conditions and partial dentures, based on the position of the spaces of the missing teeth in relation to the remaining teeth.

Kenny treatment. See **Sister Kenny's treatment.**

keno-, a combining form meaning 'empty': *kenophobia, kenotoxin, kenotron*.

kenogenesis. See **cenogenesis.**

kenophobia /kē′nō-/, the morbid fear of large and open spaces; agoraphobia. Also called **cenophobia** /sē′nō-/.

Kent bundle, an accessory pathway between atria and ventricles outside of the conduction system and found on both sides of the heart. This congenital anomaly causes Wolff-Parkinson-White syndrome. Compare **bundle of His.**

Kenya fever. See **Marseilles fever.**

kephal-. See **cephal-.**

kephir. See **kefir.**

kera-, a combining form meaning 'horn': *keracele, keraphyllocele*.

kerasin, a cerebroside, found in brain tissue, that consists of a fatty acid, galactose, and sphingosine.

kerat-, kerato-, **1.** a combining form meaning 'horny, cornified': *keratolysis, keratoma, keratonosis*. **2.** a combining form meaning 'cornea, corneal': *keratoiritis, keratoleukoma, keratome*.

keratectomy, surgical removal of a portion of the cornea, performed to excise a small, superficial lesion that does not warrant a corneal graft. Local anesthesia is used. The scar is excised, and an antibiotic is injected under the conjunctiva. A topical steroid is given, and a light pressure dressing is applied. Postoperatively, the dressings are changed daily. Corneal epithelium grows rapidly, filling a small surgical area in about 60 hours.

keratic /kərat′ik/, **1.** of or pertaining to keratin. **2.** of or pertaining to the cornea.

keratic precipitate, a group of inflammatory cells deposited on the endothelial surface of the cornea after trauma or inflammation, sometimes obscuring vision.

keratin /ker′ətin/, a fibrous, sulfur-containing protein that is the primary component of the epidermis, hair, nails, enamel of the teeth, and horny tissue of animals. The protein is insoluble in most solvents and is not dissolved by the gastric juice. For this reason, it is often used as a coating for pills that must pass through the stomach unchanged in order to be dissolved in the intestines.

keratinization, a process by which epithelial cells exposed to the external environment lose their moisture and are replaced by horny tissue.

keratinocyte, an epidermal cell that synthesizes keratin and other proteins and sterols. These cells constitute 95% of the epidermis, being formed as undifferentiated, or basal, cells at the dermal-epidermal junction. In its various successive stages keratin forms the prickle cell layer and the granular cell layer, in which the cells become flattened and slowly die to form the final layer, the stratum corneum, which gradually exfoliates.

keratitis /ker′ətī′tis/, any inflammation of the cornea. Kinds of keratitis include **dendritic keratitis, interstitial keratitis, keratoconjunctivitis sicca,** and **trachoma.** Compare **keratopathy.** **–keratic,** *adj.*

keratoacanthoma /ker′ətō•ak′anthō′mə/, *pl.* **keratoacanthomas, keratoacanthomata,** a benign, rapidly growing, flesh-colored papule of the skin with a central plug of keratin. The lesion is most common on the face or the back of the hands and arms. It disappears spontaneously in 4 to 6 months, leaving a slightly depressed scar. Biopsy is often necessary to differentiate it from a squamous carcinoma.

keratoconjunctivitis /ker′ətōkənjungk′tivī′tis/, inflammation of the cornea and the conjunctiva. Kinds of keratoconjunctivitis include **eczematous conjunctivitis, epidemic keratoconjunctivitis,** and **keratoconjunctivitis sicca.**

keratoconjunctivitis sicca, dryness of the cornea caused by a deficiency of tear secretion in which the corneal surface appears dull and rough, and the eye feels gritty and irritated. The condition may be associated with erythema multiforme, Sjögren's syndrome, trachoma, and vitamin A deficiency. Methylcellulose artificial tears may give some relief.

keratoconus /ker′ətōkō′nəs/, a noninflammatory protrusion of the central part of the cornea. More common in females, it may cause marked astigmatism; contact lenses usually restore visual acuity. The cause of the condition is unknown.

keratohyalin, a substance in the granules found in keratinocytes of the epidermis. The keratohyalin granule develops within and around the fibrillar protein, contributing in an unknown manner to the functional maturity of keratin.

keratolysis /ker′ətol′sis/,/ the loosening and shedding of the outer layer of the skin, which may occur normally by exfoliation or as a congenital condition in which the skin is shed at periodic intervals. **–keratolytic,** *adj.*

keratomalacia /ker′ətōməlā′shə/, a condition, characterized by xerosis and ulceration of the cornea, resulting from severe vitamin A deficiency. It commonly occurs as a secondary result of diseases that affect vitamin A absorption or storage, as ulcerative colitis, celiac syndrome, cystic fibrosis, or sprue. Also at risk are infants and children who are given dilute formula, who are malnourished, or who are allergic to whole milk and are fed skimmed milk, which is a poor source of vitamin A. Early symptoms include night blindness, photophobia, swelling and redness of the eyelids, and drying, roughness, pain, and wrinkling of the conjunctiva. In advanced deficiency, Bitot's spots appear, the cornea becomes dull, lusterless, and hazy, and, without adequate therapy, it eventually softens and perforates, resulting in blindness. Treatment consists of vitamin A supplements determined by the severity of the condition, although prolonged daily administration of large doses, especially to infants, may result in hypervitaminosis. An adequate diet containing whole milk and foods high in vitamin A or carotenes prevents the condition. See also **vitamin A.**

keratomycosis linguae. See **parasitic glossitis.**

keratopathy /ker′ətop′əthē/, any noninflammatory disease of the cornea. Compare **keratitis.**

keratoplasty, a procedure in ophthalmologic surgery in which an opaque portion of the cornea is excised.

keratosis /ker′ətō′sis/, any skin condition in which there is overgrowth and thickening of the cornified epithelium. Kinds of keratosis include **actinic keratosis, keratosis senilis,** and **seborrheic keratosis.** **–keratotic,** *adj.*

keratosis follicularis, a name of several skin disorders characterized by keratotic papules that coalesce to form brown or black, crusted, wartlike patches. These vegetations may spread widely, ulcerate, and become covered with a purulent exudate. Treatment includes large doses of vitamin A orally, topical vitamin A acid cream, and oral or topical corticosteroids. Also called **Darier's disease.**

keratosis seborrheica. See **seborrheic keratosis.**

kerauno-, a combining form meaning 'of or pertaining to lightning': *keraunoneurosis, keraunophobia.*

kerion /kir′ē•on/, an inflamed, boggy granuloma that develops as an immune reaction to a superficial fungus infection, generally in association with *Tinea capitis* of the scalp. The lesion heals within a short time without treatment.

KERMA, abbreviation for *kinetic energy released in the medium,* a quantity that describes the transfer of energy from a photon to a medium as the ratio of energy transferred per unit mass at each point of interaction.

kernicterus /kərnik′tərəs/, an abnormal toxic accumulation of bilirubin in central nervous system tissues caused by hyperbilirubinemia. See also **hyperbilirubinemia of the newborn.**

Kernig's sign, a diagnostic sign for meningitis marked by a loss of the ability of a seated or supine patient to completely extend the leg when the thigh is flexed on the abdomen. However, the patient usually can extend the leg completely when the thigh is not flexed on the abdomen.

kerosene poisoning, a toxic condition caused by the ingestion of kerosene or the inhalation of its fumes. Symptoms after ingestion include drowsiness, fever, a rapid heartbeat, tremors, and severe pneumonitis if the fluid is aspirated. Vomiting is not induced. Treatment for ingestion usually includes 1 or 2 ounces of vegetable oil to prevent absorption of the kerosene in the stomach and gastric lavage with copious amounts of water, a 3% sodium bicarbonate solution, or normal saline. Treatment for poisoning by inhalation includes fresh air, oxygen, and respiratory assistance if necessary. See also **petroleum distillate poisoning.**

Ketaject, a trademark for a general anesthetic (ketamine hydrochloride).

Ketalar, a trademark for a general anesthetic (ketamine hydrochloride).

ketamine hydrochloride /kē′təmēn/, a nonbarbiturate general anesthetic administered parenterally to achieve dissociative anesthesia. Because ketamine hydrochloride does not cause muscle relaxation, intubation is usually not required. Ketamine hydrochloride is particularly useful for brief, minor surgical procedures and for the induction of inhalation anesthesia in pediatric, geriatric, and disturbed patients. Hallucinations, confusion, and disorientation may occur on emergence from anesthesia. Other potential disadvantages attending use of this drug include increased blood pressure, increased cerebrospinal fluid pressure, increased intracranial pressure, and a tendency toward potentiation of the effects of alcohol, barbiturates, and narcotics. See also **dissociative anesthesia.**

keto-, a combining form indicating possession of the carbonyl (:C:O) group: *ketoheptose, ketolysis, ketonuria.*

ketoacidosis /kē′tō·as′idō′sis/, acidosis accompanied by an accumulation of ketones in the body, resulting from faulty carbohydrate metabolism. It occurs primarily as a complication of diabetes mellitus and is characterized by a fruity odor of acetone on the breath, mental confusion, dyspnea, nausea, vomiting, dehydration, weight loss, and, if untreated, coma. Emergency treatment includes the administration of insulin and IV fluids and the evaluation and correction of electrolyte imbalance. Nasogastric intubation and bladder catheterization may be required if the patient is comatose. Before discharge of the patient from the hospital, the nurse carefully reviews the diet, activity, urine testing, and insulin schedule prescribed, emphasizing to the patient that ketoacidosis may be life threatening and is largely avoidable by strict adherence to the patient's prescribed diabetic regimen. Compare **insulin shock.** See also **diabetes mellitus, ketosis.** **–ketoacidotic,** *adj.*

ketoaciduria /kē′tō·as′idŏŏr′ē·ə/, presence in the urine of excessive amounts of ketone bodies, occurring as a result of uncontrolled diabetes mellitus, starvation, or any other metabolic condition in which fats are rapidly catabolized. The condition can be diagnosed with a dipstick reagent or acetone test tablet. Also called **ketonuria.** See also **Acetest, ketosis.** **–ketoaciduric,** *adj.*

11-ketoandrosterone, a sex hormone, secreted by the testes and adrenal glands, that may be measured in the urine to assess hormonal and adrenal functions. Normal amounts in the urine of men after 24-hour collection are 0.2 to 1 mg; in women, 0.2 to 0.8 mg.

ketoconazole, an antifungal agent.

■ INDICATIONS: It is prescribed for the treatment of candidosis, coccidioidomycosis, histoplasmosis, and other fungal diseases.

■ CONTRAINDICATIONS: Known hypersensitivity to this drug prohibits its use. It should not be used for fungal meningitis.

■ ADVERSE EFFECTS: The most serious adverse reactions are liver disorders.

11-ketoetiocholanolone, a sex hormone, secreted by the testes and adrenal glands, that may be measured in the urine to assess hormonal and adrenal functions. Normal amounts in the urine of men after 24-hour collection are 0.2 to 1 mg; in women, 0.2 to 0.8 mg.

ketone alcohol /kē′tōn/, an alcohol containing the ketone group.

ketone bodies, the normal metabolic products, β-hydroxybutyric acid and aminoacetic acid, from which acetone may arise spontaneously. The two acids are products of lipid pyruvate metabolism, via acetyl-CoA in the liver, and are oxidized by the muscles. Excessive production of these bodies leads to their excretion in urine, as in diabetes mellitus. Also called **acetone bodies.**

ketonuria. See **ketoaciduria.**

ketose, the chemical form of a monosaccharide in which the carbonyl group is a ketone.

ketosis /kitō′sis/, the abnormal accumulation of ketones in the body as a result of a deficiency or inadequate utilization of carbohydrates. Fatty acids are metabolized instead, and the end products, ketones, begin to accumulate. This condition is seen in starvation, occasionally in pregnancy, if the intake of protein and carbohydrates is inadequate, and, most frequently, in diabetes mellitus. It is characterized by ketonuria, loss of potassium in the urine, and a fruity odor of acetone on the breath. Untreated, ketosis may progress to ketoacidosis, coma, and death. See also **diabetes mellitus, ketoacidosis, starvation.** **–ketotic,** *adj.*

ketosis-prone diabetes. See **insulin-dependent diabetes mellitus.**

ketosis-resistant diabetes. See **non-insulin-dependent diabetes mellitus.**

17-ketosteroid, any of the adrenal cortical hormones, or ketosteroids, that has a ketone group attached to its seventeenth carbon atom, commonly measured in the blood and urine to aid the diagnoses of Addison's disease, Cushing's syndrome, stress, and endocrine problems associated with precocious puberty, feminization in men, and excessive hair growth. Measured in patients in the morning, the normal concentration in plasma is less than 30 μg/dl; in the evening, less than 10 μg/dl. The normal amounts in the urine of men after 24-hour collection are 8 to 15 mg; in women, 6 to 11.5 mg; in children 12 to 15 years of age, 5 to 12 mg; in children less than 12 years of age, less than 5 mg. Levels of 17-ketosteroids increase 50% to 100% after an injection of ACTH.

keV, an energy unit equal to 1000 electron volts.

Kew Gardens spotted fever. See **rickettsialpox.**

keypad, a numeric keyboard consisting of the numerals 1 to 9 arranged in three ranks of three keys each and an additional key for zero, as on some calculators.

key ridge, the lowest point of the zygomaticomaxillary ridge.

kg, abbreviation for **kilogram.**

kidney, one of a pair of bean-shaped urinary organs in the dorsal part of the abdomen, one on each side of the vertebral column. The cranial extremities of the kidneys are on a level with the cranial border of the twelfth thoracic vertebra, and the caudal extremities are on a level with the third lumbar vertebra. In most individuals, the right kidney is more caudal than the left. Each kidney is about 11 cm long, 6 cm wide, and 2.5 cm thick. In men, each kidney weighs from 125 to 170 g; in women, each kidney weighs from 115 to 155 g. In the newborn, the kidneys are about three times as large in proportion to the body weight as in the adult. The kidneys produce and eliminate urine through a complex filtration network and reabsorption system comprising more than 2 million nephrons. The nephrons are composed of glomeruli and renal tubules that filter blood under high pressure, removing urea, salts, and other soluble wastes from blood plasma and returning the purified filtrate to the blood. More than 2500 pints of blood pass through the kidneys every day, entering the kidneys through the renal arteries and leaving through the renal veins. All the blood in the body passes through the kidneys about 20 times every hour but only about one fifth of the plasma is filtered by the nephrons during that period. The kidneys remove water as urine and return water that has been filtered to the blood plasma, thus helping to maintain the water balance of the body. Hormones, especially the antidiuretic hormone (ADH), produced by the pituitary gland, control the function of the kidneys in regulating the water content of the body. ADH reaches the renal tubules in the blood and stimulates the reabsorption of water from the filtrate into the blood. If water intake is inadequate to compensate for the water lost in perspiration and in respiration, the change in concentration in the blood is detected by the brain and the pituitary gland releases more ADH, thus reducing the loss of water in urine. If the blood is too dilute, the pituitary gland reduces the secretion of ADH, producing a large flow of dilute urine to restore the water balance.

kidney cancer, a malignant neoplasm of the renal parenchyma or renal pelvis. Factors associated with an increased incidence of disease are exposure to aromatic hydrocarbons or tobacco smoke and the use of drugs containing phenacetin. A long asymptomatic period may precede the onset of the characteristic symptoms, which include hematuria, flank pain, fever, and the detection of a palpable mass. Diagnostic measures include urinalysis, excretory urography, nephrotomography, ultrasonography, renal arteriography, and microscopic and cytologic studies of cells from the renal pelvis. Adenocarcinoma of the renal parenchyma accounts for 80% of kidney tumors, occurring twice as frequently in men as in women; transitional cell or squamous cell carcinomas in the renal pelvis account for approximately 15% and are equally frequent in men and women. Radical nephrectomy with lymph node dissection is usually recommended for tumors of the parenchyma; nephroureterectomy is usually recommended for operable tumors of the renal pelvis. Radiotherapy may be used preoperatively or postoperatively and as palliation for inoperable tumors. Chemotherapeutic agents that may induce temporary remission are cyclophosphamide, bleomycin, hydroxyurea, and vinblastine. See also **Wilms' tumor.**

kidney dialysis. See **hemodialysis.**

kidney disease, any one of a large group of conditions including infectious, inflammatory, obstructive, vascular, and neoplastic disorders of the kidney. Characteristics of kidney disease are hematuria, persistent proteinuria, pyuria, edema, dysuria, and pain in the flank. Specific symptoms vary with the type of disorder, for example: Hematuria with severe, colicky pain suggests obstruction by a kidney stone; hematuria without pain may indicate renal carcinoma; proteinuria is generally a sign of disease in the glomerulus, or filtration unit of the kidney; pyuria indicates infectious disease; and edema is characteristic of the nephrotic syndrome. Diagnosis of kidney disease is made after laboratory tests and other procedures have been performed. Among the special tests for kidney disorders are excretory urography, intravenous pyelography, tests of the glomerular filtration rate, biopsy, and ultrasound examination. Treatment depends upon the type of kidney disease diagnosed. Some forms of advanced kidney disease may lead to renal failure, coma, and death unless hemodialysis is started. See also **glomerulonephritis, nephrotic syndrome, renal failure, urinary calculus.**

kidney failure, *informal.* renal failure.

kidney machine. See **artificial kidney, dialyzer,** def. 1.

kidney stone. See **renal calculus.**

Kielland forceps. See **obstetric forceps.**

Kielland rotation, an obstetric operation in which Kielland forceps are used in turning the head of the fetus from an occiput posterior or occiput transverse position to an occiput anterior position. It is performed most commonly to correct an arrest in the active stage of labor. The rotation is done at the midplane of the pelvis. As it is associated with increased harm to the mother and to the baby, cesarean section is often preferred. See also **forceps delivery, obstetric forceps.**

killer cell. See **null cell.**

kilo-, a combining form meaning 'one thousand': *kilocalorie, kilogram, kilometer.*

kilobyte (K, Kb), one thousand (or, more precisely, 1024) bytes.

kilogram (kg) /kil′əgram/, a unit for the measurement of mass in the metric system. One kilogram is equal to 1000 grams or to 2.2046 pounds avoirdupois.

kilogram calorie. See **calorie.**

Kimmelstiel-Wilson disease. See **intercapillary glomerulosclerosis.**

kinase /kī′nās/, **1.** an enzyme that catalyzes the transfer of a phosphate group or another high-energy molecular group to an acceptor molecule. Each of these kinases is named for its receptor, as acetate kinase, fructokinase, or hexokinase. **2.** an enzyme that activates a preenzyme (zymogen). Each of these kinases is named for its source, as bacterial kinase, enterokinase, fibrinokinase, insulin kinase, staphylokinase, streptokinase, streptokinase-streptodornase, or urokinase.

kine-. See **kinesio-.**

kinematic face-bow, an adjustable caliper-like device, used for precisely locating the axis of rotation of a mandible through the sagittal plane.

kinematics /kin′əmat′iks, kī-′/, (in physiology) the geometry of the motion of the body without regard to the forces acting to produce the motion. Kinematics deals with the description and the measurement of body motion and the means of recording it. Recordings of body motions are defined in one-plane relationships, although natural motions of the body often occur in more than one plane. Kinematics considers the motions of all body parts relative to the segments of the part involved in the motion and not necessarily in relation to the standard anatomic position; for example, the movements of the fingers are considered in relation to the midline of the hand, not the midline of the body. The most common types of motions studied in kinematics are flexion, extension, adduction, abduction, internal rotation, and external rotation. Kinematics is especially important in orthopedics and rehabilitation medicine. Also spelled **cinematics.** Compare **kinetics.**

kinesics /kinē′siks/, the study of body position and movement in relation to communication. The observance of nonverbal interactional behavior is an integral part of nursing assessment and is used especially in mental health assessment as an objective and measurable tool for diagnosing disturbances of communication and behavioral disorders. See also **body language, communication.**

kinesio-, kine-, a combining form meaning 'of or pertaining to movement': *kinesiology, kinesioneurosis, kinesiotherapy.*

kinesiology /kinē′sē•ol′əjē, kī-/, the scientific study of muscular activity and of the anatomy, physiology, and mechanics of the movement of body parts.

-kinesis, -cinesia, -cinesis, -kinesia, 1. a combining form meaning an 'activation': *angiokinesis, lymphokinesis, thrombokinesis.* **2.** a combining form meaning a 'division (of cells)': *catakinesis, diakinesis, heterokinesis.*

kinesthetic memory, the recollection of movement, weight, resistance, and position of the body or parts of the body.

-kinetic, -cinetic, -cinetical, -kinetical, 1. a combining form meaning 'pertaining to motion': *akinetic, parakinetic, synkinetic.* **2.** a combining form meaning 'pertaining to a (specified) agent causing motion': *chemokinetic, ideokinetic, photokinetic.* **3.** a combining form meaning 'referring to kinesis': *astrokinetic, biokinetic, catakinetic.* **4.** a combining form meaning 'referring to activation of a body part by a (specified) agent': *angiokinetic, gametokinetic, gonadokinetic.*

kinetic analysis, analysis in which the change of the monitored parameter with time is related to concentration, as change of absorbance per minute.

kinetics /kinet′iks, kī-/, (in physiology) the study of the forces that produce, arrest, or modify the motions of the body. Newton's first and third laws of inertia are especially applicable to kinetics. Newton's first law states that bodies at rest tend to stay at rest and bodies in motion tend to keep moving. Newton's third law states that action and reaction are equal in magnitude but opposite in direction. These two laws are applicable to the forces produced by muscles of the body that act on joints. The reaction forces of the muscles contribute to the equilibrium and the motion of the body. Compare **kinematics.**

kineto-, a combining form meaning 'movable': *kinetochore, kinetogenic, kinetoplasm.*

kinetochore. See **centromere.**

kinetotherapeutic bath /kinet′ōthur′əpyo͞o′tik/, a bath in which underwater exercises are performed to strengthen weak or partially paralyzed muscles.

kino-, a combining form meaning 'of or pertaining to movement': *kinoplasm, kinosphere, kinotoxin.*

kinomere. See **centromere.**

kinship model family group, a family unit comprised of the biologic parents and their offspring. It is like a nuclear family but is more closely tied to an extended family. Characteristics of this family group include dominance by the maternal grandmother, who raises the children and makes most of the decisions, clearly delineated sex roles, and resistance to change.

Kirkland knife, a surgical knife with a heart-shaped blade, sharp on all edges, used for a primary gingivectomy incision.

Kirschner's wire /kursh′nərz/, a threaded or smooth metallic wire available in three diameters and 22.86 cm long. The wire is used in internal fixation of fractures or for skeletal traction.

kiting, *informal.* the improper and illegal practice of altering a drug prescription to indicate that more of a drug was prescribed than was actually ordered by the physician. Kiting may be done by a patient seeking greater quantities of drugs, especially narcotics, than the physician prescribed, or may be done by the pharmacist to increase reimbursement from a third party, as the involved insurance company.

klang association. See **clang association.**

Klebsiella /kleb′zē•el′ə/, a genus of diplococcal bacteria that appear as small, plump rods with rounded ends. Several respiratory diseases, including bronchitis, sinusitis, and some forms of pneumonia, are caused by infection by species of *Klebsiella.*

Klebs-Loeffler bacillus /klebz′lef′lər/, *Corynebacterium diphtheriae.*

kleeblattschädel deformity syndrome. See **cloverleaf skull deformity.**

Kleine-Levin syndrome /klīn′ləvēn′/, a disorder of unknown cause often associated with psychotic conditions, characterized by episodic somnolence, abnormal hunger, and hyperactivity. The episodes of sleep may last for several hours or days and are followed by confusion on awakening. There is no specific treatment. Compare **narcolepsy.**

klepto-, a combining form meaning 'of or pertaining to theft or stealing': *kleptolagnia, kleptomania.*

kleptolagnia /klep′tōlag′nē•ə/, sexual excitement or gratification produced by stealing.

kleptomania a neurosis characterized by an abnormal, uncontrollable, and recurrent urge to steal. The objects, taken not for their monetary value, immediate need, or utility but because of a symbolic meaning usually associated with some unconscious emotional conflict, are usually given away, returned surreptitiously, or kept and hidden. People who have the condition experience an increased sense of tension before committing the theft and intense gratification during the act. Afterward, they display signs of depression, guilt, and anxiety over the possibility of being apprehended and losing status in society. In less severe cases, the impulse is expressed by the continuous borrowing of objects and not returning them. Treatment consists of psychotherapy to uncover the underlying emotional problems. Also spelled **cleptomania.** **–kleptomaniac,** *n.*

Klinefelter's syndrome /klīn′feltərz/, a syndrome of gonadal defects, appearing in males, with an extra X chromosome in at least one cell line. Characteristics are small, firm testes, long legs, gynecomastia, poor social adaptation, subnormal intelligence, chronic pulmonary disease, and varicose veins. The severity of the abnormalities increases with greater numbers of X chromosomes. The most common abnormality is a 47 XXY karyotype. Men with the karyotype XXXXY have marked congenital malformations and mental retardation.

Klippel-Feil syndrome. See **congenital short neck syndrome.**

Kloehn cervical extraoral orthodontic appliance, a cervical extraoral traction appliance for correcting or improving malocclusion. It consists of a relatively light and flexible 0.045 inch (1.15 mm) inner arch rigidly attached to a long outer bow.

K-Lor, a trademark for an electrolyte replacement solution (potassium chloride).

Klorvess, a trademark for an electrolyte replenisher (potassium chloride).

K-Lyte/Cl, a trademark for an electrolyte replacement solution (potassium chloride).

kneading, a grasping, rolling, and pressing movement, as is used in massaging the muscles. See also **massage.**

knee, a joint complex that connects the thigh with the lower leg. It consists of three condyloid joints, 12 ligaments, 13 bursae, and the patella. Two of the condyloid joints comprising the knee are between the condyles of the femur and the corresponding menisci and condyles of the tibia. The third condyloid joint within the knee is a partially arthrodial joint between the patella and the femur. The motion of this joint is not a simple gliding motion, because the articular surfaces of the bones involved are not mutually adapted to each other. The ligaments of the knee include the articular capsule, the patellar ligament, the oblique popliteal ligament, the arcuate popliteal ligament, the tibial collateral ligament, the fibular collateral ligament, the anterior cruciate ligament, the posterior cruciate ligament, the medial and the lateral menisci, the transverse ligament, and the coronary ligament. Four of the bursae of the knee are located in front, four laterally, and five medially. The largest bursa is the prepatellar bursa between the patellar ligament and the skin. The painful condition "housemaid's knee" is caused by inflammation of the prepatellar bursa. The knee is relatively unprotected by surrounding muscles and is often injured by blows, sudden stops, and turns, especially those associated with sports. Ligamental tears of the knee joint are extremely common in athletes and produce a variety of signs and symptoms, as effusion surrounding the knee joint, varying degrees of edema, differences in the shape of the knee joint, tenderness on palpation, crepitation, instability of the knee joint, and possible ecchymosis. Radiographic examination may reveal varying degrees of displacement from ligamental tears, but the primary ligamentous injuries are not visible on x-ray films. Ligamental tears are a form of sprain and are treated according to the degree of trauma. Mild tears involving only a few fibers usually do not require any treatment and heal with time. Moderate ligamental tears require protective treatment, with rest essential to healing. Aspiration of excessive joint fluid and compression of the joint may be performed to control swelling. Sports injuries of this kind are commonly taped in a special way or treated with splints. Surgical intervention is often necessary to repair severe ligamentous tears, and postoperative exercises are prescribed to strengthen knee structures. Torn menisci are very common sports injuries and can cause severe pain, limping, edema, and greatly reduced motion. Surgical intervention, as a meniscectomy, may be required. Various orthopedic conditions, as arthritis, commonly affect the knee, especially in elderly individuals, and require continuing treatment and special maintenance.

knee-ankle interaction, one of the five major kinetic determinants of gait, which helps to minimize the displacement of the center of gravity of the body during the walking cycle. The knee and the foot work simultaneously to lower the center of gravity of the body. When the heel of the foot is in contact with the ground, the foot is dorsiflexed and the knee is fully extended so that the associated limb is at its maximum length with the center of gravity at its lower point. Plantar flexion of the foot with the initiation of knee flexion maintains the center of gravity in its forward progression at about the same level, also helping to minimize the vertical displacement of the center of gravity. Knee-ankle interaction is often a factor in the diagnosis and treatment of various orthopedic diseases, deformities, and abnormal conditions, and in the analysis and the correction of pathologic gaits. Compare **knee-hip flexion, lateral pelvic displacement, pelvic rotation, pelvic tilt.**

kneecap. See **patella.**

knee-chest position. See **genupectoral position.**

knee-hip flexion, one of the five major kinematic determinants of gait, which allows the passage of body weight over the supporting extremity during the walking cycle. Knee-hip flexion occurs during the stance and the swing phases of the cycle. The knee first locks into extension as the heel of the weight-bearing limb strikes the ground and is unlocked by final flexion and initiation of the swing phase in the walking cycle. Hip flexion is synchronized with these movements, which help to minimize the vertical displacement of the center of gravity of the body in the act of walking. Knee-hip flexion is often a factor in the diagnosis and treatment of various orthopedic diseases, deformities, and abnormal conditions and in the analysis and correction of pathologic gaits. Compare **knee-ankle interaction, lateral pelvic displacement, pelvic rotation, pelvic tilt.**

knee-jerk reflex. See **patellar reflex.**

knee joint, the complex, hinged joint at the knee, regarded as three articulations in one, comprising condyloid joints connecting the femur and the tibia and a partly arthrodial joint connecting the patella and the femur. The knee joint and its ligaments permit flexion, extension, and, in certain positions, medial and lateral rotation. It is a common site for sprain and dislocation. Also called **articulatio genus.**

knee replacement, the surgical insertion of a hinged prosthesis, performed to relieve pain and restore motion to a knee severely affected by osteoarthritis, rheumatoid arthritis, or trauma. Under inhalation anesthesia, the diseased surfaces are removed and a two-piece metallic hinge is cemented into the medullary cavities of the femur and tibia. Postoperatively, the knee is held in a position of maximum extension, usually with a plaster cast. Progressive exercise and whirlpool baths are prescribed through physical therapy. Possible complications include infection, fat embolism, peroneal nerve palsy, loosening of the prosthesis, and flexion contractures. To prevent contractures, the nurse cautions the patient to keep the leg extended in bed; a blanket roll along the femur prevents external rotation. The mobility and range of motion of the joint increase slowly. See also **arthroplasty, hip replacement, osteoarthritis, plastic surgery.**

knife needle, a slender surgical knife with a needle point, used in the discission of a cataract and in other ophthalmic procedures, as goniotomy and goniopuncture.

knock-knee. See **genu valgum.**

Knoop hardness test, a method of measuring surface hardness by resistance to the penetration of an indenting tool made of diamond. The test produces a diamond-shaped indentation in the material involved and is commonly used for testing the hardness of tooth structure.

knot, (in surgery) the interlacing of the ends of a ligature or suture so that they remain in place without slipping or becoming detached. The ends of the suture are passed twice around each other before being pulled taut to make a simple surgeon's knot. For additional stability, the ends may be recrossed and a second simple knot made over the first. There are many kinds of knots, some of which are interlocking.

knowledge deficit, a nursing diagnosis accepted by the Fourth National Conference on the Classification of Nursing Diagnoses. The cause of the condition may be a lack of exposure to information, a lack of ability to recall the information, a misinterpretation of the information, a cognitive or perceptual limitation in the ability to learn or to understand the information, a lack of interest in acquiring the information, or an unfamiliarity with the resources necessary to gain the information. The defining characteristics of the knowledge deficit include a statement by the person that the deficit exists, or that there is a misconception concerning the information, an observed failure on the part of the client to follow through on instructions, the observation of an inadequate performance by the client on a test, a request by the person for information, or the observation of inappropriate or exaggerated behavior on the part of the client. See also **nursing diagnosis.**

Kocher's forceps /kō′kərz/, a kind of surgical forceps that has notched jaws, interlocking teeth, and thick, curved or straight, powerful handles.

Koch's postulates /kōks/, the prerequisites for establishing that a specific microorganism causes a particular disease. The conditions are the following: (1) The microorganism must be observed in all cases of the disease; (2) the microorganism must be isolated and grown in pure culture; (3) microorganisms from the pure culture, when inoculated into a susceptible animal, must reproduce the disease; (4) the microorganism must be observed in and recovered from the experimentally diseased animal.

Koebner phenomenon /kōb′nər/, the development of isomorphic lesions at the site of an injury occurring in psoriasis, lichen nitidus, lichen planus, and verruca plana.

koilo-, a combining form meaning 'hollow or concave': *koilonychia, koilorrhachic, koilosternia.*

koilonychia /koi′lōnik′ē·ə/, spoon nails; a condition in which nails are thin and concave from side to side. It is usually familial but may occur with iron deficiency anemia and Raynaud's phenomenon.

koinoni-, a combining form meaning 'of or pertaining to a community': *koinonia, koinoniphobia.*

kolpo-. See **colpo-.**

koly-, a combining form meaning 'to hinder': *kolypeptic, kolyphrenia, kolyseptic.*

kon-, a combining form meaning 'of or pertaining to dust': *konometer, koniocortex.*

Konakion, a trademark for a vitamin K formulation (phytonadione).

Konyne, a trademark for a hemostatic (factor IX complex).

Koplik's spots /kop′liks/, small red spots with bluish-white centers on the lingual and buccal mucosa, characteristic of measles. The rash of measles usually erupts a day or two after the appearance of Koplik's spots.

kopr-, kopra-. See **copro-.**

Korotkoff sounds /kôrot′kôf/, sounds heard during the taking of blood pressure using a sphygmomanometer and stethoscope. As air is released from the cuff, pressure on the brachial artery is reduced, and the blood is heard pulsing through the vessel. See also **blood pressure, diastole, sphygmomanometer, systole.**

Korsakoff's psychosis /kôr′səkôfs/, a form of amnesia often seen in chronic alcoholics, characterized by a loss of short-term memory and an inability to learn new skills. The person is usually disoriented and confabulates to conceal the condition. The cause of the condition can often be traced to degenerative changes in the thalamus as a result of a deficiency of B complex vitamins, especially thiamine and B_{12}. Compare **Wernicke's encephalopathy.**

kosher /kō′shər/, conforming to or prepared in accordance with the dietary or ceremonial laws of Judaism.

Krabbe's disease. See **galactosyl ceramide lipidosis.**

Kraske position /kras′kə/, an anatomic position in which the patient is prone, with hips flexed and elevated, head and feet down. The position is used for renal surgery, as it enlarges the costovertebral angle, allowing the surgeon to have optimal access to the kidneys.

kraurosis /krôrō′sis/, a thickening and shriveling of the skin. See also **kraurosis vulvae.**

kraurosis vulvae, a skin disease of aged women characterized by dryness, itching, and atrophy of the external genitalia. It is a condition that exhibits a predisposition to leukoplakia and carcinoma of the vulva. See also **lichen sclerosis et atrophicus.**

Krause's corpuscles, a number of sensory end organs in the conjunctiva of the eye, mucous membranes of the lips and tongue, epineurium of nerve trunks, the penis, and the clitoris, and the synovial membranes of certain joints. Krause's corpuscles are tiny cylindric oval bodies with a capsule formed by the expansion of the connective tissue sheath of a medullated fiber. They contain a soft, semifluid core in which the axon terminates either in a bulbous extremity or in a coiled mass. Also called **end bulbs of Krause.** Compare **Golgi-Mazzoni corpuscles, Pacini's corpuscles.**

Krebs' citric acid cycle /krebz/, a sequence of enzymatic reactions involving the metabolism of carbon chains of sugars, fatty acids, and amino acids to yield carbon dioxide, water, and high-energy phosphate bonds. The cycle is initiated when pyruvate combines with coenzyme A (CoA) to form a two-carbon unit, acetyl-CoA, which enters the cycle by combining with four-carbon oxaloacetic acid to form six-carbon citric acid. In subsequent steps isocitric acid, produced from citric acid, is oxidized to oxalosuccinic acid, which loses carbon dioxide to form alpha-ketoglutaric acid. Succinic acid, resulting from the oxidative decarboxylation of alpha-ketoglutaric acid, is oxidized to fumaric acid, and its oxidation regenerates oxalacetic acid, which condenses with acetyl-CoA, closing the cycle. The Krebs' cycle provides a major source of adenosine triphosphate energy and also produces intermediate molecules that are starting points for a number of vital metabolic pathways including amino acid synthesis. Also called **tricarboxylic acid cycle.** See also **acetylcoenzyme A.**

Krebs-Henseleit cycle. See **urea cycle.**

Krukenberg's tumor /kro͞o′kənbərgz/, a neoplasm of the ovary that is a metastasis of a GI malignancy, usually stomach cancer. Cytologic examination reveals mucoid degeneration and many large cells shaped like signet rings. Also called **carcinoma mucocellulare.**

krypto-. See **crypto-.**

KUB, abbreviation for *kidney, ureter, and bladder,* a term used in a radiographic examination to determine the location and size of the kidneys.

Kulchitsky cell carcinoma. See **carcinoid.**

Kulchitsky's cell. See **argentaffin cell.**

Küntscher nail /ko͝on′chər, kin′chər/, a stainless steel nail used in orthopedic surgery for the fixation of fractures of the long bones, especially the femur. Also called **Küntscher intramedullary nail.**

Kupffer's cells /ko͝op′fərz/, specialized cells of the reticuloendothelial system lining the sinusoids of the liver. The function of Kupffer's cells is to filter bacteria and other small, foreign proteins out of the blood.

kuru /ko͞o′ro͞o/, a slow, progressive, fatal viral infection of the central nervous system seen only in natives of the New Guinea highlands. The incubation period may be 30 or more years, but death usually occurs within months of the onset of symptoms. Characteristic of kuru are ataxia and decreased coordination progressing to paralysis, dementia, slurring of speech, and visual disturbances. Transmission of the disease is probably the result of cannibalism, as brain tissue from infected people produces the disease when inoculated in primates in the laboratory and incidence of the disease has declined with the decline of cannibalism.

Kussmaul breathing /ko͝os′moul/, abnormally deep, very rapid sighing respirations characteristic of diabetic acidosis.

Kussmaul's sign, **1.** a paradoxical rise in venous pressure with distention of the jugular veins during inspiration, as seen in constrictive pericarditis or mediastinal tumor. **2.** conditions of convulsions and coma associated with a GI disorder caused by absorption of a toxic substance.

Kveim reaction, a reaction used in a diagnostic test for sarcoidosis, based on an intradermal injection of antigen derived from a lymph node known to be sarcoid. If a noncaseating granuloma appears on the skin at the test site in 4 to 8 weeks, the reaction is said to be positive evidence that the patient has sarcoidosis.

kVp, abbreviation for *kilovolts peak,* the maximum amount of voltage applied to an x-ray tube, used in making an x-ray film.

kwashiorkor /kwä'shē·ôr'kôr/, a malnutrition disease, primarily of children, caused by severe protein deficiency, usually occurring when the child is weaned from the breast. Because calorie-rich starches like breadfruit are available, the child does not lose weight as dramatically and does not look as sick as a marasmic child, who lacks protein and calories. Eventually the following symptoms occur: retarded growth, changes in skin and hair pigmentation, diarrhea, loss of appetite, nervous irritability, edema, anemia, fatty degeneration of the liver, necrosis, dermatoses, and fibrosis, often accompanied by infection and multivitamin deficiencies. Because dietary fats are poorly tolerated in kwashiorkor, a skimmed milk formula is used in initial feedings, followed by additional foods until a full, well-balanced diet is achieved. Also called **infantile pellagra, malignant malnutrition.** See also **marasmic kwashiorkor, marasmus.**

Kwell, a trademark for a pediculicide and scabicide (gamma benzene hexachloride).

Kyasanur forest disease, an arbovirus infection transmitted by the bite of a tick that is harbored by shrews and other forest animals in western tropical India. Characteristics of the infection include fever, headache, muscle ache, cough, abdominal and eye pain, and photophobia. Treatment is symptomatic.

kymo-, a combining form meaning 'of or pertaining to waves': *kymograph, kymoscope, kymotrichous.*

kymography /kēmog'rəfē/, a technique for graphically recording motions of body organs, as of the heart and the great blood vessels.

kyno-, a combining form meaning 'of or pertaining to dogs': *kynocephalus, kynophobia.*

kypho-, a combining form meaning 'of or pertaining to a hump': *kyphoscoliosis, kyphosis, kyphotone.*

kyphoscoliosis /kī'fōskō'lē·ō'sis/, an abnormal condition characterized by an anteroposterior curvature and a lateral curvature of the spine. It occurs in children and adults, often associated with cor pulmonale. Compare **kyphosis, scoliosis.** **–kyphoscoliotic,** *adj.*

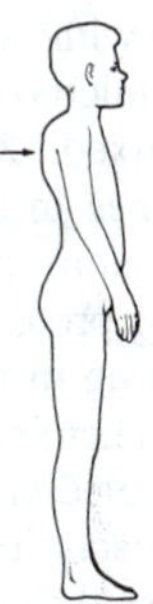

Kyphosis

kyphosis /kīfō'sis/, an abnormal condition of the vertebral column, characterized by increased convexity in the curvature of the thoracic spine as viewed from the side. Kyphosis may be caused by rickets or tuberculosis of the spine. Adolescent kyphosis is usually self-limiting and often undiagnosed, but if the curvature progresses, there may be moderate back pain. Conservative treatment consists of spine-stretching exercises and sleeping without a pillow, with a board under the mattress. A modified Milwaukee brace may be used for severe kyphosis, and, rarely, spinal fusion may be required. **–kyphotic,** *adj.*

kysth-, kystho-. See **colpo-.**

kyto-. See **cyt-.**

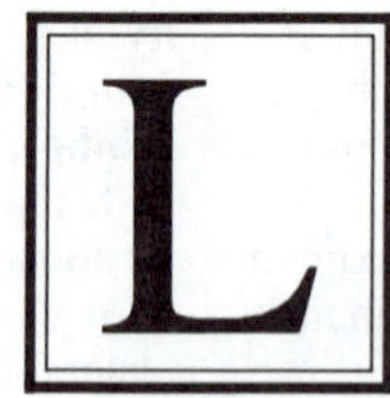

L, **1.** symbol for **liter.** **2.** symbol for **lung.**

La, symbol for **lanthanum.**

label, **1.** a substance with a special affinity for an organ, tissue, cell, or microorganism in which it may become deposited and fixed. **2.** the process of depositing and fixing a substance in an organ, tissue, cell, or microorganism. **3.** an atom or molecule attached to either a ligand or binding protein and capable of generating a signal for monitoring in the binding reaction.

labeled compound, a chemical substance in which part of the molecules are labeled with a radionuclide so that observations of the radioactivity or isotopic composition make it possible to follow the compound or its fragments through physical, chemical, or biologic processes.

labeling, **1.** the providing of information on a drug, food, device, or cosmetic to the purchaser or user. The information may be in any one of various forms, including printing on a carton, adhesive label, package insert, and monograph. Regulations for labeling are provided by the Food and Drug Administration. The label must contain directions for use, unless such directions are exempted by regulation, as well as warnings or contraindications. It must not contain false or misleading information. **2.** the assignment of a word or term to a form of behavior.

labia, *sing.* **labium,** **1.** the lips; the fleshy, liplike edges of an organ or tissue. **2.** the folds of skin at the opening of the vagina.

-labial, a combining form meaning 'of or pertaining to lips': *alveololabial, glossolabial, maxillolabial.*

labial bar, a major connector that is installed labial or buccal to the dental arch and joins bilateral parts of a mandibular removable partial denture.

labial flange, the part of a denture flange that occupies the labial vestibule of the mouth.

labial notch, a depression in the denture border that accommodates the labial frenum.

labia majora /majôr′ə/, *sing.* **labium majus** /mā′jəs/, two long lips of skin one on each side of the vaginal orifice outside the labia minora. They extend from the anterior labial commissure to the posterior labial commissure and form the lateral boundaries of the pudendal cleft. Each labium contains areolar tissue, fat, and a thin layer of nonstriated muscle. In some women the outer surface of each lip may be covered with coarse pubic hair. The embryologic derivation of the labia majora and the scrotum are homologous.

labia minora /minôr′ə/, *sing.* **labium minus** /mē′nəs/, two folds of skin between the labia majora, extending from the clitoris backward on both sides of the vaginal orifice, ending between it and the labia majora. Anteriorly, each labium divides into an upper and a lower division. The upper divisions pass above the clitoris and meet to form the preputium clitoridis; the lower divisions pass beneath the clitoris and unite to form the frenulum of the clitoris. Opposed surfaces of the labia minora contain sebaceous follicles.

LaBID, a trademark for a smooth muscle relaxant (theophylline).

labile /lā′bil/, **1.** unstable; characterized by a tendency to change or to be altered or modified. **2.** (in psychiatry) characterized by rapidly shifting or changing emotions, as in bipolar disorder and certain types of schizophrenia; emotionally unstable. **–lability,** *n.*

-labile, a combining form meaning 'unstable, subject to change': *frigolabile, siccolabile, thixolabile.*

labio-, a combining form meaning 'of or pertaining to the lips, particularly the lips of the mouth': *labiocervical, labiodental, labiomental.*

labioglossolaryngeal paralysis. See **bulbar paralysis.**

labiolingual fixed orthodontic appliance, an orthodontic appliance for correcting or improving malocclusion, characterized by anchorage to the maxillary and mandibular first permanent molars and by labial and lingual arches 0.09 to 0.10 cm in diameter. The labial arches fit into horizontal buccal tubes attached to anchor bands. The lingual arches are fastened to the lingual side of the anchor bands.

labium. See **labia.**

labium majus. See **labia majora.**

labium minus. See **labia minora.**

labor, the time and the processes that occur during parturition from the beginning of cervical dilatation to the delivery of the placenta. See also **birth, cardinal movements of labor, station.**

labor, abnormal. See **dystocia.**

laboratory, **1.** a facility, room, building, or part of a building in which scientific research, experimentation, testing, or other investigative activities are carried out. **2.** of or pertaining to a laboratory.

laboratory core. See **core.**

laboratory diagnosis, a diagnosis arrived at after study of secretions, excretions, or tissue through chemical, microsopic, or bacteriologic means or by biopsy. See also **diagnosis.**

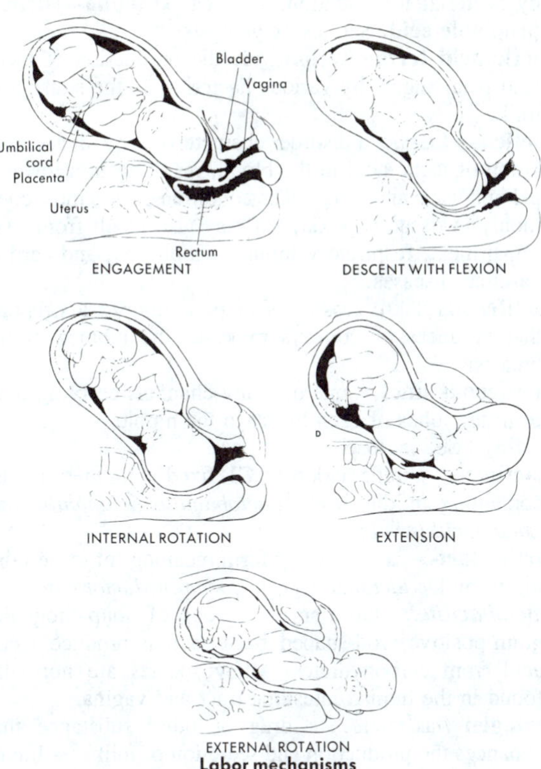

Labor mechanisms

laboratory error, any error made by the personnel in a clinical laboratory in the performance of a test, in the interpretation of the data, or in reporting or recording the results. Laboratory error must always be considered a possible explanation for findings that are at variance with the composite clinical condition of the patient or that are widely divergent from previous laboratory tests.

laboratory medicine, the branch of medicine in which specimens of tissue, fluid, or other body substance is examined outside of the person, usually in the laboratory. Some fields of laboratory medicine are **chemistry, cytology, hematology, histology,** and **pathology.**

laboratory test, a procedure, usually conducted in a laboratory, that is intended to detect, identify, or quantify one or more significant substances, evaluate organ functions, or establish the nature of a condition or disease. Laboratory tests range from quite simple to extremely sophisticated. In modern medical practice, they are commonly used to help establish or confirm a diagnosis and often aid in the management of disease.

labor coach, a person who assists a woman in labor and delivery by closely attending to her emotional needs and by encouraging her to use properly the breathing patterns, concentration techniques, body positions, and massage techniques that were taught in a program of psychophysical preparation for childbirth. The task of a labor coach is to minimize the need for pharmacologic pain relief used to decrease or eliminate the use of analgesia or anesthesia. Usually, the coach is the father of the baby or a close friend of the mother, but a professional labor coach, often a registered nurse specially trained in a method, may fill the role. See also **monitrice.**

labored breathing, abnormal respiration characterized by evidence of increased effort, including use of the accessory muscles of respiration of the chest wall, stridor, grunting, or nasal flaring.

labyrinth. See **internal ear.**

labyrinthitis, inflammation of the labyrinthine canals of the inner ear, resulting in vertigo.

labyrinthus osseus. See **osseus labyrinth.**

laceration, **1.** the act of tearing or lacerating. **2.** a torn, jagged wound. **–lacerate,** *v.*, **lacerated,** *adj.*

lachrymal. See **lacrimal.**

lachrymation. See **lacrimation.**

lacri-, lachry-, a combining form meaning 'of or pertaining to tears': *lacrimalin, lacrimator, lacrimotomy.*

lacrimal /lak′riməl/, of or pertaining to tears. Also spelled **lachrymal.**

lacrimal apparatus, a network of structures of the eye that secrete tears and drain them from the surface of the eyeball. These parts include the lacrimal glands, the lacrimal ducts, the lacrimal sacs, and the nasolacrimal ducts.

lacrimal bone, one of the smallest and most fragile bones of the face, located at the anterior part of the medial wall of the orbit. It unites with the maxilla to form the lacrimal fossa, which contains the lacrimal duct.

lacrimal canaliculi. See **lacrimal duct.**

lacrimal caruncle, the small, reddish, fleshy protuberance that fills the triangular space between the medial margins of the upper and the lower eyelids. It contains sebaceous and sudoriferous glands and secretes a whitish substance that collects in the corner of the eye.

lacrimal duct, one of two channels through which tears pass from the lacrimal lake to the lacrimal sac of each eye. Also called **lacrimal canaliculi.**

lacrimal fistula, an abnormal communication from a tear duct or sac to the surface of the eye or eyelid.

lacrimal gland, one of a pair of glands situated superior and lateral to the eye bulb in the lacrimal fossa. It is an oval structure about the size of an almond and is divided into an orbital part and a palpebral part. The orbital part is connected to the periosteum of the orbit by a few fibrous bands and rests on the tendons of the recti superioris and the recti lateralis, which separate the gland from the eye bulb. The palpebral part is separated from the orbital part by a fibrous septum and projects into the back portion of the upper eyelid. The gland has about 10 ducts that run obliquely beneath the conjunctiva and open along the upper and lateral half of the superior conjunctival fornix. The watery secretion from the gland consists of the tears, slightly alkaline and saline, that moisten the conjunctiva.

lacrimal papilla, the small conic elevation on the medial margin of each eyelid, supporting an apex pierced by the punctum lacrimale through which tears emerge to moisten the conjunctiva.

lacrimal sac, the dilated end of each of the two nasolacrimal ducts. Each sac is lodged in a deep groove formed by the lacrimal bone and the frontal process of the maxilla. The sac is oval and about 13 mm long. Its upper end is closed and rounded, its lower end continuous with the nasolacrimal duct. The lacrimal sacs fill with tears secreted by the lacrimal glands and conveyed through the lacrimal ducts.

lacrimation /lak′rimā′shən/, **1.** the normal continuous secretion of tears by the lacrimal glands. **2.** an excessive amount of tear production, as in crying or weeping. Also spelled **lachrymation.**

lact-. See **lacto-.**

lactalbumin /lak′təlbyo͞o′min/, a simple, highly nutritious protein found in milk. It is similar to serum albumin. See also **albumin, serum albumin.**

lactase, an enzyme that catalyzes the hydrolysis of lactose to glucose and galactose. Lactase is concentrated in the kidney, liver, and intestinal mucosa. Also called **beta-galactosidase.**

lactase deficiency, an inherited abnormality in which the amount of the enzyme lactase is deficient, resulting in the inability to digest lactose. The deficiency occurs in infancy in severe form and persists throughout life. In adults, a relative deficiency may appear as a natural process of aging; it occurs more frequently in persons of Asiatic and African heritage. Lactase deficiency may result from subtotal gastrectomy, any disease of the small intestine in which structural changes occur, as tropic sprue, ulcerative colitis, infectious hepatitis, and kwashiorkor, or from malnutrition. See also **lactose intolerance.**

lactate dehydrogenase (LDH), an enzyme essential in carbohydrate metabolism. See also **Duchenne's muscular dystrophy.**

lactation, the process of the synthesis and secretion of milk from the breasts in the nourishment of an infant or child. See also **breast feeding.**

lacteal /lak′tē·əl/, of or pertaining to milk.

lacteal fistula, an abnormal passage opening into a lacteal duct.

lacteal gland, one of the many central lymphatic capillaries in the villi of the small intestine. It opens into the lymphatic vessels in the submucosa. The capillary is filled with chyle that turns milky white during the absorption of fat.

lactic, referring to milk and milk products. See also **lactic acid, lactose.**

lactic acid, a three-carbon organic acid produced by anaerobic respiration. There are three forms: L-lactic acid in muscle and blood is a product of glucose and glycogen metabolism; D-lactic acid is produced by the fermentation of dextrose by a species of micrococcus; DL-lactic acid is a racemic mixture found in the stomach, in sour milk, and in certain other foods, as sauerkraut, prepared by bacterial fermentation. Also called **alpha-hydroxypropionic acid.** See also **glycolysis.**

lactic acid fermentation, 1. the production of lactic acid from sugars by various bacteria. **2.** the souring of milk.

lactic acidosis, a disorder characterized by an accumulation of lactic acid in the blood, resulting in a lowered pH in muscle and serum. The condition occurs most commonly in tissue hypoxia, but may also result from liver impairment, respiratory failure, neoplasms, and cardiovascular diseases.

lactiferous /laktif′ərəs/, of or pertaining to a structure that produces or conveys milk, as the tubules of the breasts.

lactiferous duct, one of many channels carrying milk from the lobes of each breast to the nipple.

lactin. See **lactose.**

Lactinex, a trademark for a GI, fixed-combination drug containing antidiarrheals (*Lactobacillus acidophilus* and *Lactobacillus bulgaricus*).

lacto-, lact-, a combining form meaning 'of or pertaining to milk': *lactobacillus, lactopeptin, lactotoxin.*

Lactobacillus, any one of a group of nonpathogenic, gram-positive, rod-shaped bacteria that produce lactic acid from carbohydrates. Many species are normally found in the human intestinal tract and vagina.

lactogen /lak′təjən/, a drug or other substance that enhances the production and secretion of milk. **–lactogenic,** *adj.*

lactogenic hormone. See **prolactin.**

lacto-ovo-vegetarian, one whose diet consists primarily of foods of vegetable origin and also includes some animal products, as eggs (*ovo*), milk, and cheese (*lacto*), but no meat, fish, or poultry. Also called **ovo-lacto-vegetarian.**

lactose, a disaccharide found in the milk of all mammals. On hydrolysis lactose yields the monosaccharides glucose and galactose. Lactose is used as a laxative, as a diuretic, and as a component of formulas for infants. Also called **lactin, milk sugar.** See also **sugar.**

lactose intolerance, a sensitivity disorder resulting in the inability to digest lactose because of a deficiency of or defect in the enzyme lactase. Symptoms of the disorder are bloating, flatus, nausea, diarrhea, and abdominal cramps. The diet is adjusted according to the tolerance level, restricting such foods as milk, cheese, butter, margarine, and any products containing milk, as cakes, ice cream, cream soups, and sauces. See also **lactase deficiency.**

lactosuria, the presence of lactose in the urine, a condition that may occur in late pregnancy or during lactation.

lacto-vegetarian, one whose diet consists of milk and milk products (*lacto*) in addition to foods of vegetable origin but does not include eggs, meat, fish, or poultry.

lactulose, a nonabsorbable synthetic disaccharide, 4-0-β-D-galactopyranosyl-D-fructose, $C_{12}H_{22}O_{11}$. It is hydrolyzed in the colon by bacteria, primarily to lactic acid and small amounts of formic and acetic acids, which results in increased osmotic pressure and acidification of the colonic contents. It is used as a cathartic in chronic constipation. Because the acidification causes ammonia to be removed from the blood to form ammonium ion, it is also used in the treatment of hepatic coma. Its ability to increase fecal water content, however, may also cause diarrhea.

lacuna /ləkyo͞o′nə/, *pl.* **lacunae,** **1.** a small cavity within a structure, especially bony tissue. **2.** a gap, as in the field of vision.

lacus lacrimalis /lā′kəs lak′rimā′ləs/, a triangular space separating the medial ends of the upper and the lower eyelids. It is an extension of the medial canthus and contains the lacrimal caruncle.

LADME /lad′mē/, an abbreviation for the time course of drug distribution, representing the terms *liberation, absorption, distribution, metabolism,* and *elimination.*

Laënnec's catarrh /lā′əneks′/, a form of bronchial asthma characterized by the discharge of small, round, viscous, beadlike bodies of sputum. These bodies, **Laënnec's pearls,** are formed in the bronchioles and appear in the asthmatic person's expectorated bronchial secretions.

Laetrile /lā′ətril/, a substance composed primarily of amygdalin, a cyanogenic glycoside derived from apricot pits. Laetrile has been offered as a cancer medication despite clinical studies by the National Cancer Institute that failed to show benefits from its use. It is claimed that amygdalin is hydrolyzed by enzymes in cancer cells to produce benzaldehyde and hydrogen cyanide, which kill the cancer cells. Also called **vitamin B_{17}.**

laevo-. See **levo-.**

lagen-, a combining form meaning 'flasklike': *lagena, lageniform.*

-lagnia, -lagny, a combining form meaning a 'sexual predilection': *osmolagnia, pyrolagnia, scoptolagnia.*

lagophthalmos /lag′əfthal′məs/, an abnormal condition in which an eye may not be fully closed because of a neurologic or muscular disorder. Also called **hare's eye.**

la grippe. See **influenza.**

laity, a nonprofessional segment of the population, as viewed from the perspective of a member of a particular profession. A clergyman may regard a physician as a member of the laity, and vice versa.

laked blood /lākt/, blood that is clear, red, and homogenous because of hemolysis of the red blood cells, as may occur in poisoning and severe, extensive burns.

lal-, lalio-, lalo-, a combining form meaning 'talk, babble': *laliatry, lalognosis, lalopathology.*

-lalia, a combining form meaning a 'disorder of speech': *agitolalia, eschrolalia, oxylalia.*

lalio-. See **lal-.**

laliophobia /lā′lē•ō-/, a morbid dread of talking caused by fear and anxiety that one will stammer or stutter. –**laliophobic,** *adj.*

lallation /lalā′shən/, **1.** babbling, repetitive, unintelligible utterances, like the babbling of an infant, and the mumbled speech of schizophrenics, alcoholics, and the severely mentally retarded. **2.** a speech disorder characterized by a defective pronunciation of words containing the sound "l" or by the use of the sound "l" in place of the sound "r." Compare **lambdacism, rhotacism.**

lalo-. See **lal-.**

lamarckism, the theory postulated by French naturalist Jean Baptiste de Lamarck that organic evolution results from structural changes in plants and animals that are caused by adaptation to environmental conditions and that these acquired characteristics are transmitted to offspring. Also called **lamarckianism, Lamarck's theory.** Compare **darwinism.** –**lamarckian,** *adj., n.*

Lamaze method /ləmäz′/, a method of psychophysical preparation for childbirth developed in the 1950s by a French obstetrician, Fernand Lamaze. It is based on the work of Ivan Pavlov and P.N. Nicolaiev with hypnosis and stimulus-response conditioning in Russia before 1950. The method was popularized in the United States by Marjorie Karmel who wrote the book *Thank you, Dr. Lamaze,* based on her experience delivering a child in Paris under the care of Dr. Lamaze. The first program was established at Mt. Sinai Hospital in New York City under the direction of Marjorie Karmel, Elisabeth Bing, a British physical therapist, and Dr. Alan Guttmacher. In 1960, the American Society for Psychoprophylaxis in Obstetrics was founded. The Lamaze method soon became the most often used method of natural childbirth. It requires classes, practice at home, and coaching during labor and delivery, often by a trained coach called a "monitrice." The classes, given during pregnancy, teach the physiology of pregnancy and childbirth, exercises to develop strength in the abdominal muscles and control of isolated muscles of the vagina and perineum, and techniques of breathing and relaxation to promote control and relaxation during labor. The woman is conditioned by repetition and practice to dissociate herself from the source of a stimulus by concentration on a focal point, by consciously relaxing all muscles, and by breathing in a special way at a particular rate—thereby training herself not to pay attention to the stimuli associated with labor. The kind and rate of breathing changes with the advancing stages of labor. During the early part of the first stage of labor, when the uterine cervix is dilated less than 5 cm and the contractions occur every 2 to 4 minutes, last 40 to 60 seconds, and are of mild to moderate strength, the mother does slow chest breathing during contractions. Her fingers may rest lightly on her lower ribs to feel them rise and fall. The abdominal wall does not move with respiration. She may perform an effleurage, or rhythmic fingertip massage, of her lower abdomen during the contractions. The rate of respiration is 10 or fewer breaths a minute, increasing to 12 per minute as labor intensifies. A deep "cleansing breath" is taken before and after each contraction. During the active part of the first stage of labor up to the transition to the second stage, the cervix is from 5 cm to nearly fully dilated, the interval between contractions is from 1-1/2 to 4 minutes, and the duration of contractions is from 45 to 90 seconds. (The interval decreases and the intensity and duration increase as labor progresses.) During contractions, the mother breathes quietly and shallowly in her chest. The rate of her breathing varies with the strength of the contractions, increasing during a contraction to as fast as once a second at the peak and slowing to every 6 seconds as the uterus relaxes. She is coached to concentrate on the focal point she has selected, to perform the effleurage of her abdomen, to relax her perineal and vaginal muscles, and to take a cleansing breath at the beginning and end of each contraction. At the end of the first stage of labor, when the cervix is almost completely dilated and the contractions are strong, occurring every 1-1/2 to 2 minutes and lasting 60 to 90 seconds, the mother begins to feel the urge to bear down and push during contractions. She avoids pushing before full dilatation by combining several light, shallow breaths in the chest with short puffing exhalations as the urge increases during the contractions. During the second stage of labor, the cervix is fully dilated and contractions are strong, frequent, and expulsive. The mother's head and shoulders are supported on pillows. During contractions, she is helped to draw her legs back, flexing the thighs against the abdomen, holding them behind the lower thigh with her hands. Her chin is tucked on her chest, the air is blocked from escaping from her lungs, her perineum is relaxed, and she bears down forcibly. Depending on the length of the contraction, several pushes of 10 to 15 or more seconds may be possible during the contraction. As the baby's head crowns, she is asked to pant lightly so that the head may be delivered slowly. The advantages of the method include the need for little or no analgesia for relief of pain and participation in the labor by the mother, giving her a great sense of self-satisfaction at delivery. Compare **Bradley method, Read method.**

lambdacism /lam′dəsiz′əm/, a speech disorder characterized by a defective pronunciation of words containing the sound /l/, or by the excessive use of the sound, or by the substitution of the sound /r/ for /l/. Compare **lallation, rhotacism.**

lambdoid /lam′doid/, having the shape of the Greek letter lamda. See also **lambdoidal suture.**

lambdoidal suture /lamdoi′dəl/, the serrated connection between the occipital bone and the parietal bones of the skull. It is continuous with the occipitomastoid suture between the occipital and the mastoid portions of the temporal bones.

lamella /ləmel′ə/, *pl.* **lamellae,** **1.** a thin leaf or plate, as of bone. **2.** a medicated disk, prepared from glycerin and an alkaloid, for insertion under the eyelid, where it dissolves and is absorbed.

lamellar exfoliation of the newborn, a congenital skin disorder transmitted as an autosomal recessive trait in which a parchmentlike, scaly membrane that covers the infant peels off within 24 hours of birth. Complete healing or a progressively less severe process of reforming and shedding of the scales then occurs. Also called **ichthyosis congenita, ichthyosis fetalis, lamellar desquamation of the newborn, lamellar ichthyosis of the newborn.** See also **collodion baby, lamellar ichthyosis.**

lamin-, a combining form meaning 'layer': *laminagram, laminated, laminotomy.*

lamina /lam′inə/, *pl.* **laminae,** a thin flat plate, as the lamina of the thyroid cartilage that overlays the structure on each side.

lamina dura, a sheet of compact alveolar bone that lies adjacent to the periodontal membrane.

lamina propria, a layer of connective tissue that lies just under the epithelium of the mucous membrane.

laminar flow, an airflow that is concentrated into a narrow pathway.

laminaria, a type of seaweed that swells on absorption of water.

laminaria tent, a cone of dried seaweed that swells as it absorbs water and therefore is used to dilate the cervix nontraumatically in preparation for induced abortion or induced labor.

laminated thrombus, a thrombus comprised of an aggregation of blood platelets, fibrin, clotting factors, and cellular elements, arranged in layers apparently formed at different times.

laminectomy, surgical chipping away of the bony arches of one or more vertebrae, performed to relieve compression of the spinal cord, as caused by a bone displaced in an injury or as the result of degeneration of a disk, or to reach and remove a displaced intervertebral disk. With the patient prone and under general anesthesia, the laminae are removed and the underlying problem corrected. Spinal fusion may be necessary for stability of the spine if several laminae are removed. After surgery, the bed is kept flat to hold the patient's spine in correct alignment. If the procedure was a cervical laminectomy, the patient is observed for signs of respiratory distress caused by cord edema. Motor function and sensation in the extremities are evaluated every 2 to 4 hours for 48 hours. The dressing is examined frequently for hemorrhage or leakage of cerebrospinal fluid. A sheet is used to logroll the patient without twisting the spine or hips. Ambulation often begins 3 to 5 days after surgery. **–laminectomize,** *v.*

lampbrush chromosome, an excessively large type of chromosome found in the oocytes of many lower animals. It has long, threadlike projecting loops, giving it a hairy, brushlike appearance. See also **giant chromosome.**

lampro-, a combining form meaning 'clear': *lamprophonia, lamprophonic.*

lanatoside C /lanat′əsīd/, a cardiotonic.

■ INDICATIONS: It is prescribed where digitalis action is required, as for congestive heart failure and cardiac arrhythmias.

■ CONTRAINDICATIONS: Ventricular tachycardia or known hypersensitivity to this drug prohibits its use.
■ ADVERSE EFFECTS: Among the more serious adverse reactions are irregular or slow pulse, nausea, tiredness, and loss of appetite.

lance, to incise a furuncle or an abscess to release accumulated pus. A topical anesthetic is applied, the lesion is incised, and the pus is drained. A drain is inserted if the infection is deep. The bacteria involved are most often staphylococci. The nurse uses aseptic technique; soiled dressings are wrapped in paper to be burned. An antibiotic is given systemically if the boil is facial to prevent infection from spreading into the cranial sinuses. Infected drainage is kept off surrounding skin to prevent a recurrence. The nurse teaches the patient and family stringent handwashing techniques.

Lancefield's classification, a serologic classification of streptococci based on their antigenic characteristics. The bacteria are divided into 13 groups by the identification of their pathologic action. Group A contains most of the streptococci that cause infection in humans. Groups B to T are less pathogenic and are often present without causing disease. Most are hemolytic; of those, the beta subgroup is the most likely to be the cause of infection.

Lancereaux's diabetes /lan′sərōz/, a chronic disease of carbohydrate metabolism characterized by marked emaciation. See also **diabetes mellitus.**

lancet, **1.** *obsolete.* a very small, pointed, surgical knife, sharp on both sides. **2.** a short pointed blade used to obtain a drop of blood for a capillary sample. It has a guard above the blade that prevents deep incision, and it is usually disposable.

lancinating /lan′sinā′ting/, sharply cutting or tearing, as lancinating pain.

Landau reflex /lan′dou/, a normal response of infants when held in a horizontal prone position to maintain a convex arc with the head raised and the legs slightly flexed. The reflex is poor in those with floppy infant syndrome and exaggerated in hypertonic and opisthotonic infants.

landmark position, the correct placement of the hands on the chest in cardiopulmonary resuscitation. See also **cardiopulmonary resuscitation.**

Landsteiner's classification /land′stī′nərz/, the classification of blood groups A, B, AB, and O on the basis of the presence or absence of the two agglutinogens A and B on the erythrocytes in human blood.

Langer's line. See **cleavage line.**

Langhans' layer. See **cytotrophoblast.**

language, a unified, related set of commands or instructions that a computer can accept. Also called **programing language.**

lano-, a combining form meaning 'of or pertaining to wool': *lanolin, lanonol, lanosterol.*

lanolin, a fatlike substance from the wool of sheep. It contains about 25% water as a water-in-oil emulsion and is used as an ointment base and an emollient for the skin. Also called **hydrous wool fat.**

Lanoxin, a trademark for a cardiotonic (digoxin).

lanthanum (La), a rare earth metallic element. Its atomic number is 57; its atomic weight is 138.91.

lanugo /lanyo͞o′gō/, **1.** the soft, downy hair covering a normal fetus, beginning with the fifth month of life and almost entirely shed by the ninth month. **2.** the fine, soft hair covering all parts of the body except palms, soles, and areas where other types of hair are normally found. Also called **vellus hair.**

lanulous /lan′yo͞oləs/, downy or covered with short, fine wooly hair, as the skin of a fetus. See also **lanugo.**

lapara-, laparo-, a combining form meaning 'of or pertaining to the loin or flank': *laparectomy, laparocele, laparorrhaphy.*

laparoscope /lap′əraskōp′/, a type of endoscope, consisting of an illuminated tube with an optical system, that is inserted through the abdominal wall for examining the peritoneal cavity. Also called **celioscope, peritoneoscope.** **–laparoscopic,** *adj.,* **laparascopy,** *v.*

laparoscopy /lap′əros′kəpē/, the examination of the abdominal cavity with a laparoscope through a small incision in the abdominal wall. The procedure is also used for examining the ovaries and fallopian tubes and as a gynecologic sterilization technique for fulgurating the oviducts. Also called **abdominoscopy.** See also **endoscopy, laparoscope.**

laparotomy /lap′ərot′əmē/, any surgical incision into the peritoneal cavity, usually performed under general or regional anesthesia, often on an exploratory basis. Before surgery, a complete blood count, a type and crossmatch of blood, and a urinalysis are done; the skin is shaved and cleansed from the nipple line to the pubis. A barbiturate may be given at bedtime. Food and fluids by mouth are not given after midnight. Shortly before surgery, a barbiturate or tranquilizer and a narcotic are usually given, with an anticholinergic agent such as atropine. If the intestine is to be opened, a nasogastric tube is passed. Frequent observation of vital signs and drainage systems is essential. Intake and output of fluids are recorded. The patient is turned and helped to cough and breathe deeply every hour; medication is given as needed for relief of pain. Some kinds of laparotomy are **appendectomy, cholecystectomy,** and **colostomy.** **–laparotomize,** *v.*

Laplace's law, a principle of physics that the tension on the wall of a sphere is the product of the pressure times the radius of the chamber and the tension is inversely related to the thickness of the wall. It is named for nineteenth century French physicist Marquis Pierre Simon Laplace.

-lapse, a combining form meaning 'a slip': *collapse, prolapse, relapse.*

large calorie. See **calorie.**

large for gestational age (LGA) infant, an infant whose fetal growth was accelerated and whose size and weight at birth fall above the ninetieth percentile of appropriate for gestational age infants, whether delivered prematurely, at term, or later than term. Factors other than genetic influences that cause accelerated intrauterine growth include maternal diabetes mellitus and Beckwith's syndrome. LGA infants born of diabetic mothers are generally obese and plethoric, with very pink skin and red, shiny cheeks. They are often listless and limp, feed poorly, and become hypoglycemic within the first few hours. A major problem is that preterm LGA infants, because of their size, are not recognized as high-risk neonates with immature organ system development. Often these infants develop respiratory distress syndrome because pulmonary maturation occurs later in gestation. In cases of Beckwith's syndrome, the infant is characterized by gigantism, macroglossia, omphalocele or umbilical hernia, and visceromegaly. Compare **small for gestational age infant.**

large intestine, the portion of the digestive tract comprising the cecum, appendix, the ascending, transverse, and descending colons, and the rectum. The ileocecal valve separates the cecum from the ileum.

Largon, a trademark for a sedative (propiomazine hydrochloride).

Larmor frequency, the frequency of the precession of a charged particle when its motion comes under the influence of an applied magnetic field and a central force.

Larodopa, a trademark for an antiparkinsonian (levodopa).

Larotid, a trademark for an antibiotic (amoxicillin).

larva migrans. See **cutaneous larva migrans, visceral larva migrans.**

laryng-. See **laryngo-.**

laryngeal cancer, a malignant neoplastic disease characterized by a tumor arising from the epithelium of the structures of the larynx. Laryngeal tumors are almost 20 times more common in men than in women and occur most frequently between 50 and 70 years of age. Chronic alcoholism and heavy use of tobacco increase the risk of developing the cancer. Persistent hoarseness is usually the first sign; advanced lesions may cause a sore throat, dyspnea, dysphagia, and unilateral cervical adenopathy. Diagnostic measures include direct laryngoscopy, biopsy, and radiologic examination, including tomographic studies and chest films. Malignant tumors of the larynx are epidermoid carcinomas. Radiation is generally recommended for small lesions; total laryngectomy, often combined with radiotherapy, is indicated for extensive lesions. After the operation, many persons with laryngectomies learn esophageal speech; some use an electric larynx, and a few undergo surgical reconstruction. See also **laryngectomy.**

laryngeal catheterization, the insertion of a catheter into the larynx for the purpose of removing secretions or introducing gases.

laryngeal prominence. See **Adam's apple.**

laryngectomy, surgical removal of the larynx, performed to treat cancer of the larynx. Before surgery, the patient is referred to a speech pathologist to discuss esophageal speech and prostheses. Antibiotics are usually administered to reduce the risk of infection. Under regional or general anesthesia, the trachea is sutured to the skin, as in a tracheostomy, to ensure an adequate airway. In a partial laryngectomy only the vocal cords are removed, and the tracheostomy is closed within several days. If the malignancy is extensive, the entire larynx is removed, along with the thyroid cartilage and epiglottis; the tracheostomy is permanent, and a laryngectomy tube left in place. After surgery the patient is observed for excessive coughing or any vomiting of blood, and the laryngectomy tube is kept free of mucus. A humidifier or vaporizer is useful to decrease coughing and the production of mucus. IV fluids are given, and liquid feedings may be given via nasogastric tube; oral fluids begin after 1 week. A magic slate is useful for communication between patient, staff, and family. The laryngectomy tube is removed 3 to 6 weeks after surgery. Compare **neck dissection, radical neck dissection. –laryngectomize,** *v.*

laryngismus /ler′injiz′məs/, spasm of the larynx. Laryngismus stridulus, a condition characterized by sudden laryngeal spasm with a crowing sound on inspiration and the development of cyanosis, occurs in inflammation of the larynx, in connection with rickets, and as an independent disease. The relatively small larynx of the infant and young child is susceptible to spasm when infected or irritated and readily becomes partially or totally obstructed.

laryngitis, inflammation of the mucous membrane lining the larynx, accompanied by edema of the vocal cords with hoarseness or loss of voice, occurring as an acute disorder caused by a cold, by irritating fumes, by sudden temperature changes or as a chronic condition resulting from excessive use of the voice, heavy smoking, or exposure to irritating fumes. In acute laryngitis, there may be a cough, and the throat usually feels scratchy and painful. The patient is advised to remain in an environment with an even temperature, to avoid talking and exposure to tobacco smoke, and to inhale steam containing aromatic vapors, as tincture of benzoin, oil of pine, or menthol. Acute laryngitis may cause severe respiratory distress in children under 5 years of age because the relatively small larynx of the young child is subject to spasm when irritated or infected and readily becomes partially or totally obstructed. The youngster may develop a hoarse, barking cough and an inspiratory stridor and may become restless, gasping for air. Treatment consists of the administration of copious amounts of vaporized cool mist. Chronic laryngitis may be treated by removal of irritants, avoidance of smoking, voice rest, correction of faulty voice habits, cough medication, steam inhalations, and spraying the throat with an astringent antiseptic, as hexylresorcinol.

laryngo-, laryng-, a combining form meaning 'of or pertaining to the larynx': *laryngocentesis, laryngograph.*

laryngography. See **laryngopharyngography.**

laryngopharyngitis /ləring′gōfer′injī′tis/, inflammation of the larynx and pharynx. See also **laryngitis, pharyngitis.**

laryngopharyngography /lering′gōfer′ingog′rəfē/, the radiographic examination of the larynx and the pharynx. Also called **laryngography.**

laryngopharynx /lering′gōfer′ingks/, one of the three regions of the throat, extending from the hyoid bone to the esophagus. Compare **nasopharynx, oropharynx.** –**laryngopharyngeal** /lering′gōferin′jē·əl/, *adj.*

laryngoscope, an endoscope for examining the larynx.

laryngospasm, a spasmodic closure of the larynx.

laryngostasis. See **croup.**

laryngotracheobronchitis (LTB) /lering′gōtrā′kē-ōbrongkī′tis/, an inflammation of the major respiratory passages, usually causing hoarseness, nonproductive cough, and dyspnea. Among the causes are infection by coxsackieviruses, echoviruses, *Haemophilus influenzae*, and *Corynebacterium diphtheriae*. Treatment includes steam inhalations, cough suppressants, and, for bacterial infections, appropriate antibiotics. See also **croup.**

larynx /ler′ingks/, the organ of voice that is part of the air passage connecting the pharynx with the trachea. It produces a large bump in the neck called the Adam's apple and is larger in men than in women although remaining the same size in men and women until puberty. The larynx forms the caudal portion of the anterior wall of the pharynx and is lined with mucous membrane that is continuous with that of the pharynx and the trachea. The larynx extends vertically to the fourth, fifth, and sixth cervical vertebrae and is somewhat higher in the female and during childhood. It is composed of three single cartilages and three paired cartilages, all connected together by ligaments and moved by various muscles. The single cartilages are the thyroid, cricoid, and epiglottis. The three paired cartilages are the arytenoid, corniculate, and cuneiform. The larynx is broad above and narrow and cylindric at its caudal extremity. –**laryngeal,** *adj.*

Lasan, a trademark for an antipsoriatic (anthralin).

laser /lā′zər/, abbreviation for *light amplification by stimulated emission of radiation,* a source of intense radiation of the visible, ultraviolet, or infrared portions of the spectrum. It is produced by exposing a large number of electrons to a high energy level in a gaseous, solid, or liquid medium. The electrons emit very narrow beams of light, all of one wavelength and parallel to each other. Lasers are used in surgery to divide or to cause adhesions or to destroy or to fix tissue in place. Also called **optic maser.**

Lasix, a trademark for a diuretic (furosemide).

Lassa fever /lä′sə/, a highly contagious disease caused by a virulent arenavirus. It is characterized by fever, pharyngitis, dysphagia, and ecchymoses. Pleural effusion, edema and renal involvement, mental disorientation, confusion, and death from cardiac failure often ensue. Stringent precautions are taken against the spread of infection. Supportive, symptomatic care is the only treatment available. See also **arenavirus, Argentine hemorrhagic fever, Bolivia hemorrhagic fever.**

late dyspituitary eunuchism. See **acromegalic eunuchoidism.**

latency stage, (in psychoanalysis) a period in psychosexual development occurring between early childhood and puberty when sexual motivation and expression are repressed or transferred, through sublimation, to the feelings and behavioral patterns expected as typical of the age. The manifestations are culturally influenced and vary greatly. See also **psychosexual development.**

latent, dormant; existing as a potential; for example, tuberculosis may be latent for extended periods of time and become active under certain conditions.

latent carcinoma. See **occult carcinoma.**

latent diabetes. See **impaired glucose tolerance, previous abnormality of glucose tolerance.**

latent heart failure, an abnormal condition characterized by inadequacy that is not apparent during rest but becomes evident under conditions of increased stress, as that produced by exercise, fever, and emotional excitement. During stress situations the heart affected by latent failure is unable to pump an adequate supply of blood in relation to venous return and the metabolic needs of body tissues and structures.

latent period, (in radiology) an interval of seeming inactivity between the time of exposure to an injurious dose of radiation and the response.

latent phase, the early stage of labor that is characterized by irregular, infrequent, and mild contractions and little or no dilatation of the cervix or descent of the fetus. Also called **prodromal labor.** See also **Friedman curve.**

latent schizophrenia, a form of schizophrenia characterized by the presence of mild symptoms of the disease. Latent schizophrenics have no previous history of psychotic schizophrenic episodes but do have a preexisting susceptibility to the disease in its overt form. Also called **borderline schizophrenia, pseudoneurotic schizophrenia, pseudopsychopathic schizophrenia.** See also **schizophrenia, schizotypal personality disorder.**

lateral, **1.** on the side. **2.** away from the midsagittal plane. **3.** farther from the midsagittal plane. **4.** to the right or left of the midsagittal plane.

lateral abdominal region. See **lateral region.**

lateral aortic node, a lumbar lymph node in any of three clusters of nodes serving the pelvis and abdomen. The right lateral aortic nodes are situated partly ventral to the inferior vena cava, near the termination of the renal vein, and partly dorsal to the inferior vena cava on the right crus of the diaphragm. The left lateral aortic nodes form a chain on the left side of the abdominal aorta, ventral to the origin of the psoas major and ventral to the right crus of the diaphragm. The afferents from both sides drain various structures, as the testes, ovaries, kidneys, and lateral abdominal muscles. Most of the efferents from the lateral aortic nodes converge to form the right and the left lumbar trunks, which join the cisterna chyli. Compare **preaortic node, retroaortic node.**

lateral aperture of the fourth ventricle, an opening between the end of each lateral recess of the fourth ventricle and the subarachnoid space.

lateral cerebral sulcus, a deep cleft marking the division of the temporal, frontal, and parietal lobes of brain. Also called **fissure of Sylvius.**

lateral condensation method, a technique for filling and sealing tooth root canals. A preselected gutta-percha cone is sealed into the apex of the root; other cones are forced laterally with a spreader until the canal is filled.

lateral cuneiform bone, one of the three cuneiform bones of the foot, located in the center of the front row of tarsal bones between the intermediate cuneiform bone medially, the cuboid bone laterally, the scaphoid bone posteriorly, and the third metatarsal anteriorly. It also articulates with the second and fourth metatarsals. Also called **external cuneiform bone, third cuneiform bone.**

lateral geniculate body, one of two elevations of the lateral posterior thalamus receiving visual impulses from the retina via the optic nerves and tracts and relaying the impulses to the calcarine cortex.

lateral humeral epicondylitis, inflammation of the tissue at the lower end of the humerus at the elbow joint, caused by the repetitive flexing of the wrist against resistance. It may result from athletic activity or manual manipulation of tools or other equipment. Pain radiates from the elbow joint. Treatment includes rest, correction of body mechanics, infiltration of a long-acting anesthetic, or serial injections of hydrocortisone, depending on the severity of the condition. Surgery is rarely indicated. Also called **tennis elbow.** See also **epicondylitis.**

lateral incisal guide angle, (in dentistry) the inclination of the incisal guide in the frontal plane.

laterality. See **handedness.**

lateral pectoral nerve, one of a pair of branches from the brachial plexus that, with the medial pectoral nerve, supplies the pectoral muscles. It lies lateral to the axillary artery and arises from the lateral cord of the plexus or from the anterior divisions of the superior and the middle trunks just before they unite into the cord. It passes above to the first part of the axillary artery and the axillary vein, gives a filament to the inferior pectoral branch, pierces the clavipectoral fascia, and ends on the deep surface of the clavicular and the cranial sternocostal parts of the pectoralis major. Compare **medial pectoral nerve.**

lateral pelvic displacement, one of the five major kinetic determinants of gait, which helps to synchronize the rhythmic movements of walking. It is produced by the horizontal shift of the pelvis or by relative hip abduction. It is often a factor in the diagnosis and treatment of various orthopedic diseases, deformities, and abnormal conditions, and in the analysis and the correction of dysfunctional gaits. Compare **knee-ankle interaction, knee-hip flexion, pelvic rotation, pelvic tilt.**

lateral recumbent position, the posture assumed by the patient lying on the left side with the right thigh and knee drawn up. Also called **English position, obstetric position.**

lateral region, the part of the abdomen in the middle zone on both sides of the umbilical region. Also called **external abdominal region, lateral abdominal region, lumbar region.** See also **abdominal regions.**

lateral rocking, a sideways rocking of the body used to move the body forward or backward when normal muscle action is not possible. The technique is used by some handicapped patients to move the body to or from the edge of a chair or to a different sitting position on a bed. The rocking is performed while leaning the trunk forward with the arms in front and the head in line above the knees and feet, which are pulled back.

lateral rotation, a turning away from the midline of the body. Compare **medial rotation.** See also **rotation.**

lateral umbilical fold, a fold in the peritoneum produced by a slight protrusion of the inferior epigastric artery and the interfoveolar ligament. The lateral umbilical fold is about 3 cm lateral to the middle umbilical fold. Also called **plica umbilicalis lateralis.**

latero-, a combining form meaning 'of or pertaining to the side': *laterodeviation, lateroduction, laterotorsion.*

late systolic murmur. See **systolic murmur.**

latex fixation test, a serologic test used in the diagnosis of rheumatoid arthritis in which antigen-coated latex particles agglutinate with rheumatoid factors in a slide specimen of serum or synovial fluid. If positive, the screening slide test is followed by titration. Also called **RA latex test, RF test.** See also **rheumatoid factor.**

Lathrop, Rose Hawthorne (1851–1926), an American nurse, who was a daughter of Nathaniel Hawthorne. She established a home in New York for incurable cancer patients, mostly those who were poor and who were not accepted in hospitals because of the nature of their disease. Later, she became a member of the Third Order of St. Dominic and founded the order of sisters called Servants of Relief for Incurable Cancer. The order founded hospitals wherever there was sufficient need and offered quality care to their patients.

latissimus dorsi, one of a pair of large triangular muscles on the thoracic and lumbar areas of the back. The base of the triangle inserts through lumbar aponeuroses to the spines of lumbar and sacral vertebrae and in the supraspinous ligaments, posterior iliac crest, and the lower four ribs. The fibers of the muscle twist as they pass the scapula and converge at the base of the intertubercular groove of the humerus. The latissimus dorsi extends, adducts, and rotates the arm medially, draws the shoulder back and down, and, with the pectoralis major, draws the body up when climbing. It is innervated by the thoracodorsal nerve. Compare **levator scapulae, rhomboideus major, rhomboideus minor, trapezius.**

latitude, the ability of an x-ray imaging system to produce acceptable images over a range of exposures. If a system has wide latitude, it is possible to image parts of the body that vary in thickness or density with only one exposure. A system of lesser latitude would require a lower exposure over the thin section and a greater exposure where the absorption was greater.

LATS, abbreviation for **long-acting thyroid stimulator.**

LATS-P, abbreviation for *long-acting thyroid stimulator protector*.

lattice formation, a three-dimensional cross-linked structure formed by the reaction of multivalent antigens with antibodies.

laughing gas, *informal*. nitrous oxide, a side effect of which is laughter or giggling when administered in less than anesthetizing amounts.

Laurence-Moon-Bardet-Biedl syndrome, an abnormal condition characterized by obesity, hypogenitalism, mental deficiency, polydactylism, and retinitis pigmentosa. It is an inherited disorder, transmitted as an autosomal recessive trait.

lavage /ləväzh′/, **1.** the process of washing out an organ, usually the bladder, bowel, paranasal sinuses, or stomach for therapeutic purposes. **2.** to perform a lavage. Kinds of lavage are **blood lavage, gastric lavage,** and **peritoneal dialysis.** See also **irrigation.**

law, 1. (in a field of study) a rule, standard, or principle that states a fact or a relationship between factors, as Dalton's law regarding partial pressures of gas or Koch's law regarding the specificity of a pathogen. **2.** a rule, principle, or regulation established and promulgated by a government to protect or to restrict the people affected; the field of study concerned with such laws; or the collected body of the laws of a people, derived from custom and from legislation.

law of definite composition, (in chemistry) a law stating that a given compound is always made of the same elements present in the same proportion.

law of dominance, formerly considered as a separate principle of Mendel's laws of inheritance, but in modern genetics it is incorporated as part of the first Mendelian law, the law of segregation. See also **Mendel's laws.**

law of facilitation. See **facilitation.**

law of independent assortment, law of segregation. See **Mendel's laws.**

law of universal gravitation, (in physics) a law stating that the force with which bodies are attracted to each other is directly proportional to the masses of the objects and inversely proportional to the square of the distance by which they are separated. See also **gravity, mass.**

lawrencium (Lw), a synthetic transuranic metallic element. Its atomic number is 103; its atomic weight is 257.

laxative, 1. of or pertaining to a substance that causes evacuation of the bowel by a mild action. **2.** a laxative agent that promotes bowel evacuation by increasing the bulk of the feces, by softening the stool, or by lubricating the intestinal wall. Compare **cathartic.**

lay advisers, lay persons who are influential in approving or disapproving new ideas and who may serve as consultants because of their expertise in subjects other than medicine.

lay referral system, an illness referral system through which a person passes from the first recognition of an abnormality to an announcement to the family, to members of the community, then to traditional or culturally recognized healers, and then to the regular medical system that includes nurses and physicians. Depending on the culture and the medical care available, some steps may be omitted.

lazy colon. See **atonia constipation.**

LBW, abbreviation for **low birth weight.**

LCAT, abbreviation for *lecithin-cholesterol acetyltransferase*.

LD, abbreviation for *lethal dose*.

LD50, (in toxicology) the amount of a substance sufficient to kill one half of the population of test subjects.

LDH, abbreviation for **lactate dehydrogenase.**

LDL, abbreviation for **low-density lipoprotein.**

L-dopa. See **levodopa.**

LE, abbreviation for **lupus erythematosus.** See **systemic lupus erythematosus.**

lead (Pb) /led/, a common soft, blue-gray, metallic element. Its atomic number is 82; its atomic weight is 207.19. In its metallic form, lead is used as a protective shielding against x-rays. Lead is poisonous, a characteristic that has led to a reduction in the use of lead compounds as pigments for paints and inks. Normal concentrations in whole blood are 0 to 5 μg/dl. The normal amount in urine after 24-hour collection is less the 100 μg.

lead /lēd/, an electric connection attached to the body to record electric activity, especially of the heart or brain. See also **electrocardiograph, electroencephalograph.**

lead equivalent /led/, (in radiology) the thickness of lead required to achieve the same shielding effect against radiation, under specified conditions, as that provided by a given material.

leadership, the ability to influence others to the attainment of goals. Kinds of leadership include authoritarian, democratic, participative, and permissive.

lead pipe fracture /led/, a fracture that compresses the bony tissue at the point of impact and creates a linear fracture on the opposite side of the bone involved.

lead poisoning /led/, a toxic condition caused by the ingestion or inhalation of lead or lead compounds. Many children have developed the condition as a result of eating flaked lead paint. Poisoning also occurs from the ingestion of water from lead pipes, lead salts in certain foods and wines, the use of pewter or earthenware glazed with a lead glaze, and the use of leaded gasoline. Inhalation of lead fumes is common in industry. The acute form of intoxication is characterized by a burning sensation in the mouth and esophagus, colic, constipation, or diarrhea, mental disturbances, and paralysis of the extremities, followed in severe cases by convulsions and muscular collapse. Chronic lead poisoning, which is characterized by extreme irritability, anorexia, and anemia, may progress to the acute form. If ingested, treatment commences with gastric lavage with magnesium or sodium sulfate. All cases call for fluid therapy followed by chelation with intramuscular injection of calcium disodium edetate, or for severe cases, British antilewisite. Encephalopathy must be anticipated in children with lead poisoning.

leakage radiation, radiation, exclusive of the primary beam, that is emitted through the housing of equipment used in radiation therapy.

leaky gene. See **hypomorph.**

learning, **1.** the act or process of acquiring knowledge or some skill by means of study, practice, or experience. **2.** knowledge, wisdom, or a skill acquired through systematic study or instruction. **3.** (in psychology) the modification of behavior through practice, experience, or training. See also **conditioning.**

learning disability, an abnormal condition often affecting children of normal or above-average intelligence, characterized by difficulty in learning such fundamental procedures as reading, writing, and numeric calculation. The condition may result from psychologic or organic causes and is usually related to slow development of perceptual motor skills. See also **attention deficit disorder, dysgraphia, dyslexia.**

leather-bottle stomach. See **linitis plastica.**

Leber's congenital amaurosis /lā'bərz/, a rare kind of blindness or severely impaired vision caused by a defect transmitted as an autosomal recessive trait and occurring at birth or shortly thereafter. The eyes appear normal externally, but pupillary constriction to light is sluggish or absent and retinal pigment is degenerated. Pendular nystagmus, photophobia, cataract, and keratoconus may be present, and the ophthalmic disorder may be associated with mental retardation and epilepsy. One kind of Leber's amaurosis results in complete blindness, but with a second kind the pathology does not progress and the patient has very slight vision. Also called **amaurosis congenita of Leber.**

Leboyer method of delivery /ləboiyā'/, an approach to the delivery of an infant formulated by the French obstetrician Charles Leboyer. It has four aspects: a gentle, controlled delivery in a quiet, dimly lit room, avoidance of pulling on the head, avoidance of overstimulation of the infant's sensorium, and encouragement of maternal-infant bonding. The goal of the method is to minimize the trauma of birth by gently and pleasantly introducing the newborn to life outside the womb. Unnecessary intervention in the process of birth is eschewed. After delivery, the baby is gently laid on the mother's abdomen, the back is massaged as the cord stops pulsating, and, when regular spontaneous respirations are established the baby is gently supported in a warm tub of water by the father. Many birth centers and obstetric services in the United States have found that no adverse effects result from this method. Some studies in France have suggested superior psychologic, social, and intellectual development in young children delivered by this method. Compare **Bradley method, Lamaze method, Read method.**

lecithin /les'ithin/, any of a group of phospholipids common in plants and animals. Lecithins are found in the liver, nerve tissue, semen, and in smaller amounts in bile and blood. They are essential for the metabolism of fats and are used in the processing of foods, pharmaceutic products, cosmetics, and inks. Rich dietary sources are soybeans, egg yolk, and corn. Deficiency leads to hepatic and renal disorders, high serum cholesterol levels, atherosclerosis, and arteriosclerosis. See also **choline, inositol.**

lecithin/sphingomyelin ratio, the ratio of two components of amniotic fluid, used for predicting fetal lung maturity. The normal ratio in amniotic fluid is 2:1 or greater.

lecitho-, a combining form meaning 'of or pertaining to the yolk of an egg, or to the ovum': *lecithoblast, lecithoprotein, lecithovitellin.*

lectin, a protein substance occurring in seeds and other parts of certain plants that binds with glycoproteins and glycolipids on the surface of animal cells causing agglutination. Some lectins cause agglutination of erythrocytes in specific blood groups, and others stimulate the production of T lymphocytes.

Ledercillin VK, a trademark for an antibacterial (penicillin V potassium).

Lee-White, a method of determining the length of time required for a clot to form in a test tube of venous blood. It is not specific for any coagulation disorder but is often used to monitor coagulation during heparin therapy. Because normal values and precise methodology vary, instructions are provided by most laboratories. See also **clotting time.**

LeFort I fracture. See **Guérin's fracture.**

left atrioventricular valve. See **mitral valve.**

left brachiocephalic vein, a vessel, about 6 cm long, that starts in the root of the neck at the junction of the internal jugular and the subclavian veins on the left side and runs obliquely across the thorax to join the right brachiocephalic vein and form the superior vena cava. The left brachiocephalic vein, which is longer than the right, receives various tributaries, as the vertebral vein, the internal thoracic vein, and the inferior thyroid vein. Also called **left innominate vein.** Compare **right brachiocephalic vein.**

left common carotid artery, the longer of the two common carotid arteries, springing from the aortic arch and having cervical and thoracic portions. The cervical portion passes obliquely from the level of the sternoclavicular articulation to the cranial border of the thyroid cartilage, dividing into the left internal and the left external carotid arteries. Compare **right common carotid artery.**

left coronary artery, one of a pair of branches from the ascending aorta, arising in the left posterior aortic sinus, dividing into the left interventricular artery and the circumflex branch, supplying both ventricles and the left atrium. Compare **right coronary artery.**

left-handedness, a natural tendency by some persons to favor the use of the left hand in performing certain tasks. Also called **sinistrality.** See also **cerebral dominance, handedness.**

left-heart failure, an abnormal cardiac condition characterized by the impairment of the left side of the heart and by elevated pressure and congestion in the pulmonary veins and capillaries. Left-heart failure is usually related to right-heart failure, because both sides of the heart are part of a circuit and the impairment of one side will eventually affect the other. However, research indicates that experimentally produced pure failure of one ventricle may produce significant hemodynamic and biochemical abnormalities of the opposite ventricle, even without the usual signs of failure. In "pure" left-heart failure, the body retains significant amounts of sodium and water and consequently develops peripheral edema without clinical evidence of right-heart failure. Also called **left-sided failure.** Compare **right-heart failure.**

left hepatic duct, the duct that drains the bile from the left lobe of the liver into the common bile duct.

left innominate vein. See **left brachiocephalic vein.**

left lymphatic duct. See **thoracic duct.**

left pulmonary artery, the shorter and smaller of two arteries conveying venous blood from the heart to the lungs, rising from the pulmonary trunk, connecting to the left lung, and tending to have more separate branches than the right pulmonary artery. In the fetus it is larger and more important than the right pulmonary artery because it provides the ductus arteriosus that degenerates to become a ligament after birth. Compare **right pulmonary artery.**

left subclavian artery, an artery, divided into three parts, that arises from the aortic arch dorsal to the left common carotid at the level of the fourth thoracic vertebra, ascends to the root of the neck, arches laterally to the scalenus anterior, and forms six main branches to supply the vertebral column, spinal cord, ear, and brain. The short second portion lies dorsal to the scalenus anterior and forms the arch described by the vessel. The third portion runs from the scalenus anterior to the first rib where it becomes the axillary artery. See also **subclavian artery.** Compare **right subclavian artery.**

left ventricle, the thick-walled chamber of the heart that pumps blood through the aorta and the systemic arteries, the capillaries, and back through the veins to the right atrium. It has walls about three times thicker than those of the right ventricle and contains a mitral valve with two flaps that controls the flow of blood from the left atrium. The left ventricle occupies about half the diaphragmatic surface of the heart and is longer and more conical than the right ventricle, narrowing caudally to form the apex. The chordae tendineae of the left ventricle are thicker, stronger, and less numerous than those in the right ventricle. See also **heart.**

left ventricular assist device (LVAD), a mechanic pump that temporarily and artificially aids the natural pumping action of the left ventricle.

left ventricular failure, heart failure in which the left ventricle fails to contract forcefully enough to maintain a normal cardiac output and peripheral perfusion. Pulmonary congestion and edema develop from back pressure of accumulated blood in the left ventricle. Signs include breathlessness, pallor, sweating, and peripheral vasoconstriction. The heart is usually enlarged. A prominent third heart sound (gallop), normal in children and young adults, is a sign of left ventricular failure in older adults with heart disease. Hypertension is common and may be a causative factor or a result of pulmonary edema. Treatment includes meperidine or morphine for sedation, diuretics, digitalis, and rest.

legacy, something that is handed down from the past or is intended to be bestowed on future generations.

legal, actions or conditions that are permitted or authorized by law.

legal death. See **death.**

leg cylinder cast, an orthopedic device of plaster of paris or fiberglass used to immobilize the leg in treating fractures in the legs from the ankle to the upper thigh. It is especially used for fractures and dislocations of the knee, for the soft tissue trauma around the knee, for postoperative positioning and immobilization of the knee, and for correction or maintenance of correction of deformities of the knee. The long leg cast may be used for these same conditions rather than the leg cylinder cast because it encases the foot and assures greater immobilization.

Legg-Calvé-Perthes disease. See **Perthes disease.**

Legionella pneumophila /lē′jənel′ə nōōmof′ələ/, a small, gram-negative, rod-shaped bacterium that is the causative agent in **Legionnaires' disease.**

Legionnaires' disease, an acute bacterial pneumonia caused by infection with *Legionella pneumophila* and characterized by an influenza-like illness followed within a week by high fever, chills, muscle aches, and headache. The symptoms may progress to dry cough, pleurisy, and sometimes diarrhea. Usually the disease is self-limited, but mortality has been 15% to 20% in a few localized epidemics. Contaminated air conditioning cooling towers and moist soil may be a source of organisms. Person-to-person contagion has not occurred. Risk of infection is increased by the presence of other conditions, as cardiopulmonary diseases. Treatment includes supportive care and erythromycin. Also called **legionellosis.**

leio-, lio-, a combining form meaning 'smooth': *leiodermia, leiodystonia, leiomyofibroma.*

leiomyoblastoma. See **epithelioid leiomyoma.**

leiomyofibroma /lī′ōmī′ōfībrō′mə/, *pl.* **leiomyofibromas, leiomyofibromata,** a tumor consisting of smooth muscle cells and fibrous connective tissue, commonly occurring in the uterus in middle-aged women. See also **fibroid.**

leiomyoma /lī'ōmī•ō'mə/, *pl.* **leiomyomas, leiomyomata,** a benign smooth muscle tumor most commonly occurring in the stomach, esophagus, or small intestine. Surgical resection is necessary only in the rare case in which the tumor undergoes central necrosis, causing sudden and possibly severe hemorrhage.

leiomyoma cutis, a neoplasm of the smooth muscles of the skin. The lesion is characterized by many small, tender, red nodules.

leiomyoma uteri, a benign neoplasm of the smooth muscle of the uterus. The tumor is characteristically firm, well circumscribed, round, and gray-white, and, under the microscope, shows a pattern of whorls. Multiple tumors of this kind develop most often in the myometrium and occur most frequently in women between 30 and 50 years of age. Also called **fibromyoma uteri, myoma previum,** *(informal)* **fibroids.**

leipo-. See **lipo-.**

Leishman-Donovan body /lēsh'məndon'əvən/, the resting stage of an intracellular, nonflagellated protozoan parasite (*Leishmania donovani*) that causes kala-azar, or visceral leishmaniasis as it appears in infected tissue specimens.

Leishmania /lēshmā'nē•ə/, a genus of protozoan parasites. These organisms are transmitted to humans by any of several species of sand flies.

leishmaniasis /lēsh'mənī'əsis/, infection with any species of protozoan of the genus *Leishmania*. The diseases caused by these organisms may be cutaneous or visceral. Diagnosis is made by microscopic identification of the intracellular, nonflagellated protozoan on a Giemsa-stained smear taken from a cutaneous lesion or visceral biopsy. Kinds of leishmaniasis are **American leishmaniasis, kala-azar,** and **oriental sore.** See also ***leishmania.*** **–leishmanial,** *adj.*

Lemiserp, a trademark for an antihypertensive (reserpine).

-lemma, a combining form meaning a 'confining membrane': *axiolemma, epilemma, neurolemma.*

lemo-, **1.** a combining form meaning 'of or pertaining to plague': *lemography, lemology.* **2.** a combining form meaning 'of or pertaining to the gullet': *lemoparalysis, lemostenosis.*

length of stay (LOS), the period of time a patient remains in a hospital or other health care facility as an inpatient.

lens, **1.** a curved transparent piece of plastic or glass that is shaped, molded, or ground to refract light in a specific way, as in eyeglasses, microscopes, or cameras. **2.** *informal.* the crystalline lens of the eye. **–lenticular,** *adj.*

lens capsule, the clear thin elastic capsule that surrounds the lens of the eye. Also called **capsule of the lens.**

lens implant, an artifical lens of clear polymethylmethacrylate that is usually implanted at the time of cataract extraction but may also be used for patients with extreme myopia, diplopia, ocular albinism, and certain other abnormalities. The operation may be performed with a local anesthetic, as lidocaine, but general anesthesia is often preferred, especially for patients with vitreous humor in the anterior chamber. Eyedrops containing an antibiotic, as neomycin, are applied preoperatively to prevent infection, and several times a day for a number of weeks postoperatively. After extraction of the cataract, the lens is inserted through a corneal incision; it may be held in place in the anterior chamber by extremely fine sutures to the iris, or, if the lens is implanted into the capsular sac, a miotic agent, as pilocarpine, is used to prevent the iris from dilating too widely, which would allow the implant to slip. The implanted lens does not cause the problems with abnormal peripheral vision associated with cataract spectacles, and it produces only 2% larger images on the retina than the normal lens, compared with a 24% enlargement produced by cataract spectacles and an 8% enlargement produced by contact lenses. A high rate of complications is reported in implant surgery, and the procedure is contraindicated for patients with diabetes mellitus or uveitis.

Lente Iletin, a trademark for an antidiabetic (insulin zinc suspension).

Lente Insulin, a trademark for an antidiabetic (insulin zinc suspension).

lentigo /lentī'gō/, *pl.* **lentigines** /lentij'ənēz/, a tan or brown macule on the skin brought on by sun exposure, usually in a middle-aged or older person. Another variety, called **juvenile lentigo,** is unrelated to sunlight and appears in children 2 to 5 years of age, before the onset of freckles. The melanin pigment in a lentigo is at a deeper level of the epidermis than in a freckle. Both types are benign, and no treatment is necessary. Compare **freckle.**

lentigo maligna. See **Hutchinson's freckle.**

lentigo maligna melanoma, a neoplasm developing from Hutchinson's freckle on the face or other exposed surfaces of the skin in elderly patients. It is asymptomatic, flat, and tan or brown, with irregular darker spots and frequent hypopigmentation. It is one of the three major clinical types of melanoma, occurring in about 10% to 15% of melanoma patients. See also **nodular melanoma, superficial spreading melanoma.**

lepido-, a combining form meaning 'of or pertaining to a flake or scale': *lepidoma, lepidosis.*

LE prep, abbreviation for **lupus erythematosus preparation.**

lepro-, a combining form meaning 'of or pertaining to leprosy': *leprologist, lepromatous, leprosarium.*

lepromatous leprosy. See **leprosy.**

lepromin test /leprō'min/, a skin sensitivity test used to distinguish between the lepromatous and tuberculoid forms of leprosy. The test consists of intradermal injection of lepromin, which is prepared from heat-sterilized *Mycobacterium leprae*. The appearance of a palpable nodule in 8 to 10 days is indicative of the tuberculoid form of leprosy. As no nodule appears in the lepromatous form, the test is not diagnostic of leprosy. The test is used only to follow the course of the disease. See also **leprosy.**

leprosy, a chronic, communicable disease, caused by *Mycobacterium leprae,* that may take either of two forms, depending on the degree of immunity of the host. **Tuberculoid leprosy,** seen in those with high resistance, presents as thickening of cutaneous nerves and anesthetic, saucer-shaped skin lesions. **Lepromatous leprosy,** seen in those with little resistance, involves many systems of the body, with widespread plaques and nodules in the skin, iritis, keratitis, destruction of nasal cartilage and bone, testicular atrophy, peripheral edema, and involvement of the reticuloendothelial system. Blindness may result. Death is rare unless amyloidosis or tuberculosis occurs concurrently. Contrary to traditional belief, leprosy is not very contagious, and prolonged, intimate contact is required for it to be spread between individuals. Children are more susceptible than adults. Plastic surgery, physical therapy, and psychotherapy are often necessary. Treatment with sulfones, as dapsone, continued for several years results usually in improvement of skin lesions, but recovery from nerve impairment is limited. The disease is found mostly in underdeveloped tropic and subtropic countries. In the United States, patients may be referred to the U.S. Public Health Service leprosarium in Carville, Louisiana. BCG vaccine may protect against leprosy. Also called **Hansen's disease.** See also ***Mycobacterium.*** **–lepromatous, leprotic, leprous,** *adj.*

-lepsy, -lepsia, -lepsis, a combining form meaning a 'seizure': *deolepsy, electrolepsy, pyknolepsy.*

-leptic, a combining form meaning 'pertaining to a (specified) type of seizure': *cataleptic, epileptic, hypnoleptic.*

lepto-, a combining form meaning 'thin, or delicate': *leptocephalia, leptocyte, leptosome.*

leptocyte. See **target cell.**

leptocytosis /lep'tōsītō'sis/, a hematologic condition in which target cells are present in the blood. Thalassemia, some forms of liver disease, and absence of the spleen are associated with leptocytosis.

leptomeninges /lep'tōminin'jēz/, the arachnoid membrane and the pia mater, two of the three layers covering the spinal cord. Compare **meninges.**

leptonema /lep'tənē'mə/, the threadlike chromosome formation in the leptotene stage in the first meiotic prophase of gametogenesis before the beginning of synapsis.

Leptospira, a genus of the family *Treponemataceae,* order *Spirochaetales,* tightly coiled microorganisms having spirals with hooked ends. The spirochete thrives in the urine of infected animals, especially rodents, is pathogenic to humans and other mammals, and may cause jaundice, skin hemorrhages, fever, and muscular illness. See also **leptospirosis.**

Leptospira agglutinin, an agglutinin found in the blood of patients with Weil's disease.

leptospirosis /lep'tōspīrō'sis/, an acute infectious disease caused by several serotypes of the spirochete *Leptospira interrogans,* transmitted in the urine of wild or domestic animals, especially rats and dogs. Human infections arise directly from contact with an infected animal's urine or tissues or indirectly from contact with contaminated water or soil. Clinical symptoms may include jaundice, hemorrhage into the skin, fever, chills, and muscular pain. The spirochete can be isolated from the urine or blood during the acute stage of the disease, and antibodies can be found in the patient's blood during convalescence. Treatment with antibiotics, usually penicillin or tetracycline, may be effective if they are administered during the first few days of the disease. Fluid and electrolyte replacement is essential if jaundice or other signs of severe illness are present. The disease is usually short-lived and mild, but severe infections can damage the kidneys and the liver. Blood pressure and vital signs should be monitored, and the patient's urine should be disposed of carefully to prevent spread of the organism. The most serious form of the disease is called **Weil's disease.** Also called **autumn fever.** See also **nanukayami.**

leptotene /lep'tətēn/, the initial stage in the first meiotic prophase in gametogenesis in which the chromosomes become visible as single thin filaments. See also **diakinesis, diplotene, pachytene, zygotene.**

Leriche's syndrome /lərēshs'/, a vascular disorder marked by gradual occlusion of the terminal aorta, intermittent claudication in the buttocks, thighs, or calves, absence of pulsation in femoral arteries, pallor and coldness of the legs, gangrene of the toes, and, in men, impotence. Symptoms are the result of chronic tissue hypoxia caused by inadequate arterial perfusion of the affected areas. Treatment may include endarterectomy, embolectomy, or synthetic bypass graft at the bifurcation of the aorta.

lesbian, **1.** a female homosexual. **2.** of or pertaining to the sexual preference or desire of one woman for another. **–lesbianism,** *n.*

Lesch-Nyhan syndrome /lesh'nī'han/, a hereditary disorder of purine metabolism, characterized by mental retardation, self-mutilation of the fingers and lips by biting, impaired renal function, and abnormal physical development. It is transmitted as a recessive, sex-linked trait.

lesion, **1.** a wound, injury, or pathologic change in body tissue. **2.** any visible, local abnormality of the tissues of the skin, as a wound, sore, rash, or boil. A lesion may be described as benign, cancerous, gross, occult, or primary. (Table, pages 644-645)

lesser multangular bone. See **trapezoid bone.**

lesser occipital nerve, one of a pair of cutaneous branches of the cervical plexus, arising from the second cervical nerve, curving around the sternocleidomastoideus, and ascending along the side of the head behind the ear to supply the skin. It communicates with the greater occipital and the great auricular nerves and with the posterior auricular branch of the facial nerve.

lesser omentum, a membranous extension of the peritoneum from the peritoneal layers covering the ventral

Types of skin lesions

Observed skin changes	*Differentiation*	*Term*	*Example*
Change in color or texture			
Spot	Circumscribed, flat, color change	Macule	Freckle
Discoloration, (reddish-purple)	Bleeding beneath the surface, injury to tissue	Contusion	Bruise
Soft whitening	Caused by repeated wetting of skin	Maceration	Between toes after soaking
Flake	Dry cells of surface	Scale	Dandruff
Roughness from dried fluid	Dry exudate over lesions	Crust	Eczema, impetigo
Roughness from cells	Leathery thickening of outer skin layer	Lichenification	Callus on foot
Silvery scale	Buildup of scale	Plaque	Psoriasis
Change in shape			
Solid mass, *cellular* growth	Less than 5 mm	Papule	Small mole, raised rash
	5 mm to 2 cm	Nodule	Enlarged lymph node
	Greater than 2 cm	Tumor	Benign or malignant tumor
	Excess connective tissue over scar	Keloid	Overgrown scar
Fluid-filled lesions	Less than 1 cm, clear fluid	Vesicle	Blister, chickenpox
	Greater than 1 cm, clear fluid	Bulla	Large blister, pemphigus
	Small, thick yellowish fluid (pus)	Pustule	Acne
	Semisolid	Cyst	Sebaceous cyst
Swelling of tissue	Generalized swelling; fluid between cells	Edema	Inflammation, swelling of feet
	Circumscribed surface edema, transient, some itching	Wheal	Allergic reaction

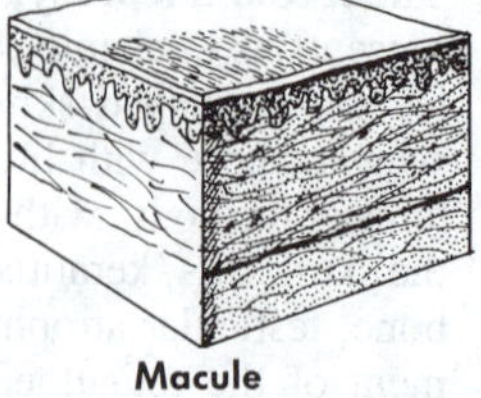

Macule

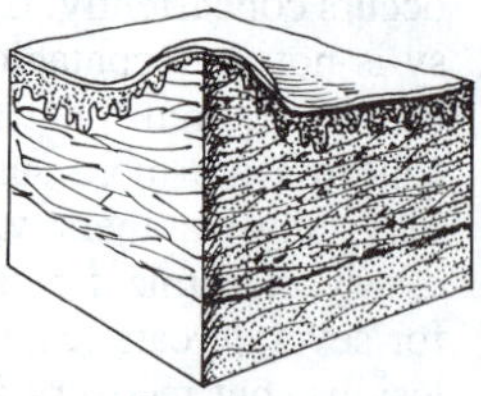

Papule

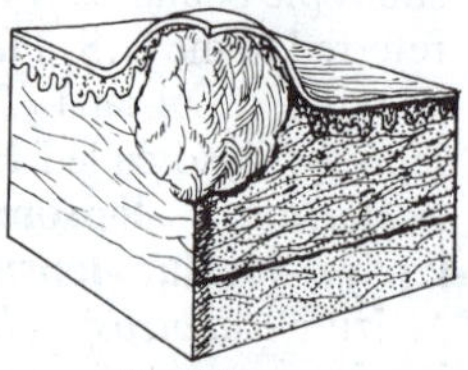

Nodule

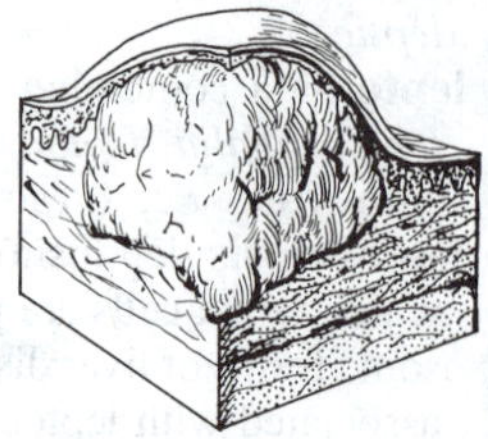

Tumor

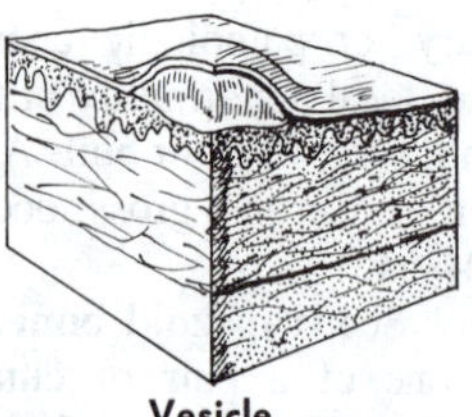
Vesicle

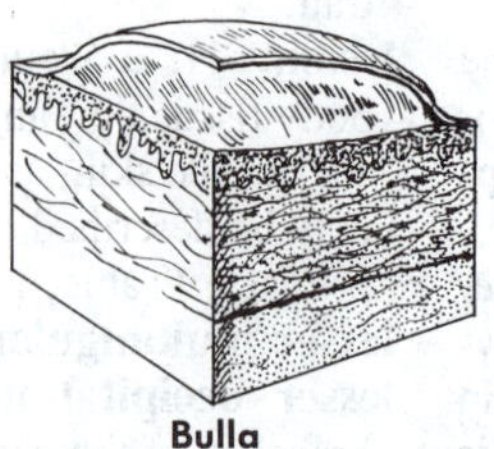
Bulla

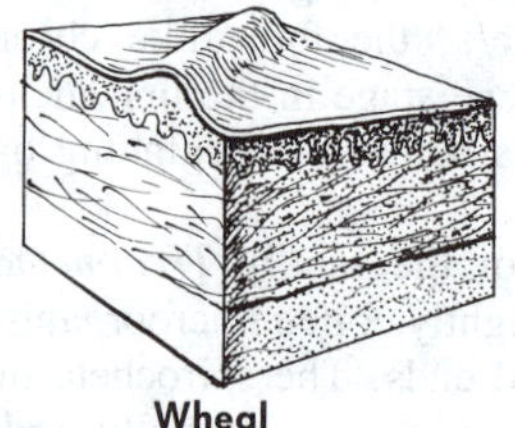
Wheal

Types of skin lesions

Observed skin changes	*Differentiation*	*Term*	*Example*
Breaks in skin surfaces			
Oozing, scraped surface	Loss of superficial surface of skin	Abrasion	"Floor burn," scrape
Linear crack or cleft	Slit or splitting of skin layers	Fissure	Athlete's foot
Scooped-out depression	Loss of deeper layers of skin	Ulcer	Decubitus, stasis ulcer
Superficial linear skin breaks	Scratch marks, frequently by fingernails	Excoriations	Scratching
Jagged cut	Tearing of skin surface	Laceration	Accidental cut by blunt object
Linear cut, edges approximated	Cutting by sharp instrument	Incision	Knife cut
Vascular lesions			
Small, flat, round, purplish-red spot	Intradermal or submucous hemorrhage	Petechia	Bleeding tendency, vitamin C deficiency
Spiderlike, red, small	Dilatation of capillaries, arterioles, or venules	Telangiectasis	Liver disease, vitamin B deficiency, sun-damaged skin
Discoloration, reddish-purple	Escape of blood into tissue	Ecchymosis	Trauma to blood vessels

Fissure

Ulcer

and the dorsal surfaces of the stomach and the first part of the duodenum. The lesser omentum extends from the portal fissure of the liver to the diaphragm where the layers separate to enclose the end of the esophagus. It also forms two ligaments, one associated with the liver, the other with the duodenum. Also called **gastrohepatic omentum, small omentum.**

lesser trochanter, one of a pair of conic projections at the base of the neck of the femur, providing insertion of the tendon of psoas major. Compare **greater trochanter.**

let-down, a sensation in the breasts of lactating women that often occurs as the milk flows into the ducts. It may occur when the infant begins to suck or when the mother hears the baby cry or even thinks of nursing the child.

let-down reflex. See **milk ejection reflex.**

lethal, capable of causing death.

lethal equivalent, any recessive gene carried in the heterozygous state that, if homozygous, would be lethal and result in the death of the individual or organism. It is estimated that any person carries from 3 to 8 lethal equivalents or any combination of genes, each with slightly deleterious effects, that are equivalent to 3 to 8 recessive genes.

lethal gene, any gene that produces a phenotypic effect that causes the death of the organism at some stage of development from fertilization of the egg to adulthood. The gene may be dominant, incompletely dominant, or recessive. In humans, examples of diseases caused by lethal genes are Huntington's chorea, which is transmitted as an autosomal dominant, and sickle cell anemia, which shows recessive lethality. Compare **sublethal gene.** See also **lethal equivalent.**

lethargic encephalitis. See **epidemic encephalitis.**

lethargy, **1.** the state or quality of being indifferent, apathetic, or sluggish. **2.** stupor or coma resulting from disease or hypnosis. Kinds of lethargy include **hysteric lethargy, induced lethargy,** and **lucid lethargy.** **–lethargic,** *adj.*

Letterer-Siwe syndrome /let′ərərzē′və/, any of a poorly classified group of malignant neoplastic diseases of unknown origin, characterized by histiocytic elements. The syndrome, which is fatal, occurs in infancy and is not familial. Anemia, hemorrhage, splenomegaly, lymphadenopathy, and localized tumefactions over bones are usually present.

letter quality printer, a printer that produces characters that resemble a typewriter in production quality.

letterword, an abbreviation that is pronounced by sounding the names of its letters, which usually are the initial letters of the full form, as in "LATS," pronounced /el′ā′tē′es′/. While a letterword is usually not treated as a word grammatically, it sometimes functions as a part of speech, as in "He MC'd the program." Compare **acronym.**

leucine (Leu) /lo͞o′sēn/, a white, crystalline amino acid essential for optimal growth in infants and nitrogen equilibrium in adults. It cannot be synthesized by the body and is obtained by the hydrolysis of protein during pancreatic digestion. An inherited defect in one of the enzymes involved in the process results in a rare disorder called maple syrup urine disease. See also **amino acid, leucinosis, maple syrup urine disease.**

leucinosis /lo͞o′sinō′sis/, a condition in which the pathways for the degradation of leucine are blocked and large amounts of the amino acid accumulate in body tissue. See also **leucine.**

leuco-. See **leuko-.**

leucocyte. See **leukocyte.**

leucovorin. See **folinic acid.**

leucovorin calcium, an antianemic.

■ INDICATIONS: It is prescribed in the treatment of an overdose of a folic acid antagonist and certain cases of megaloblastic anemia.

■ CONTRAINDICATIONS: Anemia caused by vitamin B_{12} deficiency or known hypersensitivity to this drug prohibits its use.

■ ADVERSE EFFECTS: Hypersensitivity reactions may occur.

leukapheresis, a process by which blood is withdrawn from a vein, white blood cells are selectively removed, and the remaining blood is reinfused in the donor. The white blood cells may be used for treating patients with blood deficiencies or for research. Compare **plasmapheresis, plateletpheresis.** See also **apheresis.**

leukemia, a malignant neoplasm of blood-forming organs characterized by diffuse replacement of bone marrow with proliferating leukocyte precursors, abnormal numbers and forms of immature white cells in circulation, and infiltration of lymph nodes, the spleen, liver, and other sites. Aproximateley 20,500 new cases in adults and 2500 in children are diagnosed annually in the United States, and the disease causes about 15,900 deaths a year. Males are affected twice as frequently as females. The origin of leukemia is not clear, but it may result from exposure to ionizing radiation, benzene, or other chemicals that are toxic to bone marrow. The risk of the disease is increased in individuals with Down's syndrome, Fanconi's syndrome ataxia-telangiectasia, Bloom's syndrome, or some other forms of congenital aneuploidy, and in an identical twin of a leukemia victim. Leukemia is classified according to the predominant proliferating cells, the clinical course, and the duration of the disease. Acute leukemia usually has a sudden onset and rapidly progressess from early signs, as fatigue, pallor, weight loss, and easy bruising, to fever, hemorrhages, extreme weakness, bone or joint pain, and repeated infections. Chronic leukemia develops slowly, and signs similar to those of the acute forms of the disease may not appear for years. Diagnoses of acute and chronic forms are made by blood tests and bone marrow biopsies. Involved marrow may range in color from muddy red-brown to pale gray, and changes are usually first evident in the vertebrae, ribs, sternum, and pelvis. The most effective treatment includes intensive combination chemotherapy, the use of antibiotics to prevent infections, and blood transfusions to replace red cells and platelets. See also **acute childhood leukemia, acute lymphocytic leukemia, acute myelocytic anemia.** –**leukemic,** *adj.*

-leukemia, a combining form meaning an 'increased number of leukocytes in the tissues and/or in the blood': *chloroleukemia, erythroleukemia, hypoleukemia.*

leukemia cutis, a condition in which yellow-brown, red, or purple nodular lesions and diffuse infiltrations or large accumulations of leukemic cells develop in the skin. It may be general or localized, usually in the skin of the face. Also called **lymphoderma perniciosa.**

leukemic reticuloendotheliosis. See **hairy-cell leukemia.**

leukemoid /lo͞okē′moid/, resembling leukemia.

leukemoid reaction, a clinical syndrome resembling leukemia in which the white blood cell count is elevated in response to an allergy, inflammatory disease, infection, poison, hemorrhage, burn, or other causes of severe physical stress. Compare **leukemia.**

Leukeran, a trademark for an antineoplastic (chlorambucil).

leuko-, leuco-, a combining form meaning 'of or pertaining to a white corpuscle, or white': *leukoblast, leukomaine, leukoplakia.*

leukocyte /lo͞o′kəsīt/, a white blood cell, one of the formed elements of the circulating blood system. There are five types of leukocytes, classified by the presence or absence of granules in the cytoplasm of the cell. The agranulocytes are lymphocytes and monocytes. The granulocytes are neutrophils, basophils, and eosinophils. White cells are able to squeeze through intracellular spaces by diapedesis and migrate by ameboid movements. Leukocytes are larger than erythrocytes, measuring 8 to 20 μ in diameter. A cubic millimeter of normal blood usually contains 5000 to 10,000 leukocytes. Among the most important functions of the leukocytes are phagocytosis of bacteria, fungi, and viruses, detoxification of toxic proteins that may result from allergic reactions and cellular injury, and the development of immunities. Also called **leucocyte, white blood cell, white corpuscle.** Compare **erythrocyte, platelet.** See also **complete blood count, differential white blood cell count, leukopenia, leukocytosis.** –**leukocytic,** *adj.*

leukocyte alkaline phosphatase, an enzyme that is elevated in various diseases, as cirrhosis and polycytemia, and in certain infections. It may be measured in the blood to detect these disorders and to differentiate chronic myelogenous (myelocytic) leukemia from leukemoid reactions. Normal amounts of this enzyme in a smear of fresh venous blood are 50 to 150 units. Also called **neutrophil alkaline phosphatase.**

leukocythemia. See **leukemia.**

leukocytic crystal. See **Charcot-Leyden crystal.**

leukocytopenia. See **leukopenia.**

leukocytosis /lo͞o′kōsītō′sis/, an abnormal increase in the number of circulating white blood cells. An increase often accompanies bacterial, but not usually viral, infections. The normal range is 5000 to 10,000 white cells per cubic millimeter of blood. Leukemia may be associated with a white blood cell count as high as 500,000 to 1 million per cubic millimeter of blood, the increase being either equally or disproportionately distributed among all types. Kinds of leukocytosis include **basophilia, eosinophilia,** and **neutrophilia.** Compare **leukemia, leukemoid reaction, leukopenia.** See also **leukocyte.**

leukoderma /lo͞okōdur′mə/, localized loss of skin pigment caused by any of a number of specific causes. Compare **vitiligo.**

leukoerythroblastic anemia /lo͞o′kō•erith′rōblas′tik/, an abnormal condition in which there are large numbers of immature white and red blood cells. It is characteristic of some anemias that occur as a result of the replacement of normal bone marrow with malignant tumor. See also **myeloid metaplasia, myelophthisic anemia.**

leukonychia /lo͞o′kōnik′ē•ə/, a benign, congenital condition in which white patches appear under the nails. Trauma, infection, and many systemic disorders can cause white spots or streaks on nails. A common cause is the presence of air bubbles under the nails.

leukopenia /lo͞o′kōpē′nē•ə/, an abnormal decrease in the number of white blood cells to fewer than 5000 cells per cubic millimeter. It may be caused by an adverse drug reaction, radiation poisoning, or other pathologic conditions and may affect one or all kinds of white blood cells. The two most common forms of leukopenia are neutrophilic leukopenia and lymphocytic leukopenia. Also called **leucocytopenia.** Compare **aleukia, leukocytosis.** See also **aplastic anemia, leukocyte.** –**leukopenic,** *adj.*

leukopenic leukemia. See **aleukemic leukemia.**

leukophlegmasia. See **phlegmasia alba dolens.**

leukophoresis /lo͞o′kōfərē′sis/, a laboratory procedure in which white blood cells are separated by electrophoresis for identification and an evaluation of the types of cells and their proportions.

leukoplakia /lo͞o′kōplā′kē•ə/, a precancerous, slowly developing change in a mucous membrane characterized by thickened, white, firmly attached patches that are slightly raised and sharply circumscribed. They may occur on the penis or vulva; those appearing on the lips and buccal mucosa are associated with pipe smoking. Malignant potential is evaluated by microscopic study of biopsied tissue. Compare **lichen planus.** See also **lichen sclerosis et atrophicus.**

leukopoiesis /lo͞o′kōpō•ē′sis/, the process by which white blood cells form and develop. Neutrophils, basophils, and eosinophils are produced in myeloid tissue in the bone marrow. Lymphocytes and monocytes are almost all normally derived from hemocytoblasts in lymphoid tissue, but a few develop in the marrow. –**leukopoietic,** *adj.*

leukorrhea /lo͞o′kərē′ə/, a white discharge from the vagina. Normally, vaginal discharge occurs in regular variations of amount and consistency during the course of the menstrual cycle. A greater than usual amount is normal in pregnancy and a decrease is to be expected after delivery, during lactation, and after menopause. An irritating, pruritic, copious, foul smelling, green or yellow discharge may indicate vaginal or uterine infection or other pathologic conditions of gynecologic origin. Leukorrhea is the most common reason for women to seek gynecologic care. See also **vaginal discharge.**

leukotomy. See **lobotomy.**

leukotoxin /lo͞o′kətok′sin/, a substance that can inactivate or destroy leukocytes. **–leukotoxic,** *adj.*

leukotrienes, a class of biologically active compounds that occur naturally in leukocytes and that produce allergic and inflammatory reactions. They are thought to play a role in the development of allergic and autoallergic disease, as asthma and rheumatoid arthritis.

levallorphan tartrate, a narcotic antagonist.

▪ INDICATION: It is prescribed in the treatment of severe narcotic-induced respiratory depression.

▪ CONTRAINDICATIONS: Mild respiratory depression, narcotic addiction, or known hypersensitivity to this drug prohibits its use.

▪ ADVERSE EFFECTS: Among the more serious adverse reactions are myosis, dysphoria, dizziness, respiratory depression, and, in high dosage, hallucinations and disorientation.

levamisole, a new drug used as an anthelmintic agent against a wide variety of nematodes. It has also been used in the treatment of bacterial and viral infections.

levamphetamine, an isomer of amphetamine, formerly used as an anorexiant. Also spelled **levamfetamine.**

levarterenol bitartrate. See **norepinephrine bitartrate.**

levator /livā′tər/, *pl.* **levatores** /lev′ətôr′ēz/, **1.** a muscle that raises a structure of the body, as the levator ani raises parts of the pelvic diaphragm. **2.** a surgical instrument used to lift depressed bony fragments in fractures of the skull and other bones.

levator ani, one of a pair of muscles of the pelvic diaphragm that stretches across the bottom of the pelvic cavity like a hammock, supporting the pelvic organs. It is a broad, thin muscle that separates into the pubococcygeus and the iliococcygeus. It originates from the ramus of the pubic bone, the spine of the ischium, and a band of fascia between the pubis and the ischium; it inserts into the last two segments of the coccyx, the anococcygeal raphe, the sphincter ani externus, and the central tendinous point of the perineum. The left and right levator ani muscles are divided ventrally but converge as a single sheet across the midline dorsally, forming most of the pelvic diaphragm. The levator ani is innervated by branches of the pudendal plexus, which contains fibers from the fourth sacral nerve, and it functions to support and slightly raise the pelvic floor. The pubococcygeus draws the anus toward the pubis and constricts it. Compare **coccygeus.**

levator palpebrae superioris, one of the three muscles of the eyelid, also considered a muscle of the eye. It is thin and flat and rises from the small wing of the sphenoid. It splits into three lamellae: The superficial lamella extends to the upper eyelid; the middle lamella inserts into the superior tarsus; and the deep lamella is attached to the conjunctiva. It is innervated by the oculomotor nerve, raises the upper eyelid, and is the antagonist of the orbicularis oculi. Compare **corrugator supercilii, orbicularis oculi.**

levator scapulae, a muscle of the dorsal and lateral aspects of the neck. It arises from the axis and the atlas, and it inserts in the third and fourth cervical vertebrae. It is innervated by the third and fourth cervical nerves and acts to raise the scapula and pull it toward the midline.

LeVeen shunt, a tube that is surgically implanted to connect the peritoneal cavity and the superior vena cava to drain an accumulation of fluid in the peritoneal cavity in cirrhosis of the liver, right-sided heart failure, or cancer of the abdomen. Before surgery, a sodium-restricted diet and diuretics are given to decrease sodium and water retention. Under general anesthesia, a silicone rubber tube is inserted under the subcutaneous tissue from the peritoneum to the superior vena cava. As the patient inhales, the fluid pressure in the peritoneal cavity rises and that in the blood vessel falls, allowing peritoneal fluid to enter the shunt valve. After surgery the patient is closely observed for signs of occlusion of the shunt, GI bleeding, or leakage of peritoneal fluid from the incision. Excessive dilution of the blood may lead to abnormalities of coagulation.

level of inquiry, (in nursing research) one of the levels in a rank-ordered system of classification and organization of the questions to be answered in a research study. The level of inquiry is determined by an analysis of the theory to be developed or tested and the kinds of data to be collected. Studies that describe comprise the first level whereas those that explain comprise the second level. Those that prescribe or predict are the most difficult to answer or to support.

levels of care, a classification of health care service levels by the kind of care given, the number of people served, and the people providing the care. Kinds of health care service levels are **primary health care, secondary health care, tertiary health care.**

lever, (in physiology) any one of the numerous bones and associated joints of the body that act together as a lever so that force applied to one end of the bone to lift a weight at another point tends to rotate the bone in the direction opposite from that of the applied force. The basic components of a lever are the fulcrum, the force arm, the weight arm, and the force moment. A first-class lever, as the hip, has a fulcrum between the weight and the applied force. A third-class lever, as that situated at all the joints of the upper and the lower extremities of the body, accommodates forces between the fulcrum and the weight. The body contains few second-class levers in which the force arm is longer than the weight arm. The muscles of the body produce the forces that move the levers. The body uses its third-class levers for speed and first-class levers to gain either force or speed, depending on the force applied to the weight arm. The moment of force produced by the weight of any body part involved in a lever action can be determined if the center of gravity of the part is known. Charts are available that list the center of gravity of various body parts.

Lévi-Lorain dwarf. See **pituitary dwarf.**

Levin tube /lev′in/, a #16 French, plastic catheter, used in gastric intubation, that has a closed, weighted tip and an opening on the side. Compare **Miller-Abbott tube.** See also **gastric intubation.**

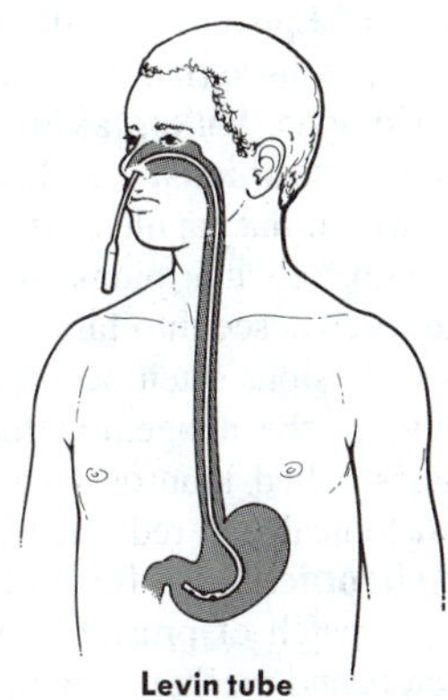

Levin tube

levitation, (in psychiatry) a hallucinatory sensation of floating or rising in the air. **–levitate,** *v.*

levo-, a combining form meaning 'left': *levocardia, levoclination, levotorsion.*

levodopa /lē′vōdō′pə/, an antiparkinsonian.

■ INDICATIONS: It is prescribed in the treatment of Parkinson's disease, juvenile forms of Huntington's disease, and chronic manganese poisoning.

■ CONTRAINDICATIONS: Narrow-angle glaucoma, concomitant use of a monoamine oxidase inhibitor, suspected melanoma, or known hypersensitivity to this drug prohibits its use.

■ ADVERSE EFFECTS: Among the more serious adverse reactions are severe GI disturbances, hypotension, various movement disorders, emotional changes, cardiac arrhythmia, and anorexia.

Levo-Dromoran, a trademark for a narcotic analgesic (levorphanol tartrate).

Levophed Bitartrate, a trademark for an adrenergic (norepinephrine bitartrate).

Levoprome, a trademark for an analgesic (methotrimeprazine).

levopropoxyphene napsylate, an antitussive.

■ INDICATION: It is prescribed for cough.

■ CONTRAINDICATIONS: Its use is prohibited during the first trimester of pregnancy, after surgery, or in cases of known hypersensitivity to this drug.

■ ADVERSE EFFECTS: Among the more serious adverse reactions are skin rash, muscle tremor, and vomiting.

levorphanol tartrate, a narcotic analgesic.

■ INDICATIONS: It is prescribed for pain and preoperative analgesia.

■ CONTRAINDICATIONS: Alcoholism, asthma, increased intracranial pressure, respiratory depression, anoxia, or known hypersensitivity to this drug prohibits its use.

■ ADVERSE EFFECTS: Among the more serious adverse reactions are drug dependence, orthostatic hypotension, cardiac arrhythmia, and retention of urine.

levothyroxine sodium, a thyroid hormone.

■ INDICATION: It is prescribed in the treatment of hypothyroidism.

■ CONTRAINDICATIONS: Recent myocardial infarction, normal thyroid function, or known hypersensitivity to this drug prohibits its use.

■ ADVERSE EFFECTS: The most serious adverse reactions are angina, tachycardia, arrhythmias, and tremors.

Levsinex, a trademark for an anticholinergic (hyoscyamine sulfate).

levulose. See **fructose.**

levulosuria. See **fructosuria.**

lewisite /lo͞o′isit/, 2-chlorovinyl arsine; a poisonous blister gas, used in World War I, that causes irritation of the lungs, dyspnea, damage to the tissues of the respiratory tract, tears, and pain.

-lexia, a combining form meaning 'reading': *alexia, bradylexia, dyslexia.*

Leyden-Moebius muscular dystrophy. See **pelvifemoral muscular dystrophy.**

Leydig cells /lī′dig/, cells of the interstitial tissue of the testes that secrete testosterone.

Leydig cell tumor, a generally benign neoplasm of interstitial cells of a testis that may cause gynecomastia in adults and precocious sexual development if the lesion occurs before puberty. The tumor is usually a circumscribed, lobulated, palpable mass.

LFT, abbreviation for **liver function test.**

LGA, abbreviation for **large for gestational age.**

LGV. See **lymphogranuloma venereum.**

LH, abbreviation for **luteinizing hormone.**

Lhermitte's sign /ler′mits/, sudden, transient, electric-like shocks spreading down the body when the head is flexed forward, occurring chiefly in multiple sclerosis but also in compression disorders of the cervical spinal cord.

Li, symbol for **lithium.**

liability, **1.** something one is obligated to do or an obligation required to be fulfilled by law, usually financial in nature. **2.** the amount of money required to fulfill a financial obligation.

liaison nursing, an arrangement with clinical specialists in psychiatric nursing whereby nurses and health professionals in other disciplines obtain consultation services in medical-surgical, parent-child, and geriatric settings.

libel, a false accusation written, printed, or typewritten, or presented in a picture or a sign that is made with malicious intent to defame the reputation of a person who is living or the memory of a person who is dead, resulting in public embarrassment, contempt, ridicule, or hatred.

liberation, the process of drug release from the dosage form.

libidinal development. See **psychosexual development.**

libidinous, **1.** pertaining to or belonging to the libido. **2.** having or characterized by sexual desire. Also **libidinal.** –**libidinize,** *v.*

libido /libē′dō, libī′dō/, **1.** the psychic energy or instinctual drive associated with sexual desire, pleasure, or creativity. **2.** (in psychoanalysis) the instinctual drives of the id. **3.** lustful desire or striving. Kinds of libido are **bisexual libido, ego libido.**

Libman-Sacks endocarditis /lib′mənsaks′/, an abnormal condition and the most common manifestation of lupus erythematosus, characterized by verrucous lesions that develop near the heart valves but rarely affect valvular action. The lesions usually are dry and granular, with a pink or tawny color, contain basophilic cellular debris, and develop in the angle of the atriventricular valves and at the base of the mitral valve. Also called **Libman-Sacks disease, Libman-Sacks syndrome.**

Librax, a trademark for a GI, fixed-combination drug containing an anticholinergic (clidinium bromide) and a sedative (chlordiazepoxide hydrochloride).

Libritabs, a trademark for an antianxiety agent (chlordiazepoxide hydrochloride).

Librium, a trademark for an antianxiety agent (chlordiazepoxide hydrochloride).

licensed practical nurse (LPN), *U.S.* a person trained in basic nursing techniques and direct patient care who practices under the supervision of a registered nurse. The course of training usually lasts 1 year. In Canada an LPN is called a nursing assistant. Also called *(U.S.)* **licensed vocational nurse.**

licensed psychologist, a person who has earned a PhD in psychology from an accredited graduate school and has completed 2 to 3 years of postgraduate training with special emphasis on the diagnosis and treatment of psychologic disorders. Also called **clinical psychologist.** See also **psychotherapist.**

licensed vocational nurse. See **licensed practical nurse.**

licensure, the granting of permission by a competent authority (usually a government agency) to an organization or individual to engage in a practice or activity that would otherwise be illegal. Kinds of licensure include the issuing of licenses for general hospitals or nursing homes, for health professionals, as physicians, and for the production or distribution of biologic products. Licensure is usually granted on the basis of education and examination rather than performance. It is usually permanent, but a periodic fee, demonstration of competence, or continuing education may be required. Licensure may be revoked by the granting agency for incompetence, criminal acts, or other reasons stipulated in the rules governing the specific area of licensure.

lichenification /līken′ifikā′shən/, thickening and hardening of the skin, often resulting from the irritation caused by repeated scratching of a pruritic lesion. –**lichenified,** *adj.*

lichen nitidus /lī′kən/, a rare skin disorder characterized by numerous flat, glistening, pale, discrete papules measuring 2 to 3 mm in diameter. Also called **Pinkus' disease.**

lichen planus, a nonmalignant, chronic, pruritic skin disease of unknown cause, characterized by small, flat, purplish papules or plaques having fine, gray lines on the surface. Common sites are flexor surfaces of wrists, forearms, ankles, abdomen, and sacrum. On mucous membranes the lesions appear gray and lacy. Nails may have longitudinal ridges. Episodes of disease activity, of which there are numerous variations, may last for months and may recur. Compare **leukoplakia.**

lichen sclerosis et atrophicus, a chronic skin disease characterized by white, flat papules with an erythematous halo and black, hard follicular plugs. In advanced cases, the papules tend to coalesce into large, white patches of thin, pruritic skin. Lesions often occur on the torso and, almost inevitably, in the anogenital regions, in which case the disease is called kraurosis vulvae. Corticosteroids are applied topically to reduce itching.

lichen simplex chronicus, a form of neurodermatitis characterized by a patch of pruritic, confluent papules. Psychogenic factors and mechanic trauma, as scratching, contribute to its chronicity. Treatment may include topical or intralesional application of corticosteroids to relieve the pruritis.

lid. See **eyelid.**

Lidaform-HC, a trademark for a topical, fixed-combination drug containing a glucocorticoid (hydrocortisone acetate), a topical antiinfective (iodochlorhydroxyquin), and a local anesthetic (lidocaine).

Lida-Mantle-HC, a trademark for a topical, fixed-combination drug containing a glucocorticoid (hydrocortisone acetate) and a local anesthetic (lidocaine).

Lidex, a trademark for a glucocorticoid (fluocinonide).

lidocaine hydrochloride /lī′dəkān/, a local anesthetic agent.

▪ INDICATIONS: It is prescribed as a local anesthetic for topical administration to skin or to mucous membrances. It is used parenterally as an antiarrhythmic agent.

▪ CONTRAINDICATIONS: Known hypersensitivity to this drug prohibits its topical use. Heart block or known hypersensitivity to this drug prohibits its systemic use.

▪ ADVERSE EFFECTS: Among the more serious adverse reactions to the systemic administration of the drug are central nervous system disturbances, hypotension, bradycardia, and cardiac arrest. A variety of hypersensitivity reactions may occur from topical administration of this drug. Eating and drinking is avoided for 1 hour after topical application of this drug to the pharynx or the esophagus.

Lidosporin, a trademark for an otic, fixed-combination drug containing an antibacterial (polymyxin B sulfate) and a local anesthetic (lidocaine hydrochloride).

lid poppers, *slang.* amphetamines.

lie, the relationship between the long axis of the fetus and the long axis of the mother. In a longitudinal lie the fetus is lying lengthwise, or vertically, in the uterus, whereas in a transverse lie the fetus is lying crosswise, or horizontally.

lie detector, an electronic device or instrument used to detect lying or anxiety in regard to specific questions. A commonly used lie detector is the polygraph recorder that senses and records pulse, respiratory rate, blood pressure, and perspiration. Some experts hold that certain patterns indicate the presence of anxiety, guilt, or fear, emotions that are likely to occur when the subject is lying.

lien. See **spleen.**

lienal vein /lē•ē′nəl/, a large vein of the lower body that unites with the superior mesenteric vein to form the portal vein. It returns blood from the spleen and arises from about six large tributaries that unite to form the single vessel passing from left to right across the superior, dorsal part of the pancreas. It receives the short gastric veins, the left gastroepiploic vein, the pancreatic veins, and the inferior mesenteric veins. Also called **splenic vein.**

lieno-, a combining form meaning 'of or pertaining to the spleen': *lienomalacia, lienomedullary, lienopathy*.

life costs, the mortality, morbidity, and suffering associated with a given disease or medical procedure.

life expectancy. See **expectation of life.**

life island, a plastic bubble enclosing a bed, used to provide a germ-free environment for a patient.

life science, the study of the laws and properties of living matter. Some kinds of life science are **anatomy, bacteriology,** and **biology.** Compare **physical science.**

life space, a term introduced by American psychologist Kurt Lewin to describe simultaneous influences that may affect individual behavior. The totality of the influences make up the life space.

life-style-induced health problems, diseases with natural histories that include conscious exposure to certain health-compromising or risk factors. An example is heart disease associated with cigarette smoking, poor dietary habits, lack of exercise, and sustaining unbuffered stress.

lifetime reserve, a lifetime total of days of inpatient hospitalization benefits that may be drawn on by a patient who has exhausted the maximum benefits allowed under Medicare for a single spell of illness.

lift assessment, the selection of the most appropriate lift method to use when moving a patient, as from the bed to a chair. The assessment involves consideration of such factors as whether the patient is conscious or unconscious, if the patient has a visual or hearing impairment, the need for special care in handling patient attachments, as IV lines or monitors, and whether the patient has full range of motion or flaccid or spastic limbs.

ligament, **1.** one of many predominantly white, shiny, flexible bands of fibrous tissue binding joints together and connecting various bones and cartilages. Such ligaments are slightly elastic and composed of parallel collagenous bundles. When part of the synovial membrane of a joint, they are covered with fibroelastic tissue that blends with surrounding connective tissue. Yellow elastic ligaments, as the ligamenta flava, connect certain parts of adjoining vertebrae. Compare **tendon. 2.** a layer of serous membrane with little or no tensile strength, extending from one visceral organ to another, as the ligaments of the peritoneum. See also **broad ligament.** Also called **ligamentum.** **–ligamentous,** *adj*.

ligamenta flava, the bands of yellow elastic tissue connecting the laminae of adjacent vertebrae from the axis to the first segment of the sacrum. They are thin, broad, and long in the cervical region, thicker in the thoracic region, and thickest in the lumbar region. They help to hold the body erect.

ligamental tear, a complete or a partial tear of a ligamentous structure connecting and surrounding the bones of a joint, caused by an injury to the joint, as by a sudden twisting motion or by a forceful blow.

■ OBSERVATIONS: Ligamental tears may occur at any joint but are most common in the knees. The pathologic features of ligamental tears of the knee are dependent on the location and severity of the injury. The most common ligaments involved in knee injuries are the medial, lateral, and posterior ligaments and the anterior and posterior cruciate ligaments. Usually, the injury involves more than one structure because of the way in which the structures connect with and support each other.

■ INTERVENTION: Treatment depends on the severity of the injury. A mild injury may cause little damage with tenderness, swelling, and pain with stress. Rest, compression, applications of heat and cold, elevation, and early use are usually recommended. Injection of an anti-inflammatory agent may be desirable. Treatment for a moderate injury in which few fibers have been completely torn is protective. In addition to the above measures, the joint is aspirated and supported. Treatment for a severe, complete tear is restorative. This may be by immobilization followed by physical therapy, or, if necessary, by surgical repair.

■ NURSING CONSIDERATIONS: Ligamental tears of the knee joint are extremely common in young adults and are associated with sports injuries. Good physical condition may help prevent many injuries, and proper care during healing is necessary to prevent permanent disability, which is often accompanied by instability, stiffness, or pain in the joint.

ligament of the neck of the rib, one of five ligaments of each costotransverse joint, consisting of short, strong fibers passing from the neck of the rib to the transverse process of the adjacent vertebra. Also called **middle costotransverse ligament.**

ligament of the tubercle of the rib, one of the five ligaments of each costotransverse joint, comprised of a short, thick fasciculus passing obliquely from the transverse process of a vertebra to the tubercle of the associated rib. Compare **ligament of the neck of the rib.**

ligamentum. See **ligament.**

ligamentum latum uteri. See **broad ligament.**

ligamentum nuchae, the fibrous membrane that reaches from the external occipital protuberance and median nuchal line to the spinous process of the seventh vertebra. A fibrous lamina from the ligament attaches to the posterior tubercle of the atlas and to the spinous processes of the cervical vertebrae, forming a septum between muscles on either side of the neck.

ligand, **1.** a molecule, ion, or group bound to the central atom of a chemical compound, as the oxygen molecule in hemoglobin, which is bound to the central iron atom. **2.** an organic molecule attached to a specific site on a surface or to a tracer element. The binding is reversible in a competitive binding assay. It may be the analyte or a cross-reactant. Examples include vitamin B_{12}, a ligand with intrinsic factor as the binding protein, and various antigens, which are ligands with antibody binding proteins.

ligases, a group of enzymes that catalyze the formation of a bond between substrate molecules coupled with the breakdown of a pyrophosphate bond in ATP or a similar donor molecule. Examples of ligases include the synthetase enzymes.

ligation /līgā′shən/, tying off of a blood vessel or duct with a suture or wire ligature performed to stop or prevent bleeding during surgery, to stop spontaneous or traumatic hemorrhage, or to prevent passage of material through a duct, as in tubal ligation or to treat varicosities. In venous ligation, the saphenous vein is tied above the varicosed portion, and the distal portions are removed. General anesthesia is used. After surgery, the nurse observes the patient's feet and legs for circulatory impairment; the foot of the bed is raised to encourage venous return. Ambulation is begun the day of surgery, with elastic bandages for firm support. Analgesics are given as necessary for pain and discomfort. See also **ligature, saphenous vein, tubal ligation, varicose veins.** **–ligate,** *v.*

ligature /lig′əchər/, **1.** a suture. **2.** a wire, as used in orthodontia.

ligature needle, a long, thin, curved needle used for passing a suture underneath an artery for ligation of the vessel.

light, **1.** electromagnetic radiation of the wavelength and frequency that stimulate visual receptor cells in the retina to produce nerve impulses that are perceived as vision. **2.** electromagnetic radiation with wavelengths shorter than ultraviolet light and longer than infrared light, the range of visible light generally in the range of 400 to 800 nm.

light bath, the exposure of the patient's uncovered skin to the sun or to actinic light rays from an artificial source for therapeutic purposes.

light chain, a subunit of an immunoglobulin molecule composed of a polypeptide chain of about 22,000 daltons, or atomic mass units. An example of a light chain is a Bence Jones protein molecule associated with multiple myeloma.

light diet, a diet suitable for convalescent or bedridden patients taking little or no exercise. It consists of simple, moderate quantities of soft-cooked and easily digested foods, including meats, potatoes, rice, eggs, pasta, some fruits, refined cereals, and breads. It avoids all highly seasoned and fried foods.

lightening, a subjective sensation reported by many women late in pregnancy as the fetus settles lower in the pelvis, leaving more space in the upper abdomen. The diaphragm, no longer restricted by the fundus of the uterus beneath it, can move down more fully during inspiration, allowing deeper breaths to be taken. The stomach, too, is less compressed, so the woman can comfortably eat more food at each meal. The profile of the abdomen changes with lightening, because the round, full uterus is visibly lower. The baby is then said to have "dropped."

light film fault, a defect in a radiograph or developed photographic film that appears as a barely distinct and inadequate image. It is caused by underexposure, underdevelopment, development in too-cold solutions, or use of the wrong film speed.

light pen, an electric device, resembling a pen, that may be used with a computer terminal to enter or modify information displayed on the screen.

light reflex, the mechanism by which the pupil of the eye becomes more or less open in response to direct or consensual pupillary stimulation. Also called **pupillary reflex.** Compare **consensual light reflex.** See also **consensual reaction to light.**

light vaginal bleeding. See **vaginal bleeding.**

ligneous /lig′nē·əs/, woody or resembling wood in texture or other characteristics.

ligneous thyroiditis. See **fibrous thyroiditis.**

lignin /lig′nin/, a polysaccharide that with cellulose and hemicellulose forms the chief part of the skeletal substances of the cell walls of plants. It provides bulk in the diet necessary for proper GI functioning. See also **dietary fiber.**

lignocaine. See **lidocaine hydrochloride.**

lilliputian hallucination /lil′ipyo͞o′shən/, one in which things seem smaller than they actually are. See also **hallucination.**

limb, **1.** an appendage or extremity of the body, as an arm or leg. **2.** a branch of an internal organ, as a loop of a nephron.

limb girdle muscular dystrophy, a form of muscular dystrophy transmitted as an autosomal recessive trait. The characteristic weakness and degeneration of the muscles begins in the shoulder girdle or in the pelvic girdle. The condition is progressive, regardless of the area in which it is first manifest. Kinds of limb girdle muscular dystrophy are **pelvifemoral muscular dystrophy, scapulohumeral muscular dystrophy.**

limbic system, a group of structures within the rhinencephalon of the brain that are associated with various emotions and feelings, as anger, fear, sexual arousal, pleasure, and sadness. The structures of the limbic system are the cingulate gyrus, the isthmus, the hippocampal gyrus, the uncis, and the hippocampus. The structures connect with various other parts of the brain, as the septum and the hypothalamus. Unless the limbic system is modulated by other cortical areas, periodic attacks of uncontrollable rage may occur in some individuals. The function of the system is poorly understood.

limb kinetic apraxia. See **ideomotor apraxia.**

lime, **1.** any of several oxides and hydroxides of calcium. The various kinds of lime have many uses, including the treatment of sewage, purification of water and refining of sugar, and the manufacture of materials such as plaster and fertilizers. **2.** a citrus fruit yielding a juice with a high ascorbic acid content. Lime juice was one of the first effective agents to be used in the treatment of scurvy. See also **ascorbic acid, scurvy.**

limited fluctuation method of dosing, a method of drug administration in which the dose is not allowed to rise or fall beyond specified maximum and minimum limits.

limo-, a combining form meaning 'of or pertaining to hunger': *limophthisis, limosis, limotherapy.*

limp, an abnormal pattern of ambulation in which the two phases of gait are markedly asymmetric. See also **stance phase of gait, swing phase of gait.**

LINAC, abbreviation for **linear accelerator.**

Lincocin, a trademark for an antibacterial (lincomycin).

Lincocin Hydrochloride, a trademark for an antibacterial (lincomycin hydrochloride).

lincomycin hydrochloride, an antibiotic.

■ INDICATIONS: It is prescribed in the treatment of certain infections.

■ CONTRAINDICATIONS: Known hypersensitivity to this drug or to clindamycin prohibits its use.

■ ADVERSE EFFECTS: Among the more serious adverse reactions are blood disorders, diarrhea and the development of life-threatening pseudomembranous colitis caused by suprainfection.

lindane /lin′dān/, gamma-benzene hexachloride.

■ INDICATIONS: It is prescribed in the treatment of pediculosis and scabies.

■ CONTRAINDICATIONS: It is not usually given to infants or pregnant women and is not applied to the face. Known hypersensitivity to this drug prohibits its use.

■ ADVERSE EFFECTS: Among the most serious adverse reactions are neurologic damage and aplastic anemia. Given topically, irritation of eyes, skin, and mucosa may occur.

Lindau-von Hippel disease. See **cerebroretinal angiomatosis.**

Lindbergh pump, a pump used to preserve an organ of the body by perfusing its tissues with oxygen and other essential nutrients, usually during the transport of an organ from a donor to a recipient. Also called **Carrel-Lindbergh pump.**

line, a stripe, streak, or narrow ridge, often imaginary, that serves to connect anatomic reference points or to separate various parts of the body, as the hairline or nipple line. Also called **linea.**

linea alba /lin′ē·ə/, the portion of the anterior abdominal aponeurosis in the middle line of the abdomen, representing the fusion of three aponeuroses into a single tendinous band extending from the xiphoid process to the symphysis pubis. It contains the umbilicus. Compare **linea semilunaris.**

linea albicantes, lines, white to pink or gray in color, that occur on the abdomen, buttocks, breasts, and thighs and are caused by the stretching of the skin and weakening or rupturing of the underlying elastic tissue. The condition is usually associated with pregnancy, excessive obesity, rapid growth during adolescence, Cushing's syndrome, or prolonged adrenal cortical hormone therapy. Also called **stria atrophica.**

linea arcuata, the curved tendinous band in the sheath of the rectus abdominis below the umbilicus. It is usually derived from the aponeurosis of the transversus abdominis or the obliquus internus, sometimes from both those muscles. It inserts into the linea alba. Compare **linea semilunaris.**

linea aspera, the posterior crest of the thigh bone, extending proximally into three ridges to which are attached various muscles, including the gluteus maximus, pectineus, and iliacus.

linea nigra, a dark line appearing longitudinally on the abdomen of a pregnant woman during the latter part of term. It usually extends from the symphysis pubis to the umbilicus.

linear accelerator (LINAC), an apparatus for accelerating charged subatomic particles used in radiotherapy, physics research, and in the production of radionuclides. In a linear accelerator a pulsed electron beam generated by an electron gun passes through a straight long vacuum tube containing alternating hollow electrodes. The electrodes are so arranged that when their high-frequency potentials are properly varied, the particles passing through the vacuum tube waveguide receive successive increments of energy. The electrons are stopped abruptly by a heavy metal target at the end of the waveguide and are directed by a collimator to deliver supervoltage x-rays to the patient receiving radiotherapy.

linear fracture, a fracture that extends parallel to the long axis of a bone but does not displace the bone tissue.

linear regression, a statistic procedure in which a straight line is established through a data set that best represents a relationship between two subsets or two methods. This mathematic technique minimizes the sum of the squares of the differences between the observed y values and the y values predicted by the regression line for a given x value.

linea semilunaris, the slightly curved line on the ventral abdominal wall, approximately parallel to the median line and lying about halfway between the median line and the side of the body. It marks the lateral border of the rectus abdominis and can be seen as a shallow groove when that muscle is tensed. Compare **linea alba.**

linea terminalis, a hypothetic line dividing the upper, or false, pelvis, from the lower, or true, pelvis.

line printer, a high-speed printer, driven by a computer, that prints an entire line of text simultaneously.

Lineweaver-Burk transformation, a method of converting experimental data from studies of enzyme activity so that they can be displayed on a linear plot. The linearized form is derived by using reciprocals of both sides of the equation.

lingu-, a combining form meaning 'of or pertaining to the tongue': *linguiform, lingulectomy, linguodental.*

lingua. See **tongue.**

lingual artery, one of a pair of arteries that arises from the external carotid arteries, divides into four branches, and supplies the tongue and surrounding muscles. The branches of the lingual artery are the suprahyoid, dorsal lingual, sublingual, and the deep lingual.

lingual bar, a major connector that is installed lingual to the dental arch and joins bilateral parts of a mandibular removable partial denture.

lingual bone. See **hyoid bone.**

lingual crib, an orthodontic appliance consisting of a wire frame suspended lingually to the maxillary incisor teeth. It is used for obstructing undesirable thumb and tongue habits that can produce malocclusions, especially in youngsters.

lingual flange, the part of a mandibular denture that occupies the space adjacent to the residual ridge and next to the mouth.

lingual frenum, a band of tissue that extends from the floor of the mouth to the inferior surface of the tongue. Also called **frenulum linguae.**

lingual goiter, a tumor at the back of the tongue formed by an enlargement of the primordial thyrolingual duct.

lingual papilla. See **papilla.**

lingual rest, a metallic extension onto the lingual surface of an anterior tooth to provide support or indirect retention for a removable partial denture.

lingual tonsil, a mass of lymphoid follicles near the root of the tongue. Each follicle forms a rounded eminence containing a small opening leading into a funnel-shaped cavity surrounded by lymphoid tissue.

lingua villosa nigra. See **parasitic glossitis.**

liniment, a preparation, usually containing an alcoholic, oily, or soapy vehicle, that is rubbed on the skin as a counterirritant.

linin, the faintly staining threads seen in the nuclei of cells, with granules of chromatin attached to the threads. See also **karyolymph.**

linitis /linī′tis/, inflammation of cellular tissue of the stomach as in linitis plastica, seen frequently in adenocarcinoma of the stomach.

linitis plastica, a diffuse fibrosis and thickening of the wall of the stomach, resulting in a rigid, inelastic organ. The layer of connective tissue of the stomach becomes fibrotic and thick, and the stomach wall becomes shrunken and rigid. Causes of this condition include infiltrating undifferentiated carcinoma, syphilis, and Crohn's disease involving the stomach. Also called **leather bottle stomach.**

linkage, **1.** (in genetics) the location of two or more genes on the same chromosome so that they do not segregate independently during meiosis but tend to be transmitted together as a unit. The closer the loci of the genes, the more likely they are to be inherited as a group and associated with a specific trait, whereas the farther apart they are, the greater the chance that they will be separated by crossing over and carried on homologous chromosomes. The concept of linkage, which opposes the independent assortment theory of mendelian genetics, led to the foundation of the modern chromosome theory of genetics. See also **synteny.** **2.** (in psychology) the association between a stimulus and the response it elicits. **3.** (in chemistry) the bond between two atoms or radicals in a chemical compound or the lines used to designate valency connections between the atoms in structural formulas.

linkage group, (in genetics) a group of genes located on the same chromosome that tends to be inherited as a unit. Theoretically, without crossing over, all of the genes on a given chromosome constitute a linkage group and are equal to the number of autosomes in the haploid cell.

linkage map. See **genetic map.**

linked genes, genes that are located on the same chromosome and whose position is close enough so that they tend to be transmitted as a linkage group.

linker, (in molecular genetics) a small segment of synthetic DNA having a place on its surface that can be ligated to DNA fragments in cloning. Some linkers are commercially available.

linoleic acid /lin′əlē′ik/, a colorless to straw-colored essential fatty acid with two unsaturated bonds, occurring in linseed and safflower oils. Commercially produced linoleic acid is used in margarine, animal feeds, emulsifying agents, soaps, and drugs.

linolenic acid, an unsaturated fatty acid essential for normal human nutrition. It occurs in glycerides of linseed and other vegetable oils.

lio-. See **leio-.**

Lioresal, a trademark for an antispastic agent (baclofen).

liothyronine sodium /lī′ōthī′rənēn/, a synthetic thyroid hormone.

■ INDICATIONS: It is prescribed in the treatment of primary hypothyroidism, myxedema, simple goiter, cretinism, and secondary hypothyroidism.

■ CONTRAINDICATIONS: Hyperthyroidism, thyrotoxicosis, acute myocardial infarction, or known hypersensitivity to this drug prohibits its use. It is used with caution in patients with diabetes mellitus or cardiovascular disease.

■ ADVERSE EFFECTS: Among the serious adverse reactions, usually caused by overdosage, are thyrotoxicosis, nausea, vomiting, hypertension, nervousness, and loss of weight.

liotrix /lī′ətriks/, a uniform mixture of the thyroid hormones T_3 and T_4.

■ INDICATION: It is prescribed in the treatment of hypothyroid conditions.

■ CONTRAINDICATIONS: Most diseases and abnormal conditions of the myocardium or known hypersensitivity to this drug prohibits its use.

■ ADVERSE EFFECTS: Among the more serious adverse reactions are symptoms of thyrotoxicosis, including tachycardia, nervousness, insomnia, and fever.

lip, **1.** either the upper or lower fleshy structure surrounding the opening of the oral cavity. **2.** any rimlike structure bordering a cavity or groove; labium.

lip-, lipo-, combining form meaning 'fat': *lipase, lipodystrophy, lipoma.*

lipase /lī′pās, lip′ās/, any of several enzymes, produced by the organs of the digestive system, that catalyze the breakdown of lipids through the hydrolysis of the linkages between fatty acids and glycerol in triglycerides and phospholipids. See also **fat, fatty acid, glycerol, phospholipid, triglyceride.**

lipectomy /lipek′təmē/, an excision of subcutaneous fat, as from the abdominal wall. Also called **adipectomy.**

lipemia /lipē′mē·ə/, a condition in which increased amounts of lipids are present in the blood, a normal occurrence after eating.

lipid, any of the free fatty acid fractions in the blood. Lipids are insoluble in water but soluble in alcohol, chloroform, ether, and other solvents. They are stored in the body and serve as an energy reserve, but are elevated in various diseases, as atherosclerosis. Kinds of lipids are **cholesterol, fatty acids, neutral fat, phospholipids, phospholipid as phosphorus,** and **triglycerides.** The normal concentrations of total lipids in serum are 400 to 800 mg/dl; cholesterol, 150 to 250 mg/dl; fatty acids, 9 to 15 mM/L; neutral fat, 0 to 200 mg/dl; phospholipids, 150 to 380 mg/dl; phospholipid as phosphorus, 9 to 16 mg/dl; triglycerides, 10 to 190 mg/dl.

lipidosis /lip′idō′sis/, a general term including several rare familial disorders of fat metabolism. The chief characteristic of these disorders is the accumulation of abnormal levels of certain lipids in the body. Kinds of lipidoses are **Gaucher's disease, Krabbe's disease, Niemann-Pick disease,** and **Tay-Sachs disease.**

lipo-. See **lip-.**

lipocele. See **adipocele.**

lipochondrodystrophy. See **Hurler's syndrome.**

lipochrome /lip′əkrōm/, any of the naturally occurring pigments that contain a lipid, and which give a yellow color to fats, as carotene.

lipodystrophia progressiva, an abnormal accumulation of fat around the buttocks and thighs and a progressive, symmetric disappearance of subcutaneous fat from areas above the pelvis and on the face. Also called **lipomatosis atrophicans.**

lipodystrophy /lip′ōdis′trəfē/, any abnormality in the metabolism or deposition of fats. Kinds of lipodystrophy are **bitrochanteric lipodystrophy, insulin lipodystrophy,** and **intestinal lipodystrophy.**

lip of hip fracture, a fracture of the posterior lip of the acetabulum, often associated with displacement of the hip.

lipogranuloma /lip′ōgran′yo͞olō′mə/, *pl.* **lipogranulomas, lipogranulomata,** a nodule of necrotic, fatty tissue associated with granulomatous inflammation or with a foreign-body reaction around a deposit of injected material containing an oily substance.

Lipo-Hepin, a trademark for an anticoagulant (heparin sodium).

lipoic acid /lipō′ik/, a bacterial growth factor found in liver and yeast.

lipoid /lip′oid/, any substance that resembles a lipid.

lipoma /lipō′mə/, *pl.* **lipomas, lipomata,** a benign tumor consisting of mature fat cells. Also called **adipose tumor.** See also **multiple lipomatosis.** **–lipomatous,** *adj.*

-lipoma, a combining form meaning a 'tumor made up of fatty tissue': *angiolipoma, fibrolipoma, osteolipoma.*

lipoma annulare colli, a diffuse, symmetric accumulation of fat around the neck, not a true lipoma. Also called **Madelung's neck.**

lipoma arborescens, a fatty tumor of a joint, characterized by a treelike distribution of fat cells.

lipoma capsulare, a benign neoplasm characterized by the abnormal presence of fat cells in the capsule of an organ.

lipoma cavernosum. See **angiolipoma.**

lipoma diffusum renis. See **lipomatous nephritis.**

lipoma dolorosa. See **lipomatosis dolorosa.**

lipoma fibrosum, a fatty tumor containing masses of fibrous tissue.

lipoma myxomatodes. See **lipomyxoma.**

lipoma sarcomatode. See **liposarcoma.**

lipomatosis /lip′ōmətō′sis/, a disorder characterized by abnormal tumorlike accumulations of fat in body tissues.

lipomatosis atrophicans. See **lipodystrophia progressiva, lipomatosis.**

lipomatosis dolorosa, a disorder characterized by the abnormal accumulation of painful or tender fat deposits. Also called **lipoma dolorosa.**

lipomatosis gigantea, a condition characterized by massive deposits of fat.

lipomatosis renis. See **lipomatous nephritis.**

lipomatous myxoma, a tumor containing fatty tissue that arises in connective tissue.

lipomatous nephritis, a rare condition in which the renal nephrons are replaced by fatty tissue. Kidney failure may result. Also called **lipoma diffusum renis, lipomatosis renis.**

lipomyxoma /lip′ōmiksō′mə/, *pl.* **lipomyxomas, lipomyxomata,** a myxoma that contains fat cells. Also called **lipoma myxomatodes.**

lipoprotein /lip′ōprō′tēn/, a conjugated protein in which lipids form an integral part of the molecule. They are synthesized primarily in the liver, contain varying amounts of triglycerides, cholesterol, phospholipids, and protein, and are classified according to their composition and density. Practically all of the plasma lipids are present as lipoprotein complexes. Kinds of lipoproteins are **chylomicrons, high-density lipoproteins, low-density lipoproteins,** and **very low-density lipoproteins.** See also **proteolipid.**

liposarcoma /lip′ōsärkō′mə/, *pl.* **liposarcomas, liposarcomata,** a malignant growth of primitive fat cells. Also called **lipoma sarcomatode.**

liposis. See **lipomatosis.**

-lipsis, -lipse, a combining form meaning 'to leave, fail, omit': *eclipsis, ellipsis, menolipsis.*

Liquaemin Sodium, a trademark for an anticoagulant (heparin sodium).

Liquamar, a trademark for an anticoagulant (phenprocoumon).

liquefaction, the process in which a solid or a gas is made liquid.

liquid, a state of matter, intermediate between solid and gas, in which the substance flows freely with little application of force and assumes the shape of the vessel in which it is contained. Compare **fluid.** See also **gas, solid.**

liquid diet, a diet consisting of foods that can be served in liquid or strained form plus custard, ice cream, pudding, tapioca, and soft-cooked eggs. It is prescribed in acute infections, in acute inflammatory conditions of the GI tract, and for patients unable to consume soft or semifluid foods, usually after surgery. See also **full liquid diet.**

liquid glucose, a thick, syrupy, odorless, and colorless or yellowish liquid obtained by the incomplete hydrolysis of starch primarily consisting of dextrose with dextrins, maltose, and water. It is used as a flavoring agent and may be used as a food, chiefly in treating dehydration.

liquor amnii. See **amniotic fluid.**

liquorice, a dried root of gummy texture from the leguminous plant *Glycyrrhiza glabra.* It has a sweet, astringent taste and is used as a flavoring agent in medicines, especially in cough syrups and laxatives, confectionery, and tobacco. Also spelled **licorice.**

Lisfranc's fracture /lisfrangks′/, a fracture dislocation of the foot in which one or all of the proximal metatarsals are displaced.

Listeria monocytogenes /mon′ōsītoj′inēz/, a common species of gram-positive, motile bacillus that causes listeriosis.

listeriosis /listir′ē·ō′sis/, an infectious disease caused by a genus of gram-positive motile bacteria that are nonsporulating. *Listeria monocytogenes* infects shellfish, birds, spiders, and mammals in all areas of the world, but infection in humans is uncommon. Transmitted by direct contact from infected animals to humans, by inhalation of dust, or by contact with mud, sewage, or soil contaminated with the organism, it is characterized by circulatory collapse, shock, endocarditis, hepatosplenomegaly, and a dark red rash over the trunk and the legs. Fever, bacteremia, malaise, and lethargy are commonly seen. Newborns and immunosuppressed, debilitated older people are more vulnerable to infection than are immunocompetent children and young or middle-aged adults. The signs of infection and the severity of the disease vary according to the site of infection and the age and condition of the person. Pregnant women characteristically experience a mild, brief episode of illness, but fetal infection acquired through the placental circulation in utero is usually fatal. Infection in the newborn apparently results from exposure to the organism in the birth canal of an infected mother. Meningitis and encephalitis occur in 75% of cases. Treatment may include ampicillin, penicillin, tetracycline, or erythromycin, given intramuscularly or intravenously. If infection is suspected in a pregnant woman, treatment is begun immediately, even before bacteriologic culture of the blood, spinal fluid, or vaginal secretions can confirm the diagnosis. All secretions from the patient may contain the organism. Also called **listerosis.**

Liston's forceps, a kind of bone cutting forceps.

lith. See **litho-.**

-lith, a combining form meaning 'a calculus': *pneumolith, ptyalith, tonsillolith.*

Lithane, a trademark for an antimanic drug (lithium carbonate).

lithiasis /lithī′əsis/, the formation of calculi in the hollow organs or ducts of the body. Calculi are formed of mineral salts and may irritate, inflame, or obstruct the organ in which they form or lodge. Lithiasis occurs most commonly in the gallbladder, kidney, and lower urinary tract. Lithiasis may be asymptomatic, but more often the condition is extremely painful. Surgery may be necessary if the stones cannot be excreted spontaneously. Lower urinary tract calculi often can be dissolved. See also **biliary calculus, cholelithiasis, renal calculus, urinary calculus.**

lithium (Li), a silvery white alkali metal occurring in various compounds, as petalite and spodumene. Its atomic number is 3; its atomic weight is 6.94. Lithium is the lightest known metal and one of the most reactive elements. Traces of lithium ion occur in animal tissue, and it abounds in many alkaline mineral spring waters. Its salts are used in the treatment of manias, but the mechanisms by which these compounds help to stabilize psychologic moods are not understood. Lithium carbonate is a salt commonly used for psychiatric purposes in the United States; it has been effective in the prevention of recurrent attacks of manic-depressive illnesses. It has helped to correct sleep disorders in manic patients, apparently by suppressing the rapid eye movement phases of sleep. Therapeutic concentrations of lithium have no observable psychotropic effects on normal individuals. In manic patients, lithium salts also produce high-voltage slow waves in the electroencephalograph, often with superimposed beta waves. An important feature of the lithium ion is its relatively small gradient of distribution across biologic membranes. Although it can replace sodium in supporting a nerve cell action potential, it cannot adequately prime the sodium pump and maintain membrane potentials. Lithium ions are quickly and almost completely absorbed from the GI tract, producing peak concentrations in plasma within 2 to 4 hours. The ion first spreads through the extracellular fluid and then gradually disperses in varying concentrations through different tissues. The ion passes slowly through the blood-brain barrier, and, when a steady state is achieved, the concentration of lithium in the cerebrospinal fluid is about 40% of the lithium concentration in the plasma. About 95% of a single dose of lithium salts is eliminated in the urine. The lithium ion has such a low therapeutic index that safe treatment requires daily determination of plasma concentrations. Intoxication may result if levels rise beyond peak concentrations, which can be 2 to 3 times higher than steady-state concentrations. Acute intoxication by lithium may cause seizure and death. Side effects may include polyuria, polydipsia, and benign enlargement of the thyroid. Mixed and inconclusive results have followed lithium treatment of disorders other than manias, as premenstrual tension, alcoholism, episodic anger, and anorexia nervosa. Patients suffering severe manic attacks are hospitalized so that they can receive proper medical maintenance; treatments start with large doses of antipsychotic drugs, which are followed by the gradual and safe introduction of lithium therapy. Ideally, lithium treatment is prescribed only for patients with normal sodium intake and normal heart and kidney function.

lithium carbonate, an antimanic agent.

■ INDICATION: It is prescribed in the treatment of manic episodes of manic-depressive disorder.

■ CONTRAINDICATIONS: It is used with caution in the presence of renal or cardiovascular disease and is not recommended for children under 12 years of age. Known hypersensitivity to this drug prohibits its use.

■ ADVERSE EFFECTS: Among the most serious adverse reactions are renal damage, polydipsia and polyuria, and impairment of mental and physical abilities. Retention of sodium and fluid may occur.

lithium fluoride (LiF), a compound commonly used for thermoluminescent dosimetry.

litho-, lith-, a combining form meaning 'of or pertaining to a stone, or to a calculus': *litholysis, lithomyl, lithophone.*

Lithonate, a trademark for an antimanic agent (lithium carbonate).

Lithonate S, a trademark for an antimanic agent (lithium carbonate).

lithopedion /lith′əpē′dē·ən/, a fetus that has died in utero and has become calcified or ossified. Also called **lithopedium, calcified fetus, ostembryon, osteopedion.**

lithotomy /lithot′əmē/, the surgical excision of a calculus, especially one from the urinary tract.

lithotomy forceps, a forceps for the extraction of a calculus, usually from the urinary tract.

lithotomy position, the posture assumed by the patient lying supine with the hips and the knees flexed and the thighs abducted and rotated externally. Also called **dorsosacral position.**

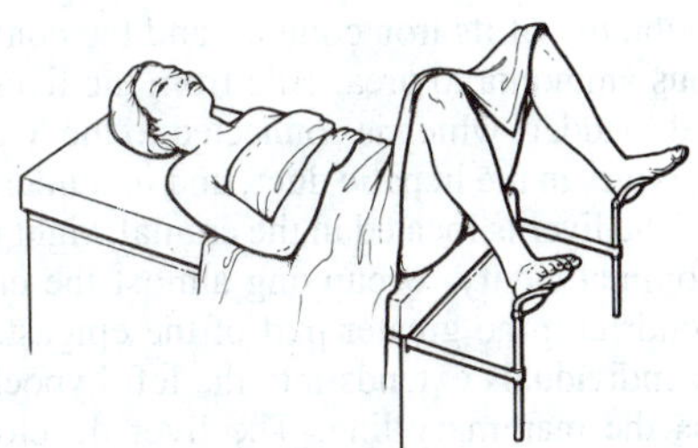

Lithotomy position

lithotrite /lith′ətrīt/, an instrument for crushing a stone in the urinary bladder. Also called **lithotriptor.** – **lithotrity,** *n.*

litigant /lit′əgənt/, (in law) a party to a lawsuit. See also **defendant, plaintiff.**

litigate, (in law) to carry on a suit or to contest.

litigious paranoia, a form of paranoia in which the person seeks legal proof or justification for systematized delusions.

litmus paper, absorbent paper coated with litmus, a blue dye, that is used to determine pH. Acid substances or solutions turn blue litmus to red. Alkaline substances or solutions do not cause a color change in blue litmus. The pH range is 4.5 (red) to 8.5 (blue).

litter, a stretcher.

Little's disease. See **cerebral palsy.**

Litzmann's obliquity. See **asynclitism.**

live birth, the birth of an infant, irrespective of the duration of gestation, that exhibits any sign of life, as respiration, heartbeat, umbilical pulsation, or movement of voluntary muscles. A live birth is not always a viable birth.

livedo /livē′dō/, a blue or reddish mottling of the skin, worse in cold weather and probably caused by arteriolar spasm. **Cutis marmorata** is a transient form of livedo. See also **livedo reticularis.**

livedo reticularis, a vasospastic disorder accentuated by exposure to cold and presenting with a characteristic reddish-blue mottling with a typical "fishnet" appearance and involving the entire leg and, less often, the arms. See also **livedo.**

livedo vasculitis. See **segmented hyalinizing vasculitis.**

liver, the largest gland of the body and one of its most complex organs: More than 500 of its functions have been identified. It is divided into four lobes, contains as many as 100,000 lobules, and is served by two distinct blood supplies. The hepatic artery conveys oxygenated blood to the liver, and the hepatic portal vein conveys nutrient-filled blood from the stomach and the intestines. At any given moment the liver holds about one pint of blood or approximately 13% of the total blood supply of the body. Some of the major functions performed by the liver are the production of bile by hepatic cells, the secretion of glucose, proteins, vitamins, fats, and most of the other compounds used by the body, the processing of hemoglobin for vital use of its iron content, and the conversion of poisonous ammonia to urea. Bile from the liver is stored in the gallbladder, which is connected to the liver by connective tissue, in the hepatic duct, and in numerous blood vessels. The liver is located in the cranial, right portion of the abdominal cavity, occupying almost the entire right hypochondrium, the greater part of the epigastrium, and in many individuals extends into the left hypochondrium as far as the mammary line. The liver develops in the embryo as a hollow projection from the ventral surface of the primitive gut, which eventually becomes the descending portion of the duodenum. The adult liver in men weighs about 1.8 kg; in women, about 1.3 kg. It has a soft, solid consistency, is shaped like an irregular hemisphere, and is dark reddish-brown in color. The right lobe of the liver is much larger than the left lobe or the caudate and the quadrate lobes. The ventral portion of the liver is separated by the diaphragm from the sixth to the tenth ribs on the right side and from the seventh and the eighth costal cartilages on the left side. It is completely covered by peritoneum except along the line of attachment of the falciform ligament. The dorsal part of the organ is wide and rounded on the right but narrow on the left, and the central section has a deep concavity that fits the vertebral column and the crura of the diaphragm. The liver attaches to the diaphragm by the coronary and the triangular ligaments. During the descent of the diaphragm in deep breathing, the liver rolls forward, shifting the inferior border downward where it can be felt through the abdominal wall. The tiny lobules of the organ are composed of polyhedral hepatic cells. These communicate with small ducts that connect with larger ducts to form the left and the right hepatic ducts that emerge on the caudal surface of the liver. The left and the right hepatic ducts converge to form the single hepatic duct, which conveys the bile to the duodenum and to the gallbladder for storage. The liver cells produce about one pint of bile daily. They also detoxify numerous ingested substances, as alcohol, nicotine, and other poisons, as well as various toxic substances produced by the intestine. See also **gallbladder.**

liver biopsy, a diagnostic procedure in which a special needle is introduced into the liver under local anesthesia to obtain a specimen for pathologic examination.

■ METHOD: Before a liver biopsy is performed by the physician, the procedure is explained to the patient, whose baseline vital signs are recorded and who is taught how to inhale and hold the breath during insertion of the needle. After the patient's possible allergy to the local anesthetic is checked and results of bleeding, clotting, and prothrombin tests are obtained, an analgesic or sedative is administered as ordered. On completion of the biopsy, pressure is applied to the site for 15 minutes; the patient is positioned on the right side for the first 2 hours and remains in a supine position in bed for the next 22 hours. The blood pressure, pulse, and respirations are checked every 15 minutes for the first hour, then every 30 minutes for the next 2 hours, and subsequently every 4 hours or as ordered. The biopsy site is observed every 30 minutes for bleeding, swelling, or increased pain; epigastric or referred shoulder pain may occur. Analgesia and vitamin K may be given as ordered, and the recumbent patient is assisted with eating and other activities as needed.

■ NURSING ORDERS: The nurse reinforces explanations of the biopsy and its purpose, provides care before and after the procedure, and closely observes the patient for postbiopsy complications, as intraperitoneal hemorrhage, shock, and pneumothorax.

■ OUTCOME CRITERIA: An uneventful liver biopsy is a valuable aid in establishing a diagnosis of hepatic disease, including primary and metastatic malignant neoplastic disease.

liver breath. See **fetor hepaticus.**

liver cancer, a malignant neoplastic disease of the liver, occurring most frequently as a metastasis from another malignancy. Primary liver cancer is common in Africa and Southeast Asia but relatively uncommon in the United States. Primary tumors are six to 10 times more prevalent in men than in women, develop most often in the sixth decade of life, and are associated with cirrhosis of the liver in 70% of the cases. Other risk factors include hemochromatosis, schistosomiasis, exposure to vinyl chloride or arsenic, and possibly nutritional deficiencies. Alcoholism may be a predisposing factor, but nonalcoholic cirrhosis is a greater risk than alcoholic cirrhosis. Aflatoxins in moldy grain and peanuts appear to be linked to high rates of hepatocellular carcinoma in parts of Africa. Characteristics of liver cancer are abdominal bloating, anorexia, weakness, dull upper abdominal pain, ascites, mild jaundice, and a tender enlarged liver; in some cases tumor nodules are palpable on the liver surface. Diagnostic procedures include radioisotope scan, needle biopsy, and various laboratory studies of liver function. An elevated level of alkaline phosphatase, increased retention of sulfobromophthalein, and the presence of alpha fetoprotein in the blood suggest liver cancer. All primary liver tumors are adenocarcinomas, classified as hepatomas when derived from hepatic cells, and cholangiomas if they originate in cells of the bile duct. They form large single nodules or satellite nodules surrounding a central lesion and are found more often in the right lobe than in the left. Primary lesions spread centrifugally in the liver, invade the portal vein and lymphatic vessels, and metastasize to lymph nodes, the lungs, brain, and other sites. Total hepatic lobectomy is the treatment of choice for primary tumors; because the liver is able to regenerate, 80% of it may be resected. Systemic chemotherapy or methotrexate and 5-fluorouracil infused through a catheter in the hepatic artery may result in temporary tumor regression. Irradiation is very destructive to liver cells and not very toxic to tumor cells in the liver.

liver cell carcinoma. See **malignant hepatoma.**

liver disease, any one of a group of disorders of the liver. The most important diseases in this group are cirrhosis, cholestasis, and viral and toxic hepatitis. Characteristics of liver disease are jaundice, anorexia, hepatomegaly, ascites, and impaired consciousness. The exact diagnosis of liver disease is made through a combination of laboratory tests and clinical findings. See also **cholestasis, cirrhosis, hepatitis.**

liver flap. See **asterixis.**

liver function test, a test used to evaluate various functions of the liver—for example, metabolism, storage, filtration, and excretion. Kinds of liver function tests include **alkaline phospatase, bromsulfalein test, prothrombin time, serum bilirubin,** and **serum glutamic pyruvic transaminase.**

liver scan, a noninvasive technique of visualizing the size, shape, and consistency of the liver by the intravenous injection of a radioactively labeled compound that is readily taken up and trapped in the Kupffer cells of the liver. The radiation emitted by the compound is recorded by a radiation detector and can be photographed with a scintillation camera or filmed with x-ray. Liver scans are most useful for diagnosing three-dimensional lesions as abscesses or tumors.

liver spot, *nontechnical.* a senile lentigo or actinic keratosis.

living-in unit, a room provided in some hospitals for mothers who want to assume immediate care of their newborn infants under the supervision of nursing personnel.

living will, a written agreement between a patient and physician to withhold heroic measures if the patient's condition is found to be irreversible.

lizard, a scaly-skinned reptile with a long body and tail and two pairs of legs. The large Gila monster of Arizona, New Mexico, and Utah, and the beaded lizard of Mexico are the only lizards known to be venomous. The symptoms of their bites and the recommended treatment are similar to those of the bites from moderately poisonous snakes.

LLD factor. See **cyanocobalamin.**

LMD. See **dextran preparation.**

L.M.D., abbreviation for *local medical doctor,* used by house staff or others to distinguish a patient's primary physician from university faculty, attending specialist physicians, or house staff. Also called **P.M.D.**

LMP, abbreviation for *last menstrual period.*

loading response stance stage, one of the five stages of the stance phase of walking or gait, specifically associated with the moment when the leg reacts to and accepts the weight of the body. The loading response stance stage is one of the factors in the diagnoses of many abnormal orthopedic conditions and is often studied in conjunction with analyses of the electromyographic activity of the muscles used in walking. Compare **initial contact stance stage, midstance, preswing stance stage, terminal stance.**

loads, *slang.* a fixed combination of a sedative hypnotic, glutethimide, and a major narcotic analgesic, codeine. The medications are taken orally by drug abusers for a euphoric effect reported to be similar to that produced by heroin, but longer lasting. Toxicity may develop, characterized by nystagmus, slurred speech, seizures, coma, pulmonary edema, or sudden apnea and death. Detoxification of an addicted person is managed under close medical supervision with methadone and phenobarbital, as sudden withdrawal can cause death.

Loa loa, a parasitic worm of western and central Africa that causes loiasis. Also called **eye worm.**

lobar bronchus, a bronchus extending from a primary bronchus to a segmental bronchus into one of the lobes of the right or left lung.

lobar pneumonia, a severe infection of one or more of the five major lobes of the lungs that, if untreated, eventually results in consolidation of lung tissue. The disease is characterized by fever, chills, cough, rusty sputum, rapid shallow breathing, cyanosis, nausea, vomiting, and pleurisy. *Streptococcus pneumoniae* is the usual cause but *Klebsiella pneumoniae, Haemophilus influenzae,* and other streptococci can produce the disease. If the diagnosis is made early, appropriate antibiotic therapy is highly successful. Complications include lung abscess, atelectasis, empyema, pericarditis, and pleural effusion. Precautions against spread of the contagious disease are important. Because the fatality rate in the elderly and those with underlying systemic illness is high, prophylactic polyvalent pneumococcal vaccine is recommended for them. Compare **bronchopneumonia.**

lobe, **1.** a roundish projection of any structure. **2.** a portion of any organ, demarcated by sulci, fissures, or connective tissue, as the lobes of the brain, liver and lungs. **–lobar, lobular,** *adj.*

-lobe, a combining form meaning a 'rounded prominence': *gonilobe, multilobe, sublobe.*

lobectomy, a type of chest surgery in which a lobe of a lung is excised, performed to remove a malignant tumor and to treat uncontrolled bronchiectasis, trauma with hemorrhage, or intractable tuberculosis. Any respiratory infection is cleared before surgery; smoking is forbidden; administration of antibiotics is begun. General anesthesia is administered via an endotracheal tube. The chest cavity is entered through a long back-to-front incision, and the diseased lobe is removed. A large caliber tube remains in the wound and is connected to a water-sealed drainage system. Oxygen is given during the first 24 hours after surgery. The vital signs are closely monitored, coughing and deep breathing are encouraged hourly, blood transfusion may be given, and IV fluids are continued. Care is taken that the chest tube remain open and that the drainage system be sealed and functional. The chest tube is removed 2 to 3 days after surgery. Some compensatory emphysema is expected as the remaining lung tissue overexpands to fill the new space. **–lobectomize,** *v.*

lobotomy, a neurosurgical procedure in which the nerve fibers in the bundle of white matter in the frontal lobe of the brain are severed to interrupt the transmission of various affective responses. Severe intractable depression and pain are among the indications for the operation. It is rarely performed, because it has many unpredictable and undesirable effects, including personality change, aggression, socially unacceptable behavior, incontinence, apathy, and lack of consideration for others. Because lobotomy is simple to perform, it was overused in the treatment of mental patients in the past. A cannula is passed through the bony orbit of the eye, and a wire loop is inserted through the cannula to the cingulum. The nerve fibers are severed with the wire loop. Also called **leukotomy.**

lobster claw deformity. See **bidactyly.**

lobular carcinoma, a neoplasm that often forms a diffuse mass and accounts for a small percentage of breast tumors.

lobule /lob′yo͞ol/, a small lobe, as the soft, lower, pendulous part of the external ear. **–lobular,** *adj.*

loc-, a combining form meaning 'place': *locomotor, locum, locus.*

local, **1.** of or pertaining to a small circumscribed area of the body. **2.** of or pertaining to a treatment or drug applied locally. **3.** *informal.* a local anesthetic.

local anesthesia, the direct administration of a local anesthetic agent to tissues to induce the absence of sensation in a small area of the body. Brief surgical or dental procedures are the most common indications for local anesthesia. The anesthetic may be applied topically to the surface of the skin or membrane or injected subcutaneously through an intradermal weal. The principal drawbacks to the use of local anesthesia are the incidence of allergic reactions to certain agents, especially the "-caine" drugs, and the occasional difficulty encountered in achieving adequate anesthesia. The advantages include low cost, ease of administration, low toxicity, and safety—a conscious patient can cooperate and does not require respiratory support or intubation. To avoid general anesthesia, major surgical procedures are occasionally performed under local anesthesia. The tissues are anesthetized layer by layer, as the surgeon approaches the deeper structures of the body. Regional anesthesia has largely replaced this procedure. In all cases, the recommended dosage of any agent is the smallest possible to achieve the desired effect, because toxicity is directly related to the total amount of drug given rather than to the initial amount or the concentration of the agent used. Each anesthetic agent also carries a recommended maximum allowable dose that is not safely exceeded. Compare **general anesthesia, regional anesthesia, topical anesthesia.**

local anesthetic, a substance used to reduce or eliminate neural sensation, specifically pain, in a limited area of the body. Local anesthetics act by blocking transmission of nerve impulses. More than 100 drugs are available for local anesthesia; they are classified as members of the alcohol-ester or the amineamide family. Differences between various trade products often may be no more than a slight chemical variation, but even these variations may cause a difference of action and effect. Principal representatives of the alcohol-ester group are phenols and benzyl, ethyl, and salicylic alcohol; these have generally been replaced by the less toxic esters (chloroprocaine, cocaine, procaine, tetracaine) and the amides (dibucaine, bupivacaine, lidocaine, mepivacaine, prilocaine, etidocaine). Specific preparations are available for use for topical administration, for infiltration, and for various kinds of regional administration, including field block, regional nerve block, epidural nerve block, and spinal nerve block. Any substance sufficiently potent to induce local anesthesia has potential for causing adverse side effects, ranging from easily reversible dermatitis to lethal anaphylaxis or simultaneous respiratory and cardiac arrest. Among the factors that are involved in an adverse reaction to a local anesthetic are hypersensitivity to the drug, the vascularity of the injection site, the speed with which the drug is given, the rapidity of action of the drug, and the presence of epinephrine in the solution. Serious adverse results have occurred when the operator has failed to notice that the local anesthetic contains epinephrine in solution. A person might be able to tolerate the local agent without adverse reaction but might be dangerously hypersensitive to the epinephrine. Some people who are sensitive to local anesthetics of the amide group, which are broken down in the liver, can tolerate local anesthetics of the ester group, which are broken down in the plasma. Vasopressors should also be at hand in case of hypotension or other forms of circulatory depression. A patient who has a severe adverse reaction to a particular local anesthetic is advised to avoid this class of drug in the future.

local control, the arrest of cancer growth at a site of treatment.

local hypothermia, the heating of a local area of tissue to therapeutic temperatures.

localization audiometry. See **audiometry.**

localization film, (in radiotherapy) a diagnostic film taken to confirm a treatment effect or to view the position of an intracavitary or interstitial implant, especially for the purpose of computing the dose delivered.

localized scleroderma. See **morphea.**

localizing symptom, local symptom. See **symptom.**

location, a specific place in the memory of a computer where a unit of information is stored.

lochia /lō′kē•ə/, the discharge that flows from the vagina after childbirth. During the first 3 or 4 days postpartum, the lochia is red (**lochia rubra**) and is made up of blood, endometrial decidua, and fetal lanugo, vernix, and sometimes meconium, small shreds of placental tissue and membranes. After the third day the amount of blood diminishes, the placental site exudes serous material and lymph, and the lochia becomes darker and thinner (**lochia fusca**), and then serous (**lochia serosa**) as evacuation of particulate material is completed. During the second week white blood cells and bacteria appear in large numbers along with fatty, mucinous decidual material, causing the lochia to appear yellow (**lochia flava** or **lochia purulenta**). During the third week and thereafter, as endometrial epithelialization progresses, the amount of lochia decreases markedly and takes on a seromucinous consistency and a gray-white color (**lochia alba**). Cessation of the flow of lochia at about 6 weeks is usual. – **lochial,** *adj.*

locked twins. See **interlocked twins.**

lock forceps. See **point forceps.**

locking point, a point on the body at which light pressure can be applied to help a weak or debilitated patient maintain a desired posture or position. A basic locking point is the body's center of gravity, at the level of the second sacral vertebra, where mild pressure can assist a patient in standing or walking erect.

lockjaw, *informal.* tetanus.

locomotor ataxia. See **tabes dorsalis.**

Locorten, a trademark for a glucocorticoid (flumethasone pivalate).

loculate /lok′yo͝olāt/, divided into small spaces or cavities.

loculus /lok′yo͝oləs/, a small chamber, pocket, or cavity, as the interior of a polyp.

locum tenens /lō′kəm ten′ənz/, a temporary substitute for a physician who is away from the practice.

locus, a specific place or position, as the locus of a particular gene on a chromosome.

locus of infection, a site in the body where an infection originates.

Lodrane, a trademark for a smooth muscle relaxant (theophylline).

Loestrin, a trademark for an oral contraceptive containing an estrogen (ethinyl estradiol) and a progestin (norethindrone acetate).

Lofenalac, a trademark for a commercial milk-substitute formula that is low in phenylalamine and used for infants with phenylketonuria. It is made from hydrolyzed casein, and is supplemented with tyrosine and fortified with added fat, carbohydrate, minerals, and vitamins to balance the formula. A common problem with the formula is diarrhea, which may appear after the first few feedings but generally disappears in a few days.

Löffler's syndrome /lef′lərz/, a benign, idiopathic disorder marked by episodes of pulmonary eosinophilia, transient opacities in the lungs, anorexia, breathlessness, fever, and weight loss. Recovery is spontaneous and prompt. See also **P.I.E.**

log-, logo-, a combining form meaning 'word, speech, thought': *logagnosia, logopathy, logorrhea.*

loga-, a combining form meaning 'of or pertaining to the whites of the eyes': *logadectomy, logaditis, logadoblennorrhea.*

-logia. See **-logy.**

logo-. See **log-.**

logotherapy, a treatment modality based on the application of humanistic and existential psychology to assist a patient in finding meaning and purpose in life and unique life experiences.

log roll, a maneuver used to turn a reclining patient from one side to the other or completely over without flexing the spinal column. The arms of the patient are folded across the chest and the legs extended. A draw sheet under the patient is manipulated by attending nursing personnel to facilitate the procedure.

-logy, -logia, a combining form meaning 'a science': *mammalogy, metabology, neonatology.*

loiasis /lō·ī′əsis/, a form of filariasis caused by the worm ***Loa loa,*** which may migrate for 10 to 15 years in subcutaneous tissue, producing localized inflammation known as Calabar swellings. Occasionally, the migrating worms may be visible beneath the conjunctiva. The disease is acquired through the bite of an infected African deer fly. Treatment with diethylcarbamazine usually results in cure and may also be successful as prophylaxis. See also **filariasis, onchocerciasis.**

loin, a part of the body on each side of the spinal column between the false ribs and the hip bones.

Lomotil, a trademark for an antidiarrheal fixed-combination drug containing an antiperistaltic (diphenoxylate hydrochloride) and an anticholinergic (atropine sulfate).

lomustine, an antineoplastic alkylating agent.

■ INDICATIONS: It is prescribed in the treatment of a variety of malignant neoplastic diseases.

■ CONTRAINDICATION: Known hypersensitivity to this drug prohibits its use.

■ ADVERSE EFFECTS: Among the more serious adverse reactions are bone marrow depression, nausea, and vomiting.

Lonalac, a trademark for a low-sodium, nutritional supplement.

long-acting drug, a pharmacologic agent with a prolonged effect because of a formulation resulting in the slow release of the active principle or the continued absorption of small amounts of the dosage of the drug over an extended period.

long-acting insulin, a preparation of the antidiabetic principle of beef pancreas or pork pancreas modified by an interaction with zinc under specific chemical conditions and supplied as a suspension with a prolonged action. An injection of the preparation takes effect within 8 hours, reaches a peak of action in 16 to 24 hours, and has a duration of action of more than 36 hours. Also called **slow-acting insulin, ultralente insulin.** See also **insulin.** Compare **intermediate-acting insulin, short-acting insulin.**

long-acting thyroid stimulator (LATS), an immunoglobulin, probably an autoantibody, that exerts a prolonged stimulatory effect on the thyroid gland, causing rapid growth of the gland and excess activity of thyroid function resulting in hyperthyroidism. It is found circulating in the blood of 50% of people affected with Graves' disease.

long-arm cast, an orthopedic cast applied to immobilize upper extremities from the hand to the upper arm. It is used in the treatment of fractures of the forearm and the elbow, fractures of the humerus, for postoperative positioning of the distal arm, the elbow, or the upper arm, and for correction or for maintenance of correction of deformities of the distal arm, the wrist, or the elbow. Compare **short-arm cast.**

longitudinal, **1.** a measurement in the direction of the long axis of an object, body, or organ, as the longitudinal arch of the foot. **2.** a scientific study that is conducted over a long period of time, as the Framingham (Massachusetts) Study of heart disease.

longitudinal diffusion, the diffusion of solute molecules in the direction of flow of the mobile phase.

longitudinal dissociation, (in cardiology) the insulation of parallel pathways of impulses from each other, usually in the AV junction.

long-leg cast, an orthopedic cast applied to immobilize the leg from the toes to the upper thigh. It is used in treating fractures and dislocations of the knee, for postoperative positioning and immobilization of the knee, distal leg, and ankle, and for correction or for maintenance of correction of the foot, distal leg, and knee. Compare **short-leg cast.**

long-leg cast with walker, an orthopedic cast applied to immobilize the lower extremities from the toes to the upper thigh in treating certain fractures of the leg. This type of cast is the same as the long-leg cast but incorporates a rubber walker, allowing the patient to walk while the leg is encased in the cast and when weight-bearing ambulation is allowed.

long-term memory, the ability to recall sensations, events, ideas, and other information for long periods of time without apparent effort.

long-term care, the provision of medical, social, and personal care services on a recurring or continuing basis to persons with chronic physical or mental disorders. The care may be provided in environments ranging from institutions to private homes. Long-term care services usually include symptomatic treatment, maintenance, and rehabilitation for patients of all age groups.

long thoracic nerve, one of a pair of supraclavicular branches from the roots of the brachial plexus. It arises by three roots, from the fifth, the sixth, and the seventh cervical nerves. Its fibers from the fifth and the sixth cervical nerves join just after they pierce the scalenus medius and are united with its fibers from the seventh cervical nerve at the level of the first rib. Compare **phrenic nerve.**

long tract signs, neurologic signs, as clonus, muscle spasticity, or bladder involvement, that usually indicate a lesion in the middle or upper portions of the spinal cord or in the brain.

Loniten, a trademark for an antihypertensive (minoxidil).

loop, **1.** a set of instructions in a computer program that causes certain commands to be executed repeatedly if specified criteria are met. **2.** *informal.* intrauterine device.

loop colostomy, a type of temporary colostomy performed as part of the surgical repair of Hirschsprung's disease. To perform the procedure, an intact segment of colon anterior to the repair is brought through an abdominal incision and sutured onto the abdomen. A loop is formed and held in position by placing a piece of glass rod between the segment and the abdomen. The two ends of the rod are connected with a piece of rubber tubing to prevent the rod from slipping. The stomal opening is made on the exterior surface of the segment. The colostomy is reversed after complete healing of the surgical repair of the megacolon, usually within a few months to 1 year. See also **colostomy irrigation, Hirschsprung's disease.**

loop diuretic. See **diuretic.**

loop of Henle /hen′lē/, the U-shaped portion of a renal tubule, consisting of a thin descending limb and a thick ascending limb.

loose association. See **loosening.**

loose fibrous tissue, a constrictive, pliable fibrous connective tissue consisting of interwoven elastic and collagenous fibers, interspersed with fluid-filled areolae. It is found in adipose tissue, areolar tissue, reticular tissue, and fibroelastic tissue. Compare **dense fibrous tissue.**

loosening, (in psychiatry) a disturbance of thinking in which the association of ideas and thought patterns become so vague, diffuse, and unfocused as to lack any logical sequences or relationship to any preceding concepts or themes. The condition is frequently a symptom of schizophrenia. Also called **loose association.**

Lo/Ovral, a trademark for an oral contraceptive containing an estrogen (ethinyl estradiol) and a progestin (norgestrel).

loperamide hydrochloride, an antiperistaltic.

■ INDICATION: It is prescribed in the treatment of diarrhea.

■ CONTRAINDICATIONS: Known hypersensitivity to this drug prohibits its use. It is not given to patients in whom constipation must be avoided.

■ ADVERSE EFFECTS: Among the most serious reactions are abdominal pain, constipation, nausea, and vomiting.

loph-, a combining form meaning 'of or pertaining to a ridge': *lophius, lophodont, lophotrichous.*

Lopid, a trademark for a lipid regulating agent (gemfibrozil).

Lopressor, a trademark for a beta-adrenergic receptor blocking agent (metoprolol tartrate).

Loprox, a trademark for an antifungal (ciclopirox olamine).

lorazepam /lôrā′zəpam/, a benzodiazepine tranquilizer.

■ INDICATIONS: It is prescribed as a minor tranquilizer in

the treatment of anxiety, nervous tension, and insomnia.

■ CONTRAINDICATIONS: Acute glaucoma, psychosis, or known hypersensitivity to this drug or to any benzodiazepine prohibits its use.

■ ADVERSE EFFECTS: Among the more serious adverse reactions are drowsiness and fatigue. Withdrawal symptoms may occur on discontinuation of the drug, especially after prolonged use or high dosage.

lordosis /lôrdō′sis/, **1.** the normal curvature of the lumbar and cervical spine, seen as an anterior concavity if the person is observed from the side. **2.** an abnormal, increased degree of curvature of any part of the back.

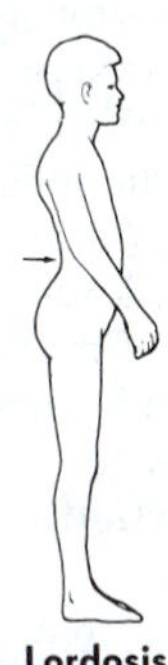

Lordosis

Lorelco, a trademark for an anticholesteremic (probucol).

Lorfan, a trademark for a narcotic antagonist (levallorphan tartrate).

Loridine, a trademark for an antibacterial (cephaloridine).

LOS, abbreviation for **length of stay.**

loss of consortium, (in law) a claim for damages sought in recompense for the loss of conjugal relations, including society, affection, and assistance, and impairment or loss of sexual relations. Loss of consortium may be charged against a person whose negligence or malfeasance caused injury to the spouse or against a person who caused a marriage to break up.

lotion, a liquid preparation applied externally to protect the skin or to treat a dermatologic disorder.

Lotrimin, a trademark for an antifungal (clotrimazole).

Lotusate, a trademark for a barbiturate (talbutal).

Lou Gehrig's disease. See **amyotrophic lateral sclerosis.**

Louis-Bar syndrome. See **ataxia-telangiectasia.**

loupe /lo͞op/, a magnifying lens mounted in a frame worn on the head, as used to examine the eyes.

louse, *pl.* **lice,** a small, wingless, parasitic insect of the order Anoplura that is the carrier of such diseases as relapsing fever and typhus. Lice are common parasites on the skin and may cause intense pruritus. See also **pediculosis.**

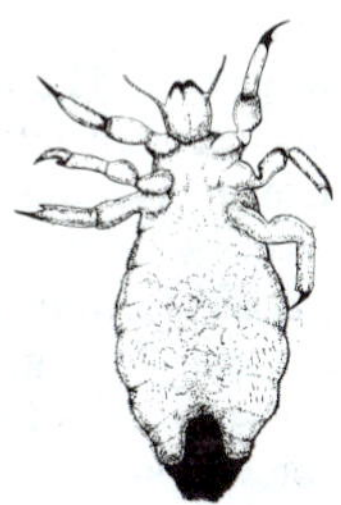

Human body louse

louse bite, a minute puncture wound produced by a louse that may transmit typhus, trench fever, and relapsing fever. Secondary infection may result from scratching the affected area. Head and body lice are the most common and are frequently found among school children. Washing and bathing, application of an approved insecticide, and the washing or cleaning of clothes and bed linens are recommended procedures for treatment and prophylaxis against spread of the infestation. See also **pediculosis.**

louse-borne typhus. See **epidemic typhus.**

low back pain, local or referred pain at the base of the spine caused by a sprain, strain, osteoarthritis, ankylosing spondylitis, a neoplasm, or a prolapsed intervertebral disk. Low back pain is a common complaint and is often associated with poor posture, obesity, sagging abdominal muscles, or sitting for prolonged periods of time.

■ OBSERVATIONS: Pain may be localized and static; it may be accompanied by muscle weakness or spasms; or it may radiate down the back of one or both legs, as in sciatica. It may be initiated or increased by coughing, sneezing, rising from a seated position, lifting, stretching, bending, or turning. To guard against the pain, the person may decrease the range of motion of the spine. If an intervertebral disk is prolapsed, deep pressure over the interspace generally causes pain, and flexion of the hip elicits sciatic pain when the knee is extended but not when the knee is flexed (Lasègue's sign).

■ INTERVENTION: The patient is placed in a semi-Fowler's position on a firm mattress with the knees flexed and supported. Analgesics, muscle relaxants, and tranquilizers may be administered, and dry or moist heat is applied. Diagnostic x-ray examinations; pelvic traction and physiotherapy, consisting of hydrotherapy, diathermy, or the application of hot paraffin; and a myelogram may be performed if a herniated disk is suspected. When the acute pain subsides, the patient may increase activity as tolerated, fatigue is avoided, and a corset or back brace may be ordered. The patient is instructed to use a straight-backed chair, not to sit with legs crossed or extended on a footstool, and to sleep on the side or back with knees flexed and a small pillow under the head. Before discharge the patient is advised to maintain a normal weight, to follow the ordered exercise program, to wear flat-heeled shoes, and to avoid constipation by using natural laxatives, if required.

■ NURSING CONSIDERATIONS: The nurse encourages the patient to follow the recommended regimen. Correct body mechanics, adequate and appropriate exercise, and the elimination of excess weight are emphasized.

low birth weight (LBW) infant, an infant whose weight at birth is less than 2500 g, regardless of gestational age. These babies are at risk for the development of hypoxia during labor, hypoglycemia after birth, and growth retardation in childhood, especially if the condition is the result of prolonged placental insufficiency, maternal malnutrition, or drug addiction. Many low birth weight infants have no problems and develop normally, their smallness being genetic or idiopathic, or the problem that caused their slowed growth being mild or brief.

low blood, *informal*. anemia.

low-calcium diet, a diet that restricts the use of calcium and that eliminates most of the dairy foods, all breads made with milk or dry skimmed milk, and deep-green leafy vegetables. It is prescribed for patients who form renal calculi. Meats, including beef, lamb, pork, veal, and poultry, fish, vegetables, legumes, and fruits are recommended.

low-caloric diet, a diet that is prescribed to limit the intake of calories, usually to cause a reduction in body weight. Such diets may be designated as 800 calorie, 1000 calorie, or other specific numbers of calories. Exchange lists may be used to allow the patient to select preferred foods from groups of foods categorized as carbohydrate, protein, and fat.

low cervical cesarean section, a method for surgically delivering a baby through a transverse incision in the thin supracervical portion of the lower uterine segment, behind the bladder and the bladder flap. This incision bleeds less during surgery and heals with a stronger scar than the higher vertical scar of the classic cesarean section. Compare **extraperitoneal cesarean section.** See also **cesarean section.**

low-cholesterol diet, a diet that restricts foods containing animal fats and saturated fatty acids, as egg yolk, cream, butter, milk, muscle and organ meats, and shellfish, and concentrates on poultry, fish, vegetables, fruits, cottage cheese, and polyunsaturated fats. The diet is indicated for persons with high serum cholesterol levels, cardiovascular disorders, obesity, hyperlipidemia, hypercholesterolemia, or hyperlipoproteinemia. Also called **low-saturated-fat diet.**

low-density lipoprotein (LDL), a plasma protein containing relatively more cholesterol and triglycerides than protein. It is derived in part, if not completely, from the intravascular breakdown of the very low-density lipoproteins. The high cholesterol content may account for its greater atherogenic potential as compared with the very low-density lipoproteins and chylomicrons.

lower extremity suspension, an orthopedic procedure used in the treatment of bone fractures and in the correction of orthopedic abnormalities of the lower limbs. The procedure uses traction equipment, including metal frames, ropes, and pulleys, to relieve the weight of the lower limb involved rather than to exert traction pull. Lower extremity suspension may be either unilateral or bilateral and is used in the postoperative, posttraumatic, or postreduction control of edema. Compare **balanced suspension, hyperextension suspension, upper extremity suspension.**

lower motor neuron paralysis, an injury to or lesion in the spinal cord that damages the cell bodies or axons, or both, of the lower motor neurons, which are located in the anterior horn cells and the spinal and peripheral nerves. If complete transection of the spinal cord occurs, voluntary muscle control is totally lost. In partial transection, function is altered in varying degrees, depending on the areas innervated by the nerves involved. In lower motor neuron paralysis the reflex arcs are permanently damaged, causing decreased muscle tone and flaccidity, diminished or absent reflexes, absence of pathologic reflexes, local twitching of muscle groups, and progressive atrophy of the atonic muscles. Compare **upper motor neuron paralysis.**

lower respiratory infection. See **respiratory tract infection.**

lower respiratory tract, one of the two divisions of the respiratory system. The lower respiratory tract includes the left and the right bronchi and the alveoli where the exchange of oxygen and carbon dioxide occurs during the respiratory cycle. The bronchi divide into smaller bronchioles in the lungs, the bronchioles into alveolar ducts, the ducts into alveolar sacs, and the sacs into alveoli. The alveolar sacs and the alveoli present a total lung surface of about 850 square feet for the exchange of oxygen and carbon dioxide, which occurs between the most internal alveolar surface and the tiny capillaries surrounding the external alveolar wall. The lower respiratory tract is a continuation of the upper respiratory tract and is a common site of infections, obstructive conditions, and neoplastic disease. Compare **upper respiratory tract.** See also **lung.**

low-fat diet, a diet containing limited amounts of fat and consisting chiefly of easily digestible foods of high carbohydrate content. It includes all vegetables, lean meats, fish, fowl, pasta, cereals, and whole wheat or enriched bread. Egg yolk and fatty meats are restricted. Cream, fried foods, foods prepared in oil, gravy, cheese, peanut butter, and olives are among the foods omitted. The diet may be indicated in gallbladder disease and malabsorption syndromes.

low-fat milk, milk containing 1% to 2% fat, making it an intermediate in fat content between whole and skimmed milk.

low forceps, an obstetric operation in which forceps are used to deliver a baby whose head is on the pelvic floor. The procedure is performed most often as an elective procedure to shorten normal labor and to control delivery, usually in conjunction with anesthesia and episiotomy. It is commonly required for the delivery of mothers whose expulsive powers have been weakened by analgesia, anesthesia, or fatigue. Also called **outlet forceps, prophylactic forceps.** Compare **high forceps, mid forceps, natural childbirth, spontaneous delivery.** See also **forceps delivery, obstetric forceps.**

low-grade fever, a temperature that is above 98.6° F but lower than 100.4° F for 24 hours.

low-level language, a computer language employing mathematic logic but requiring precise manipulation of binary numbers. Compare **high-level language.**

Lown-Ganong-Levine syndrome (LGL) /loun′gənong′ləvēn′/, a disorder of the atrioventricular (AV) conduction system, marked by ventricular preexcitation. Part or all of the AV nodal connection is bypassed by an abnormal AV connection from the atrial muscle to the bundle of His. The condition may be discovered by routine ECG or may be seen in association with paroxysmal atrial arrhythmias, supraventricular tachycardia, atrial flutter, and fibrillation. Treatments include the use of antiarrhythmic drugs, as quinidine sulfate, procainamide, and propranolol, surgical interruption of the abnormal AV pathway, and implantation of a pacemaker. Compare **Wolff-Parkinson-White syndrome.**

low-power field, the low magnification field of vision under a light microscope.

low-residue diet, a diet that will leave a minimal residue in the lower intestinal tract after digestion and absorption. It consists of tender meats, poultry, fish, eggs, white bread, pasta, simple desserts, clear soups, tea, and coffee. Omitted are highly seasoned or fried foods, all fruits and fruit juices, raw vegetables, whole grain cereals and bread, nuts, jams, and, usually, milk. The diet is prescribed in cases of diverticulosis and diverticulitis, GI irritability or inflammation, and before and after GI surgery. Because it is lacking in calcium, iron, and vitamins, it should be used only for a limited period of time.

low-salt diet. See **low-sodium diet.**

low-saturated-fat diet. See **low-cholesterol diet.**

low-sodium diet, a diet that restricts the use of sodium chloride plus other compounds containing sodium, as baking powder or soda, monosodium glutamate, sodium citrate, sodium propionate, and sodium sulfate. It is indicated in hypertension, edematous states (especially when associated with cardiovascular disease), renal or liver disease, and therapy with corticosteroids. The degree of sodium restriction depends on the severity of the condition. Foods included in the diet are eggs, skimmed milk, beef, poultry, lamb, pork, veal, fish, potatoes, green beans, broccoli, asparagus, peas, salad ingredients, and fresh fruits. Many flavoring extracts, spices, and herbs can be used to add taste to the diet. Foods to be avoided include fresh or canned shellfish, ham, bacon, frankfurters, luncheon meats, sausage, cheese, salted butter or margarine, any breads or cereals made with salt, beets, carrots, celery, sauerkraut, spinach, and most canned or frozen foods—unless prepared without sodium. Also to be avoided are many drugs, as laxatives, sedatives, and alkalizers, which contain sodium, and drinking water from a source using a water softener, because this appliance adds sodium to the water. Also called **low-salt diet, salt-free diet, sodium-restricted diet.**

loxapine, a tranquilizer.

■ INDICATION: It is prescribed in the treatment of schizophrenia.

■ CONTRAINDICATIONS: Parkinson's disease, concurrent administration of central nervous system depressants, liver or kidney dysfunction, severe hypotension, or known hypersensitivity to this drug prohibits its use.

■ ADVERSE EFFECTS: Among the more serious adverse effects are hypotension, liver toxicity, a variety of extrapyramidal reactions, and hypersensitivity reactions.

Loxitane, a trademark for a tranquilizer (loxapine succinate).

loxo-, a combining form meaning 'oblique': *loxophthalmus, loxotic, loxotomy.*

lozenge. See **troche.**

LP, abbreviation for **lumbar puncture.**

LPN, abbreviation for **licensed practical nurse.**

LPS Act, a California law named for sponsors of the legislation (Lanterman, Petris, and Short) that provides for the protection and treatment of persons judged to be "gravely disabled" and, thus, unable to provide food, clothing, or shelter for themselves. The legislation was designed to safeguard the constitutional rights of persons threatened with involuntary commitment on the basis of a psychiatric diagnosis. The LPS Act was considered a progressive measure in that it made "ability to function" the criterion for determining the need for establishing conservatorships or guardianships for senior citizens or other individuals who might appear to be mentally disordered.

Lr, symbol for **lawrencium.**

LSD. See **lysergide.**

L/S ratio, the lecithin/sphingomyelin ratio, used in a test for fetal lung maturity.

LTB, abbreviation for **laryngotracheobronchitis.** See **croup.**

Lu, symbol for **lutetium.**

luc-, a combining form meaning 'of or pertaining to light': *lucifugal, lucipetal, lucotherapy.*

-lucent, a combining form meaning 'light-admitting': *radiolucent, roentgenolucent, translucent.*

lucid /lo͞o′sid/, clear, rational, and able to be understood. See also **lucid interval.**

lucid interval, a period of relative mental clarity between periods of irrationality, especially in organic mental disorders, as delirium and dementia.

lucid lethargy, a mental state characterized by a loss of will; hence, an inability to act, even though the person is conscious and intellectual function is normal. See also **lethargy.**

Ludiomil, a trademark for an antidepressant (maprotiline hydrochloride).

Ludwig's angina /lo͞od′vigz/, acute streptococcal cellulitis of the floor of the mouth. It is treated with penicillin.

lue-, a combining form meaning 'of or pertaining to syphilis': *luetic, luetin, luetism.*

Luer-Lok syringe /lo͞o′ərlōk′/, a glass syringe for injection having a simple metal lock mechanism that securely holds the needle in place. Also called **Luer's syringe.**

lues. See **syphilis.**

-luetic, -luic, a combining form meaning 'pertaining to syphilis': *antiluetic, heredoluetic, paraluetic.*

luetic aortitis. See **syphilitic aortitis.**

Lufyllin, a trademark for a smooth muscle relaxant (dyphylline).

Lugol's solution, an aqueous solution of iodine (5%) and potassium iodide (10%).

-luic. See **-luetic.**

lukewarm bath, a bath in which the temperature of the water is between 90° and 96° F.

lumbago /lumbā′gō/, pain in the lumbar region caused by a muscle strain, rheumatoid arthritis, osteoarthritis, or a herniated intravertebral disk. Ischemic lumbago, characterized by pain in the lower back and buttocks, is caused by vascular insufficiency, as in terminal aortic occlusion. See also **low back pain.**

lumbar /lum′bər, lum′bär/, of or pertaining to the part of the body between the thorax and the pelvis.

lumbar nerves, the five pairs of spinal nerves rising in the lumbar region. They become increasingly large the more caudal their location and pass laterally and downward under the cover of the psoas major or between its fasciculi. The first three lumbar nerves and the larger part of the fourth are connected by communicating loops and, in many individuals, communicate with the twelfth thoracic nerve, forming the lumbar plexus. The ventral primary divisions of the lumbar nerves give rise to muscular branches that supply the psoas major and the quadratus lumborum before the nerves enter the lumbar plexus. The smaller section of the fourth lumbar nerve joins the fifth lumbar nerve to form the lumbosacral trunk that comprises part of the sacral plexus. Only the first two lumbar nerves extend white rami to the sympathetic trunk. All lumbar nerves receive gray rami. The lumbar ganglia follow no fixed pattern, and massive fusions of ganglia are common. When occurring independently, the lumbar ganglia lie on the body's corresponding vertebrae or intervertebral disks caudally. The ganglion on the second lumbar vertebra is the largest, the most constant, and the most easily palpated.

lumbar node, a node in one of the seven groups of parietal lymph nodes serving the abdomen and the pelvis. The lumbar nodes are very numerous and are divided into the lateral aortic nodes, the preaortic nodes, and the retroaortic nodes. They receive the afferents from many different structures, as the kidneys, the internal reproductive organs, the lateral abdominal muscles, and certain vertebrae, and pass efferents that form lymphatic trunks. Compare **sacral node.** See also **lymph, lymphatic system, lymph node.**

lumbar plexus, a network of nerves formed by the ventral primary divisions of the first three and the greater part of the fourth lumbar nerves. It is located on the inside of the posterior abdominal wall, either dorsal to the psoas major or among its fibers and ventral to the transverse processes of the lumbar vertebrae. The plexus develops from the splitting of various lumbar nerves. The first lumbar nerve splits into the cranial and the caudal branches. The cranial branch forms the iliohypogastric and the ilioinguinal nerves. The caudal branch unites with a branch from the second lumbar nerve to form the genitofemoral nerve. The rest of the second nerve and the third and the fourth nerves each split into a small ventral and a large dorsal section. The ventral portions unite to form the obturator nerve. The dorsal portions of the second and the third nerves each divide into two smaller branches to form the lateral femoral cutaneous nerve and two larger branches that join the dorsal portion of the fourth lumbar nerve to form the femoral nerve. Part of the fourth lumbar nerve joins the fifth lumbar nerve in the lumbosacral trunk. The branches of the lumbar plexus are the iliohypogastric nerve, the ilioinguinal nerve, the genitofemoral nerve, the lateral femoral cutaneous nerve, the obturator nerve, the accessory obturator nerve, and the femoral nerve. The iliohypogastric, the ilioinguinal, and the genitofemoral nerves supply the caudal part of the abdominal wall. The lateral femoral cutaneous, the obturator, the accessory obturator, and the femoral nerves supply the anterior thigh and the middle of the leg. The accessory obturator nerve is present in only 20% of individuals and comes from the third and the fourth lumbar nerves. Compare **sacral plexus.**

lumbar puncture (LP), the introduction of a hollow needle and stylet into the subarachnoid space of the lumbar portion of the spinal canal. With the use of strict aseptic technique, it is performed in various therapeutic and diagnostic procedures. Diagnostic indications include measuring of cerebrospinal fluid (CSF) pressure, obtaining CSF for laboratory analysis, evaluating the canal for the pressure of a tumor, and injecting air, oxygen, or a radiopaque substance for radiographic visualization of the structures of the nervous system of spinal canal and meninges and brain. Therapeutic indications for lumbar puncture include removing blood or pus from the subarachnoid space, injecting sera or drugs, withdrawing CSF to reduce intracranial pressure, introducing a local anesthetic to induce spinal anesthesia, and placing a small amount of the patient's blood in the subarachnoid space to form a clot to patch a rent or hole in the dura to prevent leak of CSF into the epidural space.

■ METHOD: The skin over the interspace of the third and fourth lumbar vertebrae is cleansed. A fenestrated sterile drape is placed over the back, the window over the puncture site. The needle is inserted through the interspace to the subarachnoid space, and the stylet is withdrawn. If the needle is in the proper place, clear, straw-colored

CSF will begin to drip out through the needle. Depending on the indication for the procedure, various techniques follow. The pressure of the CSF may be measured using a manometer attached to a catheter and stopcock, or fluid may be withdrawn, visually examined, and sent to the laboratory for chemical or bacteriologic analysis.

■ NURSING ORDERS: The nurse is often responsible for obtaining the patient's written permission for the physician to perform a lumbar puncture. The patient, if apprehensive, is given a sedative one half hour before the procedure. The techniques to be used and the treatments to be given or the information to be obtained are explained. The patient is placed in a lateral recumbent position, the back as near the edge of the bed as possible. The legs are flexed on the thighs, the thighs are flexed on the abdomen, and the head and shoulders are bent down, curving the spine convexly to afford the greatest space between the vertebrae. If the patient is hirsute, a dry shave of the lumbar area is performed before draping the area. After the procedure, significant signs to be observed by the nurse include pain, change in mentation or alertness, leakage of CSF from the puncture site, fever, and urinary retention. The patient is usually kept flat in bed, often in a prone position, for 4 to 6 hours after the procedure.

■ OUTCOME CRITERIA: Lumbar puncture is contraindicated if the procedure will not contribute to the diagnosis or treatment of the illness, if intracranial tumor is suspected and there is evidence of greatly increased intracranial pressure, if there are signs of infection at the site of puncture, or, to avoid a second puncture, if encephalography or myelography is planned in the near future. Infection, leakage of CSF, headache, nausea, vomiting, dysuria, or signs of meningeal irritation occur in approximately 25% of patients.

lumbar region. See **lateral region.**

lumbar subarachnoid peritoneostomy, a surgical procedure for draining cerebrospinal fluid in hydrocephalus, usually in the newborn. It spares the kidney but is a somewhat less effective method than a lumbar subarachnoid ureterostomy. The procedure may be used when a temporary shunt is needed. First a lumbar laminectomy is performed, then a polyethylene tube is passed from the subarachnoid space around the flank and into the peritoneum. This procedure is performed to correct a communicating type of hydrocephalus.

lumbar subarachnoid ureterostomy, a surgical procedure for draining excess cerebrospinal fluid through the ureter to the bladder in hydrocephalus, usually in the newborn. The procedure first completes a lumbar laminectomy and a left nephrectomy, after which a polyethylene tube is passed from the lumbar subarachnoid space through the paraspinal muscles and into the free ureter. The procedure is performed to correct a communicating type of hydrocephalus.

lumbar veins, four pairs of veins that collect blood by dorsal tributaries from the loins and by abdominal tributaries from the walls of the abdomen. They receive veins from the vertebral plexus, pass ventrally around the vertebrae, dorsal to the psoas major, and end in the inferior vena cava. The left lumbar veins are longer than the right and pass dorsal to the aorta. The lumbar veins are connected by the ascending lumbar vein that runs ventral to the transverse processes of the lumbar vertebrae.

lumbar vertebra, one of the five largest segments of the movable part of the vertebral column, distinguished by the absence of a foramen in the transverse process and by vertebral bodies without facets. The body of each lumbar vertebra is flattened or slightly concave superiorly and inferiorly and is deeply constricted ventrally at the sides. The spinous process of each is thick, broad, and somewhat quadrilateral. The body of the fifth lumbar vertebra is much deeper ventrally than dorsally, and in some individuals is defective, tending to weaken the spinal column. Compare **cervical vertebra, coccygeal vertebra, sacral vertebra, thoracic vertebra.**

lumbo-, a combining form meaning 'of or pertaining to the loins': *lumbocolostomy, lumbocostal, lumbosacral.*

lumbodorsal fascia. See **fascia thoracolumbalis.**

lumbosacral plexus /lum′bōsā′krəl/, the combination of all the ventral primary divisions of the lumbar, the sacral, and the coccygeal nerves. The lumbar and the sacral plexuses supply the lower limb. The sacral nerves also supply the perineum through the pudendal plexus and the coccygeal area through the coccygeal plexus. See also **lumbar plexus, sacral plexus.**

lumen /lo͞o′mən/, *pl.* **lumina, lumens, 1.** a cavity or the channel within any organ or structure of the body. **2.** a unit of luminous flux that equals the flux emitted in a unit solid angle by a point source of one candle intensity. –**lumenal, luminal,** *adj.*

lumin-, a combining form meaning 'of or pertaining to light': *luminescence, luminiferous, luminophore.*

Luminal, a trademark for an anticonvulsant and sedative-hypnotic (phenobarbital).

Luminal Sodium, a trademark for an anticonvulsant and sedative-hypnotic (phenobarbital sodium).

luminescence, the emission of light by a material after excitation by some stimulus. See also **thermoluminescent dosimetry.**

lumpectomy /lumpek′təmē/, surgical excision of a tumor without removal of large amounts of surrounding tissue or adjacent lymph nodes. See also **breast cancer.**

lumpy jaw, *nontechnical.* actinomycosis of cows, caused by infection with *Actinomyces bovis* and not communicable to humans.

lun-, a combining form meaning 'of or pertaining to the moon': *lunacy, lunate, lunatism.*

lunar month, a period of 4 weeks or 28 days, approximately the time required for the moon to revolve about the earth.

lunate bone, the carpal bone in the center of the proximal row of carpal bones between the scaphoid and triangular bones. It articulates with five bones, the radius proximally, the capitate and the hamate distally, the scaphoid laterally, and the triangular medially. Also called **os lunatum, semilunar bone.**

lung, one of a pair of light, spongy organs in the thorax, constituting the main component of the respiratory system. The two highly elastic lungs are the main mechanisms in the body for inspiring air from which oxygen is extracted for the arterial blood system and for exhaling carbon dioxide dispersed from the venous system. The lungs are composed of lobes that are smooth and shiny on their surface. The right lung contains three lobes; the left lung two lobes. Each lung is composed of an external serous coat, a subserous layer of areolar tissue, and the parenchyma. The serous coat comprises the thin, visceral pleura. The subserous areolar tissue contains many elastic fibers and invests the entire surface of the organ. The parenchyma is composed of secondary lobules divided into primary lobules, each of which consists of blood vessels, lymphatics, nerves, and an alveolar duct connecting with air spaces. The color of the lungs at birth is pinkish-white, and darkens in later life. The coloring is from carbon granules deposited in the areolar tissue near the surface of the lung. The carbon deposits increase with age and are more abundant in men than women. The lungs of men are usually heavier than the lungs of women and usually have a greater capacity. The quantity of air that can be exhaled from the lungs after the deepest inspiration averages 3700 cc. Each lung is conic and has an apex, a base, three borders, and two surfaces. The apex is rounded and extends into the root of the neck about 4 cm above the first rib. The base of the lung is broad and concave, rests on the convex surface of the diaphragm, and with the diaphragm moves up during expiration and down during inspiration. The surfaces of the lungs are partially concave, with a cardiac impression that cradles the heart. The bronchial arteries supply blood to nourish the lungs and are derived from the ventral side of the thoracic aorta or from the aortic intercostal arteries. The bronchial vein is formed at the root of the lung. Most of the blood supplied by the bronchial arteries is returned by the pulmonary veins.

lung cancer, a pulmonary malignancy attributable to cigarette smoking in 75% of cases. Other predisposing factors are exposure to asbestos, acronitrile, arsenic, beryllium, chromium, chloromethyl ether, coal products, ionizing radiation, iron oxide, mustard gas, nickel, petroleum, uranium, and vinyl chloride. Lung cancer develops most often in scarred or chronically diseased lungs, and is usually far advanced when detected, because metastases may precede the detection of the primary lesion in the lung. Symptoms of lung cancer include persistent cough, dyspnea, purulent or blood-streaked sputum, chest pain, and repeated attacks of bronchitis or pneumonia. Diagnostic measures include x-ray films, fluoroscopy, tomography, bronchography, angiography, cytologic studies of sputum, bronchial washings or brushings, and needle biopsy. Epidermoid cancers and adenocarcinomas each account for approximately 30% of lung tumors, about 25% are small or oat cell carcinomas, and 15% are large-cell anaplastic cancers. Epidermoid tumors tend to remain in the thorax, but other lung lesions metastasize widely; oat cell carcinomas usually invade bone marrow, and large-cell cancers frequently metastasize to mediastinal nodes and GI mucosa. Surgery is the most effective treatment, but only one half of the cases are operable at the time of diagnosis and of these 50% are not resectable. Thoracotomy is contraindicated if metastases are found in contralateral or scalene lymph nodes. Irradiation is used to treat localized lesions and unresectable intrathoracic tumors and as palliative therapy for metastatic lesions. Radiotherapy may also be administered postoperatively to destroy remaining tumor cells and may be combined with chemotherapy. Cures and remissions are obtained in some cases treated with chemotherapeutic agents, as cyclophosphamide, procarbazine, methotrexate, doxorubicin hydrochloride, and bleomycin. Chemotherapy is especially indicated for oat cell carcinoma. Postoperatively, bacillus Calmette-Guérin vaccine, an antituberculosis drug that stimulates the immune system, is administered to some patients with early stage lung cancer.

lung compliance, a measure of the ease of expansion by the lungs and thorax during respiratory movements. It is determined by pulmonary volume and elasticity, a high degree of compliance indicating a loss of elastic recoil of the lungs, as in old age or emphysema. Decreased compliance of the lungs occurs in conditions when greater pressure is needed for changes of volume, as in atelectasis, edema, fibrosis, pneumonia, or absence of surfactant. Dyspnea on exertion is the main symptom of diminished lung compliance. See also **respiration, expiratory reserve volume, residual volume, vital capacity.**

lung scan, a radiographic examination of a lung and its function.

lunula, *pl.* **lunulae,** a semilunar structure, as the crescent-shaped pale area at the base of the nail of a finger or toe.

lupoid. See **lupus.**

lupoid hepatitis. See **hepatitis.**

lupus, **1.** *nontechnical.* lupus erythematosus. **2.** *obsolete.* any chronic skin condition in which ulcerative lesions spread over the body over a long period of time. **–lupoid,** *adj.*

lupus erythematosus. See **systemic lupus erythematosus.**

lupus erythematosus preparation (LE prep), a laboratory test for lupus erythematosus in which normal neutrophils are incubated with a specimen of the patient's serum resulting in the appearance of large, spheric, phagocytized inclusions within the neutrophils if the patient has lupus erythematosus.

lupus vulgaris, a rare cutaneous form of tuberculosis in which areas of the skin become ulcerated and heal slowly, leaving deeply scarred tissue. The disease is not related to lupus erythematosus.

Luride, a trademark for a chemical prophylactic (sodium fluoride) that reduces dental caries.

lusus naturae /lo͞o′səs/, a congenital anomaly; teratism.

luteal /lo͞o′tē·əl/, of or pertaining to the corpus luteum or its functions or effects.

luteal phase. See **secretory phase.**

lutein /lo͞o′tē·in/, a yellow-red, crystalline, carotenoid pigment found in plants with carotenes and chlorophylls and also in animal fats, egg yolk, the corpus luteum, or any lipochrome.

luteinizing hormone (LH), a glycoprotein hormone, produced by the anterior pituitary, that stimulates the secretion of sex hormones by the ovary and the testes and is involved in the maturation of spermatozoa and ova. In men, it induces the secretion of testosterone by the interstitial cells of the testes. Testosterone, together with follicle stimulating hormone (FSH), induces the maturation of seminiferous tubules and stimulates them to produce sperm. In females, LH, working together with FSH, stimulates the growing follicle in the ovary to secrete estrogen. High concentrations of estrogen stimulate the release of a surge of LH, which stimulates ovulation. LH then induces the development of the ruptured follicle into the corpus luteum, which continues to secrete estrogen and progesterone. The normal LH concentration in the plasma of men is less than 11 mIU/ml. In women, it is, premenopausal, less than 25 mIU/ml; at midcycle peak, greater than three times the baseline concentration; postmenopausal, more than 25 mIU/ml. See also **ICSH, menstrual cycle.**

luteoma /lo͞o′tē·ō′mə/, *pl.* **luteomas, luteomata,** **1.** a granulosa or theca cell tumor whose cells resemble those of the corpus luteum. **2.** also called **pregnancy luteoma.** a unilateral or bilateral nodular hyperplasia of ovarian lutein cells, occasionally developing during the last trimester of pregnancy.

luteotropin. See **prolactin.**

lutetium (Lu), a rare earth metallic element. Its atomic number is 71; and its atomic weight is 174.97.

LVAD, abbreviation for **left ventricular assist device.**

LVN, abbreviation for **licensed vocational nurse.** See **licensed practical nurse.**

lyases /lē′āsis/, a group of enzymes that reversibly split carbon bonds with carbon, nitrogen, or oxygen without hydrolysis or oxygen reduction reactions. The activity results in two subunits in which one or both may contain a double-bonded carbon. An example of a lyase is deaminase.

lyco-, a combining form meaning 'of or pertaining to a wolf ': *lycomania, lycorexia.*

lycopene /lī′kəpin/, a red, crystalline, unsaturated hydrocarbon that is the carotenoid pigment in tomatoes and various berries and fruits. It is considered the primary substance from which all natural carotenoid pigments are derived.

lying-in, **1.** designating the time before, during, and after childbirth. **2.** designating a hospital that provides care for women in childbirth and the puerperium. **3.** the condition of being in confinement, or childbed.

Lyme arthritis, an acute, recurrent inflammatory disease, involving one or a few joints, believed to be transmitted by a tickborne virus. The condition was originally described in the community of Lyme, Connecticut, but has also been reported in other parts of the northeastern United States and, sporadically, in other countries. Knees, other large joints, and temperomandibular joints are most commonly involved, with local inflammation and swelling. Chills, fever, headache, malaise, and erythema chronicum migrans, an expanding annular, erythematous skin eruption, often precede the joint manifestations. Occasionally cardiac conduction abnormalities, aseptic meningitis, or Bell's palsy are associated conditions. Symptoms appear in recurrent episodes, lasting usually about 1 week, at intervals of from 1 to several weeks, declining in severity over a 2- or 3-year period. There is no significant permanent joint damage. Treatment includes salicylates for joint symptoms and corticosteroids to reduce cardiac and neurologic manifestations.

lymph, a thin opalescent fluid originating in many organs and tissues of the body that is circulated through the lymphatic vessels and filtered by the lymph nodes. Lymph enters the bloodstream at the junction of the internal jugular and subclavian veins. It contains chyle, a few erythrocytes, and variable numbers of leukocytes, most of which are lymphocytes. It is otherwise similar to plasma. See also **chyle.**

lymph-. See **lympho-.**

-lymph, a combining form meaning a 'clear body fluid': *hemolymph, neurolymph, perilymph.*

lymphadenitis /limfad′inī′tis, lim′fəd-/, an inflammatory condition of the lymph nodes, usually the result of systemic neoplastic disease, bacterial infection, or other inflammatory condition. The nodes may be enlarged, hard, smooth or irregular, red, and may feel hot. The location of the affected node is indicative of the site or origin of disease.

lymphangiectasia /limfan′jē·ektā′zhə/, dilatation of the smaller lymphatic vessels, characterized by diarrhea, steatorrhea, and protein malabsorption. It usually results from obstruction in the larger vessels, as in pelvic tuberculosis, mesenteric node metastases, and certain protozoan diseases.

lymphangiography, the x-ray examination of lymph glands and lymphatic vessels after an injection of contrast medium. Also called **lymphography.**

lymphangioma /limfan′jē·ō′mə/, *pl.* **lymphangiomas, lymphangiomata,** a benign, yellowish-tan tumor on the skin, composed of a mass of dilated lymph vessels. It is often removed by excision or electrocoagulation for cosmetic reasons. Also called **angioma lymphaticum.** Compare **hemangioma.**

lymphangioma cavernosum, a tumor formed by dilated lymphatic vessels and filled with lymph that is often mixed with coagulated blood. The lesion, which is often congenital, may cause extensive enlargement of the affected tissue, especially of the tongue and lips. Also called **cavernous lymphangioma.**

lymphangioma circumscriptum, a benign skin lesion that develops from superficial hypertrophic lymph vessels. Most commonly seen in young children, it is characteristically pigmented and may grow to several centimeters in diameter.

lymphangioma cysticum. See **cystic lymphangioma.**

lymphangioma simplex, a growth formed by moderately dilated lymph vessels in a circumscribed area, chiefly on the skin.

lymphangitis /lim′fanjī′tis/, an inflammation of one or more lymphatic vessels, usually resulting from an acute streptococcal infection of one of the extremities. It is characterized by fine red streaks extending from the infected area to the axilla or groin, and by fever, chills, headache, and myalgia. The infection may spread to the bloodstream. Penicillin and hot soaks are usually prescribed; aseptic technique is important to avoid contagion.

lymphatic /limfat′ik/, **1.** of or pertaining to the lymphatic system of the body, consisting of a vast network of tubes transporting lymph. **2.** any one of the vessels associated with the lymphatic network.

lymphatic capillary plexus, one of the numerous networks of lymphatic capillaries that collect lymph from the intercellular fluid and constitute the beginning of the lymphatic system. The lymphatic vessels arise from the capillary plexuses, which vary in size and number in different regions and organs of the body. The capillary networks do not contain lymphatic valves as do the vessels. The plexuses are especially abundant in the dermis of the skin but also lace many other areas as the mucous membranes of the repiratory and digestive systems, testes, ovaries, liver, kidneys, and heart. See also **lymphatic system.**

lymphatic leukemia. See **acute lymphocytic leukemia, chronic lymphocytic leukemia.**

lymphatic nodule. See **malpighian body.**

lymphatic system, a vast, complex network of capillaries, thin vessels, valves, ducts, nodes, and organs that helps to protect and maintain the internal fluid environment of the entire body by producing, filtering, and conveying lymph and by producing various blood cells. The lymphatic network also transports fats, proteins, and other substances to the blood system and restores 60% of the fluid that filters out of the blood capillaries into interstitial spaces during normal metabolism. The peripheral parts of the lymphatic complex do not directly communicate with the venous system into which the lymph flows, but the endothelium of the veins at the junction of the blood and the lymphatic networks is continuous with the endothelium of the lymphatic vessels. Small semilunar valves throughout the lymphatic network help to control the flow of lymph and, at the junction with the venous system, prevent venous blood from flowing into the lymphatic vessels. The lymph collected from throughout the body drains into the blood through two ducts situated in the neck. Various body dynamics, as respiratory pressure changes, muscular contractions, and movements of organs surrounding lymphatic vessels combine to pump the lymph through the lymphatic system. The thoracic duct that rises into the left side of the neck is the major vessel of the lymphatic system and conveys lymph from the whole body, except for the right quadrant, which is served by the right lymphatic duct. Lymphatics have a beaded appearance because of sinuses associated with the many valves in the vessels. They resemble veins but have more valves, thinner walls, and contain lymph nodes. The lymphatics are so thin and transparent that the lymph they contain can be seen moving through these delicate tubules in a living body. Special techniques are required, however, to examine the lymphatic system closely. The lymphatic capillaries, which are the beginning of the system, abound in the dermis of the skin, forming a continuous network over the entire body, except for the cornea. The system also includes specialized lymphatic organs, as the tonsils, the thymus, and the spleen. The lymphatics of the intestine contain a special substance, especially during the digestion of fatty foods. Lymph flows into the general circulation through the thoracic duct at a rate of about 125 ml per hour during routine exertion. The rate may jump to as high as 1800 ml per hour during vigorous exercise. See also **lymph, lymph node, spleen, thymus,** and see the Color Atlas of Human Anatomy.

lymphedema /lim′fidē′mə/, a primary or secondary disorder characterized by the accumulation of lymph in soft tissue and swelling, caused by inflammation, obstruction, or removal of lymph channels. Congenital lymphedema (Milroy's disease) is a hereditary disorder characterized by chronic lymphatic obstruction. Lymphedema praecox occurs in adolescence, chiefly in females, and causes puffiness and swelling of the lower limbs, apparently because of hyperplastic development of lymph vessels. Secondary lymphedema may follow surgical removal of lymph channels in mastectomy, obstruction of lymph drainage caused by malignant tumors, or the infestation of lymph vessels with adult filarial parasites. Lymphedema of the lower extremities begins with mild swelling of the foot, gradually extends to the entire limb, and is aggravated by prolonged standing, pregnancy, obesity, warm weather, and the menstrual period. There is no cure for the disorder, but lymph drainage from the extremity can be improved if the patient sleeps with the foot of the bed elevated 4 to 8 inches, wears elastic stockings, and takes moderate exercise regularly. Light massage in the direction of the lymph flow and thiazide diuretics may be prescribed; constricting clothing and salty or spicy foods that increase thirst are contraindicated. Surgery may be performed to remove hypertrophied lymph channels and disfiguring tissue. **–lymphedematous, lymphedematose,** *adj.*

lymph node, one of the many small oval structures that filter the lymph and fight infection, and in which there are formed lymphocytes, monocytes, and plasma cells. The lymph nodes are of different sizes, some as small as pinheads, others as large as lima beans. Each node is enclosed in a capsule, is composed of a lighter colored cortical portion and a darker medullary portion, and consists of closely packed lymphocytes, reticular connective tissue laced by trabeculae, and three kinds of sinuses, subcapsular, cortical, and medullary. Lymph flows into the node through afferent lymphatic vessels that open into the subcapsular sinuses. Efferent lymphatic vessels arise from the medullary sinuses of the node and emerge through a small peripheral hilum that also receives blood vessels. The sinuses and meshes of reticular fibers retard the flow of lymph to which lymphocytes are added from germinal centers within the node that multiply those cells by mitosis. Most lymph nodes are clustered in (specific) areas, as the mouth, the neck, the lower arm, the axilla, and the groin. The lymphatic network and nodes of the breast are especially crucial in the diagnosis and treatment of breast cancer in women. Cancer cells from a ''primary'' breast tumor often spread through the lymphatic system to other parts of the body. Also called **lymph gland.**

lympho-, lymph-, a combining form meaning 'of or pertaining to the lymph': *lymphoduct, lymphography, lymphomatous.*

lymphoblastic lymphoma, lymphoblastic lymphosarcoma, lymphoblastoma. See **poorly differentiated lymphocytic malignant lymphoma.**

lymphocyte /lim′fəsīt/, one of two kinds of small, agranulocytic leukocytes, originating from fetal stem cells and developing in the bone marrow. Lymphocytes normally comprise 25% of the total white blood cell count but increase in number in response to infection. They occur in two forms: **B cells** and **T cells.** Each develops uniquely, and each has its own function. B cells circulate in an immature form and synthesize antibodies for insertion into their own cytoplasmic membranes. They reproduce mitotically, each of the clones displaying identical antibodies on their surface membranes. When an immature B cell is exposed to a specific antigen, the cell is activated, traveling to the spleen or to the lymph nodes, differentiating, and rapidly producing **plasma cells** and **memory cells.** Plasma cells synthesize and secrete copious amounts of antibody. Memory cells do not secrete antibody, but if reexposure to the specific antigen occurs, they develop into antibody-secreting plasma cells. The function of the B cell is to search out, identify, and bind with specific antigens. T cells are lymphocytes that have circulated through the thymus gland and have differentiated to become thymocytes. When exposed to an antigen, they divide rapidly and produce large numbers of new T cells sensitized to that antigen. T cells are often called ''killer cells'' because they secrete immunologically essential chemical compounds and assist B cells in destroying foreign protein. T cells also appear to play a significant role in the body's resistance to the proliferation of cancer cells. See also **lymphokine.**

lymphocytic choriomeningitis, an arenavirus infection of the meninges and the cerebrospinal fluid, caused by the lymphocytic choriomeningitis virus and characterized by fever, headache, and stiff neck. The infection occurs primarily in young adults, most often in the fall and winter months. Recovery usually takes place within 2 weeks.

lymphocytic leukemia. See **acute lymphocytic leukemia, chronic lymphocytic leukemia.**

lymphocytic lymphoma, lymphocytic lymphosarcoma. See **well-differentiated lymphocytic malignant lymphoma.**

lymphocytic thyroiditis. See **Hashimoto's disease.**

lymphocytoma. See **well-differentiated lymphocytic malignant lymphoma.**

lymphocytopenia /lim′fōsī′təpē′nē·ə/, a smaller than normal number of lymphocytes in the peripheral circulation, occurring as a primary hematologic disorder or in association with nutritional deficiency, malignancy, or infectious mononucleosis. Compare **alymphocytosis.** See also **agranulocyte.**

lymphoderma perniciosa. See **leukemia cutis.**

lymphoepithelioma /lim′fō·ep′ithē′lē·ō′mə/, a poorly differentiated neoplasm developing from the epithelium overlying lymphoid tissue in the nasopharynx. It occurs most frequently in young Oriental people. Also called **lymphoepithelial carcinoma.**

lymphogenous leukemia. See **acute lymphocytic leukemia, chronic lymphocytic leukemia.**

lymphogranuloma venereum (LGV), a sexually transmitted disease caused by a strain of the bacterium *Chlamydia trachomatis*. It is characterized by ulcerative genital lesions, marked swelling of the lymph nodes in the groin, headache, fever, and malaise. Ulcerations of the rectal wall occur less commonly. The disease is diagnosed by isolating the organism from an infected node, demonstrating LGV antibodies by serologic blood test or by a Frei intradermal test. Tetracycline is usually prescribed for the patient and for any person with whom there has been sexual contact. When changing dressings, aseptic technique is used. Also called **lymphopathia venereum.** See also ***Chlamydia.***

lymphography. See **lymphangiography.**

lymphoid leukemia. See **acute lymphocytic leukemia, chronic lymphocytic leukemia.**

lymphoidocytic leukemia. See **stem cell leukemia.**

lymphokine /lim′fōkīn/, one of the chemical factors produced and released by T lymphocytes that attract macrophages to the site of infection or inflammation and prepare them for attack. Kinds of lymphokines include **chemotactic factor, lymphotoxin, migration inhibiting factor,** and **mitogenic factor.**

lympholysis /limfol′əsis/, cellular destruction of lymphocytes, especially of certain lymphocytes in the process of an immune response. **–lympholytic,** *adj.*

lymphoma /limfō′mə/, *pl.* **lymphomas, lymphomata,** a neoplasm of lymphoid tissue that is usually malignant but, in rare cases, may be benign. The various lymphomas differ in degree of cellular differentiation and content, but the manifestations are similar in all types. Characteristically, the appearance of a painless, enlarged lymph node or nodes in the neck is followed by weakness, fever, weight loss, and anemia. With widespread involvement of lymphoid tissue, the spleen and liver usually enlarge, and GI disturbances, malabsorption, and bone lesions frequently develop. Men are more likely than women to develop lymphoid tumors. Treatment for lymphoma includes intensive radiotherapy and chemotherapy. Kinds of lymphoma include **Burkitt's lymphoma, giant follicular lymphoma, histiocytic malignant lymphoma, Hodgkin's disease, mixed cell malignant lymphoma.** **–lymphomatoid,** *adj.*

-lymphoma, a combining form meaning a 'tumor or neoplastic disorder of lymphoid tissue': *adenolymphoma, angiolymphoma, cystadenolymphoma.*

lymphoma staging, a system for classifying lymphomas according to the stage of the disease for the purpose of appropriate treatment. Stage I is characterized by the involvement of a single lymph node region or one extralymphatic organ or site and Stage II by the involvement of two or more lymph node regions on the same side of the diaphragm or a localized involvement of an extralymphatic organ or site plus one or more node regions on the same side of the diaphragm. In Stage III lymph nodes on both sides of the diaphragm are affected, and there may be involvement of the spleen or localized involvement of an extralymphatic organ or site. Stage IV is typified by diffuse or disseminated involvement of one or more extralymphatic organs or sites with or without associated lymph node involvement.

lymphopathia venereum. See **lymphogranuloma venereum.**

lymphopenia. See **lymphocytopenia.**

lymphoreticulosis, subacute granulomatous inflammation of lymphoid tissue with proliferation of reticuloendothelial cells, occurring most commonly as the result of a cat scratch. No causative agent is known. The disorder is characterized by the formation of an ulcerated papule at the site of the scratch, and by fever and tender lymphadenopathy, sometimes progressing to suppuration. Also called **cat scratch fever.**

lymphosarcoma. See **non-Hodgkin's lymphoma.**

lymphosarcoma cell leukemia, a malignancy of blood-forming tissues characterized by many lymphosarcoma cells in the peripheral circulation that tend to infiltrate surrounding tissues. These cells are extremely immature and larger and more reticulated than lymphocytes. The disease may accompany lymphoma or exist as a separate entity with more bone marrow involvement than is found in lymphoma.

lyo-, a combining form meaning 'dissolved': *lyogel, lyophobe, lyotropic.*

Lyon hypothesis, (in genetics) a hypothesis stating that only one of the two X chromosomes in a female is functional, the other having become inactive early in development. A female is mosaic in regard to X chromosomes; some are from her father, some from her mother. Sex-linked genes may therefore appear on some of her cells and not on others.

lyonization, the process of random inactivation of one of the X chromosomes in the female gamate to compensate for the presence of the double X gene complement. See also **Lyon hypothesis.**

lypressin /līpres′in/, an antidiuretic and vasoconstrictor.

■ INDICATION: It is prescribed in diabetes insipidus to decrease urinary water loss.

■ CONTRAINDICATIONS: Vascular disease or known hypersensitivity to this drug prohibits its use.

■ ADVERSE EFFECTS: Among the most serious adverse reactions are angina in people with cardiovascular disease, nausea, cramping, and marked facial pallor.

Lys, abbreviation for **lysine.**

-lyse. See **-lyze.**

lysergide /līsur′jīd/, a psychotomimetic, semisynthetic derivate of ergot that acts at multiple sites in the central nervous system from the cortex to the spinal cord. In susceptible individuals, as little as 20 to 25 μg of the potent drug may cause pupillary dilatation, increased blood pressure, hyperreflexia, tremor, muscle weakness, piloerection, and increased body temperature. Larger doses also produce dizziness, drowsiness, paresthesia, euphoria or dysphoria, and synesthesias; colors may be heard, sounds visualized, and time is felt to pass slowly. Psychologic dependence may develop, and use of lysergide is associated with significant hazards, as panic, serious depression, paranoid behavior, and prolonged psychotic episodes. Treatment of lysergide intoxication involves "talking down" the patient and administering antianxiety agents or barbiturates. It has been proposed but not approved for use as an adjunct to psychotherapy, in the treatment of alcoholism, and to relieve pain in terminal cancer patients. Also called **LSD** (an abbreviation of the original German name, *Lyserg-Säure-Diäthylamid),* **lysergic acid diethylamide,** *(slang)* **acid.** See also **hallucinogen.**

-lysin, a combining form meaning a 'cell-dissolving antibody': *antilysin, betalysin, paralysin.*

lysine (Lys) /lī′sēn, lī′sin/, an essential amino acid needed for proper growth in infants and for maintenance of nitrogen balance in adults. See also **amino acid, protein.**

lysine intolerance, a congenital disorder resulting in the inability to use the essential amino acid lysine because of an enzyme deficiency or defect. The disorder is characterized by weakness, vomiting, and coma and is treated by adjusting the protein content of the diet, restricting those foods especially high in lysine. See also **lysinemia.**

lysinemia /lī′sinē′mē·ə/, a condition caused by an inborn error of metabolism and resulting in the inability to use the essential amino acid lysine because of an enzyme defect or deficiency. It is characterized by muscle weakness and mental retardation. Treatment consists of a diet that controls the intake of lysine by reducing proteins and including such foods as fruits, vegetables, and rice.

lysine monohydrochloride, a salt of the amino acid lysine, used as a dietary supplement to increase the use of vegetable proteins, as corn, rice, and wheat.

lysis /lī′sis/, **1.** destruction or dissolution of a cell or molecule through the action of a specific agent. Cell lysis is frequently caused by a lysin. **2.** gradual diminution in the symptoms of a disease. Compare **crisis.**

-lysis, a combining form meaning a 'breaking down or detachment': *cytolysis, dialysis, osteolysis.*

lysis of adhesions, surgery performed to free adhesions of tissues.

lyso-, a combining form meaning 'of or pertaining to dissolution': *lysocephalin, lysotype, lysozyme.*

Lysodren, a trademark for an antineoplastic (mitotane).

lysosome /lī′səsōm/, a cytoplasmic, membrane-bound particle that contains hydrolytic enzymes that function in intracellular digestive processes. The organelles are found in most cells but are particularly prominent in leukocytes and in the cells of the liver and kidney. If the hydrolytic enzymes are released into the cytoplasm, they cause self-digestion of the cell so that lysosomes may play an important role in certain self-destructive diseases characterized by the wasting of tissue, as muscular dystrophy.

lysozyme, an enzyme with antiseptic actions that destroys some foreign organisms. It is found in granulocytic and monocytic blood cells and is normally present in saliva, sweat, breast milk, and tears.

lysso-, a combining form meaning 'of or pertaining to rabies, or hydrophobia': *lyssodexis, lyssoid, lyssophobia.*

-lyte, a combining form meaning a 'substance capable of or resulting from decomposition': *ampholyte, cytolyte, sarcolyte.*

lytes /līts/, an informal abbreviation of *electrolytes,* especially the levels of potassium, sodium, phosphorus, magnesium, and calcium in the blood, as determined by laboratory testing.

-lytic, a combining form meaning 'pertaining to or effecting decomposition': *fibrillolytic, leukolytic, myelolytic.*

lytic cocktail /lit′ik/, an informal name for an anesthetic compound of chlorpromazine, meperidine, and promethazine that blocks the autonomic nervous system, depresses the circulatory system, and induces neuroplegia.

Lytren, a trademark for a nutritional supplement containing various electrolytes.

-lyze, -lyse, a combining form meaning 'to produce decomposition': *bacteriolyze, hemolyze, paralyze.*

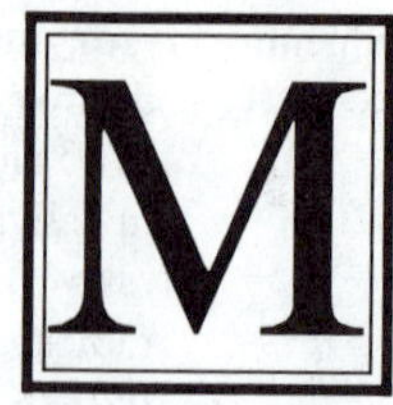

m, abbreviation for **meter.**

M, abbreviation for **metastasis** in the TNM (tumor, node, metastasis) system for staging malignant neoplastic disease. See also **cancer staging.**

ma, abbreviation for **milliampere.**

MA, abbreviation for **mental age.**

Maass, Clara (1876–1901), an American nurse. After training and working at the Newark German Hospital, which has since been renamed for her, she volunteered for military service at the outbreak of the Spanish-American War. After working at Army camps where soldiers were dying of yellow fever, she volunteered to go to Havana to participate in the experiments being done to determine the cause of that disease. She was bitten by a mosquito and died 10 days later of yellow fever. She was one of the first nurses to be inducted into the Hall of Fame of the American Nurses' Association.

MAC, abbreviation for **minimum alveolar concentration.**

MAC AWAKE, the time at which a patient recovering from general anesthesia is able to respond rationally to questions and verbal instructions.

macerate /mas′ərāt/, to soften something solid by soaking. **–maceration,** *n.*

machine language, a low-level computer language employing binary numbers.

Machupo. See **Bolivian hemorrhagic fever.**

macrencephaly /mak′rənsef′əlē/, a congenital anomaly characterized by abnormal largeness of the brain. Also called **macroencephaly.** See also **macrocephaly.** **–macrencephalic, macroencephalic,** *adj.*

macro-, makro-, a combining form meaning 'large, or abnormal size': *macrobiosis, macrocardius, macrophage.*

macroblepharia /mak′rōblifer′ē•ə/, the condition of having abnormally large eyelids.

macrocephaly /mak′rōsef′əlē/, a congenital anomaly characterized by abnormal largeness of the head and brain in relation to the rest of the body, resulting in some degree of mental and growth retardation. The head is more than two standard deviations above the average circumference size for age, sex, race, and period of gestation, with excessively wide fontanelles; the facial features are usually normal. The condition may be caused by some defect in formation during embryonic development, or it may be the result of progressive degeneration processes, as Schilder's disease, Greenfield's disease, or congenital lipoidosis. In macrocephaly there is symmetric overgrowth at the head without increased intracranial pressure, as differentiated from hydrocephalus in which the lateral, asymmetric growth of the head is caused by excessive accumulation of cerebrospinal fluid, usually under increased pressure. Specific diagnostic tests may be necessary to differentiate the two conditions. Treatment is primarily symptomatic, with nursing care concentrated specifically on helping parents learn to care for a brain-damaged child. Also called **macrocephalia, megalocephaly.** Compare **microcephaly.** See also **hydrocephalus.** **–macrocephalic, macrocephalous,** *adj.*, **macrocephalus,** *n.*

macrocyte /mak′rəsīt/, an abnormally large, mature erythrocyte usually exceeding 9 μm in diameter. It is most commonly seen in megaloblastic anemia. Compare **microcyte.** See also **macrocytic anemia.**

macrocytic /mak′rōsit′ik/, (of a cell) larger than normal, as the erythrocytes in macrocytic anemia.

macrocytic anemia, a disorder of the blood characterized by impaired erythropoiesis and the abnormal presence of large, fragile, red blood cells in the circulation. Macrocytic anemia is most often the result of a deficiency of folic acid and vitamin B_{12}. Compare **microcytic anemia.**

macrocytosis /mak′rōsītō′sis/, an abnormal proliferation of macrocytes in the peripheral blood. Compare **poikilocytosis.** See also **anisocytosis.**

Macrodantin, a trademark for a urinary antibacterial (nitrofurantoin).

Macrodex, a trademark for a plasma expander (dextran).

macrodrip, (in intravenous therapy) an apparatus that is used to deliver measured amounts of IV solutions at specific flow rates based on the size of drops of the solution. The size of the drops is controlled by the fixed diameter of a plastic delivery tube. The drops delivered by a macrodrip are larger than those delivered by a microdrip. Different macrodrips deliver 10, 15, or 20 drops per milliliter of solution. Macrodrips are not usually used to deliver a small amount of IV solution or to keep a vein open, because the time between drips is so long that a clot may form at the tip of the IV catheter. Compare **microdrip.**

macroelement. See **macronutrient.**

macroencephaly. See **macrencephaly.**

macrogamete, a large, nonmotile female gamete of certain thallophytes and sporozoa, specifically the malarial parasite *Plasmodium.* It corresponds to the ovum of the higher animals and is fertilized by the smaller, motile male gamete. See also **microgamete.**

macrogametocyte, an enlarged merozoite that undergoes meiosis to form the mature female gamete during the sexual phase of the life cycle of certain thallophytes and sporozoa, specifically the malarial parasite *Plasmodium.* Macrogametocytes are found in the red blood cells of a person infected with the malarial parasite, but they must be ingested by a female *Anopheles* mosquito to complete the maturation process and develop into a macrogamete.

macrogenitosomia /mak'rōjen'itōsō'mē·ə/, a congenital condition in which the genitalia are abnormal because of an excess of androgen during fetal development. It is characterized in boys by enlarged external genitalia and in girls by pseudohermaphroditism.

macroglobulinemia /mak'rōglob'yo͞olinē'mē·ə/, a form of monoclonal gammopathy in which a large immunoglobulin (IgM) is vastly overproduced by the clones of a plasma B cell in response to an antigenic signal. Increased viscosity of the blood may result in circulatory impairment, weakness, neurologic disorders, and fatigue. Normal immunoglobulin synthesis is decreased, and the person is susceptible to infection, particularly bacterial pneumonia and septicemia. Also called **Waldenström's macroglobulinemia.** See also **multiple myeloma.**

macroglossia /mak'rōglos'ē·ə/, a congenital anomaly characterized by excessive size of the tongue, as seen in certain syndromes of congenital defects, including Down's syndrome.

macrognathia /mak'rōnā'thē·ə/, an abnormally large growth of the jaw. Compare **micrognathia.** **–macrognathic,** *adj.*

macromolecule, a molecule of colloidal size, as proteins, nucleic acids, or polysaccharides.

macronucleus, **1.** a large nucleus. **2.** (in protozoa) the larger of two nuclei in each cell; it governs cell metabolism and growth as opposed to the micronucleus, which functions in sexual reproduction.

macronutrient, a chemical element required in relatively large quantities for the normal physiologic processes of the body. Macronutrients include carbon, hydrogen, oxygen, nitrogen, potassium, sodium, calcium, chloride, magnesium, phosphorus, and sulfur. Also called **macroelement, major element.** Compare **micronutrient.**

macrophage /mak'rəfāj/, any phagocytic cell of the reticuloendothelial system including Kupffer cell in the liver, splenocyte in the spleen, and histocyte in the loose connective tissue. See also **phagocyte, reticuloendothelial system.**

macroreentry, (in cardiology) reactivation of a tissue involving a large circuit, as involvement of both bundle branches.

macroscopic anatomy. See **gross anatomy.**

macrosomia. See **gigantism.**

macula /mak'yo͞olə/, *pl.* **maculae,** **1.** a small pigmented area or a spot that appears separate or different from the surrounding tissue. **2.** See **macula lutea.**

macula cerulea. See **blue spot,** def. 1.

macula lutea, an oval yellow spot at the center of the retina 2 mm from the optic nerve. It contains a pit, no blood vessels, and the fovea centralis. Central vision occurs when an image is focused directly on the fovea centralis of the macula lutea. Also called *(informal)* **macula.**

macule /mak'yo͞ol/, **1.** a small, flat blemish or discoloration that is flush with the skin surface. Examples are freckles and the rashes of measles and roseola. Compare **papule.** **2.** a gray scar on the cornea that is visible without magnification. **–macular,** *adj.*

Madelung's neck. See **lipoma annulare colli.**

mad hatter's disease. See **mercurialism.**

Madura foot /maj'o͝orə/, a progressive, destructive, tropical fungal infection of the foot, named for a district in India. Also called **maduromycosis.**

mafenide acetate, a topical antiinfective.

■ INDICATION: It is prescribed in the treatment of burns.

■ CONTRAINDICATIONS: Known hypersensitivity to this drug or to sulfonamide prohibits its use.

■ ADVERSE EFFECTS: Among the more serious adverse effects are hypersensitivity reactions and suprainfections particularly by *Candida albicans.*

Maffucci's syndrome /mafo͞o'chēz/, a condition characterized by enchondromatosis and multiple cutaneous or visceral hemangiomas.

magaldrate, an antiacid.

■ INDICATIONS: It is prescribed in the treatment of hypersensitivity and stomach upset associated with heartburn, sour stomach, or acid indigestion.

■ CONTRAINDICATIONS: It may alter the absorption of several drugs, as tetracyclines.

■ ADVERSE EFFECTS: There may be a change in bowel function.

Magendie's law. See **Bell's law.**

magic-bullet approach, **1.** a therapeutic or diagnostic method that makes use of a specific mechanistic connection between a drug and a disease or organ. **2.** (in clinical medicine) the administration of a specific drug to cure or ameliorate a given disease or condition. **3.** (in traditional diagnostic radiology) the administration of a specific dye to facilitate the visualization by x-ray of a given organ, as the intravenous injection of a specific dye for renal studies. **4.** (in nuclear medicine) the administration of a specific radionuclide tagged to an appropriate carrier to provide a scintillation camera image of a given organ or structure, as the use of a substance containing phosphate and technetium for bone scanning.

magnesemia, the presence of magnesium in the blood.

magnesia magma. See **milk of magnesia.**

magnesium (Mg), a silver-white mineral element. Its atomic number is 12; its atomic weight is 24.32. Magnesium occurs abundantly in nature, always in combination with other elements, in sea water, bones, seeds, in the chlorophyll in the green parts of plants, and in minerals, as magnesite, dolomite, and carnalite. It is obtained chiefly by the electrolysis of fused salts containing magnesium chloride or by the thermal reduction of magnesia and is used in photography, metallurgy, and various medicines, as magnesium sulfate. Magnesium is the second most abundant cation of the intracellular fluids in the body and is essential for many enzyme activities. It also is important to neurochemical transmissions and muscular excitability. The body of the average 145-pound adult contains about 2000 mEq of magnesium, about 50% of which is in the bones, 45% existing as intracellular cations, and about 5% in the extracellular fluid. Intracellular concentrations of magnesium range from 5 to 30 mEq per kilogram, depending on the type of tissue. The concentration of magnesium in plasma is 1.5 to 2.2 mEq per liter, with about two thirds as free cation and one third bound to plasma proteins. Very little is known about the exchange of magnesium between the plasma, the intracellular capsule, and the bone. About 30% of the magnesium in the skeleton represents an exchangeable pool. The average adult in the United States ingests between 20 and 40 mEq of magnesium daily, and about one third of the quantity ingested is absorbed from the GI tract. Absorption occurs in the upper small bowel by means of an active process closely related to the transport system for calcium. Magnesium is excreted mainly by the kidney and 3% to 5% of the magnesium is excreted in the urine. Most of the reabsorption of magnesium takes place in the proximal tubules of the kidney. Renal excretion of magnesium increases during diuresis induced by ammonium chloride, glucose, and organic mercurials. Diuretic therapy can cause hypomagnesemia. Small amounts of magnesium are excreted in milk and in the saliva. The element influences many enzymes in the body and is a cofactor of all enzymes participating in phosphate transfer reactions involving adenosine triphosphate and other nucleotide triphosphates as substrates. It is also essential to the interaction of intracellular particles and the binding of macromolecules to subcellular organelles, as the binding of messenger RNA to ribosomes. Magnesium affects the central nervous, neuromuscular, and cardiovascular systems. Hypomagnesemia increases central nervous system irritability and may cause disorientation, convulsions, and psychosis. Some researchers report abnormally high concentrations of magnesium in the plasma of manic-depressive and schizophrenic individuals and abnormally low magnesium concentrations in the plasma of patients with endogenous and neurotic depressions. Magnesium tends to depress the action of skeletal muscle, and excessive magnesium inhibits the release of acetylcholine by motor nerve impulses. Insufficient magnesium in extracellular fluid increases the release of acetylcholine, increases muscular excitability, and can cause tetany. Excess magnesium in the body can slow the heartbeat, and concentrations of magnesium greater than 15 mEq per liter can produce cardiac arrest in diastole. Excess magnesium also causes vasodilatation by directly affecting the blood vessels and by ganglionic blockade. Hypomagnesemia can cause changes in cardiac muscles and skeletal muscle and can cause nephrocalcinosis. Some of the abnormal conditions that can produce hypomagnesemia are diarrhea, steatorrhea, chronic alcoholism, and diabetes mellitus. Hypomagnesemia may also be associated with newborns and infants who are fed cow's milk or artificial formulas, apparently because of the high phosphate-magnesium ratio in such diets. Hypomagnesemia is often treated with parenteral fluids containing magnesium sulfate or magnesium chloride. Hypermagnesemia is usually caused by renal insufficiency and is manifested by hypotension, electrocardiogram changes, muscle weakness, sedation, and a confused mental state.

magnesium sulfate, a salt of magnesium. Also called **Epsom salts.**

▪ INDICATIONS: It is prescribed parenterally to prevent seizures, especially in preeclampsia, and orally to treat constipation and heartburn and to correct deficiency of magnesium in the body.

▪ CONTRAINDICATIONS: It is used with caution with renal impairment or hypersensitivity to the drug. Respiratory depression, severe cardiac myopathy, heart block, or symptoms of appendicitis or fecal impaction prohibits its use.

▪ ADVERSE EFFECTS: The most serious adverse reaction is circulatory collapse from excessive serum concentrations of magnesium. Respiratory depression, confusion, and muscle weakness also may occur.

magnetic moment, a measure of the net magnetic field produced by an elementary particle or an atomic nucleus spinning about its own axis. These fields are similar to those produced by a bar magnet.

magnetic resonance imaging (MRI), medical imaging that uses nuclear magnetic resonance as its source of energy. See also **nuclear magnetic resonance.**

magnetic susceptibility, a measure of the ability of a substance to become magnetized.

magnetic tape. See **mag tape.**

magnetization, the magnetic polarization of a material produced by a magnetic field (magnetic moment per unit volume).,

mag tape, *informal.* a ribbon of plastic tape coated with an electromagnetic compound that allows for the coding of information in the form of positive and negative charges. Also called **electromagnetic tape, magnetic tape, tape.**

magnet reflex, a pathologic reflex seen in an animal that has had its cerebellum removed. If the animal is placed on its back and its head is strongly flexed, all four limbs will flex. Then light pressure by a finger on a toepad causes contraction of limb extensor muscles so that if the finger is slowly removed the limb appears to follow the finger.

magnetron, a source of microwave energy used in medical linear accelerators to accelerate electrons to the therapeutic energies.

Mahaim fibers, conductive tracts in cardiac tissue running between the AV node or His bundle and the muscle of the ventricular septum. They conduct early excitation impulses.

Mahoney, Mary Eliza (1845–1926), the first American black nurse. She did private nursing in the Boston area and was active in furthering intergroup relationships and in improving the role of the black nurse in the community. A medal in her name, established after her death, was first presented in 1936; it is given to a black nurse in recognition of an outstanding contribution to the profession.

main en griffe. See **clawhand.**

mainframe computer, a large general-purpose computer system for high-volume data processing tasks. Compare **microcomputer, minicomputer.**

main memory, the memory of a computer contained in its circuitry.

maintenance dose, the amount of drug required to keep a desired mean steady-state concentration in the tissues.

Majocchi's granuloma, a rare type of tinea corporis, mainly affecting the lower legs. It is caused by the fungus *Trichophyton,* which infects the hairs of the affected site and raises spongy granulomas. The lesions persist for 3 to 4 months and are gradually absorbed, or they necrose, often leaving deep scars. Also called **trichophytic granuloma.**

major affective disorder, any of a group of psychotic disorders characterized by severe and inappropriate emotional responses, by prolonged and persistent disturbances of mood and related thought distortions, and by other symptoms associated with either depressed or manic states, as occurs in bipolar disorder, depression, and involutional melancholia. The disorder is usually episodic but may be chronic or cyclic, as in the case of bipolar disorder; it is not caused by any organic dysfunction of the brain.

major connector, a metal plate or bar, used for joining the components of one side of a removable partial denture to those on the opposite side of the dental arch.

major depressive episode. See **endogenous depression.**

major element. See **macronutrient.**

major medical insurance, insurance coverage designed to offset the costs of prolonged or catastrophic illness and injury. Most major medical insurance policies are written to pay a certain percentage of costs up to predetermined figure, beyond which payment is in full up to a maximum amount, at which payment ceases. Many require the insured to pay a specified initial, or deductible, amount.

major renal calyx. See **renal calyx.**

major surgery, any surgical procedure that requires general anesthesia or respiratory assistance. Compare **minor surgery.**

makro-. See **macro-.**

mal /mal, mäl/, an illness or disease, as grand mal or petit mal.

mal-, a combining form meaning 'abnormal': *maladjustment, malalignment, malignant.*

malabsorption, impaired absorption of nutrients from the GI tract. It occurs in celiac disease, sprue, dysentery, diarrhea, and other disorders and may result from an inborn error of metabolism, malnutrition, or any chemical or anatomic condition of the digestive system that prevents normal absorption. See **inborn error of metabolism, malnutrition.**

malabsorption syndrome, a complex of symptoms resulting from disorders in the intestinal absorption of nutrients, characterized by anorexia, weight loss, bloating of the abdomen, muscle cramps, bone pain, and steatorrhea. Anemia, weakness, and fatigue occur because iron, folic acid, and vitamin B_{12} are not absorbed in sufficient amounts. Among the many conditions causing this syndrome are gastric or small bowel resection, celiac disease, tropical sprue, Whipple's disease, intestinal lymphangiectasia, and cystic fibrosis. Treatment and prognosis are determined by the underlying condition. See also **celiac disease, cystic fibrosis, hypoproteinemia, tropical sprue.**

malacia /məlā′shə/, **1.** a morbid softening or a sponginess in any part or any tissue of the body. **2.** a craving for spicy foods, as mustard, hot peppers, or pickles. –**malacic,** *adj.*

-malacia, a combining form meaning the 'softening of tissue': *cardiomalacia, esophagomalacia, tracheomalacia.*

malaco-, a combining form meaning 'a condition of abnormal softness': *malacoplakia, malacosarcosis.*

maladaptation, faulty intrapersonal adaptation to stress or change. It may involve a failure to make necessary changes in the desires, values, needs, and attitudes or an inability to make necessary adjustments in the external world. Illness often provokes maladaptive behavior that increases the problems accompanying the illness.

malaise, a vague feeling of bodily weakness or discomfort, often marking the onset of disease.

malalignment, a failure of parts of the body to align normally, as the teeth in the dental arch.

malar /mā′lər/, of or pertaining to the cheek or the cheek bone.

malaria /məler′ē·ə/, a serious infectious illness caused by one or more of at least four species of the protozoan genus *Plasmodium,* characterized by chills, fever, anemia, an enlarged spleen, and a tendency to recur. The disease is transmitted from human to human by a bite from an infected *Anopheles* mosquito. Malarial infection can also be spread by blood transfusion from an infected patient or by the use of an infected hypodermic needle. Although the endemic disease is limited largely to tropic areas of South and Central America, Africa, and Asia, a number of new cases are brought to the United States by refugees, military personnel, and travelers returning from malarial areas. *Plasmodium* parasites penetrate the erythrocytes of the human host, where they mature, reproduce, and burst out periodically. Malarial paroxysms occur at regular intervals, coinciding with the development of a new generation of parasites in the body. Because the life cycle of the infecting parasite varies according to species, the clinical patterns of chills and fever differ as do the course and severity of the disease. Bouts of malaria usually last from 1 to 4 weeks, with attacks occurring less frequently as the disease progresses. Relapse is common, and the disease can persist for years. Diagnosis is made by demonstrating the *Plasmodium* parasite in a blood smear. The organism is most likely to be seen in the blood during an acute attack. The exact species of *Plasmodium* must be identified, because the treatment and prognosis will vary according to the strain found. Chloroquine, given orally or intramuscularly, is the drug of choice for all but those strains of *Plasmodium* resistant to chloroquine, which are treated with a combination of quinine, pyrimethamine, and one of the sulfonamides or sulfones. Modern antimalarial drugs can suppress symptoms or cure malaria completely. Symptoms of headache, nausea, muscle ache, and high fever can be relieved with cold compresses, aspirin, and fluids. Through the use of insecticides and by destroying the swampy habitat of *Anopheles,* the disease has been eliminated from many parts of the world where it has been endemic. Worldwide eradication of the disease has not been possible, however, and insecticide-resistant mosquitoes and drug-resistant protozoa have arisen. Prophylaxis with antimalarial drugs is still important for those visiting endemic areas. The use of netting and mosquito repellent is also encouraged. See also **antimalaria, biduotertian fever, blackwater fever, falciparum malaria, *Plasmodium,* quartan malaria, tertian malaria.** **–malarial,** *adj.*

malarial hemoglobinuria. See **blackwater fever.**

Malassezia, a genus of fungi. *M. furfur* causes tinea versicolor (previous name: *Pityrosporum oviculare*). *M. ovalis* is a nonpathogenic organism found in sebaceous areas (previous name: *Pityrosporum ovale*).

malathion poisoning, a toxic condition caused by the ingestion or absorption through the skin of malathion, an organophosphorus insecticide. Symptoms include vomiting, nausea, abdominal cramps, headache, dizziness, weakness, confusion, convulsions, and respiratory difficulties. Treatment includes immediate intravenous administration of atropine, followed by pralidoxime chloride, gastric lavage, a saline cathartic, respiratory assistance, and oxygen. Malathion is much less toxic than parathion and is the only organophosphorus insecticide approved for household use.

malaxation. See **pétrissage.**

Malayan pit viper venom. See **ancrod.**

mal del pinto. See **pinta.**

mal de mer. See **motion sickness.**

male, **1.** of or pertaining to the sex that produces sperm cells and fertilizes the female to beget children; masculine. **2.** a male person.

male dietary allowance. See **dietary allowances,** and see the table of recommended daily dietary allowances in the Appendix.

male reproductive system assessment, an evaluation of the condition of the patient's genitalia, reproductive history, and past and present genitourinary infections and disorders.

■ METHOD: In a relaxed, professional interview the procedures to be conducted are explained and the patient is reassured that his privacy will be scrupulously maintained. He is questioned about his offspring, sexual activity, the existence of nocturia, urgency, frequency, dysuria, urethral discharge, hernia, genital sores, discomfort or pain in the groin, lower back, or legs, and past treatment for epididymitis, gonorrhea, herpes genitalis, hydrocele, nonspecific urethritis, orchitis, prostatitis, syphilis, and varicocele. The examiner, while inspecting the genitalia, wears rubber gloves to prevent infection. The penis is examined for swelling, inflammation, and lesions, as herpes vesicles or a syphilitic sore, chancre, or scar. Anomalies that may be noted include hypospadias or epispadias, resulting from failed closure of the urethra, elongation of the foreskin constricting the urinary meatus, or swelling of the glans caused by a retracted, tight foreskin. The urethral orifice is inspected for a purulent or bloody discharge, and the scrotum is observed for symmetry and shape; in elderly or debilitated men the scrotum may be elongated and flat. The normally smooth testes, epididymes, and spermatic cords are palpated for the presence of beading, varicosities, and the size, location, and consistency of any scrotal mass; fluid felt around the testes may be seen by darkening the room and illuminating the scrotum with a flashlight. The patient is asked to cough or bear down to reveal a hernia, and the abdomen is palpated above the symphysis pubis to determine if the bladder is distended. The inguinal lymph nodes are palpated, and the amount and distribution of pubic hair is observed. The prostate may be examined with the patient in the Sims' knee-chest position or lithotomy position, but, when possible, it is preferable for the patient to stand bent at a right angle over a table as the examiner's well-lubricated gloved forefinger sweeps the rectal circumference and palpates the lobes and medial sulcus of the gland. The size, consistency, and any localized nodule suggesting a neoplasm of the normally smooth, firm prostate are carefully noted, and the findings are recorded as on a clock dial with the symphysis pubis representing 12 o'clock. When additional studies are indicated, a smear is prepared from the first urine voided after massage of the prostate. Enzyme tests showing elevated phosphatase levels in serum suggest prostate cancer, but a diagnosis is usually established by a biopsy. Tissue may be obtained by a perineal, transurethral, or transrectal needle biopsy, but the most accurate method is an open perineal biopsy, which permits identification of the suspect lesion and the removal of multiple specimens. The assessment includes laboratory studies of discharge from the penis. A gram-stained smear usually confirms or rules out a diagnosis of gonorrhea, and a fluorescent-tagged antibody method may be required if the result is equivocal. Cultures may be needed to determine whether nonspecific urethritis is caused by *Escherichia coli, Pseudomonas, Staphylococcus, Streptococcus,* or organisms of other pathogenic genera. Syphilis may be diagnosed by the Veneral Disease Research Laboratory serologic test, but the Fluorescent Treponemal Antibody-Absorption test is the most sensitive and specific diagnostic measure. If infertility is a problem, examinations of multiple semen samples are conducted; each specimen collected after 3 days of abstinence is inspected in the laboratory to determine if the volume of the ejaculate approximates the normal 3.5 ml average and if the semen has a pH of 7.7 and a sperm count of 60 to 150 million per milliliter.

■ NURSING ORDERS: The nurse conducts the interview and examination, assembles the results of laboratory studies, and urges the patient to inform his sex partner, or partners, if an infectious disease is diagnosed. Throughout the assessment the nurse recognizes that the patient may be reluctant to discuss his symptoms and activities and be sensitive about the necessary procedures.

■ OUTCOME CRITERIA: A careful, understanding evaluation of the male patient's reproductive system helps to establish the diagnosis and plan the treatment and aids in allaying the patient's anxiety. The assessment also serves as a public health measure by encouraging the reporting of a sexually transmitted disease to the patient's contacts and proper authorities.

male sexual dysfunction, impaired or inadequate ability of a man to carry on his sex life to his own satisfaction. Symptoms, often psychologic in origin, include difficulties in starting and maintaining an erection, premature ejaculation, inability to ejaculate, and even loss of desire. Men are often so ashamed of the problem that they ask the physician to treat a "prostate problem," hoping that the covert message becomes clear. Compare **female sexual dysfunction.** See also **impotence, premature ejaculation, sexual dysfunction.**

malfeasance /malfē′zəns/, performance of an unlawful, wrongful act. Compare **misfeasance, nonfeasance.**

malformation, an anomalous structure in the body. See also **birth defect, congenital anomaly.**

Malgaigne's fracture of pelvis /malgā′nyəz/, trauma involving multiple pelvic fractures, including fracture of the wing of the ilium or sacrum and fracture of the ipsilateral pubic rami, with associated upper displacement of the hemipelvis.

malicious prosecution, (in law) a suit begun in malice and pursued without sufficient cause. It is usually an action for damages. Malicious prosecution is a wrongful civil proceeding, and a person who takes an active part in initiating or continuing it is subject to liability.

malignant /məlig′nənt/, **1.** also **virulent.** tending to become worse and cause death. **2.** (describing a cancer) anaplastic, invasive, and metastatic. –**malignancy,** *n.*

malignant ependymoma. See **ependymoblastoma.**

malignant hemangioendothelioma. See **hemangiosarcoma.**

malignant hepatoma, a malignant tumor of the liver. Primary liver cancer is relatively rare in the United States, occurring one sixth to one fifth as often as in Africa and the Far East. The only effective treatment is surgical excision of the tumor. This is often not feasible, because the tumors grow rapidly and spread through both lobes of the liver. The prognosis is poor. Also called **hepatocarcinoma, hepatocellular carcinoma, liver cell carcinoma.**

malignant hypertension, an abnormal condition and the most lethal form of both essential hypertension and secondary hypertension. It is a fulminating condition, characterized by severely elevated blood pressure, that commonly damages the intima of small vessels, the brain, retina, heart, and kidneys. It affects more blacks than whites and may be caused by a variety of factors, as stress, genetic predisposition, obesity, the use of tobacco, the use of oral contraceptives, high intake of sodium chloride, a sedentary life-style, and aging. Many patients with this condition exhibit signs of hypokalemia, alkalosis, and aldosterone secretion rates even higher than those associated with primary aldosteronism. See also **essential hypertension.**

malignant hyperthermia (MH), an autosomal dominant trait characterized by often fatal hyperthermia with rigidity of the muscles occurring in affected people exposed to certain anesthetic agents, particularly halothane, succinylcholine, and methoxyflurane. Treatment includes the administration of dantrolene or 100% oxygen, cooling procedures, and the correction of acidosis and hyperkalemia. Patients who have malignant hyperthermia are informed of their condition and advised that one half of their first-degree relatives are likely to have the trait.

malignant malnutrition. See **kwashiorkor.**

malignant melanoma. See **melanoma.**

malignant mesenchymoma, a sarcoma that contains mesenchymal elements.

malignant mole. See **melanoma.**

malignant neoplasm, a tumor that tends to grow, invade, and metastasize. It usually has an irregular shape and is composed of poorly differentiated cells. If untreated, it may result in the death of the organism. The degree to which a neoplasm is malignant varies with the kind of tumor and the condition of the patient.

malignant neuroma. See **neurosarcoma.**

malignant pustule. See **anthrax.**

malignant tumor, a neoplasm that characteristically invades surrounding tissue, metastasizes to distant sites, and contains anaplastic cells. A malignant tumor may result in the death of the host if remission or treatment do not intervene.

malingering, a willful and deliberate feigning of the symptoms of a disease or injury to gain some consciously desired end. Compare **compensation neurosis.** –**malinger,** *v.*, **malingerer,** *n.*

malleolus /məlē′ələs/, *pl.* **malleoli,** a rounded bony process, as the protuberance on each side of the ankle.

mallet fracture, avulsion fracture of the dorsal base of a distal phalanx of the hand or foot, involving the associated extensor apparatus and causing dropped flexion of the distal segment.

malleus /mal′ē·əs/, *pl.* **mallei,** one of the three ossicles in the middle ear, resembling a hammer with a head, neck, and three processes. It is connected to the tympanic membrane and transmits sound vibrations to the incus, which communicates with the stapes. Compare **incus, stapes.** See also **middle ear.**

Mallory bodies, an eosinophilic cytoplasmic inclusion, alcoholic hyalin, found in the liver cells. It is typically, but not always, associated with acute alcoholic liver injury. See also **cirrhosis.**

Mallory-Weiss syndrome, a condition characterized by massive bleeding after a tear in the mucous membrane at the junction of the esophagus and the stomach. The laceration is usually caused by protracted vomiting, most commonly in alcoholics or in persons whose pylorus is obstructed. The esophageal tear is located by esophagoscopy or arteriography. Surgery is usually necessary to stop the bleeding. After repair, the prognosis is excellent.

malnutrition, any disorder concerning nutrition. It may result from an unbalanced, insufficient, or excessive diet or to the impaired absorption, assimilation, or use of foods. Compare **deficiency disease.**

malocclusion /mal′əklo͞o′zhən/, abnormal contact of the teeth of the upper jaw with the teeth of the lower jaw. See also **occlusion.**

malonic acid /məlō′nik/, a white, crystalline, highly toxic substance used as an intermediate compound in the production of barbiturates.

malpighian body /malpig′ē·ən/, **1.** the renal corpuscle, which includes a glomerulus with Bowman's capsule. **2.** also called **lymphatic nodule.** lymphoid tissue surrounding the arteries of the spleen.

malpighian corpuscle, one of a number of small, round, deep-red bodies in the cortex of the kidney, each communicating with a renal tubule. Malpighian corpuscles average about 0.2 mm in diameter, each capsule composed of two parts: a central glomerulus and a glomerular capsule. The corpuscles are thought to be part of a filter system through which nonprotein components of blood plasma enter the tubules for urinary excretion. Also called **malpighian body, renal corpuscle.**

malpractice, (in law) professional negligence that is the proximate cause of injury or harm to a patient, resulting from a lack of professional knowledge, experience, or skill that can be expected in others in the profession or from a failure to exercise reasonable care or judgment in the application of professional knowledge, experience, or skill.

Malta fever. See **brucellosis.**

malt worker's lung, a respiratory disorder acquired by occupational exposure to fungi-laden particles of moldy barley grain or malt. See also **organic dust.**

malunion /malyo͞o′nyən/, an imperfect union of previously fragmented bone or other tissue.

mamm-, a combining form meaning 'of or pertaining to the breast': *mammectomy, mammogram, mammotropic.*

mammary duct. See **lactiferous duct.**

mammary gland, one of two discoid, hemispheric glands on the chest of mature females, present in rudimentary form in children and in males. Glandular tissue forms a radius of lobes containing alveoli, each lobe having a system of ducts for the passage of milk from the alveoli to the nipple. The central portion of the breast is filled with glandular tissue; the periphery is made up mostly of adipose tissue. The left breast is usually larger than the right. Also called **breast, mamma.** See also **lactation.**

mammary papilla. See **nipple.**

mammillary body, either of the two small round masses of gray matter in the hypothalamus located close to one another in the interpeduncular space.

mammogram, an x-ray film of the soft tissues of the breast.

mammography, radiography of the soft tissues of the breast to allow identification of various benign and malignant neoplastic processes.

mammoplasty, plastic reshaping of the breasts, performed to reduce or lift enlarged or sagging breasts, to enlarge small breasts, or to reconstruct a breast after removal of a tumor. Antibiotic therapy is started before surgery. General anesthesia is used for all types of mammoplasty. To reduce the size of the breasts and raise them, excess tissue is removed from the underside of the breasts; the breast is then lifted and the nipple brought through an opening in an overhanging skin flap. To enlarge a breast, a thin plastic sac of silicone fluid is inserted in a pouch formed beneath the breast on the chest wall. The complications after surgery are infection and, with the use of implants, rejection reaction of tissues to the foreign body. The nurse observes the nipples for signs of vascular insufficiency or congestion, applies a firm supporting breast binder, and instructs the patient not to use her arms to lift herself. The patient stays prone in semi-Fowler's position, with elbows at her sides. Pain may be severe in the first days after surgery.

mammothermography, a diagnostic procedure in which thermography is used for examining the breast to detect abnormal growths. Compare **mammography.** See also **thermography.**

man-, a combining form meaning 'of or referring to the hand': *manoptoscope, manual, manudynamometer.*

-mancy, -mantia, a combining form meaning 'divination in, through, or by': *hidromancy, labiomancy, uromancy.*

Mandelamine, a trademark for an antibacterial (methenamine mandelate).

mandible /man′dibəl/, a large bone constituting the lower jaw. It contains the lower teeth and consists of a horizontal portion, a body, and two perpendicular rami that join the body at almost right angles. The body of the mandible is curved, somewhat resembling a horseshoe, and has two surfaces and two borders. The external surface is marked by the symphysis menti, indicating the junction of the two halves of the mandible in the fetus. Each ramus is topped by the anterior coronoid process and the posterior condyle, prominences separated by the mandibular notch. The superior border of the mandible contains sockets for the 16 lower teeth. The inferior border provides a groove for the facial artery. The mandible and its rami provide attachment for various muscles, as the masseter, temporalis, pterygoideus lateralis, digastricus, mentalis, genioglossi, geniohyoidei, and mylohyoideus. Also called **inferior maxillary bone.** Compare **maxilla.** –**mandibular,** *adj.*

mandibular canal, (in dentistry) a passage or channel that extends from the mandibular foramen on the medial surface of the ramus of the mandible to the mental foramen. It holds mandibular blood vessels and a portion of the mandibular branch of the trigeminal nerve.

mandibular notch, a depression in the inferior border of the mandible, anterior to the attachments of the masseter muscle, where the external facial muscles cross the lower border of the mandible. It is a landmark that may be accentuated by arrested condylar growth and developmental disturbances of the mandible.

mandibular sling, the connection between the mandible and the maxilla, formed by the masseter and the pterygoideus at the angle of the mandible. When the mouth is opened and closed, the mandible moves around a center of rotation formed by the mandibular sling and the sphenomandibular ligament.

mandibulofacial dysostosis, an abnormal hereditary condition characterized by antimongoloid slant of the palpebral fissures, colomboma of the lower lid, micrognathia and hypoplasia of the zygomatic arches, and microtia. Evidence indicates that this disorder is transmitted as an autosomal dominant trait. The condition occurs in the complete form as Franceschetti's syndrome and in the incomplete form as Treacher Collins' syndrome. See also **dysostosis.**

Mandol, a trademark for a cephalosporin antibiotic (cefamandole nafate).

mandrel, a shaft secured in a handpiece or lathe to support an object to be rotated, as a dental polishing disk or cutting device.

maneuver, **1.** an adroit or skillful manipulation or procedure. **2.** (in obstetrics) a manipulation of the fetus performed to aid in delivery.

manganese (Mn), a common metallic element found in trace amounts in tissues of the body where it aids in the functions of various enzymes. Its atomic number is 25; its atomic weight is 54.938.

mani-, a combining form meaning 'mental aberration': *mania, maniaphobia, manigraphy.*

mania, a mood disorder characterized by an expansive emotional state, extreme excitement, excessive elation, hyperactivity, agitation, overtalkativeness, flight of ideas, increased psychomotor activity, fleeting attention, and sometimes violent, destructive, or self-destructive behavior. It is manifested in the major affective disorders, specifically as the manic phase of bipolar disorder, and in certain organic mental disorders, as delirium and dementia. Kinds of mania include **Bell's mania, dancing mania, epileptic mania, hysteric mania, periodic mania, puerperal mania,** and **religious mania.** –**maniac,** *n., adj.,* **maniacal,** *adj.*

-mania, a combining form meaning a '(specified) state of mental disorder': *desanimania, enosimania, tristimania.*

-maniac, **1.** a combining form meaning a 'person exhibiting a type of psychosis': *kleptomaniac, narcomaniac, toxicomaniac.* **2.** a combining form meaning a 'person revealing an inordinate interest in something': *ergomaniac, nymphomaniac, opiomaniac.*

-manic, **1.** a combining form meaning a '(specified) psychosis': *choromanic, melomanic, poriomanic.* **2.** a combining form meaning a 'mental state like mania': *hyomanic, melomanic, submanic.*

manic depressive, a person with or exhibiting the symptoms of bipolar disorder.

manic-depressive psychosis. See **bipolar disorder.**

manipulation, the skillful use of the hands in therapeutic or diagnostic procedures, as palpation, reducing a dislocation, turning the position of the fetus, or various treatments in physical therapy and osteopathy. A kind of manipulation is **conjoined manipulation.** See also **massage.**

mannitol, a poorly metabolized sugar used as an osmotic diuretic and in kidney function tests.

■ INDICATIONS: It is prescribed to promote diuresis, to decrease intraocular and intracranial pressure, to promote the excretion of poisons and other toxic wastes, and to evaluate renal function.

■ CONTRAINDICATIONS: Pulmonary edema, dehydration, or known hypersensitivity to this drug prohibits its use.

■ ADVERSE EFFECTS: Among the more serious adverse reactions are pulmonary edema, heart failure, hyponatremia, headache, vomiting, and confusion.

manometer /mənom′ətər/, a device for measuring the pressure of a fluid, consisting of a tube marked with a scale and containing a relatively incompressible fluid, as mercury. The level of the fluid in the tube varies with the pressure of the fluid being measured. Kinds of manometer are **aneroid manometer** and **sphygmomanometer.**

Mantadil, a trademark for a topical, fixed-combination drug containing a glucocorticoid (hydrocortisone acetate) and an antihistaminic (chlorcyclizine hydrochloride).

-mantia. See **-mancy.**

Mantoux test /mantōō′/, a tuberculin skin test that consists of intradermal injection of a purified protein derivative of the tubercle bacillus. A hardened, raised red area of 8 to 10 mm, appearing 24 to 72 hours after injection, is a positive reaction. This method is the most reliable means of testing tuberculin sensitivity. See also **tuberculin test.**

manual rotation, an obstetric maneuver in which a baby's head is turned by hand from a transverse to an anteroposterior position in the birth canal to facilitate delivery. Compare **forceps rotation.**

manubriosternal articulation /mənōō′brē•ōstur′nəl/, the fibrocartilaginous connection between manubrium and the body of the sternum. This joint usually closes by the age of 25 years. Compare **xiphisternal articulation.**

manubrium /mənōō′brē•əm/, one of the three bones of the sternum, presenting a broad quadrangular shape that narrows caudally at its articulation with the superior end of the body of the sternum. The pectoralis major and the sternocleidomastoideus are attached to the manubrium. Compare **xiphoid process.** **–manubrial,** *adj.*

manus. See **hand.**

many-tailed bandage, **1.** a broad, evenly shaped bandage with both ends split into strips of equal size and number. As the bandage is placed on the abdomen, chest, or limb, the ends may be overlapped. **2.** an irregularly shaped bandage with torn or cut ends that are tied together. See also **Scultetus bandage.**

MAO, abbreviation for **monoamine oxidase.**

MAO inhibitor, abbreviation for **monoamine oxidase inhibitor.**

Maolate, a trademark for a skeletal muscle relaxant (chlorphenesin carbamate).

MAP, abbreviation for **mean arterial pressure.**

map distance. See **map unit.**

maple bark disease, a hypersensitivity pneumonitis caused by exposure to the mold *Cryptostroma corticale,* found in the bark of maple trees. In the susceptible person, the condition may be acute, accompanied by fever, cough, dyspnea, and vomiting, or it may be chronic, characterized by fatigue, weight loss, dyspnea on exertion, and a productive cough. Although differential diagnosis may be difficult, a good occupational history may reveal the cause and the source of exposure. In an acute or severe case, a short course of prednisone may be used to control the symptoms; avoiding exposure to the bark prevents further reaction.

maple syrup urine disease, an inherited metabolic disorder in which an enzyme necessary for the breakdown of the amino acids valine, leucine, and isoleucine is lacking. The disease is usually diagnosed in infancy, being recognized by the characteristic maple syrup odor of the urine and by hyperreflexia. Stress, fever, infection, and the ingestion of lysine, leucine, or isoleucine aggravate the condition. Treatment includes a diet avoiding these amino acids and, rarely, dialysis or transfusion. Also called **branched chain ketoaciduria.**

mapping, (in genetics) the process of locating the relative position of genes on a chromosome through the analysis of genetic recombination. Distances between genes in a linkage group are expressed in map or morgan units. Also called **chromosome mapping.**

maprotiline hydrochloride, an antidepressant similar to the tricyclics.

▪ INDICATION: It is prescribed for the treatment of mental depression.

▪ CONTRAINDICATIONS: It is used with caution in conditions where anticholinergics are contraindicated, in seizure disorders, and in patients with cardiovascular disorders. Concomitant administration of monoamine oxidase inhibitors, recent myocardial infarction, or known hypersensitivity to this drug prohibits its use.

▪ ADVERSE EFFECTS: Among the more serious adverse reactions are sedation and anticholinergic side effects. A variety of GI, cardiovascular, and neurologic reactions (including convulsions) may occur. The drug, like the tricyclics, is involved in many potential drug interactions.

map unit, (in genetics) an arbitrary unit of measure used to designate the distance between genes on a chromosome. It is calculated from the percentage of recombinations that occur between specific genes so that 1% of crossing over represents one unit on a genetic map or approximately the number of new combinations that can be detected. The measurement is accurate only for small distances, because double crossovers do not appear as new recombinations. Also called **map distance.** See also **morgan.**

marasmic kwashiorkor, a malnutrition disease, primarily of children, resulting from the deficiency of both calories and protein. The condition is characterized by severe tissue wasting, dehydration, loss of subcutaneous fat, lethargy, and growth retardation.

marasmic thrombus, an aggregation of blood platelets, fibrin, clotting factors, and cellular elements formed in infants with marasmus. Marasmic thrombus is often a terminal event in cachexia.

marasmus /məraz′məs/, a condition of extreme malnutrition and emaciation, occurring chiefly in young children, that is characterized by progressive wasting of subcutaneous tissue and muscle. It results from a lack of adequate calories and proteins and is seen in failure to thrive children and in starvation. Less commonly, marasmus occurs as a result of an inability to assimilate or use protein because of a defect in metabolism. Care of the marasmic child involves the reestablishment of fluid and electrolyte balance, followed by the slow and gradual addition of foods as they are tolerated. Stimulation appropriate to the developmental age should be provided. As much of the care of the child as possible should be given consistently by one person, because it must be assumed that the physically starved child has also been emotionally deprived. See also **failure to thrive, kwashiorkor.**

marathon encounter group, an intensive group experience that accelerates self-awareness and promotes personal growth and behavioral change through the continuous interaction of group members for a period ranging from 16 to more than 40 hours. See also **encounter group.**

Marax, a trademark for a respiratory, fixed-combination drug containing a smooth muscle relaxant (theophylline), an adrenergic (ephedrine sulfate), and a tranquilizer (hydroxyzine hydrochloride).

marble bones. See **osteopetrosis.**

Marburg-Ebola virus disease /mär′bərgeb′ələ/, a serious febrile disease characterized by rash and severe GI hemorrhages. An epidemic in Marburg, Germany, in 1967, was apparently contracted from imported African green monkeys. In 1976, in the Ebola River District of Zaire and Sudan, an explosive epidemic occurred with a mortality of 85%. This disease may be transmitted to hospital personnel by improper handling of contaminated needles or from hemorrhagic lesions of patients. The diagnosis is made by serologic abnormalities. There is no effective treatment. Also called **hemorrhagic fever.**

Marcaine Hydrochloride, a trademark for a local anesthetic (bupivacaine hydrochloride).

march foot, an abnormal condition of the foot caused by excessive use, as in a long march. The forefoot is swollen and painful, and one or more of the metatarsal bones may be broken. See also **stress fracture.**

march fracture. See **metatarsal stress fracture.**

march hemoglobinuria, a rare, abnormal condition, characterized by the presence of hemoglobin in the urine, that occurs after strenuous physical exertion or prolonged exercise, as marching or distance running. See also **hemolysis.**

Marchiafava-Micheli disease /mär′kyəfä′vəmikā′lē/, a rare disorder of unknown origin characterized by episodic hemoglobinuria, occurring usually, but not always, at night.

Marchi's method /mär′kēz/, a laboratory staining procedure for demonstrating degenerated nerve fibers. The tissue specimen is first fixed in a solution of potassium bichromate (Mueller's fluid), which prevents normal nerve fibers from being stained with osmic acid; osmic acid is then applied as a definitive black stain for abnormal nerve fibers.

Marcus Gunn pupil sign, paradoxical dilatation of the pupils in an ophthalmologic examination in response to afferent visual stimuli. In a dark room a beam of light is moved from one eye to the other. Normal miosis is caused by the consensual pupil reaction when the normal eye is illuminated; but as the light is moved to the opposite, abnormal eye, the direct reaction to light is weaker than the consensual reaction; hence both pupils dilate.

Marezine Hydrochloride, a trademark for an antiemetic (cyclizine hydrochloride).

Marfan's syndrome /märfäNz′/, an abnormal condition characterized by elongation of the bones, often with associated abnormalities of the eyes and the cardiovascular system. Marfan's syndrome is inherited as an autosomal-dominant trait. The disease causes major pathologic musculoskeletal disturbances, as muscular underdevelopment, ligamentous laxity, joint hypermobility, and bone elongation. With Marfan's syndrome pathologic alterations of the cardiovascular system appear to produce fragmentation of the elastic fibers in the media of the aorta, which may lead to aneurysm. Ocular changes associated with the disease include a variety of disorders, including dislocation of the lens. Cardiac and ocular involvement occurs in approximately one half of the patients affected. The disease affects men and women equally, elongating the limbs so that most adult patients with the disease are over 6 feet tall. The extremities of individuals with Marfan's syndrome are very long and spiderlike, with greatly extended metacarpals, metatarsals, and phalanges. The skulls of such patients are usually asymmetric. Pectus excavatum is common, and a lateral curvature of the spine may develop and increase during years of rapid vertebral growth with kyphoscoliosis developing to varying degrees. The severe ligamental laxity and the joint hypermobility associated with Marfan's syndrome may be seen by radiographic examination and often results in pes valgus and genu recurvatum. No specific treatment is advocated for Marfan's syndrome, and symptomatic management of the associated problems is the usual alternative. Resulting deformities, as kyphoscoliosis, may be treated with orthoses or other surgical procedures, as indicated.

marginal peptic ulcer, an ulcer that develops postoperatively at the surgical anastomosis of the stomach and jejunum. See also **peptic ulcer.**

marginal placenta previa, placenta previa in which the placenta is implanted in the lower uterine segment, with its margin touching or spreading to some degree over the internal os of the uterine cervix. During labor, as the cervix dilates, bleeding may occur from the separation of the edge of the placenta from the uterus beneath it. Bleeding may be so scant as to pose no clinical problem. In some cases frank severe hemorrhage may occur, but the pressure of the presenting part of the baby is often sufficient to act as a tamponade, arresting the hemorrhage. Diagnosis of marginal placenta previa may be suggested by the apparent location of the placenta on ultrasonic visualization. Cesarean section is not usually necessary. See also **placenta previa.**

marginal rale. See **atelectatic rale.**

marginal ridge, an elevation of enamel that forms the proximal boundary of the occlusal surface of a tooth.

Marie's hypertrophy, chronic enlargement of the joints caused by periostitis. Also called **hypertrophic pulmonary osteopathy.**

Marie-Strümpell disease. See **ankylosing spondylitis.**

marijuana. See **cannabis.**

mark, any nevus or birthmark.

marker gene. See **genetic marker.**

markers, body language movements that serve as indicators and punctuation marks in interpersonal communication.

Marplan, a trademark for an antidepressant (isocarboxazid).

marrow. See **bone marrow.**

Marseilles fever, a disease endemic around the Mediterranean, in Africa, in the Crimea, and in India, caused by *Rickettsia conorii* transmitted by the brown dog tick (*Rhipicephalus sanguineus*). Characteristic symptoms are chills, fever, an ulcer covered with a black crust at the site of the tick bite, and a rash appearing on the second to fourth day. Also called **boutonneuse fever, Bruch's disease, Conor's disease, escharonodulaire, Indian tick fever, Kenya fever.**

Marshall-Marchetti operation, a surgical procedure performed to correct a condition of stress incontinence. The procedure, a vesicourethropexy, involves a retropubic incision and suturing of the urethra, vesicle neck, and bladder to the posterior surface of the pubic bone. Also called **Marshall-Marchetti-Krantz operation.**

marsupialize, to form a pouch surgically to treat a cyst when simple removal would not be effective, as in a pancreatic or a pilonidal cyst. Under general or local anesthesia, the cyst sac is opened and emptied. Its edges are sutured to adjacent tissues, and a drain is left in place. Secretions decrease over a period of several months and may eventually cease.

Martorell's syndrome. See **Takayasu's arteritis.**

masculine, having the characteristics of a male.

masculinization, the normal development or induction of male sex characteristics. See also **virilization.** – **masculinize,** *v.*

mask, **1.** to obscure, as in symptomatic treatment that may mask the development of a disease. **2.** to cover, as does a skin-toned cosmetic that may mask a pigmented nevus. **3.** a cover worn over the nose and mouth to prevent inhalation of toxic or irritating materials, to control delivery of oxygen or anesthetic gas, or (by medical personnel) to shield a patient during aseptic procedures from pathogenic organisms normally exhaled from the respiratory tract.

masking, **1.** the covering or concealing of a disorder by a second condition, as when a person begins a weight-loss diet while an undiagnosed wasting disease such as cancer has developed. The loss of body weight is attributed to the diet, masking the disease and delaying diagnosis and treatment. **2.** the unconscious display of a personality trait that conceals a behavioral aberration.

masking agent, a cosmetic preparation for covering nevi, surgical scars, and other blemishes. Masking agents are generally composed of a flesh-colored pigment in a lotion or cream base.

mask of pregnancy. See **chloasma.**

Maslow's hierarchy of need, (in psychology) a hierarchic categorization of the basic needs of humans. The most basic needs on the scale are the physiologic or biologic, as the need for air, food, or water. Of second priority are the safety needs, including protection and freedom from fear and anxiety. The subsequent order of needs in the hierarchic progression are the need to belong, to love, and to be loved; the need for self-esteem; and ultimately, the need for self-actualization. To progress from one need to another, the more basic need must first be satisfied.

masochism /mas′ōkiz′əm/, pleasure or gratification derived from receiving physical, mental, or emotional abuse. The maltreatment may be inflicted by another person or by oneself. Also called **passive algolagnia.** Compare **sadism.** See also **algolagnia, sadomasochism.** – **masochistic,** *adj.*

masochist, a person deriving pleasure or gratification from masochistic acts or abuse. See also **masochism.**

mass, **1.** the physical property of matter that gives it weight and inertia. **2.** (in pharmacology) a mixture from which pills are formed. **3.** an aggregate of cells clumped together as a tumor. Compare **weight.** See also **inertia.**

massage, the manipulation of the soft tissue of the body through stroking, rubbing, kneading, or tapping, to increase circulation, to improve muscle tone, and to relax the patient. The procedure is performed either with the bare hands or through some mechanical means, as a vibrator. The most common sites for massage are the back, knees, elbows, and heels. Care is taken not to massage inflamed areas, particularly of the extremities, because of the danger of loosening blood clots; open wounds and areas of rash, tumor, or excessive sensitivity are avoided. The procedure is performed with the patient prone or on the side, comfortably positioned, with an emollient lotion or cream applied to the area to be massaged. The nurse's hands are warm, and excessive pressure is avoided so as not to cause pain or injury. Kinds of massage are **cardiac massage, effleurage, flagellation, friction, frôlement, pétrissage, tapotement,** and **vibration.**

-massage, a combining form meaning a 'therapeutic kneading of the body': *electromassage, hydromassage, phonomassage.*

masseter /masē′tər/, the thick, rectangular muscle in the cheek that functions to close the jaw. It is one of the four muscles of mastication and consists of a superficial portion and a deep portion, each arising from the zygomatic arch and inserting into the mandible. The deep portion is the smaller and more muscular of the two parts. The masseter is innervated by the masseteric nerve from the mandibular division of the trigeminal nerve.

mass fragment, a degraded portion of a molecule containing one or more charges.

mass number (A), the sum of the number of protons and neutrons in the nucleus of an atom or isotope. See also **atomic number, atomic weight.**

mass reflex, an abnormal condition, seen in patients with transection of the spinal cord, characterized by a widespread nerve discharge, resulting in flexor muscle spasms, incontinence of urine and feces, priapism, hypertension, and profuse sweating.

■ OBSERVATIONS: A mass reflex may be triggered by scratching or other painful stimulus to the skin, overdistention of the bladder or intestines, cold weather, prolonged sitting, or emotional stress. Muscle spasms may be so violent as to throw the patient off a bed or stretcher.

▪ INTERVENTION: Medications to reduce mass reflexes include diazepam, dantraline, chlordiazepoxide, and meprobamate. Hubbard baths and exercises in warm water also help. Occasionally chordotomy, rhizotomy, peripheral nerve transaction, or tenotomy may be necessary.

▪ NURSING CONSIDERATIONS: Nurses should avoid stimulating areas that trigger mass reflexes and should be prepared to accept them when they occur and to explain the cause to the patient. It is important to prevent decubitus ulcers and bladder infections in paraplegic and quadriplegic patients because they may also serve as triggers to initiate mass reflexes. Siderails should be kept up on the bed and restraining straps secured to transportation stretchers and Stryker frames. Psychotherapeutic counseling may also help reduce stress and the frequency of mass reflexes.

mass spectrometer, an analytic instrument for identifying a substance by sorting a stream of charged particles (ions) according to their mass. The sorting is usually accomplished by deflecting a stream of charged particles into a semicircular path as it enters a magnetic field and ultimately strikes a photographic plate or a photomultiplier tube sensor.

mass spectrometry, (in chemistry) a technique for the analysis of a substance in which the constituents are identified and quantified using a mass spectrometer. See also **spectrometry, spectrophotometry.**

mass storage device, a secondary memory device capable of storing large amounts of data.

mass transfer, the movement of mass from one phase to another.

mast-. See **masto.**

mastalgia /mastal′jə/, pain in the breast caused by congestion or ''caking'' during lactation, an infection, fibrocystic disease, especially during or before menstruation, or advanced cancer. The early stages of breast cancer are rarely accompanied by pain. **–mastalgic,** *adj.*

mast cell, a constituent of connective tissue containing large basophilic granules that bear heparin, serotonin, bradykinin, and histamine. These substances are freed from the mast cell in response to injury and infection.

mast cell leukemia, a malignant neoplasm of leukocytes characterized by many connective tissue mast cells in circulating blood.

mastectomy /mastek′təmē/, the surgical removal of one or both breasts, performed to remove a malignant tumor. In a simple mastectomy, only breast tissue is removed. In a radical mastectomy, some of the muscles of the chest are removed with the breast with all lymph nodes in the axilla. In a modified radical mastectomy, the large muscles of the chest that move the arm are preserved. Under general anesthesia, a biopsy of tissue taken from the tumor is performed if this was not previously done. If the specimen shows a malignancy, the tumor and adjacent tissues are removed in one piece. After surgery, a drainage catheter is placed in the wound. The nurse inspects the wound for swelling or excessive bleeding and encourages the patient to take deep breaths and to cough at frequent intervals. The affected arm is positioned with the hand pointed upwards or on pillows so that the hand is higher than the lower arm, with the lower arm above heart level. Hand and wrist movements and flexion and extension of the elbow are begun within 24 hours and performed regularly. No abduction or external rotation of the upper arm is permitted before the tenth day. An elastic bandage and, later, a pressure gradient elastic sleeve are used to reduce edema of the arm. The patient is fitted with a prosthesis when the wound is completely healed. Emotional support and counseling are essential. See also **breast cancer, modified radical mastectomy, radical mastectomy, simple mastectomy. –mastectomize,** *v.* (Figure, page 686)

master problem list, a list of a patient's problems that serves as an index to the patient's record. Each problem, the date the problem was first noted, the treatment, and the outcome are added to the master problem list as each becomes known. Thus, the master problem list provides an ongoing guide for reviewing the health status of the patient and for planning care for the patient.

master's degree program in nursing, a postgraduate program in a school of nursing, based in a university setting, that grants the degree Master of Science in Nursing to successful candidates. Most programs include theory of nursing and techniques in nursing research as integral parts of the curriculum. The degree may be awarded for work in maternal-newborn nursing, medical-surgical nursing, pediatric nursing, psychiatric nursing, or in other fields of nursing. Nurses with this degree often work in leadership roles in clinical nursing, as consultants in various settings, in faculty positions in schools of nursing, and as nurse practitioners in the various specialties.

mastery, being in command or control of a situation, as in learning accomplishment.

-mastia. See **-mazia.**

mastication, chewing, tearing, or grinding food with the teeth while it becomes mixed with saliva. See also **bolus, digestion, ptyalin.**

masticatory system, the combination of organs, structures, and nerves involved in chewing. It includes but is not limited to the jaws, the teeth and their supporting structures, the mandibular musculature, the mandible, the maxillae, the temperomandibular joints, the tongue, the lips, the cheeks, the oral mucosa, and cranial nerves. Also called masticatory apparatus. Compare **stomatognathic system.**

mastitis /mastī′tis/, an inflammatory condition of the breast, usually caused by streptococcal or staphylococcal infection. **Acute mastitis,** most common in the first 2 months of lactation, is characterized by pain, swelling, redness, axillary lymphadenopathy, fever, and malaise. If untreated or inadequately treated, abscesses may form. Antibiotics, rest, analgesia, and warm soaks are usually prescribed. Usually, breast feeding may continue,

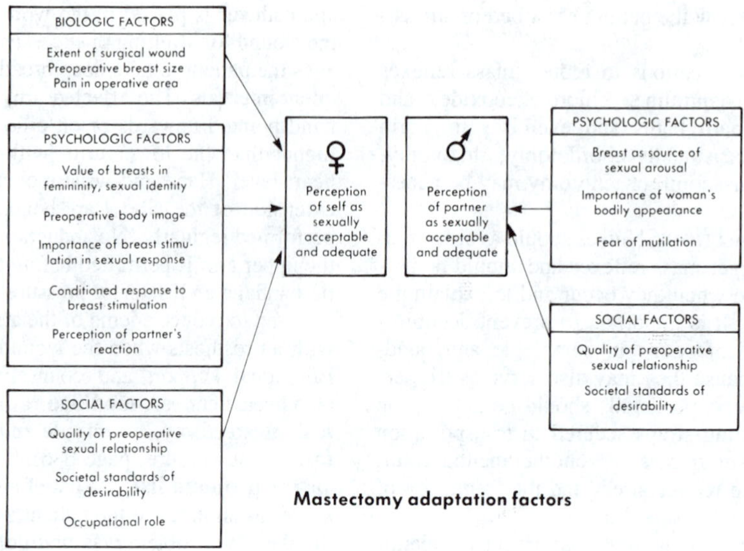

Mastectomy adaptation factors

Chronic tuberculous mastitis is rare; when it occurs, it represents extension of tuberculosis from the lungs and ribs beneath the breast.

masto-, mast-, a combining form meaning 'of or pertaining to the breast': *mastochondroma, mastologist, mastoplasia.*

mastocytosis, local or systemic overproduction of mast cells, which, in rare instances, may infiltrate liver, spleen, bones, the GI system, and skin. Systemic mastocytosis may precede mast cell leukemia.

mastoid /mas′toid/, **1.** of or pertaining to the mastoid process of the temporal bone. **2.** breast-shaped.

mastoidectomy, surgical excision of a portion of the mastoid part of the temporal bone, performed to treat chronic suppurative otitis media or mastoiditis when systemic antibiotics are ineffective. Entry is made through the ear canal or from behind the ear. In a simple mastoidectomy, under general anesthesia, infected bone cells are removed and the eardrum is incised to drain the middle ear. Topical antibiotics are then instilled in the ear. In a radical procedure, the eardrum and most middle ear structures are removed; the stapes is left intact so that a hearing aid may be used. The opening to the eustachian tube is plugged. In a modified radical procedure, the eardrum and the middle ear structures are saved, and the patient will hear better than after a radical mastoidectomy. After surgery any bright red blood on the dressing may indicate hemorrhage. A stiff neck or disorientation may signal the onset of meningitis. Dizziness is usual and may be expected to last for several days.

mastoiditis /mas′toidī′tis/, an infection of one of the mastoid bones, usually an extension of a middle ear infection, characterized by earache, fever, headache, and malaise. The infection is difficult to treat, often requiring antibiotics administered intravenously for several days. Children are most often affected. Residual hearing loss may follow the infection.

mastoid process, the conic projection of the caudal, posterior portion of the temporal bone, serving as the attachment for various muscles, including the sternocleidomastoideus, splenius capitis, and longissimus capitis. A hollow section of the process contains air cells that are distinguished from a large, irregular tympanic antrum in the superior anterior portion of the process. See also **temporal bone.**

masturbation, sexual activity in which the penis or clitoris is stimulated, usually to orgasm, by means other than coitus. It is performed, at least occasionally, by most people and is considered to be normal and harmless. Also called, in men, **onanism.** –**masturbate,** *v,* **masturbatic, masturbatory,** *adj.*

-masty. See **-mazia.**

matched group. See **group.**

materia /mətir′ē·ə/, matter or material, as materia medica.

material fact, (in law) a fact that establishes or refutes an element essential to the complaint, or charge, or to the defense. The presence of a material fact in a case being tried precludes granting of a summary judgment.

materia medica, **1.** the study of drugs and other substances used in medicine, their origins, preparation, uses, and effects. **2.** a substance or a drug used in medical treatment.

Materna 1.60, a trademark for an antenatal multivitamin supplement with calcium and iron.

maternal and child health (MCH) services, various facilities and programs organized for the purpose of providing medical and social services for mothers and children. Medical services include prenatal, postnatal, family planning care, and pediatric care in infancy.

maternal-child attachment. See **maternal-infant bonding.**

maternal-child separation syndrome. See **separation anxiety.**

maternal deprivation syndrome, a condition characterized by developmental retardation that occurs as a result of physical or emotional deprivation. It is seen primarily in infants. Typical symptoms include lack of physical growth, with weight below the third percentile for age and size, malnutrition, pronounced withdrawal, silence, apathy, and irritability, and a characteristic posture and body language, featuring unnatural stiffness and rigidity with a slow response reaction to others. Causes of the syndrome are usually multiple and complex, involving such factors as parental indifference, emotional instability or insecurity of the mother, lack of or delayed development of the mother-child attachment process, unrealistic expectations or disappointment concerning the sex, appearance, or adaptability of the child, or unfavorable socioeconomic conditions within the family. Treatment often requires hospitalization, especially in cases of severe malnutrition. Care includes assessment of the family situation, and treatment often involves psychotherapy, counseling, or special nursing instruction to help the parents learn to deal with and provide for the child. The nature and extent of the effects of the condition on later physical, emotional, intellectual, and social development vary considerably and depend on the age at which deprivation occurs, the degree and duration of the situation, the constitutional makeup of the child, and the substituted care that is provided. Emotionally deprived children often remain below normal in intellectual development, fail to learn acceptable social behavior, and are unable to form trusting, meaningful relationships with others. In severe cases of early and prolonged deprivation, the damage to an infant may be irreversible. See also **failure to thrive.**

maternal effect. See **maternal inheritance.**

maternal-infant bonding, the complex process of attachment of a mother to her newborn baby. Disastrous effects of the disruption or absence of this attachment have long been known. The specific steps in its development and the factors that disturb or encourage it have been identified and described by anthropologists, pediatricians, psychologists, nurses, midwives, and sociologists. The process begins before birth as the parents plan for the pregnancy and then discover that the mother is pregnant. The mother feels fetal movement, begins to accept the fetus as an individual, and makes plans for the baby after birth. In the first minutes and hours after birth, a sensitive period occurs during which the baby and the mother become intimately involved with each other through behaviors and stimuli that are complementary and that provoke further interactions. The mother touches the baby and holds it en face to achieve eye-to-eye contact. The infant looks back eye to eye. The mother speaks in a quiet, high-pitched voice. The mother and the baby move in turn to the voice and sounds of the other, a process known as entrainment; it can be likened to a dance. The infant's movements constitute a response to the mother's voice, and she is encouraged to continue the process. The secretion of oxytocin and prolactin by the maternal pituitary gland is stimulated by the baby's sucking or licking of the mother's breasts; T and B lymphocytes and macrophages are given to the baby in the mother's milk, promoting resistance to infection. The child is also colonized by the normal flora of the mother's skin and nasal passages, improving the baby's ability to fend off infection. Physically, the mother provides her body heat for the baby's warmth and comfort. Thus, the extended contact in the newborn period satisfies physical and emotional needs of the mother and baby. Experts have made the following recommendations to enhance the development of maternal-infant bonding: The special needs of the mother are assessed before delivery, the parents are given classes to prepare them for labor, delivery, and the puerperium, and discussions are held regarding the stresses of pregnancy and the postpartum period. In labor and delivery, a companion is encouraged to stay with the mother. After the baby is born, silver nitrate drops are not placed in the baby's eyes until the mother and the baby have had time to be together en face, with eye contact for an extended period of time, because the drops cause a film to form over the eyes, dimming vision. During the first hour after birth the parents and the infant are not separated and are given as much privacy as possible. Skin-to-skin contact is encouraged; various methods may be used to maintain an ambient temperature adequate to maintain the baby's temperature. On the postpartum unit the mother and the baby are kept together for at least 5 hours a day, but optimally for 24 hours a day in a 24-hour rooming-in unit. The entire family is allowed to visit. The mother has responsibility for the care of her baby, with consultation available from a midwife or a nurse. The staff does not criticize the mother's performance, because it is to the baby's inestimable benefit that the mother believes her baby is the best, most beautiful, perfect baby in the world and that she feels able to care for her baby. Many changes in facilities, in staff training, and in hospital policy are needed to give every mother and infant the chance to bond fully in the early days of their life together.

maternal inheritance, the transmission of traits or conditions controlled by cytoplasmic factors within the ovum that are not self-replicating and are determined by genes within the nucleus. An example of such a characteristic is the direction of coiling in the shells of snails. Also called **maternal effect.**

maternity cycle, the antepartal, intrapartal, and postpartal periods of pregnancy and the puerperium, from conception to 6 weeks after birth.

maternity nursing, nursing care of women and their families during pregnancy, during parturition, and through the first days of the puerperium. Increasingly, postpartum maternity nursing includes the supervision of the mothers' care of their newborns in rooming-in units and may include care of normal newborns in the nursery when they are not with their mothers. Maternity nursing requires extensive instruction of the mothers in the usual behavior and needs of a newborn, expected patterns of growth and development of the infant during the first week, and in details of care needed by the mother during the first weeks after birth. Breast-feeding, bottle-feeding, baby baths, perineal care, nutrition, and danger signs of the puerperium are usually taught by the maternity nurse. Observation for abnormal conditions, as thrombophlebitis, mastitis and other infections, and preeclampsia are daily ongoing concerns of the maternity nurse on the postpartum unit. Intrapartum maternity nursing involves the care of mothers in labor and delivery, as well as high-risk technical nursing, emotional support in labor and delivery, and the customary ongoing observation for abnormal signs or symptoms. Often, pregnant women with medical problems associated with pregnancy are cared for on a special high-risk antepartum unit by specially trained maternity nurses.

mat gold, a noncohesive form of pure gold, which is prepared by electrodeposition and may be used in the base of some dental restorations, then veneered or overlaid with cohesive foil. Also called **crystal gold, sponge gold.**

matrifocal family /mat′rifō′kəl/, a family unit comprised of a mother and her children. Biologic fathers have a temporary place in the family during the first years of the children's lives, but they maintain a more permanent position in their own original families. Common characteristics of this kind of family include living at a subsistence level, because of irregular employment of the fathers and unreliable economic support from them, and child care by older female relatives so that the mother of the children is free to work.

matrix, 1. an intercellular substance, **2.** also called **ground substance.** a basic substance from which a specific organ or kind of tissue develops. **3.** a form used in shaping a tooth surface in dental procedures.

matrix retainer, a mechanic device used to secure the ends of a matrix around a tooth and help compact a restoration in a tooth cavity. Also called **matrix holder.** See also **retainer.**

matter, 1. anything that has mass and occupies space. **2.** any substance not otherwise identified as to its constituents, as gray matter, pus, or serum exuding from a wound.

Matulane, a trademark for an antineoplastic (procarbazine hydrochloride).

maturation, 1. the process or condition of attaining complete development. In humans it is the unfolding of full physical, emotional, and intellectual capacities that enable a person to function at a higher level of competency and adaptability within the environment. **2.** the final stages in the meiotic formation of germ cells in which the number of chromosomes in each cell is reduced to the haploid number characteristic of the species. See also **meiosis, oogenesis, spermatogenesis. 3.** suppuration. **–maturate,** *v.*

mature, 1. to become fully developed; to ripen. **2.** fully developed or ripened.

mature cell leukemia. See **polymorphocytic leukemia.**

maturity, 1. a state of complete growth or development, usually designated as the period of life between adolescence and old age. **2.** the stage at which an organism is capable of reproduction.

maturity-onset diabetes. See **non-insulin-dependent diabetes mellitus**

Maxibolin, a trademark for an anabolic (ethylestrenol).

Maxidex, a trademark for a glucocorticoid (dexamethasone).

maxilla /maksil′ə/, *pl.* **maxillae,** one of a pair of large bones that form the upper jaw, consisting of a pyramidal body and four processes: the zygomatic, frontal, alveolar, and palatine.

-maxilla, a combining form meaning the 'upper jaw or the bones composing it': *intermaxilla, submaxilla, supermaxilla.*

maxillary artery, either of two larger terminal branches of the external carotid arteries that rise from the neck of the mandible near the parotid gland and divide into three branches, supplying the deep structures of the face.

maxillary fossa. See **canine fossa.**

maxillary sinus, one of the pair of large air cells forming a pyramidal cavity in the body of the maxilla. The apex of each sinus extends into the zygomatic arch, and its floor, formed by the alveolar process, is usually 1 to 10 mm below the floor of the nose. In the adult the volume of the sinus averages 14.75 cc. The mucous membrane of the sinus is continuous with that of the nasal cavity; an opening in the medial wall of the sinus communicates with the middle meatus. In the fourth month of gestation the embryonic sinus appears as a shallow groove on the medial surface of the bone but does not reach full size until after the second teething. Compare **ethmoidal air cell, frontal sinus, sphenoidal sinus.**

maxillary vein, one of a pair of deep veins of the face, accompanying the maxillary artery and passing between the condyle of the mandible and the sphenomandibular ligament. Each maxillary vein is formed by the confluence of veins in the pterygoid plexus and joins the superficial temporal vein to form the retromandibular vein. Each maxillary vein is a tributary of the internal jugular and the external jugular veins.

maxillofacial prosthesis, a prosthetic replacement for part, or all, of the upper jaw, nose, or cheek. It is applied when surgical repair alone is inadequate.

maxillomandibular fixation /maksil′ōmandib′yo͞olər/, stabilization of fractures of the face or jaw by temporarily connecting the maxilla and mandible by wires, elastic bands, or metal splints. See also **elastic band fixation, nasomandibular fixation.**

maximal breathing capacity (MBC), the amount of gas exchanged per minute with maximal rate and depth of respiration.

maximal diastolic membrane potential, (in cardiology) the greatest degree of negative transmembrane potential achieved by a cell during diastole.

maximal expiratory flow rate (MEFR), the rate of the most rapid flow of gas from the lungs during the expiratory phase of respiration.

maximum diastolic potential. See **maximal diastolic membrane potential.**

maximum inspiratory pressure (MIP), the maximum pressure within the alveoli of the lungs that occurs during the inspiratory phase of respiration.

maximum oxygen uptake, the greatest amount of oxygen that can be transported from the lungs to the working muscle tissue. Also called **aerobic capacity.**

maximum permissible dose equivalent, (in radiotherapy) the greatest amount of radiation that a person or a specific body part is allowed to receive in a given period of time.

Maxitrol, a trademark for an ophthalmic, fixed-combination drug containing a glucocorticoid (dexamethasone) and antibacterials (neomycin sulfate and polymyxin B sulfate).

Mayer's reflex /mā′ərz/, a normal reflex elicited by grasping the ring finger and flexing it at the metacarpophalangeal joint of a person whose hand is relaxed with thumb abducted. The normal response is adduction and apposition of the thumb. The reflex is absent in disease of the pyramidal system.

May-Hegglin anomaly, an inherited hematologic condition characterized by leukopenia, giant platelets, and Döhle bodies. The condition is usually benign but may be associated with a decreased ability of the blood to coagulate. Compare **Pelger-Huët anomaly.**

Mayo scissors. See **scissors.**

-mazia, -mastia, -masty, a combining form meaning '(condition of the) breasts': *macromazia, pleomazia, polymazia.*

mazindol /mā′zindōl/, an anorectic.

▪ INDICATION: It is prescribed to decrease the appetite in the treatment of exogenous obesity.

▪ CONTRAINDICATIONS: Glaucoma, history of drug abuse, concomitant use of a monoamine oxidase inhibitor, or known hypersensitivity to this drug prohibits its use.

▪ ADVERSE EFFECTS: Among the more serious adverse reactions are insomnia, palpitation, dizziness, dry mouth, tachycardia, and hypersensitivity reactions.

mazo-, a combining form meaning 'of or pertaining to the breast': *mazodynia, mazology, mazopexy.*

MBC, abbreviation for **maximal breathing capacity.**

MBD, abbreviation for **minimal brain dysfunction.** See **attention deficit disorder.**

mc, abbreviation for **millicurie.**

mC, abbreviation for **millicoulomb.**

McArdle's disease /məkär′dəlz/, an inherited metabolic disease marked by an absence of myophosphorylase B and abnormally large amounts of glycogen in skeletal muscle. It is milder than other glycogen storage diseases, characterized only by muscle weakness and cramping after exercise. There is no known treatment. Also called **glycogen storage disease, type V.** See also **glycogen storage disease.**

MCAT, abbreviation for **Medical College Aptitude Test.**

McBurney's point, a site of extreme sensitivity in acute appendicitis, situated in the normal area of the appendix about 2 inches from the right anterior superior spine of the ilium, on a line between that spine and the umbilicus. See also **appendicitis.**

McBurney's sign, a reaction of the patient indicating severe pain and extreme tenderness when McBurney's point is palpated. Such a reaction indicates appendicitis.

McCall's festoon, (in dentistry) any one of the enlargements of the gingival margins that may be associated with occlusal trauma.

mcg, abbreviation for **microgram.**

MCH, 1. abbreviation for **maternal and child health.** 2. abbreviation for **mean corpuscular hemoglobin.**

MCHC, abbreviation for **mean corpuscular hemoglobin concentration.**

mCi, abbreviation for **millicurie.**

McManus, R. Louise (1885–), an American nurse and writer who established the first national testing service for the nursing profession, currently the second largest educational testing program in the nation. She was also instrumental in developing a means of evaluating the nursing programs of community and junior colleges, and she established a center for training in research in nursing at Teachers College, Columbia University.

McMurray's sign, an audible click heard when rotating the tibia on the femur, indicating injury to meniscal structures.

McShirley's electromallet. See **electromallet condenser.**

MCTD, abbreviation for **mixed connective tissue disease.**

MCV, abbreviation for **mean corpuscular volume.**

Md, symbol for **mendelevium.**

M.D., abbreviation for *Doctor of Medicine.* See **physician.**

Me, abbreviation for the methyl radical CH_3-.

Meals on Wheels, a program designed to deliver hot meals to elderly, physically disabled, or other persons who lack the resources to provide themselves with nutritionally adequate warm meals on a daily basis.

mean, occupying a position midway between two extremes of a set of values or data. The **arithmetic mean** is a value that is derived by dividing the total of a set of values by the number of items in the set. The **geometric**

mean is a value that is between the first and last of a set of values organized in a geometric progression.

mean arterial pressure (MAP), the arithmetic mean of the blood pressure in the arterial portion of the circulation.

mean corpuscular hemoglobin (MCH), an estimate of the amount of hemoglobin in an average erythrocyte, derived from the ratio between the amount of hemoglobin and the number of erythrocytes present in a specimen. The normal MCH is between 28 and 32 picograms of hemoglobin per red blood cell. See also **hypochromic anemia, iron deficiency anemia.**

mean corpuscular hemoglobin concentration (MCHC), an estimation of the concentration of hemoglobin in grams per 100 ml of packed red blood cells, derived from the ratio of the hemoglobin to the hematocrit. The normal MCHC is between 32% and 36%.

mean corpuscular volume (MCV), an evaluation of the average volume of each red cell, derived from the ratio of the volume of packed red cells (the hematocrit) to the total number of red blood cells. The normal MCV is between 82 and 92 μm^3.

measles, an acute, highly contagious, viral disease involving the respiratory tract and characterized by a spreading maculopapular cutaneous rash that occurs primarily in young children who have not been immunized. Measles is caused by a paramyxovirus and is transmitted by direct contact with droplets spread from the nose, throat, and mouth of infected persons, usually in the prodromal stage of the disease. Indirect transmission by uninfected persons or by contaminated articles is unusual. Diagnosis is confirmed by the identification of Koplik's spots on the buccal mucosa and by bacteriologic culture or serologic examination. Also called **morbilli, rubeola.** See also **roseola infantum, rubella.**

■ OBSERVATIONS: An incubation period of 7 to 14 days is followed by the prodromal stage, characterized by fever, malaise, coryza, cough, conjunctivitis, photophobia, anorexia, and the pathognomonic Koplik's spots, which appear 1 to 2 days before onset of the rash. Pharyngitis and inflammation of the laryngeal and tracheobronchial mucosa develop, the temperature may rise to 103° or 104° F and there is marked granulocytic leukopenia. The papules of the rash first appear as irregular brownish-pink spots around the hairline, the ears, and the neck, then spread rapidly, within 24 to 48 hours, to the trunk and extremities, becoming red, maculopapular, and dense, giving a blotchy appearance. Within 3 to 5 days, the fever subsides, and the lesions flatten, turn a brownish color, and begin to fade, causing a fine desquamation, especially over heavily affected areas.

■ INTERVENTION: Routine treatment consists of bed rest, antipyretics, antibiotics to control secondary bacterial infection, and, when necessary, application of calamine lotion, corn starch solution, or cool water to relieve itching. Preventive measures include active immunization with measles virus vaccine after the infant is 1 year old. Passive immunization with immune serum globulin is recommended for unvaccinated individuals exposed to the disease. One attack of the disease confers lifelong immunity.

■ NURSING CONSIDERATIONS: Bed rest, isolation, and quiet activity are recommended as long as fever and rash persist. Aspirin, fluids, cool sponge baths, nose drops, and cough medication may be necessary to counteract fever and respiratory symptoms. Bright sunlight may be irritating to the eyes. Special attention is given to the care and cleansing of the eyes and skin, especially in cases of severe papular eruption. An important nursing function is instruction of the parents in the proper home care of the child, because most cases are not serious enough to require hospitalization. The disease is usually benign, and mortality is rare. Complications sometimes occur, the most common of which are otitis media, pneumonia, bronchiolitis, obstructive laryngitis, laryngotracheitis, and, occasionally, encephalitis and appendicitis. Rarely, but most gravely, the virus causes subacute sclerosing panencephalitis several years after the acute attack of measles has occurred.

measles and rubella virus vaccine live, an active immunizing agent.

■ INDICATIONS: It is prescribed for immunization against measles and rubella.

■ CONTRAINDICATIONS: Immunosuppression, concomitant administration of corticosteroids, tuberculosis, known or suspected pregnancy, hypersensitivity to neomycin, neoplasms of the lymphatic system or bone marrow, or active infection prohibits its use. It should not be given for 3 months after the use of whole blood, plasma, or immune serum globulin, or for 1 month before or after immunization with other live virus vaccines, except mumps vaccine.

■ ADVERSE EFFECT: The most serious adverse reaction is anaphylaxis.

measles immune globulin. See **immune globulin.**

measles, mumps, and rubella virus vaccine live (MMR), an active immunizing agent.

■ INDICATION: It is prescribed for simultaneous immunization against measles, mumps, and rubella.

■ CONTRAINDICATIONS: Immunosuppression, concomitant administration of corticosteroids, tuberculosis, hypersensitivity to neomycin, neoplasms of the lymphatic system or bone marrow, known or suspected pregnancy, or acute infection prohibits its use. It is not given for 3 months after the use of whole blood, plasma, or immune serum globulin, and it is not given for 1 month before or after immunization with other live virus vaccines.

■ ADVERSE EFFECTS: The most serious adverse reaction is anaphylaxis.

measurement, the determination, expressed numerically, of the extent or quantity of a substance, energy, or time. See also **international unit, metric system.**

meatorrhaphy /mē′ətôr′əfē/, the suturing of the cut end of the urethra to the glans penis after surgery to enlarge the urethral meatus.

meatoscopy /mē′ətos′kəpē/, the visual examination of any meatus, especially the urethra, usually performed with the aid of a speculum.

meatus /mē·ā′təs/, *pl.* **meatuses, meatus,** an opening or tunnel through any part of the body, as the external acoustic meatus that leads from the external ear to the tympanic membrane.

Mebaral, a trademark for an anticonvulsant and sedative (mephobarbital).

mebendazole, an anthelmintic.
▪ INDICATIONS: It is prescribed in the treatment of pinworm, whipworm, roundworm, and hookworm infestations.
▪ CONTRAINDICATIONS: Pregnancy or known hypersensitivity to this drug prohibits its use.
▪ ADVERSE EFFECTS: Among the most serious adverse reactions are abdominal pain and diarrhea.

MEC, abbreviation for *minimum effective concentration,* or the minimum inhibitory concentration for a drug to be active. The drug is effective at any level above this threshold value.

mecamylamine hydrochloride, a ganglionic blocking agent.
▪ INDICATION: It is prescribed in the management of hypertensive cardiac disease.
▪ CONTRAINDICATIONS: Coronary or cerebrovascular insufficiency, recent myocardial infarction, uremia, pyelonephritis, glaucoma, or known hypersensitivity to this drug prohibits its use.
▪ ADVERSE EFFECTS: Among the most serious adverse reactions are orthostatic hypotension, paralytic ileus, urinary retention, and cycloplegia. The incidence of side effects is very high because the drug reduces all autonomic activity.

mechanic advantage, (in physiology) the ratio of the output force developed by the muscles to the input force applied to the body structures that the muscles move, especially the ratio of these forces associated with the body structures that act as levers. Variations in the sizes of muscles and the lengths of bones in different individuals partially account for the different mechanic advantages from one body type to another and their different physical capabilities, as speed and strength.

mechanic condenser, a device that delivers automatically controlled impacts for condensing restorative material in the filling of tooth cavities. It may be spring activated, pneumatic, or electrically controlled. Also called **automatic mallet condenser.**

mechanic vector. See **vector.**

mechanism of labor. See **cardinal movements of labor.**

mechano-, a combining form meaning 'mechanic': *mechanocyte, mechanotherapy, mechanothermy.*

mechanoreceptor, any sensory nerve ending that responds to mechanic stimuli, as touch, pressure, sound, and muscular contractions. See also **proprioceptor.**

mechlorethamine hydrochloride, an antineoplastic alkylating agent. Also called **nitrogen mustard.**
▪ INDICATIONS: It is prescribed in the treatment of a variety of neoplasms.
▪ CONTRAINDICATIONS: Bone marrow depression, pregnancy, infection, or known hypersensitivity to this drug prohibits its use.
▪ ADVERSE EFFECTS: Among the most serious adverse reactions are bone marrow depression and inflammation caused by extravasation at the site of injection. Nausea, vomiting, and alopecia also may occur.

Meckel's diverticulum, an anomalous sac protruding from the wall of the ileum between 30 and 90 cm from the ileocecal sphincter. It is congenital, resulting from the incomplete closure of the yolk stalk, and occurs in 1% to 2% of the population. The diverticulum is usually asymptomatic, but the condition is suggested by signs of appendicitis in infancy, by sudden and painless bleeding, usually in childhood, or by symptoms of intestinal obstruction. Symptomatic diverticula are most commonly resected. Surgical resection of asymptomatic diverticula is also recommended to avoid diverticulitis, obstruction, and blood loss, which may occur. Many Meckel's diverticula are discovered incidentally during surgery for other causes and on postmortem examination.

Meclan, a trademark for an antibacterial (meclocycline sulfosalicylate).

meclizine hydrochloride, an antihistamine.
▪ INDICATION: It is prescribed in the prevention and treatment of motion sickness.
▪ CONTRAINDICATIONS: Newborn infants and lactating mothers are not given this drug. Asthma or known hypersensitivity to this drug prohibits its use.
▪ ADVERSE EFFECTS: Among the more serious adverse effects are drowsiness, skin rash [illegible] nsitivity reactions, dry mouth [illegible] ness.

meclo[illegible] tory agent.
▪ IND[illegible] ent of rheumatoid [illegible]
▪ CONT[illegible] ity to aspirin or to [illegible] prohibits its use. It i[illegible] upper GI disease [illegible]
▪ ADVER[illegible] s adverse reactions [illegible] dizziness, rashes, and tinni[illegible] interacts with many other drugs.

Meclomen, a trademark for an antiinflammatory agent (meclofenamate sodium).

mecocephaly. See **scaphocephaly.**

meconium /mikō′nē·əm/, a material that collects in the intestines of a fetus and forms the first stools of a newborn. It is thick and sticky in consistency, usually greenish to black in color, and composed of secretions of the intestinal glands, some amniotic fluid, and intrauterine debris, as bile pigments, fatty acids, epithelial cells, mucus, lanugo, and blood. With ingestion of breast milk or formula and the proper functioning of the GI tract, the color, consistency, and frequency of the stools change by the third or fourth day after the initiation of feedings. The presence of meconium in the amniotic fluid during labor may indicate fetal distress.

meconium aspiration, the inhalation of meconium by the fetus or newborn, which can block the air passages and result in failure of the lungs to expand or cause other pulmonary dysfunction, as pneumonia or emphysema.

meconium ileus, obstruction of the small intestine in the newborn caused by impaction of thick, dry, tenacious meconium, usually at or near the ileocecal valve. Symptoms include abdominal distention, vomiting, failure to pass meconium within the first 24 to 48 hours after birth, and rapid dehydration with associated electrolyte imbalance. The condition results from a deficiency in pancreatic enzymes and is the earliest manifestation of cystic fibrosis. In uncomplicated cases in which perforation, volvulus, or atresia does not occur, the obstruction may be relieved by giving enemas with a contrast medium, as a hypertonic solution of meglumine diatrizoate and sodium diatrizoate, under fluoroscopy. Fluid loss is replaced intravenously to prevent dehydration. If two or three enemas do not dislodge the obstruction, surgery is necessary. See also **meconium plug syndrome.**

meconium plug syndrome, obstruction of the large intestine in the newborn caused by thick, rubbery meconium that may fill the entire colon and part of the terminal ileum. Symptoms include failure to pass meconium within the first 24 to 48 hours after birth, abdominal distention, and vomiting if complete intestinal blockage occurs. A barium enema will indicate the plug and in most cases will dislodge it from the bowel wall. Subsequent gentle saline enemas may be needed to expel the plug. The condition may be an indication of Hirschsprung's disease or cystic fibrosis. See also **meconium ileus.**

MED, abbreviation for *minimal effective dose* or *minimal erythema dose*.

medcard, (in nursing) a small card listing the name, dose, and schedule of administration of each patient's medications, used in dispensing medication to each patient.

MEDEX /med′eks/, **1.** an educational program accredited by the AMA for training military personnel with *medical experience* to become physician's assistants. **2.** a physician's assistant who has gained *medical experience* during military service and further training in a physician's assistant program.

medi-, a combining form meaning 'middle': *medialecithal, medicinerea, mediotarsal*.

medial, **1.** situated or oriented toward the midline of the body. **2.** pertaining to the tunica media, the middle layer of a blood vessel wall. Also **mesial.**

medial antebrachial cutaneous nerve, a nerve of the arm that arises from the medial cord of the brachial plexus, medial to the axillary artery. Near the axilla it passes a filament to supply the skin over the biceps almost as far as the elbow. It descends on the ulnar side of the arm medial to the brachial artery, pierces the deep fascia with the basilic vein about the middle of the arm, and divides into the anterior branch and the ulnar branch. The anterior branch is the larger of the two branches and continues on the anterior part of the ulnar side of the arm, distributes filaments to the skin as far as the wrist, and communicates with the palmar cutaneous branch of the ulnar nerve. The ulnar branch descends on the medial side of the basilic nerve as far as the wrist, innervates the skin, and communicates with branches of the ulnar nerve. Compare **medial brachial cutaneous nerve.**

medial arteriosclerosis. See **Mönckeberg's arteriosclerosis.**

medial brachial cutaneous nerve, a nerve of the arm arising from the medial cord of the brachial plexus and distributed to the medial side of the arm. It passes through the axilla, pierces the deep fascia in the middle of the arm, and supplies the skin of the arm as far as the olecranon. Compare **medial antebrachial cutaneous nerve.**

medial cuneiform bone, the largest of three cuneiform bones of the foot, situated on the medial side of the tarsus, between the scaphoid bone and the first metatarsal. It serves as the attachment for various ligaments, the tendons of the tibialis anterior, and the peroneus longus. It articulates with the scaphoid, the intermediate cuneiform, and the first and second metatarsals. Also called **internal cuneiform bone.**

medial geniculate body, either of the two areas on the posterior dorsal thalamus, relaying auditory impulses from the lateral lemniscus to the auditory cortex.

medial pectoral nerve, a branch of the brachial plexus that, with the lateral pectoral nerve, supplies the pectoral muscles. It arises from the medial cord of the plexus, medial to the axillary artery, passes between the axillary artery and the axillary vein, and joins the lateral pectoral nerve to form a loop around the artery before ending deep in the pectoralis minor. The loop branches to supply the pectoralis minor and the pectoralis major. Compare **lateral pectoral nerve.**

medial rotation, a turning toward the midline of the body. Compare **lateral rotation.** See also **rotation.**

median, (in statistics) the number representing the middle value of the scores in a sample. In an odd number of scores arrayed in ascending order, it is the middle score; in an even number of scores so arrayed, it is the average of the two central scores.

median antebrachial vein /an′tēbrā′kē·əl/, one of the superficial veins of the upper limb that drains the venous plexus on the palmar surface of the hand. It ascends on the ulnar side of the anterior forearm and, at its terminus, joins the median cubital vein. In many individuals it divides into two vessels, one joining the basilic vein, the other joining the cephalic vein distal to the elbow. One of the veins of the median cubital complex commonly anastomoses with the deep veins of the forearm. The anastomosis holds the superficial vein in place and makes it a practical choice for venipuncture. Compare **basilic vein, cephalic vein, dorsal digital vein.**

median aperture of fourth ventricle, an opening between the lower part of the roof of the fourth ventricle and the subarachnoid space.

median atlantoaxial joint, one of three points of articulation of the atlas and the axis. The median atlantoaxial joint is a pivot articulation between the dens and ring of the atlas and involves five ligaments. It allows rotation of the axis and the skull, the extent of rotation limited by the alar ligaments.

median basilic vein, one of the superficial veins of the upper limb, often formed as one of two branches from the median cubital vein. The median basilic vein courses across the palmar surface of the forearm near the elbow and is commonly used for venipuncture, phlebotomy, or intravenous infusion. Compare **basilic vein.**

median effective dose (ED_{50}), the dose of a drug that may be expected to cause a specific intensity of effect in one half of the patients to whom it is given.

median glossitis. See **median rhomboid glossitis.**

median jaw relation, (in dentistry) any jaw relation that exists when the mandible is in the median sagittal plane.

median lethal dose (MLD, LD_{50}), (in radiotherapy) the amount of radiation that kills 50% of the individuals in a large group of animals or organisms within a specified period of time.

median nerve, one of the terminal branches of the brachial plexus that extends along the radial portions of the forearm and the hand and supplies various muscles and the skin of these parts. It arises from the brachial plexus by two large roots, one from the lateral and one from the medial cord. The roots unite to form the trunk of the nerve that courses down the arm with the brachial artery. In the forearm it passes between the two heads of the pronator teres and passes through the flexor retinaculum into the palm of the hand, where it is covered only by the skin and the palmar aponeurosis. Emerging from the retinaculum it is enlarged and flattened and splits into digital and muscular branches. The median nerve usually has no branches above the elbow, but in some individuals the nerve to the pronator teres arises there. The median nerve gives off a few articular branches to the elbow joint and muscular branches to the forearm, the anterior interosseous nerve, the palmar branch, the muscular branch in the hand, the first, second, and third palmar digital nerves, and the proper digital nerves. Compare **musculocutaneous nerve, radial nerve, ulnar nerve.**

median palatine suture, the line of junction between the horizontal portions of the palatine bones that extends from both sides of the skull to form the posterior part of the hard palate.

median plane, a vertical plane that divides the body into right and left halves and passes approximately through the sagittal suture of the skull. Also called **cardinal sagittal plane, midsagittal plane.** Compare **frontal plane, sagittal plane, transverse plane.**

median rhomboid glossitis, a red, depressed, diamond-shaped area on the dorsum of the tongue, frequently irritated by alcohol, hot drinks, or spicy foods. The condition is most often seen in adult men and may be caused by candidiasis.

median toxic dose (TD_{50}), the dosage that may be expected to cause a toxic effect in one half of the patients to whom it is given.

mediastinitis, an inflammation of the mediastinum.

mediastinum /mē′dē•əstī′nəm/, *pl.* **mediastina,** a portion of the thoracic cavity in the middle of the thorax, between the pleural sacs containing the two lungs. It extends from the sternum to the vertebral column and contains all the thoracic viscera, except the lungs. It is enclosed in a thick extension of the thoracic subserous fascia and is divided into the cranial portion and the caudal portion by a plane extending from the sternal angle to the caudal border of the fourth thoracic vertebra. The caudal portion is divided into the anterior mediastinum, ventral to the pericardium, the middle mediastinum, containing the pericardium, and the posterior mediastinum, dorsal to the pericardium. **–mediastinal,** *adj.*

mediate, **1.** to cause a change to occur, as in stimulation by a hormone. **2.** to settle a dispute, as in collective bargaining. **3.** situated between two places, things, parts, or terms. **4.** (in psychology) an event that follows one process or event and precedes another; for example, in the process of cognition, perception follows stimulation and precedes thinking. **–mediating,** *adj.,* **mediator,** *n.*

Mediatric, a trademark for a nutritional supplement containing multivitamins, minerals, hormones, and a central nervous system stimulant (methamphetamine hydrochloride).

Medicaid, a federally funded, state operated program of medical assistance to people with low incomes, authorized by Title XIX of the Social Security Act. Under broad federal guidelines, the individual states determine benefits, eligibility, rates of payment, and methods of administration.

Medicaid mill, *informal.* a health program or facility that solely or primarily serves persons eligible for Medicaid. Such facilities are found mainly in depressed areas where there are few other health services.

medical assistant, a person who, under the direction of a physician, performs various routine administrative and nontechnical clinical tasks in a hospital, clinic, or similar facility.

medical care, the provision by a physician of services related to the maintenance of health, prevention of illness, and treatment of illness or injury.

medical center, **1.** a health care facility. **2.** a hospital, especially one staffed and equipped to care for many patients and for a large number of kinds of diseases and dysfunctions using sophisticated technology.

Medical College Aptitude Test (MCAT), an examination taken by persons applying to medical school, the score on this examination being an important criterion for acceptance. Basic science, intellectual ability, and mathematic and verbal aptitude and knowledge are tested.

medical consultation, a procedure whereby, on request by one physician, another physician reviews a patient's medical history, examines the patient, and makes recommendations as to care and treatment. The medical consultant often is a specialist with expertise in a particular field of medicine.

medical decision level, a concentration of analyte at which some medical action is indicated for proper patient care. There may be several medical decision levels for a given analyte.

medical director, a physician who is usually employed by a hospital to serve in a medical and administrative capacity as head of the organized medical staff. The medical director may also serve as liaison for the medical staff with the hospital's administration and governing board.

medical engineering, a field of study that involves biomedical engineering and technologic concepts to develop equipment and instruments required in health care delivery.

medical examiner. See **coroner.**

medical genetics. See **clinical genetics.**

medical history. See **health history.**

medical illustrator, an artist qualified by special training in preparing illustrations of organs, tissues, and medical phenomena in normal and abnormal states.

medical indigency /in′dijen′sē/, the lack of financial reserves adequate to pay for medical care, especially a person or family able to manage other basic living expenses.

medical induction of labor. See **induction of labor.**

medical laboratory technician, a person who, under the supervision of a medical technologist or physician, performs microscopic and bacteriologic tests of human blood, tissue, and fluids for diagnostic and research purposes.

medical model, the traditional approach to the diagnosis and treatment of illness as practiced by physicians in the Western world since the time of Koch and Pasteur. The physician focuses on the defect, or dysfunction, within the patient, using a problem-solving approach. The medical history and the physical examination and diagnostic tests provide the basis for the identification and treatment of a specific illness. The medical model is thus focused on the physical and biologic aspects of specific diseases and conditions. Nursing differs from the medical model in that the patient is perceived primarily as a social person relating to the environment; nursing care is formulated on the basis of a nursing assessment that assumes multiple causes for the problems experienced by the patient.

medical record administrator, a person who maintains records of patients' medical histories, diagnoses, treatment, and outcome, in a condition that meets medical, administrative, legal, ethical, regulatory, and institutional requirements.

medical secretary, a person who prepares and maintains medical records and performs related secretarial duties.

medical staff, all physicians, dentists, and health professionals responsible for providing health care in a hospital or other health care facility. Medical staff personnel may be full-time or part-time, employed by the facility, or simply affiliated, that is, not employees.

medical staff, courtesy, physicians and dentists who meet certain qualifications of the medical staff of a hospital but who admit patients only occasionally or act as consultants. They are ineligible to participate in medical staff activities.

medical staff, honorary, physicians and dentists, usually retired, who are recognized by the hospital medical staff for their noteworthy contributions but who may not admit patients to the hospital or participate in medical staff activities.

medical-surgical nursing, the nursing care of patients whose conditions or disorders are treated pharmacologically or surgically.

medical technologist, a person who, under the direction of a pathologist or other physician or medical scientist, performs specialized chemical, microscopic, and bacteriologic tests of blood, tissue, and fluids. A medical technologist who has successfully completed an examination by the Board of Registry of the American Society of Clinical Pathologists, or a similar professional body, may be designated a certified medical technologist.

Medical Women's International Association (M.W.I.A.), an international professional organization of women physicians.

Medicare, a federally funded national health insurance for certain persons over 65 years of age. The program is administered in two parts. Part A provides basic protection against costs of medical, surgical, and psychiatric hospital care. Part B is a voluntary medical insurance program financed in part from federal funds and in part from premiums contributed by persons enrolled in the program. Medicare enrollment is offered to persons 65 years of age or older who are entitled to receive Social Security or railroad retirement benefits. Other persons over 65, as federal employees and aliens, may not be eligible. Medicare was authorized by Title XVIII of the Social Security Act of 1965.

medicated bougie, **1.** a bougie containing a medicated agent. **2.** *obsolete.* a suppository.

medicated tub bath, a therapeutic bath in which medication is dispersed in water, usually in the treatment of dermatologic disorders.

▪ METHOD: The amount of medication and the amount and temperature of the water are specified in the order for the bath. The water is run, the medication is added, and the solution is stirred with a bath thermometer to disperse the medication in the water while testing the temperature. The temperature is usually between 35.6° C (96° F) and 37.8° C (100° F) but may be as high as 39.4° C (103° F), as in the treatment of psoriasis vulgaris. Most medicated baths are prescribed as half-hour treatments. A folded towel or waterproof pillow is placed behind the head, and a towel is draped over the shoulders to add to the patient's comfort. In certain conditions, the patient may be asked to scrub affected areas with a brush and washcloth; in others, the patient is instructed not to scrub at all. After the bath the skin is patted dry and any ointment, cream, or other topical prescription is applied.

■ NURSING ORDERS: The reason for the treatment is explained to the patient, and instructions are given not to get out of the tub without assistance and not to add water without calling the nurse. If the patient is to scrub the affected areas, the necessary equipment is brought to the bath. The tub is thoroughly scrubbed and rinsed before and after the treatment.

■ OUTCOME CRITERIA: The medicated bath is usually soothing, relaxing, and comforting for the patient. Close attention to instructing the patient fully and to assuring comfort during the procedure improves the patient's compliance with the treatment.

medication, **1.** a drug or other substance that is used as a medicine. **2.** the administration of a medicine.

medication order, a written order by a physician, dentist, or other designated health professional for a medication to be dispensed by a hospital pharmacy for administration to an inpatient.

medicinal treatment, therapy of disorders based chiefly on the use of appropriate pharmacologic agents.

medicine, **1.** a drug or a remedy for illness. **2.** the art and science of the diagnosis, treatment, and prevention of disease and the maintenance of good health. **3.** the art or technique of treating disease without surgery. Two major divisions of medicine are academic medicine and clinical medicine. Some of the many branches of medicine include **environmental medicine, family medicine, forensic medicine, internal medicine,** and **physical medicine.** **–medical,** *adj.*

medicolegal, of or pertaining to both medicine and law. Medicolegal considerations are a significant part of the process of making many patient care decisions and in determining definitions and policies regarding the treatment of mentally incompetent people and minors, the performance of sterilization or therapeutic abortion, and the care of terminally ill patients. Medicolegal considerations, decisions, definitions, and policies provide the framework for informed consent, professional liability, and many other aspects of current practice in the health care field.

Medihaler-Epi, a trademark for an adrenergic (epinephrine bitartrate).

Medihaler-Ergotamine Aerosol, a trademark for an analgesic (ergotamine tartrate).

meditation, a state of consciousness in which the individual eliminates environmental stimuli from awareness so the mind can focus on a single thing, producing a state of relaxation and relief from stress. A wide variety of techniques are used to clear the mind of stressful outside interferences.

meditation therapy, a method of achieving relaxation and consciouness expansion by focusing on a mantra, or a key word, sound, or image while eliminating outside stimuli from one's awareness.

Mediterranean anemia. See **thalassemia.**

Mediterranean fever. See **brucellosis.**

medium, *pl.* **media,** a substance through which something moves or through which it acts. A **contrast medium** is a substance that has a density different from that of body tissues, permitting visual comparison of structures when used with imaging techniques such as x-ray film. A **culture medium** is a substance that provides a nutritional environment for the growth of microorganisms or cells. A **dispersion medium** is the substance in which a colloid is dispersed. A **refractory medium** is the transparent tissues and fluid of the eye that refract light.

MEDLARS /med′lärs/, abbreviation for *Medical Literature Analysis and Retrieval System,* a computerized literature retrieval service of the National Library of Medicine in Bethesda, Maryland. MEDLARS contains more than 4,500,000 references to medical articles found in professional journals and books published since 1966. The references are made available on request to more than 1000 hospitals, universities, government agencies, and other interested parties throughout the world by means of a network of computer terminals. The references are filed in 15 data bases, including MEDLINE, TOXLINE, CHEMLINE, RTECS, CANCERLIT, and EPILEPSYLINE. See also **MEDLINE.**

MEDLINE /med′līn/, a National Library of Medicine computer data base that covers approximately 600,000 references to biomedical journal articles published in the current and 2 preceding years. The files duplicate the contents of the monthly and annual volumes of the ***Unabridged Index Medicus,*** also published by the National Library of Medicine, which indexes medical reports from 3000 professional journals in more than 70 countries. See also **MEDLARS.**

Medrol, a trademark for a glucocorticoid (methylprednisolone disodium phosphate).

Medrol Acetate, a trademark for a glucocorticoid (methylprednisolone acetate).

medroxyprogesterone acetate, a progestin.

■ INDICATION: It is prescribed in the treatment of menstrual disorders caused by hormone imbalance.

■ CONTRAINDICATIONS: Known or suspected pregnancy, thrombophlebitis, embolism, stroke, liver dysfunction, cancer of the breast or genitals, abnormal vaginal bleeding, missed abortion, or known hypersensitivity to this drug prohibits its use.

■ ADVERSE EFFECTS: Among the more serious adverse reactions are thrombophlebitis, pulmonary embolism, stroke, hepatitis, and cerebral thrombosis.

medrysone, an ophthalmic glucocorticoid.

■ INDICATIONS: It is prescribed for various inflammatory conditions of the eye, as allergic conjunctivitis.

■ CONTRAINDICATIONS: Concurrent viral, fungal, or

tubercular infections of the eye or known hypersensitivity to this drug prohibits its use.

■ ADVERSE EFFECTS: Among the more serious adverse reactions are aggravation of glaucoma, damage to the optic nerve, and exacerbation of viral or fungal infections of the eye.

medulla /mədul′ə/, *pl.* **medullas, medullae, 1.** the most internal part of a structure or organ, as the spinal medulla. See also **marrow. 2.** *informal.* medulla oblongata.

medulla oblongata, the most vital part of the entire brain, continuing as the bulbous portion of the spinal cord just above the foramen magnum and separated from the pons by a horizontal groove. It is one of three parts of the brainstem and contains mostly white substance with some mixture of gray substance. The medulla contains the cardiac, the vasomotor, and the respiratory centers of the brain, and medullary injury or disease often proves fatal. Compare **mesencephalon, pons.**

medullary /med′əler′ē, mədul′erē, med′yəler′ē/, **1.** of or pertaining to the medulla of the brain. **2.** of or pertaining to the bone marrow. **3.** of or pertaining to the spinal cord and central nervous system. Also **medullar.**

medullary carcinoma, a soft, malignant neoplasm of the epithelium containing little or no fibrous tissue. A small percentage of breast and thyroid tumors are medullary carcinomas. Also called **carcinoma medullare, carcinoma molle, encephaloid carcinoma.**

medullary cystic disease, a chronic familial disease of the kidney, characterized by the slow onset of uremia. The disease appears in young children or adolescents, who pass large volumes of dilute urine with greater than normal amounts of sodium. Hemodialysis is the usual treatment for the disease as the uremia progresses and becomes severe. See also **uremia.**

medullary fold. See **neural fold.**

medullary groove. See **neural groove.**

medullary plate. See **neural plate.**

medullary sponge kidney, a congenital defect of the kidney, leading to cystic dilatation of the collecting tubules. Persons with this defect often develop a kidney stone or an infection of the kidney caused by urinary stasis. The condition is diagnosed using urographic techniques. Treatment includes drugs to acidify the urine and a diet low in calcium and high in fluids to discourage formation of stones.

medullary tube. See **neural tube.**

medulla spinalis. See **spinal cord.**

medullated neuroma. See **fascicular neuroma.**

medulloblastoma /mədul′ōblastō′mə/, a poorly differentiated malignant neoplasm composed of tightly packed cells of spongioblastic and neuroblastic lineage. The tumor usually arises in the cerebellum, occurs most frequently between 5 and 9 years of age, and affects more boys than girls. Although medulloblastomas are extremely radiosensitive, they grow rapidly, and radiotherapy usually prolongs life for only 1 or 2 years.

medulloepithelioma. See **neurocytoma.**

mefenamic acid /mef′ənam′ik/, a nonsteroidal antiinflammatory agent and analgesic.

■ INDICATION: It is prescribed in the treatment of mild to moderate pain.

■ CONTRAINDICATIONS: GI ulceration or inflammation, impaired renal function, or known hypersensitivity to this drug prohibits its use. It is used with caution in patients with athma.

■ ADVERSE EFFECTS: Dyspepsia and diarrhea are the most common adverse effects. Other GI symptoms, dizziness, drowsiness, or skin rash occasionally occur. Rarely, serious blood dyscrasias occur.

mefloquine /mef′ləkēn/, an antimalarial that has been shown to be effective in the prophylaxis and treatment of chloroquine-resistant falciparum and vivax malaria.

Mefoxin, a trademark for a cephalosporin antibiotic (cefoxitin sodium).

MEFR, abbreviation for **maximal expiratory flow rate.**

mega-, megalo-, mego-, a combining form meaning 'great or huge': *megacardia, megacoccus, megadyne.*

megabladder. See **megalocystis.**

megabyte (Mb), one million bytes, or 1000 kilobytes.

megacaryocyte /meg′əker′ē·əsīt′/, an extremely large bone marrow cell measuring between 35 and 160 μ in diameter and having a nucleus with many lobes. Megacaryocytes are essential for the production and proliferation of platelets in the marrow and are normally not present in the circulation blood. Also spelled **megakaryocyte.** See also **platelet.** –**megacaryocytic,** *adj.*

Megace, a trademark for an antineoplastic progestational agent (megestrol acetate).

megacolon /meg′əkō′lən/, massive, abnormal dilatation of the colon that may be congenital, toxic, or acquired. **Congenital megacolon** (Hirschsprung's disease) is caused by the absence of autonomic ganglia in the smooth muscle wall of the colon. **Toxic megacolon** is a grave complication of ulcerative colitis and may result in perforation of the colon, septicemia, and death. Surgery is the usual treatment for toxic and congenital megacolon. **Acquired megacolon** is the result of a chronic refusal to defecate, usually occurring in children who are psychotic or mentally retarded. The colon becomes dilated by an accumulation of impacted feces. Laxatives, enemas, and psychiatric treatment are often necessary. See also **Hirschsprung's disease.**

megaesophagus /meg′ə·isof′əgəs/, abnormal dilatation of the lower segments of the esophagus caused by distention resulting from the failure of the cardiac sphincter to relax and allow the passage of food into the stomach. See also **achalasia.**

megakaryocytic leukemia /meg′əker′ē·ōsit′ik/, a rare malignancy of blood-forming tissue in which megakaryocytes proliferate abnormally in the bone marrow and circulate in the blood in relatively large numbers.

megalencephaly /meg′əlensef′əlē/, a condition characterized by pathologic parenchymal overgrowth of the brain. In some cases generalized cerebral hyperplasia is associated with mental retardation or a brain disorder, as epilepsy. Also called **macrencephaly, macroencephaly.** –**megalencephalic, megalencephalous,** *adj*.

-megalia. See **-megaly.**

megalo-. See **mega-.**

megaloblast /meg′əlōblast′/, an abnormally large nucleated immature erythrocyte that develops in large numbers in the bone marrow and is plentiful in the circulation in many anemias associated with deficiency of vitamin B_{12}, folic acid, or intrinsic factor. Effective treatment is the intramuscular injection of vitamin B_{12}. –**megaloblastic,** *adj*.

megaloblastic anemia, a hematologic disorder characterized by the production and peripheral proliferation of immature, large, and dysfunctional erythrocytes. Megaloblasts are usually associated with severe pernicious anemia or folic acid deficiency anemia. See also **nutritional anemia.**

megalocephaly. See **macrocephaly.**

megalocystis /meg′əlōsis′tis/, an abnormal condition occurring primarily in girls, characterized by an enlarged and thin-walled bladder. Reduction of the size of the bladder or diversion of the flow of urine through the ileum may be surgically performed to correct this condition. Also called **megabladder.**

megalomania /meg′əlōmā′nē·ə/, an abnormal mental state characterized by delusions of grandeur in which one believes oneself to be a person of great importance, power, fame, or wealth. See also **mania.**

megaloureter /meg′əlōyŏŏrē′tər/, an abnormal condition characterized by marked dilatation of one or both ureters, resulting from dysfunctional peristaltic action of the smooth muscle in the ureters. Treatment may include surgical resection.

-megaly, -megalia, a combining form meaning an 'enlargement of a (specified) body part': *cardiomegaly, dactylomegaly, gastromegaly*.

megestrol acetate /məjes′trōl/, an antineoplastic progestational agent.

■ INDICATIONS: It is prescribed to treat endometrial cancer and, more commonly, to palliate advanced endometrial and breast cancer.

■ CONTRAINDICATION: Hypersensitivity to the drug prohibits its use.

■ ADVERSE EFFECTS: There are no known serious adverse reactions.

mego-. See **mega.**

megrim. See **migraine.**

meibomian cyst. See **chalazion.**

meibomian gland /mēbō′mē·ən/, one of several sebaceous glands that secrete sebum from their ducts on the posterior margin of each eyelid. The glands are embedded in the tarsal plate of each eyelid. Also called **tarsal gland, palpebral gland.**

Meigs' syndrome /megz/, ascites and hydrothorax associated with a fibroma of the ovaries or other pelvic tumor.

meio-. See **mio-.**

meiocyte /mī′əsīt/, any cell undergoing meiosis.

meiogenic /mī′əjen′ik/, producing or causing meiosis.

meiosis /mī·ō′sis/, the division of a sex cell, as it matures, into two, then four gametes, the nucleus of each receiving one half of the number of chromosomes present in the somatic cells of the species. Also called **meiotic division.** Compare **mitosis.** See also **anaphase, metaphase, oogenesis, prophase, telophase.** –**meiotic** /mī·ot′ik/, *adj*.

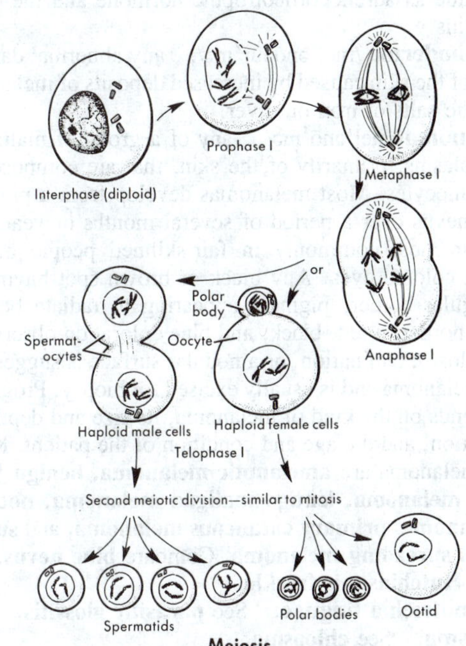

Meiosis

Meissner's corpuscle. See **tactile corpuscle.**

mel-, 1. a combining form meaning 'limb, member': *melalgia, melomelus, melosalgia*. **2.** See **melano-.**

melan-. See **melano-.**

melancholia /mel′angkō′lē·ə/, **1.** extreme sadness; melancholy. **2.** *obsolete*. the major affective depressive disorder. See also **bipolar disorder, depression.**

melancholia agitata, *obsolete*. a state of depression in which psychomotor excitement is a prominent symptom. See also **agitated depression, bipolar disorder.**

melancholia simplex, *obsolete*. a mild state of depression. See also **bipolar disorder.**

melancholia stuporosa, *obsolete*. a state of depression in which stupor in varying degrees is often accompanied by hallucinations. See also **bipolar disorder, stupor.**

melanin /mel′ənin/, a black or dark brown pigment that occurs naturally in the hair, skin, and in the iris and choroid of the eye. See also **melanocyte.**

melano-, melan-, mel-, a combining form meaning 'black': *melanoderm, melanoleukoderma, melanophore.*

melanocyte /mel′ənōsīt′, məlen′ōsīt/, a body cell capable of producing melanin. Such cells are distributed throughout the basal cell layer of the epidermis and form melanin pigment from tyrosine, an amino acid. Melanin granules are then transferred to adjacent basal cells and to hair. Melanocyte stimulating hormone from the pituitary controls the amount of melanin produced.

melanocyte stimulating hormone (MSH), a polypeptide hormone, secreted by the anterior pituitary gland, that controls the intensity of pigmentation in pigmented cells. It is synthesized on the same large precursor polypeptide as adrenocorticotrophic hormone and the enkephalins.

melanoderma /mel′ənōdur′mə/, any abnormal darkening of the skin caused by increased deposits of melanin or by the salts of iron or silver.

melanoma /mel′ənō′mə/, any of a group of malignant neoplasms, primarily of the skin, that are composed of melanocytes. Most melanomas develop from a pigmented nevus over a period of several months or years and occur most commonly in fair-skinned people having light-colored eyes. Any black or brown spot having an irregular border, pigment appearing to radiate beyond that border, a red, black, and blue coloration observable on close examination, or a nodular surface is suggestible of melanoma and is usually excised for biopsy. Prognosis depends on the kind of melanoma, its size and depth, its location, and the age and condition of the patient. Kinds of melanoma are **amelanotic melanoma, benign juvenile melanoma, lentigo maligna melanoma, nodular melanoma, primary cutaneous melanoma,** and **superficial spreading melanoma.** Compare **blue nevus.** See also **Hutchinson's freckle.**

melanotrichia linguae. See **parasitic glossitis.**

melasma. See **chloasma.**

melatonin /mel′ətō′nin/, the only hormone secreted into the bloodstream by the pineal gland. It has marked diurnal rhythm; blood levels are up to 10 times greater at night than during the day. The hormone appears to inhibit numerous endocrine functions, including the gonadotropic hormones, and to decrease the pigmentation of the skin. When injected, exogenous melatonin causes drowsiness. Decreased secretion of melatonin occurs when calcification or tumor formation destroys or damages the pineal gland. A marked decrease results in precocious puberty, especially in boys, and in diabetes insipidus, hypogonadism, and optic atrophy.

melena /məlē′nə/, abnormal, black, tarry stool containing digested blood. It usually results from bleeding in the upper GI tract and is often a sign of peptic ulcer or small bowel disease. See also **gastrointestinal bleeding.**

meli-, a combining form meaning 'sweet, or related to honey': *melicera, melitagra, melitoptyalism.*

-melia, a combining form meaning '(condition of the) limbs': *acromelia, dolichomelia, phocomelia.*

melioidosis /mel′ē•oidō′sis/, an infection uncommon in humans caused by the gram-negative bacillus ***Malleomyces pseudomallei.*** **Acute melioidasis** is fulminant and usually characterized by pneumonia, empyema, lung abscess, septicemia, and liver or spleen involvement. **Chronic melioidosis** is associated with osteomyelitis, multiple abscesses of the internal organs, and the development of fistulas from the abscesses. The disease, most commonly seen in China and Southeast Asia, is acquired by direct contact with infected animals. Human-to-human transmission is unlikely. Treatment using chloramphenicol, sulfonamides, or tetracycline for several months is usually successful.

Mellaril, a trademark for a tranquilizer (thioridazine).

melphalan /mel′fəlan/, an antineoplastic alkylating agent.

■ INDICATIONS: It is prescribed in the treatment of malignant neoplastic diseases, including multiple myeloma.

■ CONTRAINDICATIONS: Pregnancy, recent exposure to antineoplastic medication or to radiation, or known hypersensitivity to this drug prohibits its use.

■ ADVERSE EFFECTS: Among the more serious adverse reactions are bone marrow depression, nausea, and vomiting.

membrana tectoria, **1.** also called **occipitoaxial ligament.** the broad, strong ligament covering the dens and helping to connect the axis to the occipital bone of the skull. Compare **alar ligament, apical dental ligament.** **2.** a spiral membrane projecting from the vestibular lip of the cochlea over the organ of Corti.

membrana tympani. See **tympanic membrane.**

membrane, a thin layer of tissue that covers a surface, lines a cavity, or divides a space, as the abdominal membrane that lines the abdominal wall and Descemet's membrane between the substantia propria and the endothelium of the cornea. The principal kinds of membranes are **mucous membrane, serous membrane, synovial membrane,** and **cutaneous membrane.**

membrane conductance, (in cardiology) the degree of permeability of a cellular membrane to certain ions.

membrane responsiveness, (in cardiology) the relationship between the membrane potential at the time of stimulation and the maximal rate of depolarization of the action potential.

membranous labyrinth, a network of three fluid-filled, membranous, semicircular ducts suspended within the bony semicircular canals of the inner ear, associated with the sense of balance. The ducts, which contain endolymph, follow the contours of the bony canals and are about one fourth the of diameter of the canals.

membranous stomatitis. See **pseudomembranous stomatitis.**

memory, **1.** the mental faculty or power that enables one to retain and to recall, through unconscious associative processes, previously experienced sensations, impressions, ideas, concepts, and all information that has been consciously learned. **2.** the reservoir of all past experiences and knowledge that may be recollected or recalled at will. **3.** the recollection of a past event, ideas, sensations, or previously learned knowledge. Kinds of memory include **affect memory, anterograde memory, kinesthetic memory, long-term memory, screen memory, short-term memory,** and **visual memory.** See also **amnesia, déjà vu.**

memory cell. See **lymphocyte.**

memory image, a sensation, impression, or sense perception as it is recalled in the memory.

-men, a combining form meaning a 'condition or result of a (specified) action': *flumen, lumen, semen.*

menadiol sodium diphosphate, a water-soluble analog of vitamin K. See **menadione.**

menadione /men'ədī'ōn/, an analog of vitamin K. Also called **menaphthone** /mənaf'thōn/.

■ INDICATIONS: It is prescribed in the treatment of vitamin K deficiency and hypoprothrombinemia (other than the hereditary type).

■ CONTRAINDICATIONS: It is not indicated in pregnancy, for anticoagulant overdose, or to counteract heparin. Known hypersensitivity to this drug prohibits its use.

■ ADVERSE EFFECTS: Among the most serious adverse reactions are kernicterus in the newborn and hemolytic anemia in glucose-6-phosphate dehydrogenase deficient individuals. GI upset, rashes, and headaches also may occur.

menadione sodium bisulfite, an analog of vitamin K. See also **menadione.**

menaphthone. See **menadione.**

menarche /menär'kē/, the first menstruation and the commencement of cyclic menstrual function. It usually occurs between 9 and 17 years of age. See also **pubarche.**

mendelevium (Md), a synthetic element in the actinide group. Its atomic number is 101. The atomic weight of its most stable isotope is 256. It is the ninth transuranic element.

mendelian genetics. See **Mendel's laws.**

mendelism /men'dəliz'əm/, the concept of inheritance derived from the application of Mendel's laws. Also called **mendelianism.** –**mendelian,** *adj.*

Mendel's laws, the basic principles of inheritance based on the breeding experiments of garden peas by the nineteenth century Austrian monk Gregor Mendel. These are usually stated as two laws, commonly called the law of segregation and the law of independent assortment. According to the first, each characteristic of a species is represented in the somatic cells by a pair of units, now known as genes, which separate during meiosis so that each gamete receives only one gene for each trait. In any monohybrid crossing, the possible ratio for the phenotypic expression of a particular dominant characteristic is 3:1, whereas the ratio of pure dominants to dominant hybrids to pure recessives is 1:2:1. According to the second law, the members of a gene pair on different chromosomes segregate independently from other pairs during meiosis, so that the gametes show all possible combinations of factors. Genes on the same chromosome are affected by linkage and segregate in blocks according to the amount of crossing over that occurs, a discovery made after Mendel. Also called **mendelian laws, mendelian genetics.** See also **chromosome, crossing over, dominant gene, linkage, meiosis, recessive gene.**

Mendelson's syndrome, a respiratory condition caused by the chemical pneumonia resulting from the aspiration of acid gastric contents into the lungs. It usually occurs when a person vomits when inebriated, when stuporous from anesthesia, or when unconscious, as during a seizure. Also called **pulmonary acid aspiration syndrome.**

Menest, a trademark for esterified estrogens.

Ménétrier's disease. See **giant hypertrophic gastritis.**

-menia, a combining form meaning '(condition of) menstrual activity': *catamenia, ischomenia, pausimenia.*

Ménière's disease /mānē•erz'/, a chronic disease of the inner ear characterized by recurrent episodes of vertigo, progressive unilateral nerve deafness, and tinnitus. Also called **Ménière's syndrome, paroxysmal labyrinthine vertigo.**

■ OBSERVATIONS: The cause is unknown although occasionally the condition follows middle ear infection or trauma to the head. There also may be associated nausea, vomiting, and profuse sweating. Attacks last from a few minutes to several hours.

■ INTERVENTION: Treatment includes a low-salt diet and the administration of dimenhydrinate, diphenhydramine, or atropine sulfate. In severe cases, surgery on the labyrinth or vestibular nerve or ultrasonic labyrinthectomy may be necessary.

■ NURSING CONSIDERATIONS: Because sudden movements often aggravate the vertigo, the patient will usually prefer to move at a self-determined rate, although walking without assistance should not be undertaken. Siderails should be in place on the bed at all times.

meningeal hydrops. See **pseudotumor cerebri.**

meninges /minin'jēz/, *sing.* **meninx** /mē'ningks, men'-/, any one of the three membranes that enclose the brain and the spinal cord, comprising the dura mater, the pia mater, and the arachnoid. The pia mater and the arachnoid can become inflamed by bacterial meningitis, causing serious complications that may be life threatening. –**meningeal,** *adj.*

meningioma /minin'jē•ō'mə/, *pl.* **meningiomas, meningiomata,** a mesenchymal fibroblastic tumor of the membranes enveloping the brain and spinal cord. Meningiomas often grow slowly, are usually vascular, and occur most commonly near the superior longitudinal transverse and cavernous sinuses of the dura mater of the brain. The tumors may be nodular, plaquelike, or diffuse lesions that invade the skull, causing bone erosion and compression of brain tissue. Meningiomas usually occur in adults, in some cases after a head injury.

meningism /minin'jizəm/, an abnormal condition characterized by irritation of the brain and the spinal cord and by symptoms that mimic those of meningitis. In meningism, however, there is no actual inflammation of the meninges.

meningitis /min'inji'tis/, *pl.* **meningitides,** any infection or inflammation of the membranes covering the brain and spinal cord. It is usually purulent and involves the fluid in the subarachnoid space. A kind of meningitis is **tuberculous meningitis.** Compare **encephalitis.**

■ OBSERVATIONS: It is characterized by severe headache, vomiting, and pain and stiffness in the neck. The most common causes are bacterial infection with *Streptococcus pneumoniae, Neisseria meningitidis,* or *Haemophilus influenzae*. Aseptic meningitis may be caused by other kinds of bacteria, by chemical irritation, by neoplasm, or by viruses. Many of these diseases are benign and self-limited, as meningitis caused by strains of coxsackievirus or echovirus. Others are more severe, as those involving arboviruses, herpesviruses, or poliomyelitis viruses. Yeasts such as *Candida* and fungi such as *Cryptococcus* may cause a severe, often fatal, meningitis. Tuberculous meningitis, invariably fatal if untreated, may result in a variety of neurologic abnormalities even with the best treatment available.

■ INTERVENTION: Bacterial meningitis is treated promptly with antibiotics specific for the causative organism; they are administered intravenously or intrathecally. Except for adenine arabinoside, recommended for herpes simplex meningitis, there is no specific therapy available for viral infections of the meninges. Antifungal medications, such as amphotericin B, given intravenously or intrathecally for several weeks, may prevent death from fungal meningitis, but serious neurologic sequelae may occur.

■ NURSING CONSIDERATIONS: Constant skilled nursing attention is necessary to ensure early recognition of rising intracranial pressure, to prevent aspiration in the event of convulsive seizures, and to avoid airway obstruction. Except for the first day or two of meningococcal disease, strict isolation procedures are unnecessary. Intravenous fluids and nasogastric tube feeding may be necessary for a prolonged period. Sedatives and narcotic analgesics may obscure important neurologic signs in addition to depressing vital functions.

meningo-, a combining form meaning 'pertaining to membranes covering the brain or spinal cord or to other membranes': *meningocele, meningococcus, meningopathy.*

meningocele /mining'gōsēl'/, a saclike protrusion of either the cerebral or spinal meninges through a congenital defect in the skull or the vertebral column. It forms a hernial cyst that is filled with cerebrospinal fluid but does not contain neural tissue. The anomaly is designated a cranial meningocele or spinal meningocele, depending on the site of the defect; it can be easily repaired by surgery. See also **myelomeningocele, neural tube defect.**

meningococcal polysaccharide vaccine, either of two active immunizing agents against group A and group C meningococcal organisms.

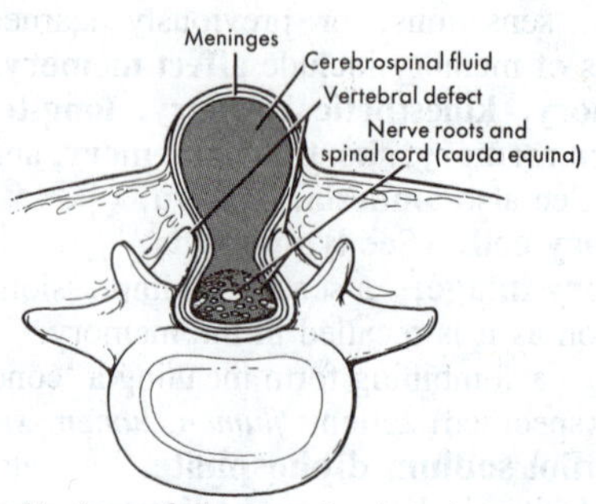

Meningocele (cross-sectional view)

■ INDICATION: It is prescribed for immunization against meningococcal meningitis.

■ CONTRAINDICATIONS: Immunosuppression or acute infection prohibits its use.

■ ADVERSE EFFECTS: The most serious adverse reaction is anaphylaxis.

meningococcemia /mining'gōkoksē'mē·ə/, a disease caused by *Neisseria meningitidis* in the bloodstream. Onset is sudden, with chills, pain in the muscles and joints, headache, petechiae, sore throat, and severe prostration. Tachycardia is present, respirations and pulse rate are increased, and fever is intermittent. Treatment of choice is penicillin G; peripheral circulatory collapse or Waterhouse-Friderichsen syndrome may occur, which is fatal if not aggressively treated.

meningococcus /mining'gōkok'əs/, *pl.* **meningococci** /-kok'sī/, a bacterium of the genus *Neisseria meningitidis,* a nonmotile, gram-negative diplococcus, frequently found in the nasopharynx of asymptomatic carriers, that may cause septicemia or epidemic cerebrospinal meningitis. Meningococcal infections are not highly communicable; however, crowded conditions, as may be found in army camps, concentrate the number of carriers and reduce individual resistance to the organism. Hemorrhagic skin lesions are significant clues to the diagnosis. Stained smears of these lesions or of cerebrospinal fluid must be examined quickly because meningococci are fragile and lyse easily. Early treatment with appropriate antibiotics, as penicillin G, is essential for cure. Several meningococcal vaccines are available. See also **meningitis.** **–meningococcal,** *adj.*

meningoencephalocele /mining'gō·ensef'əlōsēl'/, a saclike cyst containing brain tissue, cerebrospinal fluid, and meninges that protrudes through a congenital defect in the skull. The anomaly may or may not contain portions of the ventricular system and is commonly associated with defects in the brain. Also called **encephalomeningocele.** See also **neural tube defect.**

meningomyelocele. See **myelomeningocele.**

meniscectomy /men'isek'təmē/, surgical excision of one of the crescent-shaped cartilages of the knee joint, performed when a torn cartilage results in chronic pain and in instability or locking of the joint. Under low spinal or general anesthesia, the torn cartilage is freed and removed, and an elastic compression bandage is applied. After surgery, the leg is kept elevated to reduce swelling and exercises are performed to maintain muscle strength. Crutch walking usually begins about the fourth day and full ambulation about the twelfth day.

meniscocystosis. See **sickle cell anemia.**

meniscus /minis′kəs/, **1.** the interface between a liquid and air. **2.** a lens with both convex and concave aspects. **3.** a curved, fibrous cartilage in the knees and other joints. See also **meniscectomy.**

Menke's kinky hair syndrome /men′kēz/, a familial disorder affecting the normal absorption of copper from the intestine, characterized by the growth of sparse, kinky hair. Infants with the syndrome suffer cerebral degeneration, retarded growth, and early death. Early diagnosis and intravenous administration of copper may prevent irreversible damage.

meno-, a combining form meaning 'of or related to the menses': *menolipsis, menopause, menorrhea.*

menometrorrhagia /men′ōmet′rōrā′jē·ə/, excessive menstrual and uterine bleeding other than that caused by menstruation. It is a combination of metrorrhagia and menorrhagia and may be a sign of a urogenital malignancy, especially cancer of the cervix.

menopause /men′əpôz/, strictly, the cessation of menses, but commonly used to refer to the period of the female climacteric. Menses stop naturally with the decline of cyclic hormonal production and function between 45 and 60 years of age but may stop earlier in life as a result of illness or the surgical removal of the uterus or both ovaries. As the production of ovarian estrogen and pituitary gonadotropins decreases, ovulation and menstruation become less frequent and eventually stop. Fluctuations in the circulating levels of these hormones occur as the levels decline. Hot flashes are the only nearly universal symptom of the menopause. They can often be controlled with estrogen but are seldom so severe as to require therapy and will cease in time without hormonal treatment. Occasionally, heavy irregular bleeding occurs at this time, usually associated with myomata (fibroids) or other uterine pathologic condition. Estrogens given in large parenteral doses may be effective, but hysterectomy is sometimes required for control of the bleeding. Formerly—and incorrectly—emotional and psychologic turmoil was expected with the menopause and attributed to it. Symptoms of this sort that are coincidental with the cessation of the menses are unusual and are not attributable to it. The nurse can be of help to patients, menopausal or not, by encouraging them to identify properly the source of their discomfort, by counseling, and by referral to an appropriate specialist.

menorrhagia /men′ərā′jē·ə/, abnormally heavy or long menstrual periods. Menorrhagia occurs occasionally during the reproductive years of most women's lives. If the condition becomes chronic, anemia from recurrent excessive blood loss may result. Abnormal bleeding after menopause always warrants investigation to rule out malignancy. Menorrhagia is a relatively common complication of benign uterine fibromyomata; it may be so severe, or intractable, as to require hysterectomy. Also called **hypermenorrhea.** Compare **metrorrhagia, oligomenorrhea.** **–menorrhagic,** *adj.*

menorrhea /men′ôrē′ə/, the normal discharge of blood and tissue from the uterus. See also **menorrhagia, menstruation.**

menostasis /minos′təsis/, an abnormal condition in which the products of menstruation cannot escape the uterus or vagina because of stenosis, an occlusion of the cervix, or the introitus of the vagina. An imperforate hymen is a rare cause of menostasis. **–menostatic,** *adj.*

menotropins, a preparation of gonadotropic hormones from the urine of postmenopausal women.

■ INDICATION: It is prescribed with chorionic gonadotropin to induce ovulation.

■ CONTRAINDICATIONS: Elevated gonadotropin levels in the urine, thyroid or adrenal dysfunction, pituitary tumor, abnormal bleeding, ovarian cysts, pregnancy, or known hypersensitivity to this drug prohibits its use.

■ ADVERSE EFFECTS: Among the more serious adverse reactions are ovarian hyperstimulation syndrome, hemoperitoneum, arterial thromboembolism, multiple gestation, and possible birth defects.

menoxenia, any abnormality relating to menstruation.

Menrium, a trademark for a fixed-combination drug for menopausal symptoms, containing esterified estrogens and a sedative (chlordiazepoxide).

menses /men′sēz/, the normal flow of blood and decidua that occurs during menstruation. The first day of the flow of the menses is the first day of the menstrual cycle. Also called **catamenia.**

menstrual age, the age of an embryo or fetus as calculated from the first day of the last menstrual period.

menstrual cycle, the recurring cycle of change in the endometrium during which the decidual layer of the endometrium is shed, then regrows, proliferates, is maintained for several days, and sheds again at menstruation. The average length of the cycle, from the first day of bleeding of one cycle to the first of another, is 28 days. The length, duration, and character vary greatly among women. Menstrual cycles begin at menarche and end with menopause. The three phases of the cycle are the **proliferative phase, secretory phase,** and **menstrual phase.** See also **oogenesis.**

menstrual phase, the final of the three phases of the menstrual cycle, the one in which menstruation occurs. The necrotic mucosa of the endometrium is shed, leaving the stratum basale; bleeding, primarily from the spiral arteries, occurs. The average blood loss is 30 ml. For convenience, the days of the menstrual cycle are counted from the first day of the menstrual phase. Compare **proliferative phase, secretory phase.**

menstrual sponge, a small natural sponge or a piece of a sponge of synthetic material to which a loop of string is attached. It is inserted in the vagina to absorb the menstrual flow and is removed by pulling the string. It may be washed, squeezed dry, and reused as necessary through menstruation. Menstrual sponges are not commonly used and are not easily available.

menstruation, the periodic discharge through the vagina of a bloody secretion containing tissue debris from the shedding of the endometrium from the nonpregnant uterus. The average duration of menstruation is 4 to 5 days and it recurs at approximately 4-week intervals throughout the reproductive life of nonpregnant women. Kinds of menstruation are **anovular menstruation, retrograde menstruation,** and **vicarious menstruation.** See also **menstrual cycle.** **–menstruate,** *v.*

ment-, a combining form meaning 'mind': *mental, menticide, mentimeter.*

mental[1], **1.** of, relating to, or characteristic of the mind or psyche. **2.** existing in the mind; performed or accomplished by the mind. **3.** of, relating to, or characterized by a disorder of the mind.

mental[2], of or pertaining to the chin.

mental age (MA), the age level at which one functions intellectually, as determined by standardized psychologic and intelligence tests and expressed as the age at which that level is average. Compare **achievement age.** See also **developmental age.**

mental deficiency. See **mental retardation.**

mental disorder, any disturbance of emotional equilibrium, as manifested in maladaptive behavior and impaired functioning, caused by genetic, physical, chemical, biologic, psychologic, or social and cultural factors. Also called **emotional illness, mental illness, psychiatric disorder.**

mental handicap, any mental defect or characteristic resulting from a congenital abnormality, traumatic injury, or disease that impairs normal intellectual functioning and prevents a person from participating normally in activities appropriate for a particular age group. See also **mental retardation.**

mental health, a relative state of mind in which a person who is healthy is able to cope with and adjust to the recurrent stresses of everyday living in an acceptable way.

Mental Health Association (MHA), a voluntary, nonprofessional agency dedicated to the improvement of mental health facilities and services in community clinics and hospitals, the recruitment and training of volunteers, and the promotion of mental health legislation. Formerly called the **National Association for Mental Health.**

mental health nursing. See **psychiatric nursing.**

mental health service, any one of a group of government, professional, or lay organizations operating at a community, state, national, or international level to aid in the prevention and treatment of mental disorders. See also **community mental health center.**

mental hygiene, the study concerned with the development of healthy mental and emotional habits, attitudes, and behavior and with the prevention of mental illness. Also called **psychophylaxis.**

mental illness. See **mental disorder.**

mental image, any concept or sensation produced in the mind through memory or imagination.

mentality, **1.** the functional power and the capacity of the mind. **2.** intellectual character.

mental retardation, a disorder characterized by subaverage general intellectual function with deficits or impairments in the ability to learn and to adapt socially. The cause may be genetic, biologic, psychosocial, or sociocultural. The disorder, which is twice as prevalent among men as among women, is classified according to the intelligence quotient: borderline, IQ 71 to 84; mild, IQ 50 to 70; moderate, IQ 35 to 49; severe, IQ 20 to 34; and profound, IQ below 20. Treatment consists of educational programs and training specific to the level of retardation. Emphasis is placed on preventive measures, such as genetic counseling, amniocentesis, and general health care for pregnant women and for the baby after delivery, especially for the socially disadvantaged and other high-risk groups. Also called *(obsolete)* **feeblemindedness, mental deficiency.** See also **Down's syndrome, Hurler's syndrome, phenylketonuria, Tay-Sachs disease.**

mental ridge, (in dentistry) a dense elevation that extends from the symphysis to the premolar area on the anterolateral aspect of the body of the mandible.

mental status, the degree of competence shown by a person in intellectual, emotional, psychologic, and personality functioning as measured by psychologic testing with reference to a statistic norm. See also **mental status examination.**

mental status examination, a diagnostic procedure for determining the mental status of a person. The trained interviewer poses certain questions in a carefully standardized manner and evaluates the verbal responses and behavioral reactions.

mentation /mentā′shən/, any mental activity, including conscious and unconscious processes.

menthol, a topical antipruritic with a cooling effect that relieves itching. It is an ingredient in many topical creams and ointments.

mentholated camphor, a mixture of equal parts of camphor and menthol, used as a local counterirritant.

-mentia, a combining form meaning '(condition of the) mind': *dementia, moramentia, pseudodementia.*

menton, the most inferior point on the chin in the lateral view. It is a cephalometric landmark.

mentor, an older, trusted adviser or counselor who offers helpful guidance to younger colleagues.

mentum /men′təm/, the chin, especially of the fetus.

menu, a list of optional computer applications displayed for selection by the operator, who indicates the next action to be taken by signaling through the keyboard or another device a choice of the options.

mepenzolate bromide, an anticholinergic agent.

■ INDICATIONS: It is prescribed in the treatment of GI hypermotility and as an adjunct in treating peptic ulcer.

■ CONTRAINDICATIONS: Narrow-angle glaucoma, asthma, obstruction of the genitourinary or GI tract, severe

ulcerative colitis, or known hypersensitivity to this drug prohibits its use.
■ ADVERSE EFFECTS: Blurred vision, central nervous system effects, tachycardia, dry mouth, decreased sweating, or hypersensitivity reactions may occur.

Mepergan, a trademark for a central nervous system fixed-combination drug containing a narcotic analgesic (meperidine hydrochloride) and an antihistaminic (promethazine hydrochloride).

meperidine hydrochloride, a narcotic analgesic.
■ INDICATIONS: It is used to treat moderate to severe pain and as preoperative medication to relieve pain and allay anxiety.
■ CONTRAINDICATIONS: It is used with caution in many conditions, including head injuries, asthma, impaired renal or hepatic function, or unstable cardiovascular status. Concomitant use of a monoamine oxidase inhibitor or known hypersensitivity to this drug prohibits its use.
■ ADVERSE EFFECTS: Among the most serious adverse reactions are drowsiness, dizziness, nausea, constipation, sweating, respiratory and circulatory depression, and drug addiction.

mephenesin /mifen′isin/, a curare-like skeletal muscle relaxant sometimes prescribed in the relief of muscle spasm.

mephenytoin /mifen′ətō′in/, an anticonvulsant.
■ INDICATION: It is prescribed for the control of seizures in epilepsy when less toxic medications have not been effective.
■ CONTRAINDICATIONS: It is not usually recommended in pregnancy. Known hypersensitivity to this drug or to any hydantoin prohibits its use.
■ ADVERSE EFFECTS: Among the most serious adverse reactions are morbilliform rash, fever, hepatotoxicity, and various blood dyscrasias. The frequent occurrence of adverse reactions limits the use of this drug.

mephobarbital /mef′ōbär′bitol/, an anticonvulsant and sedative.
■ INDICATIONS: It is prescribed in the treatment of anxiety, nervous tension, insomnia, and epilepsy.
■ CONTRAINDICATIONS: Porphyria or known hypersensitivity to this drug or to barbiturates prohibits its use.
■ ADVERSE EFFECTS: Among the more serious adverse reactions are drug dependence, deficiency in vitamin D, paradoxical excitement, skin rash, and GI disturbance.

Mephyton, a trademark for a vitamin K product (phytonadione).

meprednisone, an oral glucocorticoid prescribed in the treatment of a large number of inflammatory conditions.

meprobamate /miprō′bəmāt/, a sedative.
■ INDICATIONS: It is prescribed in the treatment of anxiety and tension and as a muscle relaxant.
■ CONTRAINDICATIONS: Intermittent porphyria or known hypersensitivity to this drug or to the chemically related drugs tybamate, mebutamate, and carisoprodol prohibits its use.
■ ADVERSE EFFECTS: Among the most serious adverse reactions are exacerbation of intermittent porphyria, augmentation of effects of other central nervous system depressants, and various allergic reactions. Drowsiness and ataxia commonly occur.

mEq, abbreviation for **milliequivalent.**

-mer, -mere, a combining form meaning 'part, portion': *isomer, monomer*.

meralgia /miral′jə/, the presence of pain in the thigh.

meralgia paresthetica /per′esthet′ikə/, a condition characterized by pain, paresthesia, and numbness on the lateral surface of the thigh in the region supplied by the lateral femoral cutaneous nerve. The cause of the condition is ischemia of the nerve caused by its entrapped position in the inguinal ligament.

mercaptomerin sodium /mur′kaptom′ərin/, a rarely used diuretic.

mercaptopurine, an antineoplastic and immunosuppressive.
■ INDICATIONS: It is prescribed in the treatment of a variety of malignant neoplastic diseases, including acute lymphocytic leukemia.
■ CONTRAINDICATIONS: Known hypersensitivity to this drug prohibits its use.
■ ADVERSE EFFECTS: Among the more severe adverse reactions are bone marrow depression and acute GI disturbances, including nausea, vomiting, diarrhea, and stomatitis.

mercurial /mərkyŏŏr′ē•əl/, **1.** of or pertaining to mercury, particularly a medicine containing the element mercury. **2.** an adverse effect associated with the administration of a mercurial medication, as a mercurial tremor caused by mercury poisoning.

mercurial diuretic, any one of several diuretic agents that contain mercury in an organic chemical form. Mercurial diuretics inhibit tubular reabsorption of sodium and chloride and the excretion of potassium but do not produce diuresis in patients who are in metabolic alkalosis. The principal use for the drugs is in treating edema of cardiac origin, ascites associated with cirrhosis, or oliguria in the nephrotic stage of glomerulonephritis. Response usually begins within 1 to 2 hours and lasts for 12 hours. Immediate fatal reactions have occurred, usually because of ventricular failure after intravascular injection and transient high concentration of mercury in the blood. Flushing, urticaria, fever, and nausea and vomiting are common side effects. Thrombocytopenia, neutropenia, agranulocytosis, systemic mercury poisoning, and severe hypersensitivity reactions are among the more serious adverse effects of the mercurial diuretics: the drugs are contraindicated for use in the presence of renal insufficiency or acute nephritis. Because of the toxicity of these drugs, current practice usually recommends their replacement with more convenient and less toxic diuretics.

mercurialism. See **mercury poisoning.**

-mercuric, a combining form meaning 'molecules of bivalent mercury or its compounds': *phenylmercuric, potassiomercuric, trimercuric.*

mercury (Hg), a metallic element. Its atomic number is 80; its atomic weight is 200.6. It is the only common metal that is liquid at room temperature, and it occurs in nature almost entirely in the form of its sulfide, cinnabar. Mercury is produced commercially and is used in dental amalgams, thermometers, barometers, and other measuring instruments. It forms many poisonous compounds. The air, soil, and water in many areas of the world have become contaminated by mercury because of the burning of fossil fuels that contain the element and because of the greater use of mercury in industry and agriculture. The major toxic forms of this metal are mercury vapor, mercuric salts, and organic mercurials. Elemental mercury is only mildly toxic when ingested, because it is poorly absorbed. The vapor of elemental mercury, however, is readily absorbed through the lungs and enters the brain before it is oxidized. The kidneys retain mercury longer than any of the other body tissues.

mercury poisoning, a toxic condition caused by the ingestion or inhalation of mercury or a mercury compound. The chronic form, resulting from inhalation of the vapors or dust of mercurial compounds or from repeated ingestion of very small amounts, is characterized by irritability, excessive saliva, loosened teeth, gum disorders, slurred speech, tremors, and staggering. Symptoms of acute mercury poisoning appear in a few to 30 minutes and include a metallic taste in the mouth, thirst, nausea, vomiting, severe abdominal pain, bloody diarrhea, and renal failure that may result in death. The presence of mercury in the body is determined by a urine test. Treatment may include gastric lavage with milk and egg white or sodium bicarbonate, chelation with British antilewisite (BAL), and fluid therapy. Free mercury, as in thermometers, is not absorbed in the GI tract, but because it is very volatile, hazardous vapors may penetrate ordinary toxic dust respirators, causing poisoning by inhalation. Mercury compounds are found in agricultural fungicides and in certain antiseptics and pigments; they are used extensively in industry. Industrial wastes containing mercury have been identified in some areas, and seafood from contaminated waters have caused serious public health problems. Also called **hydrargyrism, mercurialism.** See also **Minamata disease.**

mercy killing. See **euthanasia.**

merergasia /mer′ərgā′zhə/, a mild mental incapacity characterized by some emotional instability and some anxiety. –**merergastic,** *adj.*

merethoxylline procaine, a diuretic.

-meria, a combining form meaning '(condition of) parts': *platymeria, polymeria.*

merisis /mer′isis/, an increase in size as a result of cell division and the addition of new material rather than of cell expansion. Also called **multiplicative growth.** Compare **auxesis.** See also **hyperplasia.**

mero-, a combining form meaning 'part': *meroacrania, merocyte, meropia.*

meroblastic /mer′əblas′tik/, pertaining to or characterizing an ovum that contains a large amount of yolk and in which cleavage is restricted to a part of the cytoplasm. Compare **holoblastic.**

meromelia /mer′əmē′lyə/, a general designation for the congenital absence of any part of a limb. It is used in reference to such conditions as adactyly, hemimelia, or phocomelia. Compare **amelia.**

merozoite /mer′əzō′īt/, an organism produced from segmentation of a schizont during the asexual reproductive phase of the life cycle of a sporozoan, specifically the malarial parasite *Plasmodium*. Merozoites can either continue the asexual phase of the life cycle by developing into trophozoites and repeating the process of schizogony, or differentiate into male and female gametes and enter the sexual stage. See also ***Plasmodium.***

Merrifield's knife, a surgical knife with a long, narrow, triangular blade set into a shank, used for gingivectomy incisions.

mersalyl and theophylline, a mercurial diuretic.

■ INDICATION: It is prescribed in the treatment of edema.

■ CONTRAINDICATIONS: Nephritis, ulcerative colitis, dehydration, severe liver disease, or known hypersensitivity to mercury or theophylline prohibits its use.

■ ADVERSE EFFECTS: Among the most serious adverse reactions are renal failure and hemorrhagic colitis after prolonged use. GI symptoms, rashes and other allergic reactions, and electrolyte disturbances also may occur.

■ NOTE: It is not to be given subcutaneously.

Merthiolate, a trademark for a topical antiinfective (thimerosal).

Meruvax, a trademark for an active immunizing agent (live rubella virus vaccine).

Mesantoin, a trademark for an anticonvulsant (mephenytoin).

mescaline /mes′kəlēn, -lin/, a psychoactive, poisonous alkaloid derived from a colorless alkaline oil in the flowering heads of the cactus *Lophophora williamsii*. Closely related chemically to epinephrine, mescaline causes heart palpitations, diaphoresis, pupillary dilatation, and anxiety. The drug, taken in capsules or dissolved in a drink, produces visual hallucinations, as color patterns and spatial distortions, but it does not ordinarily induce disorientation. Several Native American nations of North America used mescaline in religious ceremonies to produce euphoria and a feeling of ecstasy. Also called **peyote.**

mesencephalon /mes′ensef′əlon/, one of the three parts of the brainstem, lying just below the cerebrum and just above the pons. It consists primarily of white substance with some gray substance around the cerebral aqueduct. A red nucleus lies within the reticular formation of the mesencephalon and contains the terminations of fibers from the cerebellum and the frontal lobe of the cerebral cortex. The ventral part of the mesencephalon is formed by the cerebral peduncles; the dorsal part is formed by the corpora quadrigemina. The cerebral peduncles are two twisted masses of white substance that extend from the pons to the undersurface of the cerebral hemispheres. Deep within the mesencephalon are nuclei of the third and the fourth cranial nerves and the anterior part of the fifth cranial nerve. The mesencephalon also contains nuclei for certain auditory and certain visual reflexes. Also called **midbrain.** **–mesencephalic** /mes′ensi-fal′ik/, *adj.*

mesenchymal chondrosarcoma /meseng′kəməl/, a malignant cartilaginous tumor that develops in many sites.

mesenchyme /mes′engkīm/, a diffuse network of tissue derived from the embryonic mesoderm. It consists of stellate cells embedded in gelatinous ground substance with reticular fibers.

mesenchymoma /mes′engkimō′mə/, a mixed mesenchymal neoplasm composed of two or more cellular elements not usually associated and fibrous tissue. See also **benign mesenchymoma, malignant mesenchymoma.**

mesenteric adenitis. See **adenitis.**

mesenteric node, a node in one of three groups of superior mesenteric lymph glands serving parts of the intestine. An average of 125 mesenteric nodes in three different groups lie between the layers of the mesentery. The first group lies close to the wall of the small intestine, among the terminal twigs of the superior mesenteric artery. The second group is located in relation to the loops and primary branches of the artery. The third group lies along the trunk of the artery. The mesenteric nodes receive afferents from the jejunum, ileum, cecum, vermiform appendix, ascending colon, and transverse colon. Their efferents pass to the preaortic nodes. Compare **ileocolic node, mesocolic node.**

mesentery proper, a broad, fan-shaped fold of peritoneum connecting the jejunum and the ileum with the dorsal wall of the abdomen. The root of the mesentery proper is about 15 cm long and is connected to certain structures ventral to the vertebral column. The intestinal border of the mesentery proper is about 6 m long and separates to enclose the intestine. The cranial part of the mesentery is narrow but widens to about 20 cm and suspends the small intestine and various nerves and arteries. Compare **sigmoid mesocolon, transverse mesocolon.**

mesial. See **medial.**

mesiocclusion, an occlusal relationship in which the lower teeth are positioned mesially.

mesiodens, a supernumerary erupted or unerupted tooth that develops between two maxillary central incisors.

mesioversion, **1.** a condition in which one or more teeth are closer than normal to the midline. **2.** a condition in which the maxillae or mandible is postioned more anteriorly than normal.

meso-, **1.** a combining form meaning 'middle': *mesocardium, mesocecum, mesoderm.* **2.** a combining form meaning 'inactive or without effect on polarized light': *mesomerism, meson, mesoporphyrin.*

mesocolic node /mes′ōkol′ik/, a node in one of three groups of superior mesenteric lymph glands, proliferating between the layers of the transverse mesocolon, close to the transverse colon. They are best developed near the right and the left colic flexures and receive afferents from the jejunum, ileum, cecum, vermiform appendix, ascending colon, and transverse colon. Their efferents pass to the preaortic nodes. Compare **mesenteric node.**

mesocolopexy /mes′ōkō′ləpek′sē/, suspension or fixation of the mesocolon.

mesoderm /mes′ōdurm/, (in embryology) the middle of the three cell layers of the developing embryo. It lies between the ectoderm and the endoderm. Bone, connective tissue, muscle, blood, vascular and lymphatic tissue, and the pleurae of the pericardium and peritoneum are all derived from the mesoderm.

mesoglia. See **microglia.**

mesometritis. See **myometritis.**

mesomorph /mes′əmôrf′/, a person whose physique is characterized by a predominance of muscle, bone, and connective tissue, structures that develop from the mesodermal layer of the embryo. Compare **ectomorph, endomorph.** See also **athletic habitus.**

mesonephric duct, (in embryology) a duct that, in the male, gives rise to the ducts of the reproductive system (ductus epididymidis, ductus deferens, seminal vesicle, ejaculatory duct). In the female, it persists vestigially as **Gartner's duct.** Also called **wolffian duct.**

mesonephric tubule, any of the embryonic renal tubules comprising the mesonephros. They function as excretory structures during the early embryonic development of humans and other mammals but are later incorporated into the reproductive system. In males the tubules give rise to the efferent and aberrant ductules of the testes, the appendix epididymis, and paradidymis, and in females to the epoophoron, paroophoron, and vesicular appendices. All of the structures are vestigial except the efferent ductules of the testes.

mesonephros, *pl.* **mesonephroi, mesonephra,** the second type of excretory organ to develop in the vertebrate embryo. It consists of a series of twisting tubules that arise from the nephrogenic cord caudal to the pronephros and that at one end form the glomerulus and at the other connect with the excretory mesonephric duct. The organ is the permanent kidney in lower animals, but in humans and various other mammals it is functional only during early embryonic development and is later replaced by the metanephros, although the duct system is retained and incorporated into the male reproductive system. Also called **mesonephron, middle kidney, wolffian body.** See also **metanephros, pronephros.** **–mesonephric, mesonephroid,** *adj.*

mesoridazine besylate, a phenothiazine tranquilizer.
■ INDICATIONS: It is prescribed in the treatment of psychotic disorders, behavioral problems in mental deficiency, and alcoholism.

■ CONTRAINDICATIONS: Parkinson's disease, concurrent administration of central nervous system depressants, liver or renal dysfunction, severe hypotension, or known hypersensitivity to this drug or to other phenothiazine medications prohibits its use.

■ ADVERSE EFFECTS: Among the more serious adverse effects are hypotension, liver toxicity, a variety of extrapyramidal reactions, persistent tardive dyskinesia, blood dyscrasias, and hypersensitivity reactions.

mesosalpinx /mes′ōsal′pingks/, the cephalic, free border of the broad ligament in which the uterine tubes lie.

mesothelioma /mes′ōthē′lē·ō′mə/, *pl.* **mesotheliomas, mesotheliomata,** a rare, malignant tumor of the mesothelium of the pleura or peritoneum, associated with earlier exposure to asbestos. The lesion, composed of spindle cells or fibrous tissue, may form thick sheets covering the viscera. The prognosis is poor. Also called **celothelioma.**

mesothelium /mes′ōthē′lē·əm/, a layer of cells that lines the body cavities of the embryo and continues as a layer of squamous epithelial cells covering the serous membranes of the adult.

messenger RNA (mRNA), (in molecular genetics) an RNA fraction that transmits information from DNA to the protein-synthesizing ribosomes of cells.

Mestinon, a trademark for a neuromuscular blocking agent (pyridostigmine), used as an adjunct to anesthesia and in the treatment of myasthenia gravis.

mestranol /mes′trənōl/, an estrogen prescribed in fixed-combination drugs with a progestin as an oral contraceptive.

Met, abbreviation for **methionine.**

MET, abbreviation for **metabolic equivalent.**

meta-, **1.** a combining form meaning 'change or exchange': *metabasis, metallaxis, metamorphosis*. **2.** a combining form meaning 'after or next': *metachemical, metapneumonic, metapsychics*. **3.** a combining form meaning 'the 1, 3 position in derivative of benzine': *metacetone, metachloridine, metacresol*.

metabolic /met′əbol′ik/, of or pertaining to **metabolism.**

metabolic acidosis, acidosis in which excess acid is added to the body fluids or bicarbonate is lost from them. In starvation and in uncontrolled diabetes mellitus, glucose is not present or is not available for oxidation for cellular nutrition. The plasma bicarbonate of the body is used up in neutralizing the ketones that result from the breakdown of body fat for energy that occurs in compensation for the lack of glucose. Metabolic acidosis also occurs when oxidation takes place without adequate oxygen, as in heart failure or shock. Severe diarrhea, renal failure, and lactic acidosis also may result in metabolic acidosis. Hyperkalemia often accompanies the condition.

metabolic alkalosis, an abnormal condition characterized by the significant loss of acid in the body or by increased levels of base bicarbonate. The reduction of acid may be caused by excessive vomiting, insufficient replacement of electrolytes, hyperadrenocorticism, and Cushing's disease. A decrease in base bicarbonate may be caused by various problems, as the ingestion of excessive bicarbonate of soda and other antacids during the treatment of peptic ulcers, and by the administration of excessive intravenous fluids containing high concentrations of bicarbonate. Severe, untreated metabolic alkalosis can lead to coma and death. Compare **respiratory alkalosis.** See also **metabolic acidosis, respiratory acidosis.**

■ OBSERVATIONS: Signs and symptoms of metabolic alkalosis may include apnea, headache, lethargy, irritability, nausea, vomiting, and atrial tachycardia. Confirmation of the diagnosis is commonly based on laboratory findings that show a blood pH level greater than 7.45, a carbonic acid concentration greater than 29 mEq/L, and alkaline urine. The electrocardiogram of a patient with this condition may show atrial tachycardia with a low T wave merging with a P wave.

■ INTERVENTION: Treatment seeks to eliminate the underlying cause of alkalosis and may include the intravenous administration of ammonium chloride to release hydrogen chloride and restore chloride levels. Potassium chloride and normal saline solutions usually replace fluid losses from gastric drainage but are contraindicated in patients with associated congestive heart failure.

■ NURSING CONSIDERATIONS: Nurses closely monitor the status of the patient and cautiously administer any prescribed intravenous solutions. The intravenous administration of ammonium chloride is usually contraindicated in patients with liver or kidney disease. Too rapid infusion of ammonium chloride may hemolyze the red blood cells, and excessive dosage may overcorrect alkalosis and cause acidosis. The fluid intake and output of the patient are carefully noted, and the respiration rate is regularly checked. Decreased respiratory rate indicates an effort to compensate for alkalosis.

metabolic component, the bicarbonate component of plasma.

metabolic disorder, any pathophysiologic dysfunction that results in a loss of metabolic control of homeostasis in the body.

metabolic equivalent (MET), the amount of oxygen consumed per kilogram of body weight per minute when an individual is at rest.

metabolic rate, the amount of energy liberated or expended in a given unit of time. Energy is stored in the body in energy-rich phosphate compounds (adenosine triphosphate, adenosine monophosphate, and adenosine diphosphate) and in proteins, fats, and complex carbohydrates. See also **basal metabolic rate.**

metabolic respiratory quotient (R), the ratio of production of CO_2 to the corresponding consumption of O_2. The values of R change according to the fuel being burned; thus, because fat contains relatively little O_2 compared with glucose, the R of fat is lower than that of glucose, whereas the R of protein is between that of glucose and fat.

metabolism, the aggregate of all chemical processes that take place in living organisms, resulting in growth, generation of energy, elimination of wastes, and other bodily functions as they relate to the distribution of nutrients in the blood after digestion. Metabolism takes place in two steps: anabolism, the constructive phase, in which smaller molecules (as amino acids) are converted to larger molecules (as proteins); and catabolism, the destructive phase, in which larger molecules (as glycogen) are converted to smaller molecules (as pyruvic acid). Exercise, elevated body temperature, hormonal activity, and digestion can increase the metabolic rate, which is the rate determined when a person is at complete rest, physically and mentally. The metabolic rate is customarily expressed (in calories) as the heat liberated in the course of metabolism. See also **acid-base metabolism, anabolism, basal metabolism, catabolism.**

metabolite /mitab′əlīt/, a substance produced by metabolic action or necessary for a metabolic process. An essential metabolite is one required for a vital metabolic process.

metacarpus /met′əkär′pəs/, the middle portion of the hand, consisting of five slender bones numbered from the thumb side, metacarpals I through V. Each metacarpal consists of a body and two extremities. **–metacarpal,** *adj., n.*

metacentric /met′əsen′trik/, pertaining to a chromosome in which the centromere is located near the center so that the arms of the chromatids are of approximately equal length. Compare **acrocentric, submetacentric, telocentric.**

metacommunication, communication that indicates how verbal communication should be interpreted. It may support or contradict verbal communication.

metagenesis /met′əjen′əsis/, the regular alternation of sexual with asexual methods of reproduction within the same species. **–metagenetic, metagenic,** *adj.*

Metahydrin, a trademark for a diuretic and antihypertensive (trichlormethiazide).

metal, any element that conducts heat and electricity, is malleable and ductile, and forms positively charged ions (cations) in solution.

metal fume fever, an occupational disorder caused by the inhalation of fumes of metallic oxides and characterized by symptoms similar to those of influenza. The condition occurs among workers engaged in welding, metal fabrication, casting, and other occupations dealing with the manipulation of metals. Access to fresh air and treatment of the symptoms usually alleviate the condition. Also called **brass founder's ague, zinc chill.** Compare **siderosis.**

metamorphopsia /met′əmôrfop′sē·ə/, a defect in vision in which objects are seen as distorted in shape, resulting from disease of the retina or imperfection of the media.

metamorphosis /met′əmôr′fəsis/, a change in shape or structure, especially a change from one stage of development to another, as the transition from the larval to the adult stage.

metamyelocyte /met′əmī′əlōsīt′/, a stage in the development of the granulocyte series of leukocytes. It is intermediate between the myelocyte stage and the mature granulocyte. See also **leukocyte, myeloblast, myelocyte.**

Metandren, a trademark for an androgen (methyltestosterone).

metanephrine /met′ənef′rin/, one of the two principal urinary metabolites of epinephrine and norepinephrine in the urine, the other being vanillylmandelic acid. The 24-hour normal value for total metanephrine is 1.3 mg. Normally, less than 1.3 mg of metanephrine is excreted in 24 hours.

metanephrogenic /met′ənef′rəjen′ik/, capable of forming the metanephros, or fetal kidney.

metanephros, *pl.* **metanephroi, metanephra,** the third, and permanent, excretory organ to develop in the vertebrate embryo. It consists of a complex structure of secretory and collecting tubules that develop into the kidney and are formed later than the mesonephros from the caudal end of the nephrogenic cord and the mesonephric duct. In most mammals there is limited functional use of the metanephric kidney during fetal life, because waste materials are transferred across the placenta to the mother for elimination. Also called **metanephron, hind kidney.** See also **kidney, mesonephros, pronephros.**

metaphase /met′əfāz/, the second of the four stages of nuclear division in mitosis and in each of the two divisions of meiosis, during which the chromosomes become arranged in the equatorial plane of the spindle to form the equatorial plate, with the centromeres attached to the spindle fibers in preparation for separation. See also **anaphase, interphase, meiosis, mitosis, prophase, telophase.**

metaphyseal dysostosis /mətaf′izē′əl, met′əfiz′ē·əl/, an abnormal condition that affects the skeletal system and is characterized by a disturbance of the mineralization of the metaphyseal area of the bones, resulting in dwarfism. Metaphyseal dysostosis is classified as the Gansen type, Schmidt type, Spahar-Hartmann type, or cartilage-hair hypoplasia. The Gansen type is characterized by metaphyseal alterations similar to those of achondroplasia but not involving the skull or the epiphyses of the long bones. The Schmidt type of metaphyseal dysostosis is characterized by developmental changes from the weight-bearing age to approximately 5 years of age. The metaphyseal alterations associated with the Schmidt type are similar to those of achondroplasia, resulting in moderate dwarfism. The Spahar-Hartmann type is characterized by skeletal changes and severe genu varum. Cartilage-hair hypoplasia is characterized by severe dwarfism and hair that is sparse, short, and brittle. Mental retardation is not usually associated with metaphyseal dysostosis. Radiographic examination of all types of the disease reveals characteristic widening of the metaphyses of the tubular bones, with normal diaphyseal and epiphyseal ossification centers. Treatment is supportive and symptomatic with no specific modality.

metaphyseal dysplasia, an abnormal condition characterized by disordered modeling of the cylindric bones. The involvement of this disease is limited to the long bones and displays a characteristic radiographic image of the ''Erlenmeyer flask'' deformity in which the metaphyseal circumference is enlarged and the medullary area of the affected bone is reduced. Metaphyseal dysplasia most often affects the distal femur or the proximal tibia.

metaphysis /mətaf'əsis/, a region of bone in which diaphysis and epiphysis converge.

Metaprel, a trademark for a bronchodilator (metaproterenol sulfate).

metaproterenol sulfate /met'əprōter'inôl/, a beta-adrenergic bronchodilator.

■ INDICATION: It is prescribed in the treatment of bronchial asthma.

■ CONTRAINDICATIONS: Arrhythmias associated with tachycardia or known hypersensitivity to this drug prohibits its use.

■ ADVERSE EFFECTS: Among the more serious adverse reactions are tachycardia, hypertension, and cardiac arrest.

metaraminol bitartrate, an adrenergic vasopressor.

■ INDICATION: It is prescribed in the treatment of hypotension and shock.

■ CONTRAINDICATIONS: Known hypersensitivity to this drug prohibits its use. It is not used with cyclopropane or halothane anesthesia or as the sole drug for hypovolemic hypotension.

■ ADVERSE EFFECTS: Among the more serious adverse reactions are cardiac arrhythmia, tissue necrosis at the site of injection, hypertension, tremors, and nausea.

metaruricyte, a red blood cell possessing a nucleus. Such cells, usually normoblasts in their final stage, are not normally found in the blood of adults.

metastasis /mətas'təsis/, *pl.* **metastases** /-sēz/, **1.** the process by which tumor cells are spread to distant parts of the body. Because malignant tumors have no enclosing capsule, cells may escape, become emboli, and be transported by the lymphatic circulation or the bloodstream to implant on lymph nodes and other organs far from the primary tumor. **2.** a tumor that develops in this way. Compare **anaplasia.** –**metastatic,** *adj.*, **metastasize,** *v.*

metastasizing mole. See **chorioadenoma destruens.**

metastatic calcification, the pathologic process whereby calcium salts accumulate in previously healthy tissues. It is caused by excessive levels of blood calcium, as in hyperparathyroidism.

metastatic ophthalmia. See **sympathetic ophthalmia.**

metatarsal /met'ətär'səl/, **1.** of or pertaining to the metatarsus of the foot. **2.** any one of the five bones comprising the metatarsus.

metatarsalgia /met'ətärsal'jə/, a painful condition around the metatarsal bones caused by an abnormality of the foot or recalcification of degenerated heads of metatarsal bones. Also called **Morton's foot, Morton's neuroma, Morton's toe.**

metatarsal stress fracture, a break or rupture of a metatarsal bone, resulting from prolonged running or walking. The condition is often difficult to diagnose with x-ray films. Also called **fatigue fracture, march fracture.**

metatarsus, a part of the foot, consisting of five bones numbered I to V, from the medial side. Each bone has a long, slender body, a wedge-shaped proximal end, a convex distal end, and flattened, grooved sides for the attachment of ligaments. The metatarsal bones articulate with the tarsus proximally and the first row of phalanges distally. Kinds of metatarsus include **metatarsus valgus** and **metatarsus varus.** –**metatarsal,** *adj.*

metatarsus adductus. See metatarsus varus.

metatarsus valgus, a congenital deformity of the foot in which the forepart rotates outward away from the midline of the body and the heel remains straight. Also called **duck walk, toeing out.**

metatarsus varus, a congenital deformity of the foot in which the forepart rotates inward toward the midline of the body and the heel remains straight. Also called **intoe, metatarsus adductus, pigeon-toed, toeing in.**

Metatensin, a trademark for a cardiovascular, fixed-combination drug containing a diuretic (trichlormethiazide) and an antihypertensive (reserpine).

metathalamus /met'əthal'əməs/, one of five parts of the diencephalon. It is composed of a medial geniculate body and a lateral geniculate body on each side. The medial geniculate body acts as a relay station for nerve impulses between the inferior brachium and the auditory cortex. The lateral geniculate body is an oval bulge at the posterior end of the thalamus, which accommodates the terminal ends of the fibers of the optic tract. Compare **epithalamus, hypothalamus, subthalamus.** –**metathalamic,** *adj.*

metaxalone, a skeletal muscle relaxant.

■ INDICATION: It is prescribed as an adjunct in the treatment of acute skeletal muscle spasm.

■ CONTRAINDICATIONS: Significantly impaired renal or hepatic function, susceptibility to drug-induced hemolytic anemia, or known hypersensitivity to this drug prohibits its use.

■ ADVERSE EFFECTS: Among the more serious adverse reactions are hemolytic anemia, leukopenia, and liver dysfunction. GI disturbances, dizziness, and nervousness may occur.

metazoa, a category of multicellular animals whose cells have become differentiated into tissues and organs, particularly those possessing a digestive tract.

Metchnikoff's theory, a theory that living cells ingest microorganisms. The theory proved correct, as seen in the process of phagocytosis and the ingestion of injurious microbes by leukocytes.

meteorism, accumulation of gas in the abdomen or the intestine, usually with distention.

meteorotropism /mē'tē•ərətrō'pizəm/, a reaction to meteorologic influences shown by various biologic occurrences, as sudden death, attacks of arthritis, and angina. –**meteorotropic,** *adj.*

meter (m) /mē'tər/, a metric unit of length equal to 39.37 inches. Also spelled **metre.**

-meter, -metre **1.** /-m'ətər/ a combining form meaning a 'measuring instrument': *anesthesimeter, ionometer, scopometer.* **2.** /-mē'tər/ a combining form meaning 'length or measure': *centimeter, kilometer, millimeter.*

methacycline hydrochloride, a tetracycline antibiotic.

■ INDICATIONS: It is prescribed in the treatment of a variety of infections.

■ CONTRAINDICATIONS: Renal or liver dysfunction, pregnancy, early childhood, or known hypersensitivity to this drug or to other tetracycline medications prohibits its use.

■ ADVERSE EFFECTS: Among the more serious adverse reactions are GI disturbances, phototoxicity, potentially serious suprainfections, and hypersensitivity reactions. Discoloration of teeth may occur in children exposed to the drug in utero or before 8 years of age.

methadone, a synthetic narcotic analgesic.

■ INDICATIONS: It is prescribed for relief of severe pain, for treatment in detoxification, and in treatment programs for opiate-addicted patients.

■ CONTRAINDICATIONS: It is used with caution in many conditions, including head injuries, asthma, impaired renal or hepatic function, or unstable cardiovascular status. Known hypersensitivity to this drug prohibits its use.

■ ADVERSE EFFECTS: Among the more serious adverse reactions are drowsiness, dizziness, nausea, constipation, respiratory and circulatory depression, and drug addiction.

methadone hydrochloride, a narcotic analgesic used for anesthesia or as a substitute for heroin, permitting withdrawal without development of acute abstinence syndrome. Methadone does not produce marked euphoria, sedation, or narcosis. It is not given to pregnant women or to patients with liver disease.

methamphetamine sulfate, a central nervous system stimulant.

■ INDICATIONS: It is prescribed in the treatment of narcolepsy and hyperkinesis and to reduce the appetite in exogenous obesity.

■ CONTRAINDICATIONS: Glaucoma, arteriosclerosis, cardiovascular disease, hypertension, hyperthyroidism, history of drug abuse, concomitant use of a monoamine oxidase inhibitor, or known hypersensitivity to this drug or to other sympathomimetic drugs prohibits its use.

■ ADVERSE EFFECTS: Among the more serious adverse reactions are various manifestations of central nervous system excitation, increase in blood pressure, arrhythmia and other cardiovascular effects, nausea, and drug dependence.

methampyrone. See **dipyrone.**

methandriol, an anabolic hormone used as adjunctive therapy in senile and postmenopausal osteoporosis.

methandrostenolone /methan'drōsten'əlōn/, an androgen.

■ INDICATION: It is prescribed primarily in the treatment of osteoporosis.

■ CONTRAINDICATIONS: Cancer of the male breast or prostate, cardiac, renal, or hepatic disease, nephrosis, pregnancy, or known hypersensitivity to this drug prohibits its use.

■ ADVERSE EFFECTS: Among the more serious adverse reactions are various endocrine effects, depending on age of the patient. Hirsutism and masculinization are seen in women, and nausea and jaundice are common.

methanol, a clear, colorless, toxic, liquid distillate of wood miscible with water, alcohol, and ether. It is widely used as a solvent and in the production of formaldehyde. Ingestion of methanol paralyzes the optic nerve and may cause death. Also called **wood alcohol.**

methanol extractable residue, an immunotherapeutic substance, prepared from a methanol extracted fraction of the bacillus Calmette-Guérin (BCG). It is given to prevent or delay recurrences of Stage II malignant melanoma after surgery and to prolong drug-induced remissions in acute myelocytic leukemia.

methantheline bromide, an anticholinergic.

■ INDICATIONS: It is prescribed in the treatment of peptic ulcer and a wide variety of other GI disorders.

■ CONTRAINDICATIONS: Narrow-angle glaucoma, asthma, obstruction of the genitourinary or the GI tract, severe ulcerative colitis, or known hypersensitivity to this drug prohibits its use.

■ ADVERSE EFFECTS: Among the more serious adverse effects are blurred vision, central nervous system disturbances, tachycardia, dry mouth, decreased sweating, and hypersensitivity reactions.

methaqualone /methak'wəlōn/, a sedative-hypnotic.

■ INDICATIONS: It is prescribed in the treatment of anxiety and insomnia.

■ CONTRAINDICATIONS: It is not given to children or to pregnant women. Known hypersensitivity to this drug prohibits its use.

■ ADVERSE EFFECTS: Among the more serious adverse reactions are GI distress, drug hangover, peripheral neuropathy, loss of inhibition, and drug dependence.

metharbital, an anticonvulsant.

■ INDICATION: It is prescribed in the treatment of epilepsy.

■ CONTRAINDICATIONS: Porphyria or known hypersensitivity to barbiturates prohibits its use. It is prescribed with caution in pregnancy or hepatic impairment.

■ ADVERSE EFFECTS: Among the more serious adverse reactions are ataxia, irritability in children, and confusion in elderly patients. Rashes and other allergic reactions also may occur.

methazolamide, a carbonic anhydrase inhibitor.

■ INDICATION: It is prescribed in the treatment of glaucoma.

■ CONTRAINDICATIONS: Hyponatremia, hypokalemia, Addison's disease, severe pulmonary obstruction, adrenocortical insufficiency, or known hypersensitivity to this drug prohibits its use.

■ ADVERSE EFFECTS: Among the more serious adverse effects are aplastic anemia, drowsiness, paresthesia, hypersensitivity reactions, and acidosis.

methdilazine /methdil′əzēn/, a phenothiazine antihistamine.

■ INDICATION: It is prescribed to relieve itching.

■ CONTRAINDICATIONS: Asthma, glaucoma, or known hypersensitivity to this drug or to phenothiazine medications prohibits its use. It is not given to newborn infants or lactating mothers.

■ ADVERSE EFFECTS: Among the more serious adverse reactions are bone marrow depression and extrapyramidal reactions. Dry mouth and sedation commonly occur.

methemoglobin /met′hēməglō′bin, met•he′məglō′bin/, a form of hemoglobin in which the iron component has been oxidized from the ferrous to the ferric state. Methemoglobin cannot carry oxygen and so contributes nothing to the oxygen transporting capacity of the blood. Methemoglobin is a product of the various oxidative reactions that constitute normal metabolic activity. Normally present in only trace amounts (about 1%) in the blood, it is maintained at this level by an active enzymatic reducing capability, the NADH-methemoglobin reductase system present in normal red cells. See also **hemoglobin.**

methenamine, a urinary antibacterial.

■ INDICATION: It is prescribed in the treatment of urinary tract infections.

■ CONTRAINDICATIONS: Liver or kidney dysfunction or known hypersensitivity to this drug or to mandelic acid prohibits its use.

■ ADVERSE EFFECTS: Among the most serious adverse reactions are severe GI disturbances and rashes.

Methergine, a trademark for an oxytocic (methylergonovine maleate).

methicillin sodium, a penicillinase-resistant penicillin antibiotic.

■ INDICATION: It is prescribed primarily in the treatment of severe penicillinase-producing staphylococcal infection.

■ CONTRAINDICATIONS: Known hypersensitivity to this drug or to any penicillin prohibits its use.

■ ADVERSE EFFECTS: Among the more serious adverse reactions are phlebitis at the site of injection, nephritis, and allergic reactions.

methimazole, an inhibitor of thyroid hormone synthesis.

■ INDICATIONS: It is prescribed in the treatment of hyperthyroidism, in preparation for subtotal thyroidectomy, or for radioactive iodine therapy.

■ CONTRAINDICATION: Known hypersensitivity to this drug prohibits its use.

■ ADVERSE EFFECTS: Among the more serious adverse reactions are blood dyscrasias (particularly granulocytopenia) and hypersensitivity reactions resembling lupus erythematosus. Skin rash, pruritus, and GI distress commonly occur.

methionine (Met), an essential amino acid needed for proper growth in infants and for maintenance of nitrogen balance in adults. It is a source for methyl groups and sulfur in the body. It is also administered as adjunctive treatment in liver diseases. See also **amino acid, protein.**

methixene hydrochloride, an anticholinergic agent.

■ INDICATIONS: It is prescribed in the treatment of hypermotility or spasms of the GI tract.

■ CONTRAINDICATIONS: Narrow-angle glaucoma, asthma, obstruction of the genitourinary or GI tract, severe ulcerative colitis, or known hypersensitivity to this drug prohibits its use.

■ ADVERSE EFFECTS: Among the more serious adverse reactions are blurred vision, central nervous system effects, tachycardia, dry mouth, decreased sweating, and hypersensitivity reactions.

methocarbamol, a skeletal muscle relaxant.

■ INDICATION: It is prescribed in the treatment of skeletal muscle spasm.

■ CONTRAINDICATIONS: Renal dysfunction, central nervous system depression, or known hypersensitivity to this drug prohibits its use.

■ ADVERSE EFFECTS: Among the more serious adverse reactions are hypotension and tachycardia. Drowsiness, dizziness, vertigo, and nausea may occur.

method, a technique or procedure for producing a desired effect, as a surgical procedure, a laboratory test, or a diagnostic technique.

methodology, **1.** a system of principles or methods of procedure in any discipline, as education, research, diagnosis, or treatment. **–methodologic,** *adj.* **2.** the section of a research proposal in which the methods to be used are described. The research design, the population to be studied, and the research instruments, or tools, to be used are discussed in the methodology.

methohexital sodium /meth′ōhek′sitôl/, an intravenous barbiturate.

■ INDICATION: It is prescribed for the induction of anesthesia in short surgical procedures as a supplement to other anesthetics.

■ CONTRAINDICATIONS: Porphyria, status asthmaticus, or known hypersensitivity to this drug or to any barbiturate prohibits its use.

■ ADVERSE EFFECTS: Among the more serious adverse reactions are respiratory depression, skin rash, and cardiovascular dysfunction.

methotrexate, an antineoplastic antimetabolite.

■ INDICATIONS: It is prescribed in the treatment of severe psoriasis and a variety of malignant neoplastic diseases.

■ CONTRAINDICATIONS: Blood dyscrasias, severe renal or hepatic impairment, or known hypersensitivity to this drug prohibits its use.

■ ADVERSE EFFECTS: Among the more serious adverse reactions are diarrhea, ulcerative stomatis, bone marrow depression, hepatotoxicity, and skin rash.

methotrimeprazine /meth′ōtrīmep′rəzēn/, a phenothiazine analgesic.

■ INDICATION: It is prescribed for the relief of moderate to severe pain in bedridden patients.

■ CONTRAINDICATIONS: Concurrent administration of antihypertensives, hypotension, renal or hepatic disease, or known hypersensitivity to this drug or to phenothiazine medications prohibits its use.

■ ADVERSE EFFECTS: Among the more serious adverse reactions are orthostatic hypotension, dizziness, dry mouth, and mental confusion.

methoxamine hydrochloride, an adrenergic that acts as a vasoconstrictor.

■ INDICATION: It is prescribed for use during anesthesia to maintain blood pressure and in the treatment of paroxysmal supraventricular tachycardia.

■ CONTRAINDICATIONS: It is not recommended for use as a vasoconstrictor with local anesthetics. Known hypersensitivity to this drug prohibits its use.

■ ADVERSE EFFECTS: Among the most serious adverse reactions are hypertension, bradycardia, cardiac depression, severe headache, and vomiting.

methoxsalen, a pigmentation agent.

■ INDICATIONS: It is used topically to enhance pigmentation or for repigmentation in vitiligo.

■ CONTRAINDICATIONS: Liver impairment, concomitant use of a drug that may cause photosensitization, or known hypersensitivity to this drug prohibits its use.

■ ADVERSE EFFECTS: Among the most serious adverse reactions are central nervous system effects and burns. GI discomfort and allergic reactions also may occur.

3-methoxy-4-hydroxymandelic acid, a product of metabolism that may be measured in the urine to determine the levels of the catecholamines (adrenaline and noradrenaline). Increased concentrations of this acid may raise the blood pressure or indicate the presence of tumors of the adrenal glands or nervous system, muscular dystrophy, and myesthenia gravis, or may be caused by stress, exercise, or certain drugs or foods. Normal amounts in the urine of adults after 24-hour collection are 1.5 to 7.5 mg; in the urine of infants, 83 μg/kg of body weight.

methoxyphenamine hydrochloride, a beta-adrenergic agent.

■ INDICATIONS: It is prescribed in the treatment of bronchial asthma and hypersensitivity reactions.

■ CONTRAINDICATIONS: Cardiac arrhythmias, concomitant administration of monoamine oxidase inhibitors, coronary artery disease, or known hypersensitivity to this drug prohibits its use.

■ ADVERSE EFFECTS: Among the more serious adverse reactions are tachycardia and cardiac arrhythmias.

methscopolamine bromide, an anticholinergic.

■ INDICATIONS: It is prescribed in the treatment of hypermotility of the GI tract and as an adjunct in treating peptic ulcer.

■ CONTRAINDICATIONS: Narrow-angle glaucoma, asthma, obstruction of the genitourinary or GI tract, severe ulcerative colitis, or known hypersensitivity to this drug prohibits its use.

■ ADVERSE EFFECTS: Blurred vision, central nervous system effects, tachycardia, dry mouth, decreased sweating, or hypersensitivity reactions may occur.

methsuximide /methsuk′simīd/, an anticonvulsant.

■ INDICATION: It is prescribed in the treatment of refractory petit mal epilepsy.

■ CONTRAINDICATIONS: Known hypersensitivity to this drug or to any succinimide prohibits its use.

■ ADVERSE EFFECTS: Among the more serious adverse reactions are blood dyscrasias, liver and kidney damage, and systemic lupus erythematosus.

methyclothiazide /meth′əklōthī′əzīd/, a diuretic and antihypertensive.

■ INDICATIONS: It is prescribed in the treatment of hypertension and edema.

■ CONTRAINDICATIONS: Anemia, renal or urinary disorders, or known hypersensitivity to this drug, to other thiazide medications, or to sulfonamide derivatives prohibits its use.

■ ADVERSE EFFECTS: Among the more serious adverse reactions are hypokalemia, hyperglycemia, hyperuricemia, hypotension, and hypersensitivity reactions.

methyl (Me), the chemical radical $-CH_3$.

methyl alcohol. See **methanol.**

methylbenzethonium chloride, a topical antiinfective.

■ INDICATIONS: It is prescribed for the prevention and treatment of diaper rash and other dermatoses.

■ CONTRAINDICATION: Known hypersensitivity to this drug is the only contraindication.

■ ADVERSE EFFECTS: There are no known adverse reactions. Local skin irritation may occur.

methylcellulose, a bulk-forming laxative.

■ INDICATION: It is prescribed in the treatment of constipation.

■ CONTRAINDICATIONS: Appendicitis, acute surgical abdomen, intestinal adhesions, obstruction or ulceration, or known hypersensitivity to this drug prohibits its use.

■ ADVERSE EFFECTS: The most serious adverse reactions are intestinal obstruction and fecal impaction if insufficient fluids are ingested.

methyldopa, an antihypertensive.

■ INDICATION: It is prescribed for the reduction of high blood pressure.

■ CONTRAINDICATIONS: Use of monoamine oxidase

inhibitors, liver dysfunction, or known hypersensitivity to this drug prohibits its use.

■ ADVERSE EFFECTS: Among the more serious adverse reactions are liver toxicity and blood dyscrasias. Sedation, dry mouth, nasal stuffiness, and postural hypotension may occur.

methylene blue, a bluish-green crystalline substance used as a histologic stain and as a laboratory indicator. It is also used in the treatment of cyanide poisoning and methemoglobinemia.

methylergonovine maleate, a synthetic ergot alkaloid.

■ INDICATIONS: It is prescribed as an oxytocic to prevent or to treat postpartum uterine atony, hemorrhage, or subinvolution.

■ CONTRAINDICATIONS: It is not prescribed during pregnancy or given intravenously, except in life-threatening situations. Hypertension, toxemia, or known hypersensitivity to ergot alkaloids prohibits its use.

■ ADVERSE EFFECTS: Among the most serious adverse reactions are convulsions and death. Hypertension, nausea, blurred vision, and headaches also may occur. Adverse effects are more common after IV administration.

methylphenidate hydrochloride, a central nervous system stimulant.

■ INDICATIONS: It is prescribed in the treatment of hyperkinesis in children and in the treatment of narcolepsy in adults.

■ CONTRAINDICATIONS: Glaucoma, severe anxiety, tension, mental depression, or known hypersensitivity to this drug prohibits its use. It is not given to children under 6 years of age.

■ ADVERSE EFFECTS: Among the more serious adverse reactions are nervousness, insomnia, and anorexia. Hypersensitivity reactions and tachycardia may occur.

methylprednisolone, a glucocorticoid.

■ INDICATIONS: It is prescribed in the treatment of inflammatory conditions, including rheumatic fever and rheumatoid arthritis.

■ CONTRAINDICATIONS: Fungal infections or known hypersensitivity to this drug prohibits its systemic use. Viral or fungal infections of the skin, impaired circulation, or known hypersensitivity to this drug prohibits its topical use.

■ ADVERSE EFFECTS: Among the more serious adverse reactions to the systemic administration of the drug are GI, endocrine, neurologic, fluid, and electrolyte disturbances. A variety of skin reactions may occur from topical administration of this drug.

methylrosaniline chloride. See **gentian violet.**

methyl salicylate, a counterirritant and analgesic balm.

■ INDICATION: It is prescribed externally for minor pain of muscles and joints.

■ CONTRAINDICATIONS: It is not recommended for children. Known hypersensitivity to salicylates prohibits its use.

■ ADVERSE EFFECTS: Among the more serious adverse reactions are minor skin reactions and possible systemic salicylate poisoning from absorption of the drug when applied externally.

methyltestosterone /meth′iltəstos′tərōn/, an androgen.

■ INDICATIONS: It is prescribed in the treatment of testosterone deficiency, osteoporosis, and female breast cancer, and to stimulate growth, weight gain, and red blood cell production.

■ CONTRAINDICATIONS: Cancer of the male breast or prostate, cardiac, renal, or hepatic disease, hypercalcemia, known or suspected pregnancy, lactation, or known hypersensitivity to this drug prohibits its use.

■ ADVERSE EFFECTS: Among the more serious adverse reactions are hypercalcemia, edema, irreversible masculinization of female patients, and jaundice.

methyprylon /meth′əprī′lon/, a sedative and hypnotic.

■ INDICATION: It is prescribed in the treatment of insomnia.

■ CONTRAINDICATIONS: It is not given to children under 3 months of age. Intermittent porphyria or known hypersensitivity to this drug prohibits its use.

■ ADVERSE EFFECTS: Among the most serious adverse reactions are physical dependence and paradoxical excitement. Dizziness, headache, rash, and GI upset also may occur.

methysergide maleate /meth′isur′jīd/, a vasoconstrictor.

■ INDICATION: It is prescribed for relief of migraine headache.

■ CONTRAINDICATIONS: Pregnancy, severe infection, liver or kidney dysfunction, cardiovascular or lung disease, or known hypersensitivity to this drug prohibits its use. It is not recommended for use in children.

■ ADVERSE EFFECTS: Among the more serious adverse reactions are retroperitoneal fibrosis, hallucinations, abnormally low white cell count, pulmonary and cardiac complications, hemolytic anemia, leg cramps, and pain in the chest, abdomen, back, hands, or feet.

Meticortelone Acetate, a trademark for a glucocorticoid (prednisolone acetate).

Meticorten, a trademark for a glucocorticoid (prednisone).

metoclopramide hydrochloride /met′əklō′prəmīd/, a GI stimulant.

■ INDICATIONS: It is prescribed to stimulate motility and to increase the tone of gastric contractions of the upper GI tract and as an antiemetic.

■ CONTRAINDICATIONS: Epilepsy, concomitant use of drugs that cause extrapyramidal reactions, pheochromocytoma, GI hemorrhage, obstruction, or perforation, or known hypersensitivity to this drug prohibits its use.

■ ADVERSE EFFECTS: Among the more serious adverse reactions are extrapyramidal reactions, usually in children, and GI disturbances. Drowsiness and allergic reactions with a rash also may occur.

metocurine iodide, a potent neuromuscular blocking agent. Also called **dimethyl tubocurarine iodide.**

■ INDICATIONS: It is given to produce flaccid paralysis as an adjunct to anesthesia, to reduce muscle spasm in tetanus, and to assist controlled ventilation.

■ CONTRAINDICATIONS: Asthma or known hypersensitivity to this drug or to iodides prohibits its use. It is given only by medical personnel trained and equipped to maintain assisted mechanic ventilation.

■ ADVERSE EFFECTS: Among the more serious adverse reactions are hypotension, respiratory or circulatory depression, and bronchospasm.

metolazone /mətō′ləzōn/, a diuretic and antihypertensive.

■ INDICATIONS: It is prescribed for the treatment of edema and high blood pressure.

■ CONTRAINDICATIONS: Anuria or known hypersensitivity to this drug, to thiazides, or to sulfonamide drugs prohibits its use.

■ ADVERSE EFFECTS: Among the more serious adverse reactions are hypokalemia, hyperglycemia, hyperuricemia, and various allergic reactions.

"me-too" drug, *informal.* a drug product that is similar, identical, or closely related to a drug for which a manufacturer has obtained a new drug application. The drug is placed on the market by a company or companies other than the holder of the new drug application. On the assumption that the new drug has been recognized as safe and effective, clinical trials required of the original manufacturer are not required of the new supplier, but information regarding the manufacture, bioavailability, and labeling of the product is required to complete the abbreviated procedure for approval by the Food and Drug Administration.

metopic /mətō′pik/, of or pertaining to the forehead.

metopo-, a combining form meaning 'of or related to the forehead': *metopodynia, metopopagus, metopoplasty.*

metoprolol tartrate, an antiadrenergic (beta-receptor).

■ INDICATION: It is prescribed in the treatment of hypertension.

■ CONTRAINDICATIONS: Bradycardia, cardiogenic shock, overt cardiac failure, bronchospastic disease, or known hypersensitivity to this drug prohibits its use.

■ ADVERSE EFFECTS: Among the more serious adverse reactions are fatigue, bradycardia, bronchospasms, and GI upset.

metr-, a combining form meaning 'measure': *metrechoscopy, metric, metrology.*

metra-. See **metro-.**

metralgia /mətral′jə/, tenderness or pain in the uterus. Also called **metrodynia.**

Metrazol, a trademark for a central nervous system stimulant (pentylenetetrazol).

Metreton, a trademark for a glucocorticoid (prednisolone sodium phosphate).

-metria[1], a combining form meaning '(condition of the) ability to measure muscular acts': *dysmetria, hypermetria, hypometria.*

-metria[2], a combining form meaning '(condition of the) uterus': *ametria, atretometria, dimetria.*

metric, of or pertaining to a system of measurement that uses the meter as a basis. See also **metric system.**

metric equivalent, any value in metric units of measurement that equals the same value in English units, as 2.54 cm equal 1 inch or 1 L equals 1.0567 quarts.

metric system, a decimal system of measurement based on the meter (39.37 inches) as the unit of length, on the gram (15.432 grains) as the unit of weight or mass, and, as a derived unit, on the liter (0.908 U.S. dry quart or 1.0567 U.S. liquid quart) as the unit of volume.

metritis /mətrī′tis/, inflammation of the walls of the uterus. Kinds of metritis are **endometritis** and **parametritis.** Also called **uteritis.** See also **puerperal metritis.**

metro-, metra-, a combining form meaning 'of or related to the uterus': *metrocele, metrofibroma, metromalacoma.*

metrodynia. See **metralgia.**

metronidazole, an antimicrobial.

■ INDICATIONS: It is prescribed in the treatment of amebiasis, trichomonas, and certain bacterial infections.

■ CONTRAINDICATIONS: First trimester of pregnancy, blood dyscrasias, organic disease, central nervous system disorders, or known hypersensitivity to this drug prohibits its use.

■ ADVERSE EFFECTS: Among the more serious adverse reactions are severe GI distress, dizziness, neutropenia, and neurologic disturbances. A metallic taste in the mouth is commonly noted.

-metropia, -metropy, a combining form meaning '(condition of the) refraction of the eye': *allometropia, antimetropia, isometropia.*

metrorrhagia /met′rōrā′jē·ə/, uterine bleeding other than that caused by menstruation. It may be caused by uterine lesions and may be a sign of a urogenital malignancy, especially cervical cancer.

-metry, -metria, a combining form meaning the 'process of measuring something' specified: *oncometry, pelvimetry, symmetry.*

Metubine, a trademark for a neuromuscular blocking agent (metocurine iodide), used as an adjunct to anesthesia.

Metycaine Hydrochloride, a trademark for a local anesthetic (piperocaine hydrochloride).

metyrapone, a diagnostic test drug.

■ INDICATION: It is used to test hypothalamicopituitary function.

■ CONTRAINDICATIONS: Adrenal cortical insufficiency or hypersensitivity prohibits its use.

■ ADVERSE EFFECTS: Among the most serious adverse reactions are nausea, dizziness, and allergic rash.

metyrosine /mətir′əsēn/, an antihypertensive.

■ INDICATION: It is prescribed in the treatment of pheochromocytoma.

■ CONTRAINDICATION: Known hypersensitivity to this drug prohibits its use.

■ ADVERSE EFFECTS: Among the more serious adverse reactions are extrapyramidal reactions, including tremor, drooling, and crystalluria. Sedation is common, and diarrhea and anxiety may occur.

Metzenbaum scissors. See **scissors.**

Meuse fever. See **trench fever.**

mev, MeV, abbreviation for *million electron volts*, the equivalent of 3.82×10^{-14} small calories, or 1.6×10^{-6} ergs.

mevalonate kinase, an enzyme in the liver and in yeast that catalyzes the transfer of a phosphate group from adenosine triphosphate to produce adenosine diphosphate and 5-phosphomevalonate.

Meynet's node /mānāz′/, any one of the numerous nodules that may develop within the capsules surrounding joints and in tendons affected by rheumatic diseases, especially in children.

Mezlin, a trademark for a semisynthetic penicillin antibiotic (mezlocillin sodium).

mezlocillin sodium, a semisynthetic penicillin antibiotic.

■ INDICATIONS: It is prescribed for lower respiratory tract, intraabdominal, urinary tract, gynecologic, and skin infections and bacterial septicemia caused by susceptible strains of multiple microorganisms.

■ CONTRAINDICATION: Hypersensitivity to any of the penicillins prohibits its use.

■ ADVERSE EFFECTS: The most serious adverse reactions are anaphylactic reactions, convulsive seizures, epigastric pain, reduction in blood elements, and elevation in hepatic and renal parameters.

mfd, abbreviation for **microfarad.**

M.F.D., abbreviation for *minimal fatal dose*.

mg, abbreviation for **milligram.**

Mg, symbol for **magnesium.**

MH, abbreviation for **malignant hyperthermia.**

MHA, abbreviation for **Mental Health Association.**

MI, abbreviation for **myocardial infarction.**

MIC, abbreviation for **minimal inhibitory concentration.**

Michaelis-Menton kinetics, a method of transforming drug plasma levels into a linear relationship using the parameters of drug concentration and a constant, K_m, which is a measure of enzyme-substrate affinity.

miconazole nitrate /mīkon′əzōl/, an antifungal.

■ INDICATIONS: It is used topically in the treatment of certain fungal infections of the skin and vagina and parenterally to treat systemic fungal infections.

■ CONTRAINDICATION: Known hypersensitivity to this drug prohibits its use.

■ ADVERSE EFFECTS: Among the more serious adverse reactions to topical or vaginal application are irritation, burning, and maceration of the skin. When used systemically, nausea, pruritus, phlebitis, and anemia may occur.

micr-. See **micro-.**

micrencephalia. See **microcephaly.**

micrencephalon /mī′krənsef′əlon/, **1.** an abnormally small brain. See also **microcephaly. 2.** *obsolete.* the cerebellum. **–micrencephalic,** *adj., n.*

micrencephaly. See **microcephaly.**

micro-, micr-, mikro-, a combining form meaning 'small': *microadenopathy, microanalysis, microglossia.*

microaerophile, a microorganism that requires free oxygen for growth but at a lower concentration than that contained in the atmosphere. Compare **aerobe, anaerobe. –microaerophilic,** *adj.*

microaerotonometer, an instrument for measuring the volume of gases in the blood or other fluids.

microaggregate recipient set, a device composed of plastic components for the intravenous delivery of large volumes of stored whole blood or of packed blood cells. The components of the set include the plastic tubing, the roller clamp, and the special filter that prevents the microaggregates or deteriorated red blood cells of stored whole blood from entering and clogging the circulatory system of the patient. The plastic tubing of this device has a larger lumen than the tubing of most other intravenous sets, which allows the blood to be delivered more rapidly. Compare **component drip set, component syringe set, straight line blood set, Y set.**

microampere, one millionth of an ampere.

microaneurysm, a microscopic aneurysm characteristic of thrombotic purpura.

microangiopathy, a disease of the small blood vessels, as diabetic microangiopathy, in which the basement membrane of capillaries thickens, or thrombotic microangiopathy, in which thrombi form in the arterioles and the capillaries.

microbe, a microorganism. **–microbial,** *adj.*

-microbe, a combining form meaning a 'small living organism': *aeromicrobe, inframicrobe, ultramicrobe.*

-microbic, a combining form meaning 'referring to or consisting of microbes': *amicrobic, monomicrobic, polymicrobic.*

microbiology, the branch of biology concerned with the study of microorganisms, including algae, bacteria, viruses, protozoa, fungi, and rickettsiae.

microbiology technologist, a medical technologist who specializes in the identification of bacteria and other microorganisms found in patient tissues and other specimens.

microbrachia /mī′krōbrā′kē·ə/, a developmental defect characterized by abnormal smallness of the arms. **–microbrachius,** *n.*

microcentrum. See **centrosome.**

microcephaly /mī′krōsef′əlē/, a congenital anomaly characterized by abnormal smallness of the head in relation to the rest of the body and by underdevelopment of the brain, resulting in some degree of mental retardation. The head is more than two standard deviations below the average circumference size for age, sex, race, and period of gestation, and it has a narrow, receding forehead, a flattened occiput, and a pointed vertex. The facial features are generally normal. The condition may be caused by an autosomal recessive disorder, a chromosomal abnormality, a toxic stimulus, as irradiation, chemical agents, or maternal infection during prenatal development, or any trauma, especially during the third trimester of pregnancy or early infancy. There is no treatment, and nursing care is primarily supportive and educational, helping parents learn to care for a brain-damaged child. Also called **microcephalia, microcephalism.** Compare **macrocephaly. –microcephalic, microcephalous,** *adj.*, **microcephalic, microcephalus,** *n.*

microcheiria /mī′krōkī′rē·ə/, a developmental defect characterized by abnormal smallness of the hands. The condition is usually associated with other congenital malformations or with bone and muscle disorders. Also spelled **microchiria.**

microcirculation, the flow of blood throughout the system of smaller vessels of the body, those with a diameter of 100 μm or less.

microcomputer, a complete multiuse electronic digital computer system consisting of a central processing unit, storage facilities, I/O ports, and a chip with 64,000 to 256,000 bits of high-speed internal storage. Compare **mainframe computer, minicomputer.**

microcurie (μCi, μc), a unit of radiation equal to one millionth (10^{-6}) of a curie.

microcyte /mī′krəsīt/, an abnormally small erythrocyte with a mean corpuscular volume less than 80 μm^3, often occurring in iron deficiency and other anemias.

microcytic /mī′krōsit′ik/, (of a cell) smaller than normal, as the erythrocytes in microcytic anemia.

microcytic anemia, a hematologic disorder characterized by abnormally small erythrocytes, usually associated with chronic blood loss or a nutritional anemia, as iron deficiency anemia. Compare **macrocytic anemia.**

microcytosis /mī′krōsītō′sis/, a hematologic condition characterized by erythrocytes that are smaller than normal. Microcytosis and hypochromatosis are usual in iron deficiency anemia. Compare **poikilocytosis.** See also **anisocytosis. –microcytic,** *adj.*

microdactyly /mī′krōdak′təlē/, a developmental defect characterized by abnormal smallness of the fingers and toes. The condition is usually associated with bone and muscle disorders, as progressive myositis ossificans.

microdrip /mī′krōdrip′/, (in intravenous therapy) an apparatus for delivering relatively small, measured amounts of intravenous solutions at specific flow rates. The microdrip device usually consists of plastic tubing designed to allow small drops of solution to pass into the primary intravenous tubing through a clear plastic housing. A microdrip is usually used to deliver small volumes of solution over a long time. With a microdrip, 60 drops deliver 1 ml of solution. Compare **macrodrip.**

microelement. See **micronutrient.**

microencapsulation, a laboratory technique used in the bioassay of hormones in which certain antibodies are encapsulated with a perforated membrane. The antibodies cannot escape through the tiny perforations, but hormones that bind with the antibodies may enter the structure to bind with them. Technicians then can measure the amount of hormone present in the specimen. The technique is used for encapsulating unstable enzymes and in the preparation of some drugs in slow- or timed-release forms.

microfarad (mfd), a unit of capacitance that equals one millionth of a farad.

microfiche /mī′krōfēsh′/, a sheet of microfilm that contains several separate photographic reproductions. The sheet is a convenient size for filing and enables large amounts of data to be stored in a relatively small space. See also **microfilm.**

microfilament, any of the submicroscopic cellular filaments, as the tonofibrils, found in the cytoplasm of most cells, that function primarily as a supportive system.

microfilaria /mī′krōfiler′ē·ə/, *pl.* **microfilariae,** the prelarval form of any filarial worm. Certain blood-sucking insects ingest these forms from an infected host, and the microfilariae then develop in the body of the insect and become infective larvae. See also **dracontiasis, filariasis, loiasis, onchocerciasis, *Wuchereria.***

microfilm, a strip of 16 mm or 35 mm film that contains photographic reproductions of pages of books, documents, or other library or medical records in greatly reduced size. The film is viewed through special machines that enlarge the photographic images to normal reading size.

microfluorometry. See **cytophotometry.**

microgamete, the small, motile male gamete of certain thallophytes and sporozoa, specifically the malarial parasite *Plasmodium*. It corresponds to the sperm of the higher animals and unites in conjugation with the larger, nonmotile female gamete. See also **macrogamete.**

microgametocyte, an enlarged merozoite that undergoes meiosis to form the mature male gamete during the sexual phase of the life cycle of certain thallophytes and sporozoa, specifically the malarial parasite *Plasmodium*. Microgametocytes are found in the red blood cells of a person infected with the malarial parasite, but they must be ingested by a female *Anopheles* mosquito to complete the maturation process and develop into a microgamete.

microgenitalia, a condition characterized by abnormally small external genitalia.

microglia /mīkrog′lē·ə/, small migratory interstitial cells that form part of the central nervous system. They have various forms and slender, branched processes. Microglia serve as phagocytes that collect waste products of the nerve tissue of the body. Also called **Hortega cells, mesoglia.**

micrognathia /mī′krōnā′thē·ə/, underdevelopment of the jaw, especially the mandible. Compare **macrognathia. –micrognathic,** *adj.*

microgram (mg, μg), a unit of measurement of mass equal to one millionth (10^{-6}) of a gram. See also **gram.**

microgyria /mī′krōjī′rē·ə/, a developmental defect of the brain in which the convolutions are abnormally small, resulting in structural malformation of the cortex. The condition is usually associated with mental retardation and physical defects. Also called **polymicrogyria.**

microgyrus /mī′krōjī′rəs/, *pl.* **microgyri,** an underdeveloped, malformed convolution of the brain.

microhm, a unit of electric resistance equal to one millionth of an ohm.

microinvasive carcinoma, a squamous epithelial neoplasm that has penetrated the basement membrane, the first stage in invasive cancer. It is most frequently diagnosed in the uterine cervix, but the lesion is difficult to demonstrate. Some oncologists often prefer to designate the lesion as either invasive or in situ. See also **carcinoma in situ.**

microlevel interventions, health-generating changes performed at the individual level, as in conditioning or stimulus control therapies.

microliter (μL), a unit of liquid volume equal to one millionth of a liter.

microlith, a small rounded mass of mineral matter or calcified stone.

micromelic dwarf, a dwarf whose limbs are abnormally short.

micrometer, **1.** /mīkrom′ətər/, an instrument used for measuring small angles or distances on objects being observed through a microscope or telescope. **2.** /mī′krōmē′tər/, a unit of measurement, commonly referred to as a *micron,* that is, one thousandth (10^{-3}) of a millimeter.

micromicro- (μμ), a combining form meaning '10^{-12}': *micromicron.*

micromyeloblastic leukemia /mī′krōmī′əlōblas′tik/, a malignant neoplasm of blood-forming tissues, characterized by the proliferation of small myeloblasts distinguishable from lymphocytes only by special staining techniques and microscopic examination.

micron (μ, mu) /mī′kron/, **1.** a metric unit of length equal to one millionth of a meter; micrometer (def. 2). **2.** (in physical chemistry), a colloidal particle with a diameter of between 0.2 and 10 microns.

Micronor, a trademark for an oral contraceptive containing a progestin (norethindrone).

micronucleus, **1.** a small or minute nucleus. **2.** (in protozoa) the smaller of two nuclei in each cell; it functions in sexual reproduction as opposed to the macronucleus, which governs cell metabolism and growth. **3.** See **nucleolus.**

micronutrient, an organic compound, as a vitamin, or a chemical element, as zinc or iodine, essential only in minute amounts for the normal physiologic processes of the body. Also called **microelement, minor element, trace element.**

microorganism, any tiny, usually microscopic entity capable of carrying on living processes. It may be pathogenic. Kinds of microorganisms include **bacteria, fungi, protozoa,** and **viruses.**

micropenis. See **microphallus.**

microphage /mī′krəfāj/, a neutrophil capable of ingesting small things, as bacteria. Compare **macrophage.** –**microphagic,** *adj.*

microphallus, an abnormally small penis. When observed in the newborn, the nurse examines the child for other signs of ambiguous genitalia. Also called **micropenis.** See also **ambiguous genitalia.**

microphthalmos /mī′krəfthal′məs/, a developmental anomaly characterized by abnormal smallness of one or both eyes. When the condition occurs in the absence of other ocular defects, it is called pure microphthalmos or nanophthalmos. Also spelled **microphthalmus.** Also called **microphthalmia.** –**microphthalmic,** *adj.*

microplasia. See **dwarfism.**

micropodia, a developmental anomaly characterized by abnormal smallness of the feet. The condition is often associated with other congenital malformations or with bone and skeletal disorders.

microprosopus /mī′krōprō′səpəs, -prəsō′pəs/, a fetus in which the face is abnormally small or underdeveloped.

micropsia /mīkrop′sē·ə/, a condition of vision by which a person perceives objects as smaller than they really are. –**microptic,** *adj.*

microreentry, (in cardiology) an impulse reentry involving a very small circuit, as within Purkinje fibers.

microscopic, **1.** of or pertaining to a microscope. **2.** very small; visible only when magnified and illuminated by a microscope. Compare **gross.**

microscopic anatomy, the study of the microscopic structure of the tissues and cells. Kinds of microscopic anatomy are **cytology** and **histology.**

microscopy /mīkros′kəpē/, a technique for observing minute materials using a microscope. Kinds of microscopy include **darkfield microscopy, electron microscopy,** and **immunofluorescent microscopy.**

microshock, the passage of current directly into the cardiac tissue.

microsomia, the condition of having an abnormally small and underdeveloped yet otherwise perfectly formed body with normal proportionate relationships of the various parts. See also **primordial dwarf.**

Microsporum, a genus of dermatophytes of the family Moniliaceae. The spores are multiseptate, variable in shape, and have thin or thick walls. The type species is *M. audouinii,* which causes epidemic tinea capitis in children. Formerly called ***Microsporon.***

microthermy, a form of therapy in which heat generated by radio wave conversion is used in physical therapy.

microtome /mī′krətōm/, a device that cuts specimens of tissue prepared in paraffin blocks into extremely thin slices for microscopic study by a surgical pathologist.

microwaves, electromagnetic radiation in the frequency range of 300 to 2450 MHz.

microwave thermography, measurement of temperature through the detection of microwave radiation emitted from heated tissue.

micturate, micturition. See **urination.**

micturition reflex, a normal reaction to a rise in pressure within the bladder, resulting in contraction of the bladder wall and relaxation of the urethral sphincter. Voluntary inhibition normally prevents incontinence, with urination occurring on withdrawal of this inhibition.

Midamor, a trademark for a diuretic (amiloride hydrochloride).

midbrain. See **mesencephalon.**

midclavicular line /mid'kləvik'yo͞olər/, (in anatomy) an imaginary line that extends downward over the trunk from the midpoint of the clavicle, dividing each side of the anterior chest into two parts. The left midclavicular line is an important marker in describing the location of various cardiac phenomena, including the point of maximum impulse.

middle adult, an individual in the transitional age span between young adult and elderly, whose psychologic task is generativity versus stagnation.

middle cardiac vein, one of the five tributaries of the coronary sinus that drains blood from the capillary bed of the myocardium. It starts at the apex of the heart, rises in the posterior interventricular sulcus, receives tributaries from both ventricles, and ends in the right extremity of the coronary sinus. Compare **great cardiac vein, small cardiac vein.**

middle costotransverse ligament. See **ligament of the neck of the rib.**

middle cuneiform bone. See **intermediate cuneiform bone.**

middle ear, the tympanic cavity and the auditory ossicles contained in an irregular space in the temporal bone. It is separated from the external ear by the tympanic membrane and from the inner ear by the oval window. The auditory tube carries air from the posterior pharynx into the middle ear. Compare **external ear, internal ear.**

middle kidney. See **mesonephros.**

middle lobe syndrome, localized atelectasis of the middle lobe of the right lung, characterized by chronic infection, cough, dyspnea, wheezing, and obstructive pneumonitis. Asymptomatic obstruction of the bronchus may occur. The condition is caused by enlargement of the surrounding cuff of lymphatic glands, because of nonspecific or tuberculous inflammation during childhood. The middle lobe bronchus is thus compressed, with bronchiectasis developing in the obstructed part of the lung. Treatment includes antituberculosis chemotherapy, corticosteroids, or surgical excision. See also **atelectasis.**

middle mediastinum, the widest part of the mediastinum containing the heart, ascending aorta, lower half of the superior vena cava, pulmonary trunk, and phrenic nerves. It is one of three caudal portions of the mediastinum. Compare **anterior mediastinum, posterior mediastinum, superior mediastinum.**

middle plate. See **nephrotome.**

middle sacral artery, a small, visceral branch of the abdominal aorta, descending to the fourth and fifth lumbar vertebrae, the sacrum, and the coccyx. Minute branches are said to supply the posterior surface of the rectum.

middle suprarenal artery, one of a pair of small, visceral branches of the abdominal aorta, arising opposite the superior mesenteric artery, and supplying the suprarenal gland.

middle temporal artery, one of the branches of the superficial temporal artery on each side of the head. It arises just above the zygomatic arch, pierces the temporal fascia, branches to the temporalis, and anastomoses with the deep temporal branches of the maxillary artery. Compare **deep temporal artery, superficial temporal artery.**

middle umbilical fold, the fold of peritoneum over the urachal remnant within the abdomen. Approximately 3 cm lateral to the middle umbilical fold is the lateral umbilical fold. Between the lateral and the middle folds is the medial umbilical fold. Also called **plica umbilicalis mediana.**

mid forceps, an obstetric operation in which forceps are applied to the head of the baby when the head has reached the midplane of the mother's pelvis. An episiotomy is usually performed, and local, regional, or inhalation anesthesia is provided. In some cases, as severe fetal distress, mid forceps may be the most rapid and the safest means of delivery, but astute selection of cases, skill, and experience are essential. Difficult mid forceps delivery is likely to be more traumatic to the baby and the mother than cesarean section. Compare **high forceps, low forceps.** See also **failed forceps, forceps delivery, obstetric forceps, trial forceps.**

midgut, the middle portion of the embryonic alimentary canal. It consists of endodermal tissue, is connected to the yolk sac during early prenatal development, and eventually gives rise to some of the small intestine and part of the large intestine. Compare **foregut, hindgut.**

midline, an imaginary line that divides the body into right and left halves.

midline episiotomy. See **episiotomy.**

midpelvic contraction. See **contraction.**

Midrin, a trademark for a central nervous system, fixed-combination drug containing an adrenergic (isometheptene mucate), a hypnotic (dichloralphenazone), and an analgesic (acetaminophen), used in the treatment of migraine headaches.

midsagittal plane. See **median plane.**

midstance, one of the five stages in the stance phase of walking, or gait, directly associated with the period of single-leg support of body weight or the period during which the body advances over the stationary foot. During midstance the tibialis posterior and the flexor hallucis longus display their greatest activity. The midstance phase is considered in the diagnosis of many abnormal orthopedic conditions and in the analysis of the associated weaknesses of certain muscles and muscle groups. Compare **initial contact stance stage, loading response stance stage, preswing stance stage, terminal stance.** See also **swing phase of gait.**

midstream catch urine specimen, a urine specimen collected during the middle of a flow of urine, after the urinary opening has been carefully cleaned.

midwife, **1.** also called **obstetrix.** (in traditional use) a (female) person who assists women in childbirth. **2.** (according to the International Confederation of Midwives, World Health Organization, and Federation of International Gynecologists and Obstetricians) "a person who, having been regularly admitted to a midwifery educational program fully recognized in the country in which it is located, has successfully completed the prescribed course of studies in midwifery and has acquired the requisite qualifications to be registered and/or legally licensed to practice midwifery." Among the responsibilities of the midwife are supervision of the woman's pregnancy, labor, delivery, and puerperium. The midwife conducts the delivery independently, cares for the newborn, procures medical assistance when necessary, executes emergency measures as required, and may practice in a hospital, clinic, maternity home, or in a woman's home. The midwife, whose practice may include well-child care, family planning, and some aspects of gynecology, is often an important source of health counseling in the community. **3.** a lay midwife. **4.** a nurse midwife or Certified Nurse Midwife.

migraine, a recurring vascular headache characterized by a prodromal aura, unilateral onset, and severe pain, photophobia, and autonomic disturbances during the acute phase, which may last for hours or days. The disorder occurs more frequently in women than in men, and a predisposition to migraine may be inherited. The exact mechanism responsible for the disorder is not known, but the head pain is related to dilatation of extracranial blood vessels, which may be the result of chemical changes that cause spasms of intracranial vessels. A greatly increased amount of a vasodilating polypeptide related to bradykinin is found in tissue fluid of patients during migraine attacks. Allergic reactions, excess carbohydrates, iodine-rich foods, alcohol, bright lights, or loud noises may trigger attacks, which often occur during a period of relaxation after physical or psychic stress. An impending attack may be heralded by visual disturbances, as flashing lights or wavy lines, or by a strange taste or odor, numbness, tingling, vertigo, tinnitus, or a feeling that part of the body is distorted in size or shape. The acute phase may be accompanied by nausea, vomiting, chills, polyuria, sweating, facial edema, irritability, and extreme fatigue. After an attack the individual often has dull head and neck pains and a great need for sleep. Aspirin seldom provides relief during an attack, but ergotamine tartrate preparations that constrict cranial arteries can usually prevent the headache from developing if administered early in the onset as an injection, suppository, or tablet. Ergotamine tartrate is also available combined with other drugs, as caffeine, phenobarbital, and belladonna; migraine patients unable to tolerate ergot preparations may use other analgesics, including acetaminophen, phenacetin, and propoxyphene. Also called **hemicrania, megrim.**

migrainous cranial neuralgia /mīgrā′nəs/, a variant of migraine, characterized by closely spaced episodes of excruciating, throbbing, unilateral headaches often accompanied by dilatation of temporal blood vessels, flushing, sweating, lacrimation, nasal congestion or rhinorrhea, ptosis, and facial edema. Repeated episodes usually occur in clusters within a few days or weeks and may be followed by a relatively long remission period. A typical attack begins abruptly without prodromal signs, as a burning sensation in an orbit or temple, and the resulting radiating intense pain may last 1 hour or 2. Histamine diphosphate injected subcutaneously in persons subject to these headaches produces symptoms identical to those occurring in a spontaneous attack. The pain may be relieved by antihistamines, and ergotamine tartrate preparations may be helpful if administered at the onset of an attack. Also called **cluster headache, histamine headache, Horton's headache.** See also **migraine.**

migration, the passage of the ovum from the ovary into a fallopian tube and then into the uterus.

migratory gonorrheal polyarthritis. See **migratory polyarthritis.**

migratory ophthalmia. See **sympathetic ophthalmia.**

migratory polyarthritis, arthritis progressively affecting a number of joints and finally settling in one or more, occurring in patients with gonorrhea and developing a few days to a few weeks after the onset of gonorrheal urethritis. The patient usually has a moderate fever and 1 to 5 days of migratory polyarthralgia with variable signs of inflammation. In more prolonged episodes, initially arthritic sites may clear as new areas are affected, but persistently involved joints are usually severely inflamed and swollen. Large joints are most affected; after the swelling subsides, the overlying skin may peel. Treatment with penicillin or tetracycline generally produces some response in 24 to 72 hours. Also called **migratory gonorrheal polyarthritis.**

migratory thrombophlebitis, an abnormal condition in which multiple thromboses appear in both superficial and deep veins. It may be associated with malignancy, especially carcinoma of the pancreas, often preceding other evidence of cancer by several months. Pulmonary embolism is uncommon with this condition. Also called **thrombophlebitis migrans.** See also **thrombophlebitis.**

mikro-. See **micro-.**

Mikulicz's syndrome /mik′yo͞olich′ēz/, an abnormal bilateral enlargement of the salivary and lacrimal glands, found in a variety of diseases, including leukemia, tuberculosis, and sarcoidosis. Also called **Mikulicz's disease.** Compare **Sjögren's disease.**

mild, gentle, subtle, or of low intensity, as a mild infection.

milia neonatorum, a nonpathologic dermatologic condition characterized by minute epidermal cysts consisting of keratinous debris that occur on the face and, occasionally, the trunk of the newborn. They are eliminated by normal desquamation of the skin within a few weeks after birth and leave no scars.

miliaria /mil'ē•er'ē•ə/, minute vesicles and papules, often with surrounding erythema, caused by occlusion of sweat ducts during times of exposure to heat and high humidity. Backup pressure may cause sweat to escape into adjacent tissue producing itching and prickling. Prevention and treatment include cool environment, ventilation, colloidal baths, and dusting powders. Also called **prickly heat.**

miliary /mil'ē•er'ē/, describing a condition marked by the appearance of very small lesions the size of millet seeds, as miliary tuberculosis, which is characterized by tiny tubercules throughout the body.

miliary carcinosis, a condition characterized by the presence of numerous cancerous nodules resembling miliary tubercles.

miliary tuberculosis, extensive dissemination by the bloodstream of tubercle bacilli. In children it is associated with high fever, night sweats, and, often, meningitis, pleural effusions, or peritonitis. A similar illness may occur in adults but with a less abrupt onset and, occasionally, with weeks or months of nonspecific symptoms, as weight loss, weakness, and low-grade fever. Multiple small opacities resembling millet seeds may be evident on chest x-ray films. The liver, spleen, bone marrow, and meninges are often affected. The tuberculin test may be negative, and diagnosis is made by biopsy of the infected tissue or organ. Combined drug therapy with isoniazid and rifampin or with isoniazid and streptomycin is usually successful if the diagnosis is not delayed. Concurrent tuberculous meningitis makes the prognosis less favorable. See also ***Mycobacterium*, tuberculosis.**

milieu /milyœ', milyo͞o'/, *pl.* **milieus, milieux,** the environment, surroundings, or setting. Kinds of milieus are **milieu extérieur** and **milieu intérieur.**

milieu extérieur /eksterē•œr'/, the external or physical surroundings of an organism, including the social environment, especially the home, school, and recreational facilities, that plays a dominant role in personality development.

milieu intérieur /aNterē•œr'/, the basic concept in physiology, originated by Claude Bernard, that multicellular organisms exist in an aqueous internal environment composed of the blood, lymph, and interstitial fluid that bathes all cells and provides a medium for the elementary exchange of nutrients and waste material. All fundamental processes necessary for the maintenance and life of the tissue elements are dependent on the stability and balance of this environment.

milieu therapy, a type of psychotherapy in which the total environment is used in treating mental and behavioral disorders. It is primarily conducted in a hospital or other institutional setting where the entire facility acts as a therapeutic community. The emphasis is on providing pleasant physical surroundings, structured activities, and a stable social environment where behavioral modification and personal growth are promoted through patient-group interaction, staff support and understanding, and a total, humanistic approach. Individual daily routines and treatment modalities, such as drug therapy, occupational therapy, and sensitivity training, are determined by the patient's emotional and interpersonal needs. Also called **situation therapy.**

milium, *pl.* **milia** /mil'ē•ə/, a minute, white cyst of the epidermis caused by obstruction of hair follicles and eccrine sweat glands. One variety is seen in newborn infants and disappears within a few weeks. Another type is found primarily on the faces of middle-aged women. Milia may be treated with an abrasive cleanser or by incision and drainage. Also called **whitehead.** Compare **comedo, miliaria.**

milk, a liquid secreted by the mammary glands or udders of animals that suckle their young. After breast feeding, people consume the milk of the cow, as well as that of many other animals, including the goat, camel, mare, reindeer, llama, and yak. Milk is a basic food containing carbohydrate (in the form of lactose), protein (mainly casein, with small amounts of lactalbumin, and lactoglobulin), suspended fat, the minerals calcium and phosphorus, the vitamins A, riboflavin, niacin, thiamine, and, when the milk is fortified, vitamin D. It is a valuable nutrient for adults and nearly a complete food for infants, especially breast milk. Milk does not contain a significant amount of iron; its ascorbic acid content depends on the amount ingested by the mother or by the animal producing the milk. Some individuals show a sensitivity reaction to milk caused by a deficiency of the enzyme lactase. See also **breast milk.**

milk baby, an infant with iron deficiency anemia caused by ingestion of excessive amounts of milk and the delayed or inadequate addition of iron-rich foods to the diet. Milk babies are overweight, have pale skin and poor muscle development, and are highly susceptible to infection. See also **anemia.**

milk bath, a bath taken in milk for cosmetic or emollient reasons.

milk ejection reflex, a normal reflex in a lactating woman elicited by tactile stimulation of the nipple, resulting in release of milk from the glands of the breast. This reflex requires intact nerve connections from nipple to hypothalamus and the release of the hormone, oxytocin, from the posterior pituitary into the bloodstream. Also called **let-down reflex.** See also **oxytocin.**

milker's nodule, a smooth, brownish-red papilloma of the fingers or palm that begins as a macule and progresses through a vesicular stage to become a nodule. The disease is acquired from pustular lesions on the udder of a cow infected with poxvirus. No treatment is necessary because immunity is produced after primary infection.

milk fever, *nontechnical.* postpartum fever that begins with the onset of lactation. It was formerly considered a normal reaction to lactation. Maternal temperature during the puerperium does not normally exceed 99° F; higher elevations usually indicate infection.

milk globule, a spheric droplet of fat in milk that tends to separate out as cream.

milking, a procedure used to express the contents of a duct or tube, to test for tenderness, or to obtain a specimen for study. The examiner compresses the structure with a finger and moves the finger firmly along the duct or tube to its opening. Also called **stripping.**

milk leg. See **phlegmasia alba dolens.**

milk of magnesia, a laxative and antacid containing magnesium hydroxide.

▪ INDICATIONS: It is prescribed to relieve constipation and acid indigestion.

▪ CONTRAINDICATIONS: Renal impairment, symptoms of appendicitis, or known hypersensitivity to the drug prohibits its use.

▪ ADVERSE EFFECTS: Among the most serious adverse reactions are diarrhea and hypermagnesemia, usually occuring in patients who have impaired renal function.

milkpox. See **alastrim.**

milk sugar. See **lactose.**

milk therapy, a nutritional treatment used in the therapy of Curling's ulcer in patients who have been severely burned. Cool, homogenized milk is administered in doses of 1 to 2 ounces every hour through a nasogastric tube. After instillation the tube is clamped for 5 minutes and then unclamped. Milk remaining in the stomach is allowed to flow into a basin. As the milk is better absorbed and tolerated, feedings are increased to 150 ml of milk per kilogram of body weight daily. The interval between feedings is gradually lengthened to 4 hours. As the condition improves, the nasogastric tube is withdrawn, and milk may be continued by mouth.

milk tooth. See **deciduous tooth.**

milky ascites. See **chylous ascites.**

Miller-Abbott tube, a long, small-caliber, double-lumen catheter, used in intestinal intubation for decompression. It has several openings on the side of its tip and a balloon above the tip. Compare **Harris tube.** See also **gastric intubation.**

milli-, a combining form meaning '1/1000 part': *milliampere, millibar, milliliter.*

milliampere (ma), a unit of electric current that is one thousandth of an ampere.

milliampere seconds (mAs), the product obtained by multiplying the electric quantity in milliamperes by the time in seconds. It is a a term used to describe the exposure setting of an x-ray machine.

millicoulomb (mC), a unit of electric charge that is one thousandth of a coulomb.

millicurie (mCi, mc), a unit of radioactivity that is equal to one thousandth of a curie, or 3.70×10^7 disintegrations per second.

milliequivalent (mEq), **1.** the number of grams of solute dissolved in 1 ml of a normal solution. **2.** one thousandth of a gram equivalent.

milligram (mg), a metric unit of weight equal to one thousandth (10^{-3}) of a gram.

milliliter (ml), a metric unit of volume that is one thousandth (10^{-3}) of a liter.

millimeter (mm), a metric unit of length equal to one thousandth (10^{-3}) of a meter.

millimicro- (mμ), a combining form meaning 'billionth (10^{-9})': *millimicrogram, millimicroliter.* This combining form is now generally replaced by **nano-.**

millimole (mmol), a unit of metric measurement of mass that is equal to one thousandth (10^{-3}) of a mole.

milliosmol /mil′ē•oz′mōl/, a unit of measure representing the concentration of an ion in a solution, expressed in milligrams per liter divided by atomic weight. See also **osmol, osmolality, osmolarity.** **–milliosmolar,** *adj.*

millipede /mil′ipēd′/, a many-legged, wormlike arthropod. Certain species squirt irritating fluids that may cause dermatitis.

millirad, one thousandth (10^{-3}) of a rad, a unit of measurement of absorbed dose of ionizing radiation.

milliroentgen (mR, mr) /mil′irent′gən, -jən/, a unit of radiation that is equal to one thousandth (10^{-3}) of a roentgen.

millivolt (mV, mv), a unit of electromotive force equal to one thousandth of a volt.

Milontin, a trademark for an anticonvulsant (phensuximide).

Milpath, a trademark for a GI, fixed-combination drug containing an anticholinergic (tridihexethyl chloride) and a sedative (meprobamate).

Milprem, a trademark for a hormonal, fixed-combination drug containing conjugated estrogens and a sedative (meprobamate).

Miltown, a trademark for a sedative (meprobamate).

Miltrate, a trademark for a cardiovascular, fixed-combination drug containing a vasodilator (pentaerythritol tetranitrate) and a sedative (meprobamate).

Milwaukee brace, an orthotic device that helps immobilize the torso and the neck of a patient in the treatment or correction of scoliosis, lordosis, or kyphosis. It is usually constructed of strong but light metal and fiberglass supports lined with rubber to protect against abrasion. Milwaukee braces, which may be employed in the treatment of orthopedic bed patients or ambulatory patients, commonly connect cervical supports, rib supports, and hip supports with rigid bars of metal that hold the trunk and the neck erect while controlling cervical flexion and hip movements.

-mimesis, a combining form meaning 'simulation, imitation': *necromimesis, neuromimesis, pathomimesis.*

-mimetic, a combining form meaning 'pertaining to simulation of (specified) effects': *andromimetic, neuromimetic, vagomimetic.*

-mimia, a combining form meaning '(condition of) ability to express thought through gestures': *macromimia, paramimia, pathomimia.*

mimic spasm, involuntary, stereotyped movements of a small group of muscles, as of the face. The spasm is usually psychogenic and may be aggravated by stress or anxiety but is generally controllable momentarily. Multiple grimacing and blinking mimic spasms occur in Gilles de la Tourette's syndrome. Also called **tic.**

min, abbreviation for **minim.**

Minamata disease /min'əmä'tə/, a severe, degenerative, neurologic disorder caused by the ingestion of seed grain heated with alkyl compounds of mercury or of seafood taken from waters polluted with industrial wastes contaminated by soluble mercuric salts. The term is derived from a tragedy involving Japanese who ate seafood from Minamata Bay. Mercury passes the placental barrier, causing the congenital form of the disease. Symptoms may not appear for several weeks or months; they include paresthesia of the mouth and extremities, tunnel vision, difficulties with speech, hearing, muscular coordination, and concentration, weakness, emotional instability, and stupor. Continued ingestion causes serious damage to the renal tubules and corrosion of the GI tract. Acute cases may result in coma and death. See also **mercury poisoning.**

mind, **1.** the part of the brain that is the seat of mental activity and that enables one to know, reason, understand, remember, think, feel, and to react and adapt to surroundings and all external and internal stimuli. **2.** the totality of all conscious and unconscious processes of the individual that influence and direct mental and physical behavior. **3.** the faculty of the intellect or understanding in contrast to emotion and will. See also **brain, intellect, psyche.**

mine damp. See **damp.**

mineral, **1.** an inorganic substance occurring naturally in the earth's crust, having a characteristic chemical composition and (usually) crystalline structure. **2.** (in nutrition) a mineral usually referred to by the name of a metal, nonmetal, radical, or phosphate rather than by the name of the compound of which it is a part, and which is ingested as a compound, as sodium chloride (table salt), rather than as a free element. Minerals play a vital role in regulating many bodily functions.

mineral deficiency, the inability to use one or more of the mineral elements essential in human nutrition because of a genetic defect, malabsorption dysfunction, or the lack of that mineral in the diet. The symptoms and manifestations vary, depending on the specific function or functions of the element in promoting growth and maintaining body health. Minerals are constituents of all the body tissues and fluids, and they are important factors in maintaining physiologic processes. They act as catalysts in nerve response, muscle contraction, and the metabolism of nutrients in foods, they regulate electrolyte balance and hormonal production, and they strengthen skeletal structures. All mineral deficiencies are treated by adding the specific element to the diet, either in supplementary form or in the appropriate foods. See also specific minerals.

mineralization, the addition of any mineral to the body.

mineralocorticoid, a hormone, secreted by the adrenal cortex, that maintains normal blood volume, promotes sodium and water retention, and increases urinary excretion of potassium and hydrogen ions. Aldosterone, the most potent mineralocorticoid in regard to electrolyte balance, and corticosterone, a glucocorticoid and a mineralocorticoid, act on the distal tubules of the kidneys to enhance the reabsorption of sodium into the plasma. Aldosterone secretion is stimulated by angiotensin, the polypeptide formed by the action of renin, which is released by juxtaglomerular cells of the kidneys when serum sodium levels fall. Hypersecretion of aldosterone causes expansion of extracellular fluid, hypertension, hypokalemia, alkalosis, and a slight increase in plasma sodium. Hyposecretion of the hormone results in hypotension, circulatory collapse, hyperkalemia, and severe sodium loss; without aldosterone an adult may secrete as much as 25 g of sodium a day. Trauma and stress increase mineralocorticoid secretion. The synthetic mineralocorticoids desoxycorticosterone, which does not influence carbohydrate metabolism, and fluorocortisone, which also has glucocorticoid activity, are used in treating the salt-losing adrenogenital syndrome and the severe corticoid deficiency characteristic of Addison's disease. See also **glucocorticoid.**

mineral oil, a laxative, stool softener, emollient, and pharmaceutic aid used as a solvent.

■ INDICATIONS: It is prescribed to prevent constipation, to treat mild constipation, to prepare the bowel for surgery or examination, and as a solvent for various preparations.

■ CONTRAINDICATIONS: Symptoms of appendicitis, fecal impaction, obstruction or perforation of the intestinal tract, pregnancy, or known hypersensitivity to this drug prohibits its use.

■ ADVERSE EFFECTS: Among the more serious adverse reactions are laxative dependence, lipid pneumonitis, fat-soluble vitamin deficiency, and abdominal cramps.

miner's cramp. See **heat cramp.**

miner's elbow, an inflammation of the olecranon bursa, caused by resting the weight of the body on the elbow, as in some coal mining activities. The condition is sometimes seen in school children who lean on their elbows. Compare **lateral humeral epicondylitis.** See also **bursitis.**

miner's pneumoconiosis. See **anthracosis.**

Minerva cast /minur'və/, an orthopedic cast applied to the trunk and the head, with spaces cut out for the face area and the ears. The section encasing the trunk extends to the sternum and the distal rib border anteriorly and across the distal rib border posteriorly. The cast is used for immobilizing the head and part of the trunk in the treatment of torticollis, cervical and thoracic injuries, and cervical spinal infections. It is not used as frequently as it once was because of advancement in the field of orthotics. Also called **Minerva jacket.**

minicomputer, a medium-sized computer, intermediate in size and processing capacity between a microcomputer and a mainframe computer. Compare **mainframe computer, microcomputer.**

minim (min), a measurement of volume in the apothecaries' system, originally one drop (of water). Sixty minims equal 1 fluid dram. One minim equals 0.06 ml.

minimal bactericidal concentration. See **minimal inhibitory concentration.**

minimal brain dysfunction. See **attention deficit disorder.**

minimal care unit, a unit for the treatment of inpatients who are ambulatory and able to meet many of their own daily living needs but require minimal nursing care.

minimal inhibitory concentration (MIC), the lowest concentration of an antibiotic medication in the blood that is effective against an infection, determined by injecting infected venous blood into a culture medium containing various concentrations of a proposed antibiotic. The lowest antibiotic concentration that stops microbial growth may be used in further treatment of the patient. Typical antibiotic test concentrations in the culture medium range from 0.195 to 100 μg/ml. Also called **minimal bactericidal concentration.**

minimal occlusive volume (MOV), the volume of endotracheal cuff inflation that still permits a minimum airway leak during the inspiratory phase of ventilation.

minimum alveolar concentration (MAC), the smallest amount of a gas detected and measured in the alveoli of the lungs.

Minipress, a trademark for an antihypertensive (prazosin hydrochloride).

Minnesota Multiphasic Personality Inventory (MMPI), a psychologic test that includes 550 statements for interpretation by the subject, used clinically for evaluating personality and for detecting various disorders, as depression and schizophrenia.

Minocin, a trademark for an antibacterial (minocycline hydrochloride).

minocycline hydrochloride /min'əsī'klēn/, a tetracycline antibiotic active against bacteria, rickettsia, and other organisms.

■ INDICATIONS: It is prescribed in the treatment of a variety of infections.

■ CONTRAINDICATIONS: It must be used with caution with renal or hepatic dysfunction. Known hypersensitivity to this or other tetracyclines prohibits its use.

■ ADVERSE EFFECTS: Among the more serious adverse reactions are GI disturbances, phototoxicity, vestibular toxicity, potentially serious suprainfections, and various allergic reactions. Use during pregnancy or in children under 8 years of age may result in discoloration of teeth.

minor, (in law) a person not of legal age; a person beneath the age of majority. Minors usually cannot consent to their own medical treatment unless they are substantially independent from their parents, are married, support themselves, or satisfy other requirements as provided by statute. A kind of minor is **emancipated minor.**

minor connector, (in dentistry) a device that links the major connector or base of a removable partial denture to other denture units, as rests and direct and indirect retainers.

minor element. See **micronutrient.**

minor renal calyx. See **renal calyx.**

minor surgery, any surgical procedure that does not require general anesthesia or respiratory assistance.

minoxidil, a vasodilator.

■ INDICATION: It is prescribed in the treatment of severe refractory hypertension.

■ CONTRAINDICATIONS: Pheochromocytoma or known hypersensitivity to this drug prohibits its use.

■ ADVERSE EFFECTS: Among the most serious adverse reactions are tachycardia, pericardial effusion, cardiac tamponade, salt and water retention, and excessive hair growth. GI disturbances also may occur.

Mintezol, a trademark for an anthelmintic (thiabendazole).

minute ventilation, the total ventilation per minute measured by expired gas collection for a period of 1 to 3 minutes.

mio-, meio-, a combining form meaning 'less': *miolecithal, mioplasmia, miosphygmia.*

Miochol, a trademark for a parasympathetic blocking agent (acetylcholine chloride).

miosis /mī•ō'sis/, **1.** contraction of the sphincter muscle of the iris, causing the pupil to become smaller. Certain drugs and stimulation of the pupillary light reflex by an increase in light result in miosis. **2.** an abnormal condition characterized by excessive constriction of the sphincter muscle of the iris, resulting in very small, pinpoint pupils. Compare **mydriasis.**

Miostat, a trademark for a cholinergic (carbachol).

miotic /mē•ot'ik/, **1.** of or pertaining to miosis. **2.** causing constriction of the pupil of the eye. **3.** any substance or pharmaceutic, as pilocarpine, that causes constriction of the pupil of the eye. Such agents are used in the treatment of glaucoma.

MIP, abbreviation for **maximum inspiratory pressure.**

miracidium /mir'əsid'ē•əm/, *pl.* **miracidia,** the ciliated larva of a parasitic trematode that hatches from an egg and can survive only by penetrating and further developing within a host snail, whereupon the larva further develops into a maternal sporocyte that produces more larvae.

Miradon, a trademark for an anticoagulant (anisindione).

mirage /miräzh′/, an optic illusion caused by the refraction of light through air layers of different temperatures, as the illusionary sheets of water that seem to shimmer over stretches of hot sand and pavement. This phenomenon is caused by horizontal light waves being bent upwards from the layer of heated air directly over the hot surface. Wind rippling the air layers may produce surprising changes in the shapes and sizes of such mirages. Individuals under severe stress are especially susceptible to interpreting these optic phenomena in bizarre, unrealistic ways.

mirror speech, abnormal speech characterized by the reversal of the order of syllables in a word.

miscarriage. See **spontaneous abortion.**

miscible /mis′ibəl/, able to be mixed or mingled with another substance. Compare **immiscible.**

misdemeanor, (in criminal law) an offense that is considered less serious than a felony and carries with it a lesser penalty, usually a fine or imprisonment for less than 1 year. Conviction for a misdemeanor does not prohibit the person from holding public office or from practicing a licensed occupation.

misfeasance /misfē′zəns/, an improper performance of a lawful act, especially in a way that might cause damage or injury. Compare **malfeasance, nonfeasance.**

miso-, a combining form meaning 'hatred of': *misocainia, misogyny, misopedia.*

misogamy /misog′əmē/, an aversion to marriage. –**misogamic, misogamous,** *adj.*, **misogamist,** *n.*

misogyny /misoj′inē/, an aversion to women. –**misogynist,** *n.*, **misogynistic,** *adj.*

misopedia /mis′ōpē′dē•ə/, an aversion to children. –**misopedic,** *adj.*, **misopedist,** *n.*

misophobia. See **mysophobia.**

missed abortion, a condition in which a dead, immature embryo or fetus is not expelled from the uterus for 2 or more months. The uterus diminishes in size, and symptoms of pregnancy abate; infection and disorders of the clotting of the mother's blood may follow. The fetus and placenta may become necrotic, or, less commonly, the fetus becomes calcified and the rest of the products of conception are resorbed.

missile fracture, a penetration fracture caused by a projectile, as a bullet or a piece of shrapnel.

mistura , any of a number of mixtures of drugs, usually containing suspensions of insoluble substances intended for internal use. Examples include **mistura kaolini et morphinae,** a mixture of kaolin and morphine, and **mistura cretae pro infantibus,** a mixture of chalk, tragacanth, chloroform water, and other ingredients formulated for the treatment of GI disorders in infants.

mite, a minute arachnid with a flat, almost transparent body and four pairs of legs. Many species of these relatives of ticks and spiders are parasitic, including the chigger and *Sarcoptes scabiei,* which cause localized pruritus and inflammation. Some female mites burrow into the skin and lay eggs that hatch into larvae; the movements of the larvae cause intense itching. See also **scabies.**

mite typhus. See **scrub typhus.**

Mithracin, a trademark for an antineoplastic (plicamycin).

mithramycin. See **plicamycin.**

mithridatism. See **tachyphylaxis.**

mito-, a combining form meaning 'threadlike': *mitochondria, mitokinetic, mitoplasm.*

mitochondrion /mī′tōkon′drē•on/, *pl.* **mitochondria,** a small rodlike, threadlike, or granular organelle, within the cytoplasm, that functions in cellular metabolism and respiration and occurs in varying numbers in all living cells except bacteria, viruses, blue-green algae, and mature erythrocytes. It consists of two sets of membranes, a smooth outer one and a convoluted inner one, arranged in folds to form projections, or cristae, that extend into the matrix. Mitochondria provide the principal source of cellular energy through oxidative phosphorylation and adenosine triphosphate synthesis. They also contain the enzymes involved with electron transport and the citric and fatty acid cycles. Mitochondria are self-replicating and contain an extranuclear source of DNA, RNA polymerase, transfer RNA, and ribosomes. Also called **chondriosome.** –**mitochondrial,** *adj.*

mitogen /mī′təjən, mit′-/, an agent that triggers mitosis. –**mitogenic,** *adj.*

mitogenesia /mī′tōjənē′zhə/, the production by or formation resulting from mitosis.

mitogenesis /mī′tōjen′əsis/, the induction of mitosis in a cell. –**mitogenetic,** *adj.*

mitogenetic radiation, the force or specific energy that is supposedly given off by cells undergoing division. It may, in turn, stimulate the process of mitosis in other cells. Also called **mitogenic radiation, Gurvich radiation.**

mitogenic factor, a kind of lymphokine that is released from activated T lymphocytes and stimulates the production of normal unsensitized lymphocytes.

mitogenic radiation. See **mitogenetic radiation.**

mitolactol /mī′təlak′tôl/, an antineoplastic currently used investigationally for a variety of neoplasms, including Hodgkin's disease. It may be used in combination with doxorubicin. Also called **dibromodulcitol.**

mitome /mī′tōm/, the reticular network sometimes observed within the cytoplasm and nucleoplasm of fixed cells. See also **cytomitome, karyomitome.**

mitomycin, an antineoplastic antibiotic.

■ INDICATIONS: It is prescribed in the treatment of a variety of malignant neoplastic diseases.

■ CONTRAINDICATIONS: Clotting deficiency, thrombocytopenia, or known hypersensitivity to this drug prohibits its use.

■ ADVERSE EFFECTS: The most serious adverse reaction is bone marrow depression. GI disturbances, alopecia, and skin reactions commonly occur.

mitosis /mītō′sis, mit-/, a type of cell division that occurs in somatic cells and results in the formation of two genetically identical daughter cells containing the diploid number of chromosomes characteristic of the species. It consists of the division of the nucleus through the four stages of prophase, metaphase, anaphase, and telophase, during which the two chromatids of the chromosomes separate and migrate to opposite ends of the cell, followed by the division of the cytoplasm. Mitosis is the process by which the body produces new cells for both growth and repair of injured tissue. Kinds of mitosis are **heterotypic mitosis, homeotypic mitosis, multipolar mitosis,** and **pathologic mitosis.** Also called **indirect division.** Compare **meiosis.** See also **anaphase, interphase, metaphase, prophase, telophase.** **–mitotic,** *adj.*

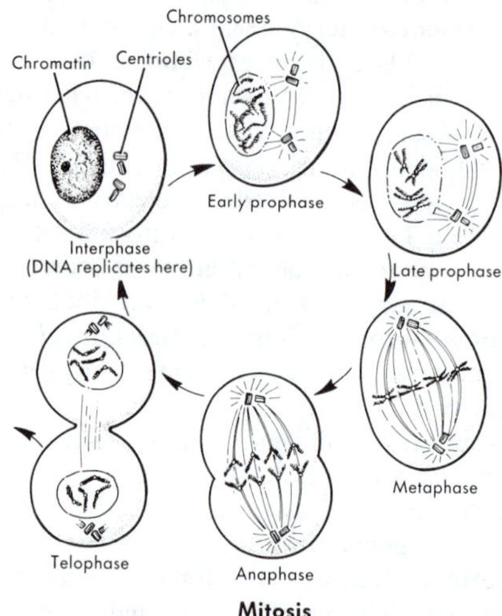

Mitosis

mitotane /mī′tətān/, an antineoplastic that destroys normal and neoplastic adrenal cortical cells.

■ INDICATION: It is prescribed in the treatment of carcinoma of the adrenal cortex.

■ CONTRAINDICATION: Known hypersensitivity to this drug is the only contraindication.

■ ADVERSE EFFECTS: Among the more serious adverse reactions are GI symptoms, lethargy, and adrenal insufficiency.

mitotic figure, any chromosome or chromosome aggregation during any of the stages of mitosis.

mitotic index, the number of cells per unit (usually 1000) undergoing mitosis during a given time. The ratio is used primarily as an estimation of the rate of tissue growth.

mitral /mī′trəl/, **1.** of or pertaining to the mitral valve of the heart. **2.** shaped like a miter.

mitral gradient, the difference in pressure in the left atrium and left ventricle during diastole.

mitral regurgitation, a lesion of the mitral valve that allows the flow of blood from the left ventricle into the left atrium. The condition may result from congenital valve abnormalities, rheumatic fever, mitral valve prolapse, endocardial fibroelastosis, dilatation of the left ventricle because of severe anemia, myocarditis, or myocardiopathy. Symptoms include dyspnea, fatigue, intolerance to exercise, and heart palpitations. Congestive heart failure may ultimately occur. Treatment depends on the severity of the condition. Surgery may be necessary in cases of refractory congestive heart failure, progressive cardiomegaly, and pulmonary hypertension. Also called **mitral insufficiency.** See also **valvular heart disease.**

mitral stenosis. See **mitral valve stenosis.**

mitral valve, one of the four valves of the heart, situated between the left atrium and the left ventricle; the only valve with two, rather than three cusps. The mitral valve allows blood to flow from the left atrium into the left ventricle but prevents blood from flowing back into the atrium. Ventricular contraction in systole forces the blood against the valve, closing the two cusps and assuring the flow of blood from the ventricle into the the aorta. The ventral cusp of the mitral valve is longer than the dorsal cusp. Also called **bicuspid valve, left atrioventricular valve.** Compare **aortic valve, pulmonary valve, semilunar valve, tricuspid valve.**

mitral valve prolapse (MVP), protrusion of one or both cusps of the mitral valve back into the left atrium during ventricular systole, resulting in incomplete closure of the valve and the backflow of blood. The condition is caused by pleating or scalloplike folds of extraneous mitral cusp tissue, frequently with myxomatous degeneration, that form along the surface of the valve. The lesions may be primary, occurring in patients with Marfan's syndrome or as an associated anomaly with atrial septal defect, or they may be secondary to previous rheumatic fever, ischemic heart disease, cardiomyopathy, or ruptured chordae tendinae. Most patients are asymptomatic, although some may experience chest pain, palpitations, fatigue, or dyspnea. The condition may lead to progressive mitral regurgitation, resulting in enlargement of the left atrium and ventricle. See also **valvular heart disease.**

mitral valve stenosis, an obstructive lesion in the mitral valve of the heart caused by adhesions on the leaflets of the valve, usually the result of recurrent episodes of rheumatic endocarditis. Hypertrophy of the left atrium develops and may be followed by right-sided heart failure and pulmonary edema (cor pulmonale). Reduced cardiac output characteristically produces fatigue, dyspnea, orthopnea, and cyanosis. Surgical correction of the defective valve may be necessary. The valve may be freed of the adhesions in a commissurotomy, or it may be replaced by a prosthetic valve. See also **atrioventricular valve, valvular heart disease, valvular stenosis.**

mittelschmerz /mit′əlshmerts/, abdominal pain in the region of an ovary during ovulation, which usually occurs midway through the menstrual cycle (German, for "middle pain"). Present in many women, mittelschmerz is useful for identifying ovulation, thus pinpointing the fertile period of the cycle.

mixed anesthesia. See **balanced anesthesia.**

mixed aneurysm. See **compound aneurysm.**

mixed cell malignant lymphoma, a lymphoid neoplasm containing lymphocytes and histiocytes (macrophages).

mixed cell sarcoma, a tumor consisting of two or more cellular elements, excluding fibrous tissue. Also called **malignant mesenchymoma.**

mixed connective tissue disease (MCTD), a systemic disease characterized by the combined symptoms of various collagen diseases, as synovitis, polymyositis, scleroderma, and systemic lupus erythematosus. This condition involves a high concentration of antibodies of ribonucleoprotein and may produce arthralgia, inflammation of the muscles, nondeforming arthritis, swollen hands, esophageal hypomotility, and reduced diffusing capacity of the lungs. Treatment often includes the administration of corticosteroids. Recurrence is common when the steroid medication is discontinued.

mixed culture, a laboratory culture that contains two or more different strains of organisms.

mixed dentition, a phase of dentition during which some of the teeth are permanent and some are deciduous.

mixed glioma, a tumor, composed of glial cells, that contains more than one kind of cell, the most common being nonneural cells of ectodermal origin.

mixed infection, an infection by several microorganisms, as in some abscesses, pneumonia, and infections of wounds. Numerous combinations of bacteria, viruses, and fungi may be involved. Compare **endogenous infection, germinal infection, retrograde infection, secondary infection.**

mixed leukemia, a malignancy of blood-forming tissues characterized by the proliferation of eosinophilic, neutrophilic, and basophilic granulocytes, in contrast to one predominant cell line, as in lymphocytic or monocytic leukemia.

mixed lymphocyte culture (MLC) reaction, an assay of the function of the T cell lymphocytes, primarily used for histocompatibility testing before grafting.

mixed porphyria. See **variegate porphyria.**

mixed tumor, a growth composed of more than one kind of neoplastic tissue, especially a complex embryonal tumor of local origin.

-mixis, -mixia, -mixie, -mixy, a combining form meaning a '(specified) means of conjugation': *amphimixis, automixis, endomixis.*

mixture, **1.** a substance composed of ingredients that are not chemically combined and do not necessarily occur in a fixed proportion. **2.** (in pharmacology) a liquid containing one or more medications in suspension. The proportions of the ingredients are specific to each mixture. Compare **compound, solution.** See also **mistura.**

-mixy. See **-mixis.**

ml, abbreviation for **milliliter.**

MLC, abbreviation for **mixed lymphocyte culture.** See **mixed lymphocyte culture reaction.**

MLD, abbreviation for **minimum lethal dose.**

mm, abbreviation for **millimeter.**

MMEF, abbreviation for *maximal midexpiratory flow.*

M-mode, abbreviation for *motion mode,* a variation of B-mode ultrasound scanning. It is used in echocardiography. See also **B-mode.**

mmol, abbreviation for **millimole.**

MMPI, abbreviation for **Minnesota Multiphasic Personality Inventory.**

MMR, abbreviation for **measles, mumps, and rubella virus vaccine live.**

Mn, symbol for **manganese.**

mne-, a combining form meaning 'of or pertaining to memory': *mnemic, mnemism, mnemonic.*

-mnesia, a combining form meaning '(condition or type of) memory': *acousmatamnesia, ecmnesia, logamnesia.*

-mnestic, -mnesic, a combining form meaning 'pertaining to memory': *amnestic, anamnestic, catamnestic.*

Mo, symbol for **molybdenum.**

Moban, a trademark for an antipsychotic agent (molindone).

Mobidin, a trademark for an analgesic (magnesium salicylate).

mobility, the velocity a particle or ion attains for a given applied voltage and a relative measure of how quickly an ion may move in an electric field.

-mobility. See **-motility.**

mobility, impaired physical, a nursing diagnosis accepted by the Fourth National Conference on the Classification of Nursing Diagnoses. The cause of the condition may be a decrease in the person's strength or endurance, the presence of pain or discomfort, impaired cognition or perception, depression or severe anxiety, or impaired neuromuscular or musculoskeletal function. The defining characteristics of the condition include an inability to achieve a functional level of mobility in the environment, a reluctance to move, a limited range of motion of the limbs or extremities, a decrease in the strength or control of the musculoskeletal system, abnormal or impaired ability to coordinate movements, or any of a large number of imposed restrictions on movement, as medically required bed rest or traction. It is suggested that the limitation of injury be ranked from 0, "completely independent," to 4, "dependent, does not participate in any activity." See also **nursing diagnosis.**

Mobitz I heart block, second degree or partial atrioventricular (AV) block in which the PR interval increases progressively until the propagation of an atrial impulse does not occur and the corresponding ventricular beat drops out. After the pause, the progressive shortening of the PR interval begins again. Symptoms include fatigue, dizziness, and, in some cases, syncope. Mobitz I heart block is caused by abnormal conduction of the cardiac impulse in the AV node and may be precipitated by increased vagal tone, occurring spontaneously, after carotid sinus pressure, or after digitalis therapy. It may be a complication of inferior myocardial infarction but is usually a transitory condition requiring no treatment. Also called **Wenchebach heart block.**

Mobitz II heart block, second degree or partial atrioventricular block, characterized by the sudden nonconduction of an atrial impulse and a periodic dropped beat without prior lengthening of the PR interval. This kind of block usually results from impaired conduction in the bundle branches and may be caused by anterior myocardial infarction, myocarditis, drug toxicity, electrolyte disturbances, rheumatoid nodules, and various degenerative diseases. Syncopal attacks, occurring without warning when the patient is upright or recumbent, are common in Mobitz II block, which may be transient or suddenly progress to complete block. Long-term therapy requires the implantation of a pacemaker.

Möbius' syndrome /mē′bē·əs/, a rare developmental disorder characterized by congenital bilateral facial palsy usually associated with oculomotor or other neurologic dysfunctions, speech disorders, and various anomalies of the extremities. The condition is caused by a developmental defect involving the motor nuclei of the cranial nerves. Also called **congenital facial diplegia, congenital oculofacial paralysis, nuclear agenesis.**

MOD, abbreviation for **maturity-onset diabetes.** See **non-insulin-dependent diabetes mellitus.**

mode, a value or term in a set of data that occurs more frequently than other values or terms.

model, (in nursing research) a symbolic representation of the interrelations exhibited by a phenomenon within a system or a process. The model is presented as a conceptual framework or a theory that explains a phenomenon and allows predictions to be made about a patient or a process. An equation is analagous to a model in mathematics. Nursing models usually describe person, environment, health, and nursing.

modeling, a technique used in behavior therapy in which a person learns a desired response by observing it performed.

modem, MODEM /mō′dəm/, abbreviation for *modulate/demodulate*. It is a device for transforming serial binary numbers into an audible tone, and vice versa, for transmission over a telephone line to another computer. Common rates of data transfer are 300 and 1200 baud.

moderator band, a thick bundle of muscle in the central part of the right ventricle of the heart. Missing in some individuals and varying in size in different persons, it usually contains part of the atrioventricular conduction bundle. Also called **trabecula septomarginalis.**

Moderil, a trademark for an antihypertensive (rescinnamine).

Modicon, a trademark for an oral contraceptive containing an estrogen (ethinyl estradiol) and a progestin (norethindrone).

modified milk, cow's milk in which the protein content has been reduced and the fat content increased to correspond to the composition of breast milk. See also **formula, infant.**

modified radical mastectomy, a surgical procedure in which a breast is completely removed with the underlying pectoralis minor and some of the adjacent lymph nodes. The pectoralis major is not excised. The operation is performed in treating early and well-localized malignant neoplasms of the breast. It appears to be as curative as the more extensive radical mastectomy when the tumor meets these criteria. Care of the woman before and after a modified radical mastectomy is similar to that for a radical mastectomy. Compare **radical mastectomy, simple mastectomy.** See also **mastectomy.**

modulation transfer function (MTF), a quantitative measure of the ability of an imaging system to reproduce patterns that vary in spatial frequency. The MTF is useful in predicting image degradation in a series of radiographic components.

Moeller's glossitis /mel′ərz/, a form of chronic glossitis, characterized by burning or pain in the tongue and an increased sensitivity to hot or spicy foods. Also called **glossodynia exfoliativa.** See also **glossitis.**

mogi-, a combining form meaning 'difficult, or with difficulty': *mogiarthria, mogigraphia, mogilalia.*

moiety /moi′itē/, a part of a molecule that exhibits a particular set of chemical and pharmacologic characteristics.

moist gangrene. See **gangrene.**

mol. See **mole^2.**

molality, the numbers of moles of solute per kilogram of water or other solvent.

molar, **1.** any one of the 12 molar teeth, six in each dental arch, three located posterior to the premolar teeth. The crown of each molar is nearly cubical, convex on its buccal surface and its lingual surface and flattened on its surfaces of contact. It is surmounted by four or five cusps separated by cruciate depressions and has a large rounded neck. Each of the upper molars has three roots, two of which are buccal, the other being lingual. The roots of the third upper molar are more or less fused. The lower molars are larger than the upper, and each has two roots, an anterior, almost vertical root and a posterior root directed almost obliquely backward. The roots of the third lower molar tend to fuse. **2.** of or pertaining to the gram molecular weight of a substance. See also **mole^2.**

molarity, the number of moles of solute per liter of water or other solvent.

molar pregnancy, pregnancy in which a hydatid mole develops from the trophoblastic tissue of the early embryonic stage of development. The signs of pregnancy are all exaggerated: the uterus grows more rapidly than is normal, morning sickness is often severe and constant, blood pressure is likely to be elevated, and blood levels of chorionic gonadotropins are extremely high. The uterus must be evacuated, because the mole may develop into a malignant trophoblastic disease, choriocarcinoma. See also **hydatid mole.**

molar solution, a solution that contains one mole of solute per liter of solution.

mold[1], **1.** a fungus. **2.** a growth of fungi.

mold[2], a hollow form for casting or shaping an object, as a prosthesis.

molding, the natural process by which a baby's head is shaped during labor as it is squeezed into and through the birth passage by the forces of labor. The head often becomes quite elongated, and the bones of the skull may be caused to overlap slightly at the suture lines. The biparietal diameter of the head may be compressed as much as 0.5 cm without intracranial damage. Most of the changes caused by molding resolve themselves during the first few days of life. Compare **caput succedaneum.** See also **cephalhematoma.**

mole[1], *informal.* **1.** a pigmented nevus. **2.** (in obstetrics) a hydatidiform mole.

mole[2], the standard unit used to measure the amount of a substance. A mole of a substance is the amount containing the same number of elementary particles (atoms, electrons, ions, molecules, or other particles) as there are atoms in 12 g of carbon 12. Also spelled **mol.** **–molar,** *adj.*

molecular genetics, the branch of genetics that focuses on the chemical structure and the functions, replication, and mutations of the molecules involved in the transmission of genetic information, as DNA and RNA. Molecular genetics is concerned with the arrangement of genes on DNA, the double helix molecule's replication and transcription into RNA, and the way RNA directs the formation of proteins. See also **recombinant DNA.**

molecular weight, the total of the atomic weights of the atoms in a molecule. See also **atom, atomic weight, molecule.**

molecule, the smallest unit that exhibits the properties of an element or compound. A molecule is composed of two or more atoms that are chemically combined. See also **atom, compound.**

molindone hydrochloride, an antipsychotic agent.

■ INDICATION: It is prescribed in the treatment of schizophrenia.

■ CONTRAINDICATIONS: Severe central nervous system depression or known hypersensitivity to this drug prohibits its use.

■ ADVERSE EFFECTS: Among the most serious adverse reactions are extrapyramidal reactions, hypotension, sedation, and other reactions characteristic of the phenothiazine antipsychotics.

molluscum /məlus′kəm/, any skin disease having soft, rounded masses or nodules. See also **molluscum contagiosum.**

molluscum contagiosum, a disease of the skin and mucous membranes, caused by a poxvirus and found all over the world. It is characterized by scattered white papules. Palms of the hands and soles of the feet are not affected. The disease most frequently occurs in children and in adults with an impaired immune response. It is transmitted from person to person by direct or indirect contact and lasts up to 3 years, although individual lesions persist for only 6 to 8 weeks. Diagnosis is easily made by electron microscopy. Curettage or electric or chemical dessication helps to clear the lesions, but untreated lesions eventually resolve spontaneously without scarring.

molybdenum (Mo), a grayish metallic element. Its atomic number is 42; its atomic weight is 95.94. Molybdenum is poisonous if ingested in large quantities.

molybdenum 99, the radionuclide that is the parent of technetium 99, and as such is present as a generator in all nuclear medicine departments.

Mönckeberg's arteriosclerosis /meng′kəbərgz/, a form of arteriosclerosis in which extensive calcium deposits are found in the media of the artery with little obstruction of the lumen. Also called **medial arteriosclerosis.**

Mondane, a trademark for a stimulant laxative (danthron).

Monday morning fever. See **byssinosis.**

Mongolian spot, a benign, bluish-black macule, between 2 and 8 cm, occurring over the sacrum and on the buttocks of some newborns. It is especially common in blacks, Native Americans, southern Europeans, and Orientals, and usually disappears during early childhood.

mongolism, mongoloid idiocy. See **Down's syndrome.**

Monilia. See ***Candida albicans.***

monilial vulvovaginitis, moniliasis. See **candidiasis.**

Monistat, a trademark for an antifungal (miconazole nitrate).

monitor, **1.** to observe and evaluate a function of the body closely and constantly. **2.** a mechanic device that provides a visual or audible signal or a graphic record of a particular function, as a cardiac monitor or a fetal monitor.

monitrice, a labor coach, usually a registered nurse, who is specially trained in the Lamaze method of childbirth. The coach provides emotional support and leads the mother through labor and delivery, using the specific techniques for breathing, concentration, and massage taught by the Lamaze method in classes for the psychophysical preparation for childbirth.

mono-, a combining form meaning 'one': *monobacillary, monodal, mononeuritis.*

monoamine, an amine containing one amine group.

monoamine oxidase (MAO), an enzyme that catalyzes the oxidation of amines. Also called **amino oxidase.** See also **monoamine oxidase inhibitor.**

monoamine oxidase (MAO) inhibitor, any of a chemically heterogeneous group of drugs used primarily in the treatment of depression. These drugs also exert an antianxiety effect, especially anxiety associated with phobia. The effects of the drugs vary greatly from patient to patient, and their specific actions leading to clinical benefits are poorly understood. Among the most common adverse effects are drowsiness, dry mouth, orthostatic hypotension, and constipation. Overdosage may cause tremor, euphoria, or manic behavior. MAO inhibitors interact with many drugs and with foods containing large amounts of the amino acid tyromine. Ingestion of these foods by a person taking a MAO inhibitor is likely to cause a severe hypertensive episode associated with headache, palpitations, and nausea. Among these foods are cheeses, red wine, smoked or pickled herring, beer, and yogurt. Patients taking MAO inhibitors are given a list of foods to avoid. Among the drugs that interact with MAO inhibitors are dopamine, meperidine, and the indirect acting sympathemimetics, one of which, ephedrine, is an ingredient in many common cold remedies. MAO inhibitors are also sometimes used in the treatment of migraine headache and hypertension. See also **amine pump.**

monobasic acid /mon′ōbā′sik/, an acid with only one replaceable hydrogen atom, as hydrochloric acid (HCl).

monobenzone, a depigmenting agent.

■ INDICATIONS: It is prescribed in the treatment of abnormal skin pigmentation, as in disseminated vitiligo. It is not to be used for more trivial conditions, as freckles.

■ CONTRAINDICATION: Known hypersensitivity to this drug prohibits its use.

■ ADVERSE EFFECTS: The most serious adverse reaction is excessive and irreversible hypopigmentation. Common reactions are irritation and allergic reactions of the skin.

monoblast /mon′əblast/, a large, immature monocyte. Certain of the leukemias are characterized by greatly increased production of monoblasts in the marrow and by the abnormal presence of these forms in the peripheral circulation. Compare **megaloblast, myeloblast.** See also **bone marrow, leukocyte.** **–monoblastic,** *adj.*

monoblastic leukemia, a progressive malignancy of blood-forming organs, characterized by the proliferation of monoblasts and monocytes. The disease occurs in children and adults and develops late in the course of a small but significant number of cases of plasma cell myeloma. Also called **monocytic leukemia, Schilling's leukemia.**

monocephalus. See **syncephalus.**

monochorial twins, monochorionic twins. See **monozygotic twins.**

monoclonal /mon′əklō′nəl/, of, pertaining to, or designating a group of identical cells or organisms derived from a single cell.

monoclonal gammopathy. See **gammopathy.**

monocyte /mon′əsīt/, a large mononuclear leukocyte, 13 to 25 μ in diameter with an ovoid or kidney-shaped nucleus, containing lacy, linear chromatin material and abundant gray-blue cytoplasm filled with fine, reddish, and azurophilic granules. See also **monocytosis.**

monocytic leukemia /mon′əsit′ik/, a malignancy of blood-forming tissues in which the predominant cells are monocytes. The disease has an erratic course characterized by malaise, fatigue, fever, anorexia, weight loss, splenomegaly, bleeding gums, dermal petechiae, anemia, and unresponsiveness to therapy. There are two forms: **Schilling's leukemia,** in which most of the cells are monocytes that probably arise from the reticuloendothelial system, and the more common **Naegeli's leukemia,** in which a large number of the cells resemble myeloblasts. Also called **histiocytic leukemia.**

monocytosis /mon′ōsītō′sis/, an increased proportion of monocytic white blood cells in the circulation.

monoethanolamine, an amino alcohol formed by the decarboxylation of serine. It is a component of certain cephalins and phospholipids and is used as a surfactant in pharmaceutic products.

monofactorial inheritance, the acquisition or expression of a trait or condition that is dependent on the transmission of a single specific gene. Compare **multifactorial inheritance.**

monohybrid, pertaining to or describing an individual, organism, or strain that is heterozygous for only one specific trait or that is heterozygous for the single trait or gene locus under consideration.

monohybrid cross, the mating of two individuals, organisms, or strains that have different gene pairs for only one specific trait or in which only one particular characteristic or gene locus is being followed.

monohydric alcohol, an alcohol containing one hydroxyl group.

monomer /mon′əmər/, a molecule that repeats itself to form a polymer, as the molecules of fibrin monomer that polymerize to form fibrin in the blood-clotting process. **–monomeric,** *adj.*

monomphalus /mənom′fələs/, conjoined twins that are united at the umbilicus. Also called **omphalopagus.**

mononeuritis multiplex. See **multiple mononeuropathy.**

mononeuropathy, any disease or disorder that affects a single nerve trunk. Some common causes of disorders involving single nerve trunks are electric shock, radiation, and fractured bones that may compress or lacerate nerve fibers. Casts and tourniquets that are too tight may also damage a nerve by compression or by ischemia. Accidental injection of penicillin and other medications into the sciatic nerve can seriously injure the nerve, especially if the injected medication is an oil-based drug. The peripheral nerve trunks are especially vulnerable to compression and entrapment.

mononuclear cell, a leukocyte, including lymphocytes and monocytes, with a round or oval nucleus.

mononucleosis /mon′ōno͞o′klē·ō′sis/, **1.** an abnormal increase in the number of mononuclear leukocytes in the blood. **2.** See **infectious mononucleosis.**

monoovular. See **uniovulvar.**

monophasic, having one phase, part, aspect, or stage.

monoploid /mon′əploid/, haploid. Also **monoploidic.**

monopodial symmelia. See **sympus monopus.**

monopus /mon′əpəs/, a fetus or individual with the congenital absence of a foot or leg.
monorchid /monôr′kid/, a male who has monorchism.
monorchism /mon′ôrkiz′əm/, a condition in which only one testicle has descended into the scrotum. Also called **monorchidism.** See also **cryptorchidism.** –**monorchidic,** *adj.*
monosaccharide a carbohydrate consisting of a single basic unit with the general formula $C_n(H_2O)_n$, with n ranging from 3 to 8.
monosome /mon′əsōm/, **1.** also called **accessory chromosome.** an unpaired X or Y sex chromosome. **2.** the single, unpaired chromosome in monosomy.
monosomy /mon′əsō′mē/, a chromosomal aberration characterized by the absence of one chromosome from the normal diploid complement. In humans, the monosomic cell contains 45 chromosomes and is designated $2n-1$, as occurs in the XO condition in Turner's syndrome. Compare **trisomy.** See also **aneuploidy.** –**monosomic,** *adj.*
monosomy X. See **Turner's syndrome.**
monospecific, an antibody that will react with only one type of antigen.
monotropy /mənot′rəpē/, a concept named by J. Bowlby, describing the phenomenon in which a mother appears to be able to bond with only one infant at a time. The concept is used by Marshall Klaus and John Kennell in their studies of maternal-infant bonding in mothers of twins. When one twin is taken home from the hospital earlier than the other, the mother often reports that she does not feel that the baby discharged later is hers. The second baby to reach the home is much more likely to fail to thrive or to be neglected or abused. Nurses working in intensive care nurseries and adoption homes are also known to become attached to only one child at a time. Monotropy may also explain a mother's common tendency to dress twins alike, in effect making them one. –**monotropic,** *adj.*
monounsaturated fatty acid. See **unsaturated fatty acid.**
monovular. See **uniovular.**
monovulatory /mənō′vyələtôr′ē/, routinely releasing one ovum during each ovarian cycle. Compare **diovulatory.**
monozygotic (MZ), pertaining to or developed from a single fertilized ovum, or zygote, as occurs in identical twins. Compare **dizygotic.** –**monozygosity,** *n.,* **monozygous,** *adj.*
monozygotic twins, two offspring born of the same pregnancy and developed from a single fertilized ovum that splits into equal halves during an early cleavage phase in embryonic development, giving rise to separate fetuses. Such twins are always of the same sex, have the same genetic constitution, possess identical blood groups, and closely resemble each other in physical, psychologic, and mental characteristics. Monozygotic twins may have single or separate placentas and membranes, depending on the time during development when division occurred. Monozygotic twinning occurs with relatively uniform frequency in all races, is unaffected by heredity, and represents approximately one third of all twin births. Also called **enzygotic twins, identical twins, true twins, uniovular twins.** Compare **dizygotic twins.** See also **Siamese twins.**
Monson curve, the curve of occlusion in which each tooth cusp and incisal edge conform to a segment of the surface of a sphere 8 inches (20 cm) in diameter, with its center in the region of the glabella.
monster, a fetus that is grossly malformed and usually nonviable. Kinds of monsters include **compound monster, double monster,** and **single monster.**
monstrosity, **1.** the state or condition of having severe congenital defects. **2.** anything that deviates greatly from the normal; a monster or teras.
mons veneris, a pad of fatty tissue and coarse skin that overlies the symphysis pubis in the woman. After puberty, it is covered with pubic hair. Also called **mons pubis.**
Monteggia's fracture /montej′əz/, fracture of the proximal third of the proximal half of the ulna, associated with radial dislocation or rupture of the annular ligament and resulting in the angulation or overriding of ulnar fragments.
Montercaux fracture /mont′ərkō′/, a fracture of the neck of the fibula associated with the diastasis of ankle mortise.
Montgomery's gland. See **Montgomery's tubercle.**
Montgomery straps, bands of adhesive tape that are used to secure dressings that must be changed frequently. Also called **Montgomery tapes.**
Montgomery's tubercle, one of several sebaceous glands on the areolae of the breasts. The tubercles normally enlarge during pregnancy. The sebaceous material that is secreted from the ducts of the glands to the skin of each areola serves to lubricate and protect the breast from infection and trauma during breast feeding. Also called **Montgomery's gland.**
Montgomery tapes. See **Montgomery straps.**
mood-congruent psychotic features, the characteristics of a psychosis in which the content of hallucinations or delusions is consistent with an elevated, expansive mood or with a depression.
moon face, a condition characterized by a rounded, puffy face, occurring in people treated with large doses of corticosteroids, as those with rheumatoid arthritis or acute childhood leukemia. The features return to normal when the medication is stopped.
moor bath, a bath taken in water containing earth from a swamp.
Moore's fracture, a fracture of the distal radius with associated dislocation of the ulnar head, resulting in the securement of the styloid process under the annular ligaments of the wrist.
MOPP /mop/, an abbreviation for a combination drug regimen used in the treatment of cancer, containing three antineoplastics, Mustargen (mechlorethamine), Oncovin

(vincristine sulfate), Matulane (procarbazine hydrochloride), and prednisone (a glucocorticoid). MOPP is prescribed in the treatment of Hodgkin's disease.

morbid anatomy. See **pathologic anatomy.**

morbidity **1.** an illness or an abnormal condition or quality. **2.** (in statistics) the rate at which an illness or abnormality occurs, calculated by dividing the entire number of people in a group by the number in that group who are affected with the illness or abnormality. **3.** the rate at which an illness occurs in a particular area or population.

morbid physiology. See **pathologic physiology.**

morbilli. See **measles.**

morbilliform /môrbil′ifôrm/, describing a skin condition that resembles the erythematous, maculopapular rash of measles.

Morgagni's globule /môrgan′yēz/, a minute opaque sphere that may form from fluid coagulation between the eye lens and its capsule, especially in cataract.

Morgagni's tubercle, one of several small, soft nodules on the surface of each of the areola in women. The tubercles are produced by large sebaceous glands just under the surface of the areolae. They secrete a bacteriostatic, lubricating substance during pregnancy and lactation.

morgan, (in genetics) a unit of measure used in mapping the relative distances between genes on a chromosome. The measurement, named after the biologist Thomas Hunt Morgan, uses the total crossover value as the basic unit so that one morgan equals 100% crossing over or one centimorgan equals 1% recombination. One centimorgan is also equal to one map unit.

morgue, a unit of a hospital with facilities for the storage and autopsy of dead persons.

-moria, a combining form meaning '(condition of) dementia': *monomoria, phantasmatomoria*.

morning after pill, *informal*. A large dose of an estrogen given orally, over a short period of time, to a woman within 24 to 72 hours after sexual intercourse to prevent conception, most commonly in an emergency situation such as rape or incest. The woman is warned that the medication may cause the formation of clots, severe nausea and vomiting, and teratogenic and carcinogenic effects on the fetus if pregnancy already exists or if contraception fails. See also **diethystilbestrol.**

morning sickness. See **nausea and vomiting of pregnancy.**

moron, *obsolete*. a retarded person having an IQ between 50 and 70 and incapable of developing beyond the mental age of 12 years. Compare **idiot, imbecile.** See also **mental retardation.**

moronism, *obsolete*. the condition of being a moron. Also called **moronity.**

Moro reflex /môr′ō/, a normal mass reflex in a young infant elicited by a sudden loud noise, as by striking the table next to the child, resulting in flexion of the legs, an embracing posture of the arms, and usually a brief cry. Also called **startle reflex.**

morph-, a combining form meaning 'form or shape': *morphallaxis, morphea, morphogenesis*.

-morph, a combining form meaning 'something possessing a (specified) form': *endomorph, hypomorph, neomorph*.

morphea /môr′fē·ə/, localized scleroderma consisting of patches of yellowish or ivory-colored, rigid, dry, smooth skin. It is more common in females and rarely progresses to a generalized or systemic form of sclerosis. Also called **Addison's keloid, circumscribed scleroderma, localized scleroderma.**

-morphia, -morphy, a combining form meaning a 'condition of form': *pantamorphia, prosopodysmorphia, theromorphia*.

morphine sulfate, a narcotic analgesic.

■ INDICATION: It is prescribed to reduce pain.

■ CONTRAINDICATIONS: Drug dependence or known hypersensitivity to this drug prohibits its use.

■ ADVERSE EFFECTS: Among the more serious adverse reactions are increased intracranial pressure, cardiovascular disturbances, respiratory depression, and drug dependence.

-morphism, a combining form meaning the 'condition of having a (specified) shape': *amorphism, isomorphism, pedomorphism*.

morphogenesis /môr′fəjen′əsis/, the development and differentiation of the structures and the form of an organism, specifically the changes that occur in the cells and tissue during embryonic development. Also called **morphogeny** /môrfoj′ənē/.

morphogenetic, (in embryology) of or pertaining to a substance or hormone that acts as an evocator in differentiation. Also **morphogenic.**

morphogeny. See **morphogenesis.**

morphology, the study of the physical shape and size of a specimen, plant, or animal. (The term was coined by Goethe.) See also **anisopoikilocytosis.** **–morphologic,** *adj*.

-morphosis, a combining form meaning a 'development or change': *chemomorphosis, epimorphosis, heteromorphosis*.

Morquio's disease /môrkē′ōz/, a familial form of mucopolysaccharidosis that results in abnormal musculoskeletal development in childhood. Dwarfism, hunchback, enlarged sternum, and knock-knees may occur. The disease may first be evident as the child, learning to walk, displays an abnormal, waddling gait. Also called **MPS IV.** See also **mucopolysaccharidosis.**

mortality, **1.** the condition of being subject to death. **2.** the death rate, which reflects the number of deaths per unit of population in any specific region, age group, disease, or other classification, usually expressed as deaths per 1000, 10,000, or 100,000.

mortar, a cup-shaped vessel in which materials are ground or crushed by a pestle in the preparation of drugs.

Morton's foot. See **metatarsalgia.**

Morton's neuroma. See **metatarsalgia.**

Morton's plantar neuralgia, a severe throbbing pain that affects the anastomotic nerve branch between the medial and the lateral plantar nerves. Also called *(obsolete)* **Morton's plantar neuroma.**

Morton's toe. See **metatarsalgia.**

morula /môr′ələ/, *pl.* **morulas, morulae,** a solid, spheric mass of cells resulting from the cleavage of the fertilized ovum in the early stages of embryonic development. It represents an intermediate stage between the zygote and the blastocyst and consists of blastomeres that are uniform in size, shape, and physiologic capabilities. –**morular,** *adj.*

-morula, a combining form meaning a 'clump of blastomeres formed by cleavage of a fertilized ovum': *amphimorula, archimorula, pseudomorula.*

mosaic /mōzā′ik/, **1.** (in genetics) an individual or organism that developed from a single zygote but that has two or more kinds of genetically different cell populations. Such a condition results from a mutation, crossing-over, or, more commonly in humans, nondisjunction of the chromosomes during early embryogenesis, which causes a variation in the number of chromosomes in the cells. The type of chromosomal aberration and its ratio depend on whether nondisjunction occurred in the first or later mitotic divisions of the zygote. Because monosomic cells are nonviable, except in X monosomic conditions, most mosaic conditions in humans represent a mixture of normal and trisomic cells, regardless of whether an autosome or the sex chromosomes are involved. The degree of clinical involvement depends on the type of tissue containing the abnormality and may vary from near normal to full manifestation of a syndrome, as Down's syndrome or Turner's syndrome. Compare **chimera.** See also **monosomy, sex chromosome mosaic, trisomy. 2.** (in embryology) a fertilized ovum that undergoes determinate cleavage. See also **mosaic development.**

mosaic bone, bone tissue appearing to be made up of many tiny pieces cemented together, as seen on microscopic examination of an x-ray film of the affected bone. It is characteristic of Paget's disease of the bone.

mosaic cleavage. See **determinate cleavage.**

mosaic development, a kind of embryonic development occurring in the blastocyst. The fertilized ovum undergoes determinate cleavage, developing according to a precise, unalterable plan in which each blastomere has a characteristic position, limited developmental potency, and is a precursor of a definite part of the embryo. Damage to or destruction of these cells results in a defective organism. Compare **regulative development.**

mosaicism /mōzā′isiz′əm/, (in genetics) a condition in which an individual or an organism that develops from a single zygote has two or more cell populations that differ in genetic constitution. Most commonly seen in humans is a variation in the number of chromosomes in the cells, which may involve either a particular autosome, as in Down's syndrome, or the sex chromosomes, as in Turner's syndrome and Kleinfelter's syndrome. See also **mosaic, sex chromosome mosaic.**

mosaic wart, a group of contiguous plantar warts.

mosquito bite, a bite of a bloodsucking arthropod of the subfamily Culicidae that may result in a systemic allergic reaction in a hypersensitive person, an infection, or, most often, a pruritic wheal. Mosquitoes, which are attracted to hosts by moisture, carbon dioxide, estrogens, sweat, or warmth, are vectors of many infectious diseases.

mosquito forceps, a small hemostatic forceps. See also **Halsted's forceps,** def. 1.

Mössbauer spectrometer /mes′bou•ər, mœs′bou•ər/, an instrument that can detect small changes between an atomic nucleus and its environment, as caused by changes in temperature, pressure, or chemical state. The device is used in chemical and physical research with applications in medicine.

mot-, a combining form meaning 'of or related to movement': *motoneuron, motorgraphic, motoricity.*

mother fixation, an arrest in psychosexual development characterized by an abnormally persistent, close, and often paralyzing emotional attachment to one's mother. Compare **father fixation.** See also **freudian fixation.**

motile /mō′til/, capable of spontaneous but unconscious or involuntary movement. –**motility,** *n.*

-motility, -mobility, a combining form meaning the 'condition of being capable of movement': *cardiomotility, hypermotility, supermotility.*

motion sickness, a condition caused by erratic or rhythmic motions in any combination of directions, as in a boat or a car. Severe cases are characterized by nausea, vomiting, vertigo, and headache, mild cases by headache and general discomfort. Various antihistamines are used prophylactically. Kinds of motion sickness are air sickness, car sickness, and seasickness (mal de mer).

motivational conflict, a conflict resulting from the arousal of two or more motives that direct behavior toward incompatible goals. Kinds of motivational conflict include **approach-approach conflict, approach-avoidance conflict,** and **avoidance-avoidance conflict.** See also **motivation.**

motor, 1. of or pertaining to motion, the body apparatus involved in movement, or the brain functions that direct purposeful activities. **2.** of or pertaining to a muscle, nerve, or brain center that produces or subserves motion.

-motor, a combining form meaning 'pertaining to the effects of activity in a body part': *nervimotor, psychomotor, viscerimotor.*

motor aphasia, the inability to utter remembered words, caused by a cerebral lesion in the inferior frontal gyrus (Broca's motor speech area) of the left hemisphere in right-handed individuals. The condition most commonly is the result of a stroke. The patient knows what to say but cannot articulate the words. Patients with motor aphasia sometimes use expletives, suggesting that emotionally charged expressions may be controlled by the right hemisphere. Also called **ataxic aphasia, expressive aphasia, frontocortical aphasia, verbal aphasia.**

motor apraxia, the inability to carry out planned movements or to handle small objects, although the proper use of the object is recognized. The condition results from a lesion in the premotor frontal cortex on the opposite side of the affected limb. Also called **cortical apraxia, innervation apraxia.** See also **apraxia.**

motor area, a portion of the cerebral cortex that includes the precentral gyrus and the posterior part of the frontal gyri and that causes the contraction of the voluntary muscles on stimulation with electrodes. It corresponds to Brodmann's areas IV and VI and is characterized histologically by the absence of the granular layer in the cortex. It contains the giant pyramidal cells of Betz in layer V. Normal voluntary activity requires associations between the motor area and other parts of the cortex; removal of the motor area from one cerebral hemisphere causes paralysis of voluntary muscles, especially of the opposite side of the body. Various parts of the motor area are associated with different body structures, as the lower limb, the face, the mouth, and the hand. The parts associated with more delicate, complicated movements, as those of the hand, are larger than those associated with more general movements.

motor end plate, a broad band of terminal fibers of the motor nerves of the voluntary muscles. Motor nerves derived from the cranial and spinal nerves enter the sheaths of striated muscle fibers, lose their myelin sheaths, and ramify like the roots of a tree. In forming the motor end plate, the neurilemma of the nerve fiber merges with the sarcolemma of the muscle, and the axon synapses with the muscle fibers.

motor fiber, one of the fibers in the spinal nerves that transmit impulses to muscle fibers.

motor image, a visual concept of one's bodily movements, real or imagined.

motor nerve. See **motor neuron.**

motor neuron, one of various efferent nerve cells that transmit nerve impulses from the brain or from the spinal cord to muscular or glandular tissue. According to location, some kinds of motor neurons are the peripheral motor neurons and the upper motor neurons. Also called **motoneuron.** Compare **sensory nerve.** See also **nervous system.**

motor neuron paralysis, an injury to the spinal cord that causes damage to the motor neurons and results in various degrees of functional impairment depending on the site of the lesion. See **lower motor neuron paralysis, upper motor neuron paralysis.**

motor point, **1.** a point at which a motor nerve enters the muscle it innervates. **2.** a point at which electric stimulation will cause contraction of a muscle. Compare **motor end plate.** See also **motor neuron, nervous system.**

motor seizure, a transitory disturbance in brain function caused by abnormal neuronal discharges that arise initially in a localized motor area of the cerebral cortex. The manifestations depend on the site of the abnormal electric activity, as tonic contractures of the thumb, caused by excessive discharges in the motor area of the cortex controlling the first digit, or chewing movements resulting from discharges in the lower part of the motor strip controlling mastication. The disturbance may spread, or it may end in a shower of clonic movements or a generalized convulsion. Also called **focal motor seizure.** See also **epilepsy, focal seizure.**

motor sense, the feeling or perception enabling a person to accomplish a purposeful movement, presumably achieved by evoking a sensory engram or memory of the pattern for that specific movement. Proprioceptive signals transmitted by feedback pathways through the cerebellum and sensory areas of the motor cortex are compared with the engram and modify the movement. Experiments with animals show that a movement cannot be performed if the corresponding sensory area of the brain is removed; if the motor area is removed, the movement is accomplished by using a different group of muscles.

motor unit, a functional structure consisting of a motor neuron and the muscle fibers it innervates.

Motrin, a trademark for an antiinflammatory (ibuprofen).

mottle, an effect observed in radiologic imaging when the dose of radiation employed is reduced to a level where individual quantum effects can be seen. Instead of a uniform beam of radiation, the number of photons being produced is so low that the statistic variations in x-ray production can be visualized.

mountain fever, mountain tick fever. See **Colorado tick fever, Rocky Mountain spotted fever.**

mourning, a psychologic process of reaction activated by an individual to assist in overcoming a great personal loss. The process is finally resolved when a new object relationship is established.

mouse-tooth forceps, a kind of dressing forceps that has one or more fine sharp points on the tip of each blade. The tips turn in, and the delicate teeth interlock.

mouth, **1.** the nearly oval oral cavity at the anterior end of the digestive tube, bounded anteriorly by the lips and containing the tongue and the teeth. It consists of the vestibule and the mouth cavity proper. The vestibule, situated in front of the teeth, is bounded externally by the lips and the cheeks, internally by the gums and the teeth. The vestibule receives the secretion from the parotid salivary glands and communicates, when the jaws are closed, with the mouth cavity proper by an aperture on each side behind the molar teeth and by narrow clefts between opposing teeth. The mouth cavity proper is bounded ventrally and laterally by the alveolar arches and the teeth, communicates dorsally with the pharynx by the ischmium faucium, and is roofed by the hard and the soft palates. The tongue forms the greater part of the floor of the cavity. The rest of the floor is formed by the reflection of the mucous membrane from the sides and the bottom of the tongue to the gum lining the inner part of the mandible. The mouth cavity proper receives the secretion from the submandibular and the sublingual salivary glands. **2.** an orifice.

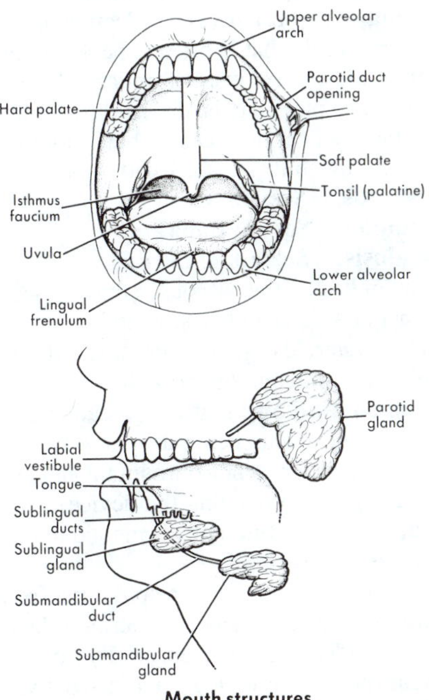

Mouth structures

mouth-to-mouth resuscitation, a procedure in artificial resuscitation, performed most often with cardiac massage. The victim's nose is sealed by pinching the nostrils closed, the head is extended, and air is breathed by the rescuer through the mouth into the lungs. See also **cardiopulmonary resuscitation.**

mouth-to-nose resuscitation, a procedure in artificial resuscitation in which the mouth of the victim is covered and held closed and air is breathed through the victim's nose. See also **mouth-to-mouth resuscitation.**

MOV, abbreviation for **minimal occlusive volume.**

moving grid, (in radiography) an x-ray grid that is continuously moved or oscillated throughout the exposure of a radiographic film.

moxalactam disodium, an antibiotic.

■ INDICATIONS: It is prescribed in the treatment of lower respiratory, intraabdominal, urinary tract, bone and joint, and skin infections and bacterial septicemia caused by a susceptible strain of a wide variety of microorganisms.

■ CONTRAINDICATION: Known sensitivity to this drug prohibits its use.

■ ADVERSE EFFECTS: Among the most serious adverse reactions are hypersensitivity reactions, eosinophilia, thrombocytopenia, reversible leukopenia, anaphylaxis, and hepatic enzyme elevations. It must be used with caution in patients allergic to penicillins.

Moxam, a trademark for an antibiotic (moxalactam).

moxibustion /mok′səbus′chən/, a method of producing analgesia or altering the function of a system of the body achieved by igniting moxa, wormwood, or other combustible, slow-burning substance and holding it as near the point on the skin as possible without causing pain or burning. It is also sometimes used in conjunction with acupuncture.

M.P.D., abbreviation for *maximum permissible dose.*

M.P.H., abbreviation for *Master of Public Health.*

MPS, abbreviation for **mucopolysaccharidosis.**

MPS I, abbreviation for *mucopolysaccharidosis I.* See **Hurler's syndrome.**

MPS II, abbreviation for *mucopolysaccharidosis II.* See **Hunter's syndrome.**

MPS IV, abbreviation for *mucopolysaccharidosis IV.* See **Morquio's disease.**

mr, mR, abbreviation for **milliroentgen.**

MS, abbreviation for **multiple sclerosis.**

M.S., **1.** abbreviation for *Master of Science.* **2.** abbreviation for *Master of Surgery.*

MSH, abbreviation for *melanocyte stimulating hormone.*

M.S.N., abbreviation for *Master of Science in Nursing.* See **master's degree program in nursing.**

M.T., abbreviation for **Medical Technologist.**

mu, symbol for **micron.**

Much's granules /mo͞oks, mo͝okhs/, granules and rods, found in tuberculosis sputum, that stain with gram stain but not by the usual methods for acid-fast bacilli.

mucin /myo͞o′sin/, a mucopolysaccharide, the chief ingredient in mucus. Mucin is present in most glands that secrete mucus and is the lubricant protecting body surfaces from friction or erosion.

mucinoid, resembling mucin. See also **mucoid,** def. 2.

mucinous adenocarcinoma. See **mucinous carcinoma.**

mucinous carcinoma, an epithelial neoplasm with a sticky gelatinous consistency caused by the copious mucin secreted by its cells. Also called **colloid carcinoma, gelatiniform carcinoma, gelatinous carcinoma.**

mucocutaneous /myo͞o′kōkyo͞otā′nē·əs/, of or pertaining to the mucous membrane and the skin.

mucocutaneous leishmaniasis. See **American leishmaniasis.**

mucocutaneous lymph node syndrome (MLNS), an acute, febrile illness, primarily of young children, characterized by inflamed mucous membranes of the mouth, "strawberry tongue," cervical lymphadenopathy, polymorphous rash on the trunk, and edema, erythema, and desquamation of the skin on the extremities. Other commonly associated findings include arthralgia, diarrhea, otitis, pneumonia, photophobia, meningitis, and electrocardiographic changes. The cause is unknown; no clear-cut environmental, seasonal, or geographic factors have been discovered, and person-to-person transmission is unproven. A genetic predisposition has been indicated.

Treatment includes aspirin in large doses, which may be prescribed over a long period of time, and supportive care. Also called **Kawasaki disease.**

mucoepidermoid carcinoma, a malignant neoplasm of glandular tissues, especially the ducts of the salivary glands. The tumor contains mucinous and epidermoid squamous cells.

mucogingival junction, the scalloped linear area of the gums that separates the gingivae from the alveolar mucosa.

mucoid /myo͞o′koid/, **1.** resembling mucus. **2.** also **mucinoid.** a group of glycoproteins, including colloid and ovomucoid, similar to the mucins, the primary difference being in solubility.

mucolytic /myo͞o′kəlit′ik/, **1.** exerting a destructive effect on the mucus. **2.** any agent that dissolves or destroys the mucus.

mucomembranous /myo͞o′kəmem′brənəs/, of or pertaining to a mucous membrane, as that of the small intestine or the bladder.

Mucomyst, a trademark for a mucolytic (acetylcysteine), used as an adjunct to anesthesia and as adjuvant therapy for patients with abnormal, viscid, or inspissated mucous secretions.

mucopolysaccharidosis (MPS) /myo͞o′kōpol′ēsak′ərido͞′sis/, *pl.* **mucopolysaccharidoses,** one of a group of genetic disorders characterized by greater than normal accumulations of mucopolysaccharides in the tissues, with other symptoms specific to each type. The disorders are numbered MPS I through MPS VII, and each type has a specific eponym. In all types, there is pronounced skeletal deformity (especially of the face), mental and physical retardation, and decreased life expectancy. The disorders may be detected before birth by testing fetal cells present in amniotic fluid. After birth, diagnosis is established through urine testing, skeletal changes observed on x-ray films, and family history. There is no successful treatment. Kinds of mucopolysaccharidosis include **Hunter's syndrome (MPS II), Hurler's syndrome (MPS I),** and **Morquio's disease (MPS IV).**

mucoprotein /myo͞o′kōprō′tēn, -tē•in/, a compound, present in all connective and supporting tissue, that contains polysaccharides combined with protein and is relatively resistant to denaturation.

mucopurulent /myo͞o′kōpyo͝or′yələnt/, characteristic of a combination of mucus and pus.

mucormycosis. See **zygomycosis.**

mucosa /myo͞okō′sə/, *pl.* **mucosae,** mucous membrane. **–mucosal,** *adj.*

mucous. See **mucus.**

-mucous, a combining form meaning 'containing or composed of mucus': *fibromucous, puromucous, seromucous.*

mucous colitis. See **irritable bowel syndrome.**

mucous membrane, any one of four major kinds of thin sheets of tissue that cover or line various parts of the body. Mucous membranes line cavities or canals of the body that open to the outside, as the linings of the mouth, the digestive tube, the respiratory passages, and the genitourinary tract. It consists of a surface layer of epithelial tissue covering a deeper layer of connective tissue and protects the underlying structure, secretes mucus, and absorbs water, salts, and other solutes. Compare **serous membrane, skin, synovial membrane.**

mucous plug, (in obstetrics) a collection of thick mucus in the uterine cervix that is often expelled at the onset of dilatation of the cervix, just before labor begins or in its early hours. The plug may be dry and firm, following the shape of the endocervical canal, but, more often, it is semifluid and mucoid, streaked with blood.

mucous shreds. See **shreds.**

mucous tumor. See **myxoma.**

mucoviscidosis. See **cystic fibrosis.**

mucus /myo͞o′kəs/, the viscous, slippery secretions of mucous membranes and glands, containing mucin, white blood cells, water, inorganic salts, and exfoliated cells. **–mucoid,** *adj.,* **mucous** /myo͞o′kəs/, *adj.*

mucus trap suction apparatus, a catheter containing a trap to prevent mucus being aspirated from the nasopharynx and trachea of a newborn infant and entering the mouth of the person operating the device.

mud bath, the application of warm mud to the body for therapeutic purposes.

Mudrane, a trademark for a respiratory, fixed-combination drug containing a smooth muscle relaxant (theophylline), an adrenergic (ephedrine hydrochloride), an expectorant (potassium iodide), and a sedative-hypnotic (phenobarbital).

mulibrey nanism /mul′ibrī/, a rare genetic disorder, transmitted as an autosomal recessive trait, characterized by dwarfism, constrictive pericarditis, muscular hypotonia, anomalies of the skull and face, and characteristic yellow dots in the ocular fundus. The name of the condition is an acronym comprised of the first two letters of the anatomic sites of the principal defects: *mus*cle, *li*ver, *br*ain, and *ey*es.

müllerian /miler′ē•ən, mYl-/, of or pertaining to the Müllerian ducts, named for Johannes Peter Müller.

müllerian duct, one of a pair of embryonic ducts that become the fallopian tubes, uterus, and vagina in females and that atrophy in males.

multi-, a combining form meaning 'many': *multicapsular, multifamilial, multipara.*

multicentric mitosis. See **multipolar mitosis.**

multifactorial, of, pertaining to, or characteristic of any condition or disease resulting from the interaction of many factors, specifically the interaction of several genes, usually polygenes, with or without the involvement of environmental factors. Many disorders, as spina bifida, neural tube defects, and Hirschsprung's disease, are considered to be multifactorial.

multifactorial inheritance, the tendency to develop a physical appearance, disease, or condition that is a condition of many genetic and environmental factors, as stature and blood pressure. See also **polygene.**

multifocal, an action, as the transmission of an impulse, that arises from more than two foci.

multiform, an organ, tissue, or other object that may appear in more than one shape.

multigravida /mul'tigrav'idə/, a woman who has been pregnant more than once. Compare **multipara, primagravida.**

multihospital system, a group of two or more hospitals owned, sponsored, or managed by a central organization.

multiinfarct dementia, a form of organic brain disease characterized by the rapid deterioration of intellectual functioning, caused by vascular disease. Symptoms include emotional lability, disturbances in memory, abstract thinking, judgment, and impulse control, and focal neurologic impairment, as gait abnormalities, pseudobulbar palsy, and paresthesia. The condition is more prevalent in men than in women and may be caused by a cerebrovascular accident with cerebrovascular insufficiency or by intracerebral hemorrhage. See also **dementia, senile psychosis.**

multilocular cyst, one of three kinds of follicular cyst, containing many spaces and not associated with a tooth. Compare **dentigerous cyst, primordial cyst.**

multipara /multip'ərə/, *pl.* **multiparae,** a woman who has been delivered of more than one viable infant. Compare **multigravida, nullipara, primipara.**

multipenniform, (of a bodily structure) having a shape resembling a pattern of many feathers, especially the pattern formed by the muscular fasciculi that converge to several tendons. Compare **bipenniform, penniform.**

multiphasic screening, a technique of screening populations for diseases in which there is combined use of a battery of screening tests. The technique serves to identify any of several diseases being screened for in a population that is apparently healthy.

multiple benign cystic epithelioma. See **trichoepithelioma.**

multiple cartilaginous exostoses. See **diaphyseal aclasis.**

multiple enchondromatosis. See **enchondromatosis.**

multiple endocrine adenomatosis. See **adenomatosis.**

multiple factor. See **polygene.**

multiple fission, cell division in which the nucleus first divides into several equal parts followed by the division of the cytoplasm into as many cells as there are nuclei. It is the common form of asexual reproduction in certain unicellular organisms. Compare **binary fission.**

multiple fracture, **1.** a fracture extending several fracture lines in one bone. **2.** the fracture of several bones at one time or from the same injury.

multiple gene. See **polygene.**

multiple idiopathic hemorrhagic sarcoma. See **Kaposi's sarcoma.**

multiple lipomatosis, a rare, inherited disorder characterized by discrete, localized, subcutaneous deposits of fat in the tissues of the body. This fat is not available for metabolic use, even in starvation.

multiple mononeuropathy, an abnormal condition characterized by dysfunction of several individual nerve trunks. It may be caused by various diseases, as necrotizing angiopathy, uremia, diabetes mellitus, and some inflammatory immunologic disorders. Also called *(obsolete)* **mononeuritis multiplex.**

multiple myeloma, a malignant neoplasm of the bone marrow. The tumor, composed of plasma cells, destroys osseous tissue, especially in flat bones, causing pain, fractures, and skeletal deformities, including spinal curvature. Characteristically, there are abnormal proteins in the plasma and urine, anemia, weight loss, pulmonary complications secondary to rib fractures, and kidney failure. Also called **multiple plasmacytoma of bone, myelomatosis, plasma cell myeloma.**

multiple myositis. See **polymyositis.**

multiple neuroma. See **neuromatosis.**

multiple peripheral neuritis, acute or subacute disseminated inflammation or degeneration of symmetrically distributed peripheral nerves, characterized initially by numbness, tingling in the extremities, hot and cold sensations, and slight fever, progressing to pain, weakness, diminished reflexes, and in some cases flaccid paralysis. The disorder may be caused by toxic substances, as antimony, arsenic, carbon monoxide, copper, lead, mercury, nitrobenzol, organophosphates, and thallium, or various drugs, including diphenylhydantoin, isoniazid, nitrofurantoin, thalidomide, and vincristine. Multiple peripheral neuritis may occur in alcoholism, arteriosclerosis, beriberi, chronic GI disease, diabetes, leprosy, pellagra, porphyria, rheumatoid arthritis, systemic lupus erythematosus, and many infectious diseases. Therapy consists of removal of the toxic agent or treatment of the causative disease, rest, and medication for pain. Guillain-Barré syndrome sometimes occurs after an influenza vaccination. Also called **peripheral polyneuritis, peripheral polyneuropathy.** See also **Guillain-Barré syndrome.**

multiple personality, an abnormal condition in which the organization of the personality is fragmented. It is characterized by the presence of two or more distinct subpersonalities. Also called **split personality.**

multiple personality disorder, a dissociative disorder characterized by the existence of two or more distinct, clearly differentiated personality structures within the same individual, any of which may dominate at a particular time. Each personality is a complex unit with separate, well-developed emotional and thought processes, behavior patterns, and social relationships. The various subpersonalities are usually dramatically different from one another and may or may not be aware of the existence of the others. Often, complex interrelationships exist between the personalities, with one functioning on a conscious level and the other or others on a subconscious level. Transition from one subpersonality to another is usually sudden and associated with psychosocial stress. The dominance of a particular subpersonality may last from a few minutes to several years. The condition, most often diagnosed in female adolescents or young adults, primarily results from intrapsychic conflicts that are so deep-seated that the only solution is to separate the conflicting parts of the psyche into separate autonomous personality systems. Classic examples of the disorder are extremely rare; various symptoms, but not the complete entity, are apparent in some schizophrenic patients. Treatment may include hypnosis or psychotropic medication and long-term psychotherapy aimed at uncovering the emotional conflicts that precipitated the development and maintenance of the various subpersonalities. See also **dissociative disorder, hysteric neurosis.**

multiple plasmacytoma of bone. See **multiple myeloma.**

multiple pregnancy, a pregnancy in which there is more than one fetus in the uterus at the same time.

multiple sclerosis (MS), a progressive disease characterized by disseminated demyelination of nerve fibers of the brain and spinal cord. It begins slowly, usually in young adulthood, and continues throughout life with periods of exacerbation and remission. The first signs are paresthesias, or abnormal sensations in the extremities or on one side of the face. Other early signs are muscle weakness, vertigo, and visual disturbances, as nystagmus, diplopia (double vision), and partial blindness. Later in the course of disease, there may be extreme emotional lability, ataxia, abnormal reflexes, and difficulty in urinating. Because many other conditions affect the nervous system and produce similar symptoms, the diagnosis of MS is difficult to make. A history of exacerbation and remission of symptoms and the presence of greater than normal amounts of protein in cerebrospinal fluid are characteristic. As the disease progresses, the intervals between exacerbations grow shorter, and disability becomes greater. There is no specific treatment for the disease; corticosteroids and other drugs are used to treat the symptoms accompanying acute episodes. Physical therapy may help to postpone or prevent specific disabilities. The patient is encouraged to live as normal and active a life as possible. Also called **disseminated multiple sclerosis.**

multiple self-healing squamous epithelioma. See **keratoacanthoma.**

multiplicative growth. See **merisis.**

multipolar mitosis, cell division in which the spindle has three or more poles and results in the formation of a corresponding number of daughter cells. Also called **multicentric mitosis, pluripolar mitosis.** See also **trisomy.**

multisource drug, a drug that can be purchased under any of several trademarks from different manufacturers or distributors. See also **generic equivalent, generic name.**

multisynaptic, pertaining to a nervous process or system of nerve cells requiring a series of synapses.

multivalent /mul′tivā′lənt/, **1.** (in chemistry) denoting the capacity of an element to combine with three or more univalent atoms. **2.** (in immunology) able to act against more than one strain of organism. Compare **valence.**

mummification, a dried-up state, as occurs in dry gangrene or a dead fetus in utero.

mummified fetus, a fetus that has died in utero and has shriveled and dried up.

mumps, an acute viral disease, characterized by a swelling of the parotid glands, caused by a paramyxovirus. It is most likely to affect children between 5 and 15 years of age, but it may occur at any age. In adulthood the infection may be severe. Passive immunity from maternal antibodies usually prevents this disease in children under 1 year of age. The incidence of mumps is highest during the late winter and early spring. The mumps paramyxovirus lives in the saliva of the affected individual and is transmitted in droplets or by direct contact. The virus is present in the saliva from 6 days before to 9 days after the onset of the swelling of the parotid gland. The time of maximum communicability is believed to be the 48-hour period immediately before the start of parotid swelling. The prognosis in mumps is good, but the disease sometimes involves complications, as arthritis, pancreatitis, myocarditis, oophoritis, and nephritis. About one half of the men with mumps-induced orchitis suffer some atrophy of the testicles, but because the condition is usually unilateral, sterility rarely results. Also called **epidemic parotitis, infectious parotitis.**

■ OBSERVATIONS: The common symptoms of mumps usually last for about 24 hours and include anorexia, headache, malaise, and low-grade fever. These signs are commonly followed by earache, parotid gland swelling and a temperature of 101° to 104° F (38.3° to 40° C). The patient also experiences pain when drinking acidic liquids or when chewing. The salivary glands may also become swollen. Complications, as epididymoorchitis and mumps meningitis, may develop. About 25% of the postpubertal men who contract mumps develop epididymoorchitis with associated testicular swelling and tenderness that may persist for several weeks. Mumps meningitis develops in 10% of the patients with mumps and occurs in three to five times as many males as females. Diagnosis of mumps is usually based on typical symptoms, especially parotid gland swelling. If the parotid gland is not swollen, confirming diagnosis may be based on serologic antibody tests.

■ INTERVENTION: The treatment of mumps commonly includes the respiratory isolation of the patient and the administration of analgesics, antipyretics, and a fluid intake adequate to prevent dehydration associated with fever and anorexia. Intravenous fluids may be administered to the patient who can't swallow as the result of severe parotitis.

■ NURSING CONSIDERATIONS: The patient is confined to bed and may be given antipyretics and tepid sponge baths to reduce fever. Patients with mumps are also encouraged to drink fluids and to avoid spicy foods and those that require considerable chewing. During the acute phase of the disease, the nurse is especially alert to any signs of central nervous system involvement, as nuchal rigidity and altered consciousness. All cases of mumps are routinely reported to local health authorities. Nurses aid public health education by stressing the importance of immunization with live attenuated mumps virus for children at 15 months of age and for susceptible persons, especially males who are approaching puberty or who are past puberty. Immunization within 24 hours of exposure may prevent the disease or may minimize its effects.

MUMPS /mumps/, abbreviation for *Massachusetts General Hospital Utility Multi-Programming System,* a high-level interactive computer language with health care applications.

Mumpsvax, a trademark for an active immunizing agent (live mumps virus vaccine).

mumps virus vaccine live, an active immunizing agent.

■ INDICATION: It is prescribed for immunization against mumps.

■ CONTRAINDICATIONS: Immunosuppression, concomitant use of corticosteroids, acute infection, pregnancy, or known hypersensitivity to chicken proteins, neomycin, or this drug prohibits its use.

■ ADVERSE EFFECTS: Among the most serious adverse effects are fevers, parotitis, and allergic reactions.

Munchausen's syndrome /mun′chousənz/, an unusual condition characterized by habitual pleas for treatment and hospitalization for a symptomatic but imaginary acute illness. The affected person may logically and convincingly present the symptoms and history of a real disease. Symptoms resolve with treatment, but the person may seek further treatment for another imaginary disease. Also called **pathomimicry.**

mural, something that is found on or against the wall of a cavity, as a mural thrombus on an interior wall of the heart.

Murchison fever. See **Pel-Ebstein fever.**

murine typhus, an acute arbovirus infection caused by *Rickettsia typhi* and transmitted by the bite of an infected flea. The disease is similar to epidemic typhus but less severe. It is characterized by headache, chills, fever, myalgia, and rash. After an 8- to 16-day incubation period, fever develops and lasts about 12 days. A dull-red, maculopapular rash, mainly on the trunk, appears about the fifth day and lasts for 4 to 8 days. Recovery is usually rapid and complete, but death has occurred in elderly or debilitated people. Weil-Felix and complement fixation tests aid in the diagnosis. Chloramphenicol or tetracycline is usually prescribed in treatment. Prevention involves the elimination of the rodents that are the natural host of the organism and the use of appropriate insecticides to control fleas. Also called **endemic typhus, flea-borne typhus, New World typhus, rat typhus, urban typhus.** Compare **epidemic typhus, Rocky Mountain spotted fever.** See also **Brill-Zinsser disease.**

murmur, a low-pitched fluttering or humming sound, as a heart murmur.

Murocoll, a trademark for an ophthalmic drug.

Murray Valley encephalitis, an acute inflammatory disease of the brain, once epidemic in Australia's Murray Valley, characterized by convulsions, muscle rigidity, high fever, mental confusion, and coma. It is believed related to Australian X disease, which is caused by a neurotropic herpeslike virus.

muscae volitantes. See **floater.**

muscarinic /mus′kərin′ik/, stimulating the postganglionic parasympathetic receptor.

muscle, a kind of tissue comprised of fibers that are able to contract, causing and allowing movement of the parts and organs of the body. Muscle fibers are richly vascular, irritable, conductive, and elastic. There are two basic kinds, striated muscle and smooth muscle. Striated muscle, which comprises all skeletal muscles except for the myocardium, is long and voluntary; it responds very quickly to stimulation and is paralyzed by interruption of its innervation. Smooth muscle, which comprises all visceral muscles, is short and involuntary; it reacts slowly to all stimuli and does not entirely lose its tone if innervation is interrupted. The myocardium is sometimes classified as a third (cardiac) kind of muscle, but it is basically a striated muscle that does not contract as quickly as the striated muscle of the rest of the body, and it is not completely paralyzed if it loses its neural stimuli. See also **cardiac muscle, smooth muscle, striated muscle.**

muscle albumin, albumin present in muscle.

muscle of expression. See **facial muscle.**

muscle relaxant, a chemotherapeutic agent that reduces the contractility of muscle fibers. Curare derivatives and succinylcholine compete with acetylcholine and block neural transmission at the myoneural junction. These drugs are used during anesthesia, in the management of patients undergoing mechanic ventilation, and in shock therapy, to reduce muscle contractions in pharmacologically or electrically induced seizures. Quinine sulfate, prescribed for the prevention and treatment of nocturnal leg cramps, reduces muscle tension by increasing the refractory period of muscle fibers and by decreasing the excitability of the motor end plate. Several drugs that relieve muscle spasms act at various levels in the central nervous system: Baclofen inhibits monosynaptic and polysynaptic reflexes at the spinal level; cyclobenzaprine acts primarily in the brainstem; chlorzoxazone inhibits multisynaptic arcs in the spinal cord and subcortical areas of the brain; and the benzodiazepines reduce muscle tension, chiefly by acting on reticular neuronal mechanisms that control muscle tone. Dantrolene acts directly on muscles in reducing contraction and apparently achieves its effect by interfering with the release of calcium from the sarcoplasmic reticulum.

muscle-setting exercise, a method of maintaining muscle strength and tonality by alternately contracting and relaxing a skeletal muscle or any group of muscles without moving the associated part of the body. Such activity is useful in preventing atrophy of the muscles, especially in patients with conditions involving the joints.

muscular, 1. of or pertaining to a muscle. 2. characteristic of well-developed musculature.

muscular atrophy, a condition of motor unit dysfunction, usually the result of a loss of efferent innervation.

muscular branch of the deep brachial artery, one of several similar branches of the deep brachial artery, supplying certain arm muscles, as the coracobrachialis, biceps brachii, and brachialis.

muscular dystrophy, a group of genetically transmitted diseases characterized by progressive atrophy of symmetric groups of skeletal muscles without evidence of involvement or degeneration of neural tissue. In all forms of muscular dystrophy there is an insidious loss of strength with increasing disability and deformity, although each type differs in the groups of muscles affected, the age of onset, the rate of progression, and the mode of genetic inheritance. The basic cause is unknown but appears to be an inborn error of metabolism. Serum creatine phosphokinase is increased in affected individuals and acts as a diagnostic aid, especially in asymptomatic children in families at risk. Diagnostic confirmation is made by muscle biopsy, electromyography, and genetic pedigree. Treatment of the muscular dystrophies consists primarily of supportive measures, as physical therapy and orthopedic procedures to minimize deformity. The main types of the disease are pseudohypertrophic (Duchenne) muscular dystrophy, limb-girdle muscular dystrophy, and facioscapulohumeral (Landouzy-Déjérine) muscular dystrophy. Rarer forms include Becker's muscular dystrophy, distal muscular dystrophy, ocular myopathy, and myotonic muscular dystrophy. See also **myotonic myopathy.**

muscular sarcoidosis, sarcoidosis of the skeletal muscles in which there is interstitial inflammation, fibrosis, atrophy, and damage of the muscle fibers as sarcoid tubercles form within and replace normal muscle cells. See also **sarcoidosis.**

muscular system, all of the muscles of the body, including the smooth, cardiac, and striated muscles, considered as an interrelated structural group. See also the Color Atlas of Human Anatomy.

muscular tumor. See **myoma.**

musculocutaneous nerve /mus′kyo͞olōyo͞otā′nē•əs/, one of the terminal branches of the brachial plexus. It is formed on each side by division of the lateral cord of the plexus into two branches. It pierces the coracobrachialis and crosses to the lateral side of the arm, where it pierces the deep fascia just above the elbow and continues into the forearm as the lateral antebrachial cutaneous nerve. Various branches and filaments supply different structures, as the biceps, the brachialis, the humerus, and the skin of the forearm. The branches of the musculocutaneous nerve are the coracobrachialis branch, the muscular branches, an articular filament to the elbow joint, a filament to the humerus, the lateral antebrachial cutaneous nerve, the anterior branch, and the dorsal branch. Compare **median nerve, radial nerve, ulnar nerve.**

musculoskeletal /mus′kyo͞olōskel′ətəl/, of or pertaining to the muscles and the skeleton.

musculoskeletal system, all of the muscles, bones, joints, and related structures, as the tendons and connective tissue, that function in the movement of the parts and organs of the body. See also the Color Atlas of Human Anatomy.

musculoskeletal system assessment, an evaluation of the condition and functioning of the patient's muscles, joints, and bones and of factors that may contribute to abnormalities in these body structures.

■ METHOD: The patient is questioned about any pain and edema in muscles, joints, and bones, weakness in extremities, limitations in movements and activities, unsteadiness on the feet, fatigability, insomnia, anorexia, weight loss, and feelings of frustration. The individual's general appearance, age, blood pressure, pulse, respirations, body alignment, ability or inability to move in bed, gait, need for assistance in walking, handgrip, range of motion, and internal and external rotation of extremities are observed. The presence of contractures, deformities, paralysis, contusions, lacerations, wounds, footdrop, wristdrop, paralysis, crutches, brace, cast, prosthesis, cane, walker, decubiti, allergies, skin rash, or tenseness is noted. It is ascertained whether the patient can perform activities of daily living, is able to sit up, turn, and use the trapeze in bed, if constipation is a complaint, and if the individual is independent or dependent. Concurrent diseases or conditions investigated include injury to the spinal cord, nerve impairment, cerebrovascular accident, rheumatoid arthritis, osteoarthritis, bursitis, polyneuritis, multiple sclerosis, muscular dystrophy, myasthenia gravis, fracture, ruptured disk, Ménière's disease, and labyrinthitis. It is determined if the patient previously had orthopedic or spinal surgery, poliomyelitis, hemiplegia, cerebral palsy, parkinsonism, a cerebrovascular accident, ataxia, syphilis, hyperparathyroidism, osteoporosis, rickets, osteomalacia, tuberculosis, alcoholism, and impaired vision or hearing. A family history of carcinoma, diabetes, or tuberculosis, the patient's involvement in a hazardous job or recreation, history of previous accidents, and the use of tobacco or medications, as steroids, sedatives, tranquilizers, analgesics, antimalarials, acetylsalicylic acid, or indomethacin, are determined. Laboratory studies important for the assessment are assays of serum and urine calcium and phosphorus and of alkaline phosphatase serum level. Diagnostic procedures that may be required include x-ray films of bones, arthrograms, myelograms, arteriograms, arthroscopy, biopsies of bone or muscle, incision and drainage of joints, and electromyograms of muscles.

■ NURSING ORDERS: The nurse conducts the interview to obtain subjective data, makes the necessary observations of the patient, and assembles the information on concurrent and previous disorders, the family history, the patient's social and medication background, and the results of laboratory studies and diagnostic procedures.

■ OUTCOME CRITERIA: A meticulous assessment of the patient's musculoskeletal system is a valuable aid in diagnosis, in planning the course of therapy, and in predicting the prognosis.

musculospiral nerve. See **radial nerve.**

mushroom, the fruiting body of the fungus of the class Basidomycetes, especially edible members of the order Agaricales, commonly known as the field mushrooms or meadow mushrooms. Although mushrooms contain some protein and minerals, they are composed largely of water and are of limited nutritional value. Fungal poisoning is caused by ingestion of mushrooms of the genus *Amanita,* in particular *A. muscaria* and *A. phalloides.* Symptoms, caused by toxic peptides, may appear within a few minutes of ingestion and consist of severe abdominal pain, vomiting, extreme nausea, salivation, sweating, diarrhea, excessive thirst, coma, and, occasionally, convulsion. Extensive damage to the liver, kidneys, and central nervous system may occur. Some mushrooms, especially *Psilocybe mexicana,* contain substances that produce hallucinatory states.

mushroom poisoning, a toxic condition caused by the ingestion of certain mushrooms, particularly two species of the genus *Amanita.* Muscarine in *Amanita muscaria* produces intoxication in from a few minutes to 2 hours. Symptoms include lacrimation, salivation, sweating, vomiting, labored breathing, abdominal cramps, diarrhea, and, in severe cases, convulsions, coma, and circulatory failure. Atropine is usually administered in treatment. More deadly but slower acting phalloidine in *A. phalloides* and *A. verna* causes similar symptoms, as well as liver damage, renal failure, and death in 30% to 50% of the cases. Treatment includes emptying the stomach by gastric lavage with a weak solution of tannic acid or of potassium permanganate, followed by a saline purgative. Intensive care, as for kidney or liver failure, and hemodialysis may reduce mortality. In some people, the consumption of alcohol complicates mushroom poisoning, and the combination has the effect of disulfiram.

mushroom worker's lung, a type of hypersensitivity pneumonitis common among workers in the mushroom-growing industry. The antigens to which the hypersensitive reactions occur are genera of the fungi *Micropolyspora* and *Thermoactinomyces.* Spores of these fungi are found in the postspawning compost used to grow mushrooms. Symptoms of the acute form of the disease include chills, cough, fever, dyspnea, anorexia, nausea, and vomiting. The chronic form of the disease is characterized by fatigue, chronic cough, weight loss, and dyspnea on exercise.

music therapy, a form of adjunctive psychotherapy in which music is used as a means of recreation and communication, especially with autistic children, and as a means to elevate the mood of depressed and psychotic patients.

mustard gas, a poisonous gas used in chemical warfare during World War I. It causes corrosive destruction of the skin and mucous membranes, often resulting in permanent respiratory damage and death.

Mustargen Hydrochloride, a trademark for an antineoplastic (mechlorethamine hydrochloride).

mutagen /myo͞o′təjən/, any chemical or physical environmental agent that induces a genetic mutation or increases the mutation rate. **–mutagenic,** *adj.,* **mutagenicity,** *n.*

mutagenesis /myo͞o′təjen′əsis/, the induction or occurrence of a genetic mutation. See also **teratogenesis.**

Mutamycin, a trademark for an antineoplastic (mitomycin).

mutant, **1.** any individual or organism with genetic material that has undergone mutation. **2.** relating to or produced by mutation.

mutant gene, any gene that has undergone a change, as the loss, gain, or exchange of genetic material, which affects the normal transmission and expression of a trait. Such genes can become inactive or show reduced, increased, or antagonistic activity. Kinds of mutant genes are **amorph, antimorph, hypermorph, hypomorph.**

mutase, any enzyme that catalyzes the shifting of a chemical group or radical from one position to another within the same molecule or, occasionally, from one molecule to another.

mutation, an unusual change in genetic material occurring spontaneously or by induction. The alteration changes the original expression of the gene. Genes are stable units, but when a mutation occurs, it often is transmitted to future generations. **–mutate,** *v.,* **mutational,** *adj.*

mutism /myo͞o′tizəm/, the inability or refusal to speak. The condition may result from an unconscious response to emotional conflict and confusion and is most commonly observed in patients who are catatonic, stuporous, hysteric, or depressed. A kind of mutism is **akinetic mutism.**

muton /myo͞o′ton/, (in molecular genetics), the smallest DNA segment whose alteration can result in a mutation.

mutually exclusive categories, categories on a research instrument that are sufficiently precise to allow each subject, factor, or variable to be classified in only one category.

mv, mV, abbreviation for **millivolt.**

m$\dot{V}O_2$, symbol for **myocardial oxygen consumption.**

MVV, abbreviation for *maximal voluntary ventilation.* See **maximal breathing capacity.**

M.W.I.A., abbreviation for **Medical Women's International Association.**

my-. See **myo-.**

myalgia /mī·al′jə/, diffuse muscle pain, usually accompanied by malaise, occurring in many infectious diseases, as brucellosis, dengue, influenza, leptospirosis, measles, malaria, relapsing fever, rheumatic fever, salmonellosis, tick-borne hemorrhagic fevers, toxoplasmosis, trichinosis, tularemia, and poliomyelitis. Myalgia occurs in arteriosclerosis obliterans, fibrositis, fibromyositis, Guillain-

Barré syndrome, hyperparathyroidism, hypoglycemia, hypothyroidism, muscle tumor, myoglobinuria, myositis, and renal tubular acidosis. Various drugs that may cause myalgia include amphotericin B, carbenoxolone, chloroquinine, clofibrate, and corticosteroids. See also **epidemic myalgia.** –**myalgic,** *adj.*

myalgic asthenia, a condition characterized by a general feeling of fatigue and muscular pain, often resulting from or associated with psychologic stress.

Myambutol, a trademark for an antibacterial (ethambutol hydrochloride).

myasthenia /mī'əsthē'nē•ə/, a condition characterized by an abnormal weakness of a muscle or a group of muscles that may be the result of a systemic myoneural disturbance, as in myasthenia gravis, or myasthenia laryngis involving the vocal cord tensor muscles. –**myasthenic,** *adj.*

myasthenia gravis, an abnormal condition characterized by the chronic fatigability and weakness of muscles, especially in the face and throat, as a result of a defect in the conduction of nerve impulses at the myoneural junction.

■ OBSERVATIONS: Muscular fatigability in myasthenia gravis is caused by the inability of receptors at the myoneural junction to depolarize because of a deficiency of acetylcholine; hence, the diagnosis may be made by administering an anticholinesterase drug and observing improved muscle strength and stamina. The onset of symptoms is usually gradual, with ptosis of the upper eyelids, diplopia, and weakness of the facial muscles. The weakness may then extend to other muscles innervated by the cranial nerves, particularly the respiratory muscles. Muscular exertion aggravates the symptoms, which typically vary over the course of the day. The disease occurs in younger women more often than in older women and in men over 60 years of age more often than in younger men.

■ INTERVENTION: Anticholinesterase drugs are given. The edrophonium test is used to determine the optimal maintenance dose. Neostigmine or pyridostigmine is the drug most often used.

■ NURSING CONSIDERATIONS: Physical activity is restricted, and bed rest encouraged. Anticholinesterase drugs are usually administered before meals, and the patient is monitored for toxic side effects. Myasthenic crisis may require emergency respiratory assistance. The patient's diet may have to be adjusted if the ability to chew and swallow is affected.

myasthenia gravis crisis, acute exacerbation of the muscular weakness characterizing the disease, triggered by infection, surgery, emotional stress, or an overdose or insufficiency of anticholinesterase medication.

■ OBSERVATIONS: Typical signs and symptoms include respiratory distress progressing to periods of apnea, extreme fatigue, increased muscular weakness, dysphagia, dysarthria, and fever. The patient may be anxious, restless, irritable, unable to move the jaws or to raise one or both eyelids. If the condition is caused by anticholinesterase toxicity, there may be anorexia, nausea, vomiting, abdominal cramps, diarrhea, excessive salivation, sweating, lacrimation, blurred vision, vertigo, and muscle cramps and spasms, as well as general weakness, dysarthria, and respiratory distress.

■ INTERVENTION: Initial treatment is directed to maintaining patency of the airway. Oxygen with assisted or controlled ventilation is administered, as a tracheostomy may be performed and bronchoscopy may be indicated. The patient is placed in a bed in which the head is elevated 30 degrees. The withdrawal or reduction of anticholinergic drugs may be ordered, or they may be given to differentiate the kind of crisis. Respiratory secretions and saliva are suctioned, and blood pressure, pulse, and respiration are carefully observed. The chest is auscultated, and the rectal temperature is taken every 2 to 4 hours; cooling measures may be necessary. Parenteral fluids, antibiotics, nasogastric feeding, and the insertion of an indwelling catheter with closed gravity drainage may be ordered. The patient is turned every 2 hours and given mouth and skin care every 2 to 4 hours; the lips are kept well lubricated and decubiti are avoided by using an air mattress or sheepskin and by keeping the skin dry at all times. If an eyelid is affected, the eye may be covered with a patch; crusts are removed whenever required, and soothing eyedrops may be administered. To enable the patient to communicate, the call bell and a pad and pencil or magic slate are placed within reach. When the acute crisis subsides, the patient may progress from clear liquids to a soft diet but may require help in eating. Nourishment is offered between meals, and a daily intake of up to 2000 ml of fluids is encouraged. Walking as tolerated and other activities are planned at the time of the maximum effect of medication. Active or passive range of motion exercises of all extremities are performed several times a day, but rest periods are maintained to avoid fatigue and relapse.

■ NURSING CONSIDERATIONS: Before discharge the patient is instructed on the importance of taking the prescribed medication with milk, crackers, or bread at the scheduled time and of reporting toxic side effects and symptoms of recurrent or progressive disease. The nurse points out the need to maintain a regular diet, to exercise to tolerance, to rest, and to avoid infections and exposure to hot or cold weather and the use of alcohol and tobacco. The nurse's help in planning a schedule that conserves energy for essential activities can enable the patient to be relatively independent and self-sufficient.

myasthenic crisis, an acute episode of muscular weakness.

myc-. See **myco-.**

mycelium /mīsē'lē•əm/, *pl.* **mycelia,** a mass of interwoven, branched, threadlike filaments that make up most fungi. Also called **hypha.**

mycetismus /mī'sitiz'məs/, mushroom poisoning.

myceto-. See **myco-.**

mycetoma /mī′sətō′mə/, a serious fungal infection involving skin, subcutaneous tissue, fascia, and bone. One kind of mycetoma is **Madura foot.**

Mychel, a trademark for an antibacterial and antirickettsial (chloramphenicol).

Mycifradin Sulfate, a trademark for an antibacterial (neomycin sulfate).

Mycitracin, a trademark for a topical, fixed-combination drug containing antibacterials (polymyxin B sulfate, bacitracin, and neomycin sulfate).

myco-, myc-, myceto-, myko-, a combining form meaning 'related to fungus': *mycobacteriosis, mycohemia, mycophage*.

mycobacteria /mī′kōbaktir′ē•ə/, acid-fast microorganisms belonging to the genus *Mycobacterium*. **–mycobacterial,** *adj.*

mycobacteriosis /mī′kōbak′tirē•ō′sis/, a tuberculosis-like disease caused by mycobacteria other than *Mycobacterium tuberculosis*.

Mycobacterium /mī′kōbaktir′ē•əm/, a genus of rod-shaped, acid-fast bacteria having two significant pathogenic species: *Mycobacterium leprae* causes leprosy; *M. tuberculosis* causes tuberculosis.

Mycolog, a trademark for a topical fixed-combination drug containing a glucocorticoid (triamcinolone acetonide), two antibacterials (neomycin sulfate and gramicidin), and an antifungal (nystatin).

mycology /mīkol′əjē/, the study of fungi and fungoid diseases. **–mycologic, mycological,** *adj.*, **mycologist,** *n.*

mycomyringitis. See **myringomycosis.**

mycophenolic acid /mī′kōfinō′lik/, a bacteriostatic and fungistatic crystalline antibiotic obtained from *Pencillium brevi compactum* and related species.

Mycoplasma /mī′kōplaz′mə/, a genus of ultramicroscopic organisms lacking rigid cell walls and considered to be the smallest free-living organisms. Some are saprophytes, some are parasites, and many are pathogens. One species is a cause of mycoplasma pneumonia, tracheobronchitis, pharyngitis, and bullous myringitis. See also **pleuropneumonia-like organism.**

mycoplasma pneumonia, a contagious disease of children and young adults caused by *Mycoplasma pneumoniae*, characterized by a 9- to 12-day incubation period and followed by symptoms of an upper respiratory infection, dry cough, and fever. Also called **Eaton-agent pneumonia, primary atypical pneumonia, walking pneumonia. See also cold agglutinin.**

■ OBSERVATIONS: Harsh or diminished breath sounds and fine inspiratory rales are frequently heard. Pulmonary infiltrates visible on chest x-ray films may resemble bacterial or viral pneumonia and may persist for 3 weeks in untreated cases. Rarely, complications, as sinusitis, pleurisy, polyneuritis, myocarditis, or Stevens-Johnson syndrome, may follow the pneumonia. In untreated adults prolonged cough, weakness, and malaise are common. Diagnosis is suggested by physical examination and by observation of the clinical course and elevated cold agglutinins and is confirmed by a complement fixation test. Prognosis is favorable.

■ INTERVENTION: Erythromycin or tetracycline, bed rest, a high-protein diet, and an adequate intake of fluids are recommended. It is important that infants and people for whom a respiratory illness would be a particular hazard avoid or be protected from contact with patients having mycoplasma pneumonia.

mycosis /mīkō′sis/, any disease caused by a fungus. Some kinds of mycoses are **athlete's foot, candidiasis,** and **coccidioidomycosis. –mycotic,** *adj.*

mycosis fungoides /fung•goi′dēz/, a rare, chronic, lymphomatous skin malignancy resembling eczema or a cutaneous tumor that is followed by microabscesses in the epidermis and lesions simulating those of Hodgkin's disease in lymph nodes and viscera. The condition is considered a distinctive entity by some specialists and a cutaneous manifestation of a malignant lymphoma by others.

Mycostatin, a trademark for an antifungal (nystatin).

mycotic, pertaining to a disease caused by a fungus.

mycotic aneurysm, a localized dilatation in the wall of a blood vessel caused by the growth of a fungus, usually occurring as a complication of bacterial endocarditis. See also **bacterial aneurysm.**

Mydriacyl, a trademark for a cycloplegic mydriatic (tropicamide).

mydriasis /midrī′əsis/, **1.** dilatation of the pupil of the eye caused by contraction of the dilator muscle of the iris, a muscular sheath that radiates outward like the spokes of a wheel from the center of the iris around the pupil. With a decrease in light or the pharmacologic action of certain drugs the dilator acts to pull the iris outward, enlarging the pupil. **2.** an abnormal condition characterized by

Mycoplasma pathogens

Organism	*Disease, clinical manifestation*	*Reservoir*	*Method of transmission*
Mycoplasma hominis	Postpartum fever	Humans	Sexual transmission?; colonizes GU tract of sexually active individuals
Mycoplasma pneumoniae	Primary atypical pneumonia	Humans	Droplet or aerosol spread from infected individual or carrier
Ureaplasma urealyticum (T strain mycoplasma)	Possible etiologic agent of urinary tract infections	Humans	Sexual transmission?; colonizes GU tract

contraction of the dilator muscle, resulting in widely dilated pupils. Compare **miosis.** **–mydriatic** /mid′rē•at′ik/, *adj.*

mydriatic and cycloplegic agent, any one of several ophthalmic pharmaceutic preparations that dilate the pupil and paralyze the ocular muscles of accommodation. Mydriatics stimulate the sympathetic nerve fibers or block parasympathetic nerve fibers of the eye, temporarily paralyzing the iris sphincter muscle. Cycloplegics temporarily paralyze accommodation while relaxing the ciliary muscle. Some drugs may cause both mydriasis and cycloplegia, whereas others are designed to produce a single effect, as the cycloplegics. These drugs are used in diagnostic ophthalmoscopic and refractive examination of the eye, before and after various procedures in eye surgery, in some tests for glaucoma, in the treatment of anterior uveitis, and in treating certain kinds of glaucoma. Blurred vision, thirst, flushing, fever, and rash may occur. In children and elderly people, ataxia, somnolence, delirium, and hallucination may occur but are rare. Among these drugs are atropine, cyclopentolate, homatropine, scopolamine and tropicamide; they are prepared in solution for topical ophthalmic application.

myel-. See **myelo-.**

myelacephalus, a fetal monster, usually a separate monozygotic twin, whose form and parts are barely recognizable; a slightly differentiated amorphous mass. –**myelacephalous,** *adj.*

myelatelia /mī′ələtē′lē•ə/, any developmental defect involving the spinal cord.

myelauxe /mī′əlôk′sē/, a developmental anomaly characterized by hypertrophy of the spinal cord.

-myelia, a combining form meaning '(condition of the) spinal cord': *atelomyelia, hydromyelia, syringomyelia.*

myelin /mī′əlin/, a substance constituting the sheaths of various nerve fibers throughout the body. It is largely composed of fat, which gives the fibers a white, creamy color. –**myelinic,** *adj.*

myelinated /mī′əlinā′tid/, (of a nerve) having a myelin sheath.

myelination, the process of furnishing or taking on myelin.

myelin globule, a fatlike droplet found in some sputum.

myelinic, of or pertaining to myelin.

myelinic neuroma, a neuroma neoplasm composed of myelinated nerve fibers.

myelinization /mī′əlin′īzā′shən/, development of the myelin sheath around a nerve fiber. Also called **myelinogenesis.**

myelinolysis /mī′əlinol′isis/, a pathologic process that dissolves the myelin sheaths around certain nerve fibers, as those of the pons in alcoholic and undernourished people who are afflicted with central pontine myelinolysis.

myelin sheath, a segmented, fatty lamination composed of myelin that wraps the axons of many nerves in the body. In myelinated peripheral nerves, the sheaths are composed of Schwann cells. The myelin sheaths around the central nerve fibers are composed of oligodendroglia. Their lipoid content gives these coverings a whitish appearance. In the peripheral nerves the sheaths are interrupted every 1 to 2 cm by the nodes of Ranvier, which occur only rarely in the fibers of the central nervous system. The usual thickness of the myelin sheath is between 2 and 10 μm. Various diseases, as multiple sclerosis, can destroy these myelin wrappings.

myelitis /mī′əlī′tis/, an abnormal condition characterized by inflammation of the spinal cord with associated motor or sensory dysfunction. Some kinds of myelitis are **acute transverse myelitis, leukomyelitis,** and **poliomyelitis.** –**myelitic,** *adj.*

myelo-, myel-, a combining form meaning 'related to marrow': *myeloblast, myelocyte, myelomenia.*

myeloblast, one of the earliest precursors of the granulocytic leukocytes. The cytoplasm appears light blue, scanty, and nongranular when seen in a stained blood smear through a microscope. The nucleus contains distinct chromatin material in strands, together with several nucleoli. In certain leukemias, a marked increase in myeloblasts is observed in the marrow and in the peripheral blood. Compare **megaloblast, myelocyte, normoblast.** See also **myelocytic leukemia.** –**myeloblastic,** *adj.*

myeloblastemia. See **myeloblastosis.**

Mydriatic and cycloplegic drugs

Drug	Form and concentrations	Duration of effect
Mydriatric action		
Phenylephrine (Neo-Synephrine)	Eyedrops, 2.5-10%	3-6 hr
Epinephrine	Eyedrops, 1-2%	3-6 hr
Cycloplegic action		
Atropine sulfate (Atropisol, Isopto-Atropine)	Eyedrops, 0.5-1% Ointment 1%	2-4 wk
Cyclopentolate (Cyclogyl)	Eyedrops, 0.5-2%	24 hr
Homatropine (Isopto-Homatropine)	Eyedrops, 0.5-5%	1-2 days
Scopolamine hydrobromide	Eyedrops, 0.25-0.5%	1-2 days
Tropicamide (Mydriacyl)	Eyedrops, 0.5-1%	2-8 hr

myeloblastic leukemia, a malignant neoplasm of blood-forming tissues, characterized by many myeloblasts in the circulating blood and tissues. The disease may be a terminal event in the course of chronic granulocytic leukemia.

myeloblastomatosis /mī'əlōblas'tōmətō'sis/, abnormal, localized clusters of myeloblasts in the peripheral circulation.

myeloblastosis /mī'əloblastō'sis/, the abnormal presence of myeloblasts in the circulation.

myelocele /mī'əlōsēl'/, a saclike protrusion of the spinal cord through a congenital defect in the vertebral column. See also **myelomeningocele, neural tube defect.**

myeloclast /mī'əlōclast'/, a cell that breaks down the myelin sheaths of nerves of the central nervous system.

myelocyst /mī'əlōsist'/, any benign cyst that is formed from the rudimentary medullary canals that give rise to the vertebral canal during embryonic development.

myelocystocele /mī'əlōsis'təsēl'/, a protrusion of a cystic tumor containing spinal cord substance through a defect in the vertebral column. See also **myelomeningocele, neural tube defect, spina bifida.**

myelocystomeningocele /mī'əlōsis'tōməning'gōsēl/, a protrusion of a cystic tumor containing both spinal cord substance and meninges through a defect in the vertebral column. See also **myelomeningocele, neural tube defect, spina bifida.**

myelocyte /mī'əlōsīt'/, an immature white blood cell normally found in the bone marrow, being the first of the maturation stages of the granulocytic leukocytes. When stained and microscopically examined, granules typical of the granulocytic series are seen in the cytoplasm. The nuclear material of the myelocyte is denser than that of the myeloblast, but it lacks a definable membrane. The cell is flat and contains increasing numbers of granules as the maturation process progresses. These cells appear in the circulating blood only in certain forms of leukemia. Compare **myeloblast.** See also **myelocytic leukemia.** **–myelocytic,** *adj.*

myelocythemia /mī'əlōsīthē'mē·ə/, an abnormal presence of myelocytes in the circulating blood, as in myelocytic leukemia.

myelocytic leukemia /mī'əlōsit'ik/, a disorder characterized by the unregulated and excessive production of myelocytes of the granulocytic series. As many as several hundred thousand per cubic millimeter may be seen. Also called **granulocytic leukemia, myelogenous leukemia.** Compare **leukemoid reaction, acute lymphocytic leukemia, chronic lymphocytic leukemia.** See also **leukocytosis.**

myelocytoma /mī'əlōsītō'mə/, a localized cluster of myelocytes in the peripheral vasculature that may occur in myelocytic leukemia.

myelocytosis. See **myelocythemia.**

myelodiastasis /mī'əlōdī·as'təsis/, disintegration and necrosis of the spinal cord.

myelodysplasia, a general designation for the defective development of any part of the spinal cord. The term is used primarily to describe abnormalities without gross superficial defects, especially of the lower segment, specifically spina bifida occulta.

myelofibrosis. See **myeloid metaplasia.**

myelogenesis, **1.** the formation and differentiation of the nervous system during prenatal development, in particular the brain and spinal cord. See also **neural tube formation.** **2.** the development of the myelin sheath around the nerve fiber. See also **myelinization.**

myelogenous /mī'əloj'ənəs/, pertaining to the cells produced in bone marrow or to the tissue from which such cells originate. Also **myelogenetic, myelogenic.**

myelogenous leukemia. See **acute myelocytic leukemia, chronic myelocytic leukemia.**

myelogeny /mī'əloj'ənē/, the formation and differentiation of the myelin sheaths of nerve fibers during the prenatal development of the central nervous system.

myelogram /mī'əlōgram'/, **1.** an x-ray film taken after the injection of a radiopaque medium into the subarachnoid space to demonstrate any distortions of the spinal cord, spinal nerve roots, and the subarachnoid space. **2.** a graphic representation of a count of the different kinds of cells in a stained preparation of bone marrow.

myelography /mī'əlog'rəfē/, a radiographic process by which the spinal cord and the spinal subarachnoid space are viewed and photographed after the introduction of a contrast medium, as air or an absorbable contrast substance. It is used to identify and study spinal lesions caused by trauma or disease. **–myelographic,** *adj.*

myeloid /mī'əloid/, **1.** of or pertaining to the bone marrow. **2.** of or pertaining to the spinal cord. **3.** of or pertaining to myelocytic forms that do not necessarily originate in the bone marrow.

myeloid leukemia. See **acute myelocytic leukemia, chronic myelocytic leukemia.**

myeloid metaplasia, a disorder in which bone marrow tissue develops in abnormal sites. Characteristics of the condition are anemia, splenomegaly, immature blood cells in the circulation, and hematopoiesis occurring in the liver and spleen. Myeloid metaplasia may be secondary to carcinoma, leukemia, polycythemia vera, or tuberculosis. The primary form is also called **agnogenic myeloid metaplasia, myelofibrosis.**

myeloidosis /mī'əloidō'sis/, an abnormal condition characterized by general hyperplasia of the myeloid tissue. See also **Hodgkin's disease, multiple myeloma.**

myeloma /mī'əlō'mə/, an osteolytic neoplasm consisting of a profusion of cells typical of the bone marrow. It may develop simultaneously in many sites, causing extensive areas of patchy destruction of the bone. The tumor, which is usually grayish-red, occurs most frequently in the ribs, vertebrae, pelvic bones, and flat bones of the skull. Intense pain and spontaneous fractures are common. The tumor is radiosensitive, and local lesions are curable. Kinds of myeloma are **endothelial myeloma, extramedullary myeloma, giant cell myeloma, multiple myeloma,** and **osteogenic myeloma.**

-myeloma, a combining form meaning a 'tumor composed of cells normally found in bone marrow': *globomyeloma, lymphomyeloma, orchiomyeloma.*

myelomalacia /mī'əlōməlā'shə/, abnormal softening of the spinal cord, caused primarily by inadequate blood supply.

myelomatosis. See **multiple myeloma.**

myelomeningocele /mī'əlōməning'gōsēl/, a developmental defect of the central nervous system in which a hernial sac containing a portion of the spinal cord, its meninges, and cerebrospinal fluid protrudes through a congenital cleft in the vertebral column. The condition is caused primarily by the failure of the neural tube to close during embryonic development, although in some instances it may result from the reopening of the tube from an abnormal increase in cerebrospinal fluid pressure. Also called **meningomyelocele.** Compare **menigocele.** See also **neural tube defect, spina bifida cystica.**

■ OBSERVATIONS: The defect, which occurs in approximately 2 in every 1000 live births, is readily apparent and easily diagnosed at birth. Although the opening may be located at any point along the spinal column, the anomaly characteristically occurs in the lumbar, low thoracic, or sacral region and extends for three to six vertebral segments. The saclike structure may be covered with a thin layer of skin or with a fine membrane that can be easily ruptured, increasing the risk of meningeal infection. The severity of neurologic dysfunction is directly related to the amount of neural tissue involved, which can be roughly estimated by the degree of the transillumination of the mass. Usually the condition is accompanied by varying degrees of paralysis of the lower extremities, by musculoskeletal defects, as clubfoot, flexion and joint deformities, or hip dysplasia, and by anal and bladder sphincter dysfunction, which can lead to serious genitourinary disorders. Hydrocephalus, frequently related to the Arnold-Chiari malformation, is the most common anomaly associated with myelomeningocele and occurs in approximately 90% of the cases in which the spinal lesion is located in the lumbosacral region. In most cases, hydrocephalus is apparent at birth, although it may appear shortly afterward. Supplementary diagnostic procedures include x-ray film of the spine, skull, and chest to determine the extent of the vertebral defect and the presence of other malformations in other organ systems, a computerized axial tomographic (CAT) scan of the brain to establish the ventricular size and the presence of any structural congenital anomalies, and laboratory examinations, especially urine analysis, culture, blood urea nitrogen evaluation, and creatinine clearance determination. Amniocentesis is recommended for all pregnant women who have had a child with a neural tube defect.

■ INTERVENTION: Supportive care and surgery are the only treatments for myelomeningocele, and they require a multidisciplinary approach involving specialists from neurology, neurosurgery, urology, pediatrics, orthopedics, rehabilitation, and physical therapy, as well as intensive nursing care. Initial treatment involves prevention of infection and assessment of neurologic involvement. Immediate surgical repair is essential if the defect is leaking cerebrospinal fluid. However, surgical intervention may not be appropriate if neurologic involvement is extreme, if the lesion is infected, or if associated problems, as hydrocephalus, are severe. When surgical repair of the spinal defect is recommended, associated problems are managed by appropriate measures, including shunt procedures for correction of hydrocephalus, antibiotic therapy to reduce the incidence of meningitis, urinary tract infections, and pneumonia, casting, bracing, traction, and surgical techniques for correction of hip, knee, and foot deformities, and prevention and treatment of renal complications. Although improved surgical techniques and other treatment modalities have significantly increased the survival rate, these procedures cannot alter the major physical disability and deformity, mental retardation, and chronic urinary tract and pulmonary infections that may afflict these children for life, nor can they alter the financial and emotional burden on and within the family. Prognosis is determined by the severity of neurologic involvement and the number of associated anomalies. With proper care and long-term maintenance, most children can survive and do well. Early death is usually caused by central nervous system infection or by hydrocephalus, whereas mortality in later childhood is caused by urinary tract infection, renal failure, complications from shunt therapy, or pulmonary disease.

■ NURSING CONSIDERATIONS: Care of the child with a spinal defect entails both immediate and long-term nursing goals. Immediate care centers on the prevention of local infection and trauma by careful handling and positioning of the infant, applying sterile moist dressings to the membranous sac, avoiding fecal contamination and breakdown of sensitive skin areas, and maintaining warmth, proper nutrition, and adequate hydration and electrolyte balance. Gentle range of motion exercises are carried out to prevent or minimize hip and lower extremity deformity. An important function of the nurse is to involve the parents in the care of the infant as soon as possible and to teach them the essential procedures for adequate home care, including how to observe for signs of complications. The nurse also helps the parents in

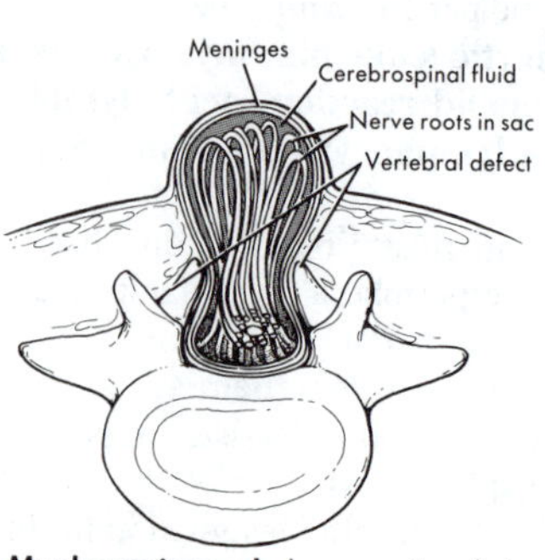

Myelomeningocele (cross-sectional view)

long-term management by planning activities appropriate to the developmental age and physical limitations of the child, by providing information for teaching all family members about the condition, and, if appropriate, by assisting with placement in schools that can accommodate the special needs of handicapped children.

myelomere /mī'əlōmir'/, any of the embryonic segments of the brain or spinal cord during prenatal development.

myelomonocytic leukemia. See **monocytic leukemia.**

myelopathic anemia. See **myelophthisic anemia.**

myelopathy /mī'əlop'əthē/, **1.** any disease of the spinal cord. **2.** any disease of the myelopoietic tissues.

myelophthisic anemia /mī'əlofthiz'ik/, a disorder attributed to several pathologic processes that displace the hemopoietic tissues of the bone marrow. It is characterized by anemia and the appearance of immature granulocytes and nucleated erythroid elements in the peripheral blood. Also called **myelopathic anemia.** Compare **hemolytic anemia, leukoerythroblastic anemia.**

myelopoiesis /mī'əlōpō·ē'sis/, the formation and development of the bone marrow or the cells that originate from it. A kind of myelopoiesis is **extramedullary myelopoiesis.** **–myelopoietic,** *adj.*

myeloradiculodysplasia /mī'əlōrədik'yəlōdisplā'zhə/, any developmental abnormality of the spinal cord and spinal nerve roots. See also **myelomeningocele, neural tube defect.**

myeloschisis /mī'əlos'kəsis/, a developmental defect characterized by a cleft spinal cord that results from the failure of the neural plate to fuse and form a complete neural tube. See also **neural tube defect, neural tube formation, myelomeningocele, rachischisis, spina bifida.**

myelosuppression, the inhibition of the process of production of blood cells and platelets in the bone marrow.

myesthesia /mī'esthē'zhə/, perception of any sensation in a muscle, as touch, direction, proprioception, contraction, relaxation, or extension.

myiasis /mī'yəsis/, infection or infestation of the body by the larvae of flies, usually through a wound or an ulcer, but, rarely, through the intact skin.

myitis. See **myositis.**

myko-. See **myco-.**

Mylaxen, a trademark for a cholinesterase inhibitor (hexafluorenium bromide), used as an adjunct to anesthesia.

Myleran, a trademark for an antineoplastic (busulfan).

Mylicon, a trademark for an antiflatulent (simethicone).

mylohyoideus /mī'lōhī·oi'dē·əs/, one of a pair of flat triangular muscles that form the floor of the cavity of the mouth. Immediately superior to the digastricus, it arises from the whole length of the mylohyoid line of the mandible and inserts into the hyoid bone. It is innervated by the mylohyoid nerve and acts to raise the hyoid bone and the tongue. Also called **mylohyoid muscle.** Compare **digastricus, geniohyoideus, stylohyoideus.**

myo-, my-, a combining form meaning 'relating to muscle': *myocardia, myocele, myolipoma.*

myocardial infarction (MI) /mī'ōkär'dē·əl/, an occlusion of a coronary artery, caused by atherosclerosis or an embolus resulting from a necrotic area in the vasculature myocardium.

■ OBSERVATIONS: The onset of MI is characterized by a crushing, viselike chest pain that may radiate to the left arm, neck, or epigastrium and sometimes simulates the sensation of acute indigestion or a gallbladder attack. The patient usually becomes ashen, clammy, short of breath, faint, and anxious and often feels that death is imminent. Typical signs are tachycardia, a barely perceptible pulse, low blood pressure, an elevated temperature, cardiac arrhythmia, and electrocardiographic evidence of elevation of the ST segment and Q wave. Laboratory studies usually show an increased sedimentation rate, leukocytosis, and elevated serum levels of creatine phosphokinase, lactic dehydrogenase, and glutamic-oxaloacetic transaminase. Potential complications in MI are pulmonary or systemic embolism, pulmonary edema, shock, and cardiac arrest.

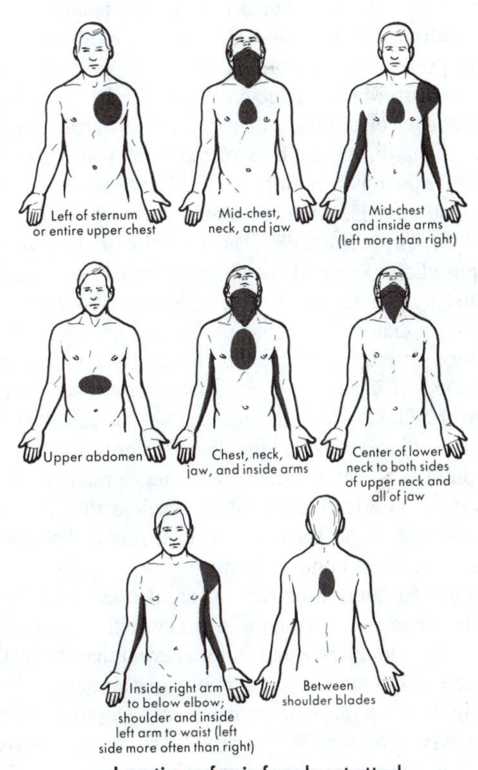

Locations of pain from heart attack

■ INTERVENTION: Emergency treatment of MI may require cardiopulmonary resuscitation before the patient is admitted to an intensive cardiac care unit and placed on a cardiac monitor. In the acute phase, oxygen, cardiotonic drugs, antiarrhythmic agents, and anticoagulants are usually administered and sedatives and analgesics may be indicated. Blood pressure, temperature, respiration, and apical pulse are checked frequently. Parenteral fluids may be administered; iced drinks and cold foods are avoided, and the patient is usually served a low-sodium, low-cholesterol diet. Stool softeners and laxatives may be indicated to prevent straining.

■ NURSING CONSIDERATIONS: The nurse's role in helping the patient and family understand the nature and treatment of the disease is extremely important. Before discharge, discussions regarding the need to adhere to the prescribed diet and medication, to limit activities, to rest at regular periods, and to avoid caffeine, nicotine, large meals, and emotional stress can facilitate the patient's convalescence.

myocardiopathy /mī′ōkär′dē·op′əthē/, any disease of the myocardium. Also called **cardiomyopathy.**

myocarditis /mī′ōkärdī′tis/, an inflammatory condition of the myocardium caused by viral, bacterial, or fungal infection, serum sickness, rheumatic fever, or chemical agent, or as a complication of a collagen disease. Myocarditis most frequently occurs in an acute viral form and is self-limited, but it may lead to acute heart failure. Management includes treatment of the cause, analgesia, oxygen, antiinflammatory agents, constant monitoring, and rest to prevent shock or heart failure.

myocardium /mī′ōkär′dē·əm/, a thick, contractile, middle layer of uniquely constructed and arranged muscle cells that forms the bulk of the heart wall. The myocardium contains a minimum of other tissue, except for the blood vessels, and is covered interiorly by the endocardium. The contractile tissue of the myocardium is composed of fibers with the characteristic cross-striations of muscular tissue. The fibers, which are about one third as large in diameter as those of skeletal muscle and contain more sarcoplasm, branch frequently and are interconnected to form a network that is continuous except where the bundles and the laminae are attached at their origins and insertions into the fibrous trigone of the heart. The bundles of myocardial fibers are spiral-shaped; the individual muscle fibers contain fibrillae that are more concentrated at the periphery of each fiber. The central cores of the fibers contain the nuclei and may also contain concentrated sarcoplasm rich in sarcosomes. Myocardial muscle fibers also contain characteristic intercalated disks. Electron microscope studies reveal that these disks represent cell boundaries and may cross an entire fiber in a straight line or may be arranged in a steplike configuration. Myocardial muscle contains less connective tissue than skeletal muscle. The fibers of the connective tissue are covered by a delicate fibrillar net with few elastic fibers. Collagenous fibers run between the muscular bundles and the associated blood vessels. Specially modified fibers of myocardial muscle constitute the conduction system of the heart, including the sinoatrial node, the atrioventricular node, the atrioventricular bundle, and the Purkinje fibers. Most of the myocardial fibers function to contract the heart. Contraction involves the action of calcium ions and sodium ions and a complex electrochemical process still not precisely understood. Defects in the kinetics of intracellular calcium may cause myocardial dysfunctions in patients with heart failure. The metabolic processes of the myocardium are almost exclusively aerobic and constantly supply the heart muscle with high-energy phosphate bonds for mechanic and chemical functions. The heart uses free fatty acids as its predominant fuel, as well as important quantities of glucose, lactate, pyruvate, and ketone bodies, and a very small amount of amino acids. Many key enzymatic reactions of the heart, as the citric acid cycle and oxidative phosphorylation, take place in the highly concentrated myocardial sarcosomes. The major anaerobic processes of glycolysis occur in the sarcoplasm. The process of oxidative phosphorylation produces adenosine triphosphate, the immediate energy source for myocardial contraction. Oxygen, which significantly affects contractibility, is the most important metabolic nutrient for the myocardium, which consumes from 6.5 to 10 ml/100 g of tissue per minute. Without this oxygen supply, myocardial contractions decrease in a few minutes. Ventricular pressure and heart rate together determine myocardial oxygen consumption. The heart normally extracts about 70% of the oxygen reaching it by the coronary arteries. This leaves only about 30% in coronary sinus blood and limits the amount of additional oxygen the heart can extract from its blood supply. In heart failure caused by hypertension, valvular heart disease, or coronary atherosclerosis, the myocardial oxygen consumption per gram of tissue is usually normal, but the total oxygen consumption per minute often increases significantly because the weight of the heart often increases with such diseases. Myocardial oxygen consumption increases in hyperthyroidism and decreases in hypothyroidism. The myocardium maintains a relatively constant level of glycogen in the form of sarcoplasmic granules. Hypoxia rapidly depletes this supply and produces lactate and hexosemonophosphate. In anemia, the total consumption of myocardial oxygen may significantly increase because of increased hemodynamic demands resulting from the disorder. Myocardial hypertrophy may develop if the anemia is chronic. Compare **epicardium.** –**myocardial,** *adj.*

Myochrysine, a trademark for an antirheumatic (gold sodium thiomalate).

myoclonus /mī′ōklō′nəs/, a spasm of a muscle or a group of muscles. –**myoclonic,** *adj.*

myodiastasis /mī′ōdī·as′təsis/, an abnormal condition in which there is separation of muscle bundles.

myoedema /mī'ō•idē'mə/, *pl.* **myoedemas, myoedemata,** muscle edema. Compare **myxedema.**

myofacial pain dysfunction syndrome. See **temporomandibular joint pain dysfunction syndrome.**

myofibril, a slender striated strand of muscle tissue. Myofibrils occur in groups of branching threads running parallel to the cellular long axis.

myogelosis /mī'ōjəlō'sis/, a condition in which there are hardened areas or nodules within muscles, especially the gluteal muscles. There are no serious consequences of this condition, and no treatment is necessary.

myogenic /mī'ōjen'ik/, pertaining to muscles, particularly cardiac and smooth muscles that do not require nerves to initiate and maintain contractions.

myoglobin /mī'ōglō'bin/, a ferrous globin complex consisting of one heme molecule containing one iron molecule attached to a single globin chain. Myoglobin is found in muscle and is responsible for the red color of that tissue and for its ability to store oxygen.

myoglobinuria, the presence of myoglobin, a respiratory pigment of muscle tissue, in the urine.

myokinase. See **adenylate kinase.**

myoma /mī•ō'mə/, *pl.* **myomas, myomata,** a common, benign fibroid tumor on the uterine muscle. It develops most frequently after 30 years of age in women, especially black women, who have never been pregnant. Menorrhagia, backache, constipation, dysmenorrhea, dyspareunia, and other symptoms develop proportionate to the size, location, and rate of growth of the tumor. Obstruction of a ureter may result if a large myoma compresses it. A myoma may be associated with sterility if it blocks the fallopian tube, with abortion if it interferes with fetal growth, or with difficult childbirth and hemorrhage if it is in or near the cervix. Also called *(informal)* **fibroid.**

myoma previum. See **leiomyoma uteri.**

myoma striocellulare. See **rhabdomyoma.**

myomere. See **myotome.**

myometritis /mī'ōmətrī'tis/, an inflammation or infection of the myometrium of the uterus.

myometrium /mī'ōmē'trē•əm/, *pl.* **myometria,** the muscular layer of the wall of the uterus. The fibers of the myometrium course around the uterus horizontally, vertically, and diagonally.

myonecrosis /mī'ōnekrō'sis/, the death of muscle fibers. **Progressive** or **clostridial myonecrosis** is caused by the anaerobic bacteria of the genus *Clostridium*. Seen in deep wound infections, progressive myonecrosis is accompanied by pain, tenderness, a brown serous exudate, and a rapid accumulation of gas within the tissue of the muscle. The affected muscle turns a blackish-green color. Treatment includes thorough wound debridement, IV administration of penicillin, and the use of hyperbaric oxygen therapy to destroy the anaerobe and to promote healing.

myoneural /mī'ōno͝or'əl/, of or pertaining to a muscle and its associated nerve, especially to nerve endings in muscles.

myoneural junction. See **neuromuscular junction.**

myopathy /mī•op'əthē/, an abnormal condition of skeletal muscle characterized by muscle weakness, wasting, and histologic changes within muscle tissue, as seen in any of the muscular dystrophies. A myopathy is distinct from a muscle disorder caused by nerve dysfunction. The specific diagnosis of any myopathy is made using tests of serum enzymes, electromyography, and muscle biopsy. See also **muscular dystrophy.** –**myopathic,** *adj.*

myope /mī'ōp/, an individual who is nearsighted or afflicted with myopia.

myophosphorylase deficiency glycogenosis. See **McArdle's disease.**

myopia /mī•ō'pē•ə/, a condition of nearsightedness caused by the elongation of the eyeball or by an error in refraction so that parallel rays are focused in front of the retina. Some kinds of myopia are **chromic myopia, curvature myopia, index myopia,** and **pathologic myopia.** Also called **nearsightedness, short sight.** See also **second sight.** –**myopic,** *adj.*

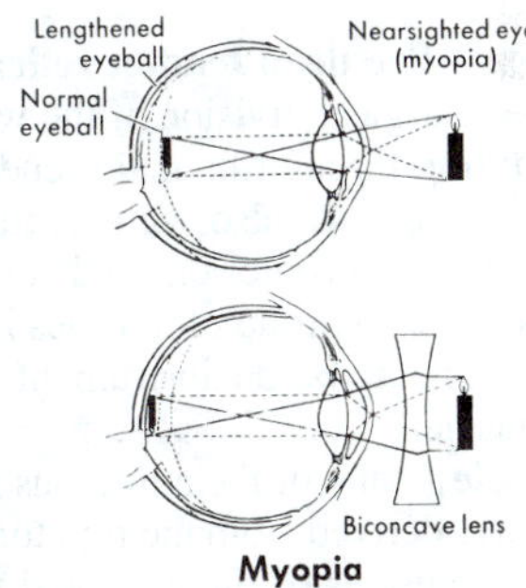

Myopia

myorrhaphy /mī•ôr'əfē/, suturing of a wound in a muscle.

myorrhexis /mī'ərek'sis/, a tearing in any muscle. –**myorrhectic,** *adj.*

myosarcoma /mī'ōsärkō'mə/, a malignant tumor of muscular tissue.

myosin /mī'əsin/, a cardiac and skeletal muscle protein that makes up close to one half of the proteins that occur in muscle tissue. The interaction of myosin and actin is essential for muscle contraction.

myositis /mī'əsī'tis/, inflammation of muscle tissue, usually of the voluntary muscles. Causes of myositis include infection, trauma, and infestation by parasites. Kinds of myositis include **epidemic myositis, interstitial myositis, parenchymatous myositis, polymyositis,** and **traumatic myositis.** Also called **myitis** /mī•ī'tis/. Compare **fibrositis.**

myositis fibrosa, an uncommon inflammation of the muscles, characterized by abnormal formation of connective tissue. Also called **interstitial myositis.** See also **myositis.**

myositis ossificans /əsif'əkanz/, a rare, inherited disease in which muscle tissue is replaced by bone. It begins in childhood, with stiffness in the neck and back and progresses to rigidity of the spine, trunk, and limbs. The administration of diphosphonates may prevent the abnormal deposition of bone, but there is no cure once it has occurred. Metabolism of calcium and phosphate remains normal throughout the course of the disease. Compare **myositis.**

myositis purulenta, any bacterial infection of muscle tissue. This condition may result in the formation of an abscess or multiple abscesses.

myositis trichinosa /trik′ənō′sə/, inflammation of the muscles resulting from infection by the parasite *Trichinella spiralis*. See also **trichinosis.**

myostasis /mī′ōstā′sis/, an abnormal condition of weakened muscle in which there is a relatively fixed length of muscle fibers in the relaxed state. In normal muscle the force of contraction is greatest at the resting length of the muscle; in myostasis the resting length is shorter than normal, and there is a shorter acting length in which the contractile force can work. **–myostatic,** *adj.*

myostroma /mī′əstrō′mə/, the framework of muscle tissue.

myotatic reflex. See **deep tendon reflex.**

myotenotomy, surgical division of the whole or part of a muscle by cutting through its main tendon.

myotome /mī′ətōm/, **1.** also called **myomere.** The muscle plate of an embryonic somite that develops into a voluntary muscle. **2.** a group of muscles innervated by a single spinal segment. **3.** an instrument for cutting or dissecting a muscle.

myotomic muscle, any of the numerous muscles of the trunk of the body, derived from the myotomes and divided into the deep muscles of the back and the thoracoabdominal muscles.

myotomy /mī•ot′əmē/, the cutting of a muscle, performed to gain access to underlying tissues or to relieve constriction in a sphincter, as in severe esophagitis or pyloric stenosis. Under general anesthesia, a longitudinal cut is made through the sphincter muscle but not through the mucosa lining the stomach. See also **abdominal surgery.**

Myotonachol, a trademark for a cholinergic (bethanechol chloride).

myotonia /mī′ətō′nē•ə/, any condition in which a muscle or a group of muscles does not readily relax after contracting. **–myotonic,** *adj.*

myotonia atrophica. See **myotonic muscular dystrophy.**

myotonia congenita /konjen′itə/, a rare, mild, and nonprogressive form of myotonic myopathy evident early in life. The only effects of the disorder are hypertrophy and stiffness of the muscles. Also called **Thomsen's disease.**

myotonic muscular dystrophy, a severe form of muscular dystrophy marked by ptosis, facial weakness, and dysarthria. Weakness of the hands and feet precedes that in the shoulders and hips. Myotonia of the hands is usually present. Electromyography is helpful in establishing the diagnosis. Although there is no specific treatment, active and passive exercises are used to alleviate symptoms. Also called **myotonia atrophica, Steinert's disease.**

myotonic myopathy, any of a group of disorders characterized by increased skeletal muscle tone and decreased relaxation of muscle after contraction. Kinds of myotonic myopathy include **myotonia congenita, myotonic muscular dystrophy.**

myria-, a combining form meaning 'a great number': *myriapod.*

myringa. See **tympanic membrane.**

myringectomy /mir′injek′təmē/, excision of the tympanic membrane.

myringitis /mir′injī′tis/, inflammation or infection of the tympanic membrane.

myringo-, a combining form meaning 'related to the tympanic membrane': *myringodectomy, myringoplasty, myringoscope.*

myringomycosis /miring′gōmīkō′sis/, a fungal infection of the tympanic membrane. Also called **mycomyringitis.**

myringoplasty /miring′gōplas′tē/, surgical repair of perforations of the eardrum with a tissue graft, performed to correct hearing loss. Under local or general anesthesia, the openings in the eardrum are enlarged, and the grafting material is sutured over them. Topical antibiotics are applied, and then a packing of absorbable gelatin sponge is applied to hold the graft in position. After surgery, an antihistamine with an ephedrine derivative is given. The nurse keeps the outer ear clean and dry. Debris is removed by gentle suctioning about 12 days after surgery. See also **myringotomy, tympanoplasty.**

myringotomy /mir′ing•got′əmē/, surgical incision of the eardrum, performed to relieve pressure and release pus from the middle ear. Antibiotics are given before surgery and continued afterwards. The drum is incised, and cultures are taken; fluid is gently suctioned from the middle ear. Ear drops may be instilled to improve drainage. The nurse cautions against putting cotton in the canal, because the ear must drain freely. The outer ear is kept clean and dry; careful handwashing is essential to prevent infection. If pain increases, the procedure may have to be repeated. Severe headache or disorientation must be reported. Also called **tympanotomy.** See also **myringoplasty.**

Mysoline, a trademark for an anticonvulsant (primidone).

mysophobia /mē′sə-/, an anxiety disorder characterized by an overreaction to the slightest uncleanliness, or an irrational fear of dirt, contamination, or defilement. Also spelled **misophobia. –mysophobic, misophobic,** *adj.*

Mytelase Chloride, a trademark for a cholinergic (ambenonium chloride).

Mytrate, a trademark for an adrenergic (epinephrine bitartrate).

myxedema, the most severe form of hypothyroidism. It is characterized by swelling of the hand, face, feet, and periorbital tissues. At this stage, the disease may lead to coma and death.

myxo-, a combining form meaning 'relating to mucus': *myxoblastoma, myxocyte, myxoma.*

myxofibroma /mik′sōfībrō′mə/, a fibrous tumor that contains myxomatous tissue. Also called **myxoma fibrosum.**

myxoid. See **mucoid,** def. 1.

myxoma /miksō′mə/, a neoplasm of the connective tissue, characteristically composed of stellate cells in a loose mucoid matrix crossed by delicate reticulum fibers. These tumors may grow to enormous size and are usually pale gray, soft, and jellylike; they may occur under the skin but are also found in bones, the genitourinary tract, and the retroperitoneal area. Some have exceeded 30 cm in diameter. –**myxomatous,** *adj.*

-myxoma, a combining form meaning a 'soft tumor made up of primitive connective tissues': *adenomyxoma, gliomyxoma, lipomyxoma.*

myxoma fibrosum. See **myxofibroma.**

myxoma sarcomatosum. See **myxosarcoma.**

myxopoiesis /mik′sōpō·ē′sis/, the production of mucus.

myxosarcoma /mik′sōsärkō′mə/, a sarcoma that contains some myxomatous tissue. Also called **myxoma sarcomatosum.**

myxovirus /mik′sōvī′rəs/, any of a group of medium-sized RNA viruses that are further divided into orthomyxoviruses and paramyxoviruses. Infection with these viruses is usually transmitted by the respiratory secretions of an infected host. Some kinds of myxoviruses are the viruses that cause influenza, mumps, and parainfluenza.

MZ, abbreviation for **monozygotic.**

n, 2n, 3n, 4n, symbols for the haploid, diploid, triploid, and tetraploid number of chromosomes in a cell, organism, strain, or individual.

N, **1.** symbol for **nitrogen. 2.** abbreviation for **normal. 3.** abbreviation for *node* in the TNM system for staging malignant neoplastic disease. See also **cancer staging.**

Na, chemical symbol for **sodium.**

NAACOG, abbreviation for **Nurses' Association of the American College of Obstetrics and Gynecology.**

nabothian cyst /nabō′thē·ən/, a cyst formed in a nabothian gland of the uterine cervix. It is a common finding on routine pelvic examination of women of reproductive age, especially in women who have borne children. The cyst, which is pearly white and firm, seldom results in adverse or pathologic effects.

nabothian gland, one of many small, mucus-secreting glands of the uterine cervix.

NADH, abbreviation for *nicotine adenine dinucleotide, reduced.*

nadolol, a beta-adrenergic blocking agent.

■ INDICATIONS: It is prescribed for long-term management of angina pectoris and for hypertension.

■ CONTRAINDICATIONS: Bronchial asthma, sinus bradycardia, and greater than first-degree conduction block, cardiogenic shock, overt cardiac failure, or known hypersensitivity to this drug prohibits its use.

■ ADVERSE EFFECTS: Among the more serious adverse reactions are bronchospasm, bradycardia, precipitation of heart failure, cardiac arrythmia, masking of signs of hypoglycemia in diabetics, fatigue, and lethargy. GI disturbances, rashes, and other allergic reactions also may occur.

NADPH, abbreviation for *nicotine adenine disphosphonucleotide, reduced.*

Naegeli's leukemia. See **monocytic leukemia.**

nafcillin sodium, an antibacterial.

■ INDICATIONS: It is prescribed in the treatment of infections caused by penicillinase-producing staphylococci.

■ CONTRAINDICATIONS: Known hypersensitivity to this drug or to other penicillins prohibits its use.

■ ADVERSE EFFECTS: Among the more serious adverse reactions are hypersensitivity reactions, nausea, and vomiting.

Nägele's obliquity. See **asynclitism.**

Nägele's rule /nā′gələz/, a method for calculating the estimated date of delivery based on a mean length of gestation. Three months are subtracted from the first day of the last normal menstrual period, and 1 year plus 7 days are added to that date. See also **estimated day of confinement.**

Nager's acrofacial dysostosis /nā′gərz/, an abnormal congenital condition characterized by limb deformities, as radioulnar synostosis, hypoplasia, and the absence of the radius or of the thumbs. Also called **dysostosis mandibularis.** Compare **cleidocranial dysostosis, craniofacial dysostosis, mandibulofacial dysostosis.**

Nahrungs-Einheit-Milch (nem) /nä′ro͝ongz īn′hīt milsh, mil*kh*/, a nutritional unit in Pirquet's system of feeding that is equivalent to 1 g of breast milk (German, for ''nutrition unit milk'').

nail, **1.** also called **unguis.** a flattened, elastic structure with a horny texture at the end of a finger or a toe. Each nail is comprised of a root, body, and free edge at the distal extremity. The root fastens the nail to the finger or the toe by fitting into a groove in the skin and is closely molded to the surface of the corium. The nail matrix beneath the body and the root projects longitudinal vascular ridges, which are easily visible through the translucent tissue of the body. The matrix firmly attaches the body of the nail to the underlying connective tissue. The whitish lunula near the root contains irregularly arranged papillae that are less firmly attached to the connective tissue than the rest of the matrix. The cuticle is attached to the surface of the nail just ahead of the root. The superficial horny part of the nail consists of the thick stratum lucidum, the thin stratum corneum, which forms the cuticle overlapping the lunula, and the stratum mucosum. The nails grow longer by proliferation of the cells in the stratum germinativum at the root. They grow thicker from proliferation of that part of the stratum germinativum underlying the lunula. **2.** any of various metallic nails used in orthopedics to fasten together bones or pieces of bone.

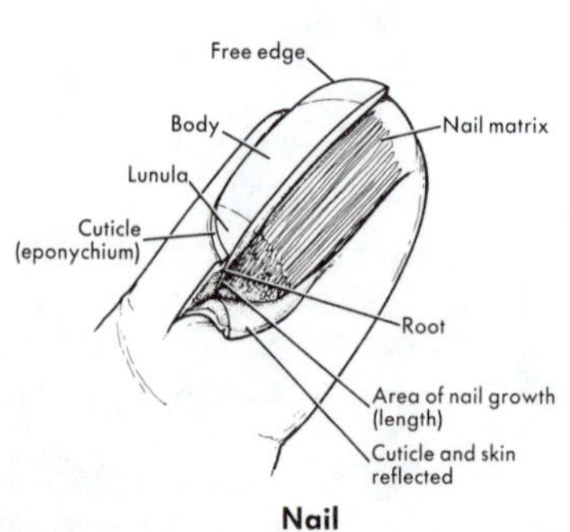

Nail

Naldecon, a trademark for a fixed-combination drug containing two adrenergics (phenylpropanolamine hydrochloride and phenylephrine hydrochloride) and two antihistamines (chlorpheniramine maleate and phenyltoloxamine citrate).

Nalfon, a trademark for an antiinflammatory agent (fenoprofen calcium).

nalidixic acid, an antibacterial.

■ INDICATIONS: It is prescribed in the treatment of certain urinary tract infections.

■ CONTRAINDICATIONS: Renal or hepatic insufficiency, a history of convulsive disorders, or known hypersensitivity to this drug prohibits its use.

■ ADVERSE EFFECTS: Among the more serious adverse reactions are mild neurologic disturbances, GI disturbances, and hemolytic anemia in glucose-6-phosphate dehydrogenase deficiency. Convulsions and increased cranial pressure may occur. Among the more serious reactions are increased intracranial pressure, seizures, hemolytic anemia in people affected with glucose-6-phosphate dehydrogenase deficiency, and GI and neurologic disturbances.

naloxone hydrochloride, a narcotic antagonist.

■ INDICATIONS: It is prescribed for reversal of narcotic depression, including narcotic depression, or for acute narcotic intoxication.

■ CONTRAINDICATION: Known hypersensitivity to this drug prohibits its use.

■ ADVERSE EFFECTS: Among the most serious adverse reactions when given to narcotic-dependent patients are side effects associated with narcotic withdrawal.

NANB, abbreviation for **non-A, non-B hepatitis.**

NANDA, abbreviation for **North American Nursing Diagnosis Association.**

nandrolone decanoate /nan′drəlōn/, an androgen.

■ INDICATIONS: It is prescribed in the treatment of testosterone deficiency, osteoporosis, and female breast cancer, and to stimulate growth, weight gain, and the production of red cells.

■ CONTRAINDICATIONS: Cancer of the male breast or prostate, liver disease, pregnancy, suspected pregnancy, or known hypersensitivity to this drug prohibits its use.

■ ADVERSE EFFECTS: Among the most serious adverse effects are various endocrine disturbances, depending on the age of the patient. Hirsutism, acne, liver toxicity, and electrolyte imbalances also occur.

nandrolone phenpropionate, an anabolic steroid with androgenic properties.

■ INDICATIONS: It is prescribed in the treatment of osteoporosis, in certain anemias, in metastatic breast cancers of women, and for protein-sparing effects in many situations.

■ CONTRAINDICATIONS: Carcinoma of the breast in males and some females, pregnancy, nephrosis, or known hypersensitivity to this drug prohibits its use.

■ ADVERSE EFFECTS: Among the more serious adverse reactions are hirsutism, acne, various endocrine effects depending on the age and sex of the patient, masculinization, liver dysfunction, hypercalcemia in women taking the drug for breast cancer, and fluid and salt retention.

nanism /nā′nizəm, nan′-/, an abnormal smallness or underdevelopment of the body; dwarfism. Kinds of nanism are **mulibrey nanism, Paltauf's nanism, pituitary nanism, renal nanism, senile nanism,** and **symptomatic nanism.** Also called **nanosomia.**

nano-, 1. a combining form meaning 'small, or related to smallness or dwarfism': *nanocephalia, nanomelia.* 2. a combining form used in measurement to mean 'billionth (10^{-9})': *nanocurie, nanogram, nanometer.*

nanocephalic dwarf. See **bird-headed dwarf.**

nanocephaly /nā′nōsef′əlē, nan′-/, a developmental defect characterized by abnormal smallness of the head. Also called **nanocephalia, nanocephalism.** **–nanocephalous,** *adj.*, **nanocephalus,** *n.*

nanocormia /nā′nōkôr′mē·ə/, abnormal disproportionate smallness of the trunk of the body in comparison to the head and limbs. **–nanocormus,** *n.*

nanocurie (nc, nC) /nā′nōkyŏŏr′ē, nan′-/, a unit of radiation equal to one billionth of a curie.

nanogram (ng), a unit of weight equal to one billionth of a gram.

nanomelia /nā′nōmē′lyə, nan′-/, a developmental defect characterized by abnormally small limbs in comparison to the size of the head and trunk. **–nanomelous,** *adj.*, **nanomelus,** *n.*

nanometer (nm) /nan′əmē′tər/, a unit of length equal to one billionth of a meter.

nanophthalmos /nā′nofthal′məs, nan′-/, the condition in which one or both eyes are abnormally small, although other ocular defects are not present. Also called **nanophthalmia.** See also **microphthalmos.**

nanosomus, a person of very short stature; a dwarf.

nanukayami /nä′nŏŏkäyä′mē/, an acute, infectious disease caused by one of the serotypes of the spirochete *Leptospira* that is indigenous to Japan. See also **leptospirosis.**

nanus, 1. a dwarf. 2. a pygmy. **–nanoid,** *adj.*

nape, the back of the neck.

naphazoline hydrochloride /nəfaz′əlēn/, an adrenergic vasoconstrictor.

■ INDICATIONS: It is prescribed in the treatment of nasal congestion and as an ophthalmic vasoconstrictor.

■ CONTRAINDICATIONS: Glaucoma or known hypersensitivity to this drug or abnormal sensitivity to sympathomimetic drugs prohibits its use.

■ ADVERSE EFFECTS: Among the most serious adverse reactions are those associated with systemic absorption, including sedation and cardiovascular effects. Irritation to mucosa and rebound congestion also may occur.

naphthalene poisoning, a toxic condition, caused by the ingestion of naphthalene or paradichlorobenzene, that may cause nausea, vomiting, headache, abdominal pain, spasm, and convulsions. Treatment may include induced emesis, lavage, a saline cathartic, and sodium bicarbonate. Blood transfusion and fluid replacement may be necessary. Diazepam is indicated for the control of involuntary muscular contractions. Naphthalene and paradichlorobenzene are common ingredients in mothballs and moth crystals; paradichlorobenzene is also used as an insecticide in agriculture.

naphthol camphor, a syrupy mixture of two parts of camphor and one part betanaphthol, used externally as an antiseptic.

naphthol poisoning. See **phenol poisoning.**

napkin ring tumor, a tumor that encircles a tubular structure of the body, usually impairing its function and constricting its lumen to some degree. These tumors are typical of colorectal cancer of the sigmoid colon.

NAP-NAP, abbreviation for **National Association of Pediatric Nurse Associates/Practitioners.**

N.A.P.N.E.S., abbreviation for **National Association for Practical Nurse Education and Services.**

napping, periods of sleep, usually during the day, which may last from 15 to 60 minutes without attaining the level of deep sleep.

Naprosyn, a trademark for a nonsteroidal antiinflammatory, antipyretic, and analgesic (naproxen).

naproxen, a nonsteroidal antiinflammatory agent.

■ INDICATION: It is prescribed for the relief of inflammatory symptoms of arthritis.

■ CONTRAINDICATIONS: Impaired renal function, GI disease, or known hypersensitivity to this drug, to aspirin, or to nonsteroidal antiinflammatory drugs prohibits its use.

■ ADVERSE EFFECTS: Among the more serious adverse reactions are GI disorders and peptic ulcers. Dizziness, rashes, and tinnitus commonly occur. This drug interacts with many other drugs.

Naqua, a trademark for a diuretic and antihypertensive (trichlormethiazide).

Naquival, a trademark for an antihypertensive, fixed-combination drug containing a diuretic (trichlormethiazide) and an antihypertensive (reserpine).

Narcan, a trademark for a narcotic antagonist (naloxone hydrochloride).

narcissism /när′sisiz′əm/, **1.** an abnormal interest in oneself, especially in one's own body and sexual characteristics; self-love. **2.** (in psychoanalysis) sexual self-interest that is a normal characteristic of the phallic stage of psychosexual development, occurring as the infantile ego acquires a libido. Narcissism in the adult is abnormal, representing fixation at this stage of development or regression to it. Compare **egotism.** See also **narcissistic personality, narcissistic personality disorder.**

narcissistic personality, a personality characterized by behavior and attitudes that indicate an abnormal love of the self. Such a person is self-centered and self-absorbed, is extremely unrealistic concerning attributes and goals, vacillates between overidealizing and devaluing others, and, in general, assumes that he or she is entitled to more than is reasonable in relationships with others. Compare **narcissism.**

narcissistic personality disorder, a condition characterized by an exaggerated sense of self-importance and uniqueness, an abnormal need for attention and admiration, preoccupation with grandiose fantasies concerning the self, and disturbances in interpersonal relationships, usually involving the exploitation of others and a lack of empathy for them. Symptoms include depression, egocentricity, self-consciousness, inconsiderateness, inconsistency, preoccupation with grooming and remaining youthful, and intense concern with psychosomatic pains and illnesses. Treatment consists of various psychotherapeutic procedures, depending on the individual and the severity of the condition. See also **histrionic personality disorder.**

narco-, a combining form meaning 'related to stupor or a stuporous state': *narcolepsy, narcomania, narcotic.*

narcoanesthesia. See **basal anesthesia.**

narcolepsy /när′kəlep′sē/, a syndrome characterized by sudden sleep attacks, cataplexy, sleep paralysis, and visual or auditory hallucinations at the onset of sleep. The syndrome begins in adolescence or young adulthood and persists throughout life. Its cause is unknown, and no pathologic lesions are found in the brain. Persons with narcolepsy experience an uncontrollable desire to sleep, sometimes many times in one day. Episodes may last from a few minutes to several hours. Momentary loss of muscle tone occurs during waking hours (cataplexy), or while the person is asleep. Narcolepsy may be difficult to diagnose because all persons with the disorder do not experience all four symptoms. EEG or other brain studies may be used to distinguish narcolepsy from an intracranial mass or encephalitis. Amphetamines and other stimulant drugs are prescribed effectively to prevent the attacks.

narcoleptic /när′kəlep′tik/, **1.** of or pertaining to a condition or substance that causes an uncontrollable desire for sleep. **2.** a narcoleptic drug. **3.** a person suffering from narcolepsy.

narcosis /närkō′sis/, a state of insensibility or stupor caused by narcotic drugs. See also **narcotic.**

narcotic, **1.** of or pertaining to a substance that produces insensibility or stupor. **2.** a narcotic drug. Narcotic analgesics, derived from opium or produced synthetically, alter perception of pain; induce euphoria, mood changes, mental clouding, and deep sleep; depress respiration and the cough reflex; constrict the pupils; and cause smooth muscle spasm, decreased peristalsis, emesis, and nausea. Repeated use of narcotics may result in physical and psychologic dependence. Among the narcotic drugs administered clinically for relief of pain are butorphanol tartrate, hydromorphone hydrochloride, morphine sulfate, pentazocine lactate, and meperidine hydrochloride. These drugs act by binding to opiate receptors in the central nervous system; narcotic antagonists, as naloxone hydrochloride, which is used in treating narcotic overdosage, apparently displace opiates from receptor sites.

-narcotic, -narcotical, a combining form meaning 'pertaining to analgesic or soporific drugs': *antinarcotic, prenarcotic, pseudonarcotic.*

narcotic analgesic. See **analgesic.**

narcotic antagonist, a drug that is used primarily in the treatment of narcotic-induced respiratory depression. The narcotic antagonists nalorphine, levallorphan, and naloxone are usually administered parenterally.

narcotic antitussive. See **antitussive.**

Nardil, a trademark for an antidepressant (phenelzine sulfate).

nares /ner′ēz/, *sing.* **naris,** the pairs of anterior openings and posterior openings in the nose that allow the passage of air from the nose to the pharynx and the lungs during respiration. See also **anterior nares, posterior nares.**

narrow-angle glaucoma. See **glaucoma.**

nas-. See **naso-.**

nasal, of or pertaining to the nose and the nasal cavity. **–nasally,** *adv.*

nasal cavity, one of a pair of cavities that open on the face through the pear-shaped anterior nasal aperture and communicate with the pharynx. Each cavity is narrower at the top than at the bottom.

nasal decongestant, a drug that provides temporary relief of nasal symptoms in acute and chronic rhinitis and sinusitis. Most are over-the-counter products compounded with a small amount of vasoconstrictor, as ephedrine or phenylephrine. An antihistamine may enhance the value of a nasal decongestant in allergic rhinitis, and a corticosteroid may reduce inflammation. Prolonged use or dosage greater than recommended on the package may cause rebound vasodilatation and severe congestion.

nasal drip, a method of slowly infusing liquid into a dehydrated infant by means of a catheter inserted through the nose down the esophagus.

nasal fossa, one of the pair of approximately equal chambers of the nasal cavity that are separated by the nasal septum and open externally through the nostrils and internally into the nasopharynx through the choanae. Each fossa is divided into an olfactory region, consisting of the superior nasal concha and part of the septum, and a respiratory region, constituting the rest of the chamber. Overhanging the three meatuses of each fossa on the lateral wall are the corresponding superior, middle, and inferior nasal conchae. The superior meatus extends obliquely about halfway along the superior border of the middle concha. The middle meatus continues into the atrium and bulges on the lateral wall at the bulla ethmoidalis. The inferior meatus courses below and lateral to the inferior nasal concha and contains the opening of the nasolacrimal duct. The olfactory region is located in the most superior part of the fossa and contains olfactory cells, olfactory nerves, and olfactory hairs. The respiratory region is lined with mucous membrane, numerous glands, nerves, a plexus of dilated veins, and blood spaces. The plexus is easily irritated, causing the membrane to swell, blocking the meatuses and the openings of sinuses.

nasal glioma, a neoplasm characterized by the ectopic growth of neural tissue in the nasal cavity.

nasal instillation of medication, the instillation of a medicated solution into the nostrils by drops from a dropper or by an atomized spray from a squeeze bottle. Drops are instilled in each nostril as the patient's neck is hyperextended and the head tilted back over the edge of the bed. The patient's mouth should remain open during the procedure, and the head should stay in the tilted back position for several minutes to allow spread of the medication through the nasal passages. Nasal spray is administered to the patient in a sitting position. The patient is asked to expectorate any solution that runs down the posterior nares into the throat.

nasalis /nāzal′is/, one of the three muscles of the nose, divided into a transverse part and an alar part. The transverse part arises from the maxilla and covers the bridge of the nose; the alar part attaches at one end to the greater alar cartilage and at the other end to the skin at the end of the nose. The transverse part serves to depress the cartilaginous portion of the nose and to draw the alar toward the septum. The alar part serves to dilate the nostril. The nasalis is innervated by buccal branches of the facial nerve. Compare **depressor septi, procerus.**

nasal septum, the partition dividing the nostrils. It is composed of bone and cartilage covered by mucous membrane.

nasal sinus, any one of the numerous cavities in various bones of the skull, lined with ciliated mucous membrane continuous with that of the nasal cavity. The membrane is very sensitive; easily irritated, it may cause swelling that blocks the sinuses. The nasal sinuses are divided into frontal sinuses, ethmoidal air cells, sphenoidal sinuses, and maxillary sinus. Also called **air cells of the nose.**

nascent, **1.** just born; beginning to exist; incipient. **2.** (in chemistry) pertaining to any substance liberated during a chemical reaction, which, because of its uncombined state, is more reactive.

nasion /nā′zē•on/, **1.** the anthropometric reference point at the front of the skull where the midsagittal plane intersects a horizontal line tangential to the highest points in the superior palpebral sulci. **2.** the depression at the root of the nose that indicates the junction of the intranasal and the frontonasal sutures.

naso-, nas-, a combining form meaning 'of or pertaining to the nose': *nasociliary, nasolabial, nasonnement.*

nasogastric feeding /nā′zōgas′trik/, the process of introducing nutrients in a liquid form directly into the stomach via a nasogastric tube. Also called **gavage feeding.** See also **nasogastric intubation.**

nasogastric intubation, the placement of a nasogastric tube through the nose into the stomach to relieve gastric distention by removing gas, gastric secretions, or food; to instil medication, food, or fluids; or to obtain a specimen for laboratory analysis. After surgery and in any condition in which the person is able to digest food but not eat it, the tube may be introduced and left in place for tube feeding until the ability to eat normally is restored.

■ METHOD: A French size 12 to 18 plastic or rubber catheter is selected. The procedure is explained to the patient.

If the catheter is rubber, it is soaked in ice water to stiffen and lubricate it. The patient is placed in an upright sitting position, and a towel or bib is placed over the chest. The necessary length of tube is marked off; it is the same as the distance from the tip of the nose to the xiphoid process. The tip of the tube may be lubricated with a water-soluble lubricating jelly, but, if a specimen is to be obtained for cytologic study, water or saline solution is preferred. The tube is grasped and held 7.5 cm from the tip and is placed in the nostril, where it is advanced forward and downward. When it has been passed 7.5 cm it is in the pharynx. The patient is then asked to bend the neck forward, to take shallow, rapid breaths, and to help advance the tube by swallowing. The placement of the tube is checked after it has been inserted the predetermined distance to be sure that the tube is in the stomach and not in the lungs. This may be done in several ways: Fluoroscopy allows visualization of the placement; gastric contents may be aspirated; or air may be injected with a syringe through the tube and heard through a stethoscope as the air enters the stomach.

■ NURSING ORDERS: In many hospitals a physician inserts the tube the first time; in most hospitals, the nurse inserts it thereafter. Oral hygiene is performed regularly, and the tube, if left in place, is carefully secured with adhesive tape to the nose and to the cheek or jaw. Orders for tube feeding usually include the amount and timing of feeding, as well as the concentration and, sometimes, the ingredients of the formula. The formula is refrigerated and then warmed in a bowl of warm water. If the person is unconscious or unresponsive, suction equipment is kept at hand. An exact record of the feedings is kept.

■ OUTCOME CRITERIA: For the patient's comfort, the tube is selected to fit well and to be suitable for the purpose of the procedure: A tight fit is irritating to the tissues, and a small tube might not allow the prescribed formula to pass through. The tube is accepted most easily with the full cooperation of the patient. Resistance, gagging, and wincing may be minimized by explaining the procedure, by a slow steady progress, and by proper lubrication of the tube and positioning of the patient.

nasogastric tube, any tube passed into the stomach through the nose. See **nasogastric intubation.**

nasolabial reflex /nā′sōlā′bē•əl/, a sudden backward movement of the head, arching of the back, and extension and stretching of the limbs that occurs in infants in response to a light touch to the tip of the nose with an upward sweeping motion. The reflex disappears by about 5 months of age.

nasolacrimal /nā′zōlak′riməl/, of or pertaining to the nasal cavity and associated lacrimal ducts.

nasolacrimal duct, a channel that carries tears from the lacrimal sac to the nasal cavity.

nasomandibular fixation /nā′sōmandib′yŏŏlər/, a type of maxillomandibular fixation to stabilize fractures of the jaw by using maxillomandibular splints connected to a wire through a hole drilled in the anterior nasal spine of the maxillary bone. It has been used particularly in edentulous patients. See also **maxillomandibular fixation.**

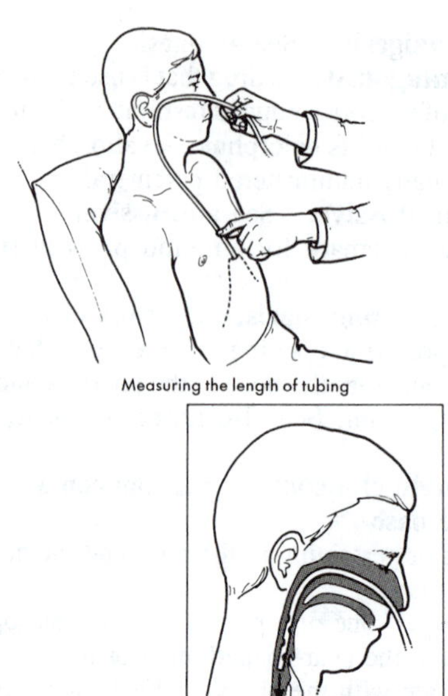

Nasogastric intubation

nasopharyngeal angiofibroma /nā′sōfərin′jē•əl/, a benign tumor of the nasopharynx, consisting of fibrous connective tissue with many vascular spaces. The tumor usually arises in puberty and is more common in boys than in girls. Typical signs are nasal and eustachian tube obstruction, adenoidal speech, and dysphagia. Also called **juvenile angiofibroma, nasopharyngeal fibroangioma.**

nasopharyngeal cancer, a malignant neoplastic disease of the nasopharynx. Depending on the site of a nasopharyngeal tumor, there may be nasal obstruction, otitis media, hearing loss, sensory or motor nerve damage, bony destruction of the skull, or deep cervical lymphadenopathy. Diagnostic measures include nasopharyngoscopy, biopsy, and radiologic examination of the skull with tomographic studies. Squamous cell and undifferentiated carcinomas are the most common lesions. Nasopharyngeal cancer occurs rarely in the United States and very frequently in southern China. Exposure to dusts of nickel, chromium, wood, and leather and to isopropyl oil increases the risk of developing nasopharyngeal cancer. High titers of antibodies to the Epstein-Barr virus are found in Chinese patients with the cancer, and there is evidence of genetic susceptibility, because a certain histocompatibility antigen is associated with the disease and multiple cases occur in some families. Radiation is the most effective therapy, and 5-fluorouracil and adriamycin are also used.

nasopharyngeal fibroangioma. See **nasopharyngeal angiofibroma.**

nasopharyngography, radiographic imaging and examination of the nasopharynx.

nasopharyngoscopy /nā'sōfer'ing•gos'kəpē/, a technique in physical examination in which the nose and throat are visually examined using a laryngoscope, a fiberoptic device, a flashlight, and a dilator for the nares. –**nasopharyngoscopic,** *adj.*

nasopharynx /nā'sōfer'ingks/, one of the three regions of the throat, situated behind the nose and extending from the posterior nares to the level of the soft palate. On the posterior wall of the nasopharynx, opposite the posterior nares, are the pharyngeal tonsils. Swollen or enlarged pharyngeal tonsils can fill the space behind the posterior nares and may completely block the passage of air from the nose into the throat. Compare **laryngopharynx, oropharynx.** See also **tonsil.** –**nasopharyngeal,** *adj.*

nasotracheal tube, a catheter inserted into the trachea through the nasal cavity and the pharynx. It is commonly used to administer oxygen and in other respiratory therapy.

natal, **1.** of or pertaining to birth. **2.** of or pertaining to the nates, or buttocks.

natamycin, an ophthalmic antifungal. Also called **pimariacin.**

■ INDICATIONS: It is prescribed in the treatment of fungal keratitis, blepharitis, and conjunctivitis.

■ CONTRAINDICATION: Known hypersensitivity to this drug prohibits its use.

■ ADVERSE EFFECTS: No adverse effects have been reported other than a rare case of conjunctival chemosis and hyperemia.

nates /nā'tēz/, *sing.* **natis,** the large fleshy protuberances at the lower posterior portion of the torso comprising fat and the gluteal muscles. Also called **buttocks.**

National Association for Mental Health. See **Mental Health Association.**

National Association of Pediatric Nurse Associates/Practitioners (NAP-NAP), a national organization of nurses who are prepared by training or experience to give primary care to pediatric patients. NAP-NAP works in conjunction with American Academy of Pediatrics.

National Association for Practical Nurse Education and Services (N.A.P.N.E.S.), a national professional organization concerned with the education of practical nurses and with the services provided by licensed practical nurses.

National Bureau of Standards (NBS), a federal agency in the Department of Commerce that sets accurate measurement standards for commerce, industry, and science in the United States. The NBS compares and coordinates its standards with those of other countries and provides research and technic service to improve computer science, materials technology, building construction, and consumer product safety. The Bureau also provides measurement services and standards for other federal agencies and for state and local governments.

National Council Licensure Examination (NCLEX), a comprehensive integrated examination, developed and administered by the National Council of State Boards of Nursing, designed to test basic competency for nursing practice. The NCLEX-RN test plan has three components including nursing behaviors grouped under nursing process categories, the process of decision making that defines nursing's role, and levels of cognitive ability.

National Eye Institute (NEI), a division of the National Institutes of Health. NEI was established in 1968 to support research in the normal functioning of the human eye and visual system, the pathology of visual disorders, and the rehabilitation of the visually handicapped. See also **eye, vision.**

National Formulary (N.F.), a publication containing the official standards for the preparation of various pharmaceutics not listed in the *United States Pharmacopoeia.* It is revised every 5 years.

national health insurance, a government-financed health insurance program providing comprehensive benefits to most or all of the population. Compare **Medicaid, Medicare.**

National Health Planning and Resources Development Act of 1974, U.S congressional legislation (PL 93-641) that established a nationwide network of health systems agencies. The act provides for the coordination and direction of national health policy through state and regional regulatory agencies.

National Health Service Corps (NHSC), a program of the United States Public Health Service (USPHS) in which health care personnel are placed in areas that are underserved. The Corps was established by the Emergency Health Personnel Act of 1970. The provisions of the Act are updated as needed. Nurses, physicians, and dentists serve in rural and urban areas, usually as employees of local health care agencies. The USPHS pays most of the salary of each corps member.

National Institute of Child Health and Human Development (N.I.C.H.H.D.), the Institute in the National Institutes of Health that is concerned with all aspects of the growth, development, and health of the children of the United States.

National Institutes of Health (N.I.H.), an agency within the United States Public Health Service made up of several institutions and constituent divisions, including the Bureau of Health Manpower Education, the National Library of Medicine, the National Cancer Institute, and several research institutes and divisions.

National Joint Practice Commission, a former organization of the American Nurses' Association and the American Medical Association established to promote collaborative efforts between medicine and nursing. The Commission was disbanded in 1981.

National League for Nursing (NLN), an organization concerned with the improvement of nursing education, nursing service, and the provision of health care in the United States. Among its many activities are accreditation of nursing programs at all levels, preadmission and achievement tests for nursing students, and compilation of statistic data on nursing personnel and on trends in health care delivery. It acts as the testing service for the

State Board Test Pool Examinations for registered and practical nurse licensure. The Research Division and the Public Affairs Office are among the other sections of NLN. A monthly refereed journal, *Nursing and Health Care,* is the official publication of the organization.

National Male Nurses' Association (NMNA), a national organization that promotes the interests and practice of male nurses.

National Society of Critical Care Nurses of Canada (NSCCN), an organization of Canadian critical care nurses, established originally in 1975 as the Toronto Chapter of the American Association of Critical-Care Nurses. The group became an independent Canadian organization in 1983. Publications include a bimonthly journal, *Critical Care Nurse,* and a newsletter, *CriticaList.*

National Student Nurses' Association (NSNA), a national organization of students in the field of nursing. Among its purposes are the improvement of nursing education to improve health care, to aid in the development of the student nurse, and to encourage optimal achievement in the professional role of the nurse and the health care of people. It publishes a journal, *Imprint,* five times a year, participates in legislative activities at all levels, and gives scholarships, awards, and career workshops.

natriuresis /nā′trēyŏŏrē′sis/, the excretion of greater than normal amounts of sodium in the urine, as from the administration of natriuretic diuretic drugs or from various metabolic or endocrine disorders.

natriuretic /nā′trēyŏŏret′ik/, **1.** of or pertaining to the process of natriuresis. **2.** a substance that inhibits the resorption of sodium ions from the glomerular filtrate in the kidneys, thus allowing more sodium to be excreted with the urine.

natural childbirth, labor and parturition accomplished by a mother with little or no medical intervention. It is generally considered the optimal way of giving birth and being born, safest for the baby and most satisfying for the mother. Prerequisites include normal gestation, an adequate birth canal, strong maternal motivation, physical and emotional preparation, and constant and intensive support of the mother during labor and birth. See also **Lamaze method.**

natural dentition, the entire array of natural teeth in the dental arch at any given time, consisting of deciduous or permanent teeth or a mixture of the two. See also **tooth.**

natural family planning method, any one of several methods of family planning that does not rely on a medication or a device for effectiveness in avoiding pregnancy. Some of the methods are also used to pinpoint the time of ovulation to increase the chance of fertilization when artificial insemination or extraction of an oocyte for in vitro fertilization is to be performed. Natural family planning methods require thorough instruction, the cooperation and self-motivation of the couple, and the diligent, accurate observation and recording of the data relevant to the method. Kinds of natural family-planning include **basal body temperature method of family planning, calendar method of family planning, ovulation method of family planning,** and **symptothermal method of family planning.**

natural immunity, a usually innate and permanent form of immunity to a specific disease. Kinds of natural immunity include **individual immunity, racial immunity,** and **species immunity.** Also called **genetic immunity, innate immunity.** Compare **acquired immunity.**

natural law, a doctrine that holds there is a natural moral order or natural moral law inherent in the structure of the universe.

naturally acquired immunity. See **acquired immunity.**

natural network, (in psychiatric nursing) a patient's natural contacts in the community, including church and social groups, friends, family, and occupation that support the person's function outside the hospital environment.

natural pacemaker, any cardiac pacing site in the heart tissues.

natural radiation, radioactivity that emanates from the soil and rocks or particles and rays that reach the earth from cosmic sources, as actinic radiation from the sun and neutrinos from beyond the solar system.

natural selection, the natural evolutionary processes by which those organisms best suited for adaptation to the environment tend to survive and propagate the species, whereas those unfit are eliminated. Compare **artificial selection.**

Naturetin, a trademark for a diuretic and antihypertensive (bendroflumethiazide).

naturopath /nā′chŏŏrəpath′, nach′-/, a person who practices naturopathy.

naturopathy /nā′chŏŏrop′əthē, nach′-/, a system of therapeutics based on natural foods, light, warmth, massage, fresh air, regular exercise, and the avoidance of medications. Advocates believe that illness can be healed by the natural processes of the body.

Nauheim bath /nou′hīm/, a bath taken in water through which carbon dioxide is bubbled, followed by systematic exercises, used in the treatment of cardiac conditions. The procedure is named after the natural waters of Bad Nauheim, Germany. Also called **Nauheim treatment.**

nausea /nô′zē·ə, nô′zhə/, a sensation often leading to the urge to vomit. Common causes are seasickness and other motion sicknesses, early pregnancy, intense pain, emotional stress, gallbladder disease, food poisoning, and various enteroviruses. **–nauseate,** *v.,* **nauseous,** *adj.*

nausea and vomiting of pregnancy, a common condition of early pregnancy, characterized by recurrent or persistent nausea, often in the morning, that may result in vomiting, weight loss, anorexia, general weakness, and malaise. The causes of the condition are poorly understood. It usually does not begin before the sixth week after the last menstrual period and ends by the twelfth to the fourteenth week of pregnancy. Symptomatic relief is often obtained by eating small, easily digested meals frequently and by not allowing the stomach to be empty. In the past, antiemetic drugs were routinely prescribed for this complaint, but this practice is currently reserved for severe cases. Nausea and vomiting after the sixteenth week is an unusual complication of pregnancy, called persistent nausea and vomiting of pregnancy. If severe and intractable, hyperemesis gravidarum may ensue. Also called *(nontechnical)* **morning sickness.**

Navane, a trademark for a tranquilizer (thiothixene).

navel. See **umbilicus.**

navicular /nəvik′yo͞olər/, having the shape of a boat, as the navicular bone in the wrist.

navicular bone. See **scaphoid bone.**

Nb, symbol for **niobium.**

NBS standard, (in nuclear medicine) a radioactive source standardized, or certified, or both, by the National Bureau of Standards.

nc, nC, abbreviation for **nanocurie.**

N-CAP, abbreviation for **Nurses' Coalition for Action in Politics.**

NCI, abbreviation for the *National Cancer Institute.* See **National Institutes of Health.**

NCLEX-RN abbreviation for **National Council Licensure Examination.**

Nd, abbreviation for **neodymium.**

Ne, symbol for **neon.**

ne-, See **neo-.**

near drowning, a pathologic state in which the victim has survived exposure to circumstances that usually cause drowning. Cardiopulmonary resuscitation is performed immediately; hospitalization is always indicated. The return of consciousness does not necessarily assure recovery. Intensive supportive therapy may be required for up to several days. Compare **drowning.** See also **hypothermia.**

nearest neighbor analysis, (in molecular genetics) a biochemical method used to estimate the frequency with which pairs of bases are located next to one another.

nearsightedness. See **myopia.**

Nebcin, a trademark for an antibacterial (tobramycin sulfate).

nebula, *pl.* **nebulae,** **1.** a slight corneal opacity or scar that seldom obstructs vision and that can be seen only by oblique illumination. **2.** a murkiness in the urine. **3.** an oily concoction that is applied with an atomizer.

nebulization, a method of administering a drug by spraying it into the respiratory passages of the patient. The medication may be given with or without oxygen to help carry it into the lungs.

nebulize, to vaporize or disperse a liquid in a fine spray.

nebulizer, a device for producing a fine spray. Intranasal medications are often administered by a nebulizer. Also called **atomizer.**

NEC, abbreviation for **necrotizing enterocolitis.**

Necator, a genus of nematode that is an intestinal parasite and causes hookworm disease. See also ***Ancylostoma.***

necatoriosis, hookworm disease, specifically that caused by *Necator americanus,* which is the most common North American hookworm. The larvae live in the soil and reach the human digestive tract through contaminated food and water or through the skin of the feet and legs. Symptoms include diarrhea, nausea, abdominal pain, and anemia in the more severe cases. Treatment consists of first correcting the anemia if present and then anthelmintic therapy, usually with pyrantel pamoate or mebendazole. Prevention includes the elimination of soil pollution and the avoidance of skin contact with the soil. See also **ancylostomiasis, hookworm.**

neck, a constricted section, as the part of the body that connects the head with the trunk. Other such constrictions are the neck of the humerus and the neck of the femur.

neck dissection, surgical removal of the cervical lymph nodes, performed to prevent the spread of malignant tumors of the head and neck. Under general anesthesia, the cervical chain of lymph nodes with their lymphatic channels is removed in one mass to prevent the spread of cancer cells. After surgery, the patient is observed closely for signs of hemorrhage and difficulty in breathing. Compare **radical neck dissection.**

neck righting reflex, **1.** an involuntary response in newborns in which turning the head to one side while the infant is supine causes rotation of the shoulders and trunk in the same direction. The reflex enables the child to roll over from the supine to prone position. Absence of the reflex or persistence beyond about 10 months of age may indicate central nervous system damage. **2.** any tonic reflex associated with the neck that maintains body orientation in relation to the head.

necro-, a combining form meaning 'of or pertaining to death or a corpse': *necrobiosis, necronectomy, necrophilia.*

necrobiosis lipoidica, a skin disease characterized by thin, shiny, yellow to red plaques on the shins or forearms. Telangiectases, crusting, and ulceration of these plaques may occur. Necrobiosis lipoidica is usually associated with diabetes mellitus and occurs most often in women. Treatment includes precise control of the diabetes and, possibly, intralesional application of corticosteroids.

necrolysis /nekrol′isis/, disintegration or exfoliation of dead tissue. Compare **necrosis.** **–necrolytic,** *adj.*

necrophilia, **1.** a morbid liking for being with dead bodies. **2.** a morbid desire to have sexual contact with a dead body, usually of men to perform a sexual act with a dead woman. **–necrophile, necrophiliac,** *n.*

necropsy, necroscopy. See **autopsy.**

necrosis /nekrō′sis/, localized tissue death that occurs in groups of cells in response to disease or injury. In **coagulation necrosis,** blood clots block the flow of blood, causing tissue ischemia distal to the clot; in **gangrenous**

necrosis, ischemia combined with bacterial action causes putrefaction to set in. See also **gangrene.**

necrotizing angiitis. See **periarteritis nodosa.**

necrotizing enteritis, acute inflammation of the small and the large intestine by the bacterium *Clostridium perfringens,* characterized by severe abdominal pain, bloody diarrhea, and vomiting. Some people recover completely, some survive with chronic bowel obstruction, and some die of perforation of the intestine, dehydration, peritonitis, or septicemia.

necrotizing enterocolitis (NEC), an acute inflammatory bowel disorder that occurs primarily in preterm or low-birth-weight neonates. It is characterized by ischemic necrosis of the GI mucosa that may lead to perforation and peritonitis. The cause of the disorder is unknown, although it appears to be a defect in host defenses with infection resulting from normal GI flora rather than from invading organisms. Also called **pseudomembranous enterocolitis.** See also **enteritis.**

■ OBSERVATIONS: Significant predisposing factors of the condition include prematurity, hypovolemia, respiratory distress syndrome, sepsis, an indwelling umbilical catheter, exchange transfusion, and feeding with hyperosmolar or high-caloric formulas. The condition results from a reflex shunting of blood away from the GI tract, which leads to convulsive vasoconstriction of the mesenteric vessels supplying the intestines. The diminished blood supply interferes with the normal production of mucus and with other bowel functions and results in severe necrosis with bacterial invasion of the bowel wall. Bottle-fed infants are more susceptible to the disorder, possibly because formula lacks the immunoglobulin A antibodies and macrophages, found in breast milk, that may protect the GI mucosa from damage and bacterial invasion. Initial symptoms, which usually develop after several days of life, include temperature instability (usually hypothermia), lethargy, poor feeding, vomiting of bile, abdominal distention, blood in the stools, and decreased or absent bowel sounds. Signs of deterioration are apnea, pallor, hyperbilirubinemia, oliguria, abdominal tenderness, erythema and edema of the anterior abdominal wall or palpable masses, with eventual respiratory failure leading to death. Diagnosis is confirmed by x-ray visualization of the intestine or by the presence of increased peritoneal fluid or pneumoperitoneum.

■ INTERVENTION: Treatment includes discontinuing oral feeding, beginning intravenous infusion, abdominal decompression by nasogastric suction, hydration, plasma or whole blood transfusion, and administration of broad-spectrum antibiotics (usually ampicillin, gentamicin, or kanamycin). With routine supportive management, improvement usually occurs within 48 to 72 hours. Oral feedings usually are not resumed for 10 days to 2 weeks. Total parenteral nutrition is necessary during that period. Surgical resection of the affected bowel segment may be necessary, especially if signs of intestinal perforation or peritonitis develop. If a large portion of bowel is affected, an ileostomy or colostomy may be necessary. Stenosis of the involved bowel segment may present later complications.

■ NURSING CONSIDERATIONS: The primary concern of the nurse is to observe high-risk, formula-fed infants for early symptoms of necrotizing enterocolitis, especially for difficulty in feeding, bile-stained regurgitation, bloody stools, temperature variations, or a distended, shiny abdomen. Once the diagnosis is confirmed, the nurse initiates nasogastric intubation for abdominal decompression and continues to monitor the baby constantly for dehydration and electrolyte balance. In addition to the ordered laboratory tests, daily weight is taken. Infants who are unable to take fluids by mouth require special oral care. Glycerin and lemon swabs reduce dryness, and a pacifier or a nipple stuffed with gauze helps to meet the infant's need to suck. Parents are encouraged to visit and are helped to meet the emotional needs of the infant and to provide tactile, auditory, and visual stimulation. The nurse explains the usual course of the disease, the medical and nursing procedures, and keeps the parents informed of the infant's progress. Frequent visits to the care unit facilitate family-infant relationships and provide the nurse with an opportunity to teach proper care techniques before discharge.

necrotizing vasculitis, an inflammatory condition of blood vessels, characterized by necrosis, fibrosis, and proliferation of the inner layer of the vascular wall, in some cases resulting in occlusion and infarction. Necrotizing vasculitis may occur in rheumatoid arthritis and is common in systemic lupus erythematosus, periarteritis nodosa, and progressive systemic sclerosis. The condition is usually treated with corticosteroids.

needle bath, a shower in which fine jets of water are sprayed over the body.

needle biopsy, the removal of a segment of living tissue for microscopic examination by inserting a hollow needle through the skin or the external surface of an organ or tumor and rotating it within the underlying cellular layers. See also **aspiration biopsy.**

needle filter, a device, usually made of plastic, used for filtering medications that are drawn into a syringe before administration. Some syringe needles are equipped with built-in filters; other filters are separate units that are attached to the needle before use. Manufacturers' instructions are usually supplied with such devices. Needle filters are commonly disposable items designed for one-time applications.

needle holder, a surgical forceps used to hold and pass a suturing needle through tissue. Also called **suture forceps.**

negative, **1.** (of a laboratory test) indicating that a substance or a reaction is not present. **2.** (of a sign) indicating on physical examination that a finding is not present, often meaning that there is no pathologic change. **3.** (of a substance) tending to carry or carrying a negative chemical charge.

negative adaptation. See **habituation.**

negative anxiety, (in psychology) an emotional and psychologic condition in which anxiety prevents a person's normal functioning and interrupts the person's ability to perform the usual activities of daily living.

negative catalysis, a decrease in the rate of any chemical reaction caused by a substance that is neither part of the process itself nor consumed nor affected by the reaction. Compare **catalysis.** See also **catalyst.**

negative feedback, **1.** (in physiology) a decrease in function in response to a stimulus; for example, the secretion of follicle stimulating hormone decreases even as the amount of circulating estrogen increases. **2.** *informal.* a critical, derogatory, or otherwise negative response from one person to what another person has communicated.

negative pi meson (pion), a form of electromagnetic radiation emitted from a proton linear accelerator.

negative pi meson (pion) radiotherapy, a form of radiotherapy using a negative pi meson (pion) beam emitted by a proton linear accelerator. In the treatment of certain tumors, negative pi meson particles are beamed at the tumor; the atomic nuclei of malignant cells take in the radioactive particles and explode, scattering intensely radioactive subatomic particles through the adjacent malignant tissue. Pion radiotherapy requires fewer rad and has a 60% greater biologic effect than conventional x-radiation techniques. It may also have less effect on normal tissue near the tumor. Some locally advanced neoplasms, especially those of the prostate, are destroyed. Gliomas and advanced cancers of the head and neck may also be well controlled with pion radiotherapy. Moderately acute toxicity occurs with treatment; chronic toxicity is minimal.

negative pressure, less than ambient atmospheric pressure, as in a vacuum, at an altitude above sea level, or in a hypobaric chamber. Some ventilators have a negative cycle that may help stimulate or cycle exhalation in controlled ventilation in IPPB therapy.

negative relationship, (in research) an inverse relationship between two variables; as one variable increases, the other decreases. Also called **inverse relationship.** Compare **positive relationship.**

negativism, a behavioral attitude characterized by opposition, resistance, the refusal to cooperate with even the most reasonable request, and the tendency to act in a contrary manner. The resulting response may be passive, as the immobile, rigid postures observed in catatonic schizophrenia, or active, as in a belligerent, impulsive, or capricious act, as lowering the arms when asked to raise them or sitting down when asked to stand.

NegGram, a trademark for an antibacterial (nalidixic acid).

negligence, (in law) the commission of an act that a prudent person would not have done or the omission of a duty that a prudent person would have fulfilled, resulting in injury or harm to another person. In particular, in a malpractice suit, a professional person is negligent if harm to a client results from such an act or such failure to act, but it must be proved that other prudent persons of the same profession would ordinarily have acted differently under the same circumstances. Thus, negligence may be misfeasance, malfeasance, or nonfeasance.

negligence per se, (in law) a finding of negligence rendered in judgment of a professional action or inaction in violation of a statute or so at odds with common sense that beyond any doubt no prudent person would have been guilty of it.

NEI, abbreviation for **National Eye Institute.**

Neisseria gonorrhoeae, a gram-negative, nonmotile, diplococcal bacterium usually seen microscopically as flattened pairs within the cytoplasm of neutrophils. It is the causative organism of gonorrhea. Also called **gonococcus.**

Neisseria meningitidis. See **meningococcus.**

NEJM, abbreviation for ***New England Journal of Medicine.***

Nelson's syndrome, an endocrine disorder that may follow adrenalectomy for Cushing's disease. It is characterized by a marked increase in the secretion of ACTH and MSH by the pituitary gland. Treatment includes irradiation to decrease pituitary function and, in some cases, hypophysectomy. See also **Cushing's disease.**

nem, abbreviation for **Nahrungs-Einheit-Milch.**

-nema, a combining form meaning a 'threadlike stage in the development of chromosomes': *chromonema, plasmonema, uronema.*

nemato-, a combining form meaning 'pertaining to a nematode, or to a threadlike structure': *nematoblast, nematocide, nematodiasis.*

nematocides, chemical pesticides that are employed to kill nematode worms.

nematode /nem′ətōd/, a multicellular, parasitic animal of the phylum Nematoda. All roundworms belong to the phylum, including *Ancylostoma duodenale, Ascaris lumbricoides, Enterobius vermicularis, Necator americanus, Strongyloides stercoralis,* and several other species.

Nembutal, a trademark for a barbiturate (pentobarbital), used as an adjunct to anesthesia.

-nemia. See **-anemia.**

neo-, ne-, a combining form meaning 'new': *neobiogenesis, neocyte, neonatal.*

neoantigen, a new specific antigen that develops in a cell infected by oncogenic virus; it appears after infection by SV40.

neobehaviorism, a school of psychology based on the general principles of behaviorism but broader and more flexible in concept. It stresses experimental research and laboratory analyses in the study of overt behavior and in various subjective phenomena that cannot be directly observed and measured, as fantasies, love, stress, empathy, trust, and personality. See also **behaviorism.**

neobehaviorist, a disciple of the school of neobehaviorism.

Neobiotic, a trademark for an antibacterial (neomycin sulfate).

neoblastic, of or pertaining to a new tissue or development within a new tissue.

Neo-Cort-Dome, a trademark for a topical, fixed-combination drug containing a glucocorticoid (hydrocortisone) and an antibacterial (neomycin sulfate).

Neo-Cortef, a trademark for a topical, fixed-combination drug containing a glucocorticoid (hydrocortisone acetate) and an antibacterial (neomycin sulfate).

NeoDecadron, a trademark for a topical, fixed-combination drug containing a glucocorticoid (dexamethasone phosphate) and an antibacterial (neomycin sulfate).

Neo-Delta-Cortef, a trademark for a topical, fixed-combination drug containing a glucocorticoid (prednisolone acetate) and an antibacterial (neomycin sulfate).

neodymium (Nd), a rare earth element. Its atomic number is 60; its atomic weight is 144.27.

neologism /nē•ol′əjiz′əm/, **1.** a newly coined word or term. **2.** (in psychiatry) a word coined by a psychotic or delirious patient that is meaningful only to the patient.

Neo-Medrol, a trademark for a topical, fixed-combination drug containing a glucocorticoid (methylprednisolone) and an antibacterial (neomycin sulfate).

Neo-Mull-Soy, a trademark for a commercial milk-substitute formula that is lactose free, used for infants with galactosemia and persons with lactose intolerance. It is made from a soy isolate base and supplemented with added nutrients, especially vitamins and minerals. See also **Nutramigen, Pro Sobee, Soyalac.**

neomycin sulfate, an aminoglycoside antibiotic.

■ INDICATIONS: It is prescribed in the treatment of infections of the intestine, in hepatic coma, and, topically, in the treatment of skin infections.

■ CONTRAINDICATIONS: Renal dysfunction, intestinal obstruction, or known hypersensitivity to this drug or to any aminoglycoside medication prohibits its use.

■ ADVERSE EFFECTS: Among the more serious adverse reactions are nausea, vomiting, diarrhea, malabsorption, or suprainfection. Prolonged treatment in patients with impaired renal function may result in the toxicities of systemic aminoglycosides. Hypersensitivity reactions may occur with topical administration of this drug.

neon (Ne), a colorless, odorless gaseous element and one of the inert gases. Its atomic number is 10; its atomic weight is 20.2. Neon has no compounds and occurs in the atmosphere in the ratio of about 18 parts per million. Some minerals and meteorites contain traces of this element. It is prepared commercially by the fractional distillation of liquefied air and is one of the first components to boil off. Neon is an excellent conductor of electricity, which ionizes the gas and causes it to emit a reddish-orange glow; this characteristic makes neon useful in devices to warn against electric current overload.

neonatal, the period of time covering the first 28 days after birth.

Neonatal Behavior Assessment Scale, a scale for evaluating and assessing an infant's alertness, motor maturity, irritability, consolability, and interaction with people. It is used as a tool for the evaluation of the neurologic condition and the behavior of a newborn infant. Using the scale, the individuality of an infant may be demonstrated for parents, and some researchers theorize that the quality of the parent-child relationship may be predicted.

neonatal breathing, respiration in newborn infants that begins when pulmonary fluid in the lungs is expelled by mechanic compression of the thorax during delivery and by resorption from the alveoli into the bloodstream and lymphatics. As air enters the lungs, the chest and lungs recoil to a resting position, but forceful inspirations are necessary to keep the lungs inflated. These forces come from changes in blood gas tension, strong Hering-Breuer reflexes, temperature, and tactile stimuli. Irregular fetal breathing movements, which occur during rapid eye movement sleep, may be observed as early as 13 weeks of gestation. At birth, the peripheral and central chemoreceptors are very active, and newborns are highly sensitive to carbon dioxide during the first weeks. However, control of rhythm is not fully developed at birth.

neonatal conjunctivitis. See **ophthalmia neonatorum.**

neonatal death, the death of a live-born infant during the first 28 days after birth. Early neonatal death is usullly considered to be one that occurs during the first 7 days. Compare **infant death, perinatal death.**

neonatal developmental profile, an evaluation of the developmental status of a newborn infant based on three examinations, a gestational age inventory, a neurologic examination, and a Neonatal Behavior Assessment score.

neonatal hyperbilirubinemia. See **hyperbilirubinemia of the newborn.**

neonatal intensive care unit (NICU), a hospital unit containing a variety of sophisticated mechanic devices and special equipment for the management and care of premature and seriously ill newborn infants. The unit is staffed by a team of nurses and neonatologists who are highly trained in the pathophysiology of the newborn. See also **intensive care unit.**

neonatal jaundice. See **hyperbilirubinemia of the newborn.**

neonatal mortality, the statistic rate of infant death during the first 28 days after live birth, expressed as the number of such deaths per 1000 live births in a specific geographic area or institution in a given time.

neonatal period, the interval from birth to 28 days of age. It represents the time of the greatest risk to the infant; approximately 65% of all deaths that occur in the first year of life happen during this 4-week period.

neonatal pustular melanosis, a transient skin condition of the neonate characterized by vesicles present at birth that become pustular. The lesions contain neutrophils rather than eosinophils as seen in erythema toxicum neonatorum, and they disappear within 72 hours, leaving dark spots that gradually fade by about 3 months of age.

neonatal thermoregulation, the regulation of the body temperature of a newborn infant, which may be affected by evaporation, conduction, radiation, and convection.

■ METHOD: To prevent the loss of body heat through evaporation, the infant is patted dry with a warm towel immediately after birth. Loss of heat by conduction is prevented by wrapping the baby in a warm blanket or wrapping a warm blanket over him as he lies on his mother's skin and by warming all equipment that is to be used to touch, cover, or examine the infant. Loss of heat by radiation can be minimized by placing the baby under a radiant heater, on a warmed, padded surface, skin-to-skin with the mother. Loss of body heat by convection is prevented by avoiding drafts, air conditioning vents, and low ambient temperatures. Infant bassinets have high sides to prevent cross drafts.

■ NURSING ORDERS: The infant is kept covered and protected from any means of heat loss. Because the surface area of the head of a newborn is proportionately large when compared with the body, heat loss from the head may be great; therefore, a cap or fold of blanket is placed around the head. Progressive family-centered maternity services, in which the practice after delivery is to place the infant skin-to-skin with the mother, often provide caps made of stockinet. An overhead radiant heater is rolled to the delivery bed to maintain a warm ambient temperature for the infant.

■ OUTCOME CRITERIA: The axillary temperature is normally between 36.5° C (97.5° F) and 37° C (98.6° F), and the rectal temperature is normally 1° higher than the axillary temperature.

eonatal tyrosinemia. See **tyrosinemia.**

eonatal unit, a unit of a hospital that provides care and treatment of newborn infants through the age of 28 days, and longer if necessary.

eonate /nē′ənāt/, an infant from birth to 4 weeks of age.

eonatology /nē′ōnətol′əjē/, the branch of medicine that concentrates on the care of the neonate and specializes in the diagnosis and treatment of the disorders of the newborn infant. –**neonatologic, neonatological,** *adj.*, **neonatologist,** *n.*

eoplasia /nē′ōplā′zhə/, the new and abnormal development of cells that may be benign or malignant. –**neoplastic,** *adj.*

eoplasm /nē′ōplaz′əm/, any abnormal growth of new tissue, benign or malignant. Also called **tumor.** See also **benign, cancer, malignant.** –**neoplastic,** *adj.*

eoplastic fracture, a fracture resulting from weakened bone tissue caused by neoplasm or by a malignant growth. Also called **pathologic fracture.**

Neosporin, a trademark for a topical, fixed-combination drug containing antibacterials (polymyxin B sulfate, neomycin sulfate, and bacitracin zinc).

eostigmine bromide /nē′ōstig′mēn/, a cholinergic.

■ INDICATION: It is prescribed in the treatment of myasthenia gravis.

■ CONTRAINDICATIONS: Bowel obstruction, urinary tract infection, or known hypersensitivity to this drug or to other bromides prohibits its use.

■ ADVERSE EFFECTS: Among the more serious adverse reactions are severe respiratory depression, ptyalism, and intestinal cramps.

Classification of neoplasms

Parent tissue	*Benign tumor*	*Malignant tumor*
Epithelium		
Skin and mucous membrane	Papilloma Polyp	Squamous cell carcinoma Basal cell carcinoma Transitional cell carcinoma
Glands	Adenoma Cystadenoma	Adenocarcinoma
Endothelium		
Blood vessels	Hemangioma	Endothelioma Hemangioendothelioma Angiosarcoma
Lymph vessels	Lymphangioma	Lymphangiosarcoma Lymphangioendothelioma
Bone marrow		Multiple myeloma Ewing's sarcoma Leukemia
Lymphoid tissue		Lymphosarcoma Reticulum cell sarcoma (difficult to classify because of cell embryology) Lymphatic leukemia
Connective tissues		
Embryonic fibrous tissue	Myxoma	Myxosarcoma
Fibrous tissue	Fibroma	Fibrosarcoma
Adipose tissue	Lipoma	Liposarcoma
Cartilage	Chondroma	Chondrosarcoma
Bone	Osteoma	Osteogenic sarcoma
Synovial membrane	Synovioma	Synovial sarcoma
Muscle tissue		
Smooth muscle	Leiomyoma	Leiomyosarcoma
Striated muscle	Rhabdomyoma	Rhabdomyosarcoma
Nerve tissue		
Nerve fibers and sheaths	Neuroma Neurinoma (neurilemoma) Neurofibroma	Neurogenic sarcoma Neurofibrosarcoma
Ganglion cells	Ganglioneuroma	Neuroblastoma
Glia cells	Glioma	Glioblastoma Spongioblastoma
Meninges	Meningioma	
Pigmented neoplasms		
Melanoblasts	Pigmented nevus	Malignant melanoma Melanocarcinoma
Miscellaneous		
Placenta	Hydatidiform mole	Chorion-epithelioma (choriocarcinoma)
	Dermoid cyst	Embryonal carcinoma Embryonal sarcoma Teratocarcinoma

Neo-Synephrine Hydrochloride, a trademark for a vasoconstrictor (phenylephrine hydrochloride).

neoteny /nē•ot′ənē/, the attainment of sexual maturity during the larval stage of development, as in certain amphibians, especially salamanders.

Neothylline, a trademark for a smooth muscle relaxant (dyphylline).

Neotrizine, a trademark for an antibacterial (trisulfapyrimidine).

nephelometer /nef′əlom′ətər/, a photometric apparatus used to determine the concentration of solids suspended in a liquid or a gas, as may be used to determine the number of bacteria in a specimen. See also **nephelometry.**

nephelometry /nef′əlom′ətrē/, a technique of determining the concentration of solids suspended in a liquid or a gas by use of a nephelometer. **–nephelometric, nephelometrical,** *adj.*

nephr-. See **nephro-.**

nephrectomy, the surgical removal of a kidney, performed to remove a tumor, drain an abcess, or treat hydronephrosis. Before surgery, the fluid intake is increased to improve the excretion of waste products. The blood is typed and crossmatched for transfusion. Under general anesthesia, the kidney is approached through either a flank or a thoracoabdominal incision and is removed. If the thoracic cavity is opened, a chest tube is inserted and connected to water-seal drainage. Hemostats may be left in place with handles extending out through the incision, preventing the patient from lying on the affected side. The nurse observes carefully for rapid pulse, restlessness, sweating, and a drop in blood pressure. The urinary output is measured hourly, and fluid intake and body weight are closely monitored. Deep breathing is difficult because the incision is close to the diaphragm; intermittent positive pressure breathing apparatus is used to drain secretions. The nurse reports at once any sudden shortness of breath, a sign of spontaneous pneumothorax that may occur if the pleura was accidentally nicked during surgery.

-nephric, a combining form meaning 'of or referring to the kidneys': *archinephric, cardionephric, splenonephric.*

nephritic calculus. See **renal calculus.**

nephritic gingivitis, a kind of stomatitis and gingivitis associated with kidney function failure, accompanied by pain, ammoniac odor, and increased salivation. Also called **uremic gingivitis.**

nephritis /nefrī′tis/, any one of a large group of diseases of the kidney characterized by inflammation and abnormal function. Kinds of nephritis include **acute nephritis, glomerulonephritis, hereditary nephritis, interstitial nephritis, parenchymatous nephritis,** and **suppurative nephritis.**

nephro-, nephr-, a combining form meaning 'of or related to the kidneys': *nephroblastoma, nephrogram, nephrorrhagia.*

nephroangiosclerosis /nef′rō•an′jē•ōsklerō′sis/, necrosis of the renal arterioles, associated with hypertension. This condition is present in a small number of hypertensive individuals between 30 and 50 years of ag Early signs of the condition are headaches, blurring vision, and a diastolic blood pressure greater than 1 mm Hg. Examination of the retina reveals hemorrhage vascular exudates, and papilledema. The heart is usual enlarged, especially the left ventricle. Proteins and r blood cells are found in the urine. Heart failure and ki ney failure may occur if the disease remains untreate Treatment includes measures to lower blood pressu using diet and antihypertensive medications. Hemodial sis is used when preventive measures have failed. Al called **malignant hypertension.** See also **hypertensio renal failure.**

nephroblastoma. See **Wilms' tumor.**

nephrocalcinosis /nef′rōkal′sinō′sis/, an abnorm condition of the kidneys in which deposits of calciu form in the parenchyma at the site of previous inflamm tion or degenerative change. Infection, hematuria, an colic, and decreased function of the kidney may occu

nephrogenic /nef′rōjen′ik/, **1.** generating kidney ti sue. **2.** originating in the kidney.

nephrogenic ascites, the abnormal presence of fluid the peritoneal cavity of patients undergoing hemodialys for renal failure. The cause of this type of ascites unknown. See also **ascites.**

nephrogenic cord, either of the paired longitudin ridges of tissue that lie along the dorsal surface of th coelom in the early developing vertebrate embryo. It formed from the fusion of the nephrotome tissue an gives rise to the structures comprising the embryonic ur genital system. See also **mesonephros, metanephro pronephros.**

nephrogenic diabetes insipidus, an abnormal cond tion in which the kidneys do not concentrate the urin resulting in polyuria, polydipsia, and very dilute urin The secretion of antidiuretic hormone (ADH) by the pit itary is normal, and all kidney function is normal exce that there is no response to ADH. See also **diabet insipidus.**

nephrogenous /nəfroj′ənəs/, of or pertaining to the fo mation and development of the kidneys.

nephrolith, a calculus formed in a kidney. **–nephr lithic,** *adj.*

nephrolithiasis /nef′rōlithī′əsis/, a disorder characte ized by the presence of calculi in the kidney. See als **renal calculus.**

nephrology, the study of the anatomy, physiology, an pathology of the kidney. **–nephrologic, nephrolog cal,** *adj.*

nephrolytic, of or pertaining to the destruction of th structure and function of a kidney.

-nephroma, a combining form meaning a 'tumor of th kidney or area of the kidney': *epinephroma, para nephroma.*

nephromere. See **nephrotome.**

nephron /nef′ron/, a structural and functional unit o the kidney, resembling a microscopic funnel with a lon stem and two convoluted sections. Each kidney contain about 1.25 million nephrons, each consisting of the renal corpuscle, the loop of Henle, and the renal tubules. Each renal corpuscle consists of the glomerulus of renal capillaries enclosed within Bowman's capsule. The renal corpuscles and the convoluted portions of the renal tubules are located in the cortex of the kidney. The renal medulla contains the loops of Henle and the collecting tubules. Urine is formed in the renal corpuscles and in the renal tubules by filtration, reabsorption, and secretion. Also called **nephrone** /nef′rōn/. See also **kidney, renal corpuscle.**

nephronophthisis. See **medullary cystic disease.**

nephropathy /nefrop′əthē/, any disorder of the kidney, including inflammatory, degenerative, and sclerotic conditions. See also **kidney disease.**

nephropexy /nef′rəpek′sē/, a surgical operation to fixate a floating or ptotic kidney.

nephroptosis /nef′rəptō′sis/, a downward displacement or dropping of a kidney.

nephrorrhaphy /nəfrôr′əfē/, an operation that sutures a floating kidney in place.

nephrosclerosis. See **nephroangiosclerosis.**

nephroscope, a fiberoptic instrument that is used specifically for the disintegration and removal of renal calculi. The nephroscope is inserted percutaneously, and the calculi are located through use of x-ray films of the renal pelvis. An ultrasonic probe emitting high-frequency sound waves breaks up the calculi, which are removed by suction through the scope.

nephrosis. See **nephrotic syndrome.**

nephrostoma, *pl.* **nephrostomas, nephrostomata,** the funnel-shaped ciliated opening of the excretory tubules into the coelom of the early developing vertebrate embryo. Also called **nephrostome.** **–nephrostomic,** *adj.*

nephrostomy, a surgical procedure in which an incision is made on the flank of the patient so that a catheter can be inserted into the kidney pelvis for the purpose of drainage.

nephrotic syndrome, an abnormal condition of the kidney characterized by marked proteinuria, hypoalbuminemia, and edema. It occurs in glomerular disease, thrombosis of a renal vein, and as a complication of many systemic diseases, diabetes mellitus, amyloidosis, systemic lupus erythematosus, and multiple myeloma. The nephrotic syndrome occurs in a severe, primary form. The presenting symptoms include anorexia, weakness, proteinuria, hypoalbuminuria, and edema. Treatment and prognosis depend on the underlying cause of disease. Patients with primary nephrotic syndrome usually respond favorably to corticosteroids. Loop diuretics are used to control symptomatic edema, and dialysis may be necessary. Also called **nephrosis.**

nephrotome, a zone of segmented mesodermal tissue in the developing vertebrate embryo lying along each side of the body dorsal to the abdominal cavity between the somite-forming dorsal mesoderm and the unsegmented lateral plate mesoderm. It is the primordial tissue for the urogenital system and gives rise to the nephrogenic cord. Also called **intermediate cell mass, intermediate mesoderm, middle plate, nephromere.** See also **mesonephros, metanephros, pronephros.**

nephrotomography, sectional radiographic examination of the kidneys.

nephrotomy, a surgical procedure in which an incision is made in the kidney.

nephrotoxic, toxic or destructive to a kidney.

nephrotoxin, a toxin with specific destructive properties for the kidneys.

Neptazane, a trademark for a carbonic anhydrase inhibitor (methazolamide).

neptunium (Np), a transuranic, metallic element. Its atomic number is 93; its atomic weight is 237. Although neptunium is considered a synthetic element, traces of natural neptunium have been found in uranium ores.

Nernst equation, (in cardiology) an expression of the relationship between the electric potential across a membrane and the concentration ratio between permeable ions on either side of the membrane.

nerve, one or more bundles of impulse-carrying fibers that connect the brain and the spinal cord with other parts of the body. Nerves transmit afferent impulses from receptor organs toward the brain and the spinal cord and efferent impulses peripherally to the effector organs. Each nerve consists of an epineurium enclosing fasciculi of nerve fibers, each fasciculus surrounded by its own sheath of connective tissue. Individual nerve fibers, which are microscopic, consist of formed elements within a matrix of protoplasm and are wrapped in a neurilemmal sheath. Inside the neurilemma are nerve fibers, also enclosed in a myelin sheath, derived from the neurilemmal cells. See also **axon, dendrite, neuroglia, neuron.**

nerve accommodation, the ability of nerve tissue to adjust to a constant source and intensity of stimulation so that some change in either intensity or duration of the stimulus is necessary to elicit a response beyond the initial reaction. Accommodation is probably caused by reduced sodium ion permeability, which results in an increased threshold intensity and subsequent stabilization of the resting membrane potential.

nerve block anesthesia. See **conduction anesthesia.**

nerve compression, a pathologic event that causes harmful pressure on one or more nerve trunks, resulting in nerve damage and muscle weakness or atrophy. Any nerve that passes over a rigid prominence is vulnerable, and the degree of damage depends on the magnitude and the duration of the compressive force. Various factors may contribute to susceptibility, as inherited predisposition, malnutrition, trauma, and disease. Various activities associated with routine occupations may unduly compress especially vulnerable nerves, as the median nerve, the radial nerve, the femoral nerve, and the plantar nerves. Rest and the cessation or modification of causative activities often heal nerve damage caused by compression. Surgery may be required to correct more severe cases. Compare **nerve entrapment.**

nerve entrapment, an abnormal condition and type of mononeuropathy, characterized by nerve damage and muscle weakness or atrophy. The peripheral nerve trunks of the body are especially vulnerable to entrapment in which repeated compression results in significant impairment. Nerves that pass over rigid prominences or through narrow bony and fascial canals are particularly prone to entrapment. The common signs of this disorder are pain and muscular weakness. Nerve damage by entrapment occurs more often when adjacent joints are affected by swelling and inflammation, as in rheumatoid arthritis, pregnancy, and acromegaly. Signs of nerve entrapment may also develop after repeated bruising of certain nerves by various activities involving repeated motions, as those associated with knitting and prolonged walking. One of the most common types of entrapment is **carpal tunnel syndrome.** Compare **nerve compression.**

nerve fiber, a slender process of a neuron, usually the axon. Each fiber is classified as myelinated or unmyelinated. Myelinated fibers are further designated as A or B fibers; C fibers are unmyelinated. The A fibers are somatic, 1 to 20 μm in diameter, and have a conduction velocity of 5 to 120 meters per second. The A alpha fibers are large fibers and transport impulses at a velocity of 60 to 100 meters per second; beta fibers are smaller and transmit pressure and temperature impulses at a velocity of 30 to 70 meters per second; gamma fibers transmit touch and pressure impulses at velocities of 15 to 40 meters per second; and delta fibers are the smallest and transmit impulses associated with sharp pain sensation. B fibers are more finely myelinated than A fibers and have a diameter up to 3 μm and a conduction rate of 3 to 15 meters per second. They are both afferent and efferent and are mainly associated with visceral innervation. The unmyelinated C fibers have a diameter of 0.3 to 1.3 μm and a conduction rate of 0.6 to 2 meters per second. They are efferent postganglionic autonomic fibers and afferent fibers that conduct impulses of prolonged, burning pain sensation from the viscera and periphery.

nerve growth factor (NGF), a protein resembling insulin whose hormonelike action affects differentiation, growth, and maintenance of neurons.

nerve impulse. See **impulse.**

nervous breakdown, *informal.* any mental condition that markedly interferes with and disrupts normal functioning.

nervous system, the extensive, intricate network of structures that activates, coordinates, and controls all the functions of the body. It is divided into the central nervous system, composed of the brain and the spinal cord, and the peripheral nervous system, which includes the cranial nerves and the spinal nerves. These morphologic subdivisions combine and communicate to innervate the somatic and the visceral parts of the body with the afferent and the efferent nerve fibers. Afferent fibers carry sensory impulses to the central nervous system; efferent fibers carry motor impulses from the central nervous system to the muscles and other organs. The somatic fibers are associated with the bones, the muscles, and the skin. The visceral fibers are associated with the internal organs, the blood vessels, and the mucous membranes. Various functions throughout the nervous system are coordinated through a vast complex of tiny structures, as neurons, axons, dendrites, and ganglia. Compare **parasympathetic nervous system, sympathetic nervous system, visceral nervous system.** See also the Color Atlas of Human Anatomy.

nervus abducens. See **abducent nerve.**

nervus accessorius. See **accessory nerve.**

nervus facialis. See **facial nerve.**

nervus glossopharyngeus. See **glossopharyngeal nerve.**

nervus hypoglossus. See **hypoglossal nerve.**

nervus oculomotorius. See **oculomotor nerve.**

nervus olfactorius. See **olfactory nerve.**

nervus opticus. See **optic nerve.**

nervus terminalis. See **terminal nerve.**

nervus trigeminus. See **trigeminal nerve.**

nervus trochlearis. See **trochlear nerve.**

nervus vagus. See **vagus nerve.**

Nesacaine, a trademark for a long-acting local anesthetic (chloroprocaine), used in regional anesthetic block.

Netromycin, a trademark for an antibiotic (netilmicin).

nettle rash, a fine, urticarial eruption resulting from skin contact with stinging nettle, a common weed with leaves containing histamine. It is characterized by stinging and itching that lasts from a few minutes to several hours.

network, a system of interconnected computer terminals and peripheral equipment in which each user has some access to others using the system while sharing data, memories, and other capabilities.

networking, **1.** (in psychiatric nursing) the process of developing a set of agencies and professional personnel that are able to create a system of communication and support for psychiatric patients, usually those newly discharged from inpatient psychiatric facilities. Kinds of networks include **natural network** and **professional network.** **2.** a network of supportive contacts or services, as the Women's Health Network.

Neufeld nail /noi′felt/, an orthopedic nail with a V-shaped tip and shank used for fixating an intertrochanteric fracture. The nail is driven into the neck of the femur until it reaches a round metal plate screwed onto the side of the femur. The nail is secured to a receptacle on the plate. Also called **Neufeld angled nail.**

neur-. See **neuro-.**

neural /no͝or′əl/, of or pertaining to nerve cells and their processes.

-neural, -neuric, a combining form meaning 'of or relating to a nerve or nerves': *epineural, epithelioneural, myoneural.*

neural canal. See **neurocoele.**

neural crest, the band of ectodermally derived cells that lies along the outer surface of each side of the neural tube in the early stages of embryonic development. The cells migrate laterally throughout the embryo and give rise to certain spinal, cranial, and sympathetic ganglia. Also called **ganglionic crest, ganglionic ridge.** See also **neural tube formation.**

neural ectoderm, the part of the embryonic ectoderm that develops into the neural tube. Also called **neuroderm.** See also **neural tube formation.**

neural fold, either of the paired longitudinal elevations resulting from the invagination of the neural plate in the early developing embryo. The folds unite to enclose the neural groove and form the neural tube. Also called **medullary fold.** See also **neural tube formation.**

neuralgia /nŏŏral′jə/, an abnormal condition characterized by severe stabbing pain, caused by a variety of disorders affecting the nervous system. –**neuralgic,** *adj.*

neural groove, the longitudinal depression that occurs between the neural folds during the invagination of the neural plate to form the neural tube in the early stages of embryonic development. Also called **medullary groove.** See also **neural tube formation.**

neural impulse. See **impulse.**

neural plate, a thick layer of ectodermal tissue that lies along the central longitudinal axis of the early developing embryo and gives rise to the neural tube and subsequently to the brain, spinal cord, and other tissues of the central nervous system. Also called **medullary plate.** See also **neural tube formation.**

neural tube, the longitudinal tube, lying along the central axis of the early developing embryo, that gives rise to the brain, spinal cord, and other neural tissue of the central nervous system. It consists of thick ectodermal tissue and is formed by the fusion of the neural folds, resulting from the invagination of the neural plate. Failure of the tube to close results in a number of congenital defects. Also called **cerebromedullary tube, medullary tube.** See also **neural tube defect, neural tube formation.**

neural tube defect, any of a group of congenital malformations involving defects in the skull and spinal column that are caused primarily by the failure of the neural tube to close during embryonic development. In some instances, the cleft results from an abnormal increase in cerebrospinal fluid pressure on the closed neural tube during the first trimester of development. The defect may occur at any point along the neural axis or extend the entire length of the spinal column, as in holorachischisis. The amount of deformity and disability depends on the degree of neural involvement, the most severe defect being complete cranioschisis, or the total absence of the skull and defective brain development. Other cerebral dysplasias resulting from the failure of the cranial end of the neural tube to fuse are meningoencephalocele and cranial meningocele. These defects, usually accompanied by severe mental and physical disorders, occur most often in the occipital region of the skull but may also occur in the frontal or basal regions. Most neural tube malformations are caused by incomplete fusion of one or more laminae of the vertebral column, with varying degrees of tissue protrusion and neural involvement. Such anomalies include rachischisis, spina bifida, myelocele, myelomeningocele, and meningocele. In all of these conditions there is constant risk of rupture of the saclike protrusion and danger of meningeal infection. Often, immediate surgical repair is necessary. Many of the major neural tube defects can be determined prenatally by ultrasonic scanning of the uterus and by the presence of elevated concentrations of alpha fetoprotein levels in the amniotic fluid. Such diagnostic tests are preferably performed during the fourteenth to sixteenth week of gestation so that termination of the pregnancy is possible. See also **anencephaly, Arnold-Chiari malformation, spina bifida cystica.**

neural tube formation, the various processes and stages involved in the embryonic development of the neural tube, which subsequently differentiates into the brain, the spinal cord, and other neural tissue of the central nervous system. The primitive tube originates from a flat, single layer of ectodermal tissue that extends longitudinally along the middorsal line of the embryonic disk from the area of the primitive streak forward to the cephalic extremity. This tissue, called the neural plate, grows rapidly and becomes striated and thickened. The rate of growth is greater along the midplane than at the margin, resulting in the invagination of the cells and formation of a hollow groove, the neural groove, bounded on either side by the elevated neural folds. With continued cell division the groove becomes deeper and the folds thicken so that they eventually meet and fuse, converting the neural groove into the neural tube. The closing of the neural tube occurs first at the midpoint and progresses both toward the caudal and the cephalic regions. At the cephalic end the tube expands into a large vesicle with three subdivisions that differentiate into the forebrain (prosencephalon), the midbrain (mesencephalon), and the hindbrain (rhombencephalon). The epithelium of the wall of the tube develops into the various tissues of the nervous system. The caudal portion of the tube subsequently forms the spinal cord. Along the outer surface of the neural tube is a thin layer of ectodermal cells that extend the entire length of the structure. These primordial cells migrate to other parts of the developing embryo and give rise to cranial and spinal ganglia and to certain cells of the autonomic nervous system. Failure of any part of the neural tube to close during early embryonic development results in a number of congenital defects. See also **neural tube defect.**

neurasthenia /nŏŏr′əsthē′nē·ə/, **1.** an abnormal condition characterized by nervous exhaustion and a vague functional fatigue that often follows depression. **2.** (in psychiatry) a stage in the recovery from a schizophrenic experience, during which the patient is listless and apparently unable to cope with routine activities and relationships. –**neurasthenic,** *adj.*

-neure, -neuron, a combining form meaning a 'nerve cell': *ganglioneure, myoneure, sporadoneure.*

neurenteric canal /nŏŏr'ənter'ik/, a tubular passage between the posterior part of the neural tube and the archenteron in the early embryonic development of lower animals. It corresponds to the notochordal canal of humans and the higher animals. Also called **archenteric canal, blastoporic canal, Braun's canal.**

-neuria, a combining form meaning a '(specified) condition involving nerves': *acystineuria, ovariodysneuria.*

neurilemma /nŏŏr'əlem'ə/, a layer of cells composed of one or more Schwann cells that encloses the segmented myelin sheaths of peripheral nerve fibers. Each myelinated nerve fiber has a neurilemma cell for each internodal segment between the nodes of Ranvier. The cell nucleus is a flattened oval that lies in a small depression in the myelin. The nerve fibers of the brain and the spinal cord are not enclosed by neurilemma. Also spelled **neurolemma.** Also called **sheath of Schwann.** –**neurilemmal, neurilemmatic, neurilemmatous,** *adj.*

neurilemoma. See **schwannoma.**

neurinoma /nŏŏr'inō'mə/, *pl.* **neurinomas, neurinomata,** **1.** a tumor of the nerve sheath. It is usually benign but may undergo malignant change. A kind of neurinoma is **acoustic neurinoma.** See also **schwannoma. 2.** a neuroma.

neuritis /nŏŏrī'tis/, *pl.* **neuritides,** an abnormal condition characterized by inflammation of a nerve. Some of the signs of this condition are neuralgia, hyperthesia, anesthesia, paralysis, muscular atrophy, and defective reflexes.

neuro-, neur-, a combining form meaning 'of or pertaining to nerves': *neuroclonic, neurohormone, neuromast.*

neuroarthropathy, a condition in which a disease of a joint is secondary to a disease of the nervous system.

neuroblast, any embryonic cell that develops into a functional neuron; an immature nerve cell. –**neuroblastic,** *adj.*

neuroblastoma /nŏŏr'ōblastō'mə/, *pl.* **neuroblastomas, neuroblastomata,** a highly malignant tumor composed of primitive ectodermal cells derived from the neural plate during embryonic life. The tumor may originate in any part of the sympathetic nervous system, but it is most common in the adrenal medulla of young children. Neuroblastomas metastasize early and widely to lymph nodes, liver, lung, and bone. Symptoms may include an abdominal mass, respiratory distress, and anemia, depending on the site of the primary tumor and metastases, and hormonally active adrenal lesions may cause irritability, flushing, sweating, hypertension, and tachycardia. Before metastasis, treatment with radical surgery, deep irradiation, and chemotherapy are often successful. Spontaneous remissions may occur with the tumor undergoing maturation and forming a benign ganglioneuroma. A kind of neuroblastoma is **Pepper's syndrome.**

neurocele. See **neurocoele.**

neurocentral, pertaining to the centrum and the developing vertebrae in the early stages of embryology.

neurocentrum, the embryonic mesodermal tissue that subsequently gives rise to the vertebrae. See also **sclerotome.**

neuro check, *nontechnical.* a brief neurologic assessment, usually performed in the triage of patients in an emergency situation or on admission to an emergency service. The level of consciousness is evaluated as alert and oriented, lethargic, stuporous, or comatose. The movements of the extremities are determined to be voluntary or involuntary. The color, temperature, and turgor of the skin are noted. The pupils of the eyes are observed for equality of dilatation, reactivity to light, and ability to accommodate. See also **neurologic assessment.**

neurocirculatory asthenia, a psychosomatic disorder characterized by nervous and circulatory irregularities, including dyspnea, palpitation, giddiness, vertigo, tremor, precordial pain, and increased susceptibility to fatigue. The symptoms often result from or are associated with psychologic stress.

neurocoele /nŏŏr'əsēl/, a system of cavities in the central nervous system of humans and other vertebrate animals. It consists of the ventricles of the brain and the central canal of the spinal cord, which originate from the neural tube during early embryonic development. Also spelled **neurocele, neurocoel.** Also called **neural canal.**

neurocytoma /nŏŏr'ōsītō'mə/, a tumor composed of undifferentiated nerve cells that are usually ganglionic. Also called **neuroma.**

neuroderm. See **neuroectoderm.**

neurodermatitis, a nonspecific, pruritic skin disorder seen in anxious, nervous individuals. Excoriations and lichenification are found on easily accessible, exposed areas of the body such as the forearms and forehead. Sometimes loosely (and incorrectly) applied to **atopic dermatitis.**

neuroectoderm, the part of the embryonic ectoderm that gives rise to the central and peripheral nervous systems, including some glial cells. –**neuroectodermal,** *adj.*

neuroepithelioma /nŏŏr'ō•ep'ithē'lē•ō'mə/, an uncommon neoplasm of neuroepithelium in a sensory nerve. Also called **neuroepithelial tumor.**

neurofibroma /nŏŏr'ōfībrō'mə/, *pl.* **neurofibromas, neurofibromata,** a fibrous tumor of nerve tissue resulting from the abnormal proliferation of Schwann cells. Multiple growths of this type in the peripheral nervous system are often associated with extensive abnormalities in other tissues. See also **neurofibromatosis.**

neurofibromatosis /nŏŏr'ōfī'brōmətō'sis/, a congenital condition transmitted as an autosomal dominant trait, characterized by numerous neurofibromas of the nerves and skin, by café-au-lait spots on the skin, and, in some cases, by developmental anomalies of the muscles, bones, and viscera. Many large, pedunculated soft-tissue tumors may develop, as exemplified by the famous case of the ''Elephant Man'' in nineteenth-century England. Bone changes may result in skeletal deformities, especially curvature of the spine. Neurofibromas may develop in the alimentary tract, bladder, endocrine glands, and cranial nerves. The disorder occurs in 1 of 2500 to 3000 live births; sometimes it is associated with meningocele, spina bifida, or epilepsy. Also called **multiple neuroma, neuromatosis, von Recklinghausen's disease.**

neurogen /nŏŏr′əjən/, a substance within the early developing embryo that stimulates the primary organizer to initiate the formation of the neural plate, which gives rise to the primary axis of the body. See also **neurotransmitter.**

neurogenesis, the development of the tissue of the nervous system. **–neurogenetic,** *adj.*

neurogenic, **1.** pertaining to the formation of nervous tissue. **2.** the stimulation of nervous energy. **3.** originating in the nervous system.

neurogenic arthropathy, an abnormal condition associated with neural damage, characterized by the gradual and usually painless degeneration of a joint. One of the major causes of this condition is believed to be a minor injury that is disregarded by the affected individual because of a lack of sensation in the injured tissue. Inadequate rest and care aggravate such injuries and prevent proper healing. See also **Charcot's joint.**

neurogenic bladder, dysfunctional urinary bladder caused by lesion of the nervous system. Treatment is aimed at enabling the bladder to empty completely and regularly, preventing infection, controlling incontinence, and preserving kidney function. Kinds of neurogenic bladder are **spastic bladder, reflex bladder,** and **flaccid bladder.** Also called **neuropathic bladder.**

neurogenic fracture, a fracture associated with the destruction of the nerve supply to a specific bone.

neurogenic shock, a form of shock that results from peripheral vascular dilatation as a result of neurologic injury.

neuroglia /nŏŏrog′lē·ə/, the supporting or connective tissue cells of the central nervous system. They perform the less specialized functions of the nerve network. Kinds of neuroglia include **astrocytes, oligodendroglia,** and **microglia.** Compare **neuron. –neuroglial,** *adj.*

neurohormonal regulation, regulation of the function of an organ or a gland by the combined effect of neurologic and hormonal activity.

neurohumor, one of the chemical substances, formed and transmitted by a neuron, that is essential for the activity of adjacent neurons or nearby organs or muscles. Kinds of neurohumoral substances are **acetylcholine, dopamine, epinephrine, norepinephrine,** and **serotonin. –neurohumoral,** *adj.*

neurohypophyseal hormone, a hormone secreted by the posterior pituitary gland. Kinds of neurohypophyseal hormones are **oxytocin** and **vasopressin.** See also **pituitary gland.**

neurohypophysis, the posterior lobe of the pituitary gland that is the source of antidiuretic hormone (ADH) and oxytocin. Nervous stimulation controls the release of both substances into the blood. The neurohypophysis releases ADH when stimulated by the hypothalamus by an increase in the osmotic pressure of extracellular fluid in the body. The hormone acts on the cells in the distal and the collecting tubules of the kidneys, making them more permeable to water and reducing the volume of urine. The neurohypophysis releases oxytocin under appropriate stimulation from the hypothalamus. Oxytocin produces powerful contractions of the pregnant uterus and causes milk to flow from lactating breasts. Stimulation of the nipples of the breast by a nursing infant triggers the release of this hormone. Also called **posterior pituitary gland.** Compare **adenohypophysis.**

neuroimmunology, the study of relationships between the immune and nervous systems, as autoimmune activity in neurologic diseases.

neurolemma. See **neurilemma.**

neurolepsis, an altered state of consciousness, as induced by a neuroleptic agent, characterized by quiescence, reduced motor activity, anxiety, and indifference to the surroundings. Sleep may occur, but usually the person can be aroused and can respond to commands. Drugs that produce neurolepsis may be administered with a narcotic analgesic to produce neuroleptanalgesia, or with an anesthetic to produce neuroleptanesthesia.

neurolept. See **neuroleptic.**

neuroleptanalgesia, a form of analgesia achieved by the concurrent administration of a neuroleptic and an analgesic. Anxiety, motor activity, and sensitivity to painful stimuli are reduced; the person is quiet and indifferent to the environment and surroundings. Sleep may or may not occur, but the patient is not unconscious and is able to respond to commands. If nitrous oxide in oxygen is also administered, neuroleptanalgesia can be converted to neuroleptanesthesia. Droperidol and fentanyl are often administered together to achieve neuroleptanesthesia.

neuroleptanesthesia, a form of anesthesia achieved by the administration of a neuroleptic agent, a narcotic analgesic, and nitrous oxide in oxygen. Induction of anesthesia is slow, but consciousness returns quickly after the inhalation of nitrous oxide is stopped.

neuroleptic, **1.** of or pertaining to neurolepsis. **2.** also called **neurolept.** a drug that causes neurolepsis, as the butyrophenone derivative, droperidol. See also **antipsychotic.**

neurologic assessment, an evaluation of the patient's neurologic status and symptoms.

■ METHOD: If alert and oriented, the patient is asked about instances of weakness, numbness, headaches, pain, tremors, nervousness, irritability, or drowsiness. Information is elicited regarding loss of memory, periods of confusion, hallucinations, and episodes of loss of consciousness. The patient's general appearance, facial expression, attention span, responses to verbal and painful stimuli, emotional status, coordination, balance, cognition, and ability to follow commands are noted. If the patient is disoriented, stuporous, or comatose, demonstrated signs of these states are recorded. Observations are made of the skin color and temperature; pupillary size, equality, dilatation, and reactions to light; the respiratory rate, rhythm, and quality; and chest movements and breath sounds. The pulse is checked; the ears and nose are examined for possible drainage; the strength of the handgrip is tested; and the extremities' sensations and voluntary and involuntary motions are assessed. The urinary output is determined for evidence of polyuria, and the patient's speech is evaluated for signs of slurring and aphasia. Included in the record are concurrent diseases, as hypertension, cancer, and coarctation of the aorta; past illnesses associated with head trauma; seizures, motor, sensory, or emotional disturbances; loss of consciousness; and neurologic, medical, or surgical procedures. Pertinent to the assessment are the patient's sleep pattern, medication, personality changes, relationships with family and friends, and a family history of seizures, stroke, mental illness, tumors, or sudden death. Diagnostic aids that may be required for a complete evaluation are a lumbar puncture, complete blood count, myelogram, echoencephalogram, brain scan, computerized tomogram, and determinations of glucose, fluid, and electrolyte levels.

■ NURSING ORDERS: The nurse may conduct the interview to obtain subjective data, examines the patient, and assembles the pertinent background information and the results of the diagnostic tests.

■ OUTCOME CRITERIA: A careful neurologic assessment is an important aid to the neurologist in establishing a diagnosis and the course of treatment.

neurologic examination, a systematic examination of the nervous system, including an assessment of mental status, of the function of each of the cranial nerves, of sensory and neuromuscular function, of the reflexes, and of proprioception and other cerebellar functions.

neurologist /no͝orol′əjist/, a physician who specializes in neurology.

neurology /no͝orol′əjē/, the field of medicine that deals with the nervous system and its disorders. –**neurologic, neurological,** *adj.* **neurologist,** *n.*

neuroma /no͝orō′mə/, *pl.* **neuromas, neuromata,** a benign neoplasm composed chiefly of neurons and nerve fibers, usually arising from a nerve tissue. It may be relatively soft or extremely hard and vary in size from 1 to 15 cm or more. Pain radiating from the lesion to the periphery of the affected nerve is usually intermittent but may become continuous and severe. Kinds of neuromas include **acoustic neuroma, cystic neuroma, false neuroma, multiple neuroma, myelinic neuroma, neuroma cutis, nevoid neuroma,** and **traumatic neuroma.**

-neuroma, a combining form meaning a 'tumor made up of nerve cells and fibers': *angiomyoneuroma, inoneuroma, myoneuroma.*

neuroma cutis, a neoplasm in the skin that contains nerve tissue and that may be extremely sensitive to painful stimuli.

neuroma telangiectodes. See **nevoid neuroma.**

neuromatosis /no͝or′ōmətō′sis/, a neoplastic disease characterized by numerous neuromas. Also called **multiple neuroma.** See also **neurofibromatosis.**

neuromuscular /no͝or′ōmus′kyo͝olər/, of or pertaining to the nerves and the muscles.

neuromuscular blocking agent, a chemical substance that interferes locally with the transmission or reception of impulses from motor nerves to skeletal muscles. Nondepolarizing agents, as metocurine, pancuronium, and tubocurarine, competitively block the transmitter action of acetylcholine at the postjunctional membrane. Depolarizing blocking agents, as succinylcholine chloride, compete with acetylcholine for cholinergic receptors of the motor end plate. Neuromuscular blocking agents are used to induce muscle relaxation in anesthesia, endotracheal intubation, and electroshock therapy and as adjuncts in the treatment of tetanus, encephalitis, and poliomyelitis. Neuromuscular blocking drugs can cause bronchospasm, hyperthermia, hypotension, or respiratory paralysis and are used with caution, especially in patients with myasthenia gravis or with renal, hepatic, or pulmonary impairment, and in elderly and debilitated individuals. See also **muscle relaxant.**

neuromuscular junction, the area of contact between the ends of a large myelinated nerve fiber and a fiber of skeletal muscle. Also called **myoneural junction.** See also **motor end plate, myelin, nerve.**

neuromuscular spindle, any one of a number of small bundles of delicate muscular fibers, enclosed by a capsule, in which sensory nerve fibers terminate. The spindles vary in length from 0.8 to 5 mm, accommodating as many as four large myelinated nerve fibers that pierce the capsule and lose their myelin sheaths. The nerve fibers end as naked axons encircling the intrafusal fibers with flattened expansions or ovoid disks.

neuromyal transmission, the passage of excitation from a motor neuron to a muscle fiber at the myoneural junction.

neuromyelitis /no͝or′ōmī′əlī′tis/, an abnormal condition characterized by inflammation of the spinal cord and peripheral nerves.

neuron /no͝or′on/, the basic nerve cell of the nervous system, containing a nucleus within a cell body and extending one or more processes. Neurons are classified according to the direction in which they conduct impulses and according to the number of processes they extend. Sensory neurons transmit nerve impulses toward the spinal cord and the brain. Motor neurons transmit nerve impulses from the brain and the spinal cord to the muscles and the glandular tissue. Multipolar neurons, the bipolar neurons, and the unipolar neurons are classified according to the number of processes they extend to the different kinds of neurons. Multipolar neurons have one axon and several dendrites, as do most of the neurons in the brain and the spinal cord. Bipolar neurons, which are less numerous than the other types, have only one axon and one dendrite. Unipolar neurons are embryonic structures that originate as bipolar bodies but fuse dendrites and axons into a single fiber that stretches for a short distance from the cell body before separating again into the two processes. All neurons have at least one axon and one or more dendrites and have a slightly gray color when clustered, as in the brain and the spinal cord. As the carriers of nerve impulses, neurons function according to electrochemical processes involving positively charged sodium and potassium ions and the changing electric potential of the extracellular and the intracellular fluid of the neuron. Also spelled **neurone.**

-neuron. See **-neure.**

neuronitis /nŏŏr′ənī′tis/, an abnormal condition characterized by inflammation of a nerve or a nerve cell, especially the cells and the roots of the spinal nerves.

neuropathic bladder. See **neurogenic bladder.**

neuropathic joint disease, a chronic, progressive, degenerative disease of one or more joints, characterized by swelling, instability of the joint, hemorrhage, heat, and atrophic and hypertrophic changes in the bone. Pain is usually less severe than would be expected by the appearance of the joint on an x-ray film. The disease is the result of an underlying neurologic disorder, as tabes dorsalis from syphilis, diabetic neuropathy, leprosy, or congenital absence or depression of pain sensation. Early recognition of the disease and prophylactic protection of the joint may prevent further damage in some cases. Surgical reconstruction is not usually effective because healing is slow. Amputation may be necessary. Also called **Charcot's joint.**

neuropathy /nŏŏrop′əthē/, any abnormal condition characterized by inflammation and degeneration of the peripheral nerves, as that associated with lead poisoning. **–neuropathic,** *adj.*

neuroplegia /nŏŏr′ōplē′jē·ə/, nerve paralysis caused by disease, injury, or the effect of neuroleptic drugs, administered to achieve **neuroleptanalgesia** or **neuroleptanesthesia.** See also **lytic cocktail.**

neuropore /nŏŏr′opôr/, the opening at each end of the neural tube during early embryonic development. The closure of these apertures as the tube grows and differentiates occurs with such precision that they are used to indicate horizons XI and XII in the systematic anatomic charting of human embryonic development. Kinds of neuropores are **anterior neuropore** and **posterior neuropore.** See also **horizon, neural tube formation.**

neurosarcoma, a malignant neoplasm composed of nerve tissue, connective tissue, and vascular tissue. Also called **malignant neuroma.**

neurosis, **1.** any faulty or inefficient way of coping with anxiety or inner conflict, usually involving the use of an unconscious defense mechanism, that may ultimately lead to a neurotic disorder. **2.** *informal.* an emotional disturbance other than psychosis. See also **neurotic disorder, neurotic process.**

-neurosis, a combining form meaning a 'disease of the nerves' or a 'mental disorder': *angioneurosis, psychoneurosis, synneurosis.*

neurosurgery, any surgery involving the brain, spinal cord, or peripheral nerves. Brain surgery is performed to treat a wound, remove a tumor or foreign body, relieve pressure in intracranial hemorrhage, excise an abcess, treat parkinsonism, or relieve pain. Before surgery skull x-ray films and a ventriculogram or an arteriogram may be taken; a diagnostic electroencephalogram, lumbar tap, or brain scan may be necessary. A blood type and crossmatch is done. Parenteral corticosteroids are given if cerebral edema is present, and urea may be given to reduce intracranial pressure. Narcotics and hypnotics are avoided, and the nurse must confirm any that are ordered. No enemas are given. Light general or local anesthesia is used, occasionally with hypothermia. After surgery, the nurse observes carefully both vital signs and changes in the level of consciousness, speech, and strength. Any yellowish drainage from the wound may be cerebrospinal fluid and is reported immediately. Sterile dressing technique is essential. Kinds of brain surgery include craniotomy, lobotomy, hypophysectomy. Surgery of the spine is performed to correct a defect, remove a tumor, repair a ruptured intervertebral disk, or relieve pain. Before surgery x-ray films are taken and a blood type and crossmatch is done. General anesthesia or a spinal block is used. After surgery, the nurse keeps the bed flat and the patient's spine in good alignment. Return of sensation and motor function are monitored carefully. Kinds of spinal surgery include fusion and laminectomy. Surgery on the peripheral nerves is performed to remove a tumor, relieve pain, or reconnect a severed nerve. Local anesthesia is used. After surgery, the nurse observes closely the return of sensation to the area. One kind of nerve surgery is **sympathectomy.**

neurosyphilis, infection of the central nervous system by syphilis organisms, which may invade the meninges and cerebrovascular system. If the brain tissue is affected, general paresis may result; if the spinal cord is infected, tabes dorsalis may result. See also **syphilis,** ***Treponema pallidum.*** **–neurosyphilitic,** *adj.*

neurotendinous spindle, a capsule containing enlarged tendon fibers, found chiefly near the junctions of tendons and muscles. One or more nerve fibers pierce the side of the capsule and lose their medullary sheaths; the axons subdivide and terminate between the tendon fibers in irregular disks or varicosities. Also called **organ of Golgi.**

neurotic, **1.** of or pertaining to neurosis or to a neurotic disorder. **2.** pertaining to the nerves. **3.** one who is afflicted with a neurosis. **4.** *informal.* an emotionally unstable person.

-neurotic, **1.** a combining form meaning 'pertaining to a (specified) abnormal condition of the nerves': *angioneurotic, aponeurotic, vasoneurotic.* **2.** a combining form meaning 'pertaining to (psycho)neurosis': *hyperneurotic, psychoneurotic, unneurotic.*

neurotic disorder, any mental disorder characterized by a symptom or group of symptoms that a person finds distressing, unacceptable, and alien to the personality, as severe anxiety, obsessional thoughts, and compulsive acts, and that produces psychologic pain or discomfort disproportionate to the reality of the situation. Although the person's ability to function may be markedly impaired, the behavior generally remains within acceptable social norms and the perception of reality is unaffected. There is no proof of organic cause. The disturbance is relatively long-lasting, cannot be considered simply a reaction to stress, and may recur if untreated. Kinds of neurotic disorders include **anxiety neurosis, obsessive-compulsive neurosis, psychosexual disorder,** and **somatoform disorder.** See also **neurosis, neurotic process.**

neurotic illness. See **neurotic disorder.**

neurotic process, (in psychology) a process in which unconscious conflicts lead to feelings of anxiety. Defense mechanisms are employed to avoid these uncomfortable feelings, and personality disturbance and the symptoms of neurosis ensue.

neurotoxic /no͝or′ōtok′sik/, having a poisonous effect on nerves and nerve cells, as when ingested lead degenerates peripheral nerves.

neurotoxin /no͝or′ōtok′sin/, a toxin that acts directly on the tissues of the central nervous system, traveling along the axis cylinders of the motor nerves to the brain. The toxin may be secreted in the venom of certain snakes, or it may be present on the spines of a shell or in the flesh of fish or shellfish; it may be produced by certain bacteria or by the cellular disintegration of certain bacteria.

neurotransmitter, any one of numerous chemicals that modify or result in the transmission of nerve impulses between synapses. Neurotransmitters are released from synaptic knobs into synaptic clefts and bridge the gap between presynaptic and postsynaptic neurons. Each vesicle within a synaptic knob stores as many as 10,000 neurotransmitter molecules. When a nerve impulse reaches a synaptic knob, thousands of neurotransmitter molecules squirt into the synaptic cleft and bind to specific receptors. This flow allows an associated diffusion of potassium and sodium ions that causes an action potential. Excitatory neurotransmitters decrease the negativity of postsynaptic membrane potentials; inhibitory neurotransmitters increase such potentials. Kinds of neurotransmitters include **acetylcholine chloride, gamma-aminobutyric acid,** and **norepinephrine.**

neurula /no͝or′ələ/, *pl.* **neurulas, neurulae,** an early embryo during the period of neurulation when the nervous system tissue begins to differentiate. The embryo at this level of growth represents a third stage in embryonic development, after the morula and blastocyst stages in humans and the higher animals and the blastula and gastrula stages in lower animals. In humans, the neurula stage occurs from about 19 to 26 days after fertilization.

neurulation, the development of the neural plate and the processes involved with its subsequent closure to form the neural tube during the early stages of embryonic development. See also **neural tube formation.**

neutral, the state exactly between two opposing values, qualities, or properties; for example, in electricity a neutral state is one in which there is neither a positive nor a negative charge, or in chemistry a neutral state is one in which a substance is neither acid nor alkaline. See also **acid, base, pH.**

neutralization, the interaction between an acid and a base that produces a solution that is neither acidic nor basic. The usual products of neutralization are a salt and water.

neutral rotation, the position of a limb that is turned neither toward nor away from the body's midline. When a person is supine and the leg is neutrally rotated, the toes should point straight up.

neutral thermal environment, an environment created by any method or apparatus to maintain the normal body temperature to minimize oxygen consumption and caloric expenditure, as in an incubator or Isolette for a premature, sick, or low-birth-weight infant. See also **incubator, Isolette.**

neutron, (in physics) an elementary particle that is a constituent of the nuclei of all elements except hydrogen. It has no electric charge and is approximately the same size as a proton. Compare **electron, proton.** See also **atom.**

neutron activation analysis, the analysis of elements in a specimen, performed by exposing it to neutron irradiation to convert many elements to a radioactive form in which they can be identified by measuring their emissions of radiation. The method is applicable, to a limited extent, to human and animal studies.

neutropenia /no͞o′trōpē′nē·ə/, an abnormal decrease in the number of neutrophils in the blood. The decrease may be relative or absolute. Neutropenia is associated with acute leukemia, infection, rheumatoid arthritis, vitamin B_{12} deficiency, and chronic splenomegaly. Compare **leukopenia.** See also **neutrophil.**

neutrophil /no͞o′trəfil/, a polymorphonuclear granular leukocyte that stains easily with neutral dyes. Its nucleus, which stains dark blue, contains three to five lobes connected by slender threads of chromatin; its cytoplasm contains fine, inconspicuous granules. Neutrophils are the circulating white blood cells essential for phagocytosis and proteolysis in which bacteria, cellular debris, and solid particles are removed and destroyed. An increase in neutrophils is the most common form of leukocytosis and may result from many causes, including acute infection, intoxication, hemorrhage, and malignant neoplastic disease. See also **basophil, eosinophil, granulocyte, polymorphonuclear leukocyte.**

neutrophil alkaline phosphatase. See **leukocyte alkaline phosphatase.**

neutrophilic leukemia. See **polymorphocytic leukemia.**

nevoid amentia. See **Sturge-Weber syndrome.**

nevoid neuroma, a tumor of nerve tissue that contains numerous small blood vessels. Also called **neuroma telangiectodes.**

nevus /nē′vəs/, a pigmented, congenital skin blemish that is usually benign but may become cancerous. Any change in color, size, or texture or any bleeding or itching of a nevus deserves investigation. Also called **birthmark, mole.** See also **blue nevus, junction nevus, nevus flammeus.**

nevus flammeus /flam′ē·əs/, a flat, capillary hemangioma that is present at birth and that varies in color from pale red to deep reddish purple. It is most commonly seen on the occiput and rarely causes any problems. If the lesion is on any other part of the body, it tends to be darker colored and, unlike the scalp lesions, does not regress spontaneously. These lesions are most often seen on the face. The depth of the color depends on whether the superficial, middle, or deep dermal vessels are involved. On the face, the lesion persists and develops a thick verrucous nodular surface. Nevus flammeus is usually unilateral, following the distribution of a cutaneous nerve. If the lesion is on the middle of the face, Sturge-Weber syndrome is suspected. Treatment is not often satisfactory. Cosmetic creams are used to cover the lesion, and electrodesication or cryotherapy is sometimes performed, especially to improve the verrucous surface appearance. Laser therapy is an experimental treatment. Also called **port-wine stain.**

nevus vascularis. See **capillary hemangioma.**

newborn, **1.** recently born. **2.** a recently born infant; a neonate.

newborn intrapartal care, care of the newborn in the delivery area during the time after birth before the mother and infant are transferred to the postpartum unit. See also **intrapartal care, postpartal care.**

■ METHOD: The nasopharynx and mouth may be suctioned to remove excess mucus as the head is born. Depending on the preference and the condition of the mother and the policies of the maternity service, the baby may then be placed on the mother's abdomen and covered with a warm, dry blanket or taken by the nurse to an infant warmer. Apgar scores are assigned at 1 minute of age and at 5 minutes of age; less commonly, another is assigned at 10 minutes of age. The baby is handled gently and quietly; bright lights are often avoided, and maternal contact is encouraged.

■ NURSING ORDERS: The nurse is usually the first person to observe and examine the baby. Most newborns are healthy and normal; if abnormal function is observed, expert assistance may be summoned and emergency measures, including tracheal suction with a DeLee mucous trap and administration of oxygen by ventilator or mask, are initiated. If there are no problems, the nurse may instill silver nitrate drops in the conjunctival sacs of the eyes, trim and clamp the umbilical cord, administer an injection of vitamin K, obtain footprints for identification, and diaper and wrap the baby. If the baby needs to be transferred to a nursery or special care facility, the nurse accompanies the infant and acts as the initial liaison for the mother with the nursery.

■ OUTCOME CRITERIA: Most infants born at term are healthy and do not need any medical intervention. Hemorrhage from the umbilical cord, difficult respiration, imperforate anus, endocrine dysfunction, and various other abnormal conditions may occur, but if a baby has good color, is alert, can cry and suck, urinate, defecate, and respond to sound and light, the nurse may reassure the mother that the baby is almost invariably healthy and normal. The individuality of each infant is remarkable and may be pointed out to the mother.

new drug, a drug for which the Food and Drug Administration requires premarketing approval. A new drug is generally regarded as one for which safety and effectiveness have not yet been demonstrated for its prescribed use.

New England Journal of Medicine (NEJM), a weekly professional medical journal that publishes findings of medical research and articles about controversial political and ethical issues in the practice of medicine.

new growth, a neoplasm or tumor.

Newman, Margaret A., a nursing theorist who contributed to the study of nursing theories and models by defining three approaches to the discovery of nursing theory. They are: "borrowing" of theories from related disciplines, analyzing nursing practice situations in search of conceptual relationships, and creating new conceptual systems from which theories can be derived. Newman's work was introduced in 1962 and received immediate federal support with funding of nurse scientist programs. In later work, Newman proposed that a holistic approach to the study of nursing problems would require the identification of patterns that reflect the whole; for example, patterns of movement, sleep, or communication might reflect the whole person. In a 1979 work, Newman noted that conceptual frameworks actually are networks within which questions, theories, and data fit together and provide a focus of inquiry.

New World leishmaniasis. See **American leishmaniasis.**

New World typhus. See **murine typhus.**

Nezelof's syndrome /nez′əlofs/, an abnormal condition characterized by absent T cell function, deficient B cell function, fairly normal immunoglobulin levels, and little or no specific antibody production. The cause of Nezelof's syndrome is unknown. It affects both male and female siblings, indicating the possibility of a genetic disorder transmitted as an autosomal recessive trait. The disease may be caused by a cytogenic dysfunction of the stem cells, resulting in deficiencies of T cells and B cells. Another theory is that the disorder is caused by underdevelopment of the thymus gland and the consequent inhibition of T cell development. Still another holds that the disease results from the failure to produce or to secrete thymic humoral factors, especially thymosin.

■ OBSERVATIONS: Nezelof's syndrome causes progressively severe, recurrent, and eventually fatal infections. Signs that often appear in infants or in children up to 4 years of age include recurrent pneumonia, otitis media, chronic fungal infections, upper respiratory tract infections, diarrhea, and hepatosplenomegaly. The disease may also enlarge the lymph nodes and the tonsils. These structures may also be totally absent in infants with the disease. Involved patients may also develop a tendency toward malignancy. Infection may cause sepsis, which is the usual cause of death. Symptoms that often suggest Nezelof's syndrome also include weight loss and poor eating habits. Definite diagnostic evidence of the disease includes defective B cell and T cell immunity despite a normal number of circulating B cells, a moderate to high rise in the number of T cells, a deficiency or an increase in one or more immunoglobulins, a nonreactive Schick test after DPT immunization, a reduced or an absent antibody reaction after specific antigen immunization, no thymus shadow on a chest x-ray film, thymus-dependent regions with abnormal lymphoid structure, and a decrease in the number of lymphocytes in the blood.

■ INTERVENTION: Initial supportive treatment of Nezelof's syndrome may include monthly injections of gamma globulin or monthly infusions of fresh frozen plasma and the heavy use of antibiotics to fight infection. The plasma infusions are especially beneficial if the patient cannot produce specific immunoglobulins. Cell-mediated immune function associated with T cells can usually be temporarily restored within weeks by a fetal thymus transplant. Repeated transplants are required to maintain the immunity. Cell-mediated immunity can be only partially restored with either transfer factor therapy or repeated injection of thymosin. Histocompatible bone marrow transplants have been used, but effective evaluation of this treatment method is incomplete.

■ NURSING CONSIDERATIONS: The nursing role in treating this disease is essentially supportive. The injection site for gamma globulin in a large muscle mass is massaged after the injection, and injection sites are rotated and recorded to prevent tissue damage. Gamma globulin doses greater than 1.5 ml are divided and injected into more than one site. The nursing role is also one of instruction and support for the parents of children affected by Nezelof's syndrome. Nurses commonly instruct parents on how to recognize the signs of infection and explain the dangers of allowing the affected child to become exposed to infection.

N.F., abbreviation for ***National Formulary***.

NGF, abbreviation for **nerve growth factor.**

NGU, abbreviation for **nongonococcal urethritis.**

NHSC, abbreviation for **National Health Service Corps.**

Ni, symbol for **nickel.**

niacin /nī′əsin/, a white, crystalline, water-soluble vitamin of the B complex group usually occurring in various plant and animal tissues as nicotinamide. It functions as a coenzyme necessary for the breakdown and use of all major nutrients and is essential for a healthy skin, normal functioning of the GI tract, maintenance of the nervous system, and synthesis of the sex hormones. It may also be effective in improving circulation and reducing high blood cholesterol levels. Rich dietary sources of both niacin and its precursor tryptophan are meats, poultry, fish, liver, kidney, eggs, nuts, peanut butter, brewer's yeast, and wheat germ. Symptoms of deficiency include muscular weakness, general fatigue, loss of appetite, various skin eruptions, halitosis, stomatitis, insomnia, irritability, nausea, vomiting, recurring headaches, tender gums, tension, and depression. Severe deficiency results in pellagra. The vitamin is not stored in the body, and any excess in the diet is excreted. Also called **nicotinic acid.** See also **pellagra.**

niacinamide, a B complex vitamin. It is closely related to niacin but has no vasodilating action. Also called **nicotinamide.**

nibble, a computer word size representing four bits, or one half of a byte.

N.I.C.H.H.D., abbreviation for **National Institute of Child Health and Human Development.**

nick, (in molecular genetics) a fissure or split in a single strand of DNA that can be made with the enzyme deoxyribonuclease or with ethidium bromide.

nickel (Ni), a silvery-white metallic element. Its atomic number is 28; its atomic weight is 58.71. Large numbers of people are allergic to nickel. Nickel causes more cases of allergic contact dermatitis than all other metals combined. Many cases occur from exposure to jewelry, coins, buckles, and snaps and to continued use of "carbonless" business forms. Nickel carbonyl, a volatile liquid, may produce serious lung damage if inhaled.

nickel dermatitis, an allergic contact dermatitis caused by the metal, nickel. Exposure comes usually from jewelry, wristwatches, metal clasps, and coins. Sweating increases the degree of rash. Treatment includes avoidance of exposure to nickel and reduction of perspiration. See also **contact dermatitis.**

nick translation, a method of labeling DNA in the laboratory by using the enzyme DNA polymerase.

Niclocide, a trademark for an anthelmintic (niclosamide).

niclosamide /niklō′səmīd/, an anthelmintic.

■ INDICATIONS: It is prescribed in the treatment of beef tapeworm and fish tapeworm infestations.

■ CONTRAINDICATIONS: Known sensitivity to this drug prohibits its use. Its safety in pregnant or nursing mothers or small children has not been established.

■ ADVERSE EFFECTS: Among the most serious adverse reactions are rectal bleeding, palpitations, alopecia, edema, nausea, and vomiting.

Nicobid, a trademark for two coenzymes (niacin and niacinamide), used as a vitamin supplement.

nicotinamide. See **niacinamide.**

nicotine, a colorless, rapidly acting toxic substance in tobacco that is one of the major contributors to the ill effects of smoking. It is used as an insecticide in agriculture and as a parasiticide in veterinary medicine. Ingestion of large amounts causes salivation, nausea, vomiting, diarrhea, headache, vertigo, slowing of the heartbeat, and, in acute cases, paralysis of respiratory muscles. Treatment includes gastric lavage with a weak solution of potassium permanganate, followed by activated charcoal, and the administration of artificial respiration and oxygen, as needed. Pentobarbital is used to control convulsions, ephedrine for hypotension, and autonomic blocking agents to control visceral symptoms.

nicotine poisoning, poisoning from intake of nicotine. Nicotine poisoning is characterized by stimulation of the central and autonomic nervous systems followed by depression of these systems. In fatal cases, death occurs from respiratory failure.

nicotinic acid. See **niacin.**

nicotinyl alcohol /nik′ətē′nil/, an alcohol used as a vasodilator, in the form of its tartrate salt, in the treatment of peripheral vascular disease, vascular spasm, varicose ulcers, decubital ulcers, chilblains, Ménière's disease, and vertigo.

NICU, abbreviation for **neonatal intensive care unit.**

nidation /nīdā′shən/, the process by which an embryo burrows into the endometrium of the uterus. Also called **implantation.** See also **placenta, uterus.**

NIDDM, abbreviation for **non-insulin-dependent diabetes mellitus.**

Niemann-Pick disease /nē′monpik′/, an inherited disorder of lipid metabolism in which there are accumulations of sphingomyelin in the bone marrow, spleen, and lymph nodes. The disease, which in the United States and Canada is most common among Jewish people, begins in infancy or childhood and is characterized by enlargement of liver and spleen, anemia, lymphadenopathy, and progressive mental and physical deterioration. There is no effective treatment, and children with the disease usually die within a few years of the onset of symptoms. Also called **sphingomyelin lipoidosis.**

nifedipine, a calcium channel blocker.

■ INDICATIONS: It is prescribed for the treatment of vasospastic and effort associated angina.

■ CONTRAINDICATION: Known hypersensitivity to this drug prohibits its use.

■ ADVERSE EFFECTS: Among the more serious adverse reactions are hypotension, peripheral edema, palpitations, dyspnea, nausea, dizziness, flushing, and headache.

night blindness. See **nyctalopia.**

nightcare program, a medical service for patients who, for therapeutic purposes, use hospital services on a regularly scheduled basis for a number of nighttime hours although fulltime inpatient care is not required.

night guard. See **bite guard.**

Nightingale, Florence (1820–1910), the founder of modern nursing. After limited formal training in nursing in Germany and Paris, she became superintendent in 1853 of a small hospital in London. Her outstanding success in reorganizing the hospital led to a request by the British government to head a mission to the Crimea, where Britain was fighting a war with Russia. She arrived in November, 1854, with 38 nurses to find 5000 men crowded into dilapidated buildings, filthy, mostly without beds, lacking adequate food and medical supplies. Through superhuman efforts, often working 20 hours on the wards and then sending off a stream of letters to England to obtain money and supplies and to mobilize the government to act, she brought order out of chaos. After her return to England, in 1856, she wrote *Notes on Hospitals* and *Notes on Nursing* and founded a training school for nurses at St. Thomas' Hospital, where she attracted well-educated, dedicated women. The graduates became matrons of the most important hospitals in Great Britain, thus raising the standards of nursing across the nation and eventually around the world. Although she was, by then, bedridden much of the time, she carried on her work on the sanitary reform of India, conducted a study of midwifery, helped establish visiting nurse services, and worked for the reform of the poor laws in which she proposed separate institutions for the sick, the insane, the incurable, and children. After Longfellow wrote *Santa Filomena,* she became known as "The Lady with The Lamp," and the Nightingale Pledge, named after her, embodies her ideals and has inspired thousands of young graduating nurses.

Nightingale ward, a kind of hospital ward, designed by Florence Nightingale, that revolutionized hospital design. The number of beds allowed in a ward of given size was limited to permit the circulation of air and for general cleanliness and the comfort of patients. Three sides of the ward were windowed to admit light and fresh air. Although multiple-bed wards are now obsolete in hospital design, the concerns and the benefits that impelled Miss Nightingale to create them remain central to hospital planning.

nightingalism, an ideology emphasizing self-sacrifice on the part of a nurse whose primary concern is the welfare of the patient, with minimum personal attention to the needs of the nurse. See also **Nightingale, Florence.**

nightmare, a dream occurring during rapid eye movement sleep that arouses feelings of intense, inescapable fear, terror, distress, or extreme anxiety and that usually awakens the sleeper. Compare **pavor nocturnus, sleep terror disorder.**

night sight. See **hemeralopia.**

night vision, a capacity to see dimly lit objects. It stems from a chemophysical phenomenon associated with the retinal rods. The rods contain the highly light-sensitive chemical rhodopsin, or visual purple, which is essential for the conduction of optic impulses in subdued light. Night vision is sharpest at the periphery of the retina because of the concentration of rods. Night vision may be diminished by a deficiency of vitamin A, an important component of rhodopsin.

nigrities linguae. See **parasitic glossitis.**

N.I.H., abbreviation for **National Institutes of Health.**

nihilistic delusion, a persistent denial of the existence of particular things or of everything, including oneself, as seen in various forms of schizophrenia. A person who has such a delusion may believe that he lives in a shadow or limbo world or that he died several years ago and that only the spirit, in a vaporous form, really exists. See also **delusion.**

nikethamide /nīketh′əmīd/, a central nervous system stimulant.

■ INDICATIONS: It is prescribed as an analeptic in the treatment of depression of the central nervous and respiratory systems.

■ CONTRAINDICATION: Known hypersensitivity to this drug prohibits its use.

■ ADVERSE EFFECTS: Among the most serious adverse reactions at high doses are tachycardia, hypertension, muscle spasm, and convulsions. Burning and itching are common.

Nikolsky's sign /nikol′skēz/, easy separation of the stratum corneum layer of the epidermis from the basal cell layer by rubbing apparently normal skin areas; found in pemphigus and a few other bullous diseases.

Nilstat, a trademark for an antifungal (nystatin).

90-90 traction. See **traction, 90-90.**

ninth nerve. See **glossopharyngeal nerve.**

niobium (Nb), a silver-gray metallic element. Its atomic number is 41; its atomic weight is 92.906. Formerly called **columbium.**

nipple, a small cylindric, pigmented structure that projects just below the center of each breast. The tip of the nipple has about 20 tiny openings to the lactiferous ducts. The skin of the nipple is surrounded by the lighter pigmented skin of the areola. The depth of pigmentation of the nipple and areola in nulliparas varies from rosy pink to brown, depending on the complexion of the individual. In pregnancy, the skin of the nipple darkens but loses some of its pigmentation when lactation is completed. Stimulation of the nipple in men and women causes the structure to become erect through the contraction of radiating smooth muscle bundles in the surrounding areola. In women the nipple enlarges somewhat and becomes more sensitive after puberty.

nipple cancer, an inflammatory malignant neoplasm of the nipple and areola that is usually associated with carcinoma in deeper breast structures. It represents only a small percentage of breast cancers and usually begins in the nipple and spreads to the areola. Also called **Paget's disease of the nipple.**

nipple discharge, spontaneous exudation of material from the nipple that may be normal, as colostrum in pregnancy, or that may be a sign of endocrinologic, neoplastic, or infectious disease.

nipple shield, a device to protect the nipples of a lactating woman. The shield is usually made of soft latex, is 4 or 5 cm wide, and has a tab on one side with which the mother may hold it. The baby nurses from a nipple at the center of the shield. It is most often used to allow sore or cracked nipples to heal while maintaining lactation. Also called **nipple protector.**

Nipride, a trademark for a direct-acting vasodilator (sodium nitroprusside), used as an adjunct to anesthesia.

niridazole /nirid′əzōl/, an antischistosomal. In the United States it is available from the Centers for Disease Control.

Nissl body /nis′əl/, any one of the large granular structures in the cytoplasm of nerve cells that stains with basic dyes and contains ribonucleoprotein.

nit, the egg of a parasitic insect, particularly a louse. It may be found attached to human or animal hair or to clothing fiber. See also **pediculosis.**

Nitoman, a trademark for a serotonin antagonist (tetrabenazine methanesulfonate), used in the treatment of Huntington's chorea and other hyperkinetic movement disorders.

nitric acid /nī′trik/, a colorless, highly corrosive liquid that may give off suffocating brown fumes of nitrogen dioxide on exposure to air. Traces of nitric acid are found in rain water during a thunderstorm. Commercially prepared nitric acid is a powerful oxidizing agent used in photoengraving and metallurgy, in the manufacture of explosives, fertilizers, dyes, and drugs, and, occasionally, as a cauterizing agent for the removal of warts.

nitrite /nī′trīt/, an ester or salt of nitrous acid, used as a vasodilator and antispasmodic. Among the most widely used nitrites in medicine are amyl, ethyl, potassium, and sodium nitrite.

nitro-, a combining form indicating presence of the group $-NO_2$: *nitrobenzol, nitrofuran, nitromethane*.

nitrobenzene poisoning, a toxic condition caused by the absorption into the body of nitrobenzene, a pale yellow, oily liquid used in the manufacture of aniline, shoe dyes, soap, perfume, and artificial flavors. Nitrobenzene, especially its vapors, is extremely toxic. Exposure in industry is usually by inhalation of the fumes or by absorption through the skin. Symptoms of acute poisoning include headache, drowsiness, nausea, ataxia, cyanosis, and in extreme cases respiratory failure. Contaminated clothing is removed, and the skin is washed with vinegar, followed by soap and water. Oxygen, blood transfusion, and, in severe cases, hemodialysis may be required. Ingestion is treated with gastric lavage with weak acetic acid, followed by the administration of liquid petrolatum, a saline cathartic, and oxygen and blood transfusion if indicated. Chronic exposure to nitrobenzene may cause headache, fatigue, loss of appetite, and anemia.

Nitrobid, a trademark for a coronary vasodilator (nitroglycerin), used as an antianginal agent.

nitrofuran, one of a group of synthetic antimicrobials used to treat infections caused by protozoa or by certain gram-positive or gram-negative bacteria. The precise mechanism by which nitrofurans exert their antimicrobial effects is not known. Three of these agents are commonly prescribed. Nitrofurazone is used topically to treat superficial wounds and infections, particularly burns. Systemic toxicity is not seen when the drug is used in this way, although allergic skin reactions may occur. Furazolidone is used to treat bacterial and protozoal diarrhea and enteritis. Nitrofurantoin is used to treat urinary tract infections caused by *Escherichia coli* and other enteric pathogens of the urinary tract. Systemic administration of nitrofurans is associated with many side effects, the most common being nausea and diarrhea. Serious side effects include polyneuropathies and several hypersensitivity reactions, including pneumonitis and blood dyscrasias. Nitrofurans can cause hemolytic anemia in patients with glucose-6-phosphate dehydrogenase deficiency.

nitrofurantoin /nī'trōfyo͞oran'tō•in/, a urinary antibacterial.

■ INDICATIONS: It is prescribed in the treatment of certain urinary tract infections.

■ CONTRAINDICATIONS: Kidney dysfunction or known hypersensitivity to this drug prohibits its use. It is not given to children under 1 month of age or to pregnant or lactating women.

■ ADVERSE EFFECTS: Among the most serious adverse reactions is hypersensitivity pneumonitis, which can lead to fibrosis, neurotoxicity, and hemolytic anemia in patients with glucose-6-phosphate dehydrogenase deficiency. GI disturbances and fever are common.

nitrofurazone, a topical antibacterial.

■ INDICATIONS: It is prescribed in the prophylaxis and treatment of infection in second- and third-degree burns and in the treatment of infections of the skin and mucous membranes.

■ CONTRAINDICATION: Known hypersensitivity to this drug prohibits its use.

■ ADVERSE EFFECTS: Among the most serious adverse reactions are severe allergic reactions and suprainfections.

nitrogen (N), a gaseous, nonmetallic element. Its atomic number is 7; its atomic weight is 14.008. Nitrogen constitutes approximately 78% of the atmosphere and is a component of all proteins and a major component of most organic substances. Nitrogen is found in mineral compounds, as saltpeter, and is the seventeenth most abundant element in the earth's crust. Compounds of nitrogen are essential constituents of all living organisms, the proteins and the nucleic acids being especially basic to all life forms. Nitrogen forms a series of oxides and oxyacids, the most important of which is nitric acid. It also unites with hydrogen to form ammonia and with many metallic elements to form nitrides. Nitrogen is essential to the synthesis of proteins that the body must have, particularly nitrogen-containing compounds or amino acids derived directly or indirectly from plant food. Nitrogen follows a cycle from atmospheric gas into nitrogen-fixing bacteria, into green vascular plants, into humans and animals, and, by decay or in excreted nitrogenous wastes, as urea, back into the soil. Denitrifying bacteria in the soil break down nitrogenous compounds and release gaseous nitrogen. During a 24-hour period in a healthy individual the nitrogen excreted in the urine, feces, and perspiration, together with the nitrogen retained in dermal structures, as the skin and hair, equals the nitrogen consumed in food and drink. The process of protein metabolism accounts for this nitrogen balance. When protein catabolism exceeds protein anabolism, the amount of nitrogen in the urine exceeds the amount of nitrogen consumed in foods, producing a negative nitrogen balance or a state of tissue wasting. A positive nitrogen balance exists in the body when the nitrogen intake in foods is greater than that excreted in urine. Conditions usually associated with positive nitrogen balance are those in which protein anabolism is proceeding faster than protein catabolism, as in conditions associated with growth, pregnancy, and convalescence from a tissue-wasting illness. Nitrogen is a component of nitrous oxide, or laughing gas, which is sometimes used as an anesthetic. Nitrous oxide is a colorless, nonflammable, sweet-tasting gas. Three liters of nitrogen may be eliminated from the lungs and tissues in the first hour of anesthesia if a nitrous oxide-oxygen mixture is inspired. Precautions are taken to exhaust this nitrogen from the breathing circuit if high concentrations of both oxygen and nitrous oxide are desired. Nitrous oxide takes effect quickly and allows a fast recovery from anesthesia but is not considered suitable for prolonged surgery or for surgery requiring deep muscle relaxation. It must be administered with oxygen or air to prevent anoxia. Nitrogen is a component of nitrogen dioxide, which is irritating to the lungs and can cause pulmonary edema. Nitrogen dioxide can be released from silage and may produce symptoms of pulmonary damage in workers who perform ensilage tasks. Some studies indicate that measurable changes in pulmonary function occur when healthy individuals are exposed to nitrous oxide concentrations of two to three parts per million. Nitrogen is also a component of nitric and nitrous acids. Organic nitrates or polyol esters of nitric acid, as nitroglycerin, and organic nitrites or esters of nitric acid, as amyl nitrite, are effective vasodilators often used in relieving angina, but exactly how they function in dilating arterial and venous smooth muscle is not yet understood.

nitrogen balance, the relationship between the nitrogen taken into the body, usually as food, and the nitrogen excreted from the body in urine and feces. Most of the body's nitrogen is incorporated into protein. Positive nitrogen balance, which occurs when the intake of nitrogen is greater than its excretion, implies tissue formation. Negative nitrogen balance, which occurs when more nitrogen is excreted than is taken in, indicates wasting or destruction of tissue.

nitrogen fixation, the process by which free nitrogen in the atmosphere is converted by biologic or chemical means to ammonia and to other forms usable by plants and animals. Biologic nitrogen fixation is the more important process and is accomplished by microorganisms in the soil, either free living or in close association with root nodules of certain plants. In contrast, chemical nitrogen fixation, as used in industry, requires extremely high temperatures and pressures.

nitrogen mustard. See **mechlorethamine hydrochloride.**

nitroglycerin, a coronary vasodilator.
■ INDICATION: It is prescribed for the prevention or relief of angina pectoris.
■ CONTRAINDICATION: Known hypersensitivity to this drug prohibits its use.
■ ADVERSE EFFECTS: Among the most serious adverse reactions are hypotension, flushing, headache, and syncope.

nitromersol, an organic mercurial antiseptic that is not a highly effective germicide, sometimes used for the disinfecting of surgical instruments and as an antiseptic on the skin and mucous membranes.

nitroprusside sodium. See **sodium nitroprusside.**

nitroso-, a combining form indicating presence of the group -N:O: *nitrosobacteria, nitrososubstitution.*

nitrosourea /nītrō′sōyo͝orē′ə/, one of a group of alkylating drugs used as an antineoplastic drug in the chemotherapy of brain tumors, multiple myeloma, Hodgkin's disease, adenocarcinomas, hepatomas, chronic leukemias, lymphomas, myelomas, and cancers of the breast and ovaries. They have been less successful in therapy for cancers of the lungs, head, neck, and GI tract. Like other alkylating agents, they have severe toxic effects, including bone marrow depression. Nausea and vomiting are almost always present. Safe use during pregnancy has not been established, and animal studies have generally shown teratogenicity and embryotoxicity. Carmustine and lomustine are typical examples of this group. See also **alkylating agent.**

Nitrospan, a trademark for a coronary vasodilator (nitroglycerin).

Nitrostat, a trademark for a coronary vasodilator (nitroglycerin).

nitrous oxide (N_2O), a gas used as an anesthetic in dentistry, surgery, and childbirth. It provides light anesthesia and is delivered in various concentrations with oxygen. Nitrous oxide alone does not provide deep enough anesthesia for major surgery, for which it is supplemented with other anesthetic agents. It is often given for induction of anesthesia, preceded by the administration of a barbiturate or an analgesic narcotic. Nitrous oxide is neither explosive nor flammable, and recovery is rapid. It is not administered to patients with hypoxemia, respiratory disease, or intestinal occlusion.

Nizoral, a trademark for an antifungal agent (ketoconazole).

NLN, abbreviation for **National League for Nursing.**

NMNA, abbreviation for **National Male Nurses' Association.**

NMR, abbreviation for **nuclear magnetic resonance.**

NMR imaging, the use of nuclear magnetic resonance (NMR) techniques in imaging the internal structure and metabolic reactions of the body. Hydrogen, the most common element in the body, appears in the complex biomolecules that are the constituents of all body tissues, as healthy brain tissue, bone tumors, or blood. In each case the nature and density of the hydrogen-bearing molecules and the local chemical environment will cause the NMR spectrum to vary slightly from that of pure hydrogen, allowing the identification of tissue types and even the monitoring of chemical activity. Spatial information can be obtained by purposely distorting the static magnetic field with extra "gradient" fields; the resultant field conditions permit resonance to occur only in a carefully defined region that, for different purposes, may be a three-dimensional volume, a plane, a line segment, or even a point. The NMR signal, encoded in this way, can be computer reconstructed into a cross-sectional image that reveals anatomic features with a spatial resolution rivaling or exceeding that obtainable with x-rays.

No, symbol for **nobelium.**

N_2O, symbol for **nitrous oxide.**

nobelium (No), a synthetic, transuranic metallic element. Its atomic number is 102. The atomic weight of its most stable isotope is 259.

noble gas. See **inert gas.**

Nocardia /nōkär′dē•ə/, a genus of gram-positive aerobic bacteria, some species of which are pathogenic, as *Nocardia asteroides* which causes maduromycosis. See also **nocardiosis.**

nocardiosis /nōkär′dē•ō′sis/, infection with *Nocardia asteroides,* an aerobic gram-positive species of actinomycetes, characterized by pneumonia, often with cavitation, and by chronic abscesses in the brain and subcutaneous tissues. The organism enters via the respiratory tract and spreads by the bloodstream, especially in Cushing's syndrome. Surgical drainage of abscesses and sulfonamide therapy for 12 to 18 months cures between 50% and 60% of the cases treated.

nociceptor, somatic and visceral free nerve endings of thinly myelinated and unmyelinated fibers. They usually react to tissue injury but may also be excited by endogenous chemical substances.

no code, a note written in the patient record and signed by a qualified, usually senior or attending physician, instructing the staff of the institution not to attempt to resuscitate a particular patient in the event of cardiac or respiratory failure. This instruction is usually given only when a patient is so gravely ill that death is imminent and inevitable. Also called **DNR.** See also **code,** def. 5.

noctambulation. See **somnambulism.**

Noctec, a trademark for a sedative-hypnotic (chloral hydrate).

nocturia /nokto͝or′ē•ə/, urination, particularly excessive urination at night. Whereas it may be a symptom of renal disease, it may occur in the absence of disease in persons who drink excessive amounts of fluids, particularly alcohol or coffee, before bedtime or in people with prostatic disease. It may occur in older patients, who may have excess fluids that are mobilized by lying down at night. Also called **nycturia.** Compare **enuresis.**

nocturnal, **1.** pertaining to or occurring during the night. **2.** describing an individual or animal that is active at night and sleeps during the day.

nocturnal emission, involuntary emission of semen during sleep, usually in association with an erotic dream. Also called **wet dream.**

nocturnal paroxysmal dyspnea, an abnormal condition of the respiratory system, characterized by sudden attacks of shortness of breath, profuse sweating, tachycardia, and wheezing that awaken the person from sleep. The paroxysms may be induced by nightmares, noises, or coughing. The condition is usually associated with heart failure or pulmonary edema. Characteristically, the attack is relieved by getting up and opening a window. See also **dyspnea.**

nod-, a combining form meaning 'knot': *nodal, nodose, nodulus.*

nodal bradycardia. See **bradycardia.**

node, **1.** a small rounded mass. **2.** a lymph node. **3.** a single computer terminal in a network of terminals and computers.

nodular, (of a structure or mass) small, firm, and knotty. See also **node, nodule.**

nodular circumscribed lipomatosis, a condition in which many circumscribed, encapsulated lipomas are distributed around the neck symmetrically, randomly, or like a collar. The adipose deposits may be painful and tender.

nodular cutaneous angiitis, an inflammatory condition of small arteries accompanied by lesions of the skin.

nodular melanoma, a melanoma that is uniformly pigmented, usually bluish-black and nodular and sometimes surrounded by an irregular halo of pale, unpigmented skin. The lesion is always raised and may be dome-shaped or polypoid. It is most often found in adults in middle age. It is one of the three major types of melanoma, occurring in 10% to 15% of patients with melanoma. See also **lentigo maligna melanoma, superficial spreading melanoma.**

nodule, **1.** a small node. **2.** a small nodelike structure.

-noia, a combining form meaning '(condition of the) mind or will': *aponoia, hypernoia, hyponoia.*

Noludar, a trademark for a sedative (methyprylon).

Nolvadex, a trademark for a nonsteroidal antiestrogen (tamoxifen).

noma /nō′mə/, an acute, necrotizing ulcerative process involving mucous membranes of mouth or genitalia. The condition is most commonly seen in children with poor nutrition and hygiene. There is rapid spreading and painless destruction of bone and soft tissue accompanied by a putrid odor. Fusospirochetal organisms have been implicated. Healing eventually occurs but often with disfiguring defects. Also called **acute necrotizing ulcerative mucositis, gangrenous stomatitis.**

-noma, a combining form meaning a 'spreading, invasive gangrene': *müllerianoma, pelidnoma.*

nomenclature /nō′mənklā′chər, nōmen′-/, a consistent, systematic method of naming used in a scientific discipline to denote classifications and to avoid ambiguities in names, as binomial nomenclature in biology and chemical nomenclature in chemistry.

-nomia, a combining form meaning 'aphasia involving names or naming ability': *anomia, paranomia, dysnomia.*

Nomina Anatomica, the book of official international nomenclature for anatomy as designated by the International Congress of Anatomists.

nominal damages. See **damages.**

nomo-, a combining form meaning 'of or relating to usage or law': *nomogenesis, nomogram, nomotopic.*

nomogram /nom′əgram, nō′mə-/, **1.** a graphic representation, by any of various systems, of a numeric relationship. **2.** a graph on which a number of variables is plotted so that the value of a dependent variable can be read on the appropriate line when the values of the other variables are given.

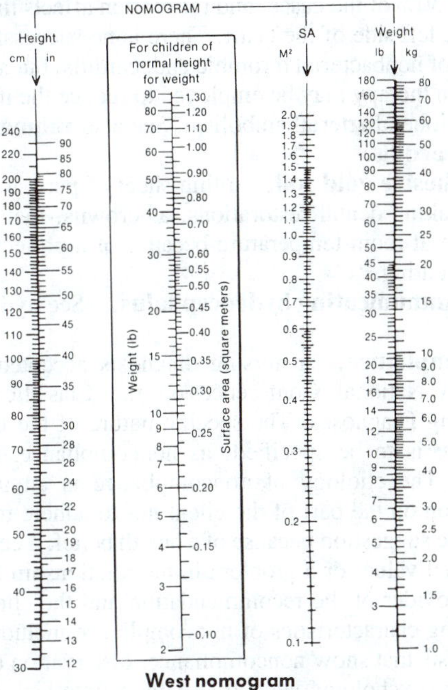

(Nomogram modified from data of E. Boyd by C.D. West; from Shirkey, H.C.: Drug therapy. In Vaughan, V.C., III, and McKay, R.J., editors: Nelson's textbook of pediatrics, ed. 10, Philadelphia, 1975, W.B. Saunders Co.)

-nomy, a combining form meaning 'received knowledge in a field': *pathonomy, physionomy, psychonomy.*

non-, a combining form meaning 'nine': *nonan, nonigravida, nonipara.*

nonadhesive skin traction, one of two kinds of skin traction in which the therapeutic pull of traction weights is applied with foam-backed traction straps that do not stick to the skin over the body structure involved. Nonadhesive skin traction straps may be easily removed to facilitate skin care and are usually used when continuous traction is not required. The straps spread the traction pull over a wide area of skin surface, thus decreasing the vulnerability of the patient to skin breakdown. Compare **adhesive skin traction.**

non-A, non-B (NANB) hepatitis, viral hepatitis that is caused by a virus antigenically separate from the serologic strains that cause hepatitis A or hepatitis B. It accounts for more than 90% of the cases of posttransfusion hepatitis in the United States, occurring primarily in patients receiving multiple transfusions. NANB hepatitis is usually milder than types A or B but is otherwise clinically indistinguishable from them. The treatment is the same as for other forms of viral hepatitis.

nonbacterial thrombic endocarditis, one of the three main types of endocarditis, characterized by various kinds of lesions that affect the heart valves. Some studies indicate that this disease may be the first step in the development of bacterial endocarditis and that the lesions involved cause peripheral arterial embolisms resulting indeath. This disease equally affects men and women between 18 and 90 years of age, causes heart murmurs in about 30% of the cases, and most often affects the valves on the left side of the heart. There is no successful treatment of nonbacterial thrombic endocarditis, but anticoagulation therapy may be employed to reduce the incidence of peripheral arterial embolism. See also **Libman-Sacks endocarditis.**

noncohesive gold foil, a thin sheet of pure gold, used for making dental restorations, as crowns, that will not cohere at room temperature because of a protective surface coating.

noncommunicating hydrocephalus. See **hydrocephalus.**

noncompliance, a nursing diagnosis accepted by the Fourth National Conference on the Classification of Nursing Diagnoses. The specific nature of the noncompliance is to be specified, as noncompliance: medications. The etiology of noncompliance is an informed decision on the part of the client not to adhere to a therapeutic suggestion because of a health belief, a cultural or spiritual value, or a problem in the relationship between the provider of the recommendation and the client. The defining characteristics of noncompliance include objective tests that show noncompliance, observation of physical or psychologic signs that demonstrate lack of compliance, or a failure to keep appointments. The critical defining characteristic, which must be present for the diagnosis to be made, is an observation of the client's failure to adhere to a recommendation or a statement by the client or knowledgeable other person that the recommendations are not being followed. See also **nursing diagnosis.**

nondirective therapy, a psychotherapeutic approach in which the psychotherapist refrains from giving advice or interpretation as the client is helped to identify conflicts and to clarify and understand feelings and values. Compare **directive therapy.** See also **client-centered therapy.**

nondisjunction, failure of homologous pairs of chromosomes to separate during the first meiotic division or of the two chromatids of a chromosome to split during anaphase of mitosis or the second meiotic division. The result is an abnormal number of chromosomes in the daughter cells. Compare **disjunction.** See also **monosomy, trisomy.**

nonfat milk. See **skimmed milk.**

nonfeasance /nonfē′zəns/, a failure to perform a task, duty, or undertaking that one has agreed to perform or that one had a legal duty to perform. Compare **malfeasance, misfeasance.** See also **negligence.**

nongonococcal urethritis (NGU), an infectious condition of the urethra in males that is characterized by mild dysuria and a scanty to moderate amount of penile discharge. The discharge may be white or clear, thin or mucoid, or, less often, purulent. The infection is often caused by the obligate intracellular parasite *Chlamydia trachomatis*. The diagnosis of NGU is made by excluding a diagnosis of gonococcal urethritis by microscopic examination and bacteriologic culture of the exudate. Untreated NGU may result in urethral stricture, epididymitis, proctitis, and chronic inflammation of the urethra. Women exposed to the exudate during coitus may develop a hyperthropic erosion of the cervix and purulent cervical mucus. An infant in passing through the cervix and vagina of a mother infected with *C. trachomatis* may develop conjunctivitis and nasopharyngeal infection in the first few days after birth and pneumonia at 3 to 4 months. Most cases of NGU are successfully treated with tetracycline or erythromycin. Sexual contacts are treated whether or not they are symptomatic. Nearly 50% of all cases of urethritis are nongonococcal.

non-Hodgkin's lymphoma, any kind of malignant lymphoma except Hodgkin's disease. Also called **lymphosarcoma.**

nonimpact printer, a computer printer that produces an image on a medium, as paper, by ink jet, or by thermal, electomagnetic, or xerographic means.

non-insulin-dependent diabetes mellitus (NIDDM), a type of diabetes mellitus in which patients are not insulin-dependent or ketosis prone although they may use insulin for correction of symptomatic or persistent hyperglycemia, and they can develop ketosis under special circumstances, as infection or stress. Usually, onset is after 40 years of age, but can occur at any age. Two subclasses are presence or absence of obesity. About 60% to 90% are obese; in these patients glucose tolerance is often improved by weight loss. Hyperinsulemia and insulin resistance characterize some patients. There are probably multiple causes for the derangement of carbohydrate metabolism. Familial aggregation implies genetic factors, and this class includes diabetes presenting in childhood and adults in whom autosomal dominant inheritance is clearly established. Environmental factors superimposed on genetic susceptibility are probably involved in onset. Previously called adult-onset diabetes, ketosis-resistant diabetes, maturity-onset diabetes, maturity-onset-type diabetes, MOD, stable diabetes. Also called **Type II diabetes mellitus.** See also **diabetes mellitus.**

noninvasive, pertaining to a diagnostic or therapeutic technique that does not require the skin to be broken or a cavity or organ of the body to be entered, as obtaining a blood pressure reading by auscultation with a stethoscope and sphygmomanometer.

nonionizing radiation, radiation for which the mechanism of action in tissue does not directly ionize atomic or molecular systems through a single interaction.

nonosteogenic fibroma /non′ostē•əjen′ik/, a common bone lesion in which there is degeneration and proliferation of the medullary and cortical tissue, usually near the ends of the diaphyses of the large long bones, especially those of the lower extremities. Frequently it does not cause any symptoms and is only discovered during x-ray examination of the skeleton for other reasons.

nonparametric test of significance, (in statistics) one of several tests that use a qualitative approach to analyze rank order data and incidence data that cannot be assumed to have a normal distribution. Kinds of nonparametric tests of significance include **chi-square, Spearman's rho.**

nonpolar, pertaining to molecules that have a hydrophobic affinity, are "water hating." Nonpolar substances tend to dissolve in nonpolar solvents.

nonproductive cough, a sudden, noisy expulsion of air from the lungs that may be caused by irritation or inflammation and does not remove sputum from the respiratory tract. Expectorants, as ammonium chloride, ammonium carbonate, sodium iodide, potassium iodide, ipecac, and terpin hydrate increase respiratory tract secretions and may result in productive coughing when administered to patients with respiratory infections. If suppression of coughing is required, antitussives that depress the cough reflex may be prescribed, including codeine or dextromethorphan. Intratracheal suctioning may be necessary when secretions cause severe respiratory difficulty and coughing is unproductive. Compare **productive cough.**

nonprotein nitrogen (NPN), the nitrogen in the blood that is not a constituent of protein, as the nitrogen associated with urea, uric acid, creatine, and polypeptides. Approximately one half of the nonprotein nitrogen in the blood is associated with urea. Measurement of NPN may aid assessment of kidney function. The normal concentrations in serum or plasma are 25 to 35 mg/dl; in whole blood, 25 to 50 mg/dl.

nonrapid eye movement. See **sleep.**

nonreflex bladder. See **flaccid bladder.**

nonreversible inhibitor, an effector substance that binds irreversibly to an active site of an enzyme, inhibiting the normal catalytic activity of the enzyme.

nonsense mutation. See **amber mutation.**

nonsexual generation. See **asexual generation.**

nonspecific urethritis (NSU), inflammation of the urethra not known to be caused by a specific organism. Onset of symptoms is often related to sexual intercourse. Its acute phase is seldom seen in women, but its chronic phase is a common urologic difficulty among them. The condition is noted by urethral discharge in men and by reddening of the urethral mucosa in women. Treatment with antibiotics is not always successful. See also **nongonococcal urethritis.**

nontoxic, not poisonous. Also **atoxic.**

nontropic sprue, a malabsorption syndrome resulting from an inborn inability to digest foods that contain gluten. See also **celiac disease.**

nonulcerative blepharitis, a form of blepharitis characterized by greasy scales on the margins of the eyelids around the lashes and hyperemia and thickening of the skin. Nonulcerative blepharitis is often associated with seborrhea of the scalp, eyebrows, and the skin behind the ears.

Noonan's syndrome, a hypergonadotropic disorder, occurring only in males, characterized by short stature, low-set ears, webbing of the neck, and cubitus valgus. Testicular function may be normal, but fertility is often decreased. The number and morphology of the chromosomes are normal. The cause is unknown. See also **Turner's syndrome.**

norepinephrine /nôr′epinef′rin/, an adrenergic hormone that acts to increase blood pressure by vasoconstriction but does not affect cardiac output. It is synthesized naturally by the adrenal medulla and is available also as a drug, levarterenol, given to maintain the blood pressure in acute hypotension secondary to trauma, heart disease, or vascular collapse.

norepinephrine bitartrate, an adrenergic vasoconstrictor.

■ INDICATIONS: It is prescribed in the treatment of cardiac arrest and in certain acute hypotensive states.

■ CONTRAINDICATIONS: Hypovolemia, vascular thrombosis, or known hypersensitivity to this drug prohibits its use. It is not used in conjunction with cyclopropane or halothane anesthesia.

■ ADVERSE EFFECTS: Among the more serious adverse reactions are local tissue necrosis at the site of injection, bradycardia, headache, and hypertension.

no response (NR), the condition for which the maximum decrease in treated tumor volume is less than 50%.

norethindrone /nôreth′indrōn/, a progestin.

■ INDICATIONS: It is prescribed in the treatment of abnormal uterine bleeding and endometriosis and is a component in oral contraceptive medications.

■ CONTRAINDICATIONS: Thrombophlebitis, liver dysfunction, unusual vaginal bleeding, breast cancer, missed abortion, or known hypersensitivity to this drug prohibits its use. It is not recommended for use during pregnancy.

■ ADVERSE EFFECTS: Among the more serious adverse reactions are breakthrough bleeding, amenorrhea, GI disturbances, breast changes, and masculinization of the female fetus.

norethindrone acetate and ethinyl estradiol, an oral contraceptive.

■ INDICATIONS: It is prescribed for contraception, endometriosis, and hypermenorrhea.

■ CONTRAINDICATIONS: Thrombophlebitis, cardiovascular disease, breast or reproductive organ cancer, unusual vaginal bleeding, gallbladder disease, liver tumor, or known hypersensitivity to this drug prohibits its use. It is not given to women over 40 years of age or during lactation, pregnancy, or suspected pregnancy. It is given with caution to women who smoke.

■ ADVERSE EFFECTS: Among the more serious adverse reactions are thrombophlebitis, uterine fibroma, porphyria, embolism, jaundice, and cerebrovascular accident.

Norflex, a trademark for a skeletal muscle relaxant and antihistamine (orphenadrine citrate).

Norgesic Forte, a trademark for a fixed-combination drug containing a muscle relaxant with anticholinergic activity (orphenadrine citrate) and APC (aspirin, phenacetin, and caffeine), used for the relief of mild to moderate pain of acute musculoskeletal disorders.

norgestrel /nôrjes′trəl/, a progestin.

■ INDICATIONS: It is prescribed alone or in combination with estrogen as a contraceptive.

■ CONTRAINDICATIONS: Thrombophlebitis, liver dysfunction, unusual vaginal bleeding, breast cancer, missed abortion, or known hypersensitivity to this drug prohibits its use.

■ ADVERSE EFFECTS: Among the more serious adverse reactions are amenorrhea, dysfunctional uterine bleeding, breast changes, and masculinization of a female fetus.

Norinyl, a trademark for an oral contraceptive containing a progestin (norethindrone) and an estrogen (mestranol).

Norisodrine Hydrochloride, a trademark for an adrenergic (isoproterenol hydrochloride).

Norlac, a trademark for a nutritional supplement containing multivitamins, calcium, and iron.

Norlestrin, a trademark for an oral contraceptive containing an estrogen (ethinyl estradiol) and a progestin (norethindrone acetate).

Norlutin, a trademark for a progestin (norethindrone).

norm, a measure of a phenomenon generally accepted as the ideal standard performance against which other measures of the phenomenon may be measured.

norma basalis, the inferior surface of the base of the skull with the mandible removed, formed by the palatine bones, the vomer, the pterygoid processes, and parts of the sphenoid and temporal bones.

normal, **1.** describing a standard, average, or typical example of a set of objects or values. **2.** describing a chemical solution in which 1 L contains 1 g of a substance or the equivalent in replaceable hydrogen ions. **3.** persons in a nondiseased population. **4.** a gaussian distribution.

-normal, a combining form meaning 'relating to a norm': *centinormal, decanormal, prenormal.*

normal dental function, the correct and healthy action of opposing teeth during mastication.

normal diet. See **regular diet.**

normal dwarf. See **primordial dwarf.**

normal human serum albumin, an isotonic preparation of pooled human serum albumin for treating hypoproteinemia, hypovolemia, and threatened or existing shock.

normal hydrogen electrode (NHE), a reference electrode that is assigned a value of 0 volts.

normal phase, a chromatographic mode in which the mobile phase is less polar than the stationary phase.

normoblast /nôr′məblast/, a nucleated cell that is the normal precursor of the adult circulating erythrocyte. The developmental stages include the pronormoblast, the basophilic normoblast, the polychromatic normoblast, and the orthochromatic normoblast. After the extrusion of the nucleus of the normoblast, the young erythrocyte becomes known as a reticulocyte. Compare **erythrocyte.** See also **reticulocyte.** **–normoblastic,** *adj.*

normochromic /nôr′məkrō′mik/, pertaining to a blood cell having normal color, usually because it contains an adequate amount of hemoglobin. Compare **hypochromic.** See also **red cell indices.**

normocyte /nôr′məsīt′/, an ordinary, normal, adult red blood cell of average size having a diameter of 7 μ. Compare **macrocyte, microcyte.** **–normocytic,** *adj.*

Normosol-M, a trademark for a balanced solution of 5% dextrose in water with electrolytes.

normotensive, pertaining to the condition of having normal blood pressure. **–normotension,** *n.*

Norpace, a trademark for an antiarrhythmic cardiac depressant (disopyramide phosphate).

Norpramin, a trademark for an antidepressant (desipramine hydrochloride).

Nor-QD, a trademark for an oral contraceptive containing a progestin (norethindrone), but no estrogen.

North American blastomycosis, an infection caused by inhaling the fungus *Blastomyces dermatitidis*. It may resemble bacterial pneumonia, and x-ray films of the chest may show cavities. Painless, well-demarcated, verrucous or ulcerated skin lesions occur on the face and hands. Occasionally, lesions of the oral mucous membrane may be mistaken for squamous cell carcinoma. The disease may progress to involve bones and the brain; many viscera are infected in fatal cases. Diagnosis is made by microscopic examination of body secretions. Treatment is amphotericin B, given intravenously, or, in severe cases, a combination of amphotericin B and sulfonamides. Also called **Gilchrist's disease.** Compare **paracoccidioidomycosis.**

North American Nursing Diagnosis Association (NANDA), a professional organization of registered nurses created in 1982. The purpose of the organization is "to develop, refine, and promote a taxonomy of nursing diagnostic terminology of general use to the professional."

North Asian tick-borne rickettsiosis, an infection, acquired in the Eastern Hemisphere, caused by *Rickettsia siberica,* transmitted by ticks, and resembling Rocky Mountain spotted fever. Usual findings include a generalized maculopapular rash involving palms and soles, fever, and lymph node enlargement. It is rarely fatal and responds quickly to treatment with chloramphenicol. No vaccine is available. See also **boutonneuse fever, relapsing fever.**

North Asian tick typhus. See **Siberian tick typhus.**

nortriptyline hydrochloride, a tricyclic antidepressant.

■ INDICATION: It is prescribed in the treatment of mental depression.

■ CONTRAINDICATIONS: Concomitant administration of monoamine oxidase inhibitors, recent myocardial infarction, or known hypersensitivity to this drug or to other tricyclic medications prohibits its use. It is used with caution in patients having a seizure disorder or a cardiovascular disease.

■ ADVERSE EFFECTS: Among the more serious adverse effects are sedation and GI, cardiovascular, and neurologic reactions. This drug interacts with many other drugs.

nose, the structure that protrudes from the anterior portion of the skull and serves as a passageway for air to and from the lungs. The nose filters the air, warming, moistening, and chemically examining it for impurities that might irritate the mucous lining of the respiratory tract. The nose also contains the organ of smell, and it aids the faculty of speech. It consists of an internal portion and an external portion. The external portion, which protrudes from the face, is considerably smaller than the internal portion, which lies over the roof of the mouth. The hollow interior portion is separated into a right cavity and a left cavity by a septum. Each cavity is divided into the superior, middle, and inferior meati by the projection of nasal conchae. The external portion of the nose is perforated by two nostrils and the internal portion by two posterior nares. The pairs of sinuses that drain into the nose are the frontal, maxillary, ethmoidal, and sphenoidal sinuses. Ciliated mucous membrane lines the nose, closely adhering to the periosteum. The mucous membrane is continuous with the skin through the nares and with the mucous membrane of the nasal part of the pharynx through the choanae. The mucous membrane contains the olfactory cells that connect with the olfactory nerves.

nosebleed, abnormal hemorrhage from the nose. Emergency responses to nosebleed include seating the patient upright with the head thrust forward to prevent swallowing of blood. Pressure with both thumbs directly under the nostril and above the lips may block the main artery supplying blood to the nose. Alternatively, pressure with both forefingers on each side of the nostril often slows bleeding by blocking the main arteries and their branches. Continued bleeding may require the insertion of cotton or other absorbent material within the nostril and reapplication of pressure. Cold compresses on the nose, lips, and the back of the head may help control hemorrhage. Continued bleeding may require cautery. Also called **epistaxis.**

noso-, a combining form meaning 'of or relating to disease': *nosochthonography, nosogeny, nosophobe.*

nosocomial /nos'əkō'mē·əl/, of or pertaining to a hospital.

nosocomial infection, an infection acquired during hospitalization, often caused by *Candida albicans, Escherichia coli,* hepatitis viruses, herpes zoster virus, *Pseudomonas,* or *Staphylococcus.* Also called **hospital-acquired infection.**

nosology /nōsol'əjē/, the science of classifying diseases. See also **nomenclature.**

nostrils. See **anterior nares.**

notch, an indentation or a depression in a bone or other organ, as the auricular notch or the cardiac notch.

notifiable, pertaining to certain conditions, diseases, and events that must, by law, be reported to a governmental agency, as birth, death, smallpox, certain other communicable diseases, and certain violations of public health regulations.

noto-, a combining form meaning 'of or related to the back': *notochord, notogenesis, notomyelitis.*

notochord, an elongated strip of mesodermal tissue that originates from the primitive node and extends along the dorsal surface of the developing embryo beneath the neural tube, forming the primary longitudinal skeletal axis of the body of all chordates. In humans and other vertebrate animals, the structure is replaced by vertebrae, although a remnant of it remains as part of the nucleus pulposus of the intervertebral disks. See also **neural tube.** **–notochordal,** *adj.*

notochordal canal, a tubular passage that extends from the primitive pit into the head process during the early stages of embryonic development in mammals. It perforates the splanchnopleure layer so that there is a temporary connection between the yolk sac and the amnion. Also called **chordal canal.**

notochordal plate. See **head process.**

notogenesis, the formation of the notochord. **–notogenetic,** *adj.*

notomelus /nətom'ələs/, a congenital malformation in which one or more accessory limbs are attached to the back.

nourish, to furnish or supply the essential foods or nutrients for maintaining life.

nourishment, **1.** the act or process of nourishing or being nourished. **2.** any substance that nourishes and supports the life and growth of living organisms.

Novahistine, a trademark for a fixed-combination drug containing an antihistamine (chlorpheniramine maleate) and an adrenergic decongestant (phenylpropanolamine).

novobiocin, an antibiotic produced by the growth of *Streptomyces niveus* and other species formerly used in the treatment of infections caused by certain cocci and other gram-positive organs. Because of the toxicity of the drug there are no current valid indications for its therapeutic use.

Novocain, a trademark for a local anesthetic (procaine hydrochloride).

Novrad, a trademark for an antitussive (levopropoxyphene napsylate).

noxious /nok′shəs/, harmful, injurious, or detrimental to health.

Np, symbol for **neptunium.**

NPH Iletin, a trademark for an insulin suspension (isophane).

NPH Insulin, a trademark for an insulin suspension (isophane).

NPN, abbreviation for **nonprotein nitrogen.**

N-propyl alcohol /en′prō′pil/, a clear, colorless liquid used as a solvent for resins.

NREM, abbreviation for **nonrapid eye movement.** See **sleep.**

NSCCN, abbreviation for **National Society of Critical Care Nurses of Canada.**

NSNA, abbreviation for **National Student Nurses' Association.**

NSU, abbreviation for **nonspecific urethritis.**

Nubain, a trademark for a synthetic analgesic (nalbuphine hydrochloride), used as an adjunct to anesthesia.

nucha /no͞o′kə/, *pl.* **nuchae,** the nape, or back of the neck. **–nuchal,** *adj.*

nuchal cord, an abnormal but common condition in which the umbilical cord is wrapped around the neck of the fetus in utero or of the baby as it is being born. It is usually possible to slip the loop or loops of cord gently over the child's head. Sometimes it is a single loose loop, and the shoulders may deliver through it. If it is tight, it may be clamped in two places and cut with sterile, blunt tipped scissors. The condition occurs in more than 25% of deliveries, more often with long cords than with short ones.

Nuck's canal, Nuck's diverticulum. See **processus vaginalis peritonei.**

nucle-. See **nucleo-.**

-nuclear, a combining form meaning 'of or referring to the nucleus': *circumnuclear, endonuclear, multinuclear.*

nuclear agenesis. See **Möbius' syndrome.**

nuclear family, a family unit consisting of the biologic parents and their offspring. The nuclear family is a relatively recent product of Western society. Dissolution of a marriage results in dissolution of the nuclear family. The nuclear family unit is less efficient than an extended family unit in providing information and vital services to family members, as in child rearing, child care, and care of older family members. Because it is most often the kind of family from which doctors, nurses, social workers, teachers, and other professional people come, it is not surprising that the nuclear family is often regarded as the norm for family style. Allowances must be made for bias in a professional's attitude toward other kinds of family units that may answer the needs and expectations of other groups of people. Compare **extended family, matrifocal family.**

nuclear fission. See **fission.**

nuclear hyaloplasm. See **karyolymph.**

nuclear isomer, one of two or more nuclides with the same number of neutrons and protons in the nucleus (the same atomic number, or Z, and the same atomic mass, or A) but existing in different energy states.

nuclear magnetic resonance (NMR), **1.** a phenomenon in which the atomic nuclei of certain materials placed in a strong, static magnetic field will absorb radio waves supplied by a transmitter at particular frequencies. The energy of the radio frequency photons promotes the nucleus from a low-energy state, in which the nuclear spin is aligned parallel to the strong magnetic field, to a higher energy state in which the nuclear spin has a component transverse or opposed to the field. These nuclei will occasionally revert to the lower energy state by emitting photons at characteristic (resonance) frequencies, providing information about the local magnetic field at the nucleus. The rate at which the nuclei revert, or relax, to the lower energy state when the source of radio waves is turned off is another important factor. See also **relaxation time.** **2.** spectra emitted by phosphorus in body tissues as measured and imaged on phosphorus nuclear magnetic resonance instruments.

nuclear medicine, a medical discipline that uses radioactive isotopes in the diagnosis and treatment of disease. The major fields of nuclear medicine are physiologic function studies, radionuclide imaging, and therapeutic techniques.

nuclear sap. See **karyolymph.**

nuclear scanning, a diagnostic technique that employs an injected or ingested radioactive material and a scanning device for determining the size, shape, location, and function of various body parts. Also called **radionuclide organ imaging.**

nuclear spin, an intrinsic form of angular momentum possessed by atomic nuclei containing an odd number of nucleons (protons or neutrons).

nucleic acid /no͞oklē′ik/, a polymeric compound of high molecular weight composed of nucleotides, each consisting of a purine or pyrimidine base, a ribose or deoxyribose sugar, and a phosphate group. Nucleic acids are involved in energy storage and release and in the determination and transmission of genetic characteristics. Kinds of nucleic acid are **deoxyribonucleic acid** and **ribonucleic acid.** See also **nucleotide.**

nucleo-, nucle-, a combining form meaning 'of or related to a nucleus': *nucleochylema, nucleokeratin, nucleolus.*

nucleocapsid /no͞o′klē·ōkap′sid/, a viral enclosure consisting of a capsid or protein coat that encloses nucleic acid. Some viruses consist solely of bare nucleocapsids; others have more complex enclosures.

nucleochylema /no͞o′klē·ōkəlī′mə/, the ground substance of the nucleus, as distinguished from that of the cytoplasm.

nucleochyme. See **karyolymph.**

nucleocytoplasmic /no͞o′klē·ōsī′tōplas′mik/, of or relating to the nucleus and cytoplasm of a cell.

nucleocytoplasmic ratio, the ratio of the volume of a nucleus of a cell to the volume of the cytoplasm. The proportion is usually constant for a specific cell type, and an increase is indicative of malignant neoplasms. Also called **karyoplasmic ratio, nucleoplasmic ratio.**

nucleohistone /no͞o′klē·ōhis′tōn/, a complex nucleoprotein that consists of deoxyribonucleic acid and a histone. It is the basic constituent of the chromatin in the cell nucleus.

nucleolar organizer, a part of the nucleus of the cell, thought to consist of heterochromatin, that is responsible for the formation of the nucleolus. Also called **nucleolar zone, nucleolus organizer.**

nucleolus /no͞oklē′ələs/, *pl.* **nucleoli,** any one of the small, dense structures composed largely of ribonucleic acid and situated within the cytoplasm of cells. Nucleoli are essential in the formation of ribosomes that synthesize cell proteins.

nucleon, a collective term applied to protons and neutrons within the nucleus.

nucleoplasm /no͞o′klē·əplaz′əm/, the protoplasm of the nucleus as contrasted with that of the cell. Also called **karyoplasm.** Compare **cytoplasm.** –**nucleoplasmic,** *adj.*

nucleoplasmic ratio. See **nucleocytoplasmic ratio.**

nucleoside monophosphate kinase, a liver enzyme that catalyzes the transfer of a phosphate group from adenosine triphosphate, producing adenosine diphosphate and a nucleoside diphosphate.

nucleosome /no͞o′klē·əsōm/, any one of the repeating nucleoprotein units consisting of histones forming a complex with deoxyribonucleic acid that appear as the bead-like structures at distinct intervals along the chromosome.

5-nucleotidase, a nonlipid enzyme, elevated in some liver disorders and measured in the blood to distinguish between certain liver and bone diseases. The normal accumulations in serum are 0.1 to 6 units.

nucleotide /no͞o′klē·ətīd′/, any one of the compounds into which nucleic acid is split by the action of nuclease. A nucleotide consists of a phosphate group, a pentose sugar, and a nitrogenous base. Chains of such structures form deoxyribonucleic acid molecules essential for life.

nucleus /no͞o′klē·əs, nyo͞o′-/, **1.** the central controlling body within a living cell, usually a spheric unit enclosed in a membrane and containing genetic codes for maintaining life systems of the organism and for issuing commands for growth and reproduction. **2.** a group of nerve cells of the central nervous system having a common function, as supporting the sense of hearing or smell. **3.** the center of an atom about which electrons rotate. **4.** the central element in an organic chemical compound or class of compounds. –**nuclear,** *adj.*

nucleus pulposus, the central portion of each intervertebral disk, consisting of a pulpy elastic substance that loses some of its resiliency with age. In elderly persons, the nucleus pulposus may be suddenly compressed by unusual exertion or by trauma and squeeze out through the annular fibrocartilage, causing a herniated disk and extreme pain.

nuclide /no͞o′klīd/, a species of atom characterized by the constitution of its nucleus, in particular by the number of protons and neutrons. Thus, Co-59 and Co-60 are both isotopes of cobalt and are each nuclides. Co-60 is a radionuclide because it undergoes radioactive decay.

Nuhn's gland, an anterior lingual gland in tissues on the inferior surface and near the apex and midline of the tongue.

null cell, a lymphocyte that develops in the bone marrow and lacks the characteristic surface markers of the B and T lymphocytes. It represents a small proportion of the lymphocyte population. Stimulated by the presence of antibody, cells of this kind can apparently attack certain cellular targets directly and are known as "killer," or K cells. Compare **B cell, T cell.** See also **cytotoxin, immune gamma globulin.**

null hypothesis (H_0), (in research) a hypothesis that predicts that no difference or relationship exists among the variables studied that could not have occurred by chance alone.

nullipara /nəlip′ərə/, *pl.* **nulliparae,** a woman who has not been delivered of a viable infant. The designation "para 0" indicates nulliparity. Compare **multipara, primapara.** –**nulliparity,** *n.,* **nulliparous,** *adj.*

numbness, a partial or total lack of sensation in a part of the body, resulting from any factor that interrupts the transmission of impulses from the sensory nerve fibers. Numbness is often accompanied by tingling.

nummular dermatitis /num′yələr/, a skin disease characterized by coin-shaped, vesicular, or scaling eczema-like lesions on the forearms and the front of the calves. The cause is unknown.

Numorphan Hydrochloride, a trademark for a narcotic analgesic (oxymorphone hydrochloride).

Nupercainal, a trademark for a local anesthetic (dibucaine hydrochloride).

Nuremberg tribunal, an international tribunal planned and implemented by the United Nations War Crimes Commission to detect, apprehend, try, and punish persons accused of war crimes. In preparation for the prosecution of World War II criminals, the War Department of the United States assigned Andrew Ivy, M.D., to devise a set of principles to govern the participation of human beings in medical research. The principle and practice of informed consent was reinforced by the precedent set in the trials in which Nazi physicians were declared guilty of crimes against humanity in performing experiments on human beings who were not volunteers and did not consent. See also **Helsinki accords.**

nurse, 1. a person educated and licensed in the practice of nursing; one who is concerned with "the diagnosis and treatment of human responses to actual or potential health problems" (American Nurses' Association). The practice of the nurse includes data collection, diagnosis, planning, treatment, and evaluation within the framework of the nurse's singular concern with the patient's response to the problem, rather than to the problem itself. The concerns of the nurse are thus broader and less discrete and circumscribed than the traditional concerns of medicine. In a cooperative participatory relationship with the client or patient, the nurse acts to promote, maintain, or restore the health of the person; wellness is the goal. A collegial collaborative relationship with other health professionals who share a mission and a common data base furthers the practice of nursing. Guided by humanitarian, ethical principles, the nurse practices in a personal, nurturing, and protective manner that promotes health in all ways. The nurse may be a generalist or a specialist and, as a professional, is ethically and legally accountable for the nursing activites performed and for the actions of others to whom the nurse has delegated responsibility. **2.** to provide nursing care. See also **five step nursing process, nursing, registered nurse.**

nurse anesthetist, a registered nurse qualified by advanced training in an accredited program in the speciality of nurse anesthesia to manage the anesthetic care of the patient in certain surgical situations.

nurse-client interaction, any process in which a nurse and a client exchange or share information, verbally or nonverbally. It is fundamental to communication and is an essential component of the nursing assessment.

nurse-client relationship, a therapeutic relationship between a nurse and a client built on a series of interactions and developing over time. All interactions do not develop into relationships but may nonetheless be therapeutic. The relationship differs from a social relationship in that it is designed to meet the needs only of the client. Its structure varies with the context, the client's needs, and the goals of the nurse and the client. Its nature varies with the context, including the setting, the kind of nursing, and the needs of the client. The relationship is dynamic and uses cognitive and affective levels of interaction. It is time-limited and goal-oriented and has three phases. During the first phase, the phase of establishment, the nurse establishes the structure, purpose, timing, and context of the relationship and expresses an interest in discussing this initial structure with the client. Data collection for the nursing care plan continues, and basic goals for the relationship are stated. During the middle, developmental, phase of the relationship, the nurse and the client get to know each other better and test the structure of the relationship to be able to trust one another. The nurse is careful to assess correctly the degree of dependency that is necessary for the particular client. Plans may be devised for improved ways of coping with problems and achieving goals. The nurse is alert to the danger of losing objectivity during this phase. The last phase, termination, ideally occurs when the goals of the relationship have been accomplished, when both the client and the nurse feel a sense of resolution and satisfaction. Often this is not possible because the nurse is transferred or the client discharged; in either case both may be left with a feeling of frustration.

nurse clinician, a nurse who is prepared to identify and diagnose problems of clients by using the expanded knowledge and skills gained by advanced study in a specific area of nursing practice. The specialist may function independently within standing orders or protocols and collaborates with associates to implement a plan of care that is focused on the client.

nurse coordinator, a registered nurse who coordinates and manages the activities of nursing personnel engaged in specific nursing services, as obstetrics or surgery, for two or more patient care units.

Nurse Corps, the branch within each of the armed services comprised of the nurses within that service, as the Army Nurse Corps. In each of the armed services, the members of the Nurse Corps have the rank, title, responsibilities, and status of officer.

nurse educator, a registered nurse whose primary area of interest, competence, and professional practice is the education of nurses.

nurse midwife, a registered nurse qualified by advanced training in obstetric and neonatal care and certified by the American College of Nurse Midwives. The nurse midwife manages the perinatal care of women having a normal pregnancy, labor, and childbirth.

nurse practice act, a statute enacted by the legislature of any of the states or by the appropriate officers of the districts or possessions. The act delineates the legal scope of the practice of nursing within the geographic boundaries of the jurisdiction.

nurse practitioner, a nurse who by advanced training and clinical experience in a branch of nursing, as in a master's degree program in nursing, has acquired expert knowledge in the special branch of practice. See specific kinds of nurse practitioner.

nursery diarrhea, diarrhea of the newborn. In nurseries, outbreaks of diarrhea caused by *Escherichia coli, Salmonella,* echoviruses, or adenoviruses are potentially life-threatening to the infant. The neonate may be infected at the time of birth by organisms from the mother's stool or infected later by organisms spread by the hands of hospital personnel. Fluid loss is the most serious aspect of the disease, leading to dehydration and electrolyte imbalance. Care includes maintaining fluid and electrolyte balance and administration of antibiotics, if appropriate. Good handwashing technique, use of disposable nursing bottles and nipples, and early isolation of infected infants reduce the possibility of such outbreaks.

nurse's aide, a person who is employed to carry out basic nonspecialized tasks in the care of a patient, as bathing and feeding, making beds, and transporting patients. Many hospitals offer extensive training and orientation programs for newly hired nurse's aides and inservice education for continued training.

Nurses' Association of the American College of Obstetrics and Gynecology (NAACOG), a national organization of nurses who work in obstetrics and gynecology. It functions in close association with the American College of Obstetrics and Gynecology.

Nurses' Coalition for Action in Politics (N-CAP), an organization that works in association with the American Nurses' Association. It raises funds for political contributions to candidates for public office at the state and national levels.

nurse's registry, an employment agency or listing service for nurses who wish to work in a specific area of nursing, usually for a short period of time or on a per diem basis.

nurses' station, an area in a clinic, unit, or ward in a health care facility that serves as the administrative center for nursing care for a particular group of patients. It is usually centrally located and may be staffed by a ward secretary or clerk who assists with paperwork and telephone and other communication. Before going on duty, nurses usually meet there to receive daily assignments, to review the patients' charts, and to update the Kardex. In a critical care unit of a large teaching hospital, the nurses' station may also contain panels of visual display terminals that allow centralized monitoring of many patients and may also have computer terminals that allow access to information in the patients' records or to a data bank of clinical information. In other parts of a hospital, the nurses' station is equipped in any of various ways appropriate to the care of the patients in that area or unit.

nurse therapist model, (in psychiatric nursing research) a theoretic framework to clarify the role of the mental health nurse. Techniques from traditional and contemporary modes of treatment, including transactional analysis and crisis intervention, may be used singly or in various combinations. The nurse therapist chooses the technique or techniques after using the model to examine the nurse-client interaction, the feedback, and the goal of the interaction.

nursing, **1.** the practice in which a nurse assists "the individual, sick or well, in the performance of those activities contributing to health or its recovery (or to a peaceful death) that he would perform unaided if he had the necessary strength, will or knowledge. And to do this in such a way as to help him gain independence as rapidly as possible." (Virginia Henderson) **2.** "the diagnosis and treatment of human responses to actual or potential health problems," (American Nurses' Association). There are four principal characteristics that further define nursing care: the phenomena that concern nurses; the use of theories to observe the need for nursing intervention and to plan nursing action; the nursing action taken; and an evaluation of the effects of the actions relative to the phenomena. This definition of nursing provides a framework for the nursing process including data collection, diagnosis, planning, treatment, and evaluation. The nursing process is supported by standards of nursing practice that are congruent with the definition and that provide more specific guidelines for practice. These standards include systematic, continuous collection of data concerning the health status of the client in recorded form that is accessible and that may be communicated. A nursing diagnosis is derived from the data collected. A plan for nursing care incorporates goals derived from the nursing diagnosis and the priorities and approaches to achieve the goals as indicated by the nursing diagnosis. Nursing actions, which are selected and performed with the client's participation, provide for the promotion, maintenance, or restoration of the health of the client and serve to maximize the health care abilities of the client. The progress or lack of progress toward the goal is mutually determined by the client and the nurse, resulting in reassessment, reordering of priorities, establishment of new goals, and revision of the plan for nursing care. Nursing touches on, intersects with, and complements other professional roles in health care, addressing itself to a wide range of health-related responses in people who are well and in those who are not. Nursing seeks to diagnose and treat the response to the problem; thus the concerns of nursing are less circumscribed and discrete than those of other health-related professions. These concerns include the following: limitations of the client's self-care ability; impaired ability to function in any fundamental area, as sleeping, breathing, eating, maintaining circulation, pain; anxiety, fear, loneliness, grief, or other physical or emotional problems related to health, illness, or treatment; impaired social or intellectual processes; impaired ability to make decisions and choices; alteration of self-image as required by the change in health; dysfunctional perception of health or health care activities; extra demands posed by such normal life processes as birth, growth, or death; and difficulty in affiliative relationships. Various concepts, principles, processes, and actions, developed and examined in nursing research, guide the steps in the nursing process, from initial observation and diagnosis through evaluation based on intrapersonal, interpersonal, and systems theories. The boundary for nursing practice is not static: it tends to move outward as the needs and capacities of society change. Collegial, collaborative practice with other health care professions further softens the boundaries of nursing practice. All health care professionals share a mission and a scientific data base, and to some degree their practices overlap. At its core, nursing is nurturative, generative, and protective; preventive care is a part of every nurse's practice. Nurses value independence and self-respect; they are guided by an ethical and humanitarian philosophy in which every human being deserves respect regardless of racial, social, cultural, sexual, economic, religious, or other factors. The nurse practices in the context of a relationship with the client, family, or group that is professional and yet close, in an interpersonal sense. The function of a nurse involves the physical intimacy of laying-on of hands; compassion and constant recognition of the person's dignity are essential. Nursing is practiced by specialists and by generalists; generalists provide most nursing care; specialists, having added to their knowledge of an organized and systematized body of knowledge and competencies, practice in specialized areas of nursing. Nursing care is given to people at all stages of life, in the home, hospital, place of employment, or school or other environment where nursing care is needed. Nurses are ethically and legally accountable for their practice and for the actions of others to whom they have delegated responsibility. **3.** the professional practice of a nurse. **4.** the process of acting as a nurse, of providing care that encourages and promotes the health of the person being served. See also **nursing process.**

nursing assessment, an identification by a nurse of the needs, preferences, and abilities of a patient. Assessment follows an interview with and observation of a patient by the nurse and considers the symptoms and signs of the condition, the patient's verbal and nonverbal communication, medical and social history, and any other information available. Among the physical aspects assessed are vital signs, skin color and condition, motor and sensory nerve function, nutrition, rest, sleep, activity, elimination, and conciousness. Among the social and emotional factors assessed are religion, occupation, attitude toward hospital and health care, mood, emotional tone, and family ties and responsibilities. Assessment is extremely important because it provides the scientific basis for a complete nursing care plan.

nursing assistant, *Canada.* a person trained in basic nursing techniques and direct patient care who practices under the supervision of a registered nurse.

nursing audit, a thorough investigation designed to identify, examine, or verify the performance of certain specified aspects of nursing care using established criteria. A **concurrent nursing audit** is performed during ongoing nursing care. A **retrospective nursing audit** is performed after discharge from the care facility, using the patient's record. Often, a nursing audit and a medical audit are performed collaboratively, resulting in a **joint audit.**

nursing bottle caries, a dental condition that occurs in children between 18 months and 3 years of age as a result of being given a bottle at bedtime, resulting in prolonged exposure of the teeth to milk or juice. Caries are formed because pools of milk or juice in the mouth break down to lactic acid and other decay-causing substances. Preventive measures include elimination of the bedtime feeding or substitution of water for milk or juice in the nighttime bottle. Also called **bottle mouth syndrome.**

nursing care plan, a plan that is based on a nursing assessment and a nursing diagnosis, devised by a nurse. It has four essential components: identification of the nursing care problems and a statement of the nursing approach to solve those problems; the statement of the expected benefit to the patient; the statement of the specific actions by the nurse that reflect the nursing approach and achieve the goals specified; and the evaluation of the patient's response to nursing care and the readjustment of that care as required. The nursing care plan is begun when the patient is admitted to the health service, and, after the initial nursing assessment, a diagnosis is formulated and nursing orders are developed. The goal of the process is to ensure that nursing care is consistent with the patient's needs and progress toward self-care. A written nursing care plan should be a part of every patient's chart; an abbreviated form should be available for quick reference, as in a Rand or Kardex file. See also **diagnosis, nursing assessment, nursing diagnosis, nursing orders, problem-solving approach to patient centered care.**

nursing diagnosis, a statement of a health problem or of a potential problem in the client's health status that a nurse is licensed and competent to treat. Four steps are required in the formulation of a nursing diagnosis: A data base is established by collecting information from all available sources, including interviews with the client and the client's family, a review of any existing records of the client's health, observation of the response of the client to any alterations in health status, a physical assessment, and a conference or consultation with others concerned in the care of the client. The data base is continually updated. The second step includes an analysis of the client's responses to the problems, healthy or unhealthy, and a classification of those responses as psychologic, physiologic, spiritual, or sociologic. The third step is the organization of the data so that a tentative diagnostic statement can be made that summarizes the pattern of problems discovered. The last step is the confirmation of the sufficiency and accuracy of the data base by evaluation of the appropriateness of the diagnosis to nursing intervention and by the assurance that, given the same information, most other qualified practitioners would arrive at the same nursing diagnosis. In use, each diagnostic category has three parts: the term that concisely describes the problem, the probable cause of the problem, and the defining characteristics of the problem. A number of nursing diagnoses have been identified and are listed as accepted by the National Group on Classification of Nursing Diagnoses, updated and refined at periodic meetings of the group. The nursing diagnoses accepted at the Fourth and the Fifth National Conferences are the following:

activity intolerance
activity intolerance: potential
airway clearance, ineffective
anxiety
bowel elimination, alteration in: constipation
bowel elimination, alteration in: diarrhea
bowel elimination, alteration in: incontinence
breathing pattern, ineffective
cardiac output, alteration in: decreased
comfort, alteration in: pain
communication, impaired: verbal
coping, family: potential for growth
coping, ineffective family: compromised
coping, ineffective family: disabling
coping, ineffective individual
diversional activity, deficit
family process, alteration in
fear
fluid volume, alteration in: excess
fluid volume deficit, actual
fluid volume deficit, potential

gas exchange, impaired
grieving, anticipatory
grieving, dysfunctional
health maintenance, alteration in
home maintenance management, impaired
injury: potential for
knowledge deficit
mobility, impaired physical
noncompliance
nutrition, alteration in: less than body requirements
nutrition, alteration in: more than body requirements
nutrition, alteration in: potential for more than body requirements
oral mucous membrane, alterations in
parenting, alteration in: actual
parenting, alteration in: potential
powerlessness
rape trauma syndrome
self-care deficit: feeding, bathing/hygiene, dressing/grooming, toileting
self-concept, disturbance in: body image, self-esteem, role performance, personal identity
sensory-perceptual alteration: visual, auditory, kinesthetic, gustatory, tactile, olfactory
sexual dysfunction
skin integrity, impairment of: actual
skin integrity, impairment of: potential
sleep pattern disturbance
social isolation
spiritual distress (distress of the human spirit)
thought processes, alteration in
tissue perfusion, alteration in: cerebral, cardiopulmonary, renal, gastrointestinal, peripheral
urinary elimination, alteration in patterns
violence, potential for: self-directed or directed at others

nursing differential, an allowance added to payments to hospitals for services rendered Medicare patients in recognition of the cost of providing nursing services to such patients that is greater than the cost to the general patient population.

nursing goal, a general goal of nursing involving activities that are desirable but difficult to measure, as self-care, good nutrition, and relaxation. Compare **nursing objective.**

nursing home. See **extended care facility.**

nursing intervention, any act by a nurse that implements the nursing care plan or any specific objective of that plan, as turning a comatose patient to avoid the development of decubitus ulcers or teaching injection technique to a patient with diabetes before discharge from the hospital. The patient may require intervention in the form of support, limitation, medication, or treatment for the current condition or to prevent the development of further stress. As stress increases, the need to adapt and the need for nursing intervention increase. See also **adaptation, stress.**

nursing intervention model, (in nursing research) a conceptual framework used to determine appropriate nursing interventions. The model is a holistic representation of the client and the health care system. The client's physiologic, psychologic, sociocultural, and developmental status, the client's stressors and ability to react to them, and the levels and patterns of available health care are observed. The goal is to learn what nursing interventions would be most effective for the particular problem within the particular health care system.

nursing objective, a specific aim planned by a nurse to decrease a person's stress, or improve the ability to adapt, or both. A nursing objective may be physical, emotional, social, or cultural and may involve the person's family, friends, and other patients. It is the purpose of any specific nursing order or nursing intervention. Some common nursing objectives are adequate understanding by the patient of certain details of the condition, adequate and comfortable daily elimination, a certain amount of rest, a balanced diet, and participation in specific items of self-care. Nursing objectives, contrasted with nursing goals, can be measured. Compare **nursing goal.**

nursing observation, an objective, holistic evaluation made by a nurse of the various aspects of a client's condition. It includes the person's general appearance, emotional affect, and nutritional status, habits, and preferences, as well as body temperature, skin condition, and any obvious abnormal processes, including those complained of by the client. The client's religious preference, ethnic background, and familial relationships are also noted. Compare **nursing assessment, nursing intervention.**

nursing orders, specific instructions for implementing the nursing care plan, including the patient's preferences, timing of activities, details of health education necessary for the particular patient, role of the family, and plans for care after discharge. Nursing orders must be signed by the professional nurse who writes them. They should not duplicate the orders of the medical staff or of other members of the health team.

nursing process, the process that serves as an organizational framework for the practice of nursing. It encompasses all of the steps taken by the nurse in caring for a patient: data collection, diagnosis, planning, treatment, and evaluation. The rationale for each step is founded in nursing theory. The process requires a systematic approach to a nursing assessment of the person's situation, including an evaluation and reconciliation of the perceptions by the person, the person's family, and the nurse. A plan for the nursing actions to be taken may then be made, and, with the participation of the person and the person's family, the plan may be set. The plan developed with the person and the person's family is then implemented. Evaluation of the outcome is performed with the person and the person's family. The steps follow each other at the start of the process but may need to be taken concurrently in some situations. The process does not reach completion with evaluation; the steps are begun again, allowing recurrent evaluation of the assessment, plan, goals, and actions. See also **five step nursing process, nursing.**

nursing process model, a conceptual framework in which the nurse-patient relationship is the basis of the nursing process. The nursing process is represented as dynamic and interpersonal, the nurse and the patient being affected by each other's behavior and by the environment around them. Each successful two-way communication is termed a ''transaction'' and can be analyzed to discover the factors that promote transactions. The constraints that the various systems in the environment (personal, interpersonal, and social) place on the development of the relationship are also examined. The nurse views the patient as a person with whom to communicate to have transactions that achieve defined adaptive objectives toward the goal of health.

nursing research, a detailed process in which a systematic study of a problem in the field of nursing is performed. One basic approach requires the following steps: formulation of the problem; review of the literature; development of a theory; formation of a hypothesis or hypotheses; definition of variables; determination of a method for weighting and counting variables; selection of a research design; choice of a population; plan for the analysis of the data; determination of interpretation; and plan for promulgation of the results. Nursing research is practice- or discipline-oriented and is essential for the continued development of the scientific aspects of professional nursing.

Nursing Research, a bimonthly refereed journal containing papers and other materials concerning nursing research. The goal of the journal is to stimulate research in nursing.

nursing rounds, chart rounds, walking rounds, teaching rounds, or grand rounds that are held specifically for nurses and that focus on nursing care problems. See also **rounds.**

nursing specialty, a nurse's particular professional field of practice, as surgical, pediatric, obstetric, or psychiatric nursing. Compare **subspecialty.**

nursing supervisor, a nurse whose function is the administrative and clinical leadership of the nursing service of a division of a health care facility, as a nursing supervisor of maternal and infant care nurses.

nursology /nursol′əjē/, a conceptual framework for the study and practice of nursing. It requires the nurse to interact with the patient in an ''authentic'' way, without aloofness and the distance of professionalism; the nurse must take the risk of caring. The patient as a person is perceived as a ''subject'' rather than an ''object''; the relationship is described as ''intersubjective,'' and the parties to the relationship as ''nurse-nursed.'' As a method, nursology requires that the nurse cut through the defenses and fears that prevent self-knowledge. The nurse tries to know the patient on an intuitive, subjective level and then, using reflection, on an objective, scientific level. The nurse recognizes that each person has an ''angular view'' of the whole truth; comparison of the views of others is necessary for a perspective that allows a synthesis, often paradoxical but closer to the truth than any one person's angular view. The nurse must then struggle with the multiple views to arrive at a final synthesis. This process is called a progression from ''we to paradoxical one.'' Nursology is intended to provide a model for nursing methods and for research. The nurse and the patient have the opportunity to grow, while the science of nursing may emerge from the ''angular'' investigations and syntheses.

Nursoy, a trademark for a hypoallergenic nutritional supplement for infants.

nutation, the act of nodding, especially involuntary nodding as occurs in some neurologic disorders.

Nutramigen, a trademark for a milk-substitute formula that is prepared from a soy isolate base and is lactose free, prescribed for infants with galactosemia and as a protein supplement for people with lactose intolerance. See also **Neo-Mull-Soy, Pro Sobee, Soyalac.**

nutri-, a combining form meaning 'of or related to nourishment': *nutriceptor, nutrient, nutritorium.*

nutrient, a substance that provides nourishment and affects the nutritive and metabolic processes of the body.

nutrient artery of the humerus, one of a pair of branches of the deep brachial arteries, arising near the middle of the arm and entering the nutrient canal of the humerus.

nutrient canal. See interdental canal.

nutriment, any substance that nourishes and aids the growth and the development of the body. See also **food.**

nutrition, **1.** nourishment. **2.** the sum of the processes involved in the taking in of nutrients and in their assimilation and use for proper body functioning and maintenance of health. The successive stages include ingestion, digestion, absorption, assimilation, and excretion. **3.** the study of food and drink as related to the growth and maintenance of living organisms.

nutritional alcoholic cerebellar degeneration. See **alcoholic nutritional cerebellar degeneration.**

nutritional anemia, a disorder characterized by the inadequate production of hemoglobin or erythrocytes caused by a nutritional deficiency of iron, folic acid, or vitamin B_{12}, or other nutritional disorders. See also **iron deficiency anemia, megaloblastic anemia, pernicious anemia.**

nutritional care, the substances, procedures, and setting involved in assuring the proper intake and assimilation of nutriments, especially for the hospitalized patient.

■ METHOD: Depending on the patient's condition, nutritional requirements may be provided by regular meals with menus selected from the ordered diet, by tube feeding, or by parenteral hyperalimentation. Meals are served on attractive trays in an environment conducive to eating; distasteful procedures are avoided before and after mealtime. Patients who are unable to feed themselves are assisted, and abnormal intake of food is recorded and reported. Supplemental nourishment when indicated and fluids are offered between meals. The nutritional assessment includes observations of the patient's appetite, food preferences, height, weight, measurements of the head, arms, abdomen, and skinfold thickness, the skin color and turgor, and the condition of the mouth, eyes, and hair. Any cutaneous lesions, thyroid enlargement, dental caries, loose teeth, ill-fitting dentures, gum problems, nausea, vomiting, dehydration, diarrhea, or constipation are noted.

■ NURSING ORDERS: The nurse sees that food is presented attractively, offers a washcloth and mouthwash before and after meals, and, when necessary, feeds the patient to maintain an adequate intake. If indicated, as in obese patients or those with disorders requiring a highly restricted diet, the nurse restricts the intake of food as ordered. Tube feedings are administered as ordered.

■ OUTCOME CRITERIA: Obvious good health, a normal weight, and the absence of GI symptoms usually indicate that the individual's nutritional requirements are being fulfilled.

nutrition, alteration in: less than body requirements, a nursing diagnosis accepted by the Fourth National Conference on Nursing Diagnoses. The cause of the condition is an inability, based on psychologic, biologic, or economic factors, to ingest or to digest food or to absorb nutrients in sufficient quantity for the maintenance of normal health. The defining characteristics of the condition may include loss of weight, reported intake of less food than is recommended, evidence or report of a lack of food, lack of interest in food, aversion to eating, alteration in the taste of food, feelings of fullness immediately after eating small quantities, abdominal pain with no other explanation, sores in the mouth, diarrhea or steatorrhea, pallor, weakness, and loss of hair. See also **nursing diagnosis.**

nutrition, alteration in: more than body requirements, a nursing diagnosis accepted by the Fourth National Conference on the Classification of Nursing Diagnoses. The cause of the condition is an excessive intake of food in relation to the metabolic needs of the body. The defining characteristics of the condition include overweight, sedentary activity level, and dysfunctional eating habits, including eating in response to internal cues other than hunger. The critical defining characteristics, one of which must be present for the diagnosis to be made, include weight gain of 20% greater than the ideal for the height and body build of the client, and triceps skin fold measurements greater than 15 mm in men and 25 mm in women. See also **nursing diagnosis.**

nutrition, alteration in: potential for more than body requirements, a nursing diagnosis accepted by the Fourth National Conference on the Classification of Nursing Diagnoses. The cause of the condition may be an inherited or familial predisposition to overweight, an excessive intake of calories during adolescence and other periods of rapid growth, frequent, closely spaced pregnancies, dysfunctional psychologic conditioning in regard to food, or membership in a lower socioeconomic group. The defining characteristics of the problem may include the use of solid foods as a significant part of the diet before 5 months of age, the use of food as a reward, an observed increase in the baseline weight at the onset of each pregnancy, or dysfunctional eating patterns, as eating in response to external cues such as social situations or the time of day. The critical defining characteristics that must be present for the diagnosis to be made include reported or observed obesity in one or both parents and rapidly increasing percentiles in measurement of the infant's or child's weight as compared with others of the same age. See also **nursing diagnosis.**

nutritionist, one who studies and applies the principles and science of nutrition.

Nutting, Mary Adelaide (1858–1947), a Canadian-born American nursing educator and reformer. As head of Johns Hopkins School of Nursing in Baltimore, beginning in 1894, she improved course content and teaching facilities, instituted the 6-months preparatory course, reduced the 12-hour day to 8 hours, and abolished the monthly payment system to students. At Teachers College, Columbia University, she created and developed the Department of Nursing and Health and became the first professor of nursing in the world. With Lavinia Dock, she wrote *History of Nursing,* a classic in nursing literature.

nyctalopia /nik'təlō'pē·ə/, poor vision at night or in dim light resulting from decreased synthesis of rhodopsin, vitamin A deficiency, retinal degeneration, or a congenital defect. Also called **day sight, night blindness.** –**nyctalopic,** *adj.*

nycto-, a combining form meaning 'pertaining to night or darkness': *nyctohemeral, nyctophilia, nyctophobia.*

nyctophobia /nik'tō-/, an anxiety reaction characterized by an obsessive, irrational fear of darkness.

nycturia. See **nocturia.**

Nydrazid, a trademark for an antibacterial (isoniazid).

nylidrin hydrochloride /nil'idrin/, a peripheral vasodilator.

■ INDICATIONS: It is prescribed in the treatment of peripheral vascular disease and circulatory disturbances of the inner ear.

■ CONTRAINDICATIONS: Acute cardiac disease, paroxysmal tachycardia, thyrotoxicosis, progressive angina pectoris, or known hypersensitivity to this drug prohibits its use.

■ ADVERSE EFFECTS: The most serious adverse reaction is hypotention with dizziness, tachycardia, nausea, and weakness.

Nylmerate, a trademark for an antimicrobial (phenylmercuric nitrate).

nympho-, a combining form meaning 'of or pertaining to the labia minora': *nymphocaruncular, nymphohymeneal, nymphoncus.*

nymphomania, a psychosexual disorder of women characterized by an insatiable desire for sexual satisfaction, often resulting from an unconscious conflict concerning personal adequacy. Compare **satyriasis.** See also **psychosexual disorder.**

nymphomaniac, **1.** a person with or displaying characteristics of nymphomania. **2.** of, pertaining to, or exhibiting nymphomania. **–nymphomaniacal,** *adj.*

Nystaform, a trademark for a topical, fixed-combination drug containing an antifungal (nystatin) and a topical antiinfective (iodochlorhydroxyquin).

nystagmus /nīstag′məs/, involuntary, rhythmic movements of the eyes; the oscillations may be horizontal, vertical, rotary, or mixed. Jerking nystagmus, characterized by faster movements in one direction than in the opposite direction, is more common than pendular nystagmus, in which the oscillations are approximately equal in rate in both directions. Jerking nystagmus occurs normally when an individual watches a moving object, but, on other occasions, it may be a sign of barbiturate intoxication or of labyrinthine vestibular, vascular,or neurologic disease. Labyrinthine vestibular nystagmus, most frequently rotary, is usually accompanied by vertigo and nausea. Vertical nystagmus is considered pathognomonic of disease of the brainstem's tegmentum, and nystagmus occurring only in the abducting eye is said to be a sign of multiple sclerosis. Seesaw nystagmus, in which one eye moves up and the other down, may be seen in bilateral hemianopia. Pendular nystagmus occurs in albinism, various diseases of the retina and refractive media, and in miners, after many years of working in darkness; in miners, the eye movements are very rapid, increase on upward gaze, and are often associated with vertigo, head tremor, and photophobia. Electronystagmography, used in testing for vestibular disease and in evaluating patients with vertigo, hearing loss, or tinnitus, records changes in the electric field around the eyes when nystagmus is induced by douching cold or warm water into the external auditory canal; this test causes nystagmus in normal individuals and a diminished or absent reaction in patients with labyrinth disorder. Also called **nystaxis.** **–nystagmic,** *adj.*

nystatin /nis′tətin/, an antifungal antibiotic.

■ INDICATIONS: It is prescribed in the treatment of fungal infections of the GI tract, vagina, and skin.

■ CONTRAINDICATION: Known hypersensitivity to this drug is the only contraindication.

■ ADVERSE EFFECTS: There are no known serious adverse reactions. Mild GI distress and mild skin reactions may occur.

nystaxis. See **nystagmus.**

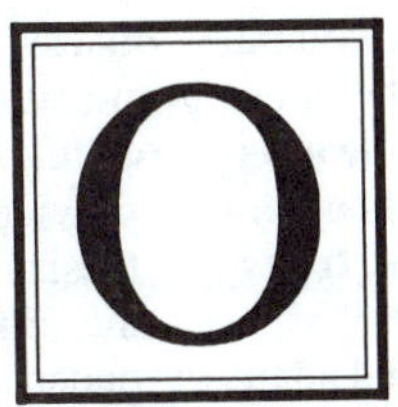

O, symbol for **oxygen atom.**

O_2, symbol for **oxygen molecule.**

oario-. See **ovario-.**

OASDHI, abbreviation for **Old Age, Survivors, Disability and Health Insurance Program.**

oat cell carcinoma, a malignant, usually bronchogenic epithelial neoplasm consisting of small, tightly packed, round, oval, or spindle-shaped epithelial cells that stain darkly and contain neurosecretory granules and little or no cytoplasm. Tumors produced by these cells do not form bulky masses but usually spread along submucosal lymphatics. One third of all malignant tumors of the lung are of this type. Usually surgical resection is not possible, and chemotherapy and radiation therapy are not effective in treatment; thus, the prognosis is poor. Also called **small cell carcinoma.**

OB, *informal.* **1.** abbreviation for **obstetrician. 2.** abbreviation for **obstetrics.**

ob-, oc-, a combining form meaning 'against, in front of': *obdormition, obduction, obtuse.*

obesity, an abnormal increase in the proportion of fat cells, mainly in the viscera and subcutaneous tissues of the body. Obesity may be exogenous or endogenous.

Obetrol, a trademark for a fixed-combination drug containing central nervous system stimulants (dextroamphetamine and amphetamine).

OBG, abbreviation for **obstetrics and gynecology.**

OB-Gyn, *informal.* abbreviation for **obstetrics and gynecology.**

objective, 1. a goal. **2.** of or pertaining to a phenomenon or clinical finding that is observed; not subjective. An objective finding is often described in health care as a sign, as distinguished from a symptom, which is a subjective finding.

objective data collection, the process in which data relating to the client's problem are obtained by an observer through direct physical examination, including observation, palpation, and auscultation, and by laboratory analyses and radiologic and other studies. Compare **subjective data collection.**

obligate /ob′ligit, -gāt/, characterized by the ability to survive only in a particular set of environmental conditions, as an obligate parasite, which can survive only within the host organism. Compare **facultative.**

obligate aerobe, an organism that cannot grow in the absence of oxygen. Compare **facultative aerobe.** See also **aerobe.**

obligate anaerobe, an organism that cannot grow in the presence of oxygen, as *Clostridium tetani, C. botulinum, and C. perfringens.* Compare **facultative anaerobe.** See also **anaerobe, anaerobic infection.**

obligate parasite. See **parasite.**

oblique, a slanting direction or any variation from the perpendicular or the horizontal.

oblique bandage, a circular bandage applied spirally in slanting turns, usually to a limb.

oblique fiber, (in dentistry) any one of the collagenous fibers that are bundled together obliquely in the periodontal ligament, insert into the cementum, and extend more occlusally in the alveolus, comprising approximately two thirds of the periodontal fibers.

oblique fissure of the lung, 1. the groove marking the division of the lower and the middle lobes in the right lung. **2.** the groove marking the division of the upper and the lower lobes in the left lung.

oblique fracture, a fracture that cracks a bone at an oblique angle.

oblique illumination. See **illumination.**

obliquus externus abdominis, one of a pair of muscles that are the largest and the most superficial of the five anterolateral muscles of the abdomen. A broad, thin, four-sided muscle that arises by eight fleshy digitations from the lower eight ribs and by the broad abdominal aponeurosis, it inserts in the iliac crest and the linea alba. It is innervated by branches of the eighth through the twelfth intercostal nerves and by the iliohypogastric and ilioinguinal nerves. It acts to compress the contents of the abdomen and assists in micturition, defecation, emesis, parturition, and forced expiration. Both sides acting together serve to flex the vertebral column, drawing the pubis toward the xiphoid process. One side alone functions to bend the vertebral column laterally and to rotate it, drawing the shoulder of the same side forward. Also called **descending oblique muscle, external oblique muscle.** Compare **obliquus internus abdominis, pyramidalis, rectus abdominis, transversus abdominis.**

obliquus internus abdominis, one of a pair of anterolateral muscles of the abdomen, lying under the obliquus externus abdominis in the lateral and ventral part of the abdominal wall. Smaller and thinner than the obliquus externus abdominis, it arises from the inguinal ligament, the iliac crest, and the lower portion of the lumbar aponeurosis. It inserts into the last three or four ribs and into the linea alba. The obliquus internus abdominis functions to compress the abdominal contents and assists in micturition, defecation, emesis, parturition, and forced expiration. Both sides acting together serve to flex the vertebral column, drawing the costal cartilages toward the pubis.

One side acting alone acts to bend the vertebral column laterally and rotate it, drawing the shoulder of the opposite side downward. Also called **ascending oblique muscle, internal oblique muscle.** Compare **obliquus externus abdominis, pyramidalis, rectus abdominis, transversus abdominis.**

observation, **1.** the act of watching carefully and attentively. **2.** a report of what is seen or noticed, as a nursing observation.

obsession, a persistent thought or idea with which the mind is continually and involuntarily preoccupied and which suggests an irrational act. The thought cannot be eliminated by logic or reason and usually gives rise to a compulsion. See also **compulsion, obsessive-compulsive neurosis.** **–obsessive,** *adj.*

obsessional personality, a type of personality in which persistent, intrusive, irrational, uncontrollable, and unwanted thoughts lead to compulsive actions. The thoughts may consist of single words, simple ideas or desires, images, ruminations, or, more commonly, a complex train of ideas referring to past events and completed actions or to anticipated events and future actions. A person with an obsessional personality is punctual, orderly, meticulous, and dependable, is dominated by feelings of inadequacy, insecurity, and guilt, and is highly vulnerable to threat, worry, indecision, overscrupulousness, and excessive anxiety.

obsessive-compulsive, **1.** characterized by or relating to the tendency to perform repetitive acts or rituals, usually as a means of releasing tension or relieving anxiety. **2.** describing a person who has an obsessive-compulsive neurosis.

obsessive-compulsive neurosis, a neurotic condition characterized by the inability to resist or stop the intrusion of persistent, irrational, and uncontrollable urges, ideas, thoughts, or fears contrary to the person's standards or judgments. The disorder usually appears after adolescence, resulting from fear, feelings of guilt, and anticipation of punishment. Treatment may consist of psychotherapy to uncover the basic fears and to help the person distinguish objective dangers from imagined dangers. Also called **psychasthenia.**

obsessive-compulsive personality, a type of personality in which there is an uncontrollable need to perform certain acts or rituals. This behavior is manifested in many forms and may range from mildly stylized personal habits, as repeating certain words or phrases before undertaking a particular act or ritually counting and touching, to more serious compulsive acts, as the continous washing of hands or changing of clothes. A person with this kind of personality is usually orderly, meticulous, punctual, dependable, and scrupulous, though with a tendency to be rigid, stubborn, and pedantic. When the acts or rituals become irrational and exaggerated, they reduce the flexibility of behavior and interfere with everyday functioning in society, becoming neurotic reactions.

obsessive-compulsive reaction. See **obsessive-compulsive neurosis.**

obstetric anesthesia, any of various procedures used to provide anesthesia for childbirth. It includes local anesthesia for episiotomy or episiotomy repair, regional anesthesia for labor or delivery, as by paracervical block or pudendal block, or, for a wider block—epidural, caudal, or saddle block. Anesthesia for cesarean section may be achieved with an epidural block or by general anesthesia. Light inhalation anesthesia with a mixture of nitrous oxide and oxygen is commonly given when forceps are required or when a difficult vaginal delivery is expected.

obstetric forceps, forceps used to assist delivery of the fetal head. They vary in weight, length, shape, and mechanism of action, but all consist of a pair of instruments comprising a handle, a shank, and a blade. The blade is curved and, sometimes, fenestrated. The shank is long enough to allow the blade to reach the fetal head. The several styles of forceps are designed to assist in various clinical situations. The station of the fetus in the pelvis, the position of the head in relation to the pelvis, the size of the fetus, and the preference of the operator all affect the choice of forceps. Kinds of obstetric forceps include **Barton forceps, Elliot forceps, Kielland forceps,** and **Simpson forceps.** See also **forceps delivery.**

obstetrician, a physician who specializes in obstetrics.

obstetric position. See **lateral recumbent position.**

obstetrics, the branch of medicine concerned with pregnancy and childbirth, including the study of the physiologic and pathologic function of the female reproductive tract and the care of the mother and fetus throughout pregnancy, childbirth, and the immediate postpartum period. **–obstetric, obstetrical,** *adj.*

obstetrix. See **midwife.**

obstipation, **1.** a condition of extreme and persistent constipation caused by obstruction in the intestinal or eliminatory system. See also **constipation.** **2.** a process of blocking. **–obstipant,** *n.,* **obstipate,** *v.*

obstruction, **1.** something that blocks or clogs. **2.** the act of blocking or preventing passage. **3.** the condition of being obstructed or clogged. **–obstruct,** *v.,* **obstructive,** *adj.*

obstructive airways disease, any clinically important obstruction of the respiratory tract that may be associated with symptoms of chronic bronchitis, abnormalities of the bronchi, and emphysema. See also **acute bronchitis, bronchial asthma, chronic obstructive pulmonary disease, cystic fibrosis.**

obstructive anuria, an abnormal urologic condition characterized by an almost complete absence of urination and caused by an obstruction of the urinary tract. See also **obstructive uropathy.**

obstructive jaundice. See **cholestasis.**

obstructive uropathy, any pathologic condition that results in obstruction of the flow of urine. The condition may lead to impairment of kidney function and an increased risk of urinary infection.

obtund /obtund′/, **1.** to deaden pain. **2.** to render insensitive to unpleasant or painful stimuli by reducing the level of consciousness, as by anesthesia or a strong narcotic analgesic. **–obtundation, obtundity,** *n.*, **obtunded, obtundent,** *adj.*

obtundation, the use of an agent that soothes and reduces irritation or pain by blocking sensibility at some level of the central nervous system, as in the preoperative use of anesthesia, the use of narcotics to control pain, and the giving of a tranquilizer as a calming agent.

obturator /ob′tərā′tər, ob′tyərā′tər/, **1.** a device used to block a passage or a canal or to fill in a space, as a prosthesis implanted to bridge the gap in the roof of the mouth in a cleft palate. **2.** *nontechnical.* an obturator muscle or membrane.

obturator externus, the flat, triangular muscle covering the outer surface of the anterior wall of the pelvis. It arises in several pelvic structures, including the rami of the pubis and the ramus of each ischium, and inserts into the trochanteric fossa of the femur. The obturator externus is innervated by a branch of the obturator nerve, which contains fibers of the third and the fourth lumbar nerves, and it functions to rotate the thigh laterally. Compare **obturator internus.**

obturator foramen, a large opening on each side of the lower portion of the hip bone, formed posteriorly by the ischium, superiorly by the illium, and anteriorly by the pubis.

obturator internus, a muscle that covers a large area of the inferior aspect of the lesser pelvis, where it surrounds the obturator foramen. It arises from the superior and the inferior rami of the pubis, the ischium, and the obturator membrane and inserts into the greater trochanter of the femur. It is innervated by a special nerve from the sacral plexus, which contains fibers from the lumbosacral trunk and the first and the second sacral nerves, and it functions to rotate the thigh laterally and to extend and abduct the thigh when it is flexed. Compare **obturator externus, piriformis.**

obturator membrane, a tough fibrous membrane that covers the obturator foramen of each side of the pelvis.

oc-. See **ob-.**

occasion of service, a specific identifiable service provided a patient, as a medical examination, test, treatment, or procedure.

occipital /oksip′itəl/, **1.** of or pertaining to the occiput. **2.** situated near the occipital bone, as the occipital lobe of the brain.

occipital artery, one of a pair of tortuous branches from the external carotid arteries that divides into six branches and supplies parts of the head and scalp. Each terminal portion at the vertex of the skull is accompanied by the greater occipital nerve.

occipital bone, the cuplike bone at the back of the skull, marked by a large opening, the foramen magnum, that communicates with the vertebral canal. Its inner surface is divided into four fossae. The occipital bone articulates with the two parietal bones, the two temporal bones, the sphenoid, and the atlas.

occipital lobe, one of the five lobes of each cerebral hemisphere, occupying a relatively small pyramidal portion of the occipital pole. The occipital lobe lies beneath the occipital bone and presents medial, lateral, and inferior surfaces. The medial surface is bounded anteriorly by the pareitooccipital sulcus and the preoccipital notch and is divided by the posterior calcarine sulcus into the wedge-shaped cuneus and the lingual gyrus. The lateral surface of the lobe is divided by the lateral sulcus into the superior and the inferior occipital gyri. An imaginary transverse line across the preoccipital notch limits the inferior surface. Compare **central lobe, frontal lobe, parietal lobe, temporal lobe.**

occipital sinus, the smallest of the cranial sinuses and one of six posterior superior venous channels associated with the dura mater. It is located in the attached margin of the falx cerebelli, courses around the foramen magnum by several small channels, communicates with the posterior internal vertebral venous plexuses, and ends in the confluence of the sinuses. Compare **inferior sagittal sinus, occipital sinus, straight sinus, superior sagittal sinus.**

occipitoaxial ligament. See **membrana tectoria.**

occipitobregmatic /oksip′itōbregmat′ik/, of or pertaining to the occiput and the bregma.

occipitofrontal /oksip′itōfrun′təl/, of or pertaining to the occiput and the frontal bone of the skull.

occipitofrontalis /oksip′itōfrəntal′is/, one of a pair of thin, broad muscles covering the top of the skull, consisting of an occipital belly and a frontal belly connected by an extensive aponeurosis. The frontal belly originates at the galea aponeurotica and inserts in the skin of the eyebrows and the nose. The occipital belly originates in the superior nuchal line of the occipital bone and inserts at the galea aponeurotica. The occipitofrontalis is innervated by the facial nerve. It is the muscle that draws the scalp and raises the eyebrows. Compare **temporoparietalis.**

occipitoparietal fissure. See **parietooccipital sulcus.**

occiput /ok′sipət/, *pl.* **occiputs, occipita** /oksip′itə/, the back part of the head. Also called **occiput cranii.**

occlusal adjustment, (in dentistry) the grinding of the occluding surfaces of teeth to improve the occlusion or relationship between opposing tooth surfaces, their supporting structures, the muscles of mastication, and the temporomandibular joints.

occlusal contouring, the modification by grinding of irregularities of occlusal tooth forms, as uneven marginal ridges, and extruded or malpositioned teeth.

occlusal form, the shape of the occluding surfaces of a tooth, a row of teeth, or any dentition.

occlusal harmony, a combination of healthy and nondisruptive occlusal relationships between the teeth and their supporting structures, the associated neuromuscular mechanisms, and the temporomandibular joints.

occlusal lug. See **occlusal rest.**

occlusal radiograph, an intraoral radiograph made with the film placed on the occlusal surfaces of one of the arches.

occlusal recontouring, the reshaping of an occlusal surface of a natural or artificial tooth.

occlusal relationship, the relationship of the mandibular teeth to the maxillary teeth when in a defined occlusal contact position.

occlusal rest, a support placed on the occlusal surface of a posterior tooth. Also called **occlusal lug.**

occlusal rest angle, (in dentistry) the angle formed by the occlusal rest with the upright minor connector. Also called **rest angle.**

occlusal spillway, a natural groove that crosses a cusp ridge or a marginal ridge of a tooth.

occlusal trauma, injury to a tooth and surrounding structures caused by malocclusive stresses, including trauma, temporomandibular joint dysfunction, and bruxism.

occlusion, **1.** (in anatomy) a blockage in a canal, vessel, or passage of the body. **2.** (in dentistry) any contact between the incising or masticating surfaces of the maxillary and mandibular teeth. –**occlude,** *v.*, **occlusive,** *adj.*

occlusion rim, an artificial dental structure with occluding surfaces attached to temporary or permanent denture bases, used for recording the relation of the maxilla to the mandible and for positioning the teeth. Also called **bite block.**

occlusive /əclo͞o′siv/, pertaining to something that effects an occlusion or closure, as an occlusive dressing.

occlusive dressing, a dressing that prevents air from reaching a wound or lesion and that retains moisture, heat, body fluids, and medication. It may consist of a sheet of thin plastic affixed with transparent tape.

occlusometer. See **gnathodynamometer.**

occult, hidden or difficult to observe directly, as occult prolapse of the umbilical cord or occult blood.

occult blood, blood that appears from a nonspecific source, with obscure signs and symptoms. It may be detected by means of a chemical test or by microscopic or spectroscopic examination. Occult blood is often present in the stools of patients with GI lesions.

occult carcinoma, a small carcinoma that does not cause overt symptoms. It may remain localized and be discovered only incidentally at autopsy after death resulting from another cause, or it may metastasize and be discovered in the diagnostic study of the resulting metastatic disease. Also called **latent carcinoma.**

occult fracture, a fracture that cannot be initially detected by radiographic examination but may be evident radiographically weeks later. It is accompanied by the usual signs of pain and trauma and may produce soft tissue edema.

occupancy, the ratio of average daily hospital census to the average number of beds maintained during the reporting period.

occupational accident, an accidental injury to an employee that occurs in the workplace. Occupational accidents account for over 95% of occupational disabilities. In most cases the injured worker is eligible for compensation.

occupational asthma, an abnormal condition of the respiratory system resulting from exposure in the workplace to allergenic or other irritating substances. The condition is most common among persons working with detergents, Western red cedar, cotton, flax, hemp, grain, flour, and stone. See also **asthma, byssinosis, occupational lung disease.**

occupational disability, a condition in which a worker is unable to perform the functions required to complete a job satisfactorily because of an occupational disease or an occupational accident.

occupational disease, a disease that results from a particular employment, usually from the effects of long-term exposure to specific substances or of continuous or repetitive physical acts.

occupational health, the ability of a worker to function at an optimum level of well-being at a worksite as reflected in terms of productivity, work attendance, disability compensation claims, and employment longevity.

occupational history, a portion of the health history in which questions are asked about the person's occupation, source of income, effects of the work on worker's health or the worker's health on the job, the duration of the job, and to what degree the occupation satisfies the person. Any adverse effects known to be associated with the work or the place of work are investigated by further questions by the interviewer; for example, a tennis player might be asked about musculoskeletal problems or a taxi driver about function of the urinary tract.

occupational lung disease, any one of a group of abnormal conditions of the lungs caused by the inhalation of dusts, fumes, gases, or vapors in an environment where a person works. See also **chronic obstructive pulmonary disease, metal fume fever, occupational asthma, silo fillers' disease.**

occupational medicine, a field of preventive medicine concerned with the medical problems and practices relating to occupations and especially to the health of workers in various industries.

occupational neurosis, a neurotic disorder in which various symptoms occur that prevent the activities required by the occupation, as in writer's cramp. The symptoms are not caused by the occupation; rather, they may be an expression of a neurotic conflict.

occupational socialization, the adaptation of an individual to a given set of job-related behaviors, particularly the expected behavior that accompanies a specific job.

occupational therapist, a person who practices occupational therapy and who may be licensed, registered, certified, or otherwise regulated by law.

occupational therapy, "the use of purposeful activity with individuals who are limited by physical injury or illness, psychosocial dysfunction, developmental or learning disabilities, poverty and cultural differences, or the aging process to maximize independence, prevent disability, and maintain health. The practice encompasses evaluation, treatment, and consultation." (American Occupational Therapy Association)

occupational therapy aid, a person who, under the supervision of an occupational therapist, performs clerical and related tasks necessary for the implementation of occupational therapy programs.

occurrence policy, a professional liability insurance policy that covers the holder during the period an alleged act of malpractice occurred. Occurrence policies are said to have a "long tail," because the statute of limitations on malpractice allegations is unlimited. Thus, an individual could be sued years after an event had taken place. If the individual held an occurrence type of malpractice policy, there would be protection under that policy; under a claims-made policy there would not be protection unless the policy were current.

ochre mutation. See **amber mutation.**

ochronosis /ō'krənō'sis/, a condition characterized by the deposition of brown-black pigment in connective tissue and cartilage, often caused by alkaptonuria or poisoning with phenol. Bluish macules may be noted on the sclera, fingers, ears, nose, genitalia, buccal mucosa, and axillae. The urine may be dark-colored. See also **alkaptonuria.**

ocontic pressure. See **colloid osmotic pressure.**

OCR, abbreviation for **optical character recognition.**

octaploid, octaploidic. See **polyploid.**

ocular /ok'yo͞olər/, **1.** of or pertaining to the eye. **2.** an eyepiece of an optic instrument.

ocular hypertelorism, a developmental defect involving the frontal region of the cranium, characterized by an abnormally widened bridge of the nose and increased distance between the eyes. The condition is often associated with other cranial and facial deformities and some degree of mental retardation. Also called **orbital hypertelorism.**

ocular hypotelorism, a developmental defect involving the frontal region of the cranium, characterized by a narrowing of the bridge of the nose and an abnormal decrease in the distance between the eyes, with resulting convergent strabismus. The condition is often associated with other cranial and facial deformities, primarily microcephaly and trigonocephaly, and some degree of mental retardation. Also called **orbital hypotelorism.**

ocular myopathy, slowly progressive weakness of ocular muscles, characterized by decreased mobility of the eye and drooping of the upper lid. The disorder may be unilateral or bilateral and may be caused by damage to the oculomotor nerve, an intracranial tumor, or a neuromuscular disease.

ocular spot, an abnormal opacity in the eye. A shower of red and black dots may be seen in the eye after hemorrhage of a retinal vessel; opacities in the crystalline lens are characteristic in cataracts. In asteroid hyalitis, often associated with diabetes, small white spherical and stellate opacities are found in the vitreous humor; these bodies consist of calcium soaps and sparkle when examined with a light.

oculo-, a combining form meaning 'of or pertaining to the eye': *oculofacial, oculomycosis, oculopathy.*

oculocephalic reflex, a test of the integrity of brainstem function. When the patient's head is quickly moved to one side and then to the other, the eyes will normally lag behind the head movement and then slowly assume the midline position. Failure of the eyes to either lag properly or revert back to the midline indicates a lesion on the ipsilateral side at the brainstem level. Also called **doll's eye maneuver.**

oculogyric crisis /ok'yo͞olōjī'rik/, a paroxysm in which the eyes are held in a fixed position, usually up and sideways, for minutes or several hours, often occurring in postencephalitic patients with signs of parkinsonism. In some cases the eyes are held down or sideways and there may be spasm or closing of the lids. Oculogyric crises may be precipitated by emotional stress, and patients with the disorder frequently show psychiatric symptoms.

oculomotor nerve, either of a pair of cranial nerves essential for eye movements, supplying certain extrinsic and intrinsic eye muscles. They pass through the superior orbital fissure, connecting to the brain in nucleus III. Also called **nervus oculomotorius, third nerve.**

Ocusert Pilo, a trademark for a cholinergic (pilocarpine).

O.D., abbreviation for *oculus dexter,* a Latin phrase meaning "right eye."

-ode[1], a combining form meaning a 'type of (specified) electric conductor': *anode, cathode, electrode.*

-ode[2], a combining form meaning 'like in form' of something specified: *cytode, icterode, sarcode.*

odontectomy, the extraction of a tooth.

-odontia, a combining form meaning a 'form, condition, or mode of treatment of the teeth': *periodontia, prosthodontia, radiodontia.*

odontiasis /ō'dontī'əsis/, the process of teething.

-odontic, **1.** a combining form meaning 'pertaining to the size of teeth': *isodontic, macrodontic, mesodontic.* **2.** a combining form meaning 'pertaining to type of dental treatment': *gerodontic, orthodontic, pedodontic.*

odontitis /ō'dontī'tis/, abnormal enlargement of a tooth, usually resulting from an inflammation of the odontoblasts (cells responsible for dentine formation) rather than of the mature, or erupted, tooth. It may be caused by infection, tumor, or trauma.

odonto-, odont-, a combining form meaning 'of or pertaining to the teeth': *odontoblast, odontopathy.*

odontodysplasia, an abnormality in the development of the teeth, characterized by deficient formation of enamel and dentin. Also called **ghost teeth.** See also **shell teeth.**

odontoid process, the toothlike projection that rises perpendicularly from the upper surface of the body of the second cervical vertebra or axis, which serves as a pivot point for the rotation of the atlas, or first cervical vertebra, enabling the head to turn. Also called **dens.**

odontogenesis imperfecta. See **dentinogenesis imperfecta.**

odontogenic /ōdon′tōjen′ik/, **1.** generating teeth. **2.** developing in tissues that produce teeth.

odontogenic fibroma, a benign neoplasm of the jaw derived from the embryonic part of the tooth germ, dental follicle, or dental papilla or developing later from the periodontal membrane.

odontogenic fibrosarcoma, a malignant neoplasm of the jaw that develops in a mesenchymal component of a tooth or tooth germ.

odontogenic myxoma, a rare tumor of the jaw; it may develop from the mesenchyme of the tooth germ.

odontoid ligament. See **alar ligament.**

odontoid vertebra. See **axis.**

odontology /ō′dontol′əjē/, the scientific study of the anatomy and physiology of the teeth and of the surrounding structures of the oral cavity.

odontoma, an anomaly of the teeth that resembles a hard tumor, as dens in dente, enamel pearl, and complex or composite ondontoma. It consists of cementum, dentin, enamel, and pulp tissue that may be arranged in the form of teeth. Also called **gestant anomaly.**

odor, a scent or smell. The sense of smell is activated when airborne molecules stimulate receptors of the first cranial nerve.

-odyne, a combining form meaning 'referring to, treating pain': *acesodyne, anodyne, biodyne.*

-odynia, a combining form meaning a 'state of pain in a (specified) location': *coccyodynia, odontodynia, uterodynia.*

odyno-, a combining form meaning 'pain': *odynolysis, odynophagia, odynopoeia.*

odynophagia /od′inōfā′jə/, a severe sensation of burning, squeezing pain while swallowing, caused by irritation of the mucosa or a muscular disorder of the esophagus, as gastroesophageal reflux, bacterial or fungal infection, tumor, achalasia, or chemical irritation.

Oedipus complex, **1.** (in psychoanalysis) a child's desire for a sexual relationship with the parent of the opposite sex, usually with strong negative feelings for the parent of the same sex. **2.** a son's desire for a sexual relationship with his mother.

oenomania. See **oinomania.**

OER, abbreviation for **oxygen enhancement ratio.**

off-line, access to computer information or equipment not part of an operating computer system, as a drive not connected to the computer, a disk not connected to the computer, a disk not mounted on a drive, or a data printout sheet. Compare **on-line.**

Ogen, a trademark for an estrogen (estropipate).

OH, symbol for **hydroxyl.**

OHF, abbreviation for **Omsk hemorrhagic fever.**

ohm, a unit of measurement of electric resistance. One ohm is the resistance of a conductor in which an electric potential of 1 V produces a current of 1 ampere. See also **ampere, Ohm's law, volt, watt.**

Ohm's law, the principle that the strength or intensity of an unvarying electric current is directly proportional to the electromotive force and inversely proportional to the resistance of the circuit.

-oi, -i, a plural-forming element in borrowings from Greek: *auloi, catanephroi, mesonephroi.*

-oid, **1.** a combining form meaning 'resembling' something specified: *alkaloid, spheroid, trochoid.* **2.** a combining form meaning 'having the form or appearance of': *cuboid, lambdoid, ovoid.*

oiko-, eco-, a combining form meaning 'house': *oikofugic, oikology, oikophobia.*

oil, any of a large number of greasy liquid substances not miscible in water. Oil may be fixed or volatile and is derived from animal, vegetable, or mineral matter.

oinomania /oi′nōmā′nē•ə/, **1.** *archaic.* a periodic, irresistible craving for alcohol, especially wine. **2.** also called **enomania, oenomania** /ē′nō-/. delirium tremens.

ointment, a semisolid, externally applied preparation, usually containing a drug. Various ointments are used as local analgesic, anesthetic, antiinfective, astringent, depigmenting, irritant, and keratolytic agents. Also called **salve, unction, unguent.**

-ol a combining form designating a member of the alcohol group: *ethanol, methanol, naphthol.*

-ol, -ole, a combining form meaning an 'oil': *benzol, furol, petrol.*

-ola, a combining form meaning, a 'singular diminutive of the noun named': *arteriola, neurovariola, taeniola.*

Old Age, Survivors, Disability and Health Insurance Program (OASDHI), a benefit program, administered by the Social Security Administration, that provides cash benefits to workers who are retired or disabled, their dependents, and survivors. This part of the program is commonly referred to as Social Security. The program also provides health insurance benefits for people over 65 and for disabled people under 65. This part of the program is commonly referred to as Medicare. See also **Medicare.**

Old World leishmaniasis. See **oriental sore.**

oleandomycin. See **troleandomycin.**

olecranon /ōlek′rənon/, a proximal projection of the ulna that forms the point of the elbow and fits into the olecranon fossa of the humerus when the forearm is extended. The anterior surface of the olecranon forms part of the trochlear notch that articulates with the humerus. Also called **olecranon process.**

olecranon bursa, the bursa of the elbow.

olecranon fossa, the depression in the posterior surface of the humerus that receives the olecranon of the ulna when the forearm is extended. Compare **coronoid fossa.**

olecranon process. See **olecranon.**

olefiant gas. See **ethylene.**

olefin, any of a group of unsaturated aliphatic hydrocarbons containing one or more double bonds in the carbon chain. The group is represented by the general formula C_nH_{2n}.

oleic acid /ōlē′ik/, a colorless, liquid, monounsaturated fatty acid occurring in almost all natural fats. Commercial oleic acid is used in soaps, cosmetics, ointments, lubricants, and food additives.

oleo-, eleo-, a combining form meaning 'of or pertaining to oil': *oleocreosote, oleodistearin, oleoresin.*

oleometer /ō′lē•om′ətər/, a device for measuring the purity of oils.

oleovitamin /ō′lē•ōvī′təmin/, a preparation of fish-liver oil or edible vegetable oil that contains one or more of the fat-soluble vitamins or their derivatives.

oleovitamin A, an oily preparation, usually fish-liver oil or fish-liver oil diluted with an edible vegetable oil, containing the natural or synthetic form of vitamin A. See also **vitamin A.**

oleovitamin D_2. See **calciferol.**

olfactory /olfak′tərē/, of or pertaining to the sense of smell. **–olfaction,** *n.*

olfactory anesthesia. See **anosmia.**

olfactory center, the part of the brain responsible for the subjective appreciation of odors, a complex group of neurons located near the junction of the temporal and parietal lobes.

olfactory foramen, one of several openings in the cribiform plate of the ethmoid bone.

olfactory nerve, one of a pair of nerves associated with the sense of smell. The olfactory nerve is cranial nerve I and is composed of numerous fine filaments that ramify in the mucous membrane of the olfactory area. The fibers of the olfactory nerve are nonmedullated and unite into fasciculi that form a plexus under the mucous membrane and rise in grooves or canals in the ethmoid bone. The fibers pass into the skull and form synapses with the dendrites of the mitral cells. The area in which the olfactory nerves arise is situated in the most superior portion of the mucous membrane that covers the superior nasal concha. The olfactory sensory endings are modified epithelial cells and the least specialized of the special senses. The olfactory nerves connect with the olfactory bulb and the olfactory tract, which are components of the portion of the brain associated with the sense of smell.

olig-. See **oligo-.**

oligemia, a condition of hypovolemia or reduced circulating intravascular volume.

oligo-, olig-, a combining form meaning 'few, little': *oligocholia, oligodontia, oligosialia.*

oligodactyly /ol′igōdak′tilē/, a congenital anomaly characterized by the absence of one or more of the fingers or toes. Also called **oligodactylism, oligodactylia.** **–oligodactylic,** *adj.*

oligodendroblastoma. See **oligodendroglioma.**

oligodendrocyte, a type of neuroglial cell with dendritic projections that coil around axons of neural cells. The projections continue as myelin sheaths over the axons.

oligodendroglioma /ol′igōden′drōglī•ō′mə/, *pl.* **oligodendrogliomas, oligodendrogliomata,** an uncommon brain tumor composed of nonneural ectodermal cells that usually form part of the supporting connective tissue around nerve cells. The lesion, a firm, reddish-gray mass with calcified spots and a distinct margin, may grow to a large size. It develops most often in frontal, parietal, and paraventricular sites but may also occur in the cerebellum. Also called **oligodendroblastoma.**

oligodontia /ol′igōdon′shə/, a genetically determined dental defect characterized by the development of fewer than the normal number of teeth.

oligogenic /ol′igōjen′ik/, of or pertaining to hereditary characteristics produced by one or only a few genes.

oligohydramnios, an abnormally small amount or absence of amniotic fluid.

oligomeganephronia /ol′igōmeg′ənefrō′nē•ə/, a type of congenital renal hypoplasia associated with chronic renal failure in children. The condition is characterized by a decreased number of functioning nephrons and hypertrophy of other renal elements without the presence of aberrant tissue. Also called **oligomeganephronic renal hypoplasia.** **–oligomeganephronic,** *adj.*

oligomenorrhea, abnormally light or infrequent menstruation. **–oligomenorrheic,** *adj.*

oligopnea, oligopnoea. See **bradypnea.**

oligospermia /ol′igōspur′mē•ə/, insufficient spermatozoa in the semen. Compare **azoospermia.**

oliguria /ol′igyŏŏr′ē•ə/, a diminished capacity to form and pass urine, less than 500 ml in every 24 hours, so that the end products of metabolism cannot be excreted efficiently. It is usually caused by imbalances in bodily fluids and electrolytes, by renal lesions, or by urinary tract obstruction. Also called **oliguresis.** Compare **anuria.** **–oliguric,** *adj.*

olivopontocerebellar /ol′ivōpon′tōsur′ibel′ər/, of or pertaining to the olivae, the middle peduncles, and the cerebellum.

Ollier's disease. See **enchondromatosis.**

Ollier's dyschondroplasia /ol′ē•āz′/, a rare disorder of bone development in which the epiphyseal tissue responsible for growth spreads through the bones, causing abnormal irregular growth and, eventually, deformity. The long bones and the ilia are most often affected. Orthopedic procedures to correct deformities may be necessary and helpful, but invalidism is the usual prognosis. A kind of dyschondroplasia is **hereditary multiple exostoses.** Also called **multiple enchondromatosis.**

oma-. See **omo-.**

-oma, a combining form meaning a 'tumor': *capsuloma, lymphadenoma, neurinoma.*

omalgia, pain in the shoulder.
omarthritis, inflammation of the shoulder joint.
ombudsman, a person who investigates and mediates patients' problems and complaints in relation to a hospital's services. Also called **patient representative.**
omental bursa, a cavity in the peritoneum behind the stomach, the lesser omentum, and the lower border of the liver and in front of the pancreas and duodenum.
omentum, *pl.* **omenta, omentums,** an extension of the peritoneum that enfolds one or more adjacent organs in the stomach. See also **greater omentum, lesser omentum.** –**omental,** *adj.*
omission, (in law) intentional or unintentional neglect to fulfill a duty required by law.
Omnipen, a trademark for an antibacterial (ampicillin).
omo-, oma-, a combining form meaning 'of or pertaining to the shoulder': *omoclavicular, omodynia, omohyoid.*
omphal-. See **omphalo-.**
omphalic, pertaining to the umbilicus.
omphalitis, an inflammation of the umbilical stump, marked by redness, swelling, and purulent exudate in severe cases.
omphalo-, omphal-, a combining form meaning 'of or related to the navel': *omphalocele, omphaloma, omphalosite.*
omphaloangiopagus. See **allantoidoangiopagus.**
omphalocele /om′fəlōsēl′/, congenital herniation of intraabdominal viscera through a defect in the abdominal wall around the umbilicus. The defect is usually closed surgically soon after birth. Compare **gastroschisis.**
omphalodidymus. See **gastrodidymus.**
omphalogenesis, the formation of the umbilicus or yolk sac during embryonic development. –**omphalogenetic,** *adj.*
omphalomesenteric artery. See **vitelline artery.**
omphalomesenteric circulation. See **vitelline circulation.**
omphalomesenteric duct. See **yolk stalk.**
omphalomesenteric vein. See **vitelline vein.**
omphalopagus. See **monomphalus.**
omphalosite, the underdeveloped parasitic member of unequal conjoined twins united by the vessels of the umbilical cord. The omphalosite has no heart, derives its blood supply from the placenta of the autosite, and is incapable of independent existence after birth. See also **allantoidoangiopagus.**
OMR, abbreviation for **optic mark recognition.**
OMS, abbreviation for **Organisation Mondiale de la Santé.** See **World Health Organization.**
Omsk hemorrhagic fever (OHF) /ômsk/, an acute infection, seen in regions of the U.S.S.R., caused by an arbovirus transmitted by the bite of an infected tick or by handling infected muskrats. The disease is characterized by fever, headache, epistaxis, GI and uterine bleeding, and other hemorrhagic manifestations. Treatment is supportive; recovery usually occurs.
-on, **1.** a combining form meaning an 'elementary atomic particle': *electron, nucleon, proton.* **2.** a combining form meaning a 'unit': *magneton, photon.* **3.** a combining form meaning a '(nonmetallic) chemical element': *carbon, krypton, silicon.*
onanism. See **masturbation.**
onchocerciasis /on′kōsərkī′əsis/, a form of filariasis common in Central and South America and in Africa, characterized by subcutaneous nodules, pruritic rash, and eye lesions. It is transmitted by the bites of black flies that deposit *Onchocera volvulus* microfilariae under the skin. The microfilariae migrate to the subcutaneous tissue and eyes, and fibrous nodules develop around the developing adult worms. Hypersensitive reactions to the dying microfilariae include extreme pruritus, a cellulitis-like rash, lichenification, depigmentation, and rarely, elephantiasis. Involvement of the eye may include keratitis, iridocyclitis, and, rarely, blindness from choroidoretinitis. Diagnosis is made by demonstrating microfilariae by skin biopsy or in the eye by slit lamp. Treatment is diethylcarbamazine for the microfilariae and surgical excision of nodules to remove adult worms. Protective clothing and control of black flies with DDT are the best preventives. Also called **river blindness.**
onco-, a combining form meaning 'of or pertaining to a swelling, tumor, or mass': *oncogenesis, oncograph, oncotomy.*
oncofetal protein, a protein produced by or associated with a tumor cell, particularly an embryologic tumor. An example of an oncofetal protein is alpha fetoprotein.
oncogene, a potential cancer-inducing gene. Under normal conditions, such genes play a role in the growth and proliferation of cells, but when altered in some way by a cancer-causing agent, as radiation, a carcinogenic chemical, or an oncogenic virus, they may cause the cell to be transformed to a malignant state. At present about 15 to 20 oncogenes have been discovered in various animals, from fruit flies to humans.
oncogenesis /ong′kōjen′əsis/, the process initiating and promoting the development of a neoplasm through the action of biologic, chemical, or physical agents. Compare **carcinogenesis, sarcomagenesis, tumorigenesis.** –**oncogenic** /ong′kōjen′ik/, *adj.*
oncogenic virus, a virus that is able to cause the development of a malignant neoplastic disease. Over 100 oncogenic viruses have been identified. In the laboratory, oncogenic viruses have been inoculated and grown in all major groups of animals, including primates. Many, especially the "slow viruses" (as the one that causes kuru), are thought to cause cancer in humans, but this is not yet proven.
oncologist /ongkol′əjist/, a physician who specializes in the study and treatment of neoplastic diseases, particularly cancer.
oncology /ongkol′əjē/, **1.** the branch of medicine concerned with the study of tumors. **2.** the study of cancerous malignancies.

Oncology Nursing Society (ONS), an organization of nurses interested or specialized in nursing of the patient with cancer. The national publication of the ONS is *Oncology Nursing Forum.*

Oncovin, a trademark for an antineoplastic (vincristine sulfate).

oncovirus /ong′kōvī′rəs/, a member of a family of viruses associated with leukemia and sarcoma in animals and, possibly, in humans.

Ondine's curse /ondēnz′/, an eponym, derived from the name of a fabled water nymph, for apnea caused by loss of automatic control of respiration. The term refers to a syndrome in patients with marked sensitivity to retained carbon dioxide. A defect in the central chemoreceptor responsiveness to carbon dioxide leaves the patient with hypercapnia and hypoxemia, although fully able to breathe voluntarily. This condition may result in the pickwickian syndrome or the sleep-apnea syndrome, and it may be one cause of sudden infant death syndrome. Ondine's curse may occur as a result of drug overdose, as with opioids; after bulbar poliomyelitis or encephalitis; or after surgery involving the brainstem or the higher segments of cervical cord, as in cervical cordotomy for intractable pain.

-one, a combining form designating organic compounds: *acetone, ketone, quinone.*

one-and-a-half spica cast, an orthopedic cast used for immobilizing the trunk of the body cranially to the nipple line, one leg caudally as far as the toes, and the other leg caudally as far as the knee. For stability, a diagonal crossbar connects the parts of the cast encasing the legs. This type of cast is used for immobilization during convalescence after healing of surgical hip repair or a fractured femur and for the correction and the maintenance of correction of a hip deformity. Compare **bilateral long leg spica cast, unilateral long leg spica cast.**

one-to-one care, a method of organizing nursing services in an inpatient care unit by which one registered nurse assumes responsibility for all nursing care provided one patient for the duration of one shift.

oneiro-, a combining form meaning 'of or related to a dream': *oneirodynia, oneirology, oneiroscopy.*

onlay, **1.** a cast type of restoration retained by friction and mechanic forces in a prepared tooth for restoring one or more cusps and adjoining occlusal surfaces of a tooth. **2.** an occlusal rest portion of a removable partial denture, extended to cover the entire occlusal surface of a tooth. Compare **inlay.**

on-line, access to information or equipment that is part of an operating computer system linked to a central processing unit.

ONS, abbreviation for **Oncology Nursing Society.**

ontogenesis. See **ontogeny.**

ontogenetic, **1.** of, relating to, or acquired during ontogeny. **2.** an association based on visible morphologic characteristics and not necessarily indicative of a natural evolutionary relationship. Also called **ontogenic.**

ontogeny /ontoj′ənē/, the life history of one organism from a single-celled ovum to the time of birth, including all phases of differentiation and growth. Compare **phylogeny.** See also **comparative anatomy.**

onych-. See **onycho-.**

onychia /ōnik′ē·ə/, inflammation of the nail bed. Compare **paronychia.**

-onychia, a combining form meaning a 'condition of the finger- or toenails': *celonychia, melanonychia, pachyonychia.*

onycho-, onych-, a combining form meaning 'of or related to the nails': *onychogenic, onychohelcosis, onychopathology.*

onychogryphosis /on′ikōgrifō′sis/, thickened, curved, clawlike overgrowth of fingernails or toenails.

onycholysis /on′ikol′isis/, separation of a nail from its bed, beginning at the free margin, associated with psoriasis, dermatitis of the hand, fungal infection, *Pseudomonas* infection, and many other conditions.

onychomycosis /on′ikōmīkō′sis/, any fungus infection of the nails.

oo-, a combining form meaning 'of or pertaining to an egg or ovum': *ooblast, oocytase, ootid.*

ooblast /ō′əblast/, the female germ cell from which the mature ovum is developed.

oocenter See **ovocenter.**

oocyesis /ō′əsī·ē′sis/, an ectopic ovarian pregnancy.

oocyst /ō′əsist/, a stage in the development of any sporozoan in which after fertilization a zygote is produced that develops about itself an enclosing cyst wall. Oocysts of malarial parasites are found in the stomachs of infected mosquitoes. Oocysts of toxoplasma organisms are excreted in the feces of infected cats. Compare **oocyte.**

oocyte /ō′əsīt/, a primordial or incompletely developed ovum.

oocytin /ō′əsī′tin/, the substance in a spermatozoon that stimulates the formation of the fertilization membrane after penetration of an ovum.

oogamy /ō·og′əmē/, **1.** sexual reproduction by the fertilization of a large, nonmotile female gamete by a smaller, actively motile male gamete, as occurs in certain algae and the malarial parasite *Plasmodium.* **2.** heterogamy. Compare **isogamy.** **–oogamous,** *adj.*

oogenesis /ō′əjen′əsis/, the process of the growth and maturation of the female gametes, or ova. Development begins during intrauterine life when the primordial germ cells within the epithelium of the fetal ovarian cortex give rise to precursor oogonia. By the time of birth, the oogonia have multiplied and developed into primary oocytes, each surrounded by a layer of epithelial cells that together form the primordial follicle. These have entered the prophase stage of the first meiotic division and remain suspended in this state until sexual maturity is reached. Then at monthly intervals one or sometimes two of the primary oocytes are stimulated simultaneously by the anterior pituitary hormones and the maturation of the follicle to continue meiotic division, forming a large secondary oocyte and a much smaller nonfunctional first polar body. The second meiotic division begins at about the time of ovulation and remains suspended in the prophase stage until fertilization stimulates the completion of the process, resulting in one large mature ovum, or ootid, and either one or three smaller secondary polar bodies that soon disintegrate. The ootid contains a pronucleus with the haploid number of maternal chromosomes that will fuse with the pronucleus of the spermatozoon to form the zygote. If fertilization does not occur, the ovum disintegrates and is discharged with the menses. The female infant is born with the entire number of primary oocytes that will function throughout reproductive life. Only a fraction of these survive until puberty and only a small percentage will be ovulated. Follicles containing the primary oocytes are found in varying stages of development in the ovary of the sexually mature woman. Egg and sperm formation differ considerably in the number and size of gametes resulting from gametogenesis, the total number of gametes produced in a lifetime, and the time sequence for the initiation of the meiotic divisions and the completion of the cycle. Also called **ovogenesis.** Compare **spermatogenesis.** See also **gametogenesis, meiosis, menstrual cycle, ovulation.** **–oogenetic,** *adj.*

oogonium /ō′əgō′nē•əm/, *pl.* **oogonia,** the precursor cell from which an oocyte develops in the fetus during intrauterine life. It is derived from primordial germ cells, multiplies rapidly during gestation, and near the time of birth enters the prophase stage of the first meiotic division to form the primary oocyte. Also called **ovogonium.** See also **oogenesis.**

ookinesis /ō′əkinē′sis/, the mitotic phenomena occurring in the nucleus of the egg cell during maturation and fertilization. Also called **ookinesia.** See also **oogenesis.** **–ookinetic,** *adj.*

ookinete /ō′əkinēt′/, the motile elongated zygote that is formed by the fertilization of the macrogamete during the sexual reproductive phase of the life cycle of a sporozoan, specifically the malarial parasite *Plasmodium.* It penetrates the lining of the stomach of the female *Anopheles* mosquito and attaches to the outer wall, where it forms an oocyst and gives rise to sporozoites.

oolemma. See **zona pellucida.**

oophor-. See **oophoro-.**

oophorectomy /ō′əfərek′təmē/, the surgical removal of one or both ovaries, performed to remove a cyst or tumor, excise an abscess, treat endometriosis, or, in breast cancer, remove the source of estrogen, which stimulates some kinds of cancer. If both ovaries are removed, sterility results and menopause is abruptly induced; in premenopausal women one ovary or a portion of one ovary may be left intact unless a malignancy is present. The operation often accompanies a hysterectomy. Regional or general anesthesia is used. Unless a malignancy is present, estrogen may be given to treat the unpleasant side effects of the abrupt onset of menopause. Also called **ovariectomy.**

oophoritis /ō′əferī′tis/, an inflammatory condition of one or both ovaries, usually occurring with salpingitis.

oophoro-, oophor-, ootheco-, a combining form meaning 'of or pertaining to the ovary': *oophorocytosis, oophorogenous, oophoroma.*

oophorosalpingectomy /ō′əfôr′əsal′pinjek′təmē/, the surgical removal of one or both ovaries and the corresponding oviducts, performed to remove a cyst or tumor, excise an abscess, or treat the condition of endometriosis. In a bilateral procedure the patient becomes sterile and menopause is induced. General anesthesia is used. Estrogen therapy may be started after bilateral surgery, unless a malignancy is present, to relieve the unpleasant side effects of the abrupt onset of menopause.

ooplasm /ō′əplaz′əm/, the cytoplasm of the egg, or ovum, including the yolk in lower animals. Also called **ovoplasm.**

oosperm /ō′əspurm/, a fertilized ovum; the cell resulting from the union of the pronuclei of the spermatozoon and the ovum after fertilization; a zygote.

ootheco-. See **oophoro-.**

ootid /ō′ətid/, the mature ovum after penetration by the spermatozoon and completion of the second meiotic division but before the fusion of the pronuclei to form the zygote. It is one of the four cells resulting from oogenesis, the other three being nonfunctional secondary polar bodies, and corresponds to the four spermatid cells derived from spermatogenesis. See also **meiosis, oogenesis.**

opacity, pertaining to an opaque quality of a substance or object, as cataract opacity.

opaque, **1.** of or pertaining to a substance or surface that neither transmits nor allows the passage of light. **2.** neither transparent nor translucent.

-ope, a combining form meaning a 'person having an eye defect': *asthenope, hyperope, protanope.*

open amputation, a kind of amputation in which a straight, guillotine cut is made without skin flaps. Open amputation is performed if an infection is probable or developing or has been recurrent. The cross section is left open for drainage, and skin traction is applied to prevent retraction. Antibiotic therapy is begun, and surgical closure is completed when the infection clears. Compare **closed amputation.** See also **gangrene.**

open-angle glaucoma. See **glaucoma.**

open bite, an abnormal dental condition in which the anterior teeth do not occlude in any mandibular position. Compare **closed bite.**

open charting, a system of medical record keeping in which the patient has access to his chart. Open charting in varying degrees is authorized in some mental health institutions.

open drainage. See **drainage.**

open-drop anesthesia, the oldest and simplest anesthetic technique. A volatile liquid anesthetic agent is dripped, one drop at a time, onto a porous cloth or mask held over the patient's face. Chloroform and ether are the major general anesthetics adaptable to open-drop administration. Some psychologists believe that open-drop anesthesia can be a traumatic experience to a child and therefore consider this form of anesthesia ill-advised in pediatric use. It is not currently used in developed countries.

open fracture. See **compound fracture.**

open operation, a surgical procedure that provides a full view of the structures or organs involved through membranous or cutaneous incisions.

operant, any act or response occurring without an identifiable stimulus. The result of the act or response determines whether or not it is repeated.

operant conditioning, a form of learning used in behavior therapy in which the person undergoing therapy is rewarded for the correct response and punished for the incorrect response. Also called **instrumental conditioning.**

operating microscope, a binocular microscope used in delicate surgery, especially surgery of the eye or ear. The standing type of operating microscope has a motorized zoom system operated by a foot pedal that quickly changes the magnification. The operating microscope that attaches to a surgeon's head has interchangeable oculars for different magnifications. Also called **surgical microscope.**

operating room (OR, O.R.), **1.** a room in a health care facility in which surgical procedures requiring anesthesia are performed. **2.** *informal.* a suite of rooms or an area in a health care facility in which patients are prepared for surgery, undergo surgical procedures, and recover from the anesthetic procedures required for the surgery.

operating system (OS), the main system programs of a computer that manage the hardware and logical resources of a system, including scheduling and file management. Also called **executive, monitor, supervisor.**

operation, any surgical procedure, as an appendectomy or a hysterectomy.

operative cholangiography, (in diagnostic radiology) a procedure for outlining the major bile ducts. It is performed during surgery by injecting a radiopaque contrast material directly into these ducts. It is usually performed to detect residual calculi in the biliary tract. See also **cholangiography.**

operator gene, (in molecular genetics) a genetic unit that regulates the transcription of structural genes in its operon. The operator gene serves as the starting point in the coding sequence and interacts with a repressor protein in controlling the activity of structural genes.

operculum /ōpur′kyo͞oləm/, *pl.* **opercula, operculums,** a lid or covering, as the mucous plug that blocks the cervix of the gravid uterus or the temporal operculum of the cerebral temporal hemisphere that overlaps the insula as an extension of the superior surface of the temporal lobe. **–opercular,** *adj.*

operon /op′əron/, (in molecular biology) a segment of DNA consisting of an operator gene and one or more structural genes with related functions controlled by the operator gene in conjunction with a regulator gene. See also **operator gene, regulator gene.**

-ophidia, a combining form meaning 'venomous snakes': *thanatophidia, toxicophidia.*

Ophthaine, a trademark for a local anesthetic (proparacaine hydrochloride) solution, used in ophthalmic procedures.

ophthalm-. See **ophthalmo-.**

ophthalmia /ofthal′mē·ə/, severe inflammation of the conjunctiva or of the deeper parts of the eye. Some kinds of ophthalmia are **ophthalmia neonatorum, sympathetic ophthalmia,** and **trachoma.**

-ophthalmia, a combining form meaning a 'pathologic or anatomic condition of the eye': *allophthalmia, echinophthalmia, polemophthalmia.*

ophthalmia neonatorum /nē′ōnətôr′əm/, a purulent conjunctivitis and keratitis of the newborn resulting from exposure of the eyes to chemical chlamydial, bacterial, or viral agents. Chemical conjunctivitis usually occurs as a result of the instillation of silver nitrate in the eyes of a newborn to prevent a gonococcal infection. Also called **neonatal conjunctivitis.** See also **conjunctivitis.**

ophthalmic /ofthal′mik/, of or pertaining to the eye.

-ophthalmic, a combining form meaning 'referring to, near, or for the eye': *exophthalmic, periophthalmic, podophthalmic.*

ophthalmic administration of medication, the administration of a drug by instillation of a cream or ointment or by drops of a liquid preparation in the conjunctival sac. The correct strength and amount of the drug are selected, and the medication is instilled in the eye or eyes as directed. The order usually specifies O.D. for right eye, O.S. for left eye, or O.U. for each eye. Ophthalmic preparations are often refrigerated for storage but are given at room temperature. Cloudiness or sedimentation in a liquid may indicate deterioration of the drug. For administration, the patient is positioned comfortably, lying back on a bed or examining table or sitting up with the neck hyperextended. The cul-de-sac of the conjunctival sac is exposed by gentle traction on the tissue just below the lower eyelid. The medication is placed in the sac as the patient is instructed to look away from the point of instillation. The dispenser is not allowed to touch the eye, and the medication is not placed directly on the cornea. The eyelid is slowly released, and the patient is asked to roll the eye around a few times to spread the medication over the entire surface of the eye.

ophthalmic herpes zoster. See **herpes zoster.**

ophthalmo-, ophthalm-, a combining form meaning 'of or pertaining to the eye': *ophthalmodynia, ophthalmolith, ophthalmostat.*

ophthalmologist /of′thalmol′əjist/, a physician who specializes in ophthalmology.

ophthalmology /of′thalmol′əjē/, the branch of medicine concerned with the study of the physiology, anatomy, and pathology of the eye and the diagnosis and treatment of disorders of the eye. **–ophthalmologic, ophthalmological,** *adj.*

ophthalmoplegia /ofthal′məplē′jē·ə/, an abnormal condition characterized by paralysis of the motor nerves of the eye. Bilateral ophthalmoplegia of rapid onset is associated with acute myasthenia gravis, acute thiamin deficiency, botulism, and acute inflammatory cranial polyneuropathy. These diseases are potentially very destructive and require prompt attention. In some patients with myopathic ophthalmoplegia structural abnormalities and biochemical disorders may be evident in limb muscles. Ophthalmoplegia is also associated with ocular dystrophy.

ophthalmoscope /of′thalmol′əskōp/, a device for examining the interior of the eye. It includes a light, a mirror with a single hole through which the examiner may look, and a dial holding several lenses of varying strengths. The lenses are selected to allow clear visualization of the structures of the eye at any depth. If the patient or the examiner ordinarily requires extensive correction of a refractive error, the examination may require that the corrective lenses normally worn be worn for the examination.

ophthalmoscopy /of′thalmos′kəpē/, the technique of using an ophthalmoscope to examine the eye.

Ophthochlor, a trademark for an ophthalmic preparation of the antibacterial and antirickettsial (chloramphenicol).

Ophthocort, a trademark for an ophthalmic, fixed-combination drug containing a glucocorticoid (hydrocortisone acetate) and antibacterials (chloramphenicol and polymyxin B sulfate).

-opia, -opy, -opsia, -opsy, a combining form meaning a '(specified) visual condition': *boopia, nonopia, senopia*.

opiate, **1.** a narcotic drug that contains opium, derivatives of opium, or any of several semisynthetic or synthetic drugs with opium-like activity. **2.** *informal.* any soporific or narcotic drug. **3.** of or pertaining to a substance that causes sleep or relief of pain. Morphine and related opiates may produce unwanted side effects, as nausea, vomiting, dizziness, and constipation. In rare instances a patient treated with an opiate may become delirious. Some patients may also develop increased sensitivity to pain after the opiate has worn off. Allergic reactions to opiates, as urticaria and other skin rashes, rarely occur, although contact dermatitis in nurses and pharmaceutic workers has been reported. Patients with reduced blood volume are more susceptible to the hypotensive effect of morphine and related drugs. Opiates are used with extreme caution in obese patients and in those with head injuries, emphysema, or other problems associated with decreased respiratory function. In patients with prostatic hypertrophy, morphine may cause acute urinary retention, requiring repeated catheterization. Also called **opioid.**

-opic, -opical, a combining form meaning 'kind of vision or visual defect': *cyclopic, hemeralopic, nyctalopic*.

opinion, **1.** (in law) a statement by the court, usually in writing, of the reasoning behind its decision or judgment in a particular case. **2.** a statement prepared for a client by an attorney that represents the attorney's understanding of the law as it pertains to a legal question posed by the client.

opistho-, a combining form meaning 'backward or relating to the back': *opisthognathism, opisthoporeia, opisthotonos*.

opisthorchiasis /ō′pisthôrkī′əsis/, infection with one of the species of *Opisthorchis* liver flukes commonly found in the Philippines, India, Thailand, and Laos. Symptoms and signs are similar to those caused by *Clonorchis sinensis*. Carcinoma of the intrahepatic bile ducts may be a late complication. Treatment is unsatisfactory. The disease is prevented by avoiding to eat raw or inadequately cooked freshwater fish.

Opisthorchis sinensis. See ***Clonorchis sinensis.***

opisthotonos /ō′pisthot′ənəs/, a prolonged severe spasm of the muscles causing the back to arch acutely, the head to bend back on the neck, the heels to bend back on the legs, and the arms and hands to flex rigidly at the joints.

opium, a milky exudate from the unripe capsules of *Papaver somniferum* and *Papaver album* yielding 9.5% or more of anhydrous morphine. It is a narcotic analgesic, a hypnotic, and an astringent. Opium contains several alkaloids, including codeine, morphine, and papaverine. See also **codeine, morphine sulfate, opium tincture, papaverine hydrochloride, paregoric.**

opium alkaloid, one of several alkaloids isolated from the milky exudate of the unripe seed pods of *Papaver somniferum,* a species of poppy indigenous to the Near East. Three of the alkaloids, codeine, papaverine, and morphine, are used clinically for the relief of pain, but their use entails the risk of physical or psychologic dependence. Morphine is the standard against which the analgesic effect of newer drugs for relief of pain are measured. The opium alkaloids and their semisynthetic derivatives, including heroin, act on the central nervous system, producing analgesia, change in mood, drowsiness, and mental slowness. The effects in a person who has pain are usually pleasant; euphoria and pain-free sleep are not uncommon, but nausea and vomiting sometimes occur. In usual doses, the analgesic effects are achieved without loss of consciousness. Morphine and its surrogates appear to relieve the discomfort of the original sensation and the person's reaction to the sensation; thus the actual pain diminishes, and what remains of it is less distressing to the patient. The opium alkaloids have several other effects on the various systems of the body: coughing is suppressed; the electric activity pattern of the brain resembles that of sleep; the pupils constrict; respiration is depressed in rate, minute volume, and tidal exchange; the secretory activity and motility of the GI tract are diminished; and biliary and pancreatic secretions are reduced. The use of morphine as an antidiarrheal preceded its use as an analgesic by hundreds of years. Prepared in a tincture, it remains the most effective constipating agent available.

opium tincture, an analgesic and antidiarrheal.
■ INDICATIONS: It is prescribed in the treatment of intestinal hyperactivity, cramping, and diarrhea.
■ CONTRAINDICATIONS: Drug dependence, the presence of toxic matter in the bowel, or known hypersensitivity to this drug prohibits its use.
■ ADVERSE EFFECTS: Among the more serious adverse reactions are drug dependence, toxic megacolon, and central nervous system depression.

Oppenheim reflex /op′ənhīm/, a variation of Babinski's reflex, elicited by firmly stroking downward on the anterior and medial surfaces of the tibia, characterized by extension of the great toe and fanning of other toes. It is a sign of pyramidal tract disease. Compare **Chaddock reflex, Gordon reflex.** See also **Babinski's reflex.**

Oppenheim's disease, a rare congenital disease of infants, characterized by flabby, atonic muscles, especially in the legs, and absent or extremely sluggish deep reflexes. The infant seems paralyzed during its first few months of life, and almost a third of the patients do not survive for a year. Also called **amyotonia congenita.** See also **myotonia congenita.**

opportunistic infection, 1. an infection caused by normally nonpathogenic organisms in a host whose resistance has been decreased by such disorders as diabetes mellitus or cancer or by a surgical procedure, as a cerebrospinal fluid shunt or a cardiac or urinary tract catheterization. **2.** an unusual infection with a common pathogen, as cellulitis, meningitis, or otitis media.

-opsia. See **-opia.**

opsonin /op′sənin/, an antibody or complement split product which, on attaching to foreign material, microorganism, or other antigen, enhances phagocytosis of that substance by leukocytes and other macrophages. – **opsonize,** *v.*

opsonization /op′sənizā′shən/, the process by which opsonins render bacteria more susceptible to phagocytosis by leukocytes.

Optef, a trademark for an ophthalmic preparation containing a glucocorticoid (hydrocortisone).

-opter, a combining form referring to 'measurement of vision': *myodiopter, oxyopter, phoropter.*

opti-. See **opto-.**

optic, of or pertaining to the eyes or to sight. Also **optical.**

-optic, -optical, a combining form meaning 'pertaining to vision': *bioptic, panoptic, preoptic.*

optic atrophy, wasting of the optic disc resulting from degeneration of fibers of the optic nerve and optic tract. In primary optic atrophy the disc is white and sharply margined, the central depression (physiologic cup) is enlarged, and the optic foramen of the sclera is clearly seen. In secondary atrophy the disc is gray, its margins are blurred, the depression is filled in, and the foramen is difficult to detect. Optic atrophy may be caused by a congenital defect, inflammation, occlusion of the central retinal artery or internal carotid artery, alcohol, arsenic, lead, tobacco, or other toxic substances. Degeneration of the disc may accompany arteriosclerosis, diabetes, glaucoma, hydrocephalus, pernicious anemia, and various neurologic disorders.

optic character recognition (OCR), any of various systems whereby graphic information is input directly into a computer by means of an optic device.

optic cup, a two-layered embryonic cavity that develops in early pregnancy. The optic cup is completed by the seventh week with the closing of the choroidal fissure. The cup initially develops from the infolding of the optic vesicle after the vesicle separates from the embryonic ectoderm. The cells of the optic cup differentiate to form the retina that first develops its layers of rods and cones in the central portion of the cup, growing as the layer gradually spreads toward the cup margin. The outer layer of the cup persists as the pigmented layer of the retina; the inner layer develops the nervous elements and the supporting fibers of the retina. Compare **optic stalk.**

optic density, a number describing the blackening of an x-ray film in any specified location. In general, the optic density is the logarithm of the ratio of incident to transmitted light through that area and is measured with a densitometer.

optic disc, the small blind spot on the surface of the retina, located about 3 mm to the nasal side of the macula. It is the only part of the retina that is insensitive to light. At its center the porus opticus marks the point of entrance of the central artery of the retina. Also called *(informal)* **blind spot, discus nervi optici.**

optic glioma, a tumor composed of glial cells. It develops slowly on the optic nerve or in the optic chiasm, causing loss of vision, and is often accompanied by secondary strabismus, exophthalmos, and ocular paralysis.

optician, a person who grinds and fits eyeglasses and contact lenses by prescription. To become an optician, a person must graduate from high school and complete a 4- or 5-year apprenticeship. In some states licensure is required.

optic mark recognition (OMR), a system whereby marks in predetermined positions on a specially prepared form are input directly into a computer by means of an optic device.

optic maser. See **laser.**

optic nerve, either of a pair of cranial nerves consisting mainly of coarse, myelinated fibers that arise in the retinal ganglionic layer, traverse the thalamus, and connect with the visual cortex. At the optic chiasm the fibers from the inner or nasal half of the retina cross to the optic tract of the opposite side. The remaining fibers from the temporal or outer half of each retina are uncrossed and pass to the visual cortex on the same side. The visual cortex functions in the perception of light and shade and in the perception of objects. Optic radiations conduct impulses from the geniculate bodies in the cerebral hemispheres to the visual cortices. The optic nerve is divided into portions within the bulb, orbit, optic canal, and cranial cavity. The intraocular portion of the nerve is about 1 mm long and contains unmyelinated fibers that become myelinated after passing through the lamina cribosa. The orbital portion of the nerve, about 3.5 mm in diameter and about 25 mm long, is invested by sheaths derived from the dura, the arachnoid, and the pia mater. The portion of the nerve within the optic canal lies superior to the ophthalmic artery, and the three sheaths are fused to each other, to the nerve, and to the periosteum of the bone, securing the nerve and preventing it from being forced back and forth in the foramen. The intracranial portion of the nerve rests on the anterior portion of the cranial sinus in close proximity to the internal carotid artery. The optic nerve is cranial nerve II and develops from a diverticulum of the lateral portion of the forebrain. The optic nerve fibers therefore correspond to a tract of fibers within the brain rather than to the other cranial nerves.

optico-. See **opto-.**

optic papilla. See **papilla.**

optics, **1.** (in physics) a field of study that deals with the electromagnetic radiation of wavelengths shorter than radio waves but longer than x-rays. **2.** (in physiology) a field of study that deals with vision and the process by which the functions of the eye and the brain are integrated in the perception of shapes, patterns, movements, spatial relationships, and color.

optic stalk, one of a pair of slender embryonic structures that become the optic nerve. In the embryo the optic stalk develops during the second week and attaches the optic vesicle to the wall of the brain. The stalk becomes complete during the seventh week of pregnancy when the choroidal fissure closes and is later converted into the optic nerve when nerve fibers fill the cavity of the stalk. Most of the fibers are centripetal and grow backward into the stalk from the nerve cells of the retina. A few fibers grow into the stalk from the brain. About the tenth week after birth, the fibers of the optic nerve receive their myelin sheaths. Compare **optic cup.**

optic system assessment, an evaluation of the patient's eyes, vision, and current and past disorders or injuries that may be responsible for abnormalities in the individual's optic system.

■ METHOD: The patient is interviewed to determine if vision is blurred; double, decreased, or absent in one or both eyes, or diminished peripherally at night or in bright light. The interviewer asks if halos or lights are seen and if the patient collides with unfamiliar objects, is unable to distinguish objects held too close or too far, if the eyes water, itch, or feel tender, painful, or fatigued, and if an injury to the eye, face, or head has occurred. Observations are made of the patient's general appearance, vital signs, kind of eyeglasses or contact lenses worn, the amount of tearing, ability to blink, tendency to rub the eyes, and visual acuity. Evidence is recorded of conjunctivitis, drainage, optic hemorrhage, edema or ptosis of the eyelids, exophthalmos, strabismus, nystagmus, scleral edema, chalazion, lacerations, contusions, or a foreign body in the eye. Carefully noted are signs of aging, glaucoma, cataract, retinal detachment, and the presence of multiple sclerosis, diabetes mellitus, myasthenia gravis, gonorrhea, thyroid dysfunction, sinus problems, or cerebral trauma or tumors. The patient's report of previous eye operations or treatments, head or face trauma, arteriosclerosis, glomerulonephritis, retinal degeneration, episodes of coma, therapy with oxygen, and drug misuse are investigated, as well as a family history of glaucoma or diabetes. Also explored are the possibility that the patient has a hazardous job or recreation (and note is made of any safety precautions taken), the individual's misuse of alcohol, and use of medication, especially antibiotics, antiemetics, miotics, mydriatics, and acetazolamide. Diagnostic aids for the evaluation include a test of visual fields, x-ray film of the orbit and skull, an ophthalmoscopic examination, tonometry, brain scan, and microscopic studies of conjunctival scrapings.

■ NURSING ORDERS: The nurse conducts the interview, makes the observations of the patient, and assembles the pertinent background data and the results of the diagnostic procedures.

■ OUTCOME CRITERIA: A careful assessment of the patient's eyes and vision and of certain aspects of the medical, family, and social history is a significant aid in establishing the diagnosis of an optic system disorder.

optic thermometer, a temperature measuring device in which the properties of transmission and reflection of visible light are temperature dependent, and whose detection can be related to tissue temperature.

Optimyd, a trademark for an ophthalmic, fixed-combination drug containing a glucocorticoid (prednisolone sodium phosphate) and an antibacterial (sulfacetamide sodium).

opto-, opti-, optico, a combining form meaning 'visible, or pertaining to vision or sight': *optoblast, optometer, optostriate.*

optometrist /optom′ətrist/, a person who practices optometry. An optometrist is awarded the degree of Doctor of Optometry (O.D.) after completion of at least 2 years of college, followed by 4 years in an approved college of optometry. A state examination and license are also required. See also **optician, optometry.**

optometry /optom′ətrē/, the practice of testing the eyes for visual acuity, prescribing corrective lenses, and recommending eye exercises. See also **optician.**

OPV, abbreviation for **oral poliovirus vaccine.**

OR, O.R., abbreviation for **operating room.**

oral, of or pertaining to the mouth. Compare **buccal, parenteral.**

oral administration of medication, the administration of a tablet, a capsule, an elixir, or a solution or other liquid form of medication by mouth. Adequate water to lubricate the solid forms or to dilute the liquid forms is given for swallowing with the medication. Preparations with a disagreeable taste may be given with something of sufficient flavor to disguise the bad taste. Substances that are harmful to the teeth are given through a straw. People who have difficulty swallowing pills or capsules may find it easier to swallow the medication if they look up as they swallow. Kinds of oral administration of medication are **buccal administration of medication** and **sublingual administration of medication.**

oral airway, a curved tubular device of rubber, plastic, or metal placed in the oropharynx during general anesthesia to maintain free passage of air and keep the tongue from falling back and obstructing the trachea. The artificial airway is not removed until the patient begins to awaken and regains pharyngeal, cough, and swallowing reflexes.

oral cancer, a malignant neoplasm on the lip or in the mouth, occurring at an average age of 60 with a frequency eight times higher in men than in women. Predisposing factors in the cause of the disease are alcoholism, heavy use of tobacco, poor oral hygiene, ill-fitting dentures, syphilis, Plummer-Vinson syndrome, betel nut chewing, and, in lip cancer, overexposure to sun and wind and the smoking of pipes. Premalignant leukoplakia or erythroplasia or a painless nonhealing ulcer may be the first sign of oral cancer; localized pain usually appears later, but lymph nodes may be involved early in the course. Diagnostic measures include digital examination, biopsy, exfoliative cytology, x-ray film of the mandible, and chest films to detect metastatic lung lesions. Almost all oral tumors are epidermoid carcinomas; adenocarcinomas occur occasionally, whereas sarcomas and metastatic lesions from other sites are rare. Small primary lesions may be treated by excision or irradiation and more extensive oral tumors by surgery, with removal of involved lymph nodes and preoperative or postoperative radiotherapy. Among chemotherapeutic agents administered palliatively for inoperable or recurrent lesions are methotrexate, 5-fluorouracil, bleomycin, and adriamycin.

oral character, (in psychoanalysis) a kind of personality exhibiting patterns of behavior originating in the oral phase of infancy, characterized by optimism, self-confidence, and carefree generosity reflecting the pleasurable aspects of the stage, or pessimism, futility, anxiety, and sadism as manifestations of frustrations or conflicts occurring during the period. See also **oral eroticism, oral stage, psychosexual development.**

oral contraceptive, oral steroid medication for contraception. The two major steroids used are progestogen and a combination of progestogen and estrogen. The steroids act by inhibiting the productivity of gonadotropin-releasing hormone by the hypothalamus, and therefore the pituitary does not secrete gonadotropins to stimulate ovulation. This results in the endometrium of the uterus being thin and the cervical mucus being thick, thus preventing the penetration of sperm. Before oral contraceptives are prescribed, the woman receives a complete physical examination and a history is taken. While on the medication, she is reexamined after 3 months and then yearly. Combination steroids are given for 3 weeks with no medication in the fourth week to allow for withdrawal bleeding. If breakthrough bleeding occurs, the estrogen dose may need to be increased. If amenorrhea develops, the progestogen may need to be decreased. Contraindications to the medication include pregnancy, diabetes mellitus, liver disease, hyperlipidemia, thrombolic complications, coronary artery disease, and sickle cell disease. Patients with depression and migraine headaches and those who are heavy cigarette smokers need to be followed up more often. Increased risk of circulatory disease occurs in women more than 35 years of age who have used oral contraceptives for more than 5 years and smoke cigarettes or who have other risk factors. Amenorrhea often occurs in women who stop taking oral contraceptives and who have had a history of oligomenorrhea or amenorrhea. The pregnancy rate when oral contraceptives are used correctly is less than 0.2% a year. See also **contraception.**

oral dosage, pertaining to the administration of a medicine by mouth.

oral eroticism, (in psychoanalysis) libidinal fixation at or regression to the oral stage of psychosexual development, often reflected in such personality traits as passivity, insecurity, and oversensitivity. Also called **oral erotism.** Compare **anal eroticism.** See also **oral character.**

oral herpes. See **herpes simplex.**

oral hygiene, the condition or practice of maintaining the tissues and structures of the mouth. Oral hygiene includes brushing the teeth to remove food particles, bacteria, and plaque; massaging the gums with a tooth brush, dental floss, or water irrigator to stimulate circulation and remove foreign matter; and cleansing of dentures and ensuring their proper fit to prevent irritation. Dependent or unconcious patients are assisted in maintaining a healthy oral condition. Such care includes lubricating the lips and cleaning the inside of the cheeks, the roof of the mouth, and the tongue. In addition, the nurse checks for loose teeth that might be swallowed or aspirated.

oral mucous membranes, alteration in, a nursing diagnosis accepted by the Fifth National Conference on the Classification of Nursing Diagnoses. The origin of the problem includes pathologic conditions within the oral cavity, as those caused by radiation to the head or neck; chemical or mechanic trauma to the oral cavity; ineffective oral hygiene; infection; malnutrition; the effect of medications; dehydration; and continuous breathing through the oral cavity. The defining characteristics include oral pain or discomfort, a coated tongue, dry mouth, oral lesions or ulcerations, a lack of or decrease in salivation, hemorrhagic gingivitis, caries, and bad breath. See also **nursing diagnosis.**

oral poliovirus vaccine (OPV), an attenuated preparation of live poliovirus that confers immunity to poliomyelitis. Also called **Sabin vaccine.**

■ INDICATION: It is routinely prescribed for immunization against poliomyelitis.

■ CONTRAINDICATIONS: Immunosuppression, concomitant use of corticosteroids, cancer, immunoglobulin abnormalities, or acute infection prohibits its use.

■ ADVERSE EFFECTS: Adverse effects are uncommon. Cases of vaccine-induced paralytic disease have occurred but are very rare.

oral sadism, (in psychoanalysis) a sadistic form of oral eroticism, manifested by such behavior as biting, chewing, and other aggressive impulses associated with eating habits. Compare **anal sadism.**

oral stage, (in psychoanalysis) the initial stage of psychosexual development, occurring in the first 12 to 18 months of life when the feeding experience and other oral activities are the predominant source of pleasurable stimulation. Experiences encountered during this stage determine to a great extent later attitudes concerning food, love, acceptance and rejection, and many other aspects of interpersonal relationships and behavioral patterns. Pleasurable experiences associated with suckling may lead to oral eroticism in adulthood, unpleasant experiences may lead to extreme aggression and such patterns as smoking, overeating, excessive talking, or sarcasm and may be a pervasive influence or underlying determinant in addictive disorders. See also **oral character, psychosexual development.**

Orap, a trademark for an antipsychotic (pimozide).

Orasone, a trademark for a glucorticoid (prednisone).

Ora-Testryl, a trademark for an androgen (fluoxymesterone).

orbicularis ciliaris /ôrbik′yo͞olär′is/, one of the two zones of the ciliary body of the eye, extending from the ora serrata of the retina to the ciliary processes at the margin of the iris. The orbicularis ciliaris is about 4 mm wide and increases in thickness as it approaches the ciliary processes.

orbicularis oculi, the muscular body of the eyelid comprising the palpebral, orbital, and lacrimal muscles. It arises from the nasal part of the frontal bone, from the frontal process of the maxilla in front of the lacrimal groove, and from the anterior surface of the medial palpebral ligament. The palpebral muscle functions to close the eyelid gently; the orbital muscle functions to close it more energetically, as in winking. Also called **orbicularis palpebrarum.** Compare **corrugator supercilii, levator palpebrae superioris.**

orbicularis oris, the muscle surrounding the mouth, consisting partly of fibers derived from other facial muscles, as the buccinator, that are inserted into the lips, and partly of fibers proper to the lips. It is innervated by buccal branches of the facial nerve and serves to close and purse the lips.

orbicularis palpebrarum. See **orbicularis oculi.**

orbicularis pupillary reflex, a normal phenomenon elicited by forceful closure of the eyelids or attempting to close them while they are held apart, resulting first in constriction and then dilatation of the pupil.

orbit, one of a pair of bony, conical cavities in the skull that accommodate the eyeballs and associated structures, as the eye muscles, the nerves, and the blood vessels. The medial walls of the orbits are approximately parallel with each other and with the middle line, but the lateral walls diverge widely. The roof of each orbit is formed by the orbital plate of the frontal bone and the small wing of the sphenoid bones. The trochlear fovea of the orbital roof accommodates the cartilaginous pulley of the obliquus superior oculi, and the lacrimal fossa in the roof cradles the lacrimal gland. The superior orbital fissure between the roof and the lateral wall of the orbit admits various nerves, as the oculomotor, trochlear, and ophthalmic division of the trigeminal and the abducent nerves. The openings that communicate with each orbit are the optic foramen, the superior and the inferior orbital fissures, the supraorbital foramen, the infraorbital canal, the anterior and the posterior ethmoidal foramina, the zygomatic foramen, and the canal for the nasolacrimal duct. –**orbital,** *adj.*

orbital aperture, an opening in the cranium to the orbit of the eye.

orbital fat, a semifluid cushion of fat that lines the bony orbit supporting the eye. Traumatic loss of the fat causes a sunken appearance of the eye. Replacement of the fat by tumor or abnormal tissue may be discovered on ophthalmologic examination. The examiner gently presses on the front of the eyes through the eyelids. Normally each eye may be displaced 0.5 cm into the socket.

orbital hypertelorism. See **ocular hypertelorism.**

orbital hypotelorism. See **ocular hypotelorism.**

orbital pseudotumor, a specific inflammatory reaction of the orbital tissues of the eye, characterized by exophthalmos and edematous congestion of the eyelids. The cause is unknown.

orbitomeatal line, a positioning line used in radiography that passes through the outer canthus of the eye and the center of the external auditory meatus.

orchi-. See **orchio-.**

orchidectomy /ôr′kidek′təmē/, a surgical procedure to remove one or both testes. It may be indicated for serious disease or injury to the testis or to control cancer of the prostate by removing a source of androgenic hormones. Also called **orchiectomy.**

orchido-. See **orchio-.**

orchiectomy. See **orchidectomy.**

orchio-, orchi-, orchido-, a combining form meaning 'of or pertaining to the testes': *orchiocatabasis, orchiopathy, orchioscirrhus.*

orchiopexy /ôr′kē•ōpek′sē/, an operation to mobilize an undescended testis, bring it into the scrotum, and attach it so that it will not retract. Sometimes a suture is attached to the lower scrotum and taped to the inner thigh. The nurse must be careful not to disturb this tension attachment.

orchis. See **testis.**

orchitis /ôrkī′tis/, inflammation of one or both of the testes, characterized by swelling and pain, often caused by mumps, syphilis, or tuberculosis. Symptomatic treatment includes support and elevation of the scrotum, cold packs, and analgesics. –**orchitic,** *adj.*

orciprenaline sulfate. See **metaproterenol sulfate.**

order of procedure, the sequence in which the required steps are taken to complete an operation, as the preparation and filling of a tooth.

Orem, Dorthea E., author of the Self-Care Nursing Model, a nursing theory introduced in 1959. The Orem theory describes the role of the nurse in giving assistance to a person experiencing inabilities in self-care. The goal of the Orem system is to meet the patient's self-care demands until the family is capable of providing care. The process is divided into three categories: Universal, which consists of self-care to meet physiologic and psychosocial needs; Developmental, the self-care required when one goes through developmental stages; and Health Deviation, the self-care required when one has a deviation from a healthy status. Assessment is made of therapeutic self-care demand, the self-care agency, and self-care deficits in the areas of knowledge, skills, motivation, and orientation. There are three systems for meeting the patient's self-care deficits. They are Wholly Compensatory, in which the patient has no active role; Partly Compensatory, in which the patient and nurse have active roles, and Educative Development, in which patients can meet their need for self-care with some assistance from the nurse.

Oretic, a trademark for a diuretic (hydrochlorothiazide).

Oreticyl, a trademark for an antihypertensive, fixed-combination drug containing a diuretic (hydrochlorothiazide) and an antihypertensive (deserpidine).

Oreton, a trademark for an androgen (testosterone).

Oreton Methyl, a trademark for an androgen (methyltestosterone).

-orexia, a combining form meaning '(condition of the) appetite': *cynorexia, dysorexia, anorexia.*

orexigenic /ôrek′sijen′ik/, a substance that increases or stimulates the appetite.

oreximania /ôrek′simā′nē·ə/, a condition characterized by a greatly increased appetite and excessive eating resulting from an unrealistic or exaggerated fear of becoming thin. Compare **anorexia nervosa.**

orexis /ôrek′sis/, **1.** desire, appetite. **2.** the aspect of the mind involving feeling and striving as contrasted with the intellectual aspect.

orf, a viral skin disease acquired from sheep, characterized by painless vesicles that may progress to red, weeping nodules and, finally, to crusting and healing. Treatment is not necessary because the condition is self-limited, and active infection results in immunity.

organ, a structural part of a system of the body that is comprised of tissues and cells that enable it to perform a particular function, as the liver, spleen, digestive organs, reproductive organs, or organs of special sense. Each one of the paired organs can function independently of the other. The liver, pancreas, spleen, and brain may maintain normal or near normal function with over 30% of the organ damaged, destroyed, or excised. Also called **organon, organum.**

organ albumin, albumin characteristic of a particular organ.

organelle /ôrgənel′/, **1.** any one of various particles of living substance bound within most cells, as the mitochondria, the Golgi complex, the endoplastic reticulum, the lysosomes, and the centrioles. **2.** any one of the tiny organs of protozoa associated with locomotion, metabolism, and other processes. Also called **organella.**

organic, 1. any chemical compound containing carbon. Compare **inorganic. 2.** of or pertaining to an organ.

-organic, a combining form meaning 'related to the internal organs of the body': *enorganic, homorganic, psychorganic.*

organic brain syndrome. See **organic mental disorder.**

organic chemistry, the branch of chemistry concerned with the composition, properties, and reactions of chemical compounds containing carbon.

organic dust, dried particles of plants, animals, fungi, or bacteria that are fine enough to be windborne. Many kinds of organic dust cause various respiratory disorders if inhaled. See also **asthma, bagassosis, byssinosis, hay fever.**

organic evolution, the theory that all existing forms of animal and plant life have descended with modification from previous, simpler forms or from a single cell; the origin and perpetuation of species.

organic mental disorder, any psychologic or behavioral abnormality associated with transient or permanent brain dysfunction caused by a disturbance of the physiologic functioning of brain tissue, as may occur with cerebral arteriosclerosis, lead poisoning, or many other pathologic conditions. Also called **organic brain syndrome.**

organic motivation. See **physiological motivation.**

Organisation Mondiale de la Santé. See **World Health Organization.**

organism, an individual living animal or plant able to carry on life functions through mutually dependent organs or organelles.

organization center, a focal point within the developing embryo from which the organism grows and differentiates. In vertebrates this point is the chordamesoderm of the dorsal lip of the blastopore.

organizer, (in embryology) any part of the embryo that induces morphologic differentiation in some other part. Those parts that are formed and in turn give rise to other parts are classified as organizers of the second degree, third degree, and so on as the embryo develops in complexity. Kinds of organizers include **nucleolar organizer, primary organizer.**

organo-, a combining form meaning 'of or pertaining to an organ or organs': *organofaction, organogenesis, organoleptic.*

organ of Giraldès. See **paradidymis.**

organ of Golgi. See **neurotendinous spindle.**

organogenesis, (in embryology) the formation and differentiation of organs and organ systems during embryonic development. In humans the period extends from approximately the end of the second week through the eighth week of gestation. During this time the embryo undergoes rapid growth and differentiation and is extremely vulnerable to environmental hazards and toxic substances. Any interference with the sequential processes involved with organogenesis causes an arrest in development and results in one or more congenital anomalies. Also called **organogeny.** See also **embryologic development, prenatal development.** **–organogenetic,** *adj.*

organoid, **1.** resembling an organ. **2.** any structure that resembles an organ in appearance or function, specifically an abnormal tumor mass. **3.** See **organelle.**

organoid neoplasm, a growth that resembles a body organ. Compare **histoid neoplasm.**

organoid tumor. See **teratoma.**

organon. See **organ.**

organotherapy, the treatment of disease by administering animal endocrine glands or their extracts. Whole glands are no longer implanted, but substances derived from animal organs are widely used. Also called **Brown-Séquard's treatment.** **–organotherapeutic,** *adj.*

organotypic growth /ôr′gənōtip′ik/, the controlled reproduction of cells, as occurs in the normal growth of tissues and organs. Compare **histiotypic growth.**

organ specificity, a substance or activity that is identified with a specific organ. The term is commonly applied to enzymes that function in particular organ systems.

organum. See **organ.**

orgasm, the sexual climax, a series of strong, involuntary contractions of the muscles of the genitalia experienced as exceedingly pleasurable, set off by sexual excitation of critical intensity. **–orgasmic,** *adj.*

orgasmic platform, congestion of the lower vagina during sexual intercourse.

orient, **1.** to make someone aware of new surroundings, including people and their roles, the layout of a facility, and its routines, rules, and services. New patients are oriented to a hospital as are new staff to a hospital unit. **2.** to help a person become aware of a situation or simply of reality, as when a patient recovers from anesthesia. **–orientation,** *n.,* **oriented,** *adj.*

oriental sore, a dermatologic disease caused by the parasite *Leishmania tropica,* transmitted to humans by the bite of the sand fly. This form of leishmaniasis, characterized by ulcerative lesions, occurs primarily in Africa, Asia, and some Mediterranean countries. Oriental sore causes no systemic symptoms, but the sores are susceptible to secondary infections. Treatment options include infrared therapy and injection of ulcers with sodium antimony gluconate. Also called **Aleppo boil, cutaneous leishmaniasis, Delhi boil, Old World leishmaniasis, tropic sore.** See also **leishmaniasis.**

orientation, **1.** (in molecular genetics) the insertion of a fragment of genetic material into a vector so that the placement of the fragment is in the same direction as the genetic map of the vector (the n orientation) or in the opposite direction (the u orientation). **2.** (in psychiatry) the awareness of one's physical environment with regard to time, place, and the identity of other persons; the ability to adapt to such an existing or new environment. Disorientation is usually a symptom of organic brain disease and most psychoses.

orifice /ôr′ifis/, the entrance or the outlet of any cavity in the body. Also called **ostium.** **–orificial,** *adj.*

ori gene /ôr′ē/, (in molecular genetics) the site or region in which DNA replication starts.

origin, the more fixed end of a muscle attachment. Compare **insertion.**

Orimune, a trademark for an active immunizing agent (live oral poliovirus vaccine).

Orinase, a trademark for an oral sulfanylurea antidiabetic (tolbutamide).

Ornade, a trademark for a fixed-combination drug containing an adrenergic decongestant (phenylpropanolamine hydrochloride), an antihistamine (chlorpheniramine maleate), and an anticholinergic (isopropamide iodide), used for the relief of symptoms of upper respiratory tract congestion.

ornithine, an amino acid, not a constituent of proteins, that is produced as an important intermediate substance in the urea cycle. It is formed by the hydrolization of arginine by arginase and is subsequently converted into citrulline. It decomposes by losing carbon dioxide, producing putrescine and a strong, foul odor characteristic of decaying animal tissue. Also called **diaminovaleric acid.**

ornithine carbamoyl transferase, an enzyme in the blood that increases in patients with liver and other diseases. Its normal concentrations in serum are 8 to 20 mIU/ml.

ornithine cycle. See **urea cycle.**

Ornithodoros /ôr′nithod′ərəs/, a genus of ticks, some species of which are vectors for the spirochetes of relapsing fevers.

ornithosis. See **psittacosis.**

oro-, **1.** a combining form meaning 'of or pertaining to the mouth': *orolingual, oromaxillary, oropharynx.* **2.** see **orrho-.**

orphan drug, any pharmaceutic product that may be available to physicians and patients in countries other than the United States but that has not been "adopted" by a domestic pharmaceutic manufacturer or distributor. An orphan drug may not be available in the United States because total sales would not justify the expense of research and development, the product may not have been approved by the Bureau of Drugs of the Food and Drug Administration, or the medication may be a natural substance that cannot be effectively protected by patent laws against competition from a similar form of the product. Many orphan drugs are pharmaceutic products developed in Europe or Asia that are available in the United States as investigational drugs. The U.S. Orphan Drug Act of 1983 offers federal financial incentives to commercial and nonprofit organizations to develop and market drugs previously unavailable in the United States.

oropharynx /ôr′ōfer′ingks/, one of the three anatomic divisions of the pharynx. It extends behind the mouth from the soft palate above to the level of the hyoid bone below and contains the palatine tonsils and the lingual tonsils. Compare **laryngopharynx, nasopharynx.** –**oropharyngeal,** *adj.*

Oroya fever. See **bartonellosis.**

orphenadrine citrate, a skeletal muscle relaxant with anticholinergic and antihistaminic activity.

■ INDICATION: It is prescribed in the treatment of severe muscle strain.

■ CONTRAINDICATIONS: Myasthenia gravis, contraindications of anticholinergic agents, or known hypersensitivity to this drug prohibits its use.

■ ADVERSE EFFECTS: Among the most serious adverse reactions are those associated with anticholinergic activity, as dry mouth and tachycardia, and allergic reactions.

orphenadrine hydrochloride, an anticholinergic and antihistaminic agent.

■ INDICATION: It is prescribed in the treatment of parkinsonism.

■ CONTRAINDICATIONS: Myasthenia gravis or another condition that contraindicates the use of anticholinergic agents or a known sensitivity to this drug prohibits its use.

■ ADVERSE EFFECTS: Among the most serious adverse reactions are anticholinergic side effects and allergic reactions.

orrho-, oro-, a combining form meaning 'of or pertaining to serum': *orrhomeningitis, orrhoreaction, orrhorrhea.*

ortho-, a combining form meaning 'straight, normal, correct': *orthobiosis, orthodontist, orthotopic.*

orthoboric acid. See **boric acid.**

orthoclase ceramic feldspar, a plentiful clay in the solid crust of the earth, used as a filler and to give body to fused dental porcelain. Compare **feldspar.**

orthodontia. See **orthodontics.**

orthodontic appliance, any device used to modify tooth position. Kinds of such appliances are fixed, movable, active, retaining, intraoral, and extraoral.

orthodontic band, a thin metal ring, usually made of stainless steel, fitted over a tooth for securing orthodontic attachments to a tooth.

orthodontics /ôr′thədon′tiks/, the specialty of dentistry concerned with the diagnosis and treatment of malocclusion and irregularities of the teeth.

orthodromic conduction /ôr′thədrom′ik/, the conduction of a neural impulse in the normal direction, from a synaptic junction or a receptor forward along an axon to its termination with depolarization. Compare **antidromic conduction.**

orthogenesis /ôr′thəjen′əsis/, the theory that evolution is controlled by intrinsic factors within the organism and progresses according to a predetermined course rather than in several directions as a result of natural selection and other environmental factors. –**orthogenetic,** *adj.*

orthogenic, **1.** of or pertaining to orthogenesis; orthogenetic. **2.** of or pertaining to the treatment and rehabilitation of children who are mentally or emotionally disturbed. See also **orthopsychiatry.**

orthogenic evolution, change within an animal or plant induced solely by an intrinsic factor, independent of any environmental elements. Also called **bathmic evolution.**

orthomyxovirus /ôr′thəmik′sōvī′rəs/, a member of a family of viruses that includes several organisms responsible for human influenza infection.

Ortho-Novum, a trademark for an oral contraceptive containing an estrogen (mestranol) and a progestin (norethindrone).

orthopantogram /ôr′thəpan′təgram/, an x-ray film showing a panoramic view of the entire dentition, alveolar bone, and other contiguous structures on a single film, taken extraorally.

orthopedic nurse, a nurse whose primary area of interest, competence, and professional practice is in orthopedic nursing.

orthopedics, the branch of medicine devoted to the study and treatment of the skeletal system, its joints, muscles, and associated structures.

orthopedic traction, a procedure in which a patient is maintained in a device attached by ropes and pulleys to weights that exert a pulling force on an extremity or body part while countertraction is maintained. Traction is applied most often to reduce and immobilize fractures, but it also is used to overcome muscle spasm, to stretch adhesions, to correct certain deformities, and to help release arthritic contractures. Traction may be applied directly to the skin by attaching the rope-pulley-weight system to bands of adhesive, moleskin, or foam rubber or to a splint affixed to the affected limb; side arm traction is a kind of skin traction used to align a fractured humerus after open reduction. Skeletal traction is exerted directly on a bone in which a wire or pin is inserted under anesthesia in the open reduction of a fracture; the ends of the pin protruding through the skin on both sides of the bone are covered with corks and attached to a metal U-shaped spreader or bow, which in turn is attached to the traction rope. Skin or skeletal traction applied to a lower extremity by a balanced suspension apparatus, as the Thomas splint and Pearson's attachment, permits the patient to move more freely in bed because the leg is balanced with countertraction and any slack in traction caused by the patient's movements is taken up by the suspension apparatus. Bryant's traction for treating fractures of the femur shaft in young children uses a suspension apparatus to hold the youngster's legs at right angles to the body. A girdle that fits over the iliac crests and pelvis is used in the application of traction to relieve low back pain, and a cervical halter is employed in applying traction to reduce neck pain; cervical traction may also be used when a fracture of the cervical spine is suspected. See specific devices and specific kinds of traction.

■ METHOD: To maintain the required constant pull, the traction ropes are kept taut, free to ride over the pulleys, and securely tied to the weights that hang free—away from the bed and off the floor. Countertraction is maintained by elevating the patient's bed under the body part to which traction is applied and exerting a pull in the opposite direction; a chest restraint sheet may be applied to the patient in side arm traction for countertraction if necessary. During the initial stages of traction, the involved extremity is checked every 2 hours for quality of the distal pulse, color, warmth, motion, sensation, and swelling. Blood pressure, temperature, pulse, and respirations are recorded every 4 hours until stable. Pain is controlled and the patient is positioned as ordered. If the patient is in balanced suspension, abduction of the leg and a 20 degree angle between the thigh and bed are maintained; the heel is kept free of the sling under the calf. A harness restraint is used to prevent a child in Bryant's traction from turning over, and the youngster's buttocks are raised slightly from the mattress. Bed linen is changed only as necessary, and an air mattress is used when required. Every 2 hours the patient is helped to cough and deep breathe; bony prominences are massaged, but vigorous rubbing is avoided. Lotion is applied to the skin, which is periodically inspected for signs of redness, abrasions, blisters, dryness, itching, excoriation, and pressure areas; special attention is given to the pin insertion sites of the patient in skeletal traction. The patient is observed every 4 hours for neurologic signs, as tingling, numbness, loss of sensation or motion, for thrombophlebitis in the involved extremity, and for evidence of a pulmonary blood clot or fat embolus, as indicated by decreased breath sounds, fever, tachypnea, diaphoresis, pallor, bloody or purulent sputum, and tachycardia. Oral hygiene is administered every 4 hours, and, unless contraindicated, a daily intake of 2500 to 3000 ml of fluids is encouraged. As the patient's condition improves, the position is changed every 4 hours; if the kind of traction permits and if the upper extremities are not involved, a trapeze is added to the bed. The patient is taught to perform range of motion exercises with the uninvolved extremities, dorsiflexion and plantar flexion of the ankles, and isometric exercises, as gluteal and abdominal contraction. A high-protein, low-carbohydrate diet is served, and vitamin and iron therapy may be ordered. The immobilized patient uses a flat, fracture bedpan and usually requires stool softeners or a mild laxative.

■ NURSING ORDERS: The patient in traction often needs extensive physical care and emotional support. The person is encouraged to verbalize feelings and concerns about prolonged hospitalization and absence from work or school. To the greatest degree possible, the nurse encourages the patient to participate in self-care and to engage in diversions, as handicrafts, reading, watching television, and listening to the radio.

■ OUTCOME CRITERIA: The healthy young adult or adolescent in traction for the treatment of a fracture usually has an uneventful recovery, but diligent attention and nursing care are necessary to avoid the formation of decubitus ulcers, infection, constipation, and other sequelae of immobility.

orthopedist, a specialist in orthopedics. Also called *(informal)* **orthopod.**

orthopnea /ôrthop′nē·ə/, an abnormal condition in which a person must sit or stand in order to breathe deeply or comfortably. It occurs in many disorders of the cardiac and respiratory systems, as asthma, pulmonary edema, emphysema, pneumonia, and angina pectoris. See also **dyspnea.** –**orthopneic,** *adj.*

orthopod. See **orthopedist.**

orthopsychiatry, the branch of psychiatry that specializes in correcting incipient and borderline mental and behavioral disorders, especially in children, and in developing preventive techniques to promote mental health and emotional growth and development. See also **mental hygiene.**

orthoptic /ôrthop′tik/, **1.** of or pertaining to normal binocular vision. **2.** of or pertaining to a procedure or technique for correcting the visual axes of eyes improperly coordinated for binocular vision.

orthoptic examination, an ophthalmoscopic examination of the binocular function of the eyes. A stereoscopic instrument presents a slightly different picture to each eye. The examiner notes the degree to which the pictures are combined by the normal process of fusion. If the person has diplopia, separate pictures are seen. If the person has suppression amblyopia, only one picture is seen. Stereoscopic training may improve binocular vision in some conditions.

orthoptist /ôrthop′tist/, a person qualified by postsecondary training and successful completion of an examination by the American Orthoptist Council who, under the supervision of an ophthalmologist, tests eye muscles and teaches exercise programs designed to correct eye coordination defects.

orthosis /ôrthō′sis/, a force system designed to control, correct, or compensate for a bone deformity, deforming forces, or forces absent from the body. Orthosis often involves the use of special braces. –**orthotic** /ôrthot′-ik/, *adj., n.*

orthostatic albuminuria. See **orthostatic proteinuria.**

orthostatic hypotension, abnormally low blood pressure occurring when an individual assumes the standing posture. Also called **postural hypotension.**

orthostatic proteinuria, presence of protein in the urine of some people, especially teenagers, who have been standing. It disappears when they recline and is of no pathologic significance. Also called **orthostatic albuminuria, postural albuminuria, postural proteinuria.**

orthotist /ôr′thətist/, a person who designs, fabricates, and fits braces or other orthopedic appliances prescribed by physicians. A certified orthotist is one who successfully completed the examination of the American Orthotist and Prosthetic Association.

orthotonos /ôrthot′ənəs/, a straight, rigid posture of the body caused by a tetanic spasm, usually resulting from strychnine poisoning or tetanus infection. The neck and all other parts of the body are in a position of extension but not as severely as in opisthotonos. Compare **emprosthotonos.**

orthovoltage, the voltage range of 100 to 350 KeV supplied by some x-ray generators used for radiation therapy. They have been replaced in many hospitals and other health facilities by equipment that operates in the megavolt range.

Ortolani's test /ôr′təlä′nēz/, a procedure used to evaluate the stability of the hip joints in newborns and infants. The baby is placed on his back, the hips and knees are flexed at right angles and abducted until the lateral aspects of the knees are touching the table. The examiner's fingers are extended along the outside of the thighs, with the thumbs grasping the insides of the knees. Internal and external rotation are attempted, and symmetry of mobility is evaluated. A click or a popping sensation (Ortolani's sign) may be felt if the joint is unstable, because the head of the femur moves out of the acetabulum under pressure from the examiner's hands during rotation and abduction. See also **congenital dislocation of the hip.**

os /os/. See **bone.**

Os, symbol for **osmium.**

OS, **1.** abbreviation for *oculus sinister,* a Latin phrase meaning "left eye." **2.** abbreviation for a computer **operating system.**

-os, a combining form signaling singular nouns: *biologos, hepatomphalos, megophthalmos.*

os calcis. See **calcaneus.**

os capitatum. See **capitate bone.**

oscheo-, a combining form meaning 'of or pertaining to the scrotum': *oscheocele, oscheolith, oscheoma.*

oscillator, an electric or other device that produces oscillations, vibrations, or fluctuations, as an alternating electric current generator.

oscilloscope, an instrument that displays a visual representation of electric variations on the fluorescent screen of a cathode ray tube. The graphic representation is produced by a beam of electrons on the screen. The beam is focused or directed by a magnetic field that is influenced in turn by a source such as an amplified current produced by heart contractions. As used in cardiology, the oscilloscope can function as a continuous electrocardiogram.

os coxae. See **innominate bone.**

os cuboideum. See **cuboid bone.**

-ose, **1.** a combining form meaning a 'carbohydrate': *cellulose, lactose, sucrose.* **2.** a combining form meaning a 'primary product of hydrolysis': *albumose, nucleose, myoproteose.*

Osgood-Schlatter disease /oz′go͝odshlat′ər/, inflammation or partial separation of the tibial tubercle caused by chronic irritation, usually as a result of overuse of the quadriceps muscle. The condition is seen primarily in muscular, athletic adolescent boys and is characterized by swelling and tenderness over the tibial tubercle that increase with exercise or any activity that extends the leg. Treatment consists primarily of preventing further irritation during the healing process and may necessitate complete immobilization of the knee in a cast. Any residual nonunion of a proximal fragment after healing may require surgical excision. Also called **Osgood's disease, Schlatter-Osgood disease, Schlatter's disease.**

os hamatum. See **hamate bone.**

os hyoideum. See **hyoid bone.**

-osis, **1.** a combining form meaning a '(specified) action, process, or result': *homeosis, narcosis, zygosis.* **2.** a combining form meaning a 'pathologic condition': *calcicosis, psittacosis, varicosis.*

Osler's disease. See **Osler-Weber-Rendu syndrome, polycythemia.**

Osler's nodes /ōs′lərz/, tender, reddish or purplish subcutaneous nodules of the soft tissue on the ends of fingers or toes, seen in subacute bacterial endocarditis and usually lasting only 1 or 2 days.

Osler-Weber-Rendu syndrome /ōs′lərweb′ərando͞o′/, a vascular anomaly, inherited as an autosomal dominant trait, characterized by hemorrhagic telangiectasia of skin and mucosa. Small red-to-violet lesions are found on the lips, the oral and nasal mucosa, the tongue, and the tips of fingers and toes. The thin, dilated vessels may bleed spontaneously or as a result of only minor trauma, and this condition becomes progressively more severe. Bleeding from superficial lesions is often profuse and may result in severe anemia. No specific treatment is known, but accessible, bleeding lesions may be treated with pressure, styptics, and topical hemostatics. Transfusions may be indicated for acute hemorrhage, and iron deficiency anemia may require continuous treatment. Also called **hereditary hemorrhagic telangiectasia, Rendu-Osler-Weber syndrome.** See also **hemorrhagic familial angiomatosis.**

os lunatum. See **lunate bone.**

os magnum. See **capitate bone.**

osmethesia, the ability to perceive and distinguish odors; the sense of smell.

-osmia, a combining form meaning '(condition of the) sense of smell': *dysosmia, hemianosmia, merosmia.*

Osmitrol, a trademark for a diagnostic aid and osmotic diuretic (mannitol).

osmium (Os), a hard, grayish, pungent-smelling metallic element. Its atomic number is 76; its atomic weight is 190.2. Used to produce alloys of extreme hardness, it is highly toxic.

osmo-, **1.** a combining form meaning 'of or pertaining to odors': *osmoceptor, osmodysphoria, osmonosology.* **2.** a combining form meaning 'pertaining to an impulse, or to osmosis': *osmophilic, osmosology, osmotaxis.*

osmoceptors, receptors in the hypothalamus that respond to osmotic pressure, thereby regulating production of the antidiuretic hormone.

osmolal gap, a difference between the observed and calculated osmolalities in serum analysis. The calculated osmolar values include sodium concentration multiplied by 2, plus glucose and blood urea nitrogen.

osmolality /oz′mōlal′itē/, the osmotic pressure of a solution expressed in osmols or milliosmols per kilogram of water. Compare **osmolarity.**

osmolar /osmō′lər/, of or pertaining to the osmotic characteristics of a solution of one or more molecular substances, ionic substances, or both, expressed in osmols or milliosmols.

osmolarity /oz′mōler′itē/, the osmotic pressure of a solution expressed in osmols or milliosmols per kilogram of the solution. Compare **osmolality.**

osmole /os′mōl/, the quantity of a substance in solution in the form of molecules, ions, or both (usually expressed in grams) that has the same osmotic pressure as one mole of an ideal nonelectrolyte. **–osmolal,** *adj.*

osmometry, a field of study that deals with the phenomenon of osmosis and the measurement of osmotic forces. **–osmometric,** *adj.*

osmosis /ozmō′sis, os-/, the movement of a pure solvent, as water, through a semipermeable membrane from a solution that has a lower solute concentration to one that has a higher solute concentration. The membrane is impermeable to the solute but is permeable to the solvent. The rate of osmosis depends on the concentration of solute, the temperature of the solution, the electric charge of the solute, and the difference between the osmotic pressures exerted by the solutions. Movement across the membrane continues until the concentrations of the solutions equalize.

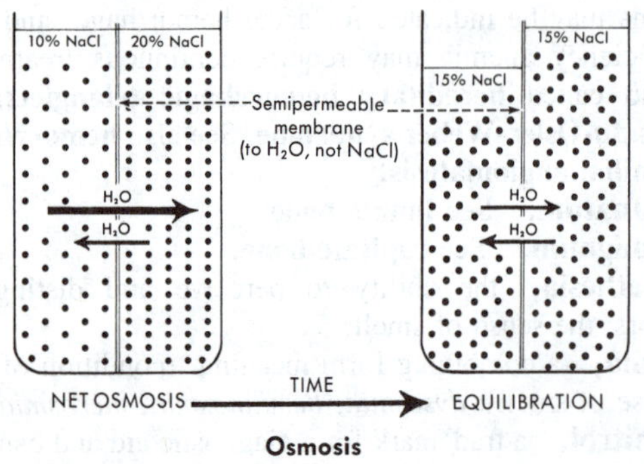

Osmosis

osmotic diuresis, diuresis resulting from the presence of certain nonabsorbable substances in tubules of the kidney, as mannitol, urea, or glucose.

osmotic fragility, a sensitivity to change in osmotic pressure characteristic of red blood cells. Exposed to a hypotonic concentration of sodium in a solution, red cells take in increasing quantities of water, swell until the capacity of the cell membrane is exceeded, and burst. Exposed to a hypertonic concentration of sodium in a solution, red cells give up intracellular fluid, shrink, and break up. Laboratory findings of exceptional fragility or resistance may be diagnostic of certain conditions. Hemolysis of normal cells begins in 0.39% to 0.45% salt solution and is complete in 0.30% to 0.33% salt solution in 24 hours at 37° C.

osmotic pressure, 1. the pressure exerted on a semipermeable membrane separating a solution from a solvent, the membrane being impermeable to the solutes in the solution and permeable only to the solvent. **2.** the pressure exerted on a semipermeable membrane by a solution containing one or more solutes that cannot penetrate the membrane, which is permeable only by the solvent surrounding it. See also **osmosis.**

os naviculares pedis. See **scaphoid bone.**

-osphresia, -osphrasia, a combining form meaning a 'condition of the sense of smell': *anosphresia, hyperosphresia, oxyosphresia.*

osphresis, olfaction; the sense of smell.

osphresio-, a combining form meaning 'of or pertaining to odors': *osphresiolagnia, osphresiology, osphresiophilia.*

oss-, a combining form meaning 'of or pertaining to bone': *osseocartilaginous, ossicle, ossific.*

osseous labyrinth, the bony portion of the internal ear, composed of three cavities: the vestibule, the semicircular canals, and the cochlea, transmitting sound vibrations from the middle ear to the acoustic nerve. All three cavities contain perilymph, in which a membranous labyrinth is suspended. Also called **labyrinthus osseus.** Compare **membranous labyrinth.**

ossicle /os′ikəl/, a small bone, as the malleus, the incus, or the stapes, ossicles of the inner ear. **–ossicular,** *adj.*

ossification /os′ifikā′shən/, the development of bone. **Intramembranous ossification** is that preceded by membrane, as in the process initially forming the roof and the sides of the skull. **Intracartilaginous ossification** is that preceded by rods of cartilage, as that forming the bones of the limbs.

ossifying fibroma, a slow-growing, benign neoplasm of bone, occurring most often in the jaws, especially the mandible. The tumor is composed of bone that develops within fibrous connective tissue.

ostealgia, any pain that is associated with an abnormal condition within a bone, as osteomyelitis. **–ostealgic,** *adj.*

osteanagenesis. See **osteoanagenesis.**

osteitis /os′tē·ī′tis/, an inflammation of bone, caused by infection, degeneration, or trauma. Swelling, tenderness, dull aching pain, and redness in the skin over the affected bone are characteristic of the condition. Some kinds of osteitis are **osteitis deformans** and **osteitis fibrosa cystica.** See also **osteomyelitis, Paget's disease.**

osteitis fibrosa cystica, an inflammatory degenerative condition in which normal bone is replaced by cysts and fibrous tissue. It is usually associated with hyperparathyroidism.

osteitis fibrosa disseminata. See **Albright's syndrome.**

ostembryon. See **lithopedion.**

osteo-, a combining form meaning 'of or pertaining to bone': *osteoanesthesia, osteocele, osteopathy.*

osteoanagenesis /os'tē•ō•an'əjen'əsis/, the regeneration or formation of bone tissue. Also called **osteanagenesis.**

osteoarthritis /os'tē•ō•ärthrī'tis/, a form of arthritis in which one or many joints undergo degenerative changes, including subchondral bony sclerosis, loss of articular cartilage, and proliferation of bone and cartilage in the joint, forming osteophytes. Inflammation of the synovial membrane of the joint is common late in the disease. The most common form of arthritis, its cause is unknown but may include chemical, mechanic, genetic, metabolic, and endocrine factors. Emotional stress often aggravates the condition. The condition usually begins with pain after exercise or use of the joint. Stiffness, tenderness to the touch, crepitus, and enlargement develop, and deformity, subluxation, and synovial effusion may eventually occur. Involvement of the hip, knee, or the spine causes more disability than osteoarthritis of other areas. Treatment includes rest of the involved joints, heat, and antiinflammatory drugs. Systemic corticosteroids are contraindicated, but intraarticular injections of corticosteroids may give relief. Surgical treatment is sometimes necessary and may reduce pain and greatly improve the function of a joint. Hip replacement, joint debridement, fusion, and decompression laminectomy are some of the surgical procedures used in treating advanced osteoarthritis. Compare **rheumatoid arthritis.**

osteoblast, a cell that originates in the embryonic mesenchyme and, during the early development of the skeleton, differentiates from a fibroblast to function in the formation of bone tissue. Osteoblasts synthesize the collagen and glycoproteins to form the matrix and, with growth, develop into osteocytes. Also called **osteoplast.** See also **ossification.** –**osteoblastic,** *adj.*

osteoblastoma /os'tē•ōblastō'mə/, *pl.* **osteoblastomas, osteoblastomata,** a small, benign, fairly vascular tumor of poorly formed bone and fibrous tissue, occurring most frequently in the vertebrae, femur, tibia, or bones of the upper extremities in children and young adults. The lesion causes pain, erosion, and resorption of native bone. When feasible, excision is the preferred treatment. Also called **osteoid osteoma.**

osteochondrodystrophy. See **Morquio's disease.**

osteochondroma /os'tē•ōkondrō'mə/, a benign tumor made of bone and cartilage.

osteochondrosis /os'tē•ōkondrō'sis/, a disease affecting the ossification centers of bone in children, initially characterized by degeneration and necrosis, followed by regeneration and recalcification. Kinds of osteochondrosis include **Legg-Calvé-Perthes disease, Osgood-Schlatter disease,** and **Scheuermann's disease.**

osteoclasia /os'tē•ōklā'zhə/, **1.** the destruction and absorption of bony tissue by osteoclasts, as during growth or the healing of fractures. **2.** the degeneration of bone through disease. See also **osteolysis.**

osteoclasis /os'tē•ok'ləsis/, the intentional surgical fracture of a bone to correct a deformity. Also called **osteoclasty.** –**osteoclastic,** *adj.*

osteoclast, 1. also called **osteophage.** a large type of multinucleated bone cell that functions in the development and periods of growth or repair, as the breakdown and resorption of osseous tissue. During bone healing of fractures, or during certain disease processes, osteoclasts excavate passages through the surrounding tissue by enzymatic action. Osteoclasts become activated in the presence of parathyroid hormone and also in a lymphokine substance produced by lymphocytes in such diseases as multiple myeloma and malignant lymphomas. See also **ossification. 2.** a surgical instrument used in the fracturing or refracturing of bones for therapeutic purposes, as correction of a deformity.

osteoclastic, 1. pertaining to or of the nature of osteoclasts. **2.** destructive to bone.

osteoclastoma /os'tē•ōklastō'mə/, *pl.* **osteoclastomas, osteoclastomata,** a giant cell tumor of the bone, occurring most frequently at the end of a long bone and appearing as a mass surrounded by a thin shell of new, periosteal bone. The lesion may be benign but is more often malignant. It causes local pain, loss of function, and, in some cases, weakness followed by pathologic fracture. Also called **giant cell myeloma, giant cell tumor of bone.**

osteoclasty. See **osteoclasis.**

osteocyte, a bone cell; a mature osteoblast that has become embedded in the bone matrix. It occupies a small cavity and sends out protoplasmic projections that anastomose with those of other osteoblasts to form a system of minute canals within the bone matrix. –**osteocytic,** *adj.*

osteodystrophy, any generalized defect in bone development, usually associated with disturbances in calcium and phosphorus metabolism and renal insufficiency, as in renal osteodystrophy. Also called **osteodystrophia.**

osteogenesis, the origin and development of bone tissue. Also called **osteogeny** /os'tē•oj'ənē/. See also **ossification.** –**osteogenetic, osteogenic,** *adj.*

osteogenesis imperfecta, a genetic disorder involving defective development of the connective tissue. It is inherited as an autosomal dominant trait and is characterized by abnormally brittle and fragile bones that are easily fractured by the slightest trauma. Also called **brittle bones, fragilitas ossium, hypoplasia of the mesenchyme, osteopsathyrosis.**

■ OBSERVATIONS: In its most severe form, the disease may be apparent at birth, when it is known as **osteogenesis imperfecta congenita.** The newborn has multiple fractures that have occurred in utero and is usually severely deformed, because of imperfect formation and mineralization of bone. Most infants die shortly after birth, although a few survive as deformed dwarfs with normal mental development if no head trauma has occurred. If the disease has a later onset, it is called **osteogenesis imperfecta tarda** and usually runs a milder course. Symptoms generally appear when the child begins to walk, but they become less severe with age and the tendency to fracture decreases and often disappears after puberty. Other manifestations of the condition include blue sclerae, translucent skin, hyperextensibility of ligaments, hypoplasia of the teeth, recurrent epistaxis, excess diaphoresis, mild hyperpyrexia, and a tendency to bruise easily and to develop otosclerosis with hearing loss. There is a broad expressivity of the disease so that the number and extent of pathologic features may range from minimal to severe involvement.

■ INTERVENTION: There is no known cure for the disease. Treatment is predominantly supportive; extreme care must be taken in handling patients, especially infants who are severely affected, to prevent fractures. In many children oral administration of magnesium oxide may decrease the fracture rate, as well as the diaphoresis, hyperpyrexia, and constipation associated with the condition.

■ NURSING CONSIDERATIONS: The primary function of the nurse is to educate the parents about the disease, especially the extent of the child's limitations, and to help them plan suitable activities that will promote optimum growth and development and, at the same time, protect the child from harm. Genetic counseling is also part of the goals of long-term care.

osteogenic, composed of or originating from any tissue involved in the development, growth, or repair of bone. Also **osteogenous** /os′tē•oj′ənəs/.

osteogenic sarcoma. See **osteosarcoma.**

osteogeny. See **osteogenesis.**

osteoid /os′tē•oid/, of, pertaining to, or resembling bone.

osteoid osteoma. See **osteoblastoma.**

osteolysis /os′tē•ol′isis/, the degeneration and dissolution of bone, caused by disease, infection, or ischemia. The condition commonly affects the terminal bones of the hands and feet, as in acroosteolysis, and is seen in disorders involving blood vessels, as in Raynaud's disease, scleroderma, and systemic lupus erythematosus. –**osteolytic,** *adj.*

osteoma /os′tē•ō′mə/, *pl.* **osteomas, osteomata,** a tumor of bone tissue.

-osteoma, a combining form meaning a 'tumor composed of bone tissue, usually benign': *endosteoma, myosteoma, periosteoma.*

osteomalacia /os′tē•ōməlā′shə/, an abnormal condition of the lamellar bone, characterized by a loss of calcification of the matrix resulting in softening of the bone, accompanied by weakness, fracture, pain, anorexia, and weight loss. The condition is the result of an inadequate amount of phosphorus and calcium available in the blood for mineralization of the bones. This deficiency may be caused by a diet lacking these minerals or vitamin D, or by a lack of exposure to sunlight, hence an inability to synthesize vitamin D, or by a metabolic disorder causing malabsorption. Osteomalacia results from and also complicates many diseases and conditions. Treatment usually includes the administration of the necessary vitamins and minerals and therapy appropriate for the underlying disorder. See also **adult rickets, hyperparathyroidism, Paget's disease, rickets.**

osteomyelitis /os′tē•ōmī•əlī′tis/, local or generalized infection of bone and bone marrow, usually caused by bacteria introduced by trauma or surgery, by direct extension from a nearby infection, or via the bloodstream. Staphylococci are the most common causative agents.

■ OBSERVATIONS: The long bones in children and the vertebrae in adults are the commonest sites of infection as a result of hematogenous spread. Persistent, severe, and increasing bone pain, tenderness, guarding on movement, regional muscle spasm, and fever suggest this diagnosis. Draining sinus tracts may accompany posttraumatic osteomyelitis or osteomyelitis from a contiguous infection. Specific diagnosis and selection of therapy depend on bacterial examination of bone, tissue, or pus.

■ INTERVENTION: Treatment includes bed rest and parenteral antibiotics for several weeks. Surgery may be necessary to remove necrotic bone and tissue, to obliterate cavities, to remove infected prosthetic appliances, and to apply prostheses to stabilize affected parts. Chronic osteomyelitis may persist for years with exacerbations and remissions despite treatment.

■ NURSING CONSIDERATIONS: Any drainage is disposed of with the usual precautions against contamination. Absolute rest of the affected part may be necessary, with a careful positioning using pillows and sandbags for good alignment. During the early phase of infection, pain is extremely severe and extraordinary gentleness in moving and manipulating the infected part is essential. –**osteomyelitic,** *adj.*

osteon /os′tē•on/, the basic structural unit of compact bone, consisting of the haversian canal and its concentric rings of 4 to 20 lamellae. Most of the units run with the long axis of the bone.

-osteon, -osteum, a combining form meaning 'bone': *melacosteon, otosteon, pleurosteon.*

osteonecrosis /os′tē•ōnəkrō′sis/, the destruction and death of bone tissue, as from ischemia, infection, malignant neoplastic disease, or trauma. –**osteonecrotic,** *adj.*

osteopath /os′tē•ōpath′/, a physician who specializes in osteopathy. Also called **osteopathist.**

osteopathy /os′tē•op′əthē/, a therapeutic approach to the practice of medicine that uses all the usual forms of medical therapy and diagnosis, including drugs, surgery, and radiation, but that places greater emphasis on the role of the relationship of the organs and the musculoskeletal system than is done in medicine. Osteopathic physicians recognize and correct structural problems using manipulation. The process is important in both the diagnosis and the treatment of health problems. See also **Doctor of Osteopathy.** –**osteopathic,** *adj.*

osteopedion. See **lithopedion.**

osteopenia, a condition of subnormally mineralized bone, usually the result of a failure of the rate of bone matrix synthesis to compensate for the rate of bone lysis.

osteopetrosis, an inherited disorder characterized by a generalized increase in bone density, probably caused by faulty bone resorption resulting from a deficiency of osteoclasts. In its most severe form, transmitted as an autosomal recessive condition, there is obliteration of the bone marrow cavity, causing severe anemia, marked deformities of the skull, and compression of the cranial nerves, which may result in deafness and blindness and lead to an early death. A milder, benign form, transmitted as an autosomal dominant trait, is characterized by short stature, fragile bones that fracture easily, and a proneness to develop osteomyelitis. Also called **Albers-Schönberg disease, ivory bones, marble bones, osteosclerosis fragilis.** **–osteopetrotic,** *adj.*

osteophage. See **osteoclast.**

osteoplast. See **osteoblast.**

osteopoikilosis, an inherited condition of the bones, transmitted as an autosomal dominant trait, characterized by multiple areas of dense calcification throughout the osseous tissue, producing a mottled appearance on x-ray examination. It is a benign condition, usually without symptoms, and of unknown cause. Also called **osteosclerosis fragilis congenita.** **–osteopoikilotic,** *adj.*

osteoporosis, a disorder characterized by abnormal rarefaction of bone, occurring most frequently in postmenopausal women, in sedentary or immobilized individuals, and in patients on long-term steroid therapy. The disorder may cause pain, especially in the lower back, pathologic fractures, loss of stature, and various deformities. Osteoporosis may be idiopathic or secondary to other disorders, as thyrotoxicosis or the bone demineralization caused by hyperparathyroidism. Estrogen therapy is often used for the prevention and management of postmenopausal osteoporosis, but use of the hormone carries the risk of endometrial cancer.

osteopsathyrosis. See **osteogenesis imperfecta.**

osteosarcoma /os′tē·ōsärkō′mə/, a malignant bone tumor composed of anaplastic cells derived from mesenchyme. Also called **osteogenic sarcoma.**

osteosclerosis, an abnormal increase in the density of bone tissue. The condition occurs in a variety of disease states, is commonly associated with ischemia, chronic infection, and tumor formation, and may be caused by faulty bone resorption as a result of some abnormality involving the osteoclasts. See also **achondroplasia, osteopetrosis, osteopoikilosis.** **–osteosclerotic,** *adj.*

osteosclerosis fragilis. See **osteopetrosis.**

osteosclerosis fragilis congenita. See **osteopoikilosis.**

osteotome, a surgical instrument for cutting through bone.

osteotomy, the sawing or cutting of a bone. Kinds of osteotomy include block osteotomy, in which a section of bone is excised, cuneiform osteotomy to remove a bone wedge, and displacement osteotomy, in which a bone is redesigned surgically to alter the alignment or weight-bearing stress areas.

-osteum. See **-osteon.**

ostium. See **orifice.**

ostium primum defect, ostium secundum defect. See **atrial septal defect.**

ostomate /os′təmāt/, a patient who has undergone an ostomy.

ostomy /os′təmē/, *informal.* a surgical procedure in which an opening is made to allow the passage of urine from the bladder or of intestinal contents from the bowel to an incision or stoma surgically created in the wall of the abdomen. An ostomy procedure may be performed to correct an anatomic defect, to relieve an obstruction in or to permit treatment of a severe infection or injury of the urinary or intestional tract. Each procedure is named for the anatomic location of the ostomy, as a colostomy, cecostomy, or cystostomy. (Table, page 816)

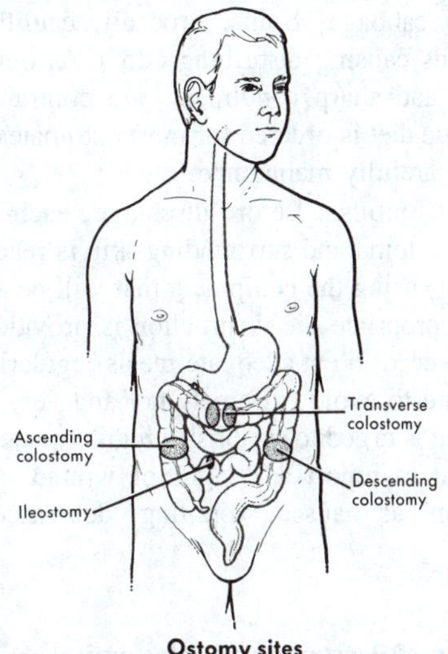

Ostomy sites

ostomy care, the management and support of a patient with a surgical opening created in the bladder, ileum, or colon for the temporary or permanent passage of urine or feces, necessitated by carcinoma, intestinal obstruction, trauma, or severe ulceration distal to the site of the incision. In most cases the opening is covered with a temporary disposable bag in the operating room.

■ METHOD: The patient with a colostomy or an ileostomy is helped to accept the stoma and the change in body image that frequently causes grief, or, in some instances, denial. Discussions of the person's feelings are encouraged, and questions regarding the procedure and possible changes in the person's life style are answered in a positive manner. The disposable bag is changed whenever necessary, and the character, color, and amount of drainage are observed; mucus secretion from the stoma usually begins within 48 hours after the operation, fecal drainage within 72 hours. The stoma is inspected periodically for color, bleeding, stricture, retraction, and infection and is measured every other day to determine the size of the permanent appliance that is to be used as soon as the condition of the opening permits. Each time the temporary or permanent appliance is changed, the skin around the stoma is washed with soap and water, rinsed thoroughly, and patted dry with a clean towel. If the skin is irritated or excoriated, karaya powder, alone or mixed with an ointment, is spread over the area before the appliance is reinstalled. An adhesive substance may be used to maintain a tight seal with the appliance, and deodorant drops, aspirin, or various bismuth or chlorophyll preparations are added to the ostomy bag to control odor. The diet is planned according to the kind of ostomy; ileostomates require food high in sodium and potassium, as bananas, citrus juices, molasses, and cola, and are advised to avoid fried, highly seasoned, and rich foods, nuts, raisins, raw fruits other than bananas, and anything that produces gas or causes diarrhea. Gas-producing foods, as cabbage, beans, broccoli, cauliflower, and corn, foods causing disturbing odors, as onions, eggs, and fish, and sharp condiments are contraindicated; a low-residue diet is ordered for most ostomates. The fluid intake is carefully maintained.

■ NURSING ORDERS: Before discharge, each step in the care of the stoma and surrounding skin is rehearsed with the patient, using the equipment that will be available at home. Appropriate diet instruction is provided, emphasizing the need to eat adequate meals regularly, to chew slowly, and to avoid extremely hot and very cold food. The patient is urged to establish a regular pattern of evacuation and to report any signs of wound infection or obstruction, as nausea, vomiting, decreased drainage from the stoma, abdominal distention, and cramps. Normal daily activity is encouraged.

■ OUTCOME CRITERIA: The ability of the patient to adjust to the ostomy procedures and equipment is greatly affected by the nursing care received in the days after surgery. A positive, patient, and matter of fact approach, sensitive emotional support, and thorough teaching of self-care measures are essential aspects of ostomy nursing care.

ostomy irrigation, a procedure for cleansing, stimulating, and regulating evacuation of an artificially created orifice. Fluids used in irrigation include tap water and saline or medicated solutions. Necessary equipment includes properly sized irrigator tips, catheters, drainage bags that allow for insertion of the catheter, an irrigation container, and shields to prevent leakage. Loop and double-barrel colostomies require a sequential irrigation of the proximal loop, distal loop, and rectum to prevent the accumulation of discharge.

os trapezium. See **trapezium.**

os trapezoideum. See **trapezoid bone.**

os triquetrum. See **triangular bone.**

OT, abbreviation for **occupational therapist, occupational therapy.**

ot-. See **oto-.**

otalgia /ōtal′jə/, pain in the ear. Also called **otodynia, otoneuralgia.**

OTC, abbreviation for *over the counter,* describing a drug available without a prescription from a physician.

Othello syndrome, a psychopathologic condition, characterized by suspicion of a spouse's infidelity and by morbid jealousy. This condition may be accompanied by rage and violence and is frequently associated with paranoia.

Comparison of ileostomy and colostomies

	Ileostomy	*Ascending colostomy*	*Transverse colostomy*	*Sigmoid colostomy*
Location	Ileum (terminal end of small intestine)	Ascending colon	Transverse colon	Sigmoid colon
Type of drainage	Initial: liquid; 3-6 mo: "toothpaste" consistency	Liquid to soft	Soft	Formed
Bowel regulation	No	No	No	Yes
Fluid and electrolyte imbalance	Occurs frequently with illness and diagnostic procedures	Same as for ileostomy	Less possibility than with ileostomy but may occur more readily than normal	No different from a person with intact colon
Skin irritation	Irritation occurs easily from digestive enzymes	Same as for ileostomy	Some skin irritation from constant moisture	Irritation may occur occasionally
Other complications	Stricture or inversion of stoma; diarrhea with antibiotic therapy; food blockage	Stricture or inversion of stoma	Stricture or inversion of stoma	Stricture or inversion of stoma

other type of diabetes, a condition that is secondary to other syndromes, as pancreatic or endocrine or drug-induced diseases, insulin receptor anomalies, or genetic conditions. Previously called **secondary diabetes.** See also **diabetes mellitus.**

-otia, a combining form meaning '(condition of the) ear': *melotia, microtia, synotia.*

otic /ō′tik, ot′ik/, of or pertaining to the ear. Also **auricular.**

-otic[1], **1.** a combining form meaning 'pertaining to part of the ear': *entotic, epitotic, prootic.* **2.** a combining form meaning 'pertaining to an area spatially related to the ear': *opisthotic, parotic, periotic.* **3.** a combining form meaning 'pertaining to a bone spatially related to the ear': *basiotic, prootic, sphenotic.*

-otic[2], **1.** a combining form meaning 'pertaining to a (specified) action or condition': *antidotic, biotic, osmotic.* **2.** a combining form meaning pertaining to a disease condition': *anthracotic, mycotic, neurotic.* **3.** a combining form meaning 'pertaining to an increase (of something specified)': *hematotic, morphotic, zymotic.*

otics /ō′tiks, ot′iks/, a group of drugs used locally to treat inflammation of the external ear canal or to remove excess cerumen.

otitic barotrauma. See **barotrauma.**

otitis /ōtī′tis/, inflammation or infection of the ear. Kinds of otitis are **otitis externa** and **otitis media.**

otitis externa, inflammation or infection of the external canal or the auricle of the external ear. Major causes are allergy, bacteria, fungi, viruses, and trauma. Allergy to nickel or chromium in earrings and to chemicals in hair sprays, cosmetics, hearing aids, and medications, particularly sulfonamides and neomycin, is common. *Staphylococcus aureus, Pseudomonas aeruginosa,* and *Streptococcus pyogenes* are common bacterial causes. Herpes simplex and herpes zoster viruses are frequently implicated. Eczema, psoriasis, and seborrheic dermatitis also may affect the external ear. Abrasions of the ear canal may become infected, and excessive swimming may wash out protective cerumen, remove skin lipids, and lead to secondary infection. Otitis externa is more prevalent during hot, humid weather. Folliculitis is particularly painful in the external auditory meatus and is a common occupational hazard in nurses, caused by irritation from the earpieces of stethoscopes. Treatment includes oral analgesics, thorough local cleansing, topical antimicrobials to treat infection, or topical corticosteroids to reduce inflammation. Prevention includes measures to reduce maceration of the skin and to avoid trauma.

otitis interna. See **labyrinthitis.**

otitis media, inflammation or infection of the middle ear, a common affliction of childhood. Acute otitis media is most often caused by *Haemophilus influenzae* or *Streptococcus pneumoniae.* Chronic otitis media is usually caused by gram-negative bacteria, as *Proteus, Klebsiella,* and *Pseudomonas.* Allergy, *Mycoplasma,* and several viruses also may be causative factors. Otitis media is often preceded by an upper respiratory infection.

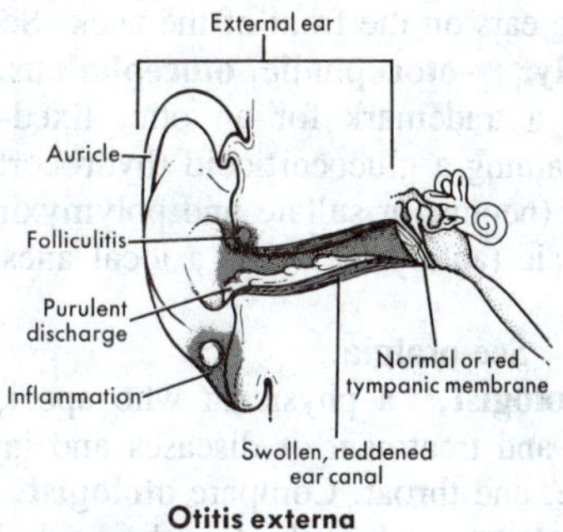

Otitis externa

■ OBSERVATIONS: Organisms gain entry to the middle ear through the eustachian tube. The small diameter and horizontal orientation of the tube in infants predisposes them to infection. Obstruction of the eustachian tube and accumulation of exudate may increase pressure within the middle ear, forcing infection into the mastoid bone or rupturing the tympanic membrane. Symptoms of acute otitis media include a sense of fullness in the ear, diminished hearing, pain, and fever. Usually, only one ear is affected. Squamous epithelium may grow in the middle ear through a rupture in the tympanic membrane, and development of a cholesteatoma and deafness may occur if repeated infections cause an opening to persist. Pneumococcal otitis media may spread to the meninges.

■ INTERVENTION: Accurate diagnosis of the causative microorganism is important for selection of effective antimicrobial therapy. Treatment also includes analgesics, local heat, nasal decongestants, needle aspiration of secretions collected behind the membrane, and myringotomy.

■ NURSING OBSERVATIONS: Parents are taught to recognize and watch for early warning signs of otitis media. The use of vaporizers and decongestants is often recommended during an upper respiratory tract infection as prophylaxis against otitis media.

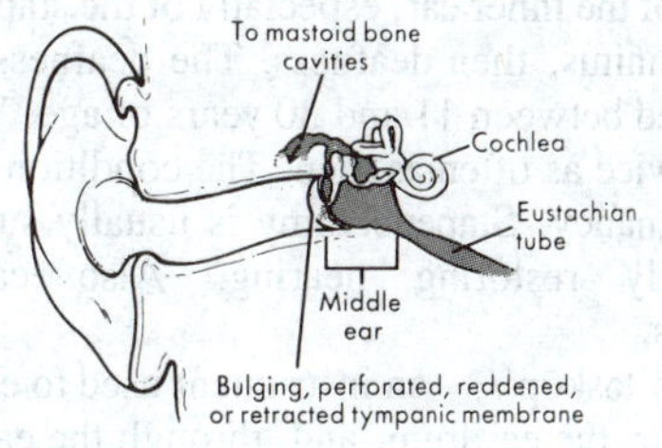

Otitis media

oto-, ot-, a combining form meaning 'of or pertaining to the ear': *otoantritis, otoblennorrhea, otocyst.*

otocephalus /ō′tōsef′ələs/, a fetus with otocephaly.

otocephaly /ō′tōsef′əlē/, a congenital malformation characterized by the absence of the lower jaw, defective formation of the mouth, and union or close approximation of the ears on the front of the neck. See also **agnathocephaly.** **–otocephalic, otocephalous,** *adj.*

Otocort, a trademark for an otic, fixed-combination drug containing a glucocorticoid (hydrocortisone), antibacterials (neomycin sulfate and polymyxin B sulfate), an analgesic (antipyrine), and a local anesthetic (dibucaine).

otodynia. See **otalgia.**

otolaryngologist, a physician who specializes in the diagnosis and treatment of diseases and injuries of the ears, nose, and throat. Compare **otologist.**

otolaryngology, a branch of medicine dealing with the diagnosis and treatment of diseases and disorders of the ears, nose, and throat, and adjacent structures of the head and neck.

otolith righting reflex /ō′təlith/, an involuntary response in newborns in which tilting of the body when the infant is in an erect position causes the head to return to the upright position. The reflex enables the infant to raise the head and is important for development of later gross motor skills. Absence of the reflex may indicate central nervous system damage.

otologist /ōtol′əjist/, a physician trained in the diagnosis and treatment of diseases and other disorders of the ear. Compare **otolaryngologist.**

otoneuralgia. See **otalgia.**

otoplasty /ō′təplas′tē/, a common procedure in reconstructive plastic surgery in which, for cosmetic reasons, some of the cartilage in the ears is removed to bring the auricle and pinna closer to the head.

Otoreid-HC, a trademark for an otic, fixed-combination drug containing a glucocorticoid (hydrocortisone) and antibacterials (neomycin sulfate and polymyxin B sulfate).

otorrhea /ō′tərē′ə/, any discharge from the external ear. Otorrhea may be serous, sanguinous, purulent, or contain cerebrospinal fluid. **–otorrheal, otorrheic, otorrhetic,** *adj.*

otosclerosis /ō′tōsklərō′sis/, a hereditary condition of unknown cause in which irregular ossification in the bony labyrinth of the inner ear, especially of the stapes, occurs, causing tinnitus, then deafness. The deafness is usually first noticed between 11 and 30 years of age. Women are affected twice as often as men. The condition may worsen in pregnancy. Stapedectomy is usually successful in permanently restoring hearing. Also called **otospongiosis.**

otoscope /ō′təskōp′/, an instrument used to examine the external ear, the eardrum, and, through the eardrum, the ossicles of the middle ear. It consists of a light, a magnifying lens, and a device for insufflation.

ototoxic /ō′tōtok′sik/, (of a substance) having a harmful effect on the eighth cranial nerve or the organs of hearing and balance. Common ototoxic drugs include the aminoglycoside antibiotics, aspirin, furosemide, and quinine.

OTR, abbreviation for *occupational therapist, registered.*

Otrivin, a trademark for an adrenergic vasoconstrictor (xylometazoline hydrochloride), used as a nasal decongestant.

OU, abbreviation for *oculus uterque,* a Latin phrase meaning "each eye."

ouabain /wəbā′in/, a cardiotonic.

■ INDICATIONS: It is prescribed in the treatment of congestive heart failure and certain atrial arrhythmias.

■ CONTRAINDICATIONS: Arrhythmias or known hypersensitivity to this drug prohibits its use.

■ ADVERSE EFFECTS: Among the more serious adverse reactions are nausea, vomiting, visual disturbances, and arrhythmias.

Ouchterlony double diffusion, a form of gel diffusion technique in which antigen and antibody in separate cells are allowed to diffuse toward each other.

ounce (oz), a unit of weight equal to 1/16 of a pound avoirdupois.

-ous, -eous, a combining form meaning an 'element or compound with a valence lower than the corresponding one ending in *-ic*': *cuprous, ferrous, hypochlorous.*

outbreeding, the production of offspring by the mating of unrelated individuals, organisms, or plants, which can lead to superior hybrid traits or strains. Compare **inbreeding.** See also **heterosis.**

outcome, the condition of a client at the end of therapy or of a disease process, including the degree of wellness and the need for continuing care, medication, support, counseling, or education.

outcome data, data collected to evaluate the capacity of a client to function at a level described in the outcome statement of a nursing care plan or in standards for client care.

outcome measure, a measure of the quality of medical care, the standard on which is made the assessment of the expected end result of the intervention employed.

outlet, an opening through which something can exit, as the pelvic outlet.

outlet contraction. See **contraction.**

outlet contracture, an abnormally small pelvic outlet. It may be anteroposterior or transverse and is of significance in childbirth because it may impede or prevent the passage of a baby through the birth canal. Anteroposterior contracture caused by fixation of the coccyx may sometimes be overcome by the force of labor, freeing the bones and allowing them to move back. Significant narrowing of the space between the ischial tuberosities is unlikely to be overcome and is most commonly associated with a heavy, android type of pelvis.

outlet forceps. See **low forceps.**

outline form, the shape of the cavosurface of a prepared tooth cavity.

outpatient, **1.** a patient, not hospitalized, who is being treated in an office, clinic, or other ambulatory care facility. **2.** of or pertaining to a health care facility for patients who are not hospitalized or to the treatment or care of such a patient. Compare **inpatient.**

output device, any device that converts information from a computer into a form that is readable by humans or another machine, as a printer or CRT.

ova and parasites test, a microscopic examination of feces for detecting parasites, as amebas or worms and their ova, that are indicators of parasitic disorders.

ovale malaria. See **tertian malaria.**

ovalocytosis. See **elliptocytosis.**

ovari-. See **ovario-.**

-ovaria, a combining form meaning '(condition of the) ovary or ovarial activity': *anovaria, hyperovaria, hypoovaria.*

ovarian, of or pertaining to the ovary.

ovarian artery, a slender branch of the abdominal aorta, arising caudal to the renal arteries, and supplying an ovary. Compare **testicular artery.**

ovarian cancer, a malignant neoplastic disease of the ovary, occurring most frequently in women between 40 and 60 years of age and occasionally in young adolescents. See also **ovarian carcinoma.**

ovarian carcinoma, a malignant neoplasm of the ovaries rarely detected in the early stage and usually far advanced when diagnosed. It occurs frequently in the fifth decade of life. The most common gynecologic tumor, ovarian cancer appears to be increasing in the United States. Risk factors of the disease are infertility, nulliparity, or low parity, delayed childbearing, repeated spontaneous abortion, endometriosis, Group A blood type, previous irradiation of pelvic organs, and exposure to chemical carcinogens, as asbestos and talc. After an insidious onset and asymptomatic period, the tumor may become evident as a palpable abdominal or pelvic mass accompanied by irregular or excessive menses or postmenopausal bleeding. In advanced cases the patient may have ascites, edema of the legs, and pain in the abdomen and the backs of the legs. Regular yearly pelvic examinations after 40 years of age contribute significantly to early diagnosis and the possibility of curative treatment. Characteristic of the disease as it advances are abdominal swelling and discomfort, abnormal vaginal bleeding, weight loss, dysuria or abnormal frequency of urination, constipation, and a palpable ovarian mass, especially in postmenopausal women. A pap smear may show malignant cells if the tumor is advanced; an ultrasonic examination can demonstrate an ovarian mass but does not distinguish between a benign and malignant lesion. A CAT scan may be useful in detecting ovarian cancer, but a definitive diagnosis requires surgical exploration. Most ovarian carcinomas are papillary or serous, followed in frequency by mucinous, endometroid, and undifferentiated cancers. In many cases the cancer spreads over the surface of the peritoneum, and, early in the course of the lesion, tumor cells invade the lymphatic vessels under the diaphragm and the paraaortic nodes. Many kinds of tumors may arise in the ovary. About 85% are epithelial in origin, with papillary serous tumors the most common, followed by mucinous, endometroid, and undifferentiated solid cancers. The surgery recommended for ovarian cancer is total abdominal hysterectomy and bilateral salpingo-oophorectomy with omentectomy. Approximately one half of the tumors diagnosed are inoperable. Treatment of resectable lesions consists of total abdominal hysterectomy, removal of both ovaries and tubes, omentectomy, and biopsies of any suspicious sites, especially in the liver and diaphragm. Postoperative supervoltage irradiation of the pelvis and paraaortic lymph nodes is recommended; the instillation of radioisotopes is used in some cases. Chemotherapeutic agents that may be administered postoperatively include chlorambucil, cyclophosphamide, melphalen, and thiotepa.

ovarian cyst, a globular sac filled with fluid or semisolid material that develops in or on the ovary. It may be transient and physiologic or pathologic. Kinds of ovarian cysts include **chocolate cyst, corpus luteum cyst,** and **dermoid cyst.**

ovarian pregnancy, a rare type of ectopic pregnancy in which the conceptus is implanted within the ovary.

ovarian seminoma. See **dysgerminoma.**

ovarian varicocele, a varicose swelling of the veins of the uterine broad ligament. Also called **pelvic varicocele.**

ovarian vein, one of a pair of veins that emerge from convoluted plexuses in the broad ligament near the ovaries and the uterine tubes. The veins from each plexus ascend and unite to form single veins. The right ovarian vein opens into the inferior vena cava, the left ovarian vein into the renal vein. In some individuals the ovarian veins contain valves and greatly enlarge during pregnancy. Compare **testicular vein.**

ovariectomy. See **oophorectomy.**

ovario-, ovari-, oario-, ootheco-, a combining form meaning 'of or pertaining to the ovary': *ovariocentesis, ovariosteresis, ovariotubal.*

ovary, one of the pair of female gonads found on each side of the lower abdomen, beside the uterus, in a fold of the broad ligament. At ovulation, an egg is extruded from a follicle on the surface of the ovary under the stimulation of the gonadotrophic hormones, follicle stimulating hormone (FSH), and luteinizing hormone (LH). The mature ovarian follicle secretes the hormones estrogen and progesterone that regulate the menstrual cycle by a negative feedback system in which an increase in estrogen decreases the secretion of FSH by the pituitary gland and an increase in progesterone decreases the secretion of LH. Each ovary is normally firm and smooth and resembles an almond in size and shape. The ovaries are homologous to the testes.

Ovcon, a trademark for an oral contraceptive containing an estrogen (ethinyl estradiol) and a progestin (norethindrone acetate).

overbite, vertical overlapping of lower teeth by upper teeth, usually measured perpendicular to the occlusal plane. Compare **overclosure, overjet.**

overclosure, an abnormal condition in which the mandible rises too far before the teeth make contact, caused by the loss of occlusal vertical dimension.

overcompensation, an exaggerated attempt to overcome a real or imagined physical or psychologic deficit. The attempt may be conscious or unconscious. See also **compensation.**

overdenture, a complete or partial removable denture supported by retained roots to provide improved support, stability, and tactile and proprioceptive sensation and to reduce ridge resorption.

overdrive suppression, the inhibitory effect of a faster cardiac pacemaker on a slower one.

overdriving, the delivery of excess compressed air to an artificial heart's ventricle during systole.

overhang, an excess of dental filling material that projects beyond the margin of the associated tooth cavity.

overinclusiveness, a type of association disorder observed in some schizophrenia patients. The individual is unable to think in a precise manner because of an inability to keep irrelevant elements outside perceptual boundaries.

overjet, a horizontal projection of upper teeth beyond the lower teeth, usually measured parallel to the occlusal plane. Also called **horizontal overlap.** Compare **overbite, overclosure.**

overload, **1.** a burden greater than the capacity of the system designed to move or process it. **2.** (in physiology) any factor or influence that stresses the body beyond its natural limits and may impair its health.

overoxygenation, an abnormal condition in which the oxygen concentration in the blood and other tissues of the body is greater than normal, and the carbon dioxide concentration is less than normal. The condition is characterized by a fall in blood pressure, decreased vital capacity, fatigue, errors in judgment, paresthesia of the hands and feet, anorexia, nausea and vomiting, and hyperemia.

over the counter (OTC), (of a drug) available to the consumer without a prescription.

overweight, more than normal in body weight after adjustment for height, body build, and age.

ovi-. See **ovo-.**

oviduct. See **fallopian tube.**

oviferous /ōvif′ərəs/, bearing or capable of producing ova (egg cells).

oviparous /ōvip′ərəs/, giving birth to young by laying eggs. Compare **ovoviviparous, viviparous.**

oviposition /ō′vipəsish′ən/, the act of laying or depositing eggs by the female member of oviparous animals.

ovipositor /ō′vipos′itər/, a specialized organ, found primarily in insects, for depositing eggs on plants or in the soil.

ovo-, ovi-, a combining form meaning 'of or pertaining to an egg, or to ova': *ovoglobulin, ovoplasm, ovotestis*.

ovocenter /ō′vəsen′tər/, the centrosome of a fertilized ovum. Also called **oocenter** /ō′əsen′tər/.

ovoflavin /ō′vəflā′vin/, a riboflavin derived from the yolk of eggs.

ovogenesis. See **oogenesis.**

ovoglobulin /ō′vəglob′yo͝olin/, a globulin derived from the white of eggs.

ovogonium. See **oogonium.**

ovoid arch, a dental arch that curves smoothly from the molars on one side to those on the opposite side to form half an oval.

ovo-lacto-vegetarian. See **lacto-vegetarian.**

ovomucin /ō′vəmyo͞o′sin/, a glycoprotein derived from the white of eggs.

ovomucoid /ō′vəmyo͞o′koid/, of or pertaining to a glycoprotein, similar to mucin, derived from the white of eggs.

ovoplasm. See **ooplasm.**

ovotestis /ō′vətes′tis/, a gonad that contains both ovarian and testicular tissue; a hermaphroditic gonad. **–ovotesticular,** *adj.*

ovovitellin. See **vitellin.**

ovoviviparous /ō′vəvip′ərəs/, bearing young in eggs that are hatched within the body, as some reptiles and fishes. Compare **oviparous, viviparous.**

Ovral, a trademark for an oral contraceptive containing a progestin (norgestrel) and an estrogen (ethinyl estradiol).

Ovrette, a trademark for an oral contraceptive containing a progestin (norgestrel).

ovulation, expulsion of an ovum from the ovary on spontaneous rupture of a mature follicle as a result of cyclic ovarian and pituitary endocrine function. It usually occurs on the fourteenth day after the first day of the last menstrual period and often causes brief, sharp lower abdominal pain on the side of the ovulating ovary. See also **oogenesis.** **–ovulate,** *v.*

ovulation method of family planning, a natural method of family planning that uses observation of changes in the character and quantity of cervical mucus as a means of determining the time of ovulation during the menstrual cycle. Because pregnancy occurs with fertilization of an ovum extruded from the ovary at ovulation, the method is used to increase or decrease the woman's chance of becoming pregnant by causing or avoiding insemination by spontaneous or artificial means during the fertile period associated with ovulation. The cyclic changes in gonadotropic hormones, especially estrogen, cause changes in the quantity and character of cervical mucus. In the first days after menstruation, scant thick mucus is secreted by the cervix. These "dry days" are "safe days," with ovulation several days away. The quantity of mucus then increases; it is pearly-white and sticky, becoming clearer and less sticky as ovulation approaches; these "wet days" are "unsafe days." During and just after ovulation the mucus is clear, slippery, and elastic; it resembles the uncooked white of an egg. The day on which this sign is most apparent is the "peak day," probably the day before ovulation. The four days after the "peak day" are "unsafe": Fertilization might occur. By the end of the four days, the mucus becomes pearly-white and sticky again and progressively decreases in quantity until menstruation supervenes to begin a new cycle. Essential to the effectiveness of this method are thorough instruction by a family planning counselor and strong self-motivation in the couple. During the first cycle, abstinence may be necessary to allow observation of the mucus without the confusing addition of semen or contraceptive foam, cream, or jelly, if being used. Daily close monitoring of the mucus is necessary even after several cycles because the length of the "safe" and "unsafe" periods and the time of ovulation vary from cycle to cycle, as they do from woman to woman. Postpartally, and during lactation, the method is not effective until the menses have become regular. Effectiveness of the method in identifying the most fertile days of the cycle is augmented by using the basal body temperature method. This combined method is called the symptothermal method of planning. Proponents of the ovulation method claim the benefits of low cost, naturalness, and effectiveness. Detractors emphasize a limited public health application of the method, stating that it requires extensive teaching and self-motivation and that its effectiveness is limited by the ability of the user to observe correctly and diligently the changes in the cervical mucus. Abstinence may be necessary for up to 10 days by a woman whose menstrual cycles are long or are of irregular length. Also called **cervical mucus method of family planning.**

Ovulen, a trademark for an oral contraceptive containing an estrogen (mestranol) and a progestin (ethynodiol diacetate).

ovum, *pl.* **ova,** **1.** an egg. **2.** a female germ cell extruded from the ovary at ovulation.

oxacillin sodium, a penicillinase resistant penicillin antibiotic.

■ INDICATION: It is prescribed in the treatment of severe infections caused by penicillinase-producing staphylococci.

■ CONTRAINDICATIONS: Known hypersensitivity to this drug or to any other penicillin prohibits its use.

■ ADVERSE EFFECTS: Among the most serious effects are anaphylaxis and other less severe allergic reactions, GI disturbances, and pruritus ani and vulvae.

Oxaine, a trademark for a topical anesthetic (oxethazaine).

Oxalid, a trademark for an antiinflammatory and antirheumatic (oxyphenbutazone).

oxaluric acid /ok′səlo͝or′ik/, a compound derived from uric acid or from parabonic acid, which occurs in normal urine.

oxamniquine /oksam′nəkwēn/, an antischistosomal.

■ INDICATION: It is prescribed in the treatment of infection caused by *Schistosoma mansoni*.

■ CONTRAINDICATIONS: Renal failure, congestive heart failure, or known hypersensitivity to this drug prohibits its use.

■ ADVERSE EFFECTS: Among the more serious adverse reactions are dizziness, drowsiness, and convulsions, particularly in patients with a history of epilepsy.

oxandrolone, an androgen.

■ INDICATIONS: It is prescribed in the treatment of testosterone deficiency, osteoporosis, and female breast cancer and for the stimulation of growth, weight gain, and red blood cell production.

■ CONTRAINDICATIONS: Cancer of the male breast or prostate, liver disease, pregnancy or suspected pregnancy, or known hypersensitivity to this drug prohibits its use.

■ ADVERSE EFFECTS: Among the more serious adverse reactions are hirsutism, acne, liver toxicity, electrolyte imbalances, and various endocrine effects in some patients.

oxazepam /oksā′zəpam/, a minor tranquilizer.

■ INDICATIONS: It is prescribed to relieve anxiety and nervous tension.

■ CONTRAINDICATIONS: Acute narrow-angle glaucoma, psychotic disorders, or known hypersensitivity to this drug prohibits its use.

■ ADVERSE EFFECTS: Among the more serious adverse reactions are withdrawal symptoms resulting from discontinuation of treatment. Dizziness and fatigue commonly occur.

-oxemia, a combining form meaning a '(specified) state of oxygen in the blood': *anoxemia, hyperoxemia, hypoxemia.*

-oxia, a combining form meaning '(condition of) oxygenation': *anoxia, asthenoxia, hypoxia.*

oxidation, **1.** any process in which the oxygen content of a compound is increased. **2.** any reaction in which the positive valence of a compound or a radical is increased because of a loss of electrons. **–oxidize,** *v.*

oxidative phosphorylation, an ATP generating process in which oxygen serves as the final electron acceptor. The process occurs in mitochondria and is the major source of ATP generation in aerobic organisms. Also called **respirations.**

oxidative water, water produced by the oxidation of molecules of food substances, as the conversion of glucose to water and carbon dioxide.

oxidize, (of an element or compound) to combine or cause to combine with oxygen, to remove hydrogen, or to increase the valence of an element through the loss of electrons. **–oxidation,** *n.,* **oxidizing,** *adj.*

oxidizing agent, a compound that readily gives up oxygen and attracts hydrogen from another compound. In chemical reactions an oxidizing agent acts as an acceptor of electrons, thereby increasing the valence of an element.

oxidoreductase, an enzyme that catalyzes a reaction in which one substance is oxidized while another is reduced. An example is alcohol dehydrogenase.

Oxsoralen, a trademark for a pigmentation agent (methoxsalen).

oxtriphylline /oks′trəfil′ēn/, a bronchodilator.

■ INDICATIONS: It is prescribed in the treatment of bronchial asthma, bronchitis, and emphysema.

■ CONTRAINDICATIONS: Known hypersensitivity to this drug or other xanthine derivatives prohibits its use. It is used with caution in patients with ulcer or with coronary disease for whom cardiac stimulation might be harmful.

■ ADVERSE EFFECTS: Among the more common adverse reactions are GI distress, palpitations, nervousness, and insomnia.

oxy-, **1.** a combining form meaning 'sharp, quick, or sour': *oxyblepsia, oxycephalia, oxyecoia*. **2.** a combining form indicating the presence of oxygen in a compound: *oxyacanthine, oxycamphor, oxyquinoline*.

oxybenzene. See **carbolic acid.**

oxybutynin chloride, an anticholinergic.

■ INDICATION: It is prescribed in the treatment of neurogenic bladder.

■ CONTRAINDICATIONS: Glaucoma, obstruction of the GI or urinary tract, ulcerative colitis, paralytic ileus, toxic megacolon, or known hypersensitivity to this drug or to other anticholinergics prohibits its use.

■ ADVERSE EFFECTS: Among the more serious adverse effects are decreased sweating, urinary retention, blurred vision, tachycardia, and severe allergic reactions.

Oxycel, a trademark for a local hemostatic (oxidized cellulose).

oxycephaly /ok'sisef'əlē/, a congenital malformation of the skull in which premature closure of the coronal and sagittal sutures results in accelerated upward growth of the head, giving it a long, narrow appearance with the top pointed or conic in shape. The cephalic index is over 75. Also called **acrocephaly, hypsicephaly, oxycephalia, steeple head, tower head, tower skull, turricephaly.** See also **craniostenosis.** **–oxycephalus,** *n.*, **oxycephalous,** *adj.*

oxycodone hydrochloride, a narcotic analgesic.

■ INDICATION: It is used to treat moderate to severe pain.

■ CONTRAINDICATIONS: It is used with caution in many conditions, including head injuries, asthma, impaired renal or hepatic function, or unstable cardiovascular status. Known hypersensitivity to this drug prohibits its use.

■ ADVERSE EFFECTS: Among the most serious adverse reactions are drowsiness, dizziness, nausea, constipation, respiratory and circulatory depression, and drug addiction.

Oxy-5, a trademark for a keratolytic (benzoyl peroxide).

oxygen (O), a tasteless, odorless, colorless gas essential for human respiration. Its atomic weight is 16; its atomic number is 8. In anesthesia, oxygen functions as a carrier gas for the delivery of anesthetic agents to the tissues of the body. It is given by mask at a rate of flow and concentration appropriate to the physical status of the patient, the surgical procedure, and the anesthetic agent being administered. In respiratory therapy, oxygen is administered to increase its amount and thus to decrease the amount of other gases circulating in the blood. Overdose of oxygen can cause irreversible toxicity in people with pulmonary abnormalities, especially when complicated by chronic carbon dioxide retention. Prolonged administration of high concentrations of oxygen may cause irreversible damage to infants' eyes. Oxygen itself is not flammable or explosive, but because an oxygen-rich environment is favorable to fire and explosion, flame or electric spark must be avoided when oxygen is being administered. See also **oxygen toxicity.**

oxygenation, the process of combining or treating with oxygen. **–oxygenate,** *v.*

oxygen consumption, the amount of oxygen in milliliters per minute required by the body for normal aerobic metabolism.

oxygen enhancement ratio (OER), a measure of tumor sensitivity to the presence or absence of oxygen, expressed as the ratio of radiation dose required to produce a given effect with no oxygen present to the dose required to produce the same effect in one atmosphere of air. This is an important effect in radiation therapy where tumor cells may exist in a state of hypoxia.

oxygen mask, a device used to administer oxygen. It is shaped to fit snugly over the mouth and nose and may be secured in place with a strap or held with the hand. The mask has inspiratory and expiratory valves allowing oxygen to be inhaled or pumped into the respiratory tract and carbon dioxide to be exhaled into the environment. Oxygen flows at a prescribed rate through a catheter to the mask, often through a soft rubber bag that can be pumped by hand.

oxygen saturation, the fraction of a total hemoglobin (HB) in the form of HbO_2 at a defined Po_2.

oxygen tension, the force with which oxygen molecules that are physically dissolved in blood are constantly trying to escape, expressed as partial pressure (Po_2). The tension at any instant is related to the amount of oxygen physically dissolved in plasma; the larger amount carried in chemical combination with hemoglobin serves as a reservoir that releases oxygen molecules to physical solution when the tension decreases and that stores additional molecules of the gas when the tension increases.

oxygen therapy, any procedure in which oxygen is administered to a patient to relieve hypoxia.

■ METHOD: Of the many methods for providing oxygen therapy, the one selected depends on the condition of the patient and the cause of hypoxia. Low or moderate amounts of oxygen may be supplied to postoperative patients by a nasal catheter or cannula. Low concentrations, precisely measured, may be delivered to patients with chronic obstructive lung disease by a Venturi mask. If hypoxia is the result of impaired cardiac function, a high concentration of oxygen may be delivered by a nonrebreathing or partial rebreathing mask. Humidity and drugs in aerosol form may be given with oxygen using a variety of devices, as an aerosol face mask, Croupette, or T-piece.

■ NURSING CONSIDERATIONS: Thorough and careful observation of the patient's need for oxygen and response to therapy are important. The concentration of oxygen received by the patient must not be assumed by the rate and concentration at which it is delivered: A person whose respirations are rapid and shallow receives more oxygen than does a person breathing deeply and slowly. Many clinical situations require frequent laboratory evaluations of the levels of arterial blood gases. The adverse effects of oxygen therapy include respiratory depression, absorption atelectasis, alveolar collapse, alveolar edema, pulmonary congestion, intraalveolar hemorrhage, hyaline membrane formation, pain, retrolental fibroplasia, and disturbance of the central nervous system with seizures and, possibly, death. Thorough knowledge of the equipment used and of the condition being treated enables the nurse to care safely and effectively for the patient who requires oxygen.

■ OUTCOME CRITERIA: Oxygen therapy may be used in the treatment of any condition that results in hypoxia. Although there are several kinds of hypoxia, all result in hypoxemia. The administration of oxygen may relieve hypotension, cardiac arrythmias, tachypnea, headache, disorientation, nausea, and agitation characteristic of hypoxia, as well as restore the ability of the cells of the body to carry on normal metabolic function.

oxygen toxicity, a condition of oxygen overdosage that can result in pathologic tissue changes, as retrolental fibroplasia or bronchopulmonary dysplasia.

oxygen transport, the process by which oxygen is absorbed in the lungs by the hemoglobin in circulating deoxygenated red cells and carried to the peripheral tissues. This process is made possible by a special characteristic of hemoglobin, that is, the ability to combine with large quantities of oxygen present at a high concentration, as in the lungs, and to release this oxygen when the concentration is low, as in the peripheral tissues. See also **hemoglobin.**

oxyhemoglobin /ok′sēhē′məglō′bin, -hem′-/, the product of the combining of hemoglobin with oxygen. It is a loosely bound complex that dissociates easily when there is a low concentration of oxygen.

Oxylone, a trademark for a glucocorticoid (fluorometholone).

oxymetazoline hydrochloride /ok′sēmətaz′əlēn/, a decongestant.

■ INDICATION: It is prescribed in the treatment of nasal congestion.

■ CONTRAINDICATIONS: Hyperthyroidism, diabetes, use of a monoamine oxidase inhibitor within 14 days, or known hypersensitivity to this drug prohibits its use.

■ ADVERSE EFFECTS: Among the more serious adverse reactions are rebound congestion, central nervous system stimulation, and, in children, a severe shocklike syndrome with coma, hypotension, and bradycardia.

oxymetholone, an androgen.

■ INDICATIONS: It is prescribed in the treatment of testosterone deficiency, osteoporosis, and female breast cancer and for the stimulation of growth, weight gain, and red blood cell production.

■ CONTRAINDICATIONS: Cancer of the male breast or prostate, liver disease, pregnancy or suspected pregnancy, or known hypersensitivity to this drug prohibits its use.

■ ADVERSE EFFECTS: Among the more serious adverse reactions are hirsutism, acne, liver toxicity, electrolyte imbalances, and, depending on the age of the patient, various endocrine effects.

oxymorphone hydrochloride, a narcotic analgesic.

■ INDICATIONS: It is prescribed to reduce moderate to severe pain, as a preoperative medication, and to support anesthesia.

■ CONTRAINDICATION: Drug dependence or known hypersensitivity to this drug prohibits its use.

■ ADVERSE EFFECTS: Among the more serious adverse reactions are drug dependence, urinary retention, and respiratory or circulatory depression.

oxyopia /ok′sē•ō′pē•ə/, unusual acuteness of vision. A person with normal (20/20) vision when standing 20 feet from the standard Snellen eye chart can read the seventh line of letters, each of which is an eighth of an inch high, while an individual with oxyopia can read smaller letters at that distance. Also called **oxyopy** /ok′sē•ō′pē/.

oxyphenbutazone, a nonsteroidal antiinflammatory agent and antirheumatic.

■ INDICATIONS: It is prescribed in the treatment of arthritis, bursitis, gout, and other inflammatory conditions.

■ CONTRAINDICATIONS: Impaired hepatic or renal function, a history of gastric ulcer, blood dyscrasias, stomatitis, hypertension, and edema, or known hypersensitivity to this drug or to other phenylbutazone medications prohibits its use.

■ ADVERSE EFFECTS: Among the more serious adverse reactions are fluid retention and blood dyscrasias. GI irritation and nausea commonly occur. This drug interacts with many other drugs.

oxyphencyclimine hydrochloride, an anticholinergic.

■ INDICATION: It is prescribed in the treatment of peptic ulcer.

■ CONTRAINDICATIONS: Glaucoma, obstruction of the GI or urinary tract, ulcerative colitis, paralytic ileus, toxic megacolon, or known hypersensitivity to this drug or to other anticholinergics prohibits its use.

■ ADVERSE EFFECTS: Among the more serious adverse effects are decreased sweating, urinary retention, circulatory or respiratory depression, and severe hypersensitivity reactions.

oxyphenonium bromide, an anticholinergic.

■ INDICATION: It is prescribed in the treatment of peptic ulcer.

■ CONTRAINDICATIONS: Glaucoma, obstruction of the GI or urinary tract, ulcerative colitis, paralytic ileus, toxic megacolon, or known hypersensitivity to this drug or to other anticholinergics prohibits its use.

■ ADVERSE EFFECTS: Among the more serious adverse effects are decreased sweating, urinary retention, tachycardia, blurred vision, and severe hypersensitivity reactions.

oxytetracycline, a tetracycline antibiotic.

■ INDICATIONS: It is prescribed in the treatment of bacterial and rickettsial infections.

■ CONTRAINDICATIONS: Pregnancy, early childhood, or known hypersensitivity to this or to other tetracyclines prohibits its use. The drug is used with caution in patients who have renal or liver dysfunction.

■ ADVERSE EFFECTS: Among the more serious adverse reactions are GI disturbances, phototoxicity, potentially serious suprainfections, and various hypersensitivity reactions. Discoloration of teeth may occur in children exposed to the drug in utero or before 8 years of age.

oxytetracycline calcium, a tetracycline antibiotic.

oxytocic /ok′sitō′sik/, **1.** of or pertaining to a substance that is similar to the hormone oxytocin. **2.** any one of numerous drugs that stimulate the smooth muscle of the uterus to contract. The administration of an oxytocic can initiate and enhance rhythmic uterine contraction at any time, but relatively high doses are required for such responses in early pregnancy. These drugs are often used to initiate labor at term. Oxytocic agents commonly used include oxytocin, certain prostaglandins, and the ergot alkaloids. These drugs are used to induce or augment labor, control postpartum hemorrhage, correct postpartum uterine atony, produce uterine contractions after cesarean section or other uterine surgery, and induce therapeutic abortion. Considerable controversy surrounds the use of oxytocics to induce labor. The U.S. Food and Drug Administration has ruled that oxytocin is not indicated for elective termination of pregnancy and should be used only in cases where continued pregnancy is seen as a greater risk to the mother or to the fetus than the risk of drug-induced labor. These drugs are used with extreme caution in parturients with severe hypotension and hypertension, partial placenta previa, cephalopelvic disproportion, or grand multiparity. The risk of using these agents is much higher in mothers who have undergone recent uterine surgery or who have suffered recent sepsis or trauma. The most serious adverse reaction is sustained tetanic contraction of the uterus resulting in fetal hypoxia or in rupture of the uterus.

oxytocin /ok′sitō′sin/, an oxytocic.

■ INDICATIONS: It is prescribed to stimulate contractions in inducing or augmenting labor, and to contract the uterus to control postpartum bleeding.

■ CONTRAINDICATIONS: Cephalopelvic disproportion, unfavorable fetal position, or known hypersensitivity to this drug prohibits its use.

■ ADVERSE EFFECTS: Among the more serious adverse reactions are tetanic contraction, jaundice, uterine rupture, and fetal anoxia.

oxytocin challenge test, a stress test for the assessment of intrauterine function of the fetus and the placenta. It is performed to evaluate the ability of the fetus to tolerate continuation of pregnancy or the anticipated stress of labor and delivery. A dilute intravenous infusion of oxytocin is begun, monitored by a meter or regulated by an infusion pump. The uterine activity is monitored with a tocodynamometer, and the fetal heart rate is monitored with an ultrasonic sensor as the uterus is stimulated to contract by the oxytocin. The amount of solution infused is increased as necessary to cause the uterus to contract for 30 to 40 seconds three times every 10 minutes. The fetal heart rate is observed for variability and for the timing of any marked variation from the normal in relation to uterine contractions. Decelerations of the fetal heart rate in certain repeating patterns may indicate fetal distress. One quarter of the infants diagnosed by this method as being in distress are normal; therefore, other tests of fetal well-being are recommended before performing an emergency cesarean section or induction of labor.

oxyuriasis. See **enterobiasis.**

Oxyuris vermicularis. See ***Enterobius vermicularis.***

ozena /ōzē′nə/, a condition of the nose characterized by atrophy of the nasal chonchae and mucous membranes. Symptoms include crusting of nasal secretions, discharge, and, especially, a very offensive odor. Ozena may follow chronic inflammation of the nasal mucosa.

ozone, a form of oxygen characterized by molecules having three atoms. Ozone is formed when oxygen is electrically charged, as might occur in a lightning storm. Ozone is used as a bleaching, cleaning, and oxidizing agent and has a faint, chlorinelike odor.

ozone shield, the layer of ozone that hangs in the atmosphere from 20 to 40 miles above the surface of the earth and protects the earth from excessive ultraviolet radiation. Some experts claim that the manufacture of various chemicals, as chlorofluorocarbons used as propellants in aerosol sprays and the effects of high-flying jet aircraft are destroying this protective layer and allowing excessive amounts of ultraviolet radiation to penetrate the earth's atmosphere, thus subjecting humans to increased dangers of skin cancer and other health problems. Some chemistry experts and federal health officials also claim that an additional threat comes from nitrous oxide in nitrogenous fertilizers rising into the atmosphere and reacting unfavorably with the ozone shield. Other experts say the depletion of the ozone layer by chlorofluorocarbons may be offset by the release of carbon dioxide into the atmosphere from the combustion of fuels. One study indicates that ozone concentration has actually increased 6% since monitoring was begun more than 50 years ago. The ozone shield is implicated in certain health problems that affect some air travelers. See also **ozone sickness.**

ozone sickness, an abnormal condition caused by the inhalation of ozone that may seep into jet aircraft at altitudes over 40,000 feet. It is characterized by headaches, chest pains, itchy eyes, and sleepiness. Exactly why and how ozone causes this condition is not known. It is more prevalent early in the year and occurs more often over the Pacific Ocean.

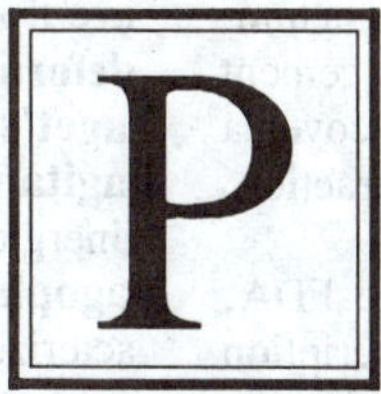

P, **1.** symbol for **phosphorus.** **2.** symbol for *gas partial pressure*. See **partial pressure.**

P_1, (in genetics) symbol for **parental generation.**

P_{50}, the partial pressure of oxygen at which hemoglobin is half saturated with bound oxygen.

P1E1, P2E1, P3E1, P4E1, P6E1, trademarks for ophthalmic fixed-combination drugs containing a cholinergic (pilocarpine hydrochloride) and an adrenergic (epinephrine bitartrate). The numbers indicate the percent of each ingredient in the solution; for example, P2E1 contains 2% pilocarpine HCl and 1% epinephrine bitartrate.

PA, abbreviation for **physician's assistant.**

PABA, abbreviation for **paraaminobenzoic acid.**

Pabanol, a trademark for an ultraviolet screen (paraaminobenzoic acid).

pabulum /pab′yələm/, any substance that is food or nutrient.

pacemaker, **1.** the sinoatrial node of specialized nervous tissue located at the junction of the superior vena cava and the right atrium. It originates the contractions of the atria, which transmit the impulse on to the atrioventricular node, thereby initiating the contraction of the ventricles. An ectopic or indioventricular pacemaker may cause contractions in cases of abnormal heart functions. **2.** also called **cardiac pacemaker.** an electric apparatus used for maintaining a normal sinus rhythm of myocardial contraction by electrically stimulating the heart muscle. A pacemaker may be permanent, emitting the stimulus at a constant and fixed rate, or it may fire only on demand, when the heart does not spontaneously contract at a minimum rate.

pacemaker current, a time-dependent decrease in outward potassium current that is peculiar to the pacemaking cell and causes it to reach threshhold potential.

pacemaker installation fluoroscopy, the fluoroscopic monitoring of the insertion of an artificial pacemaker, used as an aid for correct installation of the device.

pachometer. See **pachymeter.**

pachy-, a combining form meaning 'thick': *pachyaria, pachycephaly, pachymucosa*.

pachycephaly /pak′ēsef′əlē/, an abnormal thickness of the skull, as in acromegaly. Also called **pachycephalia.** **–pachycephalic, pachycephalous,** *adj.*

pachydactyly /pak′ēdak′tilē/, an abnormal thickening of the fingers or the toes. **–pachydactylic, pachydactylous,** *adj.*

pachyderma alba, an abnormal state of the buccal mucosa in which the appearance is suggestive of whitened elephant hide.

pachyderma oralis, an abnormal state of the buccal mucosa in which the appearance is suggestive of elephant hide. Compare **pachyderma alba.**

pachymeter /pakim′ətər/, an instrument used to measure thickness, especially of thin structures, as a membrane or a tissue. Also called **pachometer.**

pachynema /pak′inē′mə/, the postsynaptic tetradic chromosome formation that occurs in the pachytene stage of the first meiotic prophase of gametogenesis.

pachyonychia congenita /pak′ē·ōnik′ē·ə/, a congenital deformity characterized by abnormal thickening and raising of the nails on the fingers and the toes, and hyperkeratosis of the palms of the hands and the soles of the feet. The papillae of the tongue also atrophy, causing a whitish coating over the lingual surface.

pachytene /pak′itēn/, the third stage in the first meiotic prophase of gametogenesis in which the paired homologous chromosomes form tetrads. The bivalent pairs become short and thick and intertwine so that four chromatids are visible. See also **diakinesis, diplotene, leptotene, zygotene.**

pacifier, **1.** an agent that soothes or comforts. **2.** a nipple-shaped object used by infants and children for sucking. Such devices can be dangerous if they are too small or poorly constructed, because the entire object or part of it can be aspirated or lodged in the pharynx or trachea and obstruct the passage of air. The safest pacifiers are constructed in one piece, are large enough so that only the nipple fits into the mouth, and have a handle that can be easily grasped.

Pacini's corpuscles /päsē′nēz/, a number of special sensory end organs resembling tiny white bulbs, each attached to the end of a single nerve fiber in the subcutaneous, submucous, and subserous connective tissue of many parts of the body, especially the palm of the hand, sole of the foot, genital organs, joints, and in the pancreas. They average about 3 mm in diameter, are pressure sensitive, contain numerous concentric layers around a central core, and in cross section resemble an onion. Also called **pacinian corpuscles.** Compare **Golgi-Mazzoni corpuscles, Krause's corpuscles.**

pack, **1.** a treatment in which the entire body or a portion of it is wrapped in wet or dry towels or in ice for various therapeutic purposes, as with cold packs for the reduction of high temperatures and swellings or for inducing hypothermia during certain surgical procedures, especially heart surgery and organ transplants. **2.** a tampon. **3.** the act of applying a dressing or dental cement to a surgical wound. **4.** a surgical dressing to cover a wound or to fill the cavity left from a tooth extraction, especially an extraction of a wisdom tooth.

package insert, a leaflet that, by order of the FDA, must be placed inside the package of every prescription drug. In it, the manufacturer is required to describe the drug, to state its generic name, and to give the applicable indications, contraindications, warnings, precautions, adverse effects, form, dosage, and administration.

packed cells, a preparation of blood cells separated from liquid plasma, often administered in severe anemia to restore adequate levels of hemoglobin and red cells without overloading the vascular system with excess fluids. See also **bank blood, component therapy, pooled plasma.**

$Paco_2$, abbreviation for *partial pressure of carbon dioxide in arterial blood.*

pad, **1.** a mass of soft material used to cushion shock, prevent wear, or absorb moisture, as the abdominal pads used to absorb discharges from abdominal wounds or to separate viscera and improve accessibility during abdominal surgery. **2.** (in anatomy) a mass of fat that cushions various structures, as the infrapatellar pad lying below the patella between the patellar ligament, the head of the tibia, and the femoral condyles.

paedogenesis. See **pedogenesis.**

Paget's disease /paj′əts/, a common, nonmetabolic disease of bone of unknown cause, usually affecting middle-aged and elderly people, characterized by excessive bone destruction and unorganized bone repair.

■ OBSERVATIONS: Most cases are asymptomatic or mild; however, bone pain may be the first symptom. Bowed tibias (saber shins), kyphosis, and frequent fractures are caused by the soft, abnormal bone in this condition. Enlargement of the head, headaches, and warmth over involved areas caused by increased vascularity are additional features. The serum alkaline phosphatase is often markedly elevated and there is increased urinary calcium and hydroxyproline. The x-ray picture of areas of decreased bone density adjacent to sites of increased density is characteristic. Radioactive bone scans help locate regions of active disease. Complications include fractures, kidney stones if the patient is immobilized, heart failure, deafness or blindness caused by pressure from bony overgrowth, and osteosarcoma.

■ INTERVENTION: No treatment is necessary for mild cases. A high-protein, high-calcium diet, unless the patient is immobilized, is recommended. Parenteral synthetic salmon calcitonin may help the patient temporarily. Diphosphonates and mithramycin are also effective but require close monitoring for side effects.

■ NURSING CONSIDERATIONS: Immobilization of the patient is avoided, if possible, to prevent hypercalcemia and kidney stones. Observation for neurologic signs and symptoms and prompt reporting of changes may help to avert irreversible nerve damage. Also called **osteitis deformans.**

Paget's disease of the nipple. See **nipple cancer.**

Pagitane Hydrochloride, a trademark for an anticholinergic (cycrimine hydrochloride).

pagophagia /pā′gōfā′jē·ə/, an abnormal condition characterized by a craving to eat enormous quantities of ice. It is associated with a lack of nutrient iron. –**pagophagic, pagophagous,** *adj.*

-pagus, a combining form meaning 'conjoined twins': *craniopagus, pyropagus, thoracopagus.*

PAHA, abbreviation for **paraaminohippuric acid.**

PAHA sodium clearance test, a test for detecting kidney damage or certain muscle diseases. The test uses the sodium salt of paraaminohippuric acid for determining the rate at which the kidneys remove this salt from the blood and urine. The normal clearance rates in serum and 24-hour urine specimens are 600 to 750 ml/minute.

pain, an unpleasant sensation caused by noxious stimulation of the sensory nerve endings. It is a cardinal symptom of inflammation and is valuable in the diagnosis of many disorders and conditions. Pain may be mild or severe, chronic, acute, lancinating, burning, dull, or sharp, precisely or poorly localized, or referred. See also **referred pain.**

pain and suffering, (in law) an element in a claim for damages that allows recovery for the mental and physical pain, suffering, distress, and trauma that an individual has endured as a result of injury.

pain assessment, an evaluation of the factors that alleviate or exacerbate a patient's pain, used as an aid in the diagnosis and the treatment of disease and trauma. Responses to pain vary widely among individuals and depend on many different physical and psychologic factors, as specific diseases and injuries and the health, pain threshold, fear and anxiety, and the cultural background of the individual involved, as well as the way different individuals express their pain experiences. See also **pain intervention, pain mechanism.**

■ METHOD: The patient is asked to describe the cause of the pain, if known, its intensity, location, and duration, the events preceding it, and the pattern usually followed for handling pain. Severe pain causes pallor, cold perspiration, piloerection; dilated pupils, and increases in the pulse, respiratory rate, blood pressure, and muscle tension. When brief, intense pain subsides, the pulse may be slower and the blood pressure lower than before the pain began. If pain occurs frequently or is prolonged, the pulse rate and blood pressure may not increase markedly, and, if pain persists for many days, there may be an increased production of eosinophils and 17-ketosteroids and greater susceptibility to infections. The patient's statements regarding pain, the tone of voice, speed of speech, cries, groans, or other vocalizations, facial expressions, body movements, or tendency to withdraw are all noted. Pertinent background information in the assessment includes a record of the patient's chronic conditions, previous surgery, and any illnesses that caused pain, the patient's experiences with relatives and friends in pain, the role or position of the patient in the family structure, and the patient's use of alcohol and medications. Key aspects in evaluating pain intensity are the size of the pain area, the tenderness within the pain area, and the effects of movement and pressure on the pain. Duration of pain is considered in terms of hours, days, weeks, months, or years. Pain patterns are associated with various sensations as burning, pricking, aching, rhythmic throbbing, and the effects on the sympathetic and the parasympathetic nervous systems. Evaluation includes the meanings the individual may attach to pain, as a test of character, a penance, or as a sign of worsening illness. Such interpretations may affect the intensity of pain and mask its significance.

■ NURSING ORDERS: The nurse establishes a relationship with the patient and uses individual counseling or group situations to teach the person about pain and how to modify the anxiety associated with it. Analgesics ordered for the patient are administered by the nurse before the pain becomes intense, for this increases their effectiveness. In addition to helping promote rest and relaxation, the nurse decreases noxious stimuli, provides other pleasant sensory input, and helps to distract the patient by using guided imagery, walking, watching television, or reading. If the patient believes that certain acceptable measures alleviate pain, the nurse uses them.

■ OUTCOME CRITERIA: Dramatic relief of intense or chronic pain is often difficult to accomplish, but the patient can be helped to learn to handle pain effectively and to function fairly normally.

pain intervention, the relief of the painful sensations experienced in suffering the physiologic and the psychologic effects of disease and trauma. Effective pain intervention depends on proper evaluation of the type of pain the patient is experiencing, the physical and the psychologic origins of the pain, and the behavioral patterns commonly associated with different kinds of pain. The most common method of pain intervention is the administration of narcotics, as morphine, but many authorities believe that the exclusive use of pain killing drugs without consideration and implementation of psychologic aids is too narrow an approach. There are few patients without a psychogenic overlay on the physical experience of pain, and comprehensive pain intervention employs methods and procedures that incorporate both psychologic and physical measures. Methods of pain intervention for acute pain are different from those for chronic pain. Acute pain, occurring in the first 24 to 48 hours after surgery, is often difficult to relieve, and narcotics seldom relieve all such pain. Some authorities believe that the individual who has undergone repeated surgical operations has a decreased tolerance for pain. The type of pain intervention usually depends on the description of the pain by the individual experiencing it. Mild pain may best be relieved by comfort measures and the distraction afforded by television, visitors, reading, and other passive activities. Moderate pain may best be relieved by a combination of comfort measures and drugs. Cognitive dissonance, often employed to dampen moderate pain, encourages the patient to reflect on pleasant experiences and describe them to health care personnel. Intervention to relieve severe pain often includes the administration of narcotics, purposeful interaction between the patient and attending hospital personnel, reduction of environmental stimuli, increased comfort measures, and "waking imagined analgesia," in which the patient is encouraged to concentrate on and become distracted by former pleasant experiences, as relaxing on a beach surrounded by cool ocean water. In the alleviation of all types of pain, dampening or decreasing stimuli that create pain is the chief goal. Pain often increases in a cold room because the muscles of the patient tend to contract; but the local application of cold, as with an ice pack, often alleviates pain by reducing swelling. Pain intervention seeks to reduce the effects of other factors that compound pain, as fatigue and anxiety. Coping with pain becomes increasingly difficult as the patient becomes more tired. Sensory restriction may increase pain, because it blocks otherwise effective distraction; overstimulation may cause fatigue and anxiety, thus increasing pain. Religious beliefs may be effective in helping the patient to decrease pain or increase tolerance if the pain is viewed by the patient as requiring self-discipline or as a catharsis for past transgressions. Religious beliefs, however, may increase pain if the patient interprets the pain as punishment and relates the severity of the pain with the gravity of transgressions or faults. Pain intervention by the use of drugs includes the administration of mild nonnarcotic analgesics and of much more potent and potentially addictive opioids, as morphine. Opioid analgesics administered for the relief of pain, cough, or diarrhea provide only symptomatic treatment and are used cautiously in the care of patients with acute or chronic diseases. Opioids may obscure the symptoms or the progress of the disease, and repeated daily administration of any opioid will eventually produce some tolerance to the therapeutic effects of the drug and some physical dependence on the dosage. The risk of developing psychologic and physical dependency on any drug is always present, especially with opioids. In usual doses, opioids relieve suffering by altering the emotional component of the painful experience and by effecting analgesia. Some care givers are so concerned about the addictive dangers of opioids that they tend to prescribe initial doses that are too low or too infrequent to alleviate pain. A typical dose of 10 mg of morphine relieves postoperative pain in only two thirds of patients. Some patients may require considerably more than the average dose of an opioid to experience adequate pain relief. Some other patients with more rapid metabolisms may require such drugs at shorter intervals. Many drugs are appropriate substitutes for the potent opioids morphine and codeine. Some of the effective semisynthetic substitutes are hydrocodone, dihydrocodeine, and meperidine. The narcotic analgesics act on the central nervous system, but the salicylates and other nonnarcotic drugs act at the site of origin of the pain. Some nonnarcotic drugs also have antiinflammatory and antipyretic activity, as aspirin, indomethacin, ibuprofen, or naproxen. In patients who are sensitive to or are unable to take aspirin, acetaminophen is an acceptable substitute, as are the nonsteroidal antiinflammatory drugs. Pain intervention in the treatment of terminal illnesses employs numerous drugs that relieve pain and produce euphoria and tranquillity in patients who would otherwise suffer greatly. Analgesic mixtures of opioids and alcoholic solutions may be prescribed. Nerve block by the injection of alcohol, chordotomy, and other neurosurgical interventions may sometimes be employed. Other techniques include acupuncture, hypnosis, and behavior modification, in which treatment consists of reducing medication and gradually increasing mobility by exercising and any other appropriate modality, biofeedback, and transcutaneous electric nerve stimulation. The latter technique is a noninvasive and nonaddictive method of modifying pain messages to the brain. See also **pain assessment.**

pain mechanism, the psychosomatic network that communicates unpleasant sensations and the perceptions of noxious stimuli throughout the body, most commonly in association with physical disease and trauma involving tissue damage. Many studies of the pain mechanism have resulted in numerous theories as to how it functions, and such research continues; but variations in pain are so numerous and individual responses so diverse that a precise understanding of the subject still eludes health professionals. Some theories about the pain mechanism that have evolved are the gate control theories and the pattern theories. The gate control theory of pain is an attempt to explain the complexity of the nervous system. It states that pain signals reaching the nervous system excite a group of small neurons that form a "pain pool." When the total activity of these neurons reaches a minimum level, a theoretic gate opens up and allows the pain signals to proceed to higher brain centers. The areas in which the gates operate are considered to be in the spinal cord dorsal horn and the brainstem. The pattern theory holds that the intensity of a stimulus evokes a specific pattern, which is interpreted by the brain as pain. This perception is the result of the intensity and frequency of stimulation of a nonspecific end organ. One of the biggest problems in pain research is that the actual cause of pain originating at the peripheral level is poorly understood. Some authorities believe that bradykinin and histamine, two chemical substances elaborated by the body, cause pain. Recently discovered pain killers produced naturally by the body are the enkephalins and the endorphins. Some studies indicate that the enkephalins are 10 times as potent as morphine in reducing pain. It is known that once histamine and some other naturally occurring chemical substances are released in the body, pain sensations travel along fast-conducting nerve fibers and slow-conducting nerve fibers. These pain-transmitting neuropathways communicate the pain sensation to the dorsal root ganglia of the spinal cord and synapse with certain neurons in the posterior horns of the gray matter. The pain sensation is then transmitted to the reticular formation and the thalamus by neurons that form the anterolateral spinothalamic tract. It is then conveyed to various areas of the brain, as the cortex and the hypothalamus, by synapses at the thalamus. The immediate reaction to pain is transmitted over the reflex arc by sensory fibers in the dorsal horn of the spinal cord and by synapsing motor neurons in the anterior horn. This anatomic pattern of sensory and motor neurons allows the individual to move quickly at the touch of some harmful stimulus, as extreme heat or cold. Nerve impulses alerting the individual to move away from such stimuli are simultaneously sent along efferent nerve fibers from the brain. The most recent pain theories incorporate the emotional component as an important factor in the pain mechanism. Past experiences, anxiety, and motivations greatly affect the pain sensations of everyone, and the fear of pain is second only to the fear of death for most people. It is known that fear and anxiety often intensify pain.

pain receptor, any one of the many free nerve endings throughout the body that warn of potentially harmful changes in the environment, as excessive pressure or temperature. The free nerve endings constituting most of the pain receptors occur chiefly in the epidermis and in the epithelial covering of certain mucous membranes. They also appear in the stratified squamous epithelium of the cornea, in the root sheaths and in the papillae of the hairs, and around the bodies of sudoriferous glands. The terminal ends of pain receptors consist of unmyelinated nerve fibers that often anastomose into small knobs between the epithelial cells. Any kind of stimulus, if it is intense enough, can stimulate the pain receptors in the skin and the mucosa, but only radical changes in pressure and certain chemicals can stimulate the pain receptors in the viscera. Referred pain results only from stimulation of pain receptors located in deep structures, as the viscera, the joints, and the skeletal muscles, but never from pain receptors in the skin.

pain spot, any spot on the skin where a stimulus can produce pain.

paint, **1.** to apply a medicated solution to the skin, usually over a wide area. **2.** a medicated solution that is applied in this way. Kinds of paint include **antiseptics,** **germicides,** and **sporicides.**

PA interval (HBE), a measurement of intraatrial conduction time measured from the onset of the P wave on a standard ECG, or from the atrial deflection of the high right atrial electrogram to the A wave on the His bundle electrogram (HBE).

pain threshold, the point at which a stimulus, usually one associated with pressure or temperature, activates pain receptors and produces a sensation of pain. Individuals with low pain thresholds experience pain much sooner and faster than individuals with higher pain thresholds; the reaction to stimulation of pain receptors varies with individuals.

palatal, **1.** of or pertaining to the palate. **2.** of or pertaining to the lingual surface of a maxillary tooth.

palate, a structure that forms the roof of the mouth. It is divided into the hard palate and the soft palate. **–palatal, palatine** /pal′ətīn/, *adj.*

palatine arch, the vault-shaped muscular structure forming the soft palate between the mouth and the nasopharynx. An opening in the arch connects the mouth with the oropharynx; the uvula is suspended from the middle of the posterior border of the arch.

palatine bone, one of a pair of bones of the skull, forming the posterior part of the hard palate, part of the nasal cavity, and the floor of the orbit of the eye. It resembles a letter ''L'' and consists of horizontal and vertical parts and three processes.

palatine ridge, any one of the four to six transverse ridges on the anterior surface of the hard palate.

palatine suture, one of a number of thin wavy lines marking the joining of the palatine processes that form the hard palate. See also **median palatine suture, transverse palatine suture.**

palatine tonsil, one of a pair of almond-shaped masses of lymphoid tissue between the palatoglossal and the palatopharyngeal arches on each side of the fauces. They are covered with mucous membrane and contain numerous lymph follicles and various crypts.

palatitis, an inflammation of the hard palate.

palato-, a combining form meaning 'of or pertaining to the palate': *palatoglossal, palatography, palatomaxillary.*

palatomaxillary, of or pertaining to the palate and the maxilla.

palatonasal, of or pertaining to the palate and the nose.

paleo-, a combining form meaning 'old': *paleocerebellar, paleogenesis, paleostriatum.*

paleogenesis. See **palingenesis.**

paleogenetic, **1.** a trait or structure of an organism or species that originated in a previous generation. **2.** relating to the development of such a trait or structure.

pali-. See **palin-.**

palilalia, an abnormal condition characterized by the increasingly rapid repetition of the same word or phrase, usually at the end of a sentence.

palin-, pali-, a combining form meaning 'again': *palindromia, palinesthesia, palingenesis.*

palindrome /pal′indrōm′/, (in molecular genetics) a segment of DNA in which identical, or almost identical, sequences of bases run in opposite directions.

palingenesis, **1.** the regeneration of a lost part. **2.** the hereditary transmission of ancestral structural characteristics, especially abnormalities, in successive generations. Also called **paleogenesis.** Compare **cenogenesis.** **–palingenetic, palingenic,** *adj.*

Pallace, a trademark for an antineoplastic progestational agent (megestrol acetate).

palladium (Pd), a hard, silvery metallic element. Its atomic number is 46; its atomic weight is 106.4. Highly resistant to tarnish and corrosion, palladium is used in high-grade surgical instruments and in dental inlays, bridgework, and orthodontic appliances.

palliate /pal′ē·āt/, to soothe or relieve. **–palliation,** *n.*, **palliative** /pal′i·ətiv/, *adj.*

palliative treatment, therapy designed to relieve or reduce intensity of uncomfortable symptoms but not to produce a cure. Some kinds of palliative treatment are the use of narcotics to relieve pain in a patient with advanced cancer, the creation of a colostomy to bypass an inoperable obstructing lesion of the bowel, and the debridement of necrotic tissue in a patient with metastatic malignancy. Compare **definitive treatment, expectant treatment.**

pallidum. See **globus pallidus.**

pallium. See **cerebral cortex.**

pallor, an unnatural paleness or absence of color in the skin.

palm, the lower side of the hand, between the wrist and the bases of the fingers, when the hand is held horizontal with the thumb in medial position. **–palmar,** *adj.*

palmar aponeurosis, fascia surrounding the muscles of the palm. Also called **palmar fascia.**

palmar crease, a normal groove across the palm of the hand.

palmar erythema, an inflammatory redness of the palms of the hands.

palmar fascia. See **palmar aponeurosis.**

palmaris longus, a long, slender, superficial, fusiform muscle of the forearm, lying on the medial side of the flexor carpi radialis. It arises from the medial epicondyle of the humerus by a tendon from the intermuscular septa between it and the adjacent muscles and from the antebrachial fascia. It inserts by a long, thin tendon into the flexor retinaculum and into the palmar aponeurosis. A tendinous slip of the muscle is often found extending to the thumb. The palmaris longus is innervated by a branch of the median nerve, which contains fibers from the sixth and the seventh cervical nerves, and it functions to flex the hand. Compare **flexor carpi radialis, flexor carpi ulnaris.**

palmar metacarpal artery, one of several arteries arising from the deep palmar arch, supplying the fingers.

palmar reflex, a reflex that curls the fingers when the palm of the hand is tickled.

palmature, an abnormal condition in which the fingers are webbed.

palm-chin reflex. See **palmomental reflex.**

palmityl alcohol. See **cetyl alcohol.**

palmomental reflex, an abnormal neurologic sign, elicited by scratching the palm of the hand at the base of the thumb, characterized by contraction of the muscles of the chin and corner of the mouth on the same side of the body as the stimulus. It is occasionally seen in normal individuals, but an exaggerated reflex may be seen in pyramidal tract disease, latent tetany, increased intracranial pressure, and central facial paresis. Also called **palm-chin reflex.**

palpable, perceivable by touch.

palpate, to use the hands or fingers to examine.

palpation, a technique used in physical examination in which the examiner feels the texture, size, consistency, and location of certain parts of the body with the hands.

palpatory percussion, a technique in physical examination in which the vibrations produced by percussion are evaluated by using light pressure of the flat of the examiner's hand.

palpebra. See **eyelid.**

palpebral commissure. See **canthus.**

palpebral fissure, the opening between the margins of the upper and lower lids.

palpebral gland. See **meibomian gland.**

palpebra superior, *pl.* **palpebrae superiores,** the upper eyelid, larger and more movable than the lower eyelid and furnished with an elevator muscle.

palpebrate, **1.** to wink or blink. **2.** having eyelids.

palpeleral conjunctiva. See **conjunctiva.**

palpitate, to pulsate rapidly, as in the unusually fast beating of the heart under various conditions of stress and in patients with certain heart problems.

palpitation, a pounding or racing of the heart, associated with normal emotional responses or with certain heart disorders. Some people may complain of pounding hearts and display no evidence of heart disease, whereas others, with serious heart disorders, may not detect associated abnormal palpitations. Some patients complain of palpitations after receiving digitalis medication, because it increases the force of heart contractions. Many healthy individuals become concerned and describe as palpitations the normal sounds of their hearts against their pillows when they lie down to sleep.

palsy /pôl′zē/, an abnormal condition characterized by paralysis. Some kinds of palsy are **Bell's palsy, cerebral palsy,** and **Erb's palsy.**

Paltauf's dwarf. See **pituitary dwarf.**

Paltauf's nanism, dwarfism associated with excessive production or growth of lymphoid tissue.

Pamine, a trademark for an anticholinergic (methscopolamine bromide).

PAMP, abbreviation for *pulmonary arterial mean pressure*.

pampiniform, having the shape of a tendril.

pampinform body. See **epoophoron.**

pan-, a combining form meaning 'all': *panacea, pancarditis, pandemic.*

panacea /pan′əsē′ə/, **1.** a universal remedy. **2.** an ancient name for a herb or a liquid potion with healing properties.

panacinar emphysema /panas′ənər/, a form of emphysema that affects all lung areas by causing dilatation and atrophy of the alveoli and by destroying the vascular bed of the lung. Also called **panlobular emphysema.**

Panafil, a trademark for a topical, fixed-combination drug containing an enzyme (papain).

panarthritis, an abnormal condition characterized by the inflammation of many joints of the body. –**panarthritic,** *adj.*

pancake kidney, a congenital anomaly in which the left and right kidneys are fused into a single mass in the pelvis. The fused kidney has two collecting systems and two ureters and frequently becomes obstructed because of its abnormal position.

pancarditis, an abnormal condition characterized by inflammation of the entire heart, including the endocardium, myocardium, and pericardium.

Pancoast's syndrome, **1.** a combination of various signs associated with a tumor in the apex of the lung. The signs include neuritic pain in the arm, an x-ray shadow at the apex of the lung, atrophy of the muscles of the arm and the hand, and Horner's syndrome. The signs are caused by the damaging effects of the tumor on the brachial plexus. **2.** an abnormal condition caused by osteolysis in the posterior part of one or more ribs, sometimes involving associated vertebrae.

Pancoast's tumor. See **pulmonary sulcus tumor.**

pancolectomy, the excision of the entire colon, requiring also an ileostomy.

pancreas /pan′krē·əs/, a fish-shaped, grayish pink nodular gland that stretches transversely across the posterior abdominal wall in the epigastric and hypochondriac regions of the body and secretes various substances, as digestive enzymes, insulin, and glucagon. It is divided into a head, a body, and a tail. The head of the gland, divided from the body by a small constriction, is tucked into the curve of the duodenum. The tapered left extremity of the organ forms the tail. In adults, the pancreas is about 13 cm long and weighs more in a man than it does in a woman. A compound racemose gland composed of exocrine and endocrine tissue, it contains a main duct that runs the length of the organ, draining smaller ducts and emptying into the duodenum at the major duodenal papilla, the same site that accommodates the exit of the common bile duct. About 1 million cellular islets or islands of Langerhans are embedded between the exocrine units of the pancreas. Beta cells of the islands secrete insulin, which helps control carbohydrate metabolism. Alpha cells of the islets secrete glucagon that counters the action of insulin. The acinar units of the pancreas secrete digestive enzymes.

pancreas scan, an x-ray scan of the pancreas after the intravenous injection of a radioactive contrast medium, used for detecting various abnormalities, as tumors, cysts, and infections.

pancreatectomy /pan′krē·ətek′təmē/, the surgical removal of all or part of the pancreas, performed to remove a cyst or tumor, treat pancreatitis, or repair trauma. The resection is done using general anesthesia; the GI tract is reconstructed, usually with an anastomosis between the common bile duct and the upper jejunum. Drains are left in the wound. After surgery the patient is given a low-sugar, low-fat diet. If the entire pancreas is removed, a brittle type of diabetes develops, requiring precise management of both diet and insulin dosage. A frequent complication is the formation of a fistula in the pancreatic bile duct, allowing digestive enzymes to contact adjacent tissues.

-pancreatic, a combining form meaning the 'pancreas or a condition of the pancreas or adjacent organs': *hepaticopancreatic, lienopancreatic, splenopancreatic.*

pancreatic cancer /pan′krē·at′ik/, a malignant neoplastic disease of the pancreas, characterized by anorexia, flatulence, weakness, dramatic weight loss, epigastric or back pain, jaundice, pruritus, a palpable abdominal mass, the recent onset of diabetes, and clay-colored stools if the pancreatic ducts are obstructed. Insulin-secreting tumors of islet cells cause hypoglycemia, especially in the morning. Nonfunctioning islet cell lesions produce gastrin, causing symptoms of peptic ulcer, or, in some cases, acute diarrhea and hypokalemia, and achlorhydria, the result of the lesion's elaboration of secretin. Diagnostic measures include barium x-ray studies of the stomach and duodenum, transhepatic cholangiography, laboratory evaluation of liver function, celiac arteriography, and computerized axial tomography. Exploratory laparotomy is often required for a definitive diagnosis. About 90% of pancreatic tumors are adenocarcinomas; two thirds are in the head of the pancreas. Most tumors are not resectable at the time of diagnosis, but localized cancers in the pancreas may be treated by partial pancreatectomy with excision of the common bile duct, duodenum, and distal part of the stomach. Functioning islet cell lesions may be excised or treated with streptozotocin, an antibiotic toxic to beta cells of the pancreas. Total gastrectomy is recommended for nonfunctioning islet cell tumors that are accompanied by peptic ulcer disease. Radiotherapy or chemotherapy with 5-fluorouracil or mitomycin-C may offer temporary palliation, but cancer of the pancreas has a poor prognosis: few people live for more than 1 year after diagnosis. Pancreatic cancer occurs three to four times more often in men than in women. Though uncommon, it is increasing in incidence in the industrialized areas of the world. People who smoke more than 10 to 20 cigarettes a day, who have diabetes mellitus, or who have been exposed to polychlorinated biphenyl compounds are at increased risk of developing pancreatic cancer.

pancreatic diverticulum, one of a pair of membranous pouches arising from the embryonic duodenum. These two diverticula later form the pancreas and its ducts.

pancreatic dornase, an enzyme from beef pancreas that has been used as a mucolytic for upper respiratory infections and cystic fibrosis.

pancreatic duct, the primary secretory channel of the pancreas. Also called **duct of Wirsung.**

pancreatic enzyme, any one of the enzymes secreted by the pancreas in the process of digestion. The most important are trypsin, chymotrypsin, steapsin, and amylopsin. See also **pancreatic juice.**

pancreatic hormone, any one of several chemical compounds secreted by the pancreas, associated with the regulation of cellular metabolism. Major hormones secreted by the pancreas are insulin, glucagon, and pancreatic polypeptide. Insulin and glucagon are secreted by different types of cells within the alpha and beta cells of the islands of Langerhans; pancreatic polypeptide is secreted by a group of glandular cells arranged in a halo around each island of Langerhans.

pancreatic insufficiency, a condition characterized by inadequate production and secretion of pancreatic hormones or enzymes, usually occurring secondary to a disease process destructive of pancreatic tissue. Nutritional malabsorption, anorexia, poorly localized upper abdominal or epigastric pain, malaise, and severe weight loss often occur. Alcohol-induced pancreatitis is the most common form of the condition. Supportive care, specific treatment of the cause of the condition, and replacement or augmentation of the absent or lacking substances are usually recommended as therapy for pancreatic insufficiency.

pancreatic juice, the fluid secretion of the pancreas, produced by the stimulation of food in the duodenum. Pancreatic juice contains water, protein, inorganic salts, and enzymes. The juice is essential in breaking down proteins into their amino acid components, in reducing dietary fats to glycerol and fatty acids, and in converting starch to simple sugars.

pancreaticolienal node /pan′krē·at′ikōlī·ē′nəl/, a node in one of three groups of lymph glands associated with branches of the abdominal and the pelvic viscera that are supplied by branches of the celiac artery. The pancreaticolienal nodes accompany the splenic artery along the posterior surface and the upper border of the pancreas. Their afferents, which originate from the stomach, the spleen, and the pancreas, join the celiac group of preaortic nodes. Also called **splenic gland.** Compare **gastric node, hepatic node.**

pancreatin /pan′krē·ətin′/, a concentrate of pancreatic enzymes from swine or beef cattle.

■ INDICATIONS: It is prescribed as an aid to digestion to replace endogenous pancreatic enzymes in cystic fibrosis and after pancreatectomy.

■ CONTRAINDICATIONS: Known hypersensitivity to this drug or to pork or beef protein prohibits its use.

■ ADVERSE EFFECTS: There are no known serious adverse reactions. High doses may cause nausea or diarrhea.

pancreatitis /pan′krē·ətī′tis/, an inflammatory condition of the pancreas that may be acute or chronic. **Acute pancreatitis** is generally the result of damage to the biliary tract, as by alcohol, trauma, infectious disease, or certain drugs. It is characterized by severe abdominal pain radiating to the back, fever, anorexia, nausea, and vomiting. There may be jaundice if the common bile duct is obstructed. The development of pseudocysts or abscesses in pancreatic tissue is a serious complication. Treatment includes nasogastric suction to remove gastric secretions. To prevent any stimulation of the pancreas, nothing is given by mouth. Intravenous fluids and electrolytes are administered, and nonmorphine derivatives are given to relieve pain. Acute pancreatitis is associated with a mortality of 50%. The causes of **chronic pancreatitis** are similar to those of the acute form. When the cause is alcohol abuse, there may be calcification and scarring of the smaller pancreatic ducts. There is abdominal pain, nausea, and vomiting, as well as steatorrhea and creatorrhea, caused by the diminished output of pancreatic enzymes. Pancreatic insulin production may be diminished, and some patients develop diabetes mellitus. Treatment includes analgesics for pain and subtotal pancreatectomy when pain is intractable. A pancreatic extract is given orally to replace the missing enzymes; vitamin supplements are essential. Both forms of pancreatitis are diagnosed by history, physical examination, radiologic studies, endoscopy, and laboratory analysis of the amount of pancreatic enzymes in the blood.

pancreatoduodenectomy /pan′krē•ā′tōdo͞o′ōdənek′-təmē/, a surgical procedure in which the head of the pancreas and the loop of duodenum that surrounds it are excised. The operation is performed to remove the periampullary masses occurring in certain forms of biliary tract cancer.

pancreatography /pan′krē•ətog′rəfē/, visualization of the pancreas or its ducts by means of x-rays and contrast media injected into the ducts at surgery or via an endoscope or by means of ultrasonography, computerized tomography, or radionuclide imaging.

pancreatolith, a stone or calculus in the pancreas.

pancrelipase /pan′krəlip′ās/, a digestant. Also called **lipancreatin.**

■ INDICATIONS: It is prescribed in the treatment of exocrine pancreatic insufficiency as a result of chronic pancreatitis, pancreatectomy, cystic fibrosis, or obstruction caused by cancer of the the pancreas.

■ CONTRAINDICATIONS: There are no known contraindications.

■ ADVERSE EFFECTS: Among the most serious adverse reactions are nausea, abdominal cramps, and diarrhea with high doses.

pancuronium bromide, a skeletal muscle relaxant.

■ INDICATIONS: It is prescribed as an adjunct to anesthesia and mechanic ventilation.

■ CONTRAINDICATIONS: It is used with caution in patients with myasthenia gravis and renal and hepatic disease and in pregnancy. Known hypersensitivity to this drug or to other bromides prohibits its use.

■ ADVERSE EFFECTS: The most serious adverse reaction is prolonged muscle relaxation and respiratory depression.

pancytopenia /pan′sītəpē′nē•ə/, an abnormal condition characterized by a marked reduction in the number of all of the cellular elements of the blood, the red blood cells, white blood cells, and platelets. See also **anemia, aplasia.** –**pancytopenic,** *adj.*

p and a, abbreviation for *percussion and auscultation,* as noted in the patient's chart after physical examination of the chest. See **auscultation, percussion.**

pandemic, (of a disease) occurring throughout the population of a country, a people, or the world.

pandiastolic, of or pertaining to the complete diastole. Also called **holodiastolic.**

panencephalitis /pan′əsef′əlī′tis/, inflammation of the entire brain characterized by an insidious onset, a progressive course with deterioration of motor and mental functions, and evidence of a viral cause. Subacute sclerosing panencephalitis is an uncommon childhood disease thought to be caused by a "slow" latent measles virus after recovery from a previous infection. Most of the patients are younger than 11 years of age, and many more boys than girls are affected. The disease results in ataxia, myoclonus, atrophy, cortical blindness, and mental deterioration. Antiviral drugs, immunosuppressants, and interferon inducers are sometimes administered, but the disease is usually fatal. Microscopic studies of postmortem brain tissue often reveal intracellular inclusion bodies resembling the nucleocapsids of paramyxoviruses. Rubella panencephalitis, a rare disease of adolescents, follows a chronic progressive course marked by motor and mental deterioration and sometimes resembles juvenile paresis. Inclusion bodies are not found in brain cells, but the pathology is similar to the mineralization found in infantile congenital rubella, and antibodies to the virus are present.

panendoscope, a cystoscope that allows a wide view of the interior of the bladder.

panesthesia, the total of all sensations experienced by an individual at one time. Compare **cenesthesia.**

pangenesis, a darwinian theory that every cell and particle of a parent reproduces itself in progeny.

Panheprin, a trademark for an anticoagulant (heparin sodium).

panhypopituitarism /panhī′pōpito͞o′itəriz′əm/, generalized insufficiency of pituitary hormones, resulting from damage to or deficiency of the gland. **Prepubertal panhypopituitarism,** a rare disorder usually associated with a suprasellar cyst or craniopharyngioma, is characterized by dwarfism with normal body proportions, subnormal sexual development, and insufficient thyroid and adrenal function. Diabetes insipidus is frequently present; there may be bitemporal hemianopia or complete blindness; skin is often yellow and wrinkled, but mentality is usually unimpaired. X-ray pictures show delayed fusion of the epiphyses, suprasellar calcification, and, frequently, destruction of the sella turcica. The condition is treated with cortisone, thyroid and sex hormones and, if available, human growth hormone. Postpubertal panhypopituitarism may be caused by postpartum pituitary necrosis, resulting from thrombosis of pituitary circulation during or after delivery. Characteristic signs of the disorder are failure to lactate, amenorrhea, weakness, cold intolerance, lethargy, loss of libido and of axillary and pubic hair. There may be bradycardia or hypotension, and progression of the disorder leads to premature wrinkling of the skin and atrophy of the thyroid and adrenal glands. Treatment consists of the administration of ACTH, thyroid stimulating hormone, and hormones of the target organs. Also called **hypophyseal cachexia, pituitary cachexia, Simmonds' disease.**

panhysterectomy /pan'histərek'təmē/, complete surgical removal of the uterus and cervix. See also **hysterectomy.**

panic, an intense, sudden, and overwhelming fear or feeling of anxiety that produces terror and immediate physiologic changes that result in paralyzed immobility or senseless, hysteric behavior.

panic disorder. See **anxiety neurosis.**

panivorous /paniv'ərəs/, of or pertaining to the practice of subsisting exclusively on bread. **–panivore,** *n.*

panlobular emphysema. See **panacinar emphysema.**

Panmycin Hydrochloride, a trademark for an antibacterial and antiprotozoal (tetracycline hydrochloride).

panniculus, *pl.* **panniculi,** a membranous layer, the many sheets of fascia covering various structures in the body.

pannus /pan'əs/, an abnormal condition of the cornea, which has become vascularized and infiltrated with granular tissue just beneath the surface. Pannus may develop in the inflammatory stage of trachoma or after a detached retina, glaucoma, iridocylitis, or another degenerative eye disease.

panophthalmitis /pan'ofthalmī'tis/, an inflammation of the entire eye, usually caused by virulent pyogenic organisms, as strains of meningococci, pneumococci, streptococci, anthrax bacilli, and clostraidia. Initial symptoms are pain, fever, headache, drowsiness, edema, and swelling. As the infection progresses, the iris appears muddy and gray, the aqueous humor becomes turbid, and precipitates form on the posterior surface of the cornea. Treatment consists of intensive systemic and local antibiotic therapy; evisceration of the globe or excision of the eye may be required, but excision is contraindicated if surrounding tissues are infected.

Panoxyl, a trademark for a keratolytic (benzoyl peroxide).

panphobia, an anxiety disorder characterized by an irrational, vague fear or apprehension of some pervading or unknown evil; a generalized fear. Also called **panophobia, pantophobia.** **–panophobic,** *adj.*

panphobic melancholia, *obsolete.* a state of depression characterized by an irrational dread or pervading fear of everything. See also **bipolar disorder, phobia.**

pansystolic, of or pertaining to the entire systole. Also **holosystolic.**

pansystolic murmur. See **systolic murmur.**

pant-. See **panto-.**

Panteric, a trademark for an enzyme (pancreatin).

panthenol /pan'thənôl/, an alcohol converted in the body to pantothenic acid, a vitamin in the B complex.

panto-, pant-, a combining form meaning 'all, the whole': *pantophobia, pantoscopic, pantosomatous.*

pantograph, **1.** a jointed device for copying a plane figure to any desired scale. **2.** a device that incorporates a pair of face bows fixed to the jaws, used for inscribing centrically related points and arcs leading to them on segments relatable to the three craniofacial planes.

pantomography, panoramic radiography for obtaining radiographs of the maxillary and mandibular dental arches and related structures.

Pantopon, a trademark for a narcotic analgesic, fixed-combination drug containing hydrochlorides of opium alkaloids.

pantothenic acid /pan'təthen'ik/, a member of the vitamin B complex. It is widely distributed in plant and animal tissues and may be an important element in human nutrition.

pantothenyl alcohol. See **panthenol.**

Panwarfin, a trademark for an anticoagulant (warfarin sodium).

Pao_2, symbol for *arterial partial pressure of oxygen.*

papain /pəpā'ēn/, an enzyme from the fruit of *Carica papaya,* the tropic melon tree. It has been prescribed for enzymatic debridement of wounds and promotion of healing.

Papanicolaou test, a simple smear method of examining stained exfoliative cells. It is used most commonly to detect cancers of the cervix, but it may be used for tissue specimens from any organ. A smear is usually obtained during a routine pelvic examination. The technique permits early diagnosis of cancer and has contributed to a lower death rate from cervical cancer. The findings are usually reported descriptively and grouped into the following classes: Class I, only normal cells seen; Class II, atypical cells consistent with inflammation; Class III, mild dysplasia; Class IV, severe dysplasia, suspicious cells; Class V, carcinoma cells seen. Also called *(informal)* **Pap test.**

papaverine hydrochloride, a smooth muscle relaxant.

■ INDICATIONS: It is prescribed in the treatment of cardiovascular or visceral spasms.

■ CONTRAINDICATIONS: Complete atrioventricular heart block or known hypersensitivity to this drug prohibits its use.

■ ADVERSE EFFECTS: The most serious adverse reactions include jaundice, increased blood pressure, and arrhythmias.

paper chromatography, the separation of a mixture into its components by filtering it through a strip of special paper.

paper-doll fetus. See **fetus papyraceus.**

paper tape, a ribbon of paper tape into which holes are punched in certain patterns to produce information codes for reading by a paper tape reader.

paper tape punch, a computer keyboarding device for coding information by creating holes in paper tape in discrete patterns that conform to keys depressed.

paper tape reader, a device for reading the codes punched into paper tape as a series of patterns of electric impulses that may be used to actuate an electromechanic device or to transmit information to other devices for processing.

papilla /pəpil′ə/, *pl.* **papillae,** **1.** a small nipple-shaped projection, as the conoid papillae of the tongue and the papillae of the corium that extend from collagen fibers, the capillary blood vessels, and sometimes the nerves of the dermis. **2.** the optic papilla, a round white disc in the fundus oculi, which corresponds to the entrance of the optic nerve.

papilla duodeni major. See **hepatopancreatic ampulla.**

papilla of Vater. See **hepatopancreatic ampulla.**

papillary /pap′əlerē/, of or pertaining to a papilla.

papillary adenocarcinoma, a malignant neoplasm characterized by small papillae of vascular connective tissue covered by neoplastic epithelium that projects into follicles, glands, or cysts. The tumor is most common in the ovaries and thyroid gland. Also called **polypoid adenocarcinoma.**

papillary adenocystoma lymphomatosum, an unusual tumor, consisting of epithelial and lymphoid tissues, that develops in the area of the parotid and submaxillary glands. Also called **adenolymphoma, Warthin's tumor.**

papillary adenoma, a benign epithelial tumor in which the membrane lining the glandular tissue forms papillary processes that project into the alveoli or grow out of the surface of a cavity.

papillary carcinoma, a malignant neoplasm characterized by many fingerlike projections. It is the most common type of thyroid tumor.

papillary duct, any one of the thousands of straight collecting renal tubules that descend through the medulla of the kidney and join with others to form the common ducts opening into the renal papillae. Compare **Henle's loop.** See also **kidney.**

papillary muscle, any one of the rounded or conic muscular projections attached to the chordae tendineae in the ventricles of the heart. The papillary muscles vary in number, but the two main ones are the anterior papillary muscle and the posterior papillary muscle. The papillary muscles are associated with the atrioventricular valves that they help open and close. Compare **chorda tendinea, trabecula carnea.**

papillary tumor. See **papilloma.**

papillate, marked by papillae or nipplelike prominences.

papilledema, *pl.* **papilledemas, papilledemata,** swelling of the optic disc, visible on ophthalmoscopic examination of the fundus of the eye, caused by increased intracranial pressure. The meningeal sheaths that surround the optic nerves from the optic disc are continuous with the meninges of the brain; therefore, increased intracranial pressure is transmitted forward from the brain to the optic disc in the eye to cause the swelling.

papilliform, shaped like a papilla.

papillitis /pap′ilī′tis/ **1.** an abnormal condition characterized by the inflammation of a papilla, as the lacrimal papilla. **2.** an abnormal condition characterized by the inflammation of a renal papilla.

papilloma /pap′ilō′mə/, a benign epithelial neoplasm characterized by a branching or lobular tumor. Kinds of papilloma are **basal cell papilloma, cockscomb papilloma, cutaneous papilloma, fibroepithelial papilloma, hirsutoid papilloma of the penis, intracanalicular papilloma, intracystic papilloma,** and **villous papilloma.** Also called **papillary tumor.**

-papilloma, a combining form meaning an 'epithelial tumor': *fibropapilloma, myxopapilloma, polypapilloma.*

papillomatosis /pap′ilōmətō′sis/, an abnormal condition in which there is widespread development of nipple-like growths.

papillomatosis coronae penis. See **hirsutoid papilloma of the penis.**

papillomavirus /pap′ilōməvī′rəs/, the virus that causes warts in humans.

papilloretinitis /pap′ilōret′inī′tis/, an inflammatory occlusion of a retinal vein.

papovavirus /pap′əvəvī′rəs/, one of a group of small DNA viruses, some of which may be potentially cancer-producing. The human wart is caused by a kind of papovavirus, but it very rarely undergoes malignant transformation. Kinds of papovaviruses are **papilloma papovavirus, polyoma papovavirus,** and **SV-40 papovavirus.**

pappataci fever. See **phlebotomus fever.**

pappus, the first growth of beard, characterized by downy hairs.

Pap smear, *informal.* a specimen of exfoliated, epithelial cells and cervical mucus collected during a pelvic exam for cytologic evaluation according to the Papanicolaou cytologic classification.

Pap test. See **Papanicolaou test.**

papular scaling disease, any of a group of skin disorders in which there are discrete, raised, dry, scaling lesions. Some kinds of papular scaling diseases are **lichen planus, pityriasis rosea,** and **psoriasis.** Also called **papulosquamous disease.**

papulation, the development of papules.

papule /pap′yo͞ol/, a small, solid, raised skin lesion less than 1 cm in diameter, as the lesions of lichen planus and nonpustular acne. Compare **macule.** **–papular,** *adj.*

papulosquamous disease. See **papular scaling disease.**

papyraceous, having a paperlike quality.

papyraceous fetus. See **fetus papyraceus.**

Paquelin's cautery /pak′əlinz/, a cauterizing device consisting of a platinum loop through which a heated hydrocarbon is passed.

par, a pair, specifically a pair of cranial nerves, as the par nonum or the ninth pair.

PAR, abbreviation for **pulmonary arteriolar resistance.**

par-, a combining form meaning 'aside, beyond, apart from, against': *parabacteria, parotid, parumbilical.*

para-, par-, a combining form meaning 'similar, beside': *paronchia, parotid, parasympathetic.*

-para, **1.** a combining form meaning a 'woman who has given birth to children in a number of pregnancies': *bipara, nonipara, unipara.* **2.** a combining form meaning a 'female of any species producing a number or type of egg or offspring': *nymphipara, ovovipara, pipipara.*

paraaminobenzoic acid (PABA) /per′ə•amē′nōbenzō′ik/, a substance often occurring in association with the vitamin B complex, found in cereals, eggs, milk, and meat and present in detectable amounts in blood, urine, spinal fluid, and sweat. It is widely used as a sunscreen that forms a partial chemical conjugation with constituents of the horny layer and that resists removal by water and sweat. PABA is a sulfonamide antagonist and may be an effective agent for the treatment of scleroderma, dermatomyositis, and pemphigus.

paraaminohippuric acid (PAHA, PHA), the N-acetic acid of paraaminobenzoic acid. Its sodium salt is used for measuring the effective renal plasma flow and for determining kidney function.

paraaminosalicylic acid (PAS, PASA), a bacteriostatic agent.

■ INDICATIONS: It is prescribed for the treatment of pulmonary and extrapulmonary tuberculosis.

■ CONTRAINDICATIONS: Known hypersensitivity to the drug prohibits its use. It may interact with other drugs.

■ ADVERSE EFFECTS: Among the most serious reactions are nausea, vomiting, diarrhea, and abdominal pain. Fever, skin eruptions, and other kinds of hypersensitivity reactions, goiter, hypokalemia, and acidosis may occur.

parabiotic syndrome, a blood transfer condition that can occur between identical twin fetuses because of placental vascular anastomoses. One twin may become anemic and the other plethoric.

paracentesis /per′əsentē′sis/, a procedure in which fluid is withdrawn from a cavity of the body. An incision is made in the skin, and a hollow trocar, cannula, or catheter is passed through the incision into the cavity to allow outflow of fluid into a collecting device. Paracentesis is most commonly performed to remove excessive accumulations of ascitic fluid from the abdomen.

paracervical, pertaining to tissues adjacent to the cervix.

paracervical block, a form of regional anesthesia in which a local anesthetic is injected into the area on each side of the uterine cervix that contains the plexus of nerves innervating the uterine cervix. Effective anesthesia for active labor is often achieved. The duration of the anesthetic effect depends on the agent used. Transient maternal hypotension sometimes occurs after paracervical block, usually caused by inadvertent intravascular injection of the anesthetic.

paracetamol. See **acetaminophen.**

paracoccidioidomycosis /per′əkoksid′ē•oi′dōmīkō′sis/, a chronic, occasionally fatal, fungal infection caused by *Paracoccidioides brasiliensis,* characterized by ulcers of the oral cavity, larynx, and nose. Other effects include large, draining lymph nodes, cough, dyspnea, weight loss, and skin, genital, and intestinal lesions. The disease occurs in Mexico and Central and South America and is acquired by inhalation of spores of the fungus. The diagnosis is made by microscopic examination of a smear prepared from a lesion. Treatment requires several years of sulfonamides or, in severe cases, intravenous amphotericin B followed by oral sulfonamides. Also called **paracoccidioidal granuloma, South American blastomycosis.** Compare **North American blastomycosis.**

paradichlorobenzene poisoning. See **naphthalene poisoning.**

paradidymal, **1.** pertaining to the paradidymis. **2.** beside the testis.

paradidymis /per′ədid′imis/, *pl.* **paradidymides** /per′ədidim′idēz/, a rudimentary structure in the male, situated on the spermatic cord of the epididymis, that consists of vestigial remains of the caudal part of the embryonic mesonephric tubules. A similar vestigial structure, the paroophoron, is found in the female. Also called **organ of Giraldes, parepididymis.** See also **aberrant ductule, appendix epididymis.**

paradigm, a pattern that may serve as a model or example.

Paradione, a trademark for an anticonvulsant (paramethadione).

paradoxic agitation, a period of unexpected excitability that sometimes follows administration of analeptic medications.

paradoxical breathing, a condition in which a part of the lung deflates during inspiration and inflates during expiration. The condition usually is associated with a chest trauma, as an open chest wound or rib cage damage. In such cases, the paradoxical breathing that occurs spontaneously is sometimes called internal paradoxical breathing. External paradoxical breathing may be observed during deep general anesthesia.

paradoxical intention, a logotherapeutic technique that encourages a patient to do what he fears and if possible to exaggerate it to the point of humor. The technique is used in the treatment of phobias.

paradoxical pulse. See **pulsus paradoxus.**

paraffin bath, the application of heat to a specific area of the body through the use of paraffin. The part is quickly immersed in heated liquid wax and then withdrawn so that the wax solidifies to form an insulating layer. The procedure is repeated until the layer is 5 to 10 mm thick, and then the entire area is wrapped in an insulating fabric, as a loose-fitting plastic bag or paper towels. The technique is effective for heating traumatized or inflamed areas, especially the hands, feet, and wrists, and is used primarily for patients with arthritis and rheumatism or any joint condition. Also called **wax bath.**

Paraflex, a trademark for a skeletal muscle relaxant (chlorzoxazone).

parafollicular C cell, a calcitonin-secreting cell located between follicles.

Parafon Forte, a trademark for a fixed-combination drug containing an analgesic-antipyretic (acetaminophen) and a skeletal muscle relaxant (chlorzoxazone), used for the relief of painful musculoskeletal conditions.

paraganglion, *pl.* **paraganglia,** any one of the small groups of chromaffin cells associated with the ganglia of the sympathetic nerve trunk and situated outside the adrenal medulla, most often near the sympathetic ganglia along the aorta and its branches. The paraganglia are also connected with the ganglia of the celiac, renal, suprarenal, aortic, and hypogastric plexuses. The paraganglia secrete the hormones epinephrine and norepinephrine. Also called **chromaffin body.** See also **chromaffin cell.**

paragonimiasis /per'əgon'imī'əsis/, chronic infection with the lung fluke *Paragonimus westermani,* occurring most commonly in Asia. It is characterized by hemoptysis, bronchitis, and, occasionally, abdominal masses, pain and diarrhea, or cerebral involvement with paralysis, ocular pathologic conditions, or seizures. The disease is acquired by ingesting cysts in infected freshwater crabs or crayfish, the intermediate hosts. Adequate cooking of shellfish prevents the disease. Bithionol given orally is the usual treatment.

parainfluenza virus, a myxovirus with four serotypes, causing respiratory infections in infants and young children and, less commonly, in adults. Types 1 and 2 parainfluenza viruses may cause laryngotracheobronchitis or croup; type 3 is a cause of croup, tracheobronchitis, bronchiolitis, and bronchopneumonia in children; types 1, 3, and 4 are associated with pharyngitis and the common cold. Compare **influenza, rhinovirus..**

Paral, a trademark for a sedative-hypnotic (paraldehyde).

paraldehyde /peral'dəhīd/, a clear, colorless, strong-smelling liquid obtained by the polymerization of acetaldehyde with a small amount of sulfuric acid. Paraldehyde is used as a solvent and may be administered orally, intravenously, intramuscularly, or rectally to induce hypnotic states or sedation.

parallel grid, (in radiography) an x-ray grid that has lead strips oriented parallel to each other.

parallelogram condenser, (in dentistry) an instrument with a face shaped like a rectangle or parallelogram, used for compacting amalgams in filling teeth.

parallel play, a form of play among a group of children, primarily toddlers, in which each one engages in an independent activity that is similar to but not influenced by or shared with the others. Compare **cooperative play.** See also **associative play, solitary play.**

paralysis, *pl.* **paralyses,** an abnormal condition characterized by the loss of muscle function or the loss of sensation, or both. It may be caused by a variety of problems, as trauma, disease, and poisoning. Paralyses may be classified according to cause, muscle tone, distribution, or the part of the body affected. See also **flaccid paralysis, spastic paralysis.** –**paralytic,** *adj.*

paralysis agitans. See **Parkinson's disease.**

-paralytic, a combining form meaning 'pertaining to paralysis': *antiparalytic, aparalytic, subparalytic.*

paralytic dementia. See **paresis,** def. 2.

paralytic ileus, a decrease in or absence of intestinal peristalsis that may occur after abdominal surgery or peritoneal injury or in connection with severe pyelonephritis, ureteral stone, fractured ribs, myocardial infarction, extensive intestinal ulceration, heavy metal poisoning, porphyria, retroperitoneal hematomas, especially those associated with fractured vertebrae, or any severe metabolic disease. The most common overall cause of intestinal obstruction, paralytic ileus is mediated by a hormonal component of the sympathoadrenal system. Also called **adynamic ileus.**

■ OBSERVATIONS: Paralytic ileus is characterized by abdominal tenderness and distention, absence of bowel sounds, lack of flatus, and nausea and vomiting. There may be fever, decreased urinary output, electrolyte imbalance, dehydration, and respiratory distress. The loss of fluids and electrolytes may be extreme, and, unless they are replaced, the condition may lead to hemoconcentration, hypovolemia, renal insufficiency, shock, and death.

■ INTERVENTION: The patient is kept in bed in a low Fowler's position, and nothing is given by mouth. An intestinal tube is inserted as a nasogastric tube into the duodenum and connected to intermittent suction; it is not taped to the nose, and the patient is positioned to facilitate the advancement of the tube, which is checked every 30 to 60 minutes. The character of GI drainage is monitored every 2 to 4 hours, and any increase or decrease in the amount or changes in the color or consistency is reported. Bowel sounds, blood pressure, pulse, and respirations are checked every 2 to 4 hours and rectal temperature every 4 hours. Abdominal girth is measured every 2 hours, and report is made of any increase. Parenteral fluids with electrolytes and medication to promote peristalsis are administered as ordered; intake and output are measured, and if less than 30 ml of urine is excreted per hour, the physician is informed. The patient is helped to turn and deep breathe every 2 to 4 hours and is given oral hygiene every 1 to 2 hours. Active or passive range of motion exercises are performed every 4 hours. When intestinal output increases and bowel sounds return, the intestinal tube may be clamped and small amounts of warm tea or a carbonated beverage may be given. If pain, distention, or cramps do not recur, the intestinal tube may be removed, but a rectal tube or an enema may be ordered to relieve distention.

■ NURSING CONSIDERATIONS: The concerns of the nurse include monitoring and reporting the signs of paralytic ileus and its potential complications, ensuring that the patient is as comfortable as possible, and explaining to the patient the purpose of the intestinal tube. The nurse instructs the patient to avoid mouth breathing, because swallowed air can increase distention.

paralytic shellfish poisoning. See **shellfish poisoning.**

paramedic, a person who acts as an assistant to a physician or in place of a physician, especially a person in the military, trained in emergency medical procedures. –**paramedical,** *adj.*

paramedical personnel, health care workers other than physicians, dentists, podiatrists, and nurses who have special training in the performance of supportive health care tasks. Paramedical personnel includes, for example, the **Emergency Medical Technician, audiologists,** and **x-ray technologist.** Also called **allied health personnel.**

paramesonephric duct /per′əmēz′ōnef′rik/, one of a pair of embryonic ducts that develops into the uterus and the uterine tubes. Also called **müllerian duct.**

parameter /pəram′ətər/, **1.** a value or constant used to describe or measure a set of data representing a physiologic function or system, as in the use of acid-base relationships of the blood as parameters for evaluating the function of a patient's respiratory system. **2.** a statistic value of a population group. **3.** *informal.* limits or boundary.

paramethadione /per′əmeth′ədī′ōn/, an anticonvulsant.

■ INDICATION: It is prescribed for the prevention of seizures in petit mal epilepsy.

■ CONTRAINDICATIONS: Blood dyscrasias, severe renal or hepatic impairment, or known hypersensitivity to this drug prohibits its use.

■ ADVERSE EFFECTS: Among the more serious adverse reactions are exfoliative dermatitis, blood dyscrasias, and hepatitis. Sedation, hemerolopia, and moderate neutropenia may occur.

paramethasone acetate, a glucocorticoid.

■ INDICATIONS: It is prescribed in the treatment of inflammatory and allergic conditions.

■ CONTRAINDICATIONS: Systemic fungal infections or known hypersensitivity to this drug prohibits its use.

■ ADVERSE EFFECTS: Among the more serious adverse reactions are GI, endocrine, and neurologic disturbances and fluid and electrolyte imbalance.

parametric imaging, (in nuclear medicine) a diagnostic procedure in which an image of an administered radioactive tracer is derived according to a mathematic rule, as by the division of one image by another.

parametric statistics, statistics that assume a population has a symmetric, as gaussian or log normal, distribution.

parametritis /per′əmetrī′tis/, an inflammatory condition of the tissue of the structures around the uterus. See also **pelvic inflammatory disease.**

parametrium /per′əmē′trē·əm/, *pl.* **parametria,** the lateral extension of the uterine subserous connective tissue into the broad ligament. Compare **endometrium, myometrium.**

paramitome. See **hyaloplasm.**

paramnesia /per′amnē′zhə/, **1.** a perversion of memory in which one believes one remembers events and circumstances that never actually occurred. **2.** a condition in which words are remembered and used without the comprehension of their meaning. Compare **déjà vu.**

paramyxovirus, a member of a family of viruses that includes the organisms that cause parainfluenza, mumps, and some respiratory infections.

paranasal, situated near or alongside the nose, as the paranasal sinuses.

paranasal sinus, one of the air cavities in various bones around the nose, as the frontal sinus in the frontal bone lying deep to the medial part of the superciliary ridge and the maxillary sinus within the maxilla between the orbit, the nasal cavity, and the upper teeth. Compare **confluence of the sinuses, occipital sinus.**

parangi. See **yaws.**

paranoia /per′ənoi′ə/, (in psychiatry) a disorder characterized by an elaborate system of thinking with delusions of persecution and grandeur usually centered on one major theme, as a financial matter, a job situation, an unfaithful spouse, or other problem. The delusional system typically develops slowly and progressively over a period of months or years, becoming intricate, logical, and highly organized, with the result that it can be most convincing. The person appears perfectly normal in conduct, conversation, thinking patterns, and emotional responses aside from the delusions. Associated symptoms include suspiciousness, seclusion, stubbornness, resentfulness, aloofness, hostility, aggressiveness, dominating or grandiose attitudes, and unrealistic expectations. Causal factors are predominantly psychosocial in nature, as inadequate socialization during childhood, poor development of interpersonal relationships, and sexual maladjustment, and do not involve genetic or biochemical alterations. Persons with the disorder are highly resistant to available methods of treatment, although individual or group psychotherapy and behavior therapy may be effective in the early stages. Kinds of paranoia include **acute hallucinatory paranoia, alcoholic paranoia, litigious paranoia,** and **querulous paranoia.** Also called **paranoea** /per′ənē′ə/. Compare **paranoid schizophrenia.**

paranoiac /per′ənoi′ak/, **1.** a person afflicted with or exhibiting characteristics of paranoia. **2.** of or pertaining to paranoia. Also called **paranoeac.**

paranoia hallucinatoria. See **acute hallucinatory paranoia.**

paranoia quaerula. See **querulous paranoia.**

paranoid /per′ənoid/, **1.** pertaining to or resembling paranoia. **2.** a person afflicted with a paranoid disorder. **3.** *informal.* a person, or pertaining to a person, who is overly suspicious or exhibits persecutory trends or attitudes.

paranoid disorder, any of a large group of mental disorders characterized by an impaired sense of reality and persistent delusions. Kinds of paranoid disorders include **acute paranoid disorder, paranoia,** and **shared paranoid disorder.**

paranoid ideation, an exaggerated, sometimes grandiose, belief or suspicion, usually not of a delusional nature, that one is being harassed, persecuted, or treated unfairly.

paranoid personality, a personality characterized by paranoia.

paranoid personality disorder, a disorder characterized by extreme suspiciousness and distrust of others to the degree that one blames them for one's mistakes and failures and goes to abnormal lengths to validate prejudices, attitudes, or biases. Symptoms include hypersensitivity, rigidity, hostility, stubbornness, envy, exaggerated self-importance, extreme argumentativeness, tenseness, and lack of passive, sentimental, or tender feelings. The condition is more commonly diagnosed in men than in women. The disorganization of the personality in this condition is less severe than in paranoid schizophrenia.

paranoid reaction, a psychopathologic condition associated with aging and characterized by the gradual formation of delusions, usually of a persecutory nature and often accompanied by related hallucinations. Other manifestations of senile degeneration, as memory loss and confusion, do not usually accompany the reaction, and the individual maintains orientation for time, place, and person.

paranoid schizophrenia, a form of schizophrenia characterized by persistent preoccupation with illogical, absurd, and changeable delusions, usually of a persecutory, grandiose, or jealous nature, accompanied by related hallucinations. The symptoms include extreme anxiety, exaggerated suspiciousness, aggressiveness, anger, argumentativeness, hostility, and violence. The condition occurs most frequently during middle age. Current therapy is not usually effective. Also called **heboid paranoia.** Compare **paranoia.** See also **schizophrenia.**

paranoid state, a transitory abnormal mental condition characterized by illogical thought processes and generalized suspicion and distrust, with a tendency toward persecutory ideas or delusions.

paranuclear body. See **centrosome.**

parapertussis /per′əpərtus′is/, an acute bacterial respiratory infection caused by *Bordetella parapertussis,* having symptoms closely resembling those of pertussis. It is usually milder than pertussis, although it can be fatal. It is possible to be infected with both *B. parapertussis* and *B. pertussis* at the same time. A parapertussis vaccine is ailable and may be given in combination with pertussis ine.

haryngeal abscess /per′əfərin′jē·əl/, a suppura- ction of tissues adjacent to the pharynx, usually a ion of acute pharyngitis or tonsillitis. Infection to the jugular vein where it may cause throm- d septic emboli. Systemic antibiotics and surgical drainage may be required. Also called **parapharyngeal space abscess.** Compare **peritonsillar abscess, retropharyngeal abscess.** See also **tonsillitis.**

paraphilia /per′əfil′ē·ə/, sexual perversion or deviation; a condition in which the sexual instinct is expressed in ways that are socially prohibited or unacceptable or are biologically undesirable, as the use of an inanimate object for sexual arousal, sexual activity with another person that involves real or simulated suffering or humiliation, or sexual relations with a nonconsenting partner. Kinds of paraphilia include **exhibitionism, fetishism, pedophilia, transvestism, voyeurism,** and **zoophilia.** **–paraphiliac,** *adj., n.*

paraphimosis /per′əfīmō′sis/, a condition characterized by an inability to replace the foreskin in its normal position after it has been retracted behind the glans penis. Caused by a narrow or inflamed foreskin, the condition may lead to gangrene. Circumcision may be required. Compare **phimosis.**

paraplasm, any abnormal growth or malformation. Compare **hyaloplasm.** **–paraplasmic,** *adj.*

paraplastic, **1.** misshapen or malformed. **2.** showing abnormal formative power; of the nature of a paraplasm.

paraplegia /per′əplē′jē·ə/, an abnormal condition characterized by motor or sensory loss in the lower limbs. This condition may or may not involve the back and abdominal muscles and may cause either complete or incomplete paralysis. The incidence of this disorder in men is double that in women and is highest between 16 and 35 years of age. About 50% of approximately 11,000 spinal cord injuries reported each year in the United States involve paraplegia. Such injuries commonly occur as the result of automobile and motorcycle accidents, sporting accidents, falls, and gunshot wounds. Paraplegia less commonly results from nontraumatic lesions, as scoliosis, spina bifida, and alcoholism. Compare **hemiplegia, quadriplegia.** **–paraplegic,** *adj., n.*

■ OBSERVATIONS: The signs and symptoms of paraplegia may develop immediately from trauma and include the loss of sensation, motion, and reflexes below the level of the lesion. Depending on the level of the lesion and whether damage to the spinal cord is complete or incomplete, the patient may lose bladder and bowel control and develop sexual dysfunctions. An incomplete spinal cord injury does not usually inhibit circumanal sensation, voluntary toe flexion, or sphincter control. A complete spinal cord injury destroys sensation and voluntary muscle control and usually causes the permanent loss of muscle function distal to the injury. Diagnosis is based on clinical history, neurologic examination, and x-ray examinations. Various laboratory tests are performed, as a complete blood count, prothrombin time, electrolyte evaluation, and urinalysis.

■ INTERVENTION: The treatment of paraplegia seeks to restore proper spine alignment, stabilize the injured spinal area, decompress any involved neurologic structures, and rehabilitate the patient as quickly as possible. At the accident scene, when spinal cord injury is suspected, the patient must not be moved until strapped and stabilized on a board. Such stabilization helps to prevent permanent damage to any injured spinal structures. A Foley catheter is commonly inserted to ensure uninterrupted urine drainage. Treatment may also include the administration of drugs, as nitrofurantoin to prevent bladder infection and vitamin C to minimize infection by acidifying the urine. A laminectomy may be performed if bone fragments are pressing on the spinal cord. Drugs, as baclofen, may be administered to relieve any muscle spasms associated with dysfunction of the upper motor neurons.

■ NURSING CONSIDERATIONS: Nursing care in paraplegic cases commonly includes the proper positioning and maintenance of the patient on a Stryker frame or a Circolectric bed, proper wound care after a laminectomy, catheter and skin care, and meticulous monitoring of intake and output. When the paraplegic patient progresses from bed rest to a wheelchair, the nurse is alert to any signs of orthostatic hypotension. Special binders and antiembolism hose are used to help the patient adjust to the transition from bed to wheelchair. Other treatment may include the administration of a high-bulk diet and suppositories to prevent constipation. The patient and family benefit from counseling and encouragement during the rehabilitation period, especially if the patient develops psychologic problems associated with the difficult adjustment to paraplegia. Accurate assessment of paralysis is often not possible until 1 year after the injury.

parapsoriasis /per'əsərī'əsis/, a group of chronic skin diseases resembling psoriasis, characterized by maculopapular, erythematous, scaly eruptions without systemic symptoms. Parapsoriasis is resistant to all treatment.

parapsychology, a branch of psychology concerned with the study of alleged psychic phenomena, as clairvoyance, extrasensory perception, and telepathy.

paraquat poisoning /per'əkwot'/, a toxic condition caused by the ingestion of paraquat dichloride, a highly poisonous pesticide. Characteristically, progressive pulmonary fibrosis and damage to the esophagus, kidneys, and liver develop several days after ingestion. Once fibrosis begins, death is inevitable, usually within 3 weeks. The mechanism of action of the poison is unknown. Most often, poisoning results from accidental occupational exposure. There is considerable concern that the inhalation of the smoke of marijuana treated with the herbicide may cause intoxication, but no clinical syndrome resulting from such exposure has been documented.

parasite, **1.** an organism living in or on and obtaining nourishment from another organism. A **facultative parasite** may live on a host but is capable of living independently. An **obligate parasite** is one that depends entirely on its host for survival. **2.** See **parasitic fetus.** –**parasitic,** *adj.*

parasitemia /per'əsītē'mē·ə/, the presence of parasites in the blood. Compare **bacteremia, fungemia, viremia.**

parasitic fetus, the smaller, usually malformed member of conjoined, unequal, or asymmetrical twins that is attached to and dependent on the more normal fetus for growth and development. Compare **autosite.**

parasitic fibroma, a pedunculated uterine fibroid deriving part of its blood supply from the omentum.

parasitic glossitis, a mycosis of the tongue, characterized by a black or brown furry patch on the posterior dorsal surface composed of hypertrophied filiform papillae that measure about 1 cm in length and are easily broken. The condition, caused by *Cryptococcus linguaepilosasae* in symbiosis with *Nocardia lingualis,* produces no discomfort and may be treated with a simple mouthwash. The patch may disappear spontaneously and later reappear. Also called **anthracosis linguae, black hairy tongue, black tongue, glossitis parasitica, glossophytia, keratomycosis linguae, lingua villosa nigra, melanotrichia linguae, nigrities linguae.**

parasitic thrombus, an aggregation of bodies and spores of malarial parasites formed in the vessels of the brain in cerebral malaria.

parasympathetic, of or pertaining to the craniosacral division of the autonomic nervous system, consisting of the oculomotor, facial, glossopharyngeal, vagus, and pelvic nerves. The actions of the parasympathetic division are mediated by the release of acetylcholine and primarily involve the protection, conservation, and restoration of body resources. Preganglionic parasympathetic fibers, which emerge from the hypothalamus, other brain areas, and sacral segments of the spinal cord, form synapses in ganglia located near or in the walls of the organs to be innervated. Reactions to parasympathetic stimulation are highly localized and tend to counteract the adrenergic effects of sympathetic nerves. Parasympathetic fibers slow the heart, stimulate peristalsis, promote the secretion of lacrimal, salivary, and digestive glands, induce bile and insulin release, dilate peripheral and visceral blood vessels, constrict the pupils, esophagus, and bronchioles, and relax sphincters during micturition and defecation. Postganglionic parasympathetic fibers extend to the uterus, vagina, oviducts, and ovaries in females and to the prostate, seminal vesicles, and external genitalia in males, innervating blood vessels of pelvic organs in both sexes; stimulation of these nerves causes vasodilation in the clitoris and labia minora and erection of the penis.

parasympathetic nervous system. See **autonomic nervous system.**

parasympatholytic, parasympatholytic drug. See **anticholinergic.**

parasympathomimetic /per'əsim'pəthōmimet'ik/, **1.** of or pertaining to a substance producing effects similar to those caused by stimulation of a parasympathetic nerve. **2.** an agent whose effects mimic those resulting from stimulation of parasympathetic nerves, especially the effects produced by acetylcholine. The parasympathomimetic drugs include bethanechol chloride, neostigmine bromide, neostigmine methylsulfate, and pyridostigmine bromide, variously used to treat myasthenia gravis and acute postoperative and postpartum nonobstructional urinary retention and to reverse or antagonize the action of nondepolarizing muscle relaxants. Also called **cholinergic.**

parasympathomimetic drug. See **cholinergic.**

parasystole, an independent ectopic rhythm whose pacemaker cannot be discharged by impulses of the dominant, usually sinus, rhythm because of an area of depressed conduction surrounding the parasystolic focus. In the classic parasystole, the interectopic intervals are exact multiples of a common denominator reflecting the protected status of the parasystolic focus. However, more often than not, the ectopic focus is influenced by the phasic events around its protection zone. Thus, the sinus rhythm may modulate the parasystolic response so that criteria for absolute, undisturbed regularity are not fulfilled. Fusion beats are commonly seen because of the simultaneous discharge of the ventricles by both the sinus impulse and the parasystolic focus.

parataxic distortion /per′ətak′sik/, a defense mechanism in which current interpersonal relationships are perceived and judged according to a mode of reference established by an earlier experience. See also **transference.**

parataxic mode, a term introduced by H.S. Sullivan to identify a childhood perception of the physical and social environment as being illogical, disjointed, and inconsistent. The parataxic mode may persist into adulthood in some individuals.

parathion poisoning /per′əthī′on/, a toxic condition caused by the ingestion, inhalation, or absorption through the skin of the highly toxic organophosphorus insecticide parathion. Symptoms include nausea, vomiting, abdominal cramps, confusion, headache, lack of muscular control, convulsions, and dyspnea. Treatment calls for close observation and for immediate intravenous administration of atropine, followed by pralidoxime chloride and oxygen.

parathyroid gland, one of several small structures, usually four in number, attached to the dorsal surfaces of the lateral lobes of the thyroid gland. The parathyroid glands secrete parathyroid hormone, which helps maintain the level of blood calcium concentration and ensures normal neuromuscular irritability, blood clotting, and cell membrane permeability. Each parathyroid gland has the appearance of an oval, brownish-red disk and measures about 6 by 4 mm. The parathyroids are divided, according to their location, into the superior parathyroids and the inferior parathyroids. The superior parathyroids, usually two in number, are commonly situated, one on each side, on the caudal border of the cricoid cartilage beside the junction of the pharynx and the esophagus. The inferior parathyroids, also usually two in number, may be situated on the caudal edge of the lateral lobes of the thyroid gland, just caudal to the gland, or adjacent to one of the inferior thyroid veins. These glands are composed of intercommunicating columns of cells bound by connective tissue with a rich supply of capillaries. Parathyroid hypofunction usually causes tetany, which can be treated by the administration of calcium salts or parathyroid extracts.

parathyroid hormone (PH), a hormone secreted by the parathyroid glands that acts to maintain a constant concentration of calcium in the extracellular fluid. The hormone regulates absorption of calcium from the GI tract, mobilization of calcium from the bones, deposition of calcium in the bones, and excretion of calcium in the breast milk, feces, sweat, and urine. Surgical removal of the parathyroid glands, as may inadvertently occur in thyroidectomy, results in hypocalcemia, leading to anorexia, tetany, seizures, and death if not corrected. See also **hypoparathyroidism.**

parathyroid injection, bovine parathyroid hormone.

■ INDICATION: It is prescribed to regulate blood levels of calcium, especially in the treatment of hypoparathyroidism with tetany.

■ CONTRAINDICATIONS: Hypercalcemia, tetany not caused by hypoparathyroidism, hypercalciuria, or known hypersensitivity to this drug prohibits its use.

■ ADVERSE EFFECTS: Among the most serious adverse reactions are hypercalcemia and allergic reactions.

paratrooper fracture, a fracture of the distal tibia and its malleolus, commonly occurring when an individual jumps from an elevated platform, as the back of a truck, or parachutes from an airplane and lands feet first on the ground, subjecting the ankles to extreme force.

paratyphoid fever, a bacterial infection, caused by any *Salmonella* species other than *S. typhi,* characterized by symptoms resembling typhoid fever, although somewhat milder. See also **rose spots, *Salmonella,* salmonellosis, typhoid fever.**

paraurethral duct, one of two ducts that drain the bulbourethral glands into the vestibule of the vagina. Also called **Skene's duct.**

paravaccinia. See **milker's nodule.**

Paredrine, a trademark for an adrenergic (hydroxyamphetamine hydrobromide).

paregoric, a camphorated tincture of opium.

■ INDICATIONS: It is prescribed in the treatment of diarrhea and as an analgesic.

■ CONTRAINDICATIONS: Known hypersensitivity to this drug or to any opium derivative prohibits its use. It should not be used when diarrhea is caused by a toxic substance.

■ ADVERSE EFFECTS: There are usually no adverse reactions. Occasionally, GI disturbances, including constipation, occur.

parenchyma /pəreng′kimə/, the tissue of an organ as distinguished from supporting or connective tissue.

parenchymal cell, any cell that is a functional element of an organ, as a heptocyte.

parenchymatous neuritis /per'əngkim'ətəs/, any inflammation affecting the substance, axons, or myelin of the nerve. Also called **axial neuritis, central neuritis.** See also **neuritis.**

parent, a mother or father; one who bears offspring. –**parental,** *adj.*

parental generation (P_1), the initial cross between two varieties in a genetic sequence; the parents of any individual, organism, or plant belonging to an F_1 generation.

parental grief, the behavioral reactions that characterize the grieving process and result in the resolution of the loss of a child from expected or unexpected death. All persons who survive the loss of a loved one normally experience symptoms of both somatic and psychologic distress, as feelings of guilt and hostility accompanied by changes in usual patterns of conduct, depending on the individual's response to the awareness of the loss. When the death of a child is expected from terminal illness, there is time for anticipatory grieving, so that parents can evaluate their relationship with the child, set priorities for the duration of time involved, and prepare for the actual death of the child. In such cases, parental grieving begins with the discovery of the diagnosis of a life-threatening condition. Parents' adjustment to the diagnosis involves a complete cycle of reactions that extends over an indefinite period of time, depending on the severity and nature of the disease. The immediate reaction is shock and disbelief, followed by acute grief at the anticipation of losing the child. Periods of depression, anger, hope, fear, and anxiety alternate during induction therapy, remission, and maintenance of the disease as parents learn to accept and cope with the situation. Heightened anticipatory grieving recurs during episodes of relapse, and the parents experience increased fear, depression, and the final acceptance of death during the terminal stages of the illness. Although families can prepare themselves for the expected loss, at the time of death there is a period of acute grief, during which parents need to express their deep sorrow and anger. An extended phase of mourning follows, with the eventual resolution of grief and integration into society. In sudden, unexpected death, parents are denied the advantages of anticipatory grief and, because of the lack of time to prepare, usually have extreme feelings of guilt and remorse. The nurse can especially help such parents to assess their feelings so that they can work through them and progress through the resolution of grief and the mourning process, which in unexpected death takes a much longer period of time. The function of the nurse during all phases of parental grief is primarily supportive, and the degree of intervention depends on the family's strengths and weaknesses in coping with the crisis. Nurses can act directly, or they can help to find other potential sources of support for the parents, as extended family members, other parents who have lost children, or specific community services or agencies. A large part of the nursing support involves helping families explore new ways of coping, not only to meet the present crisis but to grow and change. Always an important nursing consideration is the education of the parents about all aspects of the child's illness, especially in terminal conditions. See also **death, grief reaction.**

parent-child relationship. See **maternal-infant bonding.**

parenteral /pəren'tərəl/, not in or through the digestive system. –**parenterally,** *adv.*

parenteral absorption, the taking up of substances within the body by structures other than the digestive tract.

parenteral dosage, pertaining to a medication administered by a route that bypasses the GI tract, as a drug given by injection.

parenteral fluids. See **administration of parenteral fluids.**

parenteral hyperalimentation. See **total parenteral nutrition.**

parenteral nutrition, the administration of nutrients by a route other than through the alimentary canal, as subcutaneously, intravenously, intramuscularly, or intradermally. The parenteral fluids usually consist of physiologic saline with glucose, amino acids, electrolytes, vitamins, and medications. They are not nutritionally complete but maintain fluid and electrolyte balance during the immediate postoperative period and in other conditions, as shock, coma, malnutrition, and chronic renal and hepatic failures. See also **total parenteral nutrition.**

parent figure, **1.** a parent or a substitute parent or guardian who cares for a child, providing the physical, social, and emotional requirements necessary for normal growth and development. **2.** a person who symbolically represents an ideal parent, having those attributes that one conceptualizes as necessary for forming the perfect parent-child relationship.

parent image, a conscious and unconscious concept that a child forms concerning the roles and characteristics of the personality of the mother and father. See also **imago, primordial image.**

parenting, alteration in: actual or potential, a nursing diagnosis accepted by the Fourth National Conference on the Classification of Nursing Diagnoses. This diagnosis includes any maladjustment or marked potential for maladjustment of a mother or father to the role of parent. The cause of the problem may be complex and may involve several factors, as lack of an available role model, lack of support, interruption of the process of bonding in the newborn period, unrealistic expectations for the self, the infant, or the partner, mental or physical illness, the presence of financial, legal, or cultural stressors, a lack of knowledge, limited cognitive ability, multiple pregnancies, or a death in the family concurrent with the birth or early infancy of the new baby. The defining characteristics of the condition are also multiple and may include constant complaints about the sex or the appearance of the new child; verbal self-assessment of inadequacy in the parental role; expressed disgust about the bodily functions of the child; failure to keep health care appointments for the child; inconsistent disciplinary practices; slow growth and development in the child; and an observed need on the part of the parent to receive approval from others. The critical defining characteristics, at least one of which must be present to make the diagnosis, include an observed lack of actions that demonstrate attachment to the child, inattentiveness to the needs of the child, inappropriate caretaking behavior, especially in toilet training and in sleep and feeding patterns, and a history of abuse or abandonment of the child. See also **nursing diagnosis.**

Parents Anonymous, a self-help group for parents who have abused their children or who feel that they are prone to maltreat them. The organization offers support and guidance, provides a forum for discussing mutual problems, and furnishes distressed parents with a positive mechanism for coping with anger by talking to another member rather than by releasing their emotions on the child. See also **child abuse.**

parepididymis. See **paradidymis.**

paresis /pərē′sis, per′isis/, **1.** partial paralysis related in some cases to local neuritis. **2.** also called **dementia paralytica, general paresis, paralytic dementia.** a late manifestation of neurosyphilis, characterized by generalized paralysis, tremulous incoordination, transient seizures, Argyll Robertson pupils, and progressive dementia caused by degeneration of cortical neurons. Paresis resulting from untreated syphilis usually develops in the third to fifth decades but may occur at an early age in patients with congenital syphilis. **–paretic,** *adj.*

Parest, a trademark for a sedative-hypnotic (methaqualone hydrochloride).

paresthesia, any subjective sensation, experienced as numbness, tingling, or a "pins and needles" feeling. Paresthesias often fluctuate according to such influences as posture, activity, rest, edema, congestion, or an underlying disease. When experienced in the extremities, it is sometimes identified as acroparesthesia.

paretic dementia. See **paresis.**

pareunia. See **coitus.**

pargyline hydrochloride /per′jəlēn/, a monoamine oxidase (MAO) inhibitor used as an antihypertensive.

■ INDICATION: It is prescribed in the treatment of moderate to severe hypertension.

■ CONTRAINDICATIONS: As with all MAO inhibitors, pheochromocytoma, malignant hypertension, hyperthyroidism, renal failure, concomitant use of sympathomimetic drugs, foods high in tyramine, alcoholic beverages, or hypersensitivity to this drug prohibits its use. It is not given to children under 12 years of age.

■ ADVERSE EFFECTS: Among the most serious adverse reactions are hepatotoxicity, orthostatic hypotension, hyperexcitability, constipation, and dry mouth. MAO inhibitors produce many adverse drug interactions.

paries /pā′ri•ēz/, *pl.* **parietes** /pərī′itēz/, the wall of an organ or cavity in the body.

parietal /pərī′ətəl/, **1.** of or pertaining to the outer wall of a cavity or organ. **2.** of or pertaining to the parietal bone of the skull, or the parietal lobe of the brain.

parietal bone, one of a pair of bones that form the sides of the cranium. Each parietal bone has two surfaces, four borders, and four angles and articulates with five bones: the opposite parietal, occipital, frontal, temporal, and sphenoid.

parietal lobe, a portion of each cerebral hemisphere that occupies the parts of the lateral and the medial surfaces that are covered by the parietal bone. On the lateral surface of the hemisphere the parietal lobe is separated from the frontal lobe by the central sulcus and from the temporal lobe by an imaginary line that extends from the posterior ramus of the lateral sulcus toward the occipital pole. On the parietal lobe the postcentral sulcus runs parallel with the central sulcus, so that the postcentral gyrus lies between them. The intraparietal sulcus extends posteriorly from the middle of the postcentral sulcus toward the occipital pole and joins the transverse occipital sulcus near the occipital pole. The part of the parietal lobe posterior to the postcentral sulcus is divided by the horizontal intraparietal sulcus into the superior and the inferior parietal lobules. On the medial surface of the hemisphere the parietooccipital sulcus separates the parietal and the occipital lobes. Compare **central lobe, frontal lobe, occipital lobe, temporal lobe.**

parietal lymph node, one of the small oval glands that filter the lymph coursing through the lymphatic vessels in the walls of the thorax or through the lymphatic vessels associated with the larger blood vessels of the abdomen and the pelvis. The parietal lymph nodes of the thorax include the sternal nodes, intercostal nodes, and diaphragmatic nodes. The parietal lymph nodes of the abdomen and pelvis include the common iliac nodes, epigastric nodes, external iliac nodes, iliac circumflex nodes, internal iliac nodes, lumbar nodes, and sacral nodes. See also **lymph, lymphatic system, lymph node.**

parietal pain, a sharp sensation of distress in the parietal pleura, aggravated by respiration and thoracic movements and caused by pneumonia, empyema, pneumothorax, asbestosis, tuberculosis, neoplasm, or the accumulation of fluid resulting from heart, liver, or kidney disease. Noxious stimuli do not cause pain in the visceral pleura. Pain arising from the parietal pleura lining the chest wall is perceived over the involved area, but that arising from the central part of the diaphragm is referred to the posterior shoulder area; pain from the costal portions of the diaphragm is referred to the adjacent thoracic wall.

parietal peritoneum, the portion of the largest serous membrane in the body that lines the abdominal wall. Also called **parietal pleura.** Compare **visceral peritoneum.** See also **peritoneal cavity.**

parietal pleura. See **parietal peritoneum.**

parietooccipital, of or pertaining to the parietal and the occipital bones or lobes.

parietooccipital sulcus, a groove on each cerebral hemisphere marking the division of the parietal and occipital lobes of the brain. Also called **occipitoparietal fissure.**

Parinaud's syndrome /per′ənōz/, a term often used to refer to conjunctivitis that is usually unilateral, follicular, and followed by enlargement of the preauricular lymph nodes and tenderness. The syndrome is frequently caused by infection with a species of the microorganism *Leptothrix*. It may also be associated with other infections, as tularemia, cat-scratch fever, and lymphogranuloma venereum. Also called **Parinaud's oculoglandular syndrome, Parinaud's opthalmoplegia.**

parity, **1.** (in obstetrics) the classification of a woman by the number of live-born children and stillbirths she has delivered at more than 28 weeks of gestation. Commonly, parity is noted with the total number of pregnancies and represented by the letter "P" or the word "para." A para 4 (P4) gravida 5 (G5) has had four deliveries after 28 weeks and one abortion or miscarriage before 28 weeks. Currently, a more complete system is in use in which the total number of pregnancies is followed by the number of deliveries at term, the number of premature infants, the number of abortions or miscarriages before 28 weeks' gestation, and the number of children living at present. This system may be written as TPAL. **2.** (in epidemiology) the classification of a woman by the number of live-born children she has delivered. **3.** (in computer processing) the condition of a set of items, either even or odd in number, used as a means for checking errors, as in the transmission of information between various elements of the same computer.

parkinsonism, a neurologic disorder characterized by tremor, muscle rigidity, hypokinesia, a slow shuffling gait, difficulty in chewing, swallowing, and speaking, caused by various lesions in the extrapyramidal motor system. Signs and symptoms of parkinsonism resemble those of idiopathic Parkinson's disease and may develop during or after acute encephalitis and in syphilis, malaria, poliomyelitis, and carbon monoxide poisoning. Parkinsonism frequently occurs in patients treated with antipsychotic drugs, as amitriptyline, chlorpromazine, fluphenazine, loxapine, thioridazine, and other phenothiazine derivatives. See also **Parkinson's disease.**

Parkinson's disease, a slowly progressive, degenerative, neurologic disorder characterized by resting tremor, pill rolling of the fingers, a masklike facies, shuffling gait, forward flexion of the trunk, and muscle rigidity and weakness. It is usually an idiopathic disease of persons over 60 years of age, though it may occur in younger persons, especially after acute encephalitis or carbon monoxide or metallic poisoning, particularly by reserpine or phenothiazine drugs. Typical pathologic changes are destruction of neurons in basal ganglia, loss of pigmented cells in the substantia nigra, and depletion of dopamine in the caudate nucleus, putamen, and pallidum, structures in the neostriatum that normally contain high levels of the neurotransmitter dopamine. Signs and symptoms of Parkinson's disease, which include drooling, increased appetite, intolerance to heat, oily skin, emotional instability, and defective judgment, are increased by fatigue, excitement, and frustration. Intelligence is rarely impaired. Palliative and symptomatic treatment of the disease focuses on correcting the imbalance between depleted dopamine and abundant acetylcholine in the striatum, because dopamine normally appears to inhibit excitatory cholinergic activity in this brain area. Levodopa, a dopamine precursor that crosses the blood-brain barrier, may be used, but many patients experience side effects, as nausea, vomiting, insomnia, orthostatic hypotension, and mental confusion. Carbidopa-levodopa, which contains an inhibitor of the enzyme dopa decarboxylase, limits peripheral metabolism of levodopa and thus causes fewer side effects. Anticholinergic drugs, as benztropine mesylate, biperiden, procyclidine, and trihexyphenidyl, may be used as therapeutic agents but often cause ataxia, blurred vision, constipation, dryness of the mouth, mental disturbances, slurred speech, and urinary urgency or retention. Amantadine hydrochloride, an antiviral drug with antiparkinsonian activity, promotes the accumulation of dopamine in extracellular or synaptic sites, but the therapeutic effectiveness may not last more than 3 months in some patients; side effects, as mental confusion, visual disturbances, and seizures, occur infrequently. Patients with the disease are encouraged to continue to work and remain active as long as possible and to prevent the spine from bending forward by lying prone on a firm mattress and by walking with the hands folded behind the back. Hand tremor is less apparent if the patient grasps the arms of the chair when seated. Some patients may be treated by surgical procedures in which cautery, excision, or the injection of alcohol or liquid nitrogen is used to destroy portions of the globus pallidus to relieve rigidity or of the thalamus to alleviate tremor. Also called **paralysis agitans.**

Parlodel, a trademark for a dopamine receptor agonist (bromocriptine).

Parnate, a trademark for an antidepressant (tranylcypromine sulfate).

paromomycin sulfate /per′əmōmī′sin/, an oral antiamebic aminoglycoside antibiotic.

■ INDICATION: It is prescribed in the treatment of intestinal amebiasis.

■ CONTRAINDICATIONS: Intestinal inflammation, intestinal obstruction, or known hypersensitivity to this drug prohibits its use.

■ ADVERSE EFFECTS: Among the most serious reactions are GI distress and diarrhea.

paronychia /per′ənik′ē·ə/, an infection of the fold of skin at the margin of a nail. Treatment includes hot compresses or soaks, antibiotics, and, possibly, surgical incision and drainage. Compare **onychia.**

paroophoritis /per′ō·of′ərī′tis/, **1.** inflammation of the paroophoron. **2.** inflammation of the tissues surrounding the ovary.

paroophoron /per′ō-of′əron/, a small vestigial remnant of the mesonephros, consisting of a few rudimentary tubules lying in the broad ligament between the epoophoron and the uterus. It is most evident in very young girls. A similar vestigial structure, the aberrant ductule, is found in the male. Compare **epoophoron.**

parosmia /pəroz′mē-ə/, any dysfunction or perversion concerning the sense of smell. See also **anosmia, cacosmia.**

parotid duct /pərot′id/, a tubular canal, about 7 cm long, that extends from the anterior part of the parotid gland to the mouth. It crosses the masseter after leaving the parotid gland, pierces the buccinator, runs for a short distance obliquely forward between the buccinator and the mucous membrane of the mouth, and opens on the oral surface of the cheek through a small opening opposite the second upper molar tooth. As the parotid duct crosses the masseter, it receives the duct from the accessory portion of the parotid gland. The duct, which has a thick wall, is about 4 mm in diameter over most of its length but narrows considerably at the opening into the mouth. Also called **Stensen's duct.** See also **parotid gland.**

parotid gland, one of the largest pair of salivary glands that lie at the side of the face just below and in front of the external ear. The main part of the gland is superficial, somewhat flattened and quadrilateral, and lies between the ramus of the mandible, the mastoid process, and the sternocleidomastoideus. It is wide superiorly and reaches nearly to the zygomatic arch, inferiorly tapering near the angle of the mandible. The rest of the gland is wedge-shaped and extends deeply toward the pharyngeal wall. It is enclosed in a capsule continuous with the deep cervical fascia. The parotid duct starts at the anterior part of the gland and opens on the inside of the cheek opposite the second upper molar. Compare **sublingual gland, submandibular gland.** See also **salivary gland.**

parotitis /per′ətī′tis/, inflammation or infection of one or both parotid salivary glands. See also **mumps.**

-parous, a combining form meaning 'pertaining to the quantity of offspring produced simultaneously or to the method of gestation': *quadriparous, uniparous, viviparous.*

parovarian, pertaining to residual tissues in the area near the fallopian tubes and the ovary.

parovarium. See **epoophoron.**

paroxysm /per′əksiz′əm/, **1.** a marked, usually episodic increase in symptoms. **2.** a convulsion, fit, seizure, or spasm. –**paroxysmal,** *adj.*

paroxysmal atrial tachycardia, a period of very rapid heart beats that begins suddenly and ends abruptly.

paroxysmal cold hemoglobinuria (PCH), a rare autoimmune disorder characterized by hemolysis and hematuria, associated with exposure to cold.

paroxysmal hemoglobinuria, the sudden passage of hemoglobin in urine, occurring after local or general exposure to low temperatures, as in paroxysmal cold hemoglobinuria. See also **Marchiafava-Micheli disease.**

paroxysmal labyrinthine vertigo. See **Ménière's disease.**

paroxysmal nocturnal dyspnea (PND), a disorder characterized by sudden attacks of respiratory distress, usually occurring after several hours of sleep in a reclining position, most commonly caused by pulmonary edema resulting from congestive heart failure. The attacks are often accompanied by coughing, a feeling of suffocation, cold sweat, and tachycardia with a gallop rhythm. Sleeping with the head propped up on pillows may prevent dyspneic paroxysms at night, but treatment of the underlying cause is required to prevent fluid from accumulating in the lungs.

paroxysmal nocturnal hemoglobinuria (PNH), a disorder characterized by intravascular hemolysis and hemoglobinuria. It occurs in irregular episodes of several days' duration, especially at night. The basic defect in the red blood cell is an unusual sensitivity to lysis by complement or a deficiency or absence of acetylcholinesterase. The cause of the condition is unknown, but it is seen in association with abnormalities of the function of the bone marrow. Occurring predominantly in adults between 25 and 45 years of age, it is characterized by abdominal pain, back pain, and headache. Its course may be complicated by thrombotic episodes and by iron deficiency, caused by excessive loss of hemoglobin. Therapy includes blood transfusion and the oral or parenteral administration of iron. Corticosteroids are sometimes employed and found useful; treatment of thromboses may require anticoagulant therapy.

paroxysmal supraventricular tachycardia, an ectopic rhythm in excess of 100 per minute and usually faster than 170 per minute that begins abruptly with a premature atrial or junctional beat and is supported by an AV nodal reentry mechanism or by an AV reentry mechanism involving an accessory pathway. Formerly called paroxysmal atrial (PAT) or paroxysmal junctional (PJT) tachycardia.

parrot fever. See **psittacosis.**

parry fracture. See **Monteggia's fracture.**

pars /pärs/, a part, as the pars abdominalis esophagi. See also **part.**

Parsidol, a trademark for an antiparkinsonian (ethopropazine hydrochloride).

part, a portion of a larger area, as the condylar part of the occipital bone. See also **pars.**

part-, a combining form meaning 'of or related to childbirth': *parturient, parturifacient, parturiometer.*

parthenogenesis /pär′thənōjen′əsis/, a type of nonsexual reproduction in which an organism develops from an unfertilized ovum, as in many lower animals. Initiation of the development of the unfertilized ovum may be artificially induced through mechanic or chemical stimulation. –**parthenogenetic, parthenogenic,** *adj.*

partial breech extraction. See **assisted breech.**

partial bypass, a system of blood circulation in which the heart pumps and maintains a portion of the blood flow while the remainder of the circulation depends on mechanic means.

partial cleavage, mitotic division of only part of a fertilized ovum into blastomeres, usually the activated cytoplasmic portion surrounding the nucleus; restricted division. Compare **total cleavage.** See also **meroblastic.**

partial crown, a restoration that replaces surfaces of a tooth.

partial hospitalization program, an organizational entity that provides therapeutic services to patients who use only day or night hospital services or adult day health services, rather than regular inpatient hospitalization services.

partially edentulous arch, a dental arch in which one or more but not all natural teeth are missing.

partial placenta previa, placenta previa in which the placenta is implanted in the lower uterine segment and partially covers the internal os of the uterine cervix. As the cervix dilates in labor, the portion of the placenta that lies over the cervix is separated, causing bleeding from the villous spaces of the uterine wall. Depending on the degree of separation, the bleeding may be scant or severe, resulting in hemorrhage that is life threatening to the mother and the baby. Treatment may require cesarean section if the pressure of the presenting part of the baby is not sufficient to tamponade the bleeding site, stopping the hemorrhage. Diagnosis of partial placenta previa may be made before bleeding occurs by ultrasonic visualization or digital palpation in the course of prenatal examination. See also **placenta previa.**

partial pressure, the pressure exerted by any one gas in a mixture of gases or in a liquid, with the pressure directly related to the concentration of that gas to the total pressure of the mixture. The concentration of oxygen in the atmosphere represents approximately 21% of the total atmospheric pressure, calculated at 760 mm Hg under standard conditions. Therefore, the partial pressure of atmospheric oxygen is about 160 mm Hg (760×0.21).

partial pressure of carbon dioxide, the portion of total blood gas pressure exerted by carbon dioxide. It decreases during heavy exercise, rapid breathing, or in association with severe diarrhea, uncontrolled diabetes, or diseases of the liver or kidneys. It increases in persons with chest injuries or respiratory disorders. The normal pressures of carbon dioxide in arterial blood are 35 to 45 mm Hg; in venous blood, 40 to 45 mm Hg.

partial pressure of oxygen, the part of total blood gas pressure exerted by oxygen gas. It is lower than normal in patients with asthma, obstructive lung disease, or certain blood diseases, and in healthy individuals during vigorous exercise. The normal partial pressure of oxygen in arterial blood is 95 to 100 mm Hg.

partial response, the condition in which the maximum decrease in treated tumor volume is at least 50% but less than 100%.

partial thromboplastin time (PTT), a test for detecting coagulation defects of the intrinsic system by adding activated partial thromboplastin to a sample of test plasma and to a control sample of normal plasma. The time required for the formation of a clot in test plasma is compared with that in the normal plasma. A delayed clotting time suggests an abnormality in one or more factors of the intrinsic system. If indicated, specific factor abnormalities can be identified by exposing the test plasma to a series of plasma samples with known factor deficiencies and observing for coagulation, which occurs only if the test plasma provides the missing clotting factors. Partial thromboplastin time is one of the basic tests used to measure specific factor activity and to detect hemophilias. It can also be used to monitor the activity of the anticoagulant, heparin. The normal PTT in plasma is 60 to 85 seconds after the addition to the plasma sample of partial thromboplastin reagent and ionized calcium. Compare **prothrombin time.** See also **hemostasis.**

-partite, a combining form meaning 'having the (specified) number of parts': *bipartite, tripartite, quadripartite.*

parturition /pär′tyo͞orish′ən/, the process of giving birth.

parulis. See **gumboil.**

PAS, PASA, abbreviation for **paraaminosalicylic acid.**

PASCAL /poskul′, paskal′/, a higher level computer compiler language, often used to teach programing.

Pascal's principle /poskulz′, paskalz′/, (in physics) a law stating that a confined liquid transmits pressure applied to it from an external source equally in all directions. Pascal's principle provides the basis for all hydraulic devices.

passive-aggressive personality, a personality characterized by passivity and aggression in which forceful actions or attitudes are expressed in an indirect, nonviolent manner, such as pouting, obstructionism, procrastination, inefficiency, stubbornness, and forgetfulness. Compare **aggressive personality, passive-dependent personality.** See also **passive-aggressive personality disorder.**

passive-aggressive personality disorder, a disorder characterized by the indirect expression of resistance to occupational or social demands, resulting in persistent, pervasive ineffectiveness, lack of self-confidence, poor interpersonal relationships, and pessimism that can lead, in severe cases, to major depression, alcoholism, or drug dependence. The behavior often reflects an unexpressed hostility or resentment stemming from a frustrating interpersonal or institutional relationship on which an individual is overdependent. Treatment may consist of behavior therapy or any of the various psychotherapeutic procedures, depending on the individual and the severity of the condition.

passive algolagnia. See **masochism.**

passive anaphylaxis. See **antiserum anaphylaxis.**

passive-dependent personality, a personality characterized by helplessness, indecisiveness, and a tendency to cling to and seek support from others. Compare **aggressive personality, passive-aggressive personality.**

passive euthanasia. See **euthanasia.**

passive exercise, repetitive movement of a part of the body as a result of an externally applied force or the voluntary effort of the muscles controlling another part of the body. Compare **active exercise.** See also **aerobic exercise, anaerobic exercise.**

passive immunity, a form of acquired immunity resulting from antibodies that are transmitted naturally through the placenta to a fetus or through the colostrum to an infant or artificially by injection of antiserum for treatment or prophylaxis. Passive immunity is not permanent and does not last as long as active immunity. See also **immune response.**

passive lingual arch, an orthodontic appliance that may help maintain tooth space and dental arch length when bilateral primary molars are prematurely lost.

passive movement, the moving of parts of the body by an outside force without voluntary action or resistance by the individual. Compare **active movement.**

passive play, play in which a person does not participate actively. For younger children such activity may include watching and listening to others, observing other children or animals, listening to stories, or looking at pictures. Older children are passively entertained by games and toys that require concentration and intellectual skill, as chess, reading, listening to music, or watching television. Compare **active play.**

passive smoking, the inhalation by nonsmokers of the smoke from other people's cigarettes, pipes, and cigars. The amount of such ambient smoke inhaled by a nonsmoker is small compared with that inhaled by tobacco users, but research provides increasing evidence that passive smoking can aggravate respiratory illnesses and contribute to more serious illnesses, as cancer, and can injure the health of nonsmoking spouses and of infants and unborn babies. Studies also show that individuals with chronic heart and lung diseases and allergies to tobacco can be adversely affected by passive smoking.

passive transfer test. See **Prausnitz-Küstner test.**

passive transport, the movement of small molecules across the membrane of a cell by diffusion. Passive transport occurs when the chemicals outside a cell become concentrated and start moving into the cell, changing the intracellular equilibrium. Passive transport is essential to various processes of metabolism, as the intake of digestive products by the cells lining the intestines. Compare **active transport, osmosis.**

passive tremor, an involuntary trembling occurring when the person is at rest, one of the signs of Parkinson's disease. Also called **resting tremor.**

Pasteurella /pas′tərel′ə/, a genus of gram-negative bacilli or coccobacilli, including species pathogenic to humans and domestic animals. *Pasteurella* infections may be transmitted to humans by animal bites. The plague bacillus, *Pasteurella pestis,* is now called *Yersinia pestis; P. tularensis,* which causes tularemia, has been reclassified as *Francisella tularensis.*

pasteurization, the process of applying heat, usually to milk or cheese, for a specified period of time for the purpose of killing or retarding the development of pathogenic bacteria. **–pasteurize,** *v.*

pasteurized milk, milk that has been treated by heat to destroy pathogenic bacteria. By law, pasteurization requires a temperature of 145° to 150° F for not less than 30 minutes, followed by a temperature of 161° F for 15 seconds, followed by immediate cooling.

past health, (in a health history) an overall summary of the person's general health to date, including past injuries, allergies, surgical procedures, immunizations, hospitalizations, and obstetric and psychiatric history. The past health history is obtained from the person or the person's family at the initial interview and becomes part of the permanent record.

pastoral counseling department, the hospital chaplaincy service.

Patau's syndrome. See **trisomy 13.**

patch, a small spot of surface tissue that differs from the surrounding area in color or texture or both and is not elevated above it.

patch test, a skin test for identifying allergens, especially those causing contact dermatitis. The suspected substance (food, pollen, animal fur), is applied to an adhesive patch that is placed on the patient's skin. Another patch, with nothing on it, serves as a control. After a certain period of time (usually 24 to 48 hours), both patches are removed. If the skin under the suspect patch is red and swollen and the control area is not, the test is said to be positive, and the person is probably allergic to that substance. Compare **Prausnitz-Küstner test, radioallergosorbent test.**

patella /pətel′ə/, a flat, triangular bone at the front of the knee joint, having a pointed apex that attaches to the ligamentum patellae. The convex, anterior surface of the bone is perforated for the passage of nutrient vessels and covered by an expansion from the tendon of the quadriceps femoris. Also called **knee cap.**

patellar ligament, the central portion of the common tendon of the quadriceps femoris. The ligament is a strong, flat, ligamentous band, about 8 cm long, attached proximally to the apex and the adjoining margins of the patella and distally to the tuberosity of the tibia. Its superficial fibers are continuous over the front of the patella with those of the tendon of the quadriceps femoris.

patellar reflex, a deep tendon reflex, elicited by a sharp tap on the tendon just distal to the patella, normally characterized by contraction of the quadriceps muscle and extension of the leg at the knee. The reflex is hyperactive in disease of the pyramidal tract above the level of the second lumbar vertebra. Also called **knee jerk reflex, quadriceps reflex.** See also **deep tendon reflex.**

patent, the condition of being open and unblocked, as a patent airway or a patent anus.

patent ductus arteriosus (PDA), an abnormal opening between the pulmonary artery and the aorta caused by failure of the fetal ductus arteriosus to close after birth. The defect, which is seen primarily in premature infants, allows blood from the aorta to flow into the pulmonary artery and to recirculate through the lungs where it is reoxygenated and returned to the left atrium and left ventricle, causing an increased workload on the left side of the heart and increased pulmonary vascular congestion and resistance. Clinical manifestations include cardiomegaly, especially of the left atrium and left ventricle, dilated ascending aorta, bounding pulses from increased systolic pressure, tachycardia, and a typical machinery-like murmur that is heard during all of systole and most of diastole. Characteristic auscultatory and radiologic findings are sufficient to confirm diagnosis so that cardiac catheterization is not necessary. Correction is delayed until the child is old enough to tolerate surgery and to allow time for spontaneous closure. Untreated complications include congestive heart failure, pulmonary vascular disease, calcification of the ductal site, and infective endocarditis. See also **congenital cardiac anomaly.**

paternal engrossment. See **bonding.**

Paterson-Kelly syndrome, a condition of the digestive system associated with iron deficiency anemia, characterized by the development of esophageal webs in the upper esophagus, making swallowing of solids difficult. The webs are easily ruptured during esophagoscopy and tube feeding and can produce hemorrhage. When the hemoglobin count is improved, the webs disappear. Also called **Plummer-Vinson syndrome.**

Paterson-Parker dosage system, a radiotherapy system that uses sources of specific relative loadings arranged according to defined rules, which lead to a homogenous dose in the implanted region.

path-. See **patho-.**

-path, **1.** a combining form meaning 'one suffering from a (specified) illness': *cardiopath, endocrinopath, neuropath*. **2.** a combining form meaning 'one who treats illness by a (specified) system': *dermopath, naprapath, naturopath.*

-pathetic, -pathetical, a combining form meaning 'pertaining to emotions': *antipathetic, apopathetic, sympathetic.*

Pathibamate, a trademark for a GI, fixed-combination drug containing an anticholinergic (tridihexethyl chloride) and a sedative (meprobamate).

-pathic, **1.** a combining form meaning 'referring to an illness or affected part of the body': *angiopathic, encephalopathic, hemopathic*. **2.** a combining form meaning 'referring to a form or system of treatment': *homeopathic, naturopathic, physiopathic.*

Pathilon, a trademark for an anticholinergic (tridihexethyl chloride).

Pathilon with Phenobarbital, a trademark for a GI, fixed-combination drug containing Pathilon and a sedative-hypnotic (phenobarbital).

patho-, path-, a combining form meaning 'of or related to disease': *pathocrinia, pathoformic, pathography.*

pathogen /path′əjən/, any microorganism capable of producing disease. –**pathogenic,** *adj.*

pathogenesis, the source or cause of an illness or abnormal condition.

pathogenicity, pertaining to the ability of a pathogenic agent to produce a disease.

pathogenic occlusion, an abnormal closure of the teeth, capable of producing pathologic changes in the teeth, supporting tissues, and other components of the stomatognathic system.

pathognomonic /pəthog′nəmon′ik/, (of a sign or symptom) specific to a disease or condition, as Koplik's spots on the buccal and lingual musosa, which are indicative of measles.

pathognomonic symptom. See **symptom.**

pathologic absorption, the taking up by the blood of an excretory or morbid substance.

pathologic anatomy, (in applied anatomy) the study of the structure and morphology of the tissues and cells of the body as related to disease.

pathologic diagnosis, a diagnosis arrived at by an examination of the substance and function of the tissues of the body, especially of the abnormal developmental changes in the tissues by histologic techniques of tissue examination.

pathologic fracture. See **neoplastic fracture.**

pathologic mitosis, any cell division that is atypical, asymmetrical, or multipolar and results in the unequal number of chromosomes in the nuclei of the daughter cells. It is indicative of malignancy, as occurs in cancer and the genetic anomalies.

pathologic myopia, a type of progressive nearsightedness characterized by changes in the fundus of the eye, posterior staphyloma, and deficient corrected acuity.

pathologic physiology, **1.** the study of the physical and chemical processes involved in the functioning of diseased tissues. **2.** the study of the modification of the normal functioning processes of an organism caused by disease. Also called **morbid physiology.** See also **pathophysiology.**

pathologic retraction ring, a ridge that may form around the uterus at the junction of the upper and lower uterine segments during the prolonged second stage of an obstructed labor. The lower segment is abnormally distended and thin, and the upper segment is abnormally thick. The ring, which may be seen and felt abdominally, is a warning of impending uterine rupture. Also called **Bandl's ring.** Compare **physiologic retraction ring, constriction ring.**

pathologist, a physician who specializes in the study of disease, usually in a hospital, school of medicine, or research institute or laboratory. A pathologist usually specializes in autopsy, or in clinical or surgical pathology.

pathology, the study of the characteristics, causes, and effects of disease, as observed in the structure and function of the body. **Cellular pathology** is the study of cellular changes in disease. **Clinical pathology** is the study of disease by the use of laboratory tests and methods. –**pathologic,** *adj.*

pathomimicry. See **Munchausen's syndrome.**

pathophysiology, the study of the biologic and physical manifestations of disease as they correlate with the underlying abnormalities and physiologic disturbances. Pathophysiology does not deal directly with the treatment of disease; rather, it explains the processes within the body that result in the signs and symptoms of a disease. –**pathophysiologic,** *adj.*

pathosis, a disease condition.

pathway, **1.** a network of neurons that provides a transmission route for nerve impulses from any part of the body to the spinal cord and the cerebral cortex or from the central nervous system to the muscles and organs. Neural pathways in the body are the somatic sensory pathways and the somatic motor pathways. **2.** a chain of chemical reactions that produces various compounds in critical sequence, as the Embden-Meyerhof pathway.

-pathy, **1.** a combining form meaning a 'suffering or illness' of a specified sort: *gynecopathy, nephropathy, psychopathy*. **2.** a combining form meaning a 'therapy for suffering': *homeopathy, osteopathy*.

patient, **1.** a recipient of a health care service. **2.** a health care recipient who is ill or hospitalized. **3.** a client in a health care service.

patient advocate. See **ombudsman.**

patient care committee, a hospital staff organization, composed of medical, nursing, and other health professionals, with the assigned responsibility of monitoring all patient care practices to ensure that predetermined standards are met.

patient compensation fund, a fund usually established by state law and commonly financed by a surcharge on malpractice premiums and used to pay malpractice claims.

patient day (P.D.), a unit in a system of accounting used by health care facilities and health care planners. Each day represents a unit of time during which the services of the institution or facility were used by a patient; thus 50 patients in a hospital for 1 day would represent 50 patient days.

patient interview, a systematic interview of a patient, the purpose of which is to obtain information that can be used to develop an individualized plan for care. Also called **client interview.**

patient mix, **1.** the distribution of demographic variables in a patient population, often represented by the percentage of a given race, age, sex, or ethnic derivation. **2.** the distribution of indications for admission in a patient population, as surgical, maternity, or trauma.

patient plan of care, a plan of care coordinated to include appropriate participation by each member of the health care team.

patient record, a collection of documents that provides a record of each episode in which a patient visited or sought treatment and received care or a referral for care from a health care facility. The record is confidential and is usually held by the facility, and the information in it is released only to the patient or with the patient's written permission. It contains the initial assessment of the patient's health status, the health history, laboratory reports of tests performed, notes by nurses and physicians regarding the daily condition of the patient and notes by consultants, as well as order sheets, medication sheets, admission records, discharge summaries, and other pertinent data. A problem-oriented medical record also contains a master problem list. The patient record is often a collection of papers held in a folder, but records may be computerized, making the past record available on visual display terminals or printouts. Also called *(informal)* **chart.**

patient representative. See **ombudsman.**

patient representative services, hospital services provided by designated staff members relating to the investigation and mediation of patients' complaints and the promotion and protection of patient's rights. See also **ombudsman.**

Patient's Bill of Rights, a list of patient's rights promulgated by the American Hospital Association. It offers some guidance and protection to patients by stating the responsibilities that a hospital and its staff have toward patients and their families during hospitalization, but it is not a legally binding document.

pattern logic, (in cardiology) a feature of an intraaortic ballon pump in which the QRS complex is recognized on a width basis.

pattern theory of pain. See **pain mechanism.**

patulous, pertaining to something that is open or spread apart.

Paul-Bunnell test, a blood test for heterophil antibodies, used for confirming a diagnosis of infectious mononucleosis. See also **heterophil antibody test.**

Paul's tube, a large-bore glass drainage tube with a projecting rim, used in performing an enterostomy. Also called **Paul-Mixter tube.**

Pautrier microabscess /pôtrēyā′/, an accumulation of intensely staining mononuclear cells in the epidermis, characterizing malignant lymphoma of the skin, especially mycosis fungoides. See also **mycosis fungoides.**

Pauwel's fracture /pou′əlz/, a fracture of the proximal femoral neck with varying degrees of angulation.

Pavabid, a trademark for a smooth muscle relaxant (papaverine hydrochloride).

Pavacap, a trademark for a smooth muscle relaxant (papaverine hydrochloride).

paraffin method, (in surgical pathology) a method used in preparing a selected portion of tissue for pathologic examination. The tissue is fixed, dehydrated, and infiltrated and embedded in paraffin, forming a block that is cut with a microtome into slices 8 μm thick. This method, which is more commonly used than the frozen section method, is slower and therefore not used during surgery.

pavor /pā′vôr/, a reaction to a frightening stimulus characterized by excessive terror. Kinds of pavor are **pavor diurnus** and **pavor nocturnus.**

pavor diurnus /dī·ur′nəs/, a sleep disorder occurring in children during daytime sleep in which they cry out in alarm and awaken in fear and panic. See also **sleep terror disorder.**

pavor nocturnus /noktur′nəs/, a sleep disorder occurring in children during nighttime sleep that causes them to cry out in alarm and awaken in fear and panic. See also **nightmare, sleep terror disorder.**

Pavulon, a trademark for a neuromuscular blocking agent (pancuronium bromide), used as an adjunct to anesthesia.

Payr's clamp /pī′ərz/, a heavy clamp used in GI surgery.

Pb, symbol for **lead.**

PBI, abbreviation for **protein-bound iodine.**

PC, abbreviation for **private corporation.**

PCB, abbreviation for **polychlorinated biphenyls.**

PCH, abbreviation for **paroxysmal cold hemoglobinuria.**

PCIS, abbreviation for *Patient Care Information System* of the Indian health services, an online computer system that contains full medical care data on all the residents of the Papago Indian reservation in Arizona.

P_{CO_2}, symbol for **partial pressure of carbon dioxide.** See **partial pressure.**

PCP, abbreviation for **phencyclidine hydrochloride.**

Pd, symbol for **palladium.**

P.D., abbreviation for **patient day.**

PDA, abbreviation for **patent ductus arteriosus.**

PDL, abbreviation for **periodontal ligament.**

PDR*,** abbreviation for ***Physicians' Desk Reference.

PE, abbreviation for **pulmonary embolism.**

peak, the amount of medication in the blood that represents the highest level during a drug administration cycle.

peak concentration, the maximum amount of a substance or force, as the highest concentration of a drug measured immediately after the drug has been administered.

peak level, the highest concentration, usually in the blood, that a substance reaches during the time period

A Patient's Bill of Rights*

The American Hospital Association Board of Trustees' Committee on Health Care for the Disadvantaged, which has been a consistent advocate on behalf of consumers of health care services, developed this bill of rights, which was approved by the AHA House of Delegates February 6, 1973. The following rights are affirmed:

1. The patient has the right to considerate and respectful care.
2. The patient has the right to obtain from his physician complete current information concerning his diagnosis, treatment, and prognosis in terms the patient can be reasonably expected to understand. When it is not medically advisable to give such information to the patient, the information should be made available to an appropriate person in his behalf. He has the right to know, by name, the physician responsible for coordinating his care.
3. The patient has the right to receive from his physician information necessary to give informed consent prior to the start of any procedure and/or treatment. Except in emergencies, such information for informed consent should include but not necessarily be limited to the specific procedure and/or treatment, the medically significant risks involved, and the probable duration of incapacitation. Where medically significant alternatives for care or treatment exist, or when the patient requests information concerning medical alternatives, the patient has the right to such information. The patient also has the right to know the name of the person responsible for the procedures and/or treatment.
4. The patient has the right to refuse treatment to the extent permitted by law, and to be informed of the medical consequences of his action.
5. The patient has the right to every consideration of his privacy concerning his own medical care program. Case discussion, consultation, examination, and treatment are confidential and should be conducted discreetly. Those not directly involved in his care must have the permission of the patient to be present.
6. The patient has the right to expect that all communications and records pertaining to his care should be treated as confidential.
7. The patient has the right to expect that within its capacity a hospital must make reasonable response to the request of a patient for services. The hospital must provide evaluation, service, and/or referral as indicated by the urgency of the case. When medically permissible a patient may be transferred to another facility only after he has received complete information and explanation concerning the needs for and alternatives to such a transfer. The institution to which the patient is to be transferred must first have accepted the patient for transfer.
8. The patient has the right to obtain information as to any relationship of his hospital to other health care and educational institutions insofar as his care is concerned. The patient has the right to obtain information as to the existence of any professional relationships among individuals, by name, who are treating him.
9. The patient has the right to be advised if the hospital proposes to engage in or perform human experimentation affecting his care or treatment. The patient has the right to refuse to participate in such research projects.
10. The patient has the right to expect reasonable continuity of care. He has the right to know in advance what appointment times and physicians are available and where. The patient has the right to expect that the hospital will provide a mechanism whereby he is informed by his physician or a delegate of the physician of the patient's continuing health care requirements following discharge.
11. The patient has the right to examine and receive an explanation of his bill regardless of source of payment.
12. The patient has the right to know what hospital rules and regulations apply to his conduct as a patient.

*Reprinted with the permission of the American Hospital Association, copyright 1975.

under consideration, after which the concentration declines, such as the highest blood glucose level attained during a glucose tolerance test.

peak logic, a feature of the intraaortic balloon pump in which any positive waveform may trigger the pump.

peak method of dosing, the administration of a drug dosage so that a specified maximum level is reached to produce a desired effect, such as lowering the blood pressure.

peak mucus sign, a lubricative, cloudy to clear white cervical mucus that occurs during periods of high estrogen levels, particularly at the time of ovulation. See also **spinnbarkeit.**

Péan's forceps /pē·anz′/, *obsolete*. a basic hemostatic clamp.

pearly penile papules. See **hirsutoid papillomas of the penis.**

pearly tumor. See **cholesteatoma.**

Pearson's product movement correlation, (in statistics) a statistic test of the relationship between two variables measured in interval or ratio scales. Correlations computed fall between +1.00 and −1.00.

pecilo-. See **poikilo-.**

pectin, a gelatinous carbohydrate substance found in fruits and succulent vegetables and used as the setting agent for jams and jellies and as an emulsifier and stabilizer in many foods. It also adds to the diet bulk necessary for proper GI functioning. See also **dietary fiber.**

pectineus /pektin′ē·əs/, the most anterior of the five medial femoral muscles. It arises from the pectineal line and inserts in a rough line on the femur, extending distally and caudally from the lesser trochanter to the linea aspera. The muscle is innervated by a branch of the femoral nerve containing fibers from the second, the third, and the fourth lumbar nerves, and it functions to flex and adduct the thigh and to rotate it medially. Compare **adductor brevis, adductor longus, adductor magnus, gracilis.**

pector-, a combining form meaning 'of or pertaining to the breast': *pectoralgia, pectoriloquy, pectorophony*.

pectoralis major, a large muscle of the upper chest wall that acts on the joint of the shoulder. Thick and fan-shaped, it arises from the clavicle, the sternum, the cartilages of the second to the sixth ribs, and the aponeurosis of the obliquus externus abdominis. It inserts by a flat wide tendon into the crest of the greater tubercle of the humerus. The pectoralis major is innervated by the medial and lateral pectoral nerves from the brachial plexus, which contain fibers from the fifth, sixth, seventh, and eighth cervical nerves, and by fibers from the first thoracic nerve. The pectoralis major serves to flex, adduct, and medially rotate the arm in the shoulder joint.

pectoralis minor, a thin, triangular muscle of the upper chest wall beneath the pectoralis major. The base arises from the third, fourth, and fifth ribs on their upper, outer surfaces. It inserts as a flat tendon into the corocoid process of the scapula. The pectoralis minor is innervated by the medial pectoral nerve from the brachial plexus, which contains fibers from the eighth cervical and the first thoracic nerves, and it functions to rotate the scapula, to draw it down and forward, and to raise the third, the fourth, and the fifth ribs in forced inspiration. Compare **pectoralis major, subclavius.**

ped-. See **pedo-.**

-ped, -pede, **1.** a combining form meaning a 'creature possessing feet of a (specified) sort or quantity': *biped, quadruped*. **2.** a combining form meaning 'possessing feet of a (specified) sort or quantity': *taliped*.

pedagogy, the art and science of teaching children, based on a belief that the purpose of education is the transmittal of knowledge.

-pedal. See **-pedic.**

pederosis. See **pedophilia.**

pedia-, ped-, pedo-, a combining form meaning 'of or pertaining to a child': *pediatric, pediatrician, pediatrics*.

-pedia, -paedia, a combining form meaning 'compendium of knowledge': *orthopedia, pharmacopedia, logopedia*.

Pediaflor, a trademark for a dental preparation (sodium fluoride), used as prophylaxis against dental caries in children.

Pedialyte, a trademark for a balanced solution containing various electrolytes.

Pediamycin, a trademark for an antibacterial (erythromycin ethylsuccinate).

pediatric anesthesia, a subspecialty of anesthesiology dealing with the anesthesia of neonates, infants, and children up to 12 years of age.

pediatric dosage, the determination of the correct amount, frequency, and total number of doses of a medication to be administered to a child or infant. Such variables as the age, weight, body surface area, and the ability of the child to absorb, metabolize, and excrete the medication must be considered, as well as the expected action of the drug, possible side effects, and potential toxicity. Various formulas have been devised to calculate pediatric dosage from a standard adult dose, although the most reliable method is to use the proportional amount of body surface area to body weight, based on one of the formulas. See also **Clark's rule, Cowling's rule, Young's rule.**

pediatric hospitalization, the confinement of a child or infant in a hospital for diagnostic testing or therapeutic treatment. Regardless of age or the degree of illness or injury, hospitalization constitutes a major crisis in the life of a child, and the emotional trauma elicits various behavioral reactions that the nurse must recognize and be prepared to cope with to facilitate recovery. The dominant factors influencing stress, which vary according to the child's developmental age, previous experience with illness, and the seriousness of the condition, include separation from the parents and familiar environment, disruption of routine patterns of daily life, loss of independence, and worry about bodily injury or painful experiences. The nurse can minimize stress by preparing the child and family through prehospital counseling; by encouraging active parental participation in the care of the child through rooming-in facilities or frequent visits; by maintaining as normal a daily routine as possible, especially with eating, sleeping, hygiene, and play activities; by explaining all hospital procedures and the immediate and long-term prognosis in terms that the child can easily understand; and by providing support and guidance for parents and siblings. The nurse may also use the hospital experience to foster an improved parent-child relationship and to teach other members of the family about proper health care. Emergency admission greatly increases the emotional trauma of hospitalization, making the role of the nurse in counteracting negative reactions even more significant.

pediatrician /pē′dē•ətrish′ən/, a physician who specializes in pediatrics. Also called **pediatrist** /pē′dē•at′-rist/.

pediatric nurse practitioner (PNP), a nurse practitioner who, by advanced study and clinical practice, as in a master's degree program or certificate in pediatric nursing, has gained expert knowledge in the nursing care of infants and children. See also **pediatric nursing.**

pediatric nursing, the branch of nursing concerned with the care of infants and children. Pediatric nursing requires knowledge of normal psychomotor, psychosocial, and cognitive growth and development, as well as of the health problems and needs of people in this age group. Preventive care and anticipatory guidance are integral to the practice of pediatric nursing. See also **pediatric nurse practitioner.**

pediatric nutrition, the maintenance of a proper, well-balanced diet, consisting of the essential nutrients and the adequate caloric intake necessary to promote growth and sustain the physiologic requirements at the various stages of development. Nutritional needs vary considerably with age, level of activity, and environmental conditions, and they are directly related to the rate of growth. In the prenatal period, growth is totally dependent on adequate maternal nutrition. During infancy the need for calories, especially in the form of protein, is greater than at any postnatal period because of the rapid increase in both height and weight. From toddlerhood through the preschool and middle childhood years, growth is uneven and occurs in spurts, with a subsequent fluctuation in appetite and calorie consumption. In general, the average child expends 55% of energy on metabolic maintenance, 25% on activities, 12% on growth, and 8% on excretion. The accelerated growth phase during adolescence demands greater nutritional requirements, although food habits are often influenced by emotional factors, peer pressure, and fad diets. Inadequate nutrition, especially during critical periods of growth, results in retarded development or illness, as anemia from deficiency of iron or scurvy from deficiency of vitamin C. An important function of the nurse is to give nutritional guidance and teach good eating habits. A special problem is overfeeding in the early childhood years, which may lead to obesity or hypervitaminosis. See also **dietary allowances,** and see specific vitamins.

pediatrics /pē′dē•at′triks/, a branch of medicine concerned with the development and care of children. Its specialties are the particular diseases of children and their treatment and prevention. **–pediatric,** *adj.*

pediatric surgery, the special preparation and care of the child undergoing surgical procedures for injuries, deformities, or disease. In addition to the usual fears and emotional trauma of illness and hospitalization, the child is especially concerned about being anesthetized. Younger children worry more about what will happen to them and how they will feel after awakening from anesthesia, whereas the older child fears the operation itself and possible death, the loss of control while under anesthesia, and any change in body image or mutilation of parts. The role of the nurse is to prepare the child psychologically and physically for the particular surgical procedure and any postoperative reactions, to offer support to the parents and involve them as much as possible in the care, both before and after surgery, and to explain immediate and long-term prognoses. See also **pediatric hospitalization.**

-pedic, -pedal, a combining form meaning 'referring or pertaining to the feet': *arthrosteopedic, talipedic, velocepedic.*

-pedic, -paedic, a combining form meaning 'of or pertaining to children or their treatment': *gymnopedic, orthopedic.*

pedicle clamp /ped′ikəl/, a locking surgical forceps used for compressing blood vessels or pedicles of tumors during surgery. Also called **clamp forceps.**

pedicle flap operation, a mucogingival surgical procedure for relocating or sliding gingival tissue from a donor site to an isolated defect, usually a tooth surface denuded of attached gingiva.

pediculicide /pədik′yo͝olisīd′/, any of a group of drugs that kill lice.

pediculosis /pədik′yo͝olō′sis/, infestation with blood-sucking lice. **Pediculosis capitis** is infestation of the scalp with lice. **Pediculosis corporis** is infestation of the skin of the body with lice. **Pediculosis palpebrarum** is infestation of the eyelids and eyelashes with lice. **Pediculosis pubis** is infestation of the pubic hair region with lice. See also **crab louse, louse.**

■ OBSERVATIONS: Infestation with lice causes intense itching, often resulting in excoriation of the skin and secondary bacterial infection. Frequently, only the eggs of the lice may be seen. Body lice lay eggs in the seams of clothing; crab and head lice attach their eggs to hairs. Lice are spread by direct contact with infested clothing, people, or toilet seats. Body lice may transmit certain diseases, among them relapsing fever, typhus, and trench fever.

■ INTERVENTION: Treatment includes the topical use of 1% lindane as shampoo, lotion, or cream, or of malathion 0.5% lotion. After applying the pediculocide, the eggs are combed out of the hair with a fine-toothed comb. Lice and eggs on the eyelashes require topical treatment with an ophthalmic ointment containing 0.25% physostigmine. Infestation sometimes may be prevented by avoiding contact with the organism and by washing and ironing any clothing or bedding that may be infested.

Pediculus pubis. See **crab louse.**

pedigree, **1.** line of descent; lineage; ancestry. **2.** (in genetics) a chart that shows the genetic makeup of a person's ancestors, used in the mendelian analysis of an inherited characteristic or disease in a particular family. Specific stylized symbols, usually plain and shaded or partially shaded squares and circles, are used, respectively, to designate normal males and females, those affected by the disease or trait, and those who are heterozygote carriers. The generations are numbered with Roman numerals at the left with the most recent at the bottom, and members within each generation are designated by Arabic numerals from left to right according to age, the oldest at the left. The inquiry begins with the siblings of the affected person and proceeds to the parents and grandparents and any of their immediate relatives. See also **Punnett square.**

pedo- a combining form meaning 'of or related to a child': *pedodontics, pedogenesis, pedophilia.*

pedo-, ped-, pedia-, a combining form meaning 'of or pertaining to the foot': *pedodynamometer, pedograph, pedopathy.*

pedodontics /ped′ədon′tiks/, a field of dentistry devoted to the diagnosis and the treatment of dental problems affecting children.

pedogenesis /pē′dōjen′əsis/, the production of offspring by young or larval forms of animals, often by parthenogenesis, as in certain amphibians. Also spelled **paedogenesis.** **–pedogenetic,** *adj.*

pedophilia /ped′əfil′ē·ə/, **1.** an abnormal interest in children. **2.** (in psychiatry) a psychosexual disorder in which the fantasy or act of engaging in sexual activity with prepubertal children is the preferred or exclusive means of achieving sexual excitement and gratification. It may be heterosexual or homosexual. Also spelled **paedophilia.** Also called **pederosis.** See also **paraphilia.** **–pedophilic,** *adj.*

peds, *informal.* pediatrics.

peduncle /pədung′kəl/, a stemlike connecting part, as the pineal peduncle or a peduncle graft. **–peduncular, pedunculate,** *adj.*

PEEP, abbreviation for **positive end expiratory pressure.**

Peeping Tom. See **voyeur.**

peer review, an appraisal by professional coworkers of equal status of the way an individual nurse or other health professional conducts practice, education, or research. The appraisal uses accepted standards as measures against which performance is weighed. See also **Professional Standards Review Organization.**

Peganone, a trademark for an anticonvulsant (ethotoin).

peg-shaped tooth. See **conic tooth.**

Pel-Ebstein fever /pel′eb′stēn/, a recurrent fever, occurring in cycles of several days or weeks, characteristic of Hodgkin's disease or malignant lymphoma. Also called **Murchison fever.**

Pelger-Huët anomaly /pel′gərhyo͞o′ət/, an inherited disorder characterized by granulocytes with unusually coarse nuclear material and a dumbbell-shaped or peanut-shaped nuclei. Normal nuclear segmentation does not seem to occur, but there are no associated findings. See also **band.**

pell-, a combining form meaning 'of or pertaining to the skin': *pellagra, pellicle, pellicular.*

pellagra /pəlā′grə, pəlag′rə/, a disease resulting from a deficiency of niacin or tryptophan or a metabolic defect that interferes with the conversion of the precursor tryptophan to niacin. It is frequently seen in individuals whose diet consists primarily of maize, which is deficient in tryptophan. It is characterized by scaly dermatitis, especially of the skin exposed to the sun, glossitis, inflammation of the mucous membranes, diarrhea, and mental disturbances, including depression, confusion, disorientation, hallucination, and delirium. Treatment and prophylaxis consist of administration of niacin and tryptophan, usually in conjunction with other vitamins, particularly thiamine and riboflavin, and a well-balanced diet containing foods rich in these nutrients, as liver, eggs, milk, and meat. Kinds of pellagra are **pellagra sine pellagra** and **typhoid pellagra.** Compare **kwashiorkor.** **–pellagrous,** *adj.*

pellagra sine pellagra /sī′nē, sē′nə/, a form of pellagra in which the characteristic dermatitis is not present. See **pellagra.**

pelo-, a combining form meaning 'of or pertaining to mud': *pelohemia, pelology, pelotherapy.*

pelvic, of or pertaining to the pelvis.

pelvic brim, the curved top of the bones of the hip extending from the anterior superior iliac crest in front on one side around and past the sacrum to the crest on the other side. Below the brim is the pelvis.

pelvic cellulitis, bacterial infection of the parametrium, occurring after childbirth or spontaneous therapeutic abortion. It represents an extension of infection via the blood vessels and lymphatics from a primary wound infection in the external genitalia, perineum, vagina, cervix, or uterus. It is characterized by fever, uterine subinvolution, chills and sweats, and abdominal pain that spreads laterally and, if untreated, by the formation of a large abscess and by signs of peritonitis. It is seen most commonly between the third and the ninth days after delivery or abortion. Treatment includes an antibiotic, bed rest, intravenous fluids, and drainage of any abscess that forms. Oxytocics may be given to augment involution.

pelvic classification, **1.** a process in which the anatomic and spatial relationships of the bones of the pelvis are evaluated, usually to assess the adequacy of the pelvic structures for vaginal delivery. Caldwell-Moloy's system of classification is the one most commonly used. **2.** one of the types in a classification system of the pelvis.

pelvic congestion syndrome, an abnormal gynecologic condition characterized by chronic low back pain, dysuria, dysmenorrhea, vague lower abdominal pain, vaginal discharge, and dyspareunia. The cause of the symptoms is not understood; formerly it was thought that the vascular bed of the area was distended with blood, but this has not been demonstrated. Women between 25 and 45 years of age are most often affected.

pelvic diaphragm, the caudal aspect of the body wall, stretched like a hammock across the pelvic cavity and comprised of the levator ani and the coccygeus muscles. It holds the abdominal contents, supports the pelvic viscera, and is pierced by the anal canal, the urethra, and the vagina. It is reinforced by fasciae and muscles associated with these structures and with the perineum.

pelvic examination, a diagnostic procedure in which the external and internal genitalia are physically examined using inspection, palpation, percussion, and auscultation. It should be performed regularly throughout a woman's life, usually every 1 to 3 years. See also **female reproductive system assessment.**

■ METHOD: The woman empties her bladder, disrobes, and puts on an examining gown. She is made as comfortable as possible in the dorsal lithotomy position, her feet in stirrups and her buttocks at the very edge of the foot of the examining table, and is then draped. Breast examination is often carried out at this point, before the pelvic examination, and the lower abdomen is palpated. Particular attention is paid to the suprapubic area to detect any masses extending from the pelvis above the symphysis and to the groin to detect inguinal lymphadenopathy or hernia. If a mass is felt, percussion may be performed to delineate it. If pregnancy is suspected, palpation and percussion of the uterus and auscultation of fetal heart tones are attempted. The examiner then moves to the stool at the foot of the table between the patient's legs. The labia majora are spread apart to permit inspection of the clitoris, the urethral meatus, the labia minora, and the vaginal vestibule. Any swelling, discoloration, lesion, scar, cyst, discharge, or bleeding is noted. Skene's and Bartholin's glands and ducts are palpated and milked, and any secretions expressed are evaluated and a specimen is spread on culture media. The tone of the perineal and paravaginal musculature is assessed. Cystocele, rectocele, or varying degrees of uterine descensus may be observed as the woman is asked to bear down. Because lubricating jelly interferes with cytologic and bacteriologic studies, the speculum examination is usually performed without using the jelly. The speculum is warmed, lubricated with warm water, and introduced gradually. The examiner is careful to direct the speculum along the axis of the vagina, which is at an angle of approximately 45 degrees to the axis of the table if the woman is lying flat. The speculum may need to be moved lightly from side to side to slip it over the vaginal rugae. The woman is advised that she may feel a stretching sensation; the speculum is gently opened and its position is adjusted to hold the vaginal folds out of the way to reveal the cervix. The color and condition of the vaginal epithelium are observed, and the position, size, and quality of the superficial epithelium are evaluated. Specimens for bacteriologic study are obtained before the Pap test. For the Pap test, scrapings of the endocervix and the cervix and a sample of the vaginal secretions are secured on a Pap stick and an applicator and lightly spread on labeled glass slides. The slides are immediately sprayed with a fixative or dipped in it. The speculum is then closed, rotated slightly, removed from the vagina, and rinsed or placed directly in a germicidal solution. In the bimanual part of the examination, two gloved fingers are well lubricated and inserted slowly and gently into the vagina. The examiner uses the opposite hand to apply pressure to the lower abdomen in several positions and directions to bring the uterus, tubes, and ovaries into positions in which they may be felt. The size, shape, position, mobility, and consistency of the organs and tissues are evaluated, and any tenderness or discomfort is noted. Rectal or rectovaginal examination is then performed. Before the insertion of a finger in the anus, lateral pressure is applied to the sphincter, and the woman is urged to bear down lightly to relax the muscle and minimize discomfort.

■ NURSING ORDERS: Minor unthoughtfulness or inadvertent movement may cause tension and make the examination more difficult for the woman and for the examiner. Instruments, culture materials, a light, drapes, and a gown are all made ready beforehand. The table, instruments, and drapes are clean and warm. Materials from previous examinations are not in evidence. The woman is forewarned of what to expect at each step of the examination. Gentleness and quietness are exercised at all times. On completion of the examination, the woman is helped to slide well back on the table before sitting up. Syncope after pelvic examination is uncommon but not rare; there is risk of injury should the patient faint and fall from the examining table. The woman is observed briefly after sitting up before being left alone. She is then given tissues, a sanitary napkin or tampon, and a private area in which to dress.

■ OUTCOME CRITERIA: Pelvic examination may demonstrate many pelvic abnormalities and diseases. Cytologic and bacteriologic specimens are conveniently obtained. A pelvic examination cannot be satisfactorily performed without the cooperation of the woman being examined; inadequate relaxation, obesity, extensive scarring, pelvic tenderness, and heavy vaginal discharge may also preclude an adequate examination.

pelvic exenteration, the surgical removal of all reproductive organs and adjacent tissues.

pelvic floor, the soft tissues enclosing the pelvic outlet.

pelvic inferior aperture. See **pelvic outlet.**

pelvic inflammatory disease (PID), any inflammatory condition of the female pelvic organs, especially one caused by bacterial infection. See also **endometritis.**

■ OBSERVATIONS: Characteristics of the condition include fever, foul-smelling vaginal discharge, pain in the lower abdomen, abnormal uterine bleeding, pain with coitus, and tenderness or pain in the uterus, affected ovary, or fallopian tube on bimanual pelvic examination. If an abscess has already developed, a soft, tender, fluid-filled mass may be palpated.

■ INTERVENTION: The cause of the inflammatory process is determined and treated. A specimen of cervical mucus is obtained for bacteriologic identification and antibiotic sensitivity. A sonogram may be useful in visualizing an abscess or fluid-filled fallopian tube. Bed rest and antibiotics are usually prescribed, but surgical drainage of an abscess may be required. Severe, fulminating PID may necessitate hysterectomy to avoid fatal septicemia. If the cause is infection by gonococci or chlamydiae, the woman's sexual partners are also treated with antibiotics.

■ NURSING CONSIDERATIONS: The full course of prescribed antibiotics is taken. Inadequate therapy may result in chronic PID or in the formation of an abscess. If an abscess has already developed, PID may become chronic and recurrent. Severe PID is usually very painful: the woman may be prostrate and require narcotic analgesia. Recurrent or severe PID often results in scarring of the fallopian tubes, obstruction, and infertility.

pelvic inlet, (in obstetrics) the inlet to the true pelvis, bounded by the sacral promontory, the horizontal rami of the pubic bones, and the top of the symphysis pubis. Because the infant must pass through the inlet to enter the true pelvis and to be born vaginally, the anteroposterior, transverse, and oblique dimensions of the inlet are important measurements to be made in assessing the pelvis in pregnancy. There are three anteroposterior diameters: the true conjugate, the obstetric conjugate, and the diagonal conjugate. The true conjugate can be measured only on x-ray films, because it extends from the sacral promontory to the top of the symphysis pubis. Its normal measurement is 11 cm or more. The obstetric conjugate is the shortest of the three, because it extends from the sacral promontory to the thickest part of the pubic bone. It measures 10 cm or more. The diagonal conjugate is the most easily and commonly assessed, because it extends from the lower border of the symphysis pubis to the sacral promontory. It normally measures 11.5 cm or more. The inlet is said to be contracted when any of these diameters is smaller than normal. The anteroposterior diameters are shorter than normal in the small gynecoid and platypelloid pelvis. The transverse diameter of the inlet is bounded by the inferior border of the walls of the iliac bones and is measured at the widest point. It is normally close to 13.5 cm but may be less in the small gynecoid pelvis and anthropoid pelvis. The oblique diameters of the pelvis extend from the juncture of the sacrum and ilium to the eminence on the ilium on the opposite side of the pelvis. Each oblique diameter measures nearly 13 cm. This dimension is smaller than normal in the small gynecoid and platypelloid pelves. See also **android pelvis, anthropoid pelvis, gynecoid pelvis, platypelloid pelvis.**

pelvic kidney. See **ptotic kidney.**

pelvic minilaparotomy /min′ēlap′ərot′əmē/, a surgical operation in which the lower abdomen is entered through a small, suprapubic incision, performed most often for tubal sterilization but also for diagnosis and treatment of eccyesis, ovarian cyst, endometriosis, and infertility. It may be performed as an alternative to laparoscopy, often on an outpatient basis. Compare **laparoscopy.** See also **bilateral tubal ligation, sterilization.**

■ METHOD: General, regional, or local anesthesia is administered. The patient is placed in the supine position, and the abdomen is prepared with antiseptic solution and draped with sterile drapes. Often, pelvic examination is performed, and a device with a long handle is inserted into the uterus or attached to the cervix; the handle extends from the vagina and provides a means of manipulating the uterus during surgery. An incision a few centimeters long is made, usually transversely, in the suprapubic fold of skin in the midline, and is then carried down through the fat and fascia, between the rectus abdominis muscles, and into the peritoneal cavity. Bleeders are ligated, and a small self-retaining retractor is placed in the incision. The smallness of the incision permits intraperitoneal palpation with one or, at most, two fingers. With the placement of small packs to exclude the bowel from the operative field, the various pelvic structures can usually be exposed, inspected, and palpated. A laparoscope may be used for visualization. Each uterine tube is brought up into the incision, and the sterilization or other procedure is performed. After hemostasis is ensured, each tube is replaced in its anatomic position, and the incision is closed in layers. A small, sterile dressing is applied, and the vaginal instruments are removed.

■ NURSING ORDERS: The prospect of sterilization and its effects may add to the anxiety of undergoing surgery; therefore, preoperatively and postoperatively the woman may require emotional support and information in answer to her questions. Because incisional pain in the postoperative period may mask the pain of intraperitoneal bleeding, vital signs are monitored frequently. Tachycardia and hypotension that are not alleviated by analgesia may be signs of hemorrhage or injury to the bowel. Before discharge, outpatients are carefully instructed in the postoperative danger signs and in the proper care of the incision at home. Arrangements are made for follow-up examination.

■ OUTCOME CRITERIA: Because the abdomen is entered under direct vision in minilaparotomy, the risk of injury by the trocar, inherent in laparoscopy, is reduced. Minilaparotomy can be performed in the presence of pelvic adhesions or other abnormalities that may preclude laparoscopy. Minilaparotomy affords direct rather than telescopic observation of the pelvic viscera, so there are likely to be fewer blind spots. Tissues are directly palpated, and surgery is performed in hand. The abdominal cavity need not be distended with gas, and the risks of limitation of diaphragmatic excursion and vagotonia from peritoneal distention are avoided. Often, minilaparotomy may be performed faster and less expensively than laparoscopy. Though small, the minilaparotomy incision is considerably larger than is the usual laparoscopy incision. It is, therefore, less pleasing cosmetically, as well as more painful in the postoperative period. Minilaparotomy is often performed on an outpatient basis, although some women require brief postoperative hospitalization.

pelvic outlet, the space surrounded by the bones of the lower portion of the true pelvis. In men, the shape of the pelvic outlet is narrower than in women, but this is of no clinical significance. In women, the shape and size of the pelvis varies and is of importance in childbirth. The shapes are classified by the length of the diameters as compared with each other and by the thickness of the bones. The diameters of the outlet are the anteroposterior, from the symphysis pubis to the coccyx, and the intertuberous, laterally from one to the other ischial tuberosity. See also **pelvic classification.**

pelvic pain, pain in the pelvis, as occurs in appendicitis, oophoritis, and endometritis. The character and onset of pelvic pain and any factors that alleviate or aggravate it are significant in making a diagnosis.

pelvic pole, the end of the axis at which the breech of the fetus is located.

pelvic rotation, one of the five major kinematic determinants of gait, involving the alternate rotation of the pelvis to the right and the left of the central axis of the body. The usual pelvic rotation occurring at each hip joint in most healthy individuals is approximately 4 degrees to each side of the central axis. Pelvic rotation occurs during the stance phase of gait and involves a medial to lateral circular motion. With normal locomotion or walking considered a progressive sinusoidal movement, pelvic rotation serves to minimize the vertical displacement of the center of gravity of the body during the act of walking. Analysis of pelvic rotation is often a factor in diagnosing various orthopedic diseases, deformities, and abnormal bone conditions and in the correction of pathologic gaits. Compare **knee-ankle interaction, knee-hip flexion, lateral pelvic displacement, pelvic tilt.**

pelvic tilt, one of the five major kinematic determinants of gait that lowers the pelvis on the side of the swinging lower limb during the walking cycle. Through the action of the hip joint the pelvis tilts laterally downward, adducting the lower limb in the stance phase of gait and abducting the opposite extremity in the swing phase of gait. The knee joint of the non-weight-bearing limb flexes during its swing phase to allow the pelvic tilt, which helps minimize the vertical displacement of the center of gravity of the body, thus conserving energy during walking. Pelvic tilt is often a factor in the diagnosis and treatment of various orthopedic diseases, deformities, and abnormal conditions and in the analysis and the correction of pathologic gaits. Compare **knee ankle interaction, knee hip flexion, lateral pelvic displacement, pelvic rotation.**

pelvic varicocele. See **ovarian varicocele.**

pelvifemoral, of or pertaining to the structures of the hip joint, especially the muscles and the area around the bony pelvis and the head of the femur that make up the pelvic girdle.

pelvifemoral muscular dystrophy, a form of limb-girdle muscular dystrophy that begins in the pelvic girdle. Also called **Leyden-Moebius muscular dystrophy.**

pelvimeter /pelvim′ətər/, a device for measuring the diameter and capacity of the pelvis.

pelvimetry /pelvim′ətrē/, the act or process of determining the dimensions of the bony birth canal. Kinds of pelvimetry are **clinical pelvimetry** and **x-ray pelvimetry.**

pelvis /pel′viz/, *pl.* **pelves,** the lower portion of the trunk of the body, composed of four bones, the two innominate bones laterally and ventrally and the sacrum and coccyx posteriorly. It is divided into the greater or false pelvis and the lesser or true pelvis by an oblique plane passing through the sacrum and the pubic symphysis. The greater pelvis is the expanded portion of the cavity situated cranially and ventral to the pelvic brim. The lesser pelvis is situated distal to the pelvic brim, and its bony walls are more complete than those of the greater pelvis. The inlet and outlet of the pelvis have three important diameters, anteroposterior, oblique, and transverse. The pelvis of a woman is usually less massive but wider and more circular than that of a man. **–pelvic,** *adj.*

pemoline /pem′əlēn/, a central nervous system stimulant.

■ INDICATIONS: It is prescribed in the treatment of minimal brain dysfunction and attention-deficit disorder in children.

■ CONTRAINDICATION: Known hypersensitivity to this drug prohibits its use.

■ ADVERSE EFFECTS: Some of the more serious adverse reactions are insomnia, GI disturbances, rash, convulsions, and hallucinations.

pemphigoid /pem′figoid/, a bullous disease resembling pemphigus, distinguished by thicker walled bullae arising from erythematous macules or urticarial bases. Oral lesions are uncommon. It may rarely be associated with an internal malignancy. Spontaneous remission occasionally occurs after several years. Treatment is usually with oral corticosteroids. Compare **pemphigus.**

pemphigus /pem′figəs, pemfī′gəs/, an uncommon, serious disease of the skin and mucous membranes, characterized by thin-walled bullae arising from apparently normal skin or mucous membrane. The bullae rupture easily, leaving raw patches. The person loses weight, becomes weak, and is subject to major infections. Treatment with corticosteroids and other immunosuppressive medications has changed the prognosis of this disease from an almost universally fatal one to a controllable problem compatible with a nearly normal life. The cause is unknown. Compare **pemphigoid.**

pemphigus neonatorum, neonatal impetigo.

Penapar VK, a trademark for an antibacterial (penicillin V potassium).

pendular nystagmus, an undulating involuntary movement of the eyeball.

penetrance, (in genetics) a variable factor that modifies basic patterns of inheritance. It is the regularity with which an inherited trait is manifest in the person who carries the gene. If a gene always produces its effect on the phenotype, it is fully and completely penetrant. Achondroplasia is caused by a fully penetrant gene; if the gene is present, achondroplasia results. If a gene produces its effect less frequently than 100% of the time, it is not fully penetrant. Retinoblastoma develops in 90% of the children carrying the gene; in 10% of children, the gene is nonpenetrant. **–penetrant,** *adj.*

penfluridol, an antipsychotic drug, chemically similar to pimozide.

-penia, a combining form meaning a '(specified) deficiency': *glycopenia, lipopenia, thyropenia.*

penicillamine (D-penicillamine), a chelating agent.

■ INDICATIONS: It is prescribed to bind with and remove metals from the blood in the treatment of heavy metal (especially lead) poisoning, in cystinuria, and in Wilson's disease. It is also prescribed as a palliative in the treatment of sclerosis and rheumatoid arthritis when other medications have failed.

■ CONTRAINDICATIONS: Known hypersensitivity to this drug or penicillamine-related aplastic anemia prohibits its use. It is not given during pregnancy or to patients who have kidney dysfunction.

■ ADVERSE EFFECTS: Among the more serious adverse reactions are fever, rashes, and blood dyscrasias. Severe bone marrow depression and immune disorders have been associated with long-term use of this drug. D-penicillamine is less toxic than the L form, and much of the reported toxicity is caused by the use of the L or DL forms.

penicillic acid /pen′isil′ik/, an antibiotic compound isolated from various species of the fungus *Penicillium.*

penicillin /pen′isil′in/, any one of a group of antibiotics derived from cultures of species of the fungus *Penicillium* or produced semisynthetically. Various penicillins administered orally or parenterally for the treatment of bacterial infections exert their antimicrobial action by inhibiting the biosynthesis of cell wall mucopeptides during active multiplication of the organisms. Penicillin G (benzylpenicillin), a widely used therapeutic agent for meningococcal, pneumococcal, and streptococcal infections, syphilis, and a number of other diseases, is rapidly absorbed when injected intramuscularly or subcutaneously, but it is inactivated by gastric acid and hydrolyzed by penicillinase produced by most strains of *Staphylococcus aureus.* Penicillin V (phenethicillin) is also active against gram-positive cocci, with the exception of penicillinase-producing staphylococci, and, because it is resistant to gastric acid, it is effective when administered orally. Penicillins resistant to the action of the enzyme penicillinase (beta-lactamase) are cloxacillin, dicloxacillin, methicillin, nafcillin, and oxacillin. Ampicillin, carbenicillin, and hetacillin are broad spectrum penicillins that are active against gram-negative organisms, including *Escherichia coli, Haemophilus influenzae, Neisseria gonorrhoeae, Proteus mirabilis,* and species of *Pseudomonas.* Hypersensitivity reactions are common in patients receiving penicillin and may appear in the absence of prior exposure to the drug, presumably because of unrecognized exposure to a food or other substance containing traces of the antibiotic. The most common hypersensitivity reactions are rash, fever, and bronchospasm, followed in frequency by vasculitis, serum sickness, and exfoliative dermatitis. Some patients develop severe erythema multiforme accompanied by headache, fever, arthralgia, and conjunctivitis (Stevens-Johnson syndrome); the most frequent cause of anaphylactic shock is an injection of penicillin.

penicillinase /pen′əsil′ənās/, an enzyme elaborated by certain bacteria, including many strains of staphylococci, that inactivates penicillin and thereby promotes resistance to the antibiotic. A purified preparation of penicillinase, derived from cultures of saprophytic, spore-forming *Bacillus cereus,* is used in the treatment of adverse reactions to penicillin. Also called **beta-lactamase.**

penicillinase-producing staphylococci, strains of staphylococcal organisms that elaborate the penicillin-inactivating enzyme penicillinase (beta-lactamase) and thereby resist the bacteriocidal action of the antibiotic.

penicillinase-resistant antibiotic, an antimicrobial agent that is not rendered inactive by penicillinase, an enzyme produced by certain bacteria, especially by strains of staphylococci. The semisynthetic penicillins, cloxacillin sodium, dicloxacillin sodium, methicillin sodium, nafcillin sodium, and oxacillin sodium, resist the action of penicillinase and are used in treating infections caused by staphylococci that elaborate the enzyme.

penicillinase-resistant penicillin, one of the semisynthetic penicillins derived from *Penicillium,* a genus of mold. Among these drugs are cloxacillin sodium, dicloxacillin sodium, methicillin sodium, nafcillin sodium, and oxacillin sodium. They are not inactivated by the enzyme penicillinase (beta-lactamase), which is produced by certain strains of staphylococci. These resistant antibiotics are used in treating infections caused by organisms that elaborate the enzyme.

penicillin G, an antibacterial.

■ INDICATIONS: It is prescribed in the treatment of many infections, including syphilis, rheumatic fever, and glomerulonephritis.

■ CONTRAINDICATIONS: Known hypersensitivity to this drug or to any penicillin prohibits its use.

■ ADVERSE EFFECTS: Among the more serious adverse effects are allergic reactions that vary from minor skin rashes to anaphylaxis. Nausea and diarrhea occur frequently.

penicillin G benzathine, a long-acting, depot form of penicillin.

■ INDICATIONS: It is used in the treatment of group A beta-hemolytic streptococcal pharyngitis, group A beta-hemolytic streptococcal pyoderma, and syphilitic infection occurring outside the central nervous system. It is given by deep intramuscular injection to achieve steady concentrations in the plasma and to slow systemic absorption from the repository in the muscle over a period of 12 hours to several days.

■ CONTRAINDICATIONS: Hypersensitivity to this drug or to other penicillins prohibits its use.

■ ADVERSE EFFECTS: The most serious adverse reaction is anaphylaxis. The most common side effects are maculopapular rash, urticarial rash, fever, bronchospasm, vasculitis, serum sickness, and exfoliative dermatitis.

penicillin phenoxymethyl. See **penicillin V.**

penicillin V, an antibacterial.

■ INDICATION: It is prescribed in the treatment of susceptible infections.

■ CONTRAINDICATIONS: Known hypersensitivity to this drug or to any penicillin prohibits its use.

■ ADVERSE EFFECTS: Among the more serious adverse reactions are anaphylaxis and urticaria.

penicilliosis /pen′isil′ē•ō′sis/, pulmonary infection caused by fungi of the genus *Penicillium.*

Penicillium /pen′isil′ē•əm/, a genus of fungi, some species of which have been tentatively linked to disease in humans. Penicillin G is obtained from *Penicillium chrysogenum* and *P. notatum.*

penile cancer /pē′nīl/, a rare malignancy of the penis occurring in uncircumcised men and associated with genital herpesvirus infection and poor personal hygiene. Smegma may be a causative factor, but the specific substance and mechanism are unknown. Leukoplakia or the flat-topped papules of balanitis xerotica obliterans may be premalignant lesions, and the velvety, red, painful papules of Queyrat's erythroplasia are penile squamous cell carcinoma in situ. Cancer of the penis usually presents as a local mass or a bleeding ulcer and metastasizes early in its course. Surgical treatment involves partial or total amputation of the penis and excision of inguinal nodes and adjacent tissue when necessary. Radiotherapy is often used preoperatively and postoperatively. Methotrexate or bleomycin may also be administered, especially in metastatic disease.

penis, the external reproductive organ of a man, homologous with the clitoris of a woman. It is attached with ligaments to the front and sides of the pubic arch and is composed of three cylindrical masses of cavernous tissue covered with skin. The corpora cavernosa penis surround a median mass called the corpus spongiosum penis, which contains the greater part of the urethra. The subcutaneous fascia of the penis is directly continuous with that of the scrotum, which contains the testes.

-pennate, a combining form meaning 'having feathers': *bipennate, pennate, unipennate.*

penniform /pen′ifôrm/, of or pertaining to the shape of a feather, especially the patterns of muscular fasciculi that correlate with the range of motion and the power of muscles. Penniform fasciculi converge on one side of certain tendons. Muscles with more fasciculi have greater power but less range of motion than muscles with fewer fasciculi. Compare **bipenniform, multipenniform.**

pent-, penta, a combining form meaning 'five': *pentaploid, pentose, pentoside.*

pentaerythritol tetranitrate /pen′tə•erith′rətol/, a coronary vasodilator.

■ INDICATION: It is prescribed for the relief of angina pectoris.

■ CONTRAINDICATIONS: Known hypersensitivity to this drug prohibits its use. It is contraindicated in severe anemia, cerebral hemorrhage, and head injury.

■ ADVERSE EFFECTS: Among the most serious reactions are hypotension and allergic reactions. Headaches and flushing also may occur.

pentamidine, an antiprotozoal that is available only from the Centers for Disease Control. It is sometimes prescribed in the treatment of trypanosomiasis and leishmaniasis, but, because of its extreme toxicity, other agents are usually prescribed.

pentaploid. See **polyploid.**

pentazocine hydrochloride /pentā′zəsēn/, an analgesic.

■ INDICATION: It is prescribed for the relief of moderate to severe pain.

■ CONTRAINDICATIONS: Known hypersensitivity to this drug prohibits its use. It is administered with caution to patients with head injury or those with a history of drug abuse and dependency.

■ ADVERSE EFFECTS: Nausea and dizziness commonly occur. Other minor problems include constipation, hallucinations, euphoria, and drowsiness. High dosage may cause respiratory and circulatory depression. This drug can precipitate acute withdrawal symptoms in narcotic-dependent individuals.

pentazocine lactate. See **pentazocine hydrochloride.**

Penthrane, a trademark for a general anesthetic (methoxyflurane).

Pentids, a trademark for an antibacterial (penicillin G potassium).

pentobarbital, a sedative and hypnotic.

■ INDICATIONS: It is prescribed as a preoperative sedative, in the treatment of insomnia, and in the control of acute convulsive disorders.

■ CONTRAINDICATIONS: Porphyria or known hypersensitivity to this drug or to other barbiturates prohibits its use. It is used with caution in patients having impaired respiratory or liver function or a history of dependence on sedative or hypnotic drugs.

■ ADVERSE EFFECTS: Among the more serious adverse reactions are respiratory or circulatory depression, paradoxical excitement, jaundice, or various hypersensitivity reactions. Nausea and hangover-like symptoms may be seen.

pentose, a monosaccharide made of carbohydrate molecules, each containing five carbon atoms. It is produ by the body and is elevated after the ingestion of certain fruits, as plums and cherries, and in certain rare diseases. It may be measured in the urine where its normal concentrations after 24-hour collection are 2 to 5 mg/kg.

pentosuria /pen′təso͞or′ē·ə/, a rare condition in which pentose is found in the urine. Essential or idiopathic pentosuria is caused by a genetically transmitted error of metabolism.

Pentothal Sodium, a trademark for a barbiturate drug (thiopental sodium), used as a general anesthetic and as an anesthetic adjuvant.

pentylenetetrazol, a central nervous system stimulant.

■ INDICATIONS: It is prescribed as an analeptic to stimulate the respiratory, vagal, and vasomotor centers of the brain, to counter the effects of depressants, and to increase cerebral blood flow, especially in geriatric patients.

■ CONTRAINDICATIONS: Epilepsy and low convulsive threshold prohibit its use.

■ ADVERSE EFFECTS: Among the more serious adverse reactions are convulsion, confusion, and anorexia.

Pen-Vee K, a trademark for an antibacterial (penicillin V potassium).

Peplau, Hildegard E., one of the pioneers in nursing theory development and a proponent in the 1950s of the concept that nursing is an interpersonal process. Borrowing heavily from the knowledge base of psychology, Peplau proposed hypotheses based on the premise of the interpersonal process. From the early work evolved a nursing goal to foster the assumption that humans value, strive for, and have a right to independence. In a 1952 work, Peplau wrote that the nurse-patient relationship occurs in phases during which the nurse functions as a resource person, a counselor, and a surrogate. The four phases of the process were listed as orientation, identification, exploitation, and resolution. Thus the nurse assists in orientation when the patient with a need seeks help. Identification assures the patient that the nurse can understand the patient's situation. Exploitation begins when the patient uses the services available. Resolution is marked as old needs are met and newer ones emerge.

Pepper syndrome, a neuroblastoma of the adrenal glands that usually metastasizes to the liver.

pep pills, *slang*. amphetamines.

peps-, pept-, a combining form meaning 'of or pertaining to digestion': *pepsin, pepsiniferous, pepsitensin*.

-pepsia, -pepsy, a combining form meaning a 'state of the digestion': *anapepsia, colodyspepsia, oligopepsia*.

...in/pep′sin/, an enzyme secreted in the stomach that ...zes the hydrolysis of protein. Preparations of pep...ined from pork and beef stomachs are sometimes ...igestive aids. See also **enzyme, hydrolysis.**

... /pəpsin′əjən/, a zymogenic substance se...ic and gastric chief cells and converted to ...in in an acidic environment, as in the ...rochloric acid produced in the stomach.

pept-. See **peps-.**

peptic, of or pertaining to digestion or to the enzymes and secretions essential to digestion.

-peptic, **1.** a combining form meaning 'pertaining to digestion': *apeptic, kolypeptic, proteopeptic*. **2.** a combining form meaning 'pertaining to a (specified) condition of digestion': *dyspeptic, eupeptic, hyperpeptic*.

peptic ulcer, a sharply circumscribed loss of the mucous membrane of the stomach or duodenum or of any other part of the GI system exposed to gastric juices containing acid and pepsin.

■ OBSERVATIONS: Peptic ulcers may be acute or chronic. Acute lesions are almost always multiple and superficial. They may be totally asymptomatic and usually heal without scarring or other sequelae. Chronic ulcers are true ulcers: They are deep, single, persistent, and symptomatic; the muscular coat of the wall of the organ does not regenerate; a scar forms, marking the site, and the mucosa may heal completely. Peptic ulcers are caused by a combination of poorly understood factors, including an excessive secretion of gastric acid, inadequate protection of the mucous membrane, stress, heredity, and the taking of certain drugs, including the corticosteroids, certain antihypertensives, and antiinflammatory medications. Characteristically, ulcers cause a gnawing pain in the epigastrium that does not radiate to the back, is not aggravated by a change in position, and has a temporal pattern that mimics the diurnal rhythm of gastric acidity.

■ INTERVENTION: Symptomatic relief is provided with antacids and frequent, small, bland meals. The underlying cause is treated if known. Cimetidine blocks the formation of gastric acid, but it is associated with serious adverse effects. Anticholinergic medications may slow gastric motility and diminish pain in some patients. Hemorrhage caused by perforation of the muscle and blood vessels may require surgical resection of the damaged area. The diagnosis and evaluation of peptic ulcers involves serial x-ray studies using a contrast medium, endoscopy, and analysis of the contents of the stomach and duodenum. A definitive diagnosis is important because the early signs of cancer of the stomach and duodenum are like those of peptic ulcers.

■ NURSING CONSIDERATIONS: The patient is reassured that in most cases the ulcers heal completely and that the pain may be controlled with simple measures. The nurse emphasizes the correct use of antacids and the other medications that have been prescribed. It is usually recommended that the patient eat frequent small meals consisting of foods known to be nonirritating. For many, but not all patients, fatty, highly spiced, heavy, or fibrous foods are likely to provoke pain. The use of tobacco and alcohol is discouraged.

peptide /pep′tīd/, a molecular chain compound composed of two or more amino acids joined by peptide bonds. See also **amino acid, polypeptide, protein.**

per-, **1.** a combining form meaning 'throughout, or completely': *peracephalus, perfuse, permeable*. **2.** a combining form meaning 'a large amount (in chemical terms)' or to designate a combination of an element in its highest valence: *peracetate, peracid, perhydride.*

perceived severity, (in health belief model) a person's perception of the seriousness of the consequences of contracting a disease. Compare **perceived susceptibility.**

perceived susceptibility, (in health belief model) a person's perception of the likelihood of contracting a disease. Compare **perceived severity.**

percentage depth dose, (in radiotherapy) the amount of radiation delivered at a specified dose, expressed as a percentage of the skin dose.

percent systole, an amount of time of each heartbeat that is devoted to the ejection of blood from the ventricle.

percephalus, *pl.* **percephali,** a fetus or individual with a malformed head.

percept /pur′sept/, the mental impression of an object that is perceived through the use of the senses.

perception, **1.** the conscious recognition and interpretation of sensory stimuli through unconscious associations, especially memory, that serve as a basis for understanding, learning, and knowing or for the motivation of a particular action or reaction. **2.** the end result or product of the act of perceiving. Kinds of perception include **depth perception, extrasensory perception, facial perception,** and **stereognostic perception.** **–perceptive, perceptual,** *adj.*

perceptivity, the ability to receive sense impressions; perceptiveness.

perceptual constancy, in Gestalt psychology, the phenomenon in which an object is seen in the same way under varying circumstances.

perceptual defect, any of a broad group of disorders or dysfunctions of the central nervous system that interfere with the conscious mental recognition of sensory stimuli. Such conditions are caused by lesions at specific sites in the cerebral cortex that may result from any illness or trauma affecting the brain at any age or stage of development. Impairment of mental activity, cognitive processes, and emotional responses may be diffuse, as occurs in organic mental disorders, as the psychoses, delirium, and dementia, and in attention deficit disorder, or they may be manifested focally, as in aphasia, apraxia, epilepsy, disorders of memory, cerebrovascular disorders, and various intercranial neoplasms.

perceptual deprivation, the absence of or decrease in meaningful groupings of stimuli, which may result from a constant background noise or constant inadequate illumination.

perceptual monotony, a mental state characterized by a lack of variety in the normal pattern of everyday stimuli.

perchloromethane. See **carbon tetrachloride.**

Percodan, a trademark for a central nervous system, fixed-combination drug containing narcotic analgesics (oxycodone hydrochloride and oxycodone terephthalate).

Percogesic, a trademark for a respiratory, fixed-combination drug containing an antihistaminic (phenyltoloxamine citrate) and an analgesic (acetaminophen).

percolation, **1.** the act of filtering any liquid through a porous medium. **2.** (in pharmocology) the removal of the soluble parts of a crude drug by passing a liquid solvent through it.

Percorten Acetate, a trademark for an adrenocortical steroid (desoxycorticosterone acetate).

percussion, a technique in physical examination used to evaluate the size, borders, and consistency of some of the internal organs and to discover the presence and evaluate the amount of fluid in a cavity of the body. **Immediate** or **direct percussion** refers to percussion performed by striking the fingers directly on the body surface; **indirect, mediate,** or **finger percussion** involves striking a finger of one hand on a finger of the other hand as it is placed over the organ. See also **cupping and vibrating, percussor, pleximeter.** **–percuss,** *v.,* **percussable,** *adj.*

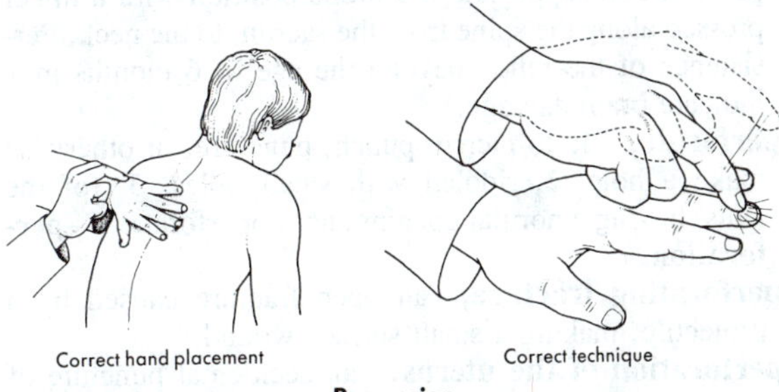

Percussion

percussor, a small, hammerlike diagnostic tool having a rubber head that is used to tap the body lightly in percussion. Also called **plexor.** See also **percussion.**

percutaneous /pur′kyo͞otā′nē·əs/, performed through the skin, such as a biopsy or the aspiration of fluid from a space below the skin using a needle, catheter, and syringe or the instillation of a fluid in a cavity or space by similar means.

percutaneous catheter placement, (in arteriography) the technique in which an intracatheter is introduced through the skin into an artery and placed at the site or structure to be studied. The puncture site is infiltrated with a local anesthetic. A special needle is inserted into the artery, and a long, flexible spring guide is passed through the needle for approximately 15 cm. The needle is then removed, the catheter is advanced to the desired position, and the guide is withdrawn. Selective angiography and other diagnostic procedures are performed using this technique. The catheter is withdrawn at the end of the procedure.

percutaneous transhepatic cholangiography, an x-ray examination of the bile duct, used for detecting obstructions. It is performed after injecting a contrast medium through the liver into the duct.

percutaneous transluminal coronary angioplasty (PTCA), a technique in the treatment of atherosclerotic coronary heart disease and angina pectoris in which one or more plaques in the arteries of the heart are flattened against the arterial walls, resulting in improved circulation. The procedure involves threading a catheter through the vessel to the atherosclerotic plaque and inflating and deflating a small balloon at the tip of the catheter several times, then removing the catheter. The procedure is performed under x-ray or ultrasonic visualization. When it is successful, the plaques remain compressed and the symptoms of heart disease, including the pain of angina, are decreased. The alternative to this treatment is coronary bypass surgery, which is more expensive and dangerous and requires longer hospitalization.

per diem rate /pər dē′əm, dī′əm/, an established rate of payment for hospital services determined by dividing the total cost of providing routine inpatient services for a given period by the total number of inpatient days of care during the period.

Perez reflex /pərez′, per′ez/, the normal response of an infant to cry, flex the limbs, and elevate the head and pelvis when supported in a prone position with a finger pressed along the spine from the sacrum to the neck. Persistence of the reflex beyond the age of 6 months may indicate brain damage.

perforate, **1.** to pierce, punch, puncture, or otherwise make a hole. **2.** riddled with small holes. **3.** (of the anus) having a normal opening; not imperforate. –**perforation,** *n.*

perforating fracture, an open fracture caused by a projectile, making a small surface wound.

perforation of the uterus, an accidental puncture of the uterus, as may occur with a curet or by an intrauterine contraceptive device.

perfusion, **1.** the passage of a fluid through a specific organ or an area of the body. **2.** a therapeutic measure whereby a drug intended for an isolated part of the body is introduced via the bloodstream.

perfusion lung scan, a radiographic examination of the lungs and their function, performed after an intravenous injection of a contrast medium, as radioactive albumin, and used to aid in the diagnosis of pulmonary embolism.

perfusion rate, the rate of blood flow through the capillaries per unit mass of tissue, expressed in ml/minute per 100 g.

perfusion scan. See **lung scan.**

perfusion technologist, a person who, under the supervision of a physician, operates a heart-lung machine used for cardiopulmonary bypass during surgery.

Pergonal, a trademark for human menopausal gonadotropin used to treat anovulation and infertility.

peri-, a combining form meaning 'around': *periaxial, pericardial, pericolitis.*

Periactin Hydrochloride, a trademark for an antihistaminic and antipruritic (cyproheptadine hydrochloride).

perianal abscess /per′ē·ā′nəl/, a focal, purulent, subcutaneous infection in the region of the anus. Treatment includes hot soaks, antibiotics, and, possibly, incision and drainage. If a rectal fistula or perianal space is found to be the cause of recurrent perianal abscesses, surgical excision is usually performed.

periapical /per′ē·ap′ikəl, per′ē·ā′pikəl/, of or pertaining to the tissues around the apex of a tooth, including the periodontal membrane and the alveolar bone.

periapical abscess, an infection around the root of a tooth, usually a result of spread from dental caries. The abscess may extend into nearby bone, causing osteomyelitis, or, more often, it may spread to soft tissues, causing cellulitis and a swollen face, or it may perforate into the oral cavity or maxillary sinus. There may be associated fever, malaise, and nausea. Treatment includes drilling into the pulp of the tooth to establish drainage and relieve pain, followed by antibiotics and later root canal therapy or tooth extraction.

periapical cyst. See **radicular cyst.**

periapical fibroma, a mass of benign connective tissue that may form at the apex of a tooth with normal pulp.

periapical infection, infection surrounding the root of a tooth, often accompanied by toothache.

periarteritis /per′ē·är′tərī′tis/, an inflammatory condition of the outer coat of one or more arteries and the tissue surrounding the vessel. Kinds of periarteritis are **periarteritis nodosa** and **syphilitic periarteritis.**

periarteritis gummosa. See **syphilitic periarteritis.**

periarteritis nodosa, a progressive, polymorphic disease of the connective tissue that is characterized by numerous large and palpable or visible nodules in clusters along segments of middle-sized arteries, particularly near points of bifurcation. This process causes occlusion of the vessel, resulting in regional ischemia, hemorrhage, necrosis, and pain. The early signs of the disease include tachycardia, fever, weight loss, and pain in the viscera. Kidney, lung, and intestinal involvement are common. Other systems and organs of the body may also be affected. Periarteritis nodosa is treated with corticosteroid medication and sometimes with cytotoxic drugs. The rate of survival 4 years after diagnosis is approximately 50%.

pericardial artery, one of several small vessels branching from the thoracic aorta, supplying the dorsal surface of the pericardium.

pericardial tamponade. See **cardiac tamponade.**

pericardiocentesis /per′ikär′dē·ōsintē′sis/, a procedure for drawing fluid in the pericardial space between the serous membranes by surgical puncture and aspiration of the pericardial sac. Also called **pericardicentesis.**

pericarditis /per′ikärdī′tis/, an inflammation of the pericardium associated with trauma, malignant neoplastic disease, infection, uremia, myocardial infarction, collagen disease, or idiopathic causes.

■ OBSERVATIONS: Two stages are observed if treatment in the first stage does not halt progress of the condition to the extremely grave second stage. The first stage is characterized by fever, substernal chest pain that radiates to the shoulder or neck, dyspnea, and a dry, nonproductive cough. On examination a rapid and forcible pulse, a pericardial friction rub, and a muffled heartbeat over the apex are noted. The patient becomes increasingly anxious, tired, and orthopneic. During the second stage, a serofibrinous effusion develops within the pericardium, restricting cardiac activity; the heart sounds become muffled, weak, and distant on auscultation. A bulge is visible on the chest over the precordial area. If the effusion is purulent, caused by bacterial infection, a high fever, sweat, chills, and prostration also occur.

■ INTERVENTION: The person is kept in bed, and the head of the bed is elevated 45 degrees to decrease dyspnea. Hypothermia treatment may be necessary to reduce the temperature. An antibiotic or antifungal and analgesic may be ordered. Oxygen and parenteral fluids are usually given, vital signs are evaluated, and the chest is auscultated frequently. Pericardiocentesis or percardiotomy may be performed to remove accumulated fluid or to make a diagnosis.

■ NURSING CONSIDERATIONS: Emotional support of a patient being treated for pericarditis requires remaining with the person if anxiety is present and explaining all procedures thoroughly. During recovery, rest periods are planned and the person is urged to avoid fatigue and exposure to upper respiratory infections. The patient is told that symptoms of recurrence, including a fever, chest pain, and dyspnea, are to be reported.

pericardium /per′ikär′dē•əm/, *pl.* **pericardia,** a fibroserous sac that surrounds the heart and the roots of the great vessels. It consists of the serous pericardium and the fibrous pericardium. The serous pericardium consists of the parietal layer, which lines the inside of the fibrous pericardium, and the visceral layer, which adheres to the surface of the heart. Between the two layers is the pericardial space containing a few drops of pericardial fluid, which lubricates opposing surfaces of the space and allows the heart to move easily during contraction. Injury or disease may cause fluid to exude into the space, causing a wide separation between the heart and the outer pericardium. The fibrous pericardium, which constitutes the outermost sac and is composed of tough, white fibrous tissue lined by the parietal layer of the serous pericardium, fits loosely around the heart and attaches to large blood vessels emerging from the top of the heart but not to the heart itself. It is relatively inelastic and protects the heart and the serous membranes. If pericardial fluid or pus accumulates in the pericardial space, the fibrous pericardium cannot stretch, causing a rapid increase of pressure around the heart. –**pericardial,** *adj.*

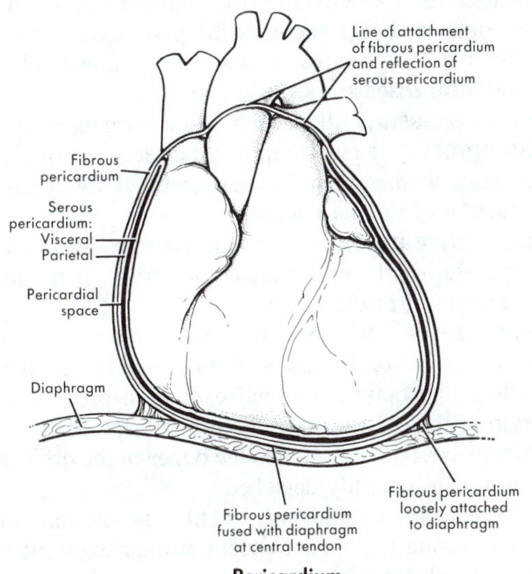

Pericardium

pericholangitis /per′əkōlanjī′tis/, an inflammatory condition of the tissues surrounding the bile ducts in the liver. Pericholangitis is a complication of ulcerative colitis and is characterized by a recurrent fever, chills, jaundice, and, possibly, portal hypertension. Treatment of the ulcerative colitis has little effect on the liver disease. See also **ulcerative colitis.**

peridural anesthesia. See **epidural anesthesia.**

perifolliculitis /per′ēfolik′yŏŏlī′tis/, inflammation of the tissue surrounding a hair follicle. Compare **folliculitis.**

perikaryon /per′iker′ē•on/, the cytoplasm of a cell body exclusive of the nucleus and any processes, specifically the cell body of a neuron. –**perikaryontic,** *adj.*

perilymph /per′ilimf/, the clear fluid separating the osseous labyrinth from the membranous labyrinth in the internal ear. Compare **endolymph.**

perimetrium /per′imē′trē•əm/, the serous membrane enveloping the uterus.

perinatal /per′inā′təl/, of or pertaining to the time and process of giving birth or being born.

perinatal death, **1.** the death of a fetus weighing more than 1000 g at 28 or more weeks of gestation. **2.** the death of an infant between birth and the end of the neonatal period.

perinatal mortality, the statistic rate of fetal and infant death, including stillbirths, from 28 weeks of gestation to the end of the neonatal period of 4 weeks after birth. Perinatal mortality is usually expressed as the number of deaths per 1000 live births in a specific geographic area or program, in a given period of time.

perinatal period, a period extending approximately from the twenty-eighth week of gestation to the twenty-eighth day after birth.

perinatal physiology, the physiology of the process of giving birth or being born.

perinatologist, a physician who specializes in the practice of perinatology.

perinatology, a branch of medicine concerned with the study of the anatomy and physiology of the mother and her unborn and newborn infant and with the diagnosis and treatment of disorders occurring in them during pregnancy, childbirth, and the puerperium. –**perinatologic, perinatological,** *adj.*

perineal care, a cleansing procedure prescribed for cleansing the perineum after various obstetric and gynecologic procedures. Sterile or clean perineal care may be prescribed. See also **postpartum perineal care.**

▪ METHOD: In the sterile procedure, the cleansing strokes always move from the vulva toward the anus and from the midline out. After each stroke, the disposable washcloth or pledget is discarded, and a new one is used for the next stroke. In sterile perineal care, a sterile basin, gloves, forceps, pledgets, and pitcher or measure containing solution are used. The draped patient is assisted into position on her back with a bedpan or on a disposable pad beneath her buttocks, and 200 to 300 ml of solution are poured over the vulva. Then pledgets moistened with the solution are used to cleanse the area more thoroughly. The pledgets are held with sterile forceps or a sterile gloved hand. The area is dried using sterile pledgets and the bedpan is removed. The patient then changes position and lies on her side for cleansing and drying of the posterior area; strokes should always move away from the perineal area. In providing clean perineal care, disposable washcloths, soap, and a basin or a squeeze bottle of warm water are used. A fresh, disposable washcloth is used for each stroke. The strokes are always from anterior to posterior. Soap may be used. A fresh pad or cloth is used to remove the soap and for each drying stroke. The patient then rolls to one side, and the posterior area is cleansed and dried in the same way.

▪ NURSING ORDERS: Perineal care is given at prescribed intervals and after urination and defecation.

▪ OUTCOME CRITERIA: Sterile and clean perineal care are practiced to remove secretions or dried blood from a wound and to avoid contaminating the urethral and vaginal areas or perineal wounds with fecal matter or urine.

perineorrhaphy /per′inē•ôr′əfē/, a surgical procedure in which an incision, tear, or defect in the perineum is repaired by suturing.

perineotomy /per′inē•ot′əmē/, a surgical incision into the perineum. See also **episiotomy.**

perineum /per′inē′əm/, the part of the body situated dorsal to the pubic arch and the arcuate ligaments, ventral to the tip of the coccyx, and lateral to the inferior rami of the pubis and the ischium and the sacrotuberus ligaments. The perineum supports and surrounds the distal portions of the urogenital and GI tracts of the body. In the female, the central fibrous perineal body is larger than in the male, and the bulbospongiosus, which is a sphincter around the orifice of the vagina and a cover over the clitoris, does not exist in the male perineum. In men and women, the muscles are innervated by the perineal branch of the pudendal nerve. **–perineal,** *adj.*

perinodal fibers, the atrial fibers surrounding the sinoatrial node.

period, *nontechnical.* menses.

periodic, (of an event or phenomenon) recurring at regular or irregular intervals. **–peridocity,** *n.*

periodic apnea of the newborn, a normal condition in the full-term newborn infant characterized by an irregular pattern of rapid breathing followed by a brief period of apnea, usually associated with rapid eye movement (REM) sleep. Apnea in the newborn not associated with REM sleep or with periodic breathing is ominous because it is symptomatic of intracranial bleeding, seizure activity, infection, pneumonia, hypoglycemia, drug depression, or various cardiac defects. See also **sudden infant death syndrome.**

periodic breathing. See **Cheyne-Stokes respiration.**

periodic deep inspiration, (in respiratory therapy) periodic deep forced inspiration of compressed gas or air in controlled ventilation. Many ventilators can be set to provide a selected number of deep respirations each hour. The process helps prevent atelectasis. Also called **sigh.**

periodic mania, *obsolete.* a mood disorder in which successive attacks of mania of various duration occur at regular intervals. See also **mania.**

periodontal /per′ē•ōdon′təl/, of or pertaining to the area around a tooth, as the peridontium.

periodontal cyst, an epithelium-lined sac that contains fluid, most often occurring at the apex of a pulp-involved tooth. Periodontal cysts that occur lateral to a tooth root are less common.

periodontal disease, disease of the tissues around a tooth, as an inflammation of the periodontal membrane or periodontal ligament.

periodontal ligament (PDL), the fibrous tissue that attaches the teeth to the alveoli, composed of many bundles of collagenous tissue arranged in groups between which is loose connective tissue interwoven with blood vessels, lymph vessels, and nerves. The periodontal ligament invests and supports the teeth.

periodontics, a branch of dentistry concerned with the diagnosis, treatment, and prevention of diseases of the periodontium. Also called **periodontia. –periodontic, periodontal,** *adj.*

periodontist, a dentist who specializes in periodontics.

periodontitis /per′ē•ōdontī′tis/, inflammation of the periodontium, which includes the periodontal ligament, the gingiva, and the alveolar bone. See also **periodontal, periodontal disease, periodontics.**

periodontoclasia, the loosening of permanent teeth.

periodontosis, a rare disease that affects young people, especially women, and is characterized by idiopathic destruction of the periodontium

perioperative nursing, nursing care provided surgery patients during the entire inpatient period, from admission to date of discharge.

periorbita /per′ē•ôr′bitə/, the periosteum of the orbit of the eye. It is continuous with the dura mater and the sheath of the optic nerve and extends a process at the margin of the orbit to form the orbital septum. The periorbita is loosely connected to the bones of the orbit, from which it can be easily detached.

periosteum /per′ē•os′tē•əm/, a fibrous vascular membrane covering the bones, except at their extremities. It consists of an outer layer of collagenous tissue containing a few fat cells and an inner layer of fine elastic fibers. Periosteum is permeated with the nerves and blood vessels that innervate and nourish underlying bone. The membrane is thick and markedly vascular over young bones but thinner and less vascular in later life. Bones that lose periosteum through injury or disease usually scale or die.

periostitis, inflammation of the periostium. The condition is caused by chronic or acute infection or trauma and is characterized by tenderness and swelling of the bone affected, pain, fever, and chills. In severe cases blood or an albuminous serous exudate forms under the membrane. In syphilitic infections, periostitis may occur as an early symptom.

peripheral, of or pertaining to the outside, surface, or surrounding area of an organ or other structure.

peripheral acrocyanosis of the newborn, a normal, transient condition of the newborn, characterized by pale cyanotic discoloration of the hands and feet, especially the fingers and toes. The blueness fades as the baby begins to breathe easily but returns if the baby is allowed to get chilled.

peripheral arteriovenography, an x-ray examination of the blood vessels in the peripheral parts of the body, as the arms and legs, after the injection of a contrast medium into these vessels.

peripheral device, any hardware device aside from the central processing unit, as a printer, CRT, or drive.

peripheral embolic phenomena, the clinical signs and symptoms of an embolus in a peripheral vessel.

peripheral glioma. See **schwannoma.**

peripheral nervous system, the motor and sensory nerves and ganglia outside the brain and spinal cord. The system consists of 12 pairs of cranial nerves, 31 pairs of spinal nerves, and their various branches in body organs. Sensory, or afferent, peripheral nerves transmitting information to the central nervous system and motor, or efferent, peripheral nerves carrying impulses from the brain usually travel together but separate at the cord level into a posterior sensory root and an anterior motor root. Fibers innervating the body wall are designated somatic; those supplying internal organs are termed visceral. The autonomic system includes the peripheral nerves involved in regulating cardiovascular, respiratory, endocrine, and other automatic body functions. Nerves in the sympathetic or thoracolumbar division of the autonomic system secrete norepinephrine and cause peripheral vasoconstriction, cardiac acceleration, coronary artery dilatation, bronchodilatation, and inhibition of peristalsis. Parasympathetic nerves, which constitute the craniosacral division of the autonomic system, secrete acetylcholine, cause peripheral vasodilatation, cardiac inhibition, and bronchoconstriction, and stimulate peristalsis. Injury to a peripheral nerve results in loss of movement and sensation in the area innervated distal to the lesion.

peripheral neuropathy, any functional or organic disorder of the peripheral nervous system. A kind of peripheral neuropathy is paresthesia.

peripheral odontogenic fibroma, a fibrous connective tissue tumor associated with the gingival margin and believed to originate from the periodontium. It is a localized form of fibromatosis gingivae and commonly contains areas of calcification.

peripheral plasma cell myeloma. See **plasmacytoma.**

peripheral polyneuritis, peripheral polyneuropathy. See **multiple peripheral neuritis.**

peripheral resistance, a resistance to the flow of blood that is determined by the tone of the vascular musculature and the diameter of the blood vessels.

peripheral vascular disease, any abnormal condition that affects the blood vessels outside the heart and the lymphatic vessels. Different kinds and degrees of peripheral vascular disease are characterized by a variety of signs and symptoms, as numbness, pain, pallor, elevated blood pressure, and impaired arterial pulsations. Various causative factors include obesity, cigarette smoking, stress, sedentary occupations, and numerous metabolic disorders. Peripheral vascular disease in association with bacterial endocarditis may involve emboli in terminal arterioles and produce gangrenous infarctions of various distal parts of the body, as the tip of the nose, the pinna of the ear, the fingers, and the toes. Large emboli may occlude peripheral vessels and cause atherosclerotic occlusive disease. Treatment of severe cases may require amputation of gangrenous body parts. Less severe peripheral vascular problems may be treated by eliminating causative factors, especially cigarette smoking, and by the administration of various drugs, as salicylates and anticoagulants. Some kinds of peripheral vascular disease are **arteriosclerosis** and **atherosclerosis.**

peripheral vision, a capacity to see objects that reflect light waves falling on areas of the retina distant from the macula.

peristalsis /per′istôl′sis, -stal′sis/, the coordinated, rhythmic, serial contraction of smooth muscle that forces food through the digestive tract, bile through the bile duct, and urine through the ureters.

peritoneal cavity /per′itōnē′əl/, the potential space between the parietal and the visceral layers of the peritoneum. Normally, the two layers are in contact. The peritoneal cavity is divided by a narrow constriction into a greater sac and a lesser sac. The greater sac is the peritoneal cavity, and the lesser sac is the omental bursa. The omental bursa is associated with the dorsal surface of the stomach and the surrounding structures. See also **epiploic foramen.**

peritoneal dialysis, a dialysis procedure performed to correct an imbalance of fluid or of electrolytes in the blood or to remove toxins, drugs, or other wastes normally excreted by the kidney. The peritoneum is used as a diffusible membrane. Peritoneal dialysis may be performed nightly for chronically ill children while they sleep and may also be carried out regularly at home. It is contraindicated in patients with extensive intraabdominal adhesions, localized peritoneal infection, and gangrenous or perforated bowels, although peritonitis may itself sometimes be treated by peritoneal lavage and antibiotics, using peritoneal dialysis.

■ METHOD: Under local anesthesia, a many-eyed catheter is sutured in place and a sterile dressing is applied. The catheter is connected to the inflow and outflow tubing with a "Y" connector, and the air in the tubing is displaced by the dialysate to avoid introducing air into the peritoneal cavity. The amount and the kind of dialysate and the length of time for each exchange cycle vary with the age, size, and condition of the patient. There are three phases in each cycle. During inflow, the dialysate is introduced into the peritoneal cavity. During equilibration, the dialysate remains in the peritoneal cavity; by means of osmosis, diffusion, and filtration, the needed electrolytes pass to the bloodstream via the vascular peritoneum to the blood vessels of the abdominal cavity, and the waste products pass from the blood vessels through the vascular peritoneum into the dialysate. During the third phase, called outflow, the dialysate is allowed to drain from the peritoneal cavity by gravity.

■ NURSING ORDERS: The fluid is warmed to body temperature before instillation, and heparin antibiotics or other additives may be added to the dialysate. The patient's fluid balance, respirations, pulse, blood pressure, temperature, and mental state are frequently evaluated, and blood glucose and electrolytes are tested regularly. The amount of fluid instilled and the amount and character of the fluid drained are noted. Bacteriologic cultures of the drainage are performed regularly, and a low-sodium, high-carbohydrate, high-fat, 20 to 40 g protein diet is usually given. Medication for pain may be necessary. The need for dialysis and the techniques, dangers, and advantages of peritoneal dialysis are explained to the patient and the patient's family.

■ OUTCOME CRITERIA: Peritoneal dialysis may result in several complications, including perforation of the bowel, peritonitis, atelectasis, pneumonia, pulmonary edema, hyperglycemia, hypovolemia, hypervolemia, and adhesions. Peritonitis, the most common problem, is usually caused by failure to use aseptic technique and is characterized by fever, cloudy dialysate, leukocytosis, and abdominal discomfort. Dialysis may usually be continued while the infection is treated with antibiotics, which are given systemically or intraperitoneally. Atelectasis and pneumonia may result from compression of the thoracic cavity, with decreased respiratory excursion and blood flow to the bases of the lungs caused by an excessive volume of dialysate in the peritoneal cavity. Dyspnea, tachypnea, rales, and tachycardia require reevaluation of the amount of dialysate, the raising of the head of the bed, and respiratory therapy to prevent atelectasis and pneumonia. Because patients with diabetes are at risk of developing hyperglycemia, serum and urine glucose levels are monitored, and, if necessary, sorbitol may be substituted for glucose in the dialsyate. If dialysate fluid is retained in the peritoneal cavity, hypervolemia may occur, predisposing the patient to pulmonary edema and congestive failure. If the dialysate is removed too rapidly or if the dialysate used is a hypotonic glucose solution, hypovolemia may result. Adhesions often develop because of local irritation to the surrounding tissues caused by the intraperitoneal catheter.

peritoneal dialysis solution, a solution of electrolytes and other substances that is introduced into the peritoneum to remove toxic substances from the body.

peritoneoscope. See **laparoscope.**

peritoneum /per′itənē′əm/, an extensive serous membrane that covers the entire abdominal wall of the body and is reflected over the contained viscera. It is divided into the parietal peritoneum and the visceral peritoneum. In men, the peritoneum is a closed membranous sac. In women, it is perforated by the free ends of the uterine tubes. The free surface of the peritoneum is smooth mesothelium, lubricated by serous fluid that permits the viscera to glide easily against the abdominal wall and against one another. The mesentery of the peritoneum fans out from the main membrane to suspend the small intestine. Other parts of the peritoneum are the transverse mesocolon, the greater omentum, and the lesser omentum. –**peritoneal,** *adj.*

peritonitis /per′itənī′tis/, an inflammation of the peritoneum produced by bacteria or irritating substances introduced into the abdominal cavity by a penetrating wound or perforation of an organ in the GI tract or the reproductive tract. Peritonitis is caused most commonly by rupture of the vermiform appendix but also occurs after perforations of intestinal diverticuli, peptic ulcers, gangrenous gallbladders, gangrenous obstructions of the small bowel, or incarcerated hernias, as well as ruptures of the spleen, liver, ovarian cyst, or fallopian tube, especially in ectopic pregnancy. In some cases peritonitis is secondary to the release of pancreatic enzyme, bile, or digestive juices of the upper GI tract, and there are reports of postoperative peritonitis caused by cornstarch used to powder surgical gloves. The bacteria most frequently identified as causative agents in peritonitis are *Escherichia coli, Bacteroides, Fusobacterium,* and anaerobic and aerobic streptococci; *Klebsiella* and *Proteus* are uncommon, and *Clostridium, Staphylococcus aureus,* and gonococci are rare. Pneumococci occasionally found in peritonitis in girls are thought to enter the abdominal cavity via the vagina and fallopian tubes. See also **appendectomy, appendicitis.**

■ OBSERVATIONS: Characteristic signs and symptoms of peritonitis include abdominal distention, rigidity and pain, rebound tenderness, decreased or absent bowel sounds, nausea, vomiting, and tachycardia. The patient has chills and fever, breathes rapidly and shallowly, is anxious, dehydrated, and unable to defecate, and may vomit fecal material. Leukocytosis, an electrolyte imbalance, and hypovolemia are usually present, and shock and heart failure may ensue.

■ INTERVENTION: The patient is placed in bed in a semi-Fowler's position with the knees flexed to facilitate breathing and localize pus in the lower abdomen. Oxygen, parenteral fluids with electrolytes, large doses of antibiotics, and emetics are administered as ordered. A nasogastric or nasointestinal tube is passed for intermittent suctioning; an indwelling catheter is inserted, and a rectal tube may be used. Measurements are made of the intake and output of fluids, and the character, color, odor, and amount of drainage are noted. Blood pressure, apical pulse, and respiration are checked every 1 to 2 hours; at similar intervals the patient is turned and instructed in coughing and deep breathing. Rectal temperature, bowel sounds, and abdominal distention are checked every 2 to 4 hours. Pain is controlled with analgesia, and the dehydrated patient, whose lips tend to be dry and cracked, receives frequent mouth care. Paracentesis may be performed to withdraw ascitic fluid that is turbid or purulent in pyogenic peritonitis. Repair of the perforation or rupture responsible for the infection may be indicated, but surgery is usually delayed until the patient is stabilized. Patients who respond to antibiotic therapy receive a liquid diet when the nasogastric tube is removed and bowel sounds return and gradually progress to a diet appropriate for the disorder that caused the peritonitis.

■ NURSING CONSIDERATIONS: The patient acutely ill with peritonitis is usually very apprehensive and needs constant care.

peritonsillar abscess, an infection of tissue between the tonsil and pharynx, usually after acute follicular tonsillitis. The symptoms include dysphagia, pain radiating to the ear, and fever. Redness and swelling of the tonsil and adjacent soft palate are present. Treatment includes penicillin, warm saline irrigation, incision and drainage with suction if there is no spontaneous rupture of the abscess, and, sometimes, tonsillectomy. Also called **quinsy.** Compare **parapharyngeal abscess, retropharyngeal abscess.** See also **tonsillitis.**

Peritrate, a trademark for a vasodilator (pentaerythritol tetranitrate).

periungual /per′ē·ung′gwəl/, of or pertaining to the area around the fingernails or the toenails.

perivascular goiter /per′ivas′kyo͞olər/, an enlargement of the thyroid gland surrounding a large blood vessel.

perivitelline /per′ivital′īn/, surrounding the vitellus or yolk mass.

perivitelline space, the space between the ovum and the zona pellucida of mammals into which the polar bodies are released at the time of maturation. In some animals it is a fluid-filled space that separates the fertilization membrane from the vitelline membrane surrounding the ovum after the penetration of the spermatozoon.

perlèche. See **cheilosis.**

permanent dentition, the eruption of the 32 permanent teeth, beginning with the appearance of the first permanent molars at about 6 years of age. The process is completed by 12 or 13 years of age except for the four wisdom teeth, which usually do not erupt until 18 to 25 years of age, or later. Also called **secondary dentition.** Compare **deciduous dentition.** See also **tooth.**

permanent tooth, one of the set of 32 teeth that appear during and after childhood and usually last until old age. In each jaw they include four incisors, two canines, four premolars, and six molars. They are divided into the permanent teeth, which replace the 20 deciduous teeth of infancy, and the superadded teeth, which include 12 molars, three on each side of the upper and lower jaws. The permanent teeth start to develop in the ninth week of fetal life with the thickening of the epithelium along the line of the future jaw. They develop from the embryonic dental lamina and dental germ tissue. As the 10 permanent teeth develop in the fetus, they recede into the substance of the gum behind the deciduous teeth. The permanent teeth start to calcify soon after birth, the teeth in the lower jaw proceeding somewhat faster than those in the upper jaw. The permanent first molar in the lower jaw calcifies just after birth; the permanent incisors and the canines, approximately 6 months later; the premolars during the second year; the second molar at about the end of the second year; and the third molar at about the twelfth year. The permanent teeth erupt first in the lower jaw; the first molars in about the sixth year; the two central incisors about the seventh year; the two lateral incisors about the eighth year; the first premolars about the ninth year; the second premolars about the tenth year; the canines between the eleventh and the twelfth years; the second molars between the twelfth and the thirteenth years; the third molars between the seventeenth and the twenty-fifth years. The eruption of each corresponding permanent tooth in the upper jaw lags only slightly behind that of the corresponding permanent tooth in the lower jaw. The third molars in many people are badly oriented or so deeply buried in bone that they must be surgically removed. In some individuals, one or all four of the third molars may not develop completely. Compare **deciduous tooth.** See also **tooth.**

Permapen, a trademark for an antibacterial (penicillin G benzathine).

permeable, a condition of being pervious so that fluids and certain other substances can pass through, as a permeable membrane. See also **osmosis.**

permissible dose, (in radiotherapy) the amount of radiation that may be received by an individual in a specified period of time with the expectation of no significantly harmful results.

Permitil, a trademark for a tranquilizer (fluphenazine hydrochloride).

pernicious anemia /pərnish′əs/, a progressive, megaloblastic, macrocytic anemia, affecting mainly older people, that results from a lack of intrinsic factor essential for the absorption of caynocobalamin. The maturation of red blood cells in bone marrow becomes disordered, the posterior and lateral columns of the spinal cord deteriorate, the white blood cell count is reduced, and the polymorphonuclear leukocytes become multilobed. Extreme weakness, numbness and tingling in the extremities, fever, pallor, anorexia, and loss of weight may occur. The condition is usually treated with cayanocobalamin injection and with folic acid and iron therapy. See also **atrophic gastritis, intrinsic factor, nutritional anemia.**

pernio. See **chilblain.**

pero-, a combining form meaning 'maimed or deformed': *perobrachius, perodactylus, peromelus*.

perobrachius /pē′rōbrā′kē·əs/, a fetus or individual with deformed arms.

perochirus /pē′rōkī′rəs/, a fetus or individual with malformed hands.

perocormus. See **perosomus.**

perodactylus /pē′rōdak′tiləs/, a fetus or an individual with a deformity of the fingers or the toes, especially the absence of one or more digits.

perodactyly /pē′rōdak′tilē/, a congenital anomaly characterized by a deformity of the digits, primarily the complete or partial absence of one or more of the fingers or toes. Also called **perodactylia.**

peromelia /pē′rōmē′lyə/, a congenital anomaly characterized by the malformation of one or more of the limbs. Also called **peromely** /pərom′əlē/. **–peromelus,** *n.*

peroneal /per′ənē′əl/, of or pertaining to the outer part of the leg, over the fibula and the peroneal nerve.

peroneal muscular atrophy, an abnormal condition characterized by the symmetric weakening or atrophy of the foot and the ankle muscles and by hammertoes. This disease is a dominantly inherited condition and occurs in a hypertrophic neuropathy form or in a neuronal form. The hypertrophic neuropathy form results in demyelination of nerve fibers and characteristic onion bulb formations. Affected individuals usually have high plantar arches and an awkward gait, caused by weak ankle muscles. In the neuronal form, this condition usually starts in the second decade of life and causes muscle weaknesses similar to those associated with the hypertrophic neuronal form. Both forms of the disease may also involve mild sensory loss in the lower limbs. Affected individuals may be helped by corrective surgery and leg braces that stabilize weak ankle joints.

peroneus brevis /per′ənē′əs/, the smaller of the two lateral muscles of the leg, lying under the peroneus longus. The peroneus brevis arises from the fibula and inserts into the fifth metatarsal bone. Innervated by a branch of the superficial peroneal nerve, it contains fibers from the fourth and the fifth lumbar and the first sacral nerves. It pronates and plantar flexes the foot. Compare **peroneus longus.**

peroneus longus, the more superficial of the two lateral muscles of the leg. It arises from the head and the body of the fibula, converges to a long tendon that crosses the sole of the foot, and inserts into the first metatarsal bone and the medial cuneiform bone. The peroneus longus is innervated by a branch of the peroneal nerve, containing fibers from the fourth and the fifth lumbar and the first sacral nerves. The muscle pronates and plantar flexes the foot. Compare **peroneus brevis.**

peronia /pərō′nē·ə/, a congenital malformation or developmental anomaly.

peropus /pərō′pəs/, a fetus or individual with malformed feet, often in association with some defect of the legs.

perosomus /pē′rōsō′məs/, a fetus or individual whose body, especially the trunk, is severely malformed. Also called **perocormus.**

perosplanchnia /pē′rōsplangk′nē·ə/, a congenital anomaly characterized by the malformation of the viscera.

peroxide. See **hydrogen peroxide.**

perphenazine, an antipsychotic.

■ INDICATIONS: It is prescribed in the treatment of psychotic disorders and in the control of severe nausea and vomiting in adults.

■ CONTRAINDICATIONS: Parkinson's disease, the concurrent administration of central nervous system depressants, liver or renal dysfunction, severe hypotension, or known hypersensitivity to any phenothiazine prohibits its use.

■ ADVERSE EFFECTS: Among the more serious adverse reactions are hypotension, liver toxicity, a variety of extrapyramidal reactions, blood dyscrasias, and various hypersensitivity reactions.

PERRLA /pur′lə/, abbreviation for *pupils equal, round, react to light, accommodation*. In the process of performing an assessment of the eyes, the size and shape of the pupils, their reaction to light, and their ability to accommodate are evaluated. If all findings are normal, the acronym is noted in the account of the physical examination.

Persadox, a trademark for a keratolytic (benzoyl peroxide).

Persa-Gel, a trademark for a keratolytic (benzoyl peroxide).

Persantine, a trademark for a coronary vasodilator (dipyridamole).

persistent cloaca, a congenital anomaly in which the intestinal, urinary, and reproductive ducts open into a common cavity resulting from the failure of the urorectal septum to form during prenatal development. Also called **congenital cloaca.**

Persistin, a trademark for a central nervous system, fixed-combination drug containing analgesics (aspirin and salicylsalicylic acid).

persona /pərsō′nə/, *pl.* **personae** /-nē/, (in analytic psychology) the personality façade or role that a person assumes and presents to the outer world to satisfy the demands of the environment or society or as an expression of some intrapsychic conflict. The persona masks the person's inner being or unconscious self (the Latin word persona literally meaning "mask"). Compare **anima.** See also **archetype.**

personal and social history, (in a health history) an account of the personal and social details of a person's life that serve to identify the person. Place of birth, religion, race, marital status, number of children, military status, occupational history, and place of residence are the usual components of this part of the history, but it may often include other information, as education, current living situation, and smoking, alcohol, and drug habits. The personal and social history is obtained at the initial interview and becomes a part of the permanent record.

personal care services, the services performed by health care workers to assist patients in meeting the requirements of daily living.

personality, **1.** the composite of the behavioral traits and attitudinal characteristics by which one is recognized as an individual. **2.** the pattern of behavior each person evolves, both consciously and unconsciously, as a means of adapting to a particular environment and its cultural, ethnic, national, and provincial standards.

personality disorder, any of a large group of mental disorders characterized by rigid, inflexible, and maladaptive behavior patterns that impair a person's ability to function in society by severely limiting adaptive potential. Such a disorder, which is generally recognized during childhood or adolescence, tends to continue through adulthood. Some kinds of personality disorders are **antisocial personality disorder, histrionic personality disorder, paranoid personality disorder, passive-aggressive personality disorder,** and **schizoid personality disorder.** Also called **character disorder.**

personality test, any of a variety of standardized tests used in the evaluation or assessment of various facets of personality structure, emotional status, and behavioral traits. Compare **achievement test, aptitude test, intelligence test, psychologic test.**

personal orientation, **1.** a continually evolving process in which a person determines and evaluates the relationships that appear to exist between the person and other people. **2.** the assessment derived by a person regarding those relationships.

personal space, the area surrounding an individual that is perceived as private by the individual, who may regard a movement into the space by another person as intrusive. Personal space boundaries vary somewhat in different cultures, but in general it is regarded as a distance of 1 m around the individual.

personal unconscious, (in analytic psychology) the thoughts, ideas, emotions, and other mental phenomena acquired and repressed during one's lifetime. Compare **collective unconscious.**

person year a statistic measure representing one person at risk of developing a disease during a period of 1 year.

perspiration, **1.** the act or process of perspiring; the excretion of fluid by the sweat glands through pores in the skin. **2.** the fluid excreted by the sweat glands. It consists of water containing sodium chloride, phosphate, urea, ammonia, and other waste products. Perspiration serves as a mechanism for excretion and for regulating body temperature. Abnormal amounts of perspiration usually result from organic causes but may also be precipitated by severe emotional stress. Kinds of perspiration are **insensible perspiration** and **sensible perspiration.** See also **diaphoresis, sweat.**

Perthes' disease /per′tās/, osteochondrosis of the head of the femur in children, characterized initially by epiphyseal necrosis or degeneration followed by regeneration or recalcification. Also called **coxa plana, Legg-Calvé-Perthes disease, pseudocoxalgia, Waldenström's disease.**

Pertofrane, a trademark for an antidepressant (desipramine hydrochloride).

pertussis /pərtus′is/, an acute, highly contagious respiratory disease characterized by paroxysmal coughing that ends in a loud whooping inspiration. It occurs primarily in infants and in children less than 4 years of age who have not been immunized. The causative organism, *Bordetella pertussis,* is a small, nonmotile, gram-negative coccobacillus. A similar organism, *B. parapertussis,* causes a less severe form of the disease called parapertussis. Also called **whooping cough.**

■ OBSERVATIONS: Transmission occurs directly by contact or by inhalation of infectious particles, usually spread by coughing and sneezing, and indirectly through freshly contaminated articles. Diagnosis consists of positive identification of the organism in nasopharyngeal secretions. The initial stages of the disease are difficult to distinguish from bronchitis or influenza. A fluorescent antibody staining technique specific for the *B. pertussis* is an accurate means of early diagnosis. The incubation period averages 7 to 14 days, followed by 6 to 8 weeks of illness divided into three distinct stages: catarrhal, paroxysmal, and convalescent. Onset of the catarrhal stage is gradual, usually beginning with coryza, sneezing, a dry cough, a slight fever, listlessness, irritability, and anorexia. The cough becomes paroxysmal after 10 to 14 days and occurs as a series of short rapid bursts during expiration followed by the characteristic whoop, a hurried, deep inhalation that has a high-pitched crowing sound. There is usually no fever, and the respiratory rate between paroxysms is normal. During the paroxysm there is marked facial redness or cyanosis and vein distention, the eyes may bulge, the tongue may protrude, and the facial expression usually indicates severe anxiety and distress. Large amounts of a viscid mucus may be expelled during or after paroxysms, which occur from four to five times a day in mild cases to as many as 40 to 50 times a day in severe cases. Vomiting frequently occurs after the paroxysms because of gagging or choking on the mucus. In infants, choking may be more common than the characteristic whoop. This stage lasts from 4 to 6 weeks, with the attacks being most frequent and severe during the first 1 to 2 weeks, then gradually declining and disappearing. During the convalescent stage, a simple persistent cough is usual. For a period of up to 2 years after the initial attack, paroxysmal coughing may accompany respiratory infections.

■ INTERVENTION: Routine treatment consists of bed rest, a good diet, and adequate amounts of fluid. Erythromycin or another antibacterial may be prescribed to reduce contagiousness or to control secondary infection. Hospitalization may be necessary for infants and children with severe or prolonged paroxysms and for those with dehydration or other complications. Oxygen may be needed to relieve dyspnea and cyanosis; intravenous therapy may be necessary when prolonged vomiting interferes with adequate nutrition. Intubation is rarely necessary but may be lifesaving in infants if the thick mucus cannot be easily suctioned from the air passages. Pertussis immune globulin is available, but its efficacy has not been established and its use is not recommended. Active immunization is recommended with pertussis vaccine, usually in combination with diphtheria and tetanus toxoids in a series of three injections. One attack of the disease usually confers immunity, although some second, usually mild episodes have occurred.

■ NURSING CONSIDERATIONS: Severe paroxysms in an infant may require oxygen, suction, and intubation. The child needs to be kept calm and protected from respiratory irritants such as dirt, smoke, or dust. Overstimulation, noise, or excitement may precipitate paroxysms. A good diet and adequate fluids are encouraged through frequent, small feedings. Common complications of the disease include bronchopneumonia; atelectasis; bronchiectasis; emphysema; otitis media; convulsions; hemorrhage, including subarachnoid, subconjunctival, and epistaxis; weight loss; dehydration; hernia; prolapsed rectum; and asphyxia, especially in infants.

pertussis immune globulin, a passive immunizing agent against whooping cough. See also **pertussis.**

■ INDICATION: It is prescribed for immunization against whooping cough.

■ CONTRAINDICATION: Known hypersensitivity to this drug prohibits its use.

■ ADVERSE EFFECTS: Among the more serious adverse reactions is anaphylaxis.

pertussis vaccine, an active immunizing agent.

■ INDICATION: It is prescribed for immunization against pertussis when the administration of diphtheria, pertussis, and tetanus vaccine is contraindicated.

■ CONTRAINDICATIONS: Thrombocytopenia or known hypersensitivity to the vaccine prohibits its use.

■ ADVERSE EFFECTS: Among the most serious adverse reactions are severe allergic reactions, pain and induration at the site of injection, and fever.

perversion, **1.** any deviation from what is considered normal or natural. **2.** the act of causing a change from what is normal or natural. **3.** *informal.* (in psychiatry) any of a number of sexual practices that deviate from what is considered normal adult behavior. See also **paraphilia.**

pervert /pur′vərt/, **1.** *informal.* a person whose sexual pleasure is derived from stimuli almost universally regarded as unnatural, as a fetishist or sadomasochist; a paraphiliac. **2.** one whose sexual behavior deviates from a social or statistic norm but is not necessarily pathologic.

pes /pēz/, *pl.* **pedes** /pē′dēz/, the foot or a footlike structure.

pes cavus, a deformity of the foot characterized by an excessively high arch with hyperextension of the toes at the metatarsophalangeal joints, flexion at the interphalangeal joints, and shortening of the Achilles tendon. The condition may be present at birth or appear later because of contractures or an imbalance of the muscles of the foot, as in neuromuscular diseases such as Friedreich's ataxia or peroneal muscular atrophy. Surgical treatment is indicated in severe cases, especially in children, although in milder forms the pain from the excessive pressure under the metatarsal heads can be relieved by sponge rubber or leather insoles fitted into the shoes. Also called **clawfoot, gampsodactyly, griffe des orteils** /grif′dezôrtā′i/, **talipes cavus.**

pes planus, an abnormal but relatively common condition characterized by the flattening out of the arch of the foot. Also called **flatfoot.**

pessary /pes′ərē/, a device inserted in the vagina to treat uterine prolapse, uterine retroversion, or cervical incompetence. It is employed in the treatment of women whose advanced age or poor general condition precludes procedures required for surgical repair. A vaginal cream containing estrogen is usually prescribed to cause the vaginal epithelium to thicken and become more resistant to irritation from the pessary. Pessaries are also used in younger women in evaluating symptomatic uterine retroversion: If pelvic pain is relieved by anteversion of the uterus with the pessary in place and returns when retroversion recurs after the pessary is removed, retroversion is demonstrated to be the cause of pain, and surgical uterine suspension can be expected to provide long-term relief. The pessary is also used in the management of cervical incompetence in pregnancy. It holds the uterus in a forward position in which intraabdominal and intrauterine pressure cause less stress on the neck of the womb. A pessary must be removed, usually daily, for cleaning. The woman may do this herself, or it may be done by someone else if she is disabled. Left in place, the pessary is likely to cause severe irritation, leading to vaginal infection. A **Smith-Hodge pessary** is a rubber- or vinyl-covered wire rectangle that fits between the pubic bone and the posterior vaginal fornix, supporting the uterus and holding the cervix in a posterior position. A **Gellhorn pessary** is an inflexible device made of lucite in the form of a large collar button. It has a canal through the stem that allows drainage of vaginal secretions. The large end of the pessary is placed deep in the vagina, the small end of the stem protruding at the introitus. A **doughnut pessary** is a permanently inflated flexible rubber doughnut that is inserted to support the uterus by blocking the canal of the vagina. An **inflatable pessary** is a collapsible rubber doughnut to which is attached a flexible stem containing a rubber valve. The pessary is inserted collapsed, inflated with a bulb similar to that of a sphygmomanometer, and deflated for removal. A **Bee cell pessary** is a soft rubber cube; in each face of the cube is a conic depression that acts as a suction cup when the pessary is in the vagina. A **diaphragm pessary** is a contraceptive diaphragm used for uterovaginal support. A similar device of somewhat heavier construction is sometimes used. A **stem pessary** is a slim curved rod that is fitted into the cervical canal for uterine positioning. It is rarely used today.

pessimism, the inclination to anticipate the worst possible results from any action or situation or to emphasize unfavorable conditions, even when progress or gain might reasonably be expected. –**pessimist,** *n.*

pesticide poisoning, a toxic condition caused by the ingestion or inhalation of a substance used for the eradication of pests. Kinds of pesticide poisoning include **malathion poisoning** and **parathion poisoning.** See also **herbicide poisoning, insecticide poisoning, rodenticide poisoning.**

pestis. See **bubonic plague.**

PET, abbreviation for **positron emission tomography.**

petalo-, a combining form meaning 'of or related to a leaf': *petalobacteria, petalococcus.*

petechiae /pētē′kē•ē/, *sing.* **petechia** /-ə/, tiny purple or red spots that appear on the skin as a result of minute hemorrhages within the dermal or submucosal layers. Petechiae range from pinpoint to pinhead size and are flush with the surface. Compare **ecchymosis.** –**petechial,** *adj.*

petechial fever /pitē′kē•əl/, any febrile illness accompanied by small petechiae on the skin, as seen in the late stage of typhoid fever.

pethidine. See **meperidine hydrochloride.**

petit mal seizure /pət′ē mal′, ptē′ mäl′/, an epileptic seizure characterized by a sudden, momentary loss of consciousness occasionally accompanied by minor myoclonus of the neck or upper extremities, slight symmetric twitching of the face, or a loss of muscle tone. The seizures usually occur many times a day without a warning aura and are most frequent in children and adolescents, especially at the time of puberty. The patient experiencing a typical seizure has a vacant facial expression and ceases all voluntary motor activity; with the rapid return of consciousness, the patient may resume conversation at the point of interruption without realizing what occurred. During and between seizures, the patient's electroencephalogram shows three cycle-per-second spike and wave discharges. Anticonvulsant drugs used to prevent petit mal attacks include clonazepam, ethosuximide, methsuximide, paramethadione, phensuximide, trimethadione, and valproic acid. See also **epilepsy.**

P.E.T.N., a trademark for a vasodilator (pentaerythritol tetranitrate).

petr-, a combining form meaning 'of or pertaining to stone': *petrifaction, petroleum, petrous.*

pétrissage /pā′trisäzh′/, a technique in massage in which the skin is gently lifted and squeezed. Pétrissage promotes circulation and relaxes the muscles. Compare **effleurage, rolling effleurage.**

Petrogalar, a trademark for a cathartic (mineral oil).

petrolatum gauze /pet′rəlā′təm/, absorbent gauze permeated with white petrolatum.

petroleum distillate poisoning, a toxic condition caused by the ingestion or inhalation of a petroleum distillate, as fuel oil, lubricating oil, glue used in making model airplanes or the like, and various solvents. Nausea, vomiting, chest pain, dizziness, and severe depression of the central nervous system characterize the condition. Severe or fatal pneumonitis may occur if the substance is aspirated; therefore induced emesis is contraindicated. Gastric lavage with water, a saline cathartic, and oxygen, if required, are recommended. See also **gasoline poisoning, kerosene poisoning.**

petrosphenoidal fissure /pet′rōsfēnoi′dəl/, a fissure on the floor of the cranial fossa between the posterior edge of the great wing of the sphenoid bone and the petrous part of the temporal bone.

Peutz-Jeghers syndrome, an inherited disorder, transmitted as an autosomal dominant trait, characterized by multiple intestinal polyps, and abnormal mucocutaneous pigmentation, usually over the lips and buccal mucosa. If obstruction or bleeding occurs, surgical removal of the polyps may be indicated.

-pexis, -pexia, -pexy, a combining form meaning 'a fixation of' something specified: *glycopexis, hemopexis, splenopexis.*

Peyer's patches /pī′ərz/, groups of lymph nodes in the terminal ileum near its junction with the colon opposite to the juncture of the mesentery. In certain infectious diseases, as typhoid fever, they become ulcerated and enlarged.

peyote /pā•ō′tē/, **1.** a cactus from which a hallucinogenic drug, mescaline, is derived. **2.** mescaline.

Peyronie's disease /pārōnēz′/, a disease of unknown cause resulting in fibrous induration of the corpora cavernosa of the penis. An association with Dupuytren's contracture of the palm has been recognized. The chief symptom of Peyronie's disease is painful erection. Palliative treatment includes radiation therapy and intralesional corticosteroid injections. There is no known cure.

Pfizerpen-AS, a trademark for an antibacterial (penicillin G procaine).

Pfizerpen G, a trademark for an antibacterial (penicillin G potassium).

PFT, abbreviation for **pulmonary function test.**

PG, abbreviation for **prostaglandin.**

PGI_2, abbreviation for **prostacyclin.**

PGY, abbreviation for *postgraduate year,* describing medical school graduates during their postgraduate training as interns (PGY-1, first year), residents (PGY-2, 3, 4), or fellows (PGY-4, 5).

pH, a scale representing the relative acidity (or alkalinity) of a solution, in which a value 7.0 is neutral, below 7.0 is acid, and above 7.0 is alkaline. The numeric pH value indicates the relative concentration of hydrogen atoms in the solution compared with that of a standard solution; it is equal to the negative log of the hydrogen ion concentration expressed in moles per liter. See also **acid, acid-base balance.**

PH, abbreviation for **parathyroid hormone.**

Ph[1]**,** symbol for **Philadelphia chromosome.**

PHA, **1.** abbreviation for **paraaminohippuric acid.** **2.** abbreviation for **phytohemagglutinin.**

phaco-, phako-, a combining form meaning 'of or related to a lens': *phacocele, phacocyst, phacoglaucoma.*

phacomalacia /fak'ōməlā'shə/, an abnormal condition of the eye in which the lens of the eye becomes soft because of the presence of a soft cataract.

phacomatosis. See **phakomatosis.**

phage. See **bacteriophage.**

-phage, -phag, a combining form meaning 'something that eats' the matter specified: *hemophage, mycophage, osteophage.*

phage typing, the identification of bacteria by testing their vulnerability to bacterial viruses.

-phagia, **1.** a combining form meaning an 'eating of a substance': *autophagia, chthonophagia, creophagia.* **2.** a combining form meaning 'desire for food': *amylophagia, monophagia, osteophagia.*

phago-, a combining form meaning 'of or pertaining to eating or ingestion': *phagocyte, phagokaryosis, phagology.*

phagocyte /fag'əsīt/, a cell that is able to surround, engulf, and digest microorganisms and cellular debris. **Fixed phagocytes,** which do not circulate, include the fixed macrophages and the cells of the reticuloendothelial system. **Free phagocytes,** which circulate in the blood stream, include the leukocytes and the free macrophages. –**phagocytic,** *adj.*

phagocytosis /fag'əsītō'sis/, the process by which certain cells engulf and dispose of microorganisms and cell debris.

-phagy, -phagia, a combining form meaning the 'practice of eating' something specified: *bacteriophagy, biophagy, coprophagy.*

-phakia, a combining form meaning a 'lens': *aphakia, microphakia, pseudophakia.*

phako-. See **phaco-.**

phakomatosis /fak'ōmətō'sis/, *pl.* **phakomatoses,** (in opthalmology) any of several hereditary syndromes characterized by benign tumorlike nodules of the eye, skin, and brain. The four disorders designated phakomatoses are neurofibromatosis (Recklinghausen's disease), tuberous sclerosis (Bourneville's disease), encephalotrigeminal angiomatosis (Sturge-Weber syndrome), and cerebroretinal angiomatosis (von Hippel-Lindau disease). Also spelled **phacomatosis.**

-phalangia, a combining form meaning a 'condition of the bones of the fingers or toes': *bradyphalangia, symphalangia, triphalangia.*

phalanx /fā'langks/, *pl.* **phalanges** /fəlan'jēz/, any one of the 14 tapering bones composing the fingers of each hand and the toes of each foot. They are arranged in three rows at the distal end of the metacarpus and the metatarsus. The fingers each have three phalanges; the thumb has two. The toes each have three phalanges; the great toe has two. The phalanges of the foot are smaller and less flexible than those of the hand.

phall-. See **phallo-.**

phallic stage, (in psychoanalysis) the period in psychosexual development occurring between 3 and 6 years of age when emerging awareness and self-manipulation of the genitals are the predominant source of pleasurable experience. Fixation at this stage may lead to extreme aggressiveness in adulthood, or it may be a precipitating factor in the development of psychosexual disorders. See also **psychosexual development.**

phallo-, phall-, a combining form meaning 'of or related to the penis': *phallocampsis, phallodynia, phalloplasty.*

phalloidine /faloi'din/, a poison present in the mushroom *Amanita phalloides.* Ingestion of phalloidine results in bloody diarrhea, vomiting, severe abdominal pain, kidney failure, and liver damage. Approximately 50% of phalloidine poisonings are fatal. Also spelled **phalloidin.**

phallus. See **penis.**

-phane, -phan, a combining form meaning a 'thing with a (specified) appearance': *diaphane, rhodophane, xanthophane.*

phanero-, a combining form meaning 'visible or apparent': *phanerogenetic, phaneromania, phaneroplasm.*

phantom, a mass of material similar to human tissue used to investigate the interaction of radiation beams with human beings. Phantom materials can range from water to complex chemical mixtures that faithfully mimic the human body as it would interact with radiation.

phantom limb syndrome, a phenomenon common after amputation of a limb in which sensation or discomfort is experienced in the missing limb. In some people severe pain persists. See also **pseudesthesia.**

phantom tumor, a swelling resembling a tumor, usually caused by muscle contraction or gaseous distention of the intestines.

phao-. See **pheo-.**

pharmaceutic, **1.** of or pertaining to pharmacy or drugs. **2.** a drug. Also called **pharmaceutical.**

pharmaceutic chemistry, the science dealing with the composition and preparation of chemical compounds used in medical diagnoses and therapies.

pharmacist, a specialist in formulating and dispensing medications. Pharmacists are licensed by the various states to practice pharmacy.

pharmaco-, a combining form meaning 'of or related to drugs or medicine': *pharmacochemistry, pharmacomania, pharmacopsychosis.*

pharmacogenetics, the study of the effect that the genetic factors belonging to a group or to an individual have on the response of the group or the individual to certain drugs.

pharmacokinetics /fär'məkōkinet'iks/, (in pharmacology) the study of the action of drugs within the body, including the routes and mechanisms of absorption and excretion, the rate at which a drug's action begins and the duration of the effect, the biotransformation of the substance in the body, and the effects and routes of excretion of the metabolites of the drug.

pharmacologic treatment. See **treatment.**

pharmacologist, a specialist in pharmacology.

pharmacology, the study of the preparation, properties, uses, and actions of drugs.

pharmacopoeia /fär′məkəpē′ə/, **1.** a compendium containing descriptions, recipes, strengths, standards of purity, and dosage forms for selected drugs. **2.** the available stock of drugs in a pharmacy. **3.** the total of all authorized drugs available within the jurisdiction of a given geographic or political area. Also spelled **pharmacopeia.** See also ***British Pharmacopoeia, United States Pharmacopeia.***

pharmacy, **1.** the study of preparing and dispensing drugs. **2.** a place for preparing and dispensing drugs.

-pharmic, a combining form meaning 'related to drugs and medicinal remedies': *alexipharmic, antipharmic, polypharmic.*

pharyng-. See **pharyngo-.**

pharyngeal aponeurosis /ferin′jē·əl/, a sheet of connective tissue just beneath the mucosa of the pharynx.

pharyngeal bursa, a blind sac at the base of the pharyngeal tonsil.

pharyngeal reflex. See **gag reflex.**

pharyngeal tonsil, one of two masses of lymphatic tissue situated on the posterior wall of the nasopharynx behind the posterior nares. During childhood these masses often swell and block the passage of air from the nasal cavity into the pharynx, preventing the child from breathing through the nose. Also called **adenoid.**

pharyngitis /fer′injī′tis/, inflammation or infection of the pharynx, usually causing symptoms of a sore throat. Some causes of pharyngitis are diphtheria, herpes simplex virus, infectious mononucleosis, and streptococcal infection. Specific treatment depends on the cause. Symptoms may be relieved by analgesic medication, drinking warm or cold liquids, or saline irrigation of the throat. See also **strep throat.**

pharyngo-, pharyng-, a combining form meaning 'of or related to the pharynx': *pharyngocele, pharyngoglossus, pharyngorrhagia.*

pharyngoconjunctival fever /fəring′gōkon′jungktī′vəl/, an adenovirus infection characterized by fever, sore throat, and conjunctivitis. An epidemic illness, particularly prevalent in summer, it is spread by droplet infection and direct contact. Contaminated water in lakes and swimming pools is a common source of infection. Also called **swimming pool conjunctivitis.** See also **adenovirus.**

pharynx /fer′inks/, the throat, a tubular structure about 13 cm long that extends from the base of the skull to the esophagus and is situated just in front of the cervical vertebrae. The pharynx serves as a passageway for the respiratory and digestive tracts and changes shape to allow the formation of various vowel sounds. The pharynx is composed of muscle, is lined with mucous membrane, and is divided into the nasopharynx, the oropharynx, and the laryngopharynx. It contains the openings of the right and the left auditory tubes, the openings of the two posterior nares, the fauces, the opening into the larynx, and the opening into the esophagus. It also contains the pharyngeal tonsils, the palatine tonsils, and the lingual tonsils. Also called **throat.** See also **larynx.**

phase, in a periodic function, such as rotational or sinusoidal motion, the position relative to a particular part of the cycle.

phase 0, (in cardiology) the upstroke of the action potential.

phase 1, (in cardiology) the initial rapid repolarization phase of the action potential.

phase 2, (in cardiology) the plateau of the action potential.

phase 3, (in cardiology) the terminal rapid repolarization phase of the action potential.

phase 3 aberration, (in cardiology) a ventricular aberration resulting from the arrival of the impulse in the ventricular fascicle during phase 3 of its action potential.

phase 4, the period of electric diastole and the last of the five phases of cardiac action potential. A plot of phase 4 shows a gradual upward slope in a pacemaker Purkinje fiber whereas the phase 4 action potential in a myocardial fiber is flat.

phase 4 aberration, (in cardiology) a ventricular aberration resulting from the arrival of the impulse in a spontaneously depolarizing ventricular fascicle late in diastole.

phase microscope, a microscope with a special condenser and objective containing a phase-shifting ring that allows the viewer to see small differences in refraction indexes as differences in image intensity or contrast. The phase microscope is used especially for examining transparent specimens, as living or unstained cells and tissues.

phase of maximum slope, the time of rapid cervical dilatation and rapid fetal descent in the active phase of labor. See **Friedman curve.**

phase one study, a clinical trial to assess the risk that might come from administering a new treatment modality. A phase two study evaluates the clinical effectiveness of the new modality, whereas a phase three study compares its effectiveness with the best existing treatment.

phases of crisis, the occurrance of a significant stressor event, onset of disequilibrium, rise in tension levels, decrease in levels of functioning, and resolution with equilibrium reestablished. See also **general adaptation syndrome.**

-phasia, a combining form meaning a 'speech disorder': *acataphasia, agitophasia, logaphasia.*

phasic /fā′zik/, referring to a process proceeding in stages or phases.

-phasic, a combining form meaning 'relating to a speech disorder': *aphasic, endophasic, paraphasic.*

-phasis, -phasia, -phasy, a combining form meaning 'speech, utterance': *allophasis, heterophasis, paraphasis.*

Phelantin, a trademark for a central nervous system, fixed-combination drug containing an anticonvulsant (phenytoin), a stimulant (methamphetamine hydrochloride), and a sedative-hypnotic (phenobarbital).

Phe-Mer-Nite, a trademark for an antimicrobial (phenylmercuric nitrate).

-phemia, a combining form meaning a '(specified) disorder of speech': *dysphemia, paraphemia, spasmophemia.*

phen-, a combining form indicating derivation from benzene: *phenacitin, phenicate, phenobarbitone.*

phenacemide /fənas′əmīd/, an anticonvulsant.

■ INDICATION: It is prescribed in the treatment of severe epilepsy, particularly mixed forms of psychomotor seizures refractory to other drugs.

■ CONTRAINDICATIONS: Pregnancy, previous personality disturbances, or known hypersensitivity to this drug prohibits its use.

■ ADVERSE EFFECTS: Among the more serious adverse reactions are aplastic anemia, acute psychosis, paranoid and depressive reactions, nephritis, and hepatitis.

phenacetin /fənas′itin/, an analgesic.

■ INDICATIONS: It is prescribed to relieve pain and to reduce fever.

■ CONTRAINDICATIONS: Known hypersensitivity to this drug prohibits its use. Repeated use is contraindicated in anemia, cardiac, pulmonary, hepatic, or renal disease.

■ ADVERSE EFFECTS: Among the more serious adverse reactions are hepatic necrosis, fever, and skin rash.

Phenaphen, a trademark for an analgesic-antipyretic (acetaminophen).

phenazopyridine hydrochloride, a urinary tract analgesic.

■ INDICATIONS: It is prescribed to reduce the pain of cystitis or other urinary tract infections..

■ CONTRAINDICATIONS: Renal insufficiency or known hypersensitivity to this drug prohibits its use.

■ ADVERSE EFFECTS: Among the more serious adverse reactions are headache and GI disturbances.

phencyclidine hydrochloride (PCP) /fensī′klidēn/, a piperidine derivative administered parenterally to achieve neuroleptic anesthesia. Because of its marked hallucinogenic and flashback properties, it is rarely used in the United States.

phendimetrazine tartrate /fen′dīmet′rəsēn/, a sympathomimetic amine used as an anorectic agent.

■ INDICATIONS: It is prescribed to decrease the appetite in the treatment of exogenous types of obesity.

■ CONTRAINDICATIONS: Cardiovascular disease, hypertension, hyperthyroidism, glaucoma, nervousness, a history of drug abuse, concomitant administration of central nervous system stimulants or monoamine oxidase inhibitors, or known hypersensitivity to this drug prohibits its use.

■ ADVERSE EFFECTS: Among the more serious adverse reactions are central nervous system stimulation, elevated blood pressure, insomnia, and dry mouth and tolerance to the drug.

-phene, -phen, a combining form denoting members of the phenol group: *camphene, phlobaphene, phosphene.*

phenelzine sulfate, a monoamine oxidase (MAO) inhibitor.

■ INDICATIONS: It is prescribed in the treatment of endogenous and other types of depression.

■ CONTRAINDICATIONS: Liver dysfunction, congestive heart failure, pheochromocytoma, concomitant use of sympathomimetic drugs or foods high in tryptophan or tyramine, or known hypersensitivity to this drug prohibits its use.

■ ADVERSE EFFECTS: Among the most serious adverse reactions are orthostatic hypotension, vertigo, constipation, blurred vision, headache, overactivity, and dryness of the mouth. MAO inhibitors produce many adverse drug interactions.

Phenergan, a trademark for a phenothiazine derivative (promethazine), used as an adjunct to anesthesia.

Phenergan Compound, a trademark for a respiratory, fixed-combination drug containing an adrenergic (pseudoephedrine hydrochloride), an antihistaminic (promethazine hydrochloride), and an analgesic (aspirin).

phenformin, phenformin hydrochloride, an oral hypoglycemic. See also **non-insulin-dependent diabetes mellitus.**

phenic acid. See **carbolic acid.**

phenindione /fənin′dē·ōn/, an anticoagulant.

■ INDICATIONS: It is prescribed for prophylaxis and treatment of thrombosis and embolism in a variety of situations.

■ CONTRAINDICATIONS: Known hypersensitivity to this drug prohibits its use. It is not used in situations where there is a risk of hemorrhage or in the presence of certain blood disorders.

■ ADVERSE EFFECTS: The most serious adverse reaction is hemorrhage. Many other drugs interact with this drug to increase or decrease its effect.

pheniramine maleate /fənir′əmēn, -min/, an antihistamine.

■ INDICATIONS: It is prescribed in the treatment of a variety of hypersensitivity reactions, including rhinitis, skin rash, and pruritus.

■ CONTRAINDICATIONS: Asthma or known hypersensitivity to this drug prohibits its use. It is not given to newborn infants or lactating mothers.

■ ADVERSE EFFECTS: Among the more serious adverse reactions are drowsiness, skin rash, and hypersensitivity reactions. Dry mouth and tachycardia commonly occur.

phenmetrazine hydrochloride, a sympathomimetic amine used as an anorectic agent.

■ INDICATIONS: It is prescribed to reduce the appetite and in the short-term treatment of exogenous obesity.

■ CONTRAINDICATIONS: Cardiovascular disease, hypertension, hyperthyroidism, glaucoma, history of drug abuse, concomitant use of a central nervous system stimulant, or a monoamine oxidase inhibitor, or known hypersensitivity to this drug or other sympathomimetic drugs prohibits its use. It is not recommended for children under 12 years of age.

■ ADVERSE EFFECTS: Among the most serious adverse reactions are central nervous system stimulation, elevated blood pressure, insomnia, dry mouth, and others common to this class of drug.

phenobarbital, a barbiturate anticonvulsant and sedative-hypnotic.

■ INDICATIONS: It is prescribed in the treatment of a variety of seizure disorders and as a long-acting sedative.

■ CONTRAINDICATIONS: Porphyria, severe pain, respiratory problems, or known hypersensitivity to this drug or other barbiturates prohibits its use.

■ ADVERSE EFFECTS: Among the most serious adverse reactions are ataxia, porphyria, paradoxical excitement, drowsiness, occasional rashes, and, rarely, blood dyscrasias. It is involved in many drug interactions.

phenobarbital-phenytoin serum levels, the concentration of phenobarbital and phenytoin in the serum, monitored to maintain concentrations sufficient to control seizures but not high enough to cause toxic reactions. The control of seizures is commonly obtained in adults with plasma concentrations of phenobarbital that average 10 mg/ml per daily dose of 1 μg/kg; in children, 5 to 7 μg/ml per daily dose of 1 μg/kg. The control of seizures is commonly obtained with plasma concentrations of phenytoin that average 10 μg/ml, whereas toxic effects, as nystagmus, typically develop with a concentration of 20 μg/ml. Ataxia may develop at a concentration of 30 μg/ml and lethargy at a concentration of 40 μg/ml.

phenocopy /fē′nōkop′ē/, a phenotypic trait or condition that is induced by environmental factors but closely resembles a phenotype usually produced by a specific genotype. The trait is neither inherited nor transmitted to offspring. Such conditions as deafness, cretinism, mental retardation, and congenital cataracts are caused by mutant genes but can also result from a number of different agents, as the rubella virus in the case of congenital cataracts. Phenocopies may present problems in genetic screening and genetic counseling so that all exogenous factors must be ruled out before any congenital trait or defect is labeled hereditary.

phenol /fē′nol/, **1.** a highly poisonous, caustic, crystalline chemical derived from coal tar or plant tar or manufactured synthetically. It has a distinctive, pungent odor and, in solution, is a powerful disinfectant, commonly called carbolic acid. **2.** Any of a large number and variety of chemical products closely related in structure to the alcohols and containing a hydroxyl group attached to a benzene ring. The phenols are components in dyes, plastics, disinfectants, and antimicrobials and other drugs, including salicylic acid.

Phenolax, a trademark for a laxative (phenolphthalein).

phenol camphor, an oily mixture of camphor and phenol, used as an antiseptic and toothache remedy.

phenol coefficient, a measure of the disinfectant activity of a given chemical in relation to carbolic acid. The activity is expressed as the ratio of a dilution of the chemical that kills in 10 minutes but not in 5 minutes to the 1:90 dilution of carbolic acid that kills in 10 minutes but not in 5 minutes.

phenolphthalein /fē′nolthal′ē•in, -thā′lēn/, **1.** a laxative that acts by stimulating the motor activity of the lower intestinal tract. **2.** an indicator of hydrogen ion in urine and gastric juice.

phenolphthalein laxative, a purgative that acts on the wall of the bowel.

■ INDICATIONS: It is prescribed in the treatment of chronic constipation and to prevent straining at the stool for postoperative patients and those afflicted with heart disease or hypertension.

■ CONTRAINDICATIONS: Symptoms of appendicitis, acute surgical abdomen, fecal impaction, intestinal obstruction or perforation, or known hypersensitivity to this drug prohibits its use.

■ ADVERSE EFFECTS: Among the most serious adverse reactions are abdominal cramping and pain, allergic reaction (particularly of the skin), dehydration, and laxative dependence.

phenol poisoning, corrosive poisoning caused by the ingestion of compounds containing phenol, as carbolic acid, creosote, creosol, guaiacol, and naphthol. Characteristic of phenol poisoning are burns of the mucous membranes, weakness, pallor, pulmonary edema, convulsion, and respiratory, circulatory, cardiac, and renal failure. In treatment, the skin around the mouth and nose is washed, as are any external burns; the mouth, throat, esophagus, and stomach are lavaged with water and charcoal. Oxygen, intravenous fluids, electrolytes, and pain medication may be necessary. Rarely, esophageal stricture may develop as a complication of extensive tissue damage.

phenolsulfonphthalein, a dye used for testing the excretory capacity of the kidney tubules. The test is performed by measuring urine levels at regular intervals after injecting 6 mg of the dye.

phenomenon, a sign that is often associated with a specific illness or condition and is, therefore, diagnostically important.

phenothiazine /fē′nōthī′əzēn/, a yellow to green crystalline compound that is a source of dyes and is used in veterinary medicine to treat infestations of threadworms and roundworms. It is too toxic for humans, but derivatives of phenothiazine are used in tranquilizers and antihistamine medications. See also **phenothiazine tranquilizers.**

phenothiazine tranquilizers, any of a group of drugs that have a three ring structure in which two benzene rings are linked by a nitrogen and a sulfur. They represent the largest group of antipsychotic compounds in clinical medicine. Of the many phenothiazines and their congeners that are used as adjuncts to general anesthesia, antiemetics, major tranquilizers (antipsychotic agents), and antihistamines the most widely used are the two prototypes, chlorpromazine and prochlorperazine; closely related are trimeprazine and triflupromazine. This group of drugs has largely revolutionized the practice of psychiatric medicine. Unlike the barbiturates, which act exclusively on the central nervous system (CNS), the phenothiazines exert significant influence on many organ systems of the body at once; for example, they exert antiadrenergic, anticholinergic, and antihistaminic activity. The effects on the CNS differ according to individual drug and patient status. All phenothiazine tranquilizers are withheld from patients with severe CNS depression or epilepsy and are given with caution to those with liver disease. These drugs are not recommended for use in pregnancy. See also specific drugs.

phenotype, **1.** the complete observable characteristics of an organism or group, including anatomic, physiologic, biochemical, and behavioral traits, as determined by the interaction of both genetic makeup and environmental factors. **2.** a group of organisms that resemble each other in appearance. Compare **genotype.** **–phenotypic,** *adj.*

Phenoxene, a trademark for an anticholinergic and antiparkinsonian (chlorphenoxamine hydrochloride).

phenoxy-, a combining form indicating the presence of a chemical group composed of phenyl and an atom of oxygen: *phenoxycaffeine.*

phenoxybenzamine hydrochloride, an antihypertensive.

■ INDICATIONS: It is prescribed in the control of hypertension and sweating in pheochromocytoma. If tachycardia is excessive, concomitant administration of propranolol may be necessary.

■ CONTRAINDICATIONS: Hypotension or known hypersensitivity to this drug prohibits its use.

■ ADVERSE EFFECTS: Among the more serious adverse reactions are severe hypotension, tachycardia, and GI irritation.

phenoxymethyl penicillin. See **penicillin V.**

phenprocoumon /fen′prōko͞o′mən/, an anticoagulant.

■ INDICATIONS: It is prescribed in the treatment and prophylaxis of thrombosis and embolism in a variety of clinical situations.

■ CONTRAINDICATIONS: Known hypersensitivity to this drug prohibits its use. It is not used in clinical situations in which there is a risk of hemorrhage.

■ ADVERSE EFFECTS: The most serious adverse reaction is hemorrhage. Many other drugs interact with this drug to either increase or decrease its effect.

phensuximide, an anticonvulsant.

■ INDICATIONS: It is prescribed to prevent and treat seizures in petit mal epilepsy.

■ CONTRAINDICATIONS: Known hypersensitivity to this drug or to any succinimide prohibits its use.

■ ADVERSE EFFECTS: Among the most serious adverse reactions are blood dyscrasias and a systemic lupuslike syndrome. Common reactions are GI disturbances and central nervous system depression with drowsiness or dizziness.

phentermine hydrochloride /fen′tərmēn/, a sympathomimetic amine used as an anorexic agent.

■ INDICATIONS: It is prescribed to decrease the appetite in the short-term treatment of exogenous obesity.

■ CONTRAINDICATIONS: Arteriosclerosis, cardiovascular disease, hypertension, glaucoma, hyperthyroidism, or known hypersensitivity to this drug or to other sympathomimetic drugs prohibits its use.

■ ADVERSE EFFECTS: Among the more serious adverse reactions are restlessness, insomnia, tachycardia, increased blood pressure, and dry mouth.

phentolamine, an antiadrenergic. It is administered as the hydrochloride form in tablets and as the mesylate form for injections.

■ INDICATIONS: It is prescribed in the control of symptoms of pheochromocytoma before and during surgery and for dermal necrosis and sloughing after extravasation of parenteral norepinephrine.

■ CONTRAINDICATIONS: History of myocardial infarction, angina, coronary artery disease, or known hypersensitivity to this drug prohibits its use.

■ ADVERSE EFFECTS: Among the more serious adverse reactions are severe hypotension, tachycardia, cardiac arrhythmias, anginal pain, and hypotension.

Phenurone, a trademark for an anticonvulsant (phenacemide).

phenylacetic acid /fen′iləsē′tik/, a metabolite of phenylalanine excreted in urine in conjugation with glutamine.

phenylalanine (Phe) /fen′ilal′ənēn/, an essential amino acid necessary for the normal growth and development of infants and children and for normal protein metabolism throughout life. The normal values of this amino acid in the serum of adults is less than 3 mg/dl; in newborns, 1.2 to 3.5 mg/dl. It is abundant in milk, eggs, and other common foods. See also **amino acid, phenylketonuria, protein.**

phenylalaninemia /fen′ilaləninē′mē·ə/, the presence of phenylalanine in the blood. See also **hyperphenylalaninemia.**

phenylbutazone, a nonsteroidal antiinflammatory agent.

■ INDICATIONS: It is prescribed in the treatment of severe symptoms of arthritis, bursitis, and other inflammatory conditions.

■ CONTRAINDICATIONS: Impaired renal or hepatic function, a history of upper GI problems, blood dyscrasia, stomatitis caused by other drugs, hypertension, edema, or known hypersensitivity to this drug or to oxyphenbutazone prohibits its use. Caution is advised in administering this drug to children or elderly persons.

■ ADVERSE EFFECTS: Among the more serious adverse reactions are fluid retention and potentially serious blood dyscrasias. GI irritation and nausea commonly occur. This drug interacts with many other drugs.

phenyl carbinol. See **benzyl alcohol.**

phenylephrine hydrochloride, an alpha-adrenergic agent.

■ INDICATIONS: It is prescribed to maintain blood pressure and is used locally as a nasal or ophthalmic vasoconstrictor.

■ CONTRAINDICATIONS: Narrow-angle glaucoma, concomitant administration of monoamine oxidase inhibitors, or known hypersensitivity to this drug prohibits its use.

■ ADVERSE EFFECTS: Among the more serious adverse reactions to the systemic administration of this drug are arrhythmias and an excessive rise in blood pressure. Anxiety, congestion, and hypersensitivity reactions may occur from local administration of this drug.

phenylethyl alcohol, a colorless, fragrant liquid with a burning taste, used as a bacteriostatic agent and preservative in medicinal solutions. Also called **benzyl carbonol.**

phenylic acid, phenylic alcohol. See **carbolic acid.**

phenylketonuria (PKU) /fen′əlkē′tōnyŏŏr′ē•ə, fē′nəl-/, abnormal presence of phenylketone and other metabolites of phenylalanine in the urine, characteristic of an inborn metabolic disorder caused by the absence or a deficiency of phenylalanine hydroxylase, the enzyme responsible for the conversion of the amino acid phenylalanine into tyrosine. Accumulation of phenylalanine is toxic to brain tissue. Untreated individuals have very fair hair, eczema, a mousy odor of the urine and skin, and progressive mental retardation. Treatment consists of a diet free of phenylalanine. Phenylketonuria occurs approximately once in 16,000 births in the United States. Most states require a screening test for all newborns. See also **Guthrie test.** –**phenylketonuric,** *adj.*

phenylmercuric nitrate, a topical antiseptic.

■ INDICATIONS: It is prescribed as an antiseptic in skin diseases and for preoperative disinfection.

■ CONTRAINDICATIONS: Known hypersensitivity to this drug or to other compounds containing mercury prohibits its use.

■ ADVERSE EFFECTS: Among the more serious adverse reactions are local hypersensitivity with rash and irritation. Systemic mercury intoxication may occur with frequent and widespread use.

phenyl methanol. See **benzyl alcohol.**

phenylpropanolamine hydrochloride /fen′əlprō′pənol′əmēn/, a sympathomimetic amine with vasoconstrictor action.

■ INDICATIONS: It is prescribed to relieve nasal congestion and related cold symptoms.

■ CONTRAINDICATIONS: Hypertension, coronary artery disease, concomitant administration of monoamine oxidase inhibitors, or known hypersensitivity to this drug prohibits its use.

■ ADVERSE EFFECTS: Among the more serious adverse reactions are nervousness, insomnia, anorexia, and increased blood pressure.

phenylpyruvic acid /fen′ilpīrōō′vik/, a product of the metabolism of phenylalanine. The presence of phenylpyruvic acid in the urine is indicative of phenylketonuria.

phenylpyruvic amentia. See **phenylketonuria.**

phenyltoloxamine citrate /fen′iltəlok′səmēn, fē′nil-/, an antihistamine usually used in a fixed-combination drug with an analgesic.

Phenylzin, a trademark for an ophthalmic, fixed-combination drug containing an adrenergic (phenylephrine hydrochloride) and an astringent (zinc sulfate).

phenytoin /fen′ətō′in/, an anticonvulsant.

■ INDICATIONS: It is prescribed as an anticonvulsant in grand mal and psychomotor seizure disorders and as an antiarrhythmic agent, particularly in digitalis-induced arrhythmias.

■ CONTRAINDICATIONS: Known hypersensitivity to this drug or to other hydantoins prohibits its use. It is used with caution in patients with a history of hepatic or hematologic abnormalities and in the presence of certain arrhythmias.

■ ADVERSE EFFECTS: Among the more serious adverse reactions are ataxia, nystagmus, hypersensitivity reactions, and gingival hyperplasia. Rarely, a variety of severe reactions occur. This drug interacts with many other drugs.

pheo-, phao-, a combining form meaning 'dusky': *pheochrome, pheochromoblast, pheophytin.*

pheochromocytoma /fē′ōkrō′mōsītō′mə/, *pl.* **pheochromocytomas, pheochromocytomata,** a vascular tumor of chromaffin tissue of the adrenal medulla or sympathetic paraganglia, characterized by hypersecretion of epinephrine and norepinephrine, causing persistent or intermittent hypertension. Typical signs include headache, palpitation, sweating, nervousness, hyperglycemia, nausea, vomiting, and syncope. There may be weight loss, myocarditis, cardiac arrhythmia, and heart failure. The tumor occurs most frequently in young people, and only a small percentage of the lesions are malignant. The diagnosis may be established by laboratory assays showing increased catecholamines and their metabolites in urine and by pressor tests; intravenously injected histamine causes a sharp increase in blood pressure of patients with pheochromocytoma, and the administration of phentolamine produces a marked decrease. Surgical excision is the usual treatment; patients with nonresectable tumors may be treated with adrenergic blocking agents or with methyl tyrosine, a drug that reduces norepinephrine production.

pheresis. See **apheresis.**

pheromone /fer′əmōn′/, a hormonal substance secreted by an organism that elicits a particular response from another individual of the same species, but usually of the opposite sex.

phil-, a combining form meaning 'having an affinity for': *philanthropist, philocatalase, philoneism.*

-phil, -philic, -philous, a combining form meaning 'of that which combines with or is stained by': *chromaphil, hydrophil, lipophil.*

Philadelphia chromosome (Ph[1]), a translocation of the long arm of chromosome 22, often seen in the abnormal myeloblasts, erythroblasts, and megakaryoblasts of patients who have chronic myelocytic leukemia.

-philia, -phily, **1.** a combining form meaning a 'tendency towards an action': *calciphelia, cryophilia, spasmophilia.* **2.** a combining form meaning 'abnormal appetite for a thing': *carcinophilia, lygophilia, necrophilia.*

-philous, a combining form meaning 'having an affinity for': *calciphilous, chromophilous, cyanophilous.* See also **-phil.**

-phily, **1.** a combining form meaning a 'fondness for something': *necrophily.* **2.** a combining form meaning an 'affinity for something': *hydrophily, photophily, xerophily.*

phimosis /fīmō'sis/, tightness of the prepuce of the penis that prevents the retraction of the foreskin over the glans. The condition is usually congenital but may be the result of infection. Circumcision is the usual treatment. An analogous condition of the clitoris occurs rarely. Compare **paraphimosis.** See also **phimosis vaginalis.**

phimosis vaginalis /vaj'inā'lis/, congenital narrowness or closure of the vaginal opening.

phi phenomenon, a sensation of apparent motion that is caused by lights that flash on and off at a certain frequency. Also called **stroboscopic illusion.**

pHisoHex, a trademark for a detergent containing a topical antiinfective (hexachlorophene).

phleb-. See **phlebo-.**

phlebitis. See **thrombophlebitis.**

phlebo-, phleb-, a combining form meaning 'of or related to a vein or veins': *phlebocarcinoma, phlebograph, phlebostenosis.*

phlebogram /fleb'əgram/, **1.** an x-ray film obtained by phlebography. **2.** a graphic representation of the venous pulse, obtained by phlebograph. Also called **venogram.**

phlebograph /fleb'əgraf'/, a device for producing a graphic record of the venous pulse.

phlebography /fləbog'rəfē/, **1.** the technique of preparing an x-ray image of veins injected with a radiopaque contrast medium. **2.** the technique of preparing a graphic record of the venous pulse by means of a phlebograph. Also called **venography.**

phlebostatic axis, the approximate location of the right atrium, found by drawing an imaginary line from the fourth intercostal space at the right side of the sternum to an intersection with the midaxillary line.

phlebothrombosis /fleb'ōthrombō'sis/, an abnormal venous condition in which a clot forms within a vein, usually caused by hemostasis, hypercoagulability, or occlusion. In contrast to thrombophlebitis, the wall of the vein is not inflamed.

phlebotomus fever, an acute, mild infection, caused by one of five distinct arboviruses transmitted to humans by the bite of an infected sandfly, characterized by rapidly developing fever, headache, eye pain, conjunctivitis, myalgia, and, occasionally, a macular or urticarial rash. Aseptic meningitis may also occur. The disease is widespread in hot, dry areas where sandflies abound, and it has been seen in Panama and Brazil. Phlebotomus fever is self-limited, no fatalities have been recorded, and no specific therapy is available. Bed rest, fluids, and aspirin are recommended. A second attack may occur a few weeks after the first. Also called **pappataci, sandfly fever, three-day fever.**

phlebotomy /fləbot'əmē/, the incision of a vein for the letting of blood, as in collecting blood from a donor. Phlebotomy is the chief treatment for polycythemia vera and may be performed every 6 months, or more frequently if required. The procedure is sometimes used to decrease the amount of circulating blood and pulmonary engorgement in acute pulmonary edema. At one time phlebotomy was practiced for almost every disorder. Also called **venesection.**

phleg-. See **phlogo-.**

phlegm /flem/, thick mucus secreted by the tissues lining the respiratory passages.

phlegmasia /flegmā'zhə/, *obsolete.* an inflammation.

phlegmasia alba dolens, thrombophlebitis of the femoral vein, resulting in edema of the leg and pain. It may occur after childbirth or after a severe febrile illness.

phlegmasia cerulea dolens, a severe form of thrombosis of a deep vein, usually the femoral vein. The condition is acute and fulminating and is usually accompanied by vast edema and cyanosis of the limb distal to the occluding thrombosis.

phlegmonous gastritis, a rare but severe form of gastritis, involving the connective tissue layer of the stomach wall. It occurs as a complication of systemic infection, peptic ulcer, cancer, surgery, or other severe stress and represents an acute abdominal emergency. Treatment includes surgery, antibiotics, and analgesics.

phlogo-, phleg-, a combining form meaning 'of or related to inflammation': *phlogocyte, phlogogen, phlogoxelotism.*

phlyctenular keratoconjunctivitis, an inflammatory condition of the cornea, characterized by tiny, ulcerating nodules, seen most often in children as a response to allergens found in tuberculin, gonococci, *Candida albicans,* or various parasites. Vitamin deficiency may be a factor. The condition responds to topical corticosteroids, but corneal scars may remain. Also called **phlyctenulosis, scrofulous keratitis.** See also **eczematous conjunctivitis.**

phob-, a combining form meaning 'of or pertaining to fear or morbid dread': *phobia, phobic, phobophobia.*

-phobe, -phobiac, -phobist, a combining form meaning 'one who fears' something specified: *dermatophobe, heliophobe, nosophobe.*

phobia /fō'bē·ə/, an anxiety disorder characterized by an obsessive, irrational, and intense fear of a specific object, as an animal or dirt, of an activity, as meeting strangers or leaving the familiar setting of the home, or of a physical situation, as heights and open or closed spaces.

Typical manifestations of phobia include faintness, fatigue, palpitations, perspiration, nausea, tremor, and panic. The fear, which is out of proportion to reality, usually results from some early painful or unpleasant experience involving the particular object or situation, or it may arise from displacing an unconscious conflict to an external object or situation to which it is symbolically related. The irrational, compelling need to avoid the feared object or situation can interfere with customary daily activities, often resulting in complex alterations in life patterns and interpersonal relationships. Although the individual usually recognizes the inappropriateness of the reaction, he is powerless to overcome the fear until the repressed conflict is recognized, usually through extensive psychotherapy. Treatment also consists of behavior therapy to reduce the maladaptive anxiety resulting from the fear by altering the behavioral response. Some kinds of phobias are **agoraphobia, algophobia, claustrophobia, erythrophobia, gynephobia, laliophobia, mysophobia, nyctophobia, photophobia, xenophobia,** and **zoophobia.** Also called **phobic disorder, phobic neurosis, phobic reaction.** Compare **compulsion.** See also **simple phobia, social phobia.** **-phobic,** *adj.*

-phobia, a combining form meaning 'abnormal fear' of the object, experience, or place specified: *agoraphobia, claustrophobia, nyctophobia.*

phobiac /fō′bē•ak/, a person who exhibits or is afflicted with a phobia.

-phobiac. See **-phobe.**

-phobic, -phobous, **1.** a combining form meaning 'exhibiting or possessing an aversion for or fear of (something)': *Anglophobic, necrophobic, zoophobic.* **2.** a combining form meaning the 'absence of a strong affinity': *chromophobic, gentianophobic, osmiophobic.*

phobic disorder, phobic neurosis, phobic reaction. See **phobia.**

phobic state, a condition characterized by extreme anxiety resulting from the excessive, irrational fear of a particular object, situation, or activity. See also **phobia.**

-phobist. See **-phobe.**

-phobous. See **-phobic.**

phocomelia /fō′kəmē′lyə/, a developmental anomaly characterized by the absence of the upper portion of one or more of the limbs so that the feet or hands or both are attached to the trunk of the body by short, irregularly shaped stumps, resembling the fins of a seal. The condition, caused by interference with the embryonic development of the long bones, is rare and is seen primarily as a side effect of the drug thalidomide taken during early pregnancy. Also called **seal limbs.** Compare **amelia.** –**phocomelic,** *adj.*

phocomelic dwarf, a dwarf in whom the long bones of any or all of the extremities are abnormally short.

phocomelus /fōkom′ələs/, an individual who has phocomelia.

phon-. See **phono-.**

-phone, **1.** a combining form meaning a 'device for transmitting sound': *auriphone, ossiphone, osteophone.* **2.** a combining form meaning a 'device for monitoring body sounds': *miophone, sphygmophone, stethophone.*

phonic, of or pertaining to voice, sounds, or speech.

-phonic, a combining form meaning 'sounds made in a (specified) part of the body': *bronchiophonic, leptophonic, organophonic.*

phono-, phon-, a combining form meaning 'of or related to sound, often specifically the sound of the voice': *phonocardiograph, phonopathy, phonopsia.*

phonocardiogram, a graphic recording obtained from a phonocardiograph.

phonocardiograph, an electroacoustic device that produces graphic heart sound recordings, used in the diagnosis and monitoring of heart disorders. This instrument produces phonocardiograms by using a system of microphones and associated recording equipment. One microphone is usually placed on the chest near the base of the heart; another is positioned on the chest over the apex of the heart. The microphone placed over the base of the heart records the timing of the aortic and the pulmonary components of the second heart sound and the loudest murmurs. The microphone placed over the apex is connected to special filters that allow the recording of low-frequency sounds, as those associated with atrial and ventricular gallops, as well as higher frequency sounds, as those associated with mitral regurgitation and ventricular septal defect. To assure an accurate recording, the examiner also uses audiophones to monitor the sounds and an oscilloscope to monitor cardiac impulses. –**phonocardiographic,** *adj.*

-phony, -phonia, **1.** a combining form meaning 'sound': *echophony, laryngophony.* **2.** a combining form meaning a 'speech disorder' of a (specified) type: *autophony, egophony, gutturophony.*

phor-, a combining form meaning 'bearing, carrying': *phoresis, phoroblast, phorology.*

-phore, -phor, a combining form meaning a 'bearer or possessor': *gluciphore, physaliphore, trochophore.*

-phoresis, a combining form meaning a 'movement in a (specified) manner or medium': *aphoresis, cataphoresis, diaphoresis.*

-phoria, **1.** a combining form meaning '(condition of the) visual axes of the eye': *anophoria, esophoria, exophoria.* **2.** a combining form meaning an 'emotional state': *adiaphoria, euphoria, ideaphoria.*

phosphatase /fos′fətāz/, an enzyme that acts as a catalyst in chemical reactions involving phosphorus. See also **catalyst, enzyme.**

phosphate, a salt of phosphoric acid. Phosphates are extremely important in living cells, particularly in the storage and use of energy and the transmission of genetic information within a cell and from one cell to another. See also **adenosine diphosphate, adenosine triphosphate, phosphorus.**

phosphatide, a phosphatidic acid from which the choline or colamine portion has been removed. It may occur as an intermediate in the biosynthesis of triglycerides and phospholipids. Also called **phosphotidate**.

phosphoglycerate kinase /fos′fōglis′ərāt/, an enzyme that catalyzes the reversible transfer of a phosphate group from adenosine triphosphate to D-3-phosphoglycerate, forming D-1,3-diphosphoglycerate. The reaction is one of the steps in glycolysis.

Phospholine Iodide, a trademark for a cholinergic (echothiophate iodide).

phospholipid /fos′fōlip′id/, one of a class of compounds, widely distributed in living cells, containing phosphoric acid, fatty acids, and a nitrogenous base. Two kinds of phospholipids are **lecithin** and **sphingomyelin.**

phosphomevalonate kinase /fos′fōməval′ənāt/, an enzyme that catalyzes the transfer of a phosphate group from adenosine triphosphate to produce adenosine diphosphate and 5-pyrophosphomevalonate.

phosphoric acid, a clear, colorless, odorless liquid that is irritating to the skin and eyes and moderately toxic if ingested. Phosphoric acid is used in the production of fertilizers, soaps, detergents, animal feeds, and certain drugs.

phosphorus (P), a nonmetallic chemical element occurring extensively in nature as a component of phosphate rock. Its atomic number is 15; its atomic weight is 30.975. Phosphorus forms a series of sulfides used commercially in the manufacture of matches. It can be prepared in yellow or white, red, and black allotropic forms. Phosphorus is essential for the metabolism of protein, calcium, and glucose. The body uses phosphorus in its combined forms, which are obtained from such nutritional sources as milk, cheese, meat, egg yolk, whole grains, legumes, and nuts. A nutritional deficiency of phosphorus can cause weight loss, anemia, and abnormal growth. Phosphorus is essential to the body for the production of adenosine triphosphate and for the process of glycolysis. Elemental white or yellow phosphorus is extremely poisonous and produces severe GI irritation. If ingested, it can produce hemorrhage, cardiovascular failure, and death. Chronic poisoning from phosphorus is characterized by anemia, cachexia, bronchitis, and necrosis of the mandible.

phosphorus poisoning, a toxic condition caused by the ingestion of white or yellow phosphorus, sometimes found in rat poisons, certain fertilizers, and fireworks. Intoxication is characterized initially by nausea, throat and stomach pain, vomiting, diarrhea, and an odor of garlic on the breath. After a few days of apparent recovery, nausea, vomiting, and diarrhea recur with renal and hepatic dysfunction. Treatment includes gastric lavage and administration of mineral oil, vitamin K, intravenous fluids, and medication to counteract shock. Physical contact with the vomitus and feces of the patient is avoided.

phot-. See **photo-.**

-photic, a combining form meaning 'pertaining to the ability to see at a (specified) light level': *euryphotic, stenophotic, sthenophotic.*

photo-, phot-, a combining form meaning 'of or pertaining to light': *photoelectric, photoreceptor, phototropism.*

photoallergic, exhibiting a delayed hypersensitivity reaction after exposure to light. Compare **phototoxic.** See also **photoallergic contact dermatitis.**

photoallergic contact dermatitis, a papulovesicular, eczematous, or exudative skin reaction occurring 24 to 48 hours after exposure to light in a previously sensitized person. The sensitizing substance concentrates in the skin and requires chemical alteration by light to become an active antigen. Among common photosensitizers are phenothiazines, hexachlorophene, oral hypoglycemic agents, and sulfanilamide. Prevention requires avoidance of the photosensitizer and sunlight. Treatment is the same as that for any other inflammatory dermatitis.

photochemotherapy, a kind of chemotherapy in which the effect of the administered drug is enhanced by exposing the patient to light, as the treatment of psoriasis with oral methoxsalen followed by exposure to ultraviolet light. See also **chemotherapy.**

photometer /fōtom′ətər/, an instrument that measures light intensity. It usually is composed of a source of radiant energy, a filter for wavelength selection, a cuvette holder, a detector, and a readout device.

photomultiplier, a device used in many radiation detection applications that converts low levels of light into electric pulses. A bank of such tubes is used in gamma cameras to view the crystal.

photon, an individual packet or quantum of electromagnetic radiation.

photophobia /fō′tō-/, **1.** abnormal sensitivity to light, especially by the eyes. The condition is prevalent in albinism and various diseases of the conjunctiva and cornea and may be a symptom of such disorders as measles, psittacosis, encephalitis, Rocky Mountain spotted fever, and Reiter's syndrome. **2.** (in psychiatry) a morbid fear of light with an irrational need to avoid light places. The anxiety disorder is seen more often in women than in men and is usually caused by a repressed intrapsychic conflict symbolically related to light. Treatment consists of psychotherapy to uncover the cause of the phobic reaction followed by behavior therapy, often using the techniques of systemic desensitization and flooding. **–photophobic,** *adj.*

photoscan, a radiograph that shows the distribution of a radiopharmaceutic in the body.

photosensitive, increased reactivity of skin to sunlight caused by a disorder, as albinism or porphyria, or more frequently resulting from the use of certain drugs. Relatively brief exposure to sunlight or to an ultraviolet lamp may cause edema, papules, urticaria, or acute burns in individuals with endogenous or acquired photosensitivity. Drugs inducing photosensitivity include phenothiazine tranquilizers, antibiotic tetracycline, antimycotic griseofulvin, antibacterial nalidixic acid, oral hypoglycemic agents, the artificial sweetener calcium cyclamate, the oral contraceptive agents mestranol and norethynodrel, and halogenated salicylanides used in antifungal soaps. Treatment involves avoidance of exposure to sunlight or the photosensitizing agent. Methoxsalen and trioxsalen are potent photosensitizers sometimes used to enhance pigmentation or increase tolerance to sunlight, but overexposure or overdosage can cause severe reactions.

photosensitivity, any abnormal response to exposure to light, specifically, a skin reaction requiring the presence of a sensitizing agent and exposure to sunlight or its equivalent. Photosensitivity includes photoallergic and phototoxic reactions.

photosynthesis /fōtōsin′thəsis/, a process by which green plants containing chlorophyll synthesize chemical substances, chiefly carbohydrates, from atmospheric carbon dioxide and water, using light for energy and liberating oxygen in the process.

phototherapy, the treatment of disorders by the use of light, especially ultraviolet light. Ultraviolet light may be employed in the therapy of acne, decubiti and other indolent ulcers, psoriasis, and hyperbilirubinemia. See also **photochemotherapy.** –**phototherapeutic,** *adj.*

phototherapy in the newborn, a treatment for hyperbilirubinemia and jaundice in the newborn that involves the exposure of an infant's bare skin to intense fluorescent light. The blue range of light accelerates the excretion of bilirubin in the skin, decomposing it by photooxidation.

■ METHOD: The infant is placed nude under the fluorescent lights with the eyes and genitalia covered. The baby is turned frequently, and the body temperature is monitored, using a skin thermistor. All vital signs are carefully noted, and details regarding position of the bulbs, time and duration of treatment, and the infant's response are charted. Adverse effects of phototherapy include dehydration: An infant may need 25% more fluid during treatment. Loose stools and "bronze baby" syndrome may occur.

■ NURSING ORDERS: The nurse performs phototherapy and may be responsible for collecting specimens for serial tests for bilirubin in the blood. The lights may scorch the nurse's hair and irritate the eyes; as protection, a cap and sunglasses may be worn. Breast feeding may be discontinued during treatment but often is not; additional water is always given. The family is encouraged to visit and to participate in caring for the infant. They may be told that the eyeshields are necessary but do not seem to bother the infant.

■ OUTCOME CRITERIA: Bilirubin levels usually decrease by 3 to 4 mg/dl in the first 8 to 12 hours of therapy; thus, simple jaundice clears rapidly. Excess bilirubin and jaundice that are the result of hemolytic disease or infection may be controlled with phototherapy, but the underlying cause is treated separately. Recovery is usually complete. The long-term safety of phototherapy has not been established; short-term efficacy and practicality of use are certain.

phototoxic, characterized by a rapidly developing, nonimmunologic reaction of the skin when it is exposed to a photosensitizing substance and light. Compare **photoallergic.** See also **phototoxic contact dermatitis.**

phototoxic contact dermatitis, a rapidly appearing, sunburnlike response of areas of skin that have been exposed to the sun after contact with a photosensitizing substance. Hyperpigmentation may follow the acute reaction. Among known photosensitizing materials are coal tar derivatives, oil of bergamot (often used in cosmetics and beverages), and many plants containing furocoumarin (cowslip, buttercup, carrot, parsnip, mustard, and yarrow). Treatment includes Burow's solution, acid mantle cream, and topical corticosteroids.

-phragma, -phragm, a combining form meaning a 'septum or musculomembranous barrier between cavities': *inophragma, mesophragma, telophragma.*

-phrasia, a combining form meaning an 'abnormal condition of speech': *aphrasia, echophrasia, embolophrasia.*

phren-, **1.** a combining form meaning 'of or related to the mind': *phrenasthenia, phrenoblabia, phrenology.* **2.** a combining form meaning 'of or related to the diaphragm': *phrenodynia, phrenogastric, phrenohepatic.*

-phrenia, a combining form meaning a 'disordered condition of mental activity': *hebephrenia, ideophrenia, kolyphrenia.*

phrenic /fren′ik/, **1.** of or pertaining to the diaphragm. **2.** of or pertaining to the mind.

-phrenic, **1.** a combining form meaning the 'diaphragm or adjacent regions of the body': *costophrenic, postphrenic, subphrenic.* **2.** a combining form meaning 'characteristic of a disorder of the mind': *hebephrenic, ideophrenic, schizophrenic.*

phrenic nerve, one of a pair of muscular branches of the cervical plexus, arising from the fourth cervical nerve. It contains about one half as many sensory as motor fibers and is generally known as the motor nerve to the diaphragm, although the lower thoracic nerves also help to innervate the diaphragm. The phrenic nerve lies on the ventral surface of the scalenus anterior, crossing from its lateral to its medial border. It continues with the scalenus anterior between the subclavian vein and the subclavian artery, enters the thorax, passes over the cupula of the pleura, along the lateral aspect of the pericardium, and reaches the diaphragm, where it divides into terminal branches. The right phrenic nerve is deeper and shorter than the left. The pleural branches of the phrenic nerve are very fine filaments supplying the mediastinal pleura. The pericardial branches are delicate filaments passing to the upper pericardium. The terminal branches diverge after passing separately through the diaphragm and are distributed on the abdominal surface of the diaphragm. On the right side, a branch near the inferior vena cava communicates with the phrenic plexus in association with a phrenic ganglion. There is no phrenic ganglion on the left side. Also called **internal respiratory nerve of Bell.** Compare **accessory phrenic nerve.**

phthi-, a combining form meaning 'decay, wasting away': *phthisiogenesis, phthisiomania, phthisis.*

Phthirus /thī′rəs/, a genus of bloodsucking lice that includes the species *Phthirus pubis,* the pubic louse, or crab.

-phthongia, a combining form meaning a 'condition of speech': *aphthongia, diphthongia, heterophthongia.*

phyco-, a combining form meaning 'of or pertaining to seaweed': *phycochrome, phycocyan, phycology.*

phychologist /fēkol′əjist/, a person who specializes in the study of algae. Also called **algologist.**

phycology /fēkol′əjē/, the branch of science that is concerned with algae. Also called **algology.**

phycomycosis /fī′kōmīkō′sis/, a fungal infection caused by a species of the order Phycomycetes. These organisms are common in the soil and are not usually pathogenic. Severe nosocomial pulmonary phycomycosis sometimes occurs with advanced diabetes mellitus that is untreated or out of control and complicated by ketoacidosis. See also **mucormycosis, zygomycosis.**

phyl-, a combining form meaning 'guarding or preservation': *phylacagogic, phylactic, phylaxis.*

-phyll, -phyl, a combining form meaning a 'coloring matter in plants': *chlorophyll, leukophyll.*

phyllo-, a combining form meaning 'of or pertaining to leaves': *phyllochlorin, phyllode, phyllosan.*

phylloquinone. See **vitamin K_1.**

phylo-, a combining form meaning 'type, kind': *phylobiology, phylogenesis, phylogeny.*

phylogenesis. See **phylogeny.**

phylogenetic /fī′lōgənet′ik/, **1.** of, relating to, or acquired during phylogeny. **2.** based on a natural evolutionary relationship, as a system of classification. Also **phylogenic.**

phylogeny /filoj′ənē/, the development of the structure of a particular race or species as it evolved from simpler forms of life. Compare **ontogeny.** See also **comparative anatomy.**

-phyma, a combining form meaning a 'swelling or tumor': *adenophyma, celiophyma, onychophyma.*

physi-. See **physio-.**

physiatrist, a physician who tests the physical functioning of a patient and supervises the patient's rehabilitation program.

-physical, a combining form meaning 'natural': *iatrophysical, medicophysical, psychophysical.*

physical abuse, one or more episodes of aggressive behavior, usually resulting in physical injury with possible damage to internal organs, sense organs, the central nervous system, or the musculoskeletal system of another person.

physical allergy, an allergic response to physical factors, as cold, heat, light, or trauma. Usually, specific antibodies are found in people having physical allergies. Common characteristics include pruritis, urticaria, and angioedema. There may be photosensitivity, caused by the use of certain cosmetics or drugs. Prophylaxis usually includes an attempt to remove the stimulus, and treatment involves the use of antihistamines or steroids. Compare **contact dermatitis.** See also **atopic.**

physical assessment, the part of the health assessment representing a synthesis of the information obtained in a physical examination.

physical chemistry, the natural science dealing with the relationship between chemical and physical properties of matter.

physical diagnosis, the diagnostic process accomplished by the study of the physical manifestations of health and illness revealed in the physical examination, as guided by the patient's complete history and supported by various laboratory tests. Physical diagnosis is to medicine what the health assessment is to nursing.

physical examination, an investigation of the body to determine its state of health, using any or all of the techniques of inspection, palpation, percussion, auscultation, and smell. The physical examination, medical history, and initial laboratory tests constitute the data base on which a diagnosis is made and on which a plan of treatment is developed.

physical fitness, the ability to carry out daily tasks with alertness and vigor, without undue fatigue, and with enough energy reserve to meet emergencies or to enjoy leisure time pursuits.

physical medicine, the use of physical therapy techniques to return physically diseased or injured patients to a useful life. See also **rehabilitation.**

physical science, the study of the laws and properties of nonliving matter. Some kinds of physical science are **chemistry, geology,** and **physics.** Compare **life science.**

physical therapist, a person who is licensed to assist in the examination, testing, and treatment of physically disabled or handicapped people through the use of special exercise, application of heat or cold, use of sonar waves, and other techniques. A physical therapist usually becomes qualified by taking a 4-year college course leading to a B.S. in physical therapy or a special 12-month certificate course after obtaining a bachelor's degree in a related field.

physical therapy, the treatment of disorders with physical agents and methods, as massage, manipulation, therapeutic exercises, cold, heat (including shortwave, microwave, and ultrasonic diathermy), hydrotherapy, electric stimulation, and light to assist in rehabilitating patients and in restoring normal function after an illness or injury. Also called **physiotherapy.**

physical therapy aide, a person who, under the supervision of a licensed physical therapist, assists in carrying out patient treatment programs and performing related clerical tasks.

physician, **1.** a health professional who has earned a degree of Doctor of Medicine (M.D.) after completing an approved course of study at an approved medical school. Satisfactory completion of National Board Examinations, usually given during both the second and the final years of medical school and after graduation, is also required.

An M.D. usually enters a hospital internship program for 1 year of postgraduate training before beginning practice or further training in a specialty. To practice medicine, an M.D. is required to obtain a license from the state in which professional services will be performed. **2.** a health professional who has earned a degree of Doctor of Osteopathy (D.O.) by satisfactorily completing a course of education in an approved college of osteopathy. Osteopathic physicians and medical physicians follow nearly identical courses of training and modes of practice, except that osteopathic medicine places special emphasis on the study of mechanic derangement of tissues as a cause of illness and on treatment that involves manipulation of body structures.

physician extender, a health care provider who is not a physician but who performs medical activities typically performed by a physician.

physician's assistant (PA), a person trained in certain aspects of the practice of medicine to provide assistance to a physician. A physician's assistant is trained by physicians and practices under the direction and supervision and within the legal license of a physician. Training programs vary in length from a few months to 2 years. Health care experience or academic preparation may be a prerequisite to admission to some programs. Most physician's assistants are prepared for the practice of primary care, but some practice subspecialities, including surgical assistance, dialysis, or radiology. National certification is available to qualified graduates of approved training programs. The national organization is the American Association of Physician's Assistants (AAPA). Also called **physician's associate.**

Physician's Desk Reference (PDR), a compendium compiled annually, containing information about drugs, primarily prescription drugs and products used in diagnostic procedures in the United States, supplied by their manufacturers.

physics, the study of the laws and properties of matter and energy, particularly as related to motion and force.

-physics, a combining form meaning the 'science of the nature of' something specified: *cytophysics, medicophysics, microphysics.*

physio-, physi-, a combining form meaning 'related to nature or to physiology': *physiochemical, physiognosis, physiotherapy.*

physiologic chemistry. See **biochemistry.**

physiologic contracture, a temporary condition in which muscles may contract and shorten for a considerable period of time. Drugs, extremes of temperature, and local accumulation of lactic acid are causes. Compare **functional contracture.**

physiologic dead space, an area in the respiratory system that includes the anatomic dead space together with the space in the alveoli occupied by air that does not contribute to the oxygen-carbon dioxide exchange. Compare **anatomic dead space.**

physiologic dwarf. See **primordial dwarf.**

physiologic hypertrophy, a temporary increase in the size of an organ or part because of normal physiologic functions, as occurs in the walls of the uterus and in the breasts during pregnancy.

physiologic motivation, a bodily need, as food or water, that initiates behavior directed toward satisfying the particular need. Also called **organic motivation.** Compare **achievement motivation, social motivation.**

physiologic occlusion, **1.** a closure of the teeth that complements and enhances the functions of the masticatory system. **2.** a closure of the teeth that produces no pathologic effects on the stomatognathic system, normally dissipating the stresses placed on the teeth and creating a balance between the stresses and the adaptive capacity of the supporting tissues. **3.** an acceptable occlusion in a healthy gnathic system.

physiologic psychology, the study of the interrelationship of physiologic and psychologic processes, especially the effects of a change from normal to abnormal.

physiologic retraction ring, a ridge around the inside of the uterus that forms during the second stage of normal labor at the junction of the thinned lower uterine segment and thickened upper segment as a result of progressive lengthening of the muscle fibers of the lower segment and concomitant shortening of the muscle fibers of the upper segment. Compare **constriction ring, pathologic retraction ring.**

physiologic third heart sound, a low-pitched extra heart sound heard early in diastole in a healthy child or young adult. It is of no clinical significance and usually disappears with age. The same sound, heard in an older person who has heart disease is an abnormal finding called a ventricular gallop. See also **gallop.**

physiology, **1.** the study of the processes and function of the human body. **2.** the study of the physical and chemical processes involved in the functioning of living organisms and their component parts. Kinds of physiology are **comparative physiology, developmental physiology, hominal physiology,** and **pathologic physiology.** Compare **anatomy.** See also the Appendix.

physiotherapy. See **physical therapy.**

-physis, a combining form meaning a 'growth or growing': *metaphysis, onychophysis, zygapophysis.*

physo-, a combining form meaning 'of or pertaining to air or gas': *physocele, physocephaly, physometra.*

physostigmine /fī'sōstig'min/, a cholinergic.

■ INDICATIONS: It is prescribed in the treatment of some forms of glaucoma and to reverse effects of neuromuscular blocking agents.

■ CONTRAINDICATIONS: Narrow-angle glaucoma, iridocyclitis, or hypersensitivity to this drug prohibits its use.

■ ADVERSE EFFECTS: Among the more serious adverse reactions are bradycardia, dyspnea, bronchospasm, anorexia, and convulsions. Also called **eserine, eserine sulfate.**

physostigmine salicylate, an anticholinergic drug inhibitor.

■ INDICATIONS: It is prescribed in the treatment of central nervous system effects caused by drugs in clinical or toxic dosages capable of producing anticholinergic poisoning.

■ CONTRAINDICATIONS: Asthma, gangrene, diabetes, cardiovascular disease, or mechanic obstruction of the intestines or urinary tract prohibits its use. It is also not administered to patients in any vagotonic state and to those receiving choline esters or depolarizing neuromuscular blocking agents.

■ ADVERSE EFFECTS: Among the most serious adverse reactions are hypersalivation, bradycardia, convulsions, and hypertensive reactions.

phytanic acid storage disease /fītan′ik/, a rare genetic disorder of lipid metabolism in which there are accumulations of phytanic acid in the plasma and tissues. The condition is characterized by ataxia, peripheral neuropathy, retinitis pigmentosa, and abnormalities of the bone and skin. Also called **Refsum's syndrome.**

-phyte, a combining form meaning a 'plant that grows in or on or produces': *epiphyte, paraphyte, pteridophyte.*

phyto-, a combining form meaning 'of or pertaining to a plant or plants': *phytobezoar, phytochemistry, phytoncide.*

phytohemagglutinin (PHA), a hemagglutinin that is derived from a plant, specifically the lectin obtained from the red kidney bean. Also called **phytolectin.**

phytohemagglutinin test, a test to identify genetic carriers of cystic fibrosis, performed by exposing white blood cells to phytohemagglutinin. A normal reaction involves a noticeable increase of cell protein.

phytolectin, See **phytohemagglutinin.**

phytonadione. See **vitamin K_1.**

P.I., (in patient records) abbreviation for *present illness.*

pia mater /pē′ə mā′tər/, the innermost of the three meninges covering the brain and the spinal cord. It is closely applied to both structures and carries a rich supply of blood vessels, which nourish the nervous tissue. The cranial pia mater covers the surface of the brain and dips deeply into the fissures and the sulci of the cerebral hemispheres. Extending into the transverse cerebral fissure, the cranial pia mater forms the tela choroidea of the third ventricle, combines with the ependyma to form the choroid plexuses of the third and the lateral ventricles, and passes over the roof of the fourth ventricle to form its tela choroidea and its choroid plexus. The spinal pia mater is thicker, firmer, and less vascular than the cranial pia mater and consists of two layers. The outer layer is composed of longitudinal collagenous fibers that are concentrated along the anterior median fissure as the linea splendens. The inner layer closely wraps the entire spinal cord and, at the end of the cord, is prolonged into the filum terminale. The pia mater also forms the denticulate ligament, which extends the entire length of the spinal cord on both sides between the dorsal and the ventral spinal nerve roots. Compare **arachnoid, dura mater.**

pian. See **yaws.**

pian bois. See **forest yaws.**

pica /pī′kə/, a craving to eat substances that are not foods, as dirt, clay, chalk, glue, ice, starch, or hair. The appetite disorder may occur with some nutritional deficiency states, with pregnancy, and in some forms of mental illness.

Pick's disease, a form of presenile dementia occurring in middle age. This disorder affects mainly the frontal and temporal lobes of the brain and characteristically produces neurotic behavior, slow disintegration of intellect, personality, and emotions, and degeneration of cognitive abilities. See also **dementia.**

pickwickian syndrome, an abnormal condition characterized by obesity, decreased pulmonary function, somnolence, and polycythemia.

pico-, a combining form meaning 'one trillionth' (10^{-12}) of the unit designated: *picogram, picoliter, picometer.*

picornavirus /pīkôr′nəvī′rəs/, a member of a group of small RNA viruses that are ether-resistant. The two main genera are *Enterovirus* and *Rhinovirus.* These viruses cause poliomyelitis, herpangina, and aseptic meningitis, encephalomyocarditis, and foot and mouth disease.

picro-, a combining form meaning 'bitter': *picroadonidin, picropyrine, picrotoxin.*

picrotoxin /pik′rōtok′sin/, a central nervous system stimulant obtained from the seeds of *Anamirta cocculus,* formerly used as an antidote for acute barbiturate poisoning.

PID, abbreviation for **pelvic inflammatory disease.**

P.I.E., abbreviation for *pulmonary infiltrate with eosinophilia,* a hypersensitivity reaction, characterized by infiltration of alveoli with eosinophils and large mononuclear cells, edema, and inflammation of the lungs. Simple pulmonary eosinophilia, in which patchy, migratory infiltrates cause minimal symptoms, is a self-limited reaction that is elicited by helminthic infections and by certain drugs, as paraaminosalicylic acid, sulfonamides, and chlorpropamide. A more prolonged illness, characterized by fever, night sweats, cough, dyspnea, weight loss, and more severe tissue reaction, occurs in certain drug allergies and bacterial, fungal, and parasitic infections. Tropical eosinophilia with paroxysmal nocturnal asthma, dyspnea, cough, low-grade fever, and malaise is related to filarial infection, and P.I.E. may occur in longstanding asthma and periarteritis nodosa. See also **Löffler's syndrome.**

piebald /pī′bôld/, having patches of white hair or skin because of an absence of melanocytes in those nonpigmented areas. It is a hereditary condition. Compare **albinism, vitiligo.**

Piedmont fracture, an oblique fracture of the distal radius, with fragments of bone pulled into the ulna.

Pierre Robin's syndrome, a complex of congenital anomalies including a small mandible, cleft lip, cleft palate, other craniofacial abnormalities, and defects of the eyes and ears, including glaucoma. Intelligence is usually normal. Plastic surgery may achieve satisfactory cosmetic repair, but speech therapy, orthodontia, and psychologic counseling and support are often necessary.

piez-, a combining form meaning 'of or related to pressure': *piezesthesia, piezallochromy, piezotherapy.*

piezoelectric effect, **1.** the generation of a voltage across a solid when a mechanic stress is applied. **2.** the dimensional change resulting from the application of a voltage.

pigeon breast, a congenital structural defect characterized by a prominent anterior projection of the xiphoid and the lower part of the sternum and by a lengthening of the costal cartilages. It may cause cardiorespiratory complications but rarely warrants surgical correction. – **pigeon-breasted,** *adj.*

pigeon breeder's lung, a respiratory disorder caused by acquired hypersensitivity to antigens in bird droppings. Also called **bird breeder's lung, hen worker's lung.**

pigeon-toed. See **metatarsus varus.**

piggyback port, a special coupling for the primary IV tubing that allows a supplementary, or piggyback, solution to run into the IV system. The piggyback port includes a backcheck valve that automatically prevents the primary IV solution from flowing while the piggyback solution is flowing. When the piggyback solution stops flowing, the backcheck valve starts the flow of the primary IV solution. Piggyback ports are part of piggyback IV sets, which are used solely for intermittent drug administration.

pigment, **1.** any organic coloring material produced in the body, as melanin. **2.** any colored, paintlike, medicinal preparation applied to the skin surface. **–pigmentary, pigmented,** *adj.,* **pigmentation,** *n.*

pigmented villonodular synovitis, a disease of the joints characterized by fingerlike proliferative growths of synovial tissue, with hemosiderin deposition within the synovial tissue. The cause of the disorder is unknown.

pigmy. See **pygmy.**

pilar cyst, an epidermoid cyst of the scalp. Its keratinized contents are firmer and less cheesy than the material in epidermoid cysts found elsewhere. The cyst originates from the middle portion of the epithelium of a hair follicle. Treatment is surgical excision. Also called **sebaceous cyst, wen.** Compare **epidermoid cyst.**

piles. See **hemorrhoids.**

pill. See **tablet.**

pillion fracture /pil′yən/, a T-shaped fracture of the distal femur with displacement of the condyles posterior to the femoral shaft, caused by a severe blow to the knee.

pilo-, a combining form meaning 'resembling or composed of hair': *pilocystic, pilomotor, pilose.*

Pilocar, a trademark for a cholinergic (pilocarpine hydrochloride).

pilocarpine /pī′lōkär′pēn/, a topical cholinergic antiglaucoma agent for ophthalmic use.

■ INDICATIONS: It is prescribed to induce miosis and to decrease intraocular pressure in chronic forms of open-angle glaucoma and in angle-closure glaucoma.

■ CONTRAINDICATIONS: It is used with caution in the presence of asthma, keratitis, conjunctivitis, and iritis. Known hypersensitivity to this drug prohibits its use.

■ ADVERSE REACTIONS: Among the more serious adverse reactions are dyspnea, wheezing, muscle tremors, diaphoresis, and hyperptyalism. Blurred vision, eye pain, and headache may occur.

pilocarpine and epinephrine, a fixed-combination drug used in the treatment of glaucoma, containing a cholinergic (pilocarpine hydrochloride) and an adrenergic vasoconstrictor (epinephrine bitartrate).

pilocarpine and physostigmine, a fixed-combination drug used in the treatment of glaucoma, containing a cholinergic (pilocarpine hydrochloride) and a short-acting cholinesterase inhibitor (physostigmine salicylate). Both ingredients reduce intraocular pressure.

pilocarpine hydrochloride, an ophthalmic cholinergic.

■ INDICATIONS: It is prescribed as a miotic in treating primary open-angle and acute-angle closure glaucoma.

■ CONTRAINDICATIONS: Acute iritis, secondary glaucoma, or known hypersensitivity to this drug prohibits its use.

■ ADVERSE EFFECTS: Among the most serious adverse reactions are ciliary spasm with pain and allergic reactions.

Pilocel, a trademark for a cholinergic (pilocarpine hydrochloride).

piloerection. See **pilomotor reflex.**

Pilomiotin, a trademark for a cholinergic (pilocarpine hydrochloride).

pilomotor reflex /pī′lōmō′tər/, erection of the hairs of the skin in response to a chilly environment, emotional stimulus, or irritation of the skin. This normal reaction is abolished below the level of a transverse spinal cord lesion and may be exaggerated on the affected side in a patient with hemiplegia. Also called **gooseflesh, horripilation, piloerection.**

pilonidal cyst /pī′lənī′dəl/, a hairy cyst that often develops in the sacral region of the skin. Pilonidal cysts may sometimes be recognized at birth by a depression, sometimes a hairy dimple, in the midline of the back, sacrococcygeal area. Usually these cysts do not cause any problems, but occasionally a sinus or fistula develops in early adulthood that communicates with the skin, resulting in infection. A fistula may also develop to the spinal tract from a pilonidal cyst. If a cyst becomes infected or inflamed, it is excised, and the space is surgically closed after the infection or inflammation has been effectively treated.

pilonidal fistula, an abnormal channel containing a tuft of hair, situated most frequently over or close to the tip of the coccyx but also occurring in other regions of the body. Also called **pilonidal sinus.**

pilosebaceous /pī′lōsibā′shəs/, of or pertaining to a hair follicle and its oil gland.

PILOT /pī′lət/, a computer interpreter language, similar to BASIC, used in computer-assisted instruction.

pilus /pē′ləs/, *pl.* **pili,** **1.** a hair or hairlike structure. **2.** (in microbiology) a fine, filamentous appendage found on certain bacteria and similar to flagellum except that it is shorter, straighter, and found in greater quantities in the organism. Pili consist solely of protein and are associated with antigenic properties of the cell surface.

Pima, a trademark for an expectorant (potassium iodide).

pimaricin. See **natamycin.**

pimelo-, a combining form meaning 'of or related to fat': *pimeloma, pimelopterygium, pimelorrhea.*

pimozide /pim′əzīd/, an investigational antipsychotic agent.

pimple, a small papule, pustule, or furuncle.

pin, **1.** (in orthopedics) to secure and immobilize fragments of bone with a nail. **2.** See **nail,** def. 2. **3.** (in dentistry) a small metal rod or peg, used as a support in rebuilding a tooth.

pin and tube fixed orthodontic appliance, an orthodontic appliance for correcting and improving malocclusion. It employs a labial arch with vertical posts that insert into tubes attached to bands on the teeth.

Pindborg tumor. See **calcifying epithelial odontogenic tumor.**

pineal body /pin′ē·əl/, a small, somewhat flattened, cone-shaped structure about 8 mm long, suspended by a stalk in the epithalamus. It consists of glial cells and pinealocytes and apparently elaborates the hormone melatonin. Also called **epiphysis cerebri.**

pineal gland, a cone-shaped structure in the brain, situated between the superior colliculi, the pulvinar, and the splenium of the corpus callosum. Its precise function has not been established. It may secrete the hormone melatonin, which appears to inhibit the secretion of luteinizing hormone. Also called **epiphysis cerebri, pineal body.**

pinealoma /pin′ē·əlō′mə/, *pl.* **pinealomas, pinealomata,** a rare neoplasm of the pineal body in the brain, characterized by hydrocephalus, pupillary changes, gait disturbances, headache, nausea, and vomiting. Precocious puberty occurs in some cases, probably caused by extension of the tumor into the hypothalamus. Also called **pinealocytoma.**

pineal tumor, a neoplasm of the pineal body. See also **pinealoma.**

pindolol, a beta-adrenergic blocker with sympathomimetic activity.

■ INDICATIONS: It is prescribed in the treatment of hypertension, alone or concomitantly with a diuretic.

■ CONTRAINDICATIONS: Bronchial asthma, overt cardiac failure, cardiogenic shock, second and third degree heart block, or severe bradycardia prohibts its use. It must be used with caution in patients with diabetes.

■ ADVERSE EFFECTS: Among the most serious adverse reactions are bradycardia, hypotension, syncope, tachycardia, aggravation of bronchospasm, and GI disturbances.

pine tar, a topical antieczematic and a rubefacient. It is a common ingredient in creams, soaps, and lotions used in the treatment of chronic skin conditions, as eczema or psoriasis.

ping-ponging, *slang.* a fraudulent practice involving passing a patient from one physician to another so that a health program or facility can charge a third party for several cursory examinations.

pinhole retention, retention developed by drilling one or more holes, 2 to 3 mm in depth, in suitable areas of a cavity preparation to supplement resistance and retention form.

pinhole test, a test performed in examining a person who has diminished visual acuity to distinguish a refractive error from organic disease. A refractive error may be corrected with glasses and is not medically dangerous. Loss of visual acuity because of organic disease is serious because it may indicate a systemic, particularly a neurologic, disease and may signal the development of avoidable blindness. The test is simple to perform. Several pinholes, 0.5 to 2 mm in diameter, are punched in a card; the patient selects one and looks through it with one eye at a time, without wearing glasses. If visual acuity is improved, the defect is refractive; if not, it is organic. The pinhole effect results from blocking peripheral light waves, those most distorted by refractive error.

pink disease. See **acrodynia.**

pinkeye. See **conjunctivitis.**

Pinkus' disease. See **lichen nitidus.**

pinna. See **auricle.**

pinocytic, pertaining to a pinocyte, particularly its ability to absorb liquids by phagocytosis in cellular metabolic processes.

pinocytosis /pī′nōsītō′sis/, the process by which extracellular fluid is taken into a cell. The cell membrane develops a saccular indentation filled with extracellular fluid, then closes around it, forming a vesicle or a vacuole of fluid within the cell.

pinta, an infection of the skin caused by *Treponema carateum,* a common organism in South and Central America. The bacterium gains entry into the body through a break in the skin. Prolonged exposure and close contact appear to be necessary for transmission. The primary lesion is a slowly enlarging papule with regional lymph node enlargement, followed in 1 to 12 months by a generalized red to slate-blue macular rash. Eventually these lesions become depigmented. Diagnosis is based on serologic tests and darkfield microscopic examination of scrapings from skin lesions. Treatment with penicillin G is effective. The major complication of the disease is social ostracism resulting from the permanently disfiguring mottling of the skin. Also called **azula, carate, mal del pinto.** Compare **yaws.**

pin track infection, an abnormal condition associated with skeletal traction and characterized by infection of superficial, deeper, or soft tissues or by osteomyelitis. These infections may develop at skeletal traction pin sites. Some of the signs of pin track infection are erythema at the pin sites, drainage and odor, pin slippage, elevated temperature, and pain. Superficial infection at the pin site is treated with antibiotics administered topically or orally. Deeper infection at the pin sites usually requires removal of the pins and antibiotic therapy.

pinworm. See ***Enterobius vermicularis.***

pio-, a combining form meaning 'of or pertaining to fat': *pionemia, piorthopnea, pioscope.*

PIo_2, the partial pressure of inspired oxygen.

pions /pī′onz/, a family of particles that can be created in nuclear reactions. Pions are unstable but can survive long enough to be formed into beams and used in certain types of medical therapy, as the treatment of brain tumors. Pions of suitable energy can penetrate the skull, spare overlying normal tissue, and then deliver most of their energy into the tumor. See also **negative pi meson.**

piperacetazine /pī′pəraset′əzēn/, a phenothiazine tranquilizer.

■ INDICATIONS: It is prescribed in the treatment of psychotic disorders and behavioral complications in mentally retarded patients.

■ CONTRAINDICATIONS: Parkinson's disease, concomitant administration of central nervous system depressants, liver or renal dysfunction, severe hypotension, or known hypersensitivity to other phenothiazine medications prohibits its use.

■ ADVERSE EFFECTS: Among the more serious adverse effects are hypotension, liver toxicity, blood dyscrasias, hypersensitivity reactions, and a variety of extrapyramidal reactions, including posttreatment tardive dyskinesia.

piperazine citrate /piper′əzēn/, an anthelmintic.

■ INDICATIONS: It is prescribed to treat infestation by pinworms or roundworms.

■ CONTRAINDICATIONS: Impaired liver or kidney function, convulsive disorders, or known hypersensitivity to this drug prohibits its use.

■ ADVERSE EFFECTS: Among the more serious adverse reactions, usually caused by overdosage, are abdominal cramps, diarrhea, vertigo, blurring of vision, and fever.

Piper forceps. See **obstetric forceps.**

piperocaine hydrochloride, a local anesthetic for the induction of spinal or caudal anesthesia.

pipette /pīpet′, pipet′/, **1.** a calibrated, transparent open-ended tube of glass or plastic used for measuring or transferring small quantities of a liquid or gas. **2.** using a pipette to dispense liquid.

pipobroman /pī′pəbrō′mən/, an antineoplastic.

■ INDICATIONS: It is prescribed in the treatment of polycythemia vera and chronic granulocytic leukemia.

■ CONTRAINDICATIONS: Bone marrow depression or known hypersensitivity to this drug prohibits its use.

■ ADVERSE EFFECTS: Among the more serious adverse reactions are nausea, abdominal cramps, and fever.

Pipracel, a trademark for an antibiotic (piperacillin).

piriform aperture, the anterior nasal opening in the skull.

piriformis /pir′ifôr′mis/, a flat, pyramidal muscle lying almost parallel with the posterior margin of the gluteus medius. It is partly within the pelvis and partly at the back of the hip joint. It arises from the sacrum, the greater sciatic foramen, and the sacrotuberous ligament, and it inserts, by a rounded tendon, into the greater trochanter of the femur. The piriformis is innervated by branches of the first and the second sacral nerves and functions to rotate the thigh laterally and to abduct and to help extend it. Compare **obturator externus, obturator internus.**

Pirquet's test /pirkāz′/, a tuberculin skin test that consists of scratching the tuberculin material onto the skin. Also called **von Pirquet's test.** See also **tuberculin test.**

pisiform bone /pē′sifôrm′/, a small, spheroidal carpal bone in the proximal row of carpal bones. It articulates with the triangular bone and is attached to the flexor retinaculum, the flexor carpi ulnaris, and the abductor digiti minimi.

pit and fissure cavity, a cavity that starts in tiny faults in tooth enamel, usually on occlusal surfaces of molars and premolars.

pitch, the quality of a tone or sound dependent on the relative rapidity of the vibrations by which it is produced.

Pitocin, a trademark for an oxytocic (oxytocin).

Pitocin Citrate, a trademark for an oxytocic (oxytocin citrate).

Pitressin, a trademark for an antidiuretic hormone (vasopressin).

pitting, **1.** small, punctate indentations in fingernails or toenails, often a result of psoriasis. **2.** an indentation that remains for a short time after pressing edematous skin with a finger. **3.** small, depressed scars in the skin or other organ of the body. **4.** the removal by the spleen of material from within erythrocytes without damage to the cells.

pituicyte, a cell of the neurohypophysis.

pituit-, a combining form meaning 'of or related to phlegm': *pituita, pituitary, pituitous.*

pituitary adamantinoma. See **craniopharyngioma.**

pituitary cachexia. See **postpubertal panhypopituitarism.**

pituitary dwarf /pito͞o′iter′ē/, a dwarf whose retarded development is caused by a deficiency of growth hormone resulting from hypofunction of the anterior lobe of the pituitary. In most cases the cause is unknown, and the defect is limited to a lack of somatotropin, although in some instances gonadotropins, adrenocorticotropic hormone, and thyroid stimulating hormone may also be deficient. The body is properly proportioned, with no facial or skeletal deformities, and there is normal mental and sexual development. The condition is usually diagnosed in childhood by radiographic examination of the bones and radioimmunoassay of levels of plasma growth hormone. Also called **hypophyseal dwarf, Lévi-Lorain dwarf, Paltauf's dwarf.**

pituitary gland, the small gland attached to the hypothalamus and couched in the sphenoid bone, supplying numerous hormones that govern many vital processes. It is divided into an anterior adenohypophysis and a smaller posterior neurohypophysis. The adenohypophysis secretes growth hormone (somatotropin), thyrotropic hormone, adrenocorticotropic hormone (ACTH), two gonadotropic hormones, follicle stimulating hormone (FSH), luteinizing hormone (LH), and prolactin, the hormone that promotes milk secretion. The neurohypophysis stores two hormones, oxytocin and vasopressin. Oxytocin stimulates the contraction of smooth muscle, especially in the uterus. Vasopressin inhibits diuresis and raises blood pressure. The pituitary gland is larger in a woman than in a man and becomes further enlarged during pregnancy. Also called **hypophysis cerebri.** See also **adenohypophysis, neurohypophysis.**

pituitary nanism, a type of dwarfism associated with hypophyseal infantilism. See also **pituitary dwarf.**

pituitary snuff lung, a type of hypersensitivity pneumonitis that sometimes occurs among takers of pituitary snuff. The antigens to which the hypersensitivity reaction occurs are found in serum proteins of cows and pigs and in pituitary tissue. Symptoms of the acute form of the disease include chills, cough, fever, dyspnea, anorexia, nausea, and vomiting. The chronic form of the disease is characterized by fatigue, chronic cough, weight loss, and dyspnea on exercise. Also called **pituitary snuff takers' disease.**

pituitary stalk, a structure that connects the pituitary gland with the hypothalamus.

Pituitrin, a trademark for an extract of the antidiuretic and oxytocic hormone of the posterior pituitary gland.

pit viper, any one of a family of venomous snakes found in the Western Hemisphere and Asia, characterized by a heat-sensitive pit between the eye and nostril on each side of the head and hollow, perforated fangs that are usually folded back in the roof of the mouth. With the exception of coral snakes, all indigenous poisonous snakes in the United States are pit vipers. See also **copperhead, cottonmouth, rattlesnake.**

pityriasis alba /pitərī′əsis/, a common idiopathic dermatosis characterized by round or oval, finely scaling patches of hypopigmentation, usually on the cheeks. The lesions are sharply demarcated, occasionally pruritic, and occur primarily in children and adolescents. The condition may recur, but spontaneous clearing is the usual prognosis. Treatment includes lubricating creams, topical corticosteroids, and, less commonly, coal tar creams. Compare **pityriasis rosea.**

pityriasis rosea, a self-limited skin disease in which a slightly scaling, pink, macular rash spreads over the trunk and other unexposed areas of the body. A characteristic feature is the **herald patch,** a larger, more scaly lesion that precedes the diffuse rash by several days. The smaller lesions tend to line up with the long axis parallel to normal lines of cleavage of the skin. Mild itching is the only symptom. The disease lasts 4 to 8 weeks and rarely recurs. It is unusual, apparently not contagious, and its cause is unknown.

Pityrosporon. See ***Malassizia.***

pivot joint, a synovial joint in which movement is limited to rotation. The joint is formed by a pivotlike process that may turn within a ring composed partly of bone and partly of ligament. The proximal radioulnar articulation is a pivot joint in which the head of the radius rotates within the ring formed by the radial notch of the ulna and the annular ligament. Also called **trochoid joint.** Compare **ball and socket joint, condyloid joint, gliding joint, hinge joint, saddle joint.**

pixel, abbreviation for *picture element,* the smallest discrete part of a digital image display.

PK, abbreviation for **psychokinesis.**

pK_a, the negative logarithm of the ionization constant of an acid that is half dissociated, used as a measure of the strength of an acid.

PKD, abbreviation for **polycystic kidney disease.**

PK test, abbreviation for **Prausnitz-Küstner test.**

PKU, abbreviation for **phenylketonuria.**

placebo /pləsē′bō/, an inactive substance, as saline, distilled water, or sugar, or a less than effective dose of a harmless substance, as a water-soluble vitamin prescribed as if it were an effective dose of a needed medication. Placebos are used in experimental drug studies to compare the effects of the inactive substance with those of the experimental drug. They are also prescribed for patients who cannot be given the medication they request or who, in the judgment of the health care provider, do not need that medication. Placebo therapy is effective in some cases, and side effects often occur as they would from the actual medication. The benefit to the patient of a placebo may occasionally outweigh the ethical, moral, and legal problems posed by its administration.

placebo effect, a physical or emotional change occurring after a substance is taken or administered that is not the result of any special property of the substance. The change may be beneficial, reflecting the expectations of the patient and, often, the expectations of the person giving the substance.

placement, the positioning of a dental prosthesis, as a removable denture in its planned site on the dental arch.

placement path, the direction of placement and removal of a removable partial denture on its supporting oral structures. The path can be varied by altering the plane to which the guiding abutment surfaces of the denture are made parallel. The choice of a placement path is considered a compromise that best fulfills five requirements: minimal torque for abutment teeth; minimal interference; maximum retention; the establishment of adequate guide plane surfaces; and acceptable esthetics.

placent-, a combining form meaning 'a cakelike mass': *placenta, placentapepton, placentogenesis.*

placenta, a highly vascular fetal organ through which the fetus absorbs oxygen, nutrients, and other substances and excretes carbon dioxide and other wastes. It begins to form on approximately the eighth day of gestation when the blastocyst touches the wall of the uterus and adheres to it. The blastocyst becomes surrounded by an outer layer of syncytiotrophoblast and an inner layer of cytotrophoblast. The trophoblast is able to digest cells of the endometrium, causing a small erosion on the uterine wall in which an embryo nidates. Under the influence of increasing amounts of progesterone, secreted by the corpus luteum of the ovary, the embryo and the placenta continue to develop. A hormone, chorionic gonadotropin, is secreted by the developing placenta and is present in the maternal blood and urine. The trophoblastic layer continues to infiltrate the maternal tissues with fingerlike projections, called chorionic villi. Separating the villi are lakes of blood in the eroded tissue. The maternal blood flows into the lakes surrounding the villi, allowing nutrients, gases, and other substances to pass into the fetal circulation by diffusion, hydrostatic pressure, and osmosis. The placenta is able to secrete large amounts of progesterone by the third month of pregnancy, enough to relieve the corpus luteum of that function. At term the normal placenta weighs one seventh to one fifth of the weight of the infant. The maternal surface is lobulated and divided into cotyledons. It has a dark red, rough, liverlike appearance. The fetal surface is smooth and shiny, covered with the fetal membranes, marked by the large white blood vessels beneath the membranes that fan out from the centrally inserted umbilical cord. The time between the delivery of the infant and the expulsion of the placenta is the third and last stage of labor.

-placenta, a combining form meaning an 'organ shaped like a flat cake': *ectoplacenta, hemiplacenta, subplacenta.*

placenta abruptio. See **abruptio placentae.**

placenta accreta, a placenta that invades the uterine muscle, making separation from the muscle difficult.

placenta battledore, a condition in which the umbilical cord is inserted into the margin of the placenta.

placental dysfunction. See **placental insufficiency.**

placental hormone, one of the several hormones produced by the placenta, including human placental lactogen, chorionic gonadotropin, estrogen, progesterone, and a thyrotropin-like hormone.

placental infarct, a localized ischemic, hard area on the fetal or maternal side of the placenta.

placental insufficiency, an abnormal condition of pregnancy, manifested clinically by retardation of the rate of fetal and uterine growth. One or more placental abnormalities cause dysfunction of maternal-placental or fetal-placental circulation sufficient to compromise fetal nutrition and oxygenation. Some of the abnormalities that can result in placental insufficiency are abnormal implantation of the placenta, multiple pregnancy, abnormal attachments of the umbilical cord or anomalies of the cord itself, and abnormalities of the placental membranes. Histopathologic abnormalities that can cause placental insufficiency include intravillous thrombi, placental infarction, and breaks in the placental membrane that result in fetal bleeding into the maternal circulation. Placental insufficiency may also result from placental senescence in postmaturity, from systemic diseases, as erythroblastosis fetalis and diabetes mellitus, or from bacterial, viral, parasitic, or fungal infections. Also called **placental dysfunction.** See also **intrauterine growth retardation, postmature infant.**

placental scan, a scan of the uterus of a pregnant woman, performed after an intravenous injection of a contrast medium, used for locating the fetus and placenta and for detecting intrauterine bleeding.

placenta previa /prē′vē·ə/, a condition of pregnancy in which the placenta is implanted abnormally in the uterus so that it impinges on or covers the internal os of the uterine cervix. It is the most common cause of painless bleeding in the third trimester of pregnancy. Its cause is unknown. The incidence of the condition increases with increased parity from approximately 1 in 1500 primiparas to approximately 1 in 20 grand multiparas. Even slight dilatation of the internal os can cause enough local separation of an abnormally implanted placenta to result in bleeding. If severe hemorrhage occurs, immediate cesarean section is usually required to stop the bleeding and to save the mother's life; it is performed regardless of the stage of fetal maturity. Before hemorrhage, placenta previa may be diagnosed by ultrasonography and treated with complete bed rest under close observation. Even at rest, sudden massive hemorrhage can occur without warning. Vaginal examination is usually contraindicated if placenta previa is present or suspected because palpation can cause local placental separation and precipitate hemorrhage. Cautious and very gentle intracervical palpation may be performed to determine the existence and exact extent of previa. Before this examination, an intravenous infusion is begun, the woman's blood is typed and crossmatched, and preparations for immediate cesarean section are made. If the placenta is next to or near, rather than touching or covering, the cervical os, labor and vaginal delivery may be attempted. Kinds of placenta previa

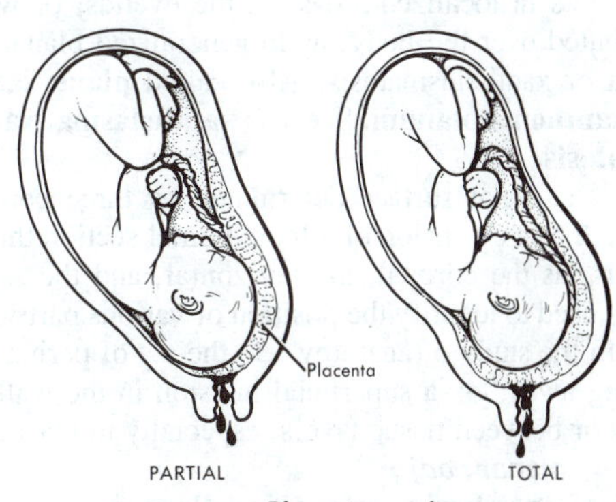

Placenta previa

are **central placenta previa, marginal placenta previa,** and **partial placenta previa.** Also called *(informal)* **previa.** Compare **abruptio placentae.**

placenta succenturiata, an accessory placenta.

Placidyl, a trademark for a sedative (ethchlorvynol).

Plafon fracture, a fracture that involves the buttress portion of the malleolus of a bone.

plagiocephaly /plā′jē·ōsef′əlē/, a congenital malformation of the skull in which premature or irregular closure of the coronal or lambdoidal sutures results in asymmetric growth of the head, giving it a twisted, lopsided appearance so that the maximum length is not along the midline but on a diagonal. Also called **plagiocephalism.** See also **craniostenosis.** –**plagiocephalic, plagiocephalous,** *adj.*

plague, an infectious disease transmitted by the bite of a flea from a rodent infected with the bacillus *Yersinia pestis*. Plague is primarily an infectious disease of rats: The rat fleas feed on humans only when their preferred rodent hosts, usually rats, have been killed by the plague in a rat epizootic; therefore, epidemics occur after rat epizootics. Kinds of plague include **bubonic plague, pneumonic plague,** and **septicemic plague.** See also ***Yersinia pestis.***

plague vaccine, an active immunizing agent prepared with killed plague bacilli.

■ INDICATIONS: It is prescribed for immunization against plague after probable exposure or as protection for travelers in endemic areas, such as Southeast Asia..

■ CONTRAINDICATIONS: Immunosuppression or acute infection prohibits its use.

■ ADVERSE EFFECTS: Among the most serious adverse reactions are allergic reactions, inflammation at the site of injection, headache, and malaise.

plaintiff, (in law) a person who files a lawsuit initiating a legal action. The plaintiff complains or sues for remedial relief and names a complainant in various civil actions. In criminal actions, the prosecution is the plaintiff, acting in behalf of the people of the jurisdiction.

-plakia, a combining form meaning 'patches on mucous membrane': *leukoplakia, malocoplakia, melanoplakia.*

planar xanthoma, a yellow or orange flat macule or slightly raised papule containing foam cells and occurring in clusters in localized areas, as the eyelids, or widely distributed over the body, as in generalized planar xanthoma or xanthelasmatosis. Also called **plane xanthoma, xanthoma planum.** See also **xanthelasma, xanthelasmatosis.**

plane, **1.** a flat surface determined by three points in space. **2.** an extension of a longitudinal section through an axis, as the coronal, the horizontal, and the sagittal planes used to identify the position of various parts of the body in the study of anatomy. **3.** the act of paring or of rubbing away. **4.** a superficial incision in the wall of a cavity or between tissue layers, especially in plastic surgery. –**planar,** *adj.*

planes of anesthesia. See **Guedel's signs.**

-plania, a combining form meaning the 'deviation from its normal location': *choloplania, pyoplania, spiloplania.*

planned change, (in psychotherapy) an alteration of the status quo by means of a carefully formulated program that follows four steps: unfreezing the present level, establishing a change relationship, moving to a new level, and freezing at the new level. The program can be implemented by collaborative, coercive, or emulative means.

planned parenthood, a philosophic framework central to the development of contraceptive methods, contraceptive counseling, and family planning programs and clinics. Advocates hold that it is the right of each woman to decide when to conceive and bear children and that contraceptive and gynecologic care and information should be available to her to help her become or avoid becoming pregnant. See also **contraceptive.**

planning, (in five step nursing process) a category of nursing behavior in which a strategy is designed for the achievement of the goals of care for an individual patient, as established in assessing and analyzing. Planning includes developing and modifying a care plan, for the patient, cooperating with other personnel, and recording relevant information. To develop the plan, the nurse anticipates the patient's needs according to established priorities; involves the patient and the patient's family and significant others in designing the plan; uses all information necessary for managing care of the patient, including recorded information from other health professionals, and the age, sex, culture, ethnicity, and religion; plans for the patient's comfort, activity, and function; and chooses nursing measures that are necessary to deliver care as planned. With the cooperation of other health personnel, the nurse coordinates care for the benefit of the patient and identifies resources in the hospital or community for social or health assistance as needed by the client or the patient's family. All information relevant to the management of the patient's care plan is recorded. Planning follows analyzing and precedes implementing in the five step nursing process. See also **analyzing, assessing, evaluating implementing, nursing process.**

plano-, a combining form meaning 'wandering': *planocyte, planotopokinesia.*

plantago seed /plantā′gō/, a bulk-forming laxative derived from *Plantago psyllium* seeds.

■ INDICATIONS: It is prescribed in the treatment of constipation and nonspecific diarrhea.

■ CONTRAINDICATIONS: Symptoms of appendicitis, intestinal obstruction, or GI ulceration prohibit its use.

■ ADVERSE EFFECTS: Among the more serious adverse effects are intestinal obstruction and allergic reactions.

plantar /plan′tər/, of or pertaining to the sole of the foot. Also called **volar.**

plantar aponeurosis, the tough fascia surrounding the muscles of the soles of the feet. Also called **plantar fascia.**

plantaris /plantä′ris/, one of three superficial muscles at the back of the leg, between the soleus and the gastrocnemius. The plantaris is a small muscle that arises from the distal part of the linea aspera of the femur and from the oblique popliteal ligament of the knee joint. It has a small fusiform belly, ending in a long, slender tendon that inserts into the calcaneus. The plantaris is innervated by a branch of the tibial nerve, containing fibers from the fourth and the fifth lumbar and the first sacral nerves. It flexes the foot and the leg. Compare **gastrocnemius, soleus.**

plantar neuroma, a neuroma of the sole of the foot.

plantar reflex, the normal response, elicited by firmly stroking the outer surface of the sole from heel to toes, characterized by flexion of the toes. Compare **Babinski's reflex.**

plantar wart, a painful verrucous lesion on the sole of the foot, primarily at points of pressure, as over the metatarsal heads and the heel. Caused by the common wart virus, it appears as a soft, central core and is surrounded by a firm, hyperkeratotic ring resembling a callus. Multiple, tiny, black spots on the surface represent bits of coagulated blood in the wart. Treatment methods include electrodesiccation, cryotherapy, topical acids, cantharidin, and even mental suggestion. See also **mosaic wart, wart.**

plantigrade /plan′tigrād′/, of, pertaining to, or characterizing the human gait; walking on the sole of the foot with the heel touching the ground.

plaque /plak/, **1.** a flat, often raised, patch on the skin or any other organ of the body. **2.** a patch of atherosclerosis. **3.** also called **dental plaque.** a thin film on the teeth made up of mucin and colloidal material found in saliva and often secondarily invaded by bacteria.

Plaquenil Sulfate, a trademark for an antimalarial, antiarthritic, and lupus erythematosus suppressant (hydroxychloroquine sulfate).

-plasia, -plastia, a combining form meaning '(condition of) formation or development': *alloplasia, anosteoplasia, cacoplasia.* See also **-plastia.**

-plasm, -plasma, a combining form meaning 'cell or tissue substance': *deutoplasm, mitoplasm, phytoplasm.* See also **-plasma.**

plasma, the watery, colorless, fluid portion of the lymph and the blood in which the leukocytes, erythrocytes, and platelets are suspended. It contains no cells and is made up of water, electrolytes, proteins, glucose, fats, bilirubin, and gases. It is essential for carrying the cellular elements of the blood through the circulation, transporting nutrients, maintaining the acid-base balance of the body, and transporting wastes from the tissues. Plasma and interstitial fluid correspond closely in content and concentration of proteins; therefore, plasma is important in maintaining the osmotic pressure and the exchange of fluids and electrolytes between the capillaries and the tissues. Compare **serum.**

plasma-, a combining form meaning 'the liquid portion of the blood': *plasmablast, plasmacyte, plasmapheresis.*

-plasma, a combining form meaning 'fluid part of cytoplasm or protoplasm': *ectoplasma, hydroplasma, ovoplasma.* See also **-plasm.**

plasma cell, a lymphoid or lymphocyte-like cell found in the bone marrow, connective tissue, and, sometimes, the blood. It contains an eccentric nucleus with deeply staining chromatin material arranged in a pattern like the spokes of a wheel or a clock face. Plasma cells are involved in the immunologic mechanism and are formed in large numbers in multiple myeloma. See also **B cell, multiple myeloma.**

plasma cell leukemia, an unusual neoplasm of blood-forming tissues in which the predominant cells in peripheral blood are plasmacytes. The disease may develop in the course of multiple myeloma or arise independently. Bence Jones proteinuria, abnormal serum globulins, hepatomegaly, and splenomegaly are usual in plasma cell leukemia. In most cases plasma cell leukemia is rapidly fatal, but some patients respond to treatment with alkylating agents and glucocorticoids.

plasma cell myeloma. See **multiple myeloma.**

plasmacytoma /plaz′məsītō′mə/, *pl.* **plasmacytomas, plasmacytomata,** a focal neoplasm containing plasma cells. It may develop in the bone marrow, as in multiple myeloma, or outside the bone marrow, as in certain tumors of the viscera and the mucosa of the nasal, oral, and pharyngeal areas. Also called **peripheral plasma cell myeloma, plasma cell tumor.**

plasma expander, a substance, usually a high molecular weight dextran, that is administered intravenously to increase the oncotic pressure of a patient.

plasma membrane. See **cell membrane.**

plasmapheresis /plaz′məfərē′sis/, the removal of plasma from withdrawn blood by centrifugation, the reconstitution of the cellular elements in an isotonic solution, and the reinfusion of this solution into the donor. Compare **leukapheresis, plateletpharesis.**

plasma protein, any one of the various proteins, including albumin, fibrinogen, prothrombin, and the gamma globulins, which constitute about 6% to 7% of the blood plasma in the body. These substances aid in the maintenance of water balance affecting osmotic pressure, increase blood viscosity, and help maintain blood pressure. Fibrinogen and prothrombin are essential to blood coagulation, and the gamma globulins are important in immunoregulation. All the plasma proteins except the gamma globulins are synthesized in the liver. See also **antibody, serum.**

plasma renin activity, the action of the enzyme renin, measured in plasma to aid in the diagnosis of adrenal disease associated with hypertension. The normal value in plasma is 0.2 to 4 ng/ml/hour, depending on salt intake and the length of time the patient is in an upright postion before a renin activity test.

plasma thromboplastin antecedent. See **factor XI.**

plasma thromboplastin component deficiency. See **hemophilia.**

plasma volume, the total volume of plasma in the body, elevated in diseases of the liver and spleen and in vitamin C deficiency, lowered in Addison's disease, dehydration, and shock. The normal plasma volume in males is 39 ml/kg of body weight; in females, 40 ml/kg.

plasmid, (in bacteriology) any type of intracellular inclusion considered to have a genetic function, especially a molecule of DNA separate from the bacterial chromosome that determines traits not essential for the viability of the organism but that in some way changes the organism's ability to adapt. R (resistance) factor is an example: A bacterium containing the factor is able to resist many antibacterial drugs that act in many different ways. Plasmid may be passed from one bacterium to another, and it is replicated in later generations of any bacterium carrying it.

plasmidotrophoblast. See **syncytiotrophoblast.**

plasmin. See **fibrinolysin.**

plasminogen. See **fibrinogen.**

plasmo-, a combining form meaning 'of or related to plasma, or to the substance of a cell': *plasmocyte, plasmodium, plasmosome.*

Plasmodium /plazmō′dē·əm/, a genus of protozoa several species of which cause malaria, transmitted to humans by the bite of an infected Anopheles mosquito. ***Plasmodium falciparum*** causes falciparum malaria, the most severe form of the disease; ***P. malariae*** causes quartan malaria; ***P. ovale*** causes mild tertian malaria with oval red blood cells; and ***P. vivax*** causes common tertian malaria. See also ***Anopheles,*** **blackwater fever, malaria.**

plasmosome /plaz′məsōm/, the true nucleolus of a cell as distinguished from the karyosomes in the nucleus. Also spelled **plasmasome.**

plast-, a combining form meaning 'formed': *plastidogenetic, plastodynamia, plastogamy.*

-plast, a combining form meaning a 'primitive cell': *chondroplast, gymnoplast, osteoplast.*

plaster, **1.** any composition of a liquid and a powder that hardens when it dries, used in shaping a cast to support a fractured bone as it heals, as plaster of paris. **2.** a home remedy consisting of a semisolid mixture applied to a part of the body as a counterirritant or for other therapeutic reasons, as a mustard plaster.

-plastia, -plasia, a combining form meaning '(condition of) cell or tissue formation or development': *ana-Plastia, macroplastia, mastplastia.* See also **-plasia.**

-plastic, a combining form meaning 'pertaining to the development of' something specified: *entoplastic, hemoplastic, rhinoplastic.*

plastic surgery, the alteration, replacement, or restoration of visible portions of the body, performed to correct a structural or cosmetic defect. In performing corrective plastic surgery, the surgeon may use tissue from the patient or from another person or an inert material that is nonirritating, has a consistency appropriate to the use, and is able to hold its shape and form indefinitely. Implants are commonly used in mammoplasty for breast augmentation. Skin grafting is the most common procedure in plastic surgery. Z-plasty and Y-plasty are simpler techniques often performed instead of a graft in areas of the body covered by skin that is loose and elastic, as the neck, axilla, throat, and inner aspect of the elbow. Dermabrasion is used to remove pockmarks, scars from acne, or signs of traumatic skin damage. Chemical peeling is another technique in corrective plastic surgery; it is used primarily for removing fine wrinkles on the face. Tattooing, in which a pigment is tattooed into the skin of a graft, is performed to change the color of the graft to resemble more closely the surrounding skin. Reconstructive plastic surgery is performed to correct birth defects, to repair structures destroyed by trauma, and to replace tissue removed in other surgical procedures. Cleft lip and cleft palate repair and other maxillofacial surgical procedures, including rhinoplasty, otoplasty, and rhytidoplasty are among these reconstructive procedures. Care of the patient before and after plastic surgery may require considerable sensitivity and tact. The patient may be exceedingly uncomfortable about the real or perceived appearance of the defect. An accepting, nonjudgmental attitude on the part of all staff members is to the patient's benefit. Optimal nutritional status helps a graft to "take" and speeds healing. Each procedure and technique involves particular kinds of care in the preoperative and postoperative periods. Instructions and assistance in self-care activities are also specific to the various procedures. Success of most of the procedures depends greatly on the patient's cooperation and fastidious nursing care. The correction of a visible abnormality may be of inestimable benefit to the patient's assurance, self-esteem, and function in society. See also specific procedures.

-plasty, a combining form meaning 'plastic surgery on a (specified) body part or by (specified) means': *bronchoplasty, cervicoplasty, uveoplasty.*

plate, **1.** a flat structure or layer, as a thin layer of bone or the frontal plate between the sides of the ethmoid cartilage and the sphenoid bone in the fetus. **2.** a single partitioning unit of a chromatographic system.

platelet, the smallest of the cells in the blood. Platelets are disk-shaped and contain no hemoglobin. They are essential for the coagulation of blood. Normally between 200,000 and 300,000 platelets are found in 1 ml^3 of blood. Compare **erythrocyte, leucocyte.** See also **thrombocytopenia, thrombocytosis.**

plateletpheresis, the removal of platelets from withdrawn blood, the remainder of the blood being reinfused into the donor. Also called **thrombapheresis, thrombotapheresis.** Compare **leukapheresis, plasmapheresis.**

platinized gold foil, a thin sheet rolled or hammered from platinum sandwiched between two sheets of gold, used for making portions of dental restorations requiring greater hardness than that obtained by using other materials, as copper amalgam.

Platinol, a trademark for an antineoplastic (cisplatin).

platinum (Pt), a silvery-white, soft metallic element. Its atomic number is 78; its atomic weight is 195.09. Platinum is used in dentistry, jewelry, and the manufacture of chemical apparatus that must withstand high temperatures.

platinum foil, a very thin sheet of rolled pure platinum that has a high fusing point, making it an ideal matrix in various soldering procedures for fabricating orthodontic appliances and dentures. It is also commonly used as the internal form of porcelain dental restorations during fabrication.

platy-, a combining form meaning 'broad or flat': *platybasia, platycephalous, platyenemic.*

Platyhelminthes, a phylum of parasitic flatworms that includes the Cestoda subclass of tapeworms and Trematoda class of flukes.

platypelloid pelvis /plat′əpel′oid/, a rare type of pelvis in which the inlet is round like the gynecoid type in the anterior section, but the posterior section is foreshortened by its flat and heavy border. The sacrum is hollow and inclines posteriorly, and the sidewalls are convergent. In the midplane, the transverse diameter is much wider than the narrowed anteroposterior diameter. Vaginal delivery is not usually possible in women who have platypelloid pelves. This type of pelvis is present in 3% of women.

platysma /plətiz′mə/, one of a pair of wide muscles at the side of the neck. It arises from the fascia covering the superior parts of the pectoralis major and the deltoideus, crosses the clavicle, and rises obliquely and medially along the side of the neck. The anterior fibers of the platysma interlace, inferior and posterior to the symphysis menti, with the fibers of the muscle of the opposite side. The posterior fibers of the platysma cross the mandible, some inserting into the bone below the oblique line, others into the skin and the subcutaneous tissue of the lower part of the face. Many of the fibers blend with the muscles at the angle and the lower part of the mouth. The platysma covers the external jugular vein as the vein descends from the angle of the mandible to the clavicle. The platysma is innervated by the cervical branch of the facial nerve and serves to draw down the lower lip and the corner of the mouth. When the platysma fully contracts, the skin over the clavicle is drawn toward the mandible, increasing the diameter of the neck.

play, any spontaneous or organized activity that provides enjoyment, entertainment, amusement, or diversion. It is essential in childhood for the development of a normal personality and as a means for developing physically, intellectually, and socially. Play provides an outlet for releasing tension and stress, as well as a means for testing and experimenting with new or fearful roles or situations. It is an indispensable part of the nursing care of children, especially in the hospital. It helps relieve the tension and anxiety of being in unfamiliar surroundings and separated from parents, and it gives the child a sense of security and a means of expressing fears and fantasies. Play also offers the nurse one of the most effective methods of communicating with and gaining the trust of the child and helping the child to understand treatments and procedures. Kinds of play include **active play, associative play, cooperative play, dramatic play, parallel play, passive play, skill play,** and **solitary play.** See also **play therapy.**

play therapy, a form of psychotherapy in which a child plays in a protected and structured environment with games and toys provided by a therapist, who observes the behavior, affect, and conversation of the child to gain insight into thoughts, feelings, and fantasies. As conflicts are discovered, the therapist often helps the child understand and work through them.

pleasure principle, (in psychoanalysis) the need for immediate gratification of instinctual drives. Compare **reality principle.**

pledget /plej′ət/, a small, flat compress made of cotton gauze, or a tuft of cotton wool, lint, or a similar synthetic material, used to wipe the skin, absorb drainage, or clean a small surface.

-plegia, a combining form meaning 'a (specified) paralysis': *colicoplegia, esophagoplegia, proctoplegia.*

-plegic, **1.** a combining form meaning 'of or pertaining to a specific paralysis': *cycloplegic, ganglionoplegic, pharyngoplegic.* **2.** a combining form meaning a 'sufferer from a specific paralysis': *diplegic, ophthalmoplegic, psychoplegic.*

Plegine, a trademark for an anorexiant (phendimetrazine tartrate).

pleiades /plē′ədēz/, *obsolete.* a mass of enlarged lymph nodes.

pleio-. See **pleo-.**

pleitropic gene, a gene that produces a complex of unrelated phenotypic effects.

pleiotropy /plī·ot′rəpē/, (in genetics) the production by a single gene of a multiple, different, and apparently unrelated manifestation of a particular disorder, as the cluster of symptoms in Marfan's syndrome, aortic aneurysm, dislocation of the optic lens, skeletal deformities, and arachnodactyly, any or all of which may be present.

pleo-, pleio-, a combining form meaning 'more': *pleochromatic, pleomastia, pleomorphism.*

plessimeter. See **pleximeter.**

plethora, a term applied to the beefy red coloration of a newborn. The "boiled lobster" hue of the infant's skin is caused by an unusually high proportion of erythrocytes per volume of blood. The term formerly was used to describe any red-faced person. **–plethoric,** *adj.*

plethysmogram /pləthiz′məgram′/, a tracing produced by a plethysmograph.

plethysmograph /pləthiz′məgraf′/, an instrument for measuring and recording changes in the sizes and volumes of extremities and organs by measuring changes in their blood volumes. **–plethysmographic,** *adj.,* **plethysmography,** *n.*

pleur-. See **pleuro-.**

pleura /plŏŏr′ə/, *pl.* **pleurae,** a delicate serous membrane enclosing the lung, composed of a single layer of flattened mesothelial cells resting on a delicate membrane of connective tissue. Beneath the membrane is a stroma of collagenous tissue containing yellow elastic fibers. The pleura divides into the visceral pleura, which covers the lung, dipping into the fissures between the lobes, and the parietal pleura, which lines the chest wall, covers the diaphragm, and reflects over the structures in the mediastinum. The parietal and visceral pleurae are separated from each other by a small amount of fluid that acts as a lubricant as the lungs expand and contract during respiration. See also **pleural cavity, pleural space.** –**pleural,** *adj.*

pleural cavity, the cavity within the thorax that contains the lungs. Between the ribs and the lungs are the visceral and parietal pleurae.

pleural effusion, an abnormal accumulation of fluid in the interstitial and air spaces of the lungs, characterized by fever, chest pain, dyspnea, and nonproductive cough. The fluid involved is an exudate or a transudate from inflamed pleural surfaces. A transudate that accumulates in pulmonary edema is commonly aspirated. An exudate may result from pulmonary infarction, trauma, tumor, or infection, as tuberculosis. The specific cause of the exudate is treated, and the exudate may be aspirated or surgically drained. Other treatment may include the administration of corticosteroids, diuretics, and vasodilators, oxygen therapy, and intermittent positive pressure breathing.

pleural space, the potential space between the visceral and parietal layers of the pleurae. The space contains a small amount of fluid that acts as a lubricant, allowing the pleurae to slide smoothly over each other as the lungs expand and contract with respiration.

pleurisy /plŏŏr′əsē/, inflammation of the parietal pleura of the lungs, characterized by dyspnea and stabbing pain, leading to restriction of ordinary breathing with spasm of the chest on the affected side. A friction rub may be heard on auscultation. Simple pleurisy with undetectable exudate is called fibrinous or dry; pleural effusion indicates extensive inflammation with considerable amounts of exudate in the pleural spaces. Common causes of pleurisy include bronchial carcinoma, lung or chest wall abscess, pneumonia, pulmonary infarction, and tuberculosis. The condition may result in permanent adhesions between the pleura and adjacent surfaces. Treatment consists of relief of pain and therapy for the primary disease. See also **pleural effusion, pleurodynia, pulmonary edema.**

pleuro-, pleur-, a combining form meaning 'of or pertaining to the pleura, to a side, or to a rib': *pleurocentrum, pleurography, pleuropulmonary.*

pleurodynia /plŏŏr′ōdin′ē·ə/, acute inflammation of the intercostal muscles and the muscular attachment of the diaphragm to the chest wall. It is characterized by sudden severe pain and tenderness, fever, headache, and anorexia. These symptoms are aggravated by movement and respiration. The lungs are not affected, and characteristically there is no cough or pleural effusion. See also **epidemic pleurodynia.**

pleuropericardial rub, an abnormal coarse friction sound heard on auscultation of the lungs during late inspiration and early expiration. It is caused by the visceral and parietal pleural surfaces rubbing against each other. The sound is not affected by coughing. A pleural rub indicates primary inflammatory, neoplastic, or traumatic pleural disease, or inflammation secondary to infection or neoplasm. See also **breath sound, Kussmaul breathing, rale, rhonchi, wheeze.**

pleuroperitoneal cavity. See **splanchnocoele.**

pleuropneumonia, **1.** a combination of pleurisy and pneumonia. **2.** an infection of cattle resulting in inflammation of both the pleura and lungs, caused by microorganisms of the *Mycoplasma* group. See also ***Mycoplasma,*** **pleuropneumonia-like organism.**

pleuropneumonia-like organism (PPLO), a group of filterable organisms of the genus *Mycoplasma* similar to *M. mycoides,* the cause of pleuropneumonia in cattle.

pleurothotonos /plŏŏr′əthot′ənəs/, an involuntary, severe, prolonged contraction of the muscles of one side of the body, resulting in an acute arch to that side. It is usually associated with tetanus infection or strychnine poisoning. Compare **emprosthotonos, opisthotonos, orthotonos.** –**pleurothotonic,** *adj.*

plex-, a combining form meaning 'a stroke or to strike': *plexalgia, pleximeter, plexor.*

-plex, -plexus, a combining form meaning a 'network': *brachiplex, cerviplex, veniplex.*

-plexia, -plexy, a combining form meaning '(condition resulting from a) stroke': *apoplexia, pagoplexia, selenoplexia.*

plexiform neuroma, a neoplasm composed of twisted bundles of nerves. Also called **Verneuil's neuroma.**

pleximeter /pleksim′ətər/, a mediating device, as a percussor or finger, used to receive light taps in percussion. Also called **plessimeter.** See also **percussion.**

plexor. See **percussor.**

plexus, *pl.* **plexuses,** a network of intersecting nerves and blood vessels or of lymphatic vessels. The body contains many plexuses, as the brachial plexus, the cardiac plexus, the cervical plexus, and the solar plexus.

-plexy. See **-plexia.**

plic-, a combining form meaning a 'fold or ridge': *plicadentin, plication, plicotomy.*

plica /plī′kə/, *pl.* **plicae** /plī′sē/, a fold of tissue within the body, as the plicae transversales of the rectum and the plicae circulares of the small intestine. –**plical,** *adj.*

plica circularis. See **circular fold.**

plicae transversales recti, semilunar, transverse folds in the rectum that support the weight of feces. Also called **Houston's valves.** See also **rectum.**

plicamycin, an antineoplastic agent. Previously called **mithramycin.**

■ INDICATIONS: It is prescribed primarily in the treatment of malignant tumors of the testis. It is also prescribed in the treatment of hypercalcemia and hypercalciuria associated with cancer.

■ CONTRAINDICATIONS: Clotting disorders, thrombocytopenia, kidney or liver dysfunction, bone marrow depression, or known hypersensitivity to this drug prohibits its use.

■ ADVERSE EFFECTS: Among the more serious adverse reactions are thrombocytopenia and clotting defects. Nausea and stomatitis commonly occur.

plica semilunaris, the semilunar fold of the conjunctiva that extends laterally from the lacrimal caruncle. It has a concave free border directed toward the cornea. In some individuals it contains smooth muscular fibers.

plica umbilicalis lateralis. See **lateral umbilical fold.**

plica umbilicalis mediana. See **middle umbilical fold.**

Plimmer's bodies, small, round, encapsulated bodies found in cancers once thought to be the causative parasites. Also called **Behla's bodies.**

-ploid, a combining form meaning 'having a (specified) number of chromosome sets': *heptaploid, octaploid, polyploid.*

ploidy /ploi′dē/, the status of a cell nucleus in regard to the number of complete chromosome sets it contains.

-ploidy, a combining form meaning the 'condition of having a (specified) number of chromosome sets': *alloploidy, haploidy, heteroploidy.*

plug, a mass of tissue cells, mucus, or other matter that blocks a normal opening or passage of the body, as a cervical plug.

Plummer's disease, goiter characterized by a hyperfunctioning nodule or adenoma and thyrotoxicosis. Also called **toxic nodular goiter.**

Plummer-Vinson syndrome /plum′ərvin′sən/, a rare disorder associated with severe and chronic iron deficiency anemia, characterized by dysphagia caused by esophageal webs at the level of the cricoid cartilage. Also called **sideropenic dysphagia.** Compare **Paterson-Kelly syndrome.**

plunging goiter. See **diving goiter.**

pluri-, a combining form meaning 'more': *pluriceptor, plurimenorrhea, pluritissular.*

pluricentric blastoma. See **blastoma.**

pluripolar mitosis. See **multipolar mitosis.**

plutonium (Pu), a synthetic transuranic metallic element. Its atomic number is 94; its atomic weight is 242. A highly toxic waste product of nuclear power plants, plutonium was used in the assembly of early nuclear weapons.

pm, abbreviation for **picometer.**

Pm, symbol for **promethium.**

P.M.D., abbreviation for *private medical doctor.* Also called **L.M.D.**

PMI, abbreviation for **point of maximum impulse.**

PMN, abbreviation for **polymorphonuclear cell.**

PMT, abbreviation for **premenstrual tension.**

PND, **1.** abbreviation for **paroxysmal nocturnal dyspnea. 2.** abbreviation for **postnasal drip.**

-pnea, -pnoea, a combining form meaning 'breath or breathing': *brachypnea, bromopnea, dyspnea.*

pneo-, a combining form meaning 'of or pertaining to the breath, or to breathing': *pneodynamics, pneograph, pneoscope.*

pneuma-. See **pneumato-.**

pneumatic condenser /no͞omat′ik/, (in dentistry) a pneumatic device, developed by George M. Hollenback, to deliver a compacting force to restorative material used in filling tooth cavities. The force is delivered by controlled pneumatic pressure and develops compacting blows that can be varied in intensity. The frequency of the blows may be up to 360 strokes/minute. Also called **Hollenback condenser.**

pneumatic heart driver, a mechanic device that regulates compressed air delivery to an artificial heart, controlling heart rate, percent systole, and delay in systole.

pneumato-, pneuma-, a combining form meaning 'of or related to air or gas, or to respiration': *pneumatology, pneumatophore, pneumatothorax.*

pneumo-, pneumono-, a combining form meaning 'of or related to the lungs, to air, or to the breath': *pneumobacillin, pneumocele, pneumolith.*

pneumococcal /no͞o′mōkok′əl/, of or pertaining to bacteria of the genus *Pneumococcus.*

pneumococcal vaccine, an active immunizing agent containing antigens of the 14 types of *Pneumococcus* associated with 80% of the cases of pneumococcal pneumonia.

■ INDICATIONS: It is prescribed for people over 2 years of age who are at high risk of developing severe pneumococcal pneumonia.

■ CONTRAINDICATIONS: Pregnancy, early childhood (under 2 years of age), or known hypersensitivity to the vaccine prohibits its use.

■ ADVERSE EFFECTS: Among the more serious adverse reactions are inflammation at the site of injection, fever, and hypersensitivity reactions.

pneumococcus /no͞o′mōkok′əs/, *pl.* **pneumococci** /no͞o′mōkok′sī/, a gram-positive diplococcal bacterium of the species *Diplococcus pneumoniae,* the most common cause of bacterial pneumonia. More than 85 subtypes of this organism are known. See also **lobar pneumonia, pneumonia.**

pneumoconiosis /no͞o′mōkōnē•ō′sis/, any disease of the lung caused by chronic inhalation of dust, usually mineral dusts of occupational or environmental origin. Some kinds of pneumoconioses are **anthracosis, asbestosis, silicosis.**

pneumocystosis /no͞o′mōsistō′sis/, infection with the parasite *Pneumocystis carinii,* usually seen in infants or debilitated or immunosuppressed people and characterized by fever, cough, tachypnea, and, frequently, cyanosis. The diagnosis is difficult to make and usually requires lung biopsy and special staining techniques.

Mortality nears 100% in untreated patients. Treatment with pentamidine isethionate or a combination of trimethoprim and sulfamethoxazole is effective. Also called **interstitial plasma cell pneumonia.**

pneumoderma. See **subcutaneous emphysema.**

pneumoencephalogram, a radiograph of the brain made during pneumoencephalography.

pneumoencephalography /n o͞o′mō•ensef′əlog′rəfē/, a procedure for the radiographic visualization of the ventricular space, basal cisterns, and subarachnoid space overlying the cerebral hemispheres of the brain. Air, helium, or oxygen is injected into the lumbar subarachnoid space after the intermittent removal of the cerebrospinal fluid by lumbar puncture. See also **encephalography, ventriculography.** –**pneumoencephalographic,** *adj.*

pneumogastric nerve. See **vagus nerve.**

pneumomediastinum /no͞o′mōmē′dē•əstī′nəm/, the presence of air or gas in the mediastinal tissues, which in infants may lead to pneumothorax or pneumopericardium, especially in those with respiratory distress syndrome or aspiration pneumonitis. In older children the condition may result from bronchitis, acute asthma, pertussis, cystic fibrosis, or bronchial rupture from cough or trauma.

pneumonectomy, the surgical removal of all or part of a lung.

pneumonia /no͞omō′nē•ə/, an acute inflammation of the lungs, usually caused by inhaled pneumococci of the species *Diplococcus pneumoniae*. The alveoli and bronchioles of the lungs become plugged with a fibrous exudate. Pneumonia may be caused by other bacteria, as well as by viruses, rickettsiae, and fungi, but in 85% of the cases, pneumococcus infection is the cause. Kinds of pneumonia are **aspiration pneumonia, bronchopneumonia, eosinophilic pneumonia, interstitial pneumonia, lobar pneumonia, mycoplasma pneumonia,** and **viral pneumonia.**

■ OBSERVATIONS: Characteristic of pneumonia are severe chills, a high fever (which may reach 105° F), headache, cough, and chest pain. Inflammation of the lower lobe of the right lung may produce a pain suggesting appendicitis. An effusion of red blood cells into the alveolar spaces, resulting from histolytic damage by the microorganism, causes a rust-colored sputum that may be a diagnostic sign of pneumococcal infection. As the disease progresses, sputum may become thicker and more purulent, and the person may experience painful attacks of coughing. Respiration usually becomes more difficult, painful, shallow, and rapid. The pulse increases in rapidity, often measuring 120 or more beats a minute. Other signs may include profuse sweating and cyanosis. GI disorders and an outbreak of herpes simplex about the face may also occur. In children, pneumonia may be accompanied by convulsion. As the alveoli become filled with exudate, the affected area of a lobe becomes increasingly firm and consolidated. A distinctive kind of rale is heard on auscultation. X-ray films are taken to evaluate consolidation; laboratory analysis of sputum and cultures of the blood help in identifying the causative organism.

■ INTERVENTION: The treatment of pneumonia includes bed rest, fluids, antibiotics, analgesics, and, if necessary, oxygen. The antibiotic prescribed is specific for the bacterium identified in the laboratory analysis of sputum or blood. Crystalline penicillin G is usually prescribed for pneumococcal pneumonia. The antibiotic is administered intramuscularly until the patient's temperature is normal for 2 days. Analgesics are given as needed for relief of chest pain. Oxygen is administered by tent, mask, or catheter to patients who are cyanotic, very weak, or delirious; the amount of oxygen to be given is determined through serial laboratory analyses of blood gases. Expectorants, postural drainage, and aspiration of the bronchi are often prescribed. Chest x-ray films are advised during the acute phase, after therapy has been completed, and on a follow-up examination 4 to 6 weeks later. Mild pneumonia is often treated without hospitalization.

■ NURSING CONSIDERATIONS: Fluid and electrolytes are often lost during prolonged high fever; intravenous replacement is often required. Ice packs or cold, wet compresses may be needed to reduce the fever. Fever, loss of fluids, and breathing through the mouth result in a need for care of the mouth and the nares, where herpes lesions frequently develop. The nurse collects samples of sputum for laboratory analysis, administers antibiotics and other medications, and notes the temperature, pulse, and respiration as often as necessary.

-pneumonia, a combining form meaning an 'inflammation of the lungs': *necropneumonia, splenopneumonia, typhopneumonia.*

-pneumonic, **1.** a combining form meaning 'related to pneumonia': *bronchopneumonic, peripneumonic, pleuropneumonic.* **2.** a combining form meaning 'related to the lungs': *gastropneumonic, hepatopneumonic.*

pneumonic plague, a highly virulent and rapidly fatal form of plague characterized by bronchopneumonia. There are two forms: **Primary pneumonic plague** results from involvement of the lungs in the course of bubonic plague; **secondary pneumonic plague** results from the inhalation of infected particles of sputum from a person having pneumonic plague. Compare **bubonic plague, septicemic plague.** See also **plague,** ***Yersinia pestis.***

pneumonitis /no͞o′mənī′tis/, *pl.* **pneumonitides,** inflammation of the lung. Pneumonitis may be caused by a virus or may be a hypersensitivity reaction to chemicals or organic dusts, as bacteria, bird droppings, or molds. It is usually an interstitial, granulomatous, fibrosing inflammation of the lung, especially of the bronchioles and alveoli. Dry cough is a common symptom. Treatment depends on the cause but includes removal of any offending agents and the administration of corticosteroids to reduce inflammation. A kind of pneumonitis is **humidifier lung.** Compare **pneumonia.**

pneumono-. See **pneumo-.**

pneumotachometer, a small cylindric device that measures the change in pressure from the exhausting air of an artificial ventricle. The pressure gradient is directly related to flow, thus allowing a computer to derive an exhaust flow curve measured in liters per minute.

pneumothorax /no͞o′mōthôr′aks/, a collection of air or gas in the pleural space causing the lung to collapse. Pneumothorax may be the result of an open chest wound that permits the entrance of air, the rupture of an emphysematous vesicle on the surface of the lung, or a severe bout of coughing, or it may occur spontaneously without apparent cause.

■ OBSERVATIONS: The onset of pneumothorax is accompanied by a sudden, sharp chest pain, followed by difficult, rapid breathing, cessation of normal chest movements on the affected side, tachycardia, a weak pulse, hypotension, diaphoresis, an elevated temperature, pallor, dizziness, and anxiety.

■ INTERVENTION: The patient is assured that the condition can be treated, is urged to remain quiet, and is placed in bed in Fowler's position. Oxygen is administered through a nasal cannula, unless contraindicated, and the air is immediately aspirated from the pleural space. A chest tube is inserted and attached to a water seal drainage system; the tube is not removed until air is no longer expelled through the underwater drainage system and an x-ray examination shows that the lung is completely expanded. Pain may be controlled by administering appropriate analgesics, but the use of respiratory depressants is avoided. Intermittent positive pressure breathing may be administered, and the patient is taught how to turn, cough, breathe deeply, and perform passive exercises and is told to avoid stretching, reaching, or making sudden movements.

■ NURSING CONSIDERATIONS: The nurse plays an important role in the patient's rehabilitation in the hospital and in preparing the individual for discharge. The patient is advised not to smoke but to drink fluids copiously, to exercise, to avoid fatigue and strenuous activity, and to report any symptoms of recurrence to the physician, as chest pain, difficult breathing, fever, or respiratory infection.

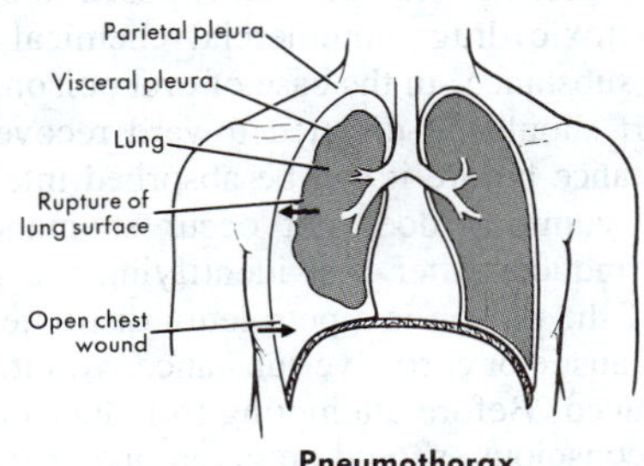

Pneumothorax

PNH, abbreviation for **paroxysmal nocturnal hemoglobinuria.**

-pnoea. See **-pnea.**

PNP, abbreviation for **pediatric nurse practitioner.**

Po, symbol for **polonium.**

Po$_2$, symbol for *partial pressure of oxygen*. See **partial pressure.**

pod-. See **podo-.**

podalic, pertaining to the feet.

podalic version, the shifting of the position of a fetus so as to bring the feet to the outlet during labor.

podiatrist. See **chiropodist.**

podiatry /pədī′ətrē/, the diagnosis and treatment of diseases and other disorders of the feet. See also **chiropody.**

-podium, a combining form meaning 'something footlike': *axiopodium, phyllopodium, pseudopodium.*

podo-, pod-, a combining form meaning 'of or related to the foot': *podogram, podology, podotrochilitis.*

podophyllotoxin, any one of a group of substances derived from the roots of *Podophyllum peltatum,* a common plant species known as mayapple, or American mandrake. Podyphillin, a resinous preparation of podophyllotoxin, is prescribed in the topical treatment of condyloma acuminatum and other types of warts. Several podophyllotoxin derivatives have been used as purgatives and studied for their antineoplastic effects, including the inhibition of mitosis. Podophyllotoxins are not recommended for use in early pregnancy.

podophyllum /pod′əfil′əm/, the dried rhizome and roots of *Podophyllum peltatum,* from which a caustic resin is derived for use in removing certain warts.

poecil-. See **poikilo-.**

-poesis. See **-poiesis.**

-poetic, -poietic, a combining form meaning 'referring to production of something specified': *cholepoetic, oenopoetic, uropoetic.*

-poiesis, -poesis, a combining form meaning 'production of': *cholanopoiesis, erythropoiesis, hemopoiesis.*

-poietic. See **-poetic.**

poikilo-, pecilo-, poecil-, a combining form meaning 'varied or irregular': *poikilocarynosis, poikiloderma, poikilothymia.*

poikilocytosis /poi′kilōsītō′sis/, an abnormal degree of variation in the shape of the erythrocytes in the blood. Compare **anisocytosis, macrocytosis, microcytosis.** See also **anisopoikilocytosis.**

poikiloderma atrophicans vasculare, an abnormal skin condition characterized by hyperpigmentation or hypopigmentation, telangiectasia, and atrophy of the epidermis. It may be symmetric or patchy, localized or widespread. It tends to be permanent.

poikiloderma of Civatte, a common benign, progressive dermatitis characterized by erythematous patches on the face and neck that become dry and scaly. As the condition progresses, pigment is deposited around the hair follicles extending down the lateral aspects of the neck. Photosensitivity is sometimes associated with this dermatitis. Also called **reticulated pigmented poikiloderma.**

poikilothermic. See **cold blooded.**

point behavior, the orientation of body parts in a certain direction within a quantum of space.

point forceps, a dental instrument used in filling root canals. It holds the filling cones during their placement.

point of maximum impulse (PMI), the place in the fifth intercostal space of the thorax, just medial to the left midclavicular line, where the apex beat of the heart is observed.

poison, any substance that impairs health or destroys life when ingested, inhaled, or absorbed by the body in relatively small amounts. Some toxicologists suggest that, depending on dosages, all substances are poisons. Many experts state that it is impossible to categorize any chemical as either safe or toxic and that the real concern is the risk or hazard associated with the use of any substance, as the high risk that may be associated with a life-saving drug that would not be acceptable as a food additive. Clinically, all poisons are divided into those that respond to specific treatments or antidotes and those for which there is no specific treatment. Research continues to develop effective antitoxins for poisons, but there are relatively few effective antidotes, and the treatment of poisoned individuals is based mainly on eliminating the toxic agent from the body before it can be absorbed. Maintaining respiration and circulation is the most important aspect of such treatment. Some substances that may be poisonous are the saps of certain plants, bacterial toxins, animal venoms, corrosives, heavy metal compounds, certain gases, various volatile and nonvolatile substances, industrial chemicals, and numerous drugs. The toxic effects of poisons may be reversible or irreversible. The capacity of body tissue to recover from poison determines the reversibility of the effect. Poisons that injure the central nervous system (CNS) create irreversible effects because CNS neurons of the brain cannot regenerate. Toxic effects of chemicals may be divided into local effects and systemic effects. Local effects, as those caused by the ingestion of caustic substances and the inhalation of irritants, involve the site of the first contact between the biologic system and the toxicant. Systemic effects depend on the absorption and the distribution of the toxicant. Systemic toxicity most often affects the central nervous system but may also affect the circulatory system, the blood and hematopoietic system, the skin, and the visceral organs, as the liver, kidneys, and lungs. The muscles and the bones are less often affected by systemic toxicity. The precise incidence of poisoning in the United States is not known, but about 150,000 cases are voluntarily reported to the National Clearinghouse for Poison Control Centers each year. Authorities, however, estimate that the real incidence is at least 10 times the number of reported cases. The total number of poisoning cases increases each year, but the incidence of poisoning in children under 5 years of age has significantly decreased, probably because of safer packaging of household drugs and products. About 60% of all poisoning involves children 1 to 2 years of age and the ingestion of chemicals other than drugs. Approximately 75% of the cases of poisoning in individuals over 15 years of age are drug related. About 4000 persons die each year in the United States from poisoning by toxic liquid and solid substances. Another 7000 persons are bitten by poisonous snakes, as the pit viper and coral snake. Such bites may cause severe pain and swelling, numbness, respiratory distress, paralysis, impaired coagulation, coma, and death. Snake bites may be treated with antivenin, tetanus toxoid, and broad spectrum antibiotics. Antihistamines and topical antipyretics are commonly used to treat toxic skin reactions from poisonous plants, as poison ivy, poison sumac, and poison oak. The saps or juices of such plants may cause severe reactions through skin contact or through ingestion. Authorities stress the importance of prompt treatment of acute poisoning from toxic chemicals and liquids. Some common treatments in such cases involve emesis and gastric lavage. Most toxic effects of drugs occur shortly after administration, but carcinogenic effects of chemicals may take 15 to 45 years to develop fully. Chemical carcinogenesis is a complex process involving the conversion of secondary carcinogens into primary carcinogens and the possible development of tumors through reactions of the toxicant with deoxyribonucleic acid. See also **poisoning treatment. –poisonous,** *adj.*

poison control center, one of a nearly worldwide network of facilities that provide information regarding all aspects of poisoning or intoxication, maintain records of their occurrence and refer patients to treatment centers.

poisoning, **1.** the act of administering a toxic substance. **2.** the condition or physical state produced by the ingestion, injection, inhalation, or exposure of a poisonous substance. Identification of the poison and the presentation of a container label are critical to expeditious diagnosis and treatment. Kinds of poisoning include **creosote poisoning, food poisoning, heavy metals poisoning, petroleum distillate poisoning,** and **salicylate poisoning.** See also **alcohol poisoning, carbon monoxide poisoning, nicotine poisoning, pesticide poisoning, poison, poisoning treatment, poison ivy, poison oak, poison sumac.**

poisoning treatment, the symptomatic and supportive care given a patient who has been exposed to or who has ingested a toxic drug, commercial chemical, or other dangerous substance. In the case of oral poisoning, a primary effort should be directed toward recovery of the toxic substance before it can be absorbed into the body tissues. If vomiting does not occur spontaneously, it should be induced after first identifying the poison, if possible. If the poison is a petroleum distillate, as kerosene, or a caustic or corrosive substance, vomiting should *not* be induced. Before attempting to induce emesis, the victim, if conscious, should be given one or two glasses of milk or water. A carbonated beverage should never be given an oral poisoning patient. Because of the danger of hypernatremia, the patient, and particularly a child, should not be given water containing salt or mustard. Syrup of ipecac can be given, if available, to induce vomiting, and the dosage can be repeated one time. But if the

Actions in selected situations with a conscious victim who has ingested poison*

Corrosive or caustic substances

Do not attempt to neutralize the substance.
Do not induce vomiting.
Offer the victim a glass of milk or water.

Noncorrosive substances

The decision on whether to induce vomiting is dependent on the substance ingested, the amount ingested, and the physical condition of the victim. In general, when pure petroleum distillates are ingested, vomiting is *not* indicated.
For other materials, vomiting may be induced. The Regional Poison Center can help in this evaluation.

Methods of inducing vomiting

1. Give 1 tbsp (15 ml) syrup of Ipecac followed by 1 glass of water. (Dose can be repeated once only if vomiting does not occur within 15 to 20 minutes.) Do not allow emetic to remain in stomach.
2. Physician's order: Apomorphine hydrochloride 0.03 mg/lb subcutaneously. (Contraindicated if respiratory depression is present or patient is comatose.) Apomorphine is rarely used. Can be reversed by the administration of naloxene.

*Information supplied by the American Association of Poison Control Centers, University of California Medical Center, San Diego.

ipecac fails to induce vomiting, vomiting should be encouraged by stimulating the patient's gag reflex at the back of the throat. Ipecac, which can be a GI irritant, should not be allowed to remain in the stomach. Ipecac should also not be given with milk or charcoal, both of which can interfere with its action. In certain cases, an antidote may be administered to render the poison inert or to prevent its absorption, as by giving a mild solution of vinegar or citrus juice to neutralize an alkali. As in other medical emergencies, a physician should be summoned to take charge of the case. If a physician is not available, the nearest Poison Control Center should be contacted for expert guidance.

poison ivy, any of several species of climbing vine of the genus *Rhus,* characterized by shiny, three-pointed leaves. It is common in North America and causes severe allergic contact dermatitis in many people. Localized vesicular eruption with itching and burning results and may be treated with antipruritic lotions, cold compresses, or topical corticosteroid ointment or cream. Severe cases may require corticosteroids given intramuscularly or orally. In people who are hypersensitive, prophylactic treatment with *Rhus* antigen may be given after contact, before symptoms develop. Careful washing of the exposed skin after suspected contact may prevent the reaction. See also **rhus dermatitis, urushiol.**

poison oak, any of several species of shrub of the genus *Rhus,* common in North America. Skin contact results in allergic dermatitis in many people. The characteristics and the treatment of the condition are similar to those of poison ivy. See also **rhus dermatitis, urushiol.**

poison sumac /so͞o′mak/, a shrub of the genus *Rhus,* common in North America. Skin contact results in allergic dermatitis in many people. The characteristics and the treatment of the condition are similar to those of poison ivy. See also **rhus dermatitis, urushiol.**

poker spine. See **bamboo spine.**

polar, **1.** See **pole, polus. 2.** pertaining to molecules that are hydrophilic, or ''water-loving.'' Polar substances tend to dissolve in polar solvents.

Polaramine, a trademark for an antihistaminic (dexchlorpheniramine maleate).

polar body, one of the small cells produced during the two meiotic divisions in the maturation process of female gametes, or ova. It is nonfunctional and incapable of being fertilized. See also **oogenesis.**

polarity /pōler′itē/, **1.** the existence or manifestation of opposing qualities, tendencies, or emotions, as pleasure and pain, love and hate, strength and weakness, dependence and independence, masculinity and femininity. The concept is central to various psychotherapeutic approaches, as client-centered therapy, in which the key to self-actualization lies in accepting polarity within oneself. **2.** (in physics) the distinction between a negative and a positive electric charge.

polarity therapy, a technique of massage based on the theory that the body has positive and negative energy patterns that must be balanced to establish physical harmony.

polarization, the concentration within a population or group of member's inerests, beliefs, and allegiances around two conflicting positions.

pole, **1.** (in biology) an end of an imaginary axis drawn through the symmetrically arranged parts of a cell, organ, ovum, or nucleus. **2.** (in anatomy) the point on a nerve cell at which a dendrite originates. –**polar,** *adj.*

policy, a principle or guideline that governs an activity and that employees or members of an institution or organization are expected to follow.

polio. See **poliomyelitis.**

polio-, a combining form meaning 'of or related to gray matter in the nervous system': *polioclastic, polioencephalitis, poliomyelitis.*

polioencephalitis /pō′lē·ō·ensef′əlī′tis/, an inflammation of the gray matter of the brain caused by infection of the brain by a poliovirus.

polioencephalomyelitis /pō′lē·ō·ensef′əlōmī′əlī′tis/, inflammation of the gray matter of the brain and the spinal cord, caused by infection by a poliovirus.

poliomyelitis /pō′lē·ōmī·əlī′tis/, an infectious disease caused by one of the three polioviruses. Asymptomatic, mild, and paralytic forms of the disease occur. Several factors influence susceptibility to the virus and the course of the disease: More boys than girls are severely affected, stress increases susceptibility, more pregnant than nonpregnant women acquire the paralytic form of the disease, and the severity of the infection increases with age. It is transmitted from person to person through fecal contamination or oropharyngeal secretions. Also called *(informal)* **polio.** See also **poliovirus.**

■ OBSERVATIONS: Asymptomatic infection has no clinical features, but it confers immunity. Abortive poliomyelitis lasts only a few hours and is characterized by minor illness with fever, malaise, headache, nausea, vomiting, and slight abdominal discomfort. Nonparalytic poliomyelitis is longer lasting and is marked by meningeal irritation with pain and stiffness in the back and by all the signs of abortive poliomyelitis. Paralytic poliomyelitis begins as abortive poliomyelitis. The symptoms abate, and for several days the person seems well. Malaise, headache, and fever recur; pain, weakness, and paralysis develop. The peak of paralysis is reached within the first week. In spinal poliomyelitis, viral replication occurs in the anterior horn cells of the spine causing inflammation, swelling, and, if severe, destruction of the neurons. The large proximal muscles of the limbs are most often affected. Bulbar poliomyelitis results from viral multiplication in the brainstem. Bulbar and spinal poliomeylitis often occur together.

■ INTERVENTION: Treatment of the abortive and nonparalytic forms of the disease is symptomatic, consisting of bed rest, good nutrition, and avoidance, for at least 2 weeks, of overexertion, stress, and fatigue. Treatment of the paralytic form includes hospitalization with observation for advance of the disease, the application of hot packs and the giving of baths, range of motion exercise, and assisted ventilation when necessary. As soon as the acute febrile stage is over, active, comprehensive rehabilitation is promptly begun.

■ NURSING CONSIDERATIONS: The more quickly function returns, the better the outcome. The pain and muscle spasm of the acute period cause the person to want to remain immobile. Such immobility enhances the tendency to deformity, and the nurse may be of great help in encouraging the person to exercise and to participate actively in the rehabilitative program. Poliomyelitis, which has not been eradicated, may be prevented by immunization. Families are encouraged to obtain the complete series for all family members, particularly before traveling in countries where the disease is endemic. Formerly, when epidemic, poliomyelitis was seen chiefly in the summer. Now the few cases occurring are sporadic rather than seasonal.

poliomyelitis vaccine. See **poliovirus vaccine.**

poliosis /pō′lē•ō′sis/, depigmentation of the hair on the scalp, eyebrows, eyelashes, mustache, beard, or body. The condition may be inherited and generalized or acquired and localized in patches. Acquired localized poliosis often occurs in alopecia areata.

poliovirus, the causative organism of poliomyelitis. There are three serologically distinct types of this very small RNA virus. Infection or immunization with one type does not protect against the others.

poliovirus vaccine, a vaccine prepared from poliovirus to confer immunity to it. TOPV, the trivalent live oral form of vaccine, is recommended for all children under 18 years of age who have no specific contraindications. The inactivated poliovirus vaccine (IPV) is recommended for infants and children who are immunodeficient and for unvaccinated adults. TOPV is called Sabin vaccine; IPV is called Salk vaccine. IPV is given subcutaneously. Rarely, vaccine-associated paralysis occurs after administration of TOPV; this reaction has not occurred with IPV.

polishing, a tendency of patients with right temporal lobe lesions to deny dysphoric affect and minimize socially disapproved behavior while exaggerating other qualities.

political nursing, the use of knowledge about power processes and strategies to influence the nature and direction of health care and professional nursing. The constituency of political nursing is patients, as communities, groups, or individuals, both diagnosed and potential.

pollakiuria /pol′əkēyo͞or′ē•ə/, an abnormal condition characterized by unduly frequent passage of urine.

pollen coryza, acute seasonal rhinitis caused by exposure to an allergenic. Also called **hay fever.** See also **coryza.**

pollinosis. See **hay fever.**

pollutant, an unwanted substance that occurs in the environment, usually with health-threatening effects. Pollutants may exist in the atmosphere as gases or fine particles that may be irritating to the lungs, eyes, and skin, as dissolved or suspended substances in drinking water, and as carcinogens or mutagens in foods or beverages.

polonium (Po), a radioactive element that is one of the disintegration products of uranium. Its atomic number is 84; its atomic weight is approximately 210.

polus /pō′ləs/, *pl.* **poli,** either of the opposite ends of any axis; the official anatomic designation for the extremity of an organ. See also **pole.** **–polar,** *adj.*

poly-, a combining form meaning ‘many or much’: *polyacid, polycholia, polydactylia.*

polyacrylamide, a polymer of acrylamide and usually some crosslinking derivative.

polyamine, any compound that contains two or more amine groups, as spermidine and spermine, which are normally occurring tissue constituents in humans. Many polyamines function as essential growth factors in microorganisms.

polyanionic, pertaining to multiple negative electric charges.

polyarteritis /pol′ē•är′tərī′tis/, an abnormal inflammatory condition of several arteries.

polyarteritis nodosa, a severe and poorly understood collagen vascular disease in which there is widespread inflammation and necrosis of small and medium-sized arteries and ischemia of the tissues they serve. Any organ or organ system may be affected. The disease attacks men and women between 20 and 50 years of age. Its cause is unknown, although immunologic factors are suspected. Polyarteritis nodosa may be acute and rapidly fatal, or chronic and wasting. It is characterized by fever, abdominal pain, weight loss, neuropathy, and, if the kidneys are affected, hypertension, edema, and uremia. Some symptoms may mimic GI or cardiac disorders. Diagnosis is based on the clinical signs, laboratory tests, and biopsy of sites affected by the disease. Mortality in polyarteritis nodosa is high, especially if there is kidney involvement. Aggressive treatment includes massive doses of corticosteroids. Immunosuppressive drugs have been used experimentally with some success. Physical therapy helps the patient to maintain muscle tone and prevents or slows the development of disability.

polychlorinated biphenyls (PCB), a group of more than 30 isomers and compounds used in plastics, insulation, and flame retardants and varying in physical form from oily liquids to crystals and resins. All are potentially toxic and carcinogenic. The toxicity varies with the type of PCB and concurrent exposure to other substances, as carbon tetrachloride. Mild exposure may cause chloracne; severe exposure may result in hepatic damage.

polychromasia. See **polychromatophilia.**

polychromatic, a light of many colors or wavelengths. The term is usually applied to white light although it may also refer to a defined portion of the spectrum

polychromatophil /pol'ēkrōmat'əfəl/, any cell that may be stained by several different dyes.

polychromatophilia /pol'ēkrō'matəfil'ē•ə/, an abnormal tendency of a cell, particularly an erythrocyte, to be dyed by a variety of laboratory stains. Also called **polychromasia.**

Polycillin, a trademark for an antibacterial (ampicillin).

Polycillin-N, a trademark for an antibacterial (ampicillin sodium).

polyclonal /pol'ēklō'nəl/, **1.** of, pertaining to, or designating a group of identical cells or organisms derived from several identical cells. **2.** of, pertaining to, or designating several groups of identical cells or organisms (clones) derived from a single cell.

polyclonal gammopathy. See **gammopathy.**

Polycose, a trademark for a nutritional supplement containing glucose polymers derived from cornstarch.

polycystic kidney disease (PKD), an abnormal condition in which the kidneys are enlarged and contain many cysts. There are three forms of the disease. **Childhood polycystic disease (CPD)** is uncommon and may be differentiated from adult or congenital polycystic disease by genetic, morphologic, and clinical facets. Death usually occurs within a few years as the result of portal hypertension and liver and kidney failure. A portacaval shunt may prolong life into the twenties. **Adult polycystic disease (APD)** may be unilateral, bilateral, acquired, or congenital. The condition is characterized by flank pain and high blood pressure. Kidney failure eventually develops, progressing to uremia and death. **Congenital polycystic disease (CPD)** is a rare congenital aplasia of the kidney involving all or only a small segment of one or both kidneys. Severe bilateral aplasia results in death shortly after birth. Minor aplasia may cause no dysfunction and may never be diagnosed.

polycystic ovary syndrome, an abnormal condition characterized by anovulation, amenorrhea, hirsutism, and infertility. It is caused by an endocrine imbalance with increased levels of testosterone, estrogen, and luteinizing hormone (LH) and decreased secretion of follicle stimulating hormone (FSH). The increased level of LH associated with this disorder may be the result of an increased sensitivity of the pituitary to stimulation by releasing hormone or of excessive stimulation by the adrenal gland. Polycystic ovary may also be associated with a variety of problems in the hypothalamic-pituitary-ovarian axis, with extragonadal sources of androgens, or with androgen-producing tumors. This condition is transmitted as an X-linked dominant or autosomal dominant trait. The depressed but continuous production of FSH associated with this disorder causes continuous partial development of ovarian follicles. Numerous follicular cysts, 2 to 6 mm in diameter, may develop. The affected ovary commonly doubles in size and is invested by a smooth, pearly-white capsule. The increased level of estrogen associated with this abnormality raises the risk of cancers of the breast and the endometrium. Depending on the severity of symptoms and whether or not the patient wants to become pregnant, treatment involves suppression of hormonal stimulation of the ovary, usually using female hormones or resection of part of one or both ovaries.

polycythemia /pol'ēsīthē'mē•ə/, an abnormal increase in the number of erythrocytes in the blood. It may be secondary to pulmonary disease or heart disease or to prolonged exposure to high altitudes. In the absence of a demonstrable cause, it is considered idiopathic. Also called **Osler's disease, polycythemia vera.** Compare **hypoplastic anemia, leukemia.** See also **altitude sickness, erythrocytosis.**

polydactyly, a congenital anomaly characterized by the presence of more than the normal number of fingers or toes. The condition is usually inherited as an autosomal dominant characteristic and can usually be corrected by surgery shortly after birth. Also called **polydactylia, polydactylism, hyperdactyly.**

polydipsia /pol'ēdip'sē•ə/, **1.** excessive thirst characteristic of several different conditions, including diabetes mellitus in which an excessive concentration of glucose in the blood osmotically increases the excretion of fluid via increased urination, which leads to hypovolemia and thirst. In diabetes insipidus, the deficiency of the pituitary antidiuretic hormone results in excretion of copious amounts of dilute urine, reduced fluid volume in the body, and polydipsia. In nephrogenic diabetes insipidus, there is also copious excretion of urine and consequent polydipsia. Polyuria resulting from other forms of renal dysfunction also leads to polydipsia. The condition may also be psychogenic in origin. **2.** *informal.* alcoholism.

polyelectrolyte, a substance with many charged or potentially charged groups.

polyesthesia, a sensory disorder involving the sense of touch in which a stimulus to one area of the skin is felt at other sites in addition to the one stimulated.

polyestradiol phosphate, an antineoplastic estrogen compound.

■ INDICATIONS: It is prescribed for cancer of the prostate and postmenopausal breast cancer.

■ CONTRAINDICATIONS: Male breast cancer, estrogen-dependent neoplasia, thrombophlebitis, or known hypersensitivity to this drug prohibits its use.

■ ADVERSE EFFECTS: Among the more serious adverse reactions are loss of libido, impotence, gynecomastia, fluid retention and edema, and, rarely, cholestatic jaundice.

polygene /pol′ējēn′/, any of a group of nonallelic genes that individually exert a small effect but together interact in a cumulative manner to produce a particular characteristic within an individual, usually of a quantitative nature, as size, weight, skin pigmentation, or degree of intelligence. Also called **cumulative gene, multiple factor, multiple gene.** See also **multifactorial inheritance.** –**polygenic,** *adj.*

polygenic inheritance. See **multifactorial inheritance.**

polyglucosan, a large molecule consisting of many anhydrous polysaccharides.

polyhybrid, (in genetics) pertaining to or describing an individual, organism, or strain that is heterozygous for more than three specific traits, that is the offspring of parents differing in more than three specific gene pairs, or that is heterozygous for more than three particular characteristics or gene loci being followed.

polyhybrid cross, (in genetics) the mating of two individuals, organisms, or strains that have different gene pairs that determine more than three specific traits or in which more than three particular characteristics or gene loci are being followed.

polyhydramnios. See **hydramnios.**

polyleptic /pol′ēlep′tik/, describing any disease or condition marked by numerous remissions and exacerbations.

polyleptic fever, a fever occurring paroxysmally, as smallpox and relapsing fever.

polymer /pol′imər/, a compound formed by combining or linking a number of monomers, or small molecules. A polymer may be composed of a variety of different monomers or from many units of the same monomer.

polymicrogyria. See **microgyria.**

polymorphism /pol′ēmôr′fizəm/, **1.** the state or quality of existing or occurring in several different forms. **2.** the state or quality of appearing in different forms at different stages of development. Kinds of polymorphism are **balanced polymorphism** and **genetic polymorphism.** –**polymorphic,** *adj.*

polymorphocytic leukemia /pol′ēmôr′fəsit′ik/, a neoplasm of blood-forming tissues in which mature, segmented granulocytes are predominant. Also called **mature cell leukemia, neutrophilic leukemia.**

polymorphonuclear /pol′ēmôr′fōno͞o′klē•ər/, having a nucleus with a number of lobules or segments connected by a fine thread.

polymorphonuclear cell (PMN), a leukocyte with a mulitlobed nucleus, as a neutrophil.

polymorphonuclear leukocyte, a white blood cell containing a segmented lobular nucleus; an eosinophil, basophil, or neutrophil. See also **granulocyte.**

polymorphous /pol′ēmôr′fəs/, occurring in many varying forms, possibly changing in structure or appearance at different stages.

polymorphous light eruption, a common, recurrent, superficial vascular reaction to sunlight or ultraviolet light in susceptible individuals. Within 1 to 4 days after exposure to the light, small, erythematous papules and vesicles appear on otherwise normal skin, then disappear within 2 weeks. A delayed allergic response is a possible cause. Tanning reduces the severity of the reaction.

Polymox, a trademark for an antibiotic (amoxicillin).

polymyalgia rheumatica, a chronic, episodic, inflammatory disease of the large arteries that usually develops in people over 60 years of age. Polymyalgia rheumatica and cranial arteritis are believed to represent the same disease process with slightly different symptoms. Polymyalgia rheumatica primarily affects the muscles, and it is characterized by pain and stiffness of the back, shoulder, or neck, usually becoming more severe on rising in the morning. There may also be a cranial headache, as in cranial arteritis, which affects the temporal and occipital arteries, causing a severe, throbbing headache. Serious complications include arterial insufficiency, coronary occlusion, stroke, or blindness. Usually, patients with polymyalgia rheumatica or cranial arteritis have marked elevations of the erythrocyte sedimentation rate. Both forms of the disease may follow a self-limited course; however, adrenocorticosteroids have proven highly effective in reducing inflammation and in speeding recovery. Both forms are probably autoimmune conditions. Also called **polymyalgia arteritica, temporal arteritis.**

polymyositis /pol′ēmī′ōsī′tis/, inflammation of many muscles, usually accompanied by deformity, edema, insomnia, pain, sweating, and tension. Some forms of polymyositis are associated with malignancy. See also **dermatomyositis.**

polymyxin, an antibiotic.

■ INDICATIONS: It is used topically and systemically in the treatment of gram-negative bacterial infections, including meningitis, corneal ulcerations, and otitis media.

■ CONTRAINDICATIONS: Hypersensitivity to this drug prohibits its use. It is used with great caution in patients with impaired renal function.

■ ADVERSE EFFECTS: Among the more serious adverse reactions when this drug is used systemically are nephrotoxicity and various neurologic alterations, including blockade of neuromuscular junction. Pain or phlebitis at the site of injection also may occur. When this drug is applied locally, irritation and allergic reactions of the skin or mucosa are sometimes seen.

polymyxin B sulfate, an antibiotic.

■ INDICATIONS: It is prescribed for infections caused by microorganisms sensitive to this drug, including urinary tract infections, septicemia, and conjunctivitis.

■ CONTRAINDICATIONS: Known hypersensitivity to this drug prohibits its use. Extreme caution is necessary when it is given systemically to people with impaired renal function.

■ ADVERSE EFFECTS: Among the more serious adverse reactions when given systemically are nephrotoxicity, neurotoxicity, and drug fever. When given topically allergies are the most common problem.

polyneuritic psychosis. See **Korsakoff's psychosis.**

polyopia, a defect of sight in which one object is perceived as many images; multiple vision. The condition can occur in one or both eyes. See also **diplopia.**

polyp, a small tumorlike growth that projects from a mucous membrane surface.

polypeptide /pol′ēpep′tīd/, a chain of amino acids joined by peptide bonds. A polypeptide has a larger molecular weight than a peptide but a smaller molecular weight than a protein. Polypeptides are formed by partial hydrolysis of proteins or by synthesis of amino acids into chains.

polyphagia /pol′ēfā′jē·ə/, eating to the point of gluttony. See also **bulimia.**

polypharmacy, a term applied to the use of a number of different drugs by a patient who may have one or several health problems.

polyploid /pol′əploid/, **1.** of or pertaining to an individual, organism, strain, or cell that has more than the two complete sets of chromosomes normal for the somatic cell. The multiple of the haploid number characteristic of the species is denoted by the appropriate prefix, as in triploid, tetraploid, pentaploid, hexaploid, heptaploid, octaploid, and so on. Polyploidy is rare in animals, producing organisms that are abnormal in appearance and usually infertile, but it is common in plants, which are generally larger, have larger cells, and are more hardy than those with the normal diploid number. **2.** such an individual, organism, strain, or cell. Also **polyploidic.** Compare **aneuploid.**

polypoid adenocarcinoma. See **papillary adenocarcinoma.**

polyploidy /pol′əploi′dē/, the state or condition of having more than two complete sets of chromosomes.

polyposis, an abnormal condition characterized by the presence of numerous polyps on a part. See also **familial polyposis.**

polyradiculitis /pol′ērədik′yo͞olī′tis/, inflammation of many nerve roots, as found in Guillain-Barré syndrome.

polyribosome. See **polysome.**

polysaccharide, a carbohydrate that contains three or more molecules of simple carbohydrates. Examples of polysaccharides include dextrins, starches, glycogens, celluloses, gums, inulin, and pentose.

polysome, (in genetics) a group of ribosomes joined together by a molecule of messenger RNA containing the genetic code. The structure is found in the cytoplasm during protein synthesis. Also called **ergosome, polyribosome.** See also **translation.**

polysomy /pol′əsō′mē/, the presence of a chromosome in at least triplicate in an otherwise diploid somatic cell as the result of chromosomal nondisjunction during meiotic division in the maturation of gametes. The chromosome may be duplicated three times (trisomy), four times (tetrasomy), or more times. In males with Klinefelter's syndrome the genotype may be XXXY or XXXXY instead of the usual XXY associated with the syndrome; among polysomic females with three, four, or five X chromosomes there may be a higher frequency of mental retardation.

Polysporin, a trademark for an ophthalmic and topical, antiinfective, fixed-combination drug containing antibacterials (polymyxin B sulfate and bacitracin).

Polytar Bath, a trademark for a fixed-combination drug containing two topical antieczematics (coal tar and pine tar).

polytene chromosome, an excessively large type of chromosome consisting of bundles of unseparated chromonemata filaments. It is found primarily in the saliva of certain insects. See also **giant chromosome.**

polythiazide, a diuretic and antihypertensive.

■ INDICATIONS: It is prescribed in the treatment of hypertension and edema.

■ CONTRAINDICATIONS: Anuria or known hypersensitivity to this drug, other thiazides, or sulfonamide derivatives prohibits its use.

■ ADVERSE EFFECTS: Among the more serious adverse reactions are hypokalemia, hyperglycemia, hyperuricemia, and various hypersensitivity reactions.

polyunsaturated fatty acid. See **unsaturated fatty acid.**

polyuria /pol′ēyo͝or′ē·ə/, the excretion of an abnormally large quantity of urine. Some causes of polyuria are diabetes insipidus, diabetes mellitus, diuretics, excessive fluid intake, hypercalcemia.

polyvalent antiserum. See **antiserum.**

Poly-Vi-Flor, a trademark for an oral, pediatric, fixed-combination drug containing several vitamins and sodium fluoride.

polyvinyl chloride (PVC), a common synthetic thermoplastic material that releases hydrochloric acid when burned and that may contain carcinogenic vinyl chloride molecules as a contaminant.

POMP /pomp/, an abbreviation for a combination drug regimen used in the treatment of cancer, containing three antineoplastics, Purinethol (mercaptopurine), Oncovin (vincristine sulfate), methotrexate, and prednisone (a glucocorticoid).

Pompe's disease, a form of muscle glycogen storage disease in which there is a generalized accumulation of glycogen, resulting from a deficiency of acid maltase (alpha-1, 4-glucosidase). It is usually fatal in infants, caused by cardiac or respiratory failure. Children with Pompe's disease appear mentally retarded and hypotonic, seldom living beyond 20 years of age. In adults muscle weakness is progressive, but the disease is not fatal. Also called **glycogen storage disease, type II.** See also **glycogen storage disease.**

pompholyx. See **dyshidrosis.**

POMR, abbreviation for **problem-oriented medical record.**

Pondimin, a trademark for an anorexiant (fenfluramine hydrochloride).

pono-, a combining form meaning 'of or related to pain': *ponograph, ponopalmosis, ponophobia.*

ponos. See **kala-azar.**

pons /ponz/, *pl.* **pontes** /pon′tēz/, **1.** any slip of tissue connecting two parts of a structure or an organ of the body. **2.** a prominence on the ventral surface of the brainstem, between the medulla oblongata and the cerebral peduncles of the midbrain. The pons consists of white matter and a few nuclei and is divided into a ventral portion and a dorsal portion. The ventral portion consists of transverse fibers separated by longitudinal bundles and small nuclei. The dorsal portion comprises the tegmentum, which is a continuation of the reticular formation of the medulla. The tegmentum contains the nucleus of the abducens nerve, the nucleus of the facial nerve, the motor nucleus of the trigeminal nerve, the sensory nuclei of the trigeminal nerve, the nucleus of the cochlear division of the eighth nerve, the superior olive, and the nuclei of the vestibular division of the eighth nerve. Also called **bridge of varolius.**

Ponstel, a trademark for an antiinflammatory and analgesic (mefenamic acid).

pont-, a combining form meaning 'bridge': *pontic, ponticulus, pontimeter.*

Pontiac fever. See **Legionnaires' disease.**

pontic, the suspended member of a fixed partial denture, as an artificial tooth, usually occupying the space previously occupied by the natural tooth crown.

Pontocaine Hydrochloride, a trademark for a local anesthetic (tetracaine hydrochloride).

pooled plasma, a liquid component of whole blood, collected and pooled to prepare various plasma products or to use directly as a plasma expander when whole blood is unavailable or is contraindicated. It is useful in surgery and in the treatment of hypovolemia because of its stability and availability in freeze-dried form. It is collected from blood banks or prepared directly from donors by plasmapheresis. It is thin and colorless or slightly yellow. Of the total volume of normal blood, 55% to 65% is plasma. See also **bank blood, component therapy, packed cells.**

poorly differentiated lymphocytic malignant lymphoma, a lymphoid neoplasm containing many cells resembling lymphoblasts that have a fine nuclear structure and one or more nucleoli. Also called **lymphoblastic lymphoma, lymphoblastic lymphosarcoma, lymphoblastoma.**

popliteal artery /pop′litē′əl/, a continuation of the femoral artery, extending from the opening in the abductor magnus, passing through the popliteal fossa at the knee, dividing into eight branches, and supplying various muscles of the thigh, leg, and foot. Its branches are the superior muscular, sural, cutaneous, medial superior genicular, lateral superior genicular, middle genicular, medial inferior genicular, and lateral inferior genicular.

popliteal node, a node in one of the groups of lymph glands in the leg. Approximately seven small popliteal nodes are imbedded in the fat of the popliteal fossa at the back of the knee. One node is near the terminal section of the saphenous vein and drains the area around the vein. Another node lying between the popliteal artery and the posterior surface of the knee joint drains that region. The other popliteal nodes lie along the popliteal vessels and receive the afferent trunks accompanying the anterior and posterior tibial vessels. Most of the efferents of the popliteal nodes course along the femoral vessels to the deep inguinal nodes. Compare **anterior tibial node, inguinal node.**

popliteal pulse, the pulse of the popliteal artery, palpated behind the knee of a person lying prone with the knee flexed.

population, **1.** (in genetics) an interbreeding group of individuals, organisms, or plants characterized by genetic continuity through several generations. **2.** a group of individuals collectively occupying a particular geographic locale. **3.** any group that is distinguished by a particular trait or situation. **4.** any group measured for some variable characteristic from which samples may be taken for statistic purposes.

population at risk, a group of people who share a characteristic that causes each member to be vulnerable to a particular event, as nonimmunized children who are exposed to poliovirus or immunosuppressed people who are exposed to herpesvirus.

population genetics, a branch of genetics that applies mendelian inheritance to groups and studies the frequency of alleles and genotypes in breeding populations. See also **Hardy-Weinberg equilibrium principle.**

por-, a combining form meaning 'passage or pore': *porencephalia, porion, porotomy.*

porcine graft, a temporary biologic heterograft made from the skin of a pig.

-pore, a combining form meaning 'passageway': *metapore, myelopore, neuropore.*

poriomania /pôr′ē·ōmā′nē·ə/, a tendency to leave home impulsively or to be a vagabond.

pork tapeworm. See ***Taenia solium.***

pork tapeworm infection, an infection of the intestine or the tissues, caused by the adult and larval forms of the tapeworm *Taenia solium*. The pork tapeworm is unique in that it can use humans as both intermediate hosts for larvae and definitive hosts for the adult worm. Humans are usually infected with the adult worm after eating contaminated, undercooked pork. The infection is rare in the United States but relatively common in South America, Asia, and Russia. See also **cysticercosis, tapeworm infection.**

poro-, a combining form meaning 'callus': *porokeratosis, poroma, porosis.*

porphobilinogen /pôr'fōbilin'əjən/, a chromogen substance that is an intermediate in the biosynthesis of heme and porphyrins. It appears in the urine of persons with porphyria, representing an error of metabolism. See also **heme, porphyria.**

porphyria /pôrfir'ē·ə/, a group of inherited disorders in which there is abnormally increased production of substances called porphyrins. Two major classifications of porphyria are **erythropoietic porphyria,** characterized by the production of large quantities of porphyrins in the blood-forming tissue of the bone marrow, and **hepatic porphyria,** in which large amounts of porphyrins are produced in the liver. Clinical signs common to both classifications of porphyria are photosensitivity, abdominal pain, and neuropathy.

porphyrin /pôr'fərin/, any iron- or magnesium-free pyrrole derivative occurring in many plant and animal tissues.

portability, a property of computer software that permits its use in a variety of compatible operating systems.

portacaval shunt, a shunt created surgically to increase the flow of blood from the portal circulation by carrying it into the vena cava.

Portagen, a trademark for a nutritional supplement containing protein, carbohydrate, and fat.

portal fissure, a fissure on the visceral surface of the liver along which the portal vein, the hepatic artery, and the hepatic ducts pass. Also called **porta hepatis.**

portal hypertension, an increased venous pressure in the portal circulation caused by compression or by occlusion in the portal or hepatic vascular system. It results in splenomegaly, large collateral veins, ascites, and, in severe cases, systemic hypertension and esophageal varices. Portal hypertension is frequently associated with alcoholic cirrhosis. Also called **renovascular hypertension.**

portal system, the network of veins that drains the blood from the abdominal portion of the digestive tract, the spleen, the pancreas, and the gallbladder and conveys blood from these viscera to the liver.

portal systemic encephalopathy. See **hepatic coma.**

portal vein, a vein that ramifies like an artery in the liver and ends in capillary-like sinusoids that convey the blood to the inferior vena cava through the hepatic veins. In the adult, the portal vein has no valves; but in the fetus and during a brief postnatal period the tributaries of the portal vein contain valves that soon atrophy and disappear. In some individuals, the valves persist as degenerate structures. About 8 cm long, the portal vein is formed at the level of the second lumbar vertebra by the junction of the superior mesenteric and the splenic veins. The portal vein passes behind the duodenum and ascends through the lesser omentum to the porta hepatis, where it divides into the right and the left branches. The vein is surrounded by the hepatic plexus of nerves and accompanied by numerous lymphatic vessels and some lymph nodes. Accompanied by corresponding branches of the hepatic artery, the right branch of the portal vein enters the right lobe of the liver and the left branch enters the left lobe. The tributaries of the portal vein are the lienal vein, the superior mesenteric vein, the coronary vein, the pyloric vein, the cystic vein, and the paraumbilical vein.

Porter-Silber reaction, a reaction, visible as a change in color to yellow, that indicates the amount of adrenal steroids (the 17-hydroxycorticosteroids) excreted per day in the urine. The test is used to evaluate adrenocortical function.

portoenterostomy, a procedure to correct biliary atresis in which the jejunum is anastomosed by a Roux-en-Y loop to the portal fissure region to establish bile flow from the bile ducts to the intestine. The operation is successful in most cases, but late mortality in a significant number of patients occurs because of chronic medical problems. Without the operation, biliary cirrhosis develops with an attendant early death. Also called **Kasai operation.**

port-wine stain. See **nevus flammeus.**

position, **1.** any one of many postures of the body, as the anatomic position, lateral recumbent position, or semi-Fowler's position. See specific positions. **2.** (in obstetrics) the relationship of an arbitrarily chosen fetal reference point, as the occiput, sacrum, chin, or scapula on the presenting part of the fetus, with respect to its location in the maternal pelvis.

-position, a combining form meaning the 'putting or setting in place': *electrodeposition, juxtaposition, reposition.*

positional behavior, the orientation of the body regions to claim a quantum of space. Positional behavior involves four body regions: head and neck, upper torso, pelvis and thighs, and lower legs and feet.

positive, **1.** (of a laboratory test) indicating that a substance or a reaction is present. **2.** (of a sign) indicating on physical examination that a finding is present, often meaning that there is pathologic change. **3.** (of a substance) tending to carry or carrying a positive chemical charge.

positive end expiratory pressure (PEEP), (in respiratory therapy) ventilation controlled by a flow of air delivered in cycles of constant pressure through the respiratory cycle. The patient is intubated, and a respirator cycles the air through an endotracheal tube. PEEP is used for the relief of respiratory distress secondary to prematurity, pancreatitis, shock, pulmonary edema, trauma, surgery, or other conditions in which spontaneous respiratory efforts are inadequate and arterial levels of oxygen are deficient. During PEEP therapy close observation is necessary; the patient often needs to be sedated to help stop resistance to the respirator. Blood gases and vital signs are monitored closely. If PEEP does not significantly improve the patient's condition, it is not continued. Compare **continuous positive airway pressure.**

positive euthanasia. See **active euthanasia.**

positive feedback, **1.** (in physiology) an increase in function in response to a stimulus; for example, micturition increases once the flow of urine has started, or the uterus contracts more frequently and with greater strength once it has begun to contract in labor. **2.** *informal.* an encouraging, favorable, or otherwise positive response from one person to what another person has communicated.

positive identification, the unconscious modeling of one's personality on that of another who is admired and esteemed. See also **identification.**

positive pressure, **1.** a greater than ambient atmospheric pressure. **2.** (in respiratory therapy) any technique in which compressed air or gas or air is delivered to the respiratory passages at greater than ambient pressure. Positive pressure techniques in respiratory therapy require a flow regulating device and a delivery system, as a cannula, mouthpiece, endotracheal tube, or tracheostomy tube.

positive pressure breathing unit. See **IPPB unit.**

positive relationship, (in research) a direct relationship between two variables; as one increases the other can be expected to increase. Also called **direct relationship.** Compare **negative relationship.**

positive signs of pregnancy, three unmistakable signs of pregnancy: fetal heart tones, heard on auscultation; fetal skeleton, seen on x-ray film or ultrasonogram; and fetal parts, felt on palpation.

positron emission tomography (PET), a computerized radiographic technique that employs radioactive substances to examine the metabolic activity of various body structures. In PET studies the patient either inhales or is injected with a biochemical, as glucose, carrying a radioactive substance that emits positively charged particles, or positrons, that combine with negatively charged electrons normally found in the cells of the body. When the positrons combine with these electrons, gamma rays are emitted. The electronic circuitry and computers of the PET device detect the gamma rays and convert them into color-coded images that indicate the intensity of the metabolic activity of the organ involved. The radioactive substances used in the PET technique are very short-lived, so that patients undergoing a PET scan are exposed to very small amounts of radiation. Researchers use PET to study blood flow and the metabolism of the heart and the blood vessels. There is also a growing application of the technique in the study and diagnosis of cancer and in studies of the biochemical activity of the brain.

post-, a combining form meaning 'after or behind': *postarbortal, postcerebellar, postdiastolic.*

postcommissurotomy syndrome, a condition of unknown cause occurring within the first few weeks after cardiac valvular surgery, characterized by intermittent episodes of pain and fever, which may last weeks or months and then resolve spontaneously.

postconcussional syndrome, a condition after head trauma, characterized by dizziness, poor concentration, headache, hypersensitivity, and anxiety. It usually resolves itself without treatment. Also called **posttraumatic syndrome.**

posterior, **1.** of or pertaining to or situated in the back part of a structure, as of the dorsal surface of the human body. **2.** the back part of something. **3.** toward the back. Compare **anterior.**

posterior asynclitism. See **asynclitism.**

posterior atlantoaxial ligament, one of five ligaments connecting the atlas to the axis. It is broad and thin and fixed to the inferior border of the anterior arch of the atlas and to the ventral surface of the body of the axis. Compare **anterior atlantoaxial ligament.**

posterior atlantooccipital membrane, one of a pair of thin, broad fibrous sheets that form part of the atlanto-occipital joint between the atlas and the occipital bone and contain an opening for the vertebral artery and the suboccipital nerve. Also called **posterior atlantooccipital ligament.** Compare **anterior atlantooccipital membrane.**

posterior auricular artery, one of a pair of small branches from the external carotid arteries, dividing into auricular and occipital branches and supplying parts of the ear, scalp, and other structures in the head.

posterior common ligament. See **posterior longitudinal ligament.**

posterior costotransverse ligament, one of the five ligaments of each costotransverse joint, comprised of a fibrous band passing from the neck of each rib to the base of the vertebra above. Compare **superior costotransverse ligament.**

posterior fontanel. See **fontanel.**

posterior fossa, a depression on the posterior surface of the humerus, above the trochlea, that lodges the olecranon of the ulna when the elbow is extended.

posterior longitudinal ligament, a thick, strong ligament attached to the dorsal surfaces of the vertebral bodies, extending from the occipital bone to the coccyx. Also called **posterior common ligament.** Compare **anterior longitudinal ligament.**

posterior mediastinal node, a node in one of three groups of thoracic visceral nodes, connected to the part of the lymphatic system that serves the esophagus, pericardium, diaphragm, and convex surface of the liver. Most of the efferents of the posterior mediastinal nodes end in the thoracic duct, but some join the tracheobronchial nodes. Compare **anterior mediastinal node.**

posterior mediastinum, the irregularly shaped caudal portion of the mediastinum, parallel with the vertebral column. It is bounded ventrally by the pericardium, caudally by the diaphragm, dorsally by the vertebral column from the fourth to the twelfth thoracic vertebra, and laterally by the mediastinal pleurae. It contains the bifurcation of the trachea, two primary bronchi, esophagus, thoracic duct, many large lymph nodes, and various vessels, as the thoracic portion of the aortic arch. Compare **anterior mediastinum, middle mediastinum, superior mediastinum.**

posterior nares, a pair of posterior openings in the nasal cavity that connect the nasal cavity with the nasopharynx and allow the inhalation and the exhalation of air. Each is an oval aperture that measures about 2.5 cm vertically and is about 1.5 cm in diameter. Also called **choana.** Compare **anterior nares.**

posterior neuropore, the opening at the caudal end of the embryonic neural tube. It closes at about the 25 somite stage, which indicates the end of horizon XII in the numeric anatomic charting of human embryonic development. Compare **anterior neuropore.** See also **horizon.**

posterior palatal seal area, the area of soft tissues along the junction of the hard and soft palates on which displacement, within the physiologic tolerance of the tissues, can be applied by a denture to aid its retention.

posterior pituitary, posterior pituitary gland. See **neurohypophysis.**

posterior tibial artery, one of the divisions of the popliteal artery, starting at the distal border of the popliteus muscle, passing behind the tibia, dividing into eight branches, and supplying various muscles of the lower leg, foot, and toes. Its eight branches are the peroneal, nutrient (tibial), muscular, posterior medial malleolar, communicating, medial calcaneal, medial plantar, and lateral plantar. Compare **anterior tibial artery.**

posterior tibialis pulse, the pulse of the posterior tibialis artery palpated on the medial aspect of the ankle, just posterior to the prominence of the ankle bone.

posterior tooth, any of the maxillary and mandibular premolars and molars of the permanent dentition, or of prostheses.

posterior vein of left ventricle, one of the five tributaries of the coronary sinus that drains blood from the capillary bed of the myocardium. It courses along the diaphragmatic surface of the left ventricle, accompanying the circumflex branch of the left coronary artery. In some individuals, it ends in the great cardiac vein. Compare **great cardiac vein, middle cardiac vein, small cardiac vein.**

postero-, a combining form meaning 'of or related to the posterior part': *posteroanterior, posteromedian, posterosuperior*.

postgastrectomy care, nursing care after the removal of all or part of the stomach. Drainage of the nasogastric tube normally changes from bright red to dark in the first 24 hours. If the tube becomes blocked, this fact is reported at once, because gastric distention strains the suture lines. Adequate medication for pain allows deeper breathing and coughing, because the incision is close to the diaphragm. When bowel sounds reappear and a small amount of water given by the ounce is retained, the nasogastric tube is removed. Small, bland meals are offered hourly as tolerated. An increase in temperature or dyspnea indicates a leakage of oral fluids around the anastomosis. The diet is changed slowly to a regular diet, with five or six dry small feedings daily. Fluids are given hourly between meals. The most common complication of gastrectomy is the dumping syndrome, with fullness and discomfort, including vertigo, sweating, palpitation, and nausea occurring 5 to 30 minutes after eating, as food enters the small bowel. Small, dry meals, eaten lying down, along with sedatives and antispasmodics, may prevent the symptoms, though they may persist up to 1 year after surgery. Other possible complications include marginal peptic ulcer, in which gastric acids come into contact with a suture line; afferent loop syndrome, in which the duodenal loop is blocked and pancreatic juices and bile flow back into the stomach; vitamin B_{12} and folic acid deficiency; reduced absorption of calcium and vitamin D; and functional hyperinsulinism, in which carbohydrates now passing directly into the small bowel cause an outpouring of insulin into the bloodstream and a resultant hypoglycemia within 2 hours.

posthepatic cirrhosis. See **cirrhosis.**

postictal /pōst′iktəl/, of or pertaining to the period following a convulsion. **–postictus,** *n.*

postinfectious, occurring after an infection.

postinfectious encephalitis. See **encephalitis.**

postinfectious glomerulonephritis, the acute form of glomerulonephritis, which may follow 1 to 6 weeks after a streptococcal infection, most often in childhood. Characteristics of the disease are hematuria, oliguria, edema, and proteinuria, especially in the form of granular casts. There may be slight impairment of renal function in adults, but most patients recover fully in 1 to 3 months. There is no specific treatment for this form of glomerulonephritis; the dietary restriction of protein and the prescription of diuretics may be necessary until kidney function returns to normal. See also **chronic glomerulonephritis, subacute glomerulonephritis.**

postmastectomy exercises, exercises essential to the prevention of shortening of the muscles and contracture of the joints following mastectomy.

■ METHOD: The woman is asked to flex and extend the fingers of the affected arm and to pronate and supinate the forearm immediately on return to her room after recovery from anesthesia and surgery. On the first postoperative day she is asked to squeeze a rubber ball in her hand. Brushing her teeth and hair are encouraged as effective exercises. Other exercises are usually taught, including four that are called climbing the wall, arm swinging, rope pulling, and elbow spreading. They are performed as follows:

Climbing the wall: The patient stands facing a wall, toes close to the wall. The elbows are bent and the palms of the hands are placed on the wall at shoulder height. The hands are moved up the wall together until the woman feels pain or pulling on the incision, then returned to the starting position.

Arm swinging: While standing, the patient bends forward from the waist, allowing both arms to relax and hang naturally. The arms are swung together from the shoulders from left to right and then in circles parallel to the floor, clockwise and counterclockwise. She straightens up slowly.

Rope pulling: A rope is attached over a shower rod or a hook. Each end of the rope is grasped, and the patient alternately pulls each end, raising one arm after the other to the height at which incisional pain or pulling is felt. The rope is shortened until the affected arm is raised almost directly overhead.

Elbow spreading: The hands are clasped behind the neck, and the elbows are slowly raised to chin level while holding the head erect. Gradually, the elbows are spread apart to the point at which incisional pain or pulling is felt.

■ NURSING ORDERS: Specific exercises may be ordered. The patient is shown how to do them and is encouraged to continue them at home.

■ OUTCOME CRITERIA: With proper exercise, full range of motion returns, both arms can be extended fully and equally high over the head. The woman benefits from having something active to do to help herself during the difficult period of adjustment after mastectomy. Many activities of daily life provide good exercise, as reaching high shelves, hanging clothes, and gardening.

postmature, 1. overly developed or matured. 2. of or pertaining to a postmature infant. See also **dysmaturity.** –**postmaturity,** *n.*

postmature infant, an infant, born after the end of the forty-second week of gestation, bearing the physical signs of placental insufficiency. Characteristically, the baby has dry, peeling skin, long fingernails and toenails, and folds of skin on the thighs and, sometimes, on the arms and buttocks. Hypoglycemia and hypokalemia are common. Postmature infants often look as if they have lost weight in utero. The newborn is fed early, and the calcium and potassium levels in the blood are monitored and corrected, if necessary, to avoid seizures and neurologic damage. To avoid the syndrome, labor may be induced as gestation approaches 42 weeks. To anticipate the problems associated with the syndrome, the fetus and the mother may be electronically monitored through labor.

postmenopausal, of or pertaining to the period of life after the menopause.

postmortem, 1. after death. 2. *informal.* also called **autopsy, necropsy.** postmortem examination.

postmyocardial infarction syndrome, a condition that may occur days or weeks after an acute myocardial infarction. It is characterized by fever, pericarditis with a friction rub, pleurisy, pleural effusion, and joint pain. It tends to recur and often provokes severe anxiety, depression, and fear that it is another heart attack. Treatment includes aspirin, reassurance, and a short course of corticosteroids. Nursing care includes close observation and emotional support, especially when debilitating anxiety and depression are present.

postnasal drip (PND), a drop-by-drop discharge of nasal mucus into the posterior pharynx, often accompanied by a feeling of obstruction, an unpleasant taste, and fetid breath, caused by rhinitis, chronic sinusitis, or hypersecretion by the nasopharyngeal mucosa. Methods of treatment include the application of drops or sprays of phenylephrine or ephedrine sulfate to constrict blood vessels and reduce hyperemia, sinus irrigation to improve drainage, and the use of appropriate antibiotics. Therapy for allergies may be indicated in some cases, and surgery may be required if the nasal passages are obstructed by polyps or a deviated septum.

postnecrotic cirrhosis, a nodular form of cirrhosis that may follow hepatitis or other inflammation of the liver. Also called **posthepatic cirrhosis.** See also **cirrhosis.**

postoperative, of or pertaining to the period of time after surgery. It begins with the patient's emergence from anesthesia and continues through the time required for the acute effects of the anesthetic or surgical procedures to abate.

postoperative atelectasis, a form of atelectasis in which collapse of lung tissue is caused by the depressant effects of anesthetic drugs. Deep breathing and coughing are encouraged at frequent intervals postoperatively to prevent this condition.

postoperative bed, a bed prepared for a patient who is weak or unconscious, as when recovering from anesthesia. The bed is in the flat position. The bottom sheet may be covered with a cotton bath blanket that is tucked tightly beneath the mattress. The top linen is fan-folded to the far side of the bed and not tucked in. The bed is made in this way to simplify transferring a patient from a stretcher into the bed.

postoperative care, the management of a patient after surgery. See also **preoperative care.**

■ METHOD: On the patient's discharge from the operating room, the surgical drapes, ground plate, and restraints are removed and a sterile dressing is applied to the incision. The patency and connections of all drainage tubes and the flow rate of parenteral infusions are checked. The patient's cleanliness and dryness are given attention, and the gown is changed, avoiding exposing the individual. Four people transfer the patient slowly and cautiously to a recovery room bed, maintaining body alignment and protecting the limbs. When indicated, an oral or nasal airway is inserted or a previously inserted endotracheal tube is suctioned; respiration may be supported with a pulmonator or intermittent positive pressure breathing (IPPB); if respiration remains impaired, the anesthesiologist is notified. The blood pressure, pulse, and respirations are initially reported to the anesthesiologist and are then checked every 15 minutes or as ordered. At similar intervals, the level of consciousness, reflexes, and movements of extremities are observed, and the incision, drainage tubes, and intravenous infusion site are inspected. Nothing is given orally; medication, blood or blood components, oxygen, and IPPB are administered as ordered, and fluid intake and output are measured. Pain is controlled by giving narcotics in one fourth, one third, or one half doses until the patient reacts fully. The patient is kept warm, dry, and positioned for optimal ventilation and comfort; if necessary, the arms are restrained. At the first sign of vomiting, the head is turned to one side and suction is applied. Oral hygiene is administered every 1 to 2 hours to keep the mouth and tongue moist. The chest is auscultated for breath sounds every 30 minutes, and the patient, when reactive, is helped to turn, cough, and deep breathe every 1 to 2 hours. The rectal or axillary temperature is taken every 1 to 4 hours. When completely awake, able to move the extremities well, and after having exhibited stable vital signs for 1 hour, the patient may be medicated for pain and transferred to the assigned room, provided the drainage tubes are functioning, the dressings show no bleeding or excessive drainage, and the anesthesiologist approves the move. The family is informed of the patient's progress and expectations in the postoperative period. The airway patency, rate, depth, and character of respirations, pulse, blood pressure, temperature, skin color, level of consciousness, and condition of dressings and drainage tubes are assessed. If respirations are noisy, the patient is assisted in coughing. A rapid, weak, thready pulse may indicate increased bleeding and is reported, especially if other signs of impending shock, as hypotension or decreased consciousness, are evident. The dressing is examined at frequent intervals, and excessive drainage is reported immediately. The patient is positioned for comfort and good ventilation with the side rails of the bed raised for safety and the head slightly elevated, except after spinal anesthesia, neurosurgery, and certain kinds of ocular surgery. A cardiac monitor may be connected. Parenteral fluids and medication for pain are administered as ordered; vitamin C may be indicated to promote the healing of a wound. Fluid intake and output are measured; range of motion exercises to extremities are performed, and ambulation, when ordered, is assisted.

■ NURSING ORDERS: The recovery room nurse performs the immediate postoperative procedures, and the clinical unit nurse provides ongoing care, emotional support, and instructions for the patient and family. Special attention is given to preventing trauma postoperatively, as may occur when confused or elderly patients fall getting out of bed. Falls by postoperative patients are second to errors in medication as the most common incidents reported by hospitals.

■ OUTCOME CRITERIA: Meticulous postoperative care prevents falls, infections, and other complications and promotes the healing of the incision and restoration of the patient to health.

postoperative cholangiography, (in diagnostic radiology) a procedure for outlining the major bile ducts. A radiopaque contrast material is injected into the common bile duct via a T-tube inserted during surgery. It is usually performed after a cholecystectomy to discover any residual calculi. See also **cholangiography.**

postpartal care, care of the mother and her newborn baby during the first few days of the puerperium. See also **antepartal care, intrapartal care, newborn intrapartal care.**

■ METHOD: The physical and physiologic changes of involution in the mother are observed for deviation from the normal. The uterus contracts after delivery, causing bleeding from the site of placental implantation to diminish. It is the size of a softball; the fundus is below the umbilicus. The lochia changes color and consistency during the first few days. Lochia rubra flows for up to 1 week, followed by straw-colored lochia serosa, and, finally, by clear, sticky lochia alba. The abdominal wall is soft, but muscle tone returns with time and exercise. On the third day the milk usually begins to fill the breasts.

■ NURSING ORDERS: Maternal-infant bonding may be augmented by increased contact between the mother and baby. The nurse is the source of most of the teaching that occurs in the postpartum phase. Breast feeding, bottle feeding, nutrition, care of the umbilical and diaper areas, baby baths, safety practices and accident prevention, and exercises for physical reconditioning are taught during the postpartum phase.

■ OUTCOME CRITERIA: During the first hours and days after delivery the nurse encourages frequent mother-infant contact. The mother's nuturing abilities are fostered and developed; many new mothers need time and contact with the baby to acquire skills of infant care and to develop feelings of love. As the mother gives to the baby, she gains satisfaction. If the baby is prevented from taking, or the mother from giving, both become frustrated. Toxemia, hemorrhage, and infection are the chief medical problems of the puerperium, but they are not common and are largely avoidable. Fatigue, breast engorgement, psychologic depression, and superficial thrombophlebitis are more common, but not usual.

postpartum /pōstpär′təm/, after childbirth.

postpartum depression, an abnormal psychiatric condition that occurs after childbirth, typically from 3 days to 6 weeks postpartum. It is characterized by symptoms that range from mild ''postpartum blues'' to an intense, suicidal, depressive psychosis. Severe postpartum depression occurs approximately once in every 2000 to 3000 pregnancies. The cause is not proven; neurochemical and psychologic influences have been implicated. Approximately one third of patients are found to have had some degree of psychiatric abnormality predating the pregnancy. The disorder recurs in subsequent pregnancies in 25% of cases. Some women at risk for postpartum depression may be identified during the prenatal period by their having made no preparations for the expected baby, by their expressing unrealistic plans for postpartum work or travel, or by their denying the reality of the responsibilities of parenthood. Depending on the severity of the disorder, psychoactive medication or psychiatric hospitalization may be necessary.

postperfusion syndrome, a cytomegalovirus (CMV) infection, occurring between 2 and 4 weeks after the transfusion of fresh blood containing CMV. It is characterized by prolonged fever, hepatitis, rash, atypical lymphocytosis, and, occasionally, jaundice. No specific treatment is yet available.

postpericardiotomy syndrome /pōst′perikär′dē·ot′əmē/, a condition that sometimes occurs days or weeks after pericardiotomy, characterized by symptoms of pericarditis, often without any fever. It appears to be an autoimmune response to damaged muscle cells of the myocardium and pericardium. See also **pericarditis.**

postpill amenorrhea, failure of normal menstrual cycles to resume within 3 months after discontinuation of oral contraception. The pathophysiology of this uncommon condition is poorly understood. Postpill amenorrhea is rarely permanent. See also **amenorrhea.**

postpolycythemic myeloid metaplasia, a common late development in polycythemia vera, characterized by anemia caused by sclerosis of the bone marrow. The production of red blood cells then occurs only in extramedullary tissue, as the liver and spleen. This condition is frequently complicated by leukemia, especially if the patient has been treated with ionizing radiation. See also **myeloid metaplasia, polycythemia.**

postprandial, after a meal.

postpubertal panhypopituitarism, insufficiency of pituitary hormones, caused by postpartum pituitary necrosis resulting from thrombosis of the circulation of the gland during or after delivery. The disorder, characterized initially by weakness, lethargy, failure to lactate, amenorrhea, loss of libido, and intolerance to cold, leads to loss of axillary and pubic hair, bradycardia, hypotension, premature wrinkling of the skin, and atrophy of the thyroid and adrenal glands. Treatment consists of the administration of ACTH, thyroid stimulating hormone, or thyroid, adrenal, and sex hormones. Also called **Simmonds' disease, hypophyseal cachexia, pituitary cachexia.**

postpuberty, a period of approximately 1 to 2 years after puberty during which skeletal growth slows and the physiologic functions of the reproductive years are established. Also called **postpubescence.** –**postpuberal, postpubertal, postpubescent,** *adj.*

postrenal anuria, cessation of urine production caused by obstruction in the ureters.

postresection filling. See **retrograde filling.**

postsynaptic, **1.** situated after a synapse. **2.** occurring after a synapse has been crossed.

postsynaptic element, any neurologic structure, as a neuron, situated distal to a synapse.

postterm infant. See **postmature infant.**

posttraumatic stress disorder, an anxiety disorder characterized by an acute emotional response to a traumatic event or situation involving severe environmental stress, as a natural disaster, airplane crash, serious automobile accident, military combat, and physical torture. Symptoms of the condition include recurrent, intrusive recollections or nightmares, diminished responsiveness to the external world, hyperalertness or an exaggerated startle response, sleep disturbances, irritability, memory impairment, difficulty in concentrating, depression, anxiety, headaches, and vertigo. Treatment usually consists of sedation in extreme cases followed by supportive psychotherapy. Also called **stress reaction, stress response syndrome.** See also **combat fatigue, shell shock.**

posttraumatic syndrome. See postconcussional syndrome.

postural albuminuria. See **orthostatic proteinuria.**

postural drainage, the use of positioning to drain secretions from specific segments of the bronchi and the lungs into the trachea. Coughing normally expels secretions from the trachea.

■ METHOD: Positions are selected that promote drainage from the affected parts of the lungs. Pillows and raised sections of the hospital bed are used to support or elevate parts of the body. The procedure is begun with the patient level, and the head is gradually lowered to a full Trendelenburg position. Inhalation through the nose and exhalation through the mouth is encouraged. Simultaneously the nurse may use cupping and vibration over the affected area of the lungs to dislodge and mobilize secretions. The person is then helped to a position conducive to coughing and is asked to breathe deeply at least three times and to cough at least twice. See also **cupping and vibrating.**

■ NURSING ORDERS: A patient who is dyspneic, or who has hemoptysis or signs of cerebral hemorrhage, increased intracerebral pressure, or lung abscess is not placed in a head down position without caution and a specific medical order. Suction is kept available in all cases in which the patient might not be able to expel the secretions that have drained into the trachea. The patient's tolerance for the procedure and the position is carefully observed; fatigue is avoided.

■ OUTCOME CRITERIA: Effectiveness of the procedure depends on positioning that allows drainage by gravity and on liquefaction, ciliary action, and effective breathing. As the secretions are cleared, the patient becomes better able to breathe, is more comfortable, and may move about more freely; thus, the respiratory passages may remain freer of obstructing secretions and regain their normal function.

postural hypotension. See **orthostatic hypotension.**

postural proteinuria. See **orthostatic proteinuria.**

postural vertigo. See **cupulolithiasis.**

posture, the position of the body with respect to the surrounding space. A posture is determined and maintained by coordination of the various muscles that move the limbs, by proprioception, and by the sense of balance.

pot-, a combining form meaning 'of or related to drinking': *potable, potocytosis, potomania.*

potassium (K), an alkali metal element, the seventh most abundant element in the earth's crust. Its atomic number is 19; its atomic weight is 39.1. Potassium occurs in a wide variety of silicate rocks; in its elemental form it is easily oxidized and extremely reactive. Potassium salts are necessary to the life of all plants and animals. Potassium in the body constitutes the predominant intracellular cation, helping to regulate neuromuscular excitability and muscle contraction. Sources of potassium in the diet are whole grains, meat, legumes, fruit, and vegetables. The average adequate daily intake for most adults is 2 to 4 g. Potassium is important in glycogen formation, protein synthesis, and in the correction of imbalances of acid-base metabolism, especially in association with the action of sodium and hydrogen ions. Most of the dietary potassium in the body is absorbed from the GI tract, and, in homeostasis, the amount of potassium excreted in the urine is essentially equal to the amount of potassium in the diet. Potassium salts are very important as therapeutic agents but are extremely dangerous if used improperly. The kidneys play an important role in controlling its secretion and absorption. Aldosterone stimulates sodium reabsorption and potassium secretion by the kidneys; the major extrarenal adaptation to this process involves the absorption of potassium by the body tissues, especially the tissues of the muscles and the liver. The intracellular concentrations of potassium and hydrogen are higher than those of the extracellular fluid of the body, and when the extracellular hydrogen ion concentration increases, as in acidosis, potassium ions move from the cells into the

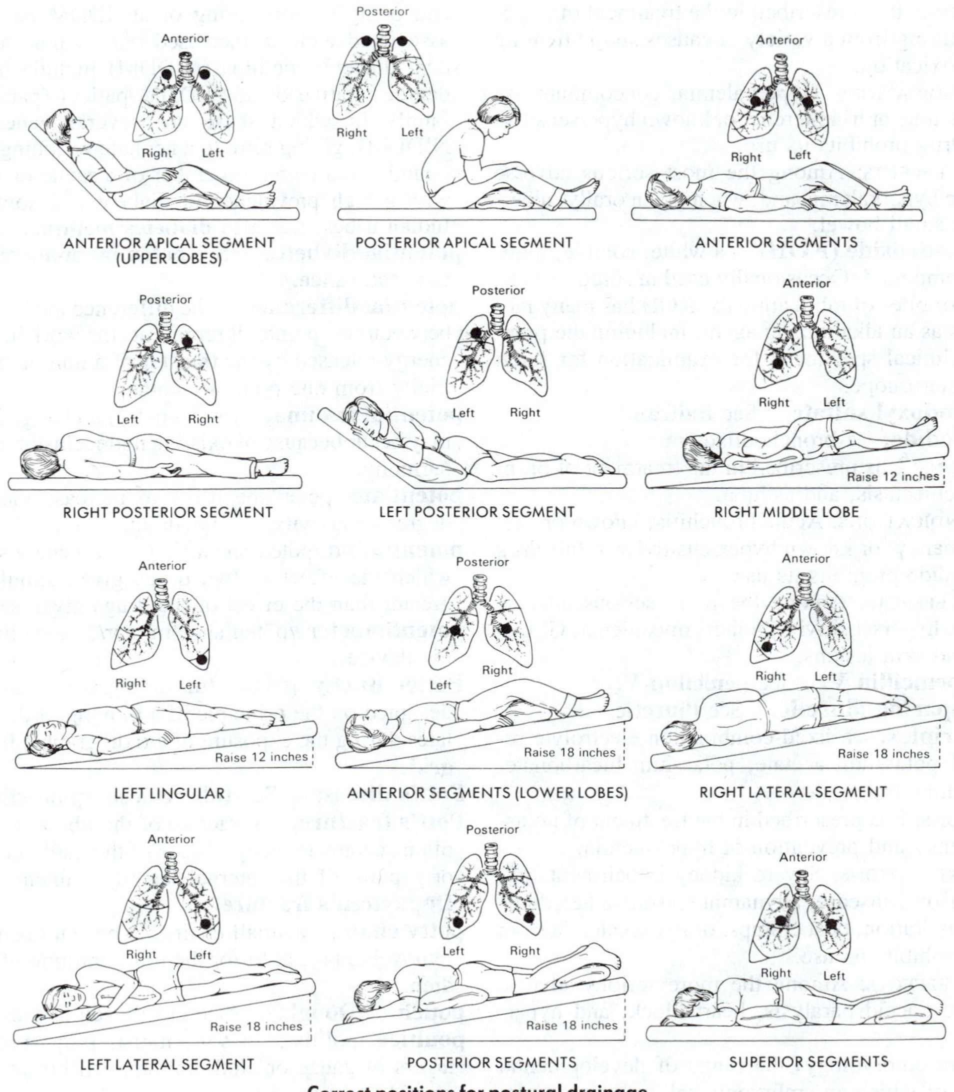

Correct positions for postural drainage

extracellular fluid. When the extracellular hydrogen ion decreases, as in alkalosis, potassium ions move from the extracellular fluid into the cells. Extracellular acidosis produces hyperkalemia. Extracellular alkalosis produces hypokalemia. Potassium is most commonly depleted in the body by an increased rate of excretion by the kidneys or the GI tract or, more rarely, by the skin. Increased renal excretion may be caused by diuretic therapy, large doses of anionic drugs, or renal disorders. Increased GI secretion of potassium may occur with the loss of GI fluid through vomiting, diarrhea, surgical drainage, or the chronic use of laxatives. Potassium loss through the skin is rare but can result from perspiring during excessive exercise in a hot environment.

potassium chloride (KCl), an electrolyte replenisher.

■ INDICATIONS: It is prescribed in the treatment of hypokalemia resulting from a variety of causes and in treating digitalis intoxication.

■ CONTRAINDICATIONS: Hyperkalemia, concomitant use of spironolactone or triamterene, or known hypersensitivity to this drug prohibits its use.

■ ADVERSE EFFECTS: Among the most serious adverse reactions are hyperkalemia and, when given orally, ulceration of the small bowel.

potassium hydroxide (KOH), a white, soluble, highly caustic compound. Occasionally used in solution as an escharotic for bites of rabid animals, KOH has many laboratory uses as an alkalinizing agent, including the preparation of clinical specimens for examination for fungi under the microscope.

potassium indoxyl sulfate. See **indican.**

potassium iodide, a bronchodilator.

■ INDICATIONS: It is prescribed in the treatment of bronchitis, bronchiectasis, and asthma.

■ CONTRAINDICATIONS: Acute bronchitis, known or suspected pregnancy, or known hypersensitivity to this drug or to any iodide prohibits its use.

■ ADVERSE EFFECTS: Among the more serious adverse reactions are hypersensitivity, goiter, myxedema, GI disturbance, and skin lesions.

potassium penicillin V. See **penicillin V.**

potassium-sparing diuretic. See **diuretic.**

potassium triplex, a fixed-combination electrolyte replenisher of potassium acetate, potassium bicarbonate, and potassium citrate.

■ INDICATIONS: It is prescribed in the treatment of potassium deficiency and prevention of hypokalemia.

■ CONTRAINDICATIONS: Severe kidney impairment, untreated Addison's disease, adynamia episodica hereditaria, acute dehydration, heat cramps, or hyperkalemia from any cause prohibits its use.

■ ADVERSE EFFECTS: Among the more serious adverse reactions are flaccid paralysis, heart block, and hyperkalemia.

potency, (in embryology) the range of developmental possibilities of which an embryonic cell or part is capable, regardless of whether the stimulus for growth or differentiation is natural, artificial, or experimental. See also **competence.**

-potent, a combining form meaning 'able to do' something specified: *pluripotent, unipotent, viripotent.*

potential, an expression of the energy involved in transfering a unit of electric charge. The gradient or slope of a potential causes the charge to move. The movement of 1 colomb of charge from a potential of V to a potential of $V-1$ volts requires 1 joule of energy.

potential abnormality of glucose tolerance, a classification that includes persons who have never had abnormal glucose tolerance but who have an increased risk of diabetes or impaired glucose tolerance. Factors associated with an increased risk of insulin-dependent diabetes mellitus (IDDM) include circulating islet cell antibodies, being a monozygotic twin or sibling of an IDDM patient, and being the off-spring of an IDDM patient. Factors associated with an increased risk of non-insulin-dependent diabetes mellitus (NIDDM) include being a first-degree relative of an NIDDM patient (particularly in a family in which there are several generations with NIDDM), giving birth to a neonate weighing more than 9 pounds, and being a member of a racial or ethnic group with a high prevalence of diabetes, as some American Indian tribes. See also **diabetes mellitus.**

potential diabetes. See **potential abnormality of glucose tolerance.**

potential difference, the difference in electric potential between two points. It represents the work involved in the energy released by the transfer of a unit quantity of electricity from one point to another.

potential trauma, (in dentistry) a change in tissue that may occur because of existing malocclusion or dental disharmony.

potentiate /pōten′shē•āt/, to increase the strength or degree of activity of something.

potentiation /pōten′shē•ā′shən/, a synergistic action in which the effect of two drugs given simultaneously is greater than the effect of the drugs given separately.

potentiometer /pōten′shē•om′ətər/, a voltage measuring device.

Potter-Bucky grid, (in radiography) an x-ray grid designed on the principle of a moving grid, which oscillates during the exposure of a radiographic film. See also **grid.**

Pott's disease. See **tuberculosis spondylitis.**

Pott's fracture, a fracture of the fibula near the ankle, often accompanied by a break of the malleolus of the tibia or rupture of the internal lateral ligament. Also called **Dupuytren's fracture.**

potty chair, a small chair that has an open seat over a removable pot, used for the toilet training of young children.

pouch of Douglas. See **cul-de-sac of Douglas.**

poultice /pōl′tis/, a soft, moist, pulp spread between layers of gauze or cloth and applied hot to a surface to provide heat or counterirritation. A kind of poultice is a **mustard poultice.**

Povan, a trademark for an anthelmintic (pyrvinium pamoate).

povidone-iodine /pō′vidōnī′ədīn/, an antiseptic microbicide.

■ INDICATIONS: It is prescribed as a topical microbicide for disinfection of wounds, as a preoperative surgical scrub, for vaginal infections, and for antiseptic treatment of burns.

■ CONTRAINDICATIONS: Known hypersensitivity to this drug or to iodine prohibits its use.

■ ADVERSE EFFECTS: Among the more serious adverse reactions are local skin irritation, redness, and swelling.

Powassan virus infection, an uncommon form of encephalitis caused by a tick-borne arbovirus found in eastern Canada and the northern United States.

powder bed, a treatment in which large areas of a patient's body are kept in contact with a powdered medication for a certain length of time. It is usually repeated three times a day, as necessary. An already made bed is prepared by placing a full-sized sheet lengthwise over the linen. The powder is spread on the sheet from a shaker. The patient lies supine on the powdered sheet. Areas of skin that are apposed are separated with gauze, and powder is shaken over the patient's body. The powdered sheet is then wrapped around the limbs and the trunk from the side to keep the powder in contact with the body. The patient is virtually helpless during treatment and requires close attention from the nurse.

powdered gold, a fine granulation of pure gold, produced by atomizing the molten metal or by chemical precipitation. It is used in some dental restorations, as prepared tooth cavities, and is available as clusters of granules or as pellets of gold powder contained in an envelope of gold foil.

powerlessness, a nursing diagnosis accepted by the Fifth National Conference on the Classification of Nursing Diagnoses. The diagnosis refers to a lack of control over a current health-related situation or problem and the client's perceived knowledge that any action by oneself will not affect the outcome of the particular situation. The cause of the condition may involve the health care environment, a regimen related to the illness, or a generalized life-style of helplessness. The defining characteristics may be of a severe, moderate, or passive nature. Severe characteristics include the client's verbal expression of having no control or influence over self-care, the particular situation, or its outcome; apathy; or depression over physical deterioration that occurs despite compliance with regimens. Moderate characteristics include the client's nonparticipation in or lack of interest in the mode of care, in decision making regarding regimens, or in monitoring progress; the client's verbal expression of dissatisfaction and frustration regarding the inability to perform previous activities; the reluctance to express true feelings, fearing alienation of others; general irritability or passivity; expressions of resentment, anger, guilt, or doubt regarding role performance. Passive characteristics involve expressions of uncertainty about fluctuating energy levels. See also **nursing diagnosis.**

power of attorney, a document authorizing one person to take legal actions in behalf of another, who acts as an agent for the grantor. The legality of a power of attorney may be challenged if the grantor can be found to have been mentally incompetent at the time the authority was granted.

power stroke, a working stroke with a dental scaling instrument, used for splitting or dislodging calculus from the surface of a tooth or tooth root.

pox, **1.** any of several vesicular or pustular exanthematous diseases. **2.** the pitlike scars of smallpox. **3.** *archaic.* syphilis.

poxvirus, a member of a family of viruses that includes the organisms that cause molluscum contagiosum, smallpox, and vaccinia.

PPD, abbreviation for **purified protein derivative,** the material used in testing for tuberculin sensitivity. Also called **PPD of Seibert, PPD-S.** See also **Mantoux test, tine test, tuberculin test, tuberculosis.**

PPLO, abbreviation for **pleuropneumonia-like organism.** See ***Mycoplasma.***

ppm, abbreviation for *parts per million.*

PPO, abbreviation for **preferred provider organization.**

PPV, abbreviation for *positive pressure ventilation.* See **positive pressure,** def. 2.

Pr, symbol for **praseodymium.**

practical anatomy. See **applied anatomy.**

practice setting, the context or environment within which nursing care is given.

practice theory, (in nursing research) a theory that describes, explains, and prescribes nursing practice in general. It serves as the basis for specific items in the curriculum of nursing education and for the development of theories in the administration of nursing and nursing education.

practicing medicine without a license, (in law) practicing activities defined under state law in the medical practice act without physician supervision, direction, or control.

practitioner, a person qualified to practice in a special professional field, as a nurse practitioner.

Prader-Willi syndrome, a metabolic condition characterized by congenital hypotonia, hyperphagia, obesity, and mental retardation. When the development of diabetes mellitus occurs with the other symptoms, the condition is called Royer's syndrome. The syndrome is associated with a less than normal secretion of gonadotropic hormones by the pituitary gland.

prae-. See **pre-.**

-pragia, a combining form meaning 'quality of action': *bradypragia, dyspragia, tachypragia.*

Pragmatar, a trademark for a topical, fixed-combination drug containing an antieczematic (cetyl alcohol-coal tar distillate), a keratolytic (salicylic acid), and a scabicide (precipitated sulfur).

pralidoxime chloride /pral′ədok′sēm/, a cholinesterase reactivator.

■ INDICATIONS: It is prescribed as an antidote for organophosphate poisoning and drug overdosage in the treatment of myasthenia gravis.

■ CONTRAINDICATION: Known hypersensitivity to this drug prohibits its use. It is contraindicated in poisoning by carbamate insecticides that react with pralixodime.

■ ADVERSE EFFECTS: Among the most serious adverse reactions are dizziness, tachycardia, hyperventilation, and muscle weakness. These reactions are most common when the drug is injected too rapidly.

Pramosone, a trademark for a topical, fixed-combination drug containing a glucocorticoid (hydrocortisone acetate) and a topical anesthetic (pramoxine hydrochloride).

pramoxine hydrochloride, a local anesthetic for the relief of pain and itching associated with dermatoses, anogenital pruritus, hemorrhoids, anal fissure, and minor burns.

prandial /pran′dē•əl/, pertaining to a meal. The term is used in relation to timing, as postprandial or preprandial. –**prandiality,** *n.*

Prantal, a trademark for an anticholinergic (diphemanil methylsulfate).

praseodymium (Pr), a rare earth metallic element. Its atomic number is 59; its atomic weight is 140.91.

Prausnitz-Küstner (PK) test /prous′nitskist′nər/, a skin test in which an allergic response is transferred to a nonallergic person who acts as a surrogate to permit identification of the allergen. After screening the allergic patient for hepatitis and other serum-borne diseases, a small amount of the patient's serum is injected intradermally into several sites on a nonallergic person (usually a relative). After 24 to 48 hours, suspected antigens are applied to these sites on the nonallergic person. A sensitive skin response (wheal and flare reaction) indicates that the suspect antigen is indeed causing hypersensitivity in the allergic patient. The Prausnitz-Küstner test is only performed when skin sensitivity testing cannot be performed directly on the allergic patient. Also called **passive transfer test, PK test.** Compare **patch test, radioallergosorbent test.** See also **anaphylaxis.**

-praxia, a combining form meaning a 'condition concerning the performance of movements': *dyspraxia, eupraxia, hypopraxia.*

-praxis, a combining form meaning a 'therapeutic treatment involving a (specified) method': *actinopraxis, echopraxis, parapraxis.*

prazepam, an antianxiety agent derived from benzodiazepine.

■ INDICATIONS: It is prescribed for the treatment of anxiety disorders or the short-term relief of symptoms of anxiety.

■ CONTRAINDICATIONS: Acute narrow-angle glaucoma or known sensitivity to this drug or other benzodiazepines prohibits its use.

■ ADVERSE EFFECTS: Among the more serious, but rare, adverse reactions are confusion, tremor, palpitations, and diaphoresis.

prazosin hydrochloride /prä′zəsin/, an antihypertensive.

■ INDICATIONS: It is prescribed in the treatment of hypertension and to decrease afterload in congestive heart disease.

■ CONTRAINDICATIONS: Known hypersensitivity to this drug prohibits its use. Concomitant use with beta blockers may result in loss of consciousness.

■ ADVERSE EFFECTS: Among the more serious adverse reactions are tachycardia, fainting, drowsiness, angina, and a sudden drop in blood pressure after the initial dose.

pre-, prae-, a combining form meaning 'before': *preataxic, precritical, pregenital.*

preagonal ascites, a rapid accumulation of fluid within the peritoneal cavity, representing the transudation of serum from the circulatory system. Preagonal ascites immediately precedes death in some cases. See also **ascites.**

preanesthetic medication. See **premedication.**

preaortic node /prē′ā•ôr′tik/, a node in one of the three sets of lumbar lymph nodes that serve various abdominal viscera supplied by the celiac, superior mesenteric, and inferior mesenteric arteries. The preaortic nodes lie ventral to the aorta and are divided into the celiac nodes, superior mesenteric nodes, and inferior mesenteric nodes. Most of the efferents from the preaortic nodes unite to form the lymphatic intestinal trunk that enters the cisterna chyli. Compare **lateral aortic node, retroaortic node.**

precancerous dermatitis. See **intraepidermal carcinoma.**

precedent, a previously adjudged decision that serves as an authority in a similar case.

preceptorship, the position of teacher or instructor, usually the headmaster or dean of a school.

precession, a comparatively slow gyration of the axis of a spinning body, so as to trace out a cone, caused by the application of a torque. The magnetic moment of a nucleus with spin will experience such a torque when inclined at an angle to the magnetic field, resulting in precession at the Larmor frequency.

precipitate /prəsip′itāt, -it/, **1.** to cause a substance to separate or to settle out of solution. **2.** a substance that has separated from or settled out of a solution. **3.** occurring hastily or unexpectedly.

precipitate delivery, childbirth that occurs with such speed or in such a situation that the usual preparations cannot be made. See also **emergency childbirth.**

precipitin /prəsip′itin/, an antibody that causes formation of an insoluble complex when combined with a specific soluble antigen. Compare **agglutinin.** See also **agglutination, antiglobulin.**

Precision, a trademark for a nutritional supplement free of lactose, cholesterol, and gluten.

precision rest, a rigid denture support consisting of two tightly fitting parts, the insert of which rests firmly against the gingival portion of the device.

precocious, pertaining to the early, often premature, development of physical or mental qualities.

precocious dentition, the abnormal acceleration of the eruption of the deciduous or permanent teeth, usually associated with an endocrine imbalance, as excess pituitary growth hormone or hyperthyroidism. Compare **retarded dentition.**

preconscious, **1.** before the development of self-consciousness and self-awareness. **2.** (in psychiatry) the mental function in which thoughts, ideas, emotions, or memories not in immediate awareness can be brought into the consciousness, usually through associations, without encountering any intrapsychic resistance or repression. **3.** the mental phenomena capable of being recalled, although not present in the conscious mind.

precordial /prēkôr′dē•əl/, of or pertaining to the precordium, which forms the region over the heart and the lower part of the thorax.

precordial movement, any motion of the anterior wall of the thorax localized in the area over the heart. Kinds of precordial movements include **apical impulse, left ventricular thrust,** and **right ventricular thrust.**

precordial thump, a cardiopulmonary resuscitation (CPR) technique used to restore circulation in cardiac arrest. The person performing precordial thumping raises a clenched fist 20 to 30 cm (8 to 12 inches) above the precordium of the patient; the fist is then brought down quickly in a single blow. Generally, if there is no response to a precordial thump, CPR chest compression and mouth-to-mouth methods are applied.

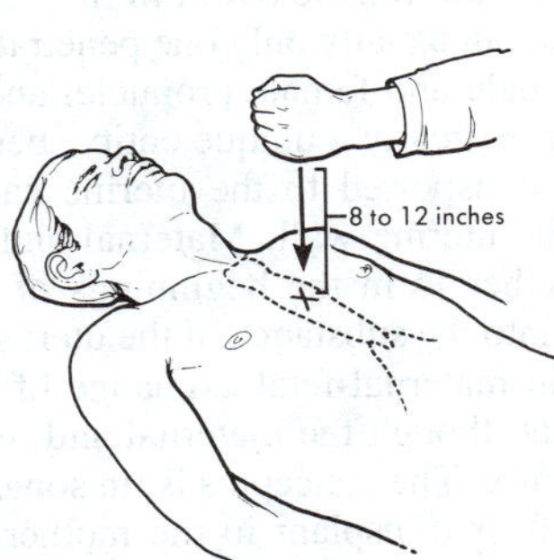

Precordial thump

precursor, a prognostic characteristic or feature of a patient's health data, as an x-ray or laboratory finding, that is associated with a higher or lower risk of death than the average.

predeciduous dentition, the epithelial structures found in the mouth of the infant preceding the eruption of the deciduous teeth. See also **deciduous dentition, teething.**

prediabetes. See **potential abnormality of glucose tolerance, previous abnormality of glucose tolerance.**

predictive hypothesis, (in research) a hypothesis that predicts the nature of a relationship among the variables to be studied.

predictive validity, validity of a test or a measurement tool that is established by demonstrating its ability to predict the results of an analysis of the same data using another test instrument or measurement tool. See also **validity.**

predictor variable. See **independent variable.**

prednisolone /prednis′əlōn/, a glucocortocoid.

■ INDICATIONS: It is prescribed as treatment for inflammation of the skin, conjuntiva, and cornea, and for immunosuppression.

■ CONTRAINDICATIONS: Fungal infections or known hypersensitivity to this drug prohibits its systemic use. Viral or fungal infections of the skin, impaired circulation, or known hypersensitivity to this drug prohibits its topical use.

■ ADVERSE EFFECTS: Among the more serious adverse reactions to the systemic administration of this drug are GI, endocrine, neurologic, fluid, and electrolyte disturbances. A variety of skin reactions may occur from topical administration of this drug.

prednisone /pred′nisōn/, a glucocorticoid.

■ INDICATIONS: It is prescribed in severe inflammation and immunosuppression.

■ CONTRAINDICATIONS: Viral or fungal infections of the skin, impaired circulation, or known hypersensitivity to this drug prohibits its use.

■ ADVERSE EFFECTS: Among the more serious adverse reactions to the systemic administration of the drug are GI, endocrine, neurologic, and fluid and electrolyte disturbances. A variety of skin reactions may occur from topical administration of this drug.

Predulose, a trademark for an ophthalmic, fixed-combination drug containing a glucocorticoid (prednisolone acetate).

preeclampsia /prē′iklamp′sē•ə/, an abnormal condition of pregnancy characterized by the onset of acute hypertension after the twenty-fourth week of gestation. The classic triad of preeclampsia is hypertension, proteinuria, and edema. The cause of the disease remains unknown despite 100 years of research by thousands of investigators. It occurs in 5% to 7% of pregnancies, most often in primigravidas, and is more common in some areas of the world than others; the incidence is particularly high in the southeastern portion of the United States. The incidence increases with increasing gestational age, and it is more common with multiple gestation, hydatidiform mole, or hydramnios. A typical lesion in the kidneys, glomeruloendotheliosis, is pathognomonic. Termination of the pregnancy results in resolution of the signs and symptoms of the disease and in healing of the renal lesion. Preeclampsia is classified as mild or severe. Mild preeclampsia is diagnosed if one or more of the following signs develop after the twenty-fourth week of gestation: systolic blood pressure of 140 mm Hg or more or a rise of 30 mm or more above the woman's usual systolic blood pressure; diastolic blood pressure of 90 mm Hg or more or a rise of 15 mm or more above the woman's usual diastolic blood pressure; proteinuria; edema. Severe preeclampsia is diagnosed if one or more of the following is present: systolic blood pressure of 160 mm Hg or more or a diastolic blood pressure of 110 mm Hg or more on two occasions 6 hours apart with the woman at bed rest; proteinuria of 5 g or more in 24 hours; oliguria of less than 400 ml in 24 hours; ocular or cerebral vascular disorders; cyanosis or pulmonary edema. Preeclampsia commonly causes abnormal metabolic function, including negative nitrogen balance, increased central nervous system irritability, hyperactive reflexes, compromised renal function, hemoconcentration, and alterations of fluid and electrolyte balance. Complications include premature separation of the placenta, hypofibrinogenemia, hemolysis, cerebral hemorrhage, ophthalmologic damage, pulmonary edema, hepatocellular changes, fetal malnutrition, and lowered birth weight. The most serious complication is eclampsia, which can result in maternal and fetal death. Healthy living conditions, including a diet high in protein, calories, and essential nutritional elements, and rest and exercise are associated with a decreased incidence of preeclampsia. Treatment includes rest, sedation, magnesium sulfate, and antihypertensives. Ultimately, if eclampsia threatens, delivery by induction of labor or cesarean section may be necessary. See also **eclampsia.** Also called **toxemia of pregnancy.**

preexcitation, activation of part of the ventricular myocardium earlier than would be expected if the activating impulses traveled only down the normal routes or had experienced a normal delay within the AV node. This may be a result of either a Kent bundle (Wolff-Parkinson-White syndrome), which is reflected on the electrocardiogram by a short PR and broad QRS, or an excessively fast intranodal pathway (Lown-Ganong-Levine syndrome), which manifests with a short PR and a normal QRS. The degree of preexcitation is determined by how fast the impulse traverses the atrial tissue and the accessory pathway or the AV node. See also **accessory pathway.**

preferential anosmia, the inability to smell certain odors. The condition is often caused by psychologic factors concerning either a particular smell or the situation in which the smell occurs.

preferred provider organization (PPO), an organization of physicians, hospitals, and pharmacists whose members discount their health care services to subscriber patients. A PPO may be organized by a group of physicians, an outside entrepreneur, an insurance company, or a company with a self-insurance plan. See also **health maintenance organization.**

prefix, a portion of a word, usually derived from Latin or Greek, occurring at the beginning of a compound word. In this dictionary, prefixes are called "combining forms." In the words *antiseptic, epidermis, hypoglycemia, periosteum, and semipermeable, anti-, epi-, hypo-, peri-,* and *semi-* are prefixes. Compare **suffix.**

preformation, an early theory in embryology in which the organism is contained in minute and complete form within the germ cell and after fertilization grows from microscopic to normal size. Compare **epigenesis.**

preformed water, the water that is contained in foods.

prefrontal lobotomy, a surgical procedure in which connecting fibers between the prefrontal lobes of the brain and the thalamus are severed. The technique is rarely used today but formerly was an accepted procedure for treating schizophrenic patients with uncontrollable, destructive behavior. After surgery, patients were often apathetic, docile, and lacking social graces. If only the white fibers are severed, the procedure is called a prefrontal leucotomy.

Pregestimil, a trademark for a hypoallergenic, nutritional supplement for infants.

pregnancy, the gestational process, comprising the growth and development within a woman of a new individual from conception through the embryonic and fetal periods to birth. Pregnancy lasts approximately 266 days (38 weeks) from the day of fertilization, but it is clinically considered to last 280 days (40 weeks; 10 lunar months; 9⅓ calendar months) from the first day of the last menstrual period. The estimated date of confinement (EDC) is calculated on the latter basis even if a woman's periods are irregular. If a woman is certain that coitus occurred only once during the month of conception and if she knows the date on which coitus occurred, the EDC may be calculated as 266 days from that date. Pregnancy begins after coitus at or near the time of ovulation (usually about 14 days before a woman's next expected menstrual period). Of the millions of ejaculated sperm cells, thousands reach the female ovum in the outer end of the fallopian tube, but usually only one penetrates the egg for union of the male and female pronuclei and conception. The zygote, genetically a unique entity, begins cell division as it is transported to the uterine cavity where it implants in the uterine wall. Maternal and embryologic elements together form the beginnings of the placenta, which grows into the substance of the uterus. The placenta functions in maternal-fetal exchange of nutrients and waste products, though the maternal and fetal bloods do not normally mix. The conceptus is, in some aspects, like a foreign graft or transplant in the mother. Though the mother normally does not activate an immune response, all of her tissues and organs undergo change, many of them profound and some of them permanent.

■ PSYCHOLOGIC CHANGES: The emotional experiences of pregnancy, as reported by pregnant women, are normal and healthy, but extraordinary. A pregnant woman is "herself," but in a very unfamiliar way. She has a sense of heightened function and expectancy. Being keenly aware of the rapid and inevitable changes her body is undergoing, she is more intensely interested in herself. Her concern for the perfection of her baby, her anticipation of the exertion of labor, and her contemplation of the new or expanded responsibilities of motherhood all serve to intensify her emotional tone.

■ CARDIOVASCULAR CHANGES: Cardiac output increases 30% to 50% in pregnancy. The increase begins at about the sixth week, reaches a maximum about the sixteenth week, declines slightly after the thirtieth week, and rapidly falls off after delivery. It returns to prepregnancy level about the sixth week postpartum. The stroke volume of the heart increases, and the pulse rate becomes more rapid: normal pulse rate in pregnancy is approximately 80 to 90 beats per minute. Blood pressure may drop slightly after the twelfth week of gestation and return to its usual level after the twenty-sixth week. The circulation of blood to the pregnant uterus near term is about one liter per minute, requiring about 20% of the total cardiac output. Total blood volume also increases in pregnancy; plasma volume increases more than red cell volume, and this results in a drop in the hematocrit, caused by dilution. The white blood cells increase: the normal WBC count in pregnancy is often over 9000/ml.

■ PULMONARY CHANGES: Though vital capacity and Po_2 remain the same in pregnancy, respiratory rate, tidal and minute volumes, and plasma pH increase. Inspiratory and expiratory reserves, residual volume and residual capacity, and plasma Pco_2 diminish.

■ RENAL CHANGES: The glomerular filtration rate (GFR) and the renal plasma flow increase approximately 30% to 50% in pregnancy; the pattern of change closely parallels that of cardiac function. A marked dilatation of the execretory tract often occurs and is called hydronephrosis of pregnancy. It is the result of the pressure exerted on the ureters by the enlarging uterus and by the influence of the hormone, progesterone. Blood urea nitrogen (BUN) normally increases as much as 10 mg/dl, and blood creatinine drops to approximately 0.7 mg/dl. Positional influences on renal function are more marked in pregnancy because of the pressure of the uterus on the great vessels. Renal function is better in the recumbent position than in the standing position and is better in the left lateral recumbent position than in the supine position.

■ GASTROINTESTINAL CHANGES: Progesterone, which is increased in pregnancy, causes some relaxation of GI smooth muscle. Heartburn may result from delayed gastric emptying and relaxation of the sphincter at the gastroesophageal junction. Decreased colonic motility and pressure on the rectum and sigmoid colon from the enlarging uterus may result in constipation. Nausea and vomiting may occur, usually early in pregnancy, probably caused by the effect of human chorionic gonadotropin. The incidence of gallbladder disease is slightly increased.

■ ENDOCRINE CHANGES: Protein binding is increased in pregnancy. Because most hormones are circulated in protein-bound forms, the function of most endocrine glands is altered. Thyroid function changes markedly in a way that mimics hyperthyroidism as indicated by a thyroid test. Adrenal hormone levels are increased and are probably responsible for stria gravidarum, which are similar to the stria of hyperadrenalism. Sugar metabolism is altered by estrogen, progesterone, and glucocorticoids; the need for insulin is increased. The placenta produces four hormones: human chorionic gonadotropin (HCG), progesterone, estrogen, and human placental lactogen (HPL). HCG prolongs the life of the corpus luteum early in pregnancy. Progesterone functions to support the modified endometrium of the uterus, called the decidua, and to stimulate the development of the breast acini. Estrogen stimulates uterine and breast growth. HPL stimulates the growth and development of breast tissue in preparation for lactation; it also has an antiinsulin effect for the sparing of maternal glucose for the benefit of the fetus.

■ BREAST CHANGES: The breasts become firm and tender early in pregnancy. This tenderness constitutes a subjective symptom of pregnancy. As the breasts enlarge and soften, the tenderness disappears. The areola around the nipple becomes more deeply pigmented, and the areolar glands become prominent. As the tubules and acini of the mammary glands develop, a clear or whitish watery material, called colostrum, begins to issue from the nipple.

■ SKIN CHANGES: Perspiration increases. Erythema of the thenar and hypothenar eminences of the palms becomes apparent. Hair growth may be stimulated. Telangiectasias are extremely common. Stria over the abdomen, breasts, and buttocks appear in some women. New deposits of the pigment melanin cause freckles to intensify; the linea nigra in the midline of the lower abdomen becomes darker and may extend nearly to the xiphoid process. There may be a darkening of the skin of the face over the nose across the malar eminences and above the eyebrows. This is called chloasma, or the ''mask of pregnancy.''

■ WEIGHT CHANGES: Normal weight gain may vary within wide limits in pregnancy. Average weight gain is 20 to 25 pounds, but greater increases are common without ill effects.

■ NUTRITIONAL CHANGES: Requirements for dietary iron, protein, and calcium increase out of proportion to the need for an overall increase in intake of calories and other nutrients.

pregnancy gingivitis, an enlargement or hyperplasia of the gingivae caused by hormonal imbalance during pregnancy.

pregnancy luteoma. See **luteoma.**

pregnancy rate, (in statistics) the ratio of pregnancies per 100 woman-years, calculated as the product of the number of pregnancies in the women observed multiplied by 1200 (months) divided by the product of the number of women observed multiplied by the number of months observed. For example, if 50 women used one contraceptive method for 12 months and 5 of them became pregnant, the pregnancy rate would be 10 per 100 woman-years.

pregnancy test. See **HCG radioreceptor assay.**

pregnanediol /pregnān′dē•ol/, a crystalline, biologically inactive compound found in the urine of women during pregnancy or the secretory phase of the menstrual cycle. A dihydroxy derivative of the saturated steroid pregnane, pregnanediol is formed by the reduction of progesterone.

preinvasive carcinoma. See **carcinoma in situ.**

preload, the initial stretch of myocardial fiber at end diastole. The ventricular end diastolic pressure and volume reflect this parameter.

Preludin, a trademark for an anorexiant (phenmetrazine hydrochloride).

premalignant fibroepithelioma, an elevated Caucasian-flesh-colored sessile neoplasm formed of interlacing ribbons of epithelial cells on a hyperplastic mesodermal stroma. The tumor occurs most often on the lower trunk of older people and may be found in association with a superficial basal cell carcinoma or may develop into a basal cell carcinoma.

Premarin, a trademark for conjugated estrogens.

Premarin with Methyltestosterone, a trademark for a hormonal, fixed-combination drug containing Premarin and an androgen (methyltestosterone).

premarket approval (P.M.A.), permission given by the federal government to equipment manufacturers to sell their devices to the medical profession.

premature, **1.** not fully developed or mature. **2.** occurring before the appropriate or usual time. **–prematurity,** *n.*

premature atrial contraction, a cardiac arrhythmia characterized by an atrial beat occurring before the expected excitation, indicated electrocardiographically as an early P wave. Premature atrial beats may occur occasionally, in a regular pattern, or several may occur in sequence. The arrhythmia may be the result of atrial enlargement or ischemia, or may be caused by stress, caffeine, or nicotine. Isolated premature atrial beats usually have no significance, but their frequent occurrence may lead to atrial tachycardia or fibrillation, and to decreased cardiac output. Also called **premature atrial beat.**

premature contraction, any contraction of either the ventricle or atrium that occurs early with respect to the dominant rhythm.

premature ejaculation, uncontrollable, untimely ejaculation of semen often caused by anxiety during sexual intercourse. Behavioral techniques can be learned by the man and his partner to extend the length of time between erection and ejaculation. See also **ejaculation, erection.**

premature impulse, any impulse that occurs early with respect to a dominant rhythm.

premature infant, any neonate, regardless of birth weight, born before 37 weeks of gestation. Because exact gestational age is often difficult to determine, low birth weight is a significant criterion for identifying the high-risk infant with incomplete organ system development. Predisposing factors associated with prematurity include multiple pregnancy, toxemia, chronic disease, acute infection, sensitization to blood incompatibility, and any severe trauma that may interfere with normal fetal development. In most instances the cause is unknown. The incidence of prematurity is highest among women from low socioeconomic circumstances for whom poor nutrition and lack of prenatal medical care are often precipitating factors. The premature infant usually appears small and scrawny, with a large head in relation to body size, and weighs less than 2500 g. The skin is bright pink, smooth, shiny, and translucent with the underlying vessels clearly visible. The arms and legs are extended, not flexed, as in the full-term infant. There is little subcutaneous fat, sparse hair, few creases on the soles and palms, and poorly developed ear cartilage. In boys, the scrotum has few rugae and the testes may be undescended; in girls, the labia gape and the clitoris is prominent. Among the common problems of the premature infant are variations of body temperature, chilling, apnea, respiratory distress, sepsis, poor sucking and swallowing reflexes, small stomach capacity, lowered tolerance of the alimentary tract that may lead to necrotizing enterocolitis, immature renal function, hepatic dysfunction often associated with hyperbilirubinemia, incomplete enzyme systems, and susceptibility to various metabolic upsets, as hypoglycemia, hyperglycemia, and hypocalcemia. The degree of complications and the rate of survival of premature infants are directly related to the state of physiologic and anatomic maturity of the various organ systems at the time of birth, the condition of the infant other than prematurity, and the quality of postnatal care. With treatment in a neonatal intensive care unit, survival rates improve yearly. Increasing numbers of very small babies develop normally, and those who do not have seizures or apneic spells in the first few days will not suffer neurologic or physical sequelae of their prematurity. Of primary concern for the nurse caring for the premature infant is the stabilization of body temperature by maintaining a neutral thermal environment, the maintenance of respiration, the prevention of infection, the provision of adequate nutrition and hydration, and the conservation of energy. Important functions of the nurse are to involve the parents in the care of the infant, to explain therapeutic procedures, and to facilitate attachment between the infant and family. Also called **preterm infant.** Compare **postmature infant.**

premature labor, labor that occurs earlier in pregnancy than normal, either before the fetus has reached a weight of 2000 to 2500 g or before the thirty-seventh or thirty-eighth week of gestation. No single measure of fetal weight or gestational age is used universally to designate premature birth; local or institutional policy dictates which of several standards is applied. Prematurity is a concomitant of 75% of births that result in neonatal mortality. It may occur spontaneously, or it may be brought about iatrogenically. The incidence of premature labor increases in inverse proportion to maternal age, weight, and socioeconomic status. Incidence is higher for

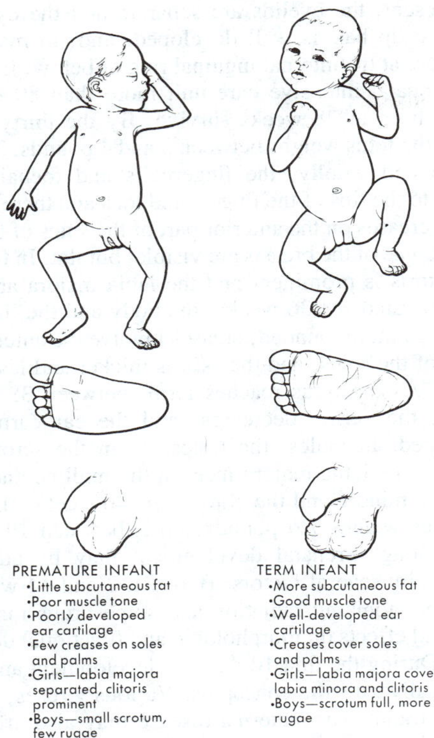
PREMATURE INFANT
•Little subcutaneous fat
•Poor muscle tone
•Poorly developed ear cartilage
•Few creases on soles and palms
•Girls—labia majora separated, clitoris prominent
•Boys—small scrotum, few rugae
TERM INFANT
•More subcutaneous fat
•Good muscle tone
•Well-developed ear cartilage
•Creases cover soles and palms
•Girls—labia majora cover labia minora and clitoris
•Boys—scrotum full, more rugae
Comparison of premature and term infants

black women, for women who have not had adequate prenatal care or whose obstetric history is abnormal, and for women who smoke or whose diets are deficient in protein or calories. Predisposing conditions include maternal infection, low weight gain, uterine bleeding, multiple gestation, polyhydramnios, uterine abnormalities, incompetent cervix, premature rupture of membranes, and intrauterine fetal growth retardation. The cause of premature labor is poorly understood; in some cases, there may be several contributing causes. In some pregnancies, premature labor may be homeostatic, resulting in the best possible outcome under the particular, abnormal conditions. If premature labor itself constitutes a threat to the fetus, the outcome of pregnancy may be improved if labor can be inhibited. Determining accurately which pregnancies are likely to benefit from the inhibition of labor and which are not is difficult. Medications used to stop labor are not always effective. Misdiagnosis of gestational age and fetal condition may lead to induction of labor that is inadvertently premature; premature babies whose births have been brought about inappropriately early account for 15% of admissions to newborn intensive care nurseries. Also called **preterm labor.** See also **small for gestational age infant.**

premature rupture of membranes, the spontaneous rupture of the amniotic sac before the onset of labor.

premature thelarche. See **thelarche.**

premature ventricular contraction (PVC), a cardiac arrhythmia characterized by a ventricular beat preceding the expected electric impulse, shown on the electrocardiogram as an early, wide QRS complex without a preceding related P wave. Premature ventricular contractions may occur occasionally, in a regular pattern, or as several in sequence. They may be caused by stress, acidosis, electrolyte imbalance, hypoxemia, hypercapnia, ventricular enlargement, or a toxic reaction to drugs, especially to digitalis or quinidine. Isolated PVCs are not clinically significant in healthy individuals, but they may produce tachycardia in persons with myocardial infarction or heart disease, and frequent occurrence of the arrhythmia indicates myocardial irritability and may be a precursor of ventricular tachycardia or fibrillation and lead to inadequate cardiac output. Agents used in treating PVCs include procainamide, lidocaine, oxygen, sodium bicarbonate, and potassium. Also called **premature ventricular beat.**

premedication, **1.** any sedative, tranquilizer, hypnotic, or anticholinergic medication administered before anesthesia. Pentobarbital, secobarbital, phenobarbital, morphine, scopolamine, and atropine are commonly used. The choice of drug depends on such variables as the patient's age and physical condition and the specific operative procedure. **2.** the administration of such medications. **–premedicate,** *v.*

premenopausal, of or pertaining to the time of life preceding the menopause.

premenstrual tension (PMT), a syndrome of nervous tension, irritability, weight gain, edema, headache, mastalgia, dysphoria, and lack of coordination occurring during the last few days of the menstrual cycle before the onset of menstruation. There are several theories that attempt to explain the cause of the syndrome, including nutritional deficiency, stress, hormonal imbalance, and various emotional disorders.

premise, a proposition that is laid down as the base of an argument, and which is usually established beforehand.

premolar /prēmō′lər/, one of eight teeth, four in each dental arch, located lateral to and posterior to the canine teeth. The premolars appear during childhood and remain until old age. They are smaller and shorter than the canine teeth. The crown of each premolar is compressed anteroposteriorly and surmounted by two cusps. The neck of the premolar is oval; the root is usually single and compressed, with an anterior and a posterior groove. The upper premolars are larger than the lower premolars. Also called **bicuspid.** Compare **canine tooth, incisor, molar.**

premonitory, an early symptom or sign of a disease. The term is commonly used to describe minor symptoms that precede a major health problem.

prenatal, prior to birth; occurring or existing before birth, referring both to the care of the woman during pregnancy and the growth and development of the fetus. Also called **antenatal.** See also **antepartal care.**

prenatal development, the entire process of growth, maturation, differentiation, and development that occurs between conception and birth. On approximately the fourteenth day before the next expected menstrual period, ovulation usually occurs. If the egg is fertilized, it immediately begins the course to fetal maturity and birth. During the first 14 days the fertilized ovum undergoes cell division several times, becoming a morula, and then a blastocyst that is able to implant in the uterine wall. From the beginning of the third to the end of the seventh week of embryonic development, implantation deepens and completes. Primitive uteroplacental circulation originates between the enlarging trophoblast and the maternal endometrial tissue of the uterus. The amniotic cavity appears as an opening between the inner cell mass and the invading trophoblast. A thin lining in the cavity becomes the amnion. At this point the embryo is a two-layered embryonic disk composed of an ectoderm and an endoderm. As the disk thickens in the middle, giving rise to the third cell layer, or mesoderm, the basic structural systems of the body begin to form. The neural tube develops as a precursor of the central nervous system in the midline of the cranial portion of the ectoderm. Primitive blood vessels and blood cells, a heart tube, and umbilical vessels are formed and begin to function. Arm and leg buds may be seen, and rudimentary gut, lungs, and kidneys form. By the fifth week, the brain has begun to grow rapidly, the heart tube is divided into chambers, the palate and the upper lip are forming, and the urogenital system is developing. By the end of the seventh week, all essential systems are present. The period of time from the eighth week to birth is called the fetal stage. From the eighth to the tenth week the fetus continues to grow and develop rapidly. The head is almost one half of its total length, and arms, legs, and face are clearly recognizable. The fetus floats in the amniotic fluid of the amniotic sac within the uterus; the umbilical vessels in the cord extend to a rapidly growing placenta. By the twelfth week the features of the face are formed and the eyelids are present but not yet closed, because they have not divided into upper and lower eyelids. The palate is fusing, there is a neck between the large head and the body, and tooth buds and nail beds have begun to form. Identification of the external genitalia is possible for the first time. From the thirteenth to the sixteenth weeks, the arms, legs, and trunk grow rapidly, and the fetus is active. Scalp hair develops. The skeleton of the fetus is calcified and may be seen on an x-ray film. Respiratory movements may sometimes be detected by a sonogram. Between the seventeenth and the twentieth weeks of pregnancy, the mother usually first feels the baby move. The fetus looks like a very small baby at this time. There are eyebrows and tiny nipples; during fetoscopic examination, the fetus has been seen and photographed sucking its thumb and grasping its own umbilical cord. At the twenty-fourth week the external ears are smooth and soft and the skin is wrinkled and translucent. The body is covered with lanugo and vernix and weighs a little more than 1 pound. At 28 weeks subcutaneous fat begins to develop, fingernails and toenails are present, the eyelids are separate and the eyes may open, scalp hair is well developed, and, in males, the testes are at the internal inguinal ring or below. In a modern neonatal intensive care unit more than 80% of the babies born at 28 weeks survive. By the thirty-second week, the fetus weighs between 3 and 4 pounds. The hair is fine and woolly, the fingernails and toenails have grown to the tips of the fingers and toes and there are one or two creases on the anterior part of the soles of the feet. The areolae of the breasts are visible, but flat. In females, the clitoris is prominent and the labia majora are small and separated. At 36 weeks, the body and the limbs are fuller and more rounded, creases involve the anterior two thirds of the soles, and the skin is thicker and less translucent. As the fetus reaches term, between 38 and 42 weeks, the vernix decreases, and the ear cartilage is developed. In males, the testes are in the scrotum; in females, the labia majora meet in the midline and cover the labia minora and the clitoris. At 40 weeks, the average fetus weighs 7¼ pounds and is between 19 and 22 inches long. Prenatal development may be adversely affected by several factors. Between 2 and 14 weeks of gestation, ionizing radiation and some drugs may have profound effects on morphologic and functional development. During the first 10 days of development any damage usually kills the conceptus. Various viruses, malnutrition, trauma, or maternal disease may also affect the morphologic development of a rapidly differentiating structure or organ during the embryologic or early fetal stage. After 14 weeks when all the organs, systems, and parts of the body have formed, any adverse effects are largely functional; major morphologic damage does not occur.

prenatal diagnosis, any of various diagnostic techniques to determine if a developing fetus in the uterus is affected with a genetic disorder or other abnormality. Such procedures as x-ray examination and ultrasound scanning can be used to follow fetal growth and detect structural abnormalities; amniocentesis enables fetal cells to be obtained from the amniotic fluid for culture and biochemical assay to detect metabolic disorders and for chromosomal analysis; fetoscopy enables fetal blood to be withdrawn from a blood vessel of the placenta and examined for disorders, as thalassemia, sickle cell anemia, and Duchenne's muscular dystrophy. If any of the tests are positive and the child is likely to be born with a severe defect or disease, the parents need support and advice from genetic counselors on whether to terminate the pregnancy. If the parents decide to have the baby, the nurse can help to educate them about the specific disorder and to prepare them for the special care required of a handicapped or genetically defective child. Also called **antenatal diagnosis.** See also **genetic counseling, genetic screening.**

preoperational thought phase, a piagetian phase of child development, during the period of 2 to 7 years of age, when the child focuses on the use of language as a tool to meet his or her needs.

preoperative, of or pertaining to the period of time preceding a surgical procedure. Commonly, the preoperative period begins with the first preparation of the patient for surgery, as when, 12 hours before scheduled procedure, fluids or food by mouth is forbidden. It ends with the induction of surgical anesthesia in the operating suite.

preoperative care, the preparation and management of a patient before surgery.

■ METHOD: The patient's nutritional and hygienic state, medical and surgical history, allergies, current medication, physical handicaps, signs of infection, and elimina-

TIMETABLE OF HUMAN PRENATAL DEVELOPMENT
1 to 6 weeks

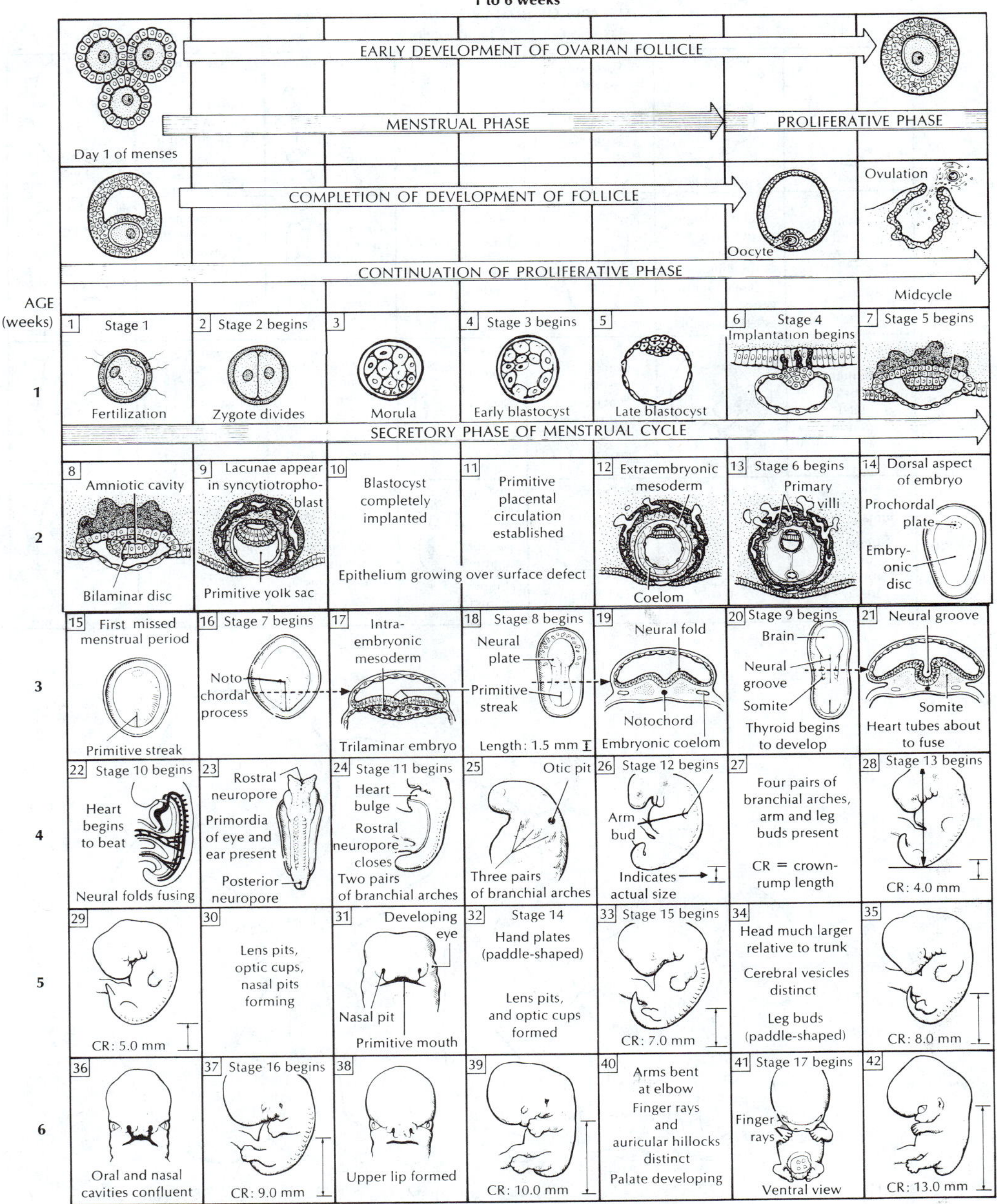

From Moore, K.L.: The developing human, ed. 3, Philadelphia, 1983, W.B. Saunders Co.

tion habits are noted and recorded. The patient's understanding of the operative, preoperative, and postoperative procedures, the patient's ability to verbalize anxieties, and the family's knowledge of the planned surgery are ascertained. The signed informed consent statement, the physician's preoperative orders, and the patient's identification bands, willingness to receive blood if necessary, and understanding of the use of the call bell and the purpose of the bed's side rails are checked. Blood pressure, temperature, pulse, and respiration are recorded, and any abnormalities are reported to the physician. The physician is also informed if the electrocardiogram, chest x-ray study, or laboratory studies show any abnormalities. On completion of the patient's blood typing, the number of matched blood units required to be held for a possible blood transfusion is determined. When ordered, an enema is given, a bowel preparation is completed, a nasogastric tube or indwelling catheter is inserted, and parenteral

TIMETABLE OF HUMAN PRENATAL DEVELOPMENT
7 to 38 weeks

AGE (weeks)							
7	43 CR: 16.0 mm	44 Stage 18 begins; Eyelids beginning	45 Tip of nose distinct; Toe rays appear; Ossification may begin; CR: 17.0 mm	46 Loss of villi; Smooth chorion forms	47 Genital tubercle; Urogenital membrane; Anal membrane; ♀ or ♂	48 Stage 19 begins; Trunk elongating and straightening	49 CR: 18 mm
8	50 Upper limbs longer and bent at elbows; Fingers distinct	51 Anal membrane perforated; Urogenital membrane degenerating; Testes and ovaries distinguishable	52 Stage 21 begins	53 Stage 21; External genitals still in sexless state but have begun to differentiate	54 Stage 22 begins; Genital tubercle; Urethral groove; Anus; ♀ or ♂	55 Beginnings of all essential external and internal structures are present	56 Stage 23; CR: 30 mm
9	57 Beginning of fetal period	58	59 Genitals show some ♀ characteristics but still easily confused with ♂	60 Phallus; Urogenital fold; Labioscrotal fold; Perineum; ♀	61 Genitals show fusion of urethral folds; Urethral groove extends into phallus	62 Phallus; Urogenital fold; Labioscrotal fold; Perineum; ♂	63 CR: 50 mm
10	64 Face has human profile; Note growth of chin compared to day 44	65	66 Face has human appearance	67 Clitoris; Labium minus; Urogenital groove; Labium majus; ♀	68 Genitals have ♀ or ♂ characteristics but still not fully formed	69 Glans penis; Urethral groove; Scrotum; ♂	70 CR: 61 mm

11 12 16 20 24 28 32 36 38 Full term

From Moore, K.L.: The developing human, ed. 3, Philadelphia, 1983, W.B. Saunders Co.

fluids are administered. Before bedtime, the patient showers, using an antibacterial soap; nothing is given orally after midnight unless ordered. After preoperative medication is administered, the side rails of the bed are raised. Before leaving for the operating room with the completed chart, the patient voids, and any dentures, contact lenses, and valuables are removed for safekeeping.

■ NURSING ORDERS: The nurse performs and explains the preoperative procedures, reinforces the physician's explanation of the operation, provides instruction and emotional support, answers the patient's questions as honestly as possible, avoiding standard clichés in responding to any anxiety, and reassures the patient that medication will be available to relieve postoperative pain. Depending on the surgical procedure, the nurse shows the patient how to turn, cough, deep breathe, and support the incision during coughing. The nurse informs the patient and the patient's family about the postoperative period in the recovery room or the intensive care unit, if indicated.

■ OUTCOME CRITERIA: The patient who is carefully prepared for an operation, psychologically and physically, experiences less anxiety and is more likely to make an uneventful recovery.

prepared cavity, a tooth cavity that has been prepared to receive and retain a restoration.

prepared childbirth. See **natural childbirth.**

prepatellar bursa, a bursa between the tendon of the quadriceps and the lower part of the femur continuous with the cavity of the knee joint.

prepayment, the payment in advance for health care services, by subscribers to a third-party insurance program, as Blue Cross.

preprandial, before a meal.

prepubertal panhypopituitarism, insufficiency of pituitary hormones, caused by damage to the gland usually associated with a suprasellar cyst or craniopharyngioma, occurring in childhood. The disorder is characterized by dwarfism with normal body proportions, subnormal sexual development, impaired thyroid and adrenal function, and yellow, wrinkled skin. Diabetes insipidus is frequently present, and there may be bitemporal hemaniopia or complete blindness, but the patient's mentality is usually normal. X-ray pictures show delayed fusion of the epiphyses, suprasellar calcification, and the sella turcica is often destroyed. The condition is treated with cortisone, thyroid and gonadotrophic hormones, and, if available, human growth hormone.

prepuberty, the period immediately preceding puberty, lasting approximately 2 years and characterized by preliminary physical changes, as accelerated growth and appearance of secondary sex characteristics, that lead to sexual maturity. –**prepuberal, prepubertal,** *adj.*

prepubescence /prē′pyo͞obes′əns/, the state of being prepubertal. –**prepubescent,** *adj.*

prepuce /prē′pyo͞os/, a fold of skin that forms a retractable cover, as the foreskin of the penis or the fold around the clitoris. –**prepucial, preputial,** *adj.*

prerenal anuria, cessation of urine production caused by the blood pressure in the kidney being too low to maintain glomerular filtration pressure.

Presamine, a trademark for an antidepressant (imipramine hydrochloride).

Pre-Sate, a trademark for an anorexiant (chlorphentermine hydrochloride).

presbycardia /prez′bikär′dē·ə/, an abnormal cardiac condition, especially affecting elderly individuals and associated with heart failure in the presence of other complications, as heart disease, fever, anemia, mild hyperthyroidism, and excess fluid administration. Presbycardia may be associated with decreased elasticity of the musculature of the heart and with mild fibrotic changes of the heart valves, but the basis for these changes and the associated pigmentation of the heart is not known. Some authorities believe that presbycardia only rarely produces heart failure but that the condition does decrease the adaptive capacity of the heart and predisposes elderly patients to heart failure in the presence of other illnesses.

presbycusis, the normal loss of hearing acuity, speech intelligibility, auditory threshold, and pitch associated with aging.

presbyopia /prez′bi·ō′pē·ə/, farsightedness resulting from a loss of elasticity of the lens of the eye. The condition commonly develops with advancing age. Compare **visual accommodation.** –**presbyopic,** *adj.*

preschizophrenic state, a period before psychosis is evident when the patient deviates from normal behavior but does not demonstrate psychotic symptoms of delusions, hallucinations, or stupor.

prescreen, **1.** to evaluate a patient or a group of patients to identify those who are at greater risk of developing a particular condition to select those who are in particular need of special diagnostic procedures or health care. **2.** *informal.* a rapid, superficial examination of a person who does not appear to be acutely ill. It may include taking a medical history.

prescribe, **1.** to write an order for a drug, treatment, or procedure. **2.** to recommend or encourage a course of action.

prescription, an order for medication, therapy, or a therapeutic device given by a properly authorized person to a person properly authorized to dispense or perform the order. A prescription is usually in written form and includes the name and address of the patient, the date, the + symbol (superscription), the medication prescribed (inscription), directions to the pharmacist or other dispenser (subscription), directions to the patient that must appear on the label, the prescriber's signature, and, in some instances, an identifying number.

prescription drug, a drug that can be dispensed to the public only with a prescription. The designation of a drug as a prescription drug is made by the Food and Drug Administration. See also **ethical drug.**

prescriptive intervention mode, a therapeutic situation in which the health professional tells the patient explicitly how to solve a problem, so that less collaboration between the consultant and patient is needed.

prescriptive theory, a theory that is comprised of a description of a specific activity, a statement of the goal of the activity, and an analysis of the elements of the activity that, together, constitute a prescription for reaching the goal.

presenile dementia. See **Alzheimer's disease.**

presentation. See **fetal presentation.**

present health, (in a health history) a chronologic, succinct account of any recent changes in the health of the patient and of the circumstances or symptoms that prompted the person to seek health care.

presenting part, the part of the fetus that lies closest to the internal os of the cervix.

presenting symptom. See **symptom.**

preservation, the involuntary, persistent repetition of the same verbal response or motor activity regardless of the stimulus or its duration. The condition occurs primarily in patients with brain damage or organic mental disorders, although it may also appear in schizophrenia as an association disturbance.

presomite embryo /prēsō′mīt/, an embryo in any stage of development before the appearance of the first pair of somites, which, in humans, usually occurs around 19 to 21 days after fertilization of the ovum.

pressor /pres′ər/, describing a substance that tends to cause a rise in blood pressure.

pressure, a force, or stress, applied to a surface by a fluid or an object, usually measured in units of mass per unit of area, as pounds per square inch.

pressure acupuncture, a system of acupuncture involving the application of pressure, as by the tip of a finger, to certain specified points of the body. See also **acupuncture.**

pressure area, an oral area that is subject to excessive displacement of soft tisue by a prosthesis.

pressure bandage, a bandage applied to stop bleeding, prevent edema, or provide support for varicose veins.

pressure dressing, a dressing firmly applied to exert pressure, usually on a wound for hemostasis.

pressure edema, **1.** edema of the lower extremities caused by pressure of a pregnant uterus against the large veins of the area. **2.** edema of the fetal scalp after cephalic presentation.

pressure point, **1.** a point over an artery where the pulse may be felt. Pressure on the point may be helpful in stopping the flow of blood from a wound distal to the point. **2.** a site that is extremely sensitive to pressure, as the phrenic pressure point along the phrenic nerve between the sternocleidomastoid and the scalenus anticus on the right side; pressure at this site may be symptomatic of gallbladder dysfunction.

pressure sore. See **decubitus ulcer.**

pressure ventilator, a ventilator in which gas delivery is limited by a predetermined pressure.

presumptive signs, manifestations that indicate a pregnancy although they are not necessarily positive. Presumptive signs may include cessation of menses and morning sickness. See also **Chadwick's sign.**

preswing stance stage, one of the five stages in the stance phase of walking or gait, involving a brief transitional period of double limb support during which one leg of the body is rapidly relieved of body-bearing weight and prepared for the swing forward. The type of preswing used by an individual is a factor in the diagnoses of many abnormal orthopedic conditions. Compare **initial contact stance stage, loading response stance stage, midstance, terminal stance.** See also **swing phase of gait.**

presymptomatic disease, an early stage of disease when physiologic changes have begun although no signs or symptoms are observed.

presynaptic, **1.** situated near or before a synapse. **2.** occurring before a synapse is crossed.

presynaptic element, any neurologic structure, as a neuron, situated proximal to a synapse.

presystolic, of or pertaining to the period preceding systole.

preterm infant. See **premature infant.**

preterm labor. See **premature labor.**

pretibial /prētib′ē•əl/, of or pertaining to the area of the leg in front of the tibia.

pretibial fever, an acute infection caused by *Leptospira autumnalis,* characterized by headache, chills, fever, enlarged spleen, myalgia, low white blood cell count, and a rash on the anterior surface of the legs. Also called **Fort Bragg fever.**

pretrial discovery. See **discovery.**

prevalence /prev′ələns/, (in epidemiology) the number of all new and old cases of a disease or occurrences of an event during a particular period of time. Prevalence is expressed as a ratio in which the number of events is the numerator and the population at risk is the denominator. See also **rate.**

prevention, (in nursing care) any action directed toward preventing illness and promoting health to avoid the need for primary, secondary, or tertiary health care. Prevention includes such nursing actions as assessment and promotion of health potential; application of prescribed measures, as immunization; health teaching; early diagnosis and treatment; and recognition of disability limitations and rehabilitation potential. In acute care nursing, many interventions are simultaneously therapeutic and preventive.

preventive, tending to slow, stop, or interrupt the course of an illness or to decrease the incidence of a disease.

preventive care, a pattern of nursing and medical care that focuses on the prevention of disease and health maintenance and includes early diagnosis of disease, discovery and identification of people at risk of developing specific problems, counseling, and other intervention to avert a health problem. Screening tests, health education, and immunization programs are common examples of preventive care.

preventive health care. See **preventive care.**

preventive treatment, a procedure, measure, substance, or program designed to prevent a disease from occurring or a mild disorder from becoming more severe. Various diseases are prevented by immunizations with vaccines, antiseptic measures, the avoidance of smoking, regular exercise, a prudent diet, adequate rest, the correction of congenital anomalies, and screening programs for the detection of preclinical signs of disorders. Also called **prophylactic treatment.**

previa. See **placenta previa.**

previllous embryo /prēvil′əs/, an embryo of a placental mammal at any stage before the development of the chorionic villi, which, in humans, begin to form between the first and second months after fertilization of the ovum.

previous abnormality of glucose tolerance, a classification that includes persons who previously had diabetic hyperglycemia or impaired glucose tolerance but whose fasting plasma glucose levels have returned to normal. Included in this category are persons who had gestational diabetes but whose plasma levels returned to normal after parturition and obese persons whose plasma levels returned to normal after losing weight. Previously called latent diabetes, prediabetes. See also **diabetes mellitus.**

previtamin. See **provitamin.**

priapism /prī′əpiz′əm/, an abnormal condition of prolonged or constant penile erection, often painful and seldom associated with sexual arousal. It may result from urinary calculi or a lesion within the penis or the central nervous system. It sometimes occurs in men who have acute leukemia.

priapitis /prī′əpī′tis/, inflammation of the penis.

priapus. See **penis.**

prickle cell layer. See **stratum spinosum.**

prickly heat. See **miliaria.**

prilocaine hydrochloride /pril′ōkān/, a local anesthetic agent of the amide family, used for nerve block, epidural, and regional anesthesia. It is not used for spinal or topical anesthesia. Prilocaine hydrochloride is about one half as toxic as lidocaine, but because methemoglobinemia is a possible reaction, prilocaine hydrochloride is not used for patients with hypoxic conditions of any kind.

prim-, a combining form meaning 'first': *primerite, primigravida, primitiae.*

primaquine phosphate /prī′məkwin/, an antimalarial.

■ INDICATIONS: It is prescribed in the treatment of malaria and prevention of relapse during recovery from the disease.

■ CONTRAINDICATIONS: Lupus erythematosus, rheumatoid arthritis, concomitant use of bone marrow depressants or hemolytic drugs, or known hypersensitivity to this drug prohibits its use.

■ ADVERSE EFFECTS: Among the more serious adverse reactions are hemolytic anemia, agranulocytosis, and abdominal distress.

primary, **1.** first in order of time, place, development, or importance. **2.** not derived from any other source or cause, specifically the original condition or set of symptoms in disease processes, as a primary infection or a primary tumor. **3.** (in chemistry) noting the first and most simple compound in a related series, formed by the substitution of one of two or more atoms or of a group in a molecule, as in amine or carboxyl radicals. Compare **secondary, tertiary.**

primary afferent fiber, a sensory nerve fiber that transmits impulses from the intrafusal fibers of the muscle spindle to the central nervous system during muscle contraction. See also **gamma efferent fiber.**

primary amenorrhea. See **amenorrhea.**

primary amputation, amputation performed after severe trauma, after the patient has recovered from shock, and before infection has set in. Compare **secondary amputation.**

primary amyloidosis. See **amyloidosis.**

primary apnea, a self-limited condition characterized by an absence of respiration. It may follow a blow to the head and is common immediately after birth in the newborn who breathes spontaneously when the carbon dioxide in the circulation reaches a certain level. Reflexes are present, and the heart is beating, but the skin color may be pale or blue and muscle tone is diminished. No treatment is necessary, but careful observation, maintenance of body temperature, and oral pharyngeal aspiration are usually performed. Within seconds the baby usually begins breathing, becomes pinker, moves the arms and legs, and cries. Compare **periodic apnea of the newborn, secondary apnea.**

primary atelectasis, failure of the lungs to expand fully at birth, most commonly seen in premature infants or those narcotized by maternal anesthesia. The infant is usually cared for in an incubator in which the temperature and humidity may be closely monitored. Nursing care includes frequent changes of position of the infant to assist respiration, suctioning to remove bronchial secretions, and very slow feedings to avoid abdominal distention.

primary atypical pneumonia. See **mycoplasma pneumonia.**

primary biliary cirrhosis, a chronic inflammatory condition of the liver. It is characterized by generalized pruritus, enlargement and hardening of the liver, weight loss, and diarrhea with pale, bulky stools. Petechiae, epistaxis, or hemorrhage resulting from hypoprothrombinemia may also be evident. Pathologic fractures and collapsed vertebrae may develop as the result of the associated malabsorption of vitamin D and calcium. Xanthomas commonly develop when the serum cholesterol level exceeds 450 mg/dl. The cause of primary biliary cirrhosis is unknown, although it is associated with autoimmune disorders. The condition most often affects women 40 to 60 years of age. The diagnosis is confirmed by liver biopsy and cholangiography. Jaundice, dark urine, pale stools, and cutaneous xanthosis may occur in the later stages of this disease. Treatment commonly includes the administration of fat-soluble vitamins A, D, E, and K to prevent and correct deficiencies caused by malabsorption. Drugs, including methyltestosterone or norethandrolene, may relieve associated pruritus. Some studies indicate that *D*-penicillamine may help correct this disorder over the long term. When treatment is begun in the early, asymptomatic stages of the condition the prognosis is excellent. The life expectancy is about 5 years for symptomatic patients after the onset of jaundice. Compare **secondary biliary cirrhosis.**

primary bronchus, one of the two main air passages that branch from the trachea and convey air to the lungs as part of the respiratory system. The right primary bronchus is about 2.5 cm long, wider and shorter than the left primary bronchus, and enters the right lung nearly opposite the fifth thoracic vertebra. The left primary bronchus is about 5 cm long, passes under the aortic arch, and courses ventral to the esophagus, the thoracic duct, and the descending aorta before dividing into bronchi for the superior and the anterior lobes of the lung. The bronchi, like the trachea, are composed of rings of hyaline cartilage, fibrous tissue, mucous membrane, and glands. The carina at the bottom of the trachea separates the two primary bronchi and is situated to the left of the midline so that the right primary bronchus is a more direct extension of the trachea than the left. Hence, foreign objects entering the trachea usually drop into the right bronchus rather than the left.

primary carcinoma, a neoplasm at its site of origin.

primary care, the first contact in a given episode of illness that leads to a decision regarding a course of action to resolve the health problem. Primary care usually is provided by a physician, but some primary care functions are also handled by nurses. See also **primary health care.**

primary constriction. See **centromere.**

primary cutaneous melanoma, a primary melanoma on the skin.

primary degenerative dementia. See **senile psychosis.**

primary dental caries, dental caries developing in the enamel of a tooth that was previously unaffected.

primary dentition. See **deciduous dentition.**

primary dysmenorrhea. See **dysmenorrhea.**

primary fissure, a fissure that marks the division of the anterior and posterior lobes of the cerebellum.

primary gain, a benefit, primarily relief from emotional conflict and freedom from anxiety, attained through the use of a defense mechanism or other psychologic process. Compare **secondary gain.**

primary health care, a basic level of health care that includes programs directed at the promotion of health, early diagnosis of disease or disability, and prevention of disease. Primary health care is provided in an ambulatory facility to limited numbers of people, often those living in a particular geographic area. In any episode of illness, it is the first patient contact with the health care system. It may be continuing health care, as provided by a family nurse practitioner, or it may be care at the point of entry into the health care system, as offered by an emergency room that provides care and referral.

primary host. See **definitive host.**

primary hypertension. See **essential hypertension.**

primary nurse, a nurse who is responsible for the planning, implementation, and evaluation of the nursing care of one or more clients 24 hours a day for the duration of the hospital stay. See also **primary nursing.**

primary nursing, a system for the distribution of nursing care in which care of one patient is managed for the entire 24-hour day by one nurse who directs and coordinates nurses and other personnel, schedules all tests, procedures, and daily activities for that patient, and cares for that patient personally when on duty. In an acute care situation, the primary care nurse might be responsible for only one patient; in an intermediate care situation, the primary care nurse might be responsible for three or more patients. Primary nursing is a new concept. Nurse midwives and other nurse practitioners practice primary nursing, and many hospital nursing services are replacing team nursing with primary nursing. Some advantages are continuity of care for the patient, accountability of the nurse for that care, patient-centered care that is comprehensive, individualized, and coordinated, and the professional satisfaction of the nurse. Compare **team nursing.**

primary organizer, the part of the dorsal lip of the blastopore that is self-differentiating and induces the formation of the neural plate that gives rise to the main axis of the embryo.

primary physician, 1. the physician who usually takes care of a patient; the physician who first sees a patient for the care of a given health problem. **2.** a family practice physician or general practitioner. See also **family medicine.**

primary prevention, a program of activities directed toward improvement of the general well-being while also involving specific protection for selected diseases, as immunization against measles.

primary proximal renal tubular acidosis. See **proximal renal tubular acidosis.**

primary relationships, relationships with intimates, close friends, and family.

primary sensation, a feeling or impression that results directly from a particular stimulus. See also **sensation,** def. 1.

primary sequestrum, a piece of dead bone that completely separates from sound bone during the process of necrosis. Compare **secondary sequestrum.**

primary shock, a state of physical collapse comparable to fainting. It may be the result of slight pain, as that produced by venipuncture, or may be caused by fright. Primary shock is usually mild, self-limited, and of short duration. Severe injury may prolong and merge primary shock with secondary shock. Compare **hemorrhagic shock.**

primary tooth. See **deciduous tooth.**

primary tuberculosis, the childhood form of tuberculosis, most commonly occurring in the lungs, the posterior pharynx, or, rarely, the skin. Infants lack resistance to the disease, being easily infected and especially vulnerable to rapid and extensive spread of the infection through their bodies. In childhood, the disease is usually brief and benign, characterized by regional lymphadenopathy, calcification of the tubercles, and residual immunity. The tuberculin test will be positive for life. See also **tuberculosis.**

prime mover, a muscle that acts directly to produce a desired movement amid other muscles acting simultaneously to produce indirectly the same movement. Most movements of the body require the combined action of numerous muscles. Compare **antagonist, fixation muscle, synergist.**

primidone /prī′mədōn/, an anticonvulsant.

■ INDICATIONS: It is prescribed in the treatment of seizure disorders, including grand mal, psychomotor, and focal epilepsy-like seizures.

■ CONTRAINDICATIONS: Porphyria or known hypersensitivity to this drug or to phenobarbital prohibits its use.

■ ADVERSE EFFECTS: The most serious adverse reaction, seen on rare occasions, is megaloblastic anemia. Drowsiness, ataxia, and dizziness are common. Other adverse effects of phenobarbital may be seen.

primigravida /prim′igrav′idə/, a woman pregnant for the first time. Also called **gravida 1.** Compare **multigravida, primipara.** –**primigravid,** *adj.*

primipara /primip′ərə/, *pl.* **primiparae,** a woman who has given birth to one viable infant, indicated by "para 1" on the patient's chart. Compare **multipara, nullipara, primagravida.**

primitive, **1.** undeveloped; undifferentiated; rudimentary; showing little or no evolution. **2.** embryonic; formed early in the course of development; existing in an early or simple form. Compare **definitive.**

primitive fold. See **primitive ridge.**

primitive groove, a furrow in the posterior region of the embryonic disk that indicates the cephalocaudal axis resulting from the active involution of cells forming the primitive streak.

primitive gut. See **archenteron.**

primitive line. See **primitive streak.**

primitive node, a knoblike accumulation of cells at the cephalic end of the primitive streak in the early stages of embryonic development in humans and the higher animals. It consists of mesoderm cells that give rise to the notochord, and it corresponds to the dorsal lip of the blastopore in lower animals. Also called **Hensen's knot, Hensen's node.**

primitive pit, a minute indentation at the anterior end of the primitive groove in the early developing embryo. It lies posterior to the primitive node and probably functions as an opening into the notochordal canal in humans and the higher animals and into the neurenteric canal in the lower animals.

primitive reflex, any reflex normal in an infant or fetus. Its presence in an adult usually indicates serious neurologic disease. Some kinds of primitive reflexes are **grasp reflex, Moro reflex,** and **sucking reflex.**

primitive ridge, a ridge that bounds the primitive groove in the early stages of embryonic development. Also called **primitive fold.** See also **primitive streak.**

primitive streak, a dense area on the central posterior region of the embryonic disk, formed by the morphogenetic movement of a rapidly proliferating mass of cells that spreads between the ectoderm and endoderm, giving rise to the mesoderm layer. This seamlike elongation indicates the cephalocaudal axis along which the embryo develops, and it corresponds to the blastopore of lower animal groups. Also called **primitive line.**

primordial /prīmôr′dē·əl/, **1.** characteristic of the most undeveloped or primitive state, specifically those cells or tissues that are formed in the early stages of embryonic development. **2.** first or original; primitive.

primordial cyst, a follicular cyst, consisting of an epithelium-lined sac that contains fluid and appears radiographically as a light area in the affected jaw. It develops from a dental enamel organ before the formation of hard tissue.

primordial dwarf, a person of extremely short stature who is otherwise perfectly formed, with the usual proportions of body parts and normal mental and sexual development. The condition may be genetically related, involving some defect in the ability to use growth hormone, or it may occur sporadically within a particular population. Also called **hypoplastic dwarf, normal dwarf, physiologic dwarf, pure dwarf, true dwarf.** See also **pituitary dwarf, pygmy.**

primordial germ cell, any of the large spheric diploid cells that are formed in the early stages of embryonic development and are precursors of the oogonia and spermatogonia. They are formed outside of the gonads and migrate to the embryonic ovaries and testes for maturation. See also **oogenesis, spermatogenesis.**

primordial image, (in analytic psychology) the archetype or original parent, representing the source of all life. It occurs in the memory as a stage preceding the differentiation of the actual mother and father. See also **collective unconscious.**

primordium /prīmôr′dē·əm/, *pl.* **primordia,** the first recognizable stage in the embryonic development and differentiation of a particular organ, tissue, or structure. Also called **anlage** /un′lägə/, **rudiment.**

principal cell. See **chief cell.**

Principen, a trademark for an antibacterial (ampicillin).

principle, **1.** a general truth or settled rule of action. **2.** a prime source or element from which anything proceeds. **3.** a law on which others are founded or from which others are derived.

PR interval, that part of the electric cardiac cycle shown on the electrocardiogram as beginning with the P wave and ending with the onset of the ventricular complex (which may not be an R wave). The PR interval is a measure of AV conduction time and is normally 0.12 to 0.20 seconds.

printout, a printed copy of information produced by a computer's printer.

Prinzmetal's angina, a form of angina pectoris in which the attacks occur during rest and are associated with an elevation of the ST segment on the electrocardiogram.

Prinzmetal's variant angina, an atypical form of angina that occurs at rest rather than with effort, and is associated with gross ST elevation in the electrocardiogram that disappears when the pain subsides. It is associated with proximal high-grade coronary artery obstructive lesions or coronary spasm, or both.

priority, actions established in order of importance or urgency to the welfare or purposes of the organization, patient, or other person at a given time.

Priscoline Hydrochloride, a trademark for a peripheral vasodilator (tolazoline hydrochloride).

-privia, a combining form meaning a '(specified) condition of loss or deprivation': *calciprivia, hormonoprivia, paraprivia.*

privileges, authority granted to a physician or dentist by a hospital governing board to provide care to the hospital's patients. Clinical privileges are limited to the individual's professional license, experience, and competence. Emergency privileges may be granted by a hospital governing board or chief executive officer in an emergency situation and without regard to the physician or dentist's regular service assignment or status. Temporary privileges may be granted a physician or dentist to provide health care to patients for a limited period or to a specific patient.

Privine Hydrochloride, a trademark for an adrenergic (naphazoline hydrochloride).

PRL, abbreviation for **prolactin.**

p.r.n., (in prescriptions) abbreviation for *pro re nata,* a Latin phrase meaning "as needed." The times of administration are determined by the needs of the patient.

Pro, abbreviation for **proline.**

pro-, a combining form meaning 'first, or in front of': *procallus, procheilon, progravid.*

proaccelerin. See **factor V.**

probable signs, clinical signs that there is a definite likelihood of pregnancy. Examples include enlargement of the abdomen, Goodell's sign, Hegar's sign, Braxton Hick's sign, and positive hormonal test results. Compare **presumptive signs.**

proband. See **propositus.**

Pro-Banthine, a trademark for an anticholinergic (propantheline bromide).

probenecid /prōben′əsid/, a uricosuric and adjunct to antibiotics.

■ INDICATIONS: It is prescribed in the treatment of gout and as an adjunct prolonging the activity of penicillin or cephalosporins in some infections, as gonorrhea..

■ CONTRAINDICATIONS: Uric acid kidney stones, blood dyscrasias, or known hypersensitivity to this drug prohibits its use. It is not initiated during acute attack of gout but is continued if an attack intervenes during treatment. It is not given to children under 2 years of age. Concomitant administration of salicylates decreases the effect of probenecid.

■ ADVERSE EFFECTS: Among the most serious adverse reactions are hemolytic anemia, GI disturbances, headache, urinary frequency, and minor allergic reactions. It is involved in many drug interactions, particularly salicylate drugs.

problem, any health care condition that requires diagnostic, therapeutic, or educational action. An active problem requires immediate action whereas an inactive problem is one of the past. A subjective problem is one reported by the patient whereas one noted by an observer is regarded as an objective problem.

problem-oriented medical record (POMR), a method of recording data about the health status of a patient in a problem-solving system. The POMR preserves the data in an easily accessible way that encourages ongoing assessment and revision of the health care plan by all members of the health care team. The particular format of the system used varies from setting to setting, but the components of the method are similar. A data base is collected before beginning the process of identifying the patient's problems. The data base consists of all information available that contributes to this end, as information collected in an interview with the patient and family or others, information from a health assessment or physical examination of the patient, and information from various laboratory tests. It is recommended that the data base be as complete as possible, limited only by potential hazard or pain or discomfort to the patient or by excessive expense of the diagnostic procedure. The interview, augmented by prior records, provides the patient's history, including the reason for contact, an identifying statement that is a descriptive profile of the person, a family illness history, a history of the current illness, a history of past illness, an account of the patient's current health practices, and a review of systems. The physical examination or health assessment comprises the second major part of the data base. The extent and depth of the examination varies from setting to setting and depends on the services offered and the condition of the patient. The next section of the POMR is the master problem list. The formulation of the problems on the list is similar to the assessment phase of the nursing process. Each problem as identified represents a conclusion or a decision resulting from examination, investigation, and analysis of the data base. A problem is defined as anything that causes concern to the patient or to the care giver, including physical abnormalities, psychologic disturbance, and socioeconomic problems. The master problem list usually includes active, inactive, temporary, and potential problems. The list serves as an index to the rest of the record and is arranged in five columns: a chronologic list of problems;

the date of onset; the action taken; the outcome of the problem (often its resolution); and its date. Problems may be added, and intervention or plans for intervention may be changed; thus, the status of each problem is available for the information of all members of the various professions involved in caring for the patient. The third major section of the POMR is the initial plan, in which each separate problem is named and described, usually written on the progress note in a SOAP format: S stands for the subjective data from the patient's point of view; O stands for the objective data acquired by inspection, percussion, auscultation, and palpation and from laboratory tests; A is an assessment of the problem that is an analysis of the subjective and objective data; and P is the plan, including further diagnostic work, therapy, and education or counseling. After an initial plan for each problem is formulated and recorded, the problems are followed in the progress notes by narrative notes in the SOAP format or by flow sheets showing the significant data in a tabular manner. A discharge summary is formulated and written, relating the overall assessment of progress during treatment and the plans for follow-up or referral. The summary allows a review of all the problems initially identified and encourages continuity of care for the patient.

problem-solving approach to patient-centered care, (in nursing) a conceptual framework that incorporates the overt physical needs of a patient with covert psychologic, emotional, and social needs. It provides a model for caring for the whole person as an individual, not as an example of a disease or a medical diagnosis. Nursing is defined within this model as a problem-solving process. The patient is viewed as a person who is in an impaired state, less than usually able to perform self-care activities. Nursing problems are conditions experienced by the patient or the patient's family in which the nurse may provide professional service. The nurse makes a nursing diagnosis that identifies the impaired state and determines the care needed to augment the patients' ability to perform self-care. The requirements for care are classified in four levels. Care given to sustain life is sustenal care; care given to assist the patient in self-care is remedial care; care that helps the patient to develop new skills and goals in self-care is restorative care; care given to guide the patient to a level of self-help beyond the normal level is preventive care. Twenty-one nursing problems are identified and sorted into four groups: problems relating to comfort, hygiene, and safety; physiologic balance; psychologic and social factors; and sociologic and community factors. See also **nursing care plan.**

probucol, an anticholesteremic.

■ INDICATIONS: It is prescribed in the treatment of primary hypercholesterolemia in patients who have not responded to diet, weight control, or other therapies.

■ CONTRAINDICATION: Known sensitivity to this drug prohibits its use.

■ ADVERSE EFFECTS: Among the most serious adverse reactions are a prolongation of the QT interval on an electrocardiogram, diarrhea, palpitations, syncope, dizziness, paresthesia, and eosinophilia.

procainamide hydrochloride /prōkān′əmīd/, an antiarrhythmic agent.

■ INDICATIONS: It is prescribed in the treatment of a variety of cardiac arrhythmias, including premature ventricular contractions, ventricular tachycardia, and atrial fibrillation.

■ CONTRAINDICATIONS: Myasthenia gravis, heart block, or known hypersensitivity to this drug, to procaine, or to related local anesthetics prohibits its use.

■ ADVERSE EFFECTS: Among the more serious adverse reactions are GI disturbances, hypersensitivity reactions, agranulocytosis, and a syndrome resembling lupus erythematosus.

procaine hydrochloride, a local anesthetic of the ester family.

■ INDICATIONS: Procaine is administered for local anesthesia by infiltration and injection and for caudal, epidural, and other regional anesthetic procedures. It is not used for topical anesthesia.

■ CONTRAINDICATIONS: Known hypersensitivity to anesthetics of the ester group prohibits its use. It is not injected into inflamed or infected tissue, and large doses are not given to patients with heart block.

■ ADVERSE EFFECTS: Among the most serious adverse reactions are potentially serious neurologic and cardiovascular reactions that result from inadvertent intravascular administration. Allergic reactions may also occur.

procarbazine hydrochloride, an antineoplastic.

■ INDICATIONS: It is prescribed in the treatment of a variety of neoplasms, including Hodgkin's disease and lymphomas.

■ CONTRAINDICATIONS: Bone marrow depression or known hypersensitivity to this drug prohibits its use.

■ ADVERSE EFFECTS: Among the most serious adverse reactions are bone marrow depression and GI disturbances, particularly nausea and vomiting.

Procardia, a trademark for a calcium channel blocker (nifedipine).

procaryon. See **prokaryon.**

procaryosis. See **prokaryosis.**

Procaryotae /prōker′ē·ō′tē/, (in bacteriology) a kingdom of plants that includes all microorganisms in which the nucleoplasm has no basic protein and is not surrounded by a nuclear membrane. The kingdom has two divisions, Cyanobacteria, which includes the blue-green bacteria, and Bacteria.

procaryote. See **prokaryote.**

procerus /prəsir′əs/, one of three muscles of the nose. Arising from the fascia of the nasal bone and the lateral nasal cartilage and inserting into the skin over the lower part of the forehead between the eyebrows, it is a small pyramidal muscle, innervated by buccal branches of the facial nerve. The procerus functions to draw down the eyebrows and wrinkle the nose. Compare **depressor septi, nasalis.**

process, **1.** a series of related events that follow in sequence from a particular state or condition to a conclusion or resolution. **2.** a natural growth that projects from a bone or other part. **3.** to put through a particular series of interdependent steps, as in preparing a chemical compound.

processor. See **central processing unit.**

process recording, (in nursing education) a system used for teaching nursing students to understand and analyze verbal and nonverbal interaction. The conversation between nurse and patient is written on special forms or in a special format. The student nurse is instructed to record observations, perceptions, thoughts, and feelings, as well as the words exchanged. The process recording is then studied by the nursing instructor to discover and to help the student nurse identify patterns of difficulty in communicating with the patient.

process schizophrenia, a form of schizophrenia caused by organic changes in the brain rather than by environmental influences. The onset of the disease is usually gradual, but it progresses rapidly or slowly to irreversible psychosis. Compare **reactive schizophrenia.** See also **schizophrenia.**

processus vaginalis peritonei, a diverticulum of the peritoneal membrane that during embryonic development extends through the inguinal canal. In males it descends into the scrotum to form the processus vaginalis testis; in females it is usually completely obliterated. Also called **Nuck's canal, Nuck's diverticulum.**

prochlorperazine, a phenothiazine antipsychotic and antiemetic.

■ INDICATIONS: It is prescribed in the treatment of psychotic disorders and for the control of nausea and vomiting.

■ CONTRAINDICATIONS: Parkinson's disease, the concurrent administration of central nervous system depressants, liver or renal dysfunction, severe hypotension, or known hypersensitivity to any phenothiazine prohibits its use.

■ ADVERSE EFFECTS: Among the more serious adverse effects are hypotension, liver toxicity, extrapyramidal reactions, blood dyscrasias, and hypersensitivity reactions.

prochlorperazine maleate. See **prochlorperazine.**

prochromosome. See **karyosome.**

procidentia, the prolapse of an organ. The term is usually applied to a prolapsed uterus.

proconvertin. See **factor VII.**

procreation, the entire reproductive process of producing offspring. **–procreate,** *v.*

proct-. See **procto-.**

-proctia, a combining form meaning '(condition of the) anus': *ankyloproctia, cacoproctia, coloproctia.*

proctitis /proktī′tis/, inflammation of the rectum and anus caused by infection, trauma, drugs, allergy, or radiation injury. Acute or chronic, it is accompanied by rectal discomfort and the repeated urge to pass feces with the inability to do so. Pus, blood, or mucus may be present in the stools, and tenesmus may be present. Also called **rectitis.**

procto-, proct-, a combining form meaning 'of or pertaining to the rectum': *proctocele, proctorrhea, proctoscopy.*

proctocele. See **rectocele.**

Proctocort, a trademark for a glucocorticoid (hydrocortisone).

proctodeum, *pl.* **proctodea,** an invagination of the ectoderm, behind the urorectal septum of the developing embryo, that forms the anus and anal canal when the cloacal membrane ruptures. Also spelled **proctodaeum** (*pl.* **proctodaea**). Compare **stomodeum. –proctodeal, proctodaeal,** *adj.*

proctologist /proktol′əjist/, a physician who specializes in proctology.

proctology /proktol′əjē/, the branch of medicine concerned with treating disorders of the colon, rectum, and anus.

proctoscope, an instrument used to examine the rectum and the distal portion of the colon. It consists of a light mounted on a tube or speculum. Compare **sigmoidoscope.**

proctoscopy, the examination of the rectum with an endoscope inserted through the anus.

procyclidine hydrochloride /prōsī′klədēn/, an anticholinergic.

■ INDICATIONS: It is prescribed in the treatment of parkinsonism, and to relieve extrapyramidal dysfuntions and to control sialorrhea that are side effects of other medications.

■ CONTRAINDICATIONS: Narrow-angle glaucoma, asthma, obstruction of the genitourinary or GI tract, severe ulcerative colitis, or known hypersensitivity to this drug prohibits its use.

■ ADVERSE EFFECTS: Among the more serious adverse effects are confusion, disorientation, blurred vision, central nervous system effects, tachycardia, dry mouth, decreased sweating, and hypersensitivity reactions.

prodromal labor, the early period in parturition before uterine contractions become forceful and frequent enough to result in progressive dilatation of the uterine cervix.

prodrome, **1.** an early sign of a developing condition or disease. **2.** the earliest phase of a developing condition or disease. **–prodromal,** *adj.*

product evaluation committee, a hospital committee composed of medical, nursing, purchasing, and administrative staff members whose purpose is to evaluate health care related products and advise on their procurement.

productive cough, a sudden, noisy expulsion of air from the lungs that effectively removes sputum from the respiratory tract and helps clear the air passages, permitting oxygen to reach the alveoli. Coughing is stimulated by irritation or by inflammation of the respiratory tract caused most frequently by infection. Deep breathing, with contraction of the diaphragm and intercostal muscles and forceful exhalation, promotes productive coughing in patients with respiratory infections. Mucolytic agents liquefy mucus in the respiratory tract so that it can be raised and expectorated more easily. Anticholinergic drugs, as atropine, decrease respiratory secretions. See also **nonproductive cough.**

professional corporation (PC), a corporation formed according to the law of a particular state for the purpose of delivering a professional service. In some states, corporations may not practice law, medicine, surgery, or dentistry, while in some states nurses may form or be partners in a professional corporation. According to the laws of the various states professional corporations may offer legal and tax benefits to the members of the corporation.

professional liability, a legal concept describing the obligation of a professional person to pay a patient or client for damages caused by the professional's act of omission, commission, or negligence. Professional liability better describes the responsibility of all professionals to their clients than does the concept of malpractice, but the idea of professional liability is central to malpractice.

professional network, (in psychiatric nursing) the network of professional resources available to support the psychiatric outpatient in the community. The network may include a therapist, a hospital day treatment program, social work agency, and other agencies.

professional organization, an organization, whose members share a professional status, created to deal with issues of concern to the professional group or groups involved.

Professional Standards Review Organization (PSRO), an organization formed under Social Security Act Amendments of 1972 to review the services provided under Medicare, Medicaid, and Maternal Child Health programs. Review is conducted by physicians to ascertain the need for the program, to ensure that it is carried out in accord with certain criteria, norms, and standards, and, in institutional situations, in a proper setting. The PSRO requires that regional organizations be formed to conduct these reviews throughout the nation.

profibrinolysin. See **fibrinogen.**

progenitive, capable of producing offspring; reproductive.

progenitor, **1.** a parent or ancestor. **2.** one who or anything that originates or precedes; precursor.

progeny /proj′ənē/, **1.** offspring; an individual or organism resulting from a particular mating. **2.** the descendants of a known or common ancestor.

progeria /prōjē′rē·ə/, an abnormal congenital condition characterized by premature aging and the appearance in childhood of gray hair and wrinkled skin and by small stature, absence of pubic and facial hair, and the posture and habitus of an aged person. Death usually occurs before 20 years of age. Compare **infantilism.**

progestagen. See **progestogen.**

Progestasert, a trademark for a progestin (progesterone).

progestational /prōjestā′shənəl/, of or pertaining to a drug with effects similar to those of progesterone, the hormone produced by the corpus luteum and adrenal cortex during the luteal phase of the menstrual cycle that prepares the uterus for reception of the fertilized ovum. Natural and synthetic preparations of progesterone and its derivative medroxyprogesterone acetate are used in the treatment of secondary amenorrhea and abnormal uterine bleeding. Progestational compounds, as norethindrone and norgestrel, are constituents of oral contraceptives. The use of progestogens to prevent habitual or threatened abortion is no longer recommended.

progestational phase. See **secretory phase.**

progesterone /prəjes′tərōn/, a natural progestational hormone.

■ INDICATIONS: It is prescribed in the treatment of various menstrual disorders, infertility associated with luteal phase dysfunction, and repeated spontaneous abortion.

■ CONTRAINDICATIONS: Thrombophlebitis, liver dysfunction, breast cancer, missed abortion, or hypersensitivity to this drug prohibits its use.

■ ADVERSE EFFECTS: Among the more serious adverse reactions are pain at the site of injection, catabolic effects, and electrolyte disturbances.

progestin **1.** progesterone. **2.** any of a group of hormones, natural or synthetic, secreted by the corpus luteum, placenta, or adrenal cortex that have progesterone-like effect on the uterus.

progestogen, any natural or synthetic progestational hormone. Also spelled **progestagen.** Also called **progestin.**

proglottid /prōglot′id/, a sexual segment of an adult tapeworm, containing both male and female reproductive organs. Each mature segment is shed and produces additional tapeworms.

prognathism /prog′nəthiz′əm/, an abnormal facial configuration in which one or both jaws project forward. It is considered real or imaginary, depending on anatomic and developmental factors involved. Real prognathism may exist when both the mandible and the maxilla increase in length or when the length of the maxilla is normal and the mandibular length increases excessively. Imaginary prognathism may exist when the maxilla is underdeveloped and the mandibular length is normal. **–prognathic,** *adj.*

prognosis, a prediction of the probable outcome of a disease based on the condition of the person and the usual course of the disease as observed in similar situations.

program, a sequence of instructions, written in computer programing language, that controls the functions of a computer.

program documentation. See **documentation.**

programer, a person skilled in writing or coding computer programs.

programing language. See **language.**

progressive, describing the course of a disease or condition in which the characteristic signs and symptoms become more prominent and severe, as progressive muscular atrophy.

progressive myonecrosis. See **myonecrosis.**

progressive patient care, a system of care in which patients are placed in units on the basis of their needs for care as determined by the degree of illness rather than in units based on a medical specialty. The usual levels or stages of progressive patient care are intensive care, intermediate care, and minimal care.

progressive relaxation, a technique for combating tension and anxiety by systematically tensing and relaxing muscle groups.

progressive resistance exercise, a method of increasing the strength of a weak or injured muscle by gradually increasing the resistance against which the muscle works, as by using graduated weights over a period of time. Also called **graduated resistance exercise.** See also **active resistance exercise.**

progressive spinal muscular atrophy of infants. See **Werdnig-Hoffmann disease.**

progressive subcortical encephalopathy. See **Schilder's disease.**

progressive systemic sclerosis (PSS), the most common form of scleroderma.

progress notes, (in the patient record) notes made by a nurse and physician that describe the patient's condition and the treatments given or planned. Progress notes may follow the problem-oriented medical record format. The physician's progress notes usually focus on the medical or therapeutic aspects of the patient's condition and care; the nurse's progress notes, although recording the medical conditions of the patient, usually focus on the objectives stated in the nursing care plan. These objectives might include the person's ability to perform activities of daily living or acceptance or understanding of a particular condition or treatment. Progress notes in an in-hospital setting are recorded daily; progress notes in a clinic or office setting are usually preceded by an episodic or an interval history and are written as an account of each visit.

projection, **1.** a protuberance; anything that thrusts or juts outward. **2.** the act of perceiving an idea or thought as an objective reality. **3.** (in psychology) an unconscious defense mechanism by which an individual attributes his or her own unacceptable traits, ideas, or impulses to another.

projectile vomiting, expulsive vomiting that is extremely forceful.

projection reconstruction imaging, the techniques used in NMR imaging to obtain a cross-sectional image of an object. Such an image is computer reconstructed from a series of projections, NMR profiles, recorded all around the object by rotating the direction of the gradient field superimposed on the static magnetic field.

projective test, a kind of diagnostic, psychologic, or personality test that uses unstructured or ambiguous stimuli, as inkblots, a series of pictures, abstract patterns, or incomplete sentences, to elicit responses that reflect a projection of various aspects of the individual's personality. See also **Rorschach test.**

prokaryocyte /prōker′ē•əsīt′/, a cell without a true nucleus and with nuclear material scattered throughout the cytoplasm. Prokaryocytic organisms include bacteria, viruses, rickettsiae, chlamydiae, mycoplasmas, actinomycetes, and certain algae. Also spelled **procaryocyte.** Compare **eukaryocyte.**

prokaryon /prōker′ē•on/, **1.** nuclear elements that are not bound by a membrane but are spread throughout the cytoplasm. **2.** an organism containing such unbound nuclear elements. Also spelled **procaryon.** Compare **eukaryon.**

prokaryosis, the condition of not containing a true nucleus surrounded by a nuclear membrane. Also spelled **procaryosis.** Compare **eukaryosis.**

prokaryote /prōker′ē•ōt/, an organism that does not contain a true nucleus surrounded by a nuclear membrane, characteristic of lower forms, as bacteria, viruses, and blue-green bacteria. Division occurs through simple fission. Also spelled **procaryote.** Compare **eukaryote.** **–prokaryotic,** *adj.*

Proketazine Maleate, a trademark for a phenothiazine tranquilizer (carphenazine maleate).

prolactin (PRL) /prōlak′tin/, a hormone produced and secreted into the bloodstream by the anterior pituitary. Prolactin, acting with estrogen, progesterone, thyroxine, insulin, growth hormone, glucocorticoids, and human placental lactogen, stimulates the development and growth of the mammary glands. After parturition, prolactin together with glucocorticoids is essential for the initiation and maintenance of milk production. Prolactin synthesis and release from the pituitary is mediated by the central nervous system in response to suckling by the infant. When suckling or its mechanic equivalent ceases, prolactin secretion slows and milk production ceases. Prolactin is similar to growth hormone in its chemical structure. It is unknown in males. Also called **lactogenic hormone, luteotropin.**

prolan, an obsolete term for human chorionic gonadotropin (HCG), a hormone produced by chorionic villi.

prolapse /prō′laps, prōlaps′/, the falling, sinking, or sliding of an organ from its normal position or location in the body, as a prolapsed uterus.

prolapsed cord, an umbilical cord that protrudes beside or ahead of the presenting part of the fetus.

proliferation, the reproduction or multiplication of similar forms. The term is usually applied to increases of cells or cysts.

proliferative phase, the phase of the menstrual cycle after menstruation. Under the influence of follicle stimulating hormone from the pituitary, the ovary produces increasing amounts of estrogen, causing the lining of the uterus to become dense and richly vascular. The phase is terminated by rupture of a mature follicle and subsequent ovulation. Compare **menstrual phase, secretory phase.**

proline (Pro), a nonessential amino acid found in many proteins of the body, particularly collagen. See also **amino acid, protein.**

Proloid, a trademark for a thyroid hormone preparation (thyroglobulin).

prolonged release, a term applied to a drug that is designed to deliver a dose of a medication over an extended period of time. The most common device for this purpose is a soft, soluble capsule containing minute pellets of the drug for release at different rates in the GI tract, depending on the thickness and nature of the oil, fat, wax, or resin coating on the pellets. Another system consists of a porous plastic carrier impregnated with the drug and a surfactant to facilitate the entry of GI fluids that slowly leach out the drug. Ion exchange resins that bind to drugs and liquids containing suspensions of slow-release drug granules are also used to provide medication over an extended period. Various mechanisms and vehicles have also been developed to prolong the release of drugs after injection.

Proloprim, a trademark for an antibacterial (trimethoprim).

Promapar, a trademark for an antiemetic and tranquilizer (chlorpromazine hydrochloride).

promethazine hydrochloride, a phenothiazine antiemetic, antihistamine, and sedative.

■ INDICATIONS: It is prescribed in the treatment of motion sickness, nausea, rhinitis, itching, and skin rash.

■ CONTRAINDICATIONS: Known hypersensitivity to this drug or to other phenothiazines prohibits its use.

■ ADVERSE EFFECTS: Drowsiness, hypotension, and dry mouth are the most common adverse reactions.

promethium (Pm), a radioactive, rare earth, metallic element. Its atomic number is 61; its atomic is weight 145.

promontory of the sacrum, the superior projecting part of the sacrum at its junction with the L5 vertebra.

promoter, (in molecular genetics) a DNA sequence that initiates RNA transcription of the genetic code.

prompt insulin zinc suspension, a fast-acting noncrystalline semilente insulin prescribed in the treatment of diabetes mellitus when a prompt, intense, and short-acting response is desired. It is only slightly slower to act than insulin injection. See also **fast-acting insulin.**

promyelocyte /prōmī′ələsīt′/, a large mononuclear blood cell not normally present in the circulating blood. It contains a single, regular, symmetric nucleus and a few undifferentiated cytoplasmic granules. It is intermediate in development between a myeloblast and a myelocyte and is indicative of leukemia.

pronation /prōnā′shən/, **1.** assumption of a prone position, one in which the ventral surface of the body faces downward. **2.** (of the arm) the rotation of the forearm so that the palm of the hand faces downward and backward. **3.** (of the foot) the lowering of the medial edge of the foot by turning it outward and abduction movements in the tarsal and metatarsal joints. –**pronate,** *v.*

pronator reflex /prōnā′tər/, a reflex elicited by holding the patient's hand vertically and tapping the distal end of the radius or ulna, resulting in pronation of the forearm. Hyperactivity of the reflex may be seen with lesions of the pyramidal system above the level of the sixth cervical nerve root. Also called **ulnar reflex.**

pronator teres, a superficial muscle of the forearm, arising from a humeral and an ulnar head. The humeral head is the larger and more superficial, originating near the medial epicondyle, from the tendon common to the superficial muscles of the forearm, from certain intermuscular septa, and from the antebrachial fascia. The ulnar head originates in the coronoid process of the ulna. Fibers from both portions of the muscle pass obliquely across the forearm, ending in a flat tendon that inserts into the radius. The pronator teres is innervated by a branch of the median nerve, which contains fibers from the sixth and the seventh cervical nerves, and it functions to pronate the hand. Compare **flexor carpi radialis, flexor carpi ulnaris, flexor digitorum superficialis, palmaris longus.**

prone, **1.** having a tendency or inclination. **2.** (of the body) being in horizontal position when lying face downward. Compare **supine.**

Pronemia, a trademark for a hematinic, fixed-combination drug containing iron, vitamin B_{12}, intrinsic factor concentrate, vitamin C, and folic acid.

proneness profile, a screening process that evaluates the probability of developmental problems occurring in the early years of a child's life. Screening ideally begins in the course of prenatal care and continues after birth. Several of the variables in the proneness profile that appear to be significant in selecting the infants who are at risk are the perinatal health status of the mother and infant, especially complications of pregnancy, delivery, the neonatal period, and the puerperium; characteristics of the mother, especially her temperament, educational level, perception of the life situation, and perception of the infant; characteristics of the infant, including alertness, activity pattern, and responsiveness; and the behaviors of the infant and caregiver as they interact. The proneness profile is followed by a developmental profile that assesses the current status of the infant and caregiver. Three areas to be considered are characteristics of the infant, including adaptation and response to the environment, the ability to give interpretable cues, and the developmental progress as compared with established norms; characteristics of the care-giver, including adaptation to the new infant, sensitivity to cues from the infant, and techniques for relieving distress; and the healthful quality of the environment, including health, safety, comfort, and stimulation.

pronephric duct, one of the paired ducts that connect the tubules of each of the pronephros with the cloaca in the early developing vertebrate embryo. They later become the functional mesonephric ducts. Also called **archinephric canal, archinephric duct.**

pronephric tubule, any of the segmentally arranged excretory units of the pronephros in the early developing vertebrate embryo. The tubules open into the pronephric duct and communicate with the coelom through a nephrostoma. In humans and the higher vertebrates the tubules are present only in vestigial form; in lower animals, they are functional.

pronephros, *pl.* **pronephroi,** the primordial excretory organ in the developing vertebrate embryo. It consists of a series of pronephric tubules that arise along the anterior portion of the nephrotome and empty into the cloaca by way of the pronephric duct. In humans and other mammals the structure is nonfunctional, representing the first of three excretory systems that are formed one after the other in an anterior to posterior sequence and that disappear with the formation of the mesonephros. The organ is functional in certain primitive fishes, as lampreys, and serves as a provisional kidney in some fishes and amphibians. Also called **pronephron** (*pl.* **pronephra**), **archinephron, head kidney.** See also **mesonephros, metanephros.** –**pronephric,** *adj.*

Pronestyl, a trademark for a cardiac depressant (procainamide hydrochloride).

pronucleus, *pl.* **pronuclei,** the nucleus of the ovum or the spermatozoon after fertilization but before the fusion of the chromosomes to form the nucleus of the zygote. Each contains the haploid number of chromosomes, is larger than the normal nucleus, and is diffuse in appearance. The female pronucleus of the mature ovum is formed only after penetration by the sperm and the completion of the second mitotic division and polar body formation. The nucleus then loses its nuclear envelope to release the chromosomes so that synapsis can occur with the chromosomes of the male pronucleus, which is contained in the head of the spermatozoon. Also called **germinal nucleus, germ nucleus.** See also **oogenesis, spermatogenesis.**

Propadrine Hydrochloride, a trademark for an adrenergic (phenylpropanolamine hydrochloride).

propantheline bromide, an anticholinergic.

■ INDICATION: It is prescribed as an adjunct in peptic ulcer therapy.

■ CONTRAINDICATIONS: Narrow-angle glaucoma, asthma, obstruction of the genitourinary or GI tract, severe ulcerative colitis, or known hypersensitivity to this drug prohibits its use.

■ ADVERSE EFFECTS: Among the more serious adverse reactions are blurred vision, central nervous system effects, tachycardia, dry mouth, decreased sweating, and hypersensitivity reactions.

proparacaine hydrochloride /prōper′əkān/, a rapid-acting, topical anesthetic of the amide family used for ophthalmologic procedures. It is used for tonometry, gonioscopy, removal of foreign objects from the eye, and other minor optic procedures, and preoperatively for major eye surgery. One drop gives 15 minutes of optic anesthesia. Prolonged use may injure the eye. Proparacaine hydrochloride is not administered to individuals with cardiac disease, hyperthyroidism, or multiple allergies. People given the drug should be warned not to touch their eyes until the anesthetic has worn off. Adverse optic reactions may occur with proparacaine, but systemic reactions are rare. Also called **proxymetacaine.**

prophase /prō′fāz/, the first of four stages of nuclear division in mitosis and in each of the two divisions of meiosis. In mitosis, the chromosomes progressively shorten and thicken to form individually recognizable elongated double structures composed of two chromatids held together by a centromere; the nucleolus and nuclear membrane disappear, the spindle and polar bodies are formed, and the chromosomes begin to migrate toward the midplane of the developing spindle. In the first meiotic division, prophase is complex and subdivided into five stages: leptotene, zygotene, pachytene, diplotene, and diakinesis. In the second meiotic division, the same processes occur as in mitotic prophase. See also **anaphase, interphase, meiosis, metaphase, mitosis, telophase.**

prophylactic /prō′filak′tik/, **1.** preventing the spread of disease. **2.** an agent that prevents the spread of disease. See also **condom.** –**prophylactically,** *adv.*

prophylactic forceps. See **low forceps.**

prophylactic odontomy, (in dentistry) the surgical removal of harmful pits and fissures in the posterior primary and permanent molars.

prophylactic treatment. See **preventive treatment.**

prophylaxis /prō′filak′sis/, prevention of or protection against disease, often involving the use of a biologic, chemical, or mechanic agent to destroy or prevent the entry of infectious organisms.

Propine, a trademark for an ophthalmic adrenergic (dipivefrin hydrochloride).

Propionibacterium, a genus of nonmotile, anaerobic, gram-positive bacteria found on the skin of humans, in the intestinal tract of humans and animals, and in dairy products. ***P. acne*** is common in acne pustules (formerly called ***Corynebacterium acne***).

propionicacidemia /prō′pē·on′ikas′idē′mē·ə/, a rare inherited metabolic defect caused by the failure of the body to metabolize the amino acids threonine, isoleucine, and methionone, characterized by lethargy and mental and physical retardation. Acidosis occurs as a result of the accumulation of propionic acid in the body. A diet low in these amino acids is difficult to achieve but is the only treatment. –**propionicacidemic,** *adj.*

propionic fermentation, the production of propionic acid by the action of certain bacteria on sugars or lactic acid.

Proplex, a trademark for human clotting factor IX.

proportional mortality, a statistic method of relating the number of deaths from a particular condition to all deaths within the same population group for the same time period.

proposition, **1.** a statement of a truth to be demonstrated or an operation to be performed. **2.** to bring forward or offer for consideration, acceptance, or adoption.

propositus /prōpoz′itəs/, a person from whom a genealogic lineage is traced, as is done to discover the pattern of inheritance of a familial disease or a physical trait.

propoxyphene /prōpok′səfēn/, a mild centrally acting narcotic analgesic.

■ INDICATION: It is prescribed to relieve mild to moderate pain.

■ CONTRAINDICATIONS: Concurrent administration of tranquilizers or antidepressant drugs, current alcohol or drug abuse, or known hypersensitivity to aspirin or to this drug prohibits its use. It is not recommended for use by people who are suicidal or prone to alcohol or drug addiction or by women who are pregnant, because neonatal withdrawal symptoms have been observed.

■ ADVERSE EFFECTS: Among the more serious reactions are hepatic dysfunction and severe depression of the central nervous system occurring with overdose or drug interraction. A small number of people may experience nausea, dizziness, sedation, or vomiting when correctly taking a usual, prescribed dosage.

propoxyphene hydrochloride, an analgesic.

■ INDICATION: It is prescribed for the relief of mild to moderate pain.

■ CONTRAINDICATIONS: Known hypersensitivity to this drug or known narcotic addiction prohibits its use.

■ ADVERSE EFFECTS: Among the more serious adverse reactions are respiratory depression, paradoxical excitement, and convulsions.

propranolol hydrochloride, a beta-adrenergic blocking agent.

■ INDICATIONS: It is prescribed in the treatment of angina pectoris, cardiac arrhythmias, and hypertension.

■ CONTRAINDICATIONS: Asthma, certain arrhythmias, congestive heart failure, concomitant use of monamine oxidase inhibitors, or known hypersensitivity to this drug prohibits its use.

■ ADVERSE EFFECTS: Among the more serious adverse reactions are heart failure, heart block, increased airway resistance, augmentation of hypoglycemic response, GI disturbances, and hypersensitivity reactions. Withdrawal syndrome has been observed in some patients.

proprietary, **1.** of or pertaining to an institution or other organization that is operated for profit. **2.** of or pertaining to a product, as a drug or device, that is made for profit.

proprietary hospital, a hospital operated as a profit-making organization. Many proprietary hospitals are owned by physicians who operate the hospital primarily for their own patients but also accept patients from other physicians. Some proprietary hospitals are owned by investor groups or large corporations.

proprietary medicine, any pharmaceutic preparation or medicinal substance that is protected from commercial competition because its ingredients or method of manufacture are kept secret or are protected by trademark or copyright.

proprioception /prō′prē•əsep′shən/, sensation pertaining to stimuli originating from within the body regarding spatial position and muscular activity or to the sensory receptors that they activate. Compare **exteroceptive, interoceptive.** See also **autopagnosia.**

proprioceptive reflex /prō′prē•əsep′tiv/, any reflex initiated by stimulation of proprioceptive receptors, as the increase in respiratory rate and volume induced by impulses arising from muscles and joints during exercise.

proprioceptor /prō′prē•əsep′tər/, any sensory nerve ending, as those located in muscles, tendons, joints, and the vestibular apparatus, that responds to stimuli originating from within the body regarding movement and spatial position. Compare **exteroceptor, interoceptor.** See also **mechanoreceptor.**

proptosis /proptō′sis/, bulging, protrusion, or forward displacement of a body organ or area.

propylformic acid. See **butyric acid.**

propylthiouracil, an inhibitor of thyroid hormone biosynthesis.

■ INDICATIONS: It is prescribed in the treatment of hyperthyroidism, thyrotoxic crisis, and preparation for thyroidectomy.

■ CONTRAINDICATIONS: Mental depression, cold intolerance, or known hypersensitivity to this drug prohibits its use. Caution is recommended in pregnancy.

■ ADVERSE EFFECTS: Among the more serious adverse reactions are GI distress, pruritus, and rashes. Rarely, blood dyscrasia occurs.

proscribe, to forbid. **–proscriptive,** *adj.*

prosector, a person who, under the supervision of a pathologist, performs gross dissections and prepares autopsy specimens for pathologic examination.

prosencephalon /pros′ensef′əlon/, the portion of the brain that includes the diencephalon and the telencephalon. It develops from the anterior of the three primary vesicles of the embryonic neural tube and contains various structures, as the thalamus and hypothalamus, that control important body functions and affect the consciousness, the appetite, and the emotions. Also called **forebrain.** Compare **mesencephalon. –prosencephalic,** *adj.*

proso-, pros-, a combining form meaning 'forward, or anterior': *prosocoele, prosodemic, prosogaster.*

Pro Sobee, a trademark for a commercial milk-substitute formula that is prepared from a soy isolate base and is lactose free, prescribed for infants with galactosemia and persons with lactose intolerance. It is supplemented with other nutrients, is fortified with vitamins and minerals, and is available in both powder and liquid forms. See also **Neo-Mull-Soy, Nutramigen, Soyalac.**

prosopalgia. See **trigeminal neuralgia.**

-prosopia, a combining form meaning '(condition of the) face': *ateloprosopia, lipoprosopia, schizoprosopia.*

prosopo-, a combining form meaning 'of or related to the face': *prosopoanoschisis, prosopodiplegia, prosoponeuralgia*.

prosoposternodidymus /pros′əpōstur′nədid′əməs/, a fetal monster consisting of conjoined twins united laterally from the head through the sternum.

prosopothoracopagus /pros′əpōthôr′əkop′əgəs/, conjoined symmetric twins who are united laterally in the frontal plane from the thorax through most of the head region.

prospective medicine, the early identification of pathologic or potentially pathologic processes and the prescription of intervention to stop the processes.

prospective reimbursement, a method of payment to an agency for health care services to be delivered based on predictions of what the agency's costs will be for the coming year.

prospective study, a study designed to determine the relationship between a condition and a characteristic shared by some members of a group. The population selected is healthy at the beginning of the study. Some of the members of the group share a particular characteristic, as cigarette smoking. The researcher follows the population group over a period of time, noting the rate at which a condition, as lung cancer, occurs in the smokers and in the nonsmokers. A prospective study may involve many variables or only two; it may seek to demonstrate a relationship that is an association or one that is causal. The kinds of data collected, the numbers of people studied, and other details of the design of the study affect the kind of analysis and the interpretation of the data. Compare **retrospective study.**

prostacyclin (PGI_2), a prostaglandin. It is a biologically active product of arachidonic acid metabolism in human vascular walls, and is a potent inhibitor of platelet aggregation. It inhibits the vasoconstrictor effect of angiotensin and stimulates renin release.

prostaglandin (PG) /pros′təglan′din/, one of several potent hormonelike unsaturated fatty acids that act in exceedingly low concentrations on local target organs. They are produced in small amounts and have a large array of significant effects. Prostaglandins given by nebulizer, in tablets, or in solutions for oral or intravenous use effect changes in vasomotor tone, capillary permeability, smooth muscle tone, aggregation of platelets, endocrine and exocrine functions, and in the autonomic and central nervous systems. Some of the pharmacologic uses for the prostaglandins are termination of pregnancy and treatment of asthma and gastric hyperacidity.

Prostaphlin, a trademark for an antibacterial (oxacillin sodium).

prostate /pros′tāt/, a gland in men that surrounds the neck of the bladder and the urethra and elaborates a secretion that liquefies coagulated semen. It is a firm structure about the size of a chestnut, composed of muscular and glandular tissue. It is located in the pelvic cavity, below the caudal part of the symphysis pubis and ventral to the rectum, through which it can be felt, especially when enlarged. A depression on its cranial border accommodates the entry of the two ejaculatory ducts and divides the posterior surface of the gland into the middle lobe above, and a larger, lower portion below. A sinus about 6 mm long runs upward and backward in the gland behind the middle lobe and is part of the urethra. The prominent lateral surfaces of the prostate are covered by a plexus of veins and by the ventral portions of the levator ani. The portion of the gland in front of the urethra is composed of dense muscular tissue. In most men the urethra lies along the junction of the anterior portion and the middle third of the prostate. The ejaculatory ducts pass obliquely through the posterior part of the gland. The prostatic secretion consists of alkaline phosphatase, citric acid, and various proteolytic enzymes.

prostatectomy /pros′tətek′təmē/, surgical removal of a portion of the prostate gland, as performed for benign prostatic hypertrophy, or the total excision of the gland, as performed for malignancy. An indwelling urinary catheter is inserted, and a type and crossmatch of blood is done to prepare for possible transfusion. Either a general or a spinal anesthetic is used. Kinds of approaches include transurethral, the most common, in which a resectoscope is inserted and through it shavings of prostatic tissue are cut off at the bladder opening with a loop, suprapubic, and retropubic. The perineal approach is used for biopsy when early cancer is suspected or for the removal of calculi. In a suprapubic approach, a large catheter is positioned into the bladder through the abdomen. Wound drains are left in place in both the perineal and the suprapubic types. After surgery, hematuria is expected for several days; on the first day the bleeding is frank, usually venous, and may be controlled by increasing the pressure in the balloon end of the urethral catheter. If arterial in nature, the bleeding will be bright red with numerous clots and increased viscosity and may lead to hemorrhagic shock, requiring transfusion and surgical intervention. The catheters are connected to a closed system of either constant or intermittent drainage. Meticulous aseptic technique is required to prevent infection when tending catheters, tubings, and collection bags, as well as when changing the dressing. Catheter patency is assured, and pain is assessed, because blockage or kinking of the drainage tubes may be the cause. Accidental removal or dislodging of catheters is avoided. Bladder spasm may occur if a catheter becomes blocked or from the irritation of the balloon of the catheter in the bladder. Antispasmodic drugs may prevent spasm but are not given in severe cardiac disease or if glaucoma is present. The nurse also assesses the patient's ability to void in adequate amounts when the urethral catheter is removed. Complications of prostatectomy include urethral stricture, especially with the transurethral approach, urinary incontinence, and impotence.

prostatic /prostat′ik/, pertaining to the prostate gland.

prostatic catheter, a catheter that is approximately 16 inches long and has an angled tip. It is used in male catheterization to pass an enlarged prostate gland obstructing the urethra.

prostatic ductule /duk′tyo͞ol/, any one of 12 to 20 tiny excretory tubes that convey the alkaline secretion of the prostate gland and open into the floor of the prostatic portion of the urethra. The ductules are joined together by areolar tissue, supported by extensions of the fibrous capsule of the prostate and its muscular stroma, and wrapped in a delicate network of capillaries.

prostatic hypertrophy. See **prostatomegaly.**

prostatic utricle, the portion of the urethra in men that forms a cul-de-sac about 6 mm long behind the middle lobe of the prostate. It is composed of fibrous tissue, muscular fibers, and mucous membrane; numerous small glands open on its inner surface. It is derived from the atrophied paramesonephric ducts and is homologous with the uterus in women. Also called **uterus masculinis.** See also **prostate.**

prostatitis /pros′tətī′tis/, acute or chronic inflammation of the prostate gland, usually the result of infection. The patient complains of burning, frequency, and urgency. Treatment consists of administration of antibiotics, sitz baths, bed rest, and fluids. Compare **benign prostatic hypertrophy.**

prostatomegaly, the hypertrophy or enlargement of the prostate gland.

prosthesis /prosthē′sis/, *pl.* **prostheses,** **1.** an artificial replacement for a missing part of the body. **2.** a device designed and applied to improve function, as a hearing aid. See also **artificial limb, maxillofacial prosthesis, Starr-Edwards prosthesis.**

prosthetic restoration. See **restoration.**

prosthetist /pros′thətist/, a person who fabricates and fits artificial limbs and similar devices prescribed by a physician. A certified prosthetist is one who has successfully completed the examination of the American Orthotic and Prosthetic Association.

prosthodontics /pros′thədon′tiks/, a branch of dentistry devoted to the construction of artificial appliances that replace missing teeth or restore parts of the face.

Prostigmin, a trademark for a neuromuscular blocking agent (neostigmine) used as an adjunct to anesthesia.

Prostin F2 Alpha, a trademark for a prostaglandin abortifacient (dinoprost tromethamine).

prostration, a condition of extreme exhaustion and inability to exert oneself further, as in heat prostration or nervous prostration.

prot-. See **proto-.**

protactinium (Pa), a radioactive element. Its atomic number is 91; its atomic weight is 231. The most long-lived isotope of protactinium is p 231, which has a half life of 34,000 years and is produced as an intermediate in the radioactive decay of uranium 235. Its own decay products are actinium and an alpha particle.

protamine sulfate /prō′təmēn/, a heparin antagonist derived from fish sperm.

■ INDICATION: It is prescribed to diminish or reverse the anticoagulant effect of heparin, particularly in cases of heparin overdosage.

■ CONTRAINDICATIONS: Pregnancy, allergy to fish, or known hypersensitivity to this drug prohibits its use.

■ ADVERSE EFFECTS: Among the more serious adverse reactions are hypotension, dyspnea, and bradycardia. Dosage greater than needed to neutralize heparin causes the toxic and anticoagulant effects of protamine itself.

protamine zinc insulin suspension, a long-acting insulin that is absorbed slowly at a steady rate. Some patients can be treated with only one injection daily, but combination therapy with regular insulin may be necessary for adequate control.

protanopia. See **daltonism.**

protease /prō′tē·ās/, an enzyme that is a catalyst in the breakdown of protein. See also **proteolytic.**

protective, describing an individual who guards another from danger or injury and provides a safe environment.

protein /prō′tē·in, prō′tēn/, any of a large group of naturally occurring, complex, organic nitrogenous compounds. Each is composed of large combinations of amino acids containing the elements carbon, hydrogen, nitrogen, oxygen, usually sulfur, and occasionally phosphorus, iron, iodine, or other essential constituents of living cells. Twenty-two amino acids have been identified as vital for proper growth, development, and maintenance of health. The body can synthesize 14 of these amino acids, called nonessential, whereas the remaining eight must be obtained from dietary sources and are termed essential. Protein is the major source of building material for muscles, blood, skin, hair, nails, and the internal organs. It is necessary for the formation of hormones, enzymes, and antibodies and as a source of heat and energy, and it functions as an essential element in proper elimination of waste materials. Rich dietary sources are meat, poultry, fish, eggs, milk, and cheese, which are classified as complete proteins because they contain the eight essential amino acids. Nuts and legumes, including navy beans, chick peas, soybeans, and split peas, are also good sources but are incomplete proteins, because they do not contain all the essential amino acids. Protein deficiency causes abnormal growth and tissue development in children, leading to kwashiorkor and marasmus, whereas in adults it results in lack of vigor and stamina, weakness, mental depression, poor resistance to infection, impaired healing of wounds, and slow recovery from disease. Excessive intake of protein may in some conditions result in fluid imbalance.

protein-bound iodine (PBI), iodine that is firmly bound to protein in serum, the measurement of which indirectly indicates the concentration of circulating thyroxine (T_4). A PBI of less than the normal range of 4 to 8 μ/ml of serum is indicative of hypothyroidism, and a PBI of more than the normal values indicates hyperthyroidism. The test is currently used less frequently because of the availability of more sensitive measurements of T_4.

protein calorie malnutrition. See **energy protein malnutrition.**

protein hydrolysate injection, a fluid and nutrient replenisher.

▪ INDICATIONS: It is prescribed to correct a negative nitrogen balance and in other clinical situations requiring parenteral nutrition.

▪ CONTRAINDICATIONS: Renal failure, anuria, severe liver disease, hepatic coma, or known hypersensitivity to one or more of the amino acids prohibits the use of this drug.

▪ ADVERSE EFFECTS: Among the more serious adverse reactions are hypotension, abdominal pain, convulsions, phlebitis, thrombosis, and edema.

protein kinase, a protein that catalyzes the transfer of a phosphate group from adenosine triphosphate to produce a phosphoprotein.

protein metabolism, the processes whereby protein foodstuffs are used by the body to make tissue proteins, together with the processes of breakdown of tissue proteins in the production of energy. Food proteins are first broken down into amino acids, then absorbed into the bloodstream, and finally used in body cells to form new proteins. Amino acids in excess of the body's needs may be converted by liver enzymes into keto acids and urea. The keto acids may be used as sources of energy via the Krebs citric acid cycle, or they may be converted into glucose or fat for storage. Urea is excreted in urine and sweat. Growth hormones and androgens stimulate protein formation, and adrenal cortical hormones tend to cause breakdown of body proteins. Diseases affecting protein metabolism include homocystinuria, liver disease, maple sugar urine disease, and phenylketonuria.

proteinuria /prō′tēnyŏŏr′ē•ə/, the presence in the urine of abnormally large quantities of protein, usually albumin. Healthy adults excrete less than 250 mg of protein per day. Persistent proteinuria is usually a sign of renal disease or renal complications of another disease, as hypertension or heart failure. However, proteinuria can result from heavy exercise or fever. Also called **albuminuria.**

proteo-, a combining form meaning 'of or pertaining to protein': *proteocrasis, proteolysis, proteopepsis.*

proteolipid /prō′tē•ōlip′id/, a type of lipoprotein in which lipid material forms more than one half of the molecule. It is insoluble in water and occurs primarily in the brain.

proteolysis /prō′tē•ol′isis/, a process in which water added to the peptide bonds of proteins breaks down the protein molecule. Numerous enzymes may catalyze this process. The action of mineral acids and heat may also induce proteolysis.

proteolytic /prō′tē•əlit′ik/, of or pertaining to any substance that promotes the breakdown of protein.

Proteus /prō′tē•əs/, a genus of motile, gram-negative bacilli often associated with nosocomial infections, normally found in feces, water, and soil. *Proteus* may cause urinary tract infections, pyelonephritis, wound infections, diarrhea, bacteremia, and endotoxic shock. Some species are sensitive to penicillin; most respond to the aminoglycoside antibiotics.

Proteus morgani, a species of bacteria associated with infectious diarrhea in infants.

Proteus vulgaris, a species of bacteria that is a frequent cause of urinary tract infections. The bacteria is found in feces, water, and soil.

prothrombin /prōthrom′bin/, a plasma protein that is the precursor to thrombin. It forms thrombin, the first step in blood clotting, when exposed to thromboplastin and calcium. It is synthesized in the liver if adequate vitamin K is present. Also called **factor II.** See also **blood coagulation.**

prothrombin time (PT), a one stage test for detecting certain plasma coagulation defects caused by a deficiency of factors V, VII, or X. Thromboplastin and calcium are added to a sample of the patient's plasma and, simultaneously, to a sample from a normal control. The length of time required for clot formation in both samples is observed. Thrombin is formed from prothrombin in the presence of adequate calcium, thromboplastin, and the essential tissue coagulation factors. A prolonged PT therefore indicates deficiency in one of the factors, as in liver disease, vitamin K deficiency, or anticoagulation therapy with the drug coumarin. Compare **partial thromboplastin time.** See also **blood clotting.**

proto-, prot-, a combining form meaning 'first': *protoblast, prototoxin, protopathic.*

protocol /prō′təkôl/, a written plan specifying the procedures to be followed in giving a particular examination, in conducting research, or in providing care for a particular condition. See also **standing orders.**

proton, a positively charged particle that is a fundamental component of the nucleus of all atoms. The number of protons in the nucleus of an atom equals the atomic number of the element. Compare **electron, neutron.** See also **atomic weight.**

Protopam Chloride, a trademark for a cholinesterase reactivator (pralidoxime chloride).

protoplasm, the living substance of a cell, usually composed of myriad molecules of water, minerals, and organic compounds.

protoplast /prō′təplast/, **1.** (in biology), the protoplasm of a cell without its containing membrane. **2.** a first entity or an original. **–protoplastic,** *adj.*

protoporphyria /prō′tōpôrfir′ē•ə/, increased levels of protoporphyrin in the blood and feces.

protoporphyrin /prō′tōpôr′firin/, a kind of porphyrin that combines with iron and protein to form a variety of important organic molecules, including catalase, hemoglobin, and myoglobin. See also **heme.**

protostoma. See **blastopore.**

prototaxic mode, a stage in infancy, according to a Sullivan theory, characterized by a lack of differentiation between the self and the environment.

protozoa /prō′təzō′ə/, *sing.* **protozoon,** single-celled microorganisms of the class Protozoa, the lowest form of animal life. Protozoa are more complex than bacteria, forming a self-contained unit with organelles that carry on such functions as locomotion, nutrition, excretion, respiration, and attachment to other objects or organisms. Approximately 30 protozoa are pathogenic to humans. **–protozoal, protozoan,** *adj.*

protozoal infection, any disease caused by single-celled organisms of the class Protozoa. Some kinds of protozoal infections are **amebic dysentery, kala-azar, malaria,** and **trichomonas vaginitis.**

protracted dose, (in radiotherapy) a low amount of radiation delivered continuously over a relatively long period of time.

protriptyline hydrochloride, a tricyclic antidepressant.

■ INDICATIONS: It is prescribed in the treatment of endogenous mental depression marked by withdrawal and anergy.

■ CONTRAINDICATIONS: Concomitant administration of monoamine oxidase inhibitors, recent myocardial infarction, or known hypersensitivity to any tricyclic medication prohibits its use. It is used with caution where anticholinergics are contraindicated, in seizure disorders, and in patients with cardiovascular disease.

■ ADVERSE EFFECTS: Among the more serious adverse reactions are sedation and anticholinergic side effects. A variety of GI, cardiovascular, and neurologic reactions may occur. This drug interacts with many other drugs.

Protropin, the trademark for a synthetic human growth hormone used to increase the growth rate of children with hypopituitary dwarfism.

protrusio bulbi. See **exophthalmia.**

protrusive incisal guide angle, (in dentistry) the inclination of the incisal guide in the sagittal plane.

proud flesh, excessive granulation tissue. See also **pyogenic granuloma.**

Proventil, a trademark for a bronchodilator (albuterol).

Provera, a trademark for a progestin (medroxyprogesterone acetate).

provider, a hospital, clinic, or health care professional, or group of health care professionals, who provide a service to patients.

Provincial Territorial Nurses' Association (PTNA), an association of Canadian nurses organized at the provincial or territorial level. The Canadian Nurses' Association is a federation of the 11 PTNAs.

provitamin /prōvī′təmin/, a precursor of a vitamin; a substance found in certain foods that in the body may be converted into a vitamin. Also called **previtamin.**

provocative diagnosis, a diagnosis in which the identity and cause of an illness are discovered by inducing an episode of the condition; for example, in immunology an allergen causing an allergic response is shown to be an etiologic factor in the patient's allergic condition.

proxemics /proksē′miks/, the study of spatial distances between people and its effect on interpersonal behavior, especially in relation to density of population, placement of people within an area, and the opportunity for privacy.

proximal /prok′siməl/, nearer to a point of reference, usually the trunk of the body, than other parts of the body. Proximal interphalangeal joints are those closest to the hand.

proximal cavity, a cavity that occurs on the mesial or distal surface of a tooth.

proximal contour, the shape or form of the medial or the distal surface of a tooth.

proximal dental caries, decay that may occur in the mesial or distal surface of a tooth.

proximal radioulnar articulation, the pivot joint between the circumference of the head of the radius and the ring formed by the radial notch of the ulna and the annular ligament. The joint allows the rotary movements of the head of the radius in pronation and supination. Also called **superior radioulnar joint.** Compare **distal radioulnar articulation.**

proximal renal tubular acidosis (proximal RTA), an abnormal condition characterized by excessive acid accumulation and bicarbonate excretion. It is caused by the defective reabsorption of bicarbonate in the proximal tubules of the kidney and the resulting flow of excessive bicarbonate into the distal tubules, which normally secrete hydrogen ions. This disruption impedes the formation of titratable acids and ammonium for excretion and ultimately leads to metabolic acidosis. Treatment is as for renal tubular acidosis. In **primary proximal RTA** the defective reabsorption of bicarbonate is the sole causative factor. In **secondary proximal RTA** the reabsorptive defect is one of several causative factors and may result from tubular cell damage produced by various disorders, as Fanconi's syndrome. Compare **distal renal tubular acidosis.**

proximate cause, a legal concept of cause and effect relationships in determining, for example, whether an injury would have resulted from a particular cause.

proximity principle, a rule that when two or more objects are close to each other they may be seen as a perceptual unit.

proxymetacaine. See **proparacaine hydrochloride.**

prurigo /pro͞orī′gō/, any of a group of chronic inflammatory conditions of the skin characterized by severe itching and multiple, dome-shaped, small papules capped by tiny vesicles. Later (as a result of repeated scratching), crusting and lichenification may occur. Some causes of prurigo are allergies, drugs, endocrine abnormalities, malignancies, and parasites. Specific treatment depends on the cause. Symptomatic therapy is the same as for pruritus. A mild form of the disease is called **prurigo mitis,** and a more severe form, **prurigo agria** or **prurigo ferox.** See also **pruritus.** **–pruriginous,** *adj.*

pruritus /pro͞orī′təs/, the symptom of itching, an uncomfortable sensation leading to the urge to scratch. Scratching often results in secondary infection. Some causes of pruritus are allergy, infection, jaundice, lymphoma, and skin irritation. Treatment is best directed at the cause; symptomatic relief may be obtained by antihistamines, starch baths, topical corticosteroids, cool water, or alcohol applications. –**pruritic,** *adj.*

pruritus ani, a common chronic condition of itching of the skin around the anus. Some causes are candidal infection, contact dermatitis, external hemorrhoids, pinworms, psoriasis, and psychogenic illness. Treatment is best directed at the specific cause; however, symptomatic relief may be obtained by careful cleansing, soothing creams or lotions, topical corticosteroids, antihistamines, and tranquilizers.

pruritus vulvae, itching of the external genitalia of a female. The condition may become chronic and result in lichenification, atrophy, and occasionally malignancy. Some causes of pruritus vulvae are contact dermatitis, lichen sclerosus et atrophicus, psychogenic pruritus, trichomoniasis, and vaginal candidiasis. Treatment of the condition depends on its cause.

Prussian blue, a chemical reagent used on microsopic preparations. It demonstrates the presence of copper by developing a bright blue color.

psammo-, a combining form meaning 'of or related to sand or to sandlike material': *psammocarcinoma, psammoma, psammosarcoma.*

psammoma /samō′mə/, *pl.* **psammomas, psammomata,** a neoplasm containing small calcified granules (psammoma bodies) that occurs in the meninges, choroid plexus, pineal body, and ovaries. Also called **sand tumor.**

psammoma body, a round, layered mass of calcareous material occurring in benign and malignant epithelial and connective tissue neoplasms and in some chronically inflamed tissue.

-pselaphesia, -pselaphesis, a combining form meaning '(condition of the) tactile sense': *apselaphesia, hyperpselaphesia, hypopselaphesia.*

pseudesthesia /sōō′desthē′zhə/, a sensation experienced without an external stimulus or a sensation that does not correspond to the causative stimulus, as phantom limb pain.

pseudo-, pseud-, a combining form meaning 'false': *pseudoangina, pseudocyst, pseudorubella.*

pseudoallele, (in genetics) one of two or more closely linked genes on a chromosome that appear to function as a single member of an allelic pair but occupy distinct, nearly corresponding loci on homologous chromosomes. Such gene pairs produce a mutant effect in the diploid state when located on homologous chromosomes but are capable of being separated by crossing over during meiosis to produce a wild-type effect when recombined on either of the homologues. –**pseudoallelic,** *adj.,* **pseudoallelism,** *n.*

pseudoanorexia, a condition in which an individual eats secretly while claiming a lack of appetite and inability to eat. Also called **false anorexia.**

pseudochylous ascites /sōō′dōkī′ləs/, the abnormal accumulation in the peritoneal cavity of a milky fluid that resembles chyle. The turbidity of the fluid is caused by cellular debris in the fluid. Pseudochylous ascites is indicative of an abdominal tumor or infection. Compare **chylous ascites.** See also **ascites.**

pseudocoxalgia. See **Perthes' disease.**

pseudocyesis /sōō′dōsī•ē′sis/, a condition in which a woman believes she is pregnant when she is not. Certain signs and symptoms suggest pregnancy, as the absence of the menses, although conception has not occurred and therefore there is no embryonic development. The condition may be psychogenic in origin or caused by a tumor or endocrine dysfunction. Also called **false pregnancy, pseudopregnancy, spurious pregnancy.**

pseudocyst, a space or cavity containing gas or liquid but without a lining membrane. Pseudocysts commonly occur after pancreatitis when digestive juices break through the normal ducts of the pancreas and collect in spaces lined by fibroblasts and surfaces of adjacent organs. Symptoms are caused by displacement of abdominal structures or fluid or to atelectasis at the base of the left lung. Ultrasound and computerized tomography are useful in diagnosis; surgical drainage is the best therapy. See also **pancreatitis.**

pseudoephedrine hydrochloride, an adrenergic that acts as a vasoconstrictor and bronchodilator.

■ INDICATIONS: It is prescribed for the relief of nasal congestion and eustachian tube congestion.

■ CONTRAINDICATIONS: Known hypersensitivity to sympathomimetic drugs prohibits its use. Interaction with monoamine oxidase inhibitors may cause hypertensive crisis. It is prescribed with caution in patients who have hypertension, glaucoma, heart disease, diabetes, or urinary retention.

■ ADVERSE EFFECTS: Among the more serious adverse reactions are central nervous system stimulation, headache, and tachycardia.

pseudoephedrine sulfate. See **pseudoephedrine hydrochloride.**

pseudogene /sōō′dōjēn′/, (in molecular genetics) a sequence of nucleotides that resembles a gene and may be derived from one but lacks a genetic function.

pseudogout. See **chondrocalcinosis.**

pseudohermaphroditism, a condition in which a person exhibits the somatic characteristics of both sexes though possessing the physical characteristics of either males (testes) or females (ovaries). Also spelled **pseudohermaphrodism.** See also **feminization,** def. 2, **hermaphroditism.**

pseudohypertrophic muscular dystrophy. See **Duchenne's muscular dystrophy.**

pseudojaundice, a yellow discoloration of the skin that is not caused by hyperbilirubinemia. The excessive ingestion of carotene results in a form of pseudojaundice.

pseudomembranous enterocolitis. See **necrotizing enterocolitis.**

pseudomembranous stomatitis, a severe inflammation of the mouth that produces a membranelike exudate. The inflammation may be caused by a variety of bacteria or by chemical irritants. It may produce dysphagia, pain, fever, and swelling of the lymph glands, or it may remain localized and mild.

pseudomonad /so͞odom′ənad/, a bacterium of the genus *Pseudomonas*.

Pseudomonas /so͞odom′ənas/, a genus of gram-negative bacteria that includes several free-living species of soil and water and some opportunistic pathogens, as *Pseudomonas aeruginosa,* isolated from wounds, burns, and infections of the urinary tract. Pseudomonads are notable for their fluorescent pigments and their resistance to disinfectants and antibiotics.

pseudomutuality, (in psychotherapy) an atmosphere maintained by family members in which there is surface harmony and a high degree of agreement with one another, but in which the atmosphere of agreement covers deep and destructive intrapsychic and interpersonal conflicts.

pseudoneurotic schizophrenia. See **latent schizophrenia.**

pseudopregnancy. See **pseudocyesis.**

pseudopsychopathic schizophrenia. See **latent schizophrenia.**

pseudorubella. See **roseola infantum.**

pseudosclerema. See **adiponecrosis subcutanea neonatorum.**

pseudotumor, a false tumor. One kind of pseudotumor is **pseudotumor cerebri.**

pseudotumor cerebri, a condition characterized by increased intracranial pressure, headache, vomiting, and papilledema without neurologic signs, except, occasionally, palsy of the sixth cranial nerve. Also called **benign intracranial hypertension, meningeal hydrops.**

pseudoxanthoma elasticum. See **Grönblad-Strandberg syndrome.**

psilocybin /sī′lōsī′bin, -sib′in/, a psychedelic drug and an active ingredient of various Mexican hallucinogenic mushrooms of the genus *Psilocybe mexicana*. It can produce altered states of mood and consciousness and has no acceptable medical use in the United States Psilocybin is controlled under Schedule I of the Comprehensive Drug Abuse Prevention and Control Act of 1970, which bans the prescription of psilocybin and numerous other drugs and allows their procurement and use only for special research projects authorized by the Drug Enforcement Administration of the U.S. Department of Justice.

psittacosis /sit′əkō′sis/, an infectious illness caused by the bacterium *Chlamydia psittaci,* characterized by respiratory, pneumonia-like symptoms and transmitted to humans by infected birds, especially parrots. The clinical manifestations of the disease are extremely variable and resemble a great number of infectious diseases, but fever, cough, anorexia, and severe headache are almost always present. A history of exposure to birds is highly suggestive, because all chlamydiae are difficult to isolate and culture. A demonstrated rise in antibody titer confirms a diagnosis. Tetracycline is usually used to treat psittacosis and is continued for 10 to 14 days after the fever subsides. Isolation is advised. Also called **ornithosis, parrot fever.** See also ***Chlamydia*.**

psoas major /sō′əs/, a long muscle originating from the transverse processes of the lumbar vertebrae and the fibrocartilages and sides of the vertebral bodies of the lower thoracic vertebrae and the lumbar vertebrae. It joins the iliacus to form the iliopsoas deep in the pelvis as it passes under the inguinal ligament and inserts in the lesser trochanter. It acts to flex and laterally rotate the thigh and to flex and laterally bend the spine.

psoas minor, a long, slender muscle of the pelvis, ventral to the psoas major. Many individuals do not have this muscle. It arises from the bodies of the twelfth thoracic and the first lumbar vertebrae and from the disk between them and ends in a long, flat tendon that inserts into the pectineal line of the pelvis and into the iliac fascia. The psoas minor is innervated by a branch of the first lumbar nerve and functions to flex the spine.

psor-, a combining form meaning 'of or related to itching': *psora, psorocomium, psorous.*

psoralen-type photosynthesizer, any one of the chemical compounds that contain photosensitizing psoralen and that react on exposure to ultraviolet light to increase the melanin in the skin. Naturally occurring psoralen photosynthesizers, as 5- and 8-methoxypsoralen, are found in buttercups, carrot greens, celery, clover, cockleburs, dill, figs, limes, parsley, and meadow grass. Some psoralen-type photosynthesizers produced as pharmaceutics are methoxsalen and trioxalen; both are used to enhance skin pigmentation or tanning in the treatment of skin diseases, as psoriasis and vitiligo. Such drugs are carefully administered to avoid oversensitization of the skin and other complications. Psoralen-type photosynthesizers are also used in the manufacture of some perfumes, colognes, and pomades. Such chemicals cause unique skin reactions, as Berlock dermatitis, in some individuals. Oil of bergamot, extracted from the peels of small oranges grown in southern France and Italy, is a photosynthesizing psoralen used as a tea flavoring and in perfumes.

psoriasis /sərī′əsis/, a common, chronic, inheritable skin disorder, characterized by circumscribed red patches covered by thick, dry, silvery, adherent scales that are the result of excessive development of epithelial cells. Exacerbations and remissions are typical. Lesions may be anywhere on the body but are more common on extensor surfaces, bony prominences, scalp, ears, genitalia, and the perianal area. An arthritis, particularly of distal small joints, may accompany the skin disease. Treatment includes topical and intralesional corticosteroids, ultraviolet light, tar solution baths, creams and shampoos, methotrexate, and photochemotherapy. Subcategories of psoriasis include **guttate psoriasis** and **pustular psoriasis.** See also **photochemotherapy, psoriatic arthritis.** **–psoriatic** /sôr′ē•at′ik/, *adj.*

psoriatic arthritis, a form of rheumatoid arthritis associated with psoriatic lesions of the skin and nails, particularly at the distal interphalangeal joints of the fingers and toes.

PSRO, abbreviation for **Professional Standards Review Organization.**

PSS, abbreviation for **progressive systemic sclerosis.**

PSSO, abbreviation for *peer specialist second opinion*.

psych-. See **psycho-.**

psychasthenia. See **obsessive-compulsive neurosis.**

psyche /sī′kē/, **1.** the aspect of one's mental faculty that encompasses the conscious and unconscious processes. **2.** the vital mental or spiritual entity of the individual as opposed to the body or soma. **3.** (in psychoanalysis) the total components of the id, ego, and superego, including all conscious and unconscious aspects. Compare **soma.**

psychedelic /sī′kədel′ik/, **1.** of or describing a mental state characterized by altered sensory perception and hallucination, accompanied by euphoria or fear, usually caused by the deliberate ingestion of drugs or other substances known to produce this effect. **2.** of or describing any drug or substance that causes this state, as mescaline or psilocybin. (The word psychedelic was coined by Humphry Osmond, in 1956.)

psychiatric disorder. See **mental disorder.**

psychiatric emergency service, a hospital service that provides immediate initial evaluation and treatment to acutely disturbed mental patients on a 24-hour-a-day basis.

psychiatric foster care, a service for discharged psychiatric patients who receive observation and care in an approved foster home.

psychiatric home care, a service whereby a discharged psychiatric patient is provided observation and care in his or her place of residence.

psychiatric inpatient unit, a hospital ward or similar area used for the treatment of inpatients who require psychiatric care.

psychiatric nurse practioner, a nurse practitioner who, by advanced study and clinical practice, as in a master's program in psychiatric nursing, has gained expert knowledge in the care and prevention of mental disorders. See also **psychiatric nursing.**

psychiatric nursing, the branch of nursing concerned with the prevention and cure of mental disorders and their sequelae. It employs theories of human behavior as its scientific framework and requires the use of the self as its art or expression in nursing practice. Some of the activities of the psychiatric nurse include the provision of a safe therapeutic milieu; working with patients, or clients, concerning the real day-to-day problems that they face; identifying and caring for the physical aspects of the patient's problems, including drug reactions; assuming the role of social agent or parent for the patient in various recreational, occupational, and social situations; conducting psychotherapy; and providing leadership and clinical assistance for other nurses and health care workers. Psychiatric nurses work in many settings; their responsibilities vary with the setting and with the level of expertise, experience, and training of the individual nurse. Also called **mental health nursing.**

psychiatric social worker. See **psychotherapist, social worker.**

psychiatry, the branch of medical science that deals with the causes, treatment, and prevention of mental, emotional, and behavioral disorders. Some kinds of psychiatry are **community psychiatry, descriptive psychiatry, dynamic psychiatry, existential psychiatry, forensic psychiatry,** and **orthopsychiatry. –psychiatric,** *adj.*

-psychic, a combining form meaning 'relating to the relation between mind and body': *allopsychic, biopsychic, physiopsychic*.

psychic infection /sī′kik/, the spread of neurotic or psychic effects or influences on others on a small scale, as in folie à deux, or on a large scale, as in the dance and witch manias of the Middle Ages or the spread of hysteric or panic reactions in a crowd. Also called **psychic contagion.** See also **sympathy.**

psychic suicide, the termination of one's own life without the use of physical means or agents, as by an older person, widowed after many years of marriage, who becomes sufficiently depressed to lose "the will to live."

psychic trauma, an emotional shock or injury or a distressful situation that produces a lasting impression, especially on the subconscious mind. Common causes of psychic trauma are abuse or neglect in childhood, rape, and loss of a loved one. Psychotherapeutic sessions in which the injured person can ventilate feelings can help alleviate psychic trauma.

psycho-, psych-, a combining form meaning 'of or related to the mind': *psychoauditory, psychodynamics, psycholepsy*.

psychoanalysis, a branch of psychiatry founded by Sigmund Freud devoted to the study of the psychology of human development and behavior. From its systematized method for investigating the processes of the mind evolved a system of psychotherapy based on the concepts of a dynamic unconscious, using such techniques as free association, dream interpretation, and the analysis of defense mechanisms, especially resistance and transference. Through these devices, emotions and behavior are traced to the influence of repressed instinctual drives in the unconscious. Treatment consists of helping the individual become aware of the existence of repressed emotional conflicts, analyzing their origin, and through the process of insight bringing them into the consciousness so that irrational and maladaptive behavior can be altered. See also **psychosexual development.**

psychoanalyst, a psychotherapist, usually a psychiatrist, who has had special training in psychoanalysis and who applies the techniques of psychoanalytic theory. A primary requisite for training is that the candidate also undergo psychoanalysis.

psychoanalytic, **1.** of or pertaining to psychoanalysis.

2. using the techniques or principles of psychoanalysis.

psychobiology, **1.** the study of personality development and functioning in terms of the interaction of the body and the mind. **2.** a school of psychiatric thought introduced by Adolf Meyer that stresses total life experience, including biologic, emotional, and sociocultural factors in assessing the psychologic makeup or mental status of an individual. Mental disorders are interpreted as dynamic adaptive reactions of the individual to stress or conflict, with little or no emphasis placed on unconscious factors. Also called **biopsychology.** See also **distributive analysis and synthesis.**

psychocatharsis. See **catharsis.**

psychodrama, a form of group therapy, originated by J. L. Moreno, in which people act out their emotional problems through dramatization and role playing. Also called **role playing therapy.**

psychogenesis /sī′kōjen′əsis/, **1.** the development of the mind or of a mental function or process. **2.** the development or production of a physical symptom or disease from mental or psychic origins rather than organic factors. **3.** the development of emotional states, either normal or abnormal, from the interaction of conscious and unconscious psychologic forces. Compare **somatogenesis.**

psychogenic /sī′kōjen′ik/, **1.** originating within the mind. **2.** referring to any physical symptom, disease process, or emotional state that is of psychologic rather than physical origin. Also **psychogenetic.** Compare **somatogenic.** See also **psychosomatic.**

psychogenic pain disorder, a disorder characterized by persistent and severe pain for which there is no apparent organic cause. The condition is often accompanied by other sensory or motor dysfunction, as paresthesia or muscle spasm. The cause may be one or many unresolved needs or conflicts. Treatment consists of immediate alleviation of the symptoms followed by long-term psychotherapy aimed at uncovering the unconscious emotional conflicts that influenced the development and maintenance of the pain. See also **psychogenesis.**

psychokinesia /sī′kōkinē′zhə, -kīnē′zhə/, **1.** impulsive, maniacal behavior resulting from deficient or defective inhibitions. **2.** (in parapsychology) psychokinesis.

psychokinesis (PK) /sī′kōkinē′sis, -kīnē′sis/, the alleged direct influence of the mind or will on matter that would result in the production of motion in objects without the intervention of the physical senses or a physical force.

psychokinetics /sī′kōkinet′iks, -kīnet′iks/, the study of psychokinesis.

psychologic test, any of a group of standardized tests designed to measure or ascertain such characteristics of an individual as intellectual capacity, motivation, perception, role behavior, values, level of anxiety or depression, coping mechanisms, and general personality integration. Compare **achievement test, aptitude test, intelligence test, personality test.**

psychologist, a person who specializes in the study of the structure and function of the brain and related mental processes of animals and humans. A clinical psychologist is one who is qualified by graduate degree in psychology and training in clinical psychology and who provides testing and counseling services to patients with mental and emotional disorders.

psychology, **1.** the study of behavior and of the functions and processes of the mind, especially as related to the social and physical environment. **2.** a profession that involves the practical applications of knowledge, skills, and techniques in the understanding of, prevention of, or solution to individual or social problems, especially in regard to the interaction between the individual and the physical and social environment. **3.** the mental, motivational, and behavioral characteristics and attitudes of an individual or group of individuals. Kinds of psychology include **analytic psychology, animal psychology, behaviorism, clinical psychology, cognitive psychology, experimental psychology, humanistic psychology,** and **social psychology.** **–psychologic, psychological,** *adj.*, **psychologically,** *adv.*

psychometrics /sī′kōmet′riks/, the development, administration, or interpretation of psychologic and intelligence tests. Also called **psychometry** /sīkom′ətrē/.

psychomotor, pertaining to or causing voluntary movements usually associated with neural activity.

psychomotor development, the progressive attainment by the child of skills that involve both mental and muscular activity, as the ability of the infant to turn over, sit, or crawl at will and of the toddler to walk, talk, control bladder and bowel functions, and begin solving cognitive problems. The mean chronologic ages at which certain psychomotor skills are attained by most children follow.

12 weeks	looks at own hand.
20 weeks	able to grasp objects voluntarily.
24 weeks	able to roll from back to front at will.
44 weeks	creeps with abdomen off the floor and imitates speech sounds.
15 months	able to walk without help.
24 months	has a vocabulary of 300 or more words and uses pronouns.
30 months	able to jump with both feet.
3 years	able to ride a tricycle and to feed self well.
4 years	able to hop and skip on one foot, catch and throw a ball; is independent, boasts, tattles, and shows off.
5 years	able to tie shoelaces, cut with scissors, tries to please, interested in facts about world, gets along more easily with parents.

psychomotor domain, the area of observable performance of skills that require some degree of neuromuscular coordination.

psychomotor seizure, a temporary impairment of consciousness, often associated with temporal lobe disease and characterized by psychic symptoms, loss of judgment, automatic behavior, and abnormal acts. No apparent convulsions occur, but there may be loss of consciousness or amnesia for the episode. During the seizure the individual may appear drowsy, intoxicated, or violent; asocial acts or crimes may be committed, but normal activities, as driving a car, typing, or eating, may continue at an automatic level. Psychic symptoms, including visual and auditory hallucinations, a sense of unreality, and déjà vu may be present and may be accompanied by visceral symptoms, as chest pain, transient respiratory arrest, tachycardia, and GI discomfort, and by abnormal sensations of smell and taste. Also called **psychomotor epilepsy.**

psychoneurosis. See **neurosis.**

psychoneurotic. See **neurotic.**

psychoneurotic disorder. See **neurotic disorder.**

psychopath /sī′kōpath/, a person who has an antisocial personality disorder. Also called **sociopath.**

psychopathia. See **psychopathy.**

psychopathia sexualis /sī′kōpā′thē·ə sek′sho͞o·al′is/, a mental disease characterized by sexual perversion.

psychopathic /sī′kōpath′ik/, of or pertaining to antisocial behavior. Also **sociopathic.** See also **antisocial personality, antisocial personality disorder.**

psychopathic personality. See **antisocial personality.**

psychopathologist, one who specializes in the study and treatment of mental disorders. **–psychopathology,** *n.*

psychopathology, **1.** the study of the causes, processes, and manifestations of mental disorders. **2.** the behavioral manifestation of any mental disorder.

psychopathy /sīkop′əthē/, any disease of the mind, congenital or acquired, not necessarily associated with subnormal intelligence. Also called **psychopathia.**

psychopharmacology, the scientific study of the effects of drugs on behavior and normal and abnormal mental functions.

psychophylaxis. See **mental hygiene.**

psychophysical preparation for childbirth, a program that prepares women for giving birth by teaching them the physiology of the process, by teaching them exercises to improve muscle tone and physical stamina, and by teaching them various techniques of breathing and relaxation to promote control and comfort during labor and delivery. There are several methods of psychophysical preparation for childbirth. Among the goals of all of the methods are a decrease in the mother's fear and pain, a decrease in or elimination of the use of analgesia and anesthesia in childbirth, and an increase in the mother's participation and cooperation, thus requiring less obstetric intervention. Methods of psychophysical preparation for childbirth include **Bradley method, Lamaze method,** and **Read method.**

psychophysics, the branch of psychology concerned with the relationships between physical stimuli and sensory responses.

psychophysiologic, **1.** of or pertaining to psychophysiology. **2.** having physical symptoms resulting from psychogenic origins; psychosomatic.

psychophysiologic disorder, any of a large group of mental disorders characterized by the dysfunction of an organ or organ system controlled by the autonomic nervous system, as a peptic ulcer, which may be caused or aggravated by emotional factors. The disorders are named and classified according to the organ system involved, such as cardiovascular, respiratory, musculoskeletal, and GI. Also called **psychosomatic illness, psychosomatic reaction.**

psychophysiology, **1.** the study of physiology as it relates to various aspects of psychologic or behavioral function. See also **psychophysiologic disorder.** **2.** the study of mental activity by physical examination and observation.

psychoprophylactic preparation for childbirth, a system of prenatal education for giving birth using the Lamaze method of natural childbirth. See also **psychophysical preparation for childbirth.**

psychosexual, of or pertaining to the psychologic and emotional aspects of sex. See also **psychosexual development, psychosexual disorder.** **–psychosexuality,** *n.*

psychosexual development, (in psychoanalysis) the emergence of the personality through a series of stages from infancy to adulthood, each stage relatively fixed in time and characterized by a dominant mode of achieving libidinal pleasure through the interaction of the person's biologic drives and the restraints of the environment. Resolution of the conflicts encountered at each of the stages theoretically leads to a balanced, heterosexual adjustment and normal development, whereas a lack of resolution results in personality disturbances, fixated at the stage during which the unresolved conflicts occurred. Such disturbances may be latent or may result in various behavioral or personality disorders. The stages of development are the oral stage, anal stage, phallic stage, latency stage, genital stage. Also called **libidinal development.** See also **anal character, oral character, psychomotor development.**

psychosexual disorder, any condition characterized by abnormal sexual attitudes, desires, or activities resulting from psychologic rather than organic causes. See also **gender identity disorder, paraphilia, psychosexual dysfunction.**

psychosexual dysfunction, any of a large group of sexual maladjustments or disorders caused by an emotional or psychologic problem.

psychosis /sīkō′sis/, *pl.* **psychoses,** any major mental disorder of organic or emotional origin characterized by extreme derangement or disorganization of the personality, often accompanied by severe depression, agitation, regressive behavior, illusions, delusions, and hallucinations that so greatly impair perception, thinking, emotional response, and personal orientation that the individual loses touch with reality, is incapable of functioning normally in society, and usually requires hospitalization. Kinds of psychoses include **affective psychosis, alcoholic psychosis, bipolar disorder, Korsakoff's psychosis, paranoia, schizophrenia,** and **senile psychosis.** See also **major affective disorder, organic mental disorder.**

-psychosis, a combining form meaning a 'serious mental disorder': *autopsychosis, encephalopsychosis, pharmacopsychosis*.

psychosocial assessment, an evaluation of a person's mental health, social status, and functional capacity within the community. See also Appendix 10: Mental Health.

■ METHOD: The person's physical status, appearance, and modes of behavior are observed for factors that may indicate or contribute to emotional distress or mental illness. Posture, facial expressions, manner of dress, speech and thought patterns, degree of motor activity, and level of consciousness are noted. The person is questioned concerning patterns of daily living, including work schedule and social and leisure activites. Pertinent background data include a history of any previous psychiatric problems, the person's response to and methods of coping with stress, relationships, cultural orientation, and any significant life changes, such as serious illnesses, unemployment or change of employment, change of residence, marriage, divorce, or death of a loved one. Various guides for assessing mental health, the family process, and group process are available for determining the person's psychocultural perceptions and orientations concerning health and illness and for evaluating self-image and self-esteem, goals, values, beliefs, and relationships.

■ NURSING ORDERS: The nurse may conduct the interview to obtain the pertinent background information and subjective data necessary for assessing the status of the person's mental health.

■ OUTCOME CRITERIA: A careful assessment of mental health and psychosocial development is an important aid for identifying high-risk factors that may contribute to or precipitate the development of mental illness and for determining the need for intervention when such factors are present.

psychosocial development, (in child development) a description devised by Erik Erikson of the normal serial development of trust, autonomy, identity, and intimacy; the development begins in infancy and progresses as the infantile ego interacts with the environment. For the child to reach a new stage, the preceding one must be fully realized. The sequence and chronology of the stages coincide with the psychosexual stages of development as described by Freud.

psychosomatic /sī'kōsəmat'ik/, **1.** of or pertaining to psychosomatic medicine. **2.** relating to, characterized by, or resulting from the interaction of the mind or psyche and the body. **3.** the expression of an emotional conflict through physical symptoms. See also **psychogenic, psychophysiologic disorder.**

psychosomatic approach, the interdisciplinary or holistic study of physical and mental disease from a biologic, psychosocial, and sociocultural point of view.

psychosomatic illness. See **psychophysiological disorder.**

psychosomatic medicine, the branch of medicine concerned with the interrelationships between mental and emotional reactions and somatic processes, in particular the manner in which intrapsychic conflicts influence physical symptoms. It maintains that the body and mind are one inseparable entity and that both physiologic and psychologic techniques should be applied in the study and treatment of illness. Also called **psychosomatics.**

psychosomatic reaction. See **psychophysiologic disorder.**

psychosomatics. See **psychosomatic medicine.**

psychosomatogenic, pertaining to factors that cause or lead to the development of psychophysiologic coping measures as learned responses to stressors.

psychosurgery, surgical interruption of certain nerve pathways in the brain, performed to treat selected cases of chronic, unremitting anxiety, agitation, or obsessional neuroses when the condition is severe and when alternative treatments, as psychotherapy, drugs, and electroshock, have proven ineffective. The procedure may be a limited prefrontal lobotomy, in which connecting fibers in the frontal region are cut, or a modified bifrontal tractotomy, in which nerve tracts of the brainstem are severed. Light general anesthesia is given. Postoperative nursing care includes observation for signs of leakage of cerebrospinal fluid. A marked alteration of personality is unavoidable. Various cognitive and affective functions are also affected, depending on the location of the induced lesion, the extent of destruction of nerve tissue, and the age, sex, and condition of the patient. Modern psychotherapeutic drugs have replaced psychosurgery in most cases.

psychotherapeutics, the treatment of personality disorders by means of psychotherapy.

psychotherapist, one who practices psychotherapy, including psychiatrists, licensed psychologists, psychiatric nurses, psychiatric social workers, and persons trained in counseling. The specific requirements for education and training differ markedly in content, breadth, and duration, depending on the form of psychotherapy practiced. Licensing procedures and definitions of practice vary from state to state. Compare **psychoanalyst.**

psychotherapy, any of a large number of related methods of treating mental and emotional disorders by psychologic techniques rather than by physical means. Included among these techniques, which are used either with individuals or with groups, are reinforcement, persuasion, suggestion, reassurance, support, and abreaction. Some of the aims of psychotherapy are to change maladaptive behavioral patterns, improve interpersonal relationships, resolve inner conflicts that cause personal distress, modify inaccurate assumptions about the self and the environment, and foster a definite sense of self-identity to promote individual growth leading to a more meaningful and fulfilling existence. Kinds of psychotherapy are **behavior therapy, group therapy, humanistic existential therapy, interpersonal therapy,** and **psychoanalysis.**

psychotic /sīkot′ik/, **1.** of or pertaining to psychosis. **2.** a person exhibiting the characteristics of a psychosis.

psychotic disorder. See **psychosis.**

psychotic insight, a stage in the development of a psychosis that follows an intitial experience of confusion, bizarreness, and apprehension. At this point, an insight is reached that enables the patient to interpret the external world in terms of a delusional system of thinking. With the new insight, the factors that had previously been confusing become a part of the systematized pattern of the delusion, which, although irrational to an observer, is perceived by the patient as the attainment of exceptionally lucid thinking.

psychotic reaction. See **psychosis.**

psychotropic, exerting an effect on the mind or modifying mental activity.

psychotropic drugs, drugs that affect the psychic functions, behavior, or experience of a person using them.

psychro-, a combining form meaning 'of or pertaining to cold': *psychrometer, psychrophilic, psychrophore.*

psyllium seed. See **plantago seed.**

Pt, symbol for **platinum.**

PT, 1. abbreviation for **physical therapist. 2.** abbreviation for **physical therapy. 3.** abbreviation for **prothrombin time.**

PTA, abbreviation for **plasma thromboplastin antecedent.**

PTCA, abbreviation for **percutaneous transluminal coronary angioplasty.**

pteroylglutamic acid. See **folic acid.**

pterygium /tərij′ē·əm/, a thick, triangular bit of pale tissue that extends medially from the nasal border of the cornea to the inner canthus of the eye.

-pterygium, a combining form meaning a '(specified) abnormality of the conjunctiva': *loxopterygium, pimelopterygium, symblepharopterygium.*

pterygoideus lateralis /ter′igoi′dē·əs/, one of the four muscles of mastication. Extending almost horizontally from the infratemporal fossa and the condyle of the mandible, it is a short, thick, somewhat conical muscle, arising by two heads from the great wing of the sphenoid, the infratemporal crest, and the lateral pterygoid plate. It inserts into the condyle of the mandible and into the articular disk of the temporomandibular articulation. The pterygoideus lateralis is innervated by the lateral pterygoid nerve and functions to open the jaws, protrude the mandible, and move the mandible from side to side. Also called **external pterygoid muscle.** Compare **masseter, pterygoideus medialis, temporalis.**

pterygoideus medialis, one of the four muscles of mastication. Arising from the pyramidal process of the palatine bone and from the tuberosity of the maxilla and inserting into the medial surface of the ramus of the mandible, it is innervated by the medial pterygoid nerve and acts to close the jaws. Also called **internal pterygoid muscle.** Compare **masseter, pterygoideus lateralis, temporalis.**

pterygoid plexus /tur′igoid/, one of a pair of extensive networks of veins between the temporalis and the pterygoideus lateralis, extending between surrounding structures in the infratemporal fossa. The plexus receives deoxygenated blood from various tributaries that correspond with branches of the maxillary artery; it communicates with the cavernous sinus through the foramen of Vesalius and with the facial vein through the deep facial and angular veins. Compare **maxillary vein.**

pterygomaxillary notch, a fissure at the junction of the maxilla and the pterygoid process of the sphenoid bone.

PTNA, abbreviation for **Provincial Territorial Nurses' Association.**

ptoma-, a combining form meaning 'of or related to a corpse': *ptomaine, ptomatopsia, ptomatopsy.*

ptomaine /tō′mān/, an imprecise term introduced in the nineteenth century to identify a group of nitrogenous substances found in putrified proteins. Because injection of the substances produced toxic reactions, the amines were once regarded as poisonous. Later studies showed the same substances were produced by the normal digestion of proteins in the human intestine without toxic effects.

ptosis /tō′sis/, an abnormal condition of one or both upper eyelids in which the eyelid droops because of a congenital or acquired weakness of the levator muscle or paralysis of the third cranial nerve. Partial ptosis and a small pupil may be caused by an unusual hemologic disorder of the sympathetic portion of the autonomic nervous system. The condition may be treated surgically by shortening the levator muscle.

-ptosis, a combining form meaning a 'prolapse of an organ': *esophagoptosis, hepatoptosis, uvulaptosis.*

ptotic kidney /tō′tik/, a kidney that is abnormally situated in the pelvis, usually over the sacral promontory behind the peritoneum. The condition of having a ptotic kidney may be either congenital or secondary to trauma. It is usually asymptomatic, but pregnancy may result in obstruction of the flow of urine from the kidney.

PTT. See **partial thromboplastin time.**

ptyalin /tī′əlin/, a starch-digesting enzyme present in saliva. Also called **amylase.**

ptyalism /tī′əliz′əm/, excessive salivation, as sometimes occurs in the early months of pregnancy. It is also a clinical sign of mercury poisoning. Also called **hyperptyalism.** See also **sialorrhea.**

ptyalo-, a combining form meaning 'of or related to the saliva': *ptyalocele, ptyalogenic, ptyalography.*

-ptysis, a combining form meaning a 'spitting of matter': *albuminoptysis, hemoptysis, plasmoptysis.*

Pu, symbol for **plutonium.**

pub-, pubo-, a combining form meaning 'adult': *puberal, puberty, pubescence.*

pubarche /pyōōbär′kē, pyōō′bärkē/, the onset of puberty, marked by the beginning of the development of secondary sexual characteristics.

puberty, the period of life at which the ability to reproduce begins.

puberulic acid /pyōōber′yōōlik/, an antibiotic isolated from the mold *Penicillium puberulum* that prevents the replication of gram-positive bacteria.

-pubic, a combining form meaning 'of, referring, or relating to the frontal part of the pelvis': *iliopubic, retropubic, vesicopubic.*

pubic bone. See **pubis.**

pubic region, the most inferior part of the abdomen in the lower zone between the right and left inguinal regions and below the umbilical region. Also called **hypogastric region, hypogastrium.** See also **abdominal regions.**

pubic symphysis, the slightly movable interpubic joint of the pelvis, consisting of two pubic bones separated by a disk of fibrocartilage and connected by two ligaments. Also called **symphysis pubis.**

pubis /pyōō′bis/, *pl.* **pubes,** one of a pair of pubic bones that, with the ischium and the ilium, form the hip bone and join the pubic bone from the opposite side at the pubic symphysis. The pubis forms one fifth of the acetabulum and is divisible into the body, the superior ramus, and the inferior ramus. The external surface of the pubis is rough and serves as the origin of the adductor longus, the obturator externus, the adductor brevis, and the proximal part of the gracilis. The internal surface of the pubis is smooth; it forms part of the anterior wall of the pelvis, giving origin to the levator ani and the obturator internus, and attachment to the puboprostatic ligaments and a few muscular fibers from the bladder. The pubic crest affords attachment to the rectus abdominis, the pyramidalis, and the inguinal falx. The lateral portion of the superior ramus of the pubis presents the superior, the inferior, and the dorsal surfaces. The superior surface presents the iliopectineal line, and the inferior ramus gives origin to the gracilis, a portion of the obturator externus, the adductor brevis, the adductor magnus, the obturator internus, and the constrictor urethrae. Compare **ilium, ischium.**

public health, a field of medicine that deals with the physical and mental health of the community, particularly in such areas as water supply, waste disposal, air pollution, and food safety. In the United States, there are more than 3000 state, county, or city public health agencies. The U.S. Public Health Service was organized originally in 1798 to provide hospital care for American merchant seamen. Subsequent legislation has expanded the role of the federal agency to include such services as the Food and Drug Administration, the National Library of Medicine, and health care for Native Americans and Alaska Natives, protection against impure and unsafe foods, drugs, cosmetics and medical devices, control of alcohol and drug abuse, and protection against unsafe radiation-producing projects.

public health nursing, a field of nursing that is concerned with the health needs of the community as a whole. Public health nurses may work with families in the home, in schools, at the workplace, in government agencies, and at major health facilities. A home care nursing service is provided by nurses who have special training in public health and are employed by such voluntary agencies as the Visiting Nurses Association or Visiting Nurse Service. Public health nurses enter practice through a baccalaureate program accredited by the National League for Nursing, which prepares the nurse to work as a generalist. Additional recognition is offered through a certification program sponsored by the Division of Community Health Nursing of the American Nurses' Association (ANA).

publish or perish, *informal.* a practice followed in many academic institutions in which a contract for employment is renewed at the same or higher rank only if a candidate has demonstrated scholarship and professional status by having had work published in a book or in a reputable, usually national, professional journal. This work is in addition to whatever obligations for teaching or professional practice are entailed by the position.

pubococcygeus exercises /pyōō′bōkoksij′ē·əs/, a regimen of isometric exercises in which a woman executes a series of voluntary contractions of the muscles of her pelvic diaphragm and perineum in an effort to increase the contractility of her vaginal introitus or to improve her retention of urine. Also called **Kegel exercises.**

■ METHOD: The exercise involves the familiar muscular squeezing action that is required to stop the urinary stream while voiding; that action is performed in an intensive, repetitive, and systematic way throughout each day.

■ NURSING ORDERS: The woman is instructed in how to duplicate the squeezing, pulling-up action. A woman whose muscles are particularly attenuated may have difficulty understanding or feeling the muscular action involved. It is often helpful for her to be told that the action is exactly the same as that required to stop the flow of urine. When the woman can effect the contraction required, she is asked to hold the contraction for 6 to 10 seconds, allowing the muscles to relax completely between contractions. She is then advised to perform four to six repetitions of the contraction in a series and to repeat the series three to four times each day. She is further advised that the physiology of muscular exercise is such that weakened muscles may make gains in strength during the early phases of an exercise program, and that, with diligence, she can expect to notice significant improvement in control that will continue as she maintains the regimen of exercise.

■ OUTCOME CRITERIA: Laxity and weakness of the pubococcygeus muscles, often a result of childbirth, may predispose certain women to looseness of the vaginal introitus and to stress incontinence. These problems may be ameliorated as the strength and tone of the muscles are increased through exercise. The rapidity with which a woman can, during voiding, close off the urinary stream is taken as a measure of the strength and tone of her pubococcygeus muscles. Ideally, she should be able to perform the action completely and almost instantly.

pudendal. See **pudendum.**

pudendal block, a form of regional anesthetic block administered to relieve the discomfort of the expulsive second stage of labor. The pudendal nerves are anesthetized by the injection of a local anesthetic in the trunk of each nerve as it passes over the sacrospinous ligament, just below the ischial spine. A 10 ml syringe, a long needle, and a guide are used in the procedure. The injection is most easily performed transvaginally; the transperitoneal approach is technically more difficult and is more uncomfortable for the woman. Pudendal block anesthetizes the perineum, vulva, clitoris, labia majora, and the perirectal area without affecting the muscular contractions of the uterus. When the block is properly administered, the risk is minimal.

pudendal canal. See **Alcock's canal.**

pudendal nerve, one of the branches of the pudendal plexus that arises from the second, third, and fourth sacral nerves, passes between the piriformis and coccygeus, and leaves the pelvis through the greater sciatic foramen. It crosses the spine of the ischium and reenters the pelvis through the lesser sciatic foramen. It accompanies the internal pudendal vessels through a fascial tunnel along the lateral wall of the ischiorectal fossa and divides into two terminal branches near the urogenital diaphragm. The branches of the pudendal nerve are the inferior rectal nerve, perineal nerve, and dorsal nerve of the penis or of the clitoris. See also **pudendal plexus.**

pudendal plexus, a network of motor and sensory nerves formed by the anterior branches of the second, the third, and all of the fourth sacral nerves. It is often considered part of the sacral plexus. The pudendal plexus lies in the posterior hollow of the pelvis, on the ventral surface of the piriformis. The branches of the plexus are the visceral branches, the muscular branches, and the pudendal nerve. The visceral branches arise from the second, third, and fourth sacral nerves and supply the bladder, prostate, seminal vesicles, uterus, external genitalia, and some of the intestinal tract. The muscular branches arise from the fourth, and, sometimes, the third and fifth sacral nerves and supply the levator ani, sphincter ani, and coccygeus. The pudendal nerve arises from the second, third, and fourth sacral nerves and divides into five branches supplying the genital structures and the pelvic region. Compare **lumbar plexus, sacral plexus.**

pudendum /pyo͞oden′dəm/, *pl.* **pudenda,** the external genitalia, especially of women. In a woman it comprises the mons veneris, the labia majora, the labia minora, the vestibule of the vagina, and the vestibular glands. In a man it comprises the penis, scrotum, and testes. –**pudendal,** *adj.*

puer-, a combining form meaning 'child': *puericulture, puerilism, puerperium.*

puericulture /pyo͞o′ərikul′chər/, the rearing and training of children. –**puericulturist,** *n.*

puerile /pyo͞o′əril, -īl/, of or pertaining to children or childhood; juvenile. –**puerility,** *n.*

puerperal /pyo͞o·ur′pərəl/, **1.** of or pertaining to the period immediately after childbirth. **2.** of or pertaining to a woman (puerpera) who has just given birth to an infant.

puerperal endometritis. See **puerperal fever.**

puerperal fever, a syndrome associated with systemic bacterial infection and septicemia that occurs after childbirth, usually as a result of unsterile obstetric technique. It is characterized by endometritis, fever, tachycardia, uterine tenderness, and foul lochia; if untreated, prostration, renal failure, bacteremic shock, and death may occur. The causative organism is most often one of the hemolytic streptococci. Puerperal fever was little known before hospital childbirth became common, early in the nineteenth century; but then it became an endemic and frequently epidemic scourge that resulted in the deaths of many thousands of mothers and infants. Maternal mortality rates of 20% and higher were common in parts of the world where childbirth occurred in hospitals. Ignaz Philipp Semmelweis, in Vienna, noted that women attended by midwives were much less likely to contract the disease than those attended by physicians and medical students. Midwives did not perform frequent vaginal examinations during labor and did not participate in autopsies. Though the germ theory of disease had not yet been elaborated, Semmelweis deduced that the causative agent of the disease was being transmitted by doctors and students from the infected cadavers in the autopsy room to women in labor on the maternity wards. By instituting a policy requiring that the hands and instruments of obstetric attendants be disinfected, maternal mortality in his clinic dropped dramatically. His work was widely ignored or discredited for almost half a century because physicians were unwilling to believe that they were the agents of transmission. Late in the nineteenth century, after Pasteur's discovery of microbes, Semmelweis was posthumously vindicated. Sterile techniques were gradually instituted, but not until the fourth decade of the twentieth century did puerperal fever cease to be the leading cause of maternal death. Postpartum uterine infection is common but is effectively treated with massive parenteral doses of antibiotics before it becomes a systemic illness. Also called **childbed fever, puerperal sepsis.**

puerperal mania, a rare, acute mood disorder that sometimes occurs in women after childbirth, characterized by a severe manic reaction. See also **mania.**

puerperal metritis. See **puerperal fever.**

puerperal sepsis, an infection acquired during the puerperium.

puerperium /pyo͞o′ərpir′ē·əm/, the time after childbirth, lasting approximately 6 weeks, during which the anatomic and physiologic changes brought about by pregnancy resolve, and a woman adjusts to the new or expanded responsibilities of motherhood and nonpregnant life.

Pulex /pyōō′leks/, a genus of fleas some species of which transmit arthropod-borne infections, as plague and epidemic typhus.

pulmo-, pulmon-, a combining form meaning 'of or pertaining to the lungs': *pulmogram, pulmolith, pulmometer*.

pulmonary /pŏŏl′məner′ē/, of or pertaining to the lungs or the respiratory system. Also **pulmonic** /pŏŏlmon′ik/.

pulmonary acid aspiration syndrome. See **Mendelson's syndrome.**

pulmonary alveolus, one of the numerous terminal air sacs in the lungs in which oxygen and carbon monoxide are exchanged.

pulmonary anthrax. See **woolsorter's disease.**

pulmonary arteriolar resistance (PAR), pressure loss per unit of blood flow from the pulmonary artery to a pulmonary vein.

pulmonary atrium, any of the spaces at the end of an alveolar duct into which alveoli open.

pulmonary carcinosis. See **alveolar cell carcinoma.**

pulmonary compliance, a measure of the elasticity or expansibility of the lungs.

pulmonary disease, an abnormal condition of the respiratory system, characterized by cough, chest pain, dyspnea, hemoptysis, sputum production, stridor, and wheezing. Less common symptoms may be anxiety, arm and shoulder pain, tenderness in the calf of the leg, erythema nodosum, swelling of the face, headache, hoarseness, pain in the joints, and somnolence. Diagnostic procedures used for pulmonary diseases include bronchoscopy, cytologic, serologic, and biochemical examination of bronchial secretions, laryngoscopy, pulmonary function tests, and radiography. Pulmonary diseases are either obstructive or restrictive. Obstructive respiratory diseases are the result of an obstacle in the airway that impedes the flow of air, especially during expiration. Such obstructions may be bronchospasm, edema of the bronchial mucosa, loss of lung elasticity, or thick bronchial secretions. Obstructive diseases are characterized by reduced expiratory flow rates and increased total lung capacities. Acute obstructive respiratory diseases include asthma, bronchitis, and bronchiolitis; chronic conditions are combinations of emphysema and bronchitis. Patients with obstructive diseases may have acute failure from any respiratory stress, as infections or general anesthesia. Restrictive respiratory diseases are caused by conditions that limit lung expansion by an actual reduction of the volume of inspired air, as fibrothorax, a neuromuscular disorder, kyphosis, scoliosis, spondylitis, or surgical removal of lung tissue. Characteristic features of restrictive respiratory diseases are decreased forced vital capacity and total lung capacity, with increased work of breathing and inefficient exchange of gases. Acute restrictive conditions are the most common pulmonary cause of acute respiratory failure.

pulmonary edema, the accumulation of extravascular fluid in lung tissues and alveoli, caused most commonly by congestive heart failure and also occurring in barbiturate and opiate poisoning, diffuse infections, hemorrhagic pancreatitis, renal failure, and after a stroke, skull fracture, near drowning, the inhalation of irritating gases, and the rapid administration of whole blood, plasma, serum albumin, or intravenous fluids. In congestive heart disease serous fluid is pushed back through the pulmonary capillaries into alveoli and quickly enters bronchioles and bronchi.

■ OBSERVATIONS: The patient with pulmonary edema breathes rapidly and shallowly with difficulty, is usually restless, apprehensive, hoarse, pale, or cyanotic, and may cough up frothy, pink sputum. The peripheral and neck veins are usually engorged; the blood pressure and heart rate are increased; and the pulse may be full and pounding or weak and thready. There may be edema of the extremities, rales in the lungs, respiratory acidosis, and profuse diaphoresis.

■ INTERVENTION: Acute pulmonary edema is an emergency requiring prompt treatment. The patient is placed in bed in a high Fowler's position, and the immediate administration of intravenous morphine sulfate is usually ordered to relieve pain, to quiet breathing, and to allay apprehension. A cardiotonic, often digitalis, a fast-acting diuretic, often furosemide or ethacrynic acid, and a bronchodilator, often aminophylline, may be given, and intermittent positive pressure breathing (IPPB) of humidified oxygen may be ordered. IPPB decreases the passage of fluid in the alveoli by exerting counterpressure on alveolar capillaries and decreases venous return to the heart by increasing pleural pressure. The use of rotating tourniquets may be ordered to pool blood in the extremities to reduce the load on the heart. The tourniquets usually are placed on three extremities at one time and are so rotated that each of the four extremities is occluded for 45 minutes of every hour in which this kind of therapy is given. While the patient is acutely ill, the blood pressure, respiration, apical pulse, and breath sounds are checked every hour or continually monitored. Parenteral fluids, if indicated, are infused slowly in limited quantities; a low-sodium diet is served; and the patient's intake and output of fluids are measured. The patient is weighed daily, and any sudden gain is noted and reported.

■ NURSING CONSIDERATIONS: In addition to providing continued care and emotional support, the nurse teaches the patient to exercise to tolerance, plan frequent rest periods, report any symptoms, avoid smoking, and follow the regimen ordered for medication, diet, and return checkups.

pulmonary embolism (PE), the blockage of a pulmonary artery by foreign matter as fat, air, tumor tissue, or a thrombus that usually arises from a peripheral vein. Predisposing factors include an alteration of blood constituents with increased coagulation, damage to blood vessel walls, and stagnation or immobilization, especially when associated with childbirth, congestive heart failure, polycythemia vera, or surgery. Pulmonary embolism is difficult to distinguish from myocardial infarction and pneumonia. It is characterized by dyspnea, sudden chest pain, shock, and cyanosis. Pulmonary infarction, which often occurs within 6 to 24 hours after the formation of a pulmonary embolus, is further characterized by pleural effusion, hemoptysis, leukocytosis, fever, tachycardia and atrial arrhythmias, and a striking distention of the neck veins. Analysis of blood gases reveals arterial hypoxia and reduced arterial carbon dioxide tension. Pulmonary embolism is detected by chest x-ray films, pulmonary angiography, and radioscanning of the lung fields. Two thirds of patients with a massive pulmonary embolus die within 2 hours. Initial resuscitative measures include external cardiac massage, oxygen, vasopressor drugs, embolectomy, and correction of acidosis. The formation of further emboli is prevented by the use of anticoagulants, and, sometimes, streptokinase or urokinase. Ambulation, exercise, and electric stimulation of the calf muscles are also recommended.

pulmonary emphysema, a chronic obstructive disease of the lungs, marked by an overdistention of the alveoli.

pulmonary function laboratory, an area of a hospital or other health facility used for examination and evaluation of patients' respiratory functions, using electromechanic and other devices.

pulmonary function test (PFT), a procedure for determining the capacity of the lungs to exchange oxygen and carbon dioxide efficiently. There are two general kinds of respiratory function tests. One measures ventilation, or the ability of the bellows action of the chest and lungs to move gas in and out of alveoli; the other kind measures the diffusion of gas across the alveolar capillary membrane and the perfusion of the lungs by blood. Efficient gas exchange in the lungs requires a balanced ventilation-perfusion ratio, with areas receiving ventilation well perfused and areas receiving blood flow capable of ventilation. Basic ventilation studies are performed with a spirometer and recording device as the patient breathes through a mouthpiece and connecting tube; a nose clip prevents nasal breathing. Measurements or calculations are made of the tidal volume (TV), or gas inspired and expired in a normal breath; the inspiratory reserve volume (IRV), or the maximal volume that can be inspired after a normal respiration; the expiratory reserve volume (ERV), or the maximal volume that can be expired forcefully after a normal expiration; the residual volume (RV), or the gas remaining in the lungs after maximal expiration; and the minute volume, or the gas inspired and expired in 1 minute of normal breathing. The vital capacity of the lungs is equal to TV + IRV + ERV and the total lung capacity to TV + IRV + ERV + RV. The forced expiratory volume (FEV), or the amount of air forcibly expelled in the first second after a maximal inspiration, and the maximal breathing capacity (MBC), or the amount of gas exchanged per minute with maximal rate and depth of respiration, have special clinical significance. Bronchospirometric measurements of the ventilation and oxygen consumption of each lung separately are performed using a specially constructed double-lumen catheter with two balloons; one balloon is inflated to seal off the contralateral lung when the other lung is tested. Arterial blood gas studies, including determinations of the acidity, partial pressure of carbon dioxide and of oxygen, and the oxyhemoglobin saturation, provide information on the diffusion of gas across the alveolar capillary membrane and the adequacy of oxygenation of tissues.

pulmonary infiltrate with eosinophilia. See **P.I.E.**

pulmonary hypertension, a condition of abnormally high pressure within the pulmonary circulation.

pulmonary stenosis, an abnormal cardiac condition, generally characterized by concentric hypertrophy of the right ventricle with relatively little increase in diastolic volume. When the ventricular septum is intact, this condition may be caused by valvular stenosis, by infundibular stenosis, or by both; it produces a pressure difference during systole between the right ventricular cavity and the pulmonary artery. Pulmonary stenosis is most often congenital but may also be produced after birth by any of a number of types of lesions. Severe pulmonary stenosis may result in heart failure and death, but mild to moderate forms of this disorder are relatively well tolerated by some individuals. Also called **pulmonic stenosis.** See also **congenital cardiac anomaly, valvular heart disease, valvular stenosis.**

pulmonary sulcus tumor, a destructive, invasive neoplasm that develops at the apex of the lung and infiltrates the ribs, vertebrae, and the brachial plexus. Also called **Pancoast's tumor.**

pulmonary surfactant, a surfactant agent found in the lungs that functions to reduce the surface tension of the fluid on the surface of the cells of the lower respiratory system, enhancing the elasticity of the alveoli and bronchioles and thus the exchange of gases in the lungs.

pulmonary trunk, the short, wide vessel that conveys venous blood from the right ventricle of the heart to the lungs. It is approximately 5 cm long and 3 cm in diameter, and it ascends obliquely, dividing into right and left branches.

pulmonary tuberculosis. See **tuberculosis.**

pulmonary valve, a cardiac structure composed of three semilunar cusps that close during each heartbeat to prevent blood from flowing back into the right ventricle from the pulmonary artery. The cusps are separated by sinuses that resemble tiny buckets when they are closed and filled with blood. These flaps grow from the lining of the pulmonary artery and, when they collapse from the inflow of ventricular blood, open the valve and allow deoxygenated blood to flow through the pulmonary artery and on to the lungs. Compare **aortic valve, mitral valve, tricuspid valve.**

pulmonary vascular resistance (PVR), the resistance in the pulmonary vascular bed against which the right ventricle must eject blood.

pulmonary vein, one of a pair of large vessels that return oxygenated blood from each lung to the left atrium of the heart. The right pulmonary veins pass dorsal to the right atrium and the superior vena cava. The left pulmonary veins pass ventral to the descending thoracic aorta. Compare **pulmonary trunk.**

pulmonary wedge pressure (PWP), the pressure produced by an inflated latex balloon against a pulmonary artery, as part of a procedure used in the diagnosis of congestive heart failure, myocardial infarction, and other conditions. A Swan-Ganz catheter, or similar balloon-tipped catheter, is inserted through a subclavian, jugular, or femoral vein to the vena cava and on through the right atrium and ventricle to the pulmonary artery. When the balloon is inflated, it can continuously measure pulmonary pressure, which is recorded by bedside instruments.

pulmonary Wegener's granulomatosis, a rare, fatal disease of young or middle-aged men, characterized by granulomatous lesions of the respiratory tract, focal necrotizing arteritis, and, finally, widespread inflammation of body organs. Pulmonary infarction and glomerulonephritis may occur.

pulmonic. See **pulmonary.**

-pulmonic. a combining form meaning 'relating to the lungs': *apulmonic, gastropulmonic, intrapulmonic*.

pulmonic stenosis. See **pulmonary stenosis.**

pulp, any soft, spongy tissue, as that contained within the spleen, the pulp chamber of the tooth, or the distal phalanges of the fingers and the toes. **–pulpy,** *adj.*

pulp canal, the space occupied by the pulp in the radicular portion of the tooth. Also called **root canal.**

pulp cavity, the space in a tooth bounded by the dentin and containing the dental pulp. It is divided into the pulp chamber and the pulp or root canal.

pulpitis /pulpī′tis/, infection or inflammation of the dental pulp. See also **caries.**

pulpless tooth, a tooth in which the dental pulp is necrotic or has been removed. Also called **devital tooth,**

pulp stone. See **denticle.**

pulsatile, pertaining to an activity characterized by a rhythmic pulsation.

pulsatile assist device (PAD), a flexible valveless balloon conduit contained within a rigid plastic cylinder that is inserted into the arterial circulation to provide pulsatile cardiopulmonary bypass perfusion.

pulse, **1.** a rhythmic beating or vibrating movement. **2.** a brief electromagnetic wave. **3.** the regular, recurrent expansion and contraction of an artery produced by waves of pressure caused by the ejection of blood from the left ventricle of the heart as it contracts. The phenomenon is easily detected on superficial arteries, as the radial and carotid arteries, and corresponds to each beat of the heart. The normal number of pulse beats per minute in the average adult varies from 60 to 80, with fluctuations occurring with exercise, injury, illness, and emotional reactions. The average pulse rate for a newborn is 120 beats per minute, which slows throughout childhood and adolescence. Girls, beginning about 12 years of age, and women have a higher rate than boys and men.

pulse deficit, a condition that exists when the radial pulse is less than the ventricular rate as auscultated at the apex or seen on the electrocardiogram. The condition indicates a lack of peripheral perfusion for some of the heart contractions.

pulseless disease. See **Takayasu's arteritis.**

pulse NMR, NMR techniques that use radiofrequency pulses and Fourier transformation of the NMR signal. Pulse NMR has largely replaced the older continuous wave techniques.

pulse point, any one of the sites on the surface of the body where arterial pulsations can be easily palpated. The most commonly used pulse point is over the radial artery at the wrist. Other pulse points are over the temporal artery in front of the ear, over the common carotid artery at the lower level of the thyroid cartilage, and over the facial artery at the lower margin of the jaw.

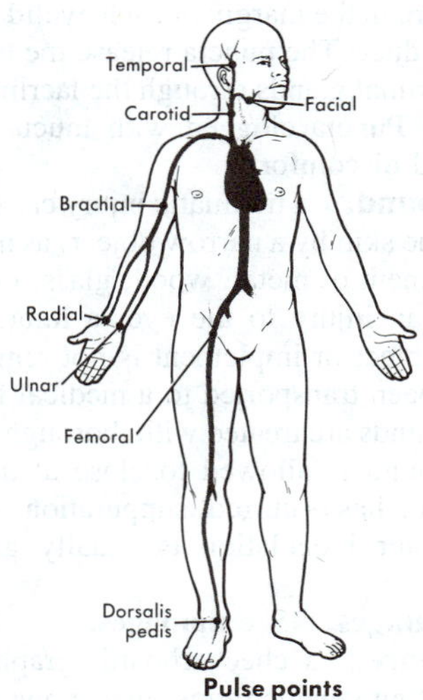

Pulse points

pulse pressure, the difference between the systolic and diastolic pressures, normally 30 to 40 mm Hg.

-pulsion, a combining form meaning the 'action or condition of pushing': *compulsion, lateropulsion, retropulsion*.

pulsus alternans /pul′səs ôl′tərnanz/, a pulse characterized by a regular alternation of weak and strong beats without changes in the length of the cycle. Also called **alternating pulse.**

pulsus paradoxus, an abnormal decrease in systolic pressure and pulse wave amplitude during inspiration. The normal fall in pressure is less than 10 mm Hg, and an excessive decline may be a sign of precardial tamponade, adhesive pericarditis, severe lung disease, advanced heart failure, and other conditions. Also called **paradoxical pulse.**

pulvule, a proprietary capsule containing a dose of a drug in powder form.

pump, **1.** an apparatus used to move fluids or gases by suction or by positive pressure, as an infusion pump or stomach pump. **2.** a physiologic mechanism by which a substance is moved, usually by active transport across a cell membrane, as a sodium pump. **3.** to move a liquid or gas by suction or positive pressure.

pump lung. See **congestive atelectasis.**

punch biopsy, the removal of living tissue for microscopic examination, usually bone marrow from the sternum, by means of a punch.

punch forceps, a surgical instrument used to cut out a disk of dense or resistant tissue, as bone and cartilage. The ends of the blades of the punch forceps are perforated to grip the involved tissue. There are several varieties of this instrument, with blades and tips specially designed for different surgical needs.

punct-, a combining form meaning 'a point, or like a point': *punctate, punctiform, punctograph.*

punctum lacrimale /pungk′təm/, *pl.* **puncta lacrimalia,** a tiny aperture in the margin of each eyelid that opens into the lacrimal duct. The puncta release the tears that travel from the lacrimal glands through the lacrimal ducts to the conjunctiva. Puncta clogged with mucus or dirt cause irritation and discomfort.

puncture wound, a traumatic injury caused by the penetration of the skin by a narrow object, as a knife, nail, or slender fragment of metal, wood, glass, or other material. In such an injury to the eye, a lung, or a visceral organ, the object or implement is not removed until the person has been transported to a medical facility. Minor puncture wounds are treated with thorough cleansing. If a puncture wound is allowed to close at the skin before deeper healing has occurred, suppuration often results. A tetanus booster inoculation is usually given for such wounds.

punitive damages. See **damages.**

Punnett square, a checkerboard, graphlike diagram, used in charting genetic ratios, that shows all of the possible combinations of male and female gametes when one or more pairs of independent alleles are crossed. Letters representing the male gametes are placed along the Y-axis and those of the female along the X-axis, with the results of the various crossings occupying the squares in a geometric pattern. See also **pedigree.**

pupil, a circular opening in the iris of the eye, located slightly to the nasal side of the center of the iris. The pupil lies behind the anterior chamber of the eye and the cornea and in front of the lens. Its diameter changes with contraction and relaxation of the muscular fibers of the iris as the eye responds to changes in light, emotional states, and other kinds of stimulation. The pupil is the window of the eye through which light passes to the lens and the retina. See also **dilatator pupillae, sphincter pupillae.** **–pupillary,** *adj.*

pupill-. See **pupillo-.**

pupillary reflex. See **accommodation reflex, light reflex.**

pupillary skin reflex. See **ciliospinal reflex.**

pupillo-, pupill-, a combining form meaning 'of or pertaining to the pupil': *pupillometer, pupilloplegia, pupillostatometer.*

pur-, a combining form meaning 'of or related to pus': *puric, puriform, purohepatitis.*

pure dwarf. See **primordial dwarf.**

pure science. See **science.**

pure tone audiometry. See **audiometry.**

pure vegetarian. See **strict vegetarian.**

purgation. See **catharsis.**

purgative, a strong medication usually administered by mouth to promote evacuation of the bowel or several bowel movements.

purge, **1.** to evacuate the bowels, as with a cathartic. **2.** a cathartic. **3.** to make free of an unwanted substance. **–purgative,** *n., adj.*

purified protein derivative (PPD), a dried form of tuberculin used in testing for past or present infection with tubercle bacilli. This product is usually introduced into the skin during such tests and may produce a tuberculin reaction within 48 to 72 hours.

purine /pyŏŏr′ēn, -in/, any one of a large group of nitrogenous compounds. Purines are produced as end products in the digestion of certain proteins in the diet, but some are synthesized in the body. Purines are also present in many medications and other substances, including caffeine, theophylline, and various diuretics, muscle relaxants, and myocardial stimulants. Hyperuricemia may develop in some people as a result of an inability to metabolize and excrete purines. A low-purine diet or a purine-free diet may be required. Foods that are high in purines include anchovies and sardines, sweetbreads, liver, kidneys, and other organ meats, legumes, and poultry. The foods lowest in purine content include vegetables other than legumes, eggs, fruit, cheese, nuts, sugar, and gelatin.

Purinethol, a trademark for an antineoplastic (mercaptopurine).

Purkinje's fibers /pərkin′jəs/, myocardial fibers that are a continuation of the bundle of His and extend into the muscle walls of the ventricles. See also **Purkinje's network.**

Purkinje's network /pərkin′jēz, pur′kinjēz, -jāz/, a complex network of muscle fibers that spread through the right and the left ventricles of the heart and carry the impulses that contract those chambers almost simultaneously. Purkinje's fibers ramify from cardiac muscle fibers spreading into the right ventricle and are continuous with the muscle of the right ventricle. The fibers that connect with Purkinje's fibers start in the atrioventricular (AV) node in the right atrium of the heart, along the lower part of the interatrial septum. Impulses generated in the sinoatrial (SA) node travel swiftly through the muscle fibers of both atria of the heart, starting atrial contraction. As the impulse enters the AV node from the right atrium, it slows and allows both atria to contract completely before traveling into the ventricles. The velocity of the impulse increases after the impulse leaves the AV node and spreads via the bundle of His to Purkinje's fibers. Purkinje's fibers, which can be identified only with the aid of a microscope, are larger in diameter than ordinary cardiac muscle fibers and contain relatively few peripheral myofibrillae. They have abundant sarcoplasm and larger central nuclei than ordinary cardiac muscle. See also **cardiac cycle, intraventricular heart block.**

Purodigin, a trademark for a cardiotonic (digitoxin).

purpur-, a combining form meaning 'purple': *purpuriferous, purpuriparous, purpurogenous.*

purpura /pur′pyo͝orə/, any of several bleeding disorders characterized by hemorrhage into the tissues, particularly beneath the skin or mucous membranes, producing ecchymoses or petechiae. The two major kinds of purpura are **thrombocytopenic purpura** and **nonthrombocytopenic purpura.** –**purpuric,** *adj.*

purulent /pyo͝or′o͝oləntl/, producing or containing pus.

pus, a creamy, viscous, pale yellow or yellow-green fluid exudate that is the result of liquefaction necrosis. Its main constituent is an abundance of polymorphonuclear leukocytes. Bacterial infection is its most common cause. The character of the pus, including its color, consistency, quantity, or odor, may be of diagnostic significance.

pustular psoriasis, a severe form of psoriasis consisting of bright red patches and sterile pustules all over the body. Crops of lesions lasting 4 to 7 days occur every few days in cycles over weeks or months. Recurrences are inevitable. Fever, leukocytosis, and hypoalbuminemia are associated. In rare cases, hypovolemia and kidney failure occur. Hospitalization may be necessary for fluid replacement, steroid therapy, and sedation. Compare **guttate psoriasis.** See also **psoriasis.**

pustule /pus′cho͞ol/, a small, circumscribed elevation of the skin containing fluid that is usually purulent. –**pustular,** *adj.*

putrefaction, the decay of enzymes, especially proteins, that produces foul-smelling compounds, as ammonia, hydrogen sulfide, and mercaptans. –**putrefactive,** *adj.*

putrefy, to decay, with the production of foul-smelling substances, especially putrescine and mercaptans associated with the decomposition of animal tissues and proteins.

putrescine, a foul-smelling, toxic ptomaine produced by the decomposition of the amino acid ornithine during the decay of animal tissues, bacillus cultures, and fecal bacteria.

putromaine, any toxin produced by the decay of food within a living body.

P value, (in research) the statistic probability attached to the occurrence of a given finding by chance alone in comparison with the known distribution of possible findings, considering the kinds of data, the technique of analysis, and the number of observations. The P value may be noted as a decimal: $p<.01$ means that the likelihood of the phenomena tested occurring by chance alone is less than 1%.

PVC, **1.** abbreviation for **polyvinyl chloride. 2.** abbreviation for **premature ventricular contraction.**

P.V. Carpine, a trademark for a cholinergic (pilocarpine nitrate).

PVR, abbreviation for **pulmonary vascular resistance.**

P wave, the component of the cardiac cycle shown on an electrocardiogram as an inverted U-shaped curve that follows the end of the T wave and precedes the spike of the QRS complex. It represents atrial depolarization, during which the atria contract, pumping blood into the ventricles from the superior vena cava and the pulmonary vein.

P′ wave (P prime wave), a P wave that is generated from other than the sinus node; an ectopic P wave.

PWP, abbreviation for **pulmonary wedge pressure.**

pyel-. See **pyelo-.**

pyelitis /pī′əlī′tis/, *obsolete.* an inflammation of the pelvis of the kidney. See **pyelonephritis.**

pyelo-, pyel-, a combining form meaning 'of or pertaining to the pelvis or the kidney': *pyelocaliectasis, pyelocystitis, pyelograph.*

pyelogram /pī′əlōgram′/, an x-ray picture of the kidneys and ureters. An intravenous pyelogram (IVP), taken after the injection of a radiopaque dye, shows the size and location of the kidneys, the outline of the ureters and bladder, the filling of the renal pelves, the patency of the urinary tract, and any cysts or tumors within the kidneys. Preparation for an IVP includes bowel cleansing, withholding of fluids for 8 hours, and testing for sensitivity to the iodine in the radiopaque dye; persons with known sensitivity are not tested lest anaphylaxis occur. Patients able to tolerate the dye may feel warm and experience a salty taste when the material is injected. Retrograde pyelograms, which demonstrate filling of the renal collecting structures, are taken after the contrast medium is injected into the ureters by means of catheters in a cystoscope introduced through the urethra into the bladder. Also called **urogram.**

pyelography. See **intravenous pyelography.**

pyelolithotomy, a surgical procedure in which renal calculi are removed from the pelvis of the ureter.

pyelonephritis /pī′əlōnəfrī′tis/, a diffuse pyogenic infection of the pelvis and parenchyma of the kidney. **Acute pyelonephritis** is usually the result of an infection that ascends from the lower urinary tract to the kidney. *Escherichia coli* contamination of the urethral meatus is a common cause in females. Infection may spread to the kidney from other locations in the body. The onset of acute pyelonephritis is rapid, characterized by fever, chills, pain in the flank, nausea, and urinary frequency. A urinalysis reveals the presence of bacteria and white blood cells. Antimicrobial treatment is continued for 10 days to 2 weeks. Relapse or reinfection is common. **Chronic pyelonephritis** develops slowly after bacterial infection of the kidney and may progress to renal failure. Most cases are associated with some form of obstruction, as a stone or a stricture of the ureter. Treatment includes removal of the cause of obstruction and long-term antimicrobial therapy.

pygmalianism /pigmā′lē•əniz′əm/, a psychosexual abnormality in which the individual directs erotic fantasies toward an object that he has created.

pygmy, an extremely small person whose bodily parts are proportioned accordingly; a primordial dwarf. Also spelled **pigmy.**

pygo-, a combining form meaning 'of or pertaining to the buttocks': *pygoamorphus, pygodidymus, pygopagus.*

pygoamorphus /pī′gō•əmôr′fəs/, asymmetric, conjoined twins in which the parasitic member is represented by an undifferentiated amorphous mass attached to the autosite in the sacral region.

pygodidymus /pī′gōdid′əməs/, **1.** a malformed fetus that has a double pelvis and hips. **2.** conjoined twins that are fused in the cephalothoracic region but separated at the pelvis.

pygomelus /pīgom′ələs/, a malformed fetus that has an extra limb or limbs attached to the buttock. Also called **epipygus.**

pygopagus /pīgop′əgəs/, conjoined twins consisting of two fully formed or nearly formed fetuses that are united in the sacral region so that they are back to back.

pyknic /pik′nik/, describing a body structure characterized by short, round limbs, a full face, a short neck, stockiness, and a tendency toward obesity. Compare **asthenic habitus, athletic habitus.** See also **endomorph.**

pykno-, a combining form meaning 'thick, compact, or dense': *pyknocardia, pyknohemia, pyknomorphous.*

pyle-, a combining form meaning 'of or related to the portal vein': *pylemphraxis, pylephlebectasis, pylephlebitis.*

pyloric orifice /pīlôr′ik/, the opening of the stomach into the duodenum lying to the right of the middle line at the level of the cranial border of the first lumbar vertebra. The orifice is usually indicated on the surface of the stomach by the circular, duodenopyloric constriction.

pyloric spasm. See **pylorospasm.**

pyloric sphincter, a thickened muscular ring in the stomach, separating the pylorus from the duodenum. Also called **pyloric valve.**

pyloric stenosis, a narrowing of the pyloric sphincter at the outlet of the stomach, causing an obstruction that blocks the flow of food into the small intestine. The condition occurs as a congenital defect in one of 200 newborns and, occasionally, in older adults secondary to an ulcer or fibrosis at the outlet. Diagnosis is made in infants by the presence of forceful projectile vomiting and palpation of a hard, prominent pylorus and in infants and adults by x-ray examinations after a barium meal. Surgical correction is done using light general anesthesia, after the stomach is emptied. The muscle fibers of the outlet are cut, without severing the mucosa, to widen the opening. After surgery in adults, a stomach tube remains in place and observation is maintained for signs of hemorrhage or of blockage of the tube. See also **pyloromyotomy.**

pyloric ulcer. See **peptic ulcer.**

pyloro-, a combining form meaning 'of or related to the pylorus': *pylorodilator, pyloroplasty, pyloroptosis.*

pyloromyotomy, the incision of the longitudinal and circular muscle of the pylorus, which leaves the mucosa intact but separates the incised muscle fibers. It is the treatment of choice for hypertrophic pyloric stenosis. Also called **Fredet-Ramstedt operation.** See also **pyloric stenosis.**

pyloroplasty /pīlôr′əplas′tē/, a surgical procedure performed to relieve pyloric stenosis. Before surgery, any electrolyte imbalances or fluid deficiencies are corrected; sodium chloride and potassium chloride solutions may be given to correct ion losses from vomiting, which is characteristic of the condition. Under light general anesthesia, the passageway is dilated. As treatment for the duodenal ulcer, the operation allows the alkaline secretions of the duodenum to flow back into the stomach. Branches of the vagus nerve that supply the acid-secreting portion of the stomach may be cut, reducing the acidity of the stomach contents. Diarrhea is a common postoperative complication.

pylorospasm /pīlôr′əspaz′əm/, a spasm of the pyloric sphincter of the stomach, as occurs in pyloric stenosis.

pylorus /pīlôr′əs/, *pl.* **pylori, pyloruses,** a tubular portion of the stomach that angles to the right from the body of the stomach toward the duodenum. The most common position of the pylorus is about 3 cm to the right of the sagittal axis. It is distinctively marked by the thickening of the pyloric sphincter, and its lining is composed of an intestinal kind of epithelium rather than the gastric kind common to the body of the stomach. **–pyloric,** *adj.*

pyo-, a combining form meaning 'of or related to pus': *pyocalyx, pyocele, pyocyte.*

Pyocidin Otic, a trademark for an otic, fixed-combination drug containing a glucocorticoid (hydrocortisone) and an antibacterial (polymyxin B sulfate).

pyoderma /pī′ōdur′mə/, any purulent skin disease, as impetigo.

pyogenic /pī′əjen′ik/, pus-producing.

pyogenic granuloma, a small, nonmalignant mass of excessive granulation tissue, usually found at the site of an injury. Most often a dull red color, it contains numerous capillaries, bleeds easily, and is very tender; it may be attached by a narrow stalk. Treatment is with electrocautery or topical silver nitrate. Also called **telangiectatic granuloma.** See also **granuloma.**

Pyopen, a trademark for an antibacterial (carbenicillin disodium).

pyorrhea /pī′ərē′ə/, **1.** a discharge of pus. **2.** a purulent inflammation of the tissues surrounding the teeth. –**pyorrheal,** *adj.*

pyosalpinx /pī′ōsal′pingks/, an accumulation of pus in a fallopian tube. See also **salpingitis.**

pyramidal /piram′idəl/, of or pertaining to the shape of a pyramid.

pyramidalis /piram′idā′lis/, one of a pair of anterolateral muscles of the abdomen, contained in the lower end of the sheath of the rectus abdominis. It is a small, triangular muscle that arises from the pubis and inserts into the linea alba. It is innervated by a branch of the twelfth thoracic nerve and functions to tense the linea alba. Compare **obliquus externus abdominis, obliquus internus abdominis, rectus abdominis, transversus abdominis.**

pyramidal tract, a pathway composed of groups of nerve fibers in the white matter of the spinal cord through which motor impulses are conducted to the anterior horn cells from the opposite side of the brain. These descending fibers, the nerve cells of which are found in the precentral cortex, regulate the voluntary and reflex activity of the muscles through the anterior horn cells.

pyrantel pamoate, an anthelmintic.

■ INDICATIONS: It is prescribed in the treatment of infestation by roundworms or pinworms.

■ CONTRAINDICATION: Known hypersensitivity to this drug prohibits its use. Caution should be used in anemia or severe malnutrition.

■ ADVERSE EFFECTS: Among the more serious adverse reactions are nausea, abdominal cramps, diarrhea, dizziness, and skin rash.

pyrazinamide /pī′rəzin′əmīd/, an antimycobacterial.

■ INDICATIONS: It is prescribed in combination chemotherapy in the treatment of tuberculosis of hospitalized patients who fail to respond to other medications.

■ CONTRAINDICATIONS: Severe liver damage or known hypersensitivity to this drug prohibits its use.

■ ADVERSE EFFECTS: Among the more serious adverse reactions are hepatotoxicity and hyperuricemia.

pyrethrin and piperonyl butoxide, a fixed-combination scabicide and pediculocide.

■ INDICATIONS: It is prescribed in the treatment of infestations of head, body, and pubic lice.

■ CONTRAINDICATIONS: Known hypersensitivity to ragweed or to this drug prohibits its use.

■ ADVERSE EFFECTS: Among the more serious adverse reactions are irritation of the skin and the mucous membranes.

pyreto-, a combining form meaning 'of or pertaining to fever': *pyretogen, pyretography, pyretotherapy.*

pyrexia. See **fever.**

-pyrexia, a combining form meaning a 'febrile condition': *apyrexia, electropyrexia, physiopyrexia.*

Pyribenzamine Hydrochloride, a trademark for an antihistaminic (tripelennamine hydrochloride).

Pyridium, a trademark for an analgesic (phenazopyridine hydrochloride).

pyridostigmine bromide /pir′idōstig′mēn/, a cholinergic.

■ INDICATIONS: It is prescribed in the treatment of myasthenia gravis and is used as an antagonist to nondepolarizing muscle relaxants, as curare.

■ CONTRAINDICATIONS: Intestinal or urinary obstruction, bradycardia, hypotension, or known hypersensitivity to this drug or to other anticholinesterases prohibits its use.

■ ADVERSE EFFECTS: Among the more serious adverse reactions are nausea, diarrhea, abdominal cramps, muscle cramps, and weakness.

pyridoxal phosphate /pir′ədok′səl/, an enzyme in the body that acts with pyridoxamine phosphate and transaminase to catalyze the reversible transfer of an amino group from an alpha-amino acid to an alpha-keto acid, especially alpha-ketoglutaric acid. Such processes are essential to metabolism.

pyridoxamine phosphate /pir′ədok′səmēn/, an enzyme that participates with pyridoxal phosphate and transaminase in the reversible transfer of an amino group from an alpha-amino acid to an alpha-keto acid.

pyridoxine /pir′idok′sēn/, a water-soluble, white, crystalline vitamin that is part of the B complex group, derived from pyridine, and converted in the body to pyridoxal and pyridoxamine for synthesis. It functions as a coenzyme essential for the synthesis and breakdown of amino acids, the conversion of tryptophan to niacin, the breakdown of glycogen to glucose 1-phosphate, the production of antibodies, the formation of heme in hemoglobin, the formation of hormones important in brain function, the proper absorption of vitamin B_{12}, the production of hydrochloric acid and magnesium, and the maintenance of the balance of sodium and potassium, which regulates body fluids and the functioning of the nervous and musculoskeletal systems. Rich dietary sources are meats, especially organ meats, whole-grain cereals, soybeans, peanuts, wheat germ, and brewer's yeast; milk and green vegetables supply smaller amounts. The most common symptoms of deficiency are seborrheic dermatitis about the eyes, nose, mouth, and behind the ears, cheilosis, glossitis and stomatitis, nervousness, depression, peripheral neuropathy, and lymphopenia, leading to convulsions in infants and anemia in adults. Treatment and prophylaxis consist of administration of the vitamin and a diet rich in foods containing it. Several drugs interfere with the use of pyridoxine, notably isoniazid and penicillamine, and supplements of the vitamin are recommended with their use. The need for increased amounts of pyridoxine occurs during pregnancy, lactation, exposure to radiation, cardiac failure, aging, and use of oral contraceptives. The vitamin is considered nontoxic. Also called **vitamin B_6.**

pyridoxine hydrochloride. See **pyridoxine.**

pyrilamine maleate, an antihistamine.

■ INDICATIONS: It is prescribed in the treatment of a variety of hypersensitivity reactions, including rhinitis, skin rash, and pruritus.

■ CONTRAINDICATIONS: Asthma or known hypersensitivity to this drug prohibits its use. It is not given to newborn infants or lactating mothers.

■ ADVERSE EFFECTS: Drowsiness, skin rash, hypersensitivity reactions, dry mouth, and tachycardia commonly occur.

pyrimethamine /pir′əmeth′əmēn/, an antimalarial.

■ INDICATIONS: It is prescribed in the treatment of malaria and toxoplasmosis.

■ CONTRAINDICATIONS: Use in chloroguanide-resistant malaria is contraindicated. Caution is recommended in use of the drug to treat toxoplasmosis because dosages needed may be at toxic level.

■ ADVERSE EFFECTS: Among the more serious adverse reactions, primarily with large doses, are megaloblastic anemia, atrophic glossitis, leukopenia, and convulsions.

pyrimethamine and sulfadoxine, an antimalarial fixed-combination drug.

■ INDICATIONS: It is prescribed for prophylaxis and attacks of malaria.

■ CONTRAINDICATIONS: Megaloblastic anemia, infant age of less than 2 months, pregnancy at term and during the nursing period, or hypersensitivity to pyrimethamine or the sulfonamides prohibits its use.

■ ADVERSE EFFECTS: The most serious adverse reactions are hypersensitivity reactions, pancreatitis, mental depression, convulsions, hallucinations, and several blood dyscrasias.

pyrimidine /pərim′ədēn/, an organic compound of heterocyclic nitrogen found in nucleic acids and in many drugs, including the antiviral drugs acyclovir, ribavirin, and trifluridine.

pyro-, a combining form meaning 'of or related to fire or heat, or produced by heating': *pyrocatechin, pyrodextrin, pyromania.*

pyrogallol triacetate. See **acetpyrogall.**

pyrogen /pī′rəjən/, any substance or agent that tends to cause a rise in body temperature, as some bacterial toxins. See also **fever.** **–pyrogenic,** *adj.*

pyrolagnia /pī′rōlag′nē•ə/, sexual stimulation or gratification from watching or setting fires.

pyromania /pī′rōmā′nē•ə/, an impulse neurosis characterized by an uncontrollable urge to set fires. The condition is found predominantly in men and is usually associated with alcohol intoxication, chronic personal frustrations, resentment of authority figures, or some other psychologic disturbance or psychosexual dysfunction. Those with the condition experience an increased sense of tension before setting the fire and intense gratification while watching it burn; they may often display satisfaction from the resulting destruction, although many show signs of depression, anxiety, and guilt over the possibility of being apprehended. Treatment consists of psychotherapy to uncover the causative emotional problems and often institutionalization for the protection of the person and of society.

pyromaniac /pī′rōmā′nē•ak/, **1.** a person with or displaying characteristics of pyromania. **2.** of, pertaining to, or exhibiting pyromania. **–pyromaniacal,** *adj.*

pyrosis. See **heartburn.**

pyrrole /pirōl′, pir′ōl/, a heterocyclic substance occurring naturally in many compounds in the body. Heme and porphyrin are pyrrole derivatives.

Pyrroxate, a trademark for a respiratory, fixed-combination drug containing an adrenergic (methoxyphenamine hydrochloride), an antihistaminic (chlorpheniramine maleate), analgesics (aspirin and phenacetin), and a stimulant (caffeine).

pyruvate kinase, an enzyme essential for anaerobic glycolysis in red blood cells. It catalyzes the transfer of a phosphate group from adenosine triphosphate to produce adenosine diphosphate.

pyruvate kinase deficiency, a congenital hemolytic disorder transmitted as an autosomal recessive trait. The homozygous condition is characterized by severe chronic hemolysis. The heterozygous form may occur with a mild to severe anemia but is usually asymptomatic and of no clinical significance.

pyruvic acid /pīro͞o′vik/, a compound formed as an end product of glycolysis, the anaerobic stage of glucose metabolism. Exposed to oxygen and acetylcoenzyme A at the entrance to the Krebs citric acid cycle, the compound is changed to citric acid.

pyrvinium pamoate /pirvin′ē•əm pam′ō•āt/, an anthelmintic.

■ INDICATION: It is prescribed in the treatment of enterobiasis, particularly for infestation by pinworms.

■ CONTRAINDICATIONS: Pregnancy or known hypersensitivity to this drug prohibits its use.

■ ADVERSE EFFECTS: Among the more serious adverse effects are nausea, cramping, diarrhea, and hypersensitivity reactions. Stools and any vomitus will be stained a bright red.

pyuria /pīyo͝or′ē•ə/, the presence of white blood cells in the urine, usually a sign of an infection of the urinary tract. Pyuria occurs most often in cystitis, pyelonephritis, urethritis, and tuberculosis of the kidney. The presence of from one to four leukocytes per high-power field count during a laboratory urine examination is considered to be within the normal range for a male or female patient. Excessive leukocytes suggest a bacterial or other infection. Abacterial pyuria usually is caused by a viral infection of the bladder and urethra. Miliary pyuria is characterized by the presence of blood cells, pus cells, and epithelial cells, in addition to bacteria. See also **bacteriuria.**

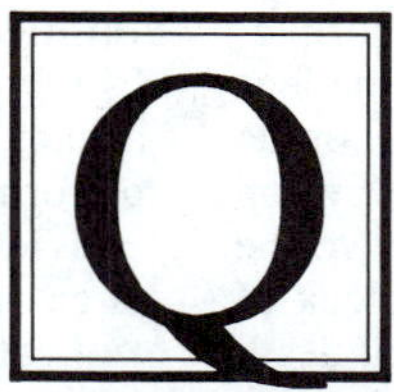

Q, **1.** symbol for **blood volume.** **2.** symbol for **quantity.**

Q̇, symbol for **rate of blood flow.**

QAP, abbreviation for **quality assurance program.**

q.d., (in prescriptions) abbreviation for *quaque die* /dē′ā/, a Latin phrase meaning "every day." Also called **quotid.**

Q fever, an acute febrile illness, usually respiratory, caused by the rickettsia, *Coxiella burnetii (Rickettsia burnetii).* The disease is spread through contact with infected domestic animals, either by inhaling the rickettsiae from their hides, drinking their contaminated milk, or being bitten by a tick harboring the organism. Onset is abrupt, and high fever may persist for 3 weeks or more. The illness is especially common among those who work with sheep, goats, and cattle. Treatment with tetracycline is usually effective in 36 to 48 hours. People who are regularly exposed to domestic animals can be vaccinated against Q fever. Also called **Australian Q fever.** Compare **scrub typhus.**

q.h., (in prescriptions) abbreviation for *quaque hora,* a Latin phrase meaning "every hour."

q.2h., (in prescriptions) abbreviation for *quaque secunda hora,* a Latin phrase meaning "every 2 hours."

q.3h., (in prescriptions) abbreviation for *quaque tertia hora,* a Latin phrase meaning "every 3 hours."

q.4h., (in prescriptions) abbreviation for *quaque quarta hora,* a Latin phrase meaning "every 4 hours."

q.6h., (in prescriptions) abbreviation for *quaque sex hora,* a Latin phrase meaning "every 6 hours."

q.8h., (in prescriptions) abbreviation for *quaque octa hora,* a Latin phrase meaning "every 8 hours."

q.i.d., (in prescriptions) abbreviation for *quater in die* /dē′ā/, a Latin phrase meaning "four times a day."

QRS complex, the components of the ventricular electric events of the cardiac cycle shown on an electrocardiogram as a sharp, angular complex normally less than 0.1 seconds in duration, reflecting the time it takes for the ventricular myocardium to depolarize. The term, when used in upper case letters, indicates any ventricular complex, regardless of its shape. Upper and lower case letters are used to describe the complex more precisely and to indicate relative size of components; anything positive (above the isoelectric line) is an R or r; anything negative (below the isoelectric line) is either a q or Q, or an s or S. When there are two of one letter the second is designated prime (′). The Q wave precedes an R, whereas the S wave follows it. If there is no R wave, a totally negative complex is designated QS. Some variations of the QRS complex are rS, qR, RS, rSR′, qRs, and QR.

q.s., (in prescriptions) abbreviation for *quantum sufficit,* a Latin phrase meaning "quantity required."

Q's test. See **Queckenstedt's test.**

QT interval, the portion on an electrocardiogram from the beginning of the QRS complex to the end of the T wave, reflecting the length of the refractory period of the heart. An excessively long QT interval is known to cause the life threatening ventricular tachycardia known as torsades des pointes.

Quaalude, a trademark for a sedative-hypnotic (methaqualone).

quack. See **charlatan.**

quadr-, a combining form meaning 'four': *quadrangular, quadribasic, quadrivalent.*

quadratus labii superioris. See **zygomaticus minor.**

quadriceps femoris, the great extensor muscle of the anterior thigh, composed of the rectus femoris, the vastus lateralis, the vastus medialis, and the vastus intermedius. The quadriceps forms a large dense mass covering the front and sides of the femur. Tendons of the four parts of the muscle unite at the distal part of the thigh, forming a single strong tendon that inserts into the patella. The quadriceps is innervated by branches of the femoral nerve, which contains fibers from the second, third, and fourth lumbar nerves. The muscle functions to extend the leg.

quadriceps reflex. See **patellar reflex.**

quadrigeminal /kwod′rijem′inəl/, **1.** in four parts. **2.** a fourfold increase in size or frequency.

quadrigeminal pulse, a pulse in which a pause occurs after every fourth beat.

Quadrinal, a trademark for a respiratory, fixed-combination drug containing a smooth muscle relaxant (theophylline calcium salicylate), an adrenergic (ephedrine hydrochloride), an expectorant (potassium iodide), and a sedative-hypnotic (phenobarbital).

quadriplegia /kwod′rəplē′jē·ə/, an abnormal condition characterized by paralysis of the arms, the legs, and the trunk of the body below the level of an associated injury to the spinal cord. This disorder may be caused by spinal cord injury, especially in the area of the fifth to the seventh vertebrae. Automobile accidents and sporting mishaps are common causes. This condition affects about 150,000 Americans, the majority of whom are men between 20 and 40 years of age.

■ OBSERVATIONS: The signs and symptoms of quadriplegia commonly include flaccidity of the arms and the legs and the loss of power and sensation below the level of the injury. Cardiovascular complications may also develop from any injury that damages the spinal cord above the fifth cervical vertebra because of an associated block of the sympathetic nervous system. A major cause of death from such injury is respiratory failure. Other symptoms may include low body temperature, bradycardia, impaired peristalsis, and autonomic dysreflexia. Diagnosis is based on a complete physical and neurologic examination with x-ray pictures of the head, chest, and abdomen to rule out underlying injuries. Extensive laboratory tests assess other body conditions, as CBC, electrolytes, urine creatinine clearance, and prothrombin time. Spinal x-ray examinations and myelography show any fractures and spinal cord blockages.

■ INTERVENTION: Treatment starts at the accident scene, where the neck and the spine of the patient are immobilized. Additional immobilization at the hospital commonly includes the use of halo traction and Stryker frame, the insertion of a Foley catheter, aggressive respiratory therapy, and the administration of diuretics to decrease spinal cord edema. After an appropriate period of therapy, surgery is commonly performed to fuse unstable spinal sections and remove bone fragments.

■ NURSING CONSIDERATIONS: Maintaining adequate respiration and the integrity of the GI system is very important in quadriplegia. Complications, as hypothermia, bradycardia, catheter obstruction, and fecal impaction, require immediate nursing attention. A quadriplegic patient who suffers hypothermia is wrapped in blankets instead of being warmed with hotwater bottles or electromechanic devices because such devices can burn the skin of the patient experiencing severe sensory loss. Abdominal binders and antiembolism hose are used when placing the patient in an upright position. Patients who develop bradycardia are commonly connected to a cardiac monitor and intravenously administered an antimuscarinic drug, as atropine. Fecal impaction may cause hypertension and is always a possible complication. Manipulation of the rectum to free such impaction may aggravate the associated hypertension. A common precaution in removing an obstructive fecal mass is first to apply a topical anesthetic ointment, as tetracaine. Throughout the therapy for quadriplegia, constant psychologic support from attending nurses benefits the patient and family and encourages healthy communication. Compare **hemiplegia, paraplegia.**

quadruplet /kwod′ro͞oplit, kwodro͞o′plit/, any one of four offspring born of the same gestation period during a single pregnancy. See also **Hellin's law.**

quale /kwā′lē/, *pl.* **qualia** /kwā′lē·ə/, **1.** the quality of a particular thing. **2.** a quality considered as an independent entity. **3.** (in psychology) a feeling, sensation, or other conscious process that has its unique, particular quality regardless of its external meaning or frame of reference.

qualified, pertaining to a health professional or health facility that is formally recognized by an appropriate agency or organization as meeting certain standards of performance related to the professional competence of an individual or the eligibility of an institution to participate in an approved health care program.

qualitative, of or pertaining to the quality, value, or nature of something.

qualitative melanin test, a test for detecting melanin in the urine of patients with malignant melanomas.

qualitative test, a test that determines the presence or absence of a substance.

quality, (in radiotherapy) specification of the penetrating ability of a beam of x-rays. Beam quality is expressed in terms of half-value layer where greater penetrating ability characterizes a beam as ''harder'' whereas less energy results in a beam being described as ''softer.''

quality assurance, (in health care) any evaluation of services provided and the results achieved as compared with accepted standards. In one form of quality assurance, various attributes of health care, as cost, place, accessibility, treatment, and benefits, are scored in a two-part process. First, the actual results are compared with standard results; then, any deficiencies noted or identified serve to prompt recommendations for improvement.

quality assurance program, a system of review of selected hospital medical records by medical staff members, performed for the purposes of evaluating the quality and effectiveness of medical care in relation to accepted standards.

quality factor, (in radiotherapy) evaluation of the biologic damage that radiation can produce. It is observed that identical doses of different types of radiation can produce differing levels of damage. In the field of radiation protection, biologically equivalent doses are set equal to one another by multiplying the actual absorbed dose by a number called the quality factor. The resulting quantity is called dose equivalent, measured in sieverts or rems.

quantitative inheritance. See **multifactorial inheritance.**

quantitative test, a test that determines the amount of a substance per unit volume or unit weight.

quantum mechanics. See **quantum theory.**

quantum mottle. See mottle.

quantum theory, (in physics) a theory dealing with the interaction of matter and electromagnetic radiation, particularly at the atomic and subatomic levels, according to which radiation consists of small units of energy called quanta. Radiation can be absorbed only in whole quanta, and the energy content of a quantum is inversely proportional to its wavelength. Also called **quantum mechanics.**

quarantine, **1.** isolation of people with communicable disease or of those exposed to communicable disease during the contagious period in an attempt to prevent spread of the illness. **2.** the practice of detaining travelers or vessels coming from places of epidemic disease, originally for 40 days, for the purpose of inspection or disinfection.

quartan /kwôr′tən/, recurring on the fourth day, or at about 72-hour intervals. See also **quartan malaria.**

quartan malaria, a form of malaria, caused by the protozoan *Plasmodium malariae,* characterized by febrile paroxysms that occur every 72 hours. Also called **quartan fever.** Compare **falciparum malaria, tertian malaria.** See also **malaria.**

quarti-, a combining form meaning 'fourth': *quartipara, quartisect, quartisternal.*

quartz silicosis. See **silicosis.**

Queckenstedt's test /kwek′ənstets/, a test for an obstruction in the spinal canal in which the jugular veins on each side of the neck are compressed alternately. The pressure of the spinal fluid is measured by a manometer connected to a lumbar puncture needle or catheter. Normally, occlusion of the veins of the neck causes an immediate rise in spinal fluid pressure; if the vertebral canal is blocked, no rise occurs. If increased intracranial pressure is suspected, this test should not be performed. See also **spinal canal.**

Queensland tick typhus, an infection caused by *Rickettsia australis,* occurring in Australia, transmitted by ticks, and resembling mild Rocky Mountain spotted fever. Treatment includes the administration of chloramphenicol or tetracycline. Prevention depends on avoiding tick bites and on the prompt removal of attached ticks. Compare **boutonneuse fever, North Asian tick-borne rickettsiosis, Rocky Mountain spotted fever.**

Quelicin, a trademark for a depolarizing agent (succinylcholine chloride), used as an adjunct to anesthesia.

Quelidrine, a trademark for a respiratory, fixed-combination drug containing adrenergics (phenylephrine hydrochloride and ephedrine hydrochloride), an antihistaminic (chlorpheniramine maleate), an antitussive (dextromethorphan hydrobromide), and an expectorant (ammonium chloride).

quellung reaction /kwel′ung/, the swelling of the capsule of a bacterium, seen in the laboratory when the organism is exposed to specific antisera. This phenomenon is used to identify the genera, species, or subspecies of the bacteria causing a disease, including *Haemophilus influenzae, Neisseria meningitides,* and many kinds of streptococci. Also called **Neufeld capsular swelling test.**

Quengle cast /kwen′gəl/, a two-section, hinged orthopedic cast for immobilizing the lower extremities from the foot or ankle to below the knee and the upper thigh to a level just above the knee. The two parts of the cast are connected by special hinges at knee level, medially and laterally. The Quengle cast is used for the gradual correction of knee contractures.

quercetin /kwur′sitin/, a yellow, crystalline, flavonoid pigment found in oak bark, the juice of lemons, asparagus, and other plants. It is used to reduce abnormal capillary fragility.

querulous paranoia /kwer′yo͞oləs/, a form of paranoia characterized by extreme discontent and habitual complaining, usually about imagined slights by others. Also called **paranoia querulans.**

Questran, a trademark for an ion exchange resin (cholestyramine resin).

queue /kyo͞o/, **1.** (in computer time sharing) to await one's turn for data processing to be done by a time sharing computer. **2.** to await one's turn for the use of peripheral computer equipment, as a printer. **3.** all of those who are queueing.

Quibron, a trademark for a respiratory, fixed-combination drug containing a smooth muscle relaxant (theophylline) and an expectorant (guaifenesin).

quick connect, a plastic or similar connecting device that is attached to or implanted in a patient who will be joined to an electromechanic or other apparatus. A patient whose circulatory system is supported by an artificial heart, for example, may have a push-fit connector sewn to the natural atria, aorta, and pulmonary artery; a plastic lip on the artificial ventricle can then be securely snapped onto the quick connect device.

quickening, the first feeling by a pregnant woman of movement of her baby in utero, usually occurring between 16 and 20 weeks of gestation.

Quide, a trademark for a tranquilizer (piperacetazine).

quin-, a combining form meaning 'of or related to quinine': *quiniretin, quinometry, quinotoxin.*

-quin, -quine, a combining form naming antimalarial medicinal compounds from quinine: *aminoquin, diodoquin, Floraquin.*

quinacrine hydrochloride, an anthelmintic and an antimalarial.

■ INDICATIONS: It is prescribed in the treatment of giardiasis and cestodiasis and in the treatment and suppression of malaria.

■ CONTRAINDICATIONS: Pregnancy, concomitant administration of primaquine, or known hypersensitivity to this drug prohibits its use. It is used with caution in patients having a history of psychosis and in patients over 60 years of age.

■ ADVERSE EFFECTS: Among the more serious adverse reactions are severe psoriasis, aplastic anemia, acute hepatic necrosis, nausea, vomiting, and jaundice.

Quinaglute, a trademark for a cardiac depressant (quinidine gluconate).

Quincke's pulse /kwing′kēz/, an abnormal alternate blanching and reddening of the skin that may be observed in several ways, as by pressing the front edge of the fingernail and watching the blood in the nail bed recede and return. This pulsation is characteristic of aortic insufficiency and other abnormal conditions but may also occur in otherwise normal individuals. Formerly, it was thought to be caused by pulsation of the capillaries, but study has shown it is caused by pulsation of subpapillary arteriolar and venous plexuses. Also called **capillary pulse.**

quinethazone /kwəneth′əzōn/, a diuretic and antihypertensive.

■ INDICATIONS: It is prescribed in the treatment of hypertension and edema.

■ CONTRAINDICATIONS: Known hypersensitivity to this drug, to other thiazide medication, or to sulfonamide derivatives prohibits its use.

■ ADVERSE EFFECTS: Among the more serious adverse effects are hypokalemia, hyperglycemia, hyperuricemia, and hypersensitivity reactions.

Quinidex, a trademark for a cardiac depressant (quinidine sulfate).

quinidine /kwin′ədēn, -din/, an antiarrhythmic agent used as a bisulfate, gluconate, polygalacturonate, or sulfate.

■ INDICATIONS: It is prescribed in the treatment of atrial flutter, atrial fibrillation, premature ventricular contractions, and tachycardias.

■ CONTRAINDICATIONS: Known hypersensitivity to this drug prohibits its use. It is contraindicated in some arrhythmias, particularly those associated with heart block.

■ ADVERSE EFFECTS: Among the most serious adverse reactions are cardiac arrhythmia, hypertension, and cinchonism. Rare, but potentially fatal hypersensitivity reactions, as anaphylaxis and thrombocytopenia, may occur. Diarrhea, nausea, and vomiting are common.

quinidine gluconate. See **quinidine.**

quinine /kwī′nīn/, a white, bitter crystalline alkaloid, made from cinchona bark, used in antimalarial medications.

quinine dihydrochloride, an antimalarial. See **quinine sulfate.**

quinine sulfate, an antimalarial with antipyretic, analgesic, and muscle relaxant activity.

■ INDICATIONS: It is prescribed in the treatment of malaria, particularly malaria caused by *Plasmodium falciparum,* and nocturnal leg cramps.

■ CONTRAINDICATIONS: Glucose 6-phosphate dehydrogenase deficiency and certain cardiac disorders prohibit its use.

■ ADVERSE EFFECTS: Among the more serious adverse reactions are symptoms of cinchonism or known hypersensitivity to this drug, including tinnitus, headache, and visual, hearing, and GI disturbances. Hemolysis, blood dyscrasia, and various hypersensitivity reactions also may occur.

Quinora, a trademark for a cardiac depressant (quinidine sulfate).

quinque-, a combining form meaning 'five': *quinquecuspid, quinquetubercular, quinquevalent.*

quinsy. See **peritonsillar abscess.**

quint-, a combining form meaning 'fifth or fivefold': *quintessence, quintipara, quintuplet.*

quintan /kwin′tən/, recurring on the fifth day, or at about 96-hour intervals. See also **trench fever.**

quintana fever. See **trench fever.**

quintuplet /kwin′to͝oplit, kwinto͞o′plit/, any one of five offspring born of the same gestation period during a single pregnancy. See also **Hellin's law.**

quotid. See **q.d.**

Q wave, the component of the cardiac cycle shown on an electrocardiogram as a short abrupt downward line from the end of the tail of the P wave before the sudden sharp ascent of the R wave. It represents the first part of the QRS complex. See also **QRS complex.**

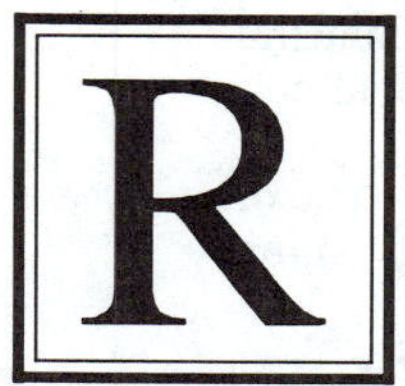

R, 1. abbreviation for **metabolic respiratory quotient.** 2. abbreviation for **resolution.** 3. abbreviation for **respiratory exchange ratio.**

R_f, symbol for a ratio used in paper chromatography and thin-layer chromatography, representing the distance from the origin to the center of the separated zone divided by the distance from the origin to the solvent front.

Ra, symbol for **radium.**

rabbit fever. See **tularemia.**

rabbit test. See **Friedman's test.**

rabies /rā′bēz/, an acute, usually fatal viral disease of the central nervous system of animals. It is transmitted from animals to people by infected blood, tissue, or, most commonly, saliva. Also called *(obsolete)* **hydrophobia.** –**rabid** /rab′id/, *adj.*

■ OBSERVATIONS: The reservoir of the virus is chiefly wild animals, including skunks, bats, foxes, dogs, raccoons, and cats. After introduction into the human body, often by a bite of an infected animal, the virus travels along nerve pathways to the brain and, later, to other organs. An incubation period ranges from 10 days to 1 year and is followed by a prodromal period characterized by fever, malaise, headache, paresthesia, and myalgia. After several days, severe encephalitis, delirium, agonizingly painful muscular spasms, seizures, paralysis, coma, and death ensue.

■ INTERVENTION: Few nonfatal cases have been documented in humans; survival in those cases has been the result of intensive supportive nursing and medical care. There is no treatment once the virus has reached the tissue of the nervous system. Local treatment of wounds inflicted by rabid animals may prevent the disease. The wound is cleansed with soap, water, and a disinfectant. A deep wound may be cauterized and rabies immune globulin (RIG) injected directly into the base of the wound. For active immunization, a series of five intramuscular injections with a human diploid cell rabies vaccine (HDCV) or duck embryo vaccine is begun. If HDCV is administered, the injections are given on the day of exposure and on days 3, 7, 14, 28, and 90. Great effort is made to locate and examine the animal. The animal that is suspected of being rabid is not immediately killed but put in isolation and carefully observed. If the animal is well in 10 days, there is little danger of rabies developing from the bite. Tissue from the animal's brain may be examined microscopically or by fluorescent antibody screening techniques.

■ NURSING CONSIDERATIONS: Rabies virus infection can be eradicated from most communities by prophylactic immunization of domestic animals, stringent measures for the control of domestic animals, and the elimination of any wild animals acting as reservoirs of infection. The nurse and other health workers may encourage compliance with such efforts and teach the necessity of avoiding direct contact with wild animals and the importance of immediate first aid for any animal bite.

rabies immune globulin (RIG), a solution of antirabies immune globulin.

■ INDICATIONS: It is used in conjunction with rabies duck embryo vaccine for possible protection against rabies in persons suspected of exposure to rabies.

■ CONTRAINDICATIONS: Previous administration of this preparation or known hypersensitivity to this solution, to gamma globulin, or to thimerosal prohibits its use.

■ ADVERSE EFFECTS: Among the more serious adverse reactions are soreness at the site of injection, fever, and hypersensitivity reactions.

rabies vaccine (DEV), a sterile suspension of killed rabies virus prepared from duck embryo.

■ INDICATIONS: It is prescribed for immunization and postexposure prophylaxis against rabies.

■ CONTRAINDICATIONS: A history of allergic reaction to chicken or duck eggs or to protein prohibits its use.

■ ADVERSE EFFECTS: Among the most serious adverse reactions are severe hypersensitivity reactions and pain and inflammation at the site of injection.

race, a vague, unscientific term for a group of genetically related people who share certain physical characteristics.

racemic, pertaining to a compound made up of levorotatory isomers, rendering it optically inactive under polarized light.

racemose /ras′əmōs′/, like a bunch of grapes. The term is used in describing a structure in which many branches terminate in nodular, cystlike forms, as pulmonary alveoli.

racemose aneurysm, a pronounced dilatation of lengthened and tortuous blood vessels, some of which may be distended to 20 times their normal size. Also called **cirsoid aneurysm.**

Racet, a trademark for a topical fixed-combination drug containing a glucocorticoid (hydrocortisone) and a topical antiinfective (iodochlorhydroxyquin).

rachio-, rachi-, rhachi-, a combining form meaning 'of or related to the spine': *rachiocampsis, rachiotome, rachiotomy.*

rachiopagus /rā′kē•op′əgəs/, conjoined symmetric twins that are united back to back along the spinal column. Also called **rachipagus.**

rachischisis /rəkis′kəsis/, a congenital fissure of one or more vertebrae. See also **neural tube defect, spina bifida.**

rachischisis totalis. See **complete rachischisis.**

rachitic /rəkit′ik/, **1.** of or pertaining to rickets. **2.** resembling or suggesting the condition of one afflicted with rickets.

rachitic dwarf, a person whose retarded growth is caused by rickets. See also **Fanconi's syndrome.**

rachitis /rəkī′tis/, **1.** rickets. **2.** an inflammatory disease of the vertebral column.

racial immunity, a form of natural immunity shared by most of the members of a genetically related population. Compare **individual immunity, species immunity.**

racial unconscious. See **collective unconscious.**

rad /rad/, abbreviation for *radiation absorbed dose*; the basic unit of absorbed dose of ionizing radiation. One rad is equal to the absorption of 100 ergs of radiation energy per gram of matter, and therefore differs from the roentgen. See also **absorbed dose, rem.**

radarkymography, a radar technique for showing the size and outline of the heart, using a radar tracking device and a fluoroscopic screen to display images produced by electric impulses passed over the chest surface.

radi-, a combining form meaning 'root': *radiciform, radicotomy, radiectomy.*

radial artery, an artery in the forearm, starting at the bifurcation of the brachial artery and passing in 12 branches to the forearm, wrist, and hand. In the forearm, it extends from the neck of the radius to the forepart of the styloid process; in the wrist, from the styloid process to the carpus; in the hand, from the carpus, across the palm, to the little finger. In the forearm, the branches of the radial artery are the radial recurrent, muscular, palmar carpal, and superficial palmar; in the wrist, the branches are the dorsal carpal and the first dorsal metacarpal. In the hand, the branches are the princeps pollicis, radialis indicis, deep palmar arch, palmar metacarpal, perforating, and recurrent.

radial keratotomy, a surgical procedure in which a series of tiny shallow incisions are made on the cornea, causing it to bulge slightly to correct for nearsightedness. The operation is performed using local anesthesia and requires only 30 minutes. Hospitalization is not necessary. Radial keratotomy usually corrects mild to moderate myopia.

radial nerve, the largest branch of the brachial plexus, arising on each side as a continuation of the posterior cord. It supplies the skin of the arm and forearm and their extensor muscles. It crosses the tendon of the latissimus dorsi beneath the axillary artery, passes the inferior border of the teres major, and winds around the medial side of the humerus to enter the triceps between the medial and the long heads of that muscle. It spirals down the arm close to the humerus in the groove separating the origins of the medial and the long heads of the triceps, accompanied by the deep brachial artery. On the lateral side of the arm it pierces the lateral intermuscular septum, runs between the brachialis and the brachioradialis, and divides into the superficial and the deep branches. The branches of the radial nerve are the medial muscular branches, the posterior brachial cutaneous nerve, the posterior muscular branches, the posterior antebrachial cutaneous nerve, the lateral muscular branches, the superficial branch, and the deep branch. Also called **musculospiral nerve.** Compare **median nerve, musculocutaneous nerve, ulnar nerve.**

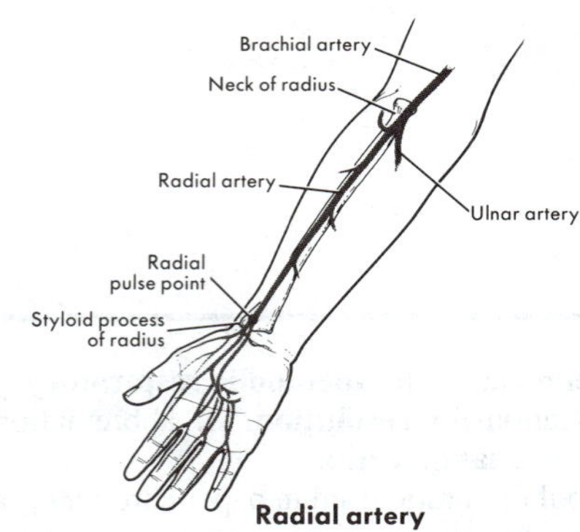

Radial artery

radial notch of ulna, the narrow, lateral depression in the coronoid process of the ulna that receives the head of the radius.

radial pulse, the pulse of the radial artery palpated at the wrist over the radius. The radial pulse is the one most often taken, because of the ease with which it is palpated.

radial recurrent artery, a branch of the radial artery, arising just distal to the elbow, ascending between the branches of the radial nerve, and supplying several muscles of the arm and the elbow.

radial reflex, a normal reflex elicited by tapping over the distal radius, with the response being flexion of the forearm. Flexion of the fingers may also occur if the reflex is hyperactive.

radiant energy, the energy emitted by electromagnetic radiation, as radio waves, visible light, x-rays, and gamma rays.

radiate, to diverge or spread from a common point.

radiate ligament, a ligament that connects the head of a rib with a vertebra and an associated intervertebral disk. Each of the 24 radiate ligaments consists of three flat fasciculi attached to the head of a rib. The superior fasciculus connects with the vertebra above, the inferior fasciculus connects with the vertebra below, and the middle fasciculus connects to the disk between the two vertebrae. Radiate ligaments to the tenth, eleventh, and twelfth ribs have only two fasciculi.

radiation, **1.** the emission of energy, rays, or waves.

2. (in medicine) the use of a radioactive substance in the diagnosis or treatment of disease.

radiation caries, tooth decay caused by ionizing radiation of the oral and maxillary structure. Radiation caries is often a side effect of treatment for oral malignancies. See also **dental caries.**

radiation detector, a device for converting radiant energy to an observable form, used for detecting the presence and sometimes the amount of radiation. A Geiger-Müller detector counts and registers the number of particles reaching it from a radioactive source and can be designed with sufficient sensitivity to detect cosmic radiation. An ionization chamber detects exposure to radiation by collecting the ion pairs formed by the passage of radiation through the device.

radiation exposure, a measure of the ionization produced in air by x-rays or gamma rays. It is the sum of the electric charges on all ions of one sign that are produced when all electrons liberated by photons in a volume of air are completely stopped, divided by the mass of air in the volume element. The unit of exposure is the roentgen. See also **acute radiation exposure.**

radiation hygiene, the art and science of protecting human beings from injury by radiation by seeking to reduce clinical exposure from external radiation through protective barriers of radiation-absorbing material, ensuring safe distances between people and radiation sources, reducing radiation exposure times, or employing combinations of all these measures. To protect against the dangers of internal radiation, precautions seek to restrict inhalation, ingestion, and other modes of entry of radioactive substances into the body.

radiation oncology, the treatment of cancer using radiation.

radiation sensitivity, a measure of the response of tissue to ionizing radiation.

radiation sickness, an abnormal condition resulting from exposure to ionizing radiation. The severity of the condition is determined by the volume of radiation, the length of time of exposure, and the area of the body affected. Moderate exposure may cause headache, nausea, vomiting, anorexia, and diarrhea; long-term exposure may result in sterility, damage to the fetus in pregnant women, leukemia or other forms of cancer, alopecia, and cataracts.

radiation syndrome. See **radiation sickness.**

radiation therapy. See **radiotherapy.**

radical, **1.** a group of atoms that acts together and forms a component of a compound. The group tends to remain bound together when a chemical reaction removes it from a compound and attaches it to another. A radical does not exist freely in nature. **2.** pertaining to drastic therapy, as the surgical removal of an organ, limb, or other part of the body.

radical dissection, the surgical removal of tissue in an extensive area surrounding the operative site. Most often it is performed to identify and excise all tissue that may possibly be malignant to decrease the chance of recurrence.

radical mastectomy, surgical removal of an entire breast, pectoral muscles, axillary lymph nodes, and all fat, fascia, and adjacent tissues. It is performed in the treatment of cancer of the breast. Preoperatively, in addition to giving usual preoperative care, the staff encourages verbalization of the patient's fears of the disease, of the surgery, and of the loss of her breast. Her self-image is usually severely threatened, and she characteristically grieves in anticipation of a loss of femininity. The postoperative period is physically and emotionally painful; the woman is best warned by supportive but realistic explanations before surgery. Edema of the arm on the affected side is the rule, because the axillary lymphatic structures that drain the lymph from the arm are removed during surgery. Atelectasis may develop if deep breathing and coughing are not regularly performed. The incision is painful but may be expected to become less so during the first few days; it should not become more inflamed or painfully swollen. A pressure dressing is usually applied and left in place until bleeding and drainage have decreased. A drain is usually left in the wound for several days. The woman may be anxious, depressed, angry, or withdrawn, or she may reflect hopelessness. In addition to the usual postoperative measures, the nurse elevates the affected arm above the level of the right atrium; checks the color, sensation, and motion of the fingers; checks the graft site if a graft was performed; and applies reinforcement to the pressure dressing as necessary. Later in the postoperative period, the patient is assisted in range of motion exercises for all extremities and is taught, with assistance, to perform gradually increasing arm and shoulder exercises. In discussion and in providing physical care, the loss of the breast is dealt with frankly; to avoid the fact is not helpful to the patient. Slowly the patient is involved in caring for herself more completely, a process that continues as she gradually resumes her normal daily activities. On discharge, she is encouraged to shower daily, to apply an emollient, like cocoa butter, to the incision, and to examine the remaining breast monthly. Reach to Recovery may be involved in counseling and support before and after a mastectomy. Chemotherapy and radiation therapy may continue after surgery. The woman is told never to allow blood to be drawn from the affected arm; intravenous injection is also to be avoided in that arm. Blood pressure measurement, vaccination, and other injections are best performed on the other arm. Compare **modified radical mastectomy, simple mastectomy.** See also **mastectomy.**

radical neck dissection, dissection and removal of all lymph nodes and removable tissues under the skin of the neck, performed to prevent the spread of malignant tumors of the head and neck that have a reasonable chance of being controlled. Before surgery, thorough mouth hygiene is given and antibiotics are begun. Under general anesthesia, a tracheostomy is done; the tumor, surrounding tissues, and the lymph nodes on the affected side are then removed in one mass from the angle of the jaw to the clavicle, forward to midline, and back to the angle of the jaw. A total laryngectomy may be done as part of the surgery. After surgery, the nurse suctions the tracheostomy as necessary and observes vital signs for indications of hemorrhage or difficulty in breathing. A humidifier or vaporizer will ease coughing and production of mucus. IV fluids are continued in the arm not used for writing. Extensive work with a speech pathologist may be necessary to learn esophageal speech. Radiation of the tumor site may be begun, and chemotherapy may continue. Compare **neck dissection.**

radical therapy, **1.** a treatment intended to cure, not palliate. **2.** a definitive, extreme treatment; not conservative, as radical mastectomy rather than simple or partial mastectomy.

radical vulvectomy. See **vulvectomy.**

radicular cyst, (in dentistry) a cyst with a wall of fibrous connective tissue and a lining of stratified squamous epithelium that is attached to the apex of the root of a tooth with dead pulp or a defective root canal filling.

radicular retainer, a type of retainer that lies within the body of a tooth, usually in the root portion, as a dowel crown. The retention or resistance to displacement and shear is developed by extending an attached dowel into the root canal of the tooth involved.

radicular retention, retention developed by placing metal projections into the root canals of pulpless teeth.

radio-, a combining form meaning 'of or related to radiation,' sometimes specifically to emission of radiant energy, to radium, or to the radius: *radioactive, radiobiology, radiohumeral.*

radioactive, giving off radiation as the result of the disintegration of the nucleus of an atom.

radioactive contamination, the undesirable addition of radioactive material to the body or part of the environment, as clothing or equipment. Beta radiation contamination of the body of health care personnel is only possible through the ingestion, inhalation, or absorption of the source, as when the skin is contaminated with a beta emitter contained in an absorbable chemical form. Instruments, drapes, surgical gloves, and clothing that come in contact with serous fluids, blood, and urine of patients containing beta or gamma radiation emitters may be contaminated. The severity of the contamination is directly related to the elapsed time between the administration of the isotope and surgery; on completion of the procedure, possibly contaminated material is isolated and checked; if found to be contaminated, it is disposed of according to institutional or federal standards for the disposal of radioactive waste.

radioactive contrast media, a solution or colloid containing material of high atomic number, used for visualizing soft tissue structures. Radiopharmaceutics indicate their positions or distribution in the body by their gamma ray emissions.

radioactive decay, the disintegration of the nucleus of an unstable nuclide by the spontaneous emission of charged particles, photons, or both.

radioactive element, an element subject to spontaneous degeneration of its nucleus accompanied by the emission of alpha particles, beta particles, or gamma rays. All elements with atomic numbers greater than 83 are radioactive. Several radioactive elements not found in nature have been produced by the bombardment of stable elements with atomic particles in a cyclotron. Some kinds of radioactive elements are radium, thorium, uranium. Compare **stable element.** See also **radioactivity.**

radioactive iodine (RAI), a radioactive isotope of iodine, used as a tracer in biology and medicine.

radioactive iodine excretion, the elimination by the body of radioactive iodine (RAI) administered in a test of thyroid function and in the treatment of hyperthyroidism. Most RAI is excreted in urine, but small amounts may be found in sputum, perspiration, feces, and vomitus.

radioactive iodine excretion test, a method of evaluating thyroid function by measuring the amount of radioactive iodine (RAI) in urine after the patient is given an oral tracer dose of the radioisotope ^{131}I. Normally, 5% to 35% of the dose is absorbed by the thyroid, but absorption is increased in hyperthyroidism and decreased in hypothyroidism, and the amount excreted in urine is inversely proportional to the uptake of RAI. After administration of the tracer, a scintillation detector is placed over the patient's neck at 2, 6, and 24 hours to measure the RAI accumulated by the thyroid, and the amount excreted is assayed in urine collected for 24 hours after the oral dose. Diarrhea can result in low values of RAI in urine; renal failure, by decreasing excretion, can cause high readings. See also **radioactive iodine uptake.**

radioactive iodine uptake (RAIU), the absorption and incorporation by the thyroid of radioactive iodine (RAI), administered orally as a tracer dose in a test of thyroid function and as larger doses for the treatment of hyperthyroidism. The radioisotope ^{131}I is rapidly absorbed in the stomach and is concentrated in the thyroid. Patients receiving a large therapeutic dose of RAI may require hospitalization for several days. See also **radioactive iodine excretion test.**

radioactivity, the emission of corpuscular or electromagnetic radiations as a consequence of nuclear disintegration. Natural radioactivity is a property exhibited by all chemical elements with an atomic number greater than 83; artificial or induced radioactivity is created through the bombardment of naturally occurring isotopes with subatomic particles or high levels of gamma or x-radiation.

radioallergosorbent test (RAST) /rā′dē·ō·alur′gō·sôr′bənt/, a test in which a technique of radioimmunoassay is used to identify and quantify IgE in serum that has been mixed with any of 45 known allergens. If an atopic allergy to a substance exists, an antigen-antibody reaction occurs with characteristic conjugation and clumping. The test is an in vitro method of demonstrating allergic reactions. Compare **patch test, Prausnitz-Küstner test.**

radiobiology, the branch of the natural sciences dealing with the effects of radiation on biologic systems. –**radiobiologic, radiobiological,** *adj.*

radiocarpal articulation, the condyloid joint at the wrist that connects the radius and distal surface of an articular disk with the scaphoid, the lunate, and the triangular bones. The joint involves four ligaments and allows all movements but rotation. Also called **wrist joint.**

radiochemistry, the branch of chemistry that deals with the properties and behavior of radioactive materials and the use of radionuclides in the study of chemical and biologic problems.

radiofrequency (rf), that portion of the electromagnetic spectrum with frequencies lower than about 10^{10} Hz.

radiograph, an x-ray picture.

radiographic magnification, visualization of small areas through magnification achieved with a small x-ray tube having a small focal point. It is a common diagnostic tool in orthopedics.

radiographic grid, a clear plastic device with horizontal and vertical wires crossing at intervals of 1 mm, used in x-ray techniques for measuring distances and relationships.

radiography /rā′dē•og′rəfē/, the production of shadow images on photographic emulsion through the action of ionizing radiation. The image is the result of the differential attenuation of the radiation in its passage through the object being radiographed. –**radiographic,** *adj.*

radioimmunoassay (RIA) /rā′dē•ō•imyōō′nō•as′ā/, a technique in radiology used to determine the concentration of an antigen, antibody, or other protein in the serum. A radioactively labeled substance known to react in a certain way with the suspected protein is injected, and any reaction is monitored.

radioimmunosorbent assay test, a test that uses serum immunoglobulin E to detect allergies to various substances, as certain cosmetics, animal fur, dust, and grasses.

radioiodine /rā′dē•ō•ī′ədīn/, a radioactive isotope of iodine used in radiotherapy. It is used especially in the treatment of some thyroid conditions and in diagnostic radiology by various scanning techniques. A common form of radioiodine is ^{131}I.

radioisotope /rā′dē•ō•ī′sətōp/, a radioactive isotope of an element, used for therapeutic and diagnostic purposes.

radioisotope scan, a two-dimensional representation of the gamma rays emitted by a radioisotope, showing its concentration in a body site, as the thyroid gland, brain, or kidney. Radioisotopes used in diagnostic scanning may be administered intravenously or orally.

radiologic anatomy, (in applied anatomy) the study of the structure and morphology of the tissues and organs of the body based on their x-ray visualization.

radiologic technologist, a person who, under the supervision of a physician radiologist, operates radiologic equipment and assists radiologists and other health professionals, and whose competence has been tested and approved by the American Registry of Radiologic Technologists. Also called **x-ray technician.**

radiologist, a physician who specializes in radiology. A certified radiologist is one whose competence has been tested and approved by the American Board of Radiology.

radiology, the branch of medicine concerned with radioactive substances and, using various techniques of visualization, with the diagnosis and treatment of disease using any of the various sources of radiant energy. Three subbranches of radiology are **diagnostic radiology,** which concerns itself with imaging using external sources of radiation; **nuclear medicine,** which is involved with imaging radioactive materials that are placed into body organs; and **therapeutic radiology,** which is concerned with the treatment of cancer using radiation. –**radiologic, radiological,** *adj.* (Table, page 964)

radiolucency, a characteristic of materials of relatively low atomic number that attenuates x-rays passing through them and produces relatively dark images. –**radiolucent,** *adj.*

radionuclide /-nōō′klīd/, **1.** an isotope (or nuclide) that undergoes radioactive decay. **2.** any of the radioactive isotopes of cobalt, iodine, phosphorus, strontium, and other elements, used in nuclear medicine for treatment of tumors and cancers and for nuclear imaging of internal parts of the body. See also **nuclear scanning.**

radionuclide angiocardiography, the radiographic examination of cardiac blood vessels after an intravenous injection of a radiopharmaceutic.

radionuclide imaging, the noninvasive examination of various parts of the body, especially the heart, using a radiopharmaceutic, as thallium 201, and a detection device, as a gamma camera, rectilinear scanner, or positron camera. See also **cardiac radionuclide imaging.**

radionuclide organ imaging. See **nuclear scanning.**

radiopaque /-pāk′/, not permitting the passage of x-rays or other radiant energy. Bones are relatively radiopaque and therefore show as white areas on an exposed x-ray film. Lead is markedly radiopaque and therefore is widely used to shield x-ray equipment and atomic power sources. See also **radioactive element, radioactivity, radiopaque dye.** –**radiopacity,** *n.*

radiopaque dye, a chemical substance that does not permit the passage of x-rays. Various radiopaque iodine compounds are used to outline the interior of hollow organs such as heart chambers, blood vessels, respiratory passages, and the biliary tract in x-ray or fluoroscopic pictures. Compare **radiolucency.**

radiopharmaceutic, a drug that exhibits spontaneous disintegration of unstable nuclei with the emission of nuclear particles or photons. Kinds of radiopharmaceutics are **diagnostic radiopharmaceutic, research radiopharmaceutic,** and **therapeutic radiopharmaceutic.**

radiopharmacist, a trained professional responsible for the formulation and dispensing of prescribed radioactive tracers and for the clinical aspects of radiopharmacy. Radiopharmacists are required to receive training in radioactive tracer techniques, in the safe handling of radioactive materials, in the preparation and quality control of drugs for administration to humans, and in the basic principles of nuclear medicine. Some states require that radioactive drugs be dispensed by licensed pharmacists only; others recognize radiopharmaceutic specialists who are not necessarily graduates of a school of pharmacy.

radiopharmacy, a facility for the preparation and dispensing of radioactive drugs and for the storage of radioactive materials, inventory records, and prescriptions of radioactive substances. The radiopharmacy is usually the correlation point for radioactive wastes, the unit responsible for waste disposal or storage, and a center for clinical investigations employing radioactive tracers. It may also be a center for research and for the training of students and residents in radiology and nuclear medicine.

radioresistance, the relative resistance of cells, tissues, organs, organisms, chemical compounds, or any other substances to the effects of radiation. Compare **radiosensitivity.**

radioresistant, unchanged by or protected against damage by radioactive emissions such as x-rays, alpha particles, or gamma rays. Compare **radiosensitive.** See also **radioactivity.**

radiosensitive, capable of being changed by or reacting to radioactive emissions such as x-rays, alpha particles, or gamma rays. Compare **radioresistant.** See also **radioactivity.**

radiosensitivity, the relative susceptibility of cells, tissues, organs, organisms, or any other living substances to the effects of radiation. Cells of self-renewing systems, as those in the crypts of the intestine, are the most radiosensitive. Cells that divide regularly but mature between divisions, as spermatogonia and spermatocytes, are next in radiosusceptibility. Long-lived cells that usually do not undergo mitosis unless there is a suitable stimulus include the less radiosensitive liver, kidney, and thyroid cells. Least sensitive are fixed postmitotic cells that have lost the ability to divide, as neurons. Connective tissue and blood vessels are intermediate in radiosensitivity; parenchymal cells are affected by moderate doses of radiation that do not damage connective tissue.

radiosensitizers, drugs that enhance the killing effect of radiation on cells. If radiosensitizers can be selectively introduced in the cells of a tumor while being absent from the surrounding normal tissue, the effect of irradiating the tumor will be increased, presumably leading to improved survival for the patient.

radiotherapy, the treatment of neoplastic disease by using x-rays or gamma rays, usually from a cobalt source, to deter the proliferation of malignant cells by decreasing the rate of mitosis or impairing DNA synthesis.

■ METHOD: Before radiotherapy, the procedure, its purpose, duration, painlessness, and the need to remain

Characteristics and uses of some commonly used radioactive substances

Radiation source	*Half-life (where applicable)*	*Rays emitted*	*Appearance or form*	*Method of administration*
X-ray	—	γ	Invisible rays	X-ray machine
Radium (^{226}Ra)	1600 yr	α β γ	In needles, plaques, molds	Interstitial (needles) Intracavitary (plaques, mold)
Radon (^{221}Rn)	25 minutes	α β γ (low intensity)	In seeds, needles	Interstitial (seeds, needles)
Cesium (^{137}Cs)	30 yrs	β γ	In needles, capsules	Interstitial (needles) Intracavitary (capsules)
Cobalt (^{60}Co)	5 yr	β γ	External (cobalt unit) Internal (needles, seeds, molds)	Machine (teletherapy) Interstitial (needles, seeds)
Iodine (^{131}I)	8 days	β γ (low intensity)	Clear liquid	By mouth
Phosphorus (^{32}P)	14 days	β	Clear liquid	By mouth, intracavitary, intravenous
Gold (^{198}Au)	3 days	β γ	Purple liquid	Intracavitary
Iridium (^{192}Ir)	74 days	β γ (low intensity)	In needles, wires, seeds	Interstitial
Yttrium (^{90}Y)	3 days	β	Beads, needles	Interstitial

completely still during irradiation are explained to the patient. Potential sequelae, as erythema, edema, desquamation, hyperpigmentation, atrophy, pruritus or skin pain, altered taste, anorexia, nausea, vomiting, headache, hair loss, malaise, tachycardia, and increased susceptibility to infection may be discussed in response to specific questions raised by the patient. A preliminary visit to the radiology department may be arranged so that the equipment and the room in which the patient will be positioned on a table can be seen. From this position the patient is able to communicate with the radiotherapist in an adjoining booth. Daily hygiene measures are completed before treatment; on returning from irradiation, the patient is placed in a noninfectious environment or, if necessary, in protective isolation; friends, family, other patients and staff members with infections, especially upper respiratory tract infections, are not permitted to visit. Skin care is administered after irradiation and every 4 hours thereafter, but the ink markings placed by the radiologist on the skin to mark the focus of treatment are not removed between treatments, and the treated area is not washed with water; sterile mineral oil, lanolin, or petroleum jelly may be applied if the radiologist approves. The patient wears loose garments and rests on an air mattress, foam or gel pad, or sheepskin; a footboard or bed cradle is used to elevate the top sheet and blanket. Cosmetics are avoided, and underarm deodorants or antiperspirants are contraindicated if the axillary area is irradiated. If hair loss occurs, the patient may wear a wig, scarf, cap, or toupee. High-protein supplements, soothing gelatins, and ice cream are provided, and other food is served when desired by the patient; six small, bland feedings may be tolerated more easily than regular meals. Quiet periods are maintained before and after meals. Antiemetics and vitamins are administered as ordered, and tube feedings or total parenteral nutrition may be indicated if the patient's food intake is severely decreased. Oral hygiene, using a soft-bristled brush and dilute mouthwash, or, if needed, foam or sponge swabs and a saline rinse, is administered whenever required, and a fluid intake of 2000 to 3000 ml daily is maintained unless contraindicated. In preparation for discharge, the patient is instructed to follow the hospital practices for skin care, oral hygiene, fluid intake, and a high-protein, nutritious diet but to avoid eating immediately before and after irradiation. The patient is told to avoid tight clothing, extremes of temperature, exposure to sunlight, tub baths or showers until ordered, and persons with infections and to report to the physician any symptom of infection, inability to eat, severe diarrhea, increasing headache, and fatigue, or increasing redness, swelling, itching, or pain at the site of therapy.

■ NURSING ORDERS: The nurse offers thorough explanation of the radiotherapy, provides care after treatment, and prepares the patient for discharge and, if indicated, continued therapy on an outpatient basis.

■ OUTCOME CRITERIA: Radiotherapy can control or arrest the development of a number of forms of cancer and provide palliation in some inoperable tumors; the maintenance of adequate nutrition and meticulous care of the skin may allow the person to avoid the most serious and unpleasant side effects of radiotherapy.

radioulnar articulation, the articulation of the radius and the ulna, consisting of a proximal articulation, a distal articulation, and three sets of ligaments.

radium (Ra), a radioactive metallic element of the alkaline earth group. Its atomic number is 88. Four radium isotopes occur naturally and have different atomic weights: 223, 224, 226, and 228. The isotope with atomic weight 226 is the most abundant. It is formed by the disintegration of uranium 238, has a half-life of 1620 years, and decays by alpha emission to form radon 222. Radium occurs in the uranium minerals carnotite and pitchblende, which contain about 3×10^{-7} g of radium per g of uranium. Radium salts have been used extensively as radiation sources in the treatment of cancer but are gradually being replaced in such therapy by cobalt and cesium.

radium insertion, the introduction of metallic radium (Ra) into a body area, as the uterus or cervix, to treat cancer.

radium 226, a radioactive substance used for most of this century to fill the needles and tubes required for brachytherapy. Radium use is now being replaced by cesium 137 and cobalt 60, which have similar energy characteristics and are not subject to hazardous leakage as radium sources sometimes are.

radius, *pl.* **radii** /rā′dē·ī/, one of the bones of the forearm, lying parallel to the ulna. Its proximal end is small and forms a part of the elbow joint. The distal end is large and forms a part of the wrist joint. The radius receives the insertions of various muscles and articulates with the humerus, ulna, scaphoid, and lunate bones.

radix. See **root.**

radon (Rn), a radioactive, inert, gaseous, nonmetallic element. Its atomic number is 86; its atomic weight is 222. Radon, a decay product of radium, is used in radiation cancer therapy.

radon seed, a small sealed tube of glass or gold containing radon, and visible radiographically, for insertion into body tissues in the treatment of malignancies.

radon 222, the radioactive daughter of radium 226 that has been used to fill seeds for permanent implantation into tumors. This material is being replaced by the more manageable radionuclide iodine 125.

RAI, abbreviation for **radioactive iodine.**

RAIU, abbreviation for **radioactive iodine uptake.**

RA latex test, abbreviation for *rheumatoid arthritis latex test.* See **latex fixation test.**

rale, a common abnormal respiratory sound heard on auscultation of the chest during inspiration, characterized by discontinuous bubbling noises. Fine rales have a crackling sound produced by air entering distal bronchioles or alveoli that contain serous secretions, as in congestive heart failure, pneumonia, or early tuberculosis. Coarse rales originate in the larger bronchi or trachea and have a lower pitch. Kinds of rales are **sibilant rale** and **sonorous rale.** Compare **rhonchus, wheeze.**

RAM /ram, är′ā′em′/, abbreviation for *random access memory,* the part of a computer's memory available to execute programs and store data. The memory to which the operator has random access usually can be used for both reading and writing.

rami-, a combining form meaning 'branch': *ramicotomy, ramification, ramisection.*

Ramsay Hunt's syndrome, a neurologic condition resulting from invasion of the seventh nerve ganglia and the geniculate ganglion by varicella zoster virus, characterized by severe ear pain, facial nerve paralysis, vertigo, hearing loss, and, often, mild, generalized encephalitis. The vertigo may last days or weeks but usually resolves itself. The facial paralysis may be permanent, and the hearing loss, which is rarely permanent, may be partial or total. Treatment usually includes the prescription of corticosteroid drugs. Also called **herpes zoster oticus.**

ramus /rā′məs/, *pl.* **rami,** a small, branchlike structure extending from a larger one or dividing into two or more parts, as a branch of a nerve or artery or one of the rami of the pubis. –**ramification,** *n.* **ramify,** *v.*

random access memory. See **RAM.**

random genetic drift. See **genetic drift.**

range of motion exercise, any body action involving the muscles, the joints, and natural directional movements, as abduction, extension, flexion, pronation, and rotation. Such exercises are usually applied actively or passively in the treatment of orthopedic deformities, in the assessment of injuries and deformities, and in athletic conditioning.

ranitidine, a histamine H_2 receptor anatgonist.

■ INDICATIONS: It is prescribed in the treatment of duodenal and gastric ulcers and gastric hypersecretory conditions.

■ CONTRAINDICATIONS: Known sensitivity to this drug prohibits its use. The drug should be used in pregnancy only if clearly needed.

■ ADVERSE EFFECTS: Among the most serious adverse reactions are headaches and rashes.

ranula /ran′yo͞olə/, *pl.* **ranulae,** a large mucocele in the floor of the mouth, usually caused by obstruction of the ducts of the sublingual salivary glands and less commonly by obstruction of the ducts of the submandibular salivary glands.

Ranvier's nodes /ränvē•āz′, räN-/, constrictions in the medullary substance of a nerve fiber at more or less regular intervals.

rape, a sexual assault, homosexual or heterosexual, the legal definitions for which vary from state to state. Rape is a crime of violence or one committed under the threat of violence, and its victims are treated for medical and psychologic trauma. See also **statutory rape.**

■ OBSERVATIONS: Characteristically, the victim is frightened and feels vulnerable, humiliated, and personally violated. General physical examination may reveal cuts, bruises, and other injuries. Pelvic or genital examination may show traumatic injury to the internal or external genitalia or anus.

■ INTERVENTION: Careful physical examination is performed and a detailed history obtained. Specimens are obtained as indicated. Ideally, counseling is available and offered immediately to all victims of rape. In the case of a woman who has been raped by a man, a pregnancy test is performed and specific injuries are treated. If the test is positive, prophylaxis against conception may be administered. Usually, antibiotics are given to prevent the development of venereal disease. Arrangements for ongoing emotional support are made.

■ NURSING CONSIDERATIONS: A trained, sympathetic nurse of the same sex is assigned to stay with the victim. Privacy for the history, examination, and police interview is ensured. The victim may or may not choose to talk to the police, but the police must be informed in every case. The victim must sign a special form to allow specimens to be released to a law enforcement agency. In general, it is the role of the nurse and other medical workers to examine, to treat, and to collect specimens as necessary, not to decide that rape has occurred. Before discharge, it should be ascertained that someone can be with the victim, because depression, anger, guilt, and fear are common after rape.

Rape preventive measures

Prevention of attack

Set house lights to go on and off by timer
Keep light on at all entrances
Place safety locks on windows and doors
Have key ready before reaching door of house or car
Look in car before entering
Insist on identification before letting a stranger in house; check identification with agency if suspicious
Do not list first name on mailbox or in telephone directory
Make arrangements with neighbor for needed assistance
Be alert when walking in street; walk in lighted areas
Walk down center of street if possible
Avoid lonely or enclosed areas

If attacked

Run toward a lighted house; yell "Fire"
Spit in rapist's face; act bizarre; vomit
Rip off rapist's glasses
Step hard on his foot (instep)
Aim at eyes—try to gouge eyes, scrape face
Hit throat at Adam's apple (larynx)
Use fighting and screaming with caution; this may scare some rapists, encourage others
Try talking to avoid rape
If powerless, make close observations about rapist, car, location

rape counseling, counseling by a trained person provided to a victim of rape. Rape counseling ideally begins at the time the crime is first reported, as in an emergency room. Initially, the counselor offers sensitive support for the victim by accepting the victim in a nonprejudicial, noncritical way. The victim's response to the trauma of the assault is empathetically elicited, and three basic statements are made: The counselor is sorry that the rape happened, is glad that the injuries are not worse, and does not think that the victim was wrong or did anything wrong. Counseling personnel may provide supportive services and advocacy and liaison between the victim and medical, legal, and law enforcement authorities. This involves staying with the victim during medical examination, police or district attorney's questioning, and throughout the criminal justice process.

rape trauma syndrome, a nursing diagnosis accepted by the Fourth National Conference on the Classification of Nursing Diagnoses. The syndrome results from the experience of being raped and includes an acute phase of disorganization and a longer phase of reorganization in the victim's life. The cause of the syndrome is the trauma of the rape. The defining characteristics are divided into three subcomponents: rape trauma, compound reaction, and silent reaction. The defining characteristics of rape trauma in the acute phase are emotional reactions of anger, guilt, and embarrassment, fear of physical violence and death, humiliation, wish for revenge, and multiple physical complaints, including GI distress, genitourinary discomfort, tension, and disturbance of the normal patterns of sleep, activity, and rest. The long-term phase of rape trauma is characterized by changes in the usual patterns of daily life (even a change in residence), nightmares and phobias, and a need for support from friends and family. The compound reaction is characterized by all of the defining characteristics of rape trauma, reliance on alcohol or drugs, or the recurrence of the symptoms of previous conditions, including psychiatric illness. The silent reaction sometimes occurs in place of the rape trauma or compound reaction. The defining characteristics of the silent reaction are an abrupt change in the victim's usual sexual relationships, an increase in nightmares, an increasing anxiety during the interview about the rape incident, a marked change in sexual behavior, denial of the rape or refusal to discuss it, and the sudden development of phobic reactions. See also **nursing diagnosis.**

raphe /rā′fē/, a line of union of the halves of various symmetric parts, as the abdominal raphe of the linea alba or the raphe penis, which appears as a narrow, dark streak on the inferior surface of the penis. Also spelled **rhaphe.**

rapid-acting insulin. See **short-acting insulin.**

rapid eye movement. See **sleep.**

rapport /rapôr′/, a sense of mutuality and understanding; harmony, accord, confidence, and respect underlying a relationship between two persons, an essential bond between a therapist and patient in psychotherapy.

raptus /rap′təs/, **1.** a state of intense emotional or mental excitement, often characterized by uncontrollable activity or behavior resulting from an irresistible impulse; ecstasy; rapture. **2.** any sudden or violent seizure or attack. Kinds of raptus include **raptus haemorrhagicus, raptus maniacus, raptus melancholicus,** and **raptus nervorum.**

raptus haemorrhagicus /hem′ôrā′jikəs/, a sudden, massive hemorrhage.

raptus maniacus /manī′əkəs/, a sudden violent attack of mania. See also **mania.**

raptus melancholicus /mel′ənkō′likəs/, an attack of extreme agitation or frenzy that occurs during the course of depression.

raptus nervorum /nervôr′əm/, a sudden, violent attack of nervousness that may be marked by cramps.

rare earth element, a metallic element having an atomic number between 57 to 71, inclusively. These closely related substances are classified in three groups: the cerium metals are lanthanum, cerium, praseodymium, neodymium, promethium, and samarium; the terbium metals are europium, gadolinium, and terbium; the yttrium metals are dysprosium, holmium, erbium, thulium, yttrium, ytterbium, and lutetium. Also called **rare earth metal.**

rare earth screen, a fluorescent material, as calcium tungstate, used as the basis of x-ray intensifying screens. In recent years, new materials including the rare earths yttrium and gadolinium also have found application in such devices. These rare earths enable lower radiation doses to be used while producing acceptable film densities.

RAS, abbreviation for **reticular activating system.**

rash, a skin eruption. Kinds of rashes include **butterfly rash, diaper rash, drug rash,** and **heat rash.**

Rashkind procedure /rash′kind/, the enlargement of an opening in the cardiac septum between the right and left atria, performed to relieve congestive heart failure in newborns with certain congenital heart defects by improving the oxygenation of the blood. The procedure allows more mixing between oxygenated blood from the lungs and systemic blood without the risk of surgery, sustaining life until the infant is 2 to 3 years of age and a shunt can be created to carry systemic blood to the lungs. Preoperatively, a cardiac catheterization is done to pinpoint the defect. Under light general anesthesia, a deflated balloon is passed pervenously through the foramen ovale into the left atrium. The balloon is inflated and pulled across the septum to enlarge the opening. Postoperatively, the infant is observed carefully for respiratory difficulty, signs of hypoxia, or decreasing cardiac output. Humidified oxygen is administered. Fluids and electrolytes are closely monitored. Also called **balloon septostomy.**

Rasmussen's aneurysm /ras′mo͞osənz/, a localized dilatation of a blood vessel in a tuberculous cavity that causes hemorrhage when it ruptures.

RAST. See **radioallergosorbent test.**

rat-bite fever, either of two distinct infections transmitted to humans by the bite of a rat or mouse, characterized by fever, headache, malaise, nausea, vomiting, and rash. In the United States, the disease is more commonly caused by *Streptobacillus moniliformis,* and its unique features are rash on palms and soles, painful joints, prompt healing of the wound, and a duration of 2 weeks. In the Far East, rat-bite fever is usually caused by *Spirillum minus* and is associated with an asymmetric rash on the extremities, no joint symptoms, a relapsing fever, swelling at the site of the wound, regional lymphadenopathy, and a duration of from 4 to 8 weeks. Relapse is common. Penicillin administered intramuscularly is effective in treating either form of the disease. Rat-bite fever resulting from infection caused by *Streptobacillus moniliformis* is also called **Haverhill fever;** infection caused by *Spirillum minus* is also called **sodoku.**

rate, a numeric ratio, often used in the compilation of data concerning the prevalence and incidence of events, in which the number of actual occurrences appears as the numerator and the number of possible occurrences appears as the denominator, as when 1 person in 15 fails an examination the failure rate is said to be 1/15 (or "one in fifteen"). Standard rates are stated in conventional units of population, as neonatal mortality per 1000 or maternal mortality per 100,000.

Rathke's pouch tumor. See **craniopharyngioma.**

ratio, the relationship of one quantity to one or more other quantities expressed as a proportion of one to the others, and written either as a fraction (8/3) or linearly (8:3).

rational, **1.** of or pertaining to a measure, method, or procedure based on reason. **2.** of or pertaining to a therapeutic method based on an understanding of the cause and mechanisms of a specific disease and the potential effects of the drugs or procedures used in treating the disorder. **3.** sane; capable of normal reasoning or behavior.

rationale /rash′ənal′/, a system of reasoning or a statement of the reasons used in explaining data or phenomena.

rational emotive therapy (RET), a form of psychotherapy, originated by Albert Ellis, that emphasizes a reorganization of one's cognitive and emotional functions, a redefinition of one's problems, and a change in one's attitudes to develop more effective and suitable patterns of behavior. RET is conducted with individuals or with groups.

rationalization, a process of constructing plausible reasons to explain and justify one's behavior.

rational treatment. See **treatment.**

rattle, an abnormal sound heard by auscultation of the lungs in some forms of pulmonary disease. It consists of a coarse vibration caused by the movement of moisture and the separation of the walls of small air passages during respiration.

rattlesnake, a poisonous pit viper with a series of loosely connected, horny segments at the end of the tail that make a noise like a rattle when shaken. More than 25 species of rattlesnakes are found in the Americas, including many parts of the United States. They have a hematoxin in their venom, and they are responsible for most of the poisonous snake bites in the United States. See **snakebite.**

rat typhus. See **murine typhus.**

Raudixin, a trademark for an antihypertensive (purified *Rauwolfia serpentina*).

Rau-Sed, a trademark for an antihypertensive (reserpine).

Rauwiloid, a trademark for an antihypertensive (alseroxylon).

rauwolfia /rôwol′fē·ə, rou-, rä-/, the dried roots of *Rauwolfia serpentina* that provide the extracts for hypotensive agents and tranquilizing alkaloid drugs, like reserpine.

rauwolfia alkaloid, any one of more than 20 alkaloids derived from the root of a climbing shrub, *Rauwolfia serpentina,* indigenous to India and the surrounding area. Formerly used as an antipsychotic agent, it is today confined to the treatment of hypertension. Numerous trademark formulations of the principal alkaloid reserpine are available.

rauwolfia serpentina, the dried root from *Rauwolfia serpentina,* used as an antihypertensive.

■ INDICATIONS: It is prescribed in the treatment of mild hypertension and hypertensive emergencies.

■ CONTRAINDICATIONS: Mental depression, peptic ulcer, ulcerative colitis, electroconvulsive therapy, or known hypersensitivity to this drug prohibits its use. It can interact adversely with monoamine oxidase inhibitors.

■ ADVERSE EFFECTS: Among the more serious adverse reactions are symptoms resembling parkinsonism, glaucoma, cardiac arrhythmias, and GI bleeding.

Rauzide, a trademark for a cardiovascular, fixed-combination drug containing a diuretic (bendroflumethiazide) and an antihypertensive (rauwolfia serpentina).

ray, a beam of radiation, as heat or light, moving away from a source.

Raynaud's phenomenon /rānōz′/, intermittent attacks of ischemia of the extremities of the body, especially the fingers, toes, ears, and nose, caused by exposure to cold or by emotional stimuli. The attacks are characterized by severe blanching of the extremities, followed by cyanosis, then redness; they are usually accompanied by numbness, tingling, burning, and often pain. Normal color and sensation are restored by heat. The attacks usually occur secondary to such conditions as scleroderma, rheumatoid arthritis, systemic lupus erythematosus, thoracic outlet syndrome, drug intoxications, dysproteinemia, myxedema, primary pulmonary hypertension, and trauma. The condition is called **Raynaud's disease** when there is a history of symptoms for at least 2 years with no progression of symptoms and no evidence of an underlying cause. Therapy for the secondary form depends on recognition and treatment of the underlying disease. Idiopathic forms, which occur most frequently in young women 18 to 30 years of age, may be controlled by protecting the body and extremities from the cold and by the use of mild sedatives and vasodilators.

Raynaud's sign. See **acrocyanosis.**

razoxane /rəzok′sān/, an antineoplastic drug approved for use in the management of certain neoplasms.

Rb, symbol for **rubidium.**

RBC, abbreviation for *red blood cell.* See **erythrocyte.**

RBE, abbreviation for **relative biologic effectiveness.**

R.C.P., abbreviation for **Royal College of Physicians.**

RCPSC, abbreviation for **Royal College of Physicians and Surgeons of Canada.**

R.C.S., abbreviation for **Royal College of Surgeons.**

RD, abbreviation for **registered dietician.**

RDA, abbreviation for **recommended daily allowance.**

RDS, abbreviation for *respiratory distress syndrome.* See **respiratory distress syndrome of the newborn.**

Re, symbol for **rhenium.**

re-, a combining form meaning 'back, again, contrary': *reaction, recombination, recurrent.*

Reach to Recovery, a national volunteer organization that offers counseling and support to women who have breast cancer and to their families. Many of the members have had mastectomies themselves.

reaction, a response in opposition to a substance, treatment, or other stimulus, as an antigen-antibody reaction in immunology, a hypersensitivity reaction in allergy, or an adverse reaction in pharmacology. **–react,** *v.,* **reactive,** *adj.*

reaction formation, a defense mechanism in which a person avoids anxiety through overt behavior and attitudes that are the opposite of repressed impulses and drives and that serve to conceal those unacceptable feelings.

reactive depression, an emotional disorder characterized by an acute feeling of despondency, sadness, and depressive dysphoria, which varies in intensity and duration. The condition is caused by an unrealistic and inappropriate reaction to some identifiable external situation or intrapsychic conflict and is relieved when the circumstance is altered or the conflict understood and resolved. Also called **exogenous depression, situational depression.** Compare **endogenous depression.** See also **depression.**

reactive schizophrenia, a form of schizophrenia caused by environmental factors rather than by organic changes in the brain. The onset of the disease is usually rapid; symptoms are of brief duration, and the affected individual appears well immediately before and after the schizophrenic episode. Compare **process schizophrenia.** See also **schizophrenia, schizophreniform disorder.**

read, (of a computer) to accept data from some storage location or medium, as a disk.

reading, (in molecular genetics) the linear process in which the genetic information contained in a nucleotide sequence is decoded, as in the translation of the messenger RNA directives for the sequence of the amino acids in a polypeptide.

Read method, a method of psychophysical preparation for childbirth designed by Dr. Grantly Dick-Read. It was the first ''natural childbirth'' program, a term coined by Dr. Read. Basically, Read held that childbirth is a normal, physiologic procedure and that the pain of labor and delivery is of psychologic origin—the fear tension pain syndrome. He countered women's fears with education about the physiologic process, encouraged a positive, welcoming attitude, corrected false information, and led tours of the hospital before birth. To decrease tension, he developed a series of breathing exercises for use during the various stages of labor. To foster relaxation and optimal physical function in labor and in recovery after delivery, he incorporated a series of physical exercises to be performed regularly in classes and in practice at home during pregnancy. The woman is helped to manage labor and delivery using the Read method in the following way: During the early and mid-first stage of labor, before cervical dilatation has reached 7 cm, contractions are 2 to 5 minutes apart and last for 30 to 40 seconds. The mother lies on her back with her knees bent. Abdominal breathing is used during contractions. Her hands are placed over her lower abdomen, fingers touching. She breathes deeply and slowly—in through her nose and out through her mouth. The abdominal wall rises with each inhalation, which she can feel with her hands. The rate of breathing is no more than six breaths in 30 seconds, or 12 to 18 in one contraction. During the late part of the first stage of labor, after 7 cm of cervical dilatation, the contractions are 1½ to 2 minutes apart and last for 40 to 60 seconds. Costal or diaphragmatic breathing is used during contractions. Her hands are placed on her sides, over the ribs. She breathes in more shallowly, feeling her ribs move sideways against her hands. Each breath is drawn in through her nose and exhaled through her mouth. The abdominal wall does not rise and fall with this kind of breathing. The rate of breathing is no more than six breaths in 30 seconds, or 12 to 18 in one contraction. At the end of the first stage of labor, near full dilatation, contractions may be very strong, occurring every 1½ to 2 minutes and lasting 60 to 90 seconds. The mother lies on her back with her knees bent. Panting respirations are used during the contractions. The mother holds one of her hands on her sternum, which rises and falls as she pants lightly and rapidly through her mouth. Panting continues through the end of the first stage to full dilatation as the urge to push grows. Panting helps the woman to avoid pushing. During the second, or expulsive, stage of labor after full dilatation of the cervix, the contractions occur every 1½ to 2 minutes, last 60 to 90 seconds, and are accompanied with an urge to bear down and push. The woman lies back, head and shoulders supported in a semisitting position. She is helped to draw her legs up, holding them with her hands behind the lower thighs, thighs on her abdomen and spread apart. As each contraction begins, she raises her head, takes a deep breath, tucks her chin on her chest, blocks the escape of air from her lungs, and bears down. During each contraction she may need to blow the air out, refill her lungs and push again two or three times. Throughout labor she is helped to understand what is occurring and to participate and accept the experience in anticipation of the birth of the baby. Currently, many authorities who advocate use of other aspects of the Read method strongly recommend that a woman in labor not lie on her back. Supine hypotension is frequently the result of this position, because the uterus can fall back, occluding the vena cava and decreasing the volume of blood returned to the heart, thus reducing the volume of the cardiac output. Maternal hypotension follows, resulting in decreased placental perfusion and an inadequate supply of oxygen to the fetus. Today, the woman using the Read method spends most of labor lying on her side or in a semisitting position with her knees, back, and head well supported. Compare **Bradley method, Lamaze method.**

read-only memory. See **ROM.**

readthrough, (in molecular genetics) transcription of RNA beyond the normal termination sequence in the DNA template, caused by the occasional failure of RNA polymerase to respond to the end point signal.

reagent /rē·ā′jənt/, a chemical substance known to react in a specific way. A reagent is used to detect or synthesize another substance in a chemical reaction.

reagin /rē′ājin/, **1.** an antibody associated with human atopy, as asthma and hay fever. It attaches to mast cells and basophils and sensitizes the skin and other tissues. In antigen-antibody reactions it triggers the release of histamine and other mediators that cause atopic symptoms. **2.** a nonspecific, nontreponemal antibody-like substance found in the serum of individuals with syphilis. It can combine with an antigen prepared as a lipid extract of normal tissue, a phenomenon that constitutes the basis of the serologic tests for syphilis. **–reaginic,** *adj.*

reaginic antibody, an IgE immunoglobulin that is elevated in hypersensitive individuals. See also **reagin, reagin-mediated disorder.**

reagin-mediated disorder, a hypersensitivity reaction, as hay fever or an allergic response to an insect sting, produced by reaginic antibodies (IgE immunoglobulins), causing degranulation and the release of histamine, bradykinin, serotonin, and other vasoactive amines. An initial sensitizing dose of the antigen induces the formation of specific IgE antibodies, and their attachment to mast cells and basophils results in hypersensitivity to a subsequent challenging dose of the antigen. Reactions range from a simple wheal and flare on the skin to life-threatening anaphylactic shock, depending on the amount and route of entrance of the sensitizing dose and challenging dose, the amount and distribution of IgE antibodies, the responsiveness of the host, the timing of exposure to the allergen, and the tissues in which the antigen-antibody reaction occurs. The abundance of mast cells in the skin, nose, and lungs makes those areas susceptible to IgE-mediated reactions. Allergens that commonly cause these reactions include plant spores, pollens, animal danders, stings, serum proteins, foods, and certain drugs. See also **allergy, generalized anaphylaxis, hay fever.**

reality, the culturally constructed world of perception, meaning, and behavior that members of a culture regard as an absolute..

reality orientation, an activity that uses specific approaches to assist confused or disoriented persons toward an awareness of reality, as by emphasizing the hour, day, month, and weather.

reality principle, an awareness of the demands of the environment and the need for an adjustment of behavior to meet those demands, expressed primarily by the renunciation of immediate gratification of instinctual pleasures to obtain long-term and future goals. In psychoanalysis, this function is held to be performed by the ego. Compare **pleasure principle.**

reality testing, a process of evaluating the physical and social aspects of one's environment so as to differentiate between external reality and any inner imaginative world and to behave in a manner that exhibits an awareness of accepted norms and customs. Distortion of reality is indicative of a disturbance in ego functioning that may lead to psychosis.

reality therapy, a form of psychotherapy in which the aims are to help define and assess basic values within the framework of a current situation and to evaluate the person's present behavior and future plans in relation to those values. The emphasis in treatment is on the present rather than the past; it focuses on responsible behavior as a means of personal fulfillment.

real time, an application of computerized equipment that allows data to be processed with relation to ongoing external events, so that the operators can make immediate diagnostic or other decisions based on the current data output. Ultrasound scanning uses real time control systems, making results available almost simultaneously with the generation of the input data.

real-time scanning, the scanning or imaging of an entire object, or a cross-sectional slice of the object, at a single moment. To produce such a "snapshot" image, scanning data must be recorded quickly over a very short time rather than by accumulation over a longer period.

reamer, **1.** a tool with a straight or spiral cutting edge, used in a rotating motion to enlarge a hole or clear an opening. **2.** (in dentistry) an instrument with a tapered and loosely spiraled metal shaft, used for enlarging and cleaning root canals.

reapproximate /rē′əprok′simāt/, to rejoin tissues separated by surgery or trauma so that their anatomic relationship is restored. **–reapproximation,** *n.*

reasonable care, the degree of skill and knowledge used by a competent health practitioner in treating and caring for the sick and injured.

reasonable person, (in law) a hypothetical person who possesses the qualities that are used as an objective standard on which to judge a defendant's action in a negligence suit. In such suits, it must be decided whether or not a reasonable person, under the same circumstances, would have acted in the same way as the defendant.

reasonably prudent person doctrine, a concept that a person of ordinary sense will use ordinary care and skill in meeting the health care needs of a patient.

rebase, a process of refitting a denture by replacing its base material without changing the occlusal relationships of the teeth.

rebound, **1.** recovery from illness. **2.** a sudden contraction of muscle after a period of relaxation, often seen in conditions in which inhibitory reflexes are lost.

rebound tenderness, a sign of inflammation of the peritoneum in which pain is elicited by the sudden release of a hand pressing on the abdomen. See also **appendicitis, peritonitis.**

rebreathing bag, (in anesthesia) a flexible bag attached to a mask. The rebreathing bag may function as a reservoir for anesthetic gases during surgery or for oxygen during resuscitation. It may be squeezed to pump the gas or air into the lungs.

recannulate, to make a new opening through an organ or tissue, as opening a passage through an occluded blood vessel.

recapitulation theory, the theory, formulated by German naturalist Ernst Heinrich Haeckel, that an organism during the course of embryonic development passes through stages that resemble the structural form of several ancestral types of the species as it evolved from a lower to a higher form of life. It is summarized by the statement "Ontogeny recapitulates phylogeny." Also called **biogenetic law, Haeckel's law.**

receiver, (in communication theory) the person or persons to whom a message is sent.

receptive aphasia, a form of sensory aphasia marked by impaired comprehension of language.

receptor, **1.** a chemical structure on the surface of a cell that combines with an antigen to produce a discrete immunologic component. **2.** a sensory nerve ending that responds to various kinds of stimulation. **3.** a specific cellular protein that must first bind a hormone before cellular response can be elicited. The protein may be in the cytoplasm or in the cell membrane.

recess, a small hollow cavity, as the epitympanic recess in the tympanic cavity of the inner ear or the retrocecal recess extending as a small pocket behind the cecum.

recessive, of, pertaining to, or describing a gene the effect of which is masked or hidden if there is a dominant gene at the same locus. If both genes are recessive and produce the same trait, the trait is expressed in the individual. See also **autosomal-recessive inheritance, dominance.**

recessive gene, the member of a pair of genes that lacks the ability to express itself in the presence of its more dominant allele; it is expressed only in the homozygous state. Compare **dominant gene.**

recessive trait, a genetically determined characteristic that is expressed only when present in the homozygotic state.

reciprocal /rəsip′rəkəl/, a type of body movement that aids in communication, as body language that indicates affiliation between people.

reciprocal gene. See **complementary gene.**

reciprocal inhibition, the theory in behavior therapy that if an anxiety-producing stimulus occurs simultaneously with a response that diminishes anxiety, the stimulus may cause less anxiety, as deep chest or abdominal breathing and relaxation of the deep muscles appear to diminish anxiety and pain in childbirth. See also **systemic desensitization.**

reciprocal translocation, the mutual exchange of genetic material between two nonhomologous chromosomes. Also called **interchange.** Compare **balanced translocation, robertsonian translocation.**

Recklinghausen's canal /rek′linghou′sənz/, the small lymph space in the connective tissues of the body.

Recklinghausen's disease. See **neurofibromatosis.**

Recklinghausen's tumor, a benign tumor, derived from smooth muscle containing connective tissue and epithelial elements, that occurs in the wall of the oviduct or posterior uterine wall. Also called **adenomyosis of the uterus.**

reclining, leaning backward. **–recline,** *v.*

recluse spider. See **brown spider.**

recombinant /rēkom′binənt/, **1.** the cell or organism that results from the recombination of genes within the DNA molecule, regardless of whether naturally or artificially induced. **2.** of or pertaining to such an organism or cell. See also **recombinant DNA.**

recombinant DNA, a DNA molecule in which rearrangement of the genes has been artificially induced. Enzymes are used to break isolated DNA molecules into fragments that are then rearranged in the desired sequence. Portions of DNA material from another organism of the same or a different species may also be introduced into the molecule, which is then replicated, resulting in both genotypic and phenotypic alterations in the organism. See also **genetic engineering.**

recombination, **1.** (in genetics) the formation of new combinations and arrangements of genes within the chromosome as a result of independent assortment of unlinked genes, crossing over of linked genes, or intracistronic crossing over of nucleotides. See also **recombinant DNA.** **2.** a method of measurement of radiation by ionimetric techniques in which it is necessary to collect the liberated charges to arrive at a value of total charge per unit mass of air. Recombination of ions will lower the value collected and will cause an underestimation of dose, particularly in intense fields. A technique for determining the magnitude of ionic recombination is routinely applied in accurate dosimetry.

recommended daily allowance (RDA), the amount of nutrients, particularly vitamins, recommended as a necessary part of one's daily food intake to maintain normal health.

recon /rē'kon/, (in molecular genetics) the smallest genetic unit that is capable of recombination, thought to be a triplet of nucleotides.

reconstitution, the continuous repair of tissue damage.

recovery room (RR, R.R.), an area adjoining the operating room to which surgical patients are taken while still under anesthesia, before being returned to their rooms. Vital signs and adequacy of ventilation are carefully observed as the patient recovers conciousness. The recovery room has equipment and a specially trained nursing staff with a nurse anesthetist or anesthesiologist available. See also **postoperative care.**

recreational therapy, a form of adjunctive psychotherapy in which games or other group activities are used as a means of modifying maladaptive behavior, awakening social interests, or improving the ability to communicate in depressed, withdrawn people.

recrudescence, a return of symptoms of a disease during a period of recovery.

recrudescent hepatitis, a form of acute viral hepatitis marked by a relapse during the period of recovery. A minority of patients experience it, and the prognosis for ultimate recovery is rarely affected.

recrudescent typhus. See **Brill-Zinsser disease.**

rectal anesthesia, general anesthesia achieved by the insertion, injection, or infusion of an anesthetic agent into the rectum; this procedure is performed rarely because of the unpredictability of absorption of the drug into the blood.

rectal cancer. See **colorectal cancer.**

rectal instillation of medication, the instillation of a medicated suppository, cream, or gel into the rectum. Some conditions treated by this method are constipation, pruritus ani, and hemorrhoids. The patient lies on the side, with the lower leg extended and the upper leg flexed. The nurse or physician unwraps the suppository and, wearing a glove, raises the upper buttock, exposing the anus. The suppository may be self-lubricating, or it may need to be lubricated with a water-soluble lubricant. The suppository is then gently inserted past the anal sphincter. Occasionally, a drug may be given in a medicated enema. See also **enema.**

Rectal Medicone, a trademark for a rectal, fixed-combination drug containing a topical anesthetic (benzocaine), an antiseptic (oxyquinoline sulfate), an astringent (zinc oxide), and a protectant (Peruvian balsam).

rectal reflex, the normal response (defecation) to the presence of an accumulation of feces in the rectum. Also called **defecation reflex.**

rectitis. See **proctitis.**

rectocele /rek'təsēl'/, a protrusion of the rectum and the posterior wall of the vagina into the vagina. The condition, which occurs after the muscles of the vagina and pelvic floor have been weakened by childbearing, old age, or surgery, may reflect a congenital weakness in the wall and may, if severe, result in dyspareunia and difficulty in evacuating the bowel. Reconstructive surgery is often helpful and is combined with any other necessary perineal, pelvic, or vaginal repair. Also called **proctocele.** Compare **cystocele.**

rectosigmoid, a portion of the anatomy that includes the lower portion of the sigmoid and the upper portion of the rectum.

rectouterine excavation, rectouterine pouch. See **cul-de-sac of Douglas.**

rectum /rek'təm/, *pl.* **rectums, recta,** the portion of the large intestine, about 12 cm long, continuous with the descending sigmoid colon, just proximal to the anal canal. It follows the sacrococcygeal curve, ends in the anal canal, and usually contains three transverse semilunar folds: one situated proximally on the right side, a second one extending inward from the left side, and the third and largest fold projecting caudally. Each fold is about 12 mm wide. The folds overlap when the intestine is empty. **–rectal,** *adj.*

rectus abdominis, one of a pair of anterolateral muscles of the abdomen, extending the whole length of the ventral aspect of the abdomen. The pair is separated by the linea alba. Each rectus arises in a lateral tendon from the crest of the pubis and is interlaced by a medial tendon with that of the opposite side. The rectus abdominis inserts into the fifth, the sixth, and the seventh ribs. It is innervated by branches of the seventh through the twelfth intercostal nerves and functions to flex the vertebral column, tense the anterior abdominal wall, and assist in compressing the abdominal contents. Compare **obliquus externus abdominis, obliquus internus abdominis, pyramidalis, transversus abdominis.**

rectus femoris, a fusiform muscle of the anterior thigh, one of the four parts of the quadriceps femoris. It arises in an anterior tendon originating in the iliac spine and in a posterior tendon originating in the brim of the acetabulum. The two tendons unite and spread into a broad, thick aponeurosis that extends downward over the thigh in the center of the quadriceps femoris. The aponeurosis narrows into a flattened tendon that inserts into the base of the patella. The rectus femoris is innervated by branches of the femoral nerve, which contain fibers from the second, third, and fourth lumbar nerves, and it functions to flex the leg. Compare **vastus intermedius, vastus lateralis, vastus medialis.** See also **quadriceps femoris.**

rectus muscle, a muscle of the body that has a relatively straight form. Some rectus muscles are **rectus abdominis, rectus capitis anterior,** and **rectus capitis lateralis.**

recumbent /rikum'bənt/, lying down or leaning backward. See also **reclining. –recumbency,** *n.*

recurrent bandage, a bandage that is wrapped several times around itself, usually applied to the head or an amputated stump.

recurrent fever. See **relapsing fever.**

recurvatum /rē′kərvā′təm/, backward thrust of the knee caused by weakness of the quadriceps or a joint disorder.

red blood cell. See **erythrocyte.**

red blood cell count, a count of the erythrocytes in a specimen of whole blood, commonly made with an electronic counting device. The normal concentrations of red blood cells in the whole blood of males are 4.6 to 6.2 million/mm^3; in females, the concentrations are 4.2 to 5.4 million/mm^3.

Red Book of the American Academy of Pediatrics, a book that serves as the standard reference source of immunization procedures for children and adults. It is published by the American Academy of Pediatrics, Inc., Evanston, Illinois.

red bug. See **chigger.**

red cell. See **erythrocyte.**

red cell indexes, a series of relationships that characterize the red cell population in terms of size, hemoglobin content, and hemoglobin concentration. Derived mathematically from the red cell count and the hemoglobin and hematocrit values, the indexes are useful in making differential diagnoses of several kinds of anemia. The values reported are the mean corpuscular hemoglobin (MCH), the mean corpuscular hemoglobin concentration (MCHC), and the mean corpuscular volume (MCV). Also called **red cell indices.** See also **iron deficiency anemia.**

red corpuscle. See **erythrocyte.**

Red Cross. See **American Red Cross, International Red Cross Society.**

red fever. See **dengue fever.**

red hepatization. See **hepatization.**

red infarct, a pathologic change that occurs in brain tissue that has been rendered ischemic by lack of blood. With restricted blood flow, diapedesis of red blood cells occurs into the parenchyma of the brain without actually producing a well-formed hematoma but only infiltration of erythrocytes.

red marrow, the red vascular substance consisting of connective tissue and blood vessels containing primitive blood cells, macrophages, megakaryocytes, and fat cells. It is found in the cavities of many bones, including the flat and the short bones, the bodies of the vertebrae, the sternum, the ribs, and the articulating ends of the long bones. Red marrow manufactures and releases leukocytes and erythrocytes into the bloodstream. Compare **yellow marrow.**

redon, the smallest unit of the DNA molecule capable of recombination; it may be as small as one deoxyribonucleotide pair. Compare **cistron, muton.**

reduce, **1.** (in surgery) the restoration of a part to its original position after displacement, as in the reduction of a fractured bone by bringing ends or fragments back into alignment or of a hernia by returning the bowel to its normal position. A fracture may be reduced using local or general anesthesia. If performed by outside manipulation alone, the reduction is said to be closed; if surgery is necessary, it is said to be open. See also **fracture, hernia, invagination, traction.** **2.** to decrease the amount, size, extent, or number of something, as of body weight.

reduction, **1.** also called **hydrogenation.** the addition of hydrogen to a substance. **2.** the removal of oxygen from a substance. **3.** the decrease in the valence of the electronegative part of a compound. **4.** the addition of one or more electrons to a molecule or atom of a substance. **5.** the correction of a fracture, hernia, or luxation. **6.** the reduction of data, as in converting interval data to an ordinal or nominal scale of measurement.

reduction diet, a diet that is low in calories, used for reduction of body weight. The diet must supply fewer calories than the individual expends each day while supplying all the essential nutrients for maintaining health. A diet of this type may provide 1200 calories per day from the basic food groups. Meats are usually broiled, roasted, stewed, or sautéed; vegetables are steamed or eaten raw; starches and fats are limited; and fresh fruits replace desserts. Foods to be avoided are sweetened carbonated beverages, fried foods, pastries, and most snack foods. Vitamin and mineral deficiencies may result if such a diet is not carefully planned. Also called **low-caloric diet, reducing diet.**

reduction division. See **meiosis.**

reductionism, an approach that tries to explain a form of behavior or an event in terms of a specific category of phenomena, as biologic, psychologic, or cultural, negating the possibility of an interrelation of causal phenomena.

Reed-Sternberg cell, one of a number of large, abnormal, multinucleated reticuloendothelial cells in the lymphatic system in Hodgkin's disease. The number and proportion of Reed-Sternberg cells identified are the basis for the histopathologic classification of Hodgkin's disease.

reefer. See **cannabis.**

reentry, (in cardiology) the reactivation of myocardial tissue for the second or subsequent time by the same impulse. Reentry is one of the most common arrhythmogenic mechanisms. It is the mechanism of paroxysmal supraventricular tachycardia caused by SA nodal reentry, AV nodal reentry, and AV reentry using the AV node and an accessory pathway, as well as some forms of ventricular tachycardia and extrasystoles. An atrial microreentry circuit is also thought to be the mechanism of atrial flutter. AV and AV nodal mechanisms can be terminated by a vagal maneuver.

refereed journal, a professional or literary journal in which articles or papers are selected for publication by a panel of referees who are experts in the field. They read and evaluate each of the articles submitted for publication. The important national professional journals in medicine and nursing are refereed.

reference electrode, an electrode that has an established potential and is used as a reference against which other potentials may be measured.

reference group, a group with which a person identifies or wishes to belong.

referential idea. See **idea of reference.**

referral, a process whereby a patient or the patient's family is introduced to additional health resources in the community, as in helping a patient find an appropriate community health nurse after discharge from a hospital.

referred pain, pain felt at a site different from that of an injured or diseased organ or part of the body. Angina, the pain of coronary artery insufficiency, may be felt in the left shoulder, arm, or jaw. In disease of the gallbladder, pain may be felt in the right shoulder or scapular region.

referred sensation, a feeling or impression that occurs at a site other than at which the stimulus is initiated. Also called **reflex sensation.** See also **sensation,** def. 1.

refined birth rate, the ratio of total births to the total female population, considered during a period of 1 year. Compare **birth rate, crude birth rate, true birth rate.**

reflection, (in cardiology) a form of reentry in which, after encountering delay in one fiber, an impulse enters a parallel fiber and returns retrogradely to its source.

reflex, **1.** a backward or return flow of energy or of an image, as a reflection. **2.** a reflected action, particularly an involuntary action or movement.

reflex action, the involuntary functioning or movement of any organ or part of the body in response to a particular stimulus. The function or action occurs immediately, without the involvement of the will or consciousness.

reflex apnea, involuntary cessation of respiration caused by irritating, noxious vapors or gases.

reflex bladder. See **spastic bladder.**

reflex dyspepsia, an abnormal condition characterized by impaired digestion associated with the disease of an organ not directly involved with digestion. See also **dyspepsia.**

reflexology, a system of treating certain disorders by massaging the soles of the feet, using principles similar to those of acupuncture.

reflex sensation. See **referred sensation.**

reflux /rē′fluks/, an abnormal backward or return flow of a fluid. Kinds of reflux include **gastroesophageal reflux, hepatojugular reflux,** and **vesicoureteral reflux.**

refracting medium. See **medium.**

refraction, **1.** the change of direction of energy as it passes from one medium to another of different density. **2.** an examination to determine and to correct refractive errors of the eye.

refractive index, a numeric expression of the refractive power of a medium, as compared with that of air, which has a refractive index value of 1. The refractive index is related to the number, charge, and mass of vibrating particles in the material through which light is passing and may be used as a measure of the total solids in a solution.

refractometer, an instrument for measuring the refractive index of a substance and used primarily for measuring the refractivity of solutions.

refractory, pertaining to a disorder that is resistant to treatment.

refractory period, the interval after the excitation of a neuron or the contraction of a muscle during which repolarization of the cell membrane occurs. The period is divided into two phases: the absolute refractory period and the relative refractory period. During the absolute stage the cell is incapable of responding to any stimulus, regardless of its strength, because of total depolarization. During the relative phase, as repolarization is underway, a stimulus intensity above the threshold may elicit a response even though the normal resting potential of the cell has not been reached.

Refsum's syndrome /ref′so͞omz/, a rare, hereditary disorder of lipid metabolism in which phytanic acid cannot be broken down. The syndrome is characterized by ataxia, abnormalities of the bones and skin, peripheral neuropathy, and retinitis pigmentosa. Foods containing phytanic acid must be avoided to prevent progressive deterioration. Also called **phytanic acid storage disease.**

regimen, a strictly regulated therapeutic program, as a diet or exercise schedule.

regional, of or pertaining to a geographic area, as a regional medical facility, or to a part of the body, as regional anesthesia.

regional anatomy, the study of the structural relationships within the organs and the parts of the body. Kinds of regional anatomy are **surface anatomy** and **cross-sectional anatomy.**

regional anesthesia, anesthesia of an area of the body by injecting a local anesthetic to block a group of sensory nerve fibers. Kinds of regional anesthesia include **brachial plexus anesthesia, caudal anesthesia, epidural anesthesia, intercostal anesthesia, paracervical block, pudendal block,** and **spinal anesthesia.** Compare **general anesthesia, local anesthesia, topical anesthesia.** See also **anesthesia.**

regional control, the control of cancer in sites that represent the first stages of spread from the local origin.

regional enteritis. See **Crohn's disease.**

regional hyperthermia, the elevation of temperature over an extended volume of tissue.

regionalization, (in health care planning) the organization of a system for the delivery of health care within a region to avoid costly duplication of services and to ensure availability of essential services. Hospitals are classified as primary, secondary, and tertiary health centers, depending on the facilities and personnel available, the population served, the number of beds in the institution, and other criteria.

regional medical program (RMP), a program of community health planning that includes all the medical resources available in a region that may be mobilized to meet a specific medical objective. The RMP was authorized by the Health, Disease, Cancer and Stroke Amendments passed by the U.S. Congress in 1965. See also **regionalization.**

registered nurse (RN), **1.** *U.S.* a professional nurse who has completed a course of study at a state approved school of nursing and passed the National Council Licensure Examination (NCLEX-RN). A registered nurse may use the initials RN after the signature. RNs are licensed to practice by individual states. **2.** *Canada.* a professional nurse who has completed a course of study at an approved school of nursing and who has taken and passed an examination administered by the Canadian Nurses Association Testing Service, called the Comprehensive Examination for Nurse Registration Licensure. See also **nurse, nursing.**

registered record administrator (RRA), a medical record administrator who has successfully completed the credentialing examination conducted by the American Medical Record Association.

Registered Technologist (R.T.), a title awarded by the American Registry of Radiologic Technologists as certification of qualification to act as an x-ray technologist. See also **radiologic technologist.**

registrar, an administrative officer whose responsibility is to maintain the records of an institution.

registry, **1.** an office or agency in which lists of nurses and records pertaining to nurses seeking employment are maintained. **2.** (in epidemiology) a listing service for incidence data pertaining to the occurrence of specific diseases or disorders, as a tumor registry.

Regitine Hydrochloride, a trademark for an alpha-adrenergic blocking agent (phentolamine hydrochloride).

Regonol, a trademark for a neuromuscular blocking agent (pyridostigmine), used as an adjunct to anesthesia.

regression, **1.** a retreat or backward movement in conditions, signs, or symptoms. **2.** a return to an earlier, more primitive form of behavior. **3.** a tendency in physical development to become more typical of the population than of the parents, as a child who attains a height closer to the average than that of tall or short parents. –**regress,** *v.*

Regroton, a trademark for a cardiovascular, fixed-combination drug containing a diuretic (chlorthalidone) and an antihypertensive (reserpine).

regular diet, a full, well-balanced diet containing all of the essential nutrients needed for optimal growth, repair of the tissues, and normal functioning of the organs. Such a diet contains foods rich in proteins, carbohydrates, fats, minerals, and vitamins in proportions that meet the specific caloric requirements of the individual. Also called **full diet, normal diet.**

Regular Iletin II, a trademark for insulin injection (crystalline zinc insulin).

regular insulin. See **insulin injection.**

regulative cleavage. See **indeterminate cleavage.**

regulative development, a type of embryonic development in which the fertilized ovum undergoes indeterminate cleavage, producing blastomeres that have similar developmental potencies and are each capable of giving rise to a single embryo. Determination of the particular organs and parts of the embryo occurs during later stages of development and is influenced by inductors and intercellular interaction. Damage or destruction of various cells during the early stages of development results in readjustments and substitutions so that a normal organism is formed. Compare **mosaic development.**

regulator gene, (in molecular genetics) a genetic unit that regulates or suppresses the activity of one or more structural genes. Also called **repressor gene.**

regulatory sequence, (in molecular genetics) a series of DNA nucleotides that regulate the expression of a gene.

regurgitant menstruation. See **retrograde menstruation.**

regurgitation, **1.** the return of swallowed food into the mouth. **2.** the backward flow of blood through a defective heart valve, named for the affected valve, as in **aortic regurgitation.**

rehabilitation, the restoration of an individual or a part to normal or near normal function after a disabling disease, injury, addiction, or incarceration. –**rehabilitate,** *v.*

rehabilitation center, a facility providing therapy and training for rehabilitation. The center may offer occupational therapy, physical therapy, vocational training, and special training, as speech therapy. See also **rehabilitation.**

Rehfuss stomach tube /rā′fəs/, a specially designed gastric tube with a graduated syringe, used for withdrawing specimens of the contents of the stomach for study after a test meal.

Reid's base line, the base line of the skull, a hypothetic line extending from the infraorbital point to the superior border of the external auditory meatus. Also called **anthropologic base line, Frankfurt line.**

Reifenstein's syndrome /rī′fənstīnz/, male hypogonadism of unknown origin, marked by azoospermia, undescended testes, gynecomastia, testosterone deficiency, and elevated gonadotropin titers. The condition appears to be inherited as an x-linked recessive trait, but no chromosomal abnormality has been identified.

reimbursement, a method of payment, usually by a third-party payer, for medical treatment or hospital costs. Cost-based reimbursement covers payment for all allowable costs incurred in the provision of services to patients included in a contract. Prospective reimbursement provides for additional payment by which costs incurred in providing services to patients are based on actual costs determined at the end of a fiscal period.

reinforcement, (in psychology) a process in which a response is strengthened by the fear of punishment or the anticipation of reward.

Reiter's syndrome /rī′tərz/, an arthritic disorder of adult males, believed to result from a myxovirus or *Mycoplasma* infection. The syndrome most often affects the ankles, feet, and sacroiliac joints and is usually associated with conjunctivitis and urethritis. The onset may be marked by unexplained diarrhea and low-grade fever, followed in 2 to 4 weeks by conjunctivitis. Lesions that become superficial ulcers may form on the palms and the soles. Arthritis usually persists after the conjunctivitis and urethritis subside, but it may become episodic. Treatment includes a short course of tetracycline to treat the infection and phenylbutazone to relieve pain and inflammation in the joint. Recovery is expected, but recurrent arthritic symptoms may continue for several years.

rejection, **1.** (in medicine) an immunologic response to organisms or substances that the system recognizes as foreign, including grafts or transplants. **2.** (in psychiatry) the act of excluding or denying affection to another person.

Rela, a trademark for a skeletal muscle relaxant (carisoprodol).

relapse, **1.** to exhibit again the symptoms of a disease from which a patient appears to have recovered. **2.** the recurrence of a disease after apparent recovery.

relapsing fever, any one of several acute infectious diseases, marked by recurrent febrile episodes, caused by various strains of the spirochete *Borrelia*. The disease is transmitted by both lice and ticks and is often seen during wars and famines. It has occurred in several western states of the United States but is more commonly found in South America, Asia, and Africa. The first episode usually starts with a sudden high fever (104° to 105° F), accompanied by chills, headache, neuromuscular pains, and nausea. A rash may appear over the trunk and extremities, and jaundice is common during the later stages. Each attack lasts 2 or 3 days and culminates in a crisis of high fever, profuse sweating, and a rise in heart and respiratory rate. This is followed by an abrupt drop in temperature and a return to normal blood pressure. People typically relapse after 7 to 10 days of normal temperature and eventually recover completely. In louse-borne disease, there is usually only a single relapse; in tick-borne disease, several successively milder relapses may occur. For a diagnosis to be made, the spirochete must be seen on a blood smear obtained during an attack. Treatment is with a long-acting penicillin, tetracycline, or chloramphenicol. Antimicrobial therapy may induce a Herxheimer reaction, therefore treatment is withheld during a febrile crisis. Bed rest, sponge baths, and aspirin alleviate the symptoms. Disinfection of clothing and bedding is necessary to destroy any lice or ticks. Also called **African tick fever, famine fever, recurrent fever, spirillum fever, tick fever.**

relapsing polychondritis, a rare disease of unknown cause resulting in inflammation and destruction of cartilage with replacement by fibrous tissue. Autoimmunity may be involved in this condition. Most commonly the ears and noses of middle-aged people are affected with episodes of tender swelling, often accompanied by fever, arthralgias, and episcleritis. Consequences include floppy ears, collapsed nose, hearing loss, or hoarseness and airway obstruction because of laryngeal and tracheal cartilage involvement. Corticosteroids suppress the activity of the disease.

relation searching, (in nursing research) a study design used to discover and describe relationships between and among variables. It may be used to describe various nursing situations to examine the efficacy of certain aspects of nursing care.

relationship therapy, a therapy that is based on a totality of patient-therapist relationship and encourages the growth of self in the patient. It has been described as "an experience in living that takes place within a relationship with another person."

relative biologic effectiveness (RBE), (in radiotherapy) a measure of the cell-killing ability of a particular radiation compared with a reference radiation. The reference is 250 keV x-rays. The ratio of cells killed with the test radiation over that of the 250 keV radiation is the RBE.

relative centrifugal force (RCF), a method of comparing the force generated by various centrifuges based on the speeds of rotation and distances from the center of rotation.

relative cephalopelvic disproportion. See **cephalopelvic disproportion.**

relative growth, the comparison of the various increases in size of similar organisms, tissues, or structures at different time intervals.

relative refractory period. See **refractory period.**

relative risk, an assessment of the degree or incidence of adverse effects that may be expected in the presence of a particular factor or event as compared with the expected adverse effects in the absence of the factor or event.

relative value unit, a comparable service measure used by hospitals to permit comparison of the amounts of resources required to perform various services within a single department or between departments. It is determined by assigning weight to such factors as personnel time, level of skill, and sophistication of equipment required to render patient services.

relativism, an attitude or belief that all cultures are logically consistent and viable and should be understood in terms of their own standards, attitudes, values, and beliefs. Relativism is the opposite of ethnocentrism.

relaxation, **1.** a reducing of tension, as when a muscle relaxes between contractions. **2.** a lessening of pain.

relaxation therapy, treatment in which patients are taught to perform breathing and relaxation exercises and to concentrate on a pleasant situation when a noxious stimulus is applied. An integral part of the Lamaze method of childbirth, relaxation therapy is also used to relieve various kinds of pain and physical manifestations of stress. Various yoga exercises and aspects of hypnotherapy may be included in the treatment program, and biofeedback techniques may be used to demonstrate actions that induce relaxation. Some patients learn through relaxation therapy to relax taut muscles at will, to abort migraine attacks, or to reduce their blood pressure. See also **Lamaze method.**

relaxation time, (in radiotherapy) the characteristic time it takes for a sample of atoms, whose nuclei have first been aligned along a static magnetic field and then excited to a higher energy (NMR) state by a radiofrequency signal, to return to a lower energy equilibrium state. Two time parameters are used to describe the return, or relaxation, to the equilibrium state once the rf source is turned off. T_1 describes the relaxation of the system of spins into a condition of thermal equilibrium with its surroundings, whereas T_2 describes the relaxation of the energy that is traded within the system itself. Maps or "images" of the values of T_1 or T_2 as a function of position in the cross-sectional view can be made.

releasing hormone (RH), one of several peptides produced by the hypothalamus and secreted directly into the anterior pituitary via a connecting vein. Each of the releasing hormones stimulates the pituitary to secrete a specific tropic hormone; thus, corticotropic releasing hormone stimulates the pituitary to secrete adrenocorticotropic hormone, whereas growth hormone releasing hormone stimulates the secretion of growth hormone. Also called **releasing factor.**

reliability, (in research) the extent to which a test measurement or a device produces the same results with different investigators, observers, or administration of the test over time. If repeated use of the same measurement tool on the same sample produces the same consistent results, the measurement is considered reliable.

relief area, the portion of the tissue surface under prosthesis on which pressures are reduced or eliminated.

religiosity, a psychiatric symptom characterized by the demonstration of excessive or affected piety.

reline, the resurfacing of the tissue side of a denture with new base material.

rem /rem, är′ē′em′/, abbreviation for *roentgen equivalent man.* A dose of ionizing radiation that produces in humans the same effect as one roentgen of x-radiation or gamma radiation. See also **sievert.**

REM /rem, är′ē′em′/, abbreviation for **rapid eye movement.** See also **sleep.**

reminiscence, the recollection of past personal experiences and significant events.

remission, the partial or complete disappearance of the clinical and subjective characteristics of a chronic or malignant disease. Remission may be spontaneous or the result of therapy. In some cases remission is permanent and the disease is cured. Compare **cure.**

remittent fever, diurnal variations of an elevated temperature with exacerbations and remissions but never a return to normal.

remnant radiation, the measurable radiation that passes through an object and can produce an image on radiographic film.

remote afterloading, (in radiotherapy) a technique in which an applicator, as an acrylic mold of an area to be irradiated, is placed in or on the patient and then loaded from a safe source with a high-activity radioisotope. The mold or applicator contains grooves for the insertion of nylon tubes into which the radioactive material can be introduced. Remote afterloading is used in the treatment of head, neck, vaginal, and cervical tumors.

remotivation, the use of special techniques that stimulate patients to become motivated to learn and interact.

remotivation group, a treatment group that is organized with the purpose of stimulating the interest, awareness, and communication of withdrawn and institutionalized mental patients.

removable lingual arch, an orthodontic arch wire designed to fit the lingual surface of the teeth and aid orthodontic movement of the dentition involved. Two posts soldered to each end of the wire fit snugly into the vertical tubes of the associated molar anchor bands.

removable orthodontic appliance, a device placed inside the mouth to correct or alleviate malocclusion and designed to be removed or replaced by the patient.

Remsed, a trademark for an antiemetic and antihistaminic (promethazine hydrochloride).

ren-, a combining form meaning 'of or pertaining to the kidneys': *renicardiac, reniform, renocortical.*

renal /rē′nəl/, of or pertaining to the kidney.

renal adenocarcinoma. See **renal cell carcinoma.**

renal angiography, a radiographic examination of the renal artery and associated blood vessels, after the injection of a contrast medium.

renal anuria, cessation of urine production caused by intrinsic renal disease.

renal artery, one of a pair of large, visceral branches of the abdominal aorta, arising caudal to the superior mesenteric artery at the level of the disk between the first and second lumbar vertebrae. The left renal artery is somewhat more cranial than the right. Before reaching the kidney, each divides into four branches. The renal arteries supply the kidneys, suprarenal glands, and the ureters.

renal biopsy, the removal of kidney tissue for microscopic examination, conducted to establish the diagnosis of a renal disorder and to aid in determining the stage of the disease, the appropriate therapy, and the prognosis. An open biopsy involves an incision, permits better visualization of the kidney, and carries a lower risk of hemorrhage; a closed or percutaneous biopsy performed by aspirating a specimen of tissue with a needle requires a shorter period of recovery and is less likely to cause infection.

■ METHOD: Before biopsy, the procedure is explained and the patient is medically evaluated and tested for bleeding or coagulation time. The patient's blood is usually typed and crossmatched with two units of donor blood that are held for a possible transfusion until there is no threat of bleeding after the procedure. An open biopsy is generally carried out in the operating room, but the percutaneous procedure may be performed in the radiology department or in the patient's room. The location of the kidney, determined by a plain x-ray film, dye contrast study, or fluoroscopic examination, is marked on the patient's skin in ink for a needle biopsy. The patient is then placed prone over a sandbag and soft pillow with the body bent at the level of the diaphragm, the shoulders on the bed, and the spine in straight alignment. A local anesthetic is injected, and the physician inserts the biopsy needle in the lower pole of the kidney, because this area contains the smallest number of large renal vessels. The needle is quickly withdrawn, and, after pressure is applied to the site for 20 minutes, a pressure bandage is applied; the patient is turned and kept supine and motionless for the next 4 hours. The dressing, blood pressure, and pulse are checked every 15 to 60 minutes for 2 hours, the temperature every 4 hours for 24 hours; excessive drainage, decreased blood pressure, tachycardia, or elevated temperature is reported to the physician. Fluids are forced to the maximum allotted for the patient's condition; the amount and character of urinary output are noted, and the physician is informed if hematuria occurs. The patient is kept in bed for at least 24 hours and is cautioned not to lift any heavy objects for 10 days.

■ NURSING ORDERS: The nurse offers an explanation of the procedure, prepares and positions the patient for the percutaneous procedure, and, on its completion, provides care and emotional support.

■ OUTCOME CRITERIA: A biopsy is the most accurate measure for determining the nature and stage of a renal pathologic condition.

renal calculus, a concretion occurring in the kidney. If the stone is large enough to block the ureter and stop the flow of urine from the kidney, it must be removed by either major surgical or radiologic fluoroscopy procedures. Also called **kidney stone, nephritic calculus.** See also **nephroscope.**

renal calyx, the first unit in the system of ducts in the kidney carrying urine from the renal pyramid of the cortex to the renal pelvis for excretion through the ureters. There are two divisions: The **minor calyx,** with several others, drains into a larger **major calyx,** which in turn joins other major calyces to form the renal pelvis.

renal cell carcinoma, a malignant neoplasm of the kidney, composed predominantly of large cells with clear cytoplasm that originate in tubular epithelium. The tumor may develop in any part of the kidney, becoming a large mass that may grow into the tributaries of the renal vein. Hematuria and pain are usually present. Metastasis, especially to the lungs and bones, may occur early in the course of development. Treatment includes surgery and radiotherapy. Also called **adenocarcinoma of the kidney, clear cell carcinoma of the kidney.** See also **Wilms' tumor.**

renal colic, sharp, severe pain in the lower back over the kidney, radiating forward into the groin. Renal colic usually accompanies forcible dilatation of a ureter followed by spasm as a stone is lodged or passed through it. See also **urinary calculus.**

renal corpuscle. See **malpighian corpuscle.**

renal cortex, the soft, granular, outer layer of the kidney, containing approximately 1.25 million renal tubules, which remove body wastes in the form of urine.

renal diet, a diet prescribed in chronic renal failure and designed to control the intake of protein, potassium, sodium, phosphorus, and fluids, depending on individual conditions. Carbohydrates and fats are the principal sources of energy. Protein is limited; the amount is determined by the patient's condition and is usually supplied from milk, eggs, and meat. Cereals, bread, rice, and pasta are the primary sources of calories. Some vegetables and fruits are included, depending on the degree of restriction of potassium and phosphorus. Special commercial flours and breads have been developed that are protein-free and low in potassium and sodium. The low potassium level of the diet also makes it useful in hyperkalemia. The diet is nutritionally inadequate and should be supplemented with vitamins and electrolytes. See also **Giordano-Giovannetti diet.**

renal dwarf, a dwarf whose retarded growth is caused by renal failure.

renal failure, inability of the kidneys to excrete wastes, concentrate urine, and conserve electrolytes. The condition may be acute or chronic. **Acute renal failure** is characterized by oliguria and by the rapid accumulation of nitrogenous wastes in the blood. It is caused by hemorrhage, trauma, burn, toxic injury to the kidney, acute pyelonephritis or glomerulonephritis, or lower urinary tract obstruction. Many forms of acute renal failure are reversible after the underlying cause has been identified. Treatment includes restricted intake of fluids and of all substances that require excretion by the kidney. Antibiotics and diuretics are also used. **Chronic renal failure** may result from many other diseases. The early signs include sluggishness, fatigue, and mental dullness. Later, anuria, convulsions, GI bleeding, malnutrition, and various neuropathies may occur. The skin may turn yellow-brown and become covered with uremic frost. Congestive heart failure and hypertension are frequent complications, the results of hypervolemia. Urinalysis reveals greater than normal amounts of urea and creatinine, waxy casts, and a constant volume of urine regardless of variations in water intake. Anemia frequently occurs. The prognosis depends on the underlying cause. Treatment usually includes restricted water and protein intake and the use of diuretics. When medical measures have been exhausted, long-term hemodialysis is often begun, and kidney transplantation is considered.

renal hypertension, hypertension resulting from kidney disease, including chronic glomerulonephritis, chronic pyelonephritis, renal carcinoma, and renal calculi. Analgesic abuse and certain drug reactions may also result in renal hypertension. Therapy depends on the cause and may include administration of antibiotics or diuretics or surgery. Untreated renal hypertension is likely to result in kidney damage and cardiovascular disease.

renal nanism, dwarfism associated with infantile renal osteodystrophy.

renal osteodystrophy, a condition resulting from chronic renal failure and characterized by uneven bone growth and demineralization. See also **renal nanism, renal rickets.**

renal papilla. See **papilla.**

renal rickets, a condition characterized by rachitic changes in the skeleton and caused by chronic nephritis. See also **renal osteodystrophy.**

renal scan, a scan of the kidneys to determine their size, shape, and exact position, used to aid in the diagnosis of a tumor or other abnormalities and performed after the intravenous injection of a radioactive substance.

renal tubular acidosis (RTA), an abnormal condition associated with persistent dehydration, metabolic acidosis, hypokalemia, hyperchloremia, and nephrocalcinosis. It is caused by the inability of the kidneys to conserve bicarbonate and to adequately acidify the urine. Some forms of RTA are more prevalent in women, older children, and young adults. Prolonged RTA can cause hypercalciuria and the formation of kidney stones. Depending on treatment and the extent of renal damage, prognosis is usually good. Compare **distal renal tubular acidosis, metabolic acidosis, proximal renal tubular acidosis, respiratory acidosis.**

■ OBSERVATIONS: Some common signs and symptoms of RTA, especially in children, may include anorexia, vomiting, constipation, retarded growth, polyuria, nephrocalcinosis, and rickets. In children and adults RTA can also cause urinary tract infections and pyelonephritis. Confirming diagnosis of distal RTA is based on laboratory tests that show impaired urine acidification in association with systemic metabolic acidosis. Confirming diagnosis of proximal RTA is based on tests that show bicarbonate wasting as a result of impaired reabsorption. Other significant laboratory findings may show decreased sodium bicarbonate, pH, potassium, and phosphorus; increased serum chloride, alkaline phosphatase, urinary bicarbonate, and potassium; and urine with low specific gravity.

■ INTERVENTION: Treatment seeks to replace excessively secreted substances, especially bicarbonate, and may include the administration of sodium bicarbonate tablets, potassium to counter low potassium levels, vitamin D to preserve calcium metabolism, and antibiotics to counter pyelonephritis. Surgery may be required to excise renal calculi.

■ NURSING CONSIDERATIONS: The nurse carefully monitors all laboratory tests, especially those involving potassium levels and urine pH. The urine of the patient is strained to capture any kidney stones for analysis, and the nurse is alert to any signs of hematuria. Patients with low potassium levels are usually advised to eat potassium-rich foods, as bananas, oranges, and baked potatoes. The patient and family also benefit from advice and encouragement in seeking genetic counseling and RTA screening.

Rendu-Osler-Weber syndrome. See **Osler-Weber-Rendu syndrome.**

Renese, a trademark for a diuretic and antihypertensive (polythiazide).

renin /rē′nin/, a proteolytic enzyme, produced by and stored in the juxtaglomerular apparatus that surrounds each arteriole as it enters a glomerulus. The enzyme affects the blood pressure by catalyzing the change of angiotensinogen to angiotensin, a strong pressor. Compare **rennin.**

renin test. See **plasma renin activity.**

rennin /ren′in/, a milk-curdling enzyme that occurs in the gastric juices of infants and is also contained in the rennet produced in the stomach of calves and other ruminants. It is an endopeptidase that converts casein to paracasein and was formerly used extensively as a curdling agent by the cheese industry. An artificially produced microbial rennet, rather than the enzyme extracted from rennet in calves, is used in one half of the cheese produced in the United States today. Compare **renin.**

Renoquid, a trademark for an antibacterial (sulfacytine).

renovascular hypertension. See **portal hypertension.**

reovirus /rē′ōvī′rəs/, any one of three ubiquitous, double-stranded RNA viruses found in the respiratory and alimentary tracts in healthy and in sick people. Reoviruses have been implicated in some cases of upper respiratory tract disease and infantile gastroenteritis.

Repen-VK, a trademark for an antibacterial (penicillin V potassium).

repetition compulsion, an unconscious need to revert to and repeat earlier situations, patterns of behavior, and acts to experience previously felt emotions or relationships. See also **compulsion.**

replacement, the substitution of a missing part or substance with a similar structure or substance, as the replacement of an amputated limb with a prosthesis or the replacement of lost blood with donor blood.

replication, **1.** a process of duplicating, reproducing, or copying; literally, a folding back of a part to form a duplicate. **2.** (in research) the exact repetition of an experiment performed to confirm the initial findings. **3.** (in genetics) the duplication of the polynucleotide strands of DNA or the synthesis of DNA. The process involves the unwinding of the double helix molecule to form two single strands, each of which acts as a template for the synthesis of a complementary strand. The two resulting molecules of DNA each contain one new and one parental strand, which coil to form the double helix. **–replicate,** *v.*

replicator, (in genetics) the segment of the DNA molecule that initiates and controls the replication of the polynucleotide strands.

replicon /rep′ləkon/, (in genetics) a replication unit; the segment of the DNA molecule that is undergoing replication. The unit is regulated by a section of the molecule called the regulator, which controls replication and coordinates it with cell division.

repolarization, (in cardiology) the process by which the cell is restored to its resting potential. The repolarization process begins after phase 0 of the action potential and is completed by the end of phase 3. It encompasses the effective and the relative refractory periods and is measured by the QT interval. See also **phase 0, phase 1, phase 2, phase 3.**

report, (in nursing) the transfer of information from the nurses on one shift to the nurses on the following shift. Report is given systematically at the time of change of shift. The head nurse, team leader, or primary nurse conducts the report, summarizing the progress and status of each patient, for the nurses who will next assume responsibility for the care. The provider of the information is said to "give report" and the oncoming staff to "take report." Report may be given to the assembled oncoming staff, or it may be tape recorded so that staff members can listen to it individually or in a group on their own schedule. The Kardex and medcard of each patient are updated before report, and staff members are informed of the changes during report.

representative group, a group of individuals whose members represent all the various sectors of a community.

repression, **1.** the act of restraining, inhibiting, or suppressing. **2.** (in psychoanalysis) an unconscious defense mechanism whereby unacceptable thoughts, feelings, ideas, impulses, or memories, especially those concerning some traumatic past event, are pushed from the consciousness because of their painful guilt association or disagreeable content and are submerged in the unconscious, where they remain dormant but operant and dynamic. Such repressed emotional conflicts are the source of anxiety that may lead to any of the anxiety disorders. Compare **suppression.** **–repress,** *v,* **repressive,** *adj.*

repressor, (in molecular genetics) a protein produced by the regulator gene. It binds to a sequence of nucleotides in the operator gene, which regulates the structural gene. The repressor, when bound, blocks the transcription of the gene.

repressor gene. See **regulator gene.**

reproduction, **1.** the process by which animals and plants give rise to offspring; procreation; the sum total of the cellular and genetic phenomena involved in the transmission of organic life from one organism to successive generations similar to the parents so that the perpetuation and continuity of the species is maintained. In humans, the germ cells, the spermatozoa in the male and the ova in the female, which are produced by the testes and ovaries, unite during fertilization to form the new individual. Kinds of reproduction include **asexual reproduction, cytogenic reproduction, sexual reproduction, somatic reproduction,** and **unisexual reproduction.** See also **fertilization, oogenesis, pregnancy, spermatogenesis.** **2.** the creation of a similar structure, situation, or phenomenon; duplication; replication. **3.** (in psychology) the recalling of a former idea, impression, or something previously learned. **–reproductive,** *adj.*

reproductive system, the male and female gonads, associated ducts and glands, and the external genitalia that function in the procreation of offspring. In women these include the ovaries, fallopian tubes, uterus, vagina, clitoris, and vulva. In men these include the testes, epididymis, vas deferens, seminal vesicles, ejaculatory duct, prostate, and penis. Also called **genital tract, genitourinary system, urogenital system.** See also the Color Atlas of Human Anatomy.

repulsion, **1.** the act of repelling, disjoining. **2.** a force that separates two bodies or things. **3.** (in genetics) the situation in linked inheritance in which the alleles of two or more mutant genes are located on homologous chromosomes so that each chromosome of the pair carries one or more mutant and wild-type genes, which are located close enough to be inherited together. Compare **coupling.** See also **transconfiguration.**

request for proposal (RFP), a solicitation by a funding agency for proposals to accomplish a particular goal. The RFP lists the requirements a project must meet to receive funding.

required arch length, the sum of the mesiodistal widths of all the natural teeth in a dental arch.

RES, abbreviation for **reticuloendothelial system.**

rescinnamine /risin′əmin/, an alkaloid antihypertensive and sedative.

■ INDICATIONS: It is prescribed in the treatment of mild hypertension involving the cardiovascular or central nervous system, or both.

■ CONTRAINDICATIONS: Mental depression, electroconvulsive therapy, or known hypersensitivity to this drug prohibits its use.

■ ADVERSE EFFECTS: Among the more serious adverse reactions are GI, cardiovascular, and central nervous system disturbances.

research, the diligent inquiry or examination of data, reports, and observations in a search for facts or principles.

research instrument, a testing device for measuring a given phenomenon, as a paper and pencil test, a questionnaire, an interview, or a set of guidelines for observation.

research measurement, an evaluation of the quantity or incidence of a given variable as obtained by using a research instrument.

research radiopharmaceutic, a drug that is labeled with a small quantity of a radioactive tracer to study its biodistribution; it may later be used in a nonradioactive form.

resect, to remove tissue from the body by surgery.

resection, the cutting out of a significant portion of an organ or structure. Resection of an organ may be partial or complete. A kind of resection is a **wedge resection.**

reserpine /res′ərpēn/, an antihypertensive.
■ INDICATIONS: It is prescribed in the treatment of high blood pressure and certain neuropsychiatric disorders.
■ CONTRAINDICATIONS: Mental depression, peptic ulcer, ulcerative colitis, or known hypersensitivity to this drug prohibits its use.
■ ADVERSE EFFECTS: Among the more serious adverse reactions are mental depression, extrapyramidal reactions, impotence, aggravation of peptic ulcer, and paradoxical excitement.

reserve, a potential capacity to maintain the vital functions of the body in homeostasis by adjusting to increased need, as cardiac reserve, pulmonary reserve, and alkali reserve. See also **homeostasis.**

reserve cell carcinoma. See **oat cell carcinoma.**

reservoir bag, a component of an anesthesia machine in which gas accumulates, forming a reserve supply of gas for use when the quantity of flow is inadequate. This component also permits "bagging," or manual control of ventilation, and serves as a visible monitor of machine function.

reservoir host, a nonhuman host that serves as a means of sustaining an infectious organism as a potential source of human infection. Wild monkeys are reservoir hosts for the yellow fever virus, which can spread from the jungle to infect humans.

reservoir of infection, a continuous source of infectious disease. People, animals, and plants may be reservoirs of infection.

resident, a physician in one of the postgraduate years of clinical training after the first, or internship, year. The length of residency varies according to the specialty. See also **PGY.**

resident bacteria, bacteria living in a specific area of the body.

residential care facility, a facility that provides custodial care to persons who, because of physical, mental, or emotional disorders, are not able to live independently.

residual, pertaining to the portion of something that remains after an activity that removes the bulk of the substance.

residual cyst, an odontogenic cyst that remains in the jaw after the removal of a tooth.

residual dental caries, any decayed material left in a prepared tooth cavity.

residual ridge, the portion of the dental ridge that remains after the alveolar process has disappeared after extraction of the teeth.

residual urine, urine that remains in the bladder after urination.

residual volume, the volume of gas in the lungs at the end of a maximum expiration.

residue schizophrenia, a form of schizophrenia in which there is a history of at least one psychotic schizophrenic episode. Objective signs of the illness, marked by social withdrawal, eccentric behavior, illogical thinking, and inappropriate emotional reactions persist. The symptoms are less severe than those manifested by persons classified as psychotic. See also **schizophrenia.**

res ipsa loquitur /rās′ ip′sə lok′witŏŏr/, a Latin phrase meaning literally "the thing speaks for itself," a legal concept that is important in many malpractice suits. It describes a situation in which an injury occurred when the defendant was solely and exclusively in control and in which the injury would not have occurred had due care been exercised. Classic examples of res ipsa loquitur are a sponge left in the abdomen after abdominal surgery or the amputation of the wrong extremity.

resistance, **1.** an opposition to a force, as the resistance offered by the constriction of peripheral vessels to the blood flow in the circulatory system. **2.** the frictional force that opposes the flow of an electric charge, as measured in ohms.

resistance form, the shape given to a prepared tooth cavity to impart strength and durability to the restoration and remaining tooth structure.

resistance transfer factor. See **R factor.**

resocialization, the reintegration of a patient into family and community life after critical or long-term hospitalization.

resolution, **1.** the ability of an imaging process to distinguish adjacent structures in the object, and an important measure of image quality. **2.** the state of having made a firm determination or decision on a course of action. **3.** the ability of a chromatographic system to separate two adjacent peaks, the degree of separation between two components being abbreviated as **R.**

resolving power, the ability to separate closely migrating substances, as in electrophoresis.

resonance, an echo or other sound produced by percussion of an organ or cavity of the body during a physical examination. **–resonant,** *adj.*

resorcinated camphor /rizôr′sinā′tid/, a mixture of camphor and resorcinol, used for the treatment of pediculosis and itching.

resorcinol /rizôr′sinol/, an antiseptic substance used as a keratolytic agent in the dermatoses. It is also used in dyes, pharmaceutics, and as a chemical intermediate.

resorcinol test. See **Boas' test.**

resorption, **1.** the loss of substance or bone by physiologic or pathologic means, as the reduction of the volume and size of the residual ridge of the mandible or maxillae. **2.** the cementoclastic and dentinoclastic action that may occur on a tooth root.

Respid, a trademark for a smooth muscle relaxant (theophylline).

respiration, the process of the molecular exchange of oxygen and carbon dioxide within the body's tissues, from the lungs to cellular oxidation processes. The rate varies with the age and condition of the person. Some kinds of respiration are **Biot's respiration, Cheyne-Stokes respiration,** and **Kussmaul's respiration.**

Abnormal patterns of respiration

Respiratory patterns	*Representative settings*

Cheynes-Stokes 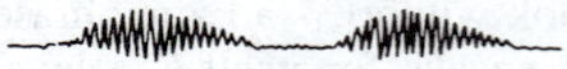	Anoxia
	Increased intracerebral pressure
	  Infections
	  Edema
	  Hydrocephalus
	  Tumor
	Cerebrovascular accidents
	  Subarachoid hemorrhage
	  Intracerebral hemorrhage
	  Cerebral thrombosis
	Cerebromedullary degeneration
	Diastolic hypotension
	  Thyrotoxicosis
	  Patent ductus arteriosis
	  Dissecting aneurysm
	Cardiac failure
	Aortic valve abnormalities
	Normal sleep of infants and elderly

Kussmaul 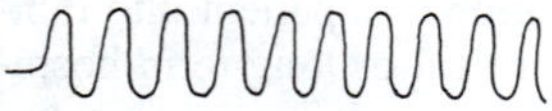	Diabetic ketoacidosis Uremia Shock Sepsis Pneumonia
Central neurogenic hyperventilation 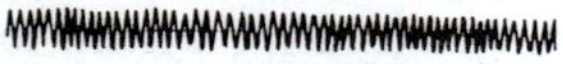	Brainstem dysfunction Transtentorial herniation
Apneustic 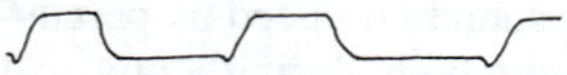	Pontine level dysfunction Pontine infarction Basilar artery occlusion Anoxia Meningitis Incipient herniation

Cluster 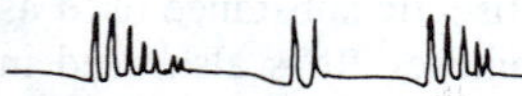	Medulla dysfunction
	Medullary glioma
	Poisonings
	  Narcotics
	  Barbiturates
	Incipient herniation

Ataxic 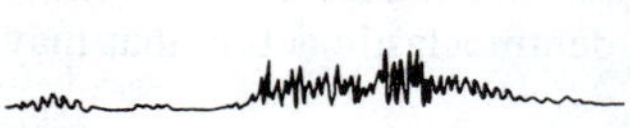	Medullary lesions Cerebellar hemorrhage Pontine hemorrhage Acute demyelinating illnesses
Shallow-breathing 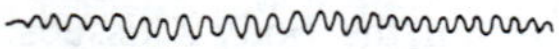	Coma
Agonal-respiration 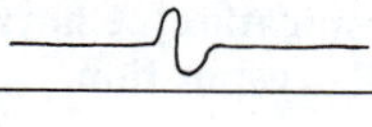	Terminal event

respirator, an apparatus used to modify air for inspiration or to improve pulmonary ventilation. See also **nebulizer, IPPB unit.**

respiratory /res′pərətôr′ē, rispī′rətôr′ē/, of or pertaining to respiration.

respiratory acidosis, an abnormal condition characterized by increased arterial P_{CO_2}, excess carbonic acid, and increased plasma hydrogen ion concentration. It is caused by reduced alveolar ventilation, which can result from various disorders, as airway obstruction, medullary trauma, neuromuscular disease, chest injuries, pneumonia, pulmonary edema, emphysema, and cardiopulmonary arrest. It may also be caused by the suppression of respiratory reflexes with narcotics, sedatives, hypnotics, or anesthetics. The hypoventilation associated with this condition inhibits the excretion of carbon dioxide, which consequently combines with water in the body to produce excessive carbonic acid and thus reduces blood pH. Compare **metabolic acidosis.** See also **metabolic alkalosis, respiratory alkalosis.**

■ OBSERVATIONS: Some common signs and symptoms of respiratory acidosis are headache, dyspnea, fine tremors, tachycardia, hypertension, and vasodilatation. Confirming diagnosis is usually based on arterial blood gas values for P_{CO_2} over the normal 45 mm/Hg and on pH values below the normal range of 7.35 to 7.45. Ineffective treatment of acute respiratory acidosis can lead to coma and death.

■ INTERVENTION: Treatment of this condition seeks to remove or to inhibit the underlying causes of associated hypoventilation. Any airway obstructions are immediately removed. Treatment may include oxygen therapy and the intravenous administration of bronchodilators and sodium bicarbonate.

■ NURSING CONSIDERATIONS: The patient with respiratory acidosis is carefully monitored for any changes in respiratory, cardiovascular, and central nervous system functions, arterial blood gas pressures, and electrolyte concentrations. In patients requiring mechanic ventilation, clear airways are maintained and tracheal tubes are regularly suctioned. Adequate hydration is also important.

respiratory alkalosis, an abnormal condition characterized by decreased P_{CO_2}, decreased hydrogen ion concentration, and increased blood pH. It is caused by pulmonary and nonpulmonary problems. Some pulmonary causes are acute asthma, pulmonary vascular disease, and pneumonia. Some nonpulmonary causes are aspirin toxicity, anxiety, fever, metabolic acidosis, inflammation of the central nervous system, gram-negative septicemia, and hepatic failure. The hyperventilation associated with respiratory alkalosis most commonly stems from extreme anxiety. Compare **metabolic alkalosis.** See also **metabolic acidosis, respiratory acidosis.**

■ OBSERVATIONS: Deep and rapid breathing at rates as high as 40 respirations per minute is a major sign of respiratory alkalosis. Other symptoms are light-headedness, dizziness, peripheral paresthesia, spasms of the hands and the feet, muscle weakness, tetany, and cardiac arrhythmia. Confirming diagnosis is often based on P_{CO_2} levels below 35 mm Hg, but the measurement of blood pH is critical in differentiating between metabolic acidosis and respiratory alkalosis. In the acute stage, blood pH rises in proportion to the fall in P_{CO_2}, but in the chronic stage it remains within the normal range of 7.35 to 7.45. The carbonic acid concentration is normal in the acute stage of this condition but below normal in the chronic stage.

■ INTERVENTION: Treatment of respiratory alkalosis concentrates on removing the underlying causes. Severe cases, especially those caused by extreme anxiety, may be treated by having the patient breathe into a paper bag and inhale exhaled carbon dioxide to compensate for the deficit being created by hyperventilation. Sedatives may also be administered to decrease the respiration rate.

■ NURSING CONSIDERATIONS: The nurse monitors neurologic, neuromuscular, and cardiovascular functions, arterial blood gases, and serum electrolytes. The patient benefits from explanations about laboratory tests and treatment.

respiratory assessment, an evaluation of the condition and function of a person's respiratory system.

■ METHOD: The nurse asks if the person coughs, wheezes, is short of breath, tires easily, or experiences chest or abdominal pain, chills, fever, excessive sweating, dizziness, or swelling of feet and hands. Signs of confusion, anxiety, restlessness, flaring nostrils, cyanotic lips, gums, earlobes, or nails, clubbing of extremities, fever, anorexia, and a tendency to sit upright are noted if present. The person's breathing is closely observed for evidence of slow, rapid, irregular, shallow, or Cheyne-Stokes respiration, hyperventilation, a long expiratory phase or periods of apnea, and for retractions in the suprasternal, supraclavicular, substernal, or intercostal areas during breathing. The presence of tachycardia, bradycardia, or sinus arrhythmia or evidence of congestive heart failure, as rales, rhonchi, edema, hepatosplenomegaly, abdominal distention, or pain, is recorded. The thorax is examined for scoliosis, kyphosis, funnel or barrel chest, or unequal shoulder height and is palpated for indications of thoracic expansion, tracheal deviation, crepitations, or fremitus. Percussion is performed to evaluate resonance, hyperresonance, tympany, and dull or flat sounds; and rales, rhonchi, wheezing, friction rubs, the transmission of spoken words through the chest wall, and decreased or absent breath sounds are detected by auscultation. Background information pertinent to the evaluation includes allergies, recent exposure to infection, immunizations, exposure to environmental irritants, previous respiratory disorders and operations, preexisting chronic conditions, medication currently taken, the person's smoking habits, and the family history. Valuable diagnostic aids are a chest x-ray examination, complete blood count, electrocardiogram, pulmonary function tests, bronchoscopy, determinations of blood gases and electrolytes, studies of sputum, throat, or nasopharyngeal cultures, and gastric washings, lung scans, and biopsies.

■ NURSING ORDERS: The nurse collects the background information and the results of diagnostic tests and may perform the examination. In a respiratory care unit, a nurse clinician or practitioner may have greatly expanded responsibilities, as interpreting data from electrocardiographic tracings, setting up and adjusting a respirator, titrating medications, and obtaining specimens for blood gas determination.

■ OUTCOME CRITERIA: An accurate and thorough assessment of respiratory function is an essential component of the physical examination and is vital to the diagnosis or ongoing care of a respiratory illness.

respiratory bronchiole. See **bronchiole.**

respiratory burn, tissue damage to the respiratory system resulting from the inhalation of a hot gas or burning particles, as may occur in a fire or explosion. Immediate hospitalization and oxygen therapy are recommended. Compare **smoke inhalation.**

respiratory center, a group of nerve cells in the pons and medulla of the brain that control the rhythm of breathing in response to changes in levels of oxygen and carbon dioxide in the blood and cerebrospinal fluid. Change in the concentration of oxygen and carbon dioxide or hydrogen ion levels in the arterial circulation and in cerebrospinal fluid activate central and peripheral chemoreceptors; these send impulses to the respiratory center, increasing or decreasing the breathing rate. This response is essential for normal breathing. In patients with retention of carbon dioxide, as in chronic bronchitis or emphysema, the respiratory center becomes insensitive to carbon dioxide, and the main stimulus to ventilation is then hypoxemia. If such patients inhale gases with a high oxygen content, breathing is depressed, leading to a further rise of blood carbon dioxide. The respiratory center is inhibited by barbiturates, anesthetics, tranquilizing agents, and morphine. See also **hyperventilation, hypoventilation, hypoxia.**

respiratory component (αP_{CO_2}), the acid component of an acid-base control system that is modified by the respiratory status.

respiratory distress syndrome of the newborn (RDS), an acute lung disease of the newborn, characterized by airless alveoli, inelastic lungs, more than 60 respirations a minute, nasal flaring, intercostal and subcostal retractions, grunting on expiration, and peripheral edema. The condition occurs most often in premature babies and in babies of diabetics. It is caused by a deficiency of pulmonary surfactant, resulting in overdistended alveoli and, at times, hyaline membrane formation, alveolar hemorrhage, severe right-to-left shunting of blood, increased pulmonary resistance, decreased cardiac output, and severe hypoxemia. The disease is self-limited; the infant dies in 3 to 5 days or completely recovers with no aftereffects. Treatment includes measures to correct shock, acidosis, and hypoxemia and use of continuous positive airway pressure especially developed for infants to prevent alveolar collapse. Also called **hyaline membrane disease.** Compare **adult respiratory distress syndrome.**

respiratory exchange ratio (R), the ratio of the net expiration of carbon dioxide to the concurrent net inspiration of oxygen, expressed by the formula $\dot{V}CO_2/\dot{V}O_2$.

respiratory failure, the inability of the cardiac and pulmonary systems to maintain an adequate exchange of oxygen and carbon dioxide in the lungs. Respiratory failure may be hypoxemic or ventilatory. Hypoxemic failure is characterized by hyperventilation and occurs in diseases that affect the alveoli or interstitial tissues of the lobes of the lungs, as alveolar edema, emphysema, fungal infections, leukemia, lobar pneumonia, lung carcinoma, various pneumoconioses, pulmonary eosinophilia, sarcoidosis, or tuberculosis. Ventilatory failure, characterized by increased arterial tension of carbon dioxide, occurs in acute conditions in which retained pulmonary secretions cause increased airway resistance and decreased lung compliance, as in bronchitis and emphysema. Ventilation may also be reduced by depression of the respiratory center by barbiturates or opiates, hypoxia, hypercarbia, intracranial diseases, trauma, or lesions of the neuromuscular system or thoracic cage. Respiratory failure in preexisting chronic lung diseases may be precipitated by added stress, as with cardiac failure, surgery, anesthesia, or upper respiratory tract infections. Treatment of respiratory failure includes clearing the airways by suction, bronchodilators, or tracheostomy, antibiotics for infections usually present, anticoagulants for pulmonary thromboemboli, and electrolyte replacement in fluid imbalance. Oxygen may be administered in some cases; in others it may further decrease the respiratory reflex by removing the stimulus of an elevated level of carbon dioxide. Respiratory failure may result in cor pulmonale with congestive heart failure and respiratory acidosis. See also **airway obstruction, carbon dioxide, hypercapnia, hyperventilation, hypoxemia, hypoxia, respiratory acidosis.**

respiratory rate, the normal rate of breathing at rest, about 14 inspirations per minute. The hydrogen ion concentration in the cerebrospinal fluid controls the rate of respiration. The rate may be more rapid in fever, acute pulmonary infection, diffuse pulmonary fibrosis, gas gangrene, left ventricular failure, thyrotoxicosis, and in states of tension. Slower breathing rates may result from head injury, coma, or narcotic overdose. See also **bradypnea, hyperpnea, hypopnea.**

respiratory rhythm, a regular oscillating cycle of inspiration and expiration, controlled by neuronal impulses transmitted between the muscles of inspiration in the chest and the respiratory centers in the brain. The normal breathing pattern may be altered by a prolonged expiratory phase in obstructive diseases of the airway, as asthma, chronic bronchitis, and emphysema, or by Cheyne-Stokes respiration in patients with raised intracranial pressure or heart failure. See also **apnea, Biot's respiration, Hering-Breuer reflexes, hyperventilation, hypoventilation, tachypnea.**

respiratory syncytial virus (RSV, RS virus), a member of a subgroup of myxoviruses that in tissue culture causes formation of giant cells or syncytia. It is a common cause of epidemics of acute bronchiolitis, bronchopneumonia, and the common cold in young children and sporadic acute bronchitis and mild upper respiratory tract infections in adults. Symptoms of infection with this virus include fever, cough, and severe malaise. Occasional fatalities occur in infants. Systemic invasion by the virus does not happen, and secondary bacterial invasion is uncommon. Treatment includes rest and the administration of aspirin and nasal decongestants. No effective vaccine for prevention is available. Compare **rhinovirus.** See also **bronchiolitis, bronchitis, bronchopneumonia, cold.**

respiratory system. See **respiratory tract.**

respiratory therapist, a person who, under the supervision of a physician, administers oxygen and other gases and provides assistance to patients with breathing difficulties. A respiratory therapist who has successfully completed the examination of the National Board for Respiratory care (NBRC) is designated as a registered respiratory therapist.

respiratory therapy (RT), 1. any treatment that maintains or improves the ventilatory function of the respiratory tract. **2.** *informal.* the department in a health care facility that provides respiratory therapy for the clients of the facility.

respiratory therapy technician, a person who, under the supervision of a physician, treats patients with cardiorespiratory disorders through the administration of oxygen and other gases. A respiratory therapy technician may be certified by successfully completing an examination of the National Board for Respiratory Care.

respiratory tract, the complex of organs and structures that performs the pulmonary ventilation of the body and the exchange of oxygen and carbon dioxide between the ambient air and the blood circulating through the lungs. It also warms the air passing into the body and assists in the speech function by providing air for the larynx and the vocal cords. Every 24 hours about 500 cubic feet of air passes through the respiratory tract of the average adult, who breathes in and out between 12 and 18 times a minute. The respiratory tract is divided into the upper respiratory tract and the lower respiratory tract. Also called **respiratory system.** See also the Color Atlas of Human Anatomy.

respiratory tract infection, any infectious disease of the upper or lower respiratory tract. **Upper respiratory tract infections** include the common cold, laryngitis, pharyngitis, rhinitis, sinusitis, and tonsillitis. **Lower respiratory tract infections** include bronchitis, bronchiolitis, pneumonia, and tracheitis.

respite time /res′pit/, relief time from responsibilities for the care of a patient.

respondeat superior /respon′dē·at/, a Latin phrase meaning literally "let the master answer," denoting the doctrine that an employer may be held liable for torts committed by employees acting within the scope of their employment.

respondent conditioning. See **classic conditioning.**

rest, an extension from a prosthesis that affords vertical support for a dental restoration.

rest angle. See **occlusal rest angle.**

rest area, a surface prepared on a tooth or fixed restoration into which the rest fits, providing support for a removable partial denture.

resting cell, a cell that is not undergoing division. See also **interphase.**

resting membrane potential, the transmembrane voltage that exists when the heart muscle is at rest.

resting tremor. See **passive tremor.**

restitution, the spontaneous turning of the fetal head to the right or left after it has extended through the vulva.

rest jaw relation, (in dentistry) the postural relation of the mandible to the maxillae when the patient is resting comfortably in the upright position. The condyles are in a neutral, unstrained position in the glenoid fossae, and the mandibular musculature is in a state of minimum tonic contraction to maintain posture.

restless legs syndrome, a benign condition of unknown origin characterized by an irritating sensation of uneasiness, tiredness, and itching deep within the muscles of the leg, especially the lower part of the limb, accompanied by twitching and, sometimes, by pain. The only relief is walking or moving the legs. The condition may be associated with various psychiatric disorders, probably as a form of extrapyramidal hyperkinesis. Also called **anxietas tibiarum, Ekbom syndrome, Wittmaack-Ekbom syndrome.**

restoration, any tooth filling, inlay, crown, partial or complete denture, or prosthesis that restores or replaces lost tooth structure, teeth, or oral tissues. Also called **prosthetic restoration.**

restoration contour, the profile of the surfaces of teeth that have been restored.

restoration of cusps, a reduction and inclusion of tooth cusps within a tooth cavity preparation and their restoration to functional occlusion with an artificial dental material.

Restoril, a trademark for a hypnotic agent (temazepam).

restraint, any one of numerous devices used in aiding the immobilization of patients, especially children in traction. Some kinds of restraints are specially designed slings, jackets, or diapers. Restraints often involve a certain amount of emotional trauma for the patient and are carefully employed. They are most effective when used consistently. Restraints that are too tight may cause skin irritation; those that fit too loosely do not serve their purpose. During the course of any therapy, restraints are usually removed every 4 hours to assess skin integrity and provide skin care, often a massage of the area involved and an alcohol rub.

restraint of trade, an illegal act that interferes with free competition in a commercial or business transaction so as to restrict the production of a product or the provision of a service, affect the cost of a product or a service, or control the market in any way to the detriment of the consumers or purchasers of the service or product. The Clayton Act and the Sherman Antitrust Act are federal statutes that embody the basic concepts of the definition and of the illegal nature of restraint of trade.

restriction endonuclease /en′dōno͞o′klē·ās/, (in molecular genetics) an enzyme that cleaves DNA at a specific site. Each of the many different endonucleases isolated from various bacteria acts at a species-specific cleavage site, making it possible for researchers to divide DNA into discrete segments.

rest seat. See **rest area.**

resuscitation, the process of sustaining the vital functions of a person in respiratory or cardiac failure while reviving him or her, using techniques of artificial respiration and cardiac massage, correcting acid-base imbalance, and treating the cause of failure. See also **cardiopulmonary resuscitation. –resuscitate,** *v.*

resuscitator /risus′itā′tər/, an apparatus for pumping air into the lungs. It consists of a mask snugly applied over the mouth and nose, a reservoir for air, and a manually or electrically powered pump. Often oxygen may be added to the air in the reservoir.

RET, abbreviation for **rational emotive therapy.**

retail dentistry, the practice of fee-for-service dentistry in an exclusively retail environment, as a shopping center or a department store, with the specific intention of attracting the customers of such retail centers and by using the marketing techniques of the retailers involved.

retained placenta, the retention of all or part of the placenta in the uterus after birth.

retainer, **1.** the part of a dental prosthesis that connects an abutment tooth with the suspended portion of a bridge. It may be an inlay, a partial crown, or a complete crown. **2.** an appliance for maintaining teeth and jaw positions gained by orthodontic procedures. **3.** the portion of a fixed prosthesis that attaches a pontic to the abutment teeth. **4.** any clasp, attachment, or device for fixing or stabilizing a dental prosthesis.

retaining orthodontic appliance, an orthodontic device for holding the teeth in place, following orthodontic tooth movement, until the occlusion is stabilized.

retarded, (of physical, intellectual, social, or emotional development) abnormally slow. **–retard,** *v.*, **retardation,** *n.*

retarded dentition, the abnormal delay of the eruption of the deciduous or permanent teeth resulting from malnutrition, malposition of the teeth, a hereditary factor, or a metabolic imbalance, as hypothyroidism. Also called **delayed dentition.** Compare **precocious dentition.**

retarded depression, the depressive phase of bipolar disorder.

retch, a strong attempt to vomit without bringing up anything. Compare **eructation, vomit.**

rete /rē′tē/, a network, especially of arteries or veins. **–retial,** *adj.*

retention, **1.** a resistance to movement or displacement. **2.** the ability of the digestive system to hold food and fluid. **3.** the inability to urinate or defecate. **4.** the ability of the mind to remember information acquired from reading, observation, or other processes. **5.** the inherent property of a dental restoration to maintain its position without displacement under axial stress. **6.** a characteristic of proper tooth cavity preparation in which provision is made for preventing vertical displacement of the cavity filling. **7.** a period of treatment during which an individual wears an appliance to maintain teeth in positions to which they have been moved by orthodontic procedures. **–retain,** *v.*

retention form, the provision made in a prepared tooth cavity to prevent displacement of the restoration.

retention groove, a depression formed by the opposing vertical constrictions in the preparation of a tooth, which improves the retention of a restoration.

retention of urine, an abnormal, involuntary accumulation of urine in the bladder as a result of a loss of muscle tone in the bladder, neurologic dysfunction or damage to the bladder, obstruction of the urethra, or the administration of a narcotic analgesic, especially morphine.

retention pin, a frictional grip of a small metal projection that extends from a dental metal casting into the dentin of a tooth to improve the retention of a tooth restoration.

retention procedure, a method established by state laws or mental health codes for committing a person to a psychiatric institution. Most states recognize four types of retention: emergency, informal, involuntary, and voluntary.

retention time (t_a), **1.** (in chromatography) the amount of elapsed time from the injection of a sample into the chromatographic system to the recording of the peak (band) maximum of the component in the chromatogram. **2.** the amount of time a compound is retained on a chromatography column.

rete peg. See **epithelial peg.**

Retet, a trademark for an antibiotic (tetracycline).

reticul-, a combining form meaning 'netlike': *recticulation, reticulocyte, reticulopod.*

reticular /ritik′yələr/, (of a tissue or surface) having a netlike pattern or structure of veins.

reticular activating system (RAS), a functional (rather than a morphologic) system in the brain essential for wakefulness, attention, concentration, and introspection. A network of nerve fibers in the thalamus, hypothalamus, brainstem, and cerebral cortex contribute to the system.

reticular formation, a small, thick cluster of neurons, nestled within the brainstem, that controls breathing, the heartbeat, the blood pressure, the level of consciousness, and other vital functions of the body. The reticular formation constantly monitors the state of the body through connections with the sensory and the motor tracts. Certain nerve cells in the formation regulate the flow of hydrochloric acid in the stomach; other cells regulate swallowing, tongue movements, and movements of the face, eyes, and tongue.

reticulation film fault, a defect in a radiograph or developed photographic film that appears as a network of corrugations. It is usually caused by film development with an excessive temperature difference between any two of the three darkroom solutions: the developer, the fixer, and the clearing agent.

reticulin, an albuminoid substance found in the connective fibers of reticular tissue.

reticulocyte /ritik′yələsīt/, an immature erythrocyte characterized by a meshlike pattern of threads and particles at the former site of the nucleus. Reticulocytes normally make up less than 1% of the circulating erythrocytes; a greater proportion reflects an increased rate of erythropoiesis. Compare **erythrocyte.** See also **normoblast.**

reticulocyte count, a count of the number of reticulocytes in a whole blood specimen, used in determining bone marrow activity. The reticulocyte count is lowered in hemolytic diseases; it is elevated after hemorrhage or during recovery from anemia. The normal concentration of reticulocytes in whole blood is 25,000 to 75,000 cells/μL.

reticuloendothelial cells, cells lining vascular and lymph vessels capable of phagocytosing bacteria, viruses, and colloidal particles or of forming immune bodies against foreign particles.

reticuloendothelial system (RES), a functional, rather than anatomic, system of the body involved primarily in defense against infection and in disposal of the products of the breakdown of cells. It is made up of macrophages, the Kupffer cells of the liver, and the reticulum cells of the lungs, bone marrow, spleen, and lymph nodes. Disorders of this system include **eosinophilic granuloma, Gaucher's disease, Hand-Schüller-Christian syndrome,** and **Niemann-Pick disease.**

reticuloendotheliosis /ritik′yəlō·en′dōthē′lē·ō′sis/, an abnormal condition characterized by increased growth and proliferation of the cells of the reticuloendothelial system. See **reticuloendothelial system.**

reticulosarcoma. See **undifferentiated malignant lymphoma.**

reticulum cell sarcoma. See **histiocytic malignant lymphoma.**

retina /ret′inə/, a 10-layered, delicate nervous tissue membrane of the eye, continuous with the optic nerve, that receives images of external objects and transmits visual impulses through the optic nerve to the brain. The retina is soft, semitransparent, and contains rhodopsin, which gives it a purple tint. The retina becomes clouded and opaque if exposed to direct sunlight. It develops from the embryonic optic cup in the eighth month of pregnancy and consists of the outer pigmented layer and the nine-layered retina proper. These nine layers, starting with the most internal, are the internal limiting membrane, the stratum opticum, the ganglion cell layer, the inner plexiform layer, the inner nuclear layer, the outer plexiform layer, the outer nuclear layer, the external limiting membrane, and the layer of rods and cones. The outer surface of the retina is in contact with the choroid; the inner surface with the vitreous body. The retina is thinner anteriorly, where it extends nearly as far as the ciliary body, and thicker posteriorly, except for a thin spot in the exact center of the posterior surface where focus is best. The nervous fibers end anteriorly in the jagged ora serrata at the ciliary body, but the membrane of the retina extends over the back of the ciliary processes and the iris. See also **Jacob's membrane, macula, optic disc.**

Retin-A, a trademark for a keratolytic (tretinoin).

retinaculum /ret′inak′yələm/, *pl.* **retinacula,** **1.** a structure that retains an organ or tissue. **2.** an instrument for retracting tissues during surgery.

retinaculum extensorum manus, the thick band of antebrachial fascia that wraps tendons of the extensor muscles of the forearm at the distal ends of the radius and the ulna. Also called **dorsal carpal ligament, extensor retinaculum of the hand.** Compare **retinaculum flexorum manus.**

retinaculum flexorum manus, the thick, fibrous band of antebrachial fascia that wraps the carpal canal surrounding the tendons of flexor muscles of the forearm at the distal ends of the radius and the ulna. Also called **flexor retinaculum of the hand, volar ligament.**

retinal /ret′inəl, ret′inal′/, **1.** an aldehyde precursor of vitamin A produced by the enzymatic dehydration of retinol. It is the active form of the vitamin necessary for night, day, and color vision. See also **retinene, vitamin A. 2.** pertaining to the retina.

retinal detachment, a separation of the retina from the choroid in the back of the eye, usually resulting from a hole in the retina that allows the vitreous humor to leak between the choroid and the retina. Severe trauma to the eye, as a contusion or penetrating wound, may be the proximate cause, but in the great majority of cases retinal detachment is the result of internal changes in the vitreous chamber associated with aging, or, less frequently, with inflammation of the interior of the eye.

■ OBSERVATIONS: In most cases retinal detachment develops slowly. The first symptom is often the sudden appearance of a large number of spots floating loosely suspended in front of the affected eye. The person may not seek help, because the number of spots tends to decrease during the days and weeks after the detachment. The person may also notice a curious sensation of flashing lights as the eye is moved. Because the retina does not contain sensory nerves that relay sensations of pain, the condition is painless. Detachment usually begins at the thin peripheral edge of the retina and extends gradually beneath the thicker, more central areas. The person perceives a shadow that begins laterally and grows in size, slowly encroaching on central vision. As long as the center of the retina is unaffected, the vision, when the person is looking straight ahead, is normal; when the center becomes affected, the eyesight is distorted, wavy, and indistinct. If the process of detachment is not halted, total blindness of the eye ultimately results. The condition does not spontaneously resolve itself.

■ INTERVENTION: Surgery is usually required to repair the hole and prevent the leakage of vitreous humor that separates the retina from its source of nourishment, the choroid. If the condition is discovered early, when the hole is small and the volume of vitreous humor lost is not large, the retinal hole may be closed by causing a scar to form on the choroid and to adhere to the retina around the hole. The scar may be produced by heat, electric current, or cold. The scar is held against the retina by local pressure achieved by a variety of surgical techniques.

■ NURSING CONSIDERATIONS: Retinal detachment requires treatment. The degree of restoration of sight depends on the extent and duration of separation; maximum vision is achieved within 3 months after surgery. Unless replaced, a detached retina slowly dies after several years of detachment. Blindness resulting from retinal detachment is irreversible.

retinene /ret′inin/, either of the two carotenoid pigments found in the rods of the retina that are precursors of vitamin A and are activated by light. See also **retinal, retinol.**

retinoblastoma /ret′inōplastō′mə/, *pl.* **retinoblastomas, retinoblastomata,** a congenital, hereditary neoplasm developing from retinal germ cells. Characteristic signs are diminished vision, strabismus, retinal detachment, and an abnormal pupillary reflex. The rapidly growing tumor may invade the brain and metastasize to distant sites. Treatment includes removal of the eye and as much of the optic nerve as possible, followed by radiation and chemotherapy. It is bilateral in about 30% of the cases; the more affected eye is enucleated, and the other eye is treated with radiation, antibiotics, cryotherapy, or photocoagulation, singly or in combination. Because nearly 20% of the cases are transmitted as an autosomal dominant trait with incomplete penetration, genetic counseling is advisable.

retinocerebral angiomatosis. See **cerebroretinal angiomatosis.**

retinol /ret′inôl/, the cis-trans form of vitamin A. It is found in the retinas of mammals. Also called **vitamin A_1.**

retinopathy /ret′inop′əthē/, a noninflammatory eye disorder resulting from changes in the retinal blood vessels.

retirement center, a facility or organized program that may be affiliated with a hospital to provide social services and activities for senior citizens who generally do not require ongoing health care.

retraction, **1.** the displacement of tissues to expose a part or structure of the body. **2.** a distal movement of the teeth. **3.** a distal or retrusive position of the teeth, dental arch, or jaw.

retraction of the chest, the visible sinking-in of the soft tissues of the chest between and around the firmer tissue of the cartilagenous and bony ribs, as occurs with increased inspiratory effort. Retraction begins in the intercostal spaces. If increased effort is needed to fill the lungs, supraclavicular and infraclavicular retraction may be seen. In infants, sternal retraction occurs with only slight increase in respiratory effort, caused by the pliability of their chests. Compare **intercostal bulging.**

retractor, an instrument for holding back the edges of tissues and organs to maintain exposure of the underlying anatomic parts, particularly during surgery, as an army retractor or a double-ended Richardson retractor.

retro-, a combining form meaning 'backward, or located behind': *retronasal, retroperitoneal, retroversion.*

retroaortic node /re′trō·ā·ôr′tik/, a node in one of three sets of lumbar lymph nodes that serve various structures in the abdomen and the pelvis. They lie below the cisterna chyli on the bodies of the third and the fourth lumbar vertebrae and receive the lymphatic trunks from the lateral aortic nodes and preaortic nodes. The efferents from the retroaortic nodes end in the cisterna chyli. Compare **lateral aortic node, preaortic node.**

retroflexion, an abnormal position of an organ in which the organ is tilted back acutely, folded over on itself.

retrognathism, a facial abnormality in which one or both jaws, usually the mandible, are posterior to their normal facial positions. Also called **bird-face retrognathism.**

retrograde, **1.** moving backward; moving in the opposite direction to that which is considered normal. **2.** degenerating; reverting to an earlier state or worse condition. **3.** catabolic.

retrograde amnesia, the loss of memory for events occurring before a particular time in a person's life, usually before the event that precipitated the amnesia. The condition may result from disease, brain injury or damage, or a traumatic emotional incident. Compare **anterograde amnesia.**

retrograde cystoscopy, a technique in radiology for examining the bladder in which a catheter is inserted through the urethra into the bladder, allowing the urine present in the bladder to pass through the catheter. A radiopaque medium is introduced, filling the bladder, and the contour of the bladder is observed, using serial x-ray films or fluoroscopy, as the contrast medium is voided. See also **cystogram, retrograde pyelography.**

retrograde filling, a filling placed in the apical portion of a tooth root to seal the apical portion of the root canal. Also called **postresection filling.**

retrograde infantilism. See **acromegalic eunuchoidism.**

retrograde infection, an infection that spreads along a tubule or duct against the flow of secretions or excretions, as in the urinary and lymphatic systems.

retrograde menstruation, a backflow of menstrual discharge through the uterine cavity and the fallopian tubes into the peritoneal cavity. Fragments of endometrium may attach to the ovaries or other organs, causing endometriosis. Also called **regurgitant menstruation.**

retrograde pyelography, a technique in radiology for examining the structures of the collecting system of the kidneys that is especially useful in locating an obstruction in the urinary tract. A radiopaque contrast medium is injected through a urinary catheter into the ureters and the calyces of the pelves of the kidneys. Rarely, severe anaphylactoid reaction to the medium may occur, because of a patient's hypersensitivity to the iodine in the medium, and infection or trauma may result from the catheterization.

retrograde urography. See **retrograde pyelography.**

retrograde Wenckenbach, a progressively lengthening conduction of impulses from the ventricles or AV junction to the atria until an impulse fails to reach the atria.

retrogression, a return to a less complex state, condition, or behavioral adaptation; degeneration; deterioration. See also **regression.**

retrolental fibroplasia, a formation of fibrous tissue behind the lens of the eye, resulting in blindness. The disorder is caused by administration of excessive concentrations of oxygen to premature infants.

retromolar pad, a mass of soft tissue, usually pear-shaped, that marks the distal termination of the mandibular residual ridge. It is composed of fibers of the buccinator muscle, the pterygomandibular raphe, the superior constrictor muscle, the temporal tendon, and mucous glands.

retromylohyoid space /ret′rōmī′lōhī′oid/, the part of the alveolingual sulcus that is distal to the distal end of the mylohyoid ridge.

retroperitoneal, of or pertaining to organs closely attached to the abdominal wall and partly covered by peritoneum, rather than suspended by that membrane.

retroperitoneal fibrosis, a chronic inflammatory process, usually of unknown cause, in which fibrous tissue surrounds the large blood vessels in the lower lumbar area. It frequently causes constriction of the midportion of the ureters, which may lead to hydronephrosis and azotemia. Occasionally the fibrosis spreads upward to involve the duodenum, bile ducts, and superior vena cava. Symptoms include low-back and abdominal pain, weakness, weight loss, fever, and, with urinary tract involvement, frequency of urination, hematuria, polyuria, or anuria. Methysergide, taken to prevent migraine headaches, is one known cause of this condition. Treatment includes stopping methysergide and instituting surgical release of the ureters from the fibrosis with transplantation laterally or intraperitoneally.

retroperitoneal lymph node dissection, surgical removal of lymph nodes behind the peritoneum, usually performed in an attempt to eliminate sites of lymphoma or metastases from malignancies originating in pelvic organs or genitalia.

retropharyngeal abscess, a collection of pus in the tissues behind the pharynx accompanied by difficulty in swallowing, fever, and pain. Occasionally, the airway becomes obstructed. Treatment includes appropriate parenteral antibiotics and surgical drainage. Tracheostomy may be necessary. Compare **parapharyngeal abscess, peritonsillar abscess.**

retroplacental, behind the placenta.

retrospective chart audit, a format for an audit developed by the Joint Commission on the Accreditation of Hospitals. The audit involves several steps that outline a procedure for evaluating the effectiveness of the care given at a particular institution and for correcting any deficiencies found by reviewing the patient's records after discharge and comparing the data with standards held to be adequate by the Commission.

retrospective nursing audit. See **nursing audit.**

retrospective study, a study in which a search is made for a relationship between one (usually current) phenomenon or condition and another that occurred in the past, as a study of the family histories of young women diagnosed as having clear cell adenomas of the vagina, which yielded a relationship between the administration of diethylstilbestrol to the mothers of the women during pregnancy and the development of the condition in the daughters.

retrouterine /re′trōyo͞o′tərin/, behind the uterus.

retroversion, 1. a common condition in which an organ is tipped backward, usually without flexion or other distortion. The uterus may be retroverted in as many as one fourth of normal women. Uterine retroversion is measured as first-, second-, or third-degree, depending on the angle of tilt with respect to the vagina. No treatment is necessary. Compare **anteversion.** See also **anteflexion, retroflexion. 2.** an abnormal condition in which the teeth or other maxillary and mandibular structures are posterior to their normal positions. Also called **retrusion. –retrovert,** *v.*

retrovirus, a member of a family of viruses that includes the oncoviruses.

retrusion. See **retroversion.**

revascularization, the restoration by surgical means of blood flow to an organ or a tissue being replaced, as in bypass surgery.

Reverdin's needle /reverdaNz′/, a surgical needle with an eye that can be opened and closed with a slide.

reverse anaphylaxis. See **inverse anaphylaxis.**

reverse Barton's fracture, a fracture of the volar articular surface of the radius with associated displacement of the carpal bones and radius.

reverse bevel. See **contra bevel.**

reverse curve, (in dentistry) a convex curve of occlusion, as viewed in the frontal plane.

reversed bandage, a roller bandage that is reversed on itself with a half twist so that it lies smoothly, conforming to the contour of the extremity. See also **roller bandage.**

reversed coarctation. See **Takayasu's arteritis.**

reversed phase, a chromatographic mode in which the mobile phase is more polar than the stationary phase.

reverse isolation, isolation procedures designed to protect a patient from infectious organisms that might be carried by the staff, other patients, or visitors or on droplets in the air or on equipment or materials. Absolute reverse isolation is rarely necessary and requires elaborate specialized equipment. Protective modified reverse isolation is less restrictive but is not prolonged needlessly, because the patient usually comes to feel lonely and sensorily deprived. Handwashing, gowning, gloving, sterilization or disinfection of materials brought into the area, and other details of housekeeping vary with the reason for the isolation and the usual practices of the hospital.

review of systems (ROS), (in a health history) a system-by-system review of the functions of the body. The ROS is begun during the initial interview with the patient and completed during the physical examination, as physical findings prompt further questions. One outline of the systems and some of the signs and symptoms that might be noted or reported are as follows:

■ SKIN: bruising, discoloration, pruritus, birthmarks, moles, ulcers, decubiti, changes in the hair or nails.

■ HEMATOPOIETIC: spontaneous or excessive bleeding, fatigue, enlarged or tender lymph nodes, pallor, history of anemia.

■ HEAD AND FACE: pain, traumatic injury, ptosis.

■ EARS: ringing in the ears, change in hearing, running or discharge from the ears, deafness, dizziness.

■ EYES: change in vision, pain, inflammation, infections, double vision, scotomata, blurring, tearing.

■ MOUTH AND THROAT: dental problems, hoarseness, dysphagia, bleeding gums, sore throat, ulcers or sores in the mouth.

■ NOSE AND SINUSES: discharge, epistaxis, sinus pain, obstruction.

■ BREASTS: pain, change in contour or skin color, lumps, discharge from the nipple.

■ RESPIRATORY TRACT: cough, sputum, change in sputum, night sweats, nocturnal dyspnea, wheezing.

■ CARDIOVASCULAR SYSTEM: chest pain, dyspnea, palpitations, weakness, intolerance of exercise, varicosities, swelling of extremities, known murmur, high blood pressure, asystole.

■ GASTROINTESTINAL SYSTEM: nausea, vomiting, diarrhea, constipation, quality of appetite, change in appetite, dysphagia, gas, heartburn, melena, change in bowel habits, use of laxatives or other drugs to alter the function of the GI tract.

■ URINARY TRACT: dysuria, change in color of urine, change in frequency of urination, pain with urgency, incontinence, edema, retention.

■ GENITAL TRACT (female): menstrual history, obstetric

history, contraceptive use, discharge, pain or discomfort, pruritus, history of venereal disease.

■ GENITAL TRACT (male): penile discharge, pain or discomfort, pruritus, skin lesions, hematuria, history of venereal disease.

■ SKELETAL SYSTEM: heat, redness, swelling, limitation of function, deformity, crepitation; pain in a joint or an extremity, the neck, or back, especially with movement.

■ NERVOUS SYSTEM: dizziness, tremor, ataxia, difficulty in speaking, change in speech, paresthesia, loss of sensation, seizures, syncope.

■ ENDOCRINE SYSTEM: tremor, palpitations, intolerance of heat or cold, polyuria, polydipsia, polyphagia, diaphoresis, exophthalmos, goiter.

■ PSYCHOLOGIC STATUS: nervousness, instability, depression, phobia, sexual disturbances, criminal behavior, insomnia, night terrors, mania, memory loss, perseveration, disorientation.

Reye's syndrome /rāz′/, a combination of acute encephalopathy and fatty infiltration of the internal organs that may follow acute viral infections. This syndrome has been associated with influenza B, chickenpox (varicella), the enteroviruses, and the Epstein-Barr virus. It usually affects people under 18 years of age, characteristically causing an exanthematous rash, vomiting, and confusion about 1 week after the onset of a viral illness. In the late stage, there may be extreme disorientation followed by coma, seizures, and respiratory arrest. Laboratory tests reveal greater than normal amounts of SGOT and SGPT, bilirubin, and ammonia in the blood. A specimen obtained by liver biopsy shows fatty degeneration and confirms the diagnosis. Mortality varies between 20% and 80%, depending on the severity of symptoms. The cause of Reye's syndrome is unknown, and there is no specific treatment available. Insulin, antibiotics, and mannitol may be given. Blood gases, blood pH, and blood pressure are monitored frequently. Intensive, supportive nursing care with meticulous monitoring of all vital functions and prompt correction of any imbalance are of extreme significance in the outcome of this syndrome.

rf, abbreviation for **radiofrequency.**

RF, abbreviation for **rheumatoid factor.**

R factor, an episome in bacteria that is responsible for drug resistance and is transmissible to progeny and to other bacterial cells by conjugation. The portion of the episome involved in replication and transmission is called **resistance transfer factor.**

RFP, abbreviation for **request for proposal.**

RF test. See **latex fixation test.**

Rh, symbol for **rhodium.**

-rh-. For combining forms containing **-rh-**, see **-(r)rh ...**; for example, **-(r)rhachia, -(r)rhage.**

rhabdo-, rhabdi-, a combining form meaning 'rod-shaped' or 'of or pertaining to a rod': *rhabdocyte, rhabdomyoma, rhabdosarcoma.*

rhabdomyoma /rab′dōmī·ō′mə/, *pl.* **rhabdomyomas, rhabdomyomata,** a tumor of striated muscle that may occur in the uterus, vagina, pharynx, or tongue, or in the heart as congenital neoplastic nodules. Also called **myoma striocellulare.**

rhabdomyosarcoma, *pl.* **rhabdomyosarcomas, rhabdomyosarcomata,** a highly malignant tumor, derived from primitive striated muscle cells, that occurs most frequently in the head and neck and is also found in the genitourinary tract, extremities, body wall, and retroperitoneum. In some cases, the onset is associated with trauma. The initial symptoms depend on the site of tumor development and indicate local tissue or organ destruction, as dysphagia, vaginal bleeding, hematuria, or obstruction of the flow of urine. Diagnostic measures may include barium x-ray studies, angiography, or tomography. Embryonal rhabdomyosarcoma occurs in the head, neck, or trunk of young children; alveolar rhabdomyosarcoma is usually seen in the extremities of adolescents; and the pleomorphic form is most common in the legs of adults. Surgical excision is rarely possible, because the tumor is poorly encapsulated and tends to spread. Amputation of an affected limb or extremity may be curative. Radiotherapy and chemotherapy with combinations of actinomycin D, adriamycin, cyclophosphamide, and vincristine may greatly increase the length of survival.

rhabdovirus, a member of a family of viruses that includes the organism causing rabies.

rhachi-. See **rachio-.**

rhagades /rag′ədēz/, cracks or fissures in skin that has lost its elasticity, especially common around the mouth. See also **cheilosis.**

rhaphe. See **raphe.**

Rh_o(D) immune globulin, a passive immunizing agent.

■ INDICATIONS: It is prescribed to prevent Rh sensitization in postabortion, postmiscarriage, postpartum, or ectopic pregnancy.

■ CONTRAINDICATIONS: It is not given to an Rh_o(D)- positive patient or to the infant or those previously immunized.

■ ADVERSE EFFECTS: The most serious adverse reaction is anaphylaxis.

rhenium (Re), a hard, brittle metallic element. Its atomic number is 75; its atomic weight is 186.2. Rhenium has a high melting point and is used in thermometers for measuring high temperatures.

rheo-, a combining form meaning 'of or pertaining to electric current, or to a flow': *rheobase, rheoscope, rheotaxis.*

Rheomacrodex, a trademark for a plasma expander (dextran 40).

Rhesus factor. See **Rh factor.**

rheumatic, of or pertaining to rheumatism.

-rheumatic, a combining form meaning 'relating to or exhibiting traits of rheumatism': *postrheumatic, prerheumatic, pseudorheumatic.*

rheumatic aortitis, an inflammatory condition of the aorta, occurring in rheumatic fever and characterized by disseminated focal lesions that may progressively form patches of fibrosis.

rheumatic arteritis, a complication of rheumatic fever characterized by generalized inflammation of arteries and arterioles. Fibrin, mixed with cellular debris, may invade, thicken, and stiffen the vessel wall, and the vessel may be surrounded by hemorrhage and exudate.

rheumatic chorea. See **Sydenham's chorea.**

rheumatic fever, an inflammatory disease that may develop as a delayed reaction to inadequately treated Group A beta-hemolytic streptococcal infection of the upper respiratory tract. This disorder usually occurs in young school-age children and may affect the brain, heart, joints, skin, or subcutaneous tissues. See also **rheumatic heart disease.**

■ OBSERVATIONS: The onset of rheumatic fever is usually sudden, often occurring in from 1 to 5 symptom-free weeks after recovery from a sore throat or from scarlet fever. Early symptoms usually include fever, joint pains, nose bleeds, abdominal pain, and vomiting. The major manifestations of this disease include migratory polyarthritis affecting numerous joints and carditis, which causes palpitations, chest pain, and, in severe cases, symptoms of cardiac failure. Sydenham's chorea, which may develop, is usually the sole, late sign of rheumatic fever and may initially be manifested as an increased awkwardness and an associated tendency to drop objects. As the chorea progresses, irregular body movements may become extensive, occasionally involving the tongue and the facial muscles, resulting in incapacitation of the affected individual. Other developments may include transient erythema marginatum with circular lesions and subcutaneous rheumatic nodules on various joints and tendons, the spine, and the back of the head. There is no specific diagnostic test for rheumatic fever. The development of serum antibodies to streptococcal antigens is a positive diagnostic sign. Affected individuals may also develop leukocytosis, moderate anemia, and proteinuria. C-reactive protein, evaluated in a specimen of blood, is abnormally high. Recurrences of rheumatic fever are common. Except for carditis, all the manifestations of this disease usually subside without any permanent effects. Mild cases may last 3 to 4 weeks. Severe cases with associated arthritis and carditis may last 2 to 3 months.

■ INTERVENTION: Management of this disease includes bed rest and severe restriction of normal activity. Penicillin is often administered, even if throat cultures are negative, and steroids or salicylates may be used, depending on the severity of any associated carditis and arthritis.

■ NURSING CONSIDERATIONS: The nurse is alert to signs of toxicity associated with salicylate and steroid therapies. Symptoms largely determine the type of nursing care. Large volumes of fluids are usually administered, and the nurse routinely helps minimize joint pains by properly positioning the patient. Throughout the course of the disease the patient benefits from emotional support and appropriate diversions.

rheumatic heart disease, damage to heart muscle and heart valves caused by episodes of rheumatic fever. When a susceptible person acquires a group A beta-hemolytic streptococcal infection, an autoimmune reaction may occur in heart tissue, resulting in permanent deformities of heart valves or chordae tendineae. Involvement of the heart may be evident during acute rheumatic fever, or it may be discovered long after the acute disease has subsided. See also **aortic stenosis, mitral stenosis, rheumatic fever.**

■ OBSERVATIONS: Rheumatic heart disease is characterized by heart murmurs resulting from stenosis or insufficiency of the valves and by compensatory alterations in the size of the chambers of the heart and the thickness of their walls. Abnormalities of pulse rate and rhythm, heart block, and congestive heart failure are also common. Deaths are usually the result of heart failure or bacterial endocarditis.

■ INTERVENTION: Episodes of acute rheumatic fever must be vigorously treated and supportive therapy given for heart failure, if needed. Chronic rheumatic heart disease may require no immediate treatment except for close observation. If signs of inefficient or decompensating heart action occur, digitalis, diuretics, and a low-sodium diet are often prescribed. In some patients, surgical commissurotomy or valve replacement is necessary. Patients with a history of rheumatic fever or evidence of rheumatic heart disease, to prevent streptococcal infection, should receive daily prophylactic penicillin by mouth or monthly intramuscular injections of benzathene penicillin, at least during childhood and adolescence. Patients with evidence of deformed heart valves should be given prophylactic antibiotics before surgical and dental procedures to prevent bacterial endocarditis.

■ NURSING CONSIDERATIONS: In addition to the care of patients with acute rheumatic fever, nurses have a responsibility to help educate them about their disease and about how to recognize the early symptoms and signs of its complications. It is especially important to stress the regular use of prophylactic penicillin to prevent streptococcal infections and the need to take special prophylactic antibiotics before surgery and all dental procedures.

rheumatism, *nontechnical.* **1.** any of a large number of inflammatory conditions of the bursae, joints, ligaments, or muscles characterized by pain, limitation of movement, and structural degeneration of single or multiple parts of the musculoskeletal system. **2.** the syndrome of pain, limitation of movement, and structural degeneration of elements in the musculoskeletal system as may occur in gout, rheumatoid arthritis, systemic lupus erythematosus, ankylosing spondylitis, and many other diseases. **–rheumatic, rheumatoid,** *adj.*

rheumatoid arthritis, a chronic, destructive, sometimes deforming, collagen disease that has an autoimmune component. Rheumatoid arthritis is characterized by symmetric inflammation of the synovium and increased synovial exudate, leading to thickening of the synovium and swelling of the joint. Rheumatoid arthritis usually first appears in early middle age, between 36 and 50 years of age, and most commonly in women. The course of the disease is variable but is most frequently marked by remissions and exacerbation. A kind of rheumatoid arthritis that occurs in younger people is **Still's disease.** Also called **arthritis deformans, atrophic arthritis.** Compare **ankylosing spondylitis.**

■ OBSERVATIONS: The medical diagnosis and prognosis of a case are based on a variety of clinical and laboratory findings. Clinical data, using mainly x-ray studies and physcical examination, classify the progress of rheumatoid arthritis into four stages. Stage I, representing early effects, is based on x-ray films showing the onset of bone changes. Stage II, moderate rheumatoid arthritis, is assigned cases in which there is evidence of some muscle atrophy and loss of mobility, in addition to x-ray findings. Stage III, severe rheumatoid arthritis, is marked by joint deformity, extensive muscle atrophy, and soft tissue lesions, as well as definite bone and cartilage destruction. Stage IV, the terminal category, includes all the Stage III clinical signs plus fibrous or bony ankylosis. Rheumatoid arthritis cases may also be classified on the basis of functional capacity: Class I, no loss of function; Class II, minor impairment of functional capacity with some pain and immobility; Class III, capacity limited to a few tasks; and Class IV, in which the patient is confined to bed or a wheelchair.

Rheumatoid arthritis may first be present with constitutional symptoms, including fatigue, weakness, and poor appetite. Other early signs include low-grade fever, anemia, and an increased erythrocyte sedimentation rate. The symptoms listed by the American Rheumatism Association include morning stiffness, joint pain or tenderness, swelling of at least two joints, subcutaneous nodules (called arthritic nodules and usually found at pressure points, as the elbows), structural changes in the joint seen on x-ray film, a positive rheumatoid factor agglutination test, decreased precipitation of mucin from synovial fluid, and characteristic histologic changes on pathologic examination of the fluid. Immune complexes are characteristically present in both the blood serum and the synovial fluid. Rheumatoid factor (RF) is present in serum and joint fluid of most persons with rheumatoid arthritis, and higher titers of rheumatoid factor are correlated with more severe forms of the disease, in particular forms with extraarticular manifestations. Antinuclear antibodies and special rheumatoid precipitins are also occasionally present. Extraarticular manifestations may include cardiac involvement, vasculitis, pulmonary disease, and proteinuria. There may also be a thickening of the synovium, called pannus formation. In long-term, severe, chronic rheumatoid arthritis, Felty's syndrome may be present.

■ INTERVENTION: The basic principles of treatment include sufficient rest, exercise to maintain joint function, medication for the relief of pain and the reduction of inflammation, orthopedic intervention to prevent or correct deformities, and excellent nutrition—with weight

Rheumatoid arthritis

Clinical stages	*Functional classification*
Stage I, early 1. X-ray films show no evidence of destructive changes. 2. X-ray films may show evidence of osteoporosis.	*Class I* No loss of functional capacity.
Stage II, moderate 1. X-ray films show evidence of osteoporosis, possibly with slight destruction of cartilage or subchondral bone. 2. Joints are not deformed, but mobility may be limited. 3. Adjacent muscles are atrophied. 4. Extraarticular soft-tissue lesions (as nodules and tenovaginitis) may be present.	*Class II* Functional capacity impaired but sufficient normal activities despite joint pain or limited mobility. *Class III* Functional capacity adequate to perform few if any occupational or self-care tasks.
Stage III, severe 1. X-ray films show cartilage and bone destruction, as well as osteoporosis. 2. Joint deformity (as subluxation, ulnar deviation, or hyperextension) exists but not fibrous or bony ankylosis. 3. Muscle atrophy is extensive. 4. Extraarticular soft-tissue lesions (as nodules and tenovaginitis) are often present.	*Class IV* Patient confined to bed or wheelchair and capable of little or no self-care.
Stage IV, terminal 1. Fibrous or bony ankylosis exists in addition to all criteria listed for stage III.	

loss, if necessary. Salicylates are usually given. If improvement is not achieved, other antiinflammatories, as indomethacin, phenylbutazone, antimalarials, gold salts, or some antineoplastic drugs may be used. Corticosteroids are prescribed with caution because of side effects, including gastric ulcer, adrenal suppression, and osteoporosis. Other treatments, including diathermy, ultrasound, warm paraffin applications, exercise under water, and applications of heat are occasionally used. ■ NURSING CONSIDERATIONS: Because rheumatoid arthritis is not always progressive, deforming, or debilitating, and early treatment may help the person to recover and perhaps to avoid future attacks, the nurse can play an important role by monitoring drug treatment so that adequate medication is taken, by noting side effects, and by adjusting treatment. Most people who have rheumatoid arthritis may continue in their jobs. The nurse encourages the person to get sufficient sleep and to rest the weight-bearing joints. Suggestions about the most effective use of heat, instruction in muscle-strengthening exercise and methods for easing pain and preventing deformities, as the proper use of pillows, splints, or molds, as well as emotional support are often given by the nurse. Because stress often precedes exacerbation of the condition, the person is counseled to avoid situations known to cause anxiety, worry, fatigue, infection, and other stressors.

rheumatoid coronary arteritis, an abnormal condition, characterized by a thickening of the tunica intima of the coronary arteries, which may produce coronary insufficiency. Rheumatoid coronary arteritis is a collagen disease that affects the connective tissue by inflammation and fibrinoid degeneration. It is commonly treated with glucocorticoids.

rheumatoid factor (RF), antiglobulin antibodies often found in the serum of patients with a clinical diagnosis of rheumatoid arthritis. Rheumatoid factors are present in about 70% of such cases, but they may also be found in such widely divergent diseases as tuberculosis, parasitic infections, leukemia, and connective tissue disorders. See also **latex fixation test.**

rheumatologist, a specialist in rheumatology.

rheumatology, the study of disorders characterized by inflammation, degeneration, or metabolic derangement of connective tissue and related structures of the body. These disorders are sometimes referred to collectively as rheumatism.

Rh factor, an antigenic substance present in the erythrocytes of most people. A person having the factor is Rh+ (Rh positive); a person lacking the factor is Rh− (Rh negative). If an Rh− person receives Rh+ blood, hemolysis and anemia occur. Rh+ infants may be exposed to antibodies to the factor produced in the Rh− mother's blood, resulting in red cell destruction and erythroblastosis fetalis. Transfusion, blood typing, and crossmatching depend on Rh+ and ABO classification. The Rh factor was first isolated and identified in the blood of a species of the rhesus (Rh) monkey. It is present in the red cells of 85% of people. See also **erythroblastosis fetalis, Rh_0(D) immune globulin.**

rhigo-, a combining form meaning 'cold': *rhigolene, rhigosis, rhigotic.*

rhin-. See **rhino-.**

Rh incompatibility, (in hematology) a lack of compatibility between two groups of blood cells that are antigenically different because of the presence of the Rh factor in one group and its absence in the other. See also **Rh factor.**

rhinencephalon /rī′nensef′əlon/, *pl.* **rhinencephala,** a portion of each cerebral hemisphere that contains the limbic system, which is associated with the emotions. The rhinencephalon develops in the embryo from a longitudinal ridge at the rostral extremity of the cerebral hemisphere. The rostral part of the ridge becomes the primitive olfactory lobe; the caudal part becomes the piriform lobe. In an adult, the caudal part of the piriform lobe is absorbed into the gyrus hippocampus. See also **limbic system.** **–rhinencephalic,** *adj.*

rhinitis /rīnī′tis/, inflammation of the mucous membranes of the nose, usually accompanied by swelling of the mucosa and a nasal discharge. It may be complicated by sinusitis. Rhinitis may be acute, allergic, atrophic, or vasomotor. Also called **coryza.**

rhino-, rhin-, a combining form meaning 'of or pertaining to the nose or to a noselike structure': *rhinocephalia, rhinolalia, rhinoplasty.*

rhinopathy /rīnop′əthē/, any disease or malformation of the nose.

rhinophyma /rī′nōfī′mə/, a form of rosacea in which there is sebaceous hyperplasia, redness, prominent vascularity, swelling, and distortion of the skin of the nose. Treatment includes dermabrasion, electrosurgery, and plastic surgery. See also **rosacea.**

rhinoplasty /rī′nəplas′tē/, a procedure in plastic surgery in which the structure of the nose is changed. Bone or cartilage may be removed, tissue grafted from another part of the body, or synthetic material implanted to alter the shape. Under local anesthesia intranasal incisions are made and the nose is reshaped. Postoperatively, any respiratory difficulty is reported immediately and the patient is kept in mid-Fowler's position. Frequent oral care is given, and ice compresses are applied to decrease the pain and edema that usually occur. Edema and discoloration around the eyes is expected to last for several days. The procedure is most frequently performed for cosmetic reasons.

rhinorrhea /rī′nôrē′ə/, **1.** the free discharge of a thin nasal mucus. **2.** the flow of cerebrospinal fluid from the nose after an injury to the head.

rhinoscope /rī′nəskōp/, an instrument for examining the nasal passages through the anterior nares or through the nasopharynx.

rhinoscopy /rīnos′kəpē/, an examination of the nasal passages to inspect the mucosa and detect inflammation, deformities, or asymmetry, as in deviation of the septum. The nasal passages may be examined anteriorally, by introducing a speculum into the anterior nares, or posteriorly, by introducing a rhinoscope through the nasopharynx. –**rhinoscopic,** *adj.*

rhinosporidiosis /rī′nōspərid′ē•ō′sis/, an infection caused by the fungus *Rhinosporidium seeberi,* characterized by fleshy red polyps on mucous membranes of nose, conjunctiva, nasopharynx, and soft palate. The disease may be acquired by swimming or bathing in infected water. The most effective treatment is electrocautery.

rhinotomy /rīnot′əmē/, a surgical procedure in which an incision is made along one side of the nose, performed to drain accumulated pus from an abscess or a sinus infection. Under local anesthesia, the flap of skin and lining of the nose are turned back to provide a full view of the nasal passages for radical sinus surgery.

rhinovirus /rī′nōvī′rəs/, any of about 100 serologically distinct, small RNA viruses that cause about 40% of acute respiratory illnesses. Infection is characterized by dry, scratchy throat, nasal congestion, malaise, and headache. Fever is minimal. Nasal discharge lasts 2 or 3 days. Children may also develop a cough. Type-specific antibodies may last for 2 to 4 years, without serious complications. The treatment is nonspecific and may include rest, analgesics, antihistamines, and nasal decongestants. Complete recovery is usual. Compare **adenovirus, parainfluenza virus, respiratory syncytial virus.** See also **cold.**

rhitid-. See **rhytid-.**

rhitidosis /rit′idō′sis/, a wrinkling, especially of the cornea. Also spelled **rhytidosis.**

rhizo-, a combining form meaning 'of or related to a root': *rhizodontropy, rhizome, rhizotomist.*

Rh negative. See **Rh factor.**

Rhodesian trypanosomiasis, an acute form of African trypanosomiasis, caused by the parasite *Trypanosoma brucei rhodesiense.* The disease may progress rapidly, causing encephalitis, coma, and death in only a few weeks. Also called **kaodzera.** Compare **Gambian trypanosomiasis.** See also **African trypanosomiasis.**

rhodium (Rh), a grayish-white metallic element. Its atomic number is 45; its atomic weight is 102.91. Rhodium is used for providing a hard lustrous coating on other metals and in the making of mirrors.

rhodo-, a combining form meaning 'red': *rhodocyte, rhodopsin, rhodotoxin.*

rhodopsin /rōdop′sin/, the purple pigmented compound in the rods of the retina, formed by a protein, opsin, and a derivative of vitamin A, retinal. Rhodopsin gives the outer segments of the rods a purple color and adapts the eye to low-density light. The compound breaks down when struck by light, and this chemical change triggers the conduction of nerve impulses. Brief periods of darkness allow the opsin and the retinal to reconstitute the rhodopsin, which accounts for the short delay a person experiences in adapting to sudden or drastic changes in lighting, as when moving out of bright sunlight into a darkened room or from darkness into bright light. Closing the eyes is a natural reflex that allows reconstitution of rhodopsin. Compare **iodopsin.**

RhoGAM, a trademark for a passive immunizing agent (Rh_o(D) immune globulin).

rhomboideus major /romboi′dē•əs/, a muscle of the upper back below and parallel to the rhomboideus minor. Arising from the spinous processes of the third, fourth, and fifth thoracic vertebrae and inserting into the lower half of the medial border of the scapula, it is innervated by the dorsal scapular nerve from the brachial plexus and, with the rhomboideus minor, functions to draw the scapula toward the vertebral column while supporting it and drawing it slightly upward. Compare **latissimus dorsi, levator scapulae, rhomboideus minor, trapezius.**

rhomboideus minor, a muscle of the upper back, above and parallel to the rhomboideus major. It arises from the ligamentum nuchae and from the spinous processes of the seventh cervical and first thoracic vertebrae. It inserts into the upper part of the medial border at the root of the spine of the scapula. It is innervated by the dorsal scapular nerve from the brachial plexus, which contains fibers from the fifth cervical nerve, and, with the rhomboideus major, acts to draw the scapula toward the vertebral column while supporting the scapula and drawing it slightly upward. Compare **latissimus dorsi, levator scapulae, rhomboideus major, trapezius.**

rhomboid glossitis. See **median rhomboid glossitis.**

rhonchi /rong′kī/, *sing.* **rhonchus,** abnormal sounds heard on auscultation of a respiratory airway obstructed by thick secretions, muscular spasm, neoplasm, or external pressure. The continuous rumbling sounds are more pronounced during expiration, and they characteristically clear on coughing, which rales do not. Rhonchi may be sibilant or sonorous. Sibilant rhonchi are high pitched and are heard in the small bronchi, as in asthma. Sonorous rhonchi are lower pitched and are heard in the large bronchi, as in tracheobronchitis. Dry rales are called rhonchi. Compare **rale, wheeze.**

rhotacism /rō′təsiz′əm/, a speech disorder characterized by a defective pronunciation of words containing the sound /r/, or by the excessive use of the sound /r/, or by the substitution of another sound for /r/. Compare **lallation, lambdacism.**

Rh positive. See **Rh factor.**

rhus dermatitis, a skin rash resulting from contact with a plant of the genus *Rhus,* as poison ivy, poison oak, or poison sumac. See also **contact dermatitis.**

rhyp-, a combining form meaning 'of or pertaining to filth': *rhyparia, rhypophagy, rhypophobia.*

rhythm, the relationship of one impulse to neighboring impulses as measured in time, movement, or regularity of action.

rhythm method. See **natural family planning method.**

rhytid-, rhitid-, a combining form meaning 'wrinkle, or wrinkled': *rhytidectomy, rhytidosis.*

rhytidoplasty /ritid′ōplas′tē/, a procedure in reconstructive plastic surgery in which the skin of the face is tightened, wrinkles are removed, and the skin is made to appear firm and smooth. An incision is made at the hairline, and excess skin is separated from the supporting tissue and excised. The edges of the remaining skin are pulled up and back and sutured at the hairline. A pressure dressing is applied and left in place for 24 to 48 hours. Postoperative medication for pain is often necessary. The sutures are removed several days after discharge in an outpatient facility or in the surgeon's office. Also spelled **rhitidoplasty.**

rhytidosis. See **rhitidosis.**

RIA. See **radioimmunoassay.**

rib, one of the 12 pairs of elastic arches of bone forming a large part of the thoracic skeleton. The first seven ribs on each side are called **true ribs** because they articulate directly with the sternum and the vertebrae. The remaining five ribs are called **false ribs,** the first three attaching ventrally to ribs above; the last two ribs are free at their ventral extremities and are called **floating ribs.**

rib fracture, a break in a bone of the thoracic skeleton caused by a blow or crushing injury or by violent coughing or sneezing. The ribs most commonly broken are the fourth to eighth, and, if the bone is splintered or the fracture is displaced, sharp fragments may pierce the lung, causing hemothorax or pneumothorax.

■ OBSERVATIONS: The patient with a fractured rib suffers pain, especially on inspiration, and usually breathes rapidly and shallowly. The site of the break is generally very tender to the touch, and the crackling of bone fragments rubbing together may be heard on auscultation. Breath sounds may be absent, decreased, or accompanied by rales and rhonchi. The location and nature of the fracture are determined by chest x-ray studies, and the patient is observed for signs of hemoptysis, hemothorax, flail chest, atelectasis, pneumothorax, and pneumonia.

■ INTERVENTION: Fractured ribs may be splinted with an elastic belt, an Ace bandage, or adhesive strapping; to prevent irritation, the area may be shaved and painted with tincture of benzoin before the adhesive tape is applied. If hospitalization is required, the patient is placed in a semi-Fowler's position, and the blood pressure, pulse, temperature, respirations, and breath sounds are checked every 2 to 4 hours. An analgesic may be ordered, but morphine sulfate is avoided. The patient is assisted in turning and is instructed in how to deep breathe, to cough, and to perform range of motion exercises of extremities. If strapping and analgesic medication fail to relieve pain, the physician may perform a regional nerve block by infiltrating the intercostal spaces above and below the fracture site with 1% procaine.

■ NURSING CONSIDERATIONS: The nurse assists in splinting the chest, administers the ordered medication, and helps the patient to turn.

riboflavin /rib'ōflā'vin/, a yellow crystalline, water-soluble pigment, one of the heat-stable components of the B vitamin complex. It combines with specific flavoproteins and functions as a coenzyme in the oxidative processes of carbohydrates, fats, and proteins. It is also important in the prevention of some visual disorders, especially cataracts. Small amounts of riboflavin are found in the liver and kidneys, but it is not stored to any great degree in the body and must be supplied regularly in the diet. Common sources are organ meats, milk, cheese, eggs, green leafy vegetables, meat, whole grains, and legumes. Deficiency of riboflavin produces cheilosis, local inflammation, desquamation, encrustation, glossitis, photophobia, corneal opacities, proliferation of corneal vessels, seborrheic dermatitis about the nose, mouth, forehead, ears, and scrotum, trembling, sluggishness, dizziness, edema, inability to urinate, and vaginal itching. There is no known toxicity of riboflavin. Also called **vitamin B_2.** See also **ariboflavinosis.**

ribonucleic acid (RNA) /rī'bōno͞oklē'ik/, a nucleic acid, found in both the nucleus and cytoplasm of cells, that transmits genetic instructions from the nucleus to the cytoplasm. In the cytoplasm, RNA functions in the assembly of proteins. See also **deoxyribonucleic acid.**

ribosome /rī'bəsōm/, a cytoplasmic organelle composed of ribonucleic acid and protein that functions in the synthesis of protein. Ribosomes interact with messenger RNA and transfer RNA to join together amino acid units into a polypeptide chain according to the sequence determined by the genetic code. The structures appear singly or in clusters as polysomes, or they may be attached to endoplasmic reticulum. See also **translation.**

rice diet, a diet consisting only of rice, fruit, fruit juices, and sugar, supplemented with vitamins and iron. Salt is strictly forbidden. It is prescribed for the treatment of hypertension, chronic renal disease, and obesity. The diet is somewhat modified after blood pressure is lowered and other symptoms are alleviated. It should not be followed for any length of time, because the severe dietary restrictions may lead to nutritional deficiencies or imbalance. Also called **Duke diet, Kempner rice-fruit diet.**

Richards, Linda (1841–1930), a nurse considered to be the first American-trained nurse, being graduated in the first class of the New England Hospital for Women and Children. She then studied at the Nightingale Training School in London and, in 1873, organized the Massachusetts General Hospital Training School on the same lines. In 1885, she was sent to Japan to develop a training school at the Charity Hospital. In 1891, she took charge of the Philadelphia Visiting Nurse Society. She is credited with being the first to keep written records on patients, a practice she started when she worked as night superintendent at Bellevue Hospital in New York under Sister Helen.

Richet's aneurysm. See **fusiform aneurysm.**

rickets, a condition caused by the deficiency of vitamin D, calcium, and, usually, phosphorus, seen primarily in infancy and childhood, and characterized by abnormal bone formation. Symptoms include soft pliable bones causing such deformities as bowlegs and knock-knees, nodular enlargements on the ends and sides of the bones, muscle pain, enlarged skull, chest deformities, spinal curvature, enlargement of the liver and spleen, profuse sweating, and general tenderness of the body when touched. Prophylaxis and treatment include a diet rich in calcium, phosphorus, and vitamin D and adequate exposure to sunlight. Kinds of rickets include **adult rickets, celiac rickets, renal rickets,** and **vitamin D resistant rickets.** See also **osteodystrophy, osteomalacia, vitamin D.**

rickettsia /riket′sē·ə/, *pl.* **rickettsiae,** any organism of the genus *Rickettsia*. Rickettsiae are small, round, or rod-shaped, specialized bacteria that live as viruslike intracellular parasites in lice, fleas, ticks, and mites. They are transmitted to humans by bites from these insects. Rickettsial diseases have been responsible for many of history's worst epidemics. The various species are distinguished on the basis of similarities in the diseases they cause: The spotted fever group includes Rocky Mountain spotted fever, rickettsialpox, and others; the typhus group includes epidemic typhus, scrub typhus, murine typhus; and a miscellaneous group includes Q fever and trench fever. Rickettsial diseases are uncommon in parts of the world where insect and rodent populations are well controlled. Tetracycline or chloramphenicol is usually prescribed in the treatment of rickettsial diseases. **–rickettsial,** *adj.*

rickettsialpox /riket′sē·əlpoks′/, a mild, acute infectious disease caused by *Rickettsia akari* and transmitted from mice to humans by mites. It is characterized by an asymptomatic, crusted primary lesion, chills, fever, headache, malaise, myalgia, and a rash resembling chickenpox. About 1 week after onset of symptoms, small, discrete, maculopapular lesions appear on any part of the body, but rarely on palms or soles. These lesions become vesicular and dry and form scabs. Eventually the scabs fall off, leaving no scars. Chloramphenicol or tetracycline will hasten recovery. Prevention involves the elimination of house mice. Also called **Kew Gardens spotted fever.** Compare **Rocky Mountain spotted fever.** See also **Rickettsia.**

rickettsiosis /riket′sē·ō′sis/, *pl.* **rickettsioses,** any of a group of infectious diseases caused by microorganisms of the genus *Rickettsia*. Kinds of rickettsioses include a spotted fever group (**boutonneuse fever, rickettsialpox, Rocky Mountain spotted fever**), a typhus group (**epidemic typhus, murine typhus, scrub typhus**), and a miscellaneous group (**Q fever, trench fever**). See also **rickettsia.**

rider's bone, a bony deposit that sometimes develops in horseback riders on the inner side of the lower end of the tendon of the adductor muscle of the thigh. Also called **cavalry bone.**

ridge, a projection or projecting structure, as the gastrocnemial ridge on the posterior surface of the femur, giving attachment to the gastrocnemius muscle.

ridge extension, an intraoral surgical operation for deepening the labial, buccal, or lingual sulci.

ridge lap, the part of an artificial tooth that is adjacent to or laps the residual ridge.

Riedel's struma, Riedel's thyroiditis. See **fibrous thyroiditis.**

Rieder's cell leukemia /rē′dərz/, a malignant neoplasm of blood-forming tissues, characterized by the presence in blood of large numbers of atypical myeloblasts with immature cytoplasm and relatively mature lobulated, indented nuclei.

Rifadin, a trademark for an antibacterial (rifampin).

rifampin, an antibacterial.

■ INDICATIONS: It is prescribed in the treatment of tuber-

Infectious pathogens of humans—rickettsiae and chlamydiae

Organism	*Disease clinical manifestation*	*Reservoir*	*Method of transmission*
Chlamydia trachomatis	Nongonococcal urethritis and cervicitis, inclusion conjunctivitis (trachoma), lymphogranuloma venereum	Humans	Sexual contact; conjunctivitis may be transmitted by hands, flies
Coxiella burnetti	Q fever	Rodents, cattle, sheep, goats	Inhalation of infectious aerosol; tick
Rickettsia akari	Rickettsialpox	Mice	Mite vector
Rickettsia australis	Queensland tick typhus	Marsupials, rodents	Tick vector
Rickettsia conorii	Boutonneuse (Mediterranean, Marseilles) fever	Dogs, rodents	Tick vector
Rickettsia rickettsii	Rocky Mountain spotted fever	Rodents, dogs, foxes, rabbits, squirrels	Tick vector
Rickettsia sibirica	Siberian tick typhus	Rodents, domestic animals, birds	Tick vector
Rickettsia tsutsugamushi	Scrub typhus	Rodents, birds	Mite (chigger) vector
Rickettsia typhi (R. mooseri)	Murine typhus (endemic typhus)	Rodents	Flea vector
Rochalimaea quintana	Trench fever	Humans	Human body louse vector

By Nickelsen, Patricia, Ph.D., Associate Director, Clinical Microbiology Laboratory, Stanford University Hospital, Stanford University Medical Center, Stanford, CA, 1984.

culosis, in meningococcal prophylaxis, and as an antileprotic.

■ CONTRAINDICATIONS: Liver dysfunction or disease or known hypersensitivity to this drug or to rifamycin prohibits its use.

■ ADVERSE EFFECTS: Among the more serious adverse reactions are liver toxicity and a syndrome resembling influenza. GI distress, aches and cramps, discoloration of urine, saliva, and sweat commonly occur. This drug interacts with many other drugs.

Rift Valley fever, an arbovirus infection of Egypt and east Africa spread by mosquitoes or by handling infected sheep and cattle. It is characterized by abrupt fever, chills, headache, and generalized aching, followed by epigastric pain, anorexia, loss of taste, and photophobia. The disease is of short duration, and recovery is usually complete. There is no specific treatment. A killed virus vaccine that provides protection for 2 years is available for those at risk, as laboratory workers and veterinarians.

RIG, abbreviation for **rabies immune globulin.**

Riga-Fede disease, an ulceration of the lingual frenum in some infants, caused by abrasion of the frenum by natal or neonatal teeth. Also called **Fede's disease.**

right atrioventricular valve. See **tricuspid valve.**

right brachiocephalic vein, a vessel, about 2.5 cm long, that starts in the root of the neck at the junction of the internal jugular and the subclavian veins on the right side and descends vertically from behind the sternal end of the clavicle to join the left brachiocephalic vein and form the superior vena cava. The right brachiocephalic vein, like the left, receives various tributaries, as the vertebral vein, the internal thoracic vein, and the inferior thyroid vein. Compare **left brachiocephalic vein.**

right bundle branch block, an abnormal cardiac condition characterized by an impaired electric signal associated with the bundle of fibers that transmit impulses from the bundle of His to the right ventricle. This dysfunction may be a complete or an incomplete block of impulses and may be caused by a lesion in the right bundle branch or a small focal lesion in the AV bundle. A right bundle branch block is often associated with right ventricular hypertrophy, especially in individuals under 40 years of age. In older individuals a right bundle branch block is commonly caused by coronary artery disease. A complete right bundle branch block commonly occurs after surgical closure of a ventricular septal defect.

right common carotid artery, the shorter of the two common carotid arteries, springing from the brachiocephalic trunk, passing obliquely from the level of the sternoclavicular articulation to the cranial border of the thyroid cartilage, and dividing into the right carotid arteries. Compare **left common carotid artery.**

right coronary artery, one of a pair of branches of the ascending aorta, arising in the right posterior aortic sinus, passing along the right side of the coronary sulcus, dividing into the right interventricular artery and a large marginal branch, supplying both ventricles, the right atrium, and the sinoatrial node. Compare **left coronary artery.**

right coronary vein. See **small cardiac vein.**

right-handedness, a natural tendency to favor the use of the right hand. Also called **dextrality.** See also **cerebral dominance, handedness.**

right-heart failure, an abnormal cardiac condition characterized by the impairment of the right side of the heart and congestion and elevated pressure in the systemic veins and capillaries. Right-heart failure is usually related to left-heart failure because both sides of the heart are part of a circuit and what affects one side will eventually affect the other. The most common cause of right-heart failure is left-heart failure. However, research indicates that experimentally induced pure failure of one ventricle may produce hemodynamic and biochemical abnormalities in the opposite ventricle without the usual signs of failure. In failure associated with either side of the heart, cardiac output may be normal, decreased, or increased. Compare **left-heart failure.**

right hepatic duct, the duct that drains bile from the right lobe of the liver into the common bile duct.

righting reflex, any reflex that tends to return an animal to its normal body position in space when it has been moved from the normal position. These reflexes involve a number of sensory receptors including the eyes, labyrinth, and muscles.

right interventricular artery. See **dorsal interventricular artery.**

right lymphatic duct, a vessel that conveys lymph from the right upper quadrant of the body into the bloodstream in the neck at the junction of the right internal jugular and the right subclavian veins. About 1.25 cm long, the duct courses over the medial border of the scalenus anterior. At its orifice are two semilunar valves that prevent venous blood from flowing backward into the duct. Lymph drains into the right lymphatic duct from numerous capillaries and vessels and from three lymphatic trunks in the right quadrant. Compare **thoracic duct.** See also **lymphatic system.**

right pulmonary artery, the longer and slightly larger of the two arteries conveying venous blood from the heart to the lungs, rising from the pulmonary trunk, bending to the right behind the aorta, and dividing into two branches at the root of the right lung. Compare **left pulmonary artery.**

right-sided failure. See **right-heart failure.**

right subclavian artery, a large artery that arises from the brachiocephalic artery. It has several important branches: the axillary, vertebral thoracic, and internal thoracic arteries and the cervical and costocervical trunks, perfusing the right side of the upper body.

right ventricle, the relatively thin-walled chamber of the heart that pumps blood received from the right atrium into the pulmonary arteries to the lungs for oxygenation. The right ventricle is shorter and rounder than the long, conical left ventricle. The chordae tendineae of the tricuspid valve of the right ventricle are finer than the coarse strands of the chordae tendineae of the left ventricle. See also **heart.**

rigidity, a condition of hardness, stiffness, or inflexibility. **–rigid,** *adj.*

rigidus /rij′idəs/, a deformity characterized by limited motion, especially dorsiflexion of the great toe. This condition causes pain and may ultimately produce degenerative changes of involved joints.

rigor, **1.** a rigid condition of the tissues of the body, as in rigor mortis. **2.** a violent attack of shivering that may be associated with chills and fever.

rigor mortis, the rigid stiffening of skeletal and cardiac muscle shortly after death.

Rimactane, a trademark for an antibacterial (rifampin).

rima glottidis. See **glottis.**

Rimso-50, a trademark for an antiinflammatory agent (dimethyl sulfoxide), used in the treatment of interstitial cystitis.

ring chromosome, a circular chromosome formed by the fusion of the two ends. It is the primary type of chromosome found in bacteria.

Ringer's lactate solution, a fluid and electrolyte replenisher.

■ INDICATIONS: It is prescribed for correction of extracellular volume and electrolyte depletion.

■ CONTRAINDICATIONS: Kidney failure, congestive heart failure, or hypoproteinemia prohibits its use.

■ ADVERSE EFFECTS: Among the more serious adverse reactions are sodium excess and fluid overload, which may lead to pulmonary and peripheral edema.

ringworm. See **tinea.**

Rinne tuning fork test /rin′ē/, a method of assessing auditory acuity, useful in distinguishing conductive from sensorineural hearing loss. The test is performed with tuning forks of 256, 512, and 1024 cycles, and while each ear is tested, the other is masked. The stem of a vibrating fork is alternately placed 0.5 inches from the external auditory meatus of the ear and on the adjacent mastoid bone until the sound is no longer heard at each of these positions. The person with normal hearing perceives the sound for a longer period when conduction is by air than by bone. If the patient has a conductive loss, the sound is heard for a longer period when conducted by bone than by air. In sensorineural loss, the sound is heard longer when conducted by air, but perception by both air and bone conduction is diminished.

Rio Grande fever. See **abortus fever.**

Riopan, a trademark for an antiacid (magaldrate).

risk factor, a factor that causes a person or a group of people to be particularly vulnerable to an unwanted, unpleasant, or unhealthful event, as immunosuppression, which increases the incidence and severity of infection, or cigarette smoking, which increases the risk of developing a respiratory or cardiovascular disease.

risk management, a function of administration of a hospital or other health facility directed toward identification, evaluation, and correction of potential risks that could lead to injury to patients, staff members, or visitors and in property loss or damage.

risorius /risôr′ē·əs/, one of the 12 muscles of the mouth. Arising in the fascia over the masseter and inserting into the skin at the corner of the mouth, it is innervated by mandibular and buccal branches of the facial nerve and acts to retract the angle of the mouth, as in a smile.

Risser cast /ris′ər/, an orthopedic device for encasing the entire trunk of the body, extending over the cervical area to the chin. In rare cases it extends over the hips to the knees. The Risser cast is of plaster of paris or fiberglass and is used to immobilize the trunk of the body in the treatment of scoliosis and in the preoperative or the postoperative correction or the maintenance of correction of scoliosis. Compare **body jacket, turnbuckle cast.**

risus sardonicus /rē′səs särdon′ikəs/, a wry, masklike grin caused by spasm of the facial muscles, as seen in tetanus.

Ritalin Hydrochloride, a trademark for a central nervous system stimulant (methylphenidate hydrochloride).

ritodrine hydrochloride, a beta-sympathomimetic agent.

■ INDICATION: It is prescribed in pregnancy management to stop the uterus from contracting in preterm labor.

■ CONTRAINDICATIONS: It is not given before the twentieth week of gestation. Known hypersensitivity to this drug prohibits its use.

■ ADVERSE EFFECTS: Among the more serious adverse reactions are tachycardia, palpitations, headache, nausea, and alterations in blood pressure. Pulmonary edema and death have occurred when it has been given concomitantly with corticosteroids to prevent the development of respiratory distress syndrome in the premature neonate.

Ritter's disease, a rare, staphylococcal infection of newborns which begins with red spots about the mouth and chin, gradually spreading over the entire body and followed by generalized exfoliation. Vesicles and yellow crusts may also be present. Ritter's disease is usually fatal unless treated with antibiotics, which should be selected on the basis of bacterial sensitivity tests. Also called **dermatitis exfoliativa neonatorum.** Compare **toxic epidermal necrolysis.**

river blindness. See **onchocerciasis.**

r-loop, (in molecular genetics) a distinctive loop formation seen under an electron microscope. It is composed of a single helical strand of DNA, wound with a hybrid strand containing another single strand of DNA with a strand of RNA.

RMSF, abbreviation for **Rocky Mountain spotted fever.**

Rn, symbol for **radon.**

RN, abbreviation for **registered nurse.**

RNA, abbreviation for **ribonucleic acid.**

RNA polymerase, (in molecular genetics) an enzyme that catalyzes the assembly of ribonucleoside triphosphates into RNA, with single-stranded DNA serving as the template. Also called **RNA nucleotidyltransferase.**

RNA splicing, (in molecular genetics) the process by which base pairs that interrupt the continuity of genetic information in DNA are removed from the precursors of messenger RNA.

Robaxin, a trademark for a skeletal muscle relaxant (methocarbamol).

Robb, Isabel Hampton (1860–1910), a Canadian-born American nursing educator and writer. She was the first to institute a systematic, step-by-step course for nursing students that integrated clinical experience and classwork and the first educator to arrange for the affiliation of her students at other hospitals for specialized training. She also helped establish university affiliation for nursing education and for postgraduate courses. When the Johns Hopkins School of Nursing was established in Baltimore, in 1889, she became its first director and while there set the high standards for both the practical and theoretic aspects of nursing education that became the base from which she worked to establish national standards. She was one of the founders of *The American Journal of Nursing* and of the forerunner of the American Nurses' Association.

robertsonian translocation, the exchange of entire chromosome arms, with the break occurring at the centromere, usually between two nonhomologous acrocentric chromosomes, to form one large metacentric chromosome and one extremely small chromosome that carries little genetic material and through successive cell divisions may be lost, leading to a reduction in total chromosome number. Compare **balanced translocation, reciprocal translocation.**

Robicillin VK, a trademark for an antibiotic (penicillin V potassium).

Ro-Bile, a trademark for a GI fixed-combination drug containing a variety of digestive enzymes.

Robimycin, a trademark for an antibacterial (erythromycin).

Robinul, a trademark for an anticholinergic (glycopyrrolate).

Robitet, a trademark for an antibiotic (tetracycline or tetracycline hydrochloride).

Robitussin, a trademark for an expectorant (guaifenesin), in various fixed-combination preparations and with an antihistamine used as a cough suppressant or a bronchodilator.

Rocaltrol, a trademark for a regulator of calcium (calcitriol).

rock fever. See **brucellosis.**

Rocky Mountain spotted fever (RMSF), a serious tick-borne infectious disease occurring throughout the temperate zones of North and South America, caused by *Rickettsia rickettsii* and characterized by chills, fever, severe headache, myalgia, mental confusion, and rash. Erythematous macules first appear on wrists and ankles, spreading rapidly over the extremities, trunk, face, and, usually, on the palms and soles. Hemorrhagic lesions, constipation, and abdominal distention are also common. The diagnosis is based on clinical examination and is confirmed by laboratory analyses, including immunofluorescent antibody screens, complement fixation test, and Weil-Felix test. Early treatment with chloramphenicol or tetracycline is important, because more than 20% of untreated patients die from shock and renal failure. A diet high in protein is important to avoid hypoproteinemia. Nursing care is especially important to avoid decubitus ulcers and hypostatic or aspiration pneumonia. Immunity follows recovery. Prevention includes the use of insect repellents, the wearing of protective clothing, frequent inspection of the body and careful removal of wood or dog ticks, and immunization with killed vaccine for those frequently exposed to ticks. Care must be taken not to crush ticks, because infection may be acquired through skin abrasions. Also called **mountain fever, mountain tick fever, spotted fever.** Compare **murine typhus, rickettsialpox.** See also **boutonneuse fever, scrub typhus, typhus.**

rod, **1.** a straight cylindric structure. **2.** one of the tiny cylindric elements arranged perpendicular to the surface of the retina. Rods contain the chemical rhodopsin, which adapts the eye to detect low-intensity light and gives the rods a purple color. Each rod is 40 to 60 μ in length and about 2 μ thick and consists of a slender, reactive outer segment and an inner granular segment. When bright light strikes a rod, rhodopsin rapidly breaks down; it reforms gradually in low-intensity light. Compare **cone.** See also **iodopsin, Jacob's membrane.**

rodenticide poisoning, a toxic condition caused by the ingestion of a substance intended for the control of rodent populations. See also **phosphorus poisoning, thallium poisoning, warfarin poisoning.**

rodent ulcer, a slowly developing serpiginous ulceration of a basal cell carcinoma of the skin. See also **basal cell carcinoma.**

roentgen (R) /rent′gən, ren′jən/, the quantity of x- or gamma radiation that creates 1 electrostatic unit of ions in 1 ml of air at 0° C and 760 mm of pressure. In radiotherapy or radiodiagnosis, the roentgen is the unit of the emitted dose. See also **rad, rem.**

roentgen fetometry, the use of radiographic techniques to measure the fetus in utero.

roentgenology, the study of the diagnostic and therapeutic uses of x-rays. See also **radiology, roentgen, x-ray.**

roentgen ray. See **x-ray.**

Rogers, Martha, author of Rogers' Science of Unitary Man, a nursing theory introduced in 1970. The Rogers theory has strong ties to the general systems theory with elements of a developmental model. It considers four "building blocks": Energy Fields, Universe of Open Systems, Pattern and Organization, and Four Dimensionality. Energy Fields refers to conceptualization of humans and their environment as matter or energy evidenced by wave patterns. Open Systems refers to views of persons as open systems who interact continuously with the environment. Pattern and Organization describes the way Energy Fields emerge, characterized by wave patterns. Four Dimensionality has been interpreted as a form of clairvoyance in which there is a "transcendence of time-space interaction," or an ability to transcend time to see into the future.

Rokitansky's disease. See **Budd-Chiari syndrome.**

Rolando's fracture /rōlan′dōz/, a fracture of the base of the first metacarpal.

role blurring, the tendency for professional roles to overlap and become indistinct.

role conflict, the presence of contradictory and often competing role expectations.

role overload, a condition in which there is insufficient time in which to carry out all of the expected role functions.

role playing, a psychotherapeutic technique in which a person acts out a real or simulated situation as a means of understanding intrapsychic conflicts.

role playing therapy. See **psychodrama.**

Rolfing. See **structural integration.**

roller bandage, a long, tightly wound strip of material that may vary in width. It is generally applied as a circular bandage.

roller clamp, a device, usually made of plastic, equipped with a small roller that may be rolled counterclockwise to close off primary intravenous tubing or clockwise to open it. The roller clamp may also be manipulated to increase and decrease the flow of the intravenous solution and is easily moved with the thumb, thus making it a one-handed convenience in the administration of intravenous therapy. Compare **screw clamp, slide clamp.**

rolling effleurage, a circular rubbing stroke used in massage to promote circulation and muscle relaxation, especially on the shoulder and buttocks. It is performed with the hand flat, the palm and closely held fingers acting as a unit. Compare **effleurage, pétrissage.**

ROM /rom, är′ō′em′/, abbreviation for *read-only memory,* the portion of a computer's memory where information is permanently stored. The operator has random access to the memory, but only for purposes of reading the contents. Special equipment is required to write or erase a read-only memory.

Romberg sign /rom′bərg/, an indication of loss of the sense of position in which the patient loses balance when standing erect, feet together, and eyes closed. Also called **Romberg test.**

Romilar, a trademark for an antitussive (dextromethorphan hydrobromide).

Rondec-DM, a trademark for a fixed-combination drug containing an antihistamine (carbinoxamine maleate), an antitussive (dextromethorphan hydrobromide), and an adrenergic decongestant and bronchodilator (pseudoephedrine hydrochloride).

Rondomycin, a trademark for an antibiotic (methacycline hydrochloride).

rongeur forceps /rônzhur′, rôNzhœr′/, a kind of biting forceps that is strong and heavy, used for cutting bone. Also called **rongeur.**

Roniacol, a trademark for a peripheral vasodilator (nicotinyl alcohol).

room, any area surrounded by four walls within a building, especially one in which a patient is housed, treated, or cared for.

rooming-in, (in a hospital) a recent practice that allows mothers and new babies to share accommodations, remaining together in the hospital as they would at home rather than being separated.

root, the lowest part of an organ or a structure by which something is firmly attached, as the anatomic root of the tooth, which is covered by cementum. Also called **radix** /rā′diks/ (*pl.* **radices**).

root amputation. See **apicectomy.**

root canal. See **pulp canal.**

root canal file, a small metal hand instrument with tightly spiraled blades, used for cleaning and shaping a root canal.

root canal filling, a material placed in the root canal system of a tooth to seal the space previously occupied by the dental pulp.

root curettage, the debridement and planing of the root surface of a tooth to remove accretions and induce the development of healthy gingival tissues.

root end cyst. See **radicular cyst.**

root furcation, the abnormal resorption of the irradicular bone in multirooted teeth, resulting from periodontal disease.

rooting reflex, a normal response in newborns when the cheek is touched or stroked along the side of the mouth to turn the head toward the stimulated side and to begin to suck. The reflex disappears by 3 to 4 months of age but in some infants may persist until 12 months of age.

root resection. See **apicectomy.**

root retention, a technique that removes the crown of a root canal treated tooth and retains enough of the root and gingival attachment to support a removable prosthesis.

root submersion, a root retention in which the tooth structure is reduced below the level of the alveolar crest and the soft tissue is allowed to heal over it. This technique is used for minimizing residual ridge resorption.

Rorschach test /rôr′shäk, rôr′shokh/, a projective personality assessment test developed by the Swiss psychiatrist Hermann Rorschach. It consists of 10 pictures of inkblots, five in black and white, three in black and red, and two multicolored, to which the subject responds by telling, in as many interpretations as is desired, what images and emotions each design evokes. Replies are evaluated according to whether the response is to the entire or only part of the image; whether color, shading, shape, or location of individual elements is significant; whether movement is seen; and the degree of complexity to which each interpretation is given. Scoring is primarily subjective and is based on both the subject's responses and the general reaction to the circumstances under which the test is administered. The test is designed to assess the degree to which intellectual and emotional factors are integrated in the subject's perception of the environment. See also **Holtzman inkblot technique.**

ROS, abbreviation for **review of systems.**

rosacea /rōzā′shē·ə/, a chronic form of acne seen in adults of all ages and associated with telangiectasia, especially of the nose, forehead, and cheeks. Also called **acne rosacea.** See also **rhinophyma.**

rose fever, a common misnomer for seasonal allergic rhinitis caused by pollen, most frequently of grasses, that is airborne at the time roses are in bloom. Roses are not the cause of common spring and summer allergic reactions; their pollen is not dispersed by the wind but is carried from flower to flower by insects.

Rosenmüller's organ. See **epoophoron.**

Rosenthal's syndrome. See **hemophilia C.**

roseola /rōzē′ələ/, any rose-colored rash. See also **roseola infantum.**

roseola infantum, a benign, presumably viral, endemic illness of infants and young children, characterized by abrupt, high sustained or spiking fever, mild pharyngitis, and lymph node enlargement. Febrile convulsions may occur. After 4 or 5 days the fever suddenly drops to normal, and a faint, pink, maculopapular rash appears on the neck, trunk, and thighs. The rash may last a few hours to 2 days. Diagnosis is based on high fever with rather mild illness and the rash. Sequelae may occur as a result of the convulsions. There is no specific therapy or vaccine. Aspirin or acetaminophen are often used to try to control fever. Anticonvulsive medication may be indicated. Also called **exanthem subitum, sixth disease, Zahorsky's disease.**

rose spots, small erythematous macules occurring on the upper abdomen and anterior thorax and lasting 2 or 3 days, characteristic of typhoid and paratyphoid fevers.

rost-, a combining form meaning 'of or pertaining to a beak': *rostellum, rostrad, rostriform.*

rostral /ros′trəl/, beak-shaped. **–rostrum,** *n.*

rot-, a combining form meaning 'turned, or to turn': *rotate, rotatory, rotexion.*

rotameter /rōtam′ətər/, a device operated by a needle valve in an anesthetic gas machine that measures gases by speed of flow, according to their viscosity and density. Also called **flowmeter.**

rotating tourniquet, one of four constricting devices used in a rotating order to pool blood in the extremities to relieve congestion in the lungs in the treatment of acute pulmonary edema.

■ METHOD: Tourniquets are applied to the upper parts of three extremities at one time. Every 15 minutes, in clockwise order, a tourniquet is placed on the nonconstricted extremity, and one tourniquet is removed; as a result of this rotation, the blood vessels of each of the four extremities are constricted for 45 minutes of each hour of the procedure. If a rotating tourniquet machine is used, blood pressure cuffs placed on all four extremities are automatically inflated and deflated in a rotating sequence. Rotating tourniquets are contraindicated for patients in shock and are not placed on an extremity receiving parenteral fluids. The patient who is to undergo the procedure is placed in a high Fowler's position. Peripheral pulses, as the brachial, radial, popliteal, and pedal, are palpated and are not occluded in applying the tourniquets. During the procedure, blood pressure, respirations, and the apical pulse are checked, and peripheral pulses are palpated every 15 minutes. The chest is auscultated for breath sounds every 30 minutes. Signs of phlebothrombosis and pulmonary embolism are watched for, and if the color of an extremity does not return to normal on release of a tourniquet, the physician is informed. At the termination of the procedure, one tourniquet is removed every 15 minutes in the rotation sequence. If pulmonary edema recurs, the tourniquets are reapplied and the physician is notified immediately.

■ NURSING ORDERS: The nurse applies the tourniquets, keeping a time schedule and rotation diagram at bedside. She explains the procedure and remains with the patient as much as possible to provide emotional support.

■ OUTCOME CRITERIA: Rotating tourniquets are beneficial in some cases but are used less frequently than in the past. Some authorities believe the effect of this therapeutic modality on patients whose condition is poor is worse than that of pulmonary edema.

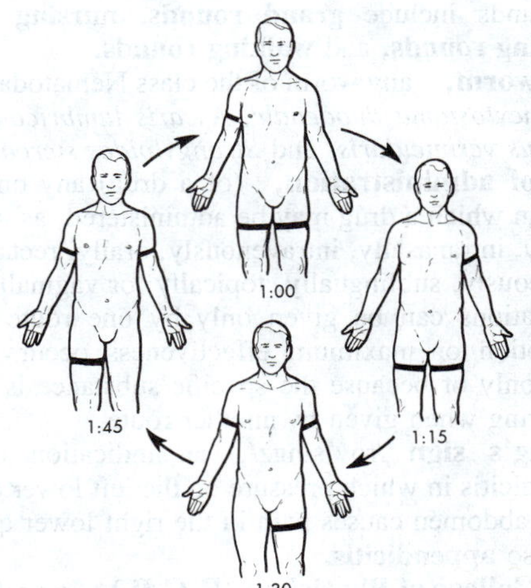

Rotating tourniquets

rotation, **1.** a turning around an axis. **2.** one of the four basic kinds of motion allowed by various joints: the rotation of a bone around its central axis, which may lie in a separate bone, as in the pivot formed by the dens of the axis around which the atlas turns. A bone, as the humerus, may also rotate around its own longitudinal axis, or the axis of rotation may not be quite parallel to the long axis of the rotating bone, as in movement of the radius on the ulna during pronation and supination of the hand. Compare **angular movement, circumduction,**

gliding. **3.** (in obstetrics) the turning of the fetal head to descend through the pelvis.

Rotor syndrome /rō′tər/, a rare condition of the liver inherited as an autosomal recessive trait. It is similar to Dubin-Johnson syndrome but can be distinguished by the normal functioning of the gallbladder and normal pigmentation of the liver. See also **Dubin-Johnson syndrome, hyperbilirubinemia of the newborn.**

rotula. See **troche.**

roughage. See **dietary fiber.**

rouleaux /ro͞olō′/, *sing.* **rouleau,** an aggregation of red cells in what looks like a stack of coins or checkers. The formation may sometimes be caused by abnormal proteins, as in multiple myeloma or macroglobulinemia, but it is most often a microscopic artifact. Compare **hemagglutination.** See also **erythrocyte sedimentation rate.**

round ligament, **1.** a curved fibrous band that is attached at one end to the fovea of the head of the femur and at the other to the transverse ligament of the acetabulum. **2.** a fibrous cord extending from the umbilicus to the anterior part of the liver. It is the remnant of the umbilical vein. **3.** in the female, a fibromuscular band that extends from the anterior surface of the uterus through the inguinal canal to the labium majus. The structure is homologous to the spermatic cord in the male.

rounds, *informal.* a teaching conference or a meeting in which the clinical problems encountered in the practice of nursing, medicine, or other service are discussed. Kinds of rounds include **grand rounds, nursing rounds, teaching rounds,** and **walking rounds.**

roundworm, any worm of the class Nematoda, including *Ancylostoma duodenale, Ascaris lumbricoides, Enterobius vermicularis,* and *Strongyloides stercoralis.*

route of administration, (of a drug) any one of the ways in which a drug may be administered, as intramuscularly, intranasally, intravenously, orally, rectally, subcutaneously, sublingually, topically, or vaginally. Some medications can be given only by one route because absorption or maximum effectiveness occurs by that route only or because the specific substance is toxic or damaging when given by another route.

Rovsing's sign /rov′singz/, an indication of acute appendicitis in which pressure on the left lower quadrant of the abdomen causes pain in the right lower quadrant. See also **appendicitis.**

Royal College of Physicians (R.C.P.), a professional organization of physicians in the United Kingdom.

Royal College of Physicians and Surgeons of Canada (RCPSC), a national Canadian organization that recognizes and confers membership on certain qualified physicians and surgeons.

Royal College of Surgeons (R.C.S.), a professional organization of surgeons in the United Kingdom.

Roy, Sister Callista, a nursing theorist who introduced the Adaptation Model of Nursing in 1970 as a conceptual framework for nursing curricula, practice, and research. In the Roy model, the human is viewed as an adaptive system. Changes occur in the system in response to stimuli. If the change promotes the integrity of the individual, it is an adaptive response. Otherwise, it is a maladaptive response. The theory provides two mechanisms for coping or adapting. One, a Regulator Mechanism, is concerned with neural, endocrine, and perception-psychomotor processes. The other, a Cognator Mechanism, is concerned with perception, learning, judgment, and emotion. Four modes for effecting adaptation of a system are physiologic needs, self-concept, role function, and interdependence. The nurse achieves the goal of promoting the patient's adaptation in situations of health and sickness by manipulating stimuli. Nursing intervention is required when the coping mechanism of the patient loses effectiveness in illness.

RPF, abbreviation for *renal plasma flow.*

RR, R.R., abbreviation for **recovery room.**

-(r)rachia, a combining form meaning a '(specified) foreign chemical substance': *calciorrhachia, glycorrhachia, polypeptidorrhachia.*

-(r)rhage, a combining form meaning a 'rupture, an excessive fluid discharge': *hemorrhage, lymphorrhage, phleborrhage.*

-(r)rhagia, a combining form meaning a 'fluid discharge of excessive quantity': *lymphorrhagia, meningorrhagia, tracheorrhagia.*

-(r)rhagic, a combining form meaning 'of, pertaining, or referring to a kind or condition of excessive fluid discharge': *haemorrhagic, lymphorrhagic, serohemorrhagic.*

-(r)rhaphy, -(r)rhaphia, a combining form meaning a 'suturing in place': *cysticorrhaphy, meningeorrhaphy, osteorrhaphy.*

-(r)rhea, -(r)rhoea, -(r)rhoeica, a combining form meaning 'fluid discharge, flow': *anarrhea, cystirrhea, laryngorrhea.*

-(r)rheic, -(r)rheal, -(r)rhetic, -(r)rhoeic, a combining form meaning 'pertaining to a fluid discharge': *cryptorrheic, diarrheic, pyorrheic.*

-(r)rhexis, a combining form meaning a 'rupture of a (specified) body part': *arteriorrhexis, cardiorrhexis, plasmarrhexis.*

-(r)rhine, a combining form meaning 'having a (specified sort of) nose': *leptorrhine, mesorrhine, platyrrhine.*

-(r)rhinia, a combining form meaning '(condition of the) nose': *arrhinia, birrhinia, microrrhinia.*

-(r)rhoeica, -(r)rhoea. See **-(r)rhea.**

-(r)rhythmia, a combining form meaning '(condition of the) heartbeat or the pulse': *bradyrrhythmia, dysrrhythmia, tachyrrhythmia.*

R-R interval, the interval from the peak of one QRS complex to the peak of the next as shown on an electrocardiogram. See also **cardiac cycle.**

RSV, RS virus, abbreviation for **respiratory syncytial virus.**

RT, abbreviation for **respiratory therapy.**

R.T., abbreviation for **Registered Technologist.**

RTA, abbreviation for **renal tubular acidosis.**

r.t.c., abbreviation for *return to clinic,* noted on the chart, usually followed by a date on which a subsequent appointment has been made for the patient.

Ru, symbol for **ruthenium.**

rub-, a combining form meaning 'red': *rubedo, ruber, rubor.*

rubber, *informal.* **condom.**

rubber dam, a thin sheet of latex rubber for isolating one or more teeth during a dental procedure.

rubber dam clamps forceps, (in dentistry) a type of forceps with beaks designed to engage holes in a rubber dam clamp to facilitate its placement.

rubbing alcohol, a disinfectant for skin and instruments. It contains 70% ethyl alcohol by volume, the remainder consisting of water and denaturants, with or without color or perfume. It may cause dryness of the skin. Rubbing alcohol is for external use only and is flammable.

rubefacient /ro͞o′bəfā′shənt/, **1.** a substance or agent that increases the reddish coloration of the skin. **2.** increasing the reddish coloration of the skin.

rubella, a contagious viral disease characterized by fever, symptoms of a mild upper respiratory tract infection, lymph node enlargement, arthralgia, and a diffuse, fine, red, maculopapular rash. The virus is spread by droplet infection, and the incubation time is from 12 to 23 days. Also called **German measles, three-day measles.** Compare **measles, scarlet fever.**

■ OBSERVATIONS: The symptoms usually last only 2 or 3 days except for arthralgia, which may persist longer or recur. One attack confers lifelong immunity. If a woman acquires rubella in the first trimester of pregnancy, fetal anomalies may result, including heart defects, cataracts, deafness, and mental retardation. An infant exposed to the virus in utero at any time during gestation may shed the virus for up to 30 months after birth. Complications of postnatal rubella are rare.

■ INTERVENTION: The illness itself is mild and needs no special treatment. Live attenuated rubella vaccine is advised for all children to reduce chances of an epidemic and thus to protect pregnant women. The vaccine is not given to women already pregnant, and it is recommended that pregnancy be avoided for 3 months after the administration of rubella vaccine. Spread of the virus from a recently vaccinated individual rarely occurs. Immune serum globulin containing rubella antibodies may help prevent fetal infection in exposed susceptible pregnant women, but ordinary gamma globulin will not protect the fetus.

■ NURSING CONSIDERATIONS: Temporary arthralgia is common after vaccination. Women of childbearing age working with children may be tested for immunity to rubella and vaccinated if not immune. The only proof of immunity is the laboratory demonstration of antibodies to the rubella virus. The rash and malaise of rubella resemble those of scarlet fever, some cases of mononucleosis, and allergic drug reactions, leading some people to think they have had rubella when they have not.

rubella and mumps virus vaccine, a suspension containing live attenuated mumps and rubella viruses.

■ INDICATIONS: It is prescribed for immunization against rubella and mumps.

■ CONTRAINDICATIONS: Acute infection or known hypersensitivity to avian proteins prohibits its use. It is not given to a patient whose immune function is compromised or to a pregnant woman. It is not given for 3 months after the use of plasma, whole blood, or an immune serum globulin. Pregnancy is avoided for 3 months after immunization.

■ ADVERSE EFFECTS: Among the more serious adverse effects are mild to severe hypersensitivity reactions.

rubella embryopathy, any congenital abnormality in an infant caused by maternal rubella in the early stages of pregnancy.

rubella panencephalitis. See **panencephalitis.**

rubella virus vaccine, a suspension containing live attenuated rubella virus.

■ INDICATION: It is prescribed for immunization against rubella.

■ CONTRAINDICATIONS: Compromised immune function, fever, acute infection, untreated tuberculosis, or hypersensitivity to proteins of the animal of the vaccine prohibits its use. It is not given to pregnant women, nor is it given for 3 months after the use of plasma, whole blood, or immune serum globulin. Pregnancy should be avoided for 3 months after immunization.

■ ADVERSE EFFECTS: Among the most serious adverse reactions are severe hypersensitivity reactions and local pain.

rubeola. See **measles.**

rubescent /ro͞obes′ənt/, reddening.

rubidium (Rb), a soft metallic element of the alkali metals group. Its atomic number is 37; its atomic weight is 85.47. Slightly radioactive, it is used in radioisotope scanning.

Rubin's test, a test performed in the process of evaluating the cause of infertility by assessing the patency of the fallopian tubes. Carbon dioxide gas (CO_2) is introduced into the tubes under pressure through a cannula inserted into the cervix. The CO_2 is passed through from a syringe connected to a manometer at pressures of up to 200 mm Hg. If the tubes are open, the gas enters the abdominal cavity and the recorded pressure falls below 180 mm Hg. A high-pitched bubbling can be heard through the abdominal wall with the stethoscope as the gas escapes from the tubes. The patient may complain of shoulder pain from diaphragmatic irritation; an x-ray film will show free gas under the diaphragm. If the tubes are blocked, gas cannot escape from the tubes into the abdominal cavity; the pressure recorded on the manometer remains at 200 mm Hg. A tracing may be made to show tubal peristalsis, any leakage in the system, tubal spasm, or partial obstruction. After the test, the patient rests for a 3-hour period. Crampy pain, dizziness, nausea, and vomiting may occur; positioning with the pelvis higher than the head, in genupectoral position or in Trendelenberg's position, allows the gas to stay in the pelvis and give some relief by avoiding diaphragmatic irritation.

rubivirus /rōō′bēvī′rəs/, a member of the togavirus family, which includes the rubella virus.

rubor /rōō′bôr/, redness, especially when accompanying inflammation.

Rubramin PC, a trademark for vitamin B_{12} (cyanocobalamin).

rubricyte, a nucleated red blood cell; the marrow stage in the normal development of an erythrocyte.

ructus. See **eructation.**

rudiment, an organ or tissue that is incompletely developed or nonfunctional. **–rudimentary,** *adj.*

Ruffini's corpuscles /rōōfē′nēz/, a variety of oval-shaped nerve endings in the subcutaneous tissue, located principally at the junction of the corium and the subcutaneous tissue. Ruffini's corpuscles consist of strong connective tissue sheaths enclosing nerve fibers with many branches that end in small knobs. Compare **Golgi-Mazzoni corpuscles, Pacini's corpuscles.**

ruga /rōō′gə/, *pl.* **rugae** /rōō′jē/, a ridge or fold, as the rugae of the stomach, which presents large folds in the mucous membrane of that organ.

rule of bigeminy, (in cardiology) the tendency of a lengthened ventricular cycle to precipitate a ventricular premature beat.

rule of confidentiality, a principle that personal information about others, particularly patients, should not be revealed to persons not authorized to receive such information.

rule of nines, a formula for estimating the amount of body surface covered by burns by assigning 9% to the head and each arm, twice 9% (18%) to each leg, and the anterior and posterior trunk, and 1% to the perineum. This is modified in infants and children because of the different body proportions.

rumination /rōō′minā′shən/, habitual regurgitation of small amounts of undigested food with little force after every feeding, a condition commonly seen in infants. It may be a symptom of overfeeding, of eating too fast, or of swallowing air. It has little or no clinical significance. More copious and forceful regurgitation may indicate a more serious condition, as an allergic intestinal reaction, an infectious disease, an obstruction of the intestinal tract, or a metabolic disorder. See also **vomit.**

rupture, **1.** a tear or break in the continuity or configuration of an organ or body tissue, including those instances when other tissue protrudes through the opening. See also **hernia.** **2.** to cause a break or tear.

ruptured intervertebral disk. See **herniated disk.**

Rural Clinics Assistance Act, an act of Congress that permitted the establishment of clinics in certain areas designated rural and underserved and in some inner cities. The clinics are designed to provide primary care through teams of physicians and nurse practitioners. The act is significant to nursing by being the first federal legislation to allow third-party reimbursement directly to nurses practicing in expanded roles.

Russell dwarf, a person affected with **Russell's syndrome,** a congenital disorder in which short stature is associated with various anomalies of the head, face, and skeleton and with varying degrees of mental retardation.

Russell's bodies, the mucoprotein inclusions found in globular plasma cells in cancer and inflammations. The bodies contain surface gamma globulins, probably derived from the condensation of internal cellular secretions. Also called **cancer bodies, fuchsin bodies.**

Russell's syndrome. See **Russell dwarf.**

Russell traction, a unilateral or a bilateral orthopedic mechanism that combines suspension and traction to immobilize, position, and align the lower extremities in the treatment of fractured femurs and hip and knee contractures and in the treatment of disease processes of the hip and the knee. Russell traction is applied as adhesive or nonadhesive skin traction and employs a sling to relieve the weight of the lower extremities subjected to traction pull. A jacket restraint is often incorporated to help immobilize the patient. Compare **split Russell traction.**

Russian bath, a hot steam bath followed by a cold plunge. Also called **Finnish bath.**

ruthenium (Ru), a hard, brittle, metallic element. Its atomic number is 44; its atomic weight is 101.07.

rutin /rōō′tin/, a bioflavonoid obtained from buckwheat and used in the treatment of capillary fragility.

RV, abbreviation for **residual volume.**

RVC, abbreviation for *responds to verbal commands.*

R wave. See **QRS complex.**

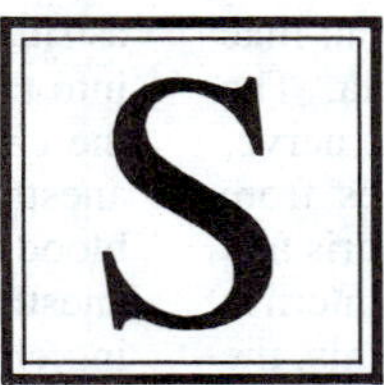

s, **1.** abbreviation for **steady state.** **2.** abbreviation for *sinister* (left).

S, **1.** symbol for **sulfur.** **2.** symbol for *saturation of hemoglobin.*

S_1, the first heart sound in the cardiac cycle occurring with ventricular systole. It is associated with closure of the mitral and tricuspid valves and is synchronous with the apical pulse. Auscultated at the apex, it is louder, longer, and lower than the second sound (S_2), which follows it.

S_2, the second heart sound in the cardiac cycle. It is associated with closure of the aortic and pulmonary valves just before ventricular diastole. Auscultated at the base of the heart, the second sound is louder than the first.

S_3, the third heart sound in the cardiac cycle. Normally, it is audible only in children and physically active young adults. In older people, it is an abnormal finding and usually indicates myocardial failure. It is heard with the bell of a stethoscope placed lightly over the apex of the heart with the patient lying down, tipped to the left.

S_4, the fourth heart sound in the cardiac cycle. It occurs late in diastole on contraction of the atria. Rarely heard in normal subjects, it indicates an abnormally increased resistance to ventricular filling, as in hypertensive cardiovascular disease, coronary artery disease, myocardiopathy, and aortic stenosis.

SA, **1.** abbreviation for **sinoatrial.** **2.** abbreviation for **surface area.** **3.** abbreviation for **surgeon's assistant.**

Sabin-Feldman dye test /sā′binfeld′mən/, a diagnostic test for toxoplasmosis that depends on the presence of specific antibodies that block the uptake of methylene blue dye by the cytoplasm of the *Toxoplasma* organisms.

Sabin Vaccine. See **oral poliovirus vaccine.**

sac, a pouch or a baglike organ, as the abdominal sac of the embryo that develops into the abdominal cavity.

sacchari-. See **saccharo-.**

saccharide /sak′ərīd′/, any of a large group of carbohydrates, including all sugars and starches. Almost all carbohydrates are saccharides. See also **carbohydrate, sugar.**

saccharin /sak′ərin/, **1.** a white, crystalline synthetic sweetener, many times sweeter than table sugar (sucrose). Saccharin is often used as a substitute for sugar. **2.** having a sweet taste, especially cloyingly sweet. Also called **saccharine** /-rīn, -rin/.

saccharo-, sacchari-, a combining form meaning 'of or pertaining to sugar': *saccharobiose, saccharorrhea, saccharosuria.*

Saccharomyces /sak′ərōmī′sēz/, a genus of yeast fungi, including brewer's and baker's yeast, as well as some pathogenic fungi, that cause such diseases as bronchitis, moniliasis, and pharyngitis.

saccharomycosis /sak′ərōmīkō′sis/, **1.** infection with yeast fungi, as the genera *Candida* or *Cryptococcus.* **2.** *obsolete.* cryptococcosis or European blastomycosis.

saccular aneurysm, a localized dilatation of an artery in which only a small area of the vessel, not the entire circumference, is distended, forming a saclike swelling or protrusion. It is usually caused by trauma. Also called **sacculated aneurysm, amullary aneurysm.** Compare **fusiform aneurysm.**

saccule /sak′yo͞ol/, a small bag or sac, as the air saccules of the lungs. See also **sacculus.** **–saccular,** *adj.*

sacculus /sak′yo͝oləs/, *pl.* **sacculi,** a little sac or bag, especially the smaller of the two divisions of the membranous labyrinth of the vestibule, which communicates with the cochlear duct through the ductus reuniens in the inner ear. See also **saccule.**

Sachs' disease. See **Tay-Sachs disease.**

SA conduction time, the conduction time for an impulse from the sinus node to the atrial musculature, measured from the SA deflection in the SA nodal electrocardiogram to the beginning of the P wave in a bipolar record, or to the beginning of the high right atrial electrogram in a unipolar record.

sacral /sā′krəl, sak′rəl/, of or pertaining to the sacrum.

sacral foramen, one of several openings between the fused segments of the sacral vertebrae in the sacrum through which the sacral nerves pass.

sacral node, a node in one of the seven groups of parietal lymph nodes of the abdomen and the pelvis, situated within the sacrum. The sacral nodes are located in relation to the middle and the lateral sacral arteries and receive lymphatics from the rectum and the posterior wall of the pelvis. Compare **lumbar node.** See also **lymph, lymphatic system, lymph node.**

sacral plexus, a network of motor and sensory nerves formed by the lumbosacral trunk from the fourth and fifth lumbar, and by the first, second, and third sacral nerves. They converge toward the caudal portion of the greater sciatic foramen and unite to become a large, flattened band, most of which continues into the thigh as the sciatic nerve. The plexus lies against the posterior, lateral wall of the pelvis between the piriformis and the internal iliac vessels embedded in the pelvic subserous fascia. The nerves of the plexus, except for the third sacral nerve, divide into ventral and dorsal portions. Branches from these divisions are the nerve to the quadratus femoris and the gemellus inferior, the nerve to the obturator internus and the gemellus superior, the nerve to the piriformis, the superior gluteal nerve, the inferior gluteal nerve, the posterior femoral cutaneous nerve, the perforating cutaneous nerve, the sciatic nerve, and the pudendal nerve. Compare **lumbar plexus.**

sacral vertebra, one of the five segments of the vertebral column that fuse in the adult to form the sacrum. The ventral border of the first sacral vertebra projects into the pelvis. The bodies of the other sacral vertebrae are smaller than that of the first and are flattened and curved ventrally, forming the convex, anterior surface of the sacrum. The rudimentary spinous processes of the first several sacral vertebrae surmount the middle sacral crest, and the transverse processes of the sacral vertebrae form the lateral sacral crests. The sacral hiatus at the caudal end of the sacral canal develops from the incomplete growth of the spinous processes of the last two sacral vertebrae. The resultant widened aperture is used by anaesthesiologists for the insertion of a needle to administer caudal analgesia. Compare **cervical vertebra, coccygeal vertebra, lumbar vertebra, thoracic vertebra.** See also **sacrum, vertebra.**

sacro-, a combining form meaning 'of or pertaining to the sacrum': *sacrococcyx, sacroiliac, sacrolumbalis.*

sacroiliac, pertaining to the part of the skeletal system that includes the sacrum and the ilium bones of the pelvis.

sacroiliac articulation, an immovable joint in the pelvis formed by the articulation of each side of the sacrum with an iliac bone.

sacrospinalis /sak′rōspīnal′is/, a large, fleshy muscle of the back that divides into a lateral iliocostalis column, an intermediate longissimus column, and a medial spinalis column. Each column consists of three parts. The sacrospinalis is sheathed in the fascia thoracolumbalis and arises in a broad, thick tendon from the sacrum, the ilium, and the lumbar vertebrae. It inserts into the ribs and into certain cervical vertebrae and is innervated by the branches of the dorsal primary divisions of the spinal nerves. It extends and flexes the vertebral column and the head, and it draws the ribs downward. Also called **erector spinae.**

sacrum /sā′krəm, sak′rəm/, the large, triangular bone at the dorsal part of the pelvis, inserted like a wedge between the two hip bones. The base of the sacrum articulates with the last lumbar vertebra, and its apex articulates with the coccyx; various muscles attach to its spinal crest. The sacrum is shorter and wider in women than in men. –**sacral,** *adj.*

saddle block anesthesia, a form of regional nerve block in which the parts of the body anesthetized are those that would touch a saddle, were the patient sitting astride one. It is performed by injecting a local anesthetic into the spinal cavity as the patient sits with the head on the chest, back curved, and legs down. As soon as the anesthetic has been injected, the patient is laid flat and the blood pressure and vital signs are noted. Saddle block anesthesia is common in some centers for anesthesia during childbirth. See also **obstetric anesthesia.**

saddle joint, a synovial joint in which surfaces of contiguous bones are reciprocally concavoconvex. A saddle joint permits no axial rotation but allows flexion, extension, adduction, and abduction, as in the carpometacarpal joint of the thumb. Also called **articulatio sellaris.** Compare **condyloid joint, pivot joint.**

sadism /sā′dizəm, sad′izəm/, **1.** abnormal pleasure derived from inflicting physical or psychologic pain or abuse on others; cruelty. **2.** also called **active algolagnia.** (in psychiatry) a psychosexual disorder characterized by the infliction of physical or psychologic pain or humiliation on another person, either a consenting or nonconsenting partner, to achieve sexual excitement or gratification. The condition is usually chronic in form, is seen predominantly in men, may result from conscious or unconscious motivations or desires, and, in severe cases, can lead to rape, torture, and murder. Kinds of sadism are **anal sadism** and **oral sadism.** Compare **masochism.** See also **algolagnia, sadomasochism.** –**sadistic,** *adj.*

sadist, a person who is afflicted with or practices sadism.

sadomasochism, a personality disorder characterized by traits of sadism and masochism. See also **algolagnia, masochism, sadism.**

SA electrogram, a direct electric recording of the SA node.

safe period. See **natural family planning method.**

safety director, a member of a hospital staff whose activities are related to safety functions, as fire prevention, environmental safety, and disaster planning activities.

sagittal /saj′ətəl/, (in anatomy) of or pertaining to a suture or an imaginary line extending from the front to the back in the midline of the body or a part of the body.

saggital axis, a hypothetic line through the mandibular condyle that serves as an axis for rotation movements of the mandible.

sagittal plane, the anterioposterior plane or the section parallel to the median plane of the body. Compare **frontal plane, median plane, transverse plane.**

sagittal suture, the serrated connection between the two parietal bones of the skull, coursing down the midline from the coronal suture to the upper part of the lambdoidal suture.

SaH, SAH, abbreviation for **subarachnoid hemorrhage.**

SAIN, abbreviation for **Society for Advancement in Nursing.**

Salamide, a trademark for an analgesic (salicylamide).

salbutamol. See **albuterol.**

salicylanilide /sal′isilan′ilīd/, a topical antifungal prescribed in the treatment of tinea capitis caused by *Microsporum audouini*. It is applied to the scalp in a 3% to 5% ointment; stonger concentrations cause skin irritation.

salicylate /səlis′əlāt/, any of several widely prescribed drugs derived from salicylic acid. Salicylates exert analgesic, antipyretic, and antiinflammatory actions. The most important is acetylsalicylic acid, or aspirin. Sodium salicylate has also been used systemically, and it exerts similar effects. Many of the actions of aspirin appear to result from its ability to inhibit cyclo-oxygenase, a rate-limiting enzyme in prostaglandin biosynthesis. Aspirin is used in a wide variety of conditions, and, in the usual analgesic dosage, it causes only mild adverse effects. Severe occult GI bleeding or gastric ulcers may occur with frequent use. Large doses taken over a long period can cause significant impairment of hemostasis. Occasionally, an asthmalike reaction is produced in hypersensitive individuals. Because of the ready availability of aspirin, accidental and intentional overdosage is common. Symptoms of salicylate intoxication include tinnitus, GI disturbances, abnormal respiration, acid-base imbalance, and central nervous system disturbances. Fatalities have occurred from ingestion of as little as 10 grains of aspirin in adults or as little as 4 ml of methyl salicylate (oil of wintergreen) in children. In addition to aspirin and sodium salicylate, which are used systemically, methyl salicylate is used topically as a counterirritant in ointments and liniments. Methyl salicylate can be absorbed through the skin in amounts capable of causing systemic toxicity. Another salicylate, salicylic acid, is too irritating to be used systemically and is used topically as a keratolytic agent, as for removing warts.

salicylate poisoning, a toxic condition caused by the ingestion of salicylate, most often in aspirin or oil of wintergreen. Intoxication is characterized by rapid breathing, vomiting, headache, irritability, ketosis, hypoglycemia, and, in severe cases, convulsions and respiratory failure. Treatment usually includes prompt induced emesis or gastric lavage with activated charcoal, the administration of a saline cathartic, a parenteral infusion of sodium bicarbonate, injection of vitamin K if bleeding is present, and correction of dehydration, hypoglycemia, and hypokalemia. Sodium bicarbonate by mouth is contraindicated.

salicylazosulfapyridine. See **sulfasalazine.**

salicylic acid /sal′isil′ik/, a keratolytic agent.

■ INDICATIONS: It is prescribed in the treatment of hyperkeratotic skin conditions and as an adjunct in fungal infections.

■ CONTRAINDICATIONS: Diabetes, impaired circulation, or known hypersensitivity to this drug prohibits its use.

■ ADVERSE EFFECTS: Among the more serious adverse reactions are skin inflammation and salicylism.

saline cathartic, one of a large group of cathartics administered to achieve prompt, complete evacuation of the bowel. A watery semifluid evacuation usually occurs within 3 to 4 hours. The most common indication for the administration of any of these agents is preparation of the bowel for diagnostic examination. Various preparations, including magnesium sulfate, sodium phosphate, sodium sulfate, and several naturally occurring mineral waters, may be used to achieve catharsis. The palatability, cost, and adverse systemic reactions of the saline cathartics depend on the particular agent used and the dose of the agent given.

saline infusion, the therapeutic introduction of a physiologic salt solution into a vein.

saline irrigation, the washing out of a body cavity or wound with a stream of salt solution, usually an isotonic aqueous solution of sodium chloride.

saline solution, a solution containing sodium chloride. Depending on the use, it may be hypotonic, isotonic, or hypertonic with body fluids.

saliva, the clear, viscous fluid secreted by the salivary and mucous glands in the mouth. Saliva contains water, mucin, organic salts, and the digestive enzyme ptyalin. It serves to moisten the oral cavity, to initiate the digestion of starches, and to aid in the chewing and swallowing of food.

salivary, of or pertaining to saliva or to the formation of saliva.

salivary duct, any one of the ducts through which saliva passes. Kinds of salivary ducts are **Bartholin's duct, duct of Rivinus, parotid duct,** and **submandibular duct.**

salivary fistula, an abnormal communication from a salivary gland or duct to an opening in the mouth or on the skin of the face or neck.

salivary gland, one of the three pairs of glands that pour their secretions into the mouth, thus aiding the digestive process. The salivary glands are the parotid, the submandibular, and the sublingual glands. They are racemose structures consisting of numerous lobes subdivided into smaller lobules connected by dense areolar tissue, vessels, and ducts. The ducts ramify inside each lobule, ending in alveoli. One kind of alveolus secretes a viscid fluid containing mucin. The other kind secretes serous fluid. The sublingual gland secretes mucus; the parotid gland, serous fluid; the submandibular gland, both mucus and serous fluid. The lobules of the salivary glands are richly supplied with blood vessels and fine plexuses of nerves. The hilum of the submandibular gland contains Langley's ganglion of nerve cells.

salivary gland cancer, a malignant neoplastic disease of a salivary gland, occurring most frequently in a parotid gland. About 75% of tumors that develop in the salivary glands are benign, characteristically slow-growing, painless, mobile masses that are cystic or rubbery in consistency. In contrast, malignant tumors are rapid-growing, hard, lumpy, fixed, and frequently tender. Pain, trismus, and facial palsy may occur. Diagnostic measures include x-ray studies, with sialographic studies and mandibular and chest films to detect metastases, and cytologic studies of saliva from Stensen's duct. Direct biopsies are not recommended. The most common malignant neoplasms are mucoepidermoid, adenoid cystic, solid, and squamous cell carcinomas. Treatment usually consists of the surgical removal of the lobe containing a benign tumor and total parotidectomy with a radical neck dissection if the lesion is advanced. Radiotherapy is administered for residual, recurrent, or inoperable cancers, and chemotherapy may be palliative.

salivation, the process of saliva secretion by the salivary glands.

Salk Vaccine. See **poliovirus vaccine.**

salmon calcitonin. See **calcitonin.**

Salmonella /sal′mənel′ə/, a genus of motile, gram-negative, rod-shaped bacteria that includes species causing typhoid fever, paratyphoid fever, and some forms of gastroenteritis. See also **salmonellosis.**

salmonellosis /sal′mənəlō′sis/, a form of gastroenteritis, caused by ingestion of food contaminated with a species of *Salmonella,* characterized by an incubation period of 6 to 48 hours followed by sudden, colicky abdominal pain, fever, and bloody, watery diarrhea. Nausea and vomiting are common, and abdominal signs may resemble acute appendicitis or cholecystitis. Symptoms usually last from 2 to 5 days, but diarrhea and fever may persist for up to 2 weeks. Dehydration may occur. There is no specific treatment. Antibiotics may prolong the excretion of *Salmonella* in stools and are usually not indicated. Adequate cooking, good refrigeration, and careful handwashing may reduce the frequency of outbreaks. See also **food poisoning.**

salol camphor /sal′ôl/, a clear, oily mixture of two parts of camphor and three parts of phenyl salicylate, used as a local antiseptic.

Salonica fever. See **trench fever.**

salpingectomy /sal′pinjek′təmē/, surgical removal of one or both fallopian tubes, performed to remove a cyst or tumor, excise an abcess, or, if both tubes are removed, as a sterilization procedure. Often the operation is done with a hysterectomy or an oophorectomy. Either spinal block or general anesthesia may be given. Postoperatively, the patient is instructed to avoid sharply flexing the thighs or the knees. Persistent low back pain or the presence of bloody or scanty urine indicates that a ureter may have been injured during surgery.

salpingitis /sal′pinjī′tis/, an inflammation or infection of the fallopian tube. See also **pelvic inflammatory disease.**

salpingo-, a combining form meaning 'of or pertaining to a tube, especially a fallopian tube': *salpingocele, salpingolysis, salpingoplasty.*

salpingostomy /sal′ping•gos′təmē/, the formation of an artificial opening in a fallopian tube, performed to restore patency in a tube whose fimbriated opening has been closed by infection or by chronic inflammation or to drain an abcess or an accumulation of fluid. Either regional or general anesthesia is used. A prosthesis may be inserted to maintain the patency of the fallopian tube and to direct the route of the ova to assist fertilization. Postoperatively, the nurse cautions the patient against sharply flexing the thighs or the knees. Low back pain or scanty or bloody urine may indicate that a ureter has been injured during the procedure, requiring surgical intervention.

salpinx /sal′pingks/, pl. **salpinges** /salpin′jēz/, a tube, as the *salpinx auditiva* or the *salpinx uterina.* **–salpingian,** *adj.*

salt, **1.** a compound formed by the chemical reaction of an acid and a base. Salts are usually composed of a metal and a nonmetal and may behave chemically as metals or nonmetals. **2.** sodium chloride (common table salt). **3.** a substance, as magnesium sulfate (Epsom salt), used as a purgative.

saltation /saltā′shən/, (in genetics) a mutation causing a significant difference in appearance between parent and offspring or an abrupt variation in the characteristics of the species. **–saltatorial, saltatoric, saltatory** /sal′tətôr′ē/, *adj.*

saltatory conduction, impulse transmission that skips from node to node.

saltatory evolution, the appearance of a sudden, abrupt change within a species, caused by mutation; the progression of a species by sudden major changes rather than by the gradual accumulation of minor changes. The phenomenon occurs predominantly in plants as a result of polyploidy. See also **emergent evolution.**

salt depletion, the loss of salt from the body through excessive elimination of body fluids by perspiration, diarrhea, vomiting, or urination, without corresponding replacement. See also **electrolyte balance, heat exhaustion.**

Salter fracture. See **epiphyseal fracture.**

salt-free diet. See **low-sodium diet.**

Saluron, a trademark for an antihypertensive and diuretic (hydroflumethiazide).

salvage therapy, therapy administered to sites at which previous therapies have failed and the disease has recurred.

salve. See **ointment.**

samarium (Sm), a rare earth, metallic element. Its atomic number is 62; its atomic weight is 150.35.

sand bath, the application of warm, dry sand or of damp sand to the body.

sand flea. See **chigoe,** def. 1.

sandfly fever. See **phlebotomus fever.**

Sandhoff's disease, a variant of Tay-Sachs disease that includes defects in both the enzymes hexosaminidase A and B. It is characterized by a progressively more rapid course and is found in the general population, not restricted as is Tay-Sachs disease. Also called **gangliosidosis type II.** See also **Tay-Sachs disease.**

Sandril, a trademark for an antihypertensive (reserpine).

sand tumor. See **psammoma.**

sangui-, a combining form meaning 'of or pertaining to blood': *sanguicolous, sanguiferous, sanguinolent.*

sanguineous /sang•gwin′ē•əs/, pertaining to blood.

sanita-, a combining form meaning 'of or pertaining to health': *sanitarium, sanitas, sanitation.*

sanitary landfill, a solid waste disposal site, usually a swamp area, ravine, or canyon where the waste is compacted by heavy machines and covered with earth.

San Joaquin fever /san′wôkēn′/, the primary stage of coccidioidomycosis.

SA node. See **sinoatrial node.**

Sanorex, a trademark for an anorexiant (mazindol).

Sansert, a trademark for a vasoconstrictor (methysergide maleate).

Santyl, a trademark for an enzyme (collagenase).

SaO_2, symbol for the percent of *saturation of arterial blood.*

saphenous nerve /səfē′nəs/, the largest and longest branch of the femoral nerve, supplying the skin of the medial side of the leg. It courses deep to the sartorius, accompanied by the femoral artery posteriorly, and crosses from the lateral to the medial side of the sartorius, within the fascial cover of the adductor canal. At the tendinous arch in the adductor magnus, it leaves the artery, pierces the fascia of the adductor canal, descends along the medial side of the knee, penetrates the fascia lata between the tendons of the sartorius and the gracilis, and becomes subcutaneous. It accompanies the great saphenous vein along the medial side of the leg, and at the medial border of the tibia in the distal third of the leg divides into two terminal branches. One branch joins the medial cutaneous and the obturator nerves to form the subsartorial plexus. A large infrapatellar branch passes to the skin over the patella and on the lateral side of the knee joins with branches of the lateral femoral cutaneous nerve to form the patellar plexus. One branch of the saphenous nerve below the knee supplies the ankle. Another branch below the knee supplies the medial side of the foot. See also **femoral nerve.**

saphenous vein. See **great saphenous vein.**

sapo-, a combining form meaning 'of or pertaining to soap': *sapogenin, saponaceous, sapotoxin.*

saponin /sap′ənin/, a soapy material found in some plants, especially soapwort (Bouncing Bet) and certain lilies. It is used in demulcent medications to provide a sudsy quality. Natural saponins, which can be hemolytic toxins, have largely been replaced by synthetic preparations.

saprophyte, an organism that lives on dead organic matter. –**saprophytic,** *adj.*

SAR, abbreviation for **structure-activity relationship.**

saralasin, a competitive antagonist of angiotensin. It is administered by intravenous injection to assess the role of the renin-angiotensin system in the maintenance of blood pressure.

-sarc, a combining form meaning '(specified type of) flesh': *ectosarc, endosarc, perisarc.*

sarco-, a combining form meaning 'of or related to the flesh': *sarcoadenoma, sarcode, sarcolyte.*

sarcoidosis /sär′koidō′sis/, a chronic disorder of unknown origin characterized by the formation of tubercles of nonnecrotizing epithelioid tissue. Common sites are the lungs, spleen, liver, skin, mucous membranes, and lacrimal and salivary glands, usually with involvement of the lymph glands. Diminished reactivity to tuberculin frequently accompanies the disorder. The lesions usually disappear over a period of months or years but progress to widespread granulomatous inflammation and fibrosis. Also called **sarcoid of Boeck.**

sarcoidosis cordis, a form of sarcoidosis in which granulomatous lesions develop in the myocardium. The number and the size of the growths vary. Mild cases with few infiltrates are asymptomatic. In severe cases the myocardium may be infiltrated with many tumors and cardiac failure may follow. See also **sarcoidosis.**

sarcoma /särkō′mə/, *pl.* **sarcomas, sarcomata,** a malignant neoplasm of the soft tissues arising in fibrous, fatty, muscular, synovial, vascular, or neural tissue, usually first presenting as a painless swelling. About 40% of sarcomas occur in the lower extremities, 20% in the upper extremities, 20% in the trunk, and the rest in the head, neck, or retroperineum. The tumor, composed of closely packed cells in a fibrillar or homogeneous matrix, tends to be vascular and is usually highly invasive. Trauma probably does not play a role in the cause, but sarcomas may arise in burn or radiation scars. Small tumors may be managed by local excision and postoperative radiotherapy, but bulky sarcomas of the extremities may require amputation followed by irradiation for local control and combination chemotherapy to eliminate small foci or neoplastic cells. See specific sarcomas.

-sarcoma, a combining form meaning a 'malignant neoplasm': *angiosarcoma, hemangiosarcoma, myelosarcoma.*

sarcoma botryoides /bot′rē•oi′dēz/, a tumor derived from primitive striated muscle cells, occurring most frequently in young children and characterized by a painful, edematous, polypoid grapelike mass in the upper vagina or on the uterine cervix or the neck of the urinary bladder. See also **rhabdomyosarcoma.**

sarcomagenesis /särkō′məjen′əsis/, the process of initiating and promoting the development of a sarcoma. Compare **carcinogenesis, oncogenesis, tumorigenesis.** –**sarcomagenetic,** *adj.*

sarcomere /sär′kōmir/, the smallest functional unit of a myofibril. Sarcomeres occur as repeating units along the length of a myofibril, occupying the region between Z disks of the myofibril.

sarcoplasmic reticulum, a network of tubules and sacs in skeletal muscles that plays an important role in muscle contraction and relaxation by releasing and storing calcium ions. This network is analogous, but not identical, to the endoplasmic reticulum of other cells.

Sarcoptes scabiei /särkop′tēz skā′bē•ī/, the genus of itch mite that causes scabies.

sartorius /särtôr′ē•əs/, the longest muscle in the body, extending from the pelvis to the calf of the leg. It is a narrow muscle that arises from the anterior superior iliac spine, passes obliquely across the proximal anterior part of the thigh from the lateral to the medial side, and inserts, by a tendon and an aponeurosis, into the tibia. It is innervated by branches of the femoral nerve. It acts to flex the thigh and rotate it laterally and to flex the leg and rotate it medially. Compare **quadriceps femoris.**

S.A.S. 500, a trademark for a sulfonamide (sulfasalazine), used to treat ulcerative colitis.

satellite clinic, a health care facility usually operated under the auspices of a large institution but situated in a location some distance from the larger health center.

saturated, **1.** having absorbed or dissolved the maximum amount of a given substance, as a solution in which no more of the solute can be dissolved. **2.** also called **saturated hydrocarbon.** an organic compound that contains the maximum number of hydrogen atoms so that only single valence bonds exist in the carbon chain, as in saturated fatty acids. Compare **unsaturated.**

saturated calomel electrode (SCE), a reference electrode commonly used in polarography.

saturated fatty acid, any of a number of glyceryl esters of certain organic acids in which all the atoms are joined by single-valence bonds. These fats are chiefly of animal origin and include beef, lamb, pork, veal, whole-milk products, butter, most cheeses, and a few plant fats such as cocoa butter, coconut oil, and palm oil. Ordinary oleomargarine and hydrogenated shortenings also contain saturated fatty acids. A diet high in saturated fatty acids may contribute to a high serum cholesterol level and, in some studies of some population groups, is associated with an increased incidence of coronary heart disease. Compare **unsaturated fatty acid.**

saturated hydrocarbon. See **saturated.**

saturated solution, a solution in which the solvent contains the maximum amount of solute it can take up. See also **solute, solvent.**

saturn-, a combining form meaning 'lead' /led/: *saturnine, saturnism, saturnotherapy*.

satyriasis /sat′irī′əsis/, excessive or uncontrollable sexual desire in the male. Also called **satyromania.** Compare **nymphomania.**

sauna bath, a bath in which hot vapor is used to induce sweating, followed by rubbing of the body, and ending with a cold shower. Also called **Finnish bath, Russian bath.**

saur-, a combining form meaning 'lizard, or reptile': *sauriasis, sauriderma, sauroid*.

Sayre's jacket /serz/, a cast applied for support and immobilization in the treatment of certain abnormalities of the spinal column.

Sb, symbol for **antimony.**

SBE, **1.** abbreviation for **self-breast examination.** **2.** abbreviation for **subacute bacterial endocarditis.**

sc, abbreviation for *sine correctione,* a Latin phrase meaning "without correction."

Sc, symbol for **scandium.**

scab. See **eschar.**

scabicide /skab′isīd/, any one of a large group of drugs that destroy the itch mite, *Sarcoptes scabiei*. These drugs are applied topically in a lotion or cream-based preparation. All are potentially toxic and irritating to the skin. They are used with caution in treating children. Kinds of scabicides include **crotamiton, lindane.**

scabies /skā′bēz/, a contagious disease caused by *Sarcoptes scabiei,* the itch mite, characterized by intense itching of the skin and excoriation from scratching. The mite, transmitted by close contact with infected humans or domestic animals, burrows into outer layers of the skin where the female lays eggs. Two to 4 months after the first infection, sensitization to the mites and their products begins, resulting in a pruritic papular rash most common on the webs of fingers, flexor surfaces of wrists, and thighs. Secondary bacterial infection may occur. Diagnosis may be made by microscopic identification of adult mites, larvae, or eggs in scrapings of the burrows. All contacts are treated simultaneously with a sulfur ointment, benzyl benzoate, or other scabicide applied locally. Oral antihistamines and salicylates reduce itching.

scag, *slang*. heroin.

scalded skin syndrome. See **toxic epidermal necrolysis.**

scale, **1.** a small, thin flake of keratinized epithelium. **2.** to remove incrusted material from the surface of a tooth.

scalp, the skin covering the head, not including the face and ears.

scalp medication, **1.** a cream, ointment, lotion, or shampoo used to treat dermatologic conditions of the scalp. **2.** the application of a medication to the scalp. If a cream, ointment, or lotion is to be applied, a shampoo is usually given first. The hair is dried, combed, and parted in the middle, and the medication is spread with the fingertips. After treatment, the medication may need to be washed off the scalp and hair with an alkaline shampoo.

scalp vein needle, a thin-gauge needle designed for use on the veins of the scalp or other small veins, especially in children.

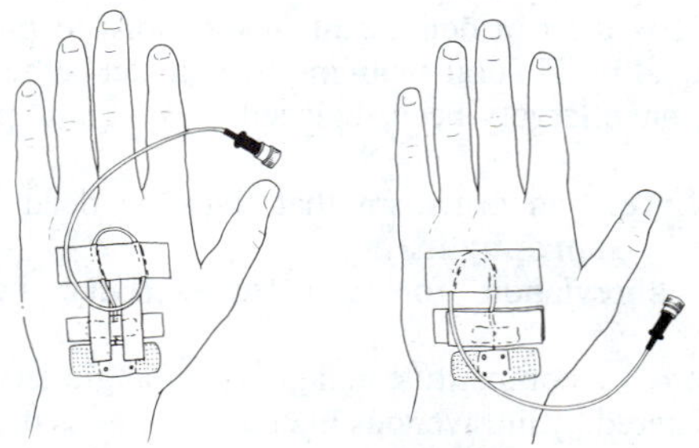

Acceptable securing methods for scalp vein needles

scamping speech, abnormal speech in which consonants or whole syllables are left out of words because of the person's inability to shape the sounds. Also called **clipped speech.**

scandium (Sc), a grayish metallic element. Its atomic number is 21; its atomic weight is 44.956.

scanning, carefully studying an area, organ, or system of the body by recording and displaying an image of the area. A concentration of a radioactive substance that has an affinity for a specific tissue may be injected to enhance the image. The liver, brain, and thyroid can be examined, tumors can be located, and function can be evaluated by various scanning techniques. See specific scanning techniques. –**scan,** *n., v.*

scanning electron microscope (SEM), an instrument similar to an electron microscope in that a beam of electrons instead of visible light is used to scan the surface of a specimen. The beam is moved in a point-to-point manner over the surface of the specimen. The number of electrons emerging from the sample is proportionate to the shape, density, and other properties of the sample. These electrons are deflected, collected, accelerated, and directed against a scintillator. The large number of photons thus created are converted into an electric signal that, in turn, modulates the beam scanning the surface of the specimen. The image produced is of less magnification than that produced by an electron microscope, but it appears to be three-dimensional and lifelike. Compare **electron microscope, transmission scanning electron microscope.**

scanning electron microscopy, the technique using a scanning electron microscope on an electrically conducting sample.

scanning speech, abnormal speech characterized by a staccato-like articulation in which the words are clipped and broken because the person pauses between syllables.

scanography /skanog′rəfē/, a method of producing a radiogram of an internal body organ or structure by using a series of parallel beams that eliminate size distortion. The technique is applied particularly in long-bone radiography.

Scanzoni rotation /skanzō′nē/, an obstetric operation in which forceps having a curved shank are applied to the fetal head while it is still high in the pelvis. The head is displaced upward and rotated to the occiput anterior position. The forceps are removed and repositioned, and the delivery is accomplished by axis traction. The operation is not often performed in modern obstetrics because cesarean section is usually safer for the mother and the baby. See also **forceps delivery, obstetric forceps.**

scapegoating, the projection of blame, hostility, or suspicion onto one member of a group by other members to avoid self-confrontation.

scapho-, a combining form meaning 'boat-shaped': *scaphocephaly, scaphohydrocephaly, scaphoid.*

scaphocephaly /skaf′ōsef′əlē/, a congenital malformation of the skull in which premature closure of the sagittal suture results in restricted lateral growth of the head, giving it an abnormally long, narrow appearance with a cephalic index of 75 or less. The condition is often associated with mental retardation. Also called **scaphocephalis, scaphocephalism, dolichocephaly, mecocephaly. See also craniostenosis.** –**scaphocephalic, scaphocephalous,** *adj.*

scaphoid bone, either of two similar bones of the hand and the foot. The scaphoid bone of the hand is slanted at the radial side of the carpus and articulates with the radius, trapezium, trapezoideum, capitate, and lunate bones. The scaphoid bone of the foot is located at the medial side of the tarsus between the talus and cuneiform bones and articulates with the talus, the three cuneiform bones, and, occasionally, with the cuboid bone. Also called **navicular bone.**

scapula /skap′ələ/, one of the pair of large, flat, triangular bones that form the dorsal part of the shoulder girdle. It has two surfaces, three borders, three angles, and a prominent dorsal spine. The acromion of the scapula forms the summit of the shoulder. The coracoid process, resembling a raven's beak, accommodates the attachment of various muscles, including the pectoralis minor, and ligaments, including the trapezoid. Also called **shoulder blade.**

-scapula, a combining form meaning a 'shoulder blade or a part of it': *mesoscapula, prescapula, proscapula.*

scapulohumeral, of or pertaining to the structures of muscles and the area around the scapula and humerus that make up the shoulder girdle.

scapulohumeral muscular dystrophy, a form of limb-girdle muscular dystrophy that begins in the shoulder girdle. Also called **Erb's muscular dystrophy.**

scapulohumeral reflex, a normal response to tapping the vertebral border of the scapula, resulting in adduction of the arm. Absence of the reflex may indicate a lesion in the region of the fifth cervical segment of the spinal cord.

scar. See **cicatrix.**

scarification /sker′ifikā′shən/, multiple superficial scratches or incisions in the skin, as are made for the introduction of a vaccine. The term is erroneously used to mean "producing a scar."

scarify /sker′əfī/, to make multiple superficial incisions into the skin; to scratch. Vaccination against smallpox is achieved by scarifying the skin under a drop of vaccine. See also **scarification.**

scarlatina. See **scarlet fever.**

scarlatiniform /skär′lətē′nifôrm/, resembling the rash of **scarlet fever.**

scarlet fever, an acute contagious disease of childhood caused by an erythrotoxin-producing strain of group A hemolytic *Streptococcus.* The infection is characterized by sore throat, fever, enlarged lymph nodes in the neck, prostration, and a diffuse bright red rash. Also called **scarlatina.**

scarlet red, an azo dye that has been used to impart color to pharmaceutic preparations.

scato-, skato, a combining form meaning 'of or related to dung, or to fecal matter': *scatophagy, scatophilia, scatoscopy.*

scattered radiation, radiation that travels in a direction other than that of its source energy, as secondary radiation and stray radiation. Also called **backscatter radiation.**

scattergram, a graph representing the distribution of two variables in a sample population. One variable is plotted on the vertical axis; the second on the horizontal axis. The scores or values of each sample unit are usually represented by dots. A scattergram demonstrates the degree or tendency to which the variables occur in association with each other.

scattering, (in radiology) a change in direction of the path of subatomic particles caused by collision or interaction with one another.

scavenging system. See **gas scavenging system.**

scel-, a combining form meaning 'leg': *scelalgia, scelotyrbe*.

-scelia, a combining form meaning '(condition of the) legs': *macroscelia, polyscelia, rhaeboscelia*.

Schedule I, a category of drugs not considered legitimate for medical use. Among the substances so classified by the Drug Enforcement Agency are mescaline, LSD, heroin, and marijuana. Special licensing procedures must be followed to use these or other Schedule I substances.

Schedule II, a category of drugs considered to have a strong potential for abuse or addiction, but which have legitimate medical use. Among the substances so classified by the Drug Enforcement Agency are morphine, cocaine, pentobarbital, oxycodone, alphaprodine, and methadone.

Schedule III, a category of drugs that have less potential for abuse or addiction than Schedule II or I drugs. Among the substances so classified by the Drug Enforcement Agency are glutethimide and various analgesic compounds containing codeine.

Schedule IV, a category of drugs that have less potential for abuse or addiction than those of Schedules I to III, Among the substances so classified by the Drug Enforcement Agency are chloral hydrate, chlordiazepoxide, meprobamate, and oxazepam.

Schedule V, a category of drugs that have a small potential for abuse or addiction. Among the substances so classified by the Drug Enforcement Agency are many commonly prescribed medications that contain small amounts of codeine or diphenoxylate. The specific drugs in Schedule V vary greatly from state to state.

Schedule of Drugs, a classification system that categorizes drugs by their potential for abuse. The schedule is divided into five groups: Schedules I to V. The assignment of drugs to the categories varies from state to state. All substances in Schedules II to V require a written prescription signed by a physician. Schedule I substances are not approved for medical use. Specific regulations for dispensing these substances vary from state to state and from institution to institution. See also specific schedules.

Scheuermann's disease /shoi′ərmonz/, an abnormal skeletal condition characterized by a fixed kyphosis that develops at puberty and is caused by wedge-shaped deformities of one or several vertebrae. The cause of the disease is unknown, but authorities have speculated that it may result from infection, inflammatory processes, aseptic necrosis, disk deterioration, mechanic influences, inadequate circulation during rapid growth, or disturbances of epiphyseal growth resulting from protrusion of the intervertebral disk through deficient or defective cartilaginous plates. The most striking pathologic feature of Scheuermann's disease is the presence of wedge-shaped vertebral bodies, seen on radiographic examination, that create an excessive curvature. Scheuermann's disease occurs most frequently in children between 12 and 16 years of age, with the onset at puberty, and the incidence is greater in girls than in boys. The onset is insidious and often associated with a history of unusual physical activity or participation in sports. The most frequent symptom is poor posture with accompanying symptoms of fatigue and pain in the involved area. Tenderness and stiffness may also affect the area involved or may affect the entire spinal column. In most affected individuals the kyphosis is within the thoracic vertebrae. If the disease is diagnosed at the onset, the associated posture may be corrected actively and passively. Otherwise, the associated posture becomes fixed within a period of 6 to 9 months. The most effective treatment of Scheuermann's disease is immobilization with a plaster cast or with a Milwaukee brace. The immobilization is continuous for 10 to 12 months, with additional immobilization at night for about the same length of time. Immobilization is usually supplemented with an exercise program that is continued after the immobilization is terminated. In adults, persistent pain in the thoracic area may indicate a degenerative alteration secondary to this disease process, and spinal arthrodesis may be required to relieve the symptoms. Also called **adolescent vertebral epiphysitis, juvenile kyphosis.**

Schick test, a skin test to determine immunity to diphtheria in which diphtheria toxin is injected intradermally. A positive reaction, indicating susceptibility, is marked by redness and swelling at the site of injection; a negative reaction, indicating immunity, is marked by absence of redness or swelling.

Schilder's disease /shil′dərz/, a group of progressive, severe, neurologic diseases beginning in childhood. All are characterized by demyelination of the white matter of the brain with muscle spasticity, optic neuritis, aphasia, deafness, adrenal insufficiency, and dementia. Many of the signs resemble those of multiple sclerosis. There is no known treatment. The cause may be viral or genetic. Also called **Schilder's encephalitis, encephalitis periaxialis diffusa, Flatau-Schilder disease, progressive subcortical encephalopathy.** See also **adrenoleukodystrophy.**

Schiller's test, a procedure for indicating areas of abnormal epithelium in the vagina or on the cervix of the uterus as a guide in selecting biopsy sites for cancer detection. A potassium iodide or aqueous iodine solution is painted on the vaginal walls and cervix under direct visualization. Normal epithelium contains glycogen and stains a deep brown color; abnormal epithelium, containing no glycogen, will not stain, and nonstaining sites may then be included in tissue biopsies. The test is not specific for malignancy, because inflammation, ulceration, and keratotic lesions also may not accept the iodine stain.

Schilling's leukemia. See **monocytic leukemia.**

Schilling test, a diagnostic test for pernicious anemia in which vitamin B_{12} tagged with radioactive cobalt is administered orally, and GI absorption is measured by determining the radioactivity of urine samples collected over a 24-hour period. In persons with pernicious anemia, the ability to absorb vitamin B_{12} is reduced, so that excretion of radioactive material in the urine is reduced.

schindylesis /skin'dilē'sis/, an articulation of certain bones of the skull in which a thin plate of one bone enters a cleft formed by the separation of two layers of another bone, as the insertion of the vomer bone into the fissure between the maxillae and the palatine bones.

Schiötz' tonometer /shē•ets'/, a tonometer used to measure intraocular pressure by observing the depth of indentation of the cornea made by the weighted plunger on the device after a topical anesthetic is applied.

schisto-, a combining form meaning 'split, or cleft': *schistocelia, schistocephalus, schistomelia.*

Schistosoma /shis'təsō'mə/, a genus of blood flukes that may cause urinary, GI, or liver disease in humans and which requires freshwater snails as intermediate hosts. *Schistosoma hematobium,* found chiefly in Africa and the Middle East, affects the bladder and pelvic organs, causing painful, frequent urination and hematuria. *S. japonicum,* found in Japan, the Philippines, and Eastern Asia, causes GI ulcerations and fibrosis of the liver. *S. mansoni,* found in Africa, the Middle East, the Caribbean, and tropic America, causes symptoms similar to those caused by *S. japonicum*. See also **schistosomiasis.**

schistosomiasis /shis'təsōmī'əsis/, a parasitic infection caused by a species of fluke of the genus *Schistosoma,* transmitted to humans, the definitive host, by contact with fresh water contaminated by human feces. A single fluke may live in one part of the body, depositing eggs frequently, for up to 20 years. The eggs are irritating to mucous membrane, causing it to thicken and become papillomatous. Symptoms depend on the part of the body infected. *Schistosoma* may be found in the bladder, rectum, liver, lungs, spleen, intestines, and portal venous system. Pain, obstruction, dysfunction of the affected organ, and anemia may result. Diagnosis requires morphologic identification of the ova or the parasite. Treatment is difficult; antimony drugs may be effective but are so toxic they seldom can be given. Inoculation with a small dose of *Klebsiella pneumoniae* has been effective experimentally in killing some species of *Schistosoma*. Prevention is more effective. Proper disposal of human waste, chlorination of water, and eradication of the intermediate host, the freshwater snail *Australorbis glabratus,* are totally effective. Second only to malaria in the number of people affected, schistosomiasis is particularly prevalent in the tropics and in the Orient. Also called **bilharziasis.** See also **blood fluke, *Schistosoma.***

schistosomicide /shis'təsō'məsīd/, a drug destructive to schistosomes, blood flukes transmitted by snails to human hosts in many parts of Africa, Brazil, and Asia. Niridazole, metrifonate, oxamniquine hycanthone hydrochloride, and various salts of antimony, including stibophen, are potent antischistosomal agents. **–schistosomicidal,** *adj.*

schizo-, a combining form meaning 'divided, or related to division': *schizocephalia, schizogenesis, schizophrenia.*

schizoaffective disorder /skit'sō-afek'tiv/, a condition that includes characteristics of schizophrenia and bipolar disorder or of other major affective disorders.

schizogenesis /skit'səjen'əsis/, reproduction by fission. **–schizogenetic, schizogenic, schizogenous,** *adj.*

schizogony /skitsog'ənē/, **1.** reproduction by multiple fission. **2.** the asexual reproductive stage of sporozoans, specifically the portion of the life cycle of the malarial parasite that occurs in the erythrocytes or liver cells. See also *Plasmodium,* **–schizogonic, schizogonous,** *adj.*

schizoid /skit'soid, skiz'oid/, **1.** characteristic of or resembling schizophrenia; schizophrenic. **2.** a person, not necessarily a schizophrenic, who exhibits the traits of a schizoid personality.

schizoid personality, a functioning but maladjusted person whose behavior is characterized by extreme shyness, oversensitivity, introversion, seclusiveness, and avoidance of close interpersonal relationships. See also **schizoid personality disorder, schizophrenia.**

schizoid personality disorder, a condition characterized by a defect in the ability to form social relationships, as shown by emotional coldness and aloofness, withdrawn and seclusive behavior, and indifference to praise, criticism, and the feelings of others. The person is unable to express hostility and ordinary aggressive feelings and reacts to disturbing experiences with apparent detachment. The condition may precede schizophrenia.

schizont /skit'sont/, the multinucleated cell stage during the sexual reproductive phase in the life cycle of a sporozoan, as the malarial parasite *Plasmodium*. It is produced by the multiple fission of the trophozoite in a cell of the vertebrate host and subsequently segments into merozoites. Also called **agamont.** Compare **sporont.** See also **schizogony.**

schizonticide /skitson'təsīd/, a substance that destroys schizonts. **–schizonticidal,** *adj.*

schizophasia /skit'səfā'zhə, skiz'ə-/, the disordered, incomprehensible speech characteristic of some forms of schizophrenia. See also **word salad.**

schizophrene /skit'səfrēn', skiz'ə-/, a person afflicted with schizophrenia.

schizophrenia /skit′səfrē′nē·ə, skiz′ə-/, any one of a large group of psychotic disorders characterized by gross distortion of reality, disturbances of language and communication, withdrawal from social interaction, and the disorganization and fragmentation of thought, perception, and emotional reaction. Apathy and confusion; delusions and hallucinations; rambling or stylized patterns of speech, as evasiveness, incoherence, and echolalia; withdrawn, regressive, and bizarre behavior; and emotional lability often occur. The condition may be mild or require prolonged hospitalization. No single cause of the disease is known; genetic, biochemical, psychologic, interpersonal, and sociocultural factors are usually involved. Treatment often requires the use of antidepressant and antianxiety drugs. Milieu therapy and group psychotherapy may be extremely helpful in providing a safe environment in which the person may test reality, develop an increased ability to communicate with other people, and learn better ways to cope with stress. Kinds of schizophrenia include **acute schizophrenia, catatonic schizophrenia, childhood schizophrenia, disorganized schizophrenia, latent schizophrenia, paranoid schizophrenia, process schizophrenia, reactive schizophrenia,** and **residual schizophrenia.** Also called **schizophrenic disorder, schizophrenic reaction.**

schizophrenic /skit′səfren′ik, skiz′ə-/, **1.** of or pertaining to schizophrenia. **2.** a person with schizophrenia.

schizophrenic disorder, schizophrenic reaction. See **schizophrenia.**

schizophreniform disorder, a condition exhibiting the same symptoms as schizophrenia but characterized by an acute onset with resolution in 2 weeks to 6 months.

schizophrenogenic /skit′səfren′əjen′ik, skiz′ə-/, tending to cause or produce schizophrenia.

Schizotrypanum cruzi. See **Chagas' disease.**

schizotypal personality disorder /skit′sōtī′pəl/, a condition characterized by oddities of thought, perception, speech, and behavior that are not severe enough to meet the clinical criteria for schizophrenia. Symptoms include magical thinking, as superstitiousness, belief in clairvoyance and telepathy, and bizarre fantasies; ideas of reference; recurrent illusions, as sensing the presence of a force or person not actually present; social isolation; peculiar speech patterns, including ideas expressed unclearly or words used deviantly; and exaggerated anxiety or hypersensitivity to real or imagined criticism. See also **schizoid personality disorder, schizophrenia.**

Schlatter-Osgood disease, Schlatter's disease. See **Osgood-Schlatter disease.**

Schlemm's canal. See **canal of Schlemm.**

Schneiderian carcinoma /shnīdir′ē·ən/, an epithelial malignancy of the nasal mucosa and paranasal sinuses.

Schönlein-Henoch purpura. See **Henoch-Schönlein purpura.**

School Nurse Practitioner (S.N.P.), a registered nurse who is qualified by a postgraduate course of study to act as a nurse practitioner in a school.

school phobia, an extreme separation anxiety disorder of children, usually in the elementary grades, characterized by a persistent, irrational fear of going to school or being in a schoollike atmosphere. Such children are usually oversensitive, shy, timid, nervous, and emotionally immature and have pervasive feelings of inadequacy. They typically try to cope with their fears by becoming overdependent on others, especially the parents. Often the fear of being separated from the parents to go to school or the emotional conflict symbolically manifested by the school atmosphere subsides with age and the development of relationships with school-age peers. In more severe cases, psychotherapy and behavior therapy, especially in structured group environments within an educational setting, may be necessary and effective.

Schultz-Charlton phenomenon, a cutaneous reaction to the intradermal injection of scarlatina antiserum in a person who has a scarletiniform rash. The rash blanches.

Schwann cells, cells of ectodermal origin that comprise the neurilemma.

schwannoma /shwänō′mə/, *pl.* **schwannomas, schwannomata,** a benign, solitary, encapsulated tumor arising in the neurilemma (Schwann's sheath) of peripheral, cranial, or autonomic nerves. Also called **Schwann cell tumor, neurilemoma.**

Schwann's sheath. See **neurilemma.**

Schwartz bed. See **hyperextension bed.**

Schwartzman-Sanarelli phenomenon, a phenomenon induced experimentally in the investigation of the role of coagulation in renal disease. Animals injected twice with a bacterial endotoxin develop massive disseminated intravascular coagulation with thrombosis of the blood vessels in the kidneys. Also called **Schwartzman phenomenon.**

scia-. See **skia-.**

sciatic /sī·at′ik/, near the ischium, as the sciatic nerve or the sciatic vein.

sciatica /sī·at′ikə/, an inflammation of the sciatic nerve, usually marked by pain and tenderness along the course of the nerve through the thigh and leg. It may result in a wasting of the muscles of the lower leg.

sciatic nerve, a long nerve originating in the sacral plexus and extending through the muscles of the thigh, leg, and foot, with numerous branches.

SCID, abbreviation for **severe combined immunodeficiency disease.**

science, a systematic attempt to establish theories to explain observed phenomena and the knowledge obtained through these efforts. **Pure science** is concerned with the gathering of information solely for the sake of obtaining new knowledge. **Applied science** is the practical application of scientific theory and laws. See also **hypothesis, law, scientific method, theory.**

scientific method, a systematic, ordered approach to the gathering of data and the solving of problems. The basic approach is the statement of the problem followed by the statement of a hypothesis. An experimental method is established to help prove or disprove the hypothesis. The results of the experiment are observed, and conclusions are drawn from observed results. The conclusions may tend to uphold or to refute the hypothesis.

scintillation detector, 1. a device that relies on the emission of light or ultraviolet radiation from a crystal subjected to ionizing radiation. The light is detected by a photomultiplier tube and converted to an electric signal that can be processed further. An array of scintillation detectors is used in a gamma camera. 2. a device used to measure the amount of radioactivity in an area of the body.

scirrho-, a combining form meaning 'hard, or related to a hard cancer or scirrhus': *scirrhoid, scirrhoma, scirrhosarca.*

scirrhous carcinoma, a hard, fibrous, particularly invasive tumor in which the malignant cells occur singly or in small clusters or strands in dense connective tissue. It is the most common form of breast cancer. Also called **carcinoma fibrosum.** See also **breast cancer.**

scissors, a sharp instrument composed of two opposing cutting blades, held together by a central pin on which the blades pivot. The most common dissecting scissors are the straight **Mayo,** for cutting sutures; the **Snowden-Pencer,** for deep, delicate tissue; the long, curved **Mayo,** for deep, heavy, or tough tissue; the short, curved **Metzenbaum,** for superficial, delicate tissue; and the long, blunt, curved **Metzenbaum,** for deep, delicate tissue.

SCL, abbreviation for **soft contact lens.**

scler-. See **sclero-.**

sclera /sklir′ə/, the tough, inelastic, opaque membrane covering the posterior five sixths of the eyebulb. It maintains the size and form of the bulb and attaches to muscles that move the bulb. Posteriorly, it is pierced by the optic nerve and, with the transparent cornea, comprises the outermost of three tunics covering the eyebulb.

scleredema /sklir′ədē′mə/, an idiopathic skin disease characterized by nonpitting induration beginning on the face or neck and spreading downward over the body, sparing the hands and feet. There also may be swelling of the tongue, restriction of the movements of the eyes, and pericardial, pleural, and peritoneal effusions. Resolution occurs after several months, but recurrences are common. The condition often follows a streptococcal infection or an exanthem of childhood. There is no specific treatment. Compare **scleroderma.**

sclerema neonatorum, a progressive generalized hardening of the skin and subcutaneous tissue of the newborn. It is usually a fatal condition that occurs as a result of severe cold stress in severely ill premature infants subject to such life-threatening conditions as metabolic acidosis, hypoglycemia, GI or respiratory infection, or gross malformation. Also called **scleredema neonatorum, sclerema adiposum.**

sclero-, scler-, a combining form meaning 'hard,' often used to show relationship to the sclera: *scleroadipose, sclerocorneal, sclerodesmia.*

sclerodactyly /kler′ōdak′tilē/, a musculoskeletal deformity affecting the hands of persons with scleroderma. The fingers are fixed in a semiflexed position, and the fingertips are pointed and ulcerated.

scleroderma /skler′ōdur′mə/, a relatively rare autoimmune disease affecting the blood vessels and connective tissue. The disease is characterized by fibrous degeneration of the connective tissue of the skin, lungs, and internal organs, especially the esophagus and kidneys. Scleroderma is most common in middle-aged women. Also called **progressive systemic sclerosis (PSS).**

■ OBSERVATIONS: The most common initial complaints are changes in the skin of the face and fingers. Raynaud's phenomenon occurs with a gradual hardening of the skin and swelling of the distal extremities. In the early stages, the disease may be confused with rheumatoid arthritis or Raynaud's disease. As the disease progresses, there is deformity of the joints and pain on movement. Skin changes include edema, then pallor; then the skin becomes firm; finally, it becomes slightly pigmented and fixed to the underlying tissues. At this stage the skin of the face is taut, shiny, and masklike, and the patient may have difficulty in chewing and swallowing. Scleroderma may occur in a mild form with the person living 30 to 50 years, or there may be early death because of cardiac, renal, pulmonary, or intestinal involvement. Localized forms of scleroderma may occur; these cases are benign and occur only as small circumscribed patches on the skin. A biopsy of the lesion may be done to diagnose the condition. X-ray examination of the lungs and GI tract may be diagnostic in the systemic form of the disease. Blood tests may reveal antinuclear antibodies.

■ INTERVENTION: There is no specific drug prescribed to cure scleroderma; however, corticosteroids may be useful in treating the symptoms of the disease, and salicylates and mild analgesics are given to ease pain in the joints. Physical therapy slows the development of muscle contracture and resultant deformity and debility.

■ NURSING CONSIDERATIONS: Severe renal disease is a major cause of death, although death may result from the involvement of other organs. The usual indication that renal disease is present is the abrupt onset of severe arterial hypertension that does not respond to medication. Nephrectomy or renal transplant may be performed. In the advanced stages of scleroderma, patients often require help to eat, and mouth and skin care are particularly important. As the patient becomes more helpless, there is a need for considerable emotional support.

-scleroma, a combining form meaning an 'induration, a hardening of the tissues': *laryngoscleroma, pharyngoscleroma, rhinoscleroma.*

scleromalacia perforans, a condition of the eyes in which devitalization and sloughing of the sclera occur as a complication of rheumatoid arthritis. The pigmented uvea becomes exposed and glaucoma, cataract formation, and detachment of the retina may result.

sclerose /sklerōz′/, to harden or to cause hardening. —**sclerotic,** *adj.*

sclerosing hemangioma, a solid, cellular tumorlike nodule of the skin or a mass of histiocytes, thought to arise from a hemangioma by the proliferation of endothelial and connective tissue cells.

sclerosing solution, a liquid containing an irritant that causes inflammation and resulting fibrosis of tissues. It may be used in cauterizing ulcers, arresting hemorrhage, and in treating hemangiomas.

sclerosis /sklerō′sis/, a condition characterized by hardening of tissue resulting from any of several causes, including inflammation, the deposit of mineral salts, and infiltration of connective tissue fibers. **–sclerotic,** *adj.*

sclerotome, (in embryology) the part of the segmented mesoderm layer in the early developing embryo that originates from the somites and gives rise to the skeletal tissue of the body, specifically, the paired segmented masses of mesodermal tissue that lie on each side of the notochord and develop into the vertebrae and ribs. See also **somite.**

scoleco-, a combining form meaning 'of or pertaining to a worm': *scolecoid, scolecoidectomy, scolecology.*

scolex /skō′leks/, *pl.* **scoleces** /skō′ləsēz/, the headlike segment or organ of an adult tapeworm that has hooks, grooves, or suckers by which it attaches itself to the wall of the intestine.

scolio-, a combining form meaning 'twisted or crooked': *scoliodontic, scoliokyphosis, scoliosiometry.*

scoliosis /skō′lē·ō′sis/, lateral curvature of the spine, a common abnormality of childhood. Causes include congenital malformations of the spine, poliomyelitis, skeletal dysplasias, spastic paralysis, and unequal leg length. Unequal heights of hips or shoulders may be a sign of this condition. Early recognition and orthopedic treatment may prevent progression of the curvature. Treatment includes braces, casts, exercises, and corrective surgery. See also **congenital scoliosis, kyphoscoliosis, kyphosis, lordosis, spinal curvature.**

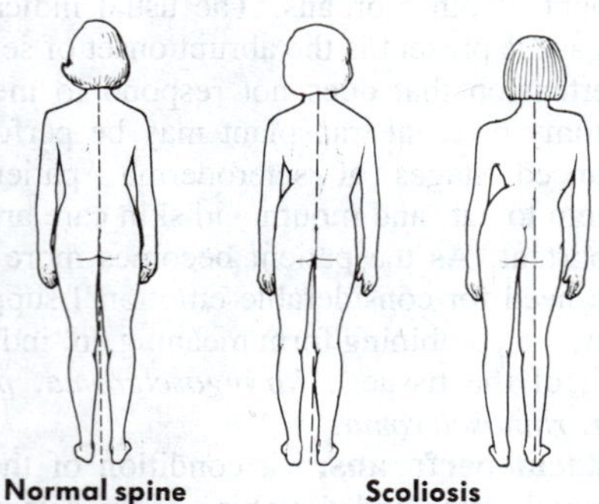

scop-, a combining form meaning 'to examine, observe': *scopograph, scopometer, scopophilia.*

scope, the breadth of opportunity to function; range of activity.

-scope, a combining form meaning an 'instrument for observation': *ciliariscope, episcope, pelviscope.*

-scopia, a combining form meaning 'observation': *aknephascopia, mixoscopia, phantasmoscopia.*

scopolamine /skōpol′əmēn/, an anticholinergic alkaloid obtained from the leaves and seeds of several solanceous plants. It is a central nervous system depressant and is used to prevent motion sickness and as an antiemetic, a sedative in obstetrics, and a cycloplegic and mydriatic. Also called **hyoscine.**

scopolamine hydrobromide, an anticholinergic.

■ INDICATIONS: It is prescribed in the treatment of nausea and vomiting, as a sedative and preanesthetic medication, and as a cycloplegic and mydriatic medication in ophthalmic procedures.

■ CONTRAINDICATIONS: Narrow-angle glaucoma, asthma, obstruction of the genitourinary or GI tracts, severe ulcerative colitis, or known hypersensitivity to this drug prohibits its use.

■ ADVERSE EFFECTS: Among the more serious adverse reactions are blurred vision, central nervous system effects, tachycardia, dry mouth, decreased sweating, and hypersensitivity reaction.

scopophilia /skō′pəfil′ē·ə, skop′-/, **1.** sexual pleasure derived from looking at sexually stimulating scenes or at another person's genitals; voyeurism. **2.** a morbid desire to be seen; exhibitionism. Also called **scotophilia.** – **scopophiliac, scopophilic, scoptophiliac, scoptophilic.** *adj., n.*

scopophobia /skō′pə-/, an anxiety disorder characterized by a morbid fear of being seen or stared at by others. The condition is commonly seen in schizophrenia. See also **phobia.**

-scopy, a combining form meaning 'observation': *bioscopy, stomachoscopy, thoracoscopy.*

-scorbic, a combining form meaning 'of or referring to the prevention or treatment of scurvy': *antiscorbic, ascorbic, glucoascorbic.*

-scorbutic, -scorbic, -scorbutical, a combining form meaning 'pertaining to scurvy': *antiscorbutic, postscorbutic, scorbutic.*

scorbutic gingivitis /skôrbyo͞o′tik/, an abnormal condition, characterized by inflamed or bleeding gums and caused by vitamin C deficiency.

scorbutic pose, the characteristic posture of a child with scurvy, with thighs and legs semiflexed and hips rotated outward. The child usually lies motionless without voluntary movements of the extremities because of the pain that accompanies any motion. See also **scurvy.**

scorbutus. See **scurvy.**

scorpion sting, a painful wound produced by a scorpion, an arachnid with a hollow stinger in its tail. The stings of many species are only slightly toxic, but some, including *Centruroides sculpturatus* of the southwestern United States, may inflict fatal injury, especially in small children. Initial pain is followed within several hours by numbness, nausea, muscle spasm, dyspnea, and convulsion. Treatment includes ice applied to the wound and intravenous calcium gluconate to control muscle spasm, if necessary. Severe cases may require oxygen and respiratory assistance. Narcotic analgesia is contraindicated. An antivenin is available in some areas.

scoto-, a combining form meaning 'of or related to darkness': *scotodinia, scotogram, scotographic.*

scratch test, a skin test for identifying an allergen, performed by placing a small quantity of a solution containing a suspected allergen on a lightly scratched area of the skin. If a wheal forms within 15 minutes, allergy to the substance is indicated.

screamer's nodule. See **vocal cord nodule.**

screening, **1.** a preliminary procedure, as a test or examination, to detect the most characteristic sign or signs of a disorder that may require further investigation. **2.** the examination of a large sample of a population to detect a specific disease or disorder, as hypertension.

screen memory, a consciously tolerable memory that replaces one that is emotionally painful to recall.

screw clamp, a device, usually made of plastic, equipped with a screw that can be manipulated to close and open the primary IV tubing for regulating the flow of intravenous solution. Turning the screw clockwise closes the tubing; turning it counterclockwise opens the tubing. Different positions of the screw between the open and the closed positions allow the intravenous fluid to flow at different rates. Compare **roller clamp, slide clamp.**

scrib-, script-, a combining form meaning 'write': *scribble, scribomania, prescription.*

Scribner shunt, a type of arteriovenous bypass, used in hemodialysis, consisting of a special tube connection outside the body.

scrofula /skrof′yələ/, *archaic.* primary tuberculosis with abscess formation, usually of the cervical lymph nodes.

scrotal cancer, an epidermoid malignancy of the scrotum, characterized initially by a small sore that may ulcerate. The lesion occurs most frequently in elderly men who have been exposed to soot, pitch, crude oil, mineral oils, polycyclic hydrocarbons, or arsenic fumes from copper smelting. Treatment involves wide surgical excision of the tumor and resection of inguinal nodes. In the eighteenth century, Sir Percival Pott associated scrotal cancer in chimney sweeps with exposure to soot. It is the first malignancy shown to be caused by an environmental carcinogen. Also called **chimney-sweeps' cancer, soot wart.**

scrotum /skrō′təm/, the pouch of skin containing the testes and parts of the spermatic cords. It is divided on the surface into two lateral portions by a ridge that continues ventrally to the undersurface of the penis and dorsally along the middle line of the perineum to the anus. In young, robust individuals the scrotum is short, corrugated, and closely wraps the testes. In older persons, debilitated individuals, and in warm environments, the scrotum becomes elongated and flaccid. The lateral left portion of the scrotum usually hangs lower than the right, corresponding with the longer length of the left spermatic cord. The two layers of the scrotum are the skin and the dartos tunic. The skin is very thin, has a brownish color and is usually wrinkled. It is supplied with sebaceous follicles that secrete a substance with a characteristic odor and has thinly scattered, kinky hairs with roots that are visible through the skin. The dartos tunic is composed of a thin layer of unstriated muscular fibers around the base of the scrotum, continuous with the two layers of the superficial fascia of the groin and the perineum. The tunic projects an internal septum that divides the pouch into two cavities for the testes, extending between the scrotal ridge and the root of the penis. The tunic is closely united to the skin but separated from subjacent parts by a distinct fascial cleft on which it glides. The scrotum is highly vascular and contains no fat. See also **testis.** **–scrotal,** *adj.*

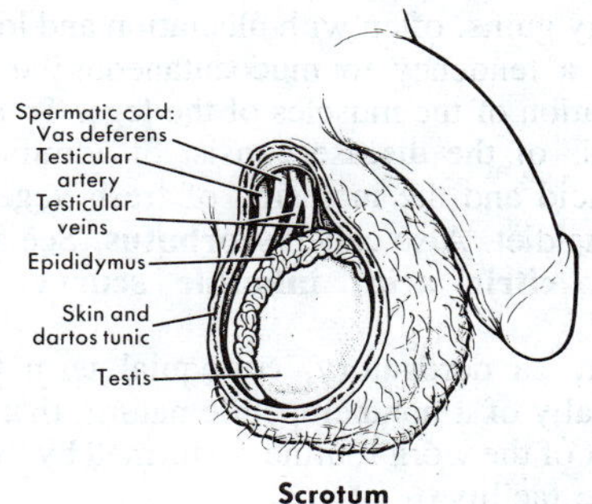

Scrotum

scrub. See **surgical scrub.**

scrub nurse, a registered nurse or operating room technician who assists surgeons during operations.

scrub room, a special hospital area where surgeons and surgical teams use disposable sterile brushes and bactericidal soaps to wash and scrub their fingernails, hands, and forearms before performing or assisting in surgical operations. Scrub rooms and meticulous washing techniques improve the sterile environment of the operating room and reduce the risk of bacterial infection.

scrub typhus, an acute, febrile disease of Asia, India, northern Australia, and the western Pacific islands, caused by several strains of the genus *Rickettsia tsutsugamushi* and transmitted from infected rodents to humans by mites. The clinical course ranges from mild to severe and is characterized by a necrotic papule or black eschar at the site of the lesion caused by the bite of the small arachnid. Tender, enlarged regional lymph nodes, fever, severe headache, eye pain, muscle aches, and a generalized rash usually occur. In severe cases, the myocardium and the central nervous system may be involved. The Weil-Felix reaction and indirect fluorescent antibody tests are useful in diagnosis. Treatment with broad spectrum antibiotics, as chloramphenicol, doxycycline, or tetracycline, has reduced mortality to nearly zero. Person-to-person transmission is not known to occur. No effective vaccine is available, and second attacks are common because of antigenic differences in various strains of rickettsiae. Prevention includes avoiding mite-infested terrain, reducing the rodent population, destroying scrub vegetation, and using insect repellents. Also called **Japanese flood fever, Japanese river fever, mite typhus, tsutsugamushi disease.** Compare **Q fever, Rocky Mountain spotted fever, typhus.**

scruple, a measure of weight in the apothecaries' system, equal to 20 grains or 1.296 g. See also **apothecaries' weight, metric system.**

Scultetus bandage /skəltē′təs/, a many-tailed bandage with an attached central piece. The tails are overlapped; the last two tied or pinned act to secure the others. A Scultetus bandage may be opened or removed without moving the bandaged part of the body.

scurvy, a condition resulting from lack of ascorbic acid in the diet. It is characterized by weakness, anemia, edema, spongy gums, often with ulceration and loosening of the teeth, a tendency to mucocutaneous hemorrhages, and induration of the muscles of the legs. Treatment and prophylaxis of the disease consist of administration of ascorbic acid and the inclusion of fresh vegetables and fruits in the diet. Also called **scorbutus.** See also **ascorbic acid, citric acid, infantile scurvy, scorbutic pose.**

scut work, a derogatory, colloquial term for menial tasks, usually of a nontherapeutic nature, that are a necessary part of the work routine performed by the staff of a health care facility.

scyt-, a combining form meaning 'skin': *scytitis, scytoblastema.*

SD, abbreviation for **standard deviation.**

Se, symbol for **selenium.**

sealed source, (in radiotherapy) a source of radiant energy in which the radioactive material is permanently encased in a container or bonding material in a manner to prevent leakage. Sealed sources, as seeds, needles, and specially designed applicators, are used in the implantation of cesium 137, iodine 125, iridium 192, radium 226, and other radionuclides for the treatment of various malignant tumors.

sealer cement, a compound used in filling a root canal. It is applied as a plastic that solidifies after insertion and fills depressions in the surface of the canal.

seal limbs. See **phocomelia.**

seasickness. See **motion sickness.**

seatworm. See ***Enterobius vermicularis.***

sea urchin sting, an injury inflicted by any of a variety of sea urchins, in which the skin is punctured and, in some species, venom released. A venomous sting is characterized by pain, muscular weakness, numbness around the mouth, and dyspnea. Immediate removal of the spines is necessary and may require the use of a local anesthetic. An antiseptic and a dressing are applied until the wound is healed. In all cases the broken spines cause local pain and irritation. Infection may result. See also **stingray.**

seawater bath, a bath taken in warm seawater or in saline solution.

sebaceous /sibā′shəs/, fatty, oily, or greasy, usually referring to the oil-secreting glands of the skin or to their secretions.

sebaceous cyst, a misnomer for epidermoid cyst or pilar cyst.

sebaceous gland, one of the many small sacculated organs in the dermis. They are located throughout the body in close association with all types of body hair but are especially abundant in the scalp, the face, the anus, the nose, the mouth, and the external ear. They are wanting in the palms of the hands and the soles of the feet. Each gland consists of a single duct that emerges from a cluster of oval alveoli. Each alveolus is composed of a transparent basement membrane enclosing epithelial cells. The outer cells are small and polyhedral and continuous with the cells lining the duct. The remainder of the alveolus is comprised of larger cells containing lipid, except in the center, where disintegrated cells leave a cavity filled with their debris and a mass of sebum cutaneum. The ducts from most sebaceous glands open into the hair follicles but some open onto the surface of the skin, as in the labia minora and the free margin of the lips. The sebum secreted by the glands oils the hair and the surrounding skin helps prevent evaporation of sweat and aids in the retention of body heat. The sebaceous glands in the nose and face are large, lobulated, and often swell with accumulated secretion. Compare **sudoriferous gland.**

seborrhea /seb′ərē′ə/, any of several common skin conditions in which there is an overproduction of sebum resulting in excessive oiliness or dry scales. See also **seborrheic blepharitis, seborrheic dermatitis. –seborrheic** /seb′ərē′ik/, *adj.*

seborrheic blepharitis, a form of seborrheic dermatitis in which the eyelids are erythematous and the margins are covered with a granular crust.

seborrheic dermatitis, a common, chronic, inflammatory skin disease characterized by dry or moist, greasy scales and yellowish crusts. Common sites are the scalp, eyelids, face, external surfaces of the ears, axillae, breasts, groin, and gluteal folds. In acute stages there may be exudate and infection resulting in secondary furunculosis. Occasionally generalized exfoliation results. In some people seborrheic dermatitis is associated with paralysis agitans, diabetes mellitus, malabsorption disorders, epilepsy, or an allergic reaction to gold or arsenic. Treatment includes selenium sulfide shampoos, topical and oral corticosteroids, topical antibiotics, proper therapy for any underlying systemic disorder, and avoidance of sweating and external irritants. Kinds of seborrheic dermatitis include **cradle cap, dandruff,** and **seborrheic blepharitis.**

seborrheic keratosis, a benign, well-circumscribed, slightly raised, tan to black, warty lesion of the skin of the face, neck, chest, or upper back. The macules are loosely covered with a greasy crust that leaves a raw pulpy base when removed. Itching is common. Treatment includes curettage or electrodesiccation or cryotherapy using local anesthesia. Also called **seborrheic wart.**

sebum /sē′bəm/, the oily secretion of the sebaceous glands of the skin, composed of keratin, fat, and cellular debris. Combined with sweat, sebum forms a moist, oily, acidic film that is mildly antibacterial and antifungal and protects the skin against drying.

Seckel's syndrome. See **bird-headed dwarf.**

seclusion, (in psychiatric nursing) the isolation of a patient in a special room to decrease stimuli that might be causing or exacerbating the patient's emotional distress.

secobarbital, a sedative and hypnotic.

■ INDICATIONS: It is prescribed in the treatment of insomnia, agitation, and as an anticonvulsant and preoperative sedative.

■ CONTRAINDICATIONS: Impaired liver function or known hypersensitivity to this drug or to any barbiturate prohibits its use.

■ ADVERSE EFFECTS: Among the more serious adverse reactions are central nervous system and respiratory depression, hypersensitivity reactions, and paradoxical excitement. Kidney damage may result from the polyethylene glycol that is used as a diluent in injectable preparations of the drug.

Seconal, a trademark for a sedative-hypnotic (secobarbital).

secondary, second in importance or in incidence or belonging to the second order of sophistication or development, as a secondary health care facility or secondary education.

secondary amenorrhea. See **amenorrhea.**

secondary amputation, amputation performed after suppuration has begun following severe trauma. An area is left open for drainage, and antibiotics are given. Compare **primary amputation.**

secondary amyloidosis. See **amyloidosis.**

secondary analysis, the study of a problem using previously compiled data.

secondary apnea, an abnormal condition in which respiration is absent and will not begin again spontaneously. Resuscitation is begun immediately with artificial respiration; oxygen, cardiac massage, analysis of blood gases, and other treatment and medication specific to the underlying cause may be necessary. Secondary apnea may result from any event that severely impedes the absorption of oxygen into the bloodstream. Compare **primary apnea.**

secondary areola, a second ring appearing around the areola of the breast during pregnancy that is more pigmented than the areola before pregnancy.

secondary biliary cirrhosis, an abnormal hepatic condition characterized by obstruction of the bile duct with or without infection. It involves periportal inflammation with progressive fibrosis, destruction of parenchymal cells, and nodular degeneration. Compare **primary biliary cirrhosis.**

secondary bronchus, a lobar or segmental bronchus. See also **bronchus, primary bronchus.**

secondary care, **1.** the provision of a specialized medical service by a physician specialist or a hospital on referral by a primary care physician. **2.** the retardation of an existing illness or other pathologic condition.

secondary dementia, dementia resulting from another, concurrent form of psychosis. See also **dementia.**

secondary dental caries, dental caries developing in a tooth already affected by the condition; often a new cavity forms adjacent to or beneath the restorative filling of an old cavity.

secondary dentition. See **permanent dentition.**

secondary diabetes. See **other types of diabetes.**

secondary dysmenorrhea. See **dysmenorrhea.**

secondary fissure, a fissure between the uvula and the pyramid of the cerebellum.

secondary fracture. See **neoplastic fracture.**

secondary gain, an indirect benefit, usually obtained through an illness or debility. Such gains may include monetary and disability benefits, personal attentions, or escape from unpleasant situations and responsibilities. Compare **primary gain.**

secondary health care, an intermediate level of health care that includes diagnosis and treatment, performed in a hospital having specialized equipment and laboratory facilities. Secondary health care is provided to a larger group of people from a larger geographic area than those served by primary care.

secondary host. See **intermediate host.**

secondary hypertension, elevated blood pressure associated with several primary diseases, as renal, pulmonary, endocrine, and vascular diseases. See also **hypertension.**

secondary hypertrophic osteoarthropathy. See **clubbing.**

secondary infection, an infection by a microorganism that follows an initial infection by another kind of organism.

secondary memory device, a peripheral computer device outside the internal memory, used for storage of computer programs and data. Also called **storage device.**

secondary nutrient, a substance that acts as a stimulant to activate the flora of the GI tract to synthesize other nutrients.

secondary occlusal traumatism, occlusal stress that affects previously weakened periodontal structures. The stress may not be excessive for normal tissues but can be damaging to the weakened structures.

secondary port, a control device for regulating the flow of a primary and a secondary intravenous solution. It consists of a Y-shaped plastic apparatus that attaches to the primary IV tubing and allows the primary and secondary IV solutions to flow separately or to flow simultaneously. Compare **piggyback port.**

secondary prevention, a level of preventive medicine that focuses on early diagnosis, use of referral services, and rapid initiation of treatment to stop the progress of disease processes or a handicapping disability.

secondary proximal renal tubular acidosis. See **proximal renal tubular acidosis.**

secondary radiation, x-ray films produced by substances that absorb primary x-rays and fluoresce as inner shell electrons of the atoms of the substance are ejected by the energy of the primary x-rays. Secondary radiation may also result from the scattering of primary x-rays. Secondary radiation often accounts for fogging of x-ray film.

secondary relationships, relationships with those who provide or accept services, or with acquaintances and friends, as distinguished from family members and intimate friends.

secondary sequestrum, a piece of dead bone that partially separates from sound bone during the process of necrosis but may be pushed back into position. Compare **primary sequestrum.**

secondary sex characteristic, any of the external physical characteristics of sexual maturity secondary to hormonal stimulation that develops in the maturing individual. These characteristics include the adult distribution of hair and the development of the penis or breasts and the labia.

secondary shock, a state of physical collapse and prostration caused by numerous traumatic and pathologic conditions. It develops over a period of time after severe tissue damage and may merge with primary shock, accompanied by various signs, as weakness, restlessness, low body temperature, low blood pressure, cold sweat, and reduced urinary output. Blood pressure drops progressively in this state, and death may occur within a relatively short time after onset unless appropriate treatment intervenes. Secondary shock is often associated with heat stroke, crushing injuries, myocardial infarction, poisoning, fulminating infections, burns, and other life-threatening conditions. The pathology of this state reflects changes in the capillaries, which become dilated and engorged with blood. Petechial hemorrhages develop in the serous membranes, edema swells the soft tissues, and the vital organs undergo degenerative changes. Compare **hemorrhagic shock, primary shock.**

secondary thrombocytosis. See **thrombocytosis.**

second cuneiform bone. See **intermediate cuneiform bone.**

second filial generation. See **F_2.**

second intention. See **intention.**

second nerve. See **optic nerve.**

second opinion, a patient privilege of requesting an examination and evaluation of a health condition by a second physician to verify or challenge the diagnosis by a first physician. The situation is most likely to arise when an examination by a first physician results in a recommendation for surgery.

second sight. See **senopia.**

secrete, to discharge a substance into a cavity, vessel, or organ or onto the surface of the skin, as a gland. **secretion,** *n.*

secretin /sikrē′tin/, a digestive hormone that is produced by certain cells lining the duodenum and jejunum when fatty acids of partially digested food enter the intestine from the stomach. It stimulates the pancreas to produce a fluid high in salts but low in enzymes. Secretin has a limited stimulating effect on the production of bile. See also **pancreas.**

secretin test, a test of pancreatic function after stimulation with a hormone, secretin. The test measures the volume and bicarbonate concentration of pancreatic secretions. A lower than normal volume suggests an obstructing malignancy. Reduced bicarbonate and amylase concentration is usually diagnostic of chronic pancreatitis.

secretory duct, (of a gland) a small duct that has a secretory function and joins with an excretory duct.

secretory phase, the phase of the menstrual cycle after the release of an ovum from a mature ovarian follicle. The corpus luteum, stimulated by luteinizing hormone (LH), develops from the ruptured follicle. It secretes progesterone, which stimulates the development of the glands and arteries of the endometrium, causing it to become thick and spongy. In a negative feedback response to the increased level of progesterone in the blood, the secretion of LH from the pituitary decreases. In the absence of an embryo and its secretion of chorionic gonadotropin, the secretory phase ends. The corpus luteum involutes, progesterone levels fall, and menstruation occurs. Also called **luteal phase, progestational phase.** Compare **menstrual phase, proliferative phase.**

secretory piece, a polypeptide chain attached to an IgA molecule. The secretory piece is necessary for secretion of the immunoglobulin molecule into mucosal spaces.

sect-, a combining form meaning 'to cut': *sectio, section, sector.*

-sect, a combining form meaning 'to cut': *dissect, medisect, quadrisect.*

sectional arch wire, a wire attached to only a few teeth, usually on one side of a dental arch or in the anterior segment of the arch to cause or guide orthodontic tooth movement.

secund-, a combining form meaning 'second, or following': *secundigravida, secundina, secundine.*

secundigravida /səkund′dəgrav′idə/, a woman who is pregnant for the second time. Also called **gravida 2.** **–secundigravid,** *adj.*

secundines /səkun′dīnz/, the placenta, umbilical cord, and membranes of afterbirth.

secundipara /sek′əndip′ərə/, a woman who has borne two viable children in separate pregnancies.

sedation, an induced state of quiet, calmness, or sleep, as by means of a sedative or hypnotic medication.

sedative, **1.** of or pertaining to a substance, procedure, or measure that has a calming effect. **2.** an agent that decreases functional activity, diminishes irritability, and allays excitement. Some sedatives have a general effect on all organs; others affect principally the activities of the heart, stomach, intestines, nerve trunks, respiratory system, or vasomotor system. Barbiturates and nonbarbiturate sedatives, as chloral hydrate, ethinamate, furazepam, glutethimide, and various minor tranquilizers, are used to induce sleep, reduce pain, facilitate the induction of anesthesia, and treat convulsive conditions, anxiety states, and irritable bowel syndrome. See also **sedative-hypnotic.**

sedative bath, the immersion of the body in water for a prolonged period of time, used especially as a calming procedure for agitated patients.

sedative-hypnotic, a drug that reversibly depresses the activity of the central nervous system, used chiefly to induce sleep and to allay anxiety. Barbiturates and many nonbarbiturate sedative-hypnotics with diverse chemical and pharmacologic properties share the ability to depress the activity of all excitable tissue, but the arousal center in the brainstem is especially sensitive to their effects. Various sedative-hypnotics and minor tranquilizers with similar effects are used in the treatment of insomnia, acute convulsive conditions, anxiety states, and to facilitate the induction of anesthesia. Although sedative-hypnotics have a soporific effect, they may interfere with rapid eye movement (REM) sleep associated with dreaming and, when administered to patients with fever, may act paradoxically and cause excitement rather than relaxation. Sedative-hypnotics may interfere with temperature regulation, depress oxygen consumption in various tissues, produce nausea and skin rashes, and, in elderly patients, may cause dizziness, confusion, and ataxia. Drugs in this group have a high potential for abuse that often results in physical and psychologic dependence; treatment of dependence involves gradual reduction of the dosage, because abrupt withdrawal frequently causes serious disorders, including convulsions. Acute reactions to an overdose of a sedative-hypnotic may be treated with an emetic, activated charcoal, gastric lavage, and measures to maintain airway patency. Among nonbarbiturate sedative-hypnotics are chloral hydrate, ethchlorvynol, ethinamate, glutethimide, methaqualone, paraldehyde, triclofos sodium, minor tranquilizers (chlordiazepoxide, flurazepam, diazepam), diphenhydramine, and meprobamate. See also **barbiturate.**

sedimentation rate. See **erythrocyte sedimentation rate.**

sed. rate, *informal.* erythrocyte sedimentation rate.

segmental bronchus, a bronchus branching from a lobar bronchus to a bronchiole.

segmental fracture, a bone break in which several large bone fragments separate from the main body of a fractured bone. The ends of such fragments may pierce the skin, as in an open fracture, or may be contained within the skin, as in a closed fracture.

segmental resection, a surgical procedure in which a part of an organ, gland, or other part of the body is excised, as a segmental resection of a part of an ovary performed to diminish the hormonal secretion of the gland by decreasing the amount of secretory tissue in the gland.

segmentation, **1.** the repetition of structured parts or the process of dividing into segments or similar parts, as the formation of somites or metameres. **2.** the division of the zygote into blastomeres; cleavage.

segmentation cavity. See **blastocoele.**

segmentation cell. See **blastomere.**

segmentation method, a technique for filling tooth root canals in which a preselected gutta-percha cone is cut into segments and the tip section sealed into the apex of a root. The other sections are usually warmed and condensed against the first piece with a plugger. More cone segments are then added until the canal is filled.

segmentation nucleus, the nucleus of the zygote resulting from the fusion of the male and female pronuclei in the fertilized ovum. It is the final stage in fertilization and initiates the first cleavage of the zygote. Also called **cleavage nucleus.**

segmented hyalinizing vasculitis, a chronic, relapsing inflammatory condition of the blood vessels of the lower legs associated with nodular or purpuric skin lesions that may become ulcerated and leave scars. Also called **livedo vasculitis.**

segmented neutrophil, a neutrophil with a filament between the lobes of its nucleus.

segregation, (in genetics) a principle stating that the pairs of chromosomes bearing genes derived from both parents are separated during meiosis. Chance alone determines which gene, maternal or paternal, will travel to which gamete. See also **dominance, independent assortment.**

seizure. See **convulsion.**

seizure threshold, the amount of stimulus necessary to produce a convulsive seizure. All humans can have seizures if the provocation is sufficient. Those who have spontaneous convulsions are said to have a ''low seizure threshold.''

selection, **1.** the act or product of choosing. **2.** (in genetics) the process by which various factors or mechanisms determine and modify the reproductive ability of a genotype within a specific population, thus influencing evolutionary change. Kinds of selection are **artificial selection, natural selection,** and **sexual selection.**

selective angiography, a graphic procedure that allows selective visualization of the aorta, the major arterial systems, or a particular vessel. It is performed using a percutaneous catheter. A few milliliters of a radiopaque substance are injected when the catheter is in place. Because the radiopaque substance is excreted quickly by the kidneys, films are taken of the fluoroscopic image, using a special camera. The patient is observed for signs of sensitivity to the radiopaque medium, including chills, tremor, or shortness of breath. After the procedure, the catheter is withdrawn, and pressure is placed on the puncture site to prevent bleeding. Blood pressure is checked every 15 minutes for 2 hours.

selective grinding, any modification of the occlusal forms of the teeth, produced by corrective grinding at selected places to improve occlusion and tooth function.

selective inattention, the screening out of unwanted stimuli, particularly the part of a message the listener does not want to hear.

selectivity, the capacity factor ratios of two substances measured under identical chromatographic conditions. Also called **chromatographic selectivity, separation factor.**

selectivity coefficient, the degree to which an ion-selective electrode (ISE) responds to a particular ion with respect to a reference ion.

selenium (Se), a metalloid element of the sulfur group. Its atomic number is 34; its atomic weight is 78.96. Selenium occurs mainly in iron, copper, lead, and nickel ores and in the form of metallic selenides. One of the chief sources commercially is the flue dust produced by the burning of pyrites to make sulfuric acid. Selenium occurs as a trace element in foods, and research continues to determine the most effective daily allowances for different age groups. Dietary experts say that the estimated safe, adequate intake of selenium for infants 6 months of age is .04 mg, for adults .05 to 0.2 mg. Although selenium deficiency can result in liver problems and degeneration of muscles in some animals, in humans its need has not yet been clearly defined. Authorities stress that all intakes of selenium and other trace elements in foods are considered safe and effective within recommended ranges, but consumption of greater amounts or smaller amounts over extended periods of time will increase the risk of marginal toxicity or marginal deficiency, respectively. The bright orange, insoluble powder selenium sulfide is used externally in the control of seborrheic dermatitis, dandruff, and other forms of dermatosis. Selenium sulfide, employed as a lotion, is used in some therapeutic shampoos containing 2.5% of selenium sulfide in a detergent vehicle; it is sold without prescription as a 1% detergent suspension in a scented detergent vehicle. Adverse effects may include conjunctivitis if the preparation enters the eyes, increased oiliness or dryness of the hair, and orange tinting of gray hair. The antidandruff effectiveness of selenium sulfide is thought to stem from its antimitotic activity and its residual adherence to the hair after shampooing. Normal skin absorbs very little of the drug, but inflamed or damaged skin absorbs it readily. Burns and dermatitis venenata may result from prolonged skin contact.

selenium sulfide, an antifungal and antiseborrheic. See also **selenium.**

■ INDICATIONS: It is prescribed for dandruff and for seborrheic dermatitis of the scalp.

■ CONTRAINDICATIONS: Acute scalp inflammation or known hypersensitivity to this drug prohibits its use.

■ ADVERSE EFFECTS: Among the more serious adverse reactions are dermatitis after prolonged skin contact or keratitis after accidental conjunctival contact.

self, *pl.* **selves, 1.** the total essence or being of a person; the individual. **2.** those affective, cognitive, and spiritual qualities that distinguish one person from another; individuality. **3.** a person's awareness of his own being or identity; consciousness; ego. See also **personality.**

self-actualization, (in humanistic psychology) the fundamental tendency toward the maximum realization and fulfillment of one's human potential.

self-alien. See **ego-dystonic.**

self-alienation. See **depersonalization.**

self-anesthesia, the self-administered inhalational anesthesia in which whiffs of anesthetic gas are inhaled from a handheld breathing device controlled by the patient. This form of anesthesia is most common in England; trilene is the usual gas.

self-breast examination (SBE), a procedure in which a woman examines her breasts and their accessory structures for evidence of change that could indicate malignant process. The SBE is usually performed 1 week to 10 days after the first day of the menstrual cycle, when the breasts are smallest and cyclic nodularity is least apparent. Self-examination is encouraged during all phases of a woman's adult life; a woman who regularly and carefully performs the examination is better able to detect small abnormalities than is a woman who is not familiar with her own breasts. The techniques are similar to those of the examination of the breast as performed in the health assessment or physical examination. Also called **breast self-examination (BSE).** See also **breast examination.**

self-care, 1. the personal and medical care performed by the patient, usually in collaboration with and after instruction by a medical professional. The need of a patient for assistance and the ability to develop a higher level of self-care must be evaluated in forming any nursing care plan. Maximal self-care appropriate to the condition and to the patient is often the ultimate goal of nursing care. Occupational therapy services also help restore, develop, or maintain the skills necessary to permit physically and mentally disabled persons to perform the daily living tasks of self-care. **2.** the medical care by laypersons of their families, friends, and themselves, including identification and evaluation of symptoms, medication, and treatment. Self-care is self-limited, voluntary, and wholly outside professional health care systems but may include consultation with a physician or other health care professional as a resource. **3.** personal care accomplished without technical assistance, as eating, washing, dressing, using the telephone, attending to one's own elimination, appearance, and hygiene. The goal of rehabilitation medicine is maximal personal self-care.

self-care deficit: feeding, bathing/hygiene, dressing/grooming, toileting, a nursing diagnosis accepted by the Fourth National Conference on the Classification of Nursing Diagnoses. The cause of the condition may be an intolerance for activity because of decreased strength or endurance, pain or discomfort, impairment of cognitive or perceptual function, depression or marked anxiety, or impairment of mobility or of neuromuscular or musculoskeletal function. The kinds of deficit are separated into functional categories and are graded from 0 (functions independently) to 4 (requires total assistance). The defining characteristics of a self-feeding deficit is an inability or a relative lack of ability to bring food to the mouth from a receptacle. The defining characteristics of a self-bathing/hygiene deficit include an inability to get or get to water for bathing and an inability to regulate properly the temperature of the water. The critical characteristic of this deficit is an inability to wash the body or parts of the body. The defining characteristics of a deficit in self-dressing or self-grooming include an impaired ability to fasten clothing, to obtain or replace articles of clothing, and to maintain a satisfactory appearance. The critical defining characteristic is an impaired ability to don or to remove necessary items of clothing. The fourth component of the deficit, self-toileting, carries the following critical defining characteristics: an inability to get to the toilet or to the commode, to sit down on or to arise from the toilet or commode, to get the necessary clothing on or off, and to perform the usual toilet hygiene. In addition, the person may not be able to flush the toilet or to empty the commode. See also **nursing diagnosis.**

self-care theory, a model, used to provide a conceptual framework for nursing care directed toward self-care by the client to the greatest degree possible. The model requires an assessment of the client's capability for self-care and need for care. The need for care includes biophysical and psychosocial needs and the specific needs that are the result of the illness.

self-catheterization, a procedure performed by a patient to empty the bladder and prevent it from becoming overdistended with urine. The patient who cannot empty the bladder completely but can retain urine for 2 to 4 hours at a time can be taught self-catheterization if the person is willing to learn and has some manual dexterity and the ability to palpate the bladder.

■ METHOD: Necessary equipment consists of a pan or toilet, two 14 French catheters, a water-soluble lubricant, soap, water, and a clean washcloth and towel; women usually require a magnifying mirror initially to identify the urethral meatus and men may prefer to perform the procedure sitting on a low stool rather than on a toilet. Women are taught to perform self-catheterization initially in a semi-Fowler's position, using a pan, but later they generally can carry out the procedure sitting on or standing over a toilet. The patient is instructed to clean the urinary meatus and labia or glans penis with soap and water, to grasp the catheter 3 or 4 inches from the tip, and to lubricate the tip before it is gently inserted in the meatus: Women insert 3 to 5 cm of the catheter and men insert 20 cm. Urine is allowed to flow into the pan or toilet until the bladder is empty. The catheter is then removed, washed in soap and water, thoroughly rinsed, dried by rolling it in a clean towel, and placed in a clean plastic or paper bag for the next self-catheterization.

■ NURSING ORDERS: The nurse teaches the procedure, ensures that the patient understands its purpose, the need to perform it at designated times, and the importance of forcing fluids up to 3000 ml daily, unless contraindicated. The nurse makes certain that the patient is able to identify the urinary meatus.

■ OUTCOME CRITERIA: Regular self-catheterization by the patient who cannot empty the bladder allows the person to work and participate in the normal activities of daily living and to prevent kidney infection and other renal pathology.

self-concept, the composite of ideas, feelings, and attitudes that a person has about his own identity, worth, capabilities, and limitations. Such factors as the values and opinions of others, especially in the formative years of early childhood, play an important part in the development of the self-concept.

self-concept, disturbance in: body image, self-esteem, role performance, personal identity, a nursing diagnosis accepted by the Fourth National Conference on the Classification of Nursing Diagnoses. The disturbance represents a disruption in the way one sees oneself. There are four subcomponents, each with its own causes and defining characteristics. The cause of a disturbance in body image may be a biophysical, cognitive, perceptual, psychosocial, cultural, or spiritual factor. The defining characteristics of the deficit include verbal or nonverbal responses to a real or perceived change in structure or function, a missing body part, personalization of the missing part by giving it a name, refusal by the client to look at a part of the body, negative feelings about the body, trauma to a nonfunctioning part, a change in general social involvement or life style, and a fear of rejection by others. The cause of a disturbance in self-esteem is to be developed at a later conference. The defining characteristics of a disturbance in self-esteem are an inability to accept praise or encouragement, a lack of participation in treatment and therapy, observed self-neglect, self-destructive behavior, or a lack of eye contact with others. The cause of a disturbance in role performance is to be developed at a later conference. The defining characteristics of a disturbance in role performance include a change in the person's perception of the role or a denial of the role, a change in the physical capacity to perform the actions of the role, and a lack of knowledge of the functions of the role. The cause and the defining characteristics of a disturbance in personal identity are to be developed at a later conference. See also **nursing diagnosis.**

self-conscious, **1.** the state of being aware of oneself as an individual entity that experiences, desires, and acts. **2.** a heightened awareness of oneself and one's actions as reflected by the observations and reactions of others; socially ill at ease. –**self-consciousness,** *n.*

self-confrontation, a technique for behavior modification that depends on a patient's recognition of and dissatisfaction with inconsistencies in his or her own values, beliefs, and behaviors, or between his or her own personal system and that of a significant other.

self-diagnosis, the diagnosis of one's own health problems, usually without direction or assistance from a physician.

self-differentiation, specialization and diversification of a tissue or part resulting solely from intrinsic factors.

self-disclosure, the process by which one person lets his or her inner being, thoughts, and emotions be known to another. It is important for psychologic growth in individual and group psychotherapy.

self-esteem, the degree of worth and competence one attributes to oneself.

self-fulfilling prophecy, a principle that states that a belief in or the expectation of a particular resolution is a factor that contributes to its fulfillment.

self-help group, a group of people who meet to improve their health through discussion and special activities. Characteristically, self-help groups are not led by a professional. A women's self-help group may be primarily supportive or it may be concerned with learning to perform basic tests, like a Pap test, or with identification and treatment of common gynecologic problems, as vaginal infections. Compare **group therapy.**

self-image, the total concept, idea, or mental image one has of oneself and of one's role in society; the person one believes oneself to be.

self-insurance, a system whereby hospitals or health professionals may, in lieu of commercial insurance, assume financial responsibility for their liability.

self-limited, (of a disease or condition) tending to end without treatment.

self-radiolysis, a process in which a compound is damaged by radioactive decay products originating in an atom within the compound.

self-retaining catheter, an indwelling urinary catheter that has a double lumen. One channel allows urine to drain from the bladder into a collecting bag; the other channel has a balloon at the bladder end and a diaphragm at the other end. Several centimeters of air or sterile water are injected through the diaphragm to fill the balloon in the bladder and hold the catheter in place. To remove the catheter, the air or water is withdrawn through the diaphragm or allowed to escape by cutting the diaphragm off the tube.

self-system, the organization of experiences that acts as a protective mechanism against anxiety.

self-theory, a personality theory that uses one's self-concept in integrating the function and organization of the personality. See also **humanistic psychology.**

self-threading pin, a threaded pin screwed into a hole drilled in tooth dentin to improve the retention of a restoration.

self-transcendence, the ability to focus attention on doing something for the sake of others, as opposed to self-actualization in which doing something for oneself is an end goal.

sella turcica /sel′ə tur′sikə/, a transverse depression crossing the midline on the superior surface of the body of the sphenoid bone and containing the pituitary gland.

Selsun, a trademark for an antifungal and antiseborrheic (selenium sulfide), used as a shampoo.

SEM. See **scanning electron microscope.**

-seme, a combining form meaning '(one) having an orbital (cephalometric) index of less than 84, more than 89, or in between' as specified by the prefix: *megaseme, mesoseme, microseme.*

semeio-, a combining form meaning 'sign, or symptom': *semeiography, semeiology, semeiotic.*

semen /sē′mən/, the thick, whitish secretion of the male reproductive organs discharged from the urethra on ejaculation. It contains various constituents, including spermatozoa in their nutrient plasma and secretions of the prostate, seminal vesicles, and various other glands. Also called **seminal fluid, sperm.** **–seminal,** *adj.*

semi-, a combining form meaning 'one half': *semicoma, semisupination, semivalent.*

semicircular canal, any of three bony, fluid-filled loops in the osseous labyrinth of the internal ear, associated with the sense of balance. The posterior, superior, and lateral canals, each about 0.8 mm in diameter, open into the cochlea. The posterior canal is the longest.

semicircular duct, one of three ducts that make up the membranous labyrinth of the inner ear. See also **membranous labyrinth.**

semicoma. See **coma.**

semi-Fowler's position, placement of the patient in an inclined position, with the upper half of the body raised by elevating the head of the bed.

semilente insulin. See **intermediate-acting insulin.**

semilunar bone. See **lunate bone.**

semilunar valve, **1.** a valve with half-moon-shaped cusps, as the aortic valve and the pulmonary valve. **2.** any one of the cusps constituting such a valve. See also **heart valve, mitral valve, tricuspid valve.**

semimembranosus /sem′ēmem′brənō′səs/, one of three posterior femoral muscles. Situated at the back and medial side of the thigh, it originates in a thick tendon attached to the tuberosity of the ischium and inserts into the horizontal groove on the medial condyle of the tibia. The tendon of insertion passes some fibers laterally and upward to insert on the lateral condyle of the femur and form part of the oblique popliteal ligament behind the knee. The tendon of insertion forms one of the two medial hamstrings. The muscle is innervated by several branches of the tibial portion of the sciatic nerve, containing fibers from the fifth lumbar and the first two sacral nerves, and functions to flex the leg, to rotate it medially after flexion and to extend the thigh. Compare **biceps femoris, hamstring muscle, semitendinosus.**

seminal duct, any duct through which semen passes, as the vas deferens or the ejaculatory duct.

seminal fluid. See **semen.**

seminal fluid test, any of several tests of semen to detect abnormalities in a male reproductive system and to determine fertility. Some common factors considered are seminal fluid liquifaction time, spermatic quantity, morphology, motility, volume, and pH. Normal values in some of these tests are: sperm count, 60 million to 150 million/ml of seminal fluid; pH, more than 7 (7.7 average); ejaculation volume, 1.5 to 5.0 ml; motility, 60% of sperm.

seminal vesicle, either of the paired, saclike glandular structures that lie behind the urinary bladder in the male and function as part of the reproductive system. Each sac is pyramidal in shape, convoluted in appearance, and at the anterior extremity becomes constricted into a narrow straight duct that joins the vas deferens to form the ejaculatory duct. The seminal vesicles produce a fluid that is added to the secretion of the testes and other glands to form the semen.

seminal vesiculitis, inflammation of a seminal vesicle.

seminarcosis. See **twilight sleep.**

semination, the introduction of semen into the female genital tract.

seminiferous /sem′inif′ərəs/, transporting or producing semen, as the tubules of the testis.

seminoma /sem′inō′mə/, *pl.* **seminomas, seminomata,** a malignant tumor of the testis. It is the most common testicular tumor and is believed to arise from the seminiferous epithelium of the mature or maturing testis. The two types are classic, or typical, and spermatocytic, with anaplastic being a variant of classic. Compare **dysgerminoma.** See also **testicular tumor.**

semipermeable membrane, a membrane barrier to the passage of substances above a specific size, but which allows the movement through the membrane of substances below that size.

semirecumbent, a reclining position.

semitendinosus /sem′iten′dinō′səs/, one of three posterior femoral muscles of the thigh, remarkable for the great length of its tendon of insertion. It is a fusiform muscle located in the posterior and medial portion of the thigh, arising from the tuberosity of the ischium. It ends just distal to the middle of the thigh in a long, round tendon that curves around the medial condyle of the tibia and inserts into the tibia. The muscle is innervated by branches of the tibial portion of the sciatic nerve, containing fibers from the fifth lumbar and the first two sacral nerves. It functions to flex the leg and rotate it medially after flexion and to extend the thigh. Compare **biceps femoris, hamstring muscle, semimembranosus.**

semustine /səmus′tēn/, an antineoplastic.

■ INDICATIONS: It is prescribed in the treatment of Lewis lung carcinoma, brain tumors, malignant melanoma, and Hodgkin's disease.

■ CONTRAINDICATIONS: Acute myelosuppression or known hypersensitivity to this drug prohibits its use. It is not given during pregnancy or to lactating mothers.

■ ADVERSE EFFECTS: Among the more serious adverse reactions are delayed bone marrow depression and thrombocytopenia.

sender, (in communication theory) the person by whom a message is encoded and sent.

senescent /sines′ənt/, aging or growing old. See also **senile.** **–senescence,** *n.*

Sengstaken-Blakemore tube, a thick catheter having a triple lumen and two balloons, used to produce pressure by balloon tamponade to arrest hemorrhaging from esophageal varices. Attached to a tube, one balloon is blown up in the stomach and exerts pressure against the upper orifice. Similarly attached, another longer and narrower balloon exerts pressure on the walls of the esophagus. The third tube is used for withdrawing gastric contents. Also called **Blakemore-Sengstaken tube.** See also **tube.**

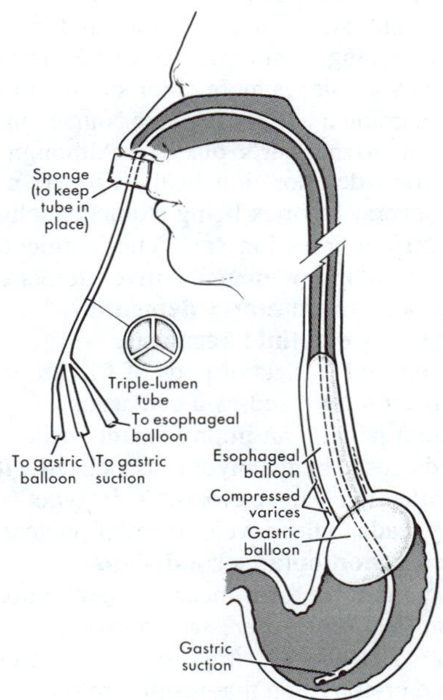

Sengstaken-Blakemore tube

senile, pertaining to, or characteristic of old age or the process of aging, especially the physical or mental deterioration accompanying aging. See also **aging.** **–senescent,** *adj.,* **senility,** *n.*

senile angioma. See **cherry angioma.**

senile cataract, a kind of cataract, associated with aging, in which a hard opacity forms in the nucleus of the lens of the eye.

senile delirium, disorientation and mental feebleness associated with extreme age and characterized by restlessness, insomnia, aimless wandering, and less commonly, hallucination. See also **delirium, senile psychosis.**

senile dementia. See **senile psychosis.**

senile dental caries, tooth decay occurring at an advanced age. Senile dental caries is usually characterized by cavity formation in or around the cementum layer and root surfaces. See also **dental caries.**

senile endometritis, *obsolete.* endometritis in a postmenopausal woman.

senile involution, a pattern of retrograde changes occurring with advancing age and resulting in the progressive shrinking and degeneration of tissues and organs.

senile keratosis. See **actinic keratosis.**

senile memory. See **anterograde memory.**

senile nanism, dwarfism associated with progeria.

senile psychosis, an organic mental disorder of the aged, resulting from the generalized atrophy of the brain with no evidence of cerebrovascular disease. Symptoms include loss of memory, impaired judgment, decreased moral and aesthetic values, inability to think abstractly, periods of confusion, confabulation, and irritability, all of which may range from mild to severe. The condition, which is irreversible, is more common in women than in men, runs a gradual and progressive course, and may be a late form of Alzheimer's disease. Although the exact cause of brain deterioration in the aged is not known, there are several theories being studied, including autoimmunity, slow infection, and cholinergic deficiency. Also called **primary degenerative dementia, senile onset.** See also **multiinfarct dementia.**

senile wart. See **actinic keratosis.**

senna, the dried leaflets or pods of *Cassia acutifolia* or *Cassia augustifolia,* used as a cathartic.

senopia /senō′pē•ə/, an improvement in the near vision of the aged caused by the myopia associated with increasing lenticular nuclear sclerosis. This type of sclerosis commonly leads to the development of nuclear cataracts. Also called **genontopia, second sight.**

sens-, a combining form meaning 'perception, or feeling': *sensation, sensimeter, sensitinogen.*

sensation, **1.** a feeling, impression, or awareness of a bodily state or condition that results from the stimulation of a sensory receptor site and transmission of the nerve impulse along an afferent fiber to the brain. Kinds of sensation include **delayed sensation, epigastric sensation, primary sensation, referred sensation,** and **subjective sensation.** **2.** a feeling or an awareness of a mental or emotional state, which may or may not result in response to an external stimulus.

sense, **1.** the faculty by which stimuli are perceived and conditions outside of and within the body are distinguished and evaluated. The major senses are sight, hearing, smell, taste, touch and pressure. Other senses include hunger, thirst, pain, temperature, proprioception, spatial, time, and visceral sensations. **2.** the ability to feel; a sensation. **3.** the capacity to understand; normal mental ability. **4.** to perceive through a sense organ.

sensible perspiration, loss of fluid from the body through the secretory activity of the sweat glands in a quantity sufficient to be observed. Compare **insensible perspiration.**

sensitive volume, (in NMR imaging) the region of the object from which an NMR signal will preferentially be acquired because of strong magnetic field inhomogeneity elsewhere. The effect can be enhanced by use of a shaped rf field that is strongest in the sensitive region.

sensitivity, **1.** capacity to feel, transmit, or react to a stimulus. **2.** susceptibility to a substance, as a drug or an antigen. See also **allergy, hypersensitivity.** **–sensitive,** *adj.*

sensitivity test, a laboratory method for testing the effectiveness of antibiotics. It is usually done on organisms known to be potentially resistant to antibiotic therapy in vitro. A report of "resistant" means the antibiotic is not effective in inhibiting the growth of a pathogen, whereas use of an effective antibiotic results in a "sensitive" report.

sensitivity training group, a group that offers members a supportive atmosphere in which to experiment with and alter behavioral patterns and interpersonal reactions. The focus of sensitivity training is on learning what occurs during group interactions, testing and refining new behavioral responses in light of the reactions they evoke, and applying those responses to situations outside the group setting. Also called **T group.** See also **encounter group, psychotherapy.**

sensitization, **1.** an acquired reaction in which specific antibodies develop in response to an antigen. This is deliberately caused in immunization by injecting a disease-causing organism that has been altered in such a way that it is no longer infectious yet remains able to cause the production of antibodies to fight the disease. Allergic reactions are hypersensitivity reactions that result from excess sensitization to a foreign protein. **2.** a photodynamic method of destroying microorganisms by inserting into a solution substances, as fluorescing dyes, that absorb visible light and emit energy at wavelengths destructive to the organism. **3.** *nontechnical.* anaphylaxis. **–sensitize,** *v.*

sensitized, pertaining to tissues that have been made susceptible to antigenic substances. See also **allergy.**

sensorimotor phase, the developmental phase of childhood, encompassing the period from birth to 2 years of age, according to piagetian psychology.

sensorineural hearing loss, a form of hearing loss in which sound is conducted through the external and middle ear in a normal way but a defect in the inner ear results in its distortion, making discrimination difficult. Amplification of the sound with a hearing aid will help some people with sensorineural hearing loss, but many have an intolerance to loud noises and will not be helped. Compare **conductive hearing loss.**

sensory apraxia. See **ideational apraxia.**

sensory deprivation, an involuntary loss of physical awareness caused by detachment from external sensory stimuli. Such deprivation often results in psychologic disorders, as panic, mental confusion, depression, and hallucinations. Sensory deprivation may be associated with various handicaps and conditions, as blindness, heavy sedation, and prolonged isolation.

sensory nerve, a nerve consisting of afferent fibers that conduct sensory impulses from the periphery of the body to the brain or spinal cord via the dorsal spinal roots. Compare **motor nerve.**

sensory-perceptual alterations: visual, auditory, kinesthetic, gustatory, tactile, olfactory perception, a nursing diagnosis accepted by the Fourth National Conference on the Classification of Nursing Diagnoses. The cause of the alteration may be excessive or insufficient environmental stimulation, involving either therapeutic restrictions, as isolation, intensive care, or traction, or those socially related, such as institutionalization, excess age, mental illness, or mental retardation; changes in the reception, transmission, or integration of stimuli, because of neurologic disease or trauma, altered status of the sense organs, the inability to communicate, sleep deprivation, or pain; endogenous or exogenous chemical alteration in the perception of stimuli, or psychologic stress or disturbance. The defining characteristics of the disturbance include disorientation, change in the ability to abstract, conceptualize, or solve problems, change in behavior and in sensory acuity, restlessness, irritability, inappropriate response to stimuli, lack of concentration, rapid mood changes, and exaggerated emotional responses, noncompliance, motor incoordination, and hallucination. Other possible defining characteristics are complaints of fatigue, changes in posture and muscular tension, and inappropriate responses. See also **nursing diagnosis.**

sensory-perceptual overload, a state in which the volume and intensity of various stimuli overcome the ability of the individual to discriminate among the varying stimuli. See also **sensory-perceptual alterations.**

SEP, abbreviation for **somatosensory evoked potential.**

separation anxiety, fear and apprehension caused by separation from familiar surroundings and significant persons. The syndrome occurs commonly in an infant when separated from its mother or from its mothering figure or when it is approached by a stranger. In a separation crisis, the child goes through three distinct states. The protest stage is marked by loud cries, which can last for several days and during which the child is inconsolable. In the second phase, the child stops crying and becomes depressed, a result of increasing hopelessness, grief, and mourning. The third stage is one of detachment or denial in which the child outwardly appears to have adjusted but actually has become resigned. See also **anxiety, anxiety neurosis.**

separation factor. See **selectivity.**

separator, an instrument for wedging teeth apart, used in the examination of proximal tooth surfaces and in finishing proximal restorations. It is stabilized against the teeth with modeling compound to prevent tissue damage.

seps-, a combining form meaning 'of or pertaining to decay': *sepsin, sepsis, sepsometer.*

sepsis /sep′sis/, infection, contamination. Compare **asepsis.** **–septic,** *adj.*

-sepsis, a combining form meaning 'decay caused by a (specified) cause or of a (specified) sort': *colisepsis, endosepsis, typhosepsis.*

sept-, **1.** a combining form meaning 'of or pertaining to the nasal septum': *septectomy, septometer, septotomy.* **2.** a combining form meaning 'seven': *septigravida, septipara, septivalent.*

septal defect, an abnormal, usually congenital defect in the wall separating two chambers of the heart. Depending on the size and the site of the defect, various amounts of oxygenated and deoxygenated blood mix, causing a decrease in the amount of oxygen carried in the blood to the peripheral tissues. Kinds of septal defects are **atrial septal defect** and **ventricular septal defect.**

septate, pertaining to a structure divided by a septum.

-septic, a combining form meaning 'referring to decay of a sort or associated with a (specified) cause': *aseptic, colyseptic, uroseptic.*

septic abortion, spontaneous or induced termination of a pregnancy in which the life of the mother may be threatened because of the invasion of germs into the endometrium, myometrium, and beyond, requiring immediate and intensive care, massive antibiotic therapy, evacuation of the uterus, and, often, emergency hysterectomy to prevent death from overwhelming infection and septic shock. Compare **infected abortion.** See also **criminal abortion, induced abortion.**

septic arthritis, an acute form of arthritis, characterized by bacterial inflammation of a joint caused by the spread of bacteria through the bloodstream from an infection elsewhere in the body or by contamination of a joint during trauma or surgery. The joint is stiff, painful, tender, warm, and swollen. The diagnosis is confirmed by bacteriologic identification of an organism in a specimen obtained by aspiration of the joint. Parenteral antibiotics are given to prevent destruction of the joint and are continued for several weeks after inflammation has resolved. Repeated aspiration of the joint or surgical incision and drainage may be performed to relieve pressure on the joint. Physical therapy as the joint heals is helpful to restore it to full range of motion. Also called **acute bacterial arthritis.**

septicemia /sep′tisē′mē·ə/, systemic infection in which pathogens are present in the circulating bloodstream, having spread from an infection in any part of the body. It is diagnosed by culture of the blood and is vigorously treated with antibiotics. Characteristically, septicemia causes fever, chill, prostration, pain, headache, nausea, or diarrhea. Also called **blood poisoning.** Compare **bacteremia.** See also **septic shock.** **–septicemic,** *adj.*

-septicemia, -septicaemia, a combining form meaning '(condition of the) blood caused by virulent microorganisms': *hemorrhagicsepticemia, pyosepticemia, streptosepticemia.*

septicemic plague, a rapidly fatal form of bubonic plague in which septicemia with meningitis occurs before buboes have had time to form. Compare **bubonic plague, pneumonic plague.** See also **plague, *Yersinia pestis*.**

septic fever, an elevation of body temperature associated with infection by pathogenic microorganisms or in response to a toxin secreted by a microorganism.

septic shock, a form of shock that occurs in septicemia when endotoxins are released from certain bacteria in the bloodstream. The endotoxins cause decreased vascular resistance, resulting in a drastic fall in the blood pressure. Fever, tachycardia, increased respirations, and confusion or coma may also occur. Septic shock is usually preceded by signs of severe infection, often of the genitourinary or GI system. The causative organism is most frequently gram-negative. Antibiotics, vasopressors, and intravenous fluids and volume expanders are usually given. In some cases an antitoxin may be available and effective. Kinds of septic shock include **toxic shock syndrome** and **bacteremic shock.** See also **shock.**

septostomy /septos′təmē/, the creation of an opening in a septum by surgery.

Septra, a trademark for the antibacterial, co-trimoxazole (a 1:5 mixture of the antibacterials trimethoprim and sulfamethoxazole.)

septum /sep′təm/, **septa,** a partition, as the interauricular septum that separates the atria of the heart.

sequela /sikwē′lə/, *pl.* **sequelae,** any abnormal condition that follows and is the result of a disease, treatment, or injury, as paralysis after poliomyelitis, deafness after treatment with an ototoxic drug, or a scar following a laceration.

sequential access memory, a computer process by which data is accessed by scanning sequential blocks of information or records.

sequential imaging, (in nuclear medicine) a diagnostic procedure in which a series of closely timed images of the rapidly changing distribution of an administered radioactive tracer is used to determine a physiologic process or processes within the body.

sequential line imaging, (in NMR imaging) techniques in which the image is built up from successive lines through the object.

sequential multiple analysis (SMA), the biochemical examination of various substances in the blood, as albumin, alkaline phosphatase, bilirubin, calcium, cholesterol, and others, using a computerized laboratory analyzer that produces a printout showing measured values of the substances tested. These analyses are commonly designated as **SMA-6, SMA-12,** or **SMA-18,** according to the number of blood constituents tested.

sequential plane imaging, (in NMR imaging) a technique in which the image of an object is built up from successive planes in the object. In various schemes, the planes are selected by oscillating gradient magnetic fields or selective excitation.

sequential point imaging, (in NMR imaging) techniques in which the image is built from successive point positions in the object.

sequester, to detach, separate, or isolate, as a patient sequestered to prevent the spread of an infection.

sequestered antigens theory, a theory of autoimmunity, stressing the relationship between antigen exposure, immunogenic cells, and body cells, maintaining that immunologic tolerance depends on a certain degree of contact between immunologic cells and body cells and on a certain degree of antigen exposure. The theory holds that certain sequestered antigens in the brain, the lenses of the eye, and spermatozoa are isolated from the circulations of the blood and the lymph and do not contact the immune system. When body tissues are damaged, the sequestered antigens are suddenly exposed to the immune system but are not recognized as such by the body, and an autoimmune reaction results. Compare **forbidden clone theory.**

sequestered edema, edema localized in the tissues surrounding a newly created surgical wound.

sequestrum /sikwes′trəm/, *pl.* **sequestra,** a fragment of dead bone that is partially or entirely detached from the surrounding or adjacent healthy bone.

sequestrum forceps, a forceps with small, powerful teeth used for extracting necrotic or sharp fragments of bone from surrounding tissue.

sequoiasis /sikwoi′əsis/, a type of hypersensitivity pneumonitis common among workers in sawmills where redwood is processed. The antigens are the fungus *Pullularia pullulans* and species of the genus *Graphium,* found in moldy redwood sawdust. Characteristics of the acute disease include chills, fever, cough, dyspnea, anorexia, nausea, and vomiting. Symptoms of the chronic disease include productive cough, dyspnea on exertion, fatigue, and weight loss.

Ser, abbreviation for **serine.**

Ser-Ap-Es, a trademark for an antihypertensive, fixed-combination drug containing a diuretic (hydrochlorothiazide) and antihypertensives (reserpine and hydralazine hydrochloride).

Serax, a trademark for a tranquilizer (oxazepam).

serendipity, the act of accidental discovery. A number of important medications have evolved through serendipity, as the discovery of antidepressant activity in a drug originally developed to treat tuberculosis.

Serentil, a trademark for a phenothiazine tranquilizer (mesoridazine).

serial determination, a laboratory test that is repeated at stated intervals, as in a series of repeated tests for cardiac enzymes in blood samples taken from a suspected myocardial infarction patient.

serial dilution, a laboratory technique in which a substance, as blood serum, is decreased in concentration in a series of proportional amounts. In antibody analysis, for example, a serum sample may be distributed in a series of tubes so that each has one half of the amount of the previous tube in the series, resulting in titers of 1:5, 1:10, 1:20, and so on.

serial extraction, the extraction of selected primary teeth over a period of years, sometimes ending with the removal of the first premolar teeth, to relieve crowding of the dental arches during eruption of the lateral incisors, canines, and premolars.

series /sir′ēs/, *pl.* **series** / sir′ēs/, a chain of objects or events arranged in a predictable order, as the series of stages through which a mature blood cell develops.

serine (Ser) /ser′ēn/, a nonessential amino acid found in many proteins in the body. It is a precursor of the amino acids, glycine and cysteine. See also **amino acid, protein.**

Sernylan, a trademark for a veterinary anesthetic (phencyclidine hydrochloride), used illicitly as a euphoric called **PCP.**

sero-, a combining form meaning 'of or pertaining to blood serum': *seroculture, serogenesis, serolin.*

serologic diagnosis /siroloj′ik/, a diagnosis that is made through laboratory examination of antigen-antibody reactions in the serum. Also called **immunodiagnosis, serum diagnosis.**

serologist, a bacteriologist or medical technologist who prepares or supervises the preparation of serums used to diagnose and treat diseases and to immunize persons against infectious diseases.

serology, the branch of laboratory medicine that studies blood serum for evidence of infection by evaluating antigen-antibody reactions in vitro. **–serologic, serological,** *adj.*

Seromycin, a trademark for a tuberculostatic (cycloserine).

serosa /sirō′sə/, any serous membrane, as the tunica serosa that lines the walls of body cavities and secretes a watery exudate.

serosanguineous /sir′ōsang·gwin′ē·əs/, (of a discharge) thin and red; composed of serum and blood. Also **serosanguinous** /sir′ōsang′gwinəs/.

serotonin /ser′ətō′nin, sir′-/, a naturally occurring derivative of tryptophan found in platelets and in cells of the brain and the intestine. Serotonin is released from platelets on damage to the blood vessel walls. It acts as a potent vasoconstrictor. Serotonin in intestinal tissue stimulates the smooth muscle to contract. In the central nervous system, it acts as a neurotransmitter. Lysergic acid diethylamide interferes with the action of serotonin in the brain. The normal concentrations of serotonin in the urine are 0.05 to 0.2 μg/ml. Also called **5-hydroxytryptamine.**

serous fluid /sir′əs/, a fluid that has the characteristics of serum.

serous membrane, one of the many thin sheets of tissue that line closed cavities of the body, as the pleura lining the thoracic cavity, the peritoneum lining the abdominal cavity, and the pericardium lining the sac that encloses the heart. Between the visceral layer of serous membrane covering various organs and the parietal layer lining the cavity containing such organs is a potential space moistened by serous fluid. The fluid reduces the friction of the structures covered by the serous membrane, as the lungs, which move against the thoracic walls in respiration. Compare **mucous membrane, skin, synovial membrane.**

Serpasil, a trademark for an antihypertensive (reserpine).

Serpasil-Apresoline, a trademark for a fixed-combination drug containing two antihypertensives (reserpine and hydralazine hydrochloride).

Serpasil-Esidrix, a trademark for an antihypertensive fixed-combination drug containing a diuretic (hydrochlorothiazide) and an antihypertensive (reserpine).

serpent ulcer, an ulceration of the skin that heals in one area while extending to another. Also called **serpiginous ulcer.**

Serratia /serā′shə/, a genus of motile, gram-negative bacilli capable of causing infection in humans, including bacteremia, pneumonia, and urinary tract infections. *Serratia* organisms are frequently acquired in hospitals. See also **nosocomial infection.**

serratus anterior /serā′təs/, a thin muscle of the chest wall extending from the ribs under the arm to the scapula. Arising from the outer surface and upper border of the first eight or nine ribs, it inserts into the medial angle, the vertebral border, and the inferior angle of the scapula. It is innervated by the long thoracic nerve of the brachial plexus that contains fibers of the fifth, the sixth, and the seventh cervical nerves. It acts to rotate the scapula and to raise the shoulder, as in full flexion and abduction of the arm. Compare **pectoralis major, pectoralis minor, subclavius.**

Sertoli-Leydig cell tumor. See **arrhenoblastoma.**

serum /sir′əm/, **1.** also called **blood serum.** any serous fluid, especially that moistening the surfaces of serous membranes. **2.** any clear, watery fluid that has been separated from its more solid elements, as the exudate from a blister. **3.** the clear, thin, and sticky fluid portion of the blood that remains after coagulation. Like plasma, it contains no blood cells or platelets; unlike plasma it contains no fibrinogen. The fibrinogen present in whole blood is consumed by the clotting process, leaving the serum separate, as can be seen in a standing tube of clotted blood. **4.** a vaccine or toxoid prepared from the serum of a hyperimmune donor for prophylaxis against a particular infection or poison.

serum albumin, a major protein in blood plasma, important in maintaining the oncotic pressure of the blood.

serum C-reactive protein. See **C-reactive protein.**

serum diagnosis. See **serologic diagnosis.**

serum glutamic oxaloacetic transaminase (SGOT), a catalytic enzyme found in various parts of the body, especially the heart, liver, and muscle tissue. Increased amounts of the enzyme occur in the serum as a result of myocardial infarction, acute liver disease, the actions of certain drugs, and any disease or condition in which cells are seriously damaged. See also **transaminase.**

serum glutamic pyruvic transaminase (SGPT), a catalytic enzyme normally found in high concentration in the liver. Greater than normal amounts in the serum indicate liver damage. See also **transaminase.**

serum hepatitis. See **hepatitis B.**

serum sickness, an immunologic disorder that may occur 2 to 3 weeks after the administration of an antiserum. It is caused by an antibody reaction to an antigen in the donor serum and is characterized by fever, splenomegaly, swollen lymph nodes, skin rash, and joint pain. Treatment is symptomatic and supportive and may include corticosteroids. See also **angioneurotic edema, antigen-antibody reaction, Arthus reaction.**

service of process, (in law) the delivery of a writ, summons, or complaint to a defendant. Once delivered or left with the party for whom it is intended, it is said to have been served. The original of the document is shown; a copy is served. Service of process gives reasonable notice to allow the person to appear, testify, and be heard in court.

sesamoid bone, any one of numerous small, round, bony masses embedded in certain tendons that may be subjected to compression and tension. The largest sesamoid bone is the patella, which is embedded in the tendon of the quadriceps femoris at the knee.

sesqui-, a combining form meaning 'one and one half': *sesquibasic, sesquibo, sesquihora.*

sessile /ses′əl/, **1.** (in biology) attached by a base rather than by a stalk or a peduncle, as a leaf that is attached directly to its stem. **2.** permanently connected.

set-, a combining form meaning 'of or related to a bristle': *setaceous, setiferous, seton.*

settlement, (in law) an agreement made between parties to a suit before a judgment is rendered by a court.

setup, **1.** an arrangement of teeth on a trial denture base. **2.** a laboratory procedure in which teeth are removed from a plaster cast and repositioned in wax, used as a diagnostic procedure or to produce a mold for a positioner appliance.

seventh cranial nerve. See **facial nerve.**

severe combined immunodeficiency disease (SCID), an abnormal condition characterized by the complete absence or by the marked deficiency of B cells and T cells with the consequent lack of humoral immunity and cell-mediated immunity. This disease occurs as an X-linked recessive disorder only in males and as an autosomal recessive disorder affecting both males and females. It results in a pronounced susceptibility to infection and is usually fatal. The precise cause of SCID is not known, but research indicates it may be caused by a cytogenic dysfunction of the embryonic stem cells in differentiating B cells and T cells. The affected individual consequently has a very small thymus and little or no protection against infection.

■ OBSERVATIONS: Pronounced susceptibility to infection usually becomes obvious in affected individuals 3 to 6 months after birth, when maternal immunoglobulin reserves are diminishing. Diagnosis is difficult because B cell immunity dysfunction is hard to detect in any individual until 5 months after birth, when immunoglobulin levels should be 1% of normal. Infants with SCID commonly fail to thrive and develop a variety of complications, as sepsis, watery diarrhea, persistent pulmonary infections, and common viral infections that are often fatal. Some infants with SCID develop mild infections and low-grade fevers that last for several months, while the infant uses maternal immunoglobulin stores, and then flare into serious, fatal conditions when maternal antibodies are totally depleted, usually within 1 year. Some of the more obvious symptoms after the infant has used most of the maternal immunoglobulin stores are cyanosis, rapid respirations, and normal chest sounds with an abnormal chest x-ray picture. Maternal IgG is persistent and gram-negative infections in the infant usually do not appear until after the sixth month of life. Normal infants less than 5 months of age have very small amounts of IgM and IgA, and normal IgG levels only reflect maternal IgG. The combination of several symptoms may confirm the diagnosis of SCID. Such symptoms include the absence or the severe reduction of T cell and B cell immunity, a lymph node biopsy that shows no lymphocytes, plasma cells, or lymphoid follicles, and no skin reaction to swabbing with dinitrochlorobenzene. Most infants with SCID die from severe infection within 1 year after birth.

■ INTERVENTION: Treatment of SCID seeks to develop the immune system and to prevent infection. The only satisfactory treatment available to correct immunodeficiency is histocompatible bone marrow transplant, but such a procedure may cause a graft-versus-host reaction, thus increasing the risk of infection and fatal consequences. Placing the infant with SCID in a completely sterile environment for a long time is a method of treatment that has prolonged the lives of some affected individuals, but this option does not prove successful if the infant involved has already had recurring infections.

■ NURSING CONSIDERATIONS: Supportive treatment is the primary approach in caring for the SCID patient. Nurses commonly try to promote an encouraging atmosphere of growth and development while providing the parents of SCID infants with spiritual and psychologic support in the face of the nearly inevitable early death of the patient. The infant must remain in strict protective isolation and benefits from frequent parental visits, gifts of toys, and frequent nursing attention. Toys brought to an infant in protective isolation should be the kind that can be easily sterilized.

Sevin, a trademark for carbaryl, a widely used carbamate insecticide that causes reversible inhibition of cholinesterase. Although less toxic than parathion, carbaryl, when concentrated, may produce skin irritation and systemic poisoning characterized by nausea, vomiting, cramps, diarrhea, diaphoresis, excessive salivation, dyspnea, weakness, loss of coordination, and slurred speech;

large doses may cause coma and death. Carbaryl on the skin is promptly removed by washing with water. Treatment of systemic poisoning includes the immediate intravenous or intramuscular injection of 1 to 4 mg of atropine sulfate, the administration of artificial respiration and oxygen, gastric lavage, and intravenous isotonic saline to correct dehydration.

sex, **1.** a classification of male or female based on many criteria, among them anatomic and chromosomal characteristics. **2.** coitus. Compare **gender.**

sex-, a combining form meaning 'six': *sexdigitate, sexivalent, sextan.*

sex chromatin, a densely staining mass within the nucleus of all nondividing cells of normal mammalian females. It represents the facultative heterochromatin of the inactivated X chromosome. Examination of cells obtained by amniocentesis for the presence or absence of sex chromatin is a technique used for determining the sex of a baby before birth. Sex chromatin is also found as a drumsticklike mass attached to one of the nuclear lobes in polymorphonuclear leukocytes in normal females. Also called **Barr body.** See also **Lyon hypothesis.**

sex chromosome, a chromosome that is responsible for the sex determination of offspring; it carries genes that transmit sex-linked traits and conditions. In humans and other mammals there are two distinct sex chromosomes, the X and the Y chromosomes, which are unequally paired and appear in females in the XX combination and in males as XY. Compare **autosome.**

sex chromosome mosaic, an individual or organism whose cells contain variant chromosomal numbers involving the X or Y chromosomes. Such variations are found in most of the syndromes associated with sex chromosome aberrations, primarily Turner's syndrome, and may be caused by nondisjunction of the chromosomes during the second meiotic division of gametogenesis or by some error in chromosome distribution during cell division of the fertilized ovum. Sex chromosome mosaics often have sexual abnormalities, but because of the sex hormones the overall phenotype is uniform and not mosaic in external characteristics, as in certain animals and insects. See also **intersexuality.**

sex-controlled. See **sex-influenced.**

sex factor. See **F factor.**

sex-influenced, of or pertaining to an autosomal genetic trait or condition, as patterned baldness or gout, that in one sex is expressed phenotypically in both homozygotes and heterozygotes, whereas in the other sex a phenotypic effect is produced in homozygotes only. Also called **sex-controlled.**

sexism, a belief that one sex is superior to the other and that the superior sex has endowments, rights, prerogatives, and status greater than those of the inferior sex. Sexism results in discrimination in all areas of life and acts as a limiting factor in educational, professional, and psychologic development. **–sexist,** *n.*

sex-limited, of or pertaining to an autosomal genetic trait or condition that is expressed phenotypically in only one sex, although the genes for them may be carried by both sexes. Such traits or conditions are typically influenced by hormonal or environmental conditions.

sex-linked, pertaining to genes or to the normal or abnormal characteristics or conditions they transmit. The genes are carried on the sex chromosomes, specifically the X chromosome. See also **sex-linked disorder, X-linked inheritance, Y-linked.** **–sex linkage,** *n.*

sex-linked disorder, any disease or abnormal condition that is determined by the sex chromosomes or a defective gene on a sex chromosome. These may involve a deviation in the number of either the X or Y chromosomes, as occurs in Turner's syndrome and Kleinfelter's syndrome, most occurrences of which are caused as a result of nondisjunction during meiosis. Such aberrations in the number of sex chromosomes do not produce the severe clinical effects that are associated with autosomal aberrations, although some degree of mental deficiency is usually apparent. Other sex-linked disorders are transmitted by single gene defects carried on the X chromosome. X-linked dominant mutants, as hypophosphatemic vitamin D resistant rickets, are rare, and males are more seriously affected than females. In inheritance patterns, X-linked dominant conditions are transmitted by affected males to all of their daughters but none of their sons, by affected heterozygous females to one half of their children regardless of sex, and by affected homozygous females to all of their children. X-linked recessive mutants are more common and are responsible for such traits and disorders as color blindness, ocular albinism, the Xg blood types, hemophilia, the Duchenne type of muscular dystrophy, and inborn errors of metabolism. Such conditions are always transmitted by females so that those predominantly affected are males, because they have only one X chromosome and all genes, whether recessive or dominant, are expressed. Affected males never transmit the condition to their sons, but all of their daughters will be carriers; they, in turn, will transmit the trait to one half of their sons. Occasionally, heterozygous females for X-linked recessive disorders show varying degrees of expression but never as severe as those of the affected male. There are no known clinically significant traits or conditions associated with the genes on the Y chromosome; its only known function is triggering the development of male characteristics.

sex-linked ichthyosis, a congenital skin disorder characterized by large, thick, dry scales that are dark in color and that cover the neck, scalp, ears, face, trunk, and flexor surfaces of the body, as the folds of the arms and the backs of the knees. It is transmitted by females as an X-linked recessive trait and appears only in males. The condition is managed by topical applications of emollients and the use of keratolytic agents to facilitate removal of the scales. Also called **X-linked ichthyosis.** See also **ichthyosis.**

sex mosaic. See **sex chromosome mosaic.**

sex role, the expectations held by society regarding what behavior is appropriate or inappropriate for each sex.

sexual, of or pertaining to sex.

sexual abuse, the sexual mistreatment of another person by fondling, rape, or forced participation in unnatural sex acts or other perverted behavior. When children are victims, they tend to experience a traumatic feeling of loss of control of themselves.

sexual dwarf, an adult dwarf whose genital organs are normally developed.

sexual dysfunction, a nursing diagnosis accepted by the Fourth National Conference on the Classification of Nursing Diagnoses. The cause of the condition may be a biologic, psychologic, or social alteration in sexuality caused by an ineffectual or absent role model, physical abuse, psychosocial abuse, as in a harmful relationship, misinformation or lack of information, a conflict in values, a lack of privacy, or an alteration in body structure or function, as may result from surgery, congenital anomalies, or trauma. The defining characteristics of the condition include a statement by the client of the perceived dysfunction, a physical alteration or limitation imposed by disease or treatment, a reported inability to achieve sexual satisfaction, an alteration in the sexual relationship with the partner, and a change in interest in the self or in others. See also **female sexual dysfunction, male sexual dysfunction, nursing diagnosis.**

sexual generation, reproduction by the union of male and female gametes.

sexual harassment, an aggressive, sexually motivated act of physical or verbal violation of a person over whom the aggressor has some power. Sexual harassment of women in the workplace is against the law, because it represents an abridgment of the victim's right to equal opportunity, privacy, and freedom from assault. Sexual harassment may be heterosexual or, as is common in prison, homosexual.

sexual history, (in a patient record) the portion of the patient's personal history concerned with sexual function and dysfunction. A sexual history is particularly important in gathering data from a patient who has a disease of the reproductive tract, who experiences sexual dysfunction, or who requests contraception, abortion, or sterilization. The extent of the history varies with the patient's age and condition and the reason for securing the history. A short sexual history is recommended as part of every complete physical examination. The therapist needs a detailed sexual history to understand the patient's complaint and to plan treatment. It may include age at onset of sexual intercourse, the kind and frequency of sexual activity, and the satisfaction derived from it.

sexual intercourse. See **coitus.**

sexuality, **1.** the sum of the physical, functional, and psychologic attributes that are expressed by one's gender identity and sexual behavior, whether or not related to the sex organs or to procreation. **2.** the genital characteristics that distinguish male from female.

sexually deviant personality, a sexual behavior that differs significantly from what is considered normal for a society. Either the quality or object of the sexual drives may be at variance with the accepted cultural norms for adults. However, the forms of sexual behavior considered as deviant for adults are often a part of normal psychosexual growth and development.

sexually transmitted disease (STD), a contagious disease usually acquired by sexual intercourse or genital contact. These diseases are the most common communicable diseases and the incidence has risen over the past 2 decades despite improved methods of diagnosis and treatment. Historically, the five venereal diseases were gonorrhea, syphilis, chancroid, granuloma inguinale, and lymphogranuloma venereum. To these have been added scabies, herpes genitalis and anorectal herpes and warts, pediculosis, trichomoniasis, genital candidiasis, molluscum contagiosum, nonspecific urethritis, chlamydial infections, cytomegalovirus, and AIDS. Also called **venereal disease.** See also specific dieseases.

sexual melancholia, *obsolete.* a state of depression in a man resulting from the belief that he is impotent. See also **bipolar disorder, depression.**

sexual psychopath, an individual whose sexual behavior is openly perverted, antisocial, and criminal. See also **antisocial personality disorder.**

sexual reassignment, a change in the gender identity of a person by legal, surgical, hormonal, or social means.

sexual reflex, (in males) a reflex in which tactile or cerebral stimulation results in penile erection, in priapism, or in ejaculation. Also called **genital reflex.**

sexual sadism. See **sadism.**

sexual selection, the theory that mates are chosen according to the attraction of or preference for certain characteristics, as coloration or behavior patterns, so that eventually only those particular traits appear in succeeding generations. The theory explains the wide variety of sexual characteristics among the various species.

SFD, abbreviation for **small for dates.** See **small for gestational age infant.**

SGA, abbreviation for **small for gestational age.** See **small for gestational age infant.**

SGOT, abbreviation for **serum glutamic oxaloacetic transaminase.**

SGPT, abbreviation for **serum glutamic pyruvic transaminase.**

shadow cells, red blood cells that have lost their hemoglobin because of exposure to urine. Also called **ghost cells.**

shadow chart, a copy of the data contained in the permanent patient record, made for use when it is important to have the information at hand and when retrieval of the record from the record room may be difficult or time-consuming.

shallow breathing, a respiration pattern marked by slow, shallow, and generally ineffective inspirations and expirations. It is usually caused by drugs and indicates depression of the medullary respiratory centers.

shaping, a procedure used for conditioning a person undergoing behavior therapy to develop new behavioral responses. Initially, any act remotely resembling the desired behavior is reinforced; gradually, the criterion is made more stringent until the desired response is attained.

shared paranoid disorder, a psychopathologic condition characterized by identical manifestations of the same mental disorder, usually ideas, in two closely associated or related persons. Also called **folie à deux** /fôlē′ädœ′, -dā′, -do͞o′/.

shared services, administrative, clinical, or other service functions that are common to two or more hospitals or other health care facilities and which are used jointly or cooperatively by them.

Sharpey's fiber, (in dentistry) any one of the many collagenous fibers that blend with the cementum of a tooth.

shaving stroke, a phase of the working stroke of a periodontal curet, used for smoothing or planing a tooth or tooth root surface.

SHCC, abbreviation for **Statewide Health Coordinating Committee.**

shearling, a sheepskin placed on a bed to help prevent decubitus ulcers.

sheath, a tubular structure that surrounds an organ or any other part of the body, as the sheath of the rectus abdominis muscle or the sheath of Schwann, which covers various nerve fibers.

Sheehan's syndrome, a postpartum condition of pituitary necrosis and hypopituitarism after circulatory collapse resulting from uterine hemorrhaging.

sheep cell test, a method that mixes human blood cells with the red blood cells of sheep to determine the absence or the deficiency of human T-lymphocytes. When mixed with human blood cells, the red blood cells of sheep cluster around the human T-lymphocytes and form characteristic rosettes. An electron microscope is used to identify the rosettes. An absence or a decrease in the number of rosettes indicates a deficiency or absence of T cells. The sheep cell test is used to diagnose several diseases, as DiGeorge's syndrome, which decreases or destroys the cellular immunity provided by T cells.

sheet bath, the application of wet sheets to the body, used primarily as an antipyretic procedure.

shellfish poisoning, a toxic, neurologic condition that results from eating clams, oysters, or mussels that have ingested the poisonous protozoa commonly called the "red tide." The characteristic symptoms appear within a few minutes and include nausea, light-headedness, vomiting, and tingling or numbness around the mouth, followed by paralysis of the extremities and, possibly, respiratory paralysis. Saxitoxin, the causative agent, is not destroyed by cooking; however, the severity of the illness is diminished if the water used in cooking is not consumed. Treatment includes an intravenous injection of a weak solution of prostigmin methylsulfate and the administration of oxygen and artificial respiration.

shell shock, any of a number of mental disorders, ranging from extreme fear to dementia, commonly attributed to the noise and concussion of exploding shells or bombs but actually resulting from a traumatic reaction to the stress of combat. See also **combat fatigue, posttraumatic stress disorder.**

shell teeth, a type of dental dysplasia characterized by large pulp chambers, insufficient coronal dentin, and, usually, no roots.

sheltered workshop, a facility or program, either for outpatients or for residents of an institution, that provides vocational experience in a controlled working environment. The workshop also offers related vocational rehabilitation services, as job interview training, to persons with physical or mental disabilities.

shield, (in radiation technology) a material for preventing or reducing the passage of charged particles or radiation. A shield may be designated by the radiation it is intended to absorb, as a gamma ray shield, or according to the kind of protection it is intended to give, as a background, biologic, or thermal shield. Lucite and aluminum can be used for beta-radiation shields, but lead is required for gamma ray shields. The amount of material needed to provide shielding is expressed as the half-value layer, which is the quantity required to reduce the radiation intensity at a point in space by one half.

shift, **1.** (in nursing) the particular hours of the day during which a nurse is scheduled to work. The day shift is usually 7:00 AM to 3:00 PM or 8:00 AM to 4:00 PM. The evening shift is usually 3:00 PM to 11:00 PM or 4:00 PM to 12:00 midnight, and the night shift the remaining hours. The evening shift is also called "relief," presumably because nurses originally worked 12-hour shifts and the evening and night shift was thought to be relief for the day nurse. Nurses are said to "work shift" when they work assigned hours. Other nurses do not "work shift" but set their own hours. Many innovations in staffing practice currently allow variations on the traditional 5-day, 40-hour week, as a nurse electing to work a shorter week, preferring longer hours for fewer days. **2.** an abrupt change in an analytic system that continues at the new level.

shift to the left, *informal.* a predominance of immature lymphocytes, noted in a differential white blood cell count. It is usually indicative of an infection or inflammation. The term derives from a graph of blood components in which immature cell frequencies appear on the left side of the graph.

shift to the right, (in hematology) a preponderence of polymorphonuclear neutrophils having three or more lobes, indicating maturity of the cell. The phenomenon is common in severe liver disease and advanced pernicious anemia. It indicates a relative lack of blood-forming activity.

Shigella /shigel′ə/, a genus of gram-negative pathogenic bacteria that causes gastroenteritis and bacterial dysentery, as *Shigella dysenteriae*. See also **shigellosis.**

shigellosis /shig′əlō′sis/, an acute bacterial infection of the bowel, characterized by diarrhea, abdominal pain, and fever, that is transmitted by hand-to-mouth contact with the feces of individuals infected with bacteria of a pathogenic species of the genus *Shigella* species. These organisms may be carried in the stools of asymptomatic people for up to several months and may be spread through contact with contaminated objects, food, or flies, especially in poor, crowded areas. The disease occurs in isolated outbreaks in the United States but is endemic in underdeveloped areas of the world. It is especially common and usually most severe in children. Diagnosis is made by isolating and identifying *Shigella* in a specimen of stool. The likelihood of encountering or engendering antibiotic-resistant organisms is very high, therefore the preferred treatment for shigellosis is supportive and the major goal is to prevent dehydration. Antimicrobials are given if the disease is severe or if the likelihood of further transmission is great. Isolation and strict handwashing precautions are instituted. Shigellosis infections must be reported to the public health department. Also called **bacillary dysentery.**

shin bone. See **tibia.**

shingles. See **herpes zoster.**

shin splints, a painful condition of the lower leg caused by strain of the long flexor muscle of the toes after strenuous athletic activity, as running. In many instances it is the result of inadequate training. Treatment usually involves rest and exercise therapy. Surgery is sometimes necessary.

Shirodkar's operation /shir′odkärz′/, a surgical procedure called a cerclage in which the cervical canal is closed by a purse-string suture embedded in the uterine cervix encircling the canal. It is performed to correct an incompetent cervix that has failed to retain previous pregnancies. Under spinal block or general anesthesia, a 5 mm wide band of nonabsorbable material is buried beneath the mucosa of the cervix and pulled in a purse-string manner to close the cervix. The band may be left in place permanently, in which case subsequent deliveries are by cesarean section. Occasionally, a temporary cerclage is done, sewing in the band and leaving the ends exposed in the vagina. The band is then removed before labor and vaginal delivery. Postoperatively, infection or vaginal fistula may occur. If labor begins with the suture in place, the suture is removed promptly or the infant is delivered by cesarean section, before rupture of the uterus occurs.

shistocytes /shis′tōsīts/, cell fragments of erythrocytes, a characteristic of hemolysis or cell fragmentation associated with severe burns and intravascular coagulation.

shock, an abnormal condition of inadequate blood flow to the body's peripheral tissues, with life-threatening cellular dysfunction, hypotension, and oliguria. The condition is usually associated with inadequate cardiac output, changes in peripheral blood flow resistance and distribution, and tissue damage. Causal factors include hemorrhage, vomiting, diarrhea, inadequate fluid intake, or excessive renal loss, resulting in hypovolemia. Kinds of shock include **anaphylactic shock, bacteremic shock, cardiogenic shock, diabetic shock, electric shock, hypovolemic shock,** and **neurogenic shock.**

■ OBSERVATIONS: The signs and symptoms of different kinds of shock are similar and are related to the condition of hypovolemia. There is decreased blood flow with a resulting reduction in the delivery of oxygen, nutrients, hormones, and electrolytes to the body's tissues and a concomitant decreased removal of metabolic wastes. Pulse and respirations are increased. There may be tachycardia. Blood pressure may decline moderately at first. The patient often shows signs of restlessness and anxiety, an effect related to decreased blood flow to the brain. There may also be weakness, lethargy, pallor, and a cool, moist skin. As shock progesses, the body temperature falls, respirations become rapid and shallow, and the pulse pressure (the difference between systolic and diastolic blood pressures) narrows. Urinary output is reduced. Hemorrhage may be apparent or concealed although other factors, as vomiting or diarrhea, may account for the deficiency of body fluids.

■ INTERVENTION: Blood volume must be restored quickly so that there can be a rapid return of oxygenated blood to the perfusion-deprived tissues. Blood volume is expanded with intravenous fluids, as a lactated Ringer's solution or a 5% dextrose in normal saline solution. Whole blood, plasma, and plasma substitutes may also be given. Nothing should be given by mouth, and sedatives, tranquilizers, or narcotics should not be administered, with the exception that morphine may be given intravenously in cases of severe pain. However, respiratory depression must be avoided because hypoventilation and hypoxemia with acidosis can lead to death. Respiratory assistance should be given with a high oxygen concentration if needed. Metabolic acidosis may be reversed by giving sodium bicarbonate. A central venous catheter is inserted for monitoring of vital signs and prevention of pulmonary edema that can result from overhydrating the patient's circulatory system.

■ NURSING CONSIDERATIONS: After vital functions are restored and diagnosis has been carried out, the shock patient must be monitored continuously until recovery is assured. The patient should remain flat in bed, but if there are no head injuries, the lower extremities can be raised slightly to improve venous return. The Trendelenburg position should be avoided because it tends to push the abdominal organs against the diaphragm, reducing effectiveness of the heart and lung functions. Position changes should be made slowly and gently. The patient must be kept warm, but external heat should be avoided. If shivering occurs, just enough covering should be added to control the shivering. Vasoactive drugs may be ordered when the blood volume is adequate. In some instances, extreme vasoconstriction may result in pain requiring analgesic medications. The patient's skin color, temperature, intravenous and oral fluid intakes, urinary output, and level of consciousness should be checked at frequent intervals and recorded in written form.

shock lung. See **acute respiratory distress syndrome.**

shock trousers, pneumatic trousers designed to counteract hypotension, associated with internal or external bleeding, and hypovolemia. Shock trousers may be contraindicated in patients with pulmonary edema, cardiogenic shock, increased intracranial pressure, or eviscerations.

■ METHOD: The shock trousers are required when the patient loses consciousness, has a decreased or falling blood pressure, and shows signs of respiratory distress, as dyspnea, rapid breathing, a cough, and pink, frothy sputum. The leg pulses may be diminished or absent, and the feet may appear pale, mottled, and cold. Before the pressurized trousers are applied, they are checked for tears or leaks and the proper functioning of their valves; any kinks or twists in the tubes connecting the trousers to the pneumatic pump are removed. The patient is placed in a flat, supine position over the open trousers and the leg sections and portion that encircles the abdomen just below the rib cage are firmly secured in place by closing the Velcro straps or zippers. The exact times at which the trousers' sections are inflated are recorded, and the inflated sections are checked every 15 minutes. The patient's blood pressure, respiration, apical and peripheral pulses are also checked every 15 minutes, and chest sounds are auscultated hourly. Parenteral fluids, whole blood, plasma protein fractions, and other plasma volume expanders are administered as ordered; the flow rate of expanders is adjusted according to central venous pressure readings. An indwelling urethral catheter is connected to a closed gravity drainage system, and fluid intake and output are measured hourly; if less than 30 ml of urine per hour are excreted, renal failure may occur. Monitoring of blood gases and intermittent suctioning through a nasogastric tube may be ordered. The trousers are not deflated or removed until the blood volume replacement is stable and the patient's physician is in attendance. As each section of the trousers, starting with the abdominal section, is gradually deflated, the patient's blood pressure, respiration, and apical pulse are checked every 5 to 10 minutes; if the blood pressure drops 4 to 6 mm Hg, deflation is stopped.

■ NURSING ORDERS: The nurse checks, applies, and inflates the shock trousers and remains with the patient during the entire procedure. The vital signs are monitored at frequent intervals, parenteral fluids and plasma volume expanders are given, measures of the intake and output are taken and recorded, and emotional support is provided.

short-acting, pertaining to or characterizing a therapeutic agent, usually a drug, with a brief period of effectiveness, generally beginning soon after the substance or measure is administered.

short-acting insulin, an aqueous preparation of the antidiabetic principle of beef pancreas or pork pancreas that begins to act within 1 hour of injection and reaches a peak of action in 2 to 4 hours. The duration of action of regular insulin is 4 to 6 hours and of crystalline zinc insulin 5 to 8 hours. Also called **rapid-acting insulin.** See also **insulin.** Compare **intermediate-acting insulin, long-acting insulin.**

shortage area, a geographic area, county as a census tract, or area designated by the federal government as being undersupplied with certain kinds of health care services, hence possibly eligible for aid under certain federal programs, including the National Health Service Corps or the Rural Clinics Assistance Act.

short-arm cast, an orthopedic cast applied to immobilize the hand or the wrist. The short-arm cast incorporates the hand below the wrist; it is used in treating fractures, for postoperative positioning, and for correction or maintenance of correction of deformities of the hand and the wrist. Compare **long-arm cast.**

shorting, the fraudulent practice of dispensing a quantity of drug less than that called for in the prescription and of charging for the quantity specified in the prescription. See also **kiting.**

short-leg cast, an orthopedic cast used for immobilizing fractures in the lower extremities from the toes to the knee. The short-leg cast is also used in severe sprains and torn soft tissue of the ankle, for postoperative positioning and immobilization of the foot and the ankle, and for correction or maintenance of correction of a deformity of the foot or the ankle. Compare **long-leg cast.**

short-leg cast with walker, an orthopedic cast applied to immobilize the lower extremities from the toes to the knee while allowing the patient to walk by incorporating a rubber walker on the bottom of the cast. The short-leg cast with walker is used when weight-bearing ambulation is desired during the period immobilization is achieved with a short-leg cast.

short-PR-normal-QRS syndrome. See **Lown-Ganong-Levine syndrome.**

short sight. See **myopia.**

short-term memory, memory of recent events.

shotgun therapy, *informal.* any treatment that has a wide range of effect and which, therefore, can be expected to correct the abnormal condition even though the particular cause is unknown. Shotgun therapy may cause more than an acceptable rate of side effects and is rarely desirable or necessary.

shoulder, the junction of the clavicle and scapula at the point where the arm attaches to the trunk of the body. See also the Color Atlas of Human Anatomy.

shoulder blade. See **scapula.**

shoulder-hand syndrome, a neuromuscular condition characterized by pain and stiffness in the shoulder and arm, limited joint motion, swelling of the hand, muscle atrophy, and decalcification of the underlying bones. The condition occurs most commonly after myocardial infarction but may be associated with other known or unknown causes.

shoulder joint, the ball and socket articulation of the humerus with the scapula. The joint includes eight bursae and five ligaments, including the glenoidal labrum that deepens the articular cavity and protects the edges of articulating bones. Also called **humeral articulation.**

shoulder spica cast, an orthopedic cast applied to immobilize the trunk of the body to the hips, the wrist, and the hand. It incorporates a diagonal shoulder support between the hip and arm portions. The shoulder spica cast is used in the treatment of shoulder dislocations and injuries or in the positioning and immobilization of the shoulder after surgery.

shoulder subluxation, the separation of the humeral head from the glenoid cavity, resulting in strain on the soft tissues surrounding the joint.

show. See **vaginal bleeding.**

shreds, glossy filaments of mucus in the urine, indicating inflammation in the urinary tract. Also called **mucous shreds.**

shunt, **1.** to redirect the flow of a body fluid from one cavity or vessel to another. **2.** a tube or device implanted in the body to redirect a body fluid from one cavity or vessel to another.

Shy-Drager syndrome /shī′drā′gər/, a rare, progressive neurologic disorder of young and middle-aged adults. It is characterized by orthostatic hypotension, bladder and bowel incontinence, atrophy of the iris, anhidrosis, tremor, rigidity, incoordination, ataxia, and muscle wasting. Treatment includes drug therapy to control motor symptoms and to maintain an adequate blood pressure. Antigravity stockings may prevent pooling of blood in the lower extremities. See also **orthostatic hypotension.**

Si, symbol for **silicon.**

SI, abbreviation for **Système International d'Unités,** the French name for the **International System of Units.**

SIADH, abbreviation for **syndrome of inappropriate antidiuretic hormone secretion.**

sial-. See **sialo-.**

-sialia, a combining form meaning '(condition of the) saliva': *asialia, oligosialia, polsialia.*

sialo-, sial- a combining form meaning 'of or related to saliva or to the salivary glands': *sialoaerophagy, sialoangitis, sialostenosis.*

sialogogue /sī·al′əgog′/, anything that stimulates the secretion of saliva.

sialography /sī·əlog′rəfē/, a technique in radiology in which a salivary gland is filmed after an opaque substance is injected into its duct. –**sialogram** /sī·al′əgram′/, *n.,* **sialographic,** *adj.*

sialolith /sī·al′əlith/, a calculus formed in a salivary gland or duct.

sialorrhea /sī·al′ərē′ə/, an excessive flow of saliva that may be associated with a variety of conditions, as acute inflammation of the mouth, mental retardation, mercurialism, pregnancy, teething, alcoholism, or malnutrition. Also called **hypersalivation, ptyalism.**

Siamese twins, conjoined, equally developed twin fetuses that were produced from the same ovum. The severity of the condition ranges from superficial fusion, as of the umbilical vessels, to that in which the heads or complete torsos are united and several internal organs are shared. With modern surgical techniques, most Siamese twins can be successfully separated. See also **conjoined twins.**

Siberian tick typhus, a mild, acute febrile illness seen in north, central, and east Asia, caused by *Rickettsia siberica,* transmitted by ticks, and characterized by a diffuse maculopapular rash, headache, conjunctival inflammation, and a small ulcer or eschar at the site of the tick bite. Treatment with chloramphenicol or tetracycline is associated with an excellent prognosis. Also called **North Asian tick-borne rickettsiosis.** See also **rickettsia, typhus.**

sibilant rale, an abnormal whistling sound that may emanate from the lungs of an individual with a respiratory disorder or disease. It is caused by the passage of air through a lumen narrowed by the accumulation of mucus or other viscid fluid.

Siblin, a trademark for a bulk laxative containing psyllium seed.

sibling, **1.** also called *(informal)* **sib.** one of two or more children who have both parents in common; a brother or sister. The number, age differences, sex, and birth order of siblings can greatly affect the childhood environment and relationships within a family. Sibling rivalry and jealousy are common in first-born children, especially when there is a 2- to 4-year difference in age. In general, sibling relationships help teach the child important social patterns and moral values, as competitiveness, loyalty, and sharing. **2.** of or pertaining to a brother or sister.

sibship, **1.** the state of being related by blood. **2.** a group of people descended from a common ancestor who are used as a basis for genetic studies. **3.** brothers and sisters considered as a group.

sicc-, a combining form meaning 'dry': *siccative, siccolabile, siccostabile.*

sickle cell, an abnormal, crescent-shaped red blood cell containing hemoglobin S, an abnormal form of hemoglobin characteristic of sickle cell anemia.

sickle cell anemia, a severe, chronic, incurable, anemic condition that occurs in people homozygous for hemoglobin S (Hb S). The abnormal hemoglobin results in distortion and fragility of the erythrocytes. Sickle cell anemia is characterized by crises of joint pain, thrombosis, and fever and by chronic anemia, with splenomegaly, lethargy, and weakness. See also **congenital nonspherocytic hemolytic anemia, elliptocytosis, hemoglobin S, sickle cell crisis.**

sickle cell crisis, an acute, episodic condition that occurs in children with sickle cell anemia. The crisis may be vasoocclusive, resulting from the aggregation of misshapen erythrocytes, or anemic, resulting from bone marrow aplasia, increased hemolysis, folate deficiency, or splenic sequestration of erythrocytes. See also **hemoglobin S, sickle cell anemia.**

■ OBSERVATIONS: Painful vasoocclusive crisis is the most common of the sickle cell crises. It is usually preceded by an upper respiratory or GI infection without an exacerbation of anemia. The clumps of sickled erythrocytes obstruct blood vessels, resulting in occlusion, ischemia, and infarction of adjacent tissue. Characteristic of this kind of crisis are leukocytosis, acute abdominal pain from visceral hypoxia, painful swelling of the soft tissue of the hands and feet (hand-foot syndrome), and migratory, recurrent, or constant joint pain, often so severe that movement of the joint is limited. Persistent headache, dizziness, convulsions, visual or auditory disturbances, facial nerve palsies, coughing, shortness of breath, and tachypnea may occur if the central nervous system or lungs are affected. Other problems associated with vasoocclusion include priapism, hematuria, and retinopathy. Anemic crisis is characterized by a dramatic, rapid drop in hemoglobin levels resulting from various causes. Aplastic crisis resulting in severe anemia occurs because red blood cell production is diminished by acute viral, bacterial, or fungal infection. Megaloblastic anemia (another form of anemic crisis) results from folic acid deficiency during periods of accelerated erythropoiesis. Severe anemia between crises is not common unless there is a generalized state of malnutrition. Hyperhemolytic crisis, characterized by anemia, jaundice, and reticulocytosis, results from glucose-6-phosphate dehydrogenase deficiency or in reaction to multiple transfusions. Acute sequestration crisis, which occurs in young children 6 months to 5 years of age, results when large quantities of blood suddenly accumulate in the spleen, causing massive splenic enlargement, severe anemia, shock, and, ultimately, death. Susceptibility to infection is a common problem of young children with sickle cell anemia and may be greatly increased during periods of crisis. Systemic infection and septicemia from pneumococcus or *Haemophilus influenzae* are not uncommon and may be rapidly fatal. In older children, local infection, especially osteomyelitis, rather than generalized septicemia is frequently a complicating factor.

■ INTERVENTION: Therapy consists of immediate transfusion of packed red cells in the acute anemic crisis and alleviation of severe abdominal and joint pain with analgesics or narcotics as needed in vasoocclusive crisis. Short-term oxygen therapy, hydration by oral or intravenous means, electrolyte replacement to counteract metabolic acidosis resulting from hypoxia, and antibiotics to treat any existing infection may be necessary. Pneumococcal and meningococcal vaccine is recommended for children between 2 and 5 years of age because they are highly susceptible to infection. Partial exchange transfusions are often mandatory in life-threatening crises, as when sickling occurs in the vessels of the brain or lungs, and may be used as a preventive technique, although multiple transfusions increase the risk of hepatitis, hemosiderosis, and transfusion reactions. Oral anticoagulants have been used to relieve the pain of vasoocclusion, but these increase the risk of bleeding. Priapism, a painful condition frequently seen in vasoocclusive crisis, may be treated by aspirating the corpora cavernosa. In children with recurrent splenic sequestration, splenectomy may be a life-saving procedure. The process is not routinely recommended because surgery increases the risk of acidosis and hypoxia from anesthesia, and, in time, the spleen usually atrophies through progressive fibrotic changes. Infarction of tissue in any organ is a potential hazard in sickle cell crisis, and special management and treatment are warranted by the specific site of damage. Typical complications include uremia (requiring renal transplantation or hemodialysis), chronic functional pulmonary impairment, aseptic necrosis of the hip, and microvascular occlusion that may lead to venous thrombosis.

■ NURSING CONSIDERATIONS: The primary concern of the nurse during a crisis is to initiate procedures that reduce sickling. Foremost is prevention of tissue deoxygenation and resulting hypoxia by maintaining bed rest to minimize energy expenditure and oxygen use, although some exercise is necessary to promote circulation. Hydration and electrolyte balance are essential. A complete record of fluid intake and output is maintained, and adequate therapy is calculated accordingly. Serum sodium is monitored closely to avoid hyponatremia. Oxygen is given in severe anoxia, although prolonged administration depresses bone marrow activity and thus aggravates anemia. Management of pain in vasoocclusion is often difficult and may require experimentation with various drugs and schedules before adequate relief is achieved. The application of warmth is often soothing; cold is contraindicated, because it enhances vasoconstriction and sickling. The nurse constantly monitors the child's condition for splenomegaly, infection, evidence of shock or cerebrovascular accident, hypervolemia, transfusion reaction, or increasing anemia. An important aspect of nursing care is the continued emotional support for parents whose child has a chronic illness that is potentially fatal.

sickle cell thalassemia, a heterozygous blood disorder in which the genes for sickle cell and for thalassemia are both inherited. A mild form and a severe form may be identified, depending on the degree of suppression of beta-chain synthesis by the thalassemia gene. In the mild form synthesis is only partially suppressed, and the red cell may contain from 25% to 35% normal hemoglobin A along with a somewhat greater concentration of hemoglobin S. The clinical course is relatively mild. When beta-chain synthesis is completely suppressed, as in the severe form, only hemoglobin S appears in the red cells, and the clinical course is generally as severe as in homozygous sickle cell anemia. See also **hemoglobinopathy, hemoglobin S, hemoglobin S-C disease, hemoglobin variant.**

sickle cell trait, the heterozygous form of sickle cell anemia, characterized by the presence of both hemoglobin S and hemoglobin A in the red blood cells. It is of little clinical significance. Anemia and the other signs of sickle cell anemia do not occur. People who have the trait are informed and counseled regarding the possibility of having an infant with sickle cell disease if both parents have the trait. See **hemoglobin S.**

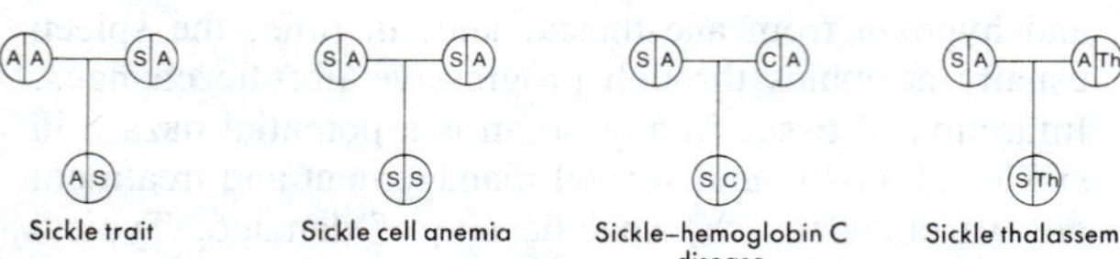

Sickle cell inheritance pattern

sick role, a pattern of behavior in which a person adopts the symptoms of a physical or mental disorder to be cared for, sympathized with, and protected from the demands and stresses of life.

sick sinus syndrome, a complex of syndromes associated with sinus node dysfunction. The condition may result from a variety of cardiac diseases, ranging from cardiomyopathies to inflammatory myocardial disease, but is most commonly related to either intermittent sinoatrial block or inadequate sinoatrial conduction. It is characterized by severe sinus bradycardia alone, sinus bradycardia alternating with tachycardia, or sinus bradycardia with atrioventricular block. The most common symptoms are lethargy, weakness, light-headedness, dizziness, and episodes of near syncope to actual loss of consciousness. The severity of symptoms is related to the duration of the asystolic period. Although many patients may be symptomatic, especially elderly patients with episodes of near syncope associated with a prior history of palpitations, accurate diagnosis can be made only with electrocardiographic documentation of sinoatrial block. At present the only treatment is by the implantation of a permanent demand pacemaker.

side effect, any reaction or consequence that results from a medication or therapy. This can be an effect carried beyond the desired limit, as hemorrhaging from an anticoagulant, or a reaction unrelated to the primary object of the therapy, as an anaphylactic reaction to an antibiotic. Usually, although not necessarily, the effect is undesirable, and may manifest itself as nausea, dry mouth, dizziness, blood dyscrasias, blurred vision, discolored urine, or tinnitus.

sidero-, a combining form meaning 'of or pertaining to iron': *siderocyte, siderofibrous, sideropenic.*

sideroblastic anemia /sid′əroblas′tik/, any one of a heterogenous group of chronic hematologic disorders characterized by normocytic or slightly macrocytic anemia, hypochromic and normochromic red blood cells, and decreased erythropoiesis and hemoglobin synthesis. The red blood cells contain a perinuclear ring of iron-stained granules. The condition may be acquired or hereditary, primary or secondary to another condition or situation. The cause of the disease is not understood. Treatment may include extract of liver, pyridoxine, folic acid, and blood transfusion. Compare **iron deficiency anemia, siderosis.**

siderocyte, an abnormal erythrocyte in which there are visible particles of nonhemoglobin iron.

sideropenic dysphagia. See **Plummer-Vinson syndrome.**

siderosis /sid′ərō′sis/, **1.** a variety of pneumoconiosis caused by the inhalation of iron dust or particles. **2.** the introduction of color in any tissue caused by the presence of excess iron. **3.** an increase in the amounts of iron in the blood. See also **hemochromatosis, hemosiderosis, sideroblastic anemia.**

SIDS, abbreviation for **sudden infant death syndrome.**

sievert (Sv), a unit dose equivalent radiation. The sievert has identical units to the gray and is arrived at by multiplying the absorbed dose by the quality factor, a number that has been determined to accurately compare the health consequences of that type of radiation to x-rays. The rem bears the same relationship to the rad as the sievert does to the gray.

sigh. See **periodic deep inspiration.**

sight, **1.** the special sense that enables the shape, size, position, and color of objects to be perceived; the faculty of vision. It is the major function of the eye. **2.** that which is seen.

Sigma Theta Tau /sig′mə thā′tə tou′/, a national honor society for nurses.

sigmoid /sig′moid/, **1.** of or pertaining to an S shape. **2.** the sigmoid colon.

sigmoid colon, the portion of the colon that extends from the end of the descending colon in the pelvis to the juncture of the rectum.

sigmoidectomy /sig′moidek′təmē/, excision of the sigmoid flexure of the colon, most commonly performed to remove a malignant tumor. A large percentage of cancers of the lower bowel occur in the sigmoid colon.

sigmoid flexure. See **sigmoid colon.**

sigmoid mesocolon /mez′ōkō′lən/, a fold of peritoneum that connects the sigmoid colon with the pelvic wall, forming a curved line of attachment, the apex of the curve located at the division of the left common iliac artery. The fold is continuous with the iliac mesocolon and ends in the median plane over the rectum at the level of the third sacral vertebra. Between the two layers of the fold are the sigmoid and the superior rectal vessels. Compare **mesentery proper, transverse mesocolon.**

sigmoid notch, a concavity on the superior surface of the mandibular ramus between the coronoid and condyloid processes.

sigmoidoscope /sigmoi′dəskōp′/, an instrument used to examine the lumen of the sigmoid colon. It consists of a tube and a light, allowing direct visualization of the mucous membrane lining the colon. Compare **proctoscope.**

sign, an objective finding as perceived by an examiner, as a fever, a rash, the whisper heard over the chest in pleural effusion, or the light band of hair seen in children after recovery from kwashiorkor. Many signs accompany symptoms, as erythema and a maculopapular rash are often seen when a patient complains of pruritus. Compare **symptom.**

signal symptom. See **symptom.**

signal-to-noise ratio (SNR), the number used to describe the relative contribution to a detected signal of the true signal and random superimposed signals or "noise."

significance, **1.** (in research) the statistic probability that a given finding is very unlikely to have occurred by chance alone. The conventional standard for attributing significance is a finding that occurs fewer than 5 times in 100 by chance alone ($p<.05$). **2.** the importance of a study in developing a practice or theory, as in nursing practice.

significant other, a person who is considered by an individual as being special and as having an impact on that individual.

sign-off, a procedure for terminating interaction between a user and a computer. **–sign off,** *v.*

sign-on, a procedure for initiating interaction between a user and a computer. **–sign on,** *v.*

silanization /sil′ənizā′shən/, (in chromatography) the chemical process of converting the SiOH moieties of a stationary form to the ester form.

silent mutation, (in molecular genetics) an alteration in a sequence of nucleotides that does not result in an amino acid change.

silicate dental cement, a relatively hard, translucent material used primarily to restore anterior teeth. Like other dental cements, it is prepared by mixing a liquid and a powder. The powder of silcate cement is acid-soluble glass prepared by fusing oxides of calcium, silicon, aluminum, and other ingredients with a fluoride flux. The liquid is a buffered phosphoric acid solution.

silicon (Si) /sil′ikon/, a nonmetallic element, second to oxygen as the most abundant of the elements. Its atomic number is 14; its atomic weight is 28. It occurs in nature as silicon dioxide and in silicates. The silicates are used as detergents, corrosion inhibitors, adhesives, and sealants. Elemental silicon is used in metallurgy and in transistors and other electronic components. About 60% of the rocks in the earth's crust contain silicon, and silica dusts are associated with many mining operations. Protracted inhalation of silica dusts can cause silicosis, which increases the susceptibility to other pulmonary diseases.

silicone /sil′ikōn/, any organic silicon polymer compound used in medicine, as an adhesive, a lubricant, or a substitute for rubber, especially in prosthetic devices.

silicosis /sil′ikō′sis/, a lung disorder caused by continued, long-term inhalation of the dust of an inorganic compound, silicon dioxide, which is found in sands, quartzes, flints, and in many other stones. Silicosis is characterized by the development of nodular fibrosis in the lungs. In advanced cases, severe dyspnea may develop. The incidence of silicosis is highest among industrial workers exposed to silica powder in manufacturing processes, in those who work with ceramics, sand, or stone, and in those who mine silica. Also called **grinder's disease, quartz silicosis.** See also **chronic obstructive pulmonary disease, inorganic dust.**

silk suture, a braided, fine, black suture material, usually used to close incisions, wounds, and cuts in the skin. It is not absorbed by the body and is removed after approximately 7 days.

silo filler's disease, a rare, acute, respiratory condition seen in agricultural workers who have inhaled nitrogen oxide as they work with fermented fodder in closed, poorly ventilated such as silos. Characteristically, symptoms of respiratory distress and pulmonary edema occur several hours after exposure. Loss of consciousness may occur. Observation in the hospital and respiratory assistance are often required. The condition is rarely fatal.

Silvadene, a trademark for an antibacterial (sulfadiazine silver).

silver (Ag), a whitish precious metal occurring mainly as a sulfide. Its atomic number is 47; its atomic weight is 107.88. It is quite soft and is usually alloyed with small amounts of copper to increase its durability. Silver dissolves readily in nitric acid and is used extensively to produce silver halides used in photographic emulsions. It is frequently associated in small amounts with the ores of zinc, copper, and lead and is used extensively as a component of amalgams of dental fillings and many medications, especially antiseptics and astringents. Some antiseptics containing silver are mild silver protein and strong silver protein, preparations that render silver colloidal in the presence of protein. Mild silver protein contains not less than 19% and not more than 23% silver. Strong silver protein contains not less than 7.5% and not more than 8.5% silver. Both preparations are used externally as antiseptics and do not have irritating properties. Silver nitrate is also used externally as an antiseptic and astringent, especially in the prevention of ophthalmia neonatorium. Silver picrate, the ionizable salt of silver, is used in the treatment of trichomoniasis and in the treatment of moniliasis of the vagina.

silver cone method, a technique for filling tooth root canals. A prefitted silver cone is sealed into the apex of a root canal, and any remaining canal space is filled with gutta-percha or sealer.

Silver dwarf, a person who has **Silver's syndrome,** a congenital disorder in which short stature is associated with lateral asymmetry, various anomalies of the head, face, and skeleton, and precocious puberty.

silver-fork fracture. See **Colles' fracture.**

Silverman-Anderson score, a system of assessing the degree of respiratory distress.

silver nitrate, a topical antiinfective.

■ INDICATIONS: A 1% solution is prescribed for the prevention of gonococcal ophthalmia in newborns and in stronger concentrations for use on wet dressings.

■ CONTRAINDICATIONS: Known sensitivity to this drug prohibits its use. It should not be used with bacitracin, which inactivates silver nitrate.

■ ADVERSE EFFECTS: Among the more serious adverse reactions are severe local inflammation, burns, and argyria.

silver salts poisoning, a toxic condition caused by the ingestion of silver nitrate, characterized by discoloration of the lips, vomiting, abdominal pain, dizziness, and convulsions. Treatment includes gastric lavage with salt water, followed by demulcents and fluid therapy. Anticonvulsant and antihypotensive therapy may be necessary.

Silver's syndrome. See **Silver dwarf.**

silver sulfadiazine, a topical antimicrobial.

■ INDICATIONS: It is prescribed to prevent or treat infection in second- and third-degree burns.

■ CONTRAINDICATIONS: Known hypersensitivity to this drug, to silver, or to sulfonamides prohibits its use. It is not given in the last weeks of pregnancy or to newborn or premature infants.

■ ADVERSE EFFECTS: Among the most serious adverse reactions are rashes, fungal infections, neutropenia, and kernicterus.

simethicone, an antiflatulent.

■ INDICATION: It is prescribed to decrease excess gas in the GI tract.

■ CONTRAINDICATIONS: There are no significant contraindications.

■ ADVERSE EFFECTS: Adverse reactions include belching and rectal flatus.

simian crease, a single crease across the palm from the fusion of proximal and distal palmar creases, seen in congenital disorders, as Down's syndrome. Also called **simian line.**

simian virus 40, a vacuolating virus isolated from the kidney tissue of rhesus monkeys.

simil-, a combining form meaning 'like': *Similac, similimum.*

Similac preparations, a trademark for a group of commercial modified milk products that are prepared especially for infant feeding. They are made from a nonfat base of cow's milk supplemented with such substances as lactose, coconut and soy oils, and mono- and disaccharides and fortified with vitamins and minerals. The ratio of the various nutrients is altered in the different preparations to accommodate infants with particular nutritional requirements, as iron or one of the other minerals, or nutritional problems, as nephrogenic diabetes insipidus. The formulas are packaged in both powder and liquid form.

similarity principle, a rule that objects similar to one another will become organized into one perceptual unit.

Simmonds' disease. See **postpubertal panhypopituitarism.**

simplate bleeding time test, a blood test for determining how quickly platelets form a plug when exposed to air. Platelet plug formation is the first step in clotting and, if slower than 8 minutes, indicates platelet deficiency or the effect of a drug, as aspirin.

simple angioma, a tumor consisting of a network of small vessels or distended capillaries surrounded by connective tissue.

simple cavity, a cavity that involves only one surface of a tooth.

simple fission. See **binary fission.**

simple fracture, an uncomplicated, closed fracture in which the bone does not break the skin. Compare **compound fracture.**

simple mastectomy, a surgical procedure in which a breast is completely removed and the underlying muscles and adjacent lymph nodes are left intact. The procedure may be performed to remove small malignant neoplasms of the breast, or it may be done as a palliative measure to remove an ulcerated carcinoma in advanced breast cancer. Postoperatively, the process of recovery from a simple mastectomy is less uncomfortable and faster than from a radical or modified radical mastectomy, but nursing care is similar. Compare **modified radical mastectomy, radical mastectomy.** See also **mastectomy.**

simple phobia, an anxiety disorder characterized by a persistent, irrational fear of specific things, as animals, dirt, light, or darkness. Compare **social phobia.** See also **phobia.**

simple protein, a protein that yields amino acids as the only or chief product on hydrolysis. The class includes albumins, globulins, glutelins, alcohol-soluble proteins, albuminoids, histones, and protamines. See **complex protein.**

simple schizophrenia, a slow, insidiously progressive form of schizophrenia characterized by apathy, withdrawal, lack of initiative, gradual depletion of emotional reactions, and an impoverishment in human relationships. See also **schizotypal personality disorder.**

simple sugar, a monosaccharide, as glucose.

simple tubular gland, one of the many multicellular glands with only one tube-shaped duct, as various glands within the epithelium of the intestine.

simple vulvectomy. See **vulvectomy.**

Simpson forceps. See **obstetric forceps.**

Sims' position, a position in which the patient lies on the left side with the right knee and thigh drawn upward toward the chest. The chest and abdomen are allowed to fall forward.

simulation, a mode of computer-assisted instruction in which a student receives basic information about a topic and then must interact with the computer to gain deeper understanding of the information and topic. Simulation enables the student to explore situations that might be too expensive, dangerous, or time consuming in real life.

sin-, a combining form meaning 'hollow, cavity': *sinography, sinus, sinusotomy.*

sinap-, a combining form meaning 'of or related to mustard': *sinapine, sinapiscopy, sinapism.*

sinciput, the anterior or upper part of the head. See also **bregma.**

Sinemet, a trademark for a central nervous system fixed-combination drug containing a decarboxylase inhibitor (carbidopa) and an antiparkinsonian (levodopa).

Sinequan, a trademark for a tricyclic antidepressant (doxepin hydrochloride).

sinew, the tendon of a muscle, as the thick, flattened tendon attached to the short head of the biceps brachii. See also **tendon.**

singer's nodule. See **vocal cord nodule.**

single-blind study, an experiment in which either the subject or the person collecting data does not know whether the subject is in the control group or the experimental group. See also **double-blind study.**

single footling breech. See **footling breech.**

single monster, a fetus with a single body and head but severely malformed or duplicated parts or organs.

single room occupant (SRO), a single person, usually an elderly individual, who lives alone in a single room of a low-cost hotel or apartment building.

singultus. See **hiccup.**

sinistrality. See **left-handedness.**

sinistro-, a combining form meaning 'left, or related to the left side': *sinistrocardia, sinistrophobia, sinistrotorsion.*

sinoatrial (SA) block /sī′nō·ā′trē·əl/, a conduction disturbance in the heart during which an impulse formed within the SA node is blocked from depolarizing the atrial myocardium. The condition is indicated on the electrocardiogram by the absence of some P waves. Causes include excessive vagal stimulation, acute infections, and atherosclerosis. SA block may also be an adverse reaction to quinidine or digitalis. Treatment for symptomatic SA block includes the use of atropine, isoproterenol, and, if these are not effective, stimulation and regulation of the heart with an electronic impulse generated by a pacemaker. See also **atrioventricular block, heart block, intraarterial block, intraventricular block.**

sinoatrial (SA) node, a cluster of hundreds of cells located in the right atrial wall of the heart, near the opening of the superior vena cava. It comprises a knot of modified heart muscle that generates impulses that travel swiftly throughout the muscle fibers of both atria, causing them to contract. Specialized pacemaker cells in the node have an intrinsic rhythm that is independent of any stimulation by nerve impulses from the brain and the spinal cord. Slender fusiform cells comprising the sinoatrial node are largely filled with sarcoplasm but contain a few striated fibrillae. The cells are irregularly grouped together and, at the edge of the node, merge with the atrial musculature. The sinoatrial node will normally ''fire'' at a rhythmic rate of 70 to 75 beats per minute. If the node fails to generate an impulse, pacemaker function will shift to another excitable component of the cardiac conduction system, as the atrioventricular node or Purkinje's fibers. Certain hormones and various autonomic impulses can affect the sinoatrial node and cause it to ''fire'' faster, as during strenuous physical activity. During a lifetime of 70 years the node generates about 2 billion impulses. Surgical implantation of an artificial pacemaker is a common procedure for individuals suffering from a defective sinoatrial node, and more than 150,000 persons are leading active lives with permanently implanted devices. Also called **Keith-Flack node, pacemaker.** Compare **atrioventricular node, Purkinje's network.**

sinus bradycardia. See **bradycardia.**

sinusitis /sīnəsī′tis/, an inflammation of one or more paranasal sinuses. It may be a complication of an upper respiratory infection, dental infection, allergy, a change in atmosphere, as in air travel or underwater swimming, or a structural defect of the nose. With swelling of nasal mucous membranes the openings from sinuses to the nose may be obstructed, resulting in an accumulation of sinus secretions, causing pressure, pain, headache, fever, and local tenderness. Complications include cavernous sinus thrombosis and spread of infection to bone, brain, or meninges. Treatment includes steam inhalations, nasal decongestants, analgesics, and, if infection is present, antibiotics. Surgery to improve drainage may be performed in the treatment of chronic sinusitis.

sinus node, an area of specialized heart tissue near the entrance of the superior vena cava that generates the cardiac electric impulse and is in turn controlled by the autonomic nervous system. Also called **sinus pacemaker.**

sinusoid, an anastomosing blood vessel, somewhat larger than a capillary, lined with reticuloendothelial cells.

sinus pacemaker. See **sinus node.**

sinus tachycardia. See **tachycardia.**

sinus venosus defect. See **atrial septal defect.**

sippy diet, a severely restricted dietary regimen for peptic ulcer patients. It consists of hourly servings of milk and cream for several days, with the gradual addition of eggs, refined cereals, puréed vegetables, crackers, and other simple foods as tolerated until the regular bland diet is reached. Because the diet restricts all fresh vegetables and fruits, supplementary iron and vitamins are indicated to prevent deficiency states. See also **bland diet.**

sireniform fetus. See **sirenomelus.**

sirenomelia /sī′rənəmē′lē·ə/, a congenital anomaly in which there is complete fusion of the lower extremities and no feet. Also called **apodial symmelia.**

sirenomelus /sī′rənom′ələs/, an infant who has sirenomelia. Also called **sireniform fetus, sympus apus.**

siriasis /sirī′əsis/, sunstroke. See also **heat hyperpyrexia.**

-sis, a combining form meaning an 'action, process, or result of': *centesis, genesis, stasis.*

Sister Kenny's treatment, poliomyelitis therapy in which the patient's limbs and back are wrapped in warm, moist woolen cloths and, after the pain subsides, the patient is taught to exercise affected muscles, especially by swimming. Equally important is passive movement of affected limbs with simultaneous stimulation at the site of muscle origins, carried out after hot packs.

-site, a combining form meaning an 'organism living inside another form from which it derives sustenance': *celiosite, hemosite, histosite*.

site visit, a visit made by designated officials to evaluate or to gather information about a department or institution. A site visit is a step in the accreditation of an institution and in the funding of many major projects.

-sitia, a combining form meaning '(condition of) appetite for food': *apositia, asitia, eusitia*.

sito-, a combining form meaning 'of or pertaining to food': *sitomania, sitophobia, sitotherapy*.

sitosterol /sītos′tərôl/, a mixture of sterols derived from plants, as wheat germ, used for treating hyperbetalipoproteinemia and hypercholesterolemia, that are unresponsive to dietary measures. Its use is controversial, for a dispersing action in the mixture tends to cause loose bowel movements and may lead to diarrhea or interfere with the absorption of concomitantly administered medications. Use in pregnancy is not recommended.

situational anxiety, a state of apprehension, discomfort, and anxiety precipitated by the experience of new or changed situations or events. Situational anxiety is not abnormal and requires no treatment; it usually disappears as the person adjusts to the new experiences. See also **anxiety, anxiety neurosis.**

situational crisis, (in psychiatry) a crisis that arises suddenly in response to an external event or a conflict concerning a specific circumstance. The symptoms are transient, and the episode is usually brief.

situational depression, (in psychiatry) an episode of emotional and psychologic depression that occurs in response to a specific set of external conditions or circumstances.

situational psychosis, (in psychiatry) a psychotic episode that results from a specific set of external circumstances.

situational therapy, (in psychiatry) a kind of psychotherapy in which the milieu is part of the treatment program. See also **milieu therapy.**

situation relating, (in nursing research) a study design used to explain or predict phenomena in nursing practice in which a relationship is thought to exist among certain practices or characteristics of the population being studied.

situation therapy. See **milieu therapy.**

situs /sī′təs/, the normal position or location of an organ or part of the body.

sitz bath /sits, zits/, literally *(German)*, "seat" bath, a bath in which only the hips and buttocks are immersed in water or saline solution. The procedure is used for patients who have had rectal or perineal surgery. Also called **hip bath.**

sixth disease. See **roseola infantum.**

sixth nerve. See **abducens nerve.**

Sjögren-Larsson syndrome /shō′grenlär′sən/, a congenital condition, inherited as an autosomal recessive trait, characterized by ichthyosis, mental deficiency, and spastic paralysis.

SK-Ampicillin, a trademark for an antibacterial (ampicillin).

skato-. See **scato-.**

SK-Bamate, a trademark for a sedative (meprobamate).

skeletal enchondromatosis. See **enchondromatosis.**

skeletal fixation, any method of holding together the fragments of a fractured bone by the attaching of wires, screws, plates, or nails. See also **external pin fixation.**

skeletal muscle. See **striated muscle.**

skeletal system, all of the bones and cartilage of the body that collectively provide the supporting framework for the muscles and organs. See also the Color Atlas of Human Anatomy.

skeletal traction, one of the two basic kinds of traction used in orthopedics for the treatment of fractured bones and the correction of orthopedic abnormalities. Skeletal traction is applied to the affected structure by a metal pin or wire inserted in the tissue of the structure and attached to traction ropes. Skeletal traction is often used when continuous traction is desired to immobilize, position, and align a fractured bone properly during the healing process. Infection of the pin tract is one of the complications that may develop with skeletal traction, and careful scrutiny of pin sites is an important precaution. Some common signs of infection of the pin tracts are erythema, drainage, noxious odor, pin slippage, temperature elevation, and pain. Superficial infection of pin tracts is often treated with antibiotic therapy. Deeper infections usually require pin removal and antibiotic therapy. Compare **skin traction.** See also **Dunlop skeletal traction.**

skeleton, the supporting framework for the body, comprising 206 bones that protect delicate structures, provide attachments for muscles, allow body movement, serve as major reservoirs of blood, and produce red blood cells. The skeleton is divided into the axial skeleton which has 74 bones, the appendicular skeleton with 126 bones, and the 6 auditory ossicles. The skeleton is derived from the mesoderm that grows from the primitive streak as skeletal cells multiply, change, and migrate into various regions and form the membranous skeleton. Most of the membranous skeleton changes to cartilaginous skeleton in which ossification centers spread to form the bony skeleton. The four types of bones comprising the skeleton are the long bones, including the humerus, the ulna, the femur, the tibia, the fibula, and the phalanges of the fingers and the toes; the short bones, including the carpals and the tarsals; the flat bones, including the frontal bone and the parietal bone of the cranium, the ribs, and the shoulder bones; and the irregular bones, including the vertebrae, the bones of the sacrum, the bones of the coccyx, and certain bones of the skull, as the sphenoid, the ethmoid, and the mandible. The skeleton changes throughout life as bone formation and bone destruction proceed concurrently. During childhood and adolescence, bone formation proceeds faster than bone destruction. Between 35 and 40 years of age, bone destruction proceeds faster than bone formation. In advanced age bone destruction increases, bones become thin and brittle, vertebrae may collapse, and height decreases. See also **bone,** and see the Color Atlas of Human Anatomy. **–skeletal,** *adj.*

Skene's duct. See **paraurethral duct.**

Skene's glands /skēnz/, the largest of the glands that open into the urethra of women. They contain ducts that open just within the urethral orifice.

skew, a deviation from a line or symmetric pattern, as data in a research study that do not follow the expected statistic curve of distribution because of the unwitting introduction of another variable.

skia-, scia-, a combining form meaning 'of or related to shadows, especially of internal structures as produced by roentgen rays': *skiabaryt, skiagenol, skiagraph.*

skilled nursing facility (SNF), an institution or part of an institution that meets criteria for accreditation established by the sections of the Social Security Act that determine the basis for Medicaid and Medicare reimbursement for skilled nursing care, including rehabilitation and various medical and nursing procedures. Written policies and protocols are formulated with appropriate professional consultation. It is required by law that these policies include a designation of which level of caregiver is responsible for implementation of each policy, that the care of every patient be under the supervision of a physician, that a physician be available on an emergency basis, that records be maintained regarding the condition and care of every patient, that nursing service be available 24 hours a day, and that at least one fulltime registered nurse be employed. Other criteria stipulate that the facility have appropriate facilities for storing and dispensing drugs and biologics, that it maintain a use review plan, that all licensing requirements of the state in which it is located be met, and that an overall budget be maintained.

Skillern's fracture /skil′ərnz/, an open fracture of the distal radius associated with a greenstick fracture of the distal ulna.

skill play, a form of play in which a child persistently repeats an action or activity until it has been mastered, as throwing or catching a ball.

skimmed milk, milk from which the fat has been removed. Most of the vitamin A is removed with the cream, although all other nutrients remain. It is available as fluid skimmed milk, fortified skimmed milk, nonfat dry milk, and a form of buttermilk. Also called **nonfat milk, skim milk.**

skimming, a practice, sometimes employed by health programs that receive their income on a prepaid or capitation basis, of seeking to enroll only relatively healthy individuals as a means of increasing profits by decreasing costs. See also **skimping.**

skimping, a practice, sometimes employed by health programs that receive their income on a prepaid or capitation basis, of delaying or denying services to enrolled members of the program as a means of increasing profits by decreasing costs. See also **skimming.**

skin, the tough, supple cutaneous membrane that covers the entire surface of the body. It is the largest organ of the body and is composed of five layers of cells. Each layer is named for its unique function, texture, or position. The deepest layer is the stratum basale. It anchors the more superficial layers to the underlying tissues, and it provides new cells to maintain the cells lost by abrasion from the outermost layer. The cells of each layer migrate upward as they mature. Above the stratum basale lies the stratum spinosum. The cells in this layer are polygonal with tiny spines on their surfaces. As the cells migrate to the next layer, the stratum granulosum, they become flat, lying parallel with the surface of the skin. Over this layer lies a clear, thin band of homogenous tissue called the stratum lucidum. The boundaries of the cells are not visible in this layer. The outermost layer, the stratum corneum, is composed of scaly, squamous plaques of dead cells that contain keratin. This horny layer is thick over areas of the body subject to abrasion, as the palms of the hands, and thin over other more protected areas. The color of the skin varies according to the amount of melanin in the epidermis. Genetic differences determine the amount of melanin. The ultraviolet rays of the sun stimulate the production of melanin, which absorbs the rays and simultaneously darkens the skin. Modified skin continues into various parts of the body as mucous membrane, as in the lining of the vagina, the bladder, the lungs, the intestines, the nose, and the mouth. Mucous membrane lacks the heavily keratinized layer of the outside skin. It secretes the mucus that lubricates and protects associated structures. The skin helps to cool the body when the temperature rises by radiating the heat of increased blood flow in expanded blood vessels and by providing a surface for the evaporation of sweat. When the temperature drops, the blood vessels constrict and the production of sweat diminishes. Also called **cutaneous membrane, integument.**

skin button, a plastic and fabric device that covers the drivelines of an artificial heart at their exit point from the skin. Its purpose is to eliminate the transmission of pumping pressure to the surrounding tissues.

skin cancer, a cutaneous neoplasm caused by ionizing radiation, certain genetic defects, or chemical carcinogens, including arsenics, petroleum, tar products, and fumes from some molten metals, or by overexposure to the sun or other sources of ultraviolet light. Skin cancers, the most common and most curable malignancies, are also the most frequent secondary lesions in patients with cancer in other sites. Risk factors are a fair complexion, xeroderma pigmentosa, vitiligo, senile and seborrheic keratitis, Bowen's disease, radiation dermatitis, and hereditary basal cell nevus syndrome. The most common skin cancers are basal cell carcinomas and squamous cell carcinomas. Tumors of the sebaceous glands or sweat glands occur infrequently and are adenocarcinomas. Basal cell carcinomas, typically raised, hard, reddish lesions with a pearly surface, do not metastasize in contrast to scaly, slightly elevated squamous cell tumors that may become exophytic, friable growths with extensive ulceration and a nonhealing scab. A definitive diagnosis may be established by incisional biopsy or by excisional biopsy, which may be the only treatment required for small lesions. Surgery is usually indicated if the lesion is large, if bone or cartilage is invaded, or if lymph nodes are involved. Radiotherapy may be preferable for some smaller facial lesions and is commonly recommended for the treatment of skin tumors without distinct margins. Because of the possibility of recurrence of cancer, surgery is favored for the treatment of younger patients. Topical zinc chloride may be used in treating fairly common recurrent skin cancers; topical 5-fluorouracil is recommended for refractory premalignant actinic keratosis and for superficial basal cell carcinomas. An immunotherapeutic method is based on the induction of delayed hypersensitivity and consists of painting the lesions with a cream containing dinitrochlorobenzene (DNCB) and triethylene-immuno-benzoquinone (TEIB). Despite the curability of skin cancer it causes many deaths because people fail to obtain treatment. Lesions caused by actinic rays may be prevented by applying a sunscreen containing paraaminobenzoic acid (PABA).

skinfold calipers, an instrument used to measure the breadth of a fold of skin, usually on the posterior aspect of the upper arm or over the lower ribs of the chest.

skin graft, a portion of skin implanted to cover areas where skin has been lost through burns or injury or by surgical removal of diseased tissue. To prevent tissue rejection of permanent grafts, the graft is taken from the patient's own body or from the body of an identical twin. Skin from another person or animal can be used as a temporary cover for large burned areas to decrease fluid loss. The area from which the graft is taken is called the donor site, that on which it is placed is called the recipient site. Various techniques are used including pinch, split-thickness, full-thickness, pedicle, and mesh grafts. In pinch grafting, ¼ inch pieces of skin are placed as small islands on the donor site that they will grow to cover. These will grow even in areas of poor blood supply and are resistant to infection. The split-thickness graft consists of sheets of superficial and some deep layers of skin. Grafts of up to 4 inches wide and 10 to 12 inches long are removed from a flat surface—abdomen, thigh, or back—with an instrument called a dermatome. The grafts are sutured into place; compression dressings may be applied for firm contact, or the area may be left exposed to the air. A split-thickness graft cannot be used for weight-bearing parts of the body or to cover those subject to friction, as the hand or foot. A full-thickness graft contains all of the layers of skin and is more durable and effective for weight-bearing and friction-prone areas. A pedicle graft is one in which a portion remains attached to the donor site whereas the remainder is transferred to the recipient site. Its own blood supply remains intact, and it is not detached until the new blood supply has fully developed. This type is often used on the face, neck, or hand. A mesh graft is composed of multiple slices of new skin. A successful new graft of any type is well established in about 72 hours and can be expected to survive unless a severe infection or trauma occurs. The procedure may be done with local anesthesia. Preoperatively, both the donor and the recipient site must be free of infection and the recipient site must have a good blood supply. Postoperatively, stretching or motion of the recipient site is prevented. Strict sterile technique is used for handling dressings, and antibiotics may be given prophylactically to prevent infection. Good nutrition with a high-protein, high-caloric diet is essential. The nurse may roll the surface of the graft regularly with a sterile applicator to express accumulated fluid to the edge of the graft, allowing better adhesion. See also **graft.**

skin integrity, impairment of: actual, a nursing diagnosis accepted by the Fourth National Conference on the Classification of Nursing Diagnoses. The cause of the condition may be environmental (external) or somatic (internal). Environmental factors that may affect the development of impaired skin integrity include heat, cold, or chemical substances; mechanic factors, as a shearing force or pressure, restraint, or laceration; radiation; physical immobilization; and humidity. Somatic factors that may result in impairment of integrity of the skin include drugs, obesity or emaciation, malnutrition, metabolic disturbance, circulatory disturbance, altered sensation or pigmentation, developmental factors, immunologic deficit, a disturbance in excretions or secretions, psychogenic factors, edema, or change in the turgor of the skin. The defining characteristics of the problem are disruption of the surface of the skin, destruction of cell layers of the skin, and invasion of structures of the body through the skin. See also **nursing diagnosis.**

skin integrity, impairment of: potential, a nursing diagnosis accepted by the Fourth National Conference on the Classification of Nursing Diagnoses. The defining characteristics of the problem are the environmental (external) or somatic (internal) risk factors that may contribute to the cause of the breakdown of the integument. Among the environmental factors are hypothermia or hyperthermia; presence of an injurious chemical substance; shearing force or pressure, restraint, or laceration; radiation; physical immobilization; presence on the skin of excretions or secretions; and an abnormally high humidity. Somatic factors include reaction to some medications; obesity or emaciation; an abnormal metabolic state; alteration in circulation, sensory function, or pigmentation; bony prominences; adverse developmental factors; decrease in normal skin turgor; and psychogenic or immunologic abnormalities. See also **nursing diagnosis.**

Skinner box, a boxlike laboratory apparatus used in operant conditioning in animals, usually containing a lever or other device that when pressed produces reinforcement by either giving a reward, as food or an escape outlet, or avoiding a punishment, as an electric shock. Also called **standard environmental chamber.** See also **operant conditioning.**

skin prep, a procedure for cleansing the skin with an antiseptic before surgery or venipuncture. Skin preps are performed to kill bacteria and pathologic organisms and to reduce the risk of infection. Various skin prep devices are available for this procedure. Such devices are commonly constructed of plastic, filled with a specific antiseptic, and equipped with an applicator. The antiseptic is applied by rubbing the device in a circular motion over the skin. Some of the most common antiseptics contained in skin prep devices are iodine, povidone-iodine, and ethyl alcohol. Each antiseptic has associated advantages and disadvantages. The iodine skin prep kills bacteria, fungi, viruses, protozoa, and yeasts and is an inexpensive and reliable device. The disadvantages of iodine, in addition to its discoloring of the skin, are that it may burn or chap the skin and may cause an allergic reaction. Povidone-iodine, which consists of water-soluble complexes of iodine and organic compounds, is less irritating than iodine tinctures or solutions and does not stain the skin as much as iodine. However, povidine-iodine is less effective than regular iodine solutions, may be absorbed through the skin during prolonged use, and may cause an allergic reaction. Ethyl alcohol, which is not effective against spore-forming organisms, viruses, and tubercle bacilli is effective as a fat solvent and a germicidal when used in concentrations of 70% to 80% and may be used as a substitute skin prep antiseptic when the patient is allergic to iodine. Some disadvantages of ethyl alcohol are that it evaporates quickly, is highly flammable, and dries the skin excessively. Most skin prep devices are prepackaged and are disposable items for onetime use. To prep the skin with such a device before a venipuncture, the device is moved in a circular motion with the applicator rubbing the skin at the intended venipuncture site. The venipuncture site is swabbed with the antiseptic for about 1 minute. The antiseptic is spread over an area about 2 inches in diameter with the venipuncture site at the center.

skin tag. See **cutaneous papilloma.**

skin test, a test to determine the reaction of the body to a substance by observing the results of injecting the substance intradermally or of applying it topically to the skin. Skin tests are used to detect allergens, to determine immunity, and to diagnose disease. Kinds of skin tests include **patch test, Schick test,** and **tuberculin test.**

skin traction, one of the two basic types of traction used in orthopedics for the treatment of fractured bones and the correction of orthopedic abnormalities. Skin traction applies pull to an affected body structure by straps attached to the skin surrounding the structure. Kinds of skin traction are **adhesive skin traction** and **nonadhesive skin traction.** Compare **skeletal traction.** See also **Dunlop skin traction.**

sklero-. See **sclero-.**

SK-Penicillin VK, a trademark for an antibacterial (penicillin V potassium).

SK-Pramine, a trademark for a tricyclic antidepressant (imipramine hydrochloride).

SK-65 Compound, a trademark for a fixed-combination drug containing analgesics (propoxyphene hydrochloride, aspirin, and phenacetin) and a stimulant (caffeine).

SK-Tetracycline, a trademark for an antibiotic (tetracycline).

skull, the bony structure of the head, consisting of the cranium and the skeleton of the face. The cranium, which contains and protects the brain, consists of eight bones. The skeleton of the face is composed of 14 bones.

SL, abbreviation for **soda lime.**

slander, any words spoken with malice that are untrue and prejudicial to the reputation, professional practice, commercial trade, office, or business of another person. Formerly, slander included published defamation, but at present it is limited to spoken accusation. To bring legal action in slander, the slandered person must be able to demonstrate real temporal damages—except for cases in which the defamation relates to the person's business or profession or in which the malicious words question the person's chastity or accuse the person of being a criminal or of having a loathsome disease. Compare **libel.**

slant of occlusal plane, (in dentistry) the inclination measured by the angle between the extended occlusal plane and the axis-orbital plane.

SLE, abbreviation for **systemic lupus erythematosus.**

sleep, a state marked by reduced consciousness, diminished activity of the skeletal muscles, and depressed metabolism. People normally experience sleep in patterns that follow four observable, progressive stages. A device such as an encephalograph is used to record the recurrent pattern of brain waves during the stages: During Stage 1, the brain waves are of the theta type, followed in Stage 2 by the appearance of distinctive sleep spindles; during Stages 3 and 4, the theta waves are replaced by delta waves. These four stages represent three fourths of a period of typical sleep and are called collectively, **nonrapid eye movement (NREM)** sleep. The remaining time is usually occupied with **rapid eye movement (REM)** sleep, which can be detected with electrodes placed on the skin around the eyes so that tiny electric discharges from contractions of the eye muscles are transmitted to recording equipment. The REM sleep periods, lasting from a few minutes to half an hour, alternate with the NREM periods. Dreaming occurs during REM time. Individual sleep patterns normally change throughout life because daily requirements for sleep gradually diminish from as much as 20 hours a day in infancy to as little as 6 hours a day in old age. Infants tend to begin a sleep period with REM sleep, whereas REM activity usually follows the four stages of NREM sleep in adults.

sleeping pill, **1.** *informal.* a sedative taken for insomnia or for postoperative sedation. **2.** an over-the-counter pill, classified pharmaceutically as an aid to sleeping. Antihistamines, as pyrilamine maleate and doxylamine succinate depend for sedative action on side effects, which may disappear with continued use of such agents. The use of all drugs that depress the central nervous system is contraindicated for pregnant and lactating women and for patients with asthma, glaucoma, or prostatic hypertrophy.

sleeping sickness. See **African trypanosomiasis.**

sleep pattern disturbance, a nursing diagnosis accepted by the Fourth National Conference on the Classification of Nursing Diagnoses. The condition is a disruption of the hours of sleep, causing discomfort or interference with normal daily activities. The cause of the problem may be change in bodily sensation, illness, psychologic disturbance, stress, or various environmental changes. Characteristics of a sleep pattern disturbance include changes in behavior and performance, as increased irritability, restlessness, disorientation, lack of energy, and fatigue. The critical defining characteristics, at least one of which must be present to make the diagnosis, are difficulty in falling asleep, wakening earlier than usual, interruption of the night's sleep by periods of wakefulness, or not feeling rested after sleep. See also **nursing diagnosis.**

sleep terror disorder, a condition occurring during stages 3 or 4 of nonrapid eye movement sleep that is characterized by repeated episodes of abrupt awakening, usually with a panicky scream, accompanied by intense anxiety, confusion, agitation, disorientation, unresponsiveness, marked motor movements, and total amnesia concerning the event. The disorder is seen usually in children, is more common in boys than in girls, and is extremely variable in frequency but is more likely to occur if the individual is fatigued, under stress, or has been given a tricyclic antidepressant or neuroleptic at bedtime. Compare **nightmare.** See also **pavor nocturnus.**

sleepwalking. See **somnambulism.**

slide clamp, a device, usually constructed of plastic, employed to regulate the flow of intravenous solution. The slide clamp has a graduated opening through which the intravenous tubing passes. Pushing the tube into the narrow end of the opening constricts the tube and reduces the flow rate of the intravenous solution. Sliding the wide end of the opening over the tube increases the flow rate. Compare **roller clamp, screw clamp.**

sliding filaments, interdigitated thick and thin filaments of a sarcomere. In muscle contraction, they slide past each other so that the sarcomere becomes shorter although the filament lengths do not change. The action of the sliding filaments contributes to the increased thickness of a muscle in contraction.

sling, a bandage or device used to support an injured part of the body.

sling restraint, a therapeutic device, usually constructed of felt, used to assist in the immobilization of patients, especially orthopedic patients in traction. The sling is placed over the pelvis to reduce pelvic motion with lower extremity traction or over the abdominal area as countertraction with Dunlop traction. With lower extremity tractions, the sling restraint is attached to both sides of the bedspring frame. With Dunlop traction the sling restraint is attached to the opposite side of the bedspring frame. If the Dunlop traction is used in association with a Bradford frame, the sling restraint is attached under the frame. The sling restraint is rarely used with balanced suspension and is not usually used with Cotrel traction, halo-femoral traction, halo-pelvic traction, or with suspension for elevation. Compare **diaper restraint, jacket restraint.**

slip-on blood pump, a plastic mesh device with an attached squeeze bulb, rubber tubing, and pressure gauge, used to help administer large amounts of blood quickly. The plastic mesh slips over the blood bag and applies pressure to the bag when the bulb is squeezed. The pressure gauge displays a danger zone, usually marked in red, and indicates pressure limits for safe blood administration. Forcing blood into the veins at excessive pressure may damage the red blood cells or may disconnect the primary intravenous line.

slipped disk. See **herniated intervertebral disk.**

slit lamp, an instrument used in ophthalmology for examining the conjunctiva, lens, vitreous humor, iris, and cornea. A high-intensity beam of light is projected through a narrow slit, and a cross section of the illuminated part of the eye is examined through a magnifying lens.

slit lamp microscope, a microscope for ophthalmic examination. It permits the viewer to examine the endothelium of the posterior surface of the cornea in a projected band of light that is shaped like a slit.

slit scan radiography, a technique for producing x-rays of body structures without length distortion by scanning a fan-shaped beam through a narrow slit collimator. The beam divergence perpendicular to the scan results in some distortion of width.

Slo-Phyllin, a trademark for a bronchodilator (theophylline).

slough /sluf/, **1.** to shed or cast off dead tissue cells of the endometrium, which are shed during menstruation. **2.** the tissue that has been shed.

slow-acting insulin. See **long-acting insulin.**

Slow-K, a trademark for a slow-release tablet of an electrolyte replacement (potassium chloride).

slow response action potential, (in cardiology) an action potential produced when one of the fast sodium channels is available for depolarization and the fiber is separated only via slower Na+/Ca+ channels, producing an action potential with a slow upstroke velocity, low amplitude, and consequent slow conduction.

slow virus, a virus that remains dormant in the body after initial infection. Years may elapse before symptoms occur. Several degenerative diseases of the central nervous system are believed to be caused by slow viruses, including subacute sclerosing panencephalitis and kuru.

slurred speech, abnormal speech in which words are not enunciated clearly or completely but are run together or partially eliminated. The condition may be caused by weakness of the muscles of articulation, damage to a motor neuron, cerebellar disease, drug usage, or carelessness.

Sm, symbol for **samarium.**

SMA, **1.** a trademark for a nutritional supplement for infants. **2.** abbreviation for **sequential multiple analysis.**

SMA-6, SMA-12, SMA-18. See **sequential multiple analysis.**

SMA 12, SMA 24, a trademark for a system that uses a small computer to perform 12 or 24 different blood chemistry tests from a single blood sample.

smack, *slang.* heroin.

small calorie. See **calorie.**

small cardiac vein, one of the five tributaries of the coronary sinus that drains blood from the myocardium. It runs through the coronary sulcus between the right atrium and the right ventricle and opens into the right side of the coronary sinus. It conveys blood from the back of the right atrium and the right ventricle and, in some individuals, is joined by the right marginal vein. Also called **right coronary vein.** Compare **great cardiac vein, middle cardiac vein, oblique vein of left atrium, posterior vein of left ventricle.**

small cell carcinoma. See **oat cell carcinoma.**

smallest cardiac vein, one of the tiny vessels that drain deoxygenated blood from the myocardium into the atria. A few of these vessels end in the ventricles. Also called **vein of Thebesius.** Compare **anterior cardiac vein.** See also **coronary vein.**

small for gestational age (SGA) infant, an infant whose weight and size at birth falls below the tenth percentile of appropriate for gestational age infants, whether delivered at term or earlier or later than term. Factors associated with smallness or retardation of intrauterine growth other than genetic influences include any disorder causing short stature, as dwarfism; malnutrition caused by placental insufficiency; and certain infectious agents, including cytomegalovirus, rubella virus, and *Toxoplasma gondii*. Other factors associated with the smallness of an SGA infant include cigarette smoking by the mother during pregnancy, her addiction to alcohol or heroin, and her having received methadone treatment. Asphyxia may be a significant risk for the SGA infant during labor and delivery if the condition is the result of placental insufficiency. Such an infant has a low Apgar score, becomes acidotic in labor and at birth, and is likely to develop hypoglycemia within the first hours or days of life. Given adequate nutrition and caloric intake, some SGA infants show phenomenal catch-up growth. Also called **small for dates (SFD) infant. Compare large for gestational age infant.** See also **dysmaturity.**

small intestine, the longest portion of the digestive tract, extending for about 7 m from the pylorus of the stomach to the iliocecal junction. It is divided into the duodenum, jejunum, and ileum. Decreasing in diameter from beginning to end, it is situated in the central and caudal part of the abdominal cavity, surrounded by large intestine. Compare **large intestine.**

small omentum. See **lesser omentum.**

smallpox, a highly contagious viral disease characterized by fever, prostation, and a vesicular, pustular rash. It is caused by one of two species of poxvirus, variola minor (alastrim) or variola major. Because human beings are the only reservoir for the virus, worldwide vaccination with vaccinia, a related poxvirus, has been effective in eradicating smallpox. For several years no natural case of the disease has been known to occur. Also called **variola.**

smallpox vaccine, a vaccine prepared from dried smallpox virus. It is indicated only for laboratory workers exposed to pox viruses.

smart terminal, a computer terminal capable of retaining a program and processing data independently of a central processing unit. See also **intelligent terminal.**

smear, a laboratory specimen for microscopic examination prepared by spreading a thin film of tissue on a glass slide. A dye, stain, reagent, diluent, or lysing agent may be applied to the specimen, depending on the purpose of the examination.

smegma /smeg′mə/, a secretion of sebaceous glands, especially the cheesy, foul-smelling secretion often found under the foreskin of the penis and at the base of the labia minora near the glans clitoris.

smell, **1.** the special sense that enables odors to be perceived through the stimulation of the olfactory nerves; olfaction. See also **anosmia.** **2.** any odor, pleasant or unpleasant.

Smith fracture, a reverse Colles' fracture of the wrist, involving volar displacement and angulation of a distal bone fragment.

Smith-Hodge pessary. See **pessary.**

Smith-Petersen nail, a three-flanged stainless steel nail used in orthopedic surgery to anchor the fractured neck of the femur to its head. It is introduced below the prominence of the greater trochanter and passed through the fractured part into the head of the femur. See also **nail, pin.**

smoke inhalation, the inhalation of noxious fumes or irritating particulate matter that may cause severe pulmonary damage. Respiratory burns are difficult to distinguish from simple smoke inhalation. Chemical pneumonitis, asphyxiation, and physical trauma to the respiratory passages may occur.

■ OBSERVATIONS: Characteristics include irritation of the upper respiratory tract, singed nasal hairs, dyspnea, hypoxia, dusty gray sputum, rhonchi, rales, restlessness, anxiety, cough, and hoarseness. Pulmonary edema may develop up to 48 hours after exposure.

■ INTERVENTION: Respiration is assisted by means of an airway and humidified oxygen, administered as necessary. Intravenous fluids, endotracheal intubation or tracheostomy, nasogastric tube, and bronchodilators may be ordered. Arterial blood gases are monitored, and corticosteroids may be given.

■ NURSING CONSIDERATIONS: The characteristics of smoke inhalation and its treatment vary with the nature of the fumes or matter inhaled and the extent of exposure; it is therefore important to know the circumstances, nature, and period of exposure and whether the person has a history of chronic respiratory or cardiac disease. Observation for at least several hours is usual; if pulmonary edema is anticipated, observation may be required for up to 48 hours.

smooth muscle, one of two kinds of muscle, composed of elongated, spindle-shaped cells in muscles not under voluntary control, as the smooth muscle of the intestines, stomach, and other visceral organs. The heart muscle is an exception because it is a striated involuntary muscle. The nucleated cells of smooth muscle are arranged parallel to one another and to the long axis of the muscle they form. Smooth muscle fibers are shorter than striated muscle fibers, have only one nucleus per fiber, and are smooth in appearance. Biofeedback devices may help many people gain partial control of contractions of involuntary smooth muscles. Also called **involuntary muscle, unstriated muscle.** Compare **striated muscle, cardiac muscle.**

smooth surface cavity, a cavity formed by decay that starts on surfaces of teeth without pits, fissures, or enamel faults.

smudge cell, a degenerated leukocyte as seen in blood smears from patients with chronic lymphatic leukemia.

Sn, symbol for **tin.**

S.N., abbreviation for **student nurse,** used in signing nursing notes.

SNA, 1. abbreviation for **State Nurses' Association.** 2. abbreviation for **Student Nurses' Association.**

snail, an invertebrate of the order Gastropoda, several species of which are intermediate hosts of the blood flukes that cause schistosomiasis in humans. See also ***Schistosoma,* schistosomiasis.**

snakebite, a wound resulting from penetration of the flesh by the fangs of a snake. Bites by snakes known to be nonvenomous are treated as puncture wounds; those produced by an unidentified or poisonous snake require immediate attention. The person is kept still, the wound is washed with soap and water, and a partially constrictive tourniquet is applied to retard the absorption of the venom. Incision of the skin through the bite marks is made and suction applied to assist bleeding and in removing the toxin. To avoid cutting muscles, nerves, or blood vessels, the incision should be only skin deep. An appropriate antivenin may be given that protects against the venom of most pit vipers, including the rattlesnakes, copperheads, and cottonmouths that are responsible for 98% of the poisonous snakebites in the United States. Bites of pit vipers are characterized by pain, redness, and edema, followed by weakness, dizziness, profuse perspiration, nausea, vomiting, or weak pulse, subcutaneous hemorrhage, and, in severe cases, shock. Treatment includes the use of analgesics and sedatives, antibiotics, and antitetanus prophylaxis to prevent infections from pathogens found in the mouths of snakes. Patients sensitive to horse serum in antivenin may require cortisone for the control of hives, urticaria, and other allergic reactions. Coral snakes rarely bite, but their venom contains a neurotoxin that can cause respiratory paralysis.

snare, a device designed for holding a wire noose, used in removing small pedunculated growths. The operator tightens the wire around the peduncle, thus removing the growth.

sneeze, a sudden, forceful, involuntary expulsion of air through the nose and mouth occurring as a result of irritation to the mucous membranes of the upper respiratory tract, as by dust, pollen, or viral inflammation. Also called **sternutation.**

Snellen chart, one of several charts used in testing visual acuity. Letters, numbers, or symbols are arranged on the chart in decreasing size from top to bottom.

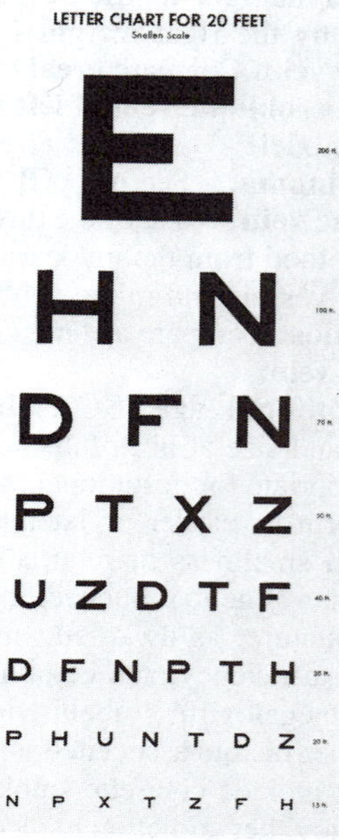

Reproduced with permission of the National Society to Prevent Blindness.

Snellen test, a test of visual acuity using a Snellen chart. The person being tested stands 20 feet from the chart and reads as many of the symbols as possible, reading each line and proceeding downward from the top. A score is assigned in the form of a ratio, comparing the subject's performance to that of a statistically normal subject's performance. A person who can read what the average person can read at 20 feet has 20/20 vision.

SNF, abbreviation for **skilled nursing facility.**

snout reflex, an abnormal sign elicited by tapping the nose, resulting in a marked facial grimace. It usually indicates bilateral corticopontine lesions.

Snowden-Pencer scissors. See **scissors.**

SNP, abbreviation for **sodium nitroprusside.**

S.N.P., abbreviation for **School Nurse Practitioner.**

snuffles, a nasal discharge in infancy characteristic of congenital syphilis. See also **syphilis.**

soap, **1.** a compound of fatty acids and an alkali. Soap cleanses because molecules of fat are attracted to molecules of soap in a water solution and are pulled off the dirty surface into the water. **2.** a metallic salt of any salt produced from an acid. Compare **detergent.**

SOAP /sōp, es′ō′ā′pē′/, (in a problem-oriented medical record) abbreviation for *subjective, objective, assessment, and plan,* the four parts of a written account of the health problem. In taking and charting the patient history and physical examination, a SOAP statement is made for each syndrome, problem, symptom, or diagnosis. Charting by this is said to be "soaped" and charts produced using it are called "soap charts." See also **problem-oriented medical record (POMR).**

social adjustment rating scale. See **social readjustment rating scale.**

social class, a grouping of persons with similar values, interests, income, education, and occupations.

social isolation, a nursing diagnosis accepted by the Fifth National Conference on the Classification of Nursing Diagnoses. The diagnosis defines a condition in which a feeling of aloneness is experienced that the client acknowledges as a negative or threatening state imposed by others. The cause of the condition involves factors that lead to unsatisfactory personal relationships, such as unacceptable social behavior or social values, the inability to engage in social situations, immature interests or inappropriate attitudes for the developmental age of the client, alterations in physical appearance or mental status, or illness. The defining characteristics may be objective or subjective, or both. Objective characteristics include the absence of family and friends; the absence of a supportive or significant personal relationship with another person; the client's withdrawal and preoccupation with his or her own thoughts and interests; meaningless actions or interests and activities inappropriate to the client's developmental age; a physical or mental handicap or illness; or unacceptable social behavior. Subjective characteristics include the verbal expression of feeling different from and rejected by others, the acknowledgment of values unacceptable to the dominant cultural group, absence of a significant purpose in life, the inability to meet the expectations of others, and the expressed feeling of insecurity in social situations. See also **nursing diagnosis.**

socialization, **1.** the process by which an individual learns to live in accordance with the expectations and standards of a group or society, acquiring the beliefs, habits, values, and accepted modes of behavior primarily through imitation, family interaction, and educational systems; the procedure by which society integrates the individual. **2.** (in psychoanalysis) the process of adjustment that begins in early childhood by which the individual becomes aware of the need to accommodate inner drives to the demands of external realty. See also **internalization.**

socialized medicine, a system for the delivery of health care in which the expense of care is borne by a governmental agency supported by taxation rather than being paid for directly by the client on a fee-for-service or contract basis.

social medicine, an approach to the prevention and treatment of disease that is based on the study of human heredity, environment, social structures, and cultural values.

social motivation, an incentive or drive resulting from a sociocultural influence that initiates behavior toward a particular goal. Compare **achievement motivation, physiologic motivation.**

social network, an interconnected group of cooperating significant others, who may or may not be related, with whom a person interacts.

social network therapy, the gathering together of patient, family, and other social contacts into group sessions for the purpose of problem solving.

social order, the manner in which a society is organized and the rules and standards required to maintain that organization.

social phobia, an anxiety disorder characterized by a compelling desire for the avoidance of and a persistent, irrational fear of situations in which the individual may be exposed to scrutiny by others, as speaking, eating, or performing in public, or using public lavatories or transportation. Compare **simple phobia.** See also **phobia.**

social psychiatry, a branch of psychiatry based on the study of social influences on the development and course of mental diseases. In treatment, social psychiatry favors the use of milieu or other situational approaches to therapy.

social psychology, the study of the effects of group membership on the behavior, attitudes, and beliefs of the individual.

social readjustment rating scale, a scale of 43 common life events associated with some degree of disruption of an individual's life. The scale was developed by psychologists T. Holmes and R.J. Raphe, who found that a number of serious physical disorders, as myocardial infarction, peptic ulcer, and infections, and a variety of psychiatric disorders, were associated with an accumulation of 200 or more points on the rating scale within a period of 1 year. Most disruptive on one's life, according to the psychologists, was the death of a spouse, an event that warrented 100 points. The lowest rated event was a minor law violation, rated at 11 points. The Holmes and Raphe scale was based on studies of hundreds of persons of different ages, cultures, and walks of life. The studies also found that one stressful event often led to another, as the death of a spouse could result in a change of residence, an altered finiancial state, or troubles with in-laws, so that within a single year a bereaved person might easily accumulate 200 or more points on the scale.

social sanctions, the measures used by a society to enforce its rules of acceptable behavior.

Social Security Act, a U.S. federal statute that provides for a national system of old age assistance, survivors' and old age insurance benefits, unemployment insurance and compensation, and other public welfare programs, including Medicare and Medicaid.

social worker, a person with special training in dealing with social, emotional, and environmental problems associated with illness or disability. A **medical social worker** usually is qualified by a master's degree and experience in counseling patients and their families in a hospital setting. A **psychiatric social worker** may specialize in counseling and advising individuals and families in dealing with social, emotional, or environmental problems resulting from mental illness.

Society for Advancement in Nursing (SAIN), a group established for advancement of the profession of nursing through higher education.

sociogenic, pertaining to personal or group activities that are motivated by social values and constraints.

sociology, the study of group behavior within a society.

sociopath. See **psychopath.**

sociopathic. See **psychopathic.**

sociopathic personality. See **antisocial personality.**

soda, a compound of sodium, particularly sodium bicarbonate, sodium carbonate, or sodium hydroxide.

soda lime (SL), a mixture of sodium and calcium hydoxides used to absorb exhaled carbon dioxide in an anesthesia rebreathing system.

sodium (Na), a soft, grayish metal of the alkaline metals group. Its atomic number is 11; its atomic weight is 22.99. Sodium is one of the most important elements in the body. Sodium ions are involved in acid-base balance, water balance, the transmission of nerve impulses, and the contraction of muscles. The recommended daily intake of sodium is 250 to 750 mg for infants 6 months to 1 year of age, 900 to 2700 mg for children 11 years of age or older, and 1100 to 3300 mg for adults. Sodium is an important component of more than 8 L of secretions produced by the body every day. These secretions include saliva, gastric and intestinal secretions, bile, and pancreatic fluid. The total daily secretion of sodium into these alimentary tract fluids averages between 1200 and 1400 mEq. A 154-pound adult has a total body pool of 2800 to 3000 mEq. Sodium is also linked to chlorine, which is the most important extracellular anion in the body. Sodium is the chief electrolyte in interstitial fluid, and its interaction with potassium as the main intracellular electrolyte is critical to survival. A decrease in the sodium concentration of the interstitial fluid immediately decreases osmotic pressure, making it hypotonic to intracellular fluid osmotic pressure. The kidney is the chief regulator of sodium levels in body fluids and will excrete sodium-free urine when the body needs to conserve sodium. In high temperatures, as those associated with fever, the body loses sodium through sweat, further diluting sodium reserves with additional water drunk by the affected individual. To avoid serious complications, depleted sodium must be replaced. Sodium salts, as sodium bicarbonate,

The social readjustment rating scale

Life event	Mean value
1. Death of spouse	100
2. Divorce	73
3. Marital separation	65
4. Jail term	63
5. Death of close family member	63
6. Personal injury or illness	53
7. Marriage	50
8. Fired at work	47
9. Marital reconciliation	45
10. Retirement	45
11. Change in health of family member	44
12. Pregnancy	40
13. Sex difficulties	39
14. Gain of new family member	39
15. Business readjustment	39
16. Change in financial state	38
17. Death of close friend	37
18. Change to different line of work	36
19. Change in number of arguments with spouse	35
20. Mortgage or loan for major purchase (home, etc.)	31
21. Foreclosure of mortgage or loan	30
22. Change in responsibilities at work	29
23. Son or daughter leaving home	29
24. Trouble with in-laws	29
25. Outstanding personal achievement	28
26. Spouse begins or stops work	26
27. Begin or end school	26
28. Change in living conditions	25
29. Revision of personal habits	24
30. Trouble with boss	23
31. Change in work hours or conditions	20
32. Change in residence	20
33. Change in schools	20
34. Change in recreation	19
35. Change in church activities	19
36. Change in social activities	18
37. Mortgage or loan for lesser purchase (car, TV, etc.)	17
38. Change in sleeping habits	16
39. Change in number of family get-togethers	15
40. Change in eating habits	15
41. Vacation	13
42. Christmas	12
43. Minor violations of the law	11

Reprinted with permission from Holmes, T.H., and Rahe, R.H.: J. Psychosom. Res. 11:213-218, 1967, Pergamon Press, Ltd.

are widely used in medications. Sodium bicarbonate has an immediate and rapid antacid action on the stomach, but any excess rapidly enters the intestine so that the substance has a shorter action than other antacids. Sodium bicarbonate, which is very effective in rendering the urine alkaline, is an ingredient in many solutions used as douches, mouthwashes, and enemas. Sodium is also important in the transport of sodium and potassium ions through the cytoplasmic membrane.

sodium acid glutamate. See **sodium glutamate.**

sodium arsenite poisoning, a toxic condition caused by the ingestion of sodium arsenite, an insecticide and weed-killer. The characteristic symptoms of arsenite poisoning are similar to those of arsenic poisoning, as is the treatment. See also **arsenic poisoning.**

sodium bicarbonate, an antacid, electroylyte, and urinary alkalinizing agent.

■ INDICATIONS: It is prescribed in the treatment of acidosis, gastric acidity, peptic ulcer, and indigestion.

■ CONTRAINDICATIONS: Pyloric obstruction, renal disease, congestive heart failure, or bleeding ulcer prohibits its use.

■ ADVERSE EFFECTS: Among the more serious adverse reactions are gastric distention, acid rebound, bicarbonate-induced alkalosis, hypernatremia, and hyperkalemia.

sodium chloride, common table salt (NaCl), used as a fluid and electrolyte replenisher, isotonic vehicle, irrigating solution, and enema.

sodium chloride and dextrose. See **dextrose and sodium chloride injection.**

sodium etidronate. See **etidronate disodium.**

sodium glutamate, a salt of glutamic acid used for the treatment of hepatic coma and the enhancement of the flavor of foods. Also called **monosodium glutamate (MSG), sodium acid glutamate.**

sodium hypochlorite solution, a 5% aqueous solution of NaOCl used as a disinfectant for utensils not harmed by its bleaching action.

sodium iodide, an iodine supplement.

■ INDICATIONS: It is prescribed in the treatment of thyrotoxic crisis, neonatal thyrotoxicosis, and in the management of hyperthyroidism before thyroidectomy.

■ CONTRAINDICATIONS: Hyperkalemia or known hypersensitivity to this drug prohibits its use.

■ ADVERSE EFFECTS: Among the more serious adverse reactions are salivary gland swelling, metallic taste, rashes, and GI disturbances. Acute poisoning may result in angioedema and pulmonary edema.

sodium lactate injection, an electrolyte replenisher that has been prescribed for metabolic acidosis.

sodium morrhuate. See **morrhuate sodium injection.**

sodium nitroprusside (SNP), a vasodilator.

■ INDICATIONS: It is prescribed primarily in the emergency treatment of hypertensive crises and in heart failure.

■ CONTRAINDICATIONS: Certain compensatory forms of hypertension, as coarctation of the aorta or impaired cerebral circulation, or known hypersensitivity to the drug prohibits its use.

■ ADVERSE EFFECTS: Among the most serious adverse reactions are a rapid fall in blood pressure or symptoms of cyanide poisoning (cyanide is produced by the metabolism of nitroprusside). Muscle spasms also may occur.

sodium perborate, an oxygen-liberating antiseptic ($NaBO_2.H_2O_2.3H_2O$) that may be used in the treatment of necrotizing ulcerative gingivitis and other kinds of gingival inflammation and for bleaching pulpless teeth. Prolonged or indiscriminate use of the compound may cause burns of the oral mucosa and blacken the tongue.

sodium phosphate, a saline cathartic.

■ INDICATIONS: It is prescribed to achieve prompt, thorough evacuation of the bowel and, in lower dosage, for laxative effect.

■ CONTRAINDICATIONS: Congestive heart failure, abdominal pain, edema, megacolon, hypovolemia, salt-restricted diet, or hypersensitivity to this drug prohibits its use. Frequent administration in any dosage is not recommended.

■ ADVERSE EFFECTS: Among the more severe adverse reactions are dehydration, hypovolemia, abdominal cramping, and electrolyte imbalance.

sodium phosphate P32, an antineoplastic, antipolycythemic, radioactive agent.

■ INDICATIONS: It is prescribed for polycythemia vera and for neoplasms, including myelocytic leukemia, and for localizing tumors of the eye.

■ CONTRAINDICATIONS: Polycythemia vera with leukopenia or decreased platelet count, chronic myelocytic leukemia with leukopenia or erythrocytopenia, concurrent administration of other alkalating agents, or hypersensitivity to this drug prohibits its use.

■ ADVERSE EFFECT: The most serious adverse reaction is radiation sickness.

sodium pump, a theoretic mechanism for transporting sodium ions across cell membranes against an opposing concentration gradient. Sodium is normally moved from a region of low concentration within a cell to the extracellular fluid that contains a much higher concentration. Energy for this transport system is obtained from the hydrolysis of adenosine triphosphate by special enzymes. See also **calcium pump, electrolyte balance.**

sodium-restricted diet. See **low-sodium diet.**

sodium salicylate, an analgesic, antipyretic, and antirheumatic.

■ INDICATIONS: It is prescribed to relieve pain and fever.

■ CONTRAINDICATIONS: GI ulceration or bleeding or known hypersensitivity to this drug or to other salicylates prohibits its use. It is not given to a newborn infant.

■ ADVERSE EFFECTS: Among the most serious adverse reactions are GI bleeding and salicylate poisoning caused by overdose. Abdominal pain, nausea, and vomiting also may occur.

sodium stibocaptate, an investigational parasiticide for certain schistosomal infections. It is available from the Center for Disease Control. Also called **stibocaptate.**

sodium sulfate, a saline cathartic for habitual constipation caused by peristaltic disorders.

■ INDICATIONS: It is prescribed to achieve prompt, thorough evacuation of the bowel and, in lower dosage, for laxative effect.

■ CONTRAINDICATIONS: Congestive heart failure, hypovolemia, or hypersensitivity to this drug prohibits its use. Frequent administration, in any dosage, is not recommended.

■ ADVERSE EFFECTS: Among the more severe adverse reactions are dehydration, hypovolemia, and electrolyte imbalance.

Sodium Versenate, a trademark for a metal chelating agent (edetate disodium).

sodoku. See **rat-bite fever.**

sodomy, **1.** anal intercourse. **2.** intercourse with an animal. **3.** a vague term for "unnatural" sexual intercourse. –**sodomite,** *n.*, **sodomize,** *v.*

soft data, health information that is mainly subjective as provided by the patient and the patient's family, including pain or other sensations, life-style habits, and family health history.

soft diet, a diet that is soft in texture, low in residue, easily digested, and well tolerated. It provides the essential nutrients in the form of liquids and semisolid foods, as milk, fruit juices, eggs, cheese, custards, tapioca and puddings, strained soups and vegetables, rice, ground beef and lamb, fowl, fish, mashed, boiled, or baked potatoes, wheat, corn, or rice cereals, and breads. Omitted are raw fruits and vegetables, coarse breads and cereals, rich desserts, strong spices, all fried foods, veal, pork, nuts, and raisins. It is commonly recommended for people who have GI disturbances or acute infections, or for anyone unable to tolerate a normal diet.

soft fibroma, a fibroma that contains many cells. Also called **fibroma molle** /mol′ē/.

soft money, *informal.* (in a university, school, or agency) income from unstable sources, as grants or contracts.

soft palate, the structure composed of mucous membrane, muscular fibers, and mucous glands, suspended from the posterior border of the hard palate forming the roof of the mouth. When the soft palate rises, as in swallowing and in sucking, it separates the nasal cavity and the nasopharynx from the posterior part of the oral cavity and the oral portion of the pharynx. The posterior border of the soft palate hangs like a curtain between the mouth and the pharynx. Suspended from the posterior border is the conic, pendulous, palatine uvula. Arching laterally from the base of the uvula are the two curved, musculomembranous pillars of the fauces. Compare **hard palate.**

soft radiation, a relatively long wavelength radiation with lower kilovolt peaks and less penetrability than short wavelength radiation.

software, the programs that control a computer and cause it to perform specific functions. Compare **firmware, hardware, wetware.**

software bug. See **bug.**

-sol, a combining form meaning a 'colloidal solution': *electrosol, nitromersol, plastisol.*

solar-, a combining form meaning 'of or pertaining to the sun': *solarium, solarization, solarize.*

solar fever. See **dengue fever, sunstroke.**

solarium /sōler′ē·əm/, a large, sunny room serving as a lounge for ambulatory patients in a hospital.

solar keratosis. See **actinic keratosis.**

solar plexus, a dense network of nerve fibers and ganglia that surrounds the roots of the celiac and the superior mesenteric arteries at the level of the first lumbar vertebra. It is one of the great autonomic plexuses of the body in which the nerve fibers of the sympathetic system and the parasympathetic system combine. The denser part of the solar plexus lies between the suprarenal glands, on the ventral surface of the crura of the diaphragm and on the abdominal aorta. The preganglionic parasympathetic fibers reach the plexus through the anterior and the posterior vagi on the stomach. The preganglionic sympathetic fibers reach the plexus through the greater and the lesser splanchnic nerves. Secondary plexuses emerging from the solar plexus are the abdominal aortic plexus, the hepatic plexus, the inferior mesenteric plexus, the phrenic plexus, the renal plexus, the spermatic plexus, the superior gastric plexus, the splenic plexus, the superior hypogastric plexus, the superior mesenteric plexus, and the suprarenal plexus. Also called **celiac plexus.**

solar radiation, the emission and diffusion of actinic rays from the sun. Overexposure may result in sunburn, keratosis, skin cancer, or lesions associated with photosensitivity.

Solatene, a trademark for an ultraviolet screen (beta-carotene), used in the treatment of erythropoietic protoporphyria.

soleus /sō′lē·əs/, one of three superficial posterior muscles of the leg. It is a broad flat muscle lying just under the gastrocnemius and arising by tendinous fibers from the head of the fibula, from the popliteal line, and from the medial border of the tibia. The fibers of the soleus merge near the middle of the leg with those of the gastrocnemius to form the tendo calcaneus, which inserts into the calcaneus of the foot. The soleus is innervated by a branch of the tibialis nerve, containing fibers from the first and the second sacral nerves. The soleus plantar flexes the foot. Compare **gastrocnemius, plantaris.**

Solfoton, a trademark for an anticonvulsant and sedative-hypnotic (phenobarbital).

Solganal, a trademark for an antirheumatic (aurothioglucose).

solid, **1.** a dense body, figure, structure, or substance that has length, breadth, and thickness, is not a liquid or a gas, contains no significant cavity or hollowness, and has no breaks or openings on its surface. **2.** describing such a body, figure, structure, or substance.

solitary play, a form of play among a group of children within the same room or area in which each child engages in an independent activity using toys that are different from the others', concentrating solely on the particular activity, and showing no interest in joining in or interfering with the play of others. Compare **cooperative play.** See also **associative play, parallel play.**

-soluble, a combining form meaning 'able to be dissolved': *acetosoluble, hydrosoluble, liposoluble.*

Solu-Cortef, a trademark for a glucocorticoid (hydrocortisone sodium succinate).

Solu-Medrol, a trademark for a glucocorticoid (methylprednisolone sodium succinate).

solute /sol′yo͞ot, sō′lo͞ot/, a substance dissolved in a solution.

solution, a mixture of one or more substances dissolved in another substance. The molecules of each of the substances disperse homogenously and do not change chemically. A solution may be a gas, a liquid, or a solid. Compare **colloid, suspension.** See also **solute, solvent.**

-solve, a combining form meaning 'to loosen': *dissolve, resolve.*

solvent, **1.** any liquid in which another substance can be dissolved. **2.** *informal.* an organic liquid, as benzene, carbon tetrachloride, and other volatile petroleum distillate that when inhaled can cause intoxication, as well as damage to mucous membranes of the nose and throat and the tissues of the kidney, liver, and brain. Repeated, prolonged exposure can result in addiction, brain damage, blindness, and other serious consequences, some of them fatal. See also **benzene poisoning, carbon tetrachloride, glue sniffing, petroleum distillate poisoning.**

soma /sō′mə/, *pl.* **somas, somata,** **1.** the body as distinguished from the mind or psyche. **2.** the body, excluding germ cells. **3.** the body of a cell. –**somatic** /sōmat′ik/, **somal,** *adj.*

Soma, a trademark for a skeletal muscle relaxant (carisoprodol).

soma-. See **somato-.**

-soma, a combining form meaning a 'body or portion of a body': *hystersoma, microsoma, prosoma.*

-somatia, a combining form meaning '(condition of the) body, especially concerning size': *diplosomatia, macrosomatia, microsomatia.*

somatic. See **soma, psychosomatic.**

-somatic, **1.** a combining form meaning the 'cause of effects on the body': *exsomatic, neurosomatic, psychosomatic.* **2.** a combining form meaning 'concerning a type of human body': *eurysomatic, leptosomatic.*

somatic cavity. See **coelom.**

somatic cell, any of the cells of body tissue that have the diploid number of chromosomes as distinguished from germ cells, which contain the haploid number. Compare **germ cell.**

somatic chromosome, any chromosome in a diploid or somatic cell, as contrasted to those in a haploid or gametic cell; an autosome.

somatic delusion, a false notion or belief concerning body image or body function. See also **delusion.**

somatist /sō′mətist/, a psychotherapist or other health professional who believes that every neurosis and psychosis has an organic cause.

somatization disorder, a disorder characterized by recurrent, multiple, physical complaints and symptoms for which there is no organic cause. The condition typically occurs in adolescence or in the early adult years and is rarely seen in men. The symptoms vary according to the individual and the underlying emotional conflict. Some common symptoms are GI dysfunction, paralysis, temporary blindness, cardiopulmonary distress, painful or irregular menstruation, sexual indifference, and pain during intercourse. Hypochondriasis may develop if the condition is untreated. Also called **Briquet's syndrome.**

somato-, soma-, a combining form meaning 'of or pertaining to the body': *somatoceptor, somatogenic, somatopleural.*

somatoform disorder, any of a group of neurotic disorders, characterized by symptoms suggesting physical illness or disease, for which there are no demonstrable organic causes or physiologic dysfunctions. The symptoms are usually the physical manifestations of some unresolved intrapsychic factor or conflict. Kinds of somatoform disorders are **conversion disorder, hypochondriasis, psychogenic pain disorder,** and **somatization disorder.**

somatogenesis /sō′matəjen′əsis/, **1.** (in embryology) the development of the body from the germ plasm. **2.** the development of a physical disease or of symptoms from an organic pathophysiologic cause. Compare **psychogenesis.** –**somatogenic, somatogenetic,** *adj.*

somatoliberin. See **growth hormone releasing factor.**

somatomedin. See **growth hormone.**

somatomegaly /sō′matōmeg′əlē/, a condition in which the body is abnormally large because of an excessive secretion of somatotropin or an inadequate secretion of somatostatin.

somatoplasm, the nonreproductive protoplasmic material of the body cells as distinguished from the reproductive material of the germ cells. Compare **germ plasm.**

somatopleure /sōmat′əplo͝or/, the tissue layer that forms the body wall of the early developing embryo. Consisting of an outer layer of ectoderm lined with somatic mesoderm, it continues as the amnion and chorion external to the embryo. Compare **splanchnopleure.** –**somatopleural,** *adj.*

somatosensory evoked potential (SEP), evoked potential elicited by repeated stimulation of the pain and touch systems. It is the least reliable of the evoked potentials studied as monitors of neurologic function during surgery.

somatosplanchnic /sōmat′ōsplangk′nik/, of or pertaining to the trunk of the body and the visceral organs.

somatostatin /sō′matōstat′in/, a hormone produced in the hypothalamus that inhibits the factor that stimulates release of somatotropin from the anterior pituitary gland. It also inhibits the release of certain hormones, including thyrotropin, adrenocorticotropic hormone, glucagon, insulin, and cholecystokinin, and of some enzymes, including pepsin, renin, secretin, and gastrin. Also called **growth hormone release inhibiting hormone.**

somatotherapy, the treatment of physcial disorders, as distinguished from psychotherapy.

somatotropic hormone, somatotropin. See **growth hormone.**

somatotype, **1.** body build or physique. **2.** the classification of individuals according to body build based on certain physical characteristics. The primary types are **ectomorph, endomorph,** and **mesomorph.**

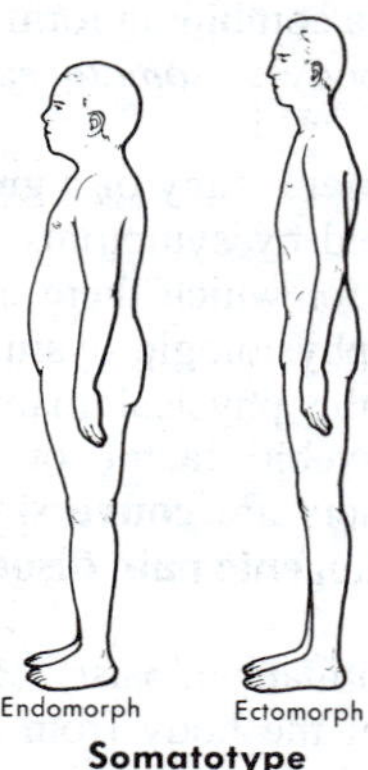

Somatotype

-some, a combining form meaning 'a body' of a specified sort: *chromosome, microsome, sarcosome.*

-somia, a combining form meaning '(condition of) possessing body': *agenosomia, diplosomia, microsomia.*

somite /sō′mīt/, any of the paired, segmented masses of mesodermal tissue that form along the length of the neural tube during the early stage of embryonic development in vertebrates. These structures give rise to the vertebrae and differentiate into various tissues of the body, including the voluntary muscle, bones, connective tissue, and the dermal layers of the skin. The first somite to appear is in the future occipital region and the formation of new somites continues in a caudal direction until 36 to 38 have developed.

somite embryo, an embryo in any stage of development between the formation of the first and the last pairs of somites, which in humans occurs in the third and fourth weeks after fertilization of the ovum.

somn-. See **somni-.**

Somnafac, a trademark for a sedative-hypnotic (methaqualone hydrochloride).

somnambulism /somnam′byəliz′əm/, **1.** also called **noctambulation, sleepwalking.** a condition occurring during stages 3 or 4 of nonrapid eye movement sleep that is characterized by complex motor activity, usually culminating in leaving the bed and walking about, with no recall of the episode on awakening. The episodes, which usually last from several minutes to half an hour or longer, are seen primarily in children, more commonly in boys than in girls, and are more likely to occur if the individual is fatigued or under stress or has taken a sedative or hypnotic medication at bedtime. Seizure disorders, central nervous system infections, and trauma may be predisposing factors, but the condition is more commonly related to anxiety. In adults, the condition is less common and is classified as a dissociative reaction. **2.** a hypnotic state in which the person has full possession of the senses but no recollection of the episode.

somni-, somn-, a combining form meaning 'of or pertaining to sleep': *somnifacient, somniferous, somnipathy.*

-somnia, a combining form meaning '(condition of or like) sleep': *asomnia, hyposomnia, hypersomnia.*

somnolent, **1.** the condition of being sleepy or drowsy. **2.** tending to cause sleepiness. **–somnolence,** *n.*

Somophyllin, a trademark for a bronchodilator (theophylline).

-somus, a combining form meaning a 'fetal monster with a body': *disomus, hemisomus, pleurosomus.*

son-, a combining form meaning 'of or pertaining to sound': *sonitus, sonometer, sonotone.*

sonogram, sonography. See **ultrasonography.**

sonorous rale, a snoring sound that may be produced by the vibration of a mass of thick secretion lodged in a bronchus. This sound is associated with various lung or respiratory disorders.

soot wart. See **scrotal cancer.**

soporific /sop′ərif′ik/, **1.** of or pertaining to a substance, condition, or procedure that causes sleep. **2.** a soporific drug. See also **hypnotic, sedative.**

sorbent, the property of a substance that allows it to interact with another compound, usually to make it bind.

sorbic acid /sôr′bik/, a compound occurring naturally in berries of the mountain ash. Commercial sorbic acid derived from acetaldehyde is used in fungicides, food preservatives, lubricants, and plasticizers.

Sorbitrate, a trademark for an antianginal (isosorbide dinitrate).

sordes /sôr′dēz/, *pl.* **sordes,** dirt or debris, especially the crusts consisting of food, microorganisms, and epithelial cells that accumulate on teeth and lips during a febrile illness or one in which the patient takes nothing by mouth. Sordes gastricae is undigested food and mucus in the stomach.

sore, **1.** a wound, ulcer, or lesion. **2.** tender or painful.

Sorrin's operation, a surgical technique for treating a periodontal abscess, used especially when the marginal gingiva appears healthy and provides no access to the abscess. A semilunar incision is made below the abscess area in the attached gingiva, leaving the gingival margin undisturbed. The tissue flap produced by the incision is raised, accessing the abscessed area for curettage, after which the wound is sutured.

s.o.s., (in prescriptions) abbreviation for *si opus sit,* a Latin phrase meaning "if necessary."

souffle /soo͞′fəl/, a soft murmur heard through a stethoscope. When detected over the uterus in a pregnant woman, it is coincident with the maternal pulse and is caused by blood circulating in the large uterine arteries.

soul food, food linked with cultural or traditional origins, especially Afro-American, that contributes emotional significance and personal satisfaction to an individual.

sound, an instrument used to locate the opening of a cavity or canal, to test the patency of a canal, to ascertain the depth of a cavity, or to reveal the contents of a canal or cavity. A sound is used to determine the depth of the uterus, to detect stones in the bladder, and, less commonly, to assist in correctly inserting a urinary catheter in the urethra through the urinary meatus.

source-image receptor distance, the distance between the focus of an x-ray beam and the x-ray film as measured along the beam. Also called **focal film distance.**

South African genetic porphyria. See **variegate porphyria.**

South American blastomycosis. See **paracoccidioidomycosis.**

South American trypanosomiasis. See **Chagas' disease.**

Southey's tube /sou′*th*ēz, *obsolete.* a small, very thin cannula introduced into edematous tissue to withdraw fluid, especially from the legs or feet, to relieve the edema of congestive heart failure. Also called **Southey-Leech tube.** See also **cannula, tube.**

sp. (*pl.* **sp., spp**), abbreviation for **species.**

space, an actual or a potential cavity of the body, as the complemental spaces in the pleural cavity that are not occupied by lung tissue and the lymph spaces occupied by lymph.

space maintainer, a fixed or movable appliance for preserving the space created by the premature loss of one or more teeth.

space obtainer, an appliance for increasing the space between adjoining teeth.

space regainer, a fixed or removable appliance for moving a displaced permanent tooth into its normal position in a dental arch.

Spanish fly. See **cantharis.**

spano-, a combining form meaning 'scanty or scarce': *spanogyny, spanomenorrhea, spanopnea.*

sparganosis /spär′gənō′sis/, an infection with larvae of the fish tapeworm of the pseudogenus Sparganum, characterized by painful subcutaneous swellings or swelling and destruction of the eye. It is acquired by ingesting larvae in contaminated water or in inadequately cooked, infected frog flesh. Treatment includes surgery and local injection of ethyl alcohol to kill the larvae.

Sparine, a trademark for a phenothiazine antipsychotic and antiemetic (promazine hydrochloride).

sparteine sulfate, an alkaloid salt used to treat cardiac disorders and formerly used as an oxytocic to reduce uterine bleeding during the third stage of labor.

spasm, **1.** an involuntary muscle contraction of sudden onset, as habit spasms, hiccups, stuttering, or a tic. **2.** a convulsion or seizure. **3.** a sudden, transient constriction of a blood vessel, bronchus, esophagus, pylorus, ureter, or other hollow organ. Compare **stricture.** See also **bronchospasm, pylorospasm.**

-spasm, a combining form meaning a 'convulsion' of a specified sort: *gastrospasm, neurospasm, vasospasm.*

spasmo-, a combining form meaning 'of or pertaining to spasm(s)': *spasmodermia, spasmophemia, spasmophilia.*

-spasmodic, -spasmodical, a combining form meaning 'of, pertaining, or referring to a convulsion': *angiospasmodic, antispasmodic, postspasmodic.*

spasmodic torticollis, a form of torticollis characterized by episodes of spasms of the neck muscles. The condition is often transient in nature, and examination seldom reveals a physical cause. In some cases, severe stress and muscular spasm may be the cause.

spastic, of or pertaining to spasms or other uncontrolled contractions of the skeletal muscles. See also **cerebral palsy.** **–spasticity,** *n.*

spastic aphonia, a condition in which a person is unable to speak because of spasmodic contraction of the abductor muscles of the throat.

spastic bladder, a form of neurogenic bladder caused by a lesion of the spinal cord above the voiding reflex center. It is marked by loss of bladder control and bladder sensation, incontinence, and automatic, interrupted, incomplete voiding. It is most often caused by trauma, but may be a result of tumor or multiple sclerosis. Also called **reflex bladder, automatic bladder.** Compare **flaccid bladder.**

spastic colon. See **irritable bowel syndrome.**

spastic entropion. See **ectropion, entropion.**

spastic hemiplegia, paralysis of one side of the body with increased tendon reflexes and uncontrolled contraction occurring in the affected muscles.

spastic paralysis, an abnormal condition characterized by the involuntary contraction of one or more muscles with associated loss of muscular function. Compare **flaccid paralysis.**

spastic pseudoparalysis. See **Creutzfeldt-Jakob disease.**

spatial dance, the body shifts or movements used by individuals as they try to adjust the distance between them. See also **spatial zones.**

spatial relationships, the relative locations of various personnel and equipment in an operating room with particular emphasis on what is sterile, clean, or contaminated. The operating room nurse must maintain an awareness of the arrangement of people, the height of personnel in relation to each other and to table level, and the proximity of sterile to nonsterile areas.

spatial summation. See **summation,** def. 2.

spatial zones, the areas of personal space in which most people interact. Four basic spatial zones are the intimate zone, in which distance between individuals is less than 18 inches; the personal zone, between 18 inches and 4 feet; the social zone, extending between 4 and 12 feet; and the public zone, beyond 12 feet.

SPE, abbreviation for **sucrose polyester.**

Spearman's rho /spir′mənz rō′/, a statistic test for correlation between two rank-ordered scales. It yields a statement of the degree of interdependence of the scores of the two scales.

special care unit, a hospital unit with the necessary specialized equipment and personnel for handling critically ill or injured patients, as an intensive care unit, burn unit, or cardiac care unit.

special gene system, a plasmid, transposon, or other genetic fragment that is able to transfer genetic information from one cell to another.

specialing, *informal.* **1.** (in psychiatric nursing) the constant attendance of a professional staff member on a disturbed patient to protect the patient from harming the self or others and to observe the patient's behavior. The patient so "specialed" is accompanied in all activities by the staff member. **2.** (in nursing) the giving of nursing care to only one person, as when acting as a private duty nurse or when caring for a patient whose needs are so great that a nurse is required at all times.

specialist, a health care professional who practices a specialty. A specialist usually has advanced clinical training and may have a postgraduate academic degree.

special sense, the sense of sight, smell, taste, touch, or hearing.

specialty, a branch of medicine or nursing in which the professional is specially qualified to practice by having attended an advanced program of study, by having passed an examination given by an organization of the members of the specialty, or by having gained experience by extensive practice in the specialty.

specialty care, specialized medical services provided by a physician specialist.

species (Sp) /spē′sēz, spē′shēz/, *pl.* **species (sp., spp)** /spē′sēz, spē′shēz/, the category of living things below genus in rank. A species includes individuals of the same genus who are similar in structure and chemical composition and who can interbreed. See also **genus.**

species immunity, a form of natural immunity shared by all members of a species. Compare **individual immunity, racial immunity.**

specific absorption rate (SAR), (in hyperthermia treatment) the rate of absorption of heat energy (W) per unit mass of tissue in units of W/kg.

specific activity, **1.** (in nuclear medicine) the radioactivity of a radioisotope per unit mass of the element or compound, expressed in microcuries per millimol or disintegrations per second per milligram. **2.** the relative activity per unit mass, expressed as counts per minute per milligram. The specific activity of potassium in the human body is the same as that of the environment or diet, and, because potassium is associated chiefly with muscle tissue, a whole body count of ^{40}K, after administration of the radioisotope, can be used to distinguish lean body mass from total body mass.

specific gravity, the ratio of the density of a substance to the density of another substance accepted as a standard. The usual standard for liquids and solids is water. Thus, a liquid or solid with a specific gravity of 4 is four times as dense as water. Hydrogen is the usual standard for gases. See also **density, mass.**

specific immune globulin, a special preparation obtained from human blood that is preselected for its high antibody count against a specific disease, as varicella zoster immune globulin.

specificity of association, the uniqueness of a relationship between a causal factor and the occurrence of a disease.

specific rates, statistic rates in which both the events in the numerator and the denominator are restricted to a specific subgroup of a population.

specific treatment. See **treatment.**

specimen /spes′imən/, a small sample of something, intended to show the nature of the whole, as a urine specimen.

Spectazole, a trademark for an antifungal (econazole nitrate).

spectinomycin hydrochloride, an antibiotic.

■ INDICATIONS: It is prescribed in the treatment of gonorrhea and certain infections in penicillin-allergic patients.

■ CONTRAINDICATION: Known hypersensitivity to this drug prohibits its use.

■ ADVERSE EFFECTS: Among the more serious adverse reactions are oliguria, urticaria, chills, fever, dizziness, and nausea.

spectr-, a combining form meaning 'image': *spectrograph, spectrophobia, spectrum.*

Spectrobid, a trademark for a semisynthetic penicillin (bacampicillin).

Spectrocin, a trademark for a topical, fixed-combination drug containing antibacterials (neomycin sulfate and gramicidin).

spectrometer /spektrom′ətər/, an instrument for measuring wavelengths of rays of the spectrum, the deviation of refracted rays, and the angles between faces of a prism. Kinds of spectrometer are **mass spectrometer** and **Mössbauer spectrometer.**

spectrometry /spektrom′ətrē/, the procedure of measuring wavelengths of light and other electromagnetic waves. See also **spectrometer.** –**spectrometric,** *adj.*

spectrophotometry /spek′trōfətom′ətrē/, the measurement of color in a solution by determining the amount of light absorbed in the ultraviolet, infrared, or visible spectrum, widely used in clinical chemistry to calculate the concentration of substances in solution. **–spectrophotometric,** *adj.*

spectrum, *pl.* **spectra,** **1.** a range of phenomena or properties occurring in increasing or decreasing magnitude. Radiant or electromagnetic energy is arranged on the basis of wavelength and frequency. Electromagnetic radiation includes spectra of radio waves, infrared, visible light, ultraviolet, x-rays, and gamma rays. **2.** the range of effectiveness of an antibiotic. A broad spectrum antibiotic is effective against a wide range of microorganisms. See also **antibiotic, electromagnetic radiation, wave.**

speculum /spek′yo͞oləm/, a retractor used to separate the walls of a cavity to make examination possible, as an ear speculum, an eye speculum, or a vaginal speculum.

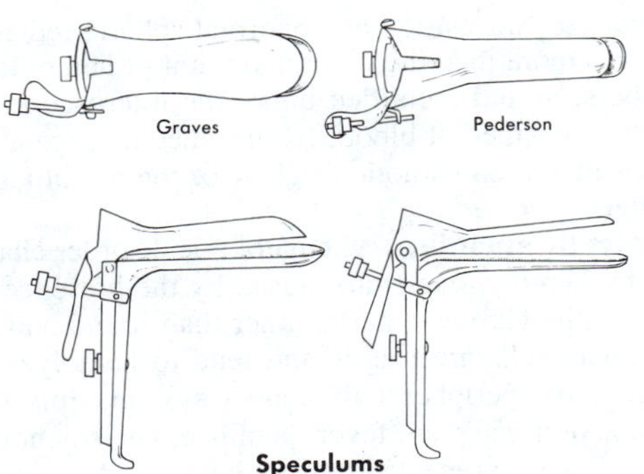

Speculums

speech, **1.** the utterance of articulate vocal sounds that form words to give expression to one's thoughts or ideas. **2.** communication by means of spoken words. **3.** the faculty of language production, which involves the complex coordination of the muscles and nerves of the organs of articulation. Any neurologic or muscular injury or defect involving these organs results in various speech impediments or dysfunctions. Kinds of dysfunctions include **ataxic speech, explosive speech, mirror speech, scamping speech, scanning speech, slurred speech,** and **staccato speech.** See also **speech dysfunction.**

speech audiometry. See **audiometry.**

speech dysfunction, any defect or abnormality of speech, including aphasia, alexia, stammering, stuttering, aphonia, and slurring. Speech problems may develop from any of a variety of causes, among them neurologic injury to the cerebral cortex, muscular paralysis because of trauma, disease, or cerebrovascular accident, structural abnormality of the organs of speech, emotional or psychologic tension, strain, or depression, hysteria, and severe mental retardation. See also **speech.**

speech pathologist. See **speech therapist.**

speech pathology, **1.** the study of abnormalities of speech or of the organs of speech. **2.** the diagnosis and treatment of abnormalities of speech as practiced by a speech pathologist or a speech therapist.

speech therapist, a person trained in speech pathology who treats people with disorders affecting normal oral communication.

speed, **1.** the rate of change of position with time. Compare **velocity. 2.** *slang.* any stimulating drug, as amphetamine. **3.** a reciprocal of the amount of radiation used to produce an image with various components of an x-ray imaging system, as screens, film, and image intensifiers. There is often a tradeoff between radiation dose to the patient and the overall image quality. Thus, a system using little radiation is "fast," whereas one requiring more radiation is "slow." **4.** the amount of exposure of film to light or x-rays needed to produce a desired image. X-ray film speed usually is indicated as the reciprocal of the exposure in roentgens necessary to produce a density of 1 above the base and fog levels.

speed shock, a sudden adverse physiologic reaction of a patient to intravenous medications or drugs that are administered too quickly. Some signs of speed shock are a flushed face, headache, a tight feeling in the chest, irregular pulse, loss of consciousness, and cardiac arrest.

spell of illness, a period regarded by Medicare rules as the number of days between the admission of an insured patient to a hospital and the day that marks the end of a 60-day period during which the insured has not been an inpatient in a hospital or a skilled nursing facility.

sperm. See **semen, spermatozoon.**

-sperm, a combining form meaning a 'seed': *gymnosperm, oosperm, zygosperm.*

spermatic cord, a structure extending from the deep inguinal ring in the abdomen to the testis, descending nearly vertically into the scrotum. The left spermatic cord is usually longer than the right, consequently the left testis usually hangs lower than the right. Each cord is comprised of arteries, veins, lymphatics, nerves, and the excretory duct of the testis.

spermatic duct. See **vas deferens.**

spermatic fistula, an abnormal passage communicating with a testis or a seminal duct.

spermatid /spur′mətid/, a male germ cell that arises from a spermatocyte and that becomes a mature spermatozoon in the last phase of the continual process of spermatogenesis.

spermato-, spermo-, a combining form meaning 'of or pertaining to seed, specifically to the male generative element': *spermatoblast, spermatocyst, spermatogenesis.*

spermatocele /spərmat′əsēl′, spur′-/, a cystic swelling, either of the epididymis or of the rete testis, that contains spermatozoa. It lies above, behind, and separate from the testis; it is usually painless and requires no therapy.

spermatocide /spərmat′əsīd, spur′-/, a chemical substance that kills spermatozoa by reducing their surface tension, causing the cell wall to break down by a bactericidal effect or by creating a highly acidic environment. Among many spermatocidal agents used in various contraceptive creams are lactic acid, phenylmercuric acetate, chloramine polyethylene glycol, benzethonium chloride, and certain quinine compounds. Also called **spermicide.**

spermatocyte /spur′mətōsīt′/, a male germ cell that arises from a spermatogonium. Each spermatocyte gives rise to two haploid secondary spermatocytes that become spermatids.

spermatocytogenesis. See **spermatogenesis.**

spermatogenesis /spərmat′əjen′əsis, spur′-/, the process of development of spermatozoa, including the first stage, called spermatogenesis, in which spermatogonia become spermatocytes that develop into spermatids, and the second stage, called spermiogenesis, in which the spermatids become spermatozoa.

spermatogonium, *pl.* **spermatogonia,** a male germ cell that gives rise to a spermatocyte early in spermatogenesis.

spermatozoon /spur′mətəzō′ən, spərmat′-/, *pl.* **spermatozoa** /-zō′ə/, a mature male germ cell that develops in the seminiferous tubules of the testes. Resembling a tadpole, it is about 50 μm (1/500 inch) long and has a head with a nucleus, a neck, and a tail that provides propulsion. Developed in vast numbers after puberty, it is the generative component of the semen, impregnating the ovum and resulting in fertilization. See **spermatogenesis.**

-spermia, -spermy, a combining form meaning '(condition of) possessing or producing seed': *aspermia, asthenospermia, necrospermia.*

spermicidal /spur′misī′dəl/, destructive to spermatozoa.

spermicide. See **spermatocide.**

spermiogenesis. See **spermatogenesis.**

spermo-. See **spermato-.**

-spermy. See **-spermia.**

sphacel-, a combining form meaning 'of or pertaining to gangrene': *sphaceloderma, sphacelotoxin, sphacelus.*

-sphaera, -sphaere. See **-sphere.**

sphaero-. See **sphero-.**

spheno-, a combining form meaning 'of or pertaining to the sphenoid bone, or to a wedge': *sphenocephaly, sphenoidotomy, sphenotemporal.*

sphenoidal fissure, a cleft between the great and small wings of the sphenoid bone.

sphenoidal sinus, one of a pair of cavities in the sphenoid bone of the skull, lined with mucous membrane that is continuous with that of the nasal cavity. Each sinus is approximately spheroidal, with a diameter of about 2 cm, but its shape and size vary from person to person. A large sphenoidal sinus may extend into the roots of the pterygoid processes, into the great wings, or into the occipital bone. The cavities are very small at birth and develop largely after puberty. Compare **ethmoidal air cells, frontal sinus, maxillary sinus.**

sphenoid bone, the bone at the base of the skull, anterior to the temporal bones and the basilar part of the occipital bone. It resembles a bat with its wings extended.

sphenomandibular ligament /sfē′nōmandib′yələr/, one of a pair of flat, thin ligaments comprising part of the temporomandibular joint between the mandible of the jaw and the temporal bone of the skull. It is attached to the spine of the sphenoid bone and becomes broader as it descends to the lingula of the mandibular foramen.

-sphere, -sphaera, -sphaere, **1.** a combining form meaning a 'spheric body': *chondriosphere, onconosphere, somosphere.* **2.** a combining form meaning a 'realm that supports life': *biosphere, vivosphere, zoosphere.*

sphero-, sphaero-, a combining form meaning 'round, or pertaining to a sphere': *spherocyte, spherolith, spherometer.*

spherocyte /sfir′əsīt/, an abnormal spheric red cell that contains more than the normal amount of hemoglobin. It can be seen and identified under the microscope on the stained specimen of blood. Its presence in large numbers causes increased osmotic fragility of the red blood cells. –**spherocytic,** *adj.*

spherocytic anemia, a hematologic disorder characterized by hemolytic anemia caused by the presence of red blood cells that are spheric rather than round and biconcave. The cells are fragile and tend to hemolyze in the oxygen-poor peripheral circulatory system. Episodic crises of abdominal pain, fever, jaundice, and splenomegaly occur. Because repeated transfusions are often needed to treat the anemia, siderosis may develop. Splenectomy may then be necessary. The condition is inherited as an autosomal dominant trait. Compare **congenital nonspherocytic hemolytic anemia.** See also **elliptocytosis.**

spherocytosis /sfir′ōsītō′sis/, the abnormal presence of spherocytes in the blood. Compare **elliptocytosis.**

spheroidea. See **ball and socket joint.**

sphincter /sfingk′tər/, a circular band of muscle fibers that constricts a passage or closes a natural opening in the body, as the hepatic sphincter in the muscular coat of the hepatic veins near their union with the superior vena cava, and the external anal sphincter, which closes the anus.

sphincter pupillae, a muscle that expands the iris, narrowing the diameter of the pupil of the eye. It is composed of circular fibers arranged in a narrow band about 1 mm wide, surrounding the margin of the pupil toward the posterior surface of the iris. The circular fibers near the free margin of the iris are closely packed; those that are near the periphery of the band are more separated and form incomplete circles. The fibers of the sphincter pupillae blend with the fibers of the dilatator pupillae near the margin of the pupil and are innervated by a motor root of the ciliary ganglion from the oculomotor nerve. Compare **dilatator pupillae.**

sphingolipid, a compound that consists of a lipid and a sphingosine. It is found in high concentrations in the brain and other tissues of the nervous system, especially membranes.

sphingomyelin /sfing'gōmī'əlin/, any of a group of sphingolipids containing phosphorus. It occurs primarily in the tissue of the nervous system, generally in membranes, and in the lipids in the blood.

sphingomyelin lipidosis, any of a group of diseases characterized by an abnormality in the ability of the body to store sphingolipids. Kinds of sphingomyelin lipidosis include **Gaucher's disease, Niemann-Pick disease,** and **Tay-Sachs disease.** See also **Fabry's disease.**

sphingosine /sfing'gōsēn/, a long-chain unsaturated amino alcohol, a major constituent of sphingolipids and sphingomyelin.

sphygm-, sphygmo-, a combining form meaning 'pulse': *sphygmodynamometer, sphygmoid, sphygmomanometer*.

-sphygmia, a combining form meaning '(condition of the) pulse': *anisosphygmia, hemisphygmia, sychnosphygmia*.

sphygmo-. See **sphygm-.**

sphygmogram /sfig'məgram/, a pulse tracing produced by a sphygmograph. A curve occurs on the tracing with each atrial pulsation. An upward, primary elevation is followed by a sudden drop to a point slightly above the baseline. The curve then gradually descends to the baseline in small decrements of amplitude. Sphygmographic abnormalities of rate, rhythm, and form may be diagnostically useful in an assessment of cardiovascular function.

sphygmograph /sfig'məgraf/, an instrument that records the force of the arterial pulse on a tracing called a sphygmogram. –**sphygmographic,** *adj.*

sphygmomanometer /sfig'mōmənom'ətər/, a device for measuring the arterial blood pressure. It consists of an arm or leg cuff with an air bladder connected to a tube and a bulb for pumping air into the bladder, and a gauge for indicating the amount of air pressure being exerted against the artery. See also **blood pressure, manometer.**

spica bandage /spī'kə/, a figure-of-eight bandage in which each turn generally overlaps the next to form a succession of V-like designs. It may be used to give support, to apply pressure, or to hold a dressing in place on the chest, limbs, thighs, or pelvis.

spica cast, an orthopedic cast applied to immobilize part or all of the trunk of the body and part or all of one or more extremities. It is used to treat various fractures, as of the hip and the femur, and in correcting or maintaining the correction of hip deformities. Kinds of spica casts are **bilateral long-leg spica cast, one-and-a-half spica cast, shoulder spica cast,** and **unilateral long-leg spica cast.**

spicule /spik'yōōl/, a sharp body with a needlelike point.

spider angioma, a form of telangiectasis characterized by a central, elevated, red dot the size of a pinhead from which small blood vessels radiate. Spider angiomas are often associated with elevated estrogen levels as occur in pregnancy or when the liver is diseased and unable to detoxify estrogens. Also called **spider nevus.** See also **telangiectasia.**

spider antivenin. See **black widow spider antivenin.**

spider bite, a puncture wound produced by the bite of a spider, an arachnid related to ticks and mites. Fewer than 100 of some 30,000 species of spiders are known to bite. Two of them, the black widow spider and the brown recluse spider, found in the United States, are poisonous.

spider nevus. See **spider angioma.**

spillway, a channel or passageway through which food normally escapes from the occlusal surfaces of the teeth during mastication.

spin, the intrinsic angular momentum of an elementary particle or a nucleus of an atom.

spina /spī'nə/, *pl.* **spinae, 1.** the spinal column. **2.** a spine or a thornlike projection, as the bony projection on the anterior border of the ilium, forming the anterior end of the iliac crest.

spina bifida /spī'nə bif'ədə, bī'fədə/, congenital neural tube defect characterized by a developmental anomaly in the posterior vertebral arch. Spina bifida is relatively common, occurring approximately 10 to 20 times per 1000 births. It may occur with only a small deformed lamina separated by a midline gap, or it may be associated with the complete absence of laminae surrounding a large area. In cases where the separation is wide enough, contents of the spinal canal protrude posteriorly, and a myelomeningocele is evident. This more serious deformity is associated with gross deficits not normally manifested in spina bifida. Neurologic deficits do not usually accompany the anomalies involving only bony deformity. Direct signs and symptoms are rarely noted in spina bifida, which is frequently diagnosed accidentally during radiographic examinations required for other reasons. Spina bifida that does not involve herniation of the meninges or the contents of the spinal canal rarely requires treatment. Also called **spinal dysrhaphis.**

spina bifida anterior, incomplete closure along the anterior surface of the vertebral column. The defect is often associated with developmental anomalies of the abdominal and thoracic viscera.

spina bifida cystica, a developmental defect of the central nervous system in which a hernial cyst containing meninges (meningocele), spinal cord (myelocele), or both (myelomeningocele) protrudes through a congenital cleft in the vertebral column. The protruding sac is encased in a layer of skin or a fine membrane that can easily rupture, causing the leakage of cerebrospinal fluid and an increased risk of meningeal infection. The severity of neurologic dysfunction and associated defects depends directly on the degree of nerve involvement. The most severe type is lumbosacral myelomeningocele, which is frequently associated with hydrocephalus and the Arnold-Chiari malformation. Compare **spina bifida occulta.** See also **myelomeningocele, neural tube defect.**

spina bifida occulta, defective closure of the laminae of the vertebral column in the lumbosacral region without hernial protrusion of the spinal cord or meninges. The defect, which is quite common, occurs in about 5% of the population and is identified externally by a skin depression or dimple, dark tufts of hair, telangiectasis, or soft, subcutaneous lipomas at the site. Because the neural tube has closed, there are usually no neurologic impairments associated with the defect. However, any abnormal adhesion of the spinal cord to the area of the malformation may lead to neuromusucular disturbances, usually problems with gait and foot weakness and with the bowel and bladder sphincters. Compare **spina bifida cystica.**

spinal, **1.** of or pertaining to a spine, especially the spinal column. **2.** *informal.* spinal anesthesia, as saddle block or caudal anesthesia.

spinal accessory nerve. See **accessory nerve.**

spinal aperture, a large opening formed by the body of a vertebra and its arch.

spinal arachnoid. See **arachnoidea spinalis.**

spinal canal, the cavity within the vertebral column.

spinal caries. See **tuberculous spondylitis.**

spinal column. See **vertebral column.**

spinal cord, a long, nearly cylindric structure lodged in the vertebral canal and extending from the foramen magnum at the base of the skull to the upper part of the lumbar region. A major component of the central nervous system, the adult cord is approximately 1 cm in diameter with an average length of 42 to 45 cm and a weight of 30 g. The cord conducts sensory and motor impulses to and from the brain and controls many reflexes. Thirty-one spinal nerves originate from the cord: 8 cervical, 12 thoracic, 5 lumbar, 5 sacral, and 1 coccygeal. It has an inner core of gray material consisting mainly of nerve cells and is enclosed by three protective membranes (meninges): the dura mater, arachnoid, and pia mater. The cord is an extension of the medulla oblongata of the brain and ends caudally between the twelve thoracic and third lumbar vertebrae, often at or adjacent to the disk between the first and second lumbar vertebrae. Until the third month of fetal life, the cord occupies the entire length of the vertebral canal. Thereafter, the canal lengthens faster than the cord. By the sixth fetal month, the caudal end of the cord reaches only as far as the upper sacrum. At birth it is on a level with the third lumbar vertebra. Originating in the ectoderm, like the entire nervous system, the cord develops from the caudal portion of the embryonic neural plate. Also called **chorda spinalis, medulla spinalis.** See also **spinal nerves.**

spinal cord compression, an abnormal and often serious condition resulting from pressure on the spinal cord. The symptoms range from temporary numbness of an extremity to permanent quadriplegia, depending on the cause, severity, and location of the pressure. Causes include spinal fracture, vertebral dislocation, tumor, hemorrhage, and edema associated with contusion. See also **herniated disk, spondylolisthesis.**

spinal cord injury, any one of the traumatic disruptions of the spinal cord, often associated with extensive musculoskeletal involvement. Common spinal cord injuries are spinal fractures and dislocations, as those commonly suffered by individuals involved in car accidents, airplane crashes, or other violent impacts. Such trauma may cause varying degrees of paraplegia and quadriplegia. Injuries to spinal structures below the first thoracic vertebra may produce paraplegia. Injuries to the spine above the first thoracic vertebra may cause quadriplegia. Injuries that completely transect the spinal cord cause permanent loss of motor and sensory functions activated by neurons below the level of the lesions involved. Spinal cord injuries produce a state of spinal shock, characterized by placid paralysis, and complete loss of skin sensation at the time of the injury. Within a few weeks the muscles affected may become spastic, and the skin sensation may return to a slight degree. The motor and the sensory losses that prevail a few weeks after the injury are usually permanent. Musculoskeletal complications are associated with the neurologic involvement of spinal cord injuries, and prevention of decubitis ulcers and the treatment of any loss of bladder and bowel control are continuing concerns. Treatment of spinal cord injuries varies considerably and involves numerous approaches, as orthopedic exercises, ambulatory techniques, and special physical and psychologic therapy.

spinal cord tumor, a neoplasm of the spinal cord of which more than 50% are extramedullary, about 25% are intramedullary, and the rest are extradural. Symptoms usually develop slowly and may progress from unilateral paresthesia and a dull ache to lancinating pain, weakness in one or both legs, abnormal deep tendon reflexes, and, in advanced cases, monoplegia, hemiplegia, or paraplegia. Function of the autonomic nervous system is sometimes disturbed, causing areas of dry, cold, bluish-pink skin or profuse sweating of the lower extremities. The diagnosis is made by x-ray and myelographic examination. About 30% of spinal cord tumors are circumscribed, encapsulated meningiomas, and 25% are schwannomas; these two kinds are found chiefly in the thoracic region. Some 20% are gliomas, and the others consist of congenital lipomas, epidermoids, and metastatic lesions. The dura is resistant to invasion, but many extradural tumors are metastatic lesions from primary cancers in the prostate, lung, breast, thyroid, and GI tract. Most extramedullary and nonmetastatic extradural tumors are surgically removed; intermedullary lesions are enucleated, whenever possible; and inoperable tumors are treated with radiotherapy and chemotherapy. Tumors of the spinal cord may arise at any age but appear most frequently in the third decade of life and are one fourth as common as brain neoplasms.

spinal curvature, any persistent, abnormal deviation of the vertebral column from its normal position. Kinds of spinal curvature are **kyphoscoliosis, kyphosis, lordosis,** and **scoliosis.**

spinal dysrhaphis. See **spina bifida.**

spinal fasciculi. See **spinal tract.**

spinal fluid. See **cerebrospinal fluid.**

spinal fusion, the fixation of an unstable segment of the spine, accomplished by skeletal traction or immobilization of the patient in a body cast but most frequently by a surgical procedure. Operative ankylosis may be performed in the treatment of spinal fractures or after discectomy or laminectomy for the correction of a herniated vertebral disk. Surgical fusion involves the stabilization of a spinal section with a bone graft introduced through a posterior incision in the lumbar region; in the less frequently fused cervical region the incision may be anterior or posterior. Also called **spondylosyndesis.**

spinal headache, a headache occurring after spinal anesthesia or lumbar puncture, caused by a loss of cerebrospinal spinal fluid (CSF) from the subarachnoid space, resulting in traction of the meninges on the pressure-sensitive intracranial structures. Severe spinal headache may be accompanied by diminished aural and visual acuity. Treatment usually includes keeping the patient flat in bed to relieve the meningeal irritation, encouraging an increased fluid intake to increase the intravascular volume to increase the production and volume of cerebrospinal fluid, and administering analgesics to reduce pain. If severe headache persists, an anesthesiologist may perform an autologous blood patch procedure in which a clot of the patient's blood is formed and planted over the leaking puncture site in the dura to prevent further loss of CSF. Meningeal irritation and backache may persist for several days. The incidence of spinal headache is greatest when a large-bore needle is used for the initial anesthetic or diagnostic procedure.

spinal manipulation, the forced passive flexion, extension, and rotation of vertebral segments, carrying the elements of articulation beyond the usual range of movement to the limit of anatomic range. Spinal manipulation may be used effectively in physiotherapy for the treatment of vertebral and sacroiliac dislocations, sprains, and adhesions.

spinal nerves, the 31 pairs of nerves without special names that are connected to the spinal cord and numbered according to the level of the cord at which they emerge. There are 8 cervical, 12 thoracic, 5 lumbar, and 5 sacral pairs, and 1 coccygeal pair. The first cervical pair of nerves emerges from the spinal cord in the space between the first cervical vertebra and the occipital bone. The rest of the cervical pairs and all the thoracic pairs emerge horizontally through the intervertebral foramen of their respective vertebrae, as the second cervical pair, which emerges through the foramina above the second cervical vertebra. The lumbar, the sacral, and the coccygeal nerve pairs descend from their points of origin at the lower end of the cord before reaching the intervertebral foramina of their respective vertebrae. Each spinal nerve attaches to the spinal cord by an anterior root and a posterior root. The posterior roots accompany a distended spinal ganglion within the vertebral foramina. Emerging from the cord, each spinal nerve divides into the anterior, the posterior, and the white rami, the anterior and the posterior rami serving the voluntary nervous system, the white rami serving the autonomic nervous system. The posterior rami subdivide into lesser nerves that extend into the muscles and the skin of the posterior surface of the head, the neck, and the trunk. The anterior rami, except for those of the thoracic nerves, subdivide and pass fibers to the skeletal muscles and the skin of the extremities. Subdivisions of the anterior rami form complex plexuses, as the brachial plexus, from which smaller nerves emerge to innervate the hand and most of the arm. The brachial plexus in the shoulder region is sometimes damaged during birth and must be treated or the injured baby may develop a withered arm. A broken neck may damage the right and the left phrenic nerves that come from the third, fourth, and fifth cervical nerves. Such damage may prevent nerve impulses from reaching the phrenic nerves, which supply the diaphragm, and thus stop respiration. The sacral plexus in the pelvic cavity is comprised of certain spinal nerve fibers from the lumbar and the sacral regions and gives rise to the great sciatic nerve in the back of the thigh, often the site of painful sciatica. See also **spinal cord.**

spinal puncture. See **lumbar puncture.**

spinal shock, a form of shock associated with acute injury to the spinal cord. See also **shock.**

spinal tract, any one of the ascending and descending pathways for motor or sensory nerve impulses that is found in the white matter of the spinal cord. Twenty-one different tracts lie within the dorsal, the ventral, and the lateral funiculi of the white substance. Ascending tracts conduct impulses up the spinal cord to the brain; descending tracts conduct impulses down the cord from the brain. The four major ascending tracts are the lateral spinothalmic, the ventral spinothalmic, the fasciculi gracilis and cuneatus, and the spinocerebellar. The four major descending tracts are the lateral corticospinal, the ventral corticospinal, the lateral reticulospinal, and the medial reticulospinal. Touch, pressure, proprioception, temperature, and pain are sensory stimuli transmitted via the spinal tracts. Reflex and voluntary motor activity are regulated by motor nerve stimulation from the brain and brainstem to the motor neurons of the spinal cord.

spindle, 1. the fusiform figure of achromatin in the cell nucleus during the late prophase and the metaphase of mitosis. It consists of tiny fibers radiating out from the centrosomes and connecting them with one another. **2.** a type of brain wave, consisting of a short series of changes in electric potential with a frequency of 14 per second. **3.** any one of the special receptor organs comprising the neurotendinous and the neuromuscular spindles distributed throughout the body. These kinds of spindles serve as special receptor organs that detect the degree of stretch in a muscle or at the junction of a muscle with its tendon and are essential in maintaining muscle tone.

spindle cell carcinoma, a rapidly growing neoplasm composed of fusiform squamous cells. It may be difficult to distinguish from a sarcoma.

spindle cell nevus. See **benign juvenile melanoma.**

spine, the vertibral column, or backbone.

spin-lattice relaxation time. See **relaxation time.**

spinnbarkeit /spin′bärkīt, shpin′-/, the clear, slippery, elastic consistency characteristic of cervical mucus during ovulation. It has the consistency of an uncooked egg white, and it is a valuable sign of the peak fertile period in a woman's menstrual cycle. Observation of spinnbarkeit is useful in natural methods of family planning, in the clinical evaluation of infertility, and in discovering the optimum time for artificial insemination. Spinnbarkeit may be evaluated by the length to which a string of mucus can be drawn between the fingers before breaking. (The literal meaning of this German word is "weavability.") See also **ovulation method of family planning.**

spino-, a combining form meaning 'of or pertaining to the spine': *spinocain, spinoglenoid, spinotransversarius.*

spinocerebellar /spī′nōser′əbel′ər/, of or pertaining to the spinal cord and the cerebellum.

spinocerebellar disorder, an inherited disorder characterized by a progressive degeneration of the spinal cord and cerebellum, often involving other parts of the nervous system as well. These disorders tend to occur within families and can be inherited as dominant or recessive traits. Onset is usually early, during childhood or adolescence. No effective treatment is known. Some kinds of spinocerebellar degeneration are **ataxia telangiectasia, Charcot-Marie-Tooth atrophy, Dejerine-Sottas disease, Friedreich's ataxia, olivopontocerebellar atrophy,** and **Refsum's syndrome.**

spinofallopian tube shunt. See **ventriculofallopian tube shunt.**

spin-spin relaxation time. See **relaxation tme.**

spinth-, a combining form meaning 'spark': *spinthariscope, spintherometer, spintheropia.*

spir-, **1.** a combining form meaning 'a coil, or coiled': *spiradenitus, spireme, spirillum.* **2.** a combining form meaning 'of or pertaining to the breath, or to breathing': *spiracle, spirogram, spirophore.*

spiral fracture, a bone break in which the disruption of bone tissue is spiral, oblique, or transverse to the long axis of the fractured bone.

spiral organ of Corti. See **Corti's organ.**

spiral reverse bandage, a spiral bandage that is turned and folded back on itself as necessary to make it fit the contour of the body more securely.

spirillary rat-bite fever, spirillum fever. See **rat-bite fever.**

spirit, **1.** any volatile liquid, particularly one that has been distilled. **2.** a volatile substance dissolved in alcohol. See also **volatile.**

spiritual distress (distress of the human spirit), a nursing diagnosis accepted by the Fourth National Conference on the Classification of Nursing Diagnoses. The cause of the condition may be separation from religious or cultural ties or a change in beliefs or value system, intense suffering, severe stress, or prolonged treatment. The defining characteristics include stated anger against the deity or questions about the meaning of the suffering being experienced. The client may joke in a macabre fashion, regard the illness as punishment, have nightmares, cry, act in a hostile or apathetic manner, express self-blame or deny all responsibility for the problem, express anger or resentment against religious figures, and cease participation in religious practices. See also **nursing diagnosis.**

spirochete /spī′rəkēt′/, any bacterium of the genus *Spirochaeta* that is motile and spiral-shaped with flexible filaments. Kinds of spirochetes include the organisms responsible for leptospirosis, relapsing fever, syphilis, and yaws. Compare **bacillus, coccus, vibrio.** **–spirochetal,** *adj.*

spirogram /spī′rōgram/, a visual record of respiratory movements made by a spirometer, used in the assessment of pulmonary function and capacity.

spirograph /spī′rəgraf/, a device for recording respiratory movements. See also **spirometer.** **–spirographic,** *adj.*

spirometer /spīrom′ətər/, an instrument that measures and records the volume of inhaled and exhaled air, used to assess pulmonary function. Volumetric information is recorded on a chart, called a spirogram. **–spirometric,** *adj.*

spirometry /spīrom′ətrē/, laboratory evaluation of the air capacity of the lungs by means of a spirometer. Compare **blood gas determination.** **–spirometric,** *adj.*

spironolactone, an aldosterone antagonist.

■ INDICATIONS: It is prescribed in the treatment of primary hyperaldosteronism, edema of congestive heart failure, cirrhosis of the liver accompanied by edema, the nephrotic syndrome, essential hypertension, and hypokalemia.

■ CONTRAINDICATIONS: Anuria, acute renal insufficiency, significant impairment of renal function, or hyperkalemia prohibits its use.

■ ADVERSE EFFECTS: Among the most serious adverse reactions are hyperkalemia, gynecomastia, mental confusion, ataxia, impotence, amenorrhea, hirsutism, and urticaria.

Spitz nevus. See **benign juvenile melanoma.**

SPL. See **Staphage Lysate.**

splanchn-. See **splanchno-.**

splanchnic /splangk′nik/, of or pertaining to the internal organs; visceral.

-splanchnic, a combining form meaning 'viscera, entrails': *somaticosplanchnic, trisplanchnic, vagosplanchnic.*

splanchno-, splanchn-, a combining form meaning 'of or pertaining to a viscus, or to the splanchnic nerve': *splanchnocele, splanchnography, splanchnoptosis.*

splanchnocele, 1. See **splanchnocoele.** 2. hernial protrusion of any abdominal viscera.

splanchnocoele /splangk′nōsēl′/, a part of the embryonic body cavity, or coelom, that gives rise to the abdominal, pericardial, and pleural cavities. Also spelled **splanchnocele.** Also called **pleuroperitoneal cavity.**

splanchnopleure /splangk′nōploo͝or′/, a layer of tissue in the early developing embryo, formed by the union of endoderm and splanchnic mesoderm. It gives rise to the embryonic gut and the visceral organs and continues external to the embryo as the yolk sac and allantois. Compare **somatopleure.** –**splanchnopleural,** *adj.*

S-plasty, a technique of plastic surgery in which an S-shaped instead of a straight line incision is made to reduce tension and improve healing in areas where the skin is loose.

spleen, a soft, highly vascular, roughly ovoid organ situated between the stomach and the diaphragm in the left hypochondriac region of the body. It is considered part of the lymphatic system, because it contains lymphatic nodules. It has a dark purple color and varies in shape in different indivuals and within the same individual at different times. The precise function of the spleen has baffled physiologists for more than 100 years, but the most recent research indicates it performs various tasks, as defense, hemopoiesis, blood storage, and the destruction of red blood cells and platelets. Macrophages lining the sinuses of the spleen destroy microorganisms by phagocytosis. The spleen also produces leukocytes, monocytes, lymphocytes, and plasma cells. It produces red cells before birth and is believed to produce red cells after birth only in extreme and hemolytic anemia. If the body suffers severe hemorrhage, the spleen can increase the blood volume from 350 ml to 550 ml in less than 60 seconds. In the adult the spleen is usually about 12 cm long, 7 cm wide, and 3 cm thick. Its weight increases from 17 g or less in the first year to about 170 g at 20 years of age, then slowly decreases to about 122 g at 75 to 80 years of age. The variation in the weight of adult spleens is 100 to 250 g and, in extreme cases, 50 to 400 g. The size of the spleen increases during and after digestion and often increases during illness. It can weigh as much as 9 kg in a victim of malarial fever. The splenic nerves are derived from the celiac plexus and are mostly unmyelinated, distributing to the blood vessels of the organ and to the smooth muscle of the splenic capsule and trabeculae. Compare **thymus.** –**splenic** /splen′ik/, *adj.*

spleen scan, the scan of the spleen after the injection of radioactive red blood cells, performed to detect a tumor, damage, or other problem.

splen-. See **spleno-.**

splenectomy /splənek′təmē/, the surgical excision of the spleen.

-splenia, a combining form meaning '(condition of the spleen': *asplenia, eusplenia, microsplenia.*

splenic. See **spleen.**

splenic flexure syndrome, a recurrent pain and abdominal distention in the left upper quadrant of the abdomen caused by a pocket of gas trapped in the large intestine below the spleen, at the flexure of the transverse and descending colon. The symptoms are relieved by defecation or passing flatus.

splenic gland. See **pancreaticolienal node.**

splenic vein. See **lienal vein.**

splenius capitis, one of a pair of deep muscles of the back. Arising from the ligamentum nuchae, the seventh cervical vertebra, and the first three or four thoracic vertebrae, it inserts in the occipital bone and the mastoid process of the temporal bone. The muscle is innervated by the lateral branches of the dorsal primary divisions of the middle and the lower cervical nerves and acts to rotate, extend, and bend the head.

splenius cervicis, one of a pair of deep muscles of the back. Arising from a narrow tendinous band from the spinous processes of the third through the sixth thoracic vertebrae, it inserts into the transverse processes of the upper two or three cervical vertebrae. The muscle is innervated by the lateral branches of the dorsal primary divisions of the middle and the lower cervical nerves. The splenius cervicis acts to rotate, bend, and extend the head and neck. Also called **splenius colli.**

spleno-, splen-, a combining form meaning 'of or pertaining to the spleen': *splenocele, splenodiagnosis, splenomalacia.*

splenomedullary leukemia. See **acute myelocytic leukemia, chronic myelocytic leukemia.**

splenomegaly /splē′nōmeg′əlē, splen′-/, an abnormal enlargement of the spleen, as associated with portal hypertension, hemolytic anemia, Niemann-Pick disease, or malaria.

splenomyelogenous leukemia. See **acute myelocytic leukemia, chronic myelocytic leukemia.**

splint, 1. an orthopedic device for immobilization, restraint, or support of any part of the body. It may be rigid (of metal, plaster, or wood) or flexible (of felt or leather). 2. (in dentistry) a device for anchoring the teeth or modifying the bite. Compare **brace, cast.**

splinter fracture, a comminuted fracture with thin, sharp bone fragments.

splinter hemorrhage, linear bleeding under a finger- or toenail, resembling a splinter. It is seen after trauma and in patients with bacterial endocarditis.

split gene, (in molecular genetics) a genetic unit whose continuity is interrupted.

split personality. See **multiple personality.**

split Russell traction, an orthopedic mechanism that combines suspension and traction to immobilize, position, and align the lower extremities in the treatment of congenital hip dislocation, hip and knee contractures, and in the correction of orthopedic deformities. Split Russell traction, usually applied as adhesive or nonadhesive skin traction, employs a sling to relieve the weight of the lower extremities. The traction weights are suspended from pulley and rope systems at the foot and the head of the patient's bed; a jacket restraint is often incorporated to help immobilize the patient. Split Russell traction may be applied as a unilateral or as a bilateral mechanism. Compare **Russell traction.**

spodo-, a combining form meaning 'of or pertaining to waste materials': *spodogenous, spodophagous, spodophorous.*

-spondylic, a combining form meaning 'referring to the vertebrae': *cyclospondylic, monospondylic, tectospondylic.*

spondylitis /spon′dəlī′tis/, an inflammation of any of the spinal vertebrae, usually characterized by stiffness and pain. The condition may follow traumatic injury to the spine, or it may be the result of infection or rheumatoid disease. See also **ankylosing spondylitis.**

spondylo-, a combining form meaning 'of or pertaining to a vertebra, or to the spinal column': *spondylocace, spondylodidymia, spondylolysis.*

spondylolisthesis /spon′dilōlisthē′sis/, the partial forward dislocation of one vertebra over the one below it, most commonly the fifth lumbar vertebra over the first sacral vertebra. See also **spinal cord compression.**

spondylosis /spon′dilō′sis/, a condition of the spine characterized by fixation or stiffness of a vertebral joint. See also **ankylosing spondylitis, spondylitis.**

spondylosyndesis. See **spinal fusion.**

sponge, **1.** a resilient, absorbent mass used to absorb fluids, to apply medication, or to cleanse. The sponge may be the internal skeleton of a certain marine animal, or it may be manufactured from cellulose, rubber, or synthetic material. **2.** *informal.* a folded gauze square used in surgery.

sponge bath, the procedure of washing the patient with a damp washcloth or sponge, used when a full bath is not necessary or as a method of reducing body temperature.

sponge contraceptive. See **vaginal sponge.**

sponge gold. See **mat gold.**

spongio-, a combining form meaning 'like a sponge, or related to a sponge': *spongioblast, spongiopilin, spongiosis.*

spongioblastoma /spun′jē·ōblastō′mə/, *pl.* **spongioblastomas, spongioblastomata,** a neoplasm composed of spongioblasts, embryonic epithelial cells that develop around the neural tube and transform into cells of the supporting connective tissue of nerve cells or cells of lining membranes of the ventricles and the spinal cord canal. A kind of spongioblastoma is **spongioblastoma unipolare.** Spongioblastoma is also called **glioblastoma, gliosarcoma, spongiocytoma.**

spongioblastoma multiforme. See **glioblastoma multiforme.**

spongioblastoma unipolare, a rare neoplasm composed of approximately parallel spongioblasts. It may occur near the third ventricle, in the pons and brainstem, in basal ganglia, or in the terminal filament of the spinal cord.

spongiocytoma. See **spongioblastoma.**

spontaneous, occurring naturally and without apparent cause, as spontaneous remission.

spontaneous abortion, a termination of pregnancy before the twentieth week of gestation as a result of abnormalities of the conceptus or maternal environment. More than 10% of pregnancies end as spontaneous abortions, almost all caused by blighted ova that have congenital defects incompatible with life. Compare **induced abortion.**

spontaneous delivery, a vaginal birth occurring without the mechanic assistance of obstetric forceps or vacuum aspirator.

spontaneous evolution, the unassisted delivery of a fetus in the transverse position. See also **Denman's spontaneous evolution.**

spontaneous fracture. See **neoplastic fracture.**

spontaneous generation, the theoretic origin of living organisms from inanimate matter; abiogenesis.

spontaneous labor, a labor beginning and progressing without mechanic or pharmacologic stimulation.

spor-. See **sporo-.**

sporadic, (of a number of events) occurring at scattered, intermittent, and apparently random intervals.

-sporangium, a combining form meaning an 'encasement of spores': *haplosporangium, oosporangium, sporangium.*

spore, **1.** a reproductive unit of some genera of fungi or protozoa. **2.** a form assumed by some bacteria that is resistant to heat, drying, and chemicals. Under proper environmental conditions the spore may revert to the actively multiplying form of the bacterium. Diseases caused by spore-forming bacteria include anthrax, botulism, gas gangrene, and tetanus.

-spore, a combining form meaning a 'reproductive element': *archespore, chlamydospore, hemispore.*

sporicide /spôr′isīd/, any agent effective in destroying spores, as compounds of chlorine and formaldehyde, and the gluteraldehydes.

sporiferous /spôrif′ərəs/, producing or bearing spores.

sporo-, spor-, a combining form meaning 'of or pertaining to a spore': *sporocyst, sporogenesis, sporogeny.*

sporoblast, any cell that gives rise to a sporozoite or spore during the sexual reproductive phase of the life cycle of a sporozoan, specifically the cells resulting from the multiple fission of the encysted zygote of the malarial parasite *Plasmodium* from which the sporozoites develop.

sporocyst, **1.** any structure containing spores or reproductive cells. **2.** a saclike structure, or oocyst, secreted by the zygote of certain protozoa before sporozoite formation. **3.** the second larval stage in the life cycle of parasitic flukes. The saclike organism develops from the miracidium, or first larval stage, in the body of a freshwater snail host and contains germinal cells that give rise either to daughter sporocysts that develop into cercariae or to rediae. See also **fluke.**

sporogenesis /spôr'ōjen'əsis/, **1.** also called **sporogeny** /spôroj'ənē/. the formation of spores. **2.** reproduction by means of spores. –**sporogenic,** *adj.*

sporogenous /spôroj'ənəs/, describing an animal or plant that reproduces by spores.

sporogeny. See **sporogenesis.**

sporogony /spôrog'ənē/, reproduction by means of spores, specifically the formation of sporozoites during the sexual stage of the life cycle of a sporozoan, primarily the malarial parasite *Plasmodium*. Fusion of the sex cells occurs in the body of the invertebrate host, the female *Anopheles* mosquito in the case of *Plasmodium,* where the encysted zygote undergoes multiple division, giving rise to the sporozoites. Compare **schizogony.**

sporont /spôr'ont/, a mature protozoan parasite in the sexual reproductive stage of its life cycle. It undergoes conjugation to form a zygote, which produces sporozoites by multiple fission. Compare **schizont.** See also **sporogony.**

sporonticide /spôron'tisīd/, any substance that destroys sporonts, as chloroquine and other antimalarial drugs. –**sporonticidal,** *adj.*

sporophore /spôr'əfôr/, the part of an organism or plant that produces spores.

sporophyte /spôr'əfīt/, the asexual, spore-bearing stage in plants that reproduce by alternation of generations.

sporotrichosis /spôr'ōtrikō'sis/, a common, chronic fungal infection caused by the species *Sporothrix schenckii,* usually characterized by skin ulcers and subcutaneous nodules along lymphatic channels. It rarely spreads to involve bones, lungs, joints, or muscles. The fungus is found in soil and decaying vegetation and usually enters the skin by accidental injury. Treatment may include amphotericin B.

Sporotrichum /spôrot'rikəm/, a genus of soil-inhabiting fungi formerly thought to cause sporotrichosis.

Sporozoa, a class of parasite in the phylum Protozoa that is characterized by the absence of any external organs of locomotion. Included in this class are the genera *Toxoplasma* and *Plasmodium*.

sporozoite /spôrəzō'it/, any of the cells resulting from the sexual union of spores during the life cycle of a sporozoan. It refers specifically to the elongated nucleated cells produced by the multiple fission of the zygote contained in the oocyst in the female *Anopheles* mosquito during the sexual reproductive stage of the life cycle of the malarial parasite *Plasmodium*. On release from the oocyst, the sporozoites migrate to the salivary glands of the mosquito where they are transmitted to humans and develop within the parenchymal cells of the liver as merozoites. Also called **falciform body.** See also **malaria, *Plasmodium*.**

sport, 1. an individual or organism that differs drastically from its parents or others of its type because of genetic mutation; a mutant. **2.** a genetic mutation. **3.** See **lusus naturae.**

sporulation /spôr'yəlā'shən/, **1.** a type of reproduction that occurs in lower plants and animals, as fungi, algae, and protozoa, and involves the formation of spores by the spontaneous division of the cell into four or more daughter cells, each of which contains a portion of the original nucleus. **2.** the formation of a refractile body, or resting spore, within certain bacteria that makes the cell resistant to unfavorable environmental conditions. The cell regains its viability when the conditions become favorable. See also **spore.**

spot, (in psychotherapy) a small quantum of space that becomes the territorial object and extension of point behavior.

spot film, a radiograph made instantly during fluoroscopy. The technique may be used to make a permanent record of a transiently observed effect or to record with definition and detail a small anatomic area.

spotted fever. See **Rocky Mountain spotted fever.**

sprain, a traumatic injury to the tendons, muscles, or ligaments around a joint, characterized by pain, swelling, and discoloration of the skin over the joint. The duration and severity of the symptoms vary with the extent of damage to the supporting tissues. Treatment requires support, rest, and alternating cold and heat. Ultrasound therapy may speed recovery. X-ray pictures are often indicated to be certain that no fracture has occurred.

sprain fracture, a fracture that results from the separation of a tendon or ligament at the point of insertion, associated with the separation of a bone at the same insertion site.

spring forceps, a kind of forceps that includes a spring mechanism, used for grasping an artery to arrest or prevent hemorrhage. Also called **bulldog forceps.**

spring lancet, a lancet with a spring-triggered blade. It may be used for collecting small specimens of blood for laboratory tests. See also **lancet.**

sprinter's fracture, a fracture of the anterior superior or the anterior inferior spine of the ilium, caused by a fragment of bone being forcibly pulled by a violent muscle spasm.

sprue, a chronic disorder resulting from malabsorption of nutrients from the small intestine and characterized by a broad range of symptoms, including diarrhea, weakness, weight loss, poor appetite, pallor, muscle cramps, bone pain, ulceration of the mucous membrane lining the digestive tract, and a smooth, shiny tongue. It occurs in both tropic and nontropic forms and affects both children and adults. Also called **catarrhal dysentery.** See also **malabsorption syndrome, nontropical sprue, tropical sprue.**

SPRX, a trademark for an anorexiant (phendimetrazine tartrate).

SPSS, (in statistics) abbreviation for *Statistical Package for the Social Sciences,* a computer program often used in research in clinical nursing for the analysis of complex data from large samples.

spurious pregnancy. See **pseudocyesis.**

sputum /spyo͞o'təm/, material coughed up from the lungs and expectorated through the mouth. It contains mucus, cellular debris, or microorganisms, and it may also contain blood or pus. The amount, color, and constituents of the sputum are important in the diagnosis of many illnesses, including tuberculosis, pneumonia, cancer of the lung, and the pneumoconioses.

squam-, a combining form meaning 'of or pertaining to scales': *squamatization, squamocellular, squamopetrosal.*

squama /skwā′mə/, *pl.* **squamae, 1.** a flattened scale from the epidermis. **2.** the thin, expanded part of a bone, especially in the cranial wall.

squamous cell /skwā′məs/, a flat, scalelike epithelial cell.

squamous cell carcinoma, a slow-growing, malignant tumor of squamous epithelium, frequently found in the lungs and skin and occurring also in the anus, cervix, larynx, nose, bladder, and other sites. The typical skin lesion, a firm, red, horny, painless nodule, ranging from less than 1 to several centimeters in size, is often the result of overexposure to the sun. The neoplastic cells characteristically resemble prickle cells and form keratin pearls on the surface of lesions. Also called **epidermoid carcinoma.**

square window, an angle of the wrist between the hypothenar prominence and forearm. It is used as a reference point for estimating the gestational age of a newborn infant.

squeeze dynamometer, a dynamometer for measuring the muscular strength of the grip of the hand.

squint. See **strabismus.**

squinting eye, the abnormal eye in a person with strabismus that cannot be focused with the fixated eye. See also **strabismus.**

Sr, symbol for **strontium.**

SRO, abbreviation for **single room occupant.**

ss, abbreviation for **steady state.**

SSKI, a trademark for an expectorant (potassium iodide).

SSSS, abbreviation for **staphylococcal scalded skin syndrome.**

S's test. See **Sulkowitch's test.**

stab, a nonsegmented neutrophil.

stab form. See **band.**

-stabile, a combining form meaning 'stable, resistant to change': *coctostabile, hydrostabile, tempostabile.*

stabile diabetes. See **non-insulin-dependent diabetes.**

stabilization, 1. the physiologic and metabolic process of attaining homeostasis. **2.** the seating of a fixed or removable denture so that it will not tilt or be displaced under pressure. **3.** the control of induced stress loads and the development of measures to counteract such forces so that the movement of the teeth or of a prosthesis does not irritate surrounding tissues.

stable element, a nonradioactive element, one not subject to spontaneous nuclear degeneration. Some kinds of stable elements are calcium, iron, lead, potassium, and sodium. Compare **radioactive element.** See also **element.**

staccato speech, abnormal speech in which the person pauses between words, breaking the rhythm of the phrase or sentence. The condition is sometimes observed in association with multiple sclerosis.

stadium, *pl.* **stadia,** a significant stage in a fever or illness, as the fastigium of a febrile illness or the prodromal stage of a viral infection.

Stadol, a trademark for an opioid analgesic (butorphanol tartrate), used as an adjunct to anesthesia.

staff, 1. the people who work toward a common goal and are employed or supervised by someone of higher rank, as the nurses in a hospital. **2.** a designation by which a staff nurse is distinguished from a head nurse or other nurse. **3.** (in nursing education) the nonprofessional employees of the institution, as librarians, technicians, secretaries, and clerks. **4.** (in nursing service administration) the units of the organization that provide service to the "line," or administratively defined hierarchy; for example, the personnel office is "staff" to the director of nursing and the nursing service administration.

staff development, (in nursing) a process that assists individual nurses in an agency or organization in attaining new skills and knowledge, gaining increasing levels of competence, and growing professionally. Various resources outside the agency employing the nurse may be used. The process may include such programs as orientation, in-service education, and continuing education. Many fields outside of nursing also develop and use programs for staff development that are specific to their needs.

staffing, the process of assigning people to fill the roles designed for an organizational structure through recruitment, selection, and placement. Centralized staffing involves a system whereby a master plan is developed at the top level of the organization. Cyclical staffing is a system in which days for work and time off for personnel are repeated in regular cycles, as every 6 weeks.

staffing pattern, (in hospital or nursing administration) the number and kinds of staff assigned to the particular units and departments of a hospital. Staffing patterns vary with the unit, department, and shift.

staff of Æsculapius, a staff carried by Æsculapius, the Greek god of medicine. It is used as the traditional symbol of the physician. A single serpent entwines the staff of Æsculapius. It is often confused with the caduceus, a staff with two serpents (which is the staff of Hermes, the Greek god of commerce and travel), symbolizing the U.S. Army Medical Corps.

-stage, a combining form meaning a '(specified) phase': *aecidiostage, multistage, uredostage.*

stages of anesthesia. See **Guedel's signs.**

stages of dying, the five emotional and behavioral stages that often occur after a person first learns of approaching death. The stages, identified and described by Elizabeth Kübler-Ross, are denial and shock, anger, bargaining, depression, and acceptance. The stages may occur in sequence or they may recur, as the person moves forward and backward—especially between denial, anger, and bargaining. Caring for a dying person requires sensitivity to the signs of each stage. At first, shock may be accompanied by signs of panic. The person may refuse care and deny the diagnosis and prognosis. Denial serves as a defense against the shock. Anger often follows this stage. It is characterized by abusive language, refusal to perform basic self-care responsibilities, negative criticism of anyone who wants to help, and other kinds of angry behavior. The third stage, bargaining, reflects the need of the person for time to accept the situation. A common observation of this period is the patient's attempt to make a bargain, "If I could live until Christmas, ..." Commonly, the person goes back and forth from anger to bargaining: sometimes silent, sometimes grieving, and sometimes apathetic, depressed, insomniac, and distant. The fourth stage is a time of depression in which the person goes through a period of grieving before death, mourning over past experiences and the anticipation of impending losses. The final stage, acceptance, is one of inner peace and resolution that death is a certainty. The person may show his or her acceptance by being disinterested in present or future events, preoccupied with past events, preferring few visitors, and wanting quiet and solitude. Nursing care includes administering adequate pain relief, ensuring privacy and dignity, and giving sensitive, honest emotional support to both patient and family. See also **emotional care of the dying patient, hospice.**

stagnant anoxia, a condition in which there is inadequate blood flow in the capillaries causing low tissue oxygen tension and reduced oxygen exchange. This state is associated with shock, cardiac standstill, and thrombosis.

stain, **1.** a pigment, dye, or substance used to impart color to microscopic objects or tissues to facilitate their examination and identification. Kinds of stains include **acid-fast stain, Gram's stain,** and **Wright's stain. 2.** to apply pigment to a substance or tissue to examine it under a microscope. **3.** an area of discoloration.

stained film fault, a defect in a radiograph or developed photographic film that appears as a streaky discoloration or abnormal opacity. It is usually caused by contaminated development solutions, improper rinsing, exhausted solutions, inadequate washing, damage to the film emulsion during processing, or film hangers contaminated with dried fixer.

-stalsis, a combining form meaning a 'contraction in the alimentary canal': *antistalsis, catastalsis, retrostalsis.*

stammering, a speech dysfunction characterized by spasmodic pauses, hesitations, and faltering utterances, as mispronunciation or the transposition of letters within a word. The term is frequently used synonymously with stuttering, especially in Great Britain.

stamp cusp, a cusp that works in a fossa, as any of the maxillary lingual cusps.

stance phase of gait, the first phase of the normal gait cycle that begins with the strike of the heel on the ground and ends with the lift of the toe at the beginning of the swing phase of gait: the brief period in which both feet are on the ground.

standard, **1.** an evaluation that serves as a basis for comparison for evaluating similar phenomena or substances, as a standard for the preparation of a pharmaceutic substance, or a standard for the practice of a profession. **2.** a pharmaceutic preparation or a chemical substance of known quantity, ingredients, and strength that is used to determine the constituents or the strength of another preparation. **3.** of known value, strength, quality, or ingredients. **4.** agreed-on criteria used to provide guidance in the operation of a health care or other facility to assure quality performance by the personnel. **–standardize,** *v.*, **standardization,** *n.*

standard air chamber, a radiation measuring device used by national and international calibration laboratories to provide exposure calibrations of ion chambers for use in the diagnostic or orthovoltage energy range. Secondary ion chambers are intercompared with a standard chamber to provide a calibration factor for the field instrument, which will make its readings traceable to the standardization laboratory.

standard death certificate, a form for a death certificate that is commonly used throughout the United States. It is the preferred form of the United States Census Bureau.

standard deviation (SD), (in statistics) a mathematic statement of the dispersion of a set of values or scores from the mean. Each sample value is subtracted from the sample mean and squared, and the squares are summed. The square root of the summed squares gives a mathematically standardized value so that sample deviations can be compared.

standard environmental chamber. See **Skinner box.**

standard error, (in statistics) the variability in scores that can be expected if measurements are made on random samples of the same size from the same universe of population, phenomena, or observations. The standard error provides a framework within which a determination of the difference between groups may be made. It is an element used in determining statistic significance by means of a wide variety of formulas and methods.

standardized death rate, the number of deaths per 1000 people of a specified population during 1 year. This rate is adjusted to avoid distortion by the age composition of the population. A standard population is used for determining this rate. Also called **adjusted death rate.**

standing orders, a written document containing rules, policies, procedures, regulations, and orders for the conduct of patient care in various stipulated clinical situations. The standing orders are usually formulated collectively by the professional members of a department in a hospital or other health care facility. Standing orders usually name the condition and prescribe the action to be taken in caring for the patient, including the dosage and route of administration for a drug or the schedule for the administration of a therapeutic procedure.

stann-, a combining form meaning 'of or pertaining to tin': *stanniferous, stanniform, stannoxyl.*

stanozolol /stənō′zəlol, -ōl/, an androgenic anabolic steroid.

■ INDICATIONS: It is prescribed in the treatment of aplastic anemia and osteoporosis.

■ CONTRAINDICATIONS: Cancer of the breast or prostate, nephrosis, pregnancy, or known hypersensitivity to this drug prohibits its use.

■ ADVERSE EFFECTS: Among the most serious adverse reactions are various androgenic effects in males and females, hypoestrogenic effects in females, and allergic reactions. GI disturbances also may occur.

stapedectomy /stā′pədek′təmē/, removal of the stapes of the middle ear and insertion of a graft and prosthesis, performed to restore hearing in the treatment of otosclerosis. The stapes that has become fixed is replaced so that vibrations again transmit sound waves through the oval window to the fluid of the inner ear. Under local anesthesia, the stapes is removed and the opening into the inner ear is covered with a graft of body tissue. One end of a small plastic tube or piece of stainless steel wire is attached to the graft; the other end is attached to the two remaining bones of the middle ear, the malleus and the incus. Headache and dizziness are expected early in the postoperative period. The patient's hearing does not improve until the edema subsides and the packing is removed. Possible complications include infection of the outer, middle, or inner ear, displacement or rejection of the graft or the prosthesis, and leaking of perilymph around the prosthesis into the middle ear, with ringing in the ear and dizziness. Compare **incudectomy.**

stapes /stā′pēz/, one of the three ossicles in the middle ear, resembling a tiny stirrup. It transmits sound vibrations from the incus to the internal ear. Compare **incus, malleus.** See also **middle ear.**

Staphage Lysat (SPL), a trademark for an active immunizing agent (staphylococcal antigen phage lysed), used in staphylococcal infection.

Staphcillin, a trademark for an antibacterial (methicillin sodium).

staphylo-, staphyl-, a combining form meaning 'resembling a bunch of grapes,' used especially to show relationship to the uvula: *staphyloangina, staphylococcide, staphylolysin.*

staphylococcal antigen phage lysed. See **Staphage Lysate.**

staphylococcal infection /staf′ilōkok′əl/, an infection caused by any one of several pathogenic species of *Staphylococcus,* commonly characterized by the formation of abscesses of the skin or other organs. Staphylococcal infections of the skin include carbuncles, folliculitis, furuncles, and hidradenitis suppurativa. Bacteremia is common and may result in endocarditis, meningitis, or osteomyelitis. Staphylococcal pneumonia often follows influenza or other viral disease and may be associated with chronic or debilitating illness. Acute gastroenteritis may result from an enterotoxin produced by certain species of staphylococci in contaminated food. Treatment usually includes bed rest, analgesics, and an antimicrobial drug that is resistant to penicillinase, an enzyme secreted by many species of *Staphylococcus.* Surgical drainage, especially of deep abscesses, is often necessary.

staphylococcal scalded skin syndrome (SSSS), an abnormal skin condition, characterized by epidermal erythema, peeling, and necrosis, that gives the skin a scalded appearance. This disorder primarily affects infants 1 to 3 months of age and other children, but it may also affect adults. It is caused by strains of *Staphylococcus aureus,* especially Group II phage types. Individuals contracting the disease may be predisposed to it by deficient immune functions and by renal insufficiency. SSSS is more common in the newborn infant because of undeveloped immunity and renal systems.

■ OBSERVATIONS: A prodromal upper respiratory tract infection with concomitant purulent conjunctivitis is commonly associated with SSSS. Epidermal complications develop in the erythemal stage, the exfoliation stage, and the desquamation stage. Erythema often spreads around the mouth and other orifices and may extend over the entire body in wide circles as the skin becomes tender and the superficial layer of the skin sloughs from friction. The exfoliation stage follows the erythema stage by 24 to 48 hours and is commonly manifested by slight crusting and erosion, which may spread from around the orifices to wider skin areas. More severe forms of SSSS may cause large, soft bullae to erupt and extend over wide skin areas. The eventual rupture of these bullae reveals areas of denuded skin. The desquamation stage of SSSS, after the exfoliation stage, is characterized by the drying up of affected areas and the formation of powdery scales. Normal skin replaces the scales within 5 to 7 days. Diagnosis is based on close observation of the development of SSSS through its three characteristic stages. Erythema multiforme and drug-induced toxic epidermal necrolysis are similar to SSSS but may be ruled out in differential diagnosis by exfoliative cytology and biopsy. Confirming diagnosis is usually made on the basis of isolation of Group II *Staphylococcus aureus* in cultures of skin lesions. The mortality in SSSS is 2% to 3%, death usually being caused by complications of fluid and electrolyte loss, sepsis, and involvement of other body systems.

■ INTERVENTION: Treatment of SSSS commonly includes the administration of systemic antibiotics to prevent secondary infections and the replacement of body fluids to maintain fluid and electrolyte balance.

■ NURSING CONSIDERATIONS: The nursing role in the treatment of this disorder focuses on special care for the neonate, as maintenance of body temperature by placing the infant in an incubator, careful monitoring of intake and output, administration of IV fluids, maintenance of skin integrity, and careful, regular checks of vital signs. Nurses caring for SSSS patients are especially alert for any sudden rise in temperature, which could be an indication of sepsis and of the immediate need for aggressive treatment. To maintain skin integrity, the nurse uses a strict aseptic technique to prevent any secondary infection. The aseptic technique in skin care is especially important during the SSSS exfoliation stage, when open lesions increase the risk of infection. The patient is loosely clothed and covered to minimize friction, which sloughs off the affected skin. Cotton is inserted between the affected fingers and toes to prevent webbing. During the recovery period, warm baths and soaks aid the healing, and gentle debridement of exfoliated areas hastens the healing process. Helpful to parents is the justifiable assurance from the nurse that complications and residual scars from SSSS rarely occur.

Staphylococcus /staf′ilōkok′əs/, a genus of nonmotile, spheric, gram-positive bacteria. Some species are normally found on the skin and in the throat; certain species cause severe, purulent infections or produce an enterotoxin, which may cause nausea, vomiting, and diarrhea. Life-threatening staphylococcal infections may arise within hospitals. *Staphylococcus aureus* is a species frequently responsible for abscesses, endocarditis, impetigo, osteomyelitis, pneumonia, and septicemia. *S. epidermidis,* formerly called *S. albus,* occasionally causes endocarditis in the presence of intracardiac prostheses. See also **staphylococcal infection.** –**staphylococcal,** *adj.*

staphylokinase /staf′ilōkī′nās/, an enzyme, produced by certain strains of staphylococci, that catalyzes the conversion of plasminogen to plasmin in various animal hosts of the microorganism.

starch, the principal molecule used for the storage of food in plants. Starch is a polysaccharide and is composed of long chains of glucose subunits. In animals, excess glucose is stored as glycogen. The molecular structure of glycogen is similar to that of starch. See also **carbohydrate, glucose, glycogen.**

Starling's law of the heart, a rule that the force of the heartbeat is determined by the length of the fibers comprising the myocardial walls.

Starr-Edwards prosthesis, an artificial cardiac valve. A caged-ball form of device, it obstructs the valve opening and prevents the backward flow of blood. See also **prosthesis.**

start codon. See **initiation codon.**

startle reflex. See **Moro reflex.**

start point, (in molecular genetics) the initial nucleotide transcribed from the DNA template in the formation of messenger RNA.

starvation, **1.** a condition resulting from the lack of essential nutrients over a long period of time and characterized by multiple physiologic and metabolic dysfunctions. **2.** the act or state of starving or being starved. See also **malnutrition.**

stas-, a combining form meaning 'stopped, or relation to standing or walking': *stasibasiphobia, stasidynic, stasis.*

-stasia, -stasis, **1.** a combining form meaning a '(specified) condition involving the ability to stand': *astasia, ananastasia, dysstasia.* **2.** a combining form meaning '(condition of) stoppage or inhibition': *cholestasia, hemostasia, menostasia.*

stasis /stā′sis, stas′is/, **1.** a disorder in which the normal flow of a fluid through a vessel of the body is slowed or halted. **2.** stillness.

-stasis. See **-stasia.**

stasis dermatitis, a common result of venous insufficiency of the legs beginning with ankle edema and progressing to tan pigmentation, patchy erythema, petechiae, and induration. Ultimately, there may be atrophy and fibrosis of the skin and subcutaneous tissue, with ulcerations that are slow to heal. The tan pigment is hemosiderin from blood leaking through capillary walls under elevated venous pressure. The involved skin is very easily irritated or sensitized to topical medications. The underlying venous insufficiency must be treated. The dermatitis is often treated by bed rest, Burow's solution for oozing lesions, antibiotics for infection, and corticosteroids to reduce inflammation. Also called **venous stasis dermatitis.** See also **stasis ulcer.**

stasis ulcer, a necrotic craterlike lesion of the skin of the lower leg caused by chronic venous congestion. The ulcer is often associated with stasis dermatitis and varicose veins. Healing is slow, and good nursing care to prevent irritation and infection is essential. Potentially sensitizing agents should not be used. Bed rest, elevation, and pressure bandages are usually ordered and appropriate antibiotics, Burow's solution compresses, Unna's paste boot, pinch grafts, and surgery to improve venous flow are useful in treatment. Also called **varicose ulcer.** See also **stasis dermatitis.**

-stat, **1.** a combining form meaning a 'device for keeping something stationary': *catheterostat, hysterostat, ophthalmostat.* **2.** a combining form meaning an 'instrument for the regulation of' something specified: *hemostat, rheostat, thermostat.* **3.** a combining form meaning an 'apparatus for the reflection of, in one direction of' something specified: *siderostat.* **4.** a combining form meaning a 'device for studying in a state of rest': *hydrostat, orbitostat, microstat.* **5.** a combining form meaning an 'agent for stopping the growth of': *bacteriostat, fungistat, mycostat.*

-state, a combining form meaning the 'result of a (specified) process': *anastate, catastate, mesostate.*

State Board Test Pool Examination (SBTPE), revised and retitled in 1982 as the NCLEX-RN, an examination prepared by the National Council of State Boards of Nursing for testing the competency of a person to perform safely as a newly licensed registered nurse. Each jurisdiction within the United States and its territories regulates entry into the practice of nursing; each requires the candidate to pass the examination. The content of the examination is planned to test the candidates' knowledge of the nursing process as applied to the broad areas of nursing practice, including maternal and child health, medical and surgical nursing, and psychiatric nursing. The process includes five steps: assessing, analyzing, planning, implementing, and evaluating. Knowledge, comprehension, application, and analysis of the nursing process are tested as they apply to decision-making situations.

state medicine. See **socialized medicine.**

State Nurses' Association (SNA), an association of nurses at the state level. The various State Nurses' Associations are constituent units of the American Nurses' Association.

Statewide Health Coordinating Committee (SHCC), a component of the national network of Health Systems Agencies.

static, without motion, at rest, in equilibrium. Compare **dynamic.**

static cardiac work, the energy transfer that occurs during the development and maintenance of ventricular pressure immediately before the opening of the aortic valve.

static electricity film fault, a defect in a radiograph or a developed photographic film, which appears as lightninglike streaks. It is caused by too rapid opening of the film packet or transfer of static electricity from the user to the film.

static imaging, (in nuclear medicine) a diagnostic procedure in which a radioactive substance is administered to a patient to visualize an internal organ or body compartment. An image or set of images is made of the fixed or slowly changing distribution of the radioactivity.

Statistical Package for the Social Sciences. See **SPSS.**

station, the level of the biparietal plane of the fetal head relative to the level of the ischial spines of the maternal pelvis. An imaginary plane at the level of the spines is designated ''zero station.'' Higher and lower stations are numbered at intervals of 1 cm; minus above, plus below. For example, ''station minus three'' is 3 cm above the spines, and ''station plus two'' is 2 cm below the spines. In breech presentation, the bitrochanteric diameter of the breech is used to determine station. See also **dilatation, effacement, labor.**

stationary grid, (in radiography) an x-ray grid that does not move or oscillate during the exposure of a radiographic film. The image of the lead strips that compose the grid appear on the radiograph.

stationary lingual arch, an orthodontic arch wire that is designed to fit the lingual surface of the teeth and is soldered to the associated anchor bands.

statistic, a number that describes a property of a set of data or other numbers.

statotonic reflex. See **attitudinal reflex.**

status, **1.** a specified state or condition, as emotional status. **2.** an unremitting state or condition, as status asthmaticus.

status asthmaticus, an acute, severe, and prolonged asthma attack. Hypoxia, cyanosis, and unconsciousness may follow. Treatment includes aminophylline given intravenously, corticosteroids, controlled positive pressure ventilation, heavy sedation, frequent bronchial hygiene therapy, and emotional support. A bronchodilator may be given by aerosol inhalation from a ventilator. See also **allergic asthma, asthma.**

status dysraphicus. See **dysraphia.**

status epilepticus, a medical emergency characterized by continual attacks of convulsive seizures occurring without intervals of consciousness. Unless convulsions are arrested, irreversible brain damage results. Status epilepticus can be precipitated by the sudden withdrawal of anticonvulsant drugs, inadequate body levels of glucose, a brain tumor, a head injury, a high fever, or poisoning. Therapy includes intravenous administration of anticonvulsant drugs, nutrients, and electrolytes, preferably given in an intensive care unit. An adequate airway is usually maintained with an oral pharyngeal or endotracheal tube.

statute of limitations, (in law) a statute that sets a limit of time during which a suit may be brought or criminal charges may be made. In a malpractice suit, dispute may arise as to whether the time set by the particular statute of limitations begins to run at the time of the injury or at the time of the discovery of the injury.

statutory rape, (in law) sexual intercourse with a female below the age of consent, which varies from state to state. See also **rape.**

STD, abbreviation for **sexually transmitted disease.**

steady state (s, ss), a basic physiologic concept implying that the various forces and processes of life are in a state of homeostasis. Living organisms are in constant flux, working to balance the internal and external environments in an effort to avoid a deficiency or an excess that might cause illness. Steady state is a complete state of well-being involving total adaptation.

steap-, stear-. See **stearo-.**

-stearic, a combining form meaning '(specified) fat or fat derivatives': *aleostearic, ketostearic, neurostearic.*

Stearns' alcoholic amentia, a form of insanity brought on by alcohol, characterized by an emotional disturbance of a less severe nature than that of delirium tremens but of longer duration and with greater mental clouding and amnesia.

stearo-, steap-, stear-, steato-, a combining form meaning 'of or pertaining to fat': *stearoconotum, stearodermia, stearopten.*

stearyl alcohol, a solid substance, prepared by the catalytic hydrogenation of stearic acid, used in various ointments.

steato-. See **stearo-.**

steatorrhea /stē′ətərē′ə/, greater than normal amounts of fat in the feces, characterized by frothy, foul-smelling fecal matter that floats, as in celiac disease, some malabsorption syndromes, and any condition in which fats are poorly absorbed by the small intestine.

Steele-Richardson-Olszewski syndrome, a rare, progressive, neurologic disorder of unknown cause, occurring in middle age, more often in men. It is characterized by paralysis of eye muscles, ataxia, neck and trunk rigidity, pseudobulbar palsy, and parkinsonian facies. Dementia and inappropriate emotional responses are also common. Treatment usually includes the antiparkinsonian drug levodopa for control of extrapyramidal symptoms. Also called **progressive supranuclear palsy.** See also **Parkinson's disease.**

steeple head. See **oxycephaly.**

Steinert's disease. See **myotonic muscular dystrophy.**

Stein-Leventhal syndrome. See **polycystic ovary syndrome.**

Stelazine, a trademark for a phenothiazine tranquilizer (trifluoperazine).

stell-, a combining form meaning 'of or pertaining to a star': *stellate, stellectomy, stellula.*

stellate /stel′it, -āt/, star-shaped or arranged in the pattern of a star.

stellate fracture, a fracture that involves the central point of impact or injury and radiates numerous fissures throughout surrounding bone tissue.

stem cell leukemia, a malignant neoplasm of blood-forming organs in which the predominant neoplastic cell is too immature to classify. The disease is extremely acute and has a rapid, relentless course. Also called **embryonal leukemia, hemoblastic leukemia, hemocytoblastic leukemia, lymphoidocytic leukemia, undifferentiated cell leukemia.**

stem cell lymphoma. See **undifferentiated malignant lymphoma.**

stem pessary. See **pessary.**

steno-, a combining form meaning 'contracted or narrow': *stenobregmate, stenocephaly, stenothorax.*

stenosis /stinō′sis/, an abnormal condition characterized by the constriction or narrowing of an opening or passageway in a body structure. Kinds of stenosis include **aortic stenosis** and **pyloric stenosis.** –**stenotic,** *adj.*

Stensen's duct. See **parotid duct.**

stent, **1.** a compound used in making dental impressions and medical molds. **2.** a mold or device made of stent, used in anchoring skin grafts and for supporting body openings and cavities during grafting or vessels and tubes of the body during surgical anastomosis.

step reflex. See **dance reflex.**

Sterane, a trademark for a glucocorticoid (prednisolone).

Sterapred, a trademark for a glucocorticoid (prednisone).

sterco-, a combining form meaning 'of or pertaining to feces': *stercobilin, stercolith, stercoremia.*

stereo-, a combining form meaning 'solid, three dimensional, or firmly established': *stereoblastula, stereograph, stereopsis.*

stereognostic perception /ster′ē·ōgnos′tik/, the ability to recognize objects by the sense of touch.

stereoisomeric specificity /ster′ē·ō·ī′sōmer′ik/, specificity of an enzyme for one form of a DL pair of compounds with an asymmetric carbon atom.

stereoradiography, a technique for producing radiograms that give a three-dimensional view of an internal body structure. The stereoradiograms are produced by combining two separate x-ray films, each made from a slightly different angle without movement of the body part being x-rayed. The developed films are then viewed through a stereoscope.

stereoscopic microscope, a microscope that produces three-dimensional images through the use of double eyepieces and double objectives. The three-dimensional image is created because the double optic systems have independent light paths. Also called **Greenough microscope.**

stereoscopic parallax. See **binocular parallax.**

stereoscopic radiograph, a composite of two radiographs, made by shifting the position of the x-ray tube a few centimeters between each of two exposures. The result is a three-dimensional presentation of the radiograph when viewed through steroscopic lenses.

stereotaxic neuroradiography, an x-ray procedure commonly performed during neurosurgery to guide the insertion of a needle into a specific area of the brain.

stereotype, a generalization about a form of behavior, an individual, or a group.

stereotypic behavior, a pattern of body movements that has autistic and symbolic meaning for an individual.

stereotypy /ster′ē·ətī′pē/, the persistent, inappropriate, mechanic repetition of actions, body postures, or speech patterns, usually occurring with a lack of variation in thought processes or ideas. It is often seen in patients with schizophrenia. –**stereotypical,** *adj.*

sterile /ster′il/, **1.** barren; unable to produce children because of a physical abnormality, often the absence of spermatogenesis in a man or blockage of the fallopian tubes in a woman. Compare **impotence.** **2.** aseptic. –**sterility,** *n.*

sterilization, **1.** a process or act that renders a person unable to produce children. See also **hysterectomy, tubal ligation, vasectomy.** **2.** a technique for destroying microorganisms using heat, water, chemicals, or gases. –**sterilize,** *v.*

-sternal, a combining form meaning 'pertaining to the sternum': *adsternal, presternal, suprasternal.*

sternal node /stur′nəl/, a node in one of the three groups of thoracic parietal lymph nodes. They are situated at the anterior ends of the intercostal spaces, adjacent to the internal thoracic artery. The afferent vessels of the sternal nodes drain the lymph from the breast, the diaphragmatic surface of the liver, and the deep, ventral thoracic wall. The efferent vessels of the sternal nodes usually form a single lymphatic trunk on each side. The trunk may open directly into the junction of the internal jugular and the subclavian veins; or the trunk on the right side may join the right lymphatic subclavian trunk, and the trunk on the left side may join the thoracic duct. Also called **internal mammary node.** Compare **diaphragmatic node, intercostal node.** See also **lymphatic system, lymph node.**

Sternheimer-Malbin stain, a crystal violet and safranin stain used in urinalyses to provide additional contrast for certain casts and cells.

-sternia, a combining form meaning '(condition of the) sternum': *asternia, koilosternia, schistosternia.*

sterno-, a combining form meaning 'of or pertaining to the sternum': *sternocleidal, sternocostal, sternopagus.*

sternoclavicular articulation, the double gliding joint between the sternum and the clavicle. It involves the sternal end of the clavicle, the superior and lateral part of the manubrium, the cartilage of the first rib, and six ligaments.

sternocostal articulation, the gliding articulation of the cartilage of each true rib and the sternum, except for the articulation of the first rib in which the cartilage is directly united with the sternum to form a synchondrosis. Each sternocostal articulation also involves five ligaments.

sternohyoideus /stur′nōhī•oi′dē•əs/, one of the four infrahyoid muscles. Arising from the medial end of the clavicle, the posterior sternoclavicular ligament, and the manubrium sterni and inserting into the inferior border of the hyoid bone, it is a thin, narrow muscle innervated by fibers from the first, second, and third cervical nerves. It acts to depress the hyoid bone. Also called **sternohyoid muscle.** Compare **omohyoideus, sternothyroideus, thyrohyoideus.**

sternothyroideus /stur′nōthīroi′dē•əs/, one of the four infrahyoid muscles. Arising from the dorsal surface of the manubrium sterni and inserting into the thyroid cartilage, it is innervated by fibers from the first, second, and third cervical nerves, through the ansa cervicalis. It acts to depress the thyroid cartilage. Also called **sternothyroid muscle.** Compare **omohyoideus, sternohyoideus, thyrohyoideus.**

sternum, the elongated, flattened bone forming the middle portion of the thorax. It supports the clavicles, articulates with the first seven pairs of ribs, and comprises the manubrium, the gladiolus (body), and the xiphoid process. It is composed of highly vascular tissue covered by a thin layer of bone and is a site for needle puncture for biopsy of bone marrow specimens. The sternum is longer in men than in women.

sternutation. See **sneeze.**

sterognosis /ster′ōgnō′sis/, **1.** the faculty of perceiving and understanding the form and nature of objects by the sense of touch. **2.** perception by the senses of the solidity of objects. –**sterognostic,** *adj.*

steroid, any of a large number of hormonal substances with a similar basic chemical structure, produced mainly in the adrenal cortex and gonads.

sterol, a large subgroup of steroids containing an OH group at position 3 and a branched aliphatic side chain of eight or more carbon atoms at position 17. Kinds of sterols include **cholesterol** and **ergosterol.**

stertorous /stur′tərəs/, pertaining to a respiratory effort that is strenuous or struggling; having a snoring sound.

stetho-, steth-, a combining form meaning 'of or pertaining to the chest': *stethometer, stethomyitis, stethospasm.*

stethoscope /steth′əskōp/, an instrument, used in mediate auscultation, consisting of two earpieces connected by means of flexible tubing to a diaphragm, which is placed against the skin of the patient's chest or back to hear heart and lung sounds.

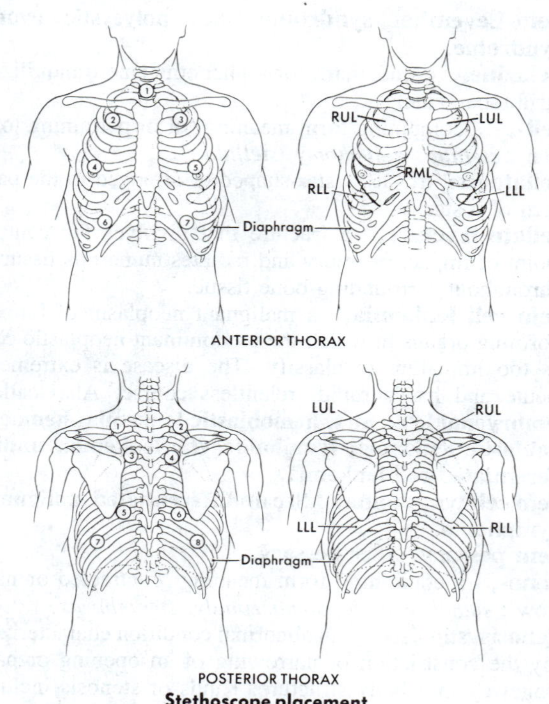

Stethoscope placement

Stevens-Johnson syndrome, a serious, sometimes fatal inflammatory disease affecting children and young adults. It is characterized by the acute onset of fever, bullae on the skin, and ulcers on the mucous membranes of the lips, eyes, mouth, nasal passage, and genitalia. Pneumonia, pain in the joints, and prostration are common. A complication may be perforation of the cornea. The syndrome may be an allergic reaction to certain drugs, or it may follow pregnancy, herpesvirus I, or other infection. It is seen rarely in association with malignancy or with radiation therapy. Treatment includes bed rest, antibiotics for pneumonia, glucocorticoids, analgesics, mouthwashes, and sedatives.

Stewart, Isabel Maitland (1878–1963), a Canadian-born American nursing educator and writer. The first nurse to receive a master's degree from Columbia University in New York, she succeeded Mary Adelaide Nutting as Professor of Nursing at Teachers College at that university. She was instrumental in upgrading the nursing curriculum and in directing educational policies and became an important figure in international nursing affairs.

sthen-. See **stheno-.**

-sthenia, a combining form meaning 'power or strength': *angiosthenia, eusthenia, hyposthenia.*

sthenic fever /sthen′ik/, high body temperature associated with thirst, dry skin, and, often, delirium.

stheno-, sthen-, a combining form meaning 'of or pertaining to strength': *sthenometer, sthenoplastic, sthenopyra.*

-sthenuria, a combining form meaning '(condition of) urination or of the specific gravity of urine': *hypersthenuria, isosthenuria, normosthenuria.*

stib-, a combining form meaning 'of or pertaining to antimony': *stibamine, stibophen, stiburea.*

stibocaptate. See **sodium stibocaptate.**

stibogluconate sodium, an antileishmanial available from the Center for Disease Control. It is a drug of choice for the visceral form of leishmaniasis and has some effect on other forms.

stibophen /stib′əfin/, a schistosomicide.

■ INDICATIONS: It is prescribed in the treatment of infestations of *Schistosoma japonicum* or *S. haematobium.*

■ CONTRAINDICATIONS: Severe hepatic, renal, or cardiac insufficiency or known hypersensitivity to this drug prohibits its use.

■ ADVERSE EFFECTS: Among the more serious adverse reactions are pain at the site of injection, GI disturbances, fever, and blood dyscrasias.

-stichia, a combining form meaning a 'condition involving rows of eyelashes': *distichia, tristichia, polystichia.*

sticky ends. See **cohesive termini.**

Stieda's fracture /stē′dəz/, a fracture of the internal condyle of the femur.

stiff lung. See **congestive atelectasis.**

stigma, *pl.* **stigmata, stigmas, 1.** a moral or physical blemish. **2.** a physical characteristic that serves to identify a disease or a condition.

stilbestrol. See **diethylstilbestrol.**

stilet, stilette. See **stylet.**

stillbirth, 1. the birth of a fetus that died before or during delivery. **2.** a fetus, born dead, that weighs more than 1000 g and would usually have been expected to live.

stillborn, 1. an infant that was born dead. **2.** of or pertaining to an infant that was born dead.

Still's disease. See **juvenile rheumatoid arthritis.**

Stilphostrol, a trademark for an estrogen (diethylstilbestrol diphosphate).

stimulant, any agent that increases the rate of activity of a body system.

stimulant cathartic, a cathartic that acts by promoting the motility of the bowel, especially the longitudinal peristalsis of the colon. Kinds of stimulant cathartics are **cascara** and **senna.**

stimulating bath, a bath taken in water that contains an aromatic substance, an astringent, or a tonic.

stimulus, *pl.* **stimuli,** anything that excites or incites an organism or part to function, become active, or respond. **–stimulate,** *v.*

stimulus control, a strategy for self-modification that depends on manipulating the antecedents of behavior to increase goals or behaviors desired by a patient while decreasing those that are undesired.

stimulus duration, the length of time a stimulus must be applied for the resulting nerve impulse to produce excitation in the receptor tissue. In general, more intense stimuli require shorter excitation times to effect cellular response. Any stimulus that acts for a period of time too brief to overcome the threshold intensity of the receptor cell will not elicit a response.

stimulus generalization, a type of conditioning in which the reaction to one stimulus is reinforced to allow transfer of the reaction to other occurrences.

sting, an injury caused by a sharp, painful penetration of the skin, often accompanied by exposure to an irritating chemical or the venom of an insect or other animal. In cases of hypersensitivity, a highly venomous sting, or multiple stings, anaphylactic shock may occur. Kinds of stings include bee, jellyfish, scorpion, sea urchin, and shellfish stings. See also **stingray, wasp.**

stingray, a flat, long-tailed fish bearing barbed spines on its back that are connected to sacs of venom. Spasm of the skeletal muscles, severe local pain, seizures, and dyspnea may occur if the skin is broken by the spines. The wound is washed with cold salt water, and the injured limb is placed in very hot water for 30 to 60 minutes; an antiseptic is applied and tetanus prophylaxis is administered. See also **sea urchin sting.**

St. Louis encephalitis, an arbovirus infection of the brain transmitted from birds to humans by the bite of an infected mosquito. It occurs most commonly in the central and southern portions of the United States and is characterized by headache, malaise, fever, stiff neck, delirium, and convulsions. Sequelae may include visual and speech disturbances, difficulty in walking, and personality changes. Convalescence may be prolonged, and death may result. Compare **California encephalitis, equine encephalitis.** See also **encephalitis.**

stoker's cramp. See **heat cramp.**

Stokes-Adams syndrome. See **Adams-Stokes syndrome.**

-stole, a combining form referring to the contraction, retraction, or dilatation of various organs: *anastole, diastole, peristole.*

stoma, *pl.* **stomas, stomata, 1.** a pore, orifice, or opening on a surface. **2.** an artificial opening of an internal organ on the surface of the body, created surgically, as for a colostomy, ileostomy, or tracheostomy. **3.** a new opening created surgically, between two body structures, as for a gastroenterostomy, pancreaticogastrostomy, pancreatoduodenostomy, or pyeloureterostomy.

-stoma, a combining form meaning a 'mouth or opening': *hypostoma, metastoma, tetrastoma.*

stomach, the major organ of digestion, located in the right upper quadrant of the abdomen and divided into a body and a pylorus. It receives and partially processes food and drink funneled from the mouth through the esophagus and moves nutritional bulk into the intestines. The stomach lies in the epigastric and left hypogastric regions bounded by the anterior abdominal wall and the diaphragm between the liver and the spleen. The shape of the stomach is modified by the amount of contents, stage of digestion, development of gastric musculature, and condition of the intestines. It is lined with a mucous coat, a submucous coat, a muscular coat, and a serous coat, all richly supplied with blood vessels and nerves, and contains fundic, cardiac, and pyloric gastric glands. Also called **gaster.**

stomach pump, a pump for withdrawing the contents of the stomach through a tube passed through the mouth or nose into the stomach.

stomadaeum, stomadeum. See **stomodeum.**

stomal peptic ulcer, a marginal peptic ulcer. See also **peptic ulcer.**

stomatitis /stō′mətī′tis/, any inflammatory condition of the mouth. It may result from infection by bacteria, viruses, or fungi, from exposure to certain chemicals or drugs, from vitamin deficiency, or from a systemic inflammatory disease. Kinds of stomatitis include **aphthous stomatitis, pseudomembranous stomatitis, thrush,** and **Vincent's infection.**

stomato-, stomo-, a combining form meaning 'of or pertaining to the mouth': *stomatodysodia, stomatogastric, stomatopathy.*

stomatognathic system /stō′mətonath′ik/, the combination of organs, structures, and nerves involved in speech and reception, mastication, and deglutition of food. This system is composed of the teeth, the jaws, the masticatory muscles, the tongue, the lips, and surrounding tissues and the nerves that control these structures.

stomatology, the study of the morphology, structure, function, and diseases of the oral cavity. **–stomatologist,** *n.,* **stomatologic, stomatological,** *adj.*

-stomia, a combining form meaning '(condition of the) mouth': *atelostomia, atretostomia, hygrostomia.*

stomion, the median point of the oral slit when the mouth is closed.

stomo-. See **stomato-.**

stomodeum /stom′ədē′əm/, *pl.* **stomodeums, stomodea,** an invagination in the ectoderm located in the foregut of the developing embryo that forms the mouth. Also spelled **stomodaeum, stomadeum, stomadaeum.** Compare **proctodeum. –stomodeal, stomodaeal, stomadeal,** *adj.*

-stomy, a combining form meaning 'surgical opening': *gastrostomy, lobostomy, tracheostomy.*

stone. See **calculus.**

-stone, a combining form meaning a 'calculus in a human organ or duct': *bilestone, gallstone, wombstone.*

stool. See **feces.**

stool softener. See **fecal softener.**

stop needle, a needle with a shoulder flange that stops it from penetrating beyond a certain distance.

storage device. See **secondary memory device.**

storing fermentation, the rapid, gaseous clotting of milk caused by *Clostridium perfringens.*

stork bite. See **telangiectatic nevus.**

Stoxil, a trademark for an antiviral (idoxuridine).

STP, *slang.* a psychedelic agent, dimethoxy-4-methylampetamine (DOM). STP is an abbreviation for *serenity, tranquility, and peace.*

STPD, abbreviation for *standard temperature, standard pressure, dry.*

strab-, a combining form meaning 'squinting': *strabismometer, strabometry, strabotomy.*

strabismus, an abnormal ocular condition in which the eyes are crossed. There are two kinds of strabismus, paralytic and nonparalytic. Paralytic strabismus results from the inability of the ocular muscles to move the eye because of neurologic deficit or muscular dysfunction. The muscle that is dysfunctional may be identified by watching as the patient attempts to move the eyes to each of the cardinal positions of gaze. If the affected eye cannot be directed to a position, the examiner infers that the associated ocular muscle is the dysfunctional one. Because this kind of strabismus may be caused by tumor, infection, or injury to the brain or the eye, an ophthalmologic examination is recommended. Nonparalytic strabismus is a defect in the position of the two eyes in relation to each other. The condition is inherited. The person cannot use the two eyes together but has to fix with one or the other. The eye that looks straight at a given time is the fixing eye. Some people have alternating strabismus, using one eye and then the other; some have monocular strabismus affecting only one eye. Visual acuity diminishes with diminished use of an eye, and suppression amblyopia may develop. Nonparalytic strabismus and suppression amblyopia are treated most successfully in early childhood. Treatment consists mainly of covering the fixing eye, forcing the child to use the deviating eye. The earlier it is begun the more rapid and effective the treatment. By 6 years of age, a deviating eye has usually become so suppressed that treatment is not effective and permanent visual loss has occurred. The eyes might be straightened by surgery, but suppression amblyopia will not be corrected. Also called **squint. –strabismal, strabismic, strabismical,** *adj.*

straight line blood set, a common device, composed of plastic components, for delivering blood infusions. It includes the plastic tubing, the clamp, the drip chamber, and the filter. Some kinds of straight-line blood sets contain filters within drip chambers; others have separate filters. The latter kind can be filled by squeezing the attached drip chamber but must not be squeezed itself or it may rupture. The former kind can be filled by squeezing the section of the blood set that contains the filter and the drip chamber. Before infusion, the filter of either kind is tapped with the fingers to dislodge any trapped air bubbles. Compare **component drip set, component syringe set, microaggregate recipient set, Y-set.**

straight sinus, one of the six posterior-superior venous channels of the dura mater, draining blood from the brain into the internal jugular vein. It has no valves and is located at the junction of the falx cerebri with the tentorium cerebelli. It is triangular in section and increases in size as it runs posteriorly from the end of the inferior sagittal sinus to the transverse sinus of the opposite side. It receives the inferior sagittal sinus, the great cerebral vein, and the superior cerebellar veins. Compare **inferior sagittal sinus, superior sagittal sinus, transverse sagittal sinus.**

straight wire fixed orthodontic appliance, an orthodontic appliance used for correcting and improving malocclusion. It is a variation of the edgewise fixed orthodontic appliance and is designed to decrease arch wire adjustments by reorienting arch wire slots.

strain, **1.** to exert physical force in a manner that may result in injury, usually muscular. **2.** to separate solids or particles from a liquid with a filter or sieve. **3.** damage, usually muscular, that results from excessive physical effort. **4.** a taxon that is a subgroup of a species. **5.** an emotional state reflecting mental pressure or fatigue.

straitjacket, a coatlike garment of canvas with long sleeves that can be tied behind the wearer's back to prevent movement of the arms. It is used for restraining violent or uncontrollable people.

strangulation, the constriction of a tubular structure of the body, as the trachea, a segment of bowel, or the blood vessels of a limb, that prevents function or impedes circulation. See also **intestinal strangulation.** **–strangulate,** *v.*, **strangulated,** *adj.*

strap, **1.** a band, as that made of adhesive plaster, that is used to hold dressings in place or to attach one thing to another. **2.** to bind securely.

strapping, the application of overlapping strips of adhesive tape to an extremity or body area to exert pressure and hold a structure in place, performed in the treatment of strains, sprains, dislocations, and certain fractures.

strati-, a combining form meaning 'layer': *stratification, stratiform, stratigraphy.*

stratiform cartilage. See **fibrocartilage.**

stratiform fibrocartilage, a structure made of fibrocartilage that forms a thin coating of osseous grooves through which tendons of certain muscles glide. Small masses of stratified fibrocartilage also develop in the tendons of some muscles that glide over bones, as in the tendons of the peroneus longus and the tibialis posterior. Compare **circumferential fibrocartilage, connecting fibrocartilage, interarticular fibrocartilage.**

stratum /strā′təm, strat′əm/, *pl.* **strata,** a uniformly thick sheet or layer, usually associated with other layers, as the stratum basale of the epidermis.

stratum basale, **1.** also called **stratum germinativum.** the deepest of the five layers of the skin, composed of tall cylindric cells. This layer provides new cells by mitotic cell division. Compare **stratum corneum, stratum granulosum, stratum lucidum, stratum spinosum.** See also **skin.** **2.** the deepest layers of the uterine decidua, containing uterine gland terminals.

stratum corneum, the horny, outermost layer of the skin, composed of dead cells converted to keratin that continually flakes away. The thickness of the layer is correlated with the normal wear of the area it covers. The stratum corneum is thick on the palms of the hands and the soles of the feet but thin over more protected areas. Also called **horny layer.** Compare **stratum basale, stratum granulosum, stratum lucidum, stratum spinosum.** See also **skin.**

stratum germinativum. See **stratum basale.**

stratum granulosum, one of the layers of the epidermis, situated just below the stratum corneum except in the palms of the hands and the soles of the feet, where it lies just under the stratum lucidum. The stratum granulosum contains visible granules in the cytoplasm of its cells, which die, become keratinized, move to the surface, and flake away. Compare **stratum basale, stratum corneum, stratum lucidum, stratum spinosum.** See also **skin.**

stratum lucidum, one of the layers of the epidermis, situated just beneath the stratum corneum and present only in the thick skin of the palms of the hands and the soles of the feet. It contains translucent eleidin that forms keratin. Also called **clear cell layer.** Compare **stratum basale, stratum corneum, stratum granulosum, stratum spinosum.** See also **skin.**

stratum spinosum, one of the layers of the epidermis, composed of several layers of polygonal cells. It lies on top of the stratum basale and beneath the stratum granulosum and contains tiny fibrils within its cellular cytoplasm. When the cells of the stratum spinsosum are pulled apart, they present minute spines at their surfaces. Also called **prickle cell layer.** Compare **stratum basale, stratum corneum, stratum granulosum, stratum lucidum.** See also **skin.**

stratum spongiosum, one of the three layers of the endometrium of the uterus, containing tortuous, dilated uterine glands and a small amount of interglandular tissue. With the stratum compactum it forms the functional part of the endometrium during pregnancy. Compare **stratum basale.** See also **decidua, placenta.**

strawberry gallbladder, a tiny, yellow gallbladder spotted with deposits on the red mucous membrane, characteristic of cholesterolosis.

strawberry hemangioma, strawberry mark. See **capillary hemangioma.**

strawberry tongue, a clinical sign of scarlet fever, characterized by a strawberry-like coloration of the inflamed tongue papillae.

stray light, radiant energy that reaches a photodetector and which consists of wavelengths other than those defined by the filter or monochromator.

stray radiation. See **leakage radiation.**

streak, a line or a stripe, as the primitive streak at the caudal end of the embryonic disk.

strength of association, the degree of relationship between a causal factor and the occurence of a disease, usually expressed in terms of a relative risk ratio.

strepho-, streph-, a combining form meaning 'twisted': *strephopodia, strephosymbolia, strephotome.*

strep throat, *informal.* an infection of the oral pharynx and tonsils caused by a hemolytic species of *Streptococcus,* usually belonging to group A. The infection is characterized by sore throat, chills, fever, swollen lymph nodes in the neck, and, sometimes, nausea and vomiting. The symptoms usually begin abruptly a few days after exposure to the organism in airborne droplets or after direct contact with an infected person. Also called **streptococcal sore throat.**

■ OBSERVATIONS: The throat is diffusely red, and tonsils often are covered with a yellow or white exudate. Diagnosis is confirmed by bacteriologic culture and identification of the streptococcal bacteria in a specimen taken from the throat. Complications of strep throat are otitis media, scarlet fever, and sinusitis; other complications include acute glomerulonephritis and acute rheumatic fever.

■ INTERVENTION: Treatment usually includes intramuscular injection of benzathene penicillin G or the administration of penicillin for 10 days. Erythromycin may be given to people allergic to penicillin. For recurrent infections, tonsillectomy may be recommended.

■ NURSING CONSIDERATIONS: Analgesics and throat irrigation with warm saline solution may give relief from pain. Family members and other contacts are observed for signs of infection, and those for whom streptococcal infection presents a special risk are treated prophylactically.

strepto-, a combining form meaning 'twisted': *streptobacilli, streptococcal, streptomicrodactyly.*

streptobacillary rat-bite fever. See **Haverhill fever.**

Streptobacillus moniliformis, a species of necklace-shaped bacteria that can cause rat-bite fever in humans.

streptococcal angina /strep′təkok′əl/, a condition in which feelings of choking, suffocation, and pain occur as the result of a streptococcal infection.

streptococcal infection, an infection caused by pathogenic bacteria of one of several species of the genus *Streptococcus* or their toxins. Almost any organ of the body may be involved. The infections occur in many forms including cellulitis, endocarditis, erysipelas, impetigo, meningitis, pneumonia, scarlet fever, tonsillitis, and urinary tract infection. See also **strep throat.**

streptococcal sore throat. See **strep throat.**

Streptococcus /strep′təkok′əs/, a genus of nonmotile, gram-positive, cocci classified by serologic types (Lancefield groups A through T), by hemolytic action (alpha, beta, gamma) when grown on blood agar, and by reaction to bacterial viruses (phage types 1 to 86). Many species cause disease in humans. *Streptococcus fecalis,* a penicillin-resistant, Group D enterococcus and normal inhabitant of the GI tract, may cause infection of the urinary tract or endocardium. *S. pneumoniae* (formerly, *Diplococcus pneumoniae*) causes 90% of the cases of bacterial pneumonia in the United States. *S. pyogenes* belongs to group A and may cause tonsillitis, respiratory, urinary, or skin infections. Some beta-hemolytic strains may lead to rheumatic fever or to glomerulonephritis. *S. viridans,* a member of the normal flora of the mouth, is the most common cause of bacterial endocarditis, especially when introduced into the bloodstream during dental procedures.

streptokinase /strep′təkī′nās/, an enzyme, produced by streptococci, that catalyzes the conversion of plasminogen to plasmin in various animal hosts of the microorganism.

streptokinase-streptodornase /-strep′tōdôr′nās/, two enzymes derived from a strain of *Streptococcus hemolyticus.*

■ INDICATIONS: It is prescribed for debridement of purulent exudates, clotted blood, radiation necrosis, or fibrinous deposits resulting from trauma or infection.

■ CONTRAINDICATIONS: Active hemorrhage, acute cellulitis, or danger of reopening bronchopleural fistulas prohibits its use.

■ ADVERSE EFFECTS: Among the more serious adverse reactions are pyrogenic reactions and irritation.

streptolysin /streptol′isis/, a filterable substance, produced by various streptococci, that liberates hemoglobin from red blood cells.

streptomycin sulfate /strep′təmī′sin/, an aminoglycoside antibiotic.

■ INDICATIONS: It is prescribed in the treatment of tuberculosis, endocarditis, and certain other infections.

■ CONTRAINDICATIONS: Labyrinthine disease or known hypersensitivity to this drug prohibits its use. It must be used with caution in impaired renal function and in the elderly.

■ ADVERSE EFFECTS: Among the most serious adverse reactions are ototoxicity, nephrotoxicity, muscle weakness, and allergic reactions.

streptozocin /strep′təzō′sin/, an investigational antineoplastic used in the treatment of a variety of neoplasms, including metastatic islet cell tumors of the pancreas. It is an antibiotic substance from *Streptomyces acromogenes.*

stress, any emotional, physical, social, economic, or other factor that requires a response or change, as dehydration, which can cause an increase in body temperature, or a separation from parents, which can cause a young child to cry. Stress may also be applied therapeutically to promote change, as implosive therapy for phobic patients, in which the patient is given support while being exposed to the situation that produces anxiety and is thereby gradually desensitized. The nature and degree of stress observed in a patient are frequently evaluated by the nurse as part of the ongoing holistic nursing assessment. See also **general adaptation syndrome.**

stress fracture, a fracture, especially of one or more of the metatarsal bones, caused by repeated, prolonged, or abnormal stress.

stress kinesic, a type of behavioral characteristic of personal conversation, as the use of body shifts or movements, that mark the flow of speech and generally coincide with linguistic stress patterns.

stressor, anything that causes wear and tear on the body's physical or mental resources. See also **general adaptation syndrome.**

stress reaction. See **general adaptation syndrome, posttraumatic stress disorder.**

stress response syndrome. See **posttraumatic stress disorder.**

stress test, a test that measures the function of a system of the body when subjected to carefully controlled amounts of stress. The data produced allow the examiner to evaluate the condition of the system being tested. Cardiopulmonary function, respiratory function, and intrauterine fetal placental function are tested with stress tests. See also **exercise electrocardiogram, oxytocin challenge test.**

stress ulcer, a gastric or duodenal ulcer that develops in previously unaffected individuals subjected to severe stress, as when severely burned. See also **Curling's ulcer.**

stretch mark. See **stria.**

stri-, a combining form meaning 'line or streak': *striation, striocellular, striomuscular*.

stria /strī′ə/, *pl.* **striae,** a streak or a linear scar that often results from rapidly developing tension in the skin, as seen on the abdomen after pregnancy. Purplish striae are one of the classic findings in hyperadrenocorticism. Also called **stretch mark.**

striae atrophica. See **linea albicantes.**

striae gravidarum, irregular depressions with red to purple colorations that appear in the skin of the abdomen, thighs, and buttocks of pregnant women.

striated muscle, muscle tissue, including all the skeletal muscles, that appears microscopically to consist of striped myofibrils. Striated muscles are composed of bundles of parallel, striated fibers under voluntary control; the heart, a striated involuntary muscle, is an exception. Each striated muscle is covered by a thin connective epimysium and divided into bundles of sheathed fibers containing smaller myofibrils. Each myofibril is comprised of thick filaments that consist of molecules of myosin and of thin filaments that consist of actin and two other protein compounds. Muscle contraction occurs when an electrochemical impulse crosses the myoneural junction, causing the thin filaments to shorten. Also called **skeletal muscle, voluntary muscle.** Compare **cardiac muscle, smooth muscle.**

stricture, an abnormal temporary or permanent narrowing of the lumen of a hollow organ, as the esophagus, pylorus of the stomach, ureter, or urethra, because of inflammation, external pressure, or scarring. Treatment varies depending on the cause. Compare **spasm.**

strict vegetarian, a vegetarian whose diet excludes the use of all foods of animal origin. Such diets, unless adequately planned, may be deficient in many essential nutrients, particularly vitamin B_{12}. Also called **pure vegetarian, vegan.**

stridor /strī′dôr/, an abnormal, high-pitched, musical respiratory sound, caused by an obstruction in the trachea or larynx. It is usually heard during inspiration. Stridor may indicate several neoplastic or inflammatory conditions, including glottic edema, asthma, diphtheria, laryngospasm, or papilloma. Compare **pleuropericardial rub, rales, rhonchi, wheeze.**

strike, an action taken by the employees of a company or institution in which they stop reporting for work in an effort to cause the employer to accede to certain demands. A strike usually follows unsuccessful negotiations between representatives of the union and management.

string carcinoma, a malignancy of the large intestine, usually of the ascending or transverse colon that, on radiologic visualization, causes the intestine to appear to be tied in segments like a string of large beads.

strip membranes, (in obstetrics) a procedure in which an examiner digitally frees the membranes of the amniotic sac from the wall of the lower segment of the uterus in the small area around the cervical os. It is done to stimulate labor, but, because infection or hemorrhage may result, it is not recommended.

stripping, **1.** *nontechnical.* a surgical procedure for the removal of the long and the short saphenous veins of the legs. See also **milking, varicose veins.** **2.** the mechanic removal of a very small amount of enamel from the mesial or distal surfaces of teeth to alleviate crowding.

stroboscopic illusion. See **phi phenomenon.**

stroke. See **cerebrovascular accident.**

-stroke, a combining form meaning a 'condition caused by or resembling an apoplectic stroke': *bloodstroke, lightstroke*.

stroke prone profile, a predictive index using a complex of risk factors that indicate susceptibility of a person to cerebrovascular accident (CVA). The factors include advanced age, hypertension, a history of transient ischemic attacks, cigarette smoking, heart disorders, associated embolism, family hisory of CVA, use of oral contraceptives, diabetes mellitus, physical inactivity, obesity, hypercholesteremia, and hyperlipidemia.

stroke volume, the amount of blood ejected by the ventricle during a ventricle contraction.

stroke volume index, the stroke volume divided by the body surface area.

stroma /strō′mə/, *pl.* **stromata,** the supporting tissue or the matrix of an organ as distinguished from its parenchyma. Some kinds of stromata are the vitreous stroma, which encloses the vitreous humor of the eye, and Rollet's stroma, which contains the hemoglobin of a red blood cell. –**stromatic,** *adj.*

stroma-, a combining form meaning 'a covering': *stromatin, stromatogenous, stromatosis.*

-stroma, a combining form meaning the 'supporting tissue of an organ': *blastostroma, mesostroma, myostroma.*

Strongyloides /stron′jiloi′dēz/, a genus of parasitic intestinal nematode. A species of *Strongyloides, S. stercoralis,* causes strongyloidiasis.

strongyloidiasis /stron′jəloidī′əsis/, infection of the small intestine by the roundworm *Strongyloides stercoralis,* acquired when larvae from the soil penetrate intact skin, incidentally causing a pruritic rash. The larvae pass to the lungs via the bloodstream, sometimes causing pneumonia. Larvae then migrate up the air passages to the pharynx, are swallowed, and develop into adult worms in the small intestine. Bloody diarrhea and intestinal malabsorption may result. Rarely, fatal disseminated strongyloidiasis occurs. Diagnosis depends on finding larvae in freshly passed feces. Treatment often includes administration of thiabendazole. Proper sanitary methods for the disposal of excrement could eliminate the disease. Wearing shoes prevents contagion from contaminated soil. Also called **threadworm infection.**

strontium (Sr), a metallic element. Its atomic number is 38; its atomic weight is 87.62. Chemically similar to calcium, it is found in bone tissue. Isotopes of strontium are used in radioisotope scanning procedures of bone. Strontium 85 (^{85}Sr) and strontium 87 (^{87}Sr) mimic calcium metabolism and are used in studies of bone physiology and disorders. These radionuclides can be counted with any standard detector or imaged at a very early stage in bone disease, whereas x-ray films of bone without the use of a radioactive tracer can show decreased density only after approximately 50% of bone is decalcified. Most ^{85}Sr or ^{87}Sr is deposited in bone within 1 hour after injection; increased deposition of these radionuclides is strongly linked to osteoblastic activity and new bone formation. In addition to four naturally occurring isotopes (^{88}Sr, ^{87}Sr, ^{86}Sr, and ^{84}Sr), 12 artificial strontium isotopes are produced by nuclear reactions. Strontium 90, the longest-lived, is the most dangerous constituent of fallout from atomic bomb tests. It can replace some of the calcium in food, become concentrated in teeth and bones, and continue to emit electrons that can cause death in the host. Cows concentrate strontium 90 in their milk.

-strophe, -strophy, a combining form meaning 'turning or twisting': *cardianastrophe, enstrophe, phallanastrophe.*

stropho-, a combining form meaning 'twisted': *strophocephalus, strophosomus.*

-strophy. See **-strophe.**

structural chemistry, the science dealing with the molecular structure of chemical substances.

structural gene, (in molecular genetics) a unit of genetic information that specifies the amino acid sequence of a polypeptide.

structural integration, a technique of deep massage intended to help in the realignment of the body by altering the length and tone of myofascial tissues. The basis of the practice is the belief that misalignment of myofascial tissues, occurring as a result of improper posture and emotional and physical traumas, may have an overall detrimental effect on a person's energy level, self-image, muscular efficiency, perceptions, and general health. Also called **Rolfing.**

structure, a part of the body, as the heart, a bone, a gland, a cell, or a limb.

structure-activity relationship (SAR), the relationship between the chemical structure of a drug and its activity.

strum-, a combining form meaning 'of or pertaining to a goiter, or to scrofula': *strumectomy, strumiform, strumitis.*

struma lymphomatosa. See **Hashimoto's disease.**

Stryker wedge frame, an orthopedic bed that allows the patient to be rotated as required to either the supine or prone position. Like the Foster bed, the Stryker wedge frame is used in the immobilization of patients with unstable spines, postoperative management of multilevel spinal fusions, and in the management of severe burn patients. Use of the Stryker wedge frame is not recommended if hyperextension of the spine is required or if lower extremity traction is needed. The Stryker wedge frame comes in only one size, the only accommodation to different body builds being an adjustable crossbar on the anterior circle of the frame. If the crossbar is properly adapted, the patient is held firmly between the frames without the addition of pillows or extra padding. The Stryker wedge frame is constructed of lightweight aluminum mounted at the head end to a base by two posts, anterior for the prone frame and posterior for the supine frame. Each frame is fastened to its corresponding post by a knurled nut. The foot ends of the frame are secured by resting on crossbars within a ring, which, when closed, secures the patient between the frames. The ring has two handles to permit turning of the patient by one person, although most hospitals usually require two staff members to turn patients confined to such frames. The ring is released for turning when the red knob or turning lock is pulled. For safety, unintentional rotation of the frames is prevented by a pin at the head end of the frames. The pin is pulled before releasing the ring by pulling a red knob. The crossbars of the frame are wedge-shaped, and the patient is always turned toward the apex of the wedge formed by the crossbars. The lower frame always locks when it is horizontal and level. The ring may then be unlocked and opened for removal of the upper frame. One half of the circle may be removed for exercises, but the circle is usually closed for added security. The Stryker wedge frame is usually equipped with armboards that may be turned up as protective siderails at night. The frame is also often equipped with a reading table. To prevent injury to the arms, the armboards and the reading table are lowered when the frame is rotated. The armboards may also be adjusted toward the head end of the frame for support when the patient is prone or toward the foot end when the patient is supine. The bedpan shelf on the frame is adjustable but must be lowered to allow free rotation of the frame. As with all horizontal turning frames, the level of the trochanters must be aligned with the bottom edge of the torso canvas to prevent hyperextension of the lumbosacral spine when the bedpan portion of the frame is open. Loose linen and catheter tubes can become entrapped in the ring during rotation of the frame unless excess top covers are removed and catheter tubing is placed between the patient's legs, with the drainage bag at the foot end of the frame. The elevation lock of the wedge is useful for elevating the head end of the anterior frame when the patient is prone. In the immediate postoperative period it is also useful for increasing pulmonary expansion by decreasing visceral pressure on the diaphragm. When a patient is in halo or tong cervical traction, the elevation lock provides countertraction up to a maximum of 7 inches. Most hospitals provide the nursing staff with charts to determine the elevation needed for countertraction according to the weight of the patient and the pull forces of traction weights. Compare **Circolectric bed, Foster bed, hyperextension bed.**

ST segment, the component of the cardiac cycle shown on an electrocardiogram as a short, gradual upward curve after the spiked QRS complex, before the ascent of the T wave. It represents the interval between complete depolarization at the end of ventricular contraction and the beginning of repolarization. Elevation or depression of the ST segment is the hallmark of myocardial ischemia or injury and coronary artery disease.

Stuartnatal 1+1, a trademark for an oral, prenatal, fixed-combination drug containing vitamins and minerals.

Stuart-Power factor. See **factor X.**

stump, the part of a limb after amputation that is proximal to the portion amputated.

stump hallucination, the sensation of the continued presence of an amputated limb. See also **hallucination, phantom limb syndrome.**

stupor, a state of lethargy and unresponsiveness in which a person seems unaware of the surroundings. The condition occurs in neurologic and psychiatric disorders. Kinds of stupor are **anergic stupor, benign stupor, delusion stupor,** and **epileptic stupor.**

Sturge-Weber syndrome /sturj′web′ər/, a congenital neurocutaneous disease marked by a port-wine-colored capillary hemangioma over a sensory dermatome of a branch of the trigeminal nerve of the face. X-ray examination of the skull reveals intracranial calcification. The cerebral cortex may atrophy, and generalized or focal seizures, angioma of the choroid, secondary glaucoma, optic atrophy, and new cutaneous hemangiomas may develop. There is no known cure. Treatment is supportive and includes anticonvulsive medication. Also called **Dimitri's disease, encephalotrigeminal angiomatosis.**

stuttering, a speech dysfunction characterized by spasmodic enunciation of words, involving excessive hesitations, stumbling, repetition of the same syllables, and prolongation of sounds. The condition may result from a cerebellar disease or a neuromuscular defect or injury of the organs of articulation, but in most cases the cause is emotional or psychologic. Hesitancy and lack of fluency in speech are normal characteristics of language development during the preschool years when a child's mental ability and level of comprehension exceed muscular coordination and vocabulary acquistion. However, if undue emphasis or stress is placed on this pattern, the child becomes conscious of the difficulties associated with acquisition and may develop a fear of speaking. Stuttering can usually be reversed until about 7 years of age. Prevention must begin early in childhood, and the nurse or physician can help parents by making them aware of the normal patterns in a child's speech and by suggesting ways that can encourage a child's speech development. If stuttering persists, treatment by a speech therapist may be necessary. See also **stammering.**

sty, a purulent infection of a meibomian or sebaceous gland of the eyelid, often caused by a staphylococcal organism. Also spelled **stye.** Also called **hordeolum.**

-style, a combining form meaning a 'bone attached to an internal structure': *cephalostyle, sarcostyle, zygostyle.*

stylet /stī′lət, stīlet′/, a thin metal probe for inserting into or passing through a needle, tube, or catheter to clean the hollow bore or for inserting in a soft, flexible catheter to make it shift as the catheter is placed in a vein or passed through an orifice of the body. Also spelled **stilet, stilette.**

stylo-, a combining form meaning 'like a stake or pole,' used especially to show relationship to the styloid process of the temporal bone: *stylomastoid, stylomyloid, stylostixis.*

stylohyoideus /stī′lōhī·oi′dē·əs/, one of four suprahyoid muscles, lying anterior and superior to the posterior belly of the digastricus. It is a slender muscle that arises from the styloid process and inserts into the hyoid bone. It is pierced near its insertion by the tendon of the digastricus. It is innervated by fibers of the mandibular branch of the facial nerve, and it serves to draw the hyoid bone up and back. Also called **stylohyoid bone.** Compare **digastricus, geniohyoideus, mylohyoideus.**

stylohyoid ligament /stī′lōhī′oid/, the ligament attached to the tip of the styloid process of the temporal bone and to the lesser cornu of the hyoid bone. It frequently contains a small cartilage in its center and is often partially ossified.

stylomandibular ligament /stī′lōmandib′yələr/, one of a pair of specialized bands of cervical fascia, forming an accessory part of the temporomandibular joint. It extends from the styloid process of the temporal bone to the ramus of the mandible between the masseter and pterygoideus muscles and separates the parotid gland from the submandibular gland. Compare **sphenomandibular ligament.**

styptic /stip′tik/, **1.** a substance used as an astringent, often to control bleeding. A chemical styptic induces coagulation of blood. A cotton pledget used as a compress to control bleeding is a mechanic styptic. **2.** acting as an astringent or agent to control bleeding.

sub-, suf-, sup-, a combining form meaning 'under, near, almost, or moderately': *subacid, subdental.*

subacromial bursa, the bursa separating the acromion and deltoid muscle from the insertion of the supraspinatus muscle and the greater tubercle of the humerus.

subacute, **1.** less than acute. **2.** of or pertaining to a disease or other abnormal condition present in a person who appears to be clinically well. The condition may be identified or discovered by means of a laboratory test or by radiologic examination.

subacute bacterial endocarditis (SBE), a chronic bacterial infection of the valves of the heart, characterized by a slow, quiet onset with fever, heart murmur, splenomegaly, and the development of clumps of abnormal tissue, called vegetations, around an intracardiac prosthesis or on the cusps of a valve. Various species of *Streptococcus* or *Staphylococcus* are commonly the cause of SBE. Dental procedures are associated with infection by *Streptococcus viridans,* surgical procedures with *Streptococcus facalis,* and self-infection (especially by drug abusers) with *Staphylococcus aureus.* See also **bacterial endocarditis, endocarditis, Janeway lesions.**

▪ OBSERVATIONS: The infected vegetations may separate from the valve or prosthesis and form emboli. Osler's nodes, petechiae, Roth's spots, and splinter hemorrhages under the fingernails are common manifestations of blood-borne metastases of these emboli. Bacteriologic examination of cultures of the blood may allow specific diagnosis and treatment.

▪ INTERVENTION: Treatment requires prolonged and regular administration of an antibiotic that is known to be effective against the causative organism. If a prosthesis has become infected, it is usually removed. Before surgery or a dental procedure, prophylactic antibiotics are given. During the acute phase of illness, the fever is treated with antipyretic medication and bed rest; adequate high-protein diet and fluids are encouraged.

▪ NURSING CONSIDERATIONS: Sometimes bed rest and hospitalization may be necessary for several weeks. Emotional and psychologic support from the nurse may help the patient adjust to the necessary inactivity and to understand that SBE is a chronic illness.

subacute glomerulonephritis, an uncommon noninfectious disease of the glomerulus of the kidney characterized by proteinuria, hematuria, decreased production of urine, and edema. Of unknown cause, the disease may progress rapidly, and renal failure may occur. Kidney transplantation and dialysis are the only treatments available. See also **chronic glomerulonephritis, postinfectious glomerulonephritis, uremia.**

subacute sclerosing panencephalitis, an uncommon, slow virus infection caused by the measles virus and characterized by diffuse inflammation of brain tissue, personality change, seizures, blindness, dementia, fever, and death. The condition occurs in children and in adolescents who have had measles at a very early age. No effective therapy is known. See also **slow virus.**

subacute thyroiditis. See **de Quervain's thyroiditis.**

subaortic, pertaining to the area of the body below the aorta.

subarachnoid /sub′ərak′noid/, situated under the arachnoid membrane and above the pia mater.

subarachnoid block anesthesia, a form of spinal anesthesia involving the injection of an anesthetic into the space between the arachnoidea and pia mater. This procedure is an especially effective form of rapid spinal anesthesia but one requiring great skill to avoid contamination or neurologic trauma. See also **obstetric anesthesia.**

subarachnoid hemorrhage (SaH, SAH), an intracranial hemorrhage into the cerebrospinal fluid-filled space between the arachnoid and pial membranes on the surface of the brain. The hemorrhage may extend into the brain if the force of the bleeding from the broken vessel is sudden and severe. The cause may be trauma, or rupture of a berry aneurysm or an arteriovenous anomaly.

▪ OBSERVATIONS: The first symptom of a subarachnoid hemorrhage is a sudden extremely severe headache that begins in one localized area and then spreads, becoming dull and throbbing. The localized pain results from vascular distortion and injury. The generalized ache is the result of meningeal irritation from blood in the subarachnoid space. Other characteristics of subarachnoid hemorrhage include dizziness, rigidity of the neck, pupillary inequality, vomiting, drowsiness, sweating and chills, stupor, and loss of consciousness. A brief period of unconsciousness immediately after the rupture is common; severe hemorrhage may result in continued unconsciousness, coma, and death. Delirium and confusion often persist through the first weeks of recovery, and permanent brain damage is common.

▪ INTERVENTION: Observation of the initial localization of the headache may be diagnosistically important. Treatment has three basic goals: preservation of the person's life, limitation of disability, and prevention of recurrence. Bed rest is recommended for as long as 4 to 6 weeks. Care for the person who is unconscious because of a subarachnoid hemorrhage is the same as for the person who is unconscious from other neurologic causes; an airway is maintained, the bladder is emptied, and fluid and electrolyte balance is maintained. The patient who is conscious needs relief from pain, especially in the first days after hemorrhage. Surgical repair of a vessel or excision of an aneurysm may be performed if the patient is conscious, relatively young, healthy, and normotensive.

■ NURSING CONSIDERATIONS: The person is given nothing by mouth for the first 24 hours. Because delirium and restlessness commonly occur, the staff tries to keep the environment around the patient quiet and nonstimulating. A family member may be encouraged to stay with the patient, and treatments, procedures, and examinations are kept to a minimum. Constipation is to be avoided, because straining to evacuate the bowel may raise intracranial pressure and cause another hemorrhage.

subarachnoid space, the space between the arachnoid and pia mater membranes.

subcapital fracture, a fracture of tissue just below the head of a bone that pivots in a ball and socket joint, as the head of the femur.

subcapsular cataract, a condition marked by opacity or cloudiness beneath the anterior or posterior capsule of the lens of the eye.

subclavian /səbklā′vē·ən/, situated under the clavicle, as the subclavian vein.

subclavian artery, one of a pair of arteries that vary in origin, course, and the height to which they rise in the neck but having six similar main branches supplying the vertebral column, spinal cord, ear, and brain. See also **left subclavian artery, right subclavian artery.**

subclavian steal syndrome, a vascular syndrome caused by an occlusion in the subclavian artery proximal to the origin of the vertebral artery. The block results in a reversal of the normal blood pressure gradient in the vertebral artery and decreased blood flow distal to the occlusion. This condition is characterized by episodes of flaccid paralysis of the arm, pain in the mastoid and occipital areas, and a diminished or absent radial pulse on the involved side. Markedly different blood pressure measurements obtained from the arms are sometimes indicative of the condition.

subclavian vein, the continuation of the axillary vein in the upper body, extending from the lateral border of the first rib to the sternal end of the clavicle, where it joins the internal jugular to form the brachiocephalic vein. It usually contains a pair of valves near its junction with the internal jugular vein. The subclavian vein receives deoxygenated blood from the external jugular vein and, on the left side, at the junction with the internal jugular vein, receives lymph from the thoracic duct. On the right side, at the corresponding junction, it receives lymph from the right lymphatic duct.

subclavius /səbklā′vē·əs/, a short muscle of the chest wall. It is a small, cylindric muscle between the clavicle and the first rib and arises in a short, thick tendon from the junction of the first rib and its cartilage. It inserts into the groove on the inferior surface of the clavicle between the costoclavicular and the conoid ligaments. The subclavius is innervated by a special nerve from the lateral trunk of the brachial plexus, which contains fibers from the fifth and sixth cervical nerves, and it acts to draw the shoulder down and forward. Compare **pectoralis major, pectoralis minor, serratus anterior.**

subclinical, of or pertaining to a disease or abnormal condition that is so mild it produces no symptoms.

subclinical diabetes. See **impaired glucose tolerance.**

subconscious, **1.** imperfectly or partially conscious. **2.** *obsolete.* (in psychiatry) the preconscious and the unconscious. **–subconsciousness,** *n.*

subconscious memory, a thought, sensation, or feeling that is not immediately available for recall to the conscious mind.

subculture, an ethnic, regional, economic, or social group with characteristic patterns of behavior and ideals that distinguish it from the rest of a culture or society.

subcutaneous /sub′kyōōtā′nē·əs/, beneath the skin.

subcutaneous fascia, a continuous layer of connective tissue over the entire body between the skin and the deep fascial investment of the specialized structures of the body, as the muscles. It is comprised of an outer, normally fatty layer, and an inner, thin elastic layer. Between the two layers lie superficial blood vessels, nerves, lymphatics, the mammary glands, most of the facial muscles, and the platysma. Compare **deep fascia, subserous fascia.**

subcutaneous fat necrosis. See **adiponecrosis subcutanea neonatorum.**

subcutaneous infusion. See **hypodermoclysis.**

subcutaneous injection, the introduction of a hypodermic needle into the subcutaneous tissue beneath the skin, usually on the upper arm, thigh, or abdomen. A 24- or 25-gauge needle 2 cm long is used. The drug is prepared and drawn into the syringe. The cleansed area of skin is held flat by the thumb and forefinger to tense and steady the injection site. The needle is inserted at an angle of 45 to 60 degrees, piercing the skin quickly and advancing steadily to minimize the pain. The barrel or plunger is withdrawn slightly to ascertain whether or not the syringe of the needle has inadvertently entered a blood vessel. If no blood is aspirated, the drug is injected slowly, the

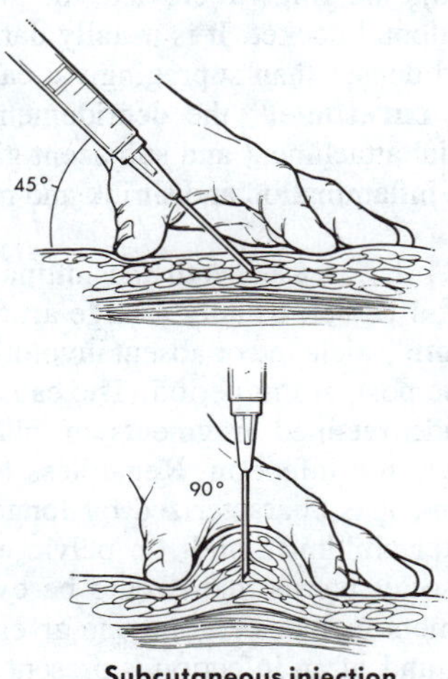

Subcutaneous injection

needle is withdrawn, and the skin is massaged gently with a sterile alcohol sponge. Certain drugs that are extremely irritating to the skin are injected into the deep subcutaneous tissues using a variation of the technique. The skin tissue overlying the injection site is grasped with the thumb and forefinger but elevated in a roll, rather than tensed and flattened. The angle of injection may be as great as 90 degrees to the skin. Heparin, insulin, and emetine are injected in this way. If subcutaneous injections are repeated, each is performed at least 5 cm from the previous site. A diagram of a plan for the rotation of injection sites helps to avoid overuse of one area of skin.

subcutaneous mastectomy, a surgical procedure in which all the breast tissue of one or both breasts is removed leaving the skin, areola, and nipple intact. The adjacent lymph nodes and the pectoralis major and pectoralis minor are not removed. It may be performed on women who are at great risk of developing breast cancer. Reconstruction of the breasts is performed, with the assistance of a plastic surgeon, through the insertion of prostheses to return the normal contour to the breasts.

subcutaneous nodule, a small, solid boss, or node, beneath the skin that can be detected by touch. Subcutaneous nodules consisting chiefly of Aschoff bodies are found in patients with rheumatic fever. Minute subcutaneous nodules formed by the perivascular infiltration of mononuclear cells occur in typhus fever.

subcutaneous test. See **intradermal test.**

subdural /səbdŏŏr′əl/, situated under the dura mater and above the arachnoid membrane.

subdural hygroma, a collection of fluid between the dura mater and arachnoid layers, resulting from a spinal fluid leak through a rupture in the arachnoid tissue.

suberosis. See **cork worker's lung.**

subgerminal cavity. See **blastocoele.**

subgingival calculus, a deposit of various mineral salts, as calcium phosphate and calcium carbonate, which accumulates with organic matter and oral debris on the teeth or within the gingival crevice, the gingival pocket, or the periodontal pocket. It is usually darker, more pigmented, and denser than supragingival calculus.

subgingival curettage, the debridement of an ulcerated epithelial attachment and subjacent gingival corium to eliminate inflammation and shrink and restore gingival tissue.

subintimal, the area beneath the intima or membrane lining a blood vessel, usually a large artery.

subinvolution, delayed or absent involution of the uterus during the postpartum period. The causes of subinvolution include retained fragments of placenta, uterine fibromyomas, and infection. Regardless of the cause of the condition, it is characterized by longer and heavier bleeding after childbirth and, on pelvic examination, a larger and softer uterus than would be expected at that time. Treatment includes ergonovine given by mouth for 2 or 3 days, and, if an infection is present, an antibiotic. The hemoglobin or hematocrit is also evaluated, and iron is given if necessary. A follow-up examination is performed 2 weeks later.

subjective, **1.** pertaining to the essential nature of an object as perceived in the mind rather than to a thing in itself. **2.** existing only in the mind. **3.** that which arises within or is perceived by the individual as contrasted with something that is modified by external circumstances or something that may be evaluated by objective standards. **4.** pertaining to a person who places excessive importance on his own moods, attitudes, or opinions; egocentric.

subjective data collection, the process in which data relating to the patient's problem are elicited from the patient. The interviewer encourages a full description of the onset, the course, and the character of the problem and any factors that aggravate or ameliorate it. Compare **objective data collection.**

subjective sensation, a feeling or impression that is not associated with or does not directly result from any external stimulus. See also **sensation,** def. 1.

sublethal gene, a gene whose presence causes abnormalities or impairs the functioning of an organism but does not cause its death. Compare **lethal gene.**

subleukemic leukemia. See **aleukemic leukemia.**

sublimate, to refine or divert instinctual impulses and energy from their immediate goal to one that can be expressed in a social, moral, or aesthetic manner acceptable to the person and to society.

sublimation, **1.** a defense mechanism by which an unacceptable instinctive drive is unconsciously diverted to and expressed through a personally approved, socially accepted means. **2.** (in psychoanalysis) the process of diverting certain components of the sex drive to a socially acceptable, nonsexual goal. Compare **displacement.**

Sublimaze Citrate, a trademark for a narcotic analgesic (fentanyl citrate).

subliminal, taking place below the threshold of sensory perception or outside the range of conscious awareness.

sublingual /səbling′gwəl/, beneath the tongue.

sublingual administration of a medication, the administration of a drug, as nitroglycerin, usually in tablet form, by placing it beneath the tongue until the tablet dissolves.

sublingual duct. See **Bartholin's duct, duct of Rivinus.**

sublingual gland, one of a pair of small salivary glands situated under the mucous membrane of the floor of the mouth, beneath the tongue. It is a narrow, almond-shaped structure, and weighs about 2 g. It is in relation, inferiorly, with the mylohyoideus; posteriorly, with the submandibular gland; laterally, with the mandible; and medially, with the genioglossus from which it is separated by the lingual nerve and the submandibular duct. It has from 8 to 20 ducts, some of which join to form the sublingual duct. The sublingual gland secretes mucus produced by its alveoli. Compare **parotid gland, submandibular gland.**

subluxation /sub′luksā′shən/. a partial dislocation.

submandibular duct, a duct through which a submandibular gland secretes saliva. Also called **submaxillary duct.**

submandibular gland, one of a pair of round, walnut-sized salivary glands in the submandibular triangle, reaching anteriorly to the anterior belly of the diagastricus and posteriorly to the stylomandibular ligament. The ligament lies between the submandibular gland and the parotid gland. The submandibular gland extends superiorly under the inferior border of the mandible and extends a deep process anteriorly above the mylohyoideus muscle. The upper portion of the superficial surface of the gland lies partly against the submandibular depression on the inner surface of the mandible and partly on the pterygoideus medialis. The lower part is covered by skin, superficial fascia, platysma, and deep cervical fascia. The submandibular duct is about 5 cm long, starts at the deep surface of the gland, runs between the sublingual gland and the genioglossus, and opens on a small papilla at the side of the frenulum linguae. The gland secretes both mucus and a thinner serous fluid, which aid the digestive process. Compare **sublingual gland, parotid gland.** See also **salivary gland.**

submaxillary duct. See **submandibular duct.**

submetacentric /sub′metəsen′trik/, pertaining to a chromosome in which the centromere is located approximately equidistant between the center and one end so that the arms of the chromatids are not equal in length. Compare **acrocentric, metacentric, telocentric.**

submentovertex, a reference point at the base of the skull used in preparing radiographic projections of the skull and its associated structures.

submucous, beneath a mucous membrane.

suboccipitobregmatic, pertaining to the smallest anteroposterior diameter of an infant's head when it is well flexed during labor.

subperiosteal fracture /sub′perē•os′tē•əl/, a fracture in a bone beneath the periosteum that does not disrupt the periosteal covering.

subphrenic, pertaining to the area beneath or under the diaphragm.

subpoena, (in law) a document from a court commanding that a person appear at a certain time and place to testify on a specific matter. Subpoenas are governed by federal rules for criminal procedure or for civil procedure.

subpoena duces tecum, (in law) a subpoena commanding a person to bring books, papers, records, or other items to the court.

subserous fascia, one of three kinds of fascia, lying between the internal layer of deep fascia and the serous membranes lining the body cavities in much the same manner as the subcutaneous fascia lies between the skin and the deep fascia. It is thin in some areas, as between the pleura and the chest wall, and thick in other areas, where it forms a pad of adipose tissue. Compare **deep fascia, subcutaneous fascia.**

subspecialty, (in nursing) a nurse's particular professional and highly specialized field of practice, as nursing in dialysis, oncology, neurology, or newborn intensive care. Compare **specialty.**

substance abuse, the overindulgence in and dependence on a stimulant, depressant, or other chemical substance, leading to effects that are detrimental to the individual's physical or mental health, or the welfare of others.

substance P, a polypeptide neurotransmitting substance that is synthesized by the body and acts to stimulate vasodilatation and contraction of intestinal and other smooth muscles. It also plays a part in salivary secretion, diuresis, and natriuresis, and it affects the function of the peripheral and central nervous systems. It has been isolated from certain cells of the GI and biliary tracts.

substantive epidemiology, the body of knowledge derived from epidemiologic studies, including for each disease the natural history of the disorder, patterns of occurrence, and risk factors for developing the disease.

substernal goiter, an enlargement of the thyroid gland, a portion of which is beneath the sternum.

substrate, a substance acted on and changed by an enzyme in any chemical reaction.

substrate depletion phase, a period during an enzyme assay when the concentration of substrate is falling and the assay is not following zero-order kinetics.

substratum, any underlying layer; a foundation.

subthalamus, a portion of the diencephalon that serves as a correlations center for optic and vestibular impulses relayed to the globus pallidus. It is a transition zone between the thalamus and the tegmentum mesencephali, squeezed between the cerebral peduncle and the mammillary area. It accommodates prolongations of the red nucleus and the substantia nigra and contains fibrous masses of the fields of Forel. Compare **epithalamus, hypothalamus, metathalamus, thalamus. –subthalamic,** *adj.*

subtle, having a low intensity; not severe and having no serious sequelae, as a mild infection or inflammation.

subungual /səbung′gwəl/, under a fingernail or toenail.

subungual hematoma, a collection of blood beneath a nail, usually resulting from trauma. The pain accompanying this condition may be quickly alleviated by burning or drilling a small hole through the nail to release the blood.

succ-, a combining form meaning 'of or pertaining to a juice': *succagogue, succorrhea, succus.*

succinic acid /suksin′ik/, a compound found in certain hydatid cysts and in lichens, amber, and fossils. Commercial succinic acid, produced by the fermentation of ammonium tartrate, is used in lacquer and dyes. Succinic acid was formerly used in the treatment of diabetic ketoacidosis.

succinylcholine chloride /suk′sinilkō′lēn/, a skeletal muscle relaxant.

■ INDICATIONS: It is prescribed as an adjunct to anesthesia or to reduce muscle contractions during surgery or mechanic ventillation, and to facilitate endotracheal intubation.

■ CONTRAINDICATIONS: Known hypersensitivity to this drug prohibits its use. Caution is used in administering this drug to patients with low pseudocholinesterase levels and in patients with myasthenia gravis or renal failure.

■ ADVERSE EFFECTS: Among the more serious adverse reactions are cardiac arrhythmia and severe respiratory depression.

succus /suk′əs/, *pl.* **succi** /suk′sī/, a juice or fluid, usually one secreted by an organ, as succus prostaticus of the prostate.

succussion splash /səkush′ən/, the sound elicited by shaking the body of an individual who has free fluid and air or gas in a hollow organ or body cavity. This sound may be present over a normal stomach but may also be heard with hydropneumothorax, large hiatal hernia, or intestinal or pyloric obstruction.

suck, **1.** to draw a liquid or semiliquid into the mouth by creating a partial vacuum through motions of the lips and tongue. **2.** to hold on the tongue and dissolve by the movements of the mouth and action of the saliva. **3.** to draw fluid into the mouth, specifically to draw milk from the breast or nursing bottle.

sucking blisters, the pale, soft pads on the upper and lower lips of a baby that look like blisters but are not. They form as soon as the baby begins to suck well, at the breast or on a bottle. They seem to augment the seal of the lips around the nipple or breast. Some babies are born with them, having sucked on their own fingers, hand, or arm before birth.

sucking reflex, involuntary sucking movements of the circumoral area in newborns in response to stimulation. The reflex continues throughout infancy and often occurs without stimulation, as during sleep. Compare **rooting reflex.**

suckle, **1.** to provide nourishment, specifically to breast feed. **2.** to take in as nourishment, especially by feeding from the breast.

suckling, an infant that has not been weaned.

Sucostrin, a trademark for a depolarizing agent (succinylcholine), used as an adjunct to anesthesia.

sucrose, sugar derived from sugar cane, sugar beets, and sorghum.

sucrose polyester (SPE), a synthetic, nonabsorbable fat that, when added to the diet, reduces plasma cholesterol levels by increasing the excretion of cholesterol in the feces. It is formulated to have the characteristic texture, taste, and consistency of regular margarine or vegetable oil and adds no calories to the diet.

suction curettage, a method of curettage in which a specimen of the endometrium or the products of conception are removed by aspiration. Under local or light general anesthesia, the cervix is dilated, a catheter is introduced into the uterus, and suction is applied. Postoperative care includes monitoring vital signs for symptoms of blood loss. Also called **vacuum aspiration.** Compare **dilatation and curettage.**

suction drainage. See **drainage.**

Sudafed, a trademark for an adrenergic vasoconstrictor (pseudoephedrine hydrochloride), used as a decongestant and bronchodilator.

sudden infant death syndrome (SIDS), the unexpected and sudden death of an apparently normal and healthy infant that occurs during sleep and with no physical or autopsic evidence of disease. It is the most common cause of death in children between 2 weeks and 1 year of age, with an incidence rate of 1 in every 300 to 350 live births. The origin is unknown but multiple causes have been proposed, including lack of biotin in the diet, abnormality of the endogenous-opioid system, mechanic suffocation, a defect in respiratory mucosal defense, prolonged apnea, an unknown virus, anatomic abnormality of the larynx, and immunoglobulin abnormalities. It is known that the condition occurs more often in infants 10 to 14 weeks of age, especially those born prematurely, in boys more often than in girls, during the winter months; and that it is seen more often among babies who have recently had a minor illness such as upper respiratory infection, or in infants born to women less than 20 years of age who have had at least one previous child, who begin prenatal care in the third trimester, or who smoke or are anemic or drug dependent. The syndrome is neither contagious nor hereditary, although there is a greater than average risk of its occurrence within the same family, which may indicate the influence of polygenic factors. Controversy exists as to whether or not home monitoring systems are of value for infants who are at risk or who have had a ''near miss'' episode. Nursing considerations consist predominantly of support and

Characteristics of SIDS

Factors	*Occurrence*
Incidence	1.5 to 2 1000 live births
Peak age	2 to 4 months; 90% occur by 6 months
Sex	Higher percentage of males affected
Time of death	Usually during nighttime
Time of year	Increased incidence in winter
Birth	Higher incidence in: Premature infants Multiple births Neonates with low Apgar scores Infants with central nervous system disturbances
Feeding habits	Not significant; breast feeding does not prevent SIDS
Siblings	Ten times greater incidence
Possible causes	CNS anomaly Cardiovascular anomaly Airway anomaly Infection Chronic hypoxia

counseling, as assessing how the parents feel about the death to help them through the resolution of grief, learning what they know about the syndrome and supplying them with whatever information and literature they need, finding out how they are coping with any guilt feelings, and how the siblings, if any, are coping with the death. The nurse can also supply information about local groups of parents who have lost a child from SIDS. Also called **cot death, crib death.** See also **parental grief.**

sudo-, a combining form meaning 'of or pertaining to sweat': *sudogram, sudokeratosis, sudorrhea.*

sudoriferous duct /so͞o′dərif′ərəs/, a duct leading from a sweat gland to the surface of the skin. Also called **sweat duct.**

sudoriferous gland, one of about 3 million tiny structures within the dermis that produce sweat. The average quantity of sweat secreted in 24 hours varies from 700 to 900 g. Most of these glands are eccrine glands, producing sweat that carries away sodium chloride, the waste products urea and lactic acid, and the breakdown products from garlic, spices, and other substances. Apocrine sweat glands associated with the coarse hair of the armpits and the pubic region are larger and secrete fluid that is much thicker than that secreted by the eccrine glands. Each sudoriferous gland consists of a single tube with a deeply coiled body and a superficial duct. In the superficial layers of the dermis the duct is straight; in the deeper layers it is convoluted. In the thick dermis of the palms of the hands and the soles of the feet the duct is spirally coiled. The number of glands per square centimeter of skin varies in different parts of the body, the sudoriferous glands being very plentiful on the palms of the hands and on the soles of the feet and least numerous in the neck and the back; they are completely absent in the deeper portions of the external auditory meatus, the prepuce, and the glans penis, and are more numerous in the fingers of Filipinos, Hindus, and black Americans than in the fingers of white Americans. Also called **sweat gland.** Compare **sebaceous gland.**

sudorific /so͞o′dərif′ik/, **1.** of or pertaining to a substance or condition, as heat or emotional tension, that promotes sweating. **2.** a sudorific agent. Sweat glands are stimulated by cholinergic drugs. The alkaloid pilocarpine is a potent sudorific drug, but it is rarely used for that purpose in modern medicine. Also called **diaphoretic.**

suf-. See **sub-.**

suffix, a portion of a word occurring at the end of a compound word. In this dictionary, a suffix is called a "combining form." In the words *appendectomy, bronchoscopy, nephrology, pharyngitis,* and *tracheotomy,* the suffixes are *-ectomy, -scopy, -logy, -itis,* and *-tomy.* Compare **prefix.**

suffocative goiter, an enlargement of the thyroid gland causing a sensation of suffocation on pressure.

sugar, any of several water-soluble carbohydrates. The two principal categories of sugars are monosaccharides and disaccharides. A monosaccharide is a single sugar, as glucose, fructose, or galactose. A disaccharide is a double sugar, as sucrose (table sugar) or lactose. See also **carbohydrate, fructose, galactose, glucose, saccharide, sucrose.**

sugar alcohol, an alcohol produced by the reduction of an aldehyde or ketone of a sugar.

suggestion, **1.** the process by which one thought or idea leads to another, as in the association of ideas. **2.** the use of persuasion, exhortation, or another device to implant an idea, thought, attitude, or belief in the mind of another as a means of influencing or altering behavior or states of mind. See also **hypnosis.** **3.** an idea, belief, or attitude implanted in the mind of another. Compare **autosuggestion.**

suicidal, of, relating to, or tending toward self-destruction.

suicidal melancholia, *obsolete.* a state of severe depression in which suicidal tendencies are prominent.

suicide, **1.** the intentional taking of one's own life. **2.** *informal.* the ruin or destruction of one's own interests. **3.** a person who commits or attempts self-destruction. Early signs of suicidal intent include depression; expressions of guilt, tension, and agitation; insomnia; loss of weight and appetite; neglect of personal appearance; and direct or indirect threats to commit suicide.

suicide gesture, (in psychiatric nursing) an apparent attempt by a patient to cause self-injury without lethal consequences and generally without actual intent to commit suicide. A suicide gesture serves to attract attention to the patient's disturbed emotional status but is not as serious as a suicide attempt.

suicidology /so͞o′isīdol′əjē/, the study of the prevention and the causes of suicide. **–suicidologist,** *n.*

Suladyne, a trademark for an antiinfective, fixed-combination drug containing antibacterials (sulfamethizole and sulfadiazine) and a urinary antiseptic (phenazopyridine hydrochloride).

sulcus /sul′kəs/, *pl.* **sulci** /sul′sī/, a shallow groove, a depression, or a furrow on the surface of an organ, as a sulcus that separates the convolutions of the cerebral hemisphere. A sulcus is usually not as deep as a fissure, but, in the terminology of anatomy, *sulcus* and *fissure* are often used interchangeably. **–sulcate,** *adj.*

sulcus centralis cerebri. See **fissure of Rolando.**

sulcus pulmonalis, a depression on each side of the vertebral bodies that accommodates the posterior portion of the lung.

sulfacetamide /sul′fəset′əmīd/, a topical antibacterial.

■ INDICATIONS: It is most commonly prescribed for the prophylaxis of infection after injury to the cornea and in the treatment of bacterial conjunctivitis, and urinary tract infections.

■ CONTRAINDICATIONS: Known hypersensitivity to the drug or to other sulfonamides or impaired kidney function prohibits its use.

■ ADVERSE EFFECTS: Among known adverse reactions are local pain, overgrowth of nonsusceptible pathogens, and hypersensitivity reaction to the drug.

Sulfacet-R, a trademark for a topical, fixed-combination drug containing a scabicide (sulfur), an antibacterial (sulfacetamide sodium), and an antiseptic and astringent (zinc oxide).

sulfachlorpyridazine /sul′fəklôr′pirid′əzēn/, a sulfonamide antibacterial.

■ INDICATION: It is prescribed in the treatment of infection, particularly of the urinary tract.

■ CONTRAINDICATIONS: Porphyria, urinary tract obstruction, or known hypersensitivity to this or to other sulfonamides prohibits its use.

■ ADVERSE EFFECTS: Among the more serious adverse reactions are crystalluria, severe allergic reactions, photosensitivity, and blood dyscrasias.

sulfacytine, a sulfonamide antibacterial.

■ INDICATIONS: It is prescribed in the treatment of infection, particularly primary pyelonephritis, and cystitis.

■ CONTRAINDICATIONS: Porphyria, urinary tract obstruction, or known hypersensitivity to sulfonamides prohibits its use.

■ ADVERSE EFFECTS: Among the more serious adverse reactions are crystalluria, photosensitivity, severe allergic reactions, and blood dyscrasias.

sulfadiazine /sul′fədī′əzēn/, a sulfonamide antibacterial.

■ INDICATIONS: It is prescribed in the treatment of infection, particularly of the urinary tract, and as a rheumatic fever prophylaxis.

■ CONTRAINDICATIONS: Porphyria, urinary tract obstruction, or known hypersensitivity to sulfonamides prohibits its use.

■ ADVERSE EFFECTS: Among the more serious adverse effects are crystalluria, photosensitivity, severe allergic reactions, and blood dyscrasias.

sulfamethizole, a sulfonamide antibacterial.

■ INDICATIONS: It is prescribed in the treatment of infection, particularly pyelonephritis, pyelitis, and cystitis.

■ CONTRAINDICATIONS: Porphyria, urinary tract obstruction, or known hypersensitivity to sulfonamides prohibits its use.

■ ADVERSE EFFECTS: Among the more serious adverse reactions are crystalluria, photosensitivity, blood dyscrasias, and severe allergic reactions.

sulfamethoxazole, a sulfonamide antibacterial.

■ INDICATIONS: It is prescribed in the treatment of otitis media, bronchitis, and certain urinary tract infections.

■ CONTRAINDICATIONS: It is not given during the last trimester of pregnancy, during lactation, or to children under 2 months of age. Known hypersensitivity to this drug or other sulfonamides prohibits its use.

■ ADVERSE EFFECTS: Among the more serious adverse reactions are crystalluria and rash, fever, and other allergic reactions.

sulfamethoxazole and trimethoprim, a fixed-combination antibacterial.

■ INDICATIONS: It is prescribed in the treatment of urinary tract infections, otitis media, and shigellosis.

■ CONTRAINDICATIONS: It is used with caution in patients with impaired renal or hepatic function, with possible folate deficiency, or with known hypersensitivity to either drug or to sulfonamides. It is not recommended for use in infants under 2 months of age or in the third trimester of pregnancy.

■ ADVERSE EFFECTS: Among the more serious adverse reactions are crystalluria and rashes, fever, and other allergic reactions.

Sulfamylon, a trademark for a topical antiinfective (mafenide acetate).

sulfanilic acid /sul′fənil′ik/, a red-tinged, white crystalline compound used in the synthesis of sulfonamides and as a reagent in tests for phenol, fecal matter in water, albumen, aldehydes, and glucose. Also called **paraaminobenzenesulfonic acid.**

sulfasalazine, a sulfonamide; salicylazosulfapyridine.

■ INDICATIONS: It is prescribed in the treatment of mild to moderate ulcerative colitis and as adjunctive therapy in severe cases.

■ CONTRAINDICATIONS: Urinary obstruction, porphyria, or known hypersensitivity to this drug, to other sulfonamide medications, or to salicylates prohibits its use. It is not given during the last trimester of pregnancy.

■ ADVERSE EFFECTS: Among the more serious adverse reactions are crystalluria, blood dyscrasias, and severe hypersensitivity reactions. GI symptoms and anorexia commonly occur.

sulfate /sul′fāt/, a salt of sulfuric acid. A sulfate is usually a combination of a metal with sulfuric acid. Natural sulfates, as sodium sulfate, calcium sulfate, and potassium sulfate, are plentiful in the body.

sulfathiazole /sul′fəthī′əzōl/, a sulfonamide antibacterial no longer commonly used.

sulfhemoglobin, a form of hemoglobin containing an irreversibly bound sulfur molecule that prevents normal oxygen binding. It is present in the blood in trace amounts.

sulfinpyrazone /sul′finpir′əzōn/, a uricosuric.

■ INDICATIONS: It is prescribed in the treatment of chronic gout and intermittent gouty arthritis.

■ CONTRAINDICATIONS: Peptic ulcer, ulcerative colitis, renal dysfunction, or known hypersensitivity to this drug or to phenylbutazone prohibits its use. It is not usually given during an acute attack of gout.

■ ADVERSE EFFECTS: Among the more serious adverse reactions are GI ulcers, blood dyscrasias, and dermatitis.

sulfisoxazole, a sulfonamide antibacterial.

■ INDICATIONS: It is prescribed in the treatment of conjunctivitis and urinary tract infections, including vaginitis, cystitis, and pyelonephritis.

■ CONTRAINDICATIONS: Porphyria, urinary tract obstruction, or known hypersensitivity to this drug or to sulfonamide medications prohibits its use. It is not given during the last trimester of pregnancy or to children under 2 months of age.

■ ADVERSE EFFECTS: Among the more serious adverse reactions are crystalluria, blood dyscrasias, and severe hypersensitivity reactions.

sulfiting agents, food preservatives composed of potassium or sodium bisulfite or potassium metabisulfite. Sulfiting agents are used in processing of beer, wine, baked goods, soup mixes, and some imported seafoods and by restaurants to impart a ''fresh'' appearance to salad fruits and vegetables. The chemicals can cause a severe allergic reaction in persons who are hypersensitive to sulfites. The reactions are marked by flushing, faintness, hives, headache, GI distress, breathing difficulty, and, in extreme cases, loss of consciousness and death.

sulfo-, a combining form naming chemical compounds, showing presence of divalent sulfur or of the group SO_2OH: *sulfonamide, sulfomethane, sulfophenol.*

sulfobromophthalein /sul′fəbrō′məfthal′ēn, -ē•in/, a substance used in its disodium salt form for evaluating the function of the liver. See also **Bromsulphalein test.**

sulfonamide /səlfon′əmīd/, one of a large group of synthetic, bacteriostatic drugs that are effective in treating infections caused by many gram-negative and gram-positive microorganisms. The drugs act by preventing the normal growth, development, and multiplication of the bacteria but do not kill mature organisms. They are bacteriostatic rather than bactericidal. Some sulfonamides are short acting, some are intermediate acting, and some are long acting, depending on the speed with which they are excreted. They are used in treating many urinary tract infections. In the past they have been used to treat gram-negative enteric infections, including those caused by species of Shigella, and as a ''bowel prep'' before and after intestinal surgery. Some people are hypersensitive to the drugs. Sulfonamides are given with caution to people who have impaired liver or kidney function, and they are not given in the last trimester of pregnancy or to young infants, because mental retardation sometimes occurs. Hemolytic anemia, agranulocytosis, thrombocytopenia, or aplastic anemia, drug fever, and jaundice may occur, particularly with long acting sulfonamides given for more than 10 days. Dosage varies with the particular drug and with the age, size, and condition of the person. Most sulfonamides are given orally.

sulfonylurea /sul′fənilyŏŏr′ē•ə/, an oral antidiabetic agent that stimulates the pancreatic production of insulin. Hypersensitivity to sulfonamides is a contraindication for using such agents, and ethanol consumption is incompatible with all sulfonylureas. The safety of these drugs for use in pregnant women has not been established, making insulin the preferred drug in treating diabetes in pregnancy. Aspirin or other salicylates taken with any sulfonylurea intensifies the hypoglycemic effect.

sulfosalicylic acid /sul′fōsalisil′ik/, a white or faintly pink crystalline substance that is highly water-soluble, used as a reagent in tests for albumin and as an intermediate compound in the manufacture of dyes and surfactants.

sulfoxone sodium, a bacteriostatic sulfone derivative.

■ INDICATIONS: It is prescribed in the treatment of leprosy and dermatitis herpetiformis.

■ CONTRAINDICATIONS: Advanced renal amyloidosis or known sensitivity to this drug prohibits its use.

■ ADVERSE EFFECTS: Among the most serious adverse reactions are hemolysis, hemolytic anemia, toxic epidermal necrolysis, and several blood dyscrasias.

Sulfoxyl, a trademark for a topical fixed-combination drug containing a disinfectant (benzoyl peroxide) and a scabicide (sulfur).

sulfur (S), a nonmetallic, multivalent, tasteless, odorless chemical element that occurs abundantly in yellow crystalline form or in masses, especially in volcanic areas. Its atomic number is 16; its atomic weight is 32.06. It is used to produce sulfuric acid and used commercially in metallurgy, rubber vulcanization, petroleum refining, and many other industrial processes. Sulfur has been used in the treatment of gout, rheumatism, and bronchitis and as a mild laxative. The sulfonamides, or sulfa drugs, are used in the treatment of various bacterial infections. Also spelled **sulphur.**

-sulfuric, -sulphuric, a combining form meaning 'compounds containing sulfur, especially in its highest valences': *hydrosulfuric, persulfuric, thiosulfuric.*

sulfuric acid, a clear, colorless, oily, highly corrosive liquid that generates great heat when mixed with water. An extremely toxic substance, sulfuric acid causes severe skin burns, blindness on contact with the eyes, serious lung damage if the vapors are inhaled, and death if it is ingested. In industry, sulfuric acid is used in the manufacture of fertilizers, dyes, glue, and other acids, in the purifying of petroleum, and in the pickling of metals. Weak solutions of sulfuric acid are used in the treatment of gastric hypoacidity and serous diarrhea. It was formerly called **oil of vitriol.**

sulindac, an antiinflammatory agent.

■ INDICATIONS: It is prescribed in the treatment of osteoarthritis, rheumatoid arthritis, and ankylosing spondylitis.

■ CONTRAINDICATIONS: Pregnancy, lactation, or known hypersensitivity to this drug, to aspirin, or to nonsteroidal antiinflammatory drugs prohibits its use. It is used with caution in patients who have upper GI tract disease or impaired renal function.

■ ADVERSE EFFECTS: Among the more serious adverse reactions are GI upset, peptic ulcer, dizziness, tinnitus, and skin rash. This drug interacts with many other drugs.

Sulkowitch's test /sul′kəwichs/, an examination of the urine for the presence of calcium. A reagent, containing oxalic acid, ammonium oxalate, and glacial acetic acid, mixed with urine, causes calcium to precipitate out of the urine. Also called **S's test.** See also **hypercalciuria.**

sulphur. See **sulfur.**

Sultrin, a trademark for a vaginal fixed-combination drug containing antibacterials (sulfathiazole, sulfacetamide, and sulfabenzamide).

summary judgment, (in law) a judgment requested by any party to a civil action to end the action when it is believed that there is no genuine issue or material fact in dispute. Summary judgment may be directed toward part or all of a claim or defense and may be based on the proceedings in court or on affadavits or other outside materials.

summation, **1.** an accumulative effect or action; a total aggregate; totality. **2.** (in neurology), the accumulation of the concentration of a neurotransmitter at a synapse, either by increasing the frequency of nerve impulses in each fiber (temporal summation) or by increasing the number of fibers stimulated (spatial summation), so that the threshold of the postsynaptic neuron is overcome and an impulse is transmitted. See also **facilitation,** def. 2.

summons, (in law) a document issued by a clerk of the court on the filing of a complaint. A sheriff, marshal, or other appointed person serves the summons, notifying a person that an action has been begun against him or her. See also **service of process.**

Sumycin, a trademark for an antibiotic (tetracycline hydrochloride).

sun bath, the exposure of the naked body to the sun.

sunDare, a trademark for an ultraviolet screen (cinoxate).

sundowning, a condition in which elderly patients tend to become confused or disoriented at the end of the day. Many of them have diminished visual acuity and varying degrees of sensorineural and conduction hearing loss. With less light, they lose visual cues that help them to compensate for their sensory impairments.

sunstroke, a morbid condition caused by overexposure to the sun and characterized by a high fever, convulsions, and coma. See also **heat hyperpyrexia.**

sup-. See **sub-.**

Supen, a trademark for an antibacterial (ampicillin).

super-, a combining form meaning 'above, or implying excess': *superduct, superfunction, supernumerary.*

superego, (in psychoanalysis) that part of the psyche, functioning mostly in the unconscious, that develops when the standards of the parents and of society are incorporated into the ego. The superego has two parts, the conscience and the ego ideal. See also **ego, ego ideal, id.**

superfecundation, the fertilization of two or more ova released during one menstrual cycle by spermatozoa from the same or different males during separate acts of sexual intercourse.

superfetation, the fertilization of a second ovum after the onset of pregnancy, resulting in the presence of two fetuses of different degrees of maturity developing within the uterus simultaneously. Also called **superimpregnation.**

superficial, **1.** of or pertaining to the skin or another surface. **2.** not grave or dangerous.

superficial fading infantile hemangioma, a superficial, transient, salmon-colored patch in the center of the forehead, face, or occiput of many newborns. It fades during the first 2 years of life, but it may temporarily deepen in color if the child becomes flushed or angry.

superficial implantation, (in embryology) the partial embedding of the blastocyst within the uterine wall so that it and, later, the chorionic sac protrude into the uterine cavity. Also called **central implantation, circumferential implantation.**

superficial inguinal node, a node in one of the two groups of inguinal lymph glands in the upper femoral triangle of the thigh. The nodes form a chain distal to the inguinal ligament and receive afferents from the skin of the penis, scrotum, perineum, buttocks, and abdominal wall below the level of the umbilicus. Compare **anterior tibial node, popliteal node.**

superficial reflex, any neural reflex initiated by stimulation of the skin. Kinds of superficial reflexes are **abdominal reflex, anal reflex,** and **cremasteric reflex.** Compare **deep tendon reflex.**

superficial sensation, the awareness or perception of feelings in the superficial layers of the skin in response to touch, pressure, temperature, and pain. Such sensations are conveyed to the brain via the spinothalamic system. Compare **deep sensation.**

superficial spreading melanoma, a melanoma that grows outward, spreading over the surface of the affected organ or tissue, most commonly on the lower legs of women and the torso of men. Occurring in late middle age, it is raised and palpable, is usually unevenly pigmented, and has an irregular shape and unclear border. It is the most common of the three types of melanoma, occurring in nearly 70% of melanoma patients. See also **lentigo-maligna melanoma, nodular melanoma.**

superficial temporal artery, an artery at each side of the head that can be easily felt in front of the ear and is often used for taking the pulse. It is the smaller of the two terminal branches of the external carotid and arises in the substance of the parotid gland. It crosses the zygomatic process of the temporal bone and about 5 cm above the process divides into the frontal branch and the parietal branch. Compare **deep temporal artery, middle temporal artery.**

superficial vein, one of the many veins between the subcutaneous fascia just under the skin. Compare **deep vein.**

superimpregnation. See **superfetation.**

superinfection, an infection occurring during antimicrobial treatment for another infection. It is usually a result of change in the normal tissue flora favoring replication of some organisms by diminishing the vitality and then the number of competing organisms, as yeast microbes flourish during penicillin therapy prescribed to cure a bacterial infection.

superior, situated above or oriented toward a higher place, as the head is superior to the torso. Compare **inferior.**

superior aperture of minor pelvis, an opening bounded by the crest and pecten of the pubic bones, the arch-shaped lines of the ilia, and the anterior margin of the base of the sacrum.

superior aperture of thorax, an elliptic opening at the summit of the thorax bounded by the first thoracic vertebra, the first ribs, and the upper margin of the sternum.

superior conjunctival fornix, the space in the fold of the conjuntiva created by the reflection of the conjunctiva covering the eyeball and the lining of the upper lid. Compare **inferior conjuctival fornix.**

superior costotransverse ligament, one of five ligaments associated with each costotransverse joint, except that of the first rib. It passes from the neck of each rib to the transverse process of the vertebra immediately above and is associated with the intercostal vessels and the intercostal nerves. The first rib has no superior costotransverse ligament. Compare **posterior costotransverse ligament.**

superior gastric node, a node in one of two sets of gastric lymph glands, accompanying the left gastric artery, and divided into the upper group of nodes on the stem of the artery, the lower group of nodes accompanying branches of the artery along the cardiac half of the lesser curvature of the stomach, and the paracardial group of nodes around the neck of the stomach. The superior gastric nodes receive their afferents from the stomach and pass their efferents to the celiac group of preaortic nodes. Compare **inferior gastric node.**

superior hemorrhagic polioencephalitis. See **Wernicke's encephalopathy.**

superior mediastinum, the cranial portion of the mediastinum in the middle of the thorax, containing the trachea, the esophagus, the aortic arch, and the origins of the sternohyoidei and the sternothyroidei. The superior mediastinum is bounded by the superior aperture of the thorax, the plane of the superior limit of the pericardium, the manubrium, the upper four thoracic vertebrae, and laterally the mediastinal aspect of the parietal pleurae of the lungs. Compare **anterior mediastinum, middle mediastinum, posterior mediastinum.**

superior mesenteric artery, a visceral branch of the abdominal aorta, arising caudal to the celiac artery, dividing into five branches, and supplying most of the small intestine and parts of the colon. The branches are the inferior pancreaticoduodenal, intestinal, ileocolic, right colic, and middle colic.

superior mesenteric node, a node in one of the three groups of visceral lymph nodes that serve the viscera of the abdomen and the pelvis. The superior mesenteric nodes are associated with branches of the superior mesenteric artery and are divided into mesenteric nodes, ileocolic nodes, and mesocolic nodes. Compare **gastric node, inferior mesenteric node.**

superior mesenteric vein, a tributary of the portal vein that drains the blood from the small intestine, the cecum, and the ascending and the transverse colons. It begins in the right iliac fossa, ascends between the two mesenteric layers to the right of the superior mesenteric artery, and joins the lienal vein to form the portal vein, dorsal to the neck of the pancreas. The tributaries of the superior mesenteric vein are the intestinal vein, the ileocolic vein, the right colic vein, the middle colic vein, the gastroepiploic vein, and the pancreaticoduodenal vein. See also **portal vein.**

superior profunda artery. See **deep brachial artery.**

superior radioulnar joint. See **proximal radioulnar articulation.**

superior sagittal sinus, one of the six venous channels in the posterior of the dura mater, draining blood from the brain into the internal jugular vein. It has no valves and presents a triangular section as the sinus courses posteriorly through a groove in the frontal bone and passes along the convex margin of the falx cerebri to the occipital protuberance, usually continuing as the right transverse sinus. The superior sagittal sinus receives the superior cerebral veins, veins from the diploe, and, near the posterior extremity of the sagittal suture, the anastomosing emissary veins from the pericranium and the veins from the dura mater. It also anastomoses with veins of the nose, the scalp, and the diploe. Compare **inferior sagittal sinus, straight sinus, transverse sinus.**

superior subscapular nerve /səbskap′yələr/, one of two small nerves on opposite sides of the body that arise from the posterior cord of the brachial plexus. It supplies the superior part of the subscapularis. Compare **inferior subscapular nerve.**

superior thyroid artery, one of a pair of arteries in the neck, usually rising from the external carotid artery, that supplies the thyroid gland and several muscles in the head.

superior ulnar collateral artery, a long, slender division of the brachial artery, arising just distal to the middle of the arm, descending to the elbow, and anastomosing with the posterior ulnar recurrent and inferior ulnar collateral arteries.

superior vena cava, the second largest vein of the body, returning deoxygenated blood from the upper half of the body to the right atrium. It is about 2 cm in diameter and 7 cm long and is formed by the junction of the two brachiocephalic veins at the level of the first intercostal space behind the sternum on the right side. The section of the superior vena cava closest to the heart comprises about one half of the vessel's length and is within the pericardial sac, covered by the serous pericardium. It has no valves and just before it enters the pericardium receives the azygous vein and several small pericardial veins. Compare **inferior vena cava.**

supernatant, the clear upper portion of any mixture after it has been centrifuged.

supernormal conduction, (in cardiology) conduction that occurs when a block is expected.

supernormal excitability, the ability of the myocardium to respond to a stimulus that would be ineffective earlier or later in the cardiac cycle.

supernormal period, a period at the end of phase 3 of the cardiac cycle when activation can be initiated with less stimulus than is required at maximal repolarization.

supernumerary nipples, an excessive number of nipples, which are usually not associated with underlying glandular tissue. They may vary in size from small pink dots to that of normal nipples.

supervisor, (in hospital or public health nursing) the midlevel management position between the director of nursing and head nurses of a division or of several units. In many hospitals "clinical director" is the preferred term. The supervisor's responsibilities are primarily administrative, although they may also include clinical leadership for the nurses working in a group of units, wards, or divisions.

supination /so͞o'pinā'shən/, **1.** one of the kinds of rotation allowed by certain skeletal joints, as the elbow and the wrist joints, which allow the palm of the hand to turn up. **2.** the position of lying on the back, face up. See also **supine.** Compare **pronation.** –**supinate,** *v.*

supinator longus. See **brachioradialis.**

supine /səpīn', so͞o'pīn/, lying horizontally on the back. Compare **prone.** See also **body position.**

supine hypotension, a fall in blood pressure that occurs when a pregnant woman is lying on her back. It is caused by impaired venous return that results from pressure of the gravid uterus on the vena cava. Also called **vena caval syndrome.**

supplemental inheritance, the acquisition or expression of a genetic trait or condition from the presence of two independent pairs of nonallelic genes that interact in such a way that one gene supplements the action of the other.

supplementary gene, one of two pairs of nonallelic genes that interact in such a way that one pair needs the presence of the other to be expressed, whereas the second pair can produce an effect independent of the first.

support, **1.** to sustain, hold up, or maintain in a desired position or condition, as in physically supporting the abdominal muscles with a Scultetus binder or emotionally supporting a client under stress. **2.** the assistance given to this end, as physical support, emotional support, or life support.

supporting area, any of the areas of maxillary or mandibular edentulous ridges that are considered best suited to bear the forces of mastication with functioning dentures.

supportive psychotherapy, a form of psychotherapy that concentrates on creating an effective means of communication with an emotionally disturbed person rather than on trying to produce psychologic insight into the underlying conflicts. Through such supportive measures as reassurance, reinforcement of the person's defenses, direction, suggestion, and persuasion, the therapist participates directly in the solution of specific problems. Compare **nondirective therapy.**

supportive treatment. See **treatment.**

suppository, an easily melted medicated mass for insertion in the rectum, urethra, or vagina. Theobroma oil, glycerinated gelatin, and high-molecular-weight polyethylene glycols are common vehicles for drugs in suppositories that are cone- or spindle-shaped for insertion in the rectum, globular or egg-shaped for use in the vagina, and pencil-shaped for insertion in the urethra. Drugs administered by rectal suppository are absorbed systemically, and this route is especially useful in babies, in uncooperative patients, and in cases of vomiting or certain digestive disorders.

suppressant /səpres'ənt/, an agent that suppresses or diminishes a physical or mental activity, as a medication that reduces hyperkinetic behavior or the excretory or secretory activity of a gland.

suppression, (in psychoanalysis) the conscious inhibition or effort to conceal unacceptable or painful thoughts, desires, impulses, feelings, or acts. Compare **repression.**

suppression amblyopia, a partial loss of vision, usually in one eye, caused by cortical suppression of central vision to avoid diplopia. It occurs commonly in strabismus in the eye that deviates and does not fixate. Early recognition of strabismus and amblyopia is essential, because occlusive therapy that forces use of the bad eye may dramatically improve the child's vision if begun early. It is ineffective after 6 years of age, and near blindness in the affected eye may result.

suppressor gene, (in molecular genetics) a genetic unit that is able to reverse the effect of a specific kind of mutation in other genes.

suppressor mutation, (in molecular genetics) a mutation that partially or completely restores a function lost by a primary mutation occurring in a different genetic site.

suppressor T cell. See **T cell.**

suppurate /sup'yərāt/, to produce purulent matter. –**suppuration,** *n.,* **suppurative** /sup'yərā'tiv/, *adj.*

supra-, a combining form meaning 'above or over': *suprabuccal, supradural, suprarenalism.*

supraclavicular, the area of the body above the clavicle, or collar bone.

supraclavicular nerve, one of a pair of cutaneous branches of the cervical plexus, arising from the third and the fourth cervical nerves, mostly from the fourth nerve. It emerges from the posterior border of the sternocleidomastoideus and crosses the posterior triangle of the neck under the deep fascia. Near the clavicle it pierces the fascia and the platysma in the anterior, the middle, and the posterior groups. The anterior group supplies the skin of the infraclavicular region, the middle group supplies the skin over the pectoralis major and the deltoideus, and the posterior group supplies the skin of the cranial and the dorsal parts of the shoulder.

supracondylar fracture /so͞o′prəkon′dilər/, a fracture involving the area between the condyles of the humerus or the femur.

supragingival calculus, a deposit composed of various mineral salts, as calcium phosphate, and calcium carbonate, which accumulates with organic matter and oral debris on the teeth occlusal or coronal to the gingival crest.

suprainfection, a secondary infection usually caused by an opportunistic pathogen, as a fungal infection after the antibiotic treatment of another infection or pneumonia in a patient debilitated by another illness.

suprapubic, located above the symphysis pubis.

suprarenal, situated above the kidney, as the suprarenal gland.

suprascapular nerve /so͞o′prəskap′yələr/, one of a pair of branches from the cords of the brachial plexus. It arises from the superior trunk, passes to the scapular notch, and, in the supraspinatous fossa, branches to the supraspinatus, the shoulder joint, the infraspinatus, and the scapula.

suprasellar cyst. See **craniopharyngioma.**

supraspinal ligament, the ligament that connects the apices of the spinous processes from the seventh cervical vertebra to the sacrum. Between the spinous processes it is continuous with the interspinal ligaments; from the seventh cervical vertebrae it continues upward to the external occipital protuberance and the medial nuchal line as the ligamentum nuchae.

supraventricular tachycardia, an impulse that originates above the ventricles but cannot be clearly identified as arising from the SA node, atria, or AV node.

suramin sodium /so͝or′əmin/, an antitrypanosomal and an antifilarial available from the Center for Disease Control. It is used primarily for treatment and prophylaxis of African trypanosomiasis and onchocerciasis.

Surfacaine, a trademark for a local anesthetic agent (cyclomethycaine sulfate).

surface anatomy, the study of the structural relationships of the external features of the body to the internal organs and parts. Compare **cross-sectional anatomy.**

surface anesthesia. See **topical anesthesia.**

surface area (SA), the total area exposed to the outside environment. The surface area of an object increases with the square of the object's linear dimensions; volume increases as the cube of the object's linear dimensions. Thus, the larger of two objects of the same shape will have less surface area per unit volume than the smaller object. Most loss of body heat takes place from the body surface.

surface biopsy, the removal of living tissue for microscopic examination by scraping the surface of a lesion. The procedure is used primarily to diagnose cancer of the uterine cervix. See also **exfoliative cytology.**

surface tension, the tendency of the surface of a liquid to minimize the area of its surface by contracting. This property causes liquids to rise in a capillary tube, affects the exchange of gases in the pulmonary alveoli, and alters the ability of various liquids to wet another surface.

surface therapy, a form of radiotherapy administered by placing one or more radioactive sources on or near an area of body surface. The resulting array of sources is called a surface mold, surface applicator, or plaque.

surface thermometer, a device that detects and indicates the temperature of the surface of any part of the body.

surfactant /sərfak′tənt/, **1.** an agent, as soap or detergent, dissolved in water to reduce its surface tension or the tension at the interface between the water and another liquid. **2.** certain lipoproteins that reduce the surface tension of pulmonary fluids, allowing the exchange of gases in the alveoli of the lungs and contributing to the elasticity of pulmonary tissue. See also **alveolus, atelectasis, surface tension.**

Surfadil, a trademark for a topical fixed-combination drug containing an antihistaminic (methapyrilene hydrochloride) and a topical anesthetic (cyclomethycaine sulfate).

Surfak, a trademark for a stool softener (docusate calcium).

surfer's nodules, nodules on the skin of the knees, ankles, feet, or toes of a surfer caused by repeated contact of the skin with an abrasive, sandy surfboard. The nodules will slowly diminish in size and disappear if surfing is discontinued. When treatment is necessary, injection of corticosteroids is usually effective.

surgeon's assistant (SA), a medical professional trained to assist in surgery and in the preoperative and postoperative periods under the supervision of a licensed medical doctor. An SA is required to attend 2 years of college studying anatomy, physiology, pharmacology, and other subjects, followed by 2 years of special clinical training and clinical experience.

surgery, a branch of medicine concerned with diseases and trauma requiring operative procedures. **–surgical,** *adj.*

-surgery, -chirurgia, a combining form meaning the 'treatment of illness or deformity': *cardiosurgery, chemosurgery, radiosurgery.*

surgical abdomen. See **acute abdomen.**

surgical anatomy, (in applied anatomy) the study of the structure and morphology of the tissues and organs of the body as they relate to surgery.

surgical anesthesia, the third stage of general anesthesia. See also **general anesthesia, Guedel's signs.**

surgical diathermy. See **electrocoagulation.**

surgical induction of labor. See **induction of labor.**

surgical ligature, the exposure of an unerupted tooth by placing a metal ligature around its cervix. The free ends of the ligature are fixed to a fine precious metal chain attached to an orthodontic appliance. These components act together to produce traction on the unerupted tooth and force it through the gum tissues.

surgical microscope. See **operating microscope.**

surgical pathology, the study of disease by the study of tissue specimens obtained during surgery. The surgical pathologist often examines specimens during surgery to determine how the operation should be modified or completed. Various techniques are used. The appearance of the specimen is first noted; then slices of the tissue are prepared by the paraffin or frozen section method and microscopically examined by a physician trained in pathology.

surgical scrub, **1.** a bactericidal soap or solution used by surgeons and surgical nurses before performing or assisting in surgery. **2.** the act of washing the fingernails, hands, and forearms with a bactericidal soap or solution before a surgical procedure.

surgical sectioning, an oral surgery procedure for dividing a tooth to facilitate its removal. A variety of instruments is used for surgical sectioning, as osteotomes and power-driven burs.

surgical suite, a group of one or more operating rooms and adjunct facilities, as sterile storage area, scrub room, and recovery room.

surgical treatment. See **treatment.**

Surital Sodium, a trademark for a barbiturate (thiamylal sodium), used as a general anesthetic.

Surmontil, a trademark for an antidepressant (trimipramine maleate).

surrogate, **1.** a substitute; a person or thing that replaces another. **2.** (in psychoanalysis) a substitute parental figure, a symbolic image or representation of another, as may occur in a dream. The identity of the person represented often remains unconscious.

sursum-, a combining form meaning 'upward': *sursumduction, sursumvergence, sursumversion.*

surveillance, supervising or observing a patient or a health condition.

surveyed height of contour, a line, scribed or marked on a cast, that designates the greatest convexity relative to a selected path of denture placement and removal.

survival curve, a curve obtained by plotting the number or percentage of organisms surviving at different intervals against doses of radiation.

susceptibility, the condition of being more than normally vulnerable to a disease or disorder. **–susceptible,** *adj.*

suspension, **1.** a liquid in which small particles of a solid are dispersed, but not dissolved, and in which the dispersal is maintained by stirring or shaking the mixture. If left standing, the solid particles settle at the bottom of the container. See also **colloid, solution.** **2.** a treatment, used primarily in spinal disorders, consisting of suspending the patient by the chin and shoulders. **3.** a temporary cessation of pain or of a vital process.

suspensory ligament of the lens. See **zonula ciliaris.**

sustained release. See **prolonged release.**

sustenance, **1.** the act or process of supporting or maintaining life or health. **2.** the food or nutrients essential for maintaining life.

sutilains /so͞o′tilānz/, a proteolytic enzyme.

■ INDICATIONS: It is prescribed for debridement of certain wounds, ulcers, and second- and third-degree burns.

■ CONTRAINDICATIONS: Wounds communicating with major body cavities, wounds containing exposed major nerves or nervous tissue, or fungating neoplastic ulcers prohibit its use. It is not given during pregnancy.

■ ADVERSE EFFECTS: Among the more serious adverse reactions are bleeding, paresthesias, and dermatitis.

sutura /so͞oto͝or′ə/, *pl.* **suturae,** an immovable, fibrous joint in which certain bones of the skull are connected by a thin layer of fibrous tissue. Compare **gomphosis, syndesmosis.**

sutura dentata, an immovable fibrous joint that is one kind of true suture in which toothlike processes interlock along the margins of connecting bones of the skull. Compare **sutura limbosa, sutura serrata.**

sutura limbosa, an immovable fibrous joint that is one kind of true suture in which beveled and serrated edges of certain connecting bones of the skull, as the parietal and temporal bones, overlap and interlock. Compare **sutura dentata, sutura serrata.**

sutura plana, a fibrous joint that is one kind of false suture in which rough, contiguous edges of certain bones of the skull, as the maxillae, form a connection. Compare **sutura squamosa.**

sutura serrata, an immovable fibrous joint that is one kind of true suture in which connecting bones interlock along serrated edges that resemble fine-toothed saws. Compare **sutura dentata, sutura limbosa.**

sutura squamosa, an immovable fibrous joint that is one kind of false suture in which overlapping, beveled edges unite certain bones of the skull, as the temporal and the parietal bone. Compare **sutura plana.**

suture /so͞o′chər/, **1.** a border or a joint, as between the bones of the cranium. **2.** to stitch together cut or torn edges of tissue with suture material. **3.** a surgical stitch taken to repair an incision, tear, or wound. **4.** material used for surgical stitches, as absorbable or nonabsorbable silk, catgut, wire, or synthetic material.

suture forceps. See **needle holder.**

Sv, abbreviation for **sievert.**

SV40, abbreviation for **simian virus 40.**

SvO_2, symbol for the percent of saturation of mixed venous blood.

swab, a stick or clamp for holding absorbent gauze or cotton, used for washing, cleansing, or drying a body surface, for collecting a specimen for laboratory examinations, or for applying a topical medication.

swamp fever. See **leptospirosis, malaria.**

Swan-Ganz catheter, a long, thin cardiac catheter with a tiny balloon at the tip. It is used during anesthesia for open heart surgery to determine left ventricular function by measuring left atrial wedge pressure.

swan neck deformity, a structural abnormality of the kidney tubules associated with rickets. The kidney tubule connecting the glomerulus with the convoluted portion of

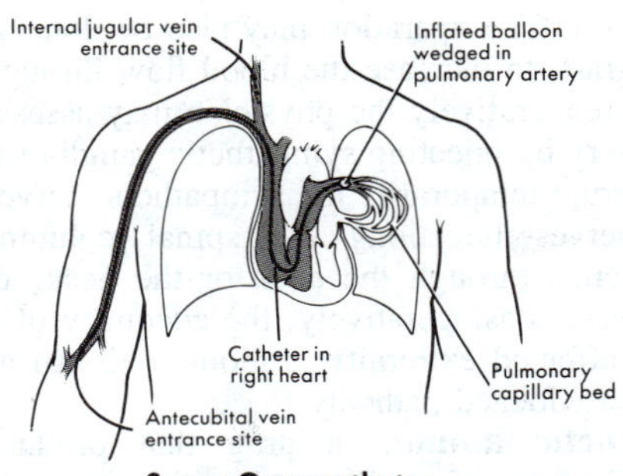

Swan-Ganz catheter

the tubule is narrowed into a configuration referred to as "swan neck." There is also a thinning and atrophy of the distal tubule and a shortening of the convoluted portion.

S wave, the component of the cardiac cycle shown on an electrocardiogram as a line slanting downward sharply from the peak of the R wave to the beginning of the upward curve of the T wave. It represents the final phase of the QRS complex.

sweat. See **perspiration.**

sweat bath, a bath given to induce sweating.

sweat duct, any one of the tiny tubules conveying sweat to the surface of the skin from about 2 million sweat glands throughout the body. Each sweat duct is the most superficial part of a coiled tube that forms the body of each sweat gland and opens onto the surface through a funnel-shaped opening. The sweat ducts in the armpits and in the groin are larger than in other parts of the body. Ducts and sweat glands abound on the palms of the hands and the soles of the feet. There are about 370 sweat ducts rising from a corresponding number of sweat glands per square centimeter on each palm. Each duct is composed of a basement membrane with two or three layers of polyhedral cells and is lined with a thin cuticle.

sweat gland. See **sudoriferous gland.**

sweating. See **diaphoresis.**

sweat test, a method for evaluating sodium and chloride excretion from the sweat glands, often the first test performed in the diagnosis of cystic fibrosis. The sweat glands are stimulated with a drug, as pilocarpine, and the perspiration produced is analyzed. The eccrine glands of patients with cystic fibrosis produce sodium and chloride concentrations that are three to six times that of the normal. Chloride levels above 60 mEq/L are considered diagnostic for the disease. The test is very reliable, and although it may be useful at any age, it is usually performed on infants from 2 weeks to 1 year of age. See also **cystic fibrosis.**

Sweet localization method, a radiographic technique for locating a foreign body in the eye by making two x-ray films of the eye while the patient's head is immobilized. A small metal ball and a cone are placed at precise distances from the center of the cornea as register marks while lateral and perpendicular x-ray views of the eye are made. A three-dimensional view of the eye is constructed from the two x-ray films, and, guided by the positions of the ball and cone, the location of the foreign body in the eye is plotted from the intersection of lines through the ball and cone.

Swift's disease. See **acrodynia.**

swimmer's ear, *informal.* otitis externa resulting from infection transmitted in the water of a swimming pool.

swimmer's itch, an allergic dermatitis caused by sensitivity to schistosome cercarias that die under the skin, leading to erythema, urticaria, and a papular rash lasting 1 or 2 days. Treatment usually includes oral antihistamines and antipruritic lotions. See also **schistosomiasis.**

swimming pool conjunctivitis. See **pharyngoconjunctival fever.**

swinging ventricular tachycardia, tachycardia in which the polarity of the wide QRS complexes swings between positive and negative. See also **torsades de pointes.**

swing phase of gait, one of the two phases in the rhythmic process of walking. The swing phase of gait follows the stance phase and is divided into the initial swing stage, the midswing stage, and the terminal swing stage. The analyses of pathologic gaits and the diagnoses of many abnormal orthopedic conditions focus on walking as a specilized function of the musculoskeletal system and the swing phase of gait as the kinetic conclusion of one complete gait cycle. By studying the two phases of stance and swing in the gait of any individual, orthopedists can often determine gait deviations associated with many abnormal conditions or deformities of the spine, hip, pelvis, legs, or feet, and weaknesses in associated muscles. Compare **stance phase of gait.**

sy-. See **syn-.**

sycosis barbae /sikō′sis/, an inflammation of hair follicles of skin that has been shaved. Treatment includes light and infrequent shaving, topical and systemic antibiotics, and daily plucking of infected hairs. Also called **barber's itch, sycosis vulgaris.**

Sydenham's chorea /sid′ənhamz/, a form of chorea associated with rheumatic fever, usually occurring during childhood. The cause is a streptococcal infection of the vascular and perivascular tissues of the brain. The choreic movements increase over the first 2 weeks, reach a plateau, and then diminish. The child is usually well within 10 weeks. With undue exertion or emotional strain, the condition may recur. Also called **chorea minor, rheumatic chorea.**

syl-. See **syn-.**

sylvatic plague, an endemic disease of wild rodents caused by *Yersinia pestis* and transmissable to humans by the bite of an infected flea. It is found on every continent except Australia. See also **bubonic plague.**

sym-. See **syn-.**

symbiosis /sim′bē·ō′sis/, **1.** (in biology) a mode of living characterized by close association between organisms of different species, usually in a mutually beneficial relationship. **2.** (in psychiatry) a state in which two mentally disturbed people are emotionally dependent on each other. **3.** pathologic inability of a child to separate from its mother emotionally and, sometimes, physically. – **symbiotic,** *adj.*

symbol, **1.** an image, object, action, or other stimulus that represents something else by reason of conscious association, convention, or other relationship. **2.** an object, mode of behavior, or feeling that disguises a repressed emotional conflict through an unconscious association rather than through an objective relationship, as in dreams and neuroses.

-symbolia, a combining form meaning '(condition involving) the ability to interpret symbols': *asymbolia, dyssymbolia, strephosymbolia.*

symbolism, **1.** the representation or evocation of one idea, action, or object by the use of another, as in systems of writing, poetic language, or dream metaphor. **2.** (in psychiatry) an unconscious mental mechanism characteristic of all human thinking in which a mental image stands for but disguises some other object, person, or thought, especially one associated with emotional conflict. The mechanism is a principal factor in the formation of dreams and in various symptoms resulting from such neurotic and psychotic conditions as conversion reactions, obsessions, and compulsions. Also called **symbolization.**

symelus. See **symmelus.**

symmelia, a fetal anomaly characterized by the fusion of the lower limbs with or without feet. Kinds of symmelia are **apodial symmelia, dipodial symmelia, monopodial symmelia,** and **tripodial symmelia.**

symmelus /sim′ələs/, a malformed fetus characterized by symmelia. Also spelled **symelus.**

Symmer's disease. See **giant follicular lymphoma.**

Symmetrel, a trademark for an antiviral (amantadine hydrochloride).

symmetric, (of the body or parts of the body) equal in size or shape; very similar in relative placement or arrangement about an axis. Also **symmetrical.** Compare **asymmetric.** –**symmetry,** *n.*

symmetric lipomatosis. See **nodular circumscribed lipomatosis.**

symmetric tonic neck reflex, a normal response in infants to assume the crawl position by extending the arms and bending the knees when the head and neck are extended. The reflex disappears when neurologic and muscular development enables independent limb movement for actual crawling. Also called **crawling reflex.** See also **tonic neck reflex.**

sympathectomy /sim′pəthek′təmē/, a surgical interruption of part of the sympathetic nerve pathways, performed for the relief of chronic pain in vascular diseases, as arteriosclerosis, claudication, Buerger's disease, and Raynaud's phenomenon. The sheath around an artery carries the sympathetic nerve fibers that control constriction of the vessel. Removal of the sheath causes the vessel to relax and expand and allows more blood to pass through it. The operation may also be done with a vascular graft, to increase the blood flow through the graft area. Preoperatively the physician may assess the effect of surgery by injecting sympathetic ganglia with alcohol to interrupt temporarily the sympathetic nerve impulses. The nerves lie along the spinal column and are approached through the back or the neck, using local anesthesia. Postoperatively, the adequacy of circulation in the affected extremity is monitored. An arteriogram shows a widened pathway.

sympathetic amine, a drug that produces effects resembling those manifested by stimulation of the sympathetic nervous system.

sympathetic nervous system. See **autonomic nervous system.**

sympathetic ophthalmia, a granulomatous inflammation of the uveal tract of both eyes occurring after an injury to the uveal tract of one eye. Corticosteroids may be helpful in treatment, but surgical enucleation of the originally injured eye may be necessary to preserve vision in the uninjured eye. Also called **metastatic ophthalmia, migratory ophthalmia.**

sympathetic trunk, one of a pair of chains of ganglia extending along the side of the vertebral column from the base of the skull to the coccyx. Each trunk is part of the sympathetic nervous system and consists of a series of ganglia connected by cords containing various types of fibers. The cranial end of the trunk is formed by the superior cervical ganglion from the internal carotid nerve of the head. In some individuals the caudal ends of both trunks merge into a single ganglion at the coccyx. Interconnection of the trunks is common but rarely occurs above the fifth lumbar nerve. In addition to the ganglia, the trunks contain the preganglionic fibers, which are small and myelinated, the postganglionic fibers, which are mostly unmyelinated, some myelinated afferent fibers, and some unmyelinated afferent fibers. The central ganglia of each trunk are irregularly shaped structures with diameters ranging from 1 to 10 mm. Each sympathetic trunk distributes branches with postganglionic fibers to the autonomic plexuses, the cranial nerves, the individual organs, the nerves accompanying arteries, and the spinal nerves.

sympathizing eye, (in sympathetic ophthalmia) the uninfected eye that becomes infected by lymphatic or blood-borne metastasis of the microorganism.

sympatholytic, sympatholytic agent. See **antiadrenergic.**

sympathomimetic /sim′pəthōmimet′ik/, denoting a pharmacologic agent that mimics the effects of stimulation of organs and structures by the sympathetic nervous system by occupying adrenergic receptor sites and acting as an agonist or by increasing the release of the neurotransmitter norepinephrine at postganglionic nerve endings. Various sympathomimetic agents are used as decongestants of nasal and ocular mucosa, as bronchodilators in the treatment of asthma, bronchitis, bronchiectasis, and emphysema and as vasopressors and cardiac stimulants in the treatment of acute hypotension and shock; they are also used for maintaining normal blood pressure during operations using spinal anesthesia. Drugs in this group include cyclopentamine, dobutamine, dopamine, ephedrine, isoproterenol, metaproterenol, metaraminol, mephentermine, methoxamine, methoxyphenamine, naphazoline, norepinephrine, phenylephrine, phenylpropanolamine, propylhexedrine, protokylol, pseudoephedrine, terbutaline sulfate, tetrahydrozoline, tuaminoheptane, xylmetazoline, and epinephrine, a synthetic isomer of the hormone secreted by the adrenal medulla. Adverse effects of sympathomimetic drugs may be nervousness, severe headache, anxiety, vertigo, nausea, vomiting, dilated pupils, glycosuria, and dysuria. Also called **adrenergic.**

sympathomimetic amine. See **adrenergic.**

sympathy, **1.** an expressed interest or concern regarding the problems, emotions, or states of mind of another. Compare **empathy.** **2.** the relation that exists between the mind and body causing the one to be affected by the other. **3.** mental contagion or the influence exerted by one individual or group on another and the effects produced, as the spread of panic, uncontrollable laughter, or yawning. **4.** the physiologic or pathologic relationship between two organs, systems, or parts of the body. –**sympathetic,** *adj.*, **sympathize,** *v.*

symphalangia /sim′fəlan′jē·ə/, **1.** a condition, usually inherited, characterized by ankylosis of the fingers or toes. **2.** a congenital anomaly in which webbing of the fingers or toes occurs in varying degrees, often in conjunction with other defects of the hands or feet. Also called **symphalangism.** See also **syndactyly.**

symphocephalus, twin fetuses joined at the head. The term is often used as a general designation for fetuses with varying degrees of the anomaly. See also **cephalothoracopagus, craniopagus, syncephalus.**

symphyseal angle /simfiz′ē·əl/, (in dentistry) the angle of the chin, which may be protruding, straight, or receding, according to type.

symphysic teratism, a congenital anomaly in which there is a fusion of normally separated parts or organs, as a horseshoe kidney, or in which parts close prematurely, as the skull bones in craniostenosis.

symphysis /sim′fəsis/, *pl.* **symphyses** /-ēz/, **1.** also called **fibrocartilaginous joint.** a line of union, especially a cartilaginous joint in which adjacent bony surfaces are firmly united by fibrocartilage. **2.** *informal.* symphysis pubis. –**symphysic,** *adj.*

symphysis pubis. See **pubic symphysis.**

sympodia /simpō′dē·ə/, a congenital developmental anomaly characterized by fusion of the lower extremities. See also **sirenomelus, sympus.**

symptom, a subjective indication of a disease or a change in condition as perceived by the patient. The halo symptom of glaucoma is the seeing by the patient of colored rings around a single light source. Many symptoms are accompanied by objective signs, as pruritus, which is often reported with erythema and a maculopapular eruption on the skin. Some symptoms may be objectively confirmed, as numbness of a body part, which may be confirmed by absence of response to a pin prick. Compare **sign.**

symptomatic nanism, dwarfism associated with defects in bone growth, tooth formation, and sexual development.

symptomatic treatment. See **treatment.**

symptom neurosis, psychologic disorders in which dysfunctional coping mechanisms appear as clinical symptoms that represent direct manifestations of anxiety.

symptothermal method of family planning, a natural method of family planning that incorporates the ovulation and basal body temperature methods of family planning. It is more effective than either method used alone and requires fewer days of abstinence, because it enables the fertile period of the menstrual cycle to be more precisely identified.

sympus /sim′pəs/, a malformed fetus in which the lower extremities are completely fused or rotated and the pelvis and genitalia are defective. Kinds of sympuses are **sirenomelus, sympus dipus,** and **sympus monopus.** See also **symmelus.**

sympus apus. See **sirenomelus.**

sympus dipus /dē′pəs/, a malformed fetus in which the lower extremities are fused and both feet are formed.

sympus monopus /mon′əpəs/, a malformed fetus in which the lower extremities are fused and one foot is formed. Also called **monopodial symmelia, uromelus.**

syn-, sy-, syl-, sym-, a combining form meaning 'union, or association': *synalgia, syncephalus, synchronous.*

synadelphus /sin′ədel′fəs/, *pl.* **synadelphi,** a conjoined twin fetal monster with a single head and trunk and eight limbs. Also called **syndelphus, cephalothoracoiliopagus.**

Synalar, a trademark for a glucocorticoid (fluocinolone acetonide).

synapse /sin′aps/, **1.** the region surrounding the point of contact between two neurons or between a neuron and an effector organ, across which nerve impulses are transmitted through the action of a neurotransmitter, as acetylcholine or norepinephrine. When an impulse reaches the terminal point of one neuron, it causes the release of the neurotransmitter, which diffuses across the gap between the two cells to bind with receptors in the other neuron, muscle, or gland, triggering electric changes that either inhibit or continue the transmission of the impulse. Synapses are polarized so that nerve impulses normally travel in only one direction; they are also subject to fatigue, oxygen deficiency, anesthetics, and other chemical agents. Kinds of synapses include **axoaxonic synapse, axodendritic synapse, axodendrosomatic synapse, axosomatic synapse,** and **dendrodendritic synapse.** Compare **ephapse.** **2.** to form a synapse or connection between neurons. **3.** (in genetics) to form a synaptic fusion between homologous chromosomes during meiosis. –**synaptic,** *adj.*

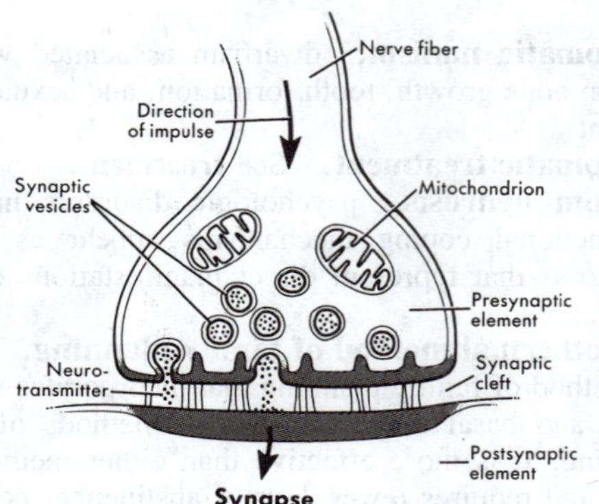

Synapse

synapsis /sinap′sis/, *pl.* **synapses,** the pairing of homologous chromosomes during the early meiotic prophase stage in gametogenesis to form double or bivalent chromosomes.

synaptic cleft, the microscopic, extracellular space at the synapse that separates the membrane of the terminal nerve endings of a presynaptic neuron and the membrane of a postsynaptic cell. Nerve impulses are transmitted across this cleft by means of a neurotransmitter. See also **myoneural junction.** Also called **synaptic gap.**

synaptic junction, the membranes of both the presynaptic neuron and the postsynaptic receptor cell together with the synaptic cleft. See also **synapse.**

synaptic transmission, the passage of a neural impulse across a synapse from one nerve fiber to another by means of a neurotransmitter. Compare **ephaptic transmission.**

synarthrosis. See **fibrous joint.**

syncephalus /sinsef′ələs/, a conjoined twin monster having a single head and two bodies. Also called **monocephalus.**

synchilia /singkē′lē·ə/, a congenital anomaly in which there is complete or partial fusion of the lips; atresia of the mouth. Also spelled **syncheilia.**

synchondrosis /sing′kondrō′sis/, *pl.* **synchondroses,** a cartilaginous joint between two immovable bones, as the synchondroses of the cranium, the pubic symphysis, the sternum, and the manubrium.

synchorial /singkôr′ē·əl/, pertaining to multiple fetuses that share a common placenta, as in monozygosity.

synclitism /sing′klitiz′əm/, **1.** (in obstetrics) a condition in which the sagittal suture of the fetal head is in line with the transverse diameter of the inlet, equidistant from the maternal symphysis pubis and sacrum. This position is usually found on examination either late in pregnancy or early in labor, as the fetal head descends into the pelvic inlet. As labor progresses, posterior asynclitism develops, and, as the head descends further, anterior asynclitism is evident because of the shape of the true pelvis below the inlet. **2.** (in hematology) the normal condition in which the nucleus and the cytoplasm of the blood cells mature simultaneously and at the same rate.

syncopal attack /sing′kəpəl/, any episode of unconsciousness or fainting, especially one associated with fear or pain. Many individuals, especially men, suffer such attacks during violent coughing spells because of associated rapid changes in arterial blood pressure. Syncopal attacks also occur as the result of any of a number of cardiovascular disorders.

syncope /sing′kəpē/, a brief lapse in consciousness caused by transient cerebral hypoxia. It is usually preceded by a sensation of light-headedness and may often be prevented by lying down or by sitting with the head between the knees. It may be caused by many different factors, including emotional stress, vagal stimulation, vascular pooling in the legs, diaphoresis, or sudden change in environmental temperature or body position.

syncretic thinking, a stage in the development of the cognitive thought processes of the child. During this phase thought is based purely on what is perceived and experienced. The child is incapable of reasoning beyond the observable or of making deductions or generalizations. Through imaginative play, questioning, interaction with others, and the increasing use of language and symbols to represent objects, the child begins to learn to make associations between ideas and to elaborate concepts. In Piaget's classification, this stage occurs between 2 and 7 years of age and is preceded by the sensorimotor stage of development when the child progresses from reflex activity to repetitive and imitative behavior. Compare **abstract thinking, concrete thinking.** –**syncresis,** *n.*

synctium, a group of cells in which the protoplasm of one cell is continuous with that of adjoining cells.

syncytiotrophoblast, the outer syncytial layer of the trophoblast of the early mammalian embryo that erodes the uterine wall during implantation and gives rise to the villi of the placenta. Also called **plasmidotrophoblast, syncytial trophoblast, syntrophoblast.** Compare **cytotrophoblast.** –**syncytiotrophoblastic,** *adj.*

syndactylus, a person with webbed fingers or toes.

syndactyly /sindak′təlē/, a congenital anomaly characterized by the fusion of the fingers or toes. It varies in degree of severity from incomplete webbing of the skin of two digits to complete union of digits and fusion of the bones and nails. Also called **syndactylia, syndactylism.** –**syndactyl, syndactylous,** *adj.*

syndelphus. See **synadelphus.**

syndesmo-, a combining form meaning 'of or pertaining to the connective tissue or particularly the ligaments': *syndesmochorial, syndesmography, syndesmoma.*

syndesmosis /sin′desmō′sis/, *pl.* **syndesmoses,** a fibrous articulation in which two bones are connected by interosseous ligaments, as the anterior and the posterior ligaments in the tibiofibular articulation. Compare **gomphosis, sutura.**

syndrome, a complex of signs and symptoms resulting from a common cause or appearing, in combination, to present a clinical picture of a disease or inherited abnormality. See also specific syndromes.

syndrome of inappropriate antidiuretic hormone secretion (SIADH), an abnormal condition characterized by the excessive release of antidiuretic hormone (ADH) that upsets the fluid and electrolytic balances of the body. It results from various malfunctions, as the inability of the body to produce and secrete dilute urine, water retention, increased extracellular fluid volume, and hyponatremia. SIADH develops in association with diseases that affect the osmoreceptors of the hypothalamus. Oat cell carcinoma of the lung is the most common cause, affecting about 80% of involved patients. Less common causes are disorders that affect the central nervous system, as brain tumors and lupus erythematosis, pulmonary diseases, as pneumonia, cancers of the pancreas and the prostate, and pathologic reactions to various drugs, as chlorpropamide, vincristine sulfate, carbamazepine, and clofibrate. Prognosis depends on the underlying disease and the response of the patient to treatment.

■ OBSERVATIONS: Common signs and symptoms of SIADH are weight gain despite anorexia, vomiting, nausea, muscle weakness, and irritability. In some patients SIADH may produce coma and convulsions. Most of the free water associated with this syndrome is intracellular, and associated edema is rare unless excess water volume exceeds 4 mosm. Confirming diagnosis is based on urine osmolality that exceeds 150 mosm/kg of water and serum osmolality of less than 280 mosm/kg of water. Normal urine osmolality is 1.5 times serum osmolality. Other significant results include less than normal concentrations of blood urea nitrogen, serum creatinine, and albumin and a concentration of sodium in the urine higher than normal.

■ INTERVENTION: Treatment of SIADH commonly includes restriction of water intake and may require administration of normal saline to raise the serum sodium level if water intoxication is severe. Furosemide may be administered to block circulatory overload, and drugs, as demeclocycline hydrochloride and lithium, may be administered to block renal response to ADH. Surgery and chemotherapy are other alternatives to remove or destroy neoplasms that may be the underlying causes of this syndrome.

■ NURSING CONSIDERATIONS: Nurses monitor the SIADH patient for any signs of hyponatremia, weight change, and fluid imbalance. The patient is carefully advised on the importance of restricted water intake to prevent water intoxication and is closely observed for any indications of restlessness, congestive heart failure, and convulsions.

synechia /sinek′ē•ə/, *pl.* **synechiae,** an adhesion, especially of the iris to the cornea or lens of the eye. It may develop from glaucoma, cataracts, uveitis, or keratitis or as a complication of surgery or trauma to the eye. Synechiae prevent or impede flow of aqueous fluid between the anterior and posterior chambers of the eye and may lead rapidly to blindness. Immediate treatment consists of dilating the pupils with a mydriatic agent, followed by treatment of the underlying cause.

Synemol, a trademark for a glucocorticoid (fluocinolone acetonide).

syneresis /siner′əsis/, the drawing together or coagulation of particles of a gel with separation from the medium in which the particles were suspended, as occurs in blood clot retraction.

synergism. See **synergy.**

synergist /sin′ərjist/, an organ, agent, or substance that augments the activity of another organ, agent, or substance.

synergy /sin′ərjē/, the process in which two organs, substances, or agents work simultaneously to enhance the function and effect of one another. Also called **synergism.** **–synergistic, synergetic,** *adj.*

syngeneic /sin′jənē′ik/, **1.** (in genetics) denoting an individual or cell type that has the same genotype as another individual or cell. **2.** (in transplantation biology) denoting tissues that are antigenically similar. Also **isogeneic.** Compare **allogeneic, xenogeneic.**

Synkayvite, a trademark for a synthetic preparation of vitamin K (menadiol sodium diphosphate).

synophthalmia. See **cyclopia.**

Synophylate, a trademark for a bronchodilator (theophylline sodium glycinate).

synotia /sīnō′shə/, a congenital malformation characterized by the union or approximation of the ears in front of the neck, often accompanied by the absence or defective development of the lower jaw. Compare **agnathia.** See also **otocephaly.**

synotus /sīnō′təs/, a fetus with synotia.

synovectomy, the excision of a synovial membrane of a joint.

synovia /sinō′vē•ə/, a transparent, viscous fluid, resembling the white of an egg, secreted by synovial membranes and acting as a lubricant for many joints, bursae, and tendons. It contains mucin, albumin, fat, and mineral salts. Also called **synovial fluid.** **–synovial,** *adj.*

synovial bursa, one of the many closed sacs filled with synovial fluid in the connective tissue between the muscles, the tendons, the ligaments, and the bones. The synovial bursae facilitate the gliding of muscles and tendons over bony and ligamentous prominences. Compare **synovial membrane, synovial tendon sheath.**

synovial chondroma, a rare cartilaginous growth developing in the connective tissue below the synovial membrane of the joints, tendon sheaths, or bursa. Foci on the surface may develop stalks and then detach, resulting in numerous loose bodies within the joint. Also called **synovial chondromatosis.**

synovial crypt, a pouch in the synovial membrane of a joint.

synovial fluid. See **synovia.**

synovial joint, a freely movable joint in which contiguous bony surfaces are covered by articular cartilage and connected by ligaments lined with synovial membrane. Kinds of synovial joints are **ball and socket joint, condyloid joint, gliding joint, hinge joint, pivot joint, saddle joint,** and **uniaxial joint.** Also called **diathrosis.** Compare **cartilaginous joint, fibrous joint.**

synovial membrane, the inner layer of an articular capsule surrounding a freely movable joint. The synovial membrane is loosely attached to the external fibrous capsule. It secretes into the joint a thick fluid that normally lubricates the joint but that may accumulate in painful amounts when the joint is injured. Compare **synovial bursa, synovial tendon sheath.**

synovial sarcoma, a malignant tumor, composed of synovioblasts, that begins as a soft swelling and often metastasizes through the bloodstream to the lung before it is discovered.

synovial sheath, any one of the membranous sacs that enclose a tendon of a muscle and facilitate the gliding of a tendon through a fibrous or a bony tunnel, as that under the flexor retinaculum of the wrist.

synovial tendon sheath, one of the many membranous sacs enclosing various tendons that glide through fibrous and bony tunnels in the body, as those under the flexor retinaculum of the wrist. One layer of the synovial sheath lines the tunnel; the other covers the tendon. The sheath secretes synovial fluid, which lubricates the tendon. Compare **synovial bursa, synovial membrane.**

synovitis /sin′əvī′tis/, an inflammatory condition of the synovial membrane of a joint as the result of an aseptic wound or a traumatic injury, as a sprain or severe strain. The knee is most commonly affected. Fluid accumulates around the capsule, the joint is swollen, tender, and painful, and motion is restricted. In most cases, the inflammation subsides, and the fluid is resorbed without medical or surgical intervention.

syntaxic mode, the ability to perceive whole, logical, coherent pictures as they occur in reality, according to the Sullivan theory of psychology.

synteny /sin′tənē/, (in genetics) the presence on the same chromosome of two or more genes that may or may not be transmitted as a linkage group but that appear to be able to undergo independent assortment during meiosis. The term is used primarily in human genetics where linked inheritance patterns are more difficult to determine. See also **linkage.**

synthesis /sin′thəsis/, a level of cognitive learning in which the individual puts together the elements of previous learning levels to create a unified whole.

-synthesis, a combining form meaning 'putting together or formation of': *narcosynthesis, psychosynthesis, velosynthesis.*

synthetic, of or pertaining to a substance that is produced by an artificial rather than a natural process or material.

synthetic chemistry, the science dealing with the formation of chemical compounds from simpler substances.

synthetic oleovitamin D. See **viosterol.**

Synthroid, a trademark for a thyroid hormone (levothyroxine sodium).

Syntocinon, a trademark for an oxytocic (oxytocin).

syntrophoblast. See **syncytiotrophoblast.**

syphilis, a sexually transmitted disease caused by the spirochete, *Treponema pallidum,* characterized by distinct stages of effects over a period of years. Any organ system may become involved. The spirochete is able to pass through the human placenta, producing congenital syphilis.

■ OBSERVATIONS: The first stage **(primary syphilis)** is marked by the appearance of a small, painless, red pustule on the skin or mucous membrane between 10 and 90 days after exposure. The lesion may appear anywhere on the body where contact with a lesion on an infected person has occurred, but is seen most often in the anogenital region. It quickly erodes, forming a painless, bloodless ulcer, called a chancre, exuding a fluid that swarms with spirochetes. The chancre may not be noticed by the patient, and many people may become infected. It heals spontaneously within 10 to 40 days, often creating the mistaken impression that the sore was not a serious event. The second stage **(secondary syphilis)** occurs about 2 months later, after the spirochetes have increased in number and spread throughout the body. This stage is characterized by general malaise, anorexia, nausea, fever, headache, alopecia, bone and joint pain, or the appearance of a morbiliform rash that does not itch, flat white sores in the mouth and throat, or condylomata lata papules on the moist areas of the skin. The disease remains highly contagious at this stage and can be spread by kissing. The symptoms usually continue for from 3 weeks to 3 months but may be recurrent over a period of 2 years. The third stage **(tertiary syphilis)** may not develop for 3 to 15 or more years. It is characterized by the appearance of soft, rubbery tumors, called gummas, that ulcerate and heal by scarring. Gummas may develop anywhere on the surface of the body and in the eye, liver, lungs, stomach, or reproductive organs. Tertiary syphilis may be painless, unnoticed except for gummas, or it may be accompanied by deep, burrowing pain. The ulceration of the gummas may result in punched-out areas of the palate, nasal septum, or larynx. Various tissues and structures of the body, including the central nervous system, myocardium, and the valves of the heart may be damaged or destroyed, leading to mental or physical disability and premature death. **Congenital syphilis** resulting from prenatal infection may result in the birth of a deformed or blind infant. In some cases, the infant appears to be well until, at several weeks of age, snuffles, sometimes with a bloodstained or mucopurulent discharge, and skin lesions are observed, particularly on the palms and soles or in the genital region. Such children may also have visual or hearing defects, and progeria and poor health may develop. Diagnosis of syphilis is made by darkfield microscopy of fluid from primary or secondary stage lesions, by bacteriologic study of blood samples, and by an examination of cerebrospinal fluid. Because of the slow development of the disease during the early stages, the various serologic tests, including the Wassermann, may not be accurate until months after exposure. Repeated tests and crosschecking with more than one test may be required in some cases. The report by a person that exposure to syphilis has occurred is often the only evidence available to the clinician.

■ INTERVENTION: Patients with primary or secondary syphilis are usually given benzathine penicillin or an equivalent in a single dose of 2.4 million units or in two doses of 1.2 million units intramuscularly. The objective is to maintain penicillin in the bloodstream for a number of days, because *Treponema pallidum* divides at an average rate of once every 33 hours, and the antibiotic is most effective during the stage of cell division. Larger doses of penicillin, of between 7.2 and 9 million units, are administered over a period of 2 to 3 weeks for tertiary syphilis. Infants and small children with congenital syphilis are usually given 50,000 units/kg intramuscularly. Treatment of an infected mother with penicillin during the first 4 months of pregnancy usually prevents the development of congenital syphilis in the fetus. Treating the mother with antibiotics later in the pregnancy usually eliminates the infection but may not protect the fetus.

■ NURSING CONSIDERATIONS: Special care and aseptic precautions are taken while handling the highly contagious fluid from syphilitic lesions used in diagnostic testing, because the infection may be acquired through a cut or break in the skin. The nurse is often the person delegated to discuss the disease and its treatment with the patient. The need for and the nearly total effectiveness of the antibiotic are stressed. The extremely contagious nature of the infection is explained, and the importance of treatment for all who may have been exposed is emphasized. Tact, patience, and understanding are required to reassure the usually upset, frightened patient, to secure the patient's cooperation in accepting treatment and in assisting in the identification and location of others needing treatment. In many states, active, serologically documented cases of syphilis must, by law, be reported to the Department of Health. See also **chancre, Hutchinson's teeth, Hutchinson's triad, snuffles.**

syphilitic aortitis, an inflammatory condition of the aorta, occurring in tertiary syphilis and characterized by diffuse dilatation with gray, wheallike plaques containing calcium on the inner coat and scars and wrinkles on the outer coat. The middle layer of the vascular wall is usually infiltrated with plasma cells and contains fragments of damaged elastic tissue and many newly formed blood vessels. There may be damage to the aortic valves, narrowing of the mouths of the coronary arteries, and the formation of thrombi. Cerebral embolism may result. Signs of syphilitic aortitis are substernal pain, dyspnea, bounding pulse, and high systolic blood pressure. Penicillin may slow the course of the disease, but it cannot reverse the structural damage to the vessels and the heart. Also called **Döhle-Heller disease, Heller-Döhle disease, luetic aortitis.**

syphilitic meningoencephalitis. See **general paresis.**

syphilitic periarteritis, an inflammatory condition of the outer coat of one or more arteries occurring in tertiary syphilis and characterized by soft gummatous perivascular lesions infiltrated with lymphocytes and plasma cells. Also called **periarteritis gummosa.** See also **syphilitic aortitis.**

syring-. See **syringo-.**

syringe, a device for withdrawing, injecting, or instilling fluids. A syringe for the injection of medication usually consists of a calibrated glass or plastic cylindric barrel having a close-fitting plunger at one end and a small opening at the other to which the head of a hollow-bore needle is fitted. Medication of the desired amount may be pulled up into the barrel by suction as the plunger is withdrawn and injected by pushing the plunger back into the barrel, forcing the liquid out through the needle. A syringe for irrigating a wound or body cavity or for extracting mucus or another body fluid from an orifice or body cavity is usually larger than the kind used for injection. It often has a rubber bulb at one end and a blunt, soft-tipped, flexible tube with an opening at the other end. The bulb is squeezed to eject a fluid and is released to withdraw one. Kinds of syringe include **asepto syringe, bulb syringe, hypodermic syringe, Luer-Lok syringe,** and **tuberculin syringe.**

syringo-, syring-, a combining form meaning 'of or pertaining to a tube or a fistula': *syringobulbia, syringocystoma, syringomyelitis.*

syringomyelocele /siring′gōmī′əlōsēl′/, a hernial protrusion of the spinal cord through a congenital defect in the vertebral column in which the cerebrospinal fluid within the central cavities of the cord is greatly increased so that the cord tissue forms a thin-walled sac that lies close to the membrane of the cavity. See also **myelomeningocele, neural tube defect, spina bifida.**

system, **1.** a collection or assemblage of parts that, unified, make a whole. Physiologic systems, as the cardiovascular or reproductive systems, are made up of structures specifically able to engage in processes that are essential for a vital function in the body. **2.** a set of computer programs and hardware that work together for some specific purpose.

systematic error, a nonrandom statistic error that affects the mean of a population of data and defines the bias between the means of two populations.

systematic heating, the elevation of the temperature of the whole body.

systematic tabulation, (in research) mechanic or manual techniques for recording and classifying data for statistic analysis.

system documentation. See **documentation.**

systemic /sistem′ik/, of or pertaining to the whole body rather than to a localized area or regional portion of the body.

systemic desensitization, a technique used in behavior therapy for eliminating maladaptive anxiety associated with phobias. The procedure involves the construction by the person of a hierarchy of anxiety-producing stimuli and the general presentation of these stimuli until they no longer elicit the initial response of fear. Also called **desensitization.** Compare **flooding.** See also **reciprocal inhibition.**

systemic lupus erythematosus (SLE), a chronic inflammatory disease affecting many systems of the body. The pathophysiology of the disease includes severe vasculitis, renal involvement, and lesions of the skin and nervous system. The primary cause of the disease has not been determined; viral infection or dysfunction of the immune system has been suggested. Adverse reaction to certain drugs may also cause a lupuslike syndrome. Four times more women than men have SLE. Also called **disseminated lupus erythematosus, lupus erythematosus.**

■ OBSERVATIONS: The initial manifestation is often arthritis. An erythematous rash over the nose and malar eminences, weakness, fatigue, and weight loss are also frequently seen early in the disease. Photosensitivity, fever, skin lesions on the neck, and alopecia where the skin lesions extend beyond the hairline may occur. The skin lesions may spread to the mucous membranes and other tissues of the body. They do not ulcerate but cause degeneration of the tissues affected. Depending on the organs involved, the patient may also have glomerulonephritis, pleuritis, pericarditis, peritonitis, neuritis, or anemia. Renal failure and severe neurologic abnormalities are among the most serious manifestations of the disease. Diagnosis of SLE is made by subjective and objective findings based on physical examination and laboratory findings, including antinuclear antibody in the cerebrospinal fluid and a positive lupus erythematosus (LE) cell reaction in a lupus erythematosus preparation (LE prep). Other laboratory examinations may be useful, depending on the organs, tissues, and systems affected by the disease.

■ INTERVENTION: In many cases SLE may be controlled with corticosteroid medication administered systemically. Care and treatment vary with the severity and nature of the disease and the body systems that are affected. Topical steroids may be applied to the rash; salicylates may be given to alleviate pain and swelling in the joints. Fatigue and stress are avoided, and all body surfaces are protected from direct sunlight. Antimalarial drugs are sometimes given to treat cutaneous lesions, but retinal damage may occur with prolonged use.

■ NURSING CONSIDERATIONS: The timing, dosage, side effects, and toxic reactions to the medications are explained before discharge. The steroids must be taken exactly as prescribed, and, in the event that the patient cannot take them, the doctor is to be consulted promptly. An identification card is carried bearing the patient's diagnosis, a list of all medications and their dosage, and the doctor's name and telephone number. As in any disease marked by chronic remission and exacerbation of many distressing symptoms, the patient may require extensive emotional and psychologic support.

systemic oxygen consumption, the amount of oxygen consumed by the body's tissues as measured during a period of 60 seconds.

systemic remedy, a medicinal substance that is given orally, parenterally, or rectally to be absorbed into the circulation for treatment of a health problem. Many remedies or medications administered locally or regionally are to some degree absorbed systemically. Medication administered systemically may have various local effects, but the intent is to treat the whole body.

systemic vascular resistance (SVR), the resistance against which the left ventricle must eject to force out its stroke volume with each beat. As the peripheral vessels constrict, the SVR increases.

systemic vein, one of a number of veins that drain deoxygenated blood from most of the body. Systemic veins arise in tiny plexuses that receive blood from the billions of capillaries lacing the body tissues and converge into trunks that increase in size as they pass toward the heart. They are larger and more numerous than the arteries, have thinner walls, and collapse when they are empty. Kinds of systemic veins are identified according to location, as deep veins, superficial veins, and venous sinuses. Groups of systemic veins include the coronary veins, the superior vena cava and its tributaries in the upper body, and the inferior vena cava and its tributaries in the lower body.

system of care, a framework within which health care is provided, comprised of health care professionals; recipients, consumers, or patients; energy resources or dynamics; organizational and political contexts or frameworks; and processes or procedures. Current theory recognizes that an analysis of the provision of health care requires knowledge of the systems of care.

system overload, an inability to cope with messages and expectations from a number of sources within a given time limit.

systems design, the art or technique of analyzing a problem, modifying it for processing or solution by data processing equipment, and determining the best means and equipment by which a solution can be reached. – **systems designer,** *n.*

systole /sis′təlē/, the contraction of the heart, driving blood into the aorta and pulmonary arteries. The occurrence of systole is indicated by the first heart sound heard on auscultation, by the palpable apex beat, and by the peripheral pulse.

-systole, a combining form referring to 'types and locations of the higher blood pressure measurement': *dyssystole, hysterosystole, tachysystole.*

systolic click /sistol′ik/, an extra sound having a click-like quality heard in mid- or late systole, and believed to originate from the abnormal notion of the mitral valve. The most frequent cause of systolic clicks is prolapse of a mitral valve leaflet, in which case there may be an associated late systolic regurgitant murmur sometimes called the click syndrome.

systolic ejection period, the amount of time spent in systole per minute.

systolic gradient, the difference in pressure in the left atrium and left ventricle during systole.

systolic murmur, cardiac murmur occurring during systole. Systolic murmurs are generally less significant than diastolic murmurs and occur in many people with no evidence of heart disease. Systolic murmurs include ejection murmurs often heard in pregnancy or in people with anemia, thyrotoxicosis, or aortic or pulmonary stenosis, pansystolic murmurs heard in people with incompetence of the mitral or tricuspid valve, and late systolic murmurs, also caused by mitral valve incompetence.

T, **1.** symbol for **temperature.** **2.** abbreviation for *tumor*. See **cancer staging.**

T_1, T_2. See **relaxation time.**

T_3, symbol for **triiodothyronine.**

T_4, symbol for **thyroxine.**

Ta, symbol for **tantalum.**

TA, abbreviation for **transactional analysis.**

ta-. See **tono-.**

tabe-, a combining form meaning 'of or pertaining to wasting (away)': *tabefaction, tabescent, tabetiform.*

tabes dorsalis, an abnormal condition characterized by the slow degeneration of all or part of the body and the progressive loss of peripheral reflexes. This disease involves the posterior columns and the posterior roots of the spinal cord and destroys the large joints of affected limbs in some individuals. It is often accompanied by incontinence and impotence and severe flashing pains in the abdomen and the extremities. The cause of tabes dorsalis is unclear, and it is believed to be an uncommon disorder. Some surveys have indicated that about 10% of individuals with late syphilis and 40% of those with clinical neurosyphilis have tabes dorsalis.

tablet, a small, solid dosage form of a medication. It may be compressed or molded in its manufacture, and it may be of almost any size, shape, weight, and color. Most tablets are intended to be swallowed whole, but some may be dissolved in the mouth, chewed, or dissolved in liquid before swallowing; some may be placed in a body cavity.

Tacaryl, a trademark for an antihistamine (methdilazine).

TACE, a trademark for an estrogen (chlorotrianisene).

tacho-, a combining form meaning 'of or pertaining to speed': *tachogram, tachography, tachometer.*

tachy-, a combining form meaning 'swift or rapid': *tachycardia, tachyphrenia, tachysystole.*

tachycardia /tak′ikär′dē·ə/, an abnormal condition in which the myocardium contracts regularly but at a rate greater than 100 beats per minute. The heart rate normally accelerates in response to fever, exercise, or nervous excitement. Pathologic tachycardia accompanies anoxia, as caused by anemia, congestive heart failure, hemorrhage, or shock. Bradycardia develops because the heart muscle becomes anoxic and cannot maintain the accelerated pace. Tachycardia acts to increase the amount of oxygen delivered to the cells of the body by increasing the amount of blood circulated through the vessels.

tachykinin. See **substance P.**

tachyphylaxis /tak′əfəlak′sis/, **1.** (in pharmacology) a phenomenon in which the repeated administration of some drugs results in a marked decrease in effectiveness. **2.** also called **mithridatism.** (in immunology) rapidly developing immunity to a toxin because of previous exposure, as from previous injection of small amounts of the toxin.

tachypnea /tak′ipnē′ə/, an abnormally rapid rate of breathing, as seen with hyperpyrexia. See also **respiratory rate.**

tact-, a combining form meaning 'of or pertaining to touch': *tactile, tactilogical, taction.*

-tactic, -tactical, -taxic, **1.** a combining form meaning 'exhibiting agent-controlled orientation or movement': *chemotactic, eosinotactic, thermotactic.* **2.** a combining form meaning 'having an arrangement of something': *cytotactic, leukotactic, phyllotactic.*

tactile /tak′təl/, of or pertaining to the sense of touch.

tactile anesthesia, the absence or lack of the sense of touch in the fingers, possibly resulting from injury or disease. This condition can be congenital or psychosomatic and may cause the patient to incur severe burns, serious cuts, contusions, or abrasions. See also **traumatic anesthesia.**

tactile corpuscle, any one of many small, oval end organs associated with the sense of touch, widely distributed throughout the body in peripheral areas, as the papillae of the corium of the hand and foot, front of the forehead, skin of the lips, mucous membrane of the tongue, palpebral conjunctivae, and skin of the mammary papillae. Each corpuscle consists of a tiny, round structure surrounded by a capsule penetrated by a nerve fiber that spirals through the interior of the capsule and ends in globular enlargements. Also called **Meissner's corpuscle.**

tactile corpuscle of Meissner. See **Wagner-Meissner corpuscle.**

tactile fremitus, a tremulous vibration of the chest wall during respiration that is palpable on physical examination. It may indicate inflammation, infection, congestion, or, most commonly, consolidation of a lung or a part of a lung.

tactile image, a mental concept of an object as perceived through the sense of touch. See also **image.**

Taenia /tē′nē·ə/, a genus of large, parasitic, intestinal flatworm of the family Taeniidae, class Cestoda, having an armed scolex and a series of segments in a chain. Taeniae are among the most common parasites infecting humans and include *Taenia saginata,* the beef tapeworm, and *T. solium,* the pork tapeworm.

taenia-. See **tenia-.**

Taenia saginata, a species of tapeworm that inhabits the tissues of cattle during its larval stage and infects the intestine of humans in its adult form. *Taenia saginata* may grow to a length of between 12 and 25 feet and is the tapeworm species that most often infects humans. Also called **beef tapeworm.** See also **tapeworm, tapeworm infection.**

taeniasis /tēnī′əsis/, an infection with a tapeworm of the genus *Taenia.* See also **tapeworm infection.**

Taenia solium, a species of tapeworm that most commonly inhabits the tissues of pigs during its larval stage and infects the intestine of humans in its adult form. Infrequently, humans will serve as the intermediate hosts for this tapeworm, and larval infestation of the muscle and brain tissue may occur. Also called **pork tapeworm.** See also **cysticercosis, tapeworm, tapeworm infection.**

Tagamet, a trademark for a histamine H_2 receptor antagonist (cimetidine).

tail bud. See **end bud.**

tail fold, a curved ridge formed at the caudal end of the early developing embryo. It consists of the tail bud, which in lower animals gives rise to the caudal appendage and in humans forms the hindgut.

tailor's bottom. See **weaver's bottom.**

tailor's bunion. See **bunionette.**

Takayasu's arteritis /tä′kəyä′so͞oz/, a disorder characterized by progressive occlusion of the innominate and the left subclavian and left common carotid arteries above their origin in the aortic arch. Signs of the disorder are absence of a pulse in both arms and in the carotid arteries, transient paraplegia, transient blindness, and atrophy of facial muscles. Also called **brachiocephalic arteritis, Martorell's syndrome, pulseless disease, reversed coarctation.**

talbutal, a barbiturate sedative-hypnotic.

■ INDICATION: It is prescribed as a hypnotic in the treatment of insomnia.

■ CONTRAINDICATIONS: Previous addiction to sedative-hypnotics, porphyria, impaired hepatic function, or known hypersensitivity to this drug or to other barbiturates prohibits its use.

■ ADVERSE EFFECTS: Among the more serious adverse effects are respiratory depression, drug hangover, allergic reactions, porphyria, and physical dependence.

talip-, a combining form meaning 'clubfooted': *taliped, talipes, talipomanus.*

talipes /tal′ipēz/, a deformity of the foot, usually congenital, in which the foot is twisted and relatively fixed in an abnormal position. Talipes refers to deformities that involve the foot and ankle, whereas pes refers only to a deformity of the foot. Kinds of talipes include and **talipes calcaneovalgus, talipes calcaneovarus,** and **talipes equinovarus.** See also **pes cavus, pes planus.**

talipes calcaneovalgus. See **clubfoot.**

talipes cavus. See **pes cavus.**

talipes equinovarus. See **clubfoot.**

talo-, a combining form meaning 'of or pertaining to the ankle': *talocalcaneal, talocrural, talofibular.*

talus /tā′ləs/, *pl.* **tali,** the second largest tarsal bone. It supports the tibia, rests on the calcaneus, and articulates with the malleoli and with the navicular bones. It consists of a body, neck, and head. Also called **ankle bone, astragalus.**

Talwin, a trademark for an analgesic (pentazocine).

tamoxifen /təmok′səfin/, a nonsteroidal antiestrogen used in the palliative treatment of advanced breast cancer in premenopausal and postmenopausal women whose tumors are estrogen-dependent.

tampon, a pack of cotton, a sponge, or other material for checking bleeding or absorbing secretions in cavities or canals or for holding displaced organs in position.

tamponade /tam′pənād′/, stoppage of the flow of blood to an organ or a part of the body by pressure, as by a tampon or a pressure dressing applied to stop a hemorrhage or by the compression of a part by an accumulation of fluid, as in cardiac tamponade.

tangentiality, an association disturbance characterized by a tendency to digress from an original topic of conversation. Tangentiality can destroy or seriously hamper the ability of people to communicate effectively.

tangible elements, objects that can be seen or touched, as distinguished from emotions, knowledge, or abstractions.

Tangier disease /tanjir′/, a rare familial deficiency of high-density lipoproteins, characterized by low blood cholesterol and an abnormal orange or yellow discoloration of the tonsils and pharynx. There may also be enlarged lymph nodes, liver, and spleen, muscle atrophy, and peripheral neuropathy. No specific treatment is known.

tannin, any of a group of astringent substances obtained from plants, used for the tanning of leather. Tannic acid, a mixture of tannins, is used in the treatment of burns.

tanning, a process in which the pigmentation of the skin deepens as a result of exposure to ultraviolet light. Skin cells containing melanin darken immediately. New melanin is formed within 2 to 3 days and moves upward rapidly, allowing the darkening process to continue.

tantalum (Ta), a silvery metallic element. Its atomic number is 73; its atomic weight is 180.95. Relatively inert chemically, tantalum is used in prosthetic devices such as skull plates and wire sutures.

tantrum, a sudden outburst or violent display of rage, frustration, and bad temper, usually occurring in a maladjusted child and certain emotionally disturbed persons. The activity is usually not directed at anyone or anything specific but toward the environment in general and is used primarily as a device for attempting to control others and the surroundings. Also called **temper tantrum.**

TAO, a trademark for an antibacterial (troleandomycin).

Tapazole, a trademark for a thyroid inhibitor (methimazole).

tapering arch, a dental arch that converges from the molars to the central incisors to such a degree that lines passing through the central grooves of the molars and premolars intersect within 1 inch (2.5 cm) anterior to the central incisors.

tapeworm, a parasitic, intestinal worm belonging to the class Cestoda and having a scolex and a ribbon-shaped body composed of segments in a chain. Humans usually acquire tapeworms by eating the undercooked meat of intermediate hosts contaminated by the cysticerus or larval form of the tapeworm. In the human alimentary canal the worm develops into an adult with an attaching head, or scolex, and numerous hermaphroditic segments, or proglottids, each of which is capable of producing eggs. Kinds of tapeworm include ***Diphyllobothrium latum, Taenia saginata,*** and ***Taenia solium.*** Also called **cestode.**

tapeworm infection, an intestinal infection by one of several species of parasitic worms, caused by eating raw or undercooked meat infested with tapeworm or its larvae. Tapeworms live as larvae in one or more vertebrate intermediate hosts and grow to adulthood in the intestine of humans. Symptoms of intestinal infection with adult worms are usually mild or absent, but diarrhea, epigastric pain, and weight loss may occur. Diagnosis is made when eggs or portions of the adult worm are passed in the stool. The drugs niclosamide and quinacrine are used to loosen and dissolve the worm so that it may be excreted. Sanitary disposal of fecal material from affected patients is necessary to prevent the passage of larvae or eggs to humans or other hosts. Certain species of tapeworm can infect humans during the larval stage, causing a serious, often cystic, condition of larval infestation. Also called **cestodiasis.** See also **cysticercosis, tapeworm.**

tapho-, a combining form meaning 'of or pertaining to the grave': *taphophilia, taphophobia.*

tapotement /täpôtmäN′/, a type of massage in which the body is tapped in a rhythmic manner with the tips of the fingers or the sides of the hands, using short, rapid, repetitive movements. The procedure is often used on the chest wall of patients with bronchitis to help loosen the mucus in the air passages. See also **massage.**

Taractan, a trademark for a tranquilizer (chlorprothixene).

Tarbonis, a trademark for a topical antieczematic containing coal tar.

Tarcortin, a trademark for a topical fixed-combination drug containing a glucocorticoid (hydrocortisone) and an antieczematic (crude coal tar).

tardive dyskinesia /tär′div/, an abnormal condition characterized by involuntary, repetitious movements of the muscles of the face, the limbs, and the trunk. This disorder most commonly affects older people who have been treated for extended periods with phenothiazine drugs to alleviate the symptoms of parkinsonism. The involuntary movements associated with the condition may slacken or disappear after weeks or months and have been significantly reduced in some individuals by the administration of large doses of choline chloride. See also **antiparkinsonian.**

tardy peroneal nerve palsy, an abnormal condition and a type of mononeuropathy in which the peroneal nerve is excessively compressed where it crosses the head of the fibula. Such compression may occur when an individual falls asleep with the legs crossed.

tardy ulnar nerve palsy, an abnormal condition characterized by atrophy of the first dorsal interosseous muscle and difficulty in the performance of fine manipulations. It may be caused by injury of the ulnar nerve at the elbow and commonly affects individuals with a shallow ulnar groove or those who persistently rest their weight on their elbows. Signs and symptoms of this disorder may include numbness of the small finger, of the contiguous half of the proximal and the middle phalanges of the ring finger, and of the ulnar border of the hand. Treatment of this condition concentrates on the prevention of further injury of the ulnar nerve. Therapy may include the use of a doughnut cushion for the elbow to relieve the pressure on the ulnar nerve. Severe cases of this disorder may be corrected by surgical procedures that mobilize and transplant the nerve to a site in front of the medial epicondyle.

target, (in radiotherapy) any object area subjected to bombardment by radioactive particles or other form of diagnostic or therapeutic radiation.

target cell, **1.** also called **leptocyte.** an abnormal red blood cell characterized, when stained and examined under a microscope, by a densely stained center surrounded by a pale unstained ring circled by a dark, irregular band. Target cells occur in the blood after splenectomy, in anemia, in hemoglobin C disease, and in thalassemia. Compare **discocyte, spherocyte. 2.** any cell having a specific receptor that reacts with a specific hormone, antigen, antibody, antibiotic, sensitized T cell, or other substance.

target organ, **1.** (in radiotherapy) an organ intended to receive a therapeutic dose of irradiation, as the kidney when high-energy x-rays or gamma rays are beamed to the renal area for the treatment of a tumor. **2.** (in nuclear medicine) an organ intended to receive the greatest concentration of a diagnostic radioactive tracer, as the liver, which accumulates ^{99}Tc sulfur colloid when it is injected intravenously to detect hepatic lesions. **3.** (in endocrinology) an organ most affected by a specific hormone, as the thyroid gland, which is the target organ of thyroid stimulating hormone secreted by the anterior pituitary gland.

tarnishing, a tendency by left foci temporal lobe epilepsy patients to make a harsh assessment of themselves by emphasizing negative qualities in their self-descriptions.

Tarpaste, a trademark for a topical fixed-combination drug containing an antieczematic (tar distillate) in a paste.

tarsal /tär′səl/, of or pertaining to the tarsus, or ankle bone.
tarsal bone, any one of seven bones comprising the tarsus of the foot, consisting of the talus, calcaneus, cuboid, navicular, and the three cuneiforms.
tarsal gland, one of numerous modified sebaceous glands on the inner surfaces of the eyelids. About 30 tarsal glands, resembling tiny, parallel strings of pearls, line each upper eyelid and somewhat fewer tarsal glands line each lower eyelid. They are embedded in grooves in the inner surfaces of the tarsi, their lengths corresponding to the width of the tarsal plates. The ducts of the tarsal glands open by tiny apertures on the free margins of the eyelids. Each gland consists of a single straight follicle with numerous lateral branches. The follicles are supported by a basement membrane and lined at their mouths by stratified epithelium. Polyhedral cells line the deeper parts of the follicles and their lateral diverticula. Acute localized bacterial infection of a tarsal gland causes a sty. Also called **meibomian gland.** Compare **ciliary gland.**
tarsal tunnel syndrome, an abnormal condition and a kind of mononeuropathy, characterized by pain and numbness in the sole of the foot. This disorder may be caused by fractures of the ankle that compress the posterior tibial nerve and may be corrected by appropriate orthopedic therapy or by surgery.
tarso-, a combining form meaning 'of or pertaining to the edge of the foot, or to the eyelid': *tarsoclasis, tarsomalacia, tarsometatarsal.*
tarsometatarsal, of or pertaining to the metatarsal bones and the tarsus of the foot, especially the articulations of the metatarsal bones with the cuneiform and cuboid bones at the instep of the foot.
tarsus, *pl.* **tarsi,** **1.** the area of articulation between the foot and the leg. **2.** also called **tarsal plate.** any one of the plates of cartilage about 2.5 cm long forming the eyelids. One tarsal plate shapes each eyelid. The superior tarsal plates form the upper eyelids. The inferior tarsal plates the lower eyelids. The superior tarsal plates are semilunar, about 10 mm wide at the center, and attach anteriorly to the levator palpebrae superioris. The inferior tarsal plates are thin, elliptic, and about 5 mm in vertical diameter. The free margins of the plates are thick and straight, the orbital margins attached to the circumference of the orbit by the orbital septum, the lateral angles attached to the zygomatic bones by the lateral palpebral raphes. The medial angles of the two plates on each side end at the lacus lacrimalis and attach to the frontal process of the maxilla by the medial palpebral ligament.
tartar /tär′tär/, **1.** a hard, gritty deposit composed of organic matter, phosphates, and carbonates that collects on the teeth and gums. An excessive accumulation of tartar may cause gum disease and other dental problems. See also **gingivitis, pyorrhea. 2.** any of several compounds containing tartrate, the salt of tartaric acid. See **antimony potassium tartrate.**
tartar emetic. See **antimony potassium tartrate.**
tartaric acid /tärter′ik/, a colorless or white powder found in various plants and prepared commercially from maleic anhydride and hydrogen peroxide. It is used in baking powder, certain beverages, and in tartar emetic.
-tas, a noun-forming combining form: *fragilitas, graviditas, infertilitas.*
task functions, behaviors that focus or direct activities toward movements with work or labor overtones.
taste, the sense of perceiving different flavors in soluble substances that contact the tongue and trigger nerve impulses to special taste centers in the cortex and the thalamus of the brain. The four basic traditional tastes are sweet, salty, sour, and bitter. The front of the tongue is most sensitive to salty and sweet substances; the sides of the tongue are most sensitive to sour substances; and the back of the tongue is most sensitive to bitter substances. The middle of the tongue produces virtually no taste sensation. Chemoreceptor cells in the taste buds of the tongue detect different substances. Adults have about 9000 taste buds, most of them situated on the upper surface of the tongue. The sense of taste is intricately linked with the sense of smell, and taste discrimination is very complex. Many experts believe the capacity to perceive different tastes involves a synthesis of chemoreactive nerve impulses and coordinating brain processes, still not completely understood.
taste bud, any one of many peripheral taste organs distributed over the tongue and the roof of the mouth. The four basic taste sensations registered by chemical stimulation of the taste buds are sweet, sour, bitter, and salty. All other tastes perceived are combinations of these four basic flavors. Each taste bud rests in a spheric pocket, which extends through the epithelium. Gustatory cells and supporting cells form each bud, which has a surface opening and an opening in the basement membrane. Also called **gustatory organ.**
TAT, abbreviation for **tetanus antitoxin.**
tattoo, a permanent coloration of the skin by the introduction of foreign pigment. A tattoo may accidentally occur when a bit of graphite from a broken pencil point is embedded in the skin. Small tattoos can be removed by surgical excision. Dermabrasion is preferred for removal of extensive areas of pigment. **–tattoo,** *v.*
tauto-, a combining form meaning 'same': *tautomenial, tautomeral, tautomerism.*
Tavist, a trademark for an antihistaminic agent (clemastine).
tax-, a combining form meaning 'order or arrangement': *taxis, taxology, taxonomy.*
-taxia, -taxis, -taxy, 1. a combining form meaning '(condition of) impaired mental or physical control': *acroataxia, cardiataxia, hypotaxia.* **2.** a combining form meaning '(condition of) internal ordering or arrangement': *cataxia, heterotaxia, prostaxia.* See also **-taxis.**
-taxic. See **-tactic.**
-taxis, -taxia, -taxy, 1. a combining form meaning a '(specified) arrangement': *biotaxis, heterotaxis, homo-*

taxis. **2.** a combining form meaning a 'movement of an organism in response to a stimulus': *aerotaxis, electrotaxis, geotaxis*. See also **-taxia.**

taxonomy /takson′əmē/, a system for classifying organisms on the basis of natural relationships and assigning them appropriate names. **–taxonomic,** *adj*.

-taxy. See **-taxia, -taxis.**

Taylor, Effie J. (1874–1970), a Canadian-born American nurse who was graduated from Johns Hopkins School of Nursing. After graduation she continued at Johns Hopkins at the Phipps Psychiatric Institute, served as a nurse in World War I, and went to Yale University School of Nursing in 1923, succeeding Annie Goodrich as Dean in 1934. She served as president of the International Council of Nurses during World War II.

Taylor brace, a padded steel brace used to support the spine. Also called **Taylor splint.**

Tay-Sachs disease /tā′saks′/, an inherited, neurodegenerative disorder of lipid metabolism caused by a deficiency of the enzyme hexosaminidase A, which results in the accumulation of sphingolipids in the brain. The condition, which is transmitted as an autosomal recessive trait, occurs predominantly in families of Eastern European Jewish origin, specifically the Ashkenazic Jews, and is characterized by progressive mental and physical retardation and early death. Symptoms first appear by 6 months of age, after which no new skills are learned and there is progressive loss of those skills already acquired. Convulsions and atrophy of the optic nerve head occur after 1 year, followed by blindness, with a cherry-red spot on each retina, spasticity, dementia, and paralysis. Most children die between 2 and 4 years of age. There is no specific therapy for the condition, and intervention is purely symptomatic and supportive. The disease can be diagnosed in utero through amniocentesis. Also called **amaurotic familial idiocy, gangliosidosis type I, infantile cerebral sphingolipidosis, Sachs' disease.** See also **Sandhoff's disease.**

Tay's spot. See **cherry-red spot.**

Tb, symbol for **terbium.**

TB, abbreviation for **tuberculosis.**

T bandage, a bandage in the shape of the letter T. It is used for the perineum and sometimes for the head. Also called **crucial bandage, Heliodorus' bandage.**

TBP, 1. abbreviation for **bithionol. 2.** abbreviation for *total bypass*.

TBT, abbreviation for **tracheobronchial tree.**

TBW, abbreviation for **total body water.**

TBZ, abbreviation for *tetrabenazine,* an anesthetic adjuvant.

t.c., abbreviation for *telephone call*.

Tc, symbol for **technetium.**

TC, abbreviation for **therapeutic community.**

T cell, a small circulating lymphocyte produced in the bone marrow that matures in the thymus or as a result of exposure to thymosin secreted by the thymus. T cells, which live for years, have several functions but primarily mediate cellular immune responses, as graft rejection and delayed hypersensitivity. One kind of T cell, the **helper cell,** affects the production of antibodies by B cells; a **suppressor T cell** suppresses B cell activity. Compare **B cell.** See also **antibody, immune response.**

Td, abbreviation for **tetanus and diptheria toxoids.**

TD, abbreviation for **toxic dose.**

TD50. See **median toxic dose.**

tDNA, abbreviation for **transfer DNA.**

Te, symbol for **tellurium.**

tea. See **cannabis.**

teacher's nodule. See **vocal cord nodule.**

teaching hospital, a hospital with accredited programs in medical, nursing, or allied health personnel education.

teaching rounds, the somewhat informal conferences held regularly, often at the beginning of the day. Various members of the department and staff may attend, including nurses, residents, interns, students, attending physicians, and faculty. Specific problems in the care of current patients are discussed. See also **nursing rounds.**

team nursing, a decentralized system in which the care of a patient is distributed among the members of a team. The charge nurse delegates authority to a team leader who must be a professional nurse. This nurse leads the team—usually of 4 to 6 members—in the care of between 15 and 25 patients. The team leader assigns tasks, schedules care, and instructs team members in details of care. A conference is held at the beginning and at the end of each shift to allow team members to exchange information, and the team leader to make changes in the nursing care plan for any patient. Compare **primary nursing.**

team practice, professional practice by a group of professionals that may include physicians, nurses, and others, as a social worker, nutritionist, or physical therapist, who manage the care of a specified number of patients as a team, usually in an outpatient setting.

teardrop fracture, an avulsion fracture of one of the short bones, as a vertebra, causing a tear-shaped disruption of bone tissue.

tear duct, any duct that carries tears, including the lacrimal ducts, nasolacrimal ducts, and the excretory ducts of the lacrimal glands.

tearing /tir′ing/, watering of the eye usually caused by excessive tear production, as by strong emotion, infection, or mechanic irritation by a foreign body. If the normal amount of fluid tears is produced but not drained into the lacrimal punctum at the nasal border of the eye, tearing will occur. If the lacrimal punctum, sac, cuniculi, or nasolacrimal duct becomes blocked, tears will also overflow. Also called **epiphora.**

technetium (Tc), a radioactive, metallic element. Its atomic number is 43; its atomic weight is 99. The first synthetic element, technetium also occurs in nature. Isotopes of technetium are used in radioisotope scanning procedures of internal organs, as the liver and spleen. Formerly called **masurium.**

technetium 99, the radionuclide most commonly used to image the body in nuclear medicine scans. It is preferred because of its short half-life and because the emitted photon has an appropriate energy for normal imaging techniques.

technic. See **technique.**

-technics, -technology, -techny, a combining form meaning 'the art or mechanics of': *balneotechnics, mnemotechnics, psychotechnics.*

technique, the method and details followed in performing a procedure, as those used in conducting a laboratory test, a physical examination, a psychiatric interview, a surgical operation, or any process requiring certain skills or an ordered sequence of actions. Also spelled **technic.**

-technique, -technic, a combining form meaning 'the skillful way in which something is done': *iatrotechnique, microtechnique, zymotechnique.*

techno-, a combining form meaning 'art': *technopsychology, technocausis, technology.*

-techny, -technics, -technology, a combining form meaning 'the art or mechanics of' a specified area: *odontotechny, zootechny, zymotechny.*

tecto-, a combining form meaning 'rooflike': *tectocephalic, tectorial, tectum.*

Tedral, a trademark for a respiratory fixed-combination drug containing a bronchodilator (theophylline), an adrenergic (ephedrine hydrochloride), and a sedative-hypnotic (phenobarbital).

teenager. See **adolescent.**

teether, an object, as a teething ring, on which an infant can bite or chew during the teething process.

teething, the physiologic process of the eruption of the deciduous teeth through the gums. It normally begins between the sixth and eighth months of life and occurs periodically until the complete set of 20 teeth has appeared at about 30 months. Discomfort and inflammation result from the pressure exerted against the periodontal tissue as the crown of the tooth breaks through the membranes. General signs of teething include excessive drooling, biting on hard objects, irritability, difficulty in sleeping, and refusal of food. Fever or diarrhea often occurs during teething but is indicative of illness rather than of teething. The pain and inflammation may usually be soothed by cold, as with a frozen teething ring, cold metal spoon, or ice wrapped in a washcloth. Use of teething powders and procedures, as rubbing or cutting the gums, are discouraged because of the possibility of infection or complications from ingestion of the medication. –**teethe,** *v.*

teething ring, a circular device, usually made of plastic or rubber, on which an infant may chew or bite during the teething process.

Teflon, a trademark for a substance (polytetrafluorethylene), used for the construction of surgical implants in restorative surgery.

teg-, a combining form meaning 'of or pertaining to a cover': *tegmen, tegmental, tegument.*

Tegopen, a trademark for an antibacterial (cloxacillin sodium).

Tegretol, a trademark for an analgesic and anticonvulsant (carbamazepine).

TEIB, abbreviation for *triethylene-immunobenzoquinone.*

tela-, a combining form meaning 'a web or weblike structure': *telalgia, telangiectasia, telangitis.*

-tela, a combining form meaning a 'weblike membrane': *aulatela, epitela, metatela.*

telangiectasia /təlan′jē·ektā′zhə/, permanent dilatation of groups of superficial capillaries and venules. Common causes are actinic damage, atrophy-producing dermatoses, rosacea, elevated estrogen levels, and collagen vascular diseases. See also **Osler-Weber-Rendu syndrome, spider angioma.**

telangiectatic epulis /təlan′jē·ektat′ik/, a benign, red tumor of the gingiva, containing prominent blood vessels. Low-grade or chronic irritation is usually associated, and the lesion is easily traumatized.

telangiectatic fibroma. See **angiofibroma.**

telangiectatic glioma, a tumor composed of glial cells and a network of blood vessels, which give the mass a vivid pink appearance.

telangiectatic granuloma. See **pyogenic granuloma.**

telangiectatic lipoma. See **angiolipoma.**

telangiectatic nevus, a common skin condition of neonates, characterized by flat, deep-pink localized areas of capillary dilatation that occur predominantly on the back of the neck, lower occiput, upper eyelids, upper lip, and bridge of the nose. The areas disappear permanently by about 2 years of age. Also called **capillary flames, stork bite.**

telangiectatic sarcoma, a malignant tumor of mesodermal cells with an unusually rich vascular network.

tele-, **1.** a combining form meaning 'of or related to the end': *telencephalon, teleneuron, telesystolic.* **2.** a combining form meaning 'operating at a distance, or far away': *telecardiogram, teleceptor, telemetry.*

telepathist /təlep′əthist/, **1.** a person who believes in telepathy. **2.** a person who claims to have telepathic powers.

telepathy /təlep′əthē/, the alleged communication of thought from one person to another by means other than the physical senses. Also called **thought transference.** See also **extrasensory perception, parapsychology.** –**telepathic,** *adj.,* **telepathize,** *v.*

teletherapy, radiation therapy administered by a machine that is positioned at some distance from the patient. Typically, a teletherapy unit can rotate around a patient and thus allow use of multiple beams that intersect at the tumor and thus lower the dose to surrounding normal tissue.

tellurium (Te), an element exhibiting metallic and nonmetallic chemical properties. Its atomic number is 52; its atomic weight is 127.60. Inhaling vapors of tellurium results in a garlicky breath.

telo-, a combining form meaning 'of or pertaining to the end': *telobiosis, telodendron, telosynapsis.*

telocentric /tel′əsen′trik/, pertaining to a chromosome in which the centromere is located at the end, so that the chromatids appear as straight filaments. Compare **acrocentric, metacentric, submetacentric.**

telogen. See **hair.**

telophase /tel′əfāz/, the final of the four stages of nuclear division in mitosis and in each of the two divisions in meiosis. The newly produced daughter chromosomes from the preceding anaphase stage assemble at the poles of the division spindle and become long and slender, the nuclear membrane forms around them, the nucleolus reappears, and the cytoplasm begins to divide. See also **anaphase, interphase, meiosis, metaphase, mitosis, prophase.**

Temaril, a trademark for an antihistamine (trimeprazine tartrate).

temazepam, a hypnotic agent.

▪ INDICATIONS: It is prescribed for the relief of transient and intermittent insomnia.

▪ CONTRAINDICATIONS: Pregnancy or lactation prohibits its use. It is not recommended for patients under 18 years of age. Patients should avoid use of alcohol while also using tenazepam.

▪ ADVERSE EFFECTS: The most serious adverse reactions are confusion, euphoria, anorexia, ataxia, palpitations, hallucinations, horizontal nystagmus, and paradoxical reactions.

temperate phage, a bacteriophage whose genome is incorporated into the host bacterium. It persists through many cell divisions of the bacterium without destroying the host, in contrast to a virulent phage that lyses and kills its host.

temperature, **1.** a relative measure of sensible heat or cold. **2.** (in physiology) a measure of sensible heat associated with the metabolism of the human body, normally maintained at a constant level of 98.6° F (37° C) by the thermotaxic nerve mechanism that balances heat gains and heat losses. **3.** *informal.* a fever.

temper tantrum. See **tantrum.**

template /tem′plit/, (in genetics) the strand of DNA that acts as a mold for the synthesis of messenger RNA. This messenger RNA contains the same sequence of nucleic acids as the DNA strand and carries the code to the ribosomes, which are located in the cytoplasm, for the synthesis of proteins.

tempo-, **1.** a combining form meaning 'of or pertaining to time': *tempolabile, temporal, tempostabile.* **2.** a combining form meaning 'of or pertaining to the temples, in the lateral regions of the head': *temporal, temporalis, temporomandibular.*

temporal arteritis, a progressive, inflammatory disorder of cranial blood vessels, principally the temporal artery, occurring most frequently in women over 70 years of age. Characteristic changes in the involved vessels include granulomatous disruption of the elastic layer and engulfment of fiber fragments by giant cells in the intimal and medial layers. Symptoms are intractable headache, difficulty in chewing, weakness, rheumatic pains, and loss of vision if the central retinal artery becomes occluded. Also called **cranial arteritis, giant cell arteritis, Horton's arteritis.**

temporal artery, any one of three arteries on each side of the head: the superficial temporal artery, the middle temporal artery, and the deep temporal artery.

temporal bone, one of a pair of large bones forming part of the lower cranium and containing various cavities and recesses associated with the ear, as the tympanic cavity and the auditory tube. Each temporal bone consists of four portions: the mastoid, the squama, the petrous, and the tympanic.

temporal bone fracture, a break of the temporal bone of the skull, sometimes characterized by bleeding from the ear. Diminished hearing, facial paralysis, or infection of the tympanic cavity leading to meningitis may occur.

temporalis /tem′pəral′is/, one of the four muscles of mastication. It is a broad, radiating muscle that arises from the whole of the temporal fossa and from the surface of the temporal fascia. It inserts into the ramus of the mandible near the last molar tooth, and it is innervated by the anterior and the posterior temporal nerves. The temporalis acts to close the jaws and retract the mandible. Also called **temporal muscle.** Compare **masseter, pterygoideus lateralis, pterygoideus medialis.**

temporal lobe, the lateral region of the cerebrum, below the lateral fissure. Within the temporal lobe of the brain is the center for smell, some association areas for memory and learning, and a region where choice is made of thoughts to express. Compare **frontal lobe, occipital lobe, parietal lobe.**

temporal lobe epilepsy. See **psychomotor seizure.**

temporal muscle. See **temporalis.**

temporal subtraction, the subtraction of two or more digitized x-ray images that were acquired at different times. The subtraction process eliminates information in the image that was static.

temporal summation. See **summation,** def. 2.

temporary stopping, a mixture of gutta-percha, zinc oxide, white wax, and coloring, used for temporarily sealing dressings in tooth cavities. It softens on heating and rehardens at room temperature but is not hard enough to be used effectively in tooth areas under occlusal stress.

temporary tooth. See **deciduous tooth.**

temporomandibular joint, one of two joints connecting the mandible of the jaw to the temporal bone of the skull. It is a combined hinge and gliding joint, formed by the anterior parts of the mandibular fossae of the temporal bone, the articular tubercles, the condyles of the mandible, and five ligaments.

temporomandibular joint pain dysfunction syndrome (TMJ), an abnormal condition characterized by facial pain and by mandibular dysfunction, apparently caused by a defective or dislocated temporomandibular joint. Some common indications of this syndrome are the clicking of the joint when the jaws move, limitation of jaw movement, subluxation, and temporomandibular dislocation. Also called **myofacial pain dysfunction syndrome.**

temporoparietalis /tem′pərōpərī′ətal′is/, one of a pair of broad, thin muscles of the scalp, divided into three parts, which fan out over the temporal fascia and insert into the galea aponeurotica. The three parts include an anterior temporal portion, a superior parietal portion, and a triangular portion in between. The temporoparietalis was formerly considered part of the superior and the inferior auricularis. On both sides, it acts in combination with the occipitofrontalis to wrinkle the forehead, to widen the eyes, and to raise the ears. It is innervated by branches of the facial nerve. Compare **occipitofrontalis.**

TEN, abbreviation for **toxic epidermal necrolysis.**

tenacious, pertaining to secretions that are sticky or adhesive or otherwise tend to hold together, as mucus and sputum.

tenaculum /tənak′yələm/, *pl.* **tenacula,** a clip or clamp with long handles used to grasp, immobilize, and hold an organ or a piece of tissue. Kinds of tenacula include the **abdominal tenaculum,** which has long arms and small hooks, the **forceps tenaculum,** which has long hooks and is used in gynecologic surgery, and the **uterine** or **cervical tenaculum,** which has short hooks or open, eye-shaped clamps used to hold the cervix.

tendinitis /ten′dənī′tis/, an inflammatory condition of a tendon, usually resulting from strain. Treatment may include rest, corticosteroid injections, and support. Also spelled **tendonitis.**

tendinous cords. See **chordae tendineae.**

tendo calcaneus, the common tendon of the soleus and gastrocnemius. It is the thickest and strongest tendon in the body and begins near the middle of the posterior part of the leg. In an adult it is about 15 cm long. The tendon becomes contracted about 4 cm above the heel and flares out again to insert into the calcaneus. Also called **Achilles tendon, tendon of Achilles.**

tendon, one of many white, glistening fibrous bands of tissue that attach muscle to bone. Except at points of attachment, tendons are sheathed in delicate fibroelastic connective tissue. Larger tendons contain a thin internal septum, a few blood vessels, and specialized sterognostic nerves. Tendons are extremely strong and flexible, inelastic, and occur in various lengths and thicknesses. Compare **ligament.** –**tendinous,** *adj.*

tendonitis. See **tendinitis.**

tendon of Achilles. See **tendo calcaneus.**

tendon reflex. See **deep tendon reflex.**

tenesmus /tənez′məs/, persistent, ineffectual spasms of the rectum or bladder, accompanied by the desire to empty the bowel or bladder. Intestinal tenesmus is a common complaint in inflammatory bowel disease and irritable bowel syndrome.

tenia-, taenia-, a combining form meaning 'ribbon, band': *taeniasis, teniafuge, taenidium.*

tennis elbow. See **lateral humeral epicondylitis.**

teno-, tenonto-, a combining form meaning 'of or pertaining to a tendon': *tenodesis, tenodynia, tenomyotomy.*

tenofibril. See **tonofibril.**

Tenon's capsule. See **fascia bulbi.**

tenonto-. See **teno-.**

Tenormin, a trademark for a beta-blocker (atenolol).

tenosynovitis /ten′ōsin′əvī′tis/, inflammation of a tendon sheath caused by calcium deposits, repeated strain or trauma, high levels of blood cholesterol, rheumatoid arthritis, gout, or gonorrhea. In some instances, movement yields crackling noise over the tendon. Most cases not associated with systemic disease respond to rest. Local injections of adrenocorticosteroids may provide relief; surgery is indicated if the condition persists.

tenotomy /tənot′əmē/, the total or partial severing of a tendon, performed to correct a muscle imbalance, as in the correction of strabismus of the eye or in clubfoot.

TENS, abbreviation for **transcutaneous electric nerve stimulation.**

Tensilon a trademark for a cholinesterase reactivator (edrophonium), used as a curare antagonist and as a diagnostic aid in myasthenia gravis.

tension, **1.** the act of pulling or straining until taut. **2.** the condition of being taut, tense, or under pressure. **3.** a state or condition resulting from the psychologic and physiologic reaction to a stressful situation, characterized physically by a general increase in muscle tonus, heart rate, respiration rate, and alertness and psychologically by feelings of strain, uneasiness, irritability, and anxiety. See also **stress.**

-tension. See **-tention.**

tension headache, a pain that affects the occipital region of the body as the result of overwork or emotional strain, tensing the body and inhibiting rest and relaxation.

tensor, any one of the muscles of the body that tenses a structure, as the tensor fasciae latae of the thigh. Compare **abductor, adductor, depressor, sphincter.**

tensor fasciae latae, one of the 10 muscles of the gluteal region, arising from the outer lip of the iliac crest, the iliac spine, and the deep fascia lata. It inserts between the two layers of fascia lata in the proximal third of the thigh. The tensor fasciae latae is innervated by a branch of the superior gluteal nerve, which contains fibers from the fourth and fifth lumbar and the first sacral nerves, and it functions to flex the thigh and to rotate it slightly medially. Also called **tensor fasciae femoris.**

tent, **1.** a transparent cover, usually of plastic, supported over the upper part of a patient by a frame. Used in the treatment of respiratory conditions, it provides a controlled environment into which steam, oxygen, vaporized medication, or droplets of cool water may be sprayed, as an oxygen tent. **2.** a cone made of various materials inserted into a cavity or orifice of the body to dilate its opening, as a laminaria tent. **3.** a pack placed in a wound to hold it open to ensure that healing progresses from the base of the wound upward to the skin.

tenth nerve. See **vagus nerve.**

tenth-value layer (TVL), the thickness of material required to attentuate a beam of radiation to one tenth of its original intensity. See also **half-value layer.**

-tention, a combining form meaning the 'condition of being held': *historetention, retention.*

-tention, -tension, a combining form meaning 'condition of being stretched': *attention, distention, intention.*

tentorial herniation, the protrusion of brain tissue into the tentorial notch, caused by increased intracranial pressure resulting from edema, hemorrhage, or a tumor. Characteristic signs are severe headache, fever, flushing, sweating, abnormal pupillary reflex, drowsiness, hypotension, and loss of consciousness. Also called **transtentorial herniation.**

tentorium /tentôr′ē·əm/, *pl.* **tentoria,** any part of the body that resembles a tent, as the tentorium of the hypophysis that covers the hypophyseal fossa.

tentorium cerebelli, one of the three extensions of the dura mater that separates the cerebellum from the occipital lobe of the cerebrum. Compare **falx cerebelli, falx cerebri.**

Tenuate, a trademark for an anorexiant (diethylpropion hydrochloride).

tenure, (in a university) a faculty appointment without a limit on the number of years it may be held; a permanent appointment usually awarded to a person who has advanced to the rank of professor and who demonstrates scholarship and excellence in a specific field of study.

Tepanil, a trademark for an anorexiant (diethylpropion hydrochloride).

tephr-, a combining form meaning 'ash-colored': *tephromalacia, tephromyelitis, tephrylometer.*

tepid, moderately warm to the touch.

teramorphous, of the nature of or characteristic of a monster.

teras /ter′əs/, *pl.* **terata,** a severely deformed fetus; a monster. **–teratic,** *adj.*

teratism, any congenital or developmental anomaly that is produced by inherited or environmental factors, or by a combination of the two; any condition in which a severely malformed fetus is produced. Kinds of teratism include **atresic teratism, ceasmic teratism, ectopic teratism, ectrogenic teratism, hypergenetic teratism,** and **symphysic teratism.** Also called **teratosis.**

terato-, a combining form meaning 'of or related to a monster': *teratoblastoma, teratogenesis, teratoma.*

teratogen /ter′ətəjen′/, any substance, agent, or process that interferes with normal prenatal development, causing the formation of one or more developmental abnormalities in the fetus. Teratogens act directly on the developing organism or indirectly, affecting such supplemental structures as the placenta or some maternal system. The type and extent of the defect are determined by the specific kind of teratogen and its mode of action, the embryonic process affected, genetic predisposition, and the stage of development at the time the exposure occurred. The period of highest vulnerability in the developing embryo is from about the third through the twelfth week of gestation, when differentiation of the major organs and systems occurs. Susceptibility to teratogenic influence decreases rapidly in the later periods of development, which are characterized by growth and elaboration. Among the known teratogens are chemical agents, including such drugs as thalidomide, alkylating agents, and alcohol; infectious agents, especially the rubella virus and cytomegalovirus; ionizing radiation, particularly x-rays; and environmental factors, as the age and general health of the mother or any intrauterine trauma that may affect the fetus, especially during the later stages of pregnancy. Compare **mutagen. –teratogenic,** *adj.*

Common teratogenic agents

Teratogens	*Effects*
Chemicals	
Alcohol	Fetal alcohol syndrome
Androgens	Masculinization of female fetus if administered to mother
Antibiotics (e.g., tetracycline)	Tooth defects Cataracts
Cancer chemotherapy (e.g., aminopterin)	Central nervous system defects
Thyroid drugs (e.g., potassium iodide)	Congenital goiter
Tranquilizers (e.g., thalidomide)	Limb and other organ defects
Microbes	
Rubella	Rubella syndrome
Cytomegalovirus	Central nervous system and ophthalmic disorders
Toxoplasma gondii	Ophthalmic disorders
Radiation	
Therapeutic and possibly diagnostic radiation	Central nervous system and skeletal system abnormalities

teratogenesis /ter′ətōjen′əsis/, the development of physical defects in the embryo. Also called **teratogeny** /ter′ətoj′ənē/. **–teratogenetic,** *adj.*

teratogenic agent. See **teratogen.**

teratogeny. See **teratogenesis.**

teratoid /ter′ətoid/, of or pertaining to abnormal physical development; resembling a monster.

teratoid tumor. See **dermoid cyst.**

teratologist, one who specializes in the science of teratology.

teratology, the study of the causes and effects of congenital malformations and developmental abnormalities. **–teratologic, teratological,** *adj.*

teratoma, *pl.* **teratomas, teratomata,** a tumor composed of different kinds of tissue, none of which normally occur together or at the site of the tumor. Teratomas are most common in the ovaries or testes.

teratosis. See **teratism.**

terbium (Tr), a rare earth metallic element. Its atomic number is 65; its atomic weight is 158.294.

terbutaline sulfate, a beta-adrenergic stimulant.

■ INDICATIONS: It is prescribed as a bronchodilator in the treatment of asthma, bronchitis, and emphysema and as a uterine relaxant to treat premature labor.

■ CONTRAINDICATIONS: Cardiac arrhythmias or known hypersensitivity to this drug prohibits its use. It may interact with monoamine oxidase inhibitors and other beta-adrenergic blockers.

■ ADVERSE EFFECTS: Among the most serious reactions are dizziness and palpitations. Nervousness and tremor are common reactions.

teres /tir′ēz, ter′ēz/, *pl.* **teretes** /ter′ətēz/, a long, cylindric muscle, as the teres minor or the teres major. –**teres,** *adj.*

teres major, a thick, flat muscle of the shoulder. Arising from the dorsal surface of the scapula and from the fibrous septa between the teres major, the teres minor, and the infraspinatus, it is innervated by a branch of the lower subscapular nerve from the brachial plexus, which contains fibers from the fifth and the sixth cervical nerves, and it functions to adduct, extend, and rotate the arm medially. Compare **teres minor.**

teres minor, a cylindric, elongated muscle of the shoulder. Arising from the dorsal surface of the scapula and from two aponeurotic laminae, one of which separates it from the teres major, the other from the infraspinatus, it is inserted into the humerus and is innervated by a branch of the axillary nerve, which contains fibers from the fifth cervical nerve. The teres minor functions to rotate the arm laterally, weakly adduct the arm, and draw the humerus toward the glenoid fossa of the scapula, strengthening the shoulder joint. Compare **teres major.**

terminal, **1.** (of a structure or process) near or approaching its end, as a terminal bronchiole or a terminal disease. **2.** an input/output (I/O) device that has two-way communication capability with a computer. A terminal usually has a keyboard and a cathode-ray or video display screen, or a text printing facility. –**terminate,** *v.*, **terminus,** *n.*

terminal bronchiole. See **bronchiole.**

terminal disinfection, the process of cleaning equipment and airing of a room after the release of a patient who has been treated for an infectious disease.

terminal drop, a rapid decline in cognitive function and coping ability that occurs 1 to 5 years before death.

terminal nerve, a small nerve originating in the cerebral hemisphere in the region of the olfactory trigone, classified by most anatomists as part of the olfactory, or first cranial, nerve. The terminal nerve courses anteriorly along the olfactory tract and passes through the ethmoid bone. Most filaments of the nerve form a single strand that passes to the membrane near the anterior superior border of the nasal septum and communicates in the nasal cavity with the ophthalmic division of the trigeminal nerve. The central connections of the terminal nerve end in the septal nuclei, the olfactory lobe, and the posterior commissural and supraoptic regions of the brain.

terminal stance, one of the five stages in the stance phase of a walking gait, directly associated with the continuation of single limb support or the period during which the body moves forward on the supporting foot. Double limb support is initiated during the latter part of terminal stance, which is often a factor in the analysis of many abnormal orthopedic conditions and the diagnosis of weaknesses that may develop in certain muscles used in walking, as the quadriceps femoris and the gluteus maximus. Compare **initial contact stance stage, loading response stance stage, midstance, preswing stance stage.** See also **swing phase of gait.**

terminal sulcus of right atrium, a shallow channel on the external surface of the right atrium between the superior and inferior venae cavae.

termination codon, (in molecular genetics) a unit in the genetic code that specifies the end of the sequence of amino acids in a polypeptide.

termination sequence, (in molecular genetics) a DNA segment at the end of a unit that is transcribed to messenger RNA from the DNA template.

term infant, any neonate, regardless of birth weight, born after the end of the thirty-seventh and before the beginning of the forty-third week of gestation. Infants delivered at term usually measure from 48 to 53 cm from head to heel and weigh between 2700 and 4000 g.

terpin hydrate and codeine elixir, a preparation of the expectorant, terpin hydrate, with sweet orange peel tincture, benzaldehyde, glycerin, alcohol, syrup, water, and the antitussive narcotic codeine. Terpin hydrate diminishes secretions and promotes healing of the mucous membrane, while codeine depresses the cough center in the medulla oblongata; prolonged use may lead to addiction.

Terra-Cortril, a trademark for a topical fixed-combination drug containing a glucocorticoid (hydrocortisone) and an antibiotic (oxytetracycline).

Terramycin, a trademark for an antibiotic (oxytetracycline).

Terrastatin, a trademark for a fixed-combination drug containing an antifungal (nystatin) and an antibiotic (oxytetracycline).

territorial, a type of body movement that aids in communication. A territorial will frame an interaction and define an individual's "territory." See also **territoriality.**

territoriality, an emotional attachment to and defense of certain areas related to one's existence. Humans and animals generally establish a claim to or occupy a defined or undefined area over which they can maintain some degree of control.

terti-, a combining form meaning 'third': *tertiary, tertigravida, tertipara.*

tertian /tur′shən/, occurring every 48 hours or 3 days, including the first day of occurrence, as vivax or tertian malaria, in which fever occurs every third day. Compare **quartan.** See also **malaria.**

tertian malaria, a form of malaria, caused by the protozoan *Plasmodium vivax* or *Plasmodium ovale,* characterized by febrile paroxysms that occur every 48 hours. **Vivax malaria,** caused by *Plasmodium vivax,* is the most common form of malaria, and although it is rarely fatal, it is the most difficult form to cure. Relapses are common. **Ovale malaria,** caused by *Plasmodium ovale,* is usually milder and causes only a few, short attacks. Both types of tertian malaria are treated with chloroquine. Compare **falciparum malaria, quartan malaria.** See also **malaria.**

tertiary /tur′shē·ərē, tursh′ərē/, third in frequency or in order of use; belonging to the third level of sophistication of development, as a tertiary health care facility.

tertiary health care, a specialized, highly technical level of health care that includes diagnosis and treatment of disease and disability in sophisticated, large research and teaching hospitals. Specialized intensive care units, advanced diagnostic support services, and highly specialized personnel are usually characteristic of tertiary health care. It offers a highly centralized care to the population of a large region; in some cases, to the world.

tertiary prevention, a level of preventive medicine that deals with the rehabilitation and return of a patient to a status of maximum usefulness with a minimum risk of recurrence of a physical or mental disorder.

tesla, a unit of magnetic flux density, defined by the International System of Units as 1 weber per square meter, the equivalent of 1 volt/second per square meter.

Teslac, a trademark for an antineoplastic (testolactone).

Tessalon, a trademark for a local anesthetic agent (benzonatate).

test, **1.** an examination or trial intended to establish a principle or determine a value. **2.** a chemical reaction or reagent that has clinical significance. **3.** to detect, identify, or conduct a trial. See also **laboratory test.**

test-, a combining form meaning 'of or pertaining to the testicles': *testicond, testitoxicosis, testosterone.*

testcross, **1.** (in genetics) the cross of a dominant phenotype with a recessive phenotype to determine either the degree of genetic linkage or whether the dominant phenotype is homozygous or heterozygous. **2.** the subject undergoing such a test.

testicle. See **testis.**

testicular /testik′yələr/, of or pertaining to the testicle.

testicular artery, one of a pair of long, slender branches of the abdominal aorta, arising caudal to the renal arteries and supplying the testis.

testicular cancer, a malignant neoplastic disease of the testis occurring most frequently in men between 20 and 35 years of age. An undescended testicle is often involved. In many cases the tumor is detected after an injury, but trauma is not considered a causative factor. Patients with early testicular cancer are often asymptomatic, and metastases may be seeded in lymph nodes, the lungs, and liver before the primary lesion is palpable. In the later stages there may be pulmonary symptoms, ureteral obstruction, gynecomastia, and an abdominal mass. Diagnostic measures include transillumination of the scrotum, excretory urography, lymphangiography, and a urine or serum test to evaluate circulating levels of luteinizing hormone. Tumors develop more often in the right than in the left testis. Seminomas are the most curable lesions and the most common, representing 40% of all testicular tumors. Embryonal carcinomas are more highly malignant and represent 15% to 20% of these tumors. Teratocarcinomas and choricarcinomas also occur. Radiotherapy and surgical excision are usually recommended to treat seminoma. Chemotherapy using combinations of drugs is recommended for nonseminomatous tumors. Chemotherapeutic agents, used in various combinations, are increasing the survival of patients with testicular cancer. Some of these drugs are actinomycin D, bleomycin, cis-platinum, cyclophosphamide, methotrexate, and vincristine.

testicular duct. See **vas deferens.**

testicular feminization. See **feminization.**

testicular vein, one of a pair of veins that emerge from convoluted venous plexuses, forming the greater mass of the spermatic cords. Veins from each plexus start from small veins at the back of the testes, ascend along the spermatic cords, anterior to the ductus deferens, and pass through the deep inguinal ring and unite to form a single vein. The right testicular vein opens into the inferior vena cava; the left testicular vein into the left renal vein. Both testicular veins contain valves. Compare **ovarian vein.**

testimony, the statement of a witness, usually made orally and given under oath, as at a court trial.

testis /tes′tis/, *pl.* **testes,** one of the pair of male gonads that produce semen. The adult testes are suspended in the scrotum by the spermatic cords; in early fetal life they are contained in the abdominal cavity behind the peritoneum. Before birth they normally descend into the scrotum and during development are covered with layers of tissue derived from the serous, the muscular, and the fibrous layers of the abdominal parietes. The coverings of the testes are the skin and the dartos tunic of the scrotum, the external spermatic fascia, the cremastic layer, the internal spermatic fascia, and the tunica virginalis. Each testis is a laterally compressed oval body about 4 cm long, 2.5 cm wide, and weighs about 12 g. It is positioned obliquely in the scrotum, with the cranial extremity directed ventrally and slightly laterally, the caudal end directed dorsally and slightly medially. The anterior border, the lateral surfaces, and the extremities of the organ are convex, free, smooth, and covered by the tunica virginalis. The convoluted epididymis lying on the posterior border of the testis is about 20 feet long and connects with the vas deferens through which spermatozoa pass during ejaculation. Each testis consists of several hundred conical lobules containing the tiny coiled seminiferous tubules, each about 75 mm long, in which spermatozoa develop. In early life the tubules are pale in color but in old age become invested with yellow fatty matter. The tubules converge to form the rete testis that is drained by the efferent ducts into the head of the epididymis. The testis, developed in the lumbar region, may be retained in the abdomen, the deep inguinal ring, or the inguinal canal. A man with both testes undescended is sterile but may not be impotent. The testes are supplied with blood by the two internal spermatic arteries that arise from the aorta, are served by the testicular veins that form the pampiniform plexuses constituting the greater part of the spermatic cords, and are innervated by the spermatic plexuses of nerves from the celiac plexuses of the autonomic nervous system. Compare **ovary.** See also **scrotum.**

test method, a method chosen for experimental testing or study by means of method evaluation.

testolactone, an antineoplastic androgen analog.

■ INDICATIONS: It is prescribed in the treatment of postmenopausal breast cancer and in premenopausal women whose ovarian function has been terminated.

■ CONTRAINDICATIONS: Pregnancy, lactation, or known hypersensitivity to this drug prohibits its use. It is not given to men.

■ ADVERSE EFFECTS: Among the more serious adverse reactions are hypercalcemia and peripheral neuropathies with numbness or tingling.

testosterone /testos′tərōn/, a naturally occurring androgenic hormone.

■ INDICATIONS: It is prescribed for androgen deficiency, female breast cancer, and for stimulation of growth, weight gain, and red blood cell production.

■ CONTRAINDICATIONS: Cancer of the male breast or prostate, liver disease, pregnancy or suspected pregnancy, or known hypersensitivity to this drug prohibits its use.

■ ADVERSE EFFECTS: Among the more serious adverse reactions are fluid retention, masculinization, acne, and erythrocythemia.

testosterone cyclopentylpropionate. See **testosterone cypionate.**

testosterone cypionate, a long-acting form of testosterone.

testosterone derivative. See **anabolic steroid.**

testosterone enanthate, a long-acting form of testosterone.

testosterone propionate, an androgen given intramuscularly. See also **testosterone.**

test tube, a tube made of transparent material having one open end. It is used in the growth of bacteriologic specimens, in the analysis of some chemical functions, and in many other common laboratory functions. See also **tube.**

-tetanic, a combining form meaning 'relating to or producing tetanus or tetany': *antitetanic, posttetanic, subtetanic.*

tetano-, a combining form meaning 'of or pertaining to tetanus': *tetanolysin, tetanometer, tetanophilic.*

tetanus /tet′ənəs/, an acute, potentially fatal infection of the central nervous system caused by an exotoxin, tetanospasmin, elaborated by an anaerobic bacillus, *Clostridium tetani.* More than 50,000 people a year die of tetanus infection worldwide. The toxin is a neurotoxin and is one of the most lethal poisons known. *C. tetani* infects only wounds that contain dead tissue. The bacillus is a common resident of the superficial layers of the soil and a normal inhabitant of the intestinal tracts of cows and horses; therefore, barnyards and fields fertilized with manure are heavily contaminated.

■ OBSERVATIONS: The bacillus may enter the body through a puncture wound, abrasion, laceration, or burn, via the uterus into the bloodstream in septic abortion or postpartum sepsis, or through the stump of the umbilical cord of the newborn. The dead tissue of the area is low in oxygen; this is the environment essential for the replication of *C. tetani.* The infection occurs in two clinical forms: one with an abrupt onset, high mortality, and a short incubation period (3 to 21 days); the other with less severe symptoms, a lower mortality, and a longer incubation period (4 to 5 weeks). Wounds of the face, head, and neck are the ones most likely to result in fatal infection, because the bacillus may travel rapidly to the brain. The disease is characterized by irritability, headache, fever, and painful spasms of the muscles resulting in lockjaw, risus sardonicus, opisthotonos, and laryngeal spasm; eventually, every muscle of the body is in tonic spasm. The motor nerves transmit the impulses from the infected central nervous system to the muscles. There is no lesion; even at autopsy no organic lesion is seen and the cerebrospinal fluid is clear and normal.

■ INTERVENTION: Prompt and thorough cleansing and debridement of the wound are essential for prophylaxis. A booster shot of tetanus toxoid is given to previously immunized people; tetanus immune globulin and a series of three injections of tetanus toxoid are given to those not immunized. People who are known to have been adequately immunized within 5 years do not usually require immunization. The treatment of people who have the infection includes maintenance of an airway, giving an antitoxin as soon as possible, sedation, control of the muscle spasms, and assuring a normal fluid balance. The room is kept quiet and benzodiazepines may be given to reduce hypertonicity; penicillin G is administered for infection; and a tracheostomy is performed and oxygen given for ventilation.

■ NURSING CONSIDERATIONS: The nurse may encourage everyone to be actively immunized against the infection. The vaccine is safe and effective. Immunization more often than required is not recommended.

tetanus and diphtheria toxoids (Td), an active immunizing agent containing detoxified tetanus and diphtheria toxoids that slowly produce an antigenic response to the diseases.

■ INDICATIONS: It is prescribed for immunization against tetanus and diphtheria in children under 7 years of age when pertussis vaccine present in the usual diphtheria, pertussis, and tetanus trivalent vaccine is contraindicated.

■ CONTRAINDICATIONS: Immunosuppression, concomitant use of corticosteroids, or acute infection prohibits its use.

■ ADVERSE EFFECTS: Among the most serious adverse reactions are allergic reactions and stinging at the site of injection.

tetanus antitoxin (TAT), a tetanus immune serum that neutralizes exotoxins in tetanus infection.

■ INDICATIONS: It is prescribed for short-term immunization against tetanus after possible exposure to the organism and in tetanus treatment.

■ CONTRAINDICATIONS: It is not given if the more effective tetanus immune globulin is available or if there is a known sensitivity to equine serum.

■ ADVERSE EFFECTS: Among the most serious adverse reactions are allergic reactions and pain and inflammation at the site of injection.

tetanus immune globulin (TIG), an injectable solution prepared from the globulin of an immune human. It is effective and much safer than tetanus antitoxin.

■ INDICATIONS: It is prescribed for short-term immunization against tetanus after possible exposure to the organism and tetanus treatment.

■ CONTRAINDICATIONS: Known hypersensitivity to this drug prohibits its use. It should not be substituted for tetanus toxoid.

■ ADVERSE EFFECTS: The most serious adverse reaction is anaphylaxis. Fever and pain and inflammation at the site of injection may occur.

tetanus toxoid, an active immunizing agent prepared from detoxified tetanus toxin that produces an antigenic response in the body, conferring permanent immunity to tetanus infection.

■ INDICATION: It is prescribed for primary active immunization against tetanus.

■ CONTRAINDICATIONS: Immunosuppression or immunoglobulin abnormalities, acute infection, or illness prohibits its use.

■ ADVERSE EFFECTS: The most serious adverse reaction is hypersensitivity. Pain and inflammation at the site of injection may occur.

tetany /tet′ənē/, a condition characterized by cramps, convulsions, twitching of the muscles, and sharp flexion of the wrist and ankle joints. These symptoms are sometimes accompanied by attacks of stridor. Tetany is a manifestation of an abnormality in calcium metabolism, which can occur in association with vitamin D deficiency, hypoparathyroidism, alkalosis, or the ingestion of alkaline salts. Kinds of tetany are **duration tetany, grass tetany, hyperventilation tetany,** and **lactation tetany.** Compare **tetanus.**

tetart-, a combining form meaning 'fourth': *tetartanopia, tetartocone, tetartoconoid.*

tetra-, tetro-, a combining form meaning 'four': *tetracycline, tetrahydric, tetranopsia.*

Tetrachel, a trademark for an antibiotic (tetracycline hydrochloride).

tetrachlormethane. See **carbon tetrachloride.**

tetracycline /tet′rəsī′klēn/, a broad spectrum antibiotic.

■ INDICATIONS: It is prescribed for the treatment of many bacterial and rickettsial infections.

■ CONTRAINDICATIONS: Significantly impaired liver or renal function or known hypersensitivity to this drug prohibits its use. Because it may cause permanent discoloration of the teeth, its use is contraindicated in the last half of pregnancy and during a child's first 8 years of life.

■ ADVERSE EFFECTS: Among the more serious adverse reactions are renal toxicity, hepatotoxicity, severe GI disturbances, enterocolitis, inflammatory lesions with monilial overgrowth in the anogenital area, hemolytic anemia, thrombocytopenia, eosinophilia, and rashes.

tetracycline hydrochloride, a tetracycline antibiotic.

■ INDICATIONS: It is prescribed in the treatment of a variety of infections.

■ CONTRAINDICATIONS: Known hypersensitivity to this drug or to other tetracyclines prohibits its use. Use during pregnancy or in children under 8 years of age may result in discoloration of the child's teeth. It is to be administered with caution with renal or liver impairment.

■ ADVERSE EFFECTS: Among the most serious reactions are potentially serious suprainfections, various allergic reactions, phototoxicity, and GI disturbances.

Tetracyn, a trademark for an antibiotic (tetracycline hydrochloride).

tetrad /tet′rad/, (in genetics) a group of four chromatids of a synapsed pair of homologous chromosomes during the first meiotic prophase stage of gametogenesis. The group is formed in preparation for the two meiotic divisions in the maturation process of gametes. **–tetradic,** *adj.*

tetrahydrocannabinol (THC), the active principle, occurring as two psychomimetic isomers, in the hemp plant *Cannabis sativa,* used in the preparation of marijuana, hashish, bhang, and ganja. THC, a rapidly metabolized beta-adrenergic antagonist, increases pulse rate, causes conjunctival reddening, a feeling of euphoria, and has variable effects on blood pressure, respiratory rate, and pupil size. The drug affects memory, cognition, and the sensorium, decreases motor coordination, and increases appetite. Propranolol blocks the peripheral effects of THC but not the psychic effects. Overdoses of THC may be treated by "talking down" the patient and administering sedative barbiturates or diazepam parenterally. Nonintoxicating doses of THC are used experimentally in the treatment of glaucoma and to relieve nausea and increase the appetite in patients receiving cancer chemotherapy. See also **cannabis.**

tetrahydrozoline hydrochloride, an adrenergic vasoconstrictor.

■ INDICATIONS: It is prescribed for the treatment of nasal and nasopharangeal congestion and as an ophthalmic vasoconstrictor.

■ CONTRAINDICATIONS: Glaucoma or known hypersensitivity to this drug or to other vasoconstrictors prohibits its use. It is used with caution in patients who have cardiovascular disease.

■ ADVERSE EFFECTS: Among the more serious adverse reactions are irritation to mucosa, rebound nasal congestion, and effects associated with systemic absorption, including sedation and alterations in cardiovascular function.

tetraiodothyronine. See **thyroxine.**

tetralogy of Fallot /falō′/, a congenital cardiac anomaly that consists of four defects: pulmonic stenosis, ventricular septal defect, malposition of the aorta so that it arises from the septal defect or the right ventricle, and right ventricular hypertrophy. The primary symptoms in the infant are cyanosis and hypoxia, usually during crying, difficulty in feeding, failure to gain weight, and poor development. In older children a typical squatting position and clubbing of the fingers and toes are evident. A pansystolic murmur is usually heard, and the second heart sound is faint or absent. Diagnosis of the condition is primarily based on the history and physical symptoms, although cardiac catheterization is performed to evaluate the severity of the defects. Treatment consists mainly of supportive measures and palliative surgical procedures, primarily systemic to pulmonary anastomoses, to decrease tissue hypoxia and prevent complications until the child is old enough to tolerate total corrective surgery. The optimal age for surgical repair is approximately 4 or 5 years. Also called **Fallot's syndrome.** See also **blue baby, trilogy of Fallot.**

tetramer /tet′rəmer/, something that is composed of four parts, as a protein composed of four polypeptide subunits.

tetraploid (4n), **1.** also **tetraploidic.** of or pertaining to an individual, organism, strain, or cell that has four complete sets of chromosomes, quadruple the normal haploid number characteristic of the species. In humans, the tetraploid number is 92 and is extremely rare, found only occasionally in abortuses and stillborn fetuses. **2.** such an individual, organism, strain, or cell. Compare **diploid, haploid, triploid.** See also **polyploid.**

tetraploidy /tet′rəploi′dē/, the state or condition of having four complete sets of chromosomes.

Tetrastatin, a trademark for an antiinfective fixed-combination drug containing an antifungal (nystatin) and an antibiotic (tetracycline hydrochloride).

Tetrex, a trademark for an antibiotic (tetracycline phosphate complex.)

tetro-. See **tetra-.**

Texacort, a trademark for a topical preparation containing a glucocorticoid (hydrocortisone).

T fracture, an intercondylar fracture in which the fracture lines are T-shaped.

TGF, abbreviation for **transforming growth factor.**

T group. See **sensitivity training group.**

Th, symbol for **thorium.**

thalamus /thal′əməs/, *pl.* **thalami,** one of a pair of large, oval organs forming most of the lateral walls of the third ventricle of the brain and part of the diencephalon. It relays sensory impulses to the cerebral cortex, measures about 4 cm long and 1.5 cm wide and consists of numerous nuclei arranged in anterior, lateral, intralaminar, medial, and posterior groups. On each side the thalamus extends caudally beyond the third ventricle, with its medial and superior surfaces exposed in the ventricle and its inferior and lateral surfaces buried against other structures. It is composed mainly of gray substance and translates impulses from appropriate receptors into crude sensations of pain, temperature, and touch. It also participates in associating sensory impulses with pleasant and unpleasant feelings, in the arousal mechanisms of the body, and in the mechanisms that produce complex reflex movements. Compare **epithalamus, hypothalamus, subthalamus.** –**thalamic,** *adj.*

thalassemia /thal′əsē′mē·ə/, hemolytic anemia characterized by microcytic, hypochromic, and short-lived red blood cells caused by deficient hemoglobin synthesis. People of Mediterranean origin are more often affected than others. It is an autosomal recessive, genetically transmitted disease occurring in two forms. **Thalassemia major (Cooley's anemia),** the homozygous form, evident in infancy, is recognized by anemia, fever, failure to thrive, and splenomegaly and confirmed by characteristic changes in the red blood cells on microscopic examination. Frequent transfusions are necessary to maintain oxygen-carrying capacity of the blood. Red cells are rapidly destroyed, freeing large amounts of iron to be deposited in the skin, which becomes bronzed and freckled. The iron is also deposited in the heart, liver, and pancreas, which become fibrotic and dysfunctional. The spleen may become so enlarged that respiratory excursion is impeded, and the abdominal organs are crowded. Headache, abdominal pain, fatigue, and anorexia often occur. There is no cure. The nurse is aware that the child is uncomfortable and that growth and sexual development are usually retarded. Rarely, a child with thalassemia major is able to function without transfusions, thereby avoiding the massive ill effects of accumulated iron deposits. **Thalassemia minor,** the heterozygous form, is characterized only by a mild anemia and minimal red blood cell changes. Thalassemia minima is a form that lacks clinical symptoms although patients show hematologic evidence of the disease. Nursing considerations in the care of thalassemia patients and their families should include observation for ill effects of transfusion, education and counseling about the disease, and referral for genetic counseling. See also **hemochromatosis, hemosiderosis.**

thalasso-, a combining form meaning 'of or pertaining to the sea': *thalassophobia, thalassotherapy.*

thalidomide /thalid′əmīd/, a sedative-hypnotic, withdrawn from general use because of its potential for teratogenic effects, particularly phocomelia, when taken during pregnancy. It is sometimes prescribed for treatment of leprosy.

thallium (Tl), a soft, bluish-white metallic element that exhibits some nonmetallic chemical properties. Its atomic number is 81; its atomic weight is 204.37. Many of its compounds are highly toxic. Thallium sulfate is widely used as a rat poison.

thallium poisoning, a toxic condition caused by the ingestion or the absorption through the skin of thallium salts, especially thallium sulfate. Characteristic of the condition are abdominal pain, vomiting, bloody diarrhea, tremor, delirium, and alopecia. Treatment may include gastric lavage, chelation with Prussian blue, and a laxative. Anticonvulsant and antihypotensive medication may be necessary. Thallium has been used in insect and rodent poisons, fireworks, and in some cosmetic hair removers, but this extremely toxic and cumulative poison was banned for use in household products in 1965.

Tham, a trademark for a buffering agent (tromethamine), used in the treatment of acid-base disturbances.

thanato-, a combining form meaning 'of or pertaining to death': *thanatobiologic, thanatognomonic, thanatology.*

thanatology /than′ətol′əjē/, the study of death and dying. **–thanatologist,** *n.*

thanatophoric dwarf /than′ətōfôr′ik/, an infant with severe micromelia, the limbs usually extending straight out from the trunk, an extremely narrow chest, and flattened vertebral bodies with wide intervertebral spaces. Death usually occurs from respiratory complications shortly after birth.

Thanatos /than′ətəs/, a freudian term for the death instinct.

thanotopsy. See **autopsy.**

THC, abbreviation for **tetrahydrocannabinol.**

the Blues, *informal.* a designation for Blue Cross (an insurance system that pays the costs of treatment by a hospital or clinic) and Blue Shield (an insurance system that pays the costs of treatment by a professional).

thec-, a combining form meaning 'of or pertaining to a sheath, as of a tendon': *thecal, thecitis, thecodont.*

theca /thē′kə/, *pl.* **thecae** /thē′sē/, a sheath or capsule, as the theca cordis or pericardium.

theca cell tumor, an uncommon, benign fibroid tumor of the ovary, composed of theca cells and usually containing granulosa (follicular) cells. These tumors, characteristically solid masses with yellow, fatty streaks, are frequently associated with excessive estrogen production and tend to develop cystic degeneration. Also called **fibroma thecocellulare xanthomatodes, thecoma.**

-thecium, a combining form meaning a 'sack or container': *bdellepithecium, epithecium, perithecium.*

thecocellulare xanthomatodes, thecoma. See **theca cell tumor.**

Theden's bandage /tā′dənz/, a roller bandage applied below the injury and continued upward over a compress, used to stop bleeding. Also called **Genga's bandage.**

thel-, a combining form meaning 'of or pertaining to the nipple': *thelalgia, theleplasty, thelitis.*

thelarche /thilär′kē/, the beginning of female pubertal breast development that normally occurs before puberty at the beginning of the phase of rapid growth between 9 and 13 years of age. **Premature thelarche** is precocious breast development in a female without other evidence of sexual maturation. Compare **menarche.**

-thelia, a combining form meaning '(condition of the) nipples': *epithelia, hyperthelia, microthelia.*

-thelioma, a combining form meaning a 'tumor in a cellular tissue': *celiothelioma, hemendothelioma, perithelioma.*

-thelium, a combining form meaning a 'layer of (specified kind of) cellular tissue': *desmepithelium, mesothelium.*

thely-, a combining form meaning 'female': *thelyblast, thelygenic, thelyplasty.*

thenar /thē′när/, **1.** the ball of the thumb. **2.** of or pertaining to the thumb side of the palm.

theo-, a combining form meaning 'of or pertaining to a god': *theomania, theophobia, theotherapy.*

Theobid, a trademark for a smooth muscle relaxant (theophylline).

Theo-Dur, a trademark for a bronchodilator (theophylline).

Theolair, a trademark for a bronchodilator (theophylline), used for the relief of acute bronchial asthma.

Theophyl, a trademark for a smooth muscle relaxant (theophylline).

theophylline, a bronchodilator.

■ INDICATIONS: It is prescribed to relax the smooth muscle of the bronchial passages in the treatment of bronchospasm in bronchial asthma, bronchitis, and emphysema.

■ CONTRAINDICATIONS: Hypertension, cardiac disease, liver disease, renal disease, or concurrent treatment with other xanthines may prohibit its use.

■ ADVERSE EFFECT: Among the most serious adverse reactions are hypersensitivity, GI bleeding, palpitations, and seizures.

theorem, **1.** a proposition to be proved by a chain of reasoning and analysis. **2.** a rule expressed by symbols or formulae.

theoretic effectiveness, (of a contraceptive method) the effectiveness of a medication, device, or method in preventing pregnancy if used consistently and exactly as intended, without error. Compare **use effectiveness.**

theoretic plate number (N), a number defining the efficiency of a chromatographic column.

theory, an abstract statement formulated to predict, explain, or describe the relationships among concepts, constructs, or events. Theory is developed and tested by observation and research, using factual data.

theotherapy /thē′ōther′əpē/, a therapeutic approach to the prevention, diagnosis, and treatment of disease and dysfunction based on religious or spiritual beliefs.

Theovent, a trademark for a smooth muscle relaxant (theophylline).

therapeutic, **1.** beneficial. **2.** pertaining to a treatment.

-therapeutic, a combining form meaning 'pertaining to medical treatment by (specified) techniques': *eutherapeutic, kinetotherapeutic, orthotherapeutic*.

therapeutic abortion, **1.** a termination of early pregnancy deemed necessary by a physician. **2.** *informal.* any legal, induced abortion. Compare **elective abortion.** See also **induced abortion.**

therapeutic communication, (in psychiatric nursing) a process in which the nurse consciously influences a client or helps the client to a better understanding through verbal or nonverbal communication.

therapeutic community (TC), (in mental health) a treatment facility in which the entire milieu is part of the treatment. The physical environment, the other clients, the staff, and the policies of the facility influence the function of the individual in the activities of daily living in the community. The concept of a therapeutic community is integral to milieu therapy.

therapeutic equivalent, a drug that has essentially the same effect in the treatment of a disease or condition as one or more other drugs. A drug that is a therapeutic equivalent may or may not be chemically equivalent, bioequivalent, or generically equivalent. See also **bioequivalent, chemical equivalent, generic equivalent.**

therapeutic exercise, any exercise planned and performed to attain a specific physical benefit, as maintenance of the range of motion, strengthening of weakened muscles, increased flexibility of a joint, or improved cardiovascular and respiratory function.

therapeutic gain, the ratio of the biologic effect of a therapy on a tumor compared with the effect on surrounding normal tissue. Higher therapeutic gains mean lower complications of therapy.

therapeutic radiopharmaceutic, a radioactive drug administered to a patient to deliver radiation to body tissues internally, as iodide 131, which is used to ablate thyroid tissue in hyperthyroid patients, or cesium 137, iridium 192, radium 226, or strontium 90, which is implanted in a sealed source for the treatment of malignancies.

therapeutic recreation specialist, a person who assists patients in their recovery or rehabilitation after physical or emotional illness or disability by planning and supervising recreation programs.

-therapeutics, a combining form meaning 'medical treatment by (specified) techniques': *hydrotherapeutics, physicotherapeutics, radiotherapeutics*.

therapeutic temperature, in hyperthermia treatment, temperatures between 42° and 45° C (107° and 113° F).

-therapia, -therapy, a combining form meaning 'medical care': *balneotherapia, odontotherapia*. See also **-therapy.**

therapist, a person with special skills, obtained through education and experience, in one or more areas of health care.

therapy, the treatment of any disease or a pathologic condition, as inhalation therapy, which administers various medicines for patients suffering from diseases of the respiratory tract.

-therapy, -therapia, **1.** a combining form meaning 'medical treatment of disease' by specified means: *chemotherapy, hypnotherapy, kinesitherapy*. **2.** a combining form meaning 'medical treatment of a (specified) disorder or body area': *cardiotherapy, sarcotherapy, urotherapy*. See also **-therapia.**

therio-, a combining form meaning 'of or pertaining to beasts': *theriomimicry, theriotherapy, theriotomy*.

therm-. See **thermo-.**

-therm, a combining form meaning an 'animal with a (specified) body temperature': *allotherm, endotherm, poikilotherm*.

thermal, of or pertaining to the production, application, or maintenance of heat. Also **thermic.**

thermal burn, tissue injury, usually of the skin, caused by exposure to extreme heat. See also **burn.**

thermal dilution, a method of cardiac output determination. A bolus of solution of known volume and temperature is added to the bloodstream, and the resultant cooling of blood temperature is detected by a thermister previously placed in the pulmonary artery with a catheter.

thermal field size, the area over which therapeutic heating is likely to be produced.

-thermia, -thermy, **1.** a combining form meaning a 'state of body temperature': *monothermia, normothermia, pantothermia*. **2.** a combining form meaning 'generation of body heat': *azothermia, diathermia, transthermia*.

thermic fever. See **heat hyperpyrexia.**

thermistor /thərmis′tər/, a kind of thermometer for measuring minute changes in temperature. The resistance of a thermistor varies with the ambient temperature, thereby enabling accurate measurements of small temperature changes. See also **temperature, thermometer.**

thermo-, therm-, a combining form meaning 'of or pertaining to heat': *thermochemistry, thermogenesis, thermopalpation*.

thermocautery /thur′mōkô′tərē/, the use of a needle or snare heated by direct flame, a heated hydrocarbon vapor, or an electric current in the destruction of tissue. See also **Paquelin's cautery.**

thermocouple, a temperature measuring device that relies on the production of a temperature-dependent voltage at the junction of two dissimilar metals.

thermogenesis /thur′mōjen′əsis/, production of heat, especially by the cells of the body. –**thermogenetic,** *adj.*

thermography /thərmog′rəfē/, a technique for sensing and recording on film hot and cold areas of the body by means of an infrared detector that reacts to blood flow. Disease states that manifest increased or decreased blood flow present thermographic patterns that can be distinguished from those of normal areas. –**thermographic,** *adj.*

thermolabile /thur′məlā′bəl/, easily destroyed or altered by heat. Also called **heat labile.** Compare **thermostable.**

thermoluminescent dosimetry, a method of measuring the ionizing radiation to which a person is exposed by a device that stores the radiant energy and releases it later as ultraviolet or visible light. The device contains a crystalline material that is altered in structure by the radiation. It stores the radiation's energy, which is later released by heating the material. The light emitted is detected by a photomultiplier tube that generates an electric signal of a magnitude that reflects the amount of ionizing radiation originally received.

thermometer, an instrument for measuring temperature. It usually consists of a sealed glass tube, marked in degrees of Celsius or Fahrenheit, containing liquid, as mercury or alcohol. The liquid rises or falls as it expands or contracts according to changes in temperature. Some kinds of thermometers are **clinical thermometer, digital thermometer,** and **electronic thermometer.**

thermoneutral environment, **1.** an environment that keeps body temperature at an optimum point at which the least amount of oxygen is consumed for metabolism. **2.** an environment that enables a neonate to maintain a body temperature of 36.5° C (97.7° F) with a minimal requirement of energy and oxygen.

thermopenetration, the use of diathermic techniques to produce warmth within the body tissues for therapeutic purposes. Also called **transthermia.**

thermoradiotherapy, a therapeutic process that applies ionizing radiation to any part of the body in which the temperature has been raised by artificial means. Thermoradiography seeks to increase the radiosensitivity of the body part being treated.

thermoregulation, the control of heat production and heat loss, specifically the maintenance of body temperature through physiologic mechanisms activated by the hypothalamus.

thermostable, unaffected by or resistant to change by an increase in temperature. Compare **thermolabile.**

thermostat, a device for the automatic control of a heating or cooling system. –**thermostatic,** *adj.*

thermotaxis, **1.** the normal adjustment and regulation of body temperature. **2.** the movement of an organism in response to heat, either toward the stimulus (positive thermotaxis) or away from the stimulus (negative thermotaxis). Also called **thermotropism.**

thermotherapeutic penetration, the depth to which heating to therapeutic temperatures is likely to extend.

thermotherapy, the treatment of disease by the application of heat. Thermotherapy may be administered as dry heat with heat lamps, diathermy machines, electric pads, or hot water bottles or as moist heat with warm compresses or immersion in warm water. Warm soaks or compresses may be used to treat local infections, to relax muscles and relieve pain in patients with motor problems, and to promote circulation in peripheral vascular disorders, as thrombophlebitis. –**thermotherapeutic,** *adj.*

thermotropism. See **thermotaxis.**

-thermy. See **-thermia.**

theta wave, one of the several types of brain waves, characterized by a relatively low frequency of 4 to 7 Hz and a low amplitude of 10 μV. Theta waves are the "drowsy waves" of the temporal lobes of the brain and are observed in electroencephalograms when the individual is awake but relaxed and sleepy. Also called **theta rhythm.** Compare **alpha wave, beta wave, delta wave.**

-thetic, -thetical, a combining form meaning 'to put, place, set': *metathetic, prosthetic, synthetic.*

thiabendazole, an anthelmintic.

■ INDICATIONS: It is prescribed in the treatment of a variety of worm infestations, including hookworms, roundworms, and pinworms.

■ CONTRAINDICATIONS: Erythema multiforme, Stevens-Johnson syndrome, and known hypersensitivity to this drug prohibits its use.

■ ADVERSE EFFECTS: Among the more serious adverse reactions are anorexia, central nervous system effects, severe GI disturbances, dizziness, and hypotension.

thiamine /thī′əmin/, a water-soluble, crystalline compound of the B complex vitamin group, essential for normal metabolism and for the health of the cardiovascular and nervous systems. Thiamine combines with pyruvic acid to form a coenzyme necessary for the breakdown of carbohydrates into glucose. Rich sources of thiamine are pork, organ meats, green leafy vegetables, legumes, sweet corn, egg yolk, corn meal, brown rice, yeast, the germ and husks of grains, berries, and nuts. It is not stored in the body and must be supplied daily. A deficiency of thiamine affects chiefly the nervous system, the circulation, and the GI tract. Symptoms include irritability, emotional disturbances, loss of appetite, multiple neuritis, increased pulse rate, dyspnea, reduced intestinal motility, and heart irregularities. Severe deficiency causes beriberi. Thiamine is not known to cause any toxic effects. Also spelled **thiamin.** Also called **antiberiberi factor, antineuritic vitamin, vitamin B_1.**

thiazide diuretic. See **diuretic.**

thiethylperazine maleate, a phenothiazine antiemetic.

■ INDICATIONS: It is prescribed to control nausea and vomiting.

■ CONTRAINDICATIONS: Parkinson's disease, central nervous system disorders, liver or renal dysfunction, severe hypotension, or known hypersensitivity to phenothiazine medications prohibits its use.

■ ADVERSE EFFECTS: Among the more serious adverse effects are hypotension, liver toxicity, a variety of extrapyramidal reactions, blood dyscrasias, and hypersensitivity reactions.

thigh, the section of the lower limb between the hip and the knee.

thigh bone. See **femur.**

thigm-, a combining form meaning 'of or pertaining to touch': *thigmesthesia, thigmocyte, thigmotropic.*

thimble printer, a character printer similar to a daisywheel printer, in which the projecting fingers bearing the character dies are bent to form a cuplike object.

thimerosal /thīmer′əsal/, an antiinfective.

■ INDICATIONS: It is prescribed as a topical and ophthalmic antiseptic and as a preoperative and postoperative skin disinfectant.

■ CONTRAINDICATIONS: Concurrent administration of permanganates, strong acids, salts of heavy metals, or known hypersensitivity to this drug or to mercury-containing compounds prohibits its use.

■ ADVERSE EFFECTS: Among the more serious adverse reactions are erythematous, vesicular, and papular eruptions at the site of application. Mercury poisoning has been reported when large doses of this drug are given.

thinking, **1.** the cognitive process of forming mental images or concepts. **2.** the process of cognitive problem solving through the sorting, organizing, and classification of facts. Kinds of thinking include **abstract thinking, concrete thinking,** and **syncretic thinking.** See also **imagination.**

thio-, a combining form designating the presence of sulfur: *thioarsenite, theocarbamide, thiocyanate.*

thioamide derivative /thī′ō·am′īd/, one of a group of antithyroid drugs prescribed in the treatment of hyperthyroidism. Thioamide drugs act by inhibiting the synthesis of thyroid hormone. The principal thioamides are propylthiouricil, methimazole, methylthiouricil, and carbamizole. Adverse reactions include agranulocytosis, hypersensitivity, and a mild transient pruritus. Because agranulocytosis may occur very rapidly, serial white blood cell counts are not useful in diagnosing that complication of treatment. Instead, the patient is requested to report immediately instances of sore throat and fever, which often herald the onset of agranulocytosis. Prompt discontinuation of the drug, before serious depletion of granulocytic white cells develops, usually results in complete recovery. Use of antithyroid medications in pregnancy may result in fetal hypothyroidism, goiter, and cretinism.

thioctic acid /thī·ok′tik/, a pyruvate oxidation factor found in liver and yeast, used in bacterial culture media.

thioester /thī′ō·es′tər/, an important group of biologic chemicals formed by the hydrosulfides and carboxylic acids and identified by an ester bond involving the -SH radical. Examples include the coenzyme A thioesters.

thioguanine /thī′ōgwä′nēn/, an antineoplastic.

■ INDICATIONS: It is prescribed in the treatment of a variety of malignant neoplastic diseases, including the acute leukemias.

■ CONTRAINDICATIONS: Known hypersensitivity or resistance to this drug prohibits its use. It is not given to pregnant women.

■ ADVERSE EFFECTS: Among the most serious adverse reactions are bone marrow depression, GI distress, and stomatitis.

Thiomerin, a trademark for a mercurial diuretic (mercaptomerin sodium).

thiopental sodium, a potent, short-acting barbiturate, used as a general anesthetic for surgical procedures that are expected to require 15 minutes or less, as an induction agent for other general anesthetics, as a hypnotic component in balanced anesthesia, and as an adjunct to regional anesthesia. It is administered intravenously in adults; in children it is occasionally given rectally. By depressing the central nervous system, thiopental sodium induces hypnotic sleep in less than 1 minute after infusion. It has no analgesic properties and therefore must be supplemented by analgesics. It is a powerful respiratory and myocardial depressant and may be habit-forming. See also **barbiturate.**

thioridazine hydrochloride, a phenothiazine antipsychotic.

■ INDICATIONS: It is prescribed in the treatment of childhood behavioral disorders, geriatric mental disorders, depression, and alcohol withdrawal.

■ CONTRAINDICATIONS: Parkinson's disease, concurrent administration of central nervous system depressants, hepatic or renal dysfunction, severe hypotension, or known hypersensitivity to this drug or to other phenothiazine medications prohibits its use.

■ ADVERSE EFFECTS: Among the more serious adverse reactions are hypotension, hepatotoxicity, a variety of extrapyramidal reactions, blood dyscrasias, and hypersensitivity reactions.

Thiosulfil, a trademark for a sulfonamide antibacterial (sulfamethizole).

thiotepa /thī′ōtep′ə/, an antineoplastic alkylating agent.

■ INDICATIONS: It is prescribed in the treatment of a variety of malignant neoplastic diseases, including adenocarcinoma of the breast and ovary, and urinary bladder carcinomas.

■ CONTRAINDICATIONS: Bone marrow depression, pregnancy, liver or kidney dysfunction, or known hypersensitivity to this drug prohibits its use.

■ ADVERSE EFFECTS: Among the most serious adverse reactions are bone marrow depression, anorexia, nausea, and headache.

thiothixene, a thioxanthene antipsychotic.

■ INDICATIONS: It is prescribed in the treatment of acute agitation and mild to severe psychotic disorders.

■ CONTRAINDICATIONS: Parkinson's disease, concurrent administration of central nervous system depressants, hepatic or renal dysfunction, severe hypotension, known hypersensitivity to this drug or to phenothiazine medications prohibits its use. It is not recommended for children under 12 years of age.

■ ADVERSE EFFECTS: Among the more serious adverse reactions are hypotension, hepatotoxicity, a variety of extrapyramidal reactions, blood dyscrasias, and hypersensitivity reactions.

thioxanthine derivative, any one of a group of antipsychotic drugs, each of which is similar to the phenothiazenes in indication, action, and adverse effects.

thiphenamil hydrochloride, an anticholinergic agent.

■ INDICATIONS: It is prescribed in the treatment of GI pain caused by hypermotility and spasm.

■ CONTRAINDICATIONS: Narrow-angle glaucoma, asthma, obstruction of the genitourinary or GI tract, severe ulcerative colitis, or known hypersensitivity to this drug prohibits its use.

■ ADVERSE EFFECTS: Among the more serious adverse reactions are blurred vision, central nervous system effects, tachycardia, dry mouth, decreased sweating, and hypersensitivity reactions.

third cranial nerve. See **oculomotor nerve.**

third cuneiform bone. See **lateral cuneiform bone.**

third-party reimbursement, reimbursement for services rendered to a person in which an entity other than the giver or receiver of the service is responsible for the payment. Third-party reimbursement for the cost of a subscriber's health care is commonly paid by insurance plans, as Blue Shield or Blue Cross.

third ventriculostomy /ventrik'yəlos'təmē/, a surgical procedure for draining cerebrospinal fluid into the cisterna chiasmatis of the subarachnoid space in hydrocephalus, usually in the newborn. The procedure is not commonly performed and is used chiefly when the cisterna magna is not available for Torkildsen's operation. The third ventriculostomy makes an opening on the anterior wall of the floor of the third ventricle into the interpeduncular cistern and is performed to correct an obstructive type of hydrocephalus.

thirst, a perceived desire for water or other fluid. The sensation of thirst is usually referred to the mouth and throat.

Thiry-Vella fistula /thī'rēvel'ə/, an artificial passage from the abdominal surface of an experimental animal to an isolated intestinal loop, created surgically for the study of intestinal secretions. The continuity of the animal's gut is restored by anastomosis of the severed sections, and the isolated loop's vascular connections and mesenteric attachment are preserved. The ends of the isolated segment are attached to two openings in the skin of the abdomen to form a closed internal loop.

Thiuretic, a trademark for a diuretic (hydrochlorothiazide).

thixo-, a combining form meaning 'of or pertaining to touch': *thixolabile, thixotropic, thixotropy.*

Thomas' splint, **1.** a rigid splint constructed of steel bars that are curved to fit the involved limb and held in place by a cast or a rigid bandage. It is used in the treatment of chronic joint diseases. **2.** also called **Thomas' ring splint.** A rigid metal splint that extends from a ring at the hip to beyond the foot. It is used in the treatment of a fractured leg and, in conjunction with various traction and suspension devices, to immobilize and position a fractured femur of the preoperative or the postoperative patient.

Thomsen's disease. See **myotonia congenita.**

thoracentesis. See **thoracocentesis.**

thoracic /thôras'ik/, of or pertaining to the thorax.

-thoracic, a combining form meaning 'of, referring, or relating to the chest': *abdominothoracic, extrathoracic, intrathoracic.*

thoracic actinomycocis. See **actinomycosis.**

thoracic aorta, the large, upper portion of the descending aorta, starting at the caudal border of the fourth thoracic vertebra, dividing into seven branches, and supplying many parts of the body, as the heart, ribs, chest muscles, and stomach. Its seven branches are the pericardial, bronchial, esophageal, mediastinal, posterior intercostal, subcostal, and superior phrenic. See also **descending aorta.** Compare **abdominal aorta.**

thoracic duct, the common trunk of all the lymphatic vessels in the body, except those on the right side of the head, the neck, and the thorax, the right upper limb, the right lung, the right side of the heart, and the diaphragmatic surface of the liver. In the adult it is 38 to 45 cm long and 3 to 5 mm in diameter. It begins high in the abdomen at the cisterna chyli, ventral to the second lumbar vertebra, enters the thorax through the aortic hiatus of the diaphragm, and ascends into the neck through the posterior mediastinum, between the aorta and the azygous vein. In the neck it arches over the clavicle and opens into the junction of the left internal jugular and the left subclavian veins. The thoracic duct contains various valves, including two at this orifice that prevent venous blood from flowing into the lymphatic system. Compare **right lymphatic duct.** See also **lymphatic system.**

thoracic fistula, an abnormal opening in the chest wall that ends blindly or that communicates with the thoracic cavity.

thoracic medicine, the branch of medicine concerned with the diagnosis and treatment of disorders of the structures and organs of the chest, especially the lungs.

thoracic nerves, the 12 spinal nerves on each side of the thorax, including 11 intercostal nerves and one subcostal nerve. They are distributed mainly to the walls of the thorax and the abdomen. The thoracic nerves do not enter a plexus but follow independent courses, making them different from other spinal nerves. The first two intercostal nerves innervate the upper limb and the thorax; the next four supply only the thorax; and the lower five supply the walls of the thorax and the abdomen. Each subcostal thoracic nerve innervates the abdominal wall and the skin of a buttock. The thoracic portion of the sympathetic trunk contains a series of ganglia often coalesced in a single mass that, when independent, corresponds approximately to the thoracic spinal nerves. The roots of the ganglia are supplied by each thoracic nerve. The first thoracic ganglion, larger than the rest, is elongated, lying in the medial end of the first intercostal space, and usually combined with the inferior cervical ganglion into a stellate ganglion. The second to the tenth ganglia lie opposite the intervertebral disk associated with but slightly lower than the corresponding thoracic nerve. In most individuals the last thoracic ganglion lies on the body of the twelfth thoracic vertebra and, by its connection to both the eleventh and the twelfth thoracic nerves, serves a dual role as a single ganglion. See also **autonomic nervous system.**

thoracic outlet syndrome, an abnormal condition and a type of mononeuropathy characterized by paresthesia of the fingers. It may be caused by a nerve root compression by a cervical disk or by carpal tunnel syndrome.

thoracic parietal node, one of the lymph glands in the thorax, associated with various lymphatic vessels and divided into sternal nodes, intercostal nodes, and diaphragmatic nodes. See also **lymphatic system, lymph node.**

thoracic vertebra, one of the 12 bony segments of the spinal column of the upper back, designated T1 to T12. T1 is just below the seventh cervical vertebra (C7) and T12 is just above the first lumbar vertebra (L1). The thoracic portion of the spine is flexible and has a concave ventral curvature. Each vertebra has a broad, thick lamina; long, obliquely directed spinous processes; and thick, strong articular facets. The vertebrae are separated from each other by intervertebral disks. The vertebrae become thicker and heavier in descending order from T1 to T12. Compare **cervical vertebra, lumbar vertebra, sacral vertebra.**

thoracic visceral node, a node in the three groups of lymph nodes connected to the part of the lymphatic system that serves certain structures within the thorax, as the thymus, pericardium, esophagus, trachea, lungs, and bronchi. The thoracic visceral nodes include the anterior mediastinal nodes, the posterior mediastinal nodes, and the tracheobronchial nodes. Compare **thoracic parietal node.** See also **lymph, lymphatic system, lymph node.**

thoraco-, a combining form meaning 'of or pertaining to the chest': *thoracobronchotomy, thoracocentesis, thoracomyodynia.*

thoracocentesis /thôr′əkōsentē′sis/, the surgical perforation of the chest wall and pleural space with a needle for the aspiration of fluid for diagnostic or therapeutic purposes or for the removal of a specimen for biopsy. The procedure is usually performed using local anesthesia, with the patient in an upright position. Thoracocentesis may be used in the treatment of pleural effusion, as may occur in bronchogenic carcinoma. Fluid samples may be examined for erythrocyte, leukocyte, and differential white cell counts, protein, glucose, and amylase concentrations and may be cultured for studies of microorganisms that may be present. Also called **thoracentesis.**

thoracodorsal nerve /thôr′əkōdôr′səl/, a branch of the brachial plexus, usually arising between the two subscapular nerves. It courses along the posterior wall of the axilla and terminates in branches that supply the latissimus dorsi.

thoracostomy /thôr′əkos′təmē/, an incision made into the chest wall to provide an opening for the purpose of drainage.

thoracotomy /thôr′əkot′əmē/, a surgical opening into the thoracic cavity.

Thoraeus filters, combinations of metals, usually tin, copper, and aluminum, used to modify the quality of orthovoltage x-ray beams to improve the penetrating ability.

thorax, *pl.* **thoraces, thoraxes,** the cage of bone and cartilage containing the principal organs of respiration and circulation and covering part of the abdominal organs. It is formed ventrally by the sternum and costal cartilages and dorsally by the 12 thoracic vertebrae and the dorsal parts of the 12 ribs. The thorax of women has less capacity, a shorter sternum, and more movable upper ribs than that of men. Also called **chest.**

Thorazine, a trademark for a phenothiazine (chlorpromazine), used as an antiemetic and tranquilizer.

thorium (Th), a heavy, grayish, radioactive, metallic element. Its atomic number is 90; its atomic weight is 232.04. Thorium is used in radiographic procedures and in radiation therapy.

thought broadcasting, a symptom of psychosis in which the patient believes that his or her thoughts are "broadcast" beyond the head so that other persons can hear them.

thought insertion, a belief by some mentally ill patients that thoughts of other persons can be inserted into their own minds.

thought processes, alterations in, a nursing diagnosis accepted by the Fourth National Conference on the Classification of Nursing Diagnoses. The cause of the condition, developed at the Fifth National Conference, may involve physiologic changes, psychologic conflicts, loss of memory, impaired judgment, or sleep deprivation. The defining characteristics of the problem include distraction, egocentrism, abnormal cognitive function, abnormal interpretations of the environment; decreased ability to grasp ideas; impaired ability to reason, solve problems, calculate, conceptualize, or make decisions; disorientation; inappropriate social behavior; altered sleep patterns; delusions or hallucinations; and attention to environmental cues that is more or less acute than might normally be expected. Another possible defining characteristic is thinking based on inappropriate concepts or unreal situations. See also **nursing diagnosis.**

thought transference. See **telepathy.**

Thr, abbreviation for **threonine.**

threadworm. See ***Enterobius vermicularis.***

threadworm infection. See **strongyloidiasis.**

thready pulse, an abnormal pulse that is weak and often fairly rapid; the artery does not feel full, and the rate may be difficult to count. It is characteristic of hypovolemia, as occurs with severe hemorrhage.

threatened abortion, a condition in pregnancy before the twentieth week of gestation characterized by uterine bleeding and cramping sufficient to suggest that miscarriage may result. A threatened abortion is generally managed with rest and observation. Compare **incomplete abortion, inevitable abortion, imminent abortion.**

three-day fever. See **phlebotomus fever.**

three-day measles. See **rubella.**

thronine (Thr), an essential amino acid needed for proper growth in infants and maintenance of nitrogen balance in adults. See also **amino acid, protein.**

threp-, a combining form meaning 'of or pertaining to nutrition': *threpsis, threpology, threptic.*

threshold, the point at which a stimulus is great enough to produce an effect; for example, a pain threshold is the point at which a person becomes aware of pain.

threshold limit values, the maximum concentration of a chemical to which workers can be exposed for a fixed period, as 8 hours per day, without developing a physical impairment.

thrill, a fine vibration, felt by an examiner's hand on the body of a patient over the site of an aneurysm or on the precordium, indicating the presence of an organic murmur of grade 4 or greater intensity. Compare **bruit, murmur.**

throat. See **pharynx.**

throb, a deep, pulsating kind of discomfort or pain. –**throbbing,** *adj., n.*

thrombapheresis. See **plateletpheresis.**

thrombasthenia /throm′basthē′nē·ə/, a rare hemorrhagic disease characterized by a defect in platelet mediated hemostasis caused by an abnormality in the membrane surface of the platelet. The platelets do not aggregate, a clot does not form, and hemorrhage ensues, often from the mucous membrane. Transfusion with platelets is usually effective in stopping the hemorrhage. The condition is an inherited autosomal recessive trait.

thrombectomy /thrombek′təmē/, the removal of a thrombus from a blood vessel, performed as emergency surgery to restore circulation to the affected part. Before surgery, anticoagulant therapy is begun, and an arteriogram is done to locate the thrombus. Under general anesthesia, a longitudinal incision is made into the blood vessel and the clot is removed. Postoperatively, the blood pressure is maintained close to its preoperative level, because a decrease would predispose to further clotting. Compare **embolectomy.**

thrombin /throm′bin/, an enzyme formed in plasma during the clotting process from prothrombin, calcium, and thromboplastin. Thrombin causes fibrinogen to change to fibrin, essential in the formation of a clot. See also **blood clot.**

thrombo-, a combining form meaning 'of or pertaining to a clot, or thrombosis': *thromboarteritis, thrombocystis, thrombolysis.*

thromboangiitis obliterans /throm′bō·an′jē·ī′tis/, an occlusive vascular condition, usually of a leg or a foot, in which the small and medium-sized arteries become inflamed and thrombotic. Early signs of the condition are burning, numbness, and tingling of the foot or leg distal to the lesion. Phlebitis and gangrene may develop as the disease progresses. Pulsation in the limb below the damaged blood vessels is often absent. The goal of therapy is to avoid all factors that decrease the blood supply to the extremity, as cigarette smoking, and to use all means possible to increase the supply. Amputation may be necessary if the condition progresses to gangrene with chronic infection and extensive tissue destruction. Men are affected 75 times more often than women; most of the affected men smoke and are between 20 and 40 years of age. Also called **Buerger's disease.**

thrombocytapheresis. See **plateletpheresis.**

thrombocyte. See **platelet.**

thrombocytopathy /throm′bōsītop′əthē/, any disorder of the blood coagulation mechanism caused by an abnormality or dysfunction of platelets. Kinds of thrombocytopathies include **thrombocytopenia** and **thrombocytosis.** –**thrombocytopathic,** *adj.*

thrombocytopenia /throm′bōsī′təpē′nē·ə/, an abnormal hematologic condition in which the number of platelets is reduced, usually by destruction of erythroid tissue in bone marrow associated with certain neoplastic diseases or an immune response to a drug. There may be decreased production of platelets, decreased survival of platelets, increased consumption of platelets, and splenomegaly. Thrombocytopenia is the most common cause of bleeding disorders. Bleeding is usually from many small capillaries. Treatment requires a specific diagnosis of the cause. All drugs are stopped because nearly any drug may cause the condition. Adrenal corticosteroids may be administered, and transfusion may be necessary.

thrombocytopenic purpura, a bleeding disorder characterized by a marked decrease in the number of platelets, resulting in multiple bruises, petechiae, and hemorrhage into the tissues. It may occur secondary to a number of causes, including infection and drug sensitivity and toxicity. Until recently it was called idiopathic thrombocytopenic purpura (ITP), a diagnosis reached only by the exclusion of other causes. Today it is considered to be a manifestation of an autoimmune response. Two distinct entities, acute and chronic thrombocytopenia, can be differentiated from clinical manifestations alone. The acute form usually occurs but not always in children between 2 and 6 years of age and is benign, with complete recovery usually apparent within 6 weeks. The chronic form usually occurs in adults between 20 and 50 years of age. Recovery is rarely spontaneous and often requires adrenocortical steroids, or, possibly, splenectomy. Compare **disseminated intravascular coagulation.**

See also **hemophilia, hemorrhagic diathesis, thrombasthenia.**

thrombocytosis /throm′bōsītō′sis/, an abnormal increase in the number of platelets in the blood. **Benign thrombocytosis,** or **secondary thrombocytosis,** is asymptomatic and usually occurs after splenectomy, inflammatory disease, hemolytic anemia, hemorrhage, or iron deficiency, as a response to exercise, or after treatment with vincristine. It may also occur in advanced carcinoma or Hodgkin's disease or in other lymphomas. **Essential thrombocythemia** is characterized by episodes of spontaneous bleeding alternating with thrombotic episodes. The platelets may reach levels exceeding 1,000,000/μL. Compare **thrombocytopenia.** See also **polycythemia.**

thromboembolism, a condition in which a blood vessel is blocked by an embolus carried in the bloodstream from the site of formation of the clot. The area supplied by an obstructed artery may tingle and become cold, numb, and cyanotic. Treatment includes quiet bed rest, warm wet packs, and anticoagulants to prevent the formation of additional thrombi. Embolectomy may be indicated, especially if the aorta or common iliac artery is obstructed. An embolus in the lungs causes a sudden, sharp, thoracic or upper abdominal pain, dyspnea, a violent cough, fever, and hemoptysis. Obstruction of the pulmonary artery or one of its branches may be rapidly fatal. Emboli in smaller pulmonary arteries may be diagnosed by x-ray films and other radiologic techniques, including lung scans and angiography.

thrombolytic, pertaining to the dissolution of blood clots.

thrombophlebitis, inflammation of a vein, often accompanied by formation of a clot. It occurs most commonly as the result of trauma to the vessel wall, hypercoagulability of the blood, infection, chemical irritation, postoperative venous stasis, prolonged sitting, standing, or immobilization, or a long period of intravenous catheterization. Also called **phlebitis.**

■ OBSERVATIONS: Thrombophlebitis of a superficial vein is generally evident; the vessel feels hard and thready or cordlike and is extremely sensitive to pressure; the surrounding area may be erythematous and warm to the touch, and the entire limb may be pale, cold, and swollen. Deep vein thrombophlebitis is characterized by aching or cramping pain, especially in the calf when the patient walks or dorsiflexes the foot (Homan's sign).

■ INTERVENTION: Thrombophlebitis of a vein of the arm or hand caused by the irritation of an intravenous catheter is usually treated by removing the catheter, elevating the arm, and applying moist heat. When the condition occurs in a vein of the leg, the person is maintained on complete bed rest in a comfortable position that does not restrict venous return. The legs are elevated, if ordered, but pillows are not used and the knees are never bent unless the foot of the bed is raised. Anticoagulant therapy and streptokinase may be administered, and moist heat is applied to the affected area; intense heat, which may burn edematous skin, is avoided. Every 4 hours the blood pressure, temperature, pulse, respiration, circulation of the affected extremity, skin condition, and pulses in all the extremities are checked; a Doppler ultrasonic sensing device may be used. The patient is kept warm and dry and is helped to turn, cough, and deep breathe every 2 hours; the chest is auscultated for breath sounds every 4 hours. Observation for signs of pulmonary embolism, myocardial infarction, cardiovascular accident, or decreased renal function is constant. The affected limb is covered with a bed cradle, is not washed or massaged, and is measured daily, with the size recorded. Active and passive range of motion exercises are performed with the unaffected extremities. Constipation is avoided, and during the acute phase the patient is lifted on and off the bedpan. When phlebography is ordered, the patient is told how the contrast medium will be injected before an x-ray study of the affected vein. As inflammation subsides, the use of support or antiembolic stockings is demonstrated, and an exercise program is initiated. The patient is instructed to alternate exercise with bed rest, never to dangle the legs, to walk 10 minutes every hour, to avoid prolonged standing, to avoid becoming overweight, and, when sitting, to elevate the legs, flex the calf muscles, and contract the quadriceps 10 minutes per hour, as well as to avoid constricting circulation in the groin or crossing the legs at the knees.

■ NURSING CONSIDERATIONS: Thrombophlebitis is a common and often avoidable complication of various treatments and conditions in the hospitalized patient. Much routine nursing care is directed toward avoiding thrombophletitis. Early postoperative and postpartum ambulation, range of motion exercises for the immobilized patient, good technique in intravenous catheterization, attention to fluid balance, and proper positioning of the patient are common nursing measures to promote good circulation and reduce venous stasis and the development of thrombophlebitis.

thrombophlebitis migrans. See **migratory thrombophlebitis.**

thrombophlebitis purulenta, an inflammation of a vein associated with the formation of a soft, purulent thrombus that infiltrates the wall of the vessel.

thromboplastin, a complex substance that initiates the clotting process by converting prothrombin to thrombin in the presence of calcium ion. It is found in most tissue cells and, in somewhat different form, in red cells and leukocytes, but both substances function as factor III in the series of blood coagulation steps. See also **blood clotting.**

thrombosis /thrombō′sis/, *pl.* **thromboses,** an abnormal vascular condition in which thrombus develops within a blood vessel of the body. See also **blood clotting.**

thrombotic phlegmasia. See **phlegmasia alba dolens.**

thrombotic thrombocytopenic purpura (TTP), a disorder characterized by thrombocytopenia, hemolytic anemia, and neurologic abnormalities. It is accompanied by a generalized purpura together with the deposition of microthrombi within the capillaries and smaller arterioles. It is seen in a chronic form and in an acute fulminating form that may be fatal in weeks. Therapy includes corticosteroids and splenectomy. Compare **disseminated intravascular coagulation.** See also **thrombocytopenic purpura.**

thrombus /throm′bəs/, *pl.* **thrombi,** an aggregation of platelets, fibrin, clotting factors, and the cellular elements of the blood attached to the interior wall of a vein or artery, sometimes occluding the lumen of the vessel. Kinds of thrombi include **agonal thrombus, hyaline thrombus, laminated thrombus, marasmic thrombus, parasitic thrombus,** and **white thrombus.** Also called **blood clot.** Compare **embolus.**

thrush, candidiasis of the tissues of the mouth.

thulium (Tm), a rare earth metallic element. Its atomic number is 69; its atomic weight is 168.93. Thulium that has been irradiated in a nuclear reactor gives off x-rays and has been used in portable x-ray devices.

thumb, the first and shortest digit of the hand, classified by some anatomists as one of the fingers because its metacarpal bone ossifies in the same manner as those of the phalanges. Other anatomists classify the thumb separately, regarding it as composed of one metacarpal bone and only two phalanges. The metacarpal bone of the thumb articulates with the trapezium of the carpus and is controlled by the thenar muscles, which occupy the radial side of the hand, and by the abductor pollicis longus, the extensor pollicis brevis, and the extensor pollicis longus. The thenar muscles include the abductor pollicis longus, the opponens pollicis, the flexor pollicis brevis, and the adductor pollicis. The nerves that innervate the various muscles controlling the thumb include branches of the radial nerve, the deep palmar branch of the ulnar nerve, and a branch of the median nerve. The metacarpal bone of the thumb, like the metacarpals of the other digits, ossifies from a center in the body of the bone and from a center at the distal end. Ossification begins in the middle of the eighth or ninth week of fetal life. About the third year of life the base extremity of the metacarpal of the thumb starts to ossify, uniting with the body of the metacarpal about the twentieth year of life. The phalanges of the thumb ossify from centers in the bodies of the phalanges and from centers at their proximal extremities. Ossification of the phalangeal body begins about the eighth week of fetal life.

thumb forceps, a surgical instrument used to grasp soft tissue, especially while suturing.

thumbsucking, the habit of sucking the thumb for oral gratification. It is normal in infants and young children as a pleasure-seeking or comforting device, especially when the child is hungry or tired. The habit reaches its peak when the child is between 18 and 20 months of age, and it normally disappears as the child develops and matures. Thumbsucking beyond 4 to 6 years of age may lead to malocclusion of the teeth and deformation of the bony tissue of the thumb. Excessive thumbsucking, especially in older children, may be indicative of some emotional problem.

-thymia, a combining form meaning '(condition of the) mind or will': *amphithymia, barythymia, poikilothymia.*

thymic /thī′mik/, of or pertaining to the thymus gland.

thymic hypoplasia, thymic parathyroid aplasia. See **DiGeorge's syndrome.**

thymo-, 1. a combining form meaning 'of or pertaining to the thymus gland': *thymocyte, thymolysis, thymoma.* **2.** a combining form meaning 'of or pertaining to the spirit or mind': *thymogenic, thymopathy, thymopsyche.*

thymol /thī′mol/, a synthetic or natural thyme oil, used as an antibacterial and antifungal, that is an ingredient in some over-the-counter preparations for the treatment of hemorrhoids, acne, and tinea pedis. It is also used as a stabilizer in various pharmaceutic preparations.

thymoma /thīmō′mə/, *pl.* **thymomas, thymomata,** a usually benign tumor of the thymus gland that may be associated with myasthenia gravis or an immune deficiency disorder.

thymosin /thī′məsin/, **1.** a naturally occurring immunologic hormone secreted by the thymus gland. It is present in greatest amounts in young children and decreases in amount throughout life. **2.** an investigational drug derived from bovine thymus extracts and prescribed as an immunomodulator in experimental treatments for certain diseases, as systemic lupus erythematosus or rheumatoid arthritis.

thymus /thī′məs/, *pl.* **thymuses, thymi,** a single, unpaired gland that is located in the mediastinum, extending superiorly into the neck to the lower edge of the thyroid gland and inferiorly as far as the fourth costal cartilage. It was once considered a minor vestigial structure, but research has established that the thymus is the primary central gland of the lymphatic system. The endocrine activity of the thymus is believed to depend on the hormone thymosin, which is composed of biologically active peptides critical to the maturation and the development of the immune system. The T cells of the cell-mediated immune response develop in this gland before migrating to the lymph nodes and the spleen. The gland consists of two lateral lobes closely bound by connective tissue, which also encloses the entire organ in a capsule. Superficial to the gland is the sternum. Lying deep to the thymus are the great vessels and the cranial portion of the pericardium. The two lobes of the gland differ in size, and, in many individuals, the right lobe overlaps the left lobe. The thymus is about 5 cm long, 4 cm wide, and 6 mm thick. The lobes are composed of numerous lobules, which vary from 0.5 to 2 mm in diameter. The lobules are separated by delicate connective tissue. Each lobule is composed of a dense cellular cortex and an inner, less dense medulla. The cortices are composed almost entirely of small lymphocytes secured by reticular tissue with relatively few reticular cells. The medullae contain far fewer lymphocytes than the cortices and are composed of reticular tissue that contains more reticular cells. The thymus develops in the embryo from the third branchial pouch and increases in size until attaining a weight of 12 to 14 g before birth. The size of the organ relative to the rest of the body is largest when the individual is about 2 years of age. The thymus usually attains its greatest absolute size at puberty, when it weighs about 35 g. After puberty, the organ undergoes involution as the small lymphocytes of the cortices disappear and the reticular tissue is compressed. Adipose tissue often replaces the receding thymic tissue, but the connective tissue capsule of the gland may persist. With aging, the gland may change in color from pinkish-gray to yellow, and in the elderly individual may appear as small islands of thymic tissue covered with fat and surrounded by the yellowish capsule. The normal involution of the thymus may be superseded by rapid accidental involution caused by starvation or by acute disease. The gland is supplied by arteries derived from the internal thoracic and from the superior and the inferior thyroids. The veins of the gland end in the left brachiocephalic vein and in the thyroid veins. The lymphatics of the thymus end in the anterior mediastinal, the tracheobronchial, and the sternal nodes. The gland is innervated by tiny nerves derived from the vagi and the sympathetic. Branches from the descendens hypoglossi and the phrenic nerve reach the thymic capsule but do not penetrate the glandular tissue. Compare **spleen.**

Thypinone, a trademark for the synthetic thyrotropin releasing hormone (protirelin), used as an adjunctive agent in the diagnostic assessment of thyroid function.

Thyrar, a trademark for thyroid hormone.

-thyrea, -thyreosis, -thyroidism, a combining form meaning a 'condition of the thyroid gland': *athyrea, hypothyrea, hyperthyrea.*

thyro-, a combining form meaning 'of or pertaining to the thyroid gland': *thyroactive, thyroidectomy, thyroiditis.*

thyrocalcitonin. See **calcitonin.**

thyrocervical trunk, one of a pair of short, thick, arterial branches, arising from the first portion of the subclavian arteries, close to the medial border of the scalenus anterior, supplying numerous muscles and bones in the head, neck, and back. Each is divided into three branches: the inferior thyroid, suprascapular, and transverse cervical.

thyroglobulin, a purified extract of porcine thyroid. See also **thyroid hormone.**

■ INDICATIONS: It is prescribed in the treatment of cretinism, myxedema, goiter, and other hypothyroid states.

■ CONTRAINDICATIONS: Cardiovascular disease, hypopituatarism, or known hypersensitivity to this drug may prohibit its use.

■ ADVERSE EFFECTS: Among the more serious adverse reactions are tremors, nervousness, palpitation and tachycardia, and arrythmias when given in excessive doses.

thyroid. See **thyroid gland, thyroid hormone.**

thyroid acropathy /thī′roid/, swelling of subcutaneous tissue of the extremities and clubbing of the digits, occurring rarely in patients with thyroid disease and usually associated with pretibial myxedema or exophthalmos.

thyroid cancer, a neoplasm of the thyroid gland, usually characterized by slow growth and a slower and more prolonged clinical course than that of other malignancies. A significant carcinogenic effect of exposure to ionizing radiation is demonstrated by the high rate of thyroid cancer in survivors of exposure to atomic bomb explosions and in individuals who have been treated with radiotherapy for an enlarged thymus in infancy or for acne or other skin disorders in adolescence. Nontoxic colloid goiters and follicular adenomas may be precursors of malignant thyroid tumors. The first sign of cancer may be an increase in size of the thyroid gland, a palpable nodule, hoarseness, dysphagia, dyspnea, or pain on pressure. Diagnostic measures include x-ray examination, transillumination of the gland, radioisotope scanning, needle biopsy, and ultrasonic examination. More than one half of thyroid malignancies are papillary carcinomas, about one third are follicular carcinomas, and the rest consist of rapidly growing invasive anaplastic carcinomas, medullary carcinomas that secrete calcitonin, and metastatic lesions from primary tumors in the breast, kidneys, or lungs. Total or subtotal thyroidectomy with excision of involved lymph nodes is usually recommended. Radioactive iodine may be administered postoperatively, and high doses of exogenous thyroid are often used to suppress thyroid stimulating hormone (TSH) in an effort to cause the regression of residual tumor dependent on TSH. Various chemotherapeutic agents, especially adriamycin, may be effective in patients with metastatic thyroid cancer that is unresponsive to conventional treatment. Cancer of the thyroid is twice as common in women as in men; although it is diagnosed most frequently in people between 30 and 50 years of age, it may occur in children and elderly individuals.

thyroid cartilage, the largest cartilage of the larynx, consisting of two laminae fused together at an acute angle in the middle line of the neck to form the Adam's apple. Immediately above this prominence the laminae are separated by the superior thyroid notch. An oblique line runs caudally from the outer surface of each lamina and serves for the attachment of the sternothyroideus, the thyrohyoideus, and the constrictor pharyngis inferior. The cranial border of the thyroid cartilage secures the thyrohyoid membrane; the caudal border holds the cricoid cartilage, and the dorsal border receives insertions of the stylopharyngeus and the pharyngopalatinus. Compare **cricoid.**

thyroid dermoid cyst, a tumor derived from embryonal tissues that is believed to have developed in the thyroid gland or in the thyrolingual duct.

thyroidectomy /thī′roidek′təmē/, the surgical removal of the thyroid gland, performed for colloid goiter, tumors, or hyperthyroidism that does not respond to iodine therapy and antithyroid drugs. All but 5% to 10% of the gland is removed; regrowth usually begins shortly after surgery, and thyroid function may return to normal. For cancer of the thyroid, the entire gland is removed, along with surrounding structures from neck to collarbone, in a radical neck dissection. Before surgery, the basal metabolism rate is lowered to normal by giving iodine and antithyroid drugs. If a tumor is present, a frozen section of the affected tissue is examined by a pathologist. If malignant cells are found, most or all of the gland is removed. After surgery the patient is most comfortable in semi-Fowler's position with continuous mist inhalation administered to liquefy oral secretions. Oral suctioning may be necessary. A tracheotomy set and oxygen are kept in the room. Postoperatively, the patient is observed for signs of hemorrhage, respiratory difficulty caused by edema of the glottis, the muscular twitching of tetany from accidental removal of a parathyroid gland, and thyroid storm.

thyroid function test, any of several laboratory tests performed to evalute the function of the thyroid gland. Often several of the tests are performed simultaneously. Thyroid function tests include protein-bound iodine, butanol-extractable iodine, T_3, T_4, free thyroxine index, thyroxin-binding globulin, thyroid stimulating hormone, long-acting thyroid stimulator, radioactive iodine uptake, and radioactive iodine excretion.

thyroid gland, a highly vascular organ at the front of the neck, usually weighing about 30 g, consisting of bilateral lobes connected in the middle by a narrow isthmus. It is slightly heavier in women than in men and enlarges during pregnancy. The thyroid gland secretes the hormone thyroxin directly into the blood and is part of the endocrine system of ductless glands. It is essential to normal body growth in infancy and childhood, and its removal greatly reduces the oxidative processes of the body, producing a lower metabolic rate characteristic of hypothyroidism. The apices of the conic lobes of the gland are directed cranially and laterally as far as the lower middle of the thyroid cartilage. The bases of the lobes are on the level with the fifth or the sixth tracheal ring. Each lobe is about 5 cm long, a maximum of 3 cm wide, and usually about 2 cm thick. The lateral surface is convex and covered by the skin, the sternocleidomastoideus, the omohyoideus, the sternohyoideus, and the sternothyroideus. The deep fascia forms a capsule for the gland. The thyroid is activated by the pituitary thyrotrophic hormone and requires iodine to elaborate thyroxine. The arteries of the thyroid are remarkably large and form numerous anastomoses. Compare **parathyroid gland.**

thyroid hormone, an iodine-containing compound secreted by the thyroid gland, predominantly as thyroxine (T_4) and in smaller amounts as four times more potent triiodothyronine (T_3). These hormones increase the rate of metabolism, affect body temperature, regulate protein, fat, and carbohydrate catabolism in all cells, maintain growth hormone secretion, skeletal maturation, the cardiac rate, force, and output, promote central nervous system development, stimulate the synthesis of many enzymes, and are necessary for muscle tone and vigor. Derivatives of thyronine, T_4 and T_3, are synthesized in the thyroid gland by a complex process involving the uptake, oxidation, and incorporation of iodide and the production of thyroglobulin; the form in which the hormones apparently are stored in thyroid follicular colloid. After the proteolysis of thyroglobulin, T_4 and T_3 are released and transported in the blood in strong, but noncovalent, association with certain plasma proteins; T_4 accounts for approximately 90% of iodine in circulation and T_3 for 5%. All phases of the production and the release of T_4 and T_3 are regulated by the thyroid stimulating hormone (TSH) secreted by the anterior pituitary gland. The production of thyroid hormones is excessive in Graves' disease and toxic nodular goiter (Plummer's disease), diminished in myxedema, and absent in cretinism. T_4's normal 6-to-7-day half-life in blood is reduced to 3 or 4 days in hyperthyroidism and extended to 9 or 10 days in myxedema. T_3 has a normal half-life of 2 days or less and, like T_4, is metabolized most actively in the liver. Pharmaceutic preparations of thyroid hormones extracted from animal glands and the synthetic compounds, levothyroxine sodium and liothyronine sodium, are used as replacement therapy in patients with hypothyroidism. The dosage is initially low and is gradually increased to the optimal level based on the patient's clinical response and tests of the basal metabolic rate, radioactive iodine uptake, protein-bound iodine, and deep tendon reflexes. Overdosage or a rapid increase in the dosage may result in signs of hyperthyroidism, as nervousness, tremor, tachycardia, cardiac arrhythmia, and menstrual irregularity.

-thyroidism. See **-thyrea.**

thyroiditis /thī'roidī'tis/, inflammation of the thyroid gland. Acute thyroiditis, caused by staphylococcal, streptococcal, or other infections, is characterized by suppuration and abscess formation and may progress to subacute, diffuse disease of the gland. Subacute thyroiditis is marked by fever, weakness, sore throat, and a painfully enlarged gland containing granulomas composed of colloid masses surrounded by giant cells and mononuclear cells. Chronic lymphocytic thyroiditis (Hashimoto's disease), characterized by lymphocyte and plasma cell infiltration of the gland and by diffuse enlargement, seems to be transmitted as a dominant trait and may be associated with various autoimmune disorders. Another chronic form of thyroiditis is Riedel's struma, a rare progressive fibrosis, usually of one lobe of the gland but sometimes involving both lobes, the trachea, and surrounding muscles, nerves, and blood vessels. Radiation thyroiditis occasionally occurs 7 to 10 days after the treatment of hyperthyroidism with radioactive iodine 131.

thyroid releasing hormone. See **thyrotropin releasing hormone.**

thyroid stimulating hormone (TSH), a substance, secreted by the anterior lobe of the pituitary gland, that controls the release of thyroid hormone and is necessary for the growth and function of the thyroid gland. The secretion of TSH is regulated by thyrotropin releasing factor, elaborated in the median eminence of the hypothalamus. Also called **thyrotropin.** See also **thyroid hormone.**

thyroid storm, a crisis in uncontrolled hyperthyroidism caused by the release into the bloodstream of increased amounts of thyroid hormones. The storm may occur spontaneously or be precipitated by infection, stress, or a thyroidectomy performed on a patient who is inadequately prepared with antithyroid drugs. Characteristic signs are fever that may reach 106° F, a rapid pulse, acute respiratory distress, apprehension, restlessness, irritability, and prostration. The patient may become delirious, lapse into a coma, and die of heart failure.

Thyrolar, a trademark for a thyroid hormone (liotrix).

thyronine. See **thyroid hormone.**

thyrotoxicosis. See **Graves' disease.**

thyrotropin. See **thyroid stimulating hormone.**

thyrotropin (systemic) /thīrot′rəpin, thī′rətrō′pin/, a preparation of bovine thyroid stimulating hormone that increases the uptake of radioactive iodine in the thyroid and the secretion of thyroxine by the thyroid.

■ INDICATIONS: It is prescribed in diagnostic tests and to enhance uptake of ^{131}I in the treatment of thyroid cancer.

■ CONTRAINDICATIONS: Coronary thrombosis or known hypersensitivity to this drug prohibits its use. It should not be given in untreated Addison's disease or after myocardial infarction.

■ ADVERSE EFFECTS: Among the most serious adverse reactions are symptoms of hyperthyroidism, allergic reactions, hypotension, and arrhythmias.

thyrotropin releasing hormone, a substance elaborated in the median eminence of the hypothalamus that stimulates the release of thyrotropin (thyroid stimulating hormone) from the anterior pituitary gland. Also called **thyrotropin releasing factor (TRF), TSH releasing factor.**

thyroxine (T_4), a hormone of the thyroid gland, derived from tyrosine, that influences metabolic rate. Also called **tetraiodothyronine.**

thyroxine-binding globulin, a plasma protein that binds with and transports thyroxine in the blood.

Thytropar, a trademark for bovine thyrotropin.

Ti, symbol for **titanium.**

TI, abbreviation for *therapeutic index.*

TIA, abbreviation for **transient ischemic attack.**

tibia, the second longest bone of the skeleton, located at the medial side of the leg. It articulates with the fibula laterally, the talus distally, and the femur proximally, forming part of the knee joint. It attaches to the ligament of the patella and to various muscles, including the popliteus and the flexor digitorum longus. Also called **shin bone.**

tibialis anterior, one of the anterior crural muscles of the leg, situated on the lateral side of the tibia. It is a thick, fleshy muscle proximally and tendinous distally, arising from various origins, as the lateral side of the tibia, and inserting into the first cuneiform bone and the first metatarsal bone. It is innervated by a branch of the deep peroneal nerve, in which there are fibers from the fourth and the fifth lumbar and the first sacral nerves, and dorsiflexes and supinates the foot. Also called **tibialis anticus.** Compare **extensor digitorum longus.**

tibial torsion, a lateral or a medial twisting rotation of the tibia on its longitudinal axis, as in the pronation of the hand because of the contraction of the pronator teres and the pronator quadratus, or the supination of the hand, caused by the contraction of the supinator muscle. Compare **femoral torsion.**

tic. See **mimic spasm.**

Ticar, a trademark for an antibiotic (ticarcillin).

ticarcillin, an antibiotic.

■ INDICATIONS: It is prescribed in the treatment of bacterial septicemia, and skin, soft tissue, and respiratory infections caused by both gram-negative and gram-positive organisms.

■ CONTRAINDICATION: A history of allergic reaction to any of the penicillins prohibits its use.

■ ADVERSE EFFECTS: Among the most serious adverse reactions are anaphylactic reactions, thrombocytopenia, leukopenia, neutropenia, esosinophilia, vein irritation, and phlebitis.

tic douloureux. See **trigeminal neuralgia.**

tick bite, a puncture wound produced by the toothed beak of a bloodsucking tick, a small, tough-skinned, arachnid. Ticks transmit several diseases to humans, and a few species carry a neurotoxin in their saliva that may cause ascending paralysis beginning in the legs. Nervousness, loss of appetite, tingling and headache, followed by muscle pain, and, in extreme cases, respiratory failure may occur. Symptoms often disappear when the attached tick is carefully removed with forceps. Placing a drop of alcohol or ether on the tick or coating it with petrolatum or nail polish facilitates removal. See also **Lyme arthritis, Q fever, relapsing fever, Rocky Mountain spotted fever, tularemia.**

tick fever. See **relapsing fever.**

tick paralysis, a rare, progressive, reversible disorder caused by several species of ticks that release a neurotoxin that causes weakness, incoordination, and paralysis. The tick must feed on the host for several days before the symptoms appear, and removal of the tick leads to rapid recovery. Because respiratory or bulbar paralysis can cause death, it is important to search for ticks, frequently hidden in scalp hair, on a patient with these symptoms.

t.i.d., (in prescriptions) abbreviation for *ter in die* /dē′ā/, a Latin phrase meaning "three times a day."

tidal drainage. See **drainage.**

tidal volume (TV), the amount of air inhaled and exhaled during normal ventilation. Inspiratory reserve volume, expiratory reserve volume, and tidal volume make up vital capacity. See also **pulmonary function test.**

tide, a variation, increase or decrease, in the concentration of a particular component of body fluids, as acid tide, fat tide. **–tidal,** *adj.*

Tietze's syndrome /tēt′sēz/, **1.** a disorder characterized by nonsuppurative swellings of one or more costal cartilages causing pain that may radiate to the neck, shoulder, or arm and mimic the pain of coronary artery disease. The syndrome may accompany chronic respiratory infections, and, if the costal swellings are extremely painful, infiltration with procaine and hydrocortisone may provide relief. **2.** albinism, except for normal eye pigment, accompanied by deaf mutism and hypoplasia of the eyebrows.

TIG, abbreviation for **tetanus immune globulin.**

Tigan, a trademark for an antiemetic (trimethobenzamide hydrochloride).

timed release. See **prolonged release.**

timolol maleate, a beta-adrenergic receptor blocking agent.

■ INDICATIONS: It is prescribed for reducing intraocular pressure in chronic open-angle, aphakic, and secondary glaucoma.

■ CONTRAINDICATIONS: Bronchial asthma, COPD, sinus bradycardia, or known hypersensitivity to this drug prohibits its use. It is used with caution in patients with contraindications to systemic use of beta-adrenergic receptor blocking agents.

■ ADVERSE EFFECTS: The most serious adverse reaction is blurring of vision. Mild eye irritation also may occur.

Timoptic, a trademark for a beta-adrenergic receptor blocking agent (timolol maleate).

tin (Sn), a whitish metallic element. Its atomic number is 50; its atomic weight is 118.69. Tin oxide is used in dentistry as a polishing agent for teeth and in some restorative procedures.

Tinactin, a trademark for an antifungal (tolnaftate).

Tindal Maleate, a trademark for a phenothiazine (acetophenazine maleate), used as a tranquilizer.

tinea /tin′ē·ə/, a group of fungal skin diseases caused by dermatophytes of several kinds, characterized by itching, scaling, and, sometimes, painful lesions. Tinea is a general term that refers to infections of various causes, which are seen on several sites; the specific type is usually designated by a modifying term. Diagnosis is made by demonstrating fungus on smear or by culture. Also called, loosely, **ringworm.**

tinea capitis, a contagious fungal disease characterized by circular, bald patches of from 1 to 6 cm in diameter with slight erythema, scaling, and crusting. Diagnosis is made by bright fluorescence of infected hairs under Wood's light, by microscopic examination of infected hairs, and by culture of the fungus. Treatment consists of 3 to 6 weeks of griseofulvin given orally. Also called **ringworm.**

tinea corporis, a superficial fungal infection of the nonhairy skin of the body, most prevalent in hot, humid climates and usually caused by species of *Trichophyton* or *Microsporum*. Topical fungicides, as miconazole, are used for moderate cases; severe infection calls for griseofulvin.

tinea cruris /kro͞o′ris/, a superficial fungal infection of the groin, caused by species of *Trichophyton* or *Epidermophyton floccosum*. It is most common in the tropics and among males. Topical antifungals, as miconazole and clotrimazole, are often prescribed. Griseofulvin is used only for severe, resistant cases. Also called **jock itch.**

tinea pedis, a chronic, superficial fungal infection of the foot, especially of the skin between the toes and on the soles. It is common worldwide and is usually caused by *Trichophyton mentagrophytes, T. rubrum,* and *Epidermophyton floccosum*. Adults are most susceptible, and the wearing of constricting footwear, as sneakers, seems to induce the infection. Drying the feet well after bathing and applying powder between the toes help prevent it. Griseofulvin is the most effective treatment, but miconazole and tolnaftate are also used. Recurrence is common. Also called **athlete's foot.**

tinea unguium, a superficial fungal infection of the nails caused by various species of *Trichophyton* and, occasionally, by *Candida albicans*. It is more common on the toes than the fingers and can cause complete crumbling and destruction of the nails. Griseofulvin is the drug of choice, but it must be continued until the nail has regrown completely.

tinea versicolor, a fungous infection of the skin characterized by finely desquamating, pale tan patches on the upper trunk and upper arms that may itch and do not tan, caused by *Malassezia furfur*. In dark-skinned persons the lesions may be depigmented. The fungus fluoresces under Wood's light and may be easily identified in scrapings viewed under a microscope. Treatment usually includes a single application of selenium sulfide left on overnight and rinsed off by thorough showering in the morning. The pale patches may persist for up to 1 year after successful treatment.

Tinel's sign /tinelz′/, an indication of irritability of a nerve, resulting in a distal tingling sensation on percussion of a damaged nerve. The sign is often present in the carpal tunnel syndrome and is produced by tapping over the median nerve on the volar aspect of the wrist.

tine test, a tuberculin skin test in which a small disposable disk with multiple tines bearing tuberculin antigen is used to puncture the skin. The method is widely used to test for sensitivity to the tuberculin antigen. Induration around the puncture site indicates previous exposure or active disease, requiring further testing. See also **tuberculin test.**

tingling, a prickly sensation in the skin or a part of the body, accompanied by diminished sensitivity to stimulation of the sensory nerves, felt by a person as the area is numbed by local anesthetic or by exposure to the cold, or as it ''goes to sleep'' from pressure on a nerve.

tinnitus /tinī′təs/, tinkling or ringing heard in one or both ears. It may be a sign of acoustic trauma, Ménière's disease, otosclerosis, or presbycusis or of an accumulation of cerumen impinging on the eardrum or occluding the external auditory canal.

tinted denture base, a denture base that simulates the coloring of natural oral tissue.

T-Ionate-P.A., a trademark for an androgen (testosterone cypionate).

tissue, a collection of similar cells that act together in the performance of a particular function.

tissue activator. See **fibrinokinase.**

tissue-base relationship, (in dentistry) the relationship of the base of a removable prosthesis to subjacent structures.

tissue committee, a group that evaluates all surgery performed in a hospital or other health care facility. The evaluation is usually made on the basis of the extent of agreement of the preoperative, postoperative, and pathologic diagnoses and on the relevance and acceptability of the diagnostic procedures. See also **tissue review.**

tissue dextrin. See **glycogen.**

tissue dose, (in radiotherapy) the amount of radiation absorbed by tissue in the region of interest, expressed in rad.

tissue fixation, a process in which a tissue specimen is placed in a fluid that preserves the cells as nearly as is possible in their natural state.

tissue fixative, a fluid that preserves cells in their natural state, so that they may be identified and examined.

tissue kinase. See **fibrinokinase.**

tissue perfusion, alteration in: cerebral, cardiopulmonary, renal, gastrointestinal, peripheral, a nursing diagnosis accepted by the Fourth National Conference on the Classification of Nursing Diagnoses. The cause of the diagnosis may be interruption of the venous or arterial circulation to the affected part of the body, hypovolemia or hypervolemia, or a condition that causes abnormal exchange of fluids and nutrients to or from the cells to the circulation. The defining characteristics of the condition include coldness of the affected extremity, paleness on elevation of the extremity, diminished arterial pulses, and changes in the arterial blood pressure when measured in the affected extremity. Claudication, gangrene, brittle nails, slowly healing ulcers or wounds, shiny skin, and lack of hair are also commonly seen. See also **nursing diagnosis.**

tissue plasminogen activator (TPA), a clot-dissolving substance produced naturally by cells in the walls of blood vessels. It is also manufactured synthetically by genetic engineering techniques. TPA activates plasminogen to dissolve clots and has been used therapeutically to remove blood clots blocking coronary arteries.

tissue response, any reaction or change in living cellular tissue when it is acted on by disease, toxin, or other external stimulus. Some kinds of tissue responses are **immune response, inflammation,** and **necrosis.**

tissue review, a review of the surgery performed in a hospital or other health care facility. The evaluation is usually made on the basis of the extent of agreement of the preoperative, postoperative, and pathologic diagnoses and on the relevance and acceptability of the diagnostic procedures. See also **tissue committee.**

tissue typing, a systematized series of tests to evaluate the intraspecies compatibility of tissues of a donor and a recipient before transplantation. This is accomplished by identifying and comparing a large series of human leukocyte antigens (HLA) in the cells of the body. See also **HLA, immune system, transplant.**

titanium (Ti), a grayish, brittle metallic element. Its atomic number is 22; its atomic weight is 47.9. An alloy of titanium is used in the manufacture of orthopedic prostheses. Titanium dioxide is the active ingredient in a number of topical ointments and lotions.

titer, **1.** a measurement of the concentration of a substance in a solution. **2.** the quantity of a substance required to produce a reaction with another substance. **3.** the smallest amount of a certain substance that indicates the presence of a colon bacillus under standard condtions. **4.** the highest dilution of a serum that causes clumping of bacteria.

title, a section of the Social Security Act that provides for the establishment, funding, and regulation of a service to a specific segment of the population, as Title XIX, which includes medical coverage under Medicaid, and Title X which awards lump-sum grants for family planning programs.

titubation /tich′o͝obā′shən/, unsteady posture characterized by a staggering or stumbling gait and a swaying head or trunk while sitting. It may be a manifestation of cerebellar disease. Compare **ataxia.**

Tl, symbol for **thallium.**

TLC, **1.** abbreviation for **total lung capacity.** **2.** *informal.* abbreviation for *tender loving care.*

T lymphocyte. See **lymphocyte, T cell.**

Tm, symbol for **thulium.**

TMJ, abbreviation for **temporomandibular joint.**

TMP/SMX, abbreviation for **trimethoprim sulfamethoxazole.**

TNM, a system for staging malignant neoplastic disease. See also **cancer staging.**

t.n.t.c., abbreviation for *too numerous to count,* usually applied to organisms or cells viewed on a slide under a microscope.

t.o., abbreviation for *telephone order.*

toadstool poisoning, a toxic condition caused by ingestion of certain varieties of poisonous mushrooms. See **mushroom poisoning.**

tobacco, a plant whose leaves are dried and used for smoking and chewing, and in snuff. See also **nicotine.**

tobacco withdrawal syndrome, a change in mood or performance associated with the cessation or reduction in exposure to nicotine. Symptoms may range from lack of concentration to anxiety and temper outbursts.

tobramycin sulfate, an aminoglycoside antibiotic.

■ INDICATIONS: It is prescribed in the treatment of external occular infection, septicemia, and lower respiratory tract and central nervous system infections.

■ CONTRAINDICATIONS: Kidney dysfunction, use of potent diuretics, or known hypersensitivity to this or other aminoglycosides prohibits its use.

■ ADVERSE EFFECTS: Among the more serious adverse reactions are ototoxicity and nephrotoxicity.

Tobruk plaster /tō′bro͝ok/, a plaster cast splint with tapes for skin traction coming through openings in the plaster and connected with Thomas' splint. It covers and immobilizes the leg from foot to groin. Also called **Tobruk splint.**

tocanide hydrochloride, an oral drug for the treatment of cardiac arrhythmias, with an action similar to that of lidocaine.

-tocia, **1.** a combining form meaning 'conditions of labor': *mogitocia, omotocia, tomotocia.* **2.** a combining form meaning the 'product of parturition': *deuterotocia, dystrophiadystocia, odontocia.*

toco-, toko-, a combining form meaning 'pertaining to childbirth or labor': *tocodynamometer, tocography, tocomania.*

tocodynamometer /tō′kōdī′nəmom′ətər/, an electronic device for monitoring and recording uterine contractions in labor. It consists of a pressure transducer that is applied to the fundus of the uterus by means of a belt, which is connected to a machine that records the duration of the contractions and the interval between them on graph paper. The relative intensity of the contractions is also indicated but cannot be quantified. The tocodynamometer is a component of external monitoring in childbirth. Also spelled **tokodynamometer.** See also **electronic fetal monitor.**

tocolytic drug, any drug used to suppress premature labor.

tocopherol. See **vitamin E.**

tocotransducer, an electronic device used to measure uterine contractions. See also **tocodynamometer.**

toddler, a child between 12 and 36 months of age. During this period of development the child acquires a sense of autonomy and independence through the mastery of various specialized tasks, as control of bodily functions, refinement of motor and language skills, and acquisition of socially acceptable behavior, especially toleration of delayed gratification and acceptance of separation from the mother or parents. The period is characterized by exploration of the environment and by rapid cognitive development as the child strives for self-assertion and personal interaction with others while struggling with parental discipline and sibling rivalry. Of primary importance for the nurse is the understanding of the dynamics of the growth and development of the toddler to help parents deal effectively with appropriate nutrition, toilet training, temper tantrums, prevention of accidental injury—primarily from falls, poisoning, burns, and childhood fears, especially anxiety as a result of separation from the parents.

toddlerhood, the state or condition of being a toddler.

toe, any one of the digits of the feet.

toeing in. See **metatarsus varus.**

toeing out. See **metatarsus valgus.**

toenail, one of the heavy ungual structures covering the terminal phalanges of the toes. Also called **unguis** /ung′gwis/.

Tofranil, a trademark for a tricyclic antidepressant (imipramine hydrochloride).

togaviruses /tō′gəvī′rəsəs/, a family of arboviruses that includes the organisms causing encephalitis, dengue, yellow fever, and rubella.

toilet training, the process of teaching a child to control the functions of the bladder and bowel. Training programs vary, but all emphasize a positive, consistent, nonpunitive, and nonpressured approach, and each program is individualized, depending on the mental and physical age and state of the child, the parent-child relationship, and readiness of the child to learn. Training often begins between 18 and 24 months of age, when voluntary control of the anal and urethral sphincters is achieved by most children. When the child has mastered some motor skills, is aware of his ability to control the body, and can communicate adequately, training is likely to be easy. Resistance occurs if the parents try to train the child before the child is physiologically and psychologically ready. Bowel training is usually accomplished before bladder training because the urge to evacuate the bowel is stronger than the urge to empty the bladder, and the need is less frequent and more regular. Nighttime bladder control may not be achieved until the child is 4 or 5 years of age or older. Behavior modification, using a system of rewards for each of the various phases of the training, has been successful with both normal and mentally retarded children. A major nursing function is to identify the readiness of the child to learn and to work with the parents, advising them in a nonauthoritarian way of the various techniques.

token economy, a technique of reinforcement used in behavior therapy in the management of a group of people, as in hospitals, institutions, or classrooms. Individuals are rewarded for specific activities or behavior with tokens they can exchange for desired objects or privileges.

toko-. See **toco-.**

tokodynamometer. See **tocodynamometer.**

tolazamide, an oral sulfonylurea antidiabetic.

■ INDICATIONS: It is prescribed in the treatment of stable or non-insulin-dependent diabetes mellitus and for some patients sensitive to other types of sulfonylureas or who have failed to respond to other similar drugs.

■ CONTRAINDICATIONS: Unstable diabetes, serious impairment of renal, hepatic, or thyroid function, pregnancy, or known hypersensitivity to this drug or to other sulfonylurea medications prohibits its use.

■ ADVERSE EFFECTS: Among the more serious adverse effects are hypoglycemia and skin reactions. Blood dyscrasias may occur.

tolazoline hydrochloride, a peripheral vasodilator.

■ INDICATIONS: It is prescribed in the treatment of spastic peripheral vascular disorders, including Buerger's disease, Raynaud's disease, and scleroderma.

■ CONTRAINDICATIONS: Coronary artery disease, cerebrovascular accident, or known hypersensitivity to this drug prohibits its use.

■ ADVERSE EFFECTS: Among the more serious adverse reactions are cardiac arrhythmia, hypertension, exacerbation of peptic ulcer, and a paradoxical response in seriously damaged limbs.

tolbutamide, an oral sulfonylurea antidiabetic.

■ INDICATIONS: It is prescribed in the treatment of stable non-insulin-dependent diabetes mellitus uncontrolled by diet alone and for some patients changing from insulin to oral therapy.

■ CONTRAINDICATIONS: Unstable diabetes, serious impairment of renal, hepatic, or thyroid function, pregnancy, or known hypersensitivity to this drug or to other sulfonylurea medications prohibits its use.

■ ADVERSE EFFECTS: Among the more serious adverse reactions are hypoglycemia and skin reactions. Blood dyscrasias may occur.

Tolectin, a trademark for a nonsteroidal antiinflammatory agent (tolmetin sodium).

tolerance, the ability to endure hardship, pain, or ordinarily injurious substances, as drugs, without apparent physiologic or psychologic injury. A kind of tolerance is **work tolerance.**

tolerance dose, (in radiotherapy) the amount of radiation that can be delivered to a body structure before irreversible damage occurs.

Toleron, a trademark for a hematinic (ferrous fumarate).

Tolinase, a trademark for an antidiabetic (tolazamide).

tolmetin sodium /tol′mətin/, a nonsteroidal antiinflammatory agent.

■ INDICATIONS: It is prescribed primarily in the treatment of rheumatoid arthritis, juvenile rheumatoid arthritis, and osteoarthritis.

■ CONTRAINDICATIONS: Impaired renal function, GI disease, or known hypersensitivity to this drug, to aspirin, or to nonsteroidal antiinflammatory medications prohibits its use.

■ ADVERSE EFFECTS: Among the more serious adverse reactions are peptic ulcer and GI distress. Dizziness, skin rash, and tinnitus commonly occur. This drug interacts with many other drugs.

tolnaftate /tolnaf′tāt/, an antifungal.

■ INDICATIONS: It is prescribed in the treatment of superficial fungus infections of the skin, including tinea pedis, tinea cruris, and tinea versicolor.

■ CONTRAINDICATION: Known hypersensitivity to this drug prohibits its use.

■ ADVERSE EFFECTS: Among the more common adverse reactions are hypersensitivity reactions and mild irritation of the skin.

-tome, **1.** a combining form meaning a 'cutting instrument': *labiotome, neurotome, thyrotome*. **2.** a combining form meaning a '(specified) segment or region': *dermomyotome, pleurotome, viscerotome*.

-tomic, -tomical, a combining form meaning 'related to incisions or sections of tissue': *dermatomic, phlebotomic, somatomic*.

tomographic DSA, the visualization of blood vessels in the body in three dimensions. See also **digital subtraction angiography (DSA).**

tomography /təmog′rəfē/, an x-ray technique that produces a film representing a detailed cross section of tissue structure at a predetermined depth. It is a valuable diagnostic tool for the discovery and identification of space occupying lesions, as might be found in the brain, liver, pancreas, and gallbladder.

-tomy, a combining form meaning a 'surgical incision': *cystotomy, oncotomy, phlebotomy*.

tone. See **tonus.**

tongue, the principal organ of the sense of taste that also assists in the mastication and the deglutition of food. It is located in the floor of the mouth within the curve of the mandible. Its root is connected to the hyoid bone posteriorly by the hypoglossi and the genioglossi muscles. It is also connected to the epiglottis by three folds of mucous membrane, to the soft palate by the glossopalatine arches, and to the pharynx by the constrictores pharyngis superiores and by the mucous membrane. The apex of the tongue rests anteriorly against the lingual surfaces of the lower incisors. The mucous membrane connecting the tongue to the mandible reflects over the floor of the mouth to the lingual surface of the gingiva and in the midline of the floor is raised into a vertical fold. The dorsum of the tongue is divided into symmetric halves by a median sulcus, which ends posteriorly in the foramen cecum. A shallow sulcus terminalis runs from this foramen laterally and forward on either side to the margin of the organ. From the sulcus, the anterior two thirds of the tongue are covered with papillae. The posterior third is smoother and contains numerous mucous glands and lymph follicles. The use of the tongue as an organ of speech is not anatomic but a secondary acquired characteristic. Also called **lingua.**

tongue-tie. See **ankyloglossia.**

-tonia, -tony, a combining form meaning '(condition or degree of) tonus of a sort or in a region of the body': *angiotonia, hemotonia, vasotonia*.

-tonic, **1.** a combining form meaning the 'quality of muscle contraction or tonus': *hypertonic, myatonic, normotonic*. **2.** a combining form meaning a 'solution with a comparative concentration': *hypertonic, hypotonic, isotonic*.

tonicity /tōnis′itē/, the quality of possessing tone, or tonus.

tonic labyrinthine reflex, a normal postural reflex in animals, abnormally accentuated in decerebrate humans, characterized by extension of all four limbs when the head is positioned in space at an angle above the horizontal in quadripeds or in the neutral, erect position in humans. Also called **decerebrate rigidity.**

tonic neck reflex, a normal response in newborns to extend the arm and the leg on the side of the body to which the head is quickly turned while the infant is supine and to flex the limbs of the opposite side. The reflex, which prevents the infant from rolling over until adequate neurologic and motor development occurs, disappears by 3 to 4 months of age to be replaced by symmetric positioning of both sides of the body. Absence or persistence of the reflex may indicate central nervous system damage. Also called **asymmetric tonic neck reflex.** See also **symmetric tonic neck reflex.**

tono-, a combining form meaning 'pertaining to tone or tension': *tonoclonic, tonoscillograph, tonoplast.*

tonofibril, a bundle of fine filaments found in the cytoplasm of epithelial cells. The individual strands, or **tonofilaments,** spread throughout the cytoplasm and extend into the intercellular bridge to converge at the desmosome. The system of fibers functions as a supportive element within the cystoskeleton. In keratinizing epithelium, the strands are the main precursor of keratin. Also called **epitheliofibril, tenofibril.** See also **keratohyalin.**

tonometer /tōnom′ətər/, an instrument used in measuring tension or pressure, especially intraocular pressure.

tonometry /tōnom′ətrē/, the measuring of intraocular pressure by determining the resistance of the eyeball to indentation by an applied force. Several kinds of tonometers are used. The air-puff tonometer, which does not touch the eye, records deflections of the cornea from a puff of pressurized air. The Schiötz impression and the aplanation tonometers record the pressure needed to indent or flatten the corneal surface.

tonsil, a small, rounded mass of tissue, especially lymphoid tissue, as that comprising the palatine tonsils in the oropharynx. Compare **intestinal tonsil, lingual tonsil, palatine tonsil, pharyngeal tonsil.**

tonsillectomy, the surgical excision of the palatine tonsils, performed to prevent recurrent streptococcal tonsillitis. Before surgery, several laboratory tests, including a bleeding and clotting time, complete blood count, and urinalysis are done. Tonsillar tissue is dissected and removed, usually using general anesthesia, and bleeding areas are sutured or cauterized. An airway remains in place until swallowing returns. An increase in pulse rate, falling blood pressure, restlessness, or frequent swallowing warns of possible hemorrhage. On recovery from anesthesia, ice chips or clear liquids without a drinking straw may be offered. Tonsillectomy is often combined with adenoidectomy.

tonsillitis, an infection or inflammation of a tonsil. Acute tonsillitis, frequently caused by streptococcus infection, is characterized by severe sore throat, fever, headache, malaise, difficulty in swallowing, earache, and enlarged, tender lymph nodes in the neck. Acute tonsillitis may accompany scarlet fever. Treatment includes systemic antibiotics, analgesics, and warm irrigations of the throat. Soft foods and ample fluids are given. Tonsillectomy is sometimes performed for recurrent tonsillitis or tonsillar abscess. See also **peritonsillar abscess, scarlet fever, strep throat.**

tonus /tō′nəs/, **1.** the normal state of balanced tension in the tissues of the body, especially the muscles. Partial contraction or alternate contraction and relaxation of neighboring fibers of a group of muscles hold the organ or the part of the body in a neutral, functional position without fatigue. Tone is essential for many normal body functions, as holding the spine erect, the eyes open, and the jaw closed. **2.** the state of the tissues of the body being strong and fit. Also called **tone.**

-tony, -tonia, a combining form meaning a 'condition of motor control': *arteriotony, neurotony, vagotony.*

tooth, *pl.* **teeth,** one of numerous dental structures that develop in the jaws as part of the digestive system and are used to cut, grind, and process food in the mouth for ingestion. Each tooth consists of a crown, which projects above the gum; two to four roots, embedded in the alveolus; and a neck, which stretches between the crown and the root. Each tooth also contains a cavity filled with pulp, richly supplied with blood vessels and nerves that enter the cavity through a small aperture at the base of each root. The solid portion of the tooth consists of dentin, enamel, and a thin layer of bone on the surface of the root. The dentin comprises the bulk of the tooth. The enamel covers the exposed portion of the crown. Two sets of teeth appear at different periods of life: the 20 deciduous teeth appear during infancy, the 32 permanent teeth during childhood and early adulthood. See also **deciduous tooth, permanent tooth.**

tooth alignment, the arrangement of the teeth in relation to their supporting bone or alveolar process, adjacent teeth, and opposing dentitions.

tooth-borne, describing a dental prosthesis or part of a prosthesis that depends entirely on abutment teeth for support.

tooth-borne base, a denture base restoring an edentulous area that has abutment teeth at each end for support. The tissue that it covers is not used for support of the base.

toothbrush, an implement of various design, with bristles fixed to a head at the end of a handle, used for brushing and cleaning the teeth and gingivae and for massaging the gingival tissues.

tooth form, the identifying curves, lines, angles, and contours of a tooth that differentiate it from other teeth.

tooth fulcrum, axis of movement of a tooth subjected to lateral forces, considered to be at the middle third of the portion of the tooth root embedded in the alveolus.

tooth germ, a primitive cell in the embryo that is the precursor of a tooth.

tooth inclination, the angle of slope of a tooth or teeth from the vertical plane, as mesially, distally, lingually, buccally, or labially inclined.

tophus /tō′fəs/, *pl.* **tophi,** a calculus, containing sodium urate deposits, that develops in periarticular fibrous tissue, typically in patients with gout.

-topia, -topy, a combining form meaning '(condition of) placement of organs in the body': *heterotopia, normotopia, skeletopia.*

topical, 1. of or pertaining to the surface of a part of the body. **2.** of or pertaining to a drug or treatment applied topically.

topical anesthesia, surface analgesia produced by application of a topical anesthetic in the form of a solution, gel, or ointment to the skin, mucous membrane, or cornea. The most common ingredients include benzocaine, butamben, cyclomethycaine, dibucaine, dimethisoquin, diperodon, dyclonine, lidocaine, piperocaine, pramoxine, hexylcaine, and tetracaine. Cocaine may be applied in solution to the mucous membranes of the nasal passages in certain otolaryngeal or maxillofacial procedures. Also called **surface anesthesia.** Compare **general anesthesia, local anesthesia, regional anesthesia.**

Topicort, a trademark for a topical glucocorticoid (desoximetasone).

topo-, a combining form meaning 'place': *topognosis, toponarcosis, topoparesthesia.*

topographic, pertaining to a freudian conceptualization of the layers of human consciousness.

Topsyn, a trademark for a glucocorticoid (fluocinonide).

TORCH /tôrch/, an abbreviation for *toxoplasmosis, other, rubella virus, cytomegalovirus, and herpes simplex viruses,* a group of agents that can infect the fetus or the newborn infant causing a constellation of morbid effects called the TORCH syndrome.

TORCH syndrome, infection of the fetus or newborn by one of the TORCH agents. The outcome of a pregnancy complicated by a TORCH agent may be abortion or stillbirth, intrauterine growth retardation, or premature delivery.

■ OBSERVATIONS: At delivery and during the first days after birth an infant infected with any one of the organisms may demonstrate various clinical manifestations, as fever, lethargy, poor feeding, petechiae on the skin, purpura, pneumonia, hepatosplenomegaly, jaundice, hemolytic and other anemias, encephalitis, microcephaly, hydrocephalus, intracranial calcifications, hearing deficits, chorioretinitis, and microophthalmia. In addition, each of the agents is associated with several other abnormal clinical findings involving abnormal immune response, cataracts, glaucoma, vesicles, ulcers, and congenital cardiac defects.

■ INTERVENTION: Before pregnancy women may be tested for susceptibility to the rubella virus and inoculated against it if not immune. There are currently no vaccines that confer immunity to the other TORCH agents, but the mother may be serologically tested for antibody levels to them. During pregnancy toxoplasmosis is asymptomatic in about 90% of cases, making diagnosis unlikely. If infection is suspected, serial paired serologic tests are performed: A high, rising titer indicates recent infection. Transplacental infection occurs in 35% of mothers infected during pregnancy. If it is contracted in the first trimester, before the placenta is fully developed, the infant may not become infected; if the infection is contracted, severe congenital manifestations of the syndrome usually occur. If the fetus is infected after the first trimester, the baby is usually born with asymptomatic or mild disease; the infection may be spread from the baby during the newborn period. Sulfadiazone, pyrimethamine, and folinic acid are sometimes given to treat the infection.

Primary cytomegalovirus infection during pregnancy is usually asymptomatic. If the infection is suspected, serologic testing may be performed to demonstrate primary infection, because infants born to mothers infected for the first time during pregnancy are much more likely to develop severe congenital anomalies than if the infection is a reactivation of previous cytomegalovirus infection. There is no specific treatment. The child is considered to be infectious, but contagion among newborns from a congenitally infected infant has not been proven.

Transplacental rubella virus infection in pregnancy during the first 8 weeks is likely to cause infection in 50% of fetuses and to result in demonstrable defects in 85% of those infected. The risk becomes less as gestation increases to 24 weeks, after which time infection has not been known to result in defects. Rubella is the only TORCH virus that is usually symptomatic, and, therefore, it is often recognized. Many mothers infected during the first trimester choose to abort the pregnancy. There is no treatment for the infection, but screening and immunization before pregnancy could prevent virtually all cases of congenital rubella.

Herpesvirus infection (HSV) in pregnancy is rarely transplacentally transmitted to the fetus. Primary infection during pregnancy sometimes results in spontaneous abortion or premature delivery. In the newborn the infection is usually systemic and life threatening. The fetus is most apt to become infected by the virus shed from an active genital lesion during vaginal delivery or as the result of vaginal examination or the placement of an intrauterine catheter or a fetal scalp electrode during labor. There is no treatment: If the mother has active, genital herpesvirus lesions, intrapartal internal monitoring is contraindicated, vaginal examinations are often omitted, regional anesthetic techniques are avoided, and the infant is delivered by cesarean section.

The TORCH infections caused by other agents are asymptomatic in pregnancy, revealing themselves by the syndrome after birth. The congenital effects are not amenable to change or to amelioration by any known treatment.

■ NURSING CONSIDERATIONS: Newborn infants who are infected with a TORCH agent or who bear the stigmata of TORCH syndrome are considered to be potential sources of neonatal spread of infection. Rubella screening and vaccination are encouraged. Only 10% of the cases of

TORCH syndrome are proven to be associated with a known agent (toxoplasmosis, rubella virus, cytomegalovirus, or herpesvirus); 90% are the result of "other" infections; therefore, pregnant women are instructed to avoid contact with people ill with infectious diseases to the greatest extent possible.

Torecan Maleate, a trademark for a phenothiazine antiemetic (thiethylperazine maleate).

Torkildsen's procedure. See **ventriculocisternostomy.**

torpid idiocy, *obsolete.* severe mental retardation associated with dullness and inactivity.

torque /tôrk/, **1.** a twisting force produced by contraction of the medial femoral muscles that tend to rotate the thigh medially. **2.** (in dentistry) a force applied to a tooth to rotate it on a mesiodistal or buccolingual axis. **3.** a rotary force applied to a denture base. Compare **torsion.**

torr /tôr/, a unit of pressure, commonly used to mean 1 mm Hg, or the amount of pressure required to raise a column of mercury 1 mm.

tors-, a combining form meaning 'twisted': *torsiometer, torsive, torsiversion.*

torsades de pointes /tôrsäd′ depô·aNt′, tôr′sād dəpoint′/, a type of ventricular tachycardia with a spirallike appearance ("twisting of the points") and complexes that at first look positive and then negative on an electrocardiogram. It is precipitated by a long QT interval, which often is drug induced (quinidine, procainamide, disopyramide, or amiodarone), but which may be the result of hypokalemia or profound bradycardia. The tachycardia may be paroxysmal and the patient conscious, causing the diagnosis to be missed. The treatment is a temporary electronic pacemaker until the offending drug can be metabolized and excreted, or drugs that shorten the Qt interval (atropine, isoproterenol) may be given.

torsion, **1.** the process of twisting in a positive (clockwise) or negative (counterclockwise) direction. **2.** the state of being turned. **3.** (in dentistry) the twisting of a tooth on its long axis.

torsion dystonia. See **dystonia musculorum deformans.**

torsion fracture, a spiral fracture, usually caused by a torsion injury.

torsion of the testis, the axial rotation of the spermatic cord that cuts off the blood supply to the testicle, epididymis, and other structures. Complete ischemia for 6 hours may result in gangrene of the testis. Partial loss of circulation may result in atrophy. Certain testes are anatomically predisposed to torsion because of inadequate connective tissue, but the condition may be caused by trauma with severe swelling. Torsion of the testis occurs more often on the left than on the right side and is most frequent in the first year of life and during puberty. Surgical correction is required in most cases; if performed within 5 hours of the onset of symptoms, the testis can usually be saved.

torsion spasm. See **dystonia musculorum deformans.**

tort, (in law) a civil wrong, other than a breach of contract. Torts include negligence, false imprisonment, assault, and battery. The elements of a tort are: a legal duty owed by the defendant to the plaintiff, a breach of duty, and damage from the breach of duty. A tort may be constitutional, in which one person deprives another of a right or immunity guaranteed by the Constitution; personal, in which a person or a person's reputation or feelings are injured; or intentional, in which the wrong is a deliberate act that is unlawful. Many other kinds of tort exist. –**tortious,** *adj.*

tort feasor, a person who commits a tort.

torticollis /tôr′tikol′is/, an abnormal condition in which the head is inclined to one side as a result of the contraction of the muscles on that side of the neck. It may be congenital or acquired. Treatment may include surgery, heat, support, or immobilization depending on the cause and the severity of the condition. Also called **wryneck.** See also **spasmodic torticollis.**

Torula histolytica. See ***Cryptococcus neoformans.***

torulopsosis /tôr′yo͞olop′səsis/, an infection with the yeast *Torulopsis glabrata,* a normal inhabitant of the oropharynx, GI tract, and skin, that causes disease in severely debilitated patients or in those with impaired immune function or, sometimes, in patients having prolonged urinary catheterization. Systemic infection is usually treated with amphotericin B.

torulosis. See **cryptococcosis.**

torus fracture. See **lead pipe fracture.**

total anomalous venous return, a rare, congenital cardiac anomaly in which the pulmonary veins attach directly to the right atrium or to various veins draining into the right atrium rather than directing flow to the left atrium. Clinical manifestations include cyanosis, pulmonary congestion, and heart failure. Other cardiac defects may also be present, as atrial septal defect, which shunts unoxygenated systemic blood to the left side of the heart and helps decompress the right atrium. Corrective surgery is indicated, usually after 1 year of age, but may be necessary at an earlier age if pulmonary venous obstruction or severe congestive heart failure is present. See also **congenital cardiac anomaly.**

total body radiation, radiation that exposes the entire body so that, theoretically, all cells in the body receive the same radiation.

total body water (TBW), all the water within the body, including intracellular and extracellular water plus the water in the GI and urinary tracts.

total cleavage, mitotic division of the fertilized ovum into blastomeres. Compare **partial cleavage.**

total iron, the total iron concentration in the blood. The normal concentrations in serum are 50 to 150 μg/dl.

total lung capacity (TLC), the volume of gas in the lungs at the end of a maximum inspiration. It equals the vital capacity plus the residual capacity.

total macroglobulins, the heavy serum macroglobulins that are elevated in various diseases, as cancer, and infections. The normal concentrations in serum are 70 to 430 mg/dl.

total nitrogen, the nitrogen content of the feces, measured to detect various disorders, as pancreatic insufficiency and impaired protein digestion. The normal amount in a 24-hour fecal specimen is 10% of intake, or 1 to 2 g.

total parenteral nutrition (TPN), the administration of a nutritionally adequate hypertonic solution consisting of glucose, protein hydrolysates, minerals, and vitamins through an indwelling catheter into the superior vena cava. The high rate of blood flow results in rapid dilution of the solution, and full nutritional requirements can be met indefinitely. The procedure is used in prolonged coma, severe uncontrolled malabsorption, extensive burns, GI fistulas, and other conditions in which feeding by mouth cannot provide adequate amounts of the essential nutrients. In infants and children it is used when feeding by way of the GI tract is impossible, inadequate, or hazardous, as in chronic intestinal obstruction from peritoneal sepsis or adhesions, inadequate intestinal length, or chronic nonremitting severe diarrhea. The hyperalimentation solution is infused through conventional tubing with an intravenous filter attached to remove any contaminates. In adults the catheter is placed directly into the subclavian vein and threaded through the right innominate vein into the superior vena cava. In infants and small children the catheter is ususally threaded to the central venous location by way of the jugular vein, which is entered through a subcutaneous tunnel beneath the scalp. Strict asepsis must be maintained because infection is a grave and present danger of this therapy. Other solutions are never instilled through this catheter. Also called **hyperalimentation, intravenous alimentation, parenteral hyperalimentation, total parenteral alimentation.**

total peripheral resistance, the maximum degree of resistance to blood flow caused by constriction of the systemic blood vessels.

total renal blood flow (TRBF), the total volume of blood that flows into the renal arteries. The average TRBF in a normal adult is 1200 ml per minute.

touch, **1.** the ability to feel objects and to distinguish their various characteristics; the tactile sense. **2.** the ability to perceive pressure when it is exerted on the skin or the mucosa of the body. **3.** to palpate or examine with the hand, as the digital examination of the abdomen, rectum, or vagina.

touch deprivation, a lack of tactile stimulation, especially in early infancy, which if continued for a sufficient length of time may lead to serious developmental and emotional disturbances, as stunted growth, personality disorders, and social regression. In severe cases, a child who is deprived of adequate physical handling and emotional stimulation may not survive infancy. See also **hospitalism.**

Tourette's syndrome. See **Gilles de la Tourette's syndrome.**

tourniquet /tur′nikit, to͞or′-/, a device used in controlling hemorrhage, consisting of a wide constricting band applied to the limb proximal to the site of bleeding. The use of a tourniquet is a drastic measure and is to be employed only if the hemorrhage is life threatening and if other, safer measures have proved ineffective. See also **hemorrhage.**

tourniquet infusion method, a technique of intraarterial regional chemotherapy used in the treatment of osteogenic sarcoma. The technique uses one or two external tourniquets, depending on the location of the tumor, which slow or interrupt the blood flow to a limb temporarily while an anticancer drug, as adriamycin, is infused into the area. The method increases the concentration of antineoplastic drug by as much as 100 times as compared with an alternative technique of injecting the drug into the circulation, without application of a tourniquet, resulting in rapid dilution of the drug by the normal blood volume.

tourniquet test, a test of capillary fragility, in which a blood pressure cuff is applied for 5 minutes to a person's arm and is inflated to a pressure halfway between the diastolic and systolic blood pressure. The number of petechiae within a circumscribed area of the skin may be counted, or the results may be reported in a range from negative (no petechiae) to +4 positive (confluent petechiae).

tower head, tower skull. See **oxycephaly.**

town-gown, of or pertaining to any aspect of the relationship between an educational institution and the community in which it is situated.

toxemia /toksē′mē•ə/, the presence of bacterial toxins in the bloodstream. Also called **blood poisoning.** See also **preeclampsia.** **–toxemic,** *adj.*

-toxemia, -toxaemia, a combining form meaning a '(specified) toxic substance in the blood': *ectotoxemia, gonotoxemia, ophiotoxemia.*

toxemia of pregnancy. See **preeclampsia.**

-toxia, a combining form meaning 'condition resulting from a poison in a (specified) region of the body': *neurotoxia, thyrotoxia, urotoxia.*

toxic, **1.** of or pertaining to a poison. **2.** (of a disease or condition) severe and progressive.

-toxic, -toxical, a combining form meaning 'pertaining to poison': *cardiotoxic, hematoxic, spermatoxic.*

toxic amblyopia, partial loss of vision because of retrooptic bulbar neuritis, caused by poisoning with quinine, lead, wood alcohol, nicotine, arsenic, or certain other poisons.

toxic dementia, dementia resulting from excessive use of or exposure to a poisonous substance. See also **dementia.**

toxic dose (TD), (in toxicology) the amount of a substance that may be expected to produce a toxic effect. See also **median toxic dose.**

toxic epidermal necrolysis (TEN), a rare skin disease, characterized by epidermal erythema, superficial necrosis, and skin erosions. This condition, which affects mainly adults, makes the skin appear scalded, often leaving scars. The cause of TEN is unknown, but it may result from toxic or hypersensitive reactions. It is commonly associated with drug reactions, as those associated with butazones, sulfonamides, penicillins, barbiturates, and hydantoins. Other drugs may be involved, and the disease has also been associated with airborne toxins, as carbon monoxide. TEN may also indicate an immune response, or it may be associated with severe physiologic stress.

■ OBSERVATIONS: Early signs of the condition include inflammation of the mucous membranes, fever, malaise, a burning sensation in the conjunctivae, and pervasive tenderness of the skin. The first phase of TEN is manifested by diffuse erythema. The second phase involves vesiculation and blistering. The third phase is marked by extensive epidermal necrolysis and desquamation. As the disease progresses, large, flaccid bullae develop and rupture, exposing wide expanses of denuded skin. Tissue fluids and electrolytes are consequently lost, resulting in extensive systemic complications, as pulmonary edema, bronchopneumonia, GI and esophageal hemorrhage, sepsis, shock, renal failure, and disseminated intravascular coagulation. These extreme conditions contribute to the high mortality associated with TEN—about 30%—especially among the infirm and the elderly. Confirming diagnosis is based on symptoms in the third phase of the disease, as skin denuded by even slight friction, affecting the areas of erythema. Diagnosis is commonly supported by bacteriologic culture and Gram's stains of lesions to determine if infection exists. The presence of leukocytosis, fluid and electrolyte imbalances, albuminuria, and elevated transaminase levels are characteristic and help confirm the diagnosis. Erythema multiforme and exfoliative dermatitis may be ruled out by exfoliative biopsy and cytology.

■ INTERVENTION: Treatment of TEN commonly involves the administration of IV fluids to replace body fluids and to maintain electrolyte balance. Frequent laboratory analyses are necessary to monitor hematocrit and hemoglobin, serum proteins, electrolytes, and blood gases.

■ NURSING CONSIDERATIONS: Nursing care of patients with TEN requires meticulous monitoring of vital signs, central venous pressure, and urinary output. Any signs of renal failure, as decreased urinary output, and of bleeding are of immediate concern. It is important to detect and quickly treat any septic infection. Temperature elevations are reported immediately, and all laboratory work, as blood cultures and sensitivity tests, are performed promptly. Ocular lesions are common with TEN, and frequent eye care is often needed to remove exudate. Protective isolation and prophylactic antibiotic therapy may be required to prevent secondary infection. Nurses also make sure that the TEN patient does not wear tight clothing and is covered loosely to minimize the friction that causes skin sloughing. A Stryker frame or a Circolectric bed may be helpful in caring for the patient. Analgesics are administered as needed, and cool, sterile compresses may be applied to relieve discomfort. Psychologic and emotional support for the patient and the family is also a key nursing concern.

toxic erythema of the newborn. See **erythema toxicum neonatorum.**

toxic gastritis. See **corrosive gastritis.**

toxic goiter, an enlargement of the thyroid gland associated with exophthalmia and systemic disease. See also **Graves' disease.**

toxic hemoglobinuria. See **hemoglobinuria.**

toxicity /toksis'itē/, **1.** the degree to which something is poisonous. **2.** a condition that results from exposure to a toxin or to toxic amounts of a substance that does not cause adverse effects in smaller amounts.

toxic nodular goiter, an enlarged thyroid gland characterized by numerous discrete nodules and hypersecretion of thyroid hormones, occurring most frequently in elderly individuals. Typical signs of thyrotoxicosis, as nervousness, tremor, weakness, fatigue, weight loss, and irritability, are usually present, but exophthalmia is rare; anorexia is more common than hyperphagia, and cardiac arrhythmia or congestive heart failure may be a predominant manifestation. When clinical findings suggest thyrotoxicosis, a therapeutic trial of antithyroid drugs, as propylthiouracil or methimazole, is indicated, but once the diagnosis is established, radioactive iodine is considered the treatment of choice, and large doses are usually required.

toxico-, toxo-, a combining form meaning 'pertaining to poison, poisonous': *toxicodendrol, toxicomucin, toxicosozin.*

toxicokinetics, the passage through the body system of a toxic agent or its metabolites, usually in an action similar to that of pharmacokinetics.

toxicologist, a specialist in toxicology.

toxicology, the scientific study of poisons, their detection, their effects, and methods of treatment for conditions they produce. –**toxicologic, toxicological,** *adj.*

toxic shock syndrome (TSS), a severe acute disease caused by infection with strains of *Staphylococcus aureus,* phage group I, that produces a unique toxin, enterotoxin F. It is most common in menstruating women using high absorbency tampons but has been seen in newborn infants, children, and men.

■ OBSERVATIONS: The onset of the syndrome is characterized by sudden high fever, headache, sore throat with swelling of the mucous membranes, diarrhea, nausea, and erythroderma. Acute renal failure, abnormal liver function, confusion, and refractory hypotension usually follow, and death may occur. It is probable that mild forms of the syndrome are not reported and, therefore, are not diagnosed. There does not appear to be any seasonal or geographic factor in the cause of the disease, and there is no evidence of contagion among household members or through sexual contacts of people who have TSS.

Bacteremia, or discernible local infection, is absent in most cases. *Staphylococcus aureus* may be cultured from many sites, including the pharynx, nares, and cervix, but the drastic effects of infection are the result of the toxin released from the organism rather than from the infection itself.

■ INTERVENTION: Aggressive volume expansion by the administration of large amounts of intravenous fluid, assisted ventilation, and administration of vasopressors may be necessary in treating severe TSS. Early recognition and active supportive treatment greatly improve the survival rates and decrease both prolonged morbidity and recurrence.

■ NURSING CONSIDERATIONS: The use of highly absorbent tampons is associated with a greater incidence of the disease than the use of regular tampons, but a few cases have occurred in women who have never used tampons. The nurse counsels women to avoid the high absorbency tampons and to report any illness occurring during the menses that is accompanied by nausea, diarrhea, and fever. Recurrence is likely; a mild, undiagnosed episode during a preceding menstrual period is often reported when severe TSS is diagnosed. Women who have had TSS are usually advised to avoid using any kind of tampons for at least several months.

toxin, a poison, usually one produced by or occurring in a plant or microorganism. See also **endotoxin, exotoxin.**

-toxin, a combining form meaning 'poison': *cynotoxin, hypnotoxin, zootoxin.*

toxo-. See **toxico-.**

toxocariasis /tok′sōkərī′əsis/, infection with the larvae of *Toxocara canis,* the common roundworm of dogs and cats. Ingestion of viable eggs, commonly found in soil, leads to the spread of tiny larvae throughout the body, resulting in respiratory symptoms, enlarged liver, skin rashes, eosinophilia, and delayed ocular lesions. Children who eat dirt are particularly subject to this disease. Specific drug therapy is not very useful; the outcome is usually good without therapy. Regular worming of pets helps prevent infection. Also called **visceral larva migrans.**

toxoid, a toxin that has been treated with chemicals or with heat to decrease its toxic effect but that retains its antigenic power. It is given to produce immunity by stimulating the creation of antibodies. See also **toxin, vaccine.**

Toxoplasma /tok′sōplaz′mə/, a genus of protozoa with only one known species, *Toxoplasma gondii,* an intracellular parasite of cats and other hosts that causes toxoplasmosis in humans.

toxoplasmosis /tok′sōplazmō′sis/, a common infection with the protozoan intracellular parasite *Toxoplasma gondii,* characterized in the congenital form by liver and brain involvement with cerebral calcification, convulsions, blindness, microcephaly or hydrocephaly, and mental retardation. The acquired form is characterized by rash, lymphadenopathy, fever, malaise, central nervous system disorders, myocarditis, and pneumonitis.

■ OBSERVATIONS: Cats acquire the organism by eating infected birds and mice. Cysts of the organism are transmitted from cat feces to humans or by human ingestion of inadequately cooked meat containing the cysts. Transplacental transmission occurs only during acute infection of the mother, but the disease is very serious in the fetus and in those with an impaired immune system. Diagnosis is made by demonstrating rising antibody titers or by immunofluorescent antibody tests. Infection confers immunity.

■ INTERVENTION: Combinations of sulfonamides with pyrimethamine are recommended as treatment, possibly reducing the severity of the illness in the fetus.

■ NURSING CONSIDERATIONS: All meat should be heated to at least 140° F (60° C) throughout to kill this parasite. Pregnant women who are not immune are advised not to handle cats, cat feces, or litter boxes.

TPA, abbreviation for **tissue plasminogen activator.**

TPAL. See **parity.**

TPN, abbreviation for **total parenteral nutrition.**

trabecula carnea /trəbek′yələ/, *pl.* **trabeculae carneae,** any one of the irregular bands and bundles of muscle that project from the inner surfaces of the ventricles, except in the arterial cone of the right ventricle. Some of these trabeculae are ridges of muscle along the ventricular walls; others are short projections into the ventricular cavities; still others form the ventricular papillary muscles. Compare **chordae tendineae.** See also **heart, left ventricle, right ventricle.**

trabeculae, (in ophthalmology) the portion of the eye in front of the canal of Schlemm and within the angle created by the iris and the cornea.

trabecula septomarginalis. See **moderator band.**

trabeculectomy, the surgical removal of a section of corneoscleral tissue to increase the outflow of aqueous humor in patients with severe glaucoma. The procedure usually involves removal of the canal of Schlemm and the trabecular meshwork.

trabeculotomy, a surgical opening in an orbital trabecula to increase the outflow of aqueous humor.

trace element, an element essential to nutrition or physiologic processes, found in such minute quantities that analysis yields a presence of virtually zero amounts.

trace gas, a gas or vapor that escapes into the atmosphere during an anesthetic procedure. Because these substances may have adverse effects on the health of personnel exposed to them, scavenging equipment is often installed in operating rooms to clean the air. See also **gas scavenging system.**

tracer, **1.** see also **radioisotope scan.** a radioactive isotope that is used in diagnostic x-ray techniques to allow a biologic process to be seen. The tracer, which is introduced into the body, binds with a specific substance and is followed with a scanner or fluoroscope as it passes through various organs or systems in the body. Kinds of tracers include **radioactive iodine (^{131}I)** and **radioactive carbon(^{14}C). 2.** a mechanic device that graphically records the outline or movements of an object, or part of the body. **3.** a dissecting instrument that is used to isolate vessels and nerves. –**trace,** *v.*

tracer depot method, (in nuclear medicine) a technique used to determine local skin or muscle blood flow, based on the rate at which a radioactive tracer deposited in a tissue is removed by diffusion into the capillaries and washed out by the local blood supply. If blood flow is diminished or absent, as in dead skin, the deposited tracer does not wash out.

trachea /trā′kē·ə/, a nearly cylindric tube in the neck, composed of cartilage and membrane, that extends from the larynx at the level of the sixth cervical vertebra to the fifth thoracic vertebra, where it divides into two bronchi. The trachea conveys air to the lungs; it is about 11 cm long and 2 cm wide. The ventral surface of the tube is covered in the neck by the isthmus of the thyroid gland and various other structures, as the sternothyroideus and the sternohyoideus. Dorsally, the trachea is in contact with the esophagus. Also called **windpipe.** See also **primary bronchus.** –**tracheal,** *adj.*

tracheal breath sound, a normal breath sound heard in auscultation of the trachea. Inspiration and expiration are equally loud, the expiratory sound being heard during the greater part of expiration, whereas the inspiratory sound stops abruptly at the height of inspiration, with a pause before the sound of expiration is heard. Compare **vesicular breath sound.**

tracheitis /trā′kē·ī′tis/, any inflammatory condition of the trachea. It may be acute or chronic, resulting from infection, allergy, or physical irritation.

trachelo-, a combining form meaning 'pertaining to the neck or a necklike structure': *trachelobregmatic, trachelocystitis, tracheloschisis.*

trachelodynia. See **cervicodynia.**

tracheo-, a combining form meaning 'pertaining to the trachea': *tracheobronchial, tracheomalacia, tracheorrhaphy.*

tracheobronchial tree (TBT), an anatomic complex that includes the trachea, the bronchi, and the bronchial tubes. It conveys air to and from the lungs and is a primary structure in respiration. See also **bronchial tree.**

tracheobronchitis /trā′kē·ōbrongkī′tis/, inflammation of the trachea and bronchi, a common form of respiratory infection.

tracheoesophageal fistula, a congenital malformation in which there is an abnormal tubelike passage between the trachea and the esophagus.

tracheostomy /trā′kē·os′təmē/, an opening through the neck into the trachea through which an indwelling tube may be inserted. After tracheostomy the patient's chest is auscultated for breath sounds indicative of pulmonary congestion, mucous membranes and fingertips are observed for cyanosis, and humidified oxygen is given via tent or directly into the tracheostomy tube. The patient is reassured that the tube is open and that air can pass through it. The tube is suctioned frequently to keep it free from tracheobronchial secretions using a suction catheter attached to a Y-connector. The catheter is inserted 6 to 8 inches into the tube. The catheter is rotated, and intermittent suction is applied for no longer than 5 seconds. The patient is taught to cough to move secretions up and out of the bronchi. The nurse holds the tube stable during intense coughing to prevent its displacement. Should the outer tube be expelled, the nurse uses a dilator or hemostat to hold the trachea open until another tube can be inserted. A fluid intake of 3000 ml per day is recommended. The dressing is changed as necessary, the area is kept dry and clean, and frequent oral care is given. Pen and paper or a magic slate is kept available for communication because the patient cannot speak. Complications of tracheostomy include pneumothorax, respiratory insufficiency, obstruction of the tracheostomy tube or its displacement from the lumen of the trachea, pulmonary infection, atelectasis, tracheoesophageal fistula, hemorrhage, and mediastinal emphysema. If the procedure was done as an emergency, the tracheostomy is closed once normal breathing is restored. If the tracheostomy is permanent, as with a laryngectomy, the patient is taught self-care. Compare **tracheotomy.**

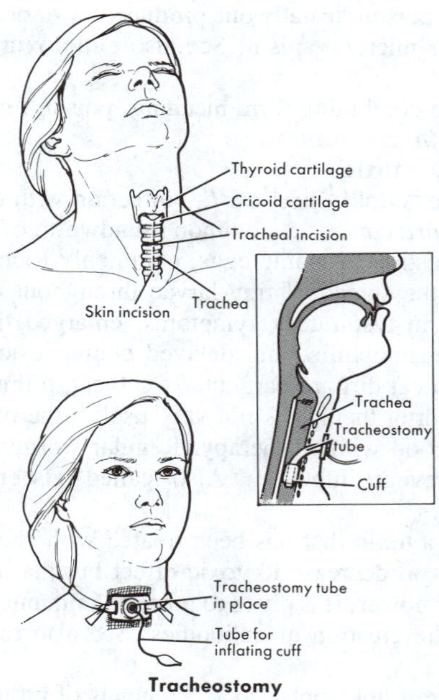

Tracheostomy

tracheotomy /trā′kē·ot′əmē/, an incision made into the trachea through the neck below the larynx, performed to gain access to the airway below a blockage with a foreign body, tumor, or edema of the glottis. The opening may be made as an emergency measure at an accident site or at a hospitalized patient's bedside or in the operating room. Local or general anesthesia may be used, if available. The patient's neck is hyperextended and an incision is made through the skin through the second, third, or fourth tracheal ring. A small hole is made in the fibrous tissue of the trachea and the opening is then dilated to allow the intake of air. In an emergency any available instrument may be used as a dilator, even the barrel of a ballpoint pen with the inner portion removed. If the blockage persists, a tracheostomy tube is inserted; if not, the incision is closed once normal respirations are established. After surgery the patient is observed for recurrent respiratory difficulty or cyanosis. Compare **tracheostomy.**

trachoma /trəkō′mə/, a chronic, infectious disease of the eye caused by the bacterium *Chlamydia trachomatis,* characterized initially by inflammation, pain, photophobia, and lacrimation. If untreated, follicles form on the upper eyelids and grow larger until the granulations invade the cornea, eventually causing blindness. Tetracycline, erythromycin, and topical sulfonamides usually provide effective treatment. Scarred eyelids may be surgically repaired. Trachoma is a significant cause of blindness and is endemic to hot, dry, poverty-ridden areas. In the United States, it is found on Native American reservations in the Southwest. Teaching an affected population about the spread of trachoma and having an adequate water supply for washing hands, towels, and handkerchiefs are important factors in eliminating the disease. Also called **Egyptian ophthalmia, granular conjunctivitis.**

tracing, a graphic record of a physical event, as an electrocardiograph tracing made by pens on a moving sheet of paper while recording the electric impulses of heart muscle contractions.

tract, **1.** an elongate group of tissues and structures that function together as a pathway, as the digestive tract or the respiratory tract. **2.** (in neurology) the neuronal axons that are grouped together to form a pathway.

traction, **1.** (in orthopedics) the process of putting a limb, bone, or group of muscles under tension by means of weights and pulleys to align or to immobilize the part or to relieve pressure on it. See also **orthopedic traction.** **2.** the process of pulling a part of the body along, through, or out of its socket or cavity, as axis traction with obstetric forceps in delivering an infant. Kinds of traction include **Bryant's traction, Buck's traction, Russell traction, skeletal traction, skin traction,** and **split Russell traction.**

traction frame, an orthopedic apparatus that supports the pulleys, the ropes, and the weights by which traction is applied to various parts of the body or by which various parts of the body are suspended. Traction frames are used in the treatment of bone fractures and dislocations, disease processes of the musculoskeletal system, in the correction of various orthopedic deformities, and in the general immobilization of specific areas of the body. The main components of a traction frame are metal uprights that attach to the bed and support an overhead metal bar. In addition to traction equipment, traction frames are often rigged with trapeze bars that the patient can grasp to help in changing positions and to exercise the muscles of the arms and the trunk. The components of a traction frame are securely clamped together when in use but can be easily disassembled and reassembled. Compare **IV-type traction frame, claw-type traction frame, Balkan traction frame.**

traction, 90-90 an orthopedic mechanism, used especially in pediatrics, that combines skeletal traction and suspension with a short-leg cast or a splint to immobilize and position the lower extremity in the treatment of a displaced fractured femur. This type of traction is usually unilateral with the opposite leg in Buck's traction or in split Russell traction for immobilization. The pin used in this kind of skeletal traction is inserted into bone in the knee area and attached to a riser running through a pulley on an overhead traction frame to a pulley and weight system fitted over the foot of the bed. The pulley and weight system at the foot of the bed also accommodates additional attachments to the short-leg cast or splint of the involved lower limb. Application of 90-90 traction may also incorporate a jacket restraint to help immobilize the patient. A variation of this type of traction is often used with adults in the treatment of low back pain.

trademark, a word, symbol, or device assigned to a product by its manufacturer and registered as a part of its identity. See also **generic name.**

tragus /trā′gəs/, *pl.* **tragi** /trā′jī/, a projection of the cartilage of the auricle at the opening of the external auditory meatus.

trained reflex. See **conditioned response.**

traineeship, a grant of money allocated to an individual for study in a given field. In nursing, many graduate students have been awarded federal traineeships that provide funds for tuition and living expenses.

training grant, a grant of money or other resources to provide training in a particular field. Many schools of nursing receive federal or state grants to provide specific educational programs. Funds may be allocated for faculty salaries, student aid, or other expenses.

trait, **1.** a characteristic mode of behavior or any mannerism or physical feature that distinguishes one individual or culture from another. **2.** any characteristic quality or condition that is genetically determined and inherited as a specific genotype. A trait is expressed in the phenotype as dominant or recessive for the particular characteristic; it is inherited in the genotype as either homozygous dominant, homozygous recessive, or heterozygous in the ratio of 1:2:1. In medicine, the term trait is used specifically to denote the heterozygous state of a recessive disorder, as the sickle cell trait. See also **dominance, gene, Mendel's laws, recessive.**

Tral, a trademark for an anticholinergic (hexocyclium methylsulfate).

trance, **1.** a sleeplike state characterized by the complete or partial suspension of consciousness and loss or diminution of motor activity, as seen in hypnosis, the dissociative form of hysteric neurosis, and various cataleptic and ecstatic states. **2.** a dazed or bewildered condition; stupor. **3.** a state of detachment from one's immediate surroundings, as in deep concentration or daydreaming. Kinds of trances are **alcoholic trance, death trance, hypnotic trance, hysteric trance,** and **induced trance.**

Trancopal, a trademark for an antianxiety agent (chlormezanone).

Tranmep, a trademark for an antianxiety agent (meprobamate).

tranquilizer, a drug prescribed to calm anxious or agitated people, ideally without decreasing their consciousness. Major tranquilizers, as derivatives of phenothiazine, butyrophenone, and thioxanthene, are generally used in the treatment of psychoses. Minor tranquilizers usually prescribed for the treatment of anxiety, irritability, tension, or psychoneurosis include chlordiazepoxide, diazepam, and hydroxyzine. Tranquilizers tend to induce drowsiness and have the potential for causing physical and psychologic dependence. See also **antipsychotic.**

trans-, a combining form meaning 'across, through, over': *transabdominal, transferase, transplacental.*

transactional analysis (TA), a form of psychotherapy developed by Eric Berne, based on a theory that three different, coherent, organized egos exist throughout life simultaneously in every person, representing the child, the adult, and the parent. Interactions between people are transactions, originating from a person in one of the ego states, received by another person who may be in a complementary or a crossed ego state. Transactions are motivated by a need for recognition and contact called "strokes." Transactions occur in six kinds of "time structure": withdrawal, rituals, pastimes, games, activities, and intimacy. The way in which a person structures time reflects internal conflicts and patterns adopted to cope with those conflicts. The goal of transactional analysis is to give the adult ego state decision-making power over the child and the parent.

transaminase /transam′inās/, an enzyme that catalyzes the transfer of an amino group from an alpha-amino acid to an alpha-keto acid, with pyridoxal phosphate and pyridoxamine phosphate acting as coenzymes. Glutamic-oxaloacetic transaminase (GOT), normally present in serum and various tissues, especially in the heart and liver, is released by damaged cells, and, as a result, a high serum level of GOT may be diagnostic in myocardial infarction or hepatic disease. Glutamic-pyruvic transaminase (GPT), a normal constituent of serum and various tissues, especially in the liver, is released by injured tissue and may be present in high concentrations in the sera of patients with acute liver disease. Also called **aminotransferase.**

transcellular water, the portion of extracellular water that is enclosed by an epithelial membrane and whose volume and composition is determined by the cellular activity of that membrane.

transcendence, the rising above one's previously perceived limits or restrictions.

transcondylar fracture /transkon′dilər/, a fracture that occurs transversally and distal to the epicondyles of any one of the long bones.

transconfiguration, **1.** (in genetics) the presence of the dominant allele of one pair of genes and the recessive allele of another pair on the same chromosome. **2.** the presence of at least one mutant gene and one wild-type gene of a pair of pseudoalleles on each chromosome of a homologous pair. Also called **transarrangement, transposition.** Compare **cis configuration.**

transcortical apraxia. See **ideomotor apraxia.**

transcortin, a diglobulin protein that binds a majority of cortisol in the plasma. Also called **corticosteroid-binding globulin.**

transcription, (in molecular genetics) the process by which RNA is formed from a DNA template in the process of manufacturing a protein. See also **anticodon, genetic code.**

transcultural nursing, a field of nursing in which the nurse transcends ethnocentricity and practices nursing in other cultural environments. Because current nursing process and theory are not culturally bound and the needs of each person are considered individually, transcultural nursing is potentially a part of all nursing practice.

transcutaneous electric nerve stimulation (TENS), a method of pain control by the application of electric impulses to the nerve endings. This is done through electrodes that are placed on the skin and attached to a stimulator by flexible wires. The electric impulses generated are similar to those of the body, but different enough to block transmission of pain signals to the brain. TENS is noninvasive and nonaddictive, with no known side effects. It is contraindicated in patients with a demand-type cardiac pacemaker.

transcutaneous nerve stimulation. See **transcutaneous electric nerve stimulation.**

transdermal delivery system, a method of applying a drug to unbroken skin. The drug is absorbed continuously through the skin and enters the systemic system. It is used particularly for the administration of nitroglycerin and scopolamine.

transducer, a device activated by some type of received energy that is then converted to a signal suitable for transmission, usually over electric circuits.

transduction, (in molecular genetics) a method of genetic recombination by which DNA is transferred from one cell to another by a viral vector. Various bacteriophages transduce genetic material from one species of bacteria to another.

transect, to sever or cut across, as in preparing a cross section of tissue.

transfection, (in molecular genetics) the process by which a cell is infected with DNA or RNA isolated from a virus or a viral vector. Acute transfection is short-term infection.

transfer agreement, a written hospital agreement between two health care institutions for the transfer of patients from one to another and for the orderly exchange of pertinent clinical information on the patients transferred.

transferase /trans′fərās/, any of a group of enzymes that catalyzes the transfer of a chemical group or radical, as the phosphate, methyl, amine, or keto groups, from one molecule to another.

transfer DNA (tDNA), (in molecular genetics) DNA transferred from its original source and present in transformed cells.

transference, **1.** the shifting of symptoms from one part of the body to another, as occurs in conversion disorder. **2.** (in psychiatry) an unconscious defense mechanism whereby feelings and attitudes originally associated with important people and events in one's early life are attributed to others in current interpersonal situations. **3.** (in psychoanalysis and psychotherapy) the feelings of a patient for the analyst to whom the patient has attributed or assigned the qualities, attitudes, and feelings of a person or persons significant in his or her emotional development, usually a figure from childhood. The phenomenon is used as a tool in understanding the emotional problems of the patient and their origins. See also **countertransference, parataxic distortion.**

transfer factor, a leukocyte extract that transfers delayed hypersensitivity from one person to another. Transfer factor has been studied for its possible use in the treatment of chronic mucocutaneous candidiasis and Wiskott-Aldrich syndrome and as a means of transferring antitumor immunity in patients with various types of cancer.

transferrin /transfer′in/, a trace protein present in the blood that is essential in the transport of iron. Its major function is to move iron from the intestine into the bloodstream, making it available to the normoblasts of the bone marrow. It may also take part in a slower exchange with ferritin, hemosiderin, and other iron forms in the tissues. See also **hemosiderin, iron transport.**

transfer RNA (tRNA), (in molecular genetics) a kind of RNA that transfers the genetic code from messenger RNA for the production of a specific amino acid. There are at least 20 different kinds of tRNA, each of which is able to combine covalently with a specific amino acid and to bond with at least one messenger RNA nucleotide triplet. Also called **adaptor RNA.**

transformation, (in molecular genetics) the process in which exogenous genes are integrated into chromosomes in a form that is recognized by the replicative and transcriptional apparatus of the host cell. Transformation occurs rarely in most cell populations.

transforming growth factor (TGF), a protein or a group of proteins produced by the cells of a tumor that, when inoculated into a normal cell culture, causes a disorderly and abnormal increase in the number of cells in the culture.

transfusion, the introduction into the bloodstream of whole blood or blood components, as plasma, platelets, or packed red cells. Whole blood may be infused into the recipient directly from a donor matched for the ABO blood group and antigenic subgroups, but more frequently the donor's blood is collected and stored by a blood bank. See also **blood transfusion.**

transfusion reaction, a systemic response by the to the administration of blood incompatible with th the recipient. The causes include red cell incompatib allergic sensitivity to the leukocytes, the platelets, o plasma protein components of the transfused blood or to the potassium or citrate preservative in the banked blood. See also **hemolysis.**

■ OBSERVATIONS: Fever is the most common transfusion reaction; urticaria is a relatively common allergic response. Asthma, vascular collapse, and renal failure occur less commonly. A hemolytic reaction from red cell incompatibility is serious and must be diagnosed and treated promptly. Symptoms develop shortly after beginning the transfusion, before 50 ml have been given, and include a throbbing headache, sudden, deep, and severe lumbar pain, precordial pain, dyspnea, and restlessness. Objective signs include ruddy facial flushing followed by cyanosis and distended neck veins, rapid, thready pulse, diaphoresis, and cold, clammy skin. Profound shock may occur within 1 hour.

■ INTERVENTION: The administration of antihistamines is usually beneficial in urticaria but offers no benefit for febrile reactions. When a hemolytic reaction is suspected, the transfusion is promptly terminated and the infusion line kept open with a normal solution of intravenous fluid for therapeutic purposes. The remaining bank blood is saved for a repeat type and crossmatch against a fresh sample of blood from the recipient. Direct and indirect antiglobulin tests are usually ordered to detect hemolytic antibodies, and a sample of urine is examined for free hemoglobin. Immediate treatment may include IV mannitol and a solution of 5% dextrose in water to maintain urine flow of more than 100 ml per hour. In the presence of oliguria, the possibility of acute renal failure is evaluated and the patient is managed accordingly. Hypovolemia is corrected with saline or plasma expanders, but the administration of more whole blood is avoided, if possible.

■ NURSING CONSIDERATIONS: The need for exceptional care to assure that typed and crossmatched blood conforms to compatibility standards is emphasized. The identifying information on the container of blood is always checked against the transfusion record. Questioning the patient about previous transfusions may elicit warning indications of possible adverse reactions. Once the transfusion is started, the patient is watched for objective signs of a transfusion reaction and is questioned for subjective symptoms. Routine temperature checks are done to detect febrile reactions that can be controlled by antipyretic drugs.

transient, pertaining to a condition that is temporary, as transient ischemic attack.

transient ischemic attack (TIA), an episode of cerebrovascular insufficiency, usually associated with a partial occlusion of an artery by an atherosclerotic plaque or an embolism. The symptoms vary with the site and the degree of occlusion. Disturbance of normal vision in one or in both eyes, dizziness, weakness, dysphasia, numbness, or unconsciousness may occur. The attack is usually brief, lasting a few minutes; rarely, symptoms continue for several hours.

transillumination, **1.** the passage of light through a solid or liquid substance. **2.** the passage of light through body tissues for the purpose of examining a structure interposed between the observer and the light source. A diaphanoscope is an instrument introduced into a body cavity to transilluminate tissues.

transition, the last phase of the first stage of labor, sometimes indicated by cervical dilatation of 8 to 10 cm.

transitional cell carcinoma, a malignant, usually papillary tumor derived from transitional stratified epithelium, occurring most frequently in the bladder, ureter, urethra, or renal pelvis. The majority of tumors in the collecting system of the kidney are of this kind. They have a better prognosis than squamous cell carcinomas in the same site.

transitional dentition. See **mixed dentition.**

transitory mania, a mood disorder characterized by the sudden onset of manic reactions that are of short duration, usually lasting from 1 hour to a few days. See also **mania.**

translation, (in molecular genetics) the process in which the genetic information carried by nucleotides in messenger RNA directs the amino acid sequence in the synthesis of a specific polypeptide. See also **anticodon, genetic code.**

translocation, (in genetics) the rearrangement of genetic material within the same chromosome or the transfer of a segment of one chromosome to another nonhomologous one. In simple translocations, one end segment of one chromosome is transferred onto the end of another nonhomologous one, involving a single break in only one of the chromosomes. Translocations in which material from the middle of one chromosome is shifted to the middle of another one are more complex and involve at least three breaks in the participating chromosomes. Such shifting of genetic material can result in serious disorders, as Down's syndrome, which is caused by a 14/21 translocation, and chronic granulocytic leukemia, in which part of the long arm of chromosome 22 is translocated to the short arm of chromosome 9. Kinds of translocations are **balanced translocation, reciprocal translocation,** and **robertsonian translocation.**

transmission, the transfer or conveyance of a thing or condition, as a neural impulse, infectious or genetic disease, or a hereditary trait, from one person or place to another. –**transmissible,** *adj.*

transmission electron microscopy. See **electron microscopy.**

transmission scanning electron microscope, an instrument that transmits a highly magnified, well-resolved, three-dimensional image on a television screen, thus combining the advantages of the electron and the scanning electron microscopes. Compare **electron microscope, scanning electron microscope.**

transmission scanning electron microscopy (TSEM), a technique using a transmission scanning electron microscope in which the atomic number of the portion of the sample being scanned is determined and used to modulate a beam of electrons in a cathode-ray tube and in the beam scanning the sample. The image produced is clear, three-dimensional, and highly magnified. Compare **electron microscopy, scanning electron microscopy.**

transmitter substance. See **neurotransmitter.**

transneuronal degeneration, degeneration of irreparably damaged nerve cells that may progress proximally or distally to involve neurons more than one synapse removed.

transovarial transmission, the transfer of pathogens to succeeding generations through invasion of the ovary and infection of the egg, as occurs in arthropods, primarily ticks and mites.

transplacental /trans′pləsen′təl/, across or through the placenta, specifically in reference to the exchange of nutrients, waste products, and other material between the developing fetus and the mother.

transplant, **1.** to transfer an organ or tissue from one person to another or from one body part to another to replace a diseased structure, to restore function, or to change appearance. Skin and kidneys are the most frequently transplanted structures; others include cartilage, bone, corneal tissue, portions of blood vessels and tendons, and recently, but infrequently, hearts and livers. Preferred donors are identical twins or persons having the same blood type and immunologic characteristics. Success of the transplant depends on overcoming the rejection of the donor tissue by the immune system of the recipient. Under local or general anesthesia, the recipient site is prepared and the donor structure is grafted in place; its oxygenation and blood supply are preserved during the procedure until the circulation can be restored at the new site. After surgery, circulation in the area is observed for signs of impairment. Antilymphocytic serum may be given, with steroids, to suppress the production of antibodies to the foreign tissue proteins. Signs of rejection reaction include fever, pain, and loss of function, usually occuring in the first 4 to 10 days after transplantation. An abscess may form if the reaction is not subdued promptly. The grafted structure may require several weeks to become established. Late rejection may occur several months or even 1 year later. **2.** any tissue or organ that is transplanted. **3.** of or pertaining to a tissue or organ that is transplanted or to a recipient of a donated tissue or organ or to a phenomenon associated with the procedure. Also called **graft, transplantation.**

transposable element, (in molecular genetics) a DNA fragment or segment that can move or be moved from one site in the genome to another.

transposase /trans′pəzās/, (in molecular genetics) an enzyme involved in the movement of a DNA fragment or segment from one site in the genome to another.

transposition, **1.** an abnormality occuring during embryonic development in which a part of the body normally on the left is found on the right or vice versa. **2.** the shifting of genetic material from one chromosome to another at some point in the reproductive process, often resulting in a congenital anomaly. –**transpose,** *v.*

transposition of the great vessels, a congenital cardiac anomaly in which the pulmonary artery arises from the left ventricle and the aorta from the right ventricle so that there is no communication between the systemic and pulmonary circulations. Life is impossible without associated cardiac defects, as septal defects or a patent ductus arteriosus, which enable the mixing of oxygenated and unoxygenated blood. The severity of the condition depends on the type and size of the associated defect. The primary symptoms are cyanosis and hypoxia, especially in infants with small septal defects, although cardiomegaly is usually evident a few weeks after birth. Signs of congestive heart failure develop rapidly, especially in infants with large ventricular septal defects. Definitive diagnosis is based on cardiac catheterization. Surgical correction of the defect is postponed, if possible, until after 6 months of age when the infant can better tolerate the procedure. Immediate palliative surgical procedures, as balloon septostomy, may be performed to decrease pulmonary vascular resistance and prevent congestive heart failure. See also **blue baby.**

transposon, a gene or a group of genes that are mobile and, like plasmids, act to transfer genetic instructions from one place to another. Transposons travel piggyback from virus to virus on bacteriophages. The genetic material is incorporated into the virus when the virus infects a bacterial cell. As the bacteria replicates itself, it also copies the genetic instructions brought by the transposon.

transseptal fiber, (in dentistry) any one of the many fibers of the gingival fiber system that extends horizontally from the supraalveolar cementum of a tooth, through the interdental attached gingiva above the septum of the alveolar bone, to the cementum of an adjacent tooth.

transtentorial herniation /trans′tentôr′ē·əl/, a bulge of brain tissue out of the cranium through the tentorial notch, caused by increased intracranial pressure. See also **tentorial herniation.**

transthermia. See **thermopenetration.**

transudate /tran′so͞odāt′/, a fluid passed through a membrane or squeezed through a tissue or into the space between the cells of a tissue. It is thin and watery and contains few blood cells or other large proteins. See also **edema.**

transudation, **1.** the passage of a substance through a membrane as a result of a difference in hydrostatic pressure. **2.** the passage of a fluid through a membrane with nearly all the solutes of the fluid remaining in solution or suspension.

transudative ascites /transyo͞o′dətiv/, an abnormal accumulation in the peritoneal cavity of a fluid that characteristically contains scant amounts of protein and cells. Ascitic fluids with protein counts of less than 2.5 g/ml are considered to be transudates. Transudative ascites is indicative of cirrhosis or congestive heart failure rather than infection, inflammation, or the presence of a tumor.

transurethral resection (TUR) /trans′yo͝orē′thrəl/, a surgical procedure through the urethra, as in transurethral prostatectomy. Compare **suprapubic.**

transverse, at right angles to the long axis of any common part, as the planes that cut the long axis of the body into upper and lower portions and are at right angles to the sagittal and frontal planes.

transverse colon, the segment of the colon that extends from the end of the ascending colon at the hepatic flexure on the right side across the midabdomen to the beginning of the descending colon at the splenic flexure on the left side.

transverse fissure, a fissure dividing the dorsal surface of the diencephalon and the ventral surface of the cerebral hemisphere. Also called **fissure of Bichat.**

transverse fracture, a fracture that occurs at right angles to the longitudinal axis of the bone involved.

transverse lie, abnormal presentation of a fetus in which the long axis of the baby's body is across the long axis of the mother's body; unless the baby turns spontaneously or is turned by means of external or internal version, vaginal delivery is impossible.

transverse ligament of the atlas, a thick, strong ligament stretched across the ring of the atlas, holding the dens against the anterior arch. As it crosses the dens, it arches cranially and caudally, forming the cruciate ligament of the atlas. The transverse ligament divides the circular opening of the atlas into posterior and anterior parts. The posterior part transmits the spinal cord and its membranes; the anterior part contains the dens.

transverse mesocolon /mez′ōkō′lən/, a broad fold of the peritoneum connecting the transverse colon to the dorsal wall of the abdomen. It is continuous with the greater omentum along the ventral surface of the transverse colon and contains between its layers the vessels that supply the transverse colon. Its two layers diverge along the anterior border of the pancreas. Compare **mesentery proper, sigmoid mesocolon.**

transverse palatine suture, the line of junction between the processes of the maxilla and the horizontal portions of the palatine bones that form the hard palate.

transverse plane, any one of the planes that cut across the body perpendicular to the sagittal and the frontal planes, dividing the body into caudal and cranial portions. Also called **cardinal horizontal plane.** Compare **frontal plane, median plane, sagittal plane.**

transverse relaxation time. See **relaxation time.**

transverse sinus, one of a pair of large venous channels in the posterior superior group of sinuses serving the dura mater. Each transverse sinus starts at the internal occipital protuberance and one, usually the right, is a direct continuation of the superior sagittal sinus, the other a continuation of the straight sinus. Each transverse sinus curves slightly to the base of the petrous portion of the temporal bone and within the margin of the tentorium. It leaves the tentorium and becomes the sigmoid sinus, which curves inferiorly and medially to the jugular foramen and ends in the internal jugular vein. The transverse sinuses are often of different size, the larger one usually formed by the superior sagittal sinus. Each transverse sinus receives the blood from the superior petrosal sinus at the base of the temporal bone; each anastomoses with the veins of the pericranium through the mastoid and the condyloid emissary veins; and each receives some of the inferior cerebral and the inferior cerebellar veins and some of the veins from the diploe. Compare **confluence of the sinuses, inferior sagittal sinus, occipital sinus, straight sinus, superior sagittal sinus.**

transversus abdominis, one of a pair of transverse abdominal muscles that are the anterolateral muscles of the abdomen, lying immediately under the obliquus internus abdominis. Arising from the inguinal ligament, the iliac crest, the thoracolumbar fascia, and the last six ribs, it inserts into the linea alba. It is innervated by branches of the seventh through the twelfth intercostal nerves and by the iliohypogastric and the ilioinguinal nerves. It serves to constrict the abdomen and, by compressing the contents, to assist in micturition, defecation, emesis, parturition, and forced expiration. Compare **obliquus externus abdominis, obliquus internus abdominis, pyramidalis, rectus abdominis.**

Tranxene, a trademark for a tranquilizer (chlorazepate dipotassium).

tranylcypromine sulfate /tran′əlsip′rəmēn/, a monoamine oxidase inhibitor that acts as an antidepressant.

■ INDICATIONS: It is prescribed in the treatment of severe reactive or endogenous mental depression.

■ CONTRAINDICATIONS: Cerebrovascular or cardiovascular diseases, paranoid schizophrenia, liver dysfunction, alcoholism, pheochromocytoma, or known hypersensitivity to this drug prohibits its use. It is not given to children under 16 years of age.

■ ADVERSE EFFECTS: Among the most serious adverse reactions are severe hypertensive episodes that can be precipitated by ingestion of foods rich in tyramine or by concurrent administration of many sympathomimetic drugs. Common side effects include headache, vertigo, dry mouth, blurred vision, and orthostatic hypotension.

trapezium /trəpē′zē·əm/, *pl.* **trapeziums, trapezia,** a carpal bone in the distal row of carpal bones. It has a deep groove on the palmar surface between the scaphoid and first metacarpal bones. The lateral surface is broad and rough for the attachment of ligaments. A deep groove in its palmar surface transmits the tendon of the flexor carpi radialis. The opponens pollicis and the abductor brevis originate on the palmar surface. The trapezium articulates with the scaphoid proximally, the first metacarpal distally, and the trapezoideum and the second metacarpal medially. Also called **greater multangular, os trapezium.**

trapezius /trəpē′zē·əs/, a large flat triangular muscle of the shoulder and upper back. It arises from the occipital bone, the ligamentum nuchae, and the spinous processes of the seventh cervical and all the thoracic vertebrae. It is innervated by the third and fourth cervical nerves and by the spinal accessory nerve. It acts to rotate the scapula, raise the shoulder, and abduct and flex the arm.

trapezoidal arch, a dental arch that has slightly less convergence than that of a tapering arch. The anterior teeth in the arch are somewhat square or abruptly rounded from tip to tip of the canines, which are at the corners of the arch.

trapezoid bone, the smallest carpal bone, located in the distal row of carpal bones between the trapezium and the capitate. It resembles a wedge with the broad end at the dorsal surface, the narrow end at the palmar surface. The trapezoid articulates with the scaphoid proximally, the second metacarpal distally, the trapezium laterally, and the capitate medially. Also called **lesser multangular bone, os trapezoideum.**

trauma /trou′mə, trô′mə/, **1.** physical injury caused by violent or disruptive action, or by the introduction into the body of a toxic substance. **2.** psychic injury resulting from a severe emotional shock. **–traumatic,** *adj.*, **traumatize,** *v.*

-trauma, a combining form meaning a 'wound or injury, psychic or physical': *arthrotrauma, barotrauma, neurotrama.*

trauma center, a service providing emergency and specialized intensive care to critically ill and injured patients.

trauma registry, a repository of data on the incidence, diagnosis, and treatment of acute trauma victims treated by emergency service personnel.

traumatic anesthesia, a total lack of normal sensation in a part of the body, resulting from injury, destruction of nerves, or interruption of nerve pathways. See also **tactile anesthesia.**

traumatic delirium, delirium after severe head injury, characterized by alertness and conciousness with disorientation, confabulation, and amnesia apparent. See also **delirium.**

traumatic fever, an elevation in body temperature secondary to mechanic trauma, particularly a crushing injury. Such fevers may last 1 or 2 days. The increased body temperature may help provide resistance to subsequent infection, and increased wound temperature may accelerate local healing.

traumatic idiocy, *obsolete.* severe mental retardation resulting from injury to the brain received at birth, during infancy, or in early childhood.

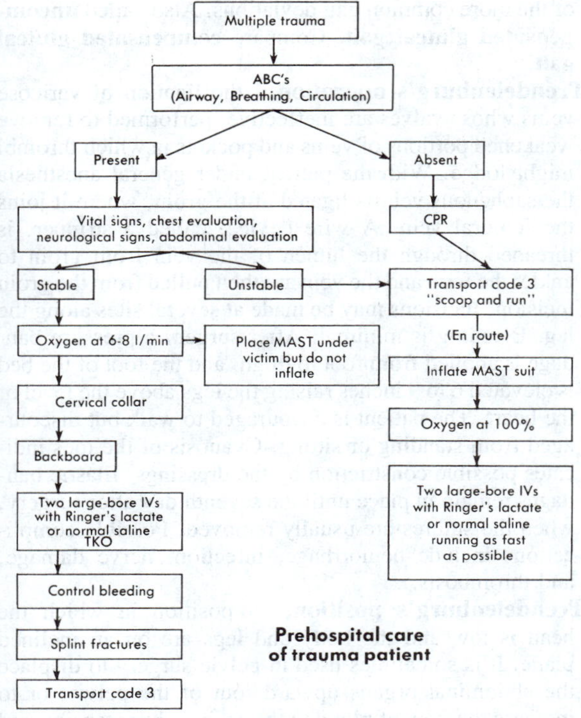

Prehospital care of trauma patient

traumatic myositis, inflammation of the muscles resulting from a wound or other trauma.

traumatic neuroma, a tangled mass of nerve elements and fibrous tissue produced by the proliferation of Schwann cells and fibroblasts after severe injury to a nerve. A kind of traumatic neuroma is **amputation neuroma.**

traumatic occlusion, a closure of the teeth that injures the teeth, the periodontal tissues, the residual ridge, or other oral structures.

traumato-, a combining form meaning 'pertaining to trauma, or to an injury or wound': *traumatogenic, traumatopnea, traumatopyra*.

traumatology /trô′mətol′əjē/, **1.** the study of wounds and injuries. **2.** a surgical specialty dealing with the treatment of wounds, injuries, and resulting disabilities. **–traumatologic, traumatological,** *adj.*

traumatopathy /trô′mətop′əthē/, a pathologic condition resulting from a wound or injury. **–traumatopathic,** *adj.*

traumatophilia /trô′mətōfil′ē·ə/, a psychologic state in which the individual derives unconscious pleasure from injuries and surgical operations. **–traumatophiliac,** *n.*, **traumatophilic,** *adj.*

traumatopnea /trô′mətop′nē·ə/, partial asphyxia with collapse of the patient, caused by a penetrating thoracic wound permitting air to enter the pleural space and compress the lungs.

traumatopyra /trô′mətōpī′rə/, an elevated temperature resulting from a wound or injury.

traumatotherapy, the medical, surgical, and psychologic treatment of wounds, injuries, and disabilities resulting from trauma. **–traumatotherapeutic,** *adj.*

traumatropism /trômat′rəpiz′əm/, the tendency of damaged tissue to attract microorganisms and to promote their growth, frequently causing infections after injuries, especially burns.

travail /trəvāl′/, **1.** physical or mental exertion, especially when distressful. **2.** (in obstetrics) the effort of labor and childbirth.

Travase, a trademark for a proteolytic enzyme (sutilains).

traveler's diarrhea, any of several diarrheal disorders commonly seen in people visiting regions of the world other than their own. Some strains of *Escherichia coli*, which produce a powerful exotoxin, are the common cause. Other causative organisms include *Giardia lamblia* and species of *Salmonella* and *Shigella*. Symptoms last for a few days and include abdominal cramps, nausea, vomiting, slight fever, and watery stools. Relapse is rare. Treatment depends on identification of the cause and includes rehydration with beverages containing electrolytes. Preventive measures include using pure or boiled water and beverages for drinking and brushing the teeth and eating only fruits and vegetables that have a skin or peel. Also called **Montezuma's revenge, turista.**

TRBF, abbreviation for **total renal blood flow.**

Treacher Collins' syndrome, an inherited disorder, characterized by mandibulofacial dysostosis. See also **Pierre Robin's syndrome.**

treatment, **1.** the care and management of a patient to combat, ameliorate, or prevent a disease, disder, or injury. **2.** a method of combating, ameliorating, or preventing a disease, disorder, or injury. Active or curative treatment is designed to cure; palliative treatment is directed to relieve pain and distress; prophylactic treatment is for the prevention of a disease or disorder; causal treatment focuses on the cause of a disorder; conservative treatment avoids radical measures and procedures; empiric treatment employs methods shown to be beneficial by experience; rational treatment is based on a knowledge of a disease process and the action of the measures used. Treatment may be pharmacologic, using drugs; surgical, involving operative procedures; or supportive, building the patient's strength. It may be specific for the disorder, or symptomatic to relieve symptoms without effecting a cure.

treatment room, a room in a patient care unit, usually in a hospital, in which various treatments or procedures requiring special equipment are performed, as removing sutures, draining a hematoma, packing a wound, or performing an examination.

Trecator-SC, a trademark for a tuberculostatic (ethionamide).

Trechona /trikon′ə/, a genus of spiders, family Dipluridae, the bite of which is toxic and irritating to humans.

tree, **1.** (in anatomy) an anatomic structure with branches that spread out like those of a tree, as the bronchial tree and the tracheobronchial tree. **2.** a pattern of searching for information in a computer data base, following a series of branching options from a general category to reach specific desired items while eliminating unwanted possibilities. MEDLINE and other computer data bases are organized in a ''logic tree'' pattern.

-trema, **1.** a combining form meaning a 'hole, orifice, opening': *gonotrema, helicotrema, peritrema.* **2.** a combining form meaning 'creatures possessing an opening': *Eurytrema, Monotrema, Troglotrema.*

trematode /trem′ətōd/, any species of flatworm of the class Trematoda, some of which are parasitic to humans, infecting the liver, the lungs, and the intestines. Kinds of trematodes include the organisms causing **clonorchiasis, fascioliasis, paragonimiasis,** and **schistosomiasis.** Also called **fluke.**

tremor, rhythmic, purposeless, quivering movements resulting from the involuntary alternating contraction and relaxation of opposing groups of skeletal muscles, occurring in some elderly individuals, in certain families, and in patients with various neurodegenerative disorders. Senile tremor is characterized by fine, quick movements, especially of the hands, rhythmic head nodding, and increased trembling during purposeful movements. Familial tremor, which may be hereditary, and the tremor occurring in multiple sclerosis also increase during voluntary movement and may be intensified by anxiety, excitement, and self-consciousness. The tremors of Graves' disease, alcoholism, mercury poisoning, and other toxicoses are usually less rhythmic, and the tremor in lead poisoning often affects the lips. The fine, quick, continuous tremor present in Parkinson's disease sometimes disappears during purposeful movements. Kinds of tremors are **continuous tremor** and **intention tremor.**

tremulous, pertaining to tremors, or involuntary muscular contractions.

trench fever, a self-limited infection, caused by *Rochalimaea quintana,* a rickettsial organism transmitted by body lice, characterized by weakness, fever, rash, and leg pains. It was common during World War I but is now rare. Also called **quintana fever.**

trench mouth. See **acute necrotizing gingivitis.**

Trendelenburg gait /trendel′ənbərg/, an abnormal gait associated with a weakness of the gluteus medius. The Trendelenburg gait is characterized by the dropping of the pelvis on the unaffected side of the body at the moment of heelstrike on the affected side. In this deviation, the pelvic drop during the walking cycle lasts until heelstrike on the unaffected side and is accompanied by an apparent lateral protrusion of the affected hip. The person with a Trendelenburg gait also shortens the step on the unaffected side and displays a lateral deviation of the entire trunk and the affected side during the stance phase of the affected lower limb. The Trendelenburg gait is one of the more common gait deviations. Also called **uncompensated gluteal gait.** Compare **compensated gluteal gait.**

Trendelenburg's operation, the ligation of varicose veins whose valves are ineffective, performed to remove weakened portions of veins and pockets in which thrombi might lodge. With the patient under general anesthesia the saphenous vein is ligated at the groin, where it joins the femoral vein. A wire device, called a stripper, is threaded through the lumen of the vein from groin to ankle; the wire and the vein are then pulled from the groin incision. Incisions may be made at several sites along the leg. Bleeding is minimal. After surgery a pressure bandage is applied from foot to thigh, and the foot of the bed is elevated 6 to 9 inches raising the legs above the level of the heart. The patient is encouraged to walk but discouraged from standing or sitting. Cyanosis of the toes indicates possible constriction by the dressings. Elastic bandages remain in place until the seventh day after surgery, when the sutures are usually removed. Possible complications include hemorrhage, infection, nerve damage, and thrombosis.

Trendelenburg's position, a position in which the head is low and the body and legs are on an inclined plane. It is sometimes used in pelvic surgery to displace the abdominal organs upward, out of the pelvis, or to increase the flow of blood to the brain in hypotension and shock.

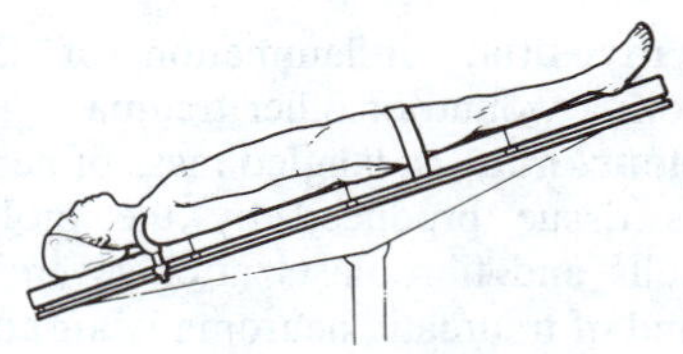

Trendelenburg's position

Trendelenburg's test, a simple test for incompetent valves in a person who has varicose veins. The person lies down and elevates the leg to empty the vein, then stands, and the vein is observed as it fills. If the valves are incompetent, the vein fills from above; if the valves are normal, they do not allow backflow of blood, and the vein fills from below.

trephine /trifīn′, trifēn′/, a circular, sawlike instrument used in removing pieces of bone or tissue, usually from the skull. Also called **trepan** /trē′pan, tripan′/.

Treponema /trep′ənē′mə/, a genus of spirochetes, including some pathogenic to humans, as the organisms causing bejel, pinta, syphilis, and yaws.

Treponema pallidum, an actively motile, slender spirochetal organism that causes syphilis.

treponematosis /trep′ənē′mətō′sis/, *pl.* **treponematoses,** any disease caused by spirochetes of the genus *Treponema.* All of these infections are effectively treated with penicillin; often one dose, given intramuscularly, results in cure. Kinds of treponematoses are **bejel, pinta, syphilis,** and **yaws.**

-tresia, a combining form meaning 'perforation': *atresia, proctotresia, sphenotresia.*

tretinoin, a keratolytic.

■ INDICATION: It is prescribed in the topical treatment of acne vulgaris.

■ CONTRAINDICATION: Known hypersensitivity to this drug prohibits its use.

■ ADVERSE EFFECTS: Among the more serious adverse reactions are red, edematous, blistered, or crusted skin.

TRF, abbreviation for **thyrotropin releasing factor.** See **thyrotropin releasing hormone.**

tri-, a combining form meaning 'three or thrice': *triage, tribrachia, tridermoma.*

triacetin /trī·as′itin/, an antifungal.

■ INDICATIONS: It is prescribed in the treatment of superficial fungus infections of the skin, including athlete's foot.

■ CONTRAINDICATIONS: There are no known contraindications.

■ ADVERSE EFFECTS: There are no known serious adverse effects.

triacetyloleandomycin. See **troleandomycin.**

triad, pertaining to a combination of three, as two parents and a child.

triage /trē·äzh′/, **1.** (in military medicine) a classification of casualties of war and other disasters according to the gravity of injuries, urgency of treatment, and place for treatment. **2.** a process in which a group of patients is sorted according to their need for care. The kind of illness or injury, the severity of the problem, and the facilities available govern the process. **3.** (in disaster medicine) a process in which a large group of patients is sorted so that care can be concentrated on those who are likely to survive.

trial forceps, an obstetric operation consisting of an attempt to deliver an infant with obstetric forceps. The forceps are applied to the baby's head, and moderate traction is applied. The delivery is continued only if the trial indicates that delivery can be accomplished safely. The procedure is abandoned if proper application of the forceps or rotation of the baby's head is not possible or if the trial indicates that completion of the delivery with forceps will require inordinately heavy traction likely to be more traumatic to mother or baby than cesarean section. Trial forceps is usually performed with a double setup so that cesarean section can be carried out immediately if necessary. Compare **failed forceps.** See also **double setup.**

triamcinolone /trī′amsin′əlōn/, a glucocorticoid.

■ INDICATIONS: It is prescribed as an antiinflammatory agent in the treatment of dermatoses, stomatitis, and lichen planus lesions.

■ CONTRAINDICATIONS: Fungal infections or known hypersensitivity to this drug prohibits its systemic use. Viral or fungal infections of the skin, impaired circulation, or known hypersensitivity to this drug prohibits its topical use.

Triage rating systems

Five-tier system (used in military triage)
Dead or will die
Life-threatening—readily correctable
Urgent—must be treated within 1 to 2 hours
Delayed—noncritical or ambulatory
No injury—no treatment necessary

Four-tier system
Immediate—seriously injured, reasonable chance of survival
Delayed—can wait for care after simple first aid
Expectant—extremely critical, moribund
Minimal—no impairment of function, can either treat self or be treated by a nonprofessional

Three-tier system
Life-threatening—readily correctable
Urgent—must be treated within 1 to 2 hours
Delayed—no injury, noncritical, or ambulatory

Two-tier system
Immediate versus delayed
Immediate—life-threatening injuries that are readily correctable on scene and those that are urgent
Delayed—no injury, noncritical injuries, ambulatory victims, moribund, and dead

■ ADVERSE EFFECTS: Among the more serious adverse reactions to the systemic administration of the drug are GI, endocrine, neurologic, fluid, and electrolyte disturbances. A variety of skin reactions may occur from topical administration of this drug.

triamterene /trī·am′tərēn/, a potassium-sparing diuretic.

■ INDICATIONS: It is usually prescribed alone or with another diuretic in the treatment of edema, hypertension, and congestive heart failure.

■ CONTRAINDICATIONS: Anuria, severe liver or kidney dysfunction, hyperkalemia, or known hypersensitivity to this drug prohibits its use.

■ ADVERSE EFFECTS: Among the most serious adverse reactions are electrolyte disturbances, particularly hyperkalemia. GI disturbances also may occur.

triangular bandage, a square of cloth folded or cut into the shape of a triangle. It may be used as a sling, a cover, or a thick pad to control bleeding.

triangular bone, the pyramidal carpal bone in the proximal row on the ulnar side of the wrist. It articulates with the lunate bone laterally, the pisiform anteriorly, the hamate distally, and with the triangular articular disk that separates it from the lower end of the ulna. Also called **cuneiform bone, os triquetrum.**

Triavil, a trademark for a central nervous system fixed-combination drug containing a phenothiazine tranquilizer (perphenazine) and a tricyclic antidepressant (amitriptyline hydrochloride).

triazolam, a hypnotic agent.

■ INDICATIONS: It is prescribed in the short-term treatment of insomnia.

■ CONTRAINDICATIONS: Known sensitivity to this drug or other benzodiazepines prohibits its use. It is not given to pregnant women, nursing mothers, or patients younger than 18 years.

■ ADVERSE EFFECTS: Among the most serious adverse reactions are anterograde amnesia, paradoxical reactions, tachycardia, depression, confusion or memory impairment, and visual disturbances.

-tribe, a combining form meaning a 'surgical instrument used to crush a body part': *cephalotribe, sphenotribe, vasotribe*.

TRIC /trik/, abbreviation for *trachoma inclusion conjunctivitis* agent, which refers to *Chlamydia trachomatis*, the organism that causes both inclusion conjunctivitis and trachoma. See also ***Chlamydia.***

tricarboxylic acid cycle. See **Krebs citric acid cycle.**

triceps brachii /trī′seps brak′ē•ī/, a large muscle that extends the entire length of the dorsal surface of the humerus. Proximally, it has a long head, a lateral head, and a medial head. The long head arises in a flattened tendon originating on the scapula; the lateral head arises from the posterior surface of the humerus, the lateral border of the humerus, and the lateral intermuscular septum; the medial head arises from the posterior body of the humerus, the medial body of the humerus, and the whole length of the medial intermuscular septum. The three portions of the muscle converge in a long tendon and insert in the posterior aspect of the olecranon. The triceps brachii is innervated by branches of the radial nerve, contains fibers from the seventh and the eighth cervical nerves, and functions to extend the forearm and to adduct the arm. Also called **triceps, triceps extensor cubiti.** Compare **biceps brachii.**

triceps reflex, a deep tendon reflex elicited by tapping sharply the triceps tendon proximal to the elbow with the forearm in a relaxed position. The response is a definite extension movement of the forearm. The reflex is accentuated by lesions of the pyramidal tract above the level of the seventh or eighth vertebra. Also called **triceps jerk.** See also **deep tendon reflex.**

triceps surae limp, an abnormal action in the walking or gait cycle, associated with a deficiency in the elevating and the propulsive factors on the affected side of the body, especially a deficiency of the triceps surae. Such a deficiency prevents the triceps surae from raising the pelvis and carrying it forward during the walking cycle. The pelvis consequently sags below its normal level and lags behind in the walking movement.

-trichia, -trichosis, **1.** a combining form meaning a 'pathologic condition of the hair': *leukotrichia, melanotrichia, sclerotrichia*. **2.** a combining form meaning a '(specified) hairiness': *glossotrichia, polytrichia*.

trichiasis /trikī′əsis/, an abnormal inversion of the eyelashes that irritates the eyeball. It usually follows infection or inflammation. Compare **ectropion.**

trichinosis /trik′inō′sis/, infestation with the parasitic roundworm *Trichinella spiralis,* transmitted by eating raw or undercooked pork or bear meat. Early symptoms of infection include abdominal pain, nausea, fever, and diarrhea; later, muscle pain, tenderness, fatigue, and eosinophilia are observed. Light infections may be asymptomatic. Also called **trichinellosis, trichiniasis.**

■ OBSERVATIONS: Encysted larvae in improperly cooked pork mature in the intestines of the host, with mature worms depositing their larvae in the intestinal wall. The larvae penetrate the intestinal mucosa and move to other parts of the body through the blood and lymphatic systems, ultimately invading skeletal muscles, especially the diaphragm and the chest muscles, where they encyst. Larval penetration of the brain or the heart may result in death. Serologic tests, skin sensitivity tests, and microscopic examination of specimens of infested muscle obtained by a biopsy often contribute to the diagnosis.

■ INTERVENTION: There is no specific treatment. Analgesics, thiabendazole, and corticosteroids may relieve symptoms. Bed rest is recommended to prevent relapse and possible death. After 2 or 3 months, the organisms are completely encysted and cause no further symptoms.

■ NURSING CONSIDERATIONS: Prevention requires cooking pork or wild game at 350° F (176° C) for 35 minutes a pound. Freezing at 10° F (−12° C) for 20 days also kills the larvae. Pork or pork products should never be eaten raw, and even smoked or salted meat may still harbor viable larvae. Routine inspection of carcasses for trichinella organisms is not performed in the United States, where the disease is on the decline.

trichlormethiazide /trī′klôrməthī′əzīd/, a thiazide diuretic and antihypertensive.

■ INDICATIONS: It is prescribed in the treatment of hypertension and edema.

■ CONTRAINDICATIONS: Anuria or known hypersensitivity to this drug, to thiazide medications, or to sulfonamide derivatives prohibits its use.

■ ADVERSE EFFECTS: Among the more serious adverse effects are hypokalemia, hyperglycemia, hyperuricemia, and various hypersensitivity reactions.

trichloroethylene /trīklôr′ō•eth′ilēn/, a general anesthetic, administered by mask with N_2O, for dentistry, minor surgery, and the first stages of labor. It is too cardiotoxic for deep anesthesia; even in light planes of anesthesia, arrhythmias may occur but may be reversed by administering oxygen and discontinuing the anesthesia. Trichloroethylene must not be given by rebreathing circuits using soda lime, because highly toxic gases may result. Its safety for use in early pregnancy has not been documented. It is contraindicated in severe cardiac disease of any kind, eclampsia, or preeclampsia and should not be combined with epinephrine.

tricho-, a combining form meaning 'pertaining to hair': *trichobezoar, trichomycosis, trichorrhea*.

trichobasalioma hyalinicum. See **cylindroma,** def. 2.

trichoepithelioma /trik′ō•ep′ithē′lē•ō′mə/, *pl.* **trichoepitheliomas, trichoepitheliomata,** a cutaneous tumor derived from the basal cells of the follicles of fine body hair. One form of trichoepithelioma is an inherited condition and usually occurs as multiple growths. Also called **acanthoma adenoides cysticum, epithelioma adenoides cysticum.**

trichoid /trik′oid/, resembling a hair.

trichologia /trik′əlō′jē•ə/, an abnormal condition in which a person pulls out his or her own hair, usually seen only in delirium.

trichomonacide, an agent destructive to *Trichomonas vaginalis,* a parasitic protozoan flagellate that causes a refractory type of vaginitis, cystitis, and urethritis. Metronidazole is used in the treatment of women with trichomoniasis and their asymptomatic partners. **–trichomonacidal,** *adj.*

Trichomonas vaginalis /trik′əmon′əs/, a motile protozoan parasite that causes vaginitis with a copious malodorous discharge and pruritus. See also **trichomoniasis.**

trichomoniasis /trik′əmənī′əsis/, a vaginal infection caused by the protozoan *Trichomonas vaginalis,* characterized by itching, burning, and frothy, pale yellow to green, malodorous vaginal discharge. With chronic infection all symptoms may disappear, although the organisms are still present. In men, infection is usually asymptomatic but may be evidenced by a persistent or recurrent urethritis. Infection is transmitted by sexual intercourse, rarely by moist washcloths or, in newborns, by passage through the birth canal. Diagnosis is by microscopic examination of fresh vaginal secretions. Treatment is by oral metronidazole. Reinfection is common if sexual partners are not treated simultaneously.

trichophytic granuloma. See **Majocchi's granuloma.**

Trichophyton /trikof′iton/, a genus of fungi that infects skin, hair, and nails. See also **dermatomycosis, dermatophyte.**

-trichosis. See **-trichia.**

trichostrongyliasis /trik′ōstron′jəlī′əsis/, infestation with *Trichostrongylus,* a genus of nematode worm. Also called **trichostrongylosis.** See also **nematode.**

Trichostrongylus /trik′ōstron′jiləs/, a genus of roundworm, some species of which are parasitic to humans, as *Trichostrongylus orientalis*. See also **trichostrongyliasis.**

trichotillomania /trik′ōtil′ōmā′nē•ə/, a morbid impulse or desire to pull out one's hair, frequently seen in cases of severe mental retardation and delirium. Also called **trichomania, hair pulling.** See also **trichologia. –trichotillomanic, trichomanic,** *adj.*

trichuriasis /trik′yŏŏrī′əsis/, infestation with the roundworm *Trichuris trichiura*. The condition is usually asymptomatic, but heavy infestation may cause nausea, abdominal pain, diarrhea, and, occasionally, anemia and rectal prolapse. It is common in tropical areas with poor sanitation. Eggs are passed in feces. Contamination of the hands, food, and water results in ingestion of the eggs that hatch in the intestines, where the adult worms embed two thirds of their length in the intestinal mucosa. The worms may live 15 to 20 years. Treatment is with mebendazole; prevention includes proper disposal of feces and good personal hygiene. Also called **trichiuriasis** /trik′ē-/.

Trichuris /trikyŏŏr′is/, a genus of parasitic roundworms of which the species *Trichuris trichiura* infects the intestinal tract. Adult worms, which are 30 to 50 mm long, resemble a whip, with a threadlike anterior and a thicker posterior. Also called **whipworm.** See also **trichuriasis.**

triclofos sodium, a sedative-hypnotic.

■ INDICATIONS: It is prescribed to treat insomnia in adults, to calm children, and to induce sleep for electroencephalography.

■ CONTRAINDICATIONS: Marked liver or kidney damage or known hypersensitivity to this drug or to chloral hydrate prohibits its use. It is not given to women in labor or to neonates.

■ ADVERSE EFFECTS: Among the most serious adverse reactions are development of drug dependence, GI disturbances, and drug hangover.

Triclos, a trademark for a sedative-hypnotic (triclofos sodium).

tricrotic pulse /trīkrot′ik/, an abnormal pulse that has three peaks of elevation on a sphygmogram, representing the pressure wave from the heart in systole followed by two pressure waves in diastole.

tricuspid /trīkus′pid/, **1.** of or pertaining to three points or cusps. **2.** of or pertaining to the tricuspid valve of the heart.

tricuspid atresia, a congenital cardiac anomaly characterized by the absence of the tricuspid valve so that there is no opening between the right atrium and right ventricle. Other cardiac defects, as atrial and ventricular septal defects, are usually present, allowing some shunting of blood into the lungs. Clinical manifestations include severe cyanosis, dyspnea, anoxia, and signs of right-sided heart failure. Definitive diagnosis is made by cardiac catheterization, although radiographic studies usually reveal a small, underdeveloped right ventricle and large atria, giving the heart a round shape, and decreased pulmonary vascularity. Immediate palliative treatment includes pulmonary to artery anastomoses to increase blood flow to the lungs and atrial septostomy if the atrial septal defect is small. Total corrective surgery has been successful in a limited number of older children.

tricuspid stenosis. See **valvular heart disease.**

tricuspid valve, a valve with three main cusps situated between the right atrium and the right ventricle of the heart. The cusps of the tricuspid valve include the ventral, dorsal, and medial cusps. The ventral cusp is the largest, the posterior cusp the smallest. The cusps are composed of strong fibrous tissue and are anchored to the papillary muscles of the right ventricle by several tendons. As the right and the left ventricles relax during the diastole phase of the heartbeat, the tricuspid valve opens, allowing blood to flow into the ventricle. In the systole phase of the heartbeat both bloodfilled ventricles contract, pumping out their contents, while the tricuspid and mitral valves close to prevent any backflow. Also called **right atrioventricular valve.** Compare **aortic valve, mitral valve, pulmonary, valve, semilunar valve.** See also **atrioventricular valve, heart valve.**

tricyclic antidepressant. See **antidepressant.**

tricyclic compound /trīsik′lik/, a chemical substance containing three rings in the molecular structure, especially a tricyclic antidepressant drug, as imipramine, amitriptyline, doxepin, and nortriptyline, used in the treatment of reactive or endogenous depression. These drugs also have anticonvulsant, antihistaminic, anticholinergic, hypotensive, and sedative effects. See also **antidepressant.**

Tridesilon, a trademark for a glucocorticoid (desonide).

tridihexethyl chloride, an anticholinergic.

■ INDICATIONS: It is prescribed in the treatment of GI muscle spasm and to reduce gastric secretion and GI motility.

■ CONTRAINDICATIONS: Narrow-angle glaucoma, asthma, obstruction of the genitourinary or GI tract, severe ulcerative colitis, or known hypersensitivity to this drug prohibits its use.

■ ADVERSE EFFECTS: Among the more serious adverse effects are blurred vision, tachycardia, dry mouth, decreased sweating, and hypersensitivity reactions. It may cause prostatic hypertrophy in elderly men.

Tridione, a trademark for an anticonvulsant (trimethadione).

triethanolamine polypeptide oleate-condensate, a ceruminolytic agent prescribed to reduce excessive earwax, used as a solution in propylene glycol. A possible serious adverse effect is severe contact dermatitis.

trifacial nerve. See **trigeminal nerve.**

trifluoperazine hydrochloride /trī′flo͞o·ōper′əzēn/, a phenothiazine tranquilizer.

■ INDICATIONS: It is prescribed in the treatment of anxiety, schizophrenia and other psychotic disorders, and as an antiemetic.

■ CONTRAINDICATIONS: Parkinson's disease, concurrent administration of central nervous system depressants, hepatic or renal dysfunction, severe hypotension, or known hypersensitivity to this drug prohibits its use.

■ ADVERSE EFFECTS: Among the more serious adverse effects are hypotension, hepatotoxicity, a variety of extrapyramidal reactions, blood dyscrasias, and hypersensitivity reactions.

trifluorothymidine /trīflo͝or′ōthī′mədēn/, an antiviral. Also called **trifluridine.**

■ INDICATIONS: It is prescribed in the treatment of keratoconjunctivitis, herpetic keratitis, and other forms of keratitis caused by herpes simplex virus.

■ CONTRAINDICATIONS: Known hypersensitivity to this drug prohibits its use. Ocular toxicity may result from continued use beyond 21 days.

■ ADVERSE EFFECTS: Among the more serious adverse effects are hypersensitivity reactions, stromal edema, and increased ocular pressure.

triflupromazine hydrochloride, a phenothiazine tranquilizer.

■ INDICATIONS: It is prescribed in the treatment of severe agitation and other psychotic disorders and for the control of severe vomiting.

■ CONTRAINDICATIONS: Parkinson's disease, concurrent administration of central nervous system depressants, liver or renal dysfunction, severe hypotension, or known hypersensitivity to this drug or to other phenothiazine medications prohibits its use.

■ ADVERSE EFFECTS: Among the more serious adverse effects are hypotension, liver toxicity, a variety of extrapyramidal reactions, blood dyscrasias, and hypersensitivity reactions.

trifluridine. See **trifluorothymidine.**

trigeminal nerve /trījem′inəl/, either of the largest pair of cranial nerves, essential for the act of chewing, general sensibility of the face, and muscular sensibility of the obliquus superior. The trigeminal nerves have sensory, motor, and intermediate roots and connect to three areas in the brain. Also called **fifth nerve, nervus trigeminus, trifacial nerve.**

trigeminal neuralgia, a neurologic condition of the trigeminal facial nerve, characterized by paroxysms of flashing, stablike pain radiating along the course of a branch of the nerve from the angle of the jaw. It is caused by degeneration of the nerve or by pressure on it. Any of the three branches of the nerve may be affected. Neuralgia of the first branch results in pain around the eyes and over the forehead; of the second branch, in pain in the upper lip, nose, and cheek; of the third branch, in pain on the side of the tongue and the lower lip. The momentary bursts of pain recur in clusters lasting many seconds; paroxysmal episodes of the pains may last for hours. Also called **prosopalgia, tic douloureux.**

trigeminal pulse, an abnormal pulse in which every third beat is absent. See also **bigeminal pulse, trigeminy.**

trigeminy /trījem′inē/, **1.** a grouping in threes. **2.** a cardiac arrhythmia characterized by the occurrence of three heartbeats, a normal beat followed by two ectopic beats in rapid succession. –**trigeminal,** *adj.*

triggered activity, rhythmic cardiac activity that results when a series of afterdepolarizations reach threshold potential.

triglyceride /trīglis′ərīd/, a compound consisting of a fatty acid (oleic, palmitic, or stearic) and glycerol. Triglycerides make up most animal and vegetable fats and are the principal lipids in the blood where they circulate, bound to a protein, forming high- and low-density lipoproteins. The total amount of triglyceride, and the amount and proportion of the kinds of lipoproteins are important in the diagnosis and treatment of many diseases and conditions including diabetes, hypertension, and heart disease. Normally the total amount of triglyceride in the blood does not exceed 200 mg to 300 mg/dl.

trigone /trī′gōn/, **1.** a triangle. **2.** the first three dominant cusps, considered collectively, of an upper molar.

trigone of the bladder. See **trigonum vesicae.**

trigonitis /trī′gənī′tis/, inflammation of the trigone of the bladder, which often accompanies urethritis.

trigonum vesicae, a triangular area of the bladder between the opening of the ureters and the orifice of the urethra. Also called **trigone of the bladder.**

trihexyphenidyl hydrochloride, an anticholinergic agent.

■ INDICATIONS: It is prescribed in the treatment of Parkinson's disease and to control drug-induced extrapyramidal reactions.

■ CONTRAINDICATIONS: Narrow-angle glaucoma, asthma, obstruction of the genitourinary or GI tract, severe ulcerative colitis, or known hypersensitivity to this drug prohibits its use.

■ ADVERSE EFFECTS: Among the more serious adverse effects are blurred vision, central nervous system effects, tachycardia, dry mouth, decreased sweating, and hypersensitivity reactions.

trihybrid, (in genetics) pertaining to or describing an individual, organism, or strain that is heterozygous for three specific traits, that is the offspring of parents differing in three specific gene pairs, or that is heterozygous for three particular characteristics or gene loci being followed.

trihybrid cross, (in genetics) the mating of two individuals, organisms, or strains that have different gene pairs that determine three specific traits or in which three particular characteristics or gene loci are being followed.

trihydric alcohol, an alcohol containing three hydroxyl groups.

triiodothyronine (T_3) /trī′ī·ō′dōthī′rənēn/, a hormone that helps regulate growth and development, helps control metabolism and body temperature, and, by a negative feedback system, acts to inhibit the secretion of thyrotropin by the pituitary. Triiodothyronine is produced mainly from the metabolism of thyroxine in the peripheral tissues but is also synthesized by and stored in the thyroid gland as an amino acid residue of the protein thyroglobulin. Triiodothyronine circulates in the plasma where it is bound mainly to thyroxine-binding globulin and thyroxine-binding prealbumin, proteins that protect the hormone from metabolism and excretion during its half-life of 2 days or less before it is degraded in the liver. The hormone acts principally by complementing thyroxine in the control of protein synthesis. It is a component of various drugs, as liotrix and liothyronine sodium, used in the treatment of hypothyroidism and simple goiter. See also **thyroid hormone.**

Trilafon, a trademark for a phenothiazine tranquilizer (perphenazine).

trilaminar blastoderm, the stage of embryonic development in which all three of the primary germ layers, the ectoderm, mesoderm, and entoderm, have formed. Compare **bilaminar blastoderm.**

trilogy of Fallot /falō′/, a congenital cardiac anomaly consisting of the combination of pulmonic stenosis, interatrial septal defect, and right ventricular hypertrophy. For discussion of diagnosis and treatment, see **tetralogy of Fallot.**

trimalleolar fracture. See **Cotton's fracture.**

trimeprazine tartrate /trīmep′rəzēn/, an antipruritic.

■ INDICATIONS: It is prescribed in the treatment of pruritis and hypersensitivity reactions of the skin.

■ CONTRAINDICATIONS: Coma, bone marrow depression, lactation, or known hypersensitivity to this drug prohibits its use. It is not given to children under 6 months of age or to patients receiving large amounts of central nervous system depressants.

■ ADVERSE EFFECTS: Among the more serious reactions are paradoxical excitement, parkinson-like problems, hepatitis, and GI disturbance.

trimester /trīmes′tər, trī′-/, one of the three periods of approximately 3 months into which pregnancy is divided. The first trimester includes the time from the first day of the last menstrual period to the end of 12 weeks. The second trimester, closer to 4 months in length than 3, extends from the twelfth to the twenty-eighth week of gestation. The third trimester begins at the twenty-eighth week and extends to the time of delivery.

trimethadione /trī′methədī′ōn/, an anticonvulsant.

■ INDICATIONS: It is prescribed to prevent seizures in petit mal epilepsy, particularly seizures that are resistant to other therapies.

■ CONTRAINDICATIONS: Severe renal or hepatic impairment, blood dyscrasias, or known hypersensitivity to this drug prohibits its use.

■ ADVERSE EFFECTS: Among the more serious adverse reactions are exfoliative dermatitis, blood dyscrasias, and aplastic anemia. Sedation and hemeralopia may occur.

trimethaphan camsylate, a ganglionic blocking agent.

■ INDICATIONS: It is prescribed to produce controlled hypotension during surgery and to lower blood pressure in hypertensive emergencies.

■ CONTRAINDICATIONS: It is not used where hypotension places a patient in undue risk or when hypersensitivity to this drug prohibits its use.

■ ADVERSE EFFECTS: The most serious adverse reaction is severe hypotension.

trimethobenzamide hydrochloride, an antiemetic.

■ INDICATION: It is prescribed for the relief of nausea and vomiting.

■ CONTRAINDICATIONS: Reye's syndrome or known hypersensitivity to this drug prohibits its use.

■ ADVERSE EFFECTS: Among the most serious adverse reactions with high doses are drowsiness, diarrhea, allergic reactions, and extrapyramidal reactions. Adverse reactions are rare at usual dosages.

trimethoprim /trīmeth′əprim/, an antibacterial.

■ INDICATIONS: It is prescribed in the treatment of various infections, particularly of the urinary tract, middle ear, and bronchi.

■ CONTRAINDICATIONS: Known hypersensitivity to this drug prohibits its use. It should not be used to treat streptococcal pharyngitis.

■ ADVERSE EFFECTS: Among the more serious adverse reactions are blood dyscrasias and allergic, GI, and central nervous system disorders.

trimethoprim and sulfamethoxazole. See **sulfamethoxazole and trimethoprim.**

trimethylene. See **cyclopropane.**

trimipramine maleate /trimip′rəmēn/, an antidepressant.

■ INDICATIONS: It is prescribed in the treatment of anxiety, depression, and insomnia.

■ CONTRAINDICATIONS: Concomitant use of a monoamine oxidase inhibitor within 14 days or known hypersensitivity to this drug prohibits its use. It is not given during recovery from myocardial infarction or to schizophrenic patients. It is not recommended for children.

■ ADVERSE EFFECTS: Among the more serious adverse reactions are tachycardia, seizures, parkinsonism, blurred vision, hypotension, and aggravation of glaucoma.

Trimox, a trademark for an antibiotic (amoxicillin trihydrate).

Trimpex, a trademark for an antibacterial (trimethoprim).

Trinsicon, a trademark for a hematinic fixed-combination drug containing iron, vitamin B_{12}, and intrinsic factor concentrate.

trioxsalen, a melanizing agent.

■ INDICATIONS: It is prescribed to enhance pigmentation, for repigmentation of the skin in idiopathic vitiligo, and to increase tolerance to sunlight.

■ CONTRAINDICATIONS: Diseases associated with photosensitivity, as porphyria, acute lupus erythematosus, or leukoderma of infectious origin, or the concomitant use of drugs having any photosensitizing activity prohibits its use.

■ ADVERSE EFFECTS: Among the most serious adverse reactions are severe burns from excessive exposure to ultraviolet light. Gastric irritation and nausea also may occur.

tripelennamine citrate. See **tripelennamine hydrochloride.**

tripelennamine hydrochloride, an antihistamine.

■ INDICATIONS: It is prescribed in the treatment of rhinitis and hypersensitivity reactions of the skin.

■ CONTRAINDICATIONS: Asthma, glaucoma, difficulty in emptying the bladder, concomitant administration of a monoamine oxidase inhibitor, or known hypersensitivity to this drug prohibits its use. It is not given to premature or newborn infants or to lactating mothers.

■ ADVERSE EFFECTS: Among the more serious adverse reactions are sedation, tachycardia, and GI upset.

triple commitment, a threefold obligation for a faculty member to teach, practice, and perform research. A triple commitment is usual for faculty appointments in schools of medicine and nursing.

triple-dye treatment, a therapy for burns in which three dyes, 6% gentian violet, 1% brilliant green, and 0.1% acriflavin base, are applied.

triple response, a triad of phenomena that occur in sequence after the intradermal injection of histamine. First, a red spot develops, spreading outward for a few millimeters, reaching its maximal size within 1 minute and then turning bluish. Next, a brighter red flush of color spreads slowly in an irregular flare around the original red spot. Finally, a wheal, filled with fluid, forms over the original spot. Also called **triple response of Lewis.**

triple sugar iron reaction, any one of several reactions seen in certain bacterial cultures growing on triple sugar iron agar, a culture medium used to aid in the identification of *Escherichia coli, Proteus, Salmonella, Shigella,* and other pathogenic enteric bacteria.

triple sulfonamides. See **trisulfapyrimidines.**

triplet, **1.** any one of three offspring born of the same gestation period during a single pregnancy. See also **Hellin's law.** **2.** (in genetics) the unit of three consecutive bases in one polynucleotide chain of DNA or RNA that codes for a specific amino acid. See also **codon, genetic code.**

triple X syndrome. See **XXX syndrome.**

triploid (3n), **1.** also **triploidic.** of or pertaining to an individual, organism, strain, or cell that has three complete sets of chromosomes, triple the normal haploid number characteristic of the species. In humans, the triploid number is 69, found in rare cases of aborted or stillborn fetuses. Of those triploid fetuses born alive, all are characterized by gross and multiple malformations; they live only for a few hours. **2.** such an individual, organism, strain, or cell. Compare **diploid, haploid, tetraploid.** See also **polyploid.**

triploidy /trip′loidē/, the state or condition of having three complete sets of chromosomes.

tripodial symmelia /trīpō′dē·əl/, a fetal anomaly characterized by the fusion of the lower extremities and the presence of three feet.

triprolidine hydrochloride, an antihistamine.

■ INDICATIONS: It is prescribed in the treatment of a variety of hypersensitivity reactions, including rhinitis, skin rash, and pruritus.

■ CONTRAINDICATIONS: Asthma or known hypersensitivity to this drug prohibits its use. It is not given to newborn infants or lactating mothers. Adverse reactions may occur in elderly patients.

■ ADVERSE EFFECTS: Drowsiness, skin rash, hypersensitivity reactions, dry mouth, and tachycardia may occur.

-tripsis, a combining form meaning a 'chafing or wearing away': *anatripsis, entripsis, syntripsis.*

-tripsy, a combining form meaning a 'crushing of a body part by a surgical instrument or other device': *basiotripsy, lithotripsy, sarcotripsy.*

trismus /triz′məs/, a prolonged tonic spasm of the muscles of the jaw. Also called *(informal)* **lockjaw.** See also **tetanus.**

trisomy /trī′səmē/, a chromosomal aberration characterized by the presence of one more than the normal number of chromosomes in a diploid complement; in humans the trisomic cell contains 47 chromosomes and is designated $2n + 1$. The additional member can join any of the normal homologous pairs, although most human trisomies involve the small chromosomes, such as those in the E or G group, or the sex chromosomes. Partial trisomy occurs when only a portion of a chromosome attaches to another. In genetic nomenclature, trisomies are indicated by the exact chromosome or karyotypic group in which the addition is made, as trisomy 13 or trisomy D. Also called **trisomia.** Compare **monosomy.** See also **aneuploidy, multipolar mitosis, trisomy syndrome.** **–trisomic,** *adj.*

trisomy C syndrome. See **trisomy 8.**

trisomy D syndrome. See **trisomy 13.**

trisomy E syndrome. See **trisomy 18.**

trisomy G syndrome. See **Down's syndrome.**

trisomy 8, a congenital condition associated with the presence of an extra chromosome 8 within the C group. Those with the condition are slender and of normal height and have a large, asymmetric head, prominent forehead, deep-set eyes, low-set prominent ears, and thick lips. There is mild to severe mental and motor retardation, often with delayed and poorly articulated speech. Skeletal anomalies and joint limitation, especially camptodactyly, may occur, and there are unusually deep palmar and plantar creases, which are diagnostically significant. Most trisomy 8 individuals are mosaic, with no abnormal or only slight clinical manifestations, or they are only partially trisomic, with part of the extra chromosome 8 missing, and show varying degrees of the clinical symptoms. In general, trisomy 8 is a less severe condition than other trisomies, especially trisomy 13 and trisomy 18, so that the mortality rate is low. Also called **trisomy C syndrome.**

trisomy 13, a congenital condition caused by the presence of an extra chromosome in the D group, predominantly chromosome 13, although in rare instances chromosome 14 or 15. It occurs in approximately 1 in 5000 births and is characterized by multiple midline anomalies and central nervous system defects, including holoprosencephaly, microcephaly, myelomeningocele, microphthalmos, and cleft lip and palate. There are also severe mental retardation, polydactyly, deafness, convulsions, and abnormalities of the heart, viscera, and genitalia. Most infants with the condition are severely affected and do not survive beyond the first 6 months of life. Also called **Patau's syndrome, trisomy D syndrome, trisomy 13-15.**

trisomy 18, a congenital condition caused by the presence of an extra chromosome 18, characterized by severe mental retardation and multiple deformities. Among the most common defects are scaphocephaly or other skull abnormalities, micrognathia, abnormal facies with low-set malformed ears and prominent occiput, cleft lip and palate, clenched fists with overlapping fingers, especially the index over the third finger, clubfeet, and syndactyly. Ventricular septal defect, patent ductus arteriosus, atrial septal defect, and renal anomalies are also common. The condition occurs in about 1 in 3000 births and predominantly in females, according to a 3:1 sex ratio, and survival for more than a few months is rare. Also called **Edwards' syndrome, trisomy E syndrome, trisomy 16-18.**

trisomy 21. See **Down's syndrome.**

trisomy 22, a congenital condition caused by the presence of an extra chromosome 22 in the G group, characterized by psychomotor retardation and various developmental anomalies. Common defects include microcephaly, micrognathia, hypotonia, hypertelorism, abnormal ears with preauricular tags or fistulas, and congenital heart disease. In partial trisomy 22, the extra chromosome is much smaller than the normal pair and causes coloboma of the iris or anal atresia, or both, as well as various other defects. See also **cat-eye syndrome.**

trisomy syndrome, any condition caused by the addition of an extra member to a normal pair of homologous autosomes or to the sex chromosomes or by the translocation of a portion of one chromosome to another. Most trisomies occur as a result of complete or partial nondisjunction of the chromosomes during cell division. The more severe conditions are related to trisomies of the autosomes rather than the sex chromosomes. The most common trisomy syndromes with clearly established clinical manifestations are trisomy 8, trisomy 13, trisomy 18, trisomy 21, and trisomy 22. See also **trisomy.**

Trisoralen, a trademark for a pigmentation agent (trioxsalen).

trisulfapyrimidines, three antibacterials in combination (sulfadiazine, sulfamerazine, and sulfamethazine), rarely prescribed today.

tritium (**^{3}H**), a low-level radioactive isotope of the hydrogen atom, used as a tracer. See also **deuterium.**

Tri-Vi-Flor, a trademark for an oral pediatric fixed-combination drug containing sodium fluoride and vitamins A, C, and D.

tRNA, abbreviation for **transfer RNA.**

Trobicin, a trademark for an antibacterial (spectinomycin hydrochloride).

trocar /trō′kär/, a sharp, pointed rod that fits inside a tube. It is used to pierce the skin and the wall of a cavity or canal in the body to aspirate fluids, to instill a medication or solution, or to guide the placement of a soft catheter. The trocar is usually removed and the catheter, tube, or instrument is left in place. See also **cannula.**

trochanter /trōkan′tər/, one of the two bony projections on the proximal end of the femur that serve for the attachment of various muscles. The two protuberances are the greater trochanter and the lesser trochanter.

troche /trō′kē/, a small oval, round, or oblong tablet containing a medicinal agent incorporated in a flavored, sweetened mucilage or fruit base that dissolves in the mouth, releasing the drug. Also called **lozenge, rotula, trochiscus.**

trochlea /trok′lē·ə/, a pulley-shaped part or structure. –**trochlear,** *adj.*

trochlear nerve, either of the smallest pair of cranial nerves, essential for eye movement and eye muscle sensibility. The trochlear nerves branch to supply the superior oblique muscle and communicate with the ophthalmic division of the trigeminal nerve, connecting with two areas in the brain. Also called **fourth nerve, nervus trochlearis.**

trochlear notch of ulna, a large depression in the ulna, formed by the olecranon and coronoid processes, that articulates with the trochlea of the humerus.

trochoid joint. See **pivot joint.**

Trocinate, a trademark for an anticholinergic (thiphenamil hydrochloride).

troleandomycin, a macrolide antibiotic.

■ INDICATIONS: It is prescribed in the treatment of certain infections, including pneumococcal pneumonia and Group A streptococcal infections of the upper respiratory tract.

■ CONTRAINDICATION: Known hypersensitivity to this drug prohibits its use.

■ ADVERSE EFFECTS: Among the more serious adverse effects are GI disturbances, mild to severe allergic reactions (including anaphylaxis), and hepatotoxicity.

trombiculosis /trombik′yo͞olō′sis/, an infestation with mites of the genus *Trombicula,* some species of which carry scrub typhus.

tromethamine, an alkalizer.

■ INDICATIONS: It is prescribed to correct acidosis, particularly metabolic acidosis in certain cardiac cases.

■ CONTRAINDICATIONS: Anuria or uremia prohibits its use. It is not given during pregnancy except in acute life-threatening situations.

■ ADVERSE EFFECTS: Among the more serious adverse reactions are hypoglycemia, respiratory depression, and local tissue damage at the site of injection.

-tron, a combining form meaning a '(specified) type of vacuum tube': *dynatron, magnetron, thyratron.*

Tronothane Hydrochloride, a trademark for a local anesthetic (pramoxine hydrochloride).

trop-, tropo-, a combining form meaning 'turn, turning' or 'tendency, affinity': *tropism, tropomyosin.* See also **tropho-,** with which this combining form is sometimes confused.

-tropal. See **-tropic.**

-trope, a combining form meaning 'influencing or influenced by': *gonadotrope, heliotrope, rheotrope.*

troph-. See **tropho-.**

-troph, 1. a combining form meaning 'that which nourishes an embryo': *embryotroph, hemotroph, histotroph.* 2. a combining form meaning an 'organism that gets nourishment from a (specified) source': *autotroph, metatroph, prototroph.*

trophectoderm. See **trophoblast.**

-trophic, a combining form meaning 'referring to a type of nutrition or nutritional requirement': *chondrotrophic, lipotrophic, viscerotrophic.*

trophic action, the stimulation of cell reproduction and enlargement, by nurturing and causing growth.

trophic fracture, a fracture resulting from the weakening of bone tissue caused by nutritional disturbances.

trophic hormones, hormones secreted by the adenohypophysis that stimulate target organs.

trophic ulcer, a decubitus ulcer caused by external trauma to a part of the body that is in poor condition resulting from disease, vascular insufficiency, or loss of afferent nerve fibers. Trophic ulcers may be painless or associated with severe causalgia. See also **decubitus ulcer.**

tropho-, troph-, a combining form meaning 'pertaining to food or nourishment': *trophoblast, trophoedema, trophoneurosis.* See also **trop-.**

trophoblast, the layer of tissue that forms the wall of the blastocyst of placental mammals in the early stages of embryonic development. It functions in the implantation of the blastocyst in the uterine wall and in supplying nutrients to the embryo. At implantation the cells differentiate into two layers, the inner cytotrophoblast, which forms the chorion, and the syncytiotrophoblast, which develops into the outer layer of the placenta. Also called **trophectoderm.** –**trophoblastic,** *adj.*

trophoblastic cancer, a malignant neoplastic disease of the uterus derived from chorionic epithelium, characterized by the production of high levels of human chorionic gonadotropin (HCG). The tumor may be an invasive hydatid mole (chorioadenoma destruens) formed by grossly enlarged, vesicular chorionic villi or a malignant uterine choriocarcinoma that arises from nonvillous chorionic epithelium. One half of the cases of choriocarcinoma follow a molar pregnancy, 25% an abortion, 22.5% a normal pregnancy, and 2.5% an ectopic pregnancy. A hydatid mole invades the myometrium and often forms extrauterine nodules that may spread to distant sites. Choriocarcinoma forms a dark red, hemorrhagic, nodular tumor on or in the uterine wall and metastasizes early in its course to the lungs, brain, liver, bones, vagina, or vulva. Initial symptoms are vaginal bleeding and a profuse, foul-smelling discharge; a persistent cough or hemoptysis signals pulmonary involvement. As the disease progresses, there may be frequent hemorrhage, weakness, and emaciation. Diagnostic measures include serial assays to determine if the HCG level in the blood is elevated and histologic examination of specimens obtained by curettage. Hysterectomy is indicated in most cases, but surgery does not eliminate the possibility of a recurrence. Chemotherapy is effective in curing a large percentage of patients with trophoblastic tumors. Single-agent chemotherapy with methotrexate or actinomycin D is recommended for low-risk patients, those with disease of less than 4 months' duration, and those with lung or vaginal metastases. Treatment of high-risk patients with more prolonged disease and liver or brain metastases is usually individualized but may include radiotherapy and a combination of methotrexate, actinomycin D, and chlorambucil. Also called **trophoblastic disease.** See also **choriocarcinoma, hydatid mole.**

trophozoite /trof′əzō′it/, an immature ameboid protozoon. Diseases in which trophozoites may be isolated by bacteriologic studies include amebic dysentery, malaria, and trichomonas vaginitis. When fully developed, a trophozite may be identified as a schizont.

-trophy, -trophia, a combining form meaning a 'condition of nutrition or growth': *cyotrophy, embryotrophy, lipotrophy*.

-tropia, a combining form meaning '(condition of) deviation in the visual axis': *cyclotropia, parectropia, talantropia*.

-tropic, -tropal, -tropous, **1.** a combining form meaning a 'turn or change in the visual axis': *anatropic, hemitropic, stereotropic*. **2.** a combining form meaning a 'tendency to have an influence on, or be influenced by': *corticotropic, pancreatropic, radiotropic*.

tropicamide, an anticholinergic mydriatic.

■ INDICATIONS: It is prescribed as a cycloplegic and mydriatic medication for diagnostic purposes in ophthalmology.

■ CONTRAINDICATIONS: Glaucoma or known hypersensitivity to this drug prohibits its use.

■ ADVERSE EFFECTS: Among the more serious adverse reactions are photophobia and tachycardia.

tropic medicine, the branch of medicine concerned with the diagnosis and treatment of diseases commonly occurring in tropic and subtropic regions of the world, generally between 30 degrees north and south of the equator.

tropic sore. See **oriental sore.**

tropic sprue, a malabsorption syndrome of unknown cause that is endemic in the tropics and subtropics. It is characterized by abnormalities in the mucosa of the small intestine resulting in protein malnutrition and multiple nutritional deficiencies, often complicated by severe infection. Symptoms include diarrhea, anorexia, and weight loss. Megaloblastic anemia may result from folic acid and vitamin B_{12} deficiency. Treatment includes administration of antibiotics, particularly tetracycline, folic acid, iron, calcium, and vitamins A, D, K, and the B complex group, as well as a balanced diet high in protein and normal in fat content. See also **nontropic sprue.**

tropic typhus. See **scrub typhus.**

-tropism. See **-tropy.**

-tropo. See **-trop.**

tropocollagen, fundamental units of collagen fibrils obtained by prolonged extraction of insoluble collagen with dilute acid.

tropomyosin, a protein component of sarcomere filaments, which, together with troponin, regulates interactions of actin and myosin in muscle contractions.

troponin, a protein in the myocardial cell ultrastructure that modulates the interaction between actin and myosin molecules. See also **tropomyosin.**

-tropous. See **-tropic.**

-tropy, -tropism, a combining form meaning 'influenced by or having an affinity for' something specified: *allotropy, ergotropy, syntropy*.

Trousseau's sign /tro͞osōz′/, a test for latent tetany in which carpal spasm is induced by inflating a sphygmomanometer cuff on the upper arm to a pressure exceeding systolic blood pressure for 3 minutes. A positive test may be seen in hypocalcemia and hypomagnesemia.

Trp, abbreviation for **tryptophan.**

true birth rate, the ratio of total births to the total female population of childbearing age, between 15 and 45 years of age. Compare **birth rate, crude birth rate, refined birth rate.**

true chondroma. See **enchondroma.**

true denticle, a calcified body, composed of irregular dentin, found in the pulp chamber of a tooth.

true dwarf. See **primordial dwarf.**

true glottis. See **glottis.**

true labor, uterine contractions that result in a change in the cervix and birth of an infant.

true neuroma, any neoplasm composed of nerve tissue.

true rib. See **rib.**

true suture, an immovable fibrous joint of the skull in which the edges of bones interlock along a series of processes and indentations. The three kinds of true sutures are the sutura dentata, the sutura limbosa, and the sutura serrata. Compare **false suture.**

true twins. See **monozygotic twins.**

true value, (in statistics) a value that is closely approximated by the definitive value and somewhat less closely by the reference value.

true vocal cord. See **vocal cord.**

truncus arteriosus, the embryonic arterial trunk that initially opens from both ventricles of the heart and later divides into the aorta and the pulmonary trunk, the two portions separated by the bulbar septum.

trunk incurvation reflex. See **Galant reflex.**

truss, an apparatus worn to prevent or retard the herniation of the intestines or other organ through an opening in the abdominal wall.

trust, a risk-taking process whereby an individual's situation depends on the future behavior of another person.

truth, a rule or statement that conforms to fact or reality.

Trypanosoma /trip′ənōsō′mə/, a genus of parasitic organisms, several species of which can cause significant diseases in humans. Most *Trypanosoma* organisms live part of their life cycle in insects and are transmitted to humans by insect bites. See also **trypanosome, trypanosomiasis.**

Trypanosoma brucei gambiense. See **Gambian trypanosomiasis.**

Trypanosoma brucei rhodesiense. See **Rhodesian trypanosomiasis.**

Trypanosoma cruzi. See **Chagas' disease.**

trypanosomal infection. See **trypanosomiasis.**

trypanosome /trip′ənōsōm′, tripan′-/, any organism of the genus *Trypanosoma.* See also **trypanosomiasis.** –**trypanosomal,** *adj.*

trypanosomiasis /trip′ənōsōmī′əsis/, an infection by an organism of the *Trypanosoma* genus. Kinds of trypanosomiasis are **African trypanosomiasis** and **Chagas' disease.**

trypanosomicide /trip′ənōsō′misīd/, a drug destructive to trypanosomes, especially the species of the protozoan parasite transmitted to humans by various insect vectors common in Africa and Central and South America. Various arsenic preparations are used to treat African sleeping sickness, caused by *Trypanosoma gambiense* and *T. rhodesiense,* and Chagas' disease, caused by *T. cruzi,* in the Americas. –**trypanosomicidal,** *adj.*

trypsin crystallized, a proteolytic enzyme from the pancreas of the ox, *Bos taurus,* that has been used as a debriding agent for open wounds and ulcers.

Tryptacin, a trademark for an amino acid (L-tryptophan), used as an antidepressant and to induce sleep.

tryptophan (Trp) /trip′təfan/, an amino acid essential for normal growth in infants and for nitrogen balance in adults. Tryptophan is the precursor of several substances, including serotonin and niacin. About 50% of the daily requirement of tryptophan is provided through the metabolism of niacin. The rest is derived from dietary protein, especially legumes, grains, and seeds. See also **amino acid, protein.**

TSEM, abbreviation for **transmission scanning electron microscopy.**

tsetse fly /tset′sē, tsē′tsē/, an insect of the genus *Glossina,* found in Africa, which carries the organisms of trypanosomiasis.

TSH, abbreviation for **thyroid stimulating hormone.**

TSH releasing factor. See **thyrotropin releasing hormone.**

TSS, abbreviation for **toxic shock syndrome.**

tsutsugamushi disease. See **scrub typhus.**

t test, a statistic test used to determine whether there are differences between two means or between a target value and a calculated mean.

TTP, abbreviation for **thrombotic thrombocytopenic purpura.**

T tube, **1.** a tubular device in the shape of a T, inserted through the skin into a cavity or a wound, used for drainage. **2.** an apparatus used to connect a source of humidified oxygen to the endotracheal tube so that a spirometer can be attached for the evaluation of tidal volume and appropriate removal of the endotracheal tube.

T tubule cholangiography, a type of biliary tract radiographic examination in which a water-soluble iodinated contrast medium is injected into the bile duct through an indwelling T-tube. The T-shaped rubber tube is inserted in the common bile duct as a routine postoperative procedure to provide drainage.

T tubule system, a system of invaginations along the surface of the myocardial cell membranes, providing an extension of the membrane into the cells. The system is believed to be a method of storing calcium ions and for the movement of substrates into the cells and the removal of metabolic end products from the cells.

tuaminoheptane /to͞o′amēnōhep′tān/, an adrenergic vasoconstrictor.

tubal abortion, a condition of pregnancy in which an embryo, ectopically implanted, is expelled from the uterine tube into the peritoneal cavity. Tubal abortion is often accompanied by significant internal bleeding causing acute abdominal and pelvic pain, but may be asymptomatic, the products of conception being resorbed. Rarely, the conceptus reimplants on the peritoneum and continues growing to become an abdominal pregnancy. See also **abdominal pregnancy, ectopic pregnancy, tubal pregnancy.**

tubal dermoid cyst, a tumor derived from embryonal tissues that develops in an oviduct.

tubal ligation, one of several sterilization procedures in which both fallopian tubes are blocked to prevent conception from occurring. Spinal or local anesthesia is used unless the procedure accompanies major surgery. Through a small abdominal incision, the fallopian tubes are ligated in two places with suture, and intervening segment is burnt, crushed, or excised. The procedure is less commonly performed vaginally. Complications of the procedure, which are rare but serious, include pulmonary embolism, hemorrhage, infection, and tubal pregnancy. The requirements for informed consent for sterilization procedures vary among states and institutions.

tubal pregnancy, an ectopic pregnancy in which the conceptus implants in the fallopian tube. Approximately 2% of all pregnancies are ectopic; of these, approximately 90% are tubal. Tubal pregnancy seldom occurs in primigravidas. The most important predisposing factor is prior tubal injury. Pelvic infection, scarring and adhesions from surgery, or IUD complications may result in damage that diminishes the motility of the tube. Transport of the ovum through the tube after fertilization is slowed, and implantation takes place before the conceptus reaches the uterine cavity. Most often the tube, which cannot long contain the growing fetus, ruptures, precipitating an intraperitoneal hemorrhage that, if not stopped, can lead rapidly to shock and, often, death. Occasionally, the conceptus does not firmly implant in the tube and is extruded from the fimbriated end of the tube as a tubal abortion. Some conceptuses apparently die and are resorbed in the tube. Diagnosis of tubal pregnancy is often difficult. With rupture of the fallopian tube, women commonly experience sudden sharp pain in one side of the lower abdomen, but signs and symptoms of tubal pregnancy are insidiously variable, and the classic triad of amenorrhea, pelvic pain, and a tender adnexal mass are present only 50% of the time. Recovery of blood from the cul-de-sac by means of culdocentesis is highly suggestive of a ruptured fallopian tube and tubal pregnancy; it requires immediate surgical exploration of the abdomen. Absence of blood on culdocentesis does not rule out the presence of an unruptured tubal pregnancy; laparoscopy or laparotomy may be required, particularly if a woman's pregnancy test is positive, the pelvic findings are suggestive, and sonography of the pelvis cannot demonstrate an intrauterine pregnancy. Because of the lethal potential of an undiagnosed tubal pregnancy, women who report any of the characteristic symptoms early in their pregnancies, particularly during the time before the existence of a normal intrauterine pregnancy can be confirmed, must be considered susceptible. In women who have a history of prior pelvic disease and in those who have symptoms or signs that are of tubal pregnancy, emergency treatment requires an immediate intravenous infusion via a large-bore intravenous catheter, type and crossmatch of blood for blood replacement, and treatment of shock as necessary. Treatment is surgical and involves laparotomy, removal of the entire products of conception and any intraperitoneal blood present, and the removal or repair of the involved tube. Conditions that predispose to a first tubal pregnancy also predispose to a second; a woman who has had one tubal pregnancy has one chance in five of having another in a subsequent pregnancy. Depending on the location of the developing embryo, the condition is classified as an ampullary, fimbrial, or interstitial tubal pregnancy.

tube, a hollow, cylindric piece of equipment or structure of the body.

tube feeding, the administration of nutritionally balanced liquefied foods through a tube inserted into the stomach or duodenum. The procedure is used after mouth or gastric surgery, in severe burns, in paralysis or obstruction of the esophagus, in severe cases of anorexia nervosa, and for unconscious patients or those unable to chew or swallow. Also called **gavage feeding, nasogastric feeding.** See also **parenteral nutrition.**

tube feeding care, the nursing care and management of a patient receiving nourishment through a nasogastric tube.

■ METHOD: The tip of a nasogastric tube is lubricated with a water-soluble lubricant, inserted into a nostril, and rapidly advanced into the stomach as the patient, if conscious, is asked to swallow hard repeatedly. Correct placement of the tube may be determined by aspirating the gastric contents, which are subsequently returned to prevent loss of electrolytes. Placement may also be checked by listening for a bubbling sound through a stethoscope placed over the stomach, as 5 ml of air is injected into the tube. If a stream of bubbles is observed when the proximal end of the tube is submerged in water or if the patient coughs forcefully when 1 or 2 ml of water is injected into the tube, it is placed in the upper respiratory tract rather than the stomach. The tube, held securely and comfortably by a tape across the nose or upper lip, may be left in place in adults and older children but usually is removed and reinserted for each feeding in infants. Before each feeding the patient is helped up to a semi-Fowler's position or is turned on the right side if unconscious. If a cuffed tracheostomy tube or endotracheal tube is in place, the cuff is inflated. The nasogastric tube is checked for proper placement and for the amount of residual formula in the stomach. Any solid medication to be given with the feeding is dissolved in water. The normal liquefied diet formula contains a mixture of milk, eggs, sugar, skim milk powder, and protein hydrolysates. A low-residue formula consists of amino acids, sugars, vitamins, and minerals. Depending on the patient's preference, the formula is at or below room temperature when administered slowly by gravity at a rate of no more than 300 ml an hour. During feeding the patient is observed for respiratory distress, nausea, vomiting, abdominal cramps, and restlessness. At the completion of the procedure, the tube is flushed with water as ordered and then clamped. The patient receives oral hygiene and lubrication and cleaning of the nares and is maintained in the same position for 30 minutes after feeding; at that time the cuff on the tracheostomy or endotracheal tube is deflated.

■ NURSING ORDERS: The nurse positions the patient for feeding, checks the tube placement, notes and replaces the amount of residual formula, and reports residual volume in excess of 100 ml. The nurse administers the feeding, ensures that the patient and family members understand the purpose of the procedure, and cautions the patient to report symptoms, as nausea, abdominal cramps, diarrhea, or constipation.

■ OUTCOME CRITERIA: A formula containing the proper proportions of protein, carbohydrate, and fat administered through a nasogastric tube can provide adequate nutrition over a short term. A high content of simple sugars may cause diarrhea. Concentrated mixtures containing too little water or large volumes administered rapidly may dehydrate the patient.

tubercle /to͞o′bərkəl/, **1.** a nodule or a small eminence, as that on a bone. **2.** a nodule, especially an elevation of the skin that is larger than a papule, as Morgagni's tubercles of the areolae of the breasts. **3.** a small rounded nodule produced by infection with *Mycobacterium tuberculosis,* consisting of a gray translucent mass of small spheric cells surrounded by connective cells.

tubercles of Montgomery, small papillae on the surface of nipples and aerolas that secrete a fatty lubricating substance.

tuberculin. See **tuberculin test, tuberculosis.**

tuberculin purified protein derivative /to͞obur′-kyo͞olin/, a solution containing a purified protein fraction derived from isolated culture filtrates of strains of *Mycobacterium tuberculosis*. It is used as an aid in the diagnosis of tuberculosis, in the Mantoux test and, for the same purpose in a dried form, in multiple puncture devices. See also **Mantoux test, Tine test.**

tuberculin test, a test to determine past or present tuberculosis infection based on a positive skin reaction, using one of several methods. A purified protein derivative (PPD) of tubercle bacilli, called **tuberculin,** is introduced into the skin by scratch, puncture, or intradermal injection. If a raised, red, or hard zone forms surrounding the tuberculin test site, the person is said to be sensitive to tuberculin, and the test is read as positive. However, a negative tuberculin reaction does not rule out a diagnosis of previous or active tuberculosis. Sputum and gastric cultures, acid-fast staining, and x-ray studies are often needed to establish a diagnosis of tuberculosis. Kinds of tuberculin tests include **Heaf test, Mantoux test, Pirquet's test,** and **tine test.**

tuberculoid leprosy. See **leprosy.**

tuberculoma /to͞obur′kyo͞olō′mə/, a rare tumorlike growth of tuberculous tissue in the central nervous system, characterized by symptoms of an expanding cerebral, cerebellar, or spinal mass. Treatment consists of the administration of antimicrobial drugs to resolve the primary growth and to prevent meningitis.

tuberculosis (TB), a chronic, granulomatous infection caused by an acid-fast bacillus, *Mycobacterium tuberculosis,* generally transmitted by the inhalation or ingestion of infected droplets and usually affecting the lungs, although infection of other organ systems by other modes of transmission occurs.

■ OBSERVATIONS: Listlessness, vague chest pain, pleurisy, anorexia, fever, and weight loss are early symptoms of pulmonary tuberculosis. Night sweats, pulmonary hemorrhage, expectoration of purulent sputum, and dyspnea develop as the disease progresses. The lung tissues react to the bacillus by producing protective cells that engulf the disease organism, forming tubercles. Untreated, the tubercles enlarge and merge to form larger tubercles that undergo caseation, eventually sloughing off into the cavities of the lungs. Hemoptysis occurs as a result of cavitary spread. Physical examination reveals apical rales, amphoric bronchial sounds, decreased respiratory excursion, and, in advanced cases, cyanosis. Laboratory examination demonstrates leukocytosis and an increased sedimentation rate, and microscopic study of a specimen of sputum stained with carbolfuchsin may be diagnostic. Culture of the tubercle bacillus is slow and requires darkness, carefully controlled temperature, and inoculation on special media. The infecting organism does not produce endotoxins or hemolysins, but **tuberculin,** a toxic substance, is released as the bacillus disintegrates. Tuberculin has no effect in people who have never been infected but produces a characteristic skin reaction when injected intradermally in people who have or have had tuberculosis. Purified protein derivative (PPD) is a stable, purified active preparation used to test for current or past infection. X-ray films of the lungs reveal infiltrates, mediastinal lymphadenopathy, caseation, pleural effusion, and calcification. Tuberculosis may spread from the lungs via the lymphatics and blood vessels; such miliary infection is characterized by tiny, seedlike tubercles in the liver, spleen, and other organs.

■ INTERVENTION: The bacillus is generally sensitive to isoniazid (INH), paraaminosalicylic acid, streptomycin, rifampin, dihydrostreptomycin, ultraviolet radiation, and heat. A combination of drugs is prescribed, with regular tests of the function of the kidneys, liver, eyes, and ears performed to discover early signs of drug toxicity. This is particularly important because drug therapy will usually continue for more than 1 year. The person is usually hospitalized for the first weeks of treatment to limit the possible spread of infection, to encourage rest and excellent nutrition, to ensure complete compliance with the prescribed drug regimen, and to observe for adverse drug effects. Samples of sputum are regularly examined. The disease is not infectious once the bacillus is no longer present in the sputum. Care of an outpatient includes continued medication, evaluation for adverse drug effects, sputum analyses, and encouragement to complete the long course of treatment. All contacts are tested periodically with PPD. People who are at increased risk of infection may be treated empirically, without a positive diagnosis having been made.

■ NURSING CONSIDERATIONS: Before discharge, the patient is taught the following: how to prevent the spread of the disease, the elements of good nutrition, the name, dose, action, and side effects of all medications prescribed, the need to take the drugs regularly, and how and where to get the next supply of drugs. Plans for follow-up are discussed; they include date, time, and place of the next laboratory tests, and a reminder that a cough, weight loss, fever, night sweats, and hemoptysis are danger signals that are to be reported immediately. See also **miliary tuberculosis, tuberculin test.**

tuberculosis vaccine. See **BCG vaccine.**

tuberculous spondylitis /to͞obur′kyələs/, a rare, grave form of tuberculosis caused by the invasion of *Mycobacterium tuberculosis* into the spinal vertebrae. The intervertebral disks may be destroyed, resulting in the collapse and wedging of affected vertebrae and the shortening and angulation of the spine. Thoracic vertebrae are more frequently involved than the vertebrae of the lumbar, the cervical, or the sacral segments of the spine. More than one area of the spine may be affected, and normal vertebrae may be evident between affected and unaffected sections. The infection characteristically dissects vertebrae anterolaterally and produces abscesses. The pressure of the abscess may cause ischemic paralysis in the subjacent spinal cord, and abscesses in the cervical area may displace or obstruct the trachea and the esophagus. Also called **Pott's disease, spinal caries.** See also **tuberculosis.**

tuberosity /to͞o′bəros′itē/, an elevation or protuberance, especially of a bone.

tuberosity of the tibia, a large oblong elevation at the proximal end of the tibia that attaches to the ligament of the patella.

tuberous carcinoma, a scirrhous carcinoma of the skin, characterized by nodular projections. Also called **carcinoma tuberosum.**

tuberous sclerosis, a familial, neurocutaneous disease characterized by epilepsy, mental deterioration, adenoma sebaceum, nodules and sclerotic patches on the cerebral cortex, retinal tumors, depigmented leaf-shaped macules on the skin, tumors of the heart or kidneys, and cerebral calcifications. There is no effective treatment. Also called **epiloia.** See also **adenoma sebaceum.**

tuberous xanthoma. See **xanthoma tuberosum.**

Tubex unit, a trademark for a unit consisting of a cartridge and needle that fits into a holder that has a plunger. The cartridge may be empty or prefilled with a standard dose of a medication. The needle is covered with a rubber protective guard and is permanently attached to the cartridge. The plunger may be unscrewed to allow the cartridge needle unit to be slipped in place. The cartridge is then twisted clockwise to secure it in the holder. The plunger is replaced and screwed onto a small projection on top of a rubber diaphragm on the cartridge. As the plunger is depressed, forcing the diaphragm into the cartridge, medication is forced out through the needle. The cartridge needle unit is sterile and disposable. The holder requires no special care and is reuseable.

tubocurarine chloride, a skeletal muscle relaxant.

■ INDICATIONS: It is prescribed as an adjunct to anesthesia and electroshock therapy and in the diagnosis of myasthenia gravis and to aid in the treatment of patients undergoing mechanic ventilation.

■ CONTRAINDICATIONS: Asthma or known hypersensitivity to this drug prohibits its use. It should not be given to patients who cannot tolerate histamine release.

■ ADVERSE EFFECTS: Among the more serious adverse effects are hypotension, hypoxia, bronchospasm (in asthmatics), and allergic reaction. Many drugs act to increase the activity of tubocurarine.

tuboplasty, a surgical procedure in which severed or damaged fallopian tubes are repaired.

tubular necrosis, the death of cells in the small tubules of the kidneys as a result of disease or injury.

tubule /to͞o′byo͞ol/, a small tube, as one of the collecting tubules in the kidneys, the seminiferous tubules of the testes, or Henle's tubules between the distal and proximal convoluted tubules. –**tubular,** *adj.*

tuft fracture, fracture of any one of the distal phalanges.

Tuinal, a trademark for a central nervous system fixed-combination drug containing two sedative-hypnotics (amobarbital sodium and secobarbital sodium).

tularemia /to͞o′lərē′mē·ə/, an infectious disease of animals caused by the bacillus *Francisella (Pasteurella) tularensis,* which may be transmitted by insect vectors or direct contact. It is characterized in humans by fever, headache, and an ulcerated skin lesion with localized lymph node enlargement, or by eye infection, GI ulcerations, or pneumonia, depending on the site of entry and the response of the host. Treatment includes streptomycin, chloramphenicol, and tetracycline. Recovery produces lifelong immunity. A vaccine is available. Also called **deerfly fever, rabbit fever.**

-tumescence, a combining form meaning a 'swelling': *detumescence, intumescence, tumescence.*

tumor, **1.** a swelling or enlargement occurring in inflammatory conditions. **2.** also called **neoplasm.** a new growth of tissue characterized by progressive, uncontrolled proliferation of cells. The tumor may be localized or invasive, benign or malignant. A tumor may be named for its location, for its cellular makeup, or for the person who first identified it.

tumor albus, a white swelling occurring in a tuberculous bone or joint.

tumoricide /to͞omôr′isīd/, a substance capable of destroying a tumor. –**tumoricidal,** *adj.*

tumorigenesis /to͞o′mərijen′əsis/, the process of initiating and promoting the development of a tumor. Compare **carcinogenesis, oncogenesis, sarcomagenesis.** –**tumorigenic,** *adj.*

tumor marker, a substance in the body that is associated with the presence of a cancer. Some authorities contend the term is misleading because the marker molecules detected in blood or other tissue samples are not specific for cancer.

tumor registry, a repository of data drawn from medical records on the incidence of cancers and personal characteristics, treatment, and treatment outcomes of cancer patients.

tungsten (W), a metallic element. Its atomic number is 74; its atomic weight is 183.85. It has the highest melting point of all metals.

tunica, an enveloping coat or covering membrane.

tunica adventitia, the outer layer or coat of an artery or other tubular structure.

tunica intima, the membrane lining an artery.

tunica media, a muscular middle coat of an artery.

tunica vaginalis testis, the serous membrane surrounding the testis and epididymis.

tunica vasculosa bulbi. See **uvea.**

tuning fork, a small metal instrument consisting of a stem and two prongs that produces a constant pitch when either prong is struck. It is used in auditory tests of nerve function and of air and bone conduction.

tunnel vision, a defect in sight in which there is a great reduction in the peripheral field of vision, as if looking through a hollow tube or tunnel. The condition occurs in advanced chronic glaucoma.

TUR, abbreviation for **transurethral resection.**

turban tumor, a benign neoplasm consisting of multiple pink or maroon nodules that may cover the entire scalp and may also occur on the trunk and extremities. The growth is apparently familial and often recurs after excision.

turbidimetry /tur′bidim′ətrē/, measurement of the turbidity (cloudiness) of a solution or suspension in which the amount of transmitted light is quantified with a spectrophotometer or estimated by visual comparison with solutions of known turbidity.

turbidity, a condition of light scattering in a liquid resulting from the presence of suspended particles in the fluid. Turbidity varies according to the concentration of particles and their shapes and sizes.

turbinate /tur′binit/, **1.** of or pertaining to a scroll shape. **2.** the concha nasalis.

turgid /tur′jid/, swollen, hard, and congested, usually as a result of an accumulation of fluid. **–turgor,** *n.*

turgor /tur′gər/, the normal resiliency of the skin caused by the outward pressure of the cells and interstitial fluid. Dehydration results in decreased skin turgor, manifested by lax skin that, when grasped and raised between two fingers, slowly returns to a position level with the adjacent tissue. Marked edema or ascites results in increased turgor manifested by smooth, taut, shiny skin that cannot be grasped and raised. An evaluation of the turgor of the skin is an essential part of physical assessment.

turista. See **traveler's diarrhea.**

turnbuckle cast, an orthopedic device used to encase and immobilize the entire trunk, one arm to the elbow, and the opposite leg to the knee. It is constructed of plaster of paris or fiberglass and incorporates hinges as part of its design in the treatment of scoliosis. The hinges are placed at the level of the apex of the curvature. Employed for preoperative and postoperative positioning, it is used less frequently than the Risser cast. An adaptation of the turnbuckle cast is used occasionally as a hyperextension cast for the treatment of kyphosis or kyphoscoliosis. Compare **Risser cast.**

Turner's sign. See **Grey Turner's sign.**

Turner's syndrome, a chromosomal anomaly seen in about 1 in 3000 live female births, characterized by the absence of one X chromosome, congenital ovarian failure, genital hypoplasia, cardiovascular anomalies, dwarfism, short metacarpals, "shield chest," extosis of tibia, and underdeveloped breasts, uterus, and vagina. Spatial disorientation and moderate degrees of learning disorders are common. Treatment includes hormone therapy (estrogens, androgens, pituitary growth hormone) and, often, surgical correction of cardiovascular anomalies and the webbing of the neck skin. Also called **Bonnevie-Ullrich syndrome, monosomy X.** See also **Noonan's syndrome.**

turnkey, a term referring to a computer system or installation that is complete on delivery and ready to operate without modification.

turricephaly. See **oxycephaly.**

-tuse, **1.** a combining form meaning 'dull or blunt': *obtuse*. **2.** a combining form meaning 'to beat or thrust': *contuse*.

Tussionex, a trademark for a fixed-combination drug containing an antitussive (hydrocodone bitartrate) and an antihistamine (phenyltoloxamine citrate).

tutorial, of or pertaining to computer-assisted instruction in which training materials are presented and relied on to direct the student to a discovery of the correct answer.

TV, abbreviation for **tidal volume.**

TVL, abbreviation for **tenth value layer.**

T wave, the component of the cardiac cycle shown on an electrocardiogram as a short, inverted, U-shaped curve following the ST segment. It represents repolarization, from phase 3 currents of the cardiac cycle as the heart recovers from contraction and prepares to begin the cycle again with atrial depolarization during the P wave.

Tweed triangle, a triangle used as a diagnostic aid, formed by the mandibular plane, the Frankfort plane, and the long axis of the lower central incisor.

twelfth cranial nerve. See **hypoglossal nerve.**

24-hour clock system, a method of designating time by using the numeric sequence from 00 to 23 for the hours and the numbers 00 to 59 for the minutes in a daily cycle beginning with 0000 (midnight) and ending with 2359 (1 minute before the following midnight). The system provides a clear distinction between prenoon and afternoon time without requiring the designations AM and PM.

twilight sleep, *obsolete*. light anesthesia obtained by the parenteral administration of a mixture of morphine and scopolamine to reduce pain and obtund recall in childbirth.

twin, either of two offspring born of the same pregnancy and developed from either a single ovum or from two ova that were released from the ovary simultaneously and fertilized at the same time. The incidence of twin births is approximately 1 in 80 pregnancies. Kinds of twins include **conjoined twins, dizygotic twins, interlocked twins, monozygotic twins, Siamese twins,** and **unequal twins.** See also **Hellin's law.**

twin monster. See **double monster.**

twinning, **1.** the development of two or more fetuses during the same pregnancy, either spontaneously or through external intervention for experimental purposes in animals. **2.** the duplication of like structures or parts by division.

twin-wire fixed orthodontic appliance, an orthodontic appliance developed by J.E. Johnson typically employing a pair of 0.01 inch (0.25 mm) wires to form the midsection of the arch wire. It is used to correct or improve malocclusion.

two-way catheter, a catheter that has a double lumen, one channel for injection of medication or fluids and the other for removal of fluid or specimens.

tybamate /tī′bəmāt/, a minor tranquilizer.

■ INDICATIONS: It is prescribed to reduce anxiety and tension in psychoneurotic disorders.

■ CONTRAINDICATIONS: Acute intermittent porphyria or known hypersensitivity to this drug or related compounds, as carisoprodol, mebutamate, or meprobamate, prohibits its use.

■ ADVERSE EFFECTS: Among the most serious effects are

drowsiness or dizziness. Rashes and other reactions also may occur.

Tylenol, a trademark for an analgesic and antipyretic (acetaminophen).

tyloxapol /tīlok′səpôl/, a respiratory tract detergent prescribed for bronchitis, emphysema, pulmonary abscess, bronchiectasis, or atelectasis.

tympanic /timpan′ik/, of or pertaining to a structure that resonates when struck; drumlike, as a **tympanic abdomen** that resonates on percussion because the intestines are distended with gas. –**tympanum** /tim′pənəm/ (*pl.* **tympana**), *n.*

tympanic antrum, a relatively large, irregular cavity in the superior anterior portion of the mastoid process of the temporal bone, communicating with the mastoid air cells and lined by the extension of the mucous membrane of the tympanic cavity. The bony tegmen tympani separates the tympanic antrum from the middle fossa of the cranial cavity, and the lateral semicircular canal of the internal ear projects into the antrum. See also **mastoid process.**

tympanic cavity. See **middle ear.**

tympanic membrane, a thin, semitransparent membrane in the middle ear that transmits sound vibrations to the internal ear by means of the auditory ossicles. It is nearly oval in form, with a vertical diameter of about 10 mm, and separates the tympanic cavity from the bottom of the external acoustic meatus. Also called **eardrum, membrana tympani.**

tympanic reflex, the reflection of a beam of light shining on the eardrum. In a normal ear a bright, wedge-shaped reflection is seen; its apex is at the end of the malleus, and its base is at the anterior inferior margin of the eardrum. In disorders of the middle ear or eardrum, this shape may be distorted. Also called **light reflex.**

tympanoplasty /timpan′əplas′tē/, any of several operative procedures on the eardrum or ossicles of the middle ear, designed to restore or improve hearing in patients with conductive deafness. These operations may be used to repair a perforated eardrum, for otosclerosis, or dislocation or necrosis of one of the small bones of the middle ear. See also **myringoplasty.**

tympanotomy. See **myringotomy.**

tympanum. See **tympanic.**

-type, a combining form meaning a 'representative form or class': *lysotype, serotype, somatotype.*

Type A personality, a behavior pattern described by Meyer Friedman and Ray Rosenman as associated with individuals who are highly competitive and work compulsively to meet deadlines. The behavior also is associated with a higher than usual incidence of coronary heart disease.

Type B personality, a form of behavior associated by Friedman and Rosenman with persons who appear free of hostility and aggression and who lack a compulsion to meet deadlines, are not highly competitive at work and play, and have a lower risk of heart attack.

Type E personality, a term introduced by Harriet Braiker to describe professional women who fit neither Type A or Type B personality categories, but who have a marked sense of insecurity and strive to convince themselves that they are worthwhile. Type E women try to be "all things to all people," according to Braiker, and tend to suffer psychologic strain.

Type I diabetes mellitus. See **insulin-dependent diabetes mellitus.**

Type II diabetes mellitus. See **non-insulin-dependent diabetes mellitus.**

type I hyperlipidemia, a familial form of primary lipoproteinemia. A rare disease transmitted as a recessive trait, it is characterized by the accumulation of triglycerides in the bloodstream, resulting in recurrent bouts of acute pancreatitis. The symptoms begin in childhood. The disease is caused by a deficiency in the activity of an enzyme, lipoprotein lipase, that normally removes triglycerides from the blood. The accumulation of triglycerides is generally proportional to the amount of dietary fat. Treatment is primarily dietary; both saturated and unsaturated fats are restricted to amounts that produce less than 500 mg/dl of blood, evaluated after an overnight fast. Also called **exogenous hyperlipemia.**

type II hyperlipoproteinemia. See **familial hypercholesterolemia.**

type I hypersensitivity. See **anaphylactic hypersensitivity.**

type II hypersensitivity. See **cytotoxic hypersensitivity.**

type III hypersensitivity. See **immune complex hypersensitivity.**

type IV hypersensitivity. See **cell-mediated immune response.**

typhlitis /tiflī′tis/, *obsolete.* appendicitis.

typhlo-, **1.** a combining form meaning 'pertaining to the cecum': *typhlocolitis, typhlostenosis, typhlostomy.* **2.** a combining form meaning 'pertaining to blindness': *typhlolexia, typhlology, typhlosis.*

-typhoid, **1.** a combining form meaning a '(specified) form of typus': *bronchotyphoid, meningotyphoid, nephrotyphoid.* **2.** a combining form meaning 'of or resembling typhus': *antityphoid, paratyphoid, posttyphoid.*

typhoid fever, a bacterial infection usually caused by *Salmonella typhi,* transmitted by contaminated milk, water, or food and characterized by headache, delirium, cough, watery diarrhea, rash, and a high fever. Also called **enteric fever.** Compare **cholera, paratyphoid fever, salmonellosis.**

■ OBSERVATIONS: The incubation period may be as long as 60 days. Characteristic maculopapular rosy spots are scattered over the skin of the abdomen. Splenomegaly and leukopenia develop first. The diagnosis is made by bacteriologic culture of blood and stool and by a rising titer of agglutinins in Widal's test. The disease is serious and may be fatal. Complications include intestinal hemorrhage or perforation and thrombophlebitis. Some people who recover from the disease continue to be carriers and excrete the organism, spreading the disease.

■ INTERVENTION: Chloramphenicol, ampicillin, amoxicillin, and trimethoprin-sulfamethoxazole are all useful in treatment. Prolonged administration of antibiotics or cholecystectomy may eliminate the carrier state. Typhoid vaccine gives some protection but requires annual booster doses for best effect.

■ NURSING CONSIDERATIONS: To lower the temperature, sponge baths are preferred to salicylates because salicylates may cause hypothermia or hypotension. Laxatives and enemas are contraindicated because of the danger of bowel perforation. Proper disposal of human wastes is essential to prevent epidemics, and carriers should not be permitted to prepare food.

typhoid pellagra, a form of pellagra in which the symptoms also include continued high temperatures.

typhoid vaccine, a bacterial vaccine prepared from an inactivated, dried strain of *Salmonella typhi*.

■ INDICATIONS: It is prescribed for primary immunization against typhoid fever for adults and children.

■ CONTRAINDICATIONS: Acute infection or concomitant use of corticosteroids prohibits its use.

■ ADVERSE EFFECTS: Among the more serious adverse reactions are anaphylaxis and pain and inflammation at the site of injection.

typhus, any of a group of acute infectious diseases caused by various species of *Rickettsia* and usually transmitted from infected rodents to humans by the bites of lice, fleas, mites, or ticks. These diseases are all characterized by headache, chills, fever, malaise, and a maculopapular rash. Kinds of typhus are **epidemic typhus, murine typhus,** and **scrub typhus.** See also **Brill-Zinsser disease, Rocky Mountain spotted fever.**

typhus vaccine, any one of three vaccines, each of which is prepared for the different rickettsial organisms that cause epidemic typhus, murine typhus, or Brill-Zinsser disease.

■ INDICATIONS: Each of the vaccines is prescribed for immunization against a form of typhus.

■ CONTRAINDICATIONS: Acute infection, debilitating disease, concomitant use of corticosteroids, or hypersensitivity to eggs prohibits its use.

■ ADVERSE EFFECTS: Among the most serious adverse reactions are anaphylaxis and various allergic reactions. Pain at the site of injection also may occur.

-typia, a combining form meaning '(condition of) conformity to type': *atypia, ectypia, zelotypia*.

typing, the process of ascertaining the classification of a specimen of blood, tissue, or other substance. See also **blood typing, tissue typing.**

Tyr, abbreviation for **tyrosine.**

tyramine, an amino acid synthesized in the body from the essential acid tyrosine. Tyramine stimulates the release of the catecholamines epinephrine and norepinephrine. It is important that people taking monoamine oxidase inhibitors avoid the ingestion of foods and beverages containing tyramine, particularly aged cheeses and meats, bananas, yeast-containing products, and alcoholic beverages. See also **adrenergic drug, amine, catecholamine, epinephrine, norepinephrine, vasoconstriction.**

tyro-, a combining form meaning 'pertaining to cheese': *tyrogenous, tyroid, tyrometosis*.

tyroma /tīrō′mə/, *pl.* **tyromas, tyromata,** a new growth or nodule with a caseous or cheesy consistency.

tyromatosis /tī′rōmətō′sis/, a process in which necrotic tissue is broken down and degenerates to a granular, amorphous, caseous mass.

tyrosine (Tyr) /tī′rəsēn/, an amino acid synthesized in the body from the essential amino acid phenylalanine. Tyrosine is found in most proteins and is a precursor of melanin and several hormones, including epinephrine and thyroxin. See also **amino acid, hormone, melanocyte.**

tyrosinemia /tī′rōsinē′mē·ə/, **1.** also called **neonatal tyrosinemia.** a benign, transient condition of the newborn, especially premature infants, in which an excessive amount of the amino acid tyrosine is found in the blood and urine. The disorder is caused by an anomaly in amino acid metabolism, usually delayed development of the enzymes necessary to metabolize tyrosine, and is controlled by dietary measures and vitamin C therapy. The metabolic defect disappears with treatment, or it may disappear spontaneously. **2.** also called **hereditary tyrosinemia.** a hereditary disorder involving an inborn error of metabolism of the amino acid tyrosine. The condition, which is transmitted as an autosomal recessive trait, is caused by an enzyme deficiency and results in liver failure or hepatic cirrhosis, renal tubular defects that can lead to renal rickets and renal glycosuria, generalized aminoaciduria, and mental retardation. Treatment consists of a diet low in tyrosine and phenylalanine and high in doses of vitamin C. In severe cases prognosis is extremely poor, and a liver transplantation may be the only lifesaving measure.

tyrosinosis /tī′rōsinō′sis/, a rare condition resulting from a defect in amino acid metabolism and transmitted as an autosomal recessive trait. It is characterized by the excretion of an excessive amount of parahydroxyphenylpyruvic acid, an intermediate product of tyrosine, in the urine. There is no known treatment. See also **tyrosinemia.**

tyrosinurea /tī′rōsino͝or′ē·ə/, the presence of tyrosine in the urine.

Tyzine, a trademark for an alpha-adrenergic drug (tetrahydrozoline hydrochloride).

Tzanck test /tsangk/, a microscopic examination of cellular material from skin lesions to help diagnose certain vesicular diseases. The tissue is scraped from the base of a vesicle, placed on a slide, and stained with Wright's or Giemsa's stain. Multinucleated giant cells are diagnostic of herpesvirus or varicella. Typical pemphigus and other cells can also be identified.

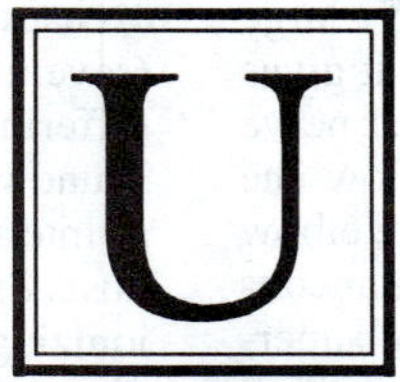

u, symbol sometimes used to stand for **micro-** (properly μ), as in "ul" or "um," representing μl or μm.

U, **1.** abbreviation for **unit.** **2.** symbol for **uranium.**

UICC, abbreviation for *International Union Against Cancer, Union internacional contra el cancer, Union internationale contre le cancer, Unio internationalis contra cancrum,* or *Unione internazionale contro il cancro.*

-ular, **1.** a combining form meaning 'pertaining to' something specified: *appendicular, molecular, pedicular.* **2.** a combining form meaning 'resembling' something specified: *circular, globular, tubular.*

ulcer, a circumscribed, craterlike lesion of the skin or mucous membrane resulting from necrosis that accompanies some inflammatory, infectious, or malignant processes. An ulcer may be shallow, involving only the epidermis, as in pemphigus, or deep, as in a rodent ulcer. Some kinds of ulcer are **decubitus ulcer, peptic ulcer,** and **serpent ulcer.** **–ulcerate,** *v.,* **ulcerative** /ul′sərā′tiv/, *adj.*

ulcerative blepharitis, a form of blepharitis in which a staphylococcal infection of the follicles of the eyelashes and glands of the eyelids results in sticky crusts forming on the lid margins. If the crusts are pulled off, the skin beneath bleeds. Tiny pustules develop in the follicles of the eyelashes and break down to form shallow ulcers. Other symptoms include burning, itching, swelling, and redness of the eyelids; a loss of eyelashes; irritation of the conjunctiva with tearing; photophobia; and gluing together of the eyelids during sleep by the dried secretions. Compare **nonulcerative blepharitis.**

ulcerative colitis, a chronic, episodic, inflammatory disease of the large intestine and rectum, characterized by profuse watery diarrhea containing varying amounts of blood, mucus, and pus. See also **Crohn's disease.**

■ OBSERVATIONS: The attacks of diarrhea are accompanied by tenesmus, severe abdominal pain, fever, chills, anemia, and weight loss. Children with the disease may suffer retarded physical growth. The debilitating symptoms often prevent persons with ulcerative colitis from carrying on the normal activities of daily living. Diagnosis of the disease is based on clinical signs, the results of barium x-ray films of the colon, and colonoscopy with biopsy. It is often difficult to differentiate between ulcerative colitis and Crohn's disease.

■ INTERVENTION: Medical treatment with corticosteroids or other antiinflammatory agents may help to control the symptoms in some persons. Those with severe disease or life-threatening complications usually require surgery. Total proctocolectomy with ileostomy is a permanent cure for ulcerative colitis.

■ NURSING CONSIDERATIONS: Some of the many systemic complications of ulcerative colitis include peripheral arthritis, ankylosing spondylitis, kidney and liver disease, and inflammation of the eyes, skin, and mouth. Persons with severe disease may develop toxic megacolon, a dangerous complication that may lead to perforation of the bowel, septicemia, and death. Ulcerative colitis also carries an increased risk of developing cancer of the colon, and periodic colonoscopy is performed to rule out this complication. A person with ulcerative colitis is suffering from a chronic, life-threatening illness and requires frequent evidence of support and understanding during prolonged hospitalization.

ule-. See **ulo-.**

-ule. See **-ulum, -ulus.**

-ulent, a combining form meaning 'full of, characterized by': *feculent, pulverulent, succulent.*

ulna, the bone on the medial or little finger side of the forearm, lying parallel with the radius. Its proximal end bulges into the olecranon and the coronoid processes and dips into the trochlear and the radial notches. The ulna articulates with the humerus and the radius. Also called **elbow bone.**

ulnar artery, a large artery branching from the brachial artery, supplying muscles in the forearm, wrist, and hand; arising near the elbow, it passes obliquely in a distal direction to become the superficial palmar arch. It has nine branches: four in the forearm, two in the wrist, and three in the hand. The forearm branches are the anterior ulnar recurrent, posterior ulnar recurrent, common interosseous, and muscular. The two branches in the wrist are the palmar carpal and dorsal carpal. The branches in the hand are the deep palmar, superficial palmar arch, and common palmar digital.

ulnar nerve, one of the terminal branches of the brachial plexus that arises on each side from the medial cord of the plexus. It receives fibers from both cervical and thoracic nerve roots and supplies the muscles and the skin on the ulnar side of the forearm and the hand. It can be easily palpated as the "funny bone" of the elbow as it courses along the groove between the olecranon process and the medial epicondyle of the humerus. It first passes medial to the axillary artery and the brachial artery to the middle of the arm, pierces the medial intermuscular septum, and follows along the medial head of the triceps to the olecranon. It descends into the forearm, and in the distal portion on the ulnar side it is covered only by the skin and the fascia. Just above the wrist it gives off a large dorsal branch and continues into the hand where it gives off the digital and the muscular branches. The ulnar nerve usually has no branches above the elbow. Below the elbow its branches are the articular branches to the elbow joint, two muscular branches, the palmar cutaneous branch, the dorsal branch, the palmar branch, the superficial branch, and the deep branch. Compare **median nerve, musculocutaneous nerve, radial nerve.**

ulo-, **1.** a combining form meaning 'pertaining to a scar or cicatrix': *ulodermatitis, uloid, ulotomy.* **2.** also **ule-.** a combining form meaning 'pertaining to the gums or gingivae': *ulocase, ulorrhagia, ulotripsis.*

ulocarcinoma /yo͞o'lōkär'sinō'mə/, *pl.* **ulocarcinomas, ulocarcinomata,** any malignant neoplastic disease of the gums that is classified as a carcinoma.

ultra-, a combining form meaning 'beyond, farther, beyond a certain limit': *ultragaseous, ultrasound, ultravirus.*

Ultracef, a trademark for a cephalosporin antibiotic (cefadroxil monohydrate).

ultracentrifuge /ul'trəsen'trifyo͞oj/, a high-speed centrifuge with a rotation rate fast enough to produce sedimentation of viruses, even in blood plasma. It is used in many kinds of biochemical analyses, including the measurement and separation of some proteins and viruses. Use of an attached microscope may make it possible to see the sediment.

ultradian, pertaining to a biorhythm that occurs in cycles of less than 24 hours.

ultrafiltrate, a solution that has passed through a special semipermeable ultrafilter membrane. It usually contains only low molecular weight solutes.

ultrafiltration, a type of filtration, sometimes conducted under pressure, through filters with very minute pores, as used by an artificial kidney. Ultrafiltration can separate large molecules from smaller molecules in body fluids.

ultra-high-speed handpiece, a device for holding rotary instruments, as drills, that permits rotational speeds of 100,000 to 300,000 rpm. It is used primarily for tooth cavity preparation.

Ultralente Iletin, a trademark for insulin zinc suspension.

ultralente insulin. See **long-acting insulin.**

ultramicroscopy. See **darkfield microscopy.**

ultrasonic cardiography. See **echocardiography.**

ultrasonography, the process of imaging deep structures of the body by measuring and recording the reflection of pulsed or continuous high-frequency sound waves. It is valuable in many medical situations, including the diagnosis of fetal abnormalities, gallstones, heart defects, and tumors. Also called **sonography.**

ultrasound, sound waves at the very high frequency of over 20,000 vibrations per second. Ultrasound has many medical applications, including fetal monitoring, imaging of internal organs, and, at an extremely high frequency, the cleaning of dental and surgical instruments.

ultrasound imaging, the use of high-frequency sound (several MHz or more) to image internal structures by the differing reflection signals produced when a beam of sound waves is projected into the body and bounces back at interfaces between those structures. Ultrasound diagnosis differs from radiologic diagnosis in that there is no ionizing radiation involved. Also called **ultrasound diagnosing.**

ultraviolet (UV), light beyond the range of human vision, at the short end of the spectrum, or that portion of the electromagnetic spectrum with wavelengths between about 10 to 400 nm. Equivalently, an ultraviolet photon has an energy between 5 and 500 eV. It occurs naturally in sunlight; it burns and tans the skin and converts precursors in the skin to vitamin D. Ultraviolet lamps are used in the control of infectious, airborne bacteria, and viruses and in the treatment of psoriasis and other skin conditions. Black light is ultraviolet light used in fluoroscopy. See also **angstrom, light, radiation, spectrum.**

ultraviolet microscopy. See **fluorescent microscopy.**

ultraviolet radiation, a range of electromagnetic waves extending from the violet or short-wavelength end of the spectrum to the beginning of the x-ray spectrum. Near-ultraviolet radiation covers a range of wavelengths from 380 to 320 mμ; middle-ultraviolet radiation covers a range from 320 to 280 mμ; and far-ultraviolet radiation extends from 280 to about 10 mμ. About 5% of the radiation from the sun is in the ultraviolet range, but little of this type of energy reaches the earth because much is absorbed by oxygen and ozone in the atmosphere. Window glass also absorbs this radiation. Artificial sources of ultraviolet radiation include the iron arc, the carbon arc, and the mercury vapor arc. For maximum transmission, quartz or fluorite envelopes, which are transparent to ultraviolet radiation, must be used instead of glass. Prisms and lenses used for work in the ultraviolet region must also be made of quartz or fluorite or of synthetic halides. In medicine, ultraviolet radiation is used in the treatment of rickets and certain skin conditions. Milk and some other foods become activated with vitamin D when exposed to this type of energy. Ultraviolet radiation also causes fluorescence and phosphorescence, a useful characteristic in such diverse applications as lighting and the identification of minerals.

-ulum, -ule, a combining form meaning 'small one': *ovulum, scutulum, speculum.*

-ulus, -ule, a combining form meaning 'small one': *homunculus, nodulus, ramulus.*

-um, a combining form marking singular nouns: *cerebellum, dextrum, quantum.*

umbilical /umbil'ikəl/, **1.** of or pertaining to the umbilicus. **2.** of or pertaining to the umbilical cord.

umbilical catheterization, a procedure in which a radiopaque catheter is passed through an umbilical artery to provide a newborn infant with parenteral fluid, to obtain blood samples, or both, or through the umbilical vein for an exchange transfusion or the emergency administration of drugs, fluids, or volume expanders.

■ METHOD: Within 1 hour of the insertion of the catheter the position of the tip is validated by x-ray examination. The infant is maintained in a neutral thermal environment as parenteral fluids are delivered by an infusion pump; the rate of flow is checked hourly, and the intravenous bottle is never allowed to empty. All connections to the umbilical line are checked every 30 to 60 minutes, and only grounded electric equipment is used on or near the infant. At hourly intervals the young patient is repositioned, and the cardiac and respiratory rates are monitored; the auxiliary temperature is taken every 2 to 3 hours, and the pedal pulses are checked every 2 to 4 hours. The condition of the cord is observed every 2 to 3 hours for signs of infection, as redness, edema, or drainage at the catheter insertion site; the intravenous tubing is retaped when required, the cord dressing is changed, and antibiotic or antiseptic ointment is applied as ordered. If the umbilical line is displaced, pressure is quickly applied to the cord with a sterile 4-by-4-inch gauze, and an associate is delegated to notify the physician immediately. Fluid intake and output are measured. The infant is observed for oliguria or anuria, signs of vasospasm, as blanching, mottling, or darkening of the legs and absence of peripheral pulses, and for evidence of sepsis, hemorrhage, or oozing from the catheter insertion site, thromboembolism, and abdominal distention and vomiting, which may indicate necrotizing enterocolitis.

■ NURSING ORDERS: The nurse provides ongoing care, monitoring the catheterized infant for any signs of complications, which are promptly reported. The family is included in the care of the infant as much as possible.

■ OUTCOME CRITERIA: Umbilical catheterization can be an effective method of administering therapeutic fluids and agents or of obtaining diagnostic blood samples from a high-risk newborn, but great care is required in inserting and monitoring the tube.

umbilical cord, a flexible structure connecting the umbilicus with the placenta in the gravid uterus and giving passage to the umbilical arteries and vein. In the newborn it is about 2 feet long and ½ inch in diameter. First formed during the fifth week of pregnancy, it contains the yolk sac and the body stalk with the enclosed allantois. Also called the **chorda umbilicalis, funiculus umbilicalis.** See also **allantois.**

umbilical duct. See **vitelline duct.**

umbilical fissure, a groove on the inferior surface of the liver that holds the ligamentum teres and separates the right and left lobes of the liver.

umbilical fistula, an abnormal passage from the umbilicus to the intestine or more frequently to the remnant of the canal in the median umbilical ligament that connects the fetal bladder with the allantois.

umbilical hernia, a soft, skin-covered protrusion of intestine and omentum through a weakness in the abdominal wall around the umbilicus. It usually closes spontaneously within 1 to 2 years, although large hernias may require surgical closure.

umbilical region, the part of the abdomen surrounding the umbilicus, in the middle zone between the right and left lateral regions. See also **abdominal regions.**

umbilical vasculitis, an inflammation of the umbilical cord and its blood vessels.

umbilical vein, one of a pair of embryonic vessels that return the blood from the placenta and fuse to form a single trunk in the body stalk. They remain separate for a short time in the embryo, opening into the sinus venosus. Development of the fetal liver breaks the connection between the umbilical veins and the sinus venosus, whereupon the right umbilical vein shrivels and disappears. The left umbilical vein remains attached to the placenta and is contained, with the fetal arteries, in the umbilical cord. After birth, the left umbilical vein and the ductus venosus atrophy and form respectively the ligamentum teres and the ligamentum venosum of the liver.

umbilical vesicle, a pear-shaped structure formed from the yolk sac at about the fourth week of prenatal development that protrudes into the cavity of the chorion and connects to the developing embryo by the yolk stalk at the region of the future midgut.

umbilicus /umbilī′kəs, umbil′ikəs/, the point on the abdomen at which the umbilical cord joined the fetal abdomen. In most adults it is marked by a depression; in some it is marked by a small protrusion of skin. It interrupts the linea alba about halfway between the infrasternal notch and the pubic symphysis. It is located at the level of the interspace of the third and the fourth lumbar vertebrae. Also called **belly button, navel.**

uncal herniation, a condition in which the medial portion of the temporal lobe protrudes over the tentorial edge as a result of increased intracranial pressure. If uncorrected, the progressive disorder causes pressure on the brainstem after first impinging on the third cranial nerve. A dilated pupil on the side of the herniation is a diagnostic sign of the disorder.

unciform bone. See **hamate bone.**

Uncinaria, a genus of nematode that causes hookworm in dogs, cats, and other carnivores.

uncompensated care, services provided by a hospital, a physician, or other health care professional for which no charge is made and for which no payment is expected.

uncompensated gluteal gait. See **Trendelenburg gait.**

uncompetitive inhibitor, an enzymatic inhibitor that appears to bond only to the enzyme substrate complex and not to free enzyme molecules.

unconditioned response, a normal, instinctive, unlearned reaction to a stimulus; one that occurs naturally and is not acquired by association and training. Also called **inborn reflex, instinctive reflex, unconditioned reflex.** Compare **conditioned response.**

unconscious, **1.** being unaware of the surrounding environment; insensible; incapable of responding to sensory stimuli. **2.** (in psychiatry) the part of the mental function in which thoughts, ideas, emotions, or memories are beyond awareness and not subject to ready recall. It contains data that have never been conscious or that were conscious at one time, usually for a brief period, and later repressed. Compare **preconscious.** See also **collective unconscious, personal unconscious.**

unconsciousness, a state of complete or partial unawareness or lack of response to sensory stimuli as a result of hypoxia, resulting from respiratory insufficiency or shock; from metabolic or chemical brain depressants, as drugs, poisons, ketones or electrolyte imbalance; or from a form of brain pathologic condition, as trauma, seizures, cerebral vasular accident, or brain tumor or infection. Various degrees of unconsciousness can occur during stupor, fugue, catalepsy, and dream states. See also **coma.**

Possible causes of unconsciousness

1. Hypoxia (decreased oxygen to brain)
   a. Respiratory insufficiency
      (1) Airway obstruction from foreign body, secretions
      (2) Pneumothorax
      (3) Spinal cord injury
   b. Shock
      (1) Cardiogenic: cardiac arrest
      (2) Hypovolemic: hemorrhage
2. Metabolic (chemical brain depressants)
   a. Extrinsic
      (1) Drugs: alcohol, narcotics, barbiturates, antihistamines, tranquilizers
      (2) Poisons: carbon monoxide, carbon tetrachloride, hydrocarbons, methane gas
   b. Intrinsic
      (1) Ketones: diabetic keroacidosis, starvation
      (2) Glucose: hypoglycemia, hyperglycemia
      (3) Ammonia: liver failure
      (4) Urea: kidney failure
      (5) Hormonal hypofunction: hypothyroidism, Addison's disease
      (6) Electrolyte imbalance: sodium, potassium, calcium, hydrogen ions
3. Brain pathologic conditions
   a. Trauma: concussion, brain stem contusion, intracranial hematoma
   b. Seizures: epilepsy, tumors, idiopathology
   c. Cerebrovascular accident: cerebral hemorrhage, thrombosis
   d. Tumors: benign, malignant
   e. Infections: meningitis, encephalitis

unction. See **ointment.**

undecylenic acid, an antifungal agent.

■ INDICATIONS: It is prescribed in the treatment of athlete's foot and ringworm.

■ CONTRAINDICATIONS: Known hypersensitivity to this drug prohibits its use. It is not used in the eyes or on mucous membranes. Caution is advised when the patient is diabetic.

■ ADVERSE EFFECTS: Among the more serious adverse effects are skin irritation and hypersensitivity reactions.

underdamping, (in cardiology) the transmission of all frequency components without a reduction in amplitude.

underdriving, a condition in artificial heart functioning in which there is insufficient compressed air during systole to eject the entire end diastolic volume of the ventricle.

underwater exercise, any physical activity performed in a pool or large tub, as a Hubbard tank, where the buoyancy of the water facilitates the movement of weak or injured muscles. See also **exercise.**

underwater seal, a seal formed by water allowed to flow over a tube that exits from the chest cavity of a patient. The water acts as a one-way valve and permits the outflow of air but denies the ingress of air. Also called **water trap.**

underweight, less than normal in body weight after adjustment for height, body build, and age.

undescended testis. See **cryptorchidism, monorchism.**

undifferentiated cell leukemia. See **stem cell leukemia.**

undifferentiated malignant lymphoma, a lymphoid neoplasm containing many large stem cells that have large nuclei, small amounts of pale cytoplasm, and borders that are not well defined. Also called **reticulosarcoma, stem cell lymphoma.**

undifferentiated schizophrenia. See **acute schizophrenia.**

undisplaced fracture, a bone break in which cracks in the osseous tissue may radiate in several directions without the separation or displacement of fragmented sections.

undoing, the performance of a specific action that is intended to negate in part a previous action or communication. According to some psychologists, undoing is related to the magical thinking of childhood.

undulant fever. See **brucellosis.**

unengaged head, the head of a floating fetus. See **engagement.** See also **ballottement.**

unequal cleavage, mitotic division of the fertilized ovum into blastomeres that are larger near the yolk portion of protoplasm, or vegetal pole, and smaller near the nucleus, or animal pole. Compare **equal cleavage.**

unequal twins, two nonjoined fetuses born of the same pregnancy in which only one of the pair is fully formed, with the other showing various degrees of developmental defects.

unfinished business, the concerns of a dying patient that require resolution before death can be accepted by the patient. Unfinished business may range from financial matters to personal relationships.

ungual phalanx. See **distal phalanx.**

unguent. See **ointment.**

unguis. See **nail.**

uni-, a combining form meaning 'one': *unibasal, uniceps, unifocal.*
uniaxial joint, a synovial joint in which movement is only in one axis, as a pivot or hinge joint.
UNICEF /yo͞o′nisef′/, abbreviation for **United Nations International Children's Emergency Fund.**
unicellular reproduction, the formation of a new organism from a female egg that has not been fertilized; parthenogenesis.
unicentric blastoma. See **blastoma.**
unidirectional block, a pathologic failure of cardiac impulse conduction in one direction while conduction is possible in the other direction.
unidose. See **unit dose.**
unification model, a theoretic framework based on the close relationship of nursing education and clinical nursing service at the University of Rochester (New York). The faculty of the school of nursing hold joint appointments to the school and the hospital, teaching nursing students and providing clinical leadership in nursing service in the hospital. See also **joint appointment.**
uniform reporting, the reporting of service and financial data by a hospital in conformance with prescribed standard definitions to permit comparisons with other health facilities.
unilateral hypertrophy, enlargement of one side or a portion of one side of the body.
unilateral long-leg spica cast, an orthopedic cast applied to immobilize one leg and the trunk of the body cranially as far as the nipple line. It is used to treat a fractured femur or for the correction or the maintenance of the correction of a hip deformity. Compare **bilateral long-leg spica cast, one-and-a-half spica cast.**
unilateral papalysis. See **hemiplegia.**
uniovular /yo͞o′nē·ov′yələr/, developing from a single ovum as in monozygotic twins as contrasted with dizygotic twins. Also **monovular.** Compare **binovular.**
uniovular twins. See **monozygotic twins.**
Unipen, a trademark for an antibacterial (nafcillin sodium).
unipolar depressive response, an affective disorder that is characterized by symptoms of depression only.
unipolar lead, **1.** an electrocardiographic conductor in which the exploring electrode is placed on the precordium or a limb while the indifferent electrode is in the central terminal. **2.** *informal.* a tracing produced by such a lead on an electrocardiograph.
unit (U), **1.** a single item. **2.** a quantity designated as a standard of measurement. **3.** an area of a hospital that is staffed and equipped for treatment of patients with a specific condition or other common characteristics.
unitary human conceptual framework, a complex theory in nursing that emphasizes the importance of holistic health care and an understanding of the human being in relation to the universal environment.
unit clerk, a person who performs routine clerical and reception tasks in a hospital inpatient care unit.
unit dose, a method of preparing medications in which individual doses of patient medications are prepared by the pharmacy and delivered in individual labeled packets to the patient's unit to be administered by the nurses on the ordered schedule. Also called **unidose.**
United Nations International Children's Emergency Fund (UNICEF) /yo͞o′nisef′/, a fund established by the General Assembly of the United Nations in 1946 to aid children in devastated areas of the world. It is funded by contributions from the member nations and acts to prevent disease, including tuberculosis, whooping cough, and diphtheria, and provides food and clothing to needy children in more than 50 countries. In 1953, UNICEF was made a permanent organization of the United Nations.
United States Pharmacopeia (USP), a compendium, recognized officially by the Federal Food, Drug, and Cosmetic Act, that contains descriptions, uses, strengths, and standards of purity for selected drugs and for all of their forms of dosage.
United States Public Health Service (USPHS), an agency of the federal government responsible for the control of the arrival from abroad of any people, goods, or substances that may affect the health of U.S. citizens. The agency sets standards for the domestic handling and processing of food and the manufacture of serums, vaccines, cosmetics, and drugs. It supports and performs research, aids localities in times of disaster and epidemics, and provides medical care for certain groups of Americans. The agency employs physicians, nurses, social workers, laboratory technicians, and many other specified health workers.
unit of service, any individual, family, aggregate, organization, or community given nursing care. The level at which service is delivered varies with the particular unit entity.
univalent /yo͞o′nivāl′ənt/, referring to a chemical valency of one, or the capacity of one atom of a chemical element to attract one atom of hydrogen or to displace one atom of hydrogen. See also **valence.**
univalent antiserum. See **antiserum.**
universal antidote, a mixture of 50% activated charcoal, 25% magnesium oxide, and 25% tannic acid, formerly thought to be useful as an antidote for most types of acid, heavy metal, alkaloid, and glycoside poisons. It is now believed that the mixture is no more effective than activated charcoal given with water.
universal donor, a person with blood of type O, Rh factor negative. Such blood may be used for emergency transfusion with minimal risk of incompatibility. See also **blood donor, blood group, transfusion.**
Unna's paste boot /o͞o′nəz/, a dressing for varicose ulcers formed by applying a layer of a gelatin-glycerin-zinc oxide paste to the leg and then a spiral bandage that is covered with successive coats of paste to produce a rigid boot.
unsaturated, **1.** describing a solution that is capable of dissolving more of the solute; not saturated. **2.** also

called **unsaturated hydrocarbon.** an organic compound in which two or more carbon atoms are united by double or triple valence bonds, as in unsaturated fatty acids. Compare **saturated.**

unsaturated alcohol, an alcohol derived from an unsaturated hydrocarbon, as an alkene or olefin.

unsaturated fatty acid, any of a number of glyceryl esters of certain organic acids in which some of the atoms are joined by double or triple valence bonds. These bonds are easily split in chemical reactions, and other substances are joined to them. Monounsaturated fatty acids have only one double or triple bond per molecule and are found in such foods as fowl, almonds, pecans, cashew nuts, peanuts, and olive oil. Polyunsaturated fatty acids have more than one double or triple bond per molecule and are found in fish, corn, walnuts, sunflower seeds, soybeans, cottonseeds, and safflower oil. Diets high in polyunsaturated fatty acids and low in saturated fatty acids have been correlated with low serum cholesterol levels in some study populations. Compare **saturated fatty acid.**

unsaturated hydrocarbon. See **unsaturated.**

unsocialized aggressive reaction, a behavior disorder of childhood characterized by overt and covert hostility, disobedience, physical and verbal aggression, vengefulness, quarrelsome behavior, and destructiveness, often manifested in acts as lying, stealing, temper tantrums, vandalism, and physical violence against others. The condition, which is more prevalent in boys than in girls, results typically from an unstable home environment that is characterized by harsh and inconsistent application of discipline, general frustration, rejection, marital discord, separation, or divorce. Punitive treatment is ineffective. Recommended psychotherapeutic techniques reinforce desirable behavioral patterns and attempt to modify unfavorable environmental conditions. If untreated, the condition may lead to antisocial personality disorder.

unstriated muscle. See **smooth muscle.**

up, referring to a condition of a computer that is serviceable or operating normally.

upper extremity suspension, an orthopedic procedure used in the treatment of bone fractures and the correction of orthopedic abnormalities of the upper limbs. The procedure uses traction equipment, including metal frames, ropes, and pulleys to relieve the weight of the upper limb involved rather than to exert traction. Upper extremity suspension is usually unilateral but may also be used bilaterally in the postoperative, posttraumatic, or postreduction control of edema. Compare **balanced suspension, hyperextension suspension, lower extremity suspension.**

upper motor neuron paralysis, an injury to or lesion in the brain or spinal cord that causes damage to the cell bodies, or axons, or both, of the upper motor neurons, which extend from the cerebral centers to the cells in the spinal column. Clinical manifestations include increased muscle tone and spasticity of the muscles involved with little or no atrophy, hyperactive deep tendon reflexes, diminished or absent superficial reflexes, the presence of pathologic reflexes, as Babinski's and Hoffmann's reflexes, and no local twitching of muscle groups. Compare **lower motor neuron paralysis.**

upper respiratory infection. See **respiratory tract infection.**

upper respiratory tract, one of the two divisions of the respiratory system. The upper respiratory tract consists of the nose, the nasal cavity, the ethmoidal air cells, the frontal sinuses, the sphenoidal sinuses, the maxillary sinus, the larynx, and the trachea. The upper respiratory tract conducts air to and from the lungs and filters and moistens and warms the air during each inspiration. Infection and irritation of the upper respiratory tract are common and often spread to the lower respiratory tract, where they may cause serious complications. See also **larynx, nose, trachea.** Compare **lower respiratory tract.**

up-time, a period during which a computer is functioning normally.

UR, abbreviation for **utilization review.**

ur-. See **uro-.**

urachus, an epithelial tube connecting the apex of the urinary bladder with the allantois. Its connective tissue forms the median umbilical ligament.

uranium (U), a heavy, radioactive metallic element. Its atomic number is 92; its atomic weight is 238.03. Uranium is the heaviest of the natural elements. Isotopes of uranium are used in nuclear power plants to provide neutrons for the nuclear reactions that result in release of energy.

urano-, a combining form meaning 'pertaining to the palate': *uranoplasty, uranoplegia, uranoschism.*

urate /yŏŏr′āt/, any salt of uric acid, as sodium urate. Urates are found in the urine, blood, and tophi or calcareous deposits in tissues. They may also be deposited as crystals in body joints. See also **gout, uric acid.**

urban typhus. See **murine typhus.**

urea /yŏŏrē′ə/, a systemic osmotic diuretic and topical keratolytic.

■ INDICATIONS: It is prescribed to reduce cerebrospinal and intraocular fluid pressure and is used topically as a keratolytic agent.

■ CONTRAINDICATIONS: Severely impaired kidney function, active intracranial bleeding, marked dehydration, or liver damage prohibits its systemic use.

■ ADVERSE EFFECTS: Among the more serious adverse reactions are pain and necrosis at the site of injection, headache, GI disturbances, and dizziness. There are no known severe reactions to topical use.

-urea, a combining form meaning a 'compound containing urea': *glycolylurea, plenylurea, solurea.*

urea cycle, a series of enzymatic reactions by which ammonia is detoxified in the liver. In the series of steps for disposing of the ammonia molecule, a waste product of protein metabolism, five enzymatic reactions occur as NH_2 radicals are combined with carbon and oxygen atoms from carbon dioxide to form urea, which is excreted. The amino acid arginine is synthesized during the same process. Also called **Krebs Henseleit cycle.**

Ureaphil, a trademark for an osmotic diuretic (urea).

Ureaplasma urealyticum, a sexually transmitted microorganism that is a common inhabitant of the urogenital systems of men and women in whom infection is asymptomatic. Neonatal death, prematurity, and perinatal morbidity are statistically associated with colonization of the chorionic surface of the placenta by *Ureaplasma urealyticum*. The mechanisms by which the unfavorable effects on pregnancy occur are not understood. There is no characteristic lesion in the fetus or newborn.

Urecholine, a trademark for a cholinergic (bethanechol chloride).

uremia /yo͞orē′mē•ə/, the presence of excessive amounts of urea and other nitrogenous waste products in the blood, as occurs in renal failure. Also called **azotemia.** See also **chronic glomerulonephritis, subacute glomerulonephritis.**

uremic frost, a pale, frostlike deposit of white crystals on the skin caused by kidney failure and uremia. Urea compounds and other waste products of metabolism that cannot be excreted by the kidneys into the urine are excreted through the small superficial capillaries into the skin, where they collect on the surface.

uremic gingivitis. See **nephritic gingivitis.**

-uret, a combining form designating a binary compound: *bromuret, phosphuret, sulphuret*.

ureter /yo͞orē′tər/, one of a pair of tubes, about 30 cm long, that carry the urine from the kidney into the bladder. They are thick-walled, vary in diameter along their length from 1 mm to 1 cm and are divided into an abdominal portion and a pelvic portion. The abdominal portion lies behind the peritoneum on the medial side of the psoas major and enters the pelvic cavity by crossing either the termination of the common iliac artery or the commencement of the external iliac artery. In men, the pelvic portion of the ureter runs caudal along the lateral wall of the pelvic cavity and reaches the lateral angle of the bladder just ventral to the upper tip of the seminal vesicle. In women, the pelvic portion of the ureter forms the posterior boundary of the ovarian fossa and runs medially and ventrally along the upper part of the vagina. The ureter enters the bladder through an oblique tunnel that functions as a valve to prevent backflow of urine into the ureter when the bladder contracts. Connecting with the kidneys, the ureters expand into funnel-shaped renal pelves that branch into calyces, each calyx containing a renal papilla. Urine draining through renal tubules drops into the papillae, passes through the calyces and the pelvis and down each ureter into the bladder. The openings of the ureters in the bladder lie at the lateral angles of the trigone, spaced about 2 cm apart when the bladder is empty, about 5 cm apart when the bladder is distended. Urine is pumped through the ureters by peristaltic waves that occur an average of three times a minute. Each ureter is composed of a fibrous, a muscular, and a mucous coat and is perfused by arterial branches of the renal, the testicular, the internal iliac, and the inferior vesical arteries. It is innervated by nerves derived from the inferior mesenteric, the testicular, and the pelvic plexi. **–ureteral** /yo͞orē′tərəl/, *adj.*

ureteral dysfunction, a disturbance of the normal peristaltic flow of urine through a ureter, resulting from dysfunction of ureteral motor nerves. See also **megaloureter.**

ureteritis /yo͞orē′tərī′tis/, an inflammatory condition of a ureter caused by infection or by the mechanic irritation of a stone.

ureterocele /yo͞orē′tərōsēl′/, a prolapse of the terminal portion of the ureter into the bladder. The condition may lead to obstruction of the flow of urine, hydronephrosis, and loss of renal function. Cystoscopy and pyelography reveal the prolapsed ureter. Surgical correction is performed to prevent permanent damage to the kidney. Compare **cystocele.**

ureterography, the radiologic imaging of a ureter, usually conducted as part of an examination of the urinary tract. The examination may involve injection of a radiopaque medium through a urinary catheter and with the aid of a ureterocystoscope (the ascending method), or by intravenous injection of a contrast medium that permits the filtering of the substance through the kidneys (the descending method) to the ureters.

ureterosigmoidostomy, a surgical procedure in which a ureter is implanted in the sigmoid flexure of the intestinal tract.

ureterotomy, an incision into a ureter.

urethra /yo͞orē′thrə/, a small tubular structure that drains urine from the bladder. In women, it is about 3 cm long and lies directly behind the symphysis pubis, anterior to the vagina. In men, it is about 20 cm long and begins at the bladder, passes through the center of the prostate gland, goes between two sheets of tissue connecting the pubic bones, and finally passes through the urinary meatus of the penis. In men, the urethra serves as a passageway for semen during ejaculation, as well as a canal for urine during voiding. See also **ureter.**

urethral /yo͞orē′thrəl/, of or pertaining to the urethra.

urethral papilla. See **papilla.**

urethritis /yo͝or′ithrī′tis/, an inflammatory condition of the urethra that is characterized by dysuria, usually the result of an infection in the bladder or kidneys. Medications, as a sulfonamide or other antibacterial, a urinary antiseptic, and an analgesic, are usually prescribed once the causative organism is identified by bacteriologic culture of a urine specimen. See also **nongonococcal urethritis.**

urethro-, a combining form meaning 'pertaining to the urethra': *urethrocele, urethrocystitis, urethrophraxis*.

urethrocele /yo͞orē′thrəsēl′/, (in women) a herniation of the urethra. It is characterized by a protusion of a segment of the urethra and the connective tissue surrounding it into the anterior wall of the vagina. The herniation may be slight and high in the vagina and only palpable on digital examination when the patient strains downward, or it may be large and low in the anterior wall with visible bulging at the vaginal introitus. A large cystocele may result in difficulty in voiding, some degree of incontinence, urinary tract infection, and dyspareunia. The condition may be congenital or acquired, secondary to obesity, parturition, and poor muscle tone. Surgical repair is the usual treatment.

urethrography, the radiologic examination of the urethra after the injection of a radiopaque agent into the urethra, usually through a catheter. The procedure may be performed as a part of a radiologic examination of the lower urinary tract.

Urex, a trademark for an antibacterial (methenamine hippurate).

-urgy, a combining form meaning the 'art of working with (specified) tools': *chemurgy, micrurgy, zymurgy.*

URI, abbreviation for **upper respiratory infection.** See **respiratory tract infection.**

-uria, **1.** a combining form meaning the 'presence of a substance in the urine': *ammoniuria, calciuria, enzymuria.* **2.** a combining form meaning '(condition of) possessing urine': *paruria, polyuria, pyuria.*

uric acid, a product of the metabolism of protein present in the blood and excreted in the urine. See also **gout, kidney, liver, purine, urine.**

uricaciduria /yŏŏr′ikas′idŏŏr′ē·ə/, a greater than normal amount of uric acid in the urine, often associated with urinary calculi or gout.

urico-, a combining form meaning 'pertaining to uric acid': *uricocholia, uricosuria, uricotelic.*

uricosuric drugs, drugs administered to relieve the pain of gout or to increase the elimination of uric acid.

urinalysis, a physical, microscopic, or chemical examination of urine. The specimen is physically examined for color, turbidity, specific gravity, and pH. Then it is spun in a centrifuge to allow collection of a small amount of sediment that is examined microscopically for blood cells, casts, crystals, pus, and bacteria. Chemical analysis may be performed for the identification and quantification of any of a large number of substances but most commonly for ketones, sugar, protein, and blood. The nurse collects the urine specimen for chemical analysis according to the directions of the specific laboratory.

urinary, of or pertaining to urine or formation of urine.

urinary bladder, the muscular membranous sac in the pelvis that stores urine for discharge through the urethra.

urinary calculus, a calculus formed in any part of the urinary tract. Calculi may be large enough to cause an obstruction in the flow of urine or small enough to be passed with the urine. Kinds of urinary calculi are **renal calculus** and **vesicle calculus.** See also **calculus.**

urinary elimination, alteration in patterns, a nursing diagnosis accepted by the Fourth National Conference on the Classification of Nursing Diagnoses. The cause of the diagnosis may involve several factors, including physical obstruction, impairment of sensory innervation or muscular function of the bladder, or mechanic trauma. Among the characteristics that define the condition are dysuria, urinary frequency, hesitancy, incontinence, nocturia, and urgency of urination. See also **nursing diagnosis.**

urinary frequency, a greater than normal frequency of the urge to void without an increase in the total daily volume of urine. The condition is characteristic of inflammation in the bladder or urethra or of diminished bladder capacity or other structural abnormalities. Burning and urgency with increased frequency herald an infection of the urinary tract. Infection requires precise diagnosis and specific antibacterial medication; structural abnormality may require surgical correction. See also **cystitis, cystocele.**

urinary hesitancy, a decrease in the force of the stream of urine, often with difficulty in beginning the flow. Hesitancy is usually the result of an obstruction or stricture between the bladder and the urethral opening; in men it may indicate an enlargement of the prostate gland, in women, stenosis of the urethral opening. Cold, stress, dehydration, and various neurogenic and psychogenic factors are common causes of this condition.

urinary incontinence, involuntary passage of urine, with the failure of voluntary control over bladder and urethral sphincters. Among the causes are neurogenic bladder dysfunction resulting from lesions of the brain and spinal cord, a neoplasm of calculus in the bladder, multiple sclerosis, obstruction of the lower urinary tract, trauma, aging, and multiparity in women. In children, incontinence may be psychogenic or the result of allergy. Treatment with medication, surgery, or psychotherapy appropriate to the underlying cause is often effective.

urinary infection. See **urinary tract infection.**

urinary meatus, the external opening of the urethra.

urinary output, the total volume of urine excreted daily, normally between 700 and 2000 ml. Various metabolic and renal diseases may change the normal urinary output, resulting in increased or decreased flow of urine. See also **anuria, oliguria, polyuria.**

urinary retention, the retention of urine in the bladder, a condition that frequently is caused by a temporary loss of muscle function.

urinary system, all of the organs involved in the secretion and elimination of urine. These include the kidneys, ureters, bladder, and urethra. See also the Color Atlas of Human Anatomy.

urinary system assessment, an evaluation of the condition and functioning of the kidneys, bladder, ureters, and urethra and an investigation of concurrent and previous disorders that may be factors in abnormalities in the urinary system.

■ METHOD: In an interview the patient is asked if dysuria, frequency or burning on urination, dribbling, a decreased urinary stream, nocturia, stress incontinence, headache, back pain, or increased thirst has occurred. The color, odor, and amount of urine voided without a catheter and with one in place are determined. The patient's vital signs, any distention of the bladder, the condition of the skin, neurologic changes, and the location, duration, and character of pain, and the presence of bladder spasms are recorded. It is determined whether or not the patient has hypertension, diabetes, a venereal disease, vaginal or urethral drainage or discharge, or a history that includes cystitis, pyelonephritis, kidney stones, prostatectomy, renal surgery, a kidney transplant, or a venereal infection. The patient's sexual activity, use of coffee, tea, cola beverages, alcohol, perfumed soaps, feminine hygiene sprays, prescribed and over-the-counter medication, and habit of bathing in a tub or shower are ascertained. A family history of polycystic kidney disease, hypertension, diabetes, or cancer is noted in the assessment, together with laboratory studies of the specific gravity, casts, protein, red and white cells in the patient's urine, and the serum creatinine level. Diagnostic procedures may include cystoscopy, excretory and intravenous urography, renal angiography, retrograde studies, and x-ray film of the kidneys, ureters, and bladder.

▪ NURSING ORDERS: The nurse interviews the patient, reports the objective data, and assembles the background information and the results of the diagnostic tests.

▪ OUTCOME CRITERIA: A comprehensive assessment of the patient's urinary system aids the urologist in establishing the diagnosis.

urinary tract, all organs and ducts involved in the secretion and elimination of urine from the body.

urinary tract infection (UTI), an infection of one or more structures in the urinary tract. Most of these infections are caused by gram-negative bacteria, most commonly *Escherichia coli* or species of *Klebsiella, Proteus, Pseudomonas,* or *Enterobacter*. The condition is more common in women than in men and may be asymptomatic. Urinary tract infection is usually characterized by urinary frequency, burning, pain with voiding, and, if the infection is severe, visible blood and pus in the urine. Diagnosis of the cause and the location of the infection is made by microscopic examination of the sediment and supernatant portion of a centrifuged urine specimen, by physical examination of the patient, by bacteriologic culture of a specimen of urine, and, if necessary, by various radiologic techniques, as retrograde pyelography, or by cystoscopy. Treatment includes antibacterial, analgesic, and urinary antiseptic drugs. Kinds of urinary tract infections include **cystitis, pyelonephritis,** and **urethritis.**

urination, the act of passing urine. Also called **micturition.**

urine, the fluid secreted by the kidneys, transported by the ureters, stored in the bladder, and voided through the urethra. Normal urine is clear, straw-colored, slightly acid, and has the characteristic odor of urea. The normal specific gravity of urine is between 1.005 and 1.03. Its normal constituents include water, urea, sodium chloride and potassium chloride, phosphates, uric acid, organic salts, and the pigment urobilin. Abnormal constituents indicative of disease include ketone bodies, protein, bacteria, blood, glucose, pus, and certain crystals. See also **bacteriuria, glycosuria, hematuria, ketoaciduria, proteinuria.**

urine osmolality, the osmotic pressure of urine. The normal values are 500 to 800 mOsm/L.

urine pH, the hydrogen ion concentration of the urine, or a measure of its acidity or alkalinity. The normal pH values for urine are 4.6 to 8.0.

urinoma /yo͝or′inō′mə/, *pl.* **urinoma, urinomatas,** a cyst filled with urine.

urinometer /yo͝or′inom′ətər/, any device for determining the specific gravity of urine, including gravitometers and hydrometers.

Urised, a trademark for a urinary fixed-combination drug containing an antibacterial (methenamine), an analgesic (phenyl salicylate), anticholinergics (atropine sulfate and hyoscyamine), an antifungal (benzoic acid), and an antiseptic (methylene blue).

Urispas, a trademark for a smooth muscle relaxant (flavoxate hydrochloride).

uro-, ur-, urono-, a combining form meaning 'pertaining to urine, the urinary tract, or urination': *urocrisia, uromancy, uropterin.*

urobilin /yo͝or′əbī′lin/, a brown pigment formed by the oxidation of urobilinogen, normally found in feces and, in small amounts, in urine.

urobilinogen /yo͝or′əbīlin′əjən/, a colorless compound formed in the intestine after the breakdown of bilirubin by bacteria. Some of this substance is excreted in feces, and some is resorbed and excreted again in bile or urine. See also **urobilin.**

Urobiotic, a trademark for a urinary fixed-combination drug containing antibacterials (oxytetracycline hydrochloride and sulfamethizole) and an analgesic (phenazopyridine hydrochloride).

urogenital /yo͝or′ōjen′itəl/, of or pertaining to the urinary and the reproductive systems. Also called **genitourinary.**

urogenital sinus, one of the elongated cavities, formed by the division of the cloaca in early embryonic development, into which open the ureter, mesonephric and paramesonephric ducts, and bladder. It also gives rise to the vestibule, urethra, and part of the vagina in the female and part of the urethra in the male.

urogenital system, the urinary and genital organs and the associated structures that develop in the fetus to form the kidneys, the ureters, the bladder, the urethra, and the genital structures of the male and female. In women these are the ovaries, the uterine tubes, the uterus, the clitoris, and the vagina. In men these are the testes, the seminal vesicles, the seminal ducts, the prostate, and the penis. Also called **genitourinary system.** See also the Color Atlas of Human Anatomy.

urogram /yo͝or′əgram′/, an x-ray film of the urinary tract, obtained by urography. See also **pyelogram.**

urography /yo͞orog′rəfē/, any of a group of x-ray techniques used to examine the urinary system. A radiopaque substance is injected, and x-ray films are taken as the substance is passed through or excreted from the part of the system being studied. Some kinds of urography are

cystoscopic urography, intravenous pyelography, and **retrograde pyelography.**

urokinase /yŏŏr′əkī′nās/, an enzyme, produced in the kidney and found in urine, that is a potent plasminogen activator of the fibrinolytic system. A pharmaceutic preparation of urokinase is administered intravenously in the treatment of pulmonary embolism.

urolithiasis. See **urinary calculus.**

urologist, a licensed physician who has completed an approved residency program and who specializes in the practice of urology.

urology, the branch of medicine concerned with the study of the anatomy and physiology, the disorders, and the care of the urinary tract in men and women and of the male genital tract.

uromelus. See **sympus monopus.**

urono-. See **uro-.**

uropathy /yŏŏrop′əthē/, any disease or abnormal condition of any structure of the urinary tract. **–uropathic,** *adj.*

uroporphyria /yŏŏr′ōpôrfir′ē·ə/, a rare, genetic disease characterized by excessive secretion of uroporphyrin in the urine, blistering dermatitis, photosensitivity, splenomegaly, and hemolytic anemia. Corticosteroid ointments may be helpful for the skin lesions; splenomegaly may be necessary to alleviate the hemolytic anemia. Most patients die from hematologic complications before middle age. See also **porphyria.**

uroporphyrin /yŏŏr′ōpôr′firin/, a porphyrin normally excreted in the urine in small amounts. See also **uroporphyria.**

urorectal septum, a ridge of mesoderm covered with endoderm that in the early developing embryo divides the endodermal cloaca into the urogenital sinus and the rectum. Also called **cloacal septum.**

ursodeoxycholic acid, a secondary bile salt. It is used in vivo to dissolve cholesterol gallstones. See also **chenodeoxycholic acid.**

urticaria /ur′tiker′ē·ə/, a pruritic skin eruption characterized by transient wheals of varying shapes and sizes with well-defined erythematous margins and pale centers, caused by capillary dilatation in the dermis that results from the release of vasoactive mediators, including histamine, kinin, and the slow, reactive substance of anaphylaxis associated with antigen-antibody reaction. Treatment includes antihistamines and removal of the stimulus or allergen. Cholinergic urticaria appears as wheals surrounded by a large axon flare. It may be caused by drugs, food, insect bites, inhalants, emotional stress, exposure to heat or cold, and exercise. Also called **hives.** See also **angioneurotic edema.** **–urticarial,** *adj.*

urticaria pigmentosa, an uncommon form of mastocytosis characterized by pigmented skin lesions that usually begin in infancy and become urticarial on mechanic or chemical irritation. Although duration of the condition is unpredictable, prognosis is good. Treatment is symptomatic and usually includes antihistamines for relief of itching. See also **mastocytosis.**

urushiol /əro͞o′shē·ôl/, a toxic resin in the sap of certain plants of the genus *Rhus,* as poison ivy, poison oak, and poison sumac, that produces allergic contact dermatitis in many people.

-us, a combining form signaling singular nouns: *echolalus, thalamus, tonus.*

USAN /yo͞o′san, yo͞o′es′ā′en′/, for *United States Adopted Names,* a list of approved drugs compiled and published by U.S. Pharmacopeial Convention, Inc.

use effectiveness, (of a contraceptive method) the actual effectiveness of a medication, device, or method in preventing pregnancy. Inconsistent use and human error usually reduce the theoretic effectiveness of any particular method of contraception. Compare **theoretic effectiveness.**

useful radiation, the portion of direct radiation that is permitted to pass from an x-ray tube housing through the tube head port, aperture, or collimator. Also called **useful beam.**

user documentation. See **documentation.**

user-friendly, pertaining to computer hardware or software designed to assist the user by presenting operating information or instructions in a form that is familiar and easy to understand.

use test, a procedure used to identify offending allergens in foods, cosmetics, or fabrics by the systematic elimination and addition of specific items associated with the life-style of the patient involved. Allergic reactions to the use test may be immediate or may be spread over a considerable period of time. Some patients undergoing the test become frustrated and discouraged, requiring regular encouragement to continue the search for sources of their allergies by this method. See also **allergy testing.**

U-shaped arch, a dental arch in which there is little difference in width between the first premolars and the last molars and the curve from canine to canine is abrupt and U-shaped.

USP. See ***United States Pharmacopeia.***

USPHS, abbreviation for **United States Public Health Service.**

uta /yo͞o′tə/, a mild cutaneous form of American leishmaniasis, occurring in the Andes of Peru and Argentina, caused by *Leishmania peruana.* The lesions are small and usually occur on the exposed surfaces of the skin, which ordinarily heal spontaneously within 1 year. The disease has been slowly disappearing because of the increased use of insecticides.

uterine anteflexion, an abnormal position of the uterus in which the uterine body is bent forward on itself at the juncture of the isthmus of the uterine cervix and the lower uterine segment.

uterine anteversion, a position of the uterus in which the body of the uterus is directed ventrally. Mild degrees of anteversion are of no clinical significance. On speculum examination of the vagina, acute anteversion of the uterus may be deduced from the location of the cervix in the posterior of the vaginal vault. Slight anteversion is the most common uterine position; on speculum examination the cervix is in the middle of the top of the vagina vault and protrudes directly downward toward the vaginal orifice.

uterine cancer, any malignancy of the uterus. It may be cervical cancer affecting the cervix or endometrial cancer affecting the lining of the body of the uterus. See also **cervical cancer, endometrial cancer.**

uterine retroflexion, a position of the uterus in which the body of the uterus is bent backward on itself at the isthmus of the cervix and the lower uterine segment. It has no clinical significance; it does not prevent conception or adversely affect pregnancy. On speculum examination of the vagina, the condition may be deduced by the location of the cervix in the anterior vaginal vault.

uterine retroversion, a position of the uterus in which the body of the uterus is directed away from the midline, toward the back. Mild degrees of retroversion are common and have no clinical significance. Severe retroversion may be accompanied by vague persistent pelvic discomfort and dyspareunia and may prevent the fitting and use of a contraceptive diaphragm. Compare **uterine anteversion.** See also **uterine retroflexion.**

uterine tenaculum. See **tenaculum.**

uterine tube. See **fallopian tube.**

uteritis. See **metritis.**

uteroglobulin. See **blastokinin.**

uteroovarian varicocele, a swelling of the veins of the pampiniform plexus of the female pelvis. Compare **ovarian varicocele, varicocele.**

uteroplacental apoplexy. See **Couvelaire uterus.**

uterovesical. See **vesicouterine.**

uterus /yo͞o′tərəs/, the hollow, pear-shaped internal female organ of reproduction in which the fertilized ovum is implanted and the fetus develops, and from which the decidua of menses flows. Its anterior surface lies on the superior surface of the bladder separated by a fold of peritoneum, the vesicouterine pouch. Its posterior surface, also covered with peritoneum, is adjacent to the sigmoid colon and some of the coils of the small intestine. The uterus is composed of three layers: the endometrium, the myometrium, and the parametrium. The endometrium lines the uterus and becomes thicker and more vascular in pregnancy and during the second half of the menstrual cycle under the influence of the hormone progesterone. The myometrium is the muscular layer of the organ. Its muscle fibers wrap around the uterus obliquely, laterally, and longitudinally. After childbirth the meshlike network of fibers contracts, creating a mass of natural ligatures that stop the flow of blood from the large blood vessels supplying the placenta. The parametrium is the outermost layer of the uterus. It is composed of serous connective tissue and extends laterally into the broad ligament. In the adult, the organ measures about 7.5 cm long and 5 cm wide at its fundus and weighs approximately 40 g. During pregnancy it is able to grow to many times its usual size, almost entirely by cellular hypertrophy. Few new cells develop. The uterus has two parts: a body and a cervix. The body extends from the fundus to the cervix, just above the isthmus. The cavity within the body is only a potential space. The walls of the body touch, unless the woman is pregnant. The cervix has a vaginal portion, protruding into the vagina, and a supravaginal portion at the juncture of the lower uterine segment. The principal ligaments of the uterus are the broad ligaments, which extend laterally from the sides of the isthmus of the cervix to the lateral wall and bottom of the pelvis; the round ligament, which crosses the pelvis between the folds of the broad ligaments; the cardinal ligament, crossing the pelvic diaphragm from the top of the cervix to the large muscles of the pelvic outlet; and the uterosacral ligament, curving back from the cervix to the sacrum around the cul-de-sac of Douglas. The body of the uterus is thus free in the abdominal cavity, fixed only at its base by the ligaments from the cervix.

uterus masculinis. See **prostatic utricle.**

UTI, abbreviation for **urinary tract infection.**

Uticillin VK, a trademark for an antibacterial (penicillin V potassium).

utilitarianism, a doctrine that the purpose of all action should be to bring about the greatest happiness for the greatest number of people and that the value of anything is determined by its utility. The philosophy is often applied in the distribution of health care resources, as in decisions regarding the expenditure of public funds for health services.

utilization review (UR), an assessment of the appropriateness and economy of an admission to a health care facility or a continued hospitalization. The length of the hospital stay is also compared with the average length of stay for similar diagnoses.

utricle /yo͞o′trikəl/, larger of two membranous pouches in the vestibule of the membranous labyrinth of the ear. It is an oblong structure that communicates with the semicircular ducts by five openings and receives utricular filaments of the acoustic nerve. Compare **saccule.**

utriculosaccular duct, a duct connecting the utricle with an endolymphatic duct of the membranous labyrinth.

uvea /yo͞o′vē·ə/, the fibrous tunic beneath the sclera that includes the iris, the ciliary body, and the choroid of the eye. Also called **tunica vasculosa bulbi, uveal tract.** –**uveal,** *adj.*

uveitis /yo͞o′vē·ī′tis/, inflammation of the uveal tract of the eye, including the iris, ciliary body, and choroid. It may be characterized by an irregularly shaped pupil, inflammation around the cornea, pus in the anterior chamber, opaque deposits on the cornea, pain, and lacrimation. Causes include allergy, infection, trauma, diabetes, collagen disease, and skin diseases. A major complication may be glaucoma. See also **chorioretinitis, choroiditis, iritis.**

uvula /yo͞o′vyo͝olə/, *pl.* **uvulae,** the small, cone-shaped process, suspended in the mouth from the middle of the posterior border of the soft palate. –**uvular,** *adj.*

uvulitis /yo͞o′vyəlī′tis/, inflammation of the uvula. Common causes are allergy and infection.

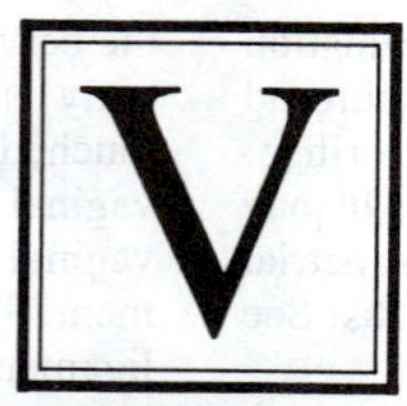

v, abbreviation for *venous blood.*
V, symbol for **vanadium.**
V̇, symbol for **rate of gas flow.**
V_{max}, the maximum rate of catalysis.
vaccination, any injection of attenuated microorganisms, as bacteria, viruses, or rickettsiae, administered to induce immunity or to reduce the effects of associated infectious diseases. Historically, the first vaccinations were administered to immunize against smallpox. Vaccinations are now available to immunize against many diseases, as typhoid, measles, and mumps. **–vaccinate,** *v.*
vaccine /vaksēn′, vak′sēn, -sin/, a suspension of attenuated or killed microorganisms administered intradermally, intramuscularly, orally, or subcutaneously to induce active immunity to infectious disease. Viruses and rickettsiae used in certain vaccines are grown in avian embryos, rabbit brain tissue, or monkey kidney tissue, and the organisms are usually inactivated by formalin, phenol, or beta-propiolactone. Bacteria for various vaccines may be inactivated by acetone, formalin, heat, or phenol. Vaccines may be used as single agents or in combinations. Compare **antiserum.**
-vaccine, a combining form meaning a 'preparation containing microorganisms for producing immunity to disease': *autovaccine, enterovaccine, heterovaccine.*
vaccinia /vaksin′ē·ə/, an infectious disease of cattle caused by a poxvirus that may be transmitted to humans by direct contact or by deliberate inoculation as a protection against smallpox. A pustule develops at the site of infection, usually followed by malaise and fever that last for several days. After 2 weeks the pustule becomes a crust that eventually drops off, leaving a scar. Satellite lesions may occur, and the virus may be spread to other sites by scratching. Individuals with eczema or other preexisting skin disease may develop generalized vaccinia. Rarely, a severe encephalitis follows vaccinia. Also called **cowpox.** Compare **smallpox.** See also **vaccination.**
vacuole /vak′yo͞o·ōl/, **1.** a clear or fluid-filled space or cavity within a cell, as when a droplet of water is ingested by the cytoplasm. **2.** a small space in the body enclosed by a membrane, usually containing fat, secretions, or cellular debris. **–vacuolar, vacuolated,** *adj.*
vacuum aspiration, a method of abortion in which the fetus and placenta are removed by suction to terminate an early pregnancy, up to the fourteenth week. Under local or light general anesthesia, the cervix is dilated and the uterus is emptied with suction. Postoperative care includes the close observation of vital signs for symptoms of blood loss. Also called **suction curettage.** Compare **dilatation and curettage.** See also **therapeutic abortion.**
vagal /vā′gəl/, of or pertaining to the vagus nerve.
vagina, the part of the female genitalia that forms a canal from the orifice through the vestibule to the uterine cervix. It is behind the bladder and in front of the rectum. In the adult woman the anterior wall of the vagina is about 7 cm long and the posterior wall is about 9 cm long. The canal is actually a potential space; the walls usually touch. The vagina widens from the vestibule upward and narrows toward the top, forming a curved vault around the protruding cervix. The vagina is lined with mucosa covering a layer of erectile tissue and muscle. The mucous membrane of the vagina forms two longitudinal columns from which transverse rugae extend around the canal. The muscular coat is composed of a strong, external longitudinal layer and an internal circular layer. The lower end of the vagina is surrounded by the erectile tissue of the bulb of the vestibule and the bulbocavernosus muscle. The muscular layer is highly vascular. The muscles of the vagina are innervated by the pudendal nerve and perfused by the vaginal artery.
vagina bulbi. See **fascia bulbi.**
vaginal bleeding, an abnormal condition in which blood is passed from the vagina, other than during the menses. It may be caused by abnormalities of the uterus or cervix; by an abnormal pregnancy; by endocrine abnormalities; by abnormalities of one or both ovaries or one or both fallopian tubes; or by an abnormality of the vagina. The following terms are commonly used in describing the approximate amount of vaginal bleeding: **heavy vaginal bleeding,** which is greater than heaviest normal menstrual flow; **moderate vaginal bleeding,** which is equal to heaviest normal menstrual flow; **light vaginal bleeding,** which is less than heaviest normal menstrual flow; **vaginal staining,** which is a very light flow of blood barely requiring the use of a sanitary napkin or tampon; **vaginal spotting,** which is the passage vaginally of a few drops of blood; **bloody show,** which is an episode of light vaginal bleeding as often occurs in early labor, during labor, and, particularly, at the time of full dilatation of the cervix at the end of the first stage of labor.
vaginal cancer, a malignancy of the vagina occurring rarely as a primary neoplasm and more often as a secondary lesion or extension of vulvar, cervical, endometrial, or ovarian cancer. Clear cell adenocarcinoma occurs in

young women exposed in utero to diethylstilbestrol, given their mother to prevent abortion, but most primary vaginal cancers arise in white women over 50 years of age. A predisposing factor is cervical carcinoma. Vaginal leukoplakia, erythematosis, erosion, or granulation of the mucosa may prove to be carcinoma in situ. Symptoms of invasive lesions are postmenopausal bleeding, purulent discharge, pain, and dysuria. Diagnostic measures include cervical, endocervical, and vaginal Pap smears, colposcopy, biopsy, and Schiller's iodine test in which malignant cells do not stain dark brown. Ninety percent of vaginal cancers are squamous cell carcinomas; others are clear cell or undifferentiated adenocarcinomas, malignant melanomas, and sarcomas. Depending on the patient's age and condition and the site and extent of the lesion, treatment may be by irradiation or vaginectomy and radical hysterectomy with lymph node dissection. Cryosurgery, topical 5-fluorouracil, and dinitrochlorobenzene (DNCB) may be used, but chemotherapy is not usually effective.

vaginal discharge, any discharge from the vagina. A clear or pearly-white discharge occurs normally. Throughout the reproductive years the amount varies greatly from woman to woman, and the amount and character vary in each woman at different times in her menstrual cycle. Before menarche and after menopause, the quantity of discharge is usually less than during the reproductive years. The discharge is largely composed of secretions of the endocervical glands. Inflammatory conditions of the vagina and cervix often cause an increase in the discharge, which may then have a foul odor and cause pruritus of the perineum and external genitalia.

vaginal fornix, a recess in the upper part of the vagina caused by the protrusion of the uterine cervix into the vagina.

vaginal instillation of medication, the instillation of a medicated cream, a suppository, or a gel into the vagina, usually performed to treat a local infection of the vagina or uterine cervix. The woman voids before the treatment. She then lies back, recumbent or semirecumbent. The nurse or physician, wearing gloves, separates the labia majora, exposing the vaginal orifice. The medication is instilled gently. A cream or gel is squeezed into an applicator from a tube and is then placed in the vagina by depressing the plunger of the applicator while withdrawing the device from the vagina. A tablet or suppository is usually placed in the vagina near the cervix with another style of applicator that holds the medication in a slotted receptacle at its tip. The woman remains recumbent after the instillation to prevent escape of the medication from the vagina. Most applicators may be washed after each instillation and reused for the same woman for the next dose. They are discarded after a course of treatment. Vaginal instillation may easily be taught to the woman.

vaginal jelly, a contraceptive product containing a spermicide in a jelly medium. It is usually used in conjunction with a contraceptive diaphragm or cervical cap. Some antimicrobial medications are also supplied in the form of a vaginal jelly.

vaginal sponge, a contraceptive sponge made of polyurethane and impregnated with the spermicide nonoxynol-9. The sponge is shaped like a mushroom and fits into the upper vagina. It is believed to work in three ways: by releasing spermicide, by absorbing semen, and by blocking the cervical opening. The sponge can be kept in place to provide protection for 24 hours. Effectiveness of the vaginal sponge contraceptive is reported as similar to that of other vaginal methods.

vaginal spotting, vaginal staining. See **vaginal bleeding.**

vaginismus /vaj′iniz′məs/, a psychophysiologic genital reaction of women, characterized by intense contraction of the perineal and paravaginal musculature tightly closing the vaginal introitus. It occurs in response to fear of painful intromission before coitus or pelvic examination. Vaginismus is considered abnormal if it occurs in the absence of genital lesions and if it conflicts with a woman's desire to participate in coition or to permit examination, but it may be a normal or physiologic response if painful genital conditions exist or if forcible or premature intromission is anticipated. Abnormal vaginismus is uncommon. Sexual adjustment can often be achieved through educative and supportive measures that lead to improved sexual self-awareness and response. In some cases, the condition is a manifestation of serious mental illness and requires formal psychiatric evaluation and treatment. Gender identity conflict, a history of trauma from rape or incest, or an intense suppression of sexuality in childhood and adolescence are factors that are often seen in association with vaginismus. See also **dyspareunia.**

vaginitis /vaj′inī′tis/, an inflammation of the vaginal tissues, as trichomonas vaginitis.

vagino-, a combining form meaning 'pertaining to the vagina': *vaginodynia, vaginolabial, vaginopexy.*

vaginography /vaj′inog′rəfē/, the radiologic examination of the vagina after injection of a radiopaque contrast medium.

Vagisec, a trademark for a vaginal douche containing polyoxyethylene nonyl phenol, edetate sodium, and dioctyl sodium sulfosuccinate, used to treat trichomoniasis.

Vagitrol, a trademark for a vaginal, fixed-combination drug containing an antibacterial (sulfanilamide) and a topical antiinfective (aminacrine hydrochloride).

vagotomy /vāgot′əmē/, the cutting of certain branches of the vagus nerve, performed with gastric surgery, to reduce the amount of gastric acid secreted and lessen the chance of recurrence of a gastric ulcer. With the patient under general anesthesia, a gastrectomy is performed and the appropriate branches of the vagus nerve are excised. Because peristalsis will be diminished, a pyloroplasty or an anastomosis of the stomach to the jejunum is done to assure proper emptying of the stomach. See also **anastomosis, gastrectomy, gastric ulcer, pyloroplasty, vagus nerve.**

vagotonus /vā'gətō'nəs/, an abnormal increase in the activity and the effects of the stimulation of the vagus nerve, especially bradycardia with decreased cardiac output, faintness, and syncope. Vagotonus may occur in suctioning the oropharynx of a newborn as the syringe, laryngoscope blade, or catheter is inadvertently pressed on the back of the throat, stimulating the nerve. It also occurs in some women after surgical treatment or simple manipulation of the uterine cervix.

vagovagal reflex /vā'gōvā'gəl/, a stimulation of the vagus nerve by reflex in which irritation of the larynx or the trachea results in slowing of the pulse rate.

vagus nerve /vā'gəs/, either of the longest pair of cranial nerves essential for speech, swallowing, and the sensibilities and functions of many parts of the body. The vagus nerves communicate through 13 main branches, connecting to four areas in the brain. Also called **nervus vagus, pneumogastric nerve, tenth cranial nerve.**

valence /vāl'əns/, **1.** (in chemistry) a numeric expression of the capability of an element to combine chemically with atoms of hydrogen or their equivalent. A negative valence indicates the number of hydrogen atoms to which one atom of a chemical element can bond. A positive valence indicates the number of hydrogen atoms that one atom of a chemical element can displace. An element is considered univalent (or monovalent) if each of its atoms can react with only one hydrogen atom or its equivalent; bivalent (or divalent) if each atom can react with two hydrogen or equivalent atoms; tervalent (or trivalent) if each atom can react with three hydrogen atoms; multivalent (or polyvalent) if each atom can react with many hydrogen atoms. **2.** (in immunology) an expression of the number of antigen-binding sites for one molecule of any given antibody or the number of antibody-binding sites for any given antigen. Most antibody molecules, and those belonging to the IgG, IgA, and IgE immunoglobulin classes have two antigen-binding sites. Most large antigen molecules are multivalent.

-valence, -valency, a combining term meaning the 'combining capacity of an atom compared with that of one hydrogen atom': *quantivalence, trivalence, univalence.*

-valent, a combining form meaning 'having a valency of a (specified) magnitude': *octavalent, pentavalent, tetravalent.*

valeric acid /vəler'ik/, an organic acid with a penetrating odor found in the roots of *Valeriana officinalis*. Commercially prepared, it is used in the production of perfumes, flavors, lubricants, and certain drugs.

valgus /val'gəs/, an abnormal position in which a part of a limb is bent or twisted outward, away from the midline, as the heel of the foot in **talipes valgus.** Compare **varus.** See also **hallux valgus.**

validity, (in research) the extent to which a test measurement or other device measures what it is intended to measure. Kinds of validity include **content validity, current validity, construct validity, face validity,** and **predictive validity.**

valine (Val), an essential amino acid needed for optimal growth in infants and for nitrogen equilibrium in adults. See also **amino acid, maple syrup urine disease, protein.**

Valisone, a trademark for a glucocorticoid (betamethasone valerate).

Valium, a trademark for an antianxiety agent (diazepam), used as an adjunct to anesthesia.

vallecula /vəlek'yŏŏlə/, **1.** any groove or furrow on the surface of an organ or structure. **2.** *See* **vallecula epiglottica.** **–vallecular,** *adj.*

vallecula epiglottica, a furrow between the glossoepiglottic folds of each side of the posterior oropharynx. Also called *(informal)* **vallecula.**

vallecular dysphagia, difficulty or pain on swallowing caused by inflammation of the vallecula epiglottica. Compare **contractile ring dysphagia, dysphagia lusoria.**

Vallestril, a trademark for an estrogen (methallenestril).

valley fever. See **coccidioidomycosis.**

Valmid, a trademark for a sedative (ethinamate).

Valpin, a trademark for an anticholinergic (anisotropine).

valproic acid, an anticonvulsant.

■ INDICATIONS: It is prescribed to prevent certain types of seizure activity, particularly complex absence and petit mal seizures.

■ CONTRAINDICATIONS: It is not recommended for use during pregnancy or lactation. Known hypersensitivity to this drug prohibits its use.

■ ADVERSE EFFECTS: Among the more severe adverse reactions are decreased platelet function and hepatotoxicity. GI disturbances are common, and alopecia, rash, headache, and insomnia may also occur.

Valsalva's maneuver /valsal'vəs/, any forced expiratory effort against a closed airway, as when an individual holds the breath and tightens the muscles in a concerted, strenuous effort to move a heavy object or to change position in bed. Most healthy individuals perform Valsalva's maneuvers during normal daily activities without any injurious consequences; but such efforts are dangerous for many patients with cardiovascular diseases, especially if they become dehydrated, increasing the viscosity of their blood and the attendant risk of blood clotting. Constipation increases the risk of cardiovascular trauma in such patients, especially if they perform Valsalva's maneuver in trying to move their bowels. On relaxing after each muscular effort with held breath, the blood of such individuals rushes to the heart, often overloading the cardiac system and causing cardiac arrest. Orthopedic patients often use Valsalva's maneuver in changing their position in bed with the aid of an overhead trapeze bar. Patients who may be endangered by performing Valsalva's maneuver are commonly instructed to exhale instead of holding their breath when they move. The exhalation decreases the risk of cardiovascular trauma.

Valsalva's test, a method for testing the patency of the eustachian tubes. With mouth and nose kept tightly closed, a forced expiratory effort is made; if the eustachian tubes are open, air will enter into the middle ear cavities and the subject will hear a popping sound. See also **Valsalva's maneuver.**

value system, the accepted mode of conduct and the set of norms, goals, and values binding any social group. Such guidelines for determining what is right or wrong, good or bad, desirable or undesirable serve as a frame of reference for the individual in reaching decisions and in achieving a meaningful life.

valve, a natural structure or artificial device in a passage or vessel that prevents reflux of the fluid contents passing through it. Valves in veins are membranous folds that prevent backflow of blood. **–valvular,** *adj.*

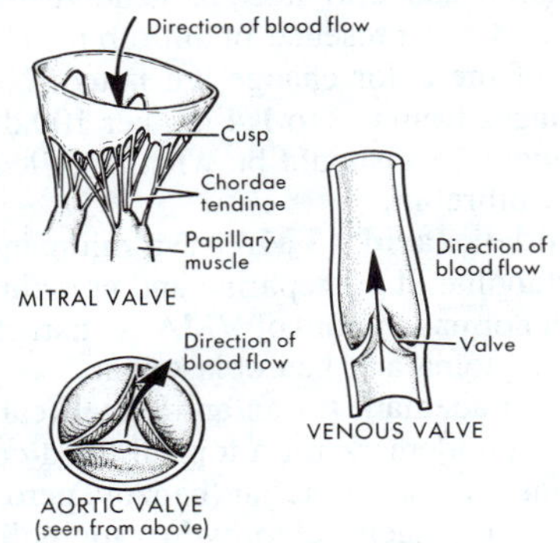

Valves

-valve, a combining form meaning 'a thing that regulates the flow of': *bivalve, pseudovalve, trivalve.*

valve of Kerkring. See **circular fold.**

valve of lymphatics, one of the tiny semilunar structures in the vessels and trunks of the lymphatic system that help regulate the flow of lymph and prevent venous blood from entering the system. There are no valves in the capillaries of the system, but there are many in the collecting vessels. The valves are attached by their convex edges to the walls of the vessels, leaving their concave edges free and directed along the course of the current of lymph. Usually, two valves of equal size are found opposite each other. They are more numerous near the lymph nodes and more prevalent in the lymphatic vessels of the neck and the arms than in the vessels of the legs. The wall of the vessel just above the attachment of each valve bulges with a small sinus that gives the vessel its beaded appearance. See also **lymphatic system.**

valvotomy /valvot'əmē/, the incision into a valve, especially one in the heart, to correct a defect and allow proper opening and closure. Before surgery a cardiac catheterization is performed. With the patient under general anesthesia, the damaged valve is repaired, if possible, or removed and a prosthetic valve suture put in its place. Complications peculiar to prosthetic valve surgery are displacement of the valve caused by broken sutures, heart block, leakage and regurgitation from chamber to chamber, infection, and embolus.

valvular heart disease, an acquired or congenital disorder of a cardiac valve, characterized by stenosis and obstructed blood flow or by valvular degeneration and regurgitation of blood. Diseases of aortic and mitral valves are most common and may be caused by congenital defects, bacterial endocarditis, syphilis, or, most frequently, rheumatic fever. Episodes of rheumatic fever often affect cardiac valves, causing them to degenerate and remain open or causing the cusps of the valves to become stiff, calcified, and constricted. Valvular dysfunction results in changes in intracardiac pressure and in pulmonary and peripheral circulation. It may lead to cardiac arrhythmia, heart failure, and cardiogenic shock.

■ OBSERVATIONS: Malaise, anorexia, embolism, pulmonary edema, and ventricular failure often accompany valvular heart disease. In moderate or severe **aortic stenosis,** pulse pressure is decreased; the carotid pulse is small and slow with a long upstroke, but the apical pulse may be strong and sustained during systole. There may be a pansystolic thrill or generally harsh heart sounds, or the second systolic sound may be diminished or absent. The patient may experience anginal pain and syncope, and the electrocardiogram may show evidence of left ventricular hypertrophy, conduction defects, or complete heart block. Characteristic signs of aortic regurgitation are dyspnea, profuse sweating, flushed skin, pounding pulsations in neck arteries, and a blowing heart murmur throughout diastole. The electrocardiogram may be normal or reveal left ventricular hypertrophy. The patient with **mitral stenosis** tires easily, is short of breath on exertion, may have paroxysmal nocturnal dyspnea, and may develop hemoptysis and systemic embolism. The first heart sound usually is increased and the second is followed by a decrescendo opening snap. There may be atrial fibrillation, right ventricular hypertrophy, and increased pressure in the left atrium, pulmonary artery, and right ventricle. Mitral regurgitation is typified by dyspnea, fatigue, intolerance of exercise, heart palpitation, and a large, laterally placed apical pulse. There may be an apical systolic murmur; a diminished first heart sound; a third heart sound; atrial arrhythmia; or elevated wedge pressure in the left atrium, pulmonary artery, or pulmonary vein. **Tricuspid stenosis** is relatively uncommon, is usually associated with lesions in other valves resulting from rheumatic fever, and, in rare cases, is caused by carcinoid heart disease or endomyocardial fibrosis. Characteristics of tricuspid stenosis are a diastolic pressure gradient between the right atrium and ventricle, jugular vein distention, pulmonary congestion, and, in severe cases, hepatic congestion and splenomegaly. Tricuspid regurgitation, usually secondary to marked dilatation of the right ventricle and the ring of the valve, commonly occurs in late stages of cardiac failure in rheumatic or congenital heart disease with severe pulmonary hypertension. Typical signs include engorged neck veins, hepatomegaly, systolic pulsations of the liver, edema, and ascites. The pulmonic valve is affected by rheumatic fever much less frequently than other cardiac valves. **Pulmonic stenosis** may cause the intraventricular septum to bulge into the right ventricular chamber, and regurgitation is a consequence of severe pulmonary hypertension, but destruction of the valve does not cause heart failure unless pulmonary hypertension is a serious problem.

■ INTERVENTION: Cardiotonics, diuretics, analgesics, sodium restriction, and antibiotics, if indicated, are used in the conservative treatment of valvular heart disease, but surgery is usually performed when the symptoms are incapacitating. A stenosed aortic valve may be repaired by removing the calcium deposits and opening the fused commissures or by removing a cusp and reconstructing the valve, or it may be replaced with a porcine or artificial valve. Defective mitral and tricuspid valves may also be replaced or repaired surgically.

■ NURSING CONSIDERATIONS: The patient undergoing cardiac valve repair or replacement may be hospitalized for from 4 to 6 weeks and requires diversional activities, as well as the standard pre- and postoperative care provided for open heart surgery.

valvular stenosis, a narrowing or constricture of any of the valves of the heart. The condition may result from a congenital defect, or it may be caused by some disease process. See also **aortic stenosis, congenital cardiac anomaly, mitral valve stenosis, pulmonic stenosis.**

valvulitis /val′vyo͞olī′tis/, an inflammatory condition of a valve, especially a cardiac valve. Inflammatory changes in the aortic, mitral, and tricuspid valves of the heart are caused most commonly by rheumatic fever and less frequently by bacterial endocarditis and syphilis. Infected valves degenerate, or their cusps become stiff and calcified, resulting in stenosis and obstructed blood flow.

VAMP /vamp/, abbreviation for a combination drug regimen, used in the treatment of cancer, containing three antineoplastics (vincristine sulfate, methotrexate, and mercaptopurine) and a glucocorticoid (prednisone).

vanadium (V), a grayish metallic element. Its atomic number is 23; its atomic weight is 50.942. Absorption of vanadium compounds results in a condition called **vanadiumism,** characterized by anemia, conjunctivitis, pneumonitis, and irritation of the respiratory tract.

van Bogaert's disease /vanbō′gərts/, a rare familial disorder of lipid metabolism in which the substance cholestanol is deposited in the nervous system, blood, and connective tissue. Persons with the disease develop progressive ataxia and dementia, premature atherosclerosis, cataracts, and xanthomas of the tendons. No effective treatment has been found. Also called **cerebrotendinous xanthomatosis.**

Vanceril, a trademark for a glucocorticoid (beclomethasone dipropionate), used for oral inhalation therapy in asthma.

Vancocin Hydrochloride, a trademark for an antibacterial (vancomycin hydrochloride).

vancomycin hydrochloride, an antibiotic.

■ INDICATIONS: It is prescribed in the treatment of infections, particularly staphylococcal infections resistant to other antibiotics.

■ CONTRAINDICATIONS: Concomitant administration of neurotoxic, nephrotoxic, or ototoxic drugs or known hypersensitivity to this drug prohibits its use.

■ ADVERSE EFFECTS: Among the more serious adverse reactions are anaphylaxis, dizziness, and tinnitus.

Van Deemter's equation, an expression of a gas chromatography relationship between the height equivalent to the theoretic plate (HEPT) to the linear velocity of the carrier gas.

van den Bergh's test /van′dənburgs′/, a test for the presence of bilirubin in the blood serum. Blood is obtained from a patient who has fasted overnight, and the diluted serum is added to diazo reagent. A blue or violet color indicates the presence of bilirubin. The rate and magnitude of the color change are noted. Normal total bilirubin ranges from 0.2 to 1.4 mg per 100 dl of serum, of which about 15% should be what is called direct, or conjugated, bilirubin.

vanillylmandelic acid (VMA) /va′nililmandel′ik/, a urinary metabolite of epinephrine and norepinephrine. A greater than normal amount of VMA is characteristic of a pheochromocytoma and neuroblastomas.

Vanobid, a trademark for an antifungal (candicidin).

Vanoxide, a trademark for a topical fixed-combination drug containing an antibacterial (benzoyl peroxide) and a keratolytic drying agent (chlorhydroxyquinoline).

Van Rensselaer /vanren′səlir/, **Euphenia** (1840–1912), an American socialite who entered the first class of the Bellevue Hospital Training School for Nurses in New York. She designed the first nurses' uniform, a blue and white seersucker dress with collar and cuffs, apron, and cap. She succeeded Sister Helen as superintendent of Bellevue and later joined the Sisters of Charity, for whom she established a mission in Nassau. She organized the Seton Hospital for Tuberculosis in New York.

Vaponefrin, a trademark for an adrenergic agent (epinephrine hydrochloride), used as a bronchodilator.

vapor bath, the exposure of the body to vapor, as steam.

vapor pressure depression, a phenomenon in which the addition of a solute molecule to a solvent will decrease the amount of solvent in equilibrium between the vapor phase and the liquid phase.

variable behavior, a response, activity, or action that may be modified by individual experience. Compare **invariable behavior.**

variable region, the N-terminal portion of an immunoglobulin polypeptide chain whose amino acid sequence can change. The region includes the antigen combining site.

variance, 1. (in statistics) a numeric representation of the dispersion of data around the mean in a given sample. It is represented by the square of the standard deviation and is used principally in performing an analysis of variance. **2.** *nontechnical.* the general range of a group of findings.

varicella. See **chickenpox.**

varicella zoster virus (VZV), a member of the herpesvirus family, which causes the diseases varicella (chickenpox) and herpes zoster (shingles). The virus has been isolated from vesicle fluid in chickenpox, is highly contagious, and may be spread by direct contact or droplets. Dried crusts of skin lesions do not contain active virus particles. Herpes zoster is produced by reactivation of latent varicella virus, usually several years after the initial infection. There is no simple test for measuring antibodies to this virus; however, zoster immune globulin (ZIG) obtained from convalescing zoster patients, if injected within 3 days of exposure, will prevent varicella in susceptible children. The temporary nature of this protection and the relative scarcity of ZIG warrant reservation of its use to children receiving immunosuppressive therapy or suffering from immune deficiency diseases. See also **chickenpox, herpesvirus hominus, herpes zoster.**

varicelliform /ver′isel′ifôrm/, resembling the rash of chickenpox.

varicocele /ver′əkōsēl′/, a dilatation of the pampiniform venous complex of the spermatic cord. The varicocele forms a soft, elastic swelling that can cause pain. It is most common in men between 15 and 25 years of age and affects the left spermatic cord more often than the right. It is usually more pronounced and painful in the standing position. Compare **ovarian varicocele, utero-ovarian varicocele.**

varicose /ver′əkōs/, **1.** (of a vein) exhibiting varicosis, or a varicosity. **2.** abnormally and permanently distended, as the bulging veins in some individuals.

varicose aneurysm, a blood-filled, saclike projection that connects an artery and one or several veins and that is formed from a localized dilatation of the adjoining vessels.

varicose ulcer. See **stasis ulcer.**

varicose vein, a tortuous, dilated vein with incompetent valves. Causes include congenitally defective valves, thrombophlebitis, pregnancy, and obesity. Varicose veins are common, especially in women. The saphenous veins of the legs are most often affected. Elevation of the legs and use of elastic stockings are frequently sufficient therapy for uncomplicated cases. Surgery (ligation and stripping) may be required in severe cases. Injection of sclerosing solutions helps prevent or treat postphlebitic syndrome.

varicosis /ver′ikō′sis/, a common condition characterized by one or more tortuous, abnormally dilated, or varicose veins, usually in the legs or the lower trunk, occurring between 30 and 60 years of age. Varicosis may be caused by congenital defects of the valves or walls of the veins or by congestion and increased intraluminal pressure resulting from prolonged standing, poor posture, pregnancy, abdominal tumor, or chronic systemic disease. Symptoms include pain and muscle cramps with a feeling of fullness and heaviness in the legs. Dilatation of superficial veins is often evident before the condition produces discomfort. Varicose veins may be treated conservatively by elevating the affected limb periodically or by wearing an elastic bandage or stocking. Ligation of the vein above the varicosity and removal of the distal portion of the vessel may be indicated for more severe cases if deeper vessels can maintain the return of venous blood.

varicosity, **1.** an abnormal condition, usually of a vein, characterized by swelling and tortuosity. **2.** a vein in this condition.

variegate /ver′ē·əgāt′/, having characteristics that vary, especially as to color.

variegate porphyria, an uncommon form of hepatic porphyria, characterized by skin lesions and photosensitivity. The condition may be congenital or acquired. The congenital form is more serious, resulting in crises of acute abdominal pain and in certain neurologic complications. See also **porphyria.**

variola, variola major. See **smallpox.**

variola minor. See **alastrim.**

varioloid /ver′ē·əloid′/, **1.** resembling smallpox. **2.** a mild form of smallpox in a vaccinated person or one who has previously had the disease.

varix /ver′iks/, *pl.* **varices** /ver′əsēz/, **1.** a tortuous, dilated vein. **2.** an enlarged, tortuous artery or a distended, twisting lymphatic.

varus /ver′əs/, an abnormal position in which a part of a limb is turned inward toward the midline, as the heel and foot in **talipes varus.** Compare **valgus.**

vas /vas/, *pl.* **vasa** /vā′sə/, any one of the many vessels of the body, especially those that convey blood, lymph, or spermatozoa.

vascular /vas′kyo͝olər/, of or pertaining to a blood vessel.

vascular hemophilia. See **Von Willebrand's disease.**

vascular insufficiency, inadequate peripheral blood flow caused by occlusion of vessels with atherosclerotic plaques, thrombi, or emboli, by damaged, diseased, or intrinsically weak vascular walls, arteriovenous fistulas, or hematologic hypercoagulability, or by heavy smoking. Signs of vascular insufficiency include pale, cyanotic, or mottled skin over the affected area, swelling of an extremity, absent or reduced tactile sensation, tingling, diminished sense of temperature, muscle pain, as intermittent claudication in the calf, and, in advanced disease, atrophy of muscles of the involved extremity. Diagnosis may be made by checking and comparing peripheral pulses in contralateral extremities, or by angiography, plethysmography, ultrasonography, and skin temperature tests. Treatment of vascular insufficiency may include a diet low in saturated fats, moderate exercise, sleeping on a firm mattress, avoidance of smoking, proper standing or sitting posture, the use of vasodilating drug, and, if indicated, surgical repair of an arteriovenous fistula or aneurysm. See also **arterial insufficiency.**

vascularization, the process by which body tissue becomes vascular and develops proliferating capillaries. It may be natural or may be induced by surgical techniques. **–vascularize,** *v.*

vascular leiomyoma, a neoplasm that has developed from smooth muscle fibers of a blood vessel.

vascular spider. See **spider angioma.**

vasculitis /vas′kyo͞olī′tis/, an inflammatory condition of the blood vessels that is characteristic of certain systemic diseases or that is caused by an allergic reaction. Kinds of vasculitis are **allergic vasculitis, necrotizing vasculitis,** and **segmented hyalinizing vasculitis.** See also **angiitis.**

vas deferens /def′ərənz/, *pl.* **vasa deferentia** /def′əren′shē·ə/, the extension of the epididymis of the testis that ascends from the scrotum and joins the seminal vesicle to form the ejaculatory duct. It is enclosed by fibrous connective tissue with blood vessels, nerves, and lymphatics and passes through the inguinal canal as part of the spermatic cord. Extending from the scrotum into the abdominal cavity, it passes over the top, then down the posterior surface of the bladder, becomes wider and convoluted, and joins the ampulla of the seminal vesicle. A vasectomy severs the vas deferens and makes a man sterile by interrupting the route spermatozoa must take to the exterior from the epididymis. Also called **deferent duct, ductus deferens, spermatic duct, testicular duct.** See also **testis.**

vasectomy /vasek′təmē/, a procedure for male sterilization involving the bilateral surgical removal of a portion of the vas deferens. Vasectomy is most commonly performed as an office procedure using local anesthesia. The procedure is also performed routinely before removal of the prostate gland to prevent inflammation of the testes and epididymides. Potency is not affected. A signed and witnessed form indicating informed consent is usually required before performance of the procedure.

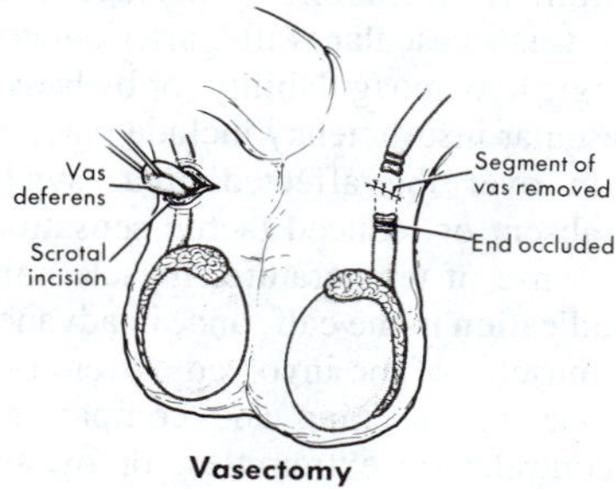

Vasectomy

vaso-, a combining form meaning 'pertaining to a vessel or duct': *vasoconstrictor, vasodilatation, vasoganglion.*

vasoactive /vā′zō·ak′tiv/, (of a drug) tending to cause vasodilation or vasoconstriction.

vasoactive intestinal polypeptide (VIP), a blood vessel dilating substance secreted by pancreatic islet cancer cells. VIP causes blood vessels throughout the body to dilate and in the intestinal tract causes secretion of fluid and salt, resulting in diarrhea. The VIP effects mimic the symptoms of Asiatic cholera and can result in death from dehydration and subsequent kidney failure if either surgery or chemotherapy is not administered at an early stage of tumor development.

vasoconstriction, a narrowing of the lumen of any blood vessel, especially the arterioles and the veins in the blood reservoirs of the skin and the abdominal viscera. It is accomplished by various mechanisms that together control blood pressure and the distribution of blood throughout the body. Vasoconstriction depends on the stimulation of the vasomotor constriction center in the medulla. Impulses from this center travel along the sympathetic nerve fibers and contract the smooth muscle layers of the arteries, the arterioles, the venules, and the veins, causing the constriction of these vessels. Vasoconstriction is also induced by vasomotor pressure reflexes, chemical reflexes, the medullary ischemic reflex, and vasomotor impulses from the cerebral cortex and the hypothalamus. Compare **vasodilatation.**

vasoconstrictor, **1.** of or pertaining to a process, condition, or substance that causes the constriction of blood vessels. **2.** an agent that promotes vasoconstriction. Cold, fear, stress, and nicotine are common exogenous vasoconstrictors. Internally secreted epinephrine and norepinephrine cause blood vessels to contract by stimulating adrenergic receptors of peripheral sympathetic nerves. Other endogenous vasoconstrictors are angiotensin, which is formed in the blood through the action of renin, and antidiuretic hormone, which is secreted by the pituitary. Adrenergic sympathomimetic drugs cause some degree of vasoconstriction, and several of these agents are used for this action in maintaining blood pressure during anesthesia and in treating pronounced hypotension resulting from hemorrhage, myocardial infarction, septicemia, sympathectomy, or drug reactions. Among these therapeutic agents are methoxamine hydrochloride, metaraminol bitartrate, and norepinephrine. Also called **vasopressor.**

Vasodilan, a trademark for a vasodilator (isoxsuprine hydrochloride).

vasodilatation /vā′zōdil′ətā′shən, -dī′lətā′shən/, widening or distention of blood vessels, particularly arterioles, usually caused by nerve impulses or certain drugs that relax smooth muscle in the walls of the blood vessels. Also called **vasodilation** /vā′zōdīlā′shən/. Compare **vasoconstriction.**

vasodilator /vā′zōdī′lātər/, **1.** a nerve or agent that causes dilatation of blood vessels. **2.** pertaining to the relaxation of the smooth muscle of the vascular system. **3.** producing dilatation of blood vessels. Vasodilators are a recent, important addition to the treatment of heart failure. Included are hydralazine, nitroglycerin, nitroprusside, and trimethaphan. They have been useful in the treatment of acute heart failure in myocardial infarction, in cases associated with severe mitral insufficiency, and in failure resulting from myocardial disease.

vasogenic shock, shock resulting from peripheral vascular dilatation produced by factors, as toxins, that directly affect the blood vessels.

vasomotor, of or pertaining to the nerves and muscles that control the caliber of the lumen of the blood vessels. Circularly arranged fibers of the muscles of arteries can contract, causing vasoconstriction, or they can relax, causing vasodilatation.

vasomotor rhinitis, chronic rhinitis and nasal obstruction, without allergy or infection, characterized by sneezing, rhinorrhea, nasal obstruction, and vascular engorgement of the mucous membranes of the nose. A vaporizer or humidifier and systemic vasoconstrictive agents are used to alleviate discomfort. Nose drops and nasal sprays are avoided, because continued use may cause further vasodilatation of the mucous membrane and aggravation of the condition. Vasomotor rhinitis is common in pregnancy.

vasomotor system, the part of the nervous system that controls the constriction and dilatation of the blood vessels. See also **vasoconstriction, vasodilatation.**

vasopressin. See **antidiuretic hormone.**

vasopressor. See **vasoconstrictor.**

Vasospan, a trademark for a smooth muscle relaxant (papaverine hydrochloride).

vasospasm, a former term for **angiospasm.**

vasospastic, **1.** relating to a spasmodic constriction of a blood vessel. **2.** any agent that produces spasms of the blood vessels.

Vasosulf, a trademark for an ophthalmic fixed-combination drug containing an antibacterial (sulfacetamide sodium) and an adrenergic (phenylephrine hydrochloride).

vasovasostomy /vā′zōvəsos′təmē/, a surgical procedure in which the function of the vas deferens on each side of the testes is restored, having been cut and ligated in a preceding vasectomy. The procedure is performed if a man wants to regain his fertility. In most cases, the patency of the canals is achieved, but in many cases fertility does not result, probably caused by circulating autoantibodies that disrupt normal sperm activity. The antibodies apparently develop after vasectomy because the developing sperm cannot be excreted through the urogenital tract.

Vasoxyl, a trademark for an alpha-adrenergic (methoxamine hydrochloride).

vastus intermedius, one of the four muscles of the quadriceps femoris, situated in the center of the thigh. It arises from the front and lateral surfaces of the femur and from the lateral intermuscular septum. Its fibers end in a superficial aponeurosis that forms the deep part of the quadriceps femoris tendon inserted into the patella. The vastus intermedius is innervated by branches of the femoral nerve, which contain fibers from the second, third, and fourth lumbar nerves, and it functions with the other three muscles of the quadriceps to extend the leg. Also called **crureus.** Compare **rectus femoris, vastus lateralis, vastus medialis.**

vastus internus. See **vastus medialis.**

vastus lateralis, the largest of the four muscles of the quadriceps femoris, situated on the lateral side of the thigh. It is a large, dense mass originating in a broad aponeurosis that is attached to the intertrochanteric line of the femur, the greater trochanter, the lateral lip of the gluteal tuberosity, and the lateral lip of the linea aspera. The fibers of the muscle are gathered to form a strong aponeurosis that converges to become a flat tendon before inserting into the patella. The vastus lateralis is innervated by branches of the femoral nerve, which contain fibers from the second, third, and fourth lumbar nerves, and it functions to help extend the leg. Compare **rectus femoris, vastus intermedius, vastus medialis.**

vastus medialis, one of the four muscles of the quadriceps femoris, situated in the medial portion of the thigh. It originates from the intertrochanteric line of the femur, the linea aspera, the medial supracondylar line, the tendons of the adductor longus and the adductor magnus, and the medial intermuscular septum. The vastus medialis extends to the lower anterior aspect of the thigh and inserts by an aponeurosis into the patella and the quadriceps femoris tendon. An expansion of the aponeurosis passes to the capsule of the knee joint. The muscle is innervated by branches of the femoral nerve, which contain fibers from the second, third, and fourth lumbar nerves, and it functions in combination with other parts of the quadriceps femoris to extend the leg. Also called **vastus internus.** Compare **rectus femoris, vastus intermedius, vastus lateralis.**

VC, abbreviation for **vital capacity.**

V-Cillin K, a trademark for an antibacterial (penicillin V potassium).

VD, abbreviation for **venereal disease.**

V deflection (HBE), a deflection on an electrocardiogram that represents ventricular activation.

VDRL test, abbreviation for *Venereal Disease Research Laboratory test,* a serologic flocculation test for syphilis. It is also positive in other treponemal diseases, as yaws. False positive and false negative results may occur. A positive test must be confirmed by further, more definitive testing.

VDT, abbreviation for **video display terminal.**

$\dot{V}$e, symbol for *expired volume.*

$\dot{V}$E, symbol for *volume expired in 1 minute.*

vector, **1.** a quantity having direction and magnitude, usually depicted by a straight arrow whose length represents magnitude and whose head represents direction. **2.** a carrier, especially one that transmits disease. A **biologic vector** is usually an arthropod in which the infecting organism completes part of its life cycle. A **mechanic vector** transmits the infecting organism from one host to another but is not essential to the life cycle of the parasite. Kinds of vectors include dogs, which carry rabies, mosquitoes, which transmit malaria, and ticks, which carry

Rocky Mountain spotted fever. **–vector,** *v.*, **vectorial,** *adj.*

VEE, abbreviation for **Venezuelan equine encephalitis.** See **equine encephalitis.**

Veetids, a trademark for an antibacterial (penicillin V potassium).

vegan. See **strict vegetarian.**

veganism /vej′əniz′əm/, the adherence to a strict vegetable diet, with the exclusion of all protein of animal origin.

vegetable albumin, albumin produced in plants.

vegetal pole, the relatively inactive part of the ovum protoplasm where the food yolk is situated, usually opposite the animal pole. Also called **vegetative pole, antigerminal pole.** Compare **animal pole.**

vegetarian /vej′əter′ē·ən/, a person whose diet is restricted to foods of vegetable origin, including fruits, grains, and nuts. Many vegetarians eat eggs and milk products but avoid all animal flesh. Kinds of vegetarians are **lacto-ovo-vegetarian, lacto-vegetarian, ovo-vegetarian,** and **strict vegetarian.**

vegetarianism, the theory or practice of restricting the diet to food substances of vegetable origin, including fruits, grains, and nuts.

vegetation, an abnormal growth of tissue around a valve, composed of fibrin, platelets, and bacteria.

vegetative /vej′ətā′tiv/, **1.** of or pertaining to nutrition and growth. **2.** of or pertaining to the plant kingdom. **3.** denoting involuntary function, as produced by the parasympathetic nervous system. **4.** resting, not active; denoting the stage of the cell cycle in which the cell is not replicating. **5.** leading a secluded, dull existence without social or intellectual activity; sluggish; lacking animation. **6.** (in psychiatry) emotionally withdrawn and passive, as may occur in schizophrenia and in the depressive phase of bipolar disorder. **–vegetate,** *v.*

vegetative nervous system. See **autonomic nervous system.**

vehicle, **1.** an inert substance with which a medication is mixed to facilitate measurement and administration or application. **2.** any fluid or structure in the body that passively conveys a stimulus.

Veillonella /vā′yənel′ə/, a genus of gram-negative anaerobic bacteria. The species *Veillonella parvula* is normally present in the alimentary tract, especially in the mouth.

Veillon tube /vāyōn′/, a transparent tube whose ends are closed with removable stoppers, one cotton and one rubber. It is used for the laboratory growth of bacteriologic cultures.

vein, one of the many vessels that convey blood from the capillaries to the heart as part of the pulmonary venous system, the systemic venous network, or the portal venous complex. Most of the veins of the body are systemic veins that convey blood from the whole body (except the lungs) to the right atrium of the heart. Each vein is a macroscopic structure enclosed in three layers of different kinds of tissue homologous with the layers of the heart. The outer tunica adventitia of each vein is homologous with the epicardium, the tunica media with the myocardium, and the tunica intima with the endocardium. Deep veins course through the more internal parts of the body, and superficial veins lie near the surface, where many of them can be seen through the skin. Veins have thinner coatings and are less elastic than arteries and collapse when cut. They also contain semilunar valves at various intervals. Compare **artery.** See also **portal vein, pulmonary vein, systemic vein.**

vein ligation and stripping, a surgical procedure consisting of the ligation of the saphenous vein and its removal from groin to ankle, performed for the treatment of recurrent thrombophlebitis or severe varicosities or for obtaining a blood vessel to graft in another site, as in a coronary bypass operation.

vein of Thebesius. See **smallest cardiac vein.**

veins of the vertebral column, the veins that drain the blood from the vertebral column, the adjacent muscles, and the meninges of the spinal cord. Along the entire vertebral column these veins form plexuses that are divided into internal and external groups, according to their locations inside or outside the vertebral canal. The plexuses and the veins of the vertebral network are the external plexus, the internal plexus, the basivertebral veins, the intervertebral veins, and the spinal cord veins.

Velban, a trademark for an antineoplastic (vinblastine sulfate).

vellus hair. See **lanugo.**

velocity, the rate of change in the position of a body moving in a particular direction. Velocity along a straight line is linear velocity. Angular velocity is that of a body in circular motion. Compare **speed.**

velopharyngeal closure /vē′lōfərin′jē·əl/, the blocking of any escape of air by the raising of the soft palate and the contraction of the posterior pharyngeal wall. Compare **closure, flask closure.**

velopharyngeal insufficiency, an abnormal condition resulting from a congenital defect in the structure of the velopharyngeal sphincter: Closure of the oral cavity beneath the nasal passages is not complete, as seen in cleft palate. Food may be regurgitated through the nose, and speech is impaired. Surgical correction is usually successful.

Velosef, a trademark for a cephalosporin antibiotic (cephradine).

Velpeau's bandage /velpōz′/, a roller bandage that immobilizes the elbow and shoulder by holding the brachium against the side and the flexed forearm on the chest. The palm of the hand rests on the clavicle of the opposite side.

vena cava /vē′nə kā′və/, *pl.* **venae cavae,** one of two large veins returning blood from the peripheral circulation to the right atrium of the heart. See also **inferior vena cava, superior vena cava.** **–vena caval,** *adj.*

vena caval syndrome. See **supine hyptension.**

vena comes /kō′mēz/, *pl.* **venae comites** /kom′itēz/, one of the deep paired veins that accompany the smaller arteries, one on each side of the artery. The three vessels are wrapped together in one sheath. Some of the arteries accompanied by such venous pairs are the brachial, the ulnar, and the tibial.

venereal /vənir′ē·əl/, pertaining to or caused by sexual intercourse or genital contact.

venereal disease. See **sexually transmitted disease.**

venereal sore. See **chancre.**

venereal wart. See **condyloma acuminatum.**

venereology /vənir′ē·ol′əjē/, the study of venereal diseases. **–venereologic, venereological,** *adj.*, **venereologist,** *n.*

venesection. See **phlebotomy.**

Venezuelan equine encephalitis. See **equine encephalitis.**

venipuncture /ven′ipungk′chər/, a technique in which a vein is punctured transcutaneously by a sharp rigid stylet or cannula carrying a flexible plastic catheter or by a steel needle attached to a syringe or catheter. The purpose of the procedure is to withdraw a specimen of blood, to perform a phlebotomy, to instill a medication, to start an intravenous infusion, or to inject a radiopaque substance for radiologic examination of a part or system of the body.

■ METHOD: The specific steps in performing a venipuncture vary with the purpose of the procedure and the equipment to be used, but in most instances it begins as follows: A convenient vein is selected, usually on the outside of the forearm, on the back of the hand, or in the antecubital fossa. The vein is palpated, and to dilate the vein a tourniquet is wrapped around the arm proximal to the intended site of puncture. The site is cleansed, and the vein is immobilized by applying traction on the skin around the puncture site. The stylet or needle is held at an angle of 30 degrees for direct venipuncture. In performing direct venipuncture the tip of the needle is pointed in the direction of the flow of blood and is advanced through the skin directly into the vein. The tip is usually inserted bevelside up, but if a large bore needle must be used in a small vein, it is preferable to insert the needle bevelside down, because it is less likely to perforate the posterior wall of the vein. After the skin is punctured, little resistance is felt as the tip passes through the subcutaneous tissue, but a sudden, slight resistance may be felt as the tip hits the wall of the vein. At this point, the tip is cautiously advanced, with the needle or stylet held nearly flush with the skin. Slight upward pressure aids in keeping the tip in the vein as it is advanced into the lumen of the intravenous space. Blood flows back into the hub of the needle or into the catheter attached to the needle or covering the stylet, and the tip of the needle can usually be felt to be in the vein. If these signs are absent, the tip is not in the vein, in which case it is usually best to remove the needle or stylet, apply pressure to the puncture site, and start the procedure again, using new equipment.

■ NURSING ORDERS: Wing-tipped "butterfly" needles, various kinds of intracatheters, and single or multiple venipuncture needles require familiarity and practice for correct insertion and stabilization. A sterile dressing and an antimicrobial ointment are applied over the insertion site. The cleansing agent used to prepare the injection site may be iodine, povidone-iodine, or ethyl alcohol. If an iodine preparation or solution is to be used, the patient is first asked about any previous allergic reaction to iodine. To aid insertion of the tip into the vein, the patient may be asked to clench the fist to further dilate the vein. If the patient is unable to do this, a second tourniquet may be placed several inches distal to the puncture site. This tourniquet is released when the needle or stylet has been placed in the vein.

■ OUTCOME CRITERIA: Aseptic technique is required to avoid infection. A quick, skillful insertion is nearly painless for the patient. Specific sequelae to venipuncture vary with the techniques and equipment used. See also **intravenous infusion, phlebotomy.**

veno-, a combining form meaning 'pertaining to a vein': *venoclysis, venopressor, venovenostomy.*

venogram. See **phlebogram.**

venography. See **phlebography.**

venom, a toxic fluid substance secreted by some snakes, arthropods, and other animals and transmitted by their stings or bites.

venom extract therapy, the administration of antivenin as prophylaxis against the toxic effects of the bite of a specific poisonous snake or spider, or other venomous animal.

venom immunotherapy, the reduction of sensitivity to the bite of a venomous insect or animal by the serial administration of gradually increasing amounts of the specific antigenic substance secreted by the insect or animal.

venous /vē′nəs/, of or pertaining to a vein.

-venous, a combining form meaning 'of or referring to veins': *endovenous, lymphovenous, perivenous.*

venous blood gas, the oxygen and carbon dioxide in venous blood measured by various methods to assess the adequacy of oxygenation and ventilation and to determine the acid-base status. The oxygen tension of venous blood normally averages 40 mm Hg; the dissolved oxygen averages 0.1% by volume, the total oxygen content 15.2%, and the oxygen saturation of venous hemoglobin 75%. The carbon dioxide tension normally averages 46 mm Hg, the dissolved carbon dioxide 2.9% by volume, and the total carbon dioxide content 50%. The normal average pH of venous plasma is 7.37. Venous blood in an extremity when analyzed for gas content provides data chiefly pertaining to that limb. Because a sample from a central venous catheter is usually an incomplete mix of venous blood from various parts of the body, a specimen of completely mixed blood may be obtained from the right ventricle or pulmonary artery for an accurate determination of venous blood gases.

venous insufficiency, an abnormal circulatory condition characterized by decreased return of the venous blood from the legs to the trunk of the body. Edema is usually the first sign of the condition; pain, varicosities, and ulceration may follow. Treatment usually consists of elevation of the legs, use of elastic hose, and correction of the underlying condition.

venous pressure, the stress exerted by circulating blood on the walls of veins, normally 60 to 120 mm of water in peripheral veins but elevated in congestive heart failure, acute or chronic constrictive pericarditis, and in venous obstruction caused by a clot or external pressure against a vein. Indications of increased pressure are continued distention of veins on the back of the hand when it is raised above the sternal notch and distention of the neck veins when the individual is sitting with the head elevated 30 to 45 degrees. Central venous pressure, normally 40 to 100 mm of water, is determined by inserting a catheter into a major vein and threading it through the superior vena cava to the right atrium. The catheter is attached by a three-way stopcock to a water manometer, and a solution, usually 5% glucose in water, is allowed to drip slowly into the vein. Before taking a reading, the stopcock is opened to fill the manometer with the intravenous solution; then the stopcock is turned to the venous opening, and the fluid level in the manometer, which fluctuates with each respiration, is allowed to stabilize. The highest level of the fluid column is used for the reading, and, as soon as it is recorded, the stopcock is turned to the solution position, and the infusion is continued.

venous pulse, the pulse of a vein usually palpated over the internal or external jugular veins in the neck. The pulse in the jugular vein is taken to evaluate the pressure of the pulse and the form of the pressure wave, especially in a person with a cardiac conduction defect or cardiac arrhythmia.

venous sinus, one of many sinuses that collect blood from the dura mater and drain it into the internal jugular vein. Each sinus is formed by the separation of the two layers of the dura mater, the outer coat of the sinus consisting of fibrous tissue, the inner coat consisting of endothelium continuous with that of the veins.

venous stasis dermatitis. See **stasis dermatitis.**

venous thrombosis, a condition characterized by the presence of a clot in a vein in which the wall of the vessel is not inflamed. Pain, swelling, and inflammation may follow if the vein is significantly occluded. Also called **phlebothrombosis.** Compare **thrombophlebitis.**

ventilate, **1.** to provide with fresh air. **2.** to provide the lungs with air from the atmosphere and to aerate or oxygenate blood in the pulmonary capillaries. **3.** (in psychiatry) to open discussion of something, as to ventilate feelings.

ventilation, the process by which gases are moved into and out of the lungs. Compare **respiration.** **–ventilatory,** *adj.*

ventilation lung scan, a radiographic examination of the lungs, performed while the patient inhales a radioactive gas as a contrast medium and the lungs are scanned to detect nonfunctional or impaired lung areas or other abnormalities.

ventilation perfusion defect, a disorder in which one or more areas of the lung receive oxygen but no blood, or blood but no oxygen.

ventilator, any of several devices used in respiratory therapy to provide assisted respiration and intensive positive pressure breathing. Kinds of ventilators are **pressure limited ventilator** and **volume ventilator.** See also **IPPB unit.**

venting, (in intravenous therapy) a method for allowing air to enter the vacuum of the intravenous bottle and displace the intravenous solution as it flows out. Glass intravenous bottles are usually equipped with a venting tube attached to the primary IV tubing or to a vent port incorporated with the bottle stopper. Venting is not required with a plastic IV bag, because the bag collapses as the fluid runs out. The air vent attached to primary IV tubing is removable to allow the injection of medication.

Ventolin a trademark for a bronchodilator (albuterol).

ventral, of or pertaining to a position toward the belly of the body; frontward; anterior. Compare **dorsal.**

-ventral, a combining form meaning 'of the stomach or abdominal region': *biventral, dorsoventral, uteroventral.*

ventral hernia. See **abdominal hernia.**

ventri-. See **ventro-.**

ventricle /ven′trikəl/, a small cavity, as one of the cavities filled with cerebrospinal fluid in the brain, or the right and the left ventricles of the heart.

ventricular /ventrik′yo͞olər/, of or pertaining to a ventricle.

ventricular aneurysm, a localized dilatation or saccular protrusion in the wall of the left ventricle, occurring most often after a myocardial infarction. Scar tissue is formed in response to the inflammatory changes of the infarction. This tissue weakens the myocardium, allowing its walls to bulge outward when the ventricle contracts. A typical sign of the lesion is a recurrent ventricular arrhythmia that does not respond to treatment with antiarrhythmic drugs, as procainamide or quinidine. Diagnostic measures are x-ray studies and cardiac catheterization. Treatment may consist of the administration of propranolol, digoxin, or procainamide but usually involves surgical removal of the scar tissue. Also called **cardiac aneurysm.**

ventricular extrasystole, an extrasystole arising from the ventricle.

ventricular fibrillation, a cardiac arrhythmia marked by rapid, disorganized depolarizations of the ventricular myocardium. The condition is characterized by a complete lack of organized electric impulse, conduction, and ventricular contraction. Blood pressure falls to zero, resulting in unconsciousness. Death may occur within 4 minutes. Defibrillation and ventilation must be initiated immediately.

ventricular gallop, an abnormal cardiac rhythm in which a low-pitched extra heart sound (S_3) is heard early in diastole on auscultation of the heart. When it is heard in an older person with heart disease, it indicates myocardial failure. The same sound heard in a healthy child or young adult is a physiologic finding (called a physiologic third heart sound) that usually disappears with age. See also **gallop.**

ventricular gradient, the algebraic sum of the areas within the QRS complex and within the T wave in the electrocardiogram.

ventricular hemiblock, an impulse blockage of only one division of the left bundle branch, as an anterior superior or posterior inferior hemiblock.

ventricular septal defect (VSD), an abnormal opening in the septum separating the ventricles, permitting blood to flow from the left ventricle to the right ventricle and to recirculate through the pulmonary artery and lungs. It is the most common congenital heart defect, with openings that may be single or multiple and may range in size from 1 to 2 mm to several centimeters. Children with small defects are usually asymptomatic, whereas those with large defects may have congestive heart failure, associated with lower respiratory tract infections, rapid breathing, poor weight gain, restlessness, and irritability. Small defects may close spontaneously; larger ones may lead to bacterial endocarditis, pulmonary vascular obstructive disease, aortic regurgitation, or congestive heart failure. Diagnosis is established by electrocardiography, cardiac catheterization, and angiography. Treatment consists of surgical repair of the defect, preferably in early childhood.

ventricular tachycardia, tachycardia that usually originates in the ventricular Purkinje system.

ventriculo-, a combining form meaning 'pertaining to a ventricle of the heart or brain': *ventriculocisternostomy, ventriculopuncture, ventriculostium.*

ventriculoatrial shunt /ventrik′yo͞olō·ā′trē·əl/, a surgically created passageway, consisting of plastic tubing and one-way valves, implanted between a cerebral ventricle and the right atrium of the heart to drain excess cerebrospinal fluid from the brain in hydrocephalus.

ventriculocisternostomy, a surgical procedure performed to treat hydrocephalus. An opening is created that allows cerebrospinal fluid to drain through a shunt from the ventricles of the brain into the cisterna magna. Also called **Torkildsen procedure, ventriculostomy.**

ventriculofallopian tube shunt, a surgical procedure with limited effectiveness for diverting cerebrospinal fluid into the peritoneal cavity. The procedure passes a polyethylene tube from the lateral ventricle or from the spinal subarachnoid space into a ligated fallopian tube and finally into the peritoneal cavity, where the shunted cerebrospinal fluid is absorbed. This procedure is used to correct both the obstructive and the communicating types of hydrocephalus. Also called **spinofallopian tube shunt.**

ventriculography /ventrik′yo͞olog′rəfē/, **1.** an x-ray examination of the head, after injection of air or another contrast medium into the cerebral ventricles. **2.** an x-ray examination of a ventricle of the heart, after injection of a radiopaque contrast medium.

ventriculoperitoneal shunt, a surgically created passageway, consisting of plastic tubing and one-way valves, between a cerebral ventricle and the peritoneum for the draining of excess cerebrospinal fluid from the brain in hydrocephalus.

ventriculoperitoneostomy /ventrik′yo͞olōper′itōnē-os′təmē/, a surgical procedure for temporarily diverting cerebrospinal fluid in hydrocephalus, usually in the newborn. In this procedure, which spares the kidney but is less efficient than a ventriculoureterostomy, a polyethylene tube is passed from the lateral ventricle subcutaneously down the dorsal spine and is reinserted into the peritoneal cavity where the diverted fluid is absorbed. This procedure is used to correct both the communicating and the obstructive types of hydrocephalus.

ventriculopleural shunt, a surgical procedure for diverting cerebrospinal fluid from engorged ventricles in hydrocephalus, usually in the newborn. In this procedure, cerebrospinal fluid is diverted from the lateral ventricle into the pleural cavity. It is used to correct both the obstructive and the communicating types of hydrocephalus.

ventriculostomy. See **ventriculocisternostomy.**

ventriculoureterostomy /ventrik′yo͞olōyo͞orē′tər-os′təmē/, a surgical procedure for directing cerebrospinal fluid into the general circulation performed in the treatment of hydrocephalus, usually in the newborn. In this procedure a polyethylene tube is passed from the lateral ventricle down the dorsal spine subcutaneously to the twelfth rib; the tube is inserted through the paraspinal muscles into a ureter. Rarely used, the method is an alternative to auriculoventriculostomy, especially if the obstruction to cerebrospinal fluid includes the basilar and the cerebral subarachnoid spaces, posterior fossa, and the spinal subarachnoid spaces. The procedure is performed to correct an obstructive type of hydrocephalus.

ventro-, ventri-, a combining form meaning 'pertaining to the belly or to the front of the body': *ventrodorsal, ventrolateral, ventroptosia.*

venule /ven′yo͞ol/, any one of the small blood vessels that gather blood from the capillary plexuses and anastomose to form the veins. –**venular,** *adj.*

VEP, abbreviation for **visual evoked potential.**

verapamil, a slow channel blocker or calcium ion antagonist.

■ INDICATIONS: It is prescribed for the treatment of vasospastic and effort-associated angina, supraventricular tachycardia, atrial fibrillation, and atrial flutter.

■ CONTRAINDICATIONS: Severe left ventricular dysfunction, hypotension, cardiogenic shock, sick sinus syndrome, or second- or third-degree atrioventricular block prohibits its use.

■ ADVERSE EFFECTS: Among the more serious adverse reactions are hypotension, peripheral edema, atrioventricular block, bradycardia, congestive heart failure, pulmonary edema, and dizziness.

Veratrum, a genus of poisonous herbs of the lily family. The dried rhizomes of the British and American hellebore provide alkaloids that are used as antihypertensive agents.

verbal aphasia. See **motor aphasia.**

verbal language, a culturally organized system of vocal sounds that communicates meaning between individuals.

Vercyte, a trademark for an antineoplastic (pipobroman).

vermicide, an agent that kills worms, particularly those in the intestine. Compare **anthelmintic, vermifuge.**

vermiform appendix, a wormlike, blunt process extending from the cecum. Its length varies from 3 to 6 inches, and its diameter is about 1/3 inch. Also called **appendix vermiformis, cecal appendix.** See also **appendicitis.**

vermifuge, an agent that causes the evacuation of parasitic worms.

vermilion border, the external pinkish to red area of the upper and lower lips, extending from the junction of the lips with the surrounding facial skin on the exterior to the labial mucosa within the mouth.

vermis /vur′mis/, *pl.* **vermes,** 1. a worm. 2. a structure resembling a worm, as the median lobe of the cerebellum. –**vermiform,** *adj.*

Vermox, a trademark for an anthelmintic (mebendazole).

vernal conjunctivitis, a chronic, bilateral form of conjunctivitis, thought to be allergic in origin, that occurs most frequently in young men under 20 years of age during the spring and summer months. Most common symptoms include intense itching and crusting discharge. Topical corticosteroids may be applied, and desensitization to pollen may be helpful. Compare **allergic conjunctivitis.**

Verneuil's neuroma. See **plexiform neuroma.**

vernix caseosa /vur′niks kas′ē·ō′sə/, a grayish-white, cheeselike substance, consisting of sebaceous gland secretions, lanugo, and desquamated epithelial cells, that covers the skin of the fetus and newborn. It acts as a protective agent during intrauterine life and is thought to have an insulating effect against heat loss.

verruca /vuro͞o′kə/, a benign, viral, warty skin lesion with a rough, papillomatous surface. It is caused by a common, contagious papovavirus. Methods of treatment include salicylic acid, cantharidin, electrodesiccation, solid carbon dioxide, liquid nitrogen, and mental suggestion. Also called **verruca vulgaris, wart.** –**verrucose, verrucous,** *adj.*

verruca plana, a small, slightly elevated, smooth, tan or flesh-colored wart, sometimes occurring in large numbers on the face, neck, back of the hands, wrists, and knees, especially in children. Also called **flat wart.**

verruca senillis. See **basal cell papilloma.**

verruca vulgaris. See **verruca.**

verrucous carcinoma, a well-differentiated squamous cell neoplasm of soft tissue of the oral cavity, larynx, or genitalia. A slow-growing tumor, it tends to displace rather than invade surrounding tissue; it does not usually metastasize.

verrucous dermatitis, any skin rash with wartlike lesions.

verruga peruana. See **bartonellosis.**

Versapen, a trademark for an antibacterial (hetacillin).

-verse, 1. a combining form meaning 'to turn': *reverse, sacrotransverse, transverse.* 2. combining form meaning 'turned, changed': *inverse, reverse.*

version, the changing of the position of the fetus in the uterus, usually done to facilitate delivery. Version may occur spontaneously as a result of uterine contractions or be performed by internal or external manipulation by the physician.

version and extraction, an obstetric operation in which a fetus presenting head first is turned and delivered feet first. It is performed by reaching deeply into the uterus, grasping the feet and pulling them down, and extracting the infant. The procedure is considered outmoded and hazardous and has been replaced by cesarean section, although it may still be done to deliver a second twin. Also called **internal podalic version and total breech extraction.** Compare **external version.** See also **breech birth.**

-vert, a combining form meaning a 'person who has turned (metaphorically)' in a specified direction: *extrovert, introvert, invert.*

vertebra, *pl.* **vertebrae,** any one of the 33 bones of the spinal column, comprising the seven cervical, 12 thoracic, five lumbar, five sacral, and four coccygeal vertebrae. The vertebrae, with the exception of the first and second cervical vertebrae, are much alike and are composed of a body, an arch, a spinous process for muscle attachment, and pairs of pedicles and processes. The first cervical vertebra is called the atlas and has no vertebral body. The second cervical vertebra is called the axis and forms the pivot on which the atlas rotates, permitting the head to turn. The body of the axis also extends into a strong, bony process.

-vertebral, a combining form referring to the spinal column: *paravertebral, pelvivertebral, subvertebral.*

vertebral artery, each of two arteries branching from the subclavian arteries, arising deep in the neck from the cranial and dorsal subclavian surfaces. Each vertebral artery divides into two cervical and five cranial branches, supplying deep neck muscles, the spinal cord and spinal membranes, and the cerebellum. The cervical branches are the spinal and the muscular. The cranial branches are the meningeal, posterior spinal, anterior spinal, posterior inferior cerebellar, and the medullary.

vertebral body, the weight-supporting, solid central portion of a vertebra. The pedicles of the arch project from its dorsolateral surfaces.

vertebral column, the flexible structure that forms the longitudinal axis of the skeleton. In the adult, it includes 26 vertebrae arranged in a straight line from the base of the skull to the coccyx. The vertebrae are separated by intervertebral disks. They provide attachment for various muscles, as the iliocostalis thoracis and the longissimus thoracis, which give the column strength and flexibility. In the adult, the five sacral and four coccygeal vertebrae fuse to form the sacrum and the coccyx. The average length of the vertebral column in men is about 71 cm. The cervical part measures about 12.5 cm, the thoracic part about 28 cm, the lumbar part about 18 cm, and the sacrum and the coccyx about 12.5 cm. The vertebral column in women measures approximately 61 cm. Several curves in the column increase its strength, as the cervical, thoracic, lumbar, and pelvic curves. The cervical curve is convex ventrally from the apex of the dens to the middle of the second thoracic vertebra and is the least marked of all the curves. The thoracic curve, concave ventrally, starts at the middle of the second and ends at the middle of the twelfth thoracic vertebra. The lumbar curve, more pronounced in women than in men, begins at the middle of the last thoracic vertebra and ends at the sacrovertebral angle. The pelvic curve starts at the sacrovertebral articulation, and it ends at the point of the coccyx. The thoracic and the sacral curves constitute primary curves, present during fetal life; the cervical and the lumbar curves constitute secondary curves, which develop after birth. The cervical curve develops when the child is able to hold up its head, usually 3 to 4 months after birth; the lumbar curve develops 12 to 18 months after birth, when the child starts to walk. The vertebral column also presents a slight lateral curve, which in most individuals presents a convexity toward the right side. The vertebral canal courses through the vertebral column and contains the spinal cord. The canal is formed by the posterior arches of the vertebrae and is large and triangular in the cervical and the lumbar sections of the column, the most flexible portions. The canal is small and rounded in the thoracic region, where motion is more restricted. Also called **spinal column, spine.** See also **vertebra.**

vertebro-, a combining form meaning 'pertaining to the vertebral column or to a vertebra': *vertebrocostal, vertebrodymus, vertebrosternal.*

vertex, **1.** the top of the head; crown. **2.** the apex or highest point of any structure.

vertex presentation, (in obstetrics) a fetal presentation in which the vertex of the fetus is the part nearest to the cervical os and can be expected to be born first. Compare **breech presentation.**

vertical angulation, (in dentistry) the measured angle within the vertical plane at which the central beam of an x-ray is projected relative to a reference in the horizontal or occlusal plane.

vertical coordination, a system of community health nurses who serve as links between their level in the organization and those above and below their level. They also serve as links between the agency and the patient.

vertical plane. See **cardinal frontal plane.**

vertical resorption, a pattern of bone loss in which the alveolar bone adjacent to the affected tooth is destroyed without simultaneous crestal loss. See also **resorption.**

vertical transmission, the transfer of a disease, condition, or trait from one generation to the next, either genetically or congenitally, as the spread of an infection through breast milk or through the placenta.

verticosubmental, a part of the skull used as a focal point for radiographic projection. It permits the central ray to pass from the vertex of the skull to its base.

vertigo. See **dizziness.**

very-low-density lipoprotein (VLDL), a plasma protein that is composed chiefly of triglycerides with small amounts of cholesterol, phospholipid, and protein. It transports triglycerides primarily from the liver to peripheral sites in the tissues for use or storage. The triglycerides are quickly converted to smaller, more soluble intermediate lipoproteins and eventually to low-density lipoproteins. See also **high-density lipoprotein (HDL).**

vesical fistula, an abnormal passage communicating with the urinary bladder. Vesical fistulae may communicate with the skin, vagina, uterus, or rectum.

vesicle /ves′ikəl/, a small bladder or blister, as a small, thin-walled, raised skin lesion containing clear fluid. Compare **bulla.** **–vesicular,** *adj.*

vesicle calculus, a concretion occurring in the bladder. Also called **bladder stone, cystolith.**

vesicle reflex, the sensation of a need to urinate when the bladder is moderately distended. See also **micturition reflex.**

vesico-, a combining form meaning 'pertaining to the bladder or to a blister': *vesicocavernous, vesicosigmoid, vesicourethral.*

vesicoureteral reflux, an abnormal backflow of urine from the bladder to the ureter, resulting from a congenital defect, obstruction of the outlet of the bladder, or infection of the lower urinary tract. Reflux increases the hydrostatic pressure in the ureters and kidneys. The condition is characterized by abdominal or flank pain, enuresis, pyuria, hematuria, proteinuria, and bacteriuria accompanied by persistent or recurrent urinary tract infections. Diagnosis is made by cystoscopy and voiding cystourethrogram. Obstruction or defective implantation of the ureter in the bladder may be surgically corrected. Antibacterial medication, urinary tract antiseptics, and analgesia are usually prescribed for any infection that causes or results from this condition.

vesicouterine /ves′ikōyo͞o′tərin, -ēn/, of or pertaining to the bladder and uterus. Also called **uterovesical.**

vesicular appendix, a cystic structure on the fimbriated end of each of the fallopian tubes. It represents a remnant of the mesonephric ducts.

vesicular breath sound, a normal sound of rustling or swishing heard with a stethoscope over the lung periphery, characteristically higher pitched during inspiration and fading rapidly during expiration. Compare **tracheal breath sound.**

vesicular mole. See **hydatid mole.**

vesiculitis /vəsik′yo͝olī′tis/, inflammation of any vesicle, particularly the seminal vesicles. Clinical manifestations of this condition are minimal; it is usually associated with prostatitis.

vesiculography, the radiologic examination of the seminal vesicles and adjacent structures, usually conducted by injecting a radiopaque medium into the deferent ducts or by catheterization of the medium into the ejaculatory ducts. The technique is used to examine the vesicles, vas deferens, and ejaculatory duct for possible tumors, cysts, or other disorders.

Vesprin, a trademark for a phenothiazine tranquilizer (triflupromazine hydrochloride) for intramuscular injection.

vessel, any one of the many tubules throughout the body that convey fluids, as blood and lymph. The main kinds of vessels are the arteries, the veins, and the lymphatic vessels.

vestibular /vestib′yo͞olər/, of or pertaining to a vestibule, as the vestibular portion of the mouth, which lies between the cheeks and the teeth.

vestibular gland, any one of four small glands, two on each side of the vaginal orifice. One pair of the small structures constitute the greater vestibular glands; the other pair constitute the lesser vestibular glands. The vestibular glands secrete a lubricating substance. Compare **Cowper's gland.** See also **Bartholin's gland.**

vestibule /ves′tibyo͞ol/, a space or a cavity that serves as the entrance to a passageway, as the vestibule of the vagina or the vestibule of the ear.

vestibulocochlear nerve. See **acoustic nerve.**

vestige, an imperfectly developed, relatively useless organ or other structure of the body that had a vital function at an earlier stage of life or in a more primitive form of life. The vermiform appendix is a vestigial organ. –**vestigial,** *adj*.

viable, capable of developing, growing, and otherwise sustaining life, as a normal human fetus at 28 weeks of gestation. –**viability,** *n*.

viable infant, an infant who at birth weighs at least 1000 g or is 28 weeks or more of gestational age.

Vibramycin Hyclate, a trademark for a tetracycline antibiotic (doxycycline hyclate).

Vibramycin Monohydrate, a trademark for a tetracycline antibiotic (doxycycline monohydrate).

vibrating. See **cupping and vibrating.**

vibration, a type of massage administered by quick tapping with the fingertips, alternating the fingers in a rhythmic manner, or by a mechanic device. See also **massage.**

vibrio /vib′rē·ō/, any bacterium that is curved and motile, as those belonging to the genus *Vibrio*. Cholera and several other epidemic forms of gastroenteritis are caused by members of the genus.

Vibrio cholerae, the species of comma-shaped, motile bacillus that is the cause of cholera.

Vibrio fetus. See ***Campylobacter.***

vibrio gastroenteritis, an infectious disease acquired from contaminated seafood and characterized by nausea, vomiting, abdominal pain, and diarrhea, caused by *Vibrio parahaemolyticus*. Headache, mild fever, and bloody stools may also be present. Spontaneous recovery usually occurs in 2 to 5 days. Compare **salmonellosis, shigellosis.**

Vibrio parahaemolyticus /per′əhē′mōlit′ikəs/, a species of microorganisms of the genus *Vibrio,* the causative agent in food poisoning associated with the ingestion of uncooked or undercooked shellfish, especially crabs and shrimp. This microorganism is a common cause of gastroenteritis in Japan, aboard cruise ships, and in the eastern and southeastern coastal areas of the United States. Thorough cooking of seafood prevents the infection associated with *Vibrio parahaemolyticus,* which causes watery diarrhea, abdominal cramps, vomiting, headache, chills, and fever. This microorganism has an incubation period of 2 to 48 hours, after which the symptoms of infection appear. The food poisoning from this agent usually subsides spontaneously within 2 days but may be more severe, even fatal, in debilitated and elderly persons. Confirming diagnosis must rule out other causes of food poisoning and acute GI disorders and requires bacteriologic examination of the vomitus, stool, and blood. Treatment usually includes bed rest and the oral replacement of fluids. Intravenous replacement of fluids is seldom required.

vicarious menstruation, discharge of blood from a site other than the uterus at the time when the menstrual flow is normally expected. Such bleeding is usually caused by the increased capillary permeability that occurs during menstruation.

vidarabine, an antiviral agent. Also called **adenine arabinoside.**

■ INDICATIONS: It is used systemically to treat herpes simplex encephalitis and locally to treat herpesvirus I keratoconjunctivitis and keratitis.

■ CONTRAINDICATIONS: It is used in pregnancy only when the risk of teratogenicity is outweighed by benefits. Known hypersensitivity to this drug prohibits its use.

■ ADVERSE EFFECTS: Among the more serious adverse reactions to systemic administration are severe nausea and other symptoms of GI distress, various central nervous system effects, and bone marrow depression. Local irritation, photophobia and corneal edema may occur in topical ophthalmic applications.

video display terminal (VDT), a cathode-ray tube device with a surface similar to a television screen, used in word processors, computer terminals, and similar equipment. Use of video display terminals has been associated with a variety of environmental health complaints, including burning and itching eyes, headaches, and back and arm pain. Published studies indicate the health effects are caused by inadequate or improper office environments, as unsuitable furniture or light levels, rather than VDT radiation.

villi. See **villus.**

villoma /vilō′mə/, *pl.* **villomas, villomata,** a villous neoplasm or papilloma, occurring chiefly in the bladder or rectum. Also called **villioma.**

villous adenoma /vil′əs/, a slow-growing, soft, spongy, potentially malignant papillary growth of the mucosa of the large intestine.

villous carcinoma, an epithelial tumor with many long, velvety papillary outgrowths. Also called **carcinoma villosum.**

villous papilloma, a benign tumor with long, slender processes, usually occurring in the bladder, breast, or a cerebral ventricle.

villus, *pl.* **villi,** one of the many tiny projections, barely visible to the naked eye, clustered over the entire mucous surface of the small intestine. The villi diffuse and transport fluids and nutrients. They are quite irregular in size and are larger in some parts of the intestine than in others, flattening out when the intestine distends. Each villus has a core of delicate areolar and reticular connective tissue supporting the epithelium, various capillaries, and usually a single lymphatic lacteal that fills with milky white chyle during the digestion of a fatty meal. **–villous,** *adj.*

vinblastine sulfate /vinblas′tēn, -tin/, an antineoplastic.

■ INDICATIONS: It is prescribed in the treatment of many neoplastic diseases, as choriocarcinoma, testicular carcinoma, Hodgkin's disease, and non-Hodgkin's lymphoma.

■ CONTRAINDICATIONS: Leukopenia, bacterial infection, or known hypersensitivity to this drug prohibits its use. It is not prescribed in pregnancy.

■ ADVERSE EFFECTS: Among the most serious adverse reactions are leukopenia and neurotoxicity. Nausea, diarrhea, stomatitis, and alopecia also may occur.

Vincent's angina, Vincent's infection. See **acute necrotizing gingivitis.**

vincristine sulfate /vinkris′tēn, -tin/, an antineoplastic.

■ INDICATIONS: It is prescribed in the treatment of many neoplastic diseases, as leukemia, neuroblastoma, lymphomas, and sarcomas.

■ CONTRAINDICATIONS: Pregnancy, leukopenia, preexisting neuromuscular disease, or known hypersensitivity to this drug prohibits its use.

■ ADVERSE EFFECTS: Among the most serious adverse reactions are neurotoxicity and leukopenia. Constipation, abdominal pain, alopecia, and inflammation at the site of injection also may occur.

vindesine sulfate, an antineoplastic agent.

■ INDICATIONS: It is prescribed in the treatment of acute lymphoblastic leukemia, breast cancer, malignant melanoma, lymphosarcoma, and non-small-cell lung carcinoma.

■ CONTRAINDICATIONS: Leukopenia, bacterial infections, or known sensitivity to this drug prohibits its use.

■ ADVERSE EFFECTS: Among the most serious adverse reactions are neurotoxicity, leukopenia, thrombocytopenia, phlebitis, and alopecia.

Vioform, a trademark for an antiamebic and topical antiinfective (iodochlorhydroxyquin).

Viokase, a trademark for an enzyme (pancreatin).

violence, potential for: self-directed or directed at others, a nursing diagnosis accepted by the Fourth National Conference on the Classification of Nursing Diagnoses. The cause of the condition may be complex and may involve an antisocial personality, mania, organic brain syndrome, panic, rage, suicidal behavior, temporal lobe epilepsy, or a toxic reaction to a medication. Characteristics of clients who are potentially violent include anxiety, fear of the self or other people, lack of verbal ability, complaining or demanding vocalization, provocative, argumentative, or overreactive behavior, poor self-esteem, or psychologic depression. Many other factors may also be present, as a history of self-destructive behavior, pacing, excitement, agitation, or the possession of a weapon. See also **nursing diagnosis.**

viosterol /vī·os′tərôl/, synthetic vitamin D_2 in an oil base. Also called **synthetic oleovitamin D.** See also **calciferol, ergosterol.**

VIP, 1. abbreviation for **vasoactive intestinal polypeptide. 2.** abbreviation for *very important person.* A VIP suite in a hospital is one reserved for such persons.

Vira-A, a trademark for an antiviral (vidarabine).

viral disease. See **viral infection.**

viral hepatitis, a viral, inflammatory disease of the liver, caused by one of the hepatitis viruses, A, B, or non-A, non-B. Transmission, speed of onset, and probable course of the illness vary with the kind and strain of virus, but the characteristics of the disease and its treatment are the same. See also **hepatitis A, hepatitis B, non-A, non-B hepatitis.**

■ OBSERVATIONS: Characteristic of viral hepatitis are anorexia, malaise, headache, pain over the liver, fever, jaundice, clay-colored stools, dark urine, nausea and vomiting, and diarrhea. Laboratory analyses reveal increased amounts of serum glutamic oxalacetic transaminase (SGOT) and bilirubin and an abnormal coagulation of the blood. Severe infection, especially with hepatitis B virus, may be prolonged and result in tissue destruction, cirrhosis, and chronic hepatitis or in hepatic coma and death.

■ INTERVENTION: Treatment of viral hepatitis is largely supportive. It includes bed rest; isolation, if necessary; fluids; a low-fat, high-protein, high-calorie diet; special skin care if pruritus is present; emotional support; vitamins B_{12}, K, and C; and monitoring of liver and kidney function. Sedatives, analgesics, antiemetics, and steroids may be ordered. However, the patient is carefully observed for adverse reaction to medication, because the liver may not be able to break down and detoxify the drugs. Decrease in the amount or frequency of administration or change of the medication may be necessary.

■ NURSING CONSIDERATIONS: The person is taught the importance of rest and of avoiding fatigue, of washing the hands carefully after urinating or defecating to avoid spreading the virus, of eating well, of following written dietary instructions after discharge, and of avoiding alcohol, usually for at least 1 year. The patient is encouraged to have certain blood tests performed periodically, including SGOT and serum bilirubin, to report any symptoms of recurrence immediately, and to avoid contact with people having infections. The person is told not to donate blood and not to take over-the-counter drugs without medical consultation.

viral infection, any of the diseases caused by one of approximately 200 viruses pathogenic to humans. Some are the most communicable and dangerous diseases known; some cause mild and transient conditions that pass virtually unnoticed. If cells are damaged by the viral attack, disease exists. The signs of the infection reflect the anatomic location of the damaged cells. Viruses are introduced into the body through a break in the skin or through a transfusion into the bloodstream, by droplet infection through the respiratory tract, or by ingestion through the digestive tract into the GI system. The pathogenicity of the particular virus depends on the rapidity of action, the enzymes released, the part of the body infected, and the particular action of the virus. The general process of viral infection reflects the life cycle of a virus. The first step in the cycle, after entry into the body, is the attachment of the virus to a susceptible cell and the cell's adsorption of the virus. This is followed by penetration of the viral nucleic acid into the parasitized cell. The dissembled virus at this point causes no symptoms and cannot be recovered from the cells in infectious form. The virus begins to mature within the cell and, carrying its own genetic information, begins to replicate itself, using chemical building blocks and energy available in the parasitized cell. The virus has now taken over the cell. After a variable period of time, masses of fully grown viruses appear, each able to survive outside the cell until more susceptible cells are found. In poliovirus infection, one parasitized cell may produce more than 100,000 poliovirus particles in a few hours. Techniques used in viral identification and immunization are based on the essential fact that viruses can multiply only inside living cells. Inoculation of susceptible animals, of tissue culture media, and of chick embryos allows cultivation of viruses for study and identification and for the preparation of vaccine. Diagnosis of the cause of viral infection is also possible using various other techniques, including serologic tests, fluorescent antibody microscopic examination, microscopic examination, and skin tests. In many viral diseases, including mumps, smallpox, and measles, one attack confers permanent immunity. In others, immunity is short-lived. The incubation period for viral infection is short, the viruses do not circulate in the bloodstream, antibodies do not form, and, most often, immunity does not develop. Exposure to a few viruses results in immunity to that virus and to other closely related viruses. Some vectors are able to spread several viruses, but only one at a time. Other mechanisms of natural resistance to viral infection are poorly understood, but susceptibility to a particular virus is somehow species-specific; for example, chickenpox, caused by the varicella zoster virus, is seen only in humans. A protective substance, interferon, is elaborated naturally in small amounts in the body. It is cell-specific and species-specific but not virus-specific. Interferon may act as a broad spectrum antiviral agent, protecting the body from the effects of many viral infections by stopping the synthesis of viral nucleic acid within the parasitized cell. See also specific viral infections.

viral pneumonia, pulmonary infection caused by a virus.

viremia /vīrē′mē•ə/, the presence of viruses in the blood. Compare **bacteremia, fungemia, parasitemia.**

virile /vir′əl/, **1.** of, pertaining to, or characteristic of an adult male; masculine; manly. **2.** possessing or exhibiting masculine strength, vigor, force, or energy. **3.** of or pertaining to the male sexual functions; capable of procreatition. Compare **virilism,** **–virility,** *n.*

virilism, **1.** See **virilization. 2.** pseudohermaphroditism in a female. **3.** premature development of masculine characteristics in the male. Kinds of virilism are **adrenal virilism** and **prosopopilary virilism.**

virilization, a process in which secondary, male sexual characteristics are acquired by a female, usually as the result of adrenal dysfunction or hormonal medication. Also called **masculinization.** See also **adrenal virilism.**

virion /vī′rē•on/, a rudimentary virus particle with a central nucleoid surrounded by a protein sheath or capsid. The complete nucleocapsid with a nucleic acid core may constitute a complete virus, as the adenoviruses and the picornaviruses, or it may be surrounded by an envelope, as in the herpesviruses and the myxoviruses. Such an envelope is a membrane that contains lipids, proteins, and carbohydrates and projects spikelike structures from its surface. See also **capsid.**

virocytes, lymphocytes altered in appearance and in staining that are seen in blood smears from patients with certain viral diseases.

virologist /vīrol′əjist, vir-/, a specialist who studies viruses and diseases caused by viruses.

virology /vīrol′əjē, vir-/, the study of viruses and viral diseases. **–virologic, virological,** *adj.*

Viroptic, a trademark for an ophthalmic antiviral (trifluridine).

virucide, any agent that destroys or inactivates a virus. **–virucidal,** *adj.*

virulence /vir′yŏŏləns/, the power of a microorganism to produce disease.

virulent /vir′yŏŏlənt/, of or pertaining to a very pathogenic or rapidly progressive condition.

virus, a minute parasitic microorganism much smaller than a bacterium that, having no independent metabolic activity, may only replicate within a cell of a living plant or animal host. A virus consists of a core of nucleic acid (DNA or RNA) surrounded by a coat of antigenic protein sometimes surrounded by an envelope of lipoprotein. The virus provides the genetic code for replication, and the host cell provides the necessary energy and raw materials. More than 200 viruses have been identified as capable of causing disease in humans. Some kinds of viruses are **adenovirus, arenavirus, enterovirus, herpesvirus,** and **rhinovirus.** See also **viral infection. –viral,** *adj.*

viscera /vis′ərə/, *sing.* **viscus** /vis′kəs/, the internal organs enclosed within a body cavity, primarily the abdominal organs.

visceral /vis′ərəl/, of or pertaining to the viscera, or internal organs in the abdominal cavity. Also **splanchnic.**

visceral afferent fibers, the nerve fibers of the visceral nervous system that receive stimuli and carry impulses toward the central nervous system and share the sensory ganglia of the cerebrospinal nerves with the somatic sensory fibers. Peripheral distribution of the visceral afferent fibers constitutes the main difference between them and the somatic afferents. The visceral afferents produce sensations different from those of the somatic afferents. The visceral efferent fibers connect with both the somatic and visceral afferents; the number and extent of the visceral afferents is not clearly established. Their peripheral processes reach the ganglia by various routes. Most of the visceral afferents accompany blood vessels for part of their course, and various afferent fibers run in the cerebrospinal nerves. Some of the parts of the body with visceral afferents are the face, scalp, nose, mouth, descending colon, lungs, abdomen, and rectum. See also **autonomic nervous system.**

visceral larva migrans, infestation with parasitic larvae or *Toxocara* or, occasionally, *Ascaris, Strongyloides,* or other nematodes. See **toxocariasis.**

visceral leishmaniasis. See **kala-azar.**

visceral lymph node, a small oval nodular gland that filters lymph circulating in the lymphatic vessels of the thoracic, abdominal, and pelvic viscera. The visceral lymph nodes of the thorax include the anterior mediastinal nodes, posterior mediastinal nodes, and tracheobronchial nodes. The visceral lymph nodes of the abdomen and pelvis include those that follow the course of the celiac artery, superior mesenteric artery, and inferior mesenteric artery. Compare **parietal lymph node.** See also **lymph, lymphatic system, lymph node.**

visceral nervous system, the visceral portion of the peripheral nervous system that comprises the whole complex of nerves, fibers, ganglia, and plexuses by which impulses travel from the central nervous system to the viscera and from the viscera to the central nervous system. It contains the usual afferent fibers that receive stimuli and carry impulses toward the central nervous system and efferent fibers that carry impulses from the appropriate centers to the active effector organs, as the nonstriated muscle, cardiac muscle, and glands of the body. Also called **involuntary nervous system.** See also **autonomic nervous system, visceral afferent fibers.**

visceral pain, abdominal pain caused by any abnormal condition of the viscera. It is characteristically severe, diffuse, and difficult to localize.

visceral peritoneum, one of two portions of the largest serous membrane in the body that invests the viscera. The free surface of the visceral peritoneum is a smooth layer of mesothelium exuding a serous fluid that lubricates the viscera and allows them to glide freely against the wall of the abdominal cavity or over each other. The attached surface of the membrane is connected to the viscera and the abdominal wall by subserous fascia. Compare **parietal peritoneum.** See also **peritoneal cavity.**

viscero-, a combining form meaning 'pertaining to the organs of the body': *viscerocranium, visceropleural, viscerosomatic.*

viscid /vis′id/, sticky or glutinous. Also **viscous** /vis′kəs/.

viscosity, pertaining to the quality of a sticky or gummy fluid, an effect caused by the adhesion of adjacent molecules.

viscous fermentation, the formation of viscous material in milk, urine, and wine by the action of various bacilli.

viscus. See **viscera.**

visible light, the radiant energy in the electromagnetic spectrum that is visible to the human eye. The wavelengths cover a range of approximately 390 to 780 nm.

vision, the capacity for sight.

visit, **1.** a meeting between a practitioner and a client or patient. In the hospital and the home, the practitioner makes a visit to the patient; in the clinic or office the patient makes a visit to the practitioner. **2.** (of a patient) to meet a practitioner to obtain professional services or (of a practitioner) to see a patient or client to render a professional service.

Visken, a trademark for a beta blocker (pindolol).

Vistaril, a trademark for a tranquilizer (hydroxyzine hydrochloride).

visual accommodation, a process by which the eye adjusts and is able to focus, producing a sharp image at various, changing distances from the object seen. The convexity of the anterior surface of the lens may be increased or decreased by contraction or relaxation of the ciliary muscle. With increasing age the lens becomes harder and less flexible, resulting in a loss of accommodation, and, usually, the ability to focus on nearby objects. Compare **presbyopia.**

visual evoked potential (VEP), an evoked potential elicited by a repeatedly flashing light. The waves produced are too variable to be reliable predictors of injury to nerve tissue. High-risk infants are monitored with VEP to evaluate visual function.

visual field defect, one or more spots or defects in the vision that move with the eye, unlike a floater. This fixed defect is usually caused by damage to the retina or visual pathways, as by chorioretinitis, traumatic injury, macular degeneration, glaucoma, or a vascular occlusion of the eye or the brain. Sudden loss of a noticeable portion of the visual field warrants ophthalmologic examination. Defects in the field of vision may be detected using an Amsler grid.

visual memory, the ability to create an eidetic image of past visual experiences. Also called **eye memory.**

visual pathway, a pathway over which a visual sensation is transmitted from the retina to the brain. A pathway consists of an optic nerve, the fibers of an optic nerve traveling through or along the sides of the optic chiasm to the lateral geniculate body of the thalamus, and an optic tract terminating in an occipital lobe. Each optic nerve contains fibers from only one retina. The optic chiasm contains fibers from the nasal portions of the retinas of both eyes; these fibers cross to the opposite side of the brain at the optic chiasm. The fibers from the temporal portion of each eye bypass the optic chiasm and pass through the lateral geniculate body on the same side of the brain continuing back to the occipital lobe. Thus the optic tracts, occipital lobe, lateral geniculate bodies of the thalamus, and optic chiasm each contain nerve fibers from both eyes. If the right optic tract were destroyed, a person would lose partial vision in both eyes—the right nasal and the left temporal fields of vision.

visual purple. See **rhodopsin.**

vita-, a combining form meaning 'pertaining to life': *vitaglass, vital, vitascope.*

vital capacity (VC), a measurement of the amount of air that can be expelled slowly after a maximum inspiration, representing the greatest possible breathing capacity. The vital capacity equals the inspiratory reserve volume plus the tidal volume plus the expiratory reserve volume. The average normal values of 4000 to 5000 ml are affected by age, physical dimensions of the chest cage, physical fitness, posture, and sex. The vital capacity may be reduced by a decrease in functioning lung tissue, resulting from atelectasis, edema, fibrosis, pneumonia, pulmonary resection, or tumors, by limited chest expansion, resulting from ascites, chest deformity, neuromuscular disease, pneumothorax, or pregnancy, or by airway obstruction. Compare **forced expiratory volume, residual volume.**

vital signs, the measurements of pulse rate, respiration rate, and body temperature. Although not strictly a vital sign, blood pressure is also customarily included. Abnormalities of vital signs are often clues to diseases, and alterations in vital signs are used to evaluate a patient's progress. See also **blood pressure, pulse, respiration, temperature.**

vital statistics, data relating to births or natality, deaths or mortality, marriages, health, and disease or morbidity.

vitamin, an organic compound essential in small quantities for normal physiologic and metabolic functioning of the body. With few exceptions, vitamins cannot be synthesized by the body and must be obtained from the diet or dietary supplements. No one food contains all the vitamins. Vitamin deficiency diseases produce specific symptoms usually alleviated by the administration of the appropriate vitamin. Vitamins are classified according to their fat or water solubility, their physiologic effects, or their chemical structures, and they are designated by alphabetic letters and chemical or other specific names. The fat-soluble vitamins are A, D, E, and K; the B complex and C vitamins are water soluble. See also **avitaminosis, hypervitaminosis, oleovitamin, provitamin,** and see the specific vitamins.

vitamin A, a fat-soluble, solid terpene alcohol essential for skeletal growth, maintenance of normal mucosal epithelium, and visual acuity. It is derived from various carotenoids, mainly carotene, and is present in leafy green vegetables, yellow fruits and vegetables, the liver oils of the cod and other fish, liver, milk, cheese, butter, and egg yolk. Deficiency leads to atrophy of epithelial tissue resulting in keratomalacia, xerophthalmia, night blindness, and lessened resistance to infection of mucous membranes. Symptoms of hypervitaminosis A are irritability, fatigue, lethargy, abdominal discomfort, painful joints, severe throbbing headache, insomnia and restlessness, night sweats, loss of body hair, brittle nails, and exophthalmus. Also called **antiinfection vitamin, antixerophthalmic vitamin.** See also **oleovitamin A.**

vitamin B_1. See **thiamine.**

vitamin B_2. See **riboflavin.**

vitamin B_6. See **pyridoxine.**

vitamin B_{12}. See **cyanocobalamin.**

vitamin B_{17}. See **Laetrile.**

vitamin B complex, a group of water soluble vitamins differing from each other structurally and in their biologic effect. All of the B vitamins are found in large quantities in liver and yeast, and they are present separately or in combination in many foods. Heat and prolonged cooking, especially cooking with water, can destroy B vitamins. See also **folic acid,** and see vitamins B_1 through B_{12}.

vitamin C. See **ascorbic acid.**

vitamin D, a fat-soluble vitamin chemically related to the steroids and essential for the normal formation of bones and teeth and for the absorption of calcium and phosphorus from the GI tract. The vitamin is present in natural foods in small amounts, and requirements are usually met by artificial enrichment of various foods, especially milk and dairy products, and exposure to sunlight. Ultraviolet rays activate a form of cholesterol in an oil of the skin and convert it to a form of the vitamin, which is then absorbed. The natural foods containing vitamin D are of animal origin and include saltwater fish, especially salmon, sardines, and herring, organ meats, fish-liver oils, and egg yolk. Deficiency of the vitamin results in rickets in children, osteomalacia, osteoporosis, and osteodystrophy. Hypervitaminosis D produces a toxicity syndrome characterized by anorexia, vomiting, headache, drowsiness, diarrhea, and calcification of the soft tissues of the heart, blood vessels, renal tubules, and lungs. Treatment consists of discontinuing the vitamin dosage and initiating a low-calcium diet until symptoms resolve. See also **calciferol, vitamin D_3.**

vitamin D_2. See **calciferol.**

vitamin D_3, an antirachitic, white, odorless, crystalline, unsaturated alcohol that is the predominant form of vitamin D of animal origin. It is found in most fish-liver oils, butter, brain, and egg yolk and is formed in the skin, fur, and feathers of animals and birds exposed to sunlight or ultraviolet rays. Also called **activated 7-dehydrocholesterol, cholecalciferol.**

vitamin deficiency, a state or condition resulting from the lack of or inability to use one or more vitamins. The symptoms and manifestations of each deficiency vary depending on the specific function of the vitamin in promoting growth and development and maintaining body health.

vitamin D resistant rickets, a disease clinically similar to rickets but resistant to treatment with large doses of vitamin D. It is caused by a congenital defect in renal tubular reabsorption of phosphate and is usually seen in men. See also **rickets.**

vitamin E, any or all of the group of fat-soluble vitamins that consist of the tocopherols and are essential for normal reproduction, muscle development, resistance of erythrocytes to hemolysis, and various other biochemical functions. It is an intracellular antioxidant and acts in maintaining the stability of polyunsaturated fatty acids and other fatlike substances, including vitamin A and hormones of the pituitary, adrenal, and sex glands. Deficiency results in muscle degeneration, abnormalities in the vascular system, megaloblastic anemia, hemolytic anemia, infertility, creatinuria, and liver and kidney damage and is associated with the aging process. The richest dietary sources are wheat germ, soybean, cottonseed, peanut, and corn oils, margarine, whole raw seeds and nuts, soybeans, eggs, butter, liver, sweet potatoes, and the leaves of many vegetables, as turnip greens. It is stored in the body for long periods of time so that severe deficiency is rare. It is considered nontoxic except in hypertensive patients and those with chronic rheumatic heart disease. Alpha-tocopherol is the most physiologically active form of the group. Also called **tocopherol.**

vitamin H. See **biotin.**

vitamin K, a group of fat-soluble vitamins known as quinones that are essential for the synthesis of prothrombin in the liver and of several related proteins involved in the clotting of blood. It is also involved with the process of phosphorylation and electron transport. The vitamin is widely distributed in foods, especially leafy green vegetables, pork liver, yogurt, egg yolk, kelp, alfalfa, fish-liver oils, and blackstrap molasses and is synthesized by the bacterial flora of the GI tract. It is also produced synthetically. Deficiency results in hypoprothrombinemia, characterized by poor coagulation of the blood and hemorrhage, and usually occurs from inadequate absorption of the vitamin from the GI tract or the inability to use it in the liver. It is used to reduce the clotting time in patients with obstructive jaundice and in hemorrhagic states associated with intestinal diseases and diseases of the liver; it is given prophylactically to infants to prevent hemorrhagic disease of the newborn. A form of the vitamin is used as a preservative to control fermentation in foods. Natural vitamin K is stored in the body and produces no toxicity. Excessive doses of synthetic vitamin K may cause anemia in newborn infants and hemolysis in persons with glucose-6-phosphate deficiency. See also **vitamin K_1, vitamin K_2, menadione.**

vitamin K_1, a yellow, viscous, oil-soluble vitamin, occurring naturally, especially in alfalfa, and produced synthetically. It is used as a prothrombinogenic agent. Also called **phylloquinone, phytonadione.**

vitamin K_2, a pale-yellow, fat-soluble crystalline vitamin of the vitamin K group that is more unsaturated than vitamin K_1 and slightly less active biologically. It is isolated from putrefied fish meal and synthesized by various bacteria in the GI tract. See also **vitamin K.**

vitamin K_3. See **menadione.**

vitaminology /vī′təminol′əjē/, the study of vitamins, including their structures, modes of action, and function in maintaining the health of the body.

vitamin P. See **bioflavonoid.**

vitellin /vitel′in/, a phosphoprotein containing lecithin, found in the yolk of eggs. Also called **ovovitellin.** –**vitelline** /-ēn/, *adj.*

vitelline artery, any of the embryonic arteries that circulate blood from the primitive aorta of the early developing embryo to the yolk sac. Also called **omphalomesenteric artery.**

vitelline circulation, the circulation of blood and nutrients between the developing embryo and the yolk sac by way of the vitelline arteries and veins. Also called **omphalomesenteric circulation.** See also **fetal circulation.**

vitelline duct, (in embryology) the narrow channel connecting the yolk sac with the intestine. Also called **umbilical duct.**

vitelline membrane, the delicate cytoplasmic membrane surrounding the ovum. Also called **yolk membrane.** See also **zona pellucida.**

vitelline sac. See **yolk sac.**

vitelline sphere. See **morula.**

vitelline vein, any of the embryonic veins that return blood from the yolk sac to the primitive heart of the early developing embryo. Also called **omphalomesenteric vein.**

vitellogenesis /vitel′ōjen′əsis/, the formation or production of yolk. –**vitellogenetic,** *adj.*

vitellus /vitel′əs, vī-/, the yolk of an ovum.

vitiligo /vit′ilē′gō/, a benign, acquired skin disease of unknown cause, consisting of irregular patches of various sizes totally lacking in pigment and often having hyperpigmented borders. Exposed areas of skin are most often affected. Treatment using 8-methoxypsoralen requires extreme care and carefully regulated sun exposure. Waterproof cosmetics are often used to cover the patches. Compare **albinism, piebald.** –**vitiliginous,** *adj.*

vitreous body. See **vitreous humor.**

vitreous cavity, the cavity posterior to the lens that contains the vitreous body and vitreous membrane and is transected by the vestigial remnants of the hyaloid canal.

vitreous hemorrhage, a hemorrhage into the vitreous humor of the eye.

vitreous humor, a transparent, semigelatinous substance contained in a thin hyoid membrane filling the cavity behind the crystalline lens of the eye. Some indications of the hyaloid canal may persist in the vitreous humor, which is not penetrated by any blood vessels and is nourished at its periphery by vessels of the retina and the ciliary processes. The vitreous humor is concave anteriorly to accommodate the crystalline lens and is closely applied to the retina around the wall of the eyeball. Also called **corpus vitreum, vitreous body.**

vitreous membrane, a membrane that lines the posterior cavity of the eye and surrounds the vitreous body.

vitriol, oil of. See **sulfuric acid.**

Vivactil, a trademark for a tricyclic antidepressant (protriptyline hydrochloride).

vivax malaria. See **tertian malaria.**

viviparous /vivip′ərəs/, bearing living offspring rather than laying eggs, as most mammals and some fishes and reptiles. Compare **oviparous, ovoviviparous.**

Vivonex, a trademark for a nutritional supplement containing protein, carbohydrate, and fat.

VLDL, abbreviation for **very-low-density lipoprotein.**

VMA, abbreviation for **vanillylmandelic acid.**

$\dot{V}O_2$, symbol for *oxygen uptake*.

vocal cord, either of two strong bands of yellow elastic tissue in the larynx enclosed by membranes called vocal folds and attached ventrally to the angle of the thyroid cartilage and dorsally to the vocal process of the arytenoid. Also called **true vocal cord, vocal ligament.** Compare **false vocal cord.**

vocal cord nodule, a small, inflammatory or fibrous growth that develops on the vocal cords of people who constantly strain their voices. Also called **screamer's nodule, singer's nodule, teacher's nodule.** See also **chorditis.**

vocal fremitus, the vibration of the chest wall as a person speaks or sings that allows the person's voice to be heard by the examiner during auscultation of the chest with a stethoscope. Vocal fremitus is decreased in emphysema, pleural effusion, pulmonary edema, or bronchial obstruction.

voice box. See **larynx.**

void, to empty, or evacuate, as urine from the bladder.

volar /vō′lər/, of or pertaining to the palm of the hand or the sole of the foot.

volar ligament. See **retinaculum flexorum manus.**

volatile, (of a liquid) having the characteristics of boiling at a low temperature or evaporating at room temperature.

volatile solvent, an easily evaporated liquid capable of dissolving a substance.

-volemia, a combining form meaning '(condition of the) volume of plasma in the body': *hypervolemia, hypovolemia, normovolemia*.

volition /vōlish′ən/, **1.** the act, power, or state of willing or choosing. **2.** the conscious impulse to perform or to abstain from an act. **–volitional,** *adj*.

Volkmann's canal /fōlk′munz/, any one of the small blood vessel canals connecting haversian canals in bone tissue. Compare **haversian canaliculus.** See also **haversian system.**

Volkmann's contracture, a serious, persistent flexion contraction of forearm and hand caused by ischemia. A pressure or crushing injury in the region of the elbow usually precedes this condition, and pressure from a cast or tight bandage about the elbow are common causes. Permanent fibrosis, muscle degeneration, and a clawlike hand may result. Nurses must watch for swelling, pallor, coldness, cyanosis, or pain distal to the injury site so that prompt loosening of constriction can restore circulation. Also called **ischemic contracture.**

Volkmann's splint, a splint that supports and immobilizes the lower leg. It has a footpiece attached to two sides that extends from the foot to the knee, allowing ambulation.

volsella forceps /volsel′ə/, a kind of forceps having a small, sharp-pointed hook at the end of each blade. Also called **volsella, volsellum forceps, vulsella forceps.**

volt, the unit of electric potential. In an electric circuit a volt is the force required to send 1 ampere of current through 1 ohm of resistance, or the difference in potential between two points on a conductor carrying a charge of 1 ampere when there is a dissipation of 1 watt between them. See also **ampere, circuit, current, ohm, watt.**

voltammetry, the measurement of an electric current as a function of potential.

voltmeter, an instrument, as a galvanometer, that measures in volts the differences in potential between different points of an electric circuit.

volume, the amount of space occupied by a body, expressed in cubic units.

volume control fluid chamber, any one of several types of transparent, plastic reservoirs with graduated volumetric markings, used to regulate the flow of intravenous solutions. These devices are components of intravenous volume control sets and accommodate the injection and the mixing of medications by means of special built-in ports. The volume control fluid chamber contains a filter that must be primed to function.

volume dose. See **integral dose.**

volume imaging, NMR imaging techniques in which NMR signals are gathered from the whole object volume to be imaged at once. Many sequential plane imaging techniques can be generalized to volume imaging, at least in principle. Advantages include potential improvement in the signal-to-noise ratio by including signals from the whole volume at once; disadvantages include a bigger computational task for image reconstruction and longer image acquistion times although the entire volume can be imaged from the one set of data.

volume ventilator, a ventilator that delivers a predetermined volume of gas with each cycle.

voluntary, referring to an action or thought originated, undertaken, controlled or accomplished as a result of a person's free will or choice.

voluntary agency, a service agency legally controlled by volunteers rather than by owners or a paid staff. Most public health nursing agencies are voluntary; most hospitals, which are legally controlled by hospital boards, are composed of lay and professional members who are not paid for their services.

voluntary hospital system, a nationwide complex of autonomous, self-established, and self-supported private not for profit and investor owned hospitals in the United States.

voluntary muscle. See **striated muscle.**

volunteer, a person who serves a hospital without pay, augmenting but not replacing paid personnel and professional staff members.

-volute, a combining form meaning 'to roll, turn around': *circumvolute, involute, revolute*.

volvulus /vol′vyŏŏləs/, a twisting of the bowel on itself, causing intestinal obstruction. The condition is frequently the result of a prolapsed segment of mesentery and occurs most often in the ileum, the cecum, or the sigmoid portions of the bowel. If it is not corrected, the obstructed bowel becomes necrotic, peritonitis and rupture of the bowel occur, and death may ensue. Severe, gripping pain, nausea and vomiting, an absence of bowel sounds, and a tense, distended abdomen suggest the diagnosis, which is confirmed by x-ray examination. Compare **intussusception.**

volvulus neonatorum, an intestinal obstruction in a newborn baby resulting from a twisting of the bowel caused by malrotation or nonfixation of the colon. Typical symptoms include abdominal distention, persistent regurgitation, often accompanied by fecal vomiting, and nonpassage of stools. Characteristic barium enema x-ray studies confirm the diagnosis. The condition requires immediate surgical correction to prevent necrosis and gangrene of the affected segment of bowel.

vomer /vō′mər/, the bone forming the posterior and inferior part of the nasal septum and having two surfaces and four borders.

vomit, **1.** to expel the contents of the stomach through the esophagus and out of the mouth. **2.** also called **emesis, vomitus.** the material expelled.

von Economo's encephalitis. See **epidemic encephalitis.**

von Gierke's disease /fôngir′kəz/, a form of glycogen storage disease in which abnormally large amounts of glycogen are deposited in the liver and kidneys. The disorder is characterized by hypoglycemia, ketoacidosis, and hyperlipemia. Biopsy of the affected organs reveals the absence of glucose-6-phosphate dehydrogenase (G-6-PD), an enzyme necessary for glycogen metabolism. There is no effective treatment for the disorder. Medical efforts are directed at preventing hypoglycemia and ketoacidosis. Also called **glycogen storage disease, type I.** See also **glycogen storage disease.**

von Hippel-Lindau disease. See **cerebroretinal angiomatosis.**

von Pirquet test. See **Pirquet test.**

von Recklinghausen's disease. See **neurofibromatosis.**

von Willebrand's disease, an inherited disorder characterized by abnormally slow coagulation of the blood and spontaneous epistaxis and gingival bleeding caused by a deficiency of factor VIII. Excessive bleeding is common postpartum, during menstruation, and after injury or surgery. Also called **angiohemophilia.** See also **hemophilia, thrombasthenia.**

-vorous, a combining form meaning 'of or referring to feeding on something': *leguminivorous, panivorous*.

vortex, *pl.* **vortexes, vortices,** a whirlpool effect produced by the whirling of a more or less cylindric mass of fluid (liquid or gas). The velocity of the motion increases as the radius of the circle described by the motion decreases; the velocity decreases as the radius increases. Tornadoes and whirlpools are examples of free vortexes.

vox /voks/, voice, as **vox cholerica,** the barely audible, hoarse voice of a patient in an advanced and severe case of cholera.

voxel /vok′səl/, abbreviation for *vo*lume element, the three-dimensional version of a pi*xel*.

voyeur /voiyur′, vô·äyœr′/, one whose sexual desire is gratified by the practice of voyeurism. Also called **Peeping Tom.**

voyeurism /voi′yəriz′əm, voiyur′izəm/, a psychosexual disorder in which a person derives sexual excitement and gratification from looking at the naked bodies and genital organs or observing the sexual acts of others, especially from a secret vantage point.

VSD, abbreviation for **ventricular septal defect.**

vulnerable period, a short period in the cardiac cycle of the atria or the ventricles during which activation may result in tachycardia or fibrillation. The ventricular vulnerable period corresponds to the apex of the T wave toward its ascending side.

vulsella forceps. See **volsella forceps.**

vulva. See **pudendum.**

vulvar /vul′vər/, of or pertaining to the vulva.

vulvectomy /vəlvek′təmē/, the surgical removal of part or all of the tissues of the vulva, performed most frequently in the treatment of malignant or premalignant neoplastic disease. **Simple vulvectomy** includes the removal of the skin of the labia minora, the labia majora, and the clitoris. **Radical vulvectomy** involves excision of the labia majora, labia minora, clitoris, surrounding tissues, and pelvic lymph nodes.

vulvocrural /vul′vōkrŏŏr′əl/, of or pertaining to the vulva and the thigh.

vulvovaginal /vul′vōvaj′inəl/, of or pertaining to the vulva and the vagina.

vulvovaginitis /vul′vōvaj′inī′tis/, an inflammation of the vulva and vagina, or of the vulvovaginal glands.

VZV, abbreviation for **varicella zoster virus.**

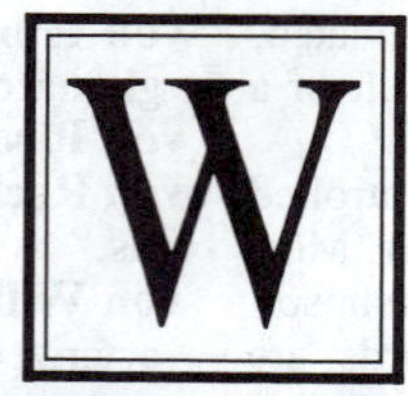

w, the amount of energy required to ionize a molecule of air, as expressed by w = 33.85 eV/ion pair. This is an important quantity for radiation dosimetry because it allows the extraction of dose from ionization measurements.

W, symbol for **tungsten.**

Wagner-Meissner corpuscle /wag′nərmīs′nər/, one of a number of small, special pressure-sensitive sensory end organs with a connective tissue capsule and tiny stacked plates in the corium of the hand and foot, the front of the forearm, the skin of the lips, the mucous membrane of the tongue, the palpebral conjunctiva, and the skin of the mammary papilla. A single nerve fiber penetrates each oval capsule, spirals through the interior, and ends as a globular mass. Also called **tactile corpuscle of Meissner.** Compare **Golgi-Mazzoni corpuscles, Krause's corpuscles.**

Wagstaffe's fracture /wag′stafs/, a fracture characterized by separation of the internal malleolus.

waking imagined analgesia (WIA), the pain relief experienced by a patient who employs the psychologic technique, usually with the help of an attending nurse or a hospital aide, of concentrating on previous pleasant personal experiences that produced tranquillity, as lying on a summer beach beside cooling ocean water or drifting down a quiet river in a canoe. The patient employing the WIA technique is encouraged to verbalize such experiences, thereby reinforcing recollection with attendant soothing biologic responses. This technique is often effective in reducing mild to moderate pain, especially when used with a mild nonnarcotic analgesic and the compassionate interaction of an attending health care professional. See also **pain evaluation, pain intervention, pain mechanism.**

Wald /wôld/, **Lillian** (1867–1940), an American public health nurse, settlement leader, and social reformer. She founded the Henry Street Settlement in New York to bring nursing care into the homes of the poor. This led to the development of the Visiting Nurse Service of New York. She was also instrumental in establishing the school nursing system, the federal government's Children's Bureau, and the Nursing Service Division of the Metropolitan Life Insurance Company. She was the first nurse to be elected into the Hall of Fame for Great Americans.

Waldenström's disease. See **Perthes' disease.**

Waldeyer's ring, the palatine, pharyngeal, and lingual tonsils that encircle the pharynx.

walker, an extremely light, movable apparatus, about waist high, made of metal tubing, used to aid a patient in walking. It has four widely placed, sturdy legs. The patient holds onto the walker and takes a step, then moves the walker forward and takes another step. Compare **crutch.**

walking pneumonia. See **mycoplasma pneumonia.**

walking rounds, rounds in which the clinician responsible leads a group of junior clinicians on a tour to visit the patients for whom they are collectively responsible. In some hospitals nurses may participate in walking rounds in lieu of or in addition to report.

wall, a limiting structure within the body, as the wall of the abdominal, the thoracic, or the pelvic cavities, or the wall of a cell.

wallerian degeneration, the fatty degeneration of a nerve fiber after it has been severed from its cell body.

wander, **1.** to move about purposelessly. **2.** to cause to move back and forth in an exploratory manner; for example, in inserting an intrauterine catheter, the tip of the inserter must usually be wandered around the fetal head in the cervix to find a space through which the catheter may be passed upward into the uterus.

wandering goiter. See **diving goiter.**

Wangensteen apparatus /wang′ənstēn/, a nasogastroduodenal catheter and a suction apparatus used for constant, gentle drainage and decompression of the stomach or duodenum. It may be used to relieve abdominal distention that often occurs postoperatively or that may complicate a GI disorder, especially an intestinal obstruction. See also **Wangensteen tube.**

Wangensteen tube, the catheter portion of a Wangensteen apparatus.

WANS, a trademark for a fixed-combination drug containing an antihistamine, antiemetic (pyrilamine maleate), and a sedative-hypnotic (pentobarbital sodium).

ward, a hospital room designed and equipped to house more than four patients.

warfarin poisoning, a toxic condition caused by the ingestion of warfarin, accidentally in the form of a rodenticide or by overdose with the substance in its pharmacologic anticoagulant form. The poison accumulates in the body and results in nosebleed, bruising, hematuria, melena, and internal hemorrhage. Treatment may include gastric lavage, a cathartic, vitamin K, and blood transfusion. The goal of therapy is to eliminate the poison and to reestablish normal coagulation.

warfarin sodium, an anticoagulant.

■ INDICATIONS: It is prescribed for the prophylaxis and treatment of thrombosis and embolism.
■ CONTRAINDICATIONS: Hemorrhage or known hypersensitivity to this drug prohibits its use.
■ ADVERSE EFFECTS: The most serious adverse reaction is hemorrhage. Many other drugs interact with this drug to increase or decrease its effects.

warm-blooded, having a relatively high and constant body temperature, as the temperatures maintained by humans, other mammals, and birds, despite changes in environmental temperatures. Heat is produced in the warm-blooded human body by the catabolism of foods in proportion to the amount of work performed by the tissues in the body. Heat is lost from the body by evaporation, radiation, conduction, and convection. About 80% of the body heat that is dissipated in humans is lost through the skin; the rest is lost through the mucous membranes of the respiratory, the digestive, and the urinary systems. The average temperature of the healthy human is 98.6° F (37° C). The human body's tolerance for change in its temperature is very small, and significant changes can have drastic, even fatal consequences. The control mechanism for temperature in the human body consists of thermal receptive neurons in the anterior portion of the hypothalamus, more than 2 million sweat glands, and the vast network of blood vessels in the skin. Reduced heat loss results from less secretion and slower evaporation of sweat and from vasoconstriction of blood vessels. Increased heat gain results from shivering, which increases the work of body tissues and, hence, increases catabolism. Fever, which raises internal body temperature, temporarily resets the thermostatic control of the hypothalamus by the action of chemical pyrogens from bacteria and viruses and by the function of the prostaglandins that the pyrogens release. The temperature control mechanisms of the body serve to restore normal heat levels during fever. Aspirin and other antipyretic drugs foil the synthesis of prostaglandins. Also called **homoiothermal, homothermal.** Compare **cold-blooded.**

war neurosis. See **combat fatigue, shell shock.**

wart. See **verruca.**

Warthin's tumor. See **papillary adenocystoma lymphomatosum.**

washout, the elimination or expulsion of one gas or volatile anesthetic agent by the administration of another.

wasp, a slender, narrow-waisted hymenopteran insect with two pairs of membranous wings that are folded lengthwise when at rest like parts of a fan. Many species of wasps may give painful stings that may have severe results in hypersensitive persons. Treatment is as for bee stings.

Wassermann test /was′ərmən, vos′ərmun/, a diagnostic blood test for syphilis based on the complement fixation reaction.

wasting, a process of deterioration marked by weight loss and decreased physical vigor, appetite, and mental activity.

water (H_2O), a chemical compound, one molecule of which contains one atom of oxygen and two atoms of hydrogen. Almost three quarters of the earth's surface is covered by water. Essential to life as it exists on this planet, water comprises more than 70% of living things. Pure water freezes at 0° C (32° F) and boils at 100° C (212° F) at sea level.

waterborne, carried by water, as a waterborne epidemic of typhoid fever.

Waterhouse-Friderichsen syndrome /wô′tərhous′-frid′ərik′sən/, overwhelming bacteremia, characterized by the sudden onset of fever, cyanosis, petechiae, and collapse from massive bilateral adrenal hemorrhage. The syndrome requires immediate emergency treatment, hospitalization, and intensive care. Emergency treatment includes vasopressor drugs, intravenous fluids, plasma, and oxygen. No sedatives or narcotics are given. Specific treatment for bacteremia is intensive antibiotic therapy, given parenterally and continued for several days after symptoms subside. Nursing management includes close observation and the maintenance of adequate provision of fluids and nutrients.

water intoxication, an increase in the volume of free water in the body, resulting in dilutional hyponatremia.

water moccasin. See **cottonmouth.**

waters. See **amniotic fluid.**

water trap. See **underwater seal.**

watt, the unit of electric power or work in the meter/kilogram/second system of notation. The watt is the product of the voltage and the amperage. One watt of power is dissipated when a current of 1 ampere flows across a difference in potential of 1 volt. See also **ampere, current, ohm, volt.**

wave, a periodic disturbance in which energy moves through a medium without permanently altering the constituents of the medium. Electromagnetic waves, as light, x-rays, and radio waves, can travel through a vacuum. Sound waves can be transmitted only through matter. See also **electromagnetic radiation, light, sound, x-ray.**

wavelength, the distance between a given point on one wave cycle and the corresponding point on the next successive wave cycle. A pure color is produced by light of a specific wavelength. Electromagnetic waves of different wavelengths account for many of the transmission characteristics of radio and television.

wax. See **cerumen.**

wax bath. See **paraffin bath.**

waxy flexibility. See **cerea flexibilitas.**

WBC, abbreviation for **white blood cell.** See **leukocyte.**

W chromosome and Z chromosome, the sex chromosomes of certain insects, birds, and fishes. Females of such species are heterogametic and have one W and one Z chromosome, whereas males are homogametic and have two Z chromosomes. The ZZ-ZW system of nomenclature was chosen to differentiate the chromosomes from the XX-XY type, which occurs in humans and various other animals and in which the female is homogametic and the male is heterogametic.

W/D, abbreviation for *well developed,* often used in the initial identifying statement in a patient record. It is used so frequently as to have lost all meaning or use in identifying or describing the patient.

wean, **1.** to induce a child to give up breast feeding and to accept other food in place of breast milk. Many children are ready for weaning during the second half of the first year; some wean themselves. **2.** to withdraw a person from something on which he is dependent.

weanling, a child who has recently been weaned.

weaver's bottom, a form of bursitis affecting the ischial bursae of the hips of people whose work requires prolonged sitting in one position. Also called *(obsolete)* **tailor's bottom.**

web, a network of fibers forming a tissue or a membrane, as the laryngeal web that spreads between the vocal cords.

Weber's tuning fork test, a method of assessing auditory acuity, especially useful in determining if defective hearing in an ear is a conductive loss caused by a middle ear problem or a sensorineural loss, resulting from a disorder in the inner ear or auditory nerve system. The test is performed by placing the stem of a vibrating 256 Hz tuning fork in the center of the person's forehead or on the maxillary incisors. The loudness of the sound is equal in both ears if hearing is normal. If the person has a sensorineural loss in one ear, the unaffected ear perceives the sound as louder. When conductive hearing loss is present, the sound is louder in the affected ear, because it does not hear ordinary background noise conducted through the air and receives only vibrations by bone conduction.

web of causation, an interrelationship of multiple factors that contribute to the occurrence of a disease.

Wechsler intelligence scales, a series of standardized tests designed to measure the intelligence at several age levels, from preschool through adult, by means of questions that examine general information, arrangement of pictures and objects, vocabulary, memory, reasoning, and other abilities.

wedge fracture, a fracture of vertebral structures with anterior compression.

wedge pressure, the capillary pressure in the left atrium, determined by measuring the pressure in a cardiac catheter wedged in the most distal segment of the pulmonary artery.

wedge resection, the surgical excision of part of an organ, as a part of an ovary containing a cyst. The segment excised may be wedge-shaped.

WEE, abbreviation for **western equine encephalitis.** See **equine encephalitis.**

weed. See **cannabis.**

weeping, **1.** crying, lacrimating. **2.** oozing or exuding fluid, as a sore or rash.

Wegener's granulomatosis /wā′gənərz/, an uncommon, chronic inflammatory process leading to the formation of nodules or tumorlike masses in the air passages, necrotizing vasculitis, and glomerulonephritis. Symptoms, depending on the organs involved, may include sinus pain, a bloody, purulent nasal discharge, saddle-nose deformity, chest discomfort and cough, weakness, anorexia, weight loss, and skin lesions. Glomerulonephritis, as a complication, was formerly fatal in a few months, but with the use of cytotoxic drugs, especially cyclophosphamide, a high percentage of patients achieve long-term remissions.

weight, the force exerted on a body by the gravity of the earth. On the surface of the earth, mass and weight are the same. As a body moves away from the earth, the weight of the body decreases, but the mass remains constant. In space, a body has mass but no weight. Weight is sometimes measured in units of force, as newtons or poundals, but it is usually expressed in pounds or kilograms, as is mass. See also **mass.**

Weil's disease. See **leptospirosis.**

weismannism /vīs′muniz′əm/, the basic concepts of heredity and development as proposed by German biologist August Weismann. These state that the vehicle of inheritance is the germ plasm, which is distinct from the somatoplasm and is transmitted from one generation to the next; that during embryonic development the hereditary components are dispersed to the somatoplasm to give rise to inherited characteristics; and that changes in somatoplasm do not affect germ plasm, so that acquired characteristics cannot be inherited. Also called **Weismann's theory, germ plasm theory.** Compare **pangenesis.** **–weismannian,** *adj., n.*

Weiss' sign. See **Chvostek's sign.**

well baby care, periodic health supervision for infants and children to promote optimal physical, emotional, and intellectual growth and development. Such health care measures include routine immunizations to prevent disease, screening procedures for early detection and treatment of illness, and parental guidance and instruction in proper nutrition, accident prevention, and specific care and rearing of the child at various stages of development. The recommended preventive health care schedule for children who are developing normally is monthly for the first 6 months of life, every 2 months until 1 year of age, every 3 months during the second year, every 6 months during the third year, followed by annual visits. Well baby care may be provided in a clinic, a convenient local meeting place, a private doctor's office, the office of a community health nursing service, or a school. Nurses or nurse practitioners frequently provide the care.

well baby clinic, a clinic that specializes in medical supervision and services for healthy infants.

well-being, achievement of a good and satisfactory existence as defined by the individual.

well-differentiated lymphocytic malignant lymphoma, a lymphoid neoplasm characterized by the predominance of mature lymphocytes. Also called **lymphocytic lymphoma, lymphocytic lymphosarcoma, lymphocytoma.**

wellness, a dynamic state of health in which an individual progresses toward a higher level of functioning, achieving an optimum balance between internal and external environments.

wen. See **pilar cyst.**

Wenckebach heart block. See **Mobitz I heart block.**

Wenckebach periodicity, a form of second-degree atrioventricular block with a progressive beat-to-beat prolongation of the PR interval, finally resulting in a nonconducting P wave. At this point, the sequence recurs. Also called **Mobitz I, Type I block, Wenckebach phenomenon.** See also **atrioventricular block.**

Werdnig-Hoffmann disease /verd′nighôf′mun/, a genetic disorder beginning in infancy or young childhood, characterized by progressive atrophy of the skeletal muscle resulting from degeneration of the cells in the anterior horn of the spinal cord and the motor nuclei in the brainstem. Onset occurs within the first year of life, with the condition usually apparent at birth. Symptoms include congenital hypotonia, absence of stretch reflexes, flaccid paralysis, especially of the trunk and limbs, lack of sucking ability, fasciculations of the tongue and sometimes of other muscles, and, often, dysphagia. Treatment is symptomatic, and death generally occurs in early childhood, often from respiratory complications. The condition is transmitted as an autosomal recessive trait and occurs more frequently in siblings than in successive generations. Also called **familial spinal muscular atrophy, Hoffmann's atrophy, infantile spinal muscular atrophy, progressive spinal muscular atrophy of infants, Werdnig-Hoffmann paralysis.** See also **floppy infant syndrome.**

Werlhof's disease. See **thrombocytopenic purpura.**

Wernicke's encephalopathy /ver′nikēz/, an inflammatory, hemorrhagic, degenerative condition of the brain, characterized by lesions in several parts of the brain including the hypothalamus, mammillary bodies, and tissues surrounding ventricles and aqueducts. The condition is characterized by double vision, involuntary and rapid movements of the eyes, lack of muscular coordination, and decreased mental function, which may be mild or severe. Wernicke's encephalopathy is caused by a thiamine deficiency and is seen in association with chronic alcoholism. It also occurs as a complication of GI tract disease and hyperemesis gravidarum associated with malabsorption and malnutrition.

West African sleeping sickness. See **Gambian trypanosomiasis.**

Westcort, a trademark for a glucocorticoid (hydrocortisone valerate).

western equine encephalitis. See **equine encephalitis.**

West nomogram, a nomogram used in estimating the body surface area. See also **nomogram.**

wet cough. See **productive cough.**

wet dream. See **nocturnal emission.**

wet dressing, a moist dressing used to relieve symptoms of some skin diseases. As the moisture evaporates, it cools and dries the skin, softens dried blood and sera, and stimulates drainage. Medication may be added if necessary.

wet lung, an abnormal condition of the lungs, characterized by a persistent cough and rales at the lung bases. It occurs in workers exposed to pulmonary irritants, as ammonia, chlorine, sulfur dioxide, volatile organic acids, dusts, and vapors of corrosive chemicals. Treatment consists of removing the person from exposure to the irritant and therapy for possible pulmonary edema. Compare **pulmonary edema.** See also **pleural effusion, pleurisy.**

wet nurse, a woman who cares for and breast-feeds another's infant.

wetware, *informal.* (in computer research) the human brain, in contrast to hardware, firmware, or software.

W/F, symbol for *white female,* often used in the initial identifying statement in a patient record.

Wharton's jelly, a gelatinous tissue that remains when the embryonic body stalk blends with the yolk sac within the umbilical cord.

wheal /wēl/, an individual lesion of urticaria.

wheat weevil disease, a hypersensitivity pneumonitis caused by allergy to weevil particles found in wheat flour.

wheelchair, a mobile chair equipped with large wheels and brakes. If long-term use of the chair is expected, a physical therapist may prescribe certain personalized requirements, as size, left- or right-hand propulsion, type of brakes, height of armrests, and special seat pads.

wheeze, **1.** a form of rhonchus, characterized by a high-pitched musical quality. It is caused by a high velocity flow of air through a narrowed airway and is heard both during inspiration and expiration. Wheezes are associated with asthma and chronic bronchitis. Unilateral wheezes are characteristic of bronchogenic carcinoma, foreign bodies, and inflammatory stenosing lesions. An asthmatoid wheeze is caused by an obstruction in the trachea or bronchus. **2.** to breathe with a wheeze. See also **rale, rhonchi.**

whiplash injury, *informal.* an injury to the cervical vertebrae or their supporting ligaments and muscles marked by pain and stiffness, usually resulting from sudden acceleration or deceleration, as in a rear-end car collision that causes violent back and forth movement of the head and neck.

Whipple's disease, a rare intestinal disease characterized by severe intestinal malabsorption, steatorrhea, anemia, weight loss, arthritis, and arthralgia. Persons with the disease are severely malnourished and have abdominal pain, chest pain, and a chronic nonproductive cough. The diagnosis is made by jejunal biopsy. Penicillin and tetracycline may alleviate the symptoms. See also **malabsorption syndrome.**

whipworm. See ***Trichuris.***

whirlpool bath, the immersion of the body or a part of the body in a tank of hot water agitated by a jet of equally hot water and air.

white blood cell. See **leukocyte.**

white cell, *informal.* white blood cell. See also **leukocyte.**

white corpuscle. See **leukocyte.**

white damp. See **damp.**

white fibrocartilage, a mixture of tough, white fibrous tissue and flexible cartilaginous tissue. It is divided into four types: interarticular fibrocartilage, connecting fibrocartilage, circumferential fibrocartilage, and stratiform fibrocartilage. Compare **hyaline cartilage, yellow cartilage.**

white gold, a gold alloy with a high content of palladium or platinum used in some dental restorations, as prepared tooth cavities and gold crowns. It has a higher fusion range, lower ductility, and greater hardness than a yellow gold alloy.

whitehead. See **milia.**

white leg. See **phlegmasia alba dolens.**

white matter. See **white substance.**

white radiation, a form of radiation that results from the rapid deceleration of high-speed electrons striking a target, as when the electron beam of a tungsten cathode strikes the tungsten or molybdenum target of the anode in an x-ray tube. Most of the x-rays emitted from a diagnostic or therapeutic x-ray unit represent white radiation. Also called **braking radiation, bremsstrahlung.**

white spots film fault, a defect in a radiograph or a developed photographic film, which appears as scattered white spots throughout the image area. It is caused by air bubbles clinging to the emulsion during development or by fixing solution splattered on the film before processing.

white substance, the tissue surrounding the gray substance of the spinal cord, consisting mainly of myelinated nerve fibers, but with some unmyelinated nerve fibers, embedded in a spongy network of neuroglia. It is subdivided in each half of the spinal cord into three funiculi: the anterior, the posterior, and the lateral white column. Each column subdivides into tracts that are closely associated in function. The anterior column divides into two ascending tracts and five descending tracts. The posterior column divides into two large ascending tracts, one small descending tract, and one intersegmental tract. The lateral column divides into six ascending tracts and four descending tracts. Also called **white matter.** Compare **gray substance.** See also **spinal cord, spinal tract.**

white thrombus, **1.** an aggregation of blood platelets, fibrin, clotting factors, and cellular elements containing few or no erythrocytes. **2.** a thrombus comprised chiefly of white blood cells. **3.** a thrombus composed primarily of blood platelets and fibrin.

whitlow /wit′lō, hwit′lō/, an inflammation of the end of a finger or toe that results in suppuration. See also **felon.**

WHO, abbreviation for **World Health Organization.**

whole blood, blood that is unmodified except for the presence of an anticoagulant. It is used for transfusion. Various components and factors may be separated from whole blood for infusion to replace or to augment a component or factor that is deficient in amount or function because of a variety of diseases and conditions.

whole body hyperthermia. See **systemic heating.**

whooping cough. See **pertussis.**

whorl /wurl, hwurl/, a spiral turn, as one of the turns of the cochlea or of the dermal ridges that form fingerprints.

WIA, abbreviation for **waking imagined analgesia.**

Widal's test /vēdäls′/, an agglutination test used to aid in the diagnosis of salmonella infections, as typhoid fever. A fourfold increase in titer of agglutinins is highly suggestive of active infection. A high titer may persist for years after the disease or after immunization against typhoid fever.

wide-angle glaucoma. See **glaucoma.**

Wiedenbach /wē′dənbak/, **Ernestine** (1900–), a German-born American nursing educator and writer. She taught maternal and newborn health nursing at Yale School of Nursing, was a leader in family-centered maternity nursing, and developed the full range of the art and science of obstetric nursing.

Wigraine, a trademark for a fixed-combination drug containing anticholinergics (belladonna alkaloids), an analgesic (phenacetin), and a vasoconstrictor (ergotamine tartrate), used to treat migraine.

wild-type gene, a normal or standard form of a gene, as contrasted with a mutant form.

will, **1.** the mental faculty that enables one consciously to choose or decide on a course of action. **2.** the act or process of exercising the power of choice. **3.** a wish, desire, or deliberate intention. **4.** a disposition or attitude toward another or others. **5.** determination or purpose; willfulness. **6.** (in law) an expression or declaration of a person's wishes as to the disposition of property, to be performed or take effect after death.

Willis' circle. See **circle of Willis.**

Willis' disease. See **diabetes mellitus.**

willow fracture. See **greenstick fracture.**

Wilms' tumor /vilms/, a malignant neoplasm of the kidney, occurring in young children, before the fifth year in 75% of the cases. The most frequent early sign of this large malignant tumor of childhood is hypertension, followed by the appearance of a palpable mass, pain, and hematuria. Diagnosis usually can be established by an excretory urogram with tomography. The tumor, an embryonal adenomyosarcoma, is well encapsulated in the early stage, but it may later extend into lymph nodes and the renal vein or vena cava and metastasize to the lungs or other sites. Prompt removal of resectable tumors by transperitoneal nephrectomy is recommended. Radiotherapy is used preoperatively or postoperatively; it may be used palliatively in inoperable cases. Cyclic chemotherapy with actinomycin-D and vincristine combined with surgery and irradiation is proving highly effective.

Wilson's disease, a rare, inherited disorder of copper metabolism, in which copper accumulates slowly in the liver and is then released and taken up in other parts of the body. Hemolysis, then hemolytic anemia occur as the copper accumulates in the red blood cells. Accumulation in the brain destroys certain tissue and may cause tremors, muscle rigidity, dysarthria, and dementia. Kidney function is diminished; the liver becomes cirrhotic. Treatment of Wilson's disease includes a reduction of copper in the diet and the prescription of copper-binding agents and penicillamine. Also called **hepatolenticular degeneration.**

Winckel's disease. See **hemoglobinuria.**

wind chill, the loss of heat from the body when it is exposed to wind of a given speed at a given temperature and humidity. The **wind chill index** is expressed in kilocalories per hour per square meter of skin surface. The **wind chill factor** is expressed in degrees Celsius or Fahrenheit as the effective temperature felt by a person exposed to the weather.

winding sheet, a shroud for wrapping a dead body.

windkessel effect /wind′kes′əl/, the stretching of the aorta during systole to accommodate the stroke volume of blood ejected. Energy that was stored propels this volume by recoil action into the peripheral artery tree during diastole.

window, a surgically created opening in the surface of a structure or an anatomically occurring opening in the surface or between the chambers of a structure. **2.** a specific time period during which a phenomenon can be observed, a reaction monitored, or a procedure initiated.

windowed, (of an orthopedic cast) having an opening, especially to relieve pressure that may irritate and inflame the skin.

Winstrol. a trademark for an androgen (stanozolol), used as an anabolic agent.

winter cough, *nontechnical.* a chronic condition characterized by a persistent cough occasioned by cold weather. See also **cough.**

wintergreen oil. See **methyl salicylate.**

winter itch, pruritus occurring in cold weather in people who have dry skin, particularly in those who have atopic dermatitis. Warmer temperature, increased humidity, and topical, antipruritic emollients may offer relief.

wiry pulse, an abnormal pulse that is strong but small.

wisdom tooth, either of the last teeth on each side of the upper and lower jaw. These are third molars and are the last teeth to erupt, usually between 17 and 21 years of age, often causing considerable pain, dental problems, and the need for extraction. Also called **dens serotinus.** See also **molar.**

wish fulfillment, **1.** the gratification of a desire. **2.** (in psychology) the satisfaction of a desire or the release of emotional tension through such processes as dreams, daydreams, and neurotic symptoms. **3.** (in psychoanalysis) one of the primary motivations for dreams in which an unconscious desire or urge, unacceptable to the ego and superego because of sociocultural restrictions or feelings of personal guilt, is given expression.

wishful thinking, the interpretation of facts or situations according to one's desires or wishes rather than as they exist in reality, usually used as an unconscious device to avoid painful or unpleasant feelings.

Wiskott-Aldrich syndrome /wis′kotôl′drich/, an immunodeficiency disorder inherited as a recessive, X-linked trait, characterized by thrombocytopenia, eczema, inadequate T and B cell function, and an increased susceptibility to viral, bacterial, and fungal infections and to cancer. Treatment includes the prescription of appropriate antibiotics for specific infectious organisms and the administration of transfer factor from activated lymphocytes to increase the resistance to infection and to clear the eczema. See also **transfer factor.**

witch hazel, **1.** a shrub, *Hamamelis virginiana,* indigenous to North America, from which an astringent extract is derived. **2.** also called **hamamelis water.** a solution comprised of the extract, alcohol, and water, used as an astringent.

witch's milk, a milklike substance secreted from the breast of the newborn, caused by circulating maternal lactating hormone. Also called **hexenmilch** /hek′-sənmilsh′/.

withdrawal, a common response to physical danger or severe stress characterized by a state of apathy, lethargy, depression, retreat into oneself, and, in grave cases, catatonia and stupor. It is pathologic if it interferes with a person's perception of reality and the ability to function in society, as in the various forms of schizophrenia. See also **schizophrenia.**

withdrawal bleeding, the passage of blood from the uterus, associated with the shedding of endometrium that has been stimulated and maintained by hormonal medication. It occurs when the medication is discontinued. In the endocrine evaluation of a woman with amenorrhea, withdrawal bleeding constitutes evidence that the woman's endometrium is reponsive to hormonal stimulation and that the cause of her amenorrhea is probably not uterine.

withdrawal method, a contraceptive technique in coitus wherein the penis is withdrawn from the vagina before ejaculation. It is not reliable because small amounts of seminal fluid carrying millions of spermatozoa may be emitted without sensation before full ejaculation. Also called **coitus interruptus.**

withdrawal symptoms, the unpleasant, sometimes life-threatening physiologic changes that occur when some drugs are withdrawn after prolonged, regular use. The effects may occur after use of a narcotic, tranquilizer, stimulant, barbiturate, alcohol, or other substance to which the person has become physiologically or psychologically dependent or addicted.

withdrawn behavior, a condition in which there is a blunting of the emotions and a lack of social responsiveness.

with spaces, spaces in which interacting persons use body parts or areas to show they share a similar spatial orientation and are thus affiliated.

Wittmaack-Ekbom syndrome. See **restless legs syndrome.**

W/M, symbol for *white male,* often used in the initial identifying statement in a patient record.

W/N, symbol for *well nourished,* often used in the initial identifying statement in a patient record. It is used so frequently as to have lost all meaning or use in identifying or describing the patient.

Wolff-Chaikoff effect, the decreased formation and release of thyroid hormone in the presence of an excess of iodine.

wolffian body. See **mesonephros.**

wolffian duct. See **mesonephric duct.**

Wolff-Parkinson-White syndrome /wôlf′pär′kinsənwīt′/, a disorder of atrioventricular conduction, characterized by two AV conduction pathways. This syndrome is often identified by a characteristic delta wave seen on an electrocardiogram at the beginning of the QRS complex. See also **Lown-Ganong-Levine syndrome.**

wolfram. See **tungsten.**

woman-year, (in statistics) 1 year in the reproductive life of a sexually active woman; a unit that represents 12 months of exposure to the risk of pregnancy. Woman-years are used in calculating a pregnancy rate in the assessment of the effectiveness of the various methods of family planning and of the adverse effect on the birth rate of various environmental factors.

womb. See **uterus.**

wood alcohol. See **methanol.**

Wood's glass, a nickel oxide filter that holds back all light except for a few violet rays of the visible spectrum and ultraviolet wavelengths of about 365 nm. It is used extensively to help diagnose fungus infections of the scalp and erythrasma and to reveal porphyrins and fluorescent materials.

Wood's light, an ultraviolet light of about 365 nm wavelength used to diagnose certain scalp and skin diseases. The light causes hairs infected with a fungus, as *tinea capitis,* to become brilliantly fluorescent. Also called **Wood's lamp, Wood's rays.**

woolsorter's disease, the pulmonary form of anthrax, so named because it is an occupational hazard to those who handle sheep's wool. Early symptoms mimic influenza, but the patient soon develops high fever, respiratory distress, and cyanosis. If the disease is not treated at this stage, it is often fatal. Also called **pulmonary anthrax.** See also **anthrax.**

word, a unit of computer information presented as a combination of bytes, usually six or eight.

word association. See **controlled association.**

word association test. See **association test.**

word processor, a system of hardware and software designed for the keyboarding, formating, correcting, and storing of correspondence, reports, manuscripts, and books or other publications.

word salad, a jumble of words and phrases that lacks logical coherence and meaning, often characteristic of disoriented individuals and schizophrenics.

working occlusion, the occlusal contacts of teeth on the side of the jaw toward which the mandible is moved.

work therapy, a therapeutic approach in which the client performs a useful activity or learns an occupation, as in occupational therapy.

work tolerance, the kind and amount of work that a physically or mentally ill person can or should perform.

work-up, the process of performing a complete evaluation of a patient, including history, physical examination, laboratory tests, and x-ray or other diagnostic procedures to acquire an accurate data base on which a diagnosis and treatment plan may be established.

World Health Organization (WHO), an agency of the United Nations, affiliated with the Food and Agricultural Organization of the UN, the International Atomic Energy Agency, the International Labor Organization, the Pan American Health Organization, and UNESCO. The WHO is primarily concerned with worldwide or regional health problems, but in emergencies it is authorized to render local assistance on request. Its functions include furnishing technical assistance, stimulating and advancing epidemiologic investigation of diseases, recommending health regulations, promoting cooperation among scientific and professional health groups, and providing information and counsel relating to health matters. Its headquarters are in Geneva, Switzerland. Its French name is **Organisation Mondiale de la Santé** /ôrgänizäsyôN′ môNdē·äl′ dəlä säNtā′/ **(OMS).**

worm, any of the soft-bodied, elongated invertebrates of the phyla Annelida, Nemathelminthes, or Platyhelminthes. Some kinds of worms parasitic for humans are **hookworm, pinworm,** and **tapeworm.** See also **fluke, roundworm.**

wormian bone /vôr′mē·ən/, any of several tiny, smooth, segmented bones that are soft, moist, and tepid to the touch, usually found as the serrated borders of the sutures between the cranial bones. Wormian bones were named for the Danish anatomist Claus Worm.

wound, **1.** any physical injury involving a break in the skin, usually caused by an act or accident rather than by a disease, as a chest wound, gunshot wound, or puncture wound. **2.** to cause an injury, especially one that breaks the skin.

wound irrigation, the rinsing of a wound or the cavity formed by a wound using a medicated solution, water, or antimicrobial liquid preparation.

■ METHOD: The dressing is removed and wrapped for disposal. The patient is assisted to an appropriate position. With the use of equipment from a sterile irrigation pack or tray, an irrigating solution is poured into a graduated measure. It is then warmed in a basin of warm water unless the solution's action depends on antibiotic or enzyme activity, which would be inhibited by warming. An emesis or kidney basin is then fitted snugly against the patient's body beneath the wound. It may be held in place by the patient or by an assistant. A catheter is held with sterile gloves or forceps and gently inserted into the wound to a prescribed depth and at a prescribed angle. A syringe filled with irrigating solution is then attached to the catheter, and the solution is gently instilled. The catheter is pinched before the empty syringe is removed to prevent aspiration of the return irrigation flow during disconnection. The syringe is filled and attached again and the wound is irrigated until the returning solution runs clear. If a catheter is not used, the solution is sprayed directly on the wound from the syringe until the wound looks clean. After irrigation is completed, the body area is dried with sterile sponges working from the wound out to the area around it, and a dry sterile dressing is applied.

■ NURSING ORDERS: Frequency of irrigation, type of solution, and amount of solution to be used are specifically prescribed. The condition of the wound, amount of irrigating solution used, and the appearance of the returned solution are noted by the nurse.

■ OUTCOME CRITERIA: Wounds are irrigated to remove secretions and dried blood and to keep the wound surface open to encourage healing from the inside out. When the irrigation solution returns clear, the wound is considered clean.

wound repair, restoration of the normal structure after an injury, especially of the skin. See also **healing, intention.**

Wright's stain, a stain containing methylene blue and eosin, used to color blood specimens for microscopic examination, as for complete blood count and, particularly, for malarial parasites.

wrist. See **carpus.**

wrist joint. See **radiocarpal articulation.**

write, to record data on a computer memory device.

writer's cramp, a painful involuntary contraction of the muscles of the hand when attempting to write. It often occurs after long periods of writing. Also called **graphospasm.**

wrongful death statute, (in law) a statute existing in all states that provides that the death of a person can give rise to a cause of legal action brought by the person's beneficiaries in a civil suit against the person whose willful or negligent acts caused the death. Before the existence of these statutes, a suit could be brought only if the injured person survived the injury.

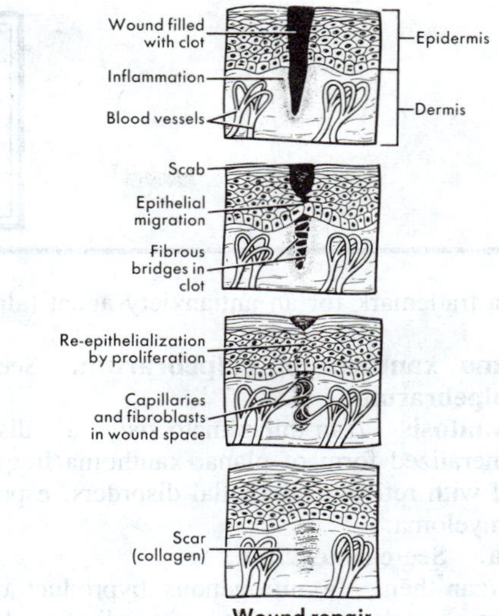

Wound repair

wrongful life action, (in law) a civil suit usually brought against a physician or health facility on the basis of negligence that resulted in the wrongful birth or life of an infant. The parents of the unwanted child seek to obtain payment from the defendant for the medical expenses of pregnancy and delivery, for pain and suffering, and for the education and upbringing of the child. Wrongful life actions have been brought and won in several situations, including malpracticed tubal ligations, vasectomies, and abortions. Failure to diagnose pregnancy in time for abortion and incorrect medical advice leading to the birth of a defective child have also led to malpractice suits for a wrongful life.

wryneck. See **torticollis.**

Wuchereria /vo͞o′kərē′rē·ə/, a genus of filarial worms found in warm, humid climates. *Wuchereria bancrofti,* transmitted by mosquitoes, is the cause of elephantiasis. See also **filariasis.**

Wyamine, a trademark for an alpha-adrenergic agent (mephentermine).

Wycillin, a trademark for an antibacterial (penicillin G procaine).

Wydase, a trademark for an enzyme (hyaluronidase).

Wymox, a trademark for an antibiotic (amoxicillin).

Wytensin, a trademark for an antihypertensive agent (guanabenz).

Wyvac, a trademark for a rabies virus vaccine (rabies human diploid cell vaccine).

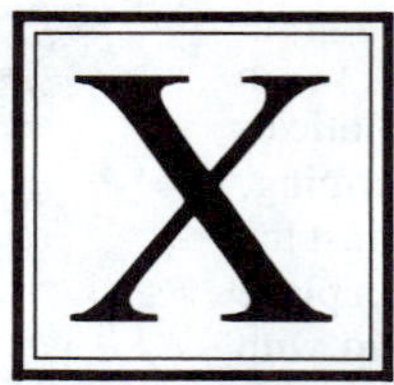

Xanax, a trademark for an antianxiety agent (alprazolam).

xanthelasma, xanthelasma palpebrarum. See **xanthoma palpebrarum.**

xanthelasmatosis /zan'thilaz'mətō'sis/, a disseminated, generalized form of planar xanthoma frequently associated with reticuloendothelial disorders, especially multiple myeloma.

xanthemia. See **carotenemia.**

xanthine /zan'thēn/, a nitrogenous byproduct of the metabolism of nucleoproteins. It is normally found in the muscles, liver, spleen, pancreas, and urine. **–xanthic,** *adj.*

xanthine derivative, any one of the closely related alkaloids caffeine, theobromine, or theophylline. They are found in plants widely distributed geographically and are variously ingested as components in different beverages, as coffee, tea, cocoa, and cola drinks. The xanthine derivatives or methylxanthines have pharmacologic properties that stimulate the central nervous system, produce diuresis, and relax smooth muscles. Theobromine has low potency and is seldom used as a pharmaceutic. Caffeine produces greater central nervous system stimulation than theophylline or theobromine. Some experiments have shown that caffeine increases the capacity for sustained intellectual effort, decreases reaction time, and improves the association of ideas. Caffeine and theophylline also affect the circulatory system, tending to dilate the systemic blood vessels but increasing cerebrovascular resistance with an associated decrease in cerebral blood flow and the oxygen tension of the brain. Some authorities believe it is this vasoconstriction that accounts for the relief of hypertensive headaches in individuals who drink beverages that contain any of the xanthine derivatives. The ability of the xanthine derivatives to relax smooth muscle is especially important in certain treatments of asthma. Theophylline is most effective in such treatment and markedly increases vital capacity. The methylxanthines reinforce the release of certain secretions of various endocrine and exocrine tissues, except for mast cells and, possibly, certain other mediators of inflammation. Caffeine can induce chromosomal abnormalities in plant cells and in mammalian cells in culture, and it strongly augments mutations of microorganisms. Such effects are apparently associated with the retardation of DNA repair mechanisms but only occur at caffeine concentrations much higher than those in xanthine beverages, and usually in life forms lacking enzymes for metabolizing xanthines. Several studies offer contradictory conclusions as to whether daily ingestion of more than five to six cups of coffee increases the susceptibility to myocardial infarction. Research continues in an effort to determine the effect of caffeine on pregnant women who ingest it in large amounts. Various studies indicate that the per capita consumption of caffeine in the United States is 200 mg daily, about 90% of which comes from coffee. One cup of coffee contains approximately 100 mg of caffeine; one cup of tea contains about 50 mg of caffeine and 1 mg of theophylline. One cup of cocoa contains about 250 mg of theobromine and 5 mg of caffeine. A 350 ml bottle of a cola beverage contains about 35 mg of caffeine. Consumption of xanthine beverages may cause various problems, including restlessness and inability to sleep, GI irritation, and excessive myocardial stimulation characterized by premature systole and tachycardia.

xanthinuria /zan'thinyŏŏr'ē·ə/, **1.** the presence of excessive quantities of xanthine in the urine. **2.** a rare disorder of purine metabolism, resulting in the excretion of large amounts of xanthine in the urine because of the absence of an enzyme, xanthine oxidase, that is necessary in xanthine metabolism. This inherited deficiency may cause the development of kidney stones made of xanthine precipitate.

xantho-, a combining form meaning 'yellow': *xanthochroia, xanthogen, xanthophore.*

xanthochromic /zan'thəkrō'mik/, having a yellowish color, as cerebrospinal fluid that contains blood or bile. Also **xanthochromatic.**

xanthochromia /zan'thəkrō'mē·ə/, a substance in cerebrospinal fluid that accounts for its yellow coloration. It is caused by the presence of hemoglobin breakdown products.

xanthogranuloma /zan'thəgran'yŏŏlō'mə/, *pl.* **xanthogranulomas, xanthogranulomata,** a tumor or nodule of granulation tissue containing lipid deposits. A kind of xanthogranuloma is **juvenile xanthogranuloma.**

xanthoma /zanthō'mə/, *pl.* **xanthomas, xanthomata,** a benign, fatty, fibrous, yellowish plaque, nodule, or tumor that develops in the subcutaneous layer of skin, often around tendons. The lesion is characterized by the intracellular accumulation of cholesterol and cholesterol esters.

xanthoma disseminatum, a benign, chronic condition in which small orange or brown papules and nodules develop on many body surfaces, especially on the mucous membrane of the oropharynx, larynx, and bronchi, and in skin folds and fissures. Also called **xanthoma multiplex.**

xanthoma eruptivum. See **eruptive xanthoma.**

xanthoma multiplex. See **xanthoma disseminatum.**

xanthoma palpebrarum, a soft, yellow spot or plaque usually occurring in groups on the eyelids. Also called **xanthelasma, xanthelasma palpebrarum.**

xanthoma planum. See **planar xanthoma.**

xanthomasarcoma /zan'thōməsärkō'mə/, *pl.* **xanthomasarcomas, xanthomasarcomata,** a giant cell sarcoma of the tendon sheaths and aponeuroses that contains xanthoma cells.

xanthoma striatum palmare, a yellow or orange flat plaque or slightly raised nodule occurring in groups on the palms of the hands.

xanthoma tendinosum, a yellow or orange elevated or flat round papule or nodule occurring in clusters on tendons, especially the extensor tendons of the hands and feet, of individuals with hereditary lipid storage disease.

xanthomatosis /zan'thōmətō'sis/, an abnormal condition in which there are deposits of yellowish fatty material in the skin, internal organs, and reticuloendothelial system. It may be associated with hyperlipoproteinemia, paraproteinemia, lipoid storage diseases, and other disorders of adipose tissue. Also called **xanthosis.** See also **lipemia, xanthoma, xanthoma palpebrarum.**

xanthoma tuberosum, a yellow or orange, flat or elevated round papule occurring in clusters on the skin of joints, especially the elbows and knees, usually in people who have a hereditary lipid storage disease, as hyperlipoproteinemia. The xanthomatous papules may also be associated with biliary cirrhosis and myxedema. Also called **tuberous xanthoma, xanthoma tuberosum multiplex.**

xanthopsia /zanthop'sē·ə/, an abnormal visual condition in which everything appears to have a yellow hue. It is sometimes associated with jaundice or digitalis toxicity.

xanthosis /zanthō'sis/, **1.** a yellowish discoloration sometimes seen in degenerating tissues of malignant diseases. **2.** See **xanthomatosis. 3.** also called **carotenosis.** a reversible yellow discoloration of the skin most commonly caused by the ingestion of large amounts of yellow vegetables containing carotene pigment. The antimalarial drug quinacrine, if taken over a prolonged period, may produce a similar skin color. Xanthosis may be differentiated clinically from jaundice because the sclerae are colored yellow in jaundice but are not discolored in xanthosis. See also **carotenemia.**

xanthureic acid /zanth'yŏŏrē'ik/, a metabolite of tryptophan that occurs in normal urine and in elevated levels in patients with vitamin B_6 deficiency.

X chromosome, a sex chromosome that in humans and many other species is present in both sexes, appearing singly in the cells of normal males and in duplicate in the cells of normal females. The chromosome is carried as a sex determinant by all of the female gametes and one half of all male gametes, is morphologically much larger than the Y chromosome, and has many sex-linked genes associated with clinically significant disorders, as hemophilia, Duchenne's muscular dystrophy, and Hunter's syndrome. Compare **Y chromosome.**

Xe, symbol for **xenon.**

xeno-, a combining form meaning 'strange or pertaining to foreign matter': *xenodiagnosis, xenogenous, xenology.*

xenobiotic, pertaining to organic substances that are foreign to the body, as drugs or organic poisons.

xenogeneic, 1. (in genetics) denoting individuals or cell types from different species and different genotypes. **2.** (in transplantation biology) denoting tissues from different species that are therefore antigenically dissimilar. Also **heterologous.** Compare **allogenic, syngeneic.**

xenogenesis /zen'əjen'əsis/, **1.** alternation of traits in successive generations; heterogenesis. **2.** the theoretic production of offspring that are totally different from both of the parents. **–xenogenetic, xenogenic,** *adj.*

xenograft /zen'əgraft'/, tissue from another species used as a temporary graft in certain cases, as in treating a severely burned patient when sufficient tissue from the patient or from a tissue bank is not available. It is quickly rejected but provides a cover for the burn for the first few days, reducing the amount of fluid loss from the open wound. Also called **heterograft.** Compare **allograft, autograft, isograft.** See also **graft.**

xenon (Xe), an inert, gaseous, nonmetallic element. Its atomic number is 54; its atomic weight is 131.30.

xenophobia /zen'ə-, zē'nə-/, an anxiety disorder characterized by a pervasive, irrational fear or uneasiness in the presence of strangers, especially foreigners, or in new surroundings.

xero-, a combining form meaning 'pertaining to dryness': *xerocheilia, xeromenia, xerophthalmia.*

xeroderma /zir'ədur'mə/, a chronic skin condition characterized by dryness and roughness.

xeroderma pigmentosum, a rare, inherited skin disease characterized by extreme sensitivity to ultraviolet light, exposure to which results in freckles, telangiectases, keratoses, papillomas, carcinoma, and, possibly, melanoma. Keratitis and tumors developing on the eyelids and cornea may result in blindness. Exposure to sunlight must be avoided.

xerogram /zē'rəgram/, an x-ray image produced by xerography.

xerophthalmia, a condition of dry and lusterless corneas and conjunctival areas, usually the result of vitamin A deficiency and associated with night blindness.

xeroradiography, a diagnostic x-ray technique in which an image is produced electrically rather than chemically, permitting lower exposure times and radiation of lower energy than that of ordinary x-rays. The latent image is made visible with a powder toner similar to that used in a copying machine. The powder image is transferred, and heat is fused to a sheet of paper. The images exhibit ''edge contrast'' because of the shape of the electric fields that pull toner onto the plate. Such edge contrast is useful for identifyling minute calcifications in the breast. Xeroradiography is used primarily for mammography.

xerosis. See **dry skin.**

xerostomia /zir′əstō′mē·ə/, dryness of the mouth caused by cessation of normal salivary secretion. The condition is a symptom of various diseases, as diabetes, acute infections, hysteria, and Sjögren's syndrome, and can be caused by paralysis of facial nerves. It is also a common adverse reaction to drugs.

X-inactivation theory. See **Lyon hypothesis.**

xiphi-. See **xipho-.**

xiphisternal articulation /zif′istur′nəl/, the cartilaginous connection between the xiphoid process and the body of the sternum. This joint usually ossifies at puberty. Compare **manubriosternal articulation.**

xiphisternum. See **xiphoid process.**

xipho-, xiphi-, a combining form meaning 'pertaining to a sword or to the xiphoid process': *xiphodymus, xiphoiditis, xiphopagus.*

xiphoid process /zif′oid/, the smallest of three parts of the sternum, articulating caudally with the body of the sternum and laterally with the seventh rib. Several muscles of the abdominal wall are attached to the xiphoid process, including the rectus abdominis and the linea alba. Also called **ensiform process, xiphisternum, xiphoid appendix.** Compare **manubrium.**

X-linked, pertaining to genes or to the characteristics or conditions they transmit that are carried on the X chromosome. Most X-linked traits and conditions, as hemophilia, are recessive and therefore occur predominantly in males, because they have only one X chromosome. Women may inherit the genes, but the recessive effects are usually masked by the normal dominant alleles carried on the second X chromosome. Compare **Y-linked.** See also **sex-linked disorder.** –**X linkage,** *n.*

X-linked dominant inheritance, a pattern of inheritance in which the transmission of a dominant gene on the X chromosome causes a characteristic to be manifested. Affected individuals all have an affected parent. All of the daughters of an affected male are affected but none of the sons. One half of the sons and one half of the daughters of an affected female are affected. Normal children of an affected parent have normal offspring. The inheritance shows a clear positive family history. Hypophosphatemic vitamin D-resistant rickets is an example of this pattern. X-linked dominant inheritance closely resembles autosomal dominant inheritance. Compare **X-linked recessive inheritance.**

X-linked ichthyosis. See **sex-linked ichthyosis.**

X-linked inheritance, a pattern of inheritance in which the transmission of traits varies according to the sex of the person, because the genes on the X chromosome have no counterparts on the Y chromosome. The inheritance pattern may be recessive or dominant. The characteristic determined by a gene on the X chromosome is always expressed in males. Transmission from father to son does not occur. Kinds of X-linked inheritance are **X-linked dominant inheritance** and **X-linked recessive inheritance.** Compare **autosomal inheritance.** See also **sex-linked.**

X-linked mucopolysaccharidosis. See **Hunter's syndrome.**

X-linked recessive inheritance, a pattern of inheritance in which transmission of an abnormal recessive gene on the X chromosome results in a carrier state in females and characteristics of the condition in males. Affected people have unaffected parents (except for the rare situation in which the father is affected and the mother is a carrier). One half of the female siblings of an affected male carry the trait. Unaffected male siblings do not carry the trait. Sons of affected males are unaffected, and daughters of affected males are carriers. Unaffected male children of a carrier female do not carry the trait. Compare **X-linked dominant inheritance.**

XO, (in genetics) the designation for the presence of only one sex chromosome; either the X or Y chromosome is missing so that each cell is monosomic and contains a total of 45 chromosomes. See also **Turner's syndrome.**

x-ray, 1. also called **roentgen ray.** electromagnetic radiation of shorter wavelength than visible light. X-rays are produced when electrons, traveling at high speed, strike certain materials, particularly heavy metals, as tungsten. They can penetrate most substances and are used to investigate the integrity of certain structures, to therapeutically destroy diseased tissue, and to make photographic images for diagnostic purposes, as in radiography and fluoroscopy. **2.** also called **x-ray film.** a radiograph made by projecting x-rays through organs or structures of the body onto a photographic plate. Because some tissue, as bone, is more radiopaque (allowing fewer x-rays to pass through) than other tissue, like skin or fat, a shadow is created on the plate that is the image of a bone or of a cavity filled with a radiopaque substance. **3.** to make a radiograph. See also **contrast medium, electron, fluoroscopy, radiopaque.** –**x-ray,** *adj.*

x-ray fluoroscopy, real-time imaging using an x-ray source that projects through the patient onto a fluorescent screen or image intensifier. Image-intensified fluoroscopy has replaced conventional fluoroscopy in current practice.

x-ray microscope, a microscope that produces images by x-rays and records them on fine-grain film or projects them as enlargements. Film images produced by x-ray microscopes may be examined at quite large magnifications with a light microscope.

x-ray pelvimetry, a radiographic examination used to determine the dimensions of the bony pelvis of a pregnant woman and, if possible, the biparietal diameter of her baby's head. It is performed when there is doubt that the head can pass safely through the pelvis in labor. Images of the pelvis and the baby are projected radiographically onto film. After the film is developed, the images are measured. The measurements are corrected for distortion, and the true dimensions of the birth canal and head are calculated. Often the cephalopelvic relationship cannot be accurately evaluated from the films because the baby's head may be positioned in such a way that the biparietal diameter cannot be visualized. Because minor degrees of cephalopelvic disproportion are often overcome safely in labor by molding of the fetal skull, and because major disproportions may be detected by clinical pelvimetry without x-rays, the value of x-ray pelvimetry is frequently judged to be insufficient to warrant the risk of radiation exposure. Other diagnostic tools, among them ultrasonography, often provide the necessary information with less apparent risk. Compare **clinical pelvimetry.** See also **cephalopelvic disproportion, contraction, dystocia.**

x-ray technician. See **radiologic technologist.**

x-ray tube, a large vacuum tube containing a tungsten filament cathode and an anode that often is a rotating tungsten disk. When heated to incandescence, the cathode emits a cloud of electrons that produce x-rays when they strike the surface of the anode at high speed. The anode is designed to deflect the x-rays toward a focal spot in the object being radiographed. X-ray tubes are produced in a variety of designs for different purposes. Low-kilovoltage x-ray tubes may contain molybdenum rather than tungsten anodes; some anodes are stationary and others rotate at high speed. Because of the intense heat generated by x-ray production, the specific design usually includes devices to help dissipate the heat.

XX, (in genetics) the designation for the normal sex chromosome complement in the human female. See also **X chromosome.**

XXX syndrome, a human sex chromosomal aberration characterized by the presence of three X chromosomes and two Barr bodies instead of the normal XX complement, so that somatic cells contain a total of 47 chromosomes. The condition occurs approximately once in every 1000 live female births and is confirmed diagnostically by the presence of the extra Barr body in the cells. Individuals with the anomaly show no significant clinical manifestations, although there is usually some degree of mental retardation. Because there is selective migration of the X chromosome during meiosis, one half of the offspring of a trisomy X female will be both chromosomally and phenotypically normal. Also called **triple X syndrome.**

XXXX, XXXXX, (in genetics) the designation for an abnormal sex chromosome complement in the human female in which there are, respectively, four or five instead of the normal two X chromosomes so that each somatic cell contains a total of 48 or 49 chromosomes. Although there is no consistent phenotype associated with such aberrations, the risk of congenital anomalies and mental retardation in the affected individual increases significantly with the increase in the number of X chromosomes.

XXXY, XXXXY, XXYY, (in genetics) the designation for an abnormal sex chromosome complement in the human male in which there are more than the normal one X chromosome resulting, respectively, in a total of 48, 49, or more chromosomes in each somatic cell. The aberration is a variant of Klinefelter's syndrome; and, in general, the more X chromosomes there are, the greater the number of congenital defects and the severity of mental retardation in the affected individual. See also **Klinefelter's syndrome.**

XXY syndrome. See **Klinefelter's syndrome.**

XY, (in genetics) the designation for the normal sex chromosome complement in the human male. See also **X chromosome, Y chromosome.**

xylitol /zī′litôl/, a sweet, crystalline pentahydroxy alcohol obtained by the reduction of xylose and used as an artificial sweetener.

xylo-, a combining form meaning 'pertaining to wood': *xyloketosuria, xylose, xylosuria.*

Xylocaine, a trademark for a local anesthetic (lidocaine).

xylometazoline hydrochloride, an adrenergic vasoconstrictor.

■ INDICATIONS: It is prescribed in the treatment of nasal congestion in colds, hay fever, sinusitis, and other upper respiratory allergies.

■ CONTRAINDICATIONS: Glaucoma or known hypersensitivity to this drug or to sympathomimetic medications prohibits its use. It is used with caution in patients having cardiovascular disease.

■ ADVERSE EFFECTS: Among the more serious adverse reactions are irritation to the mucosa, rebound nasal congestion, and effects associated with systemic absorption, including sedation and alterations in cardiovascular function.

XYY syndrome, the phenotypic manifestation of an extra Y chromosome, which tends to have a positive effect on height and may have a negative effect on mental and psychologic development. However, the anomaly also occurs in normal males. See also **trisomy.**

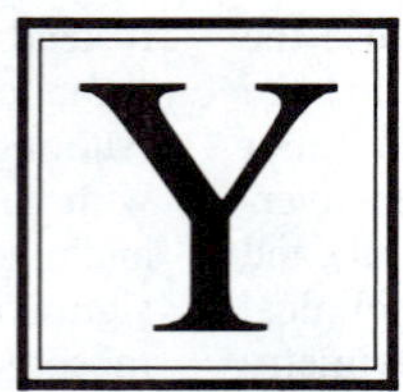

Y, symbol for **yttrium.**

yaws /yôs/, a nonvenereal infection caused by the spirochete *Treponema pertenue,* transmitted by direct contact and characterized by chronic, ulcerating sores anywhere on the body with eventual tissue and bone destruction, leading to crippling if untreated. It is a disease of unsanitary tropic living conditions and may be effectively treated with penicillin G. All serologic tests for syphilis may be positive in yaws. The infection may afford protection against syphilis. Also called **bouba, buba, frambesia, parangi, patek, pian.** Compare **bejel, pinta, syphilis.**

Yb, symbol for **ytterbium.**

Y chromosome, a sex chromosome that in humans and many other species is present only in the male, appearing singly in the normal male. It is carried as a sex determinant by one half of the male gametes and none of the female gametes, is morphologically much smaller than the X chromosome, and has genes associated with triggering the development and differentiation of male characteristics. There are no known medically significant traits or conditions associated with the genes on the Y chromosome. Compare **X chromosome.**

yeast, any unicellular, usually oval, nucleated fungus that reproduces by budding. *Candida albicans* is a kind of pathogenic yeast.

yellow cartilage, the most elastic of the three kinds of cartilage, consisting of elastic fibers in a flexible fibrous matrix. It is yellow and is located in various parts of the body, as the external ear, the auditory tube, the epiglottis, and the larynx. Also called **elastic cartilage.** Compare **hyaline cartilage, white fibrocartilage.**

yellow fever, an acute arbovirus infection transmitted by mosquitoes, characterized by headache, fever, jaundice, vomiting, and bleeding. There is no specific treatment, and mortality is about 5%. Recovery is followed by lifelong immunity. Immunization for travelers to endemic areas is advised. Nonhuman primates are a reservoir of infection.

yellow fever vaccine, a vaccine produced from live, attenuated yellow fever virus grown in chick embryos.

■ INDICATION: It is prescribed for immunization against yellow fever.

■ CONTRAINDICATIONS: Immunosuppression, pregnancy, or known hypersensitivity to chicken or egg protein prohibits its use.

■ ADVERSE EFFECTS: Among the more serious adverse effects are fever, malaise, and hypersensitivity reactions.

yellow marrow. See **bone marrow.**

Yersinia arthritis /yursin′ē·ə/, a polyarticular inflammation occurring a few days to 1 month after the onset of infection caused by *Yersinia enterocolitica* or *Y. pseudotuberculosis* and usually persisting longer than 1 month. Knees, ankles, toes, fingers, and wrists are most often affected. Cultures of synovial fluid yield no infectious organism. The clinical presentation may mimic juvenile rheumatoid arthritis, rheumatic fever, or Reiter's syndrome and may be associated with erythema nodosum or erythema multiforme. Treatment is with antibiotics.

Yersinia pestis, a small, gram-negative bacillus that causes plague. The primary host is the rat, but other small rodents also harbor the organism. A person without symptoms may be a carrier, but this happens rarely. *Yersinia pestis* is hardy, living for long periods in infected carcasses, the soil of the host's habitat, or in sputum. Also called ***Pasteurella pestis.*** See also **plague.**

Y fracture, a Y-shaped intercondylar fracture.

-yl, a combining form used in naming radicals: *benzoyl, ethyl, hydroxyl.*

Y-linked, pertaining to genes or to the characteristics or conditions they transmit that are carried on the Y chromosome. Such traits, as hypertrichosis of the pinna of the ear, can be expressed only in males. Compare **X-linked.** See also **sex-linked.** **–Y linkage,** *n.*

Yodoxin, a trademark for an antiamebic (diiodohydroxyquin).

yogurt, a slightly acid, semisolid, curdled milk preparation made from either whole or skimmed cow's milk and milk solids by fermentation with organisms from the genus *Lactobacillus.* It is rich in vitamins of the B complex group and a good source of protein. It also provides a medium in the GI tract that retards the growth of harmful bacteria and aids in the absorption of minerals.

yolk, the nutritive material, rich in fats and proteins, contained in the ovum to supply nourishment to the developing embryo. The amount and distribution of the yolk within the egg depend on the species of animal and type of reproduction and development of offspring. In humans and most mammals the yolk is absent or greatly diffused through the cell, because embryos absorb nutrients directly from the mother through the placenta. See also **deutoplasm.**

yolk membrane. See **vitelline membrane.**

yolk sac, a structure that develops in the inner cell mass of the embryo and expands into a vesicle with a thick part that becomes the primitive gut and a thin part that grows into the cavity of the chorion. The cells of the extraembryonic mesoderm differentiate to develop endothelium, primitive blood plasma, and hemoglobin. After supplying the nourishment for the embryo, the yolk sac usually disappears during the seventh week of pregnancy. See also **allantois, Meckel's diverticulum.**

yolk sphere. See **morula.**

yolk stalk, the narrow duct connecting the yolk sac with the midgut of the embryo during the early stages of prenatal development. It connects at the region of the future ileum and usually undergoes complete obliteration but occasionally may appear as a diverticulum. Also called **omphalomesenteric duct, umbilical duct, vitelline duct.** See also **Meckel's diverticulum.**

Young's rule, a method for the calculation of the appropriate dose of a drug for a child 2 years of age or more using the formula (age in years) ÷ (age + 12) × adult dose. See also **pediatric dosage.**

Y-plasty, a method of surgical revision of a scar, using a Y-shaped incision to reduce scar contractures. See also **Z-plasty.**

Y-set, a device composed of plastic components, used for delivering intravenous fluids through a primary intravenous line connected to a combination drip chamber-filter section from which two separate plastic tubes lead to fluid sources. The Y-set also includes three clamps, one for the primary intravenous line and one for each of the two separate tubes. It is often used to transfuse packed blood cells that must be diluted with saline solution to decrease their viscosity. In such a transfusion one of the tubes is connected to the container enclosing the packed cells; the other tube is connected to the receptacle containing the saline solution. During a prolonged transfusion of packed blood cells, the tubing of the Y-set must be changed every 4 hours. Compare **component drip set, component syringe set, microaggregate recipient set, straight line blood set.**

ytterbium (Yb) /itur′bē·əm/, a rare earth metallic element. Its atomic number is 70; its atomic weight is 173.04.

yttrium (Y) /it′rē·əm/, a scaly, grayish metallic element. Its atomic number is 39; its atomic weight is 88.905. Radioactive isotopes of yttrium have been used in cancer therapy.

Yutopar, a trademark for a beta-adrenergic drug (ritodrine hydrochloride), used to stop premature labor.

Z

Zahorsky's disease. See **roseola infantum.**

Zakrzewski /zakshef′skē/, **Marie** (1829–1902), a Polish-German-American midwife who studied medicine in Berlin and spent some time in Kaiserswerth, Germany, before emigrating to the United States. In New York she met Elizabeth Blackwell, who encouraged her to continue her medical studies. After receiving her medical degree in Cleveland, she worked at Blackwell's New York Infirmary before going to Boston. In 1872 she organized the first successful American school of nursing at the New England Hospital for Women and Children.

Zanosar, a trademark for an antineoplastic (streptozocin).

Zarontin, a trademark for an anticonvulsant (ethosuximide).

Zaroxolyn, a trademark for a diuretic and antihypertensive (metolazone).

Z chromosome. See **W chromosome and Z chromosome.**

Zenker's diverticulum, a circumscribed herniation of the mucous membrane of the pharynx as it joins the esophagus. Food may become trapped in the diverticulum and may be aspirated. Diagnosis is confirmed by x-ray studies. In most cases it is small, causes no dysfunction, is not diagnosed, and requires no treatment.

Zentron, a trademark for a hematinic fixed-combination drug containing iron and vitamins.

Zephiran Chloride, a trademark for a disinfectant (benzalkonium chloride).

zeranol, an estrogenic substance used to fatten livestock. Consumption of beef from zeranol-treated cattle has been associated with precocious puberty in some boys and girls.

zero order kinetics, a state at which the rate of an enzyme reaction is independent of the concentration of the substrate.

zeta potential, the potential produced by the effective charge of a macromolecule, usually measured at the boundary between what is moving in a solution with the macromolecule and the rest of the solution.

Zetar, a trademark for a topical antieczematic containing coal tar.

zeugmatography /zo͞og′mətog′rəfē/, another name for NMR imaging coined from Greek roots suggesting the role of the gradient magnetic field in joining the rf magnetic field to a desired local spatial region through nuclear magnetic resonance.

Ziehl-Neelsen test /zēl′nēl′sən/, one of the most widely used methods of acid-fast staining, commonly used in the microscopic examination of a smear of sputum suspected of containing *Mycobacterium tuberculosis*. See also **acid-fast stain.**

Ziehl's stain. See **carbol-fuchsin stain.**

ZIG, abbreviation for **zoster immune globulin.**

Zinacef, a trademark for a cephalosporin antibiotic (cefuroxime sodium).

zinc (Zn), a bluish-white crystalline metal commonly associated with lead ores. Its atomic number is 30; its atomic weight is 65.38. Zinc is ductile in its pure form and occurs abundantly in minerals such as sphalerite, zincite, and franklinite. It has many commercial uses, as a protective coating for steel and in printing plates. Zinc is an essential nutrient in the body and is used in numerous pharmaceutics, as zinc acetate, zinc oxide, zinc permanganate, and zinc stearate. Zinc acetate is used as an emetic, a styptic, and as an astringent. Zinc oxide is used internally as an antispasmodic and as a protective in ointments. Zinc permanganate is used as an astringent and in the treatment of urethritis by injection or douche in a 1:4000 solution. Zinc stearate is used as a water-repellent protective agent in the treatment of acne, eczema, and other skin diseases.

zinc chill. See **metal fume fever.**

zinc deficiency, a condition resulting from insufficient amounts of zinc in the diet, characterized by abnormal fatigue, decreased alertness, a decrease in taste and odor sensitivity, poor appetite, retarded growth, delayed sexual maturity, prolonged healing of wounds, and susceptibility to infection and injury. Other conditions that may precipitate the deficiency include alcoholic cirrhosis and other liver diseases, ulcers, myocardial infarction, Hodgkin's disease, mongolism, and cystic fibrosis. Prophylaxis and treatment consist of a diet of foods high in protein, which are also rich in zinc, including meats, eggs, liver, seafood, legumes, nuts, peanut butter, milk, and whole-grain cereals.

zinc gelatin, a topical protectant for varicosities and other lesions of the lower limbs. It is available as a smooth jelly containing zinc oxide (10%), gelatin (15%), glycerin (40%), and purified water (35%). It is also available impregnated in gauze.

zinc oxide, a topical protectant prescribed for a wide range of minor skin irritations.

zinc oxide eugenol dental cement, a luting agent consisting of a powder that is essentially zinc oxide with strengtheners and accelerators, combined with a liquid that is basically eugenol.

zinc phosphate dental cement, a material for luting of dental inlays, crowns, bridges, and orthodontic appliances and for some temporary restorations of dentitions. It is prepared by mixing a powder composed of zinc and magnesium oxides and a liquid composed of phosphoric acid, water, and buffering agents.

zinc salt poisoning, a toxic condition caused by the ingestion or inhalation of a zinc salt. Symptoms of ingestion include a burning sensation of the mouth and throat, vomiting, diarrhea, abdominal and chest pain, and, in severe cases, shock and coma. Treatment includes gastric lavage, followed by a demulcent and chelation with calcium edetate, and fluid therapy. Inhalation of zinc salts may cause metal fume fever; skin contact may produce blisters. A lethal dose of 10 g of zinc sulfate has been reported.

zinc sulfate, an ophthalmic astringent given in drops for nasal congestion or irritation of the eye, applied topically in deodorants, and given orally in tablets to promote healing and as a dietary supplement.

ZIP, abbreviation for *zoster immune plasma*. See **chickenpox.**

zirconium (Zr), a steel-gray, tetravalent metallic element. Its atomic number is 40; its atomic weight is 91.22. It occurs widely in combined form, especially in zircon and baddeleyite. It is usually extracted from sands containing zircon by heating with carbon and chlorine and passing the resulting volatile zirconium tetracholoride into hot molten magnesium or into sodium to yield a spongy form of the free metal. A component of zirconium dioxide was formerly used in some ointments for the treatment of poison ivy skin rashes, but such ointments caused skin granulomas in some individuals. Similar skin conditions developed in individuals using deodorants containing zirconium sodium lactate, and the use of zirconium compounds, except for zirconyl hydroxychloride, has been discontinued in the manufacture of skin ointments. Zirconyl hydroxychloride is still used in antiperspirants.

Zn, symbol for **zinc.**

zoanthropy /zō·an′thrəpē/, the delusion that one has assumed the form and characteristics of an animal. – **zoanthropic,** *adj.*

-zoite, a combining form meaning a 'simple organism' of a specified sort: *merozoite, saprozoite, sporozoite*.

Zollinger-Ellison syndrome /zol′injərel′isən/, a condition characterized by severe peptic ulceration, gastric hypersecretion, elevated serum gastrin, and gastrinoma of the pancreas or the duodenum. The syndrome is uncommon but not rare; it may occur in early childhood, but is seen more frequently in persons between 20 and 50 years of age. Two thirds of the tumors are malignant. Total gastrectomy may be necessary, but the administration of cimetidine in large doses may control gastric hypersecretion and allow the ulcers to heal. See also **peptic ulcer.**

Zomax, a trademark for a nonsteroidal analgesic and antiinflammatory agent (zomepirac sodium).

zomepirac sodium, an analgesic and antiinflammatory agent.

■ INDICATIONS: It is prescribed to reduce mild to moderately severe pain in rheumatoid arthritis and osteoarthritis, and related conditions.

■ CONTRAINDICATIONS: Known hypersensitivity to this drug or to any nonsteroidal antiinflammatory agent prohibits its use. It is used with caution in patients having upper GI disease. It is not given to pregnant or lactating women.

■ ADVERSE EFFECT: Among the more serious adverse reactions are GI bleeding, palpitations, depression, and skin rash.

zona /zō′nə/, *pl.* **zonae,** a zone, or girdlelike segment of a rounded or spheric structure. See also **zone.**

zona ciliaris. See **ciliary zone.**

zona fasciculata, the middle portion of the adrenal cortex, which is the site of production of glucocorticoids and sex hormones.

zona glomerulosa, the outer portion of the adrenal cortex, where mineralocorticoids are produced.

zona pellucida /pəlo͞o′sidə/, the thick, transparent, noncellular membrane that encloses the mammalian ovum. It is secreted by the ovum during its development in the ovary and is retained until near the time of implantation. Also called **oolemma** /ō′əlem′ə/. See also **vitelline membrane.**

zona radiata, a zona pellucida that has a striated appearance caused by radiating canals within the membrane. Also called **zona striata.**

zona reticularis, the innermost portion of the adrenal cortex, which borders on the adrenal medulla portion of the gland. It acts in consort with the zona fasciculata in producing various sex hormones and glucocorticoids.

zona striata. See **zona radiata.**

Zondek-Ascheim test. See **Ascheim-Zondek test.**

zone, an area with specific boundaries and characteristics, as the epigastric, the mesogastric, or the hypogastric zones of the abdomen. See also **zona.**

zone of equivalence, a region of an antibody-antigen reaction in which concentrations of both reactants are equal.

zonesthesia, a painful sensation of constriction, as of a bandage bound too tightly, especially experienced around the waist or abdomen. Also called **girdle sensation.**

zone therapy, the treatment of a disorder by mechanic stimulation and counterirritation of a body area in the same longitudinal zone as the affected organ or region.

zonography, an x-ray imaging technique used to produce films of body sections similar to those made by tomography. A very narrow exposure angle of less than 10 degrees is used in zonography, producing a focal zone of less than 1 inch in thickness.

zonula, *pl.* **zonulae,** a small zone. Also called **zonule.**

zonula ciliaris, a ligament composed of straight fibrils radiating from the ciliary body of the eye to the crystalline lens, holding the lens in place and relaxing by the contraction of the ciliary muscle. Relaxation of the ligament allows the lens to become more convex. Also called **zonule of Zinn.**

zoo-, zo-, a combining form meaning 'pertaining to an animal': *zooamylon, zoogony, zoonosis.*

zooerastia. See **bestiality.**

zoogenous /zō·oj′ənəs/, acquired from or originating in animals. See also **zoonosis.**

zoograft /zō′əgraft/, tissue of an animal transplanted to a human, as a heart valve from a pig to replace a damaged heart valve in a human.

zoology, the study of animal life.

zoomania /zō·əmā′nē·ə/, a psychopathologic state characterized by an excessive fondness for and preoccupation with animals. **–zoomaniac,** *n.*

-zoon, a combining form meaning a 'living being': *dermatozoon, entozoon, hepatozoon.*

zoonosis /zō·on′əsis, zō′ənō′sis/, a disease of animals that is transmissible to humans from its primary animal host. Some kinds of zoonoses are **equine encephalitis, leptospirosis, rabies,** and **yellow fever.**

zooparasite /zō·əper′əsīt/, any parasitic animal organism. Kinds of zooparasites are **arthropods, protozoa,** and **worms.** **–zooparasitic,** *adj.*

zoopathology, the study of the diseases of animals.

zoophilia /zō·əfil′ē·ə/, **1.** an abnormal fondness for animals. **2.** (in psychiatry) a psychosexual disorder in which sexual excitement and gratification are derived from the fondling of animals or from the fantasy or act of engaging in sexual activity with animals. Also called **zoophilism** /zō·of′iliz′əm/. See also **paraphilia.** **–zoophile,** *n.,* **zoophilic, zoophilous,** *adj.*

zoophobia /zō′ə-/, an anxiety disorder characterized by a persistent, irrational fear of animals, particularly dogs, snakes, insects, and mice. The condition is seen more often in women than in men, nearly always begins in childhood, and can typically be traced to some frightening or unpleasant experience involving an animal. Treatment consists of psychotherapy to uncover the cause of the phobic reaction followed by behavior therapy, specifically the techniques of systemic desensitization and flooding.

zoopsia /zō·op′sē·ə/, a visual hallucination of animals or insects, often occurring in delirium tremens.

zootoxin /zō′ətok′sin/, a poisonous substance from an animal, as the venom of snakes, spiders, and scorpions. **–zootoxic,** *adj.*

zoster. See **herpes zoster.**

zosteriform /zoster′ifôrm/, resembling the pocks seen in herpes zoster infection.

zoster immune globulin (ZIG), a passive immunizing agent currently in limited experimental use for preventing or attenuating herpes zoster virus infection in immunosuppressed individuals who are at great risk of severe herpes zoster virus infection.

Zovirax, a trademark for an antiviral agent (acyclovir).

Z-plasty, a method of surgical revision of a scar or closure of a wound using a Z-shaped incision to reduce contractures of the adjacent skin. See also **Y-plasty.**

Zr, symbol for **zirconium.**

zwieback, a sweetened bread that is enriched with eggs and baked, then sliced and toasted until dry and crisp. It is used as a snack food for children, especially teething infants.

zyg-, zygo-, a combining form meaning 'union or fusion, yoked or joined, pertaining to a junction, or a pair': *zygomatic, zygogenesis, zygote.*

zygogenesis /zī′gōjen′əsis/, **1.** the formation of a zygote. **2.** reproduction by the union of gametes. **–zygogenetic, zygogenic,** *adj.*

zygoma /zīgō′mə, zig-/, **1.** a long slender zygomatic process of the temporal bone, arising from the lower part of the squamous portion of the temporal bone, passing forward to join the zygomatic bone, and forming part of the zygomatic arch. **2.** the zygomatic bone that forms the prominence of the cheek.

zygomatic bone, one of the pair of bones that forms the prominence of the cheek, the lower part of the orbit of the eye, and parts of the temporal and infratemporal fossae.

zygomatic head. See **zygomaticus minor.**

zygomaticus major /zī′gōmat′ikəs/, one of the 12 muscles of the mouth. Arising from the zygomatic bone and inserting into the corner of the mouth, it is innervated by buccal branches of the facial nerve and acts to draw the angle of the mouth up and back to smile or laugh. Also called **zygomaticus.** Compare **zygomaticus minor.**

zygomaticus minor, one of the 12 muscles of the mouth. Arising from the malar surface of the zygomatic bone and inserting into the upper lip, it is innervated by buccal branches of the facial nerve and acts to deepen the nasolabial furrow in a sad facial expression. Also called **quadratus labii superioris, zygomatic head.** Compare **zygomaticus major.**

zygomaxillare. See **key ridge.**

zygomycosis /zī′gōmīkō′sis/, an acute, often fulminant and sometimes fatal fungal infection caused by a class of Phycomycetal water molds, seen primarily in patients with chronic debilitating diseases, especially uncontrolled diabetes mellitus. Characteristically, it begins with fever and with pain and discharge in the nose and paranasal sinuses that progresses to invade the eye and lower respiratory tract. The fungus may enter blood vessels and spread to the brain and other organs. Transmission is usually by inhalation. The diagnosis is confirmed by biopsy and pathologic examination of sputum. Treatment includes improved control of diabetes mellitus, extensive debridement of craniofacial lesions, and amphotericin B administered intravenously. Also called **mucormycosis.** Compare **phycomycosis.**

zygonema /zī′gənē′mə/, the synaptic chromosome formation that occurs in the zygotene stage of the first meiotic prophase of gametogenesis. **–zygonematic,** *adj.*

zygosis /zīgō′sis/, a form of sexual reproduction in unicellular organisms, consisting of the union of the two cells and fusion of the nuclei. –**zygotic** /zīgot′ik/, *adj*.

zygosity /zīgos′itē/, the characteristics or conditions of a zygote. The form occurs primarily as a suffix combining form to denote genetic makeup, referring specifically to whether the paired alleles determining a particular trait are identical (homozygosity) or different (heterozygosity) or to the condition in twins of having developed from the fertilization of one ovum (monozygosity) or two (dizygosity).

zygospore /zī′gōspôr′/, the spore resulting from the conjugation of two isogametes, as in certain fungi and algae. Also called **zygosperm.**

zygote /zī′gōt/, (in embryology) the developing ovum from the time it is fertilized until, as a blastocyst, it is implanted in the uterus.

zygotene /zī′gətēn/, the second stage in the first meiotic prophase of gametogenesis in which synapsis of homologous chromosomes occurs. See also **diakinesis, diplotene, leptotene, pachytene.**

Zyloprim, a trademark for a xanthine oxidase inhibitor (allopurinol).

-zyme, a combining form meaning a 'ferment or enzyme': *lysozyme, opzyme, serozyme*.

zymo-, a combining form meaning 'pertaining to an enzyme or to fermentation': *zymocide, zymohexase, zymophore*.

zymogenic cell. See **chief cell.**

APPENDICES

APPENDIX 1 NORMAL LABORATORY VALUES

1-1 Normal reference laboratory values

Blood, plasma, or serum values

Determination	Reference range	
	Conventional	*SI*
Acetoacetate plus acetone	0.3-2.0 mg/100 ml	3-20 mg/l
Aldolase	1.3-8.2 mU/ml	12-75 nmol · s^{-1}/l
Alpha amino nitrogen	3.0-5.5 mg/100 ml	2.1-3.9 mmol/l
Ammonia	80-110 μg/100 ml	47-65 μmol/l
Amylase	4-25 U/ml	4-25 arb. unit
Ascorbic acid	0.4-1.5 mg/100 ml	23-85 μmol/l
Barbiturate	0 Coma level: phenobarbital, approximately 10 mg/100 ml; most other drugs, 1-3 mg per 100 ml	0 μmol/l
Bilirubin (van den Bergh test)	One minute: 0.4 mg/100 ml Direct: 0.4 mg/100 ml. Total: 1.0 mg/100 ml. Indirect is total minus direct	Up to 7 μmol/l Up to 17 μmol/l
Blood volume	8.5%-9.0% of body weight in kg	80-85 ml/kg
Bromide	0 Toxic level: 17 meq/l	0 mmol/l
Bromsulfalein (BSP)	Less than 5% retention 45 min after 5 mg/kg IV	<0.05 l
Calcium	8.5-10.5 mg/100 ml (slightly higher in children)	2.1-2.6 mmol/l
Carbon dioxide content	24-30 meq/l 20-26 meq/l in infants (as HCO_3^-)	24-30 mmol/l
Carbon monoxide	Symptoms with over 20% saturation	0 (1)
Carotenoids	0.8-4.0 μg/ml	1.5-7.4 μmol/l
Ceruloplasmin	27-37 mg/100 ml	1.8-2.5 μmol/l
Chloride	100-106 meq/l	100-106 mmol/l
Cholinesterase (pseudocholinesterase)	0.5 pH U or more/h 0.7 pH U or more/h for packed cells	0.5 or more arb. unit
Copper	Total: 100-200 μg/100 ml	16-31 μmol/l
Creatine phosphokinase (CPK)	Female 5-35 mU/ml Male 5-55 mU/ml	0.08-0.58 μmol s^{-1}/l
Creatinine	0.6-1.5 mg/100 ml	60-130 μmol/l
Doriden (Glutethimide)	0 mg/100 ml	0 μmol/l
Ethanol	0.3%-0.4%, marked intoxication; 0.4%-0.5%, alcoholic stupor; 0.5% or over, alcoholic coma	65-87 mmol/l 87-109 mmol/l >109 mmol/l
Glucose	Fasting: 70-110 mg/100 ml	3.9-5.6 mmol/l
Iron	50-150 μg/100 ml (higher in males)	9.0-26.9 μmol/l
Iron-binding capacity	250-410 μg/100 ml	44.8-73.4 μmol/l
Lactic acid	0.6-1.8 meq/l	0.6-1.8 mmol/l
Lactic dehydrogenase	60-120 U/ml	1.00-2.00 μmol s^{-1}/l
Lead	50 μg/100 ml or less	Up to 2.4 μmol/l
Lipase	2 U/ml or less	Up to 2 arb. unit
Lipids		
Cholesterol	120-220 mg/100 ml	3.10-5.69 mmol/l
Cholesterol esters	60-75% of cholesterol	
Phospholipids	9-16 mg/100 ml as lipid phosphorus	2.9-5.2 mmol/l
Total fatty acids	190-420 mg/100 ml	1.9-4.2 g/l
Total lipids	450-1000 mg/100 ml	4.5-10.0 g/l
Triglycerides	40-150 mg/100 ml	0.4-1.5 g/l
Lithium	Toxic level 2 meq/l	2 mmol/l

From Kaye, D., and Rose, L.F., editors: Fundamentals of internal medicine, St. Louis, 1983, The C.V. Mosby Co. Adapted by permission from the New England Journal of Medicine, Vol. 302, pages 37-48, 1980. Abbreviations used: SI, Système international d'Unités (The SI for the Health Professions. World Health Organization, Office of Publications, Geneva, Switzerland, 1977); d, 24 hours; P, plasma; S, serum; B, blood; U, urine; l, liter; h, hour; and s, second.

Continued.

Blood, plasma or serum values—cont'd

Determination	*Reference range*	
	Conventional	*SI*
Magnesium	1.5-2.0 meq/l	0.8-1.3 mmol/l
Methanol	0	
5′Nucleotidase	0.3-3.2 Bodansky U	30-290 nmol · s^{-1}/l
Osmolality	285-295 mOsm/kg water	285-295 mmol/kg
Oxygen saturation (arterial)	96%-100%	0.96-1.001
P_{CO_2}	35-43 mm Hg	4.7-6.0 kPa
pH	7.35-7.45	Same
P_{O_2}	75-100 mm Hg (dependent on age) while breathing room air	10-0-13.3 kPa
	Above 500 mm Hg while on 100% O_2	
Phenylalanine	0-2 mg/100 ml	0-120 μmol/l
Phenytoin (Dilantin)	Therapeutic level, 5-20 μg/ml	19.8-79.5 μmol/l
Phosphatase (acid)	Male-Total: 0.13-0.63 Sigma U/ml	36-175 nmol · s^{-1}/l
	Female-Total: 0.01-0.56 Sigma U/ml	2.8-156 nmol · s^{-1}/l
	Prostatic: 0-0.7 Fishman-Lerner U/100 ml	
Phosphatase (alkaline)*	13-39 IU/l; infants and adolescents up to 104 IU/l	0.22-0.65 μmol · s^{-1}/l Up to 1.26 μmol · s^{-1}/l
Phosphorus (inorganic)	3.0-4.5 mg/100 ml (infants in 1st year up to 6.0 mg/100 ml)	1.0-1.5 mmol/l
Potassium	3.5-5.0 meq/l	3.5-5.0 mmol/l
Primidone (Mysoline)	Therapeutic level 4-12 μg/ml	18-55 μmol/l
Protein: Total	6.0-8.4 g/100 ml	60-84 g/l
Albumin	3.5-5.0 g/100 ml	35-50 g/l
Globulin	2.3-3.5 g/100 ml	23-35 g/l
Electrophoresis	% of total protein	
Albumin	52-68	0.52-0.68 l
Globulin:		
Alpha$_1$	4.2-7.2	0.042-0.072 l
Alpha$_2$	6.8-12	0.068-0.12 l
Beta	9.3-15	0.093-0.15 l
Gamma	13-23	0.13-0.23 l
Pyruvic acid	0-0.11 meq/l	0-0.11 mmol/l
Quinidine	Therapeutic: 1.5-3 μg/ml	4.6-9.2 μmol/l
	Toxic: 5-6 μg/ml	15.4-18.5 μmol/l
Salicylate:	0	
Therapeutic	20-25 mg/100 ml;	1.4-1.8 mmol/l
	25-30 mg/100 ml to age 10 yrs. 3 h post dose	1.8-2.2 mmol/l
Toxic	Over 30 mg/100 ml;	Over 2.2 mmol/l
	over 20 mg/100 ml after age 60	Over 1.4 mmol/l
Sodium	135-145 meq/l	135-145 mmol/l
Sulfate	0.5-1.5 mg/100 ml	0.05-1.2 mmol/l
Sulfonamide	0 mg/100 ml	0 mmol/l
	Therapeutic: 5-15 mg/100 ml	
Thymol:		
Flocculation	Up to 1+ in 24 hr	Up to 1+ arb. unit
Turbidity	0-4 U	0-4 arb. unit
Transaminase (SGOT) (aspartate aminotransferase)	10-40 U/ml	0.08-0.32 μmol · s^{-1}/l
Urea nitrogen (BUN)	8-25 mg/100 ml	2.9-8.9 mmol/l
Uric acid	3.0-7.0 mg/100 ml	0.18-0.42 mmol/l
Vitamin A	0.15-0.6 μg/ml	0.5-2.1 μmol/l
Vitamin A tolerance test	Rise to twice fasting level in 3 to 5 h	

*For Bodansky U, multiply IU/l by 0.15 up to 90 U; 0.13 to 256 U.

Urine values

Determination	Reference range: Conventional	Reference range: SI
Acetone plus acetoacetate (quantitative)	0	0 mg/l
Alpha amino nitrogen	64-199 mg/d; not over 1.5% of total nitrogen	4.6-14.2 mmol/d
Amylase	24-76 U/ml	24-76 arb. unit
Calcium	150 mg/d or less	3.8 or less mmol/d
Catecholamines	Epinephrine: under 20 µg/d	<55 nmol/d
	Norepinephrine: under 100 µg/d	<590 nmol/d
Chorionic gonadotropin	0	0 arb. unit
Copper	0-100 µg/d	0-1-6 µmol/d
Coproporphyrin	50-250 µg/d	80-380 nmol/d
	Children under 80 lb 0-75 µg/d	0-115 nmol/d
Creatine	Under 100 mg/d or less than 6% of creatinine. In pregnancy: up to 12%. In children under 1 yr.: may equal creatinine. In older children: up to 30% of creatinine	<0.75 mmol/d
Creatinine	15-25 mg/kg of body weight/d	0.13-0.22 mmol kg^{-1}/d
Creatinine clearance	150-180 l/d (104-125 ml/min) per 1.73 m^2 of body surface	1.7-2.1 ml/s
Cystine or cysteine	0	0
Follicle-stimulating hormone:		
Follicular phase	5-20 IU/d	Same
Mid-cycle	15-60 IU/d	
Luteal phase	5-15 IU/d	
Menopausal	50-100 IU/d	
Men	5-25 IU/d	
Hemoglobin and myoglobin	0	
Homogentisic acid	0	
5-Hydroxyindole acetic acid	2-9 mg/d (women lower than men)	10-45 µmol/d
Lead	0.08 µg/ml or 120 µg or less/d	0.39 µmol/l or less
Phenolsulfonphthalein (PSP)	At least 25% excreted by 15 min; 40% by 30 min; 60% by 120 min	0.25 l
Phenylpyruvic acid	0	0
Phosphorus (inorganic)	Varies with intake; average 1 g/d	32 mmol/d
Porphobilinogen	0	0
Protein:		
Quantitative	<150 mg/24 h	<0.15 g/d
Electrophoresis		
Steroids:		
17-Ketosteroids (per day)	*Age* — *Male* — *Female*	*µmol/d* — *µmol/d*
	10 — 1-4 mg — 1-4 mg	3-14 — 3-14
	20 — 6-21 — 4-16	21-73 — 14-56
	30 — 8-26 — 4-14	28-90 — 14-49
	50 — 5-18 — 3-9	17-62 — 10-31
	70 — 2-10 — 1-7	7-35 — 3-24
17-Hydroxysteroids	3-8 mg/d (women lower than men)	8-22 µmol/d as hydrocortisone
Sugar:		
Quantitative glucose	0	0 mmol/l
Identification of reducing substances		
Fructose	0	0 mmol/l
Pentose	0	0 mmol/l
Titratable acidity	20-40 meq/d	20-40 mmol/d
Urobilinogen	Up to 1.0 Ehrlich U	To 1.0 arb. unit
Uroporphyrin	0	0 nmol/d
Vanilmandelic acid (VMA)	Up to 9 mg/24 h	Up to 45 µmol/d

Special endocrine tests

Determination	Reference range: Conventional	Reference range: SI
Steroid hormones		
Aldosterone	Excretion: 5-19 μg/24 h	14-53 nmol/d
Fasting, at rest, 210 meq sodium diet	Supine: 48 ± 29 pg/ml	133 ± 80 pmol/l
	Upright: (2 h) 65 ± 23 pg/ml	180 ± 64 pmol/l
Fasting, at rest, 110 meq sodium diet	Supine: 107 ± 45 pg/ml	279 ± 125 pmol/l
	Upright: (2 h) 239 ± 123 pg/ml	663 ± 341 pmol/l
Fasting, at rest, 10 meq sodium diet	Supine: 175 ± 75 pg/ml	485 ± 208 pmol/l
	Upright: (2 h) 532 ± 228 pg/ml	1476 ± 632 pmol/l
Cortisol		
Fasting	8 a.m.: 5-25 μg/100 ml	0.14-0.69 μmol/l
At rest	8 p.m.: Below 10 μg/100 ml	0-0.28 μmol/l
20 U ACTH	4 h ACTH test: 30-45 μg/100 ml	0.83-1.24 μmol/l
Dexamethasone at midnight	Overnight suppression test: Below 5 μg/100 ml	<0.14 nmol/l
	Excretion: 20-70 μg/24 h	55-193 nmol/d
11-Deoxycortisol	Responsive: Over 7.5 μg/100 ml (after metyrapone)	>0.22 μmol/l
Testosterone	Adult male: 300-1100 ng/100 ml	10.4-38.1 nmol/l
	Adolescent male: Over 100 ng/100 ml	>3.5 nmol/l
	Female: 25-90 ng/100 ml	0.87-3.12 nmol/l
Unbound testosterone	Adult male: 3.06-24.0 ng/100 ml	106-832 pmol/l
	Adult female: 0.09-1.28 ng/100 ml	3.1-44.4 pmol/l
Polypeptide hormones		
Adrenocorticotropin (ACTH)	15-70 pg/ml	3.3-15.4 pmol/l
Calcitonin	Undetectable in normals.	0
	>100 pg/ml in medullary carcinoma	>29.3 pmol/l
Growth hormone		
Fasting, at rest	Below 5 ng/ml	<233 pmol/l
After exercise	Children: Over 10 ng/ml	>465 pmol/l
	Male: Below 5 ng/ml	<233 pmol/l
	Female: Up to 30 ng/ml	0-1395 pmol/l
After glucose	Male: Below 5 ng/ml	<233 pmol/l
	Female: Below 10 ng/ml	0-465 pmol/l
Polypeptide hormones—cont'd		
Insulin		
Fasting	6-26 μU/ml	43-187 pmol/l
During hypoglycemia	Below 20 μU/ml	<144 pmol/l
After glucose	Up to 150 μU/ml	0-1078 pmol/l
Luteinizing hormone	Male: 6-18 mU/ml	6-18 u/l
Pre- or postovulatory	Female: 5-22 mU/ml	5-22 u/l
Midcycle peak	30-250 mU/ml	30-250 u/l
Parathyroid hormone	<10 μl equiv/ml	<10 ml equiv/l
Prolactin	2-15 ng/ml	0.08-6.0 nmol/l
Renin activity		
Normal diet	Supine: 1.1 ± 0.8 ng/ml/h	0.9 ± 0.6 (nmol/l)h
	Upright: 1.9 ± 1.7 ng/ml/h	1.5 ± 1.3 (nmol/l)h
Low-sodium diet	Supine: 2.7 ± 1.8 ng/ml/h	2.1 ± 1.4 (nmol/l)h
	Upright: 6.6 ± 2.5 ng/ml/h	5.1 ± 1.9 (nmol/l)h
Low-sodium diet	Diuretics: 10.0 ± 3.7 ng/ml/h	7.7 ± 2.9 (nmol/l)h
Thyroid hormones		
Thyroid-stimulating hormone (TSH)	0.5-3.5 μU/ml	0.5-3.5 mU/l
Thyroxine-binding globulin capacity	15-25 μg T_4/100 ml	193-322 nmol/l
Total tri-iodothyronine by radioimmunoassay (T_3)	70-190 ng/100 ml	1.08-2.92 nmol/l
Total thyroxine by RIA (T_4)	4-12 μg/100 ml	52-154 nmol/l
T_3 resin uptake	25-35%	0.25-0.35
Free thyroxine index (FT_4I)	1-4 ng/100 ml	12.8-51.2 pmol/l

Hematologic values

Determination	Reference range: Conventional	Reference range: SI
Coagulation factors:		
Factor I (fibrinogen)	0.15-0.35 g/100 ml	4.0-10.0 μmol/l
Factor II (prothrombin)	60%-140%	0.60-1.40
Factor V (accelerator globulin)	60%-140%	0.60-1.40
Factor VII-X (proconvertin-Stuart)	70%-130%	0.70-1.30
Factor X (Stuart factor)	70%-130%	0.70-1.30
Factor VIII (antihemophilic globulin)	50%-200%	0.50-2.0
Factor IX (plasma thromboplastic cofactor)	60%-140%	0.60-1.40
Factor XI (plasma thromboplastic antecedent)	60%-140%	0.60-1.40
Factor XII (Hageman factor)	60%-140%	0.60-1.40
Coagulation screening tests:		
Bleeding time (Simplate)	3-9 min	180-540 s
Prothrombin time	Less than 2-s deviation from control	Less than 2-s deviation from control
Partial thromboplastin time (activated)	25-37 s	25-37 s
Whole-blood clot lysis	No clot lysis in 24 h	0/d
Fibrinolytic studies:		
Euglobin lysis	No lysis in 2 h	0 (in 2 h)
Fibrinogen split products:	Negative reaction at greater than 1:4 dilution	0 (at >1:4 dilution)
Thrombin time	Control ± 5 s	Control ± 5 s
"Complete" blood count:		
Hematocrit	Male: 45%-52% Female: 37%-48%	Male: 0.42-0.52 Female: 0.37-0.48
Hemoglobin	Male: 13-18 g/100 ml Female: 12-16 g/100 ml	Male: 8.1-11.2 mmol/l Female: 7.4-9.9 mmol/l
Leukocyte count	4300-10,800/mm^3	4.3-10.8 × 10^9/l
Erythrocyte count	4.2-5.9 million/mm^3	4.2-5.9 × 10^{12}/l
Mean corpuscular volume (MCV)	80-94 μm^3	80-94 fl
Mean corpuscular hemoglobin (MCH)	27-32 pg	1.7-2.0 fmol
Mean corpuscular hemoglobin concentration (MCHC)	32-36%	19-22.8 mmol/l
Erythrocyte sedimentation rate (Westergren method)	Male: 1-13 mm/h Female: 1-20 mm/h	Male: 1-13 mm/h Female:1-20mm/h
Erythrocyte enzymes:		
Glucose-6-phosphate dehydrogenase	5-15 U/gHb	5-15 U/g
Pyruvate kinase	13-17 U/gHb	13-17 U/g
Ferritin (serum)		
Iron deficiency	0-20 ng/ml	0.20 μg/l
Iron excess	Greater than 400 ng/l	>400 μg/l
Folic acid		
Normal	Greater than 1.9 ng/ml	>4.3 mmol/l
Borderline	1.0-1.9 ng/ml	2.3-4.3 mmol/l
Haptoglobin	100-300 mg/100 ml	1.0-3.0 g/l
Hemoglobin studies:		
Electrophoresis for abnormal hemoglobin		
Electrophoresis for A_2 hemoglobin	1.5-3.5%	0.015-0.035
Hemoglobin F (fetal hemoglobin)	Less than 2%	<0.02
Hemoglobin, met- and sulf-	0	0
Serum hemoglobin	2-3 mg/100 ml	1.2-1.9 μmol/l
Thermolabile hemoglobin	0	0
Lupus anticoagulant	0	0

Continued.

Hematologic values—cont'd

Determination	Reference range		Determination	Reference range	
	Conventional	SI		Conventional	SI
LE (lupus erythematosus) preparation:			Osmotic fragility of erythrocytes	Increased if hemolysis occurs in over 0.5% NaCl; decreased if hemolysis is incomplete in 0.3% NaCl	
Heparin as anticoagulant	0	0			
Defibrinated blood	0	0	Peroxide hemolysis	Less than 10%	<0.10
Leukocyte alkaline phosphatase:			Platelet count	150,000-350,000/mm^3	150-350 × 10^9/l
Quantitative method	15-40 mg of phosphorus liberated/h/10^{10} cells	15-40 mg/h	Platelet function tests:		
Qualitative method	Males: 33-188 U	33-188 U	Clot retraction	50-100%/2 h	0.50-1.00/2 h
	Females (off contraceptive pill): 30-160 U	30-160 U	Platelet aggregation	Full response to ADP, epinephrine and collagen	1.0
Muramidase	Serum, 3-7 μg/ml	3-7 mg/l	Platelet factor 3	33-57 s	33-57 s
	Urine, 0-2 μg/ml	0-2 mg/l	Reticulocyte count	0.5%-1.5% red cells	0.005-.015
			Vitamin B_{12}	90-280 pg/ml (borderline: 70-90)	66-207 pmol/l (borderline: 52-66)

Cerebrospinal fluid values

Determination	Reference range		Determination	Reference range	
	Conventional	SI		Conventional	SI
Bilirubin	0	0 μmol/l	Glucose	50-75 mg/100 ml (30%-50% less than blood)	2.8-4.2 mmol/l
Cell count	0.5 mononuclear cells				
Chloride	120-130 meq/l (20 meq/l higher than serum)		Pressure (initial)	70-180 mm of water	70-80 arb. u.
			Protein:		
Colloidal gold	0000000000-0001222111	Same	Lumbar	15-45 mg/100 ml	0.15-0.45 g/l
Albumin	Mean: 29.5 mg/100 ml	0.295 g/l	Cisternal	15-25 mg/100 ml	0.15-0.25 g/l
	±2 SD: 11-48 mg/100 ml	±2 SD: 0.11-0.48	Ventricular	5-15 mg/100 ml	0.05-0.15 g/l
IgG	Mean: 4.3 mg/100 ml	0.043 g/l			
	±2 SD: 0-8.6 mg/100 ml	±2 SD: 0-0.086			

Miscellaneous values

Determination	Reference range: Conventional	Reference range: SI
Autoantibodies in serum		
Thyroid colloid and microsomal antigens	Absent	
Stomach parietal cells	Absent	
Smooth muscle	Absent	
Kidney mitochondria	Absent	
Rebbit renal collecting ducts	Absent	
Cytoplasm of ova, theca cells, testicular interstitial cells	Absent	
Skeletal muscle	Absent	
Adrenal gland	Absent	
Carcinoembryonic antigen (CEA) in blood	0-2.5 ng/ml, 97% healthy nonsmokers	0-2.5 μg/1, 97% healthy nonsmokers
Cryoprecipitable proteins in blood	0	0 arb. unit
Digitoxin in serum	17 ± 6 ng/ml	22 ± 7.8 nmol/l
Digoxin in serum		
0.25 mg/d	1.2 ± 0.4 ng/ml	1.54 ± 0.5 nmol/l
0.5 mg/d	1.5 ± 0.4 ng/ml	1.92 ± 0.5 nmol/l
Duodenal drainage:		
pH	5.5-7.5	5.5-7.5
Amylase	Over 1200 U/total sample	>1.2 arb. u
Trypsin	Values from 35% to 160% "normal"	0.35-1.60
Viscosity	3 min or less	180 s or less
Gastric analysis	Basal:	
	Females 2.0 ± 1.8 meq/h	0.6 ± 0.5
	Males 3.0 ± 2.0 meq/h	0.8 ± 0.6 μmol/s
	Maximal: (after histalog or gastrin)	
	Females 16 ± 5 meq/h	4.4 ± 1.4 μmol/s
	Males 23 ± 5 meq/h	6.4 ± 1.4 μmol/s
Gastrin-I in blood	0-200 pg/ml	0-95 pmol/l
Immunologic tests*:		
Alpha-fetoglobulin	Abnormal if present	
Alpha 1-antitrypsin	200-400 mg/100 ml	2.0-4.0 g/l
Antinuclear antibodies	Positive if detected with serum diluted 1:10	
Anti-DNA antibodies	Less than 15 units/ml	
Immunologic tests—cont'd		
Bence-Jones protein	Abnormal if present	
Complement, total hemolytic	150-250 U/ml	
C3	Range 55-120 mg/100 ml	0.55-1.2 g/l
C4	Range 20-50 mg/100 ml	0.2-0.5 g/l
Immunoglobulins in blood:		
IgG	1140 mg/100 ml	11.4 g/l
	Range 540-1663	5.5-16.6 g/l
IgA	214 mg/100 ml	2.14 g/l
	Range 66-344	0.66-3.44 g/l
IgM	168 mg/100 ml	1.68 g/l
	Range 39-290	0.39-2.9 g/l
Viscosity	1.4-1.8 expressed as relative viscosity of serum compared to water	
Iontophoresis	Children: 0-40 meq sodium/liter. Adults: 0-60 meq sodium/l	0-40 mmol/l 0-60 mmol/l
Propranolol (includes bioactive 4-OH metabolite) in serum 4 h after last dose	100-300 ng/ml	386-1158 nmol/l
Stool fat	Less than 5 g in 24 h or less than 4% of measured fat intake in 3-d period	<5 g/d
Stool nitrogen	Less than 2 g/d or 10% of urinary nitrogen	<2 g/d
Synovial fluid:		
Glucose	Not less than 20 mg/100 ml lower than simultaneously drawn blood sugar	See blood glucose mmol/l
Mucin	Type 1 or 2 Grades as: Type 1-tight clump Type 2-soft clump Type 3-soft clump that breaks up Type 4-cloudy, no clump	1-2 arb. u
D-Xylose absorption	5-8 g/5 h in urine	33-53 mmol
	40 mg per 100 ml in blood 2 h after ingestion of 25 g of D-xylose	2.7 mmol/l

*Immunologic tests are on blood except for Bence-Jones protein on urine.

1-2 Selected pediatric reference values

Substance	*Age*	*Reference range*	
Acid phosphatase, serum	Newborn	7.4-19.4 U/L	
	2-13 yr	6.4-15.2 U/L	
Aldolase, serum	Newborn	To 4 × adult value	
	Child	To 2 × adult value	
Alkaline phosphatase, serum	Newborn	40-300 U/L	
	Child	60-270 U/L	
Alpha fetoprotein, serum	Newborn	Up to 100 mg/L	
	2 wk	Undetectable	
Amylase, serum	Newborn	Little if any activity	
	1 yr	Adult values	
Aspartate aminotransferase, serum	Newborn	16-74 U/L	
	1-3 yr	6-30 U/L	
Bilirubin, serum		*Preterm*	*Term*
	24 hr	17.1-102.8 μmol/L(10-60 mg/L)	34.2-102.8 μmol/L (20-60 mg/L)
	48 hr	102.8-137.0 μmol/L(60-80 mg/L)	102.8-119.9 μmol/L (60-70 mg/L)
	3-5 d	171.0-266.5 μmol/L (100-150 mg/L)	68.6-205.2 μmol/L (40-120 mg/L)
Calcium, serum	Preterm, first week	1.5-2.5 mmol/L (60-100 mg/L)	
	Full-term, first week	1.75-3.00 mmol/L (70-120 mg/L)	
	1-2 yr	2.5-3.0 mmol/L (100-120 mg/L)	
	2-16 yr	2.25-2.88 mmol/L (90-115 mg/L)	
Catecholamines, urine		*Norepinephrine*	*Epinephrine*
	1 yr	29.5-86.8 nmol/day (5.4-15.9 μg/day)	0.6-25.4 nmol/day (0.1-4.3 μg/day)
	1-5 yr	44.2-168.1 nmol/day (8.1-30.8 μg/day)	4.7-53.8 nmol/day (0.8-9.1 μg/day)
	6-15 yr	103.7-388.1 nmol/day (19.0-71.1 μg/day)	7.7-62.1 nmol/day (1.3-10.5 μg/day)
	>15 yr	188.8-474.8 nmol/day (34.4-87.0 μg/day)	20.7-78.0 nmol/day (3.5-13.2 μg/day)
Chloride, urine	Infant	1.7-8.5 mmol/day (1.7-8.5 mEq/24 hr)	
	Child	17-34 mmol/day (17-34 mEq/24 hr)	
Cholesterol, serum	Cord blood	1.2-2.5 mmol/L (460-980 mg/L)	
	1-2 yr	1.8-4.9 mmol/L (700-1900 mg/L)	
	2-16 yr	3.5-6.5 mmol/L (1350-2500 mg/L)	
Cortisol (free), urine	4 mo-10 yr	5.5-74.4 nmol/day (2-27 μg/day)	
	11-20 yr	1.9-151.7 nmol/day (0.7-55 μg/day)	
Creatine kinase, serum	Newborn	3 × adult values	
	3 wk-3 mo	1.5 × adult values	
	>1 yr	At adult values	
Creatinine, serum		*Upper reference value*	
	Up to 5 yr	44 μmol/L (5.0 mg/L)	
	Up to 6 yr	53 μmol/L (6.0 mg/L)	
	Up to 7 yr	62 μmol/L (7.0 mg/L)	
	Up to 8 yr	70 μmol/L (8.0 mg/L)	
	Up to 9 yr	79 μmol/L (9.0 mg/L)	
	Up to 10 yr	88 μmol/L (10.0 mg/L)	
	>10 yr	106 μmol/L (12.0 mg/L)	
Estradiol, serum	0-2 yr	0-26 pmol/L (0-7 pg/ml)	
	2-4 yr	0.26 pmol/L (0-7 pg/ml)	
	4-6 yr	0-51 pmol/L (0-14 pg/ml)	
	6-8 yr	0-37 pmol/L (0-10 pg/ml)	
	8-10 yr	0-367 pmol/L (0-100 pg/ml)	
	10-12 yr	0-367 pmol/L (0-100 pg/ml)	
	12-14 yr	0-367 pmol/L (0-100 pg/ml)	
	14-16 yr	26-285 pmol/L (7-105 pg/ml)	
	16-25 yr	26-1175 pmol/L (7-320 pg/ml)	
Fat, fecal	Preterm newborn	Up to 40% excreted	
	Full-term newborn	Up to 20% excreted	
	3 mo-1 yr	Up to 15% excreted	
	1 yr	Up to 8.5% excreted	
Fatty acids (nonesterified), plasma	Newborn	0-1845 mmol/L	
	4 mo-10 yr	300-1100 mmol/L	
Glucose, serum	Preterm newborn	1.2-3.6 mmol/L (200-656 mg/L)	
	Full-term newborn	1.1-6.0 mmol/L (200-1100 mg/L)	
	Child	3.3-5.8 mmol/L (600-1050 mg/L)	

Substance	*Age*	*Reference range*		
γ-Glutamyltransferase, serum	Preterm newborn	56-233 U/L		
	Newborn-3 wk	10-103 U/L		
	3 wk-3 mo	4-111 U/L		
	1-5 yr	2-23 U/L		
	6-15 yr	2-23 U/L		
	16 yr-adult	2-35 U/L		
Haptoglobin, serum	Newborn	Detectable haptoglobin in only 10-20s		
	1 yr and older	At adult values		
Immunoglobulins		*IgA*	*IgG*	*IgM*
	0-5 wk	None	7500-15,000 mg/L	Less than 200 mg/L
	6 mo	200-1300 mg/L	1500-7000 mg/L	300-600 mg/L
	1 yr	200-1300 mg/L	1400-10,300 mg/L	300-1600 mg/L
	5 yr	300-2000 mg/L	3700-15,000 mg/L	200-2200 mg/L
	10 yr	500-2300 mg/L	4400-15,500 mg/L	300-1700 mg/L
Inulin clearance	<1 mo	29-88 ml/min per 1.73 m^2 of body surface		
	1-6 mo	40-112 ml/min per 1.73 m^2 of body surface		
	6-12 mo	62-121 ml/min per 1.73 m^2 of body surface		
	>1 yr	78-164 ml/min per 1.73 m^2 of body surface		
17-Ketosteroids, urine	0-3 d	0-0.5 mg/day		
	1-3 yr	<2.0 mg/day		
	3-6 yr	0.5-3.0 mg/day		
	6-9 yr	0.8-4.0 mg/day		
	10-12 yr	Male: 0.7-6.0 mg/day Female: 0.7-5.0 mg/day		
	Adolescent	Male: 3-15 mg/day Female: 3-12 mg/day		
Lactic dehydrogenase, serum	1-3 d	Up to 2 × adult values		
Phosphorus (inorganic), serum		*Preterm*	*Term*	
	Newborn	1.8-2.6 mmol/L (56.0-80.0 mg/L)	1.6-2.5 mmol/L (50.0-78.0 mg/L)	
	6-10 d	2.0-3.8 mmol/L (61-117 mg/L)	1.6-2.9 mmol/L (49-89 mg/L)	
	4 mo	1.6-2.6 mmol/L (48-81 mg/L)		
	1 yr	1.25-2.1 mmol/L (39-60 mg/L)		
	2-16 yr	0.9-1.5 mmol/L (26-50 mg/L)		
Potassium, serum	Preterm newborn	4.5-7.2 mmol/L (4.5-7.2 mEq/L)		
	Full-term newborn	5.0-7.7 mmol/L (5.0-7.7 mEq/L)		
	2 days-2 wk	4.0-6.4 mmol/L (4.0-6.4 mEq/L)		
	2 wk-3 mo	4.0-6.2 mmol/L (4.0-6.2 mEq/L)		
	3 mo-1 yr	3.7-5.6 mmol/L (3.7-5.6 mEq/L)		
	1-16 yr	3.6-5.2 mmol/L (3.6-5.2 mEq/L)		
Testosterone, serum		*Male*	*Female*	
	0-2 yr	0.1-1.3 nmol/L (40-370 ng/L)	0.2-0.6 nmol/L (70-180 ng/L)	
	2-4 yr	0.2-0.6 nmol/L (50-160 ng/L)	0.2-0.7 nmol/L (70-200 ng/L)	
	4-6 yr	0.3-1.4 nmol/L (80-400 ng/L)	0.3-0.7 nmol/L (100-200 ng/L)	
	6-8 yr	0.2-1.0 nmol/L (60-280 ng/L)	0.5-1.0 nmol/L (150-300 ng/L)	
	8-10 yr	0.3-1.7 nmol/L (90-500 ng/L)	0.7-1.4 nmol/L (200-400 ng/L)	
	10-12 yr	0.3-10.1 nmol/L (80-2900 ng/L)	0.7-1.7 nmol/L (200-500 ng/L)	
	12-14 yr	0.2-24.6 nmol/L (50-7600 ng/L)	1.0-2.4 nmol/L (300-700 ng/L)	
	14-16 yr	3.1-19.5 nmol/L (900-5600 ng/L)	1.2-3.3 nmol/L (350-950 ng/L)	
	16-18 yr	9.0-25.4 nmol/L (2600-7300 ng/L)	1.4-3.3 nmol/L (400-950 ng/L)	
	18-20 yr	13.9-25.0 nmol/L (4000-7200 ng/L)	1.4-3.3 nmol/L (400-950 ng/L)	
	20-25 yr	11.8-38.9 nmol/L (3400-11,200 ng/L)	1.4-3.3 nmol/L (400-950 ng/L)	
Thyroxine, serum	1-3 days	142-296 nmol/L (11-23 μg/dl)		
	1 wk-1 mo	116-232 nmol/L (9-18 μg/dl)		
	1-4 mo	97-212 nmol/L (7.5-16.5 μg/dl)		
	4-12 mo	71-187 nmol/L (5.5-14.5 μg/dl)		
	1-6 yr	71-174 nmol/L (5.5-13.5 μg/dl)		
	6-10 yr	64-161 nmol/L (5.0-12.5 μg/dl)		

1-3 Standard laboratory values in the neonatal period

Laboratory tests

Substance	Normal neonatal value	
Hematological values		
Clotting factors	2 min	
Activated clotting time (ACT)	2 min	
Bleeding time (Ivy)	1-8 min	
Clot retraction	Complete 1-4 hr	
Clotting time		
2 tubes	5-8 min	
3 tubes	5-15 min	
Fibrinogen	150-300 mg/dl	
Fibrinolysin (plasminogen)	Lysis of clot	
Partial thromboplastin time (PTT)	<90-120 sec	
Prothrombin time, one-stage (PT)	12-21 sec	
Thromboplastin generation test (TGT)	8-24 sec in 6 min tube	
	Term	*Preterm*
Hemoglobin	17-19 g/dl	15-17 g/dl
Hematocrit	57%-58%	45%-55%
Sedimentation rate, erythrocytes (ESR)	0-2 mm/hr	1-5 mm/hr
Reticulocytes	3-7%	Up to 10%
Fetal hemoglobin	40%-70% of total	80%-90% of total
Nucleated RBC	200/mm^3 (0.05/100 RBCs)	0.2/100 RBCs
Platelet count	100-300,000/mm^3	120-180,000/mm^3
WBCs	15,000/mm^3	10,000-20,000/mm^3
Neutrophils	45%	47%
Eosinophils and basophils	3%	
Lymphocytes	30%	33%
Monocytes	5%	4%
Immature WBCs	10%	16%
Biochemical values		
Ammonia	100-150 μg/dl	
Amylase	0-1000 IU/hr	
Antistreptolysin O titer, group B		
Normal	12-100 Todd units	
Recent streptococcal infection	200-2500 Todd units	
Bilirubin, direct	0-1 mg/dl	
Bilirubin, total		
Cord blood	<2 mg/dl	
Peripheral blood		
0-1 day	6 mg/dl	
1-2 day	8 mg/dl	
3-5 day	12 mg/dl	
Blood gases		
Arterial		
pH	7.31-7.45	
P_{CO_2}	33-48 mm Hg	
P_{O_2}	50-70 mm Hg	
Venous		
pH	7.28-7.42	
P_{CO_2}	38-52 mm Hg	
P_{O_2}	20-49 mm Hg	
Calcium, ionized	2.1-2.6 mEq/L	
Calcium, total	4-7.0 mEq/L	
Catecholamines		
Neonatal		
Nonepinephrine	2-12 μg/24 hr	
Epinephrine	1-2 μg/24 hr	

Substance	*Normal neonatal value*	
Newborn		
Nonepinephrine	2-4 μg/24 hr	
Epinephrine	0-1 μg/24 hr	
Ceruloplasmin (*p*-pheylenediamine dihydrochloride, 37 C)	1-30 mg/dl	
Chloride	95-110 mEq/L	
Cholesterol, esters	42% to 71% of total	
Cholesterol, total	45-170 mg/dl	
Copper	20-70 μg/dl	
Cortisol		
AM specimen	15-25 μg/dl	
PM specimen	5-10 μg/dl	
C-reactive protein (CRP)	0	
Creatine	0.2-1 mg/dl (higher in females)	
Creatine phosphokinase (CPK) (creatine phosphate, 30 C)	10-300 IU/L	
Creatinine	0.3-1 mg/dl	
Electrophoresis	Preterm: 4.3-7.6 g/dl	
	Newborn: 4.6-7.4 g/dl	
	Term	*Preterm*
Total protein	4.6-7.4 gm/dl	4.3-7.6 gm/dl
Albumin	3.6-5.4	3.1-4.2
α_1-Globulin	0.1-0.3	0.1-0.5
α_2-Globulin	0.2-0.5	0.3-0.7
β-Globulin	0.2-0.6	0.3-1.2
α-Globulin	0.2-1.2	0.3-1.4
Fatty acids, free	0.4-1 mg/L	
α_1-fetoprotein	0	
Fibrinogen	150-300 mg/dl	
Glucose, fasting (FBS)		
Hepatitis-associated (Australia) antigen	0	
Immunoglobulin levels, serum, newborn	660-1.439 mg/dl	
IgG	654-1.244	
IgM	5-30	
IgA	0-11	
Iodine, butanol extractable (BEI)	3-13 μg/dl	
Iodine, T_4-by-column (thyroxine)	3-12 μg/dl	
Iodine, T_4 (competitive protein-binding thyroxine)	3-12 μg/dl	
Iodine, total serum organic (PBI)	4-14 μg/dl	
Iron	100-200 μg/dl	
Iron-binding capacity (IBC)	60-175 μg/dl	
17-Ketogenic steroids (17-KGS)	2.4 mg/24 hr	
17-Ketosteroids (17-KS)	0.5-2.5 mg/24 hr	
Lactic dehydrogenase (LDH) (pyruvate, 30 C)	300-1500 IU/L	
Lipids, total	170-450 mg/dl	
Lipoproteins, newborn (mg/dl)	70-180 mg/dl	
Alpha	50-160 mg/dl	
Beta	50-110 mg/dl	
Chylo	1.4-2.9 mEg/L	
Magnesium	41-68 IU/L	
Malate dehydrogenase (MDH) (oxaloacetic acid, 37 C)	10.4-16.4 IU/L	
Phosphatase, acid	50-275 IU/L	
Phosphatase, alkaline	75-170 mg/dl	
Phospholipids	3.5-8.6 mg/dl	
Phosphorus	4-7 mg/L	
Potassium	0 mg/24 hr	
Pregnanetriol	4.3-7.6 g/dl	
Protein, total	140-160 mEq/L	
Sodium		

Continued.

Laboratory tests—cont'd

Substance	*Normal neonatal value*
Transaminases, serum	
Glutamic-oxaloacetic (SGOT) (aspartate, 30 C)	5-70 IU/L
Glutamic-pyruvic (SGPT)	5-50 IU/L
Triglycerides	5-40 mg/dl
Urea nitrogen (BUN)	5-15 mg/dl
Vanillylmandelic acid (VMA)	0-1 mg/24 hr
Urinalysis	
Volume	20-40 ml excreted daily in the first few days; by 1 wk, 24 hr volume close to 200 ml
Protein	May be present first 2-4 days
Casts and WBCs	May be present first 2-4 days
Osmolarity	100-600 mOsm/L
pH	5-7
Specific gravity	1.001-1.020
Cerebrospinal fluid	
Calcium	2-3 mg/L
Cell count	0-15 WBCs/mm^3 0-500 RBCs/mm^3
Chloride	110-120 mg/L
Color	May be xanthochromic
Glucose	24-40 mg/dl
Lactic dehydrogenase (LDH)	5-80 IU/L
Magnesium	3-3.3 mg/dl
Pándy's test (For excess globulins)	Negative
pH (at 37 C)	7.33-7.42
Pressure	50-80 mm Hg
Protein, total	20-120 mg/dl
Sodium	130-165 mg/L
Specific gravity	1.007-1.009
Transaminase, glutamic-oxaloacetic (GOT)	2-10 IU/L
Volume	5 ml

Cardiorespiratory determinations

Blood pressure at birth
- Term: systolic, 78 mm Hg; diastolic, 42 mm Hg
- Preterm: systolic, 50-60 mm Hg; diastolic, 30 mm Hg

Respiratory rate: 30-60/min

Heart rate, fetus
- Baseline: 120-160/min
  - Tachycardia: $>$160 beats/min (with maternal complication)
  - Bradycardia: $<$120 beats/min (with maternal hypotension and hypoxia)
  - Acceleration: tachycardia $>$160 beats/min with uterine contraction—normal (usually)
- Beat-to-beat variability: disappears with fetal distress
- With uterine contraction
  - Early deceleration: bradycardia with onset of contraction—benign
  - Variable deceleration: bradycardia due to cord compression—usually benign
  - Late deceleration: bradycardia after lag period caused by fetal hypoxia—ominous sign

Heart rate, term infant: 140 $\pm$ 20 beats/min

Urine screening tests for inborn errors of metabolism

Benedict's test: for reducing substances in the urine—glucose, galactose, fructose, lactose; phenylketonuria, alkaptonuria, tyrosyluria, and tyrosinosis *may* give positive Benedict's test.
Ferric chloride test: an immediate, green color for phenylketonuria, histidinemia, and tyrosinuria; a gray to green color for presence of phenothiazines, isoniazid; red to purple color for presence of salicylates or ketone bodies.
Dinitrophenylhydrazine test: for phenylketonuria, maple syrup urine disease, Lowe's syndrome.
Cetyltrimethyl ammonium bromide test: for mucopolysaccharides; immediate positive reaction in gargoylism (Hurler's syndrome); delayed, moderately positive reaction for Marfan's, Morquio-Ullrich, and Murdoch syndromes.
Metachromatic stain (of urine sediment): Granules (free or as inclusion bodies in cells) are seen in metachromatic leukodystrophy; may also be seen rarely in Tay-Sachs and other lipid diseases of the central nervous system.
Amino acid chromatography: Aminoaciduria may be normal in newborns; chromatography may be helpful to detect hypophosphatasia and argininosuccinicaciduria.

Diagnostic tests for phenylketonuria

Test	*Method*	*Use*
Urine tests		
Diaper test	10% ferric chloride dropped on freshly wet diaper; green spot (positive): probable PKU	Inexpensive; useful in screening large groups of infants but not of value until infant is at least 6 wk of age
Phenistix test	Prepared test stick pressed against wet diaper or dipped in urine; green color reaction: probable PKU	Simple; more accurate than diaper test; useful in screening large groups of infants but not of value until after infant is 6 wk of age
Dinitrophenyl-hydrazine (DNPH) test	0.5-1 ml of urine placed in test tube, equal amount of DNPH solution added; immediate pale yellow-orange color reaction: negative; gradual change to opaque bright yellow: positive, indicates probable PKU	Inexpensive; accurate but more complicated than diaper test or Phenistix; most useful in clinical setting to confirm these tests
Blood/serum phenylalanine tests		
Guthrie inhibition assay methods	Drops of blood placed on filter paper; laboratory uses bacterial growth inhibition test; phenylalanine level above 8 mg/dl blood: diagnostic of PKU	Effective in newborn period; used also to monitor PKU diet; blood easily obtained by heel or finger puncture; inexpensive; used for wide-scale screening
LaDu-Michael method	5 ml of blood; serum separated and tested for phenylalanine; level above 8 mg/dl blood: PKU; in persons with PKU, phenylalanine level above 8-12 mg/dl blood: loss of dietary control	Useful diagnostic tool and to monitor PKU diet, requires blood drawn from person; laboratory method difficult (test not available in many laboratories)
McCaman and Robins fluorometric method	5 ml of blood; serum separated and tested for phenylalanine; level above 8 mg: PKU or loss of dietary control	Diagnostic and diet monitoring tool; laboratory procedure more simple than LaDu-Michael method (test not available in many laboratories)

APPENDIX 2 UNITS OF MEASUREMENT

2-1 Conversion factors

Units	Abbreviation or symbol	Conventional units		Quantity measured
To convert from		To	Multiply by	
Ångström units	Å	Centimeters	1×10^{-8}	Length
		Inches	3.9370079×10^{-9}	
		Micrometers	0.0001	
		Nanometers	0.1	
Atmospheres, standard	atm	Bars	1.01325	Pressure
		Hg (0° C)	76	
		H_2O (4° C)	1033.26	
		Feet of H_2O (39.2° F)	33.8995	
		Grams/square centimeter	1033.23	
		Inches of Hg (32° F)	29.9213	
		Kilograms/square centimeters	1.03323	
		Millimeters of Hg (0° C)	760	
		Pounds/square inch	14.6960	
		Torrs	760	
Calories	Do not abbreviate	Joules	0.23	Energy
Centigrams	cg	Grains	0.15432358	Mass
		Grams	0.01	
Centiliters	cl	Cubic centimeters	10	Volume and capacity
		Cubic inches	0.6102545	
		Liters	0.01	
		Ounces (U.S., fluid)	0.3381497	
Centimeters	cm	Ångström units	1×10^{8}	Length
		Feet	0.032808399	
		Inches	0.39370079	
		Meters	0.01	
		Microns	10,000	
		Miles (naut., int.)	5.3995680×10^{-6}	
		Miles (statute)	6.2137119×10^{-6}	
		Millimeters	10	
		Nanometers	1×10^{7}	
		Rods	0.0019883878	
		Yards	0.010936133	
Cubic centimeters	cm^3	Cubic feet	3.5314667×10^{-5}	Volume and capacity
		Cubic inches	0.061023744	
		Cubic meters	1×10^{-6}	
		Cubic yards	1.3079506×10^{-6}	
		Drams (U.S., fluid)	0.27051218	
		Gallons (Brit.)	0.0002199694	
		Gallons (U.S., dry)	0.00022702075	
		Gallons (U.S., liq.)	0.00026417205	
		Gills (Brit.)	0.007039020	
		Gills (U.S.)	0.0084535058	
		Liters	0.001	
		Ounces (Brit., fluid)	0.03519510	
		Ounces (U.S., fluid)	0.033814023	
		Pints (U.S., dry)	0.0018161660	

Modified from Weast, R.C., editor: Handbook of chemistry and physics, ed. 54, Cleveland, Ohio, 1973, CRC Press, Inc.

Units	Abbreviation or symbol	Conventional units		Quantity measured
To convert from		To	Multiply by	
		Pints (U.S., liq.)	0.0021133764	
		Quarts (Brit.)	0.0008798775	
		Quarts (U.S., dry)	0.00090808298	
		Quarts (U.S., liq.)	0.0010566882	
Cubic decimeters	dm^3	Cubic centimeters	1000	Volume and capacity
		Cubic feet	0.035316667	
		Cubic inches	61.023744	
		Cubic meters	0.001	
		Cubic yards	0.0013079506	
		Liters	1	
Cubic dekameters	dam^3	Cubic decimeters	1×10^6	Volume and capacity
		Cubic feet	35,314.667	
		Cubic inches	6.1023744×10^7	
		Cubic meters	1000	
		Liters	1,000,000	
Cubic feet	ft^3	Cubic centimeters	28,316.847	Volume and capacity
		Cubic meters	0.028316847	
		Gallons (U.S., dry)	6.4285116	
		Gallons (U.S., liq.)	7.4805195	
		Liters	28.316847	
		Ounces (Brit., fluid)	996.6143	
		Ounces (U.S., fluid)	957.50649	
		Pints (U.S., liq.)	59.844156	
		Quarts (U.S., dry)	25.714047	
		Quarts (U.S., liq.)	29.922078	
Cubic inches	in^3	Cubic centimeters	16.387064	Volume and capacity
		Cubic feet	0.00057870370	
		Cubic meters	1.6387064×10^{-5}	
		Cubic yards	2.1433470×10^{-5}	
		Drams (U.S., fluid)	4.4329004	
		Gallons (Brit.)	0.003604652	
		Gallons (U.S., dry)	0.0037202035	
		Gallons (U.S., liq.)	0.0043290043	
		Liters	0.016387064	
		Milliliters	16.387064	
		Ounces (Brit., fluid)	0.57674444	
		Ounces (U.S., fluid)	0.55411255	
		Pints (U.S., dry)	0.029761628	
		Pints (U.S., liq.)	0.034632035	
		Quarts (U.S., dry)	0.014880814	
		Quarts (U.S., liq.)	0.017316017	
Cubic meters	m^3	Cubic centimeters	1×10^6	Volume and capacity
		Cubic feet	35.314667	
		Cubic inches	61,023.74	
		Cubic yards	1.3079506	
		Gallons (Brit.)	219.9694	
		Gallons (U.S., liq.)	264.17205	
		Liters	1000	
		Pints (U.S., liq.)	2113.3764	
		Quarts (U.S., liq.)	1056.6882	
Cubic millimeters	mm^3	Cubic centimeters	0.001	Volume and capacity
		Cubic inches	6.1023744×10^{-5}	
		Cubic meters	1×10^{-9}	
		Minims (Brit.)	0.01689365	
		Minims (U.S.)	0.016230731	
Deciliters	dl	Milliliters	100	Volume and capacity
		Cubic centimeters	100	
Decimeters	dm	Centimeters	10	Length
		Feet	0.32808399	
		Inches	3.9370079	
		Meters	0.1	

Continued.

Conversion factors—cont'd

Units	*Abbreviation or symbol*	*Conventional units*		*Quantity measured*
To convert from		*To*	*Multiply by*	
Degrees Celsius	°C	Degrees Fahrenheit	9/5 (then add 32)	Temperature
Degrees Fahrenheit	°F	Degrees Celsius	5/9 (after subtracting 32)	Temperature
Dekaliters	dkl, dal	Pecks (U.S.)	1.135136	Volume and capacity
		Pints (U.S., dry)	18.16217	
Dekameters	dkm, dam	Centimeters	1000	Length
		Feet	32.808399	
		Inches	393.70079	
		Kilometers	0.01	
		Meters	10	
		Yards	10.93613	
Drams (apoth. or troy)	dr ap, ʒ	Drams (avdp.)	2.1942857	Mass
		Grains	60	
		Grams	3.8879346	
		Ounces (apoth. or troy)	0.125	
		Ounces (avdp.)	0.13714286	
		Scruples (apoth.)	3	
Drams (avdp.)	dr avdp	Drams (apoth. or troy)	0.455729166	Mass
		Grains	27.34375	
		Grams	1.7718452	
		Ounces (apoth. or troy)	0.056966146	
		Ounces (avdp.)	0.0625	
		Pennyweights	1.1393229	
		Pounds (apoth. or troy)	0.0047471788	
		Pounds (avdp.)	0.00390625	
		Scruples (apoth.)	1.3671875	
Drams (U.S., fluid)	fl dr	Cubic centimeters	3.6967162	Volume and capacity
		Cubic inches	0.22558594	
		Gills (U.S.)	0.03125	
		Milliliters	3.696588	
		Minims (U.S.)	60	
		Ounces (U.S., fluid)	0.125	
		Pints (U.S., liq.)	0.0078125	
Feet	ft	Centimeters	30.48	Length
		Inches	12	
		Meters	0.3048	
		Microns	304,800	
		Miles (naut., int.)	0.00016457883	
		Miles (statute)	0.000189393	
		Rods	0.060606	
		Yards	0.333333	
Gallons (Brit.)	gal	Barrels (Brit.)	0.027777	Volume and capacity
		Cubic centimeters	4546.087	
		Cubic feet	0.1605436	
		Cubic inches	277.4193	
		Firkins (Brit.)	0.111111	
		Gallons (U.S., liq.)	1.200949	
		Gills (Brit.)	32	
		Liters	4.545960	
		Minims (Brit.)	76,800	
		Ounces (Brit., fluid)	160	
		Ounces (U.S., fluid)	153.7215	
		Pecks (Brit.)	0.5	
		Pounds of H_2O (62° F)	10	
Gallons (U.S., dry)		Barrels (U.S., dry)	0.038095592	Volume and capacity
		Barrels (U.S., liq.)	0.036941181	
		Cubic centimeters	4404.8828	
		Cubic feet	0.15555700	
		Cubic inches	268.8025	
		Gallons (U.S., liq.)	1.16364719	
		Liters	4.404760	

Units	Abbreviation or symbol	*Conventional units*		Quantity measured
To convert from		*To*	*Multiply by*	
Gallons (U.S., liq.)	gal	Barrels (U.S., liq.)	0.031746032	Volume and capacity
		Cubic centimeters	3785.4118	
		Cubic feet	0.13368055	
		Cubic inches	231	Volume and capacity
		Cubic meters	0.0037854118	
		Cubic yards	0.0049511317	
		Gallons (Brit.)	0.8326747	
		Gallons (U.S., dry)	0.85936701	
		Gallons (wine)	1	
		Gills (U.S.)	32	
		Liters	3.7854118	
		Minims (U.S.)	61,440	
		Ounces (U.S. fluid)	128	
		Pints (U.S. liq.)	8	
		Quarts (U.S. liq.)	4	
Gills (Brit.)		Cubic centimeters	142.0652	Volume and capacity
		Gallons (Brit.)	0.03125	
		Gills (U.S.)	1.200949	
		Liters	0.1420613	
		Ounces (Brit., fluid)	5	
		Ounces (U.S., fluid)	4.803764	
		Pints (Brit.)	0.25	
Gills (U.S.)		Cubic centimeters	118.29412	Volume and capacity
		Cubic inches	7.21875	
		Drams (U.S., fluid)	32	
		Gallons (U.S., liq.)	0.03125	
		Gills (Brit.)	0.8326747	
		Liters	0.1182908	
		Minims (U.S.)	1920	
		Ounces (U.S., fluid)	4	
		Pints (U.S., liq.)	0.25	
		Quarts (U.S., liq.)	0.125	
Grains	gr	Carats (metric)	0.32399455	Mass
		Drams (apoth. or troy)	0.016666	
		Drams (avdp.)	0.036571429	
		Dynes	63.5460	
		Grams	0.06479891	
		Milligrams	64.79891	
		Ounces (apoth. or troy)	0.0020833	
		Ounces (avdp.)	0.002857143	
		Pennyweights	0.041666	
		Pounds (apoth. or troy)	0.000173611	
		Pounds (avdp.)	0.00014285714	
		Scruples (apoth.)	0.05	
Grams	g	Carats (metric)	5	Mass
		Decigrams	10	
		Dekagrams	0.1	
		Drams (apoth. or troy)	0.25720597	
		Drams (avdp.)	0.56438339	
		Grains	15.432358	
		Kilograms	0.001	
		Micrograms	1×10^6	
		Myriagrams	0.0001	
		Ounces (apoth. or troy)	0.32150737	
		Ounces (avdp.)	0.35273962	
		Pennyweights	0.64301493	
		Poundals	0.0709316	
		Pounds (apoth. or troy)	0.0026792289	
		Pounds (avdp.)	0.0022046226	
		Scruples (apoth.)	0.77161792	
		Tons (metric)	1×10^{-6}	
Hands		Centimeters	10.16	Length
		Inches	4	

Continued.

Conversion factors—cont'd

Units: To convert from	Abbreviation or symbol	Conventional units: To	Conventional units: Multiply by	Quantity measured
Hectograms	hg	Grams	100	Mass
		Poundals	7.09316	
		Pounds (apoth. or troy)	0.26792289	
		Pounds (avdp.)	0.22046226	
Hectoliters	hl	Bushels (Brit.)	2.749694	Volume and capacity
		Cubic centimeters	1.00028×10^5	
		Cubic feet	3.531566	
		Gallons (U.S., liq.)	26.41794	
		Liters	100	
		Ounces (U.S., fluid)	3381.497	
		Pecks (U.S.)	11.35136	
Hectometers	hm	Centimeters	10,000	Length
		Decimeters	1000	
		Dekameters	10	
		Feet	328.08399	
		Meters	100	
		Rods	19.883878	
		Yards	109.3613	
Inches	in	Angström units	2.54×10^8	Length
		Centimeters	2.54	
		Cubits	0.055555	
		Fathoms	0.013888	
		Feet	0.083333	
		Meters	0.0254	
		Mils	1000	
		Yards	0.027777	
Inches of Hg (32° F)		Atmospheres	0.034211	Pressure
		Bars	0.0338639	
		Feet of air (1 atm, 60° F)	926.24	
		Feet of H_2O (39.2° F)	1.132957	
		Grams/square centimeter	34.5316	
		Kilograms/square meter	345.316	
		Millimeters of Hg (60° C)	25.4	
		Ounces/square inch	7.85847	
		Pounds/square foot	70.7262	
Joules	J	Calories	4.184	Energy
Kilograms	kg	Drams (apoth. or troy)	257.20597	Mass
		Drams (avdp.)	564.38339	
		Grains	15,432.358	
		Hundredweights (long)	0.019684131	
		Hundredweights (short)	0.022046226	
		Ounces (apoth. or troy)	32.150737	
		Ounces (avdp.)	35.273962	
		Pennyweights	643.01493	
		Poundals	70.931635	
		Pounds (apoth. or troy)	2.6792289	
		Pounds (avdp.)	2.2046226	
		Scruples (apoth.)	771.61792	
		Tons (long)	0.00098420653	
		Tons (metric)	0.001	
		Tons (short)	0.0011023113	
Kiloliters	kl	Cubic centimeters	1×10^6	Volume and capacity
		Cubic feet	35.31566	
		Cubic inches	61,025.45	
		Cubic meters	1.000028	
		Cubic yards	1.307987	
		Gallons (Brit.)	219.9755	
		Gallons (U.S., dry)	227.0271	
		Gallons (U.S., liq.)	264.1794	
		Liters	1000	

Units		*Conventional units*		
To convert from	*Abbreviation or symbol*	*To*	*Multiply by*	*Quantity measured*
Kilometers	km	Centimeters	100,000	Length
		Feet	3280.8399	
		Light years	1.05702×10^{-13}	
		Meters	1000	
		Miles (naut., int.)	0.53995680	
		Miles (statute)	0.62137119	
		Rods	198.83878	
		Yards	1093.6133	
Liters	L*	Bushels (Brit.)	0.02749694	Volume and capacity
		Bushels (U.S.)	0.02837839	
		Cu centimeters	1000	
		Cubic feet	0.03531566	
		Cubic inches	61.02545	
		Cubic meters	0.001	
		Cubic yards	0.001307987	
		Drams (U.S., fluid)	270.5198	
		Gallons (Brit.)	0.2199755	
		Gallons (U.S., dry)	0.2270271	
		Gallons (U.S., liq.)	0.2641794	
		Gills (Brit.)	7.039217	
		Gills (U.S.)	8.453742	
		Minims (U.S.)	16,231.19	
		Ounces (Brit., fluid)	35.19609	
		Ounces (U.S., fluid)	33.81497	
		Pints (Brit.)	1.759804	
		Pints (U.S., dry)	1.816217	
		Pints (U.S., liq.)	2.113436	
		Quarts, (Brit.)	0.8799021	
		Quarts (U.S., dry)	0.9081084	
		Quarts (U.S., liq.)	1.056718	
Meters	m	Ångström units	1×10^{10}	Length
		Centimeters	100	
		Feet	3.2808399	
		Inches	39.370079	
		Kilometers	0.001	
		Megameters	1×10	
		Miles (naut., Brit.)	0.00053961182	
		Miles (naut., int.)	0.00053995680	
		Miles (statute)	0.00062137119	
		Millimeters	1000	
		Nanometers	1×10^{9}	
		Mils	39,370.079	
		Rods	0.19883878	
		Yards	1.0936133	
Meters of Hg (0° C)		Atmospheres	1.3157895	Pressure
		Feet of H_2O (60° F)	44.6474	
		Inches of Hg (32° F)	39.370079	
		Kilograms/square centimeters	1.35951	
		Pounds/square inch	19.3368	
Micrograms	μg	Grams	1×10^{-6}	Mass
		Milligrams	0.001	
Micrometers	μm	Ångström units	10,000	Length
		Centimeters	0.0001	
		Feet	3.2808399×10^{-6}	
		Inches	3.9370079×10^{-5}	
		Meters	1×10^{-6}	
		Millimeters	0.001	
		Nanometers	1000	

*It is recommended in the United States that the capital ''L'' be the accepted symbol for liter since most typefaces gives insufficient distinction between ''l'' and the numeral one ''1.''

Continued.

Conversion factors—cont'd

Units	Abbreviation or symbol	Conventional units		Quantity measured
To convert from		To	Multiply by	
Miles (statute)		Centimeters	160,934.4	Length
		Feet	5280	
		Inches	63,360	
		Kilometers	1.609344	
		Meters	1609.344	
		Rods	320	
		Yards	1760	
Milligrams	mg	Carats (1877)	0.004871	Mass
		Carats (metric)	0.005	
		Drams (apoth. or troy)	0.00025720597	
		Drams (advp.)	0.00056438339	
Milliliters	ml	Cubic centimeters	1	Volume and capacity
		Cubic inches	0.06102545	
		Drams (U.S., fluid)	0.2705198	
		Gills (U.S.)	0.008453742	
		Liters	0.001	
		Minims (U.S.)	16.23119	
		Ounces (Brit., fluid)	0.03519609	
		Ounces (U.S., fluid)	0.3381497	
		Pints (Brit.)	0.001759804	
		Pints (U.S., liq.)	0.002113436	
Millimeters	mm	Ångström units	1×10^{7}	
		Centimeters	0.1	
		Decimeters	0.01	
		Dekameters	0.001	
		Feet	0.0032808399	
		Inches	0.039370079	
		Meters	0.001	
		Micrometers	1000	
		Mils	39.370079	
Millimeters of Hg (0° C)	mm Hg	Atmospheres	0.0013157895	Pressure
		Bars	0.00133322	
		Dynes/square centimeter	1333.224	
		Grams/square centimeter	1.35951	
		Kilograms/square meter	13.5951	
		Pounds/square foot	2.78450	
		Pounds/square inch	0.0193368	
		Torrs	1	
Minims (Brit.)	min, ♏	Cubic centimeter	0.05919385	Volume and capacity
		Cubic inches	0.003612230	
		Milliliters	0.05919219	
		Ounces (Brit., fluid)	0.0020833333	
		Scruples (Brit., fluid)	0.05	
Minims (U.S.)	min, ♏	Cubic centimeters	0.061611520	Volume and capacity
		Cubic inches	0.0037597656	
		Drams (U.S., fluid)	0.0166666	
		Gallons (U.S., liq.)	1.6276042×10^{-5}	
		Gills (U.S.)	0.0005208333	
		Liters	6.160979×10^{-5}	
		Milliliters	0.06160979	
		Ounces (U.S., fluid)	0.002083333	
		Pints (U.S., liq.)	0.0001302083	
Nanometer	nm	Ångström units	10	Length
		Centimeters	1×10^{-7}	
		Inches	3.9370079×10^{-8}	
		Micrometers	0.001	
		Millimeters	1×10^{-6}	
Ounces (apoth. or troy)	oz, ℥	Dekagrams	1.7554286	Mass
		Drams (apoth. or troy)	8	
		Drams (avdp.)	17.554286	
		Grains	480	
		Grams	31.103486	

Units	*Abbreviation or symbol*	*Conventional units*		*Quantity measured*
To convert from		*To*	*Multiply by*	
		Milligrams	31,103.486	
		Ounces (avdp.)	1.0971429	
		Pennyweights	20	
		Pounds (apoth. or troy)	0.0833333	
		Pounds (avdp.)	0.068571429	
		Scruples (apoth.)	24	
Ounces (avdp.)	oz	Drams (apoth. or troy)	7.291666	Mass
		Drams (avdp.)	16	
		Grains	437.5	
		Grams	28.349523	
		Hundredweights (long)	0.00055803571	
		Hundredweights (short)	0.000625	
		Ounces (apoth. or troy)	0.9114583	
		Pennyweights	18.229166	
		Pounds (apoth. or troy)	0.075954861	
		Pounds (avdp.)	0.0625	
		Scuples (apoth.)	21.875	
Ounces (Brit., fluid)	oz	Cubic centimeters	28.41305	Volume and capacity
		Cubic inches	1.733870	
		Drachms (Brit., fluid)	8	
		Drams (U.S., fluid)	7.686075	
		Gallons (Brit.)	0.00625	
		Milliliters	28.41225	
		Minims (Brit.)	480	
		Ounces (U.S., fluid)	0.9607594	
Ounces (U.S., fluid)	oz	Cubic centimeters	29.573730	Volume and capacity
		Cubic inches	1.8046875	
		Cubic meters	2.9573730×10^{-5}	
		Drams (U.S., fluid)	8	
		Gallons (U.S., dry)	0.0067138047	
		Gallons (U.S., liq.)	0.0078125	
		Gills (U.S.)	0.25	
		Liters	0.029572702	
		Minims (U.S.)	480	
		Ounces (Brit., fluid)	1.040843	
		Pints (U.S., liq.)	0.0625	
		Quarts (U.S., liq.)	0.03125	
Parts per million*	ppm	Grains/gallon (Brit.)	0.07015488	Substance concentration
		Grains/gallon (U.S.)	0.058411620	
		Grams/liter	0.001	
		Milligrams/liter	1	
Pennyweights	dwt	Drams (apoth. or troy)	0.4	Mass
		Drams (avdp.)	0.87771429	
		Grains	24	
		Grams	1.55517384	
		Ounces (apoth. or troy)	0.05	
		Ounces (avdp.)	0.054857143	
		Pounds (apoth. or troy)	0.0041666	
		Pounds (avdp.)	0.0034285714	
Pints (Brit.)	pt	Cubic centimeter	568.26092	Volume and capacity
		Gallons (Brit.)	0.125	
		Gills (Brit.)	4	
		Gills (U.S.)	4.803797	
		Liters	0.5682450	
		Minims (Brit.)	9600	
		Ounces (Brit., fluid)	20	
		Pints (U.S., dry)	1.032056	
		Pints (U.S., Liq.)	1.200949	
		Quarts (Brit.)	0.5	
		Scruples (Brit., fluid)	480	

*Based on density of 1 g/ml for the solvent.

Continued.

Conversion factors—cont'd

Units	Abbreviation or symbol	Conventional units		Quantity measured
To convert from		To	Multiply by	
Pints (U.S., dry)	pt	Cubic centimeters	550.61047	Volume and capacity
		Cubic inches	33.6003125	
		Gallons (U.S., dry)	0.125	
		Gallons (U.S., liq.)	0.14545590	
		Liters	0.5505951	
		Quarts (U.S., dry)	0.5	
Pints (U.S., liq.)	pt	Cubic centimeters	473.17647	Volume and capacity
		Cubic feet	0.016710069	
		Cubic inches	28.875	
		Cubic yards	0.00061889146	
		Drams (U.S., fluid)	128	
		Gallons (U.S., liq.)	0.125	
		Gills (U.S.)	4	
		Liters	0.4731632	
		Milliliters	473.1632	
		Minims (U.S.)	7680	
		Ounces (U.S., fluid)	16	
		Pints (Brit.)	0.8326747	
		Quarts (U.S., liq.)	0.5	
Poundals		Dynes	13,825.50	Mass
		Grams	14.09808	
		Pounds (avdp.)	0.310810	
Pounds (apoth. or troy)	lb ap	Drams (apoth. or troy)	96	Mass
		Drams (avdp.)	210.65143	
		Grains	5760	
		Grams	373.24172	
		Kilograms	0.37324172	
		Ounces (apoth. or troy)	12	
		Ounces (avdp.)	13.165714	
		Pennyweights	240	
		Pounds (avdp.)	0.8228571	
		Scruples (apoth.)	288	
		Tons (long)	0.00036734694	
		Tons (metric)	0.00037324172	
		Tons (short)	0.00041142857	
Pounds (avdp.)	lb avdp.	Drams (apoth. or troy)	116.6666	Mass
		Drams (avdp.)	256	
		Grains	7000	
		Grams	453.59237	
		Kilograms	0.45359237	
		Ounces (apoth. or troy)	14.583333	
		Ounces (avdp.)	16	
		Pennyweights	291.6666	
		Poundals	32.1740	
		Pounds (apoth. or troy)	1.215277	
		Scruples (apoth.)	350	
		Slugs	0.0310810	
		Tons (long)	0.00044642857	
		Tons (metric)	0.00045359237	
		Tons (short)	0.0005	
Quarts (Brit.)	qt	Cubic centimeters	1136.522	Volume and capacity
		Cubic inches	69.35482	
		Gallons (Brit.)	0.25	
		Gallons (U.S., liq.)	0.3002373	
		Liters	1.136490	
		Quarts (U.S., dry)	1.032056	
		Quarts (U.S., liq.)	1.200949	
Quarts (U.S., dry)	qt	Bushels (U.S.)	0.03125	Volume and capacity
		Cubic centimeters	1101.2209	
		Cubic feet	0.038889251	
		Cubic inches	67.200625	

Units	*Abbreviation or symbol*	*Conventional units*		*Quantity measured*
To convert from		*To*	*Multiply by*	
		Gallons (U.S., dry)	0.25	
		Gallons (U.S., liq.)	0.29091180	
		Liters	1.1011901	
		Pints (U.S., dry)	2	
Quarts (U.S., liq.)	qt	Cubic Centimeters	946.35295	Volume and capacity
		Cubic feet	0.033420136	
		Cubic inches	57.75	
		Drams (U.S., fluid)	256	
		Gallons (U.S., dry)	0.21484175	
		Gallons (U.S., liq.)	0.25	
		Gills (U.S.)	8	
		Liters	0.9463264	
		Ounces (U.S., fluid)	32	
		Pints (U.S., liq.)	2	
		Quarts (Brit.)	0.8326747	
		Quarts (U.S., dry)	0.8593670	
Quintals (metric)		Grams	100,000	Mass
		Hundredweights (long)	1.9684131	
		Kilograms	100	
		Pounds (avdp.)	220.46226	
Scruples (apoth.)	s apoth	Drams (apoth. or troy)	0.333333	Mass
		Drams (avdp.)	0.73142857	
		Grains	20	
		Grams	1.2959782	
		Ounces (apoth. or troy)	0.041666	
		Ounces (avdp.)	0.045714286	
		Pennyweights	0.833333	
		Pounds (apoth. or troy)	0.003472222	
		Pounds (avdp.)	0.0028571429	
Scruples (Brit., fluid)		Minims (Brit.)	20	Volume and capacity
Square feet	ft^2	Square centimeters	929.0304	
		Square inches	144	
		Square meters	0.09290304	
		Square miles	3.5870064×10^{-8}	
		Square rods	0.0036730946	
		Square yards	0.111111	
Square inches	in^2	Circular mils	1,273,239.5	Surface area
		Square centimeters	6.4516	
		Square decimeters	0.064516	
		Square feet	0.0069444	
		Square meters	0.00064516	
		Square miles	$2.4909767 \times 10^{-10}$	
		Square millimeters	645.16	
		Square mils	1×10^{6}	
Square kilometers	km^2	Square feet	1.0763910×10^{7}	Surface area
		Square inches	1.5500031×10^{9}	
		Square meters	1×10^{6}	
		Square miles	0.38610216	
Square meters	m^2	Square centimeters	10,000	Surface area
		Square feet	10.763910	
		Square inches	1550.0031	
		Square kilometers	1×10^{-6}	
		Square miles	3.8610216×10^{-7}	
		Square rods	0.039536861	
Square miles	mi^2	Square feet	2.7878288×10^{7}	Surface area
		Square kilometers	2.5899881	
		Square meters	2589988.1	
		Square rods	102,400	
		Square yards	3.0976×10^{6}	

Continued.

Conversion factor—cont'd

Units		*Conventional units*		
To convert from	*Abbreviation or symbol*	*To*	*Multiply by*	*Quantity measured*
Square millimeters	mm^2	Square centimeters	0.01	Surface area
		Square inches	0.0015500031	
		Square meters	1×10^{-6}	
Suqare yards	yd^2	Square centimeters	8361.2736	Surface area
		Square feet	9	
		Square feet (U.S. survey)	8.9999640	
		Square inches	1296	
		Square meters	0.83612736	
		Square miles	$3.228305785 \times 10^{-7}$	
		Square rods	0.033057851	
Tons (long)		Kilograms	1016.0469	Mass
		Ounces (avdp.)	35,840	
		Pounds (apoth. or troy)	2722.22	
		Pounds (avdp.)	2240	
		Tons (metric)	1.0160469	
		Tons (short)	1.12	
Tons (metric)	t	Grams	1×10^6	Mass
		Hundredweights (short)	22.046226	
		Kilograms	1000	
		Ounces (avdp.)	35,273.962	
		Pounds (apoth. or troy)	2679.2289	
		Pounds (avdp.)	2204.6226	
		Tons (long)	0.98420653	
		Tons (short)	1.1023113	
Tons (short)	sh tn	Hundredweights (short)	20	Mass
		Kilograms	907.18474	
		Ounces (avdp.)	32,000	
		Pounds (apoth. or troy)	2430.555	
		Pounds (avdp.)	2000	
		Tons (long)	0.89285714	
		Tons (metric)	0.90718474	
Yards	yd	Centimeters	91.44	Length
		Chains (Gunter's)	0.454545454	
		Chains (Ramden's)	0.03	
		Cubits	2	
		Fathoms	0.5	
		Feet	3	
		Feet (U.S. survey)	2.9999940	
		Inches	36	
		Meters	0.9144	
		Quarters (Brit., linear)	4	
Years (calendar)	a	Days (mean solar)	365	Time
		Hours (mean solar)	8760	
		Minutes (mean solar)	525,600	
		Months (lunar)	12.360065	
		Months (mean calendar)	12	
		Seconds (mean solar)	3.1536×10^7	
		Weeks (mean calendar)	52.142857	
		Years (sidereal)	0.99929814	
		Years (tropical)	0.99933690	

2-2 Conversions between conventional and SI units

	Conventional units	*x*	*Factor*	=	*SI units*
Gram	g/ml		$\frac{10^{15}}{\text{mw}}$		pmol/L
	g/100 ml		10		g/L
	g/100 ml		$\frac{10}{\text{mw}}$		mol/L
	g/100 ml		$\frac{10^{4}}{\text{mw}}$		mmol/L
	g/d		$\frac{1}{\text{mw}}$		mol/d
	g/d		$\frac{10^{3}}{\text{mw}}$		mmol/d
	g/d		$\frac{10^{9}}{\text{mw}}$		nmol/d
Microgram	μg/100 ml		$\frac{10}{\text{mw}}$		μmol/L
	μg/d		$\frac{1}{\text{mw}}$		μmol/d
	μg/d		$\frac{10^{3}}{\text{mw}}$		nmol/d
Micromicrogram	μμg		$\frac{10^{3}}{\text{mw}}$		fmol
	μμg/ml		$\frac{10^{3}}{\text{mw}}$		pmol/L
Milliequivalent	mEq/L		$\frac{1}{\text{valence}}$		mmol/L
	mEq/kg		$\frac{1}{\text{valence}}$		mmol/kg
	mEq/d		$\frac{1}{\text{valence}}$		mmol/d
Milligram	mg/100 ml		10^{-2}		g/L
	mg/100 ml		$\frac{10^{-2}}{\text{mw}}$		mol/L
	mg/100 ml		$\frac{10}{\text{mw}}$		mmol/L
	mg/100 ml		$\frac{10^{4}}{\text{mw}}$		μmol/L
	mg/100 g		10		mg/kg
	mg/100 g		$\frac{10}{\text{mw}}$		mmol/kg
	mg/d		$\frac{1}{\text{mw}}$		mmol/d
	mg/d		$\frac{10^{3}}{\text{mw}}$		μmol/d
Milliliter	ml/100 g		10		ml/kg
	ml/min		1.667×10^{-2}		ml/s
Millimeters of mercury	mm Hg		1.333		mbar
	mm Hg		0.133		kPa

Continued.

Conversions between conventional and SI units—cont'd

	Conventional units	*x*	*Factor*	=	*SI units*
Minute	min		60		s
	min		0.06		ks
Percent	%		10^{-2}		1 (unity)
	% (g/100 gm)		10		g/kg
	% (g/100 gm)		10^{-2}		kg/kg
	% (g/100 ml)		10		g/L
	% (g/100 ml)		$\frac{10}{\text{mw}}$		mol/L
	% (g/100 ml)		$\frac{10^4}{\text{mw}}$		mmol/L
	% (ml/100 ml)		10^{-2}		L/L

2-3 Temperature

To *convert Centigrade or Celsius degrees to Fahrenheit degrees:* multiply the number of Centigrade degrees by $9/5$ and add 32 to the result. *To convert Fahrenheit degrees to Centigrade degrees:* Subtract 32 from the number of Fahrenheit degrees and multiply the difference by $5/9$.

Fahrenheit and Celsius equivalents: body temperature range

F°	*C°*	*F°*	*C°*	*F°*	*C°*	*F°*	*C°*	*F°*	*C°*
94.0	34.44	97.0	36.11	100.0	37.78	103.0	39.44	106.0	41.11
94.2	34.56	97.2	36.22	100.2	37.89	103.2	39.56	106.2	41.22
94.4	34.67	97.4	36.33	100.4	38.00	103.4	39.67	106.4	41.33
94.6	34.78	97.6	36.44	100.6	38.11	103.6	39.78	106.6	41.44
94.8	34.89	97.8	36.56	100.8	38.22	103.8	39.89	106.8	41.56
95.0	35.00	98.0	36.67	101.0	38.33	104.0	40.00	107.0	41.67
95.2	35.11	98.2	36.78	101.2	38.44	104.2	40.11	107.2	41.78
95.4	35.22	98.4	36.89	101.4	38.56	104.4	40.22	107.4	41.89
95.6	35.33	98.6	37.00	101.6	38.67	104.6	40.33	107.6	42.00
95.8	35.44	98.8	37.11	101.8	38.78	104.8	40.44	107.8	42.11
96.0	35.56	99.0	37.22	102.0	38.89	105.0	40.56	108.0	42.22
96.2	35.67	99.2	37.33	102.2	39.00	105.2	40.67		
96.4	35.78	99.4	37.44	102.4	39.11	105.4	40.78		
96.6	35.89	99.6	37.56	102.6	39.22	105.6	40.89		
96.8	36.00	99.8	37.67	102.8	39.33	105.8	41.00		

Fahrenheit and Celsius equivalents

F°	C°	F°	C°	F°	C°	F°	C°	F°	C°
−40	−40.0	11	−11.67	62	16.67	113	45.0	164	73.33
−39	−39.44	12	−11.11	63	17.22	114	45.56	165	73.89
−38	−38.89	13	−10.56	64	17.78	115	46.11	166	74.44
−37	−38.33	14	−10.0	65	18.33	116	46.67	167	75.0
−36	−37.78	15	−9.44	66	18.89	117	47.22	168	75.56
−35	−37.22	16	−8.89	67	19.44	118	47.78	169	76.11
−34	−36.67	17	−8.33	68	20.0	119	48.33	170	76.67
−33	−36.11	18	−7.78	69	20.56	120	48.89	171	77.22
−32	−35.56	19	−7.22	70	21.11	121	49.44	172	77.78
−31	−35.0	20	−6.67	71	21.67	122	50.0	173	78.33
−30	−34.44	21	−6.11	72	22.22	123	50.56	174	78.89
−29	−33.89	22	−5.56	73	22.78	124	51.11	175	79.44
−28	−33.33	23	−5.0	74	23.33	125	51.67	176	80.0
−27	−32.78	24	−4.44	75	23.89	126	52.22	177	80.56
−26	−32.22	25	−3.89	76	24.44	127	52.78	178	81.11
−25	−31.67	26	−3.33	77	25.0	128	53.33	179	81.67
−24	−31.11	27	−2.78	78	25.56	129	53.89	180	82.22
−23	−30.56	28	−2.22	79	26.11	130	54.44	181	82.78
−22	−30.0	29	−1.67	80	26.67	131	55.0	182	83.33
−21	−29.44	30	−1.11	81	27.22	132	55.56	183	83.89
−20	−28.89	31	−0.56	82	27.78	133	56.11	184	84.44
−19	−28.33	32	0.0	83	28.33	134	56.67	185	85.0
−18	−27.78	33	0.56	84	28.89	135	57.22	186	85.56
−17	−27.22	34	1.11	85	29.44	136	57.78	187	86.11
−16	−26.67	35	1.67	86	30.0	137	58.33	188	86.67
−15	−26.11	36	2.22	87	30.56	138	58.89	189	87.22
−14	−25.56	37	2.78	88	31.11	139	59.44	190	87.78
−13	−25.0	38	3.33	89	31.67	140	60.0	191	88.33
−12	−24.44	39	3.89	90	32.22	141	60.56	192	88.89
−11	−23.89	40	4.44	91	32.78	142	61.11	193	89.44
−10	−23.33	41	5.0	92	33.33	143	61.67	194	90.0
−9	−22.78	42	5.56	93	33.89	144	62.22	195	90.56
−8	−22.22	43	6.11	94	34.44	145	62.78	196	91.11
−7	−21.67	44	6.67	95	35.0	146	63.33	197	91.67
−6	−21.11	45	7.22	96	35.56	147	63.89	198	92.22
−5	−20.56	46	7.78	97	36.11	148	64.44	199	92.78
−4	−20.0	47	8.33	98	36.67	149	65.0	200	93.33
−3	−19.44	48	8.89	99	37.22	150	65.56	201	93.89
−2	−18.89	49	9.44	100	37.78	151	66.11	202	94.44
−1	−18.33	50	10.0	101	38.33	152	66.67	203	95.0
0	−17.78	51	10.56	102	38.89	153	67.22	204	95.56
1	−17.22	52	11.11	103	39.44	154	67.78	205	96.11
2	−16.67	53	11.67	104	40.0	155	68.33	206	96.67
3	−16.11	54	12.22	105	40.56	156	68.89	207	97.22
4	−15.56	55	12.78	106	41.11	157	69.44	208	97.78
5	−15.0	56	13.33	107	41.67	158	70.0	209	98.33
6	−14.44	57	13.89	108	42.22	159	70.56	210	98.89
7	−13.89	58	14.44	109	42.78	160	71.11	211	99.44
8	−13.33	59	15.0	110	43.33	161	71.67	212	100.0
9	−12.78	60	15.56	111	43.89	162	72.22		
10	−12.22	61	16.11	112	44.44	163	72.78		

2-4 Height and weight tables for children

Desirable weights (pounds) for persons 5 to 19 years old

Boys

Height (in)	*5 yr*	*6 yr*	*7 yr*	*8 yr*	*9 yr*	*10 yr*	*11 yr*	*12 yr*	*13 yr*	*14 yr*	*15 yr*	*16 yr*	*17 yr*	*18 yr*	*19 yr*
38	34	34													
39	35	35													
40	36	36													
41	38	38	38												
42	39	39	39	39											
43	41	41	41	41											
44	44	44	44	44											
45	46	46	46	46	46										
46	47	48	48	48	48										
47	49	50	50	50	50	50									
48		52	53	53	53	53									
49		55	55	55	55	55	55								
50		57	58	58	58	58	58	58							
51			61	61	61	61	61	61	61						
52			63	64	64	64	64	64	64						
53			66	67	67	67	67	68	68						
54				70	70	70	70	71	71	72					
55				72	72	73	73	74	74	74					
56				75	76	77	77	77	78	78	80				
57					79	80	81	81	82	83	83				
58					83	84	84	85	85	86	87				
59						87	88	89	89	90	90	90			
60						91	92	92	93	94	95	96			
61							95	96	97	99	100	103	106		
62							100	101	102	103	104	107	111	116	
63							105	106	107	108	110	113	118	123	127
64								109	111	113	115	117	121	126	130
65								114	117	118	120	122	127	131	134
66									119	122	125	128	132	136	139
67									124	128	130	134	136	139	142
68										134	134	137	141	143	147
69										137	139	143	146	149	152
70										143	144	145	148	151	155
71										148	150	151	152	154	159
72											153	155	156	158	163
73											157	160	162	164	167
74											160	164	168	170	171

Prepared by Bird T. Baldwin, Ph.D., and Thomas D. Wood, M.D. Published originally by American Child Health Association.

Girls

Height (in)	*5 yr*	*6 yr*	*7 yr*	*8 yr*	*9 yr*	*10 yr*	*11 yr*	*12 yr*	*13 yr*	*14 yr*	*15 yr*	*16 yr*	*17 yr*	*18 yr*
38	33	33												
39	34	34												
40	36	36	36											
41	37	37	37											
42	39	39	39											
43	41	41	41	41										
44	42	42	42	42										
45	45	45	45	45	45									
46	47	47	47	48	48									
47	49	50	50	50	50	50								
48		52	52	52	52	53	53							
49			54	55	55	56	56							
50			56	57	58	59	61	62						
51			59	60	61	61	63	65						
52			63	64	64	64	65	67						
53			66	67	67	68	68	69	71					
54				69	70	70	71	71	73					
55				72	74	74	74	75	77	78				
56					76	78	78	79	81	83				
57					80	82	82	82	84	88	92			
58						84	86	86	88	93	96	101		
59						87	90	90	92	96	100	103	104	
60						91	95	95	97	101	105	108	109	111
61							99	100	101	105	108	112	113	116
62							104	105	106	109	113	115	117	118
63								110	110	112	116	117	119	120
64								114	115	117	119	120	122	123
65								118	120	121	122	123	125	126
66									124	124	125	128	129	130
67									128	130	131	133	133	135
68									131	133	135	136	138	138
69										135	137	138	140	142
70										136	138	140	142	144
71										138	140	142	144	145

2-5 Height and weight tables for adults

Desirable weights for persons 25 to 29 years old (in indoor clothing*)

Men

Height (in shoes)†:				
Ft.	*In.*	*Small frame: Pounds*	*Medium frame: Pounds*	*Large frame: Pounds*
5	2	128-134	131-141	138-150
5	3	130-136	133-143	140-153
5	4	132-138	135-145	142-156
5	5	134-140	137-148	144-160
5	6	136-142	139-151	146-164
5	7	138-145	142-154	149-168
5	8	140-148	145-157	152-172
5	9	142-151	148-160	155-176
5	10	144-154	151-163	158-180
5	11	146-157	154-166	161-184
6	0	149-160	157-170	164-188
6	1	152-164	160-174	168-192
6	2	155-168	164-178	172-197
6	3	158-172	167-182	176-202
6	4	162-176	171-187	181-207

Women

Height (in shoes)†:				
Ft.	*In.*	*Small frame: Pounds*	*Medium frame: Pounds*	*Large frame: Pounds*
4	10	102-111	109-121	118-131
4	11	103-113	111-123	120-134
5	0	104-115	113-126	122-137
5	1	106-118	115-129	125-140
5	2	108-121	118-132	128-143
5	3	111-124	121-135	131-147
5	4	114-127	124-138	134-151
5	5	117-130	127-141	137-155
5	6	120-133	130-144	140-159
5	7	123-136	133-147	143-163
5	8	126-139	136-150	146-167
5	9	129-142	139-153	149-170
5	10	132-145	142-156	152-173
5	11	135-148	145-159	155-176
6	0	138-151	148-162	158-179

Source of basic data *Build Study, 1979,* Society of Actuaries and Association of Life Insurance Medical Directors of America, 1980. Copyright 1983 Metropolitan Life Insurance Company.

*Indoor clothing weighing 5 pounds for men and 3 pounds for women.

†Shoes with 1-inch heels.

2-6 Pounds to kilograms conversion*

Pounds	*0*	*1*	*2*	*3*	*4*	*5*	*6*	*7*	*8*	*9*
0	0.00	0.45	0.90	1.36	1.81	2.26	2.72	3.17	3.62	4.08
10	4.53	4.98	5.44	5.89	6.35	6.80	7.25	7.71	8.16	8.61
20	9.07	9.52	9.97	10.43	10.88	11.34	11.79	12.24	12.70	13.15
30	13.60	14.06	14.51	14.96	15.42	15.87	16.32	16.78	17.23	17.69
40	18.14	18.59	19.05	19.50	19.95	20.41	20.86	21.31	21.77	22.22
50	22.68	23.13	23.58	24.04	24.49	24.94	25.40	25.85	26.30	26.76
60	27.21	27.66	28.12	28.57	29.03	29.48	29.93	30.39	30.84	31.29
70	31.75	32.20	32.65	33.11	33.56	34.02	34.47	34.92	35.38	35.83
80	36.28	36.74	37.19	37.64	38.10	38.55	39.00	39.46	39.91	40.37
90	40.82	41.27	41.73	42.18	42.63	43.09	43.54	43.99	44.45	44.90
100	45.36	45.81	46.26	46.72	47.17	47.62	48.08	48.53	48.98	49.44
110	49.89	50.34	50.80	51.25	51.71	52.16	52.61	53.07	53.52	53.97
120	54.43	54.88	55.33	55.79	56.24	56.70	57.15	57.60	58.06	58.51
130	58.96	59.42	59.87	60.32	60.78	61.23	61.68	62.14	62.59	63.05
140	63.50	63.95	64.41	64.86	65.31	65.77	66.22	66.67	67.13	67.58
150	68.04	68.49	68.94	69.40	69.85	70.30	70.76	71.21	71.66	72.12
160	72.57	73.02	73.48	73.93	74.39	74.84	75.29	75.75	76.20	76.65
170	77.11	77.56	78.01	78.47	78.92	79.38	79.83	80.28	80.74	81.19
180	81.64	82.10	82.55	83.00	83.46	83.91	84.36	84.82	85.27	85.73
190	86.18	86.68	87.09	87.54	87.99	88.45	88.90	89.35	89.81	90.26
200	90.72	91.17	91.62	92.08	92.53	92.98	93.44	93.89	94.34	94.80

*Numbers in the farthest left column are 10-pound increments; numbers across the top row are 1-pound increments. The kilogram equivalent of weight in pounds is found at the intersection of the appropriate row and column. For example, to convert 34 pounds, read down the left column to 30 and then across that row to 4: 34 pounds = 15.42 kilograms.

2-7 Grams to pounds and ounces conversion for weight of newborns

	Ounces															
Pounds	*0*	*1*	*2*	*3*	*4*	*5*	*6*	*7*	*8*	*9*	*10*	*11*	*12*	*13*	*14*	*15*
0	—	28	57	85	113	142	170	198	227	255	283	312	430	369	397	425
1	454	482	510	539	567	595	624	652	680	709	737	765	794	822	850	879
2	907	936	964	992	1021	1049	1077	1106	1134	1162	1191	1219	1247	1276	1304	1332
3	1361	1389	1417	1446	1474	1503	1531	1559	1588	1616	1644	1673	1701	1729	1758	1786
4	1814	1843	1871	1899	1928	1956	1984	2013	2041	2070	2098	2126	2155	2183	2211	2240
5	2268	2296	2325	2353	2381	2410	2438	2466	2495	2523	2551	2580	2608	2637	2665	2693
6	2722	2750	2778	2807	2835	2863	2892	2920	2948	2977	3005	3033	3062	3090	3118	3147
7	3175	3203	3232	3260	3289	3317	3345	3374	3402	3430	3459	3487	3515	3544	3572	3600
8	3629	3657	3685	3714	3742	3770	3799	3827	3856	3884	3912	3941	3969	3997	4026	4054
9	4082	4111	4139	4167	4196	4224	4252	4281	4309	4337	4366	4394	4423	4451	4479	4508
10	4536	4564	4593	4621	4649	4678	4706	4734	4763	4791	4819	4848	4876	4904	4933	4961
11	4990	5018	5046	5075	5103	5131	5160	5188	5216	5245	5273	5301	5330	5358	5386	5415
12	5443	5471	5500	5528	5557	5585	5613	5642	5670	5698	5727	5755	5783	5812	5840	5868
13	5897	5925	5953	5982	6010	6038	6067	6095	6123	6152	6180	6290	6237	6265	6294	6322
14	6350	6379	6407	6435	6464	6492	6520	6549	6577	6605	6634	6662	6690	6719	6747	6776

1 pound = 453.59 grams. 1 ounce = 28.35 grams. Grams can be converted to pounds and tenths of a pound by multiplying the number of grams by .0022.

2-8 Physical elements*

Element	*Symbol*	*Valence*	*Atomic number*	*Atomic weight†*
Actinium	Ac	3	89	(227.0278)
Aluminum	Al	3	13	26.98154
Americium	Am	3,4,5,6	95	(243.0614)
Antimony	Sb	3,5	51	121.75
Argon	Ar	0	18	39.948
Arsenic	As	3,5	33	74.9216
Astatine	At	1,3,5,7	85	(209.987)
Barium	Ba	2	56	137.34
Berkelium	Bk	3,4	97	(247.0703)
Beryllium	Be	2	4	9.01218
Bismuth	Bi	3,5	83	208.9804
Boron	B	3	5	10.81
Bromine	Br	1,3,5,7	35	79.904
Cadmium	Cd	2	48	112.40
Calcium	Ca	2	20	40.08
Californium	Cf	3	98	(251.0796)
Carbon	C	2,4	6	12.011
Cerium	Ce	3,4	58	140.12
Cesium	Cs	1	55	132.9054
Chlorine	Cl	1,3,5,7	17	35.453
Chromium	Cr	2,3,6	24	51.996
Cobalt	Co	2,3	27	58.9332
Columbium	See:	Niobium		
Copper	Cu	1,2	29	63.546
Curium	Cm	3	96	(247.0704)
Dysprosium	Dy	3	66	162.50
Einsteinium	Es		99	(254.0881)
Erbium	Er	3	68	167.26
Europium	Eu	2,3	63	151.96
Fermium	Fm		100	(257.0951)
Fluorine	F	1	9	18.9984
Francium	Fr	1	87	(223.0198)
Gadolinium	Gd	3	64	157.25
Gallium	Ga	2,3	31	69.72
Germanium	Ge	4	32	72.59
Glucinum	See:	Beryllium		
Gold	Au	1,3	79	196.9665
Hafnium	Hf	4	72	178.49
Helium	He	0	2	4.0026
Holmium	Ho	3	67	164.9304
Hydrogen	H	1	1	1.0079
Indium	In	3	49	114.82
Iodine	I	1,3,5,7	53	126.9045
Iridium	Ir	3,4	77	192.22
Iron	Fe	2,3	26	55.847
Krypton	Kr	0	36	83.30
Lanthanum	La	3	57	138.9055
Lawrencium	Lw		103	(256.0986)
Lead	Pb	2,4	82	207.2
Lithium	Li	1	3	6.941
Lutetium	Lu	3	71	174.97
Magnesium	Mg	2	12	24.305
Manganese	Mn	2,3,4,6,7	25	54.938
Mendelevium	Md		101	(257.0956)
Mercury	Hg	1,2	80	200.59
Molybdenum	Mo	3,4,6	42	95.94
Neodymium	Nd	3	60	144.24
Neon	Ne	0	10	20.179
Neptunium	Np	4,5,6	93	237.0482
Nickel	Ni	2,3	28	58.70
Niobium	Nb	3,5	41	92.9064
Nitrogen	N	3,5	7	14.0067
Nobelium	No		102	(255.0933)
Osmium	Os	2,3,4,8	76	190.2
Oxygen	O	2	8	15.9994
Palladium	Pd	2,4,6	46	106.4
Phosphorus	P	3,5	15	30.98376
Platinum	Pt	2,4	78	195.09
Plutonium	Pu	3,4,5,6	94	(244.0642)
Polonium	Po	2,4	84	(208.9824)
Potassium	K	1	19	39.098
Praseodymium	Pr	3	59	140.9077
Promethium	Pm	3	61	(144.9128)
Protactinium	Pa		91	(231.0359)
Radium	Ra	2	88	(226.0254)
Radon	Rn	0	86	(222.0176)
Rhenium	Re		75	186.207
Rhodium	Rh	3	45	102.9055
Rubidium	Rb	1	37	85.4678
Ruthenium	Ru	3,4,6,8	44	101.07
Samarium	Sm	2,3	62	150.4
Scandium	Sc	3	21	44.9559
Selenium	Se	2,4,6	34	78.96
Silicon	Si	4	14	28.086
Silver	Ag	1	47	107.868
Sodium	Na	1	11	22.98977
Strontium	Sr	2	38	87.62
Sulfur	S	2,4,6	16	32.06
Tantalum	Ta	5	73	180.9479
Technetium	Tc	6,7	43	96.9062
Tellurium	Te	2,4,6	52	127.60
Terbium	Tb	3	65	158.9254
Thallium	Tl	1,3	81	204.37
Thorium	Th	4	90	232.0381
Thulium	Tm	3	69	168.9342
Tin	Sn	2,4	50	118.69
Titanium	Ti	3,4	22	47.90
Tungsten	W	6	74	183.85
Uranium	U	4,6	92	238.029
Vanadium	V	3,5	23	50.9414
Xenon	Xe	0	54	131.30
Ytterbium	Yb	2,3	70	173.04
Yttrium	Y	3	39	88.9059
Zinc	Zn	2	30	65.38
Zirconium	Zr	4	40	91.22

*The 103 chemical elements known at present are included in this table. Some of those recently discovered have been obtained only as unstable isotopes.
†Based on Carbon-12. Figures enclosed in parentheses represent the mass number of the most stable isotope.

2-9 Periodic chart of the elements

IA	IIA	IIIB	IVB	VB	VIB	VIIB	VIII			IB	IIB	IIIA	IVA	VA	VIA	VIIA	NOBLE GASES	
1 H 1.0079†																1 H 1.0079†	2 He 4.00260	2
3 Li 6.941†	4 Be 9.01218											5 B 10.81	6 C 12.011	7 N 14.0067	8 O 15.9994†	9 F 18.99840	10 Ne 20.179†	2 8
11 Na 22.98977	12 Mg 24.305											13 Al 26.98154	14 Si 28.086†	15 P 30.97376	16 S 32.06	17 Cl 35.453	18 Ar 39.948†	2 8 8
19 K 39.098†	20 Ca 40.08	21 Sc 44.9559	22 Ti 47.90†	23 V 50.9414†	24 Cr 51.996	25 Mn 54.9380	26 Fe 55.847†	27 Co 58.9332	28 Ni 58.70†	29 Cu 63.546†	30 Zn 65.38	31 Ga 69.72	32 Ge 72.59†	33 As 74.9216	34 Se 78.96†	35 Br 79.904	36 Kr 83.80	2 8 18 8
37 Rb 85.4678†	38 Sr 87.62	39 Y 88.9059	40 Zr 91.22	41 Nb 92.9064	42 Mo 95.94†	43 Tc 98.9062	44 Ru 101.07†	45 Rh 102.9055	46 Pd 106.4	47 Ag 107.868	48 Cd 112.40	49 In 114.82	50 Sn 118.69†	51 Sb 121.75†	52 Te 127.60†	53 I 126.9045	54 Xe 131.30	2 8 18 18 8
55 Cs 132.9054	56 Ba 137.34†	57 *La 138.9055†	72 Hf 178.49†	73 Ta 180.9479†	74 W 183.85†	75 Re 186.207	76 Os 190.2	77 Ir 192.22†	78 Pt 195.09†	79 Au 196.9665	80 Hg 200.59†	81 Tl 204.37†	82 Pb 207.2	83 Bi 208.9804	84 Po (210)	85 At (210)	86 Rn (222)	2 8 18 32 18 8
87 Fr (223)	88 Ra 226.0254	89 †Ac (227)	104 § (260)	105 § (260)														

★ Lanthanoid Series

58	59	60	61	62	63	64	65	66	67	68	69	70	71	
Ce 140.12	Pr 140.9077	Nd 144.24†	Pm (147)	Sm 150.4	Eu 151.96	Gd 157.25†	Tb 158.9254	Dy 162.50†	Ho 164.9304	Er 167.26†	Tm 168.9342	Yb 173.04†	Lu 174.97	2 8 18 32 9 2

† Actinoid Series

90	91	92	93	94	95	96	97	98	99	100	101	102	103	
Th 232.0381	Pa 231.0359	U 238.029	Np 237.0482	Pu (244)	Am (243)	Cm (247)	Bk (247)	Cf (251)	Es (254)	Fm (257)	Md (258)	No (255)	Lr (256)	2 8 18 32 32 9 2

FISHER SCIENTIFIC COMPANY
CAT. NO. 5-702-10

§The International Union for Pure and Applied Chemistry has not adopted official names or symbols for these elements.

†These weights are considered reliable to ±3 in the last place. Other weights are reliable to ±1 in the last place.

Atomic weights corrected to conform to the 1973 values of the Commission on Atomic Weights.

Used with permission of the Fisher Scientific Company, Pittsburgh, Pa.

APPENDIX P
Periodic chart of the elements

APPENDIX 3 Symbols and abbreviations

3-1 Symbols

Symbol	*Meaning*	*Symbol*	*Meaning*
ʒ	Dram	$+$	Plus; excess; acid reaction; positive
fʒ	Fluid dram	$-$	Minus; deficiency; alkaline reaction; negative
℥	Ounce	$\pm$	Plus or minus; either positive or negative; indefinite
f℥	Fluid ounce	#	Number; following a number, pounds
O	Pint	$\div$	Divided by
℔	Pound	$\times$	Multiplied by; magnification
℞	Recipe; take	$=$	Equals
Ṃ	Misce; mix	$\cong$	Approximately equals
A,Å	Angstrom unit	$\neq$	Not equal to
E_0	Electroaffinity	$>$	Greater than; from which is derived
F_1	First filial generation	$<$	Less than; derived from
F_2	Second filial generation	$\nless$	Not less than
mμ	Millimicron, micromillimeter	$\ngtr$	Not greater than
μg	Microgram	$\leqq$	Equal to or less than
mEq	Milliequivalent	$\geqq$	Equal to or greater than
mg	Milligram	$\sqrt{}$	Root; square root; radical
m%	Milligrams percent; milligrams per 100 ml	$\sqrt[2]{}$	Square root
$Q\ O_2$	Oxygen consumption	$\sqrt[3]{}$	Cube root
m-	Meta-	∞	Infinity
o-	Ortho-	:	Ratio; ''is to''
p-	Para-	°	Degree
Po_2	Partial pressure of oxygen	%	Percent
Pco_2	Partial pressure of carbon dioxide	π	3.1416—ratio of circumference of a circle to its diameter; pi
μm	Micrometer	□, ♂	Male
μ	Micron (common term for micrometer)	○, ♀	Female
μμ	Micromicron	$\rightleftharpoons$	A reversible reaction

3-2 Abbreviations

Abbreviation	*Meaning*
A	Accommodation; acetum; angström unit; anode; anterior
a	Accommodation; ampere; anterior; area
A_2	Aortic second sound
AC	Alternating current; air conduction; axiocervical; adrenal cortex
acc.	Accommodation
ACE	Adrenocortical extract
ACh	Acetylcholine
ACH	Adrenocortical hormone
ACTH	Adrenocorticotropic hormone
AD	Right ear *(auris dextra)*
add	Add to *(adde)*
ADH	Antidiuretic hormone
ADL	Activities of daily living
ADS	Antidiuretic substance
A/G; A-G ratio	Albumin-globulin ratio
Ag	Silver
ah	Hypermetropic astigmatism
AHF	Antihemophilic factor
aj	Ankle jerk
Al	Aluminum
Alb	Albumin
ALH	Combined sex hormone of the anterior lobe of the hypophysis
Am	Mixed astigmatism
a.m.a.	Against medical advice
amp.	Ampere
ana	So much of each, or $\overline{\text{aa}}$
anat	Anatomy or anatomic
AO	Anodal opening; atrioventricular value openings
AOP	Anodal opening picture
AOS	Anodal opening sound
A-P; AP; A/P	Anterior-posterior
A.P.	Anterior pituitary gland
APA	Antipernicious anemia factor
AQ	Achievement quotient
AR	Alarm reaction
ARC	Anomalous retinal correspondence
ARD	Acute respiratory disease
arg	Silver
As	Arsenic
As.	Astigmatism
AS	Left ear *(auris sinistra)*
ASD	Atrial septal defect
AsH	Hypermetropic astigmatism
AsM	Myopic astigmatism
ASS	Anterior superior spine
Ast	Astigmatism
ATS	Anxiety tension state; antitetanic serum
AU	Angström unit
Au	Gold
A-V; AV; A/V	Arteriovenous; atrioventricular
Av	Average or avoirdupois
ax	Axis
B	Boron; bacillus
Ba	Barium
BAC	Buccoaxiocervical
Bact	Bacterium
BBB	Blood-brain barrier
BBT	Basal body temperature
BE	Barium enema
Be	Beryllium
BFP	Biologically false positivity (in syphilis tests)
Bi	Bismuth
Bib	Drink
BM	Bowel movement
BMR	Basal metabolic rate
BP	Blood pressure; buccopulpal
bp	Boiling point
BPH	Benign prostatic hypertrophy
BRP	Bathroom privileges
BSA	Body surface area
BSP	Bromsulphalein
BUN	Blood urea nitrogen
C	Carbon; centigrade; Celsius
C_{alb}	Albumin clearance
C_{cr}	Creatinine clearance
C_{in}	Inulin clearance
CA	Chronologic age; cervicoaxial
Ca	Calcium, cancer
CABS	Coronary artery bypass surgery
$CaCO_3$	Calcium carbonate
Cal	Large calorie
cal	Small calorie
CBC or cbc	Complete blood count
CC	Chief complaint
cc	Cubic centimeter
CCl_4	Carbon tetrachloride
CCU	Cardiac care unit
cf	Compare or bring together
CFT	Complement-fixation test
Cg; Cgm	Centigram
CH	Crown-heel (length of fetus)
$CHCL_3$	Chloroform
CH_3COOH	Acetic acid
ChE	Cholinesterase
CHF	Congestive heart failure
$C_5H_4N_4O_3$	Uric acid
C_2H_6O	Ethyl alcohol
CH_2O	Formaldehyde
CH_4O	Methyl alcohol
Cl	Chlorine
cm	Centimeter
CMR	Cerebral metabolic rate
CNS	Central nervous system
CO	Carbon monoxide
CO_2	Carbon dioxide
Co	Cobalt
CPC	Clinicopathologic conference
CPD	Cephalopelvic disproportion
CR	Crown-rump length (length of fetus)
CSF	Cerebrospinal fluid
CSM	Cerebrospinal meningitis
Cu	Copper
$CuSO_4$	Copper sulfate
CVA	Cerebrovascular accident; costovertebral angle
cyl	Cylinder
D	Dose; vitamin D; right *(dexter)*
DAH	Disordered action of the heart
D & C	Dilation (dilatation) and curettage
DC	Direct current
DCA	Deoxycorticosterone acetate
Deg	Degeneration; degree
dg	Decigram
diff	Differential blood count
dil	Dilute or dissolve
dim	One half
DJD	Degenerative joint disease
DNA	Deoxyribonucleic acid
DOA	Dead on arrival
dr	Dram
DTR	Deep tendon reflex
Dx	Diagnosis
E	Eye
EAHF	Eczema, asthma, and hayfever
ECG	Electrocardiogram, electrocardiograph
ECT	Electroconvulsive therapy
ED	Erythema dose, effective dose
ED_{50}	Median effective dose
EDC	Estimated date of confinement
EEG	Electroencephalogram, electroencephalograph
EENT	Eye, ear, nose, and throat
EKG	Electrocardiogram, electrocardiograph

Continued.

Abbreviations—cont'd

Abbreviation	*Meaning*
Em	Emmetropia
EMB	Eosin-methylene blue
EMC	Encephalomyocarditis
EMF	Erythrocyte maturation factor
EMG	Electromyogram
EMS	Emergency medical service
ENT	Ear, nose and throat
EOM	Extraocular movement
EPR	Electrophrenic respiration
ER	Emergency room (hospital); external resistance
ERG	Electroretinogram
ERPF	Effective renal plasma flow
ESR	Erythrocyte sedimentation rate
EST	Electroshock therapy
Et	Ethyl
F	Fahrenheit; field of vision; formula
FA	Fatty acid
FANA	Fluorescent antinuclear antibody test
F & R	Force and rhythm (pulse)
FBS	Fasting blood sugar
FD	Fatal dose; focal distance
Fe	Iron
$FeCl_3$	Ferric chloride
Fl	Fluid
fld	Fluid
fl dr	Fluid dram
fl oz	Fluid ounce
FR	Flocculation reaction
FSH	Follicle-stimulating hormone
ft	Foot
FUO	Fever of undetermined origin
G; g; gm	Gram
GA	Gingivoaxial
Galv	Galvanic
GBS	Gallbladder series
GC	Gonococcus or gonorrheal
GFR	Glomerular filtration rate
GI	Gastrointestinal
GL	Greatest length (small flexed embryo)
GLA	Gingivolinguoaxial
GP	General practitioner; general paresis
gr	Grain
Grad	By degrees *(gradatim)*
Grav I, II, III, etc.	Pregnancy one, two, three, etc. *(gravida)*
GSW	Gunshot wound
gt	Drop *(gutta)*
gtt	Drops *(guttae)*
GU	Genitourinary
H	Hydrogen
H^+	Hydrogen ion
H & E	Hematoxylin and eosin stain
Hb	Hemoglobin
H_3BO_3	Boric acid
HC	Hospital corps
HCHO	Formaldehyde
HCI	Hydrochloric acid
HCN	Hydrocyanic acid
H_2CO_3	Carbonic acid
HCT	Hematocrit
HD	Hearing distance
HDLW	Distance at which a watch is heard by the left ear
HDRW	Distance at which a watch is heard by the right ear
He	Helium
HEENT	Head, eye, ear, nose, and throat
Hg	Mercury;
Hgb	Hemoglobin
HNO_3	Nitric acid
H_2O	Water
H_2O_2	Hydrogen peroxide
HOP	High oxygen pressure
H_2SO_4	Sulfuric acid
Ht	Total hyperopia
Hy	Hyperopia
I	Iodine
^{131}I	Radioactive isotope of iodine (atomic weight 131)
^{132}I	Radioactive isotope of iodine (atomic weight 132)
IB	Inclusion body
IBW	Ideal body weight
ICS	Intercostal space
ICSH	Interstitial cell-stimulating hormone
ICT	Inflammation of connective tissue
ICU	Intensive care unit
Id.	The same *(idem)*
IH	Infectious hepatitis
IM	Intramuscularly; infectious mononucleosis
IOP	Intraocular pressure
IQ	Intelligence quotient
IS	Intercostal space
IU	Immunizing unit
IV	Intravenously
IVP	Intravenous pyelogram
IVT	Intravenous transfusion
IVU	Intravenous urogram/urography
K	Potassium
k	Constant
Ka	Cathode or kathode
KBr	Potassium bromide
kc	Kilocycle
KCI	Potassium chloride
kev	Kilo electron volts
kg	Kilogram
KI	Potassium iodide
kj	Knee jerk
km	Kilometer
KOH	Potassium hydroxide
KUB	Kidney, ureter, and bladder
kv	Kilovolt
kw	Kilowatt
L	Left; liter; length; lumbar; lethal; pound
L & A	Light and accommodation
lb	Pound *(libra)*
LB	Large bowel (x-ray film)
LD	Lethal dose; perception of light difference
LE	Lupus erythematosus
l.e.s.	Local excitatory state
LFD	Least fatal dose of a toxin
LH	Luteinizing hormone
Li	Lithium
LIF	Left iliac fossa
lig	Ligament
Liq	Liquor
LLL	Left lower lobe of lung
LMP	Last menstrual period
LP	Lumbar puncture
LPF	Leukocytosis-promoting factor
LTH	Luteotrophic hormone
LUL	Left upper lobe
M	Myopia; meter; muscle; thousand
m	Meter
MA	Mental age
Mag	Large *(magnus)*
MBD	Minimal brain dysfunction
mc	Millicurie
μc	Microcurie
mcg	Microgram
MCH	Mean corpuscular hemoglobin
MCHC	Mean corpuscular hemoglobin concentration
MCV	Mean corpuscular volume
Me	Methyl
MED	Minimal erythema dose; minimal effective dose
mEq	Milliequivalent
mEq/L	Milliequivalent per liter
ME ratio	Myeloid-erythroid ratio
Mg	Magnesium
mg	Milligram
μg	Microgram
MHD	Minimal hemolytic dose
m Hg	Millimeters of mercury
MI	Myocardial infarction
MID	Minimum infective dose
ML	Midline
ml	Milliliter
MLD	Median or minimum lethal dose

Abbreviation	*Meaning*
MM	Mucous membrane
mm	Millimeter; muscles
mmm	Millimicron
mμ	Millimicron
μμ	Micromicron
Mn	Manganese
mN	Millinormal
MS	Multiple sclerosis
MSL	Midsternal line
MT	Medical technologist; membrane tympani
mu	Mouse unit
My	Myopia
N	Nitrogen
n	Normal
Na	Sodium
NaBr	Sodium bromide
NaCl	Sodium chloride
$Na_2C_2O_4$	Sodium oxalate
Na_2CO_3	Sodium carbonate
NAD	No appreciable disease
NaF	Sodium fluoride
$NaHCO_3$	Sodium bicarbonate
Na_2HPO_4	Sodium phosphate
NAI	Sodium iodide
$NaNO_3$	Sodium nitrate
Na_2O_2	Sodium peroxide
NaOH	Sodium hydroxide
Na_2SO_4	Sodium sulfate
NCA	Neurocirculatory asthenia
Ne	Neon
NH_3	Ammonia
Ni	Nickel
NPN	Nonprotein nitrogen
NPO; n.p.o.	Nothing by mouth *(non per os)*
NRC	Normal retinal correspondence
NTP	Normal temperature and pressure
NYD	Not yet diagnosed
O	Oxygen; oculus; pint
O_2	Oxygen; both eyes
O_3	Ozone
OB	Obstetrics
OD	Right eye *(oculus dexter);* optical density
OPD	Outpatient department
OR	Operating room
ORIF	Open reduction and internal fixation
OS	Left eye *(oculus sinister)*
Os	Osmium
OT	Occupational therapy
OTD	Organ tolerance dose
OU	Each eye *(oculus uterque)*
oz	Ounce
P	Phosphorus; pulse; pupil
P_2	Pulmonic second sound
P-A; P/A; PA	Posterior-anterior

Abbreviation	*Meaning*
P & A	Percussion and auscultation
PAB; PABA	Para-aminobenzoic acid
Para I, II, III, etc.	Unipara, bipara, tripara, etc.
PAS; PASA	Para-aminosalicylic acid
Pb	Lead
PBI	Protein-bound iodine
PCV	Packed cell volume
PD	Interpupillary distance
pd	Prism diopter; pupillary distance
PDA	Patent ductus arteriosus
PE	Physical examination
PEG	Pneumoencephalography
PFF	Protein-free filtrate
PGA	Pteroylglutamic acid (folic acid)
PH	Past history
pH	Hydrogen ion concentration (alkalinity and acidity in urine and blood analysis)
Pharm; Phar.	Pharmacy
PI	Previous illness; protamine insulin
PID	Pelvic inflammatory disease
PK	Psychokinesis
PKU	Phenylketonuria
PL	Light perception
PM	Postmortem; evening
PMB	Polymorphonuclear basophil leukocytes
PME	Polymorphonuclear eosinophil leukocytes
PMI	Point of maximal impulse
PMN	Polymorphonuclear neutrophil leukocytes (polys)
PN	Percussion note
PNH	Paroxysmal nocturnal hemoglobinuria
PO; p.o.	Orally *(per os)*
Pr	Presbyopia; prism
pro time	Prothrombin time
PSP	Phenolsulfonphthalein
pt	Pint
Pt	Platinum; patient
PT	Prothrombin time
PTA	Plasma thromboplastin antecedent
PTC	Plasma thromboplastin component
PTT	Partial thromboplastin time
Pu	Plutonium
PUO	Pyrexia of unknown origin

Abbreviation	*Meaning*
Px	Pneumothorax
Q	Electric quantity
qns	Quantity not sufficient
qt	Quart
Quat	Four *(quattuor)*
R	Respiration; right; Rickettsia; roentgen
Ra	Radium
rad	Unit of measurement of the absorbed dose of ionizing radiation; root
RBC; rbc	Red blood cell; red blood count
RCD	Relative cardiac dullness
RE	Right eye; reticuloendothelial tissue or cell
Re	Rhenium
Rect	Rectified
Reg umb	Umbilical region
RES	Reticuloendothelial system
Rh	Symbol of rhesus factor; symbol for rhodium
RhA	Rheumatoid arthritis
RHD	Relative hepatic dullness
RLL	Right lower lobe of lung
RM	Respiratory movement
RML	Right middle lobe of lung
Rn	Radon
RNA	Ribonucleic acid
R/O	Rule out
RPF	Renal plasma flow
RPM; rpm	Revolutions per minute
RPS	Renal pressor substance
RQ	Respiratory quotient
RT	Reading test
RU	Rat unit
RUL	Right upper lobe of lung
S	Sulfur
S.	Sacral
SAS	Sodium acetate solution
SB	Small bowel (x-ray film)
Sb	Antimony
SC	Closure of semilunar valves
Se	Selenium
SD	Skin dose
Sed rate	Sedimentation rate
SGOT	Serum glutamic oxaloacetic transaminase
SGPT	Serum glutamic pyruvic transaminase
SH	Serum hepatitis
S.I.	Soluble insulin
Si	Silicon
Sn	Tin
SOB	Shortness of breath
Sol	Solution
sp. gr.	Specific gravity
sph	Spherical
SPI	Serum precipitable iodine
spir	Spirit

Continued.

Abbreviations—cont'd

Abbreviation	Meaning	Abbreviation	Meaning	Abbreviation	Meaning
SR	Sedimentation rate	Tl	Thallium	VDM	Vasodepressor material
Sr	Strontium	Tm	Thulium; symbol for maximal tubular excretory capacity (kidneys)	VDRL	Venereal Disease Research Laboratories (sometimes used loosely to mean venereal disease report)
SSS	Specific soluble substance	TNT	Trinitrotoluene	VDS	Venereal disease—syphilis
sss	Layer upon layer *(stratum super stratum)*	TNTC	Too numerous to mention	VEM	Vasoexciter material
St	Let it stand *(stet; stent)*	TP	Tuberculin precipitation	Vf	Field of vision
Staph	*Staphylococcus*	TPI	*Treponema pallidum* immobilization test for syphilis	VHD	Valvular heart disease
Stat	Immediately *(statim)*	TPR	Temperature, pulse, and respiration	VIA	virus inactivating agent
STD	Skin test dose	Trans D	Transverse diameter	VMA	Vanillylmandelic acid
STH	Somatotrophic hormone	TRU	Turbidity reducing unit	VR	Vocal resonance
Strep	*Streptococcus*	TS	Test solution	VS	Volumetric solution
STS	Serologic test for syphilis	TSH	Thyroid-stimulating hormone	Vs	Venisection
STU	Skin test unit	TSP	Trisodium phosphate	VsB	Bleeding in arm *(venaesectio brachii)*
sv	Alcoholic spirit *(spiritus vini)*	TST	Triple sugar iron test	VSD	Ventricular septal defect
Sym	Symmetrical	TUR	Transurethral resection	VW	Vessel wall
T	Temperature; thoracic	U	Uranium; unit	W	Tungsten
t	Temporal	UBI	Ultraviolet blood irradiation	w	Watt
TA	Toxin-antitoxin	UIBC	Unsaturated iron-binding capacity	WBC; wbc	White blood cell; white blood count
Ta	Tantalum	USP	*U.S. Pharmacopeia*	WD	Well developed
T & A	Tonsillectomy and adenoidectomy	V	Vanadium; vision; visual acuity	WL	Wavelength
TAB	Vaccine against typhoid, paratyphoid A and B	v	Volt	WN	Well nourished
TAH	Total abdominal hysterectomy	VA	Visual acuity	WR	Wassermann reaction
TAM	Toxoid-antitoxoid mixture	V & T	Volume and tension	wt	Weight
TAT	Toxin-antitoxin	VC	Vital capacity	X-ray	Roentgen ray
TB	Tuberculin; tuberculosis; tubercle bacillus	VD	Venereal disease	Z	Symbol for atomic number
Tb	Terbium	VDA	Visual discriminatory acuity	Zn	Zinc
TCA	Tetrachloracetic acid	VDG	Venereal disease—gonorrhea	Zz	Ginger
Te	Tellurium; tetanus				
TEM	Triethylene melamine				
Th	Thorium				
TIBC	Total iron-binding capacity				

3-3 Common abbreviations used in writing prescriptions

Abbreviation	Derivation	Meaning
āā	ana	of each
a.c.	ante cibum	before meals
ad	ad	to, up to
ad lib.	ad libitum	freely as desired
alt. dieb.	*(alternis diebus)*	every other day
alt. hor.	*(alternis horis)*	alternate hours
alt. noct.	*(alternis noctes)*	alternate nights
aq.	aqua	water
aq. dest.	aqua destillata	distilled water
b.i.d.	bis in die	two times a day
b.i.n.	bis in noctis	two times a night
c.	cum	with
Cap.	capiat	let him take
caps.	capsula	capsule
c.m.s.	cras mane sumendus	to be taken tomorrow morning
c.n.	cras nocte	tomorrow night

Abbreviation	Derivation	Meaning
c.n.s.	cras nocte sumendus	to be taken tomorrow night
comp.	compositus	compound
Det.	*(detur)*	let it be given
Dieb. tert.	*(diebus tertiis)*	every third day
dil.	dilutus	dilute
elix.	elixir	elixir
ext.	extractum	extract
fld.	fluidus	fluid
Ft.	fiat	make
g	gramme	gram
gr	granum	grain
gt	gutta	a drop
gtt	guttae	drops
h.	hora	hour
h.d.	hora decubitus	at bedtime
h.s.	hora somni	hour of sleep (bedtime)
M.	misce	mix
m.	minimum	a minim
mist.	mistura	mixture
non rep.	non repetatur	not to be repeated
noct.	nocte	in the night
O	octarius	pint
ol.	oleum	oil
o.d.	omni die	every day
o.h.	omni hora	every hour
o.m.	omni mane	every morning
o.n.	omni nocte	every night
os	os	mouth
oz	uncia	ounce
p.c.	post cibum	after meals
per	per	through or by
pil.	pilula	pill
p.o.	per os	orally
p.r.n.	pro re nata	when required
q.d.	quaque die	every day
q.h.	quaque hora	every hour
q. 2 h.		every two hours
q. 3 h.		every three hours
q. 4 h.		every four hours
q.i.d.	quater in die	four times a day
q.l.	quantum libet	as much as desired
q.n.	quaque nocte	every night
q.p.	quantum placeat	as much as desired
q.v.	quantum vis	as much as you please
q.s.	quantum sufficit	as much as is required
℞	recipe	take
Rep.	repetatur	let it be repeated
s	sine	without
seq. luce.	sequenti luce	the following day
Sig. or S.	signa	write on label
s.o.s.	si opus sit	if necessary
sp.	spiritus	spirits
ss	semis	a half
stat.	statim	immediately
syr.	syrupus	syrup
t.d.s	ter die sumendum	to be taken three times daily
t.i.d.	ter in die	three times a day
t.i.n.	ter in nocte	three times a night
tr. or tinct.	tinctura	tincture
ung.	unguentum	ointment
ut. dict.	ut dictum	as directed
vin.	vini	wine

APPENDIX 4 TABULAR ATLAS OF HUMAN ANATOMY AND PHYSIOLOGY

4-1 Basic structures and functions of the body

Cells

Cell structures	*Functions*
Cytoplasmic membrane	Serves as the boundary of the cell, maintaining its integrity; protein molecules on outer surface of cytoplasmic membrane perform various functions; for example, they serve as markers that identify cells of each individual, receptor molecules for certain hormones and neurotransmitters provide means of communication between cells, receptor molecules for foreign proteins function to produce immunity
Endoplasmic reticulum (ER)	Serves as a cell's own circulatory system
Golgi apparatus	Synthesizes carbohydrate, combines it with protein, and packages the product as globules of glycoprotein
Mitochondria	Catabolism; ATP synthesis; a cell's "powerhouse"
Lysosomes	A cell's "digestive system"
Ribosomes	Synthesize proteins; a cell's "protein factory"
Nucleus	Dictates protein synthesis, thereby playing essential role in other cell activities, namely, active transport, metabolism, growth, and heredity
Nucleoli	Play essential role in the formation of ribosomes

Tissues

Tissue	*Location*	*Function*
Epithelial		
Simple squamous	Alveoli of lungs	Absorption by diffusion of respiratory gases between alveolar air and blood
	Lining of blood and lymphatic vessels (called endothelium; classed as connective tissue by some histologists)	Absorption by diffusion; filtration; osmosis
	Surface layer of pleura, pericardium, peritoneum (called mesothelium; classed as connective tissue by some histologists)	Absorption by diffusion; osmosis; also secretion
Stratified squamous	Surface of lining of mouth and esophagus	Protection
	Surface of skin (epidermis)	Protection
Simple columnar	Surface layer of lining of stomach, intestines, and part of respiratory tract	Protection; secretion; absorption; moving of mucus (by ciliated columnar)
Muscle		
Skeletal (striated voluntary)	Muscles that attach to bones	Movement of bones
	Extrinsic eyeball muscles	Eye movements
	Upper third of esophagus	First part of swallowing
Visceral (nonstriated involuntary or smooth)	In walls of tubular viscera of digestive, respiratory, and genitourinary tracts	Movement of substances along respective tracts
	In walls of blood vessels and large lymphatic vessels	Change diameter of blood vessels, thereby aiding in regulation of blood pressure
	In ducts of glands	Movement of substances along ducts
	Intrinsic eye muscles (iris and ciliary body)	Change diameter of pupils and shape of lens
	Arrector muscles of hairs	Erection of hairs (gooseflesh)
Cardiac (striated involuntary)	Wall of heart	Contraction of heart

Tissue	*Location*	*Function*
Connective (most widely distributed of all tissues)		
Reticular tissue	Spleen, lymph nodes, bone marrow	Defense against microbes and harmful substances by filtration from blood and lymph by reticular network; phagocytosis by reticular cells; synthesis of reticular fibers by reticular cells
Loose, ordinary (areolar)	Between other tissues and organs Superficial fascia	Connection Connection
Adipose (fat)	Under skin Padding at various points	Protection Insulation Support Reserve food
Dense fibrous	Tendons Ligaments Aponeuroses Deep fascia Dermis Scars Capsule of kidney, etc.	Flexible but strong connection
Bone	Skeleton	Support Protection
Cartilage		
Hyaline	Part of nasal septum Covering articular surfaces of bones Larynx Rings in trachea and bronchi	Firm but flexible support
Fibrous	Disks between vertebrae Symphysis pubis	
Elastic	External ear Eustachian tube	
Hemopoietic		
Myeloid (bone marrow)	Marrow spaces of bones	Formation of red blood cells, granular leukocytes, platelets; also reticuloendothelial cells and some other connective tissue cells
Lymphatic	Lymph nodes Spleen Tonsils and adenoids Thymus gland	Formation of lymphocytes and monocytes; also plasma cells and some other connective tissue cells
Blood	In blood vessels	Transportation Protection
Nervous	Brain Spinal cord Nerves	Irritability; conduction

4-2 Skeletal system

Bones of the skeleton

Part of body	*Name of bone*	*Number*	*Identification*
APPENDICULAR SKELETON (126 bones)			Bones that are appended to axial skeleton; upper and lower extremities, including shoulder and hip girdles
Upper extremities (including shoulder girdle) (64 bones)	Clavicle	2	Collar bones; shoulder girdle joined to axial skeleton by articulation of clavicles with sternum; scapula does not form joint with axial skeleton
	Scapula	2	Shoulder blades; scapulae and clavicles together comprise shoulder girdle
	Humerus	2	Long bone of upper arm
	Radius	2	Bone of thumb side of forearm
	Ulna	2	Bone of little finger side of forearm; longer than radius
	Carpals (scaphoid, lunate, triquetrum, pisiform, trapezium, trapezoid, capitate, and hamate)	16	Arranged in two rows at proximal end of hand
	Metacarpals	10	Long bones forming framework of palm of hand
	Phalanges	28	Miniature long bones of fingers, 3 in each finger, 2 in each thumb
Lower extremities (62 bones)	Ossa coxae or innominate bones	2	Large hip bones; with sacrum and coccyx, these 3 bones form basin-like pelvic cavity; lower extremities attached to axial skeleton by pelvic bones
	Femur	2	Thigh bone; largest, strongest bone of body
	Patella	2	Kneecap; largest sesamoid bone of body*; embedded in tendon of quadriceps femoris muscle
	Tibia	2	Shin bone
	Fibula	2	Long, slender bone of lateral side of lower leg
	Tarsals (calcaneus, talus, navicular, first, second, and third cuneiforms, cuboid)	14	Bones that form heel and proximal or posterior half of foot
	Metatarsals	10	Long bones of feet
	Phalanges	28	Miniature long bones of toes; 2 in each great toe, 3 in other toes
AXIAL SKELETON (80 bones)			Bones that form upright axis on body—skull, hyoid, vertebral column, sternum, and ribs
Skull (28 bones)			
Cranium (8 bones)			Cranium forms floor for brain to rest on and helmetlike covering over it
	Frontal	1	Forehead bone; also forms most of roof of orbits (eye sockets) and anterior part of cranial floor
	Parietal	2	Prominent, bulging bones behind frontal bone; form top sides of cranial cavity
	Temporal	2	Form lower sides of cranium and part of cranial floor; contain middle and inner ear structures
	Occipital	1	Forms posterior part of cranial floor and walls
	Sphenoid	1	Keystone of cranial floor; forms its midportion; resembles bat with wings outstretched and legs extended downward posteriorly; lies behind and slightly above nose and throat; forms part of floor and sidewalls of orbit

*An inconstant number of small, flat, round bones known as *sesamoid bones* (because of their resemblance to sesame seeds) is found in various tendons in which considerable pressure develops. Because the number of these bones varies greatly between individuals, only 2 of them, the patellae, have been counted among the 206 bones of the body. Generally, 2 of them can be found in each thumb (in flexor tendon near metacarpophalangeal and interphalangeal joints) and great toe plus several others in the upper and lower extremities. *Wormian bones,* the small islets of bone frequently found in some of the cranial sutures, have not been counted in this list of 206 bones because of their variable occurrence.

Part of body	Name of bone	Number	Identification
	Ethmoid	1	Complicated irregular bone that helps make up anterior portion of cranial floor, medial wall of orbits, upper parts of nasal septum, and sidewalls and part of nasal roof; lies anterior to sphenoid and posterior to nasal bones
Face (14 bones)	Nasal	2	Small bones forming upper part of bridge of nose
	Maxillary	2	Upper jaw bones; form part of floor of orbit, anterior part of roof of mouth, and floor and part of sidewalls of nose
	Zygomatic (malar)	2	Cheekbones; form part of floor and sidewall of orbit
	Mandible	1	Lower jawbone; largest, strongest bone of face
	Lacrimal	2	Thin bones about size and shape of fingernail; posterior and lateral to nasal bones in medial wall of orbit; help form sidewall of nasal cavity, often missing in dry skull
	Palatine	2	Form posterior part of hard palate floor and part of sidewalls of nasal cavity and floor of orbit
	Inferior conchae (turbinates)	2	Thin scroll of bone forming a kind of shell along inner surface of sidewall of nasal cavity; lies above roof of mouth
	Vomer	1	Forms lower and posterior part of nasal septum; shaped liked ploughshare
Ear bones (6 bones)	Malleus (hammer)	2	Tiny bones referred to as auditory ossicles in middle ear cavity in temporal bones; resemble, respectively, miniature hammer, anvil, and stirrup
	Incus (anvil)	2	
	Stapes (stirrup)	2	
Hyoid bone		1	U-shaped bone in neck between mandible and upper part of larynx; claims distinction as only bone not forming a joint with any other bone; suspended by ligaments from styloid processes of temporal bones
Sternum and ribs (25 bones)			Sternum, ribs, and thoracic vertebrae together form bony cage known as *thorax;* ribs attach posteriorly to vertebrae, slant downward anteriorly to attach to sternum (see description of false ribs below)
	Sternum	1	Breastbone; flat dagger-shaped bone
	True ribs	7 pairs	Upper seven pairs; fasten to sternum by costal cartilages
	False ribs	5 pairs	False ribs do not attach to sternum directly; upper three pairs of false ribs attach by means of costal cartilage of seventh ribs; last two pairs do not attach to sternum at all; therefore called ''floating''
Vertebral column (26 bones)			Not actually a column but a flexible segmented rod shaped like an elongated letter S; forms axis of body; head balanced above, ribs and viscera suspended in front, and lower extremities attached below; encloses spinal cord
	Cervical vertebrae	7	First, or upper, seven vertebrae
	Thoracic vertebrae	12	Next 12 vertebrae; 12 pairs of ribs attached to these
	Lumbar vertebrae	5	Next five vertebrae
	Sacrum	1	Five separate vertebrae until about 25 years of age; then fused to form one wedge-shaped bone
	Coccyx	1	Four or five separate vertebrae in child but fused into one in adult
TOTAL		206*	

Identification of bone markings

Marking	Description
SPECIAL FEATURES OF SKULL	
Sutures	Immovable joints between skull bones
Sagittal	Joint between two parietal bones
Coronal	Joint between parietal bones and frontal bone
Lambdoidal	Joint between parietal bones and occipital bone
Fontanels	"Soft spots" where ossification is incomplete at birth; allow some compression of skull during birth; also important in determining position of head before delivery; six such areas located at angles of parietal bones
Anterior (or frontal)	At intersection of sagittal and coronal sutures (juncture of parietal bones and frontal bone); diamond shaped; largest of fontanels; usually closed by 1½ years of age
Posterior (or occipital)	At intersection of sagittal and lambdoidal sutures (juncture of parietal bones and occipital bone); triangular in shape; usually closed by second month
Anterolateral (or sphenoid)	At juncture of frontal, parietal, temporal, and sphenoid bones
Posterolateral (or mastoid)	At juncture of parietal, occipital, and temporal bones; usually closed by second year
Sinuses	
Air (or bony)	Spaces or cavities within bones; those that communicate with nose called *paranasal sinuses* (frontal, sphenoidal, ethmoidal, and maxillary); mastoid cells communicate with middle ear rather than nose, therefore not included among paranasal sinuses
Blood	Veins within cranial cavity
Orbits formed by	
Frontal	Roof of orbit
Ethmoid	Medial wall
Lacrimal	Medial wall
Sphenoid	Lateral wall
Zygomatic	Lateral wall
Maxillary	Floor
Palatine	Floor
Nasal septum formed by	Partition in midline of nasal cavity; separates cavity into right and left halves
Perpendicular plate of ethmoid bone	Forms upper part of septum
Vomer bone	Forms lower, posterior part
Cartilage	Forms anterior part
Wormian bones	Small islands of bones within suture

Marking	Description
FRONTAL	
Supraorbital margin	Arched ridge just below eyebrow
Frontal sinuses	Cavities inside bone just above supraorbital margin; lined with mucosa; contain air
Frontal tuberosities	Bulge above each orbit; most prominent part of forehead
Superciliary arches	Ridges caused by projection of frontal sinuses; eyebrows lie over these ridges
Supraorbital notch (sometimes foramen)	Notch or foramen in supraorbital margin slightly mesial to its midpoint; transmits supraorbital nerve and blood vessels
Glabella	Smooth area between superciliary ridges and above nose
SPHENOID	
Body	Hollow, cubelike central portion
Greater wings	Lateral projections from body; form part of outer wall of orbit
Lesser wings	Thin, triangular projections from upper part of sphenoid body; form posterior part of roof of orbit
Sella turcica (or *Turk's saddle*)	Saddle-shaped depression on upper surface of sphenoid body; contains pituitary gland
Sphenoid sinuses	Irregular air-filled mucosa-lined spaces within central part of sphenoid
Pterygoid processes	Downward projections on either side where body and greater wing unite; comparable to extended legs of bat if entire bone is likened to this animal; form part of lateral nasal wall
Optic foramen	Opening into orbit at root of lesser wing; transmits second cranial nerve
Superior orbital fissure	Slitlike opening into orbit; lateral to optic foramen; transmits third, fourth, and part of fifth cranial nerves
Foramen rotundum	Opening in greater wing that transmits maxillary division of fifth cranial nerve
Foramen ovale	Opening in greater wing that transmits mandibular division of fifth cranial nerve
ETHMOID	
Horizontal (cribriform) plate	Olfactory nerves pass through numerous holes in this plate
Crista galli	Meninges attach to this process
Perpendicular plate	Forms upper part of nasal septum
Ethmoid sinuses	Honeycombed, mucosa-lined air spaces within lateral masses of bone
Superior and middle turbinates (conchae)	Help to form lateral walls of nose
Lateral masses	Compose sides of bone; contain many air spaces (ethmoid cells or sinuses); inner surface forms superior and middle conchae

Marking	*Description*
TEMPORAL	
Mastoid process	Protuberance just behind ear
Mastoid air cells	Air-filled mucosa-lined spaces within mastoid process
External auditory meatus (or canal)	Opening into ear and tube extending into temporal bone
Zygomatic process	Projection that articulates with malar (or zygomatic) bone
Internal auditory meatus	Fairly large opening on posterior surface of petrous portion of bone; transmits eighth cranial nerve to inner ear and seventh cranial nerve on its way to facial structures
Squamous portion	Thin, flaring upper part of bone
Mastoid portion	Rough-surfaced lower part of bone posterior to external audiotry meatus
Petrous portion	Wedge-shaped process that forms part of center section of cranial floor between sphenoid and occipital bones; name derived from Greek word for stone because of extreme hardness of this process; houses middle and inner ear structures
Mandibular fossa	Oval-shaped depression anterior to external auditory meatus; forms socket for condyle of mandible
Styloid process	Slender spike of bone extending downward and forward from undersurface of bone anterior to mastoid process; often broken off in dry skull; several neck muscles and ligaments attach to styloid process
Stylomastoid foramen	Opening between styloid and mastoid processes where facial nerve emerges from cranial cavity
Jugular fossa	Depression on undersurface of petrous portion; dilated beginning of internal jugular vein lodged here
Jugular foramen	Opening in suture between petrous portion and occipital bone; transmits lateral sinus and ninth, tenth, and eleventh cranial nerves
Carotid canal (or foramen)	Channel in petrous portion; best seen from undersurface of skull; transmits internal carotid artery
PALATINE	
Horizontal plate	Joined to palatine processes of maxillae to complete part of hard palate
MANDIBLE	
Body	Main part of bone; forms chin
Ramus	Process, one on either side, that projects upward from posterior part of body
Condyle (or head)	Part of each ramus that articulates with mandibular fossa of temporal bone
Neck	Constricted part just below condyles
Alveolar process	Teeth set into this arch
Mandibular foramen	Opening on inner surface of ramus; transmits nerves and vessels to lower teeth
Mental foramen	Opening on outer surface below space between two bicuspids; transmits terminal branches of nerves and vessels that enter bone through mandibular foramen; dentists inject anesthetics through these foramina
Coronoid process	Projection upward from anterior part of each ramus; temporal muscle inserts here
Angle	Juncture of posterior and inferior margins of ramus
MAXILLA	
Alveolar process	Arch containing teeth
Maxillary sinus or antrum of Highmore	Large air-filled mucosa-lined cavity within body of each maxilla; largest of sinuses
Palatine process	Horizontal inward projection from alveolar process; forms anterior and larger part of hard palate
Infraorbital foramen	Hole on external surface just below orbit; transmits vessels and nerves
Lacrimal groove	Groove on inner surface; joined by similar groove on lacrimal bone to form canal housing nasolacrimal duct
OCCIPITAL	
Foramen magnum	Hole through which spinal cord enters cranial cavity
Condyles	Convex, oval processes on either side of foramen magnum; articulate with depressions on first cervical vertebra
External occipital protuberance	Prominent projection on posterior surface in midline short distance above foramen magnum; can be felt as definite bump
Superior nuchal line	Curved ridge extending laterally from external occipital protuberance
Inferior nuchal line	Less well-defined ridge paralleling superior nuchal line short distance below it
Internal occipital protuberance	Projection in midline on inner surface of bone; grooves for lateral sinuses extend laterally from this process and one for sagittal sinus extends upward from it

Continued.

Identification of bone markings—cont'd

Marking	Description
VERTEBRAL COLUMN	
General features	Anterior part of vertebra (except first two cervical) consists of body; posterior part of neural arch, which in turn consists of two pedicles, two laminae, and seven processes projecting from laminae
Thoracic vertebrae	
Body	Main part; flat, round mass located anteriorly; supporting or weight-bearing part of vertebra
Pedicles	Short projections extending posteriorly from body
Laminae	Posterior part of vertebra to which pedicles join and from which porcesses project
Neural arch	Formed by pedicles and laminae; protects spinal cord posteriorly; congenital absence of one or more neural arches known as spina bifida (cord may protrude through skin)
Spinous process	Sharp process projecting inferiorly from laminae in midline
Transverse processes	Right and left lateral projections from laminae
Superior articulating processes	Project upward from laminae
Inferior articulating processes	Project downward from laminae; articulate with superior articulating processes of vertebrae below
Spinal foramen	Hole in center of vertebra formed by union of body, pedicles, and laminae; when vertebrae are superimposed one on other spinal foramina form spinal cavity that houses spinal cord
Cervical vertebrae	
General features	Foramen in each transverse process for transmission of vertebral artery, vein, and plexus of nerves; short bifurcated spinous processes except on seventh vertebra, where it is extra long and may be felt as protrusion when head is bent forward; bodies of these vertebrae small, wheras spinal foramina large and triangular
Atlas	First cervical vertebra; lacks body and spinous processes; superior articulating processes concave ovals that act as rockerlike cradles for condyles of occipital bone; named atlas because supports head as Atlas was thought to have supported the world
Axis (epistropheus)	Second cervical vertebra, named because atlas rotates about this bone in rotating movements of the head; dens, or odontoid process, projects upward like a peg from body of axis, forming pivot for rotation of atlas
Lumbar vertebrae	Strong, massive; superior articulating processes directed inward instead of upward; inferior articulating processes, outward instead of downward; short, blunt spinous process
Scaral promontory	Protuberance from anterior, upper border of sacrum into pelvis; of obstetrical importance because its size limits anteroposterior diameter of pelvic inlet
Intervertebral foramina	Opening between vertebrae through which spinal nerves emerge
Curves	Curves have great structural importance because they increase carrying strength of vertebral column, make balance possible in upright position (if column were straight, weight of viscera would pull body forward), absorb jars from walking (straight column would transmit jars straight to head), and protect column from fracture
Primary	Column curves at birth from head to sacrum with convexity posteriorly; after child stands, convexity persists only in *thoracic* and *sacral* regions, which therefore are called primary curves
Secondary	Concavities in *cervical* and *lumbar* regions; cervical concavity results from infant's attempts to hold head erect (3 to 4 months); lumbar concavity, from balancing efforts in learning to walk (10 to 18 months)
Abnormal	*Kyphosis,* exaggerated convexity in thoracic region (hunchback); *lordosis,* exaggerated concavity in lumbar region, a very common condition; *scoliosis,* lateral curvature in any region
SCAPULA	
Borders	
Superior	Upper margion
Vertebral	Margin toward vertebral column
Axillary	Lateral margin
Spine	Sharp ridge running diagonally across posterior surface of shoulder blade
Acromion process	Slightly flaring projection at lateral end of scapular spine; may be felt as tip of shoulder; articulates with clavicle
Coracoid process	Projection on anterior surface from upper border of bone; may be felt in groove between deltoid and pectoralis major muscles, about 1 inch below clavicle
Glenoid cavity	Arm socket

Marking	Description
STERNUM	
Body	Main central part of bone
Manubrium	Flaring, upper part
Xiphoid process	Projection of cartilage at lower border of bone
RIBS	
Head	Projection at posterior end of rib; articulates with corresponding thoracic vertebra and one above, except last three pairs, which join corresponding vertebrae only
Neck	Constricted portion just below head
Tubercle	Small knob just below neck; articulates with transverse process of corresponding thoracic vertebra; missing in lowest three ribs
Body or shaft	Main part of rib
Costal cartilage	Cartilage at sternal end of true ribs; attaches ribs (except floating ribs) to sternum
HUMERUS	
Head	Smooth, hemispherical enlargement at proximal end of humerus
Anatomical neck	Oblique groove just below head
Greater tubercle	Rounded projection lateral to head on anterior surface
Lesser tubercle	Prominent projection on anterior surface just below anatomical neck
Intertubercular	Deep groove between greater and lesser tubercles; long tendon of biceps muscle lodges here
Surgical neck	Region just below tubercles; so named because of its liability to fracture
Deltoid tuberosity	V-shaped, rough area about midway down shaft where deltoid muscle inserts
Radial groove	Groove running obliquely downward from deltoid tuberosity; lodges radial nerve
Epicondyles (medial and lateral)	Rough projections at both sides of distal end
Capitulum	Rounded knob below lateral epicondyle; articulates with radius; sometimes called radial head of humerus
Trochlea	Projection with deep depression through center similar to shape of pulley; articulates with ulna
Olecranon fossa	Depression on posterior surface just above trochlea; receives olecranon process of ulna when lower arm extends
Coronoid fossa	Depression of anterior surface above trochlea; receives coronoid process of ulna in flexion of lower arm

Marking	Description
ULNA	
Olecranon process	Elbow
Coronoid process	Projection on anterior surface of proximal end of ulna; trochlea of humerus fits snugly between olecranon and coronoid processes
Semilunar notch	Curved notch between olecranon and coronoid process, into which trochlea fits
Radial notch	Curved notch lateral and inferior to semilunar notch; head of radius fits into this concavity
Head	Rounded process at distal end; does not articulate with wrist bones but with fibrocartilaginous disk
Styloid process	Sharp protuberance at distal end; can be seen from outside on posterior surface
RADIUS	
Head	Disk-shaped process forming proximal end of radius; articulates with capitulum of humerus and with radial notch of ulna
Radial tuberosity	Roughened projection on ulnar side, short distance below head; biceps muscle inserts here
Styloid process	Protuberance at distal end on lateral surface (with forearm supinated as in anatomical position)
FEMUR	
Head	Rounded, upper end of bone; fits into acetabulum
Neck	Constricted portion just below head
Greater trochanter	Protuberance located inferiorly and laterally to head
Lesser trochanter	Small protuberance located inferiorly and medially to greater trochanter
Linea aspera	Prominent ridge extending lengthwise along concave posterior surface
Gluteal tubercle	Rounded projection just below greater trochanter; rudimentary third trochanter
Supracondylar ridges	Two ridges formed by division of linea aspera at its lower end; medial supracondylar ridge extends inward to inner condyle, lateral ridge to outer condyle
Condyles	Large, rounded bulges at distal end of femur; one on medial and one on lateral surface
Adductor tubercle	Small projection just above inner condyle; marks termination of medial supracondylar ridge
Trochlea	Smooth depression between condyles on anterior surface; articulates with patella
Intercondyloid notch	Deep depression between condyles on posterior surface; cruciate ligaments that help bind femur to tibia lodge in this notch

Continued.

Identification of bone markings—cont'd

Marking	Description
OS COXAE	
Ilium	Upper, flaring portion
Ischium	Lower, posterior portion
Pubic bone or pubis	Medial, anterior section
Acetabulum	Hip socket; formed by union of ilium, ischium, and pubis
Iliac crests	Upper, curving boundary of ilium
Iliac spines	
Anterior superior	Prominent projection at anterior end of iliac crest; can be felt externally as "point" of hip
Anterior inferior	Less prominent projection short distance below anterior superior spine
Posterior superior	At posterior end of iliac crest
Posterior inferior	Just below posterior superior spine
Greater sciatic notch	Large notch on posterior surface of ilium just below posterior inferior spine
Gluteal lines	Three curved lines across outer surface of ilium—posterior, anterior, inferior, respectively
Iliopectineal line	Rounded ridge extending from pubic tubercle upward and backward toward sacrum
Iliac fossa	Large, smooth, concave inner surface of ilium above iliopectineal line
Ischial tuberosity	Large, rough, quadrilateral process forming inferior part of ischium; in erect sitting position body rests on these tuberosities
Ischial spine	Pointed projection just above tuberosity
Symphysis pubis	Cartilaginous, amphiarthrotic joint between pubic bones
Superior pubic ramus	Part of pubis lying between symphysis and acetabulum; forms upper part of obturator foramen
Inferior pubic ramus	Part extending down from symphysis; unites with ischium
Pubic arch	Angle formed by two inferior rami
Pubic crest	Upper margin of superior ramus
Pubic tubercle	Rounded process at end of crest
Obturator foramen	Large hole in anterior surface of os coxa; formed by pubis and ischium; largest foramen in body
Pelvic brim (or inlet)	Boundary of aperture leading into true pelvis; formed by pubic crests, iliopectineal lines, and sacral promontory; size and shape of this inlet has great obstetrical importance, since if any of its diameters are too small, infant skull cannot enter true pelvis for natural birth
True (or lesser) pelvis	Space below pelvic brim; true "basin" with bone and muscle walls and muscle floor; pelvic organs located in this space
False (or greater) pelvis	Broad, shallow space above pelvic brim, or pelvic inlet; name "false pelvis" is misleading, since this space is actually part of abdominal cavity, not pelvic cavity
Pelvic outlet	Irregular circumference marking lower limits of true pelvis; bounded by tip of coccyx and two ischial tuberosities
Pelvic girdle (or bony pelvis)	Complete bony ring; composed of two hip bones (ossa coxae), sacrum, and coccyx; forms firm base by which trunk rests on thighs and for attachment of lower extremities to axial skeleton
TIBIA	
Condyles	Bulging prominences at proximal end of tibia; upper surfaces concave for articulation with femur
Intercondylar eminence	Upward projection on articular surface between condyles
Crest	Sharp ridge on anterior surface
Tibial tuberosity	Projection in midline on anterior surface
Popliteal line	Ridge that spirals downward and inward on posterior surface of upper third of tibial shaft
Medial malleolus	Rounded downward projection at distal end of tibia; forms prominence on inner surface of ankle
FIBULA	
Lateral malleolus	Rounded prominence at distal end of fibula; forms prominence on outer surface of ankle
TARSALS	
Calcaneus	Heel bone
Talus	Uppermost of tarsals; articulates with tibia and fibula; boxes in by medial and lateral malleoli
Longitudinal arches	Tarsals and metatarsals so arranged as to form arch from front to back of foot
Medial	Formed by calcaneus, talus, navicular, cuneiforms, and three medial metatarsals
Lateral	Formed by calcaneus, cuboid, and two lateral metatarsals
Transverse (or metatarsal) arch	Metatarsals and distal row of tarsals (cuneiforms and cuboid) so articulated as to form arch across foot; bones kept in two arched positions by means of powerful ligaments in sole of foot and by muscles and tendons

Classification of joints

Joints	*Description*	*Movement*	*Example*
Fibrous			
Sutures	Thin layer of fibrous tissue (extension of periosteum); grows between articulating surfaces of bones; fibrous connection replaced by bone in older adults	None (synarthroses)	Sutures between certain skull bones
Syndesmoses	Same as sutures, but fibrous tissue not eventually replaced by bone	None (synarthroses)	Distal tibiofibular
Cartilaginous			
Symphyses	Fibrocartilage connects articulating surfaces of bones; joint capsule present, and sometimes a joint cavity	Slight (amphiarthroses)	Symphysis pubis; joints between bodies of vertebrae
Synchondroses	Hyaline cartilage connects epiphyses to diaphysis of growing bones	Ordinarily none	In all growing long bones
Synovial			
Ball and socket (spheroidal, endarthroses)	Ball-shaped head fits into concave socket	Widest range of all joints; triaxial	Shoulder joint and hip joint
Hinge (ginglymus)	Spool-shaped surface, fits into concave surface	In one plane about single axis (uniaxial); like hinged-door movement, namely, flexion and extension	Elbow, knee, ankle, and interphalangeal joints
Pivot (trochoid)	Arch-shaped surface rotates about rounded or peglike pivot	Rotation; uniaxial	Between axis and atlas; between radius and ulna
Ellipsoidal (condyloid, ovoid)	Oval-shaped condyle fits into elliptical cavity	In two planes at right angles to each other—specifically, flexion, extension, abduction, and adduction; biaxial	Wrist joint (between radius and carpals)
Saddle	Saddle-shaped bone fits into socket that is concave-convex in opposite direction; modification of condyloid joint	Same kinds of movement as condyloid joint but freer; like rider in saddle; biaxial	Thumb, between first metacarpal and trapezium, is only saddle joint
Gliding (arthrodia)	Articulating surfaces; usually flat	Gliding—a nonaxial movement	Between carpals and between tarsals

Description of individual joints

Name	*Articulating bones*	*Type*	*Movements*
Atlantoepistropheal	Anterior arch of atlas rotates about dens of axis (epistropheus)	Diarthrotic (pivot type)	Pivoting or partial rotation of head
Vertebral	Between bodies of vertebrae	Amphiarthrotic, cartilaginous	Slight movement between any two vertebrae but considerable mobility for column as whole
	Between articular processes	Diarthrotic (gliding)	
Sternoclavicular	Medial end of clavicle with manubrium of sternum; only joint between upper extremity and trunk	Diarthrotic (gliding)	Gliding; weak joint that may be injured comparatively easily
Acromioclavicular	Distal end of clavicle with acromion of scapula	Diarthrotic (gliding)	Gliding; elevation, depression, protraction, and retraction
Thoracic	Heads of ribs with bodies of vertebrae	Diarthrotic (gliding)	Gliding
	Tubercles of ribs with transverse processes of vertebrae	Diarthrotic (gliding)	Gliding
Shoulder	Head of humerus in glenoid cavity of scapula	Diarthrotic (ball and socket type)	Flexion, extension, abduction, adduction, rotation, and circumduction of upper arm; one of most freely movable of joints
Elbow	Trochlea of humerus with semilunar notch of ulna; head of radius with capitulum of humerus	Diarthrotic (hinge type)	Flexion and extension
	Head of radius in radial notch of ulna	Diarthrotic (pivot type)	Supination and pronation of lower arm and hand; rotation of lower arm on upper as in using screwdriver
Wrist	Scaphoid, lunate, and triquetral bones articulate with radius and articular disk	Diarthrotic (condyloid)	Flexion, extension, abduction, and adduction of hand
Carpal	Between various carpals	Diarthrotic (gliding)	Gliding
Hand	Proximal end of first metacarpal with trapezium	Diarthrotic (saddle)	Flexion, extension, abduction, adduction, and circumduction of thumb and opposition to fingers; motility of this joint accounts for dexterity of human hand compared with animal forepaw
	Distal end of metacarpals with proximal end of phalanges	Diarthrotic (hinge)	Flexion, extension, limited abduction, and adduction of fingers
	Between phalanges	Diarthrotic (hinge)	Flexion and extension of finger sections
Sacroiliac	Between sacrum and two ilia	Diarthrotic (gliding); joint cavity mostly obliterated after middle life	None or slight, for example, during late months of pregnancy and during delivery
Symphysis pubis	Between two pubic bones	Synarthrotic (or amphiarthrotic), cartilaginous	Slight, particularly during pregnancy and delivery
Hip	Head of femur in acetabulum of os coxae	Diarthrotic (ball and socket)	Flexion, extension, abduction, adduction, rotation, and circumduction
Knee	Between distal end of femur and proximal end of tibia; largest joint in body	Diarthrotic (hinge type)	Flexion and extension; slight rotation of tibia
Tibiofibular	Head of fibula with lateral condyle of tibia	Diarthrotic (gliding type)	Gliding
Ankle	Distal ends of tibia and fibula with talus	Diarthrotic (hinge type)	Flexion (dorsiflexion) and extension (plantar flexion)
Foot	Between tarsals	Diarthrotic (gliding)	Gliding; inversion and eversion
	Between metatarsals and phalanges	Diarthrotic (hinge type)	Flexion, extension, slight abduction, and adduction
	Between phalanges	Diarthrotic (hinge type)	Flexion and extension

4-3 Muscular system

Muscles grouped according to location

Location	Muscles	Location	Muscles
Neck	Sternocleidomastoid	Thigh	
Back	Trapezius	Anterior surface	Quadriceps femoris group
	Latissimus dorsi		Rectus femoris
Chest	Pectoralis major		Vastus lateralis
	Serratus anterior		Vastus medialis
Abdominal wall	External oblique		Vastus intermedius
Shoulder	Deltoid	Medial surface	Gracilis
Upper arm	Biceps brachii		Adductor group (brevis, longus, magnus)
	Triceps brachii	Posterior surface	Hamstring group
	Brachialis		Biceps femoris
Forearm	Brachioradialis		Semitendinosus
	Pronator teres		Semimembranosus
Buttocks	Gluteus maximus	Leg	
	Gluteus minimus	Anterior surface	Tibialis anterior
	Gluteus medius	Posterior surface	Gastrocnemius
	Tensor fascia latae		Soleus
		Pelvic floor	Levator ani
			Levator coccygeus
			Rectococcygeus

Muscles grouped according to function

Part moved	Example of flexor	Example of extensor	Example of abductor	Example of adductor
Head	Sternocleidomastoid	Semispinalis capitis		
Upper arm	Pectoralis major	Trapezius Latissimus dorsi	Deltoid	Pectoralis major with latissimus dorsi
Forearm	With forearm supinated: biceps brachii With forearm pronated: brachialis With semisupination or semipronation: brachioradialis	Triceps brachii		
Hand	Flexor carpi radialis and ulnaris Palmaris longus	Extensor carpi radialis, longus, and brevis Extensor carpi ulnaris	Flexor carpi radialis	Flexor carpi ulnaris
Thigh	Iliopsoas Rectus femoris (of quadriceps femoris group)	Gluteus maximus	Gluteus medius and gluteus minimus	Adductor group
Leg	Hamstrings	Quadriceps femoris group		
Foot	Tibialis anterior	Gastrocnemius Soleus	Evertors Peroneus longus Peroneus brevis	Invettor Tibialis anterior
Trunk	Iliopsoas Rectus abdominis	Sacrospinalis		

Muscles that move the head

Muscle	Origin	Insertion	Function	Innervation
Sternocleidomastoid	Sternum Clavicle	Temporal bone (mastoid process)	Flexes head (prayer muscle) One muscle alone, rotates head toward opposite side; spasm of this muscle alone or associated with trapezius called torticollis or wryneck	Accessory nerve
Semispinalis capitis	Vertebrae (transverse processes of upper six thoracic, articular processes of lower four cervical)	Occipital bone (between superior and inferior nuchal lines)	Extends head; bends it laterally	First five cervical nerves
Splenius capitis	Ligamentum nuchae Vertebrae (spinous processes of upper three or four thoracic)	Temporal bone (mastoid process) Occipital bone	Extends head Bends and rotates head toward same side as contracting muscle	Second, third, and fourth cervical nerves
Longissimus capitis	Vertebrae (transverse processes of upper six thoracic, articular processes of lower four cervical)	Temporal bone (mastoid process)	Extends head Bends and rotates head toward contracting side	

Muscles of facial expression and of mastication

Muscle	Origin	Insertion	Function	Innervation
Muscles of facial expression				
Epicranius (occipitofrontalis)	Occipital bone	Tissues of eyebrows	Raises eyebrows, wrinkles forehead horizontally	Cranial nerve VII
Corrugator supercilii	Frontal bone (superciliary ridge)	Skin of eyebrow	Wrinkles forehead vertically	Cranial nerve VII
Orbicularis oculi	Encircles eyelid		Closes eye	Cranial nerve VII
Orbicularis oris	Encircles mouth		Draws lips together	Cranial nerve VII
Platysma	Fascia of upper part of deltoid and pectoralis major	Mandible (lower border) Skin around corners of mouth	Draws corners of mouth down—pouting	Cranial nerve VII
Buccinator	Maxillae	Skin of sides of mouth	Permits smiling Blowing, as in playing a trumpet	Cranial nerve VII
Muscles of mastication				
Masseter	Zygomatic arch	Mandible (external surface)	Closes jaw	Cranial nerve V
Temporal	Temporal bone	Mandible	Closes jaw	Cranial nerve V
Pterygoids (internal and external)	Undersurface of skull	Mandible (mesial surface)	Grate teeth	Cranial nerve V

Muscles that move the shoulder

Muscle	Origin	Insertion	Function	Innervation
Trapezius	Occipital bone (protuberance) Vertebrae (cervical and thoracic)	Clavicle Scapula (spine and acromion)	Raises or lowers shoulders and shrugs them Extends head when occiput acts as insertion	Spinal accessory, second, third, and fourth cervical nerves
Pectoralis minor	Ribs (second to fifth)	Scapula (coracoid)	Pulls shoulder down and forward	Medial and lateral anterior thoracic nerves
Serratus anterior	Ribs (upper eight or nine)	Scapula (anterior surface, vertebral border)	Pulls shoulder forward; abducts and rotates it upward	Long thoracic nerve

Muscles that move the upper arm

Muscle	Origin	Insertion	Function	Innervation
Pectoralis major	Clavicle (medial half) Sternum Costal cartilages of true ribs	Humerus (greater tubercle)	Flexes upper arm Adducts upper arm anteriorly; draws it across chest	Medial and lateral anterior thoracic nerves
Latissimus dorsi	Vertebrae (spines of lower thoracic, lumbar, and sacral) Ilium (crest) Lumbodorsal fascia*	Humerus (intertubercular groove)	Extends upper arm Adducts upper arm posteriorly	Thoracodorsal nerve
Deltoid	Clavicle Scapula (spine and acromion)	Humerus (lateral side about halfway down—deltoid tubercle)	Abducts upper arm Assists in flexion and extension of upper arm	Axillary nerve
Coracobrachialis	Scapula (coracoid process)	Humerus (middle third, medial surface)	Adduction; assists in flexion and medial rotation of arm	Musculocutaneous nerve
Supraspinatus	Scapula (supraspinous fossa)	Humerus (greater tubercle)	Assists in abducting arm	Suprascapular nerve
Teres major	Scapula (lower part, axillary border)	Humerus (upper part, anterior surface)	Assists in extension, adduction, and medial rotation of arm	Lower subscapular nerve
Teres minor	Scapula (axillary border)	Humerus (greater tubercle)	Rotates arm outward	Axillary nerve
Infraspinatus	Scapula (infraspinatus border)	Humerus (greater tubercle)	Rotates arm outward	Suprascapular nerve

*Lumbodorsal fascia—extension of aponeurosis of latissimus dorsi; fills in space between last rib and iliac crest.

Muscles that move the lower arm

Muscle	Origin	Insertion	Function	Innervation
Biceps brachii	Scapula (supraglenoid tuberosity)	Radius (tubercle at proximal end)	Flexes supinated forearm Supinates forearm and hand	Musculocutaneous nerve
Brachialis	Humerus (distal half, anterior surface)	Ulna (front of coronoid process)	Flexes pronated forearm	Musculocutaneous nerve
Brachioradialis	Humerus (above lateral epicondyle)	Radius (styloid process)	Flexes semipronated or semisupinated forearm; supinates forearm and hand	Radial nerve
Triceps brachii	Scapula (infraglenoid tuberosity) Humerus (posterior surface—lateral head above radial groove; medial head, below)	Ulna (olecranon process)	Extends lower arm	Radial nerve
Pronator teres	Humerus (medial epicondyle) Ulna (coronoid process)	Radius (middle third of lateral surface)	Pronates and flexes forearm	Median nerve
Pronator quadratus	Ulna (distal fourth, anterior surface)	Radius (distal fourth, anterior surface)	Pronates forearm	Median nerve
Supinator	Humerus (lateral epicondyle) Ulna (proximal fifth)	Radius (proximal third)	Supinates forearm	Radial nerve

Muscles that move the hand

Muscle	Origin	Insertion	Function	Innervation
Flexor carpi radialis	Humerus (medial epicondyle)	Second metacarpal (base of)	Flexes hand Flexes forearm	Median nerve
Palmaris longus	Humerus (medial epicondyle)	Fascia of palm	Flexes hand	Median nerve
Flexor carpi ulnaris	Humerus (medial epicondyle) Ulna (proximal two thirds)	Pisiform bone Third, fourth, and fifth metacarpals	Flexes hand Adducts hand	Ulnar nerve
Extensor carpi radialis longus	Humerus (ridge above lateral epicondyle)	Second metacarpal (base of)	Extends hand Abducts hand (moves toward thumb side when hand supinated)	Radial nerve
Extensor carpi radialis brevis	Humerus (lateral epicondyle)	Second, third metacarpals (bases of)	Extends hand	Radial nerve
Extensor carpi ulnaris	Humerus (lateral epicondyle) Ulna (proximal three fourths)	Fifth metacarpal (base of)	Extends hand Adducts hand (move toward little finger side when hand supinated)	Radial nerve

Muscles that move the trunk

Muscle	Origin	Insertion	Function	Innervation
Sacrospinalis (erector spinae)			Extend spine; maintain erect posture of trunk Acting singly, abduct and rotate trunk	Posterior rami of first cervical to fifth lumbar spinal nerves
Lateral portion				
Iliocostalis lumborum	Iliac crest, sacrum (posterior surface), and lumbar vertebrae (spinous processes)	Ribs, lower six		
Iliocostalis dorsi	Ribs, lower six	Ribs, upper six		
Iliocostalis cervicis	Ribs, upper six	Vertebrae, fourth to sixth cervical		
Medial portion				
Longissimus dorsi	Same as iliocostalis lumborum	Vertebrae, thoracic ribs		
Longissimus cervicis	Vertebrae, upper six thoracic	Vertebrae, second to sixth cervical		
Longissimus capitis	Vertebrae, upper six thoracic and last four cervical	Temporal bone, mastoid process		
Quadratus lumborum (forms part of posterior abdominal wall)	Ilium (posterior part of crest) Vertebrae (lower three lumbar)	Ribs (twelfth) Vertebrae (transverse processes of first four lumbar)	Both muscles together extend spine One muscle alone abducts trunk toward side of contracting muscle	First three or four lumbar nerves
Iliopsoas	See muscles that move the thigh		Flexes trunk	

Muscles that move the chest wall

Muscle	Origin	Insertion	Function	Innervation
External intercostals	Rib (lower border; forward fibers)	Rib (upper border of rib below origin)	Elevate ribs	Intercostal nerves
Internal intercostals	Rib (inner surface, lower border; backward fibers)	Rib (upper border of rib below origin)	Probably depress ribs	Intercostal nerves
Diaphragm	Lower circumference of thorax (of rib cage)	Central tendon of diaphragm	Enlarges thorax, causing inspiration	Phrenic nerves

Muscles that move the abdominal wall

Muscle	Origin	Insertion	Function	Innervation
External oblique	Ribs (lower eight)	Ossa coxae (iliac crest and pubis by way of inguinal ligament)* Linea alba† by way of an aponeurosis‡	Compresses abdomen Important postural function of all abdominal muscles is to pull front of pelvis upward, thereby flattening lumbar curve of spine; when these muscles lose their tone, common figure faults of protruding abdomen and lordosis develop	Lower seven intercostal nerves and iliohypogastric nerves
Internal oblique	Ossa coxae (iliac crest and inguinal ligament) Lumbodorsal fascia	Ribs (lower three) Pubic bone Linea alba	Same as external oblique	Last three intercostal nerves; iliohypogastric and ilioinguinal nerves
Transversalis	Ribs (lower six) Ossa coxae (iliac crest, inguinal ligament) Lumbodorsal fascia	Pubic bone Linea alba	Same as external oblique	Last five intercostal nerves; iliohypogastric and ilioinguinal nerves
Rectus abdominis	Ossa coxae (pubic bone and symphysis pubis)	Ribs (costal cartilage of fifth, sixth, and seventh ribs) Sternum (xiphoid process)	Same as external oblique; because abdominal muscles compress abdominal cavity, they aid in straining, defecation, forced expiration, and childbirth; abdominal muscles are antagonists of diaphragm, relaxing as it contracts and vice versa Flexes trunk	Last six intercostal nerves

*Inguinal ligament (or Poupart's)—lower edge of aponeurosis of external oblique muscle, extending between the anterior superior iliac spine and the tubercle of the pubic bone. This edge is doubled under like a hem. The inguinal ligament forms the upper boundary of the femoral triangle, a large triangular area in the thigh; its other boundaries are the adductor longus muscle medially and the sartorius muscle laterally.

†Linea alba—literally, a white line; extends from xiphoid process to symphysis pubis; formed by fibers of aponeuroses of the right abdominal muscles interlacing with fibers of aponeuroses of the left abdominal muscles; comparable to a seam up the midline of the abdominal wall, anchoring its various layers. During pregnancy the linea alba becomes pigmented and is known as the linea niger.

‡Aponeurosis—sheet of white fibrous tissue that attaches one muscle to another or attaches it to bone or other movable structures, for example, the right external oblique muscle attaches to the left external oblique muscle by means of an aponeurosis.

Muscles of the pelvic floor

Muscle	Origin	Insertion	Function	Innervation
Levator ani	Pubis (posterior surface) Ischium (spine)	Coccyx	Together form floor of pelvic cavity; support pelvic organs; if these muscles are badly torn at childbirth or become too relaxed, uterus or bladder may prolapse, that is, drop out	Pudendal nerve
Coccygeus (posterior continuation of levator ani)	Ischium (spine)	Coccyx Sacrum	Same as levator ani	Pudendal nerve

Muscles that move the thigh

Muscle	Origin	Insertion	Function	Innervation
Iliopsoas (iliacus and psoas major)	Ilium (iliac fossa) Vertebrae (bodies of twelfth thoracic to fifth lumbar)	Femur (small trochanter)	Flexes thigh Flexes trunk (when femur acts as origin)	Femoral and second to fourth lumbar nerves
Rectus femoris	Ilium (anterior, inferior spine)	Tibia (by way of patellar tendon)	Flexes thigh Extends lower leg	Femoral nerve
Gluteal group				
Maximus	Ilium (crest and posterior surface) Sacrum and coccyx (posterior surface) Sacrotuberous ligament	Femur (gluteal tuberosity) Iliotibial tract*	Extends thigh—rotates outward	Inferior gluteal nerve
Medius	Ilium (lateral surface)	Femur (greater trochanter)	Abducts thigh—rotates outward; stabilizes pelvis on femur	Superior gluteal nerve
Minimus	Ilium (lateral surface)	Femur (greater trochanter)	Abducts thigh; stabilizes pelvis on femur Rotates high medially	Superior gluteal nerve
Tensor fasciae latae	Ilium (anterior part of crest)	Tibia (by way of iliotibial tract)	Abducts thigh Tightens iliotibal tract*	Superior gluteal nerve
Piriformis	Vertebrae (front of sacrum)	Femur (medial aspect of greater trochanter)	Rotates thigh outward Abducts thigh Extends thigh	First or second sacral nerves
Adductor group				
Brevis	Pubic bone	Femur (linea aspera)	Adducts thigh	Obturator nerve
Longus	Pubic bone	Femur (linea aspera)	Adducts thigh	Obturator nerve
Magnus	Pubic bone	Femur (linea aspera)	Adducts thigh	Obturator nerve
Gracilis	Pubic bone (just below symphysis)	Tibia (medial surface behind sartorius)	Adducts thigh and flexes and adducts leg	Obturator nerve

*The iliotibial tract is part of the fascia enveloping all the thigh muscles. It consists of a wide band of dense fibrous tissue attached to the iliac crest above and the lateral condyle of the tibia below. The upper part of the tract encloses the tensor fasciae latae muscle.

Muscles that move the lower leg

Muscle	Origin	Insertion	Function	Innervation
Quadriceps femoris group				
Rectus femoris	Ilium (anterior, inferior spine)	Tibia (by way of patellar tendon)	Flexes thigh Extends leg	Femoral nerve
Vastus lateralis	Femur (linea aspera)	Tibia (by way of patellar tendon)	Extends leg	Femoral nerve
Vastus medialis	Femur	Tibia (by way of patellar tendon)	Extends leg	Femoral nerve
Vastus intermedius	Femur (anterior surface)	Tibia (by way of patellar tendon)	Extends leg	Femoral nerve
Sartorius	Os innominatum (anterior, superior iliac spines)	Tibia (medial surface of upper end of shaft)	Adducts and flexes leg Permits crossing of legs tailor fashion	Femoral nerve
Hamstring group				
Biceps femoris	Ischium (tuberosity)	Fibula (head of)	Flexes leg	Hamstring nerve (branch of sciatic nerve)
	Femur (linea aspera)	Tibia (lateral condyle)	Extends thigh	Hamstring nerve
Semitendinosus	Ischium (tuberosity)	Tibia (proximal end, medial surface)	Extends thigh	Hamstring nerve
Semimembranosus	Ischium (tuberosity)	Tibia (medial condyle)	Extends thigh	Hamstring nerve

Muscles that move the foot

Muscle	Origin	Insertion	Function	Innervation
Tibialis anterior	Tibia (lateral condyle of upper body)	Tarsal (first cuneiform) Metatarsal (base of first)	Flexes foot Inverts foot	Common and deep peroneal nerves
Gastrocnemius	Femur (condyles)	Tarsal (calcaneus by way of Achilles tendon)	Extends foot Flexes lower leg	Tibial nerve (branch of sciatic nerve)
Soleus	Tibia (underneath gastrocnemius) Fibula	Tarsal (calcaneus by way of Achilles tendon)	Extends foot (plantar flexion)	Tibial nerve
Peroneus longus	Tibia (lateral condyle) Fibula (head and shaft)	First cuneiform Base of first metatarsal	Extends foot (plantar flexion) Everts foot	Common peroneal nerve
Peroneus brevis	Fibula (lower two thirds of lateral surface of shaft)	Fifth metatarsal (tubercle, dorsal surface)	Everts foot Flexes foot	Superficial peroneal nerve
Tibialis posterior	Tibia (posterior surface) Fibula (posterior surface)	Navicular bone Cuboid bone All three cuneiforms Second and fourth metatarsals	Extends foot (plantar flexion) Inverts foot	Tibial nerve
Peroneus tertius	Fibula (distal third)	Fourth and fifth metatarsals (bases of)	Flexes foot Everts foot	Deep peroneal nerve

4-4 Circulatory system

Blood cells

Cells	Number	Function	Formation (hemopoiesis)	Destruction
Red blood cells (erythrocytes)	4.5 to 5.5 million/mm^3 (total of approximately 30 trillion in adult body)	Transport oxygen and carbon dioxide	Red marrow of bones (myeloid tissue)	Reticuloendothelial cells in lining of blood vessels in liver, spleen, and bone marrow phagocytose old red blood cells; live about 105 to 120 days in bloodstream
White blood cells (leukocytes)	Usually about 5000 to 9000/mm^3	Play important part in producing immunity; for example, phagocytosis by neutrophils and monocytes; antibody formation by lymphocytes and their descendents, plasma cells; production of heparin by basophils; detoxification by eosinophils	Granular leukocytes in red marrow; before birth and for a few months after, some lymphocytes are formed in thymus gland; later, most lymphocytes and monocytes formed in lymph nodes and other lymphatic tissues	Not known definitely; probably some destroyed by phagocytosis
Platelets (thrombocytes)	150,000 to 35,000/mm^3	Initiate blood clotting and hemostasis	Red marrow, lungs, and spleen	Unknown

Structure of blood vessels

Arteries	Veins	Capillaries
Coats Outer coat (tunica adventitia or externa) of white fibrous tissue; causes artery to stand open instead of collapsing when cut Muscle coat (tunica media) of smooth muscle, elastic, and some white fibrous tissues; this coat permits constriction and dilation Lining (tunica intima) of endothelium	Same three coats but thinner and fewer elastic fibers; veins collapse when cut; semilunar valves present at intervals	Only lining coat present; therefore walls only one cell thick

Blood supply

Endothelial lining cells supplied by blood flowing through vessels; exchange of oxygen, etc., between cells of middle coat and blood by diffusion; outer coat supplied by tiny vessels known as vasa vasorum or "vessels of vessels"

Nerve supply

Smooth muscle cells of tunica media innervated by autonomic fibers

Abnormalities

Atherosclerosis—hardening of walls of arteries (arteriosclerosis) characterized by lipid deposits in tunica intima
Aneurysm—saclike dilation of artery wall
Varicose veins—stretching of walls, particularly around semilunar valves
Phlebitis—inflammation of vein; "milk leg," phlebitis of femoral vein of women after childbirth

Coronary arteries

Right coronary artery	Left coronary artery
Divides into two main branches: Posterior descending artery—sends branches to both ventricles Marginal artery—sends branches to right ventricle and right atrium	Divides into two main branches: Anterior descending artery—sends branches to ventricles Circumflex artery—sends branches to left ventricle and left atrium

White blood cells (leukocytes)

Class	*Differential count**	
	Normal range (%)	*Typical normal (%)*
Those with granular cytoplasm and irregular nuclei		
Neutrophils (neutral staining)	65 to 75	65
Eosinophils (acid staining)	2 to 5	3
Basophils (basic staining)	½ to 1	1
Those with nongranular cytoplasm and regular nuclei		
Lymphocytes (large and small)	20 to 25	25
Monocytes	3 to 8	6
TOTAL		100

*In any differential count the sum of the percentages of the different kinds of leukocytes must, of course, total 100%.

Main arteries

Artery	*Branches (only largest ones named)*
Ascending aorta	Coronary arteries (two, to myocardium)
Aortic arch	Innominate (or brachiocephalic) artery
	Left subclavian
	Left common carotid
Innominate	Right subclavian
	Right common carotid
Subclavian (right and left)	Vertebral*
	Axillary (continuation of subclavian)
Axillary	Brachial (continuation of axillary)
Brachial	Radial
	Ulnar
Radial and ulnar	Palmer arches (superficial and deep arterial arches in hand formed by anastomosis of branches of radial and ulnar arteries; numerous branches to hand and fingers)
Common carotid (right and left)	Internal carotid (brain, eye, forehead, and nose)*
	External carotid (thyroid, tongue, tonsils, ear)
Descending thoracic aorta	Visceral branches to pericardium, bronchi, esophagus, mediastinum
	Parietal branches to chest muscles, mammary glands, and diaphragm
Descending abdominal aorta	Visceral branches:
	Celiac axis (or artery), which branches into gastric, hepatic, and splenic arteries (stomach, liver, and spleen)
	Right and left suprarenal arteries (suprarenal glands)
	Superior mesenteric artery (small intestine)
	Right and left renal arteries (kidneys)
	Right and left spermatic (or ovarian) arteries (testes or ovaries)
	Inferior mesenteric artery (large intestine)
	Parietal branches to lower surface of diaphragm, muscles and skin of back, spinal cord, and meninges
	Right and left common iliac arteries—abdominal aorta terminates in these vessels in an inverted Y formation
Right and left common iliac	Internal iliac or hypogastric (pelvic wall and viscera)
	External iliac (to leg)
External iliac (right and left)	Femoral (continuation of external iliac after it leaves abdominal cavity)
Femoral	Popliteal (continuation of femoral
Popliteal	Anterior tibial
	Posterior tibial
Anterior and posterior tibial	Plantar arch (arterial arch in sole of foot formed by anastomosis of terminal branches of anterior and posterior tibial arteries; small arteries lead from arch to toes)

*The right and left vertebral arteries extend from their origin as branches of the subclavian arteries up the neck, through foramina in the transverse processes of the cervical vertebrae, and through the foramen magnum into the cranial cavity and unite on the undersurface of the brainstem to form the *basilar artery,* which shortly branches into the right and left *posterior cerebral arteries*. The internal carotid arteries enter the cranial cavity in the midpart of the cranial floor, where they become known as the *anterior cerebral arteries*. Small vessels, the *communicating arteries,* join the anterior and posterior cerebral arteries in such a way as to form an arterial circle (the *circle of Willis*) at the base of the brain, a good example of arterial anastomosis.

4-5 Endocrine system

Production, control, and effects of pituitary hormones

Pituitary gland (hypophysis cerebri)	*Hormone*	*Source (cell type or location)*	*Control mechanism*	*Effect*
Anterior pituitary gland (adenohypophysis)	Growth hormone (GH, somatotropin [STH])	Acidophils	GRH (growth hormone–releasing hormone) from hypothalamus	Promotes body growth, protein anabolism, and mobilization and catabolism of fats; decreases glucose catabolism; increases blood glucose levels
Pars anterior	Prolactin (lactogenic or luteotropic hormone [LTH])	Acidophils	Prolactin inhibitory factor (PIF); prolactin-releasing factor (PRF) from hypothalamus and high blood levels of oxytocin	Stimulates milk secretion and development of secretory alveoli; helps maintain corpus luteum
	Thyrotropin (TH); thyroid-stimulating hormone (TSH)	Basophils	Thyrotropin-releasing hormone (TRH) from hypothalamus	Growth and maintenance of thyroid gland and stimulation of thyroid hormone secretion
	Adrenocorticotropin (ACTH)	Basophils	Corticotropin-releasing factor (CRF) from hypothalamus	Growth and maintenance of adrenal cortex and stimulation of cortisol and other glucocorticoid secretions
	Follicle-stimulating hormone (FSH)	Basophils	Follicle-stimulating hormone–releasing hormone (FSH-RH) from hypothalamus	In female—stimulates follicle growth and maturation and estrogen secretion In male—stimulates development of seminiferous tubules and maintains spermatogenesis
	Luteinizing hormone (LH in female, ICSH in male)	Basophils	Luteinizing hormone–releasing hormone (LH-RH) from hypothalamus	In female (LH)—induces ovulation and stimulates formation of corpus luteum and progesterone secretion In male (ICSH)—stimulates interstitial cell secretion of testosterone
Pars intermedia	Melanocyte-stimulating hormone (MSH); intermedin	Basophils	Unknown in humans	May cause darkening of the skin by increasing melanin production
Posterior pituitary gland (neurohypophysis)	ADH (vasopressin)	Hypothalamus, mainly supraoptic nucleus	Osmoreceptors in hypothalamus stimulated by increase in blood osmotic pressure, decrease in extracellular fluid volume, and stress	Decreased urine output
	Oxytocin	Hypothalamus, paraventricular nucleus	Nervous stimulation of hypothalamus caused by stimulation of nipples (nursing)	Contraction of uterine smooth muscle and ejection of milk into lactiferous ducts

Names and locations of endocrine glands

Name	Location
Pituitary gland (hypophysis cerebri) and hypothalamus	Cranial cavity
Anterior lobe (adenohypophysis)	
Intermediate lobe (pars intermedia)	
Posterior lobe (neurohypophysis)	
Pineal gland (epiphysis)	Cranial cavity
Thyroid gland	Neck
Parathyroid glands	Neck
Thymus	Mediastinum
Adrenal glands	Abdominal cavity (retroperitoneal)
Adrenal cortex	
Adrenal medulla	
Islands of Langerhans	Abdominal cavity (pancreas)
Gastric and intestinal mucosa	Abdominal cavity
Ovaries	Pelvic cavity
Graafian follicle	
Corpus luteum	
Testes (interstitial cells)	Scrotum
Placenta	Pregnant uterus

4-6 Nervous system

Major ascending tracts of the spinal cord

Name	Function	Location	Origin*	Termination†
Lateral spinothalamic	Pain, temperature, and crude touch opposite side	Lateral white columns	Posterior gray column opposite side	Thalamus
Ventral spinothalamic	Crude touch, pain, and temperature	Anterior white columns	Posterior gray column opposite side	Thalamus
Fasciculi gracilis and cuneatus	Discriminating touch and pressure sensations, including vibration, stereognosis, and two-point discrimination; also conscious kinesthesia	Posterior white columns	Spinal ganglia same side	Medulla
Spinocerebellar	Unconscious kinesthesia	Lateral white columns	Posterior gray column	Cerebellum

*Location of cell bodies of neurons from which axons of tract arise.
†Structure in which axons of tract terminate.

Major descending tracts of the spinal cord

Name	Function	Location	Origin*	Termination†
Lateral corticospinal (or crossed pyramidal)	Voluntary movement, contraction of individual or small groups of muscles, particularly those moving hands, fingers, feet, and toes of opposite side	Lateral white columns	Motor areas cerebral cortex (mainly areas 4 and 6) opposite side from tract location in cord	Intermediate or anterior gray columns
Ventral corticospinal (direct pyramidal)	Same as lateral corticospinal except mainly muscles of same side	Lateral white columns	Motor cortex but on same side as tract location in cord	Intermediate or anterior gray columns
Lateral reticulospinal	Mainly facilitatory influence on motoneurons to skeletal muscles	Lateral white columns	Reticular formation, midbrain, pons, and medulla	Intermediate or anterior gray columns
Medial reticulospinal	Mainly inhibitory influence on motoneurons to skeletal muscles	Anterior white columns	Reticular formation, medulla mainly	Intermediate or anterior gray columns

*Location of cell bodies of neurons from which axons of tract arise.
†Structure in which axons of tract terminate.

Spinal nerves and peripheral branches

Spinal nerves	*Plexuses formed from anterior rami*	*Spinal nerve branches from plexuses*	*Parts supplied*
Cervical 1 2 3 4	Cervical plexus	Lesser occipital Great auricular Cutaneous nerve of neck Anterior supraclavicular Middle supraclavicular Posterior supraclavicular Branches to numerous neck muscles	Sensory to back of head, front of neck, and upper part of shoulder; motor to numerous neck muscles
Cervical 5 6 7 8 Thoracic (or dorsal) 1	Brachial plexus	Phrenic (branches from cervical nerves before formation of plexus; most of its fibers from fourth cervical nerve)	Diaphragm
		Suprascapular and dorsoscapular	Superficial muscles* of scapula
		Thoracic nerves, medial and lateral branches	Pectoralis major and minor
		Long thoracic nerve	Serratus anterior
		Thoracodorsal	Latissimus dorsi
		Subscapular	Subscapular and teres major muscles
		Axillary (circumflex)	Deltoid and teres minor muscles and skin over deltoid
		Musculocutaneous	Muscles of front of arm (biceps brachii, coracobrachialis, and brachialis) and skin on outer side of forearm
		Ulnar	Flexor carpi ulnaris and part of flexor digitorum profundus; some of muscles of hand; sensory to medial side of hand, little finger, and medial half of fourth finger
		Median	Rest of muscles of front of forearm and hand; sensory to skin of palmar surface of thumb, index, and middle fingers
		Radial	Triceps muscle and muscles of back of forearm; sensory to skin of back of forearm and hand
		Medial cutaneous	Sensory to inner surface of arm and forearm
2 3 4 5 6 7 8 9 10 11 12	No plexus formed; branches run directly to intercostal muscles and skin of thorax		

*Although nerves to muscles are considered motor, they do contain some sensory fibers that transmit proprioceptive impulses.

†Sensory fibers from the tibial and peroneal nerves unite to form the *medial cutaneous* (or sural) *nerve* that supplies the calf of the leg and the lateral surface of the foot. In the thigh the tibial and common peroneal nerves are usually enclosed in a single sheath to form the *sciatic nerve*, the largest nerve in the body with a width of approximately ¾ inch. About two thirds of the way down the posterior part of the thigh, it divides into its component parts. Branches of the sciatic nerve extend into the hamstring muscles.

Spinal nerves	Plexuses formed from anterior rami	Spinal nerve branches from plexuses	Parts supplied
Lumbar 1 2 3 4 5 Sacral 1 2 3 4 5 Coccygeal 1	Lumbosacral plexus	Iliohypogastric } Sometimes fused	Sensory to anterior abdominal wall
		Ilioinguinal } Sometimes fused	Sensory to anterior abdominal wall and external genitalia; motor to muscles of abdominal wall
		Genitofemoral	Sensory to skin of external genitalia and inguinal region
		Lateral cutaneous of thigh	Sensory to outer side of thigh
		Femoral	Motor to quadriceps, sartorius, and iliacus muscles; sensory to front of thigh and medial side of lower leg (saphenous nerve)
		Obturator	Motor to adductor muscles of thigh
		Tibial† (medial popliteal)	Motor to muscles of calf of leg; sensory to skin of calf of leg and sole of foot
		Common peroneal (lateral popliteal)	Motor to evertors and dorsiflexors of foot; sensory to lateral surface of leg and dorsal surface of foot
		Nerves to hamstring muscles	Motor to muscles of back of thigh
		Gluteal nerves, superior and inferior	Motor to buttock muscles and tensor fasciae latae
		Posterior cutaneous nerve	Sensory to skin of buttocks, posterior surface of thigh, and leg
		Pudendal nerve	Motor to perineal muscles; sensory to skin of perineum

Sympathetic and parasympathetic neurons compared to location

	Sympathetic	Parasympathetic
Preganglionic neurons		
Dendrites and cell bodies	In lateral gray columns of thoracic and first four lumbar segments of spinal cord	In nuclei of brainstem and cord (in lateral gray columns of sacral segments of cord)
Axons	In anterior roots of spinal nerves, to spinal nerves (thoracic and first four lumbar), to white rami, and then in any of three following pathways: (1) ganglia; (2) through white rami to and through sympathetic ganglia, then up or down sympathetic trunk before synapsing in a sympathetic ganglion; (3) through white rami to and through sympathetic ganglia, to and through splanchnic nerves to collateral ganglia (celiac, superior, and inferior mesenteric ganglia)	From brainstem nuclei through cranial nerve III to ciliary ganglion From nuclei in pons: through cranial nerve VII to sphenopalatine or submaxillary ganglion From nuclei in medulla through cranial nerve IX to otic ganglion or through cranial nerves X and XI to cardiac and celiac ganglia, respectively
Postganglionic neurons		
Dendrites and cell bodies	In sympathetic and collateral ganglia	In parasympathetic ganglia (for example, ciliary, sphenopalatine, submaxillary, otic, cardiac, celiac) located in or near visceral effector organs
Axons	In autonomic nerves and plexuses that innervate thoracic and abdominal viscera and blood vessels in these cavities In gray rami to spinal nerves, to smooth muscle of skin blood vessels and hair follicles, and to sweat glands	In short nerves to various visceral effector organs

Cranial nerves*

Nerve†	Sensory fibers: Receptors	Sensory fibers: Cell bodies	Sensory fibers: Termination	Motor fibers: Cell bodies	Motor fibers: Termination	Functions‡
I Olfactory	*Nasal mucosa*	*Nasal mucosa*	Olfactory bulbs (new relay of neurons of olfactory cortex)			*Sense of smell*
II Optic	*Retina*	*Retina*	*Nucleus in thalamus (lateral geniculate body); some fibers terminate in superior colliculus of midbrain*			*Vision*
III Oculomotor	*External eye muscles except superior oblique and lateral rectus*	?	?	**Midbrain (oculomotor nucleus and Edinger-Westphal nucleus)**	**External eye muscles except superior oblique and lateral rectus; fibers from Edinger-Westphal nucleus terminate in ciliary ganglion and then to ciliary and iris muscles**	**Eye movements, regulation of size of pupil, accommodation,** *proprioception (muscle sense)*
IV Trochlear	*Superior oblique*	?	?	**Midbrain**	**Superior oblique muscle of eye**	**Eye movements,** *proprioception*
V Trigeminal	*Skin and mucosa of head, teeth*	*Gasserian ganglion*	*Pons (sensory nucleus)*	**Pons (motor nucleus)**	**Muscles of mastication**	*Sensations of head and face,* **chewing movements,** *muscle sense*
VI Abducens	*Lateral rectus*			**Pons**	**Lateral rectus muscle of eye**	**Abduction of eye,** *proprioception*
VII Facial	*Taste buds of anterior two thirds of tongue*	*Geniculate ganglion*	*Medulla (nucleus solitarius)*	**Pons**	**Superficial muscles of face and scalp**	**Facial expressions, secretion of saliva,** *taste*
VIII Acoustic						
1 Vestibular branch	*Semicircular canals and vestibule (utricle and saccule)*	*Vestibular ganglion*	*Pons and medulla (vestibular nuclei)*			*Balance of equilibrium sense*
2 Cochlear or auditory branch	*Organ of Corti in cochlear duct*	*Spiral ganglion*	*Pons and medulla (cochlear nuclei)*			*Hearing*

IX Glossopharyngeal	*Pharynx; taste buds and other receptors of posterior one third of tongue*	*Jugular and petrous ganglia*	*Medulla (nucleus solitarius)*	**Medulla (nucleus ambiguus)**	**Muscles of pharynx**	*Taste and other sensations of tongue*, **swallowing movements, secretion of saliva,** *aid in reflex control of blood pressure and respiration*
	Carotid sinus and carotid body	*Jugular and petrous ganglia*	*Medulla (respiratory and vasomotor centers)*	**Medulla at junction of pons (nucleus salivatorius)**	**Otic ganglion and then to parotid gland**	
X Vagus	*Pharynx, larynx, carotid body, and thoracic and abdominal viscera*	*Jugular and nodose ganglia*	*Medulla (nucleus, solitarius), pons (nucleus of fifth cranial nerve)*	**Medulla (dorsal motor nucleus)**	**Ganglia of vagal plexus and then to muscles of pharynx, larynx, and thoracic and abdominal viscera**	*Sensations and* **movements** *or organs supplied;* for example, **slows heart, increases peristalsis, and contracts muscles for voice production**
XI Spinal accessory	?	?	?	**Medulla (dorsal motor nucleus of vagus and nucleus ambiguus)**	**Muscles of thoracic and abdominal viscera and pharynx and larynx**	**Shoulder movements, turning movements of head, movements of viscera, voice productions,** *proprioception?*
				Anterior gray column of first five or six cervical segments of spinal cord	**Trapezius and sternocleidomastoid muscle**	
XII Hypoglossal	?	?	?	**Medulla (hypoglossal nucleus)**	**Muscles of tongue**	**Tongue movements,** *proprioception?*

*Italics indicate sensory fibers and functions. Boldface type indicates motor fibers and functions.

†The first letters of the words in the following sentence are the first letters of the names of the cranial nerves. Many generations of anatomy students have used this sentence as an aid to memorizing these names. "On Old Olympus Tiny Tops, A Finn and German Viewed Some Hops." (There are several slightly differing versions of this mnemonic.)

‡An aid for remembering the general function of each cranial nerve is the following 12-word saying: "Some say marry money but my brothers say bad business marry money." Words beginning with S indicate sensory function. Words beginning with M indicate motor function. Words beginning with B indicate both sensory and motor functions. For example, the first, second, and eighth words in the saying start with S, which indicates that the first, second, and eighth cranial nerves perform sensory functions.

Cranial nerves contrasted with spinal nerves

	Cranial nerves	*Spinal nerves*
Origin	Base of brain	Spinal cord
Distribution	Mainly to head and neck	Skin, skeletal muscles, joints, blood vessels, sweat glands, and mucosa except of head and neck
Structure	Some composed of sensory fibers only; some of both motor axons and sensory dendrites; some motor fibers belong to somatic nervous system, some to autonomic	All of them composed of both sensory dendrites and motor axons; some of latter, somatic, some autonomic
Function	Vision, hearing, sense of small, sense of taste, eye movements	Sensations, movements, and sweat secretion

Autonomic functions

Visceral effectors	*Sympathetic impulses*	*Parasympathetic impulses*
Cardiac muscle	Stimulate pacemaker, accelerate and strength of heartbeat	Inhibit pacemaker; decrease rate and strength of heartbeat
Smooth muscle of blood vessels		
Skin blood vessels	Stimulate; constrict	No parasympathetic fibers
Skeletal muscle blood vessels	Inhibit; dilate	No parasympathetic fibers
Coronary blood vessels	Inhibit; dilate	No parasympathetic fibers
Blood vessels in cerebrum and abdominal viscera	Stimulate; constrict	Inhibit; dilate; no parasympathetic fibers to some viscera
Blood vessels in external genitalia	Inhibit; dilate	Stimulate; constrict
Smooth muscle of hollow organs and sphincters		
Bronchi	Inhibit; dilate	Stimulate; constrict
Digestive tract, except sphincters	Inhibit; decrease peristalsis	Stimulate; increase peristalsis
Sphincters of digestive tract	Stimulate; close	Inhibit; open
Urinary bladder	Inhibit; relax	Stimulate; contract
Urinary sphincters	Stimulate; close	Inhibit; open
Eye		
Iris	Stimulate radial muscle; dilate pupil	Stimulate circular muscle; constrict pupil
Ciliary	Inhibit; accommodate for far vision	Stimulate; accommodate for near vision
Hairs (pilomotor muscles)	Stimulate; produce ''goose pimples'' (piloerection)	No parasympathetic fibers
Glands		
Sweat	Stimulate; increase sweat	No parasympathetic fibers
Digestive (salivary, gastric, etc.)	Inhibit; decrease secretion of saliva; not known for others	Stimulate; increase secretion of saliva
Pancreas, including islets	Inhibit; decrease secretion	Stimulate; increase secretion of pancreatic juice and insulin
Liver	Stimulate glycogenolysis; increase blood sugar level	No parasympathetic fibers
Adrenal medulla	Stimulate; increase epinephrine secretion	No parasympathetic fibers

4-7 Reproductive system

Female reproductive system

Organ	Location	Function
Ovary (2)	On each side of pelvic cavity; attached to posterior surface of broad ligament of the ovary, to ovarian tubes by fimbraie	Produces ova and female sex hormones
Fallopian tube (oviduct) (2)	Extends from upper angles of uterus to sides of pelvic cavity	Conveys ova toward uterus; site of fertilization; conveys fertilized ovum to uterus
Uterus	In pelvic cavity between bladder and rectum	Protects and sustains life of embryo during pregnancy
Vagina	Extends from uterus to vulva—about 7.5-10 cm (3-4 in.); placed anterior to rectum, posterior to bladder and urethra	Conveys uterine secretions to outside of body; receives erect penis during intercourse; transports fetus during birth process
Labia majora	Two folds that extend from mons pubis to within an inch of anus	Encloses and protects other external reproductive organs; maintains secretions
Labia minora	Two folds situated between labia majora	Forms margins of vestibule; protects openings of vagina and urethra
Clitoris	Small protuberance at apex of triangle formed by junction of labia minora	Glans is richly supplied with blood vessels and with endings associated with feelings of pleasure
Vestibule	Space between labia minora that includes vaginal and urethral openings	
Greater vestibular (Bartholin's) gland (2)	On each side of vagina	Secretes fluid that moistens and lubricates vestibule
Mammary gland (2)	Anterior to pectoralis muscles, extending from second to sixth ribs and from sternum into axila	Lactation

Male reproductive system

Organ	Location	Function
Testis (2)	Positioned obliquely in scrotum	
Seminiferous tubules		Produce spermatozoa
Interstitial cells		Produce and secrete male sex hormones
Epididymis (2)	Superior and posterior to testis	Storage and maturation of spermatozoa; conveys spermatozoa to vas deferens
Vas deferens (2)	Extends from scrotum into abdominal cavity, passes over the top, then down posterior surface of bladder, and joins ampulla of seminal vesicle	Conveys spermatozoa from epididymis to ejaculatory duct
Seminal vesicle (2)	Posterior to bladder	Secretes alkaline fluid containing nutrients and prostaglandins; fluid helps neutralize acidic seminal fluid
Prostate gland	Immediately inferior to internal urethral sphincter	Secretes alkaline fluid that helps neutralize acidic seminal fluid and enhances motility of spermatozoa
Bulbourethral (Cowper's) gland (2)	On each side of membranous urethra	Secretes fluid that lubricates end of penis
Scrotum	External pouch at base of penis	Encloses and protects testes
Penis	Suspended from front and sides of pubic arch	Conveys urine and seminal fluid to outside of body; inserted into vagina during intercourse; glans penis is richly supplied with sensory nerve endings associated with feelings of pleasure during sexual stimulation

4-8 Urinary system

Organ	Location	Function
Kidney (2)	Posterior part of lumbar region, behind peritoneum; on each side of spinal column, extending from upper border of twelfth thoracic to third lumbar vertebra	Excretes metabolic wastes; regulates acid-base balance; regulates osmotic pressure, electrolyte pattern, and volume of extracellular fluids; regulates renin-angiotensin system; manufactures erythropoietin
Ureter (2)	Duct connecting kidney with bladder	Conveys urine to bladder, acting as conduit
Bladder	In pelvic cavity behind pubes In male, in front of rectum In female, in front of anterior wall of vagina and neck of uterus	Serves as reservoir for urine
Urethra	Membranous canal extending from bladder to urinary meatus In male, begins at bladder, passes through prostate gland, goes between two sheets of tissue connecting pubic bones, and passes through urinary meatus of penis In female, directly behind symphysis pubis and anterior to vagina	Drains urine from bladder during voiding In male, also serves as passageway for semen during ejaculation

APPENDIX

5 MEDICAL TERMINOLOGY

The ability to break down medical terms into separate components or to recognize a complete word depends on the mastery of the combining forms (a stem or root with an "o" attached), roots or stems that appear in medical terms, and prefixes and suffixes that alter or modify meaning and usage of a term.

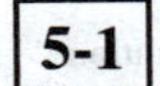

5-1 Prefixes

Prefixes, the most frequently used elements in the formation of Greek and Latin words, consist of one or more syllables (prepositions or adverbs) placed before words or roots to show various kinds of relationships. They are never used independently, but when added before verbs, adjectives, or nouns, they modify the meaning. Most prefixes are a part of words in ordinary speech and do not refer specifically to medical or scientific terminology, but many occur frequently in medical terminology. The prefixes used in medical terminology are given in Appendix 5-1.

Prefix	*Translation of Greek or Latin*	*Examples*
a-, an-	Without, lack of	Apathy (lack of feeling) Apnea (without breath) Aphasia (without speech) Anemia (lack of blood)
ab-	Away from	Abductor (leading away from) Aboral (away from mouth)
ad-	To, toward, near to	Adductor (leading toward) Adhesion (sticking to) Adnexia (structures joined to) Adrenal (near the kidney)
ambi-	Both	Ambidextrous (ability to use hands equally) Ambilateral (both sides)
amphi-	About, on both sides, both	Amphibious (living on both land and in water)
ampho-	Both	Amphogenic (producing offspring of both sexes)
ana-	Up, back, again, excessive	Anatomy (a cutting up) Anagenesis (reproduction of tissue) Anasarca (severe edema)
ante-	Before, in front of	Antecubital (in front of elbow) Anteflexion (bending forward)
anti-	Against, opposed to, reversed	Antiperistalsis (reversed peristalsis) Antisepsis (against infection)
ap-, apo-	From, separation	Apolepsis (stopping of a function) Apochromatic (free from distortion of shape or color)
bi-	Twice, double	Biarticulate (double joint) Bifocal (two foci) Bifurcation (two branches)
cata-	Down, under, lower, against	Catabolism (breaking down) Catalepsy (diminished movement)
circum-	Around, about	Circumflex (winding about) Circumference (surrounding) Circumarticular (around joint)
com-, con-	With, together	Commissure (sending or coming together) Conductor (leading together) Concentric (having a common center) Concrescence (growing together)
contra-	Against, opposite	Contralateral (opposite side) Contraception (prevention of conception) Contraindicated (not indicated)

Continued.

Prefixes—cont'd

Prefix	*Translation of Greek or Latin*	*Examples*
de-	Away from	Dehydrate (remove water) Dedentition (removal of teeth) Decompensation (failure of compensation)
dia-	Between, through, apart, across, completely	Diaphragm (wall across) Diapedesis (ooze through) Diagnosis (complete knowledge)
dis-	Reversal, apart from, separation	Disinfection (apart from infection) Disarticulation (separation at a joint) Dissect (cut apart)
e-, ex-	Out, away from	Enucleate (remove from) Eviscerate (take out viscera or bowels) Exostosis (outgrowth of bone)
ec-	Out from	Ectopic (out of place) Eccentric (away from center) Ectasia (stretching out or dilation)
ecto-	On outer side, situated on	Ectoderm (outer skin) Ectoretina (outer layer of retina)
em-, en-	In	Empyema (pus in) Encephalon (in the brain)
endo-	Within	Endocardium (within heart) Endometrium (within uterus)
epi-	Upon, on	Epidural (upon dura) Epidermis (on skin)
exo-	Upon, on, outside, on outer side, outer layer	Exogenous (originating outside) Exocolitis (inflammation of outer coat of colon)
extra-	Outside	Extracellular (outside cell) Extrapleural (outside pleura)
hyper-	Excessive, over, above	Hyperemia (excessive blood) Hypertrophy (overgrowth) Hyperplasia (excessive formation)
hypo-	Under, below, deficient	Hypotension (low blood pressure) Hypothyroidism (deficiency or underfunction of thyroid)
im-, in-	In, into	Immersion (act of dipping in) Infiltration (act of filtering in) Injection (act of forcing fluid into)
im-, in-	Not	Immature (not mature) Involuntary (not voluntary) Inability (not able)
infra-	Below	Infraorbital (below eye) Infraclavicular (below clavicle or collar bone)
inter-	Between	Intercostal (between ribs) Intervene (come between)
intra-	Within	Intracerebral (within cerebrum) Intraocular (within eye) Intraventricular (within ventricles)
intro-	Into, within	Introversion (turning inward) Introduce (lead into)
meta-	Beyond, after, change	Metamorphosis (change of form) Metastasis (beyond original position) Metacarpal (beyond wrist)
opistho-	Behind, backward	Opisthotic (behind ears) Opisthognathous (beyond jaws)
para-	Beside, beyond, near to	Paracardiac (beside the heart) Paraurethral (near the urethra)
per-	Through, excessive	Permeate (pass through) Perforate (bore through) Peracute (excessively acute)
peri-	Around	Periosteum (around bone) Periatrial (around atrium) Peribronchial (around bronchus)

Prefix	*Translation of Greek or Latin*	*Examples*
post-	After, behind	Postoperative (after operation) Postpartum (after childbirth) Postocular (behind eye)
pre-, pro-	Before, in front of	Premaxillary (in front of maxilla) Preoral (in front of mouth) Prognosis (foreknowledge) Projection (throw forward)
re-	Back, again, contrary	Reflex (bend back) Revert (turn again to) Regurgitation (backward flowing, contrary to normal)
retro-	Backward, located behind	Retrocervical (located behind cervix) Retrograde (going backward) Retrolingual (behind tongue)
sub-	Under	Subcutaneous (under skin) Subarachnoid (under arachnoid) Subungual (under nail)
super-	Above, upper, excessive	Supercilia (upper brows) Supernumerary (excessive number) Supermedial (above middle)
supra-	Above, upon	Suprarenal (above kidney) Suprasternal (above sternum) Suprascapular (on upper part of scapula)
sym-, syn-	Together, with	Symphysis (growing together) Synapsis (joining together) Synarthrosis (articulation of joints together)
trans-	Across, through, beyond	Transection (cut across) Transduodenal (through duodenum) Transmit (send beyond)
ultra-	Beyond, in excess	Ultraviolet (beyond violet end of spectrum) Ultraligation (ligation of vessel beyond point of origin) Ultrasonic (sound waves beyond the upper frequency of hearing by human ear)

5-2 Suffixes

Suffixes are the one or more syllables or elements added to the root or stem of a word (the part that indicates the essential meaning) to alter the meaning or indicate the intended part of speech.

To make a word pronounceable, the last letter or letters of the root to which the suffix is attached may be changed. The last vowel may be changed to an ''*o*'' or an ''*o*'' may be inserted if it is not already present before a suffix beginning with a consonant, as in cardiology. The final vowel in the root may be dropped before a suffix beginning with a vowel, as in neuritis.

Most suffixes are in common use in English, but some are peculiar to medical science. The suffixes most commonly used to indicate disease are *itis,* meaning inflammation; *oma,* meaning tumor; and *osis,* meaning a condition, usually morbid. The suffixes listed occur often in medical terminology, but they are also in use in ordinary language. These suffixes apply to Greek and Latin words.

Suffix	*Use*	*Examples*
ize, -ate	Add to nouns or adjectives to make verbs expressing to use, to act like, to subject to, make into	Visualize (able to see) Impersonate (act like) Hypnotize (put into state of hypnosis)
-ist, -or, -er	Add to verbs to make nouns expressing agent or person concerned or instrument	Anesthetist (one who practices the science of anesthesia) Dissector (instrument that dissects or person who dissects) Donor (one who donates)
-ent	Add to verbs to make adjectives or nouns of agency	Recipient (one who receives) Concurrent (happening at the same time)
-sia, -y, -tion	Add to verbs to make nouns expressing action, process, or condition	Anesthesia (process or condition of not feeling) Therapy (treatment) Inhalation (act of inhaling)
-ia, -ity	Add to adjectives or nouns to make nouns expressing quality or condition	Septicemia (poisoning of blood) Disparity (inequality) Acidity (condition of excess acid) Neuralgia (pain in nerves)
-ma (mata), -men (mina), -ment, -ure	Add to verbs to make nouns expressing result of action or object of action	Trauma (injury) Foramina (openings Ligament (tough fibrous band holding bone or viscera together) Fissure (groove)
-ium, -olus, -olum, -culus, -culum, -cule, -cle, -ellum	Add to nouns to make diminutive nouns	Bacterium (one-cell organism) Alveolus (air sac) Follicle (little bag) Cerebellum (little brain) Molecule (little mass) Ossicle (little bone)
-ible, -ile	Add to verbs to make adjectives expressing ability or capacity	Contractile (ability to contract) Edible (capable of being eaten) Flexible (capable of being bent)
-al, -c, -ious, -tic	Add to nouns to make adjectives expressing relationship, concern, or pertaining to	Neural (referring to nerve) Neoplastic (referring to neoplasm) Cardiac (referring to the heart) Delirious (suffering from delirium)
-id	Add to verbs or nouns to make adjectives expressing state or condition	Flaccid (state of being weak or lax) Fluid (state of being liquid)
-tic	Add to a verb to make an adjective showing relationship	Caustic (referring to burn) Acoustic (referring to sound or hearing)
-oid, -form	Add to nouns to make adjectives expressing resemblance	Polypoid (resembling polyp) Plexiform (resembling a plexus) Fusiform (resembling a fusion) Epidermoid (resembling epidermis)
-ous	Add to nouns to make adjectives expressing material	Ferrous (composed of iron) Serous (composed of serum) Mucinous (composed of mucin)

5-3 Roots and combining forms in external anatomy

The list of roots and combining forms in appendix 5-3 pertain only to external anatomy—that which can be visualized with the naked eye. Some terms are complete Latin or Greek words, and this is noted in the definition. They are arranged alphabetically, and the region of the body is indicated where applicable.

Word or combining form	*Meaning*	*Body region**
axilla (pl. axillae)	Latin for armpit	E
blepharo-, blephar-	Eyelid or eyelash	H&N
brachium	Latin for arm, mainly the arm above the elbow	E
bucca	Latin for cheek	H&N
calx	Latin for heel (Do not confuse with calyx, a recess of the pelvis of the kidney.)	E
canthus (pl. canthi), cantho-	The angle at either end of the slit between the eyelids	H&N
capillus (pl. capilli)	Latin for hair (Term can apply to hair anywhere on the body.)	H&N
caput (pl. capita)	Latin for head	H&N
carpus, carpo-	Latin for wrist; also the eight bones of the wrist collectively	E
cephalo-	Relating to the head	H&N
cervix (pl. cervices), cervico-	Latin for neck or neck-like part; (Term also used for cervix uteri, or neck-like projection of the uterus.)	H&N
cheilo-, cheil-	Greek for lip	H&N
cheiro-, chiro-, cheir-, chir-	Hand	E
cilium (pl. cilia)	Latin for eyelid or eyelash or any minute hairlike process attached to the free surface of a tissue or cell	H&N
core-, coro-	Pupil of eye	H&N
corium	Latin for true skin	
coxa	Latin for hip or hip joint (Also an internal anatomic term.)	T
cubitus	Latin for elbow, but used mainly to refer to the forearm	E
cutis	Latin for skin	
dactylo-	Digit, usually a finger but sometimes a toe	E
dento-, dent-, denta, denti, dentia	Tooth or teeth	H&N
derm-, derma-, dermato-, dermo-	Skin	
digit	Finger or toe	E
dorsum (pl. dorsa), dorso-	Latin for back	T
facio-	Face	H&N
frons, fronto-	Latin for forehead	H&N
genu	Latin for knee	E
gingiva	Gum	H&N
glosso-, gloss-	Tongue	H&N
gnatho-, gnath-	Jaw	H&N
irido-	Iris of eye (From a Greek word meaning rainbow or colored circle.)	H&N
hallux (pl. halluces)	Latin for great toe	E
inguen	Latin for groin (The "e" changes to "i" in words pertaining to the groin, e.g. inguinal.)	T
labio-	Lip, especially of the mouth	H&N
laparo-	Loin or flank; sometimes used loosely to refer to the abdomen	T
latus, latero-	Latin for side (Term may be used to denote either the side of any organ or a position)	T
lingua	Latin for tongue	H&N

*E, extremities; H&N, head and neck; T, trunk.

Continued.

Roots and combining forms in external anatomy—cont'd

Word or combining form	*Meaning*	*Body region**
lumbus	Latin for loin	T
mamma (pl. mammae)	Latin for breast, or mammary gland	T
manus	Latin for hand	E
masto-, mast-	Breast	T
melia	Greek for limbs (melos)	E
mentum	Latin for chin (Do not confuse with words beginning with *men* that refer to the mind or menses; the sense in which it is used will govern the meaning.)	H&N
naris (pl. nares)	Latin for one of the openings into the nasal cavity	H&N
naso-	Nose	H&N
nucha	Latin for back, or nape, of neck	H&N
occiput	Latin for back part of the head	H&N
oculo-	Eye	H&N
odonto-	Tooth or teeth	H&N
omo-	Shoulder	T
omphalo-	Navel (umbilicus)	T
onycho-	Nail	E
ophthalmo-, ophthalm-	Eye	H&N
orb	Latin for sphere or eyeball	H&N
orbit	Bony socket containing the eye	H&N
ora	Latin for mouth	H&N
oto-	Ear	H&N
palpebra (pl. palpebrae)	Latin for eyelid	H&N
papilla (pl. papillae)	Latin for nipple or nipple-shaped projection	T
pectus	Latin for chest, thorax, or breast	T
pes, ped-, pod-	Foot (do not confuse with Greek *paed* or *ped,* referring to a child)	E
pilo-	Hair	
plantar	Latin for sole of foot	E
pollex	Latin for thumb	E
poples	Latin for posterior surface of knee	E
rhino-, rhin-	Nose	H&N
soma, somato-	Greek for body	
sterno-	Sternum, or breastbone, as usually used, but formerly referred to chest	T
steth-, stetho-	Chest	T
stomato-, stomo-	Mouth	H&N
talus	Latin for ankle; also refers to an ankle bone	E
tarso-	Instep of the foot; also edge of eyelid	E
thele	Greek for nipple	T
thenar	Greek for palm of hand or sole of foot	E
thoraco-	Chest or thorax	T
-thrix	Suffix relating to hair	
trachelo-	Neck or neckline structure, such as the cervix	
tricho-	Hair	
unguis	Latin for nail of finger or toe	E
venter	Latin for stomach or belly, bellyshaped or hollowed part	T
ventro-	Belly; front or anterior aspect of the body	

5-4 Roots and combining forms in internal anatomy

The roots and combining forms given in appendix 5-4 pertain only to internal anatomy. Some terms are complete Latin or Greek words, and this is noted in the definition. Terms are arranged alphabetically, and the system of the body is indicated where applicable.

Word or combining form	*Meaning*	*Body system**
adeno-	Gland	E
adreno-	Adrenal gland	E
angio-, angi-	Vessel, usually a blood vessel	CVL
arterio-	Artey	CVL
arteriolo-	Arteriole	CVL
arthro-	Joint	S
articulus (pl. articuli)	Latin for joint	S
atrio-	Atrium, upper chamber of the heart	CVL
auriculo-	Ear-shaped appendage of either atrium of the heart; the pinna or flap of the ear	CVL/SS
balano-	Glans penis	GU
bronchio-, broncho-	Bronchus	R
cardio-	Heart	CVL
cerebello-	Cerebellum, a part of the brain	N
cerebro-	Cerebrum, a part of the brain	N
cholangio-	Bile duct or bile duct capillaries	GI
chole-, chol-, cholo-	Bile	GI
cholecyst, cholecysto-	Greek for gallbladder	GI
choledocho-	Common bile duct	GI
chondro-, chondr-, chrondri-, chondrio-	Cartilage	S
chordo-	Cord; may be a vocal cord or the spermatic cord	SS/GU
cleido-, cleid-	Collar bone or clavicle	S
colpo-	Vagina	GU
condyle	Latin for a rounded projection (knuckle) on a bone	S
cor	Heart (*Cor* in coronary vessel does not derive from *cor* meaning heart, but rather from *corona,* meaning crown.)	CVL
cornu	Latin for horn or hornlike projection	
corpus	Latin for body or main part of any organ, or a mass of specialized tissue	
costo-	Rib	S
cysto-	Bladder or sac, most often used in reference to the urinary bladder, but also in connection with the gallbladder	GU, GI
cyto-	Cell	
-cyte	Suffix denoting a cell; the root to which it is attached designates the type of cell, such as erythrocyte (red cell)	CVL
dacryo-	Tear	SS
duodeno-	Duodenum, a section of the intestinal tract about 12 inches long (duodenum in Latin means 12 inches)	GI
encephalo-	Brain, or sometimes the head	N
entero-	Intestine	GI
episio-	Vulva	GU
fibro-	Fiber	M

*S, skeletal system; M, muscular system; I, integumentary system; CVL, cardiovascular and lymphatic systems; R, respiratory system; GI, gastrointestinal system; GU, genitourinary system; E, endocrine system; N, nervous system; SS, special senses.

Continued.

Roots and combining forms in internal anatomy—cont'd

Word or combining form	Meaning	Body system*
gastro-, gastr-, gaster-	Stomach	GI
glio-	Glue or gluey substance, or more specifically the neuroglia, the supporting substance of the nervous system	N
hepato-, hepat-, hepatico-	Liver	GI
hystero-	Womb or uterus (This term is also used in pertaining to hysteria, a nervous reaction.)	GU
ileo-	Ileum, a part of the intestinal tract	GI
ilio-	Ilium, or flank	S
jejuno-	Jejunum, a section of the intestinal tract	GI
kerato-	Cornea, or horny tissue	SS or I
laryngo-	Larynx or voice box	R
lieno-	Spleen	CVL
lumen	Latin for light; cavity or channel within a vessel or tubular organ	
lympho-	Lymph; used to refer to lymphatic vessel or to lymphocytes	CVL
meningo-	Meninges, coverings of the brain and spinal cord	N
metra-, metro-	Uterus	GU
myelo-	Bone marrow or spinal cord	S or N
myo-, my-	Combining form for muscle	M
myringo-	Eardrum	SS
nephro-	Kidney	GU
neuro-	Nerve	N
nodus	Latin for knot or node	
oophoro-	Ovary	GU
orchio-, orchi-, orchido-	Testicle or testis	GU
os	Latin for bone; also a term for mouth or any orifice of the body	
osteo-	Bone	S
palato-	Palate or roof of mouth	GI
phalanx (pl. phalanges)	Greek for a line or array of soldiers; used in connection with fingers or toes because they somewhat resemble a line of soldiers or a battle formation	S
pharyngo-	Relating to the pharynx	R, GI
phleb-, phlebo-	Vein	CVL
phren-	Greek for diaphragm and the mind; the sense in which it is used will govern the meaning of the word or its intent	M or N
pleuro-	Pleura, side, or rib	R
pneumo-, pneumato-, pneumono-	Air, gas, or respiration and lungs	R
proct-, procto-	Anus or rectum	GI
pulmo-	Lung	R
pyel-, pyelo-	Pelvis of the kidney	GU
rachi-, rachio-	Spine	S
ren	Latin for kidney	GU
sacro-	Sacrum (The Latin *sacrum* means sacred; it has been postulated that the sacrum derived its name from the fact that it was offered in ancient sacrifices)	S
salpingo-	Fallopian tube or eustachian tube	GU,SS
sarco-	Flesh or fleshy	
splanchno-	Viscera or organs of any one of the great cavities of the body	
spondylo-	Spinal column or a vertebra	S
tendo-, teno-, tenonto-	Tendon	S
thymo-	Thymus gland	E

Word or combining form	*Meaning*	*Body system**
thyro-	Thyroid gland	E
tracheo-	Trachea	R
uretero-	Ureter, the vessel that conveys urine from the kidney to the bladder	GU
urethro-	Urethra, a tube discharging urine from the bladder	GU
vas (pl. vasa), vaso-	Latin for vessel (Vas may also be used as vas deferens, part of the genital organ in the male)	CVL/GU
vena (pl. venae), veno-	Latin for vein	CVL
ventri-, ventro-	Front (anterior aspect) of body	
vesico-	Bladder; also pertains to a blister	GU, I
viscero- (pl. viscera)	Relates to organs in the body	

5-5 Greek and Latin verbal derivatives

The verbs or combining forms of verbs listed in Appendix 5-5 are derived from either Greek or Latin. They may be attached to other roots to form words, or suffixes and prefixes may be added to them to form words. In the table the part or root of the word to which the verb is attached is italicized, and the meaning, if not clear, is given in parentheses.

Root or combining form	*Meaning*	*Examples*
-algia	Pain	*Cardi*algia (heart) *Gastr*algia (stomach) *Neur*algia (nerve)
audi-, audio-	Hear, hearing	Audio*meter* (measure) Audio*phone* (voice instrument for deaf)
bio-	Live	Bio*logy* (study of living) Bio*statistics* (vital statistics) Bio*genesis* (origin)
cau-, -caus-	Burn	Caus*tic* (suffix added to make adjective) Cau*terization* Caus*algia* (burning pain) *Electro*cautery
-centesis	Puncture, perforate	*Thoraco*centesis (chest) *Pneumo*centesis (lung) *Arthro*centesis (joint) *Entero*centesis (intestine)
-clas-	Smash, break	*Osteo*clasis (bone) *Odonto*clasis (tooth)
-duct-	Draw	Duct*al* (suffix added to make adjective) *Ovi*duct (egg—uterine tube or fallopian tube) *Peri*duct*al* (around) *Ab*duct (lead away from)
-dynia	Pain	*Masto*dynia (breast) *Pleuro*dynia (chest) *Esophago*dynia (esophagus) *Coccygo*dynia (coccyx)
-ecta-, -ectas-	Dilate	*Ven*ectasia (dilation of vein) *Cardio*ectasis (heart) Ecta*tic* (suffix added for adjective)

Continued.

Greek and Latin verbal derivatives—cont'd

Root or combining form	*Meaning*	*Examples*
-edem-	Swell	*Myo*edem*a* (muscle) *Lymph*edema (lymph) (*a* is a suffix added to make a noun)
-esthes-	Feel	Esthe*sia* (suffix added to make noun) *An*esthesia (without)
-fiss-	Split	Fiss*ure* (suffix added to make noun) Fiss*ion* (suffix added to make noun)
-flex-, -flec-	Bend	Flex*ion* (suffix added to make noun) Flex*or* *Ante*flect (before—bending forward)
flu-, flux-	Flow	Fluc*tuate* Flux*ion* *Af*fluent
geno-, -genesis	Produce, origin	Geno*type* *Homo*genesis (same origin) *Patho*genesis (disease—origin of disease) *Hetero*genesis (other—alteration of generation)
-iatro-, -iatr-	Treat, cure	*Ger*iat*rics* (old age) *Ped*iat*rics* (children)
-kine-, -kino-, -kineto-, -kinesio-	Move	Kineto*genic* (producing movement) Kine*tic* (suffix added to make adjective) Kinesi*ology* (study of motion)
-liga-	Bind	Liga*ment* (suffix added to make noun) Lig*ate* Liga*ture*
-logy	Study	*Parasito*logy (parasites) *Bacterio*logy (bacteria) *Histo*logy (tissues)
-lysis	Breaking up, dissolving	*Hemo*lysis (blood) *Glyco*lysis (sugar) *Auto*lysis (self-destruction of cells)
-morph-, -morpho-	Form	Morpho*logy* Amorph*ous* (no definite form) *Pleo*morph*ic* (more—occurring in various forms) *Poly*morph*ic* (many)
olfact-	Smell	Olfact*ophobia* (fear) Olfact*ory* (suffix added to make adjective)
-op-, -opto-	See	*Ambly*opia (dull—dimness of vision) *Presby*opia (old—impairment of vision in old age) *My*opia (shut—nearsighted)
palpit-	Flutter	Palpit*ation*
-par-, -partus-	Labor	*Post*partum (after birth) Par*turition* (act of giving birth) Para i, ii, iii, iv, etc., are symbols for numbers of births
-pep-	Digest	*Dys*pep*sia* (bad, difficult) Pep*tic* (suffix added to make adjective)
-pexy	Fix	*Masto*pexy (fixation of breast) *Nephrospleno*pexy (surgical fixation of kidney and spleen)
-phag-, -phago-	Eat	Phago*cytosis* (eating of cells) Phago*mania* (madness—mad craving for food or eating) *Dys*phag*ia* (difficult eating or swallowing)
-phan-, -phas-	Appear, visible	Phan*erosis* (act of becoming visible) Phan*tom* Phas*mophobia* (fear of ghosts)
-phas-	Speak, utter	Aphas*ia* (unable to speak) *Dys*phas*ia* (difficulty in spreading)
-phil-	Like, love	*Hemo*phil*ia* (blood—a hereditary disease characterized by delayed clotting of blood) *Acido*phil*ia* (acid stain—''liking'' or staining with acid stains) Phil*anthropy* (love of mankind)

Root or combining form	*Meaning*	*Examples*
-phobia	Fear	*Hydro*phobia (fear of water) *Photo*phobia (fear of light) *Claustro*phobia (fear of close places)
-phrag-	Fence off, wall off	*Dia*phrag*m* (across—partition separating thorax from abdomen) Phrag*moplast* (enclosed spindle where midbody forms in mitosis)
-plas-	Form, grow	*Neo*plas*m* (new growth) *Rhino*plas*ty* (nose—operation for formation of nose) *Oto*plas*ty* (common bile duct)
-plegia	Paralyze	*Para*plegia (paralysis of lower limbs) *Ophthalmo*plegia (eye) *Hemi*plegia (partial paralysis)
-pne-, -pneo-	Breathe	*Dys*pne*a* (difficult breathing) *A*pne*a* (lack of breathing) *Hyper*pne*a* (overbreathing)
-poie-	Make	*Hemato*poie*sis* (blood) *Erythro*poie*sis* (red blood cells) *Leuko*poie*sis* (white blood cells)
-ptosis	Fall	*Procto*ptosis (anus—prolapse of anus) *Splanchno*ptosis (viscera)
-rrhagia	Burst forth, pour	*Meno*rrhagia (abnormal bleeding during menstruation) *Menometro*rrhagia (abnormal uterine bleeding) *Hemo*rrhage (blood)
-rrhaphy	Suture	*Hernio*rrhaphy (suturing or repair of hernia) *Hepato*rrhaphy (liver) *Nephro*rrhaphy (kidney)
-rrhea	Flow, discharge	*Leuko*rrhea (white discharge from vagina) *Galacto*rrhea (milk discharge) *Rhino*rrhea (nasal discharge)
-rrhexis	Rupture	*Entero*rrhexis (intestines) *Meto*rrhexis (uterus)
schiz-	Split, divide	Schiz*ophrenia* (mind—split personality) Schiz*onychia* (nails) Schiz*otricha* (hair)
-scope	Examine	*Micro*scope *Cardio*scope *Endo*scope (within—an instrument for examining the interior of a hollow viscus)
-stasis	Stop, stand still	*Hemo*stasis (blood) *Epi*stasis (checking or stopping of any discharge)
-staxis	Drop	*Epi*staxis (nosebleed)
-teg-, -tect-	Cover	Teg*men* Tect*um* (rooflike structure) *In*teg*ument* (skin covering)
-therap-	Treat, cure	Therapy *Neuro*therapy (nerves) *Chemo*therapy (chemicals) *Physio*therapy
-tomy	Cut, incise	*Phlebo*tomy (incision of vein) *Arthro*tomy (joint) *Appendec*tomy (ectomy, meaning cut out—excision of appendix) *Oophorec*tomy (excision of ovary)
-topo-	Place	Topo*graphy* Topo*narcosis* (numbing—hence numbing of a part, or localized anesthesia)
-troph-, -tropho-	Nourish	*Hyper*troph*y* (enlargement or overnourishment) Atroph*y* (undernourishment) *Dys*troph*y* (difficult or bad)
-volv-	Turn	*Involution* Volv*ulus* (twisting of an organ, as in intestinal obstruction with twisting of the bowel, or twisting of the esophagus)

5-6 Greek and Latin adjectival derivatures

The roots and combining forms in appendix 5-6 are derived from Greek or Latin adjectives. Adjectives will appear most often in compounds and will be joined to either nouns or verbs. Suffixes may be added to make them into nouns. In the table the part or root of the word the adjective modifies is italicised, and the meaning, if not clear, is given in parentheses.

Root or combining form	*Meaning*	*Examples*
ankylo-	Bent or crooked	Ankylo*sis* (abnormal immobility and consolidation of a joint)
auto-	Self	Auto*infection*
		Auto*lysis*
		Auto*pathy* (disease)
		Auto*psy* (view—postmortem examination)
brachy-	Short	Brachy*cephalia* (head)
		Brachy*dactylia* (fingers)
		Brachy*chelia* (lip)
		Brachy*gnathous* (jaw)
brady-	Slow	Brady*pnea* (breath)
		Brady*cardia* (heartbeat)
		Brady*uria* (urine)
		Brady*pepsia* (digestion)
brevi-	Short	Brevity
		Brevi*flexor* (short flexor muscle)
cav-	Hollow	Cavity
		Cavernous
		vena cava (vein)
coel-	Hollow	Coel*arium* (lining membrane of body cavity)
		Coel*om* (body cavity of embryo)
cryo-	Cold	Cryo*therapy*
		Cryo*tolerant*
		Cryo*meter*
crypto-	Hidden, concealed	Crypt*orchid* (testis)
		Crypto*genic* (origin obscure or doubtful)
		Crypt*ophthalmos* (eye)
dextro-	Right	*Ambi*dextrous (using both hands with equal ease)
		Dextro*phobia* (fear of objects on right side)
		Dextro*cardia* (heart)
diplo-	Double, twice	Diplo*cephaly* (head)
		Dipl*opia* (double sight)
dolicho-	Long	Dolicho*facial* (face)
		Dolicho*cephalic* (head)
dys-	Difficult, bad, disordered, painful	Dys*arthria* (speech)
		Dys*hidrosis* (sweat)
		Dys*kinesia* (motion)
		Dys*tocia* (birth)
		Dys*phasia* (speech)
		Dys*pepsia* (digestion)
eu-	Well, good	Eu*phoria* (well-being)
		Eu*phagia*, eu*pnea* (breath)
		Eu*thyroid* (normal thyroid)
		Eu*tocia* (normal birth)
eury-	Broad, wide	Eury*cephalic* (head)
		Eury*opia* (vision)
		Eury*somatic* (body—squat, thickset body)
glyco-	Sugar, sweet	Glyco*hemia* (sugar in blood)
		Glyco*penia* (deficiency of sugar—low blood glucose level)
gravis	Heavy	Gravid*a* (pregnant woman)
		Gravid*ism* (prenancy)

Root or combining form	Meaning	Examples
haplo-	Single, simple	Haplo*id* (having a single set of chromosomes) Haplo*dermatitis* (simple inflammation of skin) Haplo*pathy* (simple uncomplicated disease)
hetero-, heter-	Other, relationship to other	Hetero*geneous* (kind—dissimilar elements) Hetero*inoculation* Heter*ology* (abnormality of structure) Hetero*intoxication*
homo-	Same	Homo*geneous* (same kind of quality throughout Homo*zygous* (possessing identical pair of genes) Homo*logous* (corresponding in structure)
hydro-	Wet, water	Hydro*nephrosis* (kidney—collection of urine in kidney pelvis) Hydro*pneumothorax* (fluid in chest) Hydro*phobia* (fear of water—water causes painful reaction in this disease, commonly called rabies)
iso-	Equal	Iso*cellular* (similar cells) Iso*dontic* (all teeth alike) Iso*cytosis* (cells of equal size) Iso*chromatic* (having same color throughout)
latus-, lat-	Broad	Lat*itude* Lat*issimus dorsi* (muscle adducting humerus)
leio-	Smooth	Leio*myosarcoma* (fleshy malignant tumor of smooth muscle) Leio*myofibroma* (tumor of muscle and fiber elements) Leio*myoma* (tumor of unstriped muscle)
lepto-	Slender	Lepto*somatic* (body) Lepto*dactylous* (fingers)
levo-	Left	Levo*cardia* (heart) Levo*rotation* (turning to left)
longus-	Long	Long*itude* *Adductor* longus (muscle of thigh)
macro-	Large, abnormal size	Macro*cephalic* (head) Macro*cheiria* (hands) Macro*mastia* (breast) Macro*nychia* (nails)
magna-	Large, great	Magn*itude* *Adductor* magnus (thigh muscle)
malaco-	Soft	Malac*ia* (softening) *Osteo*malacia (bones)
mal-	Bad	Mal*ady* Mal*aise* Mal*ignant* Mal*formation*
medi-	Middle	Medi*an* Medi*um* *Gluteus* medius (femur muscle)
mega-	Great	Mega*colon* (large colon) Mega*cephaly* (head)
megalo-	Huge	Megalo*mania* (delusion of grandeur) *Hepato*megaly (enlarged liver) *Spleno*megaly (enlarged spleen)
meso-	Middle, mid	Meso*carpal* (wrist) Meso*derm* (skin) Meso*thelium* (a membrane lining of cavities)
micro-	Small	Micro*glossia* (tongue) Micro*blepharia* (eyelids) Micro*organism* Micro*phonia* (voice)
minimus-	Smallest	*Gluteus* minimus (smallest muscle of hip) *Adductor* minimus (muscle of thigh)
mio-	Less	Mio*plasmia* (plasma—abnormal decrease in plasma in blood) Mio*pragia* (perform—decreased activity)

Continued.

Greek and Latin adjectival derivatures—cont'd

Root or combining form	*Meaning*	*Examples*
multi-	Many, much	Multi*para* (to bear—woman who has borne more than one child) Multi*lobar* (lobes) Multi*centric* (centers)
necro-	Dead	Necro*sed* Necro*sis* Necro*psy* (postmortem examination) Necro*phobia* (fear of death)
neo-	New	Neo*formation* Neo*morphism* (form) Neo*natal* (first 4 weeks of life) Neo*pathy* (disease)
oligo-	Few, scanty, little	Oligo*phrenia* (mind) Oligo*pnea* (breath) Olig*uria* (urine) Oligo*dipsia* (thirst)
ortho-	Straight, normal, correct	Ortho*dontics* (teeth—straight) Ortho*genesis* (progressive evolution in a given direction) Ortho*grade* (walk—carrying body upright) Ortho*pnea* (breath—unable to breathe unless in an upright position)
oxy-	Sharp, quick, acute	Oxy*esthesia* (feel) Oxy*opia* (vision) Oxy*osmia* (smell)
pachy-	Thick	Pachy*derm* (skin) Pachy*emia* (blood) Pachy*pleuritis* (inflammation of pleura) Pachy*cholia* (bile) Pachy*otia* (ears)
paleo-	Old	Paleo*genetic* (origin in the past) Paleo*pathology* (study of diseases in mummies)
platy-	Flat	Platy*basia* (skull base) Platy*coria* (pupil) Platy*crania* (skull)
pleo-	More	Pleo*morphism* (forms) Pleo*chromocytoma* (tumor composed of different-colored cells)
poikilo-	Varied	Poikilo*derma* (skin mottling) Poikilo*thermal* (heat—variable body temperature)
poly-	Many, much	Poly*hedral* (many bases or faces) Poly*mastia* (more than two breasts) Poly*melia* (supernumerary limbs) Poly*myalgia* (pain in many muscles)
pronus	Face down	Prone Pron*ation*
pseudo-	False, spurious	Pseudo*stratified* (layered) Pseudo*cirrhosis* (suggestive of cirrhosis of liver) Pseudo*hypertrophy*
sclero-	Hard	Sclero*sis* (hardening) *Arterio*sclerosis (artery) Scler*onychia* (nails) Sclero*dermatitis* (skin)
scolio-	Twisted, crooked	Scolio*dontic* (teeth) Scoli*osis* Scolio*kyphosis* (curvature of spine)
sinistro-	Left	Sinistro*cardia* (heart) Sinistro*manual* (left-handed) Sinistr*aural* (hearing better in left ear)
steno-	Narrow	Steno*sis* Steno*stomia* (mouth) *Mitral* steno*sis* (mitral valve in heart)
stereo-	Solid, three dimensions	Stereo*scope* Stereo*meter*

Root or combining form	Meaning	Examples
supinus	Face up	Supine Supin*ation* Supin*ator longus* (muscle in arm)
tachy-	Fast, swift	Tachy*cardia* (heart) Tachy*phrasia* (speech)
tele-	End, far away	Tele*pathy* Tele*cardiogram*
telo-	Complete	Telo*phase*
thermo-	Heat, warm	Therm*al* Thermo*meter* Thermo*biosis* (ability to live in high temperature)
trachy	Rough	Trachy*phonia* (voice) Trachy*chromatic* (deeply staining)
xero-	Dry	Xero*phagia* (eating of dry foods) Xero*stomia* (mouth) Xero*dermia* (skin)

5-7 Miscellaneous words and combining forms

Word or combining form	Definition
Body fluids	
aqua (pl. aquae)	Latin for water
chol-, chole-, cholo-	Bile
chyle	Latin for juice; a milky fluid consisting of lymph and emulsified fats that are taken up by the intestinal lymphatic glands from food and eventually mixed with the blood
dacryo-	Tears
-emia	Greek (*haima*) for blood. (*-emia* often appears as a suffix, as in anemia, deficiency of blood)
galact-, galacta-, galacto-	Milk
hem-, hema-, hemo-, hemato-	Blood
hidro	Sweat
hydr-, hydro	Water; also hydrogen
lac	Latin for milk
lacri-	Tears
lympho-	Lymph
mucus	Latin for the secretions (mucins) of the mucous membranes together with the inorganic salts, desquamated cells, and leukocytes. *Mucous* is an adjective; the mucous membrane is called *mucosa* (mu'ko'sah).
myxo-	Mucus (Greek, *myxa*)
plasma	Fluid portion of the blood in which corpuscles are suspended
pus	Latin for the liquid inflammatory product composed of leukocytes and a thin fluid
pyo-	Pus
ptyalo-	Clear, alkaline secretion from the salivary glands—submaxillary, sublingual, parotid, or other smaller mucous glands in the mouth
sangui-	Blood
serum	Latin for whey; the clear portion of animal liquid after separation from the more solid elements—especially blood serum
sialo	Saliva or salivary gland
sudor	Latin for sweat or perspiration
ur-, uro-, urono-	Urine, urinary tract, or urination

Continued.

Miscellaneous words and combining forms—cont'd

Word or combining form	*Definition*
Body substances	
adipo-	Fat
amylo	Starch
cerumen	From *cera,* Latin for wax; a waxlike secretion found within the ear (earwax)
collagen	From the Greek word *kolla;* a derivative of colla and an albuminoid substance that acts as a main supportive protein of skin, tendon, bone, cartilage, and connective tissue
ferrum	Latin for iron
glyco-	Sugar
halo-	Salt
heme	Iron; a constituent of hemoglobin (formerly called hematin)
hormone	A chemical substance produced in the body with a specific regulatory effect on certain cells or organs
hyal-, hyalo	Glassy
lapis	Latin for stone
lipos, lipo	Greek for fat
litho-	Stone or calculus
mel-, meli-	Sweet (from Greek and Latin words for honey)
natrium	Latin for sodium
oleo	Oil
petrous	Latin for resembling a rock
saccharo-	Sugar
sal	Latin for salt
sebum	Latin for suet; the secretion of the sebaceous glands
sperm	Semen, or testicular secretion
Colors	
albus	Latin for white
chloros, chloro-	Greek for green
cirrhos	From *kirrhus,* Greek for orange-yellow
cyano-	Blue
erythro-	Red
leuco-, leuko-	White
melano-	Black
polio-	Gray, particularly referring to gray matter of the nervous system
porphyro-	Purple
rhodo-	Red
ruber	Latin for red
xantho-	Yellow
Numeral combining forms	
one	mono-, mon
two	dyo-, dy-
three	tri-
four	tetra-, tetr-
five	pent-, penta-
six	hex-, hexa-
seven	hept-, hepta-
eight	octo-, octa-, oct-
nine	ennea
ten	deka-, dek-
one hundred	hecto-, hecato-, hect-
one half	hemi-
one thousand	kilo-
one and one half	
first	proto-, prot-
second	deutero-, deuto, deut-
third	trito-, trit-
fifth	
ninth	
one-hundredth part	
one-thousandth part	
twice, duplication	di-, dis-*

**di-, dis-* in Latin means separation, like Greek *dys.*

APPENDIX

6 NUTRITION

6-1 United States Recommended Daily Allowances (U.S. RDA)*

	Adults and children 4 or more years of age (For use in labeling conventional foods and also for "special dietary foods")	Infants	(For use only with "special dietary foods")	
			Children under 4 years of age	Pregnant or lactating women
Nutrients which must **be declared on the label (in the order below)**				
Protein†	45 g "high quality protein" 65 g "proteins in general"		—	—
Vitamin A	5000 IU	1500 IU	2500 IU	8000 IU
Vitamin C (or ascorbic acid)	60 mg	35 mg	40 mg	60 mg
Thiamin (or vitamin B_1)	1.5 mg	0.5 mg	0.7 mg	1.7 mg
Riboflavin (or vitamin B_2)	1.7 mg	0.6 mg	0.8 mg	2.0 mg
Niacin	20 mg	8 mg	9 mg	20 mg
Calcium	1.0 g	0.6 g	0.8 g	1.3 g
Iron	18 mg	15 mg	10 mg	18 mg
Nutrients which may **be declared on the label (in the order below)**				
Vitamin D	400 IU	400 IU	400 IU	400 IU
Vitamin E	30 IU	5 IU	10 IU	30 IU
Vitamin B_6	2.0 mg	0.4 mg	0.7 mg	2.5 mg
Folic acid (or folacin)	0.4 mg	0.1 mg	0.2 mg	0.8 mg
Vitamin B_{12}	6 μg	2 μg	3 μg	8 μg
Phosphorus	1.0 g	0.5 g	0.8 g	1.3 g
Iodine	150 μg	45 μg	70 μg	150 μg
Magnesium	400 mg	70 mg	200 mg	450 mg
Zinc‡	15 mg	5 mg	8 mg	15 mg
Copper‡	2 mg	0.5 mg	1 mg	2 mg
Biotin‡	0.3 mg	0.15 mg	0.15 mg	0.3 mg
Pantothenic acid‡	10 mg	3 mg	5 mg	10 mg

From Food and Nutrition Board: Recommended dietary allowances, Washington, D.C., 1980, National Academy of Sciences–National Research Council.

*"U.S. RDA" is a new term replacing "minimum daily requirement" (MDR). The U.S. RDA values chosen are derived from the highest value for each nutrient given in National Academy of Sciences–National Research Council tables except for calcium and phosphorus.

†"High quality protein" is defined as having a protein efficiency ratio (PER) equal to or greater than that of casein; "proteins in general" are those with a PER less than that of casein. Total protein with a PER less than 20% that of casein are considered "not a significant source of protein" and would not be expressed on the label in terms of the U.S. RDA but only as amount per serving.

‡There are no NAS-NRC RDAs for biotin, pantothenic acid, zinc, and copper.

Regulations requiring declaration of sodium content of foods were passed in July 1982.

6-2 Recommended nutrient intakes for Canadians

Average energy requirements and summary examples of recommended nutrient intakes

Age	Sex	Average height (cm)[c]	Average weight (kg)[c]	Requirements[a,b]					
				kcal/kg[c,d]	MJ/kg[d]	kcal/day[e]	MJ/day[f]	kcal/cm[g]	MJ/cm[f]
Months									
0-2	Both	55	4.5	120-100	0.50-0.42	500	2.0	9	0.04
3-5	Both	63	7.0	100-95	0.42-0.40	700	2.8	11	0.05
6-8	Both	69	8.5	95-97	0.40-0.41	800	3.4	11.5	0.05
9-11	Both	73	9.5	97-99	0.41	950	3.8	12.5	0.05
Years									
1	Both	82	11	101	0.42	1100	4.8	13.5	0.06
2-3	Both	95	14	94	0.39	1300	5.6	13.5	0.06
4-6	Both	107	18	100	0.42	1800	7.6	17	0.07
7-9	M	126	25	88	0.37	2200	9.2	17.5	0.07
	F	125	25	76	0.32	1900	8.0	15	0.06
10-12	M	141	34	73	0.30	2500	10.4	17.5	0.07
	F	143	36	61	0.25	2200	9.2	15.5	0.06
13-15	M	159	50	57	0.24	2800	12.0	17.5	0.07
	F	157	48	46	0.19	2200	9.2	14	0.06
16-18	M	172	62	51	0.21	3200	13.2	18.5	0.08
	F	160	53	40	0.17	2100	8.8	13	0.05
19-24	M	175	71	42	0.18	3000	12.4		
	F	160	58	36	0.15	2100	8.8		
25-49	M	172	74	36	0.15	2700	11.2		
	F	160	59	32	0.13	1900	8.0		
50-74	M	170	73	31	0.13	2300	9.6		
	F	158	63	29	0.12	1800	7.6		
75+	M	168	69	29	0.12	2000	8.4		
	F	155	64	23	0.10	1500	6.0		
Pregnancy (additional)[h]									
1st Trimester									
2nd Trimester									
3rd Trimester									
Lactation (additional)[h]									

[a]Recommended nutrient intakes for Canadians, 1982—Committee for the revision of the Dietary Standard for Canada, Bureau of Nutritional Sciences, Department National Health and Welfare. Recommended intakes of energy and of certain nutrients are not listed in this table because of the nature of the variables upon which they based. The figures for energy are estimates of average requirements for expected patterns of activity. For nutrients not shown, the following amounts are recommend thiamin, 0.4 mg/100 kcal (0.48 mg/5000 kJ); riboflavin, 0.5 mg/1000 kcal (0.6 mg/5000 kJ); niacin, 6.6 NE/1000 kcal (7.9 NE/5000 kJ); vitamin B_6, 15μg, pyridoxine, per gram of protein intake; phosphorus, same as calcium. Recommended intakes during periods of growth are taken as appropriate for individual rep sentative of the midpoint in each age group. All recommended intakes are designed to cover individual variations in essentially all of a healthy population subsisting upc variety of common foods available in Canada. It is emphasized that these are *examples* of the applicatoin of the RNI to particular classes of individuals and/or particu situations.

[b]Requirements can be expected to vary within a range of ±30%.

[c]Figures rounded to the closest whole number when ≥10 and to the closest 0.5 when <10.

[d]First and last figures are averages at the beginning and at the end of the 3-month period.

[e]Figures rounded to the nearest 50 when <1000 and to the nearest 100 when ≥1000.

[f]Figures include 2 decimals if value is <1 and 1 decimal if ≥1.

Protein (g/day)[i]	Fat-soluble vitamins: Vit A (RE/day)[j]	Vit D (μg/day)[k]	Vit E (mg/day)[l]	Water-soluble vitamins: Vit C (mg/day)	Folacin (μg/day)[m]	Vit B_{12} (μg/day)	Minerals: Ca (mg/day)	Mg (mg/day)	Fe (mg/day)	I (μg/day)	Zn (mg/day)
11[n]	400	10	3	20	50	0.3	350	30	0.4[o]	25	2[p]
14[n]	400	10	3	20	50	0.3	350	40	5	35	3
16[n]	400	10	3	20	50	0.3	400	45	7	40	3
18	400	10	3	20	55	0.3	400	50	7	45	3
18	400	10	3	20	65	0.3	500	55	6	55	4
20	400	5	4	20	80	0.4	500	65	6	65	4
25	500	5	5	25	90	0.5	600	90	6	85	5
31	700	2.5	7	35	125	0.8	700	110	7	110	6
29	700	2.5	6	30	125	0.8	700	110	7	95	7
38	800	2.5	8	40	170	1.0	900	150	10	125	6
39	800	2.5	7	40	170	1.0	1000	160	10	110	7
49	900	2.5	9	50	160	1.5	1100	220	12	160	9
43	800	2.5	7	45	160	1.5	800	190	13	160	8
54	1000	2.5	10	55	190	1.9	900	240	10	160	9
47	800	2.5	7	45	160	1.9	700	220	14	160	8
57	1000	2.5	10	60	210	2.0	800	240	8	160	9
41	800	2.5	7	45	165	2.0	700	190	14	160	8
57	1000	2.5	9	60	210	2.0	800	240	8	160	9
41	800	2.5	6	45	165	2.0	700	190	14[q]	160	8
57	1000	2.5	7	60	210	2.0	800	240	8	160	9
41	800	2.5	6	45	165	2.0	800	190	7	160	8
57	1000	2.5	6	60	210	2.0	800	240	8	160	9
41	800	2.5	5	45	165	2.0	800	190	7	160	8
15	100	2.5	2	0	305	1.0	500	15	6	25	0
20	100	2.5	2	20	305	1.0	500	20	6	25	1
25	100	2.5	2	20	305	1.0	500	25	6	25	2
20	400	2.5	3	30	120	0.5	500	80	0	50	6

[g]Figures rounded to the nearest 0.5.
[h]Pregnancy: Add 100 kcal during the first trimester and 300 for the second and third trimester.
Lactation: Add 450 kcal/day.
[i]The primary units are grams per kilogram of body weight. The figures shown here are only examples.
[j]One retinal equivalent (RE) corresponds to the biological activity of 1 μg of retinol, 6 μg of β-carotene or 12 μg of other carotenes.
[k]Expressed as cholecalciferol or ergocalciferol.
[l]Expressed as d-α-tocopherol equivalents, relative to which β- and γ-tocopherol and α-tocotrienol have activities of 0.5, 0.1 and 0.3 respectively.
[m]Expressed as total folate.
[n]Assumption that the protein is from breast milk or is of the same biological value as that of breast milk and that between 3 and 9 months adjustment for the quality of the protein is made.
[o]For the infant it is assumed that breast milk is the source of iron up to 2 months of age.
[p]Based on the assumption that breast milk is the source of zinc up to 2 months of age.
[q]After the menopause the recommended intake is 7 mg/day.

6-3 Recommended daily dietary allowances for selected nutrients for pregnancy and lactation

	Nonpregnant girl/woman				*Pregnant girl/woman*				*Lactation (850 ml daily)*		
Nutrients	*11-14 yr*	*15-18 yr*	*19+ yr*	*Added need*	*11-14 yr*	*15-18 yr*	*19+ yr*	*Added need*	*11-14 yr*	*15-18 yr*	*19+ yr*
Calories	2200	2100	2000	300	2500	2400	2300	500	2700	2600	2500
Protein	46	46	44	30	76	78	76	20	64	68	66
Calcium (g)	1.2	1.2	0.8	0.4	1.6	1.6	1.2	0.4	1.6	1.6	1.2
Iron (mg)	18	18	18	†	†	†	†	†	†	†	†
Vitamin A (μg RE)‡	800	800	800	200	1000	1000	1000	400	1200	1200	1200
Thiamine (mg)	1.2	1.1	1.0	0.4	1.6	1.5	1.7	0.5	1.7	1.6	1.5
Riboflavin (mg)	1.3	1.3	1.2	0.3	1.6	1.6	1.5	0.5	1.8	1.8	1.7
Niacin equivalent (mg)	15	14	13	2	17	16	15	5	20	19	18
Ascorbic acid (mg)	50	60	60	20	70	80	80	40	90	100	100
Vitamin D (μg)	10	10	5	5	15	15	15	5	15	15	15

From Food and Nutrition Board: Recommended dietary allowance, rev. ed., Washington, D.C., 1979, National Academy of Sciences–National Research Council.

†The increased requirement during pregnancy cannot be met by the iron content of habitual American diets nor by the existing iron stores of many women; therefore the use of 30-60 mg of supplemental iron is recommended. Iron needs during lactation are not substantially different from those of nonpregnant women, but continued supplementation of the mother for 2-3 mo after parturition is advisable to replenish stores depleted by pregnancy.

‡Retinol equivalent (RE) replaces international unit (IU) as the standard measures of vitamin A activity.

6-4 Daily dietary guide—the basic four food groups

Food group	*Main nutrients*	*Daily amounts**
Milk		
Milk, cheese, ice cream, or other products made with whole or skimmed milk	Calcium Protein Riboflavin	Children under 9: 2-3 cups Children 9-12: 3 or more cups Teen-agers: 4 or more cups Adults: 2 or more cups Pregnant women: 3 or more cups Nursing mothers: 4 or more cups (1 cup = 8 oz fluid milk or designated milk equivalent†)
Meats		
Beef, veal, lamb, pork, poultry, fish, eggs	Protein Iron Thiamin	2 or more servings Count as 1 serving: 2-3 oz of lean, boneless, cooked meat, poultry, or fish 2 eggs
Alternates: dry beans, dry peas, nuts, peanut butter	Niacin Riboflavin	1 cup cooked dry beans or peas 4 tbsp peanut butter
Vegetables and fruits		4 or more servings Count as 1 serving: ½ cup of vegetable or fruit or a portion such as 1 medium apple, banana, orange, potato, or ½ a medium grapefruit, melon Include:
	Vitamin A	A dark-green or deep-yellow vegetable or fruit rich in vitamin A at least every other day
	Vitamin C (ascorbic acid)	A citrus fruit or other fruit or vegetable rich in vitamin C daily
	Smaller amounts of other vitamins and minerals	Other vegetables and fruits including potatoes
Bread and cereals		4 or more servings of whole grain, enriched or restored Count as 1 serving:
	Thiamin Niacin Riboflavin Iron Protein	1 slice of bread 1 oz (1 cup) ready to eat cereal, flake or puff varieties ½-¾ cup cooked cereal ½-¾ cup cooked pastes (macaroni, spaghetti, noodles) Crackers: 5 saltines, 2 squares graham crackers

*Use additional amounts of these foods or added butter, margarine, oils, sugars, etc., as desired or needed.

†Milk equivalents: 1 oz cheddar cheese, 3 servings cottage cheese, 1 cup fluid skimmed milk, 1 cup buttermilk, ½ cup dry skimmed milk powder, 1 cup ice milk, 1⅔ cups ice cream, ½ cup evaporated milk.

6-5 Vitamins and minerals

Summary of fat-soluble vitamins

Vitamin	*Physiological functions*	*Results of deficiency*	*Requirement*	*Food sources*
A (retinol) Provitamin A (carotene)	Production of rhodopsin (visual purple) Formation and maintenance of epithelial tissue Toxic in large amounts	Xerophthalmia Night blindness Keratinization of epithelium Follicular hyperkeratosis Skin and mucous membrane infections Faulty tooth formation	Adult male: 1,000 μg RE (5,000 IU) Adult female: 800 μg RE (4,000 IU) Pregnancy: 1,000 μg RE (5,000 IU) Lactation: 1,200 μg RE (6,000 IU) Children: 400 μg RE (2,000 IU) to 800 μg RE (4,000 IU)	Liver Cream, butter, whole milk Egg yolk Green and yellow vegetables Yellow fruits Fortified margarine
D (calciferol)	Absorption of calcium and phosphorus Calcification of bones Renal phosphate clearance Toxic in large amounts	Rickets Faulty bone growth Osteomalacia in adults	Adult: 5-10 μg cholecalciferol (200-400 IU) Pregnancy and lactation: 10-12.5 μg (400-500 IU) depending on age Children: 10 μg (400 IU)	Fish oils Fortified or irradiated milk
E (tocopherol)	Related to action of selenium Antioxidant with vitamin A and unsaturated fatty acids Hemopoiesis Reproduction (in animals)	Hemolysis of red blood cells; anemia Possible protection of unsaturated fatty acids Sterility (in rats)	Adult: 8-10 mg αTE Pregnancy and lactation: 10-11 mg αTE Children: 3-10 mg αTE	Vegetable oils
K (menadione)	Blood clotting, necessary for synthesis of prothrombin Possible coenzyme in oxidation phosphorylation Toxic in large amounts	Hemorrhagic disease of the newborn Bleeding tendencies in biliary disease or surgical procedures Deficiency in intestinal malabsorption (sprue, celiac disease, colitis) Prolonged antibiotic therapy Anticoagulant therapy (dicumarol counteracts)	Unknown	Green leafy vegetables Cheese Egg yolk Liver

Summary of vitamin C (ascorbic acid)

Physiological functions	*Clinical applications*	*Requirement*	*Food sources*
Intercellular cement substance: 1. Collagen formation 2. Firm capillary walls General metabolism: 1. Makes iron available for hemoglobin and maturation of red blood cells 2. Influences conversion of folic acid to "citrovorum factor" (folinic acid)	Scurvy (deficiency) Megaloblastic anemia Wound healing; tissue formation Fevers and infections Stress reactions Growth periods	60 mg daily (adults)	Citrus fruits Tomatoes Cabbage Potatoes Strawberries Melon Chili peppers

Summary of B-complex vitamins

Vitamin	*Physiological functions*	*Clinical applications*	*Requirement*	*Food sources*
Thiamin (B_1)	Coenzyme in carbohydrate metabolism: TPP—decarboxylation TDP—transketolation	Beriberi (deficiency) GI*: anorexia, gastric atony, indigestion, deficient hydrochloric acid CNS*: fatigue, apathy, neuritis, paralysis CV*: cardiac failure, peripheral vasodilation, and edema of extremities	0.5 mg/1000 calories	Pork, beef, liver, whole or enriched grains, legumes
Riboflavin (B_2)	Coenzyme in protein of energy metabolism (flavoproteins) FMN (flavin mononucleotide) FAD (flavin-adenine dinucleotide)	Wound aggravation Cheilosis Glossitis Eye irritation; photophobia Seborrheic dermatitis	0.6 mg/1000 calories	Milk, liver, enriched calories
Niacin (nicotinic acid) (precursor—tryptophan)	Coenzyme in tissue oxidation to produce energy (ATP) NAD (nicotinamide-adenine dinucleotide) NADP (nicotinamide-adenine dinucletide phosphate)	Pellagra (deficiency) Weakness, lassitude, anorexia Skin: scaly dermatitis CNS: neuritis, confusion	14-20 mg (NE)	Meat, peanuts, enriched grains
Pyridoxine (B_6)	Coenzyme in amino acid metabolism Decarboxylation Deamination Transamination Transsulfuration Niacin formation from tryptophan Heme formation Amino acid absorption	Anemia (hypochromic microcytic) CNS: hyperirritability, convulsions, neuritis Isoniazid is an antagonist for pyridoxine Pregnancy: anemia	2 mg	Wheat, corn, meat, liver
Pantothenic acid	Coenzyme in formation of active acetate (CoA)—acetylation	Contributes to: Lipogenesis Amino acid activation Formation of cholesterol Formation of steroid hormones Formation of heme Excretion of drugs	Liver, egg, skimmed milk	
Lipoic acid (sulfur-containing fatty acid)	Coenzyme (with thiamin) in carbohydrate metabolism to reduce pyruvate to active acetate Oxidative decarboxylation	Undetermined (see thiamin)		Liver, yeast
Biotin	Coenzyme in decarboxylation (synthesis of fatty acids, amino acids, purines); deamination	Undetermined		Egg yolk, liver
Folic acid (B_9)	Coenzyme for single carbon transfer—purines, thymine, hemoglobin Transmethylation	Blood cell regeneration in pernicious anemia but not control of its neurological problems Megaloblastic anemia Macrocytic anemia of pregnancy Sprue treatment Aminopterin is antagonist	400 µg Pregnancy: 800 µg Lactation: 800 µg	Liver, green leafy vegetables, asparagus

*GI, Gastrointestinal; CNS, central nervous system; CV, cardiovascular.

Continued.

Summary of B-complex vitamins—cont'd

Vitamin	*Physiological functions*	*Clinical applications*	*Requirement*	*Food sources*
PABA (part of folic acid)		Treatment of rickettsial diseases Anemias (see folic acid)		Same as folic acid
Cobalamin (B_{12})	Coenzyme in protein synthesis Formation of nucleic acid and cell proteins—red blood cells Transmethylation	Extrinsic factor in pernicious anemia—combines with intrinsic factor of gastric secretions for absorption; forms red blood cells (with folic acid) Sprue treatment (with folic acid)	3μg	Liver, meat, milk, egg, cheese
Inositol	Lipotropic agent (?)	Undetermined		Citrus fruit, grains, meat, milk
Choline	Lipotropic agent Forms nerve mediator—acetylcholine	Fatty liver—hepatitis, cirrhosis (undetermined in human nutrition)		Meat, cereals, egg yolk

Summary of major minerals

Mineral	*Metabolism*	*Physiological functions*	*Clinical application*	*Requirement*	*Food sources*
Calcium (Ca)	Absorption according to body need, aided by vitamin D, favored by protein, lactose, acidity; hindered by excess fats and binding agents (phosphates, oxalates, phytate) Excretion chiefly in feces, 70% to 90% of amount ingested Deposition-mobilization in bone compartment constant; deposition aided by vitamin D Parathyroid hormone controls absorption and mobilization	Bone formation Teeth Blood clotting Muscle contraction and relaxation Heart action Nerve transmission Cell wall permeability Enzyme activation (ATPase)	Tetany—decrease in ionized serum calcium Rickets Renal calculi Hyperparathyroidism Hypoparathyroidism	Adults: 0.8 gm Pregnancy and lactation: 1.2 gm Infants: 360-540 mg Children: 0.8-1.2 gm	Milk Cheese Green leafy vegetables Whole grains Egg yolk Legumes, nuts
Phosphorus (P)	Absorption with calcium aided by vitamin D, hindered by excess binding agents (calcium, aluminum, iron) Excretion chiefy by kidney according to renal threshold blood level Parathyroid hormone controls renal excretion balance with blood level Deposition-mobilization in bone compartment constant	Bone formation Overall metabolism: Absorption of glucose and glycerol (phosphorylation) Transport of fatty acids Energy metabolism (enzymes, ATP) Buffer system	Growth Hypophosphatemia: Recovery state from diabetic acidosis Sprue, celiac disease (malabsorption) Bone diseases (upset Ca:P balance) Hyperphosphatemia: Renal insufficiency Hypoparathyroidism Tetany	Adults: 1½ times calcium intake Pregnancy and lactation: 1.2 gm Infants: 240-400 mg Children: 0.8-1.2 gm	Milk Cheese Meat Egg yolk Whole grains Legumes, nuts

Mineral	Metabolism	Physiological functions	Clinical application	Requirement	Food sources
Magnesium (Mg)	Absorption increased by parathyroid hormone, hindered by excess fat, phosphate, calcium Excretion regulated by kidney	In bones and teeth Activator and coenzyme in carbohydrate and protein metabolism Essential intracellular fluid (ICF) cation Muscle, nerve irritability	Tremor, spasm; low serum level following gastrointestinal losses	300-350 mg Deficiency in humans unlikely	Whole grains Nuts Meat Milk Legumes
Sodium (Na)	Readily absorbed Excretion chiefly by kidney, controlled by aldosterone, acid base balance	Major extracellular fluid (ECF) cation Water balance, osmotic pressure Acid-base balance Cell permeability; absorption of glucose Muscle irritability; transmission of electrochemical impulse and resulting contraction	Fluid shifts and control Buffer system Losses in gastrointestinal disorders	About 0.5 gm Diet usually has more: 2-6 gm	Table salt (NaCl) Milk Meat Egg Baking soda Baking powder Carrots, beets, spinach, celery
Potassium (K)	Secreted and reabsorbed in digestive juices Excretion guarded by kidney according to blood levels; increased by aldosterone	Major ICF cation Acid-base balance Regulates neuromuscular excitability and muscle contraction Glycogen formation Protein synthesis	Fluid shifts Losses in starvation, diabetic acidosis, adrenal tumors Heart action—low serum potassium (tachycardia, cardiac arrest) Treatment of diabetic acidosis (rapid glycogen production reduces serum potassium) Tissue catabolism—potassium loss	About 2-4 gm Diet adequate in protein, calcium, and iron contains adequate potassium	Whole grains Meat Legumes Fruits Vegetables
Chlorine (Cl)	Absorbed readily Excretion controlled by kidney	Major ECF anion Acid-base balance—chloride-bicarbonate shift Water balance Gastric hydrochloric acid—digestion	Hypochloremic alkalosis in prolonged vomiting, diarrhea, lube drainage	About 0.5 gm Diet usually has more: 2-6 gm	Table salt
Sulfur (S)	Absorbed as such and as constituent of sulfur-containing amino acid, methionine Excreted by kidney in relation to protein intake and tissue catabolism	Essential constituent of cell protein Activates enzymes High-energy sulfur bonds in energy metabolism Detoxification reactions	Cystine renal calculi Cystinuria	Diet adequate in protein contains adequate sulfur	Meat Egg Cheese Milk Nuts, legumes

Summary of trace minerals

Mineral	Metabolism	Physiological functions	Clinical application	Requirement	Food source
Iron (Fe)	Absorption according to body need controlled by mucosal block—ferritin mechanism, aided by vitamin C, gastric hydrochloric acid Transport—transferrin Storage—ferritin, hemosiderin Excretion from tissue in minute quantities, body conserves and reuses	Hemoglobin formation Cellular oxidation (cytochrome system producing ATP)	Growth (milk anemia) Pregnancy demands Deficiency anemia Excess hemosiderosis; hemochromatosis	Men 10 mg Women 18 mg Pregnancy 18^{+} mg Lactation; 18 mg Children: 10-18 mg	Liver Meats Egg yolk Whole grains Enriched bread and cereal Dark green vegetables Legumes, nuts
Copper (Cu)	Transported bound to an α-globulin as ceruloplasmin Stored in muscle, bone, liver, heart, kidney, and central-nervous system	Associated with iron in Enzyme systems Hemoglobin synthesis Absorption and transport of iron Involved in bone formation and maintenance of brain tissue and myelin sheath in nervous system	Hypocupremia: Nephrosis Malabsorption Wilson's disease—excess copper storage	2-2.5 mg Diet provides 2-5 mg	Liver Meat Seafood Whole grains Legumes, nuts Cocoa Raisins Food cooked in copper utensils
Iodine (I)	Absorbed as iodides, taken up by thyroid gland under control of thyroid-stimulating hormone (TSH) Excretion by kidney	Synthesis of thyroxine, the thyroid hormone, which regulates cell oxidation	Deficiency—endemic colloid goiter; cretinism	Men: 140μg Women: 100 μg Infants: 35-45 μg Children: 60-140 μg	Iodized salt Seafood
Manganese (Mn)	Absorption limited Excretion mainly by intestine	Activates reactions in Urea formation Protein metabolism Glucose oxidation Lipoprotein clearance and synthesis of fatty acids	No clinical deficiency observed in humans Inhalation toxicity in miners	2.5-7 mg (estimated) Diet provides 3-9 μg	Cereals, whole grain Soybeans Legumes, nuts Tea, coffee Vegetables Fruits
Cobalt (Co)	Absorbed chiefly as constituent of vitamin B_{12}	Constituent of vitamin B_{12}; essential factor in red blood cell formation	Deficiency associated with deficiency of vitamin B_{12}—pernicious anemia	Unknown	Supplied by preformed vitamin B_{12}
Zinc (Zn)	Transported with plasma proteins Excretion largely intestinal Stored in liver, muscle, bone, and organs	Essential enzyme constituent: Carbonic anhydrase Carboxypeptidase Lactic dehydrogenase Combined with insulin for storage of the hormone	Possible relation to liver disease Wound healing Taste and smell acuity Retarded sexual and physical development	Adults: 15 mg Children: 10 mg Infants: 3-5 mg	Widely distributed Liver Seafood, especially oysters Eggs Milk Whole grains
Molybdenum (Mo)	Minute traces in the body	Constituent of specific enzymes involved in Purine conversion to uric acid Aldehyde oxidation		450-500 μg (estimated)	Organ meats Milk Whole grains Leafy vegetables Legumes

Mineral	*Metabolism*	*Physiological functions*	*Clinical application*	*Requirement*	*Food source*
Fluorine (Fl)	Deposited in bones and teeth Excreted in urine	Associated with dental health	Small amount prevents dental caries Excess causes endemic dental fluorosis	1-3 mg (estimated)	Water (1 ppm Fl)
Selenium (Se)	Active as cofactor in cell oxidation enzyme system	Associated with fat metabolism	Constituent of "factor 3," which acts with vitamin E to prevent fatty liver	Under 100 μg (estimated)	Seafoods Meats Whole grains
Chromium (Cr)	Improves faulty uptake of glucose by body tissues	Associated with glucose metabolism; raises abnormally low fasting blood sugar levels	Infants unable to metabolize sugar, and adult diabetics show definite improvement when small amounts of chromium added to diet Possible link with cardiovascular disorders and diabetes	20-50 μg (estimated)	Animal proteins, especially meats (except fish) Whole grains
Nickel (Ni)	Binding by phytate reduces intestinal absorption	Constituent of the protein nickeloplasmin Associated with thyroid hormone High in RNA	Plasma levels decreased in cirrhosis and chronic uremia	Whole grains Legumes Vegetables Fruits	
Tin (Sn)		Structural element in protein synthesis Associated with cell enzyme systems in energy metabolism	Wound healing Tissue growth	Under 1 mg (estimated)	Meats Whole grains Legumes Vegetables Fruits Acid juices canned in tin
Silicon (Si)		Essential agent in formation of bone, cartilage, connective tissue	Bone calcification and healing	Unknown	All plant foods
Vanadium (V)		High in teeth; may have role in bone and tooth formation	Possible relation to lipid metabolism, blood lipid levels	0.1-0.3 mg (estimated)	Grains, breads Root vegetables Nuts Vegetable oils

6-6 Nutritive values of the edible part of foods

Food, approximate measure, and weight (in grams)			Food energy (calories)	Protein (g)	Fat (total lipid) (g)	Fatty acids: Saturated (total) (g)	Fatty acids: Unsaturated: Oleic (g)	Fatty acids: Unsaturated: Linoleic (g)	Carbohydrate (g)	Calcium (mg)	Iron (mg)	Vitamin A value (IU)	Thiamin (mg)	Riboflavin (mg)	Niacin (mg)	Ascorbic acid (mg)
Milk, cream, cheese (related products)																
Milk, cow's																
Fluid, whole (3.5% fat)	1 cup	244	160	9	9	5	3	Trace	12	288	0.1	350	0.08	0.42	0.1	2
Fluid, nonfat (skim)	1 cup	246	90	9	Trace	—	—	—	13	298	.1	10	.10	.44	.2	2
Buttermilk, cultured, from skim milk	1 cup	246	90	9	Trace	—	—	—	13	298	.1	10	.09	.44	.2	2
Evaporated, unsweetened, undiluted	1 cup	252	345	18	20	11	7	1	24	635	.3	820	.10	.84	.5	3
Condensed, sweetened, undiluted	1 cup	306	980	25	27	15	9	1	166	802	.3	1,090	.23	1.17	.5	3
Dry, whole	1 cup	103	515	27	28	16	9	1	39	936	.5	1,160	.30	1.50	.7	6
Dry, nonfat, instant	1 cup	70	250	25	Trace	—	—	—	36	905	.4	20	.24	1.25	.6	5
Milk, goat's																
Fluid, whole	1 cup	244	165	8	10	6	2	Trace	11	315	.2	390	.10	.27	.7	2
Cream																
Half-and-half (cream and milk)	1 cup	242	325	8	28	16	9	1	11	261	.1	1,160	.08	.38	.1	2
	1 tbsp	15	20	Trace	2	1	1	Trace	1	16	Trace	70	Trace	.02	Trace	Trace
Light, coffee or table	1 cup	240	505	7	49	27	16	1	10	245	.1	2,030	.07	.36	.1	2
	1 tbsp	15	30	Trace	3	2	1	Trace	1	15	Trace	130	Trace	.02	Trace	Trace
Whipping, unwhipped (volume about double when whipped)																
Light	1 cup	239	715	6	75	41	25	2	9	203	.1	3,070	.06	.30	.1	2
	1 tbsp	15	45	Trace	5	3	2	Trace	1	13	Trace	190	Trace	.02	Trace	Trace
Heavy	1 cup	238	840	5	89	49	29	3	7	178	.1	3,670	.05	.26	.1	2
	1 tbsp	15	55	Trace	6	3	2	Trace	Trace	11	Trace	230	Trace	.02	Trace	Trace
Cheese																
Blue or Roquefort type	1 oz	28	105	6	9	5	3	Trace	1	89	.1	350	.01	.17	.1	0
Cheddar or American																
Ungrated	1 inch cube	17	70	4	5	3	2	Trace	Trace	128	.2	220	Trace	.08	Trace	0

Grated	1 cup	112	445	28	36	20	12	1	2	840	1.1	1,470	.03	.51	.1	0
	1 tbsp	7	30	2	2	1	1	Trace	Trace	52	.1	90	Trace	.03	Trace	0
Cheddar, process	1 oz	28	105	7	9	5	3	Trace	1	219	.3	350	Trace	.12	Trace	0
Cheese foods, Cheddar	1 oz	28	90	6	7	4	2	Trace	2	162	.2	280	.01	.16	Trace	0
Cottage cheese, from skim milk																
Creamed	1 cup	225	240	31	9	5	3	Trace	7	212	0.7	380	0.07	0.56	0.2	0
	1 oz	28	30	4	1	1	Trace	Trace	1	27	.1	50	.01	.07	Trace	0
Uncreamed	1 cup	225	195	38	1	Trace	Trace	Trace	6	202	.9	20	.07	.63	.2	0
	1 oz	28	25	5	Trace	—	—	—	1	26	.1	Trace	.01	.08	Trace	0
Cream cheese	1 oz	28	105	2	11	6	4	Trace	1	18	.1	440	Trace	.07	Trace	0
	1 tbsp	15	55	1	6	3	2	Trace	Trace	9	Trace	230	Trace	.04	Trace	0
Swiss (domestic)	1 oz	28	105	8	8	4	3	Trace	1	262	.3	320	Trace	.11	Trace	0
Milk beverages																
Cocoa	1 cup	242	235	9	11	6	4	Trace	26	286	.9	390	.09	.45	.4	2
Chocolate-flavored milk drink (made with skim milk)	1 cup	250	190	8	6	3	2	Trace	27	270	.4	210	.09	.41	.2	2
Malted milk	1 cup	270	280	13	12	—	—	—	32	364	.8	670	.17	.56	.2	2
Milk desserts																
Cornstarch pudding, plain (blanc mange)	1 cup	248	275	9	10	5	3	Trace	39	290	.1	390	.07	.40	.1	2
Custard, baked	1 cup	248	285	13	14	6	5	1	28	278	1.0	870	.10	.47	.2	1
Ice cream, plain, factory packed																
Slice or cut brick, ⅛ of quart brick	1 slice or cut brick	71	145	3	9	5	3	Trace	15	87	.1	370	.03	.13	.1	1
Container	3½ fld oz	62	130	2	8	4	3	Trace	13	76	.1	320	.03	.12	.1	1
Container	8 fld oz	142	295	6	18	10	6	1	29	175	.1	740	.06	.27	.1	1
Ice milk	1 cup	187	285	9	10	6	3	Trace	42	292	.2	390	.09	.41	.2	2
Yogurt, from partially skimmed milk	1 cup	246	120	8	4	2	1	Trace	13	295	.1	170	.09	.43	.2	2
Eggs																
Eggs, large, 24 ounces per dozen																
Raw																
Whole, without shell	1 egg	50	80	6	6	2	3	Trace	Trace	27	1.1	590	.05	.15	Trace	0
White of egg	1 white	33	15	4	Trace	—	—	—	Trace	3	Trace	0	Trace	.09	Trace	0
Yolk of egg	1 yolk	17	60	3	5	2	2	Trace	Trace	24	.9	580	.04	.07	Trace	0
Cooked																
Boiled, shell removed	2 eggs	100	160	13	12	4	5	1	1	54	2.3	1,180	.09	.28	.1	0

Reprinted from Nutritive value of foods, U.S. Department of Agriculture, Home and Garden Bulletin No. 72.
Dashes show that no basis could be found for imputing a value although there was some reason to believe that a measureable amount of the constituent might be present.

Nutritive values of the edible part of foods—cont'd

Food, approximate measure, and weight (in grams)			Food energy (calories)	Protein (g)	Fat (total lipid) (g)	Fatty acids: Saturated (total) (g)	Fatty acids: Unsaturated: Oleic (g)	Fatty acids: Unsaturated: Linoleic (g)	Carbohydrate (g)	Calcium (mg)	Iron (mg)	Vitamin A value (IU)	Thiamin (mg)	Riboflavin (mg)	Niacin (mg)	Ascorbic acid (mg)
Scrambled, with milk and fat	1 egg	64	110	7	8	3	3	Trace	1	51	1.1	690	.05	.18	Trace	0
Meat, poultry, fish, shellfish (related products)																
Bacon, broiled or fried, crisp	2 slices	16	100	5	8	3	4	1	1	2	.5	0	.08	.05	.8	—
Beef, trimmed to retail basis[2], cooked																
Cuts braised, simmered, or pot-roasted																
Lean and fat	3 oz	85	245	23	16	8	7	Trace	0	10	2.9	30	.04	.18	3.5	—
Lean only	2.5 oz	72	140	22	5	2	2	Trace	0	10	2.7	10	.04	.16	3.3	—
Hamburger (ground beef), broiled																
Lean	3 oz	85	185	23	10	5	4	Trace	0	10	3.0	20	.08	.20	5.1	—
Regular	3 oz	85	245	21	17	8	8	Trace	0	9	2.7	30	.07	.18	4.6	—
Roast, oven-cooked, no liquid added																
Relatively fat, such as rib																
Lean and fat	3 oz	85	375	17	34	16	15	1	0	8	2.2	70	.05	.13	3.1	—
Lean only	1.8 oz	51	125	14	7	3	3	Trace	0	6	1.8	10	.04	.11	2.6	—
Relatively lean, such as heel of round																
Lean and fat	3 oz	85	165	25	7	3	3	Trace	0	11	3.2	10	.06	.19	4.5	—
Lean only	2.7 oz	78	125	24	3	1	1	Trace	0	10	3.0	Trace	.06	.18	4.3	—
Steak, broiled																
Relatively fat, such as sirloin																
Lean and fat	3 oz	85	330	20	27	13	12	1	0	9	2.5	50	.05	.16	4.0	—
Lean only	2.0 oz	56	115	18	4	2	2	Trace	0	7	2.2	10	.05	.14	3.6	—
Relatively lean, such as round																
Lean and fat	3 oz	85	220	24	13	6	6	Trace	0	10	3.0	20	.07	.19	4.8	—
Lean only	2.4 oz	68	130	21	4	2	2	Trace	0	9	2.5	10	.06	.16	4.1	—
Beef, canned																
Corned beef	3 oz	85	185	22	10	5	4	Trace	0	17	3.7	20	.01	.20	2.9	—
Corned beef hash	3 oz	85	155	7	10	5	4	Trace	9	11	1.7	—	.01	.08	1.8	—
Beef, dried or chipped	2 oz	57	115	19	4	2	2	Trace	0	11	2.9	—	.04	.18	2.2	—
Beef and vegetable stew	1 cup	235	210	15	10	5	4	Trace	15	28	2.8	2,310	.13	.17	4.4	15
Beef potpie, baked: individual pie, 4¼-inch diameter, weight before baking about 8 oz	1 pie	227	560	23	33	9	20	2	43	32	4.1	1,860	.25	.27	4.5	7
Chicken, cooked																
Flesh only, broiled	3 oz	85	115	20	3	1	1	1	0	8	1.4	80	0.05	0.16	7.4	—

Breast, fried ½ breast																
With bone	3.3 oz	94	155	25	5	1	2	1	1	9	1.3	70	.04	.17	11.2	—
Flesh and skin only	2.7 oz	76	155	25	5	1	2	1	1	9	1.3	70	.04	.17	11.2	—
Drumstick, fried																
With bone	2.1 oz	59	90	12	4	1	2	1	Trace	6	.9	50	.03	.15	2.7	—
Flesh and skin only	1.3 oz	38	90	12	4	1	2	1	Trace	6	.9	50	.03	.15	2.7	—
Chicken, canned, boneless	3 oz	85	170	18	10	3	4	2	0	18	1.3	200	.03	.11	3.7	3
Chicken potpie. *See* Poultry potpie																
Chile con carne, canned																
With beans	1 cup	250	335	19	15	7	7	Trace	30	80	4.2	150	.08	.18	3.2	—
Without beans	1 cup	255	510	26	38	18	17	1	15	97	3.6	380	.05	.31	5.6	—
Fish and shellfish																
Bluefish, baked or broiled	3 oz	85	135	22	4	—	—	—	0	25	.6	40	.09	.08	1.6	—
Clams																
Raw, meat only	3 oz	85	65	11	1	—	—	—	2	59	5.2	90	.08	.15	1.1	8
Canned, solids and liquid	3 oz	85	45	7	1	—	—	—	2	47	3.5	—	.01	.09	.9	—
Crabmeat, canned	3 oz	85	85	15	2	—	—	—	1	38	.7	—	.07	.07	1.6	—
Fish sticks, breaded, cooked, frozen; stick 3.8 by 1.0 by 0.5 inch	10 sticks or 8 oz package	227	400	38	20	5	4	10	15	25	.9	—	.09	.16	3.6	—
Haddock, fried	3 oz	85	140	17	5	1	3		5	34	1.0	—	0.03	0.06	2.7	2
Mackerel																
Broiled, Atlantic	3 oz	85	200	19	13	—	—	—	0	5	1.0	450	.13	.23	6.5	—
Canned, Pacific, solids and liquid[3]	3 oz	85	155	18	9	—	—	—	0	221	1.9	20	.02	.28	7.4	—
Ocean perch, breaded (egg and breadcrumbs), fried	3 oz	85	195	16	11	—	—	—	6	28	1.1	—	.08	.09	1.5	—
Oysters, meat only. Raw, 13-19 medium selects	1 cup	240	160	20	4	—	—	—	8	226	13.2	740	.33	.43	6.0	—
Oyster stew, 1 part oysters to 3 parts milk by volume, 3-4 oysters	1 cup	230	200	11	12	—	—	—	11	269	3.3	640	.13	.41	1.6	—
Salmon, pink, canned	3 oz	85	120	17	5	1	1	Trace	0	[4]167	.7	60	.03	.16	6.8	—

[2]Outer layer of fat on the cut was removed to within approximately ½ inch of the lean. Deposits of fat within the cut were not removed.
[3]Vitamin values based on drained solids.
[4]Based on total contents of can. If bones are discarded, value will be greatly reduced.

Nutritive values of the edible part of foods—cont'd

Food, approximate measure, and weight (in grams)			Food energy (calories)	Protein (g)	Fat (total lipid) (g)	Fatty acids: Saturated (total) (g)	Fatty acids: Unsaturated: Oleic (g)	Fatty acids: Unsaturated: Linoleic (g)	Carbohydrate (g)	Calcium (mg)	Iron (mg)	Vitamin A value (IU)	Thiamin (mg)	Riboflavin (mg)	Niacin (mg)	Ascorbic acid (mg)
Sardines, Atlantic, canned in oil, drained solids	3 oz	85	175	20	9	—	—	—	0	372	2.5	190	.02	.17	4.6	—
Shad, baked	3 oz	85	170	20	10	—	—	—	0	20	.5	20	.11	.22	7.3	—
Shrimp, canned, meat only	3 oz	85	100	21	1	—	—	—	1	98	2.6	50	.01	.03	1.5	—
Swordfish, broiled with butter or margarine	3 oz	85	150	24	5	—	—	—	0	23	1.1	1,780	.03	.04	9.3	—
Tuna, canned in oil, drained solids	3 oz	85	170	24	7	—	—	—	0	7	1.6	70	.04	.10	10.1	—
Heart, beef, lean, braised	3 oz	85	160	27	5	—	—	—	1	5	5.0	20	.21	1.04	6.5	1
Lamb, trimmed to retail basis,[2] cooked																
Chop, thick, with bone, broiled	1 chop, 4.8 oz	137	400	25	33	18	12	1	0	10	1.5	—	.14	.25	5.6	—
Lean and fat	4.0 oz	112	400	25	33	18	12	1	0	10	1.5	—	.14	.25	5.6	—
Lean only	2.6 oz	74	140	21	6	3	2	Trace	0	9	1.5	—	.11	.20	4.5	—
Leg, roasted																
Lean and fat	3 oz	85	235	22	16	9	6	Trace	0	9	1.4	—	.13	.23	4.7	—
Lean only	2.5 oz	71	130	20	5	3	2	Trace	0	9	1.4	—	.12	.21	4.4	—
Shoulder, roasted																
Lean and fat	3 oz	85	285	18	23	13	8	1	0	9	1.0	—	.11	.20	4.0	—
Lean only	2.3 oz	64	130	17	6	3	2	Trace	0	8	1.0	—	.10	.18	3.7	—
Liver, beef, fried	2 oz	57	130	15	6	—	—	—	3	6	5.0	30,280	.15	2.37	9.4	15
Pork, cured, cooked																
Ham, light cure, lean and fat, roasted	3 oz	85	245	18	19	7	8	2	0	8	2.2	0	.40	.16	3.1	—
Luncheon meat																
Boiled ham, sliced	2 oz	57	135	11	10	4	4	1	0	6	1.6	0	.25	.09	1.5	—
Canned, spiced or unspiced	2 oz	57	165	8	14	5	6	1	1	5	1.2	0	.18	.12	1.6	—
Pork, fresh, trimmed to retail basis,[2] cooked																
Chop, thick, with bone	1 chop, 3.5 oz	98	260	16	21	8	9	2	0	8	2.2	0	.63	.18	3.8	—

Lean and fat	2.3 oz	66	260	16	21	8	9	2	0	8	2.2	0	.63	.18	3.8	—
Lean only	1.7 oz	48	130	15	7	2	3	1	0	7	1.9	0	.54	.16	3.3	—
Roast, oven-cooked, no liquid added																
Lean and fat	3 oz	85	310	21	24	9	10	2	0	9	2.7	0	.78	.22	4.7	—
Lean only	2.4 oz	68	175	20	10	3	4	1	0	9	2.6	0	.73	.21	4.4	—
Cuts, simmered																
Lean and fat	3 oz	85	320	20	26	9	11	2	0	8	2.5	0	.46	.21	4.1	—
Lean only	2.2 oz	63	135	18	6	2	3	1	0	8	2.3	0	.42	.19	3.7	—
Poultry potpie (based on chicken potpie). Individual pie, 4¼-inch diameter, weigh before baking	1 pie	227	535	23	31	10	15	3	42	68	3.0	3,020	.25	.26	4.1	5
Sausage																
Bologna, slice, 4.1 by 0.1 inch	8 slices	227	690	27	62	—	—	—	2	16	4.1	—	.36	.49	6.0	—
Frankfurter, cooked	1	51	155	6	14	—	—	—	1	3	.8	—	.08	.10	1.3	—
Pork, links or patty, Cooked	4 oz	113	540	21	50	18	21	5	Trace	8	2.7	0	.89	.39	4.2	—
Tongue, beef, braised	3 oz	85	210	18	14	—	—	—	Trace	6	1.9	—	.04	.25	3.0	—
Turkey potpie. *See* Poultry potpie																
Veal, cooked																
Cutlet, without bone, broiled	3 oz	85	185	23	9	5	4	Trace	—	9	2.7	—	.06	.21	4.6	—
Roast, medium fat, medium done; lean and fat	3 oz	85	230	23	14	7	6	Trace	0	10	2.9	—	.11	.26	6.6	—
Mature dry beans and peas, nuts, peanuts (related products)																
Almonds, shelled	1 cup	142	850	26	77	6	52	15	28	332	6.7	0	.34	1.31	5.0	Trace
Beans, dry																
Common varieties, such as Great Northern, navy, and others, canned:																
Red	1 cup	256	230	15	1	—	—	—	42	74	4.6	Trace	.13	.10	1.5	—
White, with tomato sauce																
With pork	1 cup	261	320	16	7	3	3	1	50	141	4.7	340	.20	.08	1.5	5
Without pork	1 cup	261	310	16	1	—	—	—	60	177	5.2	160	.18	.09	1.5	5
Lima, cooked	1 cup	192	260	16	1	—	—	—	48	56	5.6	Trace	.26	.12	1.3	Trace
Brazil nuts	1 cup	140	915	20	94	19	45	24	15	260	4.8	Trace	1.34	.17	2.2	—
Cashew nuts, roasted	1 cup	135	760	23	62	10	43	4	40	51	5.1	140	.58	.33	2.4	—
Coconut																
Fresh, shredded	1 cup	97	335	3	34	29	2	Trace	9	13	1.6	0	.05	.02	.5	3
Dried, shredded sweetened	1 cup	62	340	2	24	21	2	Trace	33	10	1.2	0	.02	.02	.2	0
Cowpeas or blackeye peas, dry, cooked	1 cup	248	190	13	1	—	—	—	34	42	3.2	20	.41	.11	1.1	Trace

[2]Outer layer of fat on the cut was removed to within approximately ½ inch of the lean. Deposits of fat within the cut were not removed.

Nutritive values of the edible part of foods—cont'd

Food, approximate measure, and weight (in grams)			Food energy (calories)	Protein (g)	Fat (total lipid) (g)	Fatty acids			Carbohydrate (g)	Calcium (mg)	Iron (mg)	Vitamin A value (IU)	Thiamin (mg)	Riboflavin (mg)	Niacin (mg)	Ascorbic acid (mg)
						Saturated (total) (g)	Unsaturated									
							Oleic (g)	Linoleic (g)								
Peanuts, roasted, salted																
Halves	1 cup	144	840	37	72	16	31	21	27	107	3.0	—	.46	.19	24.7	0
Chopped	1 tbsp	9	55	2	4	1	2	1	2	7	.2	—	.03	.01	1.5	0
Peanut butter	1 tbsp	16	95	4	8	2	4	2	3	9	.3	—	.02	.02	2.4	0
Peas, split, dry, cooked	1 cup	250	290	20	1	—	—	—	52	28	4.2	100	.37	.22	2.2	—
Pecans																
Halves	1 cup	108	740	10	77	5	48	15	16	79	2.6	140	.93	.14	1.0	2
Chopped	1 tbsp	7.5	50	1	5	Trace	3	1	1	5	.2	10	.06	.01	.1	Trace
Walnuts, shelled																
Black or native, chopped	1 cup	126	790	26	75	4	26	36	19	Trace	7.6	380	.28	.14	.9	—
English or Persian																
Halves	1 cup	100	650	15	64	4	10	40	16	99	3.1	30	.33	.13	.9	3
Chopped	1 tbsp	8	50	1	5	Trace	1	3	1	8	.2	Trace	.03	.01	.1	Trace
Vegetables and vegetable products																
Asparagus																
Cooked, cut spears	1 cup	175	35	4	Trace	—	—	—	6	37	1.0	1,580	.27	.32	2.4	46
Canned spears, medium																
Green	6 spears	96	20	2	Trace	—	—	—	3	18	1.8	770	.06	.10	.8	14
Bleached	6 spears	96	20	2	Trace	—	—	—	4	15	1.0	80	.05	.06	.7	14
Beans																
Lima, immature, cooked	1 cup	160	180	12	1	—	—	—	32	75	4.0	450	.29	.16	2.0	28
Snap, green																
Cooked																
In small amount of water, short time	1 cup	125	30	2	Trace	—	—	—	7	62	.8	680	.08	.11	.6	16
In large amount of water, long time	1 cup	125	30	2	Trace	—	—	—	7	62	.8	680	0.07	0.10	0.4	13
Canned																
Solids and liquid	1 cup	239	45	2	Trace	—	—	—	10	81	2.9	690	.08	.10	.7	9
Strained or chopped (baby food)	1 oz	28	5	Trace	Trace	—	—	—	1	9	.3	110	.01	.02	.1	Trace

Bean sprouts, *See* Sprouts																
Beets, cooked, diced	1 cup	165	50	2	Trace	—	—	—	12	23	.8	40	.04	.07	.5	11
Broccoli spears, cooked	1 cup	150	40	5	Trace	—	—	—	7	132	1.2	3,750	.14	.29	1.2	135
Brussels sprouts, cooked	1 cup	130	45	5	1	—	—	—	8	42	1.4	680	.10	.18	1.1	113
Cabbage																
Raw																
Finely shredded	1 cup	100	25	1	Trace	—	—	—	5	49	.4	130	.05	.05	.3	47
Coleslaw	1 cup	120	120	1	9	2	2	5	9	52	.5	180	.06	.06	.3	35
Cooked																
In small amount of water, short time	1 cup	170	35	2	Trace	—	—	—	7	75	.5	220	.07	.07	.5	56
In large amount of water, long time	1 cup	170	30	2	Trace	—	—	—	7	71	.5	200	.04	.04	.2	40
Cabbage, celery or Chinese																
Raw, leaves and stalk, 1-inch pieces	1 cup	100	15	1	Trace	—	—	—	3	43	.6	150	.05	.04	.6	25
Cabbage, spoon (or pakchoy), cooked	1 cup	150	20	2	Trace	—	—	—	4	222	.9	4,650	.07	.12	1.1	23
Carrots																
Raw																
Whole, 5½ by 1 inch, (25 thin strips)	1	50	20	1	Trace	—	—	—	5	18	.4	5,500	.03	.03	.3	4
Grated	1 cup	110	45	1	Trace	—	—	—	11	41	.8	12,100	.06	.06	.7	9
Cooked, diced	1 cup	145	45	1	Trace	—	—	—	10	48	.9	15,220	.08	.07	.7	9
Canned, strained or chopped (baby food)	1 oz	28	10	Trace	Trace	—	—	—	2	7	.1	3,690	.01	.01	.1	1
Cauliflower, cooked, flowerbuds	1 cup	120	25	3	Trace	—	—	—	5	25	.8	70	.11	.10	.7	66
Celery, raw																
Stalk, large outer, 8 by about 1½ inches, at root end	1 stalk	40	5	Trace	Trace	—	—	—	2	16	.1	100	.01	.01	.1	4
Pieces, diced	1 cup	100	15	1	Trace	—	—	—	4	39	.3	240	.03	.03	.3	9
Collards, cooked	1 cup	190	55	5	1	—	—	—	9	289	1.1	10,260	.27	.37	2.4	87
Corn, sweet																
Cooked, ear 5 by 1¾ inches[5]	1 ear	140	70	3	1	—	—	—	16	2	.5	[6]310	.09	.08	1.0	7
Canned, solids and liquid	1 cup	256	170	5	2	—	—	—	40	10	1.0	[6]690	.07	.12	2.3	13

[5]Measure and weight apply to entire vegetable or fruit including parts not usually eaten.
[6]Based on yellow varieties; white varieties contain only a trace of cryptoxanthin and carotenes, the pigments in corn that have biological activity.

Nutritive values of the edible part of foods—cont'd

Food, approximate measure, and weight (in grams)			Food energy (calories)	Protein (g)	Fat (total lipid) (g)	Fatty acids			Carbohydrate (g)	Calcium (mg)	Iron (mg)	Vitamin A value (IU)	Thiamin (mg)	Riboflavin (mg)	Niacin (mg)	Ascorbic acid (mg)
						Saturated (total) (g)	Unsaturated									
							Oleic (g)	Linoleic (g)								
Cowpeas, cooked, immature seeds	1 cup	160	175	13	1	—	—	—	29	38	3.4	560	.49	.18	2.3	28
Cucumbers, 10 oz, 7½ by about 2 inches																
Raw, pared	1	207	30	1	Trace	—	—	—	7	35	.6	Trace	.07	.09	.4	23
Raw, pared, center slice ⅛-inch thick	6 slices	50	5	Trace	Trace	—	—	—	2	8	.2	Trace	.02	.02	.1	6
Dandelion greens, cooked	1 cup	180	60	4	1	—	—	—	12	252	3.2	21,060	.24	.29	—	32
Endive, curly (including escarole)	2 oz	57	10	1	Trace	—	—	—	2	46	1.0	1,870	.04	.08	.3	6
Kale, leaves including stems, cooked	1 cup	110	30	4	1	—	—	—	4	147	1.3	8,140	—	—	—	68
Lettuce, raw																
Butterhead, as Boston types; head, 4-inch diameter	1 head	220	30	3	Trace	—	—	—	6	77	4.4	2,130	.14	.13	.6	18
Crisphead, as Iceberg; head, 4¼-inch diameter	1 head	454	60	4	Trace	—	—	—	13	91	2.3	1,500	.29	.27	1.3	29
Looseleaf, of bunching varieties, leaves	2 large	50	10	1	Trace	—	—	—	2	34	.7	950	.03	.04	.2	9
Mushrooms, canned, solids and liquid	1 cup	244	40	5	Trace	—	—	—	6	15	1.2	Trace	.04	.60	4.8	4
Mustard greens, cooked	1 cup	140	35	3	1	—	—	—	6	193	2.5	8,120	.11	.19	.9	68
Okra, cooked, pod 3 by ⅝ inch	8 pods	85	25	3	Trace	—	—	—	5	78	.4	420	.11	.15	.8	17
Onions																
Mature																
Raw, onion 2½-inch diameter	1	110	40	2	Trace	—	—	—	10	30	0.6	40	0.04	0.04	0.2	11
Cooked	1 cup	210	60	3	Trace	—	—	—	14	50	.8	80	.06	.06	.4	14
Young green, small, without tops	6	50	20	1	Trace	—	—	—	5	20	.3	Trace	.02	.02	.2	12
Parsley, raw, chopped	1 tbsp	3.5	1	Trace	Trace	—	—	—	Trace	7	.2	300	Trace	.01	Trace	6
Parsnips, cooked	1 cup	155	100	2	1	—	—	—	23	70	.9	50	.11	.13	.2	16

Peas, green															
Cooked	1 cup	160	115	9	1	—	—	—	19	37	2.9	860	.44	.17	3.7	33
Canned, solids and liquid	1 cup	249	165	9	1	—	—	—	31	50	4.2	1,120	.23	.13	2.2	22
Canned, strained (baby food)	1 oz	28	15	1	Trace	—	—	—	3	3	.4	140	.02	.02	.4	3
Peppers, hot, red, without seeds, dried (ground chili powder, added seasonings)	1 tbsp	15	50	2	2	—	—	—	8	40	2.3	9,750	.03	.17	1.3	2
Peppers, sweet																
Raw, medium, about 6 per pound																
Green pod without stem and seeds	1 pod	62	15	1	Trace	—	—	—	3	6	.4	260	.05	.05	.3	79
Red pod without stem and seeds	1 pod	60	20	1	Trace	—	—	—	4	8	.4	2,670	.05	.05	.3	122
Canned, pimentos, medium	1 pod	38	10	Trace	Trace	—	—	—	2	3	.6	870	.01	.02	.1	36
Potatoes, medium (about 3 per pound raw)																
Baked, peeled after baking	1	99	90	3	Trace	—	—	—	21	9	.7	Trace	.10	.04	1.7	20
Boiled																
Peeled after boiling	1	136	105	3	Trace	—	—	—	23	10	.8	Trace	.13	.05	2.0	22
Peeled before boiling	1	122	80	2	Trace	—	—	—	18	7	.6	Trace	.11	.04	1.4	20
French-fried, piece 2 by ½ by ½ inch																
Cooked in deep fat	10 pieces	57	155	2	7	2	2	4	20	9	.7	Trace	.07	.04	1.8	12
Frozen, heated	10 pieces	57	125	2	5	1	1	2	19	5	1.0	Trace	.08	.01	1.5	12
Mashed																
Milk added	1 cup	195	125	4	1	—	—	—	25	47	.8	50	.16	.10	2.0	19
Milk and butter added	1 cup	195	185	4	8	4	3	Trace	24	47	.8	330	.16	.10	1.9	18
Potato chips, medium, 2-inch diameter	10 chips	20	115	1	8	3	2	4	10	8	.4	Trace	.04	.01	1.0	3
Pumpkin, canned	1 cup	228	75	2	1	—	—	—	18	57	.9	14,590	.07	.12	1.3	12
Radishes, raw, small, without tops	4	40	5	Trace	Trace	—	—	—	1	12	.4	Trace	.01	.01	.1	10
Sauerkraut, canned, solids and liquid	1 cup	235	45	2	Trace	—	—	—	9	85	1.2	120	.07	.09	.4	33
Spinach																
Cooked	1 cup	180	40	5	1	—	—	—	6	167	4.0	14,580	.13	.25	1.0	50

Nutritive values of the edible part of foods—cont'd

Food, approximate measure, and weight (in grams)			Food energy (calories)	Protein (g)	Fat (total lipid) (g)	Fatty acids: Saturated (total) (g)	Fatty acids: Unsaturated: Oleic (g)	Fatty acids: Unsaturated: Linoleic (g)	Carbohydrate (g)	Calcium (mg)	Iron (mg)	Vitamin A value (IU)	Thiamin (mg)	Riboflavin (mg)	Niacin (mg)	Ascorbic acid (mg)
Canned, drained solids	1 cup	180	45	5	1	—	—	—	6	212	4.7	14,400	.03	.21	.6	24
Canned, strained or chopped (baby food)	1 oz	28	10	1	Trace	—	—	—	2	18	.2	1,420	.01	.04	.1	2
Sprouts, raw																
Mung bean	1 cup	90	30	3	Trace	—	—	—	6	17	1.2	20	.12	.12	.7	17
Soybean	1 cup	107	40	6	2	—	—	—	4	46	.7	90	.17	.16	.8	4
Squash																
Cooked																
Summer, diced	1 cup	210	30	2	Trace	—	—	—	7	52	.8	820	.10	.16	1.6	21
Winter, baked, mashed	1 cup	205	130	4	1	—	—	—	32	57	1.6	8,610	.10	.27	1.4	27
Canned, winter, strained and chopped (baby food)	1 oz	28	10	Trace	Trace	—	—	—	2	7	.1	510	.01	.01	.1	1
Sweet potatoes																
Cooked, medium, 5 by 2 inches, weight raw about 6 oz																
Baked, peeled after baking	1	110	155	2	1	—	—	—	36	44	1.0	8,910	.10	.07	.7	24
Boiled, peeled after boiling	1	147	170	2	1	—	—	—	39	47	1.0	11,610	.13	.09	.9	25
Candied, 3½ by 2¼ inches	1	175	295	2	6	2	3	1	60	65	1.6	11,030	.10	.08	.8	17
Canned, vacuum or solid pack	1 cup	218	235	4	Trace	—	—	—	54	54	1.7	17,000	.10	.10	1.4	30
Tomatoes																
Raw, medium, 2 by 2½ inches, about 3 per pound	1	150	35	2	Trace	—	—	—	7	20	.8	1,350	.10	.06	1.0	[7]34
Canned	1 cup	242	50	2	Trace	—	—	—	10	15	1.2	2,180	.13	.07	1.7	40
Tomato juice, canned	1 cup	242	45	2	Trace	—	—	—	10	17	2.2	1,940	.13	.07	1.8	39
Tomato catsup	1 tbsp	17	15	Trace	Trace	—	—	—	4	4	.1	240	.02	.01	.3	3
Turnips, cooked, diced	1 cup	155	35	1	Trace	—	—	—	8	54	.6	Trace	.06	.08	.5	33
Turnip greens																
Cooked																

In small amount of water, short time	1 cup	145	30	3	Trace	—	—	—	5	267	1.6	9,140	.21	.36	.8	100
In large amount of water, long time	1 cup	145	25	3	Trace	—	—	—	5	252	1.4	8,260	.14	.33	.8	68
Canned, solids and liquid	1 cup	232	40	3	1	—	—	—	7	232	3.7	10,900	.04	.21	1.4	44
Fruits and fruit products																
Apples, raw, medium, 2½inch diameter, about 3 per pound[5]	1	150	70	Trace	Trace	—	—	—	18	8	.4	50	.04	.02	.1	3
Apple brown betty	1 cup	230	345	4	8	4	3	Trace	68	41	1.4	230	.13	.10	.9	3
Apple juice, bottled or canned	1 cup	249	120	Trace	Trace	—	—	—	30	15	1.5	—	.01	.04	.2	2
Applesauce, canned																
Sweetened	1 cup	254	230	1	Trace	—	—	—	60	10	1.3	100	.05	.03	.1	3
Unsweetened or artifically sweetened	1 cup	239	100	Trace	Trace	—	—	—	26	10	1.2	100	.04	.02	.1	2
Applesauce and apricots, canned, strained or junior (baby food)	1 oz	28	25	Trace	Trace	—	—	—	6	1	.1	170	Trace	Trace	Trace	1
Apricots																
Raw, about 12 per pound[5]	3 apricots	114	55	1	Trace	—	—	—	14	18	.5	2,890	.03	.04	.7	10
Canned in heavy syrup																
Halves and syrup	1 cup	259	220	2	Trace	—	—	—	57	28	.8	4,510	.05	.06	.9	10
Halves (medium) and syrup	4 halves; 2 tbsp syrup	122	105	1	Trace	—	—	—	27	13	.4	2,120	.02	.03	.4	5
Dried																
Uncooked, 40 halves, small	1 cup	150	390	8	1	—	—	—	100	100	8.2	16,350	.02	.23	4.9	19
Cooked unsweetened, fruit and liquid	1 cup	285	240	5	1	—	—	—	62	63	5.1	8,550	.01	.13	2.8	8
Apricot nector, canned	1 cup	250	140	1	Trace	—	—	—	36	22	.5	2,380	.02	.02	.5	7

[5]Measure and weight apply to entire vegetable or fruit including parts not usually eaten.
[7]Year-round average. Samples marketed from November through May average around 15 milligrams per 150-gram tomato; from June through October, around 39 milligrams.

Nutritive values of the edible part of foods—cont'd

Food, approximate measure, and weight (in grams)			Food energy (calories)	Protein (g)	Fat (total lipid) (g)	Fatty acids: Saturated (total) (g)	Fatty acids: Unsaturated: Oleic (g)	Fatty acids: Unsaturated: Linoleic (g)	Carbohydrate (g)	Calcium (mg)	Iron (mg)	Vitamin A value (IU)	Thiamin (mg)	Riboflavin (mg)	Niacin (mg)	Ascorbic acid (mg)
Avocados, raw																
California varieties, mainly Fuerte																
10-ounce avocado, about 3½ by 4¼ inches, peeled, pitted	½	108	185	2	18	4	8	2	6	11	.6	310	.12	.21	1.7	15
½-inch cubes	1 cup	152	260	3	26	5	12	3	9	15	.9	440	.16	.30	2.4	21
Florida varieties																
13 oz avocado, about 4 by 3 inches, peeled, pitted	½	123	160	2	14	3	6	2	11	12	.7	360	.13	.24	2.0	17
½-inch cubes	1 cup	152	195	2	17	3	8	2	13	15	.9	440	.16	.30	2.4	21
Bananas, raw, 6 by 1½ inches, about 3 per pound[5]	1	150	85	1	Trace	—	—	—	23	8	.7	190	.05	.06	.7	10
Blackberries, raw	1 cup	144	85	2	1	—	—	—	19	46	1.3	290	.05	.06	.5	30
Blueberries, raw	1 cup	140	85	1	1	—	—	—	21	21	1.4	140	.04	.08	.6	20
Cantaloups, raw; medium, 5-inch diameter, about 1⅔ pounds[5]	½	385	60	1	Trace	—	—	—	14	27	.8	[8]6,540	.08	.06	1.2	63
Cherries																
Raw, sweet, with stems[5]	1 cup	130	80	2	Trace	—	—	—	20	26	.5	130	.06	.07	.5	12
Canned, red, sour, pitted, heavy syrup	1 cup	260	230	2	1	—	—	—	59	36	.8	1,680	.07	.06	.4	13
Cranberry juice cocktail, canned	1 cup	250	160	Trace	Trace	—	—	—	41	12	.8	Trace	.02	.02	.1	([9])
Cranberry sauce, sweetened, canned, strained	1 cup	277	405	Trace	1	—	—	—	104	17	.6	40	.03	0.3	.1	5
Dates, domestic, natural and dry, pitted, cut	1 cup	178	490	4	1	—	—	—	130	105	5.3	90	.16	.17	3.9	0
Figs																
Raw, small, 1½-inch diameter, about 12 per pound	3 figs	114	90	1	Trace	—	—	—	23	40	.7	90	.07	.06	.5	2

Dried, large, 2 by 1 inch	1 fig	21	60	1	Trace	—	—	—	15	26	.6	20	.02	.02	.1	0
Fruit cocktail, canned in heavy syrup, solids and liquid	1 cup	256	195	1	1	—	—	—	50	23	1.0	360	.04	.03	1.1	5
Grapefruit																
Raw, medium, 4¼-inch diameter, size 64																
White[5]	½	285	55	1	Trace	—	—	—	14	22	.6	10	.05	.02	.2	52
Pink or red[5]	½	285	60	1	Trace	—	—	—	15	23	.6	640	.05	.02	.3	52
Raw sections, white	1 cup	194	75	1	Trace	—	—	—	20	31	.8	20	.07	.03	.3	72
Canned, white																
Syrup pack, solids and liquid	1 cup	249	175	1	Trace	—	—	—	44	32	.7	20	.07	.04	.5	75
Water pack, solids and liquid	1 cup	240	70	1	Trace	—	—	—	18	31	.7	20	.07	.04	.5	72
Grapefruit juice																
Fresh	1 cup	246	95	1	Trace	—	—	—	23	22	.5	([10])	.09	.04	.4	92
Canned, white																
Unsweetened	1 cup	247	100	1	Trace	—	—	—	24	20	1.0	20	.07	.04	.4	84
Sweetened	1 cup	250	130	1	Trace	—	—	—	32	20	1.0	20	.07	.04	.4	78
Frozen, concentrate, unsweetened																
Undiluted, can, 6 fluid oz	1 can	207	300	4	1	—	—	—	72	70	.8	60	.29	.12	1.4	286
Diluted with 3 parts water, by volume	1 cup	247	100	1	Trace	—	—	—	24	25	.2	20	.10	.04	.5	96
Frozen, concentrate, sweetened																
Undiluted, can 6 fluid oz	1 can	211	350	3	1	—	—	—	85	59	.6	50	.24	.11	1.2	245
Diluted with 3 parts water, by volume	1 cup	249	115	1	Trace	—	—	—	28	20	.2	20	.08	.03	.4	82
Dehydrated																
Crystals, can, net weight 4 oz	1 can	114	430	5	1	—	—	—	103	99	1.1	90	.41	.18	2.0	399
Prepared with water (1 pound yields about 1 gal)	1 cup	247	100	1	Trace	—	—	—	24	22	.2	20	.10	.05	.5	92

[5]Measure and weight apply to entire vegetable or fruit including parts not usually eaten.
[8]Value based on varieties with orange-colored flesh, for green-fleshed varieties value is about 540 IU per ½ melon.
[9]About 5 milligrams per 8 fluid ounces is from cranberries. Ascorbic acid is usually added to approximately 100 milligrams per 8 fluid ounces.
[10]For white-fleshed varieties value is about 20 IU per cup; for red-fleshed varieties, 1,080 IU per cup.

Nutritive values of the edible part of foods—cont'd

Food, approximate measure, and weight (in grams)			Food energy (calories)	Protein (g)	Fat (total lipid) (g)	Fatty acids: Saturated (total) (g)	Fatty acids: Unsaturated: Oleic (g)	Fatty acids: Unsaturated: Linoleic (g)	Carbohydrate (g)	Calcium (mg)	Iron (mg)	Vitamin A value (IU)	Thiamin (mg)	Riboflavin (mg)	Niacin (mg)	Ascorbic acid (mg)
Grapes, raw																
American type (slip skin), such as Concord, Delaware, Niagara, Catawba, and Scuppernong[5]	1 cup	153	65	1	1	—	—	—	15	15	.4	100	.05	.03	.2	3
European type (adherent skin), such as Malaga, Muscat, Thompson Seedless, Emperor, and Flame Tokay[5]	1 cup	160	95	1	Trace	—	—	—	25	17	.6	140	.07	.04	.4	6
Grape juice, bottled or canned	1 cup	254	165	1	Trace	—	—	—	42	28	.8	—	.10	.05	.6	Trace
Lemons, raw, medium, 2½-inch diameter, size 150[5]	1 lemon	106	20	1	Trace	—	—	—	6	18	.4	10	.03	.01	.1	38
Lemon juice																
Fresh	1 cup	246	60	1	Trace	—	—	—	20	17	.5	40	.08	.03	.2	113
	1 tbsp	15	5	Trace	Trace	—	—	—	1	1	Trace	Trace	Trace	Trace	Trace	7
Canned, unsweetened	1 cup	245	55	1	Trace	—	—	—	19	17	.5	40	.07	.03	.2	102
Lemonade concentrate, frozen, sweetened																
Undiluted, can, 6 fluid oz	1 can	220	430	Trace	Trace	—	—	—	112	9	.4	40	.05	.06	.7	66
Diluted with 4½ parts water, by volume	1 cup	248	110	Trace	Trace	—	—	—	28	2	.1	10	.01	.01	.2	17
Lime juice																
Fresh	1 cup	246	65	1	Trace	—	—	—	22	22	.5	30	.05	.03	.03	80
Canned	1 cup	246	65	1	Trace	—	—	—	22	22	.5	30	.05	.03	.3	52
Limeade concentrate, frozen, sweetened																
Undiluted, can, 6 fluid oz	1 can	218	410	Trace	Trace	—	—	—	108	11	.2	Trace	.02	.02	.3	26
Diluted with 4⅓ parts water, by volume	1 cup	248	105	Trace	Trace	—	—	—	27	2	Trace	Trace	Trace	Trace	Trace	6

Oranges, raw																
California, Navel (winter), 2⁴⁄₅-inch diameter, size 88[5]	1 orange	180	60	2	Trace	—	—	—	16	49	.5	240	.12	.05	.5	75
Florida, all varieties, 3-inch diameter[5]	1	210	75	1	Trace	—	—	—	19	67	.3	310	.16	.06	.6	70
Orange juice																
Fresh																
California, Valencia (summer)	1 cup	249	115	2	1	—	—	—	26	27	.7	500	.22	.06	.9	122
Florida varieties																
Early and mid-season	1 cup	247	100	1	Trace	—	—	—	23	25	.5	490	.22	.06	.9	127
Late season, Valencia	1 cup	248	110	1	Trace	—	—	—	26	25	.5	500	.22	.06	.9	92
Canned, unsweetened	1 cup	249	120	2	Trace	—	—	—	28	25	1.0	500	.17	.05	.6	100
Frozen concentrate																
Undiluted, can, 6 fluid oz	1 can	210	330	5	Trace	—	—	—	80	69	.8	1,490	.63	.10	2.4	332
Diluted with 3 parts water, by volume	1 cup	248	110	2	Trace	—	—	—	27	22	.2	500	.21	.03	.8	112
Dehydrated																
Crystals, can, net weight 4 oz	1 can	113	430	6	2	—	—	—	100	95	1.9	1,900	.76	.24	3.3	406
Prepared with water, 1 lb yield about 1 gal	1 cup	248	115	1	Trace	—	—	—	27	25	.5	500	.20	.06	.9	108
Orange and grapefruit juice																
Frozen concentrate																
Undiluted, can, 6 fluid oz	1 can	209	325	4	1	—	—	—	78	61	.8	790	.47	.06	2.3	301
Diluted with 3 parts water, by volume	1 cup	248	110	1	Trace	—	—	—	26	20	.3	270	.16	.02	.8	102
Papayas, raw, ½-inch cubes	1 cup	182	70	1	Trace	—	—	—	18	36	.5	3,190	.07	.08	.5	102
Peaches																
Raw																
Whole, medium, 2-inch diameter, about 4 per pound[5]	1	114	35	1	Trace	—	—	—	10	9	.5	[11]1,320	.02	.05	1.0	7

[5]Measure and weight apply to entire vegetable or fruit including parts not usually eaten.
[11]Based on yellow-fleshed varieties; for white-fleshed varieties value is about 50 IU per 114-gram peach and 80 IU per cup of sliced peaches.

Nutritive values of the edible part of foods—cont'd

Food, approximate measure, and weight (in grams)			Food energy (calories)	Protein (g)	Fat (total lipid) (g)	Fatty acids: Saturated (total) (g)	Fatty acids: Unsaturated: Oleic (g)	Fatty acids: Unsaturated: Linoleic (g)	Carbohydrate (g)	Calcium (mg)	Iron (mg)	Vitamin A value (IU)	Thiamin (mg)	Riboflavin (mg)	Niacin (mg)	Ascorbic acid (mg)
Sliced	1 cup	168	65	1	Trace	—	—	—	16	15	.8	[11]2,230	.03	.08	1.6	12
Canned, yellow-fleshed, solids and liquid																
Syrup pack, heavy																
Halves or slices	1 cup	257	200	1	Trace	—	—	—	52	10	.8	1,100	.02	.06	1.4	7
Halves (medium) and syrup	2 halves and 2 tbsp syrup	117	90	Trace	Trace	—	—	—	24	5	.4	500	.01	.03	.7	3
Water pack	1 cup	245	75	1	Trace	—	—	—	20	10	.7	1,100	.02	.06	1.4	7
Strained or chopped (baby food)	1 oz	28	25	Trace	Trace	—	—	—	6	2	.1	140	Trace	.01	.2	1
Dried																
Uncooked	1 cup	160	420	5	1	—	—	—	109	77	9.6	6,240	.02	.31	8.5	28
Cooked, unsweetened, 10-12 halves and 6 tbsp liquid	1 cup	270	220	3	1	—	—	—	58	41	5.1	3,290	.01	.15	4.2	6
Frozen																
Carton, 12 oz, not thawed	1 carton	340	300	1	Trace	—	—	—	77	14	1.7	2,210	.03	.14	2.4	[12]135
Can, 16 oz, not thawed	1 can	454	400	2	Trace	—	—	—	103	18	2.3	2,950	.05	.18	3.2	[12]181
Peach nectar, canned	1 cup	250	120	Trace	Trace	—	—	—	31	10	.5	1,080	.02	.05	1.0	1
Pears																
Raw, 3 by 2½-inch diameter[5]	1	182	100	1	1	—	—	—	25	13	.5	30	.04	.07	.2	7
Canned, solids and liquid																
Syrup pack, heavy																
Halves or slices	1 cup	255	195	1	1	—	—	—	50	13	.5	Trace	.03	.05	.3	4
Halves (medium) and syrup	2 halves and 2 tbsp syrup	117	90	Trace	Trace	—	—	—	23	6	.2	Trace	.01	.02	.2	2
Water pack	1 cup	243	80	Trace	Trace	—	—	—	20	12	.5	Trace	.02	.05	.3	4
Strained or chopped (baby food)	1 oz	28	20	Trace	Trace	—	—	—	5	2	.1	10	Trace	.01	.1	1
Pear nectar, canned	1 cup	250	130	1	Trace	—	—	—	33	8	.2	Trace	.01	.05	Trace	1

Persimmons, Japanese or kaki, raw, seedless, 2½-inch diameter[5]	1	125	75	1	Trace	—	—	—	20	6	.4	2,740	.01	.02	.1	11
Pineapple																
Raw, diced	1 cup	140	75	1	Trace	—	—	—	19	24	.7	100	.12	.04	.3	24
Canned, heavy syrup pack, solids and liquid																
Crushed	1 cup	260	195	1	Trace	—	—	—	50	29	.8	120	.20	.06	.5	17
Sliced, slices and juice	2 small or 1 large and 2 tbsp juice	122	90	Trace	Trace	—	—	—	24	13	.4	50	.09	.03	.2	8
Pineapple juice, canned	1 cup	249	135	1	Trace	—	—	—	34	37	.7	120	.12	.04	.5	22
Plums, all except prunes																
Raw, 2-inch diameter, about 2 ounces[5]	1	60	25	Trace	Trace	—	—	—	7	7	.3	140	.02	.02	.3	3
Canned, syrup pack (Italian prunes)																
Plums (with pits) and juice[5]	1 cup	256	205	1	Trace	—	—	—	53	22	2.2	2,970	.05	.05	.9	4
Plums (without pits) and juice	3 plums and 2 tbsp juice	122	100	Trace	Trace	—	—	—	26	11	1.1	1,470	.03	.02	.5	2
Prunes, dried, "softenized," medium																
Uncooked[5]	4	32	70	1	Trace	—	—	—	18	14	1.1	440	.02	.04	.4	1
Cooked, unsweetened, 17-18 prunes and ⅓ cup liquid[5]	1 cup	270	295	2	1	—	—	—	78	60	4.5	1,860	.08	.18	1.7	2
Prunes with tapioca, canned, strained or junior (baby food)	1 oz	28	25	Trace	Trace	—	—	—	6	2	.3	110	.01	.02	.1	1
Prune juice, canned	1 cup	256	200	1	Trace	—	—	—	49	36	10.5	—	.02	.03	1.1	4
Raisin, dried	1 cup	160	460	4	Trace	—	—	—	124	99	5.6	30	.18	.13	.9	2
Raspberries, red																
Raw	1 cup	123	70	1	1	—	—	—	17	27	1.1	160	.04	.11	1.1	31
Frozen, 10 oz carton, not thawed	1 carton	284	275	2	1	—	—	—	70	37	1.7	200	.06	.17	1.7	59
Rhubarb, cooked, sugar added	1 cup	272	385	1	Trace	—	—	—	98	212	1.6	220	.06	.15	.7	17

[5]Measure and weight apply to entire vegetable or fruit including parts not usually eaten.

[11]Based on yellow-fleshed varieties; for white-fleshed varieties value is about 50 IU per 114-gram peach and 80 IU per cup of sliced peaches.

[12]Average weighted in accordance with commercial freezing practices. For products without added ascorbic acid, value is about 37 milligrams per 12-ounce carton and 50 milligrams per 16-ounce can; for those with added ascorbic acid, 139 milligrams per 12 ounces and 186 milligrams per 16 ounces.

Nutritive values of the edible part of foods—cont'd

Food, approximate measure, and weight (in grams)			Food energy (calories)	Protein (g)	Fat (total lipid) (g)	Fatty acids			Carbohydrate (g)	Calcium (mg)	Iron (mg)	Vitamin A value (IU)	Thiamin (mg)	Riboflavin (mg)	Niacin (mg)	Ascorbic acid (mg)
						Saturated (total) (g)	Unsaturated									
							Oleic (g)	Linoleic (g)								
Strawberries																
Raw, capped	1 cup	149	55	1	1	—	—	—	13	31	1.5	90	.04	.10	1.0	88
Frozen, 10-oz carton, not thawed	1 carton	284	310	1	1	—	—	—	79	40	2.0	90	.06	.17	1.5	150
Frozen, 16-ounce can, not thawed	1 can	454	495	2	1	—	—	—	126	64	3.2	150	.09	.27	2.4	240
Tangerines, raw, medium, 2½-inch diameter, about 4 per pound[5]	1	114	40	1	Trace	—	—	—	10	34	.3	350	.05	.02	.1	26
Tangerine juice																
Canned, unsweetened	1 cup	248	105	1	Trace	—	—	—	25	45	.5	1,040	.14	.04	.3	56
Frozen concentrate																
Undiluted, can, 6 fluid oz	1 can	210	340	4	1	—	—	—	80	130	1.5	3,070	.43	.12	.9	202
Diluted with 3 parts water, by volume	1 cup	248	115	1	Trace	—	—	—	27	45	.5	1,020	.14	.04	.3	67
Watermelon, raw, wedge, 4 by 8 inches (1/16 of 10 by 16-inch melon, about 2 pounds with rind)[5]	1 wedge	925	115	2	1	—	—	—	27	30	2.1	2,510	.13	.13	.7	30
Breads and cereals																
Barley, pearled, light, uncooked	1 cup	203	710	17	2	Trace	1	1	160	32	4.1	0	.25	.17	6.3	0
Biscuits, baking powder with enriched flour, 2½-inch diameter	1	38	140	3	6	2	3	1	17	46	.6	Trace	.08	.08	.7	Trace
Bran flakes (40 percent bran) added thiamine	1 oz	28	85	3	1	—	—	—	23	20	1.2	0	.11	.05	1.7	0
Bread																
Boston brown bread, slice, 3 by ¾ inch	1 slice	48	100	3	1	—	—	—	22	43	.9	0	.05	.03	.6	0
Cracked-wheat bread																
Loaf, 1-pound, 20 slices	1 loaf	454	1,190	39	10	2	5	2	236	399	5.0	Trace	.53	.42	5.8	Trace

Slice	1	23	60	2	1	—	—	—	12	20	.3	Trace	.03	.02	.3	Trace
French or Vienna bread																
Enriched, 1-pound loaf	1 loaf	454	1,315	41	14	3	8	2	251	195	10.0	Trace	1.26	.98	11.3	Trace
Unenriched, 1-pound loaf	1 loaf	454	1,315	41	14	3	8	2	251	195	3.2	Trace	.39	.39	3.6	Trace
Italian bread																
Enriched, 1-pound loaf	1 loaf	454	1,250	41	4	Trace	1	2	256	77	10.0	0	1.31	.93	11.7	0
Unenriched, 1-pound loaf	1 loaf	454	1,250	41	4	Trace	1	2	256	77	3.2	0	.39	.27	3.6	0
Raisin bread																
Loaf, 1-pound, 20 slices	1 loaf	454	1,190	30	13	3	8	2	243	322	5.9	Trace	.24	.42	3.0	Trace
Slice	1	23	60	2	1	—	—	—	12	16	.3	Trace	.01	.02	.2	Trace
Rye bread																
American, light (⅓ rye, ⅔ wheat)																
Loaf, 1-pound, 20 slices	1 loaf	454	1,100	41	5	—	—	—	236	340	7.3	0	.81	.33	6.4	0
Slice	1	23	55	2	Trace	—	—	—	12	17	.4	0	.04	.02	.3	0
Pumpernickel, loaf, 1 pound	1 loaf	454	1,115	41	5	—	—	—	241	381	10.9	0	10.5	.63	5.4	0
White bread, enriched																
1 to 2 percent nonfat dry milk																
Loaf, 1-pound, 20 slices	1 loaf	454	1,225	39	15	3	8	2	229	318	10.9	Trace	1.13	.77	10.4	Trace
Slice	1 slice	23	60	2	1	Trace	Trace	Trace	12	16	.6	Trace	.06	.04	.5	Trace
3 to 4 percent nonfat dry milk[13]																
Loaf, 1-pound	1	454	1,225	39	15	3	8	2	229	381	11.3	Trace	1.13	.95	10.8	Trace
Slice, 20 per loaf	1	23	60	2	1	Trace	Trace	Trace	12	19	.6	Trace	.06	.05	.6	Trace
Slice, toasted	1	20	60	2	1	Trace	Trace	Trace	12	19	.6	Trace	.05	.05	.6	Trace
Slice, 26 per loaf	1	17	45	1	1	Trace	Trace	Trace	9	14	.4	Trace	.04	.04	.4	Trace
5 to 6 percent nonfat dry milk																
Loaf, 1-pound, 20 slices	1 loaf	454	1,245	41	17	4	10	2	228	435	11.3	Trace	1.22	.91	11.0	Trace
Slice	1	23	65	2	1	Trace	Trace	Trace	12	22	.6	Trace	.06	.05	.6	Trace
White bread, unenriched																
1 to 2 percent nonfat dry milk																
Loaf, 1-pound, 20 slices	1 loaf	454	1,225	39	15	3	8	2	229	318	3.2	Trace	.40	.36	5.6	Trace
Slice	1	23	60	2	1	Trace	Trace	Trace	12	16	.2	Trace	.02	.02	.3	Trace

[5]Measure and weight apply to entire vegetable or fruit including parts not usually eaten.
[13]When the amount of nonfat dry milk in commercial white bread is unknown, values for bread with 3 to 4% nonfat dry milk are suggested.

Nutritive values of the edible part of foods—cont'd

Food, approximate measure, and weight (in grams)			Food energy (calories)	Protein (g)	Fat (total lipid) (g)	Fatty acids: Saturated (total) (g)	Fatty acids: Unsaturated: Oleic (g)	Fatty acids: Unsaturated: Linoleic (g)	Carbohydrate (g)	Calcium (mg)	Iron (mg)	Vitamin A value (IU)	Thiamin (mg)	Riboflavin (mg)	Niacin (mg)	Ascorbic acid (mg)
3 to 4 percent nonfat dry milk[13]																
Loaf, 1-pound	1 loaf	454	1,225	39	15	3	8	—	228	381	3.2	Trace	.31	.39	5.0	Trace
Slice, 20 per loaf	1 slice	23	60	2	1	Trace	Trace	Trace	12	19	.2	Trace	.02	.02	.3	Trace
Slice, toasted	1	20	60	2	1	Trace	Trace	Trace	12	19	.2	Trace	.01	.02	.3	Trace
Slice, 26 per loaf	1 slice	17	45	1	1	Trace	Trace	Trace	9	14	.1	Trace	.01	.01	.2	Trace
5 to 6 percent nonfat dry milk																
Loaf, 1-pound, 20 slices	1 loaf	454	1,245	41	17	4	10	2	228	435	3.2	Trace	.32	.39	4.1	Trace
Slice	1	23	65	2	1	Trace	Trace	Trace	12	22	.2	Trace	.02	.03	.2	Trace
Whole-wheat bread, made with 2 percent nonfat dry milk																
Loaf, 1-pound, 20 slices	1 loaf	454	1,105	48	14	3	6	3	216	449	10.4	Trace	1.17	.56	12.9	Trace
Slice	1	23	55	2	1	Trace	Trace	Trace	11	23	.5	Trace	.06	.03	.7	Trace
Slice, toasted	1	19	55	2	1	Trace	Trace	Trace	11	22	.5	Trace	.05	.03	.6	Trace
Breadcrumbs, dry, grated	1 cup	88	345	11	4	1	2	1	65	107	3.2	Trace	.19	.26	3.1	Trace
Cakes[14]																
Angelfood cake; sector, 2-inch (1/12 of 8-inch-diameter cake)	1 sector	40	110	3	Trace	—	—	—	24	4	.1	0	Trace	.06	.1	0
Chocolate cake, chocolate icing; sector, 2-inch (1/16 of 10-inch-diameter layer cake)	1 sector	120	445	5	20	8	10	1	67	84	1.2	[15]190	.03	.12	.3	Trace
Fruitcake, dark (made with enriched flour); piece, 2 by 2 by ½ inch	1 piece	30	115	1	5	1	3	1	18	22	.8	[15]40	.04	.04	.2	Trace
Gingerbread (made with enriched flour); piece, 2 by 2 by 2 inches	1 piece	55	175	2	6	1	4	Trace	29	37	1.3	50	.06	.06	.5	0
Plain cake and cupcakes, without icing																
Piece, 3 by 2 by 1½ inches	1	55	200	2	8	2	5	1	31	35	.2	[15]90	.01	.05	.1	Trace

Cupcake, 2¾-inch diameter	1	40	145	2	6	1	3	Trace	22	26	.2	[15]70	.01	.03	.1	Trace
Plain cake and cupcakes, with chocolate icing																
Sector, 2-inch (1/16 of 10-inch-layer cake)	1	100	370	4	14	5	7	1	59	63	.6	[15]180	.02	.09	.2	Trace
Cupcake, 2¾-inch diameter	1	50	185	2	7	2	4	Trace	30	32	.3	[15]90	.01	.04	.1	Trace
Poundcake, old-fashioned (equal weights flour, sugar, fat, eggs); slice, 2¾ by 3 by ⅝ inch	1 slice	30	140	2	9	2	5	1	14	6	.2	[15]80	.01	.03	.1	0
Sponge cake; sector, 2-inch (1/12 of 8-inch diameter cake)	1	40	120	3	2	1	1	Trace	22	12	.5	180	.02	.06	.1	Trace
Cookies																
Plain and assorted, 3-inch diameter	1 cookie	25	120	1	5	—	—	—	18	9	.2	20	.01	.01	.1	Trace
Fig bars, small	1	16	55	1	1	—	—	—	12	12	.2	20	.01	.01	.1	Trace
Corn, rice and wheat flakes, mixed, added nutrients	1 oz	28	110	2	Trace	—	—	—	24	11	.5	0	.11	—	.9	0
Corn flakes, added nutrients																
Plain	1 oz	28	110	2	Trace	—	—	—	24	5	.4	0	.12	.02	.6	0
Sugar-covered	1 oz	28	110	1	Trace	—	—	—	26	3	.3	0	.12	.01	.5	0
Corn grits, degermed, cooked																
Enriched	1 cup	242	120	3	Trace	—	—	—	27	2	[16].7	[17]150	[16].10	[16].07	[16]1.0	0
Unenriched	1 cup	242	120	3	Trace	—	—	—	27	2	.2	[17]150	.05	.02	.5	0
Cornmeal, white or yellow, dry																
Whole ground, unbolted	1 cup	118	420	11	5	1	2	2	87	24	2.8	[17]600	.45	.13	2.4	0
Degermed, enriched	1 cup	145	525	11	2	Trace	1	1	114	9	[16]4.2	[17]640	[16].64	[16].38	[16]5.1	0

[13]When the amount of nonfat dry milk in commercial white bread is unknown, values for bread with 3 to 4% nonfat dry milk are suggested.
[14]Unenriched cake flour and vegetable cooking fat used unless otherwise specified.
[15]If the fat used in the recipe is butter or fortified margarine, the vitamin A value for chocolate cake with chocolate icing will be 490 IU per 2-inch sector; 100 IU for fruitcake; for plain cake without icing, 300 IU per piece; 220 IU per cupcake; for plain cake with icing, 440 IU per 2-inch sector; 220 IU per cupcake; and 300 IU for poundcake.
[16]Iron, thiamine, riboflavin, and niacin are based on the minimum levels of enrichment specified in standards of identity promulgated under the Federal Food, Drug, and Cosmetic Act.
[17]Vitamin A value based on yellow product. White product contains only a trace.

Nutritive values of the edible part of foods—cont'd

Food, approximate measure, and weight (in grams)			Food energy (calories)	Protein (g)	Fat (total lipid) (g)	Fatty acids: Saturated (total) (g)	Fatty acids: Unsaturated: Oleic (g)	Fatty acids: Unsaturated: Linoleic (g)	Carbohydrate (g)	Calcium (mg)	Iron (mg)	Vitamin A value (IU)	Thiamin (mg)	Riboflavin (mg)	Niacin (mg)	Ascorbic acid (mg)
Corn muffins, made with enriched degermed cornmeal and enriched flour; muffin, 2¾-inch diameter	1 muffin	48	150	3	5	2	2	Trace	23	50	.8	[18]80	.09	.11	.8	Trace
Corn, puffed, presweetened, added nutrients	1 oz	28	110	1	Trace	—	—	—	26	3	.5	0	.12	.05	.6	0
Corn, shredded, added nutrients	1 oz	28	110	2	Trace	—	—	—	25	1	.7	0	.12	.05	.6	0
Crackers																
Graham, plain	4 small or 2 medium	14	55	1	1	—	—	—	10	6	.2	0	.01	.03	.2	0
Saltines, 2 inches squares	2 crackers	8	35	1	1	—	—	—	6	2	.1	0	Trace	Trace	.1	0
Soda																
Cracker, 2½ inches square	2 crackers	11	50	1	1	Trace	1	Trace	8	2	.2	0	Trace	Trace	.1	0
Oyster crackers	10 crackers	10	45	1	1	Trace	1	Trace	7	2	.2	0	Trace	Trace	.1	0
Cracker meal	1 tbsp	10	45	1	1	Trace	1	Trace	7	2	.1	0	.01	Trace	.1	0
Doughnuts, cake type	1 doughnut	32	125	1	6	1	4	Trace	16	13	[19].4	30	[19].05	[19].05	[19].4	Trace
Farina, regular, enriched, cooked	1 cup	238	100	3	Trace	—	—	—	21	10	[16].7	0	[16].11	[16].07	[16]1.0	0
Macaroni, cooked																
Enriched																
Cooked, firm stage (8 to 10 minutes; undergoes additional cooking in a food mixture)	1 cup	130	190	6	1	—	—	—	39	14	[16]1.4	0	[16].23	[16].14	[16]1.9	0
Cooked until tender	1 cup	140	155	5	1	—	—	—	32	11	[16]1.3	0	[16].19	[16].11	[16]1.5	0

Unenriched															
Cooked, firm stage (8 to 10 minutes; undergoes additional cooking in a food mixture)	1 cup	130	190	6	1	—	—	—	39	14	.6	0	.02	.02	.5	0
Cooked until tender	1 cup	140	155	5	1	—	—	—	32	11	.6	0	.02	.02	.4	0
Macaroni (enriched) and cheese, baked	1 cup	220	470	18	24	11	10	1	44	398	2.0	950	.22	.44	2.0	Trace
Muffins, with enriched white flour; muffin, 2¾-inch diameter	1	48	140	4	5	1	3	Trace	20	50	.8	50	.08	.11	.7	Trace
Noodles (egg noodles), cooked																
Enriched	1 cup	160	200	7	2	1	1	Trace	37	16	[16]1.4	110	[16]23	[14].14	[16]1.8	0
Unenriched	1 cup	160	200	7	2	1	1	Trace	37	16	1.0	110	.04	.03	.7	0
Oats (with or without corn) puffed, added nutrients	1 oz	28	115	3	2	Trace	1	1	21	50	1.3	0	.28	.05	.5	0
Oatmeal or rolled oats, regular or quick-cooking, cooked	1 cup	236	130	5	2	Trace	1	1	23	21	1.4	0	.19	.05	.3	0
Pancakes (griddlecakes), 4-inch diameter																
Wheat, enriched flour (home recipe)	1 cake	27	60	2	2	Trace	1	Trace	9	27	.4	30	.05	.06	.3	Trace
Buckwheat (buckwheat pancake mix, made with egg and milk)	1 cake	27	55	2	2	1	1	Trace	6	59	.4	60	.03	.04	.2	Trace
Piecrust, plain, baked																
Enriched flour																
Lower crust, 9-inch shell	1	135	675	8	45	10	29	3	59	19	2.3	0	.27	.19	2.4	0
Double crust, 9-inch pie	1	270	1,350	16	90	21	58	7	118	38	4.6	0	.55	.39	4.9	0
Unenriched flour																
Lower crust, 9-inch shell	1	135	675	8	45	10	29	3	59	19	.7	0	.04	.04	.6	0
Double crust, 9-inch pie	1	270	1,350	16	90	21	58	7	118	38	1.4	0	.08	.07	1.3	0

[14]Unenriched cake flour and vegetable cooking fat used unless otherwise specified.
[16]Iron, thiamine, riboflavin, and niacin are based on the minimum levels of enrichment specified in standards of identity promulgated under the Federal Food, Drug, and Cosmetic Act.
[18]Based on recipe using white cornmeal; if yellow cornmeal is used, the vitamin A value is 140 IU per muffin.
[19]Based on product made with enriched flour. With unenriched flour, approximate values per doughnut are: Iron, 0.2 milligram; thiamine, 0.01 milligram; riboflavin, 0.03 milligram; niacin, 0.2 milligram.

Nutritive values of the edible part of foods—cont'd

Food, approximate measure, and weight (in grams)			*Food energy (calories)*	*Protein (g)*	*Fat (total lipid) (g)*	*Fatty acids*			*Carbohydrate (g)*	*Calcium (mg)*	*Iron (mg)*	*Vitamin A value (IU)*	*Thiamin (mg)*	*Riboflavin (mg)*	*Niacin (mg)*	*Ascorbic acid (mg)*
						Saturated (total) (g)	*Unsaturated*									
							Oleic (g)	*Linoleic (g)*								
Pies (piecrust made with unenriched flour); sector, 4-inch, 1/7 of 9-inch-diameter pie																
Apple	1 sector	135	345	3	15	4	9	1	51	11	.4	40	.03	.02	.5	1
Cherry	1 sector	135	355	4	15	4	10	1	52	19	.4	590	.03	.03	.6	1
Custard	1 sector	130	280	8	14	5	8	1	30	125	.8	300	.07	.21	.4	0
Lemon meringue	1 sector	120	305	4	12	4	7	1	45	17	.6	200	.04	.10	.2	4
Mince	1 sector	135	365	3	16	4	10	1	56	38	1.4	Trace	.09	.05	.5	1
Pumpkin	1 sector	130	275	5	15	5	7	1	32	66	.6	3,210	.04	.13	.6	Trace
Pizza (cheese); 5½-inch sector; ⅛ of 14-inch diameter pie	1 sector	75	185	7	6	2	3	Trace	27	107	.7	290	.04	.12	.7	4
Popcorn, popped, with added oil and salt	1 cup	14	65	1	3	2	Trace	Trace	8	1	.3	—	—	.01	.2	0
Pretzels, small stick	5 sticks	5	20	Trace	Trace	—	—	—	4	1	0	0	Trace	Trace	Trace	0
Rice, white (fully milled or polished), enriched, cooked																
Common commercial varieties, all types	1 cup	168	185	3	Trace	—	—	—	41	17	[20]1.5	0	[20].19	[20].01	[20]1.6	0
Long grain, parboiled	1 cup	176	185	4	Trace	—	—	—	41	33	[20]1.4	0	[20].19	[20].02	[20]2.0	0
Rice, puffed, added nutrients (without salt)	1 cup	14	55	1	Trace	—	—	—	13	3	.3	0	.06	.01	.6	0
Rice flakes, added nutrients	1 cup	30	115	2	Trace	—	—	—	26	9	.5	0	.10	.02	1.6	0
Rolls																
Plain, pan; 12 per 16 ounces																
Enriched	1 roll	38	115	3	2	Trace	1	Trace	20	28	.7	Trace	.11	.07	.8	Trace
Unenriched	1 roll	38	115	3	2	Trace	1	Trace	20	28	.3	Trace	.02	.03	.3	Trace
Hard, round; 12 per 22 oz	1 roll	52	160	5	2	Trace	1	Trace	31	24	.4	Trace	.03	.05	.4	Trace
Sweet, pan; 12 per 18 oz	1 roll	43	135	4	4	1	2	Trace	21	37	.3	30	.03	.06	.4	Trace
Rye wafers, whole-grain, 1⅞ by 3½ inches	2 wafers	13	45	2	Trace	—	—	—	10	7	.5	0	.04	.03	.2	0
Spaghetti																
Cooked, tender stage (14 to 20 minutes)																
Enriched	1 cup	140	155	5	1	—	—	—	32	11	[16]1.3	0	[16].19	[16].11	[16]1.5	0
Unenriched	1 cup	140	155	5	1	—	—	—	32	11	.6	0	.02	.02	.4	0

Spaghetti with meat balls in tomato sauce (home recipe)	1 cup	250	335	19	12	4	6	1	39	125	3.8	1,600	.26	.30	4.0	22
Spaghetti in tomato sauce with cheese (home recipe)	1 cup	250	260	9	9	2	5	1	37	80	2.2	1,080	.24	.18	2.4	14
Waffles, with enriched flour, ½ by 4½ by 5½ inches	1	75	210	7	7	2	4	1	28	85	1.3	250	.13	.19	1.0	Trace
Wheat, puffed																
With added nutrients (without salt)	1 oz	28	105	4	Trace	—	—	—	22	8	1.2	0	.15	.07	2.2	0
With added nutrients, with sugar and honey	1 oz	28	105	2	1	—	—	—	25	7	.9	0	.14	.05	1.8	0
Wheat, rolled; cooked	1 cup	236	175	5	1	—	—	—	40	19	1.7	0	.17	.06	2.1	0
Wheat, shredded, plain (long, round, or bite-size)	1 oz	28	100	3	1	—	—	—	23	12	1.0	0	.06	.03	1.2	0
Wheat and malted barley flakes, with added nutrients	1 oz	28	110	2	Trace	—	—	—	24	14	.7	0	.13	.03	1.1	0
Wheat flakes, with added nutrients	1 oz	28	100	3	Trace	—	—	—	23	12	1.2	0	.18	.04	1.4	0
Wheat flours																
Whole-wheat, from hard wheats, stirred	1 cup	120	400	16	2	Trace	1	1	85	49	4.0	0	.66	.14	5.2	0
All-purpose or family flour																
Enriched, sifted	1 cup	110	400	12	1	Trace	Trace	Trace	84	18	[16]3.2	0	[16].48	[16].29	[16]3.8	0
Unenriched, sifted	1 cup	110	400	12	1	Trace	Trace	Trace	84	18	.9	0	.07	.05	1.0	0
Self-rising, enriched	1 cup	110	385	10	1	Trace	Trace	Trace	82	292	[16]3.2	0	[16].49	[16].29	[16]3.9	0
Cake or pastry flour, sifted	1 cup	100	365	8	1	Trace	Trace	Trace	79	17	.5	0	.03	.03	.7	0
Wheat germ, crude, commercially milled	1 cup	68	245	18	7	1	2	4	32	49	6.4	0	1.36	.46	2.9	0

[16]Iron, thiamine, riboflavin, and niacin are based on the minimum levels of enrichment specified in standards of identity promulgated under the Federal Food, Drug, and Cosmetic Act.

[20]Iron, thiamine, and niacin are based on the minimum levels of enrichment specified in standards of identity promulgated under the Federal Food, Drug, and Cosmetic Act. Riboflavin is based on unenriched rice. When the minimum level of enrichment for riboflavin specified in the standards of identity becomes effective the value will be 0.12 milligram per cup of parboiled rice and of white rice.

Nutritive values of the edible part of foods—cont'd

Food, approximate measure, and weight (in grams)			Food energy (calories)	Protein (g)	Fat (total lipid) (g)	Fatty acids: Saturated (total) (g)	Fatty acids: Unsaturated: Oleic (g)	Fatty acids: Unsaturated: Linoleic (g)	Carbohydrate (g)	Calcium (mg)	Iron (mg)	Vitamin A value (IU)	Thiamin (mg)	Riboflavin (mg)	Niacin (mg)	Ascorbic acid (mg)
Fats, oils																
Butter, 4 sticks per pound																
Sticks, 2	1 cup	227	1,625	1	184	101	61	6	1	45	0	[21]7,500	—	—	—	0
Stick, ⅛	1 tbsp	14	100	Trace	11	6	4	Trace	Trace	3	0	[21]460	—	—	—	0
Pat or square (64 per pound)	1 pat	7	50	Trace	6	3	2	Trace	Trace	1	0	[21]230	—	—	—	0
Fats, cooking																
Lard	1 cup	220	1,985	0	220	84	101	22	0	0	0	0	0	0	0	0
Lard	1 tbsp	14	125	0	14	5	6	1	0	0	0	0	0	0	0	0
Vegetable fats	1 cup	200	1,770	0	200	46	130	14	0	0	0	—	0	0	0	0
Vegetable fats	1 tbsp	12.5	110	0	12	3	8	1	0	0	0	—	0	0	0	0
Margarine, 4 sticks per pound																
Sticks, 2	1 cup	227	1,635	1	184	37	105	33	1	45	0	[22]7,500	—	—	—	0
Stick, ⅛	1 tbsp	14	100	Trace	11	2	6	2	Trace	3	0	[22]460	—	—	—	0
Pat or square (64 per pound)	1 pat	7	50	Trace	6	1	3	1	Trace	1	0	[22]230	—	—	—	0
Oils, salad or cooking																
Corn	1 tbsp	14	125	0	14	1	4	7	0	0	0	—	0	0	0	0
Cottonseed	1 tbsp	14	125	0	14	4	3	7	0	0	0	—	0	0	0	0
Olive	1 tbsp	14	125	0	14	2	11	1	0	0	0	—	0	0	0	0
Soybean	1 tbsp	14	125	0	14	2	3	7	0	0	0	—	0	0	0	0
Salad dressings																
Blue cheese	1 tbsp	16	80	1	8	2	2	4	1	13	Trace	30	Trace	.02	Trace	Trace
Commercial mayonnaise type	1 tbsp	15	65	Trace	6	1	1	3	2	2	Trace	30	Trace	Trace	Trace	—
French	1 tbsp	15	60	Trace	6	1	1	3	3	2	.1	—	—	—	—	—
Home cooked, boiled	1 tbsp	17	30	1	2	1	1	Trace	3	15	.1	80	.01	.03	Trace	Trace
Mayonnaise	1 tbsp	15	110	Trace	12	2	3	6	Trace	3	.1	40	Trace	.01	Trace	—
Thousand Island	1 tbsp	15	75	Trace	8	1	2	4	2	2	.1	50	Trace	Trace	Trace	Trace
Sugars, sweets																
Candy																
Caramels	1 oz	28	115	1	3	2	1	Trace	22	42	.4	Trace	.01	.05	Trace	Trace
Chocolate, milk, plain	1 oz	28	150	2	9	5	3	Trace	16	65	.3	80	.02	.09	.1	Trace
Fudge, plain	1 oz	28	115	1	3	2	1	Trace	21	22	.3	Trace	.01	.03	.1	Trace
Hard candy	1 oz	28	110	0	Trace	—	—	—	28	6	.5	0	0	0	0	0
Marshmallows	1 oz	28	90	1	Trace	—	—	—	23	5	.5	0	0	Trace	Trace	0
Chocolate syrup, thin type	1 tbsp	20	50	Trace	Trace	Trace	Trace	Trace	13	3	.3	—	Trace	.01	.1	0

Honey, strained or extracted	1 tbsp	21	65	Trace	0	—	—	—	17	1	.1	0	Trace	.01	.1	Trace
Jams and preserves	1 tbsp	20	55	Trace	Trace	—	—	—	14	4	.2	Trace	Trace	.01	Trace	Trace
Jellies	1 tbsp	20	55	Trace	Trace	—	—	—	14	4	.3	Trace	Trace	.01	Trace	1
Molasses, cane																
Light (first extraction)	1 tbsp	20	50	—	—	—	—	—	13	33	.9	—	.01	.01	Trace	—
Blackstrap (third extraction)	1 tbsp	20	45	—	—	—	—	—	11	137	3.2	—	.02	.04	.4	—
Sirup, table blends (chiefly corn, light and dark)	1 tbsp	20	60	0	0	—	—	—	15	9	.8	0	0	0	0	0
Sugars (cane or beet)																
Granulated	1 cup	200	770	0	0	—	—	—	199	0	.2	0	0	0	0	0
	1 tbsp	12	45	0	0	—	—	—	12	0	Trace	0	0	0	0	0
Lump, 1⅛ by ¾ by ⅜	1 lump	6	25	0	0	—	—	—	6	0	Trace	0	0	0	0	0
Powdered, stirred before measuring	1 cup	128	495	0	0	—	—	—	127	0	.1	0	0	0	0	0
	1 tbsp	8	30	0	0	—	—	—	8	0	Trace	0	0	0	0	0
Brown, firm-packed	1 cup	220	820	0	0	—	—	—	212	187	7.5	0	.02	.07	.4	0
	1 tbsp	14	50	0	0	—	—	—	13	12	.5	0	Trace	Trace	Trace	0
Miscellaneous items																
Beer (average 3.6 percent alcohol by weight)	1 cup	240	100	1	0	—	—	—	9	12	Trace	—	.01	.07	1.6	—
Beverages, carbonated																
Cola type	1 cup	240	95	0	0	—	—	—	24	—	—	0	0	0	0	0
Ginger ale	1 cup	230	70	0	0	—	—	—	18	—	—	0	0	0	0	0
Bouillon cube, ⅝ inch	1 cube	4	5	1	Trace	—	—	—	Trace	—	—	—	—	—	—	—
Chili powder, *See* Vegetables, peppers																
Chili sauce (mainly tomatoes)	1 tbsp	17	20	Trace	Trace	—	—	—	4	3	.1	240	.02	.01	.3	3
Chocolate																
Bitter or baking	1 oz	28	145	3	15	8	6	Trace	8	22	1.9	20	.01	.07	.4	0
Sweet	1 oz	28	150	1	10	6	4	Trace	16	27	.4	Trace	.01	.04	.1	Trace
Cider, *See* Fruits, apple juice																
Gelatin, dry																
Plain	1 tbsp	10	35	9	Trace	—	—	—	—	—	—	—	—	—	—	—
Dessert powder, 3 oz package	½ cup	85	315	8	0	—	—	—	75	—	—	—	—	—	—	—

[21]Year-round average.

[22]Based on the average vitamin A content of fortified margarine. Federal specifications for fortified margarine require a minimum of 15,000 IU of vitamin A per pound.

Nutritive values of the edible part of foods—cont'd

Food, approximate measure, and weight (in grams)			*Food energy (calories)*	*Protein (g)*	*Fat (total lipid) (g)*	*Fatty acids: Saturated (total) (g)*	*Fatty acids: Unsaturated: Oleic (g)*	*Fatty acids: Unsaturated: Linoleic (g)*	*Carbohydrate (g)*	*Calcium (mg)*	*Iron (mg)*	*Vitamin A value (IU)*	*Thiamin (mg)*	*Riboflavin (mg)*	*Niacin (mg)*	*Ascorbic acid (mg)*
Gelatin dessert, ready-to-eat																
Plain	1 cup	239	140	4	0	—	—	—	34	—	—	—	—	—	—	—
With fruit	1 cup	241	160	3	Trace	—	—	—	40	—	—	—	—	—	—	—
Olives, pickled																
Green	4 medium or 3 extra large or 2 giant	16	15	Trace	2	Trace	2	Trace	Trace	8	.2	40	—	—	—	—
Ripe: Mission	3 small or 2 large	10	15	Trace	2	Trace	2	Trace	Trace	9	.1	10	Trace	Trace	—	—
Pickles, cucumber																
Dill, large, 4 by 1¾ inches	1	135	15	1	Trace	—	—	—	3	35	1.4	140	Trace	.03	Trace	8
Sweet, 2¾ by ¾ inches	1	20	30	Trace	Trace	—	—	—	7	2	.2	20	Trace	Trace	Trace	1
Popcorn, *See* Grain products																
Sherbet, orange	1 cup	193	260	2	2	—	—	—	59	31	Trace	110	.02	.06	Trace	4
Soups, canned; ready-to-serve (prepared with equal volume of water)																
Bean with pork	1 cup	250	170	8	6	1	2	2	22	62	2.2	650	.14	.07	1.0	2
Beef noodle	1 cup	250	70	4	3	1	1	1	7	8	1.0	50	.05	.06	1.1	Trace
Beef bouillon, broth, consomme	1 cup	240	30	5	0	0	0	0	3	Trace	.5	Trace	Trace	.02	1.2	—
Chicken noodle	1 cup	250	65	4	2	Trace	1	1	8	10	.5	50	.02	.02	.8	Trace
Clam chowder	1 cup	255	85	2	3	—	—	—	13	36	1.0	920	.03	.03	1.0	—
Cream soup (mushroom)	1 cup	240	135	2	10	1	3	5	10	41	.5	70	.02	.12	.7	Trace
Minestrone	1 cup	245	105	5	3	—	—	—	14	37	1.0	2,350	.07	.05	1.0	—
Pea, green	1 cup	245	130	6	2	1	1	Trace	23	44	1.0	340	.05	.05	1.0	7
Tomato	1 cup	245	90	2	2	Trace	1	1	16	15	.7	1,000	.06	.05	1.1	12
Vegetable with beef broth	1 cup	250	80	3	2	—	—	—	14	20	.8	3,250	.05	.02	1.2	—
Starch (cornstarch)	1 cup	128	465	Trace	Trace	—	—	—	112	0	0	0	0	0	0	0
	1 tbsp	8	30	Trace	Trace	—	—	—	7	0	0	0	0	0	0	0

Tapioca, quick-cooking granulated, dry, stirred before measuring	1 cup 1 tbsp	152 10	535 35	1 Trace	Trace Trace	— —	— —	— —	131 9	15 1	.6 Trace	0 0	0 0	0 0	0 0	0 0
Vinegar	1 tbsp	15	2	0	—	—	—	—	1	1	.1	—	—	—	—	—
White sauce, medium	1 cup	265	430	10	33	18	11	1	23	305	.5	1,220	.12	.44	.6	Trace
Yeast																
Baker's																
Compressed	1 oz	28	25	3	Trace	—	—	—	3	4	1.4	Trace	.20	.47	3.2	Trace
Dry active	1 oz	28	80	10	Trace	—	—	—	11	12	4.6	Trace	.66	1.53	10.4	Trace
Brewer's, dry, debittered	1 tbsp	8	25	3	Trace	—	—	—	3	17	1.4	Trace	1.25	.34	3.0	Trace
Yogurt, *See* Milk, cream; cheese, related products																

6-7 Sodium and potassium content of foods, 100 gm, edible portion[1]

Food and description	Sodium (mg)	Potassium (mg)
Almonds		
dried	4	773
roasted and salted	198	773
Apples		
raw, pared	1	110
frozen, sliced, sweetened	14	68
Apple brown betty	153	100
Apple butter	2	252
Apple juice, canned or bottled	1	101
Applesauce, canned, sweetened	2	65
Apricots		
raw	1	281
canned, syrup pack, light	1	239
dried, sulfured, cooked, fruit, and liquid	8	318
Apricot nectar, canned (approx. 40% fruit)	Trace	151
Asparagus		
cooked spears, boiled, drained	1	183
canned spears, green		
regular pack, solids and liquid	236[2]	166
special dietary pack (low-sodium), solids and liquids	3	166
frozen		
cuts and tips, cooked, boiled, drained	1	220
spears, cooked, boiled, drained	1	238
Avocados, raw, all commercial varieties	4	604
Bacon, cured, cooked, broiled or fried, drained	1021	236
Bacon, Canadian, cooked, broiled or fried, drained	2555	432
Baking powders		
home use		
straight phosphate	8220	170
special low-sodium preparations	6	10,948
Bananas, raw, common	1	370
Barbecue sauce	815	174
Bass, black sea, raw	68	256
Beans, common, mature seeds, dry white		
cooked	7	416
canned, solids and liquid, with pork and tomato sauce	463	210
red, cooked	3	340
Beans, lima		
immature seeds		
cooked, boiled, drained	1	422
Beans, lima—cont'd		
canned		
regular pack, solids and liquid	236[2]	222
special dietary pack (low-sodium), solids and liquid	4	222
frozen, thin-seeded types, commonly called baby limas, cooked, boiled, drained	129	394
mature seeds, dry, cooked	2	612
Beans, mung, sprouted seeds, cooked, boiled, drained	4	156
Beans, snap		
green		
cooked, boiled, drained	4	151
canned		
regular pack, solids and liquid	236[2]	95
special dietary pack (low sodium), solids and liquid	2	95
frozen, cut, cooked, boiled, drained	1	152
yellow or wax		
cooked, boiled, drained	3	151
canned		
regular pack, solids and liquid	236[2]	95
special dietary pack (low-sodium), solids and liquid	2	95
frozen, cut, cooked, boiled, drained	1	164
Beans and frankfurters, canned	539	262
Beef		
retail cuts, trimmed to retail level		
round	60	370
rump	60	370
hamburger, regular ground, cooked	47	450
Beef and vegetable stew, canned	411	174
Beef, corned, boneless		
cooked, medium-fat	1740	150
canned corned-beef has (with potato)	540	200
Beef, dried, cooked, creamed	716	153

[1]Numbers in parentheses denote values imputed—usually from another form of the food or from a similar food. Dashes denote lack of reliable data for a constituent believed to be present in measurable amount.
[2]Estimated average based on addition of salt in the amount of 0.6% of the finished product.

Food and description	*Sodium (mg)*	*Potassium (mg)*
Beef potpie, commercial, frozen, unheated	366	93
Beets, common, red canned		
regular pack, solids and liquid	236[2]	167
special dietary pack (low-sodium), solids and liquid	46	167
Beet greens, common, cooked, boiled, drained	76	332
Beverages, alcoholic		
beer, alcohol 4.5% by volume	7	25
(3.6% by weight)	7	25
gin, rum, vodka, whisky		
80-proof (33.4% alcohol by weight)	1	2
86-proof (36.0% alcohol by weight)	1	2
90-proof (37.9% alcohol by weight)	1	2
94-proof (39.7% alcohol by weight)	1	2
100-proof (42.5% alcohol by weight)	1	2
wines		
dessert, alcohol 18.8% by volume (15.3% by weight)	4	75
table, alcohol 12.2% by volume (9.9% by weight)	5	92
Biscuits, baking powder, made with enriched flour	626	117
Biscuit dough, commercial, frozen	910	86
Biscuit mix, with enriched flour, and biscuits baked from mix		
mix, dry form	1300	80
biscuits, made with milk	973	116
Blackberries, including dewberries, boysenberries, and youngberries, raw	1	170
Blackberries, canned, solids and liquid		
water pack, with or without artificial sweetener	1	115
syrup pack, heavy	1	109
Blueberries		
raw	1	81
frozen, not thawed, sweetened	1	66
Bluefish, cooked		
baked or boiled	104	—
fried	146	—
Boston brown bread	251	292
Bouillon cubes or powder	24,000	100
Boysenberries, frozen, not thawed, sweetened	1	105
Bran, added sugar and malt extract	1060	1070
Bran flakes (40% bran), added thiamine	925	—
Bran flakes with raisins, added thiamine	800	—
Brazil nuts	1	715
Breads		
cracked-wheat	529	134
French or vienna, enriched	580	90
Italian, enriched	585	74
raisin	365	233
rye, American (⅓ rye, ⅔ clear flour)	557	145
white, enriched, made with 3%-4% non-fat dry milk	507	105
whole-wheat, made with 2% non-fat dry milk	527	273
Bread crumbs, dry, grated	736	152
Bread stuffing mix and stuffings prepared from mix mix, dry form	1331	172
Broccoli		
cooked spears, boiled, drained	10	267
frozen, spears, cooked, boiled, drained	12	220
Brussels sprouts, frozen, cooked, boiled, drained	14	295
Buffalo fish, raw	52	293
Bulgur (parboiled wheat)		
canned, made from hard red winter wheat		
unseasoned[3]	599	87
seasoned[4]	460	112
Butter[5]	987	23
Buttermilk, fluid, cultured (made from skim milk)	130	140
Cabbage		
common varieties (Danish, domestic, and pointed types)		
raw	20	233
cooked, boiled until tender, drained, shredded, cooked in small amount of water	14	163

[3]Processed, partially debranned, whole-kernel wheat with salt added.
[4]Processed, partially debranned, whole-kernel wheat with chicken fat, chicken stock base, dehydrated onion flakes, salt, monosodium glutamate, and herbs.
[5]Values apply to salted butter. Unsalted butter contains less than 10 mg of either sodium or potassium per 100 gm. Value for vitamin A is the year-round average.

Sodium and potassium content of foods, 100 gm, edible portion—cont'd

Food and description	Sodium (mg)	Potassium (mg)
Cabbage—cont'd		
red, raw	26	268
Cabbage, Chinese (also called celery cabbage or petsai)	23	253
Cakes		
baked from home recipes		
angelfood	283	88
fruitcake, made with enriched flour, dark	158	496
gingerbread, made with enriched flour	237	454
plain cake or cupcake, without icing	300	79
pound, modified	178	78
frozen, commercial, devil's food, with chocolate	420	119
Candy		
caramels, plain or chocolate	226	192
chocolate, sweet	33	296
chocolate-coated, chocolate fudge	228	193
gum drops, starch jelly pieces	35	5
hard	32	4
marshmallows	39	6
peanut bars	10	448
Carp, raw	50	286
Carrots		
raw	47	341
canned		
regular pack, solids and liquid	236[2]	120
special dietary pack (low-sodium), solids and liquid	39	120
Cashew nuts	15[6]	464
Catfish, freshwater, raw	60	330
Cauliflower		
cooked, boiled, drained	9	206
frozen, cooked, boiled, drained	10	207
Caviar, sturgeon, granular	2200	180
Celery, all, including green and yellow varieties		
raw	126	341
cooked, boiled, drained	88	239
Chard, Swiss, cooked, boiled, drained	86	321
Cheese straws	721	63
Cheeses		
natural cheeses		
cheddar (domestic type, commonly called American)	700	82
cottage (large or small curd)		
creamed	229	85
uncreamed	290	72
cream	250	74
parmesan	734	149
Swiss (domestic)	710	104
pasteurized process cheese, American	1136[7]	80
pasteurized process cheese spread, American	1625[7]	240
Cherries		
raw, sweet	2	191
canned		
sour, red, solids and liquid, water pack	2	130
sweet, solids and liquid, syrup pack, light	1	128
frozen, not thawed, sweetened	2	130
Chicken		
all classes		
light meat without skin, cooked, roasted	64	411
dark meat without skin, cooked, roasted	86	321
Chicken potpie, commercial, frozen, unheated	411	153
Chicory, Witloof (also called French or Belgian endive), bleached head (forced), raw	7	182
Chili con carne, canned, with beans	531	233
Chocolate, bitter or baking	4	830
Chocolate syrup, fudge type	89	284
Chop suey, with meat, canned	551	138
Chow mein, chicken (without noodles), canned	290	167
Citron, candied	290	120
Clams, raw		
soft, meat only	36	235
hard or round, meat only	205	311
Clams, canned, including hard, soft, razor, and unspecified solids and liquids	—	140

[2]Estimated average based on addition of salt in the amount of 0.6% of the finished product.
[6]Applies to unsalted nuts. For salted nuts, value is approximately 200 mg per 100 gm.
[7]Values for phosphorus and sodium are based on use of 1.5% anhydrous disodium phosphate as the emulsifying agent. If emulsifying agent does not contain either phosphorus or sodium, the content of these two nutrients in milligrams per 100 gm is as follows:

	P	Na
American process cheese	444	650
Swiss process cheese	540	681
American cheese food	427	—
American cheese spread	548	1139

Food and description	Sodium (mg)	Potassium (mg)
Cocoa and chocolate-flavored beverage powders		
cocoa powder with non-fat dry milk	525	800
mix for hot chocolate	382	605
Cocoa, dry powder		
high-fat or breakfast		
plain	6	1,522
processed with alkali	717	651
Coconut cream (liquid expressed from grated coconut meat)	4	324
Coconut meat, fresh	23	256
Cod		
cooked, broiled	110	407
dehydrated, lightly salted	8100	160
Coffee, instant, water-soluble		
solids dry powder	72	3,256
beverage	1	36
Coleslaw, made with French dressing (commercial)	268	205
Collards, cooked, boiled, drained, leaves, including stems, cooked in small amount of water	25	234
Cookies		
assorted, packaged, commercial	365	67
butter, thin, rich	418	60
gingersnaps	571	462
molasses	162	138
oatmeal with raisins	162	370
sandwich type	483	38
vanilla wafer	252	72
Cookie dough, plain, chilled in roll, baked	548	48
Corn, sweet		
cooked, boiled, drained, white and yellow, kernels, cut off cob before cooking	Trace	165
canned		
regular pack, cream style, white and yellow, solids and liquid	236[2]	(97)
special dietary pack (low-sodium), cream style, white and yellow, solids and liquid	2	(97)
frozen, kernels cut off cob, cooked, boiled, drained	1	184
Corn fritters	477	133
Corn grits, degermed, enriched, dry form	1	80
Corn products used mainly as ready-to-eat breakfast cereals		
corn flakes, added nutrients	1005	120
corn, puffed, added nutrients	1060	—
corn, rice, and wheat flakes, mixed, added nutrients	950	—
Cornbread, baked from home recipes, southern style, made with degermed cornmeal, enriched	591	157
Cornbread mix and cornbread baked from mix, cornbread, made with egg, milk	744	127
Cornmeal, white or yellow, degermed, enriched, dry form	1	120
Cornstarch	Trace	Trace
Cowpeas, including blackeye peas		
immature seeds, canned, solids and liquid	236[2]	352
young pods, with seeds, cooked, boiled, drained	3	196
Crab, canned	1000	110
Crackers		
butter	1092	113
graham, plain	670	384
saltines	(1100)	(120)
sandwich type, peanut-cheese	992	226
soda	1100	120
Cranberries, raw	2	82
Cranberry juice cocktail, bottled	1	10
(approx. 33% cranberry juice)	1	10
Cranberry sauce, sweetened, canned, strained	1	30
Cream, fluid, light, coffee, or table, 20% fat	43	122
Cream substitutes, dried, containing cream, skim milk (calcium reduced), and lactose	575	—
Cream puffs with custard filling	83	121
Cress, garden, raw	14	606
Croaker, Atlantic, cooked, baked	120	323
Cucumbers, raw, pared	6	160
Custard, baked	79	146
Dates, domestic, natural and dry	1	648
Doughnuts, cake type	501	90
Duck, domesticated, raw, flesh only	74	285
Eggs, chicken		
raw		
whole, fresh and frozen	122	129
whites, fresh and frozen	146	139
yolks, fresh	52	98
Eggplant, cooked, boiled, drained	1	150
Endive (curly endive and escarole), raw	14	294

[2]Estimated average based on addition of salt in the amount of 0.6% of the finished product.

Sodium and potassium content of foods, 100 gm, edible portion—cont'd

Food and description	*Sodium (mg)*	*Potassium (mg)*
Farina		
enriched		
regular		
dry form	2	83
cooked	144	9
quick-cooking, cooked	165	10
instant-cooking, cooked	188	13
enriched, regular, dry form	2	83
Figs, canned, solids and liquid, syrup pack, light	2	152
Flatfishes (flounders, soles, and sand dabs), raw	78	342
Fruit cocktail, canned, solids and liquid, water pack, with or without artificial sweetener	5	168
Garlic, cloves, raw	19	529
Ginger root, fresh	6	264
Gizzard, chicken, all classes, cooked, simmered	57	211
Goose, domesticated, flesh only, cooked, roasted	124	605
Gooseberries, canned, solids and liquid, syrup pack, heavy	1	98
Grapefruit	1	135
raw, pulp, pink, red, white, all varieties		
canned, juice, sweetened	1	162
Grapefruit juice and orange juice blended, canned, sweetened	1	184
Grapes, raw, American type (slip skin) such as Concord, Delaware, Niagara, Catawba, and Scuppernong	3	158
Grapejuice, canned or bottled	2	116
Guavas, whole, raw, common	4	289
Haddock, cooked, fried	177	348
Hake, including Pacific hake, squirrel hake, and silver hake or whiting; raw	74	363
Halibut, Atlantic and Pacific, cooked, broiled	134	525
Ham croquette	342	83
Heart, beef, lean, cooked, braised	104	232
Herring		
raw, Pacific	74	420
smoked, hard	6231	157
Honey, strained or extracted	5	51
Horse-radish, prepared	96	290
Ice cream and frozen custard regular, approximately 10% fat	63[8]	181
Ice cream cones	232	244
Ice milk	68[8]	195
Jams and preserves	12	88
Kale, cooked, boiled, drained, leaves including stems	43	221
Kingfish; southern, gulf, and northern (whiting); raw	83	250
Lake herring (cisco), raw	47	319
Lamb, retail cuts	70	290
Lemon juice, canned or bottled, unsweetened	1	141
Lettuce, raw crisphead varieties such as iceberg, New York, and Great Lakes strains	9	175
Lime juice, canned or bottled, unsweetened	1	104
Liver, beef, cooked, fried	184	380
Lobster, northern, canned or cooked	210	180
Loganberries, canned, solids and liquid, syrup pack, light	1	111
Macadamia nuts	—	164
Macaroni, unenriched, dry form	2	197
Macaroni and cheese, canned	304	58
Margarine[9]	987	23
Marmalade, citrus	14	33
Milk, cow		
fluid (pasteurized and raw)		
whole, 3.7% fat	50	144
skim	52	145
canned, evaporated (unsweetened)	118	303
dry, skim (non-fat solids), regular	532	1745
malted		
dry powder	440	720
beverage	91	200
chocolate drink, fluid, commercial		
made with skim milk	46	142
made with whole (3.5% fat) milk	47	146
Molasses, cane		
first extraction or light	15	917
third extraction or blackstrap	96	2927
Muffin mixes, corn, and muffins baked from mixes		
muffins, made with egg, milk	479	110
muffins, made with egg, water	346	104
Mushrooms		
raw	15	414
canned, solids and liquid	400	197

8Value for product without added salt.

[9]Values apply to salted margarine. Unsalted margarine contains less than 10 mg per 100 gm of either sodium or potassium. Vitamin A value based on the minimum required to meet federal specifications for margarine with vitamin A added, namely 15,000 IU of vitamin A per pound.

Food and description	Sodium (mg)	Potassium (mg)
Muskmelons, raw, cantaloupes, other netted varieties	12	251
Mussels, Atlantic and Pacific, raw, meat only	289	315
Mustard greens, cooked, boiled, drained	18	220
Mustard, prepared		
brown	1307	130
yellow	1252	130
Nectarines, raw	6	294
New Zealand spinach, cooked, boiled, drained	92	463
Noodles, egg noodles, enriched, cooked	2	44
Oat products used mainly as hot breakfast cereals oatmeal or rolled oats		
dry form	2	352
cooked	218	61
Oat products used mainly as ready-to-eat breakfast cereals oats (with or without corn), puffed, added nutrients	1267	—
Ocean perch, Atlantic (redfish)		
raw	79	269
cooked, fried	153	284
Ocean perch, Pacific, raw	63	390
Oils, salad or cooking	0	0
Okra		
raw	3	249
cooked, boiled, drained	2	174
Olives, pickled; canned or bottled green	2400	55
ripe, Ascolano (extra large, mammoth, giant jumbo)	813	34
ripe, salt-cured, oil-coated, Greek style	3288	—
Onions, mature (dry), raw	10	157
Onions, young green (bunching varieties), raw bulb and entire top	5	231
Oranges, raw, peeled fruit, all commercial varieties	1	200
Orange juice		
raw, all commercial varieties	1	200
canned, unsweetened	1	199
frozen concentrate, unsweetened, diluted with 3 parts water, by volume	1	186
Oysters		
raw, meat only, Eastern	73	121
cooked, fried	206	203
frozen, solids and liquid	380	210
Oyster stew, commercial frozen, prepared with equal volume of milk	366	176
Pancake and waffle mixes and pancakes baked from mixes plain and buttermilk, made with egg, milk	564	154
Parsnips, cooked, boiled, drained	8	379
Peaches		
raw	1	202
canned, solids and liquid, water pack, with or without artificial sweetener	2	137
frozen, sliced, sweetened, not thawed	2	124
Peanuts		
roasted with skins	5	701
roasted and salted	418	674
Peanut butters made with small amounts of added fat, salt	607	670
Pears		
raw, including skin	2	130
canned, solids and liquid, syrup pack, light	1	85
Peas, green, immature		
cooked, boiled, drained	1	196
canned, Alaska (Early or June peas)		
regular pack, solids and liquid	236[2]	96
special dietary pack (low-sodium), solids and liquid	3	96
frozen, cooked, boiled, and drained	115	135
Peas, mature seeds, dry, whole, raw	35	1005
Peas and carrots, frozen, cooked, boiled, drained	84	157
Pecans	Trace	603
Peppers, hot, chili, mature, red, raw, pods excluding seeds	25	465
Peppers, sweet, garden varieties, immature, green, raw	13	213
Perch, yellow, raw	68	230
Pickles, cucumber, dill	1428	200
Pies		
baked, piecrust made with unenriched flour		
apple	301	80
cherry	304	105
mince	448	178
pumpkin	214	160

[2]Estimated average based on addition of salt in the amount of 0.6% of the finished product.

Sodium and potassium content of foods, 100 gm, edible portion—cont'd

Food and description	Sodium (mg)	Potassium (mg)
Piecrust or plain pastry, made with enriched flour, baked	611	50
Pike, walleye, raw	51	319
Pineapple		
raw	1	146
frozen chunks, sweetened, not thawed	2	100
Pizza, with cheese, from home recipe, baked		
with cheese topping	702	130
with sausage topping	729	168
Plate dinners, frozen, commercial, unheated		
beef pot roast, whole oven-browned potatoes, peas, and corn	259	244
chicken, fried; mashed potatoes; mixed vegetables (carrots, peas, corn, beans)	344	112
meat loaf with tomato sauce, mashed potatoes, and peas	393	115
turkey, sliced; mashed potatoes; peas	400	176
Plums		
raw, Damson	2	299
canned, solids and liquid, purple (Italian prunes), syrup pack, light	1	145
Popcorn, popped		
plain	(3)	—
oil and salt added	1940	—
Pork, fresh		
retail cuts, trimmed to retail level loin	65	390
Pork, cured, light-cure, commercial, ham, medium-fat class, separable lean, cooked, roasted	930	326
Pork, cured, canned ham, contents of can	(1100)	(340)
Potatoes		
cooked, boiled in skin	3[10]	407
dehydrated mashed		
flakes without milk		
dry form	89	1600
prepared, water, milk, table fat added	231	286
Pretzels	1680[11]	130
Prunes	3	262
dried, "softenized," cooked (fruit and liquid), with added sugar		
Pudding mixes and puddings made from mixes with starch base		
pudding made with milk, cooked	129	136
pudding made with milk, without cooking	124	129
Pumpkin, canned	2	240
Radishes, raw, common	18	322
Raisins, natural (unbleached)		
cooked, fruit and liquid, added sugar	13	355
Raspberries		
canned, solids and liquid, water pack, with or without artificial sweetener, red	1	114
frozen, red, sweetened, not thawed	1	100
Rennin products		
tablet (salts, starch, rennin enzyme)	22,300	—
dessert mixes and desserts prepared from mixes		
chocolate, dessert made with milk	52	125
other flavors (vanilla, caramel, fruit flavorings)		
mix, dry form	6	—
dessert, made with milk	46	128
Rhubarb, cooked, added sugar	2	203
Rice		
brown		
raw	9	214
cooked	282	70
white (fully milled or polished)		
enriched		
common commercial varieties, all types		
raw	5	92
cooked	374	28
Rice products used mainly as ready-to-eat breakfast cereals		
rice flakes, added nutrients	987	180
rice, puffed; added nutrients, without salt	2	100
rice, puffed or open-popped, presweetened, honey and added nutrients	706	—
Rockfish, including black, canary, yellowtail, rasphead, and bocaccio, cooked, oven-steamed	68	446
Roe, cooked, baked or broiled, cod and shad[12]	73	132

[10]Applies to product without added salt. If salt is added, an estimated average value for sodium is 236 mg per 100 gm.
[11]Sodium content is variable. For example, very thin pretzel sticks contain about twice the average amount listed.
[12]Prepared with butter or margarine, lemon juice or vinegar.

Food and description	Sodium (mg)	Potassium (mg)
Rolls and buns		
commercial		
ready-to-serve		
Danish pastry	366	112
hard rolls, enriched	625	97
plain (pan rolls), enriched	506	95
sweet rolls	389	124
Rusk	246	161
Rutabagas, cooked, boiled, drained	4	167
Rye, flour, medium	(1)	203
Rye wafers, whole-grain	882	600
Salad dressings, commercial[13]		
Blue and Roquefort cheese		
regular	1094	37
special dietary (low-calorie) low-fat (approx. 5 cal per tsp)	1108	34
French		
regular	1370	79
special dietary (low-calorie) low-fat (approx. 5 cal per tsp)	787	79
mayonnaise	597	34
Thousand island		
regular	700	113
special dietary (low-calorie, approx. 10 cal per tsp)	700	113
Salmon		
Coho (silver)		
raw	48[15]	421
canned, solids and liquid	351[14]	339
Salt pork, raw	1212	42
Salt sticks, regular type	1674	92
Sandwich spread (with chopped pickle)		
regular	626	92
special dietary (low-calorie, approx. 5 cal per tsp)	626	92
Sardines, Atlantic, canned in oil, drained solids	823	590
Sardines, Pacific, in tomato sauce, solids and liquid	400	320
Sauerkraut, canned, solids and liquid	747[16]	140
Sausage, cold cuts, and luncheon meats		
bologna, all samples	1300	230
frankfurters, raw, all samples	1100	220
Sausage, cold cuts, and luncheon meats—cont'd		
luncheon meat, pork, cured ham or shoulder, chopped, spiced or unspiced, canned	1234	222
pork sausage, links or bulk, cooked	958	269
Scallops, bay and sea, cooked, steamed	265	476
Soups, commercial, canned		
beef broth, bouillon, and consomme, prepared with equal volume of water	326	54
chicken noodle, prepared with equal volume of water	408	23
tomato		
prepared with equal volume of water	396	94
prepared with equal volume of milk	422	167
vegetable beef, prepared with equal volume of water	427	66
Soy sauce	7325	366
Spaghetti, enriched, cooked, tender stage	1	61
Spaghetti, in tomato sauce with cheese, canned	382	121
Spinach		
cooked, boiled, drained	50	324
canned		
regular pack, drained solids	236[2]	250
special dietary pack (low-sodium), solids and liquid	34	250
frozen, chopped, cooked, boiled, drained	52	333
Squash, summer, all varieties, cooked, boiled, drained	1	141
Squash, frozen		
summer, yellow crookneck, cooked, boiled, drained	3	167
winter, heated	1	207
Strawberries		
raw	1	164
frozen, sweetened, not thawed, sliced	1	112
Sturgeon, cooked, steamed	108	235
Succotash (corn and lima beans), frozen, cooked, boiled, drained	38	246
Sugars, beet or cane, brown	30	344
Sweet potatoes		
cooked, all, baked in skin	12	300

[13]Values apply to products containing salt. For those without salt, sodium content is low, ranging from less than 10 mg to 50 mg per 100 gm; the amount usually is indicated on the label.

[14]For product canned without added salt, value is approximately the same as for raw salmon.

[15]Sample dipped in brine contained 215 mg sodium per 100 gm.

[16]Values for sauerkraut and sauerkraut juice are based on salt content of 1.9% and 2.0%, respectively, in the finished products. The amounts in some samples may vary significantly from this estimate.

Sodium and potassium content of foods, 100 gm, edible portion—cont'd

Food and description	*Sodium (mg)*	*Potassium (mg)*
Sweet potatoes—cont'd		
canned, liquid pack, solids and liquid, regular pack in syrup	48	(120)
dehydrated flakes, prepared with water	45	140
Tangerines, raw (Dancy variety)	2	126
Tapioca, dry	3	18
Tapioca desserts, tapioca cream pudding	156	135
Tartar sauce, regular	707	78
Tea, instant (water-soluble solids)	—	4530
carbohydrate added dry powder beverage	—	25
Tomatoes, ripe		
raw	3	244
canned, solids and liquid, regular pack	130	217
Tomato catsup, bottled	1042[17]	363
Tomato juice		
canned or bottled		
regular pack	200	227
special dietary pack (low-sodium)	3	227
Tomato juice cocktail, canned or bottled	200	221
Tomato puree, canned		
regular pack	399	426
special dietary pack (low-sodium)	6	426
Tongue, beef, medium-fat, cooked, braised	61	164
Tuna, canned		
in oil, solids and liquid	800	301
in water, solids and liquid	41[18]	279[18]
Turkey, all classes		
light meat, cooked, roasted	82	411
dark meat, cooked, roasted	99	398
Turkey potpie, commercial, frozen, unheated	369	114
Turnips, cooked, boiled, drained	34	188
Turnip greens, leaves, including stems		
canned, solids and liquid	236[2]	243
frozen, cooked, boiled, drained	17	149
Veal, retail cuts, untrimmed	80	500
Vinegar, cider	1	100
Waffles, frozen, made with enriched flour	644	158
Walnuts		
black	3	460
Persian or English	2	450
Watercress leaves including stems, raw	52	282
Watermelon, raw	1	100
Wheat flours		
whole (from hard wheats)	3	370
patent		
all-purpose or family flour, enriched	2	95
self-rising flour, enriched (anhydrous monocalcium phosphate used as a baking aid)[19]	1079	—[20]
Wild rice, raw	7	220
Yeast		
baker's, compressed	16	610
brewer's, debittered	121	1894
Yogurt, made from whole milk	47	132
Zweiback	250	150

Estimated average based on addition of salt in the amount of 0.6% of the finished product.

[17]Applies to regular pack. For special dietary pack (low sodium), values range from 5 to 35 mg per 100 gm.

[18]One sample with salt added contained 875 mg of sodium per 100 gm and 275 mg of potassium.

[19]The acid ingredient most commonly used in self-rising flour. When sodium acid pyrophosphate in combination with either anhydrous monocalcium phosphate or calcium carbonate is used, the value for calcium is approximately 120 mg per 100 gm; for phosphorus, 540 mg; for sodium 1360 mg.

[20]90 mg of potassium per 100 gm contributed by flour. Small quantities of additional potassium may be provided by other ingredients.

6-8 Cholesterol content of foods

Item	Amount of cholesterol in		Refuse from item as purchased (%)
	100 gm edible portion[1] (mg)	Edible portion of 450 gm (1 lb) as purchased (mg)	
Beef, raw			
with bone[2]	70	270	15
without bone[2]	70	320	0
Brains, raw	>2000	>9000	0
Butter	250	1135	0
Caviar or fish roe	>300	>1300	0
Cheese			
cheddar	100	455	0
cottage, creamed	15	70	0
cream	120	545	0
other (25% to 30% fat)	85	385	0
Cheese spread	65	295	0
Chicken, flesh only, raw	60	—	0
Crab			
in shell[2]	125	270	52
meat only[2]	125	565	0
Egg, whole	550	2200	12
Egg white	0	0	0
Egg yolk			
fresh	1500	6800	0
frozen	1280	5800	0
dried	2950	13,380	0
Fish			
steak[2]	70	265	16
fillet[2]	70	320	0
Heart, raw	150	680	0
Ice cream	45	205	0
Kidney, raw	375	1700	0
Lamb, raw			
with bone[2]	70	265	16
without bone[2]	70	320	0
lard and other animal fat	95	430	0
Liver, raw	300	1360	0
Lobster			
whole[2]	200	235	74
meat only[2]	200	900	0
Margarine			
all vegetable fat	0	0	0
two-thirds animal fat, one-third vegetable fat	65	295	0
Milk			
fluid, whole	11	50	0
dried, whole	85	385	0
fluid, skim	3	15	0
Mutton			
with bone[2]	65	250	16
without bone[2]	65	295	0
Oysters			
in shell[2]	> 200	> 90	90
meat only[2]	> 200	> 900	0
Pork			
with bone[2]	70	260	18
without bone[2]	70	320	0
Shrimp			
in shell[2]	125	390	31
flesh only[2]	125	565	0
Sweetbreads (thymus)	250	1135	0
Veal			
with bone[2]	90	320	21
without bone[2]	90	410	0

[1]Data apply to 100 gm of edible portion of the item, although it may be purchased with the refuse indicated and described or implied in the first column.
[2]Designate items that have the same chemical composition for the edible portion but differ in the amount of refuse.

6-9 Examples of intentional food additives

Function	*Chemical compound*	*Common food uses*
Acids, alkalis, buffers	Sodium bicarbonate	Baking powder
	Tartaric acid	Fruit sherbets
		Cheese spreads
Antibiotics	Chlortetracycline	Dip for dressed poultry
Anticaking agents	Aluminum calcium silicate	Table salt
Antimycotics	Calcium propionate	Bread
	Sodium propionate	Bread
	Sorbic acid	Cheese
Antioxidants	Butylated hydroxyanisole (BHA)	Fats
	Butylated hydroxytoluene (BHT)	Fats
Bleaching agents	Benzoyl peroxide	Wheat flour
	Chlorine dioxide	
	Oxides of nitrogen	
Color preservative	Sodium benzoate	Green peas
		Maraschino cherries
Coloring agents	Annotto	Butter, margarine
	Carotene	
Emulsifiers	Lecithin	Bakery goods
	Monoglycerides and diglycerides	Dairy products
	Propylene glycol alginate	Confections
Flavoring agents	Amyl acetate	Soft drinks
	Benzaldehyde	Bakery goods
	Methyl salicylate	Candy; ice cream
	Essential oils; natural extractives	
	Monosodium glutamate	Canned meats
Nonnutritive sweeteners	Saccharin, calcium, and sodium cyclamates	Diet packed canned fruit
		Low-calorie soft drinks
Nutrient supplements	Potassium iodide	Iodized salt
	Vitamin C	Fruit juices
	Vitamin D	Milk
	Vitamin A	Margarine
	B vitamins, iron	Bread and cereal
Sequestrants	Sodium citrate	Dairy products
	Calcium pyrophosphoric acid	
Stabilizers and thickeners	Pectin	Jellies
	Vegetable gums (carob bean, carrageenan, guar)	Dairy desserts and chocolate milk
		Confections
	Gelatin	"Low-calorie" salad dressings
	Agar-agar	
Yeast foods and dough conditioners	Ammonium chloride	Bread rolls
	Calcium sulfate	
	Calcium phosphate	

6-10 Food exchange lists

LIST 1: MILK EXCHANGES (Includes **nonfat**, low-fat, and whole milk)

One exchange of milk contains 12 grams of carbohydrate, 8 grams of protein, a trace of fat, and 80 calories. This list shows the kinds and amounts of milk or milk products to use for one milk exchange. Those which appear in **bold type** are **nonfat.** Low-fat and whole milk contain saturated fat.

Nonfat fortified milk	
Skim or nonfat milk	1 cup
Powdered (nonfat dry, before adding liquid)	⅓ cup
Canned, evaporated—skim milk	½ cup
Buttermilk made from skim milk	1 cup
Yogurt made from skim milk (plain, unflavored)	1 cup
Low-fat fortified milk	
1% fat fortified milk (omit ½ fat exchange)	1 cup
2% fat fortified milk (omit 1 fat exchange)	1 cup
Yogurt made from 2% fortified milk (plain, unflavored) (omit 1 fat exchange)	1 cup
Whole milk (omit 2 fat exchanges)	
Whole milk	1 cup
Canned, evaporated whole milk	½ cup
Buttermilk made from whole milk	1 cup
Yogurt made from whole milk (plain, unflavored)	1 cup

LIST 2: VEGETABLE EXCHANGES

One exchange of vegetables contains about 5 grams of carbohydrate, 2 grams of protein, and 25 calories. This list shows the kinds of **vegetables** to use for one vegetable exchange. One exchange is ½ cup.

Asparagus
Bean Sprouts
Beets
Broccoli
Brussels sprouts
Cabbage
Carrots
Cauliflower
Celery
Eggplant
Green pepper
Greens:
- **Beet**
- **Chards**
- **Collards**
- **Dandelion**
- **Kale**

Greens:
- **Mustard**
- **Spinach**
- **Turnip**

Mushrooms
Okra
Onions
Rhubarb
Rutabaga
Sauerkraut
String beans, green or yellow
Summer squash
Tomatoes
Tomato juice
Turnips
Vegetable juice cocktail
Zucchini

The following **raw vegetables** may be used as desired:

Chicory
Chinese cabbage
Cucumbers
Endive
Escarole
Lettuce
Parsley
Pickles, dill
Radishes
Watercress

Starchy vegetables are found in the bread exchange list.

The exchange lists are based on material in the *Exchange Lists for Meal Planning* prepared by Committees of the American Diabetes Association, Inc. and the American Dietetic Association in cooperation with the National Institute of Arthritis, Metabolism and Digestive Diseases and the National Heart and Lung Institutes of Health, Public Health Service, U.S. Department of Health, Education and Welfare.

LIST 3: FRUIT EXCHANGES

One exchange of fruit contains 10 grams of carbohydrate and 40 calories.

This list shows the kinds and amounts of **fruits** to use for one fruit exchange.

Apple	1 small	**Mango**	½ small
Apple Juice	⅓ cup	**Melon**	
Applesauce (unsweetened)	½ cup	**Cantaloupe**	¼ small
Apricots, fresh	2 medium	**Honeydew**	⅛ medium
Apricots, dried	4 halves	**Watermelon**	1 cup
Banana	½ small	**Nectarine**	1 small
Berries		**Orange**	1 small
Blackberries	½ cup	**Orange Juice**	½ cup
Blueberries	½ cup	**Papaya**	¾ cup
Raspberries	½ cup	**Peach**	1 medium
Strawberries	¾ cup	**Pear**	1 small
Cherries	10 large	**Persimmon, native**	1 medium
Cider	⅓ cup	**Pineapple**	½ cup
Dates	2	**Pineapple Juice**	⅓ cup
Figs, fresh	1	**Plums**	2 medium
Figs, dried	1	**Prunes**	2 medium
Grapefruit	½	**Prune Juice**	¼ cup
Grapefruit Juice	½ cup	**Raisins**	2 tablespoons
Grapes	12	**Tangerine**	1 medium
Grape Juice	¼ cup		

Cranberries may be used as desired if no sugar is added.

LIST 4: BREAD EXCHANGES (includes **bread, cereal** and **starchy vegetables**)

One exchange of bread contains 15 grams of carbohydrate, 2 grams of protein and 70 calories.

This list shows the kinds and amounts of **breads, cereals, starchy vegetables** and prepared foods to use for one bread exchange. Those which appear in **bold type** are **low-fat.**

Food	Amount
Bread	
White (including French and Italian)	1 slice
Whole wheat	1 slice
Rye or pumpernickel	1 slice
Raisin	1 slice
Bagel, small	½
English muffin, small	½
Plain roll, bread	1
Frankfurter roll	½
Hamburger bun	½
Dried bread crumbs	3 Tbs.
Tortilla, 6″	1
Cereal	
Bran flakes	½ cup
Other ready-to-eat unsweetened cereal	¾ cup
Puffed cereal (unfrosted)	1 cup
Cereal (cooked)	½ cup
Grits (cooked)	½ cup
Rice or barley (cooked)	½ cup
Pasta (cooked), spaghetti, noodles, macaroni	½ cup
Popcorn (popped, no fat added, large kernel)	3 cups
Cornmeal (dry)	2 Tbs.
Flour	2½ Tbs.
Wheat germ	¼ cup
Crackers	
Arrowroot	3
Graham, 2½″ sq.	2
Matzoth, 4″ × 6″	½
Oyster	20
Pretzels, 3⅛″ long × ⅛″ dia.	25
Rye wafers, 2″ × 3½″	3
Saltines	6
Soda, 2½″ sq.	4

Food	Amount
Dried beans, peas and lentils	
Beans, peas, lentils (dried and cooked)	½ cup
Baked beans, no pork (canned)	¼ cup
Starchy vegetables	
Corn	⅓ cup
Corn on cob	1 small
Lima beans	½ cup
Parsnips	⅔ cup
Peas, green (canned or frozen)	½ cup
Potato, white	1 small
Potato (mashed)	½ cup
Pumpkin	¾ cup
Winter squash, acorn or butternut	½ cup
Yam or sweet potato	¼ cup
Prepared foods	
Biscuit 2″ dia. (omit 1 fat exchange)	1
Corn bread, 2″ × 2″ × 1″ (omit 1 fat exchange)	1
Corn muffin, 2″ dia. (omit 1 fat exchange)	1
Crackers, round butter type (omit 1 fat exchange)	5
Muffin, plain small (omit 1 fat exchange)	1
Potatoes, french fried, length 2″ to 3½″ (omit 1 fat exchange)	8
Potato or corn chips (omit 2 fat exchanges)	15
Pancake, 5″ × ½″ (omit 1 fat exchange)	1
Waffle, 5″ × ½″ (omit 1 fat exchange)	1

LIST 5: MEAT EXCHANGES—LEAN MEAT

One exchange of lean meat (1 oz.) contains 7 grams of protein, 3 grams of fat, and 55 calories. This List shows the kinds and amounts of **lean meat** and other protein-rich foods to use for one low-fat meat exchange. **Trim off all visible fat.**

Beef:	**baby beef (very lean), chipped beef, chuck, flank steak, tenderloin, plate ribs, plate skirt steak, round (bottom, top), all cuts rump, spare ribs, tripe**	1 oz.
Lamb:	**Leg, rib, sirloin, loin (roast and chops), shank, shoulder**	1 oz.
Pork:	**Leg (whole rump, center shank), ham, smoked (center slices)**	1 oz.
Veal:	**Leg, loin, rib, shank, shoulder, cutlets**	1 oz.
Poultry:	**Meat** without skin **of chicken, turkey, cornish hen, Guinea hen, pheasant**	1 oz.
Fish:	**Any fresh or frozen**	1 oz.
	Canned salmon, tuna, mackerel, crab and lobster	¼ cup
	Clams, oysters, scallops, shrimp	5 or 1 oz.
	Sardines, drained	3
Cheeses containing less than 5% butterfat		1 oz.
Cottage cheese, dry and 2% butterfat		¼ cup
Dried beans and peas (omit 1 bread exchange)		½ cup

LIST 5: MEAT EXCHANGES—MEDIUM-FAT MEAT

One exchange of medium-fat meat (1 oz.) contains 7 grams of protein, 5 grams of fat, and 75 calories. This list shows the kinds and amounts of medium-fat meat and other protein-rich foods to use for one medium-fat meat exchange. **Trim off all visible fat.**

Beef: Ground (15% fat), corned beef (canned), rib eye, round (ground commercial)	1 oz.
Pork: Loin (all cuts tenderloin), shoulder arm (picnic), shoulder blade, Boston butt, canadian bacon, boiled ham	1 oz.
Liver, heart, kidney and sweetbreads (these are high in cholesterol)	1 oz.
Cottage cheese, creamed	¼ cup
Cheese: Mozzarella, ricotta, farmer's cheese, neufchatel, parmesan	3 tbs.
Egg (high in cholesterol)	1
Peanut butter (omit 2 additional fat exchanges)	2 tbs.

LIST 5: MEAT EXCHANGES—HIGH-FAT MEAT

One exchange of high-fat meat (1 oz.) contains 7 grams of protein, 8 grams of fat, and 100 calories. This list shows the kinds and amounts of high-fat meat and other protein-rich foods to use for one high-fat meat exchange. **Trim off all visible fat.**

Beef:	Brisket, corned beef (Brisket), ground beef (more than 20% fat), hamburger (commercial), chuck (ground commercial), roasts (rib), steaks (club and rib)	1 oz.
Lamb:	Breast	1 oz.
Pork:	Spare ribs, loin (back ribs), pork (ground), country style ham, deviled ham	1 oz.
Veal:	Breast	1 oz.
Poultry:	Capon, duck (domestic), goose	1 oz.
Cheese:	Cheddar types	1 oz.
Cold cuts		4½″ × ⅛″ slice
Frankfurter		1 small

LIST 6: FAT EXCHANGES

One exchange of fat contains 5 grams of fat and 45 calories. This list shows the kinds and amounts of fat-containing foods to use for one fat exchange. To plan a diet low in saturated fat select only those exchanges which appear in **bold type.** They are **polyunsaturated.**

Margarine, soft, tub or stick*	1 teaspoon
Avocado (4″ in diameter)†	⅛
Oil, corn, cottonseed, safflower, soy, sunflower	1 teaspoon
Oil, olive†	1 teaspoon
Oil, peanut†	1 teaspoon
Olives†	5 small
Almonds†	10 whole
Pecans†	2 large whole
Peanuts†	
Spanish	20 whole
Virginia	10 whole
Walnuts	6 small
Nuts, other†	6 small
Margarine, regular stick	1 teaspoon
Butter	1 teaspoon
Bacon fat	1 teaspoon
Bacon, crisp	1 strip
Cream, light	2 tablespoons
Cream, sour	2 tablespoons
Cream, heavy	1 tablespoon
Cream cheese	1 tablespoon
French dressing‡	1 tablespoon
Italian dressing‡	1 tablespoon
Lard	1 teaspoon
Mayonnaise‡	1 teaspoon
Salad dressing, mayonnaise type‡	2 teaspoons
Salt pork	¾ inch cube

*Made with corn, cottonseed, safflower, soy or sunflower oil only.
†Fat content is primarily monounsaturated.
‡If made with corn, cottonseed, safflower, soy or sunflower oil can be used on fat-modified diet.

6-11 Food exchange lists for infants

List 1: Milk/formula exchange*

	Protein/g	CHO/g	Fat/g
Whole milk	8	12	10
Similac	3.6	17.0	8.8
Enfamil	3.6	16.8	8.8
SMA	3.6	17.3	8.6
Prosobee	6.0	16.3	8.4
isomil	4.8	16.3	8.6
2% milk	8	12	5†
Advance	6.7	14.9	4.8†

List 2: Bread exchanges for diabetic infants‡

Dry baby rice cereal	5 tablespoons
Baby oatmeal cereal	5 tablespoons
High-protein cereal	9 tablespoons
"Strained" jar = 4.75 oz (135 g)	
Strained baby rice cereal with mixed fruit (also count 1 fruit exchange)	1 jar
Baby oatmeal cereal with applesauce and banana	1 jar
High-protein cereal with applesauce and banana	1 jar
Creamed corn	1 jar
Mixed vegetables	1 jar
Sweet potatoes	1 jar
"Junior" jar = 7.75 oz (220 g)	
Junior rice with mixed fruit	1 jar
Oatmeal with applesauce and banana	1 jar
Creamed corn	1 jar
Teething biscuits, arrowroot cookies, animal cookies, and pretzels	3

List 3: Fruit exchanges for diabetic infants§

Baby apple juice	¾ can (3 oz)
Mixed fruit juice	½ can (2 oz)
Prune-orange juice	⅓ can (1½ oz)
"Baby" can = 4.2 oz	
Strained applesauce	½ jar
Bananas	⅓ jar
Peaches	⅓ jar
Plums	¼ jar
Prunes	⅓ jar
Cherry vanilla pudding	½ jar
Chocolate custard	⅓ jar
Dutch apple dessert	⅓ jar
"Strained" jar = 4.75 oz (135 g)	
Junior applesauce	⅓ jar
Bananas	¼ jar
Peaches	⅕ jar (5 tbsp)
Pears	⅓ jar (5 tbsp)
Plums	⅕ jar (5 tbsp)
Prunes	⅕ jar (5 tbsp)
"Junior" jar = 7.75 oz (220 g)	

List 4: Meat exchanges for diabetic infants‖

Strained egg yolk	1 jar
Strained chicken	½ jar
Ham	½ jar
Lamb	½ jar
Beef	½ jar
Pork	½ jar
(Above also must count 1 fat)	
1 jar = 3.33 oz (94 g)	½ jar
Junior chicken	
Ham	½ jar
Lamb	½ jar
Beef	½ jar
Pork	½ jar
Meat sticks	½ jar
1 jar = 3.5 oz (99 g)	

List 5: Vegetable exchanges for diabetic infants¶

Strained carrots	1 jar
Beets	½ jar
Creamed spinach	1 jar
Green beans	1 jar
Squash	1 jar
Peas	1 jar
"Strained" jar = 4.5 oz (128 g)	
Junior carrots	½ jar
Creamed spinach	½ jar
Green beans	½ jar
Squash	½ jar
"Junior" jar = 7.5 oz (213 g)	

List 6: Multiple exchanges for diabetic infants

Strained beef with egg noodles and vegetables	1 jar = ½ bread ½ meat
Cereal and egg yolk	1 jar = ½ bread ½ meat
Chicken and noodles	1 jar = ½ bread ½ meat
Vegetables and chicken	1 jar = ½ bread ½ meat
Macaroni and cheese	1 jar = 1 fruit ½ meat
High meat dinners	1 jar = 1 meat ½ bread
"Strained" jar = 4.5 oz (128 g)	
Junior beef with egg noodles	1 jar = 1 bread ½ meat
Cereal and egg yolk	1 jar = 1 bread 1 fat
Chicken and noodles	1 jar = 1 bread ½ meat
Vegetables and chicken	1 jar = 1 bread ½ meat
Macaroni and cheese	1 jar = 1 bread ½ meat
"Junior" jar = 7.5 oz (213 g)	

From Kohler, E.: Baby food exchanges and feeding the diabetic infant. Diabetes Care 3:553-556, 1980. Reproduced with permission from The American Diabetes Association, Inc.

*One 8-oz cup = 160 cal.

†Add 1 fat exchange.

‡Each item is 1 bread exchange (68 cal).

§Each item is 1 fruit exchange (40 cal).

‖Each item is 1 meat exchange (73 cal).

¶Each item is 1 vegetable B exchange (36 cal).

APPENDIX 7 HEALTH HISTORY: A SUBJECTIVE DATA BASE

Include laboratory data (complete blood count, electrolytes, urinalysis, other relevant values) under appropriate system.

I. Chief complaint of client
   A. Location
   B. Character
   C. Chronology
   D. Circumstances of occurrence
   E. Aggravating or alleviating factors
   F. Associated complaints
   G. Previous attempts at therapy and their effectiveness
   H. Disability resulting from this complaint
II. Social systems
   A. Social development
      1. Age
      2. Sex
      3. Developmental tasks
      4. Psychosocial personality development (Erickson's eight stages of man)
      5. Diversional, recreational interests (what to do to pass time while ill)
      6. Roles in family, community, work, and perceived performance of them
      7. Child's favorite play activity
      8. Socially oriented habits (include alcohol, drugs), frequency of use, and response to use
   B. Family or significant others
      1. Others in living group
      2. Significant others outside living group
      3. Visiting preferences and who is able to visit
      4. Marital status
      5. Alterations in family's life-style because of ill member
      6. Interaction patterns (observe this also)
      7. History of disease in other family members, especially those diseases with a familial tendency
   C. Work
      1. Occupation
      2. Source of income
      3. Insurance (hospitalization)
      4. Changes in work pattern because of illness
      5. Feelings about work and being away from productivity and routine
   D. Religion
      1. Religious affiliation
      2. Desire for chaplain visit
      3. Practices or beliefs that might affect reaction to health care (proscriptions against immunization or blood transfusion, dietary laws, beliefs about disease causation, death)
   E. Education
      1. Formal education
      2. Satisfaction and progress with school
   F. Community
      1. Type of housing
      2. Contacts or previous referrals to social agencies
      3. Availability and pattern of utilization of health care facilities (physician, dentist); frequency and reason for visits
      4. Immunizations (type, date)
   G. Ethnic-cultural system
      1. Factors that may influence reaction to hospitalization, therapy, illness
      2. Food preferences
      3. Response to stress (e.g., pain)
   H. Environment
      1. Effect of present environment on health status and developmental level (e.g., lighting, noise, activity—variation, consistency, excessive, or absent)
      2. Arrangement of environment in relation to functional abilities or disabilities
      3. Safety factors
         a. Mobility (arrangement of objects in physical environment)
         b. Use of prosthetic or supportive devices (e.g., crutches, wheelchair)
      4. Infection control
         a. Ready sources of infection
         b. Barriers to infection (isolation technique, hand-washing facility)
III. Psychologic systems
   A. Cognition
      1. Level of consciousness (response to sensory stimuli)
      2. Orientation to time, place, person
      3. Mental skills
         a. Ability to read and write
         b. Vocabulary
         c. Ability to comprehend and follow directions
         d. Attention and memory span
      4. Intellectual development relative to chronologic age (e.g., Piaget's formulation)
      5. Understanding of and reaction to health concerns and goals of medical-nursing therapy
      6. Desired information about present tests and treatment
      7. Previous experiences with and reactions to past illnesses and hospitalizations
      8. Name child or adolescent prefers
   B. Emotion
      1. Quality of mood, expression, intensity of reaction
      2. Activity level (active, sluggish, hyperactive)
      3. Effect of illness on life-style and expectation of future effects
      4. Feelings about hospitalization
      5. Coping patterns in stressful situations (describe stressful situations); availability, need for, and effectiveness of internal-external support systems
      6. Special concerns or fears
      7. Patterns of relating to others (e.g., verbal, congenial)
      8. Self-concept (body image before and in relation to current health problem)
      9. Any nervous breakdown
      10. Comfort, rest and sleep patterns (hours, time, nap periods, feeling of being rested) before and since illness
      11. Aids used to sleep
      12. Presence of pain or discomfort (location, duration, degree, character, precipitating factors, change in pattern)
      13. Use of aids to relieve pain

IV. Biologic systems
  A. General
    1. Fatigue
    2. Fever
    3. Weakness
    4. Activity tolerance
    5. Usual weight, recent weight change
  B. Gas transport and exchange
    1. Cardiovascular
      a. Past or present disease of cardiovascular system
      b. Syncope
      c. Dizziness
      d. Chest pain
        (1) Type
        (2) Pattern
        (3) Precipitating factors
        (4) Relief measures
      e. Edematous body parts
      f. Palpitations
      g. Orthopnea
      h. Medications taken to affect cardiovascular system
    2. Respiratory
      a. Past or present diseases of respiratory system
      b. Cough
        (1) Frequency
        (2) Duration
      c. Sputum
        (1) Color
        (2) Odor
        (3) Amount
      d. Shortness of breath
        (1) Precipitating factors
        (2) Frequency
        (3) Effect on activity
      e. Smoking
        (1) Pack/year history
        (2) Attempts and success at stopping
      f. Hemoptysis
      g. Frequency of colds and sore throats
      h. Medications taken to affect respiratory system
  C. Nutrition and elimination
    1. Gastrointestinal
      a. Past or present disease of gastrointestinal system
      b. Dietary habits
        (1) Amount of basic four food groups
        (2) Likes
        (3) Dislikes
        (4) Number of meals and snacks
        (5) Time of meals
        (6) Assistance needed with eating
      c. Appetite, thirst
      d. Factors related to ingestion
        (1) Nonoral intake
        (2) Chewing
        (3) Swallowing
        (4) Oral hygiene habits
      e. Factors related to digestion
        (1) Ease
        (2) Nausea
        (3) Vomiting
        (4) Belching
        (5) Pain in abdomen
      f. Bowel elimination pattern
        (1) Time and frequency of bowel movements
        (2) Degree of child's independence in toileting
        (3) Words used by child regarding elimination
        (4) Character of stools
        (5) Ease (constipation, diarrhea)
        (6) Hemorrhoids
        (7) Passage of flatus, blood
      g. Medicines taken to alter digestion and metabolism of foods
    2. Urinary
      a. Past or present diseases of urinary system
      b. Fluid intake
      c. Urination pattern
        (1) Amount
        (2) Color
        (3) Odor
        (4) Frequency, night or day urgency
        (5) Dysuria, hematuria
      d. Vaginal or urethral discharge
      e. Degree of independence in toileting
      f. Medications taken to alter urinary system
  C. Sensorimotor
    1. Musculoskeletal
      a. Past or present disease of musculoskeletal system
      b. Abnormal innervation to muscles (paralysis, weakness, spasticity)
      c. Method of ambulation
        (1) Assistance needed with dressing, hygiene
        (2) Safety measures needed
      d. Range of motion limitations
      e. Medicines taken to affect musculoskeletal subsystem
    2. Nervous
      a. Past or present diseases of nervous system
      b. Visual status
        (1) Acuity
        (2) Deficits and corrective devices
      c. Auditory status
        (1) Deficits and corrective devices
        (2) Unusual sensations (ringing, buzzing, vertigo, pain)
      d. Olfactory status
      e. Gustatory status
      f. Tactile status (ability to discriminate sharp-dull, light-firm, hot-cold sensations)
      g. Paresthesias
      h. Mobility (coordination, balance)
      i. Medicines taken to affect nervous system
  E. Protective mechanisms
    1. Integument
      a. Past or present diseases of integumentary system
      b. Factors predisposing to skin breakdown
      c. Personal hygiene
        (1) Bathing (kind, type, frequency)
        (2) Frequency, time of shaving
        (3) After bath skin care
      d. Medicines taken to affect integumentary system
    2. Immune mechanism
      a. Past or present allergy
      b. Past or present sensitivities to drugs or other agents (pollens, insect bites)
      c. Past or present high susceptibility to infection
    3. Hematologic
      a. Easy bruising
      b. Swelling in neck or groin
      c. Past transfusions
  F. Endocrine mechanisms
    1. Abnormal function of endocrine gland or glands and effects; past or present diseases
    2. Growth patterns
    3. Heat or cold intolerance

4. Excessive thirst, hunger, or urination
5. Medications taken to affect endocrine system

G. Sexuality and reproduction
1. Past or present alterations of reproduction system
2. Reproductive data
    a. Number of pregnancies
    b. Live births
    c. Living children
    d. Family planning (methods used)
    e. Menstrual pattern
    f. Menopause (age of onset and associated factors)
3. Breast self-examination routine
4. Frequency of Pap smears
5. Sexual desire and function
6. Level of sexual development
7. Attitudes toward own sexuality
8. Medicine taken to affect reproductive system

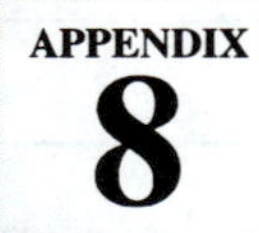

APPENDIX 8

MATERNITY AND OBSTETRICS

8-1 Relationship of drugs to breast milk and effect on infant

Drug	*Excreted in milk*	*Amount in milk after therapeutic dose*	*Effect on infant*
Analgesics and anti-inflammatory drugs (nonnarcotic)			
Acetaminopen (Datril, Tylenol)	Yes		Detoxified in liver. Avoid in immediate postdelivery period, otherwise no problems with therapeutic dose
Aspirin	Yes	1-3 mg/dl	Long history of experience shows complications rare. Can cause interference with platelet aggregation and diminished factor XII (Hageman factor) at birth. When mother requires high, continuing level of medication for arthritis, aspirin is drug of choice. Observe infant for bruisability. Platelet aggregation can be evaluated. Salicylism only seen in maternal overdosing. Mother should increase vitamin C and vitamin K intake.
Donnatal (phenobarbital, hyoscyamine sulfate, atropine sulfate, hyoscine hydrobromide)	Yes		Consider for its component parts. Can be given to children but can accumulate in neonate.
Flufenamic acid (Arlef)	Yes	0.50 μg/ml (mean)	No apparent effect on infant when maternal dosage was 200 mg, three times a day. Infant able to excrete via urine.
Indomethacin (Indocin)	Yes		Convulsions in breast-fed neonate (case report). Used to close patent ductus arteriosus. Insufficient data as to effect on other vessels. May be nephrotoxic.
Mefenamic acid (Ponstel)	Yes	Trace amounts	No apparent effect on infant at therapeutic doses; infant able to excrete via urine.
Naproxen (Naprosyn)	Yes	1% of maternal plasma; binds to plasma protein	Less toxic in adults than some other organic derivatives.
Oxyphenbutazone (Tandearil)	Yes	In milk of 2 of 55 mothers, 10% to 80% of maternal plasma level	No known effect.
Pentazocine (Talwin)	No		Withdrawal in neonatal period from ingestion during pregnancy.
Percodan (oxycodone [derived from opiate thebaine] aspirin, phenacetin, caffeine)	Yes		Consider for its component parts. In neonatal period sleepiness and failure to feed, which increase maternal engorgement and neonatal weight loss, have been observed, probably caused by oxycodone.
Phenylbutazone (Butazolidin)	Yes	0.63 mg ml 90 min after 750 mg given IM	Very potent drug; risk to infant not well defined but considerable. Not given directly to children; may accumulate in infant.
Propoxyphene (Darvon)	Yes	0.4% of maternal* dose	Only symptoms detectable would be failure to feed and drowsiness. On daily, around-the-clock dosage infant could consume 1 mg/day.

*Shown by animal experiments. Milk plasma ratio (M/P) = ½.

Continued.

Relationship of drugs to breast milk and effect on infant—cont'd

Drug	*Excreted in milk*	*Amount in milk after therapeutic dose*	*Effect on infant*
Antibiotics			
Amantadine (Symmetrel)	Yes	Not defined	Vomiting, urinary retention, rash. Contraindicated.
Ampicillin (Polycillin, Amcill, Omnipen, Penbritin)	Yes	0.07 μg/ml	Sensitivity due to repeated exposure; diarrhea or secondary candidiasis.
Carbenicillin (Pyopen, Geopen)	Yes	0.265 μg/ml 1 hr after 1 g given	Levels not significant. Drug is given to neonate.
Cefazolin (Ancef, Kefzol)	Yes	1.5 μg/ml (0.075% of dose)	Probably not significant
Cephalexin (Keflex)	No		
Cephalothin (Keflin)	No		
Chloramphenicol (Chloromycetin)	Yes	Half blood level; 2.5 mg/dl	Gray syndrome. Infant does not excrete drug well, and small amounts may accumulate. Contraindicated. May be tolerated in older infant with mature glycuronide system.
Chloroquine (Aralen)	Yes	2.7 mg in 2 days*	Can be used to treat child under 6 mo of age who is wholly breast-fed.
Colistin (Colymycin)	Yes	0.05-0.09 mg/dl	Not absorbed orally.
Demeclocycline (Declomycin)	Yes	0.2-0.3 mg/dl	Not significant in therapeutic doses. Can be given to infants.
Erythromycin (Ilosone, E-Mycin, Erythrocin)	Yes	0.05-0.1 mg/dl; 3.6-6.2 μg/ml	Higher concentrations have been reported in milk than in plasma. Should not be given under 1 mo of age because of risk of jaundice. Dose in milk higher when given IV to mother.
Gentamicin	Unknown		Not absorbed from gastrointestinal tract, may change gut flora. Drug is given to newborns directly.
Isoniazid (Nydrazid)	Yes	0.6-1.2 mg/dl†	Infant at risk for toxicity, but need for breast milk may outweigh risk.
Kanamycin (Kantrex)	Yes	18.4 μg/ml after 1 gm given IM	Infant absorbs little from gastrointestinal tract. Infants can be given drug.
Lincomycin (Lincocin)	Yes	0.5-2.4 mg/dl	Not significant in therapeutic doses to affect child.
Mandelic acid	Yes	0.3 gm/24 hr after dose of 12 gm/day	Not significant in therapeutic doses to affect child.
Methacycline (Rondomycin)	Yes	½ plasma level; 50-260 μg/dl	Same precautions as with tetracycline.
Methenamine (Hexamine)	Yes		Not significant in therapeutic doses to affect child.
Metronidazole (Flagyl)	Yes	Level comparable to serum‡	Caution should be exercised because of its high milk concentrations. Contraindicated when infant under 6 mo, may cause neurologic disorders and blood dyscrasia.
Nalidixic acid (Neggram)	Yes	0.4 mg/dl	Not significant in therapeutic doses beyond neonatal period. Hemolytic anemia in an infant attributed to nalidixic acid in G6PD deficiency or when mother has renal failure.
Nitrofurantoin (Furadantin)	Yes	Trace to 0.5 μg/ml	Not significant in therapeutic doses to affect child except in G6PD deficiency.
Novobiocin (Albamycin, cathomycin)	Yes	0.36-0.54 mg/dl	Infant can be given drug directly.
Nystatin (Mycostatin)	No	Not absorbed orally	Can be given to infant directly.
Oxacillin (Prostaphlin)	No		
Para-aminosalicylic acid	No		
Penethamate (Leocillin)	No	24-74 μg/dl	Animal study suggests it be avoided.
Penicillin G, benzathine (Bicillin)	Yes	10-12 units/dl	Clinical need should supersede possible allergic responses.

*Peaks in 6 hr.
†Same concentration in milk as in maternal serum.
‡Gives serum levels in infants of 0.05 to 0.4 μg/ml.

Drug	Excreted in milk	Amount in milk after therapeutic dose	Effect on infant
Penicillin G, potassium	Yes	Up to 6 units/dl; 1.2-3.6 μg/dl	Infant can be given penicillin directly. Parents should be told to inform physician that infant has been exposed to penicillin because of potential sensitivity.
Pyrimethamine (Daraprim)	Yes	0.3 mg/dl (3% of dose)	Significant in therapeutic doses when infant is under 6 mo and entirely breast-fed.
Quinine sulfate	Yes	0-0.1 mg/dl after maternal dose of 300-600 mg	In therapeutic doses, no effect on child except rare thrombocytopenia.
Sodium fusidate	Yes	0.02 μg/ml	Not significant in therapeutic doses to affect child.
Streptomycin	Yes	Present for long periods in slight amounts when given as dihydrostreptomycin	Not to be given more than 2 wk. Ototoxic and nephrotoxic with long use. Is given to infants directly.
Sulfanilamide	Yes	9 mg/dl after dose of 2-4 gm/24 hr	Not significant in therapeutic doses; may cause a rash or hemolytic anemia. Should be avoided for first month after delivery.
Sulfapyridine	Yes	3-13 mg/dl after dose of 3 gm/24 hr	To be avoided; has caused skin rash.
Sulfathiazole	Yes	0.5 mg/dl after dose of 3 gm/24 hr	Not significant in therapeutic doses to affect child after 1 mo of age.
Sulfisoxazole (Gantrisin)	Yes	Concentration similar to plasma level.	To be avoided during first month after delivery; may cause kernicterus.
Tetracycline HC1 (Achromycin, Panmycin, Sumycin)	Yes	0.5-2.6 μg/ml after dose of 500 mg four times a day	Not enough to treat an infection in an infant. May cause discoloration of the teeth in the infant; the antibiotic, however, may be largely bound to the milk calcium. Do not give over 10 days or repeatedly.
Anticoagulants			
Coumarin derivatives Dicumarol (bishydroxycoumarin) Warfarin (Panwarfin)	Yes	Probably little but may be cumulative*	Monitor prothrombin time. Give vitamin K to infant. Discontinue if surgery or trauma occurs. Drug of choice if mother to continue nursing.
Ethyl biscoumacetate (Tromexan)	Yes	0-0.17 mg/dl†	Hemorrhage around umbilical stump and cephalhematoma reported. Prothrombin normal in infants with hemorrhage. Vitamin K has no effect. Contraindicated while nursing.
Heparin	No		Heparin ineffective orally.
Phenindione (Hedulin) (Dindevan)	Yes		Breast milk a major route of excretion. Reports of serious hemorrhage in infant. Prothrombin times prolonged in infant. Contraindicated while nursing.
Anticonvulsants and sedatives‡			
Barbital (Veronal)	Yes	8-10 mg/L after 500 mg dose	May produce sedation in infant. In general, barbiturates pass into milk but do not sedate infant. Watch for symptoms.
Carbamazepine (Tegretol)	Yes	60% of plasma levels§	Animal studies show lack of weight gain, unkempt appearance.
Chloral hydrate (Noctec, Somnos)	Yes	Up to 1.5 mg/dl	No significant symptoms, can be given to infants directly.
Phenytoin (Dilantin)	Yes	1.5 to 2.6 μg/ml after .300 mg/24 hr dose	Once case of hemolytic reaction reported. Other infants appear to tolerate the small doses. Therapeutic plasma level 10-20 μg/ml.
Mephenytoin (Mesantoin) (hydantoin homologue of mephobarbital)	Unknown		Detoxified in liver. No information.

*Reports conflict.
†No correlation with dosage, continues in milk after plasma clear.
‡All barbitals appear in breast milk.
§When plasma 13.0 μmoles/L, 7.5 μmoles/L in milk.

Continued.

Relationship of drugs to breast milk and effect on infant—cont'd

Drug	Excreted in milk	Amount in milk after therapeutic dose	Effect on infant
Pentobarbital (Nembutal)	Yes		Depends on liver for detoxification so may accumulate in first week of life until infant able to detoxify. No problem for older infant in usual doses.
Phenobarbital (Luminal)	Yes	0.1-0.5 mg when plasma level 0.6-1.8 mg	Sleepiness and decreased sucking possible. On usual analeptic doses infant is alert and feeds well. On hypnotic doses infant is depressed and difficult to rouse.
Phensuximide (Milontin)			No specific data.
Primidone (Mysoline)	Yes		Causes drowsiness and decreased feeds. May cause bleeding due to hypoprothrombinemia. Infant needs vitamin K. Avoid drug during lactation.
Sodium bromide (Bromo-Seltzer and over-the-counter sleeping aids)	Yes	Up to 6.6 mg/dl	Drowsy, decreased crying, rash, decreased feeding.
Trimethadione (Tridione)			No specific data.
Antihistaminics			
Brompheniramine (Dimetane) Diphenhydramine (Benadryl) Methdilazine (Tacaryl) Tripelennamine (Pyribenzamine)	Yes	No specific data available. All pass into milk.	Drug is used in neonates. May cause sedation, decreased feeding, or may produce stimulation and tachycardia. Should avoid long-acting preparations, which may accumulate in infant. When combined with decongestants, may cause decrease in milk.
Autonomic drugs			
Atropine sulfate*	Yes	0.1 mg/dl	Hyperthermia, atropine toxicity, infants especially sensitive; also inhibits lactation. Infant dose 0.01 mg/kg.
Carisoprodol (Soma, Rela)	Yes	Two to four times maternal plasma	Blocks interneuronal activity in descending reticular formation and spinal cord; drowsiness, hypotonia, poor feed.
Ergot (Cafergot)	Yes	Unknown	90% of infants had symptoms of ergotism: vomiting and diarrhea to weak pulse and unstable blood pressure. Short-term therapy for migraine should not exceed 6 mg. Cafergot also contains 100 mg caffeine.
Mepenzolate bromide (Cantil)	No		Postganglionic parasympathetic inhibitor used to diminish gastric acidity and decrease spasm of colon. Oral absorption low.
Methocarbamol (Robaxin)	Yes	Minimum	Too little in milk to produce effect.
Neostigmine	No		No known harm to infant.
Propantheline bromide (Pro-Banthine)	No	Uncontrolled data indicate no measurable levels	Drug rapidly metabolized in maternal system to inactive metabolite. Moher should avoid long-acting preparations, however.
Scopolamine (hyoscine)	Yes		Usually given as single dose and of no problem to neonate. No data on repeated doses.
Cardiovascular drugs			
Diazoxide (Hyperstat)			Arteriolar dilators and antihypertensive, only given IV, not active orally.
Dibenzyline†			No data available.
Digoxin	Yes	0.96-0.61 ng/ml‡	Digoxin 20% bound to protein; infant receives <1/100 of dose. If mother at toxic level of 5 ng/ml, milk would have 4.4 ng/ml and infant would receive only 1/20 daily dose.

*Ingredients in many prescription and nonprescription drugs.

†α blocking agent.

‡Peak level occurs 4-6 hr after dose given. Maternal plasma level was higher, M/P = 0.9 and 0.8; infant's plasma level was 0.

Drug	Excreted in milk	Amount in milk after therapeutic dose	Effect on infant
Guanethidine (Ismelin)*	Yes		Not significant in therapeutic doses to affect child.
Hydralazine (Apresoline)	Yes		Jaundice, thrombocytopenia, electrolyte disturbances possible.
Methyldopa (Aldomet)*	Yes		Galactorrhea. No specific data except as affects mother's milk production.
Propranolol (Inderal)†	Yes	40 ng/ml of maternal plasma‡	Insignificant amount. Infants reported had no symptoms noted. Should watch for hypoglycemia and/or "β blocking" effects.
Quinidine	Yes		Arrhythmia may occur.
Reserpine (Serpasil)§	Yes		May produce galactorrhea, lethargy, diarrhea, or nasal stuffiness.
Cathartics			
Aloin	Yes	Low	Occasionally gave symptoms, caused colic and diarrhea in infant.
Anthraquinone laxatives such as dihydroxyanthraquinone (Dorbane and Dorbantyl)	Yes	High	Caused colic and diarrhea in infant.
Calomel	No	None	None.
Cascara	Yes	Low	Caused colic and diarrhea in infant.
Milk of magnesia	No	None	No effect.
Mineral oil	No	None	No effect.
Phenolphthalein	Unknown	Unknown‖	Reported to cause symptoms in some.
Rhubarb	Unknown	None	None in syrup form. Fresh rhubarb may give symptoms of colic and diarrhea.
Saline cathartics	No	None	No effect.
Senna	No	None	None.
Stool softeners and bulk-forming laxatives	No	None	No effect.
Suppositories (for constipation)	No	None	Not absorbed.
Diagnostic materials and proceures			
Barium	No		Not absorbed.
Iopanoic acid (Telepaque)	Yes		Not sufficient to produce problem in infant on single dose. Does contain iodine radical.
Radioactive compounds			
Radioactive sodium	Yes	0.5% to 1.3% of dose/L¶	Diminished after 24 hr; discontinue nursing 24 hr.
[^{67}Ga] citrate	Yes		Discontinue nursing until ^{67}Ga has cleared, usually 24 hr.
^{125}I, ^{131}I	Yes	M/P = 0.13 μCi/0.002 μCi#	^{131}I content in milk proportional to amount of milk. Most excreted in 24 hr. Discontinue nursing for 48 hr. or check milk before resuming feeding if under 48 hr.
^{90}Sr	Yes	M/P = 1/10	Less than in cow's milk. Bottle infant doubles stores in 1 mo.
^{99m}Tc	Yes		Reported to clear in 6-22 hr. Discontinue breast feeding 24 hr. ^{99m}Tc preferentially picked up by breast tissue.
Tuberculin test	No		Tuberculin-sensitive mothers can adoptively immunize their infants through breast milk, and that immunity may last several years.
X-ray films	No		No effect.

*Adrenergic blocking agent.
†β blocking agent.
‡Total daily dose to infant via milk is 15-20 μg.
§Adrenergic blocking agent.
‖Reports differ.
¶Peak in 2 hr; detectable for 96 hr.
#27% of dose in 48 hr.

Continued.

Relationship of drugs to breast milk and effect on infant—cont'd

Drug	*Excreted in milk*	*Amount in milk after therapeutic dose*	*Effect on infant*
Diuretics			
Acetazolamide (Diamox)	Probable	No specific data available but probably similar to sulfonamide	Acts as enzyme inhibitor on carbonic anhydrase non-bacteriostatic sulfonamide. Observe only for dehydration and electrolyte loss by monitoring urine and turgor.
Furosemide (sulfamoylanthranilic acid) (Lasix)	No		Drug is given to children under medical management.
Mercurial diuretics (Dicurin, Thiomerin)	Yes		In addition to diuretic effect, there is risk of mercury deposition. However, drug not absorbed orally.
Spironolactone (Aldactone)	Yes	Canrenone, a metabolite, appears	Acts as antagonist of aldosterone; causes sodium excretion and potassium retention. The metabolite apparently has some activity
Thiazides (Diuril, Enduron, Esidrix, Hydrodiuril, Oretic, Thiuretic tablets)	Yes	>0.1 mg/dl*	Risk of dehydration and electrolyte imbalance, especially sodium loss, which would require monitoring. Watching weight and wet diapers and taking an occasional specific gravity reading of the urine and serum sodium would indicate status of infant. Risk, however, is extremely low. May suppress lactation due to dehydration in mother.
Environmental agents			
Aldrin	Yes	Varies by location	Not a reason to wean from breast. No need to test milk unless inordinate exposure.
Benzene hexachloride (BHC)	Yes	Varies by location	Not a reason to wean from breast. No need to test milk unless inordinate exposure.
Dichlorodiphenyltrichloroethane (DDT or DDE)	Yes	Varies by location	Not a reason to wean from breast. No need to test milk unless inordinate exposure.
Dieldrin	Yes	Varies by location	Also found in permanently mothproofed garments. Avoid these. Not a reason to wean.
Hexachlorobenzene (HCB)	Yes	Varies by location	Not a reason to wean from breast. No need to test milk unless inordinate exposure.
Heptachlorepoxide	Yes	Varies by location	Not a reason to wean from breast. No need to test milk unless inordinate exposure.
Methyl mercury	Yes	500-1000 ng/ml†	Infant blood level 600 ng/ml in heavy exposure. Only in excessive exposure is testing and/or weaning necessary.
Polybrominated biphenyl (PBB)	Yes	Varies by location	If mother at high risk from the environment or the diet, milk sample should be measured. If level in milk is high, then breast feeding should be discontinued. Those at risk are (1) workers who handle PBB/PCB and (2) individuals who eat game fish from contaminated waters. Crash diets mobilize fats and should be avoided especially if PBB or PCB present.
Polychlorinated biphenyl (PCB)	Yes	Varies by location	
^{90}Sr, ^{89}Sr (strontium)	Yes	1/10 of that in maternal diet	Cow's milk has six times as much as human milk. Cow's milk-fed infant doubles amount in body in 1 mo.
Heavy metals			
Arsenic	Yes	Can be measured for given woman	Can accumulate. Check infant's blood level if there is reason to suspect exposure.
Copper	Yes		
Fluorine	Yes		Monitor for excessive dose.
Gold thiomalate (Myocrisin)	Yes	0.022 μg/ml when mother given 50 mg/wk	No proteinuria or aminoaciduria observed.
Halothane	Yes	2 ppm	Nursing mothers who work in environment with halothane should be checked.

*Linear relationship between plasma and milk. In 1 L of milk at 0.1 mg/dl there would be 1 mg/24 hr. Infant dose is 20 mg/kg/24 hr.
†M/P = 8.6% in heavy exposure.

Drug	Excreted in milk	Amount in milk after therapeutic dose	Effect on infant
Iron	Yes		
Lead	Unknown		Nursing contraindicated if maternal serum 40 μg; conflicting reports, breast milk not always cause of lead poisoning in breast-fed infant.
Magnesium	Yes		Not sufficient to be toxic.
Mercury	Yes		Hazardous to infant.
Hormones and contraceptives			
Carbimazole (neo-mercazole)	Yes		Antithyroid effect may cause goiter.
Chlorotrianisene (Tace)	Yes		Has estrogenic effect although does not change consistency of milk. May have feminizing effect on infant
Contraceptives (oral) Ethinyl estradiol Mestranol 19-Nortestosterone Norethindrone (Norlutin) Norethynodrel (Enovid)	Yes		May diminish milk supply. May decrease vitamins, protein, and fat in milk. One author showed no differences when mothers took norethindrone. Most significant concern is long-range impact of hormone on young infant, which is not certain. Reports of feminization of infant.
Corticotropin	Yes		Destroyed in gastrointestinal tract of infant. No effect.
Cortisone	Yes		Animal studies show 50% lower weight than controls and retarded sexual development and exophthalmos.
Dihydrotachysterol (Hytakerol)	Yes		May cause hypercalcemia; need monitoring of infant serum and urine calcium.
Epinephrine (adrenalin)	Yes		Destroyed in GI tract of infant.
Estrogen	Yes	0.17 μg/dl after 1 gm	Risks as with oral contraceptives.
Fluoxymesterone (Halotestin, OraTestryl, Ultandren)	Yes		Suppress lactation; masculinizing
Insulin	Unknown		Destroyed in gastrointestinal tract.
Liothyronine (Cytomel)	No		Synthetic form of natural thyroid.
Medroxyprogesterone acetate (Provera)	No		
Phenformin HCI	Yes	Minimum	Not sufficient to cause symptoms in infant. Does not cause hypoglycemia in normal infants. No case reports available.
Prednisone	Yes	0.07-0.23% dose/L after 5 mg dose*	Minimum amount not likely to cause effect on infants short course.
Pregnanediol	Yes		Unknown risk as with other female hormones over a long period of time.
Tolbutamide (Orinase)	Yes		Not recommended in the childbearing years.
Narcotics			
Codeine		0 to trace after 32 mg every 4 hr (6 doses)	No effect in therapeutic level and transient usage. Can accumulate. Individual variation. Watch for neonatal depression.
Heroin	Yes		13 of 22 infants had withdrawal. Historically breast feeding had been used to wean addict's infant. This is no longer recommended.
Marijuana *(Cannabis)*	Yes		Shown in laboratory animals to produce structural changes in nursling's brain cell; impairs DNA and RNA formation. Infant at risk of inhaling smoke during feeding or when held while smoking.
Meperidine (Dermerol)	Yes	>0.1 mg/dl†	Trace amounts may accumulate if drug taken around the clock when infant is neonate. Watch for drowsiness and poor feeding.

*0.16 μg/ml after 10 mg dose; 2.67 μg/ml after 2 hr.
†Plasma 0.07-0.1 mg/dl.

Continued.

Relationship of drugs to breast milk and effect on infant—cont'd

Drug	Excreted in milk	Amount in milk after therapeutic dose	Effect on infant
Methadone	Yes	0.03 μg/ml or 0.023-0.028 mg/24 hr*	When dosage not excessive, infant can be breast-fed and monitored for evidence of depression and failure to thrive.
Morphine	Yes	Trace amount	Single doses have minimum effect. Potential for accumulation. May be addicting to neonate. Breast feeding no longer considered appropriate means of weaning infant of an addict.
Psychotropic and mood-changing drugs			
Alcohol	Yes	Similar to plasma level	Ordinarily no problem and can be therapeutic in moderation. Infants are more susceptible to effects. Chronic drinking reported to cause obesity in one infant. Ethanol in doses of 1-2 gm/kg to mother causes depression of milk-ejection reflex (dose dependent). No acetaldehyde found in infants.
Amphetamine	Yes		Has caused stimulation in infants with jitteriness, irritability, sleeplessness. Long-acting preparations cumulative.
Benzodiazepines†			
Chlordiazepoxide HCl (Librium)	Yes		Not sufficient to affect infant first week when glucuronyl system needed for detoxification. May accumulate. Older infant, no apparent problem.
Diazepam (Valium)	Yes	90 μg/L‡	Detoxified in glucuronyl system. In first weeks of life may contribute to jaundice. Metabolite active. Effect on infant; hypoventilation, drowsiness, lethargy, and weight loss. Single doses over 10 mg contraindicated during nursing. Accumulation in infant possible.
Pineazepam	Yes	Metabolite, 5-11.2 ng/ml; pineazepam, >1.0 ng/ml§	No data, probably similar to diazepam.
Haloperidol (Haldol)	Yes	Unknown	A butyrophenone antidepressant; animal studies in nurslings show behavior abnormalities.
Lithium carbonate (Eskalith, Lithane, Lithonate)	Yes	⅓-½ maternal plasma level‖	Measurable lithium in infant's serum. Infant kidney can clear lithium; however, lithium inhibits adenosine 3′:5′-cyclic monophosphate, significant for brain growth. Also affects amine metabolism. Real effects not measurable immediately. Report on cyanosis and poor muscle tone and ECG changes in nursing infant.
Monoamine oxidase (MAO) inhibitors (Eutonyl, Nardil)			Inhibits lactation.
Meprobamate (Miltown, Equanil	Yes	2-4 times maternal plasma level	If therapy continued, infant should be followed closely.
Penfluridol¶	Yes	Unknown	Animal studies show learning abnormalities in sucklings. This is a potent long-acting oral neuroleptic drug.
Phenothiazines			
Chlorpromazine (Thorazine)	Yes	⅓ plasma level#	Can be safely nursed; minimum in milk. Increases maternal prolactin. No symptoms in infants reported; 5 yr follow-up showed infants normal.

*Mother received 50 mg/24 hr; M/P = 0.83. Peak level 4 hr after oral dose. Results obscured if addict also taking the herbal root golden seal.
†Alcohol enhances effect of this group.
‡10 mg or less yields 45 ng of diazepam/ml and 85 ng of metabolite/ml. P/M ratio is diazepam is 6.14; of metabolite is 3.64. Effect lasts about 4 days.
§Both drug and active metabolite appear for about 4 days after dose.
‖0.030 mmol/L in infant's serum, 0.56 mmole/L in infant's urine. Milk level was half of maternal serum level in one case report.
¶Neuroleptic drug.
#If dose <200 mg, milk contains bare trace. Dose of 1200 mg showed trace.

Drug	Excreted in milk	Amount in milk after therapeutic dose	Effect on infant
Mesoridazine (Serentil)	Yes	Minimum	
Piperacetazine (Quide)	Yes	Minimum	Probably no effect.
Thioridazine (Mellaril)	Yes	No information	Thioridazine is less potent in general than other phenothiazines. Probably quite safe.
Trifluoperazine (Stelazine)	Yes	Minimum	
Tricyclic antidepressants			Apparently no accumulation. No infants that have been observed showed symptoms. Watch for depression or failure to feed. Increases maternal prolactin secretion.
Amitriptyline HC1 (Elavil)	Yes	Minimum amounts	
Desipramine HC1 (Norpramin, Pertofrane)	Yes	Minimum amounts	
Imipramine HC1 (Tofranil)	Yes	0.1 mg/dl*	
Stimulants			
Caffeine	Yes	1% of dose	Accumulates when intake moderate and continual. Causes jitteriness, wakefulness, and irritability. Caffeine present in many hot and cold drinks. Consider if infant very wakeful.
Theobromine	Yes	3.7-8.2 mg/L after 240 mg dose†	No adverse symptoms observed in the infants. Chocolate most common cause of exposure.
Theophylline	Yes	10% of maternal dose‡	Irritability, fretfulness.
Thyroid and antithyroid medications			
Carbimazole (neo-mercazole)	Yes		May cause goiter.
Methimazole (Tapazole)	Yes	M/P > 1	Inhibits synthesis of thyroid hormone but does not inactivate existing thyroid. Can inhibit infant thyroid. ⅛ grain/day of thyroid can be given to infant simultaneously.
Potassium iodide	Yes	3 mg/dl§	May alter thyroid function of infant; may cause goiter in infant.
Propylthiouracil	Yes	M/P > 1;4.5-6% of dose	Risk of goiter and agranulocytosis. With present microtechniques for T_3, T_4, and TSH, close monitoring of infant is possible, as with methimazole.
Radioactive iodine ^{125}I, ^{131}I (as a treatment)	Yes	M/P > 1	*Treatment* doses are excreted via the breast for 1-3 wk. Milk can be checked by Geiger counter if there is a question. Breast feeding should be discontinued until milk is clear.
Thiouracil	Yes	9-12 mg/dl‖	Same as for propylthiouracil.
Thyroid and thyroxine	Yes		Does not produce adverse symptoms on long-range follow-up. Noted to improve milk supply of hypothyroid mothers. No contraindication.
Miscellaneous			
Cyclophosphamide	Yes	Present¶	Antineoplastic agent. Any amounts contraindicated
DPT	Yes	Minimum	Does not interfere with immunization schedule.
Methotrexate	Yes	Minor route of excretion: M/P = 0.08/1.0	Antimetabolite. Infant would receive 0.26 μg/dl. which researchers consider nontoxic for infant.
Nicotine	Yes	Mean 91 ppb (20-512 ppb)#	Decreases milk production. No apparent effect on infant—perhaps a tolerance is developed in utero. Smoking may interfere with let-down reflex if smoking started before onset of a feeding.

*Plasma level 0.2-1.3 mg/dl.
†113 gm chocolate bar.
‡M/P = 0.7
§Dose was 325-650 mg three times a day.
‖Maternal plasma level was 3.4 mg/dl after 1.0 g dose; M/P = 3.
¶Single 500 mg IV dose in milk at 1, 3, 5, and 6 hr after injection.
#At ½-1½ packs/day. Large variation from single donor.

Continued.

Relationship of drugs to breast milk and effect on infant—cont'd

Drug	*Excreted in milk*	*Amount in milk after therapeutic dose*	*Effect on infant*
Poliovirus vaccine	No		Live vaccine taken orally. Not necessary to withhold nursing 30 min before and after dose. Provide booster after infant no longer nursing.
Rb antibodies	Yes		Destroyed in gastrointestinal tract; not effective orally.
Rubella virus vaccine	Yes	Minimum	Will not confer passive immunity. Mother should not be given vaccine when at risk for pregnancy.
Smallpox vaccine	No		Exposure is by direct contact. Live virus. No longer given.

8-2 Human fetotoxic chemical agents

Maternal medication	*Reported effect on fetus or neonate*
Analgesics	
Indomethacin	Prolongs gestation (monkey)
Narcotics	70% of maternal level; death, apnea, depression, bradycardia, hypothermia
Salicylates	Death in utero; hemorrhage, methemoglobinemia, ↓ albumin-binding capacity, salicylate intoxication, difficult delivery, ? prolonged gestation
Anesthesia	
Conduction	Indirect effect of maternal hypotension; direct effect—convulsions, death, acidosis, bradycardia, myocardial depression, fetal hypotension, methemoglobinemia
General Ether Halothane (Fluothane) Trichloroethylene (Trilene)	Apnea, depression (prolonged inhalation by gravid female), ? congenital malformations, chromosome abnormality; ether has direct narcotic effect on infant
Hypnosis	Indirect effect of maternal hyperventilation and excessive bearing down
Local	
Paracervical	Methemoglobinemia, fetal acidosis, bradycardia, neurologic depression, myocardial depression
Anticoagulants	
Coumarins	Fetal death, hemorrhage, calcifications
Anticonvulsant agents	
Barbiturates	Irritability and tremulousness 4 to 5 months postdelivery; hemorrhage, enzyme inducer
Diphenylhydantoin and barbiturate	Congenital malformations, cleft lip and palate, congenital heart disease (CHD), CNS and skeletal anomalies, failure to thrive, enzyme inducer, hemorrhage
Paradione Tridione	CHD, microophthalmia, mental retardation, abortion
Antidiabetics	See hypoglycemic agents
Antimalarial	
Quinine	? Congenital anomalies of CNS and extremities, thrombocytopenia, hypoplastic optic nerve, congenital deafness

Modified from Perinatal pharmacology, Mead Johnson Symposium on Perinatal and Developmental Medicine, No. 5, Vail, Colo., 1974; and Babson, S.G., and others: Management of high-risk pregnancy and intensive care of the neonate, ed. 3, St. Louis, 1975, The C.V. Mosby Co.

Maternal medication	*Reported effect on fetus or neonate*
Antimicrobials	All antimicrobials cross placenta
Ampicillin	↓ Maternal urinary and plasma estriol levels
Cephaloridine	Blood levels maintained for hours after delivery; ? false positive direct Coombs' test
Chloramphenicol	Crosses placenta with no reported effect; interferes with biotransformation of tolbutamide, diphenylhydantoin, biohydroxycoumarin (i.e., hypoglycemia may occur if used in combination)
Chloroquine	Death, deafness, retinal hemorrhage
Erythromycin	Possible hepatic injury
Nitrofurantoin	Megaloblastic anemia, G6PD deficiency
Novobiocin	Hyperbilirubinemia
Quinine, quinidine	Possible ototoxicity, thrombocytopenia
Streptomycin	Therapeutic levels reached, nerve deafness
Sulfonamides	
Long and short acting	Icterus, hemolytic anemia, kernicterus, ? growth retardation, thrombocytopenia
Tetracycline	Placental transfer after 4 months' gestation; enamel hypoplasia, delay in bone growth, ? congenital cataract
Antituberculous	
Isoniazid	Toxic blood level in fetus; no reported effect; mother should be on pyridoxine supplement
Pyridoxine	See vitamins
Belladonna derivatives	
Atropine	Intrauterine tachycardia; dilated, nonreacting pupils
Scopolamine	? Delays labor, ? delays respiration, deleterious to premature infant
Cancer chemotherapeutic agents	
Aminopterin Busulfan Cyclophosphamide 6-Mercaptopurine Methotrexate	Abortion, congenital anomalies (first trimester); combination of drugs detrimental to fetus skeletal and cranial malformations, hydrocephalus; questionable long-term effects = slow somatic growth; ovarian agenesis; ↓ immune mechanisms
Cardiovascular agents	
Digitoxin	Placental transfer, no reported effect
Propranolol	Indirect effect of delay in cervical dilation
Cholinesterase inhibitors	Myasthenia-like symptoms for 1 week; muscle weakness in 10% to 20% of infants
Cigarette smoking	Effect equal to number of cigarettes smoked; ↑ incidence of stillbirth; low birth weight; ? effect on later somatic growth and mental development; reduction in O_2 transport to fetus
Diuretics	
Ammonium chloride Benzothiazides Chlorothiazide Thiazide	Maternal and fetal acidosis; thrombocytopenia, hemorrhage, hypoelectrolytemia, convulsions, respiratory distress, death, hemolysis
Diazoxide	Hypertrichosis lanuginosa, alopecia, ? hypoglycemia
Drugs of abuse (usually multiple drugs consumed)	
Alcohol	Blood level equal to mother's; convulsions, withdrawal syndrome, hyperactivity, crying, irritability, poor sucking reflex, low birth weight; cleft palate, ophthalmic malformation, malformation of extremities and heart; poor mental performance; microencephaly, small-for-dates, growth deficiency
Barbiturates	Withdrawal symptoms, convulsions, onset immediately after birth or at 2 weeks of age
Glutethimide	Small-for-dates, irritability
LSD (lysergic acid)	Chromosome breakage, limb and skeletal anomalies
Narcotics Heroin Methadone	Small-for-dates, 4% to 10% mortality, habituation, withdrawal symptoms, convulsions, sudden death, indirect effect on maternal complications (i.e., infection, hepatitis, venereal disease), ? permanent effect on somatic growth
Fluorine	Placental transfer—utilized for growth and development of bones and teeth of fetus

Continued.

Human fetotoxic chemical agents—cont'd

Maternal medication	*Reported effect on fetus or neonate*
Hormones	
Androgens Estrogens Progestins	Labioscrotal fusion prior to twelfth week, after 12 weeks' phallic enlargement; ? anomalies ? ↑ bilirubin, vaginal cancer; cleft lip and palate, CHD, TE fistula, anal atresia, cancer of prostate, testes, and bladder
Corticosteroids	Adrenal insufficiency, cleft palate, small-for-dates infant
Ovulatory agents	? Anencephaly, ? chromosome abnormalities in abortus, multiple pregnancy
Hypoglycemic agents	
Chlorpropamide	Higher fetal mortality, prolonged hypoglycemia, competes for albumin-binding sites
Insulin	Insulin coma, ? increased fetal damage
Tolbutamide	? Potentiates hypoglycemia in newborn, thrombocytopenia
Hypotensive agents	
Hexamethonium	Paralytic ileus, perforation, death
Reserpine	1% to 15% of infants have symptoms; nasal stuffiness, bradycardia, respiratory distress, hypothermia, abnormal muscle tone (in mice, hyperactivity and increased emotionalism)
Insecticide and pesticides	
Organochlorine	Present in fetus, ? enzyme induction, ? premature labor
Intravenous alcohol	Hypoglycemia; abnormal bone marrow morphology in premature infant
Intravenous fluids	Excessive fluids—hyponatremia, seizures
Muscle relaxants	
Curare	Paralysis in utero (prolonged use), position deformities
Narcotic antagonist	
Nalorphine (Nalline) Levallorphan (Lorfan)	Not effective unless large doses of narcotics administered to mother; act as respiratory depressant if cause of depression is other than narcotic
Oxytocin	Thrombocytopenia, fetal bradycardia, water intoxication, ? ↑ bilirubin level; abortions (ergot)
Psychotropic drugs	
Antidepressants	
Aventyl Chloropyramine Imipramine Nortriptyline	Withdrawal, coliclike syndrome, cyanosis, irritability, weight loss, hyperhydrosis, respiratory distress, craniofacial anomalies, CNS and skeletal anomalies; urinary retention
Diazepam (Valium)	High fetal levels; hypotonia, poor sucking reflex, hypothermia; ↑ low Apgar score infants; ↑ resuscitation, ↑ assisted deliveries; dose related
Lithium	Neonatal serum levels reach adult toxic range; lethargy, cyanosis for 10 days; teratogenic—dose related
Phenothiazine	? Effect on eyes; withdrawal; extrapyramidal dysfunction; delay in onset of respiration; maternal hypotension, ? prolongs labor, effective uterine contraction; ? chromosomal breakage; hypotonia, hyperactivity
Radiation	Microencephaly, mental retardation, many unknown effects; nondisjunction of chromosomes
Radiopaque media	Elevated PHI, depressed ^{131}I uptake
Sedatives	
Barbiturate	Apnea, depression, depressed EEG, poor sucking reflex, slow weight gain; concentration of drug in brain; enzyme inducer = lower bilirubin level
Bromides	Growth failure, lethargy, dilated pupils, dermatitis, hypotonia, ? effect on mental development
Magnesium sulfate	Neonatal blood level does not correlate with clinical condition; respiratory depression, hypotonia, convulsions, death; exchange transfusion may be required
Paraldehyde	Apnea, depression
Thalidomide	Administered between thirty-fourth and fiftieth day of gestation causes phocomelia, malformation of cord, angiomas of face, CHD, intestinal stenosis, eye defects, absence of appendix
Thyroid medications	
Iodine Thioureas	Normal or goitrous infants; euthyroid, hyperthyroid or hypothyroid; respiratory distress due to tracheal compression; thrombocytopenia
^{131}I	Uptake by fetal thyroid after 12 weeks' gestation; exophthalmus, arrest of brain development

Maternal medication	*Reported effect on fetus or neonate*
Toxins	
Carbon monoxide	Stillbirth, brain damage equal to anoxia
Heavy metals	
Arsenic	Concentrated in brain
Lead	Abortions, growth retardation, congenital anomalies, sterility
Mercury	Cerebral palsy, mental retardation, convulsions, involuntary movements, defective vision; mother asymptomatic
Naphthalene	Hemolysis
Vitamins	
A and D	Congenital anomalies
K (water-soluble analogues)	Icterus, anemia, kernicterus
Pyridoxine	Withdrawal seizures

8-3 Pregnancy table for expected date of delivery

Find the date of the last menstrual period in the top line (light-face type) of the pair of lines. The dark number (bold-face type) in the line below will be the expected day of delivery.

Jan.	1	2	3	4	5	6	7	8	9	10	11	12	13	14	15	16	17	18	19	20	21	22	23	24	25	26	27	28	29	30	31	
Oct.	**8**	**9**	**10**	**11**	**12**	**13**	**14**	**15**	**16**	**17**	**18**	**19**	**20**	**21**	**22**	**23**	**24**	**25**	**26**	**27**	**28**	**29**	**30**	**31**	**(1**	**2**	**3**	**4**	**5**	**6**	**7**	**Nov.**
Feb.	1	2	3	4	5	6	7	8	9	10	11	12	13	14	15	16	17	18	19	20	21	22	23	24	25	26	27	28				
Nov.	**8**	**9**	**10**	**11**	**12**	**13**	**14**	**15**	**16**	**17**	**18**	**19**	**20**	**21**	**22**	**23**	**24**	**25**	**26**	**27**	**28**	**29**	**30**	**(1**	**2**	**3**	**4**	**5**				**Dec.**
Mar.	1	2	3	4	5	6	7	8	9	10	11	12	13	14	15	16	17	18	19	20	21	22	23	24	25	26	27	28	29	30	31	
Dec.	**6**	**7**	**8**	**9**	**10**	**11**	**12**	**13**	**14**	**15**	**16**	**17**	**18**	**19**	**20**	**21**	**22**	**23**	**24**	**25**	**26**	**27**	**28**	**29**	**30**	**31**	**(1**	**2**	**3**	**4**	**5**	**Jan.**
April	1	2	3	4	5	6	7	8	9	10	11	12	13	14	15	16	17	18	19	20	21	22	23	24	25	26	27	28	29	30		
Jan.	**6**	**7**	**8**	**9**	**10**	**11**	**12**	**13**	**14**	**15**	**16**	**17**	**18**	**19**	**20**	**21**	**22**	**23**	**24**	**25**	**26**	**27**	**28**	**29**	**30**	**31**	**(1**	**2**	**3**	**4**		**Feb.**
May	1	2	3	4	5	6	7	8	9	10	11	12	13	14	15	16	17	18	19	20	21	22	23	24	25	26	27	28	29	30	31	
Feb.	**5**	**6**	**7**	**8**	**9**	**10**	**11**	**12**	**13**	**14**	**15**	**16**	**17**	**18**	**19**	**20**	**21**	**22**	**23**	**24**	**25**	**26**	**27**	**28**	**(1**	**2**	**3**	**4**	**5**	**6**	**7**	**Mar.**
June	1	2	3	4	5	6	7	8	9	10	11	12	13	14	15	16	17	18	19	20	21	22	23	24	25	26	27	28	29	30		
Mar.	**8**	**9**	**10**	**11**	**12**	**13**	**14**	**15**	**16**	**17**	**18**	**19**	**20**	**21**	**22**	**23**	**24**	**25**	**26**	**27**	**28**	**29**	**30**	**31**	**(1**	**2**	**3**	**4**	**5**	**6**		**April**
July	1	2	3	4	5	6	7	8	9	10	11	12	13	14	15	16	17	18	19	20	21	22	23	24	25	26	27	28	29	30	31	
April	**7**	**8**	**9**	**10**	**11**	**12**	**13**	**14**	**15**	**16**	**17**	**18**	**19**	**20**	**21**	**22**	**23**	**24**	**25**	**26**	**27**	**28**	**29**	**30**	**(1**	**2**	**3**	**4**	**5**	**6**	**7**	**May**
Aug.	1	2	3	4	5	6	7	8	9	10	11	12	13	14	15	16	17	18	19	20	21	22	23	24	25	26	27	28	29	30	31	
May	**8**	**9**	**10**	**11**	**12**	**13**	**14**	**15**	**16**	**17**	**18**	**19**	**20**	**21**	**22**	**23**	**24**	**25**	**26**	**27**	**28**	**29**	**30**	**31**	**(1**	**2**	**3**	**4**	**5**	**6**	**7**	**June**
Sept.	1	2	3	4	5	6	7	8	9	10	11	12	13	14	15	16	17	18	19	20	21	22	23	24	25	26	27	28	29	30		
June	**8**	**9**	**10**	**11**	**12**	**13**	**14**	**15**	**16**	**17**	**18**	**19**	**20**	**21**	**22**	**23**	**24**	**25**	**26**	**27**	**28**	**29**	**30**	**(1**	**2**	**3**	**4**	**5**	**6**	**7**		**July**
Oct.	1	2	3	4	5	6	7	8	9	10	11	12	13	14	15	16	17	18	19	20	21	22	23	24	25	26	27	28	29	30	31	
July	**8**	**9**	**10**	**11**	**12**	**13**	**14**	**15**	**16**	**17**	**18**	**19**	**20**	**21**	**22**	**23**	**24**	**25**	**26**	**27**	**28**	**29**	**30**	**31**	**(1**	**2**	**3**	**4**	**5**	**6**	**7**	**Aug.**
Nov.	1	2	3	4	5	6	7	8	9	10	11	12	13	14	15	16	17	18	19	20	21	22	23	24	25	26	27	28	29	30		
Aug.	**8**	**9**	**10**	**11**	**12**	**13**	**14**	**15**	**16**	**17**	**18**	**19**	**20**	**21**	**22**	**23**	**24**	**25**	**26**	**27**	**28**	**29**	**30**	**31**	**(1**	**2**	**3**	**4**	**5**	**6**		**Sept.**
Dec.	1	2	3	4	5	6	7	8	9	10	11	12	13	14	15	16	17	18	19	20	21	22	23	24	25	26	27	28	29	30	31	
Sept.	**7**	**8**	**9**	**10**	**11**	**12**	**13**	**14**	**15**	**16**	**17**	**18**	**19**	**20**	**21**	**22**	**23**	**24**	**25**	**26**	**27**	**28**	**29**	**30**	**(1**	**2**	**3**	**4**	**5**	**6**	**7**	**Oct.**

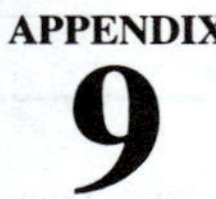

APPENDIX 9

PEDIATRICS

9-1 The Washington guide to promoting development in the young child

Motor skills

Expected tasks	*Suggested activities*
1 to 3 months	
1. Holds head up briefly when prone 2. Head erect and bobbing when supported in sitting position 3. Head erect and steady in sitting position 4. Follows object through all planes 5. Palmar grasp 6. Moro reflex	1. Place infant in prone position 2. Support in sitting position with his head erect 3. Pull infant to sitting position 4. Provide with opportunity to observe people or activity 5. Hang bright-colored objects and mobiles within reach across crib 6. Provide with opportunity to observe objects or people while in sitting position 7. Use infant seat 8. Alternate bright shiny objects with dark and light visual patterns
4 to 8 months	
1. Sits with minimal support, with stable head and back 2. Sits alone steadily 3. Plays with hands, which are open most of time 4. Grasps rattle or bottle with both hands 5. Picks up small objects, for example, cube 6. Transfers toys from one hand to other 7. Neck-righting reflex	1. Pull up to sitting position 2. Provide opportunity to sit supported or alone when head and trunk control are stabilized 3. Put bright-colored objects within reach 4. Give toys or household objects: rattles, teething ring, cloth animals or dolls, 1-inch cubes, plastic objects such as cups, rings, and balls 5. Offer small objects such as cereal to improve grasp 6. Offer a variety of patterns or textures to play with 7. Use squeak toys
9 to 12 months	
1. Rises to sitting position 2. Creeps or crawls, maybe backward at first 3. Pulls to standing position 4. Stands alone 5. Cruises 6. Uses index finger to poke 7. Finger-thumb grasp 8. Parachute reflex 9. Landau reflex	1. Provide playpen, allow child to pull himself to standing 2. Give opportunity and space to practice creeping and crawling 3. Have child practice moving on knees to improve balance prior to walking 4. Have child use walker or straddle toys 5. Play airplane with child; have child practice catching himself while rolling on large ball 6. Provide with objects such as spoons, plastic bottles, cups, ball, cubes, finger foods, saucepans, and lids
13 to 18 months	
1. Walks a few steps without support 2. Balanced when walking 3. Walks upstairs with help, creeps downstairs 4. Turns pages of book	1. Provide opportunity to practice walking, climbing stairs with help 2. Give toys that can be pushed around 3. Supervise activity with paper and large crayons 4. Provide toys such as cubes, cups, saucepans, lids, rag dolls, and other soft, cuddly toys 5. Begin introducing child to swing
19 to 30 months	
1. Runs 2. Walks up and down stairs, one at a time (not alternating feet) 3. Imitates vertical strokes 4. Imitates building tower of four or more blocks 5. Throws ball overhand 6. Jumps in place 7. Rides tricycle	1. Provide opportunity to practice and develop activities 2. Provide pattern for child while he watches and then encourage him to try 3. Provide tricycle or similar pedal toys; secure foot on pedal if necessary

Continued.

Motor skills—cont'd

Expected tasks	*Suggested activities*
31 to 48 months	
1. Walks downstairs (alternating feet) 2. Hops on one foot 3. Swings and climbs 4. Balances on one foot for 10 seconds 5. Copies circle 6. Copies cross 7. Draws person with three parts	1. Continue with blocks, combining materials, toy cars, and trains 2. Provide clay and other manipulating materials 3. Give opportunities to swing and climb 4. Provide with activities such as finger painting, chalk, and black board
49 to 52 months	
1. Balances well 2. Skips and jumps 3. Can heel-toe walk 4. Copies square 5. Catches bounced ball	1. Provide with music and games to synchronize hand and foot, tapping with music, skipping, hopping, and dancing rhythmically to improve coordination

Feeding skills

Expected tasks	*Suggested activities*
1 to 3 months	
1. Sucking reflex present 2. Rooting reflex present 3. Ability to swallow pureed foods 4. Coordinates sucking, swallowing, and breathing	1. Consider a change in nipple or posturing if there is difficulty in swallowing 2. Introduce solids, one kind at a time (use small spoon, place food well back on infant's tongue) 3. Hold in comfortable relaxed position while feeding 4. Pace feeding tempo to infant's needs
4 to 8 months	
1. Tongue used in moving food in mouth 2. Hand-to-mouth motions 3. Recognizes bottle on sight 4. Gums or mouths solid foods 5. Feeds self cracker	1. Give finger foods to develop chewing, stimulate gums, and encourage hand-to-mouth motion (cubes of cheese, bananas, dry toast, bread crust, cookies) 2. Encourage upright supported position for feeding 3. Promote bottle holding 4. Introduce junior foods
9 to 12 months	
1. Holds own bottle 2. Drinks from cup or glass with assistance 3. Finger feeds 4. Beginning to hold spoon	1. Bring child in highchair to table and include in part of or entire meal with family 2. Have child in dry comfortable position with trunk and feet supported 3. Encourage self-help in feeding; use of table foods 4. Offer spoon when interest is indicated 5. Introduce cup or glass with small amount of fluid
13 to 18 months	
1. Holds cup and handle with digital grasp 2. Lifts cup and drinks well 3. Beginning to use spoon, may turn bowl down before reaching mouth 4. Difficulty in inserting spoon into mouth 5. May refuse food	1. Continue offering finger foods (wieners, sandwiches) 2. Use nontip dishes and cups; dishes should have sides to make filling of spoon easy 3. Give opportunity for self-feeding 4. Provide fluids between meals rather than having child fill up on fluids at mealtime

Feeding skills—cont'd

Expected tasks	*Suggested activities*
19 to 30 months	
1. Drinks without spilling 2. Holds small glass in one hand 3. Inserts spoon in mouth correctly 4. Distinguishes between food and inedible material 5. Plays with food	1. Encourage self-feeding with spoon 2. Do not rush child 3. Serve foods plainly but in attractive servings 4. Small servings of food will encourage eating more than large servings
31 to 48 months	
1. Pours well from pitcher 2. Serves self at table with little spilling 3. Rarely needs assistance 4. Interest in setting table	1. Encourage self-help 2. Give opportunity for pouring (give rice and pitcher to promote pouring skills) 3. Encourage child to help set table 4. Have well-defined rules about table manners
49 to 52 months	
1. Feeds self well 2. Social and talkative during meal	1. Socialize with child at mealtime 2. Have child help with preparation, table setting, and serving 3. Include child in conversations at mealtimes by planning special times for him to tell about events, situations, or what he did during the day

Sleep

Expected tasks	*Suggested activities*
1 to 3 months	
1. Night: 4- to 10-hour intervals 2. Naps: frequent 3. Longer periods of wakefulness without crying	1. Provide separate sleeping arrangements away from parent's room 2. Reduce noise and light stimulation when placing in bed 3. Have room at comfortable temperature with no drafts or extremes in heat 4. Reverse position of crib occasionally 5. Place child in different positions from time to time for sleep 6. Alternate from back to side to stomach 7. Keep crib sides up
4 to 8 months	
1. Night: 10 to 12 hours 2. Naps: 2 to 3 (1 to 4 hours in duration) 3. Night awakenings	1. Keep crib sides up 2. Refrain from taking child into parents' room if he awakens 3. Check to determine if there is cause for awakenings: hunger, teething, pain, cold, wet, noise, or illness 4. If a baby-sitter is used, attempt to find some person with whom infant is familiar. Explain bedtime and naptime arrangements
9 to 12 months	
1. Night: 12 to 14 hours 2. Naps: one to two (1 to 4 hours in duration) 3. May begin refusing morning nap	1. Short crying periods may be source of tension release for child 2. Observe for signs of fatigue, irritability, or restlessness if naps are shorter 3. Provide familiar person to baby-sit who knows sleep routines
13 to 18 months	
1. Night: 10 to 12 hours 2. Naps: one in afternoon (1 to 3 hours in duration) 3. May awaken during night crying (associated with wetting bed) 4. As he becomes more able to move about, he may uncover himself, become cold, and awaken	1. Night terrors may be terminated by awakening infant and offering reassurance 2. Check to see that child is covered 3. Avoid hazardous devices to keep child covered, including blanket clips, pins, and garments that enclose child to neck

Continued.

Sleep—cont'd

Expected tasks	Suggested activities
19 to 30 months	
1. Night: 10 to 12 hours 2. Naps: one (1 to 3 hours duration) 3. Doesn't go to sleep at once—keeps demanding things 4. May awaken crying if wet or soiled 5. May awaken because of environmental change of temperature, change of bed, change of sleeping room, addition of sibling to room, absence of parent from home, hospitalization, trip with family, or relatives visiting	1. Quiet period of socialization prior to bedtime—reading child book or telling story 2. Holding child—talking quietly with him 3. Ritualistic behavior may be present; allow child to carry out routine; helps him overcome fear of unexpected or fear of dark, for example, child may wish to arrange toys in certain way 4. Explain bedtime ritual to baby-sitter 5. Give more reassurance, spend more time before bedtime preparation 6. Provide familiar bedtime toys or items 7. Allow crying-out period if he is safe, comfortable, and tucked in 8. Place in bed before he reaches excessive state of fatigue, excitement, or tiredness 9. Eliminate sources of stimulation or fear 10. Maintain consistent hour of bedtime
31 to 48 months	
1. Daily range: 10 to 15 hours 2. Naps: beginning to disappear 3. Prolongs process of going to bed 4. Less dependent on taking toys to bed 5. May awaken crying from dreams 6. May awaken if wet	1. Television programs may affect ability to go to sleep: avoid violent television programs 2. Anxiety about going to bed and desire to stay up with parents requires limits 3. Regularity and consistency important to promote good sleep habits 4. Reassurance—night light or leaving door ajar 5. Do not use bedtime or naptime as punishment 6. Encourage naps if signs of fatigue or irritability are evidenced
49 to 52 months	
1. Daily range: 9 to 13 hours 2. Naps: rare 3. Quieter during sleep	1. Encourage napping if excessive or strenuous activity occurs and child is overly tired 2. Explain to child if baby-sitter will be there after child is asleep

Play

Expected tasks	Suggested activities
1 to 3 months	
1. Quieted when picked up 2. Regards face of others	1. Encourage holding and touching of child by mother 2. Provide with cradle gyms and mobiles, brightly colored, visually interesting objects within arm's distance
4 to 8 months	
1. Plays with own body 2. Differentiates strangers from family 3. Seeks out objects 4. Grasps, holds, and manipulates objects 5. Repeats activities he enjoys 6. Bangs toys or objects together	1. Begin patty-cake and peekaboo 2. Provide for periods of solitary play (playpen) 3. Encourage holding and touching of child by mother 4. Provide variety of multicolored and multitextured objects that child can hold 5. Encourage exploration of body parts 6. Provide floating toys for bath
9 to 12 months	
1. Puts objects in and out of containers 2. Examines objects held in hand 3. Plays interactive games (peekaboo) 4. Extends toy to other person without releasing 5. Works to get toy out of reach	1. Continue mother-infant games 2. Give opportunity to place objects in containters and pour out 3. Provide large and small objects with which to play 4. Encourage interactive play

Play—cont'd

Expected tasks	Suggested activities
13 to 18 months	
1. Plays by himself—may play near others 2. Has preferred toys 3. Enjoys walking activities, pulling toys 4. Throws and picks up objects, throws again 5. Imitates, for example, reading newspaper, sweeping	1. Introduce to other children even though child may not play with them 2. Provide music, books, and magazines 3. Encourage imitative activities—helping with dusting, sweeping, stirring
19 to 30 months	
1. Parallel play—not interactive but plays alongside another child 2. Uses both large and small toys 3. Rough-and-tumble play 4. Play periods longer than before—interested in manipulative and constructive toys 5. Enjoys rhymes and singing (television programs)	1. Provide with new materials for manipulating and feeling—finger paints, clay, sand, stones, water, and soap Wooden toys—cars and animals Building blocks of various sizes, crayons, and paper Rhythmical tunes and equipment—swing, rocking chair, rocking horse Children's books—short, simple stories with repetition and familiar objects; enjoys simple pictures, brightly colored 2. Guide child's hand to actively participate with specific activities, for example, using crayons, hammering
31 to 48 months	
1. In playing with others, beginning to interact, sharing toys, taking turns 2. Dramatizes, expresses imagination in play 3. Combining playthings; more use of constructive materials 4. Prefers two or three children to play with; may have special friend	1. Encourage play with small groups of children 2. Encourage imaginative and dramatic play activities 3. Music: singing and experimenting with musical instruments 4. Group participation in rhymes, dancing by hopping or jumping 5. Drawing and painting (seldom recognizable)
49 to 52 months	
1. Dramatic play and interest in going on excursions 2. Fond of cutting and pasting, creative materials 3. Completes most activities	1. Painting and drawing (objects will be out of proportion; details that are most important to child are drawn largest) 2. Encourage printing of numbers and letters 3. Clay: making recognizable objects 4. Cutting and pasting 5. Provide with materials, for example, boxes, chairs, barrels, for building sturdy structures

Language

Expected tasks	Suggested activities
1 to 3 months *Receptive abilities*	
1. Movement of eyes, respiration rate, or body activity changes when bell is rung close to child's head 2. Smiles when socially stimulated 3. Has facial, vocal, and generalized bodily responses to faces 4. Reacts differently to adult voices	1. Observe facial expressions, gestures, bodily postures, and movements when vocalizations are being produced 2. Smile and talk softly in pleasant tone while holding, touching, and handling infant 3. Hold, touch, and interact frequently with infant for pleasure 4. Refrain from letting infant engage in prolonged and incessant crying
Expressive abilities	
1. Makes prelanguage vocalizations that consist of cooing, throaty sounds, for example, gu 2. Makes "pleasure" sounds that consist of soft vowels 3. Makes "sucking" sounds 4. Crying can be differentiated for discomfort, pain, and hunger as reported by mother 5. An "A" sound as in cat is commonly heard in distress crying	

Continued.

Language—cont'd

Expected tasks	*Suggested activities*
4 to 8 months *Receptive abilities* 1. Eyes locate source of sound 2. Responds to "hi, there" by looking up at face that is across and in front of him 3. Head turns to sound of cellophane held and crunched 2 feet away and at a 135-degree angle on either side of head 4. Will turn head to locate sound of "look here" when spoken at a 90-degree angle from head 2 feet away* 5. Turns head to sound of rattle 6. Responds differently to vacuum cleaner, phone, doorbell, or sound of dog barking: may cry, whimper, look toward sound, or mother may report change in body tension 7. Responds by raising arms when mother reaches toward child and says "come up" *Expressive abilities* 1. Uses different inflectional patterns: ah uh ah 2. Laughs aloud when stimulated 3. Has differential patterns of crying when hungry, in pain, or angry 4. Produces vowel sounds and chained syllables (baba, gugu, didi) 5. Makes "talking sounds" in response to others talking to him 6. Babbles to produce consonant sounds: ba, da, m-m 7. Vocalizes to toys 8. Says "da-da" or "ma-ma" but not specific to presence of parents	1. Engage in smiling eye-to-eye contact while talking to infant 2. Vocalize in response to inflectional patterns and when infant is producing babbling sounds; echo the sounds he makes 3. Observe for subtle communication clues such as eye aversion, struggling to move away, flushing of skin, tension of body, or movement of arms 4. Vocalize with infant during handling, while feeding, bathing, dressing, diapering, bedtime preparation, and holding 5. Stimulate laughing by light tickling 6. Observe child's reactions to bells, whistles, horns, phones, laughing, singing, talking, music box, noisemaking toys, and common household noises 7. While talking to infant, hold in position so that he can see your face 8. Have infant placed at position of eye level while talking to him thoughout the day 9. If crying or laughing sounds are not discerned at this stage, report to family physician, pediatrician, public health nurse, or well-child clinic
9 to 12 months *Receptive abilities* 1. Ceases activity when name is pronounced or "no-no" is said 2. Gives toys on request when accompanied by facial and bodily gestures 3. Attends to simple commands *Expressive abilities* 1. Imitates definite speech sounds such as tongue clicking, lip smacking, or coughing 2. Should have two words that are *specific* for parents: "mama," "dada," or equivalents	1. Gain child's attention when giving simple commands 2. Accompany oral directions with gestures 3. Vocalize with child during feeding, bathing, and playtimes 4. Provide sounds that child can reproduce such as lip smacking and tongue clicking 5. Repeat direction frequently and have child participate in action: open and close the drawer; move arms and legs up and down 6. Have child respond to verbal directions: stand up, sit down, close door, open door, turn around, come here
13 to 18 months *Receptive abilities* 1. Attends to person speaking to child 2. Finds "the baby" in picture when requested, for example, on baby food jar, in magazine, or in storybooks 3. Indicates wants by gestures 4. Looks toward family members or pets when named *Expressive abilities* 1. Uses three words other than mama and dada to denote *specific* objects, persons, or actions 2. Indicates wants by naming object such as cookie	1. Incorporate repetition into daily routine of home a. Feeding: name baby's food and eating utensils; ask if he is enjoying his dessert; concentrate on reviewing a day's events in simple manner b. Household duties: mother names each item as she dusts; pronounces word while cooking and preparing foods c. Playing: identify toys when using them; explain their function 2. Let child see mouthing of words 3. Encourage verbalization and expression of wants

*Do not test for localization of sound by producing sound directly behind infant's head.

Language—cont'd

Expected tasks	Suggested activities
19 to 30 months *Receptive abilities* 1. Points to one named body part 2. Follows two or three verbal directions that are not accompanied by facial or body gestures, for example, put ball on table, give it to mommy, or put toy in box *Expressive abilities* 1. Combines two different words, for example, "play ball," "want cookie" 2. Names object in picture, for example, cat, bird, dog, horse, man 3. Refers to self by pronoun rather than by name	1. Continue to present concrete objects with words; talk about activities child is involved with 2. Include child in conversations during mealtimes 3. Encourage speech by having child express wants 4. Incorporate games into bathing routine by having child name and point to body parts 5. As child gains confidence in remembering and using words appropriately, encourage less use of gestures 6. Count and name articles of clothing as they are placed on child 7. Count and name silverware as it is placed on table 8. Sort, match, and name glassware, laundry, cans, vegetables, and fruit with child 9. Have child keep scrapbook and add new picture every day to increase recognition of vocabulary words 10. Spend 15 to 20 minutes per day going through booklets and naming pictures; have child point to pictures as objects are named 11. Help child develop functional core vocabulary to express safety needs and information about neighborhood 12. Whenever possible, use word (for example, paper), show object, have child handle and use it, encourage him to watch your face while you say the words, and suggest that he repeat it; refrain from undue pressure
31 to 36 months *Receptive abilities* 1. Takes turns when asked while playing, eating 2. Attends longer to stories and television programs 3. Demonstrates understanding of two prepositions by carrying out two commands one at a time, for example, "put the block under the chair" 4. Can follow commands asking for two objects or two actions 5. Demonstrates understanding of concepts of big and little, for example, selects larger of two balls when asked for big one 6. Points to additional body parts *Expressive abilities* 1. Uses regular plurals, for example, adds "s" to apple, box, orange (does not use irregular plurals, for example, mouse to mice) 2. Gives first and last name 3. Names what he has drawn after scribbling 4. On request, tells you his sex; for example, "Are you a little boy or a little girl?" 5. Can repeat a few rhymes or songs 6. On request, tells what action is going on in picture, for example, the kitten is eating	1. Read stories with familiar content but with more detail; nonsense rhymes, humorous stories 2. Expect child to follow simple commands 3. Give child opportunity to hear and repeat his full name 4. Listen to child's explanation about pictures he draws 5. Encourage child to repeat nursery rhymes by himself and with others 6. Address child by his first name
37 to 48 months 1. Expresses appropriate responses when asked what child does when tired, cold, or hungry 2. Tells stories 3. Common expression: I don't know 4. Repeats sentence composed of twelve to thirteen syllables, for example, "I am going when daddy and I are finished playing" 5. Has mastered phonetic sounds of p, k, g, v, tf, d, z, lr, hw, j, kw, l, e, w, qe, and o	1. Provide visual stimuli while reading stories 2. Have child repeat story 3. Arrange trips to zoo, farms, seashore, stores, and movies and discuss with child 4. Give simple explanations in answering questions

Continued.

Language—cont'd

Expected tasks	*Suggested activities*
49 to 52 months *Receptive abilities* 1. Points to penny, nickel, or dime on request 2. Carries out in order command containing three parts, for example, "pick up the block, put it on the table, and bring the book to me" *Expressive abilities* 1. Names penny, nickel, or dime on request 2. Replies appropriately to questions such as, "What do you do when you are asleep?" 3. Counts three objects, pointing to each in turn 4. Defines simple words, for example, hat, ball 5. Asks questions 6. Can identify or name four colors	1. Play games in which child names colors 2. Encourage use of please and thank you 3. Encourage social-verbal interactions with other children 4. Encourage correct usage of words 5. Provide puppets or toys with movable parts that child can converse about 6. Provide group activity for child; children may stimulate each other by taking turns naming pictures 7. Allow child to make choices about games, stories, and activities 8. Have child dramatize simple stories 9. Provide child with piggy bank and encourage naming coins as they are handled or dropped into bank

Discipline

Expected tasks	*Suggested activities*
1 to 3 months	
1. Draws attention by crying	1. a. Needs should be identified and met as promptly as possible b. Every bit of fussing should not be interpreted as emergency requiring immediate attention c. Infant should not be ignored and permitted to cry for exhaustive periods
2. Infant desires whatever is pleasant and wishes to avoid unpleasant situations	2. Begin to present limit of having to wait so that infant can learn that tension and discomfort are bearable for short periods
3. Beginning to "wiggle" around	3. Place infant on surfaces that have sides to protect him from falling off
4 to 8 months	
1. Begins to respond to "no-no"	1. a. Reserve "no-no" for times when it is really needed b. Be consistent with word "no-no" for same activity and event that requires it; be friendly and firm with verbal control of limit setting
2. Infant who is left alone for long periods of time may become bored or fretful; learns that crying and whining result in attention	2. Make special efforts to attend to infant when he is quiet and amusing himself
3. Beginning to show signs of timidity and fretfulness and may whimper and cry when mother separates from him or when strangers pick him up	3. a. Gradually introduce strangers into infant's environment b. Refrain from promoting frightening situations with strangers during this stage c. Play hiding games like peekaboo in which mother disappears and reappears d. Allow infant to cling to mother and get used to persons a little at a time e. If baby-sitter is used, find person familiar to infant or introduce for brief periods before mother leaves infant in her care f. Encourage gentle handling by mother, father, and siblings. Discourage rough handling, particulary by strangers
4. Beginning to grasp objects and bring to mouth, but unable to differentiate safe from hazardous items	4. a. Provide toys that do not have small detachable parts b. Check frequently for small objects in his line of reach 5. When traveling in car, place in crib or seat with safety belts securely fastened

Discipline—cont'd

Expected tasks	*Suggested activities*
9 to 12 months	
1. Beginning to respond to simple commands, for example, "pick up the ball, put the toy in the box"	1. a. Avoid setting unreasonable number of limits b. Give simple commands one at a time c. Once limit is set, adhere to it firmly each time and connect it immediately with misbehavior d. Respond with consistency in enforcing rule e. Allow time to conform to request f. Gain child's attention
2. Ready to go places on his own and is trying out newly developing motor capacities (not to be confused with naughtiness, "spoiled," or stubbornness)	2. a. Begin setting and enforcing limits on where child is allowed to travel and explore b. Remove tempting objects c. Remove sources of danger such as light sockets, protruding pot handles, hanging table covers, sharp objects, and hanging cords d. Keep child away from fans, heaters, and certain drawers and do not place vaporizer close to infant's crib e. Keep high chair at least 2 feet away from working and cooking surfaces in kitchen f. Use gate to keep child out of kitchen when it is being used g. Be certain that pans, basins, and tubs of hot water are never left unattended h. Remove all possible poisons or substances that are not food that can be eaten or drunk off floor, low-level cabinets, and under sink i. Keep child from objects or surfaces that he may chew, for example, porch rails, windowsills, *repainted* toys or cribs that may contain lead j. Instruct baby-sitter on all safety items
3. Has emerging desires to look at, handle, and touch objects	3. a. Experiment with diversionary measures b. Provide child with own play objects
4. Explores objects by sucking, chewing, and biting	4. a. Remove household poisons, cosmetics, pins, and buttons that he could put in his mouth b. Be certain that objects that go into mouth are hygienic c. Check toys for detachable small parts
5. Beginning to test reactions to certain parental responses during feeding and may become choosy about food	5. a. Once problem behaviors are defined, plan to work on changing only one behavior at a time until child behaves or conforms to expectations b. Be certain that child understands old rules before adding new ones c. Respond with consistency in enforcing old rules: enforce each time, do not ignore next time d. Provide regular pattern of mealtimes e. Refrain from feeding throughout day f. Allow child to decide what he will eat and how much g. Introduce new foods gradually over period of time h. Continue to offer foods that may have been rejected first time i. Do not force food j. Refrain from physically punishing child for changes in eating habits
6. Beginning to test reactions to parental responses at bedtime preparation	6. a. Provide regular time for naps and bedtime b. Avoid excessive stimulation at bedtime or naptime c. Ignore fussing and crying once safety and physical needs are satisfied and usual ritual is carried out d. Keep child in own room e. Refrain from picking up and rocking and holding if needs seem satisfied

Continued.

Discipline—cont'd

Expected tasks	*Suggested activities*
13 to 18 months	
1. Understands simple commands and requests	1. a. Begin with one rule; add new ones as appropriate b. In selecting new rules, choose on the basis of being able to clearly define it to self and child, having it reasonable and enforceable at all times; demand no more than fulfillment of defined expectations c. Plan decisive limits and plan to give consistent attention to them
2. In learning mastery over impulses and self-control, child begins testing out limit setting	2. a. Immediately correct errors in behavior as they occur b. Use consistent enforcement of short-term rules (which are given as verbal commands) and long-term rules (which pertain to chores and family routines) c. Ignore temper tantrums d. Show child when you approve of his behavior and praise for obedience throughout day
3. With increasing fine motor control, child can manipulate objects that may be hazardous	3. a. Set limits regarding play with doorknobs and car door handles b. Keep away from open windows; latch screens c. Supervise around pools and ponds or drain or fence them d. Lock cabinets e. Keep open jars and bottles out of reach f. Use gate to protect child from falling down stairs
19 to 30 months	
1. Attention span increasing	1. a. Gain attention before giving simple commands, one at a time; praise for success b. Add new rules as child conforms to old ones c. Refrain from expecting *immediate* obedience
2. Begins simple reasoning—asks question why; may be repetitive	2. Make special efforts to answer questions; give simple explanations; gauge need for simplicity by number of times act is repeated or question asked
3. Interested in further exploration of environment; may lack physical control	3. a. Supervise on stair rails and waxed floors b. Set rules about crossing streets and carrying knives, sharp objects, or glass objects c. Have outdoor play area securely fenced or supervised d. When riding in car, secure child safely by seat belt or insist on his sitting in back seat; do not permit standing on car seats e. Keep matches out of reach f. Shield adult tools such as knives, lawnmowers, sharp tools
4. Negativistic behavior is expected; responds more frequently with word "no"; may show more resistance at bedtime preparation and during mealtime	4. a. Practice consistency in responding to behavior b. Allow more time to conform to expectation
5. Behavior may change if new sibling is introduced into family unit	5. a. Explain verbally or through play that new child is expected b. Exercise more patience with child c. Set special times aside for parental attention to child d. Allow child to help with special care tasks of new sibling
31 to 48 months	
1. Displays more interest in conforming	1. a. Exercise consistency in parental demands; enforce each time and avoid ignoring behavior next time b. Show concrete approval and give immediate recognition for acceptable behavior c. Refrain from use of threats that produce fearfulness
2. Shows greater understanding when simple reasoning is communicated	2. a. Give simple explanations; allow child chance to demonstrate understanding by talking about event, situation, or rule b. Eliminate unnecessary and impractical rules c. Refrain from constant verbal reprimands d. Denial of privileges should not be excessive or prolonged

Discipline—cont'd

Expected tasks	*Suggested activities*
3. Will respond to simple commands such as putting toys away	3. a. Assign simple household tasks that child can carry out each day; show approval for performance and success b. Decide if child is capable of doing what is asked by observing him c. Determine how much time is necessary to complete a chore or activity before expecting maximum performance
4. Displays a greater independence in general activities	4. a. Be extra cautious about supervising riding tricycles in streets and watching for cars in driveways b. Do not permit dashing into street while playing c. Do not allow child to follow ball into street d. Areas under swings and slides should not be paved e. Provide an imitative model that child can copy, for example, do not jaywalk f. Provide scissors that are blunt tipped
49 to 52 months	
1. Can be given two or three assignments at one time; will carry out in order 2. Complies readily with reasonable, well-defined, and consistent requirements 3. Understands reasoning	1. Give more opportunities to be independent 2. Use simple explanations and reasoning 3. Ask child to define role if he disobeys 4. Have child correct mistakes as they occur 5. Do not use punishment without warnings 6. Praise for successful performance 7. Use gold stars on chart for rewards 8. If leaving for social obligation, vacation, or visiting away from home, let child know 9. Avoid making promises that cannot be kept 10. Avoid bribing, ridicule, shaming, teasing, inflicting pain, using unfavorable comparison with other children, and exhibition of behavior by parents they are trying to stop in child 11. Remember that child may be imitating models of behavior set up by parents, brothers, sisters, a neighborhood child, or maybe a television hero 12. Recognize that there are stress periods in family or child's life that may result in changes in child's behavior including accidents, illness, moving into new neighborhood, separation from friends, death, divorce, and hospitalization of child or parents (be more patient with child's behavior, give more time to conform, show more approval for mastery of tasks, and exercise consistency in handling problems as they occur)

Dressing

Expected tasks	Suggested activities
13 to 18 months	
1. Cooperates in dressing by extending arm or leg 2. Removes socks, hat, mittens, shoes 3. Can unzip zippers 4. Tries to put shoes on	1. Encourage child to remove socks, etc. after task is initiated for him 2. Do not rush child 3. Have him practice with large buttons and with zippers
19 to 30 months	
1. Can undress 2. Can remove shoes if laces are untied 3. Helps dress 4. Tries to unbutton 5. Pulls on simple clothes	1. Provide opportunities to button with extra-large–sized buttons 2. Encourage and allow opportunity for self-help in getting drink, removing clothes with help, hand washing, unbuttoning, etc. 3. Simple clothing 4. Provide mirror at height child can observe himself for brushing teeth, etc.
31 to 48 months	
1. Greater interest and ability in dressing 2. Intent on lacing shoes (usually does incorrectly) 3. Does not know back from front 4. Washes and dries hands, brushes teeth 5. Can button	1. Provide with own dresser drawer 2. Simple garments encourage self-help; do not rush child 3. Provide large buttons, zippers, slipover clothing 4. Self hand washing but help with brushing teeth 5. Provide regular routine for dressing, either in bathroom or bedroom
49 to 52 months	
1. Dresses and undresses with care except for tying shoes and buckling belts 2. May learn to tie shoes 3. Combs hair with assistance	1. Assign regular task of placing clothes in hamper or basket 2. Continue to use simple clothing 3. Encourage self-help in dressing and undressing 4. Allow child to select clothes he will wear

Toilet training

Expected tasks	Suggested activities
9 to 12 months	
1. Beginning to show regular patterns in bladder and bowel elimination 2. Has one to two stools daily 3. Interval of dryness does not exceed 1 to 2 hours	1. Watch for clues that indicate child is wet or soiled 2. Be sure to change diapers when wet or soiled so that child begins to experience contrast between wetness and dryness
13 to 18 months	
1. Will have bowel movement if put on toilet at approximate time 2. Indicates wet pants	1. Sit child on toilet or potty chair at regular intervals for short periods of time throughout day 2. Praise child for success 3. If potty chair is used, it should be located in bathroom 4. Training should be started when social disruptions are at minimum 5. Respond promptly to signals and clues of child by taking him to bathroom or changing pants 6. Use training pants, once toilet training is commenced 7. Plan to begin training when disruptions in regular routine are minimized, that is, do not begin on vacation
19 to 30 months	
1. Anticipates need to eliminate 2. Same word for both functions 3. Daytime control (occasional accident) 4. Requires assistance (reminding, dressing, wiping)	1. Continue regular intervals of toileting 2. Reward success 3. Dress in simple clothing that child can manage 4. Remind occasionally, particularly after mealtime, juicetime, naptime, and playtime 5. Take to bathroom before bedtime 6. Bathroom should be convenient to use, easy to open door
31 to 48 months	
1. Takes responsibility for toilet if clothes are simple 2. Continues to verbalize need to go; apt to hold out too long 3. May have occasional accident 4. Needs help with wiping	1. May still need reminding 2. Dress in simple clothing that child can manage 3. Ignore accidents; refrain from shame or ridicule
49 to 52 months	
1. General independence (anticipates needs, undresses, goes, wipes, washes hands)	1. Praise child for his accomplishment

9-2 Immunization schedules

Recommended schedule for active immunization of normal infants and children

Age	*Immunization recommended*
2 months	DTP,* TOPV†
4 months	DTP, TOPV
6 months	DTP‡
1 year	Tuberculin test§
15 months	Measles, rubella, mumps‖
18 months	DTP, TOPV
4-6 years	DTP, TOPV
14-16 years	Td¶—repeat every 10 years

Modified from American Academy of Pediatrics: Report of the Committee on Infectious Diseases, III, ed. 19, 1982. Copyright 1982 American Academy of Pediatrics.

*DTP—diptheria and tetanus toxoids combined with pertussis vaccine.

†TOPV—trivalent oral poliovirus vaccine. This recommendation is suitable for breast-fed as well as bottle-fed infants.

‡A third dose of TOPV is optional but may be given in areas of high endemicity of poliomyelitis.

§Frequency of tuberculin testing depends on risk of exposure of the child and on the prevalence of tuberculosis in the population group. The initial test should be at or preceding the measles vaccine.

‖May be given at 15 months as measles-rubella or measles-mumps-rubella combined vaccines.

¶Td—combined tetanus and diphtheria toxoids (adult type) for those more than 6 years of age, in contrast to diphtheria and tetanus (DT) toxoids which contain a larger amount of diphtheria antigen.

Recommended immunization schedules for infants and children not initially immunized at usual recommended times in early infancy

Timing	*Preferred schedule*	*Alternatives**		
		No. 1	*No. 2*	*No. 3*
First visit	DTP No. 1, OPV No. 1, tuberculin test (PPD)	MMR,† PPD	DTP No. 1, OPV No. 1, PPD	DTP No. 1, OPV No. 1, MMR, PPD
1 month later	MMR	DTP No. 1, OPV No. 1	MMR, DTP No. 2	DTP No. 2
2 months later	DTP No. 2, OPV No. 2	—	DTP No. 3, OPV No. 2	DTP No. 3, OPV No. 2
3 months later	DTP No. 3‡	DTP No. 2, OPV No. 2	—	—
4 months later	DTP No. 3 (OPV No. 3)§	—	(OPV No. 3)	(OPV No. 3)
5 months later	—	DTP No. 3 (OPV No. 3)	—	—
10-16 months after last dose	DTP No. 4, OPV No. 3, or OPV No. 4	DTP No. 4, OPV No. 3, or OPV No. 4	DTP No. 4, OPV No. 3, or OPV No. 4	DTP No. 4, OPV No. 3, or OPV No. 4
Preschool‖	DTP No. 5, OPV No. 4, or OPV No. 5	DTP No. 5, OPV No. 4, or OPV No. 5	DTP No. 5, OPV No. 4, or OPV No. 5	DTP No. 5, OPV No. 4, or OPV No. 5
Age 14-16	Td¶	Td	Td	Td

Adapted from American Academy of Pediatrics: Report of the Committee on Infectious Diseases, Ill., ed. 19, 1982. Copyright American Academy of Pediatrics, 1982.

*Alternative No. 1 can be used in children more than 15 months old if measles is occurring in the community.

Alternative No. 2 allows for more rapid DTP immunization.

Alternative No. 3 should be reserved for those whose access to medical care is compromised by poor compliance.

†MMR should be given to children no younger than 15 monthws.

‡Can be given if OPV No. 3 not administered until 10-16 months.

§OPV No. 3 optional for areas likely to import polio (some southwestern states).

‖Not necessary if DTP No. 4 administered after fourth birthday.

¶Repeat every 10 years.

9-3 Possible side effects and nursing responsibilities of recommended childhood immunizations*

Immunization	*Reaction*	*Nursing responsibilities*
Diphtheria	Fever usually within 24-48 hours Soreness, redness, and swelling at site of injection	Instructions for DTP: Advise parents of possible side effects; may recommend prophylactic use of aspirin or acetaminophen if fever occurred following previous DTP immunization; recommend its use if fever occurs following present immunization; advise parents to notify physician immediately of any unusual side effects, such as those listed under pertussis
Tetanus	Same as for diphtheria but may include urticaria and malaise All may have delayed onset and last several days Lump at injection site may last for weeks, even months, but gradually disappears	
Pertussis	Same as for tetanus but may include loss of consciousness, convulsions, and thrombocytopenia	
Poliovirus (TOPV)	Essentially no side effects Vaccine-associated paralysis usually occurs within 2 months of immunization	See general comment to parents*
Measles	Anorexia, malaise, rash, and fever may occur 7 to 10 days after immunization Rarely (estimated risk 1 in 1 million doses) encephalitis may occur	Advise parents of more common side effects and use of antipyretics for fever; if a persistent high fever with other obvious signs of illness occurs, have them notify physician immediately
Mumps	Essentially no side effects other than a brief, mild fever	See general comment to parents*
Rubella	Mild rash that lasts 1 or 2 days within a few days after immunization Arthralgia, arthritis, and/or paresthesia of the hands and fingers may occur about 2 weeks after vaccination and is more frequent in older children and adults	Advise parents of side effects, especially of time delay before joint swelling and pain; assure them that these symptoms will disappear; may recommend use of mild analgesics for pain

*General comment to parents regarding each immunization: The benefit of being protected by the immunization is believed to greatly outweigh the risk from the disease.

9-4 Infectious diseases that occur during early childhood

Disease	Infectious agent	Source	Transmission	Incubation period	Period of communicability	Clinical manifestation
Chickenpox	Varicella-zoster	Primarily secretions of respiratory tract of infected person; to a lesser degree skin lesions (scabs not infectious)	Direct contact, droplet spread, and objects contaminated by contact with skin lesions and mucous membranes of infectious persons	2-3 weeks; commonly 13-17 days	Probably 1 day before eruption of lesions (prodromal period) to 6 days after first crop of vesicles when crusts have formed; most communicable in early stages of dermal eruptions	Prodromal stage: slight fever, malaise, and anorexia for first 24 hours: rash highly pruritic, begins as macule, rapidly progresses to papule and then vesicle (surrounded by erythematous base, becomes umbilicated and cloudy, breaks easily, and forms crusts); all three stages present in varying degrees at one time Distribution: centripetal, spreading to face and proximal extremities, but sparse on distal limbs Constitutional signs and symptoms: lymphadenopathy, temperature, irritability from pruritus
Diphtheria	*Corynebacterium diphtheriae*	Discharges from mucous membranes of nose and nasopharynx, from skin, and from other lesions of infected person	Direct contact with infected person, a carrier, or contaminated articles from discharge of infected person	Usually 2-5 days, possibly longer	Variable; until virulent bacili are no longer present (identified by three negative cultures); usually 2 weeks or less, but sometimes as long as 4 weeks	Varies according to anatomic location of pseudomembrane Nasal: resembles common cold, serosanguineous mucopurulent nasal discharge without constitutional symptoms; may be frank epistaxis Tonsillar/pharyngeal: malaise; anorexia; sore throat; low-grade fever; pulse increased above expected for temperature within 24 hours; smooth, adherent, white or gray membrane: lymphadenitis possibly pronounced (bull's neck); in severe cases, toxemia, septic shock, and death within 6-10 days Laryngeal: fever, hoarseness, cough, with or without signs of above; potential airway obstruction, apprehensive, dyspneic retractions, cyanosis
Erythema infectiosum (fifth disease)	Probably virus	Infected persons	Presumably direct contact by droplet infection	6-14 days	Uncertain; most outbreaks subside in 1-2 months	Rash appears in three stages: I—Erythema on face, chiefly on cheeks, "slapped face" appearance; disappears by 1-4 days II—About 1 day after rash appears on face, maculopapular red spots appear, symmetrically distributed on upper and lower extremities: rash progresses from proximal and distal surfaces and may last a week or more III—Rash subsides but reappears if skin is irritated or traumatized (sun, hot, cold, friction)

Treatment	Nursing considerations	Control measures	Complications
Specific: none Supportive: benadryl or antihistamines to relieve itching; skin care to prevent secondary bacterial infection	Administer skin care: give daily bath; change clothes and linens daily; administer topical application of calamine lotion or paste of baking soda and water; keep child's fingernails short and clean; apply mittens if child must scratch Lessen pruritus; keep child occupied Remove loose crusts that rub and irritate skin Teach child to apply pressure to pruritic area rather than scratch it If older child, reason with him regarding danger of scar formation from scratching	Immunization not available Isolation of child in home until vesicles have dried (usually 1 week after onset of disease) Isolation of high-risk children (including neonates born of mothers who contract the disease 5 days or less before delivery and infants less than 1 month of age); treatment of exposed high-risk children includes administration of immune serum globulin (ISG) or zoster immune globulin (ZIG); one attack confers permanent immunity, although second attack of herpes zoster (shingles) can occur in susceptible children or adults	Secondary bacterial infections (abscesses, cellulitis, pneumonia, sepsis) Encephalitis Varicella pneumonia Hemorrhagic varicella (tiny hemorrhages in the vesicles and numerous petechiae in the skin)
Antitoxin (usually intravenously): preceded by skin or conjunctival test to rule out sensitivity to horse serum Antibiotics (penicillin or erythromycin) Complete bed rest (prevention of myocarditis) Tracheostomy for airway obstruction	Maintain *strict* isolation Participate in sensitivity testing; have epinephrine available Administer antibiotics; observe for signs of sensitivity to penicillin Administer *complete* care to maintain bed rest Use suctioning as needed Regulate humidity for optimal liquefaction of secretions Observe respirations for signs of obstruction	Immunization during infancy and boosters every 10 years after initial series Strict isolation of all symptomatic persons Treatment of infected contacts (positive throat cultures and Schick test) and carriers (positive throat cultures but negative Schick test)	Myocarditis (second week) Neuritis
None necessary	Support parents regarding benign nature of condition	None specific, except isolation of child from other siblings	Self-limited arthritis and arthralgia

Continued.

Infectious diseases that occur during early childhood—cont'd

Disease	*Infectious agent*	*Source*	*Transmission*	*Incubation period*	*Period of communicability*	*Clinical manifestations*
Exanthem subitum (roseola)	Probably virus	Unknown	Unknown (limited virtually to children between 6 months and 2 years of age)	Unknown	Unknown	Persistent high fever for 3-4 days in child who appears well Precipitous drop in fever to normal with appearance of rash Rash: discrete rose-pink macules or maculopapules, appearing first on trunk, then spreading to neck, face, and extremities; nonpruritic, fades on pressure, lasts 1-2 days Associated signs and symptoms cervical/postauricular lymphadenopathy, injected pharynx, occasionally catarrhal otitis media
Measles (rubeola)	Virus	Respiratory tract secretions, blood, and urine of infected person	Usually by direct contact with droplets of infected person; less commonly by airborne or indirect contact with articles freshly contaminated by respiratory tract secretions	10-20 days	From 4 days before to 5 days after rash appears, mostly during catarrhal phase	Prodromal stage: fever and malaise, followed in 24 hours by coryza, cough, conjunctivitis, Koplik spots (small irregular red spots with a minute bluish white center first seen on the buccal mucosa opposite the molars) 2 days prior to rash symptoms gradually increase in severity until second day after rash appears, when they begin to subside Rash: appears 3-4 days after onset of prodromal stage: begins as erythematous maculopapular eruption on face and gradually spreads downward; more severe in earlier sites (appears confluent) and less intense in later sites (appears discrete); after 3-4 days, assumes brownish appearance and fine desquamation occurs over areas of extensive involvement Constitutional signs and symptoms: anorexia, malaise, generalized lymphadenopathy
Mumps	Virus	Saliva of infected persons	Direct contact with or droplet spread from an infected person	14-21 days	Most communicable immediately before and after swelling begins; virus present in saliva up to 7 days before and 9 days after parotid swelling	Prodromal stage: fever, headache, malaise, and anorexia for 24 hours, followed by "earache" that is aggravated by chewing Parotitis: by third day, parotid gland(s) (either unilateral or bilateral) enlarges and reaches maximal size in 1-3 days; accompanied by pain and tenderness Other manifestations: submaxillary and sublingual infection, orchitis, and meningoencephalitis

Treatment	Nursing considerations	Control measures	Complications
None specific Antipyretics to control fever Anticonvulsives for child with history of febrile seizures	Teach parents measures for lowering temperature (antipyretic drugs and tepid sponge baths) If child is prone to seizures, discuss appropriate precautions Reassure parents regarding benign nature of illness	None	Febrile seizures
Supportive: bed rest during febrile period Antipyretics Antibiotics to prevent secondary bacterial infection in high-risk children	Maintain bed rest during prodromal stage; provide quiet activity Fever: instruct parents to administer antipyretics and cool sponge bath; avoid chilling; if child is prone to seizures, institute appropriate precautions (fever spikes to 40° C [104° F] between fourth and fifth days) Eye care: dim lights if photophobia present; cleanse eyelids with warm saline solution to remove secretions or crusts; keep child from rubbing the eyes; examine cornea for signs of ulceration Coryza/cough: use cool mist vaporizer; protect skin around nares with layer of petrolatum; encourage fluids and soft bland foods Skin care: keep skin clean; use tepid baths as necessary	Immunization with measles virus vaccine at 15 months of age (if given earlier to provide protection during an epidemic, vaccine needs to be repeated at this age because of suppression of immunity by maternal antibodies) Gamma globulin may prevent or modify the illness and prevent complications in unimmunized and high-risk children One attack of measles confers lifelong immunity Isolation only necessary until fifth day of rash; if hospitalized, respiratory precautions are instituted	Otitis media Pneumonia Bronchiolitis Obstructive laryngitis and laryngotracheitis Encephalitis
Symptomatic and supportive: analgesics for pain and antipyretics for fever Intravenous fluid may be necessary for child who refuses to drink or vomits because of meningoencephalitis	Maintain bed rest during prodromal phase until swelling subsides Give analgesics for pain; if child is unwilling to chew medication, use elixir form Encourage fluids and soft bland foods; avoid foods requiring chewing Apply hot or cold compresses to neck, whichever is more comforting To relieve orchitis, provide warmth and local support by means of a nest of absorbent cotton in the diaper or tight-fitting underpants (stretch bathing suit works well)	Immunization of all infants at 15 months of age Passive protection with gamma globulin ineffective Confinement to the home recommended during period of communicability; respiratory isolation is required during hospitalization One attack of bilateral, unilateral, or inapparent infection usually confers permanent immunity	Sensorineural deafness Postinfectious encephalitis Myocarditis Arthritis Hepatitis Sterility (in adult males)

Continued.

Infectious diseases that occur during early childhood—cont'd

Disease	*Infectious agent*	*Source*	*Transmission*	*Incubation period*	*Period of communicability*	*Clinical manifestations*
Poliomyelitis	Enteroviruses: type I—most frequent cause of paralysis, both epidemic and endemic; type 2—least frequently associated with paralysis; type 3—second most frequent	Feces and oropharyngeal secretions of infected persons, especially young children	Direct contact with persons with apparent or inapparent active infection; spread is via fecal-oral and pharyngeal-oropharyngeal routes	Usually 7-14 days, with range of 5-35 days	Not exactly known; virus is present in throat and feces shortly after infection and persists for about 1 week in throat and 4-6 weeks in feces	May be manifest in three different forms: Abortive or inapparent—fever, uneasiness, sore throat, headache, anorexia, vomiting, abdominal pain; lasts a few hours to a few days Nonparalytic—same manifestations as abortive but more severe, with pain and stiffness in neck, back, and legs Paralytic—initial course similar to nonparalytic type, followed by recovery and then signs of central nervous system paralysis; acute stage (about 5-7 days) characterized by headache, vomiting, fever, stiffness of back and neck (tripod sign—unable to sit up straight unless hands are used to brace self), pain in back, limbs, and neck, and finally paralysis; any muscle groups may be involved, but demonstrates predilection for large muscles; respiratory paralysis may occur from damage to nerve cells in cervicothoracic segments of spinal cord or damage to vital centers in medulla (bulbar poliomyelitis); recovery may be complete over several months or associated with residual paralysis
Pertussis (whooping cough)	Bordetella pertussis	Discharge from respiratory tract of infected persons	Direct contact or droplet spread from infected person; indirect contact with freshly contaminated articles	5-21 days, usually 10	Greatest during catarrhal stage before onset of paroxysms and may extend to fourth week after onset of paroxysms	Catarrhal stage: begins with symptoms of upper respiratory infection, such as coryza, sneezing, lacrimation, cough, and low-grade fever, symptoms continue for 1-2 weeks, when dry hacking cough becomes more severe Paroxysmal stage: cough that most commonly occurs at night consists of a series of short rapid coughs, followed by a sudden inspiration that is associated with a high-pitched crowing sound or "whoop"; during paroxysms, cheek becomes flushed or cyanotic, eyes bulge, and tongue protrudes; paroxysm may continue until a thick mucus plus is dislodged; vomiting frequently follows an attack; stage generally lasts 4-6 weeks, followed by convalescent stage

Treatment	Nursing considerations	Control measures	Complications
No specific treatment, including antimicrobials or gamma globulin Supportive treatment; complete bed rest during acute phase Assisted respiratory ventilation in case of respiratory paralysis Physical therapy for muscles following acute stage	Maintain complete bed rest Administer mild sedatives as necessary to relieve anxiety and promote rest Participate in physiotherapy procedures (use of moist hot packs and range-of-motion exercise) Position child to maintain body alignment and prevent contractures or decubiti; use footboard Encourage child to move; administer analgesics for maximum comfort during physical activity Observe for respiratory paralysis (difficulty in talking, ineffective cough, inability to hold the breath, shallow and rapid respirations); report such signs and symptoms to physician; have tracheostomy tray at bedside	Immunization of all children with complete series of trivalent oral poliovirus vaccine Vaccination of close contacts who have not been adequately immunized During an epidemic, avoid visiting families with known cases, overexertion or chilling, eating unwashed fresh fruits or vegetables, surgical procedures in nose and oropharynx, and unnecessary injections, including vaccination other than for poliomyelitis	Permanent paralysis Respiratory arrest Hypertension Kidney stones from demineralization of bone during prolonged immobility
Antimicrobial therapy (such as erythromycin) Administration of pertussis-immune globulin Supportive treatment: hospitalization required for infants, children who are dehydrated, or those who have complications Bed rest Increased oxygen intake and humidity Adequate fluids Intubation possibly necessary	Maintain bed rest as long as fever is present Keep child occupied during the day (interest in play is associated with fewer paroxysms) Reassure parents during frightening episodes of whooping cough Provide restful environment and reduce factors that promote paroxysms (dust, smoke, sudden change in temperature, chilling, activity, excitement); keep room well-ventilated Encourage fluids: offer small frequent fluids; refeed child after vomiting Keep child in Croupette with high humidity; suction gently but often to prevent choking on secretion Observe for signs of airway obstruction (increased restlessness, apprehension, retractions, cyanosis) Involve public health nurse if child is cared for at home	Immunization during early infancy (2 months of age); no passive immunity from mother and absence of IgM antibodies Value of pertussis immune globulin in preventing illness is questionable If child is hospitalized, respiratory isolation required One attack usually confers permanent immunity	Pneumonia (usual cause of death) Atelectasis Otitis media Convulsions Hemorrhage (subarachnoid, subconjunctival, epistaxis) Weight loss and dehydration Hernia Prolapsed rectum

Continued.

Infectious diseases that occur during early childhood—cont'd

Disease	*Infectious agent*	*Source*	*Transmission*	*Incubation period*	*Period of communicability*	*Clinical manifestations*
Rubella (German measles)	Virus	Primarily nasopharyngeal secretions of persons with apparent or inapparent infection; virus also present in blood, stool, and urine	Direct contact and spread via infected person; indirectly via articles freshly contaminated with nasopharyngeal secretions, feces, or urine	14-21 days	7 days before to about 5 days after appearance of rash	Prodromal phase: absent in children, present in adults and adolescents; consists of low-grade fever, headache, malaise, anorexia, mild conjunctivitis, coryza, sore throat, cough, and lymphadenopathy; lasts for 1-5 days, subsides 1 day after appearance of rash Rash: first appears in face and rapidly spreads downward to neck, arms, trunk, and legs, by end of first day, body is covered with a discrete pinkish-red maculopapular exanthema; disappears in same order as it began and is usually gone by third day Constitutional signs and symptoms: occasionally low-grade fever, headaches, malaise, and lymphadenopathy
Congenital rubella	Primarily nasopharyngeal secretions of persons with apparent or inapparent infection; virus also present in blood, stool, and urine	Direct contact and spread via infected person; indirectly via articles freshly contaminated with nasopharyngeal secretions, feces, or urine	Transplacental	Not applicable; virus is only dangerous to fetus during first trimester	Infants may be infectious for months; virus shedding from throat disappears by 6 months of age in 80% to 90% of cases	Virtually any organ can be affected; classic rubella syndrome characterized by growth retardation, cerebral defects (mental retardation, microcephaly), deafness, eye defects (cataracts, strabismus, retinopathy), congenital heart disease (patent ductus arteriosus [PDA], ventricular septal defect; coarctation of the aorta, pulmonary stenosis), thrombocytopenic purpura, behavioral abnormalities—unusual pleasure in rocking, obsession with lights, lack of recognition of human relationships, little interest in food, difficulties with toilet training
Scarlet fever	Group A beta hemolytic streptococcus	Usually from nasopharyngeal secretions of infected persons and carriers	Direct contact with infected person or droplet spread; indirectly by contact with contaminated articles, ingestion of contaminated milk or other food	2-4 days with range of 1-7 days	During incubation period and clinical illness, approximately 10 days; during first 2 weeks of carrier phase, although may persist for months	Prodromal stage: abrupt high fever, pulse increased out of proportion to fever, vomiting, headache, chills, malaise, abdominal pain

Treatment	*Nursing considerations*	*Control measures*	*Complications*
No treatment necessary other than antipyretics for low-grade fever and analgesics for discomfort Antibiotics not indicated because secondary bacterial infection does not occur	Reassure parents of benign nature of illness Employ comfort measures as necessary Isolate child from pregnant women	Routine immunization of all children (usually at 15 months of age) and of all females before childbearing age See also measures included under congenital rubella	Complications rare (arthritis, encephalitis, or purpura); most benign of childhood communicable diseases; greatest danger is teratogenic effect on fetus
Strict isolation of neonates with rubella until throat culture is free of virus Medical treatment as indicated by various anomalies (chief causes of death are sepsis, congestive heart failure, and general debility) Rehabilitation of children who survive infancy	Identify neonates with congenital rubella and institute *strict* isolation *immediately* Select nursing personnel to care for infant who are not at high risk for rubella infection	See also preceding discussion of rubella Do not administer rubella vaccine to pregnant women (threat of contracting disease from newly vaccinated children negligible) Immunization of women of childbearing age with low hemagglutination-inhibition (HI) titer who agree to use contraception for 2 months after receiving immunization Use of immune serum globulin in pregnant women exposed to rubella who have low HI antibodies Elective therapeutic abortion for pregnant women with known (or suspected) infection during first trimester Isolate women at risk of contracting rubella from contact with infant	Same as outlined under clinical manifestations
Treatment of choice is a full course of penicillin (or erythromycin in penicillin-sensitive children); fever should subside 24 hours after beginning therapy Supportive measures: bed rest during febrile phase, analgesics for sore throat	Ensure compliance with oral antibiotic therapy (intramuscular benzathine penicillin G [Bicillin] may be given if parents' reliability in giving oral drugs is questionable) Maintain bed rest during febrile phase; provide quiet activity during convalescent period	Respiratory isolation of children with scarlet fever until 24 hours after initiation of treatment Throat cultures of children with sore throat and penicillin therapy for those with positive group A streptococci test Antibiotic therapy for newly diagnosed carriers (nose or throat cultures positive for streptococcus)	Otitis media Peritonsillar abscess Sinusitis Rheumatic fever Glomerulonephritis

Continued.

Infectious diseases that occur during early childhood—cont'd

Disease	*Infectious agent*	*Source*	*Transmission*	*Incubation period*	*Period of communicability*	*Clinical manifestations*
						Enanthema: tonsils enlarged, edematous, reddened, and covered with patches of exudate; in severe cases appearance resembles membrane seen in diphtheria; pharynx is edematous and briefly red; during first 1 or 2 days tongue is coated and papillae (become red and swollen) (white strawberry tongue); by the fourth or fifth day white coat sloughs off, leaving prominent papillae (red strawberry tongue); palate is covered with erythematous punctate lesions Exanthema: rash appears within 12 hours after prodromal signs: red pinhead-sized punctate lesions rapidly become generalized but are absent on the face, which becomes flushed; rash is more intense in folds of joints; by end of the first week, desquamation begins which may be complete by 3 weeks or longer
Smallpox (variola)	Poxvirus (variola)	Respiratory secretions and lesions of skin and mucous membranes of infected person	Prolonged direct contact with infected person; indirectly by articles freshly contaminated with crusts or secretions	12 days, with range of 7-17 days	Onset of first symptom to disappearance of all scabs, usually about 2-3 weeks	Prodromal stage: abrupt onset with chills, fever (reaches peak by end of second day), headache, backaches, and prostration; lasts 2-4 days, and symptoms begin to improve as rash develops Eruption period: painful lesions appear on mucous membranes of mouth, throat, and respiratory tract, causing symptoms of sore throat, hoarseness, and cough: macules first appear on face, forearm, trunk, (especially back), and finally lower extremities; intensity of rash is centrifugal—denser on preipheral than on central regions; within a few hours, macules become papules; by sixth day from onset of illness they become vesicles, then pustules, finally they form crusts by end of 14 days; during pustular stage constitutional signs worsen and lesions are painful; dessication of lesions is accompanied by intense pruritis and is followed by 1- to 2-week period of desquamation

Treatment	*Nursing considerations*	*Control measures*	*Complications*
	Relieve discomfort of sore throat with analgesics, gargles, lozenges, antiseptic throat sprays (Chloraseptic), and inhalation of cool mist encourage fluids during febrile phase; avoid irritating liquids (citrus juices) or rough foods; when child is able to eat, begin with soft diet Advise parents to consult physician if fever persists after beginning therapy Discuss procedures for preventing spread of infection	Prophylactic antibiotic therapy of household contacts, ideally those with cultures positive for streptococcus, regardless of associated symptoms, or an upper respiratory infection Proper food handling (use of pasteurized milk and exclusion of infected persons from handling food)	
No specific treatment available; patients are placed under strict isolation; antibiotics are used if bacterial infection is present Supportive therapy: adequate fluids, calories, and electrolytes (may require gavage feeding because oral and intravenous routes are incapacitated by presence of lesions), analgesics, antipruritics	Ensure strict isolation procedures; maintain complete bed rest; schedule analgesics to ensure optimum comfort Cleanse eyes with sterile saline solution to remove crusts, inspect cornea for evidence of infection Observe patterns of fever (peaks on second to third day and during pustular stage but is only low grade at other times; normal by tenth to twelfth day); unusual spikes may indicate bacterial infection Although no special skin care indicated, change bedclothes and linens at least daily, especially during desquamation phase Prevent child from scratching: use mittens, keep fingernails short and clean, use elbow restraints Participate in immunization procedures of close contacts or general population if epidemic is anticipated	Routine immunization no longer recommended except for groups at risk (military, health personnel, and travelers to areas where disease is endemic) Strict isolation of infected person Vaccination or revaccination of persons presumably exposed to smallpox Use of vaccines of variola immune globulin (VIG) may prevent or modify disease in exposed individuals	Secondary bacterial infection: impetigo, furuncles, cellulitis, pneumonia, septicemia, osteomyelitis, keratitis, scarring, laryngeal edema, encephalitis, psychoses, abortion in pregnant women

9-5 Contraindications to routine immunizations

Contraindication	Immunization	Rationale	Nursing considerations
Acute febrile illness or chronic debilitating diseases	All	Masks febrile reactions from the immunization, decreases body's natural defense mechanisms	Explain reason for postponing immunization to parent and reschedule it at earliest return visit. For chronic diseases, check with physician before administering any immunization.
Gastroenteritis	Live poliovirus vaccine	May interfere with colonization of the viruses in the intestines, which is essential for the immune response to occur	Explain reason for postponing immunization and reschedule it as soon as possible.
Altered immune system Immunologic disease Generalized malignancy (leukemia, lymphoma) Immunosuppressive therapy (steroids, antimetabolites, radiation)	All live viral vaccines (measles, mumps, rubella, and polio)	Depressed immune defenses may result in extreme reactions to the immunizations	Emphasize to parents the need to prevent their children from exposure to any of these childhood diseases, because they cannot be artificially protected from them.
Recently acquired passive immunity Blood transfusion or immune serum globulin within last 6 weeks Maternal antibodies during first year	Measles, mumps, and rubella vaccines	Presence of passive immunity prevents formation of antibodies to the vaccine	Inquire during the history concerning recent blood transfusions or injections of immune serum globulin; wait recommended 6 weeks before administering the immunization; follow suggested schedule for measles, mumps, and rubella (15 months).
Allergy to substances in vaccine, for example, egg protein, neomycin	Live virus vaccines grown on chick embryos, treated with neomycin	Known hypersensitivity to substance will also result in reaction to substance in vaccine	Check manufacturer's product information for specific contraindications and screen child for known allergies to potential foreign substances.
History of nervous system disorders Reaction of high fever, somnolence, or convulsions following a DTP immunization	Pertussis vaccine	Danger of serious reaction to pertussis vaccination is greatly increased	Take a detailed neurological history, including past convulsions, fainting spells, tremors, or twitching and specific reactions to DTP; report any such findings to a physician before administering the pertussis vaccine.
Pregnancy	All live virus vaccines except for poliovirus	Potential risk to fetus, especially from rubella	Take a careful history of all women of childbearing age regarding the possibility of pregnancy within the next 2 months.

APPENDIX 10 MENTAL HEALTH

10-1 Psychiatric assessment guides

The following assessment guides have been developed to:

1. Identify high-risk factors that may contribute to and/or precipitate the development of mental illness
2. Determine the need for intervention when high-risk factors are present to prevent the development or recurrence of mental illness
3. Understand the interrelationship of biological, psychological, and social factors in the maintenance of mental health and the prevention of mental illness
4. Assess mental health status
5. Assess clients' strengths and weaknesses
6. Develop nursing strategies designed to utilize strengths
7. Develop nursing strategies designed to minimize weaknesses
8. Assess psychocultural perceptions and orientations concerning health and illness
9. Establish mental health goals consistent with clients' perceptions and orientations about health and illness
10. Assess the dynamics of group and family systems
11. View individuals, families, and groups as integral subsystems of a large social system

GUIDE FOR ASSESSMENT OF MENTAL HEALTH

I. Demographic data
  - A. Name
  - B. Address
  - C. Age
  - D. Sex
  - E. Education
  - F. Ethnicity (optional)*
  - G. Religion (optional)*
  - H. Living arrangements
  - I. Marital status

II. Admission data
  - A. Date and time of admission
  - B. Manner of admission
    1. Self
    2. Relatives
    3. Police
    4. Other (describe)
  - C. Form of retention (if hospitalized)
    1. Informal retention
    2. Voluntary retention
    3. Involuntary retention
    4. Emergency
    5. Comments
  - D. Reason for admission
  - E. Client's primary complaint
  - F. Client's premorbid personality

III. History of psychiatric problems
  - A. Previous condition: date; problem
  - B. Assistance sought: native healer; therapist; agency; clergyman; other (describe)
  - C. Current levels of functioning and coping

IV. Behavioral observations
  - A. Thought patterns
    1. Delusion: grandeur; persecution; somatic; self-accusatory
    2. Obsession
    3. Ideas of reference
    4. Phobia
    5. Looseness of association
    6. Flight of ideas
    7. Fugue
    8. Impaired judgment
    9. Impaired insight
    10. Impaired orientation to time, place, or person
    11. Impaired memory
    12. No observable thought disturbance
    13. Comments
  - B. Sensory processes
    1. Hallucination: olfactory; auditory; tactile; gustatory; visual
    2. No observable sensory disturbance
    3. Comments
  - C. Speech patterns
    1. Blocking
    2. Word salad
    3. Echolalia
    4. Circumstantiality
    5. Irrelevancy
    6. Confabulation
    7. Mutism
    8. Neologism
    9. Perseveration
    10. Stuttering
    11. No observable speech disturbance
    12. Comments
  - D. Affect
    1. Elation
    2. Depression
    3. Ambivalence
    4. Apathy
    5. Anger
    6. No observable disturbance of affect
    7. Comments
  - E. Motor activity
    1. Hyperactive
    2. Hypoactive
    3. Stereotypical: persistent; aimless; repetitive
    4. Perseveration
    5. Catalepsy: stupor; waxy flexibility
    6. Compulsion
    7. No observable disturbance in motor activity
    8. Comments

*Legislation protects people from being required to reveal ethnicity and religion.

F. Level of consciousness
   1. Confusion
   2. Stupor
   3. Delirium
   4. Alert
   5. Comments

V. Physical appearance
   A. Posture
      1. Sagging
      2. Rigid
      3. Curled into fetal position
      4. Bent
      5. No observable disturbance in posture
      6. Comments
   B. Facies
      1. Drooping or sagging: deflected eyes; lusterless eyes; drooping eyelids; deep nasolabial folds
      2. Uplifted or retracted: smiling; retracted brow; wide open eyes; darting eyes
      3. Blank: staring into space; distant expression in eyes
      4. Masklike or ironed-out
      5. Facial tic
      6. No observable disturbance in facies
      7. Comments
   C. Mode of dress
      1. Overly neat
      2. Disheveled
      3. Bizarre
      4. Appropriate
      5. Comments

VI. Physical status
   A. Vital signs: pulse; temperature; respirations; blood pressure
   B. Physical condition
      1. Medical problems: acute; chronic
      2. Physical aids (describe)
      3. Medications: date and time of last dose
      4. Allergies (describe)
      5. Comments
   C. Patterns of daily living
      1. Sleep patterns: restlessness; insomnia; narcoplexy; average number of hours of sleep
      2. Eating patterns: number of meals a day; compulsive eating; anorexia
      3. Drinking patterns: beverage; quantity consumed; frequency of consumption
      4. Sexual patterns: sexual orientation or preference; attitudes about sexuality; sexual activity
      5. Elimination patterns: constipation; diarrhea; urinary frequency; urinary retention
      6. Social patterns: recreation; work; intimacy; community involvement
      7. Comments
   D. Level of self-care
      1. Personal hygiene
      2. Activities of daily living
      3. Comments

VII. Cultural orientation
   A. Place of residence: multi-ethnic neighborhood; ethnic enclave
   B. Family organization: nuclear; extended; members composing family unit; members vested with authority; members involved in child rearing; sense of obligation of family members to one another.
   C. Sex-defined roles: stereotyped male and female roles; amount of independence permitted men and women; degree of intimacy permitted between married men and women, unmarried men and women
   D. Communication patterns: language spoken at home; language spoken outside home; use of touching and/or gesturing; interpersonal spacing
   E. Type of dress: traditional ethnic dress; Western-style dress
   F. Type of food: ethnic food; American food
   G. Relationship to people: individualistic; group-oriented; egalitarian; authoritative
   H. Relationship to time: past-oriented; present-oriented; future-oriented
   I. Relationship to the world: personal control; goal directed; fatalistic
   J. Health care patterns: ideas concerning causes of mental illness; ideas concerning treatment of mental illness; people consulted for treatment of mental illness (e.g., family member, native healer, mental health therapist, other [describe])
   K. Comments

VIII. Effective social network
   A. Family
   B. Household members (if different from family)
   C. Friends
   D. Associates: employer; coworkers; neighbors; others
   E. Religious affiliates: clergyman; church elders; congregants
   F. Comments

IX. Stressors
   A. Culture shock
      1. Communication (foreign verbal, kinesic, and proxemic systems)
      2. Mechanical environment (i.e., different types of food, housing, clothing, utilities)
      3. Social isolation from family and friends
      4. Foreign customs, standards, and/or values
      5. Different or new role relationships
   B. Life Changes
      1. Affectional: marriage; birth; death; divorce; abandonment
      2. Socioeconomic: promotion; demotion; unemployment, change of employment; change of residence; increased responsiblities
      3. Biophysical: serious illness (acute or chronic); surgery; accident; loss of body part; sexual trauma (e.g., rape, incest)
   C. Other (describe)
   D. No significant stress
   E. Comments

X. Coping mechanisms
   A. Coping mechanisms used (describe)
   B. Effectiveness of coping mechanisms
   C. Client's perception of mechanisms that are effective in reducing stress
   D. Comments

XI. Resources
   A. Personal: interests; leisure time activities; physical and mental abilities; educational achievement; other
   B. Social: interpersonal networks; economic support systems (e.g., health insurance, sick leave, union benefits); food, shelter, clothing; other
   C. Comments

XII. Candidacy for active involvement in treatment program
   A. Developmental level
   B. Interactional ability
   C. Willingness to participate in treatment program

D. Areas of anticipated need for assistance from nursing staff
E. Comments

GUIDE FOR ASSESSMENT OF FAMILY PROCESS

I. Demographic data
  A. Names of members
  B. Age of members
  C. Sex of members
  D. Relationship between members: affinal; consanguineous
  E. Educational levels of members
  F. Occupations of members
  G. Ethnicity (optional)*
  H. Religion (optional)*
  I. Family members living in another household (describe relationship)
  J. Nonfamily members living in the household (describe living arrangement)
  K. Other (describe)
II. Family organization
  A. Type of family: nuclear; extended
  B. Type of system: open; closed; boundary maintaining mechanisms (describe); norms; rules
  C. Members involved in child rearing
  D. Members vested with authority
  E. Sense of obligation of family members—roles: peacemaker; protector; attacker; provider; interpreter; rescuer; other
  F. Sex-defined roles: stereotyped male-female relationships; amount of independence permitted men and women
  G. Other (describe)
III. Family world view
  A. Relationship to people: individualistic; group-oriented; egalitarian; authoritarian
  B. Relationship to time: past-oriented; present-oriented; future-oriented
  C. Relationship to the world: personal control; goal-directed; fatalistic
  D. Comments
IV. Family perceptions and definitions
  A. Family
  B. Privacy
  C. Intimacy
  D. Health (mental and physical)
  E. Illness (mental and physical)
  F. Other (describe)
V. Family health care patterns
  A. Ideas concerning causes of illness (mental and physical)
  B. Ideas concerning treatment of illness (mental and physical)
  C. People consulted in times of crisis or for treatment of mental and physical illnesses (e.g., family member; native healer; mental health therapist; pharmacist; physician; other)
  D. Comments
VI. Family living arrangements
  A. Type of residence: multifamily dwelling; single-family dwelling; one-room dwelling; other
  B. Environment of residence: urban; suburban; rural; interethnic neighborhood; ethnic enclave
  C. Time in residence: length of time in present residence; length of time in previous residences
  D. Sleeping arrangements: number of rooms serving as bedrooms (differentiate between rooms functioning solely as bedrooms and those that have other functions)
  E. Eating arrangements: family members eat together; eat alone; eat in shifts
  F. Privacy arrangements: Rooms or sections of rooms reserved for specific family members; furniture (e.g., chairs) reserved for specific family members
  G. Other (describe)
VII. Family interaction patterns
  A. Communication patterns
    1. Verbal
      a. Language spoken at home
      b. Language spoken outside home
    2. Kinesic
      a. Touching
      b. Gesturing
    3. Proxemic
      a. Interpersonal spacing
      b. Fixed and/or built space
    4. Themes
      a. Double-bind messages
      b. Manipulation
      c. Scapegoating
      d. Intellectualization
      e. Blame placing
      f. Validation
      g. Other (describe)
  B. Behavioral patterns
    1. Physical acting out
    2. Isolation
    3. Detachment
    4. Cooperation
    5. Competition
    6. Overdependency
    7. Other (describe)
  C. Social patterns
    1. Alliances
      a. Among family members
      b. Between family members and members of social network
      c. Conflict between alliances
      d. Resolution of conflict between alliances
    2. Authority
      a. Nominal authority figure(s)
      b. Actual authority figure(s)
      c. Patterns of authority
      d. Implementation of authority: direct; delegated
    3. Decision making
      a. Nominal decision-making figure(s)
      b. Actual decision-making figure(s)
      c. Patterns of decision making
      d. Implementation of decisions
    4. Dissemination of information
      a. Sources of information
      b. Pattern of communicating information
    5. Social interaction
      a. Social network: relatives; friends; employers; coworkers; neighbors; clergy; other (describe)
      b. Community involvement: school; church; union; neighborhood; other (describe)
      c. Patterns of recreation
      d. Patterns of intimacy
    6. Other (describe)

*Legislation protects people from being required to reveal ethnicity and religion.

VIII. Family stressors
  A. Culture shock
    1. Communication: foreign verbal, kinesic, and proxemic systems
    2. Mechanical environment (i.e., different types of food, housing, clothing, utilities)
    3. Social isolation from family and friends
    4. Foreign customs, standards, and/or values
    5. Different or new role relationships
  B. Life changes
    1. Affectional: marriage; birth; death; divorce; abandonment
    2. Socioeconomic: promotion; demotion; unemployment; change of employment; change of residence
    3. Biophysical: Accident or serious illness involving a family member (acute or chronic)
  C. Other (describe)
  D. No significant stress
IX. Family coping mechanisms
  A. Coping mechanisms used (indicate whether mechanisms are used only by specific family members)
  B. Effectiveness of coping mechanisms
  C. Family's perception of mechanisms that are effective in reducing stress
  D. Comments
X. Family resources
  A. Familial: interests; leisure time activities; physical and mental abilities; other
  B. Social: interpersonal networks; economic support systems (e.g., health insurance, sick leave, union benefits); food, shelter, clothing; other

GUIDE FOR ASSESSMENT OF GROUP PROCESS

I. Description of group
  A. Type of group (e.g., activity, encounter, remotivation, psychodrama)
  B. Goals of group
  C. Size of group
  D. Composition of group
    1. Age of members
    2. Sex of members
    3. Ethnic background of members (optional)*
    4. Behavior exhibited by members
    5. Educational levels of members
    6. Communicational levels of members (e.g., verbal; mute; speak a foreign language)
    7. Reality testing levels of members
    8. Other (describe)

*Legislation protects people from being required to reveal ethnic background.

II. Characteristics of group
  A. Group phase or stage (orientation, working, termination)
  B. Level of cohesiveness
  C. Level of anxiety
  D. Level of conflict
  E. Level of resistance
  F. Other (describe)
III. Patterns of group interaction
  A. Communication patterns
    1. Silence
    2. Semantic argument
    3. Intellectualization
    4. Monopolization
    5. Scapegoating
    6. Other (describe)
  B. Behavior patterns
    1. Physical activity
    2. Withdrawal
    3. Detachment
    4. Cooperation
    5. Competition
    6. Other (describe)
  C. Social patterns
    1. Group norms
    2. Group rules
    3. Roles (e.g., peacemaker, leader, protector, attacker, interpreter)
    4. Alliances among members (subgroups)
    5. Conflict between alliances
    6. Other (describe)
IV. Patterns of leadership
  A. Approach of leader(s)
    1. Laissez-faire
    2. Democratic
    3. Power struggle
    4. Authoritarian
    5. Other (describe)
  B. Competence of leader(s)
    1. Provides relaxed, nonjudgmental atmosphere
    2. Protects group members from disruptive communication patterns (scapegoating)
    3. Accepts all feelings, attitudes, and ideas as valid themes for group discussion
    4. Responds to verbal and nonverbal communication
    5. Facilitates communication and problem solving by
      a. Encouraging group members to clarify and describe feelings, attitudes, and ideas
      b. Summarizing as needed
    6. Facilitates group cohesiveness by
      a. Asking for feedback and validation
      b. Giving responsibility to the group
      c. Encouraging the group to make decisions
      d. Permitting the group to review and revise goals as indicated
      e. Developing leadership among group members
    7. Other (describe)

10-2 DSM-III classification: multiaxial evaluation

The *Diagnostic and Statistical Manual of Mental Disorders* is published by the American Psychiatric Association and is periodically revised. The third edition (DSM-III) appeared in 1980.

The *Manual* categorizes and codifies psychiatric diagnoses. A description of diagnostic criteria accompanies each diagnosis. Categories and codes are used by physicians when they make diagnoses and by institutional personnel when they compile statistics and complete insurance forms.

All official DSM-III codes and terms are included in ICD-9-CM. However, in order to differentiate those DSM-III categories that use the same ICD-9-CM codes, unofficial non-ICD-9-CM codes are provided in parentheses for use when greater specificity is necessary.

The long dashes indicate the need for a fifth-digit subtype or other qualifying term.

Axes I and II: clinical syndromes and personality disorders

DISORDERS USUALLY FIRST EVIDENT IN INFANCY, CHILDHOOD OR ADOLESCENCE

Mental retardation

Code in fifth digit: 1 = with other behavioral symptoms (requiring attention or treatment and that are not part of another disorder), 0 = without other behavioral symptoms.

317.0(x) Mild mental retardation, ________
318.0(x) Moderate mental retardation, ________
318.1(x) Severe mental retardation, ________
318.2(x) Profound mental retardation, ________
319.0(x) Unspecified mental retardation, ________

Attention deficit disorder

314.01 with hyperactivity
314.00 without hyperactivity
314.80 residual type

Conduct disorder

312.00 undersocialized, aggressive
312.10 undersocialized, nonaggressive
312.23 socialized, aggressive
312.21 socialized, nonaggressive
312.90 atypical

Anxiety disorders of childhood or adolescence

309.21 Separation anxiety disorder
313.21 Avoidant disorder of childhood or adolescence
313.00 Overanxious disorder

Other disorders of infancy, childhood or adolescence

313.89 Reactive attachment disorder of infancy
313.22 Schizoid disorder of childhood or adolescence
313.23 Elective mutism
313.81 Oppositional disorder
313.82 Identity disorder

Eating disorders

307.10 Anorexia nervosa
307.51 Bulimia
307.52 Pica
307.53 Rumination disorder of infancy
307.50 Atypical eating disorder

Stereotyped movement disorders

307.21 Transient tic disorder
307.22 Chronic motor tic disorder
307.23 Tourette's disorder
307.20 Atypical tic disorder
307.30 Atypical stereotyped movement disorder

Other disorders with physical manifestations

307.00 Stuttering
307.60 Functional enuresis
307.70 Functional encopresis
307.46 Sleepwalking disorder
307.46 Sleep terror disorder (307.49)

Pervasive developmental disorders

Code in fifth digit: 0 = full syndrome present, 1 = residual state.

299.0x Infantile autism, ________
299.9x Childhood onset pervasive developmental disorder, ________
299.8x Atypical, ________

Specific developmental disorders

NOTE: These are coded on Axis II.

315.00 Developmental reading disorder
315.10 Developmental arithmetic disorder
315.31 Developmental language disorder
315.39 Developmental articulation disorder
315.50 Mixed specific developmental disorder
315.90 Atypical specific developmental disorder

ORGANIC MENTAL DISORDERS

Section 1. Organic mental disorders whose etiology or pathophysiological process is listed below (taken from the mental disorders section of ICD-9-CM).

Dementias arising in the senium and presenium

Primary degenerative dementia, senile onset,

290.30 with delirium
290.20 with delusions
290.21 with depression
290.00 uncomplicated

Code in fifth digit: 1 = with delirium, 2 = with delusions, 3 = with depression, 0 = uncomplicated.

290.1x Primary degenerative dementia, presenile onset, ________
290.4x Multi-infarct dementia, ________

From American Psychiatric Association: Diagnostic and statistical manual of mental disorders, ed. 3, Washington, D.C., 1980, The Association.

Continued.

Axes I and II: clinical syndromes and personality disorders—cont'd

Substance-induced

Alcohol
303.00 intoxication
291.40 idiosyncratic intoxication
291.80 withdrawal
291.00 withdrawal delirium
291.30 hallucinosis
291.10 amnestic disorder
Code severity of dementia in fifth digit: 1 = mild, 2 = moderate, 3 = severe, 0 = unspecified.
291.2x Dementia associated with alcoholism, ________

Barbiturate or similarly acting sedative or hypnotic
305.40 intoxication (327.00)
292.00 withdrawal (327.01)
292.00 withdrawal delirium (327.02)
292.83 amnestic disorder (327.04)

Opioid
305.50 intoxication (327.10)
292.00 withdrawal (327.11)

Cocaine
305.60 intoxication (327.20)

Amphetamine or similarly acting sympathominetic
305.70 intoxication (327.30)
292.81 delirium (327.32)
292.11 delusional disorder (327.35)
292.00 withdrawal (327.31)

Phencyclidine (PCP) or similarly acting arylcyclohexylamine
305.90 intoxication (327.40)
292.81 delirium (327.42)
292.90 mixed organic mental disorder (327.49)

Hallucinogen
305.30 hallucinosis (327.56)
292.11 delusional disorder (327.55)
292.84 affective disorder (327.57)

Cannabis
305.20 intoxication (327.60)
292.11 delusional disorder (327.65)

Tobacco
292.00 withdrawal (327.71)

Caffeine
305.90 intoxication (327.80)

Other or unspecified substance
305.90 intoxication (327.90)
292.00 withdrawal (327.91)
292.81 delirium (327.92)
292.82 dementia (327.93)
292.83 amnestic disorder (327.94)
292.11 delusional disorder (327.95)
292.12 hallucinosis (327.96)
292.84 affective disorder (327.97)
292.89 personality disorder (327.98)
292.90 atypical or mixed organic mental disorder (327.99)

Section 2. Organic brain syndromes whose etiology or pathophysiological process is either noted as an additional diagnosis from outside the mental disorders section of ICD-9-CM or is unknown.

293.00 Delirium
294.10 Dementia
294.00 Amnestic syndrome
293.81 Organic delusional syndrome
293.82 Organic hallucinosis
293.83 Organic affective syndrome
310.10 Organic personality syndrome
294.80 Atypical or mixed organic brain syndrome

SUBSTANCE USE DISORDERS

Code in fifth digit: 1 = continuous, 2 = episodic, 3 = in remission, 0 = unspecified.
305.0x Alcohol abuse, ________
303.9x Alçohol dependence (alcoholism), ________
305.4x Barbiturate or similarly acting sedative or hypnotic abuse.
304.1x Barbiturate or similarly acting sedative or hypnotic dependence, ________
305.5x Opioid abuse, ________
304.0x Opioid dependence, ________
305.6x Cocaine abuse, ________
305.7x Amphetamine or similarly acting sympathomimetic abuse, ________
304.4x Amphetamine or similarly acting sympathomimetic dependence, ________
305.9x Phencyclidine (PCP) or similarly acting arylcyclohexylamine abuse, ________(328.4x)
305.3x Hallucinogen abuse, ________
305.2x Cannabis abuse, ________
304.3x Cannabis dependence, ________
305.1x Tobacco dependence, ________
305.9x Other, mixed or unspecified substance abuse, ________
304.6x Other specified substance dependence, ________
304.9x Unspecified substance dependence, ________
304.7x Dependence on combination of opioid and other nonalcoholic substance, ________
304.8x Dependence on combination of substances, excluding opioids and alcohol, ________

SCHIZOPHRENIC DISORDERS

Code in fifth digit: 1 = subchronic, 2 = chronic, 3 = subchronic with acute exacerbation, 4 = chronic with acute exacerbation, 5 = in remission, 0 = unspecified.
Schizophrenia,
295.1x disorganized, ________
295.2x catatonic, ________
295.3x paranoid, ________
295.9x undifferentiated, ________
295.6x residual, ________

PARANOID DISORDERS

297.10 Paranoia
297.30 Shared paranoid disorder
298.30 Acute paranoid disorder
297.90 Atypical paranoid disorder

PSYCHOTIC DISORDERS NOT ELSEWHERE CLASSIFIED

295.40 Schizophreniform disorder
298.80 Brief reactive psychosis
295.70 Schizoaffective disorder
298.90 Atypical psychosis

NEUROTIC DISORDERS

These are included in Affective, Anxiety, Somatoform, Dissociative, and Psychosexual Disorders. In order to facilitate the identification of the categories that in DSM-II were grouped together in the class of Neuroses, the DSM-II terms are included separately in parentheses after the corresponding categories. These DSM-II terms are included in ICD-9-CM and therefore are acceptable as alternatives to the recommended DSM-II terms that precede them.

AFFECTIVE DISORDERS

Major affective disorders

Code major depressive episode in fifth digit: 6 = in remission, 4 = with psychotic features (the unofficial non-ICD-9-CM fifth digit 7 may be used instead to indicate that the psychotic features are mood-incongruent), 3 = with melancholia, 2 = without melancholia, 0 = unspecified.

Code manic or mixed episode in fifth digit: 6 = in remission, 4 = with psychotic features (the unofficial non-ICD-9-CM fifth digit 7 may be used instead to indicate that the psychotic features are mood-incongruent), 2 = without psychotic features, 0 = unspecified.

Bipolar disorder,
296.6x mixed, ________
296.4x manic, ________
296.5x depressed, ________

Major depression,
296.2x single episode, ________
296.3x recurrent, ________

Other specific affective disorders

301.13 Cyclothymic disorder
300.40 Dysthymic disorder (For Depressive neurosis)

Atypical affective disorders

296.70 Atypical bipolar disorder
296.82 Atypical depression

ANXIETY DISORDERS

Phobic disorders (or Phobic neuroses)
300.21 Agoraphobia with panic attacks
300.22 Agoraphobia without panic attacks
300.23 Social phobia
300.29 Simple phobia

Anxiety states (or Anxiety neuroses)
300.01 Panic disorder
300.02 Generalized anxiety disorder
300.30 Obsessive compulsive disorder (or Obsessive compulsive neurosis)

Post-traumatic stress disorder
308.30 acute
309.81 chronic or delayed
300.00 Atypical anxiety disorder

SOMATOFORM DISORDERS

300.81 Somatization disorder
300.11 Conversion disorder (or Hysterical neurosis, conversion type)
307.80 Psychogenic pain disorder
300.70 Hypochondriasis (or Hypochondriacal neurosis)
300.70 Atypical somatoform disorder (300.71)

DISSOCIATIVE DISORDERS (OR HYSTERICAL NEUROSES, DISSOCIATIVE TYPE)

300.12 Psychogenic amnesia
300.13 Psychogenic fugue
300.14 Multiple personality
300.60 Depersonalization disorder (or Depersonalization neurosis)
300.15 Atypical dissociative disorder

PSYCHOSEXUAL DISORDERS

Gender identity disorders

Indicate sexual history in the fifth digit of Transsexualism code: 1 = asexual, 2 = homosexual, 3 = heterosexual, 0 = unspecified.
302.5x Transsexualism, ________
302.60 Gender identity disorder of childhood
302.85 Atypical gender identity disorder

Paraphilias

302.81 Fetishism
302.30 Transvestism
302.10 Zoophilia
302.20 Pedophilia
302.40 Exhibitionism
302.82 Voyeurism
302.83 Sexual masochism
302.84 Sexual sadism
302.90 Atypical paraphilia

Psychosexual dysfunctions

302.71 Inhibited sexual desire
302.72 Inhibited sexual excitement
302.73 Inhibited female orgasm
302.74 Inhibited male orgasm
302.75 Premature ejaculation
302.76 Functional dyspareunia
306.51 Functional vaginismus
302.70 Atypical psychosexual dysfunction

Other psychosexual disorders

302.00 Ego-dystonic homosexuality
302.89 Psychosexual disorder not elsewhere classified

FACTITIOUS DISORDERS

300.16 Factitious disorders with psychological symptoms
301.51 Chronic factitious disorder with physical symptoms
300.19 Atypical factitious disorder with physical symptoms

DISORDERS OF IMPULSE CONTROL NOT ELSEWHERE CLASSIFIED

312.31 Pathological gambling
312.32 Kleptomania
312.33 Pyromania
312.34 Intermittent explosive disorder
312.35 Isolated explosive disorder
312.39 Atypical impulse control disorder

Continued.

Axes I and II: clinical syndromes and personality disorders—cont'd

ADJUSTMENT DISORDER

309.00 with depressed mood
309.24 with anxious mood
309.28 with mixed emotional features
309.30 with disturbance of conduct
309.40 with mixed disturbance of emotions and conduct
309.23 with work (or academic) inhibition
309.83 with withdrawal
309.90 with atypical features

PSYCHOLOGICAL FACTORS AFFECTING PHYSICAL CONDITION

Specify physical condition on Axis III.
316.00 Psychological factors affecting physical condition

PERSONALITY DISORDERS

NOTE: These are coded on Axis II.

301.00 Paranoid
301.20 Schizoid
301.22 Schizotypal
301.50 Histrionic
301.81 Narcissistic
301.70 Antisocial
301.83 Borderline
301.82 Avoidant
301.60 Dependent
301.40 Compulsive
301.84 Passive-Aggressive
301.89 Atypical, mixed or other personality disorder

V CODES FOR CONDITIONS NOT ATTRIBUTABLE TO A MENTAL DISORDER THAT ARE A FOCUS OF ATTENTION OR TREATMENT

V65.20 Malingering
V62.89 Borderline intellectual functioning (V62.88)
V71.01 Adult antisocial behavior
V71.02 Childhood or adolescent antisocial behavior
V62.30 Academic problem
V62.20 Occupational problem
V62.82 Uncomplicated bereavement
V15.81 Noncompliance with medical treatment
V62.89 Phase of life problem or other life circumstance problem
V61.10 Marital problem
V61.20 Parent-child problem
V61.80 Other specified family circumstances
V62.81 Other interpersonal problem

ADDITIONAL CODES

300.90 Unspecified mental disorder (nonpsychotic)
V71.09 No diagnosis or condition on Axis I
799.90 Diagnosis or condition deferred on Axis I

Other

V71.09 No diagnosis on Axis II
799.90 Diagnosis deferred on Axis II

Axis III: physical disorders and conditions

Axis IV: severity of psychosocial stressors

Code	*Term*	*Adult examples*	*Child or adolescent examples*
1	None	No apparent psychosocial stressor	No apparent psychosocial stressor
2	Minimal	Minor violation of the law, small bank loan	Vacation with family
3	Mild	Argument with neighbor, change in work hours	Change in schoolteacher, new school year
4	Moderate	New career, death of close friend, pregnancy	Chronic parental fighting, change to new school, illness of close relative, birth of sibling
5	Severe	Serious illness in self or family, major financial loss, marital separation, birth of child	Death of peer, divorce of parents, arrest, hospitalization, persistent and harsh parental discipline
6	Extreme	Death of close relative, divorce	Death of parent or sibling, repeated physical or sexual abuse
7	Catastropic	Concentration camp experience, devastating natural disaster	Multiple family deaths
8	Unspecified	No information or not applicable	No information or not applicable

Axis V: highest level of adaptive functioning past year

Levels	*Adult examples*	*Child or adolescent examples*
1 SUPERIOR—Unusually effective functioning in social relations, occupational functioning and use of leisure time.	Single parent living in deteriorating neighborhood takes excellent care of children and home, has warm relations with friends, and finds time for pursuit of hobby.	A 12-year-old girl gets superior grades in school, is extremely popular among her peers, and excels in many sports. She does all of this with apparent ease and comfort.
2 VERY GOOD—Better than average functioning in social relations, occupational functioning, and use of leisure time.	A 65-year-old retired widower does some volunteer work, often sees old friends, and pursues hobbies.	An adolescent boy gets excellent grades, works part-time, has several close friends, and plays banjo in a jazz band. He admits to some distress in "keeping up with everything."
3 GOOD—No more than slight impairment in either social or occupational functioning.	A woman with many friends functions extremely well at a difficult job, but says "the strain is too much."	An 8-year-old boy does well in school, has several friends, but bullies younger children.
4 FAIR—Moderate impairment in either social relations or occupational functioning, or some impairment in both.	A lawyer has trouble carrying through assignments, has several acquaintances but hardly any close friends.	A 10-year-old girl does poorly in school but has adequate peer and family relations.
5 POOR—Marked impairment in either social relations or occupational functioning, or moderate impairment in both.	A man with one or two friends has trouble keeping a job for more than a few weeks.	A 14-year-old boy almost fails in school and has trouble getting along with his peers.
6 VERY POOR—Marked impairment in both social relations and occupational functioning.	A woman is unable to do any of her housework and has violent outbursts toward her family and neighbors.	A 6-year-old girl needs special help in all subjects and has virtually no peer relationships.
7 GROSSLY IMPAIRED—Gross impairment in virtually all areas of functioning.	An elderly man needs supervision to maintain minimal personal hygiene and is usually incoherent.	A 4-year-old boy needs constant restraint to avoid hurting himself and is almost totally lacking in skills.
0 UNSPECIFIED	No information	No information

APPENDIX 11 PHARMACOLOGY

11-1 Drug interaction guide

Disclaimer of warranty: This material is an educational service toward better health care. The creator has attempted to ensure that the drug reaction and interaction information contained herein accurately reflects published data and is in accordance with standards accepted at the time of publication. Nevertheless, this is merely a summary of information available from other sources in which specific interactions are analyzed and discussed in more detail. Therefore, the creator of this work shall not be liable for personal injury, property damage, or any consequential damages arising out of or related to the material contained herein. Creator extends no warranties whether expressed or implied as to the completeness of drug reactions or interactions.

HOW TO USE THIS APPENDIX

When the interaction of two or more prescription or over-the-counter (OTC) products is in question, look up each individual product. All prescription drugs are listed by generic name.

Column 4 of each chart lists OTC/food items that may interact with the prescription drugs listed in column 1 to produce side effects noted in the introduction to that chart. Most OTC and household remedies are listed in the charts. Chart 1 deals primarily with OTC drugs, household remedies, and their interactions.

Prescription medications primarily used in the injectable form and some anesthetics are listed in Chart 18.

Dedication and acknowledgements

The Drug Interaction Guide is dedicated to all members of the health care profession devoted to furthering the best of health. I would like to acknowledge all those associated with making the guide possible, along with Susan Mantia of Washington University Medical Center, Ben Hesselberg, R.Ph., and The C.V. Mosby Company for making this information available in the text.

Chart 1. Over-the-counter drug interactions

	Any of these OTC drugs may interact with	*any of these OTC/food items as described in introductory material.*	
This chart deals strictly with products that can be bought over the counter and points out the potentially hazardous reactions that may occur. As described in the chart, the combination of alcohol-containing products can increase the damage to the stomach lining and possibly cause blood loss. Also described in this chart is the combination of alcohol-containing OTC products that, when combined with other OTC antihistamine-containing products, may cause drowsiness. Although some cough and cold remedies cause drowsiness when taken alone, combination compounds the decrease in alertness. When selecting a product in the OTC category it is always advisable to evaluate the ingredients to avoid any further complications with other OTC products or prescription medications, as pointed out in this and following charts. The OTC products that interact with other prescription medications are described in the following charts.	Alcoholic beverages Beer Cheracol, Cheracol D Cosanyl-DM Creo-Terpin Demazin Syrup Dristan Cough Formula Histadyl E.C. Neo-Synephrine Tablets Novahistine-DH and Novahistine Expectorant Nyquil Pertussin Robitussin, Robitussin-AC, Robitussin DM Triaminic Expectorant Valadol Liquid Vicks Formula 44 Cough Mixture	A.P.C. and A.P.C. Compound A.S.A., A.S.A. Compound Alka-Seltzer Alka-2 Allerest Anacin products A.R.M. Arthritis Strength Bufferin Ascriptin Aspergum Aspirin Bayer products Bufferin Cama Chlorpheniramine products Chlor-Trimeton Compoz Comtrex Conar Contac Coricidin products Coryban-D Capsules Demazin Dormin Ecotrin Empirin compound Excedrin 4-Way Cold Tablets Histadyl E.C. Measurin Midol Neo-Synephrine Tablets Novahistine products Nyquil Nytol	PAC Pamprin Phensal Pyrilamine Robitussin-AC Sinutab Sleep-Eze Sodium salicylate Sominex Sudafed Plus Triaminic liquids Triaminicin Triaminicol Vanquish Vicks Formula 44 Cough Mixture

Chart 2. Antihistamine interactions

	Any of these prescription drugs may interact with* ➡	*any of these prescription drug groups* ➡	*and result in this interaction.*	*OTC/food items*
The drugs listed in Chart 2, column 1, are antihistamines and antihistamine combinations. The combinations listed usually contain a decongestant such as pseudoephedrine or phenylpropanolamine. Indications, depending on the type of antihistamine, include allergies, nasal congestion and drainage, and watery eyes. Antihistamines are commonly employed to aid in the treatment of nausea, vomiting, dizziness, vertigo, and insomnia. Hydroxyzine (Atarax, Vistaril) is an antihistamine but is also indicated to be useful in the management of pruritus resulting from allergic conditions and contact dermatoses. Antihistamines can potentiate other central nervous system–acting drugs, so special precautions should be exercised when these are used in conjunction, especially with narcotics, barbiturates, and alcohol. Antihistamines may cause anticholinergic effects, such as dry mouth, which could be relieved by chewing gum. Smoking tends to cause further irritation and should be avoided. If nausea or upset stomach is a problem, the medication should be taken with food or milk. The interactions denoted here between antihistamines and OTC drugs should be avoided since an increased potential for severe drowsiness or decrease in mental alertness may occur.	Azatadine (Optimine) Brompheniramine (Dimetane) Chlorpheniramine (Chlor-Trimeton, Teldrin) Clemastine (Tavist) Cyproheptadine (Periactin) Dexchlorpheniramine (Polaramine) Dimetapp Diphenhydramine (Benadryl) Disophrol Drixoral Naldecon Nolamine Novafed-A Ornade Promethazine (Phenergan) Pyribenzamine Tripelennamine (PBZ) Triprolidine (Actidil)	Acenocoumarol (Sintrom) Anisindione (Miradon) Bishydroxycoumarin (Dicumarol) Griseofulvin (Fulvicin, Grifulvin) Oral contraceptives Oxyphenbutazone (Tandearil) Phenindione (Hedulin) Phenprocoumon (Liquamar) Phenylbutazone (Azolid, Butazolidin) Phenytoin (Dilantin) Warfarin (Coumadin)	This interaction can cause a decrease in the effectiveness of the prescription drugs listed in column 2.	A.R.M. Alcoholic products Allerest Bayer Decongestant Cold Tablets Beer Cheracol, Cheracol D Coldene Compoz Comtrex Conar Contac Coricidin Coryban-D Cosanyl-DM Demazin Dormin Dristan Dristan Cough Formula Histadyl E.C. Neo-Synephrine Novahistine Nyquil Nytol Pertussin Pyrilamine Robitussin-AC & Robitussin DM Sinutab Sleep-Eze Sominex Super Anahist Triaminicin Triaminicol Vicks Formula 44 products Vicks Sinex products
		Atropine products Belladonna products (Donnatal) Dicyclomine (Bentyl) Furazolidone (Furoxone) Glycopyrrolate (Robinul) Isocarboxazid (Marplan) Pargyline (Eutonyl) Phenelzine (Nardil) Procarbazine (Matulane) Propantheline (Pro-Banthine) Tranylcypromine (Parnate) Trihexphenidyl (Artane)	The combination of these medications may cause constipation, dry mouth, blurred vision, urine retention, and possible increased heart rate. Also a possibility of decreased mental alertness may occur. See below for additional prescription drug–prescription drug interactions involving antihistamines listed in column 1.	

*Some prescription drugs listed or their active ingredients may be available OTC.

Continued.

Chart 2. Antihistamine interactions—cont'd

Any of these prescription drugs may interact with* ➡	*any of these prescription drug groups* ➡	*and result in this interaction*	*OTC/food items*
Azatadine (Optimine) Brompheniramine (Dimetane) Chlorpheniramine (Chlor-Trimeton, Teldrin) Clemastine (Tavist) Cyproheptadine (Periactin) Dexchlor-pheniramine (Polaramine) Dimetapp Diphenhydramine (Benadryl) Disophrol Drixoral Naldecon Nolamine Novafed-A Ornade Promethazine (Phenergan) Pyribenzamine Tripelennamine (PBZ) Triprolidine (Actidil)	Amobarbital (Amytal) Chloral hydrate (Noctec) Chlordiazepoxide (Librium) Chlorpromazine (Thorazine) Clonazepam (Clonopin) Clorazepate (Tranxene, Azene) Codeine-containing products Cyclobenzaprine (Flexeril) Diazepam (Valium) Esgic Ethchlorvynol (Placidyl) Fiorinal Fluphenazine (Prolixin) Flurazepam (Dalmane) Glutethimide (Doriden) Hydroxyzine (Atarax, Vistaril) Librax Limbitrol Lorazepam (Ativan) Meprobamate (Equanil, Miltown) Oxazepam (Serax) Oxybutynin (Ditropan) Pentobarbital (Nembutal) Perphenazine (Trilafon) Phenobarbital (Luminal) Prazepam (Centrax) Prochlorperazine (Compazine) Promazine (Sparine) Propoxyphene (Darvon, Darvocet) Secobarbital (Seconal) Thioridazine (Mellaril) Thiothixene (Navane) Triclofos (Triclos) Trifluoperazine (Stelazine) Tuinal	The combination of the medications listed in column 2 with the drugs in column 1 could cause an increase in the likelihood of central nervous system depression. Such a combination could result in drowsiness, dizziness, blurred vision, loss of appetite, and a decrease in mental alertness. Caution must be exercised if operating any type of machinery or driving. It is not advisable to drink alcoholic beverages while taking any of these medications as this may compound the problem of adverse side effects.	

Chart 3. Antidiabetic drug interactions

The hypoglycemic agents listed in Chart 3, column 1, aside from insulin, are sulfonamide derivatives devoid of antibacterial effects. These oral agents aid in the stimulation of synthesis of endogenous insulin in the patient with functional pancreatic beta cells.

Contraindications include fever, infections, surgery for severe trauma, ketosis, acidosis, coma, and pregnancy.

Transient side effects may include loss of appetite, nausea, and stomach upset. Prolonged discomfort, sore throat, low fever, diarrhea, or dark urine may warrant a change in dosage or discontinuation of the medication.

The OTC interactions denoted here involve the cough and cold preparations that could alter the dosage or increase the potential for nausea or stomach upset.

Alcoholic beverages should always be avoided, and aspirin or salicylate products could also lower one's blood glucose level when used in combination with these medications.

Any of these prescription drugs may interact with	*any of these prescription drug groups*	*and result in this interaction.*	*OTC/food items*
Acetohexamide (Dymelor) Chlorpropamide (Diabinese) Insulin Tolazamide (Tolinase) Tolbutamide (Orinase)	Acetazolamide (Diamox) Bendroflumethiazide (Naturetin) Benzthiazide (Exna) Chlorothiazide (Diuril) Chlorthalidone (Hygroton) Dichlorphenamide (Daranide) Ethacrynic acid (Edecrin) Ethoxyzolamide (Cardrase, Ethamide) Furosemide (Lasix) Hydrochlorothiazide (Esidrix, HydroDiuril) Methazolamide (Neptazane) Methyclothiazide (Enduron) Metolazone (Diulo, Zaroxolyn) Polythiazide (Renese) Quinethazone (Hydromox) Rifampin Steroids (Prednisone) Trichlormethiazide (Metahydrin, Naqua)	Reaction may cause an increase in blood glucose level, which could result in excessive thirst and urination (hyperglycemic effect). Drugs in column 2 may work against diabetic medication in column 1. Notify physician if loss of appetite, nausea, or vomiting is noticed. See Chart 7 for additional listing of steroids that can cause this same effect.	Alcoholic beverages Aspirin products Beer Cheracol and Cheracol D Coryban-D Cosanyl-DM Creo-Terpin Demazin Syrup Dristan Cough Formula Gemnisyn Histadyl E.C. Neo-Synephrine Elixir Novahistine-DH and Novahistine Expectorant Nyquil Pertussin Robitussin, Robitussin-AC, and Robitussin DM Triaminic Expectorant Valadol Liquid Vicks Formula 44 Cough Mixture
	Alcoholic products Clofibrate (Atromids) Dicumarol Furazolidone (Furoxone) Guanethidine (Ismelin Sulfate) Isocarboxazid (Marplan) Metoprolol (Lopressor) Nadolol (Corgard) Oxyphenbutazone (Tandearil) Pargyline (Eutonyl) Phenelzine (Nardil) Phenylbutazone (Azolid, Butazolidin) Procarbazine (Matulane) Propranolol (Inderal) Salicylates Sulfinpyrazone Sulfonamides Tranylcypromine (Parnate)	Reaction may cause a decrease in blood glucose level leading to hunger (excessive), numbness, fatigue, headache, drowsiness, or sweating (hypoglycemic effect). If this occurs use candy or lump sugar to offset this adverse reaction, and notify physician.	

Chart 4. Anticoagulant interactions

	Any of these prescription drugs may interact with ➡	*any of these prescription drug groups* ➡	*and result in this interaction.*	*OTC/food items*
The medications listed in Chart 4, column 1, are probably the most critical group to monitor in terms of interactions. Since these agents are highly but weakly bound to plasma protein (albumin), a significant potential for displacing these drugs by other drugs exists. Inhibition of hepatic metabolism is another important mechanism involved in some of the interactions listed. Even though a particular drug is known to interact with an anticoagulant, it is often difficult to predict a certain patient's response, and thus close monitoring of the patient is mandatory. The in vivo effect of depressing factors VII, IX, X, and II (prothrombin) depends on the dosage of the drug administered. Oral anticoagulants have no effect on established thrombosis and do not reverse any tissue damage. The aim of treatment is to prevent further complications. Adverse reactions range from prolonged or excessive bleeding from nose, gums, and cuts to black stools, vomiting, unusual menstrual flow, prolonged diarrhea, headaches, fever, and loss of appetite. The OTC interactions listed here are described in column 4.	Acenocoumarol (Sintrom) Anisindione (Miradon) Bishydroxycoumarin (Dicumarol) Phenindione (Hedulin) Phenprocoumon (Liquamar) Warfarin (Coumadin)	Acetohexamide (Dymelor) Allopurinol (Zyloprim) Androgens Chloral hydrate (Noctec) Chloramphenicol (Chormycetin) Chlorpropamide (Diabinese) Cimetidine (Tagamet) Clofibrate (Atromid-S) Disulfiram (Antabase) Methandrostenolone (Dianabol) Naldixic acid (NegGram) Oxymetholone (Anadrol) Oxyphenbutazone (Oxalid, Tandearil) Phenylbutazone (Azolid, Butazolidin) Salicylates Sulfinpyrazone (Anturane) Sulfonamides Thyroid preparations Tolazamide (Tolinase) Tolbutamide (Orinase)	Drug interaction may result in an increased likelihood of increasing the activity of the anticoagulant drugs listed in column 1. See Chart 16 for analgesics that may cause this same effect.	The OTC drugs listed could increase the activity of therapeutic medication and could lead to excessive bleeding. The foods listed are high in vitamin K and could *reduce* the effectiveness of an anticoagulant drug. Acetaminophen A.S.A. and A.S.A. Compound Aspirin Alka-Seltzer and Alka-Seltzer Plus Alka-2 A.P.C. Arthritis Strength Bufferin Ascriptin & Ascriptin A/D Aspergum Bayer products Bufferin Cama Coricidin products Dristan Tablets Ecotrin Empirin compound Excedrin and Excedrin PM 4-Way Cold Tablets Gemnisyn Measurin Midol PAC Pamprin Phensal Sodium salicylate Sominex Super Anahist Triaminicin Tablets Tylenol products Vanquish Leafy green vegetables, for example, cabbage, spinach, kale, cauliflower, alfalfa
		Amobarbital (Amytal) Butabarbital (Butisol) Carbamazepine (Tegretol) Cholestyramine (Questran) Ethchlorvynol (Placidyl) Glutethimide (Doriden) Griseofulvin (Fulvicin Grifulvin) Pentobarbital (Nembutal) Phenobarbital (Luminal) Rifampin (Rifadin, Rimactane) Secobarbital (Seconal) Tuinal Vitamin K (Synkayvite)	Drug interaction may result in an increased likelihood of decreasing the activity of the anticoagulant drugs listed in column 1. See the diuretics (Chart 10) and oral contraceptives (Chart 6), which may cause this same result.	
		Other prescription drugs including antihistamines (Chart 2), steroids (Chart 7), and alcoholic beverages could produce unpredictable responses to medication, and a physician should be consulted before using these drugs.		

Chart 5. Antiparkinsonism drug interactions

	Any of these prescription drugs may interact with ➧	*any of these prescription drug groups* ➧	*and result in this interaction.*	*OTC/food items*
The medications listed in Chart 5, column 1, are referred to as ''antiparkinsonism agents.'' Since the depletion of dopamine in the brain can cause the involuntary movements, levodopa products are used to cross the blood-brain barrier and then are converted to dopamine. Dopamine itself does not cross the barrier. In the combination product (Sinemet), carbidopa aids in preventing the systemic decomposition of levodopa, thus allowing more medication to reach the brain. These medications should be used with caution or not at all in patients with a history of peptic ulcers or those who are pregnant or nursing. The OTC interactions here involve reducing or reversing the beneficial effects of levodopa products when combined with foods or drugs containing pyridoxine (vitamin B_6). If a vitamin supplement is necessary, Larobec is one product formulated not to contain any pyridoxine.	Levodopa products Bendopa Bio/DOPA Dopar Larodopa L-Dopa Parda Sinemet	Furazolidone (Furoxone) Isocarboxazid (Marplan) Pargyline (Eutonyl) Phenelzine (Nardil) Procarbazine (Matulane) Tranylcypromine (Parnate)	The mixing of antidepressant or antianxiety agents with the medications listed in column 1 may cause a severe increase in blood pressure, flushing, and palpitations.	Allbee-T Beminal-500 Corn Cynal Hexa-Betalin Liver Orexin Pyridoxine tablets Stresstabs 600 Trophite Vio-Bec Vitamin B complex Vitamin B_6 tablets Yeast
		Cholorpromazine (Thorazine) Fluphenazine (Prolixin) Haloperidol (Haldol) Mesoridazine (Serentil) Perphenazine (Trilafon) Piperacetazine (Quide) Prochlorperazine (Compazine) Promazine (Sparine) Thioridazine (Mellaril) Trifluoperazine (Stelazine) Triflupromazine (Vesprin)	Various phenothiazine tranquilizers may block or diminish the effectiveness of the prescription medications in column 1. Other tranquilizers should be used with caution. Methyldopa (Aldomet) may increase dopa products' effect, while phenytoin (Dilantin) and papaverine (Pavabid) may diminish the effects. See Chart 13 for additional antianxiety agents that could also cause effects of prescription drugs in column 1.	

Chart 6. Oral contraceptive interactions

	Any of these prescription drugs may interact with ➡	*any of these prescription drug groups* ➡	*and result in this interaction.*	*OTC/food items*
The oral contraceptives suppress ovulation by increasing the level of estrogen and progestin, which inhibit the follicle-stimulating hormone and luteinizing hormone. Oral contraceptives are also employed for their supplemental effect in other conditions. These medications should not be used if any of the following conditions are present or suspected: breast cancer, history of cerebrovascular accidents, neoplasms, pregnancy, nursing, or abnormal vaginal bleeding. The individual package insert should be consulted for additional warnings and precautions. Cigarette smoking increases the risk of serious cardiovascular side effects with estrogens and should be avoided. These risks also increase with age and amount of smoking. The first group of OTC interactions denoted here involves those vitamins that may be depleted when taking contraceptives and should be corrected by supplementing diet with an OTC product containing these vitamins. The second group, vitamin A products, if taken in excess, could lead to an accumulation of vitamin A within the system.	Brevicon Demulen Enovid Loestrin ModiCon Norinyl Norlestrin Ortho-Novum Ovcon Ovral Ovulen	Ampicillin (Polycillin, Principen) Antihistamines (see Chart 2) Barbiturates Oxyphenbutazone (Tandearil) Phenylbutazone (Azolid, Butazolidin) Phenytoin (Dilantin) Rifampin (Rifadin, Rimactane)	An increased possibility of break-through bleeding or spotting and decrease in the effectiveness of the pill may occur. Another form of contraception may be advisable in these instances. When combining these interacting drugs see Chart 2, column 1, for detailed list of antihistamines that may cause the same effect.	Cyanocobalamin (vitamin B_{12}) Folic acid Pyridoxine (vitamin B_6) Vitamin C Vitamin E Vitamin A products: Adabee Cod liver oil concentrate Dayalets Mi-Cebrin Myadec Optilets-500 Super-D products Theragran Vitamin A
		Acenocoumarol (Sintrom) Anisindione (Miradon) Bishydroxycoumarin (Dicumarol) Phenindione (Hedulin) Phenprocoumon (Liquamar) Warfarin (Coumadin)	The blood-thinning drugs listed in column 2 may be decreased in their effectiveness. Onset and cessation of bleeding should be closely minitored.	

Chart 7. Steroid interactions

	Any of these prescription drugs may interact with	*any of these prescription drug groups*	*and result in this interaction.*	*OTC/food items*
The medications listed in Chart 7, column 1, are referred to as "steroids," or more specifically, adrenocortical steroids. With the exception of fludrocortisone they are all glucocorticoids. Indications include endocrine, rheumatic, allergic, dermatologic, ophthalmic, respiratory, hematologic, and neoplastic conditions. Individual drug monographs should be consulted. Stressful situations, vaccinations, and surgery should be avoided while receiving steroid therapy. Patients predisposed to ulcers or who are pregnant or nursing require special monitoring or discontinuance of steroid medication, which is primarily completed by a gradual decrease in the dosage. Adverse reactions that may require immediate medical attention involve, but are not limited to, sodium and fluid retention, muscle weakness, nausea, persistent thirst, frequent urination, increased intraocular pressure, and blurred vision. Troleandomycin (TAO) may increase the therapeutic and toxic effects of most corticosteroids. The salicylate- or alcohol-containing OTCs listed here can complicate and increase the potential for nausea, ulceration, or decrease in the steroid effectiveness.	Betamethasone (Celestone) Cortisone (Cortone) Dexamethasone (Decadron, Hexadrol) Fludrocortisone (Florinef) Hydrocortisone (Cortef, Hydrocortone) Methylprednisolone (Medrol) Prednisolone (Delta-Cortef) Prednisone (Deltasone, Meticorten) Triamcinolone (Aristocort, Kenacort)	Acetazolamide (Diamox) Bendroflumethiazide (Naturetin) Benzthiazide (Exna) Chlorothiazide (Diuril) Chlorthalidone (Hygroton) Dichlorphenamide (Daranide) Digifortis (Pil-Digis) Digitoxin (Crystodigin, Purodigin) Digoxin (Lanoxin) Ethacrynic acid (Edecrin) Ethoxzolamide (Cardrase, Ethamide) Furosemide (Lasix) Gitalin (Gitaligin) Hydrochlorothiazide (Esidrix, HydroDiuril) Methazolamide (Neptazane) Methyclothiazide (Enduron) Metolazone (Diulo, Zaroxolyn) Polythiazide (Renese) Quinethazone (Hydromox) Trichlormethiazide (Metahydrin, Naqua)	This combination may cause an increase in the effect of the heart medications in column 2. Too much potassium may be lost, and a physician should be notified if shortness of breath, fatigue, prolonged nausea, abdominal pain, cramps, and blurred vision are noticed. The diuretics listed in column 2 may also increase loss of potassium, so it is imperative to have frequent checkups. See Charts 3 and 9 for additional steroid reactions.	A.P.C. and A.P.C. Compound A.S.A. and A.S.A. Compound Alcoholic products Alka-Seltzer Alka-2 Allerest Anacin products Arthritis Strength Bufferin Ascriptin Aspergum Aspirin Bayer products Bufferin Cama Chlorpheniramine products Chor-Trimeton Compoz Conar Contac Coricidin products Coryban-D Capsules Demazin Dormin Ecotrin Empirin compound Excedrin 4-Way Cold Tablets Gemnisyn Histadyl E.C. Measurin Midol Neo-Synephrine Tablets Novahistine products Nyquil Nytol PAC Pamprin Phensal Pyrilamine Robitussin-AC Sinutab Sleep-Eze Sodium salicylate Sominex Sudafed Plus Triaminic liquids Triaminicin Triaminicol Vanquish Vicks Formula 44 Cough Mixture
		Amobarbital (Amytal) Chloral hydrate (Noctec, Somnos) Flurazepam (Dalmane) Glutethimide (Doriden) Pentobarbital (Nembutal) Phenytoin (Dilantin) Rifampin Secobarbital (Seconal) Tuinal	Rifampin, the hydantoins (phenytoin), the sedatives or hypnotics (sleeping medications) listed in column 2 may reduce a steroid's effectiveness.	

Chart 8. Antispasmodic interactions

	Any of these prescription drugs may interact with ➡	*any of these prescription drug groups* ➡	*and result in this interaction.*	*OTC/food items*
The prescription drugs listed in Chart 8, column 1, are referred to as "antispasmodics." Most of these products are used in gastrointestinal disorders, yet some are used primarily in urinary, kidney, and allergic disorders. Since these products may cause some drowsiness, dizziness, or blurred vision, the CNS depressants should be avoided. If dryness of the mouth occurs, relief could be accomplished by chewing gum. If this persists or if a skin rash, flushing, or eye pain develops, further medical attention is necessary. Some of these drugs can decrease perspiration, which could lead to fever or heat stroke, so it is advisable to remain, when possible, in a cool environment. Antacids, if used along with any of these products, should not be taken at the same time. An hour or two should be allowed between them. The OTC interactions noted here can compound the problem of dry mouth, blurred vision, or drowsiness, and these product combinations should be avoided if possible.	Atropine products Belladonna products Benztropin mesylate (Cogentin) Dicyclomine (Bentyl) Glycopyrrolate (Robinul) Librax Propantheline (Pro-Banthine) Trihexyphenidyl (Artane)	Amitriptyline (Elavil, Endep) Chlorpromazine (Thorazine) Cyclobenzaprine (Flexeril) Desipramine (Norpramin, Pertofrane) Disopyramide (Norpace) Fluphenazine (Prolixin) Haloperidol (Haldol) Imipramine (Tofranil) Meperidine (Demerol) Mesoridazine (Serentil) Nortriptyline (Aventyl) Oxybutynin (Ditropan) Perphenazine (Trilafon) Prochlorperazine (Compazine) Promazine (Sparine) Quinidine (Cin-Quin) Thioridazine (Mellaril) Trifluoperazine (Stelazine) Triflupromazine (Vesprin)	The combination of these medications may cause constipation, dryness of mouth, blurred vision, urine retention, and possible increased heart rate. If the drugs must be used in combination, physician may need to reduce the dose of one or both drugs. Refer to Chart 2 for additional interactions of antispasmodics and antihistamines. The effectiveness of the phenothiazines listed may be decreased.	Allerest A.R.M. Bayer Decongestant Cold Tablets Chlorpheniramine Chlor-Trimeton Compoz Comtrex Conar Contac Coricidin Coryban-D Capsules Demazin Dormin Dristan Histadyl E.C. Neo-Synephrine Tablets Novahistine products Nyquil Nytol Pyrilamine Robitussin-AC Sinutab Sleep-Eze Sominex Super Anahist Triaminic liquids Triaminicin Triaminicol Vicks Formula 44 Cough Mixture Vicks Sinex products

Chart 9. Heart medication interactions

	Any of these prescription drugs may interact with	*any of these prescription drug groups* 	*and result in this interaction.*	*OTC/food items*
The medications listed in Chart 9, column 1, are referred to as "cardiac glycosides." They increase the force of myocardial contraction and the refractory period of the atrioventricular (A-V) node. Indications include congestive heart failure, atrial fibrillation, flutter, and tachycardia, but these medications are contraindicated in ventricular fibrillation. Lowered potassium levels sensitize the myocardium to the glycosides, and toxic levels may be reached even with usual dosages. Many arrhythmias for which digitalis is advised closely resemble those reflecting toxic digitalis levels. Nausea and vomiting may also be associated with toxic levels, along with a loss of appetite, weakness, diarrhea, blurred vision, and yellow or green halos around objects. The first group of OTC interactions involves antacids, which, if taken *at the same time,* could decrease the effectiveness of the glycoside. The second group of antiasthmatic products could cause or complicate arrhythmias while a patient is undergoing digitalis therapy.	Digifortis (Pil-Digis) Digitoxin (Crystodigin, Purodigin) Digoxin (Lanoxin) Gitalin (Gitaligin)	Acetazolamide (Diamox) Bendroflumethiazide (Naturetin) Benthiazide (Exna) Chlorothiazide (Diuril) Chlorthalidone (Hygroton) Dichlorphenamide (Daranide) Ethacrynic acid (Edecrin) Ethoxzolamide (Cardrase, Ethamide) Furosemide (Lasix) Hydrochlorthiazide (Esidrix, HydroDiuril) Methazolamide (Neptazane) Methyclothiazide (Enduron) Metolazone (Diulo, Zaroxolyn) Polythiazide (Renese) Quinethazone (Hydromox) Trichlormethiazide (Metahydrin, Naqua)	Although these drugs are sometimes used together, there is a possibility of a decreasing potassium level, which could lead to toxic levels of a heart pill. A physician should be notified if any of the signs explained in the introduction to Chart 9 or leg cramps are noticed. Steroids (Chart 7) and licorice may also cause a loss in potassium. See Chart 10 for more information on the diuretics listed in column 2. If any potassium supplements (KC1, Kato, K-Lyte, Kaon, Kaochlor, and so on) must be taken, checkups should be frequent to ensure that levels are not too high.	Aludrox Aluminum hydroxide Amphojel Anacin Arthritis Formula Antacids Ascriptin Camalox Dristan Gelusil Kaolin/pectin (Kaopectate) Maalox Magnesium hydroxide Magnesium trisilicate Milk of Magnesia Mylanta ——— Adrenalin Asthmanefrin Breatheasy Bronkaid Mist Epinephrine Histadyl E.C. Medihaler-EPI Primatene Mist Solution A Vaponefrin Va-Tro-Nol
		Metoprolol (Lopressor) Nadolol (Corgard) Propranolol (Inderal) Phenytoin (Dilantin) Reserpine (Serpasil) Reserpine combination (see Chart 11)	The drugs in column 2 are sometimes used together with heart medications, yet could result in irregular heartbeat. Pulse should be taken regularly and any changes in pulse or persistent dizziness should be reported to a physician. See Chart 3 for additional reactions on some of the prescription drugs in column 2.	
	See Chart 8; the anticholinergics in combination with the heart medications could lead to increased toxic/therapeutic effects.			

Chart 10. Diuretic interactions

	Any of these prescription drugs may interact with ➧	*any of these prescription drug groups* ➧	*and result in this interaction.*	*OTC/food items*
The medications listed in Chart 10, column 1, are referred to as "diuretics." The range of indication includes, but is not limited to, hypertension, edema, cardiac conditions, and renal dysfunction. The carbonic anhydrase inhibitors listed are also sometimes employed in the treatment of glaucoma. The thiazide diuretics tend to cause a depletion of potassium and sodium; thus, close monitoring of potassium levels is necessary, especially in cardiac conditions requiring digitalis therapy. Lowered potassium levels may be indicated by weakness, leg cramping, and joint or foot pain. Spironolactone (Aldactone Aldactazide) and triamterene (Dyazide, Dyrenium) are used to help conserve the loss of potassium, and additional potassium ion supplements may not be necessary or even harmful. The OTC alcoholic interactions denoted here involve products that could increase the potential for severe hypotension and drowsiness. The decongestant products listed could negate the antihypertensive effect or cause an increase in blood pressure.	Acetazolamide (Diamox) Bendroflumethiazide (Naturetin) Benzthiazide (Exna) Chlorothiazide (Diuril) Chlorthalidone (Hygroton) Dichlorphenamide (Daranide) Ethacrynic acid (Edecrin) Ethoxzolamide (Cardrase, Ethamide) Furosemide (Lasix) Hydrochlorthiazide (Esidrix, HydroDiuril) Methazolamide (Neptazane) Methyclothiazide (Enduraon) Metolazone (Diulo, Zaroxolyn) Polythiazide (Renese) Quinethazone (Hydromox) Trichlormethiazide (Metahydrin, Naqua)	Digifortis (Pil-Digis) Digitoxin (Crystodigin, Purodigin) Digoxin (Lanoxin) Gitalin (Gitaligin	Although this combination of a heart tablet (column 2 drugs) with a diuretic is often used to treat various illnesses, the diuretic could decrease the potassium level, which could lead to toxic levels of the heart pill. Frequent checkups are recommended, and a physician should be notified if any weakness, leg cramps, shortness of breath, abdominal pain, or blurred or yellow vision is noticed. See Chart 9 for other heart medication interactions. See Charts 3, 4, and 7 for diuretic interactions.	Adrenalin Afrinol Alcoholic products Alconefrin Allerest capsules and spray A.R.M. Asthmanefrin Bayer Decongestant Breatheasy Bromo-Quinine Bronkaid Caffeine Coffee Comtrex Contac Coricidin Cough Syrup and Nasal Mist Coricidin-D Coryban-D Cosanyl-DM Day Care Demazine Repetabs & Syrup Dimacol Dristan tablets, capsules, and liquid Epinephrine Fedrazil 4-Way Cold Tablets and Nasal Spray Histadyl E.C. Medihaler-EPI Neo-Synephrine products No Doz Novahistine products Nyquil Ornacol Ornex Orthoxicol Phenylephrine Phenylpropanolamine Primatene Privine Romilar Cough Syrup Sinutab Cold Tablets and Sinutab II Solution A Sudafed SuperAnahist Tea Triaminic products Triaminicol Trind Ursinus Va-Tro-Nol Vicks Inhaler
		Acenocoumarol (Sintrom) Anisindione (Miradon) Bishydroxycoumarin (Dicumarol) Phenindione (Hedulin) Phenprocoumon (Liquamar) Warfarin (Coumadin)	Drug interactions could result in an increased likelihood of decreasing the activity of the anticoagulant drugs in column 2. See Chart 4 for more anticoagulant interactions. Lithium (Eskalith) should be used with caution when combined with diuretics.	

See Chart 11 for additional prescription drugs used for high blood pressure (antihypertensives).

Chart 11. Antihypertensive interactions

	Any of these prescription drugs may interact with ➡	*any of these prescription drug groups* ➡	*and result in this interaction.*	*OTC/food items*
The medications listed in Chart 11, column 1, are referred to as "antihypertensives." The diuretic antihypertensives are discussed in Chart 10. When initiating therapy, transient drowsiness or dizziness may occur, and thus the patient should avoid sudden changes in posture and balance. If medications are changed or discontinued, it is advisable to gradually reduce the dosage over a period of days. Adverse reactions that may require further medical attention might include persistent hypotension, fever fatigue, chills, sore throat, diarrhea, or swelling. The following antihypertensives are listed in other charts: clonidine (Catapres, Combipres) (see Chart 14), metoprolol (Lopressor), nadolol (Corgard), and propranolol (Inderal) (see Charts 3 and 9). The OTC interactions denoted here involve products that could cause or complicate severe drowsiness and dizziness. OTC cold remedies that contain a decongestant should be avoided since an unpredictable response may occur. This should be explained to any patient taking reserpine products, since these naturally tend to cause nasal congestion. A saline nasal spray may be the only product necessary to control this problem without further complications.	Guanethidine (Esimil, Ismelin) Hydralazine (Apresazide, Apresoline) Methyldopa (Aldomet, Aldoril) Reserpine (Serpasil, Reserpoid) Reserpine combinations: Demi-Regroton Diupres Diutensin-R Exna-R Hydropres Hydroserpine Metatensin Naquival Regroton Salutensin Ser-Ap-Es	Furazolidone (Furoxone) Isocarboxazid (Marplan) Pargyline (Eutonyl) Phenelzine (Nardil) Procarbazine (Matulane) Tranylcypromine (Parnate) Methylphenidate (Ritalin) Phenothiazines Pseudoephedrine (Sudafed)	This combination may result in a severe increase in blood pressure, fever, convulsion, or dizziness. A physician should be notified if persistent headache, sore throat, diarrhea, or any irregular heartbeat is noticed. See also Chart 14 for other antidepressants that could cause a change in blood pressure when used in combination. Although combinations of different antihypertensive drugs are used together to aid in the control of blood pressure, certain combinations should be avoided or monitored very closely. Propranolol, metoprolol, and nadolol may interact with prazosin (Minipress) or reserpine and reserpine combinations. Hydralazine may interact with minoxidil (Loniten). These reactions could produce severe low blood pressure with resultant dizziness or produce irregular heartbeat.	Adrenalin Afrinol Alcoholic products Alconefrin Allerest capsules and spray A.R.M. Asthmanefrin Bayer Decongestant Breatheasy Bromo-Quinine Bronkaid Caffeine Coffee Comtrex Contac Coricidin Cough Syrup and Nasal Mist Coricidin-D Coryban-D Cosanyl-DM Day Care Demazine Repetabs & Syrup Dimacol Dristan tablets, capsules, and liquid Epinephrine Fedrazil 4-Way Cold Tablets and Nasal Spray Histadyl E.C. Medihaler-EPI Neo-Synephrine products No Doz Novahistine products Nyquil Ornacol Ornex Orthoxicol Phenylephrine Phenylpropanolamine Primatene Privine Romilar Cough Syrup Sinutab Cold Tablets and Sinutab II Solution A Sudafed Super Anahist Tea Triaminic products Triaminicol Trind Ursinus Va-Tro-Nol Vicks Inhaler

Chart 12. Antibiotic interactions

	Any of these prescription drugs may interact with ➡	*any of these prescription drug groups* ➡	*and result in this interaction.*	*OTC/food items*
The medications listed in Chart 12, column 1, are referred to as "tetracycline" or "tetracycline-combination antibiotics." The combination products contain an antifungal agent to help decrease or eliminate the severity of a diarrhea side effect in those susceptible. Skin sensitivity to the burning rays of the sun is a common occurrence when taking these medications; it is therefore advisable to use a sunscreen agent for protection. Avoidance of these medications is advisable if one is pregnant or nursing. They should also be avoided in infants and young children to prevent any damage to tooth enamel or discoloration of the teeth. Dosage should be taken on an empty stomach, 1 hour before a meal or 2 hours after, unless otherwise directed. A change in medication or dosage may be indicated if severe diarrhea or skin rash occurs. The OTC interactions denoted here involve products that may comply with the tetracycline product and thus result in a decrease in absorption with resultant lower therapeutic levels of the antibiotic.	Achromycin V Achrostatin V Bristacycline Cyclopar Kesso-Tetra Mysteclin-F Panmycin QID Tet Robitet SK-Tetracycline Sumycin Tetrachel Tetracycline Tetracyn Tetrex V-Tet	Ampicillin (Polycillin, Principen) Bactocill Cloxacillin (Tegopen) Dicloxacillin (Dycill, Dynapen) Oxacillin (Prostaphlin) Penicillin Penicillin G potassium (Pentids) Penicillin V potassium (Ledercillin, Pen-Vee K, V-Cillin K, Veetids)	A decrease in the effectiveness of the drugs in either column 1 or 2 may occur. The mixing of these drugs should be avoided unless otherwise directed.	Iron preparations Fer-In-Sol Ferrous sulfate Milk & dairy products Antacids & products containing calcium, aluminum, or magnesium Alka-Seltzer Plus Alka-2 Aludrox Aluminum hydroxide Amphojel Anacin Arthritis Formula Ascriptin Bufferin Calcium Calcium carbonate Cama Camalox Creamalin Dicarbosil Antacid Tablets Di-Gel Dristan Tablets Gelusil Maalox & Maalox Plus Magnesium Hydroxide Magnesium trisilicate Milk of Magnesia Mylanta and Mylanta III Rolax Titralac Triaminicin Tums Vanquish
		Acenocoumarol (Sintrom) Anisindione (Miradon) Bishydroxycoumarin (Dicumarol) Phenindione (Hedulin) Phenprocoumon (Liquamar) Warfarin (Coumadin)	An increase in the effect of the blood-thinning drugs in column 2 may occur, which could result in hemorrhage or unusual bleeding.	

Chart 13. Antianxiety medication and sedative interactions

	Any of these prescription drugs may interact with	*any of these prescription drug groups* 	*and result in this interaction.*	*OTC/food items*
Although the medications listed in Chart 13, column 1, include antianxiety drugs, sedatives, hypnotics, antipsychotics, and tranquilizers, they are grouped this way since they have similar or common interactions. The therapeutic indications of these groups involve, but are not limited to, allergic disorders, nausea, tension, insomnia, muscular disorders, and epilepsy. Other anticonvulsants may also interact in a similar manner as these agents; therefore a full package insert should be consulted. An adjustment in dosage or medication may be warranted if excessive drowsiness, fatigue, difficulty in concentrating, dizziness, nightmares, irritability, muscle spasm, or dependence develops or if the patient becomes pregnant. Combination of any of the column 1 drugs may increase central nervous system depression and should be avoided if possible. The OTC interactions involved here increase the potential for severe central nervous system depression and may still cause this effect a day or two after the prescription medication has been discontinued. Caution should be exercised when in any activity requiring mental alertness.	Amobarbital (Amytal) Chloral hydrate (Noctec) Chlordiazepoxide (Limbitrol, Librium) Chlorpromazine (Thorazine) Clonazepam (Clonopin) Clorazepate (Azene, Tranzene) Diazepam (Valium) Ethchlorvynol (Placidyl) Fluphenazine (Prolixin) Flurazepam (Dalmane) Glutethimide (Doriden) Hydroxyzine (Atarax, Vistaril) Lorazepam (Ativan) Meprobamate (Equanil, Miltown) Oxazepam (Serax) Pentobarbital (Nembutal) Perphenazine (Trilafon) Phenobarbital (Luminal) Prazepam (Centrax) Prochlorperazine (Compazine) Promazine (Sparine) Secobarbital (Seconal, Tuinal) Triclofos (Triclos) Trifluoperazine (Stelazine) Thioridazine (Mellaril) Thiothixene (Navane)	Amitriptyline (Elavil, Endep) Amoxapine (Asendin) Cimetidine (Tagamet) Cyclobenzaprine (Flexeril) Desipramine (Norpramin, Pertofrane) Doxepin (Adapin, Sinequan) Etrafon Imipramine (Tofranil) Limbitrol Maprotiline (Ludiomil) Nortriptyline (Aventyl, Pamelor) Triavil Trimipramine (Surmontil)	The combination of the drugs in column 1 with any of the medications in column 2 may increase the likelihood of central nervous system depression. This may cause confusion, depression, drowsiness, unusual weakness, slurred speech, headache, or lack of mental alertness. A person taking these medications, whether a drug in column 1, a drug in column 2, or a combination of drugs in both columns, should be familiar with his or her reaction to the medication before driving or undertaking a job requiring mental alertness. See Chart 2, column 1, drugs, the antihistamines, which could also cause severe nervous system depression and drowsiness if combined with the medications in column 1.	Alcoholic products Allerest A.R.M. Bayer Decongestant Cold Tablets Beer Cheracol & Cheracol D Coldene Compoz Comtrex Conar Contac Coridin Coryban-D Cosanyl-DM Creo-Terpin Demazin Dormin Dristan & Dristan Cough Formula Histadyl E.C. Neo-Synephrine Novahistine Nyquil Nytol Pertussin Pyrilamine Robitussin-AC & Robitussin-DM Sinutab Sleep-Eze Sominex Super Anahist Synephricol Triaminicin Triaminicol Vicks Formula 44 Cough Mixture Vicks Sinex

Chart 14. Antidepressants-I interactions

	Any of these prescription drugs may interact with ➔	*any of these prescription drug groups* ➔	*and result in this interaction.*	*OTC/food Items*
The medications listed in Chart 14, column 1, are referred to as "antidepressants." Some of these medications also have antianxiety effects. Others may be used in enuresis, and one is primarily a muscle relaxant but interacts like a tricyclic. Often these medications may require up to 4 weeks of therapy before noticeable improvement may be seen. Discontinuance of therapy should be gradual to avoid headache or nausea. Transient drowsiness or dryness of the mouth may be experienced when first beginning these medications. If a sore throat develops, further medical attention may be required to adjust or discontinue medication. Drowsiness or blurred vision may occur, which may be transient. Persons predisposed to glaucoma should be monitored closely. The OTC interactions involving alcohol-containing products may result in an increased potential for severe drowsiness and decreased mental alertness. An unpredictable response to the sympathomimetics may occur when combined with the prescription drugs in column 1.	Amitriptyline (Elavil, Endep) Amoxapine (Asendin) Cyclobenzaprine (Flexeril) Disipramine (Norpramin, Pertofrane) Doxepin (Adapin, Sinequan) Etrafon Imipramine (Tofranil) Limbitrol Maprotiline (Ludiomil) Nortriptyline (Aventyl, Pamelor) Triavil Trimipramine (Surmontil)	Clonidine (Catapres, Combipres) Guanethidine (Esimil, Ismelin)	The drug reaction here can block the blood-pressure-lowering effect of the drugs listed in column 2. A physician may need to adjust the dosage required.	Alcoholic products Allerest A.R.M. Bayer Decongestant Cold Tablets Beer Cheracol and Cheracol D Coldene Compoz Comtrex Conar Contac Coricidin Coryban-D Cosadein Cosanyl-DM Demazin Dormin Dristan & Dristan Cough Formula Histadyl E.C. Neo-Synephrine Novahistine Nyquil Nytol Penetro Pertussin Pyrilamine Robitussin-AC & Robitussin-DM Sinutab Sleep-Eze Sominex Super Anahist Synephricol Triaminicin Triaminicol 2/G DM Vicks Formula 44 Cough Mixture Vicks Sinex products
		Furazolidone (Furoxone) Isocarboxazid (Marplan) Pargyline (Eutonyl) Phenelzine (Nardil) Procarbazine (Matulane) Tranylcypromine (Parnate)	This reaction could cause a severe increase in blood pressure and lead to fever, excitement, convulsions, coma, and possible circulatory collapse. This combination of drugs should be avoided.	
		Amphetamine (Benzedrine) Benzphetamine (Didrex) Chlorphentermine (Pre-Sate) Dextroamphetamine (Dexedrine) Diethylpropion (Tenuate, Tepanil) Ephedrine products Methamphetamine (Desoxyn) Phendimetrazine (Bontril, Plegine) Phenmetrazine (Preludin) Phenteramine (Fastin, lonamin)	This combination may increase or decrease the effects of the drugs in column 2. This could lead to such varied side effects as increased blood pressure and severe headache. Caution should be exercised if these groups are combined. See Charts 13 and 15 for additional antidepressant interactions.	

Chart 15. Antidepressants-II interactions

	Any of these prescription drugs may interact with ➡	*any of these prescription drug groups* ➡	*and result in this interaction.*	*OTC/food items*
The drugs listed in Chart 15, column 1, are referred to as "monoamine oxidase (MAO) inhibitors." Although the major effects are antidepressant, some are used for anxiety or in chemotherapy procedures. Because of the potency of these drugs they require special precautions and considerations when used. Transient drowsiness, dizziness, weakness, or blurred vision may occur. If these symptoms persist or severe headaches, rash, dark urine, jaundice, sore throat, or diarrhea occurs, the dosage or drug may need to be changed. Since the effects of MAO inhibitors may last for up to 2 weeks after discontinuing use, no interacting drug should be started within this period of time. The interacting OTC and food products listed here could cause severe hypertension, fever, excitement, and convulsions if combined. Therefore it is of the utmost importance to avoid these products high in tyramine and sympathomimetics. Alcohol-containing products should also be avoided if possible.	Furazolidone (Furoxone) Isocarboxazid (Marplan) Phargyline (Eutonyl) Phenelzine (Nardil) Procarbazine (Matulane) Tranylcypromine (Parnate)	Antidepressants (see Chart 14) Ephedrine products Guanethidine (Esimil, Ismelin) Levodopa (Dopar, Larodopa) Meperidine (Demerol) Methyldopa (Aldomet, Aldoril) Methylphenidate (Ritalin) OTC diet aids (see Chart 14) Phenylephrine (Neo-Synephrine) Phenylpropanolamine (Propadrine) Pseudoephedrine (Sudafed) Reserpine (Serpasil) Reserpine-containing drugs (see Chart II) Tyramine	A combination of this type could result in a lethal reaction. Concurrent use of any of the drugs in column 2 with any of the medication in column 1 may cause sudden and severe high blood pressure, fever, excitement, and convulsions. The MAO inhibitors in column 1 should not be combined with any of these drugs, nor should they be used for 14 days after discontinuing an MAO inhibitor. See Charts 2, 3, 4, 11, and 14 for additional MAO inhibitor interactions.	Cheeses: Cheddar Emmenthaler Gruyere Stilton Brie Camembert Coffee Chocolate Cola (excessive) Fermented sausages, for example, fermented bolognas, salamis, summer sausage, pepperoni A.R.M. Adrenalin Afrinol Alconefrin Allerest capsules and spray Asthmanefrin Bayer Decongestant Cold Tablets Breatheasy Bromoquinine Bronkaid Cheracol Cold Capsules Comtrex Contac Coricidin-D Cosanyl-DM Day Care Demazin Dimacol Dristan Epinephrine

Continued.

Chart 15. Antidepressants-II interactions—cont'd

	Any of these prescription drugs may interact with ➡	*any of these prescription drug groups* ➡	*and result in this interaction.*	*OTC/food items*
	Furazolidone (Furoxone) Isocarboxazid (Marplan) Pargyline (Eutonyl) Phenelzine (Nardil) Procarbazine (Matulane) Tranylcypromine (Parnate)			Fedrazil Histadyl E.C. Medihaler-EPI Beer Red wines, for example, chianti, sherry Bananas Figs (canned) Avocados Fava or yeast extract Chicken liver Beef liver Neo-Synephrine No-Doz Nyquil Ornacol Ornex Orthoxicol OTC diet aids Phenylephrine Phenylpropanolamine Primatene Privine Romilar Cough Syrup Sinutab Solution A Sudafed Super Anahist Tea Triaminic products Triaminicol Trind Ursinus Va-Tro-Nol Vicks Sinex 4-Way cold products

Chart 16. Analgesic interactions

	Any of these prescription drugs may interact with ➧	*any of these prescription drug groups* ➧	*and result in this interaction.*	*OTC/food items*
The medications listed in Chart 16, column 1, are referred to as "analgesics." The majority are more specifically referred to as "nonsteroidal antiinflammatory agents"; these help control pain and inflammation by a reduction in prostaglandin synthesis. These medications should be taken with food or milk to minimize the potential for stomach distress or bleeding of the intestinal mucosa. Patients with a history of allergies to aspirin, bleeding problems, or ulcers may not tolerate these medications. Skin rash, tinnitus, blurred vision, swelling, or unusual weight gain may require a change in dosage or drug. Dizziness may be transient with these medications. The OTC interactions denoted here involve products containing aspirin, salicylates, or alcohol, which in combination can increase the severity of stomach distress and/or bleeding. Propoxyphene (Darvon, Darvocet) and products containing codeine may react similarly with these OTC products. Aspirin and salicylate products can decrease the effectiveness of the other prescription analgesics.	Aspirin/salicylate products Fenoprofen (Nalfon) Ibuprofen (Motrin) Indomethacin (Indocin) Meclofenamate (Meclomin) Naproxen (Anaprox, Naprosyn) Oxyphenbutazone (Oxalid, Tandearil) Phenylbutazone (Azolid, Butazolidin) Sulindac (Clinoril)	Acenocoumarol (Sintrom) Anisindione (Miradon) Bishydroxycoumarin (Dicumarol) Phenindione (Hedulin) Phenprocoumon (Liquamar) Warfarin (Coumadin)	When used in combination there is an increase in the likelihood and severity of increasing the effectiveness of the prescription drugs in column 2. This could result in bruising, increased bleeding, or hemorrhage. Some of the prescription drugs in column 1 may not have as much of an effect (for example, Zomax) but still could affect bleeding time. Probenecid (Benemid) and sulfinpyrazone (Anturane) should normally not be combined with the column 1 drugs (especially with Indocin).	Alcoholic beverages Alka-Seltzer Alka-2 Anacin A.P.C. Bufferin A.S.A. and A.S.A. compound Ascriptin Aspergum Aspirin Bayer products Beer Cama Cheracol Coricidin Coryban-D Cosanyl-DM Demazin Syrup Dristan Cough Formula and Dristan Decongestant Tablets Ecotrin Empirin Excedrin 4-Way Cold Tablets Gemnisyn Histadyl E.C. Measurin Midol Neo-Synephrine Novahistine Nyquil PAC and PAC Compound Pamprin Pepto-Bismol Pertussin Phensal Robitussin Sodium salicylate Sominex Super Anahist Triaminic Expectorant Triaminicin Vanquish Vicks Formula 44 Cough Mixture

Chart 17. Chemotherapeutic drug interactions

	Any of these prescription drugs may interact with ➧	*any of these OTC/food items as described in column 1.*	*Any of these prescription drugs may interact with* ➧	*any of these prescription drug groups* ➧	*and result in this interaction.*
The antineoplastic drugs listed in Chart 17 are primarily used in various neoplastic disorders, although methotrexate is sometimes used in psoriatic conditions. The full product description should be consulted when questioning these interactions. Persistent diarrhea, fever, chills, sore throat, unusual bleeding, bruising, or jaundice may warrant a change in dosage or drug. Nursing or pregnancy should be avoided for at least 8 weeks following therapy. The patient should avoid stressful situations and maintain a well-balanced diet. The OTC reactions noted here show that if fluorouracil is used orally, acidic foods taken at the same time could significantly decrease the effectiveness of fluorouracil. The OTC interactions regarding methotrexate point out that salicylates can increase the toxic side effects of methotrexate if the two are combined. Methotrexate can also decrease the effects of fluorouracil.	Fluorouracil (5-Fu)	Acidic foods, for example, orange juice	Azathioprine (Imuran) Cyclophosphamide (Cytoxan) Mercaptopurine (Purinethol) Procarbazine (Matulane; see Chart 15)	Allopurinol (Zyloprim)	Even though this combination of two interacting drugs may often be prescribed by the physician, it is usually with a decrease in the dosage or strength of the drugs in column 1. This is done to avoid any toxic or adverse side effects. Azathioprine and mercaptopurine may also decrease oral anticoagulant drug activity (chart 4).
	Methotrexate	Alka-2 Alka-Seltzer Anacin Products A.P.C. Arthritis Strength Bufferin A.S.A. and A.S.A. Compound Ascriptin Aspergum Aspirin Bayer products Bufferin Cama Coricidin products Dristan Ecotrin Empirin Excedrin Excedrin 4-Way Cold Tablets Measurin Midol PAC and PAC Compound Pamprin Pepto-Bismol Phensal Sodium salicylate Sominex Super Anahist Triaminicin Vanquish			

Chart 18. Injectable drug and anesthetic interactions

Any of these prescription drugs may interact with	*any of these prescription drug groups*	*and result in this interaction.*
Heparin sodium	A.S.A. and salicylates Anticoagulants (oral) (Chart 4)	An increase in the anticoagulant effect may occur; patients' protime should be monitored. Guaifenesin (Robitussin) and dipyridamole (Persantine) may react with heparin and lead to increased chance of bleeding.
Methotrimeprazine (Levoprome)	Antihypertensives (Chart 11)	An increase in antihypertensive effect resulting in severe hypotension may occur.
	CNS depressants MAO inhibitors (Chart 15)	There is an increase in central nervous system depression and severe and toxic reactions. Avoid MAO inhibitor combination.
	Anticholinergics Succinylcholine chloride (Anectine)	This combination results in decreased blood pressure and effects on the central nervous system from stimulation to delirium. Extrapyramidal symptoms or tachycardia may occur.
Muscle relaxants Depolarizing: Decamethonium (Syncurine) Succinylcholine (Anectine) Nondepolarizing: Gallamine (Flaxadil) Pancuronium (Pavulon) (Metubine) Tubocurarine	Anesthetics Lithium (Lithane, Eskalith) Lidocaine (Mylocaine) Clindamycin (Cleocin) Lincomycin (Lincocin) Quinidine (CinQuin) Procainamide (Pronestyl, Procan) Colymycin-M Polymixin B (Aerosporin)	These combinations result in prolongation in neuromuscular blockade. Respiratory depression or apnea may occur. Amphotericin B (Fungizone) and aminoglycosides react with muscle relaxants (see below).
Diazoxide (Hyperstat I.V.)	Thiazide diuretics Antidiabetic agents (Chart 3)	Enhanced hyperglycemic effect and hypotension occur. Hyperglycemic effects occur.
	Anticoagulants (Chart 4)	These combinations cause increased anticoagulant effect and possible hemorrhage.
Amphotericin B (Fungizone)	Muscle relaxants (see above) Aminoglycoside (see below) Digitalis (Chart 9)	Increased skeletal muscle effect due to potassium loss occurs. There is an increased possibility of nephrotoxicity. Hypokalemia and increased digitalis toxicity are possible.
	Steroids (Chart 7)	These combinations result in increased potassium loss and possible decrease in infectious resistance, sometimes used together to control drug reaction.

Continued.

Chart 18. Injectable drug and anesthetic interactions—cont'd

Any of these prescription drugs may interact with	*any of these prescription drug groups*	*and result in this interaction.*
Methoxyflurane (Penthrane)	Tetracyclines (Chart 12)	These combinations may cause nephrotoxicity and should be avoided.
Mercaptomerin (Thiomerin)	Digitalis (Chart 9)	These may result in hypokalemia with resultant digitalis toxicity.
Doxorubicin (Adriamycin) Dannorubiecin (Cerubidine)	Cyclophosphamide (Cytoxan)	An increase in cardiotoxicity may occur.
Aminoglycosides Amikacin (Amikin) Gentamicin (Garamycin) Neomycin Kanamycin (Kantrex) Streptomycin Tobramycin (Nebcin)	Anesthetics (see below) Muscle relaxants (see above) Ether Sodium citrate	These combinations result in a possible increase in skeletal muscle response and severe possibility of respiratory paralysis.
	Diuretics Ethacrynic acid (Edecrin) Furosemide (Lasix)	These result in ototoxicity and should be avoided if possible.
	Colistimethate (Coly-Mycin M) Polymixin B (Aerosporin) Viomycin (Viocin) Cephaloridine (Loridine)	There is an increased potential of nephrotoxicity/neurotoxicity and neuromuscular block with polypeptides. Concurrent use should be avoided if possible. Cephaloridine could increase toxicity when used with diuretics above.
Anesthetics	Metaraminol (Aramine) Epinephrine preparations Dopamine (Intropin)	Ventricular arrhythmias may occur.
	Antihistamines (Chart 2) MAO inhibitors (Chart 15) Methyldopa (Aldomet, Aldoril) *Rauwolfia* alkaloids and reserpine combinations (Chart 11)	Severe increase in hypotension/hypertension and/or central nervous system depression could occur. Physicians should allow 10 to 14 days after discontinuing MAO inhibitors and *Rauwolfia* products before administering anesthetics.
Anesthetics with vasoconstrictor, for example, lidocaine (Xylocaine) with epinephrine	MAO inhibitors (Chart 15) Tricyclic antidepressants (Chart 14) Phenothiazines	Severe hypotension and/or hypertension may occur. Sufficient time should be allowed after discontinuing drugs in column 2 before administering.

11-2 Comparison of selected effects of commonly abused drugs

Some selected effects of commonly abused drugs are summarized in the following table. This table is intended for quick reference only.

Drug category	*Physical dependence*	*Characteristics of intoxication*
Opiates	Marked	Analgesia with or without depressed sensorium; pinpoint pupils (tolerance does not develop to this action); patient may be alert and appear normal; respiratory depression with overdose
Barbiturates	Marked	Patient may appear normal with usual dose, but narrow margin between doses needed to prevent withdrawal symptoms and toxic dose is often exceeded and patient appears ''drunk,'' with drowsiness, ataxia, slurred speech, and nystagmus on lateral gaze; pupil size and reaction normal; respiratory depression with overdose
Nonbarbiturate sedatives: glutethimide (Doriden)	Marked	Pupils dilated and reactive to light; coma and respiratory depression prolonged; sudden apnea and laryngeal spasm common
Antianxiety agents (''minor tranquilizers'')	Marked	Progressive depression of sensorium as with barbiturates; pupil size and reaction normal; respiratory depression with overdose
Ethanol	Marked	Depressed sensorium, acute or chronic brain syndrome, odor on breath, pupil size and reaction normal
Amphetamines	Mild to absent	Agitation, with paranoid thought disturbance in high doses; acute organic brain syndrome after prolonged use; pupils dilated and reactive; tachycardia, elevated blood pressure, with possibility of hypertensive crisis and CVA; possibility of convulsive seizures
Cocaine	Absent	Paranoid thought disturbance in high doses, with dangerous delusions of persecution and omnipotence; tachycardia; respiratory depression with overdose
Marijuana	Absent	Milder preparations: drowsy, euphoric state with frequent inappropriate laughter and disturbance in perception of time or space (occasional acute psychotic reaction reported); stronger preparations such as hashish: frequent hallucinations or psychotic reaction; pupils normal, conjunctivas injected (marijuana preparations frequently adulterated with LSD, tryptamines, or heroin)
Psychotomimetics: LSD, STP, tryptamines, mescaline, morning glory seeds	Absent	Unpredictable disturbance in ego function, manifest by extreme lability of affect and chaotic disruption of thought, with danger of uncontrolled behavioral disturbance; pupils dilated and reactive to light
Phencyclidine	Unknown	Disinhibition, agitation, confusion, chaotic thought disturbance, unpredictable behavior, hypertension, meiosis, respiratory collapse, cardiovascular collapse, death.
Anticholinergic agents	Absent	Nonpsychotropic effects such as tachycardia, decreased salivary secretion, urinary retention, and dilated, nonreactive pupils plus depressed sensorium, confusion, disorientation, hallucinations, and delusional thinking
Inhalants*	Unknown	Depressed sensorium, hallucinations, acute brain syndrome; odor on breath; often glassy-eyed appearance

*The term inhalant is used to designate a variety of gases and highly volatile organic liquids, including the aromatic glues, paint thinners, gasoline, some anesthetic ager marijuana).

Characteristics of withdrawal	"Flashback" symptoms	Masking of symptoms of illness or injury during intoxication
ıinorrhea, lacrimation, and dilated, reactive pupils, followed by gastrointestinal disturbances, low back pain, and waves of gooseflesh; convulsions not a feature unless heroin samples were adulterated with barbiturates	Not reported	An important feature of opiate intoxication, due to analgesic action, with or without depressed sensorium
gitation, tremulousness, insomnia, gastrointestinal disturbances, hyperpyrexia, blepharoclonus (clonic blink reflex), acute brain syndrome, major convulsive seizures	Not reported	Only in presence of depressed sensorium or after onset of acute brain syndrome
milar to barbiturate withdrawal syndrome, with agitation, gastrointestinal disturbances, hyperpyrexia, and major convulsive seizures	Not reported	Same as in barbiturate intoxication
milar to barbiturate withdrawal syndrome, with danger of major convulsive seizures	Not reported	Same as in barbiturate intoxication
milar to barbiturate withdrawal syndrome, but with less likelihood of convulsive seizures	Not reported	Same as in barbiturate intoxication
ethargy, somnolence, dysphoria, and possibility of suicidal depression; brain syndrome may persist for many weeks	Infrequently reported	Drug-induced euphoria or acute brain syndrome may interfere with awareness of symptoms of illness or may remove incentive to report symptoms of illness
milar to amphetamine withdrawal	Not reported	Same as in amphetamine intoxication
o specific withdrawal symptoms	Infrequently reported	Uncommon with milder preparations; stronger preparations may interfere in same manner as psychotomimetic agents
o specific withdrawal symptoms; symptoms may persist for indefinite period after discontinuation of drug	Commonly reported as late a 1 year after last dose	Affective response or psychotic thought disturbance may remove awareness of, or incentive to report, symptoms of illness
o specific withdrawal symptoms	Occasionally reported	Same as in LSD intoxication
o specific withdrawal symptoms; mydriasis may persist for several days	Not reported	Pain may not be reported as a result of depression of sensorium, acute brain syndrome, or acute psychotic reaction
o specific withdrawal symptoms	Infrequently reported	Same as in anticholinergic intoxication

d amylnitrite. The term excludes liquids sprayed into the nasopharynx (droplet transport required) and substances that must be ignited before administration (such as

11-3 Cross-reference guide to drugs (generic and brand names)

Drugs or drug type	*Brand names*	*Generic name*
Acetaminophen (systemic)	Algophen*	Acetaminophen
	Atasol*	
	Atasol Forte*	
	Campain*	
	Datril	
	Empracet*	
	Exdol*	
	Liquiprin	
	Phenaphen	
	Robigesic*	
	Rounox*	
	SK-APAP	
	Tempra	
	Tivrin*	
	Tylenol	
	Tylenol Extra Strength	
	Valadol	
Acetaminophen and codeine (systemic)	Aceta with Codeine	
	Capital with Codeine	
	Empracet with Codeine	
	Papa-Deine	
	Pavadon	
	Phenaphen with Codeine	
	Proval	
	SK-APAP with Codeine	
	Tylenol with Codeine	
Acrisorcin (topical)	Akrinol	Acrisorcin
Adrenocorticoids (dental)	Orabase HCA	Hydrocortisone
	Kenalog in Orabase	Triamcinolone
Adrenocorticoids (ophthalmic)	Decadron	Dexamethasone
	Maxidex	
	Novadex*	
	FML Liquifilm	Fluorometholone
	Cortamed*	Hydrocortisone
	Cortisol	
	Hydrocortone	
	Optef	
	HMS Liquifilm	Medrysone
	AK-Pred	Prednisone
	AK-Tate	
	Econopred	
	Hydeltrasol	
	Inflamase	
	Metreton	
	Pred Forte	
	Pred Mild	
	Predulose	
Adrenocorticoids (otic)	Decadron	Dexamethasone
	Maxidex	
	Hydeltrasol	Prednisolone
	Metreton	
Adrenocorticoids (topical)	Cyclocort	Amcinonide
	Benisone	Betamethasone
	Betacort*	
	Betaderm*	
	Betnovate*	
	Celestoderm*	
	Celestone	
	Valisone	
	Tridesilon	Desonide
	Topicort	Desoximetasone
	Aeroseb-Dex	Dexamethasone
	Decaderm	
	Decadron	
	Decaspray	
	Hexadrol	
	Florone	Diflorasone
	Locacorten*	Flumethasone
	Locorten	
	Dermalar*	Fluocinolone
	Fluoderm*	
	Fluonid	
	Flurosyn	
	Synalar	
	Lidemol*	Fluocinonide
	Lidex	
	Topsyn	
	Oxylone	Fluorometholone
	Cordran	Flurandrenolide
	Drenison*	
	Halciderm	Halcinonide
	Halog	
	Cortaid	Hydrocortisone
	Cort-Dome	
	Cortef	
	Corticreme*	
	Cortisol	
	Cortril	
	Dermacort	
	Hyderm*	
	Hydrocortone	
	Hytone	
	Texacort	
	Medrol	Methylprednisolone
	Meti-Derm	Prednisolone
	Aristocort	Triamcinolone

*Not available in the United States.

Drugs or drug type	*Brand names*	*Generic name*
	Aristogel	
	Kenalog	
	Kenalog-E*	
	Spencort	
	Triacet	
	Triaderm*	
	Triamalone*	
	Trimacort*	
Adrenocorticoids (systemic)	Betnelan*	Betamethasone
	Betnesol*	
	Celestone	
	Cortone	Cortisone
	Decadron	Dexamethasone
	Dexasone	
	Hexadrol	
	Alphadrol	Fluprednisolone
	A-Hydrocort	Hydrocortisone
	Cortef	
	Cortenema	
	Hydrocortone	
	Solu-Cortef	
	Betapar	Meprednisone
	A-MethaPred	Methylprednisolone
	Duralone	
	Medralone	
	Medrol	
	Methylone	
	Haldrone	Paramethasone
	Delta-Cortef	Prednisolone
	Hydeltrasol	
	Meticortelone	
	Sterone	
	Predoxine	Prednisolone, Buffered
	Colisone*	Prednisone
	Deltasone	
	Meticorten	
	Orasone	
	Sterapred	
	Winpred*	
	Aristocort	Triamcinolone
	Aristospan	
	Cinonide	
	Kenacort	
	Kenalog	
	Tramacort	
	Doca	Desoxycorticosterone
	Percorten	
	Florinef	Fludrocortisone
Alcohol and acetone (topical)	Seba-Nil	
	Sebasum	
	Tyrosum	
Alcohol and sulfur (topical)	Acne Aid	
	Acnomead	
	Epi-Clear	
	Liquimat	
	Postacne	
	Transact	
	Xerac	
Allopurinol (systemic)	Lopurin	Allopurinol
	Purinol*	
	Zyloprim	
Amantadine (systemic)	Symmetrel	Amantadine
Aminocaproic acid (systemic)	Amicar	Aminocaproic acid
Aminoglycosides (systemic)	Amikin	Amikacin
	Apogen	Gentamicin
	Bristagen	
	Cidomycin*	
	Garamycin	
	U-Gencin	
	Kantrex	Kanamycin
	Klebcil	
	Mycifradin	Neomycin
		Streptomycin
	Nebcin	Tobramycin
4-Aminoquinolones (systemic)	Camoquin	Amodiaquine
	Aralen	Chloroquine
	Plaquenil	Hydroxychloroquine
Aminosalicylates (systemic)	Nemasol*	Aminosalicylic acid
	P.A.S.	
	Parasal	
	Teebacin	
Amphetamines (systemic)	Benzedrine	Amphetamine
	Dexampex	Dextroamphetamine
	Dexedrine	
	Diphylets	
	Ferndex	
	Obotan	
	Oxydess	
	Spancap	
	Desoxyn	Methamphetamine
	Methampex	
Amphotericin B (systemic)	Fungizone	Amphotericin B
Amphotericin B (topical)	Fungizone	Amphotericin B
Anthralin (topical)	Anthra-Derm	Anthralin
	Lasan	
Anticoagulants (systemic)	Miradon	Anisindione
	Dufalone*	Dicumarol
	Danilone*	Phenindione
	Hedulin	
	Liquamar	Phenprocoumon
	Marcumar*	
	Athrombin-K	Warfarin Potassium
	Coumadin	Warfarin Sodium
	Panwarfin	
	Warfilone*	
	Warnerin*	
Antidiabetics, oral (systemic)	Dimelor*	Acetohexamide
	Dymelor	
	Chloromide*	Chlorpropamide
	Chloronase*	
	Diabinese	

*Not available in the United States.

Continued.

Cross-reference guide to drugs (generic and brand names)—cont'd

Drugs or drug type	*Brand names*	*Generic name*
	Tolinase	Tolazamide
	Mobenol*	Tolbutamide
	Neo-Dibetic*	
	Novobutamide*	
	Oramide*	
	Orinase	
	Tolbutone*	
Antidyskinetics—anticholinergic agents used to treat Parkinson's disease (systemic)	Bensylate*	Benztropine
	Cogentin	
	Akineton	Biperiden
	Pagitane	Cycrimine
	Parsidol	Ethopropazine
	Parsitan*	
	Kemadrin	Procyclidine
	Aparkane*	Trihexyphenidyl
	Artane	
	Tremin	
Antiglaucoma agents, cholinergic—long-acting cholinesterase inhibitors (ophthalmic)	Humorsol	Demecarium
	Echodide	Echothiophate
	Phospholine Iodide	Isoflurophate
	Floropryl	
Antihistamines (systemic)	Idulian*	Azatadine
	Optimine	
	Ambodryl	Bromodiphenhydramine
	Deserol*	
	Bromphen	Brompheniramine
	Dimetane	
	Ilvin*	
	Puretane	
	Symptom 3	
	Allergefon*	Carbinoxamine
	Clistin	
	Chloramate	Chlorpheniramine
	Chlor-Trimeton	
	Histalon*	
	Histaspan	
	Ibioton*	
	Novopheniram*	
	Phenetron	
	Piriton*	
	Teldrin	
	Tavegil*	Clemastine
	Tavist	
	Cyprodine	Cyproheptadine
	Nuran*	
	Periactin	
	Vimicon*	
	Polaramine	Dexchlorpheniramine
	Dramamine	Dimenhydrinate
	Eldodram	
	Gravol*	
	Novodimenate*	
	Travamine*	
	Dimethpyrindene	Dimethindene
	Forhistal	
	Triten	
	Benadryl	Diphenhydramine
	Bendylate	
	Eldadryl	
	Insomnal*	
	Nautamine*	
	Valdrene	
	Diafen	Diphenylpyraline
	Hispril	
	Decapryn	Doxylamine
	Allertoc	Pyrilamine
	Mepyramine	
	Neo-Antergan*	
	Thylogen	
	Benzoxal*	Tripelennamine
	PBZ	
	Pyribenzamine	
	Pyrizil*	
	Actidil	Triprolidine
	Actidilon*	
	Pro-Actidil*	
Antipyrine, benzocaine, and glycerin (otic)	Auralgan	
	Aurasol	
Antithyroid agents (systemic)	Tapazole	Methimazole
	Thiamazole	
	Propacil	Propylthiouracil
	Propyl-Thyracil	
APC (Aspirin, phenacetin, and caffeine) (systemic)	Acetophen	
	Aidant	
	APAC	
	A.S.A. Compound	
	Asalco No. 1	
	Asphac-G	
	P-A-C Compound	
	Phencaset	
	Sal-Fayne	
	Salphenine	
	Tabloid APC	
APC and codeine (systemic)	Empirin Compound with Codeine	
	A.S.A. and Codeine Compound	
	P-A-C Compound with Codeine	
	Salatin with Codeine	
	Tabloid APC with Codeine	
Appetite suppressants (systemic)	Didrex	Benzphetamine
	Pre-State	Chlorphentermine

*Not available in the United States.

Drugs or drug type	*Brand names*	*Generic name*
	Voranil	Clortermine
	Dietec*	Diethylpropion
	Regibon*	
	Tenuate	
	Tepanil	
	Sanorex	Mazindol
	Bontril PDM	Phendimetrazine
	Phendiet	
	Plegine	
	Preludin	Phenmetrazine
	Fastin	Phentermine
	Ionamin	
Asparaginase (systemic)	Elspar	
Atropine (anticholinergics) (ophthalmic)	Atropisol	Atropine
	BufOpto Atropine	
	Isopto Atropine	
	Homatrocel	Homatropine
	Isopto Homatropine	
	Isopto Hyoscine	Scopolamine
Azathioprine (systemic)	Imuran	Azathioprine
Baclofen (systemic)	Lioresal	Baclofen
Barbiturates (systemic)	Amytal	Amobarbital
	Isobec*	
	Buticaps	Butabarbital
	Butisol	
	Sombulex	Hexobarbital
	Mebaral	Mephobarbital
	Gemonil	Metharbital
	Nembutal	Pentobarbital
	Nova-Rectal*	
	Pentogen*	
	Eskabarb*	Phenobarbital
	Gardenal*	
	Nova-Pheno*	
	Sedadrops	
	SK-Phenobarbital	
	Solfoton	
	Secogen*	Secobarbital
	Seconal	
	Seral*	
	Tuinal	Secobarbital and Amobarbital
	Lotusate	Talbutal
Beclomethasone (inhalation)	Beclovent	Beclomethasone
	Vanceril	
Belladonna alkaloids and barbiturates (systemic)	Minabel	Atropine, hyoscyamine, scopolamine, and butabarbital
	Omnibel	
	Palbar	
	Cyclo-Bell	Atropine, hyoscyamine, scopolamine, butabarbital, pentobarbital, and phenobarbital
	Barbidonna	Atropine, hyoscyamine, scopolamine, and phenobarbital
	Donna-Sed	
	Donnatal	
	Donphen	
	Hasp	
	Hybephen	
	Hyosophen	
	Kinesed	
	Sedralex	
	Setamine	
	Spalix	
	Spasmolin	
	Spasmophen	
	Spasmorel	
	Tri-Spas	
	Alised	Atropine and phenobarbital
	Antrocol	
	Atrobarb	
	Amobell	Belladonna and amobarbital
	Butibel	Belladonna and butabarbital
	Belap	Belladonna and phenobarbital
	Bellophen	
	Bello-Phen	
	Chardonna	
	Donabarb	
	Donnabarb	
	Oxoids	
	Phenobel	
	Phenobella	
	Sedajen	
	Valaspas	
	Hybar	Hyoscyamine, scopolamine, and phenobarbital
	Cystospaz-SR	Hyoscyamine and butabarbital
	Anaspaz PB	Hyoscyamine and phenobarbital
	Levsin-PB	
	Levsin w/Phenobarbital	
	Levsinex w/Phenobarbital	

*Not available in the United States.

Continued.

Cross-reference guide to drugs (generic and brand names)—cont'd

Drugs or drug type	*Brand names*	*Generic name*
Benzodiazepines (systemic)	A-poxide	Chlordiazepoxide
	C-Tran*	
	Librium	
	Nack*	
	Novopoxide*	
	Relaxil*	
	SK-Lygen	
	Tranxene	Clorazepate
	D-Tran*	Diazepam
	E-Pam*	
	Novodipam*	
	Valium	
	Vivol*	
	Dalmane	Flurazepam
	Ativan	Lorazepam
	Serax	Oxazepam
	Verstran	Prazepam
Benzoyl peroxide (topical)	Benoxyl	Benzoyl peroxide
	Benzac	
	Benzagel	
	Clear By Design	
	Dermodex	
	Desquam-X	
	Epi-Clear	
	Fostex BPO	
	Panoxyl	
	Persadox	
	Persa-Gel	
	Porox 7	
	Teen	
	Topex	
	Xerac BP	
Beta-adrenergic blocking agents (systemic)	Lopressor	Metoprolol
	Corgard	Nadolol
	Inderal	Propranolol
Bethanechol (systemic)	Duvoid	
	Myotonachol	
	Urecholine	
Bleomycin (systemic)	Blenoxane	Bleomycin
Bromocriptine (systemic)	Parlodel	Bromocriptine
Brompheniramine, giuaifenesin, phenylephrine, and phenylpropanolamine (systemic)	Dimetane expectorant	
	Midatane expectorant	
	Normatene expectorant	
	Puretane expectorant	
	Spentane expectorant	
Brompheniramine, guaifenesin, phenylephrine, phenylpropanolamine, and codeine (systemic)	Dimetane expectorant-DC	
	Midatane DC expectorant	
	Normatane DC expectorant	
	Puretane Expectorant DC	
	Spentane DC expectorant	
Brompheniramine, phenylephrine, and phenylpropanolamine (systemic)	Brompheniramine Compound	
	Bromatapp	
	Dimetapp	
	Eldatapp	
	Puretapp	
Busulfan (systemic)	Myleran	Busulfan
Butalbital and APC (systemic)	Fiorinal	
Butalbital, APC, and codeine (systemic)	Fiorinal with codeine	
Butorphanol (systemic)	Stadol	Butorphanol
Calcitonin (systemic)	Calcimar	Calcitonin
Capreomycin (systemic)	Capastat	Capreomycin
Carbachol (ophthalmic)	Carbacel	Carbachol
	Isopto Carbachol	
	Miostat	
	Murocarb	
Carboprost (systemic)	Prostin/15 M	Carboprost
Carisoprodol (systemic)	Rela	Carisoprodol
	Soma	
	Soprodol	
Carmustine (systemic)	BiCNU	Carmustine
Cephalosporins (systemic)	Ceclor	Cefaclor
	Duricef	Cefadroxil
	Ultracef	
	Mandol	Cefamandole
	Ancef	Cefazolin
	Kefzol	
	Mefoxin	Cefoxitin
	Ceporex*	Cephalexin
	Keflex	
	Kafocin	Cephaloglycin
	Ceporan*	Cephaloridine
	Loridine	

*Not available in the United States.

Drugs or drug type	Brand names	Generic name
	Ceporacin*	Cephalothin
	Keflin Neutral	
	Cefadyl	Cephapirin
	Anspor	Cephradine
	Velosef	
Charcoal, activated (oral)	Charcocaps	
	Charcodote	
	Charcotabs	
Chloral hydrate (systemic)	Aquachloral	
	Chloralex*	
	Chloralvan*	
	Cohidrate	
	Noctec	
	Novochlorhydrate*	
	Oradrate	
Chlorambucil (systemic)	Leukeran	Chlorambucil
Chloramphenicol (ophthalmic)	Chloromycetin	Chloramphenicol
	Chloroptic	
	Econochlor	
	Fenicol*	
	Ophthochlor	
	Pentamycetin*	
	Sopamycetin*	
Chloramphenicol (otic)	Chloromycetin	Chloramphenicol
Chloramphenicol (systemic)	Amphicol	Chloramphenicol
	Chloromycetin	
	Novochlorocap*	
	Pentamycetin*	
Chloramphenicol (topical)	Chloromycetin	Chloramphenicol
Chlordiazepoxide and amitriptyline (systemic)	Limbitrol	
Chlordiazepoxide and clidinium (systemic)	Librax	
Chloroxine (topical)	Capitrol	Chloroxine
Chlorpheniramine, phenylpropanolamine, and isopropamide (systemic)	Allernade	
	Capade	
	Ornade	
Chlorzoxazone (systemic)	Paraflex	Chlorzoxazone
Chlorzoxazone and acetaminophen (systemic)	Chlorofon-F	
	Chlorzone Forte	
	Lobac	
	Miflex	
	Parachlor	
	Parafon Forte	
	Tuzon	
Cholestyramine (oral)	Questran	Cholestyramine
Cimetidine (systemic)	Tagamet	Cimetidine
Cisplatin (systemic)	Platinol	Cisplatin
Clindamycin (topical)	Cleocin T	Clindamycin
Clofibrate (systemic)	Atromid-S	Clofibrate
Clomiphene (systemic)	Clomid	Clomiphene
Clonidine (systemic)	Catapres	Clonidine
Clonidine and chlorthalidone (systemic)	Combipres	
Clotrimazole (topical)	Lotrimin	Clotrimazole
	Mycelex	
Clotrimazole (vaginal)	Gyne-Lotrimin	Clotrimazole
Coal tar (topical)	DHS tar	
	Estar	
	Medotar	
	Pentrax Tar	
	Pso-Rite	
	Supertah	
	Tar Dak	
	Tarbonis	
	Tarpaste	
	Tersa-Tar	
	Ul-Tar	
	Zetar	
Colchicine (systemic)	Colsalide Improved	Colchicine
Colestipol (systemic)	Colestid	Colestipol
Colistin, neomycin, and hydrocortisone (otic)	Coly-Mycin S	
Cromolyn (inhalation)	Intal	Cromolyn
Cyclandelate (systemic)	Cyclospasmol	Cyclandelate
Cyclobenzaprine (systemic)	Flexeril	Cyclobenzaprine
Cyclopentolate (ophthalmic)	Cyclogyl	Cyclopentolate
	Mydplegic*	
Cyclophosphamide (systemic)	Cytoxan	Cyclophosphamide
	Procytox*	
Cycloserine (systemic)	Seromycin	Cycloserine
Cytarabine (systemic)	Cytosar-U	Cytarabine

*Not available in the United States.

Continued.

Cross-reference guide to drugs (generic and brand names)—cont'd

Drugs or drug type	*Brand names*	*Generic name*
Dacarbazine (systemic)	DTIC-Dome	Dacarbazine
Dactinomycin (systemic)	Cosmegen	Dactinomycin
Danazol (systemic)	Cyclomen* Danocrine	Danazol
Dantrolene (systemic)	Dantrium	Dantrolene
Dapsone (systemic)	Avlosulfon	Dapsone
Desonide and acetic acid (otic)	Tridesilon	
Dexamethasone (nasal)	Decadron	Dexamethasone
Dexbrompheniramine and pseudoephedrine (systemic)	Disophrol Drixoral	
Diazoxide (oral)	Proglycem	Diazoxide
Dicyclomine (systemic)	Bentyl Bentylol* Cyclobec* Dyspas	Dicyclomine
Digitalis medicines (systemic)	Cedilanid-D	Deslanoside
	Digifortis Pil-Digis	Digitalis
	Crystodigin Purodigin	Digitoxin
	Lanoxin	Digoxin
	Gitaligin	Gitalin
	Cedilanid	Lanatoside C
	Strophanthin-G	Ouabain
Dimethyl sulfoxide (topical)	Rimso-50	Dimethyl sulfoxide
Dinoprost (intra-amniotic)	Prostin F_2 Alpha	Dinoprost
Dinoprostone (vaginal)	Prostin E_2	Dinoprostone
Dione-type anticonvulsants (systemic)	Paradione	Paramethadione
	Tridione	Trimethadione
Diphenoxylate and atropine (systemic)	Colonil Lomotil SK-Diphenoxylate	
Dipivefrin (ophthalmic)	Propine	Dipivefrin
Dipyridamole (systemic)	Persantine	Dipyridamole
Disopyramide (systemic)	Norpace Rythmodan*	Disopyramide
Disulfiram (systemic)	Antabuse	Disulfiram
Doxapram (systemic)	Dopram	Doxapram
Doxylamine and pyridoxine (systemic)	Bendectin	
Drocode, promethazine, and APC (systemic)	Synalgos-DC	
Ephedrine (systemic)	Ectasule Minus Ephedsol	
Epinephrine (ophthalmic)	Epifrin Epitrate Glaucon Murocoll Mytrate	Epinephrine
	Epinal Eppy/N	Epinephryl Borate
Epinephrine (systemic)	Adrenalin AsthmaHaler Bronitin Bronkaid Medihaler-Epi Primatene	Epinephrine
	AsthmaNefrin microNEFRIN Vaponefrin	Racepinephrine
Ergoloid mesylates (systemic)	Hydergine	
Ergonovine (systemic)	Ergotrate	Ergonovine
	Methergine	Methylergonovine
Ergotamine (systemic)	Ergomar Ergostat Gynergen Medihaler Ergotamine	Ergotamine tartrate
Ergotamine, belladonna alkaloids, and phenobarbital (systemic)	Bellergal Bellergal-S	
Ergotamine and caffeine (systemic)	Cafergot Cafermine Cafetrate Ergocaf Ergocaffeine Lanatrate Migrastat	
Ergotamine, caffeine, belladonna alkaloids, and phenobarbital (systemic)	Cafergot-PB	

*Not available in the United States.

Drugs or drug type	*Brand names*	*Generic name*
Erythromycin (ophthalmic)	Ilotycin	Erythromycin
Erythromycin (topical)	Ilotycin	Erythromycin
Erythromycin (systemic)	E-Mycin	Erythromycin
	Erythromid*	
	Ilotycin	
	Novorythro*	
	Robimycin	
	RP-Mycin	
	Ilosone	Erythromycin estolate
	E.E.S.	Erythromycin ethylsuccinate
	E-Mycin E	
	Pediamycin	
	Wyamycin E	
	Ilotycin	Erythromycin gluceptate
	Erythrocin	Erythromycin lactobionate
	Bristamycin	Erythromycin stearate
	Erypar	
	Erythrocin	
	Ethril	
	Pfizer-E	
	SK-Erythromycin	
	Wyamycin S	
Estrogens (systemic)	TACE	Chlorotrianisene
	DES	Diethylstilbestrol
	Stilphostrol	
	Delestrogen	Estradiol
	Estrace	
	Progynon	
	Premarin	Conjugated estrogens
	Amnestrogen	Esterified estrogens
	Theelin	Estrone
	Ogen	Estropipate
	Piperazine Estrone Sulfate	
	Estinyl	Ethinyl estradiol
	Feminone	
	Estrovis	Quinestrol
Estrogens (vaginal)	DV Cream	Dienestrol
	DES	Diethylstilbestrol
	Premarin	Conjugated estrogens
	Ogen	Estropipate
	Piperazine Estrone Sulfate	
Estrogens and progestins—oral contraceptives (systemic)	Demulen	Ethynodiol diacetate and ethinyl estradiol
	Ovulen	Ethynodiol diacetate and mestranol
	Ovcon	Norethindrone and ethinyl estradiol
	Brevicon	
	Modicon	
	Norinyl	Norethindrone and mestranol
	Ortho-Novum	
	Norlestrin	Norethindrone acetate and ethinyl estradiol
	Loestrin	
	Enovid	Norethynodrel and mestranol
	Ovral	Norgestrel and ethinyl estradiol
	Lo-Ovral	
Ethacrynic acid (systemic)	Edecrin	Ethacrynic acid
Ethambutol (systemic)	Etibi*	Ethambutol
	Myambutol	
Ethchlorvynol (systemic)	Placidyl	Ethchlorvynol
Ethinamate (systemic)	Valmid	Ethinamate
Ethionamide (systemic)	Trecator-SC	Ethionamide
Ethylnorepinephrine (systemic)	Bronkephrine	Ethylnorepinephrine
Fenfluramine (systemic)	Pondimin	Fenfluramine
Fenoprofen (systemic)	Nalfon	Fenoprofen
Flucytosine (systemic)	Ancobon	Flucytosine
	Ancotil*	
Fluorouracil (systemic)	Adrucil	Fluorouracil
Fluorouracil (topical)	Efudex	Fluorouracil
	Fluoroplex	
Furosemide (systemic)	Furoside*	Furosemide
	Lasix	
	Neo-renal	
	Novosemide*	
	Uritol*	
Gentamicin (ophthalmic-otic)	Garamycin	Gentamicin
	Genoptic	
Gentamicin (topical)	Garamycin	Gentamicin
Gentian violet (vaginal)	Genapax	Gentian violet
	Hyva	
Glutethimide (systemic)	Doriden	Glutethimide
	Dormtabs	
Glycerin (systemic)	Glyrol	
	Osmoglyn	
Gold compounds (systemic)	Solganal	Aurothioglucose
	Myochrysine	Gold sodium thiomalate
Griseofulvin (systemic)	Fulvicin P/G	Griseofulvin
	Fulvicin-U/F	
	Grifulvin V	
	Grisactin	

*Not available in the United States.

Continued.

Cross-reference guide to drugs (generic and brand names)—cont'd

Drugs or drug type	*Brand names*	*Generic name*
	Grisovin-FP* grisOwen Gris-PEG	
Guaifenesin (systemic)	2/G Anti-Tuss Breonesin Genetuss Glycotuss Glytuss Hytuss Malotuss Nortussin Proco Robitussin	Guaifenesin
Guaifenesin and codeine (systemic)	Cheracol Nortussin w/ Codeine Robitussin A-C Tolu-Sed	
Guaifenesin and dextromethorpan (systemic)	Anti-Tuss DM Cheracol D Dextro-Tuss GG 2-G-DM G-Tuss DM Guaiadex Neo-Vadrin Queltuss Robitussin-DM Silexin Tolu-Sed DM Trocal Unproco	
Guanethidine (systemic)	Ismelin	Guanethidine
Guanethidine and hydrochlorothiazide (systemic)	Esimil	
Haloperidol (systemic)	Haldol	Haloperidol
Haloprogin (topical)	Halotex	Haloprogin
Heparin (systemic)	Hepalean* Heprinar Lipo-Hepin Liquaemin Panheprin	Heparin
Hydantoin-type anticonvulsants (systemic)	Peganone	Ethotoin
	Mesantoin Methoin*	Mephenytoin
	Dantoin* Dilantin Di-Phen Diphenylan Diphenylhydantoin	Phenytoin
Hydralazine (systemic)	Apresoline Rolazine*	Hydralazine
Hydrocodone (systemic)	Codone Corutol DH* Dicodid Robidone*	Hydrocodone
Hydrocodone and hematropine (systemic)	Hycodan	
Hydrocodone and phenyltoloxamine resin complexes (systemic)	Tussionex	
Hydrocodone and pseudoephedrine (systemic)	Tussend	
Hydrocodone, pseudoephedrine, and guaifenesin (systemic)	Tussend expectorant	
Hydrocortisone (rectal)	Cortifoam Cort-Dome Proctocort	Hydrocortisone
Hydrocortisone and acetic acid (otic)	VōSol HC	
Hydrocortisone, belladonna, ephedrine, zinc oxide, boric acid, bismuth, and peruvian balsam (rectal)	Wyanoids HC	
Hydrocortisone, bismuth, benzyl benzoate, peruvian balsam, and zinc oxide (rectal)	Anusol-HC	
Hydroxyurea (systemic)	Hydrea	Hydroxyurea
Hydroxyzine (systemic)	Atarax Vistaril	Hydroxyzine
Ibuprofen (systemic)	Motrin	Ibuprofen
Idoxuridine (ophthalmic)	Dendrid Herplex Stoxil	Idoxuridine
Indomethacin (systemic)	Indocid* Indocin	Indomethacin
Insulin (systemic)	Actrapid Regular Insulin Regular Iletin II (new)	Insulin injection

*Not available in the United States.

Drugs or drug type	*Brand names*	*Generic name*
	Velosulin	
	Globin Insulin	Globin zinc insulin injection
	insulatard	Isophane insulin suspension
	NPH	
	NPH Iletin II	
	Mixtard	Isophane insulin suspension and insulin injection
	Lentard	Insulin zinc suspension
	Lente Insulin	
	Lente Iletin II	
	Monotard	
	Ultralente	Extended insulin zinc suspension
	Ultralente Iletin	
	Ultratard	
	Semilente	Prompt insulin zinc suspension
	Semilente Iletin	
	Semitard	
	Protamine Zinc & Iletin II	Protamine zinc insulin suspension
	PZI	
Iodochlorhydroxyquin (topical)	Vioform	Iodochlorhydroxyquin
Iodochlorhydroxyquin and hydrocortisone (topical)	Dek-Quin	
	Domeform-HC	
	HCV	
	Mity-Quin	
	Racet	
	Vioform-HC	
Iodoquinol (systemic)	Moebiquin	Iodoquinol
	Yodoxin	
Isoetharine (systemic)	Bronkometer	Isoetharine
	Bronkosol	
Isometheptene, dichloralphenazone, and acetaminophen (systemic)	Midrin	
Isoniazid (systemic)	INH	Isoniazid
	Isotamine*	
	Nydrazid	
	Rimifon*	
Isoproterenol (systemic)	Aerolone	Isoproterenol
	Iprenol	
	Isuprel	
	Medihaler-Iso	
	Norisodrine Aerotrol	
	Proternol	
	Vapo-Iso	
Isoproterenol and phenylephrine (systemic)	Duo-Medihaler	
Isoxsuprine (systemic)	Vasodilan	Isoxsurpine
	Vasoprine	
Kanamycin (oral)	Kantrex	Kanamycin
Kaolin and pectin (oral)	Kaomead	
	Kaopectate	
	Pargel	
Kaolin, pectin, belladonna alkaloids, and opium (systemic)	Donnagel-PG	
Kaolin, pectin, and paregoric (systemic)	Parepectolin	
Laxatives, bulk-forming (oral)	Maltsupex	Malt soup extract
	Cellothyl	Methylcellulose
	Cologel	
	Hydrolose	
	Mitrolan	Polycarbophil Polycarbophil Calcium
	Effersyllium	Psyllium muciloid
	Konsyl	Psyllium seed
	L.A. Formula	Psyllium
	Metamucil	
	Modane Bulk	
	Mucilose	
	Plova	
	Serutan	
	Siblin	
Laxatives, emollient (oral)	Surfak	Docusate calcium
	Kasof	Docusate potassium
	Afko-Lube	Docusate sodium
	Colace	
	Colax	
	Comfolax	
	Dioctyl Sodium Sulfosuccinate	
	Alaxin	Poloxamer 188
	Magcyl	
Laxatives, hyperosmotic-lactulose and saline (oral)	Chronulac	Magnesium citrate
	Citrate of Magnesia	
	Adlerika	Magnesium sulfate
	Epsom Salts	
	Phospho-Soda	Sodium phosphate (or phosphates)
	Sal hepatica	Effervescent sodium phosphate

*Not available in the United States.

Continued.

Cross-reference guide to drugs (generic and brand names)—cont'd

Drugs or drug type	*Brand names*	*Generic name*
Laxatives, lubricant (oral)	Liquid petrolatum	Mineral oil
	Nujol	
	Neo-Cultol	Mineral oil (jellied)
Laxatives, stimulant (oral)	Cenalax	Bisacodyl
	Codylax	
	Dulcolax	
	Theralax	
	Cascara Sagrada	Cascara
	Cas-Evac	
	Alphanmul	Castor oil
	Neoloid	
	Dorbane	Danthron
	Modane	
	Cholan-DH	Dehydrocholic acid
	Decholin	
	Neocholan	
	Alophen	Phenolphthalein
	Espotabs	
	Evac-U-Gen	
	Evac-U-Lax	
	Ex-Lax	
	Feen-A-Mint	
	Phenolax	
	Prulet	
	Black Draught	Senna
	Casa Fru	
	Dr. Caldwell's Senna Laxative	
	Fletcher's Castoria	
	Senokot	
	Swiss Kriss	
	X-Prep	
	Glysennid	Sennosides A and B
	Senokot	
	X-Prep	
Levodopa (systemic)	Sinemet	Carbidopa and levodopa
	Bendopa	Levodopa
	Dopar	
	Larodopa	
	Levopa*	
Lime, sulfurated (topical)	Vlem-Dome	
	Vleminckx's solution	
Lincomycins (systemic)	Cleocin	Clindamycin
	Dalacin C*	
	Lincocin	Lincomycin
Lindane (topical)	GBH*	Lindane
	Kwell	
	Kwellada*	
Lithium (systemic)	Eskalith	Lithium carbonate
	Lithonate	
	Lithobid	
	Lithonate-S	
	Lithane	
Lomustine (systemic)	Cee Nu	Lomustine
Loperamide (systemic)	Imodium	Loperamide
Loxapine (systemic)	Daxolin	Loxapine
	Loxitane	
Magnesia, milk of (oral)	Magnesia	
	Magnesium hydroxide	
Mannitol (systemic)	Osmitrol	Mannitol
Mecamylamine (systemic)	Inversine	Mecamylamine
Mechlorethamine (systemic)	Mustargen	Mechlorethamine
Meclizine (systemic)	Bucladin-S	Buclizine
	Marezine	Cyclizine
	Antivert	Meclizine
	Bonine	
Meclofenamate (systemic)	Meclomen	Meclofenamate
Melphalan (systemic)	Alkeran	Melphalan
Meperidine (systemic)	Demerol	Meperidine
	Demer-Idine*	
	Pethadol	
Meprobamate (systemic)	Equanil	Meprobamate
	Lan-Dol*	
	Medi-Tran*	
	Mep-E*	
	Meprospan	
	Miltown	
	Neo-Tran*	
	Novo-Mepro*	
	Quietal*	
	SK-Bamate	
	Tranmap	
Meprobamate, ethoheptazine, and aspirin (systemic)	Equagesic	
	Heptogesic	
	Mepro Compound	
	Meprogesic	
Mercaptopurine (systemic)	Purinethol	Mercaptopurine
Metaproterenol (systemic)	Alupent	Metaproterenol
	Metaprel	
Methadone (systemic)	Dolophine	Methadone
	Westadone	
Methaqualone (systemic)	Mequelon*	Methaqualone
	Mequin	
	Parest	
	Quaalude	
	Sedalone*	
	Sopor	
	Triador*	
	Tualone*	

*Not available in the United States.

Drugs or drug type	*Brand names*	*Generic name*
Methenamine (systemic)	Hiprex Urex	Methenamine hippurate
	Mandelamine Methandine* Prov-U-Sep Sterine*	Methenamine mandelate
Methocarbamol (systemic)	Delaxin Forbaxin Marbaxin-750 Metho-500 Robamol Robaxin Spinaxin Tumol	Methocarbamol
Methotrexate (systemic)	Mexate	Methotrexate
Methoxsalen (systemic)	Oxsoralen	Methoxsalen
Methyldopa (systemic)	Aldomet Dopamet* Medimet-250* Novomedopa*	Methyldopa
Methyldopa and thiazide diuretics (systemic)	Aldoclor	Methyldopa and chlorothiazide
	Aldoril	Methyldopa and hydrochlorothiazide
Methylphenidate (systemic)	Methidate* Ritalin	Methylpenidate
Methyprylon (systemic)	Noludar	Methyprylon
Methysergide (systemic)	Sansert	Methysergide
Metronidazole (systemic)	Flagyl Neo-Tric* Novonidazole* Trikacide*	Metronidazole
Metyrosine (systemic)	Demser	Metyrosine
Miconazole (systemic)	Monistat	Miconazole
Miconazole (topical)	Micatin	Miconazole
Miconazole (vaginal)	Monistat	Miconazole
Minoxidil (systemic)	Loniten	Minoxidil
Mithramycin (systemic)	Mithracin	Mithramycin
Mitomycin (systemic)	Mutamycin	Mitomycin
Mitotane (systemic)	Lysodren	Mitotane

Drugs or drug type	*Brand names*	*Generic name*
Monoamine oxidase (MAO) inhibitors (systemic)	Marplan Nardil Parnate	Isocarboxazid Phenelzine Tranylcypromine
Nalbuphine (systemic)	Nubain	Nalbuphine
Nalidixic acid (systemic)	Neg Gram	Nalidixic acid
Naproxen (systemic)	Anaprox Naprosyn	Naproxen
Natamycin (opthalmic)	Natacyn	Natamycin
Neomycin (ophthalmic)	Myciguent	Neomycin
Neomycin (oral)	Mycifradin Neobiotic	Neomycin
Neomycin (topical)	Herisan Antibiotic* Myciguent	
Neomycin, polymyxin B, and bacitracin (ophthalmic)	Mycitracin Neo-Polycin Neosporin Polyspectrin Pyocidin	
Neomycin, polymyxin B, and bacitracin (topical)	Mycitracin Neo-Polycin Neosporin	
Neomycin, polymyxin B, and gramicidin (ophthalmic)	Neo-Polycin Neosporin	
Neomycin, polymyxin B, and hydrocortisone (ophthalmic)	Cortisporin	
Neomycin, polymyxin B, and hydrocortisone (otic)	Cortisporin Otobione	
Nicotinyl alcohol (systemic)	Roniacol	Nicotinyl alcohol
Organic nitrates (other than nitroglycerin) (systemic)	Cardilate	Erythrityl tetranitrate
	Coronex* Dilatrate-SR Iso-Bid Isordil Isotrate Sorate Sorbide Sorbitrate	Isosorbide dinitrate Duotrate Kaytrate Pentraspan Pentritol Peritrate
	Pentaerythritol tetranitrate	
Nitrofurantoin (systemic)	Cyantin Furadantin Furatine* Macrodantin Nephronex*	

*Not available in the United States.

Continued.

Cross-reference guide to drugs (generic and brand names)—cont'd

Drugs or drug type	*Brand names*	*Generic name*
	Nifuran* Novofuran*	
Nitroglycerin (systemic)	Glyceryl trinitrate Nitro-Bid Nitroglyn Nitrol Nitrong Nitrospan Nitrostat	Nitroglycerin
Nylidrin (systemic)	Arlidin	Nylidrin
Nystatin (oral)	Mycostatin Nadostine* Nilstat	Nystatin
Nystatin (topical)	Candex Mycostatin Nadostine* Nilstat Nyaderm*	Nystatin
Nystatin (vaginal)	Korostatin Mycostatin Nadostine* Nilstat	Nystatin
Nystatin, neomycin, gramicidin, and triamcinolone (topical)	Mycolog Myco Triacet Mytrex Triamcinolone NNG	
Orphenadrine (systemic)	Flexojet Flexon Marflex Myolin Neocyten Norflex Ro-Orphena Tega-Flex X-Otag	
Orphenadrine and APC (systemic)	Norgesic Norgesic Forte	
Oxolinic acid (systemic)	Utibid	Oxolinic acid
Oxtriphylline and guaifenesin (systemic)	Brondecon Brondelate	
Oxycodone and acetaminophen (systemic)	Percocet-5 Tylox	
Oxycodone and aspirin (systemic)	Percodan Percodan-Demi	
Oxymetazoline (nasal)	Afrin Duration Nafrine* St. Joseph Decongestant for Children	Oxymetazoline
Papaverine (systemic)	Cerebid Cerespan Dipav Dylate Hyobid Kavrin Myobid Orapav P-A-V Pavabid Pavacap Pavacon Pavadur Pavakey Pavased Pavasule Pavatest Pavatran Paverolan Ro-Papav Sustaverine Vasal Vasospan	Papaverine
Paraldehyde (systemic)	Paral	
Pargyline (systemic)	Eutonyl	
Pemoline (systemic)	Cylert	
Penicillamine (systemic)	Cuprimine Depen	
Penicillins (systemic)	Amoxil Larotid Novamoxin* Penamox* Polymox Robamox Sumox Trimox Utimox Wymox	Amoxicillin
	Amcill Ampicin* Omnipen Penbritin Pensyn Polycillin Principen Supen Totacillin	Ampicillin
	Geocillin Geopen Pyopen	Carbenicillin
	Bactopen* Cloxapen Novocloxin* Tegopen	Cloxacillin
	Cyclapen-W	Cyclacillin
	Dycill Dynapen	Dicloxacillin

*Not available in the United States.

Drugs or drug type	*Brand names*	*Generic name*
	Pathocil	Hetacillin
	Veracillin	
	Versapen	
	Versapen-K	Methicillin
	Azapen	
	Celbenin	Nafcillin
	Staphcillin	
	Nafcil	
	Unipen	
	Bactocil	Oxacillin
	Prostaphlin	
	Bicillin	Penicillin G
	Crystapen*	
	Crysticillin	
	Duracillin	
	Megacillin*	
	Penioral*	
	Pentids	
	Permapen	
	Wycillin	
	Betapen-VK	Penicillin V
	Novopen-V*	
	Penapar VK	
	Pen-Vee K	
	Uticillin VK	
	V-Cillin	
	Veetids	
	Ticar	Ticarcillin
Pentazocine (systemic)	Talwin	Pentazocine
Pentazocine and aspirin (systemic)	Talwin Compound	
Pentobarbital and carbromal (systemic)	Carbrital	
Perphenazine and amitriptyline (systemic)	Etrafon	
	Triavil	
Phenazopyridine (systemic)	Azo-100	Phenazopyridine
	Azodine	
	Azo-Standard	
	Di-Azo	
	Phen-Azo	
	Phenazodine	
	Pyridiate	
	Pyridium	
	Pyrodine	
Phenothiazines (systemic)	Tindal	Acetophenazine
	Repoise	Butaperizine
	Proketazine	Carphenazine
	Chloramead	Chlorpromazine
	Chlor-Promanyl*	
	Chlorprom*	
	Promapar	
	Promosol*	
	Largactil*	
	Thorazine	
	Modecate*	Fluphenazine
	Moditen*	
	Permitil	
	Prolixin	
	Serentil	Mesoridazine
	Phenazine*	Perphenazine
	Trilafon	
	Quide	Piperacetazine
	Compazine	Prochlorperazine
	Stemetil	
	Norzine*	Promazine
	Promanyl*	
	Sparine	
	Mellaril	Thioridazine
	Novoridazine*	
	Thioril*	
	Clinazine*	Trifluoperazine
	Novoflurazine*	
	Pentazine*	
	Solazine*	
	Stelazine*	
	Terfluzine*	
	Triflurin*	
	Tripazine*	
	Psyquil*	Triflupromazine
	Vesprin	
Phenoxybenzamine	Dibenzyline	
Phenylbutazone (systemic)	Oxalid	Oxyphenbutazone
	Tandearil	
	Algoverine*	Phenylbutazone
	Azolid	
	Butagesic*	
	Butazolidin	
	Intrabutazone*	
	Malgesic*	
	Nadozone*	
	Neo-Zoline*	
	Novobutazone*	
	Phenbutazone*	
	Azolid-A	Buffered phenylbutazone
	Butazolidin Alka	
	Phenylzone-A	
Phenylephrine (nasal)	Alcon-Efrin	
	Allerest	
	Contac	
	Coricidin	
	Isophrin	
	Neo-Mist	
	Neo-Synephrine	
	Pyracort-D	

*Not available in the United States.

Continued.

Cross-reference guide to drugs (generic and brand names)—cont'd

Drugs or drug type	*Brand names*	*Generic name*
	Rhinall Sinarest Super Anahist Synasal Vacon	
Phenylephrine (ophthalmic)	Efricel Isopto Frin Mydfrin Neo-Synephrine Ocusol Phenoptic Prefrin Soothe Eye Tear-Efrin	
Phenylpropanolamine (systemic)	Coffee-Break Control Delcopro Diadax Dietac Obestat Pro-Dax 21 Propadrine Rhindecon	
Phenylpropanolamine, phenylephrine, phenyltoloxamine, and chlorpheniramine (systemic)	Naldecon	
Physostigmine (ophthalmic)	Eserine Isopto Eserine	Physostigmine
Pilocarpine (ophthalmic)	Adsorbocarpine Almocarpine Isopto Carpine Miocarpine* Ocusert Pilo Pilocar Pilomiotin P. V. Carpine	Pilocarpine
Potassium iodide (systemic)	KI-N Pima	Potassium iodide
Potassium phosphates (systemic)	K-Phos Original	Monobasic potassium phosphates
	Neutra-Phos-K	Potassium phosphates
Potassium and sodium phosphates (systemic)	Uro-KP-Neutral	Dibasic potassium and sodium phosphates
	K-Phos M. F. K-Phos Neutral K-Phos No. 2	Monobasic potassium and sodium phosphates
	Neutra-Phos	Potassium and sodium phosphates
Potassium supplements (sysemic)	Potassium Triplex Tri-K Trikates	Potassium acetate, potassium bicarbonate, and potassium citrate
	K-Lyte	Potassium bicarbonate and citric acid
	KEFF	Potassium bicarbonate, potassium carbonate, and potassium chloride
	Klorvess	Potassium bicarbonate and potassium chloride
	K-Lyte/Cl	Potassium bicarbonate, potassium chloride, and citric acid
	Kaochlor-Eff	Potassium bicarbonate, potassium chloride, and potassium citrate
	Kaochlor Kaon-Cl Kato Kay-Ciel K-Lor KLOR-10% KLOR-CON Klorvess Klotrix K-Lyte/Cl Slow-K	Potassium chloride
	Kolyum	Potassium chloride and potassium gluconate
	Twin-K	Potassium citrate and potassium gluconate
	Kaon	Potassium gluconate
Prazosin (systemic)	Minipress	Prazosin
Primidone (systemic)	Mysoline	Primidone
Probenecid (systemic)	Benemid Benuryl* Probalan	Probenecid
Probucol (systemic)	Lorelco	Probucol

*Not available in the United States.

Drugs or drug type	*Brand names*	*Generic name*
Procainamide (systemic)	Procamide	Procainamide
	Procan	
	Procan SR	
	Procopan	
	Pronestyl	
	Sub-Quin	
Procarbazine (systemic)	Matulane	Procarbazine
	Natulan*	
Prochlorperazine and isopropamide (systemic)	Combid	
Progestins (systemic)	Duphaston	Dydrogesterone
	Delalutin	Hydroxyprogesterone
	Provera	Medroxyprogesterone
	Megace	Megestrol
	Micronor	Norethindrone
	Nor-Q.D.	
	Norlutin	
	Norlutate	Norethindrone acetate
	Ovrette	Norgestrel
	Proluton	Progesterone
	Lipo-Lutin	
Promethazine (systemic)	Historest	Promethazine
	Phenergan	
	Remsed	
Propantheline (systemic)	Pro-Banthine	Propantheline
Propoxyphene (systemic)	Algodex*	Propoxyphene
	Darvon	
	Depronal-SA*	
	Dolene	
	Novopropoxyn*	
	Pargesic 65	
	Pro-65*	
	Proxagesic	
	Proxene	
	SK-65	
	642*	
Propoxyphene and acetaminophen (systemic)	Darvocet-N	
	Dolacet	
	Dolene AP-65	
	SK-65-APAP	
	Wygesic	
Propoxyphene and APC (systemic)	Darvon Compound	
	Dolene Compound-65	
	SK-65 Compound	
Propoxyphene and aspirin (systemic)	Darvon with A.S.A.	
	Darvon-N with A.S.A.	
Pseudoephedrine (systemic)	Afrinol	Pseudoephedrine
	D-Feda	
	Eltor*	
	Neobid	
	Novafed	
	Pseudofrin*	
	Robindrine*	
	Ro-Fedrin	
	Sudafed	
	Sudrin	
Pyrilamine and pentobarbital (systemic)	Eme-Nil	
	Wans	
Pyrithione zinc (topical)	Danex	
	Head and Shoulders	
	Zincon	
Pyrvinium (systemic)	Pamovin*	Pyrvinium
	Povan	
	Pyr-Pam*	
	Vanquin*	
Quinidine (systemic)	Cardioquin	
	Cin-Quin	
	Duraquin	
	Quinaglute Dura-Tabs	
	Quinate*	
	Quinidex Extentabs	
	Quinora	
Quinine (systemic)	Coco-Quinine	Quinine
	Kinine*	
	Quine	
Quinine and aminophylline (systemic)	Quinamm	
	Quinite	
	Strema	
Rauwolfia alkaloids (systemic)	Harmonyl	Deserpidine
	Raunormine*	Rauwolfia serpentina
	Raudixin	
	Raulfia	
	Raupoid	
	Rauserpa	
	Rau-Sed	Reserpine
	Reserpoid	
	Sandril	
	Serpasil	
Rauwolfia alkaloids and thiazide diuretics (systemic)	Oreticyl	Deserpidine and hydrochlorothiazide
	Oreticyl Forte	
	Enduronyl	Deserpidine and methyclothiazide
	Rauzide	Rauwolfia serpentina and bendroflumethiazide

*Not available in the United States.

Continued.

Cross-reference guide to drugs (generic and brand names)—cont'd

Drugs or drug type	*Brand names*	*Generic name*
	Exna-R	Reserpine and benzthiazide
	Diupres	Reserpine and chlorothiazide
	Demi-Regroton	Reserpine and chlorthalidone
	Regroton	
	Hydropres	Reserpine and hydrochlorothiazide
	Reserpazide	
	Serpasil-Esidrix	
	Salutensin	Reserpine and hydroflumethiazide
	Salutensin-Demi	
	Diutensen-R	Reserpine and methyclothiazide
	Renese-R	Reserpine and polythiazide
	Hydromox-R	Reserpine and quinethazone
	Metatensin	Reserpine and trichlormethiazide
	Naquival	
Reserpine and hydralazine (systemic)	Serpasil-Apresoline	
Reserpine, hydralazine, and hydrochlorothiazide (systemic)	Ser-Ap-Es	
	Tri-Hydroserpine	
Resorcinol and Sulfur (topical)	Acne-Dome	
	Acnomel	
	Cenac	
	Exzit	
	pHisoAc	
	Sulforcin	
Rifampin (systemic)	Rifadin	Rifampin
	Rimactane	
	Rofact*	
Rifampin and isoniazid (systemic)	Rifamate	
Salicyclates (systemic)	Bayer Aspirin	Aspirin
	Ecotrin	
	Empirin Analgesic	
	Measurin	
	St. Joseph Aspirin	
	Ascriptin	Buffered aspirin
	Bufferin	
	CAMA Inlay-Tabs	
	Calurin	Carbaspirin
	Arthropan	Choline salicylate
	Parbocyl	Sodium salicylate
	Uracel	
Salicylic acid (topical)	Calicylic	
	Domerine	
	Fomac	
	Hydrisalic	
	Ionil	
	Keralyt	
	Mediplast	
	Saligel	
	Sebisol	
	Xseb	
Salicylic acid and sulfur (topical)	Acne-Dome	
	Acno	
	Antiseb	
	BUF	
	Exzit	
	Fostex	
	Klaron	
	Meted	
	Pernox	
	Rezamid	
	SAStid	
	Sebex	
	Sebulex	
	Therac	
	Vanseb	
Salicylic acid, sulfur, and coal tar (topical)	Antiseb-T	
	Sebex-T	
	Sebutone	
	Vanseb-T	
Selenium sulfide (topical)	Exsel	
	Iosel	
	Selsun	
	Selsun Blue	
	Sul-Blue	
Sodium fluoride (systemic)	Denta-Fl	
	Flo-Tab	
	Fluorident	
	Fluoritab	
	Fluorodex	
	Flura	
	Karidium	
	Luride	
	Luride-SF	
	Nafeen	
	Pedi-Dent	
	Pediaflor	
	Stay-Flo	
	Studaflor	
Spironolactone (systemic)	Aldactone	Spironolactone
Spironolactone and hydrochlorothiazide (systemic)	Aldactazide	
Succinimide-type anticonvulsants (systemic)	Zarontin	
	Celontin	
	Milontin	
	Ethosuximide	
	Methsuximide	
	Phensuximide	

*Not available in the United States.

Drugs or drug type	*Brand names*	*Generic name*
Sulfasalazine (systemic)	Azulfidine S.A.S.-500 Salazopyrin*	Sulfasalazine
Sulfinpyrazone (systemic)	Anturan* Anturane Zynol	Sulfinpyrazone
Sulfonamides (ophthalmic)	Bleph Cetamide Isopto Cetamide Optosulfex* Sulamyd Sulf-10	Sulfacetamide
	Gantrisin	Sulfisoxazole
Sulfonamides (systemic)	Renoquid	Sulfacytine
	Gantanol Methoxal Methoxanol	Sulfamethoxazole
	Bactrim Septra	Sulfamethoxazole and trimethoprim
	Gantrisin Lipo Gantrisin Novosoxazole* Sosol Sulfalar Sulfizin Sulfizole*	Sulfisoxazole
Sulfonamides (vaginal)	AVC Femguard Nil Tricholan Vagidine Vagimine Vagitrol	Sulfanilamide, aminacrine, and allantoin
	Sultrin Trysul	Sulfathiazole, sulfacetamide, and sulfabenzamide
	Koro-Sulf	Sulfisoxazole
	Vagilia	Sulfisoxazole, aminacrine, and allantoin
Sulfonamides and phenazopyridine (systemic)	Azo Gantanol	Sulfamethoxazole and phenazopyridine
	Azo Gantrisin Azo-Soxazole Azosul Azo-Sulfizin Suldiazo	Sulfisoxazole and phenazopyridine
Sulindac (systemic)	Clinoril	Sulindac
Tamoxifen (systemic)	Nolvadex	Tamoxifen
Terbutaline (systemic)	Brethine Bricanyl	Terbutaline
Terpin hydrate and codeine (systemic)	Cortussis	
Testolactone (systemic)	Teslac	Testolactone
Tetracyclines (ophthamic)	Aureomycin	Chlortetracycline
	Achromycin	Tetracycline
Tetracyclines (systemic)	Declomycin	Demeclocycline
	Doxychel Doxy-Tabs Vibramycin Vibra-Tabs	Doxycycline
	Rondomycin	Methacycline
	Minocin Ultramycin*	Minocycline
	Oxlopar Oxy-Kesso-Tetra Terramycin Tetramine	Oxytetracycline
	Achromycin Bio-Tetra* Bristacycline Cyclopar Medicycline* Neo-Tetrine* Novotetra* Panmycin Retet Robitet Sumycin Tetracrine* Tetracyn	Tetracycline
Tetracyclines (topical)	Aureomycin	Chlortetracycline
	Achromycin Topicycline	Tetracycline
Theophylline, ephedrine, and barbiturates (systemic)	Asminyl Asma-lief Phedral Tedfern Tedral Thalfed Thedrizem Theodrine Theofed Theofenal Theoral Theotabs	
Theophylline, ephedrine, guaifenesin, and barbiturates (systemic)	Broncholate Bronkolixir Bronkotabs Duovent Luftodil Mudrane GG Quibron Plus Verequad	
Theophylline, ephedrine, and hydroxyzine (systemic)	Asminorel E.T.H. Compound Hydrophed	

*Not available in the United States.

Continued.

Cross-reference guide to drugs (generic and brand names)—cont'd

Drug or drug type	*Brand names*	*Generic name*
	Marax	
	Theophozine	
	Theozine	
Theophylline and guaifenesin (systemic)	Asbron G	
	Asma	
	Cerylin	
	Dialixir	
	Glybron	
	Glyceryl T	
	Hylate	
	Lanophyllin-GG	
	Quibron	
	Slo-Phyllin GG	
	Synophylate-GG	
	Theo-Col	
	Theo-Guaia	
Thiazide diuretics (systemic)	Naturetin	Bendroflumethiazide
	Aquastat	Benzthiazide
	Aquatag	
	Exna	
	Hydrex	
	Diuril	Chlorothiazide
	SK-Chlorothiazide	
	Hygroton	Chlorthalidone
	Novothalidone*	
	Uridon	
	Anhydron	Cyclothiazide
	Esidrix	Hydrochlorothiazide
	Hydro-Aquil	
	HydroDIURIL	
	Novohydrazide*	
	Oretic	
	Diucardin	Hydroflumethiazide
	Saluron	
	Aquatensen	Methyclothiazide
	Duretic	
	Enduron	
	Diulo	Metolazone
	Zaroxolyn	
	Renese	Polythiazide
	Hydromox	Quinethazone
	Metahydrin	Trichlormethiazide
	Naqua	
Thioxanthenes (systemic)	Taractan	Chlorprothixene
	Tarasan*	
	Navane	Thiothixene
Thyroid hormones (systemic)	Levothroid	Levothyroxine
	L-T-S	
	Ro-Thyroxine	
	Synthroid	
	Cytomel	Liothyronine
	Ro-Thyronine	Liotrix
	Tertroxin	
	Euthroid	
	Proloid	Thyroglobulin
	S-P-T	Thyroid
	Thyrar	
	Thyrocrine	
Thyrotropin (systemic)	Thyrotron	Thyrotropin
	Thytropar	
Timolol (ophthalmic)	Timoptic	Timolol
Tolmetin (systemic)	Tolectin	Tolmetin
Tolnaftate (topical)	Aftate	Tolnaftate
	Tinactin	
Tretinoin (topical)	Retin-A	Tretinoin
Triamterene (systemic)	Dyrenium	Triamterene
Triamterene and hydrochlorothiazide (systemic)	Dyazide	
Tricyclic antidepressants (systemic)	Amitid	Amitriptyline
	Amitil	
	Elavil	
	Endep	
	Norpramin	Desipramine
	Pertofrane	
	Adapin	Doxepin
	Sinequan	
	Imavate	Imipramine
	Janimine	
	SK-Pramine	
	Tofranil	
	Aventyl	Nortriptyline
	Pamelor	
	Vivactil	Protiptyline
	Surmontil	Trimipramine
Trifluridine (ophthalmic)	Viroptic	Trifluridine
Trimethobenzamide (systemic)	Tigan	Trimethobenzamide
Triprolidine and pseudoephedrine (systemic)	Actifed	
	Allerphed	
	Tagafed	
Tropicamide (ophthalmic)	Mydriacyl	Tropicamide
Undecylenic acid$_1$ compound (topical)	Decylenes	
	Desenex	
	Medaped	
	Quinsana Plus	
Urea (systemic)	Ureaphil	
Valproic acid (systemic)	Depakene	Valproic acid
Vidarabine (ophthalmic)	Vira-A	Vidarabine

*Not available in the United States.

Drug or drug type	*Brand names*	*Generic name*
Vinblastine (systemic)	Velban	Vinblastine
	Velbe*	
Vincristine (systemic)	Oncovin	Vincristine
Vitamins and fluoride (systemic)	Vita-Flor	Multiple vitamins and fluoride
	Adeflor	
	Mulvidren-F	
	Novacebrin with Fluoride	
	Vi-Penta F	
	Poly-Vi-Flor	
	V-Daylin with Fluoride	
	Cari-Tab	Vitamins A, D, and C, and fluoride
	Tri-Vi-Flor	
(methyl)-Xanthines (systemic)	Aminodur	Aminophylline
	Aminophyl*	
	Amphylline*	
	Corophyllin*	
	Lixaminol	
	Mini-Lix	
	Somophyllin	
	Aerophylline*	Dyphylline
	Airet	
	Dilin	
	Dilor	
	Lufyllin	
	Neothylline	
	Protophylline*	
	Choledyl	Oxtriphylline
	Accurbron	Theophylline
	Aerolate	
	Asthmophylline*	
	Bronkodyl	
	Elixicon	
	Elixophyllin	
	Physpan	
	Slophyllin	
	Somophyllin-T	
	Theobid	
	Theoclear	
	Theodur	
	Theolair	
	Theolixir	
	Theophyl	
	Theospan	
Xylometazoline (nasal)	4-Way Long Acting	
	Neo-synephrine II	
	Otrivin	
	Rhinall Long Acting	
	Sine-Off Once-A-Day	
	Sinex Long-Acting	
	Sinutab Long Acting Sinus Spray	

*Not available in the United States.

APPENDIX 12 GERIATRICS

12-1 Organizations pertaining to the elderly

GENERAL ORGANIZATIONS

AFL/CIO Social Security Department*
815 16th St., N.W.
Washington, D.C. 20006

American Academy of Geriatric Dentistry
2 N. Riverside Plaza
Chicago, Ill. 60603

American Aging Association
University of Nebraska Medical Center
Omaha, Nebraska
Made up of scientists, it seeks to promote research on aging.

American Art Therapy Association
P.O. Box 11604
Pittsburgh, Pa. 15228

American Association for Geriatric Psychiatry
230 N. Michigan Ave., Suite 2400
Chicago, Ill. 60601

American Association of Homes for the Aging*
1050 17th St., N.W., Suite 770
Washington, D.C. 20036
AAHA represents the nonprofit homes for the aging—religious, municipal, trust, fraternal.

American Association of Retired Persons†
1909 K St., N.W.
Washington, D.C. 20006
Age 55 or above, retired to still employed

American Coalition of Citizens with Disabilities, Inc.
1200 15th St., N.W., Suite 201
Washington, D.C. 20005

American College of Nursing Home Administrators
4650 East-West Highway
Washington, D.C. 20014

American Dance Therapy Association
2000 Century Plaza, Suite 230
Columbia, Md. 21044

American Foundation for the Blind, Inc.
15 West 16th St.
New York, N.Y. 10011

The American Geriatrics Society
10 Columbus Circle
New York, N.Y. 10019
The American Geriatrics Society, made up of physicians, has an annual meeting.

American Nurses' Association, Inc.
Council of Nursing Home Nurses
Division on Gerontological Nursing Practice
2420 Pershing Rd.
Kansas City, Mo. 64108

American Occupational Therapy Association
6000 Executive Blvd.
Rockville, Md. 20853

American Osteopathic Association
212 E. Ohio St.
Chicago, Ill. 60611

American Personnel and Guidance Association
2 Skyline Pl., Suite 400
Falls Church, Va. 22041

American Physical Therapy Association
1740 Broadway
New York, N.Y. 10019
and
1156 15th St., N.W.
Washington D.C. 20005

American Psychiatric Association
Council on Aging
1700 18th St., N.W.
Washington, D.C. 20009

American Psychological Association
Division of Adult Development and Aging (formerly Division of Maturity and Old Age)
1200 17th St., N.W.
Washington, D.C. 20036

American Public Health Association
Section of Gerontological Health
1015 18th St., N.W.
Washington, D.C. 20036

American Public Welfare Association
1125 15th St., N.W., Suite 300
Washington, D.C. 20005

American Speech and Hearing Association
10801 Rockville Pike
Rockville, Md. 20852
3,600 audiologist members.

Asian and Pacific Coalition on Aging
1851 S.W. Moreland Ave.
Los Angeles, Calif. 90006

Asociación Nacional Pro Personas Mayores†
1730 W. Olympic Blvd., Suite 401
Los Angeles, Calif. 90015
and
1801 K St., N.W., Suite 1021
Washington, D.C. 20005
For Spanish-speaking elderly.

Association for Gerontology in Higher Education†
600 Maryland Ave., S.W.
Washington, D.C. 20024

Association for Humanistic Gerontology
1711 Solano Ave.
Berkeley, Calif. 94707

Canadian Association on Gerontology/Association Canadienne de Gérontologie
722 16th Ave., N.E.
Calgary, Alberta, T2E 6V7

Canadian Psychiatric Association
225 Lisgar St., Suite 103
Ottawa, Ontario K2P 0C6

Commission on Legal Problems of the Elderly
American Bar Association
1800 M St., N.W.
Washington, D.C. 20036

Committee to Combat Huntington's Disease
250 W. 57th St.
New York, N.Y. 10010

*Denotes steering committee members of the Leadership Council.
†Denotes General Members of the Leadership Council of Aging Organizations, 1980-1981.

Concerned Seniors for Better Government†
1346 Connecticut Ave., N.W., Suite 1213
Washington, D.C. 20036

Continental Association of Funeral and Memorial Societies
1828 L St., N.W.
Washington, D.C. 20036

Council of Home Health Agencies and Community Health Services
National League for Nursing
10 Columbus Circle
New York, N.Y. 10019

The Forum for Professionals and Executives
c/o The Washington School of Psychiatry
1610 New Hampshire Ave., N.W.
Washington, D.C. 20009
The interests of this group have ranged from contemplation to active examination of public issues, including those affecting the elderly.

The Gerontological Society of America*
1835 K St., N.W., Suite 305
Washington, D.C. 20006
This professional society has an annual meeting and an international meeting every 3 years. It is made up of four components—biological sciences, clinical medicine, psychological and social sciences and social research, and planning and practice.

Gray Panthers†
3700 Chestnut St.
Philadelphia, Pa. 19104
Activistic group of older people who resent "stereotyping."

Group for the Advancement of Psychiatry, Inc.
Committee on Aging
c/o Mental Health Materials Center
419 Park Ave., S.
New York, N.Y. 10016

Home Heath Services Association
407 N St., N.W.
Washington, D.C. 20024

The Institute of Retired Professionals
The New School of Social Research
60 W. 12th St.
New York, N.Y. 10011
This pioneering school also led the way in providing intellectual activities for retired professional people.

The Institutes of Lifetime Learning
These are educational services of the National Retired Teachers Association and the American Association of Retired Persons.

International Center for Social Gerontology
425 13th St., N.W., Suite 840
Washington, D.C. 20004

The International Federation on Aging
1909 K St., N.W.
Washington, D.C. 20006
Confederation of aging organizations of various nations.

International Senior Citizens Association, Inc.
11753 Wilshire Blvd.
Los Angeles, Calif. 90025
Endeavors to reflect older people of many nations.

Memorial Society Association of Canada
Box 96
Weston, Ontario M9N 3M6

National Association of Area Agencies on Aging†
600 Maryland Ave., S.W.
Washington, D.C. 20024

National Association of Black Social Workers, Inc.
2008 Madison Ave.
New York, N.Y. 10035

National Association of Counties
Aging Program
1735 New York Ave., N.W.
Washington, D.C. 20006

National Association of Home Health Agencies
426 C St., N.E.
Washington, D.C. 20002

National Association of Mature People†
918 16th St., N.W.
Washington, D.C. 20006

National Association of Meals Programs, Inc.
924 14th St., N.W.
Washington, D.C. 20005

National Association for Music Therapy, Inc.
P.O. Box 610
901 Kentucky St.
Lawrence, Kan. 66044

National Association of Retired Federal Employees†
1533 New Hampshire Ave., N.W.
Washington, D.C. 20036
Represents and lobbies for needs of retired civil servants.

National Association of Social Workers
1425 H St., N.W.
Washington, D.C. 20005

National Association of Spanish-Speaking (Hispanic) Elderly
National Executive Offices
1730 W. Olympic Blvd., Suite 401
Los Angeles, Calif. 90015
Research Center
1801 K St., N.W., Suite 1021
Washington, D.C. 20006
There are also regional centers in Miami and New York.

National Association of State Units on Aging*
600 Maryland Ave., S.W.
Washington, D.C. 20024
Information resources on state policies on aging. Represents and lobbies for state agencies at the federal level.

National Caucus and Center on Black Aged*
1424 K St., N.W., Suite 500
Washington, D.C. 20005
Advocates improving the quality of life for the black aged. Provides comprehensive program of coordination, information, and consultative services to meet needs of black aged.

National Citizens' Coalition for Nursing Home Reform
1424 16th St., N.W., Suite 204
Washington, D.C. 20036

National Committee on Careers for Older Americans
1414 22nd St., N.W., Room 602
Washington, D.C. 20037

National Conference of State Legislatures
444 N. Capital St., N.W.
Washington, D.C. 20001

National Council on the Aging*
600 Maryland Ave., S.W.
Washington, D.C. 20024
Research and services regarding the elderly.

National Council of Health Care Services
1200 15th St., N.W., Suite 402
Washington, D.C. 20005
Represents commercial nursing home chains.

National Council for Homemaker–Home Health Aide Services
67 Irving Pl.
New York, N.Y. 10003

National Council of Senior Citizens*
925 15th St., N.W.
Washington, D.C. 20005
Represents and lobbies for needs of the elderly. Membership at any age.

National Federation of Licensed Practical Nurses
250 W. 57th St.
New York, N.Y. 10019
Educational foundation.

National Geriatrics Society
212 W. Wisconsin Ave.
Milwaukee, Wis. 53202

National Hospice Organization
1331A Dolley Madison Blvd.
McLean, Va. 22101

National Indian Council on Aging, Inc.†
P.O. Box 2088
Albuquerque, N.M. 87103

National Institute of Senior Centers
1828 L St., N.W.
Washington, D.C. 20036

National Interfaith Coalition on Aging
P.O. Box 1904
Athens, Ga. 30603
Coordinates the involvement of religious groups in meeting the needs of the elderly.

National Pacific/Asian Resource Center on Aging
811 First Ave.
Seattle, Wash. 98104
and
927 15th St., N.W., Room 812
Washington, D.C. 20005

National Retired Teachers Association (NRTA)*
1909 K St., N.W.
Washington, D.C. 20006
Members once active in an educational system, public or private.

National Tenants Organization, Inc.
425 13th St., N.W., Suite 548
Washington, D.C. 20004
Represents older people, among others, in public housing.

National Therapeutic Recreation Society
National Recreation and Park Association
1601 N. Kent St.
Arlington, Va. 22209

National Voluntary Organizations for Independent Living for the Aging (NVOILA)
National Council on Aging
1828 L St., N.W.
Washington, D.C. 20036

The Oliver Wendell Holmes Association
381 Park Ave., S.
New York, N.Y. 10016
This group is interested in the expansion of the intellectual horizons of older people.

Retired Officers Association
1625 I St., N.W.
Washington, D.C. 20006
Represents needs of retired military officers of the United States.

Retired Professionals Action Group
200 P St., N.W., Suite 711
Washington, D.C. 20001
This action group was organized through Ralph Nader. Its efforts include investigative reports and class-action cases.

Senior Action in a Gay Environment, Inc.
Serving the Older Gay Community
487A Hudson St.
New York, N.Y. 10014

Sex Information and Education Council of the United States (SIECUS)
84 Fifth Ave., Suite 407
New York, N.Y. 10011
Part of its program is to provide sex information to older people.

Southern Gerontological Society
c/o Gerontology Center
Georgia State University
Atlanta, Ga. 30303

United Auto Workers/Retired Members Department
8731 E. Jefferson St.
Detroit, Mich. 48214

Urban Elderly Coalition
600 Maryland Ave., S.W.
Washington, D.C. 20024
Effort of municipal authorities to obtain funds for the urban elderly poor.

U.S. Conference on Mayors
Task Force on Aging
1620 I St., N.W.
Washington, D.C. 20006

Western Gerontological Society†
785 Market St., Room 1114
San Francisco, Calif. 94114
Works to promote the well-being of older Americans.

ORGANIZATIONS CONCERNED WITH OLDER WOMEN

The Gray Panthers' National Task Force on Older Women
6407 Maiden Lane
Bethesda, Md. 20034

National Action Forum for Older Women
2000 P St., N.W., Suite 508
Washington, D.C. 20036

National Organization for Women
425 13th St., N.W.
Washington, D.C. 20004

The National Women's Political Caucus
1411 K St., N.W.
Washington, D.C. 20005

Older Women's League
3800 Harrison St.
Oakland, Calif. 94611

Women's Equity Action League
805 15th St., N.W.
Washington, D.C. 20005

Women's Studies Program and Policy Center
George Washington University
2025 I St., N.W.
Washington, D.C. 20052
Has formed a coalition with the Congressional Women's Caucus to draft and promote legislation to benefit older women.

LEGAL RESOURCES FOR THE ELDERLY

National Senior Citizens Law Center (NSCLC)
1200 15th St., N.W.
Washington, D.C. 20005
and
1636 W. 8th St.
Los Angeles, Calif. 90017
The NSCLC is a national support center, specializing in the legal problems of the elderly poor, and is funded by the Legal Services Corporation, the Administration on Aging of the Department of Health and Human Services; and the Community Services Administration. Its principal function is to provide support services to legal service attorneys, and other publicly funded programs providing legal assistance to older persons, on the legal problems of their elderly clients.

ALZHEIMER'S DISEASE AND RELATED DISORDERS ASSOCIATION

32 Broadway
New York, N.Y. 10004
and
360 North Michigan Ave.
Suite 601, Chicago, Ill. 60601
Purposes of the organization include coordination, education, family support, research/prevention, public policy, advocacy, and organizational development. There are some 50 chapters in 50 cities.

NATIONAL CITIZENS' COALITION FOR NURSING HOME REFORM

Membership information, May 14, 1980: the Coalition has 73 membership groups in 25 different states.

California
ACLU Medical Complaint Center, Pacoima
Citizens for Better Nursing Home Care, Oakland
Citizens Who Care, Davis
Gray Panthers of the East Bay, Berkeley
Ombudsman Inc., Riverside
United Neighbors in Action Research Association, Oakland

Colorado
Concerned Relatives and Friends of Residents, Ft. Collins
Organization for Nursing Home Improvement, Ft. Collins

District of Columbia
Christian Communities Committed to Change
Washington Home Residents' Council

Florida
Nursing Home Hotline/Patrol, St. Petersburg

Illinois
Illinois Citizens for Better Care, Chicago
Lake View Evangelical Fellowship, Chicago

Indiana
Byron Health Care Center, Residents' Council, Fort Wayne
United Senior Action, Indiana Center for Urban Encounter, Indianapolis

Maryland
Maryland Advocates for the Aging, Baltimore

Massachusetts
Age Center of Worcester Area, Inc., Worcester
Cambridge and Summerville Legal Services, Cambridge
Cape Cod Nursing Home Council, Hyannis
Central Massachusetts Legal Services, Worcester
Consumer Advocates for Better Care, Leominster
Life is for the Elderly (LIFE), Boston
Massachusetts Health Care Coalition, Boston
Nursing Home Advocacy and Assistance Project, Holyoke
West Suburban Ministries, Newton

Michigan
Citizens for Better care (statewide); chapters: Big Rapids, Flint, Grand Rapids, Lansing, metropolitan Detroit, Port Huron, Traverse City, and Upper Peninsula
Citizens for Better Care Institute, Detroit
Metro Consumer Co-op, Detroit
United Auto Workers Retired and Older Workers Dept., Detroit

Minnesota
Friends and Relatives of Nursing Home Residents, Minneapolis
Minnesota Senior Federation, St. Paul
Nursing Home Residents Advisory Council, Minneapolis
Nursing Home Residents Advocates, Minneapolis

Mississippi
Jackson Gray Panthers, Jackson
Mississippi Mental Health Project, Jackson

Missouri
Kansas City Gray Panther Network, Kansas City
St. Louis Nursing Home Ombudsman Program, St. Louis

New York
Caring Community, New York
Coalition of Institutionalized Aged and Disabled, Bronx
Community Council of Greater New York, Ombudsman Program, New York
Friends and Relatives of the Institutionalized Aged, New York
State Communities Aid Association, Buffalo

North Carolina
Friends of Nursing Home Patients, Chapel Hill

Ohio
Lutheran Metropolitan Ministry Nursing Home Ombudsman Program, Cleveland
Toledo Area Council of Churches Metropolitan Mission, Toledo

Oregon
Benton County Nursing Home Task Force, Corvallis
Gray Panthers, Portland
Gray Panthers, Salem
Northwest Portland Gray Panthers, Portland

Pennsylvania
Coalition of Advocates for the Rights of the Infirm Elderly, Philadelphia
Community Concern for Nursing Home Residents, Mechanicsburg
Interfaith Friends, Wilkes-Barre
National Gray Panthers, Philadelphia
Northwest Interfaith Movement, Philadelphia
Pennsylvania Advocates for Better Care, Harrisburg

Rhode Island
RIsource, Providence

Tennessee
SAGA—Social Action Group on Aging, Nashville

Utah
Citizens for Quality Care in Bountiful, Lake City

Virginia
Friends and Relatives of Nursing Home Residents, Richmond

Washington
Citizens for the Improvement of Nursing Homes, Seattle
Citizens for the Improvement of Nursing Homes, Spokane

Wisconsin
Nursing Home Consumers Who Care, Madison
Nursing Home Ombudsman Program, Madison

Wyoming
Advocates for the Care of the Elderly, Laramie
Concerned Citizens for Quality Nursing Home Care, Casper

12-2 Government programs for the elderly

Program	Sponsor	Purpose	Address
Volunteer employment programs			
RSVP (Retired Senior Volunteer Program)	ACTION	Funds for volunteer programs in public and nonprofit institutions; volunteers reimbursed for travel and meal expenses	ACTION* 806 Connecticut Ave., N.W. Washington, D.C. 20525
SCORE (Service Corps of Retired Executives)	ACTION, administered by Small Business Administration	Retired businesspersons advising novices in business	ACTION 806 Connecticut Ave., N.W. Washington, D.C. 20525
VISTA (Volunteers in Service to America)	ACTION	Volunteers for 1 to 2 years in community projects in United States with small salary to cover living expenses	ACTION 806 Connecticut Ave., N.W. Washington, D.C. 20525
Peace Corps	ACTION	Overseas service	ACTION 806 Connecticut Ave., N.W. Washington, D.C. 20525
Senior Environmental Employment Program	Administration on Aging and Environmental Protection Agency	Protection of the environment	Senior Environmental Employment Program 1909 K. St., N.W. Washington, D.C. 22049
Senior Community Service Employment Program (SCSEP) ''Project Agenda''	National Association for Spanish-Speaking Elderly	Community service	Senior Community Service Employment Program 1801 K St., N.W., Suite 1021 Washington, D.C. 20006
IESC (International Executive Service Corps)	An independent organization supported by government and nongovernment funds	Overseas service by executives	International Executive Service Corps 545 Madison Ave. New York, N.Y. 10022
Low-income elderly programs†			
Foster Grandparent Program	ACTION	Provide relationship and care to orphans and mentally retarded, physically handicapped, or troubled children and teenagers in institutions for 20 hours per week at modest pay	ACTION 806 Connecticut Ave., N.W. Washington, D.C. 20525
SOS (Senior Opportunities and Services programs)	Office of Economic Opportunity	Service in programs to meet needs of older people: nutrition, consumer education, outreach, employment, information, and referral	Office of Economic Opportunity 1200 19th St., N.W. Washington, D.C. 20506

*ACTION's toll-free number is (800)424-8580.
†Only persons over 60 with incomes below OEO (Office of Economic Opportunities) guidelines are eligible.

Program	Sponsor	Purpose	Address
Operation Mainstream programs			
Green Thumb	National Farmers Union Green Thumb 1012 14th St., N.W. Washington, D.C. 20005	Conservation and landscape	Write sponsor or Department of Labor Washington, D.C.
Senior AIDES	National Council of Senior Citizens 1511 K St., N.W. Washington, D.C. 20005	Community service	Write sponsor
Senior Community Service Program	National Council on the Aging 600 Maryland Ave S.W. Washington, D.C. 20024	Community service	Write sponsor
Senior Community Service Aides	National Retired Teachers Association Senior Community Service Aides Project 1909 K St., N.W. Washington, D.C. 20006	Community service	Write sponsor

FEDERAL CONGRESSIONAL AND EXECUTIVE INVOLVEMENT WITH THE ELDERLY*

U.S. Senate Special Committee on Aging

U.S. Senate Subcommittee on Aging of the Committee of Labor and Public Welfare

U.S. House of Representatives

U.S. House of Representatives Select Committee on Aging

U.S. Department of Health and Human Services
Administration on Aging
Washington, D.C. 20201

Social Security Administration
Baltimore, Md. 21235
The Social Security Administration provides services through district and branch offices and teleservice centers. Contact any office for free publications on Social Security, Supplemental Security Income, and Medicare.

National Institute on Aging
National Institutes of Health
Bethesda, Md. 20205

Alcohol, Drug Abuse, and Mental Health Administration (ADAMHA)
A government agency within the U.S. Department of Health and Human Services repsonsible for administering federal grant programs to advance and support research, training, and service programs in the areas of alcoholism, drug abuse, and mental health.

Center for Studies of the Mental Health of the Aging
National Institute of Mental Health
National Institutes of Health
Rockville, Md. 20857

National Institute on Alcohol Abuse and Alcoholism
An institute with ADAMHA responsible for programs dealing with alcohol abuse and alcoholism.

National Institute on Drug Abuse
An institute within ADAMHA responsible for programs dealing with narcotic and drug abuse.

Federal Information Centers
With the federal government comprised of 125 different departments and agencies and with 132 different federal programs directly affecting older people, locating the correct source of assistance is difficult. Federal Information Centers (FIC) have been created to help. There are 38 FICs operating in major metropolitan areas throughout the country, and toll-free telephone connections to the nearest FIC are available in 47 other cities. In areas without local FIC access, long-distance calls or letters to the nearest FIC are welcomed. If the local telephone directory (under U.S. Government) has no listing for an area FIC, contact the Federal Information Center program, General Services Administration, 18th and F Streets, N.W., Room 6034, Washington, D.C. 21415, for a list of FICs and toll-free telephone numbers.

Other federal government agencies involved with the elderly

Administration for Native Americans
Hubert Humphrey Blvd., Room 357G
Washington, D.C. 20201

Community Services Administration
Room 556
1200 19th St., N.W.
Washington, D.C. 20506

Farmers Home Administration
U.S Department of Agriculture
South Bldg., Room 5420
Washington, D.C. 20250

Federal Council on Aging
Washington, D.C. 20201
The Federal Council on the Aging was established by the 1973 Amendments to the Older Americans Act of 1965 (P.L. 93-29, 42 U.S.C. 3015) for the purpose of advising the President, the Secretary of Health and Human Services, the Commissioner on Aging, and the Congress on matters relating to the special needs of older Americans.

Health Care Financing Administration
Project Grants Branch
Room 4200-C, Mary E. Switzer Bldg.
330 C St., S.W.
Washington, D.C. 20201

Internal Revenue Service
1111 Constitution Avenue, N.W.
Office of Public Affairs
Washington, D.C. 20224
(202)566-4743
For a determination of whether a private pension plan meets minimum government requirements, local IRS offices can be contacted.

National Center for Health Services Research
Grants Review Branch
Room 7-50A
3700 East-West Highway
Hyattsville, Md. 20782

Office of Personnel Management
(formerly Civil Service Commission)
Retirement Bureau
Washington, D.C. 20415
(202)632-7700
The Retirement Information Office of the Office of Personnel Management gives general benefit information on civil service retirement and makes referrals to appropriate offices.

Pension Benefit Guaranty Corporation
202 K St., N.W.
Washington, D.C. 20006
(202)254-4817
If a pension plan is terminated or is about to be terminated, questions regarding payment of benefits can be obtained from the Pension Benefit Guaranty Corporation at the above address.

Railroad Retirement Board
844 Rush St.
Chicago, Ill. 60611
The Railroad Retirement Board has 80 district offices to provide information and to develop and process railroad retirement claims.

Veterans Administration
Central Office
Washington, D.C. 20420
(202)389-2356
There are over 500 regional offices nationwide to provide information related to veterans. Veterans Benefit Counselors can be called toll-free.

STATE AND LOCAL GOVERNMENT INVOLVEMENT WITH THE ELDERLY

National Association of Counties
1735 New York Ave., N.W., Suite 500
Washington, D.C. 20006

U.S. Conference of Mayors
1620 I St., N.W.
Washington, D.C. 20006

---

*See pamphlet of charts compiled by the Congressional Research Service of the Library of Congress for the House of Representatives Select Committee on Aging: Federal responsibility to the elderly (executive programs and legislative jurisdiction), Washington, D.C., 1979, U.S. Government Printing Office.

APPENDIX 13 THE NURSING PROFESSION: DIRECTORY OF ORGANIZATIONS AND HEALTH CARE WORKERS

13-1 Directory of nursing organizations: International and United States

INTERNATIONAL

International Committee of Catholic Nurses and Social Assistants—Palazzo S. Calisto, 1-00120 Cittadel Vaticano, Italy.

International Council of Nurses and the Florence Nightingale International Foundation—Geneva, Switzerland.

North American Nursing Diagnosis Association—The Clearinghouse, St. Louis University Department of Nursing, St. Louis, Mo. 63104.

Pan American Health Organization—Pan American Sanitary Bureau, WHO Regional Office for the Americas, 525 23rd Street N.W., Washington, D.C. 20037.

People to People Health Foundation (Project HOPE)—Millwood, Va. 22646.

World Federation of Neurosurgical Nurses—628 Greenhill Rd. Burnside, South Australia 5066. Tel. (08)3322341; 571 South Braddock Ave., Pittsburgh, Pa. 15221. Tel. 412-624-3595.

World Health Organization—Avenue Appia, 1211 Geneva 27, Switzerland.

NATIONAL

American Nurses' Association—2420 Pershing Rd., Kansas City, Mo. 64108. Tel. 816-474-5720.

Alpha Tau Delta National Fraternity for Professional Nurses—14631 No. 2nd Dr., Phoenix, Az. 85023.

American Academy of Ambulatory Nursing Administration—N. Woodbury Rd., Box 56, Pitman, N.J. 08071. Tel. 609-582-9617.

American Association of Colleges of Nursing—Suite 430, 11 Dupont Circle, Washington, D.C. 20036.

American Association of Critical-Care Nurses—One Civic Plaza, Newport Beach, Ca. Tel. 714-644-9310.

American Association of Nephrology Nurses and Technicians—North Woodbury Rd., Box 56, Pitman, N.J. 08071.

American Association of NeuroScience Nurses—National ofc., 22 So. Washington St., Suite 203, Park Ridge, Ill. 60068. Tel. 312-823-9850.

American Association of Nurse Anesthetists—216 Higgins Rd., Park Ridge, Ill. 60068.

American Association of Occupational Health Nurses, Inc.—3500 Piedmont Rd., N.E., Atlanta, Ga. 30305. Tel. 404-262-1162.

American Cancer Society—777 Third Ave., New York, N.Y. 10017.

American College of Nurse-Midwives—Suite 1120, 1522 K St., N.W., Washington, D.C. 20005.

American Heart Association—7320 Greenville Ave., Dallas, Tex. 75231.

American Holistic Nurses' Association—P.O. Box 116, Telluride, Colo. 81435. Tel. 303-728-4575.

American Hospital Association—840 N. Lake Shore Dr., Chicago, Ill. 60611.

American Public Health Association—1015 15th St., N.W., Wash., D.C. 20005.

American Society for Nursing Service Administrators, American Hospital Association—840 N. Lakeshore Drive, Chicago, Ill. 60611. Tel. 312-280-6410.

American Urological Association Allied—6845 Lake Shore Dr., P.O. Box 9397, Raytown, Mo. 64133.

Association for the Care of Children's Health—3615 Wisconsin Ave., N.W., Washington, D.C. 20016. Tel. 202-244-1801.

Association of Operating Room Nurses—10170 E. Miss. Ave., Denver, Colo. 80231.

Association of Pediatric Oncology Nurses—Pacific Medical Center, P.O. Box 7999, San Francisco, Calif. 94120.

Association for Practitioners in Infection Control—23341 N. Milwaukee Ave., Half Day, Ill. 60069.

Association of Rehabilitation Nurses—2506 Gross Point Rd., Evanston, Ill. 60201. Tel. 312-475-7530.

Catholic Health Association of the U.S.—4455 Woodson Rd., St. Louis, Mo. 63134.

Commission on Graduates of Foreign Nursing Schools—3624 Market St., Philadelphia, Pa. 19104. Tel. 215-349-8767.

Emergency Department Nurses Association—666 North Lake Shore Dr., Suite 1131, Chicago, Ill. 60611. Tel. 312-649-0297.

International Association for Enterostomal Therapy, Inc.—One Newport Pl., Suite 970, Newport Beach, Calif. 92660.

National Association for Practical Nurse Education and Service—254 West 31st St., New York, N.Y. 10001.

National Association of Hispanic Nurses—4359 Stockdale, San Antonio, Tex. 78233.

National Association of Nurse Recruiters—111 E. Wacker Dr. #600, Chicago, Ill. 60601. Tel. 312-644-6610.

National Association of Orthopaedic Nurses, Inc.—N. Woodbury Rd., Box 56, Pitman, N.J. 08071. Tel. 609-582-0111.

National Association of Pediatric Nurse Associates and Practitioners—Box 56, N. Woodbury Rd., Pitman, N.J. 08071.

National Association of School Nurses, Inc.—7395 S. Krameria St., Englewood, Colo. 80112. Tel. 303-850-9033.

National Black Nurses Association, Inc.—P.O. Box 18358, Boston, Mass. 02118.

National Council of State Boards of Nursing—303 E. Ohio, Suite 2010, Chicago, Ill. 60611. Tel. 312-329-1282.

National Federation of Licensed Practical Nurses, Inc.—214 South Driver, P.O. Box 11038, Durham, N.C. 27703. Tel. 919-596-9609.

National Flight Nurses Association—Life Flight, St. Joseph's Hospital, 601 N. 30th St., Omaha, Neb. 68131.

National Intravenous Therapy Association, Inc.—87 Blanchard Rd., Cambridge, Ma. 02138.

National League for Nursing—10 Columbus Circle, New York, N.Y. 10019. Southern Office: 50 Executive Park South, N.E., Suite 5014, Atlanta, Ga. 30329. Midwest Office: 111 N. Wabash,

Suite 1612, Chicago, Ill. 60602. Western Office: 881 Sneath Lane, Suite 112, San Bruno, Calif. 94066.

National Nurses Society on Addictions—2506 Gross Point Rd., Evanston, Ill. 60201. Tel. 312-475-7530.

National Student Nurses' Association—10 Columbus Circle, New York, N.Y. 10019. Tel. 212-581-2211.

Nurses Alliance for the Prevention of Nuclear War—Box 319, Chestnut Hill, Ma. 02178.

Nurses Association of the American College of Obstetricians and Gynecologists—600 Maryland Ave., S.W., Suite 200 East, Washington, D.C. 20024. Tel. 202-638-0026.

Nurses Christian Fellowship—233 Langdon St., Madison, Wis. 53703.

Nurses Educational Funds, Inc.—555 W. 57th St., New York, N.Y. 10019.

Nurses House, Inc.—60 East 42nd St., Rm. 1616, New York, N.Y. 10165.

Oncology Nursing Society—3111 Banksville Rd., Pittsburgh, Pa. 15216. Tel. 412-344-3899.

Sigma Theta Tau—National Honor Society of Nursing, 610 Barnhill Dr., Indianapolis, Ind.

The Society for Nursing History—Nursing Education Dept., Box 150, Teachers College, Columbia University, New York, N.Y. 10027.

Society for Peripheral Vascular Nursing—P. O. Box 151044, Columbus, Ohio 43215.

United Nurses Associations of California (UNAC)—170 W. San Jose Ave., Suite 102, Claremont, Calif. 91711. Tel. 714-625-7931.

United Nursing Home Association—16400 Southcenter Pkwy., Suite 410, Seattle, Wash. 98188. Tel. 206-575-9422.

U.S. GOVERNMENT NURSES, EXECUTIVE BRANCH

Action/Peace Corps—Office of Recruitment, 806 Connecticut Ave., N.W., Room P-301, Washington, D.C. 20526. Tel. 800-424-8580, ext. 93.

Air Force Nurse Corps—HQ USAF/SGN, Bolling Air Force Base, Washington, D.C. 20332.

Army Nurse Corps—Office of the Surgeon General, Dept. of the Army, Washington, D.C. 20310.

Navy Nurse Corps—Office of Director, Nurse Corps (OP-093N), Office of Director, Naval Medicine, Navy Dept., Washington, D.C. 20350.

Office of Human Development Services, Office of Policy Coordination and Review—200 Independence Ave., S.W., Washington, D.C. 20201.

U.S. Office of Personnel Management—1900 E St., N.W., Washington, D.C. 20415.

U.S. Public Health Service, DHHS—Office of the Assistant Secretary for Health, Office of The Surgeon General, 5600 Fishers Lane, Rockville, Md. 20857. Office of the Chief Nurse, Rm. 18-66.

Alcohol, Drug Abuse, and Mental Health Administration, 5600 Fishers Lane, Rockville, Md. 20857.

Centers for Disease Control—1600 Clifton Road, N.E., Atlanta, Ga. 30333.

National Institute for Occupational Safety and Health—Robert A. Taft Laboratories, 4676 Columbia Parkway, Cincinnati, Ohio 45226.

Food and Drug Administration—5600 Fishers Lane, Rockville, Md. 20857.

Health Resources and Services Administration, Bureau of Health Professions—Division of Nursing, 5600 Fishers Lane, Rockville, Md. 20857.

Bureau of Health Maintenance Organizations and Resource Development—5600 Fishers Lane, Rockville, Md. 20857.

Bureau of Health Care Delivery and Assistance—5600 Fishers Lane, Rockville, Md. 20857.

Indian Health Service—Office of Professional Standards and Evaluation, 5600 Fishers Lane, Rockville, Md 20857. Rm. 5A-09.

National Institute of Child Health and Human Development—Rm. 6C08, Landow Bldg., 7910 Woodmont Ave., Bethesda, Md. 20205.

National Institute of Neurological and Communicative Disorders and Stroke—7550 Wisconsin Ave., Bethesda, Md.

National Institute on Aging—Gerontology Research Center, 4940 Eastern Ave., Baltimore, Md. 21224.

Health Care Financing Administration—DHHS Office of the Administrator, Hubert H. Humphrey Bldg., 200 Independence Ave., S.W., Washington, D.C. 20201.

Bureau of Data Management and Strategy—Meadows East Bldg., 6300 Security Blvd., Baltimore, Md. 21207.

Office of Beneficiary Services—Oak Meadows Bldg., 6325 Security Blvd., Baltimore, Md. 21207.

Office of Legislation and Policy—Hubert H. Humphrey Bldg., 200 Independence Ave., S.W., Washington, D.C. 20201.

Office of Executive Operations—East High Rise Bldg., 6401 Security Blvd., Baltimore, Md. 21207.

Office of Research and Demonstrations—Oak Meadows Bldg., 6325 Security Blvd., Baltimore, Md. 21207.

Health Standards and Quality Bureau—Dogwood East Bldg., 1849 Gwynne Oak Ave., Baltimore, Md. 21207.

Bureau of Quality Control—East Low Rise Bldg., 6401 Security Blvd., Baltimore, Md. 21207.

Bureau of Program Operations—Meadows East Bldg., 6300 Security Blvd., Baltimore, Md. 21207.

Bureau of Eligibility, Reimbursement and Coverage—East High Rise Bldg., 6401 Security Blvd., Baltimore, Md. 21207.

Bureau of Support Services—Equitable Bldg., 1705 Whitehead Rd., Baltimore, Md. 21207.

Regional Offices, DHHS—Region I, John F. Kennedy Federal Bldg., Government Center, Boston, Mass. 02203; Region II, 26 Federal Plaza, New York, N.Y. 10278; Region III, P.O. Box 13716, Philadelphia, Pa. 19101; Region IV, 101 Marietta Tower, Atlanta, Ga. 30323; Region V, 300 S. Wacker Dr., Chicago, Ill. 60606; Region VI, 1200 Main Tower Bldg., Dallas, Tex. 75202; Region VII, 601 E. 12th St., Kansas City, Mo. 64106; Region VIII, Federal Office Bldg., 1961 Stout St., Denver, Colo. 80294; Region IX, Federal Office Bldg., 50 United Nations Plaza, San Francisco, Calif. 94102; Region X, 2901 3rd Ave., Seattle, Wash. 98121.

National Association for Home Care—519 C Street, N.E., Washington, D.C. 20002.

REGIONAL

Midwest Alliance in Nursing—Rm. 108-BR, Indiana University, 1226 W. Michigan St., Indianapolis, Ind. 46223. Tel. 317-264-3255.

New England Organization for Nursing—55 Chapel St., Newton, Mass. 02160. Tel. 617-969-7100.

Southern Regional Education Board—1340 Spring St., N.W., Atlanta, Ga. 30309. Tel. 404-875-9211.

Western Interstate Commission for Higher Education—P.O. Drawer P, Boulder, Colo. 80302.

STATE

Alabama State Nurses Association—360 N. Hull St., Montgomery 36197. Tel. 205-262-8321; Board of Nursing—Suite #203, 500 East Blvd., Montgomery 36117. Tel. 205-261-4060.

Alaska Nurses Association—237 East 3rd Ave., Anchorage 99501. Tel. 907-274-0827; Board of Nursing Licensing—Dept. of Commerce & Economic Development, Pouch D., Juneau 99811. Tel. 907-465-2544.

Arizona Nurses Association—4525 N. 12th St., Phoenix 85014. Tel. 602-277-4401; Board of Nursing—Rm. 254, 1645 W. Jefferson, Phoenix 85007. Tel. 602-255-5092.

Arkansas State Nurses Association—117 S. Cedar, Little Rock 72205. Tel. 501-664-5853; Board of Nursing—4120 West Markham, Suite 308, Little Rock 77205. Tel. 501-371-2751.

California Nurses Association—1855 Folsom St., Suite 670, San Francisco 94103. Tel. 415-864-4141; Board of Registered Nursing—1020 N. St., Sacramento 95814. Tel. 916-322-3350; Board of Vocational Nurse & Psychiatric Technician Examiners—1020 N. St., Sacramento 95814. Tel. 916-445-0793.

Colorado Nurses Association—5453 E. Evans Pl., Denver 80222. Tel. 303-757-7483; Board of Nursing—1525 Sherman St., Rm. 132, Denver 80203. Tel. 303-866-2871.

Connecticut Nurses Association—1 Prestige Dr., Meriden 06450. Tel. 203-238-1207; Board of Examiners for Nursing—150 Washington St., Hartford 06106. Tel. 203-566-1038.

Delaware Nurses Association—Suite 301, 1003 Delaware Ave., Wilmington 19806. Tel. 302-655-6297; Board of Nursing—Margaret O'Neill Bldg., Federal & Court Sts., Dover 19901. Tel. 302-736-4752.

District of Columbia Nurses Association—5100 Wisconsin Ave., N.W., Suite 306, Washington 20016. Tel. 202-244-2705; Registered Nurses Examining Board—614 H St., N.W., Washington 20001. Tel. 202-727-6215; Dept. of Consumer and Regulatory Affairs, Rm. 932. Practical Nurses Examining Board—614 H St., N.W., Washington 20001. Tel. 202-727-6215. Dept. of Consumer and Regulatory Affairs, Rm. 923.

Florida Nurses Association—Box 6985, Orlando 32853. Tel. 305-896-3261; Board of Nursing—111 E. Coastline Dr., Suite 504, Jacksonville 32202. Tel. 904-359-6331.

Georgia Nurses Association—1362 West Peachtree St., N.W., Atlanta 30309. Tel. 404-876-4624; Board of Nursing—166 Pryor St., S.W., Suite 400, Atlanta 30303. Tel. 404-656-3943; Board of Licensed Practical Nurses—166 Pryor St., S.W., Atlanta 30303. Tel. 404-656-3921.

Guam Nurses Association—Box 3134, Agana 96910; Board of Nurse Examiners—Box 2816, Agana 96910.

Hawaii Nurses Association—677 Ala Moana #1014, Honolulu 96813. Tel. 808-531-1628; Board of Nursing—Box 3469, Honolulu 96801. Tel. 808-548-7471.

Idaho Nurses Association—1134 North Orchard #8, Boise 83706. Tel. 208-377-0226; Board of Nursing—Hall of Mirrors, 700 W. State, 2nd fl., Boise 83720. Tel. 208-334-3110.

Illinois Nurses Association—20 N. Wacker, Suite 2520, Chicago 60606. Tel. 312-236-9708; Department of Registration and Education—320 W. Washington St., Springfield 62786. Tel. 217-785-0800; 17 N. State St., 17th fl., Chicago 60604. Tel. 312-793-8500.

Indiana State Nurses Association—2915 North High School Rd., Indianapolis 46224. Tel. 317-299-4575; Board of Nurses Registration and Nursing Education—964 N. Pennsylvania, Indianapolis 46204. Tel. 317-232-2960.

Iowa Nurses Association—215 Shops Bldg., Des Moines 50309. Tel. 515-282-9169; Board of Nursing—1223 E. Court, Des Moines 50319. Tel. 515-281-3255.

Kansas State Nurses Association—Rm. 520, 820 Quincy St., Topeka 66612. Tel. 913-233-8638; Board of Nursing—P.O. Box 1098, 503 Kansas Ave., Suite 330, Topeka 66601. Tel. 913-296-4929.

Kentucky Nurses Association—P.O. Box 8342, Station E., 1400 S. 1st St., Louisville 40208. Tel. 502-637-2546; Board of Nursing—4010 Dupont Circle, Suite 430, Louisville 40207. Tel. 502-897-5143.

Louisiana State Nurses Association—P.O. Box 837, Metairie 70004. Tel. 504-889-1030; Board of Nursing—Rm. 907, 150 Baronne St., New Orleans 70112. Tel. 504-568-5464; Board of Practical Nurse Examiners—4201½ Canal St., New Orleans 70119. Tel. 504-483-4505.

Maine State Nurses Association—283 Water St., P.O. Box 2240, Augusta 04330. Tel. 207-622-1057; Board of Nursing—295 Water St., Augusta 04330. Tel. 207-289-2921.

Maryland Nurses Association—5820 Southwestern Blvd., Baltimore 21227. Tel. 301-242-7300; Board of Examiners of Nurses—201 W. Preston St., Baltimore 21201. Tel. 301-383-2084.

Massachusetts Nurses Association—376 Boylston St., Boston 02116. Tel. 617-482-5465; Board of Registration in Nursing—Rm. 1509, 100 Cambridge St., Boston 02202. Tel. 617-727-3076, ext. 47.

Michigan Nurses Association—120 Spartan Ave., E. Lansing 48823. Tel. 517-337-1653; Board of Nursing—P.O. Box 30018, Lansing 48909. Tel. 517-373-1600.

Minnesota Nurses Association—Rm. N-377, 1821 University Ave., St. Paul 55104. Tel. 612-646-4807; Board of Nursing—717 Delaware St., S.E., Minneapolis 55414. Tel. 612-623-5493.

Mississippi Nurses Association—135 Bounds St., Suite 100, Jackson 39206. Tel. 601-982-9182; Board of Nursing—Suite 101, 135 Bounds St., Jackson 39206. Tel. 601-354-7349.

Missouri Nurses Association—206 E. Dunklin St., P.O. Box 325, Jefferson City 65102. Tel. 314-636-4623; Board of Nursing—3523 N. Ten Mile Dr., Box 656, Jefferson City 65102-0656. Tel. 314-751-2334.

Montana Nurses Association—P.O. Box 5718, 2001 Eleventh Ave., Helena 59604. Tel. 406-442-6710; Board of Nursing—Dept. of Commerce, 1424 9th Ave., Helena 59620. Tel. 406-444-3737.

Nebraska Nurses Association—Suite 7-1, 941 "O" St., Lincoln 68508. Tel. 402-475-3859; Board of Nursing—Box 95007, State House Station, Lincoln 68509. Tel. 402-471-2001.

Nevada Nurses Association—3660 Baker Lane, Reno 89509. Tel. 702-825-3555; Board of Nursing—Suite 209, 1135 Terminal Way, Reno 89502. Tel. 702-786-2778.

New Hampshire Nurses Association—48 West St., Concord 03301. Tel. 603-225-3783; Board of Nursing Education and Nurse Registration—105 Loudon Rd., Concord 03301. Tel. 603-271-2323.

New Jersey State Nurses Association—320 West State St., Trenton 08618. Tel. 609-392-4884; Board of Nursing—1100 Raymond Blvd., Rm. 319, Newark 07102. Tel. 201-648-2490-1.

New Mexico Nurses Association—525 San Pedro, N.E., Suite 100, Albuquerque 87108. Tel. 505-268-7744; Board of Nursing—5301 Central N.E., Suite 905, Albuquerque 87108. Tel. 505-841-4620.

New York State Nurses Association—2113 Western Ave., Guilderland 12084. Tel. 518-456-5371; Board for Nursing—State Education Dept., Cultural Education Center, Albany 12230. Tel. 518-474-3843-4-5.

North Carolina Nurses Association—Box 12025, Raleigh 27605. Tel. 919-821-4250; Board of Nursing—Box 2129, Raleigh 27602. Tel. 919-828-0740.

North Dakota State Nurses Association—212 N. 4th St., Greentree Sq., Bismarck 58501. Tel. 701-223-1385; Board of Nursing—418 East Rosser Ave., Bismarck 58501. Tel. 701-224-2974.

Ohio Nurses Association—4000 E. Main St., P.O. Box 13169, Columbus 43213. Tel. 614-237-5414; Board of Nursing Education and Nurse Registration—65 South Front St., Rm. 509, Columbus 43215. Tel. 614-466-3947.

Oklahoma Nurses Association—6414 N. Santa Fe, Ste. A, Oklahoma City 73116. Tel. 405-840-3476; Board of Nurse Registration and Nursing Education—Suite 400, 4001 N. Lincoln Blvd., Oklahoma City 73105. Tel. 405-521-2363.

Oregon Nurses Association—Suite 103, 9730 S.W. Cascade Blvd., Tigard 97223. Tel. 503-620-7474; Board of Nursing—1400 S.W. 5th Ave., Rm. 904, Portland 97201. Tel. 503-229-5653.

Pennsylvania Nurses Association—2515 N. Front St., Harrisburg 17110. Tel. 717-234-7935; Board of Nurse Examiners—Box 2649, Harrisburg 17120. Tel. 717-783-7146.

Puerto Rico Board of Nurse Examiners—800 Roberto H. Todd Ave., Stop 18, Santurce 00908. Tel. 809-725-8900.

Rhode Island State Nurses Association—345 Blackstone Blvd., H.C. Hall Bldg. (South), Providence 02906. Tel. 401-421-9703; Board of Nurse Registration and Nursing Education—Cannon Health Bldg., 75 Davis St., Providence 02908. Tel. 401-277-2827.

South Carolina Nurses Association—1821 Gadsden St., Columbia 29201. Tel. 803-252-4781; Board of Nursing—1777 St. Julian Pl., Suite 102, Columbia 29204. Tel. 803-758-2611.

South Dakota Nurses Association—1505 S. Minnesota, Suite 6, Sioux Falls 57105. Tel. 605-338-1401; Board of Nursing—304 S. Phillips Ave., Suite 205, Sioux Falls 57102. Tel. 605-334-1243.

Tennessee Nurses Association—Suite 400, 1720 West End Bldg., Nashville 37203. Tel. 615-329-2511; Board of Nursing—State Office Bldg., Ben Allen Rd., Nashville 37216. Tel. 615-741-7256.

Texas Nurses Association—Suite 504, 314 Highland Mall Blvd., Austin 78752. Tel. 512-452-0645; Board of Nurse Examiners—1300 E. Anderson Lane, Bldg. C, Suite 225, Austin 78752. Tel. 512-835-4880; Board of Vocational Nurse Examiners—1300 E. Anderson Lane, Bldg. C, Suite 285, Austin 78752. Tel. 512-835-2071.

Utah Nurses Association—1058 E. 9th So., Salt Lake City 84105. Tel. 801-322-3439; Division of Registration-Board of Nursing—Heber M. Wells Bldg., 4th floor, 160 East 300 South, P.O. Box 5802, Salt Lake City 84110. Tel. 801-530-6628.

Vermont State Nurses Association—500 Dorset St., Middle School, So. Burlington 05401. Tel. 802-864-9390; Board of Nursing—Pavilion Office Bldg., 109 State St., Montpelier 05602. Tel. 802-828-2363.

Virgin Island Nurses Association—P.O. Box 2866, Charlotte Amalie, St. Thomas 00801; Board of Nurse Licensure—P.O. Box 7309. Charlotte Amalie, St. Thomas 00801. Tel. 809-774-9000.

Virginia Nurses Association—1311 High Point Ave., Richmond 23230. Tel. 804-353-7311; Board of Nursing—517 West Grace St., P.O. Box 27708, Richmond 23261. Tel. 804-786-0377.

Washington State Nurses Association—4th & Vine Bldg., 2615 Fourth Ave., Suite 380, Seattle 98121. Tel. 206-622-3613; Board of Nursing—Div. of Professional Licensing, Box 9649, Olympia 98504. Tel. 206-753-3726; Board of Practical Nursing—Div. of Professional Licensing, P.O. Box 9649, Olympia 98504. Tel. 206-753-3728.

West Virginia Nurses Association—Suite 511, Union Bldg., 723 Kanawha Blvd. E., Charleston 25301. Tel. 304-342-7978; Board of Examiners for Registered Nurses—Rm. 309, Embleton Bldg., 922 Quarrier St., Charleston 25301. Tel. 304-348-3596; Board of Examiners for Licensed Practical Nurses—Rm. 506, Embleton Bldg., 922 Quarrier St., Charleston 25301. Tel. 304-348-3572.

Wisconsin Nurses Association—206 E. Olin Ave., Madison 53713. Tel. 608-251-1462; Board of Nursing—Rm. 174, Post Office Box 8936, Madison 53708. Tel. 608-266-3735.

Wyoming Nurses Association—Majestic Bldg., Rm. 305, 1603 Capitol Ave., Cheyenne 82001. Tel. 307-635-3955; Board of Nursing—2223 Warren Ave., Suite One, Cheyenne 82002. Tel. 307-777-7601.

13-2 Directory of nursing organizations: Canada

Canadian Nurses Association

Founded in 1908, the Canadian Nurses Association is the official national organization for 180,348 professional registered nurses who are members of one of the 12 provincial/territorial professional nurses' associations. Financially supported by membership fees collected by these associations, the CNA is managed by a 36-member board of directors—nine elected officers, 12 provincial/territorial presidents and their 12 advisors, plus three public representatives. Striving to promote health and conditions conducive to the best possible patient care, the CNA is continuously concerned with:

- The quality and quantity of nurses available to the health team
- Standards of preparation and performance of professional nurses
- Social and economic welfare of nurses
- Advancement of knowledge, techniques and competence within the profession
- Promotion of understanding, unity and good professional citizenship among its members
- Representing and speaking for the organized nursing profession, both nationally and internationally
- Development of research and guidelines for ethical review of research proposals
- Code of ethics for nursing

Services are provided in both official languages and include research and advisory, library, information, labor relations, national examination preparation and liaison, both nationally and internationally.

From Banning, J.: Special groups for special nurses, Canadian Nurse **79:**27-36, 1983.

50 The Driveway
Ottawa, Ontario
K2P 1E2

NATIONAL ASSOCIATIONS

Canadian Association of Critical Care Nurses

Formerly the Niagara Association of Critical Care Nurses, the Canadian Association of Critical Care Nurses has just recently been incorporated. With 200 members from right across the country, the Niagara Founding Chapter is anticipating the formation of chapters in Ottawa, Kingston, London, Ontario and St. John's, Nfld. within the next year. Promotion of professional accountability, nursing research, continuing education, certification standards, and political activity to shape the health care delivery system as it relates to the care of the critically ill are all objectives of the CACCN. Active, associate, and international memberships are available and include a subscription to *Dimensions in Critical Care* and *Heartline*.

Canadian Association of Critical Care Nurses
P.O. Box 61
Welland, Ontario
L3B 5N9

Canadian Association for Enterostomal Therapy

With a membership exceeding 170, The Canadian Association for Enterostomal Therapy is working to provide quality nursing care to all persons requiring care of an abdominal stoma, fistula, draining wound, or related problem. The CAET is a member of the International Association of Enterostomal Therapists. Members meet annually for a spring conference and a teaching seminar is usually held in the fall. Provincial interest groups are also active.

4389 Prospect Rd.
North Vancouver, B.C.
V7N 3L8

Canadian Association of Neurological and Neurosurgical Nurses

Founded in 1969, the Canadian Association of Neurological and Neurosurgical Nurses was the first group of specialized nurses in Canada to organize on a national basis. Objectives include promotion of the highest standards of practice in the field of neurological and neurosurgical nursing, fostering of continuing professional education of members, the provision of methods of sharing this knowledge, and establishment and maintenance of lines of communication between nursing and other disciplines practising in the field of neurological sciences. With more than 300 active members, the association is awaiting official notification of associate membership in the Canadian Nurses Association. Members meet annually to present papers of interest and elect a board of directors and councilors to represent each province. Both active ($35) and associate ($25) memberships are available. Members receive *Axone,* the association newsletter.

Box 1096
Shelbourne, Nova Scotia
B0T 1W0

Canadian Association of Quality Care Coordinators

Now in its second year, the Canadian Association of Quality Care Coordinators is made up of health professionals from across Canada who are working in the field of quality assurance. The group has sponsored three annual workshops and publishes a newsletter.

Nursing Practice
Surrey Memorial Hospital
King George Highway
Surrey, British Columbia
V3V 1Z2

Canadian Association of University Schools of Nursing

In 1942, eight university schools of nursing met to organize a "provisional council of university schools and departments of nursing" in order to determine desirable standards for existing schools and to support the development of future university schools of nursing. Now this voluntary association represents 25 university schools of nursing in Canada. An associate member of the Association of Universities and Colleges of Canada, CAUSN meets on a national basis to discuss issues in higher education. Objectives include the development of criteria for university education in nursing, promotion of research in nursing, the interchange of nursing knowledge among members, the representation of views of the association to educational, professional, and other appropriate bodies, and promotion of understanding by the public that university education in nursing contributes to the development of health services in Canada. To consolidate the structure of the association and ensure continuity of activities between council meetings, Atlantic, Quebec, Ontario, and Western regional groups have been established. CAUSN is the official accreditation agency for university nursing programs in Canada.

CAUSN
1200 - 151 Slater St.
Ottawa, Ontario
K1P 5N1

Canadian Council of Cardiovascular Nurses

Founded in 1973 as a scientific council of the Canadian Heart Foundation, membership in the CCCN now stands at approximately 1300. All registered nurses interested in promoting the quality of health care as it relates to cardiovascular function are welcomed as members. The CCCN has a board of management responsible to the board of directors of the Canadian Heart Foundation and has two main standing committees: the Continuing Education committee, responsible for educational events, travelling lectureship programs, workshops, and seminars; and the Research Committee established to stimulate and coordinate nursing research as well as encourage publication and dissemination of information on current trends and results of research in the cardiovascular field. An annual membership of $20 includes the opportunity to attend joint annual meetings and scientific sessions of the Canadian Heart Foundation, the Canadian Cardiovascular Society and the Canadian Council of Cardiovascular Nurses; a nursing research fellowship for nurses at the master's or doctoral level; a quarterly bulletin, as well as subscription to the three official journals of the American Heart Foundation: *Cardiovascular Nursing, Modern Concepts of Cardiovascular Disease* and *Current Concepts of Cerebrovascular Disease.*

Canadian Council of Cardiovascular Nurses
1200 - 1 Nicholas St.
Ottawa, Ontario
K1N 7B7

Canadian Diabetes Association—Professional Health Workers Section

More than half of the 700 members of the multidisciplinary PHWS section of the Canadian Diabetes Association are nurses. Formed in 1973, this group has objectives of providing and encouraging high quality diabetic health education, information, and services; providing guidance in establishing and expanding diabetes education programs, providing a forum for interchange of knowledge and skills for health professionals, and maintaining close liaison with the clinical and scientific committees of the CDA.

Contact:
Professional Health Workers Section
Canadian Diabetes Association
601 - 123 Edward St.
Toronto, Ontario
M5G 1E2

Canadian Hospital Infection Control Association

CHICA was founded in June of 1971 to support the prevention and control of infections in health care institutions in Canada. Objectives include the initiation and development of effective communications, development of effective and rational infection control programs, standardization and critical evaluation of infection control practices, quality research practices and procedures related to infection control, creation of educational programs in infection control, and creation of regional organizations to improve the exchange of scientific information. Membership is open to all individuals involved in the practice of infection control. The CHICA newsletter is the primary means of communication among membership, which meets bienially for a national conference.

Mount Sinai Hospital
600 University Ave.
Toronto, Ont.
M5G 1X5

Canadian Intravenous Nurses Association

Founded in 1975 with the aim of promoting higher standards in intravenous therapy for better and safer care through communication, education and participation, CINA now boasts a membership of over 225. At the request of CINA, a working group was established by Health and Welfare Canada to develop guidelines for the administration of intravenous therapy. These guidelines are available through Health and Welfare Canada or CINA. In addition, a course on IV therapy is now available through Centennial College, Toronto. Two chapters are now in existence: York Toronto and Southern Alberta. Membership is $40 and offers the new member the *American Journal of IV Therapy* and/or *Clinical Nutrition* at reduced rates. In addition, a quarterly newsletter is published.

CINA
200 - 4433 Sheppard Ave. E.
Agincourt, Ontario
M1S 1V3

Canadian Nurses Foundation

More than 250 nurses have benefited from scholarships awarded by the Canadian Nurses Foundation. The only Canadian foundation that deals exclusively in supporting nursing scholars, the Canadian Nurses Foundation (CNF) was launched in 1962 with a donation from the W.K. Kellogg Foundation. CNF solicits and holds funds to provide scholarships for nurses undertaking graduate and post-RN (one scholarship for post-RN study towards a baccalaureate in each province) studies in nursing and to provide grants in aid of nursing research. The foundation has an elected voluntary board of directors chosen every two years from among its membership and has a nurse representative in each province. Membership now stands at well over 500. Fees: regular membership $10, sustaining $50; and patron $500 (initial fee). Applicants for an award must be a member of their provincial nurses association and have gained acceptance into university or graduate school. They must identify the practice area in which they wish to study and have definite career goals.

Canadian Nurses Foundation
50 The Driveway
Ottawa, Ontario
K2P 1E2

Canadian Nurses Respiratory Society

An associate member of the Canadian Nurses Association and a special interest group of the Canadian Lung Association, this group welcomes all registered nurses working with or interested in alleviating the problems associated with respiratory disease. In particular the Canadian Nurses Respiratory Society promotes nursing education and research. Membership ($12) in the association allows nurses to meet, share, and consult with their colleagues at an annual scientific conference held in association with the Canadian Lung Association. Fellowships are available to nurses wishing to study at the master's level in an approved program in respiratory nursing. Members also receive the two official publications of the Canadian Lung Association: the quarterly bulletin and the bi-monthly Canadian Lung Association newsletter.

Canadian Lung Association
908 - 75 Albert St.
Ottawa, Ontario
K1P 5E7

Canadian Orthopedic Nurses Association

An affiliate member of the Canadian Nurses Association, the Canadian Orthopedic Nurses Association now boasts more than 650 members and ten chapters from St. John's to Winnipeg. Promotion of the highest standards in the practice of orthopedic nursing through continuing education has been the prime objective of this group. To meet this objective, CONA publishes a professional quarterly journal and has a very active continuing education committee dedicated to providing nurses with a library of clinical resource material to help solve orthopedic problems. An Orthopedic Nurse of the Year is recognized each year at the association's national conference. Membership is open to all concerned nurses and health professionals actively involved in the field of orthopedics.

Canadian Orthopedic Nurses Association
43 Wellesley St.
Toronto, Ontario
M4Y 1H1

Canadian Society of Dialysis Perfusionists

With more than 140 members, the Canadian Society of Dialysis Perfusionists is dedicated to achieving the highest possible standards of care for nephrology patients. Members believe that these goals can be achieved through continuing education, research and communication of ideas. To this end the society holds a yearly two-day symposium in conjunction with the annual meeting and publishes a quarterly newsletter *DIALTEC*. Membership is open to anyone concerned with the care of patients with renal diseases. Members may also be certified by meeting the society's standards for certification and passing the appropriate exams.

Dialysis Unit
Health Sciences Centre
700 William Ave.
Winnipeg, Manitoba
R3E 0Z3

Canadian University Nursing Students Association

The promotion of professionalism among university nursing students is the aim of CUNSA, a national association which held its first conference in 1968 with representatives from five universities. In 1972, CUNSA became an official association, with representatives from 22 university schools of nursing. Affiliated with the Canadian Association of University Schools of Nursing, the association's objectives include providing a communication link between university nursing students across Canada, acting as the official voice of university nursing students, providing a medium through which students can express their opinions on issues in nursing and assisting and/or initiating nursing research. Every year CUNSA undertakes a major nursing research project through the national research coordinator. CUNSA is divided into four regions: Atlantic, Quebec, Ontario, and Western, each with a regional chairperson and representative to the national executive committee. Membership fees based on student enrolment are paid by member universities. An annual conference and a quarterly newsletter facilitate communication between members.

School of Nursing
Université de Montréal
C.P. 6128
Montréal, Québec
H3T 1J4

Dynamics of Critical Care Association of Canada

Formerly the Toronto Chapter of the American Association of Critical Care Nurses, the CNSC has been formed with the purpose of providing educational programs for critical care nurses. To date, membership stands at 350. This association sponsors the "Dynamics of Critical Care" held annual in Toronto and produces a bimonthly newsletter "CriticaList." Membership is $40.

CNSC
200 - 4433 Sheppard Ave. E.
Agincourt, Ontario
M1S 1V3

Nursing Sisters Association of Canada

After World War I, nursing sisters from across Canada formed groups to keep up the friendships which they had developed overseas and to extend assistance to those in need. In 1920, the first group was officially formed in Edmonton and following this, similar groups formed across Canada. In July 1929, at the International Congress of Nurses in Montreal, the National Association of Overseas Nursing Sisters was formed. Later the name was changed to the Nursing Sisters Association of Canada. Today, membership in the association includes nurses, home sisters, dieticians and physiotherapists who have been honorably discharged or are now serving with Her Majesty's forces. With a current membership of 950, units still exist in all provinces and a national executive is elected. Their objectives include the stimulation of friendship among members, to work for national unity and international peace, and to give aid and comfort to nurses in need. Affiliated with the National Council of Veteran Associations of Canada, the association holds biennial meetings during the biennial convention of the Canadian Nurses Association. The Agnes Campbell Neill Memorial Award, presented every two years through the Canadian Nurses Foundation, is sponsored by the Nursing Sisters Association of Canada.

307 - 60 McLeod St.
Ottawa, Ontario
K2P 0Z5

Operating Room Nurses Association of Canada

An associate member of the Canadian Nurses Association, this group is primarily concerned with continuing education for O.R. nurses, upgrading standards of O.R. care, and increasing communication between O.R. nurses. Formerly the National Conference of Operating Room Nurses, the Operating Room Nurses Association of Canada appointed a national liaison officer in 1980 and this year plans to introduce the *Canadian O.R. Nursing Journal*.

213 - 52377 Range Rd.
Sherwood Park, Alberta
T8G 1B9

Psychiatric Nurses Association of Canada

This national association had its beginnings in 1950 when representatives of British Columbia and Saskatchewan psychiatric nurses met to discuss formation of a Canadian Council of Psychiatric Nurses. Delegates from B.C., Alberta, and Saskatchewan attended the founding conference in 1951. Manitoba joined in 1960, Ontario in 1971, and Nova Scotia in 1974. The Northwest Territories was admitted as an associate member in 1977. Over the past year the Psychiatric Nurses Association of Ontario has disbanded. In 1965 the Canadian Council of Psychiatric Nurses became the Psychiatric Nurses Association of Canada and a national office was established. The association sponsors research and meetings aimed at improved national standards of psychiatric care, a national conference and a bi-monthly publication, *The Canadian Journal of Psychiatric Nursing*.

Psychiatric Nurses
Association of Canada
1854 Portage Ave.
Winnipeg, Manitoba
R3J 0G9

Registered Nurses of Canadian Indian Ancestry

In 1975, during International Women's year, 43 nurses from across Canada met to form the Registered Nurses of Canadian Indian Ancestry. This was the first assembly of Indian professionals in the history of Canada. The nurses were concerned with the poor health of their people as a group and adopted several objectives, including promoting better health for the Indian people, promoting research, compiling information, assisting government and private agencies in developing programs to improve Indian health, developing courses on Indian health and cross-cultural nursing, and encouraging Indian control and decision-making in Indian health care. Their special objective for 1983 was to encourage health careers among native people.

RNCIA
500 - 222 Queen St.
Ottawa, Ontario
K1P 5V9

TPN Nurses Association of Canada

The Total Parenteral Nutrition Nurses Association of Canada was formed to represent the interests of professional nursing personnel working with patients receiving nutritional support, to promote professional communication in nutritional support through national and regional meetings, seminars, educational bulletins, and research, and to promote professional and optimum nursing care of nutritionally supported patients. Membership, which now stands at 200, includes active members ($20) and associate members ($15) who receive the quarterly newsletter ''Food for Thought.'' An annual meeting is held each spring.

P.O. Box 62
Station K
Toronto, Ont.
M4P 2G1

INTERNATIONAL ASSOCIATIONS

Association for The Care Of Children's Health

The ACCH is a multidisciplinary, international organization that promotes the psychosocial well-being of children and families in all types of health care settings. Founded in 1965, the association has more than 3000 members, including representatives of administration, architecture, child life activities, dietetic, education, medicine, nursing, occupational therapy, psychiatry, psychology, recreation, rehabilitation, social work, as well as concerned consumers. ACCH publishes a quarterly peer review journal, a bi-monthly newsletter, bibliographies, directories, pamphlets and other educational materials. It also sponsors an annual conference and through its regional affiliates holds many local community meetings. Each year in March ACCH conducts a public education campaign entitled Children and Hospitals Week.

Canadian Institute of Child Health
202 - 17 York St.
Ottawa, Ontario
K1M 5S7

Nurses Association of The American College of Obstetricians and Gynecologists

NAACOG is a professional association of over 17,000 nurses and allied health professionals whose primary interest is in obstetric, gynecologic and neonatal nursing. The purpose of the association is the promotion of the highest standards of care to women and their newborns through quality continuing education. To this end NAACOG offers a wide variety of accredited continuing education courses, educational publications, and numerous meetings and in addition publishes the *Journal of Obstetric, Gynecologic and Neonatal Nursing*, a scientific journal written by and for nurses. Membership services include a monthly newsletter, low-cost liability insurance, and many opportunities for peer interaction. Canadian membership now stands at approximately 800.

NAACOG
200 - 600 Maryland Ave. S.W.
Washington, D.C. 20024-2589

PROVINCIAL, TERRITORIAL, AND LOCAL ASSOCIATIONS

British Columbia

B.C. Nursing Supervisors Group
(RNABC Interest Group)
5611 Lancing Rd.
Richmond, B.C.
V7C 3A4

B.C. Occupational Health Nurses Group
(RNABC Interest Group)
B.C. Occupational Health Nurses Group
RNABC
2855 Arbutus
Vancouver, B.C.
V6J 3Y8

British Columbia Operating Room Nurses Group
(RNABC Interest Group)
706 - 1420 West 11th Ave.
Vancouver, B.C.
V6H 1L2

B.C. Pediatric Nurses Group
58 - 10824 - 152nd St.
Surrey, B.C.
V3R 4H2

Community Health Nurses Interest Group
(RNABC Interest Group)
8856 Prest Rd.
Chilliwack, B.C.
V2P 6H3

Emergency Nurses Group of B.C.
(Special interest group of RNABC)
Emergency Nurses Group of B.C.
Box 302
Surrey, B.C.
V3T 5B6

Gerontological Nurses Group
Shaughnessy Manor Long Term Care Society
1125 W. 12th Ave.
Vancouver, B.C.
V6H 1L8

Holistic Health Interest Group
4030 West 10th Ave.
Vancouver, B.C.
V6R 2H1

Home Care Nurses Group
(RNABC Interest Group)
1 - 1530 West 13th Ave.
Vancouver, B.C.
V6J 2G4

Licensed Practical Nurses Association of B.C.
695 Montague Rd.
Nanaimo, B.C.
V9R 3G4

Nurse Administrators Association of British Columbia
G.F. Strong Rehabilitation Centre
4255 Laurel St.
Vancouver, B.C.
V5Z 2G9

Nursing Research Interest Group
(RNABC Interest Group)
3425 West 8th Ave.
Vancouver, B.C.
V6R 1G6

Psychiatric/Mental Health Nursing Interest Group
(RNABC Interest Group)
8 - 1390 Blackwood St.
White Rock, B.C.
V4B 3V3

Registered Psychiatric Nurses' Association of B.C.
508 Clark
Coquitlam, B.C.
V3N 1B8

Alberta

Alberta Community Health Nurses Society
(AARN Interest Group)
39 Finch Crescent
St. Albert, Alta.
T8N 1Y5

Alberta Gerontological Nurses Association
(AARN Interest Group)
9608 Palisan Place S.W.
Calgary, Alta.
T2V 3S9

Alberta Health Care Educators Interest Group
(AARN Interest Group)
Coordinator of Educational Services
Rockyview General Hospital
Calgary, Alta.
T2V 1P9

Alberta Occupational Health Nurses
(AARN Interest Group)
1703 - 10135 Saskatchewan Dr.
Edmonton, Alta.
T6E 4Y9

Calgary Infection Control Group
Infection Control
Foothills Hospital
1403 - 29th St. N.W.
Calgary, Alta.
T2N 2T9

Alberta Nursing Education Administrators
Chairman
Allied Health Department
Mount Royal College
Calgary, Alta.

Emergency Nurses Interest Group
(AARN Interest Group)
115 Bradner Village
Edmonton, Alta.
T6H 5C9

Executive Nurses Association of Alberta
Director of Nursing
University of Alberta Hospitals
112 St. & 84 Ave.
Edmonton, Alta.
T6G 2B7

Gastroenterology Interest Group
11403 - 164 Ave.
Edmonton, Alta.
T5X 3W1

Nursing Advisory Committee, Alberta Lung Association
2525 - 4th Ave. N.W.
Calgary, Alta.
T2N 0P5

Oncology Club, Edmonton Alberta Nurses
10930 - 65 Ave.
Edmonton, Alta.
T6H 4R6

Operating Room Nurses of Alberta
(AARN Interest Group)
213 - 52377 Range Rd.
Sherwood Park, Alta.
T8G 1B9

Orthopedic Nursing Interest Group
(AARN Interest Group)
86 Oatway Dr.
Stony Plain, Alta.
T0E 2G0

Psychiatric Nurses Association of Alberta
Ste. D, 8711 - 96 Ave.
Edmonton, Alta.
T6C 2B1

Rehabilitation Nurses Interest Group
1227 - 39 St.
Edmonton, Alta.
T6L 2M6

Western Nurse Midwives Association
(AARN Interest Group)
5139 Lochside Dr.
Victoria, B.C.
V8Y 2G2

Saskatchewan

Administrative Nurses' Section
(SRNA Special Interest Group)
Box 2845
426 Park Avenue
Melfort, Sask.
S0E 1A0

Occupational Health Nurses Section
(SRNA Interest Group)
c/o Saskatchewan Wheat Pool
2625 Victoria Ave.
Regina, Sask.
S4P 2Y6

Saskatchewan Emergency Nurses' Group
(SRNA Interest Group)
College of Nursing
University of Saskatchewan
Saskatoon, Sask.

Manitoba

Association for the Care of Children's Health
(Manitoba Affiliate)
61 Emily St.
Winnipeg, Man.
R3E 1Y9

Canadian Association of Neurological and Neurosurgical Nurses—Manitoba Region
Misercordia General Hospital
99 Cornish Ave.
Winnipeg, Man.
R3C 1A2

Canadian Hospital Infection Control Association—Manitoba Chapter
St. Boniface General Hospital
409 Tache Ave.
Winnipeg, Man.
R2H 2A6

Cardiovascular Nurses Interest Group
630 Cordova St.
Winnipeg, Man.
R3N 1B1

Community Health Nurses Interest Group
Winnipeg City Health Department
East District Nursing Office
405 Carlton St.
Winnipeg, Man.
R3B 2K9

Dialysis Interest Group
73 Lennox Ave.
Winnipeg, Man.
R2M 1A8

Directors of Nursing Administration
Director Nursing Services
Selkirk Mental Health Centre
Box 9600
Selkirk, Man.
R1A 2B5

Directors of Nursing Education
Director, School of Nursing
Brandon Mental Health Centre
P.O. Box 420
Brandon, Man.
R7A 5Z5

Enterostomal Therapy Group
Victorian Order of Nurses
311 - 167 Lombard
Winnipeg, Man.
R3B 0T6

Manitoba Health Care Inservice
Director—Inservice Dept.
Deer Lodge Hospital
2109 Portage Ave.
Winnipeg, Man.
R3J 0Z9

Manitoba Respiratory Nurses Interest Group
Manitoba Lung Association
629 McDermot Ave.
Winnipeg, Man.
R3A 1P6

Manitoba Urology Nurses Interest Group
6A Urology
St. Boniface Hospital
409 Tache Ave.
Winnipeg, Man.
R2H 2A6

Manitoba Indian Nurses Association
Greater Winnipeg Indian Council
650 Burrows Ave.
Winnipeg, Man.
R2W 2A8

Manitoba Nursing Research Group
Registrar, School of Nursing
St. Boniface General Hospital
431 Tache Ave.
Winnipeg, Man.
R2H 2A7

Manitoba Operating Room Study Group
Operating Room
St. Boniface General Hospital
409 Tache Ave.
Winnipeg, Man.
R2H 2A6

Manitoba Ophthalmology Nurses Interest Group
Nursing Coordinator—Ophthalmology
St. Boniface Hospital
409 Tache Ave.
Winnipeg, Man.
R2H 2A6

Manitoba Orthopedic Nurses Interest Group
St. Boniface Hospital
409 Tache Ave.
Winnipeg, Man.
R2H 2A6

Nurse Practitioners Interest Group
Norwest Co-op Health Service
61 Tyndall
Winnipeg, Man.
R2X 2T4

Nurses Christian Movement of Manitoba
220 Oak St.
Winnipeg, Man.
R3M 3R4

Nursing Administration Interest Group (Manitoba)
Special Care Areas
Winnipeg General Hospital
700 William Ave.
Winnipeg, Man.
R3E 0Z3

Occupational Health Nurses Interest Group
108 - 3050 Pembina Hwy.
Winnipeg, Man.
R3T 3Z2

Oncology Interest Group
Victoria General Hospital
2340 Pembia Hwy.
Winnipeg, Man.
R3T 2E8

Personal Care Home Directors of Nursing
317 Baltimore Rd.
Winnipeg, Man.
R3L 1J2

Phillipine Nurses Association of Manitoba
824 Cloutier Dr.
Winnipeg, Man.
R3V 1L2

Westman Personal Care Interest Group
Box 960
Minnedosa, Man.
R0J 1E0

Winnipeg Association of Critical Care Nurses
211B - 294 Beliveau Ave.
Winnipeg, Man.
R2M 1S8

Ontario

Association of Nursing Directors and Supervisors of Ontario
Official Health Agencies
Supervisor
Public Health Nursing
Halton Regional Health Unit
P.O. Box 7000
Oakville, Ontario
L6J 6E1

Association of Nursing Executives of Metropolitan Toronto
Director of Nursing
York Central Hospital
10 Trench St.
Richmond Hill, Ont.
L4C 4Z3

Canadian Association of Critical Care Nurses, Niagara Chapter
Box 61
Welland, Ont.
L3B 5N9

Canadian Hospital Infection Control Association,
Thunder Bay Chapter
Infection Control Officer
McKellar General Hospital
Thunder Bay, Ont.
P7E 1G6

Clinical Nurse Specialist Interest Group (RNAO Interest Group)
c/o RNAO
33 Price St.
Toronto, Ont.
M4W 1Z2

College of Nurses of Ontario
600 Eglinton Ave. East
Toronto, Ontario
M4P 1P4

Community Health Nurses Interest Group (RNAO Interest Group)
R.R. 2
Kemptville, Ont.
K0G 1J0

Emergency Nurses Association of Ontario
Box 100-217
2 Bloor St. W.
Toronto, Ont.
M4W 3E2

Gerontological Nursing Association (RNAO Affiliate)
89 Hazelton Ave.
Toronto, Ont.
M5R 2E4

Heads of Diploma Nursing Programs
Sault College
P.O. Box 60
Sault Ste. Marie, Ont.
L6A 5L3

Lakehead Operating Room Nurses Association
Contact: c/o Operating Room
St. Joseph's General Hospital
Thunder Bay, Ont.

Northwestern Ontario Occupational Health Nurses Association
Health Services
Confederation College
P.O. Box 398, Station F
Thunder Bay, Ont.
P7C 4W1

Nurse Childbirth Educators' Interest Group
(RNAO Interest Group)
6 - 7120 Appleby Lane, R.R. 6
Milton, Ont.
L9T 2Y1

Nurse Practitioners' Association of Ontario (RNAO Affiliate)
6 - 200 Elm St.
Toronto, Ont.
M5T 1K4

Nursing Administrators' Interest Group
(RNAO Interest Group)
Staff Development
Toronto General Hospital
101 College St.
Toronto, Ontario
M5G 1L7

Ontario Association of Addiction Nurses
Alcohol and Drug Unit
Royal Ottawa Hospital
1145 Carling Ave.
Ottawa, Ont.
K1Z 7K4

Ontario Association of Registered Nursing Assistants
112 Merton St., 3rd Floor
Toronto, Ontario
M4S 1A1

Ontario Association of Rehabilitation Nurses (London Chapter)
414 Citation Dr.
London, Ont.
N6T 1L5

Ontario Community Mental Health Nurses Association (RNAO Affiliate)
204 - 1250 Bridle Court Circle
Agincourt, Ont.
M1W 2V1

Ontario Nurse Midwives Association (RNAO Affiliate)
9 Richmond St.
Hamilton, Ont.

Ontario Lung Association, Nurses Section
Editor, OLA Report
157 Willowdale Ave.
Willowdale, Ont.
M2N 4Y7

Ontario Occupational Health Nurses Association
Port Weller Dry Docks
P.O. Box 3011
St. Catharines, Ont.
L2R 7C1

Ontario Region, Canadian Association of University Schools of Nursing (ORCAUSN)
School of Nursing
Faculty of Health Sciences
McMaster University
1200 Main Street
Hamilton, Ont.
L8S 4J9

Operating Room Nurses Association of Ontario
University Hospital
339 Windermere Rd.
Box 5339
London, Ont.
N6A 5A5

Provincial Association of College Nurse Educators
Dean, Post Secondary Programs
Canadian College
P.O. Box 5001
North Bay, Ont.
P1B 8K9

Provincial Nurse Educator Interest Group
(RNAO Interest Group)
65 - 106 Chester Le Boulevard
Scarborough, Ont.
M1W 2X9

Psychiatric Nursing Interest Group (RNAO Interest Group)
511 Harris St.
Whitby, Ont.
L1N 3C6

Southwestern Ontario Practitioners in Infection Control
Infection Control Coordinator
Kitchener-Waterloo Hospital
535 King St. W.
Kitchener, Ont.
N2G 1G3

Toronto Health Educator's Association
105 - 206 George St.
Toronto, Ont.
M5R 2N6

Toronto Practitioners in Infection Control
Infection Control Nurse
Wellesley Hospital
160 Wellesley St.
Toronto, Ont.
M4Y 1J3

Quebec

Association des infirmières et infirmiers en santé du travail du Québec, Inc.
Secrétaire, AIISTQ
C.P. 160, Succ. Delorimier
Montréal, Qué.
H2H 2N6

Corporation professionnelle des infirmières et infirmiers auxiliaires du Québec
65 ouest, rue de Castelnau, pièce 300
Montréal, Qué.
H2R 2W3

Operating Room Nurses of Québec
Operating Room Coordinator
Montreal Children's Hospital
2300 Tupper St.
Montréal, Qué.
H3H 1P3

Regroupement des infirmières et infirmiers diplômés des 2e et 3e cycles du Québec
RIID
C.P. 1578, Succursale B
Hull, Qué.
J8X 3Y5

Societé québécoise des infirmières en santé respiratoire
C.P. 1057
1369 Promenade des Anciens
Havre St. Pierre, Qué.
G0G 1P0

New Brunswick

Association of New Brunswick Registered Nursing Assistants
39 Coventry Crescent
Fredericton, N.B.
E3B 4P4

Canadian Council of Cardiovascular Nurses, N.B. Division
(NBARN Interest Group)
16 Mount Pleasant Court N.
Saint John, N.B.
E2K 3V6

New Brunswick Infection Control Practitioners Group
Infection Control Nurse
Saint John Regional Hospital
Saint John, N.B.
E2M 4L1

New Brunswick Mental Health Nurses Group
(NBARN Interest Group)
St. Stephen Mental Health Clinic
Prince William St.
St. Stephen, N.B.

New Brunswick Occupational Health Nurses Group
(NBARN Interest Group)
Irving Pulp & Paper Inc.
Box 3007, Station B
Saint John, N.B.
E2M 3H1

New Brunswick Operating Room Nurses Group
(NBARN Interest Group)
4 - 560 Tartan St.
Saint John, N.B.
E2K 2R7

Nova Scotia

Ambulatory Care Nurses Group
(Halifax-Darmouth)
Family Medicine Centre
Dalhousie University
5599 Fenwick St.
Halifax, N.S.
B3H 1R2

Canadian Association of Neurological and Neurosurgical Nurses—Nova Scotia Chapter
M.S. Clinic
Camp Hill Hospital
1763 Robie St.
Halifax, N.S.
B3H 3G2

Canadian Council of Cardiovascular Nurses—Nova Scotia Branch
1254 LeMarchant St.
Halifax, N.S.
B3H 3P7

Canadian Society of Dialysis Perfusionists, Nova Scotia Chapter
Dialysis Unit
Victoria General Hospital
1278 Tower Rd.
Halifax, N.S.
B3H 2Y9

Central Service Association of Nova Scotia
CSA of N.S.
P.O. Box 8324, Station A
Halifax, N.S.
B3K 5M1

Gerontology Association of Nova Scotia
50 Pleasant St.
P.O. Box 1312
Wolfville, N.S.
B0P 1X0

Hospital Continuing Education Association of Nova Scotia
Kings Regional Health & Rehabilitation Centre
P.O. Box 128
Waterville, N.S.
B0P 1V0

Nova Scotia Operating Room Nurses Group
85 Rockmanor Dr.
Bedford, N.S.
B4A 2Y9

Occupational Health Nurses Association of Nova Scotia
Write: 5 Clysdale Dr.
Dartmouth, N.S.
B2W 2P5

Newfoundland

Association of Occupational Health Nurses of Newfoundland and Labrador
Newfoundland Telephone
Fort William Bldg.
P.O. Box 2110
St. John's, Nfld.
A1C 5H6

Atlantic Maternal and Newborn Association/Atlantic Nurse-Midwives Association
School of Nursing
Memorial University
St. John's, Nfld.
A1C 5S7

Canadian Council of Cardiovascular Nurses, Nfld. Division
14 St. Andrew's Ave.
Glendale, Mount Pearl
Nfld. A1N 1C7

Health Care Educators Association
10 Smith Avenue
St. John's, Nfld.
A1C 5E9

Newfoundland Infection Control Association
44 Reid Street
St John's, Nfld.
A1E 2K6

Nfld. and Labrador Operating Room Nurses Association
271 Anspach St.
St. John's, Nfld.
A1E 4M5

Newfoundland Nurses Respiratory Society
P.O. Box 5250
St. John's, Nfld.
A1C 5W1

13-3 Boards of nursing

Alabama Board of Nursing
Suite 203, 500 Eastern Blvd.
Montgomery, Alabama 36117
Shirley Dykes
Acting Executive Officer
Tel: (205) 261-4060

Alaska Board of Nursing
Department of Commerce and Economic Development
Div. of Occupational Licensing
The Frontier Building
3601 C Street, Suite 722
Anchorage, Alaska 99502-0333
Gail M. McGuill
Executive Officer
Tel: (907) 561-2878

For licensing information:
Licensing Examiner, Board of Nursing
Pouch "D"
Juneau, Alaska 99811

American Samoa Health Service Regulatory Board
Pago Pago, American Samoa 96799
Elizabeth B.U. Malae
Executive Secretary
Tel: (684) 633-1222 ext. 206

Arizona State Board of Nursing
State Occupational Licensing Building
1645 W. Jefferson, Room 254
Phoenix, Arizona 85007
Shirley Rennicke
Executive Secretary
Tel: (602) 255-5092

Arkansas State Board of Nursing
Westmark Bldg., Suite 308
4120 W. Markham Street
Little Rock, Arkansas 72205
June Garner
Executive Director
Tel: (501) 371-2751

California Board of Registered Nursing
1020 N Street, Room 448
Sacramento, California 95814
Catherine Puri
Executive Officer
Tel: (916) 322-3350

California Board of Vocational Nurses and Psychiatric Technical Examiners
1020 N Street
Sacramento, California 95814
Billie Haynes
Executive Secretary
Tel: (916) 445-0793

Colorado Board of Nursing
State Services Bldg., Room 132
1525 Sherman Street
Denver, Colorado 80203
Willie Enstrom
Program Administrator
Tel: (303) 866-2871

Connecticut Board of Examiners for Nursing
150 Washington Street
Hartford, Connecticut 06106
Elaine Waudby
Executive Secretary
Tel: (203) 566-1032

Delaware Board of Nursing
Margaret O'Neill Building
P.O. Box 1401
Dover, Delaware 19901
Lois O'Shea
Executive Director
Tel: (302) 736-4752

Registered Nurses' Examining Board
614 H Street, N.W.
Washington, D.C. 20001
Barbara Hatcher
President
Tel: (202) 727-7468

Practical Nurses' Examining Board
614 H Street, N.W.
Washington, D.C. 20001
John H. Word
President
Tel: (202) 727-7468

Florida Board of Nursing
111 Coastline Drive, East
Jacksonville, Florida 32202
Judie K. Ritter
Executive Director
Tel: (904) 359-6331

Georgia Board of Nursing
166 Pryor Street, S.W.
Atlanta, Georgia 30303
Carolyn Hutcherson
Executive Director
Tel: (404) 656-3943

Georgia State Board of Licensed Practical Nurses
166 Pryor Street, S.W.
Atlanta, Georgia 30303
Patricia N. Swann
Executive Director
Tel: (404) 656-3921

For licensing information:
Georgia State Examining Boards
166 Pryor Street, S.W.
Atlanta, Georgia 30303
Michael R. Fowler
Joint Secretary
Tel: (404) 656-3900

Correspondence address:
Guam Board of Nurse Examiners
Dept. of Public Health and Social Services
P.O. Box 2816
Agana, Guam 96910
Karen Cruz
Acting Nurse Examiner/Administrator
Tel: (671) 734-2783

Shipping address:
Guam Board of Nurse Examiners
Dept. of Public Health and Social Services
Room 103, First Floor
Mangilao, Guam 96914

Hawaii Board of Nursing
P.O. Box 3469
Honolulu, Hawaii 96801
Richard S. Kuniyoshi
Executive Secretary
Tel: (808) 548-7471

Idaho Board of Nursing
Hall of Mirrors
700 West State Street
Boise, Idaho 83720
Phyllis T. Sheridan
Executive Director
Tel: (208) 334-3110

Illinois Department of Registration and Education
320 West Washington Street
3rd floor
Springfield, Illinois 62786
Judy A. Otto
Nursing Education Coordinator
Tel: (217) 782-4386

Indiana State Board of Nurses' Registration and Nursing Education
Health Professions Service Bureau
964 North Pennsylvania Street
Indianapolis, Indiana 46204
Rebecca A. Brady
President
Tel: (317) 232-2960

Iowa Board of Nursing
Executive Hills East
1223 East Court
Des Moines, Iowa 50319
Ann E. Mowery
Executive Director
Tel: (515) 281-3255

Kansas Board of Nursing
503 Kansas Avenue, Suite 330
P.O. Box 1098
Topeka, Kansas 66601
Lois Rich Scibetta
Executive Administrator
Tel: (913) 296-4929

Provided by Council of State Boards of Nursing, 303 E. Ohio Street, Suite 2010, Chicago, Illinois, 60611.

Kentucky State Board of Nursing
4010 Dupont Circle, Suite 430
Louisville, Kentucky 40207
Sharon M. Weisenbeck
Executive Director
Tel: (502) 897-5143

Louisiana State Board of Nursing
150 Baronne Street, Room 907
New Orleans, Louisiana 70112
Merlyn M. Maillian
Executive Director
Tel: (504) 568-5464

Louisiana State Board of Practical Nurse Examiners
4201½ Canal Street
New Orleans, Louisiana 70119
Terry L. DeMarcay
Executive Director
Tel: (504) 483-4505

Maine State Board of Nursing
295 Water Street
Augusta, Maine 04330
Jean C. Caron
Executive Director
Tel: (207) 289-2921

Maryland Board of Examiners of Nurses
201 West Preston Street
Baltimore, Maryland 21201
Donna M. Dorsey
Executive Director
Tel: (301) 383-2084/2085

Massachusetts Board of Registration in Nursing
Leverett Saltonstall Building
100 Cambridge Street, Room 1509
Boston, Massachusetts 02202
Eleanor Burke
Executive Secretary
Tel: (617) 727-3060

Michigan Board of Nursing
Dept. of Licensing & Regulation
Ottawa Towers North
611 West Ottawa
P.O. Box 30018
Lansing, Michigan 48909
Cathy A. Seyka
Administrative Assistant
Tel: (517) 373-1600

Minnesota Board of Nursing
717 Delaware Street, S.E.
Minneapolis, Minnesota 55414
Joyce M. Schowalter
Executive Secretary
Tel: (612) 623-5493

Mississippi Board of Nursing
135 Bounds Street, Suite 101
Jackson, Mississippi 39206
Eileen Whittemore
Executive Director
Tel: (601) 354-7349

Missouri State Board of Nursing
P.O. Box 656
3523 N. Ten Mile Drive
Jefferson City, Missouri 65102
Florence McGuire
Executive Director
Tel: (314) 751-2334

Montana State Board of Nursing
Department of Commerce
Division of Business and Professional Licensing
1424 9th Avenue
Helena, Montana 59620-0407
Phyllis McDonald
Executive Secretary
Tel: (406) 444-4279

Nebraska Board of Nursing
Bureau of Examining Boards
Department of Health
State House Station, Box 95065
Lincoln, Nebraska 68509
Darlene Mattingly
Nursing Licensure Coordinator
Tel: (402) 471-2001

Nevada State Board of Nursing
1135 Terminal Way, Suite 209
Reno, Nevada 89502
Jean T. Peavy
Executive Secretary
Tel: (702) 786-2778

New Hampshire Board of Nursing Education and Nurse Registration
State Department of Education
State Office Park South
101 Pleasant Street
Concord, New Hampshire 03301
Martha Ginty
Executive Director
Tel: (603) 271-2323

New Jersey Board of Nursing
1100 Raymond Blvd., Room 319
Newark, New Jersey 07102
Sr. Teresa Harris
Executive Director
Tel: (201) 648-2570

New Mexico Board of Nursing
5301 Central, N.E., Suite 905
Albuquerque, New Mexico 87108
Nancy Twigg
Executive Director
Tel: (505) 841-4620

New York State Board for Nursing
State Education Department
Cultural Education Center
Room 3013
Albany, New York 12230
Virginia Allen
Executive Secretary
Tel: (518) 474-3843/3844/3845

For licensing information:
Division of Professional Licensing Services
State Education Department
Cultural Education Center
Albany, New York 12230
Conrad Raup
Supervisor
Tel: (518) 474-3817

North Carolina Board of Nursing
P.O. Box 2129
Raleigh, North Carolina 27602
Carol A. Osman
Acting Executive Director
Tel: (919) 828-0740

North Dakota Board for Nursing
418 East Rosser
Bismarck, North Dakota 58501
Karen MacDonald
Executive Director
Tel: (701) 224-2974

Ohio Board of Nursing Education and Nursing Registration
65 South Front Street
Suite 509
Columbus, Ohio 43215
Rosa Lee Weinert
Executive Secretary
Tel: (614) 466-3947

Oklahoma Board of Nurse Registration and Nursing Education
4001 North Lincoln Blvd.
Suite 400
Oklahoma City, Oklahoma 73105
Jenell Hubbard
Executive Director
Tel: (405) 521-2363

Oregon State Board of Nursing
1400 S.W. 5th Avenue, Room 904
Portland, Oregon 97201
Dorothy J. Davy
Executive Director
Tel: (503) 229-5653

Pennsylvania State Board of Nurse Examiners
Department of State
P.O. Box 2649
Harrisburg, Pennsylvania 17105
Bernardine E. O'Donnell
Secretary
Tel: (717) 783-7146

Rhode Island Board of Nurse Registration and Nursing Education
Health Department Building
75 Davis Street, Room 104
Providence, Rhode Island 02908
Bertha Mugurdichian
Executive Secretary
Tel: (401) 277-2827

State Board of Nursing for South Carolina
1777 St. Julian Pl., Suite 102
Columbia, South Carolina 29204
Renatta Loquist
Executive Director
Tel: (803) 758-2611

South Dakota Board of Nursing
304 S. Phillips Ave., Suite 205
Sioux Falls, South Dakota 57102
JoEllen Koerner
Executive Secretary
Tel: (605) 334-1243

Tennessee State Board of Nursing
R.S. Gass State Office Bldg.
Ben Allen Road
Nashville, Tennessee 37216
Ruth L. Elliott
Executive Director
Tel: (615) 741-7256

Board of Nurse Examiners for the State of Texas
1300 Anderson Lane, Bldg. C
Suite 225
Austin, Texas 78752
Margaret L. Rowland
Executive Secretary
Tel: (512) 835-4880

Texas Board of Vocational Nurse Examiners
1300 Anderson Lane, Bldg. C
Suite 285
Austin, Texas 78752
Joyce A. Hammer
Executive Director
Tel: (512) 835-2071

Utah State Board of Nursing
Division of Registration
Heber M. Wells Bldg., 4th Floor
160 East 300 South
P.O. Box 5802
Salt Lake City, Utah 84110
Ann G. Petersen
Executive Secretary and Nurse Consultant
Tel: (801) 530-6638

Vermont State Board of Nursing
Redstone Building
26 Terrace Street
Montpelier, Vermont 05602
Francesca Fay
Executive Director
Tel: (802) 828-3180

Virgin Islands Board of Nurse Licensure
Div. of Professional Licensing
P.O. Box 7309
Charlotte Amalie
St. Thomas, Virgin Islands 00801
Ivy Ashwood
Chairperson
Tel: (809) 774-9000 ext. 204

Virginia State Board of Nursing
P.O. Box 27708
Richmond, Virginia 23261
Corinne F. Dorsey
Executive Secretary
Tel: (804) 786-0377

Washington State Board of Nursing
Div. of Professional Licensing
P.O. Box 9649
Olympia, Washington 98504
Constance E. Roth
Executive Secretary
Tel: (206) 753-3726

Washington State Board of Practical Nursing
P.O. Box 9649
Olympia, Washington 98504
Ruth Jacobson
Executive Secretary
Tel: (206) 753-3728

West Virginia Board of Examiners for Registered Nurses
922 Quarrier Street
Suite 309, Embleton Building
Charleston, West Virginia 25301
Garnette Thorne
Executive Secretary
Tel: (304) 348-3596

West Virginia State Board of Examiners for Practical Nurses
922 Quarrier Street
Suite 506, Embleton Building
Charleston, West Virginia 25301
Nancy R. Wilson
Executive Secretary
Tel: (304) 348-3572

Wisconsin Bureau of Nursing
Dept. of Regulation & Licensing
P.O. Box 8936
Madison, Wisconsin 53708
Paula R. Possin
Director
Tel: (608) 266-3735

Wyoming State Board of Nursing
2223 Warren Avenue
Suite 1, 2nd Floor
Cheyenne, Wyoming 82002
Joan Bouchard
Executive Director
Tel: (307) 777-7601

APPENDIX 14 DIRECTORY OF ADDRESSES

14-1 Burn care services in North America

FOREWORD

This directory includes 207 hospitals at which burn physicians in the United States and Canada have reported the presence of a specialized burn care service in 1984. Its publication is designed to enable rapid communication between physicians active in burn care, and to provide a guide to the hospitals where these physicians admit burn patients. Hospital zip codes are included to facilitate written communication.

The 183 hospitals listed for the United States include 138 that report units specifically designated for the care of burn patients. These units include 1720 beds, an average of 12.5 beds per unit.

Hospitals without such units provide burn care in settings shared with other patients. These include combined burn/trauma units, other types of intensive care units, and general medical/surgical floors. The average number of severe burn patients that can be managed in a hospital without a burn unit is listed with an asterisk (*) in the Burn Unit/Burn Service column.

Many hospitals with burn care units also use shared settings to care for some acute burn patients in periods of peak occupancy or during the late stages of a burn patient's hospitalization. Where the number of burn unit beds provides a misleadingly low indication of a hospital's acute burn care capability, the total capability is also listed with an asterisk.

The telephone numbers provided by survey respondents may be located at the hospital switchboard, the emergency department, the burn care unit itself, or the physician's office. *Those using this list to refer a patient with burns should make clear the purpose of the call, in addition to asking for the physician listed or his designee.*

About 21,000 acute inpatient admissions were reported by the 183 United States facilities on this list in 1983. This is virtually identical with the 1982 total, again representing 30% of the estimated 70,000 annual acute inpatient burn admissions in the United States. An estimated 5000 reconstructive burn admissions were also reported by 120 U.S. survey respondents. Since such admissions are managed at many hospitals by a separate plastic surgery service, total reconstructive admissions could not be determined.

This list is derived primarily from an annual survey of physician members of the American Burn Association who have previously reported the presence of a specialized burn service. The comprehensiveness of the list will be confirmed on a regular basis by queries to ABA member physicians located in areas not known to have a specialized burn service, and by data from the annual hospital surveys of the American and Canadian Hospital Associations.

None of the sources used in preparing this list addresses either the quality of burn care at a given institution or the optimum number of specialized beds and services in a given region. The inclusion of hospitals and physicians on this list therefore does not represent any direct or implied endorsement by the ABA of the burn care service they provide.

Suggested additions or deletions, and any questions related to this list, should be communicated to the Secretary of the American Burn Association. A list of organizations active in burn prevention and education is also available on request from the Secretary (Thomas Wachtel, M.D., Good Samaritan Medical Center, 1130 E. McDowell Rd., Suite B-2, Phoenix, AZ 85006).

From American Burn Association: Burn care services in North America, April 1984.

Burn care services in the United States

State	City	Hospital	Zip code	Telephone number for patient referral	Burn unit bed capacity or burn service capability*	Burn service medical director or M.D.'s most active in burn treatment
Alabama	Birmingham	Children's Hospital	35233	205/933-4000	12	Marshall Pitts
		U. of Alabama Hospitals	35233	205/934-3411	13	Alan R. Dimick
	Mobile	U. of So. Alabama Medical Center Hospital	36617	205/471-7000	7	Arnold Luterman; Mary Finn/Clifford Dasco
Alaska	Anchorage	Providence Hospital	99504	907/562-2211	10	Paul Steer; W. J. Mills (hypothermia)
	Fairbanks	Fairbanks Memorial Hospital	99701	907/452-8181	5*	William Wennen; Richard Parry
Arizona	Phoenix	Maricopa Medical Center	85008	602/267-5700	20	John M. Stein
	Tucson	St. Mary's Hospital	85703	602/795-8700	9	Philip Fleishman
Arkansas	Little Rock	Arkansas Children's Hospital	72201	501/370-1100 ext. 149	14	Fred T. Caldwell; John Crabtree
		Univ. Hospital/U. of Arkansas Medical Science Campus	72205	501/661-5000	6*	Fred T. Caldwell
California	Baldwin Park	Terrace Plaza Medical Center	91706	213/338-1101 ext. 260	9*	William T. Choctaw
	Berkeley	Alta Bates Hospital	94705	415/540-1573	6	Jerold Z. Kaplan
	Castro Valley	Eden Hospital	94546	415/537-1234	6	Eleanor Kohn; Eric Bachelor; Stanley Hegg; Ronald Iverson
	Chico	Chico Community Hospital	95926	916/345-2411 or 916/342-7513	6	Donald J. Mangus; Stanley Korock
	Culver City	Brotman Medical Center	90239	213/836-7000 ext. 3340 or 2510	17/23*	Stanley Frileck; Arthur Kahn
	Downey	Rancho Los Amigos Hospital	90242	213/922-7454	24*	G. Brody et al (reconstructive only)
	Eureka	St. Joseph's Hospital	95501	707/443-8051	*	Russel Pardoe
	Fresno	Valley Medical Center	93702	209/453-4220	6	Steven N. Parks
	Los Angeles	LAC/USC Medical Center	90033	213/226-7991	26/37*	Bruce E. Zawacki
	Orange	U. of Calif. Irvine Medical Center	92668	714/634-5304	8	Bruce M. Achauer
	Sacramento	U. of Calif. Davis Medical Center	95817	916/453-3636	8	F. William Blaisdell (Acting Director)
	San Bernardino	San Bernardino Community Hospital	92411	714/887-7047 ext. 405 or 444	6*	David Hess
		San Bernardino County Medical Center	92404	714/383-3142	9	Appannagari Gnanavez
	San Diego	Univ. Hospital/U. of Calif. Medical Center	92103	619/294-6502	14	Hugh Frank (Acting Director)
	San Francisco	San Francisco General Hospital	94110	415/821-8197	6	Anthony A. Meyer; Guy Trengove-Jones
		St. Francis Memorial Hospital	94109	415/775-4321	10	Edward Falces
	San Jose	Santa Clara Valley Medical Center	95128	408/279-5242	6	Ronald M. Sato

	San Pablo	Brookside Hospital	94806	415/235-7000	6	Robert L. Shapiro
	Sherman Oaks	Sherman Oaks Community Hospital	91403	213/981-7111	30	A. Richard Grossman
	Stockton	Dameron Hospital	95203	209/944-5550	7	Genest de L'Arbre
	Torrance	Torrance Memorial Hospital	90505	213/325-9110	10	William D. Davies
Colorado	Colorado Springs	Penrose Hospital	80917	303/630-5770	8	Ian G. Walker Claude Poliakoff
	Denver	Children's Hospital	80218	303/861-6517	8*	William Carl Bailey
		University Colorado Health Science Center	80262	303/394-8052	10	John Hansbrough
	Grand Junction	St. Mary's Hospital	81502	303/242-9127	2*	William Merkel
	Greeley	N. Colorado Medical Center	80631	303/352-4121	4*	James R. Wheeler
	Pueblo	St. Mary-Corwin Hospital	81004	303/560-4000	4*	Donald Leubke
Connecticut	Bridgeport	Bridgeport Hospital	06610	203/384-3728	22	Michael L. D'Aiuto
	Hartford	Hartford Hospital	06114	203/524-2840	5*	Philip E. Trowbridge and others
	New Haven	Yale–New Haven Hospital	06504	203/785-2573 or 203/785-2574	4*	Stephen Ariyan Charles Cuono Zeno Chicarilli Richard Stahl
District of Columbia	Washington	Children's Hospital National Medical Center	20010	202/745-5116 or 202/745-5152	12	Judson G. Randolph
		Washington Hospital Center	20010	202/541-7241 or 202/541-6662	23	Marion Jordan
Florida	Gainesville	Shands Teaching Hospital	32610	904/392-3054 or 904/392-3055	6	Hal G. Bingham
	Miami	U. of Miami Jackson Memorial Hospital	33136	305/325-7085	8	C. Gillon Ward Jeffrey Hammond Donald Buckner
	Orlando	Orlando Regional Medical Center	32806	305/841-5176	5	Juan Sauer
	Tampa	Tampa General Hospital	33606	813/253-0711 or 813/251-7617	17	C. Wayne Cruse
Georgia	Atlanta	Grady Memorial Hospital	30335	404/588-4307	30	Roger Sherman
	Augusta	Doctor's Hospital of Augusta	30910	404/863-3232	10	Alton Garrison Joseph Still
		Eugene Talmadge Memorial Hospital, Medical College of Georgia	30912	404/828-3893	6	Richard C. Treat Edward Hall
	Columbus	Medical Center	31902	404/571-1336	6*	Robert K. Worman
Hawaii	Honolulu	Straub Clinic & Hospital	96813	808/523-2311	3*	James H. Penoff Robert W. Schulz
Illinois	Chicago	Children's Memorial Hospital	60614	312/880-4094	*	Victor E. Lewis
		Cook County Hospital	60612	312/633-6564 or 312/633-6570	30	Takayoshi Matsuda Marella Hanumadass Richard Kagan
		Edgewater Hospital	60660	312/878-6000	4*	Ramesh Kharwadkar
		U. of Chicago Hospitals	60637	312/962-6112	20	Robert Parsons (Acting Director)
	Evanston	Evanston Hospital	60201	312/492-7720	8*	Charles Drueck

Continued.

Burn care services in the United States—cont'd

State	City	Hospital	Zip code	Telephone number for patient referral	Burn unit bed capacity or burn service capability*	Burn service medical director or M.D.'s most active in burn treatment
	Maywood	Foster G. McGaw Hospital, Loyola U. of Chicago	60153	312/531-3988	14	Raymond Warpeha
	Rock Island	Franciscan Medical Center	61202	309/793-3173	14	Frank E. Miller
	Rockford	St. Anthony's Hospital Medical Center	61101	815/226-2000	8	Raymond Hoffman
	Springfield	Memorial Medical Center	62708	217/788-3325	10	Elof Eriksson
Indiana	Fort Wayne	St. Joseph's Hospital	46802	219/425-3431	7	Jack Patterson
	Indianapolis	J. W. Riley Hospital	46223	317/264-3927	8	A. Michael Sadove (children)
	Indianapolis	Methodist Hospital of Indiana	46202	317/929-8056	10*	Wally Zollman Stephen Olvey
		W. N. Wishard Memorial Hospital	46202	317/630-6471	8	David J. Smith, Jr.
Iowa	Iowa City	U. of Iowa Hospitals & Clinics	52242	319/356-2496	13	Albert E. Cram
		St. Luke's Reg. Medical Center	51104	712/279-3440	8	Larry D. Foster
Kansas	Kansas City	U. of Kansas Medical Center	66103	913/588-6540	10	Mani M. Mani David W. Robinson
	Wichita	St. Francis Hospital	67201	316/268-5388	11	Thomas E. Kendall and others
		Wesley Medical Center	67214	316/688-2688	2*	Richard C. Shaw and others
Kentucky	Lexington	University Hospital	40536	606/233-5260	4	Edward Luce
	Louisville	Humana Hospital University	40217	502/562-3000	5	Hiram C. Polk, Jr.
		Kosair-Children's Hospital	40202	502/895-5466	8	John M. Whetter
Louisiana	Baton Rouge	Baton Rouge General Hospital	70821	504/387-7716	14	D. V. Cacioppo
	Marrero	West Jefferson Hospital	70072	504/347-5511	14	Frank C. DiVincenti
	Shreveport	L.S.U. Medical Center Hospital	33932	318/674-6133	16	Edwin Deitch
Maine	Portland	Maine Medical Center	04102	207/871-2991	4	Joel Johnson (Acting Director)
Maryland	Baltimore	Baltimore City Hospital	21224	301/396-8765	21	Andrew Munster
Massachusetts	Boston	Boston City Hospital	02118	617/424-5204	2*	Erwin Hirsch
		Brigham & Women's Hospital	02115	617/732-7712	10	Robert H. Demling
		Massachusetts General Hospital	02114	617/726-3354	10	John F. Burke
		Shriner's Burns Institute	02114	617/722-3000	30	John P. Remensnyder
	Worcester	Worcester City Hospital	01610	617/799-8110	4*	Felix Cataldo
Michigan	Ann Arbor	Michigan Burn Center University Hospital Chelsea Community Hospital	48109	313/995-BURN	29	Irving Feller Jai K. Prasad
	Detroit	Children's Hospital of Michigan	48201	313/494-5678	15	James R. Lloyd
		Detroit Receiving Hospital & Univ. Health Center	48201	313/494-3216 or 313/494-3218	18	Martin C. Robson David J. Smith, Jr.
	Flint	Hurley Medical Center	48502	313/257-9188	13	M.S. Haffajee
	Grand Rapids	Blodgett Memorial Medical Center	49506	616/774-7670	8	William Simpson Richard A. Wehrenberg

	Kalamazoo	Bronson Methodist Hospital	49007	616/383-6485 or 1-800/632-3403	12	Frank J. Newman Paul Fierke Michael Nave
	Lansing	Edward R. Sparrow Hospital	48909	517/483-2677	6	Errikos Constant Jorge Gomez Preecha Supanwanid William Blackburn
	Marquette	Marquette General Hospital	49855	906/228-9440	*	James Kelinger Constance N. Arnold
	Saginaw	St. Mary's Hospital	48601	517/790-5055	6	Syed Akhtar
Minnesota	Duluth	Miller-Dwan Hospital & Medical Center	55805	218/727-8762	12	John W. Wolfe
	Minneapolis	Hennepin Co. Medical Center	55415	612/347-2915	10	John Twomey
	Rochester	St. Mary's Hospital	55901	507/285-5123/5591 507/285-6691	6*	George B. Irons (adults) Robert Telander (children)
	St. Paul	St. Paul-Ramsey Medical Center	55101	612/221-3351	24	Lynn D. Solem
Mississippi	Greenville	Delta Medical Center	38701	601/378-3783	16	Robert Love
Missouri	Columbia	U. of Missouri Health Sciences Center	65212	314/882-7994	7	Boyd E. Terry
	Kansas City	Children's Mercy Hospital	64108	816/234-3520	6	Ronald J. Sharp
	St. Louis	Barnes Hospital	63110	314/362-5370	6	William W. Monafo
		St. John's Mercy Medical Center	63141	314/569-6055	17	Vatche H. Ayvazian Thomas Vitale
	Springfield	St. John's Reg. Health Center	65802	417/885-2876	9	Marc Wittmer
Montana	Billings	St. Vincent Hospital	59101	406/245-2458	4*	David F. Sloan
	Lincoln	St. Elizabeth Community Health Center	68510	402/489-7181 or 402/483-9206	10	Robert W. Gillespie
Nevada	Las Vegas	Southern Nevada Memorial	89102	702/383-2268	12	Charles A. Buerk
New Jersey	Hackensack	Hackensack Hospital	07601	201/441-2020	9*	Anthony Barbara
	Livingston	Saint Barnabas Medical Center	07039	201/533-5920	12	Frederick Fuller Esber Mansour Sylvia Petrone
New Mexico	Albuquerque	St. Joseph's Hospital	87102	505/247-2449 or 1-800/221-3664	*	John L. Coon
		U. of New Mexico Hospital	87106	505/843-2111	10	John O. Kucan
New York	Albany	Albany Medical Center	12208	518/445-3010	8	Dhiraj M. Shah
	Buffalo	Children's Hospital	14222	716/878-7301 or 716/878-7435	*	Theodore Jewett Donald R. Cooney Melvyn P. Karp
		Millard Fillmore Hospital	14209	716/887-4776 or 716/887-4649	4	Evan J. Evans
		Sheehan Emergency Hospital	14203	716/842-2200	10	Louis C. Cloutier
	East Meadow	Nassau Co. Medical Center	11554	516/542-3207	18	Roger L. Simpson
	Elmira	St. Joseph's Hospital	14902	607/733-6541	4*	James Marshall James Sonsire
	New York City Bronx	Bronx Municipal Health Center	10461	212/430-8065	11*	Stanley Levenson Mahendra Patel Steven May
	Brooklyn	Kings County Hospital	11203	212/735-3131	5	Winston Mitchell

Continued.

Burn care services in the United States—cont'd

State	City	Hospital	Zip code	Telephone number for patient referral	Burn unit bed capacity or burn service capability*	Burn service medical director or M.D.'s most active in burn treatment
	Manhattan	Harlem Hospital Center	10037	212/491-1335	5	James E. C. Norris
		N.Y. Hospital—Cornell Medical Center	10021	212/472-5132	24	Cleon W. Goodwin
		St. Vincent's Hospital	10011	212/790-8941 or 212/790-8940	6	Ronald N. Ollstein
	Rochester	Strong Memorial Hospital	14642	716/275-5475	9	R. Christie Wray, Jr.
	Syracuse	Upstate Medical Center	13210	315/473-6083	6	William Clark
	Valhalla	Westchester Co. Medical Center	10595	914/347-4909	10	Roger E. Salisbury Jane A. Petro
	West Islip	Good Samaritan Hospital	11795	516/957-4000	*	Richard A. Giery
North Carolina	Chapel Hill	No. Carolina Memorial Hospital	27514	919/966-4131	23	H. D. Peterson
	Charlotte	Charlotte Memorial Medical Center	28203	704/331-2525	4	Harold F. Hamit
	Durham	Duke University Hospital	27710	919/681-2404	7	Gregory Georgiade Joseph Moylan
	Winston-Salem	North Carolina Baptist Hospital	27103	919/748-7766	6	Jesse H. Meredith Connell Shearin
North Dakota	Fargo	St. Luke's General Hospital	58122	701/280-5504	4*	David W. Todd
Ohio	Akron	Children's Hospital Medical Center Akron Reg. Burn Center (admits adults with burns)	44308	216/379-8224	12	C. R. Boeckman R. L. Klein
	Cincinnati	U. of Cincinnati Hospital	45267	513/872-3100	10	Robert P. Hummel
		Shriner's Burns Institute	45219	513/751-3900	30	Bruce G. MacMillan
	Cleveland	Cleveland Metro General Hospital	44109	216/459-5627	16	Richard Fratianne
	Columbus	Children's Hospital	43205	614/461-2000	14	E. Thomas Boles
		Ohio State Univ. Hospital	43210	614/422-4516	6	Robert Ruberg
	Dayton	Children's Medical Center	45404	513/226-8300	6	Charles D. Goodwin
		Miami Valley Hospital	45409	513/223-6192	8	R. K. Finley Sidney Miller Larry Jones
	Toledo	St. Vincent's Medical Center	43608	419/259-4734	12	Michael Yanik
Oklahoma	Oklahoma City	Baptist Medical Center	73112	405/949-3345 or 405/949-3311	32	Paul Silverstein
		Okla. Children's Memorial Hospital	73104	405/271-4733	12	William P. Tunell
	Tulsa	Hillcrest Medical Center	74104	918/584-1351	20	Bernard Swartz
Oregon	Portland	Oregon Burn Center (at Emanuel Hospital)	97227	503/280-4233	12	Philip Parshley
Pennsylvania	Allentown	Lehigh Valley Hospital Center	18103	215/821-2058	6	Walter J. Okunski
	Chester	Crozer-Chester Medical Center	19013	215/876-0356	19	Charles E. Hartford
	Danville	Geisinger Medical Center	17821	717/271-6353 or 717/271-6591	6*	Philip C. Breen

	Erie	Hamot Medical Center	16550	814/459-0344	8	Charles R. Bales Forrest C. Mischler
	Hershey	Hershey Medical Center	17033	717/534-8521	*	William P. Graham
	Philadelphia	Saint Agnes Medical Center	19145	215/339-4339	11/20*	Frederick A. DeClement
		St. Christopher's Hospital for Children	19133	215/427-5000	4	Stuart J. Hulnick
	Pittsburgh	Mercy Hospital	15219	412/232-8225	7	Thomas Layton
		Western Penna. Hospital	15224	412/363-2876	18	John Gaisford
		York Hospital	17405	717/771-2345	6*	Robert Davis Richard W. Dabb
Rhode Island	Providence	Rhode Island Hospital	02902	401/277-4000	4*	Lawrence Bowen
South Carolina	Charleston	Medical University Hospital	29425	803/792-3681 or 803/792-3851	12	Dabney R. Yarborough (adults) H. Biemann Othersen, Jr. (children)
Tennessee	Chattanooga	Baroness Erlanger Hospital	37403	615/778-7881	6	Phil D. Craft
	Memphis	Regional Medical Center	38103	901/528-5500	*	William Hickerson Gary Reynolds
	Nashville	Vanderbilt Univ. Hospital	38232	615/322-7311	20	John B. Lynch
Texas	Austin	Brackenridge Hospital	78701	512/476-6461	*	Robert A. Ersek and others
	Beaumont	Baptist Hospital of Southeast Texas	77701	409/835-3781	10	Duane Larson Wesley Washburn
	Corpus Christi	Memorial Medical Center	78405	512/881-4360	9	Robert H. Balme
	Dallas	Parkland Memorial Hospital	75235	214/637-8546 or 211/688-2152	30	John Hunt
	El Paso	Sun Towers Hospital	79902	915/532-6281	12	Charles Lyon and others
	Ft. Sam Houston	Brooke Army Medical Center	78234	512/221-4604 or 512/221-2943	40	Basil A. Pruitt, Jr.
	Fort Worth	John Peter Smith Hospital	76104	817/921-3431	*	Charles Crenshaw and others
	Galveston	U. of Texas Medical Branch Hospitals	77550	713/761-2277	16	Sally Abston
		Shriner's Burns Institute	77550	713/761-2516	30	David N. Herndon
	Houston	Ben Taub General Hospital	77030	713/791-7000	8*	Frank Gerow
		Hermann Hospital	77030	713/797-4350	15	Donald H. Parks
	Lubbock	Lubbock General Hospital	79424	806/743-3406	6*	Richard Baker Timothy Harnar
	Pasadena	Humana Hospital Southmore	77502	713/477-0411	12	David Katrana
	San Antonio	Medical Center Hospital	78284	512/696-3030 or 512/691-6151/7473	*	A.B. Cruz, Jr.
Utah	Salt Lake City	U. of Utah Hospital	84121	801/581-2700	12	Glenn Warden Jeffrey Saffle
Vermont	Burlington	Medical Center Hospital of Vermont	05401	802/656-4545	6*	John Davis Richard Gamelli
Virginia	Charlottesville	U. of Virginia Medical Center	22908	804/924-5520	6	Richard Edlich
	Norfolk	Norfolk General Hospital	23507	804/628-3117	8	William Bethea
	Richmond	Medical College of Virginia Hospital	23298	804/786-9240	12	Boyd W. Haynes

Continued.

Burn care services in the United States—cont'd

State	*City*	*Hospital*	*Zip Code*	*Telephone number for patient referral*	*Burn unit bed capacity or burn service capability**	*Burn service medical director or M.D.'s most active in burn treatment*
Washington	Bellingham	St. Joseph's Hospital	98225	206/734-5400 ext. 2501	2*	James Hines
	Seattle	Children's Orthopedic Hospital	98105	206/526-2042	8*	Robert T. Schaller, Jr.
		Harborview Medical Center	98104	206/223-3127	40	David Heimbach Loren Engrav
	Spokane	Sacred Heart Medical Center	99220	509/455-3344	4*	Charles Miller
	Tacoma	St. Joseph's Hospital	98405	206/591-6677	10	Martin Schaeferle
West Virginia	Huntington	Cabell-Huntington Hospital	25701	304/526-2390	4	James A. Coil, Jr.
Wisconsin	Madison	U. of Wisconsin Hospital & Clinics	53792	608/263-1490/1387	7	Richard Helgerson
	Milwaukee	St. Mary's Hospital	53201	414/225-8000	20	George Collentine
Alberta	Calgary	Foothills Provincial General Hospital	T2N 2T9	403/270-1110	8	D.C. Birdsell R.L. Lindsay E. Magi
	Edmonton	U. of Alberta Hospital	T6G 2B7	403/432-6149	5	Gerald Moysa
British Columbia	Vancouver	Vancouver General Hospital	V5Z 1M9	604/875-4111	22	Charles F.T. Snelling and others
	Victoria	Royal Jubilee Hospital	V8R 1J8	604/595-9200	2	D.A. Baird; H.R. Hollis; T.A. McQueen; P. Gareau; D. Naysmith
Manitoba	Winnipeg	Health Sciences Center	R3A 1M4	204/787-3776	8*	G.A. Robertson
New Brunswick	Fredericton	Dr. Everett Chalmers Hospital	E3B 5N5	506/452-5400	2	W. Cook D. Trueman
	Moncton	The Moncton Hospital	E1C 6Z8	506/855-1600	3	Douglas Inglis G.I. Curry
	Saint John	Saint John General Hospital	E2L 4L2	506/648-2200	6*	G.L. Sparkes
Nova Scotia	Halifax	Victoria General Hospital	B3H 2Y9	902/428-2525	4	Winston Parkhill
		I.W. Killam Hospital for Children	B3J 3G9	902/424-6111	3	James Ross and others
Ontario	Hamilton	Hamilton General Hospital	L8L 2X2	416/527-0271	10	Darryl G. Truscott
	Kingston	Hotel Dieu Hospital	K7L 3H6	613/548-8871	2	A. Kenneth Wylie
	London	Victoria Hospital Corporation	N6A 4G5	519/432-5241 ext. 4171	6	Robert B. Colcleugh R. McFarlane
	Ottawa	Children's Hospital of Eastern Ontario	K1H 8L1	613/737-7600	8*	Paul Benoit
		Ottawa General Hospital	K1H 8L6	613/737-8222	5*	Paul Benoit

	Scarborough	Scarborough General Hospital	M1P 2V5	416/438-2911	4	N. Poy; M. Bederman; L. Carlsen; N. Shammas; W. Carman
	Toronto	Hospital for Sick Children	M5G 1X8	416/597-1500	11	Ronald M. Zuker Hugh G. Thomson
		The Wellesley Hospital	M4Y 1J3	416/966-6600	10	Walter Peters
	Windsor	Metropolitan General Hospital	N8W 1L9	519/254-1661	6	Chosen lau, Director Stuart Young Howard Adams
Quebec	Montreal	Montreal Children's Hospital	H3H 1P3	514/937-8511	4*	H. Bruce Williams
		Montreal General Hospital	H3G 1A4	514/937-6011	22*	H. Bruce Williams
		Hotel Dieu de Montreal	H2W 1T8	514/844-0161	10	Jacques Papillon
Saskatchewan	Regina	Regina General Hospital	S4P 0W5	306/359-4256	4	G.P. Holden
	Saskatoon	University Hospital	S7N 0X0	306/343-3759	5*	Leslie R. Chasmar D.J. Classen J.H. Zondervan

14-2 Poison control centers in the United States and Canada

UNITED STATES*

Poison control centers and state coordinators

The location and telephone numbers of poison control centers operating in the United States as of October 1982 and state poison control coordinators are listed in alphabetic order of city or town within state. The listing was compiled from information supplied to the Poisoning Surveillance and Epidemiology Branch (HFN 720) (United States Food and Drug Administration, National Center for Drugs and Biologics, Office of Drugs) by poison control centers, organizations representing them, and state public health agencies. Before they were listed in the Directory, each of the institutions identified as a poison control center was contacted by the Division of Poison Control to verify that it was active. The first poison control center began operating in Chicago in 1953 with the number increasing to over 600 nationwide in the 1960s. Services offered by poison control centers vary widely. At minimum, they assist the lay public and other health professionals in cases of known or suspected poisoning by providing information on the appropriate first aid and clinical management. They may also offer specialized poisoning treatment and consultative services, professional training, and poisoning prevention education for consumers. In recent years, the number of small centers, most of them based in local hospital emergency rooms, has been declining due to their replacement with large regional poison control centers that serve populations of several million and provide more comprehensive services.

*Provided by U.S. Department of Health and Human Services, Food and Drug Administration, Office of Drugs, Poisoning Surveillance and Epidemiology Branch, 5600 Fishers Lane, Rockville, MD 20857.

Organizations and agencies

A listing of private, professional, and public service organizations and federal agencies dealing in prevention, treatment, and control of poisoning.

Poison prevention materials

A listing of sources of poison prevention educational materials and resources compiled by the Poison Prevention Week Council.

Directory of centers

State coordinators and cities	*Address*	*Telephone*	*Comments*
Alabama			
State Coordinator	Department of Public Health Montgomery, AL 36117	(205) 832-3194 832-3935	
Birmingham	The Children's Hospital of Birmingham 1601 6th Ave., S. Birmingham, AL 35233	(205) 933-4050 (800) 292-6678 (statewide)	
Tuscaloosa	The Alabama Poison Control Center Druid City Hospital 809 University Blvd., E. Tuscaloosa, AL 34501	(205) 345-0600 (800) 462-0800 (statewide)	
Alaska			
State Coordinator	Department of Health and Social Services Juneau, AK 99811	(907) 465-3100	
Anchorage	Anchorage Poison Center Providence Hospital 3200 Providence Dr. Anchorage, AK 99504	(907) 274-6535	
Fairbanks	Fairbanks Poison Center Fairbanks Memorial Hospital 1650 Cowles Fairbanks, AK 99701	(907) 456-7182	
Arizona			
State Coordinator	Arizona Poison Control System University of Arizona College of Pharmacy Tucson, AZ 85724	(602) 626-6016 (800) 362-0101 (statewide)	
Flagstaff	Flagstaff Hospital and Medical Center of N. Arizona 1215 N. Beaver St. Flagstaff, AZ 86001	(602) 779-0555	
Phoenix	St. Lukes Hospital and Medical Center 525 N. 18th St. Phoenix, AZ 85006	(602) 253-3334	

A, Center meets the American Association of Poison Control Centers' criteria for designation as a Regional Poison Control Center. This is a voluntary program, and negative inferences about the quality and level of service offered by a center should not be drawn from the absence of regional center designation.
x, Calls to center go through hospital switchboard.

State coordinators and cities	*Address*	*Telephone*	*Comments*
Tucson	Arizona Poison and Drug Information Center Arizona Health Sciences Center University of Arizona Tucson, AZ 85724	(602) 626-6016 (800) 362-0101 (statewide)	A
Arkansas			
State Coordinator	Division of Environmental Health Protection Arkansas Department of Health Little Rock, AR 72201	(501) 661-2301	
El Dorado	Warner Brown Hospital Emergency Room 460 W. Oak St. El Dorado, AR 71730	(501) 863-2266	
Fort Smith	St. Edward Mercy Medical Center Emergency Room 7301 Rogers Ave. Fort Smith, AR 72904	(501) 452-5100 ext. 2401	x
	Sparks Regional Medical Center Emergency Room 1311 S. "I" St. Fort Smith, AR 72902	(501) 441-5011	
Harrison	Boone County Hospital Emergency Room 620 N. Willow St. Harrison, AR 72601	(501) 741-6141 ext. 275	x
Helena	Helena Hospital Emergency Room Hi-way 49 By Pass Helena, AR 72342	(501) 338-6411 ext. 340	x
Little Rock	University of Arkansas Medical Center Emergency Room 4301 W. Markham St. Little Rock, AR 72201	(501) 661-6161	
	Statewide Poison Control Drug Info. Ctr. U.A.M. Sc. College of Pharmacy Slot 522 4301 W. Markham St. Little Rock, AR 72205 Pulaski Co.	(800) 428-8948	
Osceola	Osceola Memorial Hospital Emergency Room 611 Lee Ave., W. Osceola, AR 72370	(501) 563-7182 or (501) 563-3174	
Pine Bluff	Jefferson Regional Medical Center Emergency Department 1515 W. 42nd Ave. Pine Bluff, AR 71601	(501) 541-7111 or (501) 541-7100 ext. 5350	
California			
State Coordinator	Emergency Medical Services Authority 1600 Ninth St., Room 460 Sacramento, CA 95814	(916) 322-4336	
Fresno	Central Valley Regional Poison Control Center Fresno Community Hospital Fresno & R Sts. Fresno, CA 93715	(209) 445-1222	
Los Angeles	Los Angeles County Medical Association Regional Poison Information Center 1925 Wilshire Blvd. Los Angeles, CA 90057	(213) 484-5151	
Oakland	Children's Hospital Medical Center of N. California 51st & Grove Sts. Oakland, CA 94609	(415) 428-3248	

Continued.

Directory of centers—cont'd

State coordinators and cities	*Address*	*Telephone*	*Comments*
Orange	University of California Irvine Medical Center 101 City Dr., Route 32 Orange, CA 92688	(714) 634-5988	
Sacramento	Sacramento Medical Ctr. Univ. California at Davis Poison Control Center 2315 Stockton Blvd. Sacramento, CA 95817	(916) 453-3692 (800) 852-7221 (N. CA)	A
San Diego	San Diego Regional Poison Center Univ. California at San Diego Medical Center 225 W. Dickinson St. San Diego, CA 92103	(619) 294-6000	A
San Francisco	San Francisco Bay Area Regional Poison Control Center Room 1E 86 San Francisco General Hospital 1001 Potrero Ave. San Francisco, CA 94110	(415) 666-2845 (800) 792-0720 (N. CA)	A
San Jose	Central-Coast Counties Regional Poison Control Center Santa Clara Valley Medical Center 751 S. Bascom Ave. San Jose, Ca 95128	(408) 279-5112 (800) 662-9886 (statewide)	
Colorado			
State Coordinator	Department of Health Emergency Medical Services Division 4210 E. 11th Ave. Denver, CO 80220	(303) 320-8476	
Denver	Rocky Mountain Poison Center Denver General Hospital W. 8th Ave. & Cherokee Sts. Denver, CO 80204	(303) 629-1123 (800) 332-3073	A
Connecticut			
State Coordinator	University of Connecticut Health Center Farmington, CT 06032	(203) 674-3456	
Bridgeport	Bridgeport Hospital 267 Grant St. Bridgeport, CT 06602	(203) 384-3566	
	St. Vincent's Medical Center 2800 Main St. Bridgeport, CT 06606	(203) 576-5178	
Danbury	Danbury Hospital 95 Locust Ave. Danbury, CT 06810	(203) 797-7300	
Farmington	Connecticut Poison Control Center University of Connecticut Health Center Farmington, CT 06032	(203) 674-3456	
Middletown	Middlesex Memorial Hospital 28 Crescent St. Middletown, CT 06457	(203) 344-6684	
New Haven	The Hospital of St. Raphael 1450 Chapel St. New Haven, CT 06511	(203) 789-3464	
	Yale–New Haven Hospital Emergency Service 20 York St. New Haven, CT 06510	(203) 785-8958	

State coordinators and cities	Address	Telephone	Comments
Norwalk	Department of Emergency Medicine Norwalk Hospital Maple St. Norwalk, CT 06856	(203) 852-2160	
Waterbury	St. Mary's Hospital Emergency Room 56 Franklin St. Waterbury, CT 06702	(203) 574-6011	
Delaware			
State Coordinator	Wilmington Medical Center Delaware Division Wilmington, DE 19801	(302) 655-3389	
Wilmington	Wilmington Medical Center Delaware Division 501 W. 14th St. Wilmington, DE 19899	(302) 655-3389	
District of Columbia			
Washington	National Capitol Poison Center Georgetown University Hospital 3800 Reservoir Rd. Washington, DC 20007	(202) 625-3333	A
Florida			
State Coordinator	Department of Health and Rehabilitative Services Office of Emergency Medical Services Tallahassee, FL 32301	(904) 487-1566	
Bradenton	Manatee Memorial Hospital 206 Second St., E. Bradenton, FL 33505	(813) 748-2121	
Daytona Beach	Halifax Hospital Emergency Department P.O. Box 1990 Daytona Beach, FL 32014	(904) 258-1513	
Ft. Lauderdale	Broward General Medical Center Poison Control Center 1600 S. Andrews Ave. Ft. Lauderdale, FL 33316	(305) 463-3131 ext. 1955/6	x
Fort Myers	Lee Memorial Hospital 2776 Cleveland Ave. P.O. Drawer 2218 Fort Myers, FL 33902	(813) 334-5287	
Ft. Walton Beach	General Hospital of Ft. Walton Beach 1000 Mar-Walt Dr. Ft. Walton Beach, FL 32548	(904) 862-1111 ext. 106	x
Gainesville	Shands Teaching Hospital and Clinics University of Florida Gainesville, FL 32610	(904) 392-3389	
Inverness	Citrus Memorial Hospital 502 Highland Blvd. Inverness, FL 32650	(904) 726-2800	
Jacksonville	St. Vincent's Medical Ctr. P.O. Box 2982 Jacksonville, FL 32203	(904) 387-7500 387-7499 (TTY)	
Lakeland	Lakeland Regional Medical Center Lakeland General Hospital Lakeland Hills Blvd. Lakeland, FL 33802	(813) 687-1137	
Leesburg	Leesburg Regional Medical Center 600 E. Dixie Leesburg, FL 32748	(904) 787-9900	

Continued.

Directory of centers—cont'd

State coordinators and cities	*Address*	*Telephone*	*Comments*
Melbourne	James E. Holmes Regional Medical Center Emergency Department 1350 S. Hickory St. Melbourne, FL 32901	(305) 727-7000 ext. 675	x
Naples	Naples Community Hospital 350 7th St., N. Naples, FL 33940	(813) 262-3131	x
Ocala	Munroe Regional Medical Center 131 S.W. 15th St. Ocala, FL 32670	(904) 351-7607	
Orlando	Orlando Regional Medical Center Orange Memorial Division 1414 S. Kuhl Ave. Orlando, FL 32806	(305) 841-5222	
Pensacola	Gulf Region Poison Center Baptist Hospital P.O. Box 17500 Pensacola, FL 32522	(904) 434-4611 (800) 874-1555 (out of state) (800) 342-3222 (statewide)	
Punta Gorda	Medical Center Hospital 809 E. Marion Ave. Punta Gorda, FL 33950	(813) 637-2529	
Rockledge	Wuesthoff Memorial Hospital 110 Longwood Ave. Rockledge, FL 32955	(305) 636-4357	
St. Petersburg	Bay Front Medical Center, Inc. 701 6th St., S. St. Petersburg, FL 33701	(800) 282-3171 (statewide)	
Sarasota	Memorial Hospital 1901 Arlington St. Sarasota, FL 33579	(813) 953-1332	
Tallahassee	Tallahassee Memorial Regional Medical Center 1300 Miccosukee Rd. Tallahassee, FL 32304	(904) 681-5411	
Tampa	Tampa Bay Regional Poison Control Center Tampa General Hospital Davis Island Tampa, FL 33606	(813) 251-6995 (800) 282-3171 (statewide)	
Titusville	Jess Parrish Memorial Hospital 951 N. Washington Ave. P.O. Drawer W Titusville, FL 32780	(305) 268-6260	
West Palm Beach	Good Samaritan Hospital Palm Beach Lakes Blvd. West Palm Beach, FL 33402	(305) 655-5511 ext. 4250	x
Winter Haven	Poison Control Center Winter Haven Hospital, Inc. 200 Avenue F., N.E. Winter Haven, FL 33880	(813) 299-9701	
Georgia			
State Coordinator	Department of Human Resources Emergency Health Section Atlanta, GA 30303	(404) 894-5170	
Albany	Phoebe Putney Memorial Hospital 417 Third Ave. Albany, GA 31705	(912) 888-4150	
Athens	Athens General Hospital 1199 Prince Ave. Athens, GA 30613	(404) 543-5215	

State coordinators and cities	Address	Telephone	Comments
Atlanta	Georgia Poison Control Center Grady Memorial Hospital Box 26066 80 Butler St., S.E. Atlanta, GA 30305	(404) 588-4400 (800) 282-5846 (statewide) (404) 525-3323 (TTY)	A
Augusta	University Hospital 1350 Walton Way Augusta, GA 30902	(404) 724-5050	
Columbus	The Medical Center 710 Center St. Columbus, GA 31902	(404) 571-1080	
Macon	Medical Center of Central Georgia Regional Poison Control Center 777 Hemlock St. Macon, GA 31201	(912) 744-1427	
Rome	Floyd Hospital Turner McCall Blvd. Rome, GA 31061	(404) 295-5500	x
Savannah	Savannah Regional EMS Poison Center Dept. of Emergency Medicine Memorial Medical Center P.O. Box 23089 Savannah, GA 31403	(912) 355-5228	
Thomasville	John D. Archbold Memorial Hospital 900 Gordon Ave. Thomasville, GA 31792	(912) 226-4121 ext. 169	x
Valdosta	South Georgia Medical Center P.O. Box 1727 Valdosta, GA 31603	(912) 333-1110	
Waycross	Memorial Hospital 410 Darling Ave. Waycross, GA 31501	(912) 283-3030	x
Guam			
State Coordinator	Guam Memorial Hospital P.O. Box AX Agana, Guam 96910	646-5801	
Agana	Pharmacy Service, Box 7667 U.S. Naval Regional Medical Center (Guam) FPO San Francisco, CA 96630	344-9265 9354	
Hawaii			
State Coordinator	Department of Health Honolulu, HI 96801	(808) 531-7776	
Honolulu	Kapiolani-Children's Medical Center 1319 Punahou St. Honolulu, HI 96826	(808) 941-4411 (808) 362-3585	
Idaho			
State Coordinator	Department of Health & Welfare Boise, ID 83720	(208) 334-4245	
Boise	Idaho Emergency Medical Poison Center 1055 N. Curtis Rd. Boise, ID 83706	(208) 334-2241 (800) 632-8000 (statewide)	
Idaho Falls	Consolidated Hospitals Emergency Department 900 Memorial Dr. Idaho Falls, ID 83401	(208) 522-3600	
Pocatello	Idaho Drug Information Service and Poison Control Center Pocatello Regional Medical Center 777 Hospital Way Pocatello, ID 83202	(208) 234-0777 ext. 2019 (800) 632-9490 (statewide)	x

Continued.

Directory of centers—cont'd

State coordinators and cities	*Address*	*Telephone*	*Comments*
Illinois			
State Coordinator	Division of Emergency Medical Services and Highway Safety Springfield, IL 62761	(217) 785-2080	
Chicago	Rush Presbyterian-St. Luke's Poison Center Rush Presbyterian-St. Luke's Medical Center 1753 W. Congress Pkwy. Chicago, IL 60612	(312) 942-5969 (800) 942-5969 (Chicago and N.E. Illinois)	
Peoria	Peoria Poison Center St. Francis Hospital and Medical Center 530 N.E. Glen Oak Ave. Peoria, IL 61637	(309) 672-2334 (800) 322-5330 (Northern and Central Illinois)	
Springfield	Central & Southern Illinois Poison Resource Center St. John's Hospital 800 E. Carpenter Springfield, IL 62769	(217) 753-3330 (800) 252-2022 (statewide)	A
Indiana			
State Coordinator	Indiana State Board of Health Hazardous Products Section and Division of Drug Control P.O. Box 1964 Indianapolis, IN 46206	(317) 633-0332	
Anderson	Community Hospital 1515 N. Madison Ave. Anderson, IN 46012	(317) 646-5143	
	St. John's Hickey Memorial Hospital 2015 Jackson St. Anderson, IN 46014	(317) 646-8222	
Angola	Cameron Memorial Hospital, Inc. 416 E. Maumee St. Angola, IN 46703	(219) 665-2141 ext. 146	x
Crown Point	St. Anthony Medical Center Main at Franciscan Rd. Crown Point, IN 46307	(219) 738-2100 ext. 1311	x
Evansville	Poison Control Center Deaconess Hospital, Inc. 600 Mary St. Evansville, IN 47710	(812) 426-3333	
	Welborn Memorial Baptist Hospital 401 S.E. 6th St. Evansville, IN 47713	(812) 426-8336	
Fort Wayne	Emergency Department Lutheran Hospital 3024 Fairfield Ave. Fort Wayne, IN 46807	(219) 458-2211	
	Parkview Memorial Hospital 2200 Randalia Dr. Fort Wayne, IN 46805	(219) 484-9711	
	St. Joseph's Hospital 700 Broadway Fort Wayne, IN 46802	(219) 426-8280	
Gary	Methodist Hospital of Gary, Inc. 600 Grant St. Gary, IN 46402	(219) 886-4710	
Hammond	Poison Control Center St. Margaret's Hospital 25 Douglas St. Hammond, IN 46320	(219) 931-4477	

State coordinators and cities	*Address*	*Telephone*	*Comments*
Indianapolis	Indiana Poison Center 1001 W. Tenth St. Indianapolis, IN 46202	(317) 630-7351 (800) 382-9097	A
Kokomo	Howard Community Hospital 3500 S. LaFountain St. Kokomo, IN 46901	(317) 453-8444	
Lafayette	Lafayette Home Hospital 2400 South St. Lafayette, IN 47902	(317) 447-6811	x
	Poison Control Center St. Elizabeth Hospital 1501 Hartford St. Lafayette, IN 47904	(317) 423-6699	
Lebanon	Witham Memorial Hospital 1124 N. Lebanon St. Lebanon, IN 46052	(317) 482-2700 ext. 241	x
Madison	King's Daughter's Hospital 112 Presbyterian Ave. Madison, IN 47250	(812) 265-5211 ext. 131	x
Marion	Marion General Hospital Wabash and Euclid Aves. Marion, IN 46952	(317) 662-4693	x
Muncie	Ball Memorial Hospital 2401 University Ave. Muncie, IN 47303	(317) 747-4321	
Richmond	Reid Memorial Hospital 1401 Chester Blvd. Richmond, IN 47374	(317) 983-3148	
Shelbyville	William S. Major Hospital 150 W. Washington St. Shelbyville, IN 46176	(317) 392-3211 ext. 252	x
South Bend	St. Joseph's Medical Center 811 E. Madison St. South Bend, IN 46622	(219) 237-7264	
Terre Haute	Union Hospital, Inc. 1606 N. Seventh St. Terre Haute, IN 47804	(812) 238-7000 ext. 7523	x
Valparaiso	Porter Memorial Hospital 814 LaPorte Ave. Valparaiso, IN 46383	(219) 464-8611 ext. 301	x
Vincennes	The Good Samaritan Hospital 520 S. 7th St. Vincennes, IN 47591	(812) 885-3348	
Iowa			
State Coordinator	Department of Health Des Moines, IA 50319	(515) 281-4964	
Des Moines	Variety Club Poison and Drug Information Center Iowa Methodist Medical Center 1200 Pleasant St. Des Moines, IA 50308	(515) 283-6254 (800) 362-2327 (statewide)	
Dubuque	Mercy Health Center Mercy Dr. Dubuque, IA 52001	(319) 589-9099	
Fort Dodge	Trinity Regional Hospital Kenyon Rd. Fort Dodge, IA 50501	(515) 573-3101	x
Iowa City	University of Iowa Hospitals and Clinics Poison Control Center Iowa City, IA 52242	(319) 356-2922 (800) 272-6477 (statewide)	A

Continued.

Directory of centers—cont'd

State coordinators and cities	*Address*	*Telephone*	*Comments*
Waterloo	Allen Memorial Hospital Emergency Department 1825 Logan Ave. Waterloo, IA 50703	(319) 235-3893	
Kansas			
State Coordinator	Kansas Department of Health and Environment Bureau of Food and Drugs Forbes Field Topeka, KS 66620	(913) 862-9360 ext. 541	
Atchison	Atchison Hospital 1301 N. 2nd St. Atchison, KS 66002	(913) 367-2131 ext. 111	x
Dodge City	Dodge City Regional Hospital Ross & Ave., "A" Dodge City, KS 67801	(316) 225-9050 ext. 381	x
Emporia	Newman Memorial Hospital 12th and Chestnut Sts. Emporia, KS 66801	(316) 343-6800 ext. 545	x
Fort Riley	Irwin Army Hospital Emergency Room Fort Riley, KS 66442	(913) 239-7776	
Fort Scott	Mercy Hospital 821 Burke St. Fort Scott, KS 66701	(316) 223-2200 ext. 136	x
Great Bend	Central Kansas Medical Center 3515 Broadway Great Bend, KS 67530	(316) 792-2511 ext. 115	x
Hays	Hadley Regional Medical Center 201 E. 7th St. Hays, KS 67601	(913) 628-8251 ext. 145	x
Kansas City	Mid-America Poison Center University of Kansas 39th and Rainbow Blvd. Kansas City, KS 66103	(913) 588-6633 (800) 332-6633 (statewide)	
Lawrence	Lawrence Memorial Hospital 325 Maine St. Lawrence, KS 66044	(913) 843-3680 ext. 162	x
Salina	St. John's Hospital 139 N. Penn St. Salina, KS 67401	(913) 827-3187	
Topeka	Stormont-Vail Regional Medical Center 10th & Washburn Sts. Topeka, KS 66606	(913) 354-6100	
	Northeast Kansas Poison Center St. Francis Hospital and Medical Center 1700 W. 7th St. Topeka, KS 66606	(913) 295-8094	
Wichita	Wesley Medical Center 550 N. Hillside Ave. Wichita, KS 67214	(316) 688-2277	
Kentucky			
State Coordinator	Department for Human Resources Frankfort, KY 40601	(502) 564-3970	
Fort Thomas	St. Lukes Hospital 85 N. Grand Ave. Fort Thomas, KY 41075	(606) 572-3215 (800) 352-9900 (statewide)	
Lexington	Central Baptist Hospital 1740 S. Limestone St. Lexington, KY 40503	(606) 278-3411 ext. 363	x

State coordinators and cities	*Address*	*Telephone*	*Comments*
	Drug Information Center University of Kentucky Medical Center Lexington, KY 40536	(606) 233-5320	
Louisville	Kentucky Regional Poison Center of Kosair-Children's Hospital NKC, INC. P.O. Box 35070 Louisville, KY 40232	(502) 589-8222 (800) 722-5725 (statewide)	
Murray	Murray-Calloway County Hospital 803 Popular Murray, KY 420701	(502) 753-7588	
Owensboro	Owensboro-Daviess County Hospital 811 Hospital Ct. Owensboro, KY 42301	(502) 926-3030 ext. 180	x
Paducah	Western Baptist Hospital 2501 Kentucky Ave. Paducah, KY 42001	(502) 444-5180	
Prestonburg	Poison Control Center Highlands Regional Medical Center Prestonburg, KY 41653	(606) 886-8511 ext. 132	x
Louisiana			
State Coordinator	LSU Poison Control and Drug Abuse Information Center Louisiana State University P.O. Box 33932 Shreveport, LA 71130	(318) 425-1524	
Alexandria	Rapides General Hospital Poison Control Center P.O. Box 7146 Alexandria, LA 71301	(318) 445-4665	
Layfayette	Our Lady of Lourdes Hospital 611 St. Landry St. Lafayette, LA 70501	(318) 234-7381	x
Lake Charles	Lake Charles Memorial Hospital P.O. Drawer M Lake Charles, LA 70601	(318) 478-6800	
Monroe	School of Pharmacy Northeast Louisiana University 700 University Ave. Monroe, LA 71209	(318) 342-3008	
	St. Francis Hospital P.O. Box 1901 Monroe, LA 71301	(318) 325-6454	
New Orleans	Charity Hospital 1532 Tulane Ave. New Orleans, LA 70140	(504) 568-5222	
Shreveport	Louisiana State University Poison Control and Drug Abuse Information Center LSU Medical Center P.O. Box 33932 Shreveport, LA 71130	(318) 425-1524	
Maine			
State Coordinator	Maine Poison Control Center Portland, ME 04102	(207) 871-2950	
Portland	Maine Medical Center Emergency Division 22 Bramhall St. Portland, ME 04102	(207) 871-2381 (800) 442-6305 (statewide)	

Continued.

Directory of centers—cont'd

State coordinators and cities	*Address*	*Telephone*	*Comments*
Maryland			
State Coordinator	Maryland Poison Center University of Maryland School of Pharmacy Baltimore, MD 21201	(301) 528-7604 (statewide)	
Baltimore	Maryland Poison Center University of Maryland School of Pharmacy 636 W. Lombard St. Baltimore, MD 21201	(301) 528-7701 (800) 492-2414 (statewide)	A
Cumberland	Tri-State Poison Center Sacred Heart Hospital 900 Seton Dr. Cumberland, MD 21502	(301) 722-6677	
Massachusetts			
State Coordinator	Department of Public Health Boston, MA 02111	(617) 727-2700	
Boston	Massachusetts Poison Control System 300 Longwood Ave. Boston, MA 02115	(617) 232-2120 (800) 682-9211 (statewide) (617) 277-3323 TTY (MA only)	A
Michigan			
State Coordinator	Department of Public Health Emergency Medical Services Lansing, MI 48909	(517) 373-1406	
Adrian	Poison Control Center Emma L. Bixby Hospital 818 Riverside Ave. Adrian, MI 49221	(517) 263-2412	
Ann Arbor	Poison Control Center University Hospital 1405 E. Ann St. Ann Arbor, MI 48104	(313) 764-7667	
Battle Creek	Community Hospital Pharmacy Department 183 West St. Battle Creek, MI 49016	(616) 963-5521	x
Bay City	Bay Medical Center 1900 Columbus Ave. Bay City, MI 48706	(517) 894-3131	
Coldwater	Community Health Center of Branch County 274 E. Chicago St. Coldwater, MI 49036	(517) 278-7361	
Detroit	Children's Hospital Poison Center Children's Hospital 3901 Beaubien Detroit, MI 48201	(313) 494-5711 (800) 572-1655 (statewide)	A
Flint	Poison Information Center Hurley Medical Center One Hurley Plaza Flint, MI 48502	(313) 257-9111 (800) 572-5396 (statewide)	
Grand Rapids	Western Michigan Regional Poison Center Blodgett Memorial Medical Center 1840 Wealthy, S.E. Grand Rapids, MI 49506	(616) 774-7854 (800) 632-2727 (statewide)	A
Kalamazoo	Midwest Poison Center Borgess Medical Center 1521 Gull Rd. Kalamazoo, MI 49001	(616) 383-7104 (800) 632-4177 (statewide)	
	Great Lakes Poison Center	(616) 383-6409	

State coordinators and cities	Address	Telephone	Comments
	Bronson Methodist Hospital 252 E. Lovell St. Kalamazoo, MI 49006	(800) 442-4112 (statewide)	
Lansing	St. Lawrence Hospital 1210 W. Saginaw St. Lansing, MI 48914	(517) 372-5112	
Marquette	Upper Peninsula Regional Poison Center Marquette General Hospital 420 W. Magnetic Dr. Marquette, MI 49855	(906) 228-9440 (800) 562-9781 (N. MI only)	
Pontiac	Poison Information Center St. Joseph Mercy Hospital 900 S. Woodward Ave. Pontiac, MI 48053	(313) 858-7373	
Port Huron	Port Huron Hospital Poison Control Center 1001 Kearney St. Port Huron, MI 48060	(313) 987-5555	
Saginaw	Saginaw Region Poison Center Saginaw General Hospital 1447 N. Harrison Saginaw, MI 48602	(517) 755-1111	
Traverse City	Munson Medical Center Sixth and Madison Streets Traverse City, MI 49684	(616) 947-6140 ext. 303	
Minnesota			
State Coordinator	EMS Section Minnesota Dept. of Health 717 S.E. Delaware St. Minneapolis, MN 55404	(612) 623-5284	
Duluth	St. Luke's Hospital Poison Control Center 915 E. First St. Duluth, MN 55805	(218) 726-5466	
	St. Mary's Hospital 407 E. 3rd St. Duluth, MN 55805	(218) 726-4500	
Fridley	Unity Medical Center 550 Osborne Rd. Fridley, MN 55432	(612) 786-2200 ext. 6844	x
Mankato	Immanuel-St. Joseph's Hospital Poison Control Center 325 Garden Blvd. Mankato, MN 56001	(507) 625-4031 ext. 2760	x
Minneapolis	Hennepin Poison Center Hennepin County Medical Center 701 Park Ave. Minneapolis, MN 55415	(612) 347-3141	A
Morris	Stevens County Memorial Hospital Morris, MN 56267	(612) 589-1313 ext. 231	x
Rochester	Southeastern Minnesota Poison Control Center St. Mary's Hospital 1216 Second St., S.W. Rochester, MN 55901	(507) 285-6162	x
St. Cloud	St. Cloud Hospital 1406 6th Ave., N. St. Cloud, MN 56301	(612) 255-5617	
St. Paul	St. John's Hospital 403 Maria Ave. St. Paul, MN 55106	(612) 228-3132	

Continued.

Directory of centers—cont'd

State coordinators and cities	Address	Telephone	Comments
	United and Children's Hospital 333 N. Smith St. Paul, MN 55102	(612) 298-8402	
	Minnesota Poison Information Center St. Paul-Ramsey Medical Center 640 Jackson St. St. Paul, MN 55101	(612) 221-2113	
Worthington	Worthington Regional Hospital 1016 6th Ave. Worthington, MN 56187	(507) 372-2941 ext. 109	x
Mississippi			
State Coordinator	State Board of Health Jackson, MS 39205	(601) 354-7660	
Biloxi	Gulf Coast Community Hospital 4642 W. Beach Blvd. Buloxi, MS 39531	(601) 388-1919	
	USAF Hospital Keesler Keesler Air Force Base Biloxi, MS 39534	(601) 377-6555	
Brandon	Rankin General Hospital Emergency Department 350 Crossgates Blvd. Brandon, MS 39042	(601) 825-2811 ext. 405	x
Columbia	Marion County General Hospital Sumrall Rd. Columbia, MS 39429	(601) 736-6303 ext. 1020	x
Greenwood	Greenwood-Leflore Hospital River Rd. Greenwood, MS 38930	(601) 459-2790	
Hattiesburg	Forrest County General Hospital 400 S. 28th Ave. Hattiesburg, MS 39401	(601) 264-4235	
Jackson	St. Dominic-Jackson Memorial Hospital 969 Lakeland Dr. Jackson, MS 39216	(601) 982-0121 ext. 2345	x
	University Medical Center 2500 N. State St. Jackson, MS 39216	(601) 354-7660	
Laurel	Jones County Community Hospital Jefferson St. at 13th Ave. Laurel, MS 39440	(601) 649-4000 ext. 630	x
Meridian	Meridian Regional Hospital Highway 39, N. Meridian, MS 39301	(601) 483-6211 ext. 440	x
Pascagoula	Singing River Hospital Emergency Department 2609 Denny Ave. Pascagoula, MS 39567	(601) 938-5162	
University	University of Mississippi School of Pharmacy Poison Information Center University, MS 38677	(601) 234-1522	
Missouri			
State Coordinator	Bureau of EMS Missouri Division of Health Jefferson City, MO 65102	(314) 751-2713	
Cape Girardeau	St. Francis Medical Center St. Francis Dr. Cape Girardeau, MO 63701	(314) 651-6235	

State coordinators and cities	Address	Telephone	Comments
Columbia	University of Missouri Hospital and Clinics 807 Stadium Rd. Columbia, MO 65212	(314) 882-8091	
Hannibal	St. Elizabeth's Hospital 109 Virginia St. Hannibal, MO 63401	(314) 221-0414 ext. 264	x
Jefferson City	Charles E. Still Osteopathic Hospital 1125 Madison Jefferson City, MO 65101	(314) 635-7141 ext. 215	x
Joplin	St. John's Medical Center 2727 McClelland Blvd. Joplin, MO 64801	(417) 781-2727 ext. 2305	x
Kansas City	Children's Mercy Hospital 24th at Gillham Rd. Kansas City, MO 64108	(816) 234-3000	A
Kirksville	Kirksville Osteopathic Health Center #1 Osteopathy Ave. Kirksville, MO 63501	(816) 626-2266	x
Poplar Bluff	Lucy Lee Hospital 2620 N. Westwood Blvd. Poplar Bluff, MO 63901	(314) 785-7721 ext. 264	x
Rolla	Phelps County Regional Medical Center 1000 W. 10th St. Rolla, MO 65401	(314) 364-3100 ext. 287	x
St. Joseph	Methodist Medical Center Seventh to Ninth on Faron St. St. Joseph, MO 64501	(816) 271-7580 232-8481	
St. Louis	St. Louis Regional Poison Center Cardinal Glennon Memorial Hospital for Children 1465 S. Grand Ave. St. Louis, MO 63104	(314) 772-5200	A
	St. Louis Children's Hospital 500 S. Kingshighway St. Louis, MO 63110	(314) 454-6099	
Springfield	Ozark Poison Center Lester E. Cox Medical Center 1423 N. Jefferson St. Springfield, MO 65802	(417) 831-9746	
Montana			
State Coordinator	Department of Health and Environmental Sciences Helena, MT 59620	(406) 449-3895	
Helena	Montana Poison Control System Cogswell Bldg. Helena, MT 59620	(406) 442-2480 (800) 525-5042	
Nebraska			
State Coordinator	Department of Health Lincoln, NE 68502	(402) 471-2122	
Omaha	Mid-Plains Regional Poison Center Children's Memorial Hospital 8301 Dodge Omaha, NE 68114	(402) 390-5400 (800) 642-9999 (statewide) (800) 228-9515 (surrounding states)	
Nevada			
State Coordinator	Department of Human Resources Carson City, NV 89710	(702) 885-4750	
Las Vegas	Southern Nevada Memorial Hospital 1800 W. Charleston Blvd. Las Vegas, NV 89102	(702) 385-1277	

Continued.

Directory of centers—cont'd

State coordinators and cities	*Address*	*Telephone*	*Comments*
	Sunrise Hospital Medical Center 3186 S. Maryland Pkwy. Las Vegas, NV 89109	(702) 732-4989	
Reno	St. Mary's Hospital 235 W. 6th Reno, NV 89520	(702) 789-3013	
	Washoe Medical Center 77 Pringle Way Reno, NV 89520	(702) 785-4129	
New Hampshire			
State Coordinator	New Hampshire Poison Center NH - Dartmouth Hitchcock Medical Center 2 Maynard St. Hanover, NH 03756	(603) 646-5000 (800) 562-8236 (statewide)	
Hanover	New Hampshire Poison Center Mary Hitchcock Hospital 2 Maynard St. Hanover, NH 03756	(603) 646-5000 (800) 562-8236 (statewide)	x
New Jersey			
State Coordinator	Department of Health Accident Prevention and Poison Control Program Trenton, NJ 08625	(609) 292-5666	
Atlantic City	Atlantic City Medical Center 1925 Pacific Ave. Atlantic City, NJ 08401	(609) 344-4081 ext. 2359	x
Belleville	Clara Maass Medical Center 1A Franklin Ave. Belleville, NJ 07109	(201) 450-2000 ext. 781	x
Berlin	West Jersey Hospital South Division Berlin, NJ 08009	(609) 768-6666	
Boonton	Riverside Hospital Powerville Rd. Boonton, NJ 07055	(201) 334-5000 ext. 186	x
Bridgeton	Bridgeton Hospital Irving Ave. Bridgeton, NJ 08302	(609) 451-6600 ext. 251	x
Denville	St. Clare's Hospital Pocono Rd. Denville, NJ 07834	(201) 625-6065 ext. 6063	x
East Orange	East Orange General Hospital 300 Central Ave. E. Orange, NJ 07019	(201) 672-8400 ext. 223	x
Elizabeth	St. Elizabeth's Hospital 225 Williams St. Elizabeth, NJ 07207	(201) 527-5059	
Englewood	Englewood Hospital 350 Engle St. Englewood, NJ 07631	(201) 894-3262	
Flemington	Hunterdon Medical Center Route 31 Flemington, NJ 08822	(201) 782-2121 ext. 369	x
Livingston	St. Barnabas Medical Center Old Short Hills Rd. Livingston, NJ 07039	(201) 992-5161	
Long Branch	Monmouth Medical Center Emergency Department Dunbar and 2nd Ave. Long Branch, NJ 07740	(201) 222-2210	

State coordinators and cities	Address	Telephone	Comments
Montclair	Mountainside Hospital Bay and Highland Aves. Montclair, NJ 07042	(201) 429-6202	
Mount Holly	Burlington County Memorial Hospital 175 Madison Ave. Mt. Holly, NJ 08060	(609) 267-7877	
Neptune	Jersey Shore Medical Center Fitkin Hospital 1945 Corlies Ave. Neptune, NJ 07753	(201) 775-5500 (800) 822-9761 (statewide)	
Newark	Newark Beth Israel Medical Center 201 Lyons Ave. Newark, NJ 07112	(201) 926-7240	
New Brunswick	Middlesex General Hospital 180 Somerset St. New Brunswick, NJ 08903	(201) 937-8583	
	St. Peter's Medical Center 245 Easton Ave. New Brunswick, NJ 08903	(201) 745-8527	
Newton	Newton Memorial Hospital 175 High St. Newton, NJ 07860	(201) 383-2121 ext. 270	x
Orange	Hospital Center at Orange Emergency Department 188 S. Essex Ave. Orange, NJ 07051	(201) 266-2120	
Passaic	St. Mary's Hospital 211 Pennington Ave. Passaic, NJ 07055	(201) 473-1000 ext. 441	x
Perth Amboy	Perth Amboy General Hospital 530 New Brunswick Ave. Perth Amboy, NJ 08861	(201) 442-3700 ext. 2501	x
Phillipsburg	Warren Hospital 185 Roseberry St. Phillipsburg, NJ 08865	(201) 859-1500 ext. 222	x
Point Pleasant	Point Pleasant Hospital Osborn Ave. & River Front Point Pleasant, NJ 08742	(201) 892-1100 ext. 383	x
Princeton	The Medical Center at Princeton 253 Witherspoon St. Princeton, NJ 08540	(609) 734-4554	
Saddle Brook	Saddle Brook General Hospital 300 Market St. Saddle Brook, NJ 07662	(201) 368-6025	
Somers Point	Shore Memorial Hospital Brighton & Sunny Aves. Somers Point, NJ 08244	(609) 653-3515	
Somerville	Somerset Medical Center Rehill Ave. Somerville, NJ 08876	(201) 725-4000 ext. 436	x
Summit	Overlook Hospital 193 Morris Ave. Summit, NJ 07901	(201) 522-2232	
Teaneck	Holy Name Hospital 718 Teaneck Rd. Teaneck, NJ 07666	(201) 833-3242	
Trenton	Helene Fuld Medical Center 750 Brunswick Ave. Trenton, NJ 08638	(609) 396-1077	

Continued.

Directory of centers—cont'd

State coordinators and cities	*Address*	*Telephone*	*Comments*
Union	Memorial General Hospital 1000 Galloping Hill Rd. Union, NJ 07083	(201) 687-1900 ext. 3710	x
Wayne	Greater Paterson General Hospital 224 Hamburg Turnpike Wayne, NJ 07470	(201) 942-6900 ext. 224	x
New Mexico			
State Coordinator	New Mexico Poison Drug Information & Medical Center University of New Mexico Albuquerque, NM 87131	(505) 843-2551 (800) 432-6866 (statewide)	A
New York			
State Coordinator	Department of Health Albany, NY 12237	(518) 474-3785	
Binghamton	Southern Tier Poison Center United Health Services Binghamton General Hospital Binghamton, NY 13903	(607) 723-8929	
	Our Lady of Lourdes Memorial Hospital 169 Riverside Dr. Binghamton, NY 13905	(607) 798-5231	
Buffalo	Western New York Poison Control Center Children's Hospital of Buffalo 219 Bryant St. Buffalo, NY 14222	(716) 878-7654	
Dunkirk	Brooks Memorial Hospital 10 W. 6th St. Dunkirk, NY 14048	(716) 366-1111 ext. 414	x
East Meadow	Long Island Regional Poison Control Center Nassau County Medical Center 2201 Hempstead Turnpike E. Meadow, NY 11554	(516) 542-2324 (516) 542-2323 (TTY)	A
Elmira	Arnot Ogden Memorial Hospital Roe Ave. & Grove St. Elmira, NY 14901	(607) 737-4194	
	St. Joseph's Hospital Health Center 555 E. Market St. Elmira, NY 14901	(607) 734-2662	
Endicott	Ideal Hospital 600 High Ave. Endicott, NY 13760	(607) 754-7171	x
Glens Falls	Glens Falls Hospital 100 Park St. Glens Falls, NY 12801	(518) 761-5261	
Jamestown	W.C.A. Hospital 207 Foote Ave. Jamestown, NY 14701	(716) 484-8648	
Johnson City	Wilson Memorial Hospital 33 Harrison St. Johnson City, NY 13790	(607) 773-6611	
Kingston	Kingston Hospital 396 Broadway Kingston, NY 12401	(914) 331-3313	
New York City	New York City Poison Center Department of Health Bureau of Laboratories 455 First Ave. New York City, NY 10016	(212) 340-4494 (212) 764-7667	A

State coordinators and cities	Address	Telephone	Comments
Nyack	Hudson Valley Poison Center Nyack Hospital N. Midland Ave. Nyack, NY 10960	(914) 353-1000	
Rochester	Finger Lakes Poison Center LIFELINE University of Rochester Medical Center Rochester, NY 14642	(716) 275-5151 275-2700 (TTY)	A
Schenectady	Ellis Hospital Poison Control 1101 Nott St. Schenectady, NY 12308	(518) 382-4039 382-4121	
Syracuse	Syracuse Poison Information Center 750 E. Adams St. Syracuse, NY 13210	(315) 476-7529	
Troy	St. Mary's Hospital Poison Control Center 1300 Massachusetts Ave. Troy, NY 12180	(518) 272-5792	
Utica	St. Lukes Memorial Hospital Center P.O. Box 479 Utica, NY 13502	(315) 798-6200	
Watertown	House of the Good Samaritan Hospital Washington & Pratt Sts. Watertown, NY 13602	(315) 788-8700	
North Carolina			
State Coordinator	Duke University Medical Center Durham, NC 27710	(919) 684-8111 (800) 672-1697 (statewide)	
Asheville	Western North Carolina Poison Control Center Memorial Mission Hospital 509 Biltimore Ave. Asheville, NC 28801	(704) 255-4490	
Charlotte	Mercy Hospital 2001 Vail Ave. Charlotte, NC 28207	(704) 379-5827	
Durham	Duke University Medical Center Poison Control Center P.O. Box 3007 Durham, NC 27710	(919) 684-8111	
Greensboro	Triad Poison Center Moses H. Cone Memorial Hospital 1200 N. Elm St. Greensboro, NC 27401	(919) 379-4105	
Hendersonville	Margaret R. Pardee Memorial Hospital Fleming St. Hendersonville, NC 28739	(704) 693-6522 ext. 555	x
Hickory	Catawba Memorial Hospital Fairgrove-Church Rd. Hickory, NC 28601	(704) 322-6649	
Jacksonville	Onslow Memorial Hospital Western Blvd. Jacksonville, NC 28540	(919) 577-2555	
Wilmington	New Hanover Memorial Hospital 2131 S. 17th St. Wilmington, NC 28401	(919) 343-7046	
Winston-Salem	Wake Forest University Medical Center North Carolina Baptist Hospital 300 S. Hawthorne Road Winston-Salem, NC 27103	(919) 748-4991	

Continued.

Directory of centers—cont'd

State coordinators and cities	*Address*	*Telephone*	*Comments*
North Dakota			
State Coordinator	Department of Health Bismarck, ND 58505	(701) 224-2388	
Bismarck	Bismarck Hospital Emergency Department 300 N. 7th St. Bismarck, ND 58501	(701) 223-4357	
Fargo	St. Luke's Poison Center St. Luke's Hospitals Fifth St. at Mills Ave. Fargo, ND 58122	(701) 280-5575	
Grand Forks	United Hospital 1200 S. Columbia Rd. Grand Forks, ND 58201	(701) 780-5282	x
Minot	St. Joseph's Hospital Third St. & Fourth Ave., S.E. Minot, ND 58701	(701) 857-2553	
Williston	Mercy Hospital 1301 15th Ave., W. Williston, ND 58801	(701) 572-7661	x
Ohio			
State Coordinator	Department of Health Columbus, OH 43216	(614) 466-5190	
Akron	Children's Hospital Medical Center of Akron 281 Locust St. Akron, OH 44308	(216) 379-8562 (800) 362-9922 (statewide)	
Canton	Aultman Hospital Emergency Room 2600 Sixth St., S.W. Canton, OH 44710	(216) 438-6203 452-9911	
Cincinnati	Drug & Poison Information Center Bridge Medical Science Bldg. Room 7701 231 Bethesda Ave. Cincinnati, OH 45267	(513) 872-5111	
Cleveland	Greater Cleveland Poison Control Center 2119 Abington Rd. Cleveland, OH 44106	(216) 231-4455	
Columbus	Central Ohio Poison Center Children's Hospital of Ohio 700 Children's Dr. Columbus, OH 43205	(614) 228-1323	
Dayton	Children's Medical Center One Children's Plaza Dayton, OH 45404	(513) 222-2227 (800) 762-0727 (statewide)	
Lorain	Lorain Community Hospital 3700 Kolbe Rd. Lorain, OH 44053	(216) 282-2220	
Mansfield	Mansfield General Hospital 335 Glessner Ave. Mansfield, OH 44903	(419) 522-3411 ext. 2545	x
Springfield	Community Hospital 2615 E. High St. Springfield, OH 44505	(513) 325-1255	
Toledo	Poison Information Center Medical College Hospital P.O. Box 6190 Toledo, OH 43679	(419) 381-3897	

State coordinators and cities	*Address*	*Telephone*	*Comments*
Youngstown	Mahoning Valley Poison Center St. Elizabeth Hospital Medical Center 1044 Belmont Ave. Youngstown, OH 44501	(216) 746-2222 (216) 746-5510 (TTY)	
Zanesville	Bethesda Poison Control Center Bethesda Hospital 2951 Maple Ave. Zanesville, OH 43701	(614) 454-4221	
Oklahoma			
State Coordinator	Oklahoma Poison Control Center Oklahoma Children's Memorial Hospital P.O. Box 26307 Oklahoma City, OK 73126	(405) 271-5454 (800) 522-4611 (statewide)	
Ada	Valley View Hospital 1300 E. 6th St. Ada, OK 74820	(405) 332-2323 ext. 200	x
Lawton	Comanche County Memorial Hospital 3401 Gore Blvd. Lawton, OK 73501	(405) 355-8620 ext. 296	x
McAlester	McAlester General Hospital Inc., W. P.O. Box 669 McAlester, OK 74501	(918) 426-1800 ext. 240	x
Oklahoma City	Oklahoma Poison Control Center Oklahoma Children's Memorial Center P.O. Box 26307 Oklahoma City, OK 73126	(405) 271-5454 (800) 522-4611 (statewide)	
Ponca City	St. Joseph Medical Center 14th and Hartford Ponca City, OK 74601	(405) 765-0584	x
Tulsa	Hillcrest Medical Center 1120 S. Utica Tulsa, OK 74104	(918) 560-5755	
Oregon			
State Coordinator	Oregon Poison Control and Drug Information Center University of Oregon Health Sciences Center Portland, OR 97201	(503) 225-8968 (800) 452-7165 (statewide)	
Panama			
Ancon	U.S.A. MEDDAC Panama Gorgas U.S. Army Hospital Ancon, Panama APO Miami 34004	252-7500	x
Pennsylvania			
State Coordinator	Director, Division of Drugs, Devices and Cosmetics Department of Health P.O. Box 90 Harrisburg, PA 17108	(717) 787-2307	
Allentown	Lehigh Valley Poison Center Allentown General Hospital 17th and Chew Sts. Allentown, PA 18102	(215) 433-2311	
Altoona	Keystone Region Poison Center Mercy Hospital 2500 Seventh Ave. Altoona, PA 16603	(814) 946-3711	
Bloomsburg	The Bloomsburg Hospital 549 E. Fair St. Bloomsburg, PA 17815	(717) 784-4241	

Continued.

Directory of centers—cont'd

State coordinators and cities	*Address*	*Telephone*	*Comments*
Chester	Sacred Heart General Hospital Ninth and Wilson Sts. Chester, PA 19013	(215) 494-4400	
Danville	Susquehanna Poison Center Geisinger Medical Center N. Academy Ave. Danville, PA 17821	(717) 275-6116	
Erie	Doctors Osteopathic Hospital 252 W. 11th St. Erie, PA 16502	(814) 454-2120	
	Millcreek Community Hospital 5515 Peach St. Erie, PA 16509	(814) 864-4031	x
	Hamot Medical Center 201 State St. Erie, PA 16550	(814) 452-4242	
	Saint Vincent's Health Center 232 W. 25th St. Erie, PA 16544	(814) 452-3232	
Gettysburg	Annie M. Warner Hospital S. Washington St. Gettysburg, PA 17325	(717) 334-9155	x
Hanover	Hanover General Hospital 300 Highland Ave. Hanover, PA 17331	(717) 637-3711	
Hershey	Capital Area Poison Center The Milton S. Hershey Medical Center University Dr. Hershey, PA 17033	(717) 534-6111 (treatment)	
Jersey Shore	Jersey Shore Hospital ER - Poison Center Thompson St. Jersey Shore, PA 17740	(717) 398-0100	x
Johnstown	Conemaugh Valley Memorial Hospital Poison Control Center 1086 Franklin St. Johnstown, PA 15905	(814) 535-5351	
	Laurel Highlands Poison Center 320 Main St. Johnstown, PA 15901	(814) 535-8255	
	Mercy Hospital Poison Control Center 1020 Franklin St. Johnstown, PA 15905	(814) 535-5353	
Lancaster	Lancaster General Hospital ER - Poison Control Center 555 N. Duke St. Lancaster, PA 17604	(717) 295-8322	
	St. Joseph's Hospital Poison Control Center 250 College Ave. Lancaster, PA 17604	(717) 299-4546	
Lehighton	Gnaden-Huetten Memorial Hospital 11th & Hamilton Sts. Lehighton, PA 18235	(215) 377-1300	x
Lewistown	Lewistown Hospital Poison Control Center Highland Ave. Lewistown, PA 17044	(717) 248-5411	x

State coordinators and cities	*Address*	*Telephone*	*Comments*
Nanticoke	Nanticoke State Hospital N. Washington St. Nanticoke, PA 18634	(717) 735-5000	x
Paoli	Paoli Memorial Hospital Emergency Room Paoli, PA 19301	(215) 648-1043	
Philadelphia	Philadelphia Poison Information 321 University Ave. Philadelphia, PA 19104	(215) 922-5523 922-5524	
Philipsburg	Philipsburg State General Hospital Loch Lomond Rd. Philipsburg, PA 16866	(814) 342-3320	x
Pittsburgh	Pittsburgh Poison Center Children's Hospital 125 DeSoto St. Pittsburgh, PA 15214	(412) 681-6669 647-5600	
Reading	Community General Hospital 145 N. 6th St. Reading, PA 19601	(215) 375-9115	
Sayre	The Robert Packer Hospital Guthrie Square Sayre, PA 18840	(717) 888-6666	x
Sellersville	Grandview Hospital Lawn Ave. Sellersville, PA 18960	(215) 257-3611	x
State College	Centre Community Hospital Orchard Rd. State College, PA 16801	(814) 238-4351	x
York	Memorial Osteopathic Hospital 325 S. Belmont St. York, PA 17403	(717) 843-8623 ext. 123	x
	York Hospital 1001 S. George St. York, PA 17405	(717) 771-2311	
Puerto Rico			
State Coordinator	University of Puerto Rico Rio Piedras, PR	(809) 765-4880 765-0615	
Arecibo	District Hospital of Arecibo Arecibo, PR 00613	(809) 878-3535 ext. 707 (809) 878-8212	x
Fajardo	District Hospital of Fajardo Fajardo, PR 00649	(809) 863-0505	
Mayaguez	Mayaguez Medical Center Department of Health P.O. Box 1868 Mayaguez, PR 00709	(809) 832-8686 ext. 1816 1514	x
Ponce	District Hospital of Ponce Ponce, PR 00731	(809) 842-2550	
Rio Piedras	Childrens Hospital Center of Puerto Rico Rio Piedras, PR 00936	(809) 754-8535	
San Juan	Pharmacy School Medical Sciences Campus San Juan, PR 00936	(809) 753-4849	
Rhode Island			
State Coordinator	Rhode Island Poison Center Rhode Island Hospital 593 Eddy St. Providence, RI 02902	(401) 277-5727	

Continued.

Directory of centers—cont'd

State coordinators and cities	*Address*	*Telephone*	*Comments*
Providence	Rhode Island Poison Center Rhode Island Hospital Annex Bldg. 422 593 Eddy St. Providence, RI 02902	(401) 277-5727	
South Carolina			
State Coordinator	Department of Health and Environmental Control Columbia, SC 29201	(803) 758-5654	
Charleston	National Pesticide Telecommunications Network Medical University of South Carolina 171 Ashley Ave. Charleston, SC 29403	(803) 792-4201 (800) 845-7633 (outside SC)	
Columbia	Palmetto Poison Center University of South Carolina College of Pharmacy Columbia, SC 29208	(803) 765-7359 (800) 922-1117	
South Dakota			
State Coordinator	Department of Health Pierre, SD 57501	(605) 773-3361	
Aberdeen	The Dakota Midland Poison Control Center Dakota Midland Hospital 1400 15th Ave., N.W. Aberdeen, SD 57401	(605) 225-1880 (800) 592-1889	
Rapid City	Rapid City Regional Poison Control Center 353 Fairmont Blvd. P.O. Box 6000 Rapid City, SD 57709	(605) 341-3333 (800) 742-8925	
Sioux Falls	McKennan Poison Center McKennan Hospital 800 E. 21st St. Sioux Falls, SD 57101	(605) 336-3894 (800) 952-0123 (statewide) (800) 843-0505 (NE, MN, IA)	
Tennessee			
State Coordinator	Department of Public Health Division of Emergency Services Nashville, TN 37216	(615) 741-2407	
Chattanooga	T.C. Thompson Children's Hospital 910 Blackford St. Chattanooga, TN 37403	(615) 755-6100	
Columbia	Maury County Hospital 1224 Trotwood Ave. Columbia, TN 38401	(615) 778-4500 ext. 110	x
Cookeville	Cookeville General Hospital 142 W. 5th St. Cookeville, TN 38501	(615) 526-4818	
Jackson	Jackson-Madison General Hospital 708 W. Forest Jackson, TN 38301	(901) 424-0424 ext. 525	x
Johnson City	Johnson City Medical Center Hospital Emergency Department 400 State of Franklin Rd. Johnson City, TN 37601	(615) 461-6572	
Knoxville	Memorial Research Center Hospital 1924 Alcoa Hwy. Knoxville, TN 37920	(615) 971-3261	
Memphis	Southern Poison Center LeBonheur Children's Medical Center 848 Adams Ave. Memphis, TN 38103	(901) 528-6048	

State coordinators and cities	Address	Telephone	Comments
Nashville	Vanderbilt University Hospital 21st and Garland Nashville, TN 37232	(615) 322-6435	
Texas			
State Coordinator	Texas Department of Health Div. of Occupational Health Austin, TX 78756	(512) 458-7254	
Abilene	Hendrick Hospital 19th & Hickory Sts. Abilene, TX 79601	(915) 677-7762	
Amarillo	Amarillo Emergency Receiving Center Amarillo Hospital District P.O. Box 1110 1501 Coulter Dr. Amarillo, TX 79175	(806) 376-4292	
Austin	Brackenridge Hospital 14th & Sabine Sts. Austin, TX 78701	(512) 478-4490	
Beaumont	Baptist Hospital of Southeast Texas P.O. Box 1591 College & 11th St. Beaumont, TX 77701	(713) 833-7409	
Corpus Christi	Memorial Medical Center P.O. Box 5280 2606 Hospital Blvd. Corpus Christi, TX 78405	(512) 881-4559	
El Paso	El Paso Poison Control Center R.E. Thomason General Hospital 4815 Alameda Ave. El Paso, TX 79905	(915) 533-1244	
Fort Worth	W.I. Cook Children's Hospital Cook Poison Center-Fort Worth 1212 W. Lancaster St. Fort Worth, TX 76102	(817) 336-6611	
Galveston	Southeast Texas Poison Center The University of Texas Medical Branch Eighth & Mechanic Sts. Galveston, TX 77550	(713) 765-1420	A
Harlingen	Valley Baptist Hospital P.O. Box 2588 2101 S. Commerce St. Harlingen, TX 78550	(512) 421-1859	
Houston	Southeast Texas Poison Control Center Eighth & Mechanic Sts. Galveston, TX 77550	(713) 654-1701	A
Laredo	Mercy Hospital 1515 Logan St. Laredo, TX 78040	(512) 724-6247	
Lubbock	Methodist Hospital 3615 19th St. Lubbock, TX 79410	(806) 793-4366	
Odessa	Medical Center Hospital Poison Control Center P.O. Box 7239 Odessa, TX 79760	(915) 333-1231	
Plainview	Central Plains Regional Hospital 2601 Dimmitt Rd. Plainview, TX 79072	(806) 296-9601	
San Angelo	Shannon West Texas Memorial Hospital 120 E. Harris San Angelo, TX 76901	(915) 653-6741 ext. 318	x

Continued.

Directory of centers—cont'd

State coordinators and cities	Address	Telephone	Comments
San Antonio	Department of Pediatrics University of Texas Health Science Center at San Antonio 7703 Floyd Curl Dr. San Antonio, TX 78284	(512) 223-6361 ext. 473	x
Tyler	Medical Center Hospital 1000 S. Becham St. Tyler, TX 75701	(214) 597-0351	x
Waco	Hillcrest Baptist Hospital 3000 Herring Ave. Waco, TX 76708	(817) 753-1412	x
Wichita Falls	Wichita General Hospital 1600 8th St. Wichita Falls, TX 76301	(817) 322-6771	
Utah			
State Coordinator	Utah Department of Health Division of Family Health Services Salt Lake City, UT 84113	(801) 533-6161	
Salt Lake City	Intermountain Regional Poison Control Center 50 N. Medical Dr. Salt Lake City, UT 84132	(801) 581-2151	A
Vermont			
State Coordinator	Department of Health Burlington, VT 05401	(802) 862-5701	
Burlington	Vermont Poison Center Medical Center Hospital of Vermont Burlington, VT 05401	(802) 658-3456	
Virginia			
State Coordinator	Division of Emergency Medical Services Room 1102 109 Governor St. Richmond, VA 23219	(804) 786-5188	
Alexandria	Alexandria Hospital 4320 Seminary Rd. Alexandria, VA 22314	(703) 379-3070	
Arlington	Arlington Hospital 5129 N. 16th St. Arlington, VA 22205	(703) 558-6161	
Blacksburg	Montgomery County Community Hospital Rt. 460, S. Blacksburg, VA 24060	(703) 951-1111 ext. 140	x
Charlottesville	Blue Ridge Poison Center University of Virginia Hospital Charlottesville, VA 22903	(804) 924-5543 (800) 446-9876 (TTY) (out of state) (800) 552-3723 (TTY) (statewide)	
Falls Church	Fairfax Hospital 3300 Gallows Rd. Falls Church, VA 22046	(703) 698-3600	
Hampton	Hampton General Hospital 3120 Victoria Blvd. Hampton, VA 23661	(804) 722-1131	
Harrisonburg	Rockingham Memorial Hospital Emergency Room 235 Cantrell Harrisonburg, VA 22801	(703) 433-8311	
Lexington	Stonewall Jackson Hospital Lexington, VA 22043	(703) 463-9141 ext. 219	x

State coordinators and cities	Address	Telephone	Comments
Lynchburg	Lynchburg General Marshall Lodge Hospital, Inc. Tate Springs Rd. Lynchburg, VA 24504	(804) 528-2066	
Nassawadox	Northampton-Accomack Memorial Hospital Nassawadox, VA 23413	(804) 442-8700	
Newport News	Riverside Hospital 500 J. Clyde Morris Blvd. Newport News, VA 23601	(804) 599-2050	
Norfolk	DePaul Hospital Granby St. at Kingsley La. Norfolk, VA 23505	(804) 489-5288	
Portsmouth	U.S. Naval Hospital Portsmouth, VA 23708	(804) 398-5898	
Richmond	Central Virginia Poison Center Medical College of Virginia Virginia Commonwealth University P.O. Box 522, MCV Station Richmond, VA 23298	(804) 786-9123	
Roanoke	Southwest Virginia Poison Center Roanoke Memorial Hospital Belleview at Jefferson St. P.O. Box 13367 Roanoke, VA 24033	(703) 981-7336	
Staunton	King's Daughter's Hospital P.O. Box 3000 Staunton, VA 24401	(703) 885-6848	x
Waynesboro	Waynesboro Community Hospital 501 Oak Ave. Waynesboro, VA 22980	(703) 942-4096	x
Williamsburg	Williamsburg Community Hospital 1238 Mr. Vernon Ave. P.O. Drawer H Williamsburg, VA 23185	(804) 253-6005	
Virgin Islands			
State Coordinator	Department of Health St. Thomas, VI 00801	(809) 774-6097 774-0117	
St. Croix	Charles Harwood Memorial Hospital Christiansted St. Croix, VI 00820	(809) 773-8331	
St. John	Morris F. DeCastro Clinic Cruz Bay St. John, VI 00830	(809) 776-6252	
St. Thomas	Knud-Hansen Memorial Hospital St. Thomas, VI 00801	(809) 774-9000 ext. 224/5 (809) 774-1212	x
Washington			
State Coordinator	Department of Social and Health Services Emergency Medical Services Olympia, WA 98504	(206) 522-7478	
Seattle	Seattle Poison Center Children's Orthopedic Hospital and Medical Center 4800 Sand Point Way, NE Seattle, WA 98105	(206) 634-5252 (800) 732-6985	A
Spokane	Spokane Poison Center Deaconess Hospital 800 W. 5th Ave. Spokane, WA 99210	(509) 747-1077 (800) 572-5842 (statewide) (509) 747-1077 (TTY)	A

Continued.

Directory of centers—cont'd

State coordinators and cities	Address	Telephone	Comments
Tacoma	Mary Bridge Poison Information Center Mary Bridge Children's Hospital South L St. Tacoma, WA 98405	(206) 272-1281 (800) 542-6319 (statewide)	x
Yakima	Central Washington Poison Center Yakima Valley Memorial Hospital 2811 Tieton Dr. Yakima, WA 98902	(509) 248-4400 (800) 572-9176 (statewide)	
West Virginia			
State Coordinator	The West Virginia Poison System West Virginia University School of Pharmacy 3110 Mac Corkle Ave., S.E. Charleston, WV 25304	(304) 348-4211 (800) 642-3625 (statewide)	
Wisconsin			
State Coordinator	Department of Health and Social Services Division of Health Madison, WI 53701	(608) 267-7174	
Eau Claire	Eau Claire Poison Center Luther Hospital 1225 Whipple Eau Claire, WI 54701	(715) 835-1515	
Green Bay	Green Bay Poison Center St. Vincent Hospital 835 S. Van Buren St. Green Bay, WI 54305	(414) 433-8100	
LaCrosse	St. Francis Medical Center 700 West Ave., N. LaCrosse, WI 54601	(608) 784-3971	
Madison	Madison Area Poison Center University Hospital & Clinic 600 Highland Ave. Madison, WI 53792	(608) 262-3702	
Milwaukee	Milwaukee Poison Center Milwaukee Children's Hospital 1700 W. Wisconsin Ave. Milwaukee, WI 53233	(414) 931-4114	
Wyoming			
State Coordinator	Office of Emergency Medical Services Department of Health and Social Services Cheyenne, WY 82002	(307) 777-7955	
Cheyenne	Wyoming Poison Center DePaul Hospital 2600 E. 18th St. Cheyenne, WY 82001	(307) 635-9256 (800) 442-2704	

ORGANIZATIONS INVOLVED WITH POISON PREVENTION AND CONTROL

U.S. Food and Drug Administration
Poisoning Surveillance and Epidemiology Branch (HFN-720)
5600 Fishers Lane
Rockville, Maryland 20857
(301) 443-6260

U.S. Consumer Product Safety Commission
Division of Poison Prevention and Scientific Coordination
Washington, D.C. 20207
(202) 634-7780

Poison Prevention Week Council
P.O. Box 1543
Washington, D.C. 20013
(301) 492-6477

American Association of Poison Control Centers
San Diego Regional Poison Control Center
University California at San Diego Medical Center
225 W. Dickinson Street
San Diego, California
(714) 294-6000

National Poison Center Network
Children's Hospital
125 DeSoto Street
Pittsburgh, Pennsylvania 15213
(412) 681-6669

American Board of Medical Toxicology
Children's Orthopedic Hospital and Medical Center
P.O. Box 5371
Seattle, Washington 98105
(206) 634-5252
(800) 732-6985

American College of Emergency Physicians
P.O. Box 61911
Dallas, Texas 75261
(214) 659-0911

CANADA*

Newfoundland and Labrador

St. John's
Provincial Poison Control Centre
The Dr. Charles A. Janeway Child Health Centre
Dr. J. Muzychka
(709) 722-1110

Corner Brook
Western Memorial Hospital
Mr. S. Gibbons, Director
(709) 634-7121

Gander
James Paton Memorial Hospital
Mr. J. Hoddinott, Director
(709) 651-2500

Grand Falls
Central Newfoundland Hospital
Ms. Denise O'Brien, Director
(709) 489-6661

Labrador City
Capt. Wm. Jackman Memorial Hospital
Mrs. Mary Hunt, R.N., Acting Director
(709) 944-2632

St. Anthony
Charles S. Curtis Memorial Hospital
(The International Grenfell Association)
Dr. J. H. Williams
(709) 454-3333

Prince Edward Island

Charlottetown
Queen Elizabeth Hospital
(902) 566-6250

Summerside
Prince County Hospital
(902) 436-9131

Nova Scotia

Main centre

Halifax
The Izaak Walton Killam Hospital for Children
Dr. J. P. Anderson
(902) 424-6161

Satellite centres

Amherst
Highland View Regional Hospital
(902) 667-3361, ext. 145

Antigonish
St. Martha's Hospital
(902) 863-2830, ext. 122

Bridgewater
Dawson Memorial Hospital
(902) 543-4603

Dartmouth
Dartmouth General Hospital
(902) 469-9520, ext. 238

Halifax
Victoria General Hospital
(902) 428-2043

Kentville
Valley Health Services Association
(902) 678-7381, ext. 215

New Glasgow
Aberdeen Hospital
(902) 752-8311

Sydney
Sydney City Hospital
(902) 539-6400, Ext. 118

Yarmouth
Yarmouth Regional Hospital
(902) 742-3541, Ext. 111

NEW BRUNSWICK

There is a Poison Treatment Centre in the Emergency Service of most of the active treatment hospitals in New Brunswick.

Bathurst
Chaleur General Hospital
(506) 546-4666

Campbellton
Hôtel-Dieu St. Joseph
(506) 753-5212

Edmundston
Hôtel-Dieu St. Joseph
(506) 735-7384

Fredericton
Dr. Everett Chalmers Hospital
(506) 452-5400

Moncton
Moncton City Hospital
(506) 855-1600

Saint John
Saint John General Hospital
Central Division
Dr. R. Scharf
(506) 648-7111

QUÉBEC

There is a Poison Treatment Centre in the Emergency Service of every active treatment hospital or Centre Local de Santé Communautaire in the Province of Québec.

Main centres

Montréal
Hôpital Sainte-Justine
Dr. Luc Chicoine
(514) 731-4931

Montreal Children's Hospital
Dr. Norman Eade
(514) 937-8511

Québec City
Centre Hospitalier de l'Université Laval
Dr. René Blais
(418) 656-8090

The Québec Toxicology Centre is in charge of the provincial Poison Control Program.

Québec City
Centre de Toxicologie du Québec
Centre Hospitalier de l'Université Laval
Dr. Albert Nantel
(418) 656-8326

*Provided by Canadian Pharmaceutical Association, 101-1815 Alta Vista Dr., Ottawa, Ontario K1G 3Y6. Available information on telephones and personnel supplied by Health and Welfare Canada, Health Protection Branch, Ottawa.

Ontario

Main poison control information centres

Toronto
Hospital for Sick Children
Dr. M. McGuigan
(416) 598-5900
1-800-268-9017 (toll free)*

Ottawa
Children's Hospital of Eastern Ontario
Dr. R. Peterson, Director
(613) 521-4040
1-800-267-1373 (toll free)*

Other centres

Belleville
Belleville General Hospital
(613) 968-5511

Brantford
Brantford General Hospital
Dr. Karl Korri
(519) 752-7871

Guelph
St. Joseph's Hospital Emergency Department
Mrs. Marilyn Evans, Head Nurse
(519) 824-2620, ext. 208

Kingston
Kingston General Hospital
Dr. Murray Taylor
(613) 547-2001

Kirkland Lake
Kirkland and District Hospital
Dr. R. Denton
(705) 567-5251

Kitchener
Kitchener-Waterloo Hospital
Dr. C. R. Page
(519) 742-3611

St. Mary's General Hospital
Dr. C. R. Page
(519) 744-3311

London
Victoria Hospital
Dr. Robert Anthony
(519) 432-5241
South St. Campus

St. Catharines
St. Catharines General Hospital
Dr. H. R. de Souza—Pharmacy and Therapeutics Committee
Dr. P. A. Zuliani—Chief, Emergency
(416) 684-7271

Sarnia
Sarnia General Hospital
Dr. K. R. Singh
(519) 336-6311

St. Joseph's Hospital
(519) 336-3111

*The toll free numbers do not cover area code 807. Individuals in this area may call the local numbers collect.

Sault Ste. Marie
Plummer Memorial Public Hospital
Dr. A. Balogh
(705) 254-5161

Simcoe
Norfolk General Hospital
Dr. K. R. McGavin
(519) 426-0750

Sudbury
Sudbury General Hospital
Dr. Gary Bota
(705) 674-3181

Thunder Bay
McKellar General Hospital
Dr. P. J. Neelands
(807) 623-5561

Port Arthur General Hospital
Dr. Arnot R. Hawkins
(807) 344-6621

Toronto
East General and Orthopaedic Hospital
Dr. A. Kaminker
(416) 461-8272, Ext. 200

Windsor
Hôtel-Dieu de St. Joseph
Dr. P. Dedumets
(519) 973-4400

Manitoba

Poison Treatment is available in every active hospital emergency department in Manitoba.

Provincial Poison Information centre
(204) 787-2591

Health Sciences Children's Centre
685 Bannatyne Avenue
Winnipeg, Manitoba R3E 0W1
Dr. M. Tenenbein, Director
(204) 787-2444

Saskatchewan

There is a Poison Treatment Centre in the Emergency Service of most of the active treatment hospitals in Saskatchewan.

Main centres

Regina General Hospital
Poison Control Centre
Dr. B. Kitchen, Director
(306) 359-4545

Saskatoon University Hospital
Poison Control Centre
Dr. W. A. Baker, Director
(306) 343-3323

Alberta

Poison Information centres

Calgary
Calgary General Hospital
841 Centre Ave. E.
Calgary, Alberta, T2E 0A1
(403) 262-5982

Emergency Department
Foothills General Hospital
1403-29th Street N.W.
Calgary, Alberta T2N 2T9
(403) 270-1315

Alberta Children's Hospital
1820 Richmond Road S.W.
Calgary, Alberta T2T 5C7
(403) 245-7070

Edmonton
Royal Alexandra Hospital
10240 Kingsway Avenue
Edmonton, Alberta T5H 3V9
(403) 474-3431

University of Alberta Hospital
112 Street and 84 Avenue
Edmonton, Alberta T6G 2B7
(403) 432-8410

Treatment centres

All active treatment hospitals in Alberta

British Columbia

Poison treatment is available in every active hospital emergency department in British Columbia.

Vancouver
B.C. Drug and Poison Information Centre
St. Paul's Hospital
1081 Burrard St.
(604) 682-5050

Victoria
Emergency Department
Royal Jubilee Hospital
(604) 595-9212

Northwest Territories

Fort Smith
Fort Smith Health Centre
Box 1080
Fort Smith, N.W.T.
X0E 0P0
(403) 872-2713

Frobisher Bay
Baffin Regional Hospital
Bag 200
Frobisher Bay, N.W.T.
X0A 0H0
(819) 979-5231

Hay River
H. H. Williams Memorial Hospital
P.O. Box 1280, X0E 0R0
(403) 874-6512

Inuvik
Inuvik General Hospital
Bag Service No. 2
Inuvik, N.W.T.
X0E 0T0
(403) 979-2955

Yellowknife
Stanton Yellowknife Hospital
Yellowknife, N.W.T.
X0E 1H0
(403) 920-4111

Yukon Territory

Whitehorse
Whitehorse General Hospital
Emergency Department
(403) 668-9444

APPENDIX **15**

LEADING HEALTH PROBLEMS AND COMMUNICABLE DISEASES

Two leading health problems in the United States are cardiovascular disease and cancer. Nurses and other health care professionals encounter some form of these diseases daily. The following statistics are offered in an effort to increase understanding of the magnitude of the problem and to provide a basis for developing patient teaching strategies. In this way the health care professional becomes a tool for preventive health care, an increasingly important role in today's health-conscious society.

Leading Causes of Death

United States: 1981 Estimate

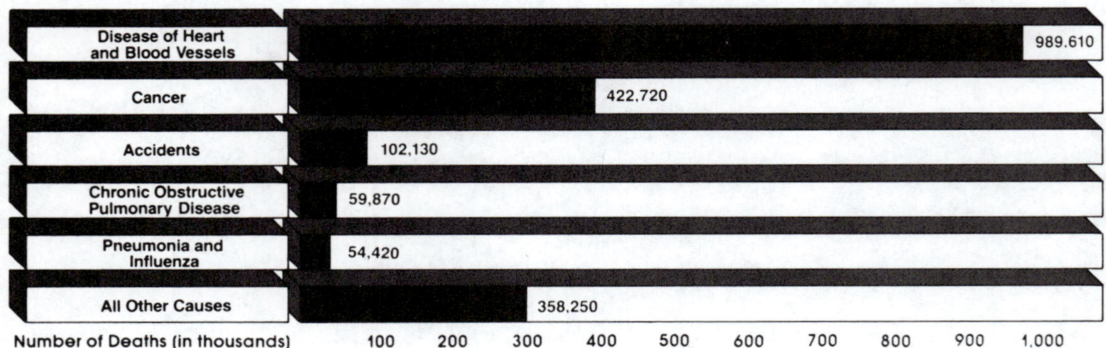

Source: National Center for Health Statistics, U.S. Public Health Service, DHHS

15-1 Cardiovascular disease

VITAL STATISTICS

- 42.75 million Americans have one or more forms of heart or blood vessel disease.
- Stroke killed 164,300 in 1981; victims of aftereffects number 1.87 million.
- As many as 1.5 million Americans may have a heart attack this year and about 550,000 of them will die.
- High blood pressure afflicts an estimated 37.33 million American adults.
- 1.91 million adults and 100,000 children in America have rheumatic heart disease.
- The economic cost of cardiovascular disease will amount to an estimated $64.4 billion in 1984 (includes physician and nursing services, hospital and nursing home services, cost of medications, and lost income due to disability).

Estimated Deaths Due to Cardiovascular Diseases by Major Type of Disorder

United States: 1981 Estimate

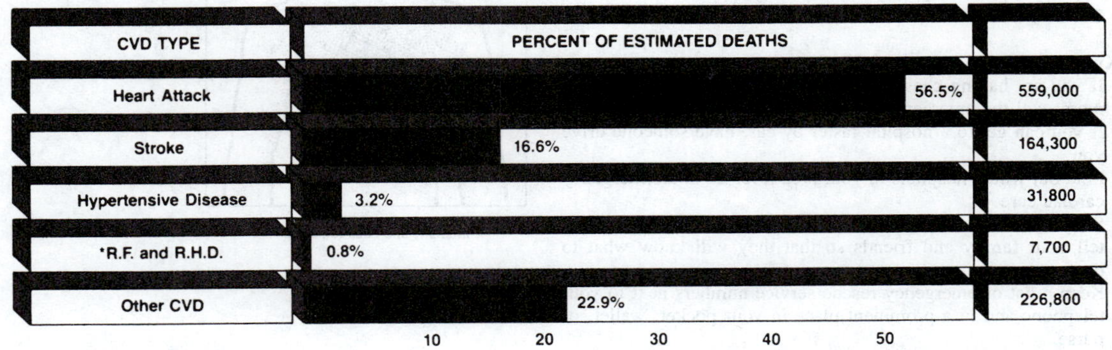

*Rheumatic Fever and Rheumatic Heart Disease

Source: National Center for Health Statistics, U.S. Public Health Service, DHHS

Estimated Economic Costs in Billions of Dollars of Cardiovascular Diseases by Type of Expenditure

United States: 1984 Estimate

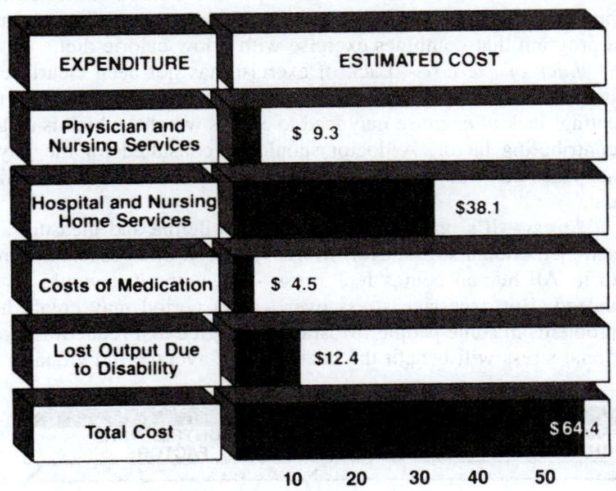

Source: American Heart Association

The costs illustrated in this chart are for physician and nursing services, hospital and nursing home facilities and medications, as well as the lost occupational output as a result of disability.

Estimated Prevalence of the Major Cardiovascular Disease

United States: 1981 Estimate

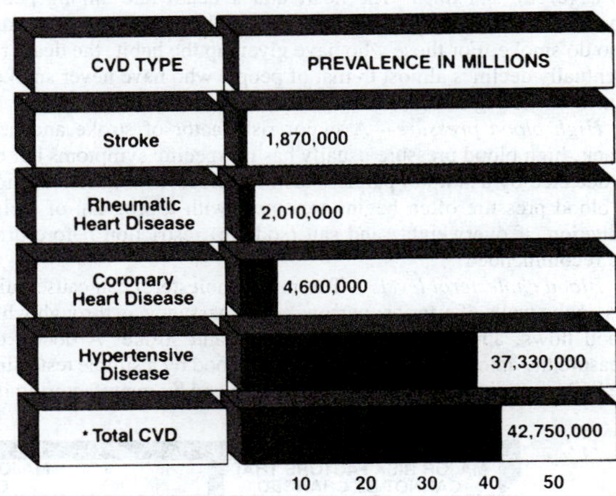

Source: American Heart Association

*The sum of the individual estimates exceeds 42,750,000 since many persons have more than one cardiovascular disorder.

HEART ATTACK—SIGNALS AND ACTION

Know the warning signals of a heart attack.

- Uncomfortable pressure, fullness, squeezing or pain in the center of your chest, lasting 2 minutes or more.
- Pain may spread to shoulders, neck, or arms.
- Severe pain, dizziness, fainting, sweating, nausea, or shortness of breath may also occur.
- Not all these signals, however, are always present. **Don't wait.** Get help immediately.

Know what to do in case of an emergency.

- If you are having chest discomfort that lasts for 2 minutes or more, call the emergency rescue service.
- If you can get to a hospital faster by car, have someone drive you.
- Find out which hospitals in your area offer 24-hour emergency cardiac care.
- Select in advance the facility nearest your home and office and tell your family and friends so that they will know what to do.
- Keep a list of emergency rescue service numbers next to your telephone and in a prominent place in your pocket, wallet, or purse.

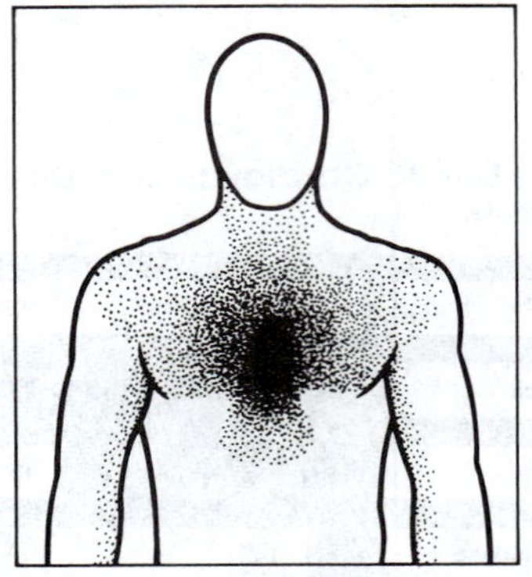

Intensity and Location of Pain

RISK FACTORS OF HEART DISEASE

Major risk factors that cannot be changed

Heredity—It appears that a tendency toward heart disease or atherosclerosis is hereditary.

Sex—Men have a greater risk of heart attack than women. Even after menopause, when women's death rate increases, it never reaches that of men.

Race—Black Americans have almost a 45% greater chance of having high blood pressure (a contributor to heart attack and stroke) than whites.

Age—Nearly one in four heart attack deaths occurs before age 65.

Major risk factors that can be changed.

Cigarette smoking—The heart attack death rate among people who do not smoke cigarettes is considerably lower than for people who do smoke. For those who have given up the habit, the death rate eventually declines almost to that of people who have never smoked. Don't smoke cigarettes.

High blood pressure—A major risk factor of stroke and heart attack, high blood pressure usually has no specific symptoms but can be detected by a simple, painless test. A person with mild elevations of blood pressure often begins treatment with a program of weight reduction, if overweight, and salt (sodium) restriction before drugs are recommended.

Blood cholesterol levels—Too much cholesterol can cause buildups on the walls of arteries, narrowing the passageway through which blood flows, and leading to heart attack and stroke. A doctor can measure the amount of cholesterol in the blood by a simple test. Since the body gets cholesterol both through diet and by manufacturing it, a diet low in saturated fat and cholesterol will help lower the level of blood cholesterol if it is too high. Medications also are available to maintain cholesterol levels within the normal range.

Diabetes—Diabetes appears most frequently during middle age, more often in people who are overweight. In its mild form, diabetes can escape detection for many years, but it can sharply increase a person's risk of heart attack, making control of other risk factors even more important. A doctor can detect diabetes and prescribe changes in eating habits, weight-control and exercise programs, and drugs, if necessary, to keep it in check.

Contributing factors

Obesity—In most cases, obesity simply results from eating too much and exercising too little. It places a heavy burden on your heart. In addition, obesity is associated with coronary heart disease primarily because of its influence on blood pressure, blood cholesterol, and precipitating diabetes. To reduce weight, doctors usually recommend a program that combines exercise with a low-calorie diet.

Lack of exercise—Lack of exercise has not been clearly established as a risk factor for heart attack. But when combined with overeating, lack of exercise may lead to excess weight, which is clearly a contributing factor. A doctor should be consulted for the physical activities that best suit the age and physical condition of the individual.

Stress—It's practically impossible to define and measure a person's emotional stress level. Moreover, each of us reacts differently to it. All human beings feel stress—life without it would be dull, indeed. But excessive stress over a long period may create health problems in some people. Most doctors agree that reduction of emotional stress will benefit the health of the average individual.

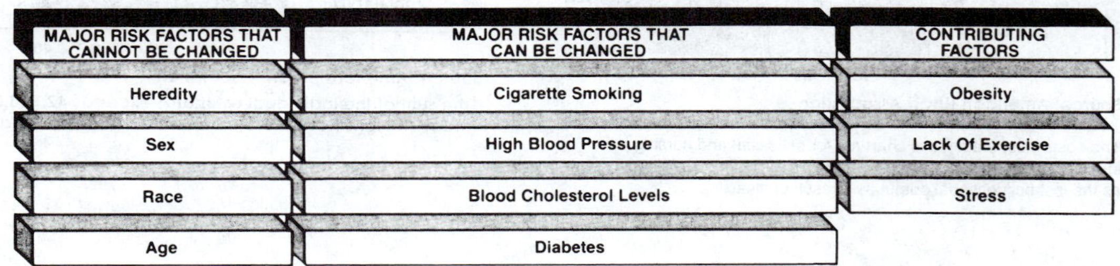

MAJOR RISK FACTORS THAT CANNOT BE CHANGED	MAJOR RISK FACTORS THAT CAN BE CHANGED	CONTRIBUTING FACTORS
Heredity	Cigarette Smoking	Obesity
Sex	High Blood Pressure	Lack Of Exercise
Race	Blood Cholesterol Levels	Stress
Age	Diabetes	

WARNING SIGNALS OF STROKE

Know the warning signals of stroke.

- Sudden, temporary weakness or numbness of the face, arm, and leg on one side of the body.
- Temporary loss of speech, or trouble in speaking or understanding speech.
- Temporary dimness or loss of vision, particularly in one eye.
- Unexplained dizziness, unsteadiness, or sudden falls.

Many major strokes are preceded by "little strokes," warning signals like the above, experienced days, weeks, or months before the more severe event.

Prompt medical or surgical attention to these symptoms may prevent a fatal or disabling stroke from occurring.

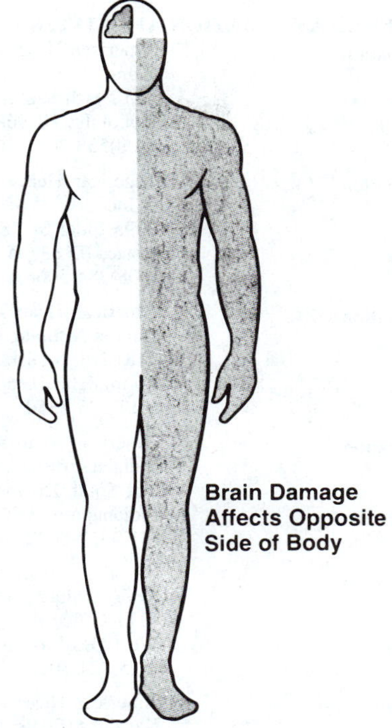

RISK FACTORS OF STROKE

Some of the factors that increase the risk of stroke are congenital, whereas others result from the hazards of life. Some of these factors can be minimized by the individual and with a doctor's help. Other factors cannot be changed.

Risk factors that cannot be changed

Sex—The risk of stroke is greater in men than in women. However, in women who take oral contraceptives the risk of stroke is slightly increased. Women who are also heavy smokers may aggravate this risk further.

Race—The risk of death and disability from stroke is much greater among black Americans than among white Americans. This may be a result of the greater prevalence of high blood pressure among blacks.

Risk factors that can be changed

High blood pressure—The control of high blood pressure will reduce the risk of stroke.

High red blood cell count—A marked increase, as well as a moderate elevation, in the red blood cell count may be a risk factor of stroke.

Heart disease—A diseased heart increases the risk of stroke in two ways: as a failing pump and as a source of emboli, clots that form in the heart and could travel to the arteries leading to the brain and cause a blockage. Good management of heart disease reduces the risk of stroke.

Diabetes mellitus—The risk of stroke is increased in diabetic individuals.

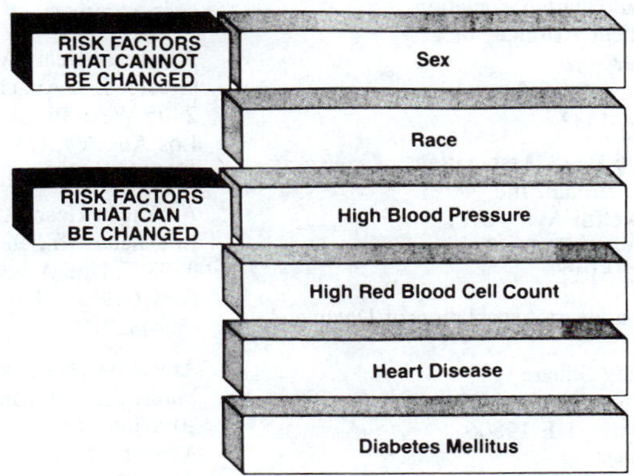

THE AMERICAN HEART ASSOCIATION AFFILIATES

American Heart Association
Alabama Affiliate, Inc.
1449 Medical Park Dr.
Birmingham, AL 35213
(205)592-7100

American Heart Association
Alaska Affiliate, Inc.
2330 East 42nd St.
Anchorage, AK 99508
(907)563-3111

American Heart Association
Arizona Affiliate, Inc.
1445 East Thomas
Phoenix, AZ 85014
(602)277-4846

American Heart Association
Arkansas Affiliate, Inc.
909 West 2nd St.
Little Rock, AR 72201
(501)375-9148

American Heart Association
California Affiliate, Inc.
805 Burlway Rd.
Burlingame, CA 94010
(415)342-5522

Chicago Heart Association
20 N. Wacker Dr.
Chicago, IL 60606
(312)346-4675

Colorado Heart Association
4521 East Virginia Ave.
Denver, CO 80222
(303)399-2131

American Heart Association
Connecticut Affiliate, Inc.
71 Parker Ave.
Meriden, CT 06450
(203)634-4532

American Heart Association
Dakota Affiliate, Inc.
1005 Twelfth Ave., S.E.
Jamestown, ND 58401
(701)252-5122

American Heart Association of Delaware, Inc.
4C Trolley Square
Delaware Ave. and DuPont St.
Wilmington, DE 19806
(302)654-5269

American Heart Association
Florida Affiliate, Inc.
810 63rd Ave., N.
St. Petersburg, FL 33702
(813)522-9477

American Heart Association
Georgia Affiliate, Inc.
Level C. Broadview Plaza
2581 Piedmont Rd., N.E.
Atlanta, GA 30324
(404)261-2260

American Heart Association of Hawaii, Inc.
245 North Kukui St.
Honolulu, HI 96817
(808)538-7021

American Heart Association of Idaho, Inc.
3295 Elder St., Suite 140
Boise, ID 83705
(208)384-5066

American Heart Association
Illinois Affiliate, Inc.
1181 North Dirksen Pkwy
Springfield, IL 62708
(217)525-1350

American Heart Association
Indiana Affiliate, Inc.
222 South Downey, Suite 222
Indianapolis, IN 46219
(317)357-8622

American Heart Association
Iowa Affiliate, Inc.
1111 Office Park Rd.
West Des Moines, IA 50265
(515)224-1025

American Heart Association
Kansas Affiliate, Inc.
5229 West 7th St.
Topeka, KA 66606
(913)272-7056

American Heart Association
Kentucky Affiliate, Inc.
207 Speed Building
Louisville, KY 40202
(502)587-8641

American Heart Association
Greater Los Angeles Affiliate, Inc.
2405 West 8th St.
Los Angeles, CA 90057
(213)385-4231

American Heart Association
Louisiana Affiliate, Inc.
3303 Tulane Ave.
New Orleans, LA 70119
(504)827-1644

American Heart Association
Maine Affiliate, Inc.
20 Winter St.
Augusta, ME 04330
(207)623-8432

American Heart Association
Maryland Affiliate, Inc.
415 N. Charles St.
Baltimore, MD 21203
(301)685-7074

American Heart Association
Massachusetts Affiliate, Inc.
33 Fourth Ave.
Needham Heights, MA 02194
(617)449-5931

American Heart Association of Michigan
16310 West Twelve Mile Rd.
Lathrup Village, MI 48076
(313)557-9500

American Heart Association
Minnesota Affiliate, Inc.
7401 West 77th St.
Minneapolis, MN 55435
(612)835-3300

American Heart Association
Mississippi Affiliate, Inc.
4830 East McWillie Circle
Jackson, MS 39236
(601)981-4721

American Heart Association
Missouri Affiliate, Inc.
105 East Ash, Suite 2
Columbia, MO 65201
(314)442-3193

American Heart Association
Montana Affiliate, Inc.
Professional Building
510 1st Ave., N.
Great Falls, MT 59401
(406)452-2362

American Heart Association
Nation's Capital Affiliate
2233 Wisconsin Ave., N.W.
Washington, DC 20007
(202)337-6400

American Heart Association
Nebraska Affiliate, Inc.
3642 Farnam
Omaha, NE 68131
(402)346-0771

American Heart Association
Nevada Affiliate, Inc.
1135 Terminal Way
Suites 104 & 105
Reno, NV 89502
(702)322-2977

American Heart Association
New Hampshire Affiliate, Inc.
2 Industrial Park Dr.
Concord, NH 03301
(603)224-7461

American Heart Association
New Jersey Affiliate, Inc.
1525 Morris Ave.
Union, NJ 07083
(201)688-4540

American Heart Association
New Mexico Affiliate, Inc.
629 Truman N.E.
Albuquerque, NM 87110
(505)268-3711

American Heart Association
New York State Affiliate, Inc.
214 South Warren St., 8th Floor
Syracuse, NY 13202
(315)478-6681

New York Heart Association, Inc.
205 East 42nd St.
New York, NY 10017
(212)661-5335

American Heart Association
North Carolina Affiliate, Inc.
One Heart Circle
Chapel Hill, NC 27514
(919)968-4453

American Heart Association
Northeast Ohio Affiliate, Inc.
1689 East 115th St.
Cleveland, OH 44106
(216)791-7500

American Heart Association
Ohio Affiliate, Inc.
6161 Busch Blvd., Suite 327
Columbus, OH 43229
(614)436-0958

American Heart Association
Oklahoma Affiliate, Inc.
2915 North Classen
Suite 220
Oklahoma City, OK 73106
(405)521-9838

American Heart Association
Oregon Affiliate, Inc.
1500 S.W. 12th Ave.
Portland, OR 97201
(503)226-2575

American Heart Association
Pennsylvania Affiliate, Inc.
2743 North Front St.
Harrisburg, PA 17110
(717)238-0895

Puerto Rico Heart Association
Cabo Alverio 554
Hato Rey
Puerto Rico 00918
(809)763-8275, (809)751-6595,
(809)751-6363

American Heart Association
Rhode Island Affiliate, Inc.
40 Broad St.
Pawtucket, RI 02860
(401)728-5300

American Heart Association
South Carolina Affiliate, Inc.
5868 Percival Rd.
Columbia, SC 29260
(803)738-9540

American Heart Association
Tennessee Affiliate, Inc.
101 23rd Ave., N.
Nashville, TN 37203
(615)320-0390

American Heart Association
Texas Affiliate, Inc.
1700 Rutherford Ln.
Austin, TX 78761
(512)836-7220

Utah Heart Association
645E-400S
Salt Lake City, UT 84102
(801)322-5601

American Heart Association
Vermont Affiliate, Inc.
2821 Shelburne Rd.
Shelburne, VT 05482
(802)985-8048

American Heart Association
Virginia Affiliate, Inc.
4217 Park Place Ct.
Glen Allen, VA 23060
(804)747-8334

American Heart Association of
Washington
4414 Woodland Park Ave., N.
Seattle, WA 98103
(206)632-6881

American Heart Association
West Virginia Affiliate, Inc.
211 35th St., S.E.
Charleston, WV 25304
(304)346-5381

American Heart Association
Wisconsin Affiliate, Inc.
795 North Van Buren St.
Milwaukee, WI 53202
(414)271-9999

American Heart Association of
Wyoming, Inc.
2015 Central Ave.
Cheyenne, WY 82001
(307)632-1746

15-2 Cancer

Cancer around the world, 1978-1979 (Age-adjusted death rates per 100,000 population for selected sites for 48 countries)*

Country	All sites		Oral		Colon and rectum	
	Male	*Female*	*Male*	*Female*	*Male*	*Female*
United States†	216.9 (18)	137.7 (19)	5.8 (14)	1.9 (7)	26.5 (15)	20.2 (15)
Argentina†	215.9 (19)	139.3 (17)	4.5 (22)	0.8 (38)	20.5 (24)	17.5 (21)
Australia	212.4 (21)	125.4 (29)	5.4 (18)	1.7 (10)	28.4 (11)	21.8 (10)
Austria	247.3 (9)	147.6 (12)	5.5 (17)	0.8 (38)	32.8 (3)	21.6 (12)
Barbados‡	179.0 (30)	136.1 (21)	9.1 (7)	1.4 (19)	5.3 (41)	14.4 (27)
Bulgaria	156.3 (38)	102.6 (37)	2.5 (38)	0.9 (34)	14.4 (31)	11.1 (33)
Canada†	214.9 (20)	136.3 (20)	6.0 (13)	1.7 (10)	29.7 (9)	23.1 (8)
Chile	191.3 (26)	148.5 (10)	3.5 (30)	0.7 (43)	9.6 (35)	9.9 (36)
Costa Rica	178.6 (31)	138.3 (18)	3.4 (31)	1.1 (27)	7.7 (37)	8.5 (38)
Cuba†	172.1 (34)	119.1 (31)	9.2 (6)	2.2 (6)	13.4 (32)	15.1 (25)
Denmark	233.3 (13)	172.3 (1)	4.0 (26)	1.9 (7)	34.0 (1)	26.1 (2)
Dominican Rep.†	53.7 (45)	48.1 (45)	1.9 (43)	1.6 (16)	4.3 (43)	3.7 (42)
Ecuador†	87.3 (42)	86.9 (40)	1.2 (46)	0.6 (45)	3.1 (44)	3.9 (41)
Egypt†	39.0 (47)	18.8 (48)	0.6 (47)	0.2 (47)	2.1 (45)	1.1 (47)
England & Wales	248.7 (8)	156.9 (5)	3.6 (29)	1.7 (10)	28.4 (11)	21.7 (11)
Fiji†	54.0 (44)	79.8 (41)	1.8 (44)	3.4 (3)	4.7 (42)	3.0 (43)
Finland†	243.9 (10)	113.9 (32)	3.7 (28)	1.4 (19)	15.7 (27)	13.3 (28)
France†	255.7 (6)	120.8 (30)	18.3 (2)	1.4 (19)	27.5 (13)	18.1 (20)
Germany, F.R.	242.0 (11)	152.0 (8)	4.1 (24)	0.9 (34)	31.3 (5)	23.9 (7)
Greece	188.3 (28)	103.6 (36)	2.2 (40)	0.8 (38)	8.3 (36)	7.7 (40)
Guatemala†	68.6 (43)	78.8 (42)	2.2 (40)	1.0 (30)	2.0 (46)	2.5 (44)
Hong Kong	235.2 (12)	125.5 (28)	20.3 (1)	7.2 (1)	19.2 (25)	12.8 (29)
Hungary	269.3 (3)	162.6 (3)	8.2 (8)	1.6 (16)	30.5 (7)	23.0 (9)
Iceland	150.7 (39)	140.7 (16)	2.0 (42)	2.6 (4)	16.2 (26)	15.1 (25)
Ireland†	219.0 (17)	158.8 (4)	5.7 (16)	1.7 (10)	32.0 (4)	26.0 (3)
Israel	174.7 (32)	145.9 (13)	1.7 (45)	0.9 (34)	22.7 (22)	18.2 (17)
Italy	228.5 (15)	126.0 (27)	7.3 (11)	1.1 (27)	23.5 (21)	17.5 (21)
Japan	190.0 (27)	109.3 (33)	2.4 (39)	0.8 (38)	15.5 (29)	11.4 (32)
Luxembourg	269.0 (4)	148.3 (11)	9.7 (5)	0.3 (46)	31.3 (5)	26.4 (4)
Mauritius	100.0 (41)	71.6 (44)	4.1 (24)	0.7 (43)	5.7 (40)	2.5 (44)
Netherlands	266.2 (5)	144.8 (14)	2.6 (36)	1.0 (30)	26.4 (16)	21.3 (14)
New Zealand	172.0 (35)	154.4 (7)	4.9 (19)	1.7 (10)	33.3 (2)	29.5 (1)
Nicaragua†	22.9 (48)	35.9 (46)	0.0 (48)	0.0 (48)	0.1 (48)	0.5 (48)
Northern Ireland†	226.0 (16)	151.7 (9)	3.3 (33)	1.8 (9)	28.5 (10)	24.1 (6)
Norway	193.8 (25)	130.4 (23)	3.1 (34)	1.1 (27)	24.0 (19)	19.7 (16)
Poland	214.2 (22)	126.2 (26)	5.8 (14)	1.3 (23)	15.2 (30)	11.7 (31)
Portugal	180.1 (29)	108.0 (34)	6.6 (12)	1.3 (23)	22.4 (23)	17.3 (24)
Puerto Rico‡	157.3 (37)	95.1 (39)	10.0 (4)	1.6 (16)	6.4 (39)	7.9 (39)
Romania†	161.7 (36)	106.0 (35)	3.8 (27)	1.0 (30)	10.2 (34)	9.0 (37)
Scotland	275.0 (1)	172.0 (2)	4.2 (23)	1.7 (10)	30.4 (8)	24.6 (4)
Singapore	249.6 (7)	130.4 (23)	16.9 (3)	5.8 (2)	23.9 (20)	18.2 (17)
Spain†	194.9 (24)	75.1 (43)	4.6 (21)	0.8 (38)	15.7 (27)	12.8 (29)
Sweden	198.0 (23)	141.2 (15)	3.4 (31)	1.4 (19)	24.2 (18)	18.2 (17)
Switzerland	230.3 (14)	134.2 (22)	7.6 (9)	1.3 (23)	25.8 (17)	17.5 (21)
Thailand	46.2 (46)	30.4 (47)	2.6 (36)	1.3 (23)	1.9 (47)	1.2 (46)
Uruguay†	271.8 (2)	156.2 (6)	7.6 (9)	1.0 (30)	27.0 (14)	21.4 (13)
Venezuela†	135.0 (40)	128.9 (25)	3.1 (34)	2.6 (4)	7.1 (38)	10.1 (35)
Yugoslavia†	172.7 (33)	102.4 (38)	4.8 (20)	0.9 (34)	13.1 (33)	10.2 (34)

*NOTE: Figures in parentheses are order of rank within site and sex group: †1978 only; ‡1979 only; NA, Not available. Source of data: World Health Statistics Annual 1980-1982.

From American Cancer Society, Inc.: Cancer Facts and Figures, 1984.

Lung		*Breast*	*Uterus*	*Stomach*		*Prostate*	*Leukemia*	
Male	*Female*	*Female*	*Female*	*Male*	*Female*	*Male*	*Male*	*Female*
70.3 (9)	19.0 (5)	27.1 (14)	8.4 (37)	8.6 (43)	4.3 (44)	22.9 (13)	8.7 (7)	5.2 (6)
54.9 (22)	9.5 (16)	24.7 (16)	14.7 (12)	23.5 (26)	11.6 (26)	18.9 (24)	6.0 (28)	4.4 (24)
62.0 (18)	11.5 (14)	23.2 (20)	7.5 (39)	14.9 (39)	7.2 (40)	22.2 (16)	7.7 (17)	4.6 (21)
66.8 (12)	9.3 (17)	23.2 (20)	14.2 (14)	36.8 (8)	18.5 (10)	22.5 (15)	7.3 (21)	4.8 (17)
12.6 (41)	5.8 (34)	27.4 (12)	30.0 (1)	33.7 (11)	12.4 (23)	41.0 (1)	8.9 (3)	1.4 (45)
43.6 (26)	7.4 (25)	15.8 (30)	9.4 (30)	33.4 (12)	20.5 (7)	9.0 (38)	5.2 (35)	4.0 (31)
65.5 (13)	14.2 (11)	27.8 (11)	8.5 (35)	14.4 (40)	6.7 (42)	21.9 (18)	8.4 (8)	5.1 (10)
24.9 (36)	6.8 (30)	14.1 (35)	21.3 (5)	61.8 (3)	28.3 (3)	16.5 (29)	4.4 (38)	4.0 (31)
15.6 (40)	7.1 (27)	9.9 (38)	18.5 (7)	62.1 (2)	33.5 (1)	14.8 (31)	7.1 (22)	6.3 (1)
50.1 (24)	16.6 (8)	17.9 (25)	17.6 (9)	13.1 (41)	7.1 (41)	23.3 (11)	5.7 (30)	4.1 (30)
68.6 (11)	17.2 (7)	30.6 (6)	14.4 (13)	18.5 (34)	10.2 (31)	23.2 (12)	9.0 (2)	5.7 (2)
5.6 (44)	3.0 (44)	4.1 (44)	8.8 (34)	4.3 (44)	2.2 (45)	8.6 (39)	2.1 (44)	1.5 (44)
5.9 (43)	2.3 (45)	6.0 (42)	23.0 (4)	31.8 (14)	20.5 (7)	10.5 (37)	2.9 (41)	2.5 (41)
2.5 (47)	1.1 (47)	3.4 (45)	2.0 (47)	1.9 (46)	1.1 (46)	1.5 (46)	2.3 (43)	1.4 (45)
95.7 (3)	20.7 (4)	33.8 (1)	10.2 (26)	24.0 (25)	11.4 (27)	18.3 (25)	7.0 (23)	4.5 (22)
4.0 (45)	5.7 (35)	7.9 (40)	28.5 (2)	9.5 (42)	4.9 (43)	3.3 (45)	2.4 (42)	5.2 (6)
86.5 (5)	6.5 (31)	17.6 (26)	8.1 (38)	30.7 (16)	15.0 (18)	24.0 (8)	8.8 (5)	4.3 (25)
51.8 (23)	4.9 (41)	21.9 (24)	10.7 (25)	18.0 (35)	8.6 (37)	22.0 (17)	8.9 (3)	5.3 (3)
36.0 (29)	7.2 (26)	25.3 (15)	11.5 (19)	30.6 (17)	16.3 (12)	23.9 (9)	7.8 (15)	5.2 (6)
58.5 (21)	8.8 (18)	16.2 (29)	7.3 (41)	17.3 (36)	9.8 (33)	11.0 (36)	8.4 (8)	4.7 (20)
2.7 (46)	2.0 (46)	2.7 (46)	12.6 (16)	21.6 (29)	18.9 (9)	4.9 (41)	1.5 (47)	1.1 (47)
68.9 (10)	30.9 (1)	10.7 (37)	8.5 (35)	19.6 (32)	9.1 (36)	3.7 (44)	5.5 (31)	3.9 (34)
72.5 (7)	12.1 (13)	24.6 (17)	18.3 (8)	44.6 (4)	20.9 (4)	24.2 (7)	7.7 (17)	5.2 (6)
28.3 (34)	16.5 (9)	27.2 (13)	6.6 (44)	26.3 (21)	12.9 (22)	14.0 (33)	9.6 (1)	3.7 (36)
60.5 (20)	17.8 (6)	32.1 (4)	7.3 (41)	21.7 (27)	14.4 (19)	23.9 (9)	6.3 (25)	4.5 (22)
32.9 (31)	10.5 (15)	28.3 (10)	6.5 (45)	15.9 (38)	9.8 (33)	13.1 (34)	8.8 (5)	4.8 (17)
61.8 (19)	7.1 (27)	22.3 (23)	11.4 (21)	31.3 (15)	15.7 (15)	15.8 (30)	8.0 (12)	5.1 (10)
31.2 (33)	8.8 (18)	6.0 (42)	9.3 (31)	66.1 (1)	31.2 (2)	3.9 (42)	4.8 (37)	3.2 (39)
87.5 (4)	8.6 (20)	24.4 (18)	13.0 (15)	26.9 (20)	12.1 (25)	20.7 (20)	7.9 (14)	5.3 (3)
21.2 (37)	5.2 (39)	6.6 (41)	10.5 (23)	21.4 (30)	9.6 (35)	5.4 (40)	1.9 (45)	1.8 (42)
101.2 (2)	6.8 (30)	31.9 (5)	9.0 (33)	25.5 (22)	11.3 (29)	24.3 (6)	8.2 (10)	5.3 (3)
64.4 (14)	16.1 (10)	30.0 (7)	9.8 (28)	16.9 (37)	7.5 (39)	22.7 (14)	7.6 (19)	5.0 (13)
1.4 (48)	0.0 (48)	0.0 (48)	0.4 (48)	0.1 (47)	0.5 (48)	0.0 (48)	1.6 (46)	1.8 (42)
74.0 (6)	14.2 (11)	32.5 (3)	7.5 (39)	24.8 (23)	14.1 (20)	19.3 (23)	8.1 (11)	4.9 (15)
31.7 (32)	6.3 (33)	23.6 (19)	10.2 (26)	21.1 (31)	10.6 (30)	31.1 (3)	7.8 (15)	4.9 (15)
63.6 (16)	7.9 (23)	16.6 (28)	15.0 (11)	41.0 (5)	16.2 (14)	12.2 (35)	6.6 (24)	4.2 (28)
25.4 (35)	4.2 (42)	17.6 (26)	12.3 (17)	40.6 (6)	20.9 (4)	21.8 (19)	6.3 (25)	4.3 (25)
19.2 (39)	5.6 (37)	9.2 (39)	7.3 (41)	NA	8.5 (38)	17.6 (26)	5.1 (36)	4.3 (25)
38.3 (28)	7.0 (29)	14.2 (34)	18.7 (6)	35.4 (9)	15.7 (15)	20.2 (21)	5.3 (33)	3.4 (38)
113.2 (1)	27.5 (2)	33.2 (2)	9.8 (28)	24.5 (24)	12.3 (24)	17.4 (27)	6.3 (25)	4.2 (28)
71.9 (8)	21.2 (3)	15.5 (32)	11.3 (22)	39.6 (7)	16.3 (12)	3.9 (42)	4.4 (38)	4.0 (31)
41.2 (27)	5.0 (40)	15.8 (30)	9.5 (29)	28.7 (18)	15.4 (17)	19.4 (22)	5.4 (32)	3.9 (34)
34.3 (30)	8.5 (21)	22.9 (22)	9.1 (32)	19.1 (33)	10.0 (32)	31.8 (2)	8.0 (12)	5.1 (10)
62.6 (17)	5.8 (34)	29.5 (8)	10.8 (24)	21.7 (27)	11.4 (27)	27.7 (4)	7.4 (20)	4.8 (17)
6.5 (42)	4.2 (42)	1.2 (47)	4.2 (46)	2.1 (45)	0.8 (47)	0.2 (47)	0.7 (48)	0.5 (48)
63.9 (15)	5.5 (38)	29.2 (9)	15.2 (10)	32.6 (13)	16.8 (11)	27.6 (5)	5.8 (29)	5.0 (13)
20.4 (38)	8.3 (22)	11.5 (36)	27.7 (3)	34.0 (10)	20.7 (6)	16.8 (28)	5.3 (33)	3.6 (37)
44.3 (25)	7.6 (24)	14.5 (33)	11.8 (18)	27.9 (19)	13.8 (21)	14.7 (32)	3.9 (40)	2.8 (40)

Estimated cancer deaths for all sites plus major sites, by state—1984

State	*All sites*		*Major sites*								
	Number of deaths	*Death rate per 100,000 population*	*Female breast*	*Colon-rectum*	*Lung*	*Oral*	*Uterus*	*Prostate*	*Stomach*	*Pancreas*	*Leukemia*
Alabama	7,600	191	500	800	2,400	125	200	425	200	375	300
Alaska	300	68	20	30	100	5	10	10	10	10	10
Arizona	5,200	174	325	600	1,500	100	50	250	125	225	175
Arkansas	4,800	210	325	550	1,600	100	100	300	150	275	225
California	45,000	176	3,700	5,600	12,300	850	900	2,400	1,500	2,400	1,700
Colorado	4,000	127	325	550	1,000	70	70	250	125	225	175
Connecticut	6,800	213	650	900	1,600	175	125	350	250	350	275
Delaware	1,300	215	80	200	325	25	20	60	30	60	40
Dist. of Columbia	1,600	261	175	200	375	75	60	100	60	100	40
Florida	27,300	244	1,900	3,400	7,800	450	400	1,600	800	1,400	850
Georgia	9,300	159	650	950	2,900	200	250	500	225	425	350
Hawaii	1,300	128	75	150	300	30	20	50	90	60	50
Idaho	1,500	151	100	150	300	25	25	90	40	70	70
Illinois	22,800	197	2,000	3,200	5,900	500	600	1,200	750	1,200	900
Indiana	10,700	198	900	1,500	3,000	200	300	550	250	500	425
Iowa	5,800	203	500	1,000	1,600	100	125	400	150	325	300
Kansas	4,700	193	425	600	1,500	100	100	300	125	250	200
Kentucky	7,200	197	475	900	2,400	175	175	400	150	375	275
Louisiana	7,800	170	550	800	2,300	175	175	450	250	400	300
Maine	2,500	217	200	350	650	50	60	150	90	125	80
Maryland	8,800	201	700	1,200	2,500	200	175	450	225	400	275
Massachusetts	12,700	217	1,200	1,900	3,200	325	275	650	500	650	450
Michigan	16,600	182	1,400	2,100	4,400	325	400	950	475	800	650
Minnesota	7,400	179	650	1,000	1,800	150	125	500	250	425	350
Mississippi	4,700	184	300	500	1,400	90	100	350	125	275	200
Missouri	10,600	212	800	1,400	2,800	200	250	600	275	475	400
Montana	1,400	173	100	175	350	30	30	125	50	80	60
Nebraska	3,300	207	275	500	800	60	70	225	125	175	175
Nevada	1,400	144	80	150	400	25	20	50	10	60	30
New Hampshire	2,000	205	150	300	425	40	40	90	40	80	70
New Jersey	16,800	224	1,600	2,400	4,300	350	375	850	650	800	550
New Mexico	1,900	136	125	200	375	25	40	90	50	100	60
New York	38,000	215	4,000	5,800	9,200	850	950	1,900	1,600	2,100	1,400
North Carolina	10,800	176	750	1,200	2,800	225	275	650	250	475	400
North Dakota	1,200	179	90	175	225	20	20	90	60	80	50
Ohio	21,900	204	1,900	3,100	5,800	425	600	1,200	650	1,100	800
Oklahoma	6,100	185	400	800	1,800	100	100	350	150	300	250
Oregon	5,200	193	375	550	1,600	100	75	325	125	275	200
Pennsylvania	27,500	232	2,400	4,300	6,600	500	700	1,400	850	1,400	950
Rhode Island	2,500	259	250	400	600	60	40	150	100	100	70
South Carolina	5,100	155	375	550	1,500	100	125	325	125	275	175
South Dakota	1,400	208	100	200	300	20	30	100	50	100	80
Tennessee	8,800	189	600	950	2,600	200	200	475	225	450	325
Texas	22,900	141	1,700	2,500	6,400	425	500	1,300	700	1,200	1,000
Utah	1,600	96	150	175	225	20	30	100	50	75	70
Vermont	1,100	208	80	150	275	20	30	70	30	50	40
Virginia	9,100	160	750	1,100	2,800	175	225	500	250	425	325
Washington	7,700	174	600	950	2,200	150	150	425	200	400	300
West Virginia	4,100	209	275	475	1,200	75	100	225	100	200	150
Wisconsin	9,200	192	900	1,300	2,100	175	175	600	325	475	375
Wyoming	700	128	50	70	175	10	10	50	15	50	30
United States	450,000	191	37,000	59,000	121,000	9,000	10,000	25,000	14,000	23,000	17,000
Puerto Rico	3,000	94	125	125	300	175	150	225	400	100	150

Estimated new cancer cases for all sites plus major sites, by state—1984*

State	All sites†	Major sites								
	Number of cases	Female breast	Colon-rectum	Lung	Oral	Uterus	Prostate	Stomach	Pancreas	Leukemia
Alabama	14,600	1,600	1,700	2,600	350	1,100	1,200	350	425	425
Alaska	600	50	50	125	15	30	25	20	10	20
Arizona	9,600	1,200	1,500	1,600	275	550	800	200	250	225
Arkansas	9,200	1,000	1,200	1,600	300	650	900	200	300	300
California	87,000	11,800	12,200	14,000	2,600	4,800	7,400	2,700	2,600	2,400
Colorado	7,800	1,000	1,200	1,100	175	400	550	200	250	250
Connecticut	13,200	2,200	2,000	1,900	450	800	1,200	400	400	400
Delaware	2,500	300	375	400	70	150	150	60	50	40
Dist. of Columbia	3,200	450	400	450	200	300	325	100	100	60
Florida	52,500	6,300	7,500	9,000	1,600	2,800	4,900	1,300	1,400	1,300
Georgia	17,500	1,900	2,100	3,200	600	1,200	1,700	400	450	500
Hawaii	2,400	325	325	375	100	125	150	200	60	70
Idaho	2,800	475	300	375	75	200	275	70	80	100
Illinois	44,000	6,000	6,800	7,000	1,500	2,700	3,600	1,400	1,300	1,200
Indiana	20,500	2,700	3,300	3,400	500	1,800	1,600	450	550	550
Iowa	11,300	1,500	2,400	1,700	300	800	1,200	300	350	400
Kansas	8,800	1,200	1,300	1,600	275	700	800	200	300	300
Kentucky	13,800	1,400	1,900	2,800	425	950	1,200	300	375	400
Louisiana	15,000	1,700	1,800	2,500	550	950	1,300	400	400	400
Maine	4,900	600	800	800	150	350	400	150	150	100
Maryland	17,000	2,500	2,500	2,700	650	1,100	1,500	400	400	400
Massachusetts	24,500	3,600	4,100	3,500	900	1,500	2,100	850	650	650
Michigan	32,500	4,300	4,700	5,200	950	2,200	3,000	900	850	900
Minnesota	14,200	2,000	2,300	1,900	375	800	1,600	500	450	475
Mississippi	9,100	850	1,100	1,600	250	600	1,100	275	300	300
Missouri	20,500	2,400	3,200	3,300	550	1,400	1,900	500	550	600
Montana	2,700	300	400	400	80	150	375	80	80	80
Nebraska	6,000	750	1,100	900	150	350	500	175	225	225
Nevada	2,700	325	325	500	60	150	150	20	60	40
New Hampshire	3,700	475	650	500	100	225	275	75	90	125
New Jersey	32,500	4,700	5,200	5,000	1,100	2,100	2,600	1,200	900	800
New Mexico	3,700	425	475	475	60	250	325	90	90	70
New York	74,500	11,600	12,600	10,800	2,600	4,800	6,100	2,800	2,400	2,000
North Carolina	21,000	2,700	2,800	3,300	650	1,400	2,100	425	600	500
North Dakota	2,500	375	425	275	50	125	300	100	80	70
Ohio	42,500	6,100	6,500	7,100	1,300	3,000	3,400	1,200	1,300	1,300
Oklahoma	11,800	1,300	1,700	2,100	375	650	1,000	300	325	325
Oregon	10,000	1,300	1,200	1,700	250	600	950	225	300	300
Pennsylvania	53,500	7,300	9,900	7,800	1,500	3,300	4,100	1,600	1,500	1,300
Rhode Island	4,800	650	900	700	200	300	400	200	150	80
South Carolina	9,900	1,200	1,200	1,600	350	800	1,000	200	300	250
South Dakota	2,600	425	450	400	50	150	300	80	90	100
Tennessee	17,500	1,900	2,300	3,100	550	1,100	1,500	350	500	475
Texas	44,500	5,400	5,600	7,600	1,500	2,700	3,800	1,300	1,200	1,400
Utah	3,100	475	425	275	60	225	300	80	80	80
Vermont	2,100	250	300	350	60	150	200	50	50	60
Virginia	17,500	2,300	2,300	3,100	550	1,100	1,500	425	475	425
Washington	14,700	2,000	2,100	2,400	450	800	1,400	375	425	450
West Virginia	7,900	850	1,000	1,300	200	600	650	200	250	200
Wisconsin	18,000	2,400	2,900	2,400	550	950	1,800	600	500	550
Wyoming	1,300	150	200	200	20	70	100	25	30	30
United States	870,000	115,000	130,000	139,000	27,000	55,000	76,000	25,000	25,000	24,000
Puerto Rico	6,000	450	450	350	425	750	400	500	100	175

*These estimates are offered as a rough guide and should not be regarded as definitive. They are calculated according to the distribution of estimated 1984 cancer deaths by state. Especially note that year-to-year changes may only represent improvements in the basic data.

†Does not include carcinoma in situ or nonmelanoma skin cancer.

Estimated new cases and deaths for major sites of cancer—1984*

Site	*Number of cases*	*Deaths*
Lung	139,000	121,000
Colon-rectum	130,000	59,000
Breast	116,000	38,000
Prostate	76,000	25,000
Uterus	55,000†	10,000
Urinary	57,000	19,000
Oral	27,000	9,000
Pancreas	25,000	23,000
Leukemia	24,000	17,000
Ovary	18,000	12,000
Skin	18,000‡	7,000

*Figures rounded to nearest 1,000.
†If carcinoma in situ is included, cases total over 99,000.
‡Estimated new cases of nonmelanoma about 400,000.
Incidence estimates are based on rates from N.C.I. SEER Program, 1973–1979.

FIVE-YEAR CANCER SURVIVAL RATES* FOR SELECTED SITES BY RACE

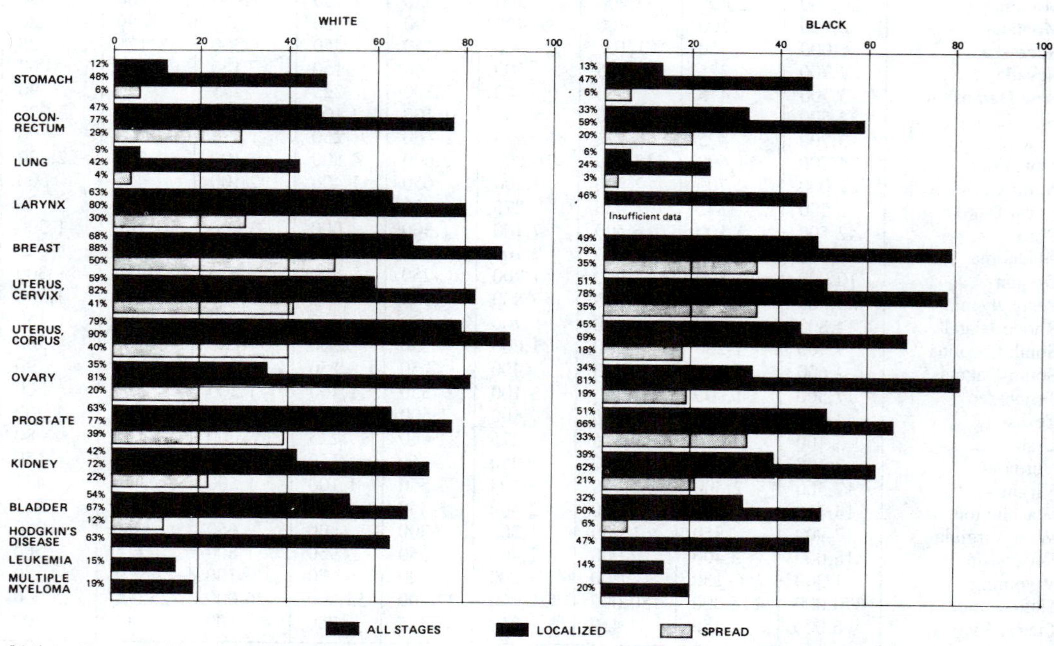

*Adjusted for normal life expectancy

Source: Biometry Branch, National Cancer Institute

Estimated new cancer cases and deaths by sex for all sites—1984*

Site	*Estimated new cases*			*Estimated deaths*		
	Total†	*Male*	*Female*	*Total*	*Male*	*Female*
All sites	870,000	429,000	441,000	450,000	244,500	205,500
Buccal cavity and pharynx **(oral)**	27,500	18,700	8,800	9,350	6,400	2,950
Lip	4,900	4,200	700	175	150	25
Tongue	4,900	3,200	1,700	2,050	1,400	650
Salivary gland }	9,800	5,800	4,000	700	450	250
Floor of mouth }				525	400	125
Other and unspecified mouth }				1,600	1,000	600
Pharynx	7,900	5,500	2,400	4,300	3,000	1,300
Digestive organs	207,000	105,100	101,900	117,300	61,450	55,850
Esophagus	9,100	6,500	2,600	8,600	6,300	2,300
Stomach	24,900	15,000	9,900	14,100	8,300	5,800
Small intestine } **(Colon-rectum)**	2,100	1,100	1,000	700	350	350
Large intestine }	90,000	41,000	49,000	50,900	24,200	26,700
Rectum	40,000	21,000	19,000	8,500	4,600	3,900
Liver and biliary passages	13,300	6,300	7,000	10,100	5,000	5,100
Pancreas	25,100	13,000	12,100	23,000	12,000	11,000
Other and unspecified digestive	2,500	1,200	1,300	1,400	700	700
Respiratory system	153,400	107,500	45,900	126,150	89,000	37,150
Larynx	11,100	9,300	1,800	3,750	3,100	650
Lung	139,000	96,000	43,000	121,000	85,000	36,000
Other and unspecified respiratory	3,300	2,200	1,100	1,400	900	500
Bone, tissue, and skin	24,500	12,500	12,000	11,150	6,400	4,750
Bone	1,900	1,100	800	1,350	800	550
Connective tissue	4,900	2,700	2,200	2,400	1,200	1,200
Skin	17,700‡	8,700	9,000	7,400‖	4,400	3,000
Breast	115,900§	900	115,000	37,600	300	37,300
Genital organs	159,300	81,600	77,700	48,150	25,950	22,200
Cervix uteri } **(Uterus)**	16,000§	—	16,000	6,800	—	6,800
Corpus, endometrium }	39,000	—	39,000	2,900	—	2,900
Ovary	18,300	—	18,300	11,500	—	11,500
Prostate	76,000	76,000	—	25,000	25,000	—
Other and unspecified genital, male	5,600	5,600	—	950	950	—
Other and unspecified genital, female	4,400	—	4,400	1,000	—	1,000
Urinary organs	57,100	39,600	17,500	19,400	12,600	6,800
Bladder	38,700	28,000	10,700	10,700	7,300	3,400
Kidney and other urinary	18,400	11,600	6,800	8,700	5,300	3,400
Eye	1,900	1,000	900	400	200	200
Brain and central nervous system	12,800	7,100	5,700	10,400	5,700	4,700
Endocrine glands	11,400	3,500	7,900	1,600	700	900
Thyroid	10,300	2,900	7,400	1,100	400	700
Other endocrine	1,100	600	500	500	300	200
Leukemia	24,400	13,200	11,200	16,700	9,300	7,400
Other blood and lymph tissues	40,600	21,100	19,500	21,600	11,300	10,300
Hodgkin's disease	7,100	4,100	3,000	1,500	900	600
Multiple myeloma	9,800	5,000	4,800	7,200	3,700	3,500
Other lymphomas	23,700	12,000	11,700	12,900	6,700	6,200
All other and unspecified sites	34,200	17,200	17,000	30,200	15,200	15,000

*NOTE: The estimates of new cancer cases are offered as a rough guide and should not be regarded as definitive. Especially note that year-to-year changes may only represent improvements in the basic data. ACS six major sites in **boldface.** Incidence estimates are based on rates from NCI SEER program 1973–1979.
†Carcinoma in situ and nonmelanoma skin cancers not included in totals. Carcinoma in situ of the uterine cervix accounts for over 45,000 new cases annually and carcinoma in situ of the female breast accounts for over 5,000 new cases annually. Nonmelanoma skin cancer accounts for about 400,000 new cases annually.
‡Melanoma only.
§Invasive cancer only.
‖Melanoma 5,500; other skin 1,900.

Trends in survival by site of cancer by race (cases diagnosed in 1960-63, in 1970-73, and in 1973-80)

Site	White			Black		
	1960-63 relative 5-year survival (%)*	*1970-73* relative 5-year survival (%)*	*1973-80† relative 5-year survival (%)*	*1960-63* relative 5-year survival (%)*	*1970-73* relative 5-year survival (%)*	*1973-80† relative 5-year survival (%)*
Prostate	50	63	68	35	55	58
Kidney	37	46	50	38	44	52
Uterine corpus	73	81	88	31	44	58
Bladder	53	61	73	24	36	48
Colon/rectum	41	48	50	31	35	42
Uterine cervix	58	64	68	47	61	62
Breast	63	68	74	46	51	62
Ovary	32	36	37	32	32	39
Brain and central nervous	18	20	21	19	19	23
Lung and bronchus	8	10	12	5	7	10
Stomach	11	13	14	8	13	14
Esophagus	4	4	5	1	4	3
Hodgkin's disease	40	67	70	‡	‡	70
Lymphocytic leukemia-acute	4	28	43			
Leukemia	14	22	32	‡	‡	27
Non-Hodgkin's lymphoma	31	41	46	‡	‡	46
Larynx	53	62	67	‡	‡	57
Melanoma of skin	60	68	79			
Testis	63	72	82	‡	‡	67
Thyroid	83	86	92	‡	‡	89

Source: Biometry Branch, National Cancer Institute.
*Rates are based on data from a series of hospital registries and one population-based registry.
†Rates are from the SEER Program and include patients diagnosed through 1980 and follow-up on all patients through 1981. They are based on data from population-based registries in Connecticut, New Mexico, Utah, Iowa, Hawaii, Atlanta, Detroit, Seattle-Puget Sound, and San Francisco-Oakland.
‡Rates could not be calculated because of insufficient number of cases.

COMPREHENSIVE CANCER CENTERS

The institutions listed have been recognized as Comprehensive Cancer Centers by the National Cancer Institute. These centers have met rigorous criteria imposed by the National Cancer Advisory Board. They receive financial support from the National Cancer Institute, the American Cancer Society and many other sources.

Alabama
University of Alabama in Birmingham Comprehensive Cancer Center
Lurleen Wallace Tumor Institute
1824 6th Avenue South
Birmingham, Alabama 35294
Phone: (205) 934-5077

California
University of Southern California Comprehensive Cancer Center
1441 Eastlake Avenue
Los Angeles, California 90033-0804
Phone: (213) 224-6416

UCLA-Jonsson Comprehensive Cancer Center
Louis Factor Health Sciences Bldg.
10833 LeConte Avenue
Los Angeles, California 90024
Phone: (213) 825-5268

Connecticut
Yale Comprehensive Cancer Center
Yale University School of Medicine
333 Cedar Street
New Haven, Connecticut 06510
Phone: (203) 785-4098

District of Columbia
Georgetown University/Howard University Comprehensive Cancer Center

Vincent T. Lombardi Cancer Research Center
Georgetown University Medical Center
3800 Reservoir Road, N.W.
Washington, D.C. 20007
Phone: (202) 625-7721

Howard University Cancer Research Center
College of Medicine
Department of Oncology
2041 Georgia Avenue, N.W.
Washington, D.C. 20060
Phone: (202) 636-7697

Florida
Comprehensive Cancer Center for the State of Florida
University of Miami School of Medicine
1475 N.W. 12th Avenue
Miami, Florida 33101
Phone: (305) 545-7707

Illinois
Illinois Cancer Council
36 South Wabash Avenue, Suite 700
Chicago, Illinois 60603
Phone: (312) 346-9813

Northwestern University Cancer Center
303 East Chicago Avenue
Chicago, Illinois 60611
Phone: (312) 266-5250

University of Chicago Cancer Research Center
950 East 59th Street
Chicago, Illinois 60637
Phone: (312) 962-6180

University of Illinois
Department of Surgery, Division of Surgical Oncology
840 South Wood Street
Chicago, Illinois 60612
Phone: (312) 996-6666

Rush Cancer Center
Suite 820
1725 West Harrison Street
Chicago, Illinois 60612
Phone: (312) 942-6028

Maryland
Johns Hopkins Oncology Center
600 North Wolfe Street
Baltimore, Maryland 21205
Phone: (301) 955-8822

Massachusetts
Dana-Farber Cancer Institute
44 Binney Street
Boston, Massachusetts 02115
Phone: (617) 732-3555

Michigan
Michigan Cancer Foundation
Meyer L Prentis Cancer Center
110 East Warren Avenue
Detroit, Michigan 48201
Phone: (313) 833-0710

Minnesota
Mayo Clinic
200 First Street, S.W.
Rochester, Minnesota 55905
Phone: (507) 284-8964

New York
Columbia University Cancer Research Center
701 West 168th Street, Rm. 1208
New York, New York 10032
Phone: (212) 694-3647

Memorial Sloan-Kettering Cancer Center
1275 York Avenue
New York, New York 10021
Phone: (212) 794-6561

Roswell Park Memorial Institute
666 Elm Street
Buffalo, New York 14263
Phone: (716) 845-5770

North Carolina
Duke Comprehensive Cancer Center
P.O. Box 3814
Duke University Medical Center
Durham, North Carolina 27710
Phone: (919) 684-2282

Ohio
Ohio State University Comprehensive Cancer Center
Suite 302
410 West 12th Avenue
Columbus, Ohio 43210
Phone: (614) 422-5022

Pennsylvania
Fox Chase/University of Pennsylvania Cancer Center

The Fox Chase Cancer Center
7701 Burholme Avenue
Philadelphia, Pennsylvania 19111
Phone: (215) 728-2781

University of Pennsylvania Cancer Center
3400 Spruce Street
7th Floor, Silverstein Pavilion
Philadelphia, Pennsylvania 19104
Phone: (215) 662-3910

Texas
The University of Texas System Cancer Center
M.D. Anderson Hospital and Tumor Institute
6723 Bertner Avenue
Houston, Texas 77030
Phone: (713) 792-6000

Washington
Fred Hutchinson Cancer Research Center
1124 Columbia Street
Seattle, Washington 98104
Phone: (206) 292-2930 or 292-7545

Wisconsin
Wisconsin Clinical Cancer Center
University of Wisconsin
Department of Human Oncology
600 Highland Avenue
Madison, Wisconsin 53792
Phone: (608)263-8610

CHARTERED DIVISIONS OF THE AMERICAN CANCER SOCIETY, INC.*

Alabama Division, Inc.
2926 Central Avenue
Birmingham, Alabama 35209
(205) 879-2242

Alaska Division, Inc.
1343 G Street
Anchorage, Alaska 99501
(907) 277-8696

Arizona Division, Inc.
634 West Indian School Road
P.O. Box 33187
Phoenix, Arizona 85067
(602) 234-3266

Arkansas Division, Inc.
5520 West Markham Street
P.O. Box 3822
Little Rock, Arkansas 72203
(501) 664-3480-1-2

California Division, Inc.
1710 Webster Street
P.O. Box 2061
Oakland, California 94604
(415) 893-7900

Colorado Division, Inc.
2255 South Oneida
P.O. Box 24669
Denver, Colorado 80224
(303) 758-2030

Connecticut Division, Inc.
Barnes Park South
14 Village Lane
P.O. Box 410
Wallingford, Connecticut 06492
(203) 265-7161

Delaware Division, Inc.
Academy of Medicine Bldg.
1708 Lovering Avenue
Suite 202
Wilmington, Delaware 19806
(302) 654-6267

District of Columbia Division, Inc.
Universal Building, South
1825 Connecticut Avenue, N.W.
Washington, D.C. 20009
(202) 483-2600

Florida Division, Inc.
1001 South MacDill Avenue
Tampa, Florida 33609
(813) 253-0541

Georgia Division, Inc.
1422 W. Peachtree Street, N.W.
Atlanta, Georgia 30309
(404) 892-0026

Hawaii Pacific Division, Inc.
Community Services Center Bldg.
200 North Vineyard Boulevard
Honolulu, Hawaii 96817
(808) 531-1662-3-4-5

Idaho Division, Inc.
1609 Abbs Street
P.O. Box 5386
Boise, Idaho 83705
(208) 343-4609

Illinois Division, Inc.
37 South Wabash Avenue
Chicago, Illinois 60603
(312) 372-0472

Indiana Division, Inc.
4755 Kingsway Drive, Suite 100
Indianapolis, Indiana 46205
(317) 257-5326

Iowa Division, Inc.
Highway #18 West
P.O. Box 980
Mason City, Iowa 50401
(515) 423-0712

Kansas Division, Inc.
3003 Van Buren Street
Topeka, Kansas 66611
(913) 267-0131

Kentucky Division, Inc.
Medical Arts Bldg.
1169 Eastern Parkway
Louisville, Kentucky 40217
(502) 459-1867

*National Headquarters: American Cancer Society, Inc., 777 Third Avenue, New York, N.Y. 10017.

Louisiana Division, Inc.
Masonic Temple Bldg., 7th Floor
333 St. Charles Avenue
New Orleans, Louisiana 70130
(504) 523-2029

Maine Division, Inc.
Federal and Green Streets
Brunswick, Maine 04011
(207) 729-3339

Maryland Division, Inc.
200 East Joppa Road
Towson, Maryland 21204
(301) 828-8890

Massachusetts Division, Inc.
247 Commonwealth Avenue
Boston, Massachusetts 02116
(617) 267-2650

Michigan Division, Inc.
1205 East Saginaw Street
Lansing, Michigan 48906
(517) 371-2920

Minnesota Division, Inc.
3316 West 66th Street
Minneapolis, Minnesota 55435
(612) 925-2772

Mississippi Division, Inc.
345 North Mart Plaza
Jackson, Mississippi 39206
(601) 362-8874

Missouri Division, Inc.
3322 American Avenue
P.O. Box 1066
Jefferson City, Missouri 65102
(314) 893-4800

Montana Division, Inc.
2820 First Avenue South
Billings, Montana 59101
(406) 252-7111

Nebraska Division, Inc.
8502 West Center Road
Omaha, Nebraska 68124
(402) 393-5800

Nevada Division, Inc.
1325 East Harmon
Las Vegas, Nevada 89109
(702) 798-6877

New Hampshire Division, Inc.
686 Mast Road
Manchester, New Hampshire 03102
(603) 669-3270

New Jersey Division, Inc.
CN2201, 2600 Route 1
North Brunswick, New Jersey 08902
(201) 297-8000

New Mexico Division, Inc.
5800 Lomas Blvd., N.E.
Albuquerque, New Mexico 87110
(505) 262-2336

New York State Division, Inc.
6725 Lyons Street, P.O. Box 7
East Syracuse, New York 13057
(315) 437-7025

☐ **Long Island Division, Inc.**
535 Broad Hollow Road
(Route 110)
Melville, New York 11747
(516) 420-1111

☐ **New York City Division, Inc.**
19 West 56th Street
New York, New York 10019
(212) 586-8700

☐ **Queens Division, Inc.**
111-15 Queens Boulevard
Forest Hills, New York 11375
(212) 263-2224

☐ **Westchester Division, Inc.**
901 North Broadway
White Plains, New York 10603
(914) 949-4800

North Carolina Division, Inc.
222 North Person Street
P.O. Box 27624
Raleigh, North Carolina 27611
(919) 834-8463

North Dakota Division, Inc.
Hotel Graver Annex Bldg.
115 Roberts Street
P.O. Box 426
Fargo, North Dakota 58102
(701) 232-1385

Ohio Division, Inc.
1375 Euclid Avenue
Suite 312
Cleveland, Ohio 44115
(216) 771-6700

Oklahoma Division, Inc.
3800 North Cromwell
Oklahoma City, Oklahoma 73112
(405) 946-5000

Oregon Division, Inc.
0330 S.W. Curry
Portland, Oregon 97201
(503) 295-6422

Pennsylvania Division, Inc.
Route 422 & Sipe Avenue
P.O. Box 416
Hershey, Pennsylvania 17033
(717) 533-6144

☐ **Philadelphia Division, Inc.**
21 South 12th Street
Philadelphia, Pennsylvania 19107
(215) 665-2900

Puerto Rico Division, Inc.
(Avenue Domenech 273 Hato Rey, P.R.)
GPO Box 6004
San Juan, Puerto Rico 00936
(809) 764-2295

Rhode Island Division, Inc.
345 Blackstone Blvd.
Providence, Rhode Island 02906
(401) 831-6970

South Carolina Division, Inc.
2442 Devine Street
Columbia, South Carolina 29205
(803) 256-0245

South Dakota Division, Inc.
1025 North Minnesota Avenue
Hillcrest Plaza
Sioux Falls, South Dakota 57104
(605) 336-0897

Tennessee Division, Inc.
713 Melpark Drive
Nashville, Tennessee 37204
(615) 383-1710

Texas Division, Inc.
3834 Spicewood Springs Road
P.O. Box 9863
Austin, Texas 78766
(512) 345-4560

Utah Division, Inc.
610 East South Temple
Salt Lake City, Utah 84102
(801) 322-0431

Vermont Division, Inc.
13 Loomis Street, Drawer C
Montpelier, Vermont 05602
(802) 223-2348

Virginia Division, Inc.
3218 West Cary Street
P.O. Box 7288
Richmond, Virginia 23221
(804) 359-0208

Washington Division, Inc.
2120 First Avenue North
Seattle, Washington 98109
(206) 283-1152

West Virginia Division, Inc.
Suite 100
240 Capitol Street
Charleston, West Virginia 25301
(304) 344-3611

Wisconsin Division, Inc.
615 North Sherman Avenue
P.O. Box 8370
Madison, Wisconsin 53708
(608) 249-0487

☐ **Milwaukee Division, Inc.**
11401 West Watertown Plank Road
Wauwatosa, Wisconsin 53226
(414) 453-4500

Wyoming Division, Inc.
Indian Hills Center
506 Shoshoni
Cheyenne, Wyoming 82009
(307) 638-3331

15-3 Communicable and infectious diseases

Name	Synopsis of symptoms	Incubation period	Mode of transmission	Period of communicability
Actinomycosis	Chronic disease most frequently localized in jaw, thorax, or abdomen; septicemic spread with generalized disease may occur. Lesions are firmly indurated areas of purulence and fibrosis.	Irregular; probably years after colonization in oral tissues, plus days or months after precipitating trauma and actual penetration of tissues.	Contact from person to person as part of normal oral flora.	Time and manner in which *A. israelii* becomes part of normal flora is unknown.
Amebiasis	Infection with a protozoan parasite that exists in two forms: the hardy, infective cyst and the more fragile, potentially invasive trophozoite; may act as a commensal or invade tissues, giving rise to intestinal or extraintestinal disease.	Variation—from a few days to several months or years. Commonly 2 to 4 weeks.	Contaminated water or food containing cysts from feces of infected persons, often as complication of another infection such as shigellosis.	During period of cyst passing, which may continue for years.
Ancylostomiasis (hookworm disease, uncinariasis, necatoriasis)	Chronic, debilitating disease with a variety of vague symptoms varying greatly, usually in proportion to degree of anemia and hypoproteinemia.	Symptoms may develop after a few weeks to many months.	Eggs in feces are deposited on ground, and under favorable environmental conditions, hatch; larvae develop to third stage, becoming infective in 7 to 10 days. Human infection occurs when infected larvae penetrate skin, usually foot.	Not transmitted from person to person, but infected persons can contaminate soil for several years in absence of treatment.
Angiostrongyliasis (eosinophilic meningoencephalitis, eosinophilic meningitis)	Disease of central nervous system caused by a nematode; may be asymptomatic or mildly symptomatic; more commonly characterized by severe headache, stiffness of neck and back, and various paresthesias. Temporary facial paralysis and low-grade fever may be present.	Usually 1 to 3 weeks.	Ingestion of raw or insufficiently cooked snails, slugs, or land planaarians, which are intermediate or transport hosts harboring infective larvae.	Not transmitted from person to person.
Anisakiasis	Disease of human gastrointestinal tract manifested by intestinal colic, fever, and eosinophilic abscesses resulting from ingesting uncooked fish containing larval nematodes of the family Anisakidae.	Stomach involvement may develop within a few hours of ingestion.	Infective larvae live in organs of fish until its death when they invade somatic muscles. When ingested by humans and liberated by digestion they penetrate gastric or intestinal mucosa.	No direct transmission from person to person.
Anthrax	Acute bacterial disease usually affecting skin but may rarely involve mediastinum or intestinal tract.	Within 7 days, usually 2 to 5 days.	Infection of skin is by contact with tissues of animals dying of the disease or contaminated animal byproducts (wool or hides).	No evidence of transmission from person to person. Articles and soil contaminated with spores may remain infective for years.

Continued.

Name	*Synopsis of symptoms*	*Incubation period*	*Mode of transmission*	*Period of communicability*
Arenaviral hemorrhagic fever	Acute febrile illnesses, duration 7 to 15 days. Onset is gradual with malaise, headache, retroorbital pain, conjunctival injection, sustained fever, and sweats, followed by prostration. An exanthem appears on thorax and flanks 3 to 5 days after onset.	Commonly 7 to 16 days.	Saliva and excreta of infected rodents contain virus. May be air-borne transmission by dust contaminated by infected rodent excreta.	Probably not often directly transmitted from person to person (although this has occurred in the Bolivia disease).
A. Arthropod-borne viral diseases (arboviral diseases)				
1. Arthropod-borne viral arthritis and rash	Acute self-limited disease characterized by arthritis, primarily in small joints of extremities that lasts from 2 days to 8 months.	10 to 11 days.	Culicine mosquitoes.	No evidence of transmission from person to person.
2. Arthropod-borne viral encephalitides a. Mosquito-borne	Group of acute inflammatory diseases of short duration. Mild cases often occur as aseptic meningitis. Severe infections are usually marked by acute onset, headache, high fever, meningeal signs, stupor, disorientation, coma, tremors, occasionally convulsions, and spastic paralysis.	Usually 5 to 15 days.	Infective mosquitoes.	Not directly transmitted from person to person. Virus is not usually demonstrable in blood of humans after onset of disease. Mosquitoes remain infective for life.
b. Tick-borne	Group of diseases resembling mosquito-borne encephalitides, except Russian spring-summer type often is associated with flaccid paralysis, particularly of the shoulder girdle.	Usually 7 to 14 days.	By infective ticks or by consuming milk from certain infected animals.	Not directly transmitted from person to person. Tick infected at any stage remains infective for life.
B. Arthropod-borne viral fevers				
1. Mosquito-borne a. Yellow fever	Acute infectious disease of short duration and varying severity. Mildest cases are clinically indeterminate; typical attacks are characterized by denguelike illness, i.e., sudden onset, fever, headache, backache, prostration, nausea, and vomiting.	3 to 6 days.	In urban and certain rural areas transmitted by infective *Aedes aegypti* mosquitoes.	Blood is infective for mosquitoes shortly before onset of fever and for first 3 to 5 days of illness. Highly communicable where many susceptible persons and abundant vector mosquitoes coexist.
b. Dengue (breakbone fever)	Characterized by sudden onset, fever for about 5 days and intense headache, retroorbital pains, joint and muscle pains, and rash.	3 to 15 days, commonly 5 to 6 days.	Infective mosquitoes.	Not directly transmitted from person to person.

c. Venezuelan equine fever	Clinical manifestations of infection are influenza-like, with abrupt onset of severe headache, chills, fever, myalgia, retroorbital pain, nausea, and vomiting.	Usually 2 to 6 days, can be as short as 1 day.	Infected mosquitoes.	Person-to-person transmission may occur but has not been demonstrated.
2. Tick-borne a. Colorado tick fever and other tick-borne fevers	Acute febrile, diphasic, denguelike disease with infrequent rash. Brief remission is usual, followed by second bout of fever lasting 2 or 3 days; neutropenia almost always occurs on fourth or fifth day of fever.	Usually 4 to 5 days.	Infective vector ticks.	Not directly transmitted from person to person except by transfusion. Virus is present during course of fever and, in Colordo tick fever, from 2 to 16 weeks or more after onset.
Ascariasis (roundworm infection)	Helminthic infection of small intestine. Symptoms are variable, often vague or absent, and ordinarily mild; live worms, passed in stools or regurgitated, are frequently first recognized sign of infection.	Worms reach maturity about 2 months after ingestion of embryonated eggs.	By ingestion of infective eggs from soil contaminated with human feces containing eggs, but not directly from person to person.	As long as mature female worms live in intestine. Maximum lifespan of adult worms is under 18 months; however, female produces up to 200,000 eggs a day that can remain viable in soil for months or years.
Aspergillosis	Variety of clinical syndromes can be produced by several *Aspergillus* species.	Probably a few days.	Inhalation of air-borne spores.	Not directly transmitted from person to person.
Babesiosis	Fever, fatigue, and hemolytic anemia lasting several days to a few months.	1 to 12 months.	During the summer months by bite of nymphal *Ixodes* ticks carried by voles or deer mice. Adult tick is normally found on deer.	Transmission from person to person is unlikely except by blood transfusion.
Balantidiasis	Disease of colon characteristically producing diarrhea or dysentery accompanied by abdominal colic, tenesmus, nausea, and vomiting.	Unknown; may be only a few days.	By ingestion of cysts from feces of infected hosts; in epidemics, mainly by fecally contaminated water.	As long as infection persists.
Blastomycosis	Chronic granulomatous mycosis primarily of lungs or skin. *Acute pulmonary blastomycosis* begins with fever and symptoms of respiratory infection and can progress gradually with fever, weight loss, cachexia, cough, and purulent sputum.	Indefinite; probably a few weeks or less to months.	Conidia, typical of the mold or saprophytic growth form, probably are inhaled in sporeladen dust.	Not transmitted directly from humans or from animals to humans.
Botulism, infant	Illness typically begins with constipation followed by lethargy, listlessness, poor feeding, ptosis, difficulty in swallowing, loss of head control, hypotonia, general-	Usually unknown, because it cannot be determined precisely when the infant ingested the botulinal spores.	By ingestion of botulinal spores. Sources of spores for infants probably are multiple.	Excretion of *C. botulinum* toxin and organisms. Continues at high levels in patient's feces for weeks to months. No instances of secondary person-to-person transmission have been documented.

Continued.

Name	Synopsis of symptoms	Incubation period	Mode of transmission	Period of communicability
	ized weakness, and in some cases, respiratory insufficiency and arrest. Wide spectrum of clinical severity ranging from mild illness to sudden infant death.			
Brucellosis (undulant fever)	Systemic disease with acute or insidious onset characterized by continued, intermittent, or irregular fever of variable duration, headache, weakness, profuse sweating, chills, arthralgia, depression, and generalized aching.	Highly variable—usually 5 to 30 days; sometimes several months.	By contact with tissues, blood, urine, vaginal discharges, aborted fetuses and especially placentas, and by ingestion of raw milk or dairy products from infected animals. Air-borne infection occurs in humans in laboratories and slaughterhouses.	No evidence of communicability from person to person.
Candidiasis (moniliasis, thrush, candidosis)	Mycosis usually confined to superficial layers of skin or mucous membranes with patient having oral thrush, intertrigo, vulvovaginitis, paronychia, or onychomycosis.	Variable, 2 to 5 days in thrush of infants.	Through contact with excretions of mouth, skin, vagina, and especially feces from patients or carriers from mother to infant during childbirth; and by indogenous spread.	Presumably for duration of lesions.
Capillariasis				
A. Intestinal capillariasis	Enteropathy with massive protein loss and a malabsorption syndrome that lead to progressive weight loss and extreme emaciation.	Unknown in humans.	Uncertain. Often obtain history of ingesting raw or inadequately cooked fish.	Not transmitted directly from person to person.
B. Hepatic capillariasis (also a pulmonary capillariasis—but only 10 documented cases of human infection recorded).	Uncommon and occasionally fatal disease in humans caused by presence of adult *Capillaria hepatica* in liver. Acute or subacute hepatitis with marked eosinophilia resembling visceral larva migrans.	3 to 4 weeks.	Ingesting liver of infected animal.	Not transmitted directly from person to person.
Carditis, Coxsackie (viral carditis, enteroviral carditis)	Acute or subacute myocarditis or pericarditis, which occurs as the only manifestation, or may occasionally be associated with other manifestations.	Usually 3 to 5 days.	Fecal-oral or respiratory droplet contact with infected person.	Apparently during acute stage of disease.
Cat-scratch disease	Subacute, self-limited infectious disease characterized by malaise, granulomatous lymphadenitis, and variable patterns of fever.	Variable; usually 3 to 14 days from innoculation to primary lesions.	90% of patients report history of scratch, bite, lick, or other exposure to healthy cat or kitten.	Unknown. Not directly transmitted from person to person.

Chancroid (ulcus molle, soft chancre)	Acute, localized, genital infection characterized by single or multiple painful necrotizing ulcers at site of innoculation, frequently accompanied by painful inflammatory swelling and suppuration of regional lymph nodes. Extragenital lesions have been reported.	From 3 to 5 days, up to 14 days.	By direct sexual contact with discharges from open lesions and pus from buboes; suggestive evidence of asymptomatic infections in women. Multiple sexual partners and uncleanliness favor transmission.	As long as infectious agent persists in original lesion or discharging regional lymph nodes; usually until healed—a matter of weeks.
Chickenpox, herpes zoster (varicella shingles)	Acute generalized viral disease with sudden onset of slight fever, mild constitutional symptoms, and a skin eruption that is maculopapular for a few hours, vesicular for 3 to 4 days, and leaves a granular scab.	From 2 to 3 weeks; commonly 13 to 17 days.	From person to person by direct contact, droplet, or airborne spread of secretion of respiratory tract of chickenpox cases or of vesicle fluid of patients with herpes zoster.	As long as 5 days but usually 1 to 2 days before onset of rash, and not more than 6 days after appearance of first crop of vesicles.
Cholera	Acute intestinal disease with sudden onset, profuse watery stools, occasional vomiting, rapid dehydration, acidosis, and circulatory collapse. Death may occur within a few hours.	From a few hours to 5 days, usually 2 to 3 days.	Through ingestion of food or water contaminated with feces or vomitus of infected persons or with feces of carriers.	Thought to be for duration of stool-positive stage, usually only a few days after recovery. Carrier stage may last for several months.
Chromoblastomycosis (chromomycosis, dermatitis verrucosa)	Chronic spreading mycosis of skin and subcutaneous tissues, usually of a lower extremity. Hematogenous spread to brain has been reported.	Unknown; probably months.	Traumatic contact with contaminated wood or other materials.	Not directly transmitted from person to person.
Clonorchiasis (Chinese or oriental liver fluke disease)	Symptoms result from local irritation of bile ducts by flukes, from toxemia and possibly from secondary bacterial invaders. Loss of appetite, diarrhea, and sensation of abdominal pressure are early common symptoms.	Unpredictable, varies with the number of worms present; flukes reach maturity within 1 month after encysted larvae are ingested.	Humans infected by eating freshwater fish containing encysted larvae *(Clonorchis sinensis)*.	Not directly transmitted from person to person, but infected individual may pass viable eggs for as long as 30 years.
Coccidioidomycosis (valley fever, desert fever, desert rheumatism, coccidiodal granuloma).	Internal mycosis that begins as respiratory infection. *Primary infection* may be entirely asymptomatic or resemble acute influenza illness with fever, chills, cough, and pleural pain.	1 to 4 weeks in primary infection.	Inhalation of spores from soil and in laboratory accidents from cultures.	Not directly transmitted from humans or animals to humans.
Conjunctivitis, acute bacterial	Clinical syndrome beginning with lacrimation, irritation, and hyperemia of the palpebral and bulbar conjunctivae of one or both eyes, followed by edema of lids, photophobia. and mucopurulent discharge.	Usually 24 to 72 hours.	Contact with discharges from conjunctivae or upper respiratory tract of infected persons through contaminated fingers, clothing, or other articles.	During course of active infection.

Continued.

Name	*Synopsis of symptoms*	*Incubation period*	*Mode of transmission*	*Period of communicability*
Conjunctivitis, epidemic hemorrhagic (Apollo 11 disease)	Virus infection with sudden onset of pain or sensation of a foreign body in eye. Disease rapidly progresses (1 to 2 days) to full case of swollen eyelids, hyperemia of the conjunctivae, often with a circumcorneal distribution, seromucous discharge, and frequent subconjunctival hemorrhages.	1 to 2 days or even shorter.	Through direct or indirect contact with discharge from infected eyes and possibly by droplet infection from those with virus in throat.	Unknown, but assumed to be for period of active disease, usually 1 to 2 weeks.
Conjunctivitis, inclusion (swimming pool conjunctivitis, paratrachoma)	In the newborn, acute papillary conjunctivitis with abundant mucopurulent discharge. In children and adults, acute follicular conjunctivitis with preauricular lymphadenopathy, often with superficial corneal involvement.	5 to 12 days.	During sexual intercourse; genital discharges of infected persons are infectious.	While genital infection persists; can be longer than 1 year in female.
Contagious pustular dermatitis	Primarily a proliferative cutaneous disease of sheep and goats transmissible to humans and usually a solitary lesion located on hands, arms, or face that is maculopapular or pustular.	Generally 3 to 6 days.	By direct contact with mucous membranes of infected animals.	Unknown. Human lesions show a decrease in number of virus particles as disease progresses.
Cryptococcosis (torulosis, European blastomycosis)	Mycosis, usually subacute or chronic meningoencephalitis. Infection of lung, kidney, prostate, bone, or liver.	Unknown. Pulmonary disease may precede brain infection by months or years.	Presumably by inhalation.	Not directory transmitted from humans or animals to humans.
Cutaneous larva migrans caused by *Ancylostoma braziliense* resulting from *Ancylostoma caninum*	Infective larvae of dog and cat hookworm that causes dermatitis in humans.	Each larva causes serpiginous track, advancing several mm to a few cm a day.	Larva, which enter skin from contact with contaminated soil, migrate intracutaneously for long periods, but eventually penetrate to deeper tissues.	Disease is self-limited, with spontaneous cure after several weeks or months.
Cytomegalovirus infections Congenital cytomegalovirus infection Cytomegalic inclusion disease	Most severe form of disease occurs in perinatal period, following congenital infection, with signs and symptoms of severe generalized infection especially involving central nervous system and liver.	Information inexact. 3 to 8 weeks following transfusion with infected blood. 3 to 12 weeks after birth.	Intimate exposure to infectious secretions or excretions. Virus is excreted in urine, saliva, cervical secretions, breast milk, and semen.	Virus is excreted in urine or saliva for months and may persist for several years following primary infection.
Dermatophytosis A. Ringworm of scalp and beard (tinea capitis, tinea kerion, favus)	Begins as small papule and spreads peripherally, leaving scaly patches of temporary baldness. Infected hairs become brittle and break off easily. Kerions sometimes develop.	10 to 14 days	Direct or indirect contact with articles infected with hair from humans or infected animals.	As long as lesions are present and viable fungus persists on contaminated materials.

B. Ringworm of nails (tinea unguium, onychomycosis)	Chronic infectious disease involving one or more nails of hands or feet. Nail thickens, becoming discolored and brittle with an accumulation of caseous-appearing material beneath nail.	Unknown.	Presumably by direct extension from skin or nail lesions of infected persons. Low rate of transmission.	Possibly as long as infected lesion is present.
C. Ringworm of groin and perianal region (dhobie itch, tinea cruris) D. Ringworm of the body (tinea corporis)	Characteristically appears as flat, spreading, ring-shaped lesions. Periphery is usually reddish, vesicular, or pustular and may be dry and scaly or moist and crusted.	4 to 10 days.	Direct or indirect contact with skin and scalp lesions of infected persons or animals.	As long as lesions are present and viable fungus persists on contaminated materials.
E. Ringworm of the foot (tinea pedis, athlete's foot)	Scaling or cracking of skin, especially between toes, or blisters containing this watery fluid are characteristic. In severe cases vesicular lesions appear on various parts of body.	Unknown.	Direct or indirect contact with skin lesions of infected persons or contaminated floors or shower stalls.	As long as lesions are present and viable spores persist on contaminated materials.
Diarrhea, acute A. Diarrhea caused by *Escherichia coli*	May be invasive, enterotoxigenic, and enteropathogenic. *Invasive*—fever and mucoid and occasionally bloody diarrhea occur. *enterotoxigenic*—profuse watery diarrhea without blood or mucous. *enteropathogenic*—associated with outbreaks of acute diarrhea disease in newborn nurseries.	12 to 72 hours.	Fecal contamination of food, water, or fomites. Persons with diarrhea excrete large numbers of organisms and constitute greatest hazard.	Not known; presumably for duration of fecal excretion, which may be several weeks or longer.
B. Diarrhea caused by *Campylobacter* (vibriosis, vibrionic enteritis)	Acute enteric disease characterized by diarrhea, abdominal pain, malaise, fever, nausea, vomiting, and constitutional complaints	Range is 1 to 10 days with a usual period of 3 to 5 days.	By ingestion of organisms in food or contaminated water; contact with contaminated animals; drinking unpasteurized milk.	Throughout course of infection from several days to several weeks.
Diphtheria	Characteristic lesion marked by patch or patches of grayish membrane with surrounding dull red inflammatory zone. Throat is moderately sore in faucial diphtheria, with cervical lymph nodes enlarged and tender; occasionally swelling and edema of neck.	2 to 5 days, sometimes longer.	Contact with patient or carrier; more rarely with articles soiled with discharges from lesions of infected persons. Raw milk has been a vehicle.	Variable, until virulent bacilli have disappeared from discharge and lesions. Usual period is 2 to 4 weeks but chronic carriers may shed organisms for 6 months or more.
Diphyllobothriasis	Symptoms commonly are trivial or absent; depending on severity, vitamin B_{12} deficiency anemia, diarrhea, and toxic symptoms may be present.	From 3 to 6 weeks from ingestion to passage of eggs in stool.	From eating raw or inadequately cooked fish.	Not directly transmitted from person to person.

Continued.

Name	Synopsis of symptoms	Incubation period	Mode of transmission	Period of communicability
Dracontiasis	Infection of subcutaneous and deeper tissues by large nematode. Blister appears, usually on a lower extremity, as gravid, meter-long adult female prepares to discharge her larvae.	About 12 months.	Humans swallow infected copepods by drinking water from contaminated stepwells and ponds.	Not directly transmitted from person to person.
Echinococcosis multilocularis infection (alveolar hydatid disease)	Disease primarily of liver caused by poorly circumscribed microvesicular larval masses of *Echinococcus multilocularis;* may be found also in lungs and other organs.	Variable from months to years, depending on number and location of cysts and how rapidly they grow.	By ingestion of infective eggs or by fecally soiled dog fur, harnesses, and environmental fomites.	Not directly transmitted from person to person or from one intermediate host to another.
Enterobiasis (pinworm disease, oxyuriasis)	Intestinal infection with mild or nonspecific symptoms, if any. May be anal itching, disturbed sleep, irritability, and local irritation with secondary infection of scratched skin.	Life cycle of *Enterobius vermicularis* is 4 to 6 weeks.	Direct transfer of infective eggs by hand from anus to mouth of the same or new host, or indirectly through materials contaminated with eggs of parasite. Dust-borne infection by inhalation is possible.	As long as gravid females are discharging eggs on perianal skin. Continuous reinfection occurs by ano-oral transfer of eggs from self or infected others.
Food poisoning A. Staphylococcal food poisoning	Intoxication (not infection) of abrupt and sometimes violent onset, with severe nausea, cramps, vomiting, usually diarrhea, and prostration; sometimes with subnormal temperature and lowered blood pressure.	Interval between eating food and onset of symptoms is 1 to 6 hours, but usually 2 to 4 hours.	By ingesting of food contacted by food-handler's hands without subsequent cooking or inadequately heated, such as pastries, custards, salads, and meat products.	Not applicable.
B. Botulism	Severe intoxication (not infection as in infant botulism) characterized by clinical manifestations relating primarily to the nervous system. Ptosis, visual difficulty, dry mouth, and sore throat are often first complaints.	Symptoms usually appear within 12 to 36 hours, sometimes several days, after eating contaminated food.	By ingestion of food in which toxin had been formed, primarily from jars or cans inadequately heated during canning, and eaten without subsequent adequate cooking.	Not applicable.
C. Clostridial food poisoning *(C. welchii)*	Intestinal disorder characterized by sudden onset of abdominal colic followed by diarrhea. Nausea is common but vomiting and fever are usually absent.	From 6 to 24 hours, usually 10 to 12 hours.	Ingestion of food contaminated by soil or feces in which conditions have permitted multiplication of organism.	Not applicable.
D. *Vibrio parahaemolyticus* food poisoning	Intestinal disorder characterized by watery diarrhea and abdominal cramps; nausea, vomiting, fever, and headache are variably present.	Usually 12 to 24 hours, but can range from 4 to 96 hours.	Ingestion of raw or inadequately cooked seafood.	Not communicable from person to person.

E. *Bacillus cereus* food poisoning	Gastrointestinal disorder characterized in some cases by sudden onset of nausea and vomiting and in others by intense abdominal colic and diarrhea.	From 1 to 5 hours in cases when vomiting is predominant symptom; from 6 to 16 hours when diarrhea is predominant.	Ingestion of food that has been kept at ambient temperatures after cooking, permitting multiplication of organisms.	Not communicable from person to person.
Gastroenteritis, viral A. Epidemic viral gastroenteritis	Usually self-limited mild disease that often occurs in outbreaks with clinical symptoms of nausea, vomiting, diarrhea, abdominal pain, myalgia, headache, malaise, low grade fever, or a combination thereof.	24 to 48 hours; in volunteer studies with Norwalk agent range was 10 to 51 hours.	Unknown; probably by fecal-oral route. Several recent outbreaks strongly suggest food-borne and water-borne transmission.	During acute stage of disease and shortly thereafter.
B. Rotavirus gastroenteritis (sporadic viral gastroenteritis of infants and children)	Sporadic severe gastroenteritis of infants and young children characterized by diarrhea and vomiting, often with severe dehydration and occasional deaths.	Approximately 48 hours.	Probably fecal-oral and possibly respiratory routes.	During acute stage of disease and later while virus shedding continues. Virus is not usually detectable after eighth day of illness.
Giardiasis (*Giardia* enteritis, lambliasis)	Protozoan infection principally of upper small bowel; often asymptomatic, it may also be associated with a variety of intestinal symptoms such as chronic diarrhea, steatorrhea, abdominal cramps, bloating, frequent loose and pale, greasy, malodorus stools, fatigue, and weight loss.	In a water-borne epidemic in United States, clinical illnesses occurred 1 to 4 weeks after exposure; average 2 weeks.	Localized outbreaks occur from contaminated water supplies. By ingestion of cysts in fecally contaminated water and occasionally by fecally contaminated food.	Entire period of infection.
Gonococcal infections A. Gonococcal infection of genitourinary tract (gonorrhea, gonococcal urethritis)	*Males*—purulent discharge from anterior urethra with dysuria appears 2 to 7 days after infecting exposure. *Females*—few days after exposure initial urethritis or cervicitis occurs, frequently so mild as to pass unnoticed. About 20% of patients have uterine invasion at the first, second, or later menstrual period with symptoms of endometritis, salpingitis, or pelvic peritonitis.	Usually 2 to 7 days, sometimes longer.	By contact with exudates from mucous membranes of infected persons, almost always result of sexual activity.	May extend for months if untreated, especially in females who frequently are asymptomatic. Specific therapy usually ends communicability within hours except with penicillin-resistant strains.
B. Gonococcal conjunctivitis neonatorum (gonorrheal ophthalmia neonatorum)	Acute redness and swelling of conjunctiva of one or both eyes, with mucopurulent or purulent discharge in which gonococci are identifiable by microscopic and cultural methods.	Usually 1 to 5 days.	Contact with infected birth canal during childbirth.	While discharge persists if untreated; for 24 hours following initiation of specific treatment.

Continued.

Name	Synopsis of symptoms	Incubation period	Mode of transmission	Period of communicability
Granuloma inguinale (donovanosis)	Mildly communicable, nonfatal, chronic and progressive, autoinoculable bacterial disease of skin and mucous membranes of external genitalia, inguinal, and anal region. Small nodule, vesicle, or papule is present.	Unknown; probably 8 to 80 days.	Presumably by direct contact with lesions during sexual activity.	Unknown and probably for duration of open lesions on skin or mucous membranes.
Hemorrhagic nephrosonephritis	Acute infectious disease characterized by abrupt onset of fever of 3 to 8 day duration, conjunctival injection, prostration, anorexia, and vomiting.	Usually 12 to 16 days, but varying from 9 to 35 days.	Unknown; transmission from rodent excreta is presumed.	Apparently not directly transmitted from person to person.
Hepatitis, viral A. Viral hepatitis A (infectious hepatitis, epidemic hepatitis, epidemic jaundice, catarrhal jaundice, Type A hepatitis)	Onset is usually abrupt with fever, malaise, anorexia, nausea, and abdominal discomfort, followed within a few days by jaundice.	From 15 to 50 days, depending on dose; average 28-30 days.	Person to person by fecal-oral route. Common-vehicle outbreaks have been related to contaminated water and food.	Studies indicate maximum infectivity during latter half of incubation period, continuing for a few days, after onset of jaundice.
B. Viral hepatitis B (Type B hepatitis, serum hepatitis)	Onset is usually insidious with anorexia, vague abdominal discomfort, nausea, and vomiting, sometimes arthralgias and rash, often progressing to jaundice. Fever may be absent or mild.	Usually 45 to 160 days, average 60 to 90 days. Variation is related in part to amount of virus in inoculum, mode of transmission, and host factors.	HB_SAG, the infectious agent, has been found in virtually all body secretions, but only blood, saliva, and semen have been shown to be infectious. Transmission usually be percutaneous inoculation of infected blood and blood products; contaminated needles, syringes, and IV equipment.	From several weeks before onset of symptoms through clinical course of disease; carrier state can last for years.
C. Hepatitis, non-A, non-B (non-B transfusion–associated hepatitis, hepatitis C)	Chronic infection may be symptomatic or asymptomatic. Differential diagnosis depends on exclusion of hepatitis types A and B.	2 weeks to 6 months, model 6 to 8 weeks.	Most common posttransfusion hepatitis in United States and is more common when paid donors are used. Percutaneous transmission documented and other modes similar to those of hepatitis B virus are suspected.	Degree of immunity following infection is not known.
Herpangina; hand-foot-and-mouth disease, acute lymphonodular pharyngitis	*Herpangina*—grayish papulovesicular pharyngeal lesions on an erythematous base. *Hand-foot-and-mouth disease*—more diffuse oral lesions on buccal surfaces of cheeks, gums, and tongue. *Acute lymphonodular phar-*	3 to 5 days for herpangina and hand-foot-and-mouth disease. 5 days for acute lymphonodular pharyngitis.	Direct contact with nose and throat discharges and feces of infected (possibly asymptomatic) persons and by droplet spread.	During acute stage of illness and longer because virus persists in stools for as long as several weeks.

	yngitis—lesions are firm, raised, discrete, whitish to yellowish nodules.			
Herpes simplex	Viral infection characterized by localized primary lesion, latency, and a tendency to localized recurrence. In perhaps 10% of primary infections overt disease may appear as illness of varying severity marked by fever and malaise lasting 1 week or more.	2 to 12 days.	HSV Type 1: Direct contact with virus in saliva of carriers. HSV Type 2: Sexual contact.	Secretion of virus in saliva has been reported for as long as 7 weeks after recovery from stomatitis. Patients with primary lesions are infective for about 7 to 12 days, with recurrent disease for 4 days to 1 week.
Histoplasmosis, histoplasma capsulatum (Darling's disease, American histoplasmosis)	Systemic mycosis of varying severity with primary lesion, usually in lung. Whereas infection is common, overt clinical disease is not. Five clinical forms are recognized.	Symptoms appear within 5 to 18 days after exposure, commonly 10 days.	Inhalation of air-borne spores.	Not transmitted from person to person.
Influenza	Acute viral disease of respiratory tract characterized by fever, chilliness, headache, myalgia, prostration, coryza, and mild sore throat. Cough is often severe and protracted.	Usually 24 to 72 hours.	By direct contact through droplet infection; probably air-borne among crowded populations in enclosed spaces.	Probably limited to 3 days from clinical onset.
Keratoconjunctivitis, epidemic	Acute viral disease of eye. Onset is sudden with pain, photophobia, blurred vision, occasionally low grade fever, headache, malaise, and tender preauricular lymphadenopathy.	Probably 5 to 12 days.	Direct contact with eye secretions of infected person or indirectly through contaminated instruments or solutions.	From late in incubation period to 14 days after onset.
Lhassa fever	Acute viral illness with duration of 7 to 31 days. Onset is gradual with malaise, fever, headache, sore throat, cough, nausea, vomiting, diarrhea, myalgia, and chest and abdominal pain; fever is persistent or intermittent-spiking.	Commonly 7 to 21 days.	Primarily through direct or indirect contact with urine of infected rodents in dust or on food.	Person-to-person infections occur during acute febrile phase when virus is present in throat. Virus may be excreted in urine of patients for 3 weeks or as long as 60 days.
Legionellosis (legionnaire's disease, legionnaire's pneumonia, Pontiac fever)	Characterized initially by anorexia, malaise, myalgia, and headache. Within 1 day is usually rapidly rising fever associated with chills. Nonproductive cough, abdominal pain, and diarrhea often occur.	Legionnaire's disease: 2 to 10 days; most often 5 to 6 days. Pontiac fever: 5 to 66 hours; most often 24 to 48 hours.	Evidence supports air-borne transmission.	Person-to-person transmission has not been documented.

Continued.

Name	*Synopsis of symptoms*	*Incubation period*	*Mode of transmission*	*Period of communicability*
Leishmaniasis, cutaneous	Polymorphic disease of skin and mucous membranes characterized by ulcerating lesions that may be single or multiple and self-limited or indolent, or multiple nodular lesions.	From a few days to many months.	Bite of infective sandfly.	As long as parasites remain in lesions; in untreated cases, 1 year or more.
Leishmaniasis, visceral	Chronic systemic infectious disease characterized by fever, hepatosplenomegaly, lymphadenopathy, anemia with leukopenia, and progressive emaciation and weakness.	Generally 2 to 4 months; range is 10 days to 2 years.	Bite of infective sandfly.	As long as parasites persist in circulating blood or skin. Transmission from person to person, and by blood transfusion, sexual contact, and bites of infected laboratory animals have been reported.
Leprosy (Hansen's disease)	Chronic bacterial disease characterized by lesions of skin and mucous membranes, by involvement and often palpable enlargement of peripheral nerves with consequent anesthesia, muscle weakness, paralysis, and trophic changes in skin, muscle, and bone.	Shortest known is 7 months. Average is probably 3 to 6 years.	Not clearly established, but household and prolonged intimate contact are important. Organisms may gain entrance through broken skin and respiratory tract.	As long as morphologically normal bacilli are demonstrable, infectiousness should be considered possible.
Listeriosis	Bacterial disease usually manifested as acute meningoencephalitis with or without associated septicemia, less frequently septicemia only; very often neonatal. Onset of meningoencephalitis is usually sudden with fever intense headache, nausea, vomiting, and signs of meningeal irritation.	Unknown; probably 4 days to 3 weeks. Fetus is usually infected within several days after maternal disease.	Largely neonatal; infection is transmitted from mother to unborn infant in utero during its passage through infected birth canal.	Mothers of infected newborn infants may shed infectious agent in vaginal discharges or urine for 7 to 10 days after delivery. Period of person-to-person communicability unknown.
Lyme disease	Characterized by distinctive skin lesion (ECM), systemic symptoms, polyarthritis, and neurological and cardiac involvement in varying combination.	From 3 to 21 days after tick exposure.	Presumably tick-borne.	No evidence of transmission from person to person.
Lymphocytic choriomeningitis (LCM, benign or serous lymphocytic meningitis)	Viral disease of animals, especially mice, transmissible to man with marked diversity of clinical manifestations. At times it begins with influenza-like attack followed by complete recovery; or after 1 to 2 weeks or remission, meningeal symptoms suddenly appear.	Probably 8 to 13 days; 15 to 20 days to meningeal symptoms.	Virus is excreted in urine, saliva, and feces of infected animals, usually mice transmission to humans, usually through contaminated food or dust.	Not known to be directly transmitted from person to person.

Lymphogranuloma venereum (lymphogranuloma inguinale, esthiomene, climatic bubo, tropical bubo)	Venereally acquired infection, beginning with painless evanescent erosion, papule, nodule, or herpetiform lesion on penis or vulva, frequently unnoticed. Regional lymph nodes undergo suppuration followed by extension of inflammatory process to adjacent tissues.	Usually 7 to 12 days, with a range of 4 to 21 days to primary lesion. If bubo is first manifestation, 10 to 30 days, sometimes several months.	Direct contact with open lesions of infected persons usually during sexual intercourse.	Variable, from weeks to years, during presence of active lesions.
Malaria	Fever, chills, sweats, and headache that may progress to icterus coagulation defects, shock, renal and liver failure, acute encephalitis, and coma are symptoms of most serious form (falciparum malaria). Symptoms difficult to differentiate in the four human malarias so laboratory confirmation is needed by demonstration of malaria parasites in blood films.	Average 12 days for *P. falciparum*, 12 days for *P. vivax* and *P. ovale*, and 30 days for *P. malariae*.	By infective female anopheline mosquito.	For infection of mosquitoes, as long as infective gametocytes are present in blood of patients; varies with species and strain of parasite and with response to therapy.
Measles (rubeola, hard measles, red measles, morbilli)	Acute, highly communicable viral disease with prodromal fever, conjunctivitis, coryza, bronchitis, and Koplik's spots on the buccal mucosa. A characteristic red blotchy rash appears on third to seventh day, beginning on face, becoming generalized, lasting 4 to 7 days and sometimes ending in branny desquamation. Leukopenia is common.	About 10 days varying from 8 to 13 days from exposure to onset of fever; about 14 days until rash appears; uncommonly longer or shorter human normal immune globulin (IG), given later than third day of incubation period for passive protection, may extend the incubation period to 21 days instead of preventing disease.	By droplet spread or direct contact with nasal or throat secretions of infected persons. Measles is one of most readily transmitted communicable diseases.	From slightly before beginning of prodromal period of 4 days after appearance of rash; communicability is minimal after second day of rash.
Melioidosis	Range of clinical manifestations from apparent infection or asymptomatic pulmonary consolidation to rapidly fatal septicemia. May simulate typhoid fever or even tuberculosis.	As short as 2 days; however, several months or years may elapse between presumed exposure and appearance of clinical disease.	Usually by contact with contaminated soil or water through overt or inapparent skin wounds, by aspiration or ingestion of contaminated water or by inhalation of dust from soil.	Person-to-person transmission and laboratory acquired infections are uncommon.
Meningitis, aseptic (viral meningitis, serous meningitis, nonbacterial or abacterial meningitis)	Common, rarely fatal, clinical syndrome with multiple causes, most commonly viral, characterized by sudden onset of febrile illness with signs and symptoms of meningeal involvement. Spinal fluid findings of pleocytosis	Varies with specific infectious agent (refer to specific diseases).	Varies with specific infectious agent (refer to specific diseases).	

Continued.

Name	Synopsis of symptoms	Incubation period	Mode of transmission	Period of communicability
	(usually mononuclear but may be polymorphonuclear in early stages), increased protein, normal sugar, and absence of bacteria. Active illness seldom exceeds 10 days.			
Meningitis, bacterial	Clinical signs and symptoms may be indistinguishable from those caused by meningococci including rash. Differentiation is based on smears and bacteriological studies.			
Meningitis, meningococcal (cerebrospinal fever, meningococcemia)	Characterized by sudden onset of fever, intense headache, nausea and often vomiting, stiff neck, and frequently a petechial rash with pink macules or, very rarely, vesicles. Delirium and coma often appear; occasional fulminating cases exhibit sudden prostration, ecchymoses, and shock at onset.	Varies from 2 to 10 days, commonly 3 to 4 days.	By direct contact, including droplets and discharges from nose and throat of infected persons, more often carriers than cases.	Until meningococci are no longer present in discharges from nose and throat. If organisms are sensitive to sulfonamides, meningococci usually disappear from nasopharynx within 24 hours after institution of treatment. They are not fully eradicated from oronasopharynx by penicillin.
Meningitis, hemophilus (meningitis caused by *Heamophilus influenzae)*	Most common bacterial meningitis in children 2 months to 3 years old in U.S. Otitis media or sinusitis may be precursor. Almost always associated with bacteremia. Onset is sudden with symptoms of fever, vomiting, lethargy, and meningeal irritation.	Probably short—within 2 to 4 days.	By droplet infection and discharges from nose and throat during infectious period. May be purulent rhinitis. Portal of entry is most commonly nasopharyngeal.	As long as organisms are present, which may be for prolonged period even without nasal discharge.
Meningitis, pneumococcal	High fatality rate is associated with this disease. Usually fulminant and occurs with bacteremia but not necessarily with another focus; although there may be otitis media or mastoiditis. Symptoms of high fever, lethargy or coma, and signs of meningeal irritation usually signal onset.			
Meningitis, neonatal	Patients exhibit symptoms of lethargy, seizures, apneic episodes, poor feeding, hypo-		Acquired from birth canal. For prevention of early onset form, ampicillin treat-	

	thermia or hyperthermia, and sometimes respiratory distress in first week of life.		ment at onset of labor has been recommended for mothers known to be infected with Group B *Streptococcus*.	
Meningoencephalitis caused by *Naegleria* and *Acanthamoeba*	*Naegleria;* Disease organisms cause a typical syndrome of fulminating pyogenic meningoencephalitis with severe frontal headache, occasional olfactory hallucinations, nausea, vomiting, high fever, nuchal rigidity, and somnolence. *Acanthamoeba:* Disease organisms invade the brain and meninges, usually without involvement of nasal and olfactory tissues, causing disease characterized by insidious onset and prolonged course.	*Naegleria:* 3 to 7 days in documented cases. *Acanthamoeba:* Much longer than in *Naegleria*.	*Naegleria:* Infection acquired by forcing infected water into nasal passages. *Naegleria* trophozoites colonize nasal tissues, then invade brain and meninges by extension along olfactory nerves. *Acanthamoebae* trophozoites reach central nervous system by metastasis from skin lesion or other site of primary colonization.	No person-to-person transmission has been observed.
Acanthamebiasis of eye, skin, and vagina	Lesions of conjunctiva, cornea, and inner structures of eye. Granulomatous lesions of the skin have been recorded. Also secondary invasion of central nervous system and occasionally of vagina.			
Molluscum contagiosum	Viral disease of skin that results in pearly pink to white papules with prominent central pore. Papules vary in size from less than 1 mm to 10 mm. Usually multiple lesions, most frequently in the genital area in adults; may occur anywhere in children. Eruption usually clears spontaneously in 6 to 9 months.	2 to 7 weeks.	Usually by direct contact, but transmission by fomites is possible. Sexual transmission occurs.	Unknown, but probably as long as lesions persist.
Mononucleosis, infectious (glandular fever, EBV mononucleosis)	Characterized by fever, sore throat (often with exudative pharyngotonsillitis), and lymphadenopathy (especially posterior cervical). Jaundice occurs in about 4% of infected young adults and splenomegaly in 50%. Duration is from 1 to several weeks.	From 4 to 6 weeks.	Person-to-person spread by oropharyngeal route via saliva. Spread may also occur via blood transfusion to susceptible recipients.	Prolonged; pharyngeal excretion may persist for 1 year after infection; 15% to 20% of healthy adults are oropharyngeal carriers.

Continued.

Name	Synopsis of symptoms	Incubation period	Mode of transmission	Period of communicability
Mumps (infectious parotitus)	Acute viral disease characterized by fever, swelling, and tenderness of one or more salivary glands, usually parotid and sometimes sublingual or submaxillary glands.	About 2 to 3 weeks, commonly 18 days.	By droplet spread and by direct contact with saliva of an infected person.	Virus has been isolated from saliva from 6 days before salivary gland involvement to as long as 9 days thereafter; but height of infectiousness occurs about 48 hours before swelling begins. Urine may be positive for as long as 14 days after onset of illness.
Mycetoma, actinomycotic (mycetomia, mycotic)	Characterized by swelling and suppuration of subcutaneous tissues, and formation of sinus tracts with visible granules in pus draining from sinus tracts. Lesions usually are on foot or lower leg.	Usually months.	Subcutaneous implantation of spores or hyphal elements from a saprophytic source by penetrating wounds (thorns, splinters).	Not transmitted from person to person.
Nocardiosis	Chronic disease often orginating in lungs, with hematogenous spread to produce abscesses of brain, subcutaneous tissue and other organs; high fatality rate.	Unknown; probably weeks.	*Nocardia* are presumed to enter body principally by inhalation of contaminated dust into lung.	Not directly transmitted from humans or animals to humans.
Onchocerciasis	Chronic, nonfatal filarial disease with fibrous nodules in subcutaneous tissues, particularly head and shoulders.	Microfilariae are found in skin usually about 1 year or more after infection.	By infected female blackflies.	Not directly transmitted from person to person; however, humans infect flies as long as living microfilariae occur in skin; i.e., for 10 to 15 years if untreated.
Ornithosis (psittacosis, parrot fever)	Acute generalized infectious disease with variable clinical presentations; fever, headache, myalgia, chills, and upper or lower respiratory tract disease are commonly present.	From 4 to 15 days, commonly 10 days.	Infection is usually acquired by inhaling agent from desiccated droppings of infected birds. Turkeys are usually involved but ducks and pigeons are occasionally responsible for human disease. Household birds are frequent source.	Person-to-person transmission is rare but can occur, especially with paroxysmal coughing.
Paracoccidioidomycosis	Chronic mycosis characterized by patchy pulmonary infiltrates or ulcerative lesions of mucosa (oral, nasal, gastrointestinal) and of skin. Lymphadenopathy is frequent. In disseminated cases all viscera may be affected; adrenal gland is especially susceptible.	Highly variable, from 1 month to many years.	Presumably acquired through inhalation of contaminated soil and dust.	Not known to be transmitted directly from person to person.
Paragonimiasis (pulmonary distomiasis, lung fluke disease)	Clinical signs depend on path of migration and organs parasitized. Lungs are most frequently involved; symptoms are cough and hemoptysis.	Flukes mature and begin to lay eggs approximately 6 weeks after humans ingest infective larvae. Interval until symptoms appear is	Infection occurs when raw or partially cooked flesh of freshwater crabs or crayfish containing infective larvae (metacercariae) are eaten.	Not directly transmitted from person to person, but eggs may be discharged by the human host for 20 years or more.

		long and variable depending on organ invaded and number of worms involved.		
Paratyphoid fever	Frequently generalized bacterial enteric infection, often with abrupt onset, continued fever, enlargement of spleen, sometimes rose spots on trunk, usually diarrhea, and involvement of lymphoid tissues of mesentery and intestines.	1 to 3 weeks for enteric fever; 1 to 10 days for gastroenteritis.	Direct or indirect contact with feces or urine of patient or carrier. Spread is by food, especially milk, milk products, and shellfish. Flies may be vectors.	As long as infectious agent persists in excreta, which is from appearance of prodromal symptoms, throughout illness, and for periods up to several weeks or months. Commonly 1 to 2 weeks after recovery.
Pediculosis (lousiness)	Infestation of head, hairy parts of body, or clothing with adult lice, larvae, or nits (eggs), which results in severe itching and excoriation of scalp or scratch marks of body.	Under optimum conditions, eggs of lice hatch in 1 week, reach sexual maturity in approximately 2 weeks.	Direct contact with infected person and indirectly by contact with personal belongings, especially clothing and headgear. Crab lice are usually transmitted through sexual contact.	Communicable as long as lice remain alive on infested person or in clothing, and until eggs in hair and clothing have been destroyed.
Pinta (carate)	Scaling papule with satellite lymphadenopathy appears within 1 to 8 weeks after infection, usually on hands, legs, or dorsum of feet. In 3 to 12 months, a maculopapular, erythematous secondary rash appears and may evolve into tertiary dyschromic macules of variable size. Organ systems are not involved.	3 to 60 days	Presumably person-to-person transmission by direct and prolonged contact with initial and early dyschromic skin lesions; location of primary lesions suggests that trauma provides portal of entry.	Unknown; potentially communicable while dyschromic skin lesions are active, sometimes for many years.
Plague (pest)	Specific zoonosis involving rodents and their fleas that transfer infection to various animals including humans. Initial response is commonly lymphadenitis in node receiving drainage from site of fleabite. Nodes become swollen and tender and fever is often present. Secondary involvement of lungs may result in severe pneumonia with mediastinitis and pleural effusion.	From 2 to 6 days; may be longer in vaccinated individuals.	Plague in humans occurs as result of intrusion into zoonotic transmission cycle or by entry of sylvatic infected animals and their infected fleas into human's habitat.	Fleas may remain infected for days, weeks, or months under suitable conditions of temperature and humidity.
Pleurodynia, epidemic	Acute viral disease characterized by sudden onset of severe pain localized in chest or abdomen that may be intensified by movement, usually accompanied by fever and frequently by headache.	Usually 3 to 5 days.	Probably fecal-oral or respiratory droplet contact with infected person or with articles freshly soiled with feces or throat discharges of infected person who may or may not have symptoms.	Apparently during acute stage of disease.

Continued.

Name	Synopsis of symptoms	Incubation period	Mode of transmission	Period of communicability
The pneumonias A. Pneumococcal pneumonia	Acute bacterial infection characterized by sudden onset with single shaking chill, fever, pleural pain, dyspnea, cough productive of "rusty" sputum and leukocytosis.	Not well determined; believed to be 1 to 3 days.	By droplet spread; by direct oral contact or indirectly, through articles freshly soiled with respiratory anisms is common.	Presumably until discharges of mouth and nose no longer contain virulent pneumococci in significant numbers. Penicillin will render patient noninfectious within 24 to 48 hours.
B. Mycoplasmal pneumonia (primary atypical pneumonia)	Predominantly afebrile lower respiratory infection. Onset is gradual with headache, malaise, cough often paroxysmal, and usually substernal pain (not pleuritic). Sputum, scant at first, may increase later.	14 to 21 days.	Probably by droplet inhalation, direct contact with infected person or with articles freshly soiled with discharges of nose and throat from acutely ill and coughing patient.	Probably less than 10 days; occasionally longer with persisting febrile illness or persistence of the organisms in convalescence (as long as 13 weeks is known).
C. Pneumocystis pneumonia (interstitial plasma-cell pneumonia)	Acute pulmonary disease occurring early in life, especially in malnourished, chronically ill, or premature infants. Characterized by progressive dyspnea, tachypnea, and cyanosis; fever may not be present.	Analysis of data from institutional outbreaks among infants indicates 1 to 2 months.	Unknown.	Unknown.
D. Chlamydial pneumonia (pertussoid eosinophilic pneumonia)	Subacute pulmonary disease occurring in early infancy, primarily in infants of mothers with infection of uterine cervix with causative organism. Characterized by insidious onset, cough, lack of fever, patchy infiltrates on chest x-ray with hyperinflation; eosinophilia, elevated IgM and IgG.	Not known, but pneumonia may occur in infants from 1 to 18 weeks of age (more commonly between 4 and 12 weeks). Nasopharyngeal infection is usually not present before 2 weeks of age.	Presumed to be vertically transmitted from infected cervix to infant during birth, with resultant nasopharyngeal infection (and occasionally conjunctival infection as inclusion conjunctivitis). Direct contact or respiratory transmission has not been established.	Unknown, but length of nasopharyngeal excretion can be at least 2 months.
Poliomyelitis (infantile paralysis)	Acute viral infection whose symptoms include fever, malaise, headache, nausea, vomiting, and stiffness of neck and back with or without paralysis.	Commonly 7 to 14 days for paralytic cases, with a range from 3 to possibly 35 days.	Direct contact through close association. In rare instances milk, foodstuffs, and other fecally-contaminated materials have been incriminated as vehicles. Fecal-oral is major route when sanitation is poor, but during epidemics and when sanitation is good, pharyngeal spread becomes relatively more important.	Not accurately known. Cases are probably most infectious during first few days after onset of symptoms.
Q fever (query fever)	Acute febrile rickettsial disease; onset may be sudden with chills, retrobulbar headache, weakness, malaise, and se-	Depends on size of the infecting dose; usually 2 to 3 weeks.	Commonly by air-borne dissemination of rickettsiae in dust from premises contaminated by placental tissues,	Direct transmission from person to person is very rare, but may occur in cases of pneumonia.

	vere sweats. Pneumonitis occurs in many cases with cough, scanty expectoration, chest pain, and minimal physical findings. Chronic endocarditis, pericarditis, hepatitis, and generalized infections have been reported.		infected animals.	
Rabies (hydrophobia, lyssa)	Almost invariably fatal acute encephalomyelitis; onset is with sense of apprehension, headache, fever, malaise, and indefintie sensory changes often referred to site of preceding animal bite wound. Disease progresses to paresis or paralysis; spasm of deglutition muscles on attempts to swallow, fear of water, and convulsions.	Usually 2 to 8 weeks, occasionally as short as 10 days or as long as 1 year or more depending on severity and site of wound.	Virus-laden saliva of a rabid animal is introduced by bite or, very rarely, through intact mucous membranes.	In dogs and most other biting animals, for 3 to 5 days before onset of clinical signs and during course of disease.
Rat-bite fever				
A. Streptobacillary fever	Abrupt onset with chills and fever, headache, and muscle pain is shortly followed by maculopapular or sometimes petechial rash. One or more joints may be swollen, red, and painful. Bacterial endocarditis and focal abscesses may occur late in untreated cases.	3 to 10 days, rarely longer.	Infection is transmitted by secretions of mouth, nose or conjunctival sac of infected animal, most frequently introduced by biting.	Not directly transmitted from person to person.
B. Spirillum fever	Symptoms rarely include arthritic symptoms, but distinctive rash of reddish or purplish plaques is evident.	1 to 3 weeks.		
Relapsing fever	Systemic spirochetal disease in which periods of fever lasting 2 to 9 days alternate with afebrile periods of 2 to 4 days; number of relapses varies from 1 to 10 or more.	5 to 15 days; usually 8 days.	Not directly transmitted from person to person.	Louse becomes infective 4 to 5 days after ingestion of blood from infected person and remains so for life (20 to 40 days).
Respiratory disease (excluding influenza)				
A. Acute febrile respiratory disease	Viral diseases of respiratory tract are characterized by fever and one or more constitutional reactions such as chills or chilliness, headache, general aching, malaise, and anorexia; in infants by occasional gastrointestinal disturbances.	From a few days to 1 week or more.	Directly by oral contact or by droplet spread, indirectly by hands or other materials soiled by respiratory discharges of infected person.	For duration of active disease; little is known about subclinical or latent infections.

Continued.

Name	Synopsis of symptoms	Incubation period	Mode of transmission	Period of communicability
B. Common cold (acute coryza)	Acute catarrhal infections of upper respiratory tract characterized by coryza, sneezing, lacrimation, irritated nasopharynx, chilliness, and malaise lasting 2 to 7 days. Fever is uncommon in children and rare in adults.		Presumably by direct oral contact or by droplet spread; indirectly by hands and articles freshly soiled by discharges of nose and throat of infected person.	
Rickettsioses, tick-borne (spotted fever group)				
A. Rocky Mountain spotted fever	Characterized by sudden onset with moderate to high fever that ordinarily persists for 2 to 3 weeks, significant malaise, deep muscle pain, severe headache, chills, and conjunctival injection. A maculopapular rash appears about the third day. Petechiae and hemorrhages are common.	From 3 to about 14 days.	Ordinarily by infected tick.	Not directly transmitted from person to person. Tick remains infective for life; commonly as long as 18 months.
B. Boutonneuse fever	Mild to moderately severe febrile illness of a few days to 2 weeks; characterized by primary lesion at site of tick bite. Lesion (tache noire), usually present at onset of fever, is small ulcer 2 mm to 5 mm in diameter with black center and red areola; regional lymph nodes are enlarged.	Usually 5 to 7 days.	By infected ticks.	Same as in Rocky Mountain spotted fever.
Also: (1) Queensland tick typhus, (2) North Asian tick fever, (3) Rickettsial pox				
Rubella (German measles)				
A. Congenital rubella	Mild febrile infectious disease with diffuse punctate and macular rash. Sometimes resembling that of measles, scarlet fever, or both. May be few or no constitutional symptoms in children but adults may experience 1 to 5 day prodrome characterized by low-grade fever, headache, malaise, mild coryza, and conjunctivitis. As many as 20% to 50% of infections may occur without evident rash; overall 50% are not recognized.	From 16 to 18 days with a range of 14 to 21 days.	Contact with nasopharyngeal secretions of infected person. Infection is by droplet spread or direct contact with patients and indirect contact.	For about 1 week before and at least 4 days after onset of rash. Highly communicable. Infants with congenital rubella syndrome may shed virus for months after birth.

B. Erythema infectiosum (fifth disease)	Mild nonfebrile erythematous eruption occurring as epidemics among children. Characterized by striking erythema of cheeks, reddening of skin, and lacelike serpiginous rash of body.			
C. Exanthema subitum (roseola infantum)	Acute illness of probable viral cause characterized by high fever that suddenly appears and lasts 3 to 5 days. A maculopapular rash on trunk and later on rest of body ordinarily follows lysis of fever.			
Salmonellosis	Commonly manifested by acute gastroenteritis. Acute infectious disease with sudden onset of abdominal pain, diarrhea, nausea, and sometimes vomiting. Dehydration may be severe. Fever is nearly always present.	6 to 72 hours, usually about 12 to 36 hours.	By ingestion of organisms in food contaminated by feces of infected person or animal.	Throughout course of infection—extremely variable.
Scabies (sarcoptic acariasis)	Infectious disease of skin caused by mite whose penetration is visible as papules or vesicles, or as tiny linear burrows containing mites and their eggs.	2 to 6 weeks before onset of itching in persons without previous exposure. Persons who have been previously infested develop symptoms 1 to 4 days after reexposure.	Transfer of parasites is by direct skin-to-skin contact and to limited extent from undergarments or soiled bedclothes freshly contaminated by infected persons; frequently acquired during sexual contact.	Until mites and eggs are destroyed by treatment, ordinarily after one or occasionally two courses of treatment 1 week apart.
Shigellosis (bacillary dysentery)	Acute bacterial disease primarily involving large intestine, characterized by diarrhea, accompanied by fever, nausea, sometimes vomiting, cramps, and tenesmus. In severe cases stools contain blood, mucous, and pus.	1 to 7 days, usually 1 to 3 days.	By direct or indirect fecal-oral transmission from patient or carrier. Infection may occur after ingestion of very few organisms.	During acute infection and until infectious agent is no longer present in feces, usually within 4 weeks of illness.
Slow virus infections of central nervous system				
A. Kuru	Signs include cerebellar ataxia, temors, rigidity, progressive wasting, and variable cranial nerve signs in patients 4 years of age or older.	8 to 9 years in childhood cases; range is 4 to more than 30 years.	Exact route of transmission not firmly established. Principally by traditional mortuary practices with intimate contact with infected tissues.	CNS tissues are infectious throughout symptomatic illness.
B. Jakob-Creutzfeldt disease	Insidious onset of confusion, progressive dementia, and variable ataxia in patients 25 years of age or older.	Unknown in most cases.	Unknown.	Same.

Continued.

Name	Synopsis of symptoms	Incubation period	Mode of transmission	Period of communicability
Smallpox	Systemic disease with usually characteristic exanthem. Onset is sudden, with fever, malaise, headache, severe backache, prostration, and occasionally abdominal pain. Rash appears after 2 to 4 days and goes through stages of macules, papules, vesicles, pustules, and finally scabs.	From 7 to 17 days; commonly 10 to 12 days to onset of illness and 2 to 4 days more to onset of rash.	Transmission normally through close contact with respiratory discharges and skin lesions of patients, and material they had recently contaminated. Air-borne spread occurs infrequently.	From a few days before development of earliest lesions to disappearance of all scabs; about 3 weeks. Most communicable during first week.
Sporotrichosis	Fungal disease, usually of skin, which begins as nodule. As nodule grows, lymphatics draining area become firm and cordlike and form series of nodules, which in turn may soften and ulcerate.	Lymphatic form may develop 1 week to 3 months after injury.	Introduction of fungus through skin following pricks by thorns or barbs, handling of sphagnum moss or by slivers from wood or lumber.	Not transmitted from person to person. Environment presumably may be contaminated for duration of active lesion.
Staphylococcal disease				
A. Staphylococcal disease in community Boils, carbuncles, furuncles Impetigo Cellutitis, abscesses Staphylococcal septicemia Staphylococcal pneumonia Osteomyelitis Endocarditis	Staphylococci produce variety of syndromes with clinical manifestations that range from single pustule to impetigo to septicemia to death. Lesion or lesions containing pus is primary clinical finding, abscess formation is typical.	Variable and indefinite. Commonly 4 to 10 days.	Major site of colonization is anterior nares. Autoinfection is responsible for at least one third of infections. Person with draining lesion or any purulent lesion or who is asymptomatic (usually nasal) carrier of pathogenic strain. Air-borne spread is rare.	As long as purulent lesions continue to drain or carrier state persists.
B. Staphylococcal disease in hospital nurseries Impetigo Abscess of breast	Characteristic lesions develop secondary to colonization of nose or umbilicus, conjunction, circumcision site, or rectum of infants with pathogenic strain.	Commonly 4 to 10 days but may occur several months after colonization.	Spread by hands of hospital personnel is primary mode of transmission within hospitals; to a lesser extent, air-borne.	Same.
C. Staphylococcal disease in medical and surgical wards of hospitals	Lesions vary from simple furuncles or stitch abscesses to extensively infected bedsores or surgical wounds, septic phlebitis, chronic osteomyelitis, fulminating pneumonia, endocarditis, or septicemia.	Variable and indefinite. Commonly 4 to 10 days.	Major site of colonization is anterior nares. Autoinfection is responsible for at least one third of infections. Person with a draining lesion or any purulent lesion or who is an asymptomatic (usually nasal) carrier of a pathogenic strain. Air-borne spread is rare.	As long as purulent lesions continue to drain or carrier state persists.

D. Toxic shock syndrome	Characterized by sudden onset of fever, vomiting, profuse watery diarrhea, and myalgia, followed by hypotension, and in severe cases, shock. An erythematous ''sunburnlike'' rash is present during acute phase.	Thought to be related to use of tampons; however, mode of transmission is still under investigation.		
Streptococcal diseases caused by group A (beta hemolytic) streptococci				
A. Streptococcal sore throat	Fever, sore throat, exudative tonsillitis or pharyngitis, and tender anterior cervical lymph nodes	Short, usually 1 to 3 days, rarely longer.	Transmission results from direct or intimate contact with patient or carrier, rarely by indirect contact through objects or hands. Nasal carriers are particularly likely to transmit diseases.	In untreated uncomplicated cases 10 to 21 days; in untreated conditions with purulent discharges, weeks or months.
B. Streptococcal skin infections	Usually superficial, may proceed through vesicular, pustular, and encrusted stages			
C. Scarlet fever	Skin rash and symptoms similar to streptococcal sore throat, enanthem, strawberry tongue, and exanthem. Rash is usually fine erythema.			
D. Erysipelas	Acute cellulitis characterized by fever, constitutional symptoms, leukocytosis, and red, tender, edematous, spreading lesion of skin with definite raised border.			
E. Streptococcal puerperal fever	Acute disease, usually febrile accompanied by local and general symptoms and signs of bacterial invasion of genital tract and sometimes bloodstream in postpartum or postabortion patient.			
Streptococcal (group B) disease of the newborn	Produces diseases of newborn infants including cases of septicemia, evidence of pulmonary involvement, and meningeal involvement.		Acquired during passage through birth canal. Some cases are acquired through environment.	
Strongyloidiasis	Helminthic infection of duodenum and upper jejunum, usually asymptomatic. Clinical manifestations include dermatitis, cough, rales, and abdominal symptoms.	From penetration of skin by filariform larvae until rhabitiform larvae appear in feces is about 2 to 3 weeks; period until symptoms appear is variable.	Infective larvae that develop in moist soil contaminated with feces penetrate skin, enter venous circulation, and are carried to lungs.	As long as living worms remain in intestine; up to 35 years.

Continued.

Name	*Synopsis of symptoms*	*Incubation period*	*Mode of transmission*	*Period of communicability*
Syphilis, venereal (lues)	Acute and chronic treponematosis characterized clinically by primary lesion, secondary eruption involving skin and mucous membranes, long periods of latency, and late lesions of skin, bone, viscerae, and central nervous and cardiovascular systems. Papule appears 3 weeks after exposure at site of initial invasion; after erosion, most common form is indurated chancre.	10 days to 10 weeks, usually 3 weeks.	By direct contact with infectious exudates form obvions or concealed moist early lesions of skin and mucous membrane, body fluids, and secretions of infected persons during sexual contact.	Variable and indefinite during primary and secondary stages and also in mucocutaneous recurrences; some cases may be intermittently communicable for 2 to 4 years.
Syphilis, nonvenereal endemic	Acute disease of limited geographical distribution, characterized clinically by eruption of skin and mucous membrane, usually without evident primary sore.	2 weeks to 3 months.	Direct or indirect contact with infectious early lesions of skin and mucous membranes. Congenital transmission does not occur.	Until moist eruptions of skin and mucous patches disappear—sometimes several weeks or months.
Taeniasis and cysticercosis *Taenia solium* infection, intesinal form (pork tapeworm) Cysticercosis (cysticerciasis, infection by *Cysticercus cellulosae*) *Taenia saginata* infection (beef tapeworm)	Taeniasis is intestinal infection with adult stage of large tapeworms. Cysticercosis is somatic infection with larvae stage of one species, *Taenia solium*. Clinical manifestations of infection with adult worm are variable and may include nervousness, insomnia, anorexia, weight loss, abdominal pain, and digestive disturbance. Cysticercosis is serious somatic disease that may involve many different organs. Eggs of tapeworm, when swallowed, hatch in small intestines and larvae migrate throughout body.	For adult tapeworm, from 8 to 14 weeks.	Ova of *Taenia saginata* passed in stool of infected person are infectious only to cattle. Infection of man follows ingestion of raw or inadequately cooked beef containing cysticerci. Ova of *Taenia solium* are infectious to both man and pigs. Human infection occurs by direct transfer of eggs in feces of person harboring adult worm to own or another's mouth, or indirectly through ingestion of food or water contaminated with eggs, resulting in somatic cysticercosis. Intestional infection of humans (taeniasis) follows ingestion of raw or inadequately cooked infected pork.	*Taenia saginata* is not directly transmitted from person to person but *Taenia solium* may be; eggs of both species are disseminated into environment as long as worm remains in intestines, sometimes more than 30 years; eggs may remain viable for months.
Tetanus (tetanus neonatorum, lockjaw)	Acute disease induced by tetanus bacillus that grows anaerobically at site of injury and produces neurotoxin. Characterized by painful muscular contractions, abdominal rigidity, and gener-	4 to 21 days, dependent on character, extent, and location of wound; average 10 days. Most cases occur within 14 days.	Tetanus spores introduced into body during injury, usually puncture wound contaminated with soil, street dust, or animal or human feces, but also through lacerations, burns,	Not directly transmitted from person to person

	alized spasms. Symptoms usually appear between fifth and twelfth day, most frequently about seventh day.		and trivial or unnoticed wounds.	
Toxocariasis (larva migrans viscervalis, *Toxocara* [Canis] [Cati] infection, visceral larva migrans syndrome)	Chronic and usually mild disease of young children caused by migration of certain nematode larvae in organs and tissues. Characterized by eosinophilia of variable duration, hepatomegaly, hyperglobulinemia, pulmonary symptoms, and fever.	Probably weeks or months, depending on intensity of infection and sensitivity of patient.	By direct or indirect transmission of infectious *Toxocara* eggs from contaminated soil to mouth; directly related to eating of dirt by young children. Eggs reach soil in feces from infected cats and dogs.	Not directly transmitted from person to person.
Toxoplasmosis (congenital toxoplasmosis)	Systemic protozoal disease. Primary infection is frequently asymptomatic; acute disease may occur with fever, lymphadenopathy, and lymphocytosis persisting for days or weeks. Rare severe manifestations include cerebral signs, pneumonitis, generalized muscle involvement, and death.	Unknown; 10 to 23 days in one outbreak larva vehicle was undercooked meat, and 5 to 20 days in an outbreak associated with infected cats.	Transplacental infection may occur in women with primary infection. Postnatal infections might be acquired by eating raw or undercooked infected meat or more often by ingesting infective oocysts. Drinking water contaminated with feces of *Felidue* has been incriminated.	Not directly transmitted from person to person except in utero.
Trachoma	Communicable keratoconjunctivitis characterized by conjunctival inflammation with papillary hyperplasia, associated with ascular invasion of cornea, and in later stages by conjunctival scarring that may eventually lead to blindness.	5 to 12 days (based on volunteer studies).	By direct contact with ocular discharges and possibly mucoid or purulent discharges of nasal mucous membranes of infected persons or materials. Flies *(Musca sorbens)* may contribute to spread of disease.	As long as active lesions are present in the conjunctivae and adnexal mucous membranes.
Trench fever (Wolhynian fever, quintan fever)	Nonfatal, febrile disease of protean manifestations characterized by headache, malaise, pain, and tenderness especially in shins; onset either sudden or slow with fever, which may be relapsing, typhoidlike, or limited to single short febrile episode lasting several days.	Generally 7 to 30 days.	Not directly transmitted from person to person. Humans infected by inoculation of organism in louse feces through a skin break from either bite of louse or other means.	Organisms may circulate in blood (by which lice can be infected) for weeks, months, or years and may recur with or without symptoms. History of trench fever is permanent contraindication to blood donation.
Trichinosis (trichiniasis, trichinellosis)	Disease caused by larvae of *Trichinella spiralis* that migrate to and become encapsulated in muscles. Clinical manifestations usually include mild febrile disease, but can range from inapparent infection to fulminating, fatal disease.	Usually about 10 to 14 days after ingestion by humans of infective meat; varies between 1 and 45 days.	Eating raw or insufficiently cooked flesh of animals containing viable encysted trichinae, chiefly pork and pork products.	Not transmitted directly from person to person. Animal hosts remain infective for months as does meat from such animals for appreciable periods unless processed to kill larvae.

Continued.

Name	Synopsis of symptoms	Incubation period	Mode of transmission	Period of communicability
Trichomoniasis	Common disease of genitourinary tract, characterized in women by vaginitis, with small petechial or sometimes punctate hemorrhagic lesions and profuse, thin, foamy, yellowish discharge with foul odor; frequently asymptomatic. In men, infectious agent invades and persists in prostate, urethra, or seminal vesicles, but rarely produces symptoms or demonstrable lesions.	4 to 20 days, average 7 days.	By contact with vaginal and urethral discharges of infected persons during sexual intercourse and possibly by contact with contaminated articles.	For duration of infection.
Trichuriasis (trichocephaliasis)	Nematode infection of large intestine, often asymptomatic. Heavy infections result in bloody stools and diarrhea. Rectal prolapse may occur in very heavily infected children.			
Trypanosomiasis, (African sleeping sickness)	In early stages chancre usually appears at primary tsetse fly bite site with fever, intense headache, insomnia, lymph node enlargement, anemia, local edema, and rash. In late stage is body wasting, somnolence, and signs referable to central nervous system.	In *T. rhodesiense* infection usually 2 to 3 weeks; in *T. gambiense* infection, usually longer and extremely variable—months or even years.	By bite of infective *Glossina*, the tsetse fly. Congenital transmission can occur in humans, as well as direct mechanical transmission by blood on proboscis of *Glossina* and other human-biting flies, or in laboratory accidents.	To tsetse fly, as long as parasite is present in blood of infected person or animal. Parasitemia is extremely variable in untreated cases and occurs in late and early stages of disease.
Trypanosomiasis, American (Chagas' disease)	Acute disease usually occurs in children; chronic manifestations generally appear later in life. Acute disease is characterized by variable fever, malaise, lymphadenopathy and hepatosplenomegaly. Inflammatory response at site of infection (chagoma) may last up to 8 weeks. Unilateral bipalpebral edema occurs in significant percentage of acute cases. Life-threatening or fatal manifestations include myocarditis and meningoencephalitis.	About 5 to 14 days after bite of insect vector; 30 to 40 days if infected by blood transfusion.	By fecal material passed while biting by infected vectors. Infection is through contamination of conjunctiva, mucous membranes, abrasions, or skin wounds by fresh infected bug feces. Transmission also may occur by blood transfusion and organisms may pass through placenta to cause congenital infection.	Organisms are present regularly in blood during acute period and may persist in very small numbers throughout life in symptomatic and asymptomatic persons. Vector becomes infective 10 to 30 days after biting an infective host and remains so for life (as long as 2 years).
Tuberculosis	Mycobacterial disease. Initial infection usually goes unno-	From infection to demonstrable primary lesion, about 4	Exposure to bacilli in airborne droplet nuclei from	As long as infectious tubercle bacilli are being discharged.

	ticed; tuberculin sensitivity appears within a few weeks; lesions commonly heal, leaving no residual changes except pulmonary or tracheobronchial lymph node calcification. May progress to pulmonary tuberculosis or, by lymphohematogenous dissemination of bacilli, to produce miliary, meningeal, or other extrapulmonary involvement.	to 12 weeks. Whereas subsequent risk of progressive pulmonary or extrapulmonary tuberculosis is greatest within 1 or 2 years after infection, it may persist for a lifetime as latent infection.	sputum of persons with infectious tuberculosis. Bovine tuberculosis results from exposure to tubercular cattle and ingestion of unpasteurized dairy products.	
Tularemia (rabbit fever, deerfly fever, Ohara's disease)	Clinical manifestations related to route of introduction and virulence of strain. Most often ulcer, often on hand, accompanied by swelling of regional lymph nodes. May be no apparent primary ulcer but only enlarged and painful lymph nodes that may suppurate.	Related to virulence of infecting strain and to size of inoculum; 2 to 10 days, usually 3 days.	Inoculation of skin, conjunctival sac, or oropharyngeal mucosa with blood or tissue while handling infected animals; or by fluids from infected flies, ticks, or other animals; or through bite of arthropods.	Not directly transmitted from person to person. Unless treated, infectious agent may be found in blood during first 2 weeks of disease, and in lesions for 1 month from onset—sometimes longer.
Typhoid fever (enteric fever, typhus abdominalis)	Systemic infectious disease characterized by sustained fever, headache, malaise, anorexia, relative bradycardia, enlargement of spleen, rose spots on trunk, nonproductive cough, constipation more commonly than diarrhea, and involvement of lymphoid tissues.	Depends on size of infecting dose; usual range 1 to 3 weeks.	By food or water contaminated by feces or urine of patient or carrier.	As long as typhoid bacilli appear in excreta; usually first week throughout convalescence; variable thereafter. About 10% of untreated patients will discharge bacilli for 3 months after onset of symptoms; 2 to 5% become permanent carriers.
Typhus fever, epidemic louse-borne (exanthematic typhus, classical typhus fever)	Onset is variable, often sudden and marked by headache, chills, prostration, fever, and general pains. Macular eruptions appears on fifth or sixth day, initially on upper trunk followed by spread to entire body but usually not to face, palms, or soles. Toxemia is usually pronounced and disease terminates by rapid lysis after about 2 weeks of fever.	From 1 to 2 weeks, commonly 12 days.	The body louse, *Pediculus humanis corporis,* is infected by feeding on blood of patient with acute typhus fever. Humans are infected by rubbing feces or crushed lice into bites of louse or other superfacial abrasions. Inhalation of infective louse feces as dust may account for some infections.	Disease is not directly transmitted from person to person. Patients are infective for lice during febrile illness and possibly for 2 or 3 days after temperature returns to normal.
Typhus fever, flea-borne (murine typhus, endemic typhus fever, shop typhus)	Course of flea-borne typhus fever resembles that of epidemic louse-borne typhus, but is milder. Fatality rate for all ages is about 2%; it increases with age.	From 1 to 2 weeks, commonly 12 days.	Infective rat fleas (usually *Xenopsylla cheopis*) defecate rickettsiae while sucking blood and contaminate bite site and other fresh skin wounds. Occasional case may follow inhalation of dried infective flea feces.	Not directly transmitted from person to person. Once infected, fleas remain so for life.

Continued.

Name	Synopsis of symptoms	Incubation period	Mode of transmission	Period of communicability
Typhus, scrub (tsutsugamushi disease, mite-borne typhus fever)	Often characterized by primary skin ulcer (eschar) corresponding to site of attachment of infected mite. Acute febrile onset follows within several days, along with headache, profuse sweating, conjunctival injection, and lymphadenopathy.	Usually 10 to 12 days; varies from 6 to 21 days.	By infected larval mites; nymphs and adults do not feed on vertebrate hosts.	Not directly transmitted from person to person.
Urethritis, chlamydial Urethritis, nongonorrheal and nonspecific	Sexually transmitted urethritis of males caused by chlamydial agent. Clinical manifestations are usually indistinguishable from gonorrhea but are often milder and include opaque discharge of moderate or scanty quantity, urethral itching, and burning on urination. Infection of women results in cervicitis and salpingitis; infections are often asymptomatic.	5 to 7 days or longer.	Sexual contact.	Unknown.
Verruca vulgaris (warts)	Viral disease manifested by variety of skin and mucous membrane lesions. Include the common wart, a circumscribed, hyperkeratotic, rough textured, painless papule varying in size from pinhead to large masses; also filiform warts, venereal warts, and plantar warts.	About 4 months; range is 1 to 20 months.	Usually by direct contact, but contaminated floors and fomites are frequently implicated. Warts may be autoinoculated. *Condyloma accuminatum* is usually sexually transmitted.	Unknown, but probably as long as visible lesions persist.
Whooping cough (pertussis)	Acute bacterial disease involving tracheobronchial tree. Initial catarrhal stage has insidions onset with irritating cough that gradually becomes paroxysmal, usually within 1 to 2 weeks, and lasts for 1 to 2 months.	Commonly 7 days; amost uniformly within 10 days, and not exceeding 21 days.	Primarily by direct contact with discharges from respiratory mucous membranes of infected persons by airborne route, probably by droplets. Frequently brought into home by older sibling.	Highly communicable in early catarrhal stage before paroxysmal cough stage. For control purposes, communicable stage extends from 7 days after exposure to 3 weeks after onset of typical paroxysms in patients not treated with antibiotics; in patients treated with erythromycin, period of infectiousness extends only 5 to 7 days after onset of therapy.
Yaws (frambesia, pian, bouba, parang)	Chronic relapsing nonvenereal treponematosis characterized by early cutaneous lesions and noncontagious late, destructive lesions. Typical initial lesion (mother yaw) is	From 2 weeks to 3 months.	Principally by direct contact with exudates of early skin lesions of infected persons. Indirect transmission by contamination from scratching, skin piercing articles,	Variable; may extend intermittently over several years while moist lesions are present. Infectious agent is not usually found in late ulcerative lesions.

	papilloma on face or extremities that persists for several weeks or months.		and by flies on open wounds is probable but of undetermined importance.	
Yersinia (pseudotuberculosis)	Acute enteric disease manifested by diarrhea, enterocolitis, acute mesenteric lymphadentitis mimicking appendicitis, low-grade fever, headache, pharyngitis, anorexia, vomiting, erythema nodosum, arthritis, cutaneous ulceration, abscesses, and septicemia.	Probably 3 to 7 days, generally less than 10 days.	Fecal-oral transmission takes place by contact with infected persons or animals (hand-to-mouth), or by eating and drinking contaminated food and water.	Fecal shedding as long as symptoms exist. Chronic carrier state probably exists.
Zygomycosis (mucormycosis, phycomycosis)	Group of mycoses usually caused by fungi of the family Mucoraceae of the class Zygomycetes. These fungi have affinity for blood vessels, causing thrombosis and infarction. In its craniofacial form is usually nasal or paranasal sinus infections, most often during ketoacidotic episodes of diabetes mellitus.	Unknown. Fungus spreads rapidly in susceptible tissues.	By inhalation or ingestion of fungus by susceptible individuals. Direct inoculation by minor trauma, intravenous catheters, and cutaneous burns are occasionally implicated.	Not directly transmitted from human or animal to human.

APPENDIX 16 DIAGNOSIS-RELATED GROUPS

16-1 Major diagnostic categories

Major diagnostic category	Group description
1	Diseases and disorders of the nervous system
2	Diseases and disorders of the eye
3	Diseases and disorders of the ear, nose, and throat
4	Diseases and disorders of the respiratory system
5	Diseases and disorders of the circulatory system
6	Diseases and disorders of the digestive system
7	Diseases and disorders of the hepatobiliary system and pancreas
8	Diseases and disorders of the musculoskeletal system and connective tissue
9	Diseases and disorders of the skin, subcutaneous tissue, and breast
10	Endocrine, nutritional, and metabolic diseases and disorders
11	Diseases and disorders of the kidney and urinary tract
12	Diseases and disorders of the male reproductive system
13	Diseases and disorders of the female reproductive system
14	Pregnancy, childbirth, and the puerperium
15	Newborns and other neonates with conditions originating in perinatal period
16	Diseases and disorders of the blood and blood-forming organs
17	Myeloproliferative disorders
18	Infectious and parasitic diseases
19	Mental diseases and disorders
20	Substance use and substance-induced organic mental disorders
21	Injuries, poisonings, and toxic effects of drugs
22	Burns
23	Factors influencing health status and other contacts with health services

From Ernest and Whinney: The revised DRGs: their importance in Medicare payment to hospitals, May 1983.

16-2 Diagnosis-related group descriptions

MDC	01	Diseases and disorders of the nervous system
001	P	Craniotomy, age ≧18 except for trauma
002	P	Craniotomy for trauma age ≧18
003*	P	Craniotomy, age <18
004	P	Spinal procedures
005	P	Extracranial vascular procedures
006	P	Carpal tunnel release
007	P	Peripheral and cranial nerve and other nervous system procedures, age ≧70 and/or C.C.
008	P	Peripheral and cranial nerve and other nervous system procedures, age <70 w/o C.C.
009	M	Spinal disorders and injuries
010	M	Nervous system neoplasms, age ≧70 and/or C.C.
011	M	Nervous system neoplasms, age <70 w/o C.C.
012	M	Degenerative nervous system disorders
013	M	Multiple sclerosis and cerebellar ataxia
014	M	Specific cerebrovascular disorders except TIA
015	M	Transient ischemic attacks
016	M	Nonspecific cerebrovascular disorders with C.C.
017	M	Nonspecific cerebrovascular disorders w/o C.C.
018	M	Cranial and peripheral nerve disorders, age ≧70 and/or C.C.
019	M	Cranial and peripheral nerve disorders, age <70 w/o C.C.
020	M	Nervous system infection except viral meningitis
021*	M	Viral meningitis
022	M	Hypertensive encephalopathy
023	M	Nontraumatic stupor and coma
024	M	Seizure and headache, age ≧70 and/or C.C.
025	M	Seizure and headache, age 18-69 w/o C.C.
026*	M	Seizure and headache, age 0-17
027*	M	Traumatic stupor and coma, coma >1 hr
028	M	Traumatic stupor and coma, coma <1 hr, age ≧70 and/or C.C.
029*	M	Traumatic stupor and coma, coma <1 hr, age 18-69 w/o C.C.
030*	M	Traumatic stupor & coma, coma <1 hr, age 0-17
031	M	Concussion, age ≧70 and/or C.C.
032	M	Concussion, age 18-69 w/o C.C.
033*	M	Concussion, age 0-17
034	M	Other disorders of nervous system, age ≧70 and/or C.C.
035	M	Other disorders of nervous system, age <70 w/o C.C.

From Yale University School of Organization and Management: The new ICD-9-CM diagnosis-related groups classification scheme, December 1981.
*DRGs excluded from calculation of case mix index because of insufficient cases.
P, Surgical case.
M, Medical case.
C.C., Comorbidity or complication.

MDC	**02**	**Diseases and disorders of the eye**
036	P	Retinal procedures
037	P	Orbital procedures
038	P	Primary iris procedures
039	P	Lens procedures
040	P	Extraocular procedures except orbit, age $\geqq$18
041*	P	Extraocular procedures except orbit, age 0-17
042	P	Intraocular procedures except retina, iris, and lens
043*	M	Hyphema
044	M	Acute major eye infections
045	M	Neurological eye disorders
046	M	Other disorders of the eye, age $\geqq$18 with C.C.
047	M	Other disorders of the eye, age $\geqq$18 w/o C.C.
048*	M	Other disorders of the eye, age 0-17

MDC	**03**	**Diseases and disorders of the ear, nose, and throat**
049	P	Major head and neck procedures
050	P	Sialodenectomy
051	P	Salivary gland procedures except sialodenectomy
052*	P	Cleft lip and palate repair
053	P	Sinus and mastoid procedures, age $\geqq$18
054*	P	Sinus and mastoid procedures, age 0-17
055	P	Miscellaneous ear, nose, and throat procedures
056	P	Rhinoplasty
057*	P	T&A procedure except tonsillectomy and/or adenoidectomy, age $\geqq$18
058*	P	T&A procedure except tonsillectomy and/or adenoidectomy, age 0-17
059*	P	Tonsillectomy and/or adenoidectomy, age $\geqq$18
060*	P	Tonsillectomy and/or adenoidectomy, age 0-17
061*	P	Myringotomy, age $\geqq$18
062*	P	Myringotomy, age 0-17
063	P	Other ear, nose, and throat O.R. procedures
064	M	Ear, nose, and throat malignancy
065	M	Dysequilibrium
066	M	Epistaxis
067*	M	Epiglottitis
068	M	Otitis media and uri, age $\geqq$70 and/or C.C.
069	M	Otitis media and uri, age 18-69 w/o C.C.
070*	M	Otitis media and uri, age 0-17
071*	M	Laryngotracheitis
072	M	Nasal trauma and deformity
073	M	Other ear, nose, and throat diagnosis, age $\geqq$18
074*	M	Other ear, nose, and throat diagnosis, age 0-17

MDC	**04**	**Diseases and disorders of the respiratory system**
075	P	Major chest procedures
076	P	O.R. procedure on respiratory system except major chest with C.C.
077	P	O.R. procedure on respiratory system except major chest w/o C.C.
078	M	Pulmonary embolism
079	M	Respiratory infections and inflammations, age $\geqq$70 and/or C.C.
080	M	Respiratory infections and inflammations, age 18-69 w/o C.C.
081*	M	Respiratory infections and inflammations, age 0-17
082	M	Respiratory neoplasms
083	M	Major chest trauma, age $\geqq$70 and/or C.C.
084*	M	Major chest trauma, age $<$70 w/o C.C.
085	M	Pleural effusion, age $\geqq$70 and/or C.C.
086	M	Pleural effusion, age $<$70 w/o C.C.
087	M	Pulmonary edema and respiratory failure
088	M	Chronic obstructive pulmonary disease
089	M	Simple pneumonia and pleurisy, age $\geqq$70 and/or C.C.
090	M	Simple pneumonia and pleurisy, age 18-69 w/o C.C.
091*	M	Simple pneumonia and pleurisy, age 0-17
092	M	Interstitial lung disease, age $\geqq$70 and/or C.C.
093	M	Interstitial lung disease, age $<$70 w/o C.C.
094	M	Pneumothorax, age $\geqq$70 and/or C.C.
095	M	Pneumothorax, age $<$70 w/o C.C.
096	M	Bronchitis and asthma, age $\geqq$70 and/or C.C.
097	M	Bronchitis and asthma, age 18-69 w/o C.C.
098*	M	Bronchitis and asthma, age 0-17
099	M	Respiratory signs and symptoms, age $\geqq$70 and/or C.C.
100	M	Respiratory signs and symptoms, age $<$70 w/o C.C.
101	M	Other respiratory diagnoses, age $\geqq$70 and/or C.C.
102	M	Other respiratory diagnoses, age $<$70

MDC	**05**	**Diseases and disorders of the circulatory system**
103*	P	Heart transplant
104	P	Cardiac valve procedure with pump and with cardiac cath
105	P	Cardiac valve procedure with pump and w/o cardiac cath
106	P	Coronary bypass with cardiac cath
107	P	Coronary bypass w/o cardiac cath
108	P	Cardiothoracic procedure, except valve and coronary bypass, with pump
109	P	Cardiothoracic procedures w/o pump
110	P	Major reconstructive vascular procedures, age $\geqq$70 and/or C.C.
111	P	Major reconstructive vascular procedures, age $<$70 w/o C.C.
112	P	Vascular procedures except major reconstruction
113	P	Amputation for circulatory system disorders except upper limb and toe
114	P	Upper limb and toe amputation for circulatory system disorders
115	P	Permanent cardiac pacemaker implant with AMI or CHF
116	P	Permanent cardiac pacemaker implant w/o AMI or CHF
117	P	Cardiac pacemaker replace and revise except pulse generator replacement only
118	P	Cardiac pacemaker pulse generator replacement only

MDC	**05**	**Diseases and disorders of the circulatory System**
119	P	Vein ligation and stripping
120	P	Other O.R. procedures on the circulatory system
121	M	Circulatory disorders with AMI and C.V. comp. disch. alive
122	M	Circulatory disorders with AMI w/o C.V. comp. disch. alive
123	M	Circulatory disorders with AMI, expired
124*	M	Circulatory disorders except AMI with cardiac cath. and complex diagnosis
125	M	Circulatory disorders except AMI with cardiac cath. w/o complex diagnosis
126	M	Acute and subacute endocarditis
127	M	Heart failure and shock
128	M	Deep vein thrombophlebitis

129	M	Cardiac arrest
130	M	Peripheral vascular disorders, age ≧ 70 and/or C.C.
131	M	Peripheral vascular disorders age < 70 w/o C.C.
132	M	Atherosclerosis, age ≧ 70 and/or C.C.
133	M	Atherosclerosis, age < 70 w/o C.C.
134	M	Hypertension
135	M	Cardiac congenital and valvular disorders, age ≧ 70 and/or C.C.
136	M	Cardiac congenital and valvular disorders, age 18-69 w/o C.C.
137*	M	Cardiac congenital and valvular disorders, age 0-17
138	M	Cardiac arrhythmia and conduction disorders, age ≧ 70 and/or C.C.
139	M	Cardiac arrhythmia and conduction disorders, age < 70 w/o C.C.
140	M	Angina pectoris
141	M	Syncope and collapse, age ≧ 70 and/or C.C.
142	M	Syncope and collapse, age < 70 w/o C.C.
143	M	Chest pain
144	M	Other circulatory diagnoses with C.C.
145	M	Other circulatory diagnoses w/o C.C.
MDC	**06**	**Diseases and disorders of the digestive system**
146	P	Rectal resection, age ≧ 70 and/or C.C.
147	P	Rectal resection, age < 70 w/o C.C.
148	P	Major small and large bowel procedures, age ≧ 70 and/or C.C.
149	P	Major small and large bowel procedures, age < 70 w/o C.C.
150	P	Peritoneal adhesiolysis, age ≧ 70 and/or C.C.
151	P	Peritoneal adhesiolysis, age < 70 w/o C.C.
152	P	Minor small and large bowel procedures, age ≧ 70 and/or C.C.
153	P	Minor small and large bowel procedures, age < 70 w/o C.C.
154	P	Stomach, esophageal, and duodenal procedures, age ≧ 70 and/or C.C.
155	P	Stomach, esophageal, and duodenal procedures, age 18-69 w/o C.C.
156*	P	Stomach, esophageal, and duodenal procedures, age 0-17
157	P	Anal procedures, age ≧ 70 and/or C.C.
158	P	Anal procedures, age < 70 w/o C.C.
159	P	Hernia procedures except inguinal and femoral, age ≧ 70 and/or C.C.
160	P	Hernia procedures except inguinal and femoral, age 18-69 w/o C.C.
161	P	Inguinal and femoral hernia procedures, age ≧ 70 and/or C.C.
162	P	Inguinal and femoral hernia procedures, age 18-69 w/o C.C.
163*	P	Hernia procedures, age 0-17
164	P	Appendectomy with complicated principal Diagnosis, age ≧ 70 and/or C.C.
165	P	Appendectomy with complicated principal Diagnosis, age < 70 w/o C.C.
166	P	Appendectomy w/o complicated principal Diagnosis, age ≧ 70 and/or C.C.
167	P	Appendectomy w/o complicated principal Diagnosis, age < 70 and/or C.C.
168	P	Procedures on the mouth, age ≧ 70 and/or C.C.
169	P	Procedures on the mouth, age < 70 w/o C.C.
170	P	Other digestive system procedures, age ≧ 70 and/or C.C.
171	P	Other digestive system procedures, age < 70 w/o C.C.
172	M	Digestive malignancy, age ≧ 70 and/or C.C.
173	M	Digestive malignancy, age < 70 w/o C.C.
174	M	G.I. hemorrhage, age ≧ 70 and/or C.C.
175	M	G.I. hemorrhage, age < 70 w/o C.C.
176	M	Complicated peptic ulcer
177	M	Uncomplicated peptic ulcer, age ≧ 70 and/or C.C.
178	M	Uncomplicated peptic ulcer, age < 70 w/o C.C.
179	M	Inflammatory bowel disease
180	M	G.I. obstruction, age ≧ 70 and/or C.C.
181	M	G.I. obstruction, age < 70 w/o C.C.
182	M	Esophagitis, gastroenteritis and miscellaneous digestive disease, age ≧ 70 and/or C.C.
183	M	Esophagitis, gastroenteritis and miscellaneous digestive disease, age 18-69 w/o C.C.
184*	M	Esophagitis, gastroenteritis and miscellaneous digestive disease, age 0-17
185	M	Dental and oral dis. Except extractions and restorations, age ≧ 18
186*	M	Dental and oral dis. Except extractions and restorations, age 0-17
187	M	Dental extractions and restorations
188	M	Other digestive system diagnoses, age ≧ 70 and/or C.C.
189	M	Other digestive system diagnoses, age 18-69 w/o C.C.
190*	M	Other digestive system diagnoses, age 0-17
MDC	**07**	**Diseases and disorders of the hepatobiliary system and pancreas**
191*	P	Major pancreas, liver, and shunt procedures
192*	P	Minor pancreas, liver, and shunt procedures
193	P	Biliary tract procedures except total cholecystectomy, age ≧ 70 and/or CC
194	P	Biliary tract procedures except total cholecystectomy, age < 70 w/o C.C.
195*	P	Total cholecystectomy with C.D.C., age ≧ 70 and/or C.C.
196*	P	Total cholecystectomy with C.D.C., age < 70 w/o C.C.
197	P	Total cholecystectomy w/o C.D.C., age ≧ 70 and/or C.C.
198	P	Total cholecystectomy w/o C.D.C., age < 70 w/o C.C.
199	P	Hepatobiliary diagnostic procedure for malignancy
200	P	Hepatobiliary diagnostic procedure for nonmalignancy
201	P	Other hepatobiliary or pancreas O.R. procedures
202	M	Cirrhosis and alcoholic hepatitis
203	M	Malignancy of hepatobiliary system or pancreas
204	M	Disorders of pancreas except malignancy
205	M	Disorders of liver except malignancy, cirrhosis, alcoholic hepatitis, age ≧ 70 and/or CC
206	M	Disorders of liver except malignancy cirrhosis, alcoholic hepatitis, age < 70 w/o C.C.
207	M	Disorders of the biliary tract, age ≧ 70 and/or C.C.
208	M	Disorders of the biliary tract, age < 70 w/o C.C.
MDC	**08**	**Diseases and disorders of the musculoskeletal system and connective tissue**
209	P	Major joint procedures
210	P	Hip and femur procedures except major joint, age ≧ 70 and/or C.C.
211	P	Hip and femur procedures except major joint. age 18-69 w/o C.C.

212*	P	Hip and femur procedures except major joint, age 0-17
213	P	Amputations for musculoskeletal system and connective tissue disorders
214	P	Back and neck procedures, age ≧ 70 and/or C.C.
215	P	Back and neck procedures, age < 70 w/o C.C.
216	P	Biopsies of musculoskeletal system and connective tissue
217	P	Wound debridement and skin graft except hand
218	P	Lower extrem. and humer. procedures except hip, foot, femur, age ≧ 70 and/or CC
219	P	Lower extrem. and humer. procedures except hip, foot, femur, age 18-69 w/o CC
220*	P	Lower extrem. and humer. procedures except hip, foot, femur, age 0-17
221	P	Knee procedures, age ≧ 70 and/or C.C.
222	P	Knee procedures, age < 70 w/o C.C.
223	P	Upper extremity procedures except humerus and hand, age ≧ 70 and/or C.C.
224	P	Upper extremity procedures except humerus and hand, age <70 w/o C.C.
225	P	Foot procedures
226	P	Soft tissue procedures, age ≧ 70 and/or C.C.
227	P	Soft tissue procedures, age <70 w/o C.C.
228	P	Ganglion (hand) procedures
229	P	Hand procedures except ganglion
230	P	Local excision and removal of internal fixation devices of hip and femur
231	P	Local excision and removal of internal fixation devices except hip and femur
232	P	Arthroscopy
233	P	Other musculoskeletal system and connective tissue O.R. procedures, age ≧ 70 and/or C.C.
234	P	Other musculoskeletal system and connective tissue O.R. procedures, age <70 w/o C.C.
235	M	Fractures of femur
236	M	Fractures of hip and pelvis
237	M	Sprains, strains, and dislocations of hip, pelvis, and thigh
238	M	Osteomyelitis
239	M	Pathological fractures and Musculoskeletal and connective tissue malignancy
240	M	Connective tissue disorders, age ≧ 70 and/or C.C.
241	M	Connective tissue disorders, age <70 w/o C.C.
242*	M	Septic arthritis
243	M	Medical back problems
244	M	Bone diseases and septic arthropathy, age ≧ 70 and/or C.C.
245	M	Bone diseases and septic arthropathy, age <70 w/o C.C.
246	M	Nonspecific arthropathies
247	M	Signs and symptoms of musculoskeletal system and connective tissue
248	M	Tendonitis, myositis, and bursitis
249	M	Aftercare
250	M	Fractures, sprains, strains, and dislocation of forearm, hand, foot, age ≧ 70 and/or CC
251	M	Fractures, sprains, strains, and dislocation of forearm, hand, foot, age 18-69 w/o CC
252*	M	Fractures, sprains, strains, and dislocation of forearm, hand, foot, age 0-17
253	M	Fractures, sprains, strains, and dislocation of upper arm, lower leg, except foot, age ≧ 70 and/or C.C.
254	M	Fractures, sprains, strains, and dislocation of upper arm, lower leg, except foot age 18-69 w/o C.C.
255*	M	Fractures, sprains, strains, and dislocation of upper arm, lower leg, except foot age 0-17
256	M	Other diagnoses of musculoskeletal system and connective tissue
MDC	**09**	**Diseases and disorders of the skin, subcutaneous tissue, and breast**
257	P	Total mastectomy for malignancy, age ≧ 70 and/or C.C.
258	P	Total mastectomy for malignancy < 70 w/o C.C.
259	P	Subtotal mastectomy for malignancy, age ≧ 70 and/or C.C.
260	P	Subtotal mastectomy for malignancy, age <70
261	P	Breast procedure for nonmalignancy except biopsy and local excision
262	P	Breast biopsy and local excision for nonmalignancy
263	P	Skin grafts for skin ulcer or cellulitis, age ≧ 70 and/or C.C.
264	P	Skin grafts for skin ulcer or cellulitis, age < 70 w/o C.C.
265*	P	Skin grafts except for skin ulcer or cellulitis with C.C.
266	P	Skin grafts except for skin ulcer or cellulitis w/o C.C.
267*	P	Perianal and pilonidal procedures
268*	P	Skin, subcutaneous tissue, and breast plastic procedures
269	P	Other skin, subcutaneous tissue and breast O.R. procedures age ≧ 70 and/or C.C.
270	P	Other skin, subcutaneous tissue and breast O.R. procedures age < 70 w/o C.C.
271	M	Skin ulcers
272	M	Major skin disorders, age ≧ 70 and/or C.C.
273	M	Major skin disorders, age < 70 w/o C.C.
274	M	Malignant breast disorders, age ≧ 70 and/or C.C.
275	M	Malignant breast disorders, age < 70 w/o C.C.
276	M	Nonmalignant breast disorders
277	M	Cellulitis, age ≧ 70 and/or C.C.
278	M	Cellulitis, age 18-69 w/o C.C.
279*	M	Cellulitis, Age 0-17
280	M	Trauma, age ≧ 70 and/or C.C.
281	M	Trauma, age 18-69 w/o C.C.
282*	M	Trauma, age 0-17
283	M	Minor skin disorders, age ≧ 70 and/or C.C.
284	M	Minor skin disorders, age < 70 w/o C.C.
MDC	**10**	**Endocrine, nutritional, and metabolic diseases and disorders**
285	P	Amputations for endocrine, nutritional, and metabolic disorders
286	P	Adrenal and pituitary procedures
287	P	Skin grafts and wound debridement
288*	P	O.R. procedures for obesity
289	P	Parathyroid procedures
290	P	Thyroid procedures
291*	P	Thyroglossal procedures
292	P	Other endocrine, nutritional and metabolic O.R. procedures, age ≧ 70 and/or C.C.
293*	P	Other endocrine, nutritional and metabolic O.R. procedures, age < 70 w/o C.C.
294	M	Diabetes, age ≧ 36
295	M	Diabetes, age 0-35

296 M Nutritional and miscellaneous metabolic disorders, age ≧ 70 and/or C.C.
297 M Nutritional and miscellaneous metabolic disorders, age 18-60 w/o C.C.
298* M Nutritional and miscellaneous metabolic disorders, age 0-17
299 M Inborn errors of metabolism
300 M Endocrine disorders, age ≧ 70 and/or C.C.
301 M Endocrine disorders, age < 70 w/o C.C.

MDC 11 Diseases and disorders of the kidney and urinary tract

302 P Kidney transplant
303 P Kidney, ureter, and major bladder procedure for malignancy
304 P Kidney, ureter, and major bladder procedure for nonmalignancy, age ≧ 70 and/or CC
305 P Kidney, ureter, and major bladder procedure for nonmalignancy, age < 70 w/o C.C.
306 P Prostatectomy, age ≧ 70 and/or C.C.
307 P Prostatectomy, age < 70 w/o C.C.
308 P Minor bladder procedures, age ≧ 70 and/or C.C.
309 P Minor bladder procedures, age < 70 w/o C.C.
310 P Transurethral procedures, age ≧ 70 and/or C.C.
311 P Transurethral procedures, age < 70 w/o C.C.
312 P Urethral procedures, age ≧ 70 and/or C.C.
313 P Urethral procedures, age 18-69 w/o C.C.
314* P Urethral procedures, age 0-17
315 P Other kidney and urinary tract O.R. procedures
316 M Renal failure w/o dialysis
317* M Renal failure with dialysis
318 M Kidney and urinary tract neoplasms age ≧ 70 and/or C.C.
319 M Kidney and urinary tract neoplasms, age < 70 w/o C.C.
320 M Kidney and urinary tract infections, age ≧ 70 and/or C.C.
321 M Kidney and urinary tract infections, age 18-69 w/o C.C.
322* M Kidney and urinary tract infections, age 0-17
323 M Urinary stones, age ≧ 70 and/or C.C.
324 M Urinary stones, age < 70 w/o C.C.
325 M Kidney and urinary tract signs and symptoms, age ≧ 70 and/or C.C.
326 M Kidney and urinary tract signs and symptoms, age 18-69 w/o C.C.
327* M Kidney and urinary tract signs and symptoms, age 0-17
328 M Urethral structure, age ≧ 70 and/or C.C.
329 M Urethral structure, age 18-69 w/o C.C.
330* M Urethral structure, age 0-17
331 M Other kidney and urinary tract diagnoses, age ≧ 70 and/or C.C.
332 M Other kidney and urinary tract diagnoses, age 18-69 w/o C.C.
333* M Other kidney and urinary tract diagnoses, age 0-17

MDC 12 Diseases and disorders of the male reproductive system

334 P Major male pelvic procedures with C.C.
335 P Major male pelvic procedures w/o C.C.
336 P Transurethral prostatectomy, age ≧ 70 and/or C.C.
337 P Transurethral prostatectomy, age < 70 w/o C.C.
338 P Testes procedures, for malignancy
339 P Testes procedures, nonmalignant, age ≧ 18
340* P Testes procedures, nonmalignant, age 0-17
341 P Penis procedures
342 P Circumcision, age ≧ 18
343* P Circumcision, age 0-17
344 P Other male reproductive system O.R. procedures for malignancy
345 P Other male reproductive system O.R. procedures except for malignancy
346 M Malignancy, age ≧ 70 and/or C.C.
347 M Malignancy, age < 70 w/o C.C.
348 M Benign prostatic hypertrophy, age ≧ 70 and/or C.C.
349 M Benign prostatic hypertrophy, age < 70 w/o C.C.
350 M Inflammation
351* M Sterilization
352 M Other male reproductive system diagnoses

MDC 13 Diseases and disorders of the female reproductive system

353 P Pelvic evisceration, radical hysterectomy, and vulvectomy
354 P Nonradical hysterectomy, age ≧ 70 and/or C.C.
355 P Nonradical hysterectomy, age < 70 w/o C.C.
356 P Female reproductive system reconstructive procedures
357 P Uterus and adenexa procedures, for malignancy
358 P Uterus and adenexa procedures for nonmalignancy except tubal interruption
359* P Tubal interruption for nonmalignancy
360 P Vagina, cervix, and vulva procedures
361* P Laparoscopy and endoscopy except tubal interruption
362* P Laparoscopic tubal interruption
363 P D&C, conization, and radioimplant, for malignancy
364 P D&C, conization except for malignancy
365 P Other female reproductive system O.R. procedures
366 M Malignancy, age ≧ 70 and/or C.C.
367 M Malignancy, age < 70 w/o C.C.
368 M Infections
369 M Menstrual and other female reproductive system disorders

MDC 14 Pregnancy, childbirth, and the puerperium

370* P Cesarean section with C.C.
371* P Cesarean section w/o C.C.
372* M Vaginal delivery with complicating diagnoses
373 M Vaginal delivery w/o complicating diagnoses
374* P Vaginal delivery with sterilization and/or D&C
375* P Vaginal delivery with O.R. procedures except sterilization and/or D&C
376* M Postpartum diagnoses w/o O.R. procedure
377* P Postpartum diagnoses with O.R. procedures
378* M Ectopic pregnancy
379* M Threatened abortion
380* M Abortion w/o D&C
381* M Abortion with D&C
382* M False labor
383* M Other anterpartum diagnoses with medical complications
384* M Other anterpartum diagnoses w/o medical complications

MDC 15 Newborns and other Neonates with condition originating in perinatal period

385* Neonates, died or transferred
386* Extreme immaturity, neonate

387*		Prematurity with major problems
388*		Prematurity w/o major problems
389*		Full-term neonate with major problems
390		Neonates with other significant problems
391*		Normal newborns
MDC	**16**	**Diseases and disorders of blood and blood-forming organs**
392	P	Splenectomy, age ≧18
393*	P	Splenectomy, age 0-17
394	P	Other O.R. procedures of the blood and blood-forming organs
395	M	Red blood cell disorders, age ≧18
396*	M	Red blood cell disorders, age 0-17
397	M	Coagulation disorders
398	M	Reticuloendothelial and immunity disorders, age ≧70 and/or C.C.
399	M	Reticuloendothelial and immunity disorders, age <70 w/o C.C.
MDC	**17**	**Myeloproliferative disorders**
400	P	Lymphoma or leukemia with major O.R. procedure
401	P	Lymphoma or leukemia with minor O.R. procedure, age ≧70 and/or C.C.
402*	P	Lymphoma or leukemia with minor O.R. procedure, age <70 w/o C.C.
403	M	Lymphoma or leukemia, age ≧70 and/or C.C.
404	M	Lymphoma or leukemia, age 18-69 w/o C.C.
405*	M	Lymphoma or leukemia, age 0-17
406	P	Myeloproliferative disorder or poorly differentiated neoplasm with major O.R. procedure & C.C.
407	P	Myeloproliferative disorder or poorly differentiated neoplasm with major O.R. procedure w/o C.C.
408	P	Myeloproliferative disorder or poorly differentiated neoplasm with minor O.R. procedure
409*	M	Radiotherapy
410	M	Chemotherapy
411	M	History of malignancy w/o endoscopy
412	M	History of malignancy with endoscopy
413	M	Other diagnoses of myeloproliferative disorder or poorly differentiated neoplasm, age ≧70 and/or CC
414	M	Other diagnoses of myeloproliferative disorder or poorly differentiated neoplasm age <70 w/o C.C.
MDC	**18**	**Infectious and parasitic diseases**
415	P	O.R. procedure
416	M	Septicemia, age ≧18
417*	M	Septicemia, age 0-17
418	M	Postoperative and posttraumatic infections
419	M	Fever of unknown origin, age ≧70 and/or C.C.
420	M	Fever of unknown origin, age 18-69 w/o C.C.
421	M	Viral illness, age ≧18
422*	M	Viral illness and fever of unknown origin, age 0-17
423	M	Other diagnoses of infections and parasitic diseases
MDC	**19**	**Mental diseases and disorders**
424	P	O.R. procedures with principal diagnosis of mental illness
425	M	Acute adjustment reaction and disturbances of psychosocial dysfunction
426	M	Depressive neuroses
427	M	Neuroses except depressive
428	M	Disorders of personality and impulse control
429	M	Organic disturbances and mental retardation
430	M	Psychoses
431*	M	Childhood mental disorders
432	M	Other diagnoses of mental disorders
MDC	**20**	**Substance use and substance-induced organic mental disorders**
433*		Substance use and substance-induced organic mental disorders, left AMA
434*		Drug dependence
435*		Drug use except dependence
436		Alcohol dependence
437*		Alcohol use except dependence
438		Alcohol and substance-induced organic mental syndrome
MDC	**21**	**Injuries, poisonings, and toxic effects of drugs**
439*	P	Skin grafts for injuries
440*	P	Wound debridements for injuries
441*	P	Hand procedures for injuries
442	P	Other O.R. procedures for injuries, age ≧70 and/or C.C.
443	P	Other O.R. procedures for injuries, age <70 w/o C.C.
444	M	Multiple trauma, age ≧70 and/or C.C.
445	M	Multiple trauma, age 18-69 w/o C.C.
446*	M	Multiple trauma, age 0-17
447	M	Allergic reactions, age ≧18
448*	M	Allergic reactions, age 0-17
449	M	Toxic effects of drugs, age ≧70 and/or C.C.
450	M	Toxic effects of drugs, age 18-69 w/o C.C.
451*	M	Toxic effects of drugs, age 0-17
452	M	Complications of treatment, age ≧70 and/or C.C.
453	M	Complications of treatment, age <70 w/o C.C.
454	M	Other diagnoses of injuries, poisonings, and toxic effects, age ≧70 and/or C.C.
455	M	Other diagnoses of injuries, poisonings, and toxic effects, age <70 w/o C.C.
MDC	**22**	**Burns**
456*		Burns, transferred to another acute care facility
457*		Extensive burns
458*	P	Nonextensive burns with skin grafts
459*	P	Nonextensive burns with wound debridement and other O.R. procedures
460	M	Nonextensive burns w/o O.R. procedure
MDC	**23**	**Factors influencing health status and other contacts with health services**
461	P	O.R. procedure with diagnoses of other contact with health services
462*	M	Rehabilitation
463	M	Signs and symptoms with C.C.
464	M	Signs and symptoms w/o C.C.
465*	M	Aftercare with history of malignancy as secondary diagnosis
466	M	Aftercare w/o history of malignancy as secondary diagnosis
467	M	Other factors influencing health status
Ungroupable records		
468		Unrelated operating procedure to a given MDC
469		Primary diagnosis invalid as discharge diagnosis
470		Invalid: record does not meet criteria for any DRG